D0853594

Jacobs & DeMott
Laboratory Test Handbook

with
Key Word Index

5th Edition

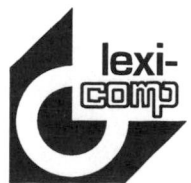

David S. Jacobs, MD
Wayne R. DeMott, MD
Dwight K. Oxley, MD

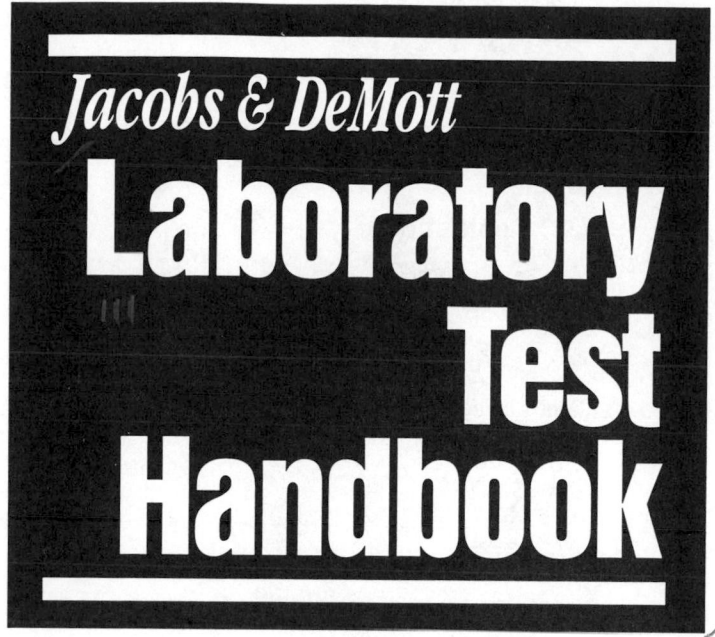

Jacobs & DeMott
Laboratory Test Handbook

with
Key Word Index

5th Edition

David S. Jacobs, MD, FACP, FCAP
Co-Editor-in-Chief
President, Pathologists Chartered
Consultant in Pathology and Laboratory Medicine
Overland Park, Kansas

Dwight K. Oxley, MD, FCAP
Co-Editor-in-Chief
Medical Director of Pathology
Wesley Medical Center
Wichita, Kansas

Wayne R. DeMott, MD, FCAP
Consultant in Pathology and Laboratory Medicine
Shawnee Mission, Kansas

LEXI-COMP, INC
Hudson (Cleveland), OH

Samford University Library

Dedication

To Judy

To Patricia

To Lee

With love and thanks

The 5th edition of the *Laboratory Test Handbook* is intended to serve as a useful reference at the time of publication, and not as a complete laboratory testing resource. No warranty is provided that the information herein is in every way accurate or complete. The explosion of information in many directions, in multiple scientific disciplines, with advances in laboratory techniques, and continuing evolution of knowledge requires constant scholarship. The publication covers common, as well as many esoteric testing procedures. The authors, editors, reviewers, contributors, and publishers cannot be responsible for the continued currency of the information or for any errors or omissions in this book or for any consequences arising therefrom, given the certainty of human error and the continuing dynamic changes in science. Because of the dynamic nature of laboratory medicine as a discipline, readers are advised that decisions regarding diagnosis and treatment must be based on the independent judgment of the clinician. The editors or authors are not responsible for any inaccuracy of quotation or for any false or misleading implication that may arise due to the text. Sources widely understood to be reliable have been used to try to provide information, but readers are encouraged to examine other sources of information (eg, footnotes, references, internet web sites), as well as other printed or electronic materials.

Copyright © 2001 by Lexi-Comp Inc. All rights reserved.

Printed in the United States of America. No part of this publication may be reproduced, stored in a retrieval system, or transmitted, in any form or by any means, electronic, mechanical, photocopying, recording, or otherwise, without the prior written permission of the publisher.

Previous editions copyrighted 1984, 1988, 1990, and 1994

This manual was produced using the Pathfinder™ Program –
a complete publishing service of Lexi-Comp Inc.

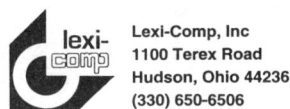

Lexi-Comp, Inc
1100 Terex Road
Hudson, Ohio 44236
(330) 650-6506

ISBN 1-930598-42-4 (case bound)

All rights reserved.

TABLE OF CONTENTS

RB
37
.L2758
2001

FOREWORD

Now in its 5th edition, the *Laboratory Test Handbook* is intended to be a resource for medical professionals who need rapid access to information about laboratory medicine. The organizational style of previous editions has been retained, presenting information about multiple aspects of each test: when to order the test, what specimen to collect, patient preparation, how the test is commonly used, how to interpret the results, and how useful the test is in practice. Readers interested in a **specific test** should first consult the Alphabetical Index which is both user-friendly and fairly encyclopedic. Readers interested in a **specific disease** should first consult the Key Word Index, in which tests linked to that disease are listed together with the pages on which they are found. Rare disease entities have sometimes been placed in the Alphabetical Index.

Methodologies are synoptically listed, but, as in previous editions, discussion of methods is truncated or deleted.

The 5th edition has been extensively revised to reflect contemporary medical practice. There are changes in a number of chapters, most notably in Coagulation. We now understand that the most prevalent coagulation disorders are those that lead to thrombosis (ie, hypercoagulable states). Most of the diagnostic tests for hypercoagulability are relatively new, and some depend on DNA-based technology. At the same time, new anticoagulant drugs have become available and require new approaches to laboratory monitoring.

A chapter called Infectious Diseases replaces the chapters called Microbiology and Virology, and parts of Immunology and Serology in previous editions. It contains information on testing across the spectrum of microbial disease: classical isolation and culture techniques, tests for serum antibodies relevant to infectious disease, and DNA-based molecular methods.

In the 3rd edition (1994), a single chapter entitled Molecular Pathology was written by one author. Presently, such topics, considerably expanded, are addressed in the 5th edition chapters of Cytogenetics, Molecular Genetic Testing, and Molecular Oncology. These three chapters are the work of eight individuals.

The present edition has divided Therapeutic Drug Monitoring from Toxicology/Drugs of Abuse, topics previously found in a single section.

Point-of-care testing is expanding. It is addressed in the revised Specimen Collection and Point-of-Care Testing chapter.

The editors, authors, and contributors are also aware that some tests are no longer useful. Rather than simply eliminating all of these, we have attempted to maintain continuity with previous editions, retained some, and written brief monographs reflecting the current state-of-the-art.

The *Laboratory Test Handbook* (LTH) is intended to overlap between the practice of medicine and the clinical laboratory. The LTH grew from the everyday world of hospital pathologists whose backgrounds included experience in direct patient care. Day-to-day problems and questions led to the development of manuals to respond to relevant needs of practicing physicians and surgeons who require sources of information about the laboratory and its results. The LTH is intended as well to address the questions of laboratory workers, who seek knowledge of the background and role of the procedures they perform. We truly hope that we have provided a helpful source of information.

ACKNOWLEDGMENTS

The editors of the *Laboratory Test Handbook with Key Word Index* wish to thank several individuals who have made this book possible. Mr Robert Kerscher, the publisher and president of Lexi-Comp Inc, is the person who saw the potential usefulness of such a book and provided the physical and financial resources required for its production to produce it, now through five editions. The unique aspects of its format, and especially the extensive cross-referencing and Key Word Index, are, in large part, due to his vision and willingness to experiment.

Barbara Kerscher, production manager of the 5th edition, has made essential administrative contributions, including the facilitation of revisions, new entries, and overall coordination among the more than 30 authors and contributors who have provided text to this edition. Despite many changes in format and content, Ms Kerscher has exhibited noteworthy patience, intelligence, flexibility, and extraordinary good humor. Assisting her have been other members of the Lexi-Comp staff: David C. Marcus, computer programming design; Matthew C. Kerscher, product manager; Kathy Smith, RN, production assistant; Alexandra J. Hart, composition specialist; and Tracey Reinecke, graphics artist.

We thank the authors and contributors who have made this volume possible. We hope that they have shared with us the sense and pride of purpose which we have seen develop as the edition evolved.

Michelle Medina-Jacobs, MD and Jonathan Todd Jacobs, MD have provided much appreciated clinical insight for several monographs.

We thank Dr Agostino Molteni for his recommendations.

Finally, we hope our readers find the *Laboratory Test Handbook*, 5th edition, a practical source of useful information to support good patient care.

Publisher's Acknowledgment and Dedication

The *Laboratory Test Handbook with Key Word Index* is the direct result of over 20 years of dedicated service by David S. Jacobs, MD and Wayne R. DeMott, MD.

Drs Jacobs and DeMott have provided clear vision and extraordinary commitment, establishing higher standards for each edition. The *Laboratory Test Handbook* was originally the effort of four community-based pathologists offering their insights on tests routinely available in a modern clinical laboratory. This 5th edition represents the culmination of contributions of over 50 medical and editorial professionals reflecting state-of-the-art offerings availabel in contemporary medical pactice.

With sincere gratitude and appreciation we henceforth rename this title, *Jacobs and DeMott Laboratory Test Handbook*.

ABOUT THE AUTHORS

Christopher D. Ackley, MD, PhD

Dr Christopher D. Ackley received his PhD in immunology from The University of Alabama at Birmingham and his MD degree from the University of South Alabama in Mobile, Alabama. Following residency training in Anatomic and Clinical Pathology at Duke University, Dr Ackley pursued a surgical and cytopathology fellowship in the Department of Pathology, Virginia Commonwealth University Health System, Medical College of Virginia Hospitals. Dr Ackley is an attending pathologist with South Texas Pathology in San Antonio, Texas.

Holly Alexander, PhD

Dr Alexander received her doctorate from the University of Connecticut Medical Center and completed a postdoctoral fellowship in Public Health and Medical Microbiology at the Califormia Department of Health Services. She is a board certified Diplomate of the American Academy of Microbiology. Dr Alexander is the Clinical Scientist at Via Christi Regional Medical Center in Wichita, Kansas. Prior to that she was the Clinical Microbiologist at Wesley Medical Center in Wichita. Dr Alexander is a member of the American Society for Microbiology, the Southwestern Society for Microbiology, and the PanAmerican Society for Clinical Virology.

Uri S. Alon, MD

Dr Alon received his MD degree from the Hebrew University, Hadassah School of Medicine in Jerusalem, Israel. Following his residency in Pediatrics he continued with Pediatric Nephrology fellowship at the Medical College of Virginia in Richmond, Virginia. Dr Alon is board certified in Pediatrics and in Pediatric Nephrology.

Dr Alon is Professor of Pediatrics at the University of Missouri Kansas City School of Medicine. He is the Director of Research and Education at the Department of Pediatric Nephrology and the Director of the Renal Laboratory at Children's Mercy Hospital in Kansas City, Missouri. Dr Alon is the Past President of the Midwest Society for Pediatric Research, he is a member of the Research Committee of the American Society of Pediatric Nephrology and Chairman of the Medical Staff Research Committee at Children's Mercy Hospital.

Leland B. Baskin, MD, MS, FCAP

Dr Baskin received a BS in bioengineering from Texas A&M University in 1974 and received an MS in civil engineering from Cornell University in Ithaca, New York in 1977. Dr Baskin worked as an engineer for EPA in research labs in Oklahoma and Georgia. He received a Master of Applied Mathematical Sciences from Rice University in Houston, Texas and received his MD from The University of Texas Medical School in San Antonio, Texas. He then completed a 4-year residency in AP/CP at The University of Texas Southwestern Medical Center in Dallas, Texas.

Dr Baskin completed a fellowship in chemical pathology at Mayo Clinic and has been on the faculty of The University of Texas Southwestern Medical Center in Dallas, Texas since 1992. He is Associate Director of Chemical Pathology at Parkland Memorial Hospital and Associate Medical Director of the Clinical Laboratory at Zale Lipshy University Hospital. Dr Baskin has been on the board of consultants of the North Texas Poison Center since 1994. Dr Baskin is the Associate Medical Director of Carter Blood Care, Texas. He is a member of AACC (2001-2002 chairman of the Texas Section) and other organizations. Dr Baskin has been on the editorial board for Medical Laboratory Observer since 2000. His main professional interests are in clinical chemistry, transfusion medicine, and in applying mathematical methods to laboratory medicine.

Malcolm L. Beck, FIMLS, FIBiol, FRCPath

Malcolm Beck received his general education and professional training in England before coming to the United States in 1965. Since then he has held positions in the Transfusion Services of Mount Sinai Hospital, New York City; the University of Michigan Medical Center (Assistant Professor, Department of Pathology) and has recently retired after serving 26 years as the Technical Director of Community Blood Center of Greater Kansas City. He has authored over 100 publications and given numerous lectures and workshops on immunohematologic topics. He served on several committees of the American Association of Blood Banks (AABB). He was the 1980 recipient of the AABB Ivor Dunsford Memorial Award as well as corecipient of the AABB 1999 Morton Grove Rasmussen Memorial Award. He was admitted to Fellowship of the Royal College of Pathology in 1993.

Jennifer A. Brainard, MD

Dr Jennifer A. Brainard received her MD degree from The Ohio State University College of Medicine. Her postgraduate training was in Anatomic and Clinical Pathology at The Cleveland Clinic Foundation, Division of Pathology and Laboratory Medicine. She is board certified in AP/CP and has completed a surgical and cytopathology fellowship in the Department of Pathology, Virginia Commonwealth University Health System, Medical College of Virginia Hospitals. She also has obtained Added Qualifications in Cytopathology by the American Board of Pathology. Dr Brainard is currently Associate Staff Pathologist at the Cleveland Clinic Foundation.

Leigh Ann Cahill, BS CT(ASCP) CMIAC

Ms Cahill is the senior cytotechnologist at the Medical College of Virginia Hospitals, Virginia Commonwealth University Health System. She received her cytology training at the Medical College of Virginia and her Bachelor of Science degree from the University of Richmond. She has served as chairman of the Cytotechnology Advisory Committee and as a member of the Long Range Planning Committee of the American Society of Cytopathology. She is currently a member of the Scientific Program Committee and Art for Advocacy Committee of the American Society of Cytopathology. She has presented platform and poster presentations as well as workshops at the national meetings of the American Society of Cytopathology and American Society of Clinical Pathologists.

Beiyun Chen, MD, PhD

Dr Chen received her medical degree from Beijing Medical University in Beijing, China in 1986. She completed her graduate study in the area of developmental biology and received her PhD degree from McGill University in Montreal, Canada in 1994. Then she entered the pathology residency program at New York Medical College in Valhalla, New York and completed a combined anatomic and clinical pathology residency in 1998. She has been a staff member at the Memorial Sloan-Kettering Cancer Center since she finished a 1 year fellowship in Molecular Genetic Pathology there in 1999. She is certified in Anatomic and Clinical Pathology. As a staff pathologist she is involved in the operation of the laboratory of diagnostic molecular pathology as well as surgical pathology.

Marilyn K. Davis-Cansler, BS SCT (ASCP) CMIAC

Ms Davis graduated with a BS in cytology from Avila College, Kansas City, Missouri. She received a certificate in cytology from the University of Kansas College of Health Sciences School of Medicine. She was certified in CT and Specialist in Cytology (SCT) by the American Society of Clinical Pathologists and CT (CMIAC) by the International Academy of Cytology.

Ms Davis received The Stata Norton Distinguished Teaching Award from the University of Kansas School of Allied Health. She is a member of Phi Theta Kappa and National Honors Fraternity. She was a previous clinical instructor with KUMC Department of Cytopathology. Ms Davis is currently employed by Kansas University Physicians, Inc (KUPI) at the University of Kansas Medical Center, since 1983, as Cytology Supervisor of the KUPI Cytology Laboratory and Technical Director of the KUMC Image Analysis Laboratory: Quantitative DNA Ploidy Analysis, Quantitative Immunohistochemical Analysis of Tumors, Tumor and Cellular Micrometry, and BLISS Tracer Slide Scanning for creation of WebSlides.

Ms Davis is a member of the American Society for Cytotechnology, Cytotechnologist Member of the American Society of Cytopathology, Associate Member of the American Society of Clinical Pathologists, and Cytotechnologist Member of the International Academy of Cytology. She has coauthored abstracts and original articles, and book chapters.

Wayne R. DeMott, MD

Dr DeMott is a graduate of the University of Oregon Medical School (1959). He completed his internship at Madigan General Hospital outside Tacoma, Washington. After service in the U.S. Air Force as a General Medical Officer, he completed the pathology residency program at the University of California San Francisco Medical Center (1967). He was certified in Anatomic and Clinical Pathology by the American Board of Pathology in 1968.

As a practicing pathologist at Providence Medical Center in Kansas City, Kansas from 1968-1994, Dr DeMott gave special attention to the areas of Hematology and Coagulation. He participated in research activities involving separation of white cells from peripheral blood, measurement of zinc levels in peripheral blood leukocytes utilizing atomic absorption spectrophotometry, and separation of neutrophil enzymes by isoelectric focusing. He was an active contributor to the Providence Medical Center (formerly Providence-St Margaret Health Center) School of Medical Technology, is a past president of the Medical Staff of Providence Medical Center, and was chairman or a member of several of the hospital professional committees, including the Cancer Committee. He directed the Cancer Conference for many years.

Dr DeMott is a Fellow of the American Society of Clinical Pathologists and College of American Pathologists, and is a member of the American Association for Clinical Chemistry, American Medical Association, Kansas Society of Pathologists, and Kansas City Society of Pathologists.

John Foxworth, PharmD

Dr Foxworth is an Associate Professor at the University of Missouri-Kansas City Medical School, where he has taught pharmacology for 15 years. He is active in the internal medicine residency program, for which he has directed the noon conference series for 10 years. He has taught a monthly journal club for the medicine residents for 6 years involving critical analysis as well as principals of evidence-based medicine. He is a member of the American Society for Clinical Pharmacology and Therapeutics and the Clinical Pharmacology Section, Department of Medicine, Truman Medical Center-Hospital Hill and UMKC School of Medicine.

Uttam Garg, PhD, DABCC, FACB

Dr Garg received his PhD from the Postgraduate Institute of Medical Education and Research, India. He did his postdoctoral training in Cell Biology and Pharmacology at the New York Medical College. He received additional training in Clinical Chemistry and Toxicology at the University of Minnesota Medical School.

Before joining his current position as Associate Professor and the Director of Clinical Chemistry and Toxicology Laboratories at the Children's Mercy Hospital and the University of Missouri School of Medicine, Kansas City, he was Assistant Professor at the University of Minnesota Medical School. He also served the New York University Medical Center as Research Assistant Professor.

Dr Garg is a recipient of a number of awards and honors including Major General Amir Chand Gold Medal for graduate excellence, American Heart Association Fellowship, FIDIA Research Foundation Award, and Outstanding Scientific Achievements Award by a young investigator by the American Association for Clinical Chemistry.

Dr Garg is a Fellow of the Academy of Clinical Biochemistry. He is on the Board of Directors of the American Board of Clinical Chemistry and serves as a member of the toxicology subcommittee. He is certified in Clinical Chemistry by the American Board of Clinical Chemistry and the American Society of Clinical Pathology. He is also certified in Clinical Toxicology by the American Board of Clinical Chemistry and the National Registry of Clinical Chemists. He has published over 50 peer-reviewed articles, which have been cited in over 1600 publications. He has been an invited reviewer for several journals including *Clinical Chemistry*, *Journal of Laboratory and Clinical Medicine*, *Life Sciences*, and *Neuroscience*. His research interests include method developments in clinical laboratory diagnosis.

Charles W. Gorodetzky, MD, PhD

After completing his undergraduate work at MIT (BS, 1958), Dr Gorodetzky earned his MD degree at Boston University School of Medicine (1962), followed by an Internal Medicine internship at Boston City Hospital, and a PhD in Pharmacology at the University of Kentucky (1975). Dr Gorodetzky spent 21 years in intramural NIH research in substance abuse at the National Institute on Drug Abuse, Addiction Research Center in Lexington, Kentucky (1963-1984). His major research interests were the human pharmacology and metabolism of drugs of abuse. He served as the director of the Lexington Center from 1979 to 1984. In 1984, Dr Gorodetzky joined the pharmaceutical industry and became Vice President of Global Therapeutic Area, CNS in the Drug Development Department at Hoechst Marion Roussel Inc in Kansas City, Missouri.

Dr Gorodetzky has authored or co-authored over 100 papers, book chapters, and books and has served on numerous government committees, including an FDA advisory committee and grant review committees. He holds or has held adjunct full professorships at the medical schools of the University of Kentucky, University of Louisville, and University of North Carolina. He served as an advisor and consultant to the Special Action Office on Drug Abuse Prevention, CDC and NIDA in the development and implementation of the Proficiency Testing Program for Drugs of Abuse. Dr Gorodetzky is currently Vice President, Medical and Scientific Services Department at Quintiles, Inc in Kansas City, Missouri.

Harold J. Grady, PhD

Dr Grady received his PhD from St Louis University in 1950 and joined the staff of University of Kansas School of Medicine as Assistant Professor and Director of Clinical Chemistry. In 1965 he became Professor of Pathology. During this period he taught in the laboratory medicine program, carried out research, and was a consultant in Clinical Chemistry for several area hospitals. He became Director of Clinical Chemistry at Baptist Medical Center in 1970. He is currently Professor of Pathology at the University of Missouri Kansas City School of Medicine and Director of Clinical Chemistry at Truman Medical Center. Dr Grady is a member of the American Association for Clinical Chemistry and has been on the Board of Directors of that organization. He was also on the Board of Directors of the American Board of Clinical Chemistry and is certified by that body in Clinical Chemistry and Toxicological Chemistry. He has authored forty scientific papers in peer reviewed journals.

Daniel R. Hinthorn, MD, FACP

Dr Hinthorn received his MD degree at the University of Kansas School of Medicine. After training in internal medicine, he spent 2 years with the Centers for Disease Control and Prevention as an Epidemic Intelligence Officer. He then completed his Infectious Diseases fellowship and joined the faculty at the University of Kansas Medical Center.

Dr Hinthorn is Professor of Internal Medicine, Pediatrics, and Family Medicine, and is the Director of the Division of Infectious Diseases at the University of Kansas Medical Center. He is board certified in Internal Medicine and Infectious Diseases. He is on the Editorial Board of Infections in Medicine, Infections in Surgery, and Complications in Surgery. He reviews manuscripts for Archives of Medicine, Clinical Infectious Diseases, Infectious Disease in Clinical Practice, and others. He is a member of the NIH Collaborative Antiviral Study Group. Besides antiviral therapy, his research interests include clinical aspects of penicillin-resistant *S. pneumoniae*. With Dr Norton Greenberger, he wrote the textbook, *Physical Diagnosis*. He is a Fellow of the American College of Physicians, the Infectious Diseases Society of America, and a member of the American Society for Microbiology.

Rebecca Horvat, PhD

Dr Horvat received her doctorate from the University of Kansas Medical Center, Department of Microbiology, and subsequently was awarded a postdoctoral fellowship from the American Cancer Society. Dr Horvat then worked as a Technical Director in the Clinical Laboratories at the University of Kansas Medical Center. In this capacity, she worked with the Microbiology, Virology, and Hematology sections to develop new diagnostic tests based on nucleic acid analysis. Dr Horvat then went on the faculty of the University of Kansas School of Medicine in the Department of Pathology and Laboratory Medicine. Her clinical responsibility included directorship of the Microbiology, Virology, and Immunology Sections of the Clinical Laboratory.

Currently, Dr Horvat is an Associate Professor and in this capacity is involved in the education and teaching of residents and medical students. She also has an active research program investigating the antibiotic resistance in gram-positive bacteria, detection of resistance using molecular analysis, and in the implications of antibiotic resistance on patient outcomes. Dr Horvat is a member of the American Association of Immunologist (AAI), the American Society for Microbiology (ASM), and the Northern Kansas Regional Director for the Southwestern Association for Clinical Microbiologist (SWACM). Dr Horvat is also active in the local Kansas City Area Society for Microbiology (KCASM).

Susan H. Hsu, PhD

Dr Hsu received her postdoctoral training from 1970-1974 in the Immunogenetics Laboratories, Division of Medical Genetics of the Johns Hopkins Medical Institution (JHMI) at Baltimore, Maryland. She has been the Assistant and subsequently the Codirector of the Immunogenetics Lab from between 1976-1986 and associate Professor in the Department of Medicine at the JHMI from 1983-1986. Since 1987 she has assumed the position of the Scientific Director and the Director of the HLA/Molecular Genetics Department of the American Red Cross, Blood Services, Penn-Jersey Region in Philadelphia, Pennsylvania.

David S. Jacobs, MD, FACP

Dr Jacobs was Director of Laboratories at Providence Medical Center in Kansas City, Kansas for 29 years, leaving that position in 1994. He served as a member of the institutional Credentials Committee for 20 years. During Dr Jacobs' tenure as Director, then Medical Director of the School of Medical Technology, 173 medical technologists graduated from 1965 to 1990.

He remains Clinical Professor at the University of Kansas and the University of Missouri-Kansas City Schools of Medicine. He is a Fellow of the American College of Physicians, the College of American Pathologists, and the American Society of Clinical Pathologists. He is a member of the International Academy of Pathology, the AMA, and the Kansas Medical Society. He was a member of the Editorial Board of *Kansas Medicine* and was Book Review Editor of that journal. Dr Jacobs is past President of the Kansas Society of Pathologists, the Kansas City Society of Pathologists, and of the Medical Staff of the Providence Medical Center (formerly Providence-St Margaret Health Center). He held a position on the Board of Directors of the Wyandotte County Medical Society for several years, and for much of his career served as an inspector for both the College of American Pathologists and for the American Association of Blood Banks.

He received his premedical education at the University of Michigan. Entering the UM Medical School in the "Letters and Medicine" program, Dr Jacobs remained at Michigan as a general rotating intern, then did his residency in Anatomic and Clinical Pathology at the same institution. Following service in the U.S. Army Medical Corps as a pathologist with 13 months residency, he returned to Ann Arbor and completed the pathology program under Drs A. J. French and M. R. Abell. He then enjoyed additional professional experience in clinical pathology in Chicago with Drs Israel Davidsohn, Douglas Huestis, and Norbert Tietz. Dr Jacobs is certified in both Anatomic and Clinical Pathology by the American Board of Pathology.

Dr Jacobs' special interests include general pathology, particularly surgical pathology, interpretation of clinical laboratory tests, and transfusion medicine. His publications address topics in surgical pathology and the clinical relevance of laboratory testing. He is active as a consultant in pathology and laboratory medicine.

Daniel H. Jacobs, MD

Daniel H. Jacobs, MD graduated from Stanford University with an AB in history in 1982 and received his medical degree from the University of Kansas School of Medicine in 1987. Dr Jacobs completed parts of his residency training at the University of Iowa (psychiatry), the Johns Hopkins University (medicine), and the University of Kansas (neurology). He completed fellowship training in Behavioral Neurology and Clinical Neuropsychology at the University of Florida in Gainesville, Florida. He served as Assistant Professor of Neurology at Tufts University from 1994-1997. Currently, Dr Jacobs is Clinical Adjunct Associate Professor of Neurology at the University of Florida School of Medicine and practices neurology in Orlando.

Michael Laposata, MD, PhD

Dr Michael Laposata is the Director of Clinical Laboratories at the Massachusetts General Hospital and Professor of Pathology at Harvard Medical School. He received his MD and PhD from Johns Hopkins University School of Medicine and completed a postdoctoral research fellowship and residency in Laboratory Medicine at Washington University School of Medicine in St Louis. He took his first faculty position at the University of Pennsylvania School of Medicine in Philadelphia in 1985, where he was an Assistant Professor and director of the hospital's coagulation laboratory. In 1989, he became Director of Clinical Laboratories at the Massachusetts General Hospital and was appointed to faculty in pathology at Harvard Medical School.

His research program, with more than 90 peer reviewed publications, has focused on fatty acids and their metabolites. His research group is focused on the study of fatty acid ethyl esters, which are esterification products of fatty acid and ethanol. He has demonstrated that these ethanol metabolites are toxic mediators of ethanol-induced cell injury and that the ethyl esters are present in the serum after ethanol intake, serving as long-term markers of ethanol intake.

Dr Laposata's clinical expertise is in the field of blood coagulation, with a special expertise in the diagnosis of hypercoagulable states.

Dr Laposata has implemented a system at MGH whereby the clinical laboratory data in coagulation, toxicology, and other areas are interpreted, with the generation of a narrative paragraph by a physician with expertise in the area. This service is essentially identical to the service provided by physicians in radiology and anatomic pathology, except that it involves clinical laboratory test results. This new program in laboratory medicine has resulted in shorter time to diagnosis and fewer laboratory tests to reach a diagnosis. Physician specialists in many areas of laboratory medicine provide expert interpretations for clinicians at various locations within the U.S. A web-based system that offers advice on test selection, as well as an interpretation of the data, is being developed to increase the scope of the service and streamline the communication between physicians. The interpretive service will be linked to a well illustrated concise teaching program that allows physicians to learn about their patients' diseases at the time they are interacting with the patient.

Dr Laposata is the recipient of 12 major teaching prizes at Harvard, the Massachusetts General Hospital, and the University of Pennsylvania School of Medicine. His recognitions include the 1989 Lindback award, a teaching prize with competition across the entire University of Pennsylvania system; the 1998 A. Clifford Barger mentorship award from Harvard Medical School; and the award – by vote of the graduating class – for the best preclinical instructor at Harvard Medical School in both 1999 and 2000.

Geralyn M. Meny, MD

Dr Meny received her BS degree in medical technology from the University of Kentucky. She received certification as a Medical Technologist and a Specialist in Blood Banking from the American Society of Clinical Pathologists. Dr Meny received her MD degree from the University of Texas Southwestern Medical Center at Dallas in 1990. She completed a pathology residency at Parkland Memorial Hospital in Dallas in 1995. She is board certified in Anatomic and Clinical Pathology and Blood Banking/Transfusion Medicine by the American Board of Pathology.

Dr Meny is currently Medical Director at the American Red Cross, Penn-Jersey Region, Philadelphia, Pennsylvania.

Phillip A. Munoz, MD

Dr Munoz received his MD degree from the University of Kansas Medical Center. He completed his first year of pathology training at Northwestern University and continued his training as a Research Associate in Immunology at the National Institutes of Health. He completed his training in Pathology at the University of Kansas Medical Center, then joined the medical faculty for the next 6 years. During that time, he developed a focus on hybridoma technology and cell marker studies applied to hematopathology and general surgical pathology. He is currently an Associate Pathologist and Director of Hematology and the Cell Marker Laboratories at Research Medical Center, Kansas City, Missouri.

In his current position, Dr Munoz oversees various laboratory aspects of an active hematology/oncology patient population in a large private hospital that serves as the center of a multihospital Kansas City based healthcare network. In addition to general surgical pathology and hematology services, he maintains an integrated immunocytochemistry and flow cytometry laboratory that serves as a reference laboratory for the healthcare system and other hospitals in the Kansas City area.

Dr Munoz is a member of the Kansas City Society of Pathologists, College of American Pathologists, American Society of Clinical Pathologists, American Pathology Foundation, and American Medical Association.

Eugene S. Olsowka, MD, PhD

Dr Olsowka is a pathologist at Covenant HealthCare, Saginaw, Michigan. He is a Fellow of the College of American Pathologists and the American Society of Clinical Pathologists.

Dr Olsowka studied mathematics as an undergraduate at the University of Chicago. He entered medical school at the University of Illinois in 1977. He received his MD degree from the University of Illinois in 1984 and a PhD in Nutritional Sciences from the University of Illinois in 1989. Dr Olsowka trained in Anatomic and Clinical Pathology at The McGaw School of Medicine, Northwestern University in Chicago, from 1986 to 1990. He was a Fellow in Surgical Pathology at Rush-Presbyterian-St Luke's Medical Center in Chicago from 1990 to 1991. He is board certified in Anatomic and Clinical Pathology.

Dr Olsowka's interests are general pathology including surgical pathology, chemistry, and cytology. He also holds the rank of 2nd Dan in Tae Kwon Do.

Dwight K. Oxley, MD

Dr Oxley received his MD degree from the University of Kansas and took his Anatomic Pathology residency at that institution; his Clinical Pathology residency was at the U.S. Naval Hospital, St Albans, New York. He took a fellowship in Nuclear Medicine at Johns Hopkins University. He is the Medical Director of Pathology at Wesley Medical Center, Wichita, Kansas, a position which he has held since 1988. Prior to 1988 he was a community pathologist in Kansas City, Missouri (St Joseph Hospital) and, before that in Rancho Mirage, California (Eisenhower Medical Center).

Dr Oxley is a Trustee of the American Board of Pathology and served as President of the Board in 1999. He is a member of the Executive Committee of the American Board of Medical Specialties. He has served on the editorial boards of the *American Journal of Clinical Pathology*, the *Archives of Pathology and Laboratory Medicine*, and *Clinica Chimica Acta*. While practicing in Kansas City he was active in the teaching of the sophomore pathology course at the University of Kansas, and he has an appointment as a Clinical Professor of Pathology at that institution.

He is a community pathologist with a major interest in clinical pathology, particularly the clinical relevance of laboratory test results. He is a Fellow of the College of American Pathologists and the American Society of Clinical Pathologists. He is a member of the American Pathology Foundation, the American Association for the History of Medicine, the Kansas Society of Pathologists, the American Medical Association, the Kansas Medical Society, and the Medical Society of Sedgwick County.

Mary Ann Pedigo BS CT(ASCP) CMIAC

Ms Pedigo is the cytology supervisor and educational coordinator at the Medical College of Virginia Hospitals, Virginia Commonwealth University Health System. She received her cytology training at the Johns Hopkins University School of Medicine and her Bachelor of Science from Virginia Commonwealth University. She is an active member of state, national, and international societies. She has presented poster presentations at the national meetings of the American Society of Cytopathology and published several articles in cytology journals.

Diane L. Persons, MD

Dr Persons received her MA in Microbiology and her MD degree at the University of Kansas. Following a residency in Anatomic Pathology at the University of Kansas Medical Center, she spent 3 years in a combined clinical and research fellowship in Cytogenetics and Molecular Cytogenetics at the Mayo Clinic in Rochester, Minnesota. She is board certified in Anatomic Pathology and Clinical Cytogenetics.

Presently, Dr Persons is the Director of the Cytogenetics Laboratory and is an Associate Professor in the Department of Pathology and Laboratory Medicine at the University of Kansas Medical Center. In addition to her clinical responsibilities, she has a basic research program that investigates the molecular mechanisms involved in sensitivity to chemotherapeutic agents.

Dr Persons is a Fellow of the College of American Pathologists and a member of the American Society of Human Genetics, American Association for Cancer Research, Association for Molecular Pathology, Association of Clinical Scientists, the Southwest Oncology Group, and American Medical Association. She is currently a member of the Editorial Board of the Annals of Clinical and Laboratory Science, a member of the Southwest Oncology Group Cytogenetics Committee, and a member of the joint Cytogenetics Resource Committee of the College of American Pathologists and the American College of Medical Genetics.

Frederick V. Plapp, MD, PhD

Dr Frederick V. Plapp received his MD and PhD degrees in a combined medical scientist program from the University of Kansas Medical Center. He completed an internship at the University of Chicago and pathology residency at the University of Kansas Medical Center. He is board certified in Clinical Pathology.

Following completion of his residency, Dr Plapp practiced pathology at the University of Kansas Medical Center for 5 years, and then became Assistant Medical Director of the Community Blood Center of Greater Kansas City. During the next 5 years, he and his colleagues developed the solid phase red cell adherence method for pretransfusion serologic testing that is now marketed as Capture P and Capture R by Immucor Inc. In 1987, Dr Plapp became a Clinical Pathologist at Saint Luke's Hospital in Kansas City, MO and has served as Medical Director of Saint Luke's Regional Laboratories since 1991.

His areas of special interest include clinical chemistry, immunoassays, and transfusion medicine. He has published more than 70 articles in these areas.

Celeste N. Powers, MD, PhD

Dr Celeste N. Powers received her PhD in Microbiology and Immunology from Baylor College of Medicine, Houston, Texas and her MD from The University of Texas Medical School at Houston. She also did her residency training in Anatomic and Clinical Pathology at UTMSH. Dr Powers completed fellowship training in Surgical and Cytopathology at the Medical College of Virginia in Richmond, Virginia. She is board certified in Anatomic and Clinical Pathology and has Added Qualifications in Cytopathology from the American Board of Pathology. Dr Powers has played an active role in several national pathology societies, including American Society of Clinical Pathologists, American Society of Cytopathology and the United States and Canadian Academy of Pathology. She has authored numerous articles and book chapters, including a book on the fine needle aspiration biopsy of the head and neck.

Dr Powers is currently Professor and Chair of the Division of Surgical and Cytopathology as well as Director of Anatomic Pathology Services for the Department of Pathology, Virginia Commonwealth University Health System, Medical College of Virginia Hospitals.

Charlotte E. Shideler, PhD

Dr Shideler earned her PhD in biochemistry from the University of Arkansas for Medical Sciences in Little Rock, Arkansas and received postdoctoral training in clinical chemistry at the University of Virginia Medical Center in Charlottesville, Virginia. Dr Shideler is certified in Clinical Chemistry by the American Board of Clinical Chemistry and National Registry in Clinical Chemistry and is employed by Wesley Pathology Consultants in Wichita, Kansas.

Dr Shideler is a member of the American Association for Clinical Chemistry, American Chemical Society, American Society of Clinical Pathologists, Association of Clinical Scientists, Clinical Laboratory Management Association, and American Association for the Advancement of Science.

Jasbir Singh, PhD

Dr Singh is the Chief of Clinical Chemistry and Toxicology at the Veterans Affairs Medical Center in Minneapolis, Minnesota and an Assistant Professor in the Department of Laboratory Medicine and Pathology, University of Minnesota. He completed his PhD in biochemistry from the University of Otago, New Zealand and his postdoctoral fellowship in Clinical Chemistry at the University of Minnesota. Dr Singh is certified in both Clinical Chemistry and Toxicological Chemistry by the American Board of Clinical Chemistry.

Barry S. Skikne, MBBCh, FACP, FCP(SA)

Dr Skikne is a Professor of Medicine in the Division of Hematology/Oncology at the University of Kansas Medical Center in Kansas City, Kansas. He received his medical degree at the University of the Witwatersrand in South Africa. After completing residency, he became a member of the clinical staff in the Hematology/Oncology Division at the University of the Witwatersrand in 1974. He did a fellowship in Hematology at the University of Kansas Medical Center in 1977. He is Director of the Hematopoietic Stem Cell Transplantation Program at that Institution.

He has extensive research experience and publications in the area of iron metabolism and disorders related to iron and hematopoiesis.

Karen Stephens, PhD

Dr Stephens is Research Associate Professor of Medicine and Laboratory Medicine, Adjunct Research Associate Professor of Pathology, and Director of the Genetics Section, Molecular Diagnosis Laboratory at the University of Washington in Seattle, Washington. She received her PhD in microbiology from Indiana University and was a Damon Runyon-Walter Winchell Fellow in the Department of Biochemistry, Stanford University. Dr Stephens' major research interests are the molecular pathogenesis of inherited disease, in particular neurofibromatosis type 1 on which she has published extensively, mechanisms of human gene mutation, and epidermal differentiation.

Dr Stephens is a member of the American Society of Human Genetics, the Society for Investigative Dermatology, and the Association for Molecular Pathology. She is a Diplomate of the American Board of Medical Genetics in Clinical Molecular Genetics.

Jonathan F. Tait, MD, PhD

Dr Tait received his MD and PhD degrees from Washington University (St Louis) in 1983. He did residency training in clinical pathology at the University of Washington (Seattle) and postdoctoral training in biochemistry at the same institution. He is currently on the faculty at the University of Washington School of Medicine, where he is Associate Professor of Laboratory Medicine with adjunct appointments in Medicine/Medical Genetics and Pathology. Dr Tait is the codirector of the Genetics Laboratory at the University of Washington Medical Center and head of the Genetics Division in the Department of Laboratory Medicine. He is board certified in clinical pathology and clinical molecular genetics, and has published about seventy research articles in the fields of laboratory medicine and biochemistry. He is a member of a number of societies, including the Academy of Clinical Laboratory Physicians and Scientists, Association for Molecular Pathology, American Society of Human Genetics, American Society for Biochemistry and Molecular Biology, and the Washington State Medical Association.

Ossama Tawfik, MD, PhD

Dr Tawfik received his MBBCh (MD) and PhD degrees from Cairo University in 1978. He completed his AP/CP residency and postdoctoral fellowship at the Kansas University Medical Center. Dr Tawfik is board certified in AP/CP and Cytopathology. Dr Tawfik is currently Director of Surgical Pathology, and Associate Professor of Pathology and Laboratory Medicine at the University of Kansas Medical Center. Dr Tawfik provides service activities in General Surgical Pathology and Cytopathology, the latter with special expertise in diseases of breast, female genital tract, and lung. Dr Tawfik is active in application of immunocytochemical markers of tumors and in image analysis. His research interests include prognostic markers in breast, prostate, and gynecologic malignancies and the immunobiology of endometriosis. He was the recipient of the Residents' Excellence in Teaching Award in 1998 and 1999.

Elizabeth M. Van Cott, MD

Dr Van Cott received her MD degree from Harvard Medical School. She completed residency training in clinical pathology at Massachusetts General Hospital. Currently, she is the Director of the Coagulation Laboratory and Assistant Pathologist in the Department of Pathology at Massachusetts General Hospital. She provides written interpretations of lab results to clinicians for about 25 complex coagulation cases a day as part of the Coagulation Service operated through the Coagulation Laboratory. She has numerous teaching responsibilities at Harvard Medical School. She is a Fellow of the College of American Pathologists and the American Society of Clinical Pathologists and a member of the International Society on Thrombosis and Haemostasis. She is certified by the American Board of Pathology in Clinical Pathology. She holds several patents in the molecular biology field and has a number of publications in the field of coagulation.

HOW TO USE THIS HANDBOOK

The *Laboratory Test Handbook with Key Word Index* is arranged alphabetically by major clinical laboratory disciplines: Anatomic Pathology, Chemistry, Clinical Microscopy, Coagulation, Cytogenetics, Cytopathology, Hematology, Immunology, Infectious Diseases, Molecular Genetic Testing, Molecular Oncology, Therapeutic Drug Monitoring, Toxicology/ Drugs of Abuse, Trace Elements, Transfusion Medicine (Blood Bank), and Urinalysis. A general section, Specimen Collection and Point-of-Care Testing precedes the individual laboratory monographs. Issues of laboratory accuracy, laboratory statistics, and "normal range" are provided in the chapter titled Maximizing the Information From Laboratory Tests - The Ulysses Syndrome. The laboratory tests are listed alphabetically within each chapter and cross-referenced with synonyms referring the user to the actual test name.

Each individual test listing is arranged in a consistent format providing specific types of information. The fields of information include the following. The **test name**; **related information** which lists other tests that may be of interest and the page number in which such tests can be found; **synonyms** or other common names for a test are noted; topics or procedures which are not exact synonyms but have similar instructions or require similar consideration are referred to under the **applies to** heading; tests **replaced by** a current procedure may be noted; a definition of procedures included within the named test is given under **test includes**; an **abstract** or overview of the test is often provided; patient **preparation** includes patient care considerations prior to the collection of specimen or performance of a test; **aftercare** includes patient care considerations following the collection of a specimen or performance of a procedure; the specific **specimen** required, the **container, sampling time**, specific **collection** instructions, specimen **storage instructions, causes for rejection** of the specimen by the laboratory, **turnaround time** when relevant, and **special instructions** indicating additional pertinent considerations relating to the specimen are listed; a discussion of basic information relevant to the clinical application of the test, including **reference** (or normal) **range, critical values,** and **possible panic ranges,** specific **use** of the test, **limitations** of the test method(s), specific test **methodology** where appropriate, **contraindications** to the test, and **additional information** which may contribute to the interpretation or utilization of the test are given.

Footnotes and References

The bibliographic information provided with test listings may include footnotes referring to specific literature citations, specific points of information, or opinions. Selected general references are provided as sources of information concerning the individual test listings. Footnotes and references are intended, as well, to expedite access to useful literature. Many are current, but the alert reader will find an important reference from 1785.

The importance of the clinicopathologic conference as a teaching tool continues to be supported by the Case Records of the Massachusetts General Hospital in the *New England Journal of Medicine*. We have inserted these exercises as references, and sometimes footnotes, in numerous monographs throughout the *Laboratory Test Handbook*. We do not think that very sharp lines can or should be drawn between anatomic and clinical pathology, and we feel that these Cabot cases provide wonderful support for that notion.

Internet Web Sites

This edition of the *Laboratory Test Handbook* includes citations to internet web sites for those seeking additional information. There are numerous citations to special interest web sites, many of which are excellent. Various governmental agencies maintain web sites, such as the Centers for Disease Control and Prevention (ww.cdc.gov) and the Food and Drug Administration (www.fda.gov). There is growing interest in on-line medical textbooks (eg, emedicine.com) which are edited by established investigators and are usually fairly complete.

The editors point out that these sites are undergoing frequent revisions. Thus, we cannot be responsible for the quality of information on each site at any given time. Information at each web site should be compared with other sites for verification.

Acronyms and Abbreviations Glossary

This glossary provides a useful listing of many acronyms and abbreviations commonly associated with laboratory medicine. We offer this glossary not as an exhaustive authoritative list, but more as a guide to assist in interpretation of frequently used terminology.

Key Word Index

The Key Word Index is not intended in any way to suggest patterns of physicians' orders, nor is it complete. Rather, it is the intent of the authors and editors to make information easier to find and utilize in order to support better patient care.

The Key Word Index provides a reference to test names based on a diagnostic property, disease entity, organ system, or syndrome for which the test may be useful. It provides lists of specific tests. Some may support possible clinical diagnoses or help to rule out other diagnostic possibilities. The Key Word Index is further refined by using symbols: the (••) symbol indicates a test regarded as essential in the diagnosis of the disease; the (•) symbol denotes a test that is frequently used in the diagnosis or management of the disease. Other tests, listed without a symbol, are those that may or may not be useful, depending on particular clinical circumstances. A negative laboratory test result can be, and frequently is, highly relevant in the practice of medicine.

Clinical diagnosis is determined following history, physical examination, and usual laboratory investigation with selected additional tests. Complete blood count (CBC) with differential, urinalysis, and a basic chemistry profile are not only good medicine, they are in fact cost effective. Thus, these basic tests are excluded from much of the Key Word Index.

A few of the entities in the Key Word Index include a very brief explanation of the process or additional information which may be helpful.

Diagnoses with *International Classification of Disease—Ninth Revision—Clinical Modification* (ICD-9-CM) codes are indicated within the [ ] symbol.

Alphabetical Index

The most expedient method for locating a given test is the Alphabetical Index in the last section of this handbook. Test names and synonyms are listed and the page number on which the test description may be found is indicated.

MAXIMIZING THE INFORMATION FROM LABORATORY TESTS — THE ULYSSES SYNDROME

TESTS IN SEARCH OF A DISEASE

Dwight K. Oxley, MD

Uttam Garg, PhD

Eugene S. Olsowka, MD, PhD

Appropriate use of laboratory testing is so difficult that it has been compared with the obstacles encountered by the Greek hero Ulysses on his return from the Trojan War.[1] In this metaphor, the patient, like Ulysses, is put at risk, here because of misleading results from tests that should not, in a more perfect world, have been ordered. However, optimizing laboratory information has not been a high priority in undergraduate or graduate medical education; as a result, students must fend for themselves. This guide, intended as an introduction to an important topic, is divided into two major parts. In the first part, we examine how to protect the patient from misinterpreted or erroneously ordered tests. This goal includes four subtasks: how a "reference range" is established, why "normal range" is a misnomer, how to assess the analytical error involved in testing, and how to measure the usefulness of a test in actual practice. In the second part, we present some statistical principles important to laboratorians and to those who use laboratory tests.

PART ONE

THE "REFERENCE RANGE" PROBLEM AND BIOLOGIC VARIATION

Every test result from an accredited laboratory is accompanied by a "reference range." For certain tests, the reference range has been determined with reasonable accuracy and is well known; examples include hemoglobin, serum calcium, serum sodium, and leukocyte count. Even with these basic tests, however, the concept of a population-wide reference range is problematic. For clinical decision-making, the population-wide data for blood hemoglobin should be partitioned into one reference range for women and another for men. In fact, population-wide data distributions for many analytes are partitioned into subsets based on age, gender, and other patient attributes (eg, pregnancy).

The term "normal range" has been frequently used in the past and is not recommended for clinical practice because it is potentially misleading; the reference population used to define the reference range is selected for specific attributes rather than "normalcy." **Reference interval** is the preferred term for a statement which comprises lower and upper boundary values against which a patient result will be compared. A test result from an accredited laboratory is always reported with such a reference interval. Results outside of this interval are often flagged by the laboratory and interpreted by physicians as being significantly different from some accepted benchmark. Consider the example total serum calcium, an analyte in which concentration is under tight homeostatic control. The population-based "reference range" for such an analyte is approximately the same as the reference interval reported by most laboratories: 8.6-10.0 mg/dL. However, if the patient is a newborn full-term infant, the appropriate interval is quite different, viz 7.6-10.4 mg/dL. And if the patient has a low concentration of serum proteins, the reference interval must be adjusted by a formula based on the protein value. Patient age and serum protein status are only two of the many variables which influence the reference interval and therefore the interpretation of this test result. Other variables include gender, ethnicity, hydration status, lean body mass, pregnancy, posture, diet, exercise, current medications, how the specimen was obtained, and how the specimen was handled and stored before reaching the analytical system. **Preanalytical variability** is the term which includes all of these effects.

Another important source of variability in test results is that due to normal physiologic fluctuations (circadian rhythms). Consider the example of serum iron. An individual's serum iron is highest in the morning. The result obtained from a specimen obtained at 2 PM may be as much as 50% less than the value obtained at 8 AM.[2] Some analytes have fluctuations with periods that are measured in days or weeks. **Biologic variability** is the term which refers to this source of variability. An encyclopedic compilation of biologic variability is available.[3] Some examples of the within-day biologic variability of common analytes are presented in the table.

Total and Analytical Variation for Serum Tests on Specimens Obtained at 8 AM and 2 PM

Constituent	Mean	Total Variation (%)	Analytical Variation (%)
Sodium (mmol/L)	141	1.9	1.8
Potassium (mmol/L)	4.4	7.1	2.8
Calcium (mg/dL)	10.8	3.2	2.7
Chloride (mmol/L)	102	3.8	3.4
Phosphate (mg/dL)	3.8	10.7	2.4
Urea N (mg/dL)	14	22.5	2.5
Creatinine (mg/dL)	1.0	14.5	6.3
Uric acid (mg/dL)	5.6	11.5	2.6
Iron (µg/dL)	116	36.6	3.4
Cholesterol (mg/dL)	193	14.8	5.7
Albumin (g/dL)	4.5	5.5	3.9
Total protein (g/dL)	7.3	4.8	1.7
Total lipids (g/L)	5.3	25.0	3.6
Aspartate aminotransferase (units/L)	9	25	6
Alanine aminotransferase (units/L)	6	56	17
Acid phosphatase (units/L)	3	15	8
Alkaline phosphatase (units/L)	63	20	3
Lactate dehydrogenase (units/L)	195	16	12

11 male subjects, age 21-27 years, studied at 8 AM, 11 AM, and 2 PM.

From Burtis CA and Ashwood ER, eds, *Tietz Textbook of Clinical Chemistry*, 3rd ed, Philadelphia, PA: WB Saunders Co, 1999, 59.

The effects of both preanalytical and biologic variability on **plasma glucose** assays have been extensively studied. Fasting plasma glucose has a reference interval often stated as 60-109 mg/dL. But, as with calcium, this interval does not apply to all age groups. Much more important than the upper boundary of 109 mg/dL is the **clinical decision limit** of 126 mg/dL.[4] This clinical decision limit applies only to the diagnosis of diabetes mellitus. The point for emphasis is that a clinical decision limit is conceptually different from a reference range. A contingency affecting the clinical decision limit for the fasting plasma glucose reference interval arises from biologic variability: as revealed by the work of Troisi et al,[5] fasting plasma glucose levels are lower in the afternoon than in the morning. Since the criterion of 126 mg/dL was based on morning specimens, applying the 126 mg/dL clinical decision limit to patients whose blood is obtained in the afternoon will miss half of the cases of undiagnosed diabetes mellitus. One way to deal with this is to use a different clinical decision limit, viz 114 mg/dL, for patients whose specimens are obtained in the afternoon; another is to use only morning specimens.

Some of the most common sources of preanalytical variability are summarized below.

1. **Pregnancy.** Many of the analytes affected by pregnancy are listed in the following table.[6] An encyclopedic source also is available.[7]

Mean Serum and Plasma Laboratory Findings During Normal Pregnancy, Expressed as a Percentage of the Nonpregnant Mean*

Analyte	12 wk	28 wk	32 wk	36 wk	Term	1 d pp†
Sodium	97	99	98	98	97	99
Potassium	95	95	95	98	100	98
Bicarbonate	85	85	85	85	81	88
Chloride	98	99	100	99	99	100
Urea nitrogen	77	63	63	63	77	72
Creatinine	71	71	74	79	81	74
Fasting glucose	98	94	94	91	94	94
Bilirubin, unconjugated	56	56	67	67	78	78
Albumin	93	78	78	78	78	71
Protein	92	83	83	83	83	77
Uric acid	68	79	92	106	120	135
Calcium	98	94	94	95	97	94
Free ionized calcium	99	102	101	102	102	100
Parathyroid hormone, intact					140	
Vitamin 1,25-$(OH)_2D_3$					400	
Phosphate	108	99	97	103	96	106
Magnesium	92	90	87	87	87	86
Alkaline phosphatase	90	131	203	274	347	284

Mean Serum and Plasma Laboratory Findings During Normal Pregnancy, Expressed as a Percentage of the Nonpregnant Mean* *(continued)*

Analyte	Time of Gestation					
	12 wk	28 wk	32 wk	36 wk	Term	1 d pp†
Creatine kinase	87	86	86	90	135	257
α₁-Antitrypsin	129	169	174	189	191	187
Transferrin	105	145	160	160	170	139
Cholesterol	100	132	144	148	156	138
HDL cholesterol	121	121	119	127	130	116
LDL cholesterol	80	118	118	150	146	121
Fasting triglycerides	141	244	300	356	349	328
Iron	112	82	94	94	94	82
Iron-binding capacity	95	129	139	142	144	128
Transferrin saturation	136	68	68	76	64	56
Zinc protoporphyrin	107	116	109	119	144	135
Ferritin	81	33	33	37	59	81
Thyroxine	103	102	107	99	100	92
Triiodothyronine	100	121	121	116	121	95
Free thyroxine	98	71	72	62	74	80
Thyroxine-binding globulin	114	177	155	155	182	150
Thyroid-stimulating hormone	111	106	122	111	139	111
Cortisol	111	284	301	292	309	238
Aldosterone					1500	
Prolactin					800	
Hemoglobin	95	89	90	93	96	89
Hematocrit	94	89	91	94	97	91
Leukocyte count	144	167	167	165	240	222
Prothrombin time	99	99	97	98	97	100
Activated partial thromboplastin time	95	94	91	92	93	92
Platelet count	98	99	96	95	100	94
Fibrinogen	119	132	154	157	165	161

*The values are the means in pregnant subjects expressed as a percentage of the means in nonpregnant controls. (Most of the values are from Lockitch G, ed, *Handbook of Diagnostic Biochemistry and Hematology in Normal Pregnancy*, Boca Raton, FL: CRC Press, 1993.)

†pp = postpartum.

From Burtis CA and Ashwood ER, eds, *Tietz Textbook of Clinical Chemistry*, 3rd ed, Philadelphia, PA: WB Saunders Co, 1999, 1741.

2. **Exercise.** Individuals who exercise regularly are apt to experience a moderate or marked increase in high density lipoprotein cholesterol (HDLC) and slight elevations of urea nitrogen (BUN), and lactate dehydrogenase (LD). Immediately after strenuous exercise there are often elevations of lactate, creatine kinase (including the MB fraction), aldolase, alanine aminotransferase (ALT), aspartate aminotransferase (AST), phosphorus, acid phosphatase, creatinine, uric acid, haptoglobin, uric acid, transferrin, catecholamines, and leukocyte count; decreases may be seen in albumin, iron, and sodium. Marathon runners may develop marked hyponatremia during a race and may present emergently with hyponatremic encephalopathy.[8]

3. **Neonatal Period and Childhood.** Reference intervals appropriate for adults often are not valid for babies and children. Pediatric reference values are available in standard textbooks.[9,10]

4. **Older Individuals.** This is a relatively new field of investigation. A compilation of geriatric reference values is available.[11]

5. **Body Weight.** Most persons who are "overweight" have increased body fat (obesity) while a much smaller subset has increased lean body mass. Obesity itself has subdivisions based on the distribution of the excess adipose tissue (central vs peripheral). The effects of obesity as a preanalytical variable are not well understood. For example, obese individuals have elevated C-reactive protein levels but we do not know whether this is a marker for systemic inflammation or a preanalytical variable.[12]

6. **Posture** affects a number of test results. When blood is drawn in the upright position, the following analytes are described as increased: total protein, albumin, calcium, hemoglobin and hematocrit, renin, catecholamines (urine), alkaline phosphatase, cholesterol, alanine aminotransferase (ALT), and iron. As a person moves from the recumbent to the upright position, plasma water enters the interstitial fluid resulting in higher plasma concentrations of substances which do not readily pass the capillary endothelium.

7. **Diet** is a major source of preanalytic variability. For many analytes, such variation is controlled by obtaining specimens in the fasting state after 2 weeks on a diet of stable composition. Some of the more common tests for which an overnight fast is recommended are plasma glucose, lipids, iron, iron-binding capacity, vitamin B_{12}, folate, insulin, and gastrin.

   Blood specimens obtained shortly after a meal are problematic for many reasons. Postprandial turbidity interferes with many analytes, especially bilirubin, total protein, uric acid, and urea nitrogen (BUN). Postprandial potassium, triglyceride, and alkaline phosphatase values are increased, while phosphorus may be decreased. Diets high in protein can result in increased urea nitrogen (BUN), ammonia, and uric acid. Diets high in purines increase uric acid levels. The serotonin metabolite, 5-hydroxyindoleacetic acid (5-HIAA), is increased by diets rich in bananas, pineapples, tomatoes, and avocados. Caffeine and theophylline elevate catecholamines.

8. **Ethanol**. The ingestion of ethyl alcohol is followed acutely by increases in the serum levels of uric acid, lactate, gamma glutamyl transferase, triglycerides, and aspartate aminotransferase (AST). Long-term alcohol abuse is associated with increases in bilirubin, alkaline phosphatase, and the ratio AST:alanine aminotransferase (ALT). See also footnote 13.

9. **Oral Contraceptives and Estrogens**. These agents increase thyroxine-binding globulin, alpha₁-antitrypsin, iron, triglycerides, alanine aminotransferase, and gamma glutamyl transferase. Albumin may be decreased. See footnote 13.

10. **Other Drugs**. The potential effects of other drugs on laboratory tests are enormous. Current encyclopedic references are very helpful in practice.[13,14]

11. **Hemolysis** is a cause for specimen rejection in most nonemergent situations. Hemolysis causes increases in lactate dehydrogenase, bilirubin, potassium, aspartate aminotransferase (AST), creatine kinase (CK), alanine aminotransferase (ALT), and magnesium. Hemolysis invalidates the results of most coagulation tests and can mask hemolyzing antibodies in the antibody screen and crossmatch.

12. **Sampling Problems**. It is prudent to avoid, when possible, obtaining blood specimens from an extremity which is also an intravenous infusion site. Such samples are apt to have artefactually lowered values due to dilutional effects; this is a major problem in the interpretation of electrolytes, glucose, urea nitrogen (BUN), glucose, and coagulation tests.

    Tourniquets cause increases in potassium and lactate, and a decrease in pH. **Capillary whole blood samples** should be reported as such and accompanied by reference values appropriate for this matrix.

    Arterial samples should be reported as such and accompanied by reference values appropriate for this matrix.

    Inappropriate blood and urine collection containers, if unrecognized, can lead to misleading results.

    Specimens containing **clots** should be rejected. When serum is in prolonged contact with clots in venipuncture tubes, glucose decreases, while lactate dehydrogenase, potassium, and iron increase.

    Other Specimen Mishandling. Exposure to sunlight causes increases in leukocyte count, platelet count, and erythrocyte sedimentation rate, while bilirubin is decreased. Any delay beyond ~5 minutes in analyzing blood gases causes significant errors.

13. **Circadian Rhythms:** Circadian (approximately 24-hour) rhythms have implications for physiology, measurement of many laboratory tests, drug excretion (eg, salicylates, sulfonamides), and responses to therapy. Levels fluctuating very significantly during the 24-hour cycle include cortisol (which has different normals for 8 AM and 8 PM), growth hormone, serum acid phosphatase, aldosterone (high 6 AM to 3 PM), transferrin (maximum 4 PM to 8 PM), ACTH, serum iron, serum creatinine (7 PM values 130% of 7 AM concentration), eosinophils (low in afternoon), lymphocytes (maximum in early AM), WBC (maximum in early AM), leukocyte function, and urine urobilinogen (maximum excretion in afternoon). Urinary excretion of potassium, LH, FSH, TSH, testosterone, and some less commonly ordered hormones have some diurnal variation. Parathyroid hormone is best drawn at 8 AM.

    Triglyceride is higher in the afternoon, as is phosphate, BUN, and the hematocrit. Bilirubin falls in the PM, but overnight fasting itself causes bilirubin to increase.

    The waves which characterize circadian rhythms may be square shaped or may occur as a series of pulses. The latter pattern is seen with plasma cortisol concentration, which begins to increase during sleep. A large difference exists between this level and that found in the evening. Still another pattern is a single daily pulse such as occurs with growth hormone secretion.

    The magnitude of the effect of circadian rhythms is greater than is generally recognized. Although only 10% variation exists for plasma potassium concentration, urinary potassium excretion can vary fivefold during the day.

    Some hormone secretion cycles are longer (infradian) – eg, the menstrual cycle.

An encyclopedic compilation of the effects of preanalytical variables is available.[15]

PROBABILITIES OF TEST RESULTS WITHIN REFERENCE RANGE ON MULTIPLE PANELS

A reference range for a particular analyte generally covers 95% of healthy or normal results. It means that 5% of results from healthy individuals will fall outside this limit. Thus, the probability of a healthy person having two test results within reference range is 0.95 x 0.95 = 0.9025 or 90.25%. This phenomenon will progress as multiple tests are ordered (see table below).

Probability That a Healthy Individual Will Have All Test Results Within Reference Range

Number of Tests Ordered	Probability (%)
1	95.0
2	90.2
5	77.4
10	59.9
20	35.8

ANALYTICAL ERROR AND THE COEFFICIENT OF VARIATION

Imprecision, also known as **random error**, refers to the distribution of results when an assay is performed repeatedly on the same specimen. Imprecision may be measured as within-run, within-day, day-to-day, or over any other time interval. In general, the longer the time interval, the larger the random error. When the distribution of repeated results is approximately Gaussian in distribution (ie, a bell-shaped curve), imprecision is expressed numerically as the **coefficient of variation (CV)**. **The CV is the standard deviation of the results divided by the mean, and expressed as a percentage**. A small CV implies good precision, while a large CV implies relatively poor precision. All laboratories can, and should, calculate the within-run and day-to-day imprecision of their assays and make the results available to interested clients.

Accuracy refers to how close a reported test result is to the true value. Proficiency testing results, both external and internal, provide a measure of accuracy. External proficiency testing programs often provide results that are obtained by, or linked to, definitive or reference methods. The difference between a particular clinical result and the result obtained by the definitive (or reference) method is proportional to the **bias** or **systematic error**. It is important to note that even reference methods can have bias when comparing results. As an example, reference methods may give a different concentration of a particular analyte when compared to gravimetrically prepared specimens. Ionicity, protein concentrations, and other environmental factors are known matrix effects in proficiency testing. Matrix effects are inherent in any analytical system. Laboratories should choose methods that minimize matrix effects.

While random error is relatively easy to calculate, and systematic error is difficult, what really counts is the combination of the two, or **total error**. Methods of calculating total error, and its components, can be found in the following section of this chapter as well as in standard references.[16] A laboratory director should furnish information on total error performance to interested physicians and other scientists.

DECISION ANALYSIS — PREDICTIVE VALUE THEORY — WHAT DOES THIS RESULT MEAN?

The ability of a laboratory test to identify a particular disease is quantified by two measurements: **sensitivity** and **specificity**.

Sensitivity is the frequency of a positive (abnormal) test result among all patients with a particular disease ("positivity in disease" is a commonly used descriptive that is easy to remember). In other words sensitivity of a test indicates its ability to generate a true positive (TP), not false negative (FN), result when a diseased individual is tested. It is calculated by testing a population of patients who have been found to have a particular disease by some gold standard method. Mathematically it is expressed as:

$$\text{Sensitivity} = \frac{TP}{TP + FN} \times 100\%$$

Specificity is the frequency of a negative (normal) test result among all persons who do not have disease ("negativity in health" is a commonly used descriptive that is easy to remember). In other words specificity of a test indicates its ability to generate a true negative (TN), not false positive (FP), result when a healthy individual is tested. It is calculated by testing a group of persons who do not have a particular disease in question. Mathematically it is expressed as:

$$\text{Specificity} = \frac{TN}{TN + FP} \times 100\%$$

Example: A method is evaluated for its sensitivity and specificity for disease XYZ. 100 healthy individuals and 100 individuals with disease XYZ are tested with this test. The following results are obtained:

Test Result	DISEASE XYZ Present	Absent	Total
Positive	95 (TP)	10 (FP)	105
Negative	5 (FN)	90 (TN)	95
Total	100 (TP + FN)	100 (FP + TN)	200

Sensitivity and specificity of the test are:

$$\text{Sensitivity} = \frac{95}{95 + 5} \times 100\% = 95\%$$

$$\text{Specificity} = \frac{90}{90 + 10} \times 100\% = 90\%$$

Other statistics, which are used to assess the diagnostic value of a test, are **predictive value** and **efficiency** of a test. Predictive value of a positive or negative result relates to the number of correct positive or negative results respectively. Efficiency relates to the total number of correct results. Mathematically these terms are defined as:

$$\textbf{Predictive value (positive result)} = \frac{TP}{TP + FP} \times 100\%$$

$$\textbf{Predictive value (negative result)} = \frac{TN}{TN + FN} \times 100\%$$

$$\textbf{Efficiency} = \frac{TP + TN}{TP + FP + TN + FN} \times 100\%$$

What will be the predictive value of the above test for the diagnosis of disease XYZ? To answer that question we must know one more statistic: the prevalence of disease XYZ in the population under study. Illustrated below is the performance of the test where the prevalence of XYZ is 50%. In actual practice, what we really need to know is how predictive a positive (or negative) test result is for the presence (or absence) of disease XYZ in a particular patient. To determine the predictive value we calculate as follows:

Test Result	DISEASE XYZ (PREVALENCE 50%) Present	Absent	Total	
Positive	95	10	105	PV positive = 95/105 = 90.4%
Negative	5	90	95	PV negative = 90/95 = 94.7%
Total	100	100	200	

The **predictive value (PV)** of a positive test result is the frequency of disease XYZ among all persons with a positive (abnormal) test result. As illustrated above, the predictive value of a positive test in this situation is ~90%; this means that 90% of persons with the disease will have a positive test, and 10% will have a negative test (false negative). The PV of a negative test result is the frequency of disease XYZ absence among all persons with a negative test result. Approximately 95% of persons free of disease XYZ will have a negative (normal) result, while ~5% of such persons will have a false positive result.

The following table illustrates the effect of disease prevalence on predictive values.

Test Result	DISEASE XYZ (PREVALENCE 10%) Present	Absent	Total	
Positive	95	90	185	PV positive = 95/185 = 51.3%
Negative	5	810	815	PV negative = 810/815 = 99.3%
Total	100	900	1000	

A point for emphasis is the marked decrease in the predictive value of a positive test when the prevalence changes from high to low. In the low prevalence situation only about 50% of the positive tests are true positives, while in the high prevalence situation ~90% of positive results are true positives. In many clinical scenarios, the disease prevalence may be ~1%, or even lower; in such situations false positives may outnumber true positives by factors of 100 or 1000. A corollary of this is that, to function as a good screening test – a test applied across an entire population of asymptomatic persons – test sensitivity must approach 100%.

RECEIVER OPERATING CHARACTERISTIC (ROC) CURVES

The statistics of sensitivity, specificity, and predictive values can be formatted in many ways. One of the more popular ways is the construction of receiver operating characteristic (ROC) curves. Whereas the tables shown allow one to determine the predictive values at one decision limit, ROC curve analysis portrays, in graphic fashion, the trade-off between true positives and false positives.

ROC curves were developed during World War II. Radar receiver operators detected blips that may have represented hostile aircraft. Many a receptor squadron scrambled on the basis of such blips to find a flock of wild geese instead of hostile aircraft. It was recognized that there was a trade-off between sensitivity and specificity. As sensitivity increased so did the false-positive interpretations.

The principle of ROC states that for any given test system, the false-positive rate (1-specificity) is a function of sensitivity. As sensitivity increases, the false-positive rate increases linearly – up to a point. After this point, the false-positive rate rises disproportionately high. Thus, there is a limit to the sensitivity of any test system. When the limit is exceeded, the false-positive rate may become unacceptable. A laboratory test becomes unacceptable when desired sensitivity cannot be attained because of a large number of false positives. The limitation of the ROC curve analysis is that it depends on a gold standard (independent criterion) for the presence of clinical disease. The analysis will not be very good if the gold standard is a poor one. ROC analysis should be used in conjunction with clinical decision analysis by clinicians who have an understanding of the benefits and risks of the therapeutic and diagnostic procedures that may follow from the results of a particular laboratory test.

Figure 1 presents a prototypic ROC curve. The dashed diagonal line represents a test with a sensitivity of 50% and a specificity of 50% – equivalent to a coin toss. A good test will have an ROC curve that lies to the left of the dashed diagonal; the farther to the left, the better the combination of sensitivity and specificity and the better the performance in practice. The curve denoted as a nonideal test performs only slightly better than a coin toss, and the curve denoted ideal is typical of many clinically useful tests. The curve denoted "Brand X" is typical of tests which, while perhaps adequate for limited purposes, do not perform well and, over time, are replaced by better ones.

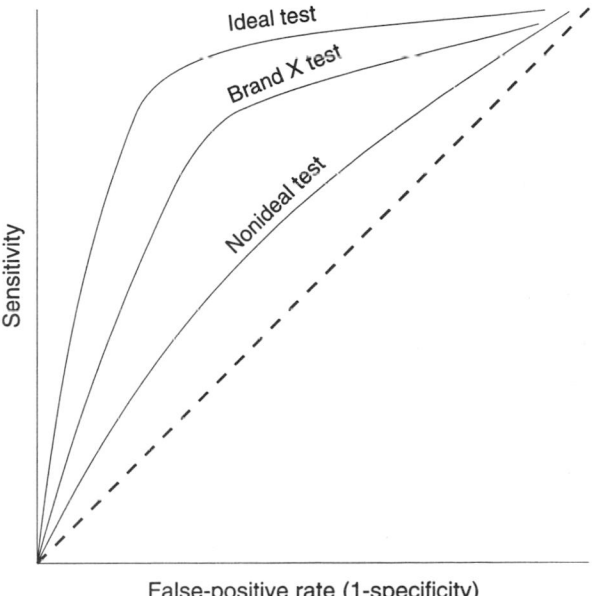

Figure 1. Typical receiver operating curve

A laboratory director must decide what numerical **clinical decision limit** (cutoff value) is best for a given test. The selection of such a decision limit involves an inevitable trade-off between sensitivity and specificity. Thus, selection of a very high (or stringent) limit will usually reduce sensitivity and increase specificity – more false negatives and fewer false positives. A less stringent decision limit has the opposite effects – increased sensitivity and decreased specificity.

Figure 2[17] illustrates two ROC curves, one for prostate-specific antigen (PSA) and one for prostatic acid phosphatase (PAP) in the detection of prostate carcinoma.

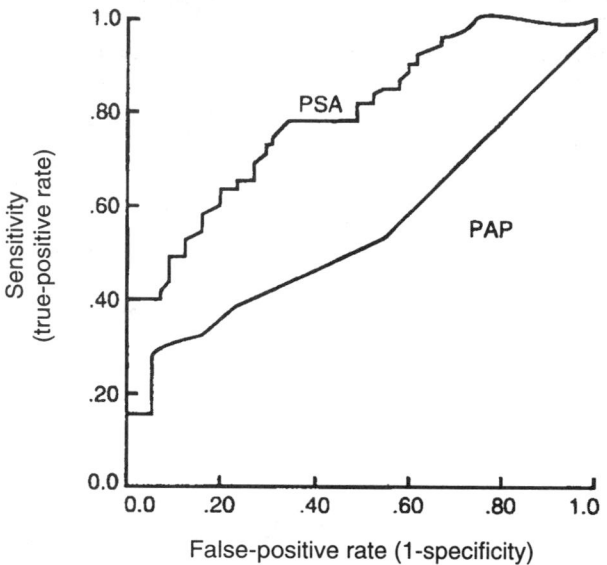

Figure 2. Receiver operating characteristic curves of prostatic acid phosphatase (PAP) and prostate-specific antigen (PSA) assays for patients with benign hyperplasia and carcinoma of prostate. Because the PSA assay curve is above the PAP assay curve at all points, the better assay for the patients tested is the PSA assay.

Adapted from *Tietz Textbook of Clinical Chemistry*, 3rd ed, Burtis CA and Ashwood ER, eds, Philadelphia, PA: WB Saunders Co, 1999, 314.

Note that the true-positive rate is on the vertical axis and the false-positive rate is on the horizontal axis. Moving upward on the vertical axis, and moving to the right on the horizontal axis, corresponds to lowering the cutoff value associated with a positive test. Diagnostic accuracy is approximately proportional to the area under the ROC curve. The fact that the PSA curve lies to the left of the PAP curve means that the area under the PSA curve is greater than the area under the PAP curve, and, therefore, that the PSA test performs better.

Another example of ROC analysis is in the evaluation of new tests. Bender et al[18] have compared two tests for fetal lung maturity: the conventional lecithin:sphingomyelin ratio (L:S ratio) and a fluorescence polarization immunoassay, the surfactant:albumin ratio (S:A ratio). They reported that, between 29 and 37 weeks gestation, a wide range of values is observed at every interval, and this indicates that gestational age accounts for only a small fraction of the total variation in test results for both tests. They found a wide divergence between the L:S ratio results and S:A ratio results, which suggests either a nonlinear relationship between the two tests, or that one (or both) test(s) is/are affected by nonsurfactant substances in amniotic fluid. Their ROC curves are presented in Figure 3. It is important to note that the ROC curve for the S:A ratio (heavy line) lies to the left of the ROC curve for the L:S test; stated another way, the area under the S:A curve (0.869) is slightly larger than the area under the L:S curve (0.847). The clinically important implication from the Figure 3 is that there is no statistically significant difference between the area under the two ROC curves. Stated another way, once the result from one of the tests is known, determining the other result appears to provide no additional information.

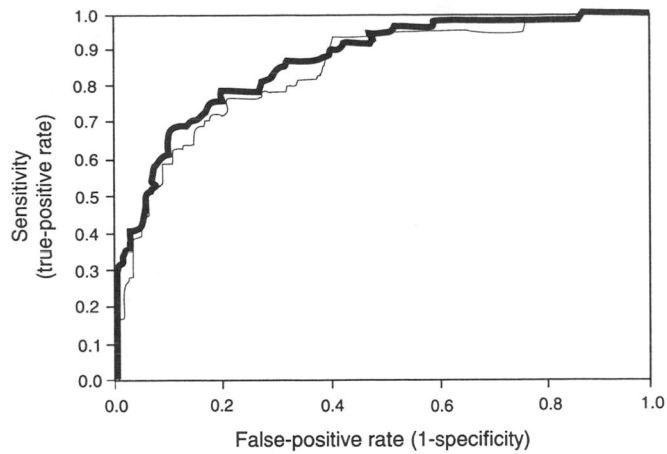

Figure 3. ROC curves comparing L/S (thin line) and S/A (heavy line). The area defined by the L/S curve is 0.847 (SE 0.0438); that for the S/A curve, 0.869 (SE 0.0406). The Z score for difference in areas was 0.729 (P >0.05).

Adapted from Bender TM, Stone LR, and Amenta JS, "Diagnostic Power of Lecithin/Sphingomyelin Ratio and Fluorescence Polarization Assays for Respiratory Distress Syndrome Compared by Relative Operating Characteristic Curves," *Clin Chemistry*, 1994, 40(4):543.

CONCURRENT DISEASE PROCESSES

While most physicians of a certain age were indoctrinated in medical school with the goal of finding one grand unifying diagnosis to explain all of a patient's symptoms, signs, laboratory results and imaging findings, the reality is that many people have multiple disease processes at once. Quite obviously, concurrent diseases will also modify test results and alter the significance of certain reference intervals. A useful listing of how these concurrent diseases affect test results is available.[19]

ULYSSES REACHES HOME AT LAST

Sources of variation, preanalytical and biologic, and sources of analytic error are so numerous that, at the current state-of-the-art, no test result should be interpreted without consideration of the entire clinical picture. Even with computer-based decision support systems,[20] test interpretation remains a complex process, and patients are still at risk from unintended consequences of well-intentioned diagnostic evaluations. We began this chapter by referring to an analogy between the Greek hero Ulysses and the patient at risk. We conclude by turning to the lessons taught in Homer's masterpiece. Recall that Ulysses finally reached his home in Ithaca only after overcoming a host of obstacles and injuries, many of which could have been predicted and, therefore, avoided. During his long arduous journey of self-discovery, Ulysses received help from a number of people, but most significantly from the beautiful Phaeacian princess, Nausicaä. The astute clinician models an error-avoidance strategy after the wily Ulysses, and adopts a skeptical attitude toward test results, especially results which do not fit clinically. A successful outcome will be even more likely if the clinician's pathologist follows the model of Nausicaä, who showed Ulysses how to resist the temptation of the moment and stay the homeward course.

PART TWO

LABORATORY STATISTICS

Statistics is a branch of mathematics often much maligned by many current day savants. One often hears the incorrect expression, "You can say anything you like by using statistics." Substitution of the word "using" for the more accurate "misusing" corrects an incorrect expression. It is by the misuse of statistics (intentional or otherwise) that facts may be misconstrued. More colloquially, "statistics don't lie, people do." As our common everyday statistics and hypothesis testing are ultimately derived from probabilistic equations, discussion of statistics must necessarily include a discussion of probability. Following are some of the more common definitions and equations that are used daily in laboratory medicine, often hidden from conscious thought.

Sample Space: A collection of objects or outcomes of interest. As an example, in an unbiased single coin toss the sample space consists of the outcome heads or tails.

Relative Frequency: The ratio of the number of times an event occurs to the total number of observations. Relative frequencies are unstable for a small number of observations. For example, the relative frequency of obtaining a heads or a tails in an unbiased coin toss is 50% for a large number of tosses. It may be different for a limited number of tosses – say four.

Probability: The stable (over a large number of observations) relative frequency associated with an event. The probability of event A is usually denoted by the symbol $P(A)$.

Random Variable: Given a sample space S with elements s and a function X, X is called a random variable if it assigns to each element s in the sample space S one and only one real number. Put mathematically, the random function X acting on sample space S is defined by the set of real numbers [x: x=X(s), s is an element of S]. One of the major problems for applied statisticians is to define such functions. As an example: to determine the effect of a diet on development of an animal, we may choose to look at total body weight gain, bone or organ growth, or times to maturation or senescence.

Statistic: A function of the elements of a random sample that does not depend upon any unknown parameters of the sample. Mean, median, mode, range, and variance of a given sample are all statistics.

Median: The middle most number in a data set (when the data set is arranged in ascending or descending order).

Mode: Most frequently occurring result or measurement in a data set.

Population Mean: Usually denoted by the symbol μ.

Population Variance: Usually denoted by the symbol σ^2. Typically μ and σ^2 are unknown and are estimated from $\overline{X}$ and S^2 – the sample mean and variance.

Mean of a Sample: Denoted by:

$$\overline{X} = 1/n \left(\sum_{i=1}^{n} X_i \right)$$

Variance of a Sample: Denoted by:

$$S^2 = (1/n) \sum_{i=1}^{n} (X_i - \overline{X})^2$$

or

$$S^2 = \left((1/n) \sum_{i=1}^{n} X_i^2 \right) - \overline{X}^2$$

Note: Using 1/n yields the variance of the empirical (sample) distribution. Use of 1/n-1 yields the unbiased estimator of σ^2. 1/n+1 yields the minimum mean square error estimator of σ^2. Standard deviation σ is the square root of the variance σ^2.

Coefficient of Variation (CV): Standard deviation expressed as percent of mean. Mathematically, it can be calculated by dividing standard deviation by the mean and multiplying by 100%. Mathematically it is defined as:

$$CV = \frac{\text{standard deviation}}{\text{mean}} \times 100\%$$

Standard Deviation (S): It is a measure of the spread or dispersion within a set of sample data. Mathematically it is the **square root of variance**.

Standard Error (SE): The standard error, or standard error of the mean, is an estimate of the standard deviation of the sampling distribution of means, based on the data from one or more random samples from population being tested. Mathematically it is defined as:

$$SE = \frac{standard\ deviation}{\sqrt{n}}$$

Confidence Interval: Limits in which a specified portion of a population is expected to lie or limits with probability of including true value, 95% confidence intervals are mean ± 2SE.

Example: A glucose control was repeated in a laboratory, with the following values (mg/dL) arranged in descending order. Calculate the mean, median, mode, variance, standard deviation, coefficient of variation, standard error, and 95% confidence interval.

Value (mg/dL)	$(X_i-\overline{X})$	$(X_i-\overline{X})^2$
104	5	25
103	4	16
102	3	9
102	3	9
101	2	4
101	2	4
101	2	4
100	1	1
100	1	1
100	1	1
100	1	1
99	0	0
99	0	0
99	0	0
99	0	0
99	0	0
98	-1	1
98	-1	1
98	-1	1
98	-1	1
97	-2	4
97	-2	4
97	-2	4
96	-3	9
96	-3	9
95	-4	16
94	-5	25

Using above equations:

Mean ($\overline{X}$) = 99 mg/dL

Median = 99 mg/dL; the middle value when values are arranged in ascending or descending order

Mode = 99 mg/dL; the most frequent value

Note: The data is normally distributed and thus has same mean, median, and mode

Variance (S^2) = 5.76 mg/dL

Standard deviation (S) = 2.40 mg/dL

Coefficient of variation (CV) = S x 100% / mean = 2.43%

$$Standard\ error\ of\ mean\ (SE) = \frac{SD}{\sqrt{n}} = \frac{2.4}{\sqrt{27}} = 0.46\ mg/dL$$

95% confidence interval: (mean − 2 x SE) to (mean + 2 x SE) = 98.1- 99.9 mg/dL

There is 95% probability that mean glucose value is between 98.1-99.9 mg/dL

Biased Statistic: A statistic is said to be biased if it is not equal to the parameter it is intended to measure. For example, if the mean $\overline{X}$ of a sampling distribution is not equal to the population mean μ, then the mean $\overline{X}$ is said to be biased. Conversely, if the mean $\overline{X}$ equals the parameter μ, then $\overline{X}$ is said to be unbiased.

Binomial Probability Function: Let p be a probability of success for a certain event. Then the probability of failure of the event is q = 1 − p. If n = total number of trials and x = the number of successes, the probability (p) of the number of successes in n trials is:

$$P(x) = (n!/x!(n-x)!) \; p^x q^{n-x}$$

Example: If each assay in a particular laboratory has a 1 in 100 chance of being erroneous, find the probability of finding 3 erroneous results in a batch of 10. Here n = 10, x = 3, p = 0.01, and q = 1 - 0.01 = 0.99. Probability of 3 erroneous results in a batch of 10 in this laboratory is given by:

$P(3) = (10!/3! \; (7)!) \; 0.01^3 \; 0.99^7$

$P(3) = (3628800/6 \; (5040)) \; 10^{-6} \; 0.9321$

$P(3) = 120 \; (9.321 \times 10^{-7})$

$P(3) = 0.000112$

Example: Under the above error rate assumptions, find the probability of an error with 5 replicated tests being made. Here the 10 tests consist of 5 tests with replication. With 10 tests, there is a total of 45 pairs of tests that could be in error; (10!/2! 8!) however, we are constrained to 5 combinations of replicate tests. The probability is given by:

$P(error) = 5 \; (0.01^2) \; 0.99^8 = 5 \; (10^{-4}) \; 0.9227$

$P(error) = 5 \; (9.23 \times 10^{-5}) = 0.0046$

Poisson Distribution: A special adaptation of the binomial distribution, given by the formula:

$$P \; (X=x) = \lambda^x e^{-\lambda}/x!$$

or

$$P(X \leq x) = \sum_{k=0}^{x} (\lambda^k e^{-\lambda}/k!)$$

where λ is equal to both the mean and the variance of the Poisson distribution (the probability of a given event occurring in a short time h must be λh). This distribution may be used to calculate the probabilities of the number of times particular events occur in a given time or on a given object. For example, this distribution may be used to calculate the probability of obtaining defective cuvettes over a period of time in a manufacturing process. If a manufacturer of cuvettes expects two bad cuvettes every 5 minutes, what is the probability of five or more bad cuvettes in 15 minutes? Here, the average number of bad cuvettes in 15 minutes is six (ie, $\lambda = 6$). If we assume a Poisson process then

$$P(X \geq 5) = 1 - P(X=4) = \sum_{i=0}^{4} 6^i e^{-6}$$

$$= 1 - 0.285 = 0.715 \text{ or } 71\%$$

Normal (Bell-Shaped) Distribution: Let μ = mean of the normal random variable, x, σ = standard deviation, π = 3.1416, and e = 2.71828, then the probability density function of a normal distribution is given by the equation:

$$f(x) = (1/\sigma \sqrt{2\pi}) \; e^{-((x-\mu)^2/2\sigma^2)}$$

The z score gives the distance between a measurement and the mean in units equal to the standard deviation (ie, $z = (x - \mu)/\sigma$). The distribution of z scores, also known as a standard normal distribution, always has a mean of 0 and a standard deviation of 1.

Student's t Distribution: Let Z be a random variable that is normally distributed with mean 0 and variance 1, and let U be a random variable that is chi-square distributed with r degrees of freedom. If Z and U are independent, then

$$T = Z/\sqrt{U/r}$$

has a t distribution with r degrees of freedom. The probability density function is a rather complicated gamma function and the interested reader is encouraged to seek it in more specialized statistical textbooks. Figure 4 compares a normal distribution with mean 0 and variance 1 with a t distribution with 4 degrees of freedom. Note that the t distribution has more extreme probability than the normal distribution.

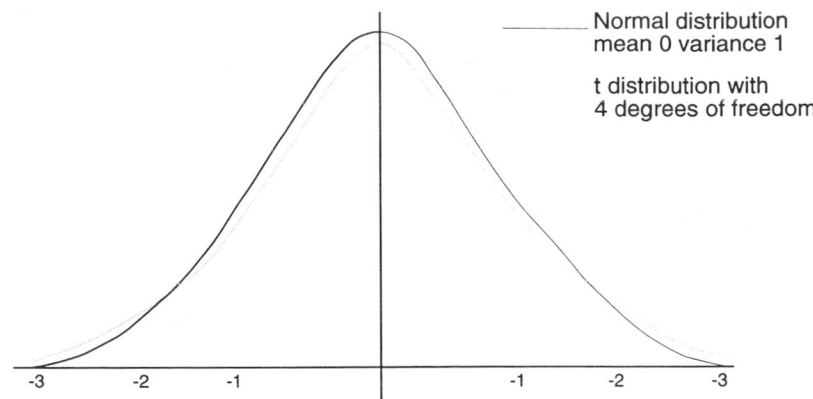

Figure 4. t distribution with 4 degrees of freedom compared with
a normal distribution of mean 0 and variance 1

The Gamma Distribution: The random variable X is said to have a gamma distribution if its probability density function is defined by the equation

$$F(x) = \begin{cases} \dfrac{1}{\Upsilon(\alpha)\theta^{\alpha}} X\alpha^{-1}e^{-x/\theta} & 0 \le x < \infty \\ 0 & x < 0 \end{cases}$$

where the gamma function is defined as:

$$\Upsilon(t) = \int_{0}^{\infty} y^{t-1}e^{-y}dy \qquad\qquad t > 0$$

The Chi-Square Distribution: Let X have a gamma distribution with $\theta = 2$ and $\alpha = r/2$ where r is a positive integer called the "degrees of freedom". X is chi-square distributed if its probability density function is given by:

$$f(x) = \begin{cases} \dfrac{1}{\Upsilon(r/2)2^{r/2}} X^{r/2-1}e^{-x/2} & 0 \le x < \infty \\ 0 & x < 0 \end{cases}$$

The mean and variance of a chi-square distribution are

$$u = \alpha\theta = r \qquad \text{and} \qquad \sigma^2 = \alpha\theta^2 = 2r$$

(ie, the mean is equal to the number of degrees of freedom and the variance is equal to twice the number of the degrees of freedom).

The F Distribution: Let U and V be independent chi-square variables with r1 and r2 degrees of freedom. Then F is said to have an F distribution with r1 and r2 degrees of freedom when defined as:

$$F = \frac{U/r1}{V/r2}$$

The probability density function is complicated and the reader is encouraged to seek out advanced statistical textbooks. Graphs of some typical F distributions are seen in Figure 5. Note that this distribution is asymmetric and skewed. F distributions have many uses. They may be used to test equality of variances and linearity in regression analysis, among other uses.

The F Test: Let MST be the mean square for a group of k treatments (sum of squares/k-1). Let MSE be the mean square for error given by sum of squares for error/n-k, where n = number of measurements. Then to compare the two sources of variability – source of variability among treatment means with that due to differences within samples, one may use the statistic:

$$F = MST/MSE$$

with k-1 and n-k degrees of freedom. This test assumes that all k populations are normally distributed, the k population variances are equal, and samples are randomly and independently selected. In the case of determining linearity in a single variable regression, the error may be partitioned into that of the regression and residual. An F test defined as:

$$F = MS \text{ (regression)}/MS \text{ (residual)}$$

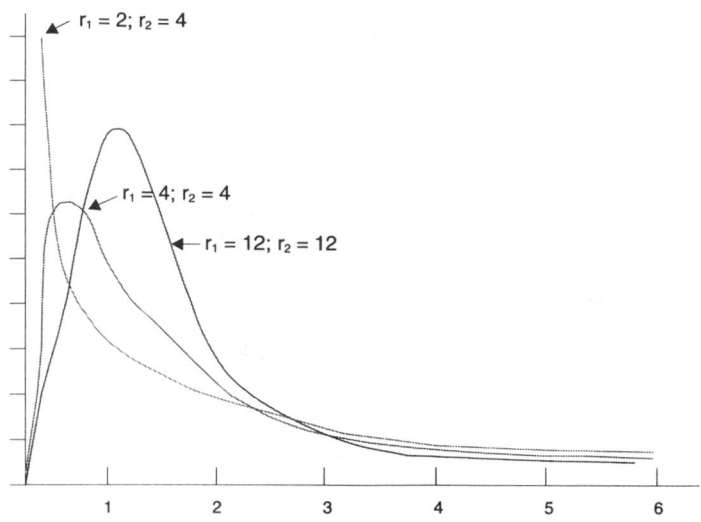

Figure 5. F distribution with r_1 and r_2 degrees of freedom

may be used to determine whether there is a true linear effect. Note that as assays become more precise, mean square residual error decreases which tends to increase the ratio. Thus, as assays become more precise, the F test may appear to magnify subtle departures from linearity. This helps to explain the observation that with very precise assays a clinically acceptable linear assay may not pass a statistical test of linearity. As the F test typically involves a comparison of two sources of variance, procedures utilizing F tests may be referred to as "analysis of variance."

The F test may be used to test for equal variances. Assay variance is also termed "imprecision" or "precision". The larger the variance (hence, standard deviation and coefficient of variability), the less precise the assay is said to be. One may then use the F test to determine if one assay is as imprecise as another.

Example: Assay 1 was compared with assay 2 for 21 days. The variance (S^2) of a series of measurements was 1432 for assay 1 and 3500 for assay 2. Is the imprecision of each assay comparable?

Answer: The test statistic here is denoted by:

$$F = \frac{\text{larger sample variance}}{\text{smaller sample variance}} = \frac{3500}{1432} = 2.44$$

From published tables, the critical value of $F_{0.5}$ with 20 degrees of freedom in the numerator and denominator is 2.12 and $F_{0.01}$ is 2.94. Thus, at the $\alpha=0.05$ significance level, we conclude that assay 1 is more precise (less imprecise) than assay 2. If we were held to more stringent significance levels, say $\alpha=0.01$, we could not conclude that the variances of the two assays were different (null hypothesis: $S_1^2 - S_2^2 = 0$).

Completely random design:

Let:

  N = total number of observations

  b = number of blocks

  K = number of treatments

  T_i = treatment total for a given block

  B_i = block totals

Assume:

  1. Distribution are normal

  2. Variances are equal

An example is taken from McClove and Dietrich[21] with figures representing serum creatinine and blocks representing laboratories rather than supermarkets. The different treatments represent different assay methods. Here there are four treatments and ten blocks.

Serum Creatinine (mg/dL)

Lab	A	B	C	D	Total
1	2.43	2.47	2.47	2.41	9.78
2	2.48	2.52	2.53	2.48	10.01
3	2.38	2.44	2.42	2.35	9.59
4	2.40	2.47	2.46	2.39	9.72
5	2.35	2.42	2.44	2.32	9.53
6	2.43	2.49	2.47	2.42	9.81
7	2.55	2.62	2.64	2.56	10.37
8	2.41	2.49	2.47	2.39	9.76
9	2.53	2.60	2.59	2.49	10.21
10	2.35	2.43	2.44	2.36	9.58
Total	24.31	24.95	24.93	24.17	98.36

Then:

SS(Total) = Total sum of squares

$$= \Sigma x^2 - \frac{(\Sigma x)^2}{N}$$

SST = Sum of squares for treatments

$$= \frac{\Sigma (\text{treatment totals})^2}{b} = \frac{T_i^2 + \ldots + T_k^2}{b} = SS(\text{Total})$$

SSB = Sum of squares for blocks

$$= \frac{\Sigma (Bi)^2}{K} - SS(\text{Total})$$

SSE = Sum of squares for error

$$= SS(\text{Total}) - SST - SSB$$

Mean square for treatments $= MST = \dfrac{SST}{K-1}$

Mean square for blocks $= MSE = \dfrac{SSE}{(b-1)(K-1)}$

Then: $F = \dfrac{MST}{MSE}$

Is there a difference in the assay values from a standard serum creatinine among the assay methods A to D?

SS(Total) = 0.22936
SST = 0.05000
SSB = 0.17451
SSE = SS(Total) - SST - SSB = 0.00485

$$MST = \frac{SST}{K-1} = \frac{0.05}{3} = 0.01667$$

$$MSB = \frac{SSB}{b-1} = \frac{0.17451}{9} = 0.01939$$

$$MSE = \frac{SSE}{(b-1)(K-1)} = \frac{0.00485}{(9)(3)} = \frac{0.00485}{27} = 0.00017963$$

$$\text{Then } F = \frac{MST}{MSE} = \frac{0.01667}{0.00017963} = 92.8$$

Here the critical F for an $\alpha=0.05$ is 2.96

Thus, F = 92.8 > 2.96, and we conclude that at least two of the assay means are different.

29

t-Test: A statistical test to determine if two means are different or if experimental mean is different from the target value. t-Test may be unpaired (means derived from independent populations) or paired (means derived from the same population). Depending on whether variances of two data sets are equal or not, unpaired t-test is divided into unpaired t-test for equal or unequal variances. The following equations are used:

$$t \text{ (unpaired equal variance)} = \frac{\overline{X}_1 - \overline{X}_2}{Sp^2 \sqrt{(1/n_1 + 1/n_2)}}$$

where $\overline{X}_1 - \overline{X}_2$ are means of two data sets, and n_1 and n_2 are number of observations of two data sets respectively. Sp^2 is the pooled variance and is calculated as follows:

$$Sp^2 = \frac{(n_1 - 1) S_1^2 + (n_2 - 1) S_2^2}{n_1 + n_2 - 2}$$

$$t \text{ (unpaired unequal variance)} = \frac{\overline{X}_1 - \overline{X}_2}{\sqrt{S_1^2/n_1 + S_2^2/n_2}}$$

where S_1 and S_2 are standard deviations of two data sets.

$$t \text{ (paired)} = \frac{\overline{X}_1 - \overline{X}_2}{S_d/\sqrt{n}}$$

where S_d is the standard deviation of differences between the paired values and n is the number of samples.

Example (unpaired t-test):[22] A laboratory receives samples for serum immunoglobulin A from two different regions. The laboratory wants to know if immunoglobulin A levels in healthy individuals from these two regions are the same. The following data (mg/L) is obtained from healthy individuals. As the data is derived from two independent populations, unpaired t-test should be used.

	Region A	Region B
Mean	2260	2650
Standard deviation	584	473
N	33	29

First, F-test must be used to find out whether variances of two data sets are same or not.

$$F = \frac{\text{larger variance}}{\text{smaller variance}} = \frac{(584)^2}{(473)^2} = 1.52$$

Critical value for F, at $p = 0.05$ is 1.84 (from F-table). It means that difference between two variances is not significant with $p < 0.05$. Therefore, t-test for equal variances must be used. To calculate t value, Sp^2 must be calculated. Using following equations:

$$Sp^2 = \frac{(33 - 1) \times (584)^2 + (29 - 1) \times (473)^2}{33 + 29 - 2} = 535$$

$$t = \frac{2260 - 2650}{(535)^2 \times \sqrt{(1/33) + (1/29)}} = -2.86$$

Critical value for t at $p = 0.05$ is 2.00 (from t-table). It means the difference between two means is significant with $p < 0.05$.

If variances would have been significantly different, then t-test for unpaired unequal variances must be used.

Example (paired t-test): A laboratory evaluated a new method for glucose assay by comparing with old method. Following results were obtained (in mg/dL). Are means of these two assays significantly different?

Old Method (X)	New Method (Y)	X-Y
45	42	3
102	105	-3
89	92	-3
109	112	-3
202	193	9
57	53	4
152	144	8
85	89	-4
56	52	4
89	95	-6
154	153	1
83	81	2
110	115	-5
175	168	7
125	121	4
67	63	4
49	52	-3
78	83	-5
133	142	-9
169	159	10

Bias = (mean of X) − (mean of Y) = 0.75
Standard deviation of differences (X-Y) = 5.52

Using above formula for paired t-test:

$$t = \frac{0.75}{5.52 / \sqrt{20}} = 0.61$$

The critical t value for p = 0.05 at 19 degrees of freedom is 1.72 (from t-table). As the calculated t value is less than the critical value, there is no significant difference between the two methods.

Linear Regression or Least Square Analysis and Correlation Statistics: Simple regression is a method of estimating the numerical relationship between two variables. Correlation coefficient (r) provides an index of the degree to which the paired measures co-vary. Least square analysis is used to estimate this relationship. In clinical laboratories, regression analysis is frequently used to compare methods.

The equation of a straight line relationship between variables X and Y is given as:

$$Y = a + bX$$

where X and Y are two variables, a is intercept and b is slope. Intercept and slope are calculated from the following equations:

$$a = \bar{Y} - b\bar{X}$$

Where $\bar{Y}$ and $\bar{X}$ are means of two variables:

$$b = \frac{n\Sigma xy - \Sigma x\Sigma y}{n\Sigma x^2 - (\Sigma x)^2}$$

Correlation coefficient is calculated from the following equation:

$$r = \frac{n\Sigma xy - \Sigma x\Sigma y}{\sqrt{[n\Sigma x^2 - (\Sigma x)^2][n\Sigma y^2 - (\Sigma y)^2]}}$$

The other regression statistics, which is frequently used in method comparison is standard deviation about the regression line ($SD_{y/x}$) and is calculated as:

$$SD_{y/x} = \sqrt{\frac{\Sigma(y-\hat{y})^2}{n-2}}$$

Where Y is the observed value at each X and $\hat{Y}$ is calculated value from regression equation.

Ideally when test method is compared with a reference method, slope = 1.00; Y-intercept = 0 and $SD_{x/y}$ = 0. **Deviation from these values are due to different kinds of analytical errors. Slope, Y-intercept and $SD_{y/x}$ represent proportional, constant, and random errors respectively**.

Example: Using above example of paired t-test data for glucose analysis by two methods, calculate slope, intercept, correlation coefficient, and standard deviation about regression line.

Old Method (X)	New Method (Y)	X^2	Y^2	XY	$\hat{Y}$	$(Y-\hat{Y})^2$
45	42	2025	1764	1890	47.4	28.6
102	105	10404	11025	10710	101.5	12.3
89	92	7921	8464	8188	89.2	8.1
109	112	11881	12544	12208	108.2	14.8
202	193	40804	37249	38986	196.5	12.2
57	53	3249	2809	3021	58.8	33.1
152	144	23104	20736	21888	149.0	25.0
85	89	7225	7921	7565	85.4	13.3
56	52	3136	2704	2912	57.8	33.6
89	95	7921	9025	8455	89.2	34.2
154	153	23716	23409	23562	150.9	4.4
83	81	6889	6561	6723	83.5	6.0
110	115	12100	13225	12650	109.1	34.8
175	168	30625	28224	29400	170.9	8.1
125	121	15625	14641	15125	123.4	5.5
67	63	4489	3969	4221	68.3	27.6
49	52	2401	2704	2548	51.2	0.7
78	83	6084	6889	6474	78.7	18.5
133	142	17689	20164	18886	131.0	122.1
169	159	28561	25281	26871	165.2	37.8
Average 106.4	105.7					
Sum 2129	2114	265849	259308	262283		480.9

Using equations given above:

$$\text{Slope (b)} = \frac{20 \times 262283 - 2129 \times 2114}{20 \times 265849 - (2129)^2} = 0.95$$

$$\text{Intercept (a)} = 105.7 - 0.95 \times 106.4 = 4.6$$

$$\text{Correlation coefficient (r)} = \frac{20 \times 262283 - 2129 \times 2114}{\sqrt{[20 \times 265849 - (2129)^2][20 \times 259308 - (2114)^2]}} = 0.99$$

$$SD_{y/x} = \sqrt{\frac{480.9}{20-2}} = 5.2$$

This data shows that proportional analytical error is 5%, constant error is 4.6 mg/dL, and standard deviation about regression line is 5.2 mg/dL.

Footnotes

1. Rang M, "The Ulysses Syndrome," *Can Med Assoc J*, 1972, 106(2):122-3.
2. Young DS and Bermes EW, "Specimen Collecting and Processing: Sources of Biological Variation," *Tietz Textbook of Clinical Chemistry*, 3rd ed, Burtis CA and Ashwood ER, eds, Philadelphia, PA: WB Saunders Co, 1999, 42-72.
3. Fraser CG, "Biological Variation in Clinical Chemistry," *Am J Clin Pathol*, 1992, 116(9):916-23.
4. "Report of the Expert Committee on the Diagnosis and Classification of Diabetes Mellitus," *Diabetes Care*, 1997, 20(7):1183-97.
5. Troisi RJ, Cowie CC, and Harris MI, "Diurnal Variation in Fasting Plasma Glucose: Implications for Diagnosis of Diabetes Patients Examined in the Afternoon," *JAMA*, 2000, 284(24):3157-9.
6. Ashwood ER, "Clinical Chemistry of Pregnancy," *Tietz Textbook of Clinical Chemistry*, 3rd ed, Burtis CA and Ashwood ER, eds, Philadelphia, PA: WB Saunders Co, 1999, 1736-75.
7. Ramsay MM, James DK, Weiner CP, et al, *Normal Values in Pregnancy*, London, England: WB Saunders Co, 1996.
8. Ayus JC, Varon J, and Arieff AI, "Hyponatremia, Cerebral Edema, and Noncardiogenic Pulmonary Edema in Marathon Runners," *Ann Intern Med*, 2000, 132(9):711-4.
9. Soldin SJ, Brugnara C, and Hicks JM, eds, *Pediatric Reference Ranges*, 3rd ed, Washington, DC: AACC Press, 1999.
10. Nicholson JF and Pesce MA, "Reference Ranges for Laboratory Tests and Procedures," *Nelson Textbook of Pediatrics*, 16th ed, Behrman RE, Kliegman RM, and Jenson HB, eds, Philadelphia, PA: WB Saunders Co, 2000, 2181-229.
11. Faulkner WR, ed, *Geriatric Clinical Chemistry Reference Values*, Washington, DC: AACC Press, 1994.
12. Visser M, Bouter LM, McQuillan GM, et al, "Elevated C-Reactive Protein Levels in Overweight and Obese Adults," *JAMA*, 1999, 282(22):2131-5.

13. Young DS, *Effects of Drugs on Clinical Laboratory Tests*, 5th ed, Volume One: Listing by Test, Washington, DC: AACC Press, 2000.

14. Young DS, *Effects of Drugs on Clinical Laboratory Tests*, 5th ed, Volume Two: Listing by Drug, Washington, DC: AACC Press, 2000.

15. Young DS, *Effects of Preanalytical Variables on Clinical Laboratory Tests*, 2nd ed, Washington, DC: AACC Press, 1997.

16. Koch DD and Peters T, "Selection and Evaluation of Methods," *Tietz Textbook of Clinical Chemistry*, 3rd ed, Burtis CA and Ashwood ER, eds, Philadelphia, PA: WB Saunders Co, 1999, 320-35.

17. Shultz EK, "Selection and Interpretation of Laboratory Procedures," *Tietz Textbook of Clinical Chemistry*, 3rd ed, Burtis CA and Ashwood ER, eds, Philadelphia, PA: WB Saunders Co, 1999, 314.

18. Bender TM, Stone LR, and Amenta JS, "Diagnostic Power of Lecithin/Sphingomyelin Ratio and Fluorescence Polarization Assays for Respiratory Distress Syndrome Compared by Relative Operating Characteristic Curves," *Clin Chem*, 1994, 40(4):541-5.

19. Friedman RB, Effects of Disease in Clinical Laboratory Tests, 3rd ed, Washington, DC: AACC Press, 1997.

20. van Wijk MA, van der Lei J, Mooseveld M, et al, "Assessment of Decision Support for Blood Test Ordering in Primary Care," *Ann Intern Med*, 2001, 134(4):274-81.

21. McClove JT and Detrich FH 2nd, "Analysis of Variance: Comparing More From Two Means," *Statistics*, Chapter 9, San Francisco, CA: Dellen Publishing Co, 1985, 421-3.

22. Kahn SE and Jondreski MA, "Laboratory Statistics," *Clinical Chemistry: Theory, Analysis and Correlation*, Kablan LA and Pesce AJ, eds, St Louis, MO: Mosby, 1996, 342-64.

References

Bland M, *An Introduction to Medical Statistics*, Oxford University Press, 1995.

Kringle RO and Bogovich M, "Statistical Procedure," *Tietz Textbook of Clinical Chemistry*, 3rd ed, Burtis CA and Ashwood ER, eds, Philadelphia, PA: WB Saunders Co, 1999, 265-309.

SPECIMEN COLLECTION AND POINT-OF-CARE TESTING

Eugene S. Olsowka, MD, PhD

Uttam Garg, PhD

Proper specimen collection is pivotal for provision of meaningful clinical laboratory information.

Although rigorous laboratory quality assurance procedures are required to assure technically accurate results, such techniques cannot safeguard against incorrectly labeled tubes or improperly drawn specimens. If the specimen is not representative or has been compromised by improper collection or inappropriate handling, results may be misleading or potentially dangerous. As an example, a study reported that preanalytical sources of variation from behavioral, clinical, and sampling sources constituted about 60% of the total variation in a reported lipid measurement of an individual.[1] **The laboratory must have an optimum, properly labeled specimen**.

This section includes general information pertaining to the collection of laboratory specimens. Listings for common methods of blood and urine collection are outlined as general considerations. Specimen collection information specific for each individual test is provided with the detailed discussion of the test within the sections of the text. A discussion of the special requirements for collection of specimens for detection of **drugs of abuse and therapeutic drug levels** is presented in the introduction to Therapeutic Drug Monitoring *on page 731* and Toxicology/Drugs of Abuse *on page 773*, and a typical **chain-of-custody** form is illustrated in the Toxicology/Drugs of Abuse Introduction *on page 773*. The unique considerations required for the collection of specimens for **trace element** testing are discussed in the Introduction to Trace Elements *on page 811* chapter. Specifically, specimens submitted for trace elements must be submitted in heavy metal-free containers or metal-free Vacutainers®. The contaminating role of air in the procurement of blood samples for trace metals analysis has been discussed.[2] **Transfusion Service** needs are addressed in the introduction of that chapter *on page 827*. Special requirements exist for **coagulation** testing, as described in that chapter.

OVERVIEW AND REGULATORY CONSIDERATIONS

Every healthcare employee, from nurse to housekeeper, has some (albeit small) risk of exposure to HIV and other viral agents such as hepatitis B and Jakob-Creutzfeldt agent. The incidence of HIV-1 transmission associated with a percutaneous exposure to blood from an HIV-1 infected patient is approximately 0.3% per exposure.[3,4] Exposure management should include preexposure education and immediate postexposure care and counseling. Chemoprophylaxis, despite its questionable effectiveness, is widely used.[4] Each year, approximately 6500-9000 healthcare workers in the United States are exposed to infectious body fluids.[5] Exposure to tuberculosis and hepatitis C by healthcare workers is also significant. The risk to healthcare workers of becoming infected after exposure from a needlestick, infected by hepatitis C, is 1.2% to 10%.[6] An understanding of the appropriate procedures, responsibilities, and risks inherent in the collection and handling of patient specimens is necessary and is required by Occupational Safety and Health Administration (OSHA) regulations.

The Occupational Safety and Health Administration published its "Final Rule on Occupational Exposure to Bloodborne Pathogens" in the Federal Register on December 6, 1991. OSHA has chosen to follow the Centers for Disease Control (CDC) definition of universal precautions. The Final Rule provides full legal force to universal precautions and requires employers and employees to treat blood and certain body fluids as if they were infectious. The Final Rule mandates that healthcare workers must avoid parenteral contact and must avoid splattering blood or other potentially infectious material on their skin, hair, eyes, mouth, mucous membranes, or on their personal clothing. Hazard abatement strategies must be used to protect workers. Such plans typically include, but are not limited to, the following:

- safe handling of sharp items ("sharps") and disposal of such into puncture resistant containers
- gloves required for employees handling items soiled with blood or equipment contaminated by blood or other body fluids
- provisions of protective clothing when more extensive contact with blood or body fluids may be anticipated (eg, surgery, autopsy, or deliveries)
- resuscitation equipment to reduce necessity for mouth to mouth resuscitation
- restriction of HIV-1 or hepatitis B-exposed employees to noninvasive procedures

OSHA has specifically defined the following terms: **Occupational exposure** means reasonably anticipated skin, eye, mucous membrane, or parenteral contact with blood or other potentially infectious materials that may result from the performance of an employee's duties. **Other potentially infectious materials** are human body fluids including semen, vaginal secretions, cerebrospinal fluid, synovial fluid, pleural fluid, pericardial fluid, peritoneal fluid, amniotic fluid, saliva in dental procedures, and body fluids that are visibly contaminated with blood, and all body fluids in situations in which it is difficult or impossible to differentiate between body fluids; any unfixed tissue or organ (other than intact skin) from a human (living or dead); and HIV-containing cell or tissue cultures, organ cultures, and HIV- or hepatitis B virus (HBV)-containing culture medium or other solutions, and blood, organs, or other tissues from experimental animals infected with HIV or HBV. An **exposure incident** involves specific eye, mouth, other mucous membrane, nonintact skin, or parenteral contact with blood or other potentially infectious materials that results from the performance of an employee's duties.[7] It is important to understand that some exposures may go unrecognized despite the strictest precautions. Two simple techniques that decrease the risk of infection while obtaining blood for hematocrit and bilirubin measurements in neonates have been proposed.[8]

A written Exposure Control Plan is required. Employers must provide copies of the plan to employees and to OSHA upon request. Compliance with OSHA rules may be accomplished by the following methods.

- **Universal precautions (UPs)** means that all human blood and certain body fluids are treated as if known to be infectious for HIV, HBV, and other bloodborne pathogens. UPs do not apply to feces, nasal secretions, sputum, sweat, tears, urine, or vomitus unless they contain visible blood.

- **Engineering controls (ECs)** are physical devices which reduce or remove hazards from the workplace by eliminating or minimizing hazards or by isolating the worker from exposure. Engineering control devices include sharps disposal containers, self-resheathing syringes, etc.

- **Work practice controls (WPCs)** are practices and procedures that reduce the likelihood of exposure to hazards by altering the way in which a task is performed. Specific examples are the prohibition of two-handed recapping of needles, prohibition of storing food alongside potentially contaminated material, discouragement of pipetting fluids by mouth, encouraging handwashing after removal of gloves, safe handling of contaminated sharps, and appropriate use of sharps containers.

- **Personal protective equipment (PPE)** is specialized clothing or equipment worn to provide protection from occupational exposure. PPE includes gloves, gowns, laboratory coats (the type and characteristics will depend upon the task and degree of exposure anticipated), face shields or masks, and eye protection. Surgical caps or hoods and/or shoe covers or boots are required in instances in which gross contamination can reasonably be anticipated (eg, autopsies, orthopedic surgery). If PPE is penetrated by blood or any contaminated material, the item must be removed immediately or as soon as feasible. **The employer must provide and launder or dispose of all PPE at no cost to the employee.** Gloves must be worn when there is a reasonable anticipation of hand contact with potentially infectious material, including a patient's mucous membranes or nonintact skin. Disposable gloves must be changed as soon as possible after they become torn or punctured. Hands must be washed after gloves are removed.

- **Regulated Waste:** Liquid or semiliquid blood, items contaminated with blood, dry-blood, pathological and micro-biological wastes are "regulated wastes." They must be contained in certified containers and must be disposed in accordance with applicable regulations.

Housekeeping protocols: OSHA requires that all bins, cans, and similar receptacles, intended for reuse which have a reasonable likelihood for becoming contaminated, be inspected and decontaminated immediately or as soon as feasible upon visible contamination and on a regularly scheduled basis. Broken glass that may be contaminated must not be picked up directly with the hands. Mechanical means (eg, brush, dust pan, tongs, or forceps) must be used. Broken glass must be placed in a proper sharps container.

Employers are responsible for teaching appropriate clean-up procedures for the work area and personal protective equipment. A 1:10 dilution of household bleach is a popular and effective disinfectant. It is necessary for employers to maintain signatures or initials of employees who have been properly educated. If one does not have written proof of education of universal precautions teaching, then by OSHA standards, such education never happened.

Pre-exposure and postexposure protocols: OSHA's Final Rule includes the provision that employees, who are exposed to contamination, be offered the hepatitis B vaccine at no cost to the employee. Employees may decline; however, a declination form must be signed. The employee must be offered free vaccine if he/she changes his/her mind. Vaccination to prevent the transmission of hepatitis B in the healthcare setting is widely regarded as sound practice.[9] In the event of exposure, a confidential medical evaluation and follow-up must be offered at no cost to the employee. Follow-up must include collection and testing of blood from the source individual for HBV and HIV if permitted by state law if a blood sample is available. If a postexposure specimen must be specially drawn, the individual's consent is usually required. Some states may not require consent for testing of patient blood after accidental exposure. One must refer to state and/or local regulations for proper guidance.

The employee follow-up must also include appropriate postexposure prophylaxis, counseling, and evaluation of reported illnesses. The employee has the right to decline baseline blood collection and/or testing. If the employee gives consent for the collection but not the testing, the sample must be preserved for 90 days in the event that the employee changes his/her mind within that time. Confidentiality related to blood testing must be ensured. **The employer does not have the right to know the results** of the testing of either the source individual or the exposed employee.[7]

COMMUNICATION OF HAZARDS

Communication regarding the dangers of bloodborne infections through the use of labels, signs, information, and education is required. Storage locations (eg, refrigerators and freezers, waste containers) that are used to store, dispose of, transport, or ship blood or other potentially infectious materials require labels. The label background must be red or bright orange with the biohazard design and the word biohazard in a contrasting color. The label must be part of the container or affixed to the container by permanent means.

Education provided by a qualified and knowledgeable instructor is mandated. The sessions for employees must include:[7]

- accessible copies of the regulation
- general epidemiology of bloodborne diseases
- modes of bloodborne pathogen transmission
- an explanation of the exposure control plan and a means to obtain copies of the written plan
- an explanation of the tasks and activities that may involve exposure
- the use of exposure prevention methods and their limitations (eg, engineering controls, work practices, personal protective equipment)
- information on the types, proper use, location, removal, handling, decontamination, and disposal of personal protective equipment)
- an explanation of the basis for selection of personal protective equipment
- information on the HBV vaccine, including information on its efficacy, safety, and method of administration and the benefits of being vaccinated (ie, the employee must understand that the vaccine and vaccination will be offered free of charge)
- information on the appropriate actions to take and persons to contact in an emergency involving exposure to blood or other potentially infectious materials
- an explanation of the procedure to follow if an exposure incident occurs, including the method of reporting the incident
- information on the postexposure evaluation and follow-up that the employer is required to provide for the employee following an exposure incident
- an explanation of the signs, labels, and color coding
- an interactive question-and-answer period

RECORD KEEPING

The OSHA Final Rule requires that the employer maintain both education and medical records. Medical records must be kept confidential and be maintained for the duration of employment plus 30 years. They must contain a copy of the employee's HBV vaccination status and postexposure incident information. The training record must contain dates of training, the content or summary of training sessions, and the names, qualifications, and job titles of trainers. Education records must be maintained for 3 years from the date the program was given.

OSHA has the authority to conduct inspections without notice. Penalties for cited violation may be assessed as follows.[7]

Serious violations. In this situation, there is a substantial probability of death or serious physical harm, and the employer knew, or should have known, of the hazard. A violation of this type carries a mandatory penalty of up to $7000 for each violation.

Other-than-serious violations. The violation is unlikely to result in death or serious physical harm. This type of violation carries a discretionary penalty of up to $7000 for each violation.

Willful violations. These are violations committed knowingly or intentionally by the employer and have penalties of up to $70,000 per violation with a minimum of $5000 per violation. If an employee dies as a result of a willful violation, the responsible party, if convicted, may receive a personal fine of up to $250,000 and/or a 6-month jail term. A corporation may be fined $500,000.

Large fines frequently follow visits to laboratories, physicians' offices, and healthcare facilities by OSHA Compliance Safety and Health Offices (CSHOs). Regulations are vigorously enforced. A working knowledge of the final rule and implementation of appropriate policies and practices is imperative for all those involved in the collection and analysis of medical specimens.

COMPLIANCE WITH SAFETY PROTOCOLS

Although percutaneous exposure to HIV-infected blood results in an infection rate that is estimated at 0.3%,[10,11] low compliance with certain parts of the standards mandated by OSHA have been recognized. Compliance with universal precautions by laboratory professionals is relatively high in general compliance, including properly disposing of contaminated materials, taking special precautions with sharp objects and scalpels, not consuming food within potentially contaminated areas, and washing hands after removing of gloves.[12] Compliance tends to fall in use of personal protective equipment. In particular, laboratorians are less compliant in the wearing of protective eye shields or disposable facemasks whenever a chance of splashes or splatter to the face or mouth exists.[12] Laboratorians tend to have a high degree of knowledge about universal precautions. The lower levels of compliance for personal protective equipment may relate more to the safety climate of the organization and the perceived risk of exposure rather than to training and to knowledge. McGovern[11] also found an inverse relationship between level of education and compliance with the use of personal protective devices. Men were approximately 50% as likely as women to comply with personal protective procedures. In 1976, approximately 70% of laboratory acquired infections resulted from splashes, needlesticks, and cuts from sharp objects.[13] Such accidents are likely to occur less frequently today than in the past because of use of personal protective equipment and procedural changes.

Today, blood collection, specimen handling, and specimen processing pose the greater risk for the acquisition of bloodborne infections.[13] Significant risk factors for the transmission of HIV after percutaneous exposure are the volume of blood a person is exposed to and the titer of HIV in the source patient's blood.[14] Longitudinal study of percutaneous exposure to body fluids in medical students has identified the emergency department as a high-risk location for serious body fluid exposures. Fatigue and stress impede the learning and safe practice of medical procedures.[15] Phlebotomists suffer fewer needlesticks per number of percutaneous punctures than those individuals who perform these procedures infrequently, but have a higher absolute number of injuries due to the volume of needlesticks that they perform.[16,17]

Various safety devices have come to market. The most effective safety device is the capping block which allows for one-handed recapping of needles[15,16] Mayo Medical Laboratories reports that care is taken to evaluate new products thoroughly as a new device may solve one problem only to create another. Phlebotomists report concern for some of the newer safety devices which tend to be larger, heavier, and more difficult to manipulate.[18] Butterfly needles are an example of a device which solves one problem but creates another. Butterfly needles with tubing have reduced the number of accidental percutaneous exposures associated with difficult phlebotomies, but increased the number of accidental percutaneous exposures associated with disposal: the lightweight tubing attached to the butterfly needle allows for rebound during disposal, and allows the butterfly to scratch or to stick to the technician.[17] Attaching the butterfly to the cork of a vacuum collection tube with the vacuum expelled allows for easier disposal .

PATIENT SATISFACTION ISSUES

The healthcare climate, in the new millenium, is one of apparently contradictory goals. Reimbursement reductions both from medicare and managed care contracts have forced institutions to implement cost-saving strategies while attempting to keep the quality of medical care services high. It is not surprising that medical laboratories, as part of these same medical care institutions, have also been operating under the same pressures. Laboratorians, who in the past have been isolated from direct patient care, have been finding themselves accountable for both quality services and patient satisfaction. The Joint Commission on Accreditation of Healthcare Organizations (JCAHO) has recognized patient satisfaction issues as an important indicator of quality and requires its members to collect data regarding patient satisfaction.[19] The phlebotomy service is typically the major segment of the laboratory that has direct patient contact., although in the current climate of healthcare, phlebotomy services are sometimes taken over by nursing staff. The patient's level of satisfaction with the laboratory often revolves around the phlebotomy experience. Recent articles have begun to address patient satisfaction issues.[20,21] Factors that are associated with patient dissatisfaction include discourteous treatment, large bruises (>25 mm), more discomfort than expected, a wait of longer than 30 minutes, and a bruise of any size. The factor most strongly associated with patient dissatisfaction is discourteous treatment.[20] It is interesting that the factor that can be controlled best has the most profound impact on the patient's level of satisfaction.

Footnotes

1. Cooper GR, Myers GL, Smith SJ, et al, "Blood Lipid Measurements. Variations and Practical Utility," *JAMA*, 1992, 268:985-6.
2. Chappuis P, Pineau A, Guillard O, et al, "Practical Advice Concerning Biological Fluids for Analysis of Trace-Elements," *Ann Biol Clin*, 1994, 52(2):103-9.
3. Henderson D, Fahey BJ, Willy M, et al, "Risk for Occupational Transmission of Human Immunodeficiency Virus Type 1 (HIV-1) Associated With Clinical Exposures. A Prospective Evaluation," *Ann Intern Med*, 1990, 113(10):740-6.
4. Fraser VJ and Powderly WG, "Risks of HIV Infection in the Health Care Setting," *Annu Rev Med*, 1995, 46:203-11.
5. Corser WD, "Occupational Exposure of Health Care Workers to Bloodbourne Pathogens. A Proposal for a Systematic Intervention Approach," *AAOHN J*, 1998, 46(5):246-52.
6. Dillman CM, "Hepatitis C: A Danger to Healthcare Workers," *Nurs Forum*, 1999, 34(2):23-8.
7. Bruning LM, "The Bloodbourne Pathogens Final Rule – Understanding the Regulation," *AORN Journal*, 1993, 57(2):439-40.
8. Leistikow EA, Mack WN, de Sierra TM, et al, "Reducing Risk of Infection When Obtaining Hematocrit and Bilirubin Determinations: Beyond Universal Precautions," *J Perinatol*, 1995, 15(1):7-9.
9. Schaffner W, Gardner P, and Gross PA, "Hepatitis B Immunization Strategies: Expanding the Target," *Ann Intern Med*, 1993, 118(4):308-9.
10. Ipolito G, "The Risk of Occupational Human Immunodeficiency Virus Infection in Healthcare Workers," *Arch Int Med*, 1993, 153:1451-8.
11. McGovern PM, Kochevar LK, Vesley D, et al, "Laboratory Professionals' Compliance With Universal Precautions," *Lab Med*, 1997, 28(11):725-30.
12. Sewell DL, "Laboratorians at Risk: The Threat of Exposure to Infectious Agents and the Role of the Biosafety Program," *Lab Med*, 1996, 27(10):673-8.
13. Cardo DM, Culver DH, Ciesielski CA, et al, "A Case-Control Study of HIV Seroconversion in Healthcare Workers After Percutaneous Exposure," *N Engl J Med*, 1997, 337(21):1485-90.
14. Osburn EHS, Papadakis MA, and Gerberding JL, "Occupational Exposures to Body Fluids Among Medical Students: A Seven Year Longitudinal Study," *Ann Intern Med*, 1999, 130(1):45-51.
15. Pruett S, "Needlestick Safety for Phlebotomists," *Lab Med*, 1998, 29(12):754-60.
16. Bush VJ, Leonard L, and Szamosi D, "Advancements in Blood Collection Devices," *Lab Med*, 1998, 29(10):616-22.
17. "Accidental Needlesticks in the Phlebotomy Service of the Department of Laboratory Medicine and Pathology at Mayo Clinic Rochester," *Communique*, 1998, 23(5):1-5.
18. Joint Commission on Accreditation of Healthcare Organizations (JCAHO), Accreditation Manual for Hospital Standards, Oak Brook Terrace, IL, 1996:39
19. Dale JC and Howanitz PJ, "Patient Satisfaction in Phlebotomy: A College of American Pathologist's Q-Probes Study," *Lab Med*, 1996, 27(3):188-192.
20. Lindsay RL, "Professional Perspectives: Minimizing the Trauma of Phlebotomy," *Lab Med*, 1996, 27(10):645-7.
21. Klosinski DD, "Collecting Specimens From the Elderly Patient," *Lab Med*, 1997, 28(8):518-20.

References

Bailey EM, "Exposure to Bloodborne Pathogens," *Am J Nurs*, 1998, 98(3):67-8.

Brown JW and Blackwell H, "Complying With the New OSHA Regs, Part 1: Teaching Your Staff About Biosafety," *MLO*, 1992, 24(4):24-8. Part 2: "Safety Protocols No Lab Can Ignore," 1992, 24(5):27-9. Part 3: "Compiling Employee Safety Records That Will Satisfy OSHA," 1992, 24(6):45-8.

Bryce EA, Ford J, Chase L, et al, "Sharps Injuries: Defining Prevention Priorities," *Am J Infect Control*, 1999, 27(5):447-52.

Buehler JW and Ward JW, "A New Definition for AIDS Surveillance," *Ann Intern Med*, 1993, 118(5):390-2.

Cuny EJ and Carpenter WM, "Occupational Exposure to Blood and Body Fluids: New Postexposure Prophylaxis Recommendations. United States Occupational Safety and Health Administration," *J Calif Dent Assoc*, 1998, 26(4):261-7, 269-71.

Cuny EJ, Fredekind R, and Budenz AW, "Safety Needles. New Requirements of the Occupational Safety and Health Administration Bloodbourne Pathogens Rule," *J Calif Dent Assoc*, 1999, 27(7):525-30.

Department of Labor, Occupational Safety and Health Administration, "Occupational Exposure to Bloodborne Pathogens; Final Rule (29 CFR Part 1910.1030)," *Federal Register*, December 6, 1991, 64004-182.

Gold JW, "HIV-1 Infection: Diagnosis and Management," *Med Clin North Am*, 1992, 76(1):1-18.

Griffith DE, Hardeman JL, Zhang Y, et al, "Tuberculosis Outbreak Among Healthcare Workers in a Community Hospital," *Am J Respir Crit Care Med*, 1995, 152(2):808-11.

"Hepatitis B Virus: A Comprehensive Strategy for Eliminating Transmission in the United States Through Universal Childhood Vaccination," *MMWR Morb Mortal Wkly Rep*, 1991, 40(RR-13):1-25.

Hibberd PL, "Patients, Needles, and Healthcare Workers: Understanding the Epidemiology, Pathophysiology, and Transmission of the Human Immunodeficiency Virus, Hepatitis B and C, and Cytomegalovirus," *J Intraven Nurs*, 1995, 18(6 Suppl):S22-31.

Malone N and Larson E, "Factors Associated With a Significant Reduction in Hospital-Wide Infection Rates," *Am J Infect Control*, 1996, 124(3):180-5.

"Nosocomial Transmission of Hepatitis B Virus Associated With a Spring-Loaded Fingerstick Device – California", *MMWR Morb Mortal Wkly Rep*, 1990, 39(35):610-3.

Polish LB, Shapiro CN, Bauer F, et al, "Nosocomial Transmission of Hepatitis B Virus Associated With the Use of a Spring-Loaded Fingerstick Device," *N Engl J Med*, 1992, 326(11):721-5.

"Recommendations for Preventing Transmission of Human Immunodeficiency Virus and Hepatitis B Virus to Patients During Exposure-Prone Invasive Procedures," *MMWR Morb Mortal Wkly Rep*, 1991, 40(RR-8):1-9.

"Update: Acquired Immunodeficiency Syndrome – United States," *MMWR Morb Mortal Wkly Rep*, 1992, 41(26):463-8.

Wong ES, Stotka JL, Chinchili VM, et al, "Are Universal Precautions Effective in Reducing the Number of Occupational Exposures Among Healthcare Workers?" *JAMA*, 1991, 265:1123-8.

Web Sites

http:/www.osha.gov

♦ **Acquired Immunodeficiency Syndrome Precautions, Specimen Collection** see Blood and Fluid Precautions, Specimen Collection on page 40

♦ **Allen Test** see Arterial Blood Collection on page 40

♦ **Alternate Site Testing** see Point-of-Care Testing on page 43

♦ **Ancillary Testing** see Point-of-Care Testing on page 43

Arterial Blood Collection

Related Information
Blood and Fluid Precautions, Specimen Collection on page 40
Blood Gases and pH, Arterial on page 119
Oxygen Saturation, Blood on page 240
pCO_2, Blood on page 246
pH, Blood on page 247
Specimen Identification Requirements on page 46

Synonyms Arterial Puncture

Applies to Allen Test

Test Includes Brachial, radial, or femoral artery puncture by trained personnel to obtain arterial blood, most frequently for blood gas analysis

Patient Preparation The patient should be resting for 20-30 minutes before collection of the specimen.

Aftercare Direct pressure must be applied to the arterial puncture site and should be maintained for a minimum of 10 minutes. Patients with bleeding tendency due to anticoagulation, platelet deficiency, factor deficiency, or liver disease may bleed excessively and form a hematoma. Such patients should be monitored carefully after the procedure to be sure bleeding has been controlled. Arterial spasm preventing aspiration of the specimen and thrombosis of the punctured artery can occur.

Specimen Arterial blood

Container Heparinized syringe with 21- or 23-gauge needle. Alternatively, a 21- or 23-gauge Butterfly® infusion set may be used. Glass syringes are preferred over plastic syringes, as gases can dissolve in plastic.

Collection The experienced arterial puncturist should carefully select an appropriate artery. If the radial artery is used, **Allen's test** to assure collateral circulation to the hand from the ulnar artery is performed: the hand is closed tightly by the patient or by an assistant to form a fist. Pressure is then applied at the wrist, compressing and obstructing both the radial and ulnar arteries. The hand is then opened (but not fully extended), revealing a blanched palm and fingers. The obstructing pressure is next removed from only the ulnar artery while the palm and fingers, including thumb, are observed; they should become flushed within 15 seconds as the blood from the ulnar artery refills the empty capillary bed. If the ulnar artery does not adequately supply the entire hand (a negative Allen test), the radial artery should not be used as a puncture site; an alternate artery should be selected.[1] Recent studies have confirmed the efficacy and usefulness of this test.[2,3]

Careful preparation of the puncture site is performed with 70% alcohol (isopropanol) using a circular motion working out from the site. Dry with gauze or let air dry. The artery is stabilized by holding with a finger. Take care not to contaminate the puncture site. The artery is punctured at a 30° angle for the radial artery, 45° angle for the brachial, 45° or 90° angle for the femoral. The bevel of the needle or Butterfly® should be pointed toward the direction of blood flow. The syringe should fill spontaneously. Small bore needles or plastic syringes may require gentle slow suction. Be sure no air bubbles are aspirated into the syringe. After adequate sample volume is obtained, quickly remove the needle and apply pressure. See Aftercare. The detailed technique for arterial puncture is described in NCCLS Standard H11-A2.[1] Place specimen on ice after sealing the needle into a piece of hard rubber or plastic. Deliver to the laboratory within 15 minutes of collection.

Storage Instructions Keep the specimen air tight and water tight in a container of ice. This slows the metabolic rate of white cells in the specimen and reduces oxygen consumption. The specimen must be analyzed rapidly. Results are often needed urgently.

Causes for Rejection Clots in specimen, specimen left at room temperature for more than 10 minutes (if collected for blood gas analysis)

Special Instructions Provide patient's temperature on the laboratory requisition if specimen is collected for blood gases.

Use Obtain arterial blood for analysis. See Blood Gases and pH, Arterial on page 119.

Limitations Arterial puncture should be performed by persons familiar with the procedure and the potential complications. For example, forearm compartment syndrome occurs after percutaneous arterial blood sampling and is usually associated with anticoagulation therapy. This syndrome has occurred once in a young woman with Goodpasture syndrome.[4] Liquid sodium heparin should be used sparingly only to fill the needle and dead space. Excess heparin in the sample will lower the pCO_2. pO_2 may be variably affected, and acid base calculations will be erroneous. Air bubbles in the syringe can greatly alter pO_2.

Additional Information The evaluation of alveolar pO_2 is routinely done by assuming that the respiratory gas exchange ratio is equal to 0.8. A study of the respiratory gas exchange ratio in patients undergoing arterial puncture revealed that in ~25% of cases, there is a transient change in alveolar ventilation associated with arterial puncture that may cause a change in the gas exchange ratio and lead to at least a 10 mm Hg error in estimating alveolar pO_2.[5] Evidently, some patients respond to arterial puncture by transient breath holding or by taking rapid shallow breaths. Arterialized capillary blood is addressed in Skin Puncture Blood Collection on page 45.

Footnotes
1. National Committee for Clinical Laboratory Standards, "Percutaneous Collection of Arterial Blood for Laboratory Analysis," Approved Standard, H11-A2, 2nd ed, Wayne, PA: National Committee for Clinical Laboratory Standards, 1992.
2. Fuhrman TM, Reilley TE, and Pippin WD, "Comparison of Digital Blood Pressure, Plethysmography, and the Modified Allen's Test as Means of Evaluating the Collateral Circulation to the Hand," *Anaesthesia*, 1992, 47(11):959-61.
3. Choudhury RP and Cleator SJ, "An Examination of Needlestick Injury Rates, Hepatitis B Vaccination Uptake and Instruction on "Sharps" Technique Among Medical Students," *J Hosp Infect*, 1992, 22(2):143-8.
4. Safran MR, Bernstein A, and Lesavoy MA, "Forearm Compartment Syndrome Following Brachial Arterial Puncture in Uremia," *Ann Plast Surg*, 1994, 32(5):535-8.
5. Cinel D, Markwell K, Lee R, et al, "Variability of the Respiratory Gas Exchange Ratio During Arterial Puncture," *Am Rev Respir Dis*, 1991, 143(2):217-8.

♦ **Arterialized Capillary Blood** see Skin Puncture Blood Collection on page 45

♦ **Arterial Puncture** see Arterial Blood Collection on page 40

♦ **AST** see Point-of-Care Testing on page 43

♦ **Bacteriology Specimen Identification** see Specimen Identification Requirements on page 46

♦ **Bedside Testing** see Point-of-Care Testing on page 43

Blood and Fluid Precautions, Specimen Collection

Related Information
Arterial Blood Collection on page 40
Hepatitis B Surface Antigen on page 625
Phlebotomist Procedures on page 43
Skin Puncture Blood Collection on page 45
Venous Blood Collection on page 47

Synonyms Acquired Immunodeficiency Syndrome Precautions, Specimen Collection; Isolation Patients, Precautions for Specimen Collection; Precautions, Specimen Collection

Abstract It has been well documented that exposure to blood and body fluid-borne pathogens can be significantly reduced by following universal precautions.[1,2] It is also well known that universal precautions are not strictly followed among all healthcare workers.[3,4]

Patient Preparation The **Occupational Safety and Health Administration (OSHA)** Final Rule requires that the risk to healthcare workers of accidental exposure to infection be minimized. By careful planning and thoughtful attention to detail, an appropriate and representative specimen can be safely collected. See Overview and Regulatory Considerations, discussed in the Specimen Collection Introduction on page 35.

Before entering the isolation room or drawing area:
- Check orders and assemble the equipment needed for this patient.
- Read the isolation sign on the door or patient's chart. It will explain the type of isolation and what you must wear and do. **Follow these directions carefully.**
- Find out if it is necessary to take a tourniquet and/or a plastic holder into the room. Many times these items will be there already.
- Take in the minimum equipment needed: tourniquet; plastic holder; evacuated tube needle; alcohol sponges; evacuated blood collection tubes or blood culture media; glass slides (if a blood smear is to be made).

In the room:
- Ask the patient to state his/her name to confirm patient identification. Check wristband.
- Put on gloves.
- Place paper towels on table and place your equipment on these towels.
- Obtain blood samples in the usual manner, avoiding any unnecessary contact with the patient and the bed.
- After obtaining blood samples, leave tourniquet and plastic holder in room and discard needle in proper container.
- Place several clean paper towels on the table, one on top of the other. If the outside of the tubes is contaminated, follow established laboratory decontamination procedures.
- If blood smears were made, place smears on two clean paper towels. When ready to leave, wrap smears and tubes in the top paper towel and discard the bottom paper towel.
- Label specimens for proper identification (see Specimen Identification Requirements on page 46) as directed by institutional policy. Label specimens for infectious hazards in a distinctive manner as required by institutional policy. Since the implementation of universal blood and body fluid precautions for **all** patients, special labeling for specific patients may be eliminated, depending upon institutional policies and local regulations. In any case, **universal precautions must be observed.**
- Wash hands.
- Bring specimens to the laboratory.[5]

Collection All specimens of blood and body fluids should be put in a well-constructed container with a secure lid to prevent leaking during transport. Care should be taken when collecting each specimen to avoid contamination of the outside of the container and of the laboratory form accompanying the specimen.

Special Instructions

Precautions for laboratories: Universal precautions should be followed at all times. Blood and other body fluids from **all** patients should be considered infective. To supplement universal blood and body fluid precautions, the following precautions are recommended for healthcare workers in clinical laboratories.

All persons collecting and processing blood and body fluid specimens should wear gloves. Masks, protective eyewear, and laboratory coats or gowns should be worn if contact with blood or body fluids is anticipated. Gloves should be changed and hands washed after completion of specimen processing.

For routine procedures, such as histologic and pathologic studies or microbiologic culturing, a biological safety cabinet is not necessary. However, biological safety cabinets (class I or II) should be used whenever procedures are conducted that have a high potential for generating droplets. These include activities such as blending, sonicating, and vigorous mixing. Mechanical pipetting devices must be used for manipulating all liquids in the laboratory. **Mouth pipetting must not be done.**

Use of needles and syringes should be limited to situations in which there is no alternative, and the recommendations for preventing injuries with needles outlined under universal precautions must be followed.

Laboratory work surfaces should be decontaminated with an appropriate chemical germicide after a spill of blood or other body fluids and when work activities are completed.

Contaminated materials used in laboratory tests should be decontaminated before reprocessing or be placed in bags and disposed in accordance with institutional policies for disposal of infective waste.

Scientific equipment that has been contaminated with blood or other body fluids should be decontaminated and cleaned before being repaired in the laboratory or transported to the manufacturer.

All persons must wash their hands after completing laboratory activities and should remove personal protective equipment before leaving the laboratory.

Implementation of universal blood and body fluid precautions for **all** patients eliminates the need for warning labels on specimens, since blood and other body fluids from all patients should be considered infective. OSHA rules require "Biohazard" labeling or color coding of containers of regulated waste, refrigerators and freezers containing blood or other potentially infectious material, and containers used to store, transport, or ship such materials.

Additional Information Human immunodeficiency virus (HIV), the virus that causes acquired immunodeficiency syndrome (AIDS), is transmitted through sexual contact, exposure to infected blood or blood components, and perinatally from mother to neonate. HIV has been isolated from blood, semen, vaginal secretions, saliva, tears, breast milk, cerebrospinal fluid, amniotic fluid, and urine and is likely to be isolated from other body fluids, secretions, and excretions. However, epidemiologic evidence has implicated only blood, semen, vaginal secretions, and possibly breast milk in transmission.

The increasing prevalence of HIV infection increases the risk that healthcare workers will be exposed to blood from patients infected with HIV, especially when blood and body fluid precautions are not followed for all patients.[6] Thus, the Centers for Disease Control (CDC) in its recommendations for prevention of HIV transmission in healthcare settings[7] emphasizes the need for healthcare workers to consider **all** patients as potentially infected with HIV and/or other blood-borne pathogens and to adhere rigorously to infection control precautions for minimizing the risk of exposure to blood and body fluids of all patients.

The CDC universal precaution recommendations and the OSHA Final Rule regulations[7,8] have been developed for use in healthcare settings and emphasize the need to treat blood and other body fluids from **all** patients as potentially infective. These same prudent precautions also should be taken in other settings in which persons may be exposed to blood or other body fluids.

Precautions to Prevent Transmission of HIV - Universal Precautions: Since medical history and examination cannot reliably identify all patients infected with HIV or other blood-borne pathogens, blood and body fluid precautions should be consistently used for **all** patients. This approach, recommended by CDC and referred to as "universal blood and body fluid precautions" or "universal precautions," must be used in the care of **all** patients as a result of OSHA's Final Rule.[8]

All healthcare workers must routinely use appropriate barrier precautions to prevent skin and mucous membrane exposure when contact with blood or other body fluids of any patient is anticipated. Gloves should be worn for touching blood and body fluids, mucous membranes, or nonintact skin of all patients, for handling items on surfaces soiled with blood or body fluids, and for performing venipuncture and other vascular access procedures. Gloves should be changed after contact with each patient. Masks and protective eyewear or face shields should be worn during procedures that are likely to

generate droplets of blood or other body fluids to prevent exposure of mucous membranes of the mouth, nose, and eyes. Laboratory coats, gowns, or aprons should be worn during procedures that are likely to generate splashes of blood or other body fluids.

Hands and other skin surfaces should be washed immediately and thoroughly if contaminated with blood or other body fluids. Hands should be washed immediately after gloves are removed.

All healthcare workers must take precautions to prevent injuries caused by needles, scalpels, and other sharp instruments or devices during procedures; when cleaning used instruments; during disposal of used needles; and when handling sharp instruments after procedures. To prevent needlestick injuries, needles must not be recapped, purposely bent or broken by hand, removed from disposable syringes, or otherwise manipulated by hand. After they are used, disposable syringes and needles, scalpel blades, and other sharp items must be placed in puncture-resistant containers for disposal; the puncture-resistant containers should be located as close as possible to the area of use. Large-bore reusable needles should be placed in a puncture-resistant container for transport to the reprocessing area. Recapping of syringes, if absolutely necessary, may be done by a one-handed method which employs the use of a recapping block.[9]

Two simple procedures are described to decrease the risk of exposure while obtaining specimens for hematocrit and bilirubin measurement.[10]

Although saliva has not been implicated in HIV transmission, to minimize the need for emergency mouth-to-mouth resuscitation, mouthpieces, resuscitation bags, or other ventilation devices should be available for use in areas in which the need for resuscitation is predictable.

Healthcare workers who have exudative lesions or weeping dermatitis should refrain from all direct patient care and from handling patient care equipment until the condition resolves.

Pregnant healthcare workers are not known to be at greater risk of contracting HIV infection than healthcare workers who are not pregnant; however, if a healthcare worker develops HIV infection during pregnancy, the infant is at risk of infection resulting from perinatal transmission. Because of this risk, **pregnant healthcare workers should be especially familiar with and strictly adhere to precautions to minimize the risk of HIV transmission.**

Implementation of universal blood and body fluid precautions for **all** patients eliminates the need for use of the isolation category of "Blood and Body Fluid Precautions" previously recommended by CDC for patients known or suspected to be infected with blood-borne pathogens. Isolation precautions (eg, enteric, AFB) should be used as necessary if associated conditions, such as infectious diarrhea or tuberculosis, are diagnosed or suspected.

Environmental Considerations for HIV Transmission: No environmentally mediated mode of HIV transmission has been documented. Nevertheless, the precautions described should be taken routinely in the care of **all** patients.

Sterilization and Disinfection: Standard sterilization and disinfection procedures for patient care equipment currently recommended for use in a variety of healthcare settings, including hospitals, medical and dental clinics and offices, hemodialysis centers, emergency care facilities, and long-term nursing care facilities, are adequate to sterilize or disinfect instruments, devices, or other items contaminated with blood or other body fluids from persons infected with blood-borne pathogens including HIV.

Cleaning and Decontaminating Spills of Blood or Other Body Fluids: Chemical germicides that are approved for use as "hospital disinfectants" and are tuberculocidal when used at recommended dilutions can be used to decontaminate spills of blood and other body fluids. Strategies for decontaminating spills of blood and other body fluids in a patient care setting are different than for spills of cultures or other materials in clinical, public health, or research laboratories. In patient care areas, visible material should first be removed and then the area should be decontaminated. With large spills of cultured or concentrated infectious agents in the laboratory, the contaminated area should be flooded with a liquid germicide before cleaning, then decontaminated with fresh germicidal agent. In both settings, gloves should be worn during the cleaning and decontaminating procedures.

Studies have shown that HIV is inactivated rapidly after being exposed to commonly used chemical germicides at concentrations that are much lower than used in practice. Embalming fluids (formalin preparations) are similar to the types of chemical germicides that have been tested and found to completely inactivate HIV. Formalin may not rapidly inactivate hepatitis B virus nor quickly kill bacteria. It is a slow-acting antiseptic agent requiring 18 hours or more to kill microorganisms. In addition to commercially available chemical germicides, a solution of sodium hypochlorite (household bleach) prepared daily is an inexpensive and effective germicide. Concentrations ranging from ~500 ppm (1:100 dilution of household bleach) sodium hypochlorite to 5000 ppm (1:10 dilution of household bleach) are effective depending on the amount of organic material (eg, blood, mucus) present on the surface to be cleaned and disinfected. Disinfecting surfaces in cases of known Jakob-Creutzfeld agent may require full strength bleach. Commercially available chemical germicides may be more compatible with certain medical devices that might be corroded by repeated exposure to sodium hypochlorite.

(Continued)

Blood and Fluid Precautions, Specimen Collection

(Continued)

Housekeeping: Environmental surfaces such as walls, floors, and other surfaces are not associated with transmission of infections to patients or healthcare workers. Therefore, extraordinary attempts to disinfect or sterilize these environmental surfaces are not necessary. However, cleaning and removal of soil should be done routinely.

Cleaning schedules and methods vary according to the area of the hospital or institution, type of surface to be cleaned, and the amount and type of soil present. Horizontal surfaces (eg, bedside tables and hard-surfaced flooring) in patient care areas are usually cleaned on a regular basis, when soiling or spills occur, and when a patient is discharged. Cleaning of walls, blinds, and curtains is recommended only if visibly soiled. Disinfectant fogging is an unsatisfactory method of decontaminating air and surfaces and is not recommended.

Disinfectant detergent formulations registered by EPA may be used for cleaning environmental surfaces, but the actual physical removal of micro-organisms by scrubbing is probably as important as any antimicrobial effect of the cleaning agent. Therefore, cost, safety, and acceptability by house-keepers can be the main criteria for selecting any such registered agent. The manufacturers' instructions for appropriate use should be followed.

Laundry: Although soiled linen has been identified as a source of large numbers of certain pathogenic microorganisms, the risk of actual disease transmission is negligible. Rather than rigid procedures and specifications, hygienic and common sense storage and processing of clean and soiled linen are recommended. Soiled linen should be handled as little as possible with minimum agitation to prevent gross microbial contamination of the air and persons handling the linen. All soiled linen should be bagged at the location where it was used; it should not be sorted or rinsed in patient care areas. Linen soiled with blood or body fluids must be placed and transported in bags that prevent leakage.

Infective Waste: There is no epidemiologic evidence to suggest that most hospital waste is any more infective than residential waste. Moreover, there is no epidemiologic evidence that hospital waste has caused disease in the community as a result of improper disposal. Therefore, identifying wastes for which special precautions are indicated is largely a matter of judgment about the relative risk of disease transmission. The most practical approach to the management of infective waste is to identify those wastes with the potential for causing infection during handling and disposal and for which some special precautions appear prudent. Hospital wastes for which special precautions are required include microbiology laboratory waste, pathology waste, blood specimens or blood products, and other potentially infectious material. Any item that has had contact with blood, exudates, or secretions may be potentially infective. Infective waste, in general, should either be incinerated or should be autoclaved before disposal in a sanitary landfill. Bulk blood, suctioned fluids, excretions, and secretions may be carefully poured down a drain connected to a sanitary sewer. Sanitary sewers may also be used to dispose of other infectious wastes capable of being ground and flushed into the sewer.

Survival of HIV in the Environment: The most extensive study on the survival of HIV after drying involved greatly concentrated HIV samples (ie, 10 million tissue culture infectious doses/mL). This concentration is at least 100,000 times greater than that typically found in the blood or serum of patients with HIV infection. HIV was detectable by tissue culture techniques 1-3 days after drying, but the rate of inactivation was rapid. Studies performed at CDC have also shown that drying HIV causes a rapid (within several hours) 1-2 log (90% to 99%) reduction in HIV concentration. In tissue culture fluid, cell-free HIV could be detected up to 15 days at room temperature, up to 11 days at 37°C (98.6°F), and up to 1 day if the HIV was cell-associated. HIV can be isolated from peripheral blood mononuclear cells and plasma for up to 48 hours after sample collection.[11]

When considered in the context of environmental conditions in healthcare facilities, these results do not require any changes in currently recommended sterilization, disinfection, or housekeeping strategies. When medical devices are contaminated with blood or other body fluids, existing recommendations include the cleaning of these instruments followed by disinfection or sterilization, depending on the type of medical device. These protocols assume "worst case" conditions of extreme virologic and microbiologic contamination and whether or not viruses have been inactivated after drying plays no role in formulating these strategies. Consequently, no changes in the published procedures for cleaning, disinfecting, or sterilizing need to be made.

Risk to Healthcare Workers of Acquiring HIV in Healthcare Settings: Healthcare workers with documented percutaneous or mucous membrane exposures to blood or body fluids of HIV-infected patients have been prospectively evaluated to determine the risk of infection after such exposures. The risk of HIV-1 transmission associated with a percutaneous exposure to blood from an HIV-1 infected patient is ~0.3% per exposure (95% confidence intervals, 0.13% to 0.70%). The risks associated with occupational mucous membrane and cutaneous exposures are likely to be substantially smaller.

The risk of healthcare workers being infected from needlestick contaminated with hepatitis C is 1.2% to 10%.[12]

Footnotes

1. Perry C and Barnett J, "Principles of Universal Precautions," *Emerg Nurse*, 1998, 6(6):25-8.
2. Diekema DJ, Schuldt SS, Albanese MA, et al, "Universal Precautions Training of Preclinical Students: Impact on Knowledge, Attitudes, and Compliance," *Prev Med*, 1995, 24(6):580-5.
3. Kim LE, Evanoff BA, Parks RL, et al, "Compliance With Universal Precautions Among Emergency Department Personnel: Implications for Prevention Programs," *Am J Infect Control*, 1999, 27(5):453-5.
4. Michalsen A, Delclos GL, Felknor SA, et al, "Compliance With Universal Precautions Among Physicians," *J Occup Environ Med*, 1997, 39(2):130-7.
5. Bennett BD, Cox RS, Davis CM, et al, eds, *So You're Going to Collect a Blood Specimen: An Introduction to Phlebotomy*, 5th ed, Northfield, IL: College of American Pathologists, 1992.
6. Fraser VJ and Powderly WG, "Risks of HIV Infection in the Health Care Setting," *Ann Rev Med*, 1995, 46:203-11.
7. "Leads From the *MMWR*. Update: Universal Precautions for Prevention of Transmission of Human Immunodeficiency Virus, Hepatitis B Virus, and Other Blood-Borne Pathogens in Healthcare Settings," *JAMA*, 1988, 260(4):462-5.
8. Department of Labor, Occupational Safety and Health Administration, "Occupational Exposure to Blood-Borne Pathogens; Final Rule (29 CFR Part 1910.1030)," *Fed Regist*, 1991, 64004-182.
9. Pruett S, "Needlestick Safety for Phlebotomists," *Lab Med*, 1998, 29(12):754-60.
10. Leistikow EA, Mach WN, de Sierra, et al, "Reducing Risk of Infection When Obtaining Hematocrit and Bilirubin Determinations: Beyond Universal Precautions," *J Perinatol*, 1995, 15(1):7-9.
11. O'Shea S, Rostron T, Mullen JE, et al, "Stability of Infectious HIV in Clincial Samples and Isolation From Small Volumes of Whole Blood," *J Clin Pathol*, 1999, 47(2):152-4.
12. Dillman CM, "Hepatitis C: A Danger to Healthcare Workers," *Nurs Forum*, 1999, 34(2):23-8.

Internet Web Sites

www.osha.gov

Blood Collection Tube Information

Related Information

Chain-of-Custody Protocol *on page 785*
Phlebotomist Procedures *on page 43*
Venous Blood Collection *on page 47*

Synonyms Blood Container Description; Tubes for Blood Collection; Vacutainer® Tube Description

Special Instructions See individual listings throughout this book for particular test requirements.

Additional Information The table describes most commonly used color codes, optimum and minimum volumes required, and additives contained in common vacuum draw tubes. In the last 5-10 years, due to advent of different anticoagulant combinations and other additives, tube color codes have changed and are becoming increasingly confusing. International Standard Organization (ISO), along with blood collection tube manufacturers is making efforts to standardize color codes. **It is important to be certain that a tube is filled with the prescribed minimum volume in order to avoid spurious results due to an inappropriate anticoagulant to specimen ratio.**

Tube Codes

Color	Optimum Volume/ Minimum Volume	Additive
Blue	4.5 mL/4.5 mL	Sodium citrate
Blue/navy	7 mL/3 mL	No additive (for trace metals) Heparin (for trace metals)
Culture (yellow)	8.3 mL/8.3 mL	SPS
FSP (blue)	2 mL/2 mL	Thrombin, trypsin inhibitor
Gray	5 mL/5 mL 7 mL/7 mL	Potassium oxalate, sodium fluoride
Green	10 mL/3.5 mL	Heparin
Lavender	7 mL/2 mL	EDTA
Orange	10 mL/NA	Thrombin
Red	10 mL/NA	None
Red/gray (gel)	10 mL/NA	Inert barrier material; clot activator
Yellow	5 mL/NA	ACD
Yellow/black	7 mL	Thrombin
Pediatric Tubes		
Blue	2.7 mL/2.7 mL	Sodium citrate
Culture (yellow)	3.3 mL/3.3 mL	SPS
Green	2 mL/2 mL	Heparin
Lavender	2 mL/0.6 mL 3 mL/0.9 mL 4 mL/1 mL	EDTA
Red	2 mL/NA 3 mL/NA 4 mL/NA	None

Special needs exist for specimens for coagulation testing. See the Coagulation Introduction *on page 327*.

See Transfusion Service Introduction *on page 827* for specimen requirements.

The Trace Metals Introduction *on page 811* provides information for specimens drawn for those substances.

See the Therapeutic Drug Monitoring Introduction *on page 731* and the Toxicology Drugs of Abuse Introduction *on page 773* for appropriate specimen requirements. It addresses anticonvulsants (antiepileptic drugs), antibiotic and cardiac drug levels, peaks and troughs, as well as collections for drugs of abuse. See Toxicology/Drugs of Abuse Introduction *on page 773* for Chain-of-Custody form and Chain-of-Custody Protocol *on page 785*.

- ◆ **Blood Collection, Venous** *see* Venous Blood Collection *on page 47*
- ◆ **Blood Container Description** *see* Blood Collection Tube Information *on page 42*
- ◆ **Blood Specimen Identification** *see* Specimen Identification Requirements *on page 46*
- ◆ **Body Fluid Identification** *see* Specimen Identification Requirements *on page 46*
- ◆ **Capillary Blood Collection** *see* Skin Puncture Blood Collection *on page 45*
- ◆ **Cytology Smear Identification** *see* Specimen Identification Requirements *on page 46*
- ◆ **Decentralized Testing** *see* Point-of-Care Testing *on page 43*
- ◆ **Fingerstick Blood Collection** *see* Skin Puncture Blood Collection *on page 45*
- ◆ **Heelstick Blood Collection** *see* Skin Puncture Blood Collection *on page 45*
- ◆ **Identification Requirements, Specimen** *see* Specimen Identification Requirements *on page 46*
- ◆ **Isolation Patients, Precautions for Specimen Collection** *see* Blood and Fluid Precautions, Specimen Collection *on page 40*
- ◆ **Near Patient Testing** *see* Point-of-Care Testing *on page 43*
- ◆ **NPT** *see* Point-of-Care Testing *on page 43*
- ◆ **Off-Site Testing** *see* Point-of-Care Testing *on page 43*
- ◆ **Pathology Specimen Identification** *see* Specimen Identification Requirements *on page 46*
- ◆ **Peripheral Blood Smear Preparation** *see* Skin Puncture Blood Collection *on page 45*

Phlebotomist Procedures

Related Information
Blood and Fluid Precautions, Specimen Collection *on page 40*
Blood Collection Tube Information *on page 42*
Skin Puncture Blood Collection *on page 45*
Specimen Identification Requirements *on page 46*
Venous Blood Collection *on page 47*

Synonyms Specimen Collection Policy, Phlebotomist

Collection Phlebotomists are generally required to adhere to the following procedures. Phlebotomists are only allowed to obtain samples from patients who have been positively identified. See Specimen Identification Requirements *on page 46*. Phlebotomists are limited to attempting venipunctures in upper extremities unless so ordered by the physician. **Phlebotomists may not perform a venipuncture above an I.V. site or in an arm with a heparin lock or shunt.** Only by a physician's order may a trained phlebotomist collect a sample from a fistula or shunt. Phlebotomists should not collect a sample from an arm which is on the same side as a recent mastectomy. Phlebotomists are generally limited to two attempts to obtain a blood sample. After two unsuccessful tries, the phlebotomist must call another phlebotomist or supervisor. If the second phlebotomist is unsuccessful, the physician or responsible nurse will be notified. Phlebotomists are not allowed to force a patient to have blood drawn. If a patient refuses, the phlebotomist will notify the responsible nurse or physician. The phlebotomist will perform skin punctures when ordered by the physician (with some exceptions) or if venipuncture is unsuccessful or prohibited (due to I.V., etc), provided the procedure requested can be performed on a skin puncture specimen. (Dependent on the policy and equipment available in laboratory receiving the specimen.) See Skin Puncture Blood Collection *on page 45*.

Special Instructions The perception of pain associated with venipuncture in children increases with anxiety and is inversely correlated with the patient's age.[1] Strategies to reduce the child's and parents' distress during venipuncture are important considerations.[2,3] Use of topical anesthetics has also been suggested.[4,5] Pain on venipuncture, cost, and convenience of four analgesic agents (lidocaine, brilocaine, dichlorotetrafluoroethane, and benzyl alcohol) has been compared. 0.9% benzyl alcohol was found to be best.[6] Approximately 30% of adult patients report needle discomfort greater than expected, which is one factor associated with patient dissatisfaction.[7]

Every effort should be made to improve patient satisfaction by reducing discomfort from phlebotomy procedures.

Additional Information See Sampling Problems in Maximizing the Information From Laboratory Tests - The Ulysses Syndrome *on page 15*.

Footnotes

1. Lander J, Fowler-Kerry S, and Oberle S, "Children's Venipuncture Pain: Influence of Technical Factors," *J Pain Symptom Manage*, 1992, 7(6):343-9.
2. Manne SL, Redd WH, Jacobsen PB, et al, "Behavioral Intervention to Reduce Child and Parent Distress During Venipuncture," *J Consult Clin Psychol*, 1990, 58(5):565-72.
3. Harrison A, "Preparing Children for Venous Blood Sampling," *Pain*, 1991, 45(3):299-306.
4. Woolfson AD, McCafferty DF, and Boston V, "Clinical Experiences With a Novel Percutaneous Amethocaine Preparation: Prevention of Pain Due to Venipuncture in Children," *Br J Clin Pharmacol*, 1990, 30(2):273-9.
5. Joyce TH 3d, "Topical Anesthesia and Pain Management Before Venipuncture," *J Pediatr*, 1993, 122(5 Pt 2):S24-9.
6. Patterson P, Hussa AA, Fedele KA, et al, "Comparison of 4 Analgesic Agents for Venipuncture," *AANA J*, 2000, 68(1):43-51.
7. Dale JC and Howanitz PJ, "Patient Satisfaction in Phlebotomy: A College of American Pathologist's Q-Probes Study," *Lab Med*, 1996, 27(3):188-92.

References
Bennett BD, Cox RS, Davis CM, et al, eds, *So You're Going to Collect a Blood Specimen: An Introduction to Phlebotomy*, 5th ed, Northfield, IL: College of American Pathologists, 1992.
Love G, "Easing the Discomfort of Venipuncture," *Nursing*, 1998, 28(3):30.
Roth D, "Venipuncture Tips for Geriatric Patients," *Nursing*, 1997, 27(10):69.
Scholz MJ, "Minimizing the Pain of Venipuncture," *RN*, 1996, 59(5):78.
Wray D and Wells G, "Procedures in Phlebotomy," *Arch Pathol Lab Med*, 2000, 124(4):641.

- ◆ **Phlebotomy, Venous** *see* Venous Blood Collection *on page 47*
- ◆ **POCT** *see* Point-of-Care Testing *on page 43*

Point-of-Care Testing

Related Information
Carboxyhemoglobin, Blood *on page 784*
Fibronectin, Fetal, Cervicovaginal Secretions *on page 174*
Glucose, Fasting, Plasma *on page 183*
Glucose, Noninvasive *on page 185*
Glucose, Random, Plasma *on page 186*
Glucose, Whole Blood *on page 188*

Synonyms Alternate Site Testing; Ancillary Testing; AST; Bedside Testing; Decentralized Testing; Near Patient Testing; NPT; Off-Site Testing; POCT

Applies to Pulse Oximetry

Test Includes Point-of-care assays may include hematocrit, hemoglobin, hemoglobin A_{1c}, glucose,[1] beta-hCG, CK-MB, blood gases (pH, pCO_2, pO_2, SO_2%), electrolytes (Na^+, K^+, Cl^-, ionized calcium, ionized magnesium), lactate, blood urea nitrogen, creatinine, ethanol, drugs of abuse, activated clotting time, troponin T, myoglobin, PTT, aPTT,[2] bilirubin, and other assays.

Abstract Development of diagnosis-related groups (DRGs), manufacturer's incentives to provide instrumentation to less regulated sites (eg, physicians' office laboratories prior to CLIA '88),[3] advancing technology[3] including development of biosensors with improved electronics,[4] and evolving requirements for abbreviated turnaround times have driven interest in near patient testing. Point-of-care testing (POCT) is finding a niche in terms of clinical utility. It has been proven practicable and some aspects desirable. Growth in POCT has been climbing at a rate of about 18% compared to the overall growth of diagnostic testing of 4% to 5% per year.[5] Its shortcomings include use by individuals with limited training in medical technology and quality control needs.

Specimen Whole blood, urine, saliva; small sample volume requirements by many of the new instruments provide enhancement of patient care.[1]

Turnaround Time Minutes

Reference Interval See reference range for each particular analyte. Ranges may differ from those of the laboratory hospital or reference laboratory depending on the specimen utilized, (ie, whole blood versus plasma or serum).

Critical Values See each analyte listing for critical values and panic ranges.

Use Bedside glucose monitoring to guide dosage of insulin administration; intensive care, emergency departments, and surgical theaters and other settings in which need for rapid turnaround times is great or desirable. Physician offices with on-site availability of results can avoid patient revisits and provide early treatment. The major use of POCT glucose testing at bedside or home is to monitor individuals with diabetes mellitus, not to establish that diagnosis.

Limitations Point-of-care testing generally is more expensive than analysis of specimens in a centralized laboratory. Expense is related in part to volume of testing and the number of personnel involved in such testing; handheld bedside-type devices tend to be less precise than larger instruments in centralized laboratories, although technological changes in microminaturization may soon challenge this advantage.[6] Assay range is generally lower than that of central laboratory instruments. Information handling, storage, and billing may be problematic if POCT instruments are not linked to laboratory or hospital information systems. Such challenges (Continued)

Point-of-Care Testing *(Continued)*

may be overcome by incorporation of radiofrequency and infrared links to the central laboratory as part of the point-of-care testing devices.

Preanalytical problems may exist when POCT programs are run and operated by staff unaware of appropriate sampling procedures. Some observe that such devices are used by personnel who may not be fully trained to use them, nor have they backgrounds which support a quality improvement mind-set. One report of critical limit protocol assessment revealed that while split sample control specimens showed good correlation of glucose data with the central laboratory results, only 18% of high/low critical limit glucose meter readings were confirmed by drawing a central lab specimen within the required time limits; the users thought it less urgent to confirm a sequence of such results. This led to a modification of the critical limit protocol in which patients with an initial critical high/low limit glucose meter reading were followed by laboratory testing until glucose values went to other predefined limits (eleven follow-up results showed a >50% discordance between the central lab and the glucose meters).[7]

Inspection and accreditation requirements, quality assurance and proficiency testing, supervision and management for POCT continue to evolve. Difficulties include as well needs to monitor such programs and requirements to maintain standards[8] with training and competency requirements.[9] Only 34.2% of hospitals in one series had a multidisciplinary POCT team, yet 88.7% of glucose testing, 41% of electrolyte testing, 58.3% of coagulation testing, 45.5% of hematocrit, and 47.7% of blood gas testing was performed at the bedside.[10]

Maintaining adequate quality control of POCT instruments, in a hospital setting, is a major concern. The main laboratory may be held responsible for quality of results, without direct laboratory staff involvement or authority in testing.

Pulse oximetry, a practical example of POCT, has been unable to distinguish carboxyhemoglobin from oxyhemoglobin at the wavelengths used by most oximeters. See Carboxyhemoglobin, Blood *on page 784.*

Most POCT devices calculate hematocrit by conductivity. Measurement of hematocrit by conductivity in seriously sick patients can lead to incorrect results.[11]

Methodology Methodology ranges from reflectance measurements of glucose oxidase strips for some of the simplest bedside glucometers to microelectrode technology for some of the most sophisticated devices measuring electrolytes and blood gases. The technology is ever-evolving and newer devices are being developed with technology that parallels central laboratory methodology but which may be more robust. Some bedside devices for example measure cardiac troponin T by a biotinylated antitroponin T antibody/streptavidin methodology much as do some central laboratory methods.[6] Immunoassays for proteins, such as beta-hCG, and for drugs of abuse are becoming available. Methods include ion-selective electrodes, substrate-specific electrodes, electrical conductance sensors, and analyte-specific optical sensors.[1]

Additional Information Point-of-care testing (POCT) or alternate site testing (AST) is an area in which laboratory tests are performed outside of the central laboratory, usually by nonlaboratory personnel with little or no formal training in laboratory technology, nor exposure to the concepts of quality control or continuous quality improvement. Laboratory testing has until recently been delivered by increasingly large centralized entities, predominantly sophisticated laboratories including those in hospitals. Assay equipment for most of the recent past was composed of ever-increasingly complex large automated instruments with interfaced information systems. This complex of large machines with an associated cadre of highly-trained professional personnel has created laboratories with ability to generate large amounts of test data at a relatively low cost per test. Bachner[12] relates that the growth of large central laboratories has been a direct result of the linkage of technological development and the increase in the number and size of American hospitals. Recently, the advent of microminiature electronics and very powerful microprocessors has led to a new generation of compact portable instruments that are relatively easy to use and reported to be capable of reasonable precision even in the hands of relatively inexperienced users. Such devices are not inexpensive, nor are they foolproof. In many ways, technological trends have driven instrumentation to a central location and then recently, have begun to move to more peripheral (hopefully essential) sites.

The concept of POCT, however controversial, is one that is continually evolving, being driven in part by the ability to manufacture microsensor systems capable of ever-accurate and precise measurement of various analytes. Proponents argue that the need for decreased turnaround times in areas such as anticoagulation during balloon angioplasty, bedside coagulation monitoring, and bedside glucose testing to guide insulin therapy has driven the site of testing from the central laboratory to the bedside, at which turnaround times may be as little as 3 minutes.[13] Tests felt to be the most critical in managing unstable and critically ill patients include blood gas measurements, electrolytes, and coagulation and hematology tests.[5] Use of POCT for cardiac markers and drugs of abuse is increasing in emergency departments.

While point-of-care testing tends to be more expensive than centralized laboratory testing, some have pointed out that cost analyses may not include the "costs of failure", which include such items as the loss of ability

to make timely clinical decisions, unnecessary stat orders induced by slow specimen transport to the laboratory, and poor communication between laboratory and clinical care providers.[14] Laposata et al[15] studied costs for bedside glucose monitoring and reported that increased POCT costs relate to the volume of alternate site testing performed and the number of healthcare workers performing such tests. Reagent and instrument costs also are relevant. Limiting POCT to units in which glucose testing is performed five times or more per day and limiting the number of personnel doing such testing minimizes the expense of bedside glucose monitoring. However, such limits preclude POCT application in many community hospital settings. Limitations of POCT to more active services supports enhancement of competence by those performing bedside testing. A method for monitoring the continuous quality improvement of point-of-care testing by comparing the natural duplications of results of point-of-care data with central laboratory results offers promise as a method to monitor the quality of point-of-care testing without complex quality assurance procedures.[16]

Other issues that likely will remain controversial include selection of performance standards for POCT, definition of acceptable reproducibility (precision), information handling, reporting and billing issues, responsibility for POCT programs in hospitals, and definition of realistic turnaround times. A report on timeliness of clinical laboratory tests[17] makes it clear that the perception of reasonable turnaround time is much different for clinical care providers than for laboratory staff.

An important paper provides recommendations for bedside glucose monitoring programs, essentially outlining organizational structure and requirements for successful programs. First among these is specific designation of responsible individual(s) and whenever possible, involvement of laboratory personnel in administration and quality assurance. Written procedures, organized training programs, defined maintenance, regular quality control testing with two levels of control material, and standards for acceptable performance are needed. Orchestrated, regular comparisons of POC results with corresponding specimens analyzed in the clinical laboratory and with performance standards are recommended. Participation in external proficiency testing programs, recognition of glucose concentration limits of POC instruments, specified out-of-limits requirements for central laboratory glucose assays, and acknowledgment of effects of the hematocrit, appropriate clinical restrictions, and determination of instrument bias are needed.[18] A significant amount of institutional point-of-care testing did not fall within current standards for accuracy or for quality control in a 1998 publication.[19]

In the past, glucose values obtained by POCT analyzers were lower due to whole blood glucose values. Currently, most of the glucose meters are adjusted to give plasma equivalent values. Thus, glucose values obtained by glucose meters match well with main laboratory chemistry analyzers. However, the upper limit of result reporting is still limited. (Most of the instruments do not provide glucose values more than ~600 mg/dL). Difficulties include variation in hematocrit, mannitol interference, and the need for completion within 30 minutes. See Glucose, Whole Blood *on page 188.*

POCT devices for coagulation and infectious disease testing are becoming available. Due to the number of different reagents and technologies in use, comparisons with main lab results are critical.

Use of anticoagulated samples versus capillary specimens, and use of different anticoagulants between central laboratory and point-of-care procedures may create confusion, possibly harming patient care.

Vital to the effective administration of any point-of-care testing program is the realization that someone must be designated as responsible for point-of-care testing service. Responsibilities would include, but not be limited to, the following:[20]

- knowing which point-of-care tests are being performed, by whom and in which locations
- appropriate administrative responsibilities for delegation of the program
- monitoring quality control documentation
- evaluation and selection of appropriate equipment
- troubleshooting all aspects of the point-of-care testing program
- coordination of training
- serving as a liaison between the nursing service, other units such as emergency department, operating rooms, and the laboratory

It is recommended that any institution with point-of-care testing have a standing committee to ensure appropriate oversight. Such a committee would be composed of representatives from the laboratory, nursing service, medical staff, and the quality assurance officer. The committee should have the authority to approve the methodology to be used and control the purchasing of point-of-care devices.

COST BENEFIT ISSUES

The literature is filled with opinions of the costs and effectiveness of point-of-care testing. Extreme forms of point-of-care testing ("Patient Focused Care") have been advocated[21] which seem to imply expensive reduplication of capital investments for laboratory equipment despite lack of proof of cost-effective performance.[22] Cost studies and cost-effectiveness studies are extraordinarily complicated and expensive undertakings that might apply only to the particular institution doing the study. Baer[23] reviewed the issues of cost analysis for point-of-care testing. His summary of the deficiencies in published cost analyses include the following.

- Only incremental costs of labor and consumables are included with many assumptions about the costs of nonlaboratory personnel.
- Studies do not differentiate the differences between fixed and incremental costs as they impact the central laboratory and point-of-care testing.
- They do not consider the cost of the episode of care or the patient's long-term follow-up costs.

Keffer[24] makes the following assertions.

- Testing at the point-of-care is arguably more expensive than batches by volume testing in the central laboratory.
- Pneumatic tube transport of specimens can optimize delivery of specimens to the central laboratory with minimal delays (if operating ideally).
- The assignment of costs for centralized testing is frequently underestimated. Some of the hidden costs include training, certification, quality assurance, quality control, method duplication, instrumentation, and proficiency testing.
- Not assessed in studies of costs solely focused on the centralized analytical test are additional "negative and positive" costs associated with the use of point-of-care testing including cost of performing a cost-efficiency assessment, analytic costs, quality costs including training, retraining, quality assurance, duplicate testing, preventative maintenance, service contracts, and dilution of samples yielding high values.

It is important to recognize that assessment of the costs of point-of-care testing should include potential savings to the institution as decreased inpatient days, more efficient care leading to decreased utilization of services, and reduced numbers of follow-up visits to the clinic. There are other costs which may be hard to quantify such as the savings of a diabetic patient remaining in good control and thus avoiding or delaying the onset of microangiopathy. Other benefits from point-of-care testing include:[24]

- improved turnaround time
- improved patient management
- improved patient satisfaction and compliance
- improved throughput of the clinic/institution
- improved clinic/laboratory relations
- improved job satisfaction of physician and nurse empowerment
- improved clinic reputation
- decreased transfusions in surgery and decreased re-explorations
- decreased operating room time
- improved morbidity and mortality
- decreased dietetic services awaiting early morning glucose testing
- small sample volume
- reduced pre- and postanalytical errors

It is clear that decisions must be made daily, even in the absence of hard data. In most cases, cost must be weighed against quality impact of point-of-care methods.

A current editorial notes that a major disadvantage of POCT is lack of bidirectional communication between information systems and POCT devices.[25]

Footnotes

1. Louie RF, Tang Z, Shelby DG, et al, "Point-of-Care Glucose Testing: Millenium Technology for Critical Care," *Lab Med*, 2000, 31:402-8.
2. Koepke JA, "Point-of-Care Coagulation Testing," *Lab Med*, 2000, 31:343-6.
3. Handorf CR, "Background-Setting the Stage for Alternate-Site Laboratory Testing," *Clin Lab Med*, 1994, 14(3):451-8.
4. Woo J and Henry JB, "The Advance of Technology as a Preclude to the Laboratory of the Twenty-First Century," *Clin Lab Med*, 1994, 14(3):459-71.
5. Paxton A, "Point-of-Care Testing: How Much Growth Lies Ahead," *CAP Today*, 1998, 12(4):40-4.
6. Wilding P and Ciaverelli C, "Hand Held Sensor Systems," *Point of Care Testing*, Price CP and Hicks JM, eds, AACC Press: Washington, DC, 1999, 41-66.
7. Lum G, "Assessment of a Critical Limit Protocol for Point-of-Care Glucose Testing," *Am J Clin Pathol*, 1996, 106(3):390-5.
8. Travers EM, Wolke JC, and Stitak MM, "Consolidating Ancillary Testing in Multihospital Systems," *Clin Lab Med*, 1994, 14(3):493-524.
9. Allred TJ and Stelner L, "Alternate-Site Testing. Consider the Analyst," *Clin Lab Med*, 1994, 14(3):569-604.
10. Titus K, "Nurses At the Point of Care Whether or Not Labs Are There," *CAP Today*, 1996, 25.
11. Stott RA, Hortin GL, Wilhite TR, et al, "Analytical Artifacts in Hematocrit Measurements by Whole-Blood Chemistry Analyzers," *Clin Chem*, 1995, 41(2):306-11.
12. Bachner P, "Alternate Site Testing. The Old and New Paradigm or the Past Is Prologue," *Arch Pathol Lab Med*, 1995, 119(10):881-5.
13. Becker RC, "Exploring the Medical Need for Alternate Site Testing. A Clinician's Perspective," *Arch Pathol Lab Med*, 1995, 119(10):894-7.
14. Fuhrman SA, Travers FM, and Handorf CR, "The Mobile Laboratory in Alternative Site Testing," *Arch Pathol Lab Med*, 1995, 119(10):939-42.
15. Laposata M and Lewandrowski KB, "Near Patient Blood Glucose Monitoring," *Arch Pathol Lab Med*, 1995, 119(10):926-8.
16. Kilgore ML, Steindel SJ, and Smith JA, "Continuous Quality Improvement for Point-of-Care Testing Using Background Monitoring of Duplicate Specimens," *Arch Pathol Lab Med*, 1999, 123(9):824-28.
17. Steindel SJ, "Timeliness of Clinical Laboratory Tests. A Discussion Based on Five College of American Pathologists Q-Probe Studies," *Arch Pathol Lab Med*, 1995, 119(10):918-23.
18. Jones BA, Bachner P, and Howanitz PJ, "Bedside Glucose Monitoring: A College of American Pathologists Q-Probes Study of the Program Characteristics and Performance in 605 Institutions," *Arch Pathol Lab Med*, 1993, 117(11):1080-7.

19. Novis DA and Jones BA, "Interinstitutional Comparison of Bedside Blood Glucose Monitoring Program Characteristics, Accuracy, Performance and Quality Control Documentation," *Arch Pathol Lab Med*, 1998, 122(11):495-502.
20. Chapman B, "Glucose Tests at the Point of Care," *CAP Today*, 1998, 12(4):24-6, 28, 31 passim.
21. Jenner EA, "A Case Study Analysis of Nurses' Roles, Education, and Training Needs Associated With Patient-Focused Care," *J Adv Nurs*, 1998, 27(5):1087-95.
22. Heymann TD and Culling W, "The Patient-Focused Approach: A Better Way to Run a Hospital?" *J Royal Coll Physicians Lond*, 1996, 30(2):142-4.
23. Baer DM, "Point-of-Care Testing Versus Lab Costs," *MLO*, 1998, 30(9):46-56.
24. Keffer JH, "Point of Care Testing Update," The 6th Annual Progress in Clinical Pathology (Workshop), March 4-6, 1999, Dallas, Texas.
25. Kost GJ, "Connectivity - The Millenium Challenge for Point-of-Care Testing," *Arch Pathol Lab Med*, 2000, 124(8):1108-10.

References

Auerbach DM, "Alternate Site Testing - Information Handling and Reporting Issues," *Arch Pathol Lab Med*, 1995, 119(10):924-5.

Belanger AC, "Alternate Site Testing - The Regulatory Perspective," *Arch Pathol Lab Med*, 1995, 119(10):902-6.

Bennett J, Cervantes C, and Pacheco S, "Point-of-Care Testing: Inspection Preparedness," *Perfusion*, 2000, 15(2):137-42.

Chance, JJ, Li DJ, Jones AA, et al, "Technical Evaluation of Five Glucose Meters With Data," *Am J Clin Pathol*, 1999, 111(4):547-56.

"Coagulation at the Point of Care," *CAP Today*, October 2000, 80-2, 86-7, 90.

Foubister V, "POC Checklist a Road Map for Bedside Testing," *CAP Today*, October 2000, 36-40.

Fraser CG and Petersen PH, "Desirable Performance Standards for Imprecision and Bias in Alternate Sites - The Views of Laboratory Professionals," *Arch Pathol Lab Med*, 1995, 119(10):909-13.

Gallichan M, "Self Monitoring of Glucose by People With Diabetes: Evidence Based Practice," *BMJ*, 1997, 314(7085):964-7.

Gonzales Y and Kampa IS, "The Effect of Various Storage Environments on Reagent Strips," *Lab Med*, 1999, 28(2):136-7.

Green M, "Successful Alternatives to Alternate Site Testing - Use of a Pneumatic Tube System to the Central Laboratory," *Arch Pathol Lab Med*, 1995, 119(10):943-7.

Greendyke RM and Gifford FR, "Testing Blood Glucose at the Bedside in a Chronic Care Hospital," *Lab Med*, 1997, 28(1):63-5.

Hirschl M, Herkner H, Laggner AN, et al, "Analytical and Clinical Performance of an Improved Qualitative Troponin T Rapid Test in Laboratories and Critical Care Units," *Arch Pathol Lab Med*, 2000, 124(4):583-7.

Kost GJ, Nguyen TH, and Tang Z, "Whole-Blood Glucose and Lactate. Trilayer Biosensors, Drug Interference, Metabolism, and Practice Guidelines," *Arch Pathol Lab Med*, 2000, 124(8):1128-34.

Lamb LS Jr, "Responsibilities in Point-of-Care Testing - An Institutional Perspective," *Arch Pathol Lab Med*, 1995, 119(10):886-9.

Maln RI and Kiechle FL, "Point-of-Care Testing: Administration Within a Health System," *Lab Med*, 2000, 31(8):453-9.

Mohammed AA, Summers H, Burchfield JE, et al, "STAT Turnaround Time; Satellite and Point-to-Point Testing," *Lab Med*, 1996, 27(10):684-7.

Ng VL, Kraemer R, Hogan C, et al, "The Rise and Fall of i-STAT Point-of-Care Blood Gas Testing in an Acute Care Hospital," *Am J Clin Pathol*, 2000, 114(1):128-38.

Peredy TR and Powers RD, "Bedside Diagnostic Testing of Body Fluids," *Am J Emerg Med*, 1997, 15(4):400-7.

Quality Point-of-Care Testing: A Joint Commission Handbook, Oakbrook Terrace, IL: Joint Commission on Accreditation of Healthcare Organizations, 1999, 140.

Sandrick K, "Moving Blood Gas Testing to the Point of Care," *CAP Today*, 2000, 14(8):37-42.

St Louis P, "Status of Point-of-Care Testing: Promise, Realities, and Possibilities," *Clin Biochem*, 2000, 33(6):427-40.

Tang Z, Lee JH, Louie RF, et al, "Effects of Different Hematocrit Levels on Glucose Measurements With Handheld Meters for Point-of-Care Testing," *Arch Pathol Lab Med*, 2000, 124(8):1135-40.

Voss EM, Bina DM, McNeil LD, et al, "Determining Acceptability of Blood Glucose Meters. Statistical Methods for Determining Error," *Lab Med*, 1996, 27(9):601-6.

Voss EM, Bina DM, McNeil LD, et al, "Determining Acceptability of Blood Glucose Meters. Evaluating a Blood Glucose Testing System," *Lab Med*, 1996, 27(10):679-82.

Watts NB, "Reproducibility (Precision) in Alternate Site Testing, a Clinician's Perspective," *Arch Pathol Lab Med*, 1995, 119:(10)914-7.

Wilson F, "Minimally Invasive Testing Expands Beyond Glucose," *Lab Med*, 2000, 31(8):436-41.

♦ **Precautions, Specimen Collection** *see* Blood and Fluid Precautions, Specimen Collection *on page 40*

♦ **Pulse Oximetry** *see* Point-of-Care Testing *on page 43*

♦ **Rejection Criteria, Specimen** *see* Specimen Rejection Criteria *on page 47*

♦ **Requisition Information** *see* Specimen Identification Requirements *on page 46*

Skin Puncture Blood Collection

Related Information

Blood and Fluid Precautions, Specimen Collection *on page 40*
Phlebotomist Procedures *on page 43*
Specimen Identification Requirements *on page 46*

Synonyms Capillary Blood Collection; Fingerstick Blood Collection; Heelstick Blood Collection

Applies to Arterialized Capillary Blood; Peripheral Blood Smear Preparation
(Continued)

Skin Puncture Blood Collection *(Continued)*

Test Includes Obtaining capillary blood from finger tip of an adult or heel in infants

Abstract If only a small volume of blood is required, skin puncture may be the optimal method of blood collection, particularly in infants and children. It is also an ideal way of collecting blood for home testing (eg, glucose testing).

Patient Preparation

Heel puncture: Select a site on the medial or lateral portion of the plantar surface of the foot. Do not puncture greater than 2.4 mm. Do not puncture the posterior curvature of the heel.[1] Do not repuncture previous puncture sites because of the possibility of infection.

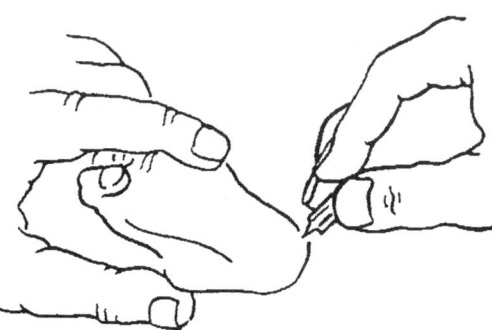

Gloves should be worn when collecting capillary blood specimens.
From JD Bauer, *Clinical Laboratory Methods*, 9th ed, St. Louis, MO: Mosby-Year Book Inc, 1982, with permission.

Finger puncture: Select a site on the palmar aspect on the center of distal phalanx. Do not puncture the side or tip of the phalanx because the skin is much thinner.

Skin preparation: The skin site selected should be cleaned with 70% isopropyl alcohol (isopropanol) and dried with sterile gauze. Infection is a frequent complication of fingersticks. Prepare the skin site carefully. Do not use iodine, which interferes with many assays.

Arterialized blood: Warming the site with a moist towel at temperatures not to exceed 42°C produces an increase in blood flow and **arterializes the capillary blood**. pH and blood gas determinations are usually performed on arterialized capillary blood in infants and children.

Aftercare Elevate the site above the body and apply direct pressure to the puncture site with sterile gauze until bleeding stops. Bandaids or bandages are generally not applied because of the risk of skin sensitization to tape and the risk of aspiration, should the bandage come loose.

Specimen Capillary blood or arterialized capillary blood

Container Capillary tube or microtube

Collection Patient identification: Confirm that the patient being drawn is the correct one by comparing the requisition with the identification wristband. After preparation of the selected site, the skin should be punctured at a slight angle. A disposable skin puncture lancet should be used rather than a surgical blade because a surgical blade may make too deep an incision and damage underlying tissues. The first drop should be wiped away as it may be diluted by tissue fluid. Blood flow will be increased by holding the site downward. Slight pressure may be applied to the surrounding tissue. **Squeezing or milking the puncture site should not be done.** Tubes should be sealed quickly to avoid exposure to atmospheric oxygen. The specimen should be labeled with the patient's name, hospital number, room number, date and time of collection, and initials or identification of the person collecting the specimen.

Special Instructions Avoid injury to the calcaneus (heel bone). Be aware of the volume of specimens being collected from newborns. The limited blood volumes of neonates makes extensive testing hazardous and sometimes necessitates transfusion if the volume of blood required for testing is significant. Such caution includes specimens for blood gas analysis.

Use Obtain capillary or arterialized capillary blood for analysis. Collection of blood from infants and children, patients who have had repeated venipunctures or whose veins are damaged or inadequate. Procedure of choice for preparing peripheral blood smears for morphologic examinations.

Limitations Technically, a specimen obtained by skin puncture consists of a mixture of arterial, capillary and venous blood, and tissue fluid. Specimen volume is limited. Repeat determinations often require repeat blood collection. Finger tips are sensitive; the procedure may be painful. Infection, particularly in debilitated hosts, may occur. Cell counts (ie, RBC, WBC, and platelets) are not accurate on capillary specimens. There is greater risk of infection than venipuncture.

Contraindications Use of surgical blades may create a wound deeper and larger than necessary and are contraindicated. **Finger punctures should not be performed on infants because the distance from the skin to the bone is less than 1.5 mm.**

Additional Information In recent years, blood collection by skin puncture has become more convenient and standardized due to availability of spring-loaded lancets. A cut of standard width and depth can be made with these lancets.

Footnotes

1. Blumenfeld TA, Turi GK, and Blanc WA, "Recommended Site and Depth of Newborn Heel Skin Punctures Based on Anatomical Measurements and Histopathology," *Lancet*, 1979, 1(8110):230-3.

References

National Committee for Clinical Laboratory Standards, *Procedures for the Collection of Diagnostic Blood Specimens by Skin Puncture*, 3rd ed, Approved Standard, NCCLS Publication H4-A3, Wayne, PA: National Committee for Clinical Laboratory Standards, 1991.

♦ **Specimen Collection Policy, Phlebotomist** *see* Phlebotomist Procedures *on page 43*

Specimen Identification Requirements

Related Information

Arterial Blood Collection *on page 40*
Phlebotomist Procedures *on page 43*
Skin Puncture Blood Collection *on page 45*
Venous Blood Collection *on page 47*

Synonyms Identification Requirements, Specimen

Applies to Bacteriology Specimen Identification; Blood Specimen Identification; Body Fluid Identification; Cytology Smear Identification; Pathology Specimen Identification; Requisition Information; Spinal Fluid Identification; Urine Specimen Identification

Abstract Regulatory agencies require that each laboratory has a written policy for specimen identification.

Causes for Rejection Laboratories reserve the right to refuse improperly labeled specimens. Accurate specimen identification is critical to the provision of accurate results. Specimens must be provided in appropriate containers with correct preservatives; see individual test listings.

Special Instructions Patient identification: Inpatient: Compare the information on the request form with the patient's identification band and room and bed number. Confirm identification by asking the patient to state his/her full name. If the patient cannot state his/her name, ask a nurse or patient's relative to confirm the patient's identity. Confirm that the specimen label information is identical to the wristband and request form information. Label specimens as indicated below. Outpatient: Confirm identification by asking the patient to state his/her full name. If the patient cannot state his/her name, ask a nurse or patient's relative to confirm the patient's identity. Confirm the specimen label information is identical to the wristband and request form information. The requirements for labeling specimens and requisitions are as follows.

Blood specimens: All blood specimens received by the laboratory must have a permanently attached label with the following information written in black indelible ink: patient's name, hospital number, date and time of collection, initials of person drawing the specimen. Person obtaining blood sample must perform the proper identification check. Draw the sample of blood. Label all the tubes at the patient's bedside. Certain blood tests require special or immediate handling after collection. Consult the individual test listings for specific information and also the Transfusion Service (Blood Bank) Introduction *on page 827* for specifics on Blood Bank patient identification.

Urine specimens: All urine specimens received by the laboratory must have the following information fixed to the container (not cover): patient's name, hospital number, date and time of collection. Urine specimens delivered to the laboratory usually must be placed in the specimen refrigerator. Certain urine tests require special or immediate handling after collection; eg, crystalluria is best evaluated on a fresh, warm specimen. Consult the individual test listings for specific information.

Cerebrospinal fluids: Each tube submitted must be labeled with the patient's name, hospital number, source of specimen, date and time of collection, tube identification number (#1, #2, #3 according to the order of collection). Spinal fluid tests are usually considered to be stat procedures because spinal fluid constituents are unstable and cells degrade quickly, and because some may be samples from patients with meningitis. Consequently, spinal fluid must be taken to the laboratory immediately after collection and handed to a technologist or receptionist. Consult the individual test listings for specific information; most such listings in this book bear designations beginning "Cerebrospinal Fluid...".

Body fluids: All body fluids must be labeled with the patient's name, hospital number, date and time of collection, source of fluid. Body fluid constituents are unstable, and thus, expeditious handling is required. Some may derive from patients with medical emergencies or catastrophies. Consult individual test listings for specific information; many in this book bear designations beginning "Body Fluid...".

Cytology smears: All slides for cytologic examination should be appropriately and immediately fixed, labeled with the patient's name, and placed in a cardboard folder with the cytology requisition slip containing patient's name, patient information, and physician's name wrapped around it. Further information is provided in the Cytopathology Introduction *on page 369*.

Bacteriology specimens: All specimens for bacteriology testing must be labeled with the patient's name, hospital number, date and time of collection, source of material. Bacteriology specimens should be delivered to the laboratory as soon after collection as possible to preserve the viability of bacteria or viruses and to provide optimal patient care.

Pathology (surgical) specimens: All specimens for pathology must be labeled with the patient's name, hospital number, name of physician, name of surgeon, and source of specimen. Further information is available in the Anatomic Pathology Introduction *on page 49*. For many but not all specimens, the listing Histopathology provides detailed information. Consult individual test listings for specific information pertinent to specimens requiring special handling.

Chain-of-custody specimens: Specimens for drugs of abuse screening and specimens which may be used as legal evidence (eg, bullets removed surgically) must be collected according to a chain-of-custody protocol. For further information, see Toxicology/Drugs of Abuse Introduction *on page 773* for Chain-of-Custody form, and also see Chain-of-Custody Protocol *on page 785*.

Specimen Rejection Criteria

Synonyms Rejection Criteria, Specimen; Unsatisfactory Specimens Criteria

Causes for Rejection Criteria for specimen rejection are dependent on individual tests. Generally, specimens received by a laboratory are not discarded until the physician ordering the test or responsible nursing unit is notified. Events which may lead to the rejection of a specimen include specimen improperly labeled or unlabeled, specimen improperly collected and/or preserved, specimen sample volume not sufficient for requirement of test protocol, outside of container contaminated by specimen (ie, infectious hazard), or patient not properly prepared for test requirements. An example of the latter includes a nonfasting state for assays in which fasting is needed.

Some information is provided under Causes for Rejection in individual test listings, but most requirements are provided under appropriate fields such as Preparation.

It is ultimately the responsibility of the ordering physician to make certain that the laboratory is provided with a properly collected and identified specimen for analysis. Communications regarding less than optimal specimens generally should be oriented toward concern for patient welfare rather than nonavailability or unwillingness to provide laboratory service.

♦ **Spinal Fluid Identification** *see* Specimen Identification Requirements *on page 46*

♦ **Timed Urine Collection** *see* Urine Collection, 24-Hour *on page 47*

♦ **Tubes for Blood Collection** *see* Blood Collection Tube Information *on page 42*

♦ **Twenty-Four Hour Urine Collection** *see* Urine Collection, 24-Hour *on page 47*

♦ **Unsatisfactory Specimens Criteria** *see* Specimen Rejection Criteria *on page 47*

♦ **Urine Collection, 12-Hour, 2-Hour, and Timed** *see* Urine Collection, 24-Hour *on page 47*

Urine Collection, 24-Hour

Related Information
Aldosterone, Urine *on page 91*
Arsenic, Urine *on page 781*
Beta₂-Microglobulin, Serum or Urine *on page 509*
Cadmium, Urine *on page 783*
Calcium, Urine *on page 133*
Catecholamines, Fractionation, Urine *on page 139*
Chromium, Urine *on page 816*
Citrate, Serum, Plasma, or Urine *on page 149*
Copper, Urine *on page 818*
Cortisol, Free, Urine *on page 154*
Creatinine, 12- or 24-Hour Urine *on page 159*
Creatinine Clearance *on page 160*
Delta (5)-Aminolevulinic Acid, Urine *on page 165*
Follicle Stimulating Hormone, Serum, Plasma, or Urine *on page 175*
Glucose, Quantitative, Urine *on page 874*
Heavy Metal Screen, Urine *on page 792*
Homovanillic Acid, Urine *on page 195*
17-Hydroxycorticosteroids, Urine *on page 196*
5-Hydroxyindoleacetic Acid, Quantitative, Urine *on page 197*
Hydroxyproline, Total, Urine *on page 199*
Lactose Tolerance Test *on page 209*
Lead, Urine *on page 795*
Luteinizing Hormone, Blood or Urine *on page 219*
Lysozyme, Blood and Urine *on page 457*
Magnesium, Urine *on page 222*
Manganese, Urine *on page 820*

Mercury, Urine *on page 798*
Metanephrines, Urine or Plasma *on page 223*
Microalbuminuria *on page 879*
Mucopolysaccharides, Urine *on page 226*
N-Telopeptides, Urine *on page 233*
Oxalate, Urine *on page 238*
Porphyrins, Quantitative, Urine *on page 255*
Potassium, Urine *on page 259*
Pregnanetriol, Urine *on page 261*
Protein, Quantitative, Urine *on page 883*
Selenium, Urine *on page 823*
Thallium, Urine or Blood *on page 807*
Uric Acid, Urine *on page 295*
Vanillylmandelic Acid, Urine *on page 297*
Zinc, Urine *on page 825*

Synonyms Twenty-Four Hour Urine Collection

Applies to Timed Urine Collection; Urine Collection, 12-Hour, 2-Hour, and Timed

Abstract Proper instruction of the patient is critically important. The individuals who provide collection materials are situated ideally to review appropriate procedures. If several tests are needed, using different preservatives, explanation is desirable.

Patient Preparation Fasting the evening before urine collection is requested by some laboratories for some determinations (eg, amylase). Deletion of alcoholic beverages may be requested (eg, before collection for uric acid). Deletion of over-the-counter substances before testing may be needed (eg, ascorbic acid during collection for urinary oxalate).

Specimen The patient should understand whether or not refrigeration of the specimen during collection is needed or contraindicated.

Collection Twenty-four hour urine collections are often a problem for both patient and laboratory. A good collection regimen is as follows: Discard first morning specimen on day one. Collect all specimens during the remainder of the day and evening. Collect the first morning specimen on day two. Stop collection. Label specimen with patient's name, hospital number, room number, and date and time of collection. This presumes that time of arising is the same on day one and day two. Alternate regimen: Patient is to empty his/her bladder completely at a designated time (eg, 8 AM). This specimen is discarded. All urine is saved throughout the day and evening. Patient is to empty his/her bladder at the same time on day two as in step 1 above (eg, 8 AM). This specimen is combined with the rest of the collection for the previous 24 hours. Stop collection. Label specimen with patient's name, hospital number, room number, date and time of collection. Urines must be kept chilled at 5°C if bacteriologic activity will adversely affect results (eg, Schilling's test).

Normal fluid intake is allowed during 24-hour urine collections. Dietary restrictions are required for some procedures and are specified in the individual test listing. Since results are based on total volume, it is critical that the volume be measured accurately and the information included with the paper or electronic test requisition. Clearance tests require an estimate of body surface area; patient's height and weight must be available to the laboratory or provided to the laboratory when a clearance is requested.

For other timed collection (eg, 12-hour, etc), similar directions, as for 24-hour urine collection, should be followed.

Causes for Rejection A number of laboratories reject the sample, if >10% is lost in collection.

Special Instructions See instructions in the particular listings listed above under Related Information for urine collections for trace metals. See specific instructions elsewhere in this book under specific listings for collection procedures for other substances. For information on urine collection procedures for drugs of abuse testing, see the Toxicology/Drugs of Abuse Introduction *on page 773*.

Limitations Some tests require a critical minimal volume for accuracy. For example, some Schilling test protocols require a minimum of 500 mL/24 hours, and are unreliable for reduced urine volumes. Consult individual test listings for information on critical urine volumes.

Additional Information The procedure may be followed for other timed collections (ie, 12-hour, etc) as follows: Discard the initial specimen. Record time. Collect all specimens voided within the requested time frame. Label the specimen with patient's name, hospital number, room number, and date and time of collection.

Due to difficulties in 24-hour urine collection, particularly in children, an increasing number of test results (eg, organic acids, amino acids, HVA, VMA, etc) are normalized to creatinine on randomly collected urine.

♦ **Urine Specimen Identification** *see* Specimen Identification Requirements *on page 46*

♦ **Vacutainer® Tube Description** *see* Blood Collection Tube Information *on page 42*

♦ **Venipuncture, Venous** *see* Venous Blood Collection *on page 47*

Venous Blood Collection

Related Information
Blood and Fluid Precautions, Specimen Collection *on page 40*
Blood Collection Tube Information *on page 42*
(Continued)

Venous Blood Collection *(Continued)*

Synonyms Blood Collection, Venous; Phlebotomy, Venous; Venipuncture, Venous

Test Includes Routine method for obtaining blood when anticoagulants or larger volumes than can be obtained by capillary blood collection are required

Patient Preparation Select a suitable site for venipuncture. Prepare the site by scrubbing with 70% isopropyl alcohol (isopropanol) using a circular motion working out from the site. Dry with gauze or let air dry. Do not touch site after cleansing until blood drawing is complete. Special requirements exist for alcohol levels; see Ethanol, Blood, Urine, and Other Sources *on page 789*. Avoid hand pumping.

Aftercare Apply pressure to the venipuncture site and elevate the arm until bleeding stops. If bleeding persists, apply a pressure dressing to the site.

Specimen Venous blood

Container Syringe with a 20- or 21-gauge needle for volumes up to 10 mL, 18-gauge for larger volumes to assure adequate blood flow. Use a Vacutainer® or similar system for multiple specimens or anticoagulants. A 20- or 21-gauge Butterfly® infusion set may be used for difficult draws or blood cultures with multiple tubes.

Sampling Time Some samples for analytes that exhibit diurnal variation should be drawn at specific times of the day. See individual test listings.

Collection Before collecting blood, the phlebotomist should verify that the patient is fasting, if fasting is indicated. The patient should be comfortably seated or supine for a few minutes before blood collection. If one must be used at all, apply tourniquet 4-6 inches above drawing site. Do not leave tourniquet applied for more than 1 minute. Cleanly puncture the vein, loosen the tourniquet, and apply gentle suction or insert Vacutainer® tube into holder to fill tubes. Remove the needle and fill the tubes without delay.

If blood is being drawn for venous pH, pCO₂, lactic acid, or electrolytes, it is best to draw blood without a tourniquet. If one is needed, leave it in place while the sample is drawn. Alternatively, if a tourniquet must be used, sample blood 1-2 minutes after the hand is relaxed and the tourniquet removed. **Avoid hand clenching for these tests, especially for potassium and lactic acid determinations.** The first aliquot is best for pH.

Gently invert tubes 10 times to assure mixing of anticoagulants.

Causes for Rejection Samples collected for coagulation studies which have <90% of the expected fill should be rejected. Samples collected for coagulation studies may require additional anticoagulant if the hematocrit is low. Grossly hemolyzed specimens may be rejected depending on tests requested. Specimens that are not properly identified cannot be accepted.

Use Obtain venous blood for analysis

Limitations Venipuncture is technically difficult in obese patients, infants, children, patients with collapsed veins such as those in shock, and occasionally, other subjects as well. Hemolysis may occur as a result of excessive suction during collection, violent mixing of the specimen, or vigorous transfer of the specimen from syringe to tube.

Contraindications Fist clenching will alter potassium, pH and pCO₂ studies. If a tourniquet is applied but released before blood is aspirated, K⁺ and lactic acid are washed out resulting in erroneous and misleading results.[1]

Additional Information Draw EDTA tube last. Hematology tubes contain K-EDTA. Any contamination can raise potassium and decrease pH.

See individual test listings for specific specimen collection requirements. To avoid contamination with tissue thromboplastins released by the venipuncture, a two-syringe or two-tube collection technique, in which the first tube is discarded, is required for coagulation specimens (eg, prothrombin time, activated partial thromboplastin time, etc). Blood collection for cytokine measurements needs particular attention to prevent possible contamination by endotoxins which can trigger cytokine production after sampling.[2] Strategies to reduce pain, particularly in children and geriatric patients have been published.[3,4,5]

Footnotes

1. Gambino R, "The Correct Way to Draw Venous Blood - Does Stasis Matter?" *Lab Rep*, 1996, 18(1):1-3.
2. Bienvenu J, Doche C, and Gutowski MC, "Methods for Studying Cytokines in Biologic Media," *Allerg Immunol* 1995, 27(4):116, 119-22.
3. Love G, "Easing the Discomfort of Venipuncture," *Nursing*, 1998, 28(3):30.
4. Farber V, "Venipunctures on the Elderly: Handle With Care," *Adv Med Lab Professionals*, 2001, 13:9-11.
5. Scholz MJ, "Minimizing the Pain of Venipuncture," *RN*, 1996, 59(5):78.

References

Bennett BD, Cox RS, Davis CM, et al, eds, *So You're Going to Collect a Blood Specimen: An Introduction to Phlebotomy*, 5th ed, Northfield, IL: College of American Pathologists, 1992.

Flynn JC Jr, *Procedures in Phlebotomy*, 2nd ed, Philadelphia, PA: WB Saunders Co, 1999.

National Committee for Clinical Laboratory Standards, *Procedures for the Handling and Processing of Blood Specimens, Approved Guideline*, NCCLS Publication H18-A, Villanova, PA: National Committee for Clinical Laboratory Standards, 1990.

National Committee for Clinical Laboratory Standards, *Procedures for the Collection of Diagnostic Blood Specimens by Venipuncture*, 3rd ed, Approved Standard, H3-A3, Villanova, PA: NCCLS, 1991.

Wray D and Wells G, "Procedures in Phlebotomy," *Arch Pathol Lab Med*, 2000, 124(4):641.

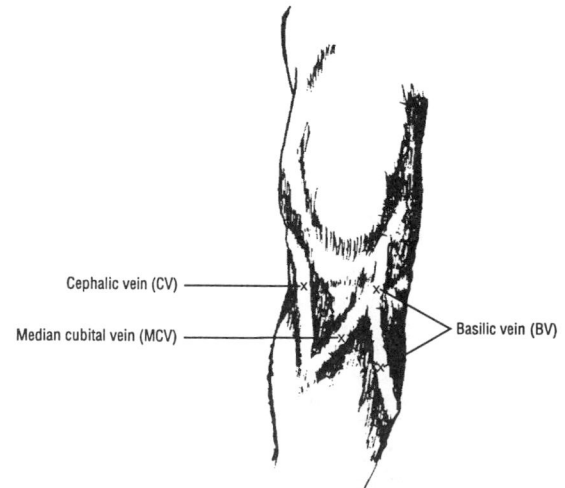

Cephalic vein (CV)

Median cubital vein (MCV)

Basilic vein (BV)

From JD Bauer, *Clinical Laboratory Methods*, 9th ed, St. Louis, MO: Mosby-Year Book Inc, 1982, with permission.

ANATOMIC PATHOLOGY

Phillip A. Munoz, MD

David S. Jacobs, MD

Contributors:

Ossoma W. Tawfik, MD, PhD

Marilyn K. Davis-Cansler, BS SCT (ASCP) CMIAC

Uri S. Alon, MD

Dwight K. Oxley, MD

Beiyen Chen, MD

Wayne R. DeMott, MD

Diane L. Persons, MD

The specialty of anatomic pathology is deeply rooted in the history of modern medicine. Its foundation is based on astute observations of anatomical changes induced by disease at the gross and microscopic levels. For the pathologist, the journey to mastering this discipline begins at the autopsy table, at which the sum of a lifetime of disease is dissected, classified, and placed in a perspective appropriate for the case at hand. The autopsy is the ultimate quality control procedure in the care of patients. It remains the validator or the invalidator of the results of many of the more recent diagnostic modalities.

For most pathologists, the journey continues in the surgical pathology laboratory, where tissue diagnoses based on gross, microscopic, and sometimes ultrastructural studies form critical junctures for the clinical decision-making process. With increasing emphasis on minimally invasive procedures, the journey is carried into the cytology laboratory, where minute fragments of tissue and individual cells are morphologically interrogated to yield clues addressing the underlying disease process. Such is a thumbnail history of diagnostic anatomic pathology.

Today, a morphologic diagnosis is often just the first step to complete a pathologic evaluation. With increasing frequency, we are called on to augment morphologic diagnoses with critical descriptors of phenotype, genotype, and fundamental pathology at the molecular level. Faced with the challenge of completing this task in an appropriate, cost-effective, and timely fashion, we are compelled to continually update our fund of knowledge and convey our collective experience in a venue that meets the needs of a broad range of clinical specialties.

We are indebted to the many contributors who have shaped this chapter through its previous editions. We especially recognize the contribution of the late Dr John G. Gruhn, a true scholar, physician, and gentleman.

- ♦ **Alpha Fetoprotein** *see* Immunoperoxidase Procedures *on page 60*
- ♦ **Aneuploidy** *see* Cell Cycle Analysis by Flow Cytometry *on page 53*
- ♦ **Automated Cytophotometry** *see* Image Analysis *on page 59*

Autopsy

Synonyms Necropsy; Postmortem Examination

Applies to Cause of Death; Coroner's Case; Death Certificate; Disease Reporting; Medical Examiner's Case; Quality Assurance in the Practice of Medicine; Vital Statistics

Abstract The expression **"autopsy"** means to see for oneself, or to see with one's own eyes. The procedure provides analysis of cause of death; the nature, extent, and type of disease(s); the effects of therapy; and indications of genetic influences. It determines primary site of tumor, source of bleeding, and major and minor findings which may or may not have been anticipated, may or may not have required treatment, and may or may not have contributed to the patient's demise.

Special Instructions Consent: A properly signed autopsy permit is usually required before a hospital necropsy can be performed. A valid permit must contain the signature of the highest ranking survivor in the next-of-kin lineage. A commonly used decreasing order of responsibility: spouse, adult children, parents, adult brothers and sisters, relatives, and then anyone who will accept responsibility for the body for purposes of burial. (State laws are not uniform.) Permits include name of decedent, date of birth, hospital number, date and time of death, authorizing signature(s) with relationship to the decedent, date and time permission given, and extent (complete autopsy or specific designated restrictions). Clinical information is always desirable, including the major clinical diagnoses, surgical procedures, recognized complications, a summary of the clinical cause and terminal episode. Compliance with appropriate state laws is, of course, necessary.[1] Witnesses are often required to sign autopsy permits. It is usually the responsibility of the attending physician to obtain permission for the autopsy from the next-of-kin.

It is desirable as well as courteous for the attending physician to discuss the clinical particulars with the pathologist before the dissection is begun. In regard to physician attendance at autopsy, some of the most important clinicopathologic correlations and in-depth investigations occur in autopsies at which clinicians attend. Topics are often discussed which are not in the medical record, and morphologic findings may provide immediate feedback to a clinician in a way unavailable to him/her from even a lengthy autopsy report. Clinician attendance at autopsy is always rewarding to everyone involved. Particularly in autopsies on individuals who are not hospital inpatients, critical clinical facts are likely to be unavailable, fragmentary, or completely unknown. The presence of the attending physician at such autopsies compensates to some degree for the lack of a well worked up chart. Except in Coroner's cases, it is usually the responsibility of the attending physician to complete the death certificate.

Use A teaching instrument of great value, the autopsy remains a component of good medical care. A vital clinical quality control measure,[2] it is a definitive monitor of quality of care given to the patient or by the medical system;[3] *vide infra.* The autopsy supports recognition of emerging medical entities, such as acquired immunodeficiency syndrome (AIDS), hantavirus infection, and Ebola virus infection, and provides recognition of changes taking place in old ones.

Validated for over a century, the autopsy is a great deal more than an educational tool. It determines the cause and manner of death, determines severity of disease, represents an effort to preserve the quality of medical practice and to support excellence in medicine (quality assurance). It enhances medical knowledge, provides insight to understand pathogenesis and recognition of hereditary/familial diseases relevant to genetic counseling and possibly pertinent to surviving relatives, and permits diagnosis of contagious diseases and exposure to toxic entities. The autopsy provides valid comparisons between premortem and postmortem diagnoses. It produces valid statistics not otherwise available. Autopsies provide information on certain environmental or occupational exposures, provide data relevant to the public health and vital statistics, yield information on the success or failure of therapy, and provide data for evaluation of new procedures and new drugs not obtained by other means.

Autopsies support communication between the attending physician and the decedent's family and diminish family grief over unanswered questions.

Limitations Autopsies may be time-consuming, often are expensive but are not regularly reimbursed. The need for relevance has been expressed and emphasis on partial autopsies has been emphasized.[4]

Contraindications Improperly completed written permission

Methodology Gross organ examination, often with microscopy, with subsequent special procedures as indicated. A useful guide to format is available, providing practical definitions.[5] Extensive methods, procedures, and techniques are available. Heart blood cultures are often done in hospital necropsies. Toxicology, DNA investigation, additional microbiologic studies, and many other procedures are performed as indicated.

Additional Information

THE AUTOPSY MAY SUPPORT RISK MANAGEMENT

It may eliminate suspicion and provide reassurance to families; it may provide facts instead of conjecture, and support malpractice defense and reduce medicolegal claims as well as improve the quality of care.[6,7]

QUALITY ASSURANCE AND THE AUTOPSY

Overreliance on contemporary procedures including imaging techniques occasionally leads to missed diagnoses. Of 176 autopsies in a recently published series, 44.9% uncovered one or more undiagnosed causes of death. The most often misdiagnosed or missed entities included infections, infarcts, and malignancies.[7] The most frequently overlooked immediate causes of death in another study included pulmonary embolism and gastrointestinal hemorrhage.[8] In a Belgian paper, the most frequent class I missed major diagnoses were fungal infections, cardiac tamponade, abdominal hemorrhage, and myocardial infarct.[9]

Discrepancies between antemortem and postmortem diagnoses lead to skepticism about critical health statistics which are not based on autopsy findings. Cabot had questioned the accuracy of death certificates in 1912; such questions have persisted in the United Kingdom, in the United States, and in a number of other Western countries for good reasons. The vast inaccuracy of death certificates, can lead to wrong priorities and wrong policies derived from faulty statistics.

It is not currently possible to predict which autopsy cases will have high yields.[7,10,11] Overwhelming data document the need for the autopsy in quality assurance.[12] Ideally cases to be autopsied should be randomly selected to exclude bias.

Guidelines for request for postmortem examination somewhat overlap forensic considerations and may include:

- unanticipated death
- obscure cause of death
- death occurring while the patient is being treated with a new therapy
- intraoperative or intraprocedural death
- death occurring within 48 hours after surgery or an invasive diagnostic procedure
- death related to pregnancy or within 7 days of delivery
- death during a psychiatric admission
- death in admitted infants and children

MEDICAL EXAMINER AND CORONER SYSTEMS; FORENSIC PATHOLOGY[13]

In possible medical legal cases, the Medical Examiner or Coroner should be contacted before any suggestion regarding autopsy permission is made to the family of the deceased. Cases falling under the jurisdiction of the Medical Examiner or Coroner usually include all unnatural deaths including sudden unexpected or unexplained death, death due to accident and violence (death following injury immediately or delayed for an indefinite time), cases of suspected homicide or suicide, unusual or suspicious circumstances including poisoning, and cases falling in the public interest (ie, possible threat to public health such as meningitis or other contagious diseases). The Medical Examiner's or Coroner's Office should be notified in the event of all deaths in which a physician was not recently attending the patient (usually defined as the 48 hours prior to death) or in which the personal physician is unwilling to sign the death certificate. The Medical Examiner's or Coroner's office should be notified of unexpected deaths of infants and children and of all drug deaths, save for anesthetic deaths in most jurisdictions, or complications of diagnostic or therapeutic procedures. Deaths in custody (jail, psychiatric facilities, and other custodial situations) should elicit notification. Deaths due to unlawful termination of pregnancy, whether self-induced or otherwise, require notification. Deaths related to disease, injury, or toxins related to employment require notification. Such deaths need not be immediate. Investigation may be indicated for a body to be cremated or buried at sea, for unclaimed bodies, for deaths of operators of public conveyances while performing their duties, and for unexplained deaths of public officials. Persons who have knowledge of such deaths are usually required to notify the medical examiner or Coroner. Failure to do so may be a misdemeanor. Transfer of a body from another jurisdiction without medical death certification may be illegal, depending on local statutes and regulations.[14]

The autopsy may resolve insurance questions, including addressing diagnoses of suicide or homicide.

HAZARDS OF THE AUTOPSY

Hazards of necropsies include tuberculosis, hepatitis B, acquired immune deficiency syndrome (AIDS), and Jakob-Creutzfeldt disease.[15,16] Formalin does not kill the etiologic agent of Jakob-Creutzfeldt disease, and it may not kill mycobacteria promptly.

Footnotes

1. Zarbo RJ, Baker PB, and Howanitz PJ, "Quality Assurance of Autopsy Permit Form Information, Timeliness of Performance, and Issuance of Preliminary Report," *Arch Pathol Lab Med*, 1996, 120(4):346-52.
2. Scottolini AG and Weinstein SR, "The Autopsy in Clinical Quality Control," *JAMA*, 1983, 250:1192-4.
3. Lundberg GD, "Medical Students, Truth, and Autopsies," *JAMA*, 1983, 250:1199-1200.
4. Rosai J, "The Posthumous Analysis (PHA): An Alternative to the Conventional Autopsy," *Am J Clin Pathol*, 1996, 106(Suppl 1):S15-S17.
5. Hutchins GM, Berman JJ, Moore GW, et al, "Practice Guidelines for Autopsy Pathology," *Arch Pathol Lab Med*, 1999, 123(11):1085-92.

6. Valaske MJ, "Loss Control/Risk Management. A Survey of the Contribution of Autopsy Examination," *Arch Pathol Lab Med*, 1984, 108(6):462-8.

7. Nichols L, Aronica P, and Babe C, "Are Autopsies Obsolete?" *Am J Clin Pathol*, 1998, 110(2):210-18.

8. Stevanovic G, Tucakovic G, Dotlic R, et al, "Correlation of Clinical Diagnosis With Autopsy Findings: A Retrospective Study of 2145 Consecutive Autopsies," *Hum Pathol*, 1986, 17(12):1225-30.

9. Roosen J, Frans E, Wilmer A, et al, "Comparison of Premortem Clinical Diagnoses in Critically Ill Patients and Subsequent Autopsy Findings," *Mayo Clin Proc*, 2000, 75(6):562-7.

10. Friederici HH and Sebastian M, "Autopsies in a Modern Teaching Hospital. A Review of 2,537 Cases," *Arch Pathol Lab Med*, 1984, 108(6):518-21.

11. Lundberg GD, "Now Is the Time to Emphasize the Autopsy in Quality Assurance," *JAMA*, 1988, 260(23):3488.

12. Landefeld CS, Chren MM, Myers A, et al, "Diagnostic Yield of the Autopsy in a University Hospital and a Community Hospital," *N Engl J Med*, 1988, 318(19):1249-54.

13. Hanzlick R and Combs D, "Medical Examiner and Coroner Systems: History and Trends," *JAMA*, 1998, 279(11):870-4.

14. Randall BB, Fierro MF, and Froede RC, "Practice Guideline for Forensic Pathology," *Arch Pathol Lab Med*, 1998, 122(12):1056-64.

15. Orenstein JM, "Guidelines for High Risk or Potentially High Risk Autopsy Cases," *Pathologist*, 1984, 33-4.

16. Johnson MD, Schaffner W, Atkinson J, et al, "Autopsy Risk and Acquisition of Human Immunodeficiency Virus Infection: A Case Report and Reappraisal," *Arch Pathol Lab Med*, 1997, 121(1):64-6.

References

Arch Pathol Lab Med, 1996, 120(8): Please refer to this entire issue which focuses on facets of the autopsy and provides a wealth of further information.

Burke MC, Aghababian RV, and Blackbourne B, "Use of Autopsy Results in the Emergency Department Quality Assurance Plan," *Ann Emerg Med*, 1990, 19(4):363-6.

Friederici HH, "Reflections on the Postmortem Audit," *JAMA*, 1988, 260(23):3461-5.

Froede RC, "Forensic Pathology, Part II," *Clinics in Laboratory Medicine*, Volume 18, Philadelphia, PA: WB Saunders Co, 1998.

Geller SA, "Religious Attitudes and the Autopsy," *Arch Pathol Lab Med*, 1984, 108(6):494-6.

Hill RB and Anderson RE, "The Recent History of the Autopsy," *Arch Pathol Lab Med*, 1996, 120(8):702-12.

Hirsch CS, "Talking to the Family After an Autopsy," *Arch Pathol Lab Med*, 1984, 108(6):513-4.

Lundberg GD, "Medicine Without the Autopsy," *Arch Pathol Lab Med*, 1984, 108(6):449-54.

Moore GW and Hutchins GM, "The Persistent Importance of Autopsies," Mayo Clinic Proceedings, *Mayo Clin Proc*, 2000, 75(6):557-8.

Nemetz PN, Leibson C, Naessens JM, et al, "Determinants of the Autopsy Decision: A Statistical Analysis," *Am J Clin Pathol*, 1997, 108(2):175-83.

Palmer KP, Hayes PC, and Forrest JAH, "Gastrointestinal Bleeding," *Diseases of the Gastrointestinal Tract and Liver*, 3rd ed, Shearman DJC, Finlayson N, Camilleri M, et al, eds, New York, NY: Churchill Livingstone, 1997.

Sarode VR, Datta BN, Banerjee AK, et al, "Autopsy Findings and Clinical Diagnoses: A Review of 1000 Cases," *Hum Pathol*, 1993, 24(2):194-8.

Schwartz DA and Herman CJ, "The Importance of the Autopsy in Emerging and Reemerging Infectious Diseases," *Clin Infect Dig*, 1996, 23(2):248-54.

Stehbens WE, "An Appraisal of the Epidemic Rise of Coronary Heart Disease and Its Decline," *Lancet*, 1987, 1(8533):606-11.

Stothert JC Jr, Gbaanador GB, and Herndon DN, "The Role of Autopsy in Death Resulting From Trauma," *J Trauma*, 1990, 30(8):1021-5.

Wagner BM, "Mortality Statistics Without Autopsies: Wonderland Revisited," *Hum Pathol*, 1987, 18(9):875-6.

Zarbo RJ, Baker PB, and Howanitz PJ, "The Autopsy as a Performance Measurement Tool - Diagnostic Discrepancies and Unresolved Clinical Questions," *Arch Pathol Lab Med*, 1999, 123(3):191-8.

♦ **Basement Membrane Zone Antibodies** *see* Skin Biopsy, Immunofluorescence *on page 72*

♦ **Biopsy** *see* Histopathology *on page 59*

♦ **B-Lymphocyte Analysis by Flow Cytometry** *see* Immunophenotypic Analysis of Tissues by Flow Cytometry *on page 62*

♦ **Brain Biopsy** *see* Electron Microscopy *on page 54*

♦ **BRCA1** *see* Breast Biopsy *on page 51*

♦ **BRCA2** *see* Breast Biopsy *on page 51*

Breast Biopsy

Related Information

Applies to BRCA1; BRCA2; DNA Ploidy; Flow Cytometry; Gross Cystic Disease Fluid Protein-15 (GCDFP-15); Lumpectomy; Ploidy; Segmental Resection of Breast; S Phase; Tylectomy

Abstract Breast biopsies are performed to evaluate the pathologic nature of mammographically detected or palpable abnormalities. Breast lesions may be sampled by fine needle aspiration, skinny needle biopsy, mammotome suction biopsy, and open surgical biopsy.

Patient Preparation Pertinent history and physical findings should accompany the biopsy. A strong personal or family history of breast or ovarian cancer, concurrent pregnancy, exogenous estrogenic hormone therapy, and trauma history is relevant. Suspicious mammographic abnormalities include spiculated masses, stellate microcalcifications, or significant interval change of a previous abnormality. Physical findings suspicious for malignancy include a fixed indurated mass, skin retraction, nipple discharge, peau d'orange, palpable axillary mass, and findings suspicious for metastatic disease. Location of the tumor in relation to the nipple is critical to the final evaluation.

Specimen Needle biopsies are usually submitted in neutral buffered formalin for routine histologic preparation. Open breast biopsies are often submitted fresh for immediate evaluation.

Container Fresh specimens of breast tissue should be sent in a clean, dry, labeled container and placed in the hands of a pathologist or histotechnologist. When lesions are initially detected by mammography, the excised tissue is commonly radiographed to confirm the presence of lesional tissue. Such specimens are often submitted in a device with radiopaque grids, permitting the coordinates of the abnormality to be precisely documented for histopathologic correlation. The radiographs should accompany the specimen to the Pathology Laboratory.

Special Instructions When relevant, the specimen is oriented by the surgeon to identify surgical margins in three dimensions for histopathologic correlation.

Use The primary intent of breast biopsy is to determine the presence of cancer and, for open biopsies, evaluate the adequacy of excision. The information derived from the biopsy has profound implications on the subsequent management of malignant disease.

Limitations Diagnostic limitations are conferred by the adequacy of sampling, tissue fixation, or processing. Needle biopsies are susceptible to crush artifact. Evaluation of margins is complicated or rendered impossible by tissue fragmentation.

Additional Information Upon receipt of the specimen, dimensions, consistency of tissues, and gross abnormalities are recorded. Margins are inked by the surgical pathologist with insoluble dyes, sometimes using several colors to identify specific margins histologically. The relationship of gross abnormalities to surgical margins is carefully noted.

Pathologic diagnosis encompasses a wide variety of benign and malignant disorders. Some benign lesions carry no associated increased risk of malignancy while others (eg, atypical ductal hyperplasia) carry a significantly increased risk for the eventual development of cancer.[1] Malignant tumors include in situ carcinoma, infiltrating carcinoma, combinations thereof, and some phylloides tumors. Rarely, stromal tumors and lymphomas are documented. The proximity of malignant tumors to the surgical margins plays a pivotal role in the subsequent management of neoplastic disease.

In cases in which microcalcifications are mammographically detected, histopathologic confirmation of their presence is imperative. A high percentage of such cases demonstrates significant breast disease in fibrous tissue adjacent to benign tissues containing microcalcifications.[2] Calcium oxalate is often rendered inconspicuous by routine tissue processing, but is readily found using polarized microscopy.

The role of frozen section examination for the intraoperative management of breast conservation therapy is controversial. If mastectomy is planned to immediately follow a biopsy diagnosis of malignancy, frozen section examination is indicated. Frozen section exam, touch imprint cytology, or scrape preparation cytology is useful for to establish a working diagnosis of malignancy to triage the specimen for ancillary studies (vide infra). Frozen section examination of nonpalpable breast lesions is contraindicated.[3] Frozen section examination to evaluate surgical margins of specimens with grossly discernible tumor is not clearly indicated. Connolly et al conclude that frozen section evaluation of margins grossly free of tumor has no significant role in intraoperative management and may compromise margin evaluation in permanent section.[4]

Margins are best evaluated in intact segmental resections.[5] Positive margins, defined as neoplastic cells on inked margins, often require re-excision or mastectomy. Surgical margins clear by <1 mm carry an increased risk for local recurrence.[6] Margins clear by >1 mm carry a relatively low risk of local recurrence when followed by adjuvant radiotherapy. This risk decreases with greater margins of clearance.

Alternate methods are sometimes employed in the final evaluation of surgical margins. Biopsy sampling of the surgical cavity is useful to evaluate margins, even in frozen section setting, but is subject to sampling error.[7] Circumferential shave margins from the segmental resection can be made. Using this method, any neoplasm identified in this tissue represents a positive margin with clinical implications.[8] Cytologic evaluation of biopsy bed washings have found some use.[9] Imprint cytology from the surface of the breast biopsy has also been employed with variable success.[10]

(Continued)

Breast Biopsy (Continued)

Histologic classification and grading are important in the final management of epithelial breast cancers. The most commonly used histologic grading system was described by Bloom and Scharff and subsequently modified in the following table.

Nottingham Modification for the Bloom-Richardson System

Tubule Formation
- 1 point: tubules in >75% of tumor
- 2 points: tubules in 10% to 75% of tumor
- 3 points: tubules in <10% of tumor

Nuclear Pleomorphism
- 1 point: nuclei with minimal variation in size and shape
- 2 points: nuclei with moderate variation in size and shape
- 3 points: nuclei with marked variation in size and shape

Mitotic Count (actual counts vary somewhat based on microscope field size)
- 1 point: 0-4/40x field
- 2 points: 6-10/40x field
- 3 points: >11/40x field

In addition to routine histologic classification, grading, and staging information, the pathologist is also a central resource for a variety of ancillary studies. In broad terms, these studies are divided into those with predictive and those with prognostic value. Predictive studies are those that assess the likelihood of response to a particular therapeutic modality. Prognostic studies estimate the likelihood of disease recurrence. Hormone receptor and HER-2/neu are both predictive and prognostic markers in breast cancer.

Numerous prognostic factors have been studied in the setting of breast cancer. Recently published guidelines detail the current status of prognostic markers in breast cancer.[11,12]

Estrogen and progesterone receptor studies are routinely obtained on epithelial carcinomas of the breast. Approximately 1 cc of fresh or fresh frozen tissue is necessary to obtain quantitative assays for hormone receptors. Alternatively, hormone receptor status is better determined by immunohistochemical techniques using paraffin embedded tissue. These assays are discussed in greater detail in Estrogen and Progesterone Receptor Assay on page 55.

The frequency of estrogen receptor (ER) positivity increases with age, as does the degree of ER expression. Progesterone receptor (PR) expression is estrogen inducible and is thought to reflect functional integrity of estrogen regulatory pathways.[13] Despite some conflicting data, there is a consensus that ER positivity correlates with longer disease-free and overall survival, at least during the first 5 years. Survival curves tend to merge with longer follow-up. Stage-matched patients with higher expression of ER tend to follow a more favorable course than do patients with low levels of expression. Generally, both ER and PR expression tend to reflect tumor growth rate rather than metastatic potential. Patterns of metastases may differ in receptor-positive and receptor-negative patients. Patients with ER-negative tumors have higher rates of visceral involvement while patients with ER-positive tumors have a predilection for bony metastases.[14]

ER expression is highly correlated with response to endocrine therapy. Antiestrogen therapy produces a tumor static response generally in direct proportion to the degree of ER expression, especially when PR is coexpressed.

HER-2/neu expression also confers both predictive and prognostic value.[15] Intraductal carcinoma expressing HER-2/neu is associated with high nuclear grade and comedocarcinoma architecture. HER-2/neu overexpression is correlated with increased local recurrence rate. In cases of infiltrating ductal carcinoma, HER-2/neu expression is correlated with decreased disease-free and overall survival, particularly in those with lymph node positive disease. HER-2/neu overexpression may also predict patients with increased resistance to cyclophosphamide therapy and enhanced sensitivity to chemotherapeutic regimens containing Adriamycin®.[16] Recently, a monoclonal antibody directed against HER-2/neu received FDA approval for use in patients with metastatic disease. Documentation of HER-2/neu overexpression is mandatory in patients considered for this therapy. For more information, please see HER-2/neu on page 57.

Flow cytometric determination of DNA ploidy and S-phase fraction (SPF) have gained wide acceptance in the evaluation of breast cancer. Most reference laboratories can obtain DNA ploidy and S-phase determinations from the same tissue sample submitted for hormone receptor assays. These studies can also be obtained from paraffin-embedded tissue.[17] Approximately 66% of breast cancers are aneuploid and 30% to 40% are regarded as high SPF tumors. Several studies have demonstrated shorter disease-free and shorter overall survival in patients with aneuploid tumors or with high SPF. When considered separately, tetraploid tumors behave more like diploid tumors than other aneuploid tumors.[18] Aneuploidy and high SPF cancers correlate with high nuclear grade and are more commonly hormone receptor-negative.

Other prognostic markers under active investigation include p53, bcl-2, and proliferation markers PCNA and Ki-67 (MIB-1 protein). Studies attempting to quantitate neoangiogenesis have also yielded intriguing data.

The risk of local recurrence is dependent on tumor size, adequacy of resection, histologic grade with mitotic count, and presence of extensive intraductal carcinoma.[6] Age and presence of certain phenotypic markers also have a bearing on local recurrence. Local recurrence is significantly reduced with adjuvant radiotherapy.[19]

The risk of regional and distant metastasis is associated with a number of factors. The single most important factor for distant metastasis is the presence of axillary lymph node metastases.[12] Recent advances in the identification and biopsy of sentinel lymph node are hoped to promote the identification of patients at risk for developing distant metastases (see Sentinel Lymph Node Biopsy on page 70).

As mammographic techniques improve and public awareness grows, increasing numbers of smaller breast carcinomas are being detected. Nonetheless, approximately 20% of stage 1 carcinomas develop metastatic disease by 10 years. Careful attention to biopsy findings and subsequent staging procedures, in conjunction with prudent application of prognostic and predictive studies, will hopefully promote a cost-effective strategy for the management of patients with breast cancer.

Footnotes

1. Page DL, "The Woman at High Risk for Breast Cancer. Importance of Hyperplasia," Surg Clin North Am, 1996, 76(2):221-30.
2. Owings DV, Hann L, and Schnitt SJ, "How Thoroughly Should Needle Localization Breast Biopsies Be Sampled for Microscopic Examination? A Prospective Mammographic/Pathologic Correlative Study," Am J Surg Pathol, 1990, 14(6):578-83.
3. Powell DE, and Stelling CE, The Diagnosis and Detection of Breast Disease, 1st ed, St Louis, MO: CV Mosby, 1994.
4. Connolly J and Schnitt S, "Evaluation of Breast Biopsy Specimens in Patients Considered for Treatment by Conservative Surgery and Radiation Therapy for Early Breast Cancer," Pathol Annu, 1988, (23 Pt 1):1-23.
5. Schnitt SJ and Connolly JL, "Processing and Evaluation of Breast Excision Specimens. A Clinically Oriented Approach," Am J Clin Pathol, 1992. 98(1):125-37.
6. Schnitt SJ, Abner A, Gelman R, et al, "The Relationship Between Microscopic Margins of Resection and the Risk of Local Recurrence in Patients With Breast Cancer Treated With Breast-Conserving Surgery and Radiation Therapy," Cancer, 1994, 74(6):1746-51.
7. Weber S, Storm FK, Stitt J, et al, "The Role of Frozen Section Analysis of Margins During Breast Conservation Surgery," Cancer J Sci Am, 1997, 3(5):173-7.
8. Guidi AJ, Connolly JL, Harris JR, et al, "The Relationship Between Shaved Margin and Inked Margin Status in Breast Excision Specimens," Cancer, 1997. 79(8):1568-73.
9. Motomura K, Koyama H, Noguchi S, et al, "Malignant Seeding of the Lumpectomy Cavity Upon Breast-Conserving Surgery," Oncology, 1999, 57(2):121-6.
10. Cox CE, Hyacinthe M, Gonzalez RJ, et al, "Cytologic Evaluation of Lumpectomy Margins in Patients With Ductal Carcinoma In Situ: Clinical Outcome," Ann Surg Oncol, 1997, 4(8):644-9.
11. Henson DE, Fielding LP, Grignon DJ, et al, "College of American Pathologists Conference XXVI on Clinical Relevance of Prognostic Markers in Solid Tumors. Summary," Members of the Cancer Committee, Arch Pathol Lab Med, 1995. 119(12):1109-12.
12. Fitzgibbons PL, Page DL, Weaver D, et al, "Prognostic Factors in Breast Cancer," College of American Pathologists Consensus Statement 1999, Arch Pathol Lab Med, 2000. 124(7):966-78.
13. Osborne C, "Receptors," Breast Diseases, J Harris, et al, eds, Philadelphia, PA: JB Lippincott, 1991, 301-25.
14. Clark G, Sledge G, and Osborne G, "Survival From the First Recurrence: Relative Importance of Prognostic Factors in 1015 Breast Cancer Patients," J Clin Oncol, 1988. 37:221-6.
15. Ross J. and Fletcher J, "HER-2/neu (c-erb-B2) Gene and Protein in Breast Cancer," Am J Clin Pathol, 1999. 122(Suppl 1):S53-S67.
16. Sjogren S, Inganas M, and Lindgren A, "Prognostic and Predictive Value of c-erbB-2 Overexpression in Primary Breast Cancer, Alone and in Combination With Other Prognostic Markers," J Clin Oncol, 1998, 16(2):462-9.
17. Dressler LG, Geradts J, Burroughs M, et al, "Policy Guidelines for the Utilization of Formalin-Fixed, Paraffin-Embedded Tissue Sections: The UNC SPORE Experience." University of North Carolina Specialized Program of Research Excellence," Breast Cancer Res Treat, 1999, 58(1):31-9.
18. Witzig TE, Gonchoroff NJ, Thernear T, et al, "DNA Content Flow Cytometry as a Prognostic Factor for Node-Positive Breast Cancer. The Role of Multiparameter Ploidy Analysis and Specimen Sonication," Cancer, 1991, 68(8):1781-8.
19. Fisher B, Dignam J, Wolmark N, et al, "Lumpectomy and Radiation Therapy for the Treatment of Intraductal Breast Cancer: Findings From National Surgical Adjuvant Breast and Bowel Project B-17," J Clin Oncol, 1998. 16(2):441-52.

Cell Cycle Analysis by Flow Cytometry

Related Information

Synonyms Cell Cycle Analysis; Ploidy Analysis; S-Phase Analysis

Applies to Aneuploidy; DNA Content; DNA Synthesis Phase; G_1 Phase; G_2M; G_o Phase; Ploidy; Proliferative Indices; S Phase; Thymidine Labeling Index

Test Includes Measurement of nuclear DNA content to identify aneuploidy clones; estimation of percentage of cells in S phase (S phase fraction, SPF)

Abstract Assessment of ploidy and SPF may be helpful to estimate prognosis and to plan therapy for patients with limited stage neoplastic disease.

Specimen Portion of fresh tissue, fresh frozen tissue, or adequately cellular body fluid; needle aspirates of neoplasm. Paraffin-embedded tissue may also be used.

Storage Instructions Fresh tissues require immediate processing. Frozen and paraffin-embedded tissues are suitable for months to years.

Causes for Rejection Extensive tumor necrosis, poor fixation, or other factors which severely limits histogram analysis

Reference Interval Diploid cell population with low S-phase fraction

Use DNA analysis by flow cytometry generates information of prognostic importance, particularly in tumors of limited stage. Major applications are in carcinomas of breast, colon, prostate, and bladder.

Limitations This assay is not capable of differentiating a benign from a malignant disorder. Results are relevant only in context of an established tissue diagnosis and must be interpreted with caution and experience. Necrotic tissues often yield poor or uninterpretable results. Flow cytometry from paraffin blocks may lack sufficient sensitivity to detect minor abnormalities when compared to parallel studies performed on fresh tissue[1] Poor tissue fixation, improperly stored paraffin blocks, or the use of certain fixatives (eg, B5, Zenker's) may significantly compromise results[2,3] The presence of normal tissue may obscure abnormalities of a neoplastic population. When using paraffin-embedded tissue, it may be possible to separate normal from abnormal tissue and focus analysis on the neoplastic population. The application of other phenotypic markers to distinguish neoplastic from normal tissues may also be used. Finally, DNA content measurements by flow cytometry are intrinsically insensitive. The gain or loss of several chromosomes may go undetected using conventional flow cytometric methods.

Methodology When using fresh or frozen tissue, a single cell suspension is prepared and the cells rendered permeable to a fluorescent dye that binds stoichiometrically to DNA. When paraffin-embedded tissues are used, nuclei are isolated from thick deparaffinized tissue sections and stained in a similar fashion.[4,5] Suspensions are analyzed by flow cytometry and fluorescence intensity is quantitated for each nucleus passing through the laser beam. Typically, at least 10,000 nuclei are evaluated and a histogram is generated depicting cell number versus fluorescence intensity. The histogram is computer analyzed using a specialized program that mathematically models the data set and generates clinically useful information (see diagram). In routine clinical applications, SPF is calculated, not directly measured.

Additional Information Non-neoplastic tissues characteristically contain a dominant population of diploid cells containing a stainable amount of DNA defined as "2C" (see figure).

This tissue will also contain a smaller population of cells actively synthesizing DNA, defined as the S-phase fraction. Another small population of cells will be in either premitotic or mitotic phase with a stainable DNA content twice that of the diploid population, designated "4C". The proportions of these populations will vary with the tissue source. DNA analysis by either flow cytometry or image analysis generally shows high concordance, but disparate results do occur.[6,7]

The characterization of DNA content by flow cytometry represents an attempt to standardize and quantitate the subjective impression that a tumor "looks bad". Nuclear hyperchromasia, anisocytosis, and polylobations are just a few morphologic correlates of DNA aneuploidy. The presence of nucleoli and mitoses are counterparts of an increased S-phase fraction. However, such correlations are imperfect. Neoplasms that appear low grade or well differentiated may display aneuploid DNA content or high SPF. Converse exceptions also occur but with less frequency.

The predictive value of ploidy and SPF determinations is most comprehensively studied in breast cancer. Cancers of the colon, prostate, urinary bladder, and lung have also been extensively investigated. In general, tumor aneuploidy or increased SPF is associated with worse overall outcome. Notable exceptions include childhood acute lymphoblastic leukemia and neuroblastoma in which aneuploidy is associated with a more favorable outcome.

In limited stage breast cancer, both DNA ploidy and SPF are prognostically relevant.[8,9,10] When evaluated as independent prognostic variables, high SPF is a statistically significant poor prognostic finding. However, the prognostic value of SPF is offset by numerous technical limitations affecting standardization, quality control and outcome validated reference points.[11] Recent College of American Pathologists guidelines for the interpretation of prognostic findings in breast cancer consider documentation of proliferation status a desirable goal but minimize the importance of DNA ploidy.[12] Similar approaches have been recommended for the interpretation of ploidy and SPF in carcinoma of the colon[13] and prostate.[14,15]

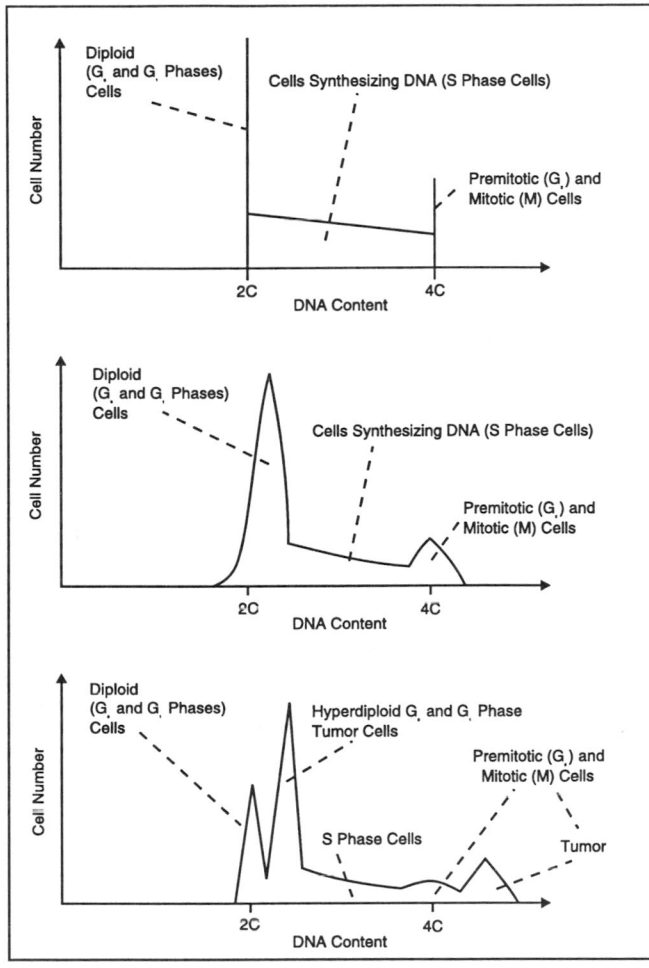

Top: An ideal distribution of DNA content in a cell population. Center: A distribution more typical of those actually obtained by flow cytometry. Bottom: A distribution such as is obtained from a tumor exhibiting DNA aneuploidy.
From Shapiro HM, "Flow Cytometry of DNA Content and Other Indicators of Proliferative Activity," *Arch Pathol Lab Med*, 1989, 113:591-7, with permission.

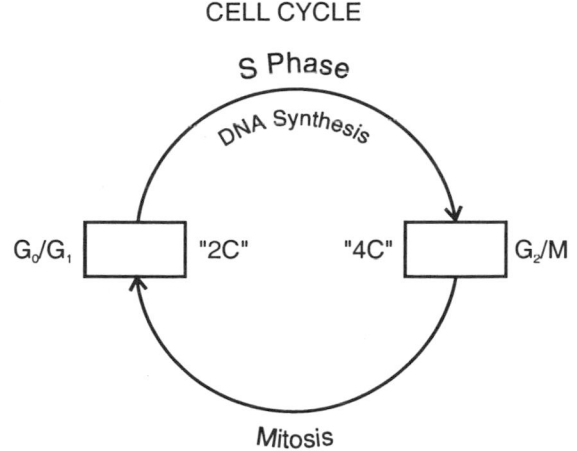

(Continued)

Cell Cycle Analysis by Flow Cytometry *(Continued)*

Footnotes

1. Frierson HF, "Flow Cytometric Analysis of Ploidy in Solid Neoplasms: Comparison of Fresh Tissues With Formalin-Fixed Paraffin-Embedded Specimens," *Hum Pathol*, 1988, 19(3):290-4.
2. Esteban JM, Sheibani K, Owens M, et al, "Effects of Various Fixatives and Fixation Conditions on DNA Ploidy Analysis. A Need for Strict Internal DNA Standards," *Am J Clin Pathol*, 1991, 95(4):460-6.
3. Herbert DJ, Nishiyama RH, Bagwell CB, et al, "Effects of Several Commonly Used Fixatives on DNA and Total Nuclear Protein Analysis by Flow Cytometry," *Am J Clin Pathol*, 1989, 91(5):535-41.
4. Schultz DS and Zarbo RJ, "Comparison of Eight Modifications of Hedley's Method for Flow Cytometric DNA Ploidy Analysis of Paraffin-Embedded Tissue," *Am J Clin Pathol*, 1992, 98(3):291-5.
5. Babiak J and Poppema S, "Automated Procedure for Dewaxing and Rehydration of Paraffin-Embedded Tissue Sections for DNA Flow Cytometric Analysis of Breast Tumors," *Am J Clin Pathol*, 1991, 96(1):64-9.
6. Elsheikh TM, Silverman JF, McCool JW, et al, "Comparative DNA Analysis of Solid Tumors by Flow Cytometric and Image Analyses of Touch Imprints and Flow Cell Suspensions," *Am J Clin Pathol*, 1992, 98(3):296-304.
7. Ghali VS, Liau S, Teplitz C, et al, "A Comparative Study of DNA Ploidy in 115 Fresh-Frozen Breast Carcinomas by Image Analysis Versus Flow Cytometry," *Cancer*, 1992, 70(11):2668-72.
8. Dressler LG, Seamer LC, Owens MA, et al, "DNA Flow Cytometry and Prognostic Factors in 1331 Frozen Breast Cancer Specimens," *Cancer*, 1988, 61(3):420-7.
9. Clark GM, Dressler LG, Owens MA, et al, "Prediction of Relapse or Survival in Patients With Node-Negative Breast Cancer by DNA Flow Cytometry," *N Engl J Med*, 1989, 320(10):627-33.
10. Clark GM, Mathieu MC, Owens MA, et al, "Prognostic Significance of S-Phase Fraction in Good-Risk, Node-Negative Breast Cancer Patients," *J Clin Oncol*, 1992, 10(3):428-32.
11. Wenger CR and Clark GM, "S-Phase Fraction and Breast Cancer - a Decade of Experience," *Breast Cancer Res Treat*, 1998, 51(3):255-65.
12. Fitzgibbons PL, Page DL, Weaver D, et al, "Prognostic Factors in Breast Cancer. College of American Pathologists Consensus Statement 1999," *Arch Pathol Lab Med*, 2000, 124(7):966-78.
13. Fielding LP and Pettigrew N, "College of American Pathologists Conference XXVI on Clinical Relevance of Prognostic Markers in Solid Tumors. Report of the Colorectal Cancer Working Group," *Arch Pathol Lab Med*, 1995, 119(12):1115-21.
14. Grignon DJ and Hammond EH, "College of American Pathologists Conference XXVI on Clinical Relevance of Prognostic Markers in Solid Tumors. Report of the Prostate Cancer Working Group," *Arch Pathol Lab Med*, 1995, 119(12):1122-6.
15. Bostwick DG and Foster CS, "Predictive Factors in Prostate Cancer: Current Concepts From the 1999 College of American Pathologists Conference on Solid Tumor Prognostic Factors and the 1999 World Health Organization Second International Consultation on Prostate Cancer," *Semin Urol Oncol*, 1999, 17(4):222-72.

References

Bauer KD, Bagwell CB, Giaretti W, et al, "Consensus Review of the Clinical Utility of DNA Flow Cytometry in Colorectal Cancer," *Cytometry*, 1993, 14(5):486-91.
Duque RE, Andreeff M, Braylan RC, et al, "Consensus Review of the Clinical Utility of DNA Flow Cytometry in Neoplastic Hematopathology," *Cytometry*, 1993, 14(5):492-6.
Fitzgibbons PL, Page DK, Weaver D, et al, "Prognostic Factors in Breast Cancer. College of American Pathologists Consensus Statement 1999," *Arch Pathol Lab Med*, 2000, 124(7):966-78.
Hedley DW, Shankey TV, and Wheeless LL, "DNA Cytometry Consensus Conference," *Cytometry*, 1993, 14(5):471.
Shankey TV, Kallioniemi OP, Koslowski JM, et al, "Consensus Review of the Clinical Utility of DNA Content Cytometry in Prostate Cancer," *Cytometry*, 1993, 14(5):497-500.

♦ **Cell Measurement/Micrometry** *see* Image Analysis *on page 59*

♦ **c-erbB-2** *see* HER-2/neu *on page 57*

♦ **Chromogranin** *see* Immunoperoxidase Procedures *on page 60*

♦ **Computerized Interactive Morphometry** *see* Image Analysis *on page 59*

♦ **Copper, Hepatic** *see* Liver Biopsy *on page 65*

♦ **Coroner's Case** *see* Autopsy *on page 50*

♦ **Cyclins** *see* Image Analysis *on page 59*

♦ **Cytokeratin** *see* Sentinel Lymph Node Biopsy *on page 70*

♦ **Cytokeratins** *see* Immunoperoxidase Procedures *on page 60*

♦ **Cytosol Hormone Receptors** *see* Estrogen and Progesterone Receptor Assay *on page 55*

♦ **Death Certificate** *see* Autopsy *on page 50*

♦ **Dermatitis Herpetiformis Antibodies** *see* Skin Biopsy, Immunofluorescence *on page 72*

♦ **Desmin** *see* Immunoperoxidase Procedures *on page 60*

♦ **Disease Reporting** *see* Autopsy *on page 50*

♦ **DNA Content** *see* Cell Cycle Analysis by Flow Cytometry *on page 53*

♦ **DNA Content** *see* Image Analysis *on page 59*

♦ **DNA Index** *see* Image Analysis *on page 59*

♦ **DNA Ploidy** *see* Breast Biopsy *on page 51*

♦ **DNA Ploidy Interpretation** *see* Image Analysis *on page 59*

♦ **DNA Ploidy Studies** *see* Immunophenotypic Analysis of Tissues by Flow Cytometry *on page 62*

♦ **DNA Synthesis Phase** *see* Cell Cycle Analysis by Flow Cytometry *on page 53*

♦ **Dystrophin** *see* Muscle Biopsy *on page 69*

Electron Microscopy

Related Information

Electron Microscopic Examination for Viruses, Stool *on page 603*
Fine Needle Aspiration, Deep Masses *on page 381*
Fine Needle Aspiration, Superficial Masses (Palpable) *on page 382*
Kidney Biopsy *on page 64*
Microsporidia Diagnostic Procedures *on page 652*
Muscle Biopsy *on page 69*
Skin Biopsy *on page 71*

Synonyms EM; Transmission Electron Microscopy; Ultrastructural Study

Applies to Brain Biopsy; Cardiac Biopsy; Viral Diseases by EM

Abstract A major application of electron microscopy (EM) is to delineate histogenesis of poorly differentiated neoplasms when light microscopy is equivocal and when proper therapy and prognosis depend on precise diagnosis. Although applications have diminished with development of immunoperoxidase methods, EM remains useful and provides information which otherwise cannot be obtained.

Specimen Fresh unfixed tissue, blood, bone marrow aspirate

Container Vial containing glutaraldehyde or other appropriate fixative, depending upon institution or reference laboratory. Blood and bone marrow aspirate may be collected in heparinized or EDTA tubes and submitted immediately.

Collection Specimen obtained by surgical biopsy should be cut within minutes of excision, minced into cubes 1 mm or less, and placed in glutaraldehyde, paraformaldehyde, or other special fixative. (See Kidney Biopsy *on page 64*.) Two percent to 4% phosphate or cacodylate-buffered glutaraldehyde is recommended. Formaldehyde-fixed tissue may be used if glutaraldehyde is not available. All EM fixatives, particularly glutaraldehyde, should be refrigerated until used to retard oxidative damage to fixative. Discard if a precipitate forms.

Causes for Rejection Poor tissue preservation owing to delayed fixation or use of wrong fixative; sampling artifact resulting in lack of tissue or tumor in question

Use The distinction between poorly differentiated carcinoma, amelanotic melanoma, and lymphoma can be reliably established by electron microscopy. Poorly differentiated carcinomas characteristically demonstrate desmosomes or tight junctions and may show other features of epithelial differentiation, such as intracytoplasmic mucin vacuoles, microvilli, or tonofilaments. Such findings are characteristically absent in melanomas, but the observation of premelanosomes is highly specific for melanocytic differentiation. Lymphomas are ultrastructurally simple, typically showing free ribosomes, simple rough endoplasmic reticulum, and simple Golgi structure. Neuroendocrine neoplasms contain neurosecretory granules. Small cell carcinomas contain few neurosecretory granules while more differentiated tumors, such as carcinoids and islet cell tumors, are rich in them. Mesotheliomas are differentiated from adenocarcinomas by elongated, delicate microvilli. Birbeck granules characterize the Langerhans cells of eosinophilic granuloma and other forms of Langerhans histiocytoses.[1] Electron microscopic demonstration of platelet peroxidase in the nuclear envelope of leukemic blasts establishes a key diagnostic feature of megakaryoblastic leukemia (FAB M7).[2] When limited material is available, such as in fine needle aspiration biopsies, electron microscopy may allow a more precise classification in selected cases.[3,4]

Electron microscopy is useful in certain viral and other infectious diseases. In AIDS encephalopathy, EM of brain biopsies helps to determine the responsible agent (ie, HIV, CMV, herpes, Jakob Creutzfeldt, progressive multifocal leukoencephalopathy, and so forth). EM may be invaluable in the evaluation of muscle biopsies (eg, mitochondrial myopathies) and peripheral nerve biopsies. Storage/metabolic diseases sometimes are well evaluated with EM. Ceroid lipofuscinoses and Pompe type II glycogenosis bear characteristic inclusions in peripheral blood lymphocytes by EM. Many other lysosomal storage diseases can be identified by EM of skin, conjunctival, or gum biopsies.[5] The immotile cilia syndrome is diagnosed by the absence of one or both dynein arms in cross sections of ciliary microtubules in nasal or bronchial biopsies.[6] Some liver biopsies have lesions in which EM may be useful (eg, Dubin-Johnson syndrome, Rotor disease). With heart biopsy, EM can reveal Adriamycin® cardiotoxicity.

Limitations EM is labor intensive and limited by cost and sampling errors. This method is usually not useful to distinguish benign from malignant neoplasms. Utility is diminished by poor fixation, crush or drying artifact. The role of EM has recently been eroded by rapid advances in immunocytochemistry for the differential diagnosis of tumors and infectious agents. For instance immunodiagnostic methods are definitive and rapid for herpes encephalitis, but EM supports diagnosis.

Methodology Properly fixed tissues are embedded in a high density plastic polymer from which thick sections (1 micron) are cut and stained to select the best areas for ultrastructural studies. Thin sections are subsequently prepared and stained with electron dense materials such as uranyl acetate. The specimens are then ready to examine in a transmission electron microscope.

Additional Information Concomitant light microscopic evaluation is usually required for ultrastructural correlation. Often light microscopic findings lead to a decision of whether or not EM is indicated (eg, tumors). EM is not a substitute for light microscopy. When renal biopsies are obtained, immunofluorescence studies are often performed, as well as light microscopy. Immunofluorescence and EM are mutually complementary. Applications in immunoelectron microscopy are invaluable tools for research scientists.[7]

Footnotes

1. Lieberman PH, Jones CR, Steinman RM, et al, "Langerhans Cell (Eosinophilic) Granulomatosis - A Clinicopathologic Study Encompassing 50 Years," *Am J Surg Pathol*, 1996, 20(5):519-552.
2. Koike T, "Megakaryoblastic Leukemia: The Characterization and Identification of Megakaryoblasts," *Blood*, 1984, 64(3):683-92.
3. Strausbauch P, Neill J, Dabbs DJ, et al, "The Impact of Fine Needle Aspiration Biopsy on a Diagnostic Electron Microscopy Laboratory," *Arch Pathol Lab Med*, 1989, 113(12):1354-6.
4. Yazdi HM and Dardick I, "Techniques for Specimen Processing," *Guides to Clinical Aspiration Biopsy, Diagnostic Immunocytochemistry, and Electron Microscopy*, New York, NY: Igaku-Shoin, 1991, 11-25.
5. Dolman CL, "Diagnosis of Neurometabolic Disorders by Examination of Skin Biopsies and Lymphocytes," *Semin Diag Pathol*, 1984, 1(2):82-97.
6. Afzelius BA, "The Immotile-Cilia Syndrome and Other Ciliary Diseases," *Int Rev Exp Pathol*, 1979, 19:1-43.
7. Herrera GA, Lowery MC, and Turbat-Herrera EA, "Immunoelectron Microscopy in the Age of Molecular Pathology," *Appl Immunohistochem Molecul Morphol*, 2000, 8(2):87-97.

References

Dvorak AM, *Diagnostic Ultrastructural Pathology*, Volume I, Boca Raton, FL: CRC Press, Inc, 1992.

Erlandson RA, *Diagnostic Transmission Electron Microscopy of Human Tumors With Clinicopathological, Immunohistochemical, and Cytogenetic Correlations*, New York, NY: Raven Press, 1994.

♦ **EM** *see* Electron Microscopy *on page 54*

♦ **Endoscopic Biopsy** *see* Histopathology *on page 59*

♦ **Epithelial Membrane Antigen (EMA)** *see* Immunoperoxidase Procedures *on page 60*

Estrogen and Progesterone Receptor Assay

Related Information

Breast Biopsy *on page 51*
Breast Cancer, Hereditary, BRCA1, BRCA2 *on page 722*
Histopathology *on page 59*
Image Analysis *on page 59*
Immunoperoxidase Procedures *on page 60*

Applies to Breast Cancer; Cytosol Hormone Receptors; Ovarian Cancer; Tamoxifen

Abstract Estrogen receptor (ER) and progesterone receptor (PR) analysis provides invaluable predictive and prognostic information in patients with breast cancer and with certain gynecologic malignancies.

Specimen Fresh or fresh frozen tissue is required for cytosol assays for either estrogen receptor (ER) or progesterone receptor (PR). Paraffin-embedded tissue or alcohol-fixed cytology specimens are suitable substrates for immunohistochemical procedures.

Storage Instructions The sensitivity of detecting ER and other prognostic or predictive markers using paraffin sections stored for a long period of time may decrease.[1] However, freshly cut sections from paraffin blocks stored for many years are generally suitable.

Causes for Rejection Lack of tumor in sampled tissues

Use Detection of ER and PR is used primarily to determine the potential responsiveness of breast cancer or some gynecologic tumors to estrogen receptor antagonists. Secondarily, expression of ER or PR has prognostic value in breast cancer.

Limitations Quantitation of cytosol hormone receptors may result in significant false-positive and false-negative results. In these assays, hormone receptor activity is standardized to the amount of protein in the extract. Typical scirrhous infiltrating carcinomas are protein rich but may have an exceedingly low density of receptor-positive tumor cells. **Thus, a hormone receptor-positive tumor may be reported as negative. Conversely, hormone receptor-negative tumors may be contaminated with receptor-positive normal epithelium and be falsely reported as positive. Such artifacts have profound impact on therapeutic decisions.**

Methodology Historically, estrogen and progesterone receptors have been assayed using cytosol extracts in a competitive ligand-binding assay.[2] Fresh or frozen tissue is homogenized and the cytosol fraction is isolated on a sucrose density gradient. A competitive radioimmunoassay is used to accurately quantitate hormone receptor activity. Drawbacks to this approach include relatively large tissue requirements, extreme thermolability caused by short delays in freezing tissues, sensitivity to exposure to fixatives, low tumor cell density, contamination by normal breast tissue, and interference by endogenous hormone levels or exogenous hormone therapy.

Subsequently, enzyme-linked immunoassays supplanted the more fastidious competitive radioimmunoassays.[3,4] These assays utilize monoclonal antibodies to accurately measure hormone-binding epitopes without relying on functional activity. These assays require less tissue, are not subject to aberrations conferred by exogenous hormone therapy and are not as thermosensitive as their predecessor. Intrinsic to the use of homogenates, these assays also require fresh or frozen tissue and are adversely influenced by normal tissue contamination or low tumor cell density.

More recently, immunohistochemical procedures have gained favor as the assay of choice. Currently available monoclonal antibodies and antigen retrieval techniques allow accurate detection of ER and PR activity on routinely processed histologic and cytologic materials.[5,6,7] Immunohistochemical procedures correlate well with ligand-binding assays.[8] Small amounts of neoplastic tissue can be assayed without interference by normal tissue. Results are reported using either qualitative assessment[9,10] or quantitative measures aided by image cytometry.[6,11,12] A recently published study of 1982 breast cancers concluded that immunohistochemistry was superior to the traditional ligand-binding assay in prediction of response to endocrine therapy.[13] These authors also demonstrated that low levels of ER expression defined a population of patients with potential responsiveness that may be considered ER negative in other assay systems.

Additional Information Proliferation of breast cancer cells is often highly estrogen dependent. Antiestrogen therapy has been shown effective in both the adjuvant and metastatic disease settings.[14] Additionally, antiestrogens have been shown to have protective effects in patients at risk for developing breast cancer.[15] These agents down-regulate tumor growth and may promote programmed cell death but do not have direct cytotoxic properties. ER expression is the most important predictive factor for a beneficial response to endocrine therapy.[16]

The frequency of hormone receptor phenotype in pre- and postmenopausal women is depicted in the following table.[17]

	Premenopausal Receptor Status	Postmenopausal Receptor Status
ER[+], PR[+]	45%	63%
ER[+], PR[-]	12%	15%
ER[-], PR[-]	28%	17%
ER[-], PR[+]	15%	5%

Progesterone receptor is one of many estrogen inducible proteins. Hence, PR expression is most commonly seen in parallel with ER expression.

Overall, approximately 33% of patients with ER positive, metastatic breast cancer will show a beneficial clinical response to tamoxifen for a period of approximately 12-18 months. Postmenopausal patients with tumors expressing high levels of ER and PR benefit the most, whereas patients with receptor negative tumors rarely benefit from antiestrogen therapy.[18] Approximately 5% of breast cancers are PR-positive but ER-negative. Patients with metastatic disease and this phenotype may benefit from antiestrogen therapy.[19] Antiestrogen therapy is also beneficial in men with metastatic breast cancer.

Estrogen receptor activity can fluctuate during the course of disease.[20,21] Most commonly, hormone receptor positive tumors recur with similar patterns of hormone receptor expression. Approximately 30% to 35% of tumors will recur with a different pattern of hormone receptor expression. Most common phenotypic changes are loss of ER, loss of PR, or loss of both receptors. Conversely, a small percentage of tumors initially ER-negative recur as ER-positive tumors. Conversion to receptor-negativity tends to occur in tumors that relapse within 12 months and are associated with a poor response to endocrine therapy and worse overall survival.

Response to one form of endocrine therapy predicts responsiveness to second-line therapy. Occasionally, tamoxifen induces tumor growth. Eventually, refractiveness to endocrine therapy develops. Mechanisms by which resistance occurs includes absence or loss of estrogen receptors, mutation in the estrogen receptor genes, altered expression of receptor interacting proteins, and cross-talk among growth factor signaling pathways.[19]

Footnotes

1. Jacobs TW, Prioleau JE, Stillman IE, et al, "Loss of Tumor Marker-Immunostaining Intensity on Stored Paraffin Slides of Breast Cancer," *J Natl Cancer Inst*, 1996, 88(15):1054-9.
2. Osborne C, "Receptors," *Breast Diseases*, Harris J, et al, eds, Philadelphia PA: JB Lippincott, 1991, 301-25.
3. De Negri F, Campani D, Sarnelli R, et al, "Comparison of Monoclonal Immunocytochemical and Immunoenzymatic Methods for Steroid Receptor Evaluation in Breast Cancer," *Am J Clin Pathol*, 1991, 96(1):53-8.
4. Delage V, Teulon JM, Bellanger L, et al, "Microtiter Plate Immunoenzymometric Assay for Estrogen Receptor," *Clin Chem*, 1996, 42(12):1955-60.
5. Goulding H, Pinder S, Cannon P, et al, "A New Immunohistochemical Antibody for the Assessment of Estrogen Receptor Status on Routine Formalin-Fixed Tissue Samples," *Hum Pathol*, 1995, 26(3):291-4.
6. Nichols GE, Frierson HF Jr, Boyd JC, et al, "Automated Immunohistochemical Assay for Estrogen Receptor Status in Breast Cancer Using Monoclonal Antibody CC4-5 on the Ventana ES," *Am J Clin Pathol*, 1996, 106(3):332-8.
7. Schmitt FC, Bento MJ, and Amendoeira I, "Estimation of Estrogen Receptor Content in Fine-Needle Aspirates From Breast Cancer Using the Monoclonal Antibody 1D5 and Microwave Oven Processing: Correlation With Paraffin Embedded and Frozen Sections Determinations," *Diagn Cytopathol*, 1995, 13(4):347-51.

(Continued)

Estrogen and Progesterone Receptor Assay
(Continued)

8. Alberts SR, Ingle JN, Roche PR, et al, "Comparison of Estrogen Receptor Determinations by a Biochemical Ligand-Binding Assay and Immunohistochemical Staining With Monoclonal Antibody ER1D5 in Females With Lymph Node Positive Breast Carcinoma Entered on Two Prospective Clinical Trials," *Cancer*, 1996, 78(4):764-72.

9. Benitez-Bribiesca L, Guevara R, Ruiz MT, et al, "A Simplified Histoscore for the Estrogen Receptor Assay in Breast Cancer," *Pathol Res Pract*, 1992, 188(4-5):461-5.

10. Detre S, Saclani Jotti G, and Dowsett M, "A Quickscore Method for Immunohistochemical Semiquantitation: Validation for Oestrogen Receptor in Breast Carcinomas," *J Clin Pathol*, 1995, 48(9):876-8.

11. Esteban JM, Kandalaft PL, Mehta P, et al, "Improvement of the Quantification of Estrogen and Progesterone Receptors in Paraffin-Embedded Tumors by Image Analysis," *Am J Clin Pathol*, 1993, 99(1):32-8.

12. Esteban JM, Ahn C, Mehta P, et al, "Biologic Significance of Quantitative Estrogen Receptor Immunohistochemical Assay by Image Analysis in Breast Cancer," *Am J Clin Pathol*, 1994, 102(2):158-62.

13. Harvey JM, Clark GM, Osborne CK, et al, "Estrogen Receptor Status by Immunohistochemistry Is Superior to the Ligand-Binding Assay for Predicting Response to Adjuvant Endocrine Therapy in Breast Cancer," *J Clin Oncol*, 1999, 17(5):1474-81.

14. Fisher B, Costantino JP, Redmond C, et al, "A Randomized Clinical Trial Evaluating Tamoxifen in the Treatment of Patients With Node-Negative Breast Cancer Who Have Estrogen-Receptor-Positive Tumors," *N Engl J Med*, 1989, 320(8):479-84.

15. Fisher B and Costantino JP, for Prevention of Breast Cancer: Report of the National Surgical Adjuvant Breast and Bowel Project P-1 Study," *J Natl Cancer Inst*, 1998, 90(18):1371-88.

16. Bezwoda WR, Esser JD, Dansey R, et al, "The Value of Estrogen and Progesterone Receptor Determinations in Advanced Breast Cancer. Estrogen Receptor Level but Not Progesterone Receptor Level Correlates With Response to Tamoxifen," *Cancer*, 1991, 68(4):867-72.

17. Wittliff J, "Hormone and Growth Factor Receptors," *Cancer of the Breast*, Donegan W and Spratt J eds, Philadelphia, PA: WB Saunders Co, 1995.

18. Osborne CK, Zhao H, and Fuqua S, "Selective Estrogen Receptor Modulators: Structure, Function and Clinical Use," *J Clin Oncol*, 2000, 18(17):3172-86.

19. Osborne CK, "Tamoxifen in the Treatment of Breast Cancer, *N Engl J Med*, 1998, 339(22):1609-18.

20. Kuukasjarvi T, Kononen J, Helin H, et al, "Loss of Estrogen Receptor in Recurrent Breast Cancer Is Associated With Poor Response to Endocrine Therapy," *J Clin Oncol*, 1996, 14(9):2584-9.

21. Spataro V, Price K, Goldhirsch A, et al, "Sequential Estrogen Receptor Determinations From Primary Breast Cancer and at Relapse: Prognostic and Therapeutic Relevance. The International Breast Cancer Study Group (formerly Ludwig Group)," *Ann Oncol*, 1992, 3(9):733-40.

♦ **Factor VIII Related Antigen** *see* Immunoperoxidase Procedures *on page 60*

♦ **FISH Assays** *see* HER-2/*neu on page 57*

♦ **Flow Cytometry** *see* Breast Biopsy *on page 51*

♦ **Flow Cytometry** *see* Immunophenotypic Analysis of Tissues by Flow Cytometry *on page 62*

♦ **Fluorescein-Tagged Antibodies** *see* Kidney Biopsy *on page 64*

♦ **Fluorescence Activated Cell Sorting** *see* Immunophenotypic Analysis of Tissues by Flow Cytometry *on page 62*

Frozen Section

Related Information
Breast Biopsy *on page 51*
Histopathology *on page 59*
Lymph Node Biopsy *on page 67*
Virus, Direct Detection by Fluorescent Antibody *on page 696*

Synonyms FS; Intraoperative Consultation, Pathology; Pathology Operating Room Consultation; Surgical Pathology Consultation

Test Includes Gross examination by a pathologist with specimen evaluation and possible frozen section (FS) with interpretation, followed by histopathology report. Imprints and smears may be made from fresh tissue. Further studies may be initiated depending on clinical information, gross observations, and frozen section and/or cytologic findings.

Abstract Immediate intraoperative consultation to establish or confirm diagnosis, to provide support for determination of type or extent of operation[1] (ie, provision of immediate intraoperative diagnosis when consultation is needed to enhance patient care). Intraoperative consultation may not require a frozen section at all. It is the pathologist's responsibility to do that which is in the best interest of the patient. Tissue freezing may actually be contraindicated. When patient care is not enhanced, a frozen section is often not indicated, especially if the specimen may be compromised. More sampling limitations and technical problems exist than with fixed, paraffin sections.[2]

Patient Preparation Pertinent clinical history should be provided to the pathologist.

Specimen Fresh tissue with **no** added fixative or fluid, **rapidly** brought to the Surgical Pathology Laboratory.

Container Sterile towel, Petri dish, or sterile jar with appropriate attention to biohazard containment

Collection Container must be labeled with patient's name, date, operating room, and name of the surgeon requesting frozen section.

Causes for Rejection Specimen in fixative, dense bone without soft tissue. See Limitations and Contraindications.

Turnaround Time Delays may take place when FS is not scheduled, when earlier slides must be retrieved and reviewed, when other FS specimens simultaneously arrive from the same or another surgeon, when technical problems arise, and when additional pathologists or residents participate.[3]

Use Establish rapid histopathologic diagnosis of the presence and nature of a pathologic process;[4] provision of rapid intraoperative diagnosis to support immediate intraoperative decisions.[5] The frozen section diagnosis should respond to a clear, unambiguous surgical question.[2] FS is used to ascertain whether or not the specimen is adequate for diagnosis, even if diagnosis on FS must be deferred (ie, to establish whether or not additional sampling is needed). FS may be used to ascertain if cultures are indicated and, if so, to provide indication of the type of cultures needed; procure tissue for fat stains; procure tissue for direct immunofluorescent examination (eg, products of immune activation, viral antigens); rapid evaluation for direction of fresh tissues for possible subsequent special studies such as lymphocyte markers, flow cytometry, receptor assays, and/or electron microscopy. Determination of extent of disease may be accomplished with frozen sections in selected settings; for instance, evaluation of margins of resection. Surgeons sometimes request frozen sections to evaluate unanticipated findings (eg, a nodule in the liver) which are relevant to immediate surgical decisions.

Limitations Surgeons, pathologists, and other physicians should be aware of the limitations and pitfalls of FS diagnosis, a potentially high-risk procedure.

Limitations are imposed by the type and size of tissue, intrinsic difficulties associated with certain types of diseases, and extent of examination required within a limited time frame. Bone or heavily calcified tissue often cannot be cut. Tissues dominated by fat are technically difficult and may not be amenable to frozen section. Fixed tissues are technically difficult to manage for frozen section. Small biopsies pose technical difficulties and may significantly compromise evaluation of corresponding paraffin sections.

Some lesions require paraffin sections for definitive diagnosis, such as many lymphoid lesions and occasional problematic breast lesions (eg, papillary lesions, instances of lobular and intraductal proliferation). Frozen sections are more useful to provide diagnosis of a visible lesion than to rule out a possibility of an entity of microscopic proportions. The problems of frozen section for thyroid surgery include the differential diagnosis between instances of follicular adenoma versus carcinoma,[6] as well as identification of the occasional relatively small papillary carcinoma. Differential diagnosis between reactive gliosis and low grade glioma has been a problem for many experienced surgical pathologists and may continue to pose difficulties in high quality paraffin sections. In these setting, false-negative responses are more frequent than false-positive ones. Sufficient nonfrozen tissue for routine processing and ancillary studies is desirable.

Sampling errors are important pitfalls in application of frozen sections.[5,7,8,9] Patients usually should not be kept anesthetized while multiple frozen section blocks are processed, cut, stained, and examined when paraffin sections would serve as well, or better.

Frozen sections are used to assess adequacy of resection. **Margins** of specimens in resections for cancer may be a problem for which surgeons may request frozen section support. Negative margins in tumor resections may be of very limited value, especially when such margins are of substantial size, by virtue of sampling problems. Special problems in the breast are touched upon in the listing Breast Biopsy *on page 51*. The presence of fat, the geometry of multiple irregular surfaces in specimens, multiplicity of specimens in some cases, and time limitation while the patient remains under anesthesia all limit the significance of a negative frozen section report of margins. Absence of positive margins does not guarantee local control of the tumor, nor is it in any way a reliable guide to tumor behavior. Luna's head and neck series shows a relationship between **positive** margins and patient survival. If frozen section margins were positive, only 1 of 20 patients lived 2 years.[10]

False-negative frozen section diagnoses relate to the limited sampling possible within the abbreviated time available. Pathologists recognize the potential gravity of false-positive frozen section diagnosis of cancer. In some series, a zero incidence of false positives is reported.[8] The poorest accuracy reported from George Washington University was associated with thyroid and parathyroid glands, related in the former to the ease with which microscopic foci of papillary carcinoma or the presence of capsular or vascular invasion can be missed.[7] Intraoperative consultation on diseases of the parathyroid glands may be challenging.[11] Published results of frozen section examinations (false positives, false negatives, deferrals) often originate from institutions which have a great deal of experience with the technique.

In addition to sampling errors, Luna recognizes three other types of errors: interpretive, communicative, and technical.[10] Misinterpretation as a cause of diagnostic error at the Mayo Clinic involved mostly false-negative errors, but false-positive errors occurred as well.[5] Lack of proper clinical information (eg, history of prior irradiation) can lead to interpretive error.

Reasons to defer diagnosis at frozen section include need for more extensive sampling, lack of adequate epithelium lining cysts, twisted and infarcted lesions,[8] and need for special stains, immunohistochemistry, and optimal sections. In some cases, diagnosis must be delayed for permanent sections. The need for deferral in some cases is widely known; the frequency of false-positive diagnoses relates inversely to that of deferral of diagnosis.[7] In a series of 18,532 FS diagnoses, 4.6% were deferred.[12]

Contraindications Tissue is consumed in the process of frozen section. Tiny critical specimens (for example, possible breast carcinomas less than 5 mm in diameter) are best not risked. Breast specimens not grossly suspicious should not be frozen.[2] A substantial study concluded that FS examination of breast specimens should be limited to cases with distinct lesions >1.0 cm.[13] The freezing process may distort lymphoid as well as other tissues. Therefore, for suspected lymphoma, it is advisable to await proper fixation of the lymph node and paraffin sections for definitive diagnosis, but frozen sections are commonly utilized for immunohistochemical evaluation of lymphoid lesions. See Lymph Node Biopsy *on page 67* for further details. Frozen section artifact in paraffin sections subsequently processed may preclude definitive diagnosis. Frozen sections are considered contraindicated when the patient is known to be HIV positive, to avoid contamination of the cryostat.[7] In such instances, imprints and smears can sometimes replace frozen sections.[14] Luna and others include small melanocytic lesions among contraindications to frozen section.[10,14]

Methodology Gross examination by a pathologist is indicated. Freezing tissues in liquid nitrogen is widely utilized. vacuum bottle containing liquid nitrogen may be kept in the frozen section room. A slice of the specimen on an object holder, placed onto O.C.T.® compound, is lowered into the vacuum bottle with a metal clamp. Cryobaths with a refrigerant such as 2-methyl butane chilled to -70°C also give satisfactory results. Rapid H&E stains are commonly used and often preferred. Some cases are adequately evaluated with a single rapid supravital dye such as toluidine blue.

Additional Information Direct communication between pathologist and surgeon must take place at the time of frozen section diagnosis, according to requirements both of regulatory agencies and of good patient care.

Imprints may be stained with H&E, Diff-Quik®, Wright stain, or by other methods. They sometimes are extremely helpful in interpretation of frozen sections. Occasionally, imprints are more diagnostic than the frozen section. They are especially helpful with lymphoid specimens, occasional breast specimens, and in diagnosis of meningioma.

Pathology intraoperative consultations resulted in changed surgical procedures in 39% of cases in a large multi-institutional study.[1]

Footnotes

1. Zarbo RJ, Schmidt WA, Bachner P, et al, "Indications and Immediate Patient Outcomes of Pathology Intraoperative Consultations: A College of American Pathologists/Centers for Disease Control and Prevention Outcomes Working Group Study," *Arch Pathol Lab Med*, 1996, 120(1):19-25.

2. Page DL and Gray GF Jr, "Intraoperative Consultations by Pathologists at the Mayo Clinic: A Unique Experience," *Mayo Clin Proc*, 1995, 70(12):1222-3.

3. Novis DA and Zarbo RJ, "Interinstitutional Comparison of Frozen Section Turnaround Time: A College of American Pathologists Q-Probes Study of 32,868 Frozen Sections in 700 Hospitals," *Arch Pathol Lab Med*, 1997, 121(6):559-67.

4. Sawady J, Berner JJ, and Siegler EE, "Accuracy of and Reasons for Frozen Sections: A Correlative, Retrospective Study," *Hum Pathol*, 1988, 19(9):1019-23.

5. Ferreiro JA, Myers JL, and Bostwick DG, "Accuracy of Frozen Section Diagnosis in Surgical Pathology: Review of a 1-Year Experience With 24,880 Cases at Mayo Clinic Rochester," *Mayo Clin Proc*, 1995, 70(12):1137-41.

6. Shaha A, Gleich L, DiMaio T, et al, "Accuracy and Pitfalls of Frozen Section During Thyroid Surgery," *J Surg Oncol*, 1990, 44(2):84-92.

7. Oneson RH, Minke JA, and Silverberg SG, "Intraoperative Pathologic Consultation. An Audit of 1000 Recent Consecutive Cases," *Am J Surg Pathol*, 1989, 13(3):237-43.

8. Obiakor I, Maiman M, Mittal K, et al, "The Accuracy of Frozen Section in the Diagnosis of Ovarian Neoplasms," *Gynecol Oncol*, 1991, 43(1):61-3.

9. Prey MU, Vitale T, and Martin SA, "Guidelines for Practical Utilization of Intraoperative Frozen Sections," *Arch Surg*, 1989, 124(3):331-5.

10. Luna MA, "Uses, Abuses, and Pitfalls of Frozen Section Diagnoses of Diseases of the Head and Neck," *Surgical Pathology of the Head and Neck*, Volume 1, Barnes L, ed, New York, NY: Marcel Dekker Inc, 1985, 7-22.

11. LiVolsi VA and Hamilton R, "Intraoperative Assessment of Parathyroid Gland Pathology. A Common View From the Surgeon and the Pathologist," *Am J Clin Pathol*, 1994, 102(3):365-73.

12. Novis DA, Gephardt GN, and Zarbo RJ, "Interinstitutional Comparison of Frozen Section Consultation in Small Hospitals: A College of American Pathologists Q-Probes Study of 18,532 Frozen Section Consultation Diagnoses in 233 Small Hospitals," *Arch Pathol Lab Med*, 1996, 120:1087-93.

13. Niemann TH, Lucas JG, and Marsh WL Jr, "To Freeze or Not to Freeze: A Comparison of Methods for the Handling of Breast Biopsies With no Palpable Abnormality," *Am J Clin Pathol*, 1996, 106(2):225-8.

14. Reyes MG, Homsi MF, McDonald LW, et al, "Imprints, Smears, and Frozen Sections of Brain Tumors," *Neurosurgery*, 1991, 29(4):575-9.

References

Fechner RE, "Frozen Section (Intraoperative Consultation)," *Hum Pathol*, 1988, 19(9):999-1000.

Ranchod M, "Intraoperative Consultations in Surgical Pathology," *Pathology*, State of the Art Reviews, Volume 3(2), Philadelphia, PA: Hanley & Belfus, Inc, 1996.

Rosai J, *Ackerman's Surgical Pathology*, 8th ed, Volume 1, Chapter 1, St Louis, MO: CV Mosby Co, 1996, 7-9.

◆ **FS** *see* Frozen Section *on page 56*

◆ **G₁ Phase** *see* Cell Cycle Analysis by Flow Cytometry *on page 53*

◆ **G₂M** *see* Cell Cycle Analysis by Flow Cytometry *on page 53*

◆ **GCDFP-15** *see* Immunoperoxidase Procedures *on page 60*

◆ **Glial Fibrillary Acidic Protein** *see* Immunoperoxidase Procedures *on page 60*

◆ **G₀ Phase** *see* Cell Cycle Analysis by Flow Cytometry *on page 53*

◆ **Grocott's-Methenamine Silver Stain** *see* Skin Biopsy *on page 71*

◆ **Gross and Microscopic Pathology** *see* Histopathology *on page 59*

◆ **Gross Cystic Disease Fluid Protein-15** *see* Immunoperoxidase Procedures *on page 60*

◆ **Gross Cystic Disease Fluid Protein-15 (GCDFP-15)** *see* Breast Biopsy *on page 51*

◆ **hCG** *see* Immunoperoxidase Procedures *on page 60*

◆ **β-hCG** *see* Immunoperoxidase Procedures *on page 60*

◆ **Hepatic Iron Index** *see* Liver Biopsy *on page 65*

HER-2/*neu*

Related Information

Breast Biopsy *on page 51*
Fluorescence *In Situ* Hybridization *on page 367*
Immunoperoxidase Procedures *on page 60*

Synonyms c-*erb*B-2; *H*uman *E*pidermal *G*rowth *F*actor *R*eceptor Gene

Applies to FISH Assays

Abstract HER-2/*neu* is intimately associated with cellular proliferative capacity. Numerous studies have demonstrated an adverse effect of oncoprotein overexpression on prognosis, particularly in breast and ovarian cancer. More recently, this protein has been targeted for monoclonal antibody therapy in patients with metastatic breast carcinoma.

Specimen The HER-2/*neu* proto-oncogene is commonly evaluated by immunoperoxidase techniques using paraffin-embedded tissue. Paraffin-embedded tissue is also suitable for fluorescence *in situ* hybridization (FISH) assays. Fresh or frozen tissues are required for Southern, Northern, Western, or dot blot analysis.

Storage Instructions Routinely stored paraffin blocks are suitable for use over many years. Unstained slides may lose immunoreactivity for some antigens over time.[1]

Causes for Rejection Lack of demonstrable tumor in paraffin section, extensive tissue necrosis

Limitations Immunoperoxidase methods are limited by tumor necrosis or sample size. Fluorescence *in situ* hybridization (FISH) techniques may not be performed by all laboratories and are more costly than immunoperoxidase procedures. Suboptimal tissue fixation or processing can adversely affect all immunostaining and probe techniques.

Methodology Immunoperoxidase staining procedures are most commonly used to determine HER-2/*neu* overexpression. Production of consistent staining results was initially challenging. Various staining patterns were produced by different antibodies and were influenced by different fixatives.[2] Improved antigen retrieval methodologies, enhanced detection systems, and automated staining procedures have circumvented many of the early technical difficulties. However, interpretation of results, in some cases, may be problematic. Staining of non-neoplastic epithelium may complicate interpretation and must be considered.[3] It is uncertain if the extent of HER-2/*neu* protein overexpression has different implications for prognosis, resistance or sensitivity to certain chemotherapeutic protocols, or responsiveness to monoclonal antibody therapy.

Other methods to detect HER-2/*neu* protein overexpression include Western blot and enzyme-linked immunoassay. Enzyme-linked immunoassays for HER-2/*neu* in cytosol extracts have also been highly correlated with patient outcome.[4,5] Western blot assays also provide useful information. Both methods are limited by the requirement for fresh or frozen tissues.

Molecular techniques may be utilized. FISH has proven reliable for the determination of HER-2/*neu* gene amplification. Recent instrumentation allows for significant automation of the process. Tissues are fixed in formalin, optimally for 24-48 hours, and embedded in paraffin. Sections of 4-5 microns thick are deparaffinized, treated with protease, denatured, and hybridized with fluorescent-labeled DNA probes. A color-coded fluorescent probe specific for the HER-2/*neu* gene and a second color-coded fluorescent probe specific for the centromeric region of chromosome 17 are used. The slides are then washed, counterstained, and examined using a fluorescent microscope for hybridization signals in the nuclei of neoplastic cells. The microscopist can distinguish benign epithelium, *in situ* carcinoma, and invasive carcinoma and record the ratio of HER-2/*neu* signal to chromosome 17 signal. A ratio ≥2 is interpreted as positive for HER-2/*neu* gene amplification. An alternate (also commercially available) system provides data as an average number of HER-2/*neu* signals per cell. Recent studies using FISH have shown independent prognostic significance in multivariate analysis.[6] Immunoassay and FISH results correlate well in most cases.[7] Considerable controversy has arisen as to which method (immunohistochemistry vs FISH) should be employed for decisions concerning

(Continued)

HER-2/neu (Continued)

therapy.[3,8,9] Footnotes and references, as provided herein, may assist individual laboratories with their choice. A decision based upon cost consideration alone may not be advantageous to all patients. In attempts to provide optimum therapy, false-positive and false-negative results may have financial consequences.[8] The College of American Pathologists Consensus Statement of 1999 notes that there is a current lack of standardization and comparability data.[9] A specific method for c-erbB-2 (HER-2/neu) testing "cannot yet" be recommended. The CAP statement refers to erbB-2 testing as a "work in progress."[9] Future recommendations will likely relate to the results of large multicenter outcome-based trials comparing FISH and immunohistochemical methods (currently in progress). FISH-based assays have won FDA approval for breast cancer prognosis (Inform; Ventana Medical Systems, Tucson, AZ) and for predicting response to docetaxel (Path Vysion; Vysis, Downers Grove, IL).

Southern blot assays detecting tumor DNA have more value in a research setting than in the clinical environment. Use of extract preparations avoids many of the technical and interpretive problems of immunostaining methods, but also introduces dilutional effects (of normal breast epithelium and/or stroma) when attempting to obtain quantitative results.

Additional Information HER-2/neu is a protein encoded by chromosome 17 and expressed as a 185 kd transmembrane receptor with tyrosine kinase activity.[10] HER-2/neu shares close structural and functional similarities with the epidermal growth factor family of proteins, of which four are currently known.[11] These membrane protein receptors transduce signals conferred by peptides in the extracellular milieu to promote cellular proliferation and differentiation by initiating a complex cascade of intracellular pathways. However, the specific ligand for HER-2/neu is unknown.

HER-2/neu protein expression is closely related to gene copy number.[12] Normal cells have little or no demonstrable surface expression of HER-2/neu by immunohistochemical methods. On a molecular basis, gene overexpression in breast cancer is most commonly related to gene amplification. FISH studies typically show 6-20 signals when HER-2/neu protein is detected.[7] A less common mechanism is aneuploidy of chromosome 17. Increased gene copy numbers do not necessarily correlate with surface protein overexpression, probably owing to post-transcriptional defects. The clinical significance of this observation is unclear.

Mechanisms by which HER-2/neu confers increased proliferative capacity include point mutation or sequence deletions promoting unregulated tyrosine kinase activity (animal studies). Gene amplification is the primary mechanism by which HER-2/neu is overexpressed in human tumors. Formation of abnormal heterodimers with epidermal growth factor and HER-2/neu represents one of the more common abnormalities found in experimental settings. In experimental tumor models, transfection of target cells with HER-2/neu gene leads to enhanced metastatic potential.[10]

HER-2/neu is most studied in breast carcinoma, in which overexpression is detected in approximately 25% to 30% of neoplasms. Most early studies focused on the prognostic role of HER-2/neu overexpression, while more recent studies have emphasized its predictive attributes. Protein overexpression is highly correlated with high nuclear grade, negative hormone receptor status, high S-phase fraction, and tumor aneuploidy. Despite these associations, HER-2/neu expression has been shown in many studies to represent an independent adverse prognostic finding. Other studies have confirmed its negative impact on prognosis but failed to validate its value as an independent prognostic factor. Excellent reviews addressing the prognostic and predictive values of HER-2/neu overexpression have been recently published.[13,14,15]

HER-2/neu protein overexpression has gained special significance since the 1998 FDA approval of trastuzumab (Herceptin®; Genentech, San Francisco, CA) for the therapy of metastatic breast cancer. This humanized monoclonal antibody is directed against HER-2/neu protein and has shown significant response rates in patients with stage IV breast cancer.[16] The role of Herceptin® in the adjuvant setting is currently under investigation. As a prerequisite for Herceptin® therapy, the demonstration of HER-2/neu expression is mandatory.

HER-2/neu protein over-expression also has predictive value for other therapeutic modalities. HER-2/neu overexpression is thought to predict increased resistance to cyclophosphamide therapy and enhanced sensitivity to chemotherapeutic regimens containing Adriamycin®.[17]

In synchrony with the release of Herceptin®, the FDA approved the use of HercepTest® (DAKO Corporation, Carpinteria, CA), an immunoperoxidase kit for detection of HER-2/neu. Use of this kit offers interpretive guidelines restricted for use in patients being considered for trastuzumab therapy. While the sensitivity of this test appears high, its low specificity results in false-positive or equivocal reactions. Interpretive standards remain problematic.[3] Application of these guidelines to other immunostaining procedures using different antibodies in a setting in which prognostic attributes of HER-2/neu overexpression are questioned have not been established.

HER-2/neu protein overexpression is also detected with some frequency in ovarian carcinoma,[18] prostatic adenocarcinoma,[19,20] nonsmall cell carcinoma of lung,[21,22] pancreatic adenocarcinoma,[23] gastric adenocarcinoma, oral carcinomas, and salivary gland adenocarcinoma.[10]

Future strategies targeting the mechanisms of HER-2/neu overexpression may utilize antisense DNA constructs or techniques designed to enhance promoter region deactivation with the goal of normalizing cell proliferation.

Footnotes

1. Jacobs TW, Prioleau JE, Stillman IE, et al, "Loss of Tumor Marker-Immunostaining Intensity on Stored Paraffin Slides of Breast Cancer," *J Natl Cancer Inst*, 1996, 88(15):1054-9.
2. Ross JS and Fletcher JA, "HER-2/neu (c-erb-B2) Gene and Protein in Breast Cancer," *Am J Clin Pathol*, 1999, 112(1 Suppl 1):S53-67.
3. Jacobs TW, Gown AM, Yaziji H, et al, "Specificity of HercepTest in Determining HER-2/neu Status of Breast Cancers Using the United States Food and Drug Administration-Approved Scoring System," *J Clin Oncol*, 1999, 17(7):1983-7.
4. Valeron P, Chirino R, and Vega V, "Quantitative Analysis of p185 (HER-2/neu) Protein in Breast Cancer and Its Association With Other Prognostic Factors," *Int J Cancer*, 1997, 74(2):175-9.
5. Koscielny S, Terrier P, and Daver A, "Quantitative Determination of c-erbB-2 in Human Breast Tumours: Potential Prognostic Significance of Low Values," *Eur J Cancer*, 1998, 34(4):476-81.
6. Press M, Bernstein L, and Thomas P, "HER-2/neu Gene Amplification Characterized by Fluorescence In Situ Hybridization: Poor Prognosis in Node-Negative Breast Carcinomas," *J Clin Oncol*, 1997, 15(8):2894-904.
7. Jacobs TW, Gown AM, Yaziji H, et al, "Comparison of Fluorescence In Situ Hybridization and Immunohistochemistry for the Evaluation of HER-2/neu in Breast Cancer," *J Clin Oncol*, 1999. 17(7):1974-82.
8. Seelig S, "Fluorescence In Situ Hybridization Versus Immunohistochemistry: Importance of Clinical Outcome," *J Clin Oncol*, 1999, 17(11):3690-2.
9. Fitzgibbons PL, Page DL, Weaver D, et al, "Prognostic Factors in Breast Cancer. College of American Pathologists Consensus Statement 1999," *Arch Pathol Lab Med*, 2000, 124(7):966-78.
10. Hung MC and Lau YK, "Basic Science of HER-2/neu: A Review," *Semin Oncol*, 1999, 26(4 Suppl 12):51-9.
11. Bacus SS, Zelnick CR, Plowman G, et al, "Expression of the erbB-2 Family of Growth Factor Receptors and Their Ligands in Breast Cancers. Implication for Tumor Biology and Clinical Behavior," *Am J Clin Pathol*, 1994, 102(4 Suppl 1):S13-24.
12. Slamon D, Godolphin W, and Jones L, "Studies of the HER-2/neu Proto-oncogene in Human Breast and Ovarian Cancer," *Science*, 1989, 244(4905):707-12.
13. Ross J and Fletcher J, "HER-2/neu (c-erb-B2) Gene and Protein in Breast Cancer," *Am J Clin Pathol*, 1999, 122(Suppl 1):S53-S67.
14. Allred D and Swanson P, "Testing for erbB-2 by Immunohistochemistry in Breast Cancer," *Am J Clin Pathol*, 2000, 113(2):171-5.
15. Pauletti G, Dandekar S, Rong H, et al, "Assessment of Methods for Tissue-Based Detection of the HER-2/neu Alteration in Human Breast Cancer: A Direct Comparison of Fluorescence In Situ Hybridization and Immunohistochemistry," *J Clin Oncol*, 2000, 18(21):3651-64.
16. Pegram M, Lipton A, and Hayes D, "Phase II Study of Receptor-Enhanced Chemosensitivity Using Recombinant Humanized Anti-p185HER-2/neu Monoclonal Antibody Plus Cisplatin in Patients With HER-2/neu-Overexpressing Metastatic Breast Cancer Refractory to Chemotherapy Treatment," *J Clin Oncol*, 1998, 16(8):2659-71.
17. Muss H, Thor A, and Berry D, "C-erbB-2 Expression and Response to Adjuvant Therapy in Node-Positive Early Breast Cancer," *N Engl J Med*, 1994, 330(18):1260-6.
18. Matias-Guiu X and Prat J, "Molecular Pathology of Ovarian Carcinomas," *Virchows Arch*, 1998, 433(2):103-11.
19. Mydlo JH, Kral JG, Volpe M, et al, "An Analysis of Microvessel Density, Androgen Receptor, p53 and HER-2/neu Expression and Gleason Score in Prostate Cancer. Preliminary Results and Therapeutic Implications," *Eur Urol*, 1998, 34(5):426-32.
20. Visakorpi T, Kallioniemi OP, Koivula T, et al, "Expression of Epidermal Growth Factor Receptor and erb-2 (HER-2/neu) Oncoprotein in Prostatic Carcinomas," *Mod Pathol*, 1992, 5(6):643-8.
21. Hsieh CC, Chow KC, Fahn HJ, et al, "Prognostic Significance of HER-2/neu Overexpression in Stage I Adenocarcinoma of Lung," *Ann Thorac Surg*, 1998, 66(4):1159-63 (discussion 1163-4).
22. Smit EF, Groen HJ, Splinter TA, et al, "New Prognostic Factors in Resectable Nonsmall Cell Lung Cancer," *Thorax*, 1996, 51(6):638-46.
23. Day JD, Digiuseppe JA, Yeo C, et al, "Immunohistochemical Evaluation of HER-2/neu Expression in Pancreatic Adenocarcinoma and Pancreatic Intraepithelial Neoplasms," *Hum Pathol*, 1996, 27(2):119-24.

References

Hoang MP, Sahin AA, Ordonez NG, et al, "HER-2/neu Gene Amplification Compared With HER-2/neu Protein Overexpression and Interobserver Reproducibility in Invasive Breast Carcinoma," *Am J Clin Pathol*, 2000, 113(6):852-9.

Masood S, Bui MM, Yung JF, et al, "Reproducibility of LSI HER-2/neu SpectrumOrange and CEP 17 SpectrumGreen Dual Color Deoxyribonucleic acid Probe Kit. For Enumeration of Gene Amplification in Paraffin-Embedded Specimens: A Multicenter Clinical Validation Study," *Ann Clin Lab Sci*, 1998, 28(4):215-23.

Menard S, Tagliabue E, Campiglio M, et al, "Role of HER-2 Gene Overexpression in Breast Carcinoma," *J Cell Physiol*, 2000, 182(2):150-62.

Nelson NJ, "Experts Debate Value of HER2 Testing Methods," *J Natl Cancer Inst*, 2000, 92(4):292-4.

O'Malley FP, Parkes R, Latta E, et al, "Comparison of HER-2/neu Status Assessed by Quantitative Polymerase Chain Reaction and Immunohistochemistry," *Am J Clin Pathol*, 2001, 115(4):504-11.

Pegram MD, Pauletti G, and Slamon DJ, "HER-2/neu as a Predictive Marker of Response to Breast Cancer Therapy," *Breast Cancer Res Treat*, 1998, 52(1-3):65-77.

Persons DL, Bui MM, Lowery MC, et al, "Fluorescence In Situ Hybridization (FISH) for Detection of HER-2/neu Amplification in Breast Cancer: A Multicenter Portability Study," *Ann Clin Lab Sci*, 2000, 30(1):41-8.

Histopathology

Related Information

Synonyms Biopsy; Gross and Microscopic Pathology; Pathologic Examination; Surgical Pathology; Tissue Examination

Applies to Bronchial Biopsy; Endoscopic Biopsy; Lung Biopsy; Medical Legal Specimens

Test Includes Gross and microscopic examination and diagnosis with comments, notes, prognostic and other information in selected cases. Imprints may be made if the tissue is fresh and unfixed and if indications for imprints exist. Additional studies are done as indicated.

Abstract Surgical pathology has been defined as the discipline which deals with the anatomic pathology of tissues removed from living patients. Smears, aspirates, special stains, histochemistry, immunocytochemistry, flow cytometry, electron microscopy, and/or molecular pathology may be needed.

Patient Preparation Each specimen should be accompanied by an adequate description of what it is thought to represent, as well as an appropriate clinical history. The appearances of disease processes may be seriously misleading out of context.[1]

Specimen Fresh tissue, tissue fixed in phosphate-buffered formalin or other appropriate fixative. Each specimen container must be labeled to include source as well as patient's name. Each specimen from a different anatomic site must be placed in a separate, correctly labeled container, designated "left," "right," "proximal," "distal," "ventral," "dorsal," and so forth. Crushed or damaged specimens may lead to incorrect interpretations.

Container Jars of assorted sizes, containing formalin or another appropriate fixative; the neck of the container should not be smaller than its diameter. Fresh specimens should be submitted on a sterile gauze pad moistened with sterile saline and should not be left on countertops; they must be placed in the hands of a responsible person.

Collection Small biopsy specimens should be placed immediately in fixative, unless special needs such as frozen section exist. Use approximately 5-20 times as much fixative solution as the bulk of the tissue. Small tissues such as those from bronchoscopic biopsy, bladder biopsy, and endometrium can be ruined in a very short time by drying out.

Storage Instructions Fixation in formalin solution or other appropriate fixative

Causes for Rejection Mislabeled specimen container, unlabeled specimen

Turnaround Time Biopsy reports commonly require a day or more. Delays are caused by need for proper fixation, clinical information, deeper sections, decalcification, immunochemistry or other special stains.

Special Instructions See specific handling instructions in test listings such as Muscle Biopsy *on page 69*, Estrogen and Progesterone Receptor Assay *on page 55*, Frozen Section *on page 56*, Kidney Biopsy *on page 64*, and Liver Biopsy *on page 65*. Consult the Pathology Department prior to beginning the procedure for specific instructions. Requisition should state operative diagnosis and source of specimen, as well as patient's name, age, sex, room or location, name of surgeon, and names of other physicians who will need a copy of the pathology report.

Use Histopathologic diagnosis; distinguish benign from malignant entities when possible; evaluate extent of lesions, adequacy of resection, provision of classification and, when appropriate, grading in the case of tumors

Limitations Tissue fixed in formalin **cannot** be used for microbial culture, certain types of histochemistry, frozen sections, gene rearrangement, or optimal electron microscopy.

The practice of surgical pathology often depends on the clinical input of other physicians, including surgeons. Miracles of extrapolation cannot consistently be provided from incomplete clinical information and/or inadequate biopsies.[1] Medicolegal activity may follow inadequate sampling by surgeon or pathologist.

Additional Information A major advantage of conventional over frozen sections is that extensive sampling of the entire specimen can take place.

Cultures of tissue are best taken in the O.R., where a sterile field exists. A piece of tissue (eg, a curetting of a fistulous tract) should be placed in an appropriate sterile tube with requests for smear, culture, anaerobic culture, AFB, and fungus culture if appropriate. It should be immediately taken to the Microbiology Laboratory. See Infectious Diseases listings.

Routine tissues are brought in fixative. Fixatives should be picked up prior to the biopsy. Commonly used fixatives include modified Zenker's fluid (for tiny specimens, eg, endometrial curettage, liver, and other needle biopsies, **not** skin), and formalin (for specimens thicker than 3 mm).

Bullets, shotgun pellets, and other metallic objects require special handling, but no fixative is needed. Of major importance in handling bullets and other specimens of possible forensic significance, including vaginal swabs obtained in rape cases, is the scrupulous maintenance of a chain-of-custody. Specimens must be accurately labeled, and transfer and receipt must be documented. Specimens must be kept under safeguards in the laboratory until turned over to law enforcement officials. See Chain-of-Custody Protocol *on page 785*.

Bone biopsy for metabolic bone disease requires special handling.

Materials sometimes not sent for histopathologic examination, depending on the institution, include bullets, shotgun pellets, neonatal foreskins, grossly unremarkable placentas from uneventful deliveries, and orthopedic appliances. If a specimen is not sent to the Pathology Department, the surgeon should carefully describe the specimen in the operative report.

The surgical pathology report includes clinical information provided by the physician or surgeon; description of the gross examination; a microscopic description; or diagnosis and, in selected cases, a comment or note. The last may include discussion of the differential diagnosis and/or may provide prognostic or therapeutic recommendations. References may be provided in appropriate cases. If a frozen section was done, it is addressed.

Third party payors commonly use surgical pathology reports to validate CPT codes.

Footnotes

1. Rosai K, *Ackerman's Surgical Pathology*, 8th ed, Volume 1, Chapter 1, St Louis, MO: CV Mosby Co, 1996, 1-12.

Image Analysis

Related Information

Synonyms Automated Cytophotometry; Computerized Interactive Morphometry; Image Cytometry; Image Morphometry; Quantitative Image Analysis; Static Image Analysis

Applies to Cell Measurement/Micrometry; Cyclins; DNA Content; DNA Index; DNA Ploidy Interpretation; Ki-67; PCNA; Pixels; Proliferation Index (MIB-1 Quantitation); Quantitative Histomorphometry; Quantitative Immunohistochemistry; Quantitative Nuclear Morphometry; S Phase

Test Includes Use of computerized imaging systems to contribute information which may be useful in determination of tumor prognosis and therapy. Such factors may include quantitative analysis of DNA ploidy/index, ER/PR (hormone receptors); cellular proliferative proteins; oncogene protein content, in addition to nuclear morphology and Markovian textures.

Abstract This is a means of quantifying microscopic images by digital conversion and computer analysis. Systems can selectively measure neoplastic cell populations. Such information from optical physics and engineering appears in pathology journals.[1,2,3]

Computer-based image analysis applies digital technology to quantitative measurements in cyto- and histopathology. Cell images are digitized into pixels (picture elements). The most widespread applications of this technology are in the quantitation of DNA content and in quantitation of immunohistochemical stained biomarkers. The image analysis system consists of a modified optical microscope, a video camera with digitizer, and a high-speed computer workstation. The image is converted to numerical data. Affordable memory devices with microprocessors and quality cameras make image processing and statistical image analysis practical. The availability of image processing instruments allows the pathologist direct visualization of the cell population being studied for DNA measurement, providing simultaneous correlation between DNA studies and morphology. Quantitative immunohistochemistry allows for an automated assessment of the degree of reactivity of immunologic markers based on summation of optical density measurements with a particular chromagen. The image analysis (Continued)

Image Analysis (Continued)

method can be used to quantitate various immunohistochemical measurements of cell proliferation, including Ki-67, PCNA, and the cyclins. In addition, cytoplasmic antigen quantification can also be performed.[4]

Specimen DNA ploidy is best analyzed from touch preps or tissue smears/scrapes prepared from freshly excised tissues. Tissue sections from frozen or paraffin-embedded tissues may also be used but complicate statistical analysis owing to considerations attributable to "sliced nuclei". Quantitation of immunohistochemical markers may be performed on any source of tissue suitable for staining and is most commonly performed on paraffin-embedded tissues.

Turnaround Time From the time of surgery to completion of report, typically takes from 2-5 days. This includes routine tissue or cytology processing, completion of special stains, analysis, and interpretation. Technical and interpretive expertise are concentrated in medical centers, large hospitals, and large reference laboratories.

Reference Interval For DNA index, normal is 0.9-1.1 or the diploid state. The following values reflect the DNA index for:

- hypodiploid (aneuploid): <0.9
- diploid: 0.9-1.1
- hyperdiploid (aneuploid): >1.1 to <1.9
- tetraploid: 1.9-21.
- hypertetraploid: >2.1
- multiploid: variable → multiple aneuploid peaks

Normal proliferation index (Ki-67 positivity of tumor cells) is <10%; S phase should be <7%.

Use Image analysis is an emerging method which is used to evaluate tumor aggressiveness and patient prognosis. The concept of image analysis holds that the further dedifferentiated a tumor becomes, the further it deviates from the normal diploid state. This may be expressed as a tetraploid or aneuploid state according to the amount of DNA in the Feulgen-stained nuclei. In terms of ploidy, this is expressed as a DNA index between 1.0 and 2.0. The fraction of cells in the S phase of the cell cycle is also a parameter that can be measured by image analysis. In general, the more cells in S phase (DNA synthesis phase), the more aggressive the tumor.

Image analysis, in combination with immunohistochemistry, may be used to study antigens expressed by tumor cells that are important in cancer prognosis. Estrogen and progesterone receptors[2] may be semiquantitated with immunochemical staining of breast cancer cells with subsequent study by image analysis.

Other biomarkers (eg, HER-2/neu, p53, bcl-2, EGFR, proliferation markers including Ki-67, PCNA, cyclin A, and markers for apoptosis) have been helpful in tumor diagnosis, prognosis, prediction of response to therapy, assessment of tumor proliferation and progression, and assessment of tumor invasion and metastasis.[5] MIB-1 antibody reacts with the antigen Ki-67, which is a proliferation marker.

Limitations While flow cytometry assays 10,000-50,000 or more nuclei, in image analysis only a few hundred nuclei are counted.[3] Image analysis is labor intensive and the process is enhanced when the operator has a background in cytology or histopathology to allow for the advantages of simultaneous morphologic assessment and DNA analysis.[4] Studies based on image analysis cannot reliably distinguish benign from malignant tumors.

Methodology Essentially, a computer is used to analyze digitized microscopic images. Reproducibility can be achieved with presently available equipment. Commercial systems are available and personally compiled systems are described.[1]

Additional Information Analysis can be restricted to counting only cells of interest (eg, keratin-positive cells in instances of epithelial tumors)[3] and rejecting the nontumor cells or artifactually distorted ones.

Much less tissue is needed than that required for flow cytometry. Correlation between these methods depends upon the amount of tumor in the specimen; the greater the percentage of tumor cells, the better the correlation. Digital image analysis provides more sensitive measurement of ploidy and of proliferation when only small volumes of tumor or low percentages of neoplastic cells are available in a specimen. Very small populations of neoplastic cells can be overlooked by flow cytometry.

Footnotes

1. Wells WA, Rainer RO, and Memoli VA, "Basic Principles of Image Processing," Am J Clin Pathol, 1992, 98(5):493-501.
2. El-Badawy N, Cohen C, Derose PB, et al, "Immunohistochemical Progesterone Receptor Assay, Measurement by Image Analysis," Am J Clin Pathol, 1991, 96(6):704-10.
3. Robinson RA, "Defining the Limits of DNA Cytometry," Am J Clin Pathol, 1992, 98(3):275-7.
4. Ross JS, DNA Ploidy and Cell Cycle Analysis in Pathology, New York, NY: Igaku-Shoin, 1996.
5. Eissa S, Tumor Markers, London, UK: Chapman & Hall, 1998.

References

Baak JPA, Manual of Quantitative Pathology in Cancer Diagnosis and Prognosis, Berlin, Germany: Springer-Verlag, 1991.

Balis UJ, "Imaging in the Clinical Laboratory," Clinics in Laboratory Medicine, Volume 17, Philadelphia, PA: WB Saunders Co, 1997.

Bejar J, Sabo E, Misselevich I, et al, "Comparative Study of Computer-Assisted Image Analysis Light-Microscopically Determined Estrogen Receptor Status of Breast Carcinomas," Arch Pathol Lab Med, 1998, 122(4):346-52.

Bosari S, Wiley BD, Hamilton WM, et al, "DNA Measurement by Image Analysis of Paraffin-Embedded Breast Carcinoma Tissue - A Comparative Investigation," Am J Clin Pathol, 1991, 96(6):698-703.

Elsheikh TM, Silverman JF, McCool JW, et al, "Comparative DNA Analysis of Solid Tumors by Flow Cytometric and Image Analyses of Touch Imprints and Flow Cell Suspensions," Am J Clin Pathol, 1992, 98(3):296-304.

Gschwendtner A, Neher A, Kreczy A, et al, "DNA Ploidy Determination of Early Molar Pregnancies by Image Analysis," Arch Pathol Lab Med, 1998, 122(11):1000-4.

Marchevsky AM and Bartels PH, Image Analysis. A Primer for Pathologists, New York, NY: Raven Press, 1994.

Martin-Reay DG, Kamentsky LA, Weinberg DS, et al, "Evaluation of a New Slide-Based Laser Scanning Cytometer for DNA Analysis of Tumors. Comparison With Flow Cytometry and Image Analysis," Am J Clin Pathol, 1994, 102(4):432-8.

Salmon I and Kiss R, "Relationship Between Proliferative Activity and Ploidy Level in a Series of 530 Human Brain Tumors, Including Astrocytomas, Meningiomas, Schwannomas, and Metastases," Hum Pathol, 1993, 24(3):329-35.

Wu J and Nakamura R, Human Circulating Tumor Markers: Current Concepts and Clinical Applications, Chicago, IL: ASCP Press, 1997.

- **Image Cytometry** see Image Analysis on page 59

- **Image Morphometry** see Image Analysis on page 59

- **Immunocytochemistry** see Immunoperoxidase Procedures on page 60

- **Immunocytochemistry** see Sentinel Lymph Node Biopsy on page 70

- **Immunofluorescence** see Immunoperoxidase Procedures on page 60

- **Immunofluorescence Skin Biopsy** see Skin Biopsy, Immunofluorescence on page 72

- **Immunohistochemistry** see Immunoperoxidase Procedures on page 60

- **Immunomicroscopy** see Immunoperoxidase Procedures on page 60

Immunoperoxidase Procedures

Related Information

Body Cavity Fluid Cytology on page 372
Bone Marrow on page 410
Breast Biopsy on page 51
CA 19-9, Serum on page 128
CA 125, Serum on page 126
Calcitonin, Serum or Plasma on page 129
Carcinoembryonic Antigen, Serum on page 135
Cerebrospinal Fluid Cytology on page 376
Cystic Fibrosis DNA Detection on page 705
Fine Needle Aspiration, Deep Masses on page 381
Fine Needle Aspiration, Superficial Masses (Palpable) on page 382
Fluorescence In Situ Hybridization on page 367
Gene Rearrangement for Leukemia and Lymphoma on page 725
Immunophenotypic Analysis of Tissues by Flow Cytometry on page 62
Kidney Biopsy on page 64
Lymph Node Biopsy on page 67
p53, Functional Assay/Sequencing on page 728
Prostate Specific Antigen, Serum on page 263
Skin Biopsy on page 71
Viral Culture, Tissue on page 695

Synonyms Immunocytochemistry; Immunohistochemistry; Immunomicroscopy; Immunostains

Applies to Alpha Fetoprotein; CA-125; Chromogranin; Cytokeratins; Desmin; Epithelial Membrane Antigen (EMA); Factor VIII Related Antigen; GCDFP-15; Glial Fibrillary Acidic Protein; Gross Cystic Disease Fluid Protein-15; hCG; β-hCG; HMB-45; Immunofluorescence; In Situ Hybridization; Intermediate Filaments; Kappa Light Chains; Ki-67; Lambda Light Chains; Lectins; Leukocyte Common Antigen; Leu M1; Light Chains; Lysozyme; MIB-1; Monoclonal Immunoglobulins; Myoglobin; Myosin; PCNA; Peptide Hormones; Prostate Specific Acid Phosphatase; S-100; Synaptophysin; Thyroglobulin; Tissue Antigens; T Lymphocytes; TTF-1; Vimentin

Test Includes Histology, frozen section, immunofluorescence. Immunostains are often used in conjunction with flow cytometry in the characterization of hematopoietic and lymphoid neoplasms.

Abstract Immunohistochemical procedures provide important diagnostic tools in all disciplines of surgical pathology. Results of such tests often document lineage of poorly differentiated neoplasms, offer insights to the origin of carcinomas of unknown primary site, document expression of biomarkers of prognostic and predictive importance, and document phenotypic evidence of clonal lymphoid proliferation. Additionally, it is possible to identify and characterize infectious agents using these methods.

Specimen Routine surgical biopsies or excisions submitted in formalin are suitable for the majority of immunohistochemical procedures.

Container Suitable for safe handling of tissues and formalin or similar fixatives. Sterile Petri dish is ideal for submitting fresh tissue for lymphoma evaluation.

Causes for Rejection Improperly labeled specimen; desiccation, extensive necrosis, and inadequate fixation will significantly compromise final evaluation.

Special Instructions Special fixatives are useful for documenting expression of some antigens, particularly for those of hematopoietic origin. When the diagnosis of lymphoma is a serious consideration, submission of fresh tissue is necessary to fully characterize the process. See Lymph Node Biopsy *on page 67*.

Use Immunoperoxidase techniques are used to localize antigens in tissues. One such important application is to establish the lineage of a poorly differentiated neoplasm. This is most reliably done by use of a panel of immunostains selected to provide complimentary positive and negative results. Use of overly restricted panels may lead to false interpretive results (eg, S100 positive carcinoma, as in breast). A commonly used panel for a poorly differentiated neoplasm generally includes pan-cytokeratin, CD45 (leukocyte common antigen), S100 protein, and vimentin. See Table 1.

Carcinoma of unknown primary is a common diagnostic challenge, particularly in today's era of image guided needle biopsy. Immunohistochemical stains often provide significant clues as to the site of origin.[1] Although such an approach may not firmly establish the site of origin, correlation with clinical and radiographic findings will often allow a working diagnosis with reasonable medical certainty.

Cytokeratins 7 and 20 have proven extremely useful in this regard.[2,3] The majority of adenocarcinomas show a CK7+/CK20- phenotype. Neoplasms which are CK7+/CK20+, CK7-/CK20+, or CK7-/CK20- form a select group of tumors whose inclusion or exclusion may have a significant impact on the final diagnosis. See Table 2.

Thyroid transcript factor 1 (TTF-1) is a recently characterized marker with extreme utility in diagnostic surgical pathology.[4,5] Distribution of the marker is limited and is among the first clinically useful markers for adenocarcinoma of lung origin. TTF-1 is also useful in differentiating small cell carcinoma of lung origin from Merkel cell carcinoma,[6,7] but not in discriminating small cell carcinoma of lung from extrapulmonary small cell carcinoma.[8] TTF-1 is also useful in distinguishing pulmonary adenocarcinoma from malignant mesothelioma.[9]

Gross cystic disease fluid protein-15 (GCDFP-15) is useful in identifying carcinoma of breast origin.[10] Apart from breast cancer, salivary gland tumors and sweat gland tumors are commonly immunoreactive.[11,12] Many sweat gland carcinomas also express estrogen receptors.[13] Appropriate caution is necessary when considering this differential diagnosis.

Other tissue selective antigens useful for addressing primary site of origin include prostate specific antigen, prostatic acid phosphatase, thyroglobulin, CA-125 (ovary), and placental alkaline phosphatase (gynecologic and germ cell tumors).

Markers of potential prognostic and predictive value have been extensively studied in a variety of neoplasms. Suffice it to say that only a few markers have achieved recognized utility in clinical practice. These include HER-2/neu (see HER-2/neu *on page 57*) and estrogen and progesterone receptors (see Estrogen and Progesterone Receptor Assay *on page 55*). Proliferative markers such as MIB-1 are under intense investigation and are considered useful in certain malignancies by the College of American Pathologists.[14,15]

Immunohistochemical stains are also extremely useful in the diagnosis and characterization of hematopoietic and lymphoid neoplasms. In recent years, a number of useful commercially available antibodies with activity in paraffin embedded tissue have been characterized.[16,17,18] The availability of these markers often circumvents the need for fresh frozen tissue. Nonetheless, documentation of light chain restriction is still best achieved by frozen section immunohistochemistry. Furthermore, frozen tissue blocks can be utilized for molecular genetic studies if needed. See Lymph Node Biopsy *on page 67*.

Table 2. Distinguishing Phenotypic Features of Selected Carcinoma*

	Pan-CK	CK7	CK20	TTF-1	GCDFP-15	PSA
Lung						
Adenoca	+	+	–	+	–	–
Small cell	+	–/+	–	+	–	–
Squamous	+	–	–	–	–	–
Breast	+	+	–	–	+	–
Colon	+	–	+	–	–	–
Pancreas	+	+	+/–	–	–	–
Liver	+	–	–	–	–	–
Kidney	+	–	–	–	–	–
Prostate	+	–	–	–	+	+
Bladder	+	+	+/–	–	–	–
Ovary	+	+	–	–	–	–

Abbreviations: Pan-CK = pan cytokeratin, CK7 = cytokeratin 7, CK20 = cytokeratin 20, TTF-1 = thyroid transcription factor 1, GCDFP-15 = gross cystic disease fluid protein 15, PSA = prostate specific antigen.

Reactions: (+) characteristically positive; (+/–) characteristically positive but sometimes negative; (–) characteristically negative; (–/+) characteristically negative but sometimes positive.

*There are many exceptions to the indicated reactions. The phenotypic findings must always be put in perspective with light microscopic and other clinical findings.

Limitations Appropriate application and interpretation of immunohistochemical procedures is the result of a long and steep learning curve. Inadequate tissue sampling and deficient basic histology are among the most commonly encountered problems limiting interpretation of immunostains. Variation in tissue fixation and processing, selection of most appropriate antigen retrieval techniques, and variable antibody reactivities supplied by different vendors are a few of the confounding factors that highlight the need for vigilant quality control and skilled technical personnel. Relative to routine histochemical procedures, immunostains are costly. Finally, intrinsic variability of antigen expression owing to the neoplastic state creates the potential for significant interpretive errors.

Methodology There are many modifications based on the following theme (see figure).

- Intrinsic tissue enzyme activity specific for the detection system is blocked.
- The primary antibody, which conveys the specificity of the stain, is applied to tissue sections, incubated, and unbound antibody is washed free.
- An enzyme-linked detection system specific for the primary antibody is applied to the tissues, incubated, and unbound reagents washed free.
- A substrate for the enzyme detection system is incubated, allowing the reaction product to form an insoluble precipitate, localizing the primary antibody, which is then visualized by light microscopy.

Primary antibodies of diagnostic importance are available from a variety of commercial sources. Monoclonal antibodies are derived from mouse or rat, and polyclonal antibodies are usually derived from rabbits or goats. The most commonly used detection system uses a biotin and avidin or streptavidin complex to introduce the detection enzyme into the complex. See figure on following page.

Table 1. Characteristic Phenotypic Profile of Neoplasms Based on Histogenesis*

	Intermediate Filaments					CD45 (LCA)	S100	Synapto	Chromo A
	CK	**Vim**	**Des**	**NF**	**GFAP**				
Carcinoma†									
NOS	+	–/+	–	–	–	–	–/+	–	–
Neuroendocrine‡	+/–	–/+	–	–/+	–	–	–	+	+
Lymphoma¶	–	–/+	–	–	–	+	–	–	–
Melanoma§	–	+	–	–	–	–	+	–	–
Soft tissue tumors									
Fibrous histiocytoma	–/+	+	–	–	–	–	–	–	–
Nerve sheath	–	+	–	–	–	–	+	–	–
Muscle	–	+	+	–	–	–	–	–	–
Vascular#	–	+	–	–	–	–	–	–	–
Glioma	–	+	–	–	+	–	+	–	–

Abbreviations: CK = cytokeratin, Vim = vimentin, Des = desmin, NF = neurofilament, GFAP = glial acid fibrillary protein, LCA = leukocyte common antigen, Synapto = synaptophysin, Chromo A = chromogranin A.

Reactions: (+) characteristically positive; (+/–) characteristically positive but sometimes negative; (–) characteristically negative; (–/+) characteristically negative but sometimes positive.

*There are many exceptions to the indicated reactions. The phenotypic findings must always be put in perspective with light microscopic and other clinical findings.

†Cytokeratin profile and expression of other tissue-associated antigens often help identify origin of metastatic neoplasms.

‡Expression of various peptide hormones may further aid in the classification of the neoplasm.

¶For additional information, see listings Lymph Node Biopsy and Immunophenotypic Analysis of Tissue by Flow Cytometry in this chapter.

§Expression of melanoma-associated antigen HMB-45 may help distinguish from nerve sheath tumors.

#Many vascular tumors express factor VIII-related antigen, CD31 and CD34.

(Continued)

Immunoperoxidase Procedures *(Continued)*

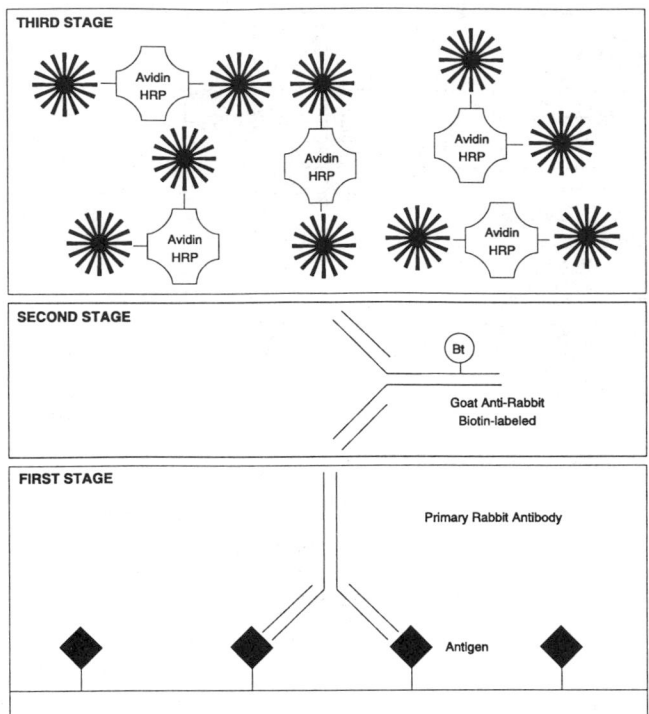

General scheme for performing immunoperoxidase stains: Tissue sections are deparaffinized and blocked to suppress endogenous peroxidase activity and nonspecific protein binding. For some stains (eg, cytokeratin), antigenic determinants are unmasked by protease digestion or microwave techniques. The first stage, incubation with the primary antibody, confers the specificity of the stain. The second stage antibody is covalently labeled with biotin for which avidin has an extraordinarily high affinity. Horse radish peroxidase (HRP) may be covalently coupled to avidin and after incubation with an appropriate substrate, antigens are localized.

Specificity and sensitivity of the primary antibody and the detection system should always be verified by testing on a limited library of tissues, which include known positives and negatives. When validated for diagnostic testing, careful attention must be continuously rendered to appropriately fixed control tissues and to internal controls which may be present in the test tissues. A valid positive immunostain will have a clean background and discrete reaction. A negative reaction is equally valid if properly controlled and if it complements a positive reaction for another mutually exclusive antigen.

Automated immunostainers have gained wide acceptance in the clinical laboratory.[19] Some platforms are now incorporating routine histochemical stains and *in situ* hybridization with the same intention of improving quality, consistency and turnaround time.[20]

Additional Information Immunofluorescent procedures address similar issues, but require a relatively expensive fluorescence microscope, are less sensitive, lack the resolution afforded by light microscopy, and do not produce an archivable slide. However, immunofluorescence is the method of choice for the localization of immunoglobulins, complement, and fibrin in the evaluation of renal biopsies and inflammatory dermatoses. Lectins, plant proteins with specificity for given carbohydrate moieties, are useful for antigen localization and can be used much like a primary antibody. More recently, *in situ* hybridization has been employed to identify nucleic acid sequences in cells.[21,22,23] Following procedures generally similar to immunoperoxidase stains, biotin-labeled, genetically-engineered sequences of nucleic acids localize complementary gene sequences to detect viral genes and oncogenes of potential diagnostic significance.

Footnotes

1. DeYoung BR and Wick MR, "Immunohistologic Evaluation of Metastatic Carcinomas of Unknown Origin: An Algorithmic Approach," *Semin Diagn Pathol*, 2000, 17(3):184-93.

2. Blumenfeld W, Turi GK, Harrison G, et al, "Utility of Cytokeratin 7 and 20 Subset Analysis as an Aid in the Identification of Primary Site of Origin of Malignancy in Cytologic Specimens," *Diagn Cytopathol*, 1999, 20(2):63-6.

3. Chu P, Wu E, and Weiss LM, "Cytokeratin 7 and Cytokeratin 20 Expression in Epithelial Neoplasms: A Survey of 435 Cases," *Mod Pathol*, 2000, 13(9):962-72.

4. Ordonez NG, "Thyroid Transcription Factor-1 Is a Marker of Lung and Thyroid Carcinomas," *Adv Anat Pathol*, 2000, 7(2):123-7.

5. Kaufmann O and Dietel M, "Thyroid Transcription Factor-1 Is the Superior Immunohistochemical Marker for Pulmonary Adenocarcinomas and Large Cell Carcinomas Compared to Surfactant Proteins A and B," *Histopathology*, 2000, 36(1):8-16.

6. Hanly AJ, Elgart GW, Jorda M, et al, "Analysis of Thyroid Transcription Factor-1 and Cytokeratin 20 Separates Merkel Cell Carcinoma From Small Cell Carcinoma of Lung," *J Cutan Pathol*, 2000, 27(3):118-20.

7. Byrd-Gloster AL, Khoor A, Glass LF, et al, "Differential Expression of Thyroid Transcription Factor 1 in Small Cell Lung Carcinoma and Merkel Cell Tumor," *Hum Pathol*, 2000, 31(1):58-62.

8. Kaufmann O and Dietel M, "Expression of Thyroid Transcription Factor-1 in Pulmonary and Extrapulmonary Small Cell Carcinomas and Other Neuroendocrine Carcinomas of Various Primary Sites," *Histopathology*, 2000, 36(5):415-20.

9. Ordonez NG, "Value of Thyroid Transcription Factor-1, E-Cadherin, BG8, WT1, and CD44S Immunostaining in Distinguishing Epithelial Pleural Mesothelioma From Pulmonary and Nonpulmonary Adenocarcinoma," *Am J Surg Pathol*, 2000, 24(4):598-606.

10. Wick MR, Lillemoe TJ, Copland GT, et al, "Gross Cystic Disease Fluid Protein-15 as a Marker for Breast Cancer: Immunohistochemical Analysis of 690 Human Neoplasms and Comparison With Alpha-Lactalbumin," *Hum Pathol*, 1989, 20(3):281-7.

11. Swanson PE, Pettinato G, Lillemoe TJ, et al, "Gross Cystic Disease Fluid Protein-15 in Salivary Gland Tumors," *Arch Pathol Lab Med*, 1991, 115(2):158-63.

12. Wick MR, Ockner DM, Mills SE, et al, "Homologous Carcinomas of the Breasts, Skin, and Salivary Glands. A Histologic and Immunohistochemical Comparison of Ductal Mammary Carcinoma, Ductal Sweat Gland Carcinoma, and Salivary Duct Carcinoma," *Am J Clin Pathol*, 1998, 109(1):75-84.

13. Swanson PE, Mazoujian G, Mills SE, et al, "Immunoreactivity for Estrogen Receptor Protein in Sweat Gland Tumors," *Am J Surg Pathol*, 1991, 15(9):835-41.

14. Hammond ME, Fitzgibbons PL, Compton CC, et al, "College of American Pathologists Conference XXXV: Solid Tumor Prognostic Factors - Which, How and So What? Summary Document and Recommendations for Implementation," Cancer Committee and Conference Participants, *Arch Pathol Lab Med*, 2000, 124(7):958-65.

15. Fitzgibbons PL, Page DL, Weaver D, et al, "Prognostic Factors in Breast Cancer," College of American Pathologists Consensus Statement 1999, *Arch Pathol Lab Med*, 2000, 124(7):966-78.

16. Abbondanzo SL, "Paraffin Immunohistochemistry as an Adjunct to Hematopathology," *Ann Diagn Pathol*, 1999, 3(5):318-27.

17. Ritter JH, Adesokan PN, Fitzgibbon JF, et al, "Paraffin Section Immunohistochemistry as an Adjunct to Morphologic Analysis in the Diagnosis of Cutaneous Lymphoid Infiltrates," *J Cutan Pathol*, 1994, 21(6):481-93.

18. Kurtin PJ, Hobday KS, Ziesmer S, et al, "Demonstration of Distinct Antigenic Profiles of Small B-Cell Lymphomas by Paraffin Section Immunohistochemistry," *Am J Clin Pathol*, 1999, 112(3):319-29.

19. Grogan TM, "Automated Immunohistochemical Analysis," *Am J Clin Pathol*, 1992, 98(4 Suppl 1):S35-8.

20. Grogan TM, Reinhardt K, Jaramillo M, et al, "An Update on Special Stain Histochemistry With Emphasis on Automation," *Adv Anat Pathol*, 2000, 7(2):110-22.

21. Fletcher JA, "DNA *In Situ* Hybridization as an Adjunct in Tumor Diagnosis," *Am J Clin Pathol*, 1999, 112(1 Suppl 1):S11-8.

22. Jin L and Lloyd RV, "*In Situ* Hybridization: Methods and Applications," *J Clin Lab Anal*, 1997, 11(1):2-9.

23. Capodieci P, Magi-Galluzzi C, Moreira G, et al, "Automated *In Situ* Hybridization: Diagnostic and Research Applications," *Diagn Mol Pathol*, 1998, 7(2):69-75.

References

Colvin RB, Bhan AK, and McCluskey RT, *Diagnostic Immunopathology*, 2nd ed, New York, NY: Raven Press, 1995.

De Lellis RA and Kwan P, "Technical Considerations in the Immunohistochemical Demonstration of Intermediate Filaments," *Am J Surg Pathol*, 1988, 12(Suppl 1):17-23.

Grogan TM, Casey TT, Miller PC, et al, "Automation of Immunohistochemistry," *Advances in Pathology and Laboratory Medicine*, Volume 6, St Louis, MO: CV Mosby Co, 1993, 253-83.

Nagle RB, "Intermediate Filaments: A Review of the Basic Biology," *Am J Surg Pathol*, 1988, 12(Suppl 1):4-16.

Raab SS, "The Cost-Effectiveness of Immunohistochemistry," *Arch Pathol Lab Med*, 2000, 124(8):1185-91.

Taylor CR, "The Total Test Approach to Standardization of Immunohistochemistry," *Arch Pathol Lab Med*, 2000, 124(7):945-51.

Immunophenotypic Analysis of Tissues by Flow Cytometry

Related Information

Synonyms Flow Cytometry; Fluorescence Activated Cell Sorting; Lymphocyte Immunophenotyping

Applies to B-Lymphocyte Analysis by Flow Cytometry; DNA Ploidy Studies; Kappa Light Chain Analysis by Flow Cytometry; Lambda Light Chain Analysis by Flow Cytometry; Leukemia Analysis by Flow Cytometry; Light Chain

Analysis by Flow Cytometry; Lymphocyte Analysis by Flow Cytometry; Lymphocyte Markers; Lymphoma Analysis by Flow Cytometry; Solid Tumors Analysis by Flow Cytometry; T-Lymphocyte Analysis by Flow Cytometry

Abstract Flow cytometry provides important immunophenotypic and DNA cycle information of both diagnostic and prognostic interest in hematopathology, cytopathology, and general surgical pathology.

Specimen Fresh tissues, fresh frozen tissues, body fluids; formalin-fixed paraffin-embedded tissue may be used for DNA studies

Container Fresh tissues are best submitted in a Petri dish, test tube, or jar containing saline or tissue culture media. Frozen tissue submitted for DNA ploidy studies should not be embedded in O.C.T.®

Storage Instructions Fresh tissues submitted for immunophenotypic studies are sufficiently stable to be transported by overnight courier on ice pack to a reference laboratory. Frozen tissue submitted for DNA ploidy studies should be maintained frozen during transport to a reference laboratory.

Reference Interval Flow cytometry provides immunophenotypic data and/or DNA cell cycle data, depending on the desired information and processing methodologies. More information on DNA cell cycle studies is available in the listing Cell Cycle Analysis by Flow Cytometry *on page 53.* Immunophenotypic studies are most useful in evaluation of hematologic or lymphoid tissues. Individual cell populations may be selected based on size or antigen expression to minimize preparatory steps. For example, information relating to cell size (forward light scatter) and internal complexity (90° light scatter) can be used to evaluate a population of interest. In a lymph node containing small and large lymphoid cells, independent analysis may show a reactive population of small T cells and a monoclonal population of large B cells. Flow cytometry is not well suited for evaluation of nonhematopoietic neoplasms, but lack of CD45 (leukocyte common antigen) expression on a cellular population should be regarded as suspicious for involvement by another process.

Approximately 90% of non-Hodgkin lymphomas are derived from monoclonal B cells. Characteristically, B-cell lymphomas will express pan B-cell antigens and express either kappa or lambda immunoglobulin light chains, proving clonality.[1] B-cell lymphomas never express both kappa and lambda light chains, but approximately 5% to 10% of lymphomas are surface immunoglobulin negative.[2] The presence of a significant population of surface immunoglobulin negative B cells is also substantial proof of clonality. Loss of normal pan B-cell antigen expression or acquisition of T-cell antigen expression represents phenotypic aberrancy and satisfies minor criteria for malignancy. B-cell lymphomas which coexpress the T-cell associated antigen CD5 characterize lymphomas of small lymphocytic and mantle cell lymphocytic varieties. Expression of CD10 is commonly documented in follicular lymphomas. B-cell lymphomas lacking HLA-DR expression are thought to represent a poor prognostic group.

Approximately 8% to 10% of non-Hodgkin lymphomas are derived from T cells. For these neoplasms, proof of clonality is more challenging. Clonality may be inferred by documenting abnormal pan T-cell antigen expression, abnormal T-cell subset antigen expression, or expression of thymocyte antigens.[3] For atypical T-cell lymphoproliferative disorders in which flow cytometry cannot prove clonality, use of gene rearrangement studies may be invaluable; see Gene Rearrangement for Leukemia and Lymphoma *on page 725.*

Flow cytometric studies of cases of Hodgkin disease are generally nondiagnostic. Typically, the majority of cells are reactive mature T cells with variable numbers of polyclonal B cells. This pattern cannot be distinguished from a totally benign reactive hyperplasia. Immunophenotypic verification of Hodgkin disease is best accomplished in paraffin section using an appropriate panel of antibodies correlated with morphological features of the neoplastic cells.

When considering the possibility of a neoplasm of granulocytic/monocytic precursors, expression of CD13, CD14, or CD33 is usually documented. Additionally, expression of CD45 is characteristically weaker than that typically seen in lymphoid neoplasms. Lack of reactivity for other markers of T- or B-cell lineage is also expected. A panel of commonly utilized lymphocyte markers for the evaluation of lymphoma and leukemia is listed in the table.

See also a tabular presentation of CD antigens in the Introduction to Hematology *on page 391.*

Limitations Flow cytometry is of limited use when nonlymphoid or nonhematopoietic neoplasms are evaluated. The nature of the tissue may also confer severe limitations. Generally, endoscopic biopsies are too small to extract sufficient cells for a meaningful evaluation. However, blood, bone marrow, and body fluids are readily suitable for flow cytometric studies. Tissues which are fibrotic or sclerotic, such as skin, are frequently too difficult to dissociate and extract enough viable cells for evaluation. Additionally, necrotic tissues frequently produce poor results. Finally, important diagnostic morphologic and architectural features are lost when single cell suspensions are made. Therefore, the suitability of each biopsy needs to be individually considered before tissues are allocated for special studies beyond that of conventional histopathology. Interpretation of the phenotypic profile must always be correlated with pathological features of individual cases.[4] In those cases in which flow cytometry fails to demonstrate clonality, the use of gene rearrangement studies may be helpful.

Methodology A single cell suspension is required for flow cytometric evaluation. When using tissues, cells are isolated from stromal elements by gentle mechanical dissociation.[5] Most lymphoid tissues release lymphocytes with relative ease while other tissues, such as skin, pose significant difficulties in extracting viable lymphocytes. Isolated lymphocytes are washed and viability may be enriched by density gradient centrifugation. In some specimens, overnight culture is useful to decrease nonspecific staining caused by cytophilic antibody binding mediated by immunoglobulin Fc receptors expressed by lymphoid and other inflammatory cells. However, necrotic tissues and those with high grade neoplasm often lose viable tumor cells and become enriched by reactive T cells. Therefore, discretion is necessary to optimize the preparatory aspects of tissue processing. Ultimately, the single cell suspension is stained with fluorochrome conjugated antibodies, washed, and analyzed on the flow cytometer. Panels of antibodies are utilized to quantitate the numbers of B cells, T cells, and myelomonocytic cells. B-cell clonality is assessed with immunoglobulin light chains while T-cell clonality is inferred by abnormal expression of T-cell antigens.

Footnotes

1. Huh YO and Andreeff M, "Flow Cytometry. Clinical and Research Applications in Hematologic Malignancies," *Hematol Oncol Clin North Am,* 1994, 8(4):703-23.
2. Little JV, Foucar K, Horvath A, et al, "Flow Cytometric Analysis of Lymphoma and Lymphoma-Like Conditions," *Semin Diagn Pathol,* 1989, 6(1):37-54.
3. Picker LJ, Weiss LM, Medeiros LJ, et al, "Immunophenotypic Criteria for the Diagnosis of non-Hodgkin's Lymphoma," *Am J Pathol,* 1987, 128(1):181-201.
4. Foucar K, Chen IM, and Crago S, "Organization and Operation of a Flow Cytometric Immunophenotyping Laboratory," *Semin Diagn Pathol,* 1989, 6(1):13-36.
5. Visscher DW and Crissman JD, "Dissociation of Intact Cells From Tumors and Normal Tissues," *Methods Cell Biol,* 1994, 41:1-13.

References

Coon JS and Weinstein RS, *Diagnostic Flow Cytometry,* Baltimore, MD: Lippincott Williams & Wilkins, 1991.

Finn WG, Peterson LC, James C, et al, "Enhanced Detection of Malignant Lymphoma in Cerebrospinal Fluid by Multiparameter Flow Cytometry," *Am J Clin Pathol,* 1998, 110(3):341-6.

Johnson RL, "Flow Cytometry. From Research to Clinical Laboratory Applications," *Clin Lab Med,* 1993, 13(4):831-52.

Kipps TJ, Meisenholder G, and Robbins BA, "New Developments in Flow Cytometric Analysis of Lymphocyte Markers," *Clin Lab Med,* 1992, 12(2):237-75.

Knowles DM, *Neoplastic Hematopathology,* Baltimore, MD: Lippincott Williams & Wilkins, 1992.

Risberg B, Davidson B, Dong HP, et al, "Flow Cytometric Immunophenotyping of Serous Effusions and Peritoneal Washings: Comparison With Immunocytochemistry and Morphological Findings," *J Clin Pathol,* 2000, 53(7):513-7.

(Continued)

Frequently Used Lymphocyte Differentiation Antigens for Flow Cytometry

Lineage Association	Antigenic Specificity/ Predominate Antigen Distribution
B-cell associated markers	
CD19	Pan B cell
CD20	Pan B cell
CD21	C3d and EBV receptor, resting B cell
CD10	CALLA, follicular center cells
Kappa, lambda	Mature B cells
Ig heavy chains	Mature B cells
T-cell associated antigens	
CD2	Sheep erythrocyte receptor, pan T cell
CD3	T-cell antigen receptor complex, pan T cell
CD5	Pan T cell, B-CLL, B-cell small lymphocytic lymphoma, B-cell mantle cell lymphoma
CD7	Pan T cell
CD4	Helper/inducer subset
CD8	Cytotoxic, suppressor subset
CD1	Cortical thymocyte
Myeloid/monocytic antigens	
CD13	Predominately myeloid
CD15	Predominately myeloid, Reed-Sternberg cells
CD14	Predominately monocytic
CD33	Predominately monocytic
Miscellaneous antigens	
CD11c	Predominately granulocytic/monocytic; hairy cell leukemia, some CLL
CD25	IL-2 receptor, activated T cells, hairy cell leukemia
HLA-Dr	Immune response associated antigen, most B cells, activated T cells, early granulocytic and most monocytic cells
Glycophorin A	Erythroid precursors
CDw41	GPIIb/IIIa complex, megakaryocytes

See also the table, Cluster of Differentiation (CD) Antigens, at the end of the introduction to the Hematology chapter. CD indicates cluster designations.

Immunophenotypic Analysis of Tissues by Flow Cytometry *(Continued)*

Stelzer GT, Marti G, Hurley A, et al, "U.S.-Canadian Consensus Recommendations on the Immunophenotypic Analysis of Hematologic Neoplasia by Flow Cytometry: Standardization and Validation of Laboratory Procedures," *Cytometry*, 1997, 30(5):214-30.

- ◆ **Immunostains** *see* Immunoperoxidase Procedures *on page 60*

- ◆ **In Situ Hybridization** *see* Immunoperoxidase Procedures *on page 60*

- ◆ **Intercellular Substance Antibodies** *see* Skin Biopsy, Immunofluorescence *on page 72*

- ◆ **Intermediate Filaments** *see* Immunoperoxidase Procedures *on page 60*

- ◆ **Intraoperative Consultation, Pathology** *see* Frozen Section *on page 56*

- ◆ **Iron, Hepatic** *see* Liver Biopsy *on page 65*

- ◆ **Isosulfan Blue** *see* Sentinel Lymph Node Biopsy *on page 70*

- ◆ **Jones Stain** *see* Kidney Biopsy *on page 64*

- ◆ **Kappa Light Chain Analysis by Flow Cytometry** *see* Immunophenotypic Analysis of Tissues by Flow Cytometry *on page 62*

- ◆ **Kappa Light Chains** *see* Immunoperoxidase Procedures *on page 60*

- ◆ **Ki-67** *see* Image Analysis *on page 59*

- ◆ **Ki-67** *see* Immunoperoxidase Procedures *on page 60*

Kidney Biopsy

Related Information
Antineutrophil Cytoplasmic Antibody *on page 507*
Antinuclear Antibody *on page 507*
Autosomal Dominant Polycystic Kidney Disease DNA Detection *on page 704*
Creatinine Clearance *on page 160*
Electron Microscopy *on page 54*
Fat, Urine *on page 874*
Glomerular Basement Membrane Antibody *on page 526*
Hemoglobin, Qualitative, Urine *on page 875*
Immunoperoxidase Procedures *on page 60*
Protein, Quantitative, Urine *on page 883*
Protein, Semiquantitative, Urine *on page 885*
Topoisomerase I Antibody *on page 546*
Urea Nitrogen, Serum or Plasma *on page 293*
Urinalysis *on page 887*

Synonyms Renal Biopsy

Applies to Fluorescein-Tagged Antibodies; Jones Stain; Michael's Solution; PAS Stain; Zeus Fixative

Test Includes Light microscopy: H&E, PAS, methenamine silver, trichrome, congo red, and other stains; immunofluorescent studies; electron microscopy

Abstract Renal biopsy provides evaluation of type and extent of renal disease.

Patient Preparation CBC, prothrombin time, activated thromboplastin time, and urine Gram stain are prerequisite, with appropriate imaging and sometimes with a template bleeding time.[1]

Specimen Fresh kidney tissue obtained by percutaneous needle biopsy or open surgery.

Specimen handling: The core(s) of renal tissue or a wedge obtained by open biopsy is(are) immediately placed in a Petri dish containing physiologic saline solution or sterile culture media to prevent drying. An alternative is wrapping the specimen(s) in saline-moistened gauze. The specimen(s) should be sent to the laboratory within 5-10 minutes. If the specimen(s) cannot be sent to the laboratory within this time frame, it(they) should be divided into three parts and prepared in the appropriate fixative for light microscopy, electron microscopy, and immunofluorescence. Avoid compression of the specimen. A single core may be divided:

Specimen separation: When dividing the specimen, each part must contain glomeruli. A suggested method is:

A. If an open biopsy or three or more tissue cores are obtained, one core or fragment of the wedge biopsy is submitted for immunofluorescence, one for electron microscopy, and the remainder for light microscopy.

B. If two tissue cores are obtained, one is submitted for light microscopy, and the second core is divided as follows.
- Cut four 1-2 mm fragments with a sharp razor blade. Two from each end of the core to avoid lack of cortex for ultrastructural examination.
- Submit two fragments for electron microscopy and the other two for immunofluorescence. The central portion of the core is submitted for light microscopy (see illustration).

C. If only one tissue core is obtained and it is small (<8 mm), submit it for light microscopy. If it is larger than 8 mm, divide it and submit as B. When

dividing a small biopsy, priority usually is given to: 1) light microscopy, 2) immunofluorescence, and 3) electron microscopy in this order, or at the discretion of the clinician depending on the clinical situation. A hand lens or a dissecting scope can be useful in recognizing the difference between renal cortex and medulla (glomeruli in the cortex appears as red dots, cortex is darker than medulla and is proximal within the needle used for biopsy).

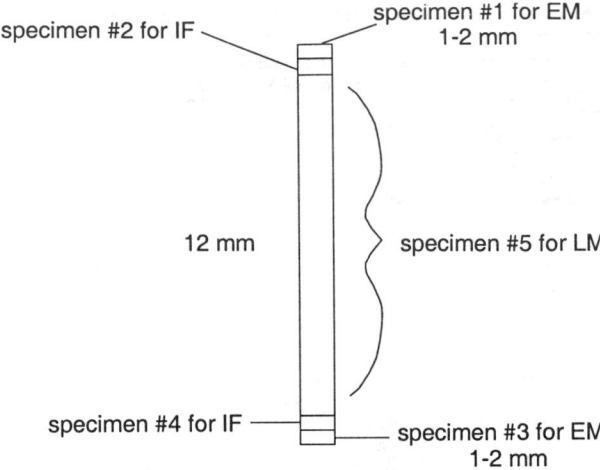

Specimen preparation: Several means of collection may be used. For immunofluorescence studies, one core or portion of a wedge (open biopsy) is placed in a foil or plastic bag, snap-frozen in liquid nitrogen or in a cryostat, shipped on dry ice to the laboratory, and stored at -76°C until processed. The frozen state must be maintained. An alternative method is to immerse the biopsy in a half-saturated ammonium sulfate buffer at room temperature. Michael's solution is used to transport the specimen to another institution. Zeus fixative is sometimes used. The tissue should not be held in this fixative for more than 5 days, preferably less. For **light microscopy**, the second core or fragment is commonly fixed in 4% formaldehyde that is 10 times the volume of the tissue, but a variety of fixatives are in use. For **electron microscopy**, the third core or fragment is fixed in 2.5% glutaraldehyde fixative.

Possible problems:
- Drying of the specimen. In order to avoid drying, place the specimen, immediately after the biopsy is obtained, in normal saline. Keep it in saline until it is frozen or placed in fixative.
- Absence of cortex. If glomeruli are not identified in the tissue, a repeat biopsy is necessary. If glomeruli are only present in the specimen submitted for immunofluorescence or electron microscopy, the remaining tissue may be cut and slides made for light microscopy.
- Too few glomeruli present in the biopsy. A minimum of 8-10 glomeruli is considered to be adequate for proper evaluation of a renal biopsy. This is particularly important in focal glomerular disease. The probability of finding abnormal glomeruli is closely related to the total number of glomeruli present. For evaluation of severity of disease, an adequate number of glomeruli is necessary.[2]

Causes for Rejection Drying of specimen due to lack of fixative

Special Instructions Adequate clinical history, differential diagnosis, and laboratory findings are essential for proper interpretation of renal biopsies and should be received with the specimen.

Use There are no absolute indications for renal biopsy. Clinical judgment is required to determine necessity of biopsy. A single disease can lead to different patterns of abnormality, and several disease entities can cause similar clinical presentations. In general, renal biopsy is useful to establish diagnosis in subjects with renal dysfunction, ascertain prognosis, evaluate disease severity and extent,[1] and guide therapy[3] in conditions which include the following:
- acute renal failure in cases in which clinical diagnosis cannot be established and/or which are unresponsive
- asymptomatic non-nephrotic progressive proteinuria
- nephrotic syndrome in adults, especially including SLE; selected diabetic patients
- nephrotic syndrome in children older than 6 years of age, and children of any age who do not respond to therapy as anticipated[4]
- acute nephritic syndrome; characteristics of acute nephritic syndrome include acute onset of hematuria with red cell casts, hypertension, edema, and proteinuria often with deteriorating renal function. Causes include postinfectious glomerulonephritis, antiglomerular basement membrane disease, membranoproliferative glomerulonephritis, IgA nephropathy, hemolytic uremic syndrome, Henoch-Schönlein purpura, SLE, and vasculitis.[1]
- hematuria of uncertain etiology, selected cases
- systemic diseases with renal involvement
- drug toxicity
- candidacy for renal transplantation in patients in chronic renal failure
- evaluation of dysfunction in recipients of renal allografts; transplantation reactions, rejection, or failure

Contraindications

- Bleeding diathesis
- Neoplasm
- Cystic disease, large cysts
- Obstructive uropathy
- Acute pyelonephritis
- Abscess
- Uncontrolled hypertension
- Anatomic abnormalities
- Pregnancy
- Chronic renal disease with very small kidneys
- Renal arterial aneurysm

This list of contraindications is more relative than absolute. In several of these situations, the patient may be considered for biopsy after receiving appropriate therapy. In some cases, an open biopsy may be performed.

Methodology Light microscopy: Specimen is embedded in paraffin, sections are cut at 2-4 microns and stained with H&E, Gomori or Masson's trichrome, PAS, and silver methenamine (Jones stain). Additional stains such as amyloid, fibrin, and so forth are occasionally needed. In the H&E and PAS stain, the basic pattern of the disease process is determined, and the extent and distribution of morphologic change is noted. Glomeruli, tubules, interstitium, and blood vessels are examined separately and any abnormality noted. The degrees of glomerular sclerosis, interstitial fibrosis, tubular atrophy, and vascular changes are quantitatively estimated. Such parameters are important in determination of the degree of activity and chronicity, severity of the renal disease, and overall prognosis. The **PAS stain** is helpful in studying glomerular and tubular basement membranes and the mesangium. PAS stain highlights hyaline and fibrinoid changes, and the presence of glomerular and arterial sclerosis (all stain red). It supports diagnoses of mesangial proliferative glomerulonephritis, focal segmental glomerulosclerosis, and diabetic nephropathy, and usually reacts with light chains.[1] The **trichrome stain** is used to determine the presence of interstitial fibrosis and glomerular and vascular sclerosis. It may show immune deposits and fibrin (the collagen stains blue; muscle, immune deposits, and fibrin stain red). The **silver stain (Jones stain)** is used especially to study glomerular and tubular basement membranes. It also brings out the mesangium and demonstrates the presence of glomerular sclerosis (all appear black). **Congo red** for amyloid is often used. **Phosphotungstic acid hematoxylin (PTAH)** is used for fibrin.

Immunofluorescence: The specimen is snap frozen and sectioned. A battery of fluorescein-tagged antibodies against different immunoglobulins and complement are used. The most commonly used are IgG, IgM, IgA, C3, C4, C1q, properdin, fibrinogen, albumin, and kappa and lambda light chains. Sections are then examined under fluorescence microscopy. Intensity, pattern, and distribution of immunoglobulins are noted. Normal renal biopsy usually shows no immunoglobulin depositions. Immunofluorescence allows for classification of renal disease, demonstrating immune complex deposition in glomerular diseases. One may ascertain the degree of immunologic activity in immune diseases, suggest systemic entities (eg, SLE) and establish certain diagnoses (eg, IgA nephropathy).

Electron microscopy (EM): The specimen is embedded in plastic. Ultra-thin sections are treated with osmium. Electron microscopy is useful for localization and quantitation of immune deposits. Abnormalities of the basement membrane, the presence of cellular inclusions, and fusion of foot processes may be detected. Survey sections 1 µm thick are stained with 1% toluidine blue. EM is necessary to establish some diagnoses (eg, Alport's syndrome, thin basement membrane nephritis, and fibrillary glomerulonephritis).

Light microscopy, immunofluorescence, and electron microscopy are complementary and necessary in most cases. EM is essential in about 25% of cases and helpful in half.[1] In patients with suspected kidney transplant rejection, light microscopy is usually sufficient.

Additional Information Complications of renal biopsy:

- Hematuria: Microscopic hematuria is a common complication seen in most patients. It resolves spontaneously. Gross hematuria is seen in 5% to 9% of the cases and is more common in patients with uncontrolled hypertension or uremia. It usually resolves spontaneously in 2-3 days. In 0.5% of the patients, hematuria will persist for 2-3 weeks, occasionally occurring a few days after the biopsy. Blood transfusions are only necessary in about 1% to 3% of the cases, and medical or surgical nephrectomy for massive or persistent bleeding is necessary in only 1 of 2000-5000 cases.
- Perinephric hematoma is not uncommon, however, only 1% to 2% of patients develop a local mass, hypotension, or diminution in hematocrit. The hematoma usually resolves within a few months.
- Arteriovenous fistula is considered frequent in arteriographic studies. Most cases are clinically silent and resolve spontaneously within 2 years.
- Flank pain may last 2-3 days and responds to pain medications.
- A large blood clot may form in the bladder, causing obstruction and requiring an indwelling catheter for a few days.
- Other complications: Postbiopsy aneurysm appears in <1% of patients. Other rare complications that have been described include infection; ileus; lacerations of the liver, spleen, pancreas, gallbladder, intestine, visceral and subcostal arteries; pancreatitis; pneumothorax; and dissemination of carcinoma. Death has occurred in 0.12% of patients.[1]

Comparison to previous biopsies is customary.

In summary, renal biopsy is relatively safe and useful in diagnosis and management of significant renal disease.

Footnotes

1. Radford MG Jr, Donadio JV Jr, Holley KE, et al, "Renal Biopsy in Clinical Practice," *Mayo Clin Proc*, 1994, 69(10):983-4.
2. Madaio MP, "Renal Biopsy," *Kidney Int*, 1990, 38(3):529-43.
3. Vidt DG, "Recognition and Management of Reversible Renal Failure," *South Med J*, 1994, 87(10):1018-27.
4. Srivastava T, Simon SD, and Alon US, "High Incidence of Focal Sequential Glomerulosclerosis in Nephrotic Syndrome of Childhood," *Pediatr Nephrol*, 1999, 13(1):13-8.

References

Alon US, "Hemorrhagic Complications of Kidney Biopsy," *Clin Pediatr (Phila)*, 1991, 30(6):391.

Espinel CH, "Diagnosis of Acute and Chronic Renal Failure," *Clin Lab Med*, 1993, 13(1):89-102.

Feneberg R, Schaeffer F, Zieger B, et al, "Percutaneous Renal Biopsy in Children: A 27-Year Experience," *Nephron*, 1998, 79(4):438-46.

Jennette JC, Olson JL, Schwartz MM, et al, *Heptinstall's Pathology of the Kidney*, Baltimore, MD: Lippincott Williams & Wilkins, 1998.

Kern W, Silva F, Laszik Z, et al, *Atlas of Renal Pathology*, Philadelphia, PA: WB Saunders Company, 1999.

Khajehdehi P, Junaid SM, Salinas-Madrigal L, et al, "Percutaneous Renal Biopsy in the 1990s: Safety, Value, and Implications for Early Hospital Discharge," *Am J Kidney Dis*, 1999, 34(1):92-7.

Menon SK and Kirchner KA, "The Role of Percutaneous Renal Biopsy in Clinical Nephrology," *Curr Opin Nephrol Hypertens*, 1993, 2(6):968-73.

Seifter JL and Nickeleit V, "A 67-Year-Old Woman With Vomiting, Bloody Diarrhea, and Azotemia," Case Records of the Massachusetts General Hospital, Case 17-1997, Scully RE, Mark EJ, McNeely WF, et al, eds, *N Engl J Med*, 1997, 336(22):1587-94.

Striker G, Striker LJ, and D'Agati V, "Major Problems in Pathology," *The Renal Biopsy*, Philadelphia, PA: WB Saunders Company, 1997.

Internet Web Sites

www.ajkd.org
www.kidneyatlas.org

- ◆ **Lambda Light Chain Analysis by Flow Cytometry** *see* Immunophenotypic Analysis of Tissues by Flow Cytometry *on page 62*
- ◆ **Lambda Light Chains** *see* Immunoperoxidase Procedures *on page 60*
- ◆ **LE Antibodies** *see* Skin Biopsy, Immunofluorescence *on page 72*
- ◆ **Lectins** *see* Immunoperoxidase Procedures *on page 60*
- ◆ **Leukemia** *see* Lymph Node Biopsy *on page 67*
- ◆ **Leukemia Analysis by Flow Cytometry** *see* Immunophenotypic Analysis of Tissues by Flow Cytometry *on page 62*
- ◆ **Leukocyte Common Antigen** *see* Immunoperoxidase Procedures *on page 60*
- ◆ **Leu M1** *see* Immunoperoxidase Procedures *on page 60*
- ◆ **Light Chain Analysis by Flow Cytometry** *see* Immunophenotypic Analysis of Tissues by Flow Cytometry *on page 62*
- ◆ **Light Chains** *see* Immunoperoxidase Procedures *on page 60*

Liver Biopsy

Related Information

Acetaminophen, Serum *on page 778*
Alanine Aminotransferase, Serum *on page 87*
Albumin, Serum *on page 88*
Alkaline Phosphatase, Serum *on page 93*
Alpha$_1$-Antitrypsin Phenotyping *on page 95*
Alpha$_1$-Fetoprotein, Serum *on page 97*
Amiodarone, Serum *on page 735*
Antimitochondrial Antibody *on page 505*
Antinuclear Antibody *on page 507*
Aspartate Aminotransferase, Serum *on page 112*
Bilirubin, Total, Serum *on page 118*
Ceruloplasmin, Serum *on page 143*
Copper, Serum *on page 816*
Copper, Urine *on page 818*
Electron Microscopy *on page 54*
Ethanol, Blood, Urine, and Other Sources *on page 789*
Ferritin, Serum *on page 173*
Fine Needle Aspiration Culture *on page 609*
Fine Needle Aspiration, Deep Masses *on page 381*
Gamma-Glutamyl Transferase, Serum *on page 179*
Hepatitis B Core Antibody *on page 622*
Hepatitis B$_e$ Antigen *on page 624*
Hepatitis B Surface Antibody *on page 625*
Hepatitis B Surface Antigen *on page 625*
Hepatitis C Virus RNA Detection and Quantitation *on page 626*
Hepatitis C Virus Serology *on page 627*
Hepatitis: Laboratory Assessment, Overview *on page 629*
Hereditary Hemochromatosis DNA Test *on page 709*
(Continued)

Liver Biopsy (Continued)

Synonyms Needle Biopsy of Liver

Applies to Copper, Hepatic; Hepatic Iron Index; Iron, Hepatic; Toxic Reactions, Liver; Transjugular Needle Biopsy of Liver

Test Includes Needle biopsies of the liver may be acquired by percutaneous or transjugular routes. Investigation includes light microscopy, commonly with a number of special stains. Immunohistochemistry is often helpful. Electron microscopy is occasionally needed. In situ hybridization techniques may be helpful. Liver concentrations of copper or iron can be provided for evaluation of Wilson disease or hemochromatosis, respectively. Microbiologic culture may be required.

Abstract Liver biopsy is often needed in patients who have persistent/unexplained abnormalities of liver function tests. Liver biopsy remains a vital diagnostic modality. Its interpretation commonly requires, and is supported by, clinical laboratory investigation. Results of history, physical examination, clinical evaluation, and testing must be provided to the histopathologist who works up and holds responsibility for interpretation of the liver biopsy. Liver biopsy is a valuable and time-honored means for diagnosis of diffuse liver parenchymal disease as well as disseminated focal disease.

Patient Preparation Procedures and risks of the procedure are explained and consent is required. All aspirin products and nonsteroidal agents must be discontinued at least 7 days beforehand. If taking oral anticoagulants (Coumadin®), hospitalization is required to convert to heparin therapy before biopsy. Screening laboratory studies ordered 24-48 hours in advance commonly include CBC (with platelet count), PT/PTT, BUN, bleeding time, type and screen or type and crossmatch for possible transfusion, additional to careful history and physical examination. Patients with diffuse liver disease and at significant risk for bleeding complications may be candidates for transjugular needle biopsy. See table in listing Bilirubin, Total, Serum on page 118 and diagrams in listings Alkaline Phosphatase, Serum on page 93 and Aspartate Aminotransferase, Serum on page 112. Electrolytes are usually optional. If pneumonia or pleural effusion is suspected, PA and lateral chest x-ray is obtained.

Aftercare In general, patient is monitored in a recovery area with frequent vital signs postbiopsy. If hypotension, tachycardia, fever, rigidity of abdomen, or uncontrolled pain occurs, physician should be notified immediately and an intravenous line placed. Some physicians recheck hematocrit 24 hours after the procedure.

Specimen At least two to three liver cores, each >2 cm in length are desirable.

Collection Tissue fixation for light microscopy: specimen is usually fixed in 10% buffered formalin within 1 minute; alternatives include Zenker's fluid or a Zenker modification. A specimen from subjects with cystinosis should be separately alcohol-fixed and so labeled. For transmission electron microscopy, 1 mm cubes of specimen are fixed immediately in glutaraldehyde, but EM is not often needed. Management of specimens for evaluation for Wilson disease has been published. Copper concentrations can be assayed.[1]

Use This procedure, by nature, is invasive. In most cases, noninvasive imaging studies such as CT scan or ultrasound are obtained first. **Indications for liver biopsy include:**

- persistent elevations of AST and ALT concentrations to > twice the upper limits of reference range, abnormalities of other liver-related chemistry assays
- chronic hepatitis, with or without cirrhosis, to identify cases of autoimmune hepatitis, and the entities included in its differential diagnosis; evaluation of nonalcoholic steatohepatitis (NASH); grading and staging of disease severity (eg, chronic hepatitis B,C). Patients with positive results for hepatitis B virus DNA and hepatitis B$_e$ antigen should be considered for liver biopsy. Chronic hepatitis is itself defined as a necroinflammatory disease lasting longer than 6 months.
- suspected cases of hepatic cirrhosis, to confirm and grade the diagnosis and, if possible, establish etiology (eg, chronic hepatitis C infection, alcohol, alpha$_1$-antitrypsin deficiency, primary biliary cirrhosis vs primary sclerosing cholangitis); assess and stage level of activity; assess complications
- liver biopsy is essential in diagnosis of hemochromatosis and Wilson disease; quantitative estimation of iron and copper respectively
- portal hypertension
- cholestasis of unknown etiology in which other studies of biliary obstruction are negative; liver biopsy, needed for staging of primary biliary cirrhosis and primary sclerosing cholangitis, is unnecessary in extrahepatic cholestasis
- instances of disorders of bilirubin metabolism (eg, Dubin-Johnson syndrome)
- selected cases of fever of unknown origin (eg, tuberculosis, brucellosis); a portion of biopsy can be cultured for appropriate organisms[2]

- suspected liver disease in the known alcoholic patient, to confirm alcoholic liver disease, exclude alternative causes of liver disease, stage and assess disease activity
- diagnosis of benign and malignant tumors (eg, hepatoma, metastatic neoplasms)
- recognition and staging of lymphoma
- suspected multisystem and/or infiltrative disease with liver involvement in which other diagnostic techniques have not been fruitful (eg, sarcoidosis, amyloidosis, tuberculosis, glycogen storage disease)
- unexplained hepatomegaly
- selected cases of hepatitis of unknown etiology, in order to try to differentiate viral from drug-induced etiologies (not always possible) or to assess complications, such as cholestasis; differential diagnosis of drug-induced hepatic disease;[3,4] see tables.

Table 1. Types of Toxic Reactions Occurring in the Liver

Type of Reaction	Examples of Agents
Direct reaction	Acetaminophen, carbon tetrachloride, mushrooms, phosphorus
Idiosyncratic reaction	Isoniazid, disulfiram, propylthiouracil*
Toxic-allergic reaction	Halothane, isoflurane, ticrynafen
Allergic hepatitis	Phenytoin, amoxicillin-clavulanic acid, sulfonamides
Cholestatic reaction	Chlorpromazine, erythromycin estolate, estradiol, captopril, sulfonamides
Granulomatous reaction	Diltiazem, quinidine, phenytoin, procainamide
Chronic hepatitis	Nitrofurantoin, methyldopa, isoniazid, trazodone
Alcoholic hepatitis-like reaction	Amiodarone, perhexiline maleate, valproic acid
Microvesicular steatosis	Tetracyclines, aspirin, zidovudine, didanosine, fialuridine
Fibrosis or cirrhosis alone	Methotrexate, vitamin A, methyldopa
Veno-occlusive disease	Cyclophosphamide, other chemotherapeutic agents, herbal teas
Ischemic damage	Cocaine, sustained-release nicotinic acid, methylenedioxyamphetamine

*There are hundreds of other agents that can cause idiosyncratic reactions.

Adapted from Lee WM, "Drug-Induced Hepatotoxicity," N Engl J Med, 1995, 333(17):1121.

Table 2. Relative Degree of Increase of Aminotransferases in Toxic Hepatic Injury

Toxicant	Lesion		Degree of Increase in Serum Enzyme Levels	
	Zonal Necrosis	Steatosis	AST	ALT
CCl$_4$	+	+	4+	3+
Thioacetamide	+	−	4+	3+
Tetracycline	−	+	2	+
Ethionine	−	+	+	−
Phosphorous	±	+	1-2+	1-2+

ALT = alanine aminotransferase; AST = aspartate aminotransferase; CCl$_4$ = carbon tetrachloride; 4+ refers to relative degree of increase.

Modified from Zimmerman HJ, Hepatotoxicity: The Adverse Effects of Drugs and Other Chemicals on the Liver, 2nd ed, Philadelphia, PA: Lippincott Williams and Wilkins, 1999.

- acute hepatitis without explained etiology; in protracted cases
- infectious disease (eg, Q fever); extrapulmonary P. carinii infection is reported in liver and spleen in immunocompromised individuals[5]
- evaluation of efficacy of or adverse response to treatment (eg, patients on methotrexate)
- following bone marrow or liver transplantation
- investigate inborn error of metabolism (eg, Wilson disease, α$_1$-antitrypsin deficiency, glycogen storage disease, Gaucher disease, other storage diseases)
- instances of certain vascular abnormalities (eg, veno-occlusive disease)

Liver biopsy is less useful in:
- acute hepatitis A or B infection, unless the diagnosis is in question
- extrahepatic biliary obstruction in which percutaneous transhepatic cholangiography and endoscopic retrograde cholangiopancreatography (ERCP) are considered first-line procedures
- fluid-filled liver cysts (with the exception of echinococcal cysts) detected on ultrasound or CT scan, probably more amenable to guided thin needle aspiration first

Limitations Mahal et al (1979) noted that failure to heed accepted contraindications led directly to 22 bleeding episodes in 3800 percutaneous liver biopsies.[6]

Contraindications to percutaneous liver biopsy include:

- if AST and ALT are not > twice the upper limit of reference range and a chronic liver disease has not been found, observation may be the best course.
- impaired hemostasis, accepted as prothrombin time more than 3 seconds over control, PTT more than 20 seconds over control, thrombocytopenia <50,000/mm^3, or markedly prolonged bleeding time (≥10 minutes)
- history of bleeding which has gone without diagnosis
- severe anemia (Hb <9.5 g/dL)
- local infection near needle entry site, such as right-sided empyema, right lower lobe pneumonia, right subphrenic abscess, local cellulitis, infected ascites or peritonitis
- tense ascites (low yield technically, risk of leakage)
- high-grade extrahepatic biliary obstruction with jaundice (increased risk of bile peritonitis)
- septic cholangitis
- possible hemangioma, other vascular tumors
- possible echinococcal (hydatid) cyst
- lack of adequate facilities for blood transfusion, lack of appropriate blood
- uncooperative patient
- liver biopsy is more hazardous when performed on outpatients who have cirrhosis or neoplasms, since these are the categories associated with mortality (from hemoperitoneum)
- relative contraindications include morbid obesity, hemophilia

Complications: Significant morbidity has been estimated at 1%. Fatality rate of up to 0.1% is recognized with thick needle biopsy. More commonly seen complications include:

- pain
- hemorrhage - minor episodes are common. Significant hemorrhage is infrequent but is the most common cause of death from liver biopsy. Several series have estimated an incidence of ~0.2%, but Sherlock (1984) reported 40 patients out of 6379 who required transfusion for intraperitoneal bleeding. Specific sites include the abdominal cavity (hemoperitoneum), liver capsule (capsular hematoma), liver parenchyma (intrahepatic hematoma), biliary tree (hemobilia), or into the pleural space. Postulated risk factors include cirrhosis, coagulopathy, amyloid liver, hepatocellular injury, hemangioma and vascularized tumor. However, bleeding may be massive even when no risk factors are present.
- bile leakage with peritonitis - associated with severe obstruction of the larger bile ducts.
- laceration of internal organs and viscera - right kidney, gallbladder, colon, pancreas, and others
- others: right-sided pneumothorax, bacteremia, sepsis, arteriovenous fistula, drug toxicity

Contraindications Frozen section is usually contraindicated for needle biopsy material except for recognition of tumor in the course of open surgical procedures.

Methodology Several biopsy needles are available: Menghini needle, "Trucut" needle, Vim-Silverman needle.

- Tissue stains including: **H&E** for general histopathology; **reticulin** preparation; **Masson's trichrome** - fibrosis, cirrhosis in concert with a reticulin preparation; **pentachrome** may be helpful; **iron stain** (eg, Perls' stain) - useful for hemosiderosis, hemochromatosis, and to distinguish these from hemofuchsin and bile pigments; **PAS stain** with and without diastase - useful for alpha$_1$-antitrypsin globules, bile ducts; **orcein** - for hepatitis B surface antigen; stains for amyloid and various stains for organisms; other stains occasionally needed as well. Immunohistochemistry is sometimes needed (eg, CEA).
- Cytologic preparation - fluid from aspirating syringe may be smeared on clean microscope slide, fixed, and sent to Cytology Laboratory
- Microbiological culture - send specimen without fixative in sterile container. Special stains (AFB, KOH, etc) and cultures (tuberculosis, viral, Brucella, parasites, fungi) as needed. See Bacterial Culture, Abscess on page 562;[2] Entamoeba histolytica Serology on page 605;[1] Bacterial Culture, Biopsy or Body Fluid on page 565; Fungal Culture, Biopsy or Body Fluid on page 610; Mycobacterial Culture, Biopsy or Body Fluid on page 655. Liver biopsies are most likely to contain acid-fast organisms in HIV-positive subjects when the patient is febrile, AIDS is longstanding and serum alkaline phosphatase is very high.[7]
- Hepatic copper is assayed by graphite furnace atomic absorption spectrometry or neutron activation.[8]

Additional Information Although **fine needle aspiration** is useful for the diagnosis of carcinoma, it is not usually adequate for evaluation of other hepatic disease entities. Fine needle aspiration is used to confirm malignant tumors with less morbidity and mortality than is encountered with thick needle biopsies. Guided (by imaging techniques) biopsies bear increased diagnostic yield both for thick and thin needle aspirations.

In Wilson disease, **tissue copper** values are >250 µg/g (4 µmol/g) dry weight, while in other entities characterized by increased copper (chronic cholestatic liver diseases including primary biliary cirrhosis and primary sclerosing cholangitis) liver copper concentration is <80 µg/g (1.26 µmol/g) dry weight. Normal range is reported as 20-50 µg/g.[8] The only other entity with very high copper levels, Indian childhood cirrhosis, is extremely rare in

the U.S. If copper levels are needed, specific paraffins are required to embed the needle biopsy.[1] See Copper, Serum on page 816; Copper, Urine on page 818; and Ceruloplasmin, Serum on page 143.

The hepatic **iron index** is the ratio of liver concentration of iron to patient age:

hepatic iron (µg/g dry weight) / 56 x age of patient

A result >2.0 is diagnostic of genetic **hemochromatosis**.[9]

Footnotes

1. Ludwig J, Moyer TP, and Rakela J, "The Liver Biopsy Diagnosis of Wilson's Disease. Methods in Pathology," Am J Clin Pathol, 1994, 102(4):443-6.
2. Pitt HA, "Surgical Management of Hepatic Abscesses," World J Surg, 1990, 14(4):498-504.
3. Lee WM, "Drug-Induced Hepatotoxicity," N Engl J Med, 1995, 333(17):1118-27.
4. Zimmerman HJ, Hepatotoxicity: The Adverse Effects of Drugs and Other Chemicals on the Liver, 2nd ed, Baltimore, MD: Lippincott Williams & Wilkins, 1999.
5. "A 29-Year-Old Man With AIDS and Multiple Splenic Abscesses," Case Records of the Massachusetts General Hospital, Case 3-1995, Scully RE, Mark EJ, McNeely WF, et al, eds, N Engl J Med, 1995, 332(4):249-57.
6. Mahal AS, Knauer CM, and Gregory PB, "Bleeding After Liver Biopsy," West J Med, 1981, 134(1):11-4.
7. Christie JD and Callihan DR, "The Laboratory Diagnosis of Mycobacterial Diseases. Challenges and Common Sense," Clin Lab Med, 1995, 15(2):279-306.
8. Gahl WA, "Wilson Disease," Cecil Textbook of Medicine, 21st ed, Goldman L and Bennett JC, eds, Philadelphia, PA: WB Saunders Co, 2000, 1130-32.
9. Kamath PS, "Clinical Approach to the Patient With Abnormal Liver Test Results," Mayo Clin Proc, 1996, 71(11):1089-95.

References

"A 68-Year-Old Woman With Hepatic Encephalopathy," Case Records of the Massachusetts General Hospital, Case 10-1997, Scully RE, Mark EJ, McNeely WF, et al, eds, N Engl J Med, 1997, 336(13):939-47.

Bird GL, "Investigation of Alcoholic Liver Disease," Baillieres Clin Gastroenterol, 1993, 7(3):663-82.

Bravo AA, Sheth SG, and Chopra S, "Liver Biopsy," N Engl J Med, 2001, 344(7):495-500.

Burgart LJ, Batts KP, Ludwig J, et al, "Recent-Onset Autoimmune Hepatitis. Biopsy Findings and Clinical Correlations," Am J Surg Pathol, 1995, 19(6):699-708.

Ferrell L, "Liver Pathology: Cirrhosis, Hepatitis, and Primary Liver Tumors. Update and Diagnostic Problems," Mod Pathol, 2000, 13(6):679-704.

Froehlich F, Lamy O, Fried M, et al, "Practice and Complications of Liver Biopsy. Results of a Nationwide Survey in Switzerland," Dig Dis Sci, 1993, 38(8):1480-4.

Iezzoni JC, Gaffey MJ, Stacy EK, et al, "Hepatocytic Globules in End-Stage Hepatic Disease," Am J Clin Pathol, 1997, 107(6):692-7.

Ishak KG, "Pathologic Features of Chronic Hepatitis: A Review and Update," Am J Clin Pathol, 2000, 113(1):40-55.

James O and Day C, "Nonalcoholic Steatohepatitis; Another Disease of Affluence," Lancet, 1999, 353(9165):1634-6.

John TG and Garden OJ, "Needle Track Seeding of Primary and Secondary Liver Carcinoma After Percutaneous Liver Biopsy," HPB Surg, 1993, 6(3):199-204.

McGill DB, Rakela J, Zinsmeister AR, et al, "A 21-Year Experience With Major Hemorrhage After Percutaneous Liver Biopsy," Gastroenterology, 1990, 99(5):1396-400.

Perrault J, McGill DB, Ott BJ, et al, "Liver Biopsy: Complications in 1000 Inpatients and Outpatients," Gastroenterology, 1978, 78(1):103-6.

Piccinino F, Sagnelli E, Pasquale G, et al, "Complications Following Percutaneous Liver Biopsy," J Hepatol, 1986, 2(2):165-73.

Pratt DS and Kaplan MM, "Evaluation of Abnormal Liver-Enzyme Results in Asymptomatic Patients," N Engl J Med, 2000, 342(17):1266-71.

Van Thiel DH, Gavaler JS, Wright H, et al, "Liver Biopsy. Its Safety and Complications as Seen at a Liver Transplant Center," Transplantation, 1993, 55(5):1087-90.

Zamcheck N and Klausenstock O, "Liver Biopsy. II. The Risk of Needle Biopsy," N Engl J Med, 1953, 249(26):1062-3.

Zucker SD and Flieder A, "A 23-Year-Old Man With Fulminant Hepatorenal Failure of Uncertain Cause," Case Records of the Massachusetts General Hospital, Case 1-1997, Scully RE, Mark EJ, McNeely WF, et al, eds, N Engl J Med, 1997, 336(2):118-25 (published erratum appears in N Engl J Med, 1997, 336(7):523).

♦ **Lumpectomy** see Breast Biopsy on page 51

♦ **Lung Biopsy** see Histopathology on page 59

♦ **Lupus Band Test** see Skin Biopsy on page 71

♦ **Lupus Band Test** see Skin Biopsy, Immunofluorescence on page 72

Lymph Node Biopsy

Related Information

Bone Marrow on page 410
Buffy Coat Smear Study of Peripheral Blood on page 412
Carbamazepine, Serum on page 741
Chromosome Analysis, Blood on page 361
Chromosome Analysis, Bone Marrow on page 362
Chromosome Analysis, Lymph Node and Solid Tumor on page 364
Complete Blood Count on page 419
Epstein-Barr Virus Culture on page 607
Fluorescence In Situ Hybridization on page 367
Frozen Section on page 56
Gene Rearrangement for Leukemia and Lymphoma on page 725
Gold, Serum on page 751
Histopathology on page 59
Immunofixation Electrophoresis, Serum or Urine on page 530
Immunoperoxidase Procedures on page 60
(Continued)

Lymph Node Biopsy *(Continued)*

Applies to Hodgkin Disease; Leukemia; non-Hodgkin Lymphoma

Test Includes Histopathology, frozen section, imprint cytology, immunoperoxidase procedures, flow cytometry, cytogenetics, molecular genetics

Abstract Lymph nodes are commonly involved in a variety of infectious, inflammatory, neoplastic, and other infiltrative disorders and are commonly biopsied to establish a diagnosis. The diagnosis of lymphoma and related disorders necessitates special processing to optimize diagnostic studies.

Specimen Lymph node or other tissues suspected of harboring lymphoma, ideally submitted fresh within minutes of the biopsy

Container Petri dish with sterile saline-moistened gauze

Collection Indications for lymph node biopsy have been recently reviewed.[1] Important clinical considerations include age, location, duration, and associated manifestations. Larger nodes are more likely diagnostic than smaller ones, especially if smaller ones are superficial to deeper large nodes. Needle aspiration and biopsy can yield diagnostic information but is suboptimal for initial lymphoma classification. Excisional biopsy is preferred.

Initial triage can usually be confidently directed by imprint cytology. If a frozen section evaluation is necessary to initiate a "lymphoma protocol", the tissues used for this rapid diagnosis are often unsuitable for immunophenotypic analysis. If the size of biopsy is limiting, a routine frozen section evaluation should be discouraged as freezing distorts lymphoid tissue and may result in errors in final interpretation.

Ideally, sufficient tissue must be available for both permanent sections and snap frozen for possible immunophenotypic analysis. Flow cytometry is ideally suited for characterization of most lymphomas, particularly small cell variants. Tissues should also be snap frozen for possible frozen section immunohistochemistry. Snap freezing small, thin slices of tissue using liquid nitrogen-cooled isopentane yields tissues free of freezing artifacts. Frozen tissues are also suitable for genotypic studies if necessary. If tissues are to be sent to a reference laboratory for immunotyping, three basic options are available. First, the tissues may be snap frozen and stored at -70°C or colder until such time as immunotyping is considered necessary. If facilities for proper snap freezing and storage are not available, this option should be discouraged. Second, the tissues may be delivered in carrier media or saline-soaked gauze on ice immediately by courier to the reference laboratory, where experienced personnel will process the tissue. Third, tissues may be placed in a carrier media that may circumvent the need for immediate action for 24 hours without significantly compromising the immunologic studies. Primary and reference laboratories should establish a standing agreement upon such options.

Routine histopathologic study remains the gold standard in diagnostic hematopathology and optimal histology begins with prompt and proper fixation. Fine nuclear detail is best achieved using B5, zinc formalin, or a Zenker-like fixative. These fixatives are also best for cell marker analysis in paraffin section. Deficient basic histology is a common cause of interpretive error in hematopathology.[2]

Storage Instructions Snap frozen tissues should be maintained at -70°C or colder until immunophenotypic analysis can be performed. If frozen tissues are to be transported to a reference laboratory, they should be shipped on dry ice, using an overnight courier if necessary. Tissues placed in carrier media should be maintained on wet ice or at room temperature and packaged in insulated containers to avoid large fluctuations in temperature, if sent to a reference laboratory.

Causes for Rejection Desiccated specimen, formalin exposure, excessive freezing artifact

Special Instructions Lymph node biopsies should be immediately delivered to the Histology Laboratory uncut in a small sterile jar or Petri dish. The specimen should not be placed in fixative if it can be delivered immediately to the laboratory. All such specimens should be brought to the immediate attention of a pathologist.

Use Diagnose various lymphadenopathies, including malignant lymphoma and metastatic neoplasia

Limitations Formalin-fixed tissue cannot be used for culture or imprints and is suboptimal for electron microscopy. Classification of lymphoma is complicated by small sample size. Drug reactions may cause confusion with other entities.

Additional Information A multiparameter approach is essential in the accurate diagnosis and classification of lymphoid and hematopoietic neoplasms.[3] Previous lymphoma classification schemes have relied exclusively on morphologic features. Since 1995, criteria set forth in the Revised European American Lymphoma classification have emphasized the need for immunophenotypic and genetic studies.[4] This approach has been validated in the proposed WHO classification and extended to include myeloid malignancies.[5]

At times, sufficient fresh tissue may not be available for flow cytometric studies or frozen section immunohistochemistry. However, an ever-expanding selection of antibodies is useful for establishing lineage of hematopoietic cells in paraffin section. Recent studies have documented the utility of these markers in the paraffin section evaluation of small B-cell lymphoid malignancies.[6,7,8] T-cell malignancies,[9,10] Hodgkin disease,[11,12] and blastic hematopoietic neoplasms.[13,14] Nonetheless, phenotypic indicators of clonal proliferation are most reliably established by flow cytometry or frozen section immunohistochemistry. As molecular techniques continue to improve, reliance on fresh or frozen tissue will continue to wan.[15,16,17]

Footnotes

1. Habermann TM and Steensma DP, "Lymphadenopathy," *Mayo Clin Proc*, 2000, 75(7):723-32.
2. Warnke RA and Rouse RV, "Limitations Encountered in the Application of Tissue Section Immunodiagnosis to the Study of Lymphomas and Related Disorders," *Hum Pathol*, 1985, 16(4):326-31.
3. Jaffe ES, "Hematopathology: Integration of Morphologic Features and Biologic Markers for Diagnosis," *Mod Pathol*, 1999, 12(2):109-15.
4. Chan JK, Banks PM, Cleary ML, et al, "A Revised European-American Classification of Lymphoid Neoplasms Proposed by the International Lymphoma Study Group. A Summary Version," *Am J Clin Pathol*, 1995, 103(5):543-60.
5. Harris NL, Jaffe ES, Diebold J, et al, "The World Health Organization Classification of Hematological Malignancies Report of the Clinical Advisory Committee Meeting, Airlie House, Virginia, November 1997," *Mod Pathol*, 2000, 13(2):193-207.
6. Kurtin PJ, Hobday KS, Ziesmer S, et al, "Demonstration of Distinct Antigenic Profiles of Small B-Cell Lymphomas by Paraffin Section Immunohistochemistry," *Am J Clin Pathol*, 1999, 112(3):319-29.
7. Chen CC, Raikow RB, Sonmez-Alpan E, et al, "Classification of Small B-Cell Lymphoid Neoplasms Using a Paraffin Section Immunohistochemical Panel," *Appl Immunohistochem Molecul Morphol*, 2000, 8(1):1-11.
8. de Leon ED, Alkan S, Huang JC, et al, "Usefulness of an Immunohistochemical Panel in Paraffin-Embedded Tissues for the Differentiation of B-Cell non-Hodgkin's Lymphomas of Small Lymphocytes," *Mod Pathol*, 1998, 11(11):1046-51.
9. Izban KF, Hsi Ed, and Alkan S, "Immunohistochemical Analysis of Mycosis Fungoides on Paraffin-Embedded Tissue Sections," *Mod Pathol*, 1998, 11(10):978-82.
10. Kurtin PJ and Roche PC, "Immunoperoxidase Staining of non-Hodgkin's Lymphomas for T-Cell Lineage Associated Antigens in Paraffin Sections. Comparison of the Performance Characteristics of Four Commercially Available Antibody Preparations," *Am J Surg Pathol*, 1993, 17(9):898-904.
11. Abbondanzo SL, "Paraffin Immunohistochemistry as an Adjunct to Hematopathology," *Ann Diagn Pathol*, 1999, 3(5):318-27.
12. Rudiger T, Ott G, Ott MM, et al, "Differential Diagnosis Between Classic Hodgkin's Lymphoma, T-Cell-Rich B-Cell Lymphoma, and Paragranuloma by Paraffin Immunohistochemistry," *Am J Surg Pathol*, 1998, 22(10):1184-91.
13. Ritter JH, Goldstein NS, Argenyi Z, et al, "Granulocytic Sarcoma: An Immunohistologic Comparison With Peripheral T-Cell Lymphoma in Paraffin Sections," *J Cutan Pathol*, 1994, 21(3):207-16.
14. Soslow RA, Bhargava V, and Warnke RA, "MIC2, TdT, bcl-2, and CD34 Expression in Paraffin-Embedded High-Grade Lymphoma/Acute Lymphoblastic Leukemia Distinguishes Between Distinct Clinicopathologic Entities," *Hum Pathol*, 1997, 28(10):1158-65.
15. Lim LC, Segal GH, and Wittwer CT, "Detection of bcl-1 Gene Rearrangement and B-Cell Clonality in Mantle Cell Lymphoma Using Formalin-Fixed, Paraffin-Embedded Tissues," *Am J Clin Pathol*, 1995, 104(6):689-95.
16. El-Zimaity HM, El-Zaatari FA, Dore MP, et al, "The Differential Diagnosis of Early Gastric Mucosa-Associated Lymphoma: Polymerase Chain Reaction and Paraffin Section Immunophenotyping," *Mod Pathol*, 1999, 12(9):885-93.
17. Cataldo KA, Jalal SM, Law ME, et al, "Detection of t(2;5) in Anaplastic Large Cell Lymphoma: Comparison of Immunohistochemical Studies, FISH, and RT-PCR in Paraffin-Embedded Tissue," *Am J Surg Pathol*, 1999, 23(11):1386-92.

References

Jaffe ES, "Surgical Pathology of the Lymph Nodes and Related Organs," *Major Problems in Pathology*, Volume 16, Philadelphia, PA: WB Saunders Co, 1995.
Knowles DM, *Neoplastic Hematopathology*, Baltimore, MD: Lippincott Williams & Wilkins, 1992.
Warnke RA, Weiss LM, Chan JKC, et al, "Tumors of the Lymph Nodes and Spleen," *Atlas of Tumor Pathology*, 3rd Series, Fascicle 14, Washington, DC: Armed Forces Institute of Pathology, 1995.

♦ **Lymph Node Mapping** *see* Sentinel Lymph Node Biopsy *on page 70*

♦ **Lymphocyte Analysis by Flow Cytometry** *see* Immunophenotypic Analysis of Tissues by Flow Cytometry *on page 62*

♦ **Lymphocyte Immunophenotyping** *see* Immunophenotypic Analysis of Tissues by Flow Cytometry *on page 62*

♦ **Lymphocyte Markers** *see* Immunophenotypic Analysis of Tissues by Flow Cytometry *on page 62*

♦ **Lymphoma Analysis by Flow Cytometry** *see* Immunophenotypic Analysis of Tissues by Flow Cytometry *on page 62*

♦ **Lymphoscintigraphy** *see* Sentinel Lymph Node Biopsy *on page 70*

♦ **Lysozyme** *see* Immunoperoxidase Procedures *on page 60*

♦ **MART-1** *see* Sentinel Lymph Node Biopsy *on page 70*

♦ **Medical Examiner's Case** *see* Autopsy *on page 50*

♦ **Medical Legal Specimens** *see* Histopathology *on page 59*

♦ **MIB-1** *see* Immunoperoxidase Procedures *on page 60*

♦ **Michael's Solution** *see* Kidney Biopsy *on page 64*

♦ **Monoclonal Immunoglobulins** *see* Immunoperoxidase Procedures *on page 60*

Muscle Biopsy

Related Information
Aldolase, Plasma or Serum *on page 89*
Cerebrospinal Fluid Analysis: Overview *on page 416*
Creatine Kinase, Serum *on page 158*
Duchenne/Becker Muscular Dystrophy DNA Detection *on page 706*
Electron Microscopy *on page 54*
Histopathology *on page 59*
Inherited Diseases of Metabolism and Cell Structure *on page 449*
Jo-1 Antibody *on page 538*
Mucopolysaccharides, Urine *on page 226*
Myoglobin, Blood, Serum, or Plasma *on page 228*
Myoglobin, Qualitative, Urine *on page 880*
Myotonic Dystrophy DNA Test *on page 712*
Potassium, Serum or Plasma *on page 258*
Thyroid Stimulating Hormone, Serum *on page 282*
Trichinosis Serology *on page 684*

Synonyms Skeletal Muscle Biopsy

Applies to Dystrophin

Abstract Diagnosis and classification of muscle disease includes medical history, examination, laboratory assessment, electromyogram with nerve conduction studies, and muscle biopsy. The most important and specific diagnostic procedure for study of muscle is the muscle biopsy.[1]

Patient Preparation Clinical data is required and should include the patient's age and sex; the pattern, severity, duration, and tempo of the muscle involvement; relevant laboratory results (eg, aldolase, creatine kinase, lactate dehydrogenase, LDH isoenzymes, aspartate aminotransferase, erythrocyte sedimentation rate, antinuclear antibodies, and rheumatoid factor); nerve conduction and electromyographic (EMG) findings; and the presence of significant related conditions (ie, dermatitis, neoplasm, AIDS); all current medications, and particularly any exposure to corticosteroids during the previous 3 months; and the site of muscle biopsy. Family history may be essential.

Specimen Most pathologists who undertake muscle biopsies have specific protocols which should be followed.

Sampling Time The biopsy should be performed early in the day as the specimen will immediately require special handling and should arrive when histotechnical personnel are available. The requisition should provide a brief clinical history, pertinent laboratory findings, and the location of the biopsy site.

Collection Selection of muscle biopsy site: The site for muscle biopsy should be one that bears well characterized features (ie, quadriceps femoris or biceps brachii (preferred) or gastrocnemius).[2] Unusual muscle groups such as oculomotor or pharyngeal muscles should be avoided, as they have several unique and potentially confusing features. Biopsy should be from an accessible muscle that is involved by the disease but has not reached "end-stage" atrophy. If more distal muscles are involved, a more distal biopsy site may be required. EMG or injection sites and sites near the myotendinous junction should be avoided, as these biopsies commonly exhibit artifactual changes. It is the muscle belly that should be sampled, not the tendon insertion. Needle biopsies of muscle provide inferior specimens.[1]

Surgical technique: Except for children or exceptional adult cases, the procedure is done with local anesthesia. The biopsy should be approximately 750 mg and measure 1.5 x 1.5 x 1.0 cm, to allow histochemistry, immunomicroscopy, electron microscopy, and biochemical studies. Some muscle pathologists believe that it is best to use a surgical muscle clamp that prevents contraction. However, other authorities prefer that no clamp be used.[3] A small piece may be placed in 1% glutaraldehyde in those cases in which electron microscopy is needed. Deliver on a saline-moistened gauze pad immediately to the Pathology Department. Moistened gauze is used to prevent drying. The specimen must not become saturated as this will cause severe ice crystal artifact during snap freezing. **The tissue should not be placed in fixative and should ideally reach the Pathology Laboratory as quickly as possible.** The tissue should be frozen in isopentane which is cooled (to at least -150°C) in liquid nitrogen. After the tissue is frozen, cryostat sections may be prepared, or the tissue may be sent unsectioned to a specialty muscle laboratory.

Use Evaluate neurogenic atrophy, muscular dystrophies, myositis (infectious and "idiopathic," or autoimmune), hereditary and acquired metabolic and endocrine myopathies, ischemic, traumatic, and drug-induced problems, acquired diseases of the neuromuscular junction, and congenital/hereditary myopathies and enzyme deficiencies. Very rarely, muscle biopsy may shed light on a systemic condition such as systemic vasculitis in the absence of overt clinical muscle disease.

Limitations Normal morphometric features vary with age, sex, and the muscle biopsied.[2] The electromyogram (EMG) is especially important in myasthenia gravis.

Methodology A portion of the clamped muscle is oriented, frozen in isopentane/liquid nitrogen, and transverse sections are obtained for H&E, trichrome, and various histochemical preparations, some of which are listed below.

- Adenosine triphosphate (ATPase): At differing pHs, used to differentiate type I, IIa, and IIb myofibers and reveal abnormal fiber type distributions and diseases that selectively involve certain myofiber types.
- Succinate dehydrogenase (SDH): Stains mitochondria and shows abnormal aggregates or loss. SDH studies are particularly helpful in identifying patients with respiratory-chain enzyme defects.[4] Nicotinamide adenine dinucleotide-tetrazolium reductase (NADH-TR) may be used, but it is less sensitive.
- Oil red O: Stains lipids to detect abnormal accumulations.
- Periodic acid-Schiff (PAS): Used to detect glycogen in glycogenoses (ie, McArdle disease, Pompe disease, etc).
- Dystrophin, which is usually prominent in sarcolemmal membranes, can be demonstrated by immunostains and is markedly reduced or absent in patients with Duchenne muscular dystrophy.[5]

Extra frozen sections should be obtained and held in case additional more specific, enzyme preparations are needed (ie, cytochrome C oxidase, phosphofructokinase, phosphorylase). The remaining muscle tissue is formalin-fixed, paraffin-embedded, and stained with H&E and trichrome. Such preparations are used to detect small foci of myositis or vasculitis which may be missed on cryostat-cut sections, which are, of necessity, much smaller.

Additional Information See the Key Word Index entries for Dermatomyositis, Duchene Muscular Dystrophy, Guillain-Barré Syndrome, Muscle Disease, Muscular Dystrophy, Myasthenia Gravis, and Myositis.

Footnotes
1. Sarnat HB, "Neuromuscular Disorders, Evaluation and Investigation" *Nelson Textbook of Pediatrics*, 16th ed, Chapter 614, Behrman RE, Kliegman RM, and Jenson HB, eds, Philadelphia, PA: WB Saunders Co, 2000, 1867-9.
2. Pearl GS and Ghatak NR, "Muscle Biopsy," *Arch Pathol Lab Med*, 1995, 119(4):303-6.
3. Mayo Medical Laboratories, *2001 Test Catalogue*, Rochester, MN, 388.
4. Vladutiu GD and Heffner RR, "Succinate Dehydrogenase Deficiency," *Arch Pathol Lab Med*, 2000, 124(12):1755-8.
5. Ohlendieck K, Matsumura K, Ionasecu VV, et al, "Duchenne Muscular Dystrophy: Deficiency of Dystrophin-Associated Proteins in the Sarcolemma," *Neurology*, 1993, 43(4):795-800.

References
Brooke MH, "Disorders of Skeletal Muscle," *Neurology in Clinical Practice*, Bradley WG, Daroff RB, Fenichel GM, et al, eds, Boston, MA: Butterworth-Heinemann, 1991, 1843-86.
Carpenter S, "Light-Microscopic Pathology of Skeletal Muscle," *Disorders of Voluntary Muscle*, 6th ed, Walton J, Karpati G, Hilton-Jones D, eds, Edinburgh, England: Churchill Livingstone, 1994, 233-59.
Cullen MF, Hudgson P, and Mastaglia FL, "Ultrastructural Studies of Diseased Muscle," *Disorders of Voluntary Muscle*, 6th ed, Walton J, Karpati G, Hilton-Jones D, eds, Edinburgh, England: Churchill Livingstone, 1994, 319-80.
Dalakas MC, Illa I, Dambrosia JM, et al, "A Controlled Trial of High-Dose Intravenous Immune Globulin Infusions as Treatment for Dermatomyositis," *N Engl J Med*, 1993, 329(27):1993-2000.
Heffner RR Jr, "Muscle Biopsy in Neuromuscular Diseases," *Diagnostic Surgical Pathology*, Sternberg SS, ed, 3rd ed, Philadelphia, PA: Lippincott and Williams, 1999, 109-29.
Heffner RR Jr, "Skeletal Muscle," *Histology for Pathologists*, 2nd ed, Sternberg SS, ed, New York, NY: Raven Press, 1997, 197-220.
Hoffman EP, Fischbeck KH, Brown RH, et al, "Characterization of Dystrophin in Muscle-Biopsy Specimens From Patients With Duchenne's or Becker's Muscular Dystrophy," *N Engl J Med*, 1988, 318(21):1363-8.
Plotz PH, "Not Myositis: A Series of Chance Encounters," *JAMA*, 1992, 268(15):2074-7.
Sewry CA and Dubowitz V, "Histochemical and Immunocytochemical Studies in Neuromuscular Diseases," *Disorders of Voluntary Muscle*, 6th ed, Walton J, Karpati G, Hilton-Jones D, eds, Edinburgh, England: Churchill Livingstone, 1994, 261-318.
Varga J, Uitto J, and Jimenez SA, "The Cause and Pathogenesis of the Eosinophilia-Myalgia Syndrome," *Ann Intern Med*, 1992, 116(2):140-7.

♦ **Myoglobin** *see* Immunoperoxidase Procedures *on page 60*

♦ **Myosin** *see* Immunoperoxidase Procedures *on page 60*

♦ **Necropsy** *see* Autopsy *on page 50*

♦ **Needle Biopsy of Liver** *see* Liver Biopsy *on page 65*

♦ **non-Hodgkin Lymphoma** *see* Lymph Node Biopsy *on page 67*

♦ **Ovarian Cancer** *see* Estrogen and Progesterone Receptor Assay *on page 55*

♦ **PAS Stain** *see* Kidney Biopsy *on page 64*

♦ **PAS Stain** *see* Skin Biopsy *on page 71*

♦ **Pathologic Examination** *see* Histopathology *on page 59*

♦ **Pathology Operating Room Consultation** *see* Frozen Section *on page 56*

♦ **PCNA** *see* Image Analysis *on page 59*

♦ **PCNA** *see* Immunoperoxidase Procedures *on page 60*

♦ **Peptide Hormones** *see* Immunoperoxidase Procedures *on page 60*

Sentinel Lymph Node Biopsy

Related Information
Synonyms Lymph Node Mapping

Applies to Cytokeratin; HMB-45; Immunocytochemistry; Isosulfan Blue; Lymphoscintigraphy; MART-1; Regional Lymph Node Dissection; Tyrosinase

Test Includes Surgical biopsy, lymph node biopsy, immunohistology

Abstract Sentinel lymph node (SLN) mapping is a technique designed to identify the first lymph node or nodes in the lymphatic drainage of a tumor bed, which represents highest risk for metastatic disease. The procedure is considered a standard of care for patients at risk for metastatic melanoma and is gaining wide acceptance for selected patients with breast cancer. Early studies suggest that this procedure may spare a significant population from postoperative morbidity related to lymphedema.

Specimen Lymph nodes may be submitted in neutral buffered formalin or other suitable fixative or submitted fresh. Appropriate labeling for radioactive materials is necessary. Delays in processing may be required to allow radioactivity to decay to permissible levels. The half-life of ^{99}Tc is approximately 6 hours.

Limitations Identification of SLNs is performed with a high success rate. Technical aspects limiting their identification are discussed below. Surgeons must undergo appropriate training and acknowledge a significant learning curve.[1] Even though pathologic examination is more intense than for most cases, a portion of submitted tissue remains unexamined. Use of molecular methods which tremendously amplify genetic markers of metastatic disease are still experimental and may be subject to a high false-positive rate.[2]

Contraindications Patients undergoing mastectomy or those with palpable adenopathy are generally not suitable for SLN biopsy procedures. SLN identification is sometimes more difficult following excisional biopsy.

Methodology Pathologic examination is designed to optimize the chance of finding micrometastatic disease.[3,4] Although protocols at individual institutions vary, commonly each lymph node is thinly sectioned and separately submitted *in toto*. Eight to 12 cut surfaces are microscopically examined from at least three different levels. If the routine sections are morphologically negative, additional sections are subjected to immunohistochemical stains. In patients with breast cancer, stains for cytokeratin provide a high degree of sensitivity and specificity for malignant cells.[5] In patients with melanoma, a cocktail of HMB-45 and MART-1 may provide the highest degree of sensitivity and specificity. The role of melanoma markers (eg, tyrosinase) detected by reverse transcriptase polymerase chain reaction poses intriguing questions currently under investigation.[6]

Additional Information Numerous multicenter studies have demonstrated the powerful prognostic implications of lymph node involvement in patients with either melanoma or breast cancer. Furthermore, approximately 25% of node-negative patients with either breast cancer or melanoma eventually develop metastatic disease. While some of these recurrences no doubt reflect initial hematologic dissemination, many cases probably reflect intrinsic limitations of regional lymph node examination. Historically, lymph node staging for these diseases is performed by pathologic examination of multiple lymph nodes isolated from a regional dissection. Microscopic examination is commonly limited to 1 or 2 cut surfaces of a lymph node at one level and typically does not include special studies to detect micrometastatic disease. This traditional approach limits microscopic examination to approximately 1% to 5% of available tissue and is thought to miss metastatic disease 25% to 50% of the time.[7] This limitation is a practical and economic reality of examining multiple lymph nodes in a regional dissection.

SLNs are thought to represent the first lymph nodes encountered within the lymphatic drainage bed of a neoplasm and, thus, represent the highest risk for early metastatic involvement. Selective excisional biopsy of SLNs allows for concentrated pathologic examination of one or several lymph nodes for metastatic disease. Examination is commonly performed on multiple cut surfaces at multiple levels and may employ immunohistochemical or molecular techniques to identify micrometastatic disease not detected with routine hematoxylin and eosin stains.

If SLNs are negative for metastatic disease, then the patient may be spared from regional lymph node dissection and subsequent morbidity related to lymphedema. In contrast, SLN involvement justifies full regional node dissection.

The technique to identify the SLN is generally similar in patients with either melanoma or breast cancer. The tumor bed is carefully infiltrated with radiolabeled ^{99}Tc filtered colloid 2-6 hours prior to surgery. Lymphoscintigraphy is helpful for locating SLNs and may reveal unexpected lymphatic drainage patterns. Approximately 5-10 minutes prior to lymph node biopsy, the tumor bed is infiltrated with isosulfan blue (Lymphazurin Blue™) which rapidly gains access to the lymphatic channels surrounding the neoplasm. At the time of surgery, a gamma probe aids in the percutaneous localization of "hot spots". A small incision is made over a hot spot and soft tissues are dissected until the lymph node is located. Optimally, the blue dye will often highlight lymphatic channels leading into a blue stained lymph node. Confirmation is established with the gamma probe and all lymph nodes are separately excised and submitted for pathologic examination. Lymphatic bed counts confirm that all SLNs are sampled. A successful mapping produces an average of two SLNs. In breast cancer patients initially diagnosed by excisional biopsy, approximately 25% will have three or more SLNs.[8] For technical reasons, SLN mapping is generally easier for melanoma than for breast cancer.

Critical factors for a successful mapping procedure include timing and placement of radiolabeled colloid and blue dye, and tumor bed massage. Reported success rates are generally in the 90% to 95% range for experienced surgeons and institutions. Occasionally, SLNs are not found despite optimal localization techniques. A limited series of patients with breast cancer subjected to complete axillary node dissection failed to identify metastatic disease in 25 consecutive patients. These preliminary observations raise the possibility that these patients represent a unique subgroup warranting special consideration.[8]

Most commonly, patients with melanoma undergo SLN mapping at the time of wide local excision. Patients with melanoma >1.0 mm in thickness are regarded as candidates for SLN mapping and biopsy.[7] Recent studies have suggested that some patients with melanoma 0.67 mm in thickness may also benefit from this approach. This may be especially true with ulcerated melanomas. Multicenter trials are currently underway to establish the role of SLN biopsy in the management and outcome of patients with melanoma.

The role of SLN mapping and biopsy in patients with breast cancer is under active investigation. Most commonly, patients with breast cancer undergo SLN mapping at the time of segmental resection for breast conservation surgery. Some protocols require the intraoperative evaluation of SLNs to determine the need to proceed with complete axillary lymph node dissection. While frozen section evaluation with rapid immunohistochemical staining for cytokeratin has been described in some settings, other protocols require intraoperative cytologic evaluation based on imprint or scrape preparation cytology. Approximately 10% of patients with infiltrating mammary carcinoma histologically negative for metastatic disease are upgraded following more extensive sectioning and staining for cytokeratin.[5] Typically, axillary node sampling is not performed for patients with ductal carcinoma *in situ* (DCIS). However, recent studies in patients with comedo DCIS suggest that up to 6% of these patients have positive SLN biopsies.[9]

As a consequence of detailed pathologic staging studies afforded by SLN biopsy, new questions addressing the clinical significance of micrometastatic, submicroscopic, and molecular metastatic disease are being addressed in multicenter clinical trials. While the best applications of this new procedure are still under investigation, SLN biopsy offers a new gateway to the ultra staging of patients with selected malignancies.

Footnotes

1. Bass S, Cox C, and Reintgen D, "Learning Curves and Certification for Breast Cancer Lymphatic Mapping," *Surg Oncol Clin North Am*, 1999, 8(3):497-509.
2. Shivers S, Stall A, Goscin C, et al, "Molecular Staging for Melanoma and Breast Cancer," *Surg Oncol Clin North Am*, 1999, 8(3):515-26.
3. Meyer JS, "Sentinel Lymph Node Biopsy: Strategies for Pathologic Examination of the Specimen," *J Surg Oncol*, 1998, 69(4):212-8.
4. Messina J, Glass LF, Cruse CW, et al, "Pathologic Examination of the Sentinel Lymph Node in Malignant Melanoma," *Am J Surg Pathol*, 1999, 23(6):686-90.
5. Pendas S, Dauway E, Cox CE, et al, "Sentinel Node Biopsy and Cytokeratin Staining for the Accurate Staging of 478 Breast Cancer Patients," *Am J Surg*, 1999, 65(6):500-5.
6. Shivers S, Wang X, Li W, et al, "Molecular Staging of Malignant Melanoma: Correlation With Clinical Outcome," *JAMA*, 1998, 280(16):1410-5.

7. Reintgen D and Brobeil A, "Lymphatic Mapping and Selective Lymphadenectomy as an Alternative to Elective Lymph Node Dissection in Patients With Melanoma," *Hematol Oncol Clin N Am*, 1998, 12(3):807-21.
8. Dauway E, Giuliano R, Haddad F, et al, "Lymphatic Mapping in Breast Cancer," *Hematol Oncol Clin N Am*, 1999, 13(2):349-71.
9. Pendas S, Dauway E, Giuliano R, et al, "Sentinel Node Biopsy in Ductal Carcinoma *In Situ* Patients," *Ann Surg Oncol*, 2000, 7(1):15-20.

♦ **Skeletal Muscle Biopsy** *see* Muscle Biopsy *on page 69*

Skin Biopsy

Related Information

Applies to Grocott's-Methenamine Silver Stain; Lupus Band Test; PAS Stain

Abstract Inflammatory and neoplastic disorders of the skin are among the most commonly encountered disorders in clinical medicine. Biopsy of the skin is often central to the diagnosis and subsequent management of the disorder. This section deals with the biopsy techniques for a selected group of skin disorders.

Container 10% neutral formalin is satisfactory for submission of most specimens, but there are special requirements for immunofluorescence and electron microscopy. See also listings Histopathology *on page 59*, Electron Microscopy *on page 54*, and Immunoperoxidase Procedures *on page 60*.

Collection Several techniques for skin biopsy are commonly employed. The selection of biopsy technique should be based on a fundamental understanding of the suspected pathology, thus, affording the most acceptable diagnostic, therapeutic, and cosmetic result. Indications and techniques for skin biopsy have been recently reviewed.[1,2]

Shave biopsy: A technique for obtaining superficial samples of predominantly epidermal or projecting lesions (eg, seborrheic keratoses, verrucae) by cutting them flush with adjacent skin is illustrated in Figure 1. This technique is usually used for nonmalignant lesions but may be useful for the patch phase of mycosis fungoides. **Since shave biopsy provides the most limited specimen, a serious potential for histopathologic misdiagnosis exists, especially in regard to melanocytic lesions.**

Figure 1. Shave Biopsy

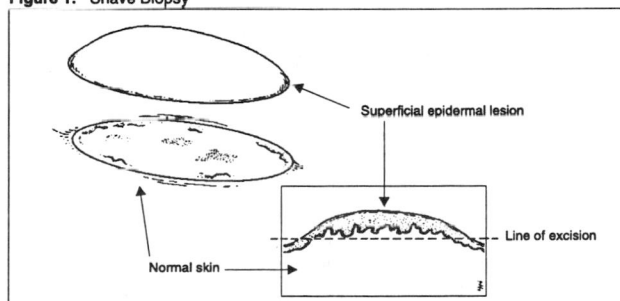

Punch biopsy: Very popular with dermatologists because it can be done easily, quickly, and repetitively at low cost in office practice. Biopsy punches, illustrated in Figure 2, range from 3-6 mm in size. 4 mm is adequate for many purposes. 3 mm punches may be used on the face. The punch is pressed into the skin and rotated. It yields a plug or core of tissue which is cut from its base by scissors as the punch is withdrawn. Punch biopsy may limit one's ability to evaluate adjacent skin and subcutaneous tissue to fully characterize some disorders. Very early lesions should be

sampled in cases of ulcers, pustular lesions, and vesiculobullous disorders. Avoid crushing.

Figure 2. Punch Biopsy

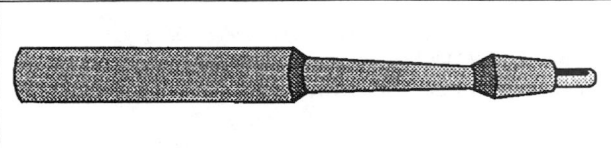

Excisional biopsy: This usually implies total removal of a skin lesion, most commonly a tumor, with a scalpel as illustrated in Figure 3. It is the preferred technique for removal of pigmented lesions and tumors.

Figure 3. Excisional Biopsy by Scalpel

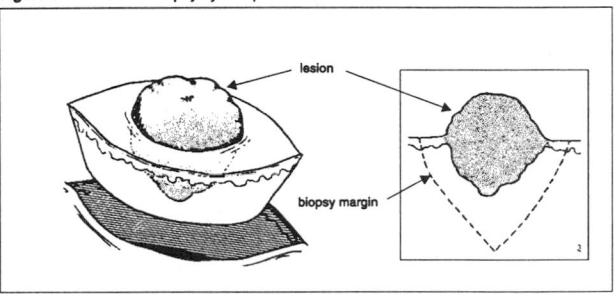

Incisional biopsy: Removal of a portion of a lesion by scalpel is illustrated in Figure 4. It is performed when a non-neoplastic lesion (eg, necrobiosis lipoidica) is too large to be totally excised but definitive diagnosis mandates a large sample to evaluate overall architectural detail. It may be used selectively in the case of tumors for which complete excision would require extensive surgery and/or would produce cosmetic deformity that would not be warranted, until accurate histopathologic diagnosis is established.

Figure 4. Incisional Biopsy by Scalpel

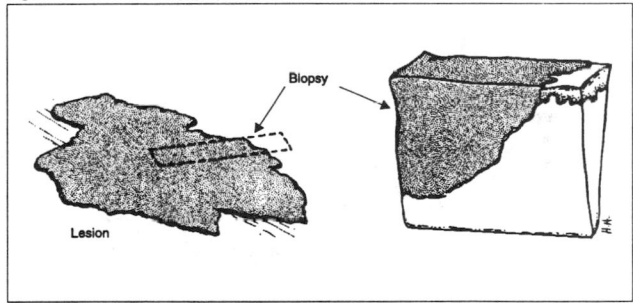

Smears and/or aspirates: Wright or Giemsa type stains may suffice to demonstrate polymorphonuclear leukocytes or eosinophils (as in toxic erythema or pustular melanosis of newborns). Gram, acid-fast, PAS, and Grocott methenamine-silver (GMS) stains, and cultures are used to study bacterial or fungal organisms. Finding appropriate multinucleated giant cells in smears in a proper clinical context suggests herpes or related viral infection;[3] see Herpesvirus Cytology *on page 383*. Smears of *Molluscum contagiosum* may be diagnostic. Aspirates may be adequate for cultures for bacteria, fungi, and viruses. Scrapings are often utilized to evaluate dermatophytoses. Negative KOH examination does not exclude the diagnosis of fungal infection. Cytologic techniques (Tzanck smears) are rarely used in practice to evaluate acantholytic processes or tumors.

Curettings: Most frequently used when nodular basal cell carcinoma is suspected, and used as well for actinic and seborrheic keratoses. **Contraindicated for suspicious melanotic lesions.**

Storage Instructions See Histopathology *on page 59*.

Special Instructions Detailed clinical information with clinical differential diagnosis may be pivotal to correct histopathologic diagnosis.

Use Diagnosis of dermatologic disease

Limitations Shave biopsies are contraindicated for lesions which may be melanoma. Differential diagnosis cannot be established between squamous cell carcinoma and keratoacanthoma in shave biopsy specimens. Shave biopsies of acral skin may not even reach the basal layer.

Curettage specimens sometimes cannot be evaluated. They are irregular, scanty, superficial, without architectural relationships, and often crushed.

Contraindications Anti-inflammatory agents and other therapy may alter histopathologic appearances. It is best to biopsy lesions prior to such treatment.

(Continued)

Skin Biopsy *(Continued)*

Avoid old, entirely scarred areas in scarring alopecia: select an area of erythema in which hair shafts are visible.

When the low dermis and subcutaneum are not included in the biopsy, characteristic features of some disease entities will be lost.

Additional Information

Selected Problems in Dermatopathology:

A. Tumors and Pigmented Lesions of the Skin

1. Tumors and pigmented lesions should be excised with careful attention to margins. The pathologists will commonly identify surgical margins with ink for proper microscopic evaluation. Pigmented lesions should not be aspirated, curetted, shaved, or punched. In a general practice, benign nevi, seborrheic keratoses, actinic keratoses, cysts, and dermatofibromas are most commonly encountered.[1] In the diagnosis of malignant melanoma, important prognostic information includes tumor size, Clark level, Breslow depth of invasion, adequacy of margins, presence of satellite lesions, and hemolymphatic invasion.[4]

B. Specimens of Vesiculobullous Lesions

1. If the diagnostic impression is pemphigus or pemphigoid, fresh lesions are preferred. Figure 5 illustrates appropriate biopsy technique.

Figure 5. Punch Biopsy Pemphigus or Pemphigoid

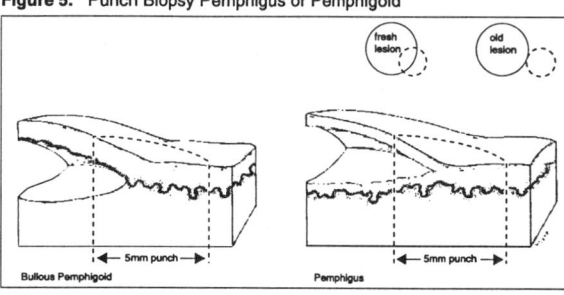

2. If the diagnostic impression is dermatitis herpetiformis, take the biopsy at the edge of the lesion (to study the change in dermal papillae) as shown in Figure 6, rather than the lesion itself.

Figure 6. Punch Biopsy: Dermatitis Herpetiformis

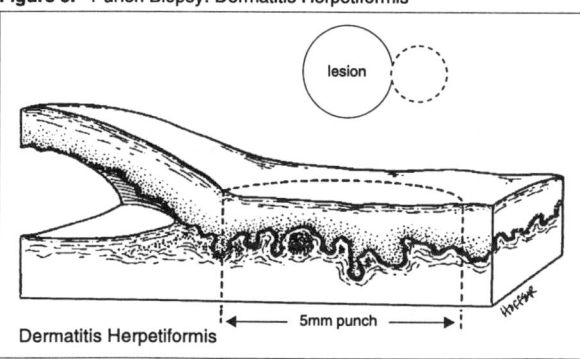

3. If the diagnostic impression is epidermolysis bullosa, the clinician should be aware of availability of four special regional reference centers in the USA for special studies of vesiculobullous lesions. The Epidermolysis Registry Center is located in Chapel Hill, North Carolina (see Websites).

4. Immunofluorescent studies of vesiculobullous lesions: Vesiculobullous lesions which require biopsy should be considered for immunofluorescent studies (IF). In many laboratories, skin samples for immunofluorescent studies are separately submitted in vials of isopentane prior to snap freezing in liquid nitrogen by the laboratory. Some reference laboratories provide special solutions such as Michael's solution or Zeus fixative to store specimens for their analysis. See Skin Biopsy, Immunofluorescence *on page 72.*

C. Specimens for Lupus Erythematosus (LE)

1. Direct immunofluorescence was first utilized on cutaneous biopsies in LE. The procedure (lupus band test) was widely utilized to study systemic lupus erythematosus (SLE), discoid lupus erythematosus (DLE), and mixed connective tissue disorder (MCTD). Recent data suggests the band test is much less specific and sensitive than previously thought. It is not clinically useful in discrimination of SLE from other connective tissue (CT) disorders or in predicting which patients with undifferentiated CT disease would develop SLE. Serologic evaluation is more sensitive, efficient, and cost-effective in discriminating DLE and SLE.[5] Specimens for the lupus band test should be taken from sun-protected skin; false positives result from specimens obtained from sun-exposed areas.

D. Special Studies for Hematopoietic Disorders

1. Special studies for T and B cells and lymphocyte markers are considered elsewhere. See Lymph Node Biopsy *on page 67* and Immunoperoxidase Procedures *on page 60.*

Pitfalls and artifacts to avoid: The biopsy technique should provide adequate and representative lesional tissue. Specimens should be handled gently without crushing by forceps. Cautery of lesions may burn or coagulate tissue, making pathologic diagnosis impossible. If specimens are mailed to a reference laboratory in freezing weather, they may freeze after fixation. Formation of ice crystals may render interpretation hazardous if not impossible. Send in Lillie's "winter fixative" (acetic acid alcohol and formaldehyde).[6]

Footnotes

1. Jones TP, Boiko PE, and Piepkorn MW, "Skin Biopsy Indications in Primary Care Practice: A Population-Based Study," *J Am Board Fam Pract*, 1996, 9(6):397-404.
2. Alguire PC and Mathes BM, "Skin Biopsy Techniques for the Internist," *J Gen Intern Med*, 1998, 13(1):46-54.
3. Cohen LM, Images in Clinical Medicine, "Positive Tzanck Smear," *N Engl J Med*, 1997, 337(8):535.
4. Stadelmann WK and Reintgen DS, "Prognosis in Malignant Melanoma," *Hematol Oncol Clin North Am*, 1998, 12(4):767-96.
5. Harrist T, *Selected Topics in Cutaneous Immunofluorescence*, Boston, MA: International Academy of Pathology, 1990.
6. Lillie RD, *Histopathologic Technique and Practical Histochemistry*, Blakiston Co, 1954.

References

Elder DE and Murphy GF, "Melanocytic Tumors of the Skin," *Atlas of Tumor Pathology*, Washington, DC: Armed Forces Institute of Pathology, 1990.

Elenitsas R and Halpern AC, "Biopsy Techniques," *Lever's Histopathology of the Skin*, 8th ed, Chapter 2, Elder D, Elenitsas R, Jaworsky C, et al, eds, Philadelphia, PA: JB Lippincott Raven, 1997, 3-4.

Logan RA, Bhogal B, Das AK, et al, "Localization of Bullous Pemphigoid Antibody - An Indirect Immunofluorescence Study of 228 Cases Using a Split-Skin Technique," *Br J Dermatol*, 1987, 117(4):471-8.

Murphy GF and Elder DE, "Nonmelanocytic Tumors of the Skin," *Atlas of Tumor Pathology*, Washington, DC: Armed Forces Institute of Pathology, 1991.

Internet Web Sites

www.med.unc.edu/derm/nebr_site/index.htm

♦ **Skin Biopsy Antibodies** *see* Skin Biopsy, Immunofluorescence *on page 72*

♦ **Skin Biopsy For Bullous or Collagen Disease** *see* Skin Biopsy, Immunofluorescence *on page 72*

♦ **Skin Biopsy For Pemphigus/Pemphigoid** *see* Skin Biopsy, Immunofluorescence *on page 72*

Skin Biopsy, Immunofluorescence

Related Information

Endomysial Antibodies *on page 525*
Oral Cavity Cytology *on page 386*
Pemphigus-Like Antibodies *on page 541*
Skin Biopsy *on page 71*
Viral Culture *on page 689*
Viral Culture, Dermatological Symptoms *on page 693*

Synonyms Immunofluorescence Skin Biopsy

Applies to Basement Membrane Zone Antibodies; Dermatitis Herpetiformis Antibodies; Intercellular Substance Antibodies; LE Antibodies; Lupus Band Test; Skin Biopsy Antibodies; Skin Biopsy For Bullous or Collagen Disease; Skin Biopsy For Pemphigus/Pemphigoid

Test Includes Anti-IgG, anti-IgA, anti-IgM, anti-C3, antifibrin immunofluorescence

Abstract Two methods of immunofluorescence are commonly used in the evaluation of skin biopsies. The most common is direct immunofluorescence (DFA) when the patient's skin is tested for autoantibodies or indicators of inflammation. The second method is indirect immunofluorescence (IFA) when the patient's serum is tested for the presence of antibodies to epidermal antigens on a test substrate such as monkey or guinea pig esophagus. Both methods provide valuable information in the differential diagnosis of certain inflammatory diseases of the skin.

Specimen 3 mm³ skin punch biopsy and patient serum

Container Covered Petri dish, or screw-cap glass vial; red top tube for blood

Collection Take biopsies from the following sites: If **pemphigus** or **bullous pemphigoid** is suspected, take a perilesional biopsy. If **dermatitis herpetiformis** is suspected, take biopsy of uninvolved area, 0.5-1.0 cm from lesion. Repeated biopsies are sometimes necessary to confirm dermatitis herpetiformis. If **systemic lupus erythematosus** or **discoid LE** is suspected, take biopsy of involved skin for diagnosis. Uninvolved skin, preferably of the wrist, is indicated to distinguish between discoid and systemic LE. Biopsies from lesions may be positive in both SLE and discoid LE while normal appearing sun-exposed skin yields positive findings in SLE only. Lesions older than 6 weeks should be biopsied in suspected SLE. Nonexposed skin may be biopsied to **rule out** SLE. In **vasculitis**, biopsy of lesion less than 24 hours old is recommended.

Consult your laboratory prior to biopsy for the best way to submit tissue for immunofluorescent antibody tests. The biopsy should not be fixed in formalin or similar aldehyde fixatives. The biopsy may be submitted on saline-soaked gauze and delivered on ice immediately to the laboratory. Alternatively, the biopsy may be placed directly into a transport/holding media (eg, Michael's media or Zeus fixative).

Storage Instructions If received fresh, the biopsy may be snap frozen directly, then stored at -20°C or colder. If received in transport media containing N-ethylmaleimide, the biopsy must be washed prior to freezing.

Causes for Rejection Specimen in fixative, drying out of specimen

Use Useful in differential diagnosis of bullous skin diseases including epidermolysis bullosa acquisita, SLE, DLE, pemphigus, bullous pemphigoid, herpes gestationis and dermatitis herpetiformis, other skin entities, and for small vessel vasculitis

Limitations Steroid therapy can convert findings to negative in previously positive patients. Many skin lesions which may clinically resemble SLE and DLE also have deposits of immunoglobulins at the basement membrane. These include psoriasis, polymorphous light eruption, and drug eruptions. Low titer anti-intercellular substance antibodies must be interpreted cautiously in the diagnosis of pemphigus. This is a complex subject which is difficult even to summarize. For instance, electron microscopy may be needed for diagnosis of **epidermolysis bullosa**. In the blistering disease **porphyria cutanea tarda**, uroporphyrinogen, uroporphyrin, and coproporphyrin urinary excretion is increased.

Contraindications Specimen should not be taken from heavily keratinized body areas if possible. Failure to demonstrate IgG in some biopsies may be due to a secondary change in the tissue due to infection and inflammatory reaction.

Methodology Direct immunofluorescence is performed on frozen sections from the **skin biopsy** (see Frozen Section *on page 56*). Frozen sections are washed and then stained with fluorescein-labeled antibody to IgG, IgA, IgM, fibrin, and complement components and subsequently examined under a fluorescence microscope. The presence and distribution of fluorescence is noted and correlated with findings by conventional light microscopy.

Indirect immunofluorescence antibody testing uses the **patient's serum** on a substrate (eg, monkey esophagus) to determine the presence of antibodies to skin. Saline-split preparations of human skin are used to distinguish between bullous pemphigoid and epidermolysis bullosa acquisita.[1]

Additional Information Distinctive patterns of IgG, IgA, IgM, fibrin, and complement components in epidermis, basement membrane, and dermal vessels may contribute to the differential diagnosis of bullous skin diseases, discoid and systemic lupus erythematosus, and other entities.

Serum antibodies to skin components can be demonstrated, using a tissue substrate (usually monkey or guinea pig esophagus). Such observations must be correlated with clinical and histopathologic facets as well as findings on direct immunofluorescence. In bullous disease, antibody levels often reflect disease activity and rising titers may foretell clinical relapse, but such correlation is imperfect.

See Endomysial Antibodies *on page 525*, relevant to dermatitis herpetiformis and celiac disease. See Antinuclear Antibody *on page 507*, relevant to systemic lupus erythematosus and related diseases.

Immunoglobulins or complement deposition in vessels may be found in skin biopsies in instances of vasculitis.

Footnotes

1. Wick MR, Ritter JH, Humphrey PA, et al, "Immunopathology of Non-neoplastic Skin Disease. A Brief Review," *Am J Clin Pathol*, 1996, 105(4):417-29.

References

Cardinali C, Caproni M, and Fabbri P, "The Utility of the Lupus Band Test on Sun-Protected Nonlesional Skin for the Diagnosis of Systemic Lupus Erythematosus," *Clin Exp Rheumatol*, 1999, 17(4):427-32.

Dabelsteen E, "Molecular Biological Aspects of Acquired Bullous Diseases," *Crit Rev Oral Biol Med*, 1998, 9(2):162-78.

David-Bajar KM and Davis BM, "Pathology, Immunopathology, and Immunohistochemistry in Cutaneous Lupus Erythematosus," *Lupus*, 1997, 6(2):145-57.

Elenitsas R, Van Belle P, and Elder D, "Laboratory Methods," *Lever's Histopathology of the Skin*, 8th ed, Chapter 4, Elder D, Elenitsas R, Jaworsky C, et al, eds, Philadelphia, PA: Lippincott-Raven, 1997, 51-60.

Gammon WR, Kowalewski C, Chorzelski TP, et al, "Direct Immunofluorescence Studies of Sodium Chloride-Separated Skin in the Differential Diagnosis of Bullous Pemphigoid and Epidermolysis Bullosa Acquisita," *J Am Acad Dermatol*, 1990, 22(4):664-70.

Magro CM and Crowson AN, "The Immunofluorescent Profile of Dermatomyositis: A Comparative Study With Lupus Erythematosus," *J Cutan Pathol*, 1997, 24(9):543-52.

Mutasim DF, Pelc NJ, and Supapannachart N, "Established Methods in the Investigation of Bullous Diseases," *Dermatol Clin*, 1993, 11(3):399-418.

Udey MC and Stanley JR, "Pemphigus - Diseases of Antidesmosomal Autoimmunity," *JAMA*, 1999, 282(6):572-6.

Vaughn Jones SA, Palmer I, Bhogal BS, et al, "The Use of Michel's Transport Medium for Immunofluorescence and Immunoelectron Microscopy in Autoimmune Bullous Diseases," *J Cutan Pathol*, 1995, 22(4):365-70.

Yancey KB and Hintner H, "Advances in the Diagnosis of Subepidermal Bullous Diseases," *Arch Dermatol*, 1996, 132(2):220-2.

CHEMISTRY

David S. Jacobs, MD

Uttam Garg, PhD

Dwight K. Oxley, MD

Charlotte Shideler, PhD

Harold J. Grady, PhD

Wayne R. DeMott, MD

Eugene S. Olsowka, MD, PhD

Leland Baskin, MD

Uri Alon, MD

Major advances in analytical methods, reagents, and instrumentation have markedly improved the scope and efficiency of clinical chemistry laboratories. Most analytical techniques in such laboratories are presently performed by automated or semiautomated analyzers, which have large test menus as well as stat-interrupt capability, rapid turnaround time and high through-put. Single instruments that are capable of standard spectrophotometric methods as well as immunoassay techniques have become available, saving on instrument cost, space, and personnel requirements by decreasing the number of workstations required. As such systems have become more sophisticated, their accuracy and precision have also improved. Coefficients of variation (imprecision) for most tests are <5% and for nearly all tests, <10%. Bias (inaccuracy) is usually <5%.

Such contemporary systems are typically coupled to laboratory information systems (LIS) which use computers and computer techniques to track and record the patient sample from order entry to the final printout of the analytical result at the site of data use. Many computer systems also furnish automatic alerts for out-of-range sample results, "panic" values, and warnings of unacceptable control values. All control values are stored, and detailed control histories are available for inspection by technologists, supervisors, and directors. All must sign such reports to satisfy requirements of accrediting and government agencies. These systems also warn of the need for restandardization because of time expiration or the introduction of new reagent lots.

Many of the above chemical techniques are used for other tests found in this book in several other chapters. Use of point-of-care testing (POCT) is increasing in attempts to shorten turnaround time and decrease sample handling. Automated systems (many of them hand-held) for POCT, with a limited menu, have been designed for this purpose. Such instruments, capable of analysis of whole blood, minimize the patient's blood loss for laboratory samples and save sample-handling time, but create other problems. Decrease in sample volume requirement is especially important for pediatric testing. A long monograph on POCT testing is included in the chapter, Specimen Collection and Point-of-Care Testing.

Turnaround time is often not discussed under the test entries in much of this book because it can be quite variable. It depends upon instrumentation, availability of sample volume, staff, geographic location, and laboratory organization. In many modern laboratories, results from the usual orders are available within 2 hours and from stats within 15-60 minutes. Most of this time is devoted to specimen procurement, transport, and preparation. The use of plasma rather than serum as the sample saves time (clotting time) and avoids interference from fibrin. Results from tests sent to reference laboratories will often be available the next day (for tests done every day) or in 2-3 days (for tests done only several times per week).

Some terminology has been changed to meet current standards of acceptance. The ambiguous term "normal range" has been replaced with "reference range," a term which can be used for any population, provided a description of that population is furnished. CLIA regulations require that all laboratories acquire the data set that justifies the applicability of their reference ranges to the population they serve.

For most analytes, SI units are given after conventional units. If SI units are widely used, then only the SI units are given. A review of many of the factors involved in the decision as to whether or not a result is within the "normal" or "reference" range for a given patient is found in the chapter entitled Maximizing the Information From Laboratory Tests – the Ulysses Syndrome on page 15.

Because of restrictions in funding, control and direction of laboratory utilization has become extremely important. Scientists in charge of clinical laboratories are aware of efforts to increase the efficiency and productivity of these areas. See References.

It is hazardous to interpret a set of test results without clinical information, and even more hazardous to interpret a single test result without knowing the clinical context in which the need for the test arose. Therefore, we try to stress relationships between clinical context and test results. The revisions and new entries in this chapter, as well as in all other chapters, reflect the rapid increase in knowledge and expertise of laboratory medicine and the dedication of laboratory scientists to implementation of contemporary advances.

The editors and authors wish to acknowledge and express appreciation to those who have written this chapter in prior editions. We especially note the contributions of the late Dr Paul R. Finley, leading author of Chemistry in the 3rd edition of the *Laboratory Test Handbook*, 1994. Dr Finley was an outstanding physician and clinical chemist.

References

Burtis C and Ashwood E, *Tietz Textbook of Clinical Chemistry*, 3rd ed, Philadelphia, PA: WB Saunders, 1999.

Innis M, "Clinical Problem Solving - The Role of Expert Laboratory Systems", *Med Inf*, 1997, 22:251-62.

Kaplan L and Pesce A, *Clinical Chemistry: Theory, Analysis, and Correlation*, 3rd ed, St Louis, MO: Mosby, 1996.

Peters M, "Decision Support Systems in Pathology," *Br J Hosp Med*, 1996, 56:502-3.

Peters and Broughton P, "The Role of Expert Systems in Improving the Test-Requesting Patterns of Clinicians," *Ann Clin Biochem*, 1993, 30:52-9.

Rainey P, "Outcomes Assessment for Point-of-Care Testing," *Clin Chem*, 1998, 44:1595-6, (editorial).

Smith B and McNeely M, "The Influence of an Expert System for Test Ordering and Interpretation on Laboratory Investigations," *Clin Chem*, 1999, 45:1168-175.

van Walraven C and Naylor C, "Do We Know What Inappropriate Laboratory Utilization Is? A Systematic Review of Laboratory Clinical Audits," *JAMA*, 1998, 280:550-8.

INTERNATIONAL UNIT (SI UNIT) CONVERSION TABLE

Analyte	Conventional Units	Conventional to SI (multiply by)	SI Units	SI to Conventional (multiply by)
Acetaminophen (Datril®, Tylenol®)	µg/mL	6.62	µmol/L	0.151
Acid phosphatase	units/L	NA	units/L	NA
Adrenocorticotropic hormone (ACTH)	pg/mL	1	ng/L	1
Albumin, serum	g/dL	10	g/L	0.10
Aldolase, serum	units/L	NA	units/L	NA
Aldosterone				
blood	ng/dL	0.0277	nmol/L	36.10
urine	µg/24 h	2.77	nmol/d	0.361
Alkaline phosphatase	units/L	NA	units/L	NA
Alpha$_1$-antitrypsin	mg/dL	0.01	g/L	100
Alpha$_1$-fetoprotein				
amniotic fluid	ng/mL	1	µg/L	1
serum	ng/mL	1	µg/L	1
Alanine aminotransferase (ALT)	units/L	NA	units/L	NA
Aluminum, serum	ng/mL	0.0371	µmol/L	26.95
Amikacin	µg/mL	1.71	µmol/L	0.585
Ammonia, blood	µg/dL	0.714	µmol/L	1.4
Amylase, serum	units/L	NA	units/L	NA
Androstenedione	ng/dL	0.0349	nmol/L	28.7
Angiotensin	ng/dL	10	ng/L	0.1
Angiotensin converting enzyme (ACE)	nmol/min/mL	1	units/L	1
Anion gap	mEq/L	1	mmol/L	1
Antidiuretic hormone (ADH) (vasopressin)	pg/mL	1	ng/L	1
Arsenic				
serum	µg/dL	0.133	µmol/L	7.52
urine	µg/L	0.0133	µmol/d	75.2
Ascorbic acid, blood	mg/dL	56.78	µmol/L	0.018
Aspartate aminotransferase (AST)	units/L	NA	units/L	NA
Base excess	mEq/L	1	mmol/L	1
Bicarbonate (HCO$_3^-$)	mEq/L	1	mmol/L	1
Bilirubin, serum				
direct	mg/dL	17.1	µmol/L	0.0584
total	mg/dL	17.1	µmol/L	0.0584
CA 15-3	units/mL	1	kU/L	1
CA 125	units/mL	1	kU/L	1
Cadmium	µg/L	8.897	nmol/L	0.112
Caffeine	µg/mL	5.15	µmol/L	0.194
Calcitonin	pg/mL	1	ng/L	1
Calcium				
ionized	mg/dL	0.25	mmol/L	4
serum	mg/dL	0.25	mmol/L	4
urine	mg/24 h	0.025	mmol/d	40
Carbamazepine (Tegretol®)	µg/mL	4.23	µmol/L	0.236
Carbon dioxide	mEq/L	1	mmol/L	1
Carboxyhemoglobin	%	NA	%	NA
Carcinoembryonic antigen (CEA)	ng/mL	1	µg/L	1
Carotene, serum	µg/dL	0.0186	µmol/L	53.7
Catecholamines, fractionation, urine	µg/24 h	5.91	nmol/d	0.169
Ceruloplasmin	mg/dL	10	µmol/L	0.10
Chloramphenicol	µg/mL	3.09	µmol/L	0.323
Chlordiazepoxide (Librium®)	µg/mL	3.33	µmol/L	0.30
Chloride				
serum	mEq/L	1	mmol/L	1
sweat	mEq/L	1	nmol/L	1
urine	mmol/24 h	1	mmol/d	1
Cholesterol	mg/dL	0.0259	mmol/L	38.61
HDL	mg/dL	0.0259	mmol/L	38.61
LDL	mg/dL	0.0259	mmol/L	38.61
Cholinesterase, serum	units/mL	1	kU/L	1
Chromium, serum	ng/mL	19.23	nmol/L	0.052
Clonazepam (Klonopin™)	ng/mL	3.17	nmol/L	0.316
Codeine	ng/mL	3.34	nmol/L	0.299
Compound S (11-deoxycortisol)	µg/dL	0.029	µmol/L	34.5
Copper				
serum	µg/dL	0.157	µmol/L	6.37
urine	µg/24 h	0.0157	µmol/d	63.69
Coproporphyrins (I and III)				
blood	µg/dL	15	nmol/L	0.067

Analyte	Conventional Units	Conventional to SI (multiply by)	SI Units	SI to Conventional (multiply by)
fluid	μg/g	1.5	nmol/g	0.67
urine	μg/24 h	1.5	nmol/d	0.67
Cortisol				
blood	μg/dL	27.6	nmol/L	0.036
urine	μg/24 h	2.76	nmol/d	0.362
C-Peptide	ng/mL	0.33	nmol/L	3.03
Creatine kinase (CK)	units/L	NA	units/L	NA
Creatinine				
serum	mg/dL	88.4	μmol/L	0.0113
urine	mg/kg/24 h	8.84	μmol/kg/d	0.113
Creatinine Clearance	mL/minute/1.73 m²	0.0166	mL/second/1.73 m²	60
Cyanide, blood	mg/24 h	0.0088	μmol/d	113.1
	mg/L	38.4	μmol/L	0.026
Cyclic AMP				
plasma	ng/mL	3.04	nmol/L	0.329
urine	μg/L	3.04	μmol/L	0.329
Cystine, urine	mg/24 h	8.32	μmol/24 h	0.120
Delta aminolevulinic acid, urine	mg/24 h	7.626	μmol/d	0.131
DHEA	ng/mL	3.47	nmol/L	0.288
DHEA sulfate	μg/mL	2.6	μmol/L	0.38
Diazepam (Valium®)	ng/mL	0.0035	μmol/L	0.286
Digitoxin	ng/mL	1.31	nmol/L	0.765
Digoxin (Lanoxin®)	ng/mL	1.28	nmol/L	0.781
Diphenylhydantoin (Dilantin®)	μg/mL	3.96	μmol/L	0.253
Disopyramide (Norpace®)	μg/mL	2.95	μmol/L	0.339
Doxepin (Sinequan®)	ng/mL	3.58	nmol/L	0.279
d-Xylose	mg/dL	0.066	mmol/L	15.01
Erythropoietin, serum	mIU/mL	1	IU/L	1
Estradiol (E₂), serum	pg/mL	3.67	pmol/L	0.272
Estriol (E₃), serum	μg/L	3.47	nmol/L	0.288
Estrone (E₁), serum	ng/dL	37	pmol/L	0.027
Ethanol	mg/dL	0.217	mmol/L	4.61
Ethchlorvynol (Placidyl®)	μg/mL	6.92	μmol/L	0.145
Ethosuximide (Zarontin®)	μg/mL	7.08	μmol/L	0.141
Ethylene glycol	mg/L	16.1	μmol/L	0.0621
Factor B (properdin)	mg/dL	10	mg/L	0.10
Fatty acids, free, serum	mg/dL	0.0354	mmol/L	28.25
Fecal fat	g/24 h	1	g/d	1
Ferritin, serum	ng/mL	1	μg/L	1
Folate				
red cell	ng/mL	2.265	nmol/L	0.442
serum	ng/mL	2.265	nmol/L	0.442
Follicle stimulating hormone (FSH)	mIU/mL	1	IU/L	1
Gamma glutamyl transferase (GGT)	units/L	NA	units/L	NA
Gastrin, serum	pg/mL	1	ng/L	1
Gentamicin	μg/mL	2.09	μmol/L	0.478
Glucagon, plasma	pg/mL	1	ng/L	1
Glucose				
blood	mg/dL	0.0555	mmol/L	18.02
CSF	mg/dL	0.0555	mmol/L	18.02
urine	mg/dL	0.0555	mmol/L	18.02
Glutamine, CSF	mg/dL	68.5	μmol/L	0.0146
Glutethimide (Doriden®)	μg/mL	4.60	μmol/L	0.217
Glycated hemoglobin	% of total Hb	0.01	Fraction of total Hb	100
Gold	μg/dL	0.0508	μmol/L	19.68
Growth hormone (GH)	ng/mL	1	μg/L	1
Haloperidol (Haldol®)	ng/mL	2.66	nmol/L	0.376
Haptoglobin, serum	mg/dL	10	mg/L	0.10
Homovanillic acid (HVA), urine	mg/24 h	5.49	μmol/d	0.182
	μg/mg of creatinine	0.621	mmol/mol of creatinine	1.61
Human chorionic gonadotropin (hCG), serum	mIU/mL	1	IU/L	1
17-Hydroxycorticosteroids (17-OHCS), urine	mg/24 h	2.76	μmol/d	0.362
5-Hydroxyindoleacetic acid (5-HIAA), urine	mg/24 h	5.2	μmol/d	0.19
17-Hydroxyprogesterone	ng/dL	0.030	nmol/L	33.3
Imipramine (Tofranil®)	ng/mL	3.57	nmol/L	0.280

78

Analyte	Conventional Units	Conventional to SI (multiply by)	SI Units	SI to Conventional (multiply by)
Insulin, blood	μIU/mL	1	mIU/L	1
Iron	μg/dL	0.179	μmol/L	5.587
Iron binding capacity, total (TIBC)	μg/dL	0.179	μmol/L	5.587
Isopropanol	mg/L	0.0166	mmol/L	60.1
17-Ketogenic steroids, urine	mg/24 h	3.467	μmol/d	0.288
17-Ketosteroids	mg/24 h	3.467	μmol/d	0.288
Lactate dehydrogenase (LDH)	units/L	NA	units/L	NA
Lactic acid				
blood	mg/dL	0.111	mmol/L	9.01
CSF	mg/dL	0.111	mmol/L	9.01
Lead				
serum	μg/dL	0.0483	μmol/L	20.70
urine	μg/24 h	0.00483	μmol/d	207.04
Leucine aminopeptidase (LAP)	units/L	NA	units/L	NA
Lidocaine (Xylocaine®)	μg/mL	4.27	μmol/L	0.234
Lipase, serum	units/L	NA	units/L	NA
Lipids, total	mg/dL	0.01	g/L	100
Lithium	mEq/L	1	mmol/L	1
Lorazepam	ng/mL	3.11	nmol/L	0.321
Luteinizing hormone (LH)	mIU/mL	1	IU/L	1
Lysergic acid diethylamide (LSD)	μg/mL	3.09	μmol/L	0.323
Magnesium				
serum	mEq/L	0.50	mmol/L	2
urine	mEq/24 h	0.50	mmol/d	2
Manganese				
serum	μg/L	18.2	nmol/L	0.055
urine	μg/L	18.2	nmol/L	0.055
Mercury				
blood	μg/dL	0.0499	μmol/L	20.0
urine	μg/L	0.00499	μmol/d	200
Meperidine (Demerol®)	μg/mL	4.04	nmol/L	0.247
Meprobamate	μg/mL	4.58	μmol/L	0.218
Metanephrines, urine	mg/24 h	5.07	μmol/d	0.197
Methadone	ng/mL	0.00323	μmol/L	309
Methanol	mg/dL	0.312	mmol/L	3.2
Methsuximide (Celontin®)	μg/mL	5.29	μmol/L	0.189
Methyldopa (Aldomet®)	μg/mL	4.73	μmol/L	0.211
Methyprylon (Noludar®)	μg/mL	5.46	μmol/L	0.183
Myoglobin, blood	μg/L	NA	μg/L	NA
N-Acetylprocainamide (NAPA)	μg/mL	3.61	μmol/L	0.277
Nortriptyline (Aventyl®)	ng/mL	3.80	nmol/L	0.263
5' Nucleotidase	units/L	NA	units/L	NA
Osmolality				
serum	mOsm/kg	NA	mmol/kg	NA
urine	mOsm/kg	NA	mmol/kg	NA
Oxalate, urine	mg/24 h	11.4	μmol/d	0.088
Oxazepam (Serax®)	μg/mL	3.49	μmol/L	0.287
Pancreatic polypeptide, human	pg/mL	1	mmol/L	1
Parathyroid hormone	pg/mL	1	ng/L	1
Pentobarbital (Nembutal®)	μg/mL	4.42	μmol/L	0.266
Phencyclidine (PCP)	ng/mL	4.11	nmol/L	0.243
Phenobarbital	μg/mL	4.31	μmol/L	0.232
Phenylalanine, blood	mg/dL	60.5	μmol/L	0.016
Phenytoin (Dilantin®)				
free	μg/mL	3.96	μmol/L	0.253
total	μg/mL	3.96	μmol/L	0.253
Phosphorus				
serum	mg/dL	0.323	mmol/L	3.10
urine	g/24 h	32.3	mmol/d	0.031
Porphobilinogen (PBG), urine	mg/24 h	4.42	μmol/d	0.226
Potassium				
blood	mEq/L	1	mmol/L	1
urine	mEq/24 h	1	mmol/d	1
Pregnanediol, urine	mg/24 h	3.12	μmol/24 h	0.321
Pregnanetriol, urine	mg/24 h	2.97	μmol/24 h	0.337
Primidone (Mysoline®)	μg/mL	4.58	μmol/L	0.218
Procainamide (Pronestyl®)	μg/mL	4.23	μmol/L	0.236
Progesterone	ng/mL	3.18	nmol/L	0.314
Prolactin	ng/mL	1	μg/L	1

Analyte	Conventional Units	Conventional to SI (multiply by)	SI Units	SI to Conventional (multiply by)
Propoxyphene (Darvon®)	µg/mL	2.95	µmol/L	0.339
Propranolol (Inderal®)	ng/mL	3.86	nmol/L	0.259
Protein				
CSF	mg/dL	10	mg/L	0.10
serum	g/dL	10	g/L	0.10
urine	mg/24 h	0.001	g/d	1000
Protoporphyrin, free erythrocyte	µg/dL	0.0178	µmol/L	56.18
Protoporphyrin, zinc (ZPP)	µg/dL	0.016	µmol/L	62.5
Quinidine	µg/mL	3.08	µmol/L	0.250
Renin, plasma	ng/mL/h	0.77	nmol/L/h	1.30
Salicylate	mg/dL	0.0724	mmol/L	13.81
Secobarbital (Seconal™)	µg/mL	4.20	µmol/L	0.238
Serotonin	ng/mL	0.00568	µmol/L	176
Sodium				
blood	mEq/L	1	mmol/L	1
urine	mEq/24 h	1	mmol/d	1
T_3 uptake (T_3U)	%	0.01	Fraction of total	100
Testosterone	ng/dL	0.0347	nmol/L	28.8
Theophylline	µg/mL	5.55	µmol/L	0.18
Thiocyanate	µg/mL	0.0172	mmol/L	58.0
Thyroglobulin	ng/mL	1	µg/L	1
Thyroid stimulating hormone (TSH)	µIU/mL	1	mIU/L	1
Thyrotropin-releasing hormone (TRH)	pg/mL	1	ng/L	1
Thyroxine binding globulin (TBG)	mg/dL	10	mg/L	0.10
Thyroxine (T_4)	µg/dL	12.9	nmol/L	0.0075
Thyroxine, free (FT_4)	ng/dL	12.9	pmol/L	0.0075
Tobramycin	µg/mL	2.14	µmol/L	0.467
Transferrin	mg/dL	0.01	g/L	100
Triglycerides	mg/dL	0.0113	mmol/L	88.5
Triiodothyronine (T_3)	ng/dL	0.0154	nmol/L	65.1
Troponin	µg/L	NA	µg/L	NA
Urea nitrogen, blood (BUN)	mg/dL	0.357	mmol/L	2.80
Uric acid				
serum	mg/dL	0.059	mmol/L	16.9
urine	mg/24 h	0.0059	mmol/d	169
Valproic acid (Depakene®)	µg/mL	6.93	µmol/L	0.144
Vancomycin	µg/mL	0.690	µmol/L	1.45
Vanillylmandelic acid (VMA), urine	mg/24 h	5.05	µmol/d	0.198
Vasoactive intestinal polypeptide	pg/mL	1	ng/L	1
Vitamin				
A	µg/dL	0.0349	µmol/L	28.65
B_6	ng/mL	4.046	nmol/L	0.247
B_{12}	pg/mL	0.738	pmol/L	1.355
D_3 (calcitriol, 1,25-dihydroxy)	pg/mL	2.4	pmol/L	0.417
E	mg/dL	23.22	µmol/L	0.043
Warfarin (Coumadin®)	µg/mL	3.24	µmol/L	0.308
Zinc				
blood	µg/dL	0.153	µmol/L	6.54
urine	µg/24 h	0.0153	µmol/d	65.36

NA = not applicable.

- **A₁AT** *see* Alpha₁-Antitrypsin, Serum *on page 96*

- **βA4 Peptide** *see* Apolipoprotein E, Plasma *on page 110*

- **ABGs** *see* Blood Gases and pH, Arterial *on page 119*

- **ACE** *see* Angiotensin Converting Enzyme, Serum *on page 105*

- **Acetaminophen** *see* Liver Disease: Laboratory Assessment, Overview *on page 216*

- **Acetaminophen Hepatotoxicity** *see* Aspartate Aminotransferase, Serum *on page 112*

- **Acetoacetate** *see* Ketone Bodies, Blood *on page 205*

- **Acetone** *see* Ketone Bodies, Blood *on page 205*

Acetylcholinesterase, Amniotic Fluid

Related Information
Acetylcholinesterase, Red Cell *on page 81*
Alpha₁-Fetoprotein, Amniotic Fluid *on page 96*

Synonyms AChE

Abstract An enzyme with MW of 300,000, not filtered by the glomerulus, not freely diffusible through membranes, normally absent in amniotic fluid. Along with alpha-fetoprotein, amniotic fluid AChE is used in the diagnosis of neural tube and ventral wall fetal defect.

Specimen Amniotic fluid

Sampling Time Amniotic fluid acetylcholinesterase is independent of gestational age.

Causes for Rejection Fetal blood in the specimen invalidates results; AChE is present in fetal blood.

Use Used with amniotic fluid alpha-fetoprotein to detect open neural tube and open ventral wall defects; AChE correctly identifies most false positives and almost all true positives. AChE has high specificity. Its sensitivity for anencephaly is 97%, and for open spina bifida 99%. Visible AChE bands are found about 95% of the instances of gastroschisis but much less frequently with omphalocaele.

AChE is not detected in cases of congenital nephrosis, a disease consistently associated with increased amniotic fluid AFP. Amniotic AChE and AFP both are associated with fetal death.

Limitations AChE cannot be measured for this purpose in maternal serum.

Both AFP and AChE are likely to be found in increased concentrations following substantial fetal hemorrhage into amniotic fluid.

Methodology Polyacrylamide gel electrophoresis followed by an inhibitor of AChE. While normal amniotic fluid includes a single cholinesterase, that from pregnancies with open neural tube and abdominal wall defects has a more rapidly migrating second cholinesterase.

Additional Information The ratio between AChE and pseudocholinesterase densities permits differentiation between open neural tube and open ventral wall defects. Typically, AChE:pseudocholinesterase ratio is <0.10 in ventral wall defects and >0.15 in open neural tube defects.

Neural tissue is the source of amniotic fluid AChE until day 28 of fetal development. AChE persists in amniotic fluid until about the 11th week of fetal development. The presence of amniotic fluid AChE throughout pregnancy indicates that the neural tube is not closed.

References
Ashwood ER, "Clinical Chemistry of Pregnancy," *Tietz Textbook of Clinical Chemistry*, 3rd ed, Chapter 48, Burtis CA and Ashwood ER, eds, Philadelphia, PA: WB Saunders Co, 1999, 1736-75.

Baskin LB, "Pregnancy and Prenatal Testing," *The Handbook of Clinical Pathology*, 2nd ed, Chapter 21, McKenna RW and Keffer JH, eds, Chicago, IL: American Society of Clinical Pathologists, 2000, 281-92.

Haddow JE and Palomaki GE, "Biochemical Markers of Fetal Disorders in Maternal Serum and Amniotic Fluid," *Medicine of the Fetus and Mother*, 2nd ed, Chapter 40, Reece EA and Hobbins JC, eds, Philadelphia, PA: Lippincott-Raven, 1999, 689-706.

Acetylcholinesterase, Red Cell

Related Information
Acetylcholinesterase, Amniotic Fluid *on page 81*
Dibucaine Number, Serum or Plasma *on page 166*
Organophosphate Pesticides, Urine, Blood, or Serum *on page 804*
Pseudocholinesterase, Serum *on page 270*

Synonyms AChE Activity; Cholinesterase, Erythrocytic; Cholinesterase I; Erythrocyte Cholinesterase; True Cholinesterase

Applies to Carbamate Toxicity; Organophosphate Toxicity; Sarin Exposure; Succinylcholine Sensitivity

Abstract The **red cell** enzyme (**true cholinesterase**) is specific for the substrate acetylcholine. Red cell acetylcholinesterase is most often used to detect past exposure to organophosphate and carbamate insecticides. The **serum** enzyme (**pseudocholinesterase**) hydrolyzes other choline esters.

Specimen Red blood cells

Container Green top (heparin) tube or heparinized capillary tubes

Storage Instructions Stable at 4°C to 25°C for 1 week.

Reference Interval Not well established, varies with method, age, sex, and use of oral contraceptives. Typical value: 30-50 units/g Hb. Normally absent in amniotic fluid.

Use Erythrocyte cholinesterase is measured to diagnose organophosphate and carbamate toxicity and to detect atypical forms of the enzyme, although most frequently the serum enzyme (pseudocholinesterase) is used for these purposes. Cholinesterase is irreversibly inhibited by organophosphate insecticides and reversibly inhibited by carbamate insecticides. Serum or plasma pseudocholinesterase is commonly used to measure acute toxicity, while erythrocyte levels are better for chronic exposure. (Serum level returns to normal before red cell levels.) Half-life of pseudocholinesterase is ~8 days, whereas that of acetylcholinesterase in red blood cells is 3 months. Persons with an atypical form of the enzyme (with low enzyme activity) exhibit prolonged apnea following the use of certain suxamethonium-type muscle relaxants in anesthesia (succinylcholine sensitivity - AA phenotype). These atypical forms may be detected by the use of fluoride or dibucaine inhibition. Again, the serum enzyme (pseudocholinesterase) is the one usually used for this purpose.

The assay was used to evaluate sarin toxicity (*vide infra*).

Its presence in amniotic fluid in conjunction with increased alpha-fetoprotein is evidence for neural tube and ventral wall fetal defects.

Limitations Values decrease as erythrocytes become senescent. Values are higher in younger red blood cells and reticulocytosis, and may mask the effect of acetylcholinesterase inhibition. Activity in red blood cells may not always provide a good index of intoxication with acetylcholine inhibitors.[1]

Pseudocholinesterase in serum is the indicated test for succinylcholine sensitivity.

High resolution ultrasonography may prove to be more cost-effective and accurate than alpha-fetoprotein and acetylcholinesterase at second trimester amniocentesis in detection of congenital anomalies.[2]

Methodology Methods are based on determination of the rate of hydrolysis of an ester catalyzed by the enzyme acetylcholinesterase and include colorimetry, fluorometry, spectrophotometry based systems. An improved method was recently published.[3] Polyacrylamide gel electrophoresis is used for the qualitative demonstration of acetylcholinesterase in amniotic fluid. Screening methods are available.

Additional Information The cholinesterase activity in human red cells is highly, but not exclusively specific, for acetylcholine. It is referred to as true or specific cholinesterase. Cholinesterase present in the serum/plasma hydrolyses both choline and aliphatic esters, has a broader range of esterolytic activity and is referred to as "pseudo-" or "nonspecific" cholinesterase. It hydrolyses acetylcholine only slowly. The systematic name for acetylcholinesterase is acetylcholine acetylhydrolase. Systematic name for cholinesterase (serum/plasma) is acylcholine acylhydrolase. The different nature of the cholinesterases was first described in 1940. The plasma enzyme is synthesized by the liver, the red cell enzyme during erythropoiesis.

Cholinesterase activity is low at birth and higher in adult males than females. The enzyme is a large complex protein. There is evidence that it has a multiple subunit structure, four peptide chains that form two dimers. Because of the many constituent amino acids, many molecular variants are possible. The RBC level is **increased** in hemolytic states such as the thalassemias, spherocytosis, hemoglobin SS, and acquired hemolytic anemias. It is **decreased** in paroxysmal nocturnal hemoglobinuria and in relapse of megaloblastic anemia and it returns to normal with therapy. It is not widely regarded as useful as a test for paroxysmal nocturnal hemoglobinuria.

Potent inhibitors of cholinesterase may present important clinical toxicological problems. Systemic insecticides (eg, organophosphates or carbamates) are examples. Both RBC acetylcholinesterase and plasma cholinesterase are usually inhibited. The effect on the plasma enzyme is more marked, however, and serum levels are usually utilized in diagnosis and assessment of recovery. Recovery is best determined by looking for a plateau in erythrocyte cholinesterase activity. Toxic potency may vary, plasma versus red cell cholinesterase, such that in some cases erythrocyte levels may be needed for diagnosis and/or monitoring. If there is suspicion that a decrease in cholinesterase activity may not relate to the inhibitor effect of an organophosphate, then red cell level of acetylcholinesterase should be obtained. If both serum and RBC levels are significantly decreased, findings are those of exogenous toxic effect.

AchE activity use was studied following a terrorist attack in Tokyo subways in which terrorists used sarin. Systemic poisoning was apparently less likely to evolve when pupil size was normal on arrival. Miosis was perceived as a more sensitive index of exposure to sarin vapor then RBC AChE.[4]

True cholinesterase (acetylcholinesterase-RBC cholinesterase) is not normally present in amniotic fluid. Presence of acetylcholinesterase activity and increased levels of alpha-fetoprotein in amniotic fluid are presumptive evidence of an open neural tube defect (eg, anencephaly, open spina bifida, or omphalocele) or ventral wall defect in the fetus. See Acetylcholinesterase, Amniotic Fluid *on page 81*.

Footnotes
1. Igisu H, Matsumura H, and Matsuoka M, "Acetylcholinesterase in the Erythrocyte Membrane," *Sangyo Ika Daigaku Zasshi*, 1994, 16(3):253-62.

2. Sepulveda W, Donaldson A, Johnson RD, et al, "Are Routine Alpha-Fetoprotein and Acetylcholinesterase Determinations Still Necessary at Second-Trimester Amniocentesis? Impact of High-Resolution Ultrasonography," *Obstet Gynecol*, 1995, 85(1):107-12.

(Continued)

Acetylcholinesterase, Red Cell (Continued)

3. Worek F, Mast U, Kiderlen D, et al, "Improved Determination of Acetylcholinesterase Activity in Human Whole Blood," Clin Chim Acta, 1999, 288(1-2):73-90.
4. Nozaki H, Hori S, Shinozawa Y, et al, "Relationship Between Pupil Size and Acetylcholinesterase Activity in Patients Exposed to Sarin Vapor," Intensive Care Med, 1997, 23(9):1005-7.

References

Boschetti N, Brodbeck U, Jensen SP, et al, "Monoclonal Antibodies Against a C-Terminal Peptide of Human Brain Acetylcholinesterase Distinguish Between Erythrocyte and Brain Acetylcholinesterases," Clin Chem, 1996, 42(1):19-23.

Boyle N and Talesa V, "Synthesis and Study of Thiocarbonate Derivatives of Choline as Potential Inhibitors of Acetylcholinesterase," J Med Chem, 1997, 40(19):3009-13.

Burtis CA and Ashwood ER, Tietz Textbook of Clinical Chemistry, 3rd ed, Philadelphia, PA: WB Saunders Co, 1999, 708.

Carlock LL and Chen WL, "Regulating and Assessing Risks of Cholinesterase-Inhibiting Pesticides," J Toxicol Environ Health, 1999, 2(2):105-60.

Datta C, Gupta J, and Sengupta D, "Interaction of Organophosphorus Insecticides Phosphamidon and Malathion on Lipid Profile and Acetylcholinesterase Activity in Human Erythrocyte Membrane," Indian J Med Res, 1994, 100:87-9.

Mason HJ, "The Recovery of Plasma Cholinesterase and Erythrocyte Acetylcholinesterase Activity in Workers After Overexposure to Dichlorvos," Occp Med (Lond), 2000, 50(5):543-7.

♦ **AChE** see Acetylcholinesterase, Amniotic Fluid on page 81

♦ **AChE Activity** see Acetylcholinesterase, Red Cell on page 81

♦ **Acid-Base Regulation** see Base Excess, Blood on page 114

♦ **Acid-Base Status** see pCO_2, Blood on page 246

♦ **Acid-Base Status Evaluation** see Carbon Dioxide, Total, Blood on page 135

Acid Phosphatase, Plasma

Related Information
Prostate Specific Antigen, Serum on page 263

Synonyms o-Phosphoric-Monoester Phosphohydrolase; PAP; Phosphatase, Acid; Prostatic Acid Phosphatase

Applies to Tartrate-Resistant Acid Phosphatase

Abstract Several acid phosphatases are present in serum from various sources. Acid phosphatase from the prostate is of most interest, but attention is turning to tartrate-resistant acid phosphatases as potential markers of bone metastasis from breast cancer and as collagen-related marker for assessing bone turnover. The interested reader is referred to a moderately recent review of the acid phosphatases.[1]

Patient Preparation Do not order immediately after rectal examination of the prostate, after TUR, or after prostatic massage. Fasting specimen is preferred, as lipemia may interfere.

Specimen Serum or plasma

Container Lavender top (EDTA) tube is preferred; red top tube may be acceptable.

Collection Morning collection is recommended, since diurnal variation (circadian rhythms) exist.[2] The sample should be drawn in EDTA anticoagulant to provide proper pH for stabilizing acid phosphatase. Due to the unstable nature of the enzyme, the test should be performed as soon as possible. Serum (red top tube) may also be used although it is possible to lose acid phosphatase activity within 1 hour.

Storage Instructions Separate sample and store on ice. Acidify and freeze sample if it cannot be run immediately. For acidification 50 μL of acetic acid (5 M) per mL of serum is added. Crystalline disodium citrate monohydrate at a level of 10 mg/mL of serum can be used as an alternative. Stable frozen at -20°C for 6 months, or at -70°C indefinitely.

Reference Interval Method dependent.
- Male: enzymatic, total: 2-12 units/L; enzymatic, prostatic: 0.2-3.5 units/L; RIA, prostatic: 2.5-3.7 ng/mL
- Female: enzymatic, total: 0.3-9.2 units/L; prostatic: 0-0.8 units/L

Use Staging of carcinoma of prostate, with other parameters. Helpful in diagnosis of metastatic adenocarcinoma of prostate and/or extension beyond prostatic capsule; monitor therapy and follow patient's response to treatment. **Not a screening test** for prostatic adenocarcinoma. Used on vaginal material in work-up of alleged rape.[3] Used in immunocytochemistry. A direct two-site immunoassay for serum tartrate-resistant acid phosphatase has been proposed as a potentially useful method for determining bone resorption rates.[4]

Limitations Specimens stored for any length of time, even at 4°C, will lose activity, especially if exposed to air. Acidification to pH 6 will stabilize the enzyme for 1 week at 4°C. When adenocarcinoma is confined within the prostate, acid phosphatase is usually normal. Occasionally, in patients with extensive carcinoma of prostate, acid phosphatase levels may be within normal limits. Even immunoassay methods do not detect early carcinomas consistently and in enzyme methods, there may be false positives. Acid phosphatase may be **increased** in diseases other than adenocarcinoma of prostate (eg, in infarct). Increased serum PAP with normal serum PSA may provide indication of significant extraprostatic (nonprostatic) disease[5] and has been rarely elevated in other cancers not metastatic to bone.[6] Moderate elevations of total acid phosphatase have been observed also with malignant invasion of bone from nonprostatic primaries, as well as with myelocytic leukemia, Gaucher disease, and Niemann-Pick disease. However, the thymolphthalein monophosphate method is said to be more specific for prostatic acid phosphatase than are some other chemical substrates. Specimens drawn after recent rectal digital examination, TUR, bladder catheterization, and/or other manipulation of the prostate may have elevated values. The enzyme may be increased with prostatitis and may be increased with urinary retention. Acid phosphatase is increased by radioimmunoassay in up to 27% of patients with benign hypertrophy.[7] When using nonspecific substrates (eg, 4-nitrophenyl phosphate), the tartrate inhibition is measured. The inhibited fraction is considered to be of prostatic origin. In males, approximately half of the normal total acid phosphatase is of prostatic origin. Tartrate inhibition is not entirely specific. High serum bilirubin (>2.0 mg/dL) almost totally interferes with determination of serum tartrate-resistant acid phosphatase.[8] Normal results do not consistently distinguish between localized and more extensive neoplasm. As use of PSA has increased in the past several years, use of PAP has diminished.

Methodology Immunoassays: radioimmunoassay (RIA), enzyme immunoassay (EIA), counterimmunoelectrophoresis (CIE); chemical methods: hydrolysis of thymolphthalein monophosphate, alpha naphthylphosphate, other enzymatic methods; tartrate inhibition. An improved method for the kinetic measurement of tartrate-resistant acid phosphatase is described.[9]

Additional Information The acid phosphatases form a family of genetically distinct isoenzymes with post-translational modifications. Erythrocytic and lysosomal forms show widespread distribution in most cells. Prostatic and macrophagic forms have more limited expression and distribution. Erythrocytic and macrophagic forms comprise the tartrate-resistant group and are linked with miscellaneous disorders such as increased osteolysis, Gaucher disease, and hairy cell leukemia.[1] Exacerbations and remissions of adenocarcinoma of prostate are not always correlated with acid phosphatase levels. A recent study found that serum PSA was the best marker for differentiating clinical stages while serum alkaline phosphatase showed the most significant differences regarding the extent of bone metastases.[10] However, prostatic acid phosphatase may be of value in predicting the first PSA recurrence and appeared to be an independent predictor of recurrence[11] and a more accurate indicator of micrometastatic disease.[12]

Prostate-specific antigen is more sensitive than prostatic acid phosphatase, but neither test is specific for adenocarcinoma of prostate.[13] Neither is 100% sensitive. See Prostate Specific Antigen, Serum on page 263. Benign prostatic hyperplasia causes definite increase in PAP, whereas in intracapsular prostate cancer normal PAP levels are found.[14] Tartrate-resistant acid phosphatase is a potential marker of bone metastasis from breast cancer[15] and appears to be increased in proportion to the number of bone metastases.[16]

Footnotes

1. Moss DW, Raymond FD, and Wile DB, "Clinical and Biological Aspects of Acid Phosphatase," Crit Rev Clin Lab Sci, 1995, 32(4):431-67.
2. Brenckman WD, Lastinger LB, and Sedor F, "Unpredictable Fluctuations in Serum Acid Phosphatase Activity in Prostatic Cancer," JAMA, 1981, 245:2501-4.
3. Gomez RR, Wunsch CD, Davis JH, et al, "Qualitative and Quantitative Determinations of Acid Phosphatase Activity in Vaginal Washings," Am J Clin Pathol, 1975, 64(4):423-32.
4. Halleen JM, Hentunen TA, Karp M, et al, "Characterization of Serum Tartrate-Resistant Acid Phosphatase and Development of a Direct Two-Site Immunoassay," J Bone Miner Res, 1998, 13(4):683-7.
5. Gambino R, "An Elevated Prostatic Acid Phosphatase (PAP) Level, in the Presence of a Normal Prostate-Specific Antigen (PSA) Level, Usually Indicates Serious Nonprostatic Disease," Lab Rep, 1994, 16(9):70-1.
6. Kaneko Y, Motoi N, Matsui A, et al, "Neuroendocrine Tumors of the Liver and Pancreas Associated With Elevated Serum Prostatic Acid Phosphatase, Intern Med, 1995, 34(9):886-91.
7. Gittes RF, "Serum Acid Phosphatase and Screening for Carcinoma of the Prostate," N Engl J Med, 1983, 309:852-3.
8. Alvarez L, Peris P, Bedini JL, et al, "High Bilirubin Levels Interfere With Serum Tartrate-Resistant Acid Phosphatase Determination: Relevance as a Marker of Bone Resorption in Jaundiced Patients," Calcif Tissue Int, 1999, 64(4):301-3.
9. Akimoto S, Furuya Y, Akakura K, et al, "Relationship Between Prostate-Specific Antigen, Clinical Stage, and Degree of Bone Metastasis in Patients With Prostate Cancer: Comparison With Prostatic Acid Phosphatase and Alkaline Phosphatase," Int J Urol, 1997, 4(6):572-5.
10. Nakanishi M, Yoh K, Uchida K, et al, "Improved Method for Measuring Tartrate-Resistant Acid Phosphatase Activity in Serum," Clin Chem, 1998, 44(2):221-5.
11. Moul JW, Connelly RR, Perahia B, et al, "The Contemporary Value of Pretreatment Prostatic Acid Phosphatase to Predict Pathological Stage and Recurrence in Radical Prostatectomy Cases," J Urol, 1998, 159(3):935-40.
12. Dattoli M, Wallner K, True L, et al, "Prognostic Role of Serum Prostatic Acid Phosphatase for 103 Pd-Based Radiation for Prostatic Carcinoma," Int J Radiat Oncol Biol Phys, 1999, 45(4):853-6.
13. Stamey TA, Yang N, Hay AR, et al, "Prostate-Specific Antigen as a Serum Marker for Adenocarcinoma of the Prostate," N Engl J Med, 1987, 317(15):909-16.
14. Salo JO, Rannikko S, and Haapiainen R, "Serum Acid Phosphatase in Patients With Localized Prostatic Cancer, Benign Prostatic Hyperplasia or Normal Prostates," Br J Urol, 1990, 66(2):188-92.
15. Agbedana EO and Ebesunun MO, "Abnormal Serum Alkaline and Acid Phosphatase Isoenzymes in Female Breast Cancer Patients," Afr J Med & Med Sci, 1998, 27(1-2):65-9.
16. Wada N, Ishii S, Ikeda T, et al, "Serum Tartrate Resistant Acid Phosphatase as a Potential Marker of Bone Metastasis From Breast Cancer," Anticancer Res, 1999, 19(5C):4515-21.

References

Bull H, Choy M, Manyonda I, et al, "Reactivity and Assay Restriction Profiles of Monoclonal and Polyclonal Antibodies to Acid Phosphatases: A Preliminary Study," *Immunol Lett*, 1999, 70(3):143-9.

Halleen JM, Karp M, Viloma S, et al, "Two-Site Immunoassays for Osteoclastic Tartrate-Resistant Acid Phosphatase Based on Characterization of Six Monoclonal Antibodies," *J Bone Miner Res*, 1999, 14(3):464-9.

Kim ED, Smith ND, and Grayhack JT, "Total Protein and Acid Phosphatase Concentrations in Prostatic Fluid From Patients With BPH Compared to Carcinoma," *Int Urol Nephrol*, 1998, 30(4):471-9.

Kroll MH and Nipper H, "Rapid Rise of Serum Acid Phosphatase After Irradiation of Metastatic Carcinoma of Prostate," *Urology*, 1987, 29:650-2.

Nakasato YR, Janckila AJ, Halleen JM, et al, "Clinical Significance of Immunoassays for Type-5 Tartrate-Resistant Acid Phosphatase," *Clin Chem*, 1999, 45(12):2150-7.

Nakanishi M, Yoh K, Uchida K, et al, "Clinical Usefulness of Serum Tartrate-resistant Fluoride-Sensitive Acid Phosphatase Activity in Evaluating Bone Turnover," *J Bone Miner Metab*, 1999, 17(2):125-30.

Panara F, Guiderdone S, Pellegrini M, et al, "Acid Phosphatase and Zinc Ion-Dependent Acid Phosphatase Expression in Normal Human Liver and in Hep G2 (Human Hepatocellular Carcinoma) Cell Line," *Cytobios*, 1998, 94(376):111-9.

Romas NA and Kwan DJ, "Prostatic Acid Phosphatase. Biomolecular Features and Assays for Serum Determination," *Urol Clin North Am*, 1993, 20(4):581-8.

♦ **ACTH** *see* Adrenocorticotropic Hormone, Plasma *on page 86*

♦ **ACTH Infusion Test** *replaced by* Corticotropin Stimulation Test (Rapid) *on page 153*

♦ **Acute Phase Reactant** *see* Alpha$_1$-Antitrypsin, Serum *on page 96*

♦ **Acylcholine Acylhydrolase** *see* Pseudocholinesterase, Serum *on page 270*

AD7c Neural Thread Protein, CSF or Urine

Related Information
Apolipoprotein E, Plasma *on page 110*
Cerebrospinal Fluid and Plasma β-Amyloid$_{(1-42)}$ *on page 513*

Synonyms NTP

Applies to Neuronal Thread Proteins

Abstract AD7c-neural thread protein (AD7c-NTP) is a protein present in certain neurons. Its production is increased in the brains[1,2] and CSF[3] of patients with Alzheimer disease (AD). The protein in CSF is 41-kD in size, and its concentration in CSF correlates with the severity of dementia.[4] The same protein is excreted in the urine, and preliminary studies report a higher concentration of AD7c-NTP in urine of AD patients compared with non-AD controls.[5]

Specimen Cerebrospinal fluid or urine

Collection Collect CSF by lumbar puncture; the CSF specimen should be clear and free of blood. Use a first morning, midstream urine collection.

Storage Instructions Freeze at -20°C or colder until analysis.

Reference Interval CSF: ≤2.0 ng/mL; urine: ≤1.5 ng/mL

Use The test is a presumptive diagnostic aid that can be used along with other relevant clinical information to diagnose Alzheimer disease.

Limitations Both the CSF and urinary tests are relatively new and only a few published clinical studies are presently available.

Methodology Enzyme-linked sandwich immunoassay (ELISA), microparticle enzyme immunoasay (MEIA)

Additional Information The test in CSF is reported to have sensitivities of 83% in patients with probable/possible AD and 89% in patients with early AD[4,6] The specificities of the CSF test in non-AD dementia controls and normal controls are 94% and 89%, respectively.[4,6] Preliminary studies suggest that the urine test is approximately 80% to 85% sensitive and 91% specific.[5] However, these levels of sensitivity and specificity have not yet been independently confirmed.

Footnotes
1. de la Monte SM and Wands JR, "Neuronal Thread Protein Over-Expression in Brains With Alzheimer's Disease Lesions," *J Neurol Sci*, 1992, 113(2):152-64.
2. de la Monte SM, Carlson RI, Brown NV, et al, "Profiles of Neuronal Thread Protein Expression in Alzheimer's Disease," *J Neuropathol Exp Neurol*, 1996, 55(10):1038-50.
3. Monte SM, Volicer L, Hauser SL, et al, "Increased Levels of Neuronal Thread Protein in Cerebrospinal Fluid of Patients With Alzheimer's Disease," *Ann Neurol*, 1992, 32(6):733-42.
4. Monte SM, Ghanbari K, Frey WH, et al, "Characterization of the AD7c-NTP cDNA Expression in Alzheimer's Disease and Measurement of a 41-kD Protein in Cerebrospinal Fluid," *J Clin Invest*, 1997, 100(12):3093-104.
5. Ghanbari HA, Ghanbari K, Beheshti I, et al, "Biochemical Assay for AD7c-NTP in Urine as an Alzheimer's Disease Marker," *J Clin Lab Anal*, 1998, 12(5):285-8.
6. Ghanbari HA, Ghanbari K, Munzar M, et al, "Specificity of AD7c-NTP as a Biochemical Marker for Alzheimer's Disease," *J Contemp Neurol*, 1998, 4A:2-6.

References
Chong JK, Cantrell L, Husain M, et al, "Automated Microparticle Enzyme Immunoassay for Neuronal Thread Protein in Cerebrospinal Fluid From Alzheimer's Disease Patients," *J Clin Lab Anal*, 1992, 6(6):379-83.

de la Monte SM, Xu YY, and Wands JR, "Modulation of Neuronal Thread Protein Expression With Neuritic Sprouting: Relevance to Alzheimer's Disease," *J Neurol Sci*, 1996, 138(1-2):26-35.

Ghanbari K and Ghanbari HA, "A Sandwich Enzyme Immunoassay for Measuring AD7c-NTP as an Alzheimer's Disease Marker: AD7c Test," *J Clin Lab Anal*, 1998, 12(4):223-6.

Mulder C, Scheltens P, Visser JJ, et al, "Genetic and Biochemical Markers for Alzheimer's Disease: Recent Developments," *Ann Clin Biochem*, 2000, 37(Pt 5):593-607.

Stephenson J, "Alzheimer Disease Experts Advise a 'Wait for the Data' Response to New Diagnostic Test," *JAMA*, 1997, 277(11):870.

Internet Web Sites
www.nymox.com

Adenosine Deaminase, CSF, Pleural Fluid, Pericardial Fluid, Peritoneal Fluid

Related Information
Mycobacterial Culture, Biopsy or Body Fluid *on page 655*
Mycobacterial Culture, Cerebrospinal Fluid *on page 656*

Abstract Adenosine deaminase (ADA) is a purine catabolic enzyme that catalyzes the conversion of adenosine or deoxyadenosine to inosine or deoxyinosine. It has a broad tissue distribution and exists in at least three isoforms (ADA$_1$, ADA$_{1+CP}$, and ADA$_2$). It appears to be involved in the proliferation and differentiation of lymphocytes associated with the immune response.

Specimen Cerebrospinal fluid, pleural fluid, pericardial fluid, or peritoneal fluid

Storage Instructions Centrifuge specimen at ambient temperature. Store supernatant at -20°C until analysis.

Causes for Rejection Specimen unfrozen

Reference Interval
- CSF: <6 units/L[1]
- Pleural fluid: ≤47 units/L[2]
- Pericardial fluid: ≤50 units/L[3]
- Peritoneal fluid: ≤32 units/L[4,5]

Use Elevated body fluid adenosine deaminase (ADA) activity has been used as an indirect marker for diagnosing tuberculous meningitis (CSF), tuberculous pleural effusion (pleural fluid), tuberculous pericarditis (pericardial fluid), and tuberculous peritonitis (peritoneal or ascitic fluid). Values are higher in tuberculosis than in carcinomatosis.

Limitations Patients with both tuberculous pleuritis and human immunodeficiency virus have a high frequency of false-negative pleural fluid ADA levels. Interferon gamma has been suggested as a better marker for this patient population.[6] The authors of a recent publication, which included a review of the literature in addition to a report of two cases of pseudochylothorax secondary to tuberculosis, concluded that pleural fluid ADA testing is inadequate for diagnostic or therapeutic decisions.[7]

Methodology Kinetic spectrophotometric

Additional Information Polymerase chain reaction (PCR) methods for detection of mycobacterial tuberculosis DNA in body fluids are available and have the potential for more effective diagnosis of tuberculous meningitis/effusions.

CSF: A recent study showed that an ADA cutoff ≥6 units/L was 90.9% sensitive and 94% specific in detection of tuberculous meningitis and useful to differentiate this disorder from aseptic meningitis and normal individuals. However, significant overlap was observed between patients with tuberculous meningitis and those with cryptococcal meningitis or acute bacterial meningitis. Improved differentiation among these groups was achieved by measurement of the ADA$_2$ isoenzyme.[1]

Pleural fluid: 253 of 254 patients (99.6%) with known tuberculous pleural effusions had pleural fluid ADA activities >47 units/L. Most ADA activity in these patients was due to the ADA$_2$ isoenzyme.[2]

Pericardial fluid: An ADA cutoff of 50 units/L was 100% sensitive and 83% specific for the diagnosis of tuberculous effusion in a study that included subjects with tuberculous pericarditis, malignant pericardial effusion, uremic pericarditis, purulent pericarditis, and no pericardial disease. This same study found no correlation between serum and pericardial ADA activity.[3]

Peritoneal (ascites) fluid: Voigt et al,[4] using an ADA cutoff of 32.3 units/L, conducted retrospective and prospective studies and reported, respectively, sensitivities of 95% and 100% and specificities of 98% and 96% in distinguishing patients with tuberculous peritonitis from patients with ascites of other causes.

A discussion in a 1998 Case Records of the Massachusetts General Hospital exercise observed a reported high sensitivity and excellent specificity of this analyte for detection of *M. tuberculosis* in pleural or peritoneal fluid, and noted that some authorities predicted that the current gold standard for diagnosis (a peritoneal biopsy) may eventually be replaced by this test.[8]

Footnotes
1. Eintracht S, Silber E, Sonnenberg P, et al, "Analysis of Adenosine Deaminase Isoenzyme-2 (ADA2) in Cerebrospinal Fluid in the Diagnosis of Tuberculosis Meningitis," *J Neurol Neurosurg Psychiatry*, 2000, 69(1):137-8.
2. Valdes L, Alvarez D, San Jose E, et al, "Tuberculous Pleurisy: A Study of 254 Patients," *Arch Intern Med*, 1998, 158(18):2017-21.
3. Dogan R, Demircin M, Sarigul A, et al, "Diagnostic Value of Adenosine Deaminase Activity in Pericardial Fluids," *J Cardiovasc Surg (Torino)*, 1999, 40(4):501-4.
4. Voigt MD, Kalvaria I, Trey C, et al, "Diagnostic Value of Ascites Adenosine Deaminase in Tuberculous Peritonitis," *Lancet*, 1989, 1(8641):751-4.

(Continued)

Adenosine Deaminase, CSF, Pleural Fluid, Pericardial Fluid, Peritoneal Fluid (Continued)

5. Fernandez-Rodriguez CM, Perez-Arguelles BS, Ledo L, et al, "Ascites Adenosine Deaminase Activity I Decreased in Tuberculous Ascites With Low Protein Content," *Gastroenterology*, 1991, 86(10):1500-3.
6. Villena V, Lopez-Encuentra A, Echave-Sustaeta J, et al, "Interferon-Gamma in 388 Immunocompromised and Immunocompetent Patients for Diagnosing Pleural Tuberculosis," *Eur Respir J*, 1996, 9(12):2635-9.
7. Garcia-Zamalloa A, Ruiz-Irastorza G, Aguayo FJ, et al, "Pseudochylothorax. Report of 2 Cases and Review of the Literature," *Medicine*, 1999, 78(3):200-7.
8. Sheets EE and Smith RN, "A 31-Year-Old Woman With a Pleural Effusion, Ascites, and Persistent Fever Spikes," Case Records of the Massachusetts General Hospital, Case 3-1998, Scully RE, Mark EJ, McNeely WF, et al, eds, *N Engl J Med*, 1998, 338(4):248-54.

References

Kjeldsberg CR and Knight JA, *Body Fluids - Laboratory Examination of Amniotic, Cerebrospinal, Seminal, Serous, and Synovial Fluids*, 3rd ed, Chicago, IL: ASCP Press, American Society of Clinical Pathologists, 1993, 65-253.

Light RW, "Establishing the Diagnosis of Tuberculous Pleuritis," *Arch Intern Med*, 1998, 158(18):1967-8.

Querrol JM, Minguez J, Garcia-Sanchez E, et al, "Rapid Diagnosis of Pleural Tuberculosis by Polymerase Chain Reaction," *Am J Respir Crit Care Med*, 1995, 152(6 Pt 1):1977-81.

Villena V, Navarro-Gonzalvez JA, Garcia-Benayas C, et al, "Rapid Automated Determination of Adenosine Deaminase and Lysozyme for Differentiating Tuberculous and Nontuberculous Pleural Effusions," *Clin Chem*, 1996, 42(2):218-21.

Villena V, Rebollo MJ, Aguado JM, et al, "Polymerase Chain Reaction for the Diagnosis of Pleural Tuberculosis in Immunocompromised and Immunocompetent Patients," *Clin Infect Dis*, 1998, 26:212-4.

Adenosine Deaminase, Erythrocyte

Abstract Adenosine deaminase (ADA) is an enzyme of the purine salvage pathway that catalyzes the deamination of adenosine and deoxyadenosine to inosine and deoxyinosine. It is deficient in certain forms of severe combined immunodeficiency (SCID).

Specimen Whole blood

Container Lavender top (EDTA) tube

Storage Instructions Stable at 4°C for 1 week.

Special Instructions Specimens must be sent to a specialized referral laboratory.

Reference Interval 0.8-1.3 units/g Hb

Use Activities are decreased in patients with ADA-deficient SCID. Usually these patients present at birth with severe lymphopenia (absolute lymphocyte count <500/mm^3) and develop repeated infections and failure to thrive.

Limitations Recent transfusion may obscure the presence of abnormality.

Methodology Spectrophotometric, kinetic assay; fluorometric

Additional Information ADA deficiency is due to an autosomal-recessive, single-gene defect that is responsible for approximately 15% to 25% of SCID cases. Over 50 mutations have been identified in the ADA gene. ADA deficiency causes an accumulation of cytotoxic purine intermediates with subsequent T- and B-cell damage and lethal loss of immune protection. This disorder was the first human genetic disease to be treated by gene transfer techniques with limited success. Enzyme replacement with polyethylene-glycol (PEG) modified ADA has been shown to be effective and safe, but expensive.

References

Bartlett JS, "Gene Therapy," *Molecular Diagnostics for the Clinical Laboratorian*, Chapter 9, Coleman WB and Tsongalis GJ, eds, Totowa, NJ: Humana Press, 1997, 193-214.

Buckley RH, "Combined B- and T-Cell Diseases," *Nelson Textbook of Pediatrics*, 16th ed, Chapter 126, Behrman RE, Kliegman RM, and Jenson HB, eds, Philadelphia, PA: WB Saunders Co, 2000, 601-6.

Grabowski GA and Whitsett JA, "Gene Therapy," *Nelson Textbook of Pediatrics*, 16th ed, Chapter 79, Behrman RE, Kliegman RM, and Jenson HB, eds, Philadelphia, PA: WB Saunders Co, 2000, 333-41.

Hershfield MS, "Adenosine Deaminase Deficiency: Clinical Expression, Molecular Basis, and Therapy," *Semin Hematol*, 1998, 35(4):291-8.

Insel RA and Quaidoo EA, "Disorders of Lymphocyte Function," *Hematology: Basic Principles and Practice*, 3rd ed, Chapter 42, Hoffman R, Benz EJ, et al, eds, New York, NY: Churchill Livingstone, 2000, 782.

◆ **ADH** *see* Antidiuretic Hormone, Plasma *on page 107*

Adrenal Cortex: Laboratory Assessments Overview

Related Information

Adrenocorticotropic Hormone, Plasma *on page 86*
Aldosterone, Serum or Plasma *on page 90*
Aldosterone, Urine *on page 91*
Corticotropin-Releasing Hormone Stimulation Test *on page 152*
Corticotropin Stimulation Test (Rapid) *on page 153*
Cortisol, Free, Urine *on page 154*
Cortisol, Serum or Plasma *on page 154*
Follicle Stimulating Hormone, Serum, Plasma, or Urine *on page 175*
21-Hydroxylase Antibodies, Serum *on page 530*
17-Hydroxyprogesterone, Serum or Plasma *on page 197*
Insulin Tolerance Test *on page 202*
Metyrapone Stimulation Test, Serum *on page 225*
Potassium, Serum or Plasma *on page 258*
Potassium, Urine *on page 259*
Renin Activity, Plasma *on page 273*
Testosterone, Total and Free, Serum or Plasma *on page 280*
Urinary Cortisol/Creatinine Increment *on page 296*

Applies to Dexamethasone Suppression Test; Loperamide Inhibition Test; Naloxone Stimulation Test

Abstract Many adrenal cortical disorders are caused by an excess or deficiency of either cortisol or aldosterone, or one of their secretagogues. The interpretation of an isolated serum cortisol or aldosterone value, however, is often impossible because hormone secretion fluctuates over a broad and unpredictable range, both in patients with adrenal disease and in acutely ill patients with normal adrenals. The solution to the resulting clinical problems usually requires specialized tests, especially tests which evaluate the dynamics of the negative feedback systems that control the secretion of cortisol and aldosterone.

The primary stimulants of the adrenal cortex are corticotropin (ACTH) and angiotensin II. Other factors exert regulatory roles as well.

Clinically relevant information includes presence or absence of virilization or feminization, change in body habitus, hypertension, endocrine syndromes, and family history (eg, multiple endocrine neoplasia).

Use

CORTISOL-RELATED DISORDERS

Cushing Syndrome (CS)

CS may include various combinations of weight gain, hypertension, glucose intolerance, oligomenorrhea, amenorrhea, decreased libido, easy bruisability, truncal obesity, moon facies, enlarged cervical/dorsal fat pad, plethoric appearance, lower abdominal striae, depression, and hirsutism. The biochemical hallmark of CS is increased cortisol secretion, most readily identified by the 24-hour **urine free cortisol** (see Cortisol, Free, Urine *on page 154*). **Serum cortisol** values, especially when drawn at midnight, are often, but not invariably, elevated. Cortisol values drawn at 0800 are usually resistant to suppression by a 1 mg dose of dexamethasone; for some patients a multiple-dose dexamethasone suppression protocol is required (see Cortisol, Serum or Plasma *on page 154*). Once CS has been biochemically confirmed, the underlying cause must be identified. This process may require specialized laboratory testing and a variety of imaging studies. The differential diagnosis of CS includes the following.

1. Corticotropin (ACTH)-secreting basophilic pituitary adenoma, classically known as **Cushing disease** (CD) - 65% to 70% of CS cases
2. **Adrenal adenoma** or **carcinoma** - 15% to 20% of CS cases
3. The **ectopic corticotropin syndrome** (ECS) - 10% to 15% of CS cases. The most common nonpituitary corticotropin-producing neoplasm is small cell carcinoma of lung.
4. **Pseudo-Cushing syndrome**
5. **Ectopic corticotropin-releasing hormone (CRH) syndrome**
6. **Food-dependent CS**
7. **Iatrogenic** (therapy in asthma and rheumatoid arthritis)

Diagnoses 1 and 3 are collectively referred to as **corticotropin-dependent CS**. Patients typically have elevated serum ACTH (see Adrenocorticotropic Hormone, Plasma *on page 86*) and hyperplastic adrenals. Specialized tests include Corticotropin-Releasing Hormone Stimulation Test *on page 152*, in which patients with CD have an exaggerated cortisol and ACTH response; Metyrapone Stimulation Test, Serum *on page 225*, in which patients with CD will have a marked increase in serum 11-deoxycortisol and ACTH; and the **high-dose dexamethasone suppression test** in which approximately 60% to 70% of patients with CD will have a diagnostic decrease in urine free cortisol.

The **ectopic corticotropin syndrome** (ECS), with elevated cortisol and ACTH levels, occurs in patients with various neuroendocrine neoplasms. Classically, the very elevated ACTH levels are resistant to **high-dose dexamethasone suppression testing**, and the **metyrapone stimulation test** demonstrates no significant increase in serum 11-deoxycortisol. Small cell lung carcinoma accounts for 75% to 80% of ECS cases, and these patients usually present with an acute syndrome (hypokalemia, edema, glucose intolerance, and hypertension) that is not a diagnostic problem. The other 20% to 25% of patients have carcinoid tumors, or other neuroendocrine neoplasms, and a clinical presentation much like CD. When the differential is ECS vs CD, a very effective procedure is to measure the basal and the CRH-stimulated serum ACTH gradient (ratio) between the inferior petrosal sinuses and a peripheral vein; patients with CD have a twofold or higher basal gradient, and a threefold or higher stimulated gradient.[1] (See Corticotropin-Releasing Hormone Stimulation Test *on page 152*.) Other useful procedures are the Metyrapone Stimulation Test, Serum *on page 225*, the low-dose and high-dose dexamethasone suppression test, or a protocol that combines metyrapone and dexamethasone testing.[2,3,4]

Diagnoses 2, 5, and 6 are collectively referred to as **corticotropin-independent CS**. Patients with adrenal adenoma or carcinoma have elevated serum cortisol and low or absent serum ACTH. These patients classically show no suppression of cortisol secretion in the **high-dose dexamethasone suppression test**.

Food-dependent CS, a member of the promiscuous receptor disease family, is a very rare entity in which the diurnal rhythm of cortisol secretion is inverted: low in the early morning, with marked increases following food ingestion. These patients have low or absent serum ACTH and macronodular adrenal hyperplasia. Food-dependent CS appears to be due to an inappropriately heightened sensitivity of adrenal cortical cells to normal postprandial increases in gastric inhibitory polypeptide.[5,6,7]

The **ectopic CRH syndrome** clinically resembles the ectopic corticotropin syndrome. Serum ACTH is elevated and, in typical cases, suppressed in the high-dose dexamethasone suppression test. The anatomic substrate is usually a bronchial carcinoid.

Pseudo-CS is a heterogeneous grouping which includes patients with one or more of the following putatively nonendocrine disorders: depression, chronic alcoholism, severe obesity, eating disorder, hypertension, and hirsutism. The biochemical diagnosis of pseudo-CS, an exercise in exclusion, is facilitated by one or more of the following tests:

- midnight serum cortisol (values >7.5 µg/dL (SI: >207 nmol/L) suggest CD)
- sequential CRH-dexamethasone stimulation test (pseudo-CS patients have markedly decreased cortisol after dexamethasone, and CS patients have a markedly increased response to CRH)[8]
- naloxone stimulation test (CS patients release less ACTH and cortisol in response to the opioid antagonist, naloxone)[9]
- loperamide inhibition test (pseudo-CS patients have a marked decrease in serum cortisol following loperamide hydrochloride, an opiate agonist)[10,11]
- insulin tolerance test (serum cortisol increases in pseudo-CS, but not in CS)[3]

Adrenal Insufficiency (AI)

Adrenal insufficiency (AI) refers to any disorder in which the adrenal secretion of cortisol is insufficient for metabolic needs. AI is a potentially life-threatening condition. Successful diagnosis and management requires an experienced clinician who can integrate both clinical and laboratory information. Reliance on only one category of information can lead to disastrous consequences for the patient. Anatomically, AI may be primary (disease in the adrenals) or secondary (disease in the pituitary or hypothalamus). The clinical onset may be abrupt (acute AI) or gradual (chronic AI).[12]

Chronic primary AI (Addison disease) refers to destruction of the adrenals by neoplasm, infection (including AIDS, tuberculosis, and histoplasmosis), autoimmune disease, amyloidosis, postbilateral adrenalectomy, or a metabolic process (adrenomyeloneuropathy and adrenoleukodystrophy). Patients have increased **serum ACTH** and hyperpigmentation of the skin. 21-hydroxylase autoantibodies are markers for autoimmune Addison disease.[13,14] See 21-Hydroxylase Antibodies, Serum *on page 530*.

The disorders grouped as **congenital adrenal hyperplasia** include 21-hydroxylase deficiency and others, recently reviewed and tabulated by Levine and DiGeorge. They include abnormalities of ACTH, corticosteroids, renin, 17-OH progesterone, androgens, potassium, and other assays.[15] These autosomal recessive diseases are included here since adrenocortical insufficiency is present in some. See 17-Hydroxyprogesterone, Serum or Plasma *on page 197* and the Key Word Index.

Acute primary AI is usually due to adrenal hemorrhage and/or necrosis; the differential diagnosis includes meningococcemia, anticoagulant therapy, thrombosis due to a thrombophilic state, and (very rarely) a procoagulant defect. The **serum cortisol** is low and the **ACTH** high.

Chronic secondary AI is caused by cessation of long-term glucocorticoid therapy, neoplasms involving the pituitary or hypothalamus, surgical procedures in the pituitary region, and involvement of the pituitary by granulomatous disease, autoimmune inflammation, and Langerhans cell histiocytosis. Findings are similar to those in chronic primary AI, except that serum ACTH is low and there is no hyperpigmentation.

Acute secondary AI is usually caused by hemorrhage or necrosis involving the pituitary/hypothalamic region. The differential diagnosis includes anticoagulant therapy, thrombosis due to a thrombophilic state, surgical procedures in the pituitary or hypothalamus, and (very rarely) a procoagulant defect. The serum cortisol and ACTH are low.

The diagnosis of AI is confirmed if the **basal morning serum cortisol** is <5.0 µg/dL (SI: 140 nmol/L).[16] Some authorities use a more conservative value of <3.1 µg/dL (SI: <86 nmol/L).[12] If the AI is primary, **serum ACTH** is >100 pg/mL (SI: 22 pmol/L).[12] A random serum cortisol >20 µg/dL (SI: >550 nmol/L) excludes the diagnosis of AI, **but only in an "unstressed" patient.** Increased secretion of cortisol is a normal response to the metabolic requirements imposed by sepsis, trauma, systemic neoplasm, and surgical procedures (collectively referred to as stress).[17] Therefore, in a patient whose basal morning cortisol is >3.1 µg/dL (SI: >86 nmol/L), or who is stressed (as defined above), a dynamic test is required to make a biochemical diagnosis of AI.

The most commonly used dynamic test to evaluate AI is the Corticotropin Stimulation Test (Rapid) *on page 153*. There are two protocols: a high-dose protocol (using a pharmacologic dose),[18] and a low-dose protocol (using a physiologic dose).[19,20,21,22] The high-dose test correctly identifies patients with primary AI, but false-negative results are a problem in patients with secondary AI. The low-dose test is the more sensitive procedure and is preferred. Additional dynamic tests include the Metyrapone Stimulation Test, Serum *on page 225* and the Insulin Tolerance Test *on page 202*.

A recently described test for AI is the Urinary Cortisol/Creatinine Increment *on page 296*. This procedure, which is noninvasive and performed at home, uses sleep as a stimulus for ACTH release.[23]

The **insulin tolerance test (ITT)** is usually regarded as the gold standard for evaluation of the hypothalamic-pituitary axis (HPA).[24] In this procedure, insulin-induced hypoglycemia stimulates hypothalamic corticotropin-releasing hormone (CRH), and this produces increases in ACTH and cortisol.

Metyrapone is a testing agent which metabolically inhibits the synthesis of cortisol at the 11-deoxycortisol step. When this agent is given to a person whose HPA is functionally intact, the serum ACTH and 11-deoxycortisol increase, and the serum cortisol decreases. An impaired response to the metyrapone stimulation test is seen in patients with pituitary or hypothalamic disease, as well as some cases of Cushing syndrome. When testing patients for secondary AI, the ITT is less sensitive than the metyrapone stimulation test.

ALDOSTERONE-RELATED DISORDERS

Primary Hyperaldosteronism (PH)

PH (Conn syndrome) refers to a group of disorders which share characteristic features: hypertension, hypokalemia, urine potassium >30 mmol/day, metabolic alkalosis, elevated serum aldosterone, and low serum renin. Despite such unifying features, PH has significant clinical and biochemical diversity. It is important to avoid basing a diagnostic conclusion on one or two findings. In PH, increased aldosterone secretion is autonomous and at least partially independent of the renin-angiotensin system. Helpful diagnostic algorithms are found in Footnotes 25, 26, 27, and 28. PH includes the following differential diagnoses:

- aldosterone-producing adenoma (APA) of the adrenal cortex (65%)
- idiopathic adrenal hyperplasia (IAH) (30%)
- glucocorticoid-remediable aldosteronism (GRA) (rare)
- adrenal carcinoma (very rare)
- ectopic aldosterone-secreting tumor (very rare)[29,30]

Biochemical confirmation of diagnoses 1, 2, and 4 may be obtained from several different dynamic tests, each of which involves manipulating the renin-angiotensin system and using serum aldosterone as the end point. Maneuvers that normally increase renin (eg, upright posture, sodium restriction, furosemide diuresis, or infusion of angiotensin II) fail to increase aldosterone in patients with PH. Maneuvers that normally decrease renin (eg, supine posture, saline infusion) fail to suppress aldosterone in PH. The **ratio of serum aldosterone to plasma renin** is >50 in PH patients.[26] A ratio >30 deserves further evaluation.[29]

Patients with PH, after 3 days of a high sodium diet (urine Na >250 mmol/day), have 24-hour urine aldosterone values >14 µg/day (SI: >38.9 nmol/day).[26]

It is important to emphasize that as many as 20% of total APA cases have a normal aldosterone response to angiotensin II, but otherwise are typical.[29] The biochemical findings of PH can be closely simulated in patients who are taking thiazide diuretics.[26] Confounding test results also occur in patients taking angiotensin-converting enzyme inhibitors and calcium channel blockers. It is recommended that antihypertensive medications be discontinued for at least 2, and preferably 4, weeks before biochemical testing for PH.[26]

IAH is a poorly defined diagnostic category. Classical patients with IAH may have findings similar to classical APA, but others (78% in one recent series)[30] have increased aldosterone in response to angiotensin II. Many, or even most, patients with IAH may actually have essential hypertension.[31]

The diagnosis and treatment of **GRA**, an autosomal dominant inherited condition, requires recognition that the hyperaldosteronism is produced by ACTH and responds to treatment with dexamethasone.[25,27]

Secondary hyperaldosteronism is not a disease entity but a physiological adaption to a variety of disease processes which have decreased "effective" blood volume as a common denominator. Examples include diseases associated with edema formation: congestive heart failure, cirrhosis, and nephrotic syndrome. In addition, secondary hyperaldosteronism occurs in patients with renal artery stenosis and renin-secreting tumors, possibly reflecting situations in which blood volume "seems" reduced at the level of the juxtaglomerular apparatus and afferent arteriole, even though actual blood volume is normal. In none of these diseases is aldosterone the primary abnormality. Moreover, the clinical and biochemical alterations, apart from elevated aldosterone, are completely different from PH.

Additional Information Chromosomal markers are recognized in several familial adrenal syndromes, including multiple endocrine neoplasia type 1 and glucocorticoid-remediable hyperaldosteronism.[32]

Footnotes

1. Oldfield EH, Doppman JL, Nieman LK, et al, "Petrosal Sinus Sampling With and Without Corticotropin-Releasing Hormone for the Differential Diagnosis of Cushing's Syndrome," *N Engl J Med*, 1991, 325:897-905 (published erratum *N Engl J Med*, 1992, 326:1172).
2. Avgerinos PC, Yanovski JA, Oldfield EH, et al, "The Metyrapone and Dexamethasone Suppression Tests for the Differential Diagnosis of the Adrenocorticotropin-Dependent Cushing Syndrome: A Comparison," *Ann Intern Med*, 1994, 121(5):318-27.
3. Orth DN, "The Cushing Syndrome: Quest for the Holy Grail," *Ann Intern Med*, 1994, 121(5):377-8.

(Continued)

Adrenal Cortex: Laboratory Assessments Overview
(Continued)

4. Avgerinos PC and Cutler GB, "The Cushing Syndrome," *Ann Intern Med*, 1995, 122(12):959-60.
5. Lacroix A, Bolte E, Tremblay J, et al, "Gastric Inhibitory Polypeptide-Dependent Cortisol Hypersecretion - A New Cause of Cushing's Syndrome," *N Engl J Med*, 1992, 327:974-80.
6. Reznik Y, Allali-Zerah V, Chayvialle JA, et al, "Food-Dependent Cushing's Syndrome Mediated by Aberrant Adrenal Sensitivity to Gastric Inhibitory Polypeptide," *N Engl J Med*, 1992, 327:981-6.
7. Bertagna X, "New Causes of Cushing's Syndrome," *N Engl J Med*, 1992, 327:1024-5.
8. Yanovski JA, Cutler GB, Chrousos GP, et al, "Corticotropin-Releasing Hormone Stimulation Following Low-Dose Dexamethasone Administration," *JAMA*, 1993, 269:2232-8.
9. Jackson RV, Grice JE, Jackson AJ, et al, "Naloxone-Induced ACTH Release in Man Is Inhibited by Clonidine," *Clin Exp Pharmacol Physiol*, 1990, 17(3):179-84.
10. Ambrosi B, Bochicchio D, Ferrario R, et al, "Effects of the Opiate Agonist Loperamide on Pituitary-Adrenal Function in Patients With Suspected Hypercortisolism," *J Endocrinol Invest*, 1989, 12:31-5.
11. Ambrosi B, Bochicchio D, Colombo P, et al, "Loperamide to Diagnose Cushing's Syndrome," *JAMA*, 1993, 270:2301-2.
12. Oelkers W, "Adrenal Insufficiency," *N Engl J Med*, 1996, 335(16):1206-12.
13. Mayo Medical Laboratories, "21-Hydroxylase Antibodies, Serum," *Mayo Reference Services*, Rochester, MN, 2000.
14. Tanaka H, Perez M, Powell M, et al, "Steroid 21-Hydroxylase Autoantibodies: Measurements With a New Immunoprecipitation Assay," *J Clin Endocrinol Metab*, 1997, 82(5):1440-6.
15. Levine LS and DiGeorge AM, "Disorders of the Adrenal Glands," *Nelson Textbook of Pediatrics*, 16th ed, Behrman RE, Kliegman RM, and Jenson HB, eds, Philadelphia, PA: WB Saunders Co, 2000, 1722-43.
16. Thorner MO, Vance ML, Laws ER Jr, et al, "The Anterior Pituitary," *Williams Textbook of Endocrinology*, 9th ed, Wilson JD, Foster DW, Kronenberg HM, et al, eds, Philadelphia, PA: WB Saunders Co, 1998, 280.
17. Streeten DH, Anderson GH Jr, and Bonaventura MM, "The Potential for Serious Consequences From Misinterpreting Normal Responses to the Rapid Adrenocorticotropin Test," *J Clin Endocrinol Metab*, 1996, 81(1):285-90.
18. Demers LM and Whitley RJ, "Function of the Adrenal Cortex," *Tietz Textbook of Clinical Chemistry*, 3rd ed, Burtis CA and Ashwood ER, eds, Philadelphia, PA: WB Saunders Co, 1999, 1530-69.
19. Tordjman K, Jaffe A, Grazas N, et al, "The Role of Low Dose (1 µg) Adrenocorticotropin Test in the Evaluation of Patients With Pituitary Diseases," *J Clin Endocrinol Metab*, 1995, 80(4):1301-5.
20. Broide J, Soferman R, Kivity S, et al, "Low-Dose Adrenocorticotropin Test Reveals Impaired Adrenal Function in Patients Taking Inhaled Corticosteroids," *J Clin Endocrinol Metab*, 1995, 80(4):1243-6.
21. Thaler LM and Blevins LS, "The Low Dose (1 µg) Adrenocorticotropin Stimulation Test in the Evaluation of Patients With Suspected Central Adrenal Insufficiency," *J Clin Endocrinol Metab*, 1998, 83(8):2726-9.
22. Henzen C, Suter A, Lerch E, et al, "Suppression and Recovery of Adrenal Response After Short-Term, High-Dose Glucocorticoid Treatment," *Lancet*, 2000, 355(9203):542-5.
23. Kong WM, Alaghband-Zadeh J, Jones J, et al, "The Midnight to Morning Urinary Cortisol Increment Is an Accurate, Noninvasive Method for Assessment of the Hypothalamic-Pituitary-Adrenal Axis," *J Clin Endocrinol Metab*, 1999, 84:3093-8.
24. Plumpton FS and Besser GM, "The Adrenocortical Response to Surgery and Insulin-Induced Hypoglycemia in Corticosteroid-Treated and Normal Subjects," *Br J Surg*, 1969, 56(3):216-9.
25. Stewart PM, "Mineralocorticoid Hypertension," *Lancet*, 1999, 353(9161):1341-7.
26. Blumenfeld JD, Sealey JE, Schlussel Y, et al, "Diagnosis and Treatment of Primary Hyperaldosteronism," *Ann Intern Med*, 1994, 121(11):877-85.
27. Dluhy RG and Williams GH, "Endocrine Hypertension," *Williams Textbook of Endocrinology*, 9th ed, Wilson JD, Foster DW, Kronenberg HM, et al, eds, Philadelphia, PA: WB Saunders Co, 1998, 740-4.
28. Desai SP and Isa-Pratt S, "Adrenal Cortical Function Tests," *Clinician's Guide to Laboratory Medicine*, Cleveland, OH: Lexi-Comp, 2000, 334-7.
29. Ganguly A, "Primary Aldosteronism," *N Engl J Med*, 1998, 339(25):1828-34.
30. Abdelhamid S, Muller-Lobeck H, Pahl S, et al, "Prevalence of Adrenal and Extraadrenal Conn Syndrome in Hypertensive Patients," *Arch Intern Med*, 1996, 156(11):1190-5.
31. "Idiopathic Aldosteronism: A Diagnostic Artifact?" *Lancet*, 1979, 2:1221-2.
32. Bornstein SR, Stratakis CA, and Chrousos GP, "Adrenocortical Tumors: Recent Advances in Basic Concepts and Clinical Management," *Ann Intern Med*, 1999, 130(9):759-71.

References

Arioglu E, Doppman J, Gomes M, et al, "Cushing's Syndrome Caused by Corticotropin Secretion by Pulmonary Tumorlets," *N Engl J Med*, 1998, 339(13):883-6.
Brandt LJ and Mark EJ, "A 64-Year-Old Man With Cushing's Syndrome and a Pancreatic Mass," Case Records of the Massachusetts General Hospital, Case 4-2000, Scully RE, Mark EJ, McNeely WF, et al, eds, *N Engl J Med*, 2000, 342(6):414-20.
Brosnan PG, Brosnan CA, Kemp SF, et al, "Effect of Newborn Screening for Congenital Adrenal Hyperplasia," *Arch Pediatr Adolesc Med*, 1999, 153(12):1272-8.
Krasner AS, "Glucocorticoid-Induced Adrenal Insufficiency," *JAMA*, 1999, 282(7):671-6.
Lack EE, Askin FB, Dehner LP, et al, Association of Directors of Anatomic and Surgical Pathology, "Recommendations for Reporting of Tumors of the Adrenal Cortex and Medulla," *Am J Clin Pathol*, 1999, 112(4):451-55.
Orth DN and Kovacs WJ, "The Adrenal Cortex," *Williams Textbook of Endocrinology*, 9th ed, Wilson JD, Foster DW, Kronenberg HM, et al, eds, Philadelphia, PA: WB Saunders Co, 1998, 517-664.
White PC, "Disorders of Aldosterone Biosynthesis and Action," *N Engl J Med*, 1994, 331:250-8.

Adrenocorticotropic Hormone, Plasma

Related Information

Adrenal Cortex: Laboratory Assessments Overview *on page 84*
Corticotropin-Releasing Hormone Stimulation Test *on page 152*
Corticotropin Stimulation Test (Rapid) *on page 153*
Cortisol, Free, Urine *on page 154*
Cortisol, Serum or Plasma *on page 154*
Growth Hormone, Serum *on page 189*
Metyrapone Stimulation Test, Serum *on page 225*
Testosterone, Total and Free, Serum or Plasma *on page 280*
Urinary Cortisol/Creatinine Increment *on page 296*

Synonyms ACTH; Corticotropin

Applies to Dexamethasone Suppression

Abstract Adrenocorticotropic hormone (ACTH), secreted by the anterior pituitary, is the second step in the hypothalamic-pituitary-adrenal axis. Hypothalamic corticotropin-releasing hormone (CRH) stimulates the secretion of ACTH which, in turn, stimulates the secretion from the adrenal cortex of cortisol, adrenal androgens, and mineralocorticoids.

Specimen Plasma

Container Use chilled syringe. Use two lavender top (EDTA) tubes previously cooled in ice. (Check with laboratory for appropriate container.)

Sampling Time ACTH is normally characterized by diurnal variation. Peak values occur in the morning. Normal secretion, as well as that in Cushing disease, is pulsatile and so may require multiple samples.[1] For sequential follow-up, ACTH should always be drawn at the same time each day.

Collection Samples for demonstration of the normal circadian rhythm should be drawn between 6 AM and 10 AM and between 9 PM and midnight. Simultaneously obtained cortisol levels may be helpful. Transport specimen **immediately** to the laboratory following collection.

Storage Instructions Separate plasma in refrigerated centrifuge and freeze immediately. Store frozen at -70°C in plastic tubes. Aprotinin (Trasylol®) 500 kU/mL should be added for long-term storage.

Reference Interval
- Cord blood:[2] 50-570 pg/mL (SI: 11-125 pmol/L)
- Newborns:[2] 10-185 pg/mL (SI: 2.2-41 pmol/L)
- Adults, 8 AM:[2] <120 pg/mL (SI: <26.0 pmol/L)
- Adults, 8 AM (ICMA[3]): 10-60 pg/mL (SI: 2.2-13.2 pmol/L)

Clinical Diagnosis of Cushing Syndrome

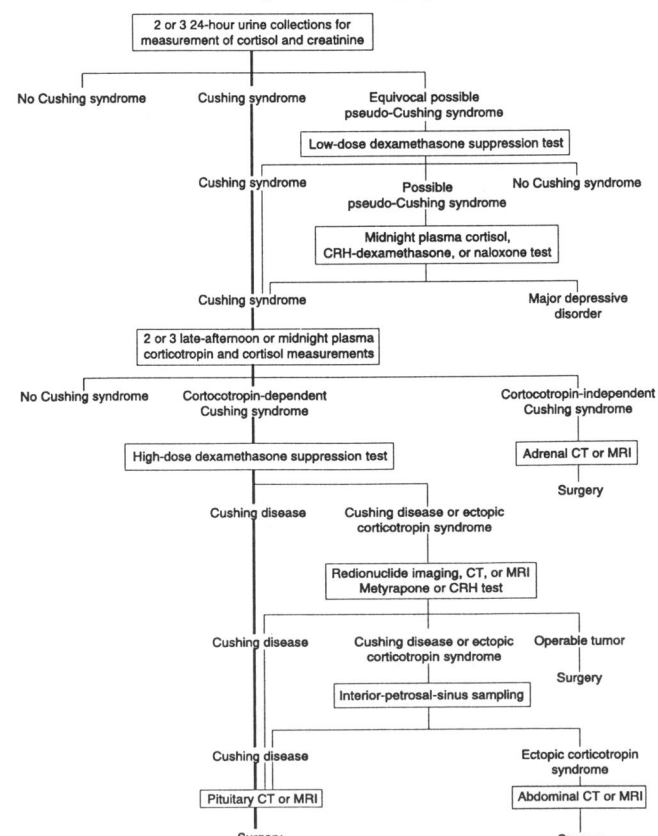

An approach to the diagnosis of Cushing syndrome and its cause. The heavy line indicates the diagnostic path for the majority of patients who have Cushing disease. CT denotes computed tomography and MRI magnetic resonance imaging.

Adapted from Orth DN, "Cushing's Syndrome," *N Engl J Med*, 1995, 332(12):795..

Use Evaluate the etiology of Cushing syndrome; differentiate pituitary from other causes of corticosteroid excess and deficiency syndromes (ie, distinguish corticotropin-dependent from corticotropin-independent Cushing syndrome); evaluate ectopic ACTH production by neoplasms; examine results of transsphenoidal surgery; follow up patients after bilateral adrenalectomy; for diagnosis of Nelson syndrome. (Nelson syndrome consists of a tumor of the anterior pituitary gland and skin pigmentation following bilateral adrenalectomy.) Evaluate secondary hypopituitarism (target gland failures secondary to lack of stimulation by a pituitary hormone like ACTH). Increased ACTH concentrations in a subject with hypocortisolism signal primary adrenocortical insufficiency. A suppressed level in a patient with Cushing syndrome or hypercortisolism is consistent with cortisol-producing adrenocortical adenoma or carcinoma, with primary adrenocortical micronodular hyperplasia, or with use of exogenous corticosteroids. A normal to increased concentration in a subject with Cushing syndrome is in keeping with ACTH-dependent Cushing syndrome, caused by ACTH production from an adenoma of the anterior pituitary or by an ectopic source of ACTH [eg, small cell carcinoma of lung, carcinoid (especially those of lung or thymus)]. Cushing syndrome sometimes coexists with gastrinoma, multiple endocrine neoplasia syndrome, and Zollinger-Ellison syndrome. Evaluate hirsutism (see Lima et al, 1997).

Limitations A single determination may be within normal limits in patients with either excessive production (Cushing disease) or borderline deficiency. ACTH level is affected by stress, which may obscure the normal diurnal and pulsatile changes. ACTH level must be correlated with cortisol levels. Rarely, in cases of the ectopic ACTH syndrome, increased ACTH can be metabolically active but not detected by the assay used.

Other useful tests include low-dose dexamethasone suppression test, high-dose dexamethasone suppression tests, metyrapone stimulation test, and petrosal venous sinus catheterization (see below and Adrenal Cortex: Laboratory Assessments Overview *on page 84*).

Methodology Radioimmunoassay (RIA) after separatory step and immunoradiometric assay (IRMA), immunochemiluminometric assay (ICMA).

Additional Information See Adrenal Cortex: Laboratory Assessments Overview *on page 84*. See algorithm on previous page for diagnosis of Cushing syndrome.

Footnotes

1. Gudmundsson A and Carnes M, "Pulsatile Adrenocorticotropic Hormone: An Overview," *Biol Psychiatry*, 1997, 41(3):342-65.
2. Painter PC, Cope JY, and Smith JL, "Reference Information for the Clinical Laboratory," *Tietz Textbook of Clinical Chemistry*, 3rd ed, Burtis CA and Ashwood ER, eds, Philadelphia, PA: WB Saunders Co, 1999.
3. Mayo Medical Laboratories, "Adrenocorticotropic Hormone Test Update," Rochester, MN, July 2000.

References

Desai SP and Isa-Pratt S, *Clinician's Guide to Laboratory Medicine*, Cleveland, OH: Lexi-Comp, 2000, Chapters 17, 20.

Gennari FJ, "Hypokalemia," *N Engl J Med*, 1998, 339(7):451-8.

Lima MF, Nunes MG, Bonduki CE, et al, "The ACTH Test in the Diagnosis of Hirsutism," *Rev Paul Med*, 1997, 115(2):1403-5.

Magiakou MA, Mastorakos G, Oldfield EH, et al, "Cushing's Syndrome in Children and Adolescents: Presentation, Diagnosis, and Therapy," *N Engl J Med*, 1994, 331(10):629-36.

Midgette AS and Aron DC, "High-Dose Dexamethasone Suppression Testing Versus Inferior Petrosal Sinus Sampling in the Differential Diagnosis of Adrenocorticotropin-Dependent Cushing's Syndrome: A Decision Analysis," *Am J Med Sci*, 1995, 309(3):162-70.

Orth DN, "The Cushing Syndrome: Quest for the Holy Grail," *Ann Intern Med*, 1994, 121(5):377-8.

Perlitz Y, Varkel J, Markovitz J, et al, "Acute Adrenal Insufficiency During Pregnancy and Puerperium: Case Report and Literature Review," *Obstet Gynecol Surv*, 1999, 54(11):717-22.

Redei E, Rittenhouse PA, Revskoy S, et al, "A Novel Endogenous Corticotropin Release Inhibiting Factor," *Ann N Y Acad Sci*, 1998, 840:456-69.

Siegel SF, Finegold DN, Lanes R, et al, "ACTH Stimulation Tests and Plasma Dehydroepiandrosterone Sulfate Levels in Women With Hirsutism," *N Engl J Med*, 1990, 323(13):849-54.

Snow K, Jiang NS, and Kao PC, "Biochemical Evaluation of Adrenal Dysfunction: The Laboratory Perspective," *Mayo Clin Proc*, 1992, 67(11):1055-65.

Thaler LM, and Blevins LS Jr, "The Low Dose (1-microgram) Adrenocorticotropin Stimulation Test in the Evaluation of Patients With Suspected Central Adrenal Insufficiency," *J Clin Endocrinol Metab*, 1998 83(8):2726-9.

Vance ML, "Hypopituitarism," *N Engl J Med*, 1994, 330(23):1651-62.

Wickus GG, Pagliara AS, and Caplan RH, "Spurious Elevation of Plasma Immunoreactive Adrenocorticotropic Hormone in Cyclic Cushing's Syndrome," *Arch Pathol Lab Med*, 1989, 113(7):797-9.

♦ **AFP** *see* Alpha₁-Fetoprotein, Serum *on page 97*

♦ **A:G Ratio** *see* Albumin:Globulin Ratio, Serum *on page 88*

♦ **ALA** *see* Delta (5)-Aminolevulinic Acid, Urine *on page 165*

♦ **ALA Dehydratase** *see* Delta (5)-Aminolevulinic Acid, Urine *on page 165*

Alanine Aminotransferase, Serum

Related Information

Synonyms ALT; Glutamic Pyruvate Transaminase; GPT; L-Alanine-2-Oxoglutarate Aminotransferase, Serum; SGPT; Transaminase

Applies to Aminotransferases; AST:ALT Ratio

Replaces Cephalin Flocculation; Isocitric Dehydrogenase; Thymol Turbidity

Abstract Of the aminotransferases, AST and ALT are important, widely used enzymes. Increases over tenfold occur in some cases of hepatitis and shock. The greatest amount of ALT is in the liver. See table in listing Bilirubin, Total, Serum *on page 118*, Table 2 in Liver Biopsy *on page 65*, and the table in Liver Disease: Laboratory Assessment, Overview *on page 216*.

Patient Preparation Strenuous exercise can cause elevation.

Specimen Serum; plasma may be used.

Container Red top tube; green top (heparin) tube for plasma

Storage Instructions Stable 1 day at 25°C and 3 days at 4°C; refrigeration is preferable to freezing.

Causes for Rejection Excessive hemolysis

Reference Interval Slightly increased ranges in infancy compared to adult normal range.

- Male: 10-40 units/L (SI: 0.17-0.68 µkat/L)
- Female: 8-35 units/L (SI: 0.14-0.6 µkat/L)

Use A liver function test, ALT is more sensitive for detection of hepatocyte injury than for biliary obstruction. ALT is more specific for liver injury than is AST (SGOT). Causes of chronic increases of aminotransferase concentrations include alcohol abuse, medications, chronic hepatitis B and C, steatosis and nonalcoholic steatohepatitis, hepatic fibrosis, cirrhosis, autoimmune hepatitis, hemochromatosis, Wilson disease in subjects 40 years of age and younger, and alpha₁-antitrypsin deficiency. AST and ALT levels are elevated before signs or symptoms of viral hepatitis appear. Increased with AST in Reye syndrome. Screening test for hepatitis; acute hepatitis A, B, and C can be confirmed serologically. Negative serological findings in the presence of hepatitis-like chemical abnormalities may suggest acute drug-induced hepatitis, an impression supported by resolution after removal of the offending agent.[1] The combination of increased AST and ALT with negative hepatitis markers occurs in a number of other entities, including infectious mononucleosis. Correlating ALT levels with liver cell necrosis in hepatitis C virus - associated cirrhosis, ALT has been proposed as a marker for risk of development of hepatocellular carcinoma in this patient group.[2]

Both AST and ALT are increased after liver cell injury but ALT elevations are more specific for liver cell damage. Increased AST and triglycerides are the most reliable markers for hepatic steatosis.[3] ALT equals or exceeds AST level in nonalcoholic steatohepatitis.[4] AST is increased after myocardial infarction but ALT usually is not. As liver function tests, the transaminases play a role in evaluation of inborn errors of metabolism.

Causes of chronic elevations not deriving from the liver include celiac sprue and inherited and acquired disorders of striated muscle.

Limitations Grossly hemolyzed samples can generate somewhat spurious results. The activity in red cells is six times that of serum. Elevations are found in trauma to striated muscle, rhabdomyolysis, polymyositis, and dermatomyositis, but CK (CK-MM fraction) is increased in such patients and is preferable for evaluation of diseases of skeletal muscle. ALT is less sensitive than is AST to alcoholic liver disease and can even be within normal range in the presence of severe alcohol abuse. Increased ALT is found with obesity. Although ALT is used to select hepatitis C virus-infected subjects for therapy and liver biopsy, high visit-to-visit variability is reported; ALT is not consistently elevated with hepatitis C.[5,6]

Drugs: A few agents can cause a decrease by some methods (eg, metronidazole). A large number of drugs can cause an increase, including acyclovir; allopurinol; antibiotics including synthetic penicillins, ciprofloxacin, nitrofurantoin, ketoconazole, fluconazole, and isoniazid; carbamazepine; carbenicillin; cefoxitin; chloramphenicol; dicumarol; diethylstilbestrol; doxorubicin; erythromycin; esterified estrogens; flutamide; furosemide; gentamicin; inhibitors of hydroxymethylglutaryl-coenzyme A reductase including simvastatin, pravastatin, lovastatin, and atorvastatin; ibuprofen; interleukin-
(Continued)

Alanine Aminotransferase, Serum *(Continued)*

2; mefenamic acid; meprobamate; methotrexate; methyldopa; methyltestosterone; naproxen; nonsteroidal anti-inflammatory drugs such as acetaminophen and aminosalicylic acid; phenobarbital; phenothiazine; phenytoin; progesterone; propranolol; pyrazinamide; rifampin; sulfa drugs; sulfonylureas for hypoglycemia (eg, glipizide); thiazides; ticarcillin; tolbutamide; trimethoprim; troleandomycin; valproic acid; zidovudine; and many others.[7]

Herbs and homeopathic treatments including Chinese herbs may cause elevations.

Drugs/substances of abuse causing increases include anabolic steroids, cocaine, "ecstasy" (see 3,4 Methylenedioxymethamphetamine, Urine *on page 801*), "angel dust" (see Phencyclidine, Qualitative, Urine *on page 804*), glues and solvents containing toluene, trichlorethylene, and chloroform.

Methodology Spectrophotometry by rate assay

Additional Information Among entities in which AST and ALT increases occur are therapeutic applications of bovine or porcine heparin. LD (LDH) abnormality with elevation of hepatic fractions has also been reported.

In children with acute lymphoblastic leukemia, high ALT activity at diagnosis is associated with rapidly progressive ALL.[8]

Acetaminophen hepatotoxicity may be potentiated in alcoholics, the alcohol-acetaminophen syndrome, in which coagulopathy and extremely abnormal ALT and AST are found.[9] The ALT and AST, about 9000 units/L in a study, distinguish the alcohol-acetaminophen syndrome from alcoholic or viral hepatitis. Such levels are found with overdose as well.[8]

AST:ALT ratios are highest in alcoholic liver disease, typically at least 2:1, but are often above unity in nonalcoholic cirrhosis. Of ratios >3:1, >96% of patients have alcoholic liver disease. AST > ALT is reported with typhoid fever.[10] AST:ALT ratios are commonly 0.5-0.8 with acute and chronic viral hepatitis.[11] (See Aspartate Aminotransferase, Serum *on page 112*.)

Footnotes

1. Frank BB and Members of the Patient Care Committee of the American Gastroenterological Association, "Clinical Evaluation of Jaundice - A Guideline of the Patient Care Committee of the American Gastroenterological Association," *JAMA*, 1989, 262(21):3031-4.
2. Tarao K, Rino Y, Ohkawa S, et al, "Association Between High Serum Alanine Aminotransferase Levels and More Rapid Development and Higher Rate of Incidence of Hepatocellular Carcinoma in Patients With Hepatitis C Virus-Associated Cirrhosis," *Cancer*, 1999, 86(4):589-95.
3. Bellentani S, Saccoccio G, Masutti F, et al, "Prevalence of and Risk Factors for Hepatic Steatosis in Northern Italy," *Ann Intern Med*, 2000, 132(2):112-7.
4. James O and Day C, "Nonalcoholic Steatohepatitis; Another Disease of Affluence," *Lancet*, 1999, 353(9165):1634-6.
5. Inglesby TV, Rai R, Astemborski J, et al, "A Prospective Community-Based Evaluation of Liver Enzymes in Individuals With Hepatitis C After Drug Use," *Hepatology*, 1999, 29(2):590-6.
6. Zylberberg H, Pol S, Thiers V, et al, "Significance of Repeatedly Normal Aminotransferase Activities in HCV-Infected Patients," *J Clin Gastroenterol*, 1999, 29(1):71-5.
7. Young DS, *Effects of Drugs on Clinical Laboratory Tests*, 5th ed, Volume 1: Listing by Test, Washington, DC: AACC Press, American Association of Clinical Chemistry, 2000, Section 3, 8-23.
8. Rautonen J and Siimes MA, "Elevated Serum Transaminase Activity at Diagnosis Is Associated With Rapidly Progressing Disease in Children With Acute Lymphoblastic Leukemia," *Cancer*, 1988, 61(4):754-7.
9. Seeff LB, Cuccherini BA, Zimmerman HJ, et al, "Acetaminophen Hepatotoxicity in Alcoholics, a Therapeutic Misadventure" *Ann Intern Med*, 1986, 104(3):399-404.
10. Kamath PS, Jalihal A, and Chakraborty A, "Differentiation of Typhoid Fever From Fulminant Hepatic Failure in Patients Presenting With Jaundice and Encephalopathy," *Mayo Clin Proc*, 2000, 75(5):462-6.
11. Williams AL and Hoofnagle JH, "Ratio of Serum Aspartate to Alanine Aminotransferase in Chronic Hepatitis. Relationship to Cirrhosis," *Gastroenterology*, 1988, 95(3):734-9.

References

Andrei VE, Schein M, Margolis M, et al, "Liver Enzymes Are Commonly Elevated Following Laparoscopic Cholecystectomy: Is Elevated Intra-abdominal Pressure the Cause?" *Dig Surg*, 1998, 15(3):256-9.

Berasain C, Betes M, Panizo A, et al, "Pathological and Virological Findings in Patients With Persistent Hypertransaminasaemia of Unknown Aetiology," *Gut*, 2000, 47(3)429-35.

Halevy A, Gold-Deutch R, Negri M, et al, "Are Elevated Liver Enzymes and Bilirubin Levels Significant After Laparoscopic Cholecystectomy in the Absence of Bile Duct Injury?" *Ann Surg*, 1994, 219(4):362-4.

Herlong HF, "Approach to the Patient With Abnormal Liver Enzymes," *Hosp Pract*, 1994, 29(11):32-8.

Mathiesen UL, Franzen LE, Fryden A, et al, "The Clinical Significance of Slightly to Moderately Increased Transaminase Values in Asymptomatic Patients," *Scand J Gastroenterol*, 1999, 34(1):85-91.

Patwardhan RV, Smith OJ, and Farmelant MH, "Serum Transaminase Levels and Cholescintigraphic Abnormalities in Acute Biliary Tract Obstruction," *Arch Intern Med*, 1987, 147(7):1249-53.

Pratt DS and Kaplan MM, "Evaluation of Abnormal Liver-Enzyme Results in Asymptomatic Patients," *N Engl J Med*, 2000, 342(17):1266-71.

♦ **Albumin, Ascites Fluid** *see* Body Fluid Chemical Analysis *on page 123*

♦ **Albumin:Globulin Ratio** *see* Albumin, Serum *on page 88*

Albumin:Globulin Ratio, Serum

Related Information
Albumin, Serum *on page 88*
Protein Electrophoresis, Capillary Zone *on page 266*
Protein Electrophoresis, Serum *on page 267*
Protein, Quantitative, Urine *on page 883*
Protein, Total, Serum *on page 269*

Synonyms A:G Ratio

Test Includes Total protein, albumin, A:G ratio

Abstract The A:G ratio is a calculation derived from total protein and albumin measurements. Principally of historic interest, it was used to detect abnormalities in serum protein composition. Information from the A:G ratio alone is rarely useful in contemporary practice.

Specimen Serum or plasma

Container Red top tube or green top (heparin) tube

Reference Interval Generally, ratios ≥1 are expected. Interpretation is confounded, however, by different analytical methods. A:G ratios are much higher by capillary zone electrophoresis than by agarose gel electrophoresis.[1]

Use Low A:G ratio is found in cirrhosis and other liver diseases, chronic glomerulonephritis and nephrotic syndromes, myeloma, macroglobulinemia of Waldenström, sarcoidosis and other granulomatous diseases, connective tissue diseases, severe infections, cachexia, burns, ulcerative colitis and other chronic inflammatory states. Elevated ratios are usually clinically insignificant.

Limitations The A:G ratio lacks specificity. Electrophoresis provides considerably more information.

Methodology Electrophoretic or chemically determined albumin divided by [total protein minus albumin]

Additional Information Total protein minus albumin equals globulins. Albumin divided by globulins equals the ratio.

Footnotes

1. Katzmann JA, Clark R, Sanders E, et al, "Prospective Study of Serum Protein Capillary Zone Electrophoresis and Immunotyping of Monoclonal Proteins by Immunosubtraction," *Am J Clin Pathol*, 1998, 110(4):503-9.

Albumin, Serum

Related Information
Albumin:Globulin Ratio, Serum *on page 88*
Anion Gap, Serum, Plasma, or Urine *on page 106*
C-Reactive Protein, Serum *on page 523*
Liver Disease: Laboratory Assessment, Overview *on page 216*
Protein Electrophoresis, Capillary Zone *on page 266*
Protein Electrophoresis, Serum *on page 267*
Protein, Quantitative, Urine *on page 883*
Protein, Total, Serum *on page 269*
Zinc, Serum *on page 824*

Applies to Albumin:Globulin Ratio

Abstract Albumin is the most abundant protein in human plasma, constituting 55% to 65% of total protein. Serum albumin is synthesized in the liver. It is lower in liver disease, malnutrition, malabsorption (decreased synthesis), and in renal disease (increased loss in urine in diseases including nephrotic syndrome, chronic glomerulonephritis, diabetes mellitus).

Specimen Serum

Container Red top tube

Reference Interval 0-1 year: 2.9-5.5 g/dL (SI: 29-55 g/L); 1-31 years: 3.5-4.8 g/dL (SI: 35-50 g/L) with A:G ratio >1. After age 40, the interval decreases. By serum protein electrophoresis in agarose gel, the interval is 3.1-4.6 g/dL. Capillary zone electrophoresis provides 3.7-5.2.[1]

Possible Panic Range <1.5 g/dL (SI: <15 g/L)

Use Evaluate nutritional status, blood oncotic pressure, liver disease, renal disease with proteinuria and other chronic illnesses. Hypoalbuminemia is reported as an independent risk factor in older subjects for mortality.[2,3] Decreased admission serum albumin in geriatric patients is a predictor of longer hospital stay and less satisfactory outcome.[4,5] Low serum albumin in preoperative patients is a negative predictor of 30-day complications, mortality, and morbidity.[6] Use of C-reactive protein as well provides somewhat better sensitivity and specificity.[7] Among patients presenting with colorectal adenocarcinoma, prognostic indicators include pretreatment serum albumin as well as Dukes' stage, histopathologic differentiation, and patient age.[8]

High albumin indicates dehydration. Look for increase in hemoglobin, hematocrit in such patients.

Low albumin is found with use of intravenous fluids, rapid hydration, overhydration; hemodilution by inappropriate secretion of antidiuretic hormone, cirrhosis, other liver disease, including chronic alcoholism; in pregnancy and with oral contraceptive use; many chronic diseases, including the nephrotic syndromes, neoplasia, protein-losing enteropathies (including Crohn disease and ulcerative colitis), peptic ulcer, thyroid disease, burns, severe skin disease, prolonged immobilization, heart failure, chronic inflammatory entities such as autoimmune diseases and other chronic catabolic states.

Starvation, malabsorption, or malnutrition: In the absence of intravenous fluid therapy and in patients without liver or renal disease, low albumin may be regarded as an indication of inadequate body protein reserves. Serum albumin has a half-life of about 18-20 days. Its half-life is decreased in patients with catabolic states: infection and with protein loss through the kidneys (eg, nephrosis), gastrointestinal tract, and skin (eg, burns). Its prognostic application is most useful in patients with weight loss, anorexia, surgical therapy, hemorrhage, and infection. Total iron binding capacity <240 µg/dL (SI: <43 µmol/L) and/or low transferrin levels would support an impression of inadequate protein reserves. In **severe malnutrition,** albumin may decrease to <2.5 g/dL (SI: <25 g/L).

Albumin levels ≤2.0-2.5 g/dL (SI: ≤20-25 g/L) may be the cause of edema (eg, nephrotic syndrome, protein-losing enteropathies).

Albumin, prealbumin, and transferrin are regarded as "negative" acute phase reactants (ie, these proteins decrease with acute inflammatory/infectious processes).

Hypoalbuminemia can mask the presence of increased anion gap.[9]

Limitations Bromcresol green (BCG) yields higher results than does bromcresol purple (BCP). Albumin concentration appears decreased in highly icteric specimens by HABA method but not by bromocresol green. Ampicillin added *in vitro* interferes with both methods. Salicylates do not interfere with BCG method.[10] Monochromatic measurement of albumin by BCG overestimates albumin in heparinized plasma owing to fibrinogen. The artifact is avoided by using bichromatic wavelengths.[11] Increased albumin-bilirubin complexes (ie, icteric sera) cause an underestimation of albumin in the bromcresol purple method but not in the bromcresol green method.[12]

Albumin levels decrease (<0.5 g/dL) in patients in supine position.

Drugs: Drugs which may cause decrease of albumin include acetaminophen (in severe poisoning), amiodarone, estrogen/progestin therapy in postmenopausal women, interleukin-2, oral contraceptives, phenytoin, prednisone, valproic acid and other agents. Drugs which may cause increase of albumin include other anticonvulsants, furosemide, phenobarbital, prednisolone, and others.[13]

Methodology Bromcresol green (BCG) and bromcresol purple (BCP) are widely used. These dyes measure some alpha-globulins and therefore provide slightly higher values than does serum protein electrophoresis. Albumin can also be measured by turbidimetry or nephelometry.

Additional Information Twenty-four hour urine collection to measure protein loss is helpful in work-up of some patients with hypoalbuminemia.

Although several studies have found correlation between admission albumin, mortality, and hospital stay, there is no evidence that administration of albumin reduces mortality in critically ill patients with hypoalbuminemia.[14,15]

Other tests useful in assessment of nutritional status include serum prealbumin, retinal binding protein, transferrin, iron, absolute lymphocyte count, and vitamin B_{12}/folate levels.

Globulin is generally provided as a calculation by the laboratory: total protein minus albumin = globulin. Total protein and albumin are commonly measured on chemistry profiling instruments. Globulins are measured by serum protein electrophoresis or immunofixation. Quantitative IgA, IgM, and IgG are also more precise.

Footnotes
1. Katzmann JA, Clark R, Sanders E, et al, "Prospective Study of Serum Protein Capillary Zone Electrophoresis and Immunotyping of Monoclonal Proteins by Immunosubtraction," *Am J Clin Pathol*, 1998, 110(4):503-9.
2. Corti MC, Guralnik JM, Salive ME, et al, "Serum Albumin Level and Physical Disability as Predictors of Mortality in Older Persons," *JAMA*, 1994, 272(13):1036-42.
3. Sullivan DH, Sun S, and Walls RC, "Protein-Energy Undernutrition Among Elderly Hospitalized Patients: A Prospective Study," *JAMA*, 1999, 281(21):2013-9.
4. Marinella MA and Markert RJ, "Admission Serum Albumin Level and Length of Hospitalization in Elderly Patients," *South Med J*, 1998, 91(9):851-4.
5. McEllistrum MC, Collins JC, and Powers JS, "Admission Serum Albumin Level as a Predictor of Outcome Among Geriatric Patients," *South Med J*, 1993, 86(12):1360-1.
6. Gibbs J, Cull W, Henderson W, et al, "Preoperative Serum Albumin Level as a Predictor of Operative Mortality and Morbidity: Results From the National VA Surgical Risk Study," *Arch Surg*, 1999, 134(1):36-42.
7. Goransson J, Jonsson S, and Lasson A, "Screening of Concentrations of C-Reactive Protein and Various Plasma Protease Inhibitors Preoperatively for the Prediction of Postoperative Complications," *Eur J Surg*, 1998, 164:89-101.
8. Heys SD, Walker LG, Deehan DJ, et al, "Serum Albumin: A Prognostic Indicator in Patients With Colorectal Cancer," *J R Coll Surg Edinb*, 1998, 43(3):163-8.
9. Figge J, Jabor A, Kaszda A, "Anion Gap and Hypoalbuminemia," *Crit Care Med*, 1998, 26(11):1807-10.
10. Beng CG and Lim KL, "An Improved Automated Method for Determination of Serum Albumin Using Bromcresol Green," *Am J Clin Pathol*, 1973, 59(1):14-21.
11. Hallbach J, Hoffmann GE, and Guder WG, "Overestimation of Albumin in Heparinized Plasma," *Clin Chem*, 1991, 37(4):566-8.
12. Ihara H, Nakamura H, Aoki Y, et al, "Effects of Serum-Isolated vs Synthetic Bilirubin-Albumin Complexes on Dye-Binding Methods for Estimating Serum Albumin," *Clin Chem*, 1991, 37(7):1269-72.
13. Young DS, *Effects of Drugs on Clinical Laboratory Tests*, 5th ed, Volume 1: Listing by Test, Washington, DC: AACC Press, American Association of Clinical Chemistry, 2000, Section 3, 23-32.
14. D'Angio RG, "Is There a Role for Albumin Administration in Nutrition Support?" *Ann Pharmacother*, 1994, 28(4):478-82.
15. Offringa M, "Excess Mortality After Human Albumin Administration in Critically Ill Patients. Clinical and Pathophysiological Evidence Suggests Albumin Is Harmful," *BMJ*, 1998, 317(7153):223-4.

References
Orth SR and Ritz E, "The Nephrotic Syndrome," *N Engl J Med*, 1998, 338(17):1202-11.

♦ **Alcoholism** *see* Carbohydrate-Deficient Transferrin, Serum *on page 134*

♦ **ALD** *see* Aldolase, Plasma or Serum *on page 89*

Aldolase, Plasma or Serum

Related Information
Creatine Kinase, Serum *on page 158*
Duchenne/Becker Muscular Dystrophy DNA Detection *on page 706*
Muscle Biopsy *on page 69*
Myoglobin, Blood, Serum, or Plasma *on page 228*

Synonyms ALD; Fructose Biphosphate Aldolase

Abstract Very high elevations of this enzyme occur in certain diseases of skeletal muscle such as muscular dystrophy and dermatomyositis but not in diseases of neurogenic origin (eg, polio, multiple sclerosis).

Specimen Serum or plasma; plasma is preferred over serum because of possible release of platelet enzyme during clotting.

Container Red top tube, SST™ tube, green top (heparin) tube

Storage Instructions Separate serum and freeze immediately. May be stored at -20°C until analysis. The addition of boric acid will stabilize aldolase.

Causes for Rejection Hemolysis (red cells contain aldolase)

Reference Interval Newborns: up to four times adult levels; age 10-24 months: 3.4-11.8 units/L, 25 months to 16 years: 1.2-8.8 units/L (method of Pinto et al[1]); adults: 1.7-4.9 units/L for assay at 30°C with patient at bedrest. Values are slightly lower for females and are lower in inactive subjects. Other reference ranges exist in reputable laboratories.

Use Evaluate muscle wasting processes. Very high levels are found in progressive Duchenne muscular dystrophy (MD), with the highest concentrations found early. Elevations occur in carriers of MD, in limb-girdle dystrophy and other dystrophies, in dermatomyositis, polymyositis, and trichinosis, but not in neurogenic atrophies (eg, myasthenia gravis, multiple sclerosis, or poliomyelitis).

Limitations As muscle mass diminishes, aldolase decreases. Serum aldolase elevation is not specific for muscle disease (see following discussion). Assay of creatine kinase (CK) is preferred for evaluation of muscle disease. It is more specific for skeletal muscle degeneration. AST and LD also reflect damage to muscle, but lack specificity.

Elevated aldolase levels may be found with hepatitis, other liver diseases, myocardial infarction, hemorrhagic pancreatitis, gangrene, delirium tremens, and in some cases of neoplasia. In cases of acute viral hepatitis, increase in serum aldolase tends to parallel ALT (SGPT) levels. A small fraction of cases of measles in young adults have been reported to have significant elevations of serum CK and aldolase.[2,3] Aldolase is an ubiquitous enzyme and has limited clinical application.

Contraindications Aldolase levels are not frequently needed or ordered. Many laboratories do not offer this test.

Methodology Ultraviolet, kinetic, coupled enzymatic[4]

Additional Information In the progressive dystrophies, aldolase levels may be 10-15 times normal when muscle mass is relatively intact as in early stages of the disease. When advanced muscle wasting is present, values decline. In the inflammatory myopathies (eg, dermatomyositis) serum aldolase (as well as CK) levels may be applied to monitor the response to steroid therapy. They are of value in guiding tapering of steroid administration.[1]

Aldolase is formed of two subunits. There are three different possible subunits designated A, B, and C, but just four isoenzymes. The molecular form AAAA is the predominant aldolase in skeletal muscle, BBBB predominates in liver, and CCCC in brain and other tissue. A hybrid isoenzyme, AAAC is present in tissues but at a lower concentration. The UV coupled enzymatic methods determine total enzyme activity and, thus, are not specific for muscle aldolase.[5]

The level of serum aldolase B (RIA method) may be decreased (<20 ng/mL) in some patients with epithelial malignancy (cases studied included esophageal, hepatic, pancreatic, lung, and breast cancers).[6] After successful surgical resection, serum aldolase B levels recovered to normal range (20-60 ng/mL).

Serum aldolase and CK may be elevated in the serum of patients who have taken L-tryptophan and develop eosinophilia-myalgia syndrome.[7]

In a recent publication, it was shown that CK is not a reliable marker for muscle damage in multiple organ failure associated with low extracellular glutathione concentrations. In these patients, serum CK was significantly low as compared to controls (p <0.001), whereas levels of myoglobin and aldolase were increased.[8]

Footnotes
1. Visnapuu LA, Karlson LK, Dubinsky EH, et al, "Pediatric Reference Ranges for Serum Aldolase," *Am J Clin Pathol*, 1989, 91(4):476-7.
2. Harjanne A, "The Kinetic Measurement of Serum Aldolase," *Clin Chim Acta*, 1979, 92(2):311-3.

(Continued)

Aldolase, Plasma or Serum *(Continued)*

3. Leibovici L, Sharir T, Kalter-Leibovici O, et al, "An Outbreak of Measles Among Young Adults: Clinical and Laboratory Features in 461 Patients," *J Adolesc Health Care*, 1988, 9(3):203-7.
4. Gavish D, Kleinman Y, Morag A, et al, "Hepatitis and Jaundice Associated With Measles in Young Adults. An Analysis of 65 Cases," *Arch Intern Med*, 1983, 143(4):674-7.
5. Moss DW and Henderson AR, "Clinical Enzymology," *Tietz Textbook of Clinical Chemistry*, 3rd ed, Burtis CA and Ashwood ER, eds, Philadelphia, PA: WB Saunders Co, 1999, 666-8.
6. Asaka M, Kimura T, Nishikawa S, et al, "Decreased Serum Aldolase B Levels in Patients With Malignant Tumors," *Cancer*, 1988, 62(12):2554-7.
7. Kilbourne EM, Swygert LA, Philen RM, et al, "Interim Guidance on the Eosinophilia-Myalgia Syndrome," *Ann Intern Med*, 1990, 112(2):85-7.
8. Gunst JJ, Langlois MR, Delanghe JR, et al, "Serum Creatine Kinase Activity Is Not a Reliable Marker for Muscle Damage in Conditions Associated With Low Extracellular Glutathione Concentration," *Clin Chem*, 1998, 44(5):939-43.

Aldosterone, Serum or Plasma

Related Information

Adrenal Cortex: Laboratory Assessments Overview *on page 84*
Aldosterone, Urine *on page 91*
Potassium, Serum or Plasma *on page 258*
Potassium, Urine *on page 259*
Renin Activity, Plasma *on page 273*

Applies to Renin

Abstract Aldosterone is a mineralocorticoid hormone produced in the zona glomerulosa of the adrenal cortex under complex control by the renin-angiotensin system and by potassium levels. Its action is on the renal distal tubule, where it increases resorption of sodium and water at the expense of increased potassium excretion. Primary hyperaldosteronism (PH) is characterized by hypokalemia (a key laboratory finding), hypersecretion of aldosterone, hypertension, and suppressed plasma renin activity. PH is found in 1% to 2% of unselected subjects with hypertension. Serum or plasma electrolytes are relevant.

Aldosterone-producing adenomas are usually not large. They varied from 0.5-2.4 cm in a recent series.[1]

Patient Preparation Preanalytic variables which must be controlled are sodium balance, posture, blood pressure medications, and time of day. Hypokalemia, if present, should be corrected before additional testing. Blood pressure medications and diuretics should be discontinued for **at least** 2 weeks (4-6 weeks is preferable) before additional testing is undertaken.

In the most common scenario, a patient with hypertension and increased urine potassium (>30 mmol/L) will be evaluated with a **screening protocol** in which the patient fasts overnight and a blood specimen for plasma renin and aldosterone is obtained the next day after 4 hours in the upright position. Some clinicians augment this protocol by giving furosemide, 40-80 mg, orally or intravenously on arising.

A patient whose plasma **aldosterone (ng/mL):renin (ng/mL/hour) ratio** is >20 on the screening evaluation can then be further evaluated by a **sodium loading protocol**, consisting of 1) a fasting, early morning blood specimen for aldosterone and renin before arising; 2) spending 2 hours in the upright position; and 3) 2 L of isotonic saline intravenously over 4 hours, at the completion of which another blood specimen for aldosterone and renin is obtained. A variation in this protocol is provided by Ganguly.[2]

The **captopril protocol** provides diagnostic information similar to the sodium loading protocol and is useful for patients who may not tolerate the sodium loading protocol. Captopril is an antihypertensive agent which inhibits the conversion of angiotensin I to angiotensin II, thus, removing the physiologic stimulus to aldosterone secretion. The patient is given 25 mg (adult dose) of captopril by mouth; blood specimens for aldosterone are obtained just before, and 2 hours after, the drug is taken. This test, however, has fallen short of expectations.[2]

Specimen Serum or plasma, peripheral blood and if indicated, percutaneous catheterization for sampling adrenal vein aldosterone and cortisol

Container Lavender top (EDTA) tube (if also to be used for renin). For aldosterone alone, use heparin, EDTA, citrate, or red top tube; consult laboratory during the assay.

Sampling Time The timing of sampling (morning) and the posture of the patient before sampling (upright) require standardization; *vide supra*.

Collection Specify time and exact source of specimen.

Storage Instructions Transport at once to the laboratory on ice. Freeze serum or plasma in a plastic vial as soon as possible after sampling.

Reference Interval Method dependent. See table.

Critical Values Ratio of plasma aldosterone to renin >30-50; a ratio >30 deserves further evaluation.[2]

Bornstein et al, with two-site immunoradiometric assays, indicate a ratio ≥20, measured while the patient is upright, to suggest the presence of an aldosterone-producing tumor. β-adrenoceptor blocking drugs and dihydropyridine calcium-channel blocking agents should be avoided for 2 weeks before testing. Loop diuretics and spirolactone should be withheld for 6 weeks. This group has published a diagnostic algorithm.[6]

	Serum Aldosterone ng/dL (SI: pmol/L)	Plasma Renin ng/mL/h	Ratio Aldosterone (ng/dL): Renin (ng/mL/h)
Screening protocol			
Normal subjects			<20[3]
1-10 y	3.5-124.0 (96.9-3434.8)[4]		
>11 y	1.0-21.0 (27.7-581.7)[4]		
18-39 y		2.9-24.0[4]	
>40 y		2.9-10.8[4]	
Sodium loading protocol			
Normal subjects (all ages)	<5 (SI: <140)[5]		
18-39 y		<0.6-4.3[4]	
≥40 y		<0.6-3.0[4]	
Primary hyperaldosteronism (PH)	>10 (>280)[5]	Very low, often undetectable	
Captopril protocol			
Normal subjects	<10 (<280)[5]		
	<15 (<420)[3]		

Use The principal use for aldosterone measurements (serum and urine) is in the diagnosis of primary hyperaldosteronism (PH), a medically important subset of patients with hypertension. Because the renin-angiotensin system responds rapidly to many physiologic stimuli, a random measurement of aldosterone has no diagnostic value, and can be misleading. **The key to the diagnosis of PH is demonstrating increased aldosterone (blood and/or urine) at the same time that plasma renin is low.**

Hypertensive patients with PH have the potential of being cured by adrenalectomy, and therefore extensive testing is warranted. The **screening protocol** (above) may be done after the patient has been off all antihypertensive and diuretic medications for 2 weeks, and after hypokalemia, if present, has been corrected. (**Note:** As many as 12% of patients with PH due to adrenal adenoma, and 50% of patients with PH due to hyperplasia may have serum potassium >3.5 mmol/L. If 4.0 mmol/L is used as the decision threshold, nearly all patients with PH will be identified, but with the usual trade-off in false positives). This screen takes advantage of the fact that the upright posture stimulates renin release; the augmented protocol adds sodium depletion - an additional renin stimulant.

In the **sodium loading protocol** and the **captopril protocol** the physiologic secretion of renin is strongly suppressed; hypertensives without PH have a proportionate decrease in aldosterone.

Limitations Hepatic blood flow is the primary determinant of aldosterone metabolism. Plasma aldosterone concentrations can reach 20 times normal levels in subjects with congestive heart failure.[7]

Methodology Two-site immunoradiometric assays, chemiluminescence immunoassay (CIA),[8] enzyme-linked immunosorbent assay (ELISA),[9] radioimmunoassay (RIA)

Additional Information In aldosterone testing, the principal pitfall to be avoided is performing the test on a patient with secondary hyperaldosteronism (see Adrenal Cortex: Laboratory Assessments Overview *on page 84*) and misinterpreting the elevated aldosterone as indicative of PH. Secondary hyperaldosteronism is a common physiologic response to several disease processes which have the common denominators of decreased effective renal plasma flow or contracted plasma volume. Examples include congestive heart failure, cirrhosis, and the nephrotic syndrome. (Volume expansion or contraction, as well as high sodium intake and sodium deficiency, act through the renin-angiotensin system to influence aldosterone secretion.) It is important to recall that patients with renal artery stenosis also have secondary hyperaldosteronism, reflecting the pathophysiology of their hypertension. The combination of elevated renin and aldosterone is also encountered in Bartter syndrome and the Gitelman syndrome. Patients on thiazide diuretics will have laboratory testing results strikingly similar to patients with PH.

Adjunctive tests, imaging, and therapy are recently reviewed.[2]

Although management of aldosterone-producing adenomas is predominantly surgical, medical management is described as an alternative in the presence of overriding comorbid conditions.[1]

Footnotes

1. Ghose RP, Hall PM, and Bravo EL, "Medical Management of Aldosterone-Producing Adenomas," *Ann Intern Med*, 1999, 131(2):105-8.
2. Ganguly A, "Primary Aldosteronism," *N Engl J Med*, 1998, 339(25):1828-34.
3. Orth DN and Kovacs WJ, "The Adrenal Cortex," *Williams Textbook of Endocrinology*, 9th ed, Philadelphia, PA: WB Saunders Co, 1998, 596.
4. Mayo Medical Laboratories, *2001 Test Catalogue*, Rochester, MN, 47, 457.
5. Demers LM and Whitley RJ, "Function of the Adrenal Cortex," *Tietz Textbook of Clinical Chemistry*, 3rd ed, Burtis CA and Ashwood ER, eds, Philadelphia, PA: WB Saunders Co, 1999, 1530-69.

6. Bornstein SR, Stratakis CA, and Chrousos GP, "Adrenocortical Tumors: Recent Advances in Basic Concepts and Clinical Management," *Ann Intern Med*, 1999, 130(9):759-71.

7. Weber KT, "Aldosterone and Spironolactone in Heart Failure," *N Engl J Med*, 1999, 341(10):753-5.

8. Stabler TV and Siegel AL, "Chemiluminescence Immunoasay of Aldosterone in Serum," *Clin Chem*, 1991, 37(11):1987-9.

9. Schwartz F and Hadas E, "Enzyme-Linked Immunosorbent Assays for Plasma Aldosterone," *J Immunoassay*, 1990, 11:215034.

References

Blumenfeld JD, Sealey JE, Schlussel Y, et al, "Diagnosis and Treatment of Primary Hyperaldosteronism," *Ann Intern Med*, 1994, 121:877-85.

Conn JW, "Presidential Address II. Primary Aldosteronism, a New Clinical Syndrome," *J Lab Clin Med*, 1955, 45:3-17.

Desai SP and Isa-Pratt S, *Clinician's Guide to Laboratory Medicine*, Cleveland, OH: Lexi-Comp, 2000, Chapter 17.

Mattingly D, Martin H, and Tyler CM, "Estimation of Urinary Aldosterone Using Thin Layer Chromatography and Fluorometry," *J Clin Pathol*, 1993, 46(12):1109-12.

Pratt JH, Rebhun JF, Zhou L, et al, "Levels of Mineralocorticoids in Whites and Blacks," *Hypertension*, 1999, 34(2):315-9.

Schrier RW and Abraham WT, "Hormones and Hemodynamics in Heart Failure," *N Engl J Med*, 1999, 341(8):577-85.

White PC, "Disorders of Aldosterone Biosynthesis and Action," *N Engl J Med*, 1994, 331(4):250-8.

Aldosterone, Urine

Related Information

Adrenal Cortex: Laboratory Assessments Overview *on page 84*
Aldosterone, Serum or Plasma *on page 90*
Potassium, Serum or Plasma *on page 258*
Potassium, Urine *on page 259*
Renin Activity, Plasma *on page 273*
Sodium, Urine *on page 278*
Urine Collection, 24-Hour *on page 47*

Applies to Renin

Abstract Aldosterone is a mineralocorticoid hormone produced in the adrenal zona glomerulosa under complex control by the renin-angiotensin system. Its action is on the renal distal tubule where it increases resorption of sodium and water at the expense of increased potassium excretion. Primary hyperaldosteronism (PH) is characterized by hypokalemia (a key laboratory finding), hypersecretion of aldosterone, hypertension, and suppressed plasma renin activity. Edema is not characteristic.[1] PH is found in 1% to 2% of unselected subjects with hypertension.

Patient Preparation Diuretics, antihypertensive drugs, cyclic progestogens, estrogens, and licorice should be terminated for at least 2 weeks (and preferably 4-6 weeks) prior to testing. Patient should be on a diet containing 135 mmol (3 g) sodium/day for at least 2 weeks and preferably 30 days prior to testing. No recent radioactive scans. Potassium deficiencies should be corrected before specimen is collected.[2]

Specimen 24-hour urine

Container Refrigerated during collection

Collection Boric acid preservative, 50% acetic acid (25 mL/24-hour specimen) added to reach pH 2-4. Consult reference laboratory.

Storage Instructions Freeze

Reference Interval There are significant interlaboratory differences.
- 0-30 days: 0.7-11.0 µg/24 hours (SI: 1.94-30.5 nmol/day)[3]
- 1-11 months: 0.7-22.0 µg/24 hours (SI: 1.94-61.0 nmol/day)[3]
- >12 months: 2.0-16.0 µg/24 hours (SI: 5.5-44.3 nmol/day)[3]

Note: Measure also the **sodium** in the urine specimen. A person with normal renin-angiotensin dynamics on a high sodium diet (urine sodium >200 mEq/24 hours), should have urine aldosterone <10 µg/24 hours (SI: <27.7 nmol/day).[3] Urinary potassium and creatinine may also be needed.[4]

Use Urine aldosterone measurements are useful in the diagnosis of primary hyperaldosteronism (PH). The key finding in PH is elevated aldosterone (serum and/or urine) simultaneous with low plasma renin. See discussions on Aldosterone, Serum or Plasma *on page 90* and Adrenal Cortex: Laboratory Assessments Overview *on page 84*.

Methodology Radioimmunoassay (RIA) following acid hydrolysis, enzyme-linked immunosorbent assay (ELISA)

Additional Information Urinary aldosterone excretion, adjunctive tests, and therapy were recently reviewed.[5]

Pseudohypoaldosteronism was recently discussed in an excellent review of the genetic disorders of renal electrolyte transport.[6]

Footnotes

1. Weber KT, "Aldosterone and Spironolactone in Heart Failure," *N Engl J Med*, 1999, 341(10):753-4.

2. Orth DN and Kovacs WJ, "The Adrenal Cortex," *Williams Textbook of Endocrinology*, 9th ed, Philadelphia, PA: WB Saunders Co, 1998, 517-664.

3. Mayo Medical Laboratories, *2001 Test Catalogue*, Rochester, MN, 47.

4. Ghose RP, Hall PM, and Bravo EL, "Medical Management of Aldosterone-Producing Adenomas," *Ann Intern Med*, 1999, 131(2):105-8.

5. Ganguly A, "Primary Aldosteronism," *N Engl J Med*, 1998, 339(25):1828-34.

6. Scheinman SJ, Guay-Woodford LM, Thakker RV, et al, "Genetic Disorders of Renal Electrolyte Transport," *N Engl J Med*, 1999, 340(15):1177-87.

References

Blumenfeld JD, Sealey JE, Schlussel Y, et al, "Diagnosis and Treatment of Primary Hyperaldosteronism," *Ann Intern Med*, 1994, 121:877-85.

Desai SP and Isa-Pratt S, *Clinician's Guide to Laboratory Medicine*, Cleveland, OH: Lexi-Comp, 2000, Chapter 17.

Mattingly D, Martin H, and Tyler CM, "Estimation of Urinary Aldosterone Using Thin Layer Chromatography and Fluorometry," *J Clin Pathol*, 1993, 46(12):1109-12.

Pratt JH, Rebhun JF, Zhou L, et al, "Levels of Mineralocorticoids in Whites and Blacks," *Hypertension*, 1999, 34(2):315-9.

White PC, "Disorders of Aldosterone Biosynthesis and Action," *N Engl J Med*, 1994, 331(4):250-8.

Alkaline Phosphatase, Heat Stable, Serum

Related Information

Alkaline Phosphatase Isoenzymes, Serum *on page 92*
Alkaline Phosphatase, Serum *on page 93*
Calcium, Serum *on page 131*
Gamma-Glutamyl Transferase, Serum *on page 179*
Hydroxyproline, Total, Urine *on page 199*
Liver Disease: Laboratory Assessment, Overview *on page 216*
N-Telopeptides, Urine *on page 233*
Osteocalcin, Serum or Plasma *on page 237*

Synonyms Fractionated Alkaline Phosphatase; Heat Stable Alkaline Phosphatase

Applies to Nagao Isoenzyme; Regan Isoenzyme

Test Includes Total alkaline phosphatase and heat stable alkaline phosphatase as a percent of total.

Abstract The placental isoenzyme is very heat stable, as is the Regan isoenzyme (a placental-like fetal form occurring in some cancers). Liver isoenzyme is more stable than the bone form. In hepatobiliary disease, GGT is often helpful and more definitive than this fractionation of alkaline phosphatase. GGT is increased with hepatobiliary disease. Assays for bone-specific alkaline phosphatase are also available.

Patient Preparation Patient should be fasting.

Specimen Serum

Container Red top tube or SST™ tube

Storage Instructions Refrigerate serum.

Causes for Rejection Hemolysis

Reference Interval In nonpregnant subjects, heating at 55°C for 15 minutes resulting in percent residual activity >25% favors hepatic origin; <10% favors bone origin. The addage "bone burns, liver lives" makes the differentiation easier to remember. If >90% of stability, probably a placental form is present.

Use Differentiate liver and bone diseases in patients with increased alkaline phosphatase. High alkaline phosphatase of bone origin is found with Paget disease of bone, in which very high concentrations may occur. High levels may be found with osteogenic sarcoma and increases occur in hyperparathyroidism, rickets, osteomalacia, Fanconi syndrome, fracture healing, and with physiologic bone growth in childhood and adolescence. Levels are normal in uncomplicated osteoporosis. **Preferred method for this purpose is separation of isoenzyme by electrophoresis.** See Alkaline Phosphatase Isoenzymes, Serum *on page 92*.

Limitations Sometimes misleading. Prolonged storage at room temperature can increase alkaline phosphatase activity. Hemolysis causes false elevation of alkaline phosphatase. If intestinal ALP or other more heat stable isozymes (eg, placental) of ALP are present, percentage of liver fraction may be falsely increased. Serum GGT, leucine aminopeptidase, and 5' nucleotidase may be more helpful in differentiating between osseous and hepatobiliary etiologies of elevated alkaline phosphatase.

Lack of standardization of maximum temperatures or duration of heating impair interlaboratory comparisons.

Contraindications Total alkaline phosphatase not elevated

Methodology Heat inhibition at 56°C. Liver fraction is more resistant to heat and urea inactivation than is the bone isoenzyme. The bone fraction is very heat labile, while placental and cancer (Regan, Nagao) isoenzymes are extremely stable to heat (90% stable).[1] Heating serum at 65°C for 5 minutes results in loss of activity of all ALP fractions with the exception of placental ALP. Heating at 55°C for 15 minutes results in 50% loss of intestinal fraction activity, 60% loss of hepatic fraction, and 90% loss of bone ALP activity. Heat inactivation, when used alone, is an inferior technique, since sharp demarcations of the heat stability of the ALP isoenzymes do not occur. The presence of very heat-stable forms (Regan) may give unusually high half-life values. Extremely close temperature control is required. The preferred method is electrophoresis in polyacrylamide gel or high resolution agarose.[2]

Additional Information Heat stable alkaline phosphatase provides an alternative to alkaline phosphatase electrophoresis. Postmenopausal females generally have slightly elevated total alkaline phosphatase and a low percentage of heat stable fraction, indicating osseous origin.

Heat stable alkaline phosphatase has been proposed as a tumor marker for head and neck squamous cell carcinoma. Enzyme activity was significantly higher prior to therapy and decreased during successful treatment.[3]

Footnotes

1. Wolf PL, "Clinical Significance of an Increased or Decreased Serum Alkaline Phosphatase Level," *Arch Pathol Lab Med*, 1978, 102(10):497-501.

2. Day AP, Saward S, Royle CM, et al, "Evaluation of Two New Methods for Routine Measurement of Alkaline Phosphatase Isoenzymes," *J Clin Pathol*, 1992, 45(1):68-71.

(Continued)

Alkaline Phosphatase, Heat Stable, Serum

(Continued)

3. Rassam MB, al-Bashir NN, al-Salihi AR, et al, "Heat-Stable Alkaline Phosphatase. A Putative Tumor Marker of Head and Neck Squamous Cell Carcinoma," *Acta Oncol*, 1995, 34(1):49-52.

References

Farley JR, Hall SL, Herring S, et al, "Reference Standards for Quantification of Skeletal Alkaline Phosphatase Activity in Serum by Heat Inactivation and Lectin Precipitation," *Clin Chem*, 1993, 39(9):1878-84.

Watts NB, "Clinical Utility of Biochemical Markers of Bone Remodeling," *Clin Chem*, 1999, 45(8B):1359-68.

Alkaline Phosphatase Isoenzymes, Serum

Related Information

Alkaline Phosphatase, Heat Stable, Serum *on page 91*
Alkaline Phosphatase, Serum *on page 93*
Calcium, Serum *on page 131*
Hydroxyproline, Total, Urine *on page 199*
Liver Disease: Laboratory Assessment, Overview *on page 216*
N-Telopeptides, Urine *on page 233*
Osteocalcin, Serum or Plasma *on page 237*
Pyridinolines (Pyridinoline and Deoxypyridinoline), Urine *on page 272*

Synonyms ALP Isoenzymes; Isoenzymes of Alkaline Phosphatase

Applies to Bone Alkaline Phosphatase; Nagao Isoenzyme; Regan Isoenzyme

Test Includes Total ALP level with or without neuraminidase and with or without pretreatment by monoclonal antibody to intestinal fraction ALP. May include combinations of heat and/or L-phenylalanine inactivation with or without electrophoretic differentiation.

Abstract Isoelectric focusing, use of selective inhibitors and enzyme immunometric techniques allows identification of the principle isoenzymes of alkaline phosphatase, which include those from bone, liver, intestine, and placenta.

Patient Preparation Patient should be fasting.

Specimen Serum

Container Red top tube or SST™ tube

Causes for Rejection Hemolysis

Turnaround Time Method dependent, ordinarily at least 2-3 days

Special Instructions Send 1 mL frozen serum in plastic container on dry ice to reference laboratory.

Use Evaluate contribution of liver, bone, placental, and Regan isoenzymes to total alkaline phosphatase. Bone fraction is increased in Paget disease of bone. In a chemistry panel, marked isolated increase of alkaline phosphatase in a nonpregnant, older patient who has no healing fracture, with other tests within normal range, is likeliest to indicate Paget disease of bone. Osteoblastic tumor can also cause increased alkaline phosphatase. Other causes of increased serum alkaline phosphatase concentrations of bone origin include hyperparathyroidism, rickets, and osteomalacia. Monitor bone mineral density response to hormonal replacement therapy and treatment of osteoporosis. Aid in detection in bone metastases from prostate and breast carcinoma. Useful as a marker of bone formation - serum bone alkaline phosphatase isoenzymes may be a predictor of effectiveness of growth hormone therapy in children with growth hormone deficiency.[1] If gamma-glutamyl transferase is elevated, the source of the elevated ALP is most likely the liver.

Limitations In the presence of liver disease, the specificity of alkaline phosphatase measurements is improved by measuring bone alkaline phosphatase. In most other clinical situations, total serum alkaline phosphatase activity may provide sufficient clinical information.[2]

Methodology Differential susceptibility of alkaline phosphatase to inhibition by L-phenylalanine (intestinal and placental ALP are inhibited by L-phenylalanine). Polyacrylamide gel electrophoresis with or without pretreatment of sample with neuraminidase and/or monoclonal antibody to isolate the intestinal fraction of ALP (I-ALP). Isoelectric focusing, lectin precipitation (wheat germ agglutinin) enzyme immunoassay, immunoradiometric assay. Partial digestion with neuraminidase enhances subsequent electrophoretic separation of bone and liver fractions. Isoelectric focusing has separated ALP isoenzymes into 17 fractions, including a fraction which may be a marker of activated T-lymphocytes.[3]

Additional Information In most cases, elevation in serum total alkaline phosphatase (T-ALP) is reasonably well defined on the basis of other already established clinical-pathologic findings. LD (LDH) isoenzyme fractionation or serum gamma-glutamyl transferase activity frequently may help to define the clinical problem sufficiently. In a minority of patients, elevation of T-ALP resists explanation. Here, application of ALP isoenzyme studies may indicate whether T-ALP is increased on the basis of contributions from liver, bone, intestinal, placental, endothelial cell, or pathologic (tumor markers Regan and Nagao) fractions.

Total liver and bone ALP are increased in hyperthyroid patients. B-ALP is most commonly and significantly increased. I-ALP is not elevated in the hyperthyroid state.[4]

T-ALP may be elevated in rheumatic diseases (30% to 50% of cases) (eg, rheumatoid arthritis and ankylosing spondylitis).[5] Osteoarthritis and inactive RA are nearly always associated with normal T-ALP. A few cases of RA have increase in liver AP. Increase in T-ALP and in bone fraction has been shown to correlate with disease activity and the number of involved joints.[5]

Cobalamin (vitamin B_{12}) deficient patients have reduced bone ALP. The degree of megaloblastic anemia has been found to correlate with the decrease in enzyme level.[6] T-ALP level, however, is usually within normal range in B_{12} deficient patients.

Newer applications for alkaline phosphatase isoenzymes include monitoring the reduction of bone turnover after alendronate therapy in postmenopausal osteoporotic women[7,8] or after hormonal replacement therapy.[9] Skeletal alkaline phosphatase may help to provide information for staging prostate cancer[10,11] and breast cancer.[12] Isoforms of bone alkaline phosphatase may provide information on bone turnover[13] as well as bone turnover within specific bone compartments.[14] Immunoassays for bone alkaline phosphatase (skeletal alkaline phosphatase) are available. Bone alkaline phosphatase, like osteocalcin, is a marker of bone formation. Bone alkaline phosphatase derives from osteoblasts. Since it is cleared by the liver, its concentrations may be elevated with diseases of the liver.[15]

A number of ALP isoenzymes have been described (rarely) in association with carcinoma. They are most commonly seen with hepatocellular cancer or carcinoma metastatic to liver. They include Regan, Magoo, Regan variant, Kashahara, fetal intestinal, and Timperley types. The Regan isoenzyme, which is similar to placental ALP, is seen in 1% to 3% of carcinomas (varying in primary site of origin) metastatic to liver.

Footnotes

1. Tobiume H, Kanzaki S, Hida, S, et al "Serum Bone Alkaline Phosphatase Isoenzyme Levels in Normal Children and Children With Growth Hormone (GH) Deficiency: A Potential Marker for Bone Formation and Response to GH Therapy," *J Clin Endocrinol Metab*, 1997, 82(7):2056-61.
2. Woitge HW, Seibel MJ, and Ziegler R, "Comparison of Total and Bone Specific Alkaline Phosphatases in Patients With Nonskeletal Disorder or Metabolic Bone Diseases," *Clin Chem*, 1996, 42(11):1796-804.
3. Wallace BH, Lott JA, Griffiths J, et al, "Isoforms of Alkaline Phosphatase Determined by Isoelectric Focusing in Patients With Chronic Liver Disorders," *Eur J Clin Chem Clin Biochem*, 1996, 34(9):711-20.
4. Tibi L, Patrick AW, Leslie P, et al, "Alkaline Phosphatase Isoenzymes in Plasma in Hyperthyroidism," *Clin Chem*, 1989, 35(7):1427-30.
5. Siede WH, Seiffert UB, Merle S, et al, "Alkaline Phosphatase Isoenzymes in Rheumatic Diseases," *Clin Biochem*, 1989, 22(2):121-4.
6. Carmel R, Lau, KH, Baylink DJ, et al, "Cobalamin and Osteoblast-Specific Proteins," *N Engl J Med*, 1988, 319(2):70-5.
7. Garnero P, Darte C, and Delmas PD, "A Model to Monitor the Efficacy of Alendronate Treatment in Women With Osteoporosis Using a Biochemical Marker of Bone Turnover," *Bone*, 1999, 24(6):603-9.
8. Kress BC, Mizrahi IA, Armour KW, et al, "Use of Bone Alkaline Phosphatase to Monitor Alendronate Therapy in Individual Postmenopausal Osteoporotic Women," *Clin Chem*, 1999 45(7):1009-17.
9. Dresner-Pollak R, Mayer M, and Hocher-Celinker D, "The Decrease in Serum Bone-Specific Alkaline Phosphatase Predicts Bone Mineral Density Response to Hormone Replacement Therapy in Early Postmenopausal Women," *Calcif Tissue Int*, 2000, 66(2):104-7.
10. Wolff JM, Ittel TH, Borchers H, et al, "Metastatic Workup of Patients With Prostate Cancer Employing Alkaline Phosphatase and Skeletal Alkaline Phosphatase," *Anticancer Res*, 1999, 19(4A):2653-5.
11. Lorente JA, Valenzuela H, Morote J, et al, "Serum Bone alkaline Phosphatase Levels Enhance the Clinical Utility of Prostate Specific Antigen in the Staging of Newly Diagnosed Prostate Cancer Patients," *Eur J Nucl Med*, 1999, 26(6):625-32.
12. Ritzke C, Steiber P, Untch M, et al, "Alkaline Phosphatase Isoenzymes in Detection and Follow Up of Breast Cancer Metastases," *Anticancer Res*, 1998, 18(2B):1243-9.
13. Broyles DL, Nielsen RG, Bussett EM, et al, "Analytical and Clinical Performance Characteristics of Tandem-MP Ostase, a New Immunoassay for Serum Bone Alkaline Phosphatase," *Clin Chem*, 1998, 14(11):1926-33.
14. Magnusson P, Larsson L, Magnusson M, et al, "Isoforms of Bone Alkaline Phosphatase: Characterization and Origin in Human Trabecular and Cortical Bone," *J Bone Miner Res*, 1999, 14(11):1926-33.
15. Watts NB, "Clinical Utility of Biochemical Markers of Bone Remodeling," *Clin Chem*, 1999, 45(8 Pt 2):1359-68.

References

Atsumi K, Kushida K, Yamazaki K, et al, "Risk Factors for Vertebral Fractures in Renal Osteodystrophy," *Am J Kidney Dis*, 1999, 33(2):287-93.

Chamberlain BR, Buttery JE, Pannall PR, "A Simple Electrophoretic Method for Separating Elevated Liver and Bone Alkaline Phosphatase Isoenzymes in Plasma After Neuraminidase Treatment," *Clin Chim Acta*, 1992, 208(3):219-24.

Delmas PD and Beaudreuil J, "Biochemical Markers of Bone Turnover in Osteoporosis," *Rev Rhum Engl Ed*, 1997, 64(6 Suppl):31S-36S.

Domar U, Danielsson A, Hirano K, et al, "Alkaline Phosphatase Isozymes in Non-Malignant Intestinal and Hepatic Diseases," *Scand J Gastroenterol*, 1988, 23(7):793-800.

Hanna AN, Waldman WJ, Lott JA, et al, "Increased Alkaline Phosphatase Isozymes in Non-Malignant Intestinal and Hepatic Diseases," *Clin Chem*, 1997, 43(8 Pt 1):1357-64.

Kisabeth PM, Mayo Medical Laboratories, *2000 Test Catalogue*, Rochester, MN.

Martin M, Van Hoof V, Couttenye M, et al, "Analytical and Clinical Evaluation of a Method to Quantify Bone Alkaline Phosphatase, a Marker of Osteoblastic Activity," *Anticancer Res*, 1997, 17(4B):3167-70.

Milligan TP, Park HR, Noonan K, et al, "Assessment of the Performance of a Capture Immunoassay for the Bone Isoform of Alkaline Phosphatase in Serum," *Clin Chim Acta*, 1997, 263(2):165-75.

Panteghini M and Pagani F, "Reference Intervals for Two Bone-Derived Enzyme Activities in Serum: Bone Isoenzyme of Alkaline Phosphatase (ALP) and Tartrate-Resistant Acid Phosphatase (TR-ACP)," *Clin Chem*, 1989, 35(1):180-1.

Price CP, Milligan TP, and Darte C, "Direct Comparison of Performance Characteristics of Two Immunoassays for Bone Isoform of Alkaline Phosphatase in Serum," *Clin Chem*, 1997, 43(11):2052-7.

Rauch F, Middelman B, cagnoli M, et al, "Comparison of Total Alkaline Phosphatase and Three Assays for Bone Specific Alkaline Phosphatase in Childhood and Adolescence," *Acta Paediatr*, 1997, 86(6):583-7.

Schreiber WE and Sadro LC, "Agarose Gel Patterns of ALkaline Phosphatase Isoenzymes Before and After Treatment With Neuraminidase," *Am J Clin Pathol*, 1988, 90(2):181-6.

Steinlauf AF, Traube M, Neitlich JD, et al, "Clostridium difficile Colitis: A Possible Cause of Unexplained Elevation of Serum Alkaline Phosphatase Levels in Patients With AIDS," *Clin Infect Dis*, 1998, 26(5):1248-9.

Walach N and Gur Y, "Leukocyte Alkaline Phosphatase, CA 15-3, CA 125, and CEA in Cancer Patients," *Tumori*, 1998, 84(3):360-3.

Withold W, Schulte U, and Reinauer H, "Method for Determination of Bone Alkaline Phosphatase Activity: Analytical Performance and Clinical Usefulness in Patients With Metabolic and Malignant Bone Disease," *Clin Chem* , 1996, 42(2):210-7.

Yamamoto T and Katsuoka Y, "Purification and Characterization of Alkaline Phosphatase From Human Seminomas," *Tokai J Exp Clin Med*, 1998, 23(4):199-207.

Alkaline Phosphatase, Serum

Related Information
Alkaline Phosphatase, Heat Stable, Serum *on page 91*
Alkaline Phosphatase Isoenzymes, Serum *on page 92*
Antimitochondrial Antibody *on page 505*
Aspartate Aminotransferase, Serum *on page 112*
Bilirubin, Total, Serum *on page 118*
Carbohydrate-Deficient Transferrin, Serum *on page 134*
Ethanol, Blood, Urine, and Other Sources *on page 789*
Gamma-Glutamyl Transferase, Serum *on page 179*
Hepatitis B Core Antibody *on page 622*
Hepatitis C Virus RNA Detection and Quantitation *on page 626*
Hepatitis: Laboratory Assessment, Overview *on page 629*
Hydroxyproline, Total, Urine *on page 199*
Immunoglobulin M *on page 537*
Kidney Stone Analysis *on page 877*
Leucine Aminopeptidase (LAP), Serum and Urine *on page 211*
Liver Biopsy *on page 65*
Liver Disease: Laboratory Assessment, Overview *on page 216*
Liver/Kidney Microsomal Type 1 Antibodies *on page 539*
5' Nucleotidase, Serum *on page 234*
Osteocalcin, Serum or Plasma *on page 237*
Smooth Muscle Antibody *on page 543*

Synonyms ALP; Phosphatase, Alkaline

Abstract A family of enzymes which catalyze hydrolysis of phosphate esters at alkaline pH; 80% of serum alkaline phosphatase (ALP) activity normally originates from liver and bone. Other sources include intestine, kidney, and placenta. Synthesized by biliary epithelium, ALP is excreted in bile. Serum total ALP level provides a useful but nonspecific indication of liver or bone disease. Increased in cholestatic, infiltrative and inflammatory liver disease, ALP is increased with obstructive biliary processes, even small secondary bile duct obstruction and, thus, may be elevated when bilirubin is normal due to compensatory bilirubin excretion by the rest of the liver. ALP may be helpful in localized obstructive problems such as hepatic metastases. With biliary tract obstruction, the rise in ALP parallels increases in serum bilirubin. Increased synthesis of ALP can take place even without increases in bilirubin.[1] Heating serum at 56°C causes significant inactivation of ALP of bone origin, but electrophoresis (see Alkaline Phosphatase Isoenzymes, Serum *on page 92*) or determination of serum gamma-glutamyl transferase are better tests for the determination of the source of elevated ALP. GGT is more readily available. See the table in Bilirubin, Total, Serum *on page 118*.

Patient Preparation Patient should be fasting.

Specimen Serum

Container Red top tube or capillary tube

Storage Instructions Refrigerate. Serum alkaline phosphatase increases slowly with storage. Increases of 5% to 10% can be expected after less than 4 hours storage at 4°C. For this reason, it is best to analyze on the day of collection.

Reference Interval Method dependent. Normal values are higher for pediatric patients and in pregnancy. Levels are two to three or more the adult range in children and are increased in puberty compared to adult range. During episodes of very rapid growth, levels as high as 1000 units/L may be normal. The high level of ALP in childhood reflects osteoblastic activity of bone growth. Postpuberty, serum ALP is mostly of liver origin. Adult normal range is approximately 50-120 units/L (IFCC reference method at 37°C). ALP is up to two times adult upper limit in pregnancy. Values in adult males are slightly higher than in adult females. With menopause and after, values in women increase, are similar to or higher than those in men, and are higher than in younger subjects.

Use Causes of **high alkaline phosphatase** include nonfasting specimen, bone growth, healing fracture, acromegaly, osteogenic sarcoma, liver or bone metastases, leukemia, myelofibrosis, mastocytosis, and rarely myeloma. Alkaline phosphatase is used as a tumor marker. Elevations occur, usually 2-4 hours after a fatty meal, especially in people who are Lewis positive secretors of blood type O or B. Standing of blood specimen before analysis; up to 30% increase with storage of serum.

In rickets and osteomalacia, serum calcium and phosphorus are low to normal, and alkaline phosphatase may be normal or increased. Hypervitaminosis D may cause elevations in alkaline phosphatase, as may vitamin D malabsorption (eg, celiac sprue).

In Paget disease of bone, there is often isolated elevation of ALP, some among the highest levels seen.

Hyperthyroidism, by its effects upon bone, may elevate alkaline phosphatase.

Hyperparathyroidism, in some patients; pseudohyperparathyroidism.

Chronic alcohol ingestion (in chronic alcoholism, alkaline phosphatase may be normal or increased, but often with high AST (SGOT) and/or high bilirubin and especially with high GGT; MCV may be high).

Biliary obstruction (eg, tenfold increase may be seen with carcinoma of head of pancreas, choledocholithiasis); cholestasis; GGT also high. Cholecystitis with cholangitis: in most patients with cholecystitis and cholangitis who do not have a common duct stone, alkaline phosphatase is within normal limits or only slightly increased. Sclerosing cholangitis (eg, with ulcerative colitis), although 3% of cases of symptomatic sclerosing cholangitis may have normal serum ALP.[2] Endoscopic retrograde cholangiography might be considered then in patients with diseases known to be associated with primary sclerosing cholangitis and with appropriate symptomatology even though ALP level is normal.

Cirrhosis, especially in primary biliary cirrhosis, in which fivefold or more increases are seen; antimitochondrial antibodies needed for evaluation of primary biliary cirrhosis. GGT and 5' nucleotidase serum levels parallel those of ALP, while AST and ALT are normal to slightly increased in primary biliary cirrhosis. Bilirubin is usually normal early.[3] Liver biopsy is used to confirm the diagnosis.

Infiltrative/granulomatous liver diseases (eg, sarcoid, TB, amyloidosis, metastatic tumor, abscess). When ALP is >1000 units/L with hepatobiliary source confirmed with increased liver fraction of ALP or with high GGT and bilirubin <1.0 mg/dL, suggested diagnoses include infiltrative/granulomatous liver disease including sarcoidosis, mycoses, tuberculosis, and lymphoma. In early primary biliary cirrhosis and primary sclerosing cholangitis, there is also increased ALP with normal bilirubin.[1]

Autoimmune cholangiopathy includes features of primary biliary cirrhosis or primary sclerosing cholangitis, pruritus with high ALP without antimitochondrial antibodies.[4]

With primary or metastatic tumor in the liver, there may be a marked increase in alkaline phosphatase and GGT. In one study, three laboratory markers were useful in screening for metastatic carcinoma of breast, prior to clinical detectability of metastases: these were alkaline phosphatase, GGT, and CEA.[5] Moderate to marked elevations of levels of ALP, bilirubin, and GGT are found with biliary tract cancer.[6]

Gilbert syndrome;[7] postoperative cholestasis, pancreatitis, carcinoma of pancreas, cystic fibrosis.

Hepatitis: Moderate increases in alkaline phosphatase occur in viral hepatitis, but greater elevations of the transaminases (AST (SGOT), ALT (SGPT)) are usually found. Increased in typhoid fever, with AST > ALT, in patients with jaundice and encephalopathy.[8]

Hepatic steatosis (fatty metamorphosis) (moderate increase occurs in acute fatty liver).

Diabetes mellitus, diabetic hepatic steatosis.

Sepsis and certain viral diseases, including infectious mononucleosis, cytomegalovirus infections, and AIDS. *Clostridium difficile* colitis in AIDS patients can also be a cause of unexplained elevation of serum alkaline phosphatase.[9]

Pulmonary infarct (1-3 weeks after embolism. Healing infarcts in other organs, including kidney, may also cause increased ALP); other situations in which angiofibroplasia occurs, such as healing in a large decubitus ulcer.

Tumors, especially renal cell carcinoma; neoplastic ectopic production (Regan, Nagao isoenzymes); lymphoma. Paraneoplastic serum alkaline phosphatase elevation in renal cell carcinoma patients portends an unfavorable prognosis. Additional paraneoplastic syndromes further worsen the prognosis. The return of serum alkaline phosphatase to normal does not guarantee cure.[10]

Fanconi syndrome, familial hyperphosphatasemia, idiopathic.

Peptic ulcer, erosion; intestinal strangulation or obstruction, or ulcerative lesion; steatorrhea, malabsorption (from bone, secondary to vitamin D deficiency); ulcerative colitis with pericholangitis, other erosive lesions of colon.

Congestive heart failure, parenteral hyperalimentation of glucose, intravenous albumin administration.

Benign familial increase of alkaline phosphatase.
(Continued)

Alkaline Phosphatase, Serum *(Continued)*

Drugs - aminoglycosides, amiodarone, anticonvulsants, aspirin (prolonged use), chlorpromazine, erythromycin, esterified estrogens, isoniazid, levothyroxine, lithium, oral hypoglycemic agents, methyltestosterone, oral contraceptives, phenothiazines, and any drug producing hypersensitivity or toxic cholestasis. Many commonly and uncommonly used drugs may elevate alkaline phosphatase, and tenfold increases may be seen with drug cholestasis.

Causes of **low alkaline phosphatase** are said to include hypothyroidism, but most hypothyroid patients have normal alkaline phosphatase.

Some cases of Wilson disease.

Pernicious anemia - in very few patients.

Hypophosphatasia: Very low ALP values are found in the presence of normocalcemia or hypocalcemia. This diagnosis may be confirmed by quantitation of urinary phosphoethanolamine.

Transient hyperphosphatasemia: Very high (sometimes in thousands) levels of alkaline phosphatase, mainly in children under 5 years of age. In these patients there is no sign of bone or liver disease. More than 400 cases have been reported. Excessive diagnostic procedures should be avoided in these patients.[11,12]

Malnutrition has been reported to relate to low values, but in practice, diseases causing malnutrition relate often to high ALP (eg, disseminated neoplasia).

Some **drugs** (alendronate, clofibrate, estrogens in postmenopausal women on estrogen replacement therapy, theophylline, and other agents) may lower serum ALP activity.

Limitations Normal ranges dependent upon methodology, age, sex, and pregnancy status. Used alone, alkaline phosphatase may be misleading.

Methodology Some original spectrophotometric methods and their modifications (eg, King-Armstrong, described in 1934 and using the substrate phenylphosphate[13]) have been largely supplanted by more recent endpoint, kinetic spectrophotometric or fluorescent procedures. Most current assays use *p*-nitrophenyl phosphate (pNPP) as substrate (eg, Bessey-Lowry-Brock or the current modification by Bowers and McComb). More recent techniques utilize chromogenic substrates (eg, methylumbelliferyl phosphate) and improved buffer systems with resultant increased sensitivity. Specific immunoassay for bone alkaline phosphatase is now available.

Additional Information Serum ALP is a member of a family of zinc metalloprotein enzymes that function to split off a terminal phosphate group from an organic phosphate ester. This enzyme functions in an alkaline environment (optimum pH of 10). Active center of ALP enzymes includes a serine residue. Magnesium and zinc ions are required for minimal activity. Enzyme activity is localized in the brush border of the proximal convoluted tubule of the kidney, intestinal mucosal epithelial cells, hepatic sinusoidal membranes, vascular endothelial cells, and osteoblasts of bone. There are distinctive forms of ALP in the placenta and small intestine; hepatic, renal, and osteoblast (bone) ALP are similar molecules.

An electrophoretically slow moving isoenzyme with high relative mass may occur in some patients with bile duct obstruction and hepatic metastases and may result in false elevation of CK-MB.[14]

Basic approach to patient with elevated alkaline phosphatase (ALP). ERCP = endoscopic retrograde cholangiopancreatography, GGT = γ-glutamyltransferase. Other relevant tasks include bilirubin, AST, ALT, antimitochondrial antibody, IgM, prothrombin time, and carbohydrate-deficient transferrin. Modified from Kamath PS, "Clinical Approach to the Patient With Abnormal Liver Test Results," *Mayo Clin Proc*, 1996, 71:1089-95.

To confirm biliary abnormality, additional useful tests include GGT, bilirubin, and occasionally 5′-nucleotidase. They are elevated in hepatobiliary disease, not in uncomplicated bone disease. In the presence of liver disease, the specificity of alkaline phosphatase measurements is improved by measuring bone alkaline phosphatase isoenzyme levels. In most other clinical situations, total serum alkaline phosphatase levels appear to provide

sufficient clinical information.[15] Serum alkaline phosphatase levels may serve as an indicator of liver function after hepatectomy but may not reflect morphological regeneration of the liver.[16]

Marked decline of the high ALP of pregnancy is seen with placental insufficiency and imminent fetal demise.

A characteristic of acute liver failure in Wilson disease is the combination of a very high bilirubin, >30 mg/dL (>513 µmol/L) with decreased serum alkaline phosphatase activity. The ratio of ALP to bilirubin <2.0 is relatively distinctive.[17]

See the following diagram.

In the presence of jaundice, see the table in Bilirubin, Total, Serum on page 118.

Footnotes

1. Kamath PS, "Clinical Approach to the Patient With Abnormal Liver Test Results," *Mayo Clin Proc*, 1996, 71(11):1089-95.
2. Cooper JF and Brand EJ, "Symptomatic Sclerosing Cholangitis in Patients With a Normal Alkaline Phosphatase: Two Case Reports and a Review of the Literature," *Am J Gastroenterol*, 1988, 83(3):308-11.
3. Kaplan MM, "Primary Biliary Cirrhosis," *N Engl J Med*, 1996, 335(21):1570-80.
4. Krawitt EL, "Autoimmune Hepatitis," *N Engl J Med*, 1996, 334(14):897-903.
5. Coombes RC, Powles TJ, Gazet JC, et al, "Screening for Metastases in Breast Cancer: An Assessment of Biochemical and Physical Methods," *Cancer*, 1981, 48(2):310-5.
6. de Groen PC, Gores GJ, LaRusso NF, et al, "Biliary Tract Cancers," *N Engl J Med*, 1999, 341:(18):1368-78.
7. Lieverse AG, van Essen GG, Beukeveld GJ, et al, "Familial Increased Serum Intestinal Alkaline Phosphatase: A New Variant Associated With Gilbert's Syndrome," *J Clin Pathol*, 1990, 43(2):125-8.
8. Kamath PS, Jalihal A, and Chakraborty A, "Differentiation of Typhoid Fever From Fulminant Hepatic Failure in Patients Presenting With Jaundice and Encephalopathy," *Mayo Clin Proc*, 2000, 75(5):462-6.
9. Steinlauf AF, Traube M, Neitlich JD, et al, "*Clostridium difficile* Colitis: A Possible Cause of Unexplained Elevation of Serum Alkaline Phosphatase Levels in Patients With AIDS," *Clin Infect Dis*, 1998, 26(5):1248-9.
10. Chuang YC, Lin AT, Chen KK, et al, "Paraneoplastic Elevation of Serum Alkaline Phosphatase in Renal Cell Carcinoma: Incidence and Implication on Prognosis," *J Urol*, 1997, 158(5):1684-7.
11. Kutilek S and Bayer M, "Transient Hyperphosphatasemia - Where Do We Stand?" *Turk J Pediatr*, 1999, 41(2):151-60.
12. Garty BZ and Nitzan M, "Benign Transient Hyperphosphatasemia," *Isr J Med Sci*, 1994, 30(1):66-9.
13. King EJ and Armstrong AR, "A Convenient Method for Determining Serum and Bile Phosphatase Activity," *Can Med Assoc J*, 1934, 31:376-81.
14. Butch AW, Goodnow TT, Brown WS, et al, "Stratus Automated Creatine Kinase - MB Assay Evaluated: Identification and Elimination of Falsely Increased Results Associated With High-Molecular-Mass Form of Alkaline Phosphatase," *Clin Chem*, 1989, 35(10):2048-53.
15. Woitge HW, Seibel MJ, and Ziegler R, "Comparison of Total and Bone-Specific Alkaline Phosphatase in Patients With Nonskeletal Disorder or Metabolic Bone Diseases," *Clin Chem*, 1996, 42(11):1796-804.
16. Nagino M, Nimura Y, Kamiya J, et al, "Serum Alkaline Phosphatase After Extensive Liver Resection: A Study in Patients With Biliary Tract Carcinoma," *Hepatogastroenterology*, 1999, 46(26):766-70.
17. Lee WM, "Acute Liver Failure," *N Engl J Med*, 1993, 329(25):1862-72.

References

Ben-Arie A, Hagay Z, Ben-Hur H, et al, "Elevated Serum Alkaline Phosphatase May Enable Early Diagnosis of Ovarian Cancer," *Eur J Obstet Gynecol Reprod Biol*, 1999, 86(1):69-71.

Gordon T, "Factors Associated With Serum Alkaline Phosphatase Level," *Arch Pathol Lab Med*, 1993, 117(2):187-90.

Kihn L, Dinwoodie A, and Stinson RA, "High-Molecular-Weight Alkaline Phosphatase in Serum Has Properties Similar to the Enzyme in Plasma Membranes of the Liver," *Am J Clin Pathol*, 1991, 96(4):470-8.

Maldonado O, Demasi R, Maldonado Y, et al, "Extremely High Levels of Alkaline Phosphatase in Hospitalized Patients," *J Clin Gastroenterol*, 1998, 27(4):342-5.

Pratt DS and Kaplan MM, "Evaluation of Abnormal Liver-Enzyme Results in Asymptomatic Patients," *N Engl J Med*, 2000, 342(17):1266-71.

Tietz NW, Burtis CA, Duncan P, et al, "A Reference Method for Measurement of Alkaline Phosphatase Activity in Human Serum," *Clin Chem*, 1983, 29:751-61.

Van Hoof VO, Hoylaerts MF, Geryl H, et al, "Age and Sex Distribution of Alkaline Phosphatase Isoenzymes by Agarose Electrophoresis," *Clin Chem*, 1990, 36(6):875-8.

Wallace BH, Lott JA, Griffiths J, et al, "Isoforms of Alkaline Phosphatase Determined by Isoelectric Focusing in Patients With Chronic Liver Disorders," *Eur J Clin Chem Clin Biochem*, 1996, 34(9):711-20.

Wilson JW, "Inherited Elevation of Alkaline Phosphatase Activity in the Absence of Disease," *N Engl J Med*, 1979, 301:983-4.

Withold W, Schulte U and Reinauer H, "Method for Determination o Bone Alkaline Phosphatase Activity: Analytical Performance and Clinical Usefulness in Patients With Metabolic and Malignant Bone Diseases," *Clin Chem*, 1996, 42(2):210-7.

Wolff JM, Ittel TH, Borchers H, et al, "Metastatic Workup of Patients with Prostate Cancer Employing ALkaline Phosphatase and Skeletal ALkaline Phosphatase," *Anticancer Res*, 1999, 19(4A):2653-5.

Young DS, *Effects of Drugs on Clinical Laboratory Tests*, 5th ed, Volume 1: Listing by Test, Washington, DC: AACC Press, American Association of Clinical Chemistry, 2000, Section 3, 36-48.

◆ **Alkalosis** *see* Chloride, Urine *on page 145*

◆ **Allen Test** *see* Blood Gases and pH, Arterial *on page 119*

◆ **ALP** *see* Alkaline Phosphatase, Serum *on page 93*

Alpha₁-Acid Glycoprotein, Serum

Related Information
Haptoglobin, Serum *on page 190*

Synonyms Orosomucoid

Abstract Alpha₁-acid glycoprotein (AAG) is a 40-kD plasma glycoprotein consisting of ~181 amino acids. It is synthesized predominantly in hepatocytes and has a plasma half-life of 3-5 days. Its small size allows its filtration through the glomerulus and reabsorption in the proximal tubule. It migrates in the alpha₁ region on electrophoresis, but does not stain well due to its high carbohydrate content (45% by weight). AAG is an acute phase reactant, appearing in plasma within 12 hours of injury and peaking at 3-5 days. AAG binds with certain basic drugs and hormones, in some cases rendering them ineffective. Markedly increased serum levels are found in inflammation, pregnancy, and certain malignancies.

Patient Preparation Patient should be fasting.

Specimen Serum

Container Red top tube

Storage Instructions Refrigerate (4°C) for up to 72 hours. After 72 hours, the specimen should be stored frozen at -20°C and thawed only once prior to analysis.

Causes for Rejection Gross hemolysis, lipemia

Reference Interval The reference interval in adults 20-60 years of age is 50-120 mg/dL.[1] Children 3-16 years of age have reference intervals ranging from 43-308 mg/dL.[2] Reference intervals for infants are as follows:[3] birth: 12-56 mg/dL, 1 month: 24-93 mg/dL, 3 months: 27-107 mg/dL, 6 months: 35-149 mg/dL.

Use Serum AAG is increased by acute-phase inflammatory conditions and glucocorticoids; it is decreased in nephrotic syndrome, protein-losing enteropathy, and estrogen therapy. In patients with suspected hemolysis, measurement of AAG has been suggested as an aid in interpretation of low haptoglobin levels (see Haptoglobin, Serum *on page 190*), since both proteins are affected similarly by inflammation, glucocorticoids, and estrogens.

Limitations Alpha₁-acid glycoprotein is a nonspecific marker of inflammation. The test does not contribute much diagnostic information to the wide array of conditions with which it is associated and, therefore, is not widely used.

Methodology Immunonephelometry, immunoturbidimetry, enzyme-linked Immunosorbent assay (ELISA), radioimmunoassay (RIA), and radial immunodiffusion (RID)

Additional Information AAG is heterogeneic with respect to the proportions of oligosaccharides bound to its glycosylation sites, and distinct glycosylation patterns have been identified in specimens from patients with tuberculosis[4] as well as other inflammatory disorders. These glycosylation patterns appear to be the result of inflammation-induced expression of sialyl Lewis X-containing glycan structures,[5] which consist of fucose residues that may have a role in the interaction between leukocytes and inflamed endothelium via binding to cell-surface selectins.[6]

Footnotes
1. Dati F, Schumann G, Thomas L, et al, "Consensus of a Group of Professional Societies and Diagnostic Companies on Guidelines for Interim Reference Ranges for 14 Proteins in Serum Based on the Standardization Against the IFCC/BCR/CAP Reference Material (CRM 470). International Federation of Clinical Chemistry. Community Bureau of Reference of the Commission of the European Communities. College of American Pathologists," *Eur J Clin Chem Clin Biochem*, 1996, 34(6):517-20.
2. Malvy DJM, Poveda JD, Debruyne M, et al, "Laser Immunonephelometry Reference Intervals for Eight Serum Proteins in Healthy Children," *Clin Chem*, 1992, 38(3):394-9.
3. Kanakoudi F, Drossou V, Tzimouli V, et al, "Serum Concentrations of 10 Acute-Phase Proteins in Healthy Term and Preterm Infants From Birth to Age 6 Months," *Clin Chem*, 1995, 41(4):605-8.
4. Fassbender K, Fassbender M, Schaberg T, "Glycosylation of α₁-Acid Glycoprotein in Bacterial Lung Infections: Distinct Pattern in Tuberculosis," *Clin Chem*, 1995, 41(3):472-3.
5. De Graaf TW, Van der Stelt ME, Anbergen MG, et al, "Inflammation-Induced Expression of Sialyl Lewis X-Containing Glycan Structures on Alpha 1-Acid Glycoprotein (Orosomucoid) in Human Sera," *J Exp Med*, 1993, 177(3):657-66.
6. Listinsky JJ, Siegal GP, and Listinsky CM, "α-L-Fucose. A Potentially Critical Molecule in Pathologic Processes Including Neoplasia," *Am J Clin Pathol*, 1998, 110(4):425-40.

References
Johnson AM, Rohlfs EM, and Silverman LM, "Proteins," *Tietz Textbook of Clinical Chemistry*, 3rd ed, Chapter 20, Burtis CA and Ashwood ER, eds, Philadelphia, PA: WB Saunders Co, 1999, 477-540.

Ryden I, Lundblad A, and Pahlsson P, "Lectin ELISA for Analysis of α-Acid Glycoprotein Fucosylation in the Acute Phase Response," *Clin Chem*, 1999, 45(11):2010-12.

Tissot B, Seta N, Durand G, et al, "Polyclonal Antibody-Based Enzyme-Linked Immunosorbent Assay of α₁-Acid Glycoprotein," *Clin Chem*, 1990, 36(4):666-8.

Alpha₁-Antitrypsin Phenotyping

Related Information
Alpha₁-Antitrypsin, Serum *on page 96*

Aspartate Aminotransferase, Serum *on page 112*
Liver Biopsy *on page 65*
Liver Disease: Laboratory Assessment, Overview *on page 216*
Protein Electrophoresis, Serum *on page 267*

Synonyms α₁-Antiprotease Phenotype; α₁-AT Phenotype

Applies to Protease Inhibitors

Test Includes Serum trypsin inhibitory capacity

Abstract Alpha₁-antitrypsin (α₁-AT) deficiency (alpha₁-protease inhibitor deficiency), characterized by varying levels of severity, is the most common genetic cause of liver disease in the pediatric population. α₁-AT is a glycoprotein which is the largest fraction (65%) in the alpha₁ globulins. Patients are detected by lack or diminution of the alpha₁ band on serum protein electrophoresis, abnormal migration of the alpha₁ band or by decreased levels determined immunochemically.

Hereditary α₁-AT deficiency accounts for 1% to 2% of emphysema cases.

Patient Preparation Fasting is preferred.

Specimen Serum

Container Red top tube, lavender top (EDTA) tube for molecular analysis

Sampling Time Misleading results can follow sampling during acute illness; *vide infra*.

Storage Instructions Separate serum and refrigerate or freeze.

Reference Interval Interpretation usually accompanies report; phenotypes are designated. Pi•MM phenotype is normal; Pi•MZ is heterozygous, intermediate deficient; and Pi•ZZ is homozygous, severely deficient. Over 70 alleles are described.[1] Biosynthesis of α₁-AT is controlled at the Pi locus by a pair of genes. There is codominant expression. The phenotype is "Pi" for protease inhibitor. α₁-AT is the most abundant protease inhibitor. It protects tissue from proteases, especially neutrophil elastase. Other proteases inhibited by α₁-AT include cathepsin G, pancreatic elastase and trypsin, chymotrypsin, and collagenases.[1] Z and S are mutant proteins. A null-null state occurs as well. In a dysfunctional type, α₁-AT is found in normal amounts but does not function normally.

Use Alpha₁-AT phenotyping provides definitive analysis of hereditary α₁-AT deficiency, which is associated with chronic obstructive pulmonary disease (COPD) (panacinar or panlobular emphysema), hepatic cirrhosis, and hepatoma. α₁-AT deficiency is not an uncommon cause of neonatal cholestasis. Cholestasis with neonatal hepatitis is found in a minority of neonates with α₁-AT deficiency. Such neonatal hepatitis leads to cirrhosis. In addition to pulmonary and hepatic manifestations, evidence exists that α₁-AT deficiency may play a role in other entities in many of which inflammation and/or immune components exist. These diseases are thought to include severe erosive rheumatoid arthritis, panniculitis, membranoproliferative glomerulonephritis, uveitis, and vascular aneurysms, including aortic, large artery (eg, colic) and intracranial ones. Pi typing of patients with aneurysms is recommended.[2,3]

Limitations α₁-AT is a positive acute phase protein because it rises whenever there is tissue injury, necrosis, inflammation, or infection. Therefore, patients with α₁-AT deficiency who suffer from bronchitis, pneumonia, or similar respiratory inflammation may have falsely normal levels during acute illness. After the acute phase of illness has passed, repeat determinations often reveal the "true" or "resting" α₁-AT level which is indicative of heterozygous phenotypic deficiency.

Serum α₁-AT may be increased in patients during normal pregnancy, chronic pulmonary diseases, hereditary angioneurotic edema, gastric diseases, liver diseases, pancreatitis, diabetes, carcinomas, renal diseases, and rheumatic diseases and may be decreased in patients with severe protein loss or with improper storage of specimen.

Methodology Isoelectric focusing[1] in a narrow range pH gradient, crossed immunoelectrophoresis. Use of high-resolution electrophoresis which would detect the slower electrophoretic migration of the Z and S variants is preferred over quantification of α₁-AT by nephelometry as a screen for this deficiency. Further, a high-resolution electrophoretic system will detect heterozygotes, which could lead to important family studies of potentially deficient first-degree relatives who may benefit from therapy.

Additional Information An M null genotype will have phenotype as MM but low serum level of α₁-AT.

α₁-AT is a glycoprotein synthesized in the liver. α₁-AT represents about 90% of serum antiprotease capacity.[4] When α₁-AT is deficient, unopposed activity of these enzymes results in emphysema. Cigarette smoke is reported to inactivate α₁-AT.[4] The age of occurrence of emphysema varies with the type of deficiency, ZZ being most severe. PiZZ is expressed in about 1 in 2500 American Caucasians. It leads to an α₁-AT which differs from M by only a single amino acid substitution (lysine for glutamic acid). Among children, severe ZZ α₁-AT deficiency most frequently presents as liver disease, cholestasis, and cirrhosis. Over 80% of individuals with ZZ ultimately develop chronic lung or liver disease.[4] Clinically, the most important phenotypes are MM, MS, SS, MZ, ZZ, and a null phenotype. These variants are associated with 100%, 80%, 60%, 57.5%, 15%, and 0% of α₁-AT activity. Severity varies with the personal habits of the individual, especially regarding smoking.

Patients with the null phenotype are more likely to develop emphysema than hepatic disease.

A possible etiologic role of α₁-AT deficiency is development of Crohn disease and ulcerative colitis in a subset of patients was recently discussed.[1]

(Continued)

Alpha₁-Antitrypsin Phenotyping (Continued)

The significance of α₁-AT deficiency bears legal, insurance, and other implications.[4]

Footnotes

1. Yang P, Tremaine WJ, Meyer RL, et al, "Alpha₁-Antitrypsin Deficiency and Inflammatory Bowel Diseases," *Mayo Clin Proc*, 2000, 75:450-5.
2. Cox DW, "Alpha₁-Antitrypsin: A Guardian of Vascular Tissue," *Mayo Clin Proc*, 1994, 69(11):1123-4.
3. Schievink WI, Björnsson J, Parisi JE, et al, "Arterial Fibromuscular Dysplasia Associated With Severe Alpha₁-Antitrypsin Deficiency," *Mayo Clin Proc*, 1994, 69(11):1040-3.
4. Wulfsberg EA, Hoffmann DE, and Cohen MM, "Alpha₁-Antitrypsin Deficiency. Impact of Genetic Discovery on Medicine and Society," *JAMA*, 1994, 271(3):217-22.

References

Buist AS, "Alpha 1-Antitrypsin Deficiency - Diagnosing Treatment and Control: Identification of Patients," *Lung*, 1990, 168(Suppl):543-51.
Crystal RG, "Alpha-1-Antitrypsin Deficiency: Pathogenesis and Treatment," *Hosp Pract (Off Ed)*, 1991, 26(2):81-4, 88-9, 93-4.
Eriksson S, Carlson J, and Velez R, "Risk of Cirrhosis and Primary Liver Cancer in Alpha₁-Antitrypsin Deficiency," *N Engl J Med*, 1986, 314(12):736-9.
Garver RI Jr, Mornex JF, Nukiwa T, et al, "Alpha₁-Antitrypsin Deficiency and Emphysema Caused by Homozygous Inheritance of Nonexpressing Alpha₁-Antitrypsin Genes," *N Engl J Med*, 1986, 314(12):762-66.
Hutchison DC, "Natural History of Alpha-1-Protease Inhibitor Deficiency," *Am J Med*, 1988, 84(6A):3-12.
Perlmutter DH, "Alpha₁-Antitrypsin Deficiency: Biochemistry and Clinical Manifestations," *Ann Med*, 1996, 28(5):385-94.
Shields RC and Su WP, "35-Year-Old Woman With Ulcerating Skin Lesions," *Mayo Clin Proc*, 1996, 71(1):59-62.
Silverman EK, Pierce JA, Province MA, et al, "Variability of Pulmonary Function in Alpha₁-Antitrypsin Deficiency: Clinical Correlates," *Ann Intern Med*, 1989, 111(12):982-91.
Snider GL, "Pulmonary Disease in Alpha₁-Antitrypsin Deficiency," *Ann Intern Med*, 1989, 111(12):957-9.

Alpha₁-Antitrypsin, Serum

Related Information

Alpha₁-Antitrypsin Phenotyping *on page 95*
Bilirubin, Total, Serum *on page 118*
C-Reactive Protein, Serum *on page 523*
Liver Biopsy *on page 65*
Liver Disease: Laboratory Assessment, Overview *on page 216*
Protein Electrophoresis, Serum *on page 267*

Synonyms A₁AT; α₁-Antiprotease; α₁-AT

Applies to Acute Phase Reactant; Protease Inhibitors

Abstract Deficiency of α₁-antitrypsin (α₁-AT) was described in 1963. It may present as emphysema, classically in smokers younger than 40 years of age. It is the most common genetic cause of liver disease in the pediatric population. α₁-antitrypsin is the most abundant proteinase inhibitor (Pi) in plasma.[1]

Specimen Serum. Prenatal diagnosis is possible.

Container Red top tube, lavender top (EDTA) tube for molecular analysis

Reference Interval 110-140 mg/dL,[2] method dependent. Levels are normally low at birth but rise soon thereafter.

Critical Values Levels <70 mg/dL (SI: <0.70 g/L) are likely to correlate with homozygous deficiency; subjects having levels <125 mg/dL (SI: <1.40 g/L) should be phenotyped.

Use Detect hereditary decreases in the production of alpha₁-antitrypsin (α₁-AT) (see Alpha₁-Antitrypsin Phenotyping *on page 95*). Decreased or nearly absent levels of α₁-AT are important in chronic obstructive lung disease and in liver disease. An increased prevalence of non-MM phenotypes is found with cirrhosis, chronic liver disease, and with hepatocellular carcinoma. Cirrhosis in a child should raise consideration of α₁-AT deficiency or Wilson disease. α₁-AT deficiency is a leading cause of childhood liver disease. However, only a minority of children with Pi•ZZ phenotype develop evidence of liver disease by adolescence.

Limitations α₁-AT is one of the alpha globulins which together are called acute phase reactants. These rise rapidly, but nonspecifically, in response to inflammatory insults. α₁-AT may be elevated into normal range in heterozygous deficient patients during concurrent infection, pregnancy, estrogen therapy, steroid therapy, cancer, and during postoperative periods. Homozygous deficient patients will not show such elevation. Normal α₁-AT levels may occur in patients with liver disease who are heterozygotes. In normals, pregnancy and contraceptive medication may elevate levels. α₁-AT is often elevated in inflammatory states (eg, rheumatoid arthritis, bacterial infection, vasculitis, neoplasia).

Contraindications If CRP is elevated, retest α₁-AT in 10-14 days.

Methodology Nephelometry, radial immunodiffusion (RID), molecular analysis by polymerase chain reaction (PCR), isoelectric focusing for phenotyping

Additional Information This assay should be run when alpha₁ globulin in serum protein electrophoresis is decreased, when two bands are seen in the alpha₁ region, when the alpha₁ region is obscured by alpha₁ lipoprotein and especially on clinical indications. Heterozygous patients (Pi•MZ phenotype) or homozygous patients with PiSS exhibit α₁-AT levels which are commonly about 60% of normal, but most of these patients do not have

clinically important liver disease. In one report, the P variant in conjunction with Z allele has been attributed to the progression of liver disease in one patient. One of the P variants, P_lowell mutation, results in alpha₁-AT that is rapidly degraded by hepatocytes.[3] Homozygous (Pi•ZZ phenotype) patients exhibit activity levels of about 10% to 18% of normal. Phenotyping is desirable on patients with low values and on all patients being worked up for α₁-AT-deficient liver disease. Most pathologic is homozygous state ZZ. Early emphysema exacerbated by smoking develops in PiZZ individuals with A₁AT concentrations <10%. However, this is a very uncommon cause of chronic obstructive pulmonary disease. Neutrophil elastase, inhibited in pulmonary parenchyma by A₁AT, leads to the emphysema of A₁AT deficiency.[4] An M null genotype will have phenotype as MM but a low serum level.

More than 100 alleles are described. Molecular methods for detection of most common PiZ or PiS mutations are available. These mutations are in blacks and Oriental populations.[5,6]

Footnotes

1. Cox DW, "α₁-Antitrypsin: A Guardian of Vascular Tissue," *Mayo Clin Proc*, 1994, 69(11):1123-4 (editorial).
2. Yang P, Tremaine WJ, Meyer RL, et al, "α₁-Antitrypsin Deficiency and Inflammatory Bowel Diseases," *Mayo Clin Proc*, 2000, 75:450-5.
3. Berg CL and Graeme-Cook FM, "A 68-Year-Old Woman With Hepatic Encephalopathy," Case Records of the Massachusetts General Hospital, Case 10-1997, Scully RE, Mark EJ, McNally WF, et al, eds, *N Engl J Med*, 1997, 336(13):939-47.
4. Barnes PJ, "Chronic Obstructive Pulmonary Disease," *N Engl J Med*, 2000, 343(4):269-80.
5. von Ahsen N, Oellerich M, and Schutz E, "Use of Two Reporter Dyes Without Interference in a Single-Tubed Rapid-Cycle PCR: Alpha(1)-Antitrypsin Genotyping by Multiplex Real-Time Fluorescence PCR With the LightCycler," *Clin Chem*, 2000, 46(2):156-61.
6. Rieger S, Riemer H, and Mannhalter C, "Multiplex PCR Assay for the Detection of Genetic Variants of α₁-Antitrypsin," *Clin Chem*, 1999, 45(5):688-90.

References

Brantly ML, Wittes JT, Vogelmeier CF, et al, "Use of a Highly Purified Alpha₁-Antitrypsin Standard to Establish Ranges for the Common Normal and Deficient Alpha₁-Antitrypsin Phenotypes," *Chest*, 1991, 100(3):703-8.
Hodges JR, Millward-Sadler GH, Barbatis C, et al, "Heterozygous MZ Alpha₁ Antitrypsin Deficiency in Adults With Chronic Active Hepatitis and Cryptogenic Cirrhosis," *N Engl J Med*, 1981, 304:557-68.
Perlmutter DH, "Alpha-1-Antitrypsin Deficiency: Biochemistry and Clinical Manifestations," *Ann Med*, 1996, 28(5):385-94.
Shin SJ and Meininger G, Images in Clinical Medicine, "Alpha₁-Antitrypsin Deficiency," *N Engl J Med*, 2000, 343(26):1933.

Alpha₁-Fetoprotein, Amniotic Fluid

Related Information

Acetylcholinesterase, Amniotic Fluid *on page 81*
Acetylcholinesterase, Red Cell *on page 81*
Alpha₁-Fetoprotein, Serum *on page 97*
Amniotic Fluid, Chromosome and Genetic Abnormality Analysis *on page 360*
Cystic Fibrosis DNA Detection *on page 705*
Duchenne/Becker Muscular Dystrophy DNA Detection *on page 706*
Fluorescence *In Situ* Hybridization *on page 367*
Kleihauer-Betke *on page 453*

Applies to Amniotic Fluid Acetylcholinesterase

Test Includes Cytogenetic studies can be initiated from the same specimen.

Abstract Alpha-fetoprotein (AFP) is a glycoprotein. Amniotic fluid AFP (AF-AFP) testing is done following positive maternal screening, but may also be done when the maternal or family history is positive for neural tube defect. A shortcoming of reliance on family history is that only 3% to 5% of annual births affected by open neural tube defects are found in families in whom high risk is recognized (anencephaly, spina bifida).[1] Prediction of neural tube defects can be projected much more accurately by amniotic fluid AFP than by serum screening.

Patient Preparation Since interpretation depends on gestational age, diagnostic ultrasound is more desirable than calculated gestational age. Nevertheless, first day of last menstrual period should be provided to the laboratory. Ultrasound may also delineate other important information (eg, twins, neural tube or ventral wall anatomic defects).

Specimen Amniotic fluid

Container Sterile syringe

Collection Concentration of AF-AFP is very high at the 8th week, decreases to the 11th week, and reaches a second, smaller peak at the 13th week.[2] Although the optimal time to collect amniotic fluid for AFP is between the 16th and 18th week of gestation, reference ranges are generally established for 14-25 weeks. Provide gestational age to the laboratory. If the amniotic fluid is traumatic (bloody), a maternal blood specimen should also be submitted. One or two drops of fetal blood in amniotic fluid can give false-positive results.

Storage Instructions Refrigerate

Causes for Rejection Sample determined not to be amniotic fluid; contamination of amniotic fluid with maternal and fetal blood; recently administered radioisotopes if RIA is used for assay. Urine urea nitrogen (UUN) may be used to distinguish maternal urine from amniotic fluid, since UUN of maternal urine is >100 g/day (that of normal amniotic fluid is much less).

Special Instructions Amniotic fluid for AFP probably should not be collected before the 14th week.[2]

Reference Interval Interlaboratory differences exist. Ranges are stratified by weeks of gestation, decreasing with increasing maturity. **It is essential that the reference ranges supplied by the laboratory performing the assay be used to interpret results,** which are expressed as "multiples of the median" (MoM) and are generally >0.5 MoM and <2.5 MoM. Most authorities, however, regard MoM >2.0 as abnormal until proven otherwise. The curves for unaffected and open spina bifida pregnancies, during the second trimester, slightly overlap. They are published.[1] MoM is **not** corrected for maternal race, maternal weight, and maternal insulin-dependent diabetes mellitus. Amniotic fluid AFP peak differs from that of maternal serum.

Possible Panic Range Median AF-AFP is ~7 MoM in open spina bifida and ~20 MoM in anencephaly.[2]

Use Analyze second trimester amniotic fluid for detection of neural tube defects: anencephaly, spina bifida (with ultrasound), myelocele, hydrocephaly.

Limitations Amniotic fluid alpha-fetoprotein may also be increased in non-neural tube anomalies (such as congenital nephrosis, esophageal atresia, duodenal atresia, ventral wall defects including gastroschisis and omphalocele), distressed or dead fetus, and fetal bleeding into the amniotic space. The Kleihauer-Betke stain can detect fetal blood contamination of the tap but requires that fetal intact red cells be present. Fetal serum contains mg/mL levels of AFP. In specimens in which AF-AFP is increased, testing for fetal hemoglobin is desirable. Closed neural tube defects are generally not detected by alpha-fetoprotein testing. When an amniotic fluid alpha-fetoprotein level is elevated, confirmatory testing, such as **high resolution ultrasonography** and measurement of **amniotic fluid acetylcholinesterase**, should be undertaken to confirm the neural tube defect. Acetylcholinesterase is independent of gestational age and is not affected by fetal blood contamination. It may also be increased with open ventral wall defects.

Unexplained AFP increases are occasionally encountered.

Measurement of AFP and acetylcholinesterase in second trimester amniotic fluid specimens appears to be low yield and may not be as effective as high resolution ultrasonography.[3]

Methodology Immunoassay, solid-phase and enzyme-labeled monoclonal antibody directed to different epitopes

Additional Information Levels of amniotic fluid AFP >2.5 MoM are generally regarded as abnormally high.

When evaluating amniotic fluid AFP and acetylcholinesterase levels in twin gestations in which only one fetus is affected, placental anatomy appears to be important.[2] With diamniotic-dichorionic twin placentas, amniotic fluid AFP and acetylcholinesterase are within normal range for the unaffected fetus, and elevated in the affected fetus. With diamniotic-monochorionic twin placentas, the unaffected twin may demonstrate elevated amniotic fluid AFP and acetylcholinesterase levels, presumably due to diffusion across the amnion bilayer membrane from the affected site.

Fetal status can be assessed by ultrasound (high-resolution) and chorionic villus sampling by the end of the first trimester. The finding that determination of AFP (coupled with "cautious" interpretation of acetylcholinesterase) has application to detection of neural tube defects during this period has important value.[4] The expected level of α-fetoprotein in amniotic fluid between 11 and 15 weeks should not be determined by extrapolation backward from medians of later gestational age.[5,6] The laboratory must establish its own database for MoMs. The calculation is based on a smoothed weighted log-linear regression. The amniotic fluid MoM usually is uncorrected, whereas the serum MoM must be corrected for weight, race, and insulin-dependent diabetes.

AFP in amniotic fluid is derived from two sources, the fetal liver and the fetal yolk sac. These two forms show varying affinity for concanavalin-A. As gestation advances, the yolk sac contribution to amniotic fluid decreases. The decrease in AFP in amniotic fluid surrounding fetuses with trisomy 21 involves proportionately equal reduction in the yolk sac subfraction and total AFP. No advantage in diagnostic efficiency has been found, therefore, in differential determination of the yolk sac subfractions.[7]

AFP levels in Down syndrome overlap normal values but amniotic fluid concentrations of AFP are lower in the presence of a fetus afflicted with Down syndrome. A large percentage of open tube neural defects can be detected by maternal serum AFP measurement. Prenatal assessment of serum AFP with unconjugated estriol, pregnancy-associated protein A, inhibin A, and β-hCG to screen for Down syndrome is outlined in other listings.

See Amniotic Fluid, Chromosome and Genetic Abnormality Analysis on page 360.

Footnotes

1. Haddow JE and Palomaki GE, "Biochemical Markers of Fetal Disorders in Maternal Serum and Amniotic Fluid," *Medicine of the Fetus and Mother*, 2nd ed, Reece EA and Hobbins JC, eds, Philadelphia, PA: Lippincott-Raven Publishers, 1999, 689-706.
2. Ashwood ER, "Clinical Chemistry of Pregnancy," *Tietz Textbook of Clinical Chemistry*, 3rd ed, Burtis CA and Ashwood ER, eds, Philadelphia, PA: WB Saunders Co, 1999, 1736-75.

3. Sepulveda W, Donaldson A, Johnson RD, et al, "Are Routine Alpha-Fetoprotein and Acetylcholinesterase Determinations Still Necessary at Second-Trimester Amniocentesis? Impact of High-Resolution Ultrasonography," *Obstet Gynecol*, 1995, 85(1):107-12.
4. Drugan A, Syner FN, Greb A, et al, "Amniotic Fluid Alpha-Fetoprotein and Acetylcholinesterase in Early Genetic Amniocentesis," *Obstet Gynecol*, 1988, 72(1):35-8.
5. Crandall BF, Hanson FW, Tennant F, et al, "Alpha-Fetoprotein Levels in Amniotic Fluid Between 11 and 15 Weeks," *Am J Obstet Gynecol*, 1989, 160(5 Pt 1):1204-6.
6. Brumfield CG, Cloud GA, Davis RO, et al, "The Relationship Between Maternal Serum and Amniotic Fluid Alpha-Fetoprotein in Women Undergoing Early Amniocentesis," *Am J Obstet Gynecol*, 1990, 163(3):903-6.
7. Jones SR, Evans SE, and Gillan L, "Amniotic Fluid Alpha-Fetoprotein Subfractions in Fetal Trisomy 21 Affected Pregnancies," *Br J Obstet Gynaecol*, 1988, 95(4):327-9.

References

Bock JL, "Current Issues in Maternal Serum Alpha-Fetoprotein Screening," *Am J Clin Pathol*, 1992, 97(4):541-54.

Cuckle HS, "Screening for Neural Tube Defects," *Ciba Found Symp*, 1994, 181:253-69.

Knight GJ, "Maternal Serum Alpha-Fetoprotein Screening," *Techniques in Diagnostic Human Biochemical Genetics*, Hommes FA, ed, New York, NY: Wiley-Liss, 1991, 491-518.

Wenk RE and Rosenbaum JM, "Examination of Amniotic Fluid," Todd-Sanford-Davidsohn Clinical Diagnosis and Management by Laboratory Methods, 19th ed, Henry JB, ed, Philadelphia, PA: WB Saunders Co, 1996, 493-506.

Alpha₁-Fetoprotein, Serum

Related Information

Acetylcholinesterase, Red Cell on page 81
Alpha₁-Fetoprotein, Amniotic Fluid on page 96
Amniotic Fluid, Chromosome and Genetic Abnormality Analysis on page 360
Body Fluid Chemical Analysis on page 123
CA 19-9, Serum on page 128
Carcinoembryonic Antigen, Serum on page 135
Chorionic Gonadotropin, Human, Serum and Urine on page 147
Cyst Fluid Cytology on page 379
Fanconi Anemia, Chromosome Breakage Study on page 365
Inhibin A, Serum on page 199
Pregnancy-Associated Protein A, Serum on page 260

Synonyms AFP

Applies to Triple Test

Abstract An oncofetal antigen, AFP is a glycoprotein of normal fetal plasma found in the alpha₁ region on electrophoresis. Very low levels of AFP are present in the serum of nonpregnant adults. It is increased in hepatic disorders attended by hepatocyte regenerative activity, in hepatoma (hepatocellular carcinoma) and in various nonseminomatous germ cell tumors.

With open fetal neural tube congenital (developmental) defects (principally spina bifida and anencephaly), AFP is elevated in amniotic fluid and therefore in the serum of the gravid woman, but not in all instances.

With certain fetal chromosomal abnormalities (Down syndrome [trisomy 21], and Edwards syndrome [trisomy 18]), it is relatively low in the maternal serum. The risk of Down syndrome increases with advancing maternal age, but 70% to 80% of children with Down syndrome are born to mothers younger than 35. Fetal chromosome analysis provides reliable diagnosis.

Specimen Serum; can also be done on cerebrospinal fluid (CSF)

Container Plain red top tube; not SST™ if intended for maternal screening.[1]

Sampling Time The optimal time to draw **maternal serum** for AFP, for prenatal screening, is at the 16th week of gestation. Maternal serum can be collected between 15th and 21st weeks. For neural tube evaluation and for Down syndrome and Edwards syndrome, recommended collection is between 16-18 weeks.[1] Maternal AFP, unconjugated estriol, and hCG represent the **triple test,** a second-trimester screen for detection of risk for Down syndrome. Down syndrome risk evaluation can be projected at 15-22 weeks.

One of the most common reasons for an abnormal result is uncorrected gestational age. Thus, confirmation of gestational age with ultrasound is helpful.

AFP levels are fairly insensitive for detection of open spina bifida in the third trimester.

Storage Instructions Freeze

Special Instructions Include maternal birth date, first day of last menstrual period, gestational age by calculation and gestation by ultrasound and by physical examination, expected date of delivery,[1] maternal weight, race, and diabetic status with request when testing is intended for prenatal screening. AFP should be used with other tests when Down syndrome risk is estimated.

Reference Interval Normal nonpregnant adults: <15.0 ng/mL serum. Interlaboratory differences exist. Maternal AFP concentrations rise by about 15% per week during the second trimester in normal singleton gestations, while amniotic fluid AFP falls.[2] The level in maternal serum increases to a maximum of 500 ng/mL (SI: 500 µg/L) during the third trimester of pregnancy. Normal values for maternal serum may vary from laboratory to laboratory. Normal is considered 0.5-2.5 **multiples of the median** (MoM) (Continued)

Alpha₁-Fetoprotein, Serum *(Continued)*

when assessing neural tube risk, although some authorities have recommended 0.5-2.0 MoM.[3] The MoM is always corrected for each week of gestation, maternal weight, and maternal race. Maternal insulin-dependent diabetes is related to average 20% lower maternal serum AFP than unaffected singleton women. Black American women have maternal serum AFP ~10% to 15% higher than white American women at all gestational ages.

Use Diagnosis, monitoring of treatment and determination of prognosis in patients with **hepatocellular carcinoma:** With sensitive procedures, elevation of AFP will occur in 90% of patients with hepatocellular carcinoma. Values >1000 ng/mL (SI: >1000 µg/L) are almost always secondary to hepatocellular carcinoma or other neoplasms in nonpregnant individuals. However, overlap with AFP elevations caused by nonmalignant chronic liver disease is widely recognized. Patients who have cirrhosis with chronic hepatitis B or chronic hepatitis C should be monitored with serum AFP and ultrasonography for their risk of hepatocellular carcinoma.[4]

In patients with chronic hepatitis C, AFP concentrations >17.8 ng/mL provide evidence for a diagnosis of cirrhosis.[5]

Gonadal and extragonadal relevant germinal tumor types include **endodermal sinus tumor (yolk sac tumor), embryonal carcinoma, teratocarcinoma, and choriocarcinoma.** AFP is increased in patients with yolk sac tumor. Both AFP and hCG are increased with embryonal carcinoma, while hCG is increased in patients with choriocarcinoma. AFP is not increased in subjects with seminoma. Neither AFP nor hCG are increased with uncomplicated teratoma. AFP increases occur as well from tumors in extragonadal locations: pineal, retroperitoneum, and mediastinum. Since pure seminomas, dysgerminomas, and teratomas do not produce AFP, increased AFP in a subject with seminoma by histopathologic sampling suggests nonseminomatous elements such as embryonal carcinoma and demands further investigation.[6] AFP is useful as an immunoperoxidase reagent in histopathologic study of such tumors.

Monitor therapy with antineoplastic drugs, in patients being treated for hepatoma or germinal neoplasm.

Differential diagnosis of **neonatal hepatitis** versus biliary atresia in newborns.

Maternal serum AFP was the first chemical assay used to screen for fetal malformations. It is useful in **intrauterine** screening with other tests, including chorionic gonadotropins, unconjugated estriol, PAPP-A, inhibin A, amniotic fluid AFP and acetylcholinesterase, and ultrasound. **Elevated values** are found in anencephaly, spina bifida (with support of ultrasound), myelomeningocele, and other open neural tube defects; intrauterine fetal death; esophageal atresia; congenital nephrosis; diagnosis of multiple pregnancy; oligohydramnios; abruptio placentae; and preeclampsia.[7] Increased maternal AFP with normal amniotic fluid AFP signal risk for low-birth-weight infants, related to intrauterine growth retardation or to prematurity. Increased values of AFP in maternal serum can result from underestimated gestational age or from contamination with fetal plasma. **Low values** are associated with chromosomal abnormalities including trisomy 21 and trisomy 18, with misdating of the gestation and with nonpregnancy. See table.

Maternal Serum: Abnormalities of Gestation Summary

	AFP	hCG	uE₃
Abortion, spontaneous or impending		Low	Low
Anencephaly	Very high		Very low
Atresia, esophagus, duodenum	High		
Encephalocoele	High		
Fetal blood contamination	High		
Fetal demise	Low	Low	Low
Gastroschisis	High		
Hemolytic disease of the newborn	High		
Herpesviral fetal liver necrosis	High		
Hydrocephalus	High		
Molar gestation	Undetectable	Very high	Very low
Molar gestation, partial	Low to normal	Very high	Low to normal
Multiple gestation	High	High	High
Myelomeningocoele	High		
Omphalocoele	High		
Preeclampsia		High	
Sulfatase deficiency (fetal)			Very low
Trisomy 13	High		
Trisomy 18	Low	Low	Very low
Trisomy 21 (Down syndrome)	Low	High	Low

Replacement of unconjugated estriol (uE₃) with inhibin A in the multiple marker screening test has been advocated for Down syndrome.

Modified from Ashwood ER, "Clinical Chemistry of Pregnancy" in *Tietz Textbook of Clinical Chemistry* 3rd ed, Burtis CA and Ashwood ER, eds, Philadelphia: WB Saunders Co, 1999.

Limitations High in some cases of nonmalignant liver disease (eg, massive hepatic necrosis, hepatitis, cirrhosis). AFP levels are usually <150 µg/L in such nonmalignant diseases.[8] American instances of hepatocellular carcinoma are not as consistently AFP rich, as many cases from overseas. Thus, overlap exists between AFP levels related to smaller and more readily resected hepatomas, and those of non-neoplastic liver disease.

AFP and hCG are often not increased in patients with stage I neoplasms.

Elevations have been described in tyrosinemia, ataxia telangiectasia, and congenital nephrotic syndrome. A low incidence of elevations occurs in a variety of tumors, especially carcinoma of stomach,[9] pancreas, and biliary tract.

Some maternal serum samples from women carrying fetuses with closed **neural tube defects** have normal levels of AFP. Maternal serum AFP detects about 75% of instances of spina bifida at 18-20 weeks.[10] False-positives for prenatal diagnosis of neural tube defects have been reported. There is a degree of overlap between the curves for unaffected gestations and those of open spina bifida, using maternal serum MoM distributions.

Increased AFP in maternal serum can occur with twins, incorrect gestational age, any blockage of fetal gastrointestinal tract, fetal death, introductions of fetal blood into the maternal circulation, and other conditions.[11] A downward slope in AFP is seen with increasing maternal weight. A formula has been proposed to adjust for this variable.[2]

AFP provides only a 33% detection rate for Down syndrome when used alone.

Elevations are reported with alcoholism.[12]

Contraindications Recently administered radioisotopes may interfere with RIA testing.

Methodology Enzyme immunoassay (EIA), monoclonal immunofluorescent assay, immunochemiluminescent assay, radioimmunoassay (RIA)

Additional Information AFP is structurally similar to albumin with molecular weight of about 65,000. In the embryo it is synthesized by the yolk sac and later by the fetal liver. AFP appears in fetal serum during the sixth week of gestation. It achieves peak concentration in fetal serum and amniotic fluid at 12-14 weeks gestation. In the maternal circulation, AFP is about 10 ng/mL (SI: 10 µg/L) at the 8th week, 60 ng/mL (SI: 60 µg/L) at 20 weeks and undergoes further rise to term.

Maternal screening for presence of open neural tube defects (eg, spina bifida) is based on the finding of elevated AFP in a maternal serum specimen ideally taken at the 16th to 18th week of gestation. The findings must be confirmed by elevated amniotic fluid acetylcholinesterase study and ultrasound study of the fetal spine to attempt to detect the possibility of false-positive results from inaccurate dating, twins, threatened abortion, congenital nephrosis, and other causes.

Unexplained increase in maternal serum AFP with second trimester oligohydramnios is associated with an especially poor prognosis. There is evidence that serial ultrasound evaluations of amniotic fluid volume can assist in predicting pregnancy outcome.[13] With severe decrease in amniotic fluid (eg, severe oligohydramnios or no amniotic fluid), the majority (essentially all) of cases will have pulmonary hypoplasia, Potter deformities, renal developmental abnormalities (such as polycystic kidney), or neonatal death. Genetic testing may be indicated in cases of low values for correct gestational age.

AFP levels may be increased in cases of hepatic parenchymal regeneration (eg, following traumatic injury, associated with the viral hepatitides, and following recovery from exposure to hepatotoxins).

Extremely high AFP levels are found with **endodermal sinus tumors** (yolk sac tumors).[6] Such neoplasms occur in testis, ovary, and in certain extragonadal sites, typically in young subjects. Patients with nonseminomatous germ cell tumors may present with increased levels of hCG, depending upon tumor stage. Approximately 7% to 18% of patients with pure seminoma present or develop an elevated hCG in the course of their disease. Assay of AFP and hCG correlate with tumor volume and are useful in prediction of prognosis and response to treatment.[6] Both AFP and β-hCG are included in the protocol for pathologic evaluation of malignant germ cell neoplasms. Elevated serum levels may indicate need for additional sections.[14] They also provide a means to monitor patients with such tumors - increase of either provides evidence of recurrence or metastasis.

Some **hepatocarcinomas** are associated with very high AFP levels (>10,000 µg/L). For size-matched cases of hepatocellular carcinoma, prognosis relates to serum AFP levels. Patients with low levels of AFP (≤20 µg/L) had two- to threefold increase in survival as compared with patients having the highest (>10,000 µg/L) levels.[15] AFP levels are increased in patients with hepatoblastoma and are used as predictors of outcome.[16]

Low serum levels of AFP and of unconjugated estriol with increased hCG are found in first and second trimesters in mothers with **Down syndrome** (trisomy 21) pregnancies. However, AFP employed alone to screen for this condition has poor predictive value and should always be used with other tests. Maternal serum AFP levels are decreased in trisomy 18. The combination of maternal serum AFP with maternal serum human chorionic gonadotropin (hCG) and unconjugated estriol (uE₃) have been advocated to improve the predictive value of screening for Down syndrome. This **"triple test"** can detect 60% to 75% of Down syndrome cases with a false-positive rate of about 6%. Some sources suggest that the uE₃ is not essential for the screen. Others have advocated the use of a free beta-hCG assay to improve predictive value. In the **second trimester**, the best detection rates have included AFP, β-hCG, inhibin A, and age. (Inhibin A is increased with Down syndrome). However, use of inhibin A failed to contribute to the detection of trisomy 18.[17]

AFP testing is useful in the detection of pregnancy complications such as intrauterine growth retardation, fetal distress, fetal demise, or in the presence of severe maternal pregnancy-induced hypertension. In all these instances, the serum AFP was increased >2.0 MOM. The use of AFP was found to be more valuable in detection of these complications than in detection of neural tube defects.[3]

Footnotes

1. Kisbeth RM, Mayo Medical Laboratories, *2000 Test Catalog*, Rochester, MN.
2. Haddow JE and Palomaki GE, "Biochemical Markers of Fetal Disorders in Maternal Serum and Amniotic Fluid," *Medicine of the Fetus and Mother*, 2nd ed, Chapter 40, Reece EA and Hobbins JC, eds, Philadelphia, PA: Lippincott-Raven, 1999, 689-706.
3. Lenke RR, Guerrieri J, Nemes JM, et al, "Elevated Maternal Serum Alpha-Fetoprotein Values: How Low Is High?" *J Reprod Med*, 1989, 34(8):511-6.
4. Ince N and Wands JR, "The Increasing Incidence of Hepatocellular Carcinoma," *N Engl J Med*, 1999, 340(10):798-9.
5. Bayati N, Silverman AL, Gordon SC, "Serum Alpha-Fetoprotein Levels and Liver Histology in Patients With Chronic Hepatitis C," *Am J Gastroenterol*, 1998, 93(12):2452-6.
6. Bajorin DF and Bosl GJ, "The Use of Serum Tumor Markers in the Prognosis and Treatment of Germ Cell Tumors," *Principles and Practice of Oncology*, 1992, 1-11.
7. Milunsky A, Jick SS, Bruell CL, et al, "Predictive Values, Relative Risks, and Overall Benefits of High and Low Maternal Serum α-Fetoprotein Screening in Singleton Pregnancies: New Epidemiologic Data," *Am J Obstet Gynecol*, 1989, 161(2):291-7.
8. Goldstein NS, Blue DE, Hankin R, et al, "Serum Alpha-Fetoprotein Levels in Patients With Chronic Hepatitis C," *Am J Clin Pathol*, 1999, 111(6):811-16.
9. Koide N, Nishio A, Igarashi J, et al, "Alpha-Fetoprotein-Producing Gastric Cancer: Histochemical Analysis of Cell Proliferation, Apoptosis and Angiogenesis," *Am J Gastroenterol*, 1999, 94(6):1658-63.
10. Cuckle HS, "Screening for Neural Tube Defects," *Ciba Found Symp*, 1994, 181:253-69.
11. Cunningham FG and Gilstrap LC, "Maternal Serum Alpha-Fetoprotein Screening," *N Engl J Med*, 1991, 325(1):55-7.
12. Christiansen M, Andersen JR, Tørning J, et al, "Serum Alpha-Fetoprotein and Alcohol Consumption," *Scand J Clin Lab Invest*, 1994, 54(3):215-20.
13. Richards DS, Seeds JW, Katz VL, et al, "Elevated Maternal Serum Alpha-Fetoprotein With Oligohydramnios: Ultrasound Evaluation and Outcome," *Obstet Gynecol*, 1988, 72(3 Pt 1):337-41.
14. Ulbright TM, "Protocol for the Examination of Specimens From Patients With Malignant Germ Cell and Sex Cord-Stromal Tumors of the Testis, Exclusive of Paratesticular Malignancies," *Arch Pathol Lab Med*, 1999, 123(1):14-19.
15. Nomura F, Ohnishi K, and Tanabe Y, "Clinical Features and Prognosis of Hepatocellular Carcinoma With Reference to Serum Alpha-Fetoprotein Levels," *Cancer*, 1989, 64(8):1700-7.
16. Van Tornout JM, Buckley JD, Quinn JJ, et al, "Timing and Magnitude of Decline in Alpha-Fetoprotein Levels in Treated Children With Unresectable or Metastatic Hepatoblastoma Are Predictors of Outcome: A Report From the Children's Cancer Group," *J Clin Oncol*, 1997, 15(3):1190-7.
17. Altken DA, Wallace EM, Crossley JA, et al, "Dimeric Inhibin A as a Marker for Down Syndrome in Early Pregnancy," *N Engl J Med*, 1996, 334(19):1231-6.

References

Baskin LB, personnel correspondence, 2000.

Benn PA, Clive JM, and Collins R, "Medians for Second-Trimester Maternal Serum Alpha-Fetoprotein, Human Chorionic Gonadotropin, and Unconjugated Estriol: Differences Between Races or Ethnic Groups," *Clin Chem*, 1997, 43(2):333-7.

Benn PA, Horne D, Briganti S, et al, "Elevated Second-Trimester Maternal Serum hCG Alone or in Combination With Elevated Alpha-Fetoprotein," *Obstet Gynecol*, 1996, 87(2):217-22.

Bidart JM, Thuillier F, Augereau C, et al, "Kinetics of Serum Tumor Marker Concentrations and Usefulness in Clinical Monitoring," *Clin Chem*, 1999, 45(10):1695-707.

Bock JL, "Current Issues in Maternal Serum Alpha-Fetoprotein Screening," *Am J Clin Pathol*, 1992, 97(4):541-54.

Curtin JP, Rubin SC, Hoskins WJ, et al, "Second-Look Laparotomy in Endodermal Sinus Tumor: A Report of Two Patients With Normal Levels of Alpha-Fetoprotein and Residual Tumor at Reexploration," *Obstet Gynecol*, 1989, 73(4):893-5.

de Wit R, Collette L, Sylvester R, et al, "Serum Alpha-Fetoprotein Surge After the Initiation of Chemotherapy for Nonseminomatous Testicular Cancer Has an Adverse Prognostic Significance," *Br J Cancer*, 1998, 78(10):1350-5.

Macri JN, "Critical Issues in Prenatal Maternal Serum Alpha-Fetoprotein Screening for Genetic Abnormalities," *Am J Obstet Gynecol*, 1986, 155(2):240-6.

Matsumura M, Shiratori Y, Niwa Y, et al, "Presence of Alpha-Fetoprotein mRNA in Blood Correlates With Outcome in Patients With Hepatocellular Carcinoma," *J Hepatol*, 1999, 31(2):332-9.

Palomaki GE and Haddow JE, "Prenatal Screening for Open Neural-Tube Defects in Maine," *N Engl J Med*, 1999, 340(13)1049-50.

Saller DN Jr, Cranick JA, Kellner LH, et al, "Maternal Serum Analyte Levels in Pregnancies With Fetal Down Syndrome Resulting From Translocations," *Am J Obstet Gynecol*, 1997, 177(4):879-81.

Sato Y, Nakata K, Kato Y, et al, "Early Recognition of Hepatocellular Carcinoma Based on Altered Profiles of Alpha-Fetoprotein," *N Engl J Med*, 1993, 328(25):1802-6.

Schefer H, Mattmann S, Joss RA, "Hereditary Persistence of Alpha-Fetoprotein," *Ann Oncol*, 1998, 9(6):667-72.

Spong CY, Ghidini A, Walker CN, et al, "Elevated Maternal Serum Midtrimester Alpha-Fetoprotein Levels Are Associated With Fetoplacental Ischemia," *Am J Obstet Gynecol*, 1997, 177(5):1085-7.

Wenstrom KD, Owen J, Chu DC, et al, "Alpha-Fetoprotein, Free Beta-Human Chorionic Gonadotropin, and Dimeric Inhibin A Produce the Best Results in a Three-Analyte, Multiple-Marker Screening Test for Fetal Down Syndrome," *Am J Obstet Gynecol*, 1997, 177(5):987-91.

Wenstrom KD, Owen J, Chu DC, et al, "Maternal Serum Alpha-Fetoprotein and Dimeric Inhibin A Detect Aneuploidies Other Than Down Syndrome," *Am J Obstet Gynecol*, 1998, 179(4):966-70.

Wong NA, D'Costa H, Barry RE, et al, "Primary Yolk Sac Tumour of the Liver in Adulthood," *J Clin Pathol*, 1998, 51(12):939-40.

Yaron Y, Cherry M, Kramer RL, et al, "Second-Trimester Maternal Serum Marker Screening: Maternal Serum Alpha-Fetoprotein, Beta-Human Chorionic Gonadotropin, Estriol, and Their Various Combinations as Predictors of Pregnancy Outcome," *Am J Obstet Gynecol*, 1999, 181(4):968-74.

◆ **Alpha₁ Lipoprotein Cholesterol** *see* High Density Lipoprotein Cholesterol, Serum *on page 192*

Alpha₂-Macroglobulin, Serum

Abstract α_2-Macroglobulin (AMG) is a very large, 725-kD glycoprotein, consisting of four identical peptides configured into two dimer subunits. It is synthesized primarily by hepatic parenchymal cells and functions as a panproteinase inhibitor using a clever trapping mechanism. The loss of AMG in the urine is prevented by its large size. Its plasma concentration increases dramatically in nephrotic syndrome due to volume shifts secondary to changes in plasma oncotic pressure and increases in synthesis compensatory to albumin loss. In humans, AMG is not an acute phase reactant. Levels are decreased in proteolytic diseases such as acute pancreatitis and peptic ulcer disease.

Patient Preparation Patient should be fasting.

Specimen Serum

Container Red top tube

Storage Instructions Refrigerate (4°C) for up to 72 hours. After 72 hours, the specimen should be stored frozen at -20°C and thawed only once prior to analysis.

Causes for Rejection Gross hemolysis, lipemia

Reference Interval The reference interval in adults 20-60 years of age is 130-300 mg/dL.[1] Since estrogen increases AMG synthesis, levels in women of childbearing age are higher than in age-matched men. Children and infants have levels higher than adults.[2] Reference intervals for infants are as follows:[3] birth: 125-392 mg/dL, 1 month: 217-439 mg/dL, 3 months: 261-466 mg/dL, 6 months: 269-503 mg/dL. In subjects 6 months to 15 years, results range from 250-640 mg/dL, peaking at 2-4 years of age.[2]

Use Measurement of AMG may be used to evaluate patients with nephrotic syndrome and patients with proteolytic conditions such as pancreatitis, or to further characterize an electrophoretic change in the α_2-zone.

Limitations Estrogen therapy, exercise, pregnancy, and any number of disease states (eg, diabetes mellitus, hepatitis, cirrhosis of the liver, α_1-antitrypsin deficiency, cerebral infarction, amyloidosis) may result in increased AMG serum levels. Decreased levels have been observed following surgery.

Methodology Immunonephelometry, immunoturbidimetry, radial immunodiffusion (RID)

Additional Information A deletion polymorphism of the human α_2-macroglobulin gene has been identified as a potential risk factor for Alzheimer disease.[4] The gene is located on chromosome 12p13.3-p12.3, and the mutation affects the proteinase trapping functionality in a way that may reverse the protection AMG normally affords against β-amyloid deposition by binding with brain amyloid and facilitating its clearance. Methods for detecting the deletion polymorphism recently have been described.[5,6]

Prostate-specific antigen (PSA) forms complexes with AMG in addition to other proteins (α_1-chymotrypsin and α_1-proteinase inhibitor), and the proportion of PSA binding to AMG is increased in patients with benign prostatic hypertrophy compared to patients with prostate cancer.[7] Pretreatment concentrations are decreased in patients with advanced carcinoma of prostate.

Footnotes

1. Dati F, Schumann G, Thomas L, et al, "Consensus of a Group of Professional Societies and Diagnostic Companies on Guidelines for Interim Reference Ranges for 14 Proteins in Serum Based on the Standardization Against the IFCC/BCR/CAP Reference Material (CRM 470). International Federation of Clinical Chemistry. Community Bureau of Reference of the Commission of the European Communities. College of American Pathologists," *Eur J Clin Chem Clin Biochem*, 1996, 34(6):517-20.
2. Geiger H and Hoffman P, "Quantitative Immunologische Bestimmung Von 16 Verschiedenen Serumproteinen Bei 260 Normalen, 0-15 Jahre Alten Kindern," *Z Kinderheilk*, 1970, 109:22-40.
3. Kanakoudi F, Drossou V, Tzimouli V, et al, "Serum Concentrations of 10 Acute-Phase Proteins in Healthy Term and Preterm Infants From Birth to Age 6 Months," *Clin Chem*, 1995, 41(4):605-8.
4. Blacker D, Wilcox MA, Laird NM, et al, "α-2 Macroglobulin Is Genetically Associated With Alzheimer Disease," *Nat Genet*, 1998, 19(4):357-60.
5. Dodel RC, Bales KR, Farlow MR, et al, "Rapid Detection of a Pentanucleotide Deletion Polymorphism in the Human α_2-Macroglobulin Gene," *Clin Chem*, 1999, 45(2):307-17.
6. Wu YY, Delgado RM, Sunderland T, et al, "Detection of a Deletion Polymorphism of the Human α_2-Macroglobulin Gene (A2M-2) by a Semiautomated PCR-Single-Stranded Conformational Polymorphism Method," *Clin Chem*, 1999, 45(9):1572-3.

(Continued)

Alpha₂-Macroglobulin, Serum (Continued)

7. Zhang WM, Finne P, Leinonen J, et al, "Characterization and Immunological Determination of the Complex Between Prostate-Specific Antigen and α₂-Macroglobulin," Clin Chem, 1998, 44(12):2471-9.

References

Borth W, "α₂-Macroglobulin, a Multifunctional Binding Protein With Targeting Characteristics," FASEB J, 1992, 6:3345-53.

Chan DW and Sokoll LJ, "Prostate-Specific Antigen: Advances and Challenges," Clin Chem, 1999, 45(4 Pt 1):755-6.

Du Y, Bales KR, Dodel RC, et al, "α₂-Macroglobulin Attenuates β-Amyloid Peptide 1-40 Fibril Formation and Associated Neurotoxicity of Cultured Fetal Rat Cortical Neurons," J Neurochem, 1998, 70(3):1182-8.

Du Y, Ni B, Glinn M, et al, "α₂-Macroglobulin as a β-Amyloid Peptide-Binding Plasma Protein," J Neurochem, 1997, 69(1):299-305.

Ganrot PO and Schersten B, "Serum α₂-Macroglobulin Concentration and Its Variation With Age and Sex," Clin Chim Acta, 1967, 15:113-20.

Johnson AM, Rohlfs EM, and Silverman LM, "Proteins," Tietz Textbook of Clinical Chemistry, 3rd ed, Chapter 20, Burtis CA and Ashwood ER, eds, Philadelphia, PA: WB Saunders Co, 1999, 477-540.

Lasson A, Berling R, Goransson J, et al, "Alpha-2-Macroglobulin Decreases Parallel to Albumin and Hemoglobin After Elective Surgery," Scand J Clin Lab Invest, 1991, 51:225-33.

Levine JJ, Udall JN, Evernden BA, et al, "Elevated Levels of α2-Macroglobulin-Protease Complexes in Infants," Biol Neonate, 1987, 51:149-55.

Qiu WQ, Borth W, Ye Z, et al, "Degradation of Amyloid β-Protein by a Serine Protease-α₂-Macroglobulin Complex," J Biol Chem, 1996, 271(14):8443-51.

♦ **Alpha-Hydroxybutyric Dehydrogenase (HBDH)** replaced by Cardiac Markers: Laboratory Assessment, Overview on page 137

♦ **Alpha-Hydroxybutyric Dehydrogenase, Serum** replaced by Lactate Dehydrogenase Isoenzymes, Serum on page 206

♦ **Alpha Tocopherol** see Vitamin E, Serum or Plasma on page 301

♦ **ALP Isoenzymes** see Alkaline Phosphatase Isoenzymes, Serum on page 92

♦ **ALT** see Alanine Aminotransferase, Serum on page 87

♦ **ALT:AST Ratio** see Liver Disease: Laboratory Assessment, Overview on page 216

♦ **Aminoacidopathies** see Amino Acids, Urine on page 101

Amino Acids, Plasma

Related Information

Amino Acids, Urine on page 101
Ammonia, Plasma on page 102
Newborn Screen for Phenylketonuria on page 229
Phenylalanine, Blood on page 248

Synonyms Inborn Errors of Metabolism Screen; Metabolic Screen for Amino Acids

Applies to Biotinidase; Carnitine; Organic Acids

Test Includes Screening and quantitation of amino acids

Reference Interval Varies significantly with age. Established by each laboratory. See table as a guide.[1] Age specific reference ranges are published.[2]

Amino Acids in Plasma
(μmol/L)

Amino Acid	Men	Women	Adolescents	Children
Alanine	146-494	218-474	242-594	120-600
α-Aminobutyrate	15-35	7-35	8-36	12-43
Arginine	28-96	28-108	1-81	12-112
Asparagine	32-92	26-74	34-94	15-83
Aspartic Acid	2-9	3-6	3-15	1-17
Citrulline	19-47	10-58	19-52	8-47
Cystine	24-54	31-49	36-58	23-68
Glutamic Acid	6-62	6-38	17-69	14-78
Glutamine	466-798	340-696	457-857	333-809
Glycine	147-299	100-384	166-330	107-343
Histidine	72-108	68-104	68-108	47-135
Isoleucine	46-90	39-67	34-106	6-122
Leucine	113-205	98-142	86-206	30-246
Lysine	135-243	119-203	116-276	66-270
Methionine	213-37	214-30	213-41	223-43
Ornithine	55-135	36-96	47-195	20-136
Phenylalanine	46-74	42-62	34-86	26-98
Proline	97-297	112-220	58-324	40-332
Serine	89-165	78-166	92-196	70-194
Taurine	27-95	18-66	20-90	20-120
Threonine	92-180	93-197	102-246	40-204
Tryptophan	25-65	17-53	—	12-69
Tyrosine	37-77	26-78	35-107	19-119
Valine	179-335	172-248	155-343	132-480

Abstract Plasma amino acids concentrations show diurnal variation and are higher after a high protein meal. Therefore, fasting samples are preferred, **except** in hyperammonemia screening. Postprandial ammonia samples are preferred since elevations are maximum in the fed state.

Patient Preparation Infants: 4-hour fast; children and adults: 12-hour fast. Protein intake does not affect diurnal variation, but it influences absolute concentrations of amino acids in blood or urine.

Specimen Plasma

Container Green top (heparin) tube

Sampling Time Fasting sample is preferred as marked circadian rhythm is exhibited with values highest in afternoon and lowest in early morning.

Collection Routine venipuncture

Storage Instructions Centrifuge. Transfer plasma to plastic vial and freeze within 1 hour of collection. Stable for 1 week at -20°C. For longer periods, deproteinize sample and store at -70°C.

Use Screen for inborn errors of metabolism of amino acids (eg, investigation of metabolic acidosis, ketosis, hyperammonemia, developmental impairment, failure to thrive)

Limitations For some of these entities, investigation should include urine organic acids, amino acids, blood ammonia, biotinidase, and carnitine.

Methodology Plasma screen by single dimension thin-layer chromatography (TLC), amino acid analyzer (ion-exchange chromatography), gas chromatography (GC), and high performance liquid chromatography (HPLC)[3,4,5]

Additional Information Amino acid concentrations show a significant circadian rhythm with intra-day plasma level variation of 30%. Values are highest in midafternoon and lowest in the early morning. A variety of inherited metabolic disorders result in aminoacidemia/aminoaciduria. Typically, the abnormal amino acids concentration exceeds 3-4 times normal, but may be >10 times normal.

Congenital Disorders of Amino Acid Metabolism

Name	Enzyme or Metabolic Pathways	Clinical Findings	Laboratory Findings
Classic phenylketonuria	Phenylalanine hydroxylase	Mental retardation, psychiatric dysfunction	Plasma phenylalanine >15 mg/dL
Benign phenylalaninemia	Phenylalanine hydroxylase	Asymptomatic	Increased plasma phenylalamine
Malignant phenylalaninemia	Dihydropteridine reductase	Mental retardation, psychiatric dysfunction	Increased plasma phenylalanine
Malignant phenylalaninemia	GTP cyclohydrolase	Mental retardation, psychiatric dysfunction	Increased plasma phenylalanine
Hereditary tyrosinemia	p-hydroxy phenyl acetic acid hydroxylase	Hepatic cirrhosis, renal tubular dysfunction	Increased plasma tyrosine
Alkaptonuria	Homogentisic acid oxidase	Ochronosis, arthritis	Increased urinary homogentisic acid
Histidinemia	Histidine-ammonia lyase	Hearing and speech defect	Increased plasma and urine histidine
Branched-chain aminoacidemia	Branched-chain amino acid oxidase	Seizures, ketosis, mental retardation	Increased urine and plasma branched-chain amino acids
Homocystinuria	Cystathionine synthase	Mental retardation, thromboembolism	Increased plasma and urine homocystine and methionine
Cystathioninuria	Cystathionase	Asymptomatic	Increased urine cystathionine
Cystinuria	Renal transport system for cystine and dibasic amino acids	Cystine stones	Increased urine cystine and dibasic amino acids
Hyperglycinemias			
Ketotic form	Propionyl-CoA-carboxylase	Ketosis, neutropenia, mental retardation	Increased urine and plasma glycine and propionic acid
Nonketotic form	Glycine decarboxylase	Developmental retardation	Increased urine and plasma glycine
Urea cycle abnormalities	Carbamoylphosphate synthase, ornithine-carbamoyltransferase, citrulline aspartate lyase, argininosuccinate arginine-lyase	Developmental retardation, vomiting, lethargy, seizures, hepatomegaly	Increased urine and plasma ammonia, glutamine, citrulline, and arginosuccinate
Glycinuria	Renal transport system for glycine and amino acids	Asymptomatic	Increased urine glycine, proline, and hydroxyproline
Hartnup disease	Renal transport system for neutral amino acids	Ataxia, retardation	Increased urine neutral amino acids
Fanconi syndrome	General renal transport deficiency	Acidosis and rickets	General aminoaciduria, glycinemia, phosphaturia

Cystinuria has an autosomal recessive mode of inheritance, is a disorder of amino acid transport involving renal tubules/GI tract and should be suspect in cases of urinary stone disease. It is characterized by the formation of radiopaque urinary stones and by the presence of characteristic hexagonal crystals in the urine. Dibasic amino acids are increased in urine (see Cystine, Urine *on page 164*).

Lysinuric protein intolerance is another disorder of membrane transport. As in some cases of cystinuria, cationic amino acids (lysine, arginine and ornithine) are involved. Lysine is present in large amounts in the urine but is normal or decreased in plasma. Patients have poor appetite, fail to thrive, develop hepatosplenomegaly, hypotonia, sparse hair, osteoporosis, mental retardation, and a variety of other problems. In **Hartnup disease**, there is impaired neutral amino acid transport involving the kidneys and small intestine. It is characterized clinically by pellagra-like features, mental retardation and/or psychotic behavior, intermittent ataxia and is inherited as an autosomal recessive. A comprehensive review of these and other amino acidurias is provided in the text edited by Scriver et al.[6] Congenital disorders of amino acids are given in the table on previous page.

The usual approach is to screen urine for amino acids. However, urinary levels are variable: plasma measurements usually have better predictive values. Quantitative tests for plasma amino acids are available. In almost all cases in which an amino acid is elevated in blood, it will also be elevated in urine.

CSF amino acids are useful in the diagnosis of nonketotic hyperglycinemia.

When urea cycle defects are suspected, plasma quantitative amino acids, urine orotic acids and organic acids should be assessed.[7] See table.

Footnotes

1. Shih VE, "Amino Acid Analysis," *Physician's Guide to the Laboratory Diagnosis of Metabolic Diseases*, Blau N, Duran M, and Blaskovics, eds, London: Chapman and Hall, 1996, 1-29.
2. Soldin SJ, Brugnara C, Hicks SJM, "Pediatric Reference Ranges," Washington, DC: AACC Press, American Association of Clinical Chemistry, 1999, 11-9.
3. Desgrès J and Padieu P, "Gas-Liquid Chromatographic Analysis of Amino Acids as Isobutyl Esters, N(O)-Heptafluorobutyrate Derivatives: Applications to Clinical Biology," *Amino Acid Analysis by Gas Chromatography*, Volume I, Chapter 5, Gehrke CW, Kuo KCT, and Zumwalt RW, eds, Boca Raton, FL: CRC Press Inc, 1987, 119-42.
4. Hancock WS and Harding DR, "Review of Separation Conditions," *CRC Handbook of HPLC for the Separation of Amino Acids, Peptides, and Proteins*, Volume I, Hancock WS, ed, Boca Raton, FL: CRC Press Inc, 1984, 235-62.
5. Slocum RH and Cummings JG, "Amino Acid Analysis of Physiological Samples," *Techniques in Diagnostic Human Biochemical Genetics*, Hommes FA, ed, New York, NY: Wiley-Liss, 1991, 87-126.
6. Scriver CR, Kaufman S, Eisensmith RC, et al, "Amino Acids," Part 5, *The Metabolic and Molecular Basis of Inherited Disease*, 7th ed, Scriver CR, Beaudet AL, Sly WS, et al, eds, New York, NY: McGraw-Hill Inc, 1995, 1015-368.
7. Lindor NM and Karnes PS, "Laboratory Medicine and Pathology: Initial Assessment of Infants and Children With Suspected Inborn Errors of Metabolism," *Mayo Clin Proc*, 1995, 70(10):987-8.

References

Burlina AB, Bonafé L, and Zacchello F, "Clinical and Biochemical Approach to the Neonate With a Suspected Inborn Error of Amino Acid and Organic Acid Metabolism," *Semin Perinatol*, 1999, 23(2):162-73.

Christenson RM and Azzazy HME, "Amino Acids," *Tietz Textbook of Clinical Chemistry*, 3rd ed, Burtis CA and Ashwood ER, eds, Philadelphia, PA: WB Saunders Co, 1999, 444-76.

Cleary MA and Wraith JE, "Antenatal Diagnosis of Inborn Errors of Metabolism," *Arch Dis Child*, 1991, 66(7 Spec No):816-22.

Elsas LJ, Longo N, and Rosenberg LE, "Inherited Disorders of Amino Acid Metabolism and Storage," *Harrison's Principles of Internal Medicine*, 14th ed, Chapter 349, Fauci AS, Braunwald E, Isselbacher KJ, et al, eds, New York, NY: McGraw-Hill Inc, 1998, 2194-203.

Forman DT, "Role of the Laboratory in Diagnosis of Organic Acidurias," *Ann Clin Lab Sci*, 1991, 21(2):85-93.

National Academy of Clinical Biochemistry 14th Annual Symposium, "Diagnosis and Treatment of Inborn Errors of Metabolism," *Clin Biochem*, 1991, 24(4):289-381.

Shih VE, "Detection of Hereditary Metabolic Disorders Involving Amino Acids and Organic Acids," *Clin Biochem*, 1991, 24(4):301-9.

Amino Acids, Urine

Related Information

Synonyms Metabolic Screen for Amino Acids

Applies to Aminoacidopathies; Beta-Amino Isobutyrate; Cystathionine; Cystine; Glycine; Homocyst(e)ine; Hydroxyproline; Isoleucine; Leucine; Methionine; Organic Acids; Ornithine; Phenylalanine; Proline; Tryptophan; Tyrosine; Valine

Test Includes Differences exist between laboratories. Urine amino acid screen may include alanine, arginine, citrulline, glutamine, beta-amino isobutyrate, cystathionine, cystine, glycine, homocyst(e)ine, hydroxyproline, isoleucine, leucine, methionine, ornithine, phenylalanine, proline, tryptophan, tyrosine, and valine.

Abstract Aminoacidurias may be primary or secondary; the former being due to inherited enzyme defect or inborn error of metabolism. Secondary aminoaciduria is due to organ failure, such as liver or renal failure. Although amino acids filtered through the renal glomerulus are normally almost entirely reabsorbed, in Fanconi syndrome they are not, in spite of the presence of normal plasma concentrations.

Patient Preparation Amphetamines, norepinephrine, levodopa, some antibiotics (particularly penicillins and cephalosporins), methyldopa, levodopa, and polythiazide have been reported to interfere chemically with this test. Amino acid concentrations in urine are physiologically increased by aspirin, bismuth, hydrocortisone, insulin, lead poisoning, triamcinolone, and valproic acid.

Specimen Urine

Collection Random specimen acceptable, no preservative. Morning urine preferred.

Storage Instructions Refrigerate; freeze for long-term storage.

Causes for Rejection Specific gravity of the urine must be ≥1.010

Reference Interval Subjective interpretation based on comparison of patient, normal, and control urines of comparable age. Interpretation is age dependent. Urinary amino acids separated by thin-layer chromatography (TLC) are not usually quantitated. If any amino acids appear to be in high concentration compared to normals or controls, quantitation can be carried out by separate methodology, such as amino acid analyzer (ion-exchange chromatography), gas chromatography (GC), and high performance liquid chromatography (HPLC). Significant differences exist between laboratories. Approximate reference ranges are published.[1]

Use This urine screen is used in investigation of failure to thrive, acidosis, hypokalemia, hypophosphatemia, and abnormalities of vitamin D metabolism.[2] It is a screen for "inborn errors of metabolism" of amino acids, Fanconi syndrome, Wilson disease, and Lowe syndrome.

Limitations Dilute urines cannot be run; concentrated urine is needed.

Methodology Screening: thin-layer chromatography (TLC); quantitation: amino acid analyzer (ion-exchange chromatography), gas chromatography (GC), and high performance liquid chromatography (HPLC)

Additional Information Excretion of certain amino acids is increased in several specific **aminoacidurias**, such as phenylketonuria and maple syrup urine disease. Dibasic amino acids (lysine, ornithine, arginine, cystine) are increased in cystinuria. **Aminoacidopathies**, with ninhydrin-positive urinary amino acids, include phenylketonuria, cystinuria, nonketotic hyperglycinemia and homocystinuria. Their investigation includes urine organic acids and amino acids, plasma amino acids, blood NH_3^+, biotinidase, and carnitine.[2] Aminoaciduria may also be seen in a variety of other disorders, including viral hepatitis, multiple myeloma, rickets, hyperparathyroidism, and chronic renal failure. A positive test should be followed up with quantitation on a 24-hour collection. See table in listing Amino Acids, Plasma *on page 100*.

The Fanconi syndrome (FS), characterized by dysfunction of the proximal renal tubule, is caused by a variety of hereditary and acquired diseases. The former include primary idiopathic FS, cystinosis, Lowe's syndrome, tyrosinemia type 1, galactosemia, hereditary fructose intolerance, glycogen storage disease, Wilson disease, and other entities. Acquired FS may be caused by aminoglycosides, outdated tetracyclines, cephalothins, valproic acid, streptozotocin, 6-mercaptopurine, azathioprine, and cis-platinum; toxins including heavy metals, toluene sniffing and paraquat. It may be found with nephrotic syndrome, myeloma, amyloidosis, antitubular basement membrane antibody, renal vein thrombosis, cancer, and following renal transplantation.[3]

Footnotes

1. Soldin SJ, Brugnara C, Hicks JM, "Pediatric Reference Ranges," Washington, DC: AACC Press, American Association of Clinical Chemistry, 1999, 20-30.
2. Lindor NM and Karnes PS, "Initial Assessment of Infants and Children With Suspected Inborn Errors of Metabolism," *Mayo Clin Proc*, 1995, 70(10):987-8.
3. Brewer ED and Powell DR, "Pan-Proximal Tubular Dysfunction (Fanconi's Syndrome)," *Oski's Pediatrics Principles and Practice*, 3rd ed, McMillan JA, DeAngelis CD, Feigin RD, et al, eds, Philadelphia, PA: JB Lippincott Co, 1999, 1613-8.

References

Asplin JR and Coe FL, "Hereditary Tubular Disorders," *Harrison's Principles of Internal Medicine*, 14th ed, Chapter 278, Fauci AS, Braunwald E, Isselbacher KJ, et al, eds, New York, NY: McGraw-Hill Inc, 1998, 1562-9.

Burlina AB, Bonafé L, and Zacchello F, "Clinical and Biochemical Approach to the Neonate With a Suspected Inborn Error of Aino Acid and Organic Acid Metabolism," *Semin Perinatol*, 1999, 23(2):162-73.

Elsas LJ, Longo N, and Rosenberg LE, "Inherited Disorders of Amino Acid Metabolism and Storage," *Harrison's Principles of Internal Medicine*, 14th ed, Chapter 349, Fauci AS, Braunwald E, Isselbacher KJ, et al, eds, New York, NY: McGraw-Hill Inc, 1998, 2194-203.

Scriver CR, Kaufman S, Eisensmith RC, et al, "Amino Acids," *The Metabolic and Molecular Basis of Inherited Disease*, 7th ed, Part 5, Scriver CR, Beaudet AL, Sly WS, et al, New York, NY: McGraw-Hill Inc, 1995, 1015-368.

Slocum RH and Cummings JG, "Amino Acid Analysis of Physiological Samples," *Techniques in Diagnostic Human Biochemical Genetics*, Hommes FA, ed, New York, NY: Wiley-Liss, 1991, 87-126.

- **Aminolevulinic Acid** *see* Delta (5)-Aminolevulinic Acid, Urine *on page 165*

- **5-Aminolevulinic Acid** *see* Delta (5)-Aminolevulinic Acid, Urine *on page 165*

- **Aminotransferases** *see* Alanine Aminotransferase, Serum *on page 87*

- **Aminotransferases** *see* Aspartate Aminotransferase, Serum *on page 112*

- **Ammonia, Cerebrospinal Fluid** *see* Ammonia, Plasma *on page 102*

Ammonia, Plasma

Related Information
Amino Acids, Plasma *on page 100*
Cerebrospinal Fluid Glutamine *on page 141*
Insulin, Serum *on page 201*
Lactic Acid, Whole Blood or Plasma *on page 208*

Synonyms NH_3, Blood

Applies to Ammonia, Cerebrospinal Fluid

Abstract May be useful for diagnosis of Reye syndrome, urea cycle metabolic abnormalities, organic acidurias, hepatic encephalopathy, and in monitoring patients on hyperalimentation therapy.

Patient Preparation Patient should avoid smoking prior to sampling. Avoid clenching of fist.

Specimen Plasma

Container Green top (sodium or lithium heparin) tube or lavender top (EDTA) tube. One author, however, suggests that heparin will produce false low results.[1]

Collection Tube must be filled completely and kept tightly stoppered at all times. Avoid hemolysis, which increases plasma ammonia. Specimen must be placed on ice immediately and rotated, then centrifuged at 4°C. Plasma should be very promptly separated from the cells. Test must be performed within 20 minutes of the venipuncture, or the plasma frozen immediately. Concentration rapidly increases on standing. Never freeze whole blood.

Storage Instructions In separated plasma, ammonia is stable for several days at -70°C.

Causes for Rejection Specimen not received on ice within 20 minutes of collection

Reference Interval Reference ranges vary among laboratories. See table for approximate ranges. Ammonia level in cerebrospinal fluid is about 33% to 50% of that in arterial blood.[2]

Plasma Ammonia

Age	μg N/dL	SI: μmol N/L
Neonates	90-150	64-107
<2 wk	79-129	56-92
Children	29-70	21-50
Adults	15-45	11-32

Note: Values are somewhat higher in capillary blood.

Use Ammonia is elevated in liver disease; urinary tract infection with distention and stasis; Reye syndrome; urea cycle disorders; HHH (hyperornithinemia, hyperammonemia-homocitrullinuria) syndrome; certain organic disorders such as propionic, methylmalonic, and isovaleric acidemias; some normal neonates (usually returning to normal in 48 hours); total parenteral nutrition; ureterosigmoidostomy; gastrointestinal bleed; and sodium valproate therapy. Ammonia determination is indicated in neonates with neurological deterioration, subjects with lethargy and/or emesis not explained, and in patients with possible encephalopathy.

Ammonia is used in the diagnosis of **urea cycle enzyme deficiencies** (to be considered in any neonate with unexplained nausea, vomiting, or neurological deterioration appearing after the first feeding). Investigation includes plasma amino acids, urine orotic and organic acids.[3]

In **Reye syndrome** there are marked elevations of ammonia, AST, ALT, and prothrombin time, while bilirubin is normal.[4] Glucose should be monitored to anticipate hypoglycemia. Acid-base and osmolal status are monitored to anticipate encephalopathy. Liver biopsy is recommended to confirm the diagnosis and exclude other metabolic and toxic liver disorders.

Limitations The correlation between blood ammonia levels and **hepatic coma** is poor. Ammonia determinations are not reliable predictors of impending hepatic coma. Ammonia levels are not always high in all patients with urea cycle disorders. High protein diet may cause increased levels. Ammonia levels may also be elevated with **gastrointestinal hemorrhage**. If portal hypertension develops with cirrhosis, hepatic blood flow is altered, leading to elevated blood ammonia levels.

Methodology Enzymatic assay, spectrophotometric endpoint, ammonia-selective electrode

Additional Information Ammonia and alpha-ketoglutarate with NADH yield glutamate; glutamate and ammonia yield glutamine. **Cerebrospinal fluid glutamine levels** are useful in hepatic encephalopathy and with Reye syndrome. In the HHH syndrome, hyperammonemia is intermittent; it presents in infancy often, but symptoms can be delayed.

Metabolic acidosis with ketosis are found in the **organic acidemias**, in which hyperammonemia is found. Plasma amino acids, urine organic acids, and amino acids are indicated with NH_3, biotinidase, and carnitine.[3]

Recently, hyperinsulinaemic hypoglycaemia with persistent hyperammonia has been described.[5,6,7] This disorder is not associated with any of the abnormalities of amino acids or organic acids observed in urea cycle enzyme defects, and is thought to be due to mutations in glutamate dehydrogenase.[8]

Footnotes
1. Dorwart WV and Saner M, "Heparinized Plasma Is an Unacceptable Specimen for Ammonia Determination," *Clin Chem*, 1992, 38(1):161.
2. Burtis CA and Ashwood ER, *Tietz Textbook of Clinical Chemistry*, 3rd ed, Philadelphia, PA: WB Saunders Co, 1999, 1146-7.
3. Lindor NM and Karnes PS, "Initial Assessment of Infants and Children With Suspected Inborn Errors of Metabolism," *Mayo Clin Proc*, 1995, 70(10):987-8.
4. Meythaler JM and Varma RR, "Reye's Syndrome in Adults: Diagnostic Considerations," *Arch Intern Med*, 1987, 147(1):61-4.
5. Yorifuji T, Muroi J, Uematsu A, et al, "Hyperinsulinism-Hyperammonemia Syndrome Caused by Mutant Glutamate Dehydrogenase Accompanied by Novel Enzyme Kinetics," *Hum Genet*, 1999, 104(6):476-9.
6. Kitaura J, Miki Y, Kato H, et al, "Hyperinsulinaemic Hypoglycaemia Associated With Persistent Hyperammonaemia," *Eur J Pediatr*, 1999, 158(5):410-3.
7. Glaser B, "Hyperinsulinism of the Newborn," *Semin Perinatol*, 2000, 24(2):150-63.
8. Stanley CA, Lieu YK, Hsu BY, et al, "Hyperinsulinism and Hyperammonemia in Infants With Regulatory Mutations of the Glutamate Dehydrogenase Gene," *N Engl J Med*, 1998, 338(19):1352-7.

References
Butterworth RF, "Effects of Hyperammonaemia on Brain Function," *J Inherit Metab Dis*, 1998, 21(Suppl 1):6-20.
Green A, "When and How Should We Measure Plasma Ammonia?" *Ann Clin Biochem*, 1988, 25(Pt 3):199-204.
Hurwitz ES, "Reye's Syndrome," *Epidemiol Rev*, 1989, 11:249-53.
Miga DE and Roth KS, "Hyperammonemia: The Silent Killer," *South Med J*, 1993, 86(7):742-7.
Treem WR, "Inherited and Acquired Syndromes of Hyperammonemia and Encephalopathy in Children," *Semin Liver Dis*, 1994, 14(3):236-58.

- **Amniotic Fluid Acetylcholinesterase** *see* Alpha₁-Fetoprotein, Amniotic Fluid *on page 96*

- **Amniotic Fluid Analysis for Erythroblastosis Fetalis** *replaced by* Bilirubin, Amniotic Fluid, Delta A450 *on page 116*

- **Amniotic Fluid Analysis for Hemolytic Disease of the Newborn** *see* Bilirubin, Amniotic Fluid, Delta A450 *on page 116*

- **Amniotic Fluid Bilirubin** *see* Bilirubin, Amniotic Fluid, Delta A450 *on page 116*

- **Amniotic Fluid Creatinine** *see* Creatinine, Amniotic Fluid *on page 160*

- **Amniotic Fluid Glucose** *see* Body Fluid Glucose *on page 124*

- **Amniotic Fluid Lecithin:Sphingomyelin Ratio** *see* Lecithin:Sphingomyelin Ratio, Amniotic Fluid *on page 210*

- **Amniotic Fluid Phosphatidylglycerol** *see* Phosphatidylglycerol, Amniotic Fluid *on page 251*

- **Amniotic Fluid Pulmonary Surfactant** *see* Pulmonary Surfactant, Amniotic Fluid *on page 271*

- **Amniotic Fluid Spectral Analysis** *see* Bilirubin, Amniotic Fluid, Delta A450 *on page 116*

- **AMP, Cyclic, Plasma** *see* Cyclic AMP, Plasma *on page 163*

- **AMP, Cyclic, Urine** *see* Cyclic AMP, Urine *on page 163*

- **Amylase, Body Fluid** *see* Body Fluid Amylase *on page 122*

- **Amylase:Creatinine Clearance Ratio** *see* Amylase, Urine *on page 104*

- **Amylase, Peritoneal Fluid** *see* Body Fluid Amylase *on page 122*

- **Amylase, Pleural Fluid** *see* Body Fluid Amylase *on page 122*

Amylase, Serum

Related Information
Amylase, Urine *on page 104*
Bile Fluid Examination *on page 304*
Bilirubin, Total, Serum *on page 118*
Body Fluid Amylase *on page 122*
Calcium, Serum *on page 131*
C-Reactive Protein, Serum *on page 523*
Lipase, Serum *on page 212*
Triglycerides, Serum or Plasma *on page 288*

Synonyms 1,4-α-D Glucanohydrolase, Serum

Applies to Interleukin-6; Trypsinogen Activation Peptide

Abstract Amylase is a group of enzymes (hydrolases) from the exocrine pancreas. Serum amylase is usually a sensitive and useful diagnostic method in those patients with acute pancreatitis who present within hours of the onset of pain. **Serum lipase** assay provides somewhat better sensitivity and specificity and is optimally used with amylase determination. Simultaneous determination of both is widely recommended for evaluation of abdominal pain.[1]

Pancreatitis is a disease which varies from mild to catastrophic.[2] Its etiologies include biliary disease, toxins (including ethanol), drugs, metabolic disorders, trauma, certain infections and infestations, penetrating duodenal ulcer, and other entities.[1]

Specimen Serum, plasma; amylase can also be determined from body fluids.

Container Red top tube, green top (heparin) tube

Sampling Time Usually elevated within 12 hours of onset of pancreatitis, serum amylase increases persist for 3-4 days. Delay in laboratory evaluation may lead to a normal amylase result with increased lipase. Since the biologic half-life of amylase is less than that of lipase, delay in laboratory evaluation may lead to a normal amylase result with increased lipase. For detection of blunt injury to the pancreas, determination more than 3 hours following trauma is advocated.[3] Serum amylase should be drawn 4 hours following endoscopic sphincterotomy to assess postprocedure pancreatitis.[4]

Collection Anticoagulants other than heparin diminish amylase activity

Storage Instructions Amylase is stable for 1 week at 25°C and 2 months at 4°C.

Special Instructions Dilution of lipemic sera may cause amylase values to increase.

Reference Interval Method dependent. Several automated methods have a reference interval of 20-300 units/L. Newborns' serum shows little amylase activity. Much of this activity is salivary. Children up to 2 years of age have virtually no pancreatic isoamylase. Markedly low values may not rise to adult values until the end of the second year of life.

Critical Values Although results greater than 3-5 times the upper limit of normal for a given method usually are considered significant increases, severity of acute pancreatitis is independent of amylase or lipase levels on admission.[5]

Use Useful in diagnosis of acute pancreatitis; desirable to support the clinical significance of elevated serum lipase.[1,6] Serum amylase is used to work up abdominal pain, epigastric tenderness, nausea, and vomiting, findings which characterize acute pancreatitis as well as acute surgical emergencies such as gastrointestinal perforation (eg, peptic ulcer with perforation) or bowel infarct. Pancreatitis in an individual may or may not be related to alcoholism. Hypercalcemia related to pancreatitis is recognized with hyperparathyroidism and other entities. About 80% of subjects with acute pancreatitis have increased serum amylase within 24 hours. Both amylase and lipase assays are recommended in organophosphate poisoning.[7] Causes of **high serum pancreatic enzymes** include acute pancreatitis, chronic pancreatitis, pancreatic pseudocyst, pancreatic ascites, pancreatic abscess, neoplasm in or adjacent to pancreas, trauma to pancreas, and common duct stones.

Limitations Poor specificity. Oxalate or citrate depress results. Lipemic sera (hypertriglyceridemia) may contain inhibitors which falsely depress results. About 20% of patients with acute pancreatitis have abnormal lipids. Normal serum amylase may occur in pancreatitis,[8] especially relapsing and chronic pancreatitis. (Subjects in whom pseudocysts complicate chronic pancreatitis often do have elevations of the pancreatic enzymes.) The entire pancreas can be destroyed in pancreatitis, including its amylase-producing cells; in such cases, serum amylase will derive from other structures (eg, salivary glands). Urinary amylase increases often persist longer than do those of serum.

Nonpancreatic causes of hyperamylasemia can confuse interpretation in some cases. They include inflammatory salivary lesions (eg, mumps), perforated peptic ulcer involving pancreas or not, intestinal obstruction and infarction, afferent loop syndrome, biliary tract disease usually including stones, but uncommonly occurring in gallbladder disease even without pancreatitis; hepatic cirrhosis; aortic aneurysm, peritonitis, acute appendicitis, cerebral trauma, burns and traumatic shock, the postoperative state (with and without pancreatitis), diabetic ketoacidosis, and extrapancreatic carcinomas (especially of esophagus, lung, ovary). Amylase levels more than 25-fold the upper limit of normal may be found when metastatic tumors produce ectopic amylase. Such levels are higher than those usually found in cases of pancreatitis. Moderate increases may be reported in normal pregnancy. Increases may be found with tubo-ovarian abscess, ruptured ectopic pregnancy, macroamylasemia, and with a substantial number of drugs, including morphine. Relationships between pancreatitis and hyperlipidemias are recognized. High levels in alcoholics, during pregnancy, and in diabetic ketoacidosis are of salivary rather than pancreatic origin. Salivary type amylase makes up about 60% of the serum enzyme, while it is the pancreatic fraction that is of clinical interest. The expression "salivary amylase" includes other nonpancreatic sources of the enzyme. Serum amylase is cleared by renal excretion. Serum amylase may increase up to three times the upper limit of normal in renal failure without diagnostic significance. In such cases, urine amylase is normal or low.

A substantial number of **drugs** cause increase in amylase levels. These include those which cause spasm of the sphincter of Oddi (eg, cholinergics, bethanechol, codeine, fentanyl, meperidine, morphine and other narcotics, pentazocine) and those which may cause pancreatitis (eg, aminosalicylic acid, amoxapine, azathioprine, chlorthalidone, cimetidine, clozapine, diazoxide, dideoxyinosine, felbamate, fluvastatin, glucocorticoids, hydantoin

derivatives, hydrochlorothiazide, hydroflumethiazide, isoniazid, mercaptopurine, minocycline, mirtazapine, pegaspargase, penicillamine, sulfamethoxazole, sulfisoxazole). Some may cause parotitis (eg, phenylbutazone, potassium iodide, procyclidine). Other drugs which may cause increased levels include cisplatin, thiazides, and valproic acid.[9]

Macroamylase is a high molecular weight material, normal amylase complexed to high molecular weight protein such as immunoglobulin. It is characterized by persistent, usually small increases of serum amylase over weeks, with low to normal urine amylase. Macroamylase occurs in normal as well as abnormal subjects. Its concentration can be assayed by some reference laboratories; testing is not often requested.

Methodology Amyloclastic, saccharogenic, chromolytic; up to 200 methods exist. Monoclonal antibody techniques are in use.

Additional Information Other tests: In **pancreatitis**, varying percentages of patients have the following other abnormalities in varying combinations: elevation of triglyceride, alkaline phosphatase, aspartate aminotransferase (AST), total bilirubin, white blood cell count (left shift). Alanine aminotransferase (ALT), increased to three times baseline or more, provides evidence of gallstone-induced etiology of pancreatitis. Calcium levels should be followed in fulminant pancreatitis, since extremely low serum calcium levels can evolve. Although C-reactive protein is elevated in many cases of acute pancreatitis, its concentration is also increased in substantial numbers of instances of nonpancreatic acute abdomen.[10] Other tests recently recommended for acute pancreatitis include interleukin-6[10] and trypsinogen activation peptide.[11] Although determination of serum methemalbumin has been advocated as a test for acute hemorrhagic pancreatitis, it is cumbersome and is not done in many American laboratories.

A list of causes of pancreatitis in children was recently published.[12] We would add one more: pinworm infestation with involvement of the pancreatic duct.

Laboratory and other factors useful to project severity have recently been discussed.[1]

Isoenzymes of amylase exist: pancreatic and salivary type, which can be separated by polyacrylamide gel or agarose film electrophoresis, isoelectric focusing, ion exchange chromatography, plant isoamylase inhibitors, and by monoclonal antibody technique on a centrifugal analyzer. Amylase isoenzymes are separated in few laboratories. Where available, the procedure is moderately expensive. Separations of amylase into its P and S isoenzymes adds little to the diagnosis of pancreatitis.[1]

Footnotes

1. Soergel KH, "Pancreatitis," *Cecil Textbook of Medicine*, 21st ed, Goldman L and Bennett JC, eds, Philadelphia PA: WB Sanders Co, 2000, 752-9.
2. Steinberg W and Tenner S, "Acute Pancreatitis," *N Engl J Med*, 1994, 330(17):1198-210.
3. Takishima T, Sugimoto K, Hirata M, et al, "Serum Amylase Level on Admission in the Diagnosis of Blunt Injury to the Pancreas: Its Significance and Limitations," *Ann Surg*, 1997, 226(1):70-6.
4. Testoni PA, Bagnolo F, Caporuscio S, et al, "Serum Amylase Measured Four Hours After Endoscopic Sphincterotomy Is a Reliable Predictor of Postprocedure Pancreatitis," *Am J Gastroenterol*, 1999, 94(5):1129-30.
5. Lankisch PG, Burchard-Reckert S, and Lehnick D, "Underestimation of Acute Pancreatitis: Patients With Only a Small Increase in Amylase/Lipase Levels Can Also Have or Develop Severe Acute Pancreatitis," *Gut*, 1999, 44(4):542-4.
6. Frank B and Gottlieb K, "Amylase Normal, Lipase Elevated: Is it Pancreatitis?" *Am J Gastroenterol*, 1999, 94(2):463-9.
7. Lee WC, Yang CC, Deng JF, et al, "The Clinical Significance of Hyperamylasemia in Organophosphate Poisoning," *J Toxicol Clin Toxicol*, 1998, 36(7):673-81.
8. Torrens JK and McWhinney PH, "Acute Pancreatitis. Normal Serum Amylase Does Not Exclude Severe Acute Pancreatitis," *BMJ*, 1998, 316(7149):1982-3.
9. Young DS, *Effects of Drugs on Clinical Laboratory Tests*, 5th ed, Volume 1: Listing by Test, Washington, DC: AACC Press, American Association of Clinical Chemistry, 2000, Section 3, 59-63.
10. Pezzilli R, Morselli-Labate AM, Miniero R, et al, "Simultaneous Serum Assays and Lipase and Interleukin-6 for Early Diagnosis and Prognosis of Acute Pancreatitis," *Clin Chem*, 1999, 45(10):1762-7.
11. Neoptolemos JP, Kemppainen EA, Mayer JM, et al, "Early Prediction of Severity in Acute Pancreatitis by Urinary Trypsinogen Activation Peptide: A Multicentre Study," *Lancet*, 2000, 355(9219):1955-60.
12. Benkow KJ and Winter HS, "A 15-Year-Old Girl With Abdominal Pain and Bloody Stools," Case Records of the Massachusetts General Hospital, Case 2-1999, Scully RE, Mark EJ, McNeely WF, et al, eds, *N Engl J Med*, 1999, 340(3):215-21.

References

Adam DJ, Milne AA, Evans SM, et al, "Serum Amylase Isoenzymes in Patients Undergoing Operation for Ruptured and Nonruptured Abdominal Aortic Aneurysm," *J Vasc Surg*, 1999, 30(2):229-35.
Andersén JM, Hedström J, Kemppainen E, et al, "The Ratio of Trypsin-2-α_1-Antitrypsin to Trypsinogen-I Discriminates Biliary and Alcohol-Induced Acute Pancreatitis," *Clin Chem*, 2001, 47(2):231-6.
Argiris A, Mathur-Wagh U, Wilets I, et al, "Abnormalities of Serum Amylase and Lipase in HIV-Positive Patients," *Am J Gastroenterol*, 1999, 94(5):1248-52.
Corsetti JP, Cox C, Schulz TJ, et al, "Combined Serum Amylase and Lipase Determinations for Diagnosis of Suspected Acute Pancreatitis," *Clin Chem*, 1993, 39(12):2495-9.
Eckfeldt JH and Kershaw MJ, "Hyperamylasemia Following Methyl Alcohol Intoxication: Source and Significance," *Arch Intern Med*, 1986, 146(1):193-4.
Heikius B, Niemela S, Lehtola J, et al, "Elevated Pancreatic Enzymes in Inflammatory Bowel Disease Are Associated With Extensive Disease," *Am J Gastroenterol*, 1999, 94(4):1062-9.
(Continued)

Amylase, Serum *(Continued)*

Justice AD, DiBenedetto RJ, and Stanford E, "Significance of Elevated Pancreatic Enzymes in Intracranial Bleeding," *South Med J*, 1994, 87(9):889-93.

Kleinman DS and O'Brien JF, "Macroamylase," *Mayo Clin Proc*, 1986, 61(8):669-70.

Kurzweil SM, Shapiro MJ, Andrus CH, et al, "Hyperbilirubinemia Without Common Bile Duct Abnormalities and Hyperamylasemia Without Pancreatitis in Patients With Gallbladder Disease," *Arch Surg*, 1994, 129(8):829-33.

Lott JA and Lu CJ, "Lipase Isoforms and Amylase Isoenzymes: Assays and Application in the Diagnosis of Acute Pancreatitis," *Clin Chem*, 1991, 37(3):361-8.

Maringhini A, Lankisch MR, Zinsmeister AR, et al, "Acute Pancreatitis in the Postpartum Period: A Population-Based Case-Control Study," *Mayo Clin Proc*, 2000, 75(4):361-4.

Mayo Reference Services, Test Update, "Amylase, Pancreatic, Serum," April 2000.

Orebaugh SL, "Normal Amylase Levels in the Presentation of Acute Pancreatitis," *Am J Emerg Med*, 1994, 12(1):21-4.

Pezzilli R, Andreone P, Morselli-Labate AM, et al, "Serum Pancreatic Enzyme Concentrations in Chronic Viral Liver Diseases," *Dig Dis Sci*, 1999, 44(2):350-5.

Simon HK, Muehlberg A, and Linakis JG, "Serum Amylase Determinations in Pediatric Patients Presenting to the ED With Acute Abdominal Pain or Trauma," *Am J Emerg Med*, 1994, 12(3):292-5.

Stimac D, Lenac T, and Marusic Z, "A Scoring System for Early Differentiation of the Etiology of Acute Pancreatitis," *Scand J Gastroenterol* , 1998, 33(2):209-11.

Uretsky G, Goldschmiedt M, and James K, "Childhood Pancreatitis," *Am Fam Phys*, 1999, 59(9):2507-12.

Windsor JA, "Search for Prognostic Markers for Acute Pancreatitis," *Lancet*, 2000, 355(9219):1924-5.

Amylase, Urine

Related Information

Amylase, Serum *on page 102*
Body Fluid Amylase *on page 122*
Lipase, Serum *on page 212*

Synonyms 1,4-α-D Glucanohydrolase, Urine

Applies to Amylase:Creatinine Clearance Ratio; Trypsin, Immunoreactive

Abstract Urine amylase is elevated early and reaches high levels in acute pancreatitis. However, diagnostic utility of the combination of serum amylase and lipase is superior.

Patient Preparation Fasting from 10 PM to 6 AM is recommended before a 24-hour urine collection.

Specimen 2-hour urine specimen is preferred, no preservative

Collection Collect timed specimen. Instruct the patient to void at the beginning of the collection period and discard the specimen. Collect all urine including the final specimen voided at the end of the collection period. Centrifugation to provide optically clear specimen is desirable.

Storage Instructions Keep refrigerated.

Special Instructions Requisition should include date and time collection started, date and time collection finished.

Reference Interval Method dependent; 1-17 units/hour[1]

Use Work up abdominal pain, epigastric tenderness, nausea, and vomiting. An enzyme with molecular weight of 45,000-55,000 daltons, the role of increased **urinary** amylase in the differential diagnosis of acute pancreatitis has diminished, save for diagnosis of macroamylasemia.[2] It is also elevated in about 25% of patients with carcinoma of pancreas. It is useful in diagnosis of pseudocyst of the pancreas, in which the urine amylase may remain elevated for weeks after the serum amylase has returned to normal, after a bout of acute pancreatitis.

Methodology Maltopentose, other methods also available

Additional Information Macroamylasemia is characterized by high serum amylase but normal urine amylase. The **amylase:creatinine clearance ratio** remains useful for the diagnosis of macroamylasemia, but its nonspecificity has otherwise left it with few other applications. It is the ratio of urinary amylase concentration over that of plasma, divided by corresponding creatinine values. In macroamylasemia the clearance is very low.[3] Unlike serum amylase, urine amylase levels are normal with renal failure. While serum amylase usually returns to normal within 3-5 days, without complications urine amylase is increased longer than serum amylase in acute pancreatitis. Two-hour collections are more practical and provide results sooner than longer collections. The major test for pancreatitis additional to serum and urine amylase is serum lipase. It has good specificity and its laboratory analysis is greatly improved from the 1960s.

Some patients with pancreatitis have very high triglyceride levels. **Immunoreactive trypsin** has not been widely available, but a urine trypsinogen-2 test strip has recently been described.[4] Further evaluation is needed.

Footnotes

1. Painter CY, Cope JY, and Smith JL, "Reference Information for the Clinical Laboratory," *Tietz Textbook of Clinical Chemistry*, 3rd ed, Burtis VA and Ashwood ER, eds, Philadelphia, PA: WB Saunders Co, 1999, 1801.

2. Steinberg W and Tenner S, "Acute Pancreatitis," *N Engl J Med*, 1994, 330(17):1198-210.

3. Eckfeldt JH and Levitt MD, "Diagnostic Enzymes for Pancreatic Disease," *Clin Lab Med*, 1989, 9(4):731-43.

4. Kylänpää-Bäck ML, Kemppainen E, Puolakkainen P, et al, "Reliable Screening for Acute Pancreatitis With Rapid Urine Trypsinogen-2 Test Strip," *Br J Surg*, 2000, 87:49-52.

References

Hedström J, Svens E, Kenkimaki P, et al, "Evaluation of a New Urinary Amylase Test Strip in the Diagnosis of Acute Pancreatitis," *Scand J Clin Lab Invest*, 1998, 58(8):611-6.

♦ **Androstenedione** *see* Dehydroepiandrosterone and Dehydroepiandrosterone Sulfate, Serum or Plasma *on page 164*

Androstenedione, Serum

Related Information

Chorionic Villus Sampling, Chromosome and Genetic Abnormality Analysis *on page 361*
Cortisol, Serum or Plasma *on page 154*
Dehydroepiandrosterone and Dehydroepiandrosterone Sulfate, Serum or Plasma *on page 164*
17-Hydroxyprogesterone, Serum or Plasma *on page 197*
Testosterone, Total and Free, Serum or Plasma *on page 280*

Abstract Androstenedione is a corticosteroid, and an intermediate in the metabolism of androgens and estrogens. It is produced from 17-hydroxyprogesterone and dehydroepiandrosterone (DHEA). It is the major steroid produced by the theca interstitial cells of the ovary. In females, androstenedione is a major source of testosterone.

Patient Preparation Fasting morning specimen is preferred. Collect 1 week before or after menstrual period.

Specimen Serum

Container Red top tube

Storage Instructions Freeze serum.

Causes for Rejection Recently administered radioisotopes

Reference Interval Variation exists between laboratories. Some representative intervals[1] are given in the following table.

Androstenedione, Serum

Age	Male		Female	
	ng/mL	nmol/L	ng/mL	nmol/L
1-5 mo	5-45	0.2-1.6	5-35	0.2-1.2
1-9 y	5-55	0.2-1.9	5-45	0.2-1.6
10-17 y	10-100	0.3-3.5	25-200	0.9-7.0
Adults	50-250	1.7-8.7	50-250	1.7-8.7

Values are higher in pregnancy and highest at delivery. A marked diurnal variation exists, with a peak around 7 AM and a nadir around 4 PM. Levels rise sharply after puberty to peak at about 20 years of age. An abrupt decline occurs after menopause. Concentrations are lower following bilateral oophorectomy.

Use This test is used to evaluate androgen production in hirsute females; it is less useful in evaluation of other aspects of virilization. Results are significantly elevated in the most common type of congenital adrenal hyperplasia due to C_{21}-hydroxylase deficiency, in which in infancy elevated 17-hydroxyprogesterone, progesterone, urinary 17-ketosteroids, renin, and ACTH with low serum cortisol are anticipated. A result >1000 ng/dL (SI: >34.9 nmol/L) suggests a virilizing tumor.

Limitations There is poor correlation of plasma levels with clinical severity.

Methodology Radioimmunoassay (RIA)

Additional Information Androstenedione is a major precursor in the biosynthesis of androgens and estrogens. It serves as a prohormone for testosterone and estrone, particularly in menopausal females. Androstenedione is a weak androgen produced in equal amounts by adrenal glands and ovaries in normal women. The predominant androgens in the female are androstenedione and dehydroepiandrosterone. Androstenedione is increased in cases of hirsutism, including Stein-Leventhal syndrome, ovarian stromal hyperplasia, congenital adrenal hyperplasia, Cushing syndrome and ectopic ACTH-producing tumor. Luteinized stromal cells produce hormones in ovarian tumors with functioning stroma. About 60% of cases of female hirsutism show elevations of androstenedione. Chronic increase of plasma luteinizing hormone causes overexpression of androstenedione.

Peripheral conversion of androstenedione to estrogen takes place in adipose tissue of obese women, who may develop endometrial hyperplasia.

Concentrations of androstenedione as well as testosterone and dihydrotestosterone were increased in a case of massive ovarian edema with virilization.[2]

Prenatal diagnosis of **congenital adrenal hyperplasia** (due to **21-hydroxylase deficiency**) includes measurement of 17-hydroxyprogesterone, androstenedione, testosterone, 21-deoxycortisol and HLA typing.[3] Early diagnosis can also be made with molecular genetic studies from chorionic villus sampling.[4]

Though congenital adrenal hyperplasia (due to 21-hydroxylase deficiency) most often presents in infancy or early childhood, the disorder occasionally presents in adulthood.[5]

Footnotes

1. Soldin SJ, Brugnara C, Gunter KC, et al, "Pediatric Reference Ranges," 3rd ed, Washington, DC: AACC Press, American Association of Clinical Chemistry, 1999, 30.
2. van den Brule F, Bourque J, Gaspard UJ, et al, "Massive Ovarian Edema With Androgen Secretion. A Pathological and Endocrine Study With Review of the Literature," *Horm Res*, 1994, 41(5-6):209-14.
3. Levine LS and Pang S, "Prenatal Diagnosis and Treatment of Congenital Adrenal Hyperplasia," *J Pediatr Endocrinol*, 1994, 7(3):193-200.
4. Forest MG, David M, and Morel Y, "Prenatal Diagnosis and Treatment of 21-Hydroxylase Deficiency," *J Steroid Biochem Mol Biol*, 1993, 45(1-3):75-82.
5. Summers RH, Herold DA, and Seely BL, "Hormonal and Genetic Analysis of a Patient With Congenital Adrenal Hyperplasia," *Clin Chem*, 1996, 42(9):1483-7.

References

Adashi EY, "The Climacteric Ovary as a Functional Gonadotropin-Driven Androgen-Producing Gland," *Fertil Steril*, 1994, 62(1):20-7.

Gompel A, Wright F, Kuttenn F, et al, "Contribution of Plasma Androstenedione to 5 Alpha-Androstanediol Glucuronide in Women With Idiopathic Hirsutism," *J Clin Endocrinol Metab*, 1986, 62(2):441-4.

Mahlck CG, Backstrom T, Kjellgren O, et al, "Plasma Progesterone and Androstenedione in Relation to Changes in Tumor Volume and Recurrence in Women With Ovarian Carcinoma," *Gynecol Obstet Invest*, 1986, 22(3):157-64.

Ylikorkala O, Stenman UH, and Halmesmaki E, "Testosterone, Androstenedione, Dehydroepiandrosterone Sulfate, and Sex-Hormone-Binding Globulin in Pregnant Alcohol Abusers," *Obstet Gynecol*, 1988, 71(5):731-5.

♦ **Androsterone** see 17-Ketosteroids Fractionation, Urine *on page 206*

♦ **Angiotensin** see Renin Activity, Plasma *on page 273*

♦ **Angiotensin Converting Enzyme, CSF** see Angiotensin Converting Enzyme, Serum *on page 105*

Angiotensin Converting Enzyme, Serum

Synonyms ACE; Angiotensin-I-Converting Enzyme

Applies to Angiotensin Converting Enzyme, CSF; Cerebrospinal Fluid Angiotensin Converting Enzyme

Abstract Angiotensin-I-converting enzyme (ACE) is a dipeptidyl carboxypeptidase. It functions to split dipeptides from the free carboxy end of a variety of polypeptides including angiotensin I and bradykinin. It is especially known for its generation of the octapeptide, angiotensin II, by releasing the dipeptide histidyl-leucine from angiotensin I. The major site of normal ACE production is the pulmonary endothelial cells.

Increased concentrations of ACE with imaging abnormalities, lymphadenopathy, and tissue biopsies characterized by noncaseating granulomas negative to appropriate special strains and cultures for organisms, and negative to polarizing microscopy, support a diagnosis of sarcoidosis.

Patient Preparation Angiotensin converting enzyme inhibiting drugs cause decreased ACE values.

Specimen Serum

Container Red top tube or SST™ tube; EDTA inhibits ACE

Storage Instructions Separate serum (or plasma) immediately. Stable 1 week at 4°C, 6 months at -20°C.

Reference Interval The reference interval is approximately 15-70 units/L,[1] though large interindividual variations exist due to differing genotypes for the insertion (I)/deletion (D) polymorphism in the ACE gene.[2] Sharma et al[1] have suggested that ACE reference intervals be related to genotype as follows to improve the diagnostic sensitivity of the test in acute sarcoidosis. See table.

Angiotensin Converting Enzyme, Serum

Genotype	ACE Reference Interval (units/L)
II	4.6-30.6
ID	10.0-47.6
DD	17.9-64.3

Reference ranges for children and adolescents may be up to 50% greater than specimens from individuals 20 years of age and older.

Use Results are elevated in sarcoidosis, more often when the disease is active and are of value in assessing the response of sarcoidosis to corticosteroid therapy. A marked decrease is found in some patients on prednisone. A falling ACE level had been considered a favorable prognostic sign. Rising levels were thought to reflect activity uncontrolled by therapy, but its prognostic value in identification of subjects with progressive disease is limited. It also is used in investigation for Gaucher disease and may be useful for monitoring noncompliance with ACE inhibitor treatment. ACE is thought to be produced by epithelioid cells and macrophages; elevations are found in a variety of granulomatous diseases.

Limitations Test lacks specificity and sensitivity for diagnosis of sarcoidosis. Elevations have been reported in about 35% to 91% of cases of sarcoidosis (see reference by Jordan et al for entry to the somewhat older literature on this subject). ACE levels are less likely to be increased with chronic sarcoidosis. Different admixtures of acute and chronic cases may explain some of

the apparent variation in reported incidence of elevation in sarcoidosis. Elevations have been found in patients with diabetes mellitus, Gaucher disease and leprosy. Twenty-five percent of 86 patients with acute histoplasmosis had elevated levels.[3] Increased levels have been observed in some patients with primary biliary cirrhosis, amyloidosis, myeloma, Melkersson-Rosenthal syndrome, some alpha$_1$-antitrypsin variants, untreated hyperthyroidism, and psoriasis. It has been found increased in some cases of hyperparathyroidism and in some instances of oncogenic hypercalcemia. Thus, it is not a specific marker for the diagnosis of sarcoidosis.[4] Positives are also reported in patients with extrinsic allergic alveolitis, coccidioidomycosis, beryllium disease, asbestosis, silicosis, and alcoholic liver disease.[5] ACE activity is decreased during starvation, independent of the level of thyroid activity (as monitored by T_3 levels).[6] ACE is physiologically decreased by administration of captopril, enalapril, and lisinopril. Hemolysis and lipemia interfere with these methods.

A small number of apparently normal adults have increased concentrations.

Methodology Spectrofluorometric or radioimmunoassay (RIA), spectrophotometric utilizing synthetic substrates

Additional Information Other abnormalities found in some sarcoidosis patients may include elevations of serum alkaline phosphatase, calcium, gamma globulin with polyclonal gammopathy, and hypercalciuria. Serum angiotensin converting enzyme is not usually elevated in cases of active tuberculosis or Hodgkin disease. Increases are less frequent when sarcoidosis is inactive.[4] Some 80% to 90% of patients with demonstrably active sarcoidosis have elevated serum ACE. Angiotensin converting enzyme activity is also increased in sarcoid lymph node homogenate. The diagnosis of sarcoidosis is a histopathologic/clinical complex. Lymph nodes, liver, skin, and lung, especially transbronchial lung biopsies, are often useful. Cultures and special strains to rule out mycobacterial and fungal infection are needed, and polarizing microscopy is utilized to identify crystaline material in granulomas in tissue sections. (Noncaseating granulomas must be proven not to be caused by histoplasmosis or other microbiologic entities.) Berylliosis is a very rare cause of such granulomas.

Thyroid hormone may modulate ACE activity. Both patients with low T_3 levels (and clinical hypothyroidism) and patients with anorexia nervosa with associated findings of hypothyroidism may have low serum ACE activity.[7,8] Monitoring of ACE levels may have application in assessing risk of pulmonary damage due to use of some antineoplastic agents, in particular bleomycin.[9] Serum ACE is decreased in some patients with carcinoma of the lung. With response to chemotherapy/radiation therapy the ACE level has been noted to normalize.[10] Cerebrospinal fluid ACE increase is described in patients with neurosarcoidosis, but there is not sufficient evidence to support the use of ACE in CSF.

Elevated serum ACE levels in a case of the uncommon entity, Melkersson-Rosenthal syndrome, probably relate to the sarcoid-like noncaseating granulomas that are found in this condition. ACE levels normalized after successful therapy with methotrexate.[11]

Serum ACE abnormality has been reported in 20% to 30% of alpha$_1$-antitrypsin variants (MZ, ZZ, and MS Pi types) but in only about 1% of individuals with normal MM Pi type.[12] There is evidence that paraquat poisoning (because of its effect on pulmonary capillary endothelium) is associated with elevated serum ACE.[13]

Serum ACE concentrations are associated with an insertion (I)/deletion (D) polymorphism within intron 16 of the ACE gene.[2] Individuals with the homozygous *DD* genotype have been reported to be at higher risk for cardiovascular disease than those having the homozygous *II* or heterozygous *DI* genotypes,[14,15] though there is controversy surrounding the strength of this association.[16,17]

Footnotes

1. Sharma P, Smith I, Maguire G, et al, "Clinical Value of ACE Genotyping in Diagnosis of Sarcoidosis," *Lancet*, 1997, 349(9065):1602-3.
2. Rigat B, Huber C, Alhenc-Gelas F, et al, "An Insertion/Deletion Polymorphism in the Angiotensin I-Converting Enzyme Gene Accounting for Half the Variance of Serum Enzyme Levels," *J Clin Invest*, 1990, 86:1343-6.
3. Ryder KW, Jay SJ, Kiblawi SO, et al, "Serum Angiotensin Converting Enzyme Activity in Patients With Histoplasmosis," *JAMA*, 1983, 249:1888-9.
4. Lufkin EG, DeRemee RA, and Rohrbach MS, "The Predictive Value of Serum Angiotensin Converting Enzyme Activity in the Differential Diagnosis of Hypercalcemia," *Mayo Clin Proc*, 1983, 58:447-51.
5. Studdy PR, Lapworth R, and Bird R, "Angiotensin Converting Enzyme and Its Clinical Significance - A Review," *J Clin Pathol*, 1983, 36:938-47.
6. Butkus NE, Burman KD, and Smallridge RC, "Angiotensin-Converting Enzyme Activity Decreases During Fasting," *Horm Metab Res*, 1987, 19(2):76-9.
7. Matsubayashi S, Tamai H, Kobayashi N, et al, "Angiotensin Converting Enzyme and Anorexia Nervosa," *Horm Metab Res*, 1988, 20(12):761-4.
8. Smallridge RC, Rogers J, and Verma PS, "Serum Angiotensin Converting Enzyme: Alterations in Hyperthyroidism, Hypothyroidism, and Subacute Thyroiditis," *JAMA*, 1983, 250:2489-93.
9. Nussinovitch N, Peleg E, Yaron A, et al, "Angiotensin Converting Enzyme in Bleomycin-Treated Patients," *Int J Clin Pharmacol Ther Toxicol*, 1988, 26(6):310-3.
10. Schweisfurth H, Schmidt M, Brugger E, et al, "Alterations of Serum Carboxypeptidases N and Angiotensin-I-Converting Enzyme in Malignant Diseases," *Clin Biochem*, 1985, 18(4):242-6.
11. Leicht S, Youngberg G, and Modica L, "Melkersson-Rosenthal Syndrome: Elevations in Serum Angiotensin Converting Enzyme and Results of Treatment With Methotrexate," *South Med J*, 1989, 82(1):74-6.

(Continued)

Angiotensin Converting Enzyme, Serum *(Continued)*

12. Lieberman J and Sastre A, "Serum Angiotensin Converting Enzyme Levels in Patients With Alpha₁-Antitrypsin Variants," *Am J Med*, 1986, 81(5):821-4.

13. Hollinger MA, Patwell SW, Zuckerman JE, et al, "Effect of Paraquat on Serum Angiotensin Converting Enzyme," *Am Rev Respir Dis*, 1980, 121(5):795-8.

14. Cambien F, Poirier O, Lecerf L, et al, "Deletion Polymorphism in the Gene for Angiotensin-Converting Enzyme Is a Potent Risk Factor for Myocardial Infarction," *Nature*, 1992, 359:641-4.

15. Raynolds MV, Bristow MR, Bush EW, et al, "Angiotensin-Converting Enzyme DD Genotype in Patients With Ischaemic or Idiopathic Dilated Cardiomyopathy," *Lancet*, 1993, 342:1073-5.

16. Lindpaintner K, Pfeffer MA, Kreutz R, et al, "A Prospective Evaluation of an Angiotensin-Converting-Enzyme Gene Polymorphism and the Risk of Ischemic Heart Disease," *N Engl J Med*, 1995, 332(11):706-11.

17. Singer DR, Missouris CG, and Jeffery S, "Angiotensin-Converting Enzyme Gene Polymorphism. What to Do About All the Confusion?" *Circulation*, 1996, 94(3):236-9.

References

Alhenc-Gelas F, Richard J, Courbon D, et al, "Distribution of Plasma Angiotensin Converting Enzyme in Healthy Men: Relationship to Environmental and Hormonal Parameters," *J Lab Clin Med*, 1991, 117(1):33-9.

"Angiotensin Converting Enzyme, Serum," *Mayo Medical Laboratories*, Rochester, MN, Test Update, 2000.

Beneteau-Burnat B, Baudin B, Morgant G, et al, "Serum Angiotensin-Converting Enzyme in Healthy and Sarcoidotic Children: Comparison With the Reference Interval for Adults," *Clin Chem*, 1990, 36(2):344-6.

Jordan DR, Anderson RL, Nerad JA, et al, "The Diagnosis of Sarcoidosis," *Can J Ophthalmol*, 1988, 23(5):203-7.

Lieberman J, "Enzymes in Sarcoidosis: Angiotensin Converting Enzyme (ACE)," *Clin Lab Med*, 1989, 9(4):745-55.

Maguire GA and Price CP, "A Continuous Monitoring Spectrophotometric Method for the Measurement of Angiotensin-Converting Enzyme in Human Serum," *Ann Clin Biochem*, 1985, 22:204-10.

Newman LS, Rose CS, and Maier LA, "Sarcoidosis," *N Engl J Med*, 1997, 336(17):1224-34.

Seidman MD, Lewandowski CA, Sarpa JR, et al, "Angioedema Related to Angiotensin-Converting Enzyme Inhibitors," *Otolaryngol Head Neck Surg*, 1990, 102(6):727-31.

Sharma OP, "Sarcoidosis," *Dis Mon*, 1990, 36(9):469-535.

Struthers AD, Anderson G, MacFadyen RJ, et al, "Nonadherence With ACE Inhibitor Treatment Is Common in Heart Failure and Can Be Detected by Routine Serum ACE Activity Assays," *Heart Lung*, 1999, 82(5):584-8.

Thompson AB, Cale WF, and Lapp NL, "Serum Angiotensin-Converting Enzyme Is Elevated in Association With Underground Coal Mining," *Chest*, 1991, 100(4):1042-5.

♦ **Angiotensin-I-Converting Enzyme** *see* Angiotensin Converting Enzyme, Serum *on page 105*

Anion Gap, Serum, Plasma, or Urine

Related Information

Base Excess, Blood *on page 114*
Bicarbonate, Blood *on page 115*
Chloride, Serum, Plasma, or Blood *on page 144*
Chloride, Urine *on page 145*
Electrolyte Panel, Serum *on page 168*
Ethylene Glycol, Serum or Plasma *on page 790*
Ibuprofen, Serum *on page 793*
Ketone Bodies, Blood *on page 205*
Ketones, Urine *on page 877*
Lactic Acid, Whole Blood or Plasma *on page 208*
Osmolality, Calculated, Serum or Plasma *on page 234*
Osmolality, Serum *on page 236*
pH, Blood *on page 247*
Phosphorus, Serum *on page 251*
Salicylate, Serum or Plasma *on page 806*
Sodium, Serum or Plasma *on page 275*
Sodium, Urine *on page 278*
Volatile Screen, Blood or Urine *on page 809*

Synonyms Electrolyte Gap; Gap; Ion Gap

Applies to Anion Gap, Urine; Base Excess; BEua; Fencl-Stewart Method

Test Includes A calculation from sodium, potassium, HCO₃⁻, and chloride to ascertain quantities of unmeasured cations and anions

Abstract The anion gap is useful in evaluation of patients with acid-base abnormalities. It is based on the principle of electroneutrality, which requires that the sum of anions and cations be equal in blood or other body fluids. This calculation (anion gap) is an estimate of unmeasured anions. Most cases of increased anion gap are caused by lactic acidosis or ketoacidosis.[1]

Aftercare Patient urinary output may be relevant in cases of increased anion gap.

Specimen Serum, plasma, urine

Container Red top tube or green top (heparin) tube, plastic urine container

Reference Interval Using ion-selective electrode technology: 3-11 mmol/L;[2,3] considerable variation has been shown among instruments, and each laboratory should establish or verify its own reference interval.[4,5] The reference interval by flame photometry is approximately 8-16 mmol/L using the following:

$$[Na^+] - [HCO_3^- + Cl^-]$$

If K is included with the cations, the reference range is 10-20 mmol/L.

Use The major clinical application of the anion gap is in the differential diagnosis of metabolic acidosis. Within the laboratory, the anion gap is often used as an internal check on the accuracy of the component measurements.

A marked elevation of anion gap suggests **metabolic acidosis**.[6] Increased anion gaps are found in states such as renal failure and toxic ingestions. A result >30 mmol/L is commonly secondary to **lactic acidosis** or **ketoacidosis** but can be caused also by rhabdomyolysis or nonketotic hyperglycemic coma. Clinical and laboratory facets of D-lactic acidosis are included in Lactic Acid, Whole Blood or Plasma *on page 208*.

Acid-base abnormalities may coexist (eg, loss of acid by vomiting and increased acid production from ketoacidosis of diabetes mellitus). See table.

Anion Gap in Metabolic Acid-Base Disorders

Mechanism	Anion Gap	Osmotic Gap	Chloride	Potassium	Other
Metabolic Acidosis					
Increased acid	↑	N*	N	↑	↑ Lactate or production ketones = anion gap
Acid precursor ingestion	↑	↑†	N	↑	Measure methanol, ethylene glycol, and salicylates, depending on history
Decreased acid excretion	↑	N	N	↑	Severe renal failure also present; usually low urine output
Increased base excretion	N	N	↑	↑ or ↓	Urine anion gap ↑ with stool losses; ↓ with renal tubular acidosis
Metabolic Alkalosis					
Dehydration	N	N	↓	↓	Urine chloride, sodium usually undetectable
Vomiting	N	N	↓	↓	Urine chloride undetectable; urine sodium usually normal
Base ingestion	N	N	↓	↓	Very high urine anion gap
Primary mineralocorticoid excess	N	N	↓	↓	Urine chloride, sodium usually measurable

↑Indicates increased; N indicates normal; ↓ indicates decreased.
*Osmotic gap may be slightly high in patients with ketoacidosis.
†Osmotic gap is normal with salicylates.

Adapted from Dufour DR, "Laboratory Recognition and Testing in Acid-Base Disorders," *Lab Med*, 1999, 30(12):776-81.

Limitations A spurious increase may follow excessive exposure of the sample to room air as well as underfilling the Vacutainer® tube.[7] All metabolic abnormalities are not detected by abnormal gaps (eg, isopropanol ingestion is accompanied by a normal gap, but ketone bodies are positive). There are a number of causes of normal anion gap acidosis associated with hyperchloremia. The anion gap is unsuitable as a quick screen for lactic acidosis due to its lack of sensitivity.[8,9,10] In fact, hyperlactatemia is in the differential diagnosis of normal anion gap acidosis.[8] The anion gap should not replace assays for lactate, ketone bodies, or osmolality. In one study, only 71% of patients with an anion gap of 20-29 mmol/L could be proven to have an organic acidosis.[11] In critically ill newborns, however, a recent study found anion gap >16 mmol/L to be highly predictive of lactic acidosis and <8 mmol/L highly predictive of absence of lactic acidosis.[12]

Methodology Most commonly, the anion gap is calculated from the electrolyte measurements as:

$$Na^+ - (Cl^- + HCO_3^-)$$

Less often, the following is used:

$$(Na^+ + K^+) - (Cl^- + HCO_3)$$

Additional Information The existence of a "gap" reflects the fact that some anions and cations are not measured in routine practice. Unmeasured cations include Ca^{2+} and Mg^{2+}. Unmeasured anions include protein, PO_4^{3-}, SO_4^{2-}, and organic acids.[13] Organic acids include lactic acid and ketoacids as well as others.

High anion gaps are caused by elevated concentrations of unmeasured anions. **When the anion gap is high and pH is low**, possible causes include uremia, ketoacidosis, lactic acidosis,[14] salicylate toxicity, methanol toxicity, ethylene glycol toxicity, paraldehyde toxicity,[6] or toluene toxicity.[15] Toluene exposure by glue sniffing can cause severe high anion gap metabolic acidosis, which can convert to hyperchloremic acidosis.[16] Metabolic acidoses with profoundly elevated anion gaps appear to be due to multifactorial causes, including renal failure, rhabdomyolysis, nonketotic hyperglycemic hyperosmolar syndrome, marked hyperphosphatemia, hemoconcentration, and identified and unidentified organic metabolic acidosis.[17] Abnormal anion gaps due to uremia are usually seen only when the creatinine is >4.0 mg/dL (SI: >354 μmol/L). Uremic acidosis is rare without hyperphosphatemia. **When both the anion gap and pH are high,**

the cause could be due to extracellular volume contraction, massive transfusion (with renal failure and/or volume contraction), carbenicillin or penicillin (in large doses), or salts of organic acids such as citrate. Common mnemonic "MUDPILES" is used to remember conditions causing increased anion gap. These are Methanol toxicity, Uremia of renal failure, Diabetes mellitus, Paraldehyde toxicity, Isoniazid/Iron toxicity, Lactic acidosis, Ethylene glycol toxicity, Salicylate toxicity.

Low anion gaps are caused by retained unmeasured anions. The most common causes are hypoalbuminemia (eg, in nephrosis or cirrhosis), dilution, hypernatremia, very marked hypercalcemia, very severe hypermagnesemia, IgG myeloma, and polyclonal gamma globulinemia.[18] Hyperviscosity, lithium toxicity, and bromism also have been associated with low anion gaps. Decreased anion gap with spurious hyperchloremia and with hyponatremia is reported in hyperlipidemia.[19] Dilution of extracellular fluid may cause a decreased gap.[20] The finding of a low anion gap is perceived as an unreliable diagnostic finding but should be strongly considered as an indication of laboratory error. Figge et al[21] have suggested use of an adjusted anion gap in cases of hypoalbuminemia.

Normal anion gaps occur with metabolic acidosis. Causes include diarrhea, renal tubular acidosis, hyperalimentation, ureteroileostomy, ureterosigmoidostomy, external drainage of pancreaticobiliary fluids, and administration of NH_4Cl and other drugs.

The urinary anion gap (Na + K - Cl) is reported to be useful in the diagnosis of hyperchloremic metabolic acidosis[22] and evaluation of renal potassium wasting.[23] Marked increase occurs following ingestion of baking soda (sodium bicarbonate) and accumulation of citrate following massive transfusions, with metabolic alkalosis. As for its role in diagnosis of metabolic acidosis, the urinary anion gap has been suggested as a replacement for the uncommonly measured urinary ammonium concentration.[22] Recent studies, however, give varying assessments with respect to its accuracy and usefulness for this purpose.[24,25]

The Fencl-Stewart Method for estimating the portion of base excess in plasma due to unmeasured anions (BEua) has been shown to be superior to the anion gap, the standard base excess calculation, and the determination of plasma lactate in predicting mortality in a population of pediatric intensive care patients.[26] The calculation is derived from the standard base excess (BE net) derived from bicarbonate levels (determined in arterial blood using blood gas instrumentation) and plasma levels of sodium, chloride, and albumin. It is given below:

BE ua = BE net - { [0.3 x (Na - 140)] + [102 - (Cl x 140/Na)] + [3.4 x (4.5 - albumin)] }

Footnotes

1. DuFour DR, "Laboratory Recognition and Testing in Acid-Base Disorders," *Lab Med*, 1999, 30(12):776-81.
2. Winter SD, Pearson JR, Gabow PA, et al, "The Fall of the Serum Anion Gap," *Arch Intern Med*, 1990, 150(2):311-3.
3. Sadjadi SA, "A New Range for the Anion Gap," *Ann Intern Med*, 1995, 123(10):807.
4. Roberts WL and Johnson RD, "The Serum Anion Gap. Has the Reference Interval Really Fallen?" *Arch Pathol Lab Med*, 1997, 121(6):568-72.
5. Paulson WD, Roberts WL, Lurie AA, et al, "Wide Variation in Serum Anion Gap Measurements by Chemistry Analyzers," *Am J Clin Pathol*, 1998, 110(6):735-42.
6. Emmett M and Narins RG, "Clinical Use of the Anion Gap," *Medicine*, 1977, 56:38-54.
7. Herr RD and Swanson T, "Pseudometabolic Acidosis Caused by Underfill of Vacutainer® Tubes," *Ann Emerg Med*, 1992, 21(2):177-80.
8. Iberti TJ, Leibowitz AB, Papadakos PJ, et al, "Low Sensitivity of the Anion Gap as a Screen to Detect Hyperlactatemia in Critically Ill Patients," *Crit Care Med*, 1990, 18(3):275-7.
9. Levraut J, Bounatirou T, Ichai C, et al, "Reliability of Anion Gap as an Indicator of Blood Lactate in Critically Ill Patients," *Intensive Care Med*, 1997, 23(4):417-22.
10. Mikulaschek A, Henry SM, Donovan R, et al, "Serum Lactate Is Not Predicted by Anion Gap or Base Excess After Trauma Resuscitation," *J Trauma*, 1996, 40(2):218-24.
11. Gabow PA, Kaehny WD, Fennessey PV, et al, "Diagnostic Importance of an Increased Serum Anion Gap," *N Engl J Med*, 1980, 303(15):854-8.
12. Lorenz JM, Kleinman LI, Markarian K, et al, "Serum Anion Gap in the Differential Diagnosis of Metabolic Acidosis in Critically Ill Newborns," *J Pediatr*, 1999, 135(6):751-5.
13. Oh MS and Carroll HJ, "The Anion Gap," *N Engl J Med*, 1977, 297:814-7.
14. Uribarri J, Oh MS, and Carroll HJ, "D-Lactic Acidosis. A Review of Clinical Presentation, Biochemical Features, and Pathophysiologic Mechanisms," *Medicine (Baltimore)*, 1998, 77(2):73-82.
15. Fischman CM and Oster JR, "Toxic Effects of Toluene: A New Cause of High Anion Gap Metabolic Acidosis," *JAMA*, 1979, 241:1713-5.
16. Adrogué HJ and Madias NE, "Management of Life-Threatening Acid-Base Disorders," First of Two Parts, *N Engl J Med*, 1998, 338(1):26-34.
17. Oster JR, Singer I, Contreras GN, et al, "Metabolic Acidosis With Extreme Elevation of Anion Gap: Case Report and Literature Review," *Am J Med Sci*, 1999, 317(1):38-49.
18. Keshgegian AA, "Anion Gap and Immunoglobulin Concentration," *Am J Clin Pathol*, 1980, 74(3):282-4.
19. Graber ML, Quigg RJ, Stempsey RJ, et al, "Spurious Hyperchloremia and Decreased Anion Gap in Hyperlipidemia," *Ann Intern Med*, 1983, 98(5 Pt 1):607-9.
20. Preuss HG, "Fundamentals of Clinical Acid-Base Evaluation," *Clin Lab Med*, 1993, 13(1):103-16.
21. Figge J, Jabor A, Kazda A, et al, "Anion Gap and Hypoalbuminemia," *Crit Care Med*, 1998, 26(11):1807-10.
22. Battle DC, Hizon M, Cohen E, et al, "The Use of the Urinary Anion Gap in the Diagnosis of Hyperchloremic Metabolic Acidosis," *N Engl J Med*, 1988, 318(10):594-9.
23. Oster JR, Perez GO, and Materson BJ, "Use of the Anion Gap in Clinical Medicine," *South Med J*, 1988, 81(2):229-37.
24. Kirschbaum B, Sica D, and Anderson FP, "Urine Electrolytes and the Urine Anion and Osmolar Gaps," *J Lab Clin Med*, 1999, 133(6):597-604.
25. Kim GH, Han JS, Kim YS, et al, "Evaluation of Urine Acidification by Urine Anion Gap and Urine Osmolal Gap in Chronic Metabolic Acidosis," *Am J Kidney Dis*, 1996, 27(1):42-7.
26. Balasubramanyan N, Havens PL, and Hoffman GM, "Unmeasured Anions Identified by the Fencl-Stewart Method Predict Mortality Better Than Base Excess, Anion Gap, and Lactate in Patients in the Pediatric Intensive Care Unit," *Crit Care Med*, 1999, 27(8):1577-81.

References

Adams SL, "Alcoholic Ketoacidosis," *Emerg Med Clin North Am*, 1990, 8(4):749-60.
Badrick T and Hickman PE, "The Anion Gap: A Reappraisal," *Am J Clin Pathol*, 1992, 98(2):249-52.
Baker RJ, "Biochemical Gaps: Osmolal and Anion," *Curr Surg*, 1987, 44(5):378-81.
Brandenburg MA and Dire DJ, "Comparison of Arterial and Venous Blood Gas Values in the Initial Emergency Department Evaluation of Patients With Diabetic Ketoacidosis," *Ann Emerg Med*, 1998, 31(4):459-65.
Cembrowski GS, Westgard JO, and Kurtycz DF, "Use of the Anion Gap for the Quality Control of Electrolyte Analyzers," *Am J Clin Pathol*, 1983, 79(6):688-96.
Hertford JA, McKenna JP, and Chamovitz BN, "Metabolic Acidosis With an Elevated Anion Gap," *Am Fam Phys*, 1989, 39(4):159-68.
Hood VL and Tannen RL, "Protection of Acid-Base Balance by pH Regulation of Acid Production," *N Engl J Med*, 1998, 339(12):819-26.
Kirschbaum B, "Hyperglobulinemia With an Increased Anion Gap," *Am J Med Sci*, 1998, 316(6):393-7.
Reilly RF and Anderson RJ, "Interpreting the Anion Gap," *Crit Care Med*, 1998, 26(11):1771-2.
Rothenberg DM, Berns AS, Barkin R, et al, "Bromide Intoxication Secondary to Pyridostigmine Bromide Therapy," *JAMA*, 1990, 263(8):1121-2.
Wrenn KD, "The Delta (Delta) Gap: An Approach to Mixed Acid-Base Disorders," *Ann Emerg Med*, 1990, 19(11):1310-3.
Wrenn KD, Slovis CM, Minion GE, et al, "The Syndrome of Alcoholic Ketoacidosis," *Am J Med*, 1991, 91(2):119-28.
Wrong OM, "Urinary Anion Gap in Hyperchloremic Metabolic Acidosis," *N Engl J Med*, 1988, 319(9):585-7.

♦ Anion Gap, Urine see Anion Gap, Serum, Plasma, or Urine on page 106

Antidiuretic Hormone, Plasma

Related Information

Concentration Test, Urine on page 872
Methadone, Urine on page 798
Osmolality, Calculated, Serum or Plasma on page 234
Osmolality, Serum on page 236
Osmolality, Urine on page 236
Sodium, Serum or Plasma on page 275
Specific Gravity, Urine on page 886

Synonyms ADH; Arginine[8]-Vasopressin; Arginine-Vasopressin; AVP; Vasopressin

Test Includes Serum osmolality, urine osmolality, serum sodium

Abstract Antidiuretic hormone (ADH) is a cyclic, 9-amino-acid peptide that is synthesized in the hypothalamus and stored and released by the posterior pituitary. ADH binds to specific receptors on the basal membranes of the renal collecting ducts and initiates a series of events resulting in water reabsorption. ADH is essential to the maintenance of water homeostasis and blood pressure, and its synthesis and release are carefully regulated by hypothalamic osmoreceptors that respond to changes in osmolality and baroreceptors that respond to changes in blood volume.

Deficiency of production or secretion of or lack of normal response to ADH results in polyuria, increased serum osmolality, hypernatremia, and decreased urine osmolality. Excess production or secretion of ADH results in oliguria, decreased serum osmolality, hyponatremia, and increased urine osmolality.

Patient Preparation Patient should avoid substances that influence ADH secretion (eg, nicotine, alcohol, caffeine, diuretics). Fasting, water deprivation, or water loading may be required, depending upon diagnostic test protocol in use.

Specimen Plasma

Container Prechilled lavender top (EDTA) tube(s)

Storage Instructions Immediately upon receipt in laboratory, centrifuge the blood in a refrigerated (4°C) centrifuge at sufficient speed and time to produce platelet-poor plasma (eg, 3600 g for 20 minutes[1]). Remove the plasma into a plastic transport tube, and freeze at -20°C until analysis. Transport to referral laboratory frozen.

Causes for Rejection Specimen not received frozen, recently administered radioisotopes

Special Instructions Following collection, place the tube in ice and deliver to the laboratory for immediate processing.

Reference Interval Basal values in normally hydrated individuals: 0.5-2.0 ng/L (SI, 0.5-1.9 pmol/L).[2] In a study of 203 children, age 1 day to 18 years, basal levels averaged 1.1 ±0.6 ng/L (SI: 1.0 ±0.6 pmol/L) with no significant differences between males and females and no age correlation within the study population.[1] This same study reported basal levels of 1.0 ±0.5 ng/L (Continued)

Antidiuretic Hormone, Plasma *(Continued)*

(SI: 0.9 ±0.5 pmol/L) in 16 adult controls.[1] Results are best interpreted with simultaneously determined plasma osmolalities. See table.[3]

Antidiuretic Hormone, Plasma

ADH ng/L (SI: pmol/L)	Osmolality (mOsm/kg)
<1.5 (<1.4)	270-280
<2.5 (<2.3)	280-285
1-5 (0.9-4.6)	285-290
2-7 (1.9-6.5)	290-295
4-12 (3.7-11.1)	295-300

Use Though serum and urine osmolality and serum sodium determinations are primarily used for diagnosis of ADH abnormalities, plasma ADH measurements are occasionally useful in the differential diagnosis of syndrome of inappropriate secretion of ADH (SIADH), diabetes insipidus (DI), chronic hyponatremia, and psychogenic water intoxication.

Limitations Assays are complex to perform and lack sensitivity and specificity. Consequently, it is important to evaluate plasma osmolality levels concurrently with ADH levels. Since ADH is contained in platelets, plasma contaminated with platelets will result in overestimation of plasma ADH.[1]

Methodology Radioimmunoassay following extraction of ADH from plasma

Additional Information Overnight water deprivation protocols[3] are useful for differentiating polyuric patients with DI from other causes of polyuria (eg, psychogenic polydipsia) and for characterizing DI as neurogenic (cranial or central) or nephrogenic (failure of kidneys to respond to ADH). After water deprivation, patients with DI have high plasma osmolalities, low urine osmolalities, and either lower than expected (neurogenic) or high (nephrogenic) plasma ADH levels. Patients with psychogenic polydipsia respond similarly to normal individuals, having plasma osmolalities within the normal range, appropriately concentrated urines, and ADH levels that correlate predictably with the plasma osmolality. Saline infusion test protocols[3] are sometimes used when overnight water deprivation studies are inconclusive. Idiopathic diabetes insipidus is the most common type, but a variety of causes of central DI exist, including trauma, autosomal dominant type of inherited disease, and pregnancy. Tumors of the hypothalamus or pituitary which can cause DI include craniopharyngioma, ependymona, germinoma, pinealoma, leukemic infiltrates, some tumors of the anterior pituitary, and metastases. Langerhans cell histiocytosis, sarcoidosis, and tuberculosis may cause DI.

SIADH is characterized by hyponatremia, low plasma osmolality, and increased plasma ADH. Water loading protocols, though hazardous, are occasionally useful for diagnosis of difficult cases of SIADH.[3]

Footnotes

1. Kluge M, Riedl S, Erhart-Hofmann B, et al, "Improved Extraction Procedure and RIA for Determination of Arginine[8]-Vasopressin in Plasma: Role of Premeasurement Sample Treatment and Reference Values in Children," *Clin Chem*, 1999, 45(1):98-103.
2. Robinson AG, "Posterior Pituitary," *Cecil Textbook of Medicine*, 21st ed, Chapter 238, Goldman L and Bennett JC, eds, Philadelphia, PA: WB Saunders Co, 2000, 1225-31.
3. Demers LM, "Pituitary Function," *Tietz Textbook of Clinical Chemistry*, 3rd ed, Chapter 41, Burtis CA and Ashwood ER, eds, Philadelphia, PA: WB Saunders Co, 1999, 1470-95.

References

Camps J, Martinez-Vea A, Perez-Ayuso RM, et al, "Radioimmunoassay for Arginine-Vasopressin in Cold Ethanol Extracts of Plasma," *Clin Chem*, 1983, 29(5):882-4.

Crawford GA and Gyory AZ, "Measuring Arginine Vasopressin in Children and Babies," *Clin Chem*, 1990, 36(9):1689.

Crawford GA, Johnson AG, Gyory AZ, et al, "Change in Arginine Vasopressin Concentrations With Age," *Clin Chem*, 1993, 39(9):2023.

Foster SV and Wians FH, "Renal Function Tests," *The Handbook of Clinical Pathology*, 2nd ed, Chapter 5, McKenna RW and Keffer JH, eds, Chicago, IL: American Society of Clinical Pathologists, 2000, 55-65.

Gavras H, "Role of Vasopressin in Clinical Hypertension and Congestive Cardiac Failure: Interaction With the Sympathetic Nervous System," *Clin Chem*, 1991, 37(10B):1828-30.

Ysewijn-Van Brussel KARN and De Leenheer AP, "Development and Evaluation of a Radioimmunoassay for Arg[8]-Vasopressin, After Extraction With Sep-Pak C18," *Clin Chem*, 1985, 31(6):861-3.

Antioxidant Concentrations, Plasma

Related Information

Ascorbic Acid, Serum or Plasma *on page 112*
Vitamin A, Serum or Plasma *on page 298*
Vitamin E, Serum or Plasma *on page 301*

Applies to Oxygen Radical Absorbance Capacity; Total Antioxidant Capacity; Total Radical Absorbin Parameter

Test Includes Measurement of total antioxidant capacity of plasma

Abstract Total antioxidant capacity: Halliwell and Gutteridge[1] defined antioxidants as any substance that delays or inhibits damage to a target molecule by an oxidant. The balance between pro-oxidant challenge and the presence of antioxidants determines net oxidative stress. Antioxidants may be present within cells, in cell membranes or extracellular fluids; may be hydrophilic or lipophilic; and may be endogenously produced or derived from the diet. Intracellular antioxidants include glutathione and enzymes such as glutathione peroxidase, superoxide dismutase, and catalase. Membrane-bound antioxidants include alpha-tocopherol, beta-carotene, and ubiquinone. Many antioxidants that are derived from the diet, including ascorbate, polyphenols, and flavinoids, are hydrophilic and carried in plasma, while the lipophilic tocopherols and carotenoids are carried by lipoproteins. Other predominantly extracellular antioxidants are bilirubin and uric acid. Some weaker antioxidants are chelating proteins, such as albumin, transferrin, lactoferrin, and ceruloplasmin. Assessment of antioxidant status employs methods to measure total antioxidant capacity.

Antioxidants include vitamins A, C, and E and many of the carotenoids.

Patient Preparation Patient must fast for a minimum of 8 hours.

Specimen Plasma

Container Green top (heparin) tube

Collection Draw in chilled tube protected from light. Keep specimen on ice until separation of plasma.

Storage Instructions Store at -20°C for 3 months or -70°C for longer periods of time.

Turnaround Time 6 hours

Reference Interval Measures as units of Trolox

Use Assess total antioxidant deficiency (eg, vitamin C or E); especially useful for water soluble antioxidant status

Methodology All published methods of estimating antioxidant capacity of a solution measure the inhibition of an artificially generated species.[2] A free radical species is generated in a solution containing an oxidation target; antioxidants in the added sample quench the target response by interaction with the reactive oxygen species. Published methods differ in the choice of free radical generator used, target, and type of measurement used to detect the oxidized product. One of the most widely adapted techniques is the total peroxyl radical-trapping antioxidant parameter (TRAP).[3] In this assay, the water-soluble compound, 2,2'-azobis(2-amidinopropane hydrochloride) (AAPH), undergoes thermal decomposition to produce peroxyl free radicals. The rate of oxygen uptake is monitored by performing the reaction in an oxygen-electrode chamber. The measurement is calibrated using Trolox, a water-soluble alpha-tocopherol analog. In an effort to improve this assay, a method has been developed for use on a centrifugal analyzer with plasma volumes as low as 3 mL.[4] In this assay, 2,2'-azinobis-(3-ethylbenzothiazoline-6-sulphonic acid) (ABTS) is incubated with metmyoglobin (this acts as a peroxidase) and hydrogen peroxide, resulting in the formation of the long-lived cation, ABTS[+]. The presence of an antioxidant in heparinized plasma reduces this radical cation, the concentration of which is measured by absorbance. The assay is calibrated using Trolox. However, its clinical utility needs to be assessed.

Another widely used method for determining total antioxidant capacity is the ORAC (oxygen radical absorbance capacity) assay based on the procedure described by Cao et al.[5] The method utilizes β-phycoerythrin (β-PE) as an indicator protein and AAPH as a peroxyl radical generator. Under appropriate conditions, the loss of β-PE fluorescence in the presence of reactive species is an index of oxidative damage of the protein. The inhibition by an antioxidant, which is reflected in the protection against the loss of β-PE fluorescence in the ORAC assay, is a measure of its antioxidant capacity.

Additional Information An inverse relationship is postulated, but unproven, between vitamin C and E and carotenoids, and cataracts and macular degeneration.[6]

Footnotes

1. Halliwell B and Gutteridge JM, "Free Radicals and Antioxidants in the Year 2000," *Ann N Y Acad Sci*, 2000, 899:136-47
2. Rice-Evans C and Miller NJ, "Total Antioxidant Status in Plasma and Body Fluids," *Methods Enzymol*, 1994, 234:279-93.
3. Wayner DD, Burton GW, Ingold KU, et al, "The Relative Contribution of Vitamin E, Urate, Asorbate and Proteins to TRAP in Human Blood Plasma," *Biochim Biophys Acta*, 1987, 924(3):408-19.
4. Miller NJ, Rice-Evans C, Davies MJ, et al, "A Novel Method for Measuring Antioxidant Capacity and its Application for Monitoring the Antioxidant Status in Premature Neonates," *Clin Sci*, 1993, 84(4):407-12.
5. Cao G and Prior RL, "Measurement of Oxygen Radical Absorbance Capacity in Biological Samples," *Methods Enzymol*, 1999, 299:50-62.
6. Mason JB, "Consequences of Altered Micronutrient Status," *Cecil Textbook of Medicine*, 21st ed, Chapter 231, Goldman L and Bennett JC, eds, Philadelphia, PA: WB Saunders Co, 2000, 1170-8.

References

Kushi LH, Folsom AR, Prineas RJ, et al, "Dietary Antioxidant Vitamins and Death From Coronary Heart Disease in Postmenopausal Women," *N Engl J Med*, 1996, 334(18):1156-62.

♦ **Antipernicious Anemia Factor** *see* Cobalamin, Serum *on page 150*

♦ **α₁-Antiprotease** *see* Alpha₁-Antitrypsin, Serum *on page 96*

♦ **α₁-Antiprotease Phenotype** *see* Alpha₁-Antitrypsin Phenotyping *on page 95*

♦ **Apo A** *see* Apolipoprotein A-I, Serum *on page 109*

♦ **Apo-A-I** *see* Lipids, Overview *on page 213*

♦ **Apo B** *see* Apolipoprotein B-100, Serum *on page 109*

♦ **Apo B-100** *see* Lipids, Overview *on page 213*

◆ **APOE** *see* Apolipoprotein E, Plasma *on page 110*

◆ **Apolipoprotein A** *see* Apolipoprotein A-I, Serum *on page 109*

◆ **Apolipoprotein A-I** *see* High Density Lipoprotein Cholesterol, Serum *on page 192*

Apolipoprotein A-I, Serum

Related Information
Apolipoprotein B-100, Serum *on page 109*
Apolipoprotein E, Plasma *on page 110*
Cholesterol, Total, Serum or Plasma *on page 146*
High Density Lipoprotein Cholesterol, Serum *on page 192*
Lipid Panel, Serum *on page 212*
Lipids, Overview *on page 213*
Low Density Lipoprotein Cholesterol *on page 218*
Triglycerides, Serum or Plasma *on page 288*

Synonyms Apo A; Apolipoprotein A

Abstract Apolipoprotein A-I (apo A-I) is the principal protein associated with the HDL particle and is a cofactor for lecithin:cholesterol acetyltransferase (LCAT). Apo A-I participates in the removal of excess cholesterol from tissues and is the primary lipoprotein in the interstitial space. Similar to HDL, serum Apo A-I is a negative risk factor for coronary heart disease (CHD) and stroke.

Patient Preparation Many laboratories require a 9- to 14-hour fast. However, no significant differences in apo-A-I result between fasting and nonfasting subjects have been reported.[1]

Specimen Serum or plasma

Container Red top tube or lavender (EDTA) top tube

Storage Instructions Separate serum or plasma and refrigerate or freeze according to the instructions provided by the individual testing laboratory.

Reference Interval For this analyte, high coronary risk is associated with low serum levels. See Lipids, Overview *on page 213* and following table.[2]

Population Distributions for Apolipoprotein A-I (mg/dL)

Age (y)	Percentile						
	5	10	25	50	75	90	95
Male							
12-20	107	121	128	142	154	169	191
22-29	102	113	116	135	150	174	184
30-39	104	110	119	134	150	161	176
40-49	103	108	119	132	146	161	171
50-59	102	107	119	131	145	159	172
60-69	100	105	116	132	150	168	183
70-79	92	104	114	128	144	175	202
Female							
12-20	97	112	127	144	166	179	188
22-29	107	117	128	137	152	177	220
30-39	107	119	132	149	160	182	199
40-49	114	121	134	149	168	191	202
50-59	116	122	135	153	174	198	211
60-69	119	124	137	152	170	193	212
70-79	116	118	140	154	173	186	189

Data for ages 12-20 obtained from African-American adolescents (Rifai et al, 1996) and data for ages 22-79 obtained from white adults (Contois et al, 1996).

Adapted from Rifai N, Bachorik PS, and Albers JS, "Lipids, Lipoproteins and Apolipoproteins," *Tietz Textbook of Clinical Chemistry*, 3rd ed, Burtis CA and Ashwood ER, eds, Philadelphia, PA: WB Saunders Co, 1999, 828.

Use Apo A-I assays are primarily of use in investigating patients with low HDL cholesterol concentrations (eg, familial apo A-I deficiency, Tangier disease, and LCAT deficiency).

Limitations Apo A-I measurement may provide no advantage over high density lipoprotein cholesterol (HDLC) measurement for prediction of coronary risk; the topic is controversial.[3] Plasma lipoproteins change significantly during cardiac catheterization and measurements shortly thereafter should be avoided.[4,5]

Methodology Analytical methods include immunonephelometry, immunoturbidimetry, enzyme-linked immunosorbent assay (ELISA), radioimmunoassay (RIA), and radical immunodiffusion (RID). Current commercial apo A-I assays are standardized with WHO-IFCC reference materials.[5,6] Automation has become available for this assay. Addition of Tween 20 has been advocated to enhance diagnostic discrimination for CHD.[3]

Additional Information Apolipoproteins are the protein components of the lipoprotein complexes. Apolipoprotein A-I is the main protein component of HDL.

Footnotes
1. Bachorik PS, Lovejoy KL, Carroll MD, et al, "Apolipoprotein B and AI Distributions in the United States, 1988-1991: Results of the National Health and Nutrition Examination Survey III (NHANES III)," *Clin Chem*, 1997, 43(12):2364-78.
2. Contois JH, McNamara JR, Lammi-Keefe CJ, et al, "Reference Intervals for Plasma Apolipoprotein A-I Determined With a Standardized Commercial Immunoturbidimetric Assay: Results From the Framingham Offspring Study," *Clin Chem*, 1996, 42(4):507-14.
3. Levinson SS and Hobbs GA, "Optimized Automated Apolipoprotein A-1 Assays as Markers for Coronary Artery Disease," *Arch Pathol Lab Med*, 1997, 121(7):678-84.
4. Contois JH, McNamara JR, Lammi-Keefe CJ, et al, "Reference Intervals for Plasma Apolipoprotein B Determined With a Standardized Commercial Immunoturbidimetric Assay: Results From the Framingham Offspring Study," *Clin Chem*, 1996, 42(4).515-23.
5. Miida T, Otsuka H, Tsuchiya A, et al, "Plasma Lipoprotein Profiles Change Significantly During Cardiac Catheterization," *Clin Chem*, 1998, 44(3):517-21.
6. Albers JJ and Marcovina SM, "Standardization of Apolipoprotein B and A-1 Measurements," *Clin Chem*, 1989, 35(7):1357-61.

References
Bhatnagar D and Durrington PN, "Measurement and Clinical Significance of Apolipoproteins A-I and B," *Handbook of Lipoprotein Testing*, Chapter 10, Rifai N, Warnick GR, and Dominiczak MH, eds, Washington, DC: AACC Press, American Association of Clinical Chemistry, 1997, 177-98.

Boerwinkle E, Brown SA, Rohrbach K, et al, "Role of Apolipoprotein E and B Gene Variation in Determining Response of Lipid, Lipoprotein, and Apolipoprotein Levels to Increased Dietary Cholesterol," *Am J Hum Genet*, 1991, 49(6):1145-54.

Genest JJ Jr, Bard JM, Fruchart JC, et al, "Plasma Apolipoprotein A-I, A-II, B, E, and C-III Containing Particles in Men With Premature Coronary Artery Disease," *Atherosclerosis*, 1991, 90(2-3):149-57.

Graziani MS, Zanolla L, Righetti G, et al, "Plasma Apolipoproteins A-I and B in Survivors of Myocardial Infarction and n a Control Group," *Clin Chem*, 1998, 44(1):134-40.

Jungner I, Marcovina SM, Walldius G, et al, "Apolipoprotein B and A-I Values in 147576 Swedish Males and Females, Standardized According to the World Health Organization-International Federation of Clinical Chemistry First International Reference Materials," *Clin Chem*, 1998, 44(8 Pt 1):1641-9.

Lamarche B, Tchernof A, Mauriege P, et al, "Fasting Insulin and Apolipoprotein B Levels and Low-Density Lipoprotein Particle Size as Risk Factors for Ischemic Heart Disease," *JAMA*, 1998, 279(24):1955-61.

Paulweber B, Friedl W, Krempler F, et al, "Association of DNA Polymorphism at the Apolipoprotein B Gene Locus With Coronary Heart Disease and Serum Very Low Density Lipoprotein Levels," *Arteriosclerosis*, 1990, 10(1):17-24.

Rifai N, Bachorik PS, and Albers JS, "Lipids, Lipoproteins and Apolipoproteins," *Tietz Textbook of Clinical Chemistry*, 3rd ed, Burtis CA and Ashwood ER, eds, Philadelphia, PA: WB Saunders Co, 1999, 809-61.

Shephard MD, Hester J, Walmsley RN, et al, "Variation in Plasma Apolipoprotein A-1 and B Concentrations Following Myocardial Infarction," *Ann Clin Biochem*, 1990, 27(Pt 1):9-14.

Sniderman AD, "Counterpoint: To (Measure Apo)B or Not to (Measure Apo)B: A Critique of Modern Medical Decision Making," *Clin Chem*, 1997, 43(8 Pt 1):1310-4.

Sniderman AD and Cianflone K, "Measurement of Apoproteins: Time to Improve the Diagnosis and Treatment of the Atherogenic Dyslipoproteinemias," *Clin Chem*, 1996, 42(4):489-91.

Walmsley TA, Grant S, and George PM, "Effect of Plasma Triglyceride Concentrations on the Accuracy of Immunoturbidimetric Assays of Apolipoprotein B," *Clin Chem*, 1991, 37(5):748-53.

Williams KJ, Petrie KA, Brocia RW, et al, "Lipoprotein Lipase Modulates Net Secretory Output of Apolipoprotein B In Vitro. A Possible Pathophysiologic Explanation for Familial Combined Hyperlipidemia," *J Clin Invest*, 1991, 88(4):1300-6.

Young SG, "Recent Progress in Understanding Apolipoprotein B," *Circulation*, 1990, 82(5):1574-94.

◆ **Apolipoprotein B** *see* Apolipoprotein B-100, Serum *on page 109*

Apolipoprotein B-100, Serum

Related Information
Apolipoprotein A-I, Serum *on page 109*
Apolipoprotein E, Plasma *on page 110*
Cholesterol, Total, Serum or Plasma *on page 146*
High Density Lipoprotein Cholesterol, Serum *on page 192*
Lipid Panel, Serum *on page 212*
Lipids, Overview *on page 213*
Lipoprotein (a), Serum *on page 215*
Low Density Lipoprotein Cholesterol *on page 218*
Triglycerides, Serum or Plasma *on page 288*

Synonyms Apo B; Apolipoprotein B

Abstract Apolipoprotein B-100 (apo B-100) is a large polypeptide of more than 4500 amino acids and is an important constituent of the following lipoproteins: VLDL, IDL, LDL, and Lp(a). Apo B-100 is synthesized in the liver and secreted into plasma as part of the VLDL particle. Apo B-100 participates in the delivery of cholesterol to the tissues and interacts directly with the LDL receptor. Serum Apo B-100 is a positive risk factor for coronary heart disease. See Lipids, Overview *on page 213*.

Patient Preparation Many laboratories require a 9- to 14-hour fast. However, no significant differences in apo-B-100 results between fasting and nonfasting subjects have been reported.[1]

Specimen Serum or plasma

Container Red top tube or lavender (EDTA) top tube

Storage Instructions Separate serum or plasma and refrigerate or freeze according to the instructions provided by the individual testing laboratory.

Reference Interval See Lipids, Overview *on page 213* and the following table.[2]

Use Apo B-100 measurement is used in the evaluation of risk for coronary heart disease and in the diagnosis of abetalipoproteinemia, hypobetalipoproteinemia, and hyperabetalipoproteinemia.

Limitations Plasma lipoproteins change significantly during cardiac catheterization and measurements shortly thereafter should be avoided.[3,4]
(Continued)

Apolipoprotein B-100, Serum *(Continued)*

Population Distributions for Apolipoprotein B-100
(mg/dL)

Age (y)	Percentile						
	5	10	25	50	75	90	95
12-20	M: 59 F: 55	M: 61 F: 60	M: 75 F: 74	M: 86 F: 90	M: 108 F: 104	M: 122 F: 121	M: 140 F: 138
22-29	M: 54 F: 59	M: 60 F: 61	M: 68 F: 69	M: 84 F: 80	M: 98 F: 97	M: 107 F: 107	M: 109 F: 114
30-39	M: 57 F: 50	M: 64 F: 57	M: 76 F: 66	M: 91 F: 75	M: 107 F: 88	M: 123 F: 99	M: 133 F: 110
40-49	M: 66 F: 58	M: 73 F: 63	M: 88 F: 73	M: 104 F: 87	M: 118 F: 103	M: 134 F: 119	M: 144 F: 130
50-59	M: 68 F: 66	M: 78 F: 72	M: 90 F: 84	M: 105 F: 99	M: 120 F: 116	M: 134 F: 137	M: 146 F: 150
60-69	M: 69 F: 72	M: 78 F: 79	M: 90 F: 90	M: 106 F: 103	M: 120 F: 120	M: 134 F: 137	M: 145 F: 145
70-79	M: 74 F: 78	M: 77 F: 79	M: 86 F: 92	M: 104 F: 106	M: 123 F: 120	M: 133 F: 136	M: 144 F: 142

Data for ages 12-20 obtained from African-American adolescents (Rifai et al 1996) and data for ages 22-79 obtained from white adults (Contois et al 1999, 43).

Adapted from Rifai N, Bachorik PS, and Albers JS, "Lipids, Lipoproteins and Apolipoproteins," *Tietz Textbook of Clinica Chemistry*, 3rd ed, Burtis CA and Ashwood ER, eds, Philadelphia, PA: WB Saunders Co, 1999, 809-61.

Methodology Analytical methods include immunonephelometry, immunoturbidimetry, enzyme-linked immunosorbent assay (ELISA), radioimmunoassay (RIA), and radical immunodifusion (RID). Current commercial apo B-100 assays are standardized with WHO-IFCC reference materials.[4,5]

Additional Information Apolipoproteins are the protein components of the lipoprotein complexes. Apolipoprotein B-100 is the major component of the low density lipoproteins (VLDL, IDL, LDL, and Lp(a)). There is one apo B-100 molecule per low density lipoprotein particle. Consequently, the plasma concentration of apo B-100 is unaffected by LDL heterogeneity and provides a rough indication of the number of atherogenic particles in plasma. Unlike the LDL cholesterol calculated by the Friedewald equation, apo B-100 measurement does not require a fasting specimen and is useful for patients with high triglyceride levels.

Point mutations in the gene coding for apolipoprotein B in the domain associated with the LDL binding site have been identified and associated with increased risk of ischemic heart disease,[6] hypercholesterolemia,[6] and decreased receptor-mediated uptake of LDL.[7]

Footnotes

1. Bachorik PS, Lovejoy KL, Carroll MD, et al, "Apolipoprotein B and AI Distributions in the United States, 1988-1991: Results of the National Health and Nutrition Examination Survey III (NHANES III)," *Clin Chem*, 1997, 43(12):2364-78.
2. Contois JH, McNamara JR, Lammi-Keefe CJ, et al, "Reference Intervals for Plasma Apolipoprotein A-I Determined With a Standardized Commercial Immunoturbidimetric Assay: Results From the Framingham Offspring Study," *Clin Chem*, 1996, 42(4):507-14.
3. Contois JH, McNamara JR, Lammi-Keefe CJ, et al, "Reference Intervals for Plasma Apolipoprotein B Determined With a Standardized Commercial Immunoturbidimetric Assay: Results From the Framingham Offspring Study," *Clin Chem*, 1996, 42(4):515-23.
4. Miida T, Otsuka H, Tsuchiya A, et al, "Plasma Lipoprotein Profiles Change Significantly During Cardiac Catheterization," *Clin Chem*, 1998, 44(3):517-21.
5. Albers JJ and Marcovina SM, "Standardization of Apolipoprotein B and A-I Measurements," *Clin Chem*, 1989, 35(7):1357-61.
6. Tybjaerg-Hansen A, Steffensen R, Meinertz H, et al, "Association of Mutations in the Apolipoprotein B Gene With Hypercholesterolemia and the Risk of Ischemic Heart Disease," *N Engl J Med*, 1998, 338(22):1577-84.
7. Fisher E, Scharnagl H, Hoffmann MM, et al, "Mutations in the Apolipoprotein (apo) B-100 Receptor-Binding Region: Detection of Apo B-100 (Arg^{3500} → Trp) Associated With Two New Haplotypes and Evidence That Apo B-100 (Glu^{3405} → Gln) Diminishes Receptor-Mediated Uptake of LDL," *Clin Chem*, 1999, 45(7):1026-38.

References

Bhatnagar D and Durrington PN, "Measurement and Clinical Significance of Apolipoproteins A-I and B," *Handbook of Lipoprotein Testing*, Chapter 10, Rifai N, Warnick GR, and Dominiczak MH, eds, Washington, DC: AACC Press, American Association of Clinical Chemistry, 1997, 177-98.

Boerwinkle E, Brown SA, Rohrbach K, et al, "Role of Apolipoprotein E and B Gene Variation in Determining Response of Lipid, Lipoprotein, and Apolipoprotein Levels to Increased Dietary Cholesterol," *Am J Hum Genet*, 1991, 49(6):1145-54.

Genest JJ Jr, Bard JM, Fruchart JC, et al, "Plasma Apolipoprotein A-I, A-II, B, E, and C-III Containing Particles in Men With Premature Coronary Artery Disease," *Atherosclerosis*, 1991, 90(2-3):149-57.

Graziani MS, Zanolla L, Righetti G, et al, "Plasma Apolipoproteins A-I and B in Survivors of Myocardial Infarction and n a Control Group," *Clin Chem*, 1998, 44(1):134-40.

Jungner I, Marcovina SM, Walldius G, et al, "Apolipoprotein B and A-I Values in 147576 Swedish Males and Females, Standardized According to the World Health Organization-International Federation of Clinical Chemistry First International Reference Materials," *Clin Chem*, 1998, 44(8 Pt 1):1641-9.

Lamarche B, Tchernof A, Mauriege P, et al, "Fasting Insulin and Apolipoprotein B Levels and Low-Density Lipoprotein Particle Size as Risk Factors for Ischemic Heart Disease," *JAMA*, 1998, 279(24):1955-61.

Ozturk IC and Killeen AA, "An Overview of Genetic Factors Influencing Plasma Lipid Levels and Coronary Artery Disease Risk," *Arch Pathol Lab Med*, 1999, 123:1219-22.

Paulweber B, Friedl W, Krempler F, et al, "Association of DNA Polymorphism at the Apolipoprotein B Gene Locus With Coronary Heart Disease and Serum Very Low Density Lipoprotein Levels," *Arteriosclerosis*, 1990, 10(1):17-24.

Rifai N, Bachorik PS, and Albers JS, "Lipids, Lipoproteins and Apolipoproteins," *Tietz Textbook of Clinical Chemistry*, 3rd ed, Burtis CA and Ashwood ER, eds, Philadelphia, PA: WB Saunders Co, 1999, 809-61.

Shephard MD, Hester J, Walmsley RN, et al, "Variation in Plasma Apolipoprotein A-1 and B Concentrations Following Myocardial Infarction," *Ann Clin Biochem*, 1990, 27(Pt 1):9-14.

Sniderman AD, "Counterpoint: To (Measure Apo)B or Not to (Measure Apo)B: A Critique of Modern Medical Decision Making," *Clin Chem*, 1997, 43(8 Pt 1):1310-4.

Sniderman AD and Cianflone K, "Measurement of Apoproteins: Time to Improve the Diagnosis and Treatment of the Atherogenic Dyslipoproteinemias," *Clin Chem*, 1996, 42(4):489-91.

Walmsley TA, Grant S, and George PM, "Effect of Plasma Triglyceride Concentrations on the Accuracy of Immunoturbidimetric Assays of Apolipoprotein B," *Clin Chem*, 1991, 37(5):748-53.

Williams KJ, Petrie KA, Brocia RW, et al, "Lipoprotein Lipase Modulates Net Secretory Output of Apolipoprotein B In Vitro. A Possible Pathophysiologic Explanation for Familial Combined Hyperlipidemia," *J Clin Invest*, 1991, 88(4):1300-6.

Young SG, "Recent Progress in Understanding Apolipoprotein B," *Circulation*, 1990, 82(5):1574-94.

Apolipoprotein E, Plasma

Related Information

AD7c Neural Thread Protein, CSF or Urine *on page 83*
Apolipoprotein A-I, Serum *on page 109*
Apolipoprotein B-100, Serum *on page 109*
Cerebrospinal Fluid and Plasma β-Amyloid$_{(1-42)}$ *on page 513*
Cerebrospinal Fluid Protein *on page 517*
Cerebrospinal Fluid Protein Electrophoresis *on page 518*
Cholesterol, Total, Serum or Plasma *on page 146*
High Density Lipoprotein Cholesterol, Serum *on page 192*
Lipid Panel, Serum *on page 212*
Lipids, Overview *on page 213*
Lipoprotein (a), Serum *on page 215*
Low Density Lipoprotein Cholesterol *on page 218*
Triglycerides, Serum or Plasma *on page 288*

Synonyms APOE; Apo E; Apoprotein E

Applies to βA4 Peptide; Clusterin (Apo J); Neurofibrillary Tangles; Tau Protein

Test Includes ε2, ε3, and ε4

Abstract Apolipoprotein E (apoE) is produced by many cell types, including hepatic cells and astrocytes. ApoE is found in most lipoproteins, but very little is present in LDL. ApoE is a ligand for the LDL and apoE receptors, and has a major role in the clearance of apoB-containing lipoproteins, especially chylomicrons, VLDL, and VLDL remnants. ApoE also participates in HDL metabolism. Elevated apoE is probably not a coronary risk factor. Deficient or defective apoE usually presents as an increase in apoB-containing lipoproteins, especially VLDL and chylomicron-containing remnants. There are multiple molecular forms of apoE. This polymorphism is expressed with the common alleles, ε2, ε3, and ε4.[1] Apoε4 predisposes to coronary artery disease (CAD) and to Alzheimer dementia.

Specimen Plasma

Container Lavender top (EDTA) tube

Storage Instructions Store at 2°C to 8°C. Do not freeze.

Causes for Rejection Hemolysis, heparinized blood collected, specimen frozen

Special Instructions Test will usually be performed by a reference laboratory. Schedule patient sample requirements, handling, and timing with laboratory.

Reference Interval Variation in methodology has resulted in wide variation of reported **mean** values in healthy individuals (30-120 mg/L), see reference by Siest et al. A reference range should be supplied by the laboratory performing the test.

Use This test is used to evaluate abnormal lipid metabolism associated with coronary artery disease, study predisposing factors to the development of Alzheimer disease (AD), and aid in the differential diagnosis of AD.

Methodology Quantitative methods for total apoE include radioimmunoassay (RIA), immunonephelometry, radial immunodiffusion (RID), and electroimmunoassay. ApoE identification (phenotyping) can be performed using polyacrylamide gel isoelectric focusing (PAGE-IEF) or PAGE-IEF of plasma followed by immunoblotting[2] or immunofixation.[3] Because of technical problems, presence of rare variants and of post-translational modifications, isoelectric focusing is less desirable than apoE genotyping for determination of apoE polymorphism. ApoE genotyping is generally performed by restriction enzyme isoform genotyping (restriction isotyping). This technique utilizes polymerase chain reaction (amplification of the genomic sequence containing the apoE polymorphic sites) followed by restriction endonuclease (Hhal) digestion and PAGE electrophoresis of the resultant fragments.[4] "MADGE" (microplate array diagonal gel electrophoresis) should allow lower cost and large scale apoE genotyping.[5]

Additional Information Apolipoprotein E (apoE) circulates in the blood as a 299 amino acid single chain protein. Isoelectric focusing (phenotypic analysis) confirmed by direct sequencing of cDNA (genotyping) has shown that apoE is present in three major isoforms, ε2, ε3, and ε4, with rarely encountered variants. The three isoforms result in six different phenotypes, ε2/2, ε3/3, ε4/4 (homozygotes) and ε2/3, ε2/4, and ε3/4 (heterozygotes). ApoE polymorphism has its structural basis in variation at amino acids 112 and 158, the alleles ε2, ε3, and ε4 encoding Cys-Cys, Cys-Arg, and Arg-Arg, respectively.

Apolipoprotein E plays a variety of roles in lipid metabolism with increasing evidence of significance in both vascular and central nervous system (Alzheimer) degenerative disease.

ApoE and Vascular Disease

ApoE mediates removal of chylomicron and very low density lipoprotein (VLDL) remnants from plasma by binding these particles to low density lipoprotein (LDL). ApoE is a ligand for the LDL receptor, a function dependent upon basic amino acids present between apoE residues 136 and 150. In this role, apoE facilitates removal of circulating VDRL and chylomicron remnant particles through a specific hepatocyte plasma membrane receptor. Fully functioning apoE (eg, apoε3) is associated with decreased plasma cholesterol levels. This in contrast to apoE forms with impaired LDL ligand function (eg, apoε4) which are associated with increased plasma cholesterol levels and development of premature athero-sclerosis.[6] ApoE isoforms affect plasma concentration of cholesterol and LDL (apoε4 being associated with elevated levels). Isoform type is perhaps the most important lipid risk factor for coronary artery disease.[7] While apoE mediates metabolism of LDL plasma cholesterol levels, other lipoproteins are involved in the absorption and assimilation of dietary cholesterol (eg, apolipoprotein A-IV).[8] Rare mutant apoE isoforms have been associated with aberrant lipid metabolism (eg, apoε3' with double pre-β very low density lipoprotein[9] and apoε7 with xanthomas of the Achilles tendon and coronary artery disease[10]).

The apoε2/ε2 phenotype (apoε3 deficient) is associated with familial dysbe-talipoproteinemia in which there is chylomicronemia, increased plasma triglyceride, cholesterol, and β-VLDL. The ε2/ε2 genotype is uncommon (about 1% of individuals) and, as additional risk factors are involved, only 2% to 5% of ε2/ε2 individuals develop type III hyperlipidemia. Presence of the amino acid cysteine at sites 112 and 158 (see above) are considered to impair binding to the LDL receptor, resulting in impaired clearance of plasma intermediate density lipoprotein. The ε4 allele is present in 10% to 15% of individuals in the population and, in contrast to the ε3 allele, is over-represented in association with coronary heart disease.[11] While the average effect of the ε2 allele is to decrease cholesterol and apolipoprotein B levels, both apoε2 and ε4 alleles may be associated with increased cholesterol and/or triglyceride levels. The lowest cholesterol levels are associated with ε3/ε3 phenotype. There is compelling evidence that apoE polymorphism is a major determinant of risk for development of atherosclerotic vascular disease and its complications.[6] Demand for apoE genotype and/or phenotype determination is likely to increase, in particular, if therapeutic modulation of the effect of apoε4 is developed.

ApoE and Alzheimer Disease

Since 1993, there have been some 90 reports worldwide confirming an association between Alzheimer disease (AD) and apoε4. The allele frequency of apoε4 is increased in patients with late-onset AD and in cases of sporadic AD.[12] In a study of elderly patients with mild cognitive impairment, many (24% by 18 months, 44% by 36 months, and 55% by 54 months) progressed to dementia with apoε4 a strong predictor of progression.[13] A reliable phenotypic marker of AD is not currently available. ApoE genotyping cannot be used for prediction of development of AD.[12] Reduced rates of glucose metabolism in certain areas of the brain (eg, posterior cingulate gyrus) have been associated with preclinical evidence of AD in homozygotes for the ε4 allele.[14]

A functional role of apoE in the pathogenesis of late-onset AD is suggested by the finding that apoE is localized (immunochemically) in senile plaques, vascular amyloid and neurofibrillary tangles (neuropathologic morphologic hallmarks of AD).[15] In addition, cerebrospinal fluid has been shown to bind synthetic βA4 peptide in vitro. βA4 peptide is the primary constituent of senile plaques.[15]

In a series of randomly selected (85 year old or older) individuals with both clinical and autopsy-based diagnosis, 28 of 33 carriers of the apoε4 allele had dementia and pathologic confirmation of AD. The other 5 carriers had no cognitive impairment, indicating that presence of apoε4, while an important risk factor for AD, does not mean that dementia is inevitable.[16] The ε4 allele frequency was 30% in subjects with AD, but only 8% in those without dementia.

Functional aspects of apoE in relation to tau protein may underlie the increased risk for AD observed among individuals who bear the apoε4 allele. Normally, apoε3 binds to tau protein and is believed to slow the initial rate of phosphorylation of tau protein and self-assembly to form paired helical filaments (PHFs) of neurofibrillary tangles (NFTs). NFTs are pathologic intracellular formations composed of PHFs made of hyperphosphorylated tau protein. Apoε4 does not bind to tau protein; however, it may allow for hyperphosphorylation of tau which is then unable to bind and stabilize microtubules.[17]

Other contenders for a role in the pathophysiology of AD include clusterin (apoJ), a multifunctional apolipoprotein which is associated with amyloid β-peptide (Aβ) in senile plaques of AD. Slowly sedimenting Aβ complexes (formed in the presence of clusterin) may contribute to the neurotoxicity of Aβ deposits.[18]

In search of a phenotypic marker of AD that could be paired with the results of apoE genotyping, it is of interest that cerebrospinal fluid (CSF) Aβ$_{42}$ levels have been reported to be significantly lower in AD patients as compared to controls.[19] Aβ$_{42}$ has been shown to preferentially deposit in the brains of AD patients. A study of Aβ$_{42}$ CSF levels, however, found no association of CSF Aβ$_{42}$ or tau protein with apoE genotype.[19] See Cerebrospinal Fluid and Plasma β-Amyloid$_{(1-42)}$ on page 513.

A current review of recent developments in markers for AD is available.[20]

Footnotes

1. Hill JS and Pritchard PH, "Improved Phenotyping of Apolipoprotein E: Application to Population Frequency Distribution," *Clin Chem*, 1990, 36(11):1871-4.
2. Kataoka S, Paidi M, and Howard BV, "Simplified Isoelectric Focusing/Immunoblotting Determination of Apoprotein E Phenotype," *Clin Chem*, 1994, 40(1):11-3.
3. Hackler R, Schafer JR, Motzny S, et al, "Rapid Determination of Apolipoprotein E Phenotypes From Whole Plasma by Automated Isoelectric Focusing Using Phast-System™ and Immunofixation," *J Lipid Res*, 1994, 35(1):153-8.
4. Hixson JE and Vermier DT, "Restriction Isotyping of Human Apolipoprotein E by Gene Amplification and Cleavage With HhaI," *J Lipid Res*, 1990, 31(3):545-8.
5. Bolla MK, Haddad L, Humphries SE, et al, "High-Throughput Methods for Determination of Apolipoprotein E Genotypes With Use of Restriction Digestion Analysis by Microplate Array Diagonal Gel Electrophoresis," *Clin Chem*, 1995, 41(11);1599-604.
6. Davignon J, Gregg RE, and Sing CF, "Apolipoprotein E Polymorphism and Atherosclerosis," *Arteriosclerosis*, 1988, 8(1):1-21.
7. Wilson PW, Myers RH, Larson MG, et al, "Apolipoprotein E Alleles, Dyslipidemia, and Coronary Heart Disease: The Framingham Offspring Study," *JAMA*, 1994, 272(21):1666-71.
8. McCombs RJ, Marcadis DE, Ellis J, et al, "Attenuated Hypercholesterolemic Response to a High-Cholesterol Diet in Subjects Heterozygous for the Apolipoprotein A-IV-2 Allele," *N Engl J Med*, 1994, 331(11):706-10.
9. Minnich A, Weisgraber KH, Newhouse Y, et al, "Identification and Characterization of a Novel Apolipoprotein E Variant, Apolipoprotein ε3' (Arg → His): Association With Mild Dyslipidemia and Double Pre-β Very Low Density Lipoproteins," *J Lipid Res*, 1995, 36(1):57-66.
10. Ueyama Y, Nozaki S, Yanagi K, et al, "Familial Hypercholesterolaemia-Like Syndrome With Apolipoprotein E-7 Associated With Marked Achilles Tendon Xanthomas and Coronary Artery Disease: A Report of Two Cases," *J Intern Med*, 1994, 235(2):169-74.
11. Luc G, Bard JM, Arveiler D, et al, "Impact of Apolipoprotein E Polymorphism on Lipoproteins and Risk of Myocardial Infarction. The ECTIM Study," *Arterioscler Thromb*, 1994, 14(9):1412-9.
12. Roses AD, "Apolipoprotein E Genotyping in the Differential Diagnosis, Not Prediction, of Alzheimer's Disease," *Ann Neurol*, 1995, 38(1):6-14.
13. Petersen RC, Smith GE, Ivnik RJ, et al, "Apolipoprotein E Status as a Predictor of the Development of Alzheimer's Disease in Memory-Impaired Individuals," *JAMA*, 1995, 273(16):1274-8.
14. Reiman EM, Caselli RJ, Yun LS, et al, "Preclinical Evidence of Alzheimer's Disease in Persons Homozygous for the ε4 Allele for Apolipoprotein E," *N Engl J Med*, 1996, 334(12):752-8.
15. Strittmatter WJ, Saunders AM, Schmechel D, et al, "Apolipoprotein E: High-Avidity Binding to β-Amyloid and Increased Frequency of Type 4 Allele in Late-Onset Familial Alzheimer Disease," *Proc Natl Acad Sci U S A*, 1993, 90(5):1977-81.
16. Hyman BT and Tanzi R, "Molecular Epidemiology of Alzheimer's Disease," *N Engl J Med*, 1995, 333(19):1283-4 (editorial).
17. Strittmatter WJ, Weisgraber KH, Goedert M, et al, "Hypothesis: Microtubule Instability and Paired Helical Filament Formation in the Alzheimer Disease Brain Are Related to Apolipoprotein E Genotype," *Exp Neurol*, 1994, 125(2):163-71.
18. Oda T, Wals P, Osterburg HH, et al, "Clusterin (ApoJ) Alters the Aggregation of Amyloid β-Peptide (Aβ$_{1-42}$) and Forms Slowly Sedimenting Aβ Complexes That Cause Oxidative Stress," *Exp Neurol*, 1995, 136(1):22-31.
19. Motter R, Vigo-Pelfrey C, Kholodenko D, et al, "Reduction of β-Amyloid Peptide$_{42}$ in the Cerebrospinal Fluid of Patients With Alzheimer's Disease," *Ann Neurol*, 1995, 38(4):643-8.
20. Mulder C, Scheltens P, Visser JJ, et al, "Genetic and Biochemical Markers for Alzheimer's Disease: Recent Developments," *Ann Clin Biochem*, 2000, 37(Pt 5):593-607.

References

Bird TD, "Apolipoprotein E Genotyping in the Diagnosis of Alzheimer's Disease: A Cautionary View," *Ann Neurol*, 1995, 38(1):2-4.
Dyer CA, Cistola DP, Parry GC, et al, "Structural Features of Synthetic Peptides of Apolipoprotein E That Bind the LDL Receptor," *J Lipid Res*, 1995, 36(1):80-8.
Ganguli M, Chandra V, Kamboh MI, et al, "Apolipoprotein E Polymorphism and Alzheimer Disease: The Indo-US Cross-National Dementia Study," *Arch Neurol*, 2000, 57(6):824-30.
Growdon JH, "Biomarkers of Alzheimer Disease," *Arch Neurol*, 1999, 56(3):281-3.
Haan MN, Shemanski L, Jagust WJ, et al, "The Role of ApoE ε4 in Modulating Effects of Other Risk Factors for Cognitive Decline in Elderly Persons," *JAMA*, 1999, 282(1):40-6.
Jordan BD, Relkin NR, Ravdin LD, et al, "Apolipoprotein E ε4 Associated With Chronic Traumatic Brain Injury in Boxing," *JAMA*, 1997, 278(2):136-40.
Kukull WA and Martin GM, "ApoE Polymorphisms and Late-Onset Alzheimer Disease: The Importance of Ethnicity," *JAMA*, 1998, 279(10):788-9.
Mayeux R, Saunders AM, Shea S, et al, "Utility of the Apolipoprotein E Genotype in the Diagnosis of Alzheimer's Disease," *N Engl J Med*, 1998, 338(8):506-11.
Mooser V, Helbecque N, Miklossy J, et al, "Interactions Between Apolipoprotein E and Apolipoprotein(a) in Patients With Late-Onset Alzheimer Disease," *Ann Intern Med*, 2000, 132(7):533-7.

(Continued)

Apolipoprotein E, Plasma *(Continued)*

O'Brien KD, Deeb SS, Ferguson M, et al, "Apolipoprotein E Localization in Human Coronary Atherosclerotic Plaques by *In Situ* Hybridization and Immunohistochemistry and Comparison With Lipoprotein Lipase," *Am J Pathol*, 1994, 144(3):538-48.

O'Donnell HC, Rosand J, Knudsen KA, et al, "Apolipoprotein E Genotype and the Risk of Recurrent Lobar Intracerebral Hemorrhage," *N Engl J Med*, 2000, 342(4):240-5.

Polvikoski T, Sulkava R, Haltia M, et al, "Apolipoprotein E, Dementia, and Cortical Deposition of β-Amyloid Protein," *N Engl J Med*, 1995, 333(19):1242-7.

Rogaeva E, Premkumar S, Song Y, et al, "Evidence for an Alzheimer Disease Susceptibility Locus on Chromosome 12 and for Further Locus Heterogeneity," *JAMA*, 1998, 280(7):614-8.

Sacco RL, "Lobar Intracerebral Hemorrhage," *N Engl J Med*, 2000, 342(4):276-9.

Siest G, Pillot T, Regis-Bailly A, et al, "Apolipoprotein E: An Important Gene and Protein to Follow in Laboratory Medicine," *Clin Chem*, 1995, 41(8 Pt 1):1068-86.

Tang MX, Stern Y, Marder K, et al, "The ApoE-ε4 Allele and the Risk of Alzheimer Disease Among African Americans, Whites, and Hispanics," *JAMA*, 1998, 279(10):751-5.

Wu LH, Wu JT, and Hopkins PN, "Apolipoprotein E: Laboratory Determinations and Clinical Significance," *Handbook of Lipoprotein Testing*, Rifai N, Warnick GR, and Dominiczak MH, eds, Washington, DC: AACC Press, American Association of Clinical Chemistry, 1997, 329-56.

Wu WS, Holmans P, Wavrant-DeVrieze F, et al, "Genetic Studies on Chromosome 12 in Late-Onset Alzheimer Disease," *JAMA*, 1998, 280(7):619-22.

Ascorbic Acid, Serum or Plasma

Related Information
Antioxidant Concentrations, Plasma *on page 108*
Oxalate, Urine *on page 238*
Urinalysis *on page 887*

Synonyms Ascorbate; Vitamin C

Abstract The functions of vitamin C, an essential micronutrient, include roles in collagen synthesis, carnitine biosynthesis, stimulation of neutrophil chemotaxis, lipid and protein metabolism, and in wound healing.[1] It also facilitates the absorption of iron. It is a reducing agent (an electron donor), an antioxidant. The principal disease associated with vitamin C deficiency is scurvy. Decreased plasma levels indicate nutritional deficiency. An individual on a diet totally deficient in vitamin C will develop scurvy in 60-90 days. If vitamin C ingestion is suddenly stopped, steady state concentrations of 55-60 µmol/L will probably serve to prevent deficiency for a month.

Patient Preparation Patient should be fasting.

Specimen Plasma or leukocytes; uncommonly, urine following a loading test

Container Green top (heparin) tube preferred; red top tube, lavender top (EDTA) tube, or gray top (sodium fluoride) tube also acceptable; check with the laboratory.

Collection Draw blood in chilled tube. Keep specimen on ice.

Storage Instructions Keep specimen refrigerated until frozen. Freeze separated plasma. Stable 30 minutes at 25°C. Stable 4 days at -20°C.

Causes for Rejection Specimen not frozen

Reference Interval Plasma: 0.6-2.0 mg/dL (SI: 34-114 µmol/L); leukocytes: 20-50 µg/10³ WBC. Lassitude (fatigue) appears at concentrations <20 µmol/L.

Critical Values <0.3 mg/dL (SI: <17 µmol/L) in plasma provides evidence for at least the risk of deficiency and <0.2 mg/dL (SI: <11 µmol/L) indicates deficiency. Clinical scurvy appears when total body stores diminish to <300 mg.[1]

Use Evaluate vitamin C deficiency. Principal clinical findings in scurvy include bleeding gums, petechiae, follicular hyperkeratosis, perifollicular hemorrhages beginning on the lower thighs, muscle aches, easy fatiguability, effusions, and emotional changes.

The metabolic product of hypervitaminosis C, oxalate, may lead to oxalate renal calculi. Safe vitamin C intake is reported to be 1 g/day.[2]

Contraindications Ascorbic acid therapy

Methodology High performance liquid chromatography (HPLC) with coulometric electrochemical detection,[2] acidic 2,4-dinitrophenylhydrazine

with photometry. HPLC is a preferred method; spectrophotometric methods tend to overestimate low concentrations.

Additional Information The recommended dietary allowance (RDA), proposed in 1999, is 120 mg/day. The tolerable upper intake is proposed to be <1 g/day.[2] Plasma or serum levels of vitamin C are an adequate measurement of clinical status, although leukocyte levels are superior but more difficult to obtain. Vitamin C is a cofactor for protocollagen hydroxylase; it promotes the conversion of tropocollagen to collagen. Low values occur in scurvy, patients with sepsis, those recovering from surgery, those with HIV infection, acute respiratory distress syndrome, and pancreatitis.[2] Smokers have lower levels than nonsmokers. The disease scurvy and its treatment, from Tierra del Fuego in 1519 to the present, represents a tapestry of naval and world history. The defeat of the French and Spanish at Trafalgar and the successful blockade of the French at Brest may have been supported by the interest in prevention and treatment of scurvy by the British Admiralty, limited as that interest may have been.[1] Vitamin C is a very important antioxidant and its possibly uncertain role in the prevention of atherogenesis is frequently cited.[3] A role in prevention of lead toxicity has also been proposed.[4] Vitamin C has a half-life of about 16 days.

Vitamin C promotes small intestinal iron absorption 1.5-10-fold.[2]

Boiling vegetables causes 50% to 80% loss of vitamin C. Consumption of at least 5 fruits and vegetables daily is recommended. A list of food sources recently published[2] fails to address limes. (When the British controlled the Caribbean, their seamen were provided with limes to prevent scurvy, leading to the expression "limey").

Vitamin C, not bound to plasma proteins, is dialyzable. Those on dialysis require replacements.

Intake ≥250 mg of vitamin C causes false-negative results on stool guaiac testing. Diets with ≥200 mg from fruits and vegetables are associated with lower carcinoma risk.[2]

Footnotes
1. Cuppage FE, *James Cook and the Conquest of Scurvy*, Westport, CT: Greenwood Press, 1994.
2. Levine M, Rumsey SC, Daruwala R, et al, "Criteria and Recommendation for Vitamin C Intake," *JAMA*, 1999, 281(15):1415-23.
3. Siow R, Sato H, Leake DS, et al, "Induction of Antioxidant Stress Proteins in Vascular Endothelial and Smooth Muscle Cells: Protective Action of Vitamin C Against Atherogenic Lipoproteins," *Free Radic Res*, 1999, 31:309-18.
4. Houston DK and Johnson MA, "Does Vitamin C Intake Protect Against Lead Toxicity?" *Nutr Rev*, 2000, 58(3 Pt 1):73-5.

References
Ausman LM, "Criteria and Recommendations of Vitamin C Intake," *Nutr Rev*, 1999, 57(7):222-4.
Dhariwal KR, Hartzell WO, and Levine M, "Ascorbic Acid and Dehydroascorbic Acid Measurements in Human Plasma and Serum," *Am J Clin Nutr*, 1991, 54(4):712-6.
Frei B, "On the Role of Vitamin C and Other Antioxidants in Atherogenesis and Vascular Dysfunction," *Proc Soc Exp Biol Med*, 1999, 222(3):196-204.
Margolis SA and Duewer DL, "Measurement of Ascorbic Acid in Human Plasma and Serum: Stability, Intralaboratory Repeatability, and Interlaboratory Reproducibility," *Clin Chem*, 1996, 42(8 Pt 1):1257-62.

Aspartate Aminotransferase, Serum

Related Information
Acetaminophen, Serum *on page 778*
Alanine Aminotransferase, Serum *on page 87*
Alkaline Phosphatase, Serum *on page 93*
Alpha₁-Antitrypsin Phenotyping *on page 95*
Antimitochondrial Antibody *on page 505*
Antinuclear Antibody *on page 507*
Bilirubin, Total, Serum *on page 118*
Ceruloplasmin, Serum *on page 143*
Copper, Serum *on page 816*
Copper, Urine *on page 818*
Ethanol, Blood, Urine, and Other Sources *on page 789*
Ferritin, Serum *on page 173*
Gamma-Glutamyl Transferase, Serum *on page 179*
Hepatitis B Core Antibody *on page 622*
Hepatitis B Surface Antigen *on page 625*
Hepatitis C Virus RNA Detection and Quantitation *on page 626*
Hepatitis E Serology *on page 628*
Hepatitis: Laboratory Assessment, Overview *on page 629*
Isoniazid, Serum or Plasma *on page 753*
Lactate Dehydrogenase, Serum *on page 207*
Liver Biopsy *on page 65*
Liver Disease: Laboratory Assessment, Overview *on page 216*

Synonyms AST; Glutamic Oxaloacetic Transaminase, Serum; GOT; SGOT; Transaminase

Applies to Acetaminophen Hepatotoxicity; Aminotransferases; AST:ALT Ratio; AST:LD Ratio; L-Aspartate-2-Oxoglutarate Aminotransferase

Replaces Cephalin Flocculation; Thymol Turbidity

Abstract AST and ALT, widely used enzymes, are increased in diseases of the liver and in many other disease entities. AST is also found in cardiac and skeletal muscle and in lesser amounts in kidneys, brain, lungs, pancreas, spleen, white cells, and erythrocytes. See Table 2 in Liver

Biopsy *on page 65* and the table in Liver Disease: Laboratory Assessment, Overview *on page 216*. The aminotransferases (transaminases) are extensively used by virtue of their ease of assay and extensive clinical experience with their levels. The sensitivity of AST is widely recognized.

Patient Preparation Strenuous exercise can cause increase.

Specimen Serum; plasma may be used.

Container Red top tube; green top (heparin) tube for plasma

Storage Instructions Stable 3 days at 25°C and 1 week at 4°C; fairly stable refrigerated or frozen.

Causes for Rejection Hemolysis in sample collected

Reference Interval Levels in infancy are two to three times those found in adults. Ranges decrease during childhood years.
- Newborns: 25-75 units/L (SI: 0.43-1.28 µkat/L)
- Infants: 15-60 units/L (SI: 0.26-1.02 µkat/L)
- Adult male: 20-40 units/L (SI: 0.34-0.68 µkat/L)
- Adult female: 15-30 units/L (SI: 0.25-0.51 µkat/L)

Use A wide range of disease entities alters AST (SGOT). When an increased AST is from the liver, it is likely to relate to disease of the **hepatocyte**. Other enzymes, including alkaline phosphatase and GGT, are more sensitive indicators of **biliary** obstruction.

Causes of low AST: uremia, vitamin B_6 deficiency.

Causes of high AST: chronic alcohol ingestion, not limited to overt chronic alcoholism; cirrhosis. In alcoholic hepatitis, AST values usually are <250 units/L. AST is distributed in both cytosol and mitochondria, while serum activity of ALT is predominantly related to cytosol. The damage from alcohol is predominantly to mitochondria; therefore, the increase of AST is greater than that of ALT. Pyridoxine deficiency is commonplace in alcoholism. ALT is more sensitive to pyridoxine deficiency than is AST; thus, the **AST:ALT ratio** is driven higher; it is >2.0.[1] AST is rarely >8 times the upper reference range in subjects with alcohol abuse. The AST:ALT ratio is generally less helpful in chronic diseases of the liver, but has a role in assessment of the patient with chronic hepatitis C, in whom AST:ALT ratio of one or more provides suggestion of cirrhosis. (Liver biopsy is the only definitive means of establishing the diagnosis of cirrhosis.)[2,3]

Most instances of toxic necrosis lead to ALT as high or higher than those of AST.[4]

In viral hepatitis, look for high **AST:LD ratio**, >3, and very high AST peaking at 500-3000 units/L in acute viral hepatitis (ie, in clinical acute viral hepatitis the transaminases may be increased 10 times or more above their upper limits of normal). See Hepatitis: Laboratory Assessment, Overview *on page 629*

AST increases are found in other types of liver disease, including earlier stages of hemochromatosis and chemical injury (eg, with drug overdose and with necrosis related to toxins such as carbon tetrachloride). Some instances of cholecystitis cause increased AST. A mean 1.8-fold increase in AST was found 24 hours following laparoscopic cholecystectomy in 73% of patients, in 82% a 2.2-fold increment in ALT.[5] AST increase, not greater than fivefold, is found early in choledocholithiasis. AST can increase 10-fold with cholangitis.

Transaminases increase abruptly and may exceed 10,000 IU/L in ischemia, as in subjects in congestive heart failure with hypotension.[1]

Transaminases can be increased with nonalcoholic steatohepatitis, which often accompanies obesity, diabetes mellitus, jejunoileal bypass, with amiodarone, total parenteral nutrition, and without recognized relationship. ALT is equal to or more than AST level in nonalcoholic steatohepatitis.

Elevated aminotransferase concentrations may be found in asymptomatic patients with Wilson disease, for which the initial screening test is serum ceruloplasmin.

AST and ALT are increased in Reye syndrome.[6,7] In infectious mononucleosis, LD is commonly considerably higher than AST. Trauma (including head trauma and surgery) and skeletal muscle diseases, including dystrophy, dermatomyositis, trichinosis, polymyositis, and gangrene cause AST increases. Both AST and ALT elevations are found with Duchenne muscular dystrophy. Look for high CK in myositis, with high LD_5 (or isomorphic pattern in some instances of polymyositis) on LD isoenzymes. CK and aldolase are at least as sensitive to diseases of skeletal muscle.

In myocardial infarction (MI) AST peaks about 24 hours after infarct and returns to normal 3-7 days later, but is no longer used in evaluation of acute MI. In acute MI without shock or heart failure, ALT is not apt to increase significantly. AST increases in congestive failure with centrilobular liver congestion, in which high LD_5 is found, and in pericarditis, myocarditis, pancreatitis, and other inflammatory states including Legionnaires' disease. In renal infarction LD is usually high, out of proportion to AST. Lung infarction and other disease entities leading to necrosis including large, necrotic tumors cause increased AST; LD is commonly also increased in such instances. Shock (LD also usually increased); hypothyroidism (LD and/or CK not infrequently increased in myxedema); hemolytic anemias (LD high with increased LD_1) and certain CNS diseases may increase AST. AST may be increased with nonbiliary sepsis.

Drugs: Some drugs may cause **decreases** in AST, including allopurinol, cyclosporine, progesterone, and others. A large number of commonly used drugs have been reported to **elevate** AST, some of them by particular chemistry methods, but many by pathophysiologic means. They include acetaminophen, aminosalicylic acid, amiodarone, amitriptyline, anabolic steroids, anticonvulsants, ascorbic acid, aspirin, carbamazepine, cephalosporins, chlorambucil, chloroform, chlorothiazide, chlorpromazine, conjugated estrogens, cyclosporine, diclofenac, erythromycin, fluconazole, gentamicin, haloperidol, halothane, hydralazine, ibuprofen, indomethacin, interferon alpha$_2$, isoniazid, isoproterenol, levodopa, lovastatin, mefenamic acid, meprobamate, methotrexate, methyldopa, methyltestosterone, metronidazole (certain methods), naproxen, niacin (large doses), nonsteroidal anti-inflammatory agents, nortriptyline, opiates, oral contraceptives, oxacillin, papaverine, penicillamine, penicillin, phenobarbital, phenothiazines, procainamide, progesterone, propylthiouracil, pyrazinamide, quinidine, rifampin, ritonavir, streptomycin, sulfonamides, tamoxifen, ticarcillin, tobramycin, tocainide, tolbutamide, valproic acid, verapamil, and other drugs.[8] See Alanine Aminotransferase, Serum *on page 87*.

Acetaminophen hepatotoxicity deserves special mention. In alcoholics, apparently moderate doses of acetaminophen have caused severe hepatotoxicity.[9] Doses of 2.6-16.5 g/24 hours are reported with total bilirubin 1.3-23.9 mg/dL (SI: 22-409 µmol/L), AST 1960-29,700 units/L, and ALT 12,000-12,550 units/L. The characteristic findings include mild to severe coagulopathy and AST greater than ALT by a considerable margin.[10]

Macroenzyme (macro-AST) causing unexplained increase of AST is found with normal levels of CK and ALT.[11] Macro-AST is complexed with an immunoglobulin, thus, not readily cleared.

See the following diagram.

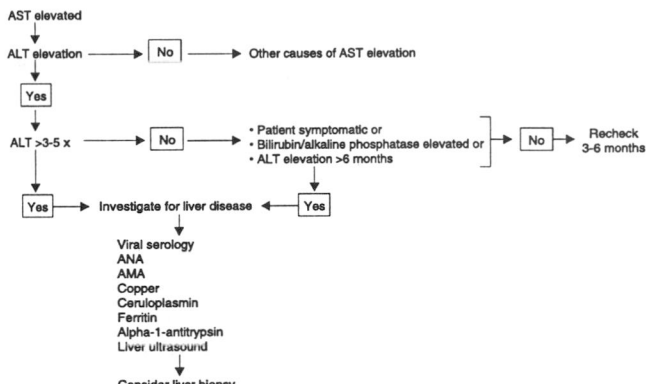

Approach to patient with elevated aspartate aminotransferase (AST).
ALT = alanine aminotransferase, AMA = antimitochondrial antibody, ANA = antinuclear antibody.
From Karnath PS, "Clinical Approach to the Patient With Abnormal Liver Test Results," *Mayo Clin Proc*, 1996, 71:1089-95.

Limitations Gross hemolysis causes falsely high values. Specific diagnoses require more specialized studies. Serum enzymes are relatively insensitive to uncomplicated hepatic steatosis. ALT is more specific for liver but both enzymes and others are useful when used together. Zimmerman is among those who recommend using several enzymes together for interpretation.[4] (See Liver Disease: Laboratory Assessment, Overview *on page 216*).

AST can be falsely low following dialysis.

Methodology Spectrophotometry, kinetic assay, malate dehydrogenase; like ALT, AST can be measured at 25°C, 30°C, 32°C, and 37°C.[12] The best assays used pyridoxal-5'-phosphate (a coenzyme) supplementation of the reaction mixture. Assay temperatures in the United States are almost always 37°C.

Additional Information AST has origin from liver, heart, skeletal muscle, kidney, brain, pancreas, spleen, lung, white cells, and erythrocytes. Very high values, >500 units/L, usually suggest hepatitis, ischemia, or other types of hepatocellular necrosis but can also be found with large necrotic tumors, congestive failure, and shock. Unexplained AST elevations should first be investigated with ALT and GGT. Mitochondrial AST (m-AST) may be useful in the diagnosis of alcoholic liver disease; it is reviewed by Rej.[12]

AST >3x the upper limit of reference range supports diagnosis of the **HELLP** syndrome.[13] (Refer to the Key Word Index.)

Laboratory findings supportive of the diagnosis of **acute liver failure** include high aminotransferase and low glucose concentrations and evidence of respiratory alkalosis.[14]

Footnotes

1. Karnath PS, "Clinical Approach to the Patient With Abnormal Liver Test Results," *Mayo Clin Proc*, 1996, 71(11):1089-95.
2. Reedy DW, Loo AT, and Levine RA, "AST/ALT Ratio ≥1 Is Not Diagnostic of Cirrhosis in Patients With Chronic Hepatitis C," *Dig Dis Sci*, 1998, 43(9):2156-9.
3. Giannini E, Botta F, Fasoli A, et al, "Progressive Liver Functional Impairment Is Associated With an AST/ALT Ratio," *Dig Dis Sci*, 1999, 44(6):1249-53.
4. Zimmerman HJ, *Hepatotoxicity: The Adverse Effects of Drugs and Other Chemicals on the Liver*, 2nd ed, Baltimore, MD: Lippincott Williams & Wilkins, 1999.
5. Halevy A, Gold-Deutch R, Negri M, et al, "Are Elevated Liver Enzymes and Bilirubin Levels Significant After Laparoscopic Cholecystectomy in the Absence of Bile Duct Injury?" *Ann Surg*, 1994, 219(4):362-4.

(Continued)

Aspartate Aminotransferase, Serum (Continued)

6. Lichtenstein PK, Heubi JE, Daugherty CC, et al, "Grade I Reye's Syndrome. A Frequent Cause of Vomiting and Liver Dysfunction After Varicella and Upper Respiratory Tract Infection," *N Engl J Med*, 1983, 309(3):133-9.
7. DeVivo DC, "How Common Is Reye's Syndrome?" *N Engl J Med*, 1983, 309(3):179-81.
8. Young DS, *Effects of Drugs on Clinical Laboratory Tests*, 5th ed, Volume 1: Listing by Test, Washington, DC: AACC Press, American Association of Clinical Chemistry, 2000, Section 3, 93-110.
9. Lee WM, "Drug-Induced Hepatotoxicity," *N Engl J Med*, 1995, 333(17):1118-27.
10. Seeff LB, Cuccherini BA, Zimmerman HJ, et al, "Acetaminophen Hepatotoxicity in Alcoholics. A Therapeutic Misadventure," *Ann Intern Med*, 1986, 104(3):399-404.
11. Litin SC, O'Brien JF, Pruett S, et al, "Macroenzyme as a Cause of Unexplained Elevation of Aspartate Aminotransferase," *Mayo Clin Proc*, 1987, 62(8):681-7.
12. Rej R, "Aminotransferase in Disease," *Clin Lab Med*, 1989, 9(4):667-87.
13. Stone JH, "HELLP Syndrome: Hemolysis, Elevated Liver Enzymes, and Low Platelets," *JAMA*, 1998, 280(6):559-62.
14. Lee WM, "Acute Liver Failure," *N Engl J Med*, 1993, 329(25):1862-72.

References

Beyeler C, Reichen J, Thomann SR, et al, "Quantitative Liver Function in Patients With Rheumatoid Arthritis Treated With Low-Dose Methotrexate: A Longitudinal Study," *Br J Rheumatol*, 1997, 36(3):338-44.

Pratt DS and Kaplan MM, "Evaluation of Abnormal Liver-Enzyme Results in Asymptomatic Patients," *N Engl J Med*, 2000, 342(17):1266-71.

Rosenthal P and Haight M, "Aminotransferase as a Prognostic Index in Infants With Liver Disease," *Clin Chem*, 1990, 36(2):346-8.

ter Borg F, ten Kate FJW, Cuypers HTM, et al, "Relation Between Laboratory Test Results and Histological Hepatitis Activity in Individuals Positive for Hepatitis B Surface Antigen and Antibodies to Hepatitis B$_e$ Antigen," *Lancet*, 1998, 351(9120):1914-8.

Whitehead MW, Hawkes ND, Hainsworth I, et al, "A Prospective Study of the Causes of Notably Raised Aspartate Aminotransferase of Liver Origin," *Gut*, 1999, 45(1):129-33.

Williams AL and Hoofnagle JH, "Ratio of Serum Aspartate to Alanine Aminotransferase in Chronic Hepatitis. Relationship to Cirrhosis," *Gastroenterology*, 1988, 95(3):734-9.

♦ **AST** *see* Aspartate Aminotransferase, Serum *on page 112*

♦ **AST:ALT Ratio** *see* Alanine Aminotransferase, Serum *on page 87*

♦ **AST:ALT Ratio** *see* Aspartate Aminotransferase, Serum *on page 112*

♦ **AST:ALT Ratio** *see* Cardiac Markers: Laboratory Assessment, Overview *on page 137*

♦ **AST:ALT Ratio** *see* Gamma-Glutamyl Transferase, Serum *on page 179*

♦ **AST:ALT Ratio** *see* Liver Disease: Laboratory Assessment, Overview *on page 216*

♦ **AST:LD Ratio** *see* Aspartate Aminotransferase, Serum *on page 112*

♦ **α_1-AT** *see* Alpha$_1$-Antitrypsin, Serum *on page 96*

♦ **α_1-AT Phenotype** *see* Alpha$_1$-Antitrypsin Phenotyping *on page 95*

♦ **AVP** *see* Antidiuretic Hormone, Plasma *on page 107*

♦ **B$_{12}$** *see* Cobalamin, Serum *on page 150*

♦ **Baby Bilirubin** *see* Bilirubin, Neonatal, Serum *on page 117*

♦ **Base Excess** *see* Anion Gap, Serum, Plasma, or Urine *on page 106*

♦ **Base Excess** *see* Blood Gases and pH, Arterial *on page 119*

Base Excess, Blood

Related Information

Anion Gap, Serum, Plasma, or Urine *on page 106*
Bicarbonate, Blood *on page 115*
Blood Gases and pH, Arterial *on page 119*
pH, Blood *on page 247*

Synonyms BE$_B$; Delta Base; *In Vitro* Base Excess

Applies to Acid-Base Regulation; Base Excess of Extracellular Fluid (BE$_{ecf}$); *In Vivo* Base Excess; Standard Base Excess

Test Includes Base excess of whole blood (BE$_B$) is calculated/derived from measured pH, pCO$_2$, and hemoglobin and calculated HCO$_3^-$. Base excess of extracellular fluid (BE$_{ecf}$) is calculated/derived from measured pH and pCO$_2$ and calculated HCO$_3^-$.

Abstract Base excess of whole blood (BE$_B$) is a calculated or graphically derived value defined as the amount of strong acid or base needed to restore the pH to 7.40 in a blood sample equilibrated at pCO$_2$ of 40 mm Hg and 37°C. BE$_B$ is an *in vitro* expression that represents deviation from normal buffer base and is affected primarily by metabolic acid-base imbalance.

Specimen Whole blood; see Blood Gases and pH, Arterial *on page 119* for collection details.

Reference Interval

Adults: -3 to +3 mmol/L
Newborns:[1] -10 to -2 mmol/L
Infants:[1] -7 to -1 mmol/L
Children:[1] -4 to +2

Critical Values -5 or +5 mmol/L

Use BE$_B$ is used to assess acid-base abnormalities and assists in estimation of the equivalents of sodium bicarbonate or ammonium chloride necessary to restore the patient's pH to normal. BE$_B$ < -3 mmol/L indicates a deficiency of base (or an excess of fixed acid). BE$_B$ >+3 mmol/L indicates an excess of base (or a deficit of fixed acid). Therapy usually is not given until ±5 mmol/L is reached.

Limitations The validity of BE$_B$ has been questioned because of its assumption that the carbon dioxide titration curve (ie, plot of pCO$_2$ versus HCO$_3^-$ or pH) of whole blood is the same *in vitro* as *in vivo*. This has led to the determination of the base excess of extracellular fluid (BE$_{ecf}$), also known as *in vivo* base excess or standard base excess (SBE). BE$_{ecf}$ is a quantity that reflects **only** the nonrespiratory component of pH disturbances. BE$_B$ should not be confused with BE$_{ecf}$. Though values for these do not differ much at pH and pCO$_2$ levels at or near 7.40 and 40 mm Hg, the values will not be the same when the deviations are more extreme. Schlichtig et al[2] suggest that the BE$_{ecf}$ and arterial pCO$_2$ be used as independent variables for evaluating, respectively, the metabolic and respiratory components of acid-base disturbances. However, an abnormal BE$_{ecf}$ (or an abnormal BE$_B$) does not necessarily mean that a metabolic acidosis/alkalosis is present. Compensatory mechanisms affect the results and interpretation.

Methodology BE$_B$ and BE$_{ecf}$ can be determined from Siggaard-Andersen curve nomograms or can be calculated from equations. Blood gas instruments with computer calculation capabilities can directly calculate these values from the measured pH, pCO$_2$, and hemoglobin levels and calculated HCO$_3^-$, as appropriate. See NCCLS Document C12-A for equations.[3]

Additional Information In acute respiratory alkalosis or acidosis, BE$_{ecf}$ is approximately zero (ie, normal). In chronic respiratory alkalosis or acidosis, in which renal compensatory mechanisms are in place, BE$_{ecf}$ is, respectively, negative or positive. Thus, BE$_{ecf}$ provides a means to differentiate acute respiratory acid-base disorders from chronic respiratory acid-base disorders in the absence of confounding mixed disturbances.[2,4]

Footnotes

1. Soldin SJ and Hicks JM, "Pediatric Reference Ranges," Washington, DC: AACC Press, American Association of Clinical Chemistry, 1995, 35.
2. Schlichtig R, Grogono AW, and Severinghaus JW, "Human PaCO$_2$ and Standard Base Excess Compensation for Acid-Base Imbalance," *Crit Care Med*, 1998, 26(7):1173-9.
3. National Committee for Clinical Laboratory Standards, *Definitions of Quantities and Conventions Related to Blood pH and Gas Analysis: Approved Standard C12-A*, Wayne, PA: NCCLS, 1994.
4. Mizock BA, "Utility of Standard Base Excess in Acid-Base Analysis," *Crit Care Med*, 1998, 26(7):1146-7.

References

Burbea ZH, Gullans SR, and Ben-Yaakov S, "Delta Alkalinity: A Simple Method to Measure Cellular Net Acid-Base Fluxes," *Am J Physiol*, 1987, 253(4 Pt 1):C525-34.

Degen BR and Moran RF, "Comparison and Assessment of Blood Gas Related Quantities Including Base Excess, the Gas Exchange Indices, and Temperature Corrected pH/pO$_2$/pCO$_2$, as Defined in Approved NCCLS Standard C12-A, Using a Computer Simulation of Input Variables," *Scand J Clin Lab Invest*, 1996, 56(Suppl 224):89-106.

♦ **Base Excess of Extracellular Fluid (BE$_{ecf}$)** *see* Base Excess, Blood *on page 114*

♦ **BE$_B$** *see* Base Excess, Blood *on page 114*

♦ **Bence Jones Protein** *replaced by* Protein Electrophoresis, Urine *on page 268*

♦ **Benzoyl Cholinesterase** *see* Pseudocholinesterase, Serum *on page 270*

♦ **Beta-Amino Isobutyrate** *see* Amino Acids, Urine *on page 101*

♦ **Beta-Cell Peptides** *see* C-Peptide, Serum *on page 156*

♦ **Beta-Gamma Bridging** *see* Protein Electrophoresis, Serum *on page 267*

Beta-Hexosaminidase, Serum, White Blood Cells

Synonyms Beta-N-Acetylglucosaminidase; Beta-N-Acetylhexosaminidase; Hexosaminidase; β-Hexosaminidase, Serum; N-Acetyl-β-Hexosaminidase A; NAG; β-NAG A

Test Includes May include isolation of isoenzyme hexosaminidase A, B, and S. Patients with Tay-Sachs disease lack hexosaminidase A, while B may be normal or elevated.

Abstract Tay-Sachs disease is a fatal autosomal recessive lysosomal sphingolipid storage disorder characterized by hypotonia, blindness, seizures, and dementia. The enzyme includes the isoenzymes, hexosaminidase A, hexosaminidase B, and hexosaminidase S. In Tay-Sachs disease, isoenzyme A is missing and B and S may be normal or increased. Deficiency of hexosaminidase A results in more than a 100-fold increase in G$_{M2}$ ganglioside in the neurons of affected children. In Sandhoff disease, even less common, A and B are absent.

Specimen Serum, white blood cells, cultured fibroblasts, amniotic fluid cells

Container Red top tube for serum, yellow top for white blood cells

Storage Instructions Store at -20°C.

Special Instructions Usually sent to reference laboratory.

Reference Interval Hexosaminidase A isoenzyme: noncarriers, 450-600 μmol/hour/mL; Tay-Sachs homozygotes: none present; heterozygotes: 200-

300 µmol/hour/mL. If isoenzyme A is <50% of total activity, carrier status is indicated.

Use Isoenzyme A is absent in serum of Tay-Sachs homozygotes. Isoenzyme A and B are absent in Sandhoff disease.

Limitations Total hexosaminidase levels are not useful for evaluation of Tay-Sachs disease. A mutant allele may prevent reliable measurement of enzyme activity when artificial substrates are employed. Serum assays are ambiguous on pregnant females.

Methodology DEAE chromatography followed by photometric or fluorometric assay of appropriate isoenzyme

Additional Information Hexosaminidase A can be measured in serum, cultured fibroblasts or leukocytes. Prenatal diagnosis of Tay-Sachs disease is done with amniocentesis or chorionic villus sampling. If females wish to be screened for carrier status of hexaminidase A deficiency by serum assays, they must be tested prior to pregnancy, as serum assays are ambiguous on pregnant females. More than 50 mutations have been reported in alpha subunit of hexaminidase A gene. DNA-based assays using PCR are available, but the enzyme assay is presently recommended as a general screen. Ultimately, molecular methods will replace the enzyme assay.

References

Kaback M, Lim-Steele J, Dabholkar D, et al, "Tay-Sachs Disease - Carrier Screening, Prenatal Diagnosis, and the Molecular Era. An International Perspective, 1970 to 1993," *JAMA*, 1993, 270(19):2307-15.

Mahuran DJ, "Biochemical Consequences of Mutations Causing the GM2 Gangliosidoses," *Biochim Biophys Acta*, 1999, 1455(2-3):105-38.

Peleg L and Goldman B, "Detection of Tay-Sachs Disease Carriers Among Individuals With Thermolabile Hexosaminidase B," *Eur J Clin Chem Clin Biochem*, 1994, 32(2):65-9.

Tanaka A, Fujimaru M, Choeh K, et al, "Novel Mutations, Including the Second Most Common in Japan, in the Beta-Hexosaminidase Alpha Subunit Gene, and a Simple Screening of Japanese Patients With Tay-Sachs Disease," *J Hum Genet*, 1999, 44(2):91-5.

Wappner RS, "Lysosomal Storage Disorders," *Oski's Pediatrics: Principles and Practice*, McMillan JA, DeAngelis CD, Feigin RD, et al, eds, Philadelphia, PA: JB Lippincott Co, 1999, 1863-83.

♦ **Beta-Hydroxybutyrate** *see* C-Peptide, Serum *on page 156*

♦ **Beta-Hydroxybutyrate** *see* Ketone Bodies, Blood *on page 205*

♦ **11-Beta-Hydroxylase** *see* 17-Hydroxyprogesterone, Serum or Plasma *on page 197*

♦ **Beta Lipoproteins** *see* Low Density Lipoprotein Cholesterol *on page 218*

♦ **Beta-N-Acetylglucosaminidase** *see* Beta-Hexosaminidase, Serum, White Blood Cells *on page 114*

♦ **Beta-N-Acetylhexosaminidase** *see* Beta-Hexosaminidase, Serum, White Blood Cells *on page 114*

♦ **Beta Subunit, hCG** *see* Chorionic Gonadotropin, Human, Serum and Urine *on page 147*

♦ **Beta Subunit Human Chorionic Gonadotropin, Urine or Serum** *see* Pregnancy Test, Serum or Urine *on page 260*

♦ **BEua** *see* Anion Gap, Serum, Plasma, or Urine *on page 106*

♦ **Beutler-Baluda Test** *see* Newborn Screening Tests for Galactosemia *on page 232*

♦ **Beutler Test** *see* Newborn Screening Tests for Galactosemia *on page 232*

♦ **BGP** *see* Osteocalcin, Serum or Plasma *on page 237*

♦ **BH₄ Cofactor Deficiencies** *see* Newborn Screen for Phenylketonuria *on page 229*

♦ **Bicarbonate** *see* Carbon Dioxide, Total, Blood *on page 135*

Bicarbonate, Blood

Related Information

Anion Gap, Serum, Plasma, or Urine *on page 106*
Base Excess, Blood *on page 114*
Blood Gases and pH, Arterial *on page 119*
Carbon Dioxide, Total, Blood *on page 135*
Chloride, Serum, Plasma, or Blood *on page 144*
Creatinine, Serum or Plasma *on page 161*
Electrolyte Panel, Serum *on page 168*
Ketone Bodies, Blood *on page 205*
Ketones, Urine *on page 877*
Osmolality, Calculated, Serum or Plasma *on page 234*
pCO₂, Blood *on page 246*
pH, Blood *on page 247*
Potassium, Serum or Plasma *on page 258*
Transfusion Reaction Work-up *on page 864*
Urea Nitrogen, Serum or Plasma *on page 293*

Synonyms Carbon Dioxide; CO₂; HCO₃⁻

Applies to Henderson-Hasselbalch Equation; TCO₂

Test Includes Test is part of blood gases panel and electrolytes panel

Abstract The two major extracellular anions are chloride and bicarbonate. Bicarbonate (HCO_3^-) makes up about 25 mmol/L of the anions found in normal plasma and is a major contributor to the bicarbonate/carbonic acid plasma-buffering system that maintains acid-base homeostasis. Its estimation is fundamental in evaluation of acid-base and electrolyte status.

Specimen Whole blood, plasma or serum

Container Heparinized blood gas syringe, green top (heparin) tube, red top tube

Reference Interval Newborns and infants: whole blood: 16-24 mmol/L; children and adults: serum or plasma: arterial: 21-28 mmol/L, venous: 22-29 mmol/L

Possible Panic Range <10 mmol/L, >40 mmol/L

Use With anion gap, HCO_3 is used as a preliminary screen for many abnormalities of acid-base balance, but additional studies are needed for some diseases (eg, acute respiratory disorders).

HCO_3^- is **increased** with metabolic alkalosis, respiratory acidosis, and compensated respiratory acidosis. Metabolic alkalosis is usually acute and often is accompanied by hypokalemia. It may be seen with dehydration, use of some diuretics, and with vomiting. Ingestion of baking soda and citrate intoxication from massive transfusions leads to increased urine anion gap. Increased cortisol or aldosterone may cause metabolic alkalosis from urinary losses of hydrogen and potassium ions.

HCO_3^- is **decreased** with metabolic acidosis (eg, low in ketoacidosis) and compensated respiratory alkalosis. Severe metabolic acidemia bears an implication of bicarbonate levels ≤8 mmol/L.[1]

The combination of decreased HCO_3^- with high chloride and normal anion gap, resulting from loss of bicarbonate, occurs with diarrhea and with renal tubular acidosis. Such disorders are called hyperchloremic or nonanion gap metabolic acidosis, but when gastrointestinal HCO_3^- losses are profuse, the anion gap can be raised. Subjects with renal tubular acidosis and hypobicarbonatemia can present with hypokalemia.[1]

Severe acidemia is treated with intravenous sodium bicarbonate, among other measures. To provide it judiciously, HCO_3^- must be followed with other studies.

Marked hypobicarbonatemia is seen in alcoholic ketoacidosis.

Limitations Excessive heparin dilution can falsely lower calculated arterial bicarbonate by as much as 10 mmol/L, and should be avoided by using only enough heparin sufficient to fill the dead space of the syringe.[2] Inadequate filling of red top evacuated collection tubes will decrease apparent serum bicarbonate concentrations.[3]

Methodology HCO_3^- is not necessarily directly measured. Instead, in whole blood specimens, pH and pCO_2 are measured using standard blood gas instrumentation, and the concentration of HCO_3^- ($cHCO_3^-$) is calculated using the Henderson-Hasselbalch equation:

$$pH = 6.103 + \log [HCO_3^- / (0.0306 \times pCO_2)].$$

Additionally, methods for measuring total carbon dioxide (TCO_2) in serum or plasma are widely used to estimate HCO_3^-. See Carbon Dioxide, Total, Blood *on page 135*.

Ion-selective electrode (ISE) and enzymatic methods are in current use.

Additional Information Under normal conditions, HCO_3^- constitutes ~95% of TCO_2. In the vast majority of clinical settings, the calculated HCO_3^- value is comparable to the measured TCO_2 for diagnostic and therapeutic considerations.[4] If only TCO_2 is measured (without pH) it is often used interchangeably with HCO_3^-. Error using this estimate is usually ≤2 mmol/L.

Most pediatric diabetic patients whose initial pH was ≥7.20 or whose HCO_3^- concentration was ≥10 mmol/L had resolution of acidosis without hospitalization, while most patients whose pH was <7.20 and HCO_3^- <10 mmol/L require hospitalization.[5] Rapid correction of metabolic acidosis in chronic renal failure patients may attenuate circulating PTH activity.[6]

Other laboratory tests used in the evaluation of diabetic ketoacidosis include the other electrolytes, plasma glucose, blood and urine ketone bodies, hematocrit, BUN, pH and osmolality.

In early infancy, higher bicarbonate and lower serum chloride provide help to distinguish infants with pyloric stenosis from those with gastroesophageal reflux. Bicarbonate concentrations ≥29 mmol/L identified infants with pyloric stenosis with sensitivity of 36%, specificity of 99%, and positive predictive value of 99%. Chloride levels ≤98 mmol/L were found in infants with pyloric stenosis with sensitivity of 50%, specificity of 99%, and positive predictive value of 97%.[7]

Footnotes

1. Adrogué HJ and Madias NE, "Management of Life-Threatening Acid-Base Disorders," First of Two Parts, *N Engl J Med*, 1998, 338(1):26-34.
2. Bloom SA, Canzanello VJ, Strom JA, et al, "Spurious Assessment of Acid-Base Status Due to Dilutional Effect of Heparin," *Am J Med*, 1985, 79(4):528-30.
3. Herr RD and Swanson T, "Serum Bicarbonate Declines With Sample Size in Vacutainer® Tubes," *Am J Clin Pathol*, 1992, 97(2):213-6.
4. Rivkees SA and Fine BP, "The Reliability of Calculated Bicarbonate in Clinical Practice," *Clin Pediatr (Phila)*, 1988, 27(5):240-2.
5. Bonadio WA, Gutzeit MF, Losek JD, et al, "Outpatient Management of Diabetic Ketoacidosis," *Am J Dis Child*, 1988, 142(4):448-50.
6. Lu KC, Shieh SD, Li BL, et al, "Rapid Correction of Metabolic Acidosis in Chronic Renal Failure: Effect on Parathyroid Hormone Activity," *Nephron*, 1994, 67(4):419-24.

(Continued)

Bicarbonate, Blood *(Continued)*

7. Smith GA, Mihalov L, and Shields BJ, "Diagnostic Aids in the Differentiation of Pyloric Stenosis From Severe Gastrointestinal Reflux During Early Infancy," *Am J Emerg Med*, 1999, 17(1):28-31.

References

Brandenburg MA and Dire DJ, "Comparison of Arterial and Venous Blood Gas Values in the Initial Emergency Department Evaluation of Patients With Diabetic Ketoacidosis," *Ann Emerg Med*, 1998, 31(4):459-65.

DuFour DR, "Laboratory Recognition and Testing in Acid-Base Disorders," *Lab Med*, 1999, 30(12):776-81.

Heusel JW, Siggaard-Andersen O, and Scott MG, "Physiology and Disorders of Water, Electrolyte, and Acid-Base Metabolism," *Tietz Textbook of Clinical Chemistry*, 3rd ed, Chapter 32, Burtis CA and Ashwood ER, eds, Philadelphia, PA: WB Saunders Co, 1999, 1095-124.

Hood VL and Tannen RL, "Protection of Acid-Base Balance by pH Regulation of Acid Production," *N Engl J Med*, 1998, 339(12):319-26.

O'Leary TD and Langton SR, "Calculated Bicarbonate or Total Carbon Dioxide?" *Clin Chem*, 1989, 35(8):1697-700.

Preuss HG, "Fundamentals of Clinical Acid-Base Evaluation," *Clin Lab Med*, 1993, 13(1):103-16.

♦ **Biliprotein** *see* Bilirubin, Direct, Serum *on page 117*

Bilirubin, Amniotic Fluid, Delta A450

Related Information

Amniotic Fluid, Chromosome and Genetic Abnormality Analysis *on page 360*

Bilirubin, Neonatal, Serum *on page 117*

Cord Blood Screen *on page 838*

Hemolytic Disease of the Newborn, Antibody Identification *on page 846*

Newborn Crossmatch and Transfusion *on page 848*

Prenatal Screen, Immunohematology *on page 855*

Rh Genotype *on page 860*

Synonyms Amniotic Fluid Analysis for Hemolytic Disease of the Newborn; Amniotic Fluid Bilirubin; Amniotic Fluid Spectral Analysis; Liley Test; OD 450 Method

Replaces Amniotic Fluid Analysis for Erythroblastosis Fetalis

Abstract The fetus affected by isoimmunization-induced hemolytic disease of the newborn (HDN) (erythroblastosis fetalis) has increased serum and amniotic fluid bilirubin.[1] The amniotic fluid bilirubin level is directly proportional to the degree of fetal anemia in HDN. The test is performed to monitor the pregnancies of women with atypical antibodies (see Hemolytic Disease of the Newborn, Antibody Identification *on page 846*). Measurement of the 450 nm peak (delta A450) by scanning spectrophotometry estimates the bilirubin level in amniotic fluid, which is directly related to the severity of disease. Each patient's delta A450 numerical result is compared to normative data which were originally developed by Liley[2,3] and later extended by Queenan et al[4] (see the following graphic). A graphic format is usual, and includes four zones, with zone 1 implying an unaffected fetus and zone 4 implying a high risk for intrauterine death from HDN.

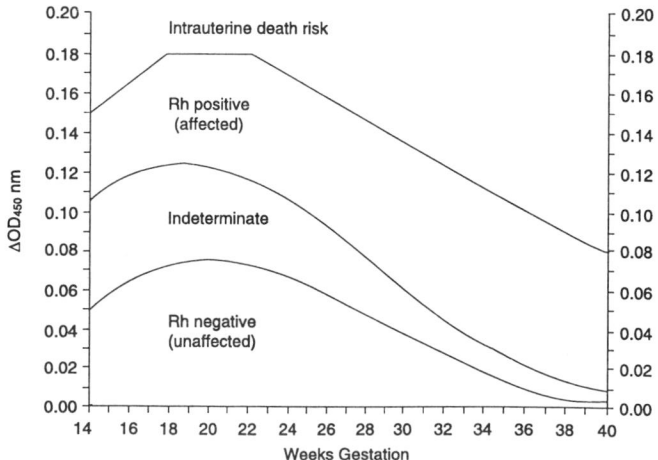

Amniotic fluid ΔOD$_{450}$ management zones

Aftercare All nonsensitized Rh-negative patients should receive anti-D immunoglobulin within 72 hours after amniocentesis.

Specimen Amniotic fluid

Collection Ultrasound-guided amniocentesis is performed by the physician, usually at 27 weeks or more gestation. Protect the specimen from light for transport to the laboratory. In the case of multiple pregnancy, each amniotic sac should be sampled and analyzed individually.

Storage Instructions Centrifuge the specimen promptly and filter the supernatant in the dark. Store the supernatant protected from light at 4 °C until analysis.

Reference Interval See Use.

Use The reference range cutoffs for zone 1, implying an unaffected fetus, vary with gestational age (see graphic). These cutoffs apply most specifically to pregnancies complicated by Rh(D) isoimmunization, and to the first such affected pregnancy. In practice, however, the same cutoffs are applied to HDN caused by other red cell antigens.

Limitations Amniocentesis is an invasive procedure and poses potential hazards to the fetus, including enhanced maternal sensitization, amnionitis, or premature rupture of membranes.[5]

Amniotic fluid contaminated with meconium and/or maternal blood can give erroneous results.[3] Maternal urine can be aspirated inadvertently instead of amniotic fluid,[3] but can be conveniently identified with urea nitrogen and creatinine measurements.

After anti-D, anti-Kell (K) antibody is the second most common antibody in HDN; it causes 10% of cases of severe HDN. Affected fetuses have more severe anemia and less severe hyperbilirubinemia than fetuses with antibodies to D; *vide infra*.[6]

Methodology Spectral analysis of centrifuged amniotic fluid is done using a scanning spectrophotometer. The peak at 450 nm corresponds to bilirubin.

Additional Information Monitoring serum antibody titers of anti-D antibodies has been reported to be superior to delta A450 determinations for predicting fetal anemia; however, the titers must be less ≤32 or ≥1000 to be useful, leaving a large gray area.[7] Consultation with clinical experts is recommended for alloantibody titrations other than anti-D.

In the past, most cases of HDN were caused by anti-D. With the widespread utilization of Rh immune globulin, the incidence of anti-D HDN has decreased. This has lead to a **relative** increase in the incidence of other antibodies, particularly other Rh antibodies and anti-Kell, as causes of HDN. Since both anti-D positive and anti-D negative patients can have these atypical antibodies, all pregnant women who have previously given birth or received blood fractions should have a prenatal antibody screen followed by appropriate titers. In cases of **Kell isoimmunizations**, delta A450 testing is probably not helpful since fetal anemia is due to erythroid suppression rather than hemolysis.[8,9] This fact, in addition to the low predictive value of anti-Kell titers in these instances, mandates aggressive surveillance of the Kell positive fetus and, if necessary, fetal umbilical blood determinations to assess disease severity.[10]

High amniotic fluid delta-OD450 is usually followed by fetal blood sampling; the management of pregnancies complicated by red cell autoimmunization is directed at evaluation of fetal anemia, then intervention if indicated. Noninvasive fetal RhD genotyping is possible in maternal plasma, beginning in the second trimester.[11] Prenatal diagnosis of fetal antigen status by molecular methods for fetal DNA in the maternal circulation bears a potential to decrease requirements for invasive testing.[12]

Footnotes

1. Weiner CP, "Human Fetal Bilirubin Levels and Fetal Hemolytic Disease," *Am J Obstet Gynecol*, 1992, 166(5):1449-54.

2. Liley AW, "Liquor Amnii Analysis in the Management of the Pregnancy Complicated by Rhesus Sensitization," *Am J Obstet Gynecol*, 1961, 82(6):1359-70.

3. Liley AW, "Errors in the Assessment of Hemolytic Disease From Amniotic Fluid," *Am J Obstet Gynecol*, 1963, 86:485-94.

4. Queenan JT, Tomai TP, Ural SH, et al, "Deviation in Amniotic Fluid Optical Density at a Wavelength of 450 nm in Rh-Immunized Pregnancies From 14 to 40 Weeks Gestation: A Proposal for Clinical Management," *Am J Obstet Gynecol*, 1993, 168(5):1370-6.

5. Weiner CP, "Fetal Hemolytic Disease," *High Risk Pregnancy Management Options*, 2nd ed, Chapter 22, James DK, Steer PJ, Weiner CP, et al, eds, London: WB Saunders Co, 1999, 343-61.

6. Luban NLC, "Hemolytic Disease of the Newborn: Progenitor Cells and Late Effects," *N Engl J Med*, 1998, 338(12):830-1.

7. Gottvall T and Hilden JO, "Concentration of Anti-D Antibodies in Rh(D) Alloimmunized Pregnant Women, as a Predictor of Anemia and/or Hyperbilirubinemia in Their Newborn Infants," *Acta Obstet Gynecol Scand*, 1997, 76(8):733-8.

8. Vaughan JI, Warwick R, Letsky E, et al, "Erythropoietic Suppression in Fetal Anemia Because of Kell Alloimmunization," *Am J Obstet Gynecol*, 1994, 171(1):247-52.

9. Vaughan JI, Manning M, Warwick RM, et al, "Inhibition of Erythroid Progenitor Cells by Anti-Kell Antibodies in Fetal Alloimmune Anemia," *N Engl J Med*, 1998, 338(12):798-803.

10. Scott JR and Branch DW, "Immunologic Disorders in Pregnancy," *Danforth's Obstetrics and Gynecology*, Chapter 24, Scott JR, Di Saia PJ, Hammond CB, et al, eds, Philadelphia, PA: Lippincott Williams & Wilkins, 1999, 369-77.

11. Lo YMD, Hjelm NM, Fidler C, et al, "Prenatal Diagnosis of Fetal RhD Status by Molecular Analysis of Maternal Plasma," *N Engl J Med*, 1998, 339(24):1734-8.

12. Saade GR, "Noninvasive Testing for Fetal Anemia," *N Engl J Med*, 2000, 342(1):52-3.

References

Ananth U and Queenan JT, "Does Midtrimester ΔOD$_{450}$ of Amniotic Fluid Reflect Severity of Rh Disease?" *Am J Obstet Gynecol*, 1989, 161(1):47-9.

Ananth U, Warsof SL, Coulehan JM, et al, "Midtrimester Amniotic Fluid Delta Optical Density at 450 nm in Normal Pregnancies," *Am J Obstet Gynecol*, 1986, 155(3):664-6.

Ashwood ER, "Clinical Chemistry of Pregnancy," *Tietz Textbook of Clinical Chemistry*, 3rd ed, Chapter 48, Burtis CA and Ashwood ER, eds, Philadelphia, PA: WB Saunders Co, 1999, 1736-75.

Bowman JM, "Hemolytic Disease (Erythroblastosis Fetalis)," *Maternal-Fetal Medicine*, 4th ed, Chapter 43, Creasy RK and Resnik R, eds, Philadelphia, PA: WB Saunders Co, 1999, 736-67.

Hadi HA, Fadel HE, Nelson GH, et al, "The Unreliability of Amniotic Fluid Bilirubin Measurements in Isoimmunized Pregnancies in Sickle Cell Disease Patients," *Obstet Gynecol*, 1985, 65(5):758-60.

Horger EO 3d and Moody LO, "Use of Indigo Carmine for Twin Amniocentesis and Its Effect on Bilirubin Analysis," *Am J Obstet Gynecol*, 1984, 150(7):858-60.

Lindsay MK and Lupo VR, "Nonpredictive Value of Measurements of Delta Optical Density at 450 nm in SS Disease," *Am J Obstet Gynecol*, 1985, 153(1):75-6.

Nicolaides KH, Rodeck CH, Mibashan RS, et al, "Have Liley Charts Outlived Their Usefulness?" *Am J Obstet Gynecol*, 1986, 155(1):90-4.

Spinnato JA, Clark AL, Ralston KK, et al, "Hemolytic Disease of the Fetus: A Comparison of the Queenan and Extended Liley Methods," *Obstet Gynecol*, 1998, 92(3):441-5.

Weiner CP and Widness JA, "Decreased Fetal Erythropoiesis and Hemolysis in Kell Hemolytic Anemia," *Am J Obstet Gynecol*, 1996, 174(2):547-51.

Weiner CP, Williamson RA, Wenstrom KD, et al, "Management of Fetal Hemolytic Disease by Cordocentesis. I. Prediction of Fetal Anemia," *Am J Obstet Gynecol*, 1991, 165(3):546-53.

♦ **Bilirubin, Conjugated** *see Bilirubin, Direct, Serum on page 117*

Bilirubin, Direct, Serum

Related Information

Bilirubin, Neonatal, Serum *on page 117*
Bilirubin, Total, Serum *on page 118*
Bilirubin, Urine *on page 870*
Hepatitis B Core Antibody *on page 622*
Hepatitis C Virus RNA Detection and Quantitation *on page 626*
Hepatitis: Laboratory Assessment, Overview *on page 629*
Liver Disease: Laboratory Assessment, Overview *on page 216*
Urobilinogen, 2-Hour Urine *on page 889*

Synonyms Bilirubin, Conjugated; Direct Bilirubin

Applies to Biliprotein; Conjugated Hyperbilirubinemia; Delta Bilirubin

Abstract The mono- and diconjugated bilirubin and some of the delta bilirubin (covalently bound to albumin) account for the "direct" value. If more than half of total bilirubin is direct-reacting, jaundice is expressed as **"conjugated hyperbilirubinemia,"** which indicates hepatocellular dysfunction or cholestasis.[1]

Specimen Serum

Container Red top tube, red top Microtainer™ for babies

Collection Pediatrics: Blood drawn from a heelstick. If blood is drawn by capillary puncture, avoid excessive squeezing or milking (to avoid hemolysis).

Storage Instructions Store in refrigerator. **Protect from light.**

Causes for Rejection Specimen not protected from light, gross hemolysis

Special Instructions Transport promptly.

Reference Interval Newborns: varies with age in days, prematurity vs maturity (see table in listing Bilirubin, Neonatal, Serum *on page 117*); adults: ≤0.4 mg/dL (SI: ≤7 µmol/L)

Use Increased direct bilirubin occurs with hepatobiliary diseases, including both intrahepatic and extrahepatic lesions. Hepatocellular causes of elevation include hepatitis, cirrhosis, and advanced neoplastic states. Increased with cholestatic drug reactions, Dubin-Johnson syndrome, and Rotor syndrome. In the latter two syndromes, the level is usually <5 mg/dL.

Infections (eg, bacterial sepsis, hepatitis B, syphilis, toxoplasmosis, rubella, CMV, herpes), drug-induced cholestasis, and parenteral nutrition-associated cholestasis are among acquired causes of increased direct bilirubin.

Genetic and metabolic disorders which may increase direct bilirubin include galactosemia, tyrosinemia, Niemann-Pick disease, and trisomy 18.

Limitations Cord blood samples may yield elevated values. Visibly hemolyzed samples may yield spurious results by some methods. **Drugs** which may cause increases include acetaminophen, aminosalicylic acid, anabolic steroids (cholestatic syndrome), chlorpromazine, interleukin-2, mephenytoin, nalidixic acid, methyldopa, oral contraceptives, phenothiazine, propylthiouracil, sulfasalazine, and other agents.[2]

Contraindications Measurement of direct bilirubin is usually not necessary when the total bilirubin is <1.2 mg/dL (SI: <21 µmol/L).

Methodology Diazo reaction with spectrophotometry, high performance liquid chromatography (HPLC), bilirubin oxidase

Additional Information Theoretically, direct bilirubin should not be increased in hemolytic anemias, in which bilirubin increase should be in the indirect bilirubin fraction in the absence of complications. In practice, some increase in the direct fraction may be encountered in patients with hemolytic anemia in whom complications have not been proven. Some methods have shown the direct bilirubin to be spuriously high. This may be due to different concentrations of sodium nitrite, which may convert some of the unconjugated bilirubin to conjugated bilirubin.[3,4] Direct bilirubin is the water soluble (conjugated) fraction. When conjugated bilirubin is increased in serum, bilirubin should become positive in urine. Physiologic jaundice, occurring 2-4 days after birth, is due to lack of liver glucuronyl transferase. Physiological jaundice does not produce conjugated (direct) bilirubin levels >1.5-2.0 mg/dL.

When bilirubin is rising in early liver disease, very little delta bilirubin (biliprotein) is present. In resolving liver disease, conjugated fractions may return to normal quickly whereas delta bilirubin may stay elevated for a long time due to long half-life (20 days) of albumin.[5]

Footnotes

1. Kamath PS, "Clinical Approach to the Patient With Abnormal Liver Test Results," *Mayo Clin Proc*, 1996, 71:1089-95.
2. Young DS, *Effects of Drugs on Clinical Laboratory Tests*, 5th ed, Volume 1: Listing by Test, Washington, DC: AACC Press, American Association of Clinical Chemistry, 2000, Section 3, 139-40.
3. Chan KM, Scott MG, Wu TW, et al, "Inaccurate Values for Direct Bilirubin With Some Commonly Used Direct Bilirubin Procedures," *Clin Chem*, 1985, 31(9):1560-3.
4. Mair B and Klempner LB, "Abnormally High Values for Direct Bilirubin in the Serum of Newborns as Measured With the Du Pont aca®," *Am J Clin Pathol*, 1987, 87(5):642-4.
5. Gordon ER, Seligson D, and Flye MW, "Serum Bilirubin Pigments Covalently Linked to Albumin," *Arch Pathol Lab Med*, 1996, 120:648-53.

References

Franquemont DW, Sutphen JL, Herold DA, et al, "Characterization of Sulfasalazine's Interference in the Measurement of Conjugated Bilirubin by the Ektachem® Slide Method," *Clin Chem*, 1989, 35(8):1760-2.

Iyanagi T, Emi Y, and Ikushiro S, "Biochemical and Molecular Aspects of Genetic Disorders of Bilirubin Metabolism," *Biochim Biophys Acta*, 1998, 1407(3):173-84.

Kurosaka K, Senba S, Tsubota H, et al, "A New Enzymatic Assay for Selectively Measuring Conjugated Bilirubin Concentration in Serum With Use of Bilirubin Oxidase," *Clin Chim Acta*, 1998, 269(2):125-36.

Newman TB, Hope S, and Stevenson DK, "Direct Bilirubin Measurements in Jaundiced Term Newborns. A Re-Evaluation," *Am J Dis Child*, 1991, 145(11):1305-9.

Rosenthal P, Keefe MT, Henton D, et al, "Total and Direct-Reacting Bilirubin Values by Automated Methods Compared With Liquid Chromatography and With Manual Methods for Determining Delta Bilirubin," *Clin Chem*, 1990, 36(5):788-91.

Shiomi S, Habu D, Kuroki T, et al, "Clinical Usefulness of Conjugated Bilirubin Levels in Patients With Acute Liver Diseases," *J Gastroenterol*, 1999, 34(1):88-93.

Bilirubin, Neonatal, Serum

Related Information

Bilirubin, Amniotic Fluid, Delta A450 *on page 116*
Bilirubin, Direct, Serum *on page 117*
Bilirubin, Total, Serum *on page 118*
Cord Blood Screen *on page 838*
Hemolytic Disease of the Newborn, Antibody Identification *on page 846*
Newborn Crossmatch and Transfusion *on page 848*

Synonyms Baby Bilirubin; Microbilirubin; Total Bilirubin, Neonatal

Applies to Transcutaneous Bilirubinometry

Abstract Neonatal bilirubin is used to monitor entities causing jaundice in the newborn (icterus neonatorum), most importantly, hemolytic disease of the newborn (HDN) (erythroblastosis fetalis) and hydrops fetalis as well as exaggerated physiologic accumulation of bilirubin. Physiologic jaundice is characterized by unconjugated hyperbilirubinemia which peaks by the third or fourth day in full-term neonates, then declines. In premature infants, bilirubin peaks on the fifth to seventh day. Pathologic jaundice usually is found within the first 24 hours;[1] bilirubin rises rapidly, often >5 mg/dL/day.[2]

Patient Preparation Clinical assessment of neonatal jaundice must be done in a well-lighted room.[1]

Specimen Serum

Container Microbilirubin tube

Collection Draw blood from heel using capillary pipette. Avoid excessive squeezing (to avoid specimen hemolysis).

Storage Instructions Protect sample from light; bilirubin is photosensitive.

Reference Interval Normal range depends on whether baby is premature or term, and age in days. See table.

Bilirubin, Neonatal Upper Reference Limit (mg/dL)

Age	Premature	Full-Term
Cord	2.9	2.5
<24 h	8.0	6.0
<48 h	12.0	10.0
3-5 d	15.0	12.0
7 d	15.0	10.0

Note: At 7 days, occasional premature infants may develop kernicterus at 10.0-12.0 mg/dL of bilirubin.

Critical Values Jaundice in the first 24 hours of life is indication for a neonatal bilirubin determination; it is generally considered pathologic, and further evaluation may be indicated.[1]

Possible Panic Range >15.0 mg/dL (SI: >257 µmol/L) in term infants, 10.0-15.0 mg/dL (SI: 171-257 µmol/L) in premature babies. Premature infants are at greater risk for bilirubin toxicity.[2] In HDN, published indications for exchange transfusion include:

- hematocrit <45%, positive direct antiglobulin test with bilirubin >4 mg/dL in cord blood
- Postnatal rise of bilirubin >1 mg/dL/hour for more than 6 hours
- Progressive anemia with rate of increase of bilirubin >0.5 mg/dL/hour
- Continuing progression of anemia
- Using bilirubin only, bilirubin >15 mg/dL for more than 48 hours
- Other criteria[3]

Use Most often used in cases of neonatal hyperbilirubinemia. Neonatal serum bilirubin is measured to monitor hemolytic disease of the newborn
(Continued)

Bilirubin, Neonatal, Serum *(Continued)*

(HDN) (erythroblastosis fetalis). HDN usually causes jaundice in the first 1-2 days of life. Blood group incompatibility, including Rh and ABO incompatibility, is a major cause of HDN and hydrops fetalis. Other etiologies of neonatal jaundice include physiologic jaundice, hematoma/hemorrhage, hypothyroidism, increased bilirubin load because of increased RBC volume or decreased RBC survival, glucose-6-phosphate deficiency, pyruvate kinase deficiency, hexokinase deficiency, sepsis, galactosemia, deficiency of glucuronyl transferase (Crigler-Najjar syndrome), Gilbert syndrome, spherocytosis, elliptocytosis, congenital erythropoietic porphyria, and cholestasis (eg, biliary atresia). Other risk factors include streptomycin, chloramphenicol, benzyl alcohol, and sulfisoxazole.[4] Dark urine or light stools are among indications for measurement of serum bilirubin.

Limitations If direct spectrophotometric method is used, only total bilirubin is measured with "neonatal bilirubin." Procedure is not utilized for patients older than 10 days of age due to formation of endogenous carotenoids. Ten percent fat emulsion has been reported to interfere with neonatal bilirubin measurement.[5]

Contraindications Spectrometric assay for bilirubin should not be used for infants older than 10 days of age, for whom usual total bilirubin is indicated.

Methodology Spectrophotometric, direct (bichromatic), bilirubin oxidase, diazo-dye binding, transcutaneous bilirubin by reflectance.

Bilirubin measurement by transcutaneous bilirubinometry has become available in recent years. Although it cannot substitute for laboratory measurement of bilirubin, it is an adjunctive screening tool which enhances patient care by reducing frequent blood draws.[6]

Additional Information In 1932, Diamond showed that hydrops fetalis and kernicterus were aspects of the same disease, in which fetal and neonatal hemolysis takes place. Kernicterus is caused by deposition of unconjugated bilirubin in the brain and leads to devastating injury.[4] HDN occurs from maternal alloimmunization to RhD, other Rh antibodies including hr'(c), ABO incompatibility (A), and antibodies involving additional blood groups including Kell (K1).

Causes of neonatal jaundice also include galactosemia, sepsis, hepatitis, syphilis, toxoplasmosis, cytomegalovirus, and rubella. Red cell enzyme problems include G6PD and pyruvate kinase deficiencies. Spherocytosis and elliptocytosis can lead to neonatal icterus.[5,7] Additional laboratory studies which may be indicated include CBC, differential smear, reticulocyte count, and hemoglobin electrophoresis. Less common causes of neonatal jaundice include Crigler-Najjar syndrome, α-thalassemia, extrahepatic obstruction, intrahepatic biliary atresia, extravascular blood, and a number of metabolic diseases including hypothyroidism and other entities.[2]

If bilirubin concentration is >15-17 mg/dL in a term infant at 25-48 hours, phototherapy may be indicated, an individual clinical judgment related to age and bilirubin level. The American Academy of Pediatrics has published a practice parameter which includes management tables, treatment options, and algorithms.[1]

Breast-feeding increases the incidence of neonatal jaundice and bears weak association with kernicterus.[8]

Drugs may displace bilirubin from albumin. It is the so-called "free" form of bilirubin, thus, displaced, which crosses the blood-brain barrier and causes neurotoxicity.[9]

Premature babies and those with HDN are often treated at lower levels of bilirubin. More aggressive therapy is advocated in instances of acidosis, asphyxia, and hypothermia. Useful tables of guidelines for initiation of exchange transfusion consider age, birth weight, and bilirubin concentrations in low-risk and high-risk infants (the latter includes premature infants and those with HDN).[1,2] Albumin concentration and drugs are important variables. Useful overviews are available.[1,10,11,12] Analysis of amniotic fluid by PCR to determine fetal RhD status has become available.[11] Fetal RhD genotyping using maternal plasma is described.[12]

Information relevant to this topic is included in Bilirubin, Amniotic Fluid, Delta A450 *on page 116* and Hemolytic Disease of the Newborn, Antibody Identification *on page 846*.

Footnotes
1. American Academy of Pediatrics, "Practice Parameter: Management of Hyperbilirubinemia in the Healthy Term Newborn," *Pediatrics*, 1994, 94(4):558-65.
2. Lasker MR and Holzman IR, "Neonatal Jaundice: When to Treat, When to Watch and Wait," *Postgrad Med*, 1996, 99(3):187-93.
3. Gourley GR, "Bilirubin Metabolism and Kernicterus," *Adv Pediatr*, 1997, 44:173-229.
4. Dennery PA, Seidman DS, and Stevenson DK, "Neonatal Hyperbilirubinemia," *N Engl J Med*, 2001, 344(8):581-90.
5. Moore JJ, Sax SM, and DeFranc S, "Liposyn® Interference With Neonatal Bilirubin Measurements," *Clin Chem*, 1982, 28(11):2334-5.
6. Dai J, Pary DM, and Krahn J, "Transcutaneous Bilirubinometry: Its Role in the Assessment of Neonatal Jaundice," *Clin Biochem*, 1997, 30(1):1-9.
7. Polesky HF, "Diagnosis, Prevention, and Therapy in Hemolytic Disease of the Newborn," *Clin Lab Med*, 1982, 2(1):107-22.
8. Johnson L and Bhutani VK, "Guidelines for Management of the Jaundiced Term and Near-Term Infant," *Clin Perinatol*, 1998, 25(3):555-74.
9. Kemper K, Forsyth B, and McCarthy P, "Jaundice, Terminating Breast Feeding, and the Vulnerable Child," *Pediatrics*, 1989, 84(5):773-8.
10. Bratlid D, "Criteria for Treatment of Neonatal Jaundice," *J Perinatol*, 1996, 16(3 Pt 2):S83-S88.
11. Bowman JM, "RhD Hemolytic Disease of the Newborn," *N Engl J Med*, 1998, 339(24):1775-7 (editorial).
12. Lo YD, Hjelm YM, Fidler C, et al, "Prenatal Diagnosis of Fetal RhD Status by Molecular Analysis of Maternal Plasma," *N Engl J Med*, 1998, 339(24):1734-8.

References
Cashore WJ, "Neonatal Hyperbilirubinemia," *N Y State J Med*, 1991, 91(11):476-7.

Dale JC and Hamrick HJ, "Neonatal Bilirubin Testing Practices. Reports From 312 Laboratories Enrolled in the College of American Pathologists Excel Proficiency Testing Program," *Arch Pathol Lab Med*, 2000, 124(10):1425-8.

Graziani LJ, Mitchell DG, Kornhauser M, et al, "Neurodevelopment of Preterm Infants: Neonatal Neurosonographic and Serum Bilirubin Studies," *Pediatrics*, 1992, 89(2):229-34.

Kaplan M, Hammerman C, Renbaum P, et al, "Gilbert's Syndrome and Hyperbilirubinaemia in ABO-Incompatible Neonates," *Lancet*, 2000, 356:652-3.

Luban NL, "Hemolytic Disease of the Newborn: Progenitor Cells and Late Effects," *N Engl J Med*, 1998, 338(12):830-1.

Newman TB and Maisels MJ, "Bilirubin and Brain Damage: What Do We Do Now?" *Pediatrics*, 1989, 83(6):1062-5.

Scheidt PC, Graubard BI, Nelson KB, et al, "Intelligence at Six Years in Relation to Neonatal Bilirubin Levels: Follow-up of the National Institute of Child Health and Human Development Clinical Trial of Phototherapy," *Pediatrics*, 1991, 87(6):797-805.

Seidman DS and Stevenson DK, "Neonatal Bilirubin," *Lancet*, 1992, 339(8784):65-6.

Bilirubin, Total, Serum

Related Information

Synonyms Total Bilirubin

Applies to Ascitic Fluid/Serum:Total Bilirubin Ratio; Fasting Bilirubin Test

Abstract Used to monitor diseases of the liver, biliary tract, and hemolytic diseases. Bilirubin is also increased in congenital hyperbilirubinemia and may be increased with malnutrition, infection, and congenital hyperthyroidism.

Specimen Serum

Container Red top tube; capillary tube for babies

Collection Pediatrics: Blood drawn from a heelstick. If sample is collected by capillary puncture, excess squeezing should be avoided (to avoid hemolysis and dilution with tissue fluids).

Storage Instructions Protect sample from light.

Causes for Rejection Gross hemolysis, specimen not protected from light

Special Instructions Transport promptly.

Reference Interval Newborns: see table in listing Bilirubin, Neonatal, Serum *on page 117*; adults: 0.3-1.0 mg/dL (SI: 5-17 μmol/L). Approximately 70% is indirect (unconjugated).

Use
Causes of **High Bilirubin**
- Hepatobiliary disease: hepatitis, cholangitis, cholecystitis, even without common duct calculi; cirrhosis, other types of liver disease (including primary or secondary neoplasia); alcoholism (usually with high AST (SGOT), GGT, MCV, or some combination of these findings); cholestasis (intrahepatic or extrahepatic); infectious mononucleosis (look also for increased LD (LDH), lymphocytosis); Dubin-Johnson syndrome; Gilbert disease[1,2] (familial hyperbilirubinemia). If >80% of total bilirubin is indirect and total bilirubin is <6.0 mg/dL hemolysis or Gilbert syndrome is suggested.[1]
- Malnutrition, anorexia, or prolonged fasting: 36 hours or more may cause moderate rise.
- Pernicious anemia, hemolytic anemias, erythroblastosis fetalis, other neonatal jaundice, hematoma and following a blood transfusion, especially if several units are given in a short time or with delayed hemolytic

transfusion reaction. The major source of bilirubin is hemoglobin catabolism from lysis of red blood cells.

- Pulmonary embolism/infarct
- Congestive heart failure
- **Drugs:** A large number of drugs can cause jaundice by *in vivo* action. Drugs which may cause cholestasis and/or hepatocellular damage include acetaminophen, aminosalicylic acid, anabolic steroids, azathioprine, chlorpromazine, clindamycin, erythromycin, esterified estrogens, gentamicin, indinavir, indomethacin, isoniazid, MAO inhibitors, methyldopa, nortriptyline, oleandomycin, oral contraceptives, penicillin, phenothiazines, procainamide, progesterone, pyrazinamide, sulfonamides, valproic acid, warfarin, drugs of abuse (eg, 3,4 methylenedioxymethamphetamine - MDMA), and many other agents. A few drugs can cause analytical decreases (eg, amikacin, high doses of ascorbic acid, theophylline) and a large number of drugs can cause analytic, physiologic, or pathologic increases.[3]

Limitations Differential diagnosis of liver diseases requires total and direct bilirubin values, as well as other tests. Visibly hemolyzed sera and lipemia can produce erroneous results. Serum alkaline phosphatase can be more sensitive to focal biliary obstruction.

Methodology Diazo reaction photometric method for adults is the most common; differential spectrophotometry for neonates (not useful for infants >10 days old); bilirubin oxidase method is also available.

Additional Information Total bilirubin is commonly found in chemistry multitest instruments, in which it is a useful test. Interpretation of increased bilirubin is greatly enhanced by other chemistry results and selectively, with other studies; see table. In acute viral hepatitis with jaundice, for instance, the transaminases ALT (SGPT) and AST (SGOT) are consistently increased, while an isolated elevation of bilirubin is seen in Gilbert disease.[2] **Obstruction** causes increases in bilirubin and alkaline phosphatase greater than and out of proportion to the transaminases. Gamma-glutamyl transferase is also increased in obstructive jaundice. Amylase and lipase are useful in differential diagnosis of obstructive jaundice. In **intrahepatic cholestasis**, the transaminases are not as increased, relative to bilirubin, as they are in hepatitis.[4]

Nicotinic acid increases the formation of bilirubin in the spleen, leading to a rise in unconjugated bilirubin. This can be used as a test for **Gilbert disease**[2] in which there is a moderate elevation of bilirubin with otherwise unremarkable chemistries. In Gilbert disease[2], decreased hepatic clearance of unconjugated bilirubin occurs with the criterion of basal total bilirubin >1.2 mg/dL. Although the indirect bilirubin level is increased in normal controls when nicotinic acid is given, the increase is greater in patients with Gilbert disease. The **fasting bilirubin test** can be used to support the diagnosis of constitutional hyperbilirubinemia. It involves fasting for 24 hours following a light breakfast, with only 100 g of sucrose and water allowed. Unconjugated bilirubin increases 1 mg/dL in subjects with Gilbert disease, or 1.5 mg/dL increase of total bilirubin.[4]

Acute liver failure in **Wilson disease** is characterized by very high bilirubin, often >30 mg/dL (513 µmol/L) with decreased alkaline phosphatase (see Copper, Serum *on page 816* and Copper, Urine *on page 818*) A ratio of alkaline phosphatase to bilirubin <2.0 is fairly distinctive.[5] In the **Crigler-Najjar** syndrome type I, the unconjugated bilirubin is >20 mg/dL. In type II, the level is <20 mg/dL.

Ascitic fluid/serum:total bilirubin ratio >6.0 supports distinction of exudate (eg, malignancy) from transudate with accuracy of 80%.[6]

Recently, it is thought that in neonates, high bilirubin levels may provide an antioxidant defense mechanism to compensate for otherwise deficient antioxidant enzymes.[7]

Footnotes
1. Kamath PS, "Clinical Approach to the Patient With Abnormal Liver Test Results," *Mayo Clin Proc*, 1996, 71:1089-95.
2. Ohkubo H and Okuda K, "The Nicotinic Acid Test in Constitutional Conjugated Hyperbilirubinemia and Effects of Corticosteroids," *Hepatology*, 1984, 4(6):1206-8.
3. Young DS, *Effects of Drugs on Clinical Laboratory Tests*, 5th ed, Volume 1: Listing by Test, Washington, DC: AACC Press, American Association for Clinical Chemistry, 2000, Section 3, 122-38.
4. Baldassare V and Ricci GL, "Specific Pattern of Unconjugated Bilirubin During Fasting Can Identify Constitutional Hyperbilirubinemia," *Ital J Gastroenterol*, 1993, 25(7):375-9.
5. Lee WM, "Acute Liver Failure," *N Engl J Med*, 1993, 329(25):1862-72.
6. Elis A, Meisel S, Tishler T, et al, "Ascitic Fluid to Serum Bilirubin Concentration Ratio for the Classification of Transudates or Exudates," *Am J Gastroenterol*, 1998, 93(3):401-3.
7. Hammermann C, Goldstein R, Kaplan M, et al, "Bilirubin in the Premature: Toxic Waste or Natural Defense?" *Clin Chem*, 1998, 44(12):2551-3.

References
Adachi Y, Katoh H, Fuchi I, et al, "Serum Bilirubin Fractions in Healthy Subjects and Patients With Unconjugated Hyperbilirubinemia," *Clin Biochem*, 1990, 23(3):247-51.
Gourley GR, "Bilirubin Metabolism and Kernicterus," *Adv Pediatr*, 1997, 44:173-229.
Iyanagi T, Emi Y, and Ikushiro S, "Biochemical and Molecular Aspects of Genetic Disorders of Bilirubin Metabolism," *Biochim Biophys Acta*, 1998, 1407(3):173-84.
Jonas MM and Graeme-Cook FM, "A 17-Year-Old Girl With Marked Jaundice and Weight Loss," Case Records of the Massachusetts General Hospital, Case 6-2001, Scully RE, Mark EJ, McNeely WF, et al, eds, *N Engl J Med*, 2001, 344(8):591-9.
Kurzweil SM, Shapiro MJ, Andrus CH, et al, "Hyperbilirubinemia Without Common Bile Duct Abnormalities and Hyperamylasemia Without Pancreatitis in Patients With Gallbladder Disease," *Arch Surg*, 1994, 129(8):829-33.
Westwood A, "The Analysis of Bilirubin in Serum," *Ann Clin Biochem*, 1991, 28(Pt 2):119-30.

- **Biopterin Cofactor Deficiency** *see* Phenylalanine, Blood *on page 248*
- **Biotin** *see* Lactic Acid, Whole Blood or Plasma *on page 208*
- **Biotinidase** *see* Amino Acids, Plasma *on page 100*
- **Bisalbuminemia** *see* Protein Electrophoresis, Capillary Zone *on page 266*

Blood Gases and pH, Arterial

Related Information
Anion Gap, Serum, Plasma, or Urine *on page 106*
Arterial Blood Collection *on page 40*
Base Excess, Blood *on page 114*
Bicarbonate, Blood *on page 115*
Blood Gases and pH, Capillary *on page 121*
Blood Gases and pH, Umbilical Cord *on page 121*
Blood Gases and pH, Venous *on page 122*
Carbon Dioxide, Total, Blood *on page 135*
Carboxyhemoglobin, Blood *on page 784*
Lactic Acid, Whole Blood or Plasma *on page 208*
Oxygen Saturation, Blood *on page 240*
P_{50}, Blood *on page 241*

Clinical Approach to the Patient With Jaundice

Diagnostic Factors	Type of Jaundice			
	Hemolytic	Hepatocellular	Intrahepatic Cholestatic	Extrahepatic Cholestatic
Symptoms	May be asymptomatic or backache, joint pain	Nausea, vomiting, fever, anorexia	Deep jaundice, dark-colored urine, light-colored stools, pruritus	Deep jaundice, dark-colored urine, light-colored stools, pruritus, cholangitis, biliary colic
Physical findings	Splenomegaly	Tender hepatomegaly, splenomegaly*	Tender hepatomegaly	Hepatomegaly, palpable gallbladder
Liver tests				
Bilirubin				
Total	<6 mg/dL	Variable	Variable, may be >30 mg/dL	<30 mg/dL
Direct	<20%	>50%	>50%	>50%
Alanine aminotransferase (ALT)	Normal	>5-fold increase	2- to 5-fold increase	<2- to 3-fold increase; >3- to 5-fold increase with cholangitis
Alkaline phosphatase	Normal	<2- to 3-fold increase	>3- to 5-fold increase	>3- to 5-fold increase
Prothrombin time	Normal	Prolonged	Prolonged	Prolonged
Corrected by vitamin K		No	Variable	Yes
Ultrasonography of liver				
Biliary dilatation	No	No	No	Yes
Endoscopic retrograde cholangiopancreatography	Not necessary	Not necessary	Usually not necessary	Usually necessary

*May or may not be present.

Modified from Kamath PS, "Clinical Approach to the Patient With Abnormal Liver Test Results," *Mayo Clin Proc*, 1996, 71:1089-95.

(Continued)

Blood Gases and pH, Arterial *(Continued)*

pCO_2, Blood *on page 246*
pH, Blood *on page 247*
Red Blood Cells *on page 857*
Uncrossmatched Blood, Emergency *on page 865*
Whole Blood *on page 866*

Synonyms ABGs; Arterial Blood Gases; Gases, Arterial

Applies to Allen Test; Base Excess; HCO_3^-; Oxygen Saturation; pCO_2; pH; pO_2; TCO_2

Test Includes Measured results include pH, pCO_2 (PaCO$_2$), and pO_2 (PaO$_2$). Calculated values include, among others, total carbon dioxide (TCO_2), bicarbonate (HCO_3^-), oxygen saturation, and base excess.

Abstract The measurement in arterial blood of pH, pCO_2, pO_2 and the calculation of HCO_3^-, TCO_2, and O_2 saturation, are used to evaluate oxygen and carbon dioxide exchange, respiratory function, and acid-base balance. Arterial blood is preferred for these determinations due to its superior uniformity throughout the body, but venous pH is extremely similar in most situations and is more easily obtained. The context in which the specimen is drawn is pivotal relevant to its significance (eg, pH 7.10 drawn in the immediate postictal state is of little consequence, but is ominous in methanol intoxication).[1]

Patient Preparation Patient should be supine, relaxed. The patient's temperature, breathing pattern, and concentration of inspired air (FiO$_2$) should be recorded to permit interpretation of results. Refer to NCCLS Approved Standard H11-A3[2] for complete guidelines.

Aftercare Observe for bleeding. Pressure must be applied to puncture site for at least 10-15 minutes; longer times are required for anticoagulated patients. See Arterial Blood Collection *on page 40*.

Specimen Whole blood (arterial)

Container Heparinized blood gas syringe (plastic or glass) or via an indwelling arterial line. Gases are capable of dissolving in plastic, which may alter results in some situations. Mahoney et al[3] reported clinically significant increases in pO_2 levels in whole blood stored in iced plastic syringes for 30 minutes. Specimens stored in iced glass syringes did not change significantly.

Collection See Arterial Blood Collection *on page 40*. Very small diameter needles are used. Specimen is drawn into air-free heparinized syringe, then stoppered. The radial artery is frequently used after the Allen test, which assesses the presence of normal collateral circulation. The brachial artery is the second choice. **The specimen should be transported to the laboratory immediately and analysis should be prompt. If testing will be delayed by more than 10-15 minutes, the specimen should be placed in a slurry of ice chips and water.** Mode of oxygen delivery (quantity of therapeutic oxygen or room air) and patient's temperature must be indicated. Rapid changes may occur if collected immediately after exercise.[4] Avoid excessive heparin. Strict anaerobiosis must be maintained.

Storage Instructions Testing should occur **immediately**; therefore, specimens should not require storage. However, if testing must be delayed more than 10-15 minutes, the specimen should be cooled to about 0°C by placing the syringe into a slurry of ice chips and water. Delay of analysis should not exceed 1 hour. Specimens for critical alveolar-arterial oxygen tension or shunt fraction samples must be analyzed immediately (within 10 minutes) to minimize changes in gas tensions. The following *in vitro* changes occur in blood gas parameters: pH decreases by <0.01 pH units/hour at 4°C,[5] pCO_2 increases by about 0.5 mm Hg/hour at 4°C,[5] and pO_2 decreases negligibly (<3 mm Hg/hour) if collected in a glass syringe and stored in an ice water slurry.[3]

Causes for Rejection Specimen **not** received correctly iced, air bubbles or clots in syringe, unsealed/open syringe

Special Instructions Sample obtained just after a change in inspired oxygen concentration (FiO$_2$) (eg, room air or quantity of therapeutic oxygen delivered) is likely to generate confusing results. Normally, arterial blood gases and pH will achieve steady-state levels within a minute or two after a change in FiO$_2$ or alveolar ventilation, but in certain disease states (eg, lung disease) the time necessary to achieve equilibrium can be as long as 20-30 minutes.[6]

Reference Interval
- Arterial pH: 7.35-7.45
- TCO_2: 23-29 mmol/L
- pCO_2: 35-45 mm Hg
- pO_2: newborns: 60-70 mm Hg, adults: 80-95 mm Hg
- O_2 saturation: 95% to 99%

Such ranges must be interpreted in light of the FiO$_2$ and other variables.

Possible Panic Range pH: <7.2, >7.55; pCO_2: <20 mm Hg, >60 mm Hg; pO_2: <40 mm Hg

Use Blood gas and pH testing are done to evaluate oxygen and carbon dioxide gas exchange, respiratory function including hypoxia and acid-base status. They are clinically indicated in a wide variety of medical and surgical situations involving cardiorespiratory, metabolic, and central nervous system disturbances. Raffin has pointed out that few studies are available to indicate how many arterial samples are actually indicated and that a complete list of clinical settings involving ill patients in whom blood gas studies might be indicated would include much of the tables of contents of general medicine texts.[7]

Acidosis and alkalosis are addressed in Anion Gap, Serum, Plasma, or Urine *on page 106*. Refer as well to the Key Word Index.

Limitations Arterial puncture is a hazardous procedure and may be extremely difficult in some individuals. Complications of arterial puncture potentially include hematoma, bleeding, arterial occlusion and insufficiency, infection, and, very rarely, gangrene. (Gangrene can complicate diseases for which gases are ordered, independent of the puncture, as well.)

The metabolic processes of markedly elevated leukocytes and/or platelets in a blood gas specimen will significantly alter blood gas and pH results regardless of specimen transport/storage methods. Point-of-care or *in vivo* methods of analysis are helpful in these situations.

By some instruments, O_2 saturation is calculated from oxyhemoglobin and total hemoglobin. The reported value may be misleading when nonfunctional hemoglobins (CoHB, MetHb, or sulfhemoglobin) are present or other hemoglobins with different dissociation curves are present. Calculations commonly assume body temperature of 37°C.

Variability of results occurs;[8,9] changes in pO_2 in isolated reports must be interpreted cautiously and in light of data trends, oxygen delivery, and the patient's clinical appearance. Such variation occurs without change in FiO$_2$ or the patient's clinical status.

Correlation of arterial gases with pulmonary function testing and with severity in asthma was reported as poor.[10]

Arterial gases and pH are of little value in treatment decisions for carbon monoxide poisoning.[11]

Although normal pO_2 diminishes the likelihood of pulmonary embolism, the former does not rule out the latter. (Alveolar-arterial gradient usually is widened in pulmonary embolism.)

Methodology Selective electrodes measuring pH, pCO_2, and pO_2

Additional Information

"Hypoxemia" can be defined as pO_2 <80 mm Hg, but other, more sophisticated definitions are available.[7]

The combination of pH values <7.25 without elevation of pCO_2, may indicate need for a lactic acid determination.

Potassium leaves the intracellular fluids in acidemia, leading to hyperkalemia.

Nonsurvivors in a group of COPD patients had lower arterial oxygen tension and higher carbon dioxide tension.[12,13]

The **acute respiratory distress syndrome (ARDS)** is usually initially characterized by respiratory alkalosis and hypoxemia. This complex response to pulmonary injury requires insight to enhance survival.[14]

Exercise testing with ABG has been advocated for patients in congestive heart failure. Hypoxemia is rare on exercise in subjects in stable congestive failure. Hypoxemia on exercise may indicate an alternative diagnosis.[15] Assessment of acid-base status of tissues in patients in circulatory failure may be misleading if only arterial blood gas data is available. Adrogué presents data supporting the need for information on **mixed venous** as well as arterial gases in care of critically ill patients.[16]

For a review of definitions and calculated values, see two outstanding *New England Journal of Medicine* review papers[1] and NCCLS Approved Standard C12-A.[17]

Footnotes
1. Adrogué HJ and Madias NE, "Management of Life-Threatening Acid-Base Disorders," First of Two Parts, *N Engl J Med*, 1998, 338(1):26-34, Second of Two Parts, *N Engl J Med*, 1998, 338(2):107-11.
2. National Committee for Clinical Laboratory Standards, *Procedures for the Collection of Arterial Blood Specimens: Approved Standard*, 3rd ed, H11-A3, Wayne, PA: NCCLS, 1999.
3. Mahoney JJ, Harvey JA, Wong RJ, et al, "Changes in Oxygen Measurements When Whole Blood Is Stored in Iced Plastic or Glass Syringes," *Clin Chem*, 1991, 37(7):1244-8.
4. Ries AL, Fedullo PF, and Clausen JL, "Rapid Changes in Arterial Blood Gas Levels After Exercise in Pulmonary Patients," *Chest*, 1983, 83(3):454-6.
5. Scott MG, Heusel JW, and LeGrys VA, et al, "Electrolytes and Blood Gases," *Tietz Textbook of Clinical Chemistry*, 3rd ed, Chapter 31, Burtis CA and Ashwood ER, eds, Philadelphia, PA: WB Saunders Co, 1999, 1056-92.
6. National Committee for Clinical Laboratory Standards, *Blood Gas Preanalytical Considerations: Specimen Collection, Calibration, and Controls: Approved Guideline C27-A*, Wayne PA: NCCLS, 1993.
7. Raffin TA, "Indications for Arterial Blood Gas Analysis," *Ann Intern Med*, 1986, 105(3):390-8.
8. Thorson SH, Marini JJ, Pierson DJ, et al, "Variability of Arterial Blood Gas Values in Stable Patients in the ICU," *Chest*, 1983, 84(1):14-8.
9. Sasse SA, Chen PA, and Mahutte CK, "Variability of Arterial Blood Gas Values Over Time in Stable Medical ICU Patients," *Chest*, 1994, 106(1):187-93.
10. Nowak RM, Tomlanovich MC, Sarkar DD, et al, "Arterial Blood Gases and Pulmonary Function Testing in Acute Bronchial Asthma. Predicting Patient Outcomes," *JAMA*, 1983, 249:2043-6.
11. Myers RA and Britten JS, "Are Arterial Blood Gases of Value in Treatment Decisions for Carbon Monoxide Poisoning?" *Crit Care Med*, 1989, 17(2):139-42.
12. Kawakami Y, Kishi F, Yamamoto H, et al, "Relation of Oxygen Delivery, Mixed Venous Oxygenation, and Pulmonary Hemodynamics to Prognosis in Chronic Obstructive Pulmonary Disease," *N Engl J Med*, 1983, 308:1045-9.
13. Bergofsky EH, "Tissue Oxygen Delivery and Cor Pulmonale in Chronic Obstructive Pulmonary Disease," *N Engl J Med*, 1983, 308:1092-4.

14. Kollef MH and Schuster DP, "The Acute Respiratory Distress Syndrome," *N Engl J Med*, 1995, 332(1):27-37.

15. Clark AL and Coats AJ, "Usefulness of Arterial Blood Gas Estimations During Exercise in Patients With Chronic Heart Failure," *Br Heart J*, 1994, 71(6):528-30.

16. Adrogué HJ, Rashad MN, Gorin AB, et al, "Assessing Acid-Base Status in Circulatory Failure: Differences Between Arterial and Central Venous Blood," *N Engl J Med*, 1989, 320(20):1312-6.

17. National Committee for Clinical Laboratory Standards, *Definitions of Quantities and Conventions Related to Blood pH and Gas Analysis: Approved Standard C12-A*, Wayne, PA: NCCLS, 1994.

References

Anderson S, "ABGs. Six Easy Steps to Interpreting Blood Gases," *Am J Nurs*, 1990, 90(8):42-5.

Brandenburg MA and Dire DJ, "Comparison of Arterial and Venous Blood Gas Values in the Initial Emergency Department Evaluation of Patients With Diabetic Ketoacidosis," *Ann Emerg Med*, 1998, 31(4):459-65.

Charan NB, Marks M, and Carvalho P, "Use of Plasma for Arterial Blood Gas Analysis in Leukemia," *Chest*, 1994, 105(3):954-5.

Courtney SE, Weber KR, Breakie LA, et al, "Capillary Blood Gases in the Neonate. A Reassessment and Review of the Literature," *Am J Dis Child*, 1990, 144(2):168-72.

Delclaux B, Orcel B, Housset B, et al, "Arterial Blood Gases in Elderly Persons With Chronic Obstructive Pulmonary Disease (COPD)," *Eur Respir J*, 1994, 7(5):856-61.

Ehrmeyer S, et al, "Performance Characteristics for Devices Measuring pO₂ and pCO₂ in Blood Samples," National Committee for Clinical Laboratory Standards (NCCLS), 1992, NCCLS Document C21-A.

Hansen JE, "Arterial Blood Gases," *Clin Chest Med*, 1989, 10(2):227-37.

Hibbard JU, Hibbard MC, and Whalen MP, "Umbilical Cord Blood Gases and Mortality and Morbidity in the Very Low Birth Weight Infant," *Obstet Gynecol*, 1991, 78(5 Pt 1):768-73.

Hood VL and Tannen RL, "Protection of Acid-Base Balance by pH Regulation of Acid Production," *N Engl J Med*, 1998, 339(12):819-26.

Meyer BA, Dickinson JE, Chambers C, et al, "The Effect of Fetal Sepsis on Umbilical Cord Blood Gases," *Am J Obstet Gynecol*, 1992, 166(2):612-7.

Pierson DJ, "Pulse Oximetry Versus Arterial Blood Gas Specimens in Long-Term Oxygen Therapy," *Lung*, 1990, 168(Suppl):782-8.

Ribbert LS, Snijders RJ, Nicolaides KH, et al, "Relation of Fetal Blood Gases and Data From Computer-Assisted Analysis of Fetal Heart Rate Patterns in Small for Gestation Fetuses," *Br J Obstet Gynaecol*, 1991, 98(8):820-3.

Blood Gases and pH, Capillary

Related Information

Bicarbonate, Blood *on page 115*
Blood Gases and pH, Arterial *on page 119*
Blood Gases and pH, Venous *on page 122*
Carbon Dioxide, Total, Blood *on page 135*
Oxygen Saturation, Blood *on page 240*
pCO₂, Blood *on page 246*
pH, Blood *on page 247*

Synonyms Capillary Blood Gases

Test Includes Measured results include pH, pCO₂, and pO₂. Calculated values include total carbon dioxide (TCO₂), bicarbonate (HCO₃⁻), oxygen saturation, and base excess.

Abstract Capillary pCO₂ and pH determinations are entirely adequate for many purposes, and are usually used for monitoring blood gases in neonates or other patients in whom traditional arterial blood collection is not practical. Arterialization of capillary blood by prewarming the puncture site yields a blood specimen similar to arterial blood with results for pH and pCO₂ that match very well those of arterial blood. Capillary pO₂ values do not correlate well with arterial pO₂ values, especially in sick patients with either abnormal peripheral vasoconstriction or vasodilation.[1]

Patient Preparation See Skin Puncture Blood Collection *on page 45*. The puncture site (eg, lateral exterior side of the foot, tip of finger or toe, earlobe) should be prewarmed to about 42°C to dilate the capillaries and increase arteriolar flow and free bleeding. The puncture should be deep enough to allow a free flow of blood. Blood is then collected in heparinized capillary tubes, which should be filled as much as possible, capped and mixed well.

Aftercare Elevate the site above the body and apply direct pressure to the puncture site with sterile gauze until bleeding stops. Bandaids or bandages are generally not applied because of the risk of skin sensitization to tape and the risk of aspiration, should the bandage come loose.

Specimen Whole blood (capillary)

Container Heparinized capillary tube(s) capped tightly with internal mixing flea

Collection See Skin Puncture Blood Collection *on page 45*. Fill capillary tubes completely excluding any air bubbles, and mix immediately with heparin to avoid clotting.

Storage Instructions Specimen should be analyzed immediately (within 10-15 minutes). If delay in analysis is unavoidable or otherwise anticipated, put specimen in a slurry of ice chips and water.

Causes for Rejection No heparin, sample clotted, specimen not received on ice

Reference Interval pH: 7.35-7.45, pCO₂: 26-41 mm Hg

Possible Panic Range pH: <7.2, >7.55; pCO₂: <20 mm Hg, >60 mm Hg

Use Testing is done to assess and monitor acid-base balance. Although capillary blood is satisfactory for most purposes for pH and pCO₂, the role of

capillary pO₂ is limited.[2] Capillary blood sampling is less likely to cause complications than is arterial puncture.

Limitations Arterialized capillary blood specimens should not be used for pO₂ determinations in patients with systolic blood pressure <95 mm Hg, in patients with vasoconstriction, for patients on O₂ therapy, for newborns during the first few hours following birth, or newborns with respiratory distress syndrome. These situations are associated with high likelihoods for venous admixture and erroneously low pO₂ results.[3]

Methodology Specific electrodes for pH, pCO₂, and pO₂

Additional Information Warming the heel, a traditional practice, made no difference in a study from Leeds.[2]

Footnotes

1. National Committee for Clinical Laboratory Standards, *Blood Gas Preanalytical Considerations: Specimen Collection, Calibration, and Controls: Approved Guideline C27-A*, Wayne, PA: NCCLS, 1993.
2. McLain BI, Evans J, Dear PR, et al, "Comparison of Capillary and Arterial Blood Gas Measurements in Neonates," *Arch Dis Child*, 1988, 63(7 Spec Issue):743-7.
3. Scott MG, Heusel JW, LeGrys VA, et al, "Electrolytes and Blood Gases," *Tietz Textbook of Clinical Chemistry*, 3rd ed, Chapter 31, Burtis CA and Ashwood ER, eds, Philadelphia, PA: WB Saunders Co, 1999, 1056-92.

References

Couriel JM, "Interpretation of Blood Gas Analysis," *Indian J Pediatr*, 1988, 55(5):656-60.

Dong SH, Liu HM, Song GW, et al, "Arterialized Capillary Blood Gases and Acid-Base Studies in Normal Individuals From 29 Days to 24 Years of Age," *Am J Dis Child*, 1985, 139(10):1019-22.

National Committee for Clinical Laboratory Standards, *Procedures for the Collection of Arterial Blood Specimens; Approved Standard - Third Edition, H11-A3*, Wayne, PA: NCCLS, 1999.

Blood Gases and pH, Umbilical Cord

Synonyms pH; pH, Umbilical Venous Blood Gases (pCO₂ and pO₂); Umbilical Arterial Blood Gases (pCO₂ and pO₂)

Test Includes Measured pH, pCO₂, and pO₂ and calculated total carbon dioxide (TCO₂), bicarbonate (HCO₃⁻), O₂ saturation, and base excess

Abstract Umbilical cord blood acid-base analysis provides a means for ruling out asphyxiation in newborns with low Apgar scores. **Asphyxia** is defined as hypoxia with metabolic acidosis.[1]

Patient Preparation Double clamping of the umbilical cord must occur immediately after delivery. Delays in clamping of as little as 20-30 seconds can significantly alter the pCO₂ and pH. The American College of Obstetricians and Gynecologists (ACOG)[1] recommends that cords be clamped for all deliveries regardless of whether cord blood pH and gas analyses are indicated.

Specimen Whole blood (umbilical cord); the umbilical arteries contain blood that is returning from the fetus to the placenta and provides the better cord blood specimen for evaluating fetal/newborn acid-base status. Blood gas and pH values analyzed in umbilical vein specimens can be normal concurrently with significantly abnormal umbilical artery values. ACOG recommends obtaining a specimen from an artery on the chorionic surface of the placenta, if a specimen cannot be obtained from the umbilical artery.[1]

Container Glass or plastic heparinized syringe

Sampling Time As soon as it has been determined that cord blood pH and gases are indicated in a given case, sampling from the clamped cord should occur. pH, pCO₂, and pO₂ values have been shown to be stable from umbilical cord segments left at room temperature for up to 60 minutes.[2]

Collection Blood is anaerobically collected into the heparinized syringe from either an umbilical artery (preferable) or umbilical vein from the clamped umbilical cord. Residual air is ejected from the syringe, and the syringe is sealed and transported immediately to the laboratory for analysis.

Storage Instructions Analysis should occur immediately. If delay beyond 10-15 minutes is unavoidable or anticipated, specimen should be placed in a slurry of ice chips and water. Delay of analysis should not exceed 1 hour.

Causes for Rejection Air bubbles in syringe, unsealed/open syringe, improperly iced syringe

Reference Interval The table gives the 5th and 95th percentiles from a study[3] of cord blood specimens from 1015 preterm infants delivered vaginally. The same study examined 3522 term infants delivered vaginally, and the ranges were similar.

	Arterial Cord Blood	Venous Cord Blood
pH	7.14-7.40	7.23-7.46
pCO₂ (mm Hg)	32-69	28-57
pO₂ (mm Hg)	8-33	15-42
HCO₃⁻ (mmol/L)	16.0-27.1	17.4-25.4
BE (mmol/L)	-7.6 to +1.3	-5.8 to +0.7
O₂ saturation (%)	5-59	14-75

Critical Values Umbilical arterial blood pH <7.00 is consistent with pathologic fetal acidemia that is of sufficient degree to be associated with birth asphyxia or hypoxia capable of subsequent neurologic abnormalities.[1]

Use Severe fetal acidemia is associated with increased perinatal mortality and increased risk for later impaired neurodevelopment. An umbilical artery blood pH <7.00 with a metabolic pattern (ie, normal pCO₂, low HCO₃⁻, and base deficit) and persistent Apgar scores ≤3 for 5 minutes or longer are (Continued)

Blood Gases and pH, Umbilical Cord *(Continued)*

consistent with a degree of birth asphyxia or hypoxia capable of subsequent neurologic abnormalities.[1]

Limitations Even with umbilical arterial pH levels below the critical threshold of 7.00, the majority of newborns will be neurologically normal with no apparent morbidity.[1]

Methodology Blood gas instrumentation with specific pH, pCO_2, and pO_2 electrodes

Additional Information ACOG[1] recommends that cord blood pH and gases be done only in cases in which serious abnormalities arise in the delivery process and/or when a problem with the neonate's condition persists beyond the first 5 minutes after birth. While ACOG[1] does not recommend that cord blood pH and gases be done for all deliveries, doubly clamping the umbilical cord immediately after each birth is recommended in the event assessment of fetal acidemia is warranted.

Footnotes

1. ACOG Technical Bulletin Number 216-November 1995 (Replaces No. 127, April 1989), "Umbilical Artery Blood Acid-Base Analysis," *Int J Gynaecol Obstet*, 1996, 52(3):305-10.
2. Duerbeck NB, Chaffin DG, and Seeds JW, "A Practical Approach to Umbilical Artery pH and Blood Gas Determinations," *Obstet Gynecol*, 1992, 79(6):959-62.
3. Riley RJ and Johnson JWC, "Collecting and Analyzing Cord Blood Gases," *Clin Obstet Gynecol*, 1993, 36(1):13-23.

References

Andres RL, Saade G, Gilstrap LC, et al, "Association Between Umbilical Blood Gas Parameters and Neonatal Morbidity and Death in Neonates With Pathologic Fetal Acidemia," *Am J Obstet Gynecol*, 1999, 181(4):867-71.

Arikan GM, Scholz HS, Haeusler MC, et al, "Low Fetal Oxygen Saturation at Birth and Acidosis," *Obstet Gynecol*, 2000, 95(4):565-71.

Brouillette RT and Waxman DH, "Evaluation of the Newborn's Blood Gas Status," *Clin Chem*, 1997, 43(1):215-21.

Goldaber KG, Gilstrap LC, Leveno KJ, et al, "Pathologic Fetal Acidemia," *Obstet Gynecol*, 1991, 78(6):1103-7

Hibbard JU, Hibbard MC, and Whalen MP, "Umbilical Cord Blood Gases and Mortality and Morbidity in the Very Low Birth Weight Infant," *Obstet Gynecol*, 78(5):768-73.

Huch A, Huch R, and Rooth G, "Guidelines for Blood Sampling and Measurement of pH and Blood Gas Values in Obstetrics," *Eur J Obstet Gynecol Reprod Biol*, 1994, 54(3):165-175.

Blood Gases and pH, Venous

Related Information

Blood Gases and pH, Arterial *on page 119*
Blood Gases and pH, Capillary *on page 121*
Carbon Dioxide, Total, Blood *on page 135*
pH, Blood *on page 247*
Venous Blood Collection *on page 47*

Synonyms Venous Blood Gases

Applies to Central Venous Blood

Test Includes Measured results include pH, pCO_2, and pO_2. Calculated values include, among others, total carbon dioxide (TCO$_2$), bicarbonate (HCO$_3^-$), oxygen saturation, and base excess.

Abstract Determination of pH and pCO_2 can be done reliably from venous blood in most clinical situations, but measurements involving oxygen are not usually useful when done on venous blood.

Patient Preparation The patient should be supine, relaxed.

Specimen Whole blood (venous)

Container Heparinized syringe, green top (heparin) tube

Collection See Venous Blood Collection *on page 47*. Draw specimen into air-free heparinized syringe or green top vacuum blood collection tube. If a vacuum blood collection tube is used, it must be completely filled and removed from needle before needle is removed from patient's arm. It is best not to use a tourniquet and to avoid hand clenching. Indicate specimen source (ie, venous) and mode of oxygen delivery or room air if applicable on requisition.

Storage Instructions Specimen should be analyzed immediately (within 10-15 minutes). If delay in analysis is unavoidable or otherwise anticipated, place specimen in a slurry of ice chips and water.

Causes for Rejection Specimen **not** received correctly iced, specimen clotted

Reference Interval Venous pH: 7.32-7.43, TCO$_2$: 23-30 mmol/L, pCO_2: 38-50 mm Hg, pO_2 should be about 40 mm Hg, O$_2$ saturation should be about 75%.

Possible Panic Range pH: <7.2, >7.55; pCO_2: <20 mm Hg, >60 mm Hg

Use The tests are used to evaluate cellular hypoxia and acid-base balance. A major use is to obtain pH without arterial puncture in infants, children, and adults in whom oxygen measurements are not needed. In many metabolic situations a venous pH is adequate and arterial puncture is unnecessary. Both arterial and central venous blood samples play a role in assessment of acid-base status in subjects in critical hemodynamic compromise. With severe hypoperfusion central venous blood better detects hypercapnia and acidemia.[1] The pO_2, pCO_2, and pH from pulmonary arterial samples correlate with central venous specimens.[2] The value of venous blood gas assays is supported in well-perfused subjects. A strong linear relationship between venous and capillary gas results exists, with the exception of pO_2.[3]

Limitations In hypotensive subjects with severe circulatory failure, Adrogué et al describe substantial differences between mean arterial and central venous pH and pCO_2.[1]

Methodology Specific electrodes for pH, pCO_2, and pO_2

Additional Information The arteriovenous pH difference is usually extremely small (0.01-0.03), except in patients in congestive heart failure and in shock. The differences in pH and pCO_2 widen only slightly with moderate cardiac failure.[1] Total CO$_2$ values are slightly higher in venous blood than in arterial blood. Arterial blood, however, must be used to accurately measure pO_2 and oxygen saturation.

Footnotes

1. Adrogué HJ, Rashad MN, Gorin AB, et al, "Assessing Acid-Base Status in Circulatory Failure: Differences Between Arterial and Central Venous Blood," *N Engl J Med*, 1989, 320(20):1312-6.
2. Eichhorn JH, "Accuracy and Comparisons in Blood Gas Measurements," *Chest*, 1988, 94(1):1-2.
3. McGillivray D, Ducharme FM, Charron Y, et al, "Clinical Decision Making Based on Venous Versus Capillary Blood Gas Values in the Well-Perfused Child," *Ann Emerg Med*, 1999, 34(1):58-63.

References

Adrogué HJ and Madias NE, "Management of Life-Threatening Acid-Base Disorders," First of Two Parts, *N Engl J Med*, 1998, 338(1):26-34, Second of Two Parts, *N Engl J Med*, 1998, 338(2):107-11.

Brandenburg MA and Dire DJ, "Comparison of Arterial and Venous Blood Gas Values in the Initial Emergency Department Evaluation of Patients With Diabetic Ketoacidosis," *Ann Emerg Med*, 1998, 31(4):459-65.

Hood VL and Tannen RL, "Protection of Acid-Base Balance by pH Regulation of Acid Production," *N Engl J Med*, 1998, 339(12):319-26.

National Committee for Clinical Laboratory Standards, *Blood Gas Preanalytical Considerations: Specimen Collection, Calibration, and Controls: Approved Guideline C27-A*, Wayne, PA: NCCLS, 1993.

Scott MG, Heusel JW, LeGrys VA, et al, "Electrolytes and Blood Gases," *Tietz Textbook of Clinical Chemistry*, 3rd ed, Chapter 31, Burtis CA and Ashwood ER, eds, Philadelphia, PA: WB Saunders Co, 1999, 1056-92.

♦ **Blood Gas P-50** *see* P$_{50}$, Blood *on page 241*

♦ **Blood Lactate** *see* Lactic Acid, Whole Blood or Plasma *on page 208*

♦ **Blood pH** *see* pH, Blood *on page 247*

♦ **Blood Spot Screen for Galactose/Galactose-1-Phosphate** *see* Newborn Screening Tests for Galactosemia *on page 232*

♦ **Blood Sugar, Fasting** *see* Glucose, Fasting, Plasma *on page 183*

♦ **Blood Urea Nitrogen** *see* Urea Nitrogen, Serum or Plasma *on page 293*

Body Fluid Amylase

Related Information

Amylase, Serum *on page 102*
Amylase, Urine *on page 104*
Body Cavity Fluid Cytology *on page 372*
Body Fluid Chemical Analysis *on page 123*
Cyst Fluid Cytology *on page 379*
Lipase, Serum *on page 212*

Synonyms Amylase, Body Fluid; Amylase, Peritoneal Fluid; Amylase, Pleural Fluid

Abstract High pleural or peritoneal fluid amylase is associated with pancreatitis (and its complications), rupture or perforation of the esophagus and occasionally with tumors, especially adenocarcinoma of lung and ovary. Pancreatitis is related to left-sided or bilateral pleural effusion. (Right-sided pleural effusions related to abdominal disease are often caused by cirrhosis, subdiaphragmatic abscess, hepatic abscess, and Meig syndrome).[1]

Specimen Body fluid (ie, ascitic fluid, pleural fluid, etc) and simultaneously drawn serum for amylase. Often, fluid for cytopathology is indicated.

Container Clean container, no preservative

Collection Peritoneal fluid may be obtained by peritoneal lavage.[2] Centrifugation is desirable.

Storage Instructions Amylase is fairly stable, at 4°C, at normal levels. If specimen is to be sent to a reference laboratory, it should be frozen in a plastic vial on dry ice.[3]

Reference Interval Body fluid (peritoneal or pleural) amylase values are usually compared to simultaneously obtained serum values. No established reference intervals exist for body fluids.

Use Pancreatitis, with or without pseudocyst formation or pancreatic pleural fistula, is the most common cause of a pleural or peritoneal fluid amylase value greater than the serum amylase. Rupture of the esophagus is the second most common cause and malignant effusion is the third.[4] Other causes include pancreatic ascites and pancreatic duct trauma. A defect in the wall of the gastrointestinal tract (eg, perforated peptic ulcer) will allow pancreatic secretion to enter the peritoneal cavity. Similarly, peritoneal fluid amylase elevations may be found in the presence of necrotic bowel.

An ascitic fluid amylase >3 times the serum amylase is strong evidence for disease in the pancreas, including pancreatitis, pancreatic pseudocyst, or trauma.

Limitations In collection of ascitic fluid, the localization of the catheter is likely to affect the chemistry result.[2] Oxalate or citrate depress results.

Lipemic sample may contain inhibitors which falsely depress results. Benign ovarian cyst fluids may have significant amylase activity. In about 10% of instances of pancreatic disease, ascitic fluid, as well as serum amylase, may be within normal limits.[5]

Methodology Absorbance following hydrolysis. For pancreatic amylase assay, after salivary amylase is inhibited by antibodies, pancreatic amylase is assayed by a coupled kinetic procedure.[3]

Additional Information Most patients with pancreatic ascites have high peritoneal fluid amylase as well as amylase and lipase elevations in serum. Pancreatitis may present with pleural effusion. Of 34 patients who had high amylase in pleural fluid associated with neoplasms, 18 had carcinoma of lung. Other tumors were gynecologic, gastrointestinal, lymphoma, breast, and malignancy of unknown origin.[6] Of these, tumors of lung and serous tumors of ovary are especially recognized as causes of hyperamylasemia with pleural effusion.

Dark, prune juice-like peritoneal fluid is described as characteristic of severe, necrotizing pancreatitis.[7]

The presence of bacteria in a foul-smelling peritoneal fluid indicates perforated viscus in the differential diagnosis of pancreatitis[7] and peritonitis.

Footnotes

1. DeMay RM, "Fluids," *The Art and Science of Cytopathology*, Chapter 8, Chicago, IL: ASCP Press, American Society of Clinical Pathologists, 1996, 257-325.
2. Robert JH, Meyer P, and Rohner A, "Can Serum and Peritoneal Amylase and Lipase Determinations Help in the Early Prognosis of Acute Pancreatitis?" *Ann Surg*, 1986, 203(2):163-8.
3. Mayo Medical Laboratories, "Amylase, Pancreatic, Body Fluid," *Mayo Reference Services*, Rochester, MN, 2000.
4. Kramer MR, Saldana MJ, Cepero RJ, et al, "High Amylase Levels in Neoplasm-Related Pleural Effusion," *Ann Intern Med*, 1989, 110(7):567-9.
5. Desai SP and Isa-Pratt S, *Clinician's Guide to Laboratory Medicine*, Hudson, OH: Lexi-Comp Inc, 2000, Chapters 23, 39.
6. Kjeldsberg CR and Knight JA, *Body Fluids - Laboratory Examination of Amniotic, Cerebrospinal, Seminal, Serous, and Synovial Fluids*, 3rd ed, Chicago, IL: American Society of Clinical Pathologists, 1993, 159-222.
7. Steinberg W and Tenner S, "Acute Pancreatitis," *N Engl J Med*, 1994, 330(17):1198-210.

References

Baer KE and Smith GP, "Serous Body Cavity Fluid Examination," *Lab Med*, 2001, 32(2):85-8.

Body Fluid Chemical Analysis

Related Information

Synonyms Ascitic Fluid Analysis; Fluid, Pericardial; Fluid, Peritoneal; Fluid, Pleural; Paracentesis Fluid Analysis; Pericardial Fluid Analysis; Peritoneal Fluid Analysis; Pleural Fluid Analysis; Thoracentesis Fluid Analysis

Applies to Albumin, Ascites Fluid; CEA, Body Fluid; Chylous Fluid; Cyst Fluid Chemistry; Lactic Acid, Body Fluid; LD, Body Fluid; Protein, Body Fluids; Rheumatoid Factor, Body Fluid; Serum-Ascites Albumin Gradient (Alb$_{s-a}$); Vascular Endothelial Growth Factor

Test Includes Tests commonly helpful in work-up of a fluid include **cell count** and differential, hemoglobin/hematocrit, **glucose, lactate dehydrogenase (LD), albumin**, specific gravity, **amylase** and **pH**. **Protein** quantitation is occasionally useful for pleural fluid but is less reliable for peritoneal fluid. **Cultures** are very commonly indicated, require sterile specimens, and generally are ordered for routine, anaerobic, TB, and sometimes fungi. **Gram and acid-fast smears** are often essential for guiding diagnosis and therapy. **Cytology** and **tumor markers** may be indicated.

Abstract The serous effusions (pleural, peritoneal, and pericardial) are fluids which may be classified either as transudates or exudates. Transudates are produced in systemic diseases (eg, congestive heart failure, hepatic cirrhosis, nephrotic syndrome) due to noninflammatory processes: increased hydrostatic pressure or decreased plasma oncotic pressure, changes at the capillary level. Exudates result from inflammatory processes (eg, infection, esophageal or other hollow viscus rupture, subphrenic or liver

abscess, rheumatoid arthritis, pancreatitis, lung embolization or infarct, trauma, systemic LE) that increase capillary permeability or decrease absorption of fluid by the lymphatic system (eg, by lymphatic obstruction). (Fluids caused by malignant diseases are classified as exudates.) Laboratory tests are done to determine whether an effusion is a transudate or an exudate. Follow-up testing is done to characterize the cause of fluid accumulation and establish its etiology.

A third type of fluid accumulation, **chylous effusion**, is also recognized. Chylous pleural effusions may be secondary to leakage and/or obstruction of the thoracic duct and are further described below.

When the explanation for a fluid accumulation is unknown, consider cirrhosis, carcinomatosis, or tuberculosis.[1] See Body Cavity Fluid Cytology *on page 372*.

While pleural transudates are apt to be bilateral, pleural exudates (pleuritis) are commonly unilateral.

Specimen Pleural, peritoneal, or pericardial fluid

Container Fluids are often aspirated using syringes anticoagulated with heparin or EDTA. Chemistry testing requires red top tube or green top (heparin) collection tubes. Check with the laboratory for requirements for hematology, microbiology, and cytology testing.

Collection Specimen is obtained surgically by the physician using sterile technique. Since testing of body fluids usually occurs in several laboratory sections, a common error is to provide the laboratory insufficient quantity of fluid for adequate examinations. 50 mL is desirable, divided into appropriate containers. A simultaneously drawn blood specimen is desirable for appropriate serum chemistry testing: protein and LD, sometimes glucose.

Special Instructions Laboratory must be made aware of the source of the specimen.

Reference Interval Since accumulations of fluid in the body cavities are abnormal, no reference intervals exist.

Use Testing is done to determine whether a fluid is a transudate or an exudate (see table). Some authors publish slightly varying figures.

	Transudate	Exudate
Fluid appearance	Clear, colorless to yellow	Cloudy, variable color (yellow, green, red)
Coaguability	Will not clot	May clot due to presence of fibrinogen
WBC/mm^3	<1000/mm^3	>1000/mm^3
Specific gravity	<1.016	>1.016
Fluid to serum total protein ratio	<0.5	>0.5
Fluid to serum LD ratio	<0.6	>0.6
Glucose	Equal to serum level	Less than or equal to serum levels - especially low in rheumatoid effusion
Cholesterol pleural	<60 mg/dL (SI: <1.55 mmol/L)	>60 mg/dL (SI: >1.55 mmol/L)
Cholesterol peritoneal	<40 mg/dL (SI: <1.19 mmol/L)	>46 mg/dL (SI: >1.19 mmol/L)
Albumin (serum-fluid)	1.6 ±0.5 g/dL	0.6 ±0.4 g/dL

Limitations Postural changes are significant in exudates but not in transudates in pleural effusions.[2]

Additional Information Vascular endothelial growth factor (VEGF) has been shown to be higher in pleural fluid from patients with malignant **pleural effusions** and may be responsible for fluid accumulation in these patients.[3] Lung and breast carcinoma are the two most common tumors causing pleural effusion. Exfoliative cytology is often critically important in diagnosing malignant effusions, though sensitivity is low. In addition to cytology, **tumor markers** in body fluids have been used, including CEA,[4,5,6,7] CA 125,[5,6,8] cytokeratin 19 fragments (CYFRA 21-1),[6,7] CA 15-3,[4,7] hCG,[4] and neuron-specific enolase (NSE).[7] CEA increases occur with many carcinomas primary in the gastrointestinal tract, breast, and lung. Increased CA 125 without elevated CEA is consistent with primary carcinoma of ovary, fallopian tube, or endometrium, but may occur with stage III or IV endometriosis.[8] CEA is commonly negative in Müllerian carcinomas but positive with mucinous cystadenocarcinoma of ovary.[9] (Adenocarcinoma primary in the endocervix is often CEA positive.) Normal CEA and CA 125 concentrations in malignant fluids suggest possible mesothelioma, melanoma, or lymphoma.[5]

Pericardial fluid specimens are often exudates. Significant palliation may be achieved with diagnosis and therapy of some malignant effusions (eg, of pericardium, in which primaries include lung, breast, esophagus, melanoma, and lymphoma).[1,10] Other causes of pericardial effusions include bacterial infection, TB, Coxsackieviruses, AIDS, uremia, myocardial infarction, radiation, hypothyroidism, fluid overload, hypoproteinemia, connective tissue diseases, and trauma. The most common cause of pericardial transudate is congestive heart failure.[1]

In descending order of frequency, the **causes of ascites** (peritoneal fluid accumulation) in the U.S. are cirrhosis, cancer, heart failure, tuberculosis, dialysis, and pancreatic disease.[11] Malignant causes include carcinomas of ovary, breast, stomach, pancreas, liver, colon and rectum, endometrium, cervix, lymphoma, and mesothelioma.[1]

(Continued)

Body Fluid Chemical Analysis *(Continued)*

Long-term dialysis is a cause of pleural, pericardial or ascitic effusions.

Other tests that are sometimes helpful include **pH**, especially in chest fluids. **Urea nitrogen (BUN)** is helpful if a question of bladder content versus ascitic fluid exists.

Green fluids may be tested for **bilirubin**; positive results are consistent with perforated intestine, peptic ulcer, or gallbladder.

Bloody fluids, if not caused by traumatic tap, are generally exudates. Trauma, TB, as well as infarct or cancer must be considered. **Hematocrit** of the fluid is useful for diagnosis of hemothorax or hemoperitoneum (eg, trauma).

Chylous fluid appears milky, may appear bloody, yellow or green, contains chylomicrons, and has very high **triglyceride** levels (>110 mg/dL). Fluid triglyceride concentrations <60 mg/dL are inconsistent with chylous effusion. For fluids having triglyceride levels of 60-110 mg/dL, lipoprotein electrophoresis is recommended to identify the presence or absence of chylomicrons.[12] Chylous effusions relate to trauma, surgical procedures,[13] lymphoma, carcinoma, and tuberculosis,[14] and an idiopathic group is recognized as well. The most common cause is lymphoma. **Pseudochylous effusions**, with triglycerides <50 mg/dL, are found with cases of rheumatoid pleuritis, tuberculosis,[15] and myxedema.[1]

High levels of **rheumatoid factor** in a pleural fluid support a diagnosis of rheumatoid effusion, while in SLE, rheumatoid factor titers are apt to be only about 1:40.[16]

Peritoneal and pleural fluid **lactic acid** levels are increased with infection. In uninfected ascites, ascitic fluid lactate was 15 ±5 mg/dL (SI: 1.7 ±0.6 mmol/L), while in bacterial peritonitis, 14 patients ranged 45 ±37 mg/dL (SI: 5.0 ±4.1 mmol/L). A cutoff >25 mg/dL (SI: >2.8 mmol/L) is suggested.[17] Lactic acid may also be increased in malignant disease in body fluids.

The differential diagnosis of ascites includes cancer and hepatic cirrhosis. The **ratio of LD** in serum to that of ascitic fluid is helpful. Ratios of less than unity occur with malignant disease, while ratios >1 are reported mostly with cirrhosis, when these two groups are compared.[18] However, a few instances of cancer have ratios greater than unity.[18] The LD of the ascitic fluid of cirrhosis is usually <60% that of serum.[19]

Since **albumin** in body fluids is the main determinant of oncotic pressure, the **serum-ascites albumin gradient (Alb$_{s-a}$)** has been used for differentiating transudates and exudates in peritoneal fluid. It is calculated by subtracting the albumin value of the fluid from that of serum and is greater in transudates than exudates.[14] It correlates with portal pressure (ie, the pressure gradient between the portal capillaries and the peritoneal cavity).[20,21] Gradients ≥1.1 g/dL (SI: 11 g/L) strongly correlate with portal hypertension. Disease states related to high gradients include cirrhosis, alcoholic hepatitis, cardiac failure, massive liver metastases, fulminant hepatic failure, Budd-Chiari syndrome, portal vein thrombosis, veno-occlusive disease, and fatty liver of pregnancy.[11] Constrictive pericarditis is usually associated with high gradients. **Low gradients** are found with peritoneal carcinomatosis and tuberculosis, pancreatic and biliary ascites, nephrotic syndrome, serositis, and bowel obstruction or infarct.[11] Other diseases reported with low gradients include SLE, certain ovarian diseases, and severe hypoalbuminemia.[19,20]

"High protein ascites," >2.5 g total protein/dL (SI: >25 g/L), is found in 15% to 20% of subjects who have hepatic disease, while a similar fraction of patients with malignant disease have **"low protein ascites."**[20]

Since **secondary peritonitis** often requires surgery, its distinction from spontaneous peritonitis is critical. Secondary peritonitis is characterized by total protein ≥1.0 g/dL, fluid LD greater than upper limit of normal for serum, glucose <50 mg/dL, and polymicrobial infection.[11] See Body Fluid Amylase *on page 122.*

Cholesterol levels have been studied in pleural[9] and ascitic[22] fluids. Discrimination between ascites of hepatocellular carcinoma and other malignant entities is supported by assays of ascitic fluid cholesterol and LD.[23] The usefulness of fluid cholesterol has been questioned.[11]

Gram stains for bacteria and Wright stains for white cell count may also be helpful.

Footnotes

1. DeMay RM, "Fluids," *The Art and Science of Cytopathology*, Chapter 8, Chicago, IL: ASCP Press, American Society of Clinical Pathologists, 1996, 257-325.
2. Brandstetter RD, Velazquez V, Viejo C, et al, "Postural Changes in Pleural Fluid Constituents," *Chest*, 1994, 105(5):1458-61.
3. Cheng DS, Rodriguez RM, Perkett EA, et al, "Vascular Endothelial Growth Factor in Pleural Fluid," *Chest*, 1999, 116(3):760-5.
4. Couch WD, "Combined Effusion Fluid Tumor Marker Assay, Carcinoembryonic Antigen (CEA) and Human Chorionic Gonadotropin (hCG), in the Detection of Malignant Tumors," *Cancer*, 1981, 48(11):2475-9.
5. Pinto MM, Bernstein LH, Brogan DA, et al, "Immunoradiometric Assay of CA 125 in Effusions: Comparison With Carcinoembryonic Antigen," *Cancer*, 1987, 59(2):218-22.
6. Ferrer J, Villarino MA, Encabo G, et al, "Diagnostic Utility of CYFRA 21-2, Carcinoembryonic Antigen, CA 125, Neuron Specific Enolase, and Squamous Cell Antigen Level Determinations in the Serum and Pleural Fluid of Patients With Pleural Effusions," *Cancer*, 1999, 86(8):1488-95.

7. Miedouge M, Rouzaud P, Salama G, et al, "Evaluation of Seven Tumour Markers in Pleural Fluid for the Diagnosis of Malignant Effusions," *Br J Cancer*, 1999, 81(5):1059-65.
8. Dawood MY, Khan-Dawood FS, and Ramos J, "Plasma and Peritoneal Fluid Levels of CA 125 in Women With Endometriosis," *Am J Obstet Gynecol*, 1988, 159(6):1526-31.
9. Hamm H, Brohan U, Bohmer R, et al, "Cholesterol in Pleural Effusions. A Diagnostic Aid," *Chest*, 1987, 92(2):296-302.
10. Wilkes JD, Fidias P, Vaickus L, et al, "Malignancy-Related Pericardial Effusion. 127 Cases From the Roswell Park Cancer Institute," *Cancer*, 1995, 76(8):1377-87.
11. Runyon BA, "Care of Patients With Ascites," *N Engl J Med*, 1994, 330(5):337-42.
12. Brunzel NA, "Pleural, Pericardial, and Peritoneal Fluid Analysis," *Fundamentals of Urine and Body Fluids*, Chapter 15, Philadelphia, PA: WB Saunders Co, 1994, 401-14.
13. Horn KD and Penchansky L, "Chylous Pleural Effusions Simulating Leukemic Infiltrate Associated With Thoracoabdominal Disease and Surgery in Infants," *Am J Clin Pathol*, 1999, 111(1):99-104.
14. Kjeldsberg CR and Knight JA, *Body Fluids - Laboratory Examination of Amniotic, Cerebrospinal, Seminal, Serous, and Synovial Fluids*, 3rd ed, Chicago, IL: American Society of Clinical Pathologists, 1993, 159-253, 186-7.
15. Meny GM and Southern PM, "Serous Effusions and Synovial Fluid," *Handbook of Clinical Pathology*, 2nd ed, Chapter 8, McKenna RW and Keffer JH, eds, Chicago, IL: American Society of Clinical Pathologists, 2000, 105-20.
16. Dines DE, "Studies on Pleural Fluid," *Mayo Clin Proc*, 1981, 56:460.
17. Garcia-Tsao G, Conn HO, and Lerner E, "The Diagnosis of Bacterial Peritonitis: Comparison of pH, Lactate Concentration and Leukocyte Count," *Hepatology*, 1985, 5(1):91-6.
18. Greene LS, Levine R, Gross MJ, et al, "Distinguishing Between Malignant and Cirrhotic Ascites by Computerized Step-Wise Discriminant Functional Analysis of Its Biochemistry," *Am J Gastroenterol*, 1978, 70(5):448-54.
19. Rector WG Jr, "An Improved Diagnostic Approach to Ascites," *Arch Intern Med*, 1987, 147(2):215.
20. Marshall JB and Vogele KA, "Serum-Ascites Albumin Differences in Tuberculous Peritonitis," *Am J Gastroenterol*, 1988, 83(11):1259-61.
21. Rector WG Jr and Reynolds TB, "Superiority of the Serum-Ascites Albumin Difference Over the Ascites Total Protein Concentration in Separation of 'Transudative' and 'Exudative' Ascites," *Am J Med*, 1984, 77(1):83-5.
22. Prieto M, Gómez-Lechón MJ, Hoyos M, et al, "Diagnosis of Malignant Ascites: Comparison of Ascitic Fibronectin, Cholesterol, and Serum-Ascites Albumin Difference," *Dig Dis Sci*, 1988, 33(7):833-8.
23. Castaldo G, Oriani G, Cimino L, et al, "Total Discrimination of Peritoneal Malignant Ascites From Cirrhosis- and Hepatocarcinoma-Associated Ascites by Assays of Ascitic Cholesterol and Lactate Dehydrogenase," *Clin Chem*, 1994, 40(3):478-83.

References

Bac DJ, Siersema PD, and Wilson JH, "Paracentesis. The Importance of Optimal Ascitic Fluid Analysis," *Neth J Med*, 1993, 43(3-4):147-55.

Baer KE and Smith GP, "Serous Body Cavity Fluid Examination," *Lab Med*, 2001, 32(2):85-8.

Erasmus JJ, Goodman PC, and Patz EF, "Management of Malignant Pleural Effusions and Pneumothorax," *Radiol Clin North Am*, 2000, 38(2):375-83.

Horowitz ML, Schiff M, Samuels J, et al, "*Pneumocystis carinii* Pleural Effusion. Pathogenesis and Pleural Fluid Analysis," *Am Rev Respir Dis*, 1993, 148(1):232-4.

Kiltz RJ, Burke MS, and Porreco RP, "Amniotic Fluid Glucose Concentration as a Marker for Intra-amniotic Infection," *Obstet Gynecol*, 1991, 78(4):619-22.

Paavonen T, Liippo K, Aronen H, et al, "Lactate Dehydrogenase, Creatine Kinase, and Their Isoenzymes in Pleural Effusions," *Clin Chem*, 1991, 37(11):1909-12.

Rocco VK and Ware AJ, "Cirrhotic Ascites," *Ann Intern Med*, 1986, 105(4):573-85.

Rodriguez-Panadero F and Lopez-Mejias J, "Low Glucose and pH Levels in Malignant Pleural Effusions. Diagnostic Significance and Prognostic Value in Respect to Pleurodesis," *Am Rev Respir Dis*, 1989, 139(3):663-7.

Sheets EE and Smith RN, "A 31-Year-Old Woman With a Pleural Effusion, Ascites, and Persistent Fever Spikes," Case Records of the Massachusetts General Hospital, Case 3-1998, Scully RE, Mark EJ, McNeely WF, et al, eds, *N Engl J Med*, 1998, 338(4):248-54.

♦ **Body Fluid Creatinine** *see* Body Fluid pH *on page 125*

♦ **Body Fluid GGT** *see* Gamma-Glutamyl Transferase, Serum *on page 179*

Body Fluid Glucose

Related Information
Body Cavity Fluid Cytology *on page 372*
Body Fluid Chemical Analysis *on page 123*
Body Fluid Lactate Dehydrogenase *on page 125*
Body Fluid pH *on page 125*
Cerebrospinal Fluid Glucose *on page 140*
Glucose, Fasting, Plasma *on page 183*
Washing Cytology *on page 390*

Synonyms Glucose, Body Fluid

Applies to Amniotic Fluid Glucose

Abstract Decreased body fluid glucose may be found in bacterial infection, tuberculosis, rheumatoid effusion and occasionally with malignant disease.

Specimen Body fluid; simultaneously drawn plasma glucose

Reference Interval Fluid glucose concentration is usually similar to plasma glucose concentration. A value <60 mg/dL, or a value 40 mg/dL less than the simultaneous plasma level is considered decreased.[1]

Use Decreased fluid glucose concentration is usually associated with septic or inflammatory processes or malignancy. Pleural fluid glucose levels <60

mg/dL indicate often grossly purulent parapneumonic effusion or rheumatoid effusion, and glucose <50 mg/dL (SI: <2.8 mmol/L) characterizes rheumatoid effusion. In contrast, fluid glucose in SLE is usually >60 mg/dL. Pericardial effusions with decreased glucose are reported with malignant disease and with bacterial endocarditis.[1] Ascitic fluid glucose is often decreased in tuberculous peritonitis and with malignant disease but is usually normal with cirrhosis or congestive failure.

Limitations Garcia-Tsao et al found ascitic fluid glucose the least reliable of the tests they evaluated for the diagnosis of bacterial peritonitis; ascitic fluid glucose in their series ranged from 0-418 mg/dL (SI: 0-23 mmol/L). They also found poor correlation with blood glucose levels. Peritoneal fluid glucose is rarely of clinical value. This group recognized the more consistent glucose decrease found in smaller, sequestered fluid collections such as those of meningitis (cerebrospinal fluid) and empyema (pleural fluid).[2]

Methodology Enzymatic with photometry

Additional Information Potts et al describe loculated effusions or empyemas with low glucose and low pH. Low glucose is found with empyema, tuberculosis, and neoplasia, as well as rheumatoid effusion.[3] In cases of malignant pleural effusions, when there is low pleural fluid glucose, <60 mg/dL (SI: <3.3 mmol/L), and pH <7.30, a probability of 90% that the cytologic yield will be positive was reported.[4]

Amniotic fluid glucose when low, is a marker for intrauterine infection in women with preterm labor. Its specificity is 94% to 100%, but it has poor sensitivity.[5] However, in a study comparing several amniotic fluid markers of intra-amniotic infection (glucose, polymorphonuclear leukocytes, Gram stain, and culture), amniotic fluid glucose levels <20 mg/dL were the most sensitive predictors of histologic chorioamnionitis.[6]

Footnotes

1. Kjeldsberg CR and Knight JA, *Body Fluids - Laboratory Examination of Amniotic, Cerebrospinal, Seminal, Serous, and Synovial Fluids*, 3rd ed, Chicago, IL: American Society of Clinical Pathologists, 1993, 159-222.
2. Garcia-Tsao G, Conn HO, and Lerner E, "The Diagnosis of Bacterial Peritonitis: Comparison of pH, Lactate Concentration and Leukocyte Count," *Hepatology*, 1985, 5(1):91-6.
3. Potts DE, Taryle DA, and Sahn SA, "The Glucose-pH Relationship in Parapneumonic Effusions," *Arch Intern Med*, 1978, 138(9):1378-80.
4. Rodriguez-Panadero F and Lopez-Mejias JL, "Low Glucose and pH Levels in Malignant Pleural Effusions. Diagnostic Significance and Prognostic Value in Respect to Pleurodesis," *Am Rev Respir Dis*, 1989, 139(3):663-7.
5. Greig PC, Ernest JM, and Teot L, "Low Amniotic Fluid Glucose Levels Are a Specific but Not a Sensitive Marker for Subclinical Intrauterine Infections in Patients in Preterm Labor With Intact Membranes," *Am J Obstet Gynecol*, 1994, 171(2):365-71.
6. Odibo AO, Rodis JF, Sanders MM, et al, "Relationship of Amniotic Fluid Markers of Intra-amniotic Infection With Histopathology in Cases of Preterm Labor With Intact Membranes," *J Perinatol*, 1999, 19(6 Pt 1):407-12.

References

Desai SP and Isa-Pratt S, *Clinician's Guide to Laboratory Medicine*, Hudson, OH: Lexi-Comp Inc, 2000, Chapters 23, 30.

Body Fluid Lactate Dehydrogenase

Related Information

Body Cavity Fluid Cytology *on page 372*
Body Fluid Chemical Analysis *on page 123*
Body Fluid Glucose *on page 124*
Body Fluid pH *on page 125*
Cerebrospinal Fluid Lactate Dehydrogenase *on page 142*
Herpesvirus 8 *on page 634*
Lactate Dehydrogenase, Serum *on page 207*

Synonyms LD, Body Fluid

Abstract Body fluid LD levels are often higher than serum levels in malignant effusions. Elevations are also found in inflammatory states, including tuberculous effusions.[1]

Specimen Body fluid; simultaneously drawn serum

Special Instructions Source of fluid must be made known to the laboratory.

Reference Interval Exudates exhibit pleural fluid to serum LD ratios >0.6, whereas transudates exhibit ratios <0.6.

Use Differential diagnosis and classification of effusions; aid in the differential diagnosis of traumatic tap vs central nervous system (CNS) hemorrhage in newborns. Analysis of serum and body fluid drawn at the same time, for LD and total protein, often provides distinction between transudates and exudates (see table in Body Fluid Chemical Analysis *on page 123*).

Limitations This test has limited usefulness due to its nonspecificity. Like use of total protein, LD fails to classify fluids accurately as transudate or exudate.[2] Though transudates and exudates are often said to be characterized by fluid LD activities <200 units/L and >200 units/L, respectively, assay methodologies give widely varying results, thus, making the fluid to serum ratio a more useful assessment.[1]

Methodology Lactate to pyruvate monitored at 340 nm

Additional Information Lactate dehydrogenase (LD) is a normal component of CSF and is increased in bacterial and viral meningitis. LD_1 and LD_2 are decreased in lavage fluid in pulmonary alveolar proteinosis.[3] With ascitic fluid cholesterol, ascitic fluid LDH is helpful in the differential diagnosis of hepatocellular carcinoma versus ascites from other malignant neoplasms.[4] See Body Fluid Chemical Analysis *on page 123* for more information.

Median concentrations of vascular endothelial growth factor (VEGF), a cytokine, are significantly higher from patients with malignant pleural effusions than from those having pleural effusions due either to congestive heart failure or coronary artery bypass grafting and seem to correlate with pleural fluid LD activities measured in these groups.[5]

Footnotes

1. Kjeldsberg CR and Knight JA, *Body Fluids - Laboratory Examination of Amniotic, Cerebrospinal, Seminal, Serous, and Synovial Fluids*, 3rd ed, Chicago, IL: American Society of Clinical Pathologists, 1993, 159-222.
2. Runyon BA, "Care of Patients With Ascites," *N Engl J Med*, 1994, 330(5):337-42.
3. Hoffman RM and Rogers RM, "Serum and Lavage Lactate Dehydrogenase Isoenzymes in Pulmonary Alveolar Proteinosis," *Am Rev Respir Dis*, 1991, 143(1):42-6.
4. Castaldo G, Oriani G, Cimino L, et al, "Total Discrimination of Peritoneal Malignant Ascites From Cirrhosis- and Hepatocarcinoma-Associated Ascites by Assays of Ascitic Cholesterol and Lactate Dehydrogenase," *Clin Chem*, 1994, 40(3):478-83.
5. Cheng D, Rodriguez RM, Perkett EA, et al, "Vascular Endothelial Growth Factor in Pleural Fluid," *Chest*, 1999, 116(3):760-5.

References

Brandstetter RD, Velazquez V, Viejo C, et al, "Postural Changes in Pleural Fluid Constituents," *Chest*, 1994, 105(5):1458-61.
Desai SP and Isa-Pratt S, *Clinician's Guide to Laboratory Medicine*, Hudson, OH: Lexi-Comp Inc, 2000, Chapters 23, 39.
Drapkin MS and Mark EJ, "A 38-Year-Old Man With Fever, Cough, and a Pleural Effusion," Case Records of the Massachusetts General Hospital, Case 25-1996, Scully RE, Mark EJ, McNeely WF, et al, eds, *N Engl J Med*, 1996, 335(7):499-505.

♦ **Body Fluid Lipase** *see Lipase, Serum on page 212*

Body Fluid pH

Related Information

Body Cavity Fluid Cytology *on page 372*
Body Fluid Chemical Analysis *on page 123*
Body Fluid Glucose *on page 124*
Body Fluid Lactate Dehydrogenase *on page 125*
Gram Stain *on page 617*
Washing Cytology *on page 390*

Synonyms pH, Body Fluid

Applies to Arterial-Ascitic Fluid pH Gradient; Body Fluid Creatinine; Creatinine, Ratio; Peritoneal Fluid pH; pH Body Fluid; Pleural Fluid pH; Rheumatoid Effusion; Thoracentesis Fluid pH

Abstract Pleural, peritoneal, or pericardial fluid pH levels have been used where appropriate in the evaluation of pneumonia, rheumatoid pleuritis, malignancy, uremia, empyema, tuberculosis, hemothorax, esophageal rupture, and cirrhosis with spontaneous bacterial peritonitis.

Specimen Pleural, peritoneal, or pericardial fluid

Container Heparinized blood gas syringe or green top (lithium heparin) tube

Collection The usual recommendation is for the sample to be collected anaerobically, directly into a heparinized blood gas syringe or green top (lithium heparin) tube to prevent clotting. "Indirect" collection recently has been shown to be acceptable as well, in which pleural fluid initially is collected into a large (30- to 60-mL) heparinized syringe followed by aliquot transfer to a heparinized blood gas syringe.[1] If the specimen is collected in a syringe, all air should be expelled and needle sealed and capped. The pH should be measured anaerobically without delay.

Storage Instructions Most recommend that the pH be measured anaerobically, keeping the specimen on ice when delay of any kind is unavoidable. A recent study, however, showed that pleural fluid pH preserved anaerobically at room temperature is stable during the first hour following thoracentesis.[2]

Causes for Rejection Purulent or viscous sample

Reference Interval Pleural fluid pH is usually about 7.6.

Use Pleural, peritoneal, and pericardial fluid pH measurements have been used in the evaluation of a variety of conditions. See Abstract and Additional Information. Low pleural fluid pH concentrations (<7.3) are considered abnormal and are usually found in exudates, including empyema, connective tissue diseases, rupture or perforation of esophagus, rheumatoid disease, and tuberculosis. In malignant disease, low pH is suggestive of positive cytopathologic findings and poor prognosis.[3] Levels ≥7.3 are considered a benign finding and are found in transudates.

Methodology Blood gas instrumentation should be used. pH meters and pH paper should not be used.[4,5]

Additional Information Pleural fluid: Low pleural fluid pH levels (<7.2-7.3) identify patients with effusions due to pneumonia, empyema or lung abscess; such conditions require aggressive treatment.[6,7] Low pleural fluid pH is accompanied by low pleural fluid glucose in these patients.[8]

pH of pleural fluid <6.0 is highly suggestive of rupture of esophagus.[6] Pleural fluid amylase is very helpful for this diagnosis as well (see Body Fluid Amylase *on page 122*).

The pleural fluid pH is often <7.2 and consistently <7.3 in rheumatoid pleural effusion, which is characterized by low glucose, high LD, and high rheumatoid factor. Effusions related to lupus erythematosus generally have pleural fluid pH levels >7.35.[6]

Low pleural fluid pH with negative cytologic examination may occur in a malignant effusion as well as tuberculosis or rheumatoid disease. Differences in survival have been shown between patients with malignant pleural effusions having low pleural fluid pH (<7.30) compared to those having pH (Continued)

Body Fluid pH (Continued)

≥7.30.[9] On the basis of these observations, recommendations exist for selecting patients for pleurodesis.[10] However, the use of pleural fluid pH for this purpose is controversial.[11,12,13]

A low, transudative, pleural fluid pH (<7.30) accompanied by a pleural fluid creatinine to serum creatinine ratio >1 is consistent with urinothorax, a condition found in some patients with obstructive uropathy.[14]

Peritoneal (ascitic) fluid: The most reliable diagnostic criteria for spontaneous bacterial peritonitis have been reported to include ascitic fluid pH <7.35 (with a mean of 7.24), ascitic fluid PMN >500/mm³, and an **arterial-ascitic fluid pH gradient** >0.10.[15] Reduction of ascitic fluid pH and in some, but not all, series increments of ascitic fluid PMN counts may be found with peritoneal metastases.[15]

Pericardial fluid: Pericardial fluid pH measurements are not widely used, though decreased (<7.30) levels are observed in rheumatic and purulent disorders, malignancy, uremia, tuberculosis, and other conditions.

Footnotes

1. Goldstein LS, McCarthy K, Mehta AC, et al, "Is Direct Collection of Pleural Fluid Into a Heparinized Syringe Important for Determination of Pleural pH?" *Chest*, 1997, 112(3):707-8.
2. Sarodia BD, Goldstein LS, Laskowski DM, et al, "Does Pleural Fluid pH Change Significantly at Room Temperature During the First Hour Following Thoracentesis?" *Chest*, 2000, 117(4):1043-8.
3. DeMay RM, "Fluids," *The Art and Science of Cytopathology*, Chapter 8, Chicago, IL: ASCP Press, 1996, 257-325.
4. Lesho EP and Roth BJ, "Is pH Paper an Acceptable, Low-Cost Alternative to the Blood Gas Analyzer for Determining Pleural Fluid pH?" *Chest*, 1997, 112(5):1291-2.
5. Cheng DS, Rodriguez M, Rogers J, et al, "Comparison of Pleural Fluid pH Values Obtained Using Blood Gas Machine, pH Meter, and pH Indicator Strip," *Chest*, 1998, 114(5):1368-72.
6. Kjeldsberg CR and Knight JA, *Body Fluids - Laboratory Examination of Amniotic, Cerebrospinal, Seminal, Serous, and Synovial Fluids*, 3rd ed, Chicago, IL: American Society of Clinical Pathologists, 1993, 186-7.
7. Dines DE, "Studies on Pleural Fluid," *Mayo Clin Proc*, 1981, 56:460.
8. Potts DE, Taryle DA, and Sahn SA, "The Glucose-pH Relationship in Parapneumonic Effusions," *Arch Intern Med*, 1978, 138(9):1378-80.
9. Sahn SA and Good JT, "Pleural Fluid pH in Malignant Effusions: Diagnostic, Prognostic, and Therapeutic Implications," *Ann Intern Med*, 1988, 108(3):345.
10. Sahn SA, "Pleurodesis for Malignant and Nonmalignant Pleural Effusions," *Clin Pulm Med*, 1999, 6:141-6.
11. Burrows CM, Mathews WC, and Colt HG, "Predicting Survival in Patients With Recurrent Symptomatic Malignant Pleural Effusions: An Assessment of the Prognostic Values of Physiologic, Morphologic, and Quality of Life Measures of Extent of Disease," *Chest*, 2000, 117(1):73-8.
12. Heffner JE, Nietert PJ, and Barbieri C, "Pleural Fluid pH as a Predictor of Survival for Patients With Malignant Pleural Effusions," *Chest*, 2000, 117(1):79-86.
13. Heffner JE, Nietert PJ, and Barbieri C, "Pleural Fluid pH as a Predictor of Pleurodesis Failure: Analysis of Primary Data," *Chest*, 2000, 117(1):87-95.
14. Miller KS, Wooten S, and Sahn SA, "Urinothorax: A Cause of Low pH Transudative Pleural Effusions," *Am J Med*, 1988, 85(3):448-9.
15. Garcia-Tsao G, Conn HO, and Lerner E, "The Diagnosis of Bacterial Peritonitis: Comparison of pH, Lactate Concentration, and Leukocyte Count," *Hepatology*, 1985, 5(1):91-6.

References

Desai SP and Isa-Pratt S, *Clinician's Guide to Laboratory Medicine*, Hudson, OH: Lexi-Comp Inc, 2000, Chapters 23, 30.

el-Touny M, Osman L, Abdelhamid T, et al, "Re-Evaluation of the Value of Ascitic Fluid pH Lactate Dehydrogenase and Total Proteins in the Diagnosis of Spontaneous Bacterial Peritonitis (SBP)," *J Trop Med Hyg*, 1989, 92(1):6-9.

Halla JT, Schrohenloher RE, and Volanakis JE, "Immune Complexes and Other Laboratory Features of Pleural Effusions: A Comparison of Rheumatoid Arthritis, Systemic Lupus Erythematosus, and Other Diseases," *Ann Intern Med*, 1980, 92:748-52.

CA 125, Serum

Related Information

Synonyms Cancer Antigen 125; Carbohydrate Antigen 125

Abstract CA 125, a glycoprotein tumor marker, is a mainstay in the management of patients with ovarian carcinoma, and has potential application in certain other malignancies (endometrium, fallopian tube, pancreas, breast, colon, and lung). CA 125 is present in the serum of normal persons at levels <35 kU/L, and, in normal persons, has a biological half-life in the serum of 4.8 days.[1] In patients with completely resected Stage I and II ovarian carcinoma, the half-life ranges from 5.1-12 days.[2] In patients with more extensive carcinoma, the half-life is often substantially longer. CA 125 may be visualized histologically in a variety of epithelia and has potential application in the evaluation of metastatic adenocarcinomas.[3]

Specimen Serum

Container Red top tube

Sampling Time Abdominal surgery, by itself, causes a temporary increase in serum CA 125, therefore, no postsurgical specimen should be obtained until **3 weeks after the procedure**.[4,5]

Storage Instructions Refrigerate within 2 hours of collection. Freeze at -20°C for long-term storage.

Reference Interval Most commonly used is <35 kU/L; however, depending on the purpose of testing, other cutoff values and other approaches (ie, half-life and other kinetic measurements) are used (see Use).

Use

Monitor the response to treatment and the probability of recurrence of ovarian carcinoma. This is the principal use for CA 125, and serial serum levels are often required in clinical trials. In general, serum levels are proportional to tumor burden, and the extent to which CA 125 values decrease after treatment reflects the effectiveness of the treatment. Some investigators measure the kinetics of serum CA 125 to monitor treatment and reach prognostic conclusions.[2] Rosman et al[6] found a low probability for recurrence in women with a minimum CA 125 <35 kU/L and a half-life of 12 days or less. Buller et al[7] derived an "ideal" exponential regression curve which yielded a serum CA 125 half-life of 10.4 days in patients whose primary tumors were completely removed. When patient values are entered into this model, the results can provide early evidence of treatment failure (within 60 days of surgery) and, thus, lead to treatment modification sooner than would otherwise be possible. Hawkins et al[8] and Hunter et al[9] have found the CA 125 half-life a useful prognostic assessment. Gadducci et al[10] have demonstrated the prognostic value of measuring the CA 125 half-life in early chemotherapy.

CA 125-based standard response criteria in ovarian carcinoma. The World Health Organization (WHO) gold standard for defining an objective response to cancer treatment requires serial measurements of tumor deposits, either directly at surgery or indirectly from a standardized imaging study.[11] This WHO consensus statement, published in 1981, specifically excludes biochemical measurements from any role in the determination of a response.[11] Rustin et al[12] undertook a study, involving a total of 403 assessable patients, to determine whether serial CA 125 values could be as accurate as the WHO gold standard. These investigators used a subset of 117 patients to derive definitions of a 50% response and a 75% response. They then tested such definitions in a subset of 186 patients and found predictive values that compare favorably with those using the gold standard. Bridgewater et al[13] have tested such criteria in 769 patients and found them equivalent in accuracy, and superior in cost and convenience, to the gold standard. The precise definitions of a 50% response and a 75% response are complex, requiring a minimum of 4 and 3 samples, respectively; they have been incorporated into a computer program, reported to be available from Dr Rustin.[12]

Screen for ovarian carcinoma. A review of twenty-five screening studies (1983-1996), yielded inconclusive results.[14] When CA 125 was used as a stand alone test, and applied across all age groups, the predictive values were too low for an effective screen.

When restricted to asymptomatic postmenopausal women, using a cutoff of 30 kU/L, Jeyarajah et al[15] found an odds ratio of 21.56 in screening for ovarian carcinoma. In this study, elevated CA 125 values were also recorded in patients who, on investigation, had other gynecologic cancers. Although women with elevated CA 125 values were more likely to have a history of breast cancer, breast cancer did not develop more frequently in the women with elevated CA 125 values. Therefore, based on these findings, asymptomatic postmenopausal women with elevated CA 125 values should be investigated for gynecologic cancer.

Another study in **postmenopausal** women[16] found a positive predictive value of 20% (one ovarian carcinoma surgically confirmed for every five women explored), using a screening cutoff of CA 125 >30 kU and performing transvaginal ultrasound on all patients with elevated values.

Screening programs for ovarian cancer are based on the premise that many ovarian carcinomas begin as cystic lesions which are readily identified by ultrasound scans. It was, therefore, surprising that in a study of >5000 subjects, the removal of persistent benign ovarian cysts was **not** associated with reduced mortality due to carcinoma of the ovary.[17,18]

Other gynecologic malignancies. CA 125 values are often elevated in patients with carcinoma of the the fallopian tube and endometrium. The magnitude of the elevation is generally proportional to total tumor burden. According to Kurihara et al,[19] a CA 125 value <20 kU/L in a postmenopausal woman with endometrial carcinoma indicates a low probability of myometrial invasion and extrauterine spread.

Therapy selection for endometrial carcinoma. One report suggests that women with endometrial carcinoma and a preoperative CA 125 <20 kU/L can be treated more conservatively than patients with higher values.[20]

Monitoring cardiac function. Nagele et al[21] have reported that CA 125 values reflect heart failure status and the response to treatment in patients with congestive heart failure.

Limitations Elevations of CA 125 are also found in carcinomas of the fallopian tube, endometrium, pancreas, lung, breast, prostate, and gastrointestinal tract.[1] Elevated values have also been reported in mesothelioma,[22] primary peritoneal carcinoma,[23] and rhabdomyosarcoma of the uterus.[24] Benign diseases in which elevations are reported[1] include endometriosis, liver disease, pregnancy, pelvic inflammatory disease, ovarian cysts, tuberculous peritonitis,[25] Meigs syndrome,[26] and pseudo-Meigs syndrome.[27]

Biologic variability: Recently reported[28] is a patient with probable pelvic endometriosis whose serum CA 125 was >1000 kU/L in a specimen obtained during the menstrual phase of her cycle. The serum CA 125 then fell markedly, but not into the normal range, during the luteal and premenstrual phases. Therefore, appropriate interpretation of CA 125 values may require knowledge of menstrual cycle status.

Methodology Enzyme immunoassay (EIA), radioimmunoassay (RIA), immunoradiometric assay (IRMA), microparticle enzyme immunoassay (MEIA)

Additional Information A newly described assay for lysophosphatidic acid may have better sensitivity than CA 125 in early ovarian cancer. See Lysophosphatidic Acid, Plasma *on page 220.*

Footnotes

1. Chan DW and Sell S, "Tumor Markers," *Tietz Textbook of Clinical Chemistry*, 3rd ed, Burtis CA and Ashwood ER, eds, Philadelphia, PA: WB Saunders Co, 1999, 738.

2. Bidart JM, Thuillier F, Augereau C, et al, "Kinetics of Serum Tumor Marker Concentrations and Usefulness in Clinical Monitoring," *Clin Chem*, 1999, 45:1695-1707.

3. Nap M, "Immunohistochemistry of CA 125. Unusual Expression in Normal Tissues, Distribution in the Human Fetus and Questions About Its Application in Diagnostic Pathology," *Int J Biol Markers*, 1998, 13(4):210-5.

4. Morgensen O, Brock A, and Nyland MH, "CA 125 Measurements in Ovarian Cancer Patients During Their First Postoperative Week," *Int J Gynecol Cancer*, 1993, 3:54-6.

5. Yedema CA, Kenemans P, Thomas CM, et al, "CA 125 Levels in the Early Postoperative Period Do Not Reflect Tumour Reduction Obtained by Cytoreductive Surgery," *Eur J Cancer*, 1993, 29A(7):966-71.

6. Rosman M, Hayden CL, Thiel RP, et al, "Prognostic Indicators for Poor Risk Epithelial Ovarian Carcinoma," *Cancer*, 1994, 74(4):1323-8.

7. Buller RE, Beman ML, Bloss JD, et al, "CA 125 Regression: A Model for Epithelial Ovarian Cancer Response," *Am J Obstet Gynecol*, 1991, 165(2):360-7.

8. Hawkins RE, Roberts K, Wiltshaw E, et al, "The Prognostic Significance of the Half-Life of Serum CA 125 in Patients Responding to Chemotherapy for Epithelial Ovarian Cancer," *Br J Obstet Gynaecol*, 1989, 96:1395-9.

9. Hunter VJ, Daly L, Helms M, et al, "The Prognostic Significance of CA 125 Half-Life in Patients With Ovarian Cancer Who Have Received Primary Chemotherapy After Surgical Cytoreduction," *Am J Obstet Gynecol*, 1990, 163(4):1164-7.

10. Gadducci A, Zola P, Landoni FT, et al, "Serum Half-Life of CA 125 During Early Chemotherapy as an Independent Prognostic Variable for Patients With Advanced Epithelial Ovarian Cancer: Results of a Multicentric Italian Study," *Gynecol Oncol*, 1995, 58(1):42-7.

11. Miller AB, Hoogstraten B, Staquet M, et al, "Reporting Results of Cancer Treatment," *Cancer*, 1981, 47(1):207-14.

12. Rustin GJ, Nelstrop AE, McClean P, et al, "Defining Response of Ovarian Carcinoma to Initial Chemotherapy According to Serum CA 125," *J Clin Oncol*, 1996, 14(5):1545-51.

13. Bridgewater JA, Nelstrop AE, Rustin GS, et al, "Comparison of Standard and CA-125 Response Criteria in Patients With Epithelial Ovarian Cancer Treated With Platinum or Paclitaxel," *J Clin Oncol*, 1999, 17(2):501-8.

14. Bell R, Petticrew M, and Sheldon T, "The Performance of Screening Tests for Ovarian Cancer: Results of a Systematic Review," *Br J Obstet Gynaecol*, 1998, 105(11):1136-47.

15. Jeyarajah AR, Ind TE, Skates S, et al, "Serum CA 125 Elevation and Risk of Clinical Detection of Cancer in Asymptomatic Postmenopausal Women," *Cancer*, 1999, 85(9):2068-72.

16. Jacobs IJ, Skates SJ, MacDonald N, et al, "Screening for Ovarian Cancer: A Pilot Randomised Controlled Trial," *Lancet*, 1999, 353(9160):1207-10.

17. Crayford TJ, Campbell S, Bourne TH, et al, "Benign Ovarian Cysts and Ovarian Cancer: A Cohort Study With Implications for Screening," *Lancet*, 2000, 355(9209):1060-3.

18. Scully RE, "Influence of Origin of Ovarian Cancer on Efficacy of Screening," *Lancet*, 2000, 355(9209):1028-9.

19. Kurihara T, Mizunuma KT, Obara N, et al, "Determination of Normal Level of Serum CA 125 in Postmenopausal Women as a Tool for Preoperative Evaluation and Postoperative Surveillance of Endometrial Carcinoma," *Gynecol Oncol*, 1998, 69(3):192-6.

20. Sood AK, Buller RE, Burger RA, et al, "Value of Preoperative CA 125 Level in the Management of Uterine Cancer and the Prediction of Clinical Outcome," *Obstet Gynecol*, 1997, 90(3):441-7.

21. Nagele H, Bahlo M, Klapdor R, et al, "CA 125 and its Relation to Cardiac Function," *Am Heart J*, 1999, 137(6):1044-9.

22. Almudevar BE, Garcia-Rostan PGM, Bragado F, et al, "Prognostic Value of High Serum Levels of CA-125 in Malignant Secretory Peritoneal Mesotheliomas Affecting Young Women. A Case Report With Differential Diagnosis and Review of the Literature," *Histopathology*, 1997, 31:267-73.

23. Whitcomb BP, Kost ER, Hines JF, et al, "Primary Peritoneal Psammocarcinoma. A Case Presenting With an Upper Abdominal Mass and Elevated CA-125," *Gynecol Oncol*, 1999, 73(2):331-4.

24. Chiarle R, Godio L, Fusi D, et al, "Pure Alveolar Rhabdomyosarcoma of the Corpus Uteri: Description of a Case With Increased Serum Level of CA-125," *Gynecol Oncol*, 1997, 66(2):320-3.

25. Ibrahim G, Gelzayd B, DeMatia F, et al, "CA 125 Tumor-Associated Antigen in a Patient With Tuberculous Peritonitis," *Soyth Med J*, 1999, 92(11):1103-4.

26. Abad A, Cazorla E, Ruiz F, et al, "Meigs' Syndrome With Elevated CA 125: Case Report and Review of Literature," *Europ J Obstet Gynecol Reprod Biol*, 1999, 82(1):97-9.

27. Dunn JS, Anderson CD, Method MW, et al, "Hydropic Degenerating Leiomyoma Presenting as Pseudo-Meigs Syndrome With Elevated CA 125," *Obstet Gynecol*, 1998, 92(4 Pt 2):648-9.

28. Imai A, Horibe S, Takagi A, et al, "Drastic Elevation of Serum CA 125, CA 72-4, and CA 19-9 Levels During Menses in a Patient With Probable Endometriosis," *Eur J Obstet Gynecol Reprod Biol*, 1998, 78(1):79-81.

References

Ozols RF, Schwartz PE, and Eifel PJ, "Ovarian Cancer, Fallopian Tube Carcinoma and Peritoneal Carcinoma," De Vita VT, Hellman S, Rosenberg SA, eds, *Cancer: Principles and Practice of Oncology*, 5th ed, Philadelphia, PA: Lippincott-Raven, 1997, 1502-11.

CA 15-3, Serum

Related Information
Body Fluid Chemical Analysis *on page 123*
Breast Biopsy *on page 51*
Breast Cancer, Hereditary, BRCA1, BRCA2 *on page 722*
CA 125, Serum *on page 126*
Carcinoembryonic Antigen, Serum *on page 135*

Synonyms Cancer Antigen 15-3; Carbohydrate Antigen 15-3; *MUC1*; Polymorphic Epithelial Mucin

Abstract CA 15-3 has been proposed as a biomarker for breast cancer. The substance actually measured in assays labeled CA 15-3 is a glycoprotein product of the *MUC1* gene, variously known as CA 15-3, polymorphic epithelial mucin (PEM), DF3 and *MUC1*[1] CA 15-3 is the designation most often found in the medical literature. This glycoprotein is normally found in most glandular epithelial cells and in normal serum. It is overexpressed in many carcinomas, including both adenocarcinomas and squamous carcinomas.[2,3,4] Such overexpression often results in increased serum levels of CA 15-3. The original CA 15-3 assays, employing radioactive and enzyme labels, use monoclonal antibodies directed against two epitopes of *MUC1*. A newer assay,[5] with a chemiluminescence label, uses a single antibody.

Specimen Serum

Container Red top tube

Storage Instructions Refrigerate serum. Stable at 4°C for 2 weeks. For long-term storage, hold frozen at -70°C.

Reference Interval Usually stated as <30 kU/L, but actually method dependent, with cutoff values ranging from <26 kU/L to <39 kU/L.[5]

Use No established usefulness at this time. There is no evidence that CA 15-3 is useful in screening, diagnosis, or staging of breast cancer. Proposals, based largely on theoretical considerations, that CA 15-3 would be useful in patients with breast cancer by 1) detecting relapse, recurrence, and metastasis, and 2) monitoring the response to therapy, have **not** been confirmed. In a prospective study of 664 patients, each with 6 months of follow-up, CA 15-3 values had a positive predictive value of only 27% and a negative predictive value of 91% in the detection of relapse.[6]

Other investigators have reported, more optimistically, that when a battery of tests (including CA 15-3 result, HER-2/neu status, and CEA result) are run, the results of the battery were the first sign of recurrence in 69.5% of patients.[7]

An earlier study of a three-marker battery (CA 15-3, CEA, and tissue polypeptide antigen (TPA)) concluded that this battery allowed the earlier detection of progressive disease,[8] but the clinical significance of this finding is not clear. Attempts to use multiple CA 15-3 measurements in kinetic models (marker half-life and doubling time) have **not** yet been shown clinically effective.[9]

According to the practice guidelines for breast cancer from the American Society of Clinical Oncology (ASCO), CA 15-3 is **not** recommended for screening, diagnosis, staging, or surveillance following primary treatment. CA 15-3 is also **not** recommended by ASCO as a stand-alone monitor of response to treatment; one potential exception is that in patients who have

(Continued)

CA 15-3, Serum (Continued)

no readily measurable disease to follow, rising levels of CA 15-3 are suggestive of treatment failure.[10,11]

Limitations Elevations occur in benign diseases of the breast and liver. See Use and footnotes 10 and 11.

Methodology Radioimmunoassay (RIA), enzyme-linked immunosorbent assay (ELISA), microparticle enzyme immunoassay (MEIA), and chemiluminescent immunoassay (CIA)[5]

Footnotes

1. Miles DW and Taylor-Papadimitriou J, "Therapeutic Aspects of Polymorphic Epithelial Mucin in Adenocarcinoma," *Pharmacol Ther*, 1999, 82(1):97-106.
2. Ikeda Y, Kuwano H, Ikebe M, et al, "Immunohistochemical Detection of CEA, CA 19-9, and DF3 in Esophageal Carcinoma Limited to the Submucosal Layer," *J Surg Oncol*, 1994, 56(1):7-12.
3. McGuckin M, Walsh M, Hohn BG, et al, "Prognostic Significance of *MUC1* Epithelial Mucin Expression in Breast Cancer," *Hum Pathol*, 1995, 26(4):432-9.
4. Nitta T, Sugihara K, Tsuyama S, et al, "Immunohistological Study of *MUC1* in Premalignant Oral Lesions and Oral Squamous Carcinoma," *Cancer*, 2000, 88(2):245-54.
5. Bon GB, von Mensdorff-Pouilly S, Kenemans P, et al, "Clinical and Technical Evaluation of ACS BR Serum Assay of *MUC1* Gene-Derived Glycoprotein in Breast Cancer, and Comparison With CA 15-3 Assays," *Clin Chem*, 1997, 43(4):585-93.
6. Sutterlin M, Bussen S, Trott S, et al, "Predictive Value of CEA and CA 15-3 in the Follow-up of Invasive Breast Cancer," *Anticancer Res*, 1999, 19(4A):2567-70.
7. Molina R, Jo J, Filella X, et al, C-erbB-2, CEA, and CA 15-3 Serum Levels in the Early Diagnosis of Recurrence of Breast Cancer Patients," *Anticancer Res*, 1999, 19(4A):2551-5.
8. Soletormos G, Nielsen D, Schioler V, et al, "Tumor Markers Cancer Antigen 15-3, Carcinoembryonic Antigen, and Tissue Polypeptide Antigen for Monitoring Metastatic Breast Cancer During First-Line Chemotherapy and Follow-up," *Clin Chem*, 1996, 42(4):564-5.
9. Bidart JM, Thuillier F, Augereau C, et al, "Kinetics of Serum Tumor Marker Concentrations and Usefulness in Clinical Monitoring," *Clin Chem*, 1999, 45:1695-1707.
10. "Clinical Practice Guidelines for the Use of Tumor Markers in Breast and Colorectal Cancer Adopted on May 17, 1996 by the American Society of Clinical Oncology," *J Clin Oncol*, 1996, 14:2843-77.
11. Smith TJ, Davidson NE, Schapira DV, et al, "American Society of Clinical Oncology 1998 Update of Recommended Breast Cancer Surveillance Guidelines," *J Clin Oncol*, 1999, 17:1080-2.

CA 19-9, Serum

Related Information

Alpha$_1$-Fetoprotein, Serum *on page 97*
Body Fluid Chemical Analysis *on page 123*
CA 15-3, Serum *on page 127*
CA 125, Serum *on page 126*
Carcinoembryonic Antigen, Serum *on page 135*
Fine Needle Aspiration, Deep Masses *on page 381*
Immunoperoxidase Procedures *on page 60*

Synonyms Cancer Antigen 19-9; Carbohydrate Antigen 19-9

Applies to CA 50; CA 242; TAG-72; Tissue Polypeptide Antigen; TPA

Abstract Proposed as a marker for pancreatic carcinoma (and occasionally for colorectal and hepatocellular carcinomas), CA 19-9 can be measured in serum and body fluids and can be localized by immunohistology. The concentration of CA 19-9 in blood and body fluids is strongly influenced by the patient's Lewis blood group phenotype, secretor genotype, and gender. CA 19-9 is synthesized by a wide range of epithelial tissues, including colonic, pancreatic, biliary, gastrointestinal, salivary, and endometrial; however, CA 19-9 is not synthesized in persons who have the Le (a-b-) phenotype.

Specimen Serum

Container Red top tube

Storage Instructions Freeze to ship.

Reference Interval

- Detection, diagnosis, and prognosis of pancreatic cancer. Most commonly reported is the arbitrary cutoff of <37 kU/L, but <35 kU/L and <40 kU/L also are used. When the patient's Lewis blood group genotype and secretor genotype are taken into account, the cutoff values range from <10.3 kU/L (in *Le/le*, *Se/Se* individuals) to <61.3 kU/L (in *Le/Le*, *se/se* individuals).[1]
- Monitoring the effectiveness of cancer treatment and the potential for recurrence. In this situation, the patient's current value(s) is usually compared with his/her previous value(s), obviating the need to resort to an arbitrary cutoff.

Use According to the 1997 update of the clinical practice guidelines of the American Society of Clinical Oncology (ASCO), CA 19-9 is **not** recommended for "screening, diagnosis, staging, surveillance, or monitoring treatment of patients with colorectal cancer."[2]

Elevated values (>37 kU/L) are reported in 75% to 80% of pancreatic carcinomas,[3,4] 67% of hepatobiliary carcinomas, and <50% of gastric and hepatocellular carcinomas. The Mayo Clinic reports that CA 19-9 values >200 kU/L in a nonjaundiced patient with a "confirming" CT scan are highly predictive of pancreatic carcinoma.[5] In addition, this group and others[6,7] use CA 19-9 values to monitor the response to therapy and to predict disease-free survival and median survival following pancreatic resection.

In a study of carcinomas of the pancreatic head and periampullary region, CA 19-9 values were useful in assessing both resectability and prognosis.[8] In this study, the cutoff value was 35 kU/L, but that difference does not appear to change the impact of the results. Similar to the results with surgical treatment, CA 19-9 is reported to be of prognostic value in patients receiving primary radiation therapy.[9] CA 19-9 can be measured in bile obtained via percutaneous stents. In this setting,[10] values of 34,379-5,000,000 kU/L of bile were associated with liver metastases, while values of 6620-239,880 kU/L were found in patients without liver metastases. The biologic variability (both intraindividual and interindividual) of CA 19-9 is high. When CA 19-9 values are used to monitor treatment, the current values are compared to previous values from the same patient. Based on data from an asymptomatic white population, sequential values should differ by at least 40% to 50% in order to conclude that a significant change has occurred.[1]

Limitations

Nonspecificity: Marked elevations of CA 19-9 are common in patients with acute liver failure, regardless of etiology.[11] Such high values are believed to reflect hepatocellular regeneration, and they should not be interpreted as a reason to delay liver transplantation in otherwise appropriate candidates.[12] Elevated CA 19-9 values have been reported in a wide variety of benign processes, including endometriosis, Sjögren syndrome, inflammatory hepatic pseudotumor, idiopathic pulmonary fibrosis, splenic cyst, bronchogenic cyst of the esophagus, cystadenoma of the hepatic duct, chronic pancreatitis, allergic bronchopulmonary aspergillosis, autoimmune hepatitis, and xanthogranulomatous cholecystitis.[13] Elevated values are also reported in a number of malignancies, further diminishing the specificity of this test.[13]

Population distribution: CA 19-9 is absent from the serum (and other body fluids) of individuals who have the Le(a-b-) phenotype. This phenotype is found in ~6% of the U.S. white population and 22% of the U.S. black population.[14] Women have higher CA 19-9 values than men.[1]

Methodology Immunoradiometric assay (IRMA), microparticle enzyme immunoassay (MEIA), and chemiluminescence enzyme immunoassay

Footnotes

1. Vestergaard EM, Hein HO, Meyer H, et al, "Reference Values and Biological Variation for Tumor Marker CA 19-9 in Serum for Different Lewis and Secretor Genotypes and Evaluation of Secretor and Lewis Genotyping in a Caucasian Population," *Clin Chem*, 1999; 45:54-61.
2. "1997 Update of Recommendations for the Use of Tumor Markers in Breast and Colorectal Cancer," Adopted November 7, 1997 by the American Society of Clinical Oncology, *J Clin Oncol*, 1998, 16(2):793-5.
3. Chan DW and Sell S, "Tumor Markers," *Tietz Textbook of Clinical Chemistry*, 3rd ed, Burtis CA and Ashwood E, eds, Philadelphia, PA: WB Saunders Co, 1999, 738-9.
4. Kim HJ, Kim MH, Myung SJ, et al, "A New Strategy for the Application of CA 19-9 in the Differentiation of Pancreaticobiliary Cancer: Analysis Using a Receiver Operating Characteristic Curve," *Am J Gastroenterol*, 1999, 94(7):1941-6.
5. Ritts RE and Pitt HA, "CA 19-9 in Pancreatic Cancer," *Surg Oncol Clin N Am*, 1998, 7(1):93-101.
6. Montgomery RC, Hoffman JP, Riley LB, et al, "Prediction of Recurrence and Survival by Postresection CA 19-9 Values in Patients With Adenocarcinoma of the Pancreas," *Ann Surg Oncol*, 1997, 4(7):551-6.
7. Safi F, Schlosser W, Falkenreck S, et al, "Prognostic Value of CA 19-9 Serum Course in Pancreatic Cancer," *Hepatogastroenterology*, 1998, 45(19):253-9.
8. Kau SY, Shyr YM, Su CH, et al, "Diagnostic and Prognostic Values of CA 19-9 and CEA in Periampullary Cancers," *J Am Coll Surg*, 1999, 188(4):415-20.
9. Katz A, Hanlon A, Lanciano R, et al, "Prognostic Value of CA 19-9 Levels in Patients With Carcinoma of the Pancreas Treated With Radiotherapy," *Int J Radiat Oncol Biol Phys*, 1998, 41(2):393-6.
10. Montgomery RC, Hoffma JP, Ross EA, et al, "Biliary CA 19-9 Values Correlate With the Risk of Hepatic Metastases in Patients With Adenocarcinoma of the Pancreas," *J Gastrointest Surg*, 1998, 2(1):28-35.
11. Maestranzi S, Przemioslo R, and Sherwood RA, "The Effect of Benign and Malignant Liver Disease on the Tumour Markers CA 19-9 and CEA," *Ann Clin Biochem*, 1998, 35(Pt 1):99-103.
12. Halme L, Karkkainen P, Isoniemi H, et al, "Carbohydrate 19-9 Antigen as a Marker of Nonmalignant Hepatocytic Ductular Transformation in Patients With Acute Liver Failure. A Comparison With Alpha-Fetoprotein and Carcinoembryonic Antigen," *Scand J Gastroenterol*, 1999, 34(4):426-31.
13. McLaughlin R, O'Hanlon D, Kerin M, et al, "Are Elevated Levels of the Tumor Marker CA 19-9 of any Clinical Significance?: An Evaluation," *Ir J Med Sci*, 1999, 168(2):124-6.
14. American Association of Blood Banks, *Technical Manual*, 13th ed, Bethesda, MD: American Association of Blood Banks Press, 1999, 286-7.

References

Nishida K, Kaneko T, Yoneda M, et al, "Doubling Time of Serum CA 19-9 in the Clinical Course of Patients With Pancreatic Cancer and its Significant Association With Prognosis," *J Surg Oncol*, 1999, 71(3):140-6.

CA 27.29, Serum

Related Information

Body Cavity Fluid Cytology *on page 372*
Breast Biopsy *on page 51*
Breast Cancer, Hereditary, BRCA1, BRCA2 *on page 722*
CA 15-3, Serum *on page 127*
Carcinoembryonic Antigen, Serum *on page 135*
Fine Needle Aspiration, Deep Masses *on page 381*
Sentinel Lymph Node Biopsy *on page 70*

Synonyms Breast Carcinoma-Associated Antigen; Cancer Antigen 27.29

Applies to *MUC1* Gene

Test Includes Long-term serial monitoring of results

Abstract CA 27.29 is a tumor marker used for detection of breast cancer recurrence. It is an antigen defined by a monoclonal antibody (B27.29) specific to the protein core of the breast-cancer-associated mucin encoded by the *MUC1* gene.

Specimen Serum

Container Red top tube

Storage Instructions Refrigerate or freeze specimen according to directions of testing laboratory.

Reference Interval ≤37.7 units/mL (SI: ≤37.7 kU/L)[1]

Use CA 27.29 is used for the monitoring of the recurrence of breast carcinoma in patients diagnosed with stage II or III disease.[1]

Limitations CA 27.29 testing is not approved for screening. In addition, according to the American Society of Clinical Oncology, there is insufficient basis to recommend use of this tumor marker for routine breast cancer surveillance.[2]

Methodology Radioimmunoassay (RIA), chemiluminescent immunoassay

Additional Information The *MUC1* gene product is a large glycoprotein known as polymorphic epithelial mucin. It is expressed on the ductal cell surface of glandular epithelia and is released into blood in increased amounts in patients with breast cancer. In addition to CA 27.29, other monoclonal-antibody-defined markers to the *MUC1* gene product exist (eg, the more extensively studied CA 15-3, Serum *on page 127*).

The CA 27.29 assay, in a multicenter study, was shown to have a sensitivity of 57.7%, specificity of 97.9%, positive predictive value of 83.3%, and negative predictive value of 92.6% for detection of breast cancer recurrence in a group of 166 patients previously diagnosed with either stage II (80.1% of study population) or III (19.9% of study population) disease.[1] A retrospective study of 275 primary breast cancer patients and 83 healthy controls showed CA 27.29 to have better discriminating power than CA 15.3 in differentiating these populations.[3]

Footnotes

1. Chan DW, Beveridge RA, Muss H, et al, "Use of the Truquant BR Radioimmunoassay for Early Detection of Breast Cancer Recurrence in Patients With Stage II and Stage III Disease," *J Clin Oncol*, 1997, 15(6):2322-8.
2. Smith TJ, Davidson NE, Schapira DV, et al, "American Society of Clinical Oncology 1998 Update of Recommended Breast Cancer Surveillance Guidelines," *J Clin Oncol*, 1999, 17(3):1080-2.
3. Gion M, Mione R, Leon AE, et al, "Comparison of the Diagnostic Accuracy of CA 27.29 and CA 15-3 in Primary Breast Cancer," *Clin Chem*, 1999, 45(5):630-7.

References

Bon GG, von Mensdorff-Pouilly S, Kenemans P, et al, "Clinical and Technical Evaluation of ACS™BR Serum Assay of *MUC1* Gene-Derived Glycoprotein in Breast Cancer, and Comparison With CA 15-3 Assays," *Clin Chem*, 1997, 43(4):585-93.

Chan DW and Sell S, "Tumor Markers," *Tietz Textbook of Clinical Chemistry*, 3rd ed, Chapter 23, Burtis CA and Ashwood ER, eds, Philadelphia, PA: WB Saunders Co, 1999, 722-49.

Cheung KL, Graves CR, and Robertson JF, "Tumour Marker Measurement in the Diagnosis and Monitoring of Breast Cancer," *Cancer Treat Rev*, 2000, 26(2):91-102.

Calcitonin, Serum or Plasma

Related Information

Synonyms Thyrocalcitonin

Applies to Calcium Stimulation Test; Chromogronin A, Serum; MEN A; MEN B; Pentagastrin Stimulation Test; Sipple Syndrome

Abstract Calcitonin is a hypocalcemic polypeptide made by the C cells (parafollicular cells) of the thyroid gland, by tumors of the C cells (medullary carcinoma of thyroid - MCT), and by certain other neoplasms (lung, breast, kidney, liver, pancreas).

Patient Preparation Patient should fast overnight. Avoid recent isotope scan or other exposure to radioactivity.

Specimen Serum or plasma

Container Red top tube or green top (heparin) tube

Collection Avoid hemolysis.

Storage Instructions Collect into chilled tube. Process within 10 minutes of collection. Separate in a refrigerated centrifuge. Separate serum (plasma) into plastic tube and freeze.

Causes for Rejection Sample not kept chilled during collection and transportation to the laboratory

Reference Interval <19 pg/mL (SI: <19 ng/L) basal for a sensitive RIA assay or column chromatography. Normal ranges for calcium/pentagastrin stimulation tests are available. For stimulation tests, values <350 pg/mL in men and <100 pg/mL in women are expected.

Possible Panic Range Elevated levels are not diagnostic of medullary carcinoma of thyroid (MCT), because elevations have been described in other circumstances.[1] However, some patients with MCT have values >500 pg/mL.

Use MCT is a distinctive type of neuroendocrine carcinoma. About 80% of cases are sporadic. Calcitonin concentrations are increased in both the sporadic and the familial types of MCT and in its precursors, C-cell hyperplasia and microscopic medullary carcinoma. Among the most significant of tumor markers, calcitonin levels roughly correlate with tumor burden[2] and the degree of tumor differentiation, and are used in postoperative patients with CEA to monitor residual, recurrent, and/or metastatic carcinoma. Recurrent or persistent postoperative elevation reliably indicates tumor persistence or relapse. Serum chromogranin A is increased as well with MCT.

Calcitonin concentrations may be returned to normal in up to 25% of selected patients with compartment-oriented lymphadenectomy in patients with primary or recurrent MCT.[3] Postoperative levels have prognostic application.

Multiple endocrine neoplasia (MEN) type 2A includes medullary carcinoma of thyroid, pheochromocytoma, and sometimes, parathyroid adenoma (Sipple syndrome). MEN type 2B includes medullary carcinoma of thyroid, pheochromocytoma, mucosal neuromas, marfanoid habitus, and intestinal ganglioneuromatosis. Medullary carcinoma is found without such other tumors in familial medullary carcinoma (FMTC). FMCT is an autosomal dominant of virtually complete penetrance.

Another important use of calcitonin assay is investigation of families to detect early, subclinical cases of C-cell hyperplasia or MCT. Indications for calcitonin assay include family history of unspecified type of thyroid cancer, amyloid-containing metastatic carcinoma of unknown primary site and the presence of mucosal neuromas.

Limitations In numbers of patients with MCT (especially those with FMCT) the baseline calcitonin may be normal; however, an abnormally large calcitonin response may follow secretagogues, provocative infusion of calcium and/or pentagastrin.[4,5,6] A combined calcium pentagastrin test is described. These tests are much more useful than random plasma levels of calcitonin for the diagnosis of MCT. Most subjects with microscopic medullary carcinoma and all with C-cell hyperplasia have normal basal calcitonin levels; provocative testing is needed. However, false-negative pentagastrin stimulation tests occur in individuals with the positive RET mutation and/or linkage analysis who have MEN IIA and FMTC. Patients from RET-negative kindreds with negative linkage analysis need pentagastrin-stimulation follow-up testing.[7] Serum calcitonin levels usually cannot differentiate between C-cell hyperplasia alone, and that complicated by emerging microscopic MCT.

Occasional spurious high results are encountered. Hemolysis can cause spurious high levels. Misleading results are recognized. The purity of standards may vary and antibodies in various assays may lack uniform specificities. Calcitonin in patients' sera lacks immunoreactive uniformity. Side effects take place.

DNA analysis identifies carriers of MEN 2A without ambiguity.[8] Molecular genetic techniques are available. See Multiple Endocrine Neoplasia/Familial Medullary Thyroid Carcinoma *on page 727*.

Methodology Radioimmunoassay (RIA), immunoradiometric assay (IRMA)[9] or enzyme immunoassay (EIA),[10] chemiluminescent enzyme immunoassay[11]

Additional Information High concentrations of calcitonin occur not only in patients with malignant parafollicular or C-cell tumors (medullary thyroid carcinoma) but may also be found in patients with small cell carcinomas of the lung; carcinoids; in some individuals with carcinoma of breast, islet cell tumors, amine precursor uptake and decarboxylation cell tumors (APUDomas), in patients with pancreatitis, thyroiditis,[12] and in renal failure. Hypergastrinemia may account for calcitonin elevations in the Zollinger-Ellison syndrome and in pernicious anemia. Medullary carcinoma arises from thyroid C cells (parafollicular cells). C-cell hyperplasia is a preneoplastic state in patients with MEN. Early diagnosis of MCT is needed; total thyroidectomy is curative if the tumor is treated early.

Calcitonin was increased in 48% of patients with small cell (oat cell) carcinoma in a study of 110 patients with lung cancer.

Calcitonin gene-related peptide (CGRP) has been suggested as a useful test together with calcitonin, as tumor markers in MEN type 2.[13]

CEA is next most useful, after calcitonin, as a marker for medullary carcinoma. CEA generates less fluctuation than calcitonin in calculation of doubling time. Histaminase is elevated in most patients with medullary carcinoma. Medullary carcinomas may produce other substances, including (Continued)

Calcitonin, Serum or Plasma (Continued)

ACTH and serotonin. Such ectopic ACTH secretion may cause Cushing syndrome.

If there are preoperative findings to suggest MCT (eg, family history of unspecified type of thyroid cancer) in a patient with a thyroid mass, then calcitonin level, metanephrines, catecholamines, and CAT scan of the adrenals for pheochromocytoma should be considered. Medullary carcinomas of the thyroid gland have a variable histologic picture. Correlation between serum calcitonin levels and immunoperoxidase staining of the neoplastic thyroid tissue for calcitonin chromogranin and CEA assist in confirmation of diagnosis in difficult cases.

The direct manifestation of high calcitonin levels is secretory diarrhea in 30% of patients with medullary thyroid carcinoma.

Increased calcitonin has been found in systemic mast cell disease.[14]

The prohormone of calcitonin is procalcitonin. This substance is considered an acute-phase protein.[15]

Footnotes

1. Lamb EJ, Heddle RM, and Ellis A, "Spuriously Elevated Plasma Calcitonin in a Patient With a Thyroid Nodule Not Associated With Medullary Thyroid Carcinoma," *Postgrad Med*, 1999, 75(883):289-90.
2. Tisell LE, Dilley WG, and Wells SA Jr, "Progression of Postoperative Residual Medullary Thyroid Carcinoma as Monitored by Plasma Calcitonin Levels," *Surgery*, 1996, 119(1):34-9.
3. Fleming JB, Lee JE, Bouvet M, et al, "Surgical Strategy for the Treatment of Medullary Thyroid Carcinoma," *Ann Surg*, 1999, 230(5):697-707.
4. Scheuba C, Kaserer K, Weinhausl A, et al, "Is Medullary Thyroid Cancer Predictable? A Prospective Study of 86 Patients With Abnormal Pentagastrin Tests," *Surgery*, 1999, 126(6):1089-95.
5. Vierhapper H, Raber W, Bieglmayer C, et al, "Routine Measurement of Plasma Calcitonin in Nodular Thyroid Diseases," *J Clin Endocrinol Metab*, 1997, 82(5):1589-93.
6. Guilloteau D, Perdrisot R, Calmettes C, et al, "Diagnosis of Medullary Carcinoma of the Thyroid (MCT) by Calcitonin Assay Using Monoclonal Antibodies: Criteria for the Pentagastrin Stimulation Test in Hereditary MCT," *J Clin Endocrinol Metab*, 1990, 71(4):1064-7.
7. Heshmati HM, Gharib H, Khosla S, et al, "Genetic Testing in Medullary Thyroid Carcinoma Syndromes: Mutation Types and Clinical Significance," <*Mayo Clin Proc*, 1997, 72(5):430-6.
8. Lips CJ, Landsvater RM, Höppener JW, et al, "Clinical Screening as Compared With DNA Analysis in Families With Multiple Endocrine Neoplasms Type 2A," *N Engl J Med*, 1994, 331(13):828-35.
9. Perdrisot R, Bigorgne JC, Guilloteau D, et al, "Monoclonal Immunoradiometric Assay of Calcitonin Improves Investigation of Familial Medullary Thyroid Carcinoma," *Clin Chem*, 1990, 36(2):381-3.
10. Seth R and Motte P, "A Sensitive and Specific Two-Site Enzyme-Immunoassay for Human Calcitonin Using Monoclonal Antibodies," *J Endocrinol*, 1988, 119:351-7.
11. Isomura M, Honda N, Kawada A, et al, "Development of a Highly Sensitive Enzyme Immunoassay for Human Calcitonin Using Solid Phase Coupled With Multiple Antibodies," *Ann Clin Biochem*, 1999, 36(Pt 5):629-35.
12. Borges MF, Abelin NM, Menezes FO, et al, "Calcitonin Deficiency in Early Stages of Chronic Autoimmune Thyroiditis," *Clin Endocrinol*, 1998, 49(1):69-75.
13. Schifter S, "Calcitonin Gene-Related Peptide and Calcitonin as Tumour Markers in MEN 2 Family Screening," *Clin Endocrinol (Oxf)*, 1989, 30(3):263-70.
14. Yocum MW, Butterfield JH, and Gharib H, "Increased Plasma Calcitonin Levels in Systemic Mast Cell Disease," *Mayo Clin Proc*, 1994, 69(10):987-90.
15. Nijsten MW, Olinga P, The TH, et al, "Procalcitonin Behaves as a Fast Responding Acute Phase Protein *In Vivo* and *In Vitro*," *Crit Care Med*, 2000, 28(2):458-61.

References

Boultwood J, Wynford-Thomas D, Richards GP, et al, "*In Situ* Analysis of Calcitonin and CGRP Expression in Medullary Thyroid Carcinoma," *Clin Endocrinol (Oxf)*, 1990, 33(3):381-90.

Carter WB, Taylor RL, Kao PC, et al, "Determination of Plasma Calcitonin Gene-Related Peptide Concentrations by a New Immunochemiluminometric Assay in Normal Persons and Patients With Medullary Thyroid Carcinoma and Other Neuroendocrine Tumors," *J Clin Endocrinol Metab*, 1991, 72(2):387-34.

Erdogan MF, Gullu S, Baskal N, et al, "Omeprazole: Calcitonin Stimulation Test for the Diagnosis Follow-up and Family Screening in Medullary Thyroid Carcinoma," *J Clin Endocrinol Metab*, 1997, 82(3):897-9.

Rosai J, Carcangiu ML, and DeLellis RA, "Tumors of the Thyroid Gland," *Atlas of Tumor Pathology*, Washington, DC: Armed Forces Institute of Pathology, 1992.

Rougier P, Calmettes C, LaPlanche A, et al, "The Values of Calcitonin and Carcinoembryonic Antigen in the Treatment and Management of Nonfamilial Medullary Thyroid Carcinoma," *Cancer*, 1983, 51:855-62.

Sanchez GJ, Venkataraman PS, Pryor RW, et al, "Hypercalcitoninemia and Hypocalcemia in Acutely Ill Children: Studies in Serum Calcium, Blood Ionized Calcium, and Calcium-Regulating Hormones," *J Pediatr*, 1989, 114(6):952-6.

♦ **Calcitriol** *see* Vitamin D, Serum *on page 300*

♦ **Calcium:Creatinine Ratio** *see* Calcium, Urine *on page 133*

Calcium, Ionized, Serum

Related Information

Calcium, Serum *on page 131*
Calcium, Urine *on page 133*
Kidney Stone Analysis *on page 877*
Parathyroid Hormone-Related Protein, Serum *on page 243*
Parathyroid Hormone, Serum *on page 243*

Synonyms Ionized Calcium

Abstract This is the physiologically active portion of serum calcium and represents about half of total serum calcium. The serum ionized calcium has a diurnal variation with minimum values at 8 PM and peak values at 10 AM. Since binding of free calcium to proteins is pH dependent, alkalosis decreases and acidosis increases ionized calcium concentrations.

Patient Preparation Patient should be recumbent for 30 minutes prior to collection.

Specimen Whole blood (preferred), serum, or plasma

Container Green top (heparin) tube if whole blood or plasma is used; red top tube for serum

Collection Collect anaerobically, leave stoppers in; do not use tourniquet. Heparin syringe is best; 1 unit of heparin/mL of blood lowers ionized calcium 0.01 mmol/L. The use of dry, electrolyte balanced heparin virtually eliminates the heparin interference.[1]

Storage Instructions Store anaerobically. Such specimens can be stored 48 hours at 4°C or 2 hours at room temperature.

Special Instructions Controversy exists over the ideal specimen for ionized calcium determination. Concern exists that ionized calcium values may be altered by clotting (serum) or by heparin binding of calcium (plasma). However, serum and plasma have been found to give generally similar values, while whole blood is 1% to 2% higher.

Most large laboratories have instrumentation (selective ion electrode) for direct measurement of ionized calcium. Adjusting pH to 7.4 is not necessary if blood is collected anaerobically.

Reference Interval See table.[2]

Calcium, Ionized, Serum

	Reference Range	
	Conventional (mg/dL)	SI (mmol/L)
Whole blood		
1 d	4.2-5.48	1.05-1.37
2-4 d	4.4-5.68	1.10-1.42
5 d	4.8-5.92	1.20-1.48
Adults	4.6-5.10	1.15-1.27
Plasma		
Adults	4.12-4.92	1.03-1.23
Serum		
1-18 y	4.8-5.52	1.20-1.38
Adults	4.64-5.28	1.16-1.32

Critical Values Replacement may begin when the ionized calcium value is <0.8 mmol/L.[3] Hypocalcemia may result in tetany or seizures.

Possible Panic Range <0.70 mmol/L[3]

Use Ionized calcium is a measure of physiologically active calcium fraction. Ionized calcium is increased in the same diseases that produce elevations in total serum calcium, of which the most important are hyperparathyroidism, cancer, and granulomatous diseases (see Calcium, Serum *on page 131*).

In a series of 60 proven cases of primary hyperparathyroidism, increased total calcium was found in only 47, but 59 cases had increased ionized calcium.[4] Ionized calcium is the more helpful test for evaluation of hyperparathyroidism and hypoparathyroidism.

Ionized calcium is measured in patients with renal failure and/or transplantation, in whom problems include secondary hyperparathyroidism. It is indicated for patients with sepsis, with magnesium deficiency, and in pancreatitis. Hypocalcemia occurs following administration of citrate (eg, liver transplantation) or infusion of other fluids during extracorporeal membrane oxygenation or surgery, and measurement of ionized calcium is needed to ascertain balance in dialysis patients.[3] Ionized calcium measurements are indicated in patients who are given rapid transfusions, as citrate present in blood or blood fractions chelates ionized calcium. In such situations, total calcium may be high and ionized calcium low. Therefore, a role for ionized calcium levels exists in patients undergoing surgery and transplantation.[5]

Ionized calcium is measured in premature infants with hypoproteinemia and acidosis. Occasionally useful when hypercalcemia coexists with abnormal protein state such as myeloma, in disturbances of acid base balance; in cirrhosis.

Low values are encountered in hypoparathyroidism, vitamin D deficiency and resistance, pseudohypoparathyroidism, and anxiety-related hyperventilation. Low or high in genetic abnormalities of the calcium-sensing receptor.

Methodology Ion-selective electrode (ISE)

Additional Information If an ionized calcium measurement is not available, it can be estimated by the following formula.[6]

Ionized Ca (mmol/L) = total Ca [TC] (mmol/L)
minus 0.00613 x TC x albumin (g/L)
minus 0.00244 x TC x globulin (g/L)
minus 0.0043 x TC x anion gap (mmol/L)
minus 0.00375 x TC x bicarbonate (mmol/L)

Measurement of serum ionized calcium provides insight into the effect of total protein and albumin on serum calcium levels. A patient can have high total calcium, with normal ionized calcium and increased total protein and/or albumin, as in dehydration or in myeloma.

Women have greater circadian variation of ionized calcium and intact PTH than men.[7]

An inverse relationship between ionized calcium and phosphate concentration exists.[8]

Footnotes

1. Toffaletti J, Ernst P, Hunt P, et al, "Dry Electrolyte-Balanced Heparinized Syringes Evaluated for Determining Ionized Calcium and Other Electrolytes in Whole Blood," *Clin Chem*, 1991, 37:(10 Pt 1)1730-3.
2. Painter PC, Cope JY, and Smith JL, "Reference Information for the Clinical Laboratory," *Tietz Textbook of Clinical Chemistry*, 3rd ed, Philadelphia, PA: WB Saunders Co, 1999, 1804.
3. Toffaletti J, "Physiology and Regulation. Ionized Calcium, Magnesium and Lactate Measurements in Critical Care Settings," *Am J Clin Pathol*, 1995, 104(4 Suppl 1):S88-94.
4. Glendenning P, Gutteridge DH, Retallack RW, et al, "High Prevalence of Normal Total Calcium and Intact PTH in 60 Patients With Proven Primary Hyperparathyroidism: A Challenge to Current Diagnostic Criteria," *Aust N Z J Med*, 1998, 28(2):173-8.
5. Diaz J, Acosta F, Parrilla P, et al, "Correlation Among Ionized Calcium, Citrate, and Total Calcium Levels During Hepatic Transplantation," *Clin Biochem*, 1995, 28(3):315-7.
6. Nordin BE, Need AG, Hartley TF, et al, "Improved Method for Calculating Calcium Fractions in Plasma: Reference Values and Effect of Menopause," *Clin Chem*, 1989, 35(1):14-7.
7. Calvo MS, Eastell R, Offord KP, et al, "Circadian Variation in Ionized Calcium and Intact Parathyroid Hormone: Evidence for Sex Differences in Calcium Homeostasis," *J Clin Endocrinol Metab*, 1991, 72(1):69-76.
8. Lehmann M and Mimouni F, "Serum Phosphate Concentration. Effect on Serum Ionized Calcium Concentration *In Vitro*," *Am J Dis Child*, 1989, 143(11):1340-1.

References

Baron J, Winer KK, Yanovski JA, et al, "Mutations in the Ca(2+)-Sensing Receptor Gene Cause Autosomal Dominant and Sporadic Hypoparathyroidism," *Hum Mol Genet*, 1996, 5(5):601-6.

Cole DE, Peltekova VD, Rubin LA, et al, "A986S Polymorphism of the Calcium-Sensing Receptor and Circulating Calcium Concentration," *Lancet*, 1999, 353(9147):112-5.

Dewitte K, Stockl D, and Thienpont LM, "pH Dependency of Serum Ionized Calcium," *Lancet*, 1999, 354(9192):1793-4.

Forman DT and Lorenzo L, "Ionized Calcium: Its Significance and Clinical Usefulness," *Ann Clin Lab Sci*, 1991, 21(5):297-304.

Goodman WG, Misra S, Veldhuis JD, et al, "Altered Diurnal Regulation of Blood Ionized Calcium and Serum Parathyroid Hormone Concentrations During Parenteral Nutrition," *Am J Clin Nutr*, 2000, 71(2):560-8.

Loughead JL, Mimouni F, and Tsang RC, "Serum Ionized Calcium Concentrations in Normal Neonates," *Am J Dis Child*, 1988, 142(5):516-8.

Rasmussen N, Frolich A, Hornnes PJ, et al, "Serum Ionized Calcium and Intact Parathyroid Hormone Levels During Pregnancy and Postpartum," *Br J Obstet Gynaecol*, 1990, 97(9):857-9.

Thode J, Holmegaard SN, Transbol I, et al, "Adjusted Ionized Calcium (at pH 7.4) and Actual Ionized Calcium (at Actual pH) in Capillary Blood Compared for Clinical Evaluation of Patients With Disorders of Calcium Metabolism," *Clin Chem*, 1990, 36(3):541-4.

◆ **Calcium Oxalate, Urine** *see* Oxalate, Urine *on page 238*

Calcium, Serum

Related Information

Aluminum, Bone and Bone Biopsy *on page 813*
Aluminum, Serum *on page 814*
Calcium, Ionized, Serum *on page 130*
Calcium, Urine *on page 133*
Concentration Test, Urine *on page 872*
Cyclic AMP, Urine *on page 163*
Hydroxyproline, Total, Urine *on page 199*
Kidney Stone Analysis *on page 877*
Magnesium, Serum *on page 221*
Magnesium, Urine *on page 222*
Multiple Endocrine Neoplasia/Familial Medullary Thyroid Carcinoma *on page 727*
Osteocalcin, Serum or Plasma *on page 237*
Parathyroid Hormone-Related Protein, Serum *on page 243*
Parathyroid Hormone, Serum *on page 243*
Phosphorus, Serum *on page 251*
Phosphorus, Urine *on page 253*
Potassium, Serum or Plasma *on page 258*
Pyridinolines (Pyridinoline and Deoxypyridinoline), Urine *on page 272*
Vitamin D, Serum *on page 300*

Synonyms Ca, Blood; Total Calcium, Serum

Applies to Chloride:Phosphorus Ratio; Parathyroid Hormone-Related Protein

Abstract Total plasma calcium has three components, protein-bound (47%), ionized (free - 43%), and complexed (10%). The extent of protein binding varies with protein concentrations and pH. The two most common causes of hypercalcemia are primary hyperparathyroidism (HPT) and malignancy.

Activation of osteoclasts by parathormone or parathyroid hormone-related protein leads to hypercalcemia through bone resorption.[1] Hypercalcemia is also a feature of certain granulomatous diseases (eg, sarcoidosis, cat-scratch disease, and lymphoma) which have in common the presence of elevated serum 1,25 dihydroxyvitamin D (1,25[OH]$_2$D). Such patients have granulomas with macrophages in which the enzyme 1-α hydroxylase (25-hydroxy-D-1 hydroxylase) facilitates the production of 1,25[OH]$_2$D.[2,3,4]

Specimen Serum

Container Red top tube

Sampling Time Morning, fasting sample is desirable. The diurnal variation has peaks at 5 PM and 4 AM.[5]

Collection Pediatrics: Blood drawn from heelstick for capillary. Since about half of serum calcium is bound to proteins, there is variation with posture. Venous stasis in sampling causes misleading results.

Storage Instructions Refrigerate in stoppered vials, not in sample cups.

Causes for Rejection Gross hemolysis

Reference Interval See table.[6]

	mg/dL	mmol/L
Cord	8.2-11.2	2.05-2.80
Premature	6.2-11.0	1.55-2.75
0-10 d	7.6-10.4	1.90-2.60
10 d to 24 mo	9.0-11.0	2.25-2.75
2-12 y	8.8-10.8	2.20-2.70
Adults	8.6-10.0	2.15-2.50
Male (>60 y)	8.8-10.2	2.20-2.55

These intervals apply to persons with normal serum albumin, since about 45% of serum calcium is bound to serum proteins. Although it is rarely necessary, the following formula may be used to adjust total serum calcium for abnormalities of albumin concentration.

adjusted calcium (mmol/L) = measured calcium (mmol/L) + 0.02 (mean normal albumin - measured albumin [g/L])[7]

Critical Values <7.0 mg/dL (SI: <1.75 mmol/L) may lead to tetany and in young children, seizures. Calcium >12.0 mg/dL (SI: >2.99 mmol/L)[8] may induce coma, although most patients tolerate higher levels. More commonly, hypercalcemia leads to polyuria, anorexia, nausea, and constipation.

Possible Panic Range Possibly life-threatening levels: ≤6.0 mg/dL (SI: ≤1.50 mmol/L); **severe hypercalcemia** is defined as ≥14.0 mg/dL (SI: ≥3.5 mmol/L). Extremely high levels may be found with primary parathyroid carcinomas in patients with malignancies and infants with Williams syndrome.

Use

Causes of High Calcium

- Primary hyperparathyroidism (HPT) - look also for high ionized calcium, measured or calculated, and hypophosphatemia. Hyperparathyroidism may coexist with other endocrine tumors (multiple endocrine adenomatosis syndromes). Individuals with hypercalcemia, elevated intact parathyroid hormone concentration, and normal renal function, with few exceptions, have primary hyperparathyroidism.[9]
- Carcinoma, with or without bone metastases.
  - Humoral hypercalcemia of malignancy (HHM), tumor-induced hypercalcemia in patients without bone metastases,[10] is seen especially in primary squamous cell carcinoma of lung, head and neck, but other important tumors include primaries in the breast, kidney, liver, bladder, and ovary. It is usually caused by **parathyroid hormone-related protein**, for which assays exist (see Parathyroid Hormone-Related Protein, Serum *on page 243*). PTH-related protein is now recognized as the cause of hypercalcemia in most solid tumors, particularly squamous and renal carcinomas.[11] A rare entity, humoral hypercalcemia of benignancy, is characterized by hypercalcemia with benign tumors associated with increased production of parathyroid hormone-related protein.[12]
  - The most common solid tumors causing bone metastases are primaries in the breast and lung. Other neoplasms may also cause hypercalcemia, especially myeloma. Differences between HPT and humoral hypercalcemia of malignancy include low 1,25[OH]$_2$D, reduced calcium absorption, and the presence of a nonparathyroid tumor. Hypercalcemia with alkaline phosphatase more than twice its upper limit is more suggestive of **cancer** than of hyperparathyroidism. Especially if there is only a brief duration of symptoms, anemia, increased LDH and alkaline phosphatase, hypoalbuminemia, and other findings suggestive of malignant disease, chloride:phosphorus ratio <29 mmol/L, chloride <100 mmol/L, high serum LD (LDH) and/or phosphorus, think first of malignant neoplasm.[13] **The chloride:phosphorus ratio** is predominantly of value when it is <29 mmol/L, to provide evidence **against** a diagnosis of primary hyperparathyroidism.[13]
- Myeloma, leukemia,[14] lymphoma; especially T-cell[15] lymphoma/leukemia and Burkitt lymphoma.
- Dehydration is an extremely common cause of slight increases of calcium.
- Sarcoidosis and other granulomatous diseases[2,3,4] All of these hypercalcemic patients have elevated 1,25[OH]$_2$D. About 50% have hypercalciuria. Other granulomatous diseases include tuberculosis,

(Continued)

Calcium, Serum (Continued)

histoplasmosis, berylliosis, silicosis, Wegener granulomatosis, Langerhans cell histiocytosis, coccidioidomycosis,[16] *Nocardia* infection,[17] leprosy, and *Pneumocystis pneumoniae*.

- Chronic hypervitaminosis D; ectopic production of 1,25-dihydroxy vitamin D_3; vitamin A intoxication, isotretinoin (a vitamin A derivative).[18]
- Prolonged immobilization (uncommon), in patient with increased bone turnover (eg, Paget disease of bone, malignancy, children).
- Milk-alkali syndrome: prolonged use of calcium-containing materials and alkali (eg, $CaCO_3$) or other absorbable alkali ulcer remedies with high milk intake (now rare).
- Idiopathic hypercalcemia of infancy, Williams syndrome (uncommon)
- Endocrine: hyperthyroidism; Addison disease; acromegaly; pheochromocytoma (rare cause of hypercalcemia); vasoactive intestinal polypeptide hormone-producing tumor
- Advanced chronic liver disease
- Bacteremia
- Familial hypocalciuric hypercalcemia[19] (dominant inheritance); the best test for familial benign hypercalciuria (FBH) is a plot of fasting serum PTH against fasting urine calcium excretion[20]
- Aluminum-induced renal osteodystrophy
- Parenteral nutrition
- Renal insufficiency
- Postrenal transplant
- Drugs: calcium salts, lithium, thiazide/chlorthalidone therapy, other diuretics; antiestrogens and estrogens (rapid increase in patients with breast carcinoma).

In any case of hypercalcemia, it is desirable to measure magnesium and potassium levels.

Causes of Low Calcium

- Low albumin and low total protein relate to common, usually slight decreases of calcium. The usual method measures **total** calcium, about 47% of which is bound to plasma proteins.
- High phosphorus: renal insufficiency, hypoparathyroidism, pseudohypoparathyroidism
- Vitamin D deficiency and resistance
- Osteomalacia (including Milkman fractures)
- Pseudovitamin D deficiency rickets[21]
- Celiac disease and other malabsorption disorders
- Renal tubular acidosis
- Pancreatitis, acute
- Dilutional: Intravenous fluids
- Bacteremia
- Hypomagnesemia
- Anticonvulsants and other common drugs, most by *in vivo* action, can depress calcium. Barbiturates in elderly may cause calcium decrease; other drugs including calcitonin, corticosteroids, gastrin, glucagon, glucose, insulin, magnesium salts, methicillin, and tetracycline in pregnancy.
  - A rare genetic disorder can cause hypocalcemia due to an abnormality in the calcium-sensing receptor.[22]

Limitations When plasma proteins are abnormal, total calcium results can be misleading. Sodium citrate, EDTA, and NaF potassium oxalate interfere. Gross hemolysis falsely elevates results. Patients receiving citrate-containing blood or blood fractions may have increased total serum calcium, despite decreased ionized calcium. In such patients, measurement of ionized calcium is indicated (see Calcium, Ionized, Serum *on page 130*). A formula to calculated corrected value can be found in Reference Range; *vide supra*.

In a series of 60 cases of proven hyperparathyroidism, increased corrected calcium concentrations were found in only 78%, but 98.3% had elevated ionized calcium.[23] The latter is the more useful test for hyperparathyroidism and hypoparathyroidism.

Methodology Spectrophotometry; atomic absorption spectrometry (AA) is not used extensively, but remains the reference method.

Additional Information In the differential diagnosis of hypercalcemia, serum calcium should be measured on at least three occasions. In **primary hyperparathyroidism**, parathyroid hormone, serum chloride, and urine calcium are increased. Rarely, in HPT the hypercalcemia is accompanied by a low-normal PTH.[24] In HPT, calcium rises, then phosphorus falls, then alkaline phosphatase rises. Alkaline phosphatase is usually not more than twice its upper limit in HPT. Measured ionized calcium and calculated ionized calcium may be helpful. Primary hyperparathyroidism and cancer with or without metastases cause 95% of instances of hypercalcemia.

Twenty-four hour urinary calcium is increased in HPT, low in **familial hypocalciuric hypercalcemia** (FHH) which is characterized by hypercalcemia and hypocalciuria. An autosomal dominant, it apparently has no complications. Ratio of renal calcium clearance to creatinine clearance <0.01 suggests this genetic disease. The calcium:creatinine clearance ratio is said to discriminate between FHH and hyperparathyroidism.[12] Family studies are highly desirable.

Hypocalcemia, rather then hypercalcemia, occur with rhabdomyolysis - induced acute renal failure.[25,26]

Footnotes

1. Bilezikian JP, "Management of Acute Hypercalcemia," *N Engl J Med*, 1992, 326(18):1196-203.
2. Bosch X, López-Soto A, Morelló A, et al, "Vitamin D Metabolite-Mediated Hypercalcemia in Wegener's Granulomatosis," *Mayo Clin Proc*, 1997, 72:440-4.
3. Bosch X, "Hypercalcemia Due to Endogenous Overproduction of Active Vitamin D in Identical Twins With Cat-Scratch Disease," *JAMA*, 1998, 279(7):532-4.
4. Seymour JF, Gagel RF, Hagemeister FB, et al, "Calcitriol Production in Hypercalcemic and Normocalcemic Patients With non-Hodgkin Lymphoma," *Ann Intern Med*, 1994, 121(9):633-40.
5. Cundy T and Reid I, "Calcium, Phosphate and Magnesium," *Clinical Biochemistry*, Marshall WJ and Bangert SK, eds, New York, NY: Churchill Livingstone, 1995, 93-4.
6. Painter PC, Cope JY, and Smith JL, "Reference Information for the Clinical Laboratory," *Tietz Textbook of Clinical Chemistry*, 3rd ed, Philadelphia, PA: WB Saunders Co, 1999, 1804.
7. Selby PL and Adams PH, "The Investigation of Hypercalcemia," *J Clin Pathol*, 1994, 47:579-84.
8. Lum G, "Evaluation of a Laboratory Critical Limit (Alert Value) Policy for Hypercalcemia," *Arch Pathol Lab Med*, 1996, 120(7):633-6.
9. Irvin GL 3rd and Carneiro DM, "Management Changes in Primary Hyperparathyroidism," *JAMA*, 2000, 284(8):934-6.
10. Crespo M, Sopena B, Orloff JJ, et al, "Immunohistochemical Detection of Parathyroid Hormone-Related Protein in a Cutaneous Squamous Cell Carcinoma Causing Humoral Hypercalcemia of Malignancy," *Arch Pathol Lab Med*, 1999, 123(8):725-30.
11. Rankin W, Grill V, and Martin TJ, "Parathyroid Hormone-Related Protein and Hypercalcemia," *Cancer*, 1997, 80(8 Suppl):1564-71.
12. Knecht TP, Behling CA, Burton DW, et al, "The Humoral Hypercalcemia of Benignancy. A Newly Appreciated Syndrome," *Am J Clin Pathol*, 1996, 105(4):487-92.
13. Wong ET and Freier EF, "The Differential Diagnosis of Hypercalcemia. An Algorithm for More Effective Use of Laboratory Tests," *JAMA*, 1982, 247:75-80.
14. Kumar S, Mow BM, and Kaufmann SH, "Hypercalcemia Complicating Leukemic Transformation of Agnogenic Myeloid Metaplasia-Myelofibrosis," *Mayo Clin Proc*, 1999, 74(12):1233-7.
15. Sirianni SR, Mora ME, Sands AM, et al, "Malignant Lymphoma Presenting With Severe Hypercalcemia," *N Y State J Med*, 1989, 89(9):533-5.
16. Westphal SA, "Disseminated Coccidioidomycosis Associated With Hypercalcemia," *Mayo Clin Proc*, 1998, 73(9):893-4.
17. Dockrell DH and Poland GA, "Hypercalcemia in a Patient With Hypoparathyroidism and *Nocardia asteroides* Infection: A Novel Observation," *Mayo Clin Proc*, 1997, 72(8):757-60.
18. Valentic JP, Elias AN, and Weinstein GD, "Hypercalcemia Associated With Oral Isotretinoin in the Treatment of Severe Acne," *JAMA*, 1983, 250:1899-900.
19. Marx SJ, "Familial Hypocalciuric Hypercalcemia," *N Engl J Med*, 1980, 303:810-1.
20. Gunn IR and Wallace JR, "Urine Calcium and Serum Ionized Calcium, Total Calcium and Parathyroid Hormone Concentrations in the Diagnosis of Primary Hyperparathyroidism and Familial Benign Hypercalcaemia," *Ann Clin Biochem*, 1992, 29(Pt 1):52-8.
21. Kitanaka S, Takeyama K, Murayama A, et al, "Inactivating Mutations in the 25-Hydroxyvitamin D_3 1α-Hydroxylase Gene in Patients With Pseudovitamin D Deficiency Rickets," *N Engl J Med*, 1998, 338:653-61.
22. Pearce SH, Williamson C, Kifor O, et al, "A Familial Syndrome of Hypocalcemia With Hypercalciuria Due to Mutations in the Calcium-Sensing Receptor," *N Engl J Med*, 1996, 335(15):1115-22.
23. Glendenning P, Gutteridge DH, Retallack RW, et al, "High Prevalence of Normal Total Calcium and Intact PTH in 60 Patients With Proven Primary Hyperparathyroidism: A Challenge to Current Diagnostic Criteria," *Aust N Z J Med*, 1998, 28(2):173-8.
24. Hollenberg AN and Arnold A, "Hypercalcemia With Low-Normal Serum Intact PTH: A Novel Presentation of Primary Hyperparathyroidism," *Am J Med*, 1991, 91(5):547-8.
25. Llach F, Felsenfeld AJ, and Haussler MR, "The Pathophysiology of Altered Calcium Metabolism in Rhabdomyolysis-Induced Acute Renal Failure, Interactions of Parathyroid Hormone, 25-Hydroxycholecalciferol, and 1,25-Dihydroxycholecalciferol," *N Engl J Med*, 1981, 305:117-23.
26. Knochel JP, "Serum Calcium Derangements in Rhabdomyolysis," *N Engl J Med*, 1981, 305:161-3.

References

Balland M and Trivin F, "Total Calcium," *Drug Effects on Laboratory Test Results Analytical Interferences and Pharmacological Effects*, Siest G and Galteau MM, eds, Littleton, MA: PSG Publishing Co Inc, 1988, 148-64.

Baron J, Winer KK, Yanovski JA, et al, "Mutations in the Ca(2+)-Sensing Receptor Gene Cause Autosomal Dominant and Sporadic Hypoparathyroidism," *Hum Mol Genet*, 1996, 5(5):601-6.

Bourke E and Delaney V, "Assessment of Hypocalcemia and Hypercalcemia," *Clin Lab Med*, 1993, 13(1):157-81.

Broadus AE, Mangin M, Ikeda K, et al, "Humoral Hypercalcemia of Cancer. Identification of a Novel Parathyroid Hormone-Like Peptide," *N Engl J Med*, 1988, 319(9):556-63.

Budayr AA, Nissenson RA, Klein RF, et al, "Increased Serum Levels of a Parathyroid Hormone-like Protein in Malignancy-Associated Hypercalcemia," *Ann Intern Med*, 1989, 111(10):807-12.

Cole DE, Peltekova VD, Rubin LA, et al, "A986S Polymorphism of the Calcium-Sensing Receptor and Circulating Calcium Concentration," *Lancet*, 1999, 353(9147):112-5.

Glendenning P, Gutteridge DH, and Retallack RW, "Treatment of Primary Hyperparathyroidism," *N Engl J Med*, 2000, 342(13):976-7.

Howanitz PJ and Cembrowski GS, "Postanalytical Quality Improvement: A College of American Pathologists Q-Probes Study of Elevated Calcium Results in 525 Institutions," *Arch Pathol Lab Med*, 2000, 124(4):504-10.

Hruska KA and Teitelbaum SL, "Renal Osteodystrophy," *N Engl J Med*, 1995, 333(3):166-74.

Jaffey P, Kahky M, and Ackerman E, "Pathologic Quiz Case: Recurrent Hypercalcemia," *Arch Pathol Lab Med*, 2000, 124(7):1087-8.

Klee GG, Kao PC, and Heath H 3d, "Hypercalcemia," *Endocrinol Metab Clin North Am*, 1988, 17(3):573-600.

Law WM Jr, Wahner HW, and Heath H ed, "Bone Mineral Density and Skeletal Fractures in Familial Benign Hypercalcemia (Hypocalciuric Hypercalcemia)," *Mayo Clin Proc*, 1984, 59(12):811-5.

Lobaugh B, Neelon FA, Oyama H, et al, "Circadian Rhythms for Calcium, Inorganic Phosphorus, and Parathyroid Hormone in Primary Hyperparathyroidism: Functional and Practical Considerations," *Surgery*, 1989, 106(6):1009-16.

Marx SJ, "Hyperparathyroid and Hypoparathyroid Disorders," *N Engl J Med*, 2000, 343(25):1863-75.

Nellen JF, Smulders YM, Frissen PH, et al, "Hypovitaminosis D in Immigrant Women: Slow to Be Diagnosed," *BMJ*, 1996, 312(7030):570-2.

Pearce S, "Extracellular "Calcistat" in Health and Disease," *Lancet*, 1999, 353(9147):83-4.

Wagner B, Begic-Karup S, Raber W, et al, "Prevalence of Primary Hyperparathyroidism in 13,387 Patients With Thyroid Diseases, Newly Diagnosed by Screening of Serum Calcium," *Exp Clin Endocrinol Diabetes*, 1999, 107(7):457-61.

♦ **Calcium Stimulation Test** *see* Calcitonin, Serum or Plasma *on page 129*

Calcium, Urine

Related Information

Calcium, Serum *on page 131*
Hydroxyproline, Total, Urine *on page 199*
Kidney Stone Analysis *on page 877*
Magnesium, Urine *on page 222*
Osteocalcin, Serum or Plasma *on page 237*
Parathyroid Hormone-Related Protein, Serum *on page 243*
Parathyroid Hormone, Serum *on page 243*
Phosphorus, Urine *on page 253*
Uric Acid, Urine *on page 295*
Urine Collection, 24-Hour *on page 47*
Vitamin D, Serum *on page 300*

Applies to Calcium:Creatinine Ratio

Abstract Urine calcium determinations are used to investigate effects of vitamin D, parathyroid hormone, and parathyroid hormone-related protein. When bone resorption is accelerated, the kidney defends against hypercalcemia by enhanced calciuria. Symptoms of hypercalciuria include polyuria, polydipsia, and sometimes nephrocalcinosis and nephrolithiasis.[1] In children, high urinary calcium can result in hematuria, dysuria, and urinary frequency.[2]

Patient Preparation In stone evaluation, urinary calcium results are more meaningful if the patient initially is on his/her usual diet for 3 days prior to urine collection. Drugs affecting mineral metabolism include antacids, phosphates, glucocorticoids, carbonic anhydrase inhibitors, anticonvulsants, and diuretics including thiazides. Thiazides are used therapeutically to lower urine calcium excretion. If the patient is on a stone prevention regime and test is for follow-up, then medications should **not** be stopped for the test.

Specimen 24-hour urine is preferred; random urine is acceptable for calcium:creatinine ratio calculations

Container Plastic urine container or acid-washed glass bottle

Reference Interval Varies with diet; based on average calcium intake of 600-800 mg/24 hours (SI: 15-20 mmol/day): excretion may be 100-250 mg/24 hours (SI: 2.5-6.2 mmol/day). On a diet of 400-800 mg/24 hours of calcium daily (SI: 10-20 mmol/day), others set the upper limit at 200 mg/24 hours of calcium (SI: 5 mmol/day) in a 24-hour urine collection. More than 4 mg/kg is associated with increased prevalence of stone formation. Low calcium diet: <150 mg/24 hours (SI: <3.7 mmol/day) excreted. High calcium diet: 250-300 mg/24 hours (SI: 6.2-7.5 mmol/day) excreted. Hypercalciuria has been defined as calcium excretion in excess of 250 mg/24 hours (SI: 6.2 mmol/day) for women, 300 mg/24 hours (SI: 7.5 mmol/day) for men.[3] Calcium excretion, like other laboratory results, must be related to the individual patient. The rate of calcium excretion can also be expressed as a calcium:creatinine ratio. In healthy individuals with constant muscle mass, urinary calcium (mg/dL):creatinine (mg/dL) is <0.14 (SI: calcium (mmol/L):creatinine (mmol/L) is <0.40). Values >0.20 (mg/dL) or >0.57 (mmol/L units) suggest hypercalciuria.

In children younger than 6 years of age, urine calcium:creatinine ratio is inversely related to age with the upper limit of normal being 0.8 mg/mg (SI: 2.25) at age 1 month.[4,5] See graphic.

Critical Values Urine calcium excretion >300 mg/24 hours (7.5 mmol/day) provides an indication for parathyroidectomy in the presence of other criteria for hyperparathyroidism.[6]

Use Reflects intake, rates of intestinal calcium absorption, bone resorption, and renal loss. Those processes relate to parathyroid hormone, parathyroid hormone-related protein, and vitamin D levels. Evaluate bone disease, calcium metabolism, renal stones (nephrolithiasis)[7] and idiopathic hypercalciuria.[8] Follow up patients on calcium therapy for osteopenia.

High in 30% to 80% of instances of primary hyperparathyroidism, but urinary calcium excretion does not consistently, reliably distinguish hyperparathyroidism from other entities. High in about 50% of patients with sarcoidosis. Increased with immobilization, with steroid therapy, with Paget disease of bone, and in primary (idiopathic) hypercalciuria.[9] Increased with entities causing high ultrafiltrable calcium: humoral hypercalcemia of malignancy, some cases of renal tubular acidosis, Fanconi syndrome, Bartter

syndrome, increased calcium intake, vitamin D intoxication, hyperthyroidism, diabetes mellitus, acromegaly, glucocorticoid excess, some cases of Crohn disease and ulcerative colitis, myeloma, some instances of leukemia and lymphoma, and carcinoma metastatic to bone. Reported relationship to hematuria in children.[2]

An association was found between dietary sodium and potassium intake and hypercalciuria.[2]

Low in familial hypocalciuric hypercalcemia, for which urine calcium measurements are mandatory; Gitelman syndrome, low with thiazide diuretics, vitamin D deficiency, renal osteodystrophy, vitamin D resistant rickets, hypoparathyroidism, pseudohypoparathyroidism and preeclampsia.[10]

Limitations Decreased in patients on oral contraceptives. Lacks specificity for hyperparathyroidism when increased. Five percent of the population have hypercalciuria.[9]

Additional tests are important in the differential diagnosis of hyperparathyroidism, including serum calcium, ionized calcium, and parathormone concentration.

Methodology Spectrophotometry, atomic absorption (AA) spectrometry

Additional Information Hypercalcemia leads to polyuria through interference with renal reabsorption of sodium and water.[1]

Twenty percent to 25% of patients who form calcium stones have hyperuricosuria. Urinary calcium reflects in part the relation between GFR and tubular reabsorption.

In the fasting state when intestinal and renal components are relatively constant, calcium excretion is used to assess the skeletal component. Values >0.16 mg (>0.04 mmol/L)/100 mL of glomerular filterate implies an increase in osteoclastic bone resorption.[11] The following equation is used to calculate calcium excretion in urine.

$$UCa \text{ (mg/100 mL glomerular filterate)} = [UCa \text{ (mg/dL)} \times \text{serum creatinine (mg/dL)}] / \text{urinary creatinine (mg/dL)}$$

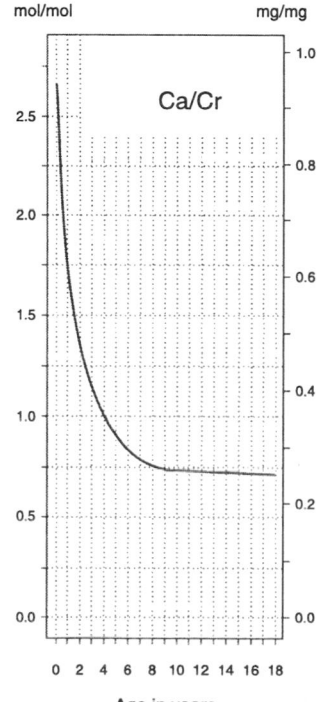

Estimated 95th percentiles for urinary Ca/Cr ratios in relation to age.

Footnotes

1. Bilezikian JP, "Management of Acute Hypercalcemia," *N Engl J Med*, 1992, 326(18):1196-1203.
2. Osorio AV and Alon US, "The Relationship Between Urinary Calcium, Sodium, and Potassium Excretion and the Role of Potassium in Treating Idiopathic Hypercalcinuria," *Pediatrics*, 1997, 100(4):675-81.
3. Palmieri GM, "Calcium, Phosphate, and Magnesium Metabolism," *The Laboratory in Clinical Medicine. Interpretation and Application*, 2nd ed, Halsted JA and Halsted CH, eds, Philadelphia, PA: WB Saunders Co, 1981, 688-96.
4. Matos V, Van Melle G, Boulat O, et al, "Urinary Phosphate/Creatinine, Calcium/Creatinine and Magnesium/Creatinine Ratios in Healthy Pediatric Populations," *J Pediatr*, 1997, 131(2):252-7.
5. Sargent JD, Stukel TA, Kresel J, et al, "Normal Values for Random Urinary Calcium to Creatinine Ratios in Infancy," *J Pediatr*, 1993, 123:393-7.
6. Irvin GL and Carneiro DM, "Management Changes in Primary Hyperparathyroidism," *JAMA*, 2000, 284(8):934-6.
7. Silverberg SJ, Shane E, Jacobs TP, et al, "Nephrolithiasis and Bone Involvement in Primary Hyperparathyroidism," *Am J Med*, 1990, 89(3):327-34.

(Continued)

Calcium, Urine *(Continued)*

8. Weisinger JR, "New Insights Into the Pathogenesis of Idiopathic Hypercalciuria: The Role of Bone," *Kidney Int*, 1996, 49(5):1507-18.

9. Erickson SB, "Hypercalciuria," *Mayo Clin Proc*, 1981, 56:579.

10. Taufield PA, Ales KL, Resnick LM, et al, "Hypocalciuria in Pre-eclampsia," *N Engl J Med*, 1987, 316(12):715-8.

11. Endres DB and Rude RK, "Mineral and Bone Metabolism," *Tietz Textbook of Clinical Chemistry*, 3rd ed, Burtis CA and Ashwood ER, eds, Philadelphia, PA: WB Saunders Co, 1999, 1395-457.

References

Gunn IR and Wallace JR, "Urine Calcium and Serum Ionized Calcium, Total Calcium and Parathyroid Hormone Concentrations in the Diagnosis of Primary Hyperparathyroidism and Familial Benign Hypercalcaemia," *Ann Clin Biochem*, 1992, 29(Pt 1):52-8.

Lemann J Jr, "Pathogenesis of Idiopathic Hypercalcinuria and Nephrolithiasis," *Disorders of Bone and Mineral Metabolism*, Coe FL and Favus MJ, eds, New York, NY: Raven Press, 1992, 685-706.

Lemann J Jr, Pleuss JA, Gray RW, et al, "Potassium Administration Reduces and Potassium Deprivation Increases Urinary Calcium Excretion in Healthy Adults," *Kidney Int*, 1991, 39(5):973-83.

Manz F, Kehrt R, Lausen B, et al, "Urinary Calcium Excretion in Healthy Children and Adolescents," *Pediatr Nephrol*, 1999, 13(9):894-9.

Sanchez-Ramos L, Jones DC, and Cullen MT, "Urinary Calcium as an Early Marker for Pre-eclampsia," *Obstet Gynecol*, 1991, 77(5):685-8.

Young DS, *Effects of Disease on Clinical Laboratory Tests*, 5th ed, Volume 1: Listing by Test, Washington, DC: AACC Press, American Association of Clinical Chemistry, 2000, Section 3, 149-59.

Carbohydrate-Deficient Transferrin, Serum

Related Information

Synonyms CDT

Applies to Alcoholism; Carbohydrate-Deficient Glycoprotein Syndrome; Congenital Disorders of Glycosylation

Abstract The transferrin isoforms found in serum are glycoproteins with varying numbers of sialic acid residues. The major serum isoform is a tetrasialotransferrin. Carbohydrate-deficient transferrin (CDT) includes the di-, mono-, and asialotransferrin isoforms. CDT is increased in alcoholics, and in patients with a group of autosomal recessive disorders of infancy and childhood, until recently known as carbohydrate-deficient glycoprotein syndrome. Presently designated "congenital disorders of glycosylation" (CDG), there is variable phenotype. Its characteristics include mental retardation, cerebellar hypoplasia, liver dysfunction, or stroke-like occurrences.[1]

Specimen Serum

Container Red top tube or SST™ tube

Storage Instructions Freeze immediately; ship on dry ice. Specimens exhibit excellent stability for up to 8 years at -20°C.[2]

Special Instructions Usually sent to reference laboratory.

Reference Interval Check with testing laboratory. Reference intervals vary according to different analytic specificities and various recovery rates of CDT assays. Values are reported either in relative (ie, percentage of total transferrin) or absolute (ie, units/L) terms.

Relative: <2.5%[3]

Absolute:
- children: <30 units/L[4]
- adult male: <20 units/L,[4] <27 units/L[5]
- adult female: <26 units/L,[4] <35 units/L[5]

Values for CDG evaluation are:[1]
- mono-oligosaccharide/di-oligosaccharide: <0.074 units/L
- indeterminate: 0.075-0.109 units/L
- α-oligosaccharide/di-oligosaccharide: <0.022 units/L

Use CDT is used as a marker for excessive alcohol consumption and for monitoring relapse or progressive abstinence in alcoholics. It is also used to diagnose carbohydrate-deficient glycoprotein syndrome, a central nervous system developmental disorder characterized by muscular weakness and hypotonia.

Limitations False-negative and false-positive CDT results occur in diagnosis of alcohol abuse; thus, the test is not recommended for screening in a general population.[6] CDT may be useful in case findings and appears to be the best single marker for alcoholism.[7] The sensitivity and/or specificity may be affected by female sex, smoking, body mass index, diastolic hypertension,[8] iron stores,[9,10] and other factors.[11,12] It is especially insensitive among women who abuse alcohol and is relatively insensitive among those without liver damage. False positives (relevant to alcohol consumption) occur in cases of nonalcoholic liver disease, women on estrogen replacement, and recipients of combined pancreas and kidney transplantation.[6] Sensitivity of 58% and 70% and specificity 82% to 98% for detection of alcohol abuse are reported.[13]

Methodology Over a dozen methods are available. They include anion-exchange chromatography with immunoassay detection or RIA, isoelectric focusing with densitometric or immunochemical detection, affinity chromatography, HPLC, turbidimetric immunoassay. Some methods measure the trisialo-isoform in addition to the disialo-, monosialo-, and asialo-isoforms, but doing so appears to offer little to no diagnostic value for evaluation of alcoholism.[3]

For evaluation for congenital disorders of glycosylation, affinity chromatography coupled to electrospray ionization/mass spectrometry has recently been introduced.[1]

Additional Information The overall clinical sensitivity and specificity of the CDT assay are estimated to be approximately 82% and 97%, respectively.[14] The combined use of CDT with gamma-glutamyl transpeptidase (GGT)[15] (see Gamma-Glutamyl Transferase, Serum *on page 179*) and mean corpuscular volume (MCV) (see Red Blood Cell Indices *on page 477*) raises the sensitivity above 90%.[16] Total bilirubin, AST:ALT ratio, and alkaline phosphatase are all relevant as well. Increased CDT has been demonstrated in patients with cystic fibrosis[10] and in a patient with achondroplasia;[9] these patients did not abuse alcohol and had no known causes otherwise of impaired glycosylation. False-positive results have occasionally been reported in patients with liver disease and in patients with genetic transferrin variants.

Though interindividual variability of CDT is considerable, intraindividual variation is minimal.[17] Thus, measurements within an individual, comparing results over time compared with initial, baseline results, provide a reliable means of monitoring success of treatment in alcohol-dependent individuals. During abstinence, serum CDT exhibits a half-life of ~2 weeks.[6,14]

Footnotes

1. Mayo Reference Services Publication, "Carbohydrate Deficient Transferrin, Serum," *New Test Announcement*, Rochester, MN: Mayo Medical Laboratories, 2000.

2. Martensson O, Schink E, and Brandt R, "Diurnal Variability and *In Vitro* Stability of Carbohydrate-Deficient Transferrin," *Clin Chem*, 1998, 44(10):2226-7.

3. Dibbelt L, "Does Trisialo-Transferrin Provide Valuable Information for the Laboratory Diagnosis of Chronically Increased Alcohol Consumption by Determination of Carbohydrate-Deficient Transferrin?" *Clin Chem*, 2000, 46(8 Pt 1):1203-5.

4. Stibler H and Jaeken J, "Carbohydrate Deficient Serum Transferrin in a New Systemic Hereditary Syndrome," *Arch Dis Child*, 1990, 65(1):107-11.

5. Lott JA, Curtis LW, Thompson A, et al, "Reported Alcohol Consumption and the Serum Carbohydrate-Deficient Transferrin Test in Third-Year Medical Students," *Clin Chim Acta*, 1998, 276(2):129-41.

6. Laposata M, "Assessment of Ethanol Intake," *Am J Clin Pathol*, 1999, 112(4):443-50.

7. Meerkerk GJ, Njoo KH, Bongers IM, et al, "Comparing the Diagnostic Accuracy of Carbohydrate-Deficient Transferrin, Gamma-Glutamyltransferase, and Mean Cell Volume in a General Practice Population," *Alcohol Clin Exp Res*, 1999, 23(6):1052-9.

8. Whitfield JB, Fletcher LM, Murphy TL, et al, "Smoking, Obesity, and Hypertension Alter the Dose-Response Curve and Test Sensitivity of Carbohydrate-Deficient Transferrin as a Marker of Alcohol Intake," *Clin Chem*, 1998, 44(12):2480-9.

9. De Feo TM, Fargion S, Duca L, et al, "Carbohydrate-Deficient Transferrin, a Sensitive Marker of Chronic Alcohol Abuse, Is Highly Influenced by Body Iron," *Hepatology*, 1999, 29(3):658-63.

10. Van Pelt J and Azimi H, "False-Positive CDTect Values in Patients With Low Ferritin Values," *Clin Chem*, 1998, 44(10):2219-20.

11. Assmann B, Hackler R, Peters V, et al, "Increased Carbohydrate-Deficient Transferrin Concentration and Abnormal Protein Glycosylation of Unknown Etiology in a Patient With Achondroplasia," *Clin Chem*, 2000, 46(4):584-6.

12. Larsson A, Flodin M, and Kollberg H, "Increased Serum Concentrations of Carbohydrate-Deficient Transferrin (CDT) in Patients With Cystic Fibrosis," *Upsala J Med Sci*, 1998, 103:231-6.

13. O'Connor PG and Schottenfeld RS, "Patients With Alcohol Problems," *N Engl J Med*, 1998, 338(9):592-602.

14. Stibler H, "Carbohydrate-Deficient Transferrin in Serum: A New Marker of Potentially Harmful Alcohol Consumption Reviewed," *Clin Chem*, 1991, 37(12):2029-37.

15. Allen JP, Sillamaukee P, and Anton R, "Contribution of Carbohydrate Deficient Transferrin to Gamma Glutamyl Transpeptidase in Evaluating Progress of Patients in Treatment for Alcoholism," *Alcohol Clin Exp Res*, 1999, 23(1):115-20.

16. Mundle G, Ackermann K, Munkes J, et al, "Influence of Age, Alcohol Consumption and Abstinence on the Sensitivity of Carbohydrate-Deficient Transferrin, γ-Glutamyltransferase and Mean Corpuscular Volume," *Alcohol and Alcoholism*, 1999, 34(5):760-6.

17. Helander A, Vabo E, Levin K, et al, "Intra- and Interindividual Variability of Carbohydrate-Deficient Transferrin, γ-Glutamyltransferase, and Mean Corpuscular Volume in Teetotalers," *Clin Chem*, 1998, 44(10):2120-5.

References

Anton RF, Stout RL, Roberts JS, et al, "The Effect of Drinking Intensity and Frequency on Serum Carbohydrate-Deficient Transferrin and Gamma-Glutamyl Transferase Levels in Outpatient Alcoholics," *Alcohol Clin Exp Res*, 1998, 22(7):1456-62.

Fagerberg B, Agewall S, Berglund A, et al, "Is Carbohydrate-Deficient Transferrin in Serum Useful for Detecting Excessive Alcohol Consumption in Hypertensive Patients?" *Clin Chem*, 1994, 40(11 Pt 1):2057-63.

Foo Y and Rosalki SB, "Carbohydrate Deficient Transferrin Measurement," *Ann Clin Biochem*, 1998, 35(Pt 3):345-50.

Hackler R, Arndt T, Helwig-Rolig A, et al, "Investigation by Isoelectric Focusing of the Initial Carbohydrate-Deficient Transferrin (CDT) and non-CDT Transferrin Isoform Fractionation Step Involved in Determination of CDT by the ChronAlcol.D. Assay," *Clin Chem*, 2000, 46(4):483-92.

Hagberg B, Blennow G, Kristiansson B, et al, "Carbohydrate-Deficient Glycoprotein Syndromes: Peculiar Group of New Disorders," *Pediatr Neurol*, 1993, 9(4):255-62.

Halm U, Tannapfel A, Mossner J, et al, "Relative Versus Absolute Carbohydrate-Deficient Transferrin as a Marker of Alcohol Consumption in Patients With Acute Alcoholic Hepatitis," *Alcohol Clin Exp Res*, 1999, 23(10):1614-8.

Helander A, "Absolute or Relative Measurement of Carbohydrate-Deficient Transferrin in Serum? Experiences With Three Immunological Assays," *Clin Chem*, 1999, 45(1):131-5.

Jaeken J and Carchon H, "The Carbohydrate-Deficient Glycoprotein Syndromes: An Overview," *J Inherit Metab Dis*, 1993, 16(5):813-20.

Keating J, Cheung C, Peters TJ, et al, "Carbohydrate Deficient Transferrin in the Assessment of Alcohol Misuse: Absolute or Relative Measurements? A Comparison of Two Methods With Regard to Total Transferrin Concentration," *Clin Chim Acta*, 1998, 272(2):159-69.

Leavelle DE, *Mayo Medical Laboratories Interpretive Handbook*, Rochester, MN: Mayo Medical Laboratories, 1997.

Nikkari ST, Koivu TA, Anttila P, et al, "Carbohydrate-Deficient Transferrin and Gamma-Glutamyltransferase Are Inversely Associated With Lipid Markers of Cardiovascular Risk," *Eur J Clin Invest*, 1998, 28(10):793-7.

Rosman AS and Lieber CS, "Diagnostic Utility of Laboratory Tests in Alcoholic Liver Disease," *Clin Chem*, 1994, 40(8):1641-51.

Iamaro G, Simeone R, Mangiarotti M, et al, "Carbohydrate-Deficient Transferrin Assay in Pediatrics and Pregnancy: Expression of Results," *Int J Clin Lab Res*, 1998, 28:140.

♦ **Carbon Dioxide** *see* Bicarbonate, Blood *on page 115*

Carbon Dioxide, Total, Blood

Related Information
Bicarbonate, Blood *on page 115*
Blood Gases and pH, Arterial *on page 119*
Blood Gases and pH, Capillary *on page 121*
Blood Gases and pH, Venous *on page 122*
Chloride, Serum, Plasma, or Blood *on page 144*
Electrolyte Panel, Serum *on page 168*
pCO_2, Blood *on page 246*
pH, Blood *on page 247*

Synonyms CO_2; CO_2 Content; $ctCO_2$; TCO_2

Applies to Acid-Base Status Evaluation; Bicarbonate; Oximeters, Pulse; Tidal Volume

Abstract Total carbon dioxide (TCO_2) consists primarily of bicarbonate (HCO_3^-), plus small to trace amounts of carbonic acid (H_2CO_3), dissolved CO_2, carbonate ions (CO_3^{2-}), and CO_2 bound amino groups (carbamino compounds). Laboratory measurement of TCO_2 is done to estimate the HCO_3^- concentration, which usually makes up all but ≤2 mmol/L of the TCO_2 concentration. The two terms, TCO_2 and HCO_3^-, are used interchangeably in routine practice. (See Bicarbonate, Blood *on page 115*.)

Specimen Whole blood; plasma or serum

Container Red top tube or green top (heparin) tube

Collection Specimen should be kept tightly closed, as CO_2 will diffuse out, causing erroneously low values. This loss may amount to 6 mmol/hour.[1] Anaerobic conditions are best.

Reference Interval Whole blood - infancy to 2 years: 18-28 mmol/L; 2 years and older: arterial: 23-29 mmol/L; venous: 22-26 mmol/L. Plasma or serum - venous: 23-29 mmol/L.

Possible Panic Range <15 mmol/L, >50 mmol/L

Use TCO_2 is used in the evaluation of acid-base and electrolyte status. High results may represent respiratory acidosis with CO_2 retention (eg, advanced pulmonary emphysema) or metabolic alkalosis (eg, prolonged vomiting). Low values may indicate respiratory alkalosis as in hyperventilation or metabolic acidosis (eg, diabetes with ketoacidosis). Hypercapnia may go unrecognized despite adequate arterial oxygen saturation measured by pulse oximetry.[2]

Limitations Interpretation requires clinical information and evaluation of other laboratory data (eg, electrolytes, blood gases, glucose). Organic acids[1,3] and nitrate[4] have been reported to interfere (positively) in one TCO_2 (direct ion-specific electrode) method.

Methodology Colorimetry, enzyme assay, pCO_2 electrode ("indirect" electrode assay), or TCO_2 electrode ("direct" ISE). TCO_2 can be calculated from blood gas measurements.

Additional Information Hypercapnia from impaired elimination of CO_2 is due to abnormalities in mechanisms controlling respiratory drive, the muscles of respiration, and the function of the lung. Elimination of CO_2 from the lung involves alveolar ventilation but not dead-space ventilation. Partitioning of these spaces is expressed as a ratio between dead space and total volume per breath: the tidal volume. The tidal volume normally is <0.30. These and other aspects of pulmonary gas exchange, ventilation and their consequences are addressed as the partial pressure of arterial carbon dioxide, $PaCO_2$, a part of arterial blood gases.[5]

Footnotes
1. Rifai N, Hyde J, Iosefsohn M, et al, "Organic Acids Interfere in the Measurement of Carbon Dioxide Concentration by the Kodak Ektachem® 700," *Ann Clin Biochem*, 1992, 29(Pt 1):105-8.

2. Ayas N, Bergstrom LR, Schwab TR, et al, "Unrecognized Severe Postoperative Hypercapnia: A Case of Apneic Oxygenation," *Mayo Clin Proc*, 1998, 23:51-4.

3. O'Leary TD and Langton SR, "Calculated Bicarbonate or Total Carbon Dioxide?" *Clin Chem*, 1989, 35(8):1697-700.

4. Daoud EW, McClellan AC, and Scott MG, "Positive Interferences With the Ektachem Total CO_2 Assay From Therapy With Topical Cerous Nitrate," *Clin Chem*, 1990, 36(8):1521-2.

5. Weinberger SE, Schwartzstein RM, and Weiss JW, "Hypercapnia," *N Engl J Med*, 1989, 321(18):1223-31.

References
McLain BI, Evans J, Dear PR, et al, "Comparison of Capillary and Arterial Blood Gas Measurements in Neonates," *Arch Dis Child*, 1988, 63(7 Spec No):743-7.

Misuri G, Lanini B, Gigliotti F, et al, "Mechanism of CO_2 Retention in Patients With Neuromuscular Disease," *Chest*, 2000, 117(2):447-53.

Scott MG, Heusel JW, LeGrys VA, et al, "Electrolytes and Blood Gases," *Tietz Textbook of Clinical Chemistry*, 3rd ed, Chapter 31, Burtis CA and Ashwood ER, eds, Philadelphia, PA: WB Saunders Co, 1999, 1056-92.

Zenger M, Brenner M, Hua P, et al, "Measuring Oxygen Uptake and Carbon Dioxide Production in Critically Ill Patients Using a Standard Blood Gas Analyzer," *Crit Care Med*, 1994, 22(5):783-8.

♦ **Carbonic Anhydrase III** *see* Myoglobin, Blood, Serum, or Plasma *on page 228*

Carcinoembryonic Antigen, Serum

Related Information
Alpha$_1$-Fetoprotein, Serum *on page 97*
Body Cavity Fluid Cytology *on page 372*
Body Fluid Analysis, Cell Count *on page 408*
Body Fluid Chemical Analysis *on page 123*
Body Fluid Glucose *on page 124*
Breast Biopsy *on page 51*
CA 15-3, Serum *on page 127*
CA 19-9, Serum *on page 128*
CA 27.29, Serum *on page 128*
CA 125, Serum *on page 126*
Colon Cancer, Hereditary Nonpolyposis Type *on page 724*
Cyst Fluid Cytology *on page 379*
Fine Needle Aspiration, Deep Masses *on page 381*
Heterophilic Antibodies *on page 191*
Homovanillic Acid, Urine *on page 195*
Immunoperoxidase Procedures *on page 60*
Liver Disease: Laboratory Assessment, Overview *on page 216*
Occult Blood, Stool *on page 315*

Synonyms CEA

Abstract One of the first tumor markers, CEA is an oncofetal glycoprotein antigen. It is not organ specific. Abnormalities are found in a wide range of tumor types, but application is widest with adenocarcinomas of the gastrointestinal tract and with CA 15-3 for primaries of breast.

CEA may be used as an adjunct to staging and as a monitor. Increasing concentrations of CEA may be the first evidence of disease progression in patients with primary carcinoma of gastrointestinal tract, breast and ovary, rising before other laboratory abnormalities or symptoms appear.

CEA is a useful reagent in immunocytochemistry as well.

Specimen Serum or plasma, usually serum; effusion fluid; bronchoalveolar lavage;[1] cerebrospinal fluid

Container Plain red top tube, SST™ tube, or lavender top (EDTA) tube; avoid heparin anticoagulant

Sampling Time Preoperative; ~4 weeks postoperative and subsequently

Storage Instructions Separate serum (or plasma) from cells and refrigerate if assayed within 24 hours. For longer storage, freeze at -20°C.

Special Instructions Transport to reference laboratory on dry ice.

Reference Interval Adults: nonsmoker: <2.5 ng/mL (SI: <2.5 µg/L), smoker: ≤5.0 ng/mL (SI: ≤5.0 µg/L); method-dependent

Use CEA remains the best tumor marker available as an independent factor to project prognosis and is most useful as a chemical monitor of recurrence (Continued)

Carcinoembryonic Antigen, Serum *(Continued)*

and of response to therapy in patients with gastrointestinal carcinomas, especially colorectal neoplasms. It is the best marker available to follow postoperative patients regardless of whether or not preoperative CEA was increased; and it is the most useful means of detection of hepatic metastases. Increase bears an implication of treatment failure or recurrence and may be a signal for second-look procedures. Detection of locally recurrent carcinoma, lung or hepatic metastasis, especially from colorectal primaries, may lead to resection of recurrent or metastatic carcinoma for cure. The highest levels occur with metastases to liver or bone. Serum CEA concentrations are often more sensitive for metastases in bone than are bone scans. Marker for monitoring effectiveness of therapy. CEA is also used for other primary carcinomas of entodermal origin, including stomach and pancreas. Significant elevations may be found with primaries of breast and lung. High CEA occurs with medullary carcinoma of thyroid. Increases have been reported with giant cell carcinomas of thyroid, with neuroblastoma, with some tumors of ovary, and with some squamous cell carcinomas of the head and neck. Work-up of effusion fluids for carcinoma.

Limitations CEA levels are modestly elevated in smokers; patients with inflammation including infections, peptic ulcer, some instances of liver disease, inflammatory bowel disease, and pancreatitis; some patients with hypothyroidism and cirrhosis may have increased concentrations. CA 15-3 is a better marker than CEA in breast cancer.[2] Many negatives occur in patients with early carcinoma. Doubtful cost-effectiveness for many patients. **CEA is negative in some patients with even metastatic colorectal and other neoplasms:** a minority of such patients do not have high CEA levels. Increased CEA concentrations are found only in 10% to 20% of subjects with surgically resectable gastric carcinoma.[3] Correlation between tumor burden and CEA level is imperfect, especially with lung primaries. Hepatotoxicity of antineoplastic drugs, as well as tumor cell necrosis or membrane damage may permit escape of CEA into the circulation and cause CEA increase; simultaneous evaluation of liver-related tests has been advocated for the former. Radiation therapy may also induce a transient rise in CEA. As patients are followed, CEA testing should be repeated by the same laboratory, by the same method, for all assays. Benign diseases usually do not cause CEA levels >5-10 ng/mL (SI: >5-10 µg/L). When longitudinal monitoring is carried out, use the same method for all samples.

Contraindications CEA is **not** a screening test for occult cancer.

Methodology Immunometric, chemiluminometric, monoclonal or polyclonal antibodies or combinations

Additional Information CEA is present in embryonic tissues and certain epithelial malignancies as described above. Chemical heterogeneity in the carbohydrate portion of the CEA molecule is the basis for a family of molecules varying in immunologic specificity. CEA may vary in different tissues and individuals. Preoperative CEA increases were correlated with increasing Dukes stage.[4] Progressive elevations of CEA may herald tumor recurrence 3-36 months before clinical evidence of metastases. A small rise may signal local recurrence, a large rise hepatic metastasis. Postoperative CEA elevation following hepatic resection of metastatic colorectal carcinoma provides indication for further therapy. Important monitors for breast and colon cancer patients include GGT, alkaline phosphatase, and CEA. CEA is not specific for any one type of cancer; however, values >20 ng/mL (SI: >20 µg/L) are most significantly correlated with metastatic disease and/or with primary pancreatic and colorectal carcinoma.

CEA is more sensitive to recurrence of **colonic** than **rectal** primaries.[5] It is positive in about 63% of patients having a colorectal carcinoma; about 20% of patients with Dukes A, 58% with Dukes B, 68% with Dukes C.[6]

Hepatic scans have become positive months after a rise in CEA; lack of sensitivity of liver scans for early, resectable metastases is widely recognized, as is their expense. Similarly, serum alkaline phosphatase has been disappointing, but its value may be enhanced in concert with GGT and CEA. Testing for these three may be desirable every 3-6 months for the first 2 years after resection, followed by progressively less frequent testing until 5 years have elapsed. However, such application of CEA testing has become controversial.

Although 37 of 118 tumor-free patients had CEA false-positive at >5 ng/mL (SI: >5 µg/L) on at least one occasion, CEA remains the most sensitive and cost-effective means to detect recurrent colon cancer.[7] CEA may be more sensitive to distant metastasis of colon cancer than to local recurrence.[8] Sites of recurrent colon cancer include liver, lung, colon, abdomen, and mixed.[7]

Preoperative level of serum CEA is reported as a prognostic indicator (of survival) in patients with Dukes B colorectal cancer.[9] Median survival rate and disease-free interval were better in those whose preoperative CEA elevations returned to normal following hepatic reaction for metastatic disease.[10] CEA monitoring may be valuable to evaluate response to chemotherapy.[11] CEA has prognostic significance for **gastric carcinoma** as well.[12]

On the other hand, an immunocytochemistry study of 180 primary **breast carcinomas** utilizing antisera to CEA and CEA/NCA-50 (nonspecific cross reacting antigen) showed no correlation between positivity of CEA immunocytochemistry and histologic grade, lymph node stage, disease-free interval or patient survival.[13] As concerns circulating levels of CA 15-3 and CEA, a study of 173 patients with advanced breast carcinoma found that elevated CEA levels correlated with extent of disease but not with survival.[14]

An exacerbation may be seen in some patients with carcinoma of breast after hormonal therapy is begun, although excellent responses may follow. Measurement of CEA levels in nipple discharge from patients with nonpalpable breast cancer has been reported to have value in separating malignant from benign disease, although cytopathology is more widely applied for nipple discharge. Cases of breast cancer generally had nipple discharge levels >100 ng/mL (SI: >100 µg/L).[15]

Preoperative CEA is a predictor of poor survival in patients with carcinoma of lung following resection.[16]

As the measurement of CEA and other oncofetal antigens has not been useful in screening for presence of colon cancer, attention is currently focused on utilization of molecular biologic techniques and genotypic markers. The familial adenomatous polyposis syndrome (Gardner syndrome) as well as some sporadic colorectal carcinomas have 5q chromosome defects (Gardner's interstitial deletion of 5q13-q22).

CEA may be measured in effusion fluids. False positives are reported with empyema and complicated parapneumonic effusions.[17]

Footnotes

1. deDiego A, Compte L, Sanchis J, et al, "Usefulness of Carcinoembryonic Antigen Determination in Bronchoalveolar Lavage Fluid. A Comparative Study Among Patients With Peripheral Lung Cancer, Pneumonia, and Healthy Individuals," *Chest*, 1991, 100(4):1060-3.
2. Safi F, Kohler I, Rottinger E, et al, "The Value of the Tumor Marker CA 15-3 in Diagnosing and Monitoring Breast Cancer. A Comparative Study With Carcinoembryonic Antigen," *Cancer*, 1991, 68(3):574-82.
3. Fuchs CS and Mayer RJ, "Gastric Carcinoma," *N Engl J Med*, 1995, 333(1):32-41.
4. Chapman MA, Buckley D, Henson DB, et al, "Preoperative Carcinoembryonic Antigen Is Related to Tumour Stage and Long-Term Survival in Colorectal Cancer," *Br J Cancer*, 1998, 78(10):1346-1349.
5. Welch CE and Malt RA, "Abdominal Surgery (Second of Three Parts)," *N Engl J Med*, 1983, 308:685-95.
6. Martin EW Jr, James KK, Hurtubise PE, et al, "The Use of CEA as an Early Indicator for Gastrointestinal Tumor Recurrence and Second-Look Procedures," *Cancer*, 1977, 39(2):440-6.
7. Graham RA, Wang S, Catalano PJ, et al, "Postsurgical Surveillance of Colon Cancer: Preliminary Cost Analysis of Physical Examination, Carcinoembryonic Antigen Testing, Chest X-ray, and Colonoscopy," *Ann Surg*, 1998, 228(1):59-63.
8. Beart RW Jr and O'Connell MJ, "Postoperative Follow-up of Patients With Carcinoma of the Colon," *Mayo Clin Proc*, 1983, 58:361-3.
9. Slentz K, Senagore A, Hibbert J, et al, "Can Preoperative and Postoperative CEA Predict Survival After Colon Cancer Resection?" *Ann Surg*, 1994, 60(7):528-31.
10. Hohenberger P, Schlag PM, Gerneth T, et al, "Pre- and Postoperative Carcinoembryonic Antigen Determinations in Hepatic Resection for Colorectal Metastases: Predictive Value and Implications for Adjuvant Treatment Based on Multivariate Analysis," *Ann Surg*, 1994, 219(2):135-43.
11. Rockall TA and McDonald PJ, "Carcinoembryonic Antigen: Its Value in the Follow-up of Patients With Colorectal Cancer," *Int J Colorectal Dis*, 1999, 14(1):73-7.
12. Nakane Y, Okamura S, Akehira K, et al, "Correlation of Preoperative Carcinoembryonic Antigen Levels and Prognosis of Gastric Cancer Patients," *Cancer*, 1994, 73(11):2703-8.
13. Robertson JFR, Ellis IO, Bell J, et al, "Carcinoembryonic Antigen Immunocytochemistry in Primary Breast Cancer," *Cancer*, 1989, 64(8):1638-45.
14. Colomer R, Ruibal A, and Salvador L, "Circulating Tumor Marker Levels in Advanced Breast Carcinoma Correlate With the Extent of Metastatic Disease," *Cancer*, 1989, 64(8):1674-81.
15. Inaji H, Yayoi E, Maeura Y, et al, "Carcinoembryonic Antigen Estimation in Nipple Discharge as an Adjunctive Tool in the Diagnosis of Early Breast Cancer," *Cancer*, 1987, 60(12):3008-13.
16. Rubins JB, Dunitz J, Rubins HB, et al, "Serum Carcinoembryonic Antigen as an Adjunct to Preoperative Staging of Lung Cancer," *J Thorac Cardiovasc Surg*, 1998, 116(3):412-16.
17. Garcia-Pachon E, Padilla-Navas I, Dosda MD, et al, "Elevated Level of Carcinoembryonic Antigen in Nonmalignant Pleural Effusions," *Chest*, 1997, 111(3):643-7.

References

Bakalakos EA, Burak WE, Young DC, et al, "Is Carcinoembryonic Antigen Useful in the Follow-up Management of Patients With Colorectal Liver Metastases?" *Am J Surg*, 1999, 177(1):2-6.

Ballesta AM, Molina R, Filella X, et al, "Carcinoembryonic Antigen in Staging and Follow-up of Patients With Solid Tumors," *Tumour Biol*, 1995, 16(1):32-41.

Bidart JM, Thuillier F, Augereau C, et al, "Kinetics of Serum Tumor Marker Concentrations and Usefulness in Clinical Monitoring," *Clin Chem*, 1999, 45(10):1695-707.

Carl J, Brunsgaard N, Kjaer M, et al, "Estimated Treatment Responses in Metastatic Colorectal Carcinoma Based on Longitudinal Carcinoembryonic Antigen Series," *Scand J Clin Lab Invest*, 1993, 53(8):829-34.

Carriquiry LA and Pineyro A, "Should Carcinoembryonic Antigen Be Used in the Management of Patients With Colorectal Cancer?" *Dis Colon Rectum*, 1999, 42(7):921-29.

Casetta G, Piana P, Cavallini A, et al, "Urinary Levels of Tumour Associated Antigens (CA 19-9, TPA and CEA) in Patients With Neoplastic and Non-neoplastic Urothelial Abnormalities," *Br J Urol*, 1993, 72(1):60-4.

Cohen AM and Paty P, "CEA for Monitoring Colon Cancer," *JAMA*, 1994, 271(5):346.

Compton CC, Fielding LP, Burgart LJ, et al, "Prognostic Factors in Colorectal Cancer. College of American Pathologists Consensus Statement 1999," *Arch Pathol Lab Med*, 2000, 124(7):979-94.

Fritsche HA, "Serum Tumor Markers for Patient Monitoring: A Case Oriented Approach Illustrated With Carcinoembryonic Antigen," *Clin Chem*, 1993, 39(11 Pt 2):2431-4.

Horie Y, Miura K, Matsui K, et al, "Marked Elevation of Plasma Carcinoembryonic Antigen and Stomach Carcinoma," *Cancer*, 1996, 77(10):1991-7.

Ikemoto S, Iimori H, Nishimoto K, et al, "Two Cases of Urothelial Tumor With High Serum Level of Carcinoembryonic Antigen and TA-4," *Urol Int*, 1993, 51(2):105-7.

Kiang DT, Greenberg LJ, and Kennedy BJ, "Tumor Marker Kinetics in the Monitoring of Breast Cancer," *Cancer*, 1990, 65(2):193-9.

Kim JC, Han MS, Lee HK, et al, "Distribution of Carcinoembryonic Antigen and Biologic Behavior in Colorectal Carcinoma," *Dis Colon Rectum*, 1999, 42(5):640-8.

Kudo R, Sasano H, Koizumi M, et al, "Immunohistochemical Comparison of New Monoclonal Antibody 1C5 and Carcinoembryonic Antigen in the Differential Diagnosis of Adenocarcinoma of the Uterine Cervix," *Int J Gynecol Pathol*, 1990, 9(4):325-36.

McCall JL, Black RB, Rich CA, et al, "The Value of Serum Carcinoembryonic Antigen in Predicting Recurrent Disease Following Curative Resection of Colorectal Cancer," *Dis Colon Rectum*, 1994, 37(9):875-81.

Norton JA, "Carcinoembryonic Antigen. New Applications for an Old Marker," *Ann Surg*, 1991, 213(2):95-7.

Pectasides D, Bourazanis J, Economides N, et al, "Squamous Cell Carcinoma Antigen (SCC), Carcinoembryonic Antigen (CEA), and Tumour-Associated Trypsin Inhibitor (TATI) for Monitoring Head and Neck Cancer," *Int J Biol Markers*, 1993, 8(2):81-7.

Rocklin MS, Senagore AJ, and Talbott TM, "Role of Carcinoembryonic Antigen and Liver Function Tests in the Detection of Recurrent Colorectal Carcinoma," *Dis Colon Rectum*, 1991, 34(9):794-7.

Wang JY, Tang R, and Chiang JM, "Value of Carcinoembryonic Antigen in the Management of Colorectal Cancer," *Dis Colon Rectum*, 1994, 37(3):272-7.

♦ **Cardiac Enzymes/Isoenzymes** *see* Cardiac Markers: Laboratory Assessment, Overview *on page 137*

♦ **Cardiac Index** *see* Creatine Kinase Isoenzymes/Isoforms, Serum *on page 157*

Cardiac Markers: Laboratory Assessment, Overview

Related Information
C-Reactive Protein, Serum *on page 523*
Creatine Kinase Isoenzymes/Isoforms, Serum *on page 157*
Creatine Kinase, Serum *on page 158*
Myoglobin, Blood, Serum, or Plasma *on page 228*
Troponins, Serum *on page 291*

Applies to AST:ALT Ratio; Cardiac Enzymes/Isoenzymes; LD Isoenzymes; Myocardial Infarct Panel

Replaces Alpha-Hydroxybutyric Dehydrogenase (HBDH)

Test Includes Myoglobin, CK with isoenzymes, troponins; occasionally LD (LDH) with the five LD isoenzymes which have been useful especially in instances when patients present late.

Abstract Measurement of these substances can detect presence of acute myocardial infarction (AMI). Diagnostic electrocardiograms for AMI are initially found in about 8% of the six million patients annually presenting to the emergency departments of the U.S. with chest pain consistent with acute coronary syndrome. **Most frequent cause of medical malpractice litigation is reported to be missed diagnosis of acute myocardial infarct.**[1] Missed diagnosis of AMI may cause significant morbidity and mortality.

Medical history, physical examination, electrocardiograms, and laboratory markers including myoglobin, CK-MB, total CK, and troponin I (TnI) are especially relevant.

The first assays to become positive are myoglobin and CK isoforms, but each is increased by damage to striated (skeletal) muscle, and each presents problems. The major markers for AMI presently are myoglobin, CK-MB with CK, and troponin I (TnI). The troponins are more specific for injury to myocardium than CK-MB, CK isoforms, and myoglobin.

Specimen Serum; plasma or anticoagulated whole blood are the specimens of choice for the stat analysis of cardiac markers.[2]

Container Red top tube, green top (lithium heparin) tube

Sampling Time The sensitivity of myoglobin is greater than that of CK-MB in the first hours following AMI; its release precedes that of CK-MB by 2-5 hours.[3] Samples are usually taken on admission, then in a sequence, depending on clinical history, initial results, perceptions of the attending physician and/or existing institutional protocols. Some suggest sampling on admission and at 6 and 12 hours, which may permit earlier diagnosis. Total CK and CK-MB have been advocated, to be measured every 6-8 hours for the first 24 hours after admission. Serial LD (LDH) isoenzymes have been supplanted by troponin I measurements in subjects who present between 24 and 72 hours following onset of symptoms. (At that interval, CK and CK isoenzymes may have returned to normal). Further information on timing is provided in the listing Creatine Kinase Isoenzymes/Isoforms, Serum *on page 157*. See Troponins *on page 291* for recommendations for sampling for this assay; cardiac troponin I (TnI) remains elevated for up to 5-7 days and provides higher sensitivity than does CK-MB or myoglobin. Its application has greatly decreased the need for LD isoenzymes, making them presently obsolete as markers of acute myocardial injury.[4]

A recently published accelerated protocol advocates testing at 0, 2, 6, and 9 hours, deleting myoglobin in the 6- and 9-hour specimens.[5]

Collection Blood samples for cardiac markers should be referenced to the time of presentation in the emergency department (eg, "T_0" would indicate arrival).[5]

Turnaround Time Stat cardiac marker testing with a target turnaround time of 1 hour or less is recommended.[2]

Reference Interval Decision limits are extensively discussed in the literature. They are method dependent. Each laboratory should evaluate its own methods and experience in concert with cardiologists and with active chart review. Problems relevant to decision limits in cardiac enzymes and isoenzymes are shared with many other laboratory tests, as problems of sensitivity versus specificity.

Use Diagnosis of acute infarct of myocardium (acute MI or AMI); evaluation of chest pain. The two most important acute coronary arterial disease entities are the poles of a spectrum which include AMI and unstable angina pectoris. The latter is the cause of more 750,000 annual hospitalizations.

Distinction of unstable angina from non-Q-wave AMI may be difficult. "High-risk unstable angina" has been defined as elevated TnI with negative CK-MB.

Goals of the cardiac markers should include preventing or minimizing loss of myocardium.[5]

Limitations At onset of acute infarction of myocardium, all enzymes and isoenzymes are normal. It is desirable to draw cardiac enzymes at onset for a baseline. LD_1:LD_2 flip (inversion) and CK-MB elevation have been reported during marathon training with increases of total LD and CK.[4] Elevations of total CK with increased CK-MB and CK-BB, was found with necrotic intestine in experimental animals.[6] Myositis, various myopathies, rhabdomyolysis, and Reye syndrome are reported to cause elevations of CK-MB. In these situations CK-MB is elevated and remains elevated for days, while the values peak in about 1 day after onset of AMI and then begin to decline. Thus, the test is not entirely specific for AMI.[7] Confirmation by troponin I is widely advocated. The negative predictive value of myoglobin early in AMI is very high, but its role as a marker exists only as a narrow window at presentation and its use may not be appropriate for some institutions.

The system for isoform testing is labor-intensive.

Methodology Immunoassays and immunoinhibition are more rapid, sensitive, and specific than electrophoresis (for CK-MB).[8] Immunochemical CK-2 is commonly used and reported in mass units. It has distinct advantages over electrophoresis, including a short turnaround time (15-20 minutes).

Additional Information Acute MI: CK and CK-MB (CK-MB2) have been widely considered to peak about 1 day following onset. However, see Sampling Time in the listing Creatine Kinase Isoenzymes/Isoforms, Serum *on page 157*. CK and CK isoenzymes can be discontinued after MB returns to normal.

Myoglobin, CK isoforms, troponins, CK-MB, total CK, LD_1, LD_1:LD_2 ratio, and total LD classically increase with acute MI, then decrease. More information is provided in the individual test listings.

Newer tests which may allow for earlier detection of acute myocardial injury include CK-MM and CK-MB isoforms,[9,10,11] and quantitation of human ventricular myosin light chains in blood. Assay of troponin I has represented the most important advance. Its combination in serial mode with myoglobin has been advocated as the best combination in one study,[12] but CK-MB is more specific than myoglobin assay for injury of myocardium. Another study has advocated using troponin I as a second-line assay in a subset of higher-risk patients in whom the CK-MB is normal and early exercise testing is not an option.[13]

The literature continues to call attention to the poor sensitivity of the ECG for acute myocardial infarction, especially when the infarct is small. In emergency room patients, the sensitivity of electrocardiograms may be as poor as 50% in evaluation of patients with acute chest pain.

Aminotransferases are no longer used in AMI work-up. Myocardial injury can generate an AST:ALT ratio ≥3.1, or a twofold increase in this ratio. Only certain kinds of hepatocellular injury can also cause such AST:ALT ratio abnormality; they include acetaminophen or ethanol toxicity, hepatoma or metastatic carcinoma to liver, marked hepatocellular congestion, cirrhosis, and severe injury to striated muscle.

Sensitivity and specificity for TnI excel those of CK-MB or myoglobin.[14]

Increased concentrations of troponin T and C-reactive protein are related to long-term (as well as short-term) risk of cardiac death.[15,16]

Cost-effectiveness has been studied.[5]

Footnotes

1. Wu AH, "Use of Cardiac Markers as Assessed by Outcomes Analysis," *Clin Biochem*, 1997, 30(4):339-50.

2. Wu AH, Apple FS, Gibler WB, et al, "National Academy of Clinical Biochemistry Standards of Laboratory Practice: Recommendations for the Use of Cardiac Markers in Coronary Artery Diseases," *Clin Chem*, 1999, 45(7):1104-21.

3. Plebani M and Zaninotto M, "Diagnostic Strategies Using Myoglobin Measurement in Myocardial Infarction," *Clin Chim Acta*, 1998, 272(1):69-77.

4. Keffer JH, "Assessment of Myocardial Injury," *The Handbook of Clinical Pathology*, 2nd ed, Chapter 17, Chicago, IL: ASCP Press, American Society of Clinical Pathologists, 2000, 235-44.

5. Caragher TE, Fernandez BB, and Barr LA, "Long-Term Experience With an Accelerated Protocol for Diagnosis of Chest Pain," *Arch Pathol Lab Med*, 2000, 124(10):1434-9.

6. Graeber GM, O'Neill JF, Wolf RE, et al, "Elevated Levels of Peripheral Serum Creatine Phosphokinase With Strangulated Small Bowel Obstruction," *Arch Surg*, 1983, 118(7):837-40.

7. Wolf PL, "Common Causes of False-Positive CK-MB Test for Acute Myocardial Infarction," *Clin Lab Med*, 1986, 6(3):577-81.

(Continued)

Cardiac Markers: Laboratory Assessment, Overview *(Continued)*

8. Gibler WB, Lewis LM, Erb RE, et al, "Early Detection of Acute Myocardial Infarction in Patients Presenting With Chest Pain and Nondiagnostic ECGs: Serial CK-MB Sampling in the Emergency Department," *Ann Emerg Med*, 1990, 19(12):1359-66.

9. Puleo PR, Meyer D, Wathen C, et al, "Use of a Rapid Assay of Subforms of Creatine Kinase MB to Diagnose or Rule Out Acute Myocardial Infarction," *N Engl J Med*, 1994, 331(9):561-6.

10. Puleo PR, Guadagno P, Scheel M, et al, "Diagnostic Accuracy of a Rapid MB-CK Subform Assay in the Early Hours of Myocardial Infarction," *Clin Chem*, 1989, 35:1119.

11. Wu AH, Gornet TG, Wu VH, et al, "Early Diagnosis of Acute Myocardial Infarction by Rapid Analysis of Creatine Kinase Isoenzyme-3 (CK-MM) Sub-Types," *Clin Chem*, 1987, 33(3):358-62.

12. Zaninotto M, Altinier S, Lachin M, et al, "Strategies for the Early Diagnosis of Acute Myocardial Infarction Using Biochemical Markers," *Am J Clin Pathol*, 1999, 111(3):399-405.

13. Polaczyk CA, Kuntz KM, Sacks DB, et al, "Emergency Department Triage Strategies for Acute Chest Pain Using Creatine Kinase-MB and Troponin I Assays: A Cost-Effectiveness Analysis," *Ann Intern Med*, 1999, 131(12):909-18.

14. Feng YJ, Chen C, Fallon JT, et al, "Comparison of Cardiac Troponin I, Creatinine Kinase-MB, and Myoglobin for Detection of Acute Ischemic Myocardial Injury in a Swine Model," *Am J Clin Pathol*, 1998, 110(1):70-7.

15. Rader DJ, "Inflammatory Markers of Coronary Risk," *N Engl J Med* , 2000, 343(16):1179-82.

16. Lindahl B, Toss H, Siegbahn A, et al, "Markers of Myocardial Damage and Inflammation in Relation to Long-Term Mortality in Unstable Coronary Artery Disease. FRISC Study Group. Fragmin During Instability in Coronary Artery Disease," *N Engl J Med*, 2000, 343(16):1139-47.

References

Adams JE 3d, Sicard GA, Allen BT, et al, "Diagnosis of Perioperative Myocardial Infarction With Measurement of Cardiac Troponin I," *N Engl J Med*, 1994, 330(10):670-4.

D'Costa M, Fleming E, and Patterson MC, "Cardiac Troponin I for the Diagnosis of Acute Myocardial Infarction in the Emergency Department," *Am J Clin Pathol*, 1997, 108(5):550-5.

Goldman L, "Assessment of Perioperative Cardiac Risk," *N Engl J Med*, 1994, 330(10):707-9.

Kahn SE, "The Challenge of Evaluating the Patient With Chest Pain," *Arch Pathol Lab Med*, 2000, 124(10):1418-9.

Kost GJ, Kirk JD, and Omand K, "A Strategy for the Use of Cardiac Injury Markers (Troponin I and T, Creatinine Kinase-MB Mass and Isoforms, and Myoglobin) in the Diagnosis of Acute Myocardial Infarction," *Arch Pathol Lab Med*, 1998, 122(3):245-51.

Mehta RH and Eagle KA, "Missed Diagnoses of Acute Coronary Syndromes in the Emergency Room - Continuing Challenges," *N Engl J Med*, 2000, 342(16):1207-10.

Pope JH, Aufderheide TP, Ruthazer R, et al, "Missed Diagnoses of Acute Cardiac Ischemia in the Emergency Department," *N Engl J Med*, 2000, 342(16):1163-70.

Thygesen K and Alpert JS, "Myocardial Infarction Redefined - A Concensus Document of The Joint European Society of Cardiology/American College of Cardiology Committee for the Redefinition of Myocardial Infarction," The Joint European Society of Cardiology/American College of Cardiology Committee, *J Am Coll Cardiol*, 2000, 36(3):959-69.

♦ **Cardiac Troponin** *see* Troponins, Serum *on page 291*

♦ **Carnitine** *see* Amino Acids, Plasma *on page 100*

♦ **Carotene** *see* Vitamin A, Serum or Plasma *on page 298*

♦ **Catecholamines** *see* Metanephrines, Urine or Plasma *on page 223*

Catecholamines, Fractionation, Plasma

Related Information

Catecholamines, Fractionation, Urine *on page 139*
Homovanillic Acid, Urine *on page 195*
Metanephrines, Urine or Plasma *on page 223*
Vanillylmandelic Acid, Urine *on page 297*

Synonyms Epinephrine, Norepinephrine, Dopamine; Pressor Amines

Applies to Chromogranin A, Plasma; Clonidine Suppression Test; Dopamine

Test Includes Epinephrine (E) and norepinephrine (N); some laboratories also report dopamine.

Abstract Epinephrine (E), norepinephrine (NE), and dopamine are the catecholamines of interest in diagnostic medicine and are synthesized in the adrenal medulla, brain, and sympathetic nervous system. Clinical interest is focused primarily on the diagnosis of pheochromocytoma, a neoplasm usually (90% of cases) occurring in the adrenal medulla. When a similar neoplasm occurs as a primary tumor outside the adrenal, predominantly in the retroperitoneum, it may be called an extra-adrenal pheochromocytoma. Comparable tumors, some of which may be functioning, are called by the more general term, paraganglioma. Pheochromocytoma (ie, a paraganglioma of the adrenal medulla), when hormonally active, secretes large quantities of E, NE, or both. Early diagnosis of pheochromocytoma is important because it is a surgically curable cause of severe hypertension, and in ~10% of cases the neoplasm is malignant. Thus, removal of the primary neoplasm before metastasis is particularly beneficial. About 90% of cases of pheochromocytoma are sporadic. Familial cases include the type 2

multiple endocrine neoplasia (MEN) syndromes, 2A and 2B, Von-Hippel Lindau disease and von Recklinghausen disease.

The catecholamines are highly labile and have very brief (~2 minute) half-life in the circulation. Their plasma levels are influenced by multiple environmental factors, foods, and drugs; a successful testing protocol must control these preanalytic variables. E, NE, and dopamine undergo complex metabolic changes and are ultimately excreted in the urine.

Patient Preparation Because of the many factors that influence catecholamine secretion, and other factors that have similar chemical properties, meticulous patient preparation is usually recommended. All of the drugs being taken by the patient (see Additional Information) must be known, and there must be a thorough dietary history. A reference laboratory should provide a list of drugs and foods which interfere with its measurement technique. At the time of specimen collection, the patient should be relaxed and at rest; emotional stress and physical activity result in elevated plasma catecholamines. Epinephrine and epinephrine-like drugs (eg, Aldomet®, Inderal®) interfere; such drugs should be stopped a week prior to testing.

Clonidine suppression protocol: The patient remains recumbent for the entire 3-hour test period. Testing is conducted in the morning after an overnight fast. After a baseline blood specimen for plasma catecholamines is obtained, clonidine, 4.3 µg/kg body weight is given by mouth with water.[1]

Specimen Plasma

Container Green top (heparin) tube or lavender top (EDTA) tube; check with reference laboratory before obtaining specimen.

Sampling Time Blood specimens are obtained in anticoagulant just before the clonidine is given, and 3 hours later.

Collection Patient should be fasting and without use of tobacco for at least 4 hours. An indwelling heparinized venous catheter is advocated, since venipuncture can cause a stress-related increase in the substances for which testing is being done. Patient should remain supine in quiet surroundings for at least 30 minutes before specimen collection. Some laboratories require a chilled, special container; invert to mix blood with preservatives and place in an ice bath.

Reference Interval Method-dependent; the following are reference intervals reported by one reference laboratory using high performance liquid chromatography.[2]

Norepinephrine:
- supine: 70-750 pg/mL
- standing: 200-1700 pg/mL

Epinephrine:
- supine: undetectable: 110 pg/mL
- standing: undetectable: 140 pg/mL

Dopamine: <30 pg/mL (does not vary with posture)

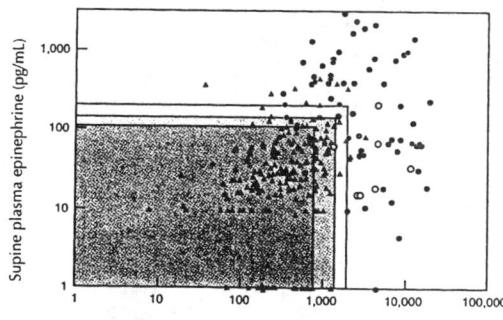

Study of ~500 Hypertensive Individuals

▲ Individuals without pheochromocytoma
o Extra-adrenal pheochromocytomas
● Surgically proven pheochromocytoma

The darkest-shaded zone represents patients with epinephrine (E) values ≤110 pg/mL and norepinephrine (NE) values ≤750 pg/mL. Concentrations outside of these limits result in sensitivities and specificities in the diagnosis of pheochromocytoma as shown in the following chart. Similarly, there is a medium-shaded area with E values ≤140 pg/mL and NE values ≤1400 pg/mL. The next lighter-shaded area has upper limits for E of 200 pg/mL and NE of 2000 pg/mL. See the following for the sensitivity and specificity figures for values falling outside of each of the areas defined above.

Adapted from *2000 Test Catalogue*, Mayo Medical Laboratories, Rochester, MN.

Limits From the Graph and Diagnostic Efficacy in Diagnosis of Pheochromocytoma

Limits	Sensitivity (%)	Specificity (%)
E: 110 pg/mL NE: 750 pg/mL	93 (66/71)	68 (130/191)
E: 140 pg/mL NE: 1400 pg/mL	90 (64/71)	90 (172/191)
E: 200 pg/mL NE: 2000 pg/mL	85 (60/71)	95 (182/191)

Adapted from Mayo Medical Laboratories, *2000 Test Catalogue*, 123-4 and 526-7.

Use Resting values: Plasma catecholamines are used to diagnose catecholamine-secreting neoplasms, most often adrenal pheochromocytomas. Some of the preanalytic variability is mitigated if specimens are always obtained after 15 minutes in the supine position in a minimally stressful environment. The interpretation of individual patient results is subject to the usual tradeoffs between sensitivity and specificity. Presented below are a graph and table containing results from ~500 hypertensive patients seen at the Mayo Clinic. The sensitivity and specificity results are shown, in the table, at three different cutoffs for E and NE.[2]

Clonidine suppression: Clonidine suppresses catecholamines in persons with essential hypertension, but not in persons with pheochromocytoma. Plasma NE should be within the reference interval at 3 hours. Levels above this threshold are consistent with pheochromocytoma.[1]

Reported Drug-Induced Changes in Catecholamine Concentrations

Increase

α-blockers (α-adrenergic antagonists)	Diuretics
Phentolamine (Regitine®)	Hydrochlorothiazide (HydroDiuril®)
Phenoxybenzamine (Dibenzyline®)	Furosemide
Prazosin (Minipres®)	Monoamine oxidase inhibitors
Antidepressants	Phenelzine (Nardil®)
Amitriptyline (Elavil®)	Stimulants
Amoxapine (Ascendin®)	Caffeine (coffee, tea)
Desipramine (Norpramin®)	Nicotine (tobacco)
Imipramine (Tofanil®)	Aminophylline
Nortriptyline (Acentyl®)	Theophylline
Antihistamines	Sympathomimetics
Diphenylhydramine (Benadryl®)	Albuterol (Proventil®)
Chlorpheniramine	Amphetamines
Promethazine (Phenergan®)	Ephedrine
Antipsychotics	Isoproterenol (Isuprel®)
Chlorpromazine (Thorazine®)	Metaproterenol (Metaprel®)
Clozapine (Clozaril®)	Pseudoephedrine (Sudafed®)
Perphenazine (Trilafon®)	Terbutaline (Brethine®)
β-blockers (β-adrenergic antagonists)	Vasodilators
Atenolol (Tenormin®)	Diazoxide (Proglycem®)
Labetalol (Normadyne®)	Hydralazine (Apresoline®)
Metoprolol (Lopressor®)	Isosorbide (Isordil®, Sorbitrate®)
Nadolol (Corgard®)	Minoxidil (Loniten®)
Findolol (Visken®)	Nitroglycerin
Propranolol (Inderal®)	Other nitrates/nitrites
Timolol (Blocadren®)	Others
Calcium channel antagonists	Cocaine
Felodipine (Plendil®)	Insulin
Nicardipine (Carden®)	Levodopa (Sinemet®)
Nifedipine (Procardia®)	Methylphenidate (Ritalin®)
Verapamil (Calan®, Isoptin®)	Metoclopramide (Reglan®)
Catecholamines/related compounds	Morphine
Epinephrine	Naloxone (Narcan®)
Norepinephrine	Pentazocine (Talwin®)
Dopamine	Prochlorperazine (Compazine®)
Methyldopa (Aldomet®)	TRH (Protirelin®)

Decrease

Antihypertensive agents	Antipsychotics
Captopril (Capoten®)	Haloperidol (Haldol®)
Clonidine (Catapres®)	Dopamine agonists
Guanabenz (Wytensin®)	Bromocriptine (Parlodel®)
Guanethidine (Ismelin®)	Others
Guanfacin (Tenex®)	Disulfiram (Antabuse®)
Reserpine (Serpasil®)	Metyrosine (Demser®)
	Octreotide (Sandostatin®)

Adapted from Rosano TG and Whitley RJ, "Catecholamines and Serotonin," *Tietz Textbook of Clinical Chemistry*, 3rd ed, Burtis CA and Ashwood ER, eds, Philadelphia, PA: WB Saunders Co, 1999, 1570-600.

Limitations There are many causes of elevated plasma catecholamines, including recent surgery, traumatic injury, upright posture, cold, anxiety, pain, clonidine withdrawal, and concurrent acute or chronic illness.[3]

Methodology High performance liquid chromatography (HPLC) with electrochemical detection is the method of choice.[1] Other methods include coupled-column liquid chromatography,[4] fluorometry, radioenzymatic assay, and radioimmunoassay (RIA). HPLC provides higher levels than do radioenzymatic methods.[5]

Additional Information A partial list of drugs which increase and decrease plasma and urine catecholamines is presented in the table.[1] New immunoassays for urinary catecholamines and metanephrines are reported to provide advantages from drug interference.[6] Using HPLC with electrochemical detection, measurement of urinary metanephrines to creatinine ratios, Héron et al reported near elimination of false positives from food or drugs.[7]

Footnotes

1. Rosano TG and Whitley RJ, "Catecholamines and Serotonin," *Tietz Textbook of Clinical Chemistry*, 3rd ed, Burtis CA and Ashwood ER, eds, Philadelphia, PA: WB Saunders Co, 1999, 1570-600.
2. Mayo Medical Laboratories, *2000 Test Catalog*, Rochester, MN, 123-4 and 526-7.
3. Desai SP and Isa-Pratt S, *Clinician's Guide to Laboratory Medicine*, Hudson, OH: Lexi-Comp, 2000, 353-60.
4. Panholzer TJ, Beyer J, and Lichtwald K, "Coupled-Column Liquid Chromatographic Analysis of Catecholamines, Serotonin, and Metabolites in Human Urine," *Clin Chem*, 1999, 45(2):262-8.
5. Bravo EL, "Plasma or Urinary Metanephrines for the Diagnosis of Pheochromocytoma? That Is the Question," *Ann Intern Med*, 1996, 125(4):331-2.
6. Wassell J, Reed P, Kane J, et al, "Freedom From Drug Interference in New Immunoassays for Urinary Catecholamines and Metanephrines," *Clin Chem*, 1999, 45(12):2216-23.
7. Héron E, Chatellier G, Billaud E, et al, "The Urinary Metanephrine-to-Creatinine Ratio for the Diagnosis of Pheochromocytoma," *Ann Intern Med*, 1996, 125(4):300-3.

References

Eisenhofer G, Lenders JW, Linehan WM, et al, "Plasma Normetanephrine and Metanephrine for Detecting Pheochromocytoma in von Hippel-Lindau Disease and Multiple Endocrine Neoplasia Type 2," *N Engl J Med*, 1999, 340(24):1872-9.

Gerlo EA and Sevens C, "Urinary and Plasma Catecholamines and Urinary Catecholamine Metabolites in Pheochromocytoma: Diagnostic Value in 19 Cases," *Clin Chem*, 1994, 40(2):250-6.

Krakoff LR, "Searching for Pheochromocytoma: A New and Better Test?" *Ann Intern Med*, 1995, 123(2):150-1.

Lenders JW, Keiser HR, Goldstein DS, et al, "Plasma Metanephrines in the Diagnosis of Pheochromocytomas," *Ann Intern Med*, 1995, 123(2):101-9.

Neumann HP, Berger DP, Sigmund G, et al, "Pheochromocytomas, Multiple Endocrine Neoplasia Type 2, and von Hippel-Lindau Disease," *N Engl J Med*, 1993, 329(21):1531-8.

Catecholamines, Fractionation, Urine

Related Information

Calcitonin, Serum or Plasma *on page 129*
Catecholamines, Fractionation, Plasma *on page 138*
Homovanillic Acid, Urine *on page 195*
Metanephrines, Urine or Plasma *on page 223*
Urine Collection, 24-Hour *on page 47*
Vanillylmandelic Acid, Urine *on page 297*

Synonyms Free Catecholamine Fractionation, Urine

Applies to Dopamine, Urine; Epinephrine, Urine; Norepinephrine, Urine

Replaces Total Urinary Catecholamines

Abstract Following their release and transmitter/hormonal activity, the catecholamines, epinephrine, norepinephrine, and dopamine are either taken back up by storage particles, converted to metabolites (eg, metanephrine, normetanephrine, methoxyhydroxyphenylglycol, vanillylmandelic acid), or excreted in the urine as free amines and as glucuronide or sulfate conjugates. Disorders associated with abnormal production of catecholamines include neurochromaffin tumors: pheochromocytoma, paraganglioma, and neuroblastoma.

Patient Preparation Avoid patient stress, exercise, smoking, and pain. Many drugs (reserpine and α-methyldopa, levodopa, monoamine oxidase inhibitors, and sympathomimetic amines) may interfere and should be discontinued 2 weeks prior to specimen collection. Nose drops, sinus and cough medicines, bronchodilators and appetite suppressants, α_2-agonists, calcium channel blockers, converting enzyme inhibitors, bromocriptine, phenothiazine, tricyclic antidepressants, alpha and beta blockers, labetalol may interfere.[1] Mandelamine® interferes, but thiazides do not. Drug effects may be difficult to anticipate. Caffeine products should be avoided before and during collection. The patient should not be subjected to hypoglycemia or exertion. Increased intracranial pressure and clonidine withdrawal can also cause false-positive results.[1]

Specimen 24-hour urine

Overnight collections for urinary metanephrines and catecholamines have been advocated for diagnosis of pheochromocytoma.[2]

Container Brown urine container with sufficient acetic acid to keep pH between 2-4. Typically, 25 mL of 50% acetic acid for an adult, and 15 mL of 50% acetic acid for a child younger than 5 years of age.[3]

Storage Instructions Refrigerate during and after collection.

Special Instructions Consult performing laboratory

Reference Interval The following ranges are from a reference laboratory employing HPLC methodology.[3,4]

Epinephrine:
- <1 year: 0.0-2.5 µg/24 hours
- 1 year: 0.0-3.5 µg/24 hours
- 2-3 years: 0.0-6.0 µg/24 hours
- 4-9 years: 0.2-10.0 µg/24 hours
- 10-15 years: 0.5-20.0 µg/24 hours

(Continued)

Catecholamines, Fractionation, Urine (Continued)

- ≥16 years: 0.0-20.0 µg/24 hours

Norepinephrine:
- <1 year: 0-10 µg/24 hours
- 1 year: 1-17 µg/24 hours
- 2-3 years: 4-29 µg/24 hours
- 4-6 years: 8-45 µg/24 hours
- 7-9 years: 13-65 µg/24 hours
- ≥10 years: 15-80 µg/24 hours

Dopamine:
- <1 year: 0-85 µg/24 hours
- 1 year: 10-140 µg/24 hours
- 2-3 years: 40-260 µg/24 hours
- ≥4 years: 65-400 µg/24 hours

Critical Values An epinephrine secretion >50 µg/24 hours (SI: >297 nmol/day) may be the only abnormality in subjects who have the multiple endocrine adenomatosis syndrome.

Use Measurement of urine catecholamines is one of the most effective biochemical tests for the diagnosis of catecholamine-secreting neoplasms. More than 90% of these are adrenal pheochromocytomas; other catecholamine-secreting neoplasms include paragangliomas and neuroblastomas. Presented in the graph and table in the listing Catecholamines, Fractionation, Plasma *on page 138* are results from ~500 hypertensive patients seen at the Mayo Clinic. Note the usual tradeoff between sensitivity and specificity.[3] See diagram.

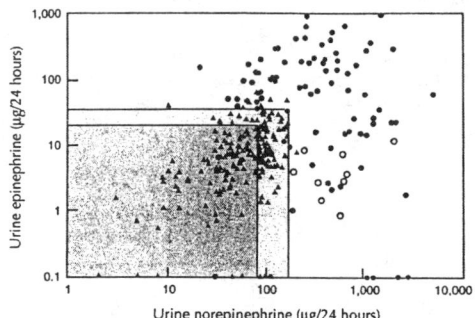

▲ Individuals without pheochromocytoma
○ Extra-adrenal pheochromocytomas
● Surgically proven pheochromocytoma

The darkest-shaded zone represents patients with epinephrine (E) values ≤ 20 µg/24 hours and norepinephrine (NE) values ≤80 µg/24 hours. Concentrations outside of these limits result in sensitivities and specificities in the diagnosis of pheochromocytoma as shown in the following chart. Similarly, the medium-shaded area has upper limits for E of 35 µg/24 hours and NE of 170 µg/24 hours. The next lighter-shaded area has upper limits for E of 200 pg/mL and NE of 2000 pg/mL. See the following for the sensitivity and specificity figures for values falling outside of each of the areas defined above.

Adapted from *2000 Test Catalogue*, Mayo Medical Laboratories, Rochester, MN.

Limits From the Graph and Their Diagnostic Efficacy in Diagnosis of Pheochromocytoma

Limits	Sensitivity (%)	Specificity (%)
E: 20 µg/24 hours NE: 80 µg/24 hours	98 (90/92)	45 (90/200)
E: 35 µg/24 hours NE: 170 µg/24 hours	97 (89/92)	95 (191/200)

Adapted from Mayo Medical Laboratories, *2000 Test Catalogue*.

Limitations There are many causes of elevated plasma catecholamines including recent surgery, traumatic injury, upright posture, cold, anxiety, pain, clonidine withdrawal, and concurrent acute or chronic illness.[4]

Methodology High performance liquid chromatography (HPLC), fluorometry, radioenzymatic assay, radioimmunoassay (RIA)

Additional Information A partial list of drugs which increase and decrease urinary catecholamines appears in the listing Catecholamines, Fractionation, Plasma *on page 138*. New immunoassays are reported to provide advantages from drug interference.[5]

See Catecholamines, Fractionation, Plasma *on page 138* and Metanephrines, Urine or Plasma *on page 223*.

Footnotes

1. Sheps SG, Jiang NS, Klee GG, et al, "Recent Developments in the Diagnosis and Treatment of Pheochromocytoma," *Mayo Clin Proc*, 1990, 65(1):88-95.
2. Peaston RT, Lennard TW, and Lai LC, "Overnight Excretion of Urinary Catecholamines and Metabolites in the Detection of Pheochromocytoma," *J Clin Endocrinol Metab*, 1996, 81(4):1378-84.
3. Mayo Medical Laboratories, *2000 Test Catalogue*, Rochester, MN, 124.
4. Desai SP and Isa-Pratt S, *Clinician's Guide to Laboratory Medicine*, Hudson, OH: Lexi-Comp, 2000, 353-60.
5. Wassell J, Reed P, Kane J, et al, "Freedom From Drug Interference in New Immunoassays for Urinary Catecholamines and Metanephrines," *Clin Chem*, 1999, 45(12):2216-23.

References

Gerlo EA and Sevens C, "Urinary and Plasma Catecholamines and Urinary Catecholamine Metabolites in Pheochromocytoma: Diagnostic Value in 19 Cases," *Clin Chem*, 1994, 40(2):250-6.

Krakoff LR, "Searching for Pheochromocytoma: A New and Better Test?" *Ann Intern Med*, 1995, 123(2):150-1.

Panholzer TJ, Beyer J, and Lichtwald K, "Coupled-Column Liquid Chromatographic Analysis of Catecholamines, Serotonin, and Metabolites in Human Urine," *Clin Chem*, 1999, 45(2):262-8.

Payne RB, "Urinary Catecholamine Excretion in Relation to Renal Function," *Ann Clin Biochem*, 2000, 37(Pt 2):228-9.

Roberts NB, Dutton J, McClelland P, et al, "Urinary Catecholamine Excretion in Relation to Renal Function," *Ann Clin Biochem*, 1999, 36(Pt 5):587-91.

Rosano TG and Whitley RJ, "Catecholamines and Serotonin," *Tietz Textbook of Clinical Chemistry*, 3rd ed, Chapter 14, Burtis CA and Ashwood ER, eds, Philadelphia, PA: WB Saunders Co, 1999, 1570-600.

Rosano TG, Swift TA, and Hayes LW, "Advances in Catecholamine and Metabolite Measurements for Diagnosis of Pheochromocytoma," *Clin Chem*, 1991, 37(10 Pt 2):1854-67.

Tzontcheva A and Denikova N, "Analytical Interference of Drugs on the Fluorimetric Determination of Urinary Catecholamines," *Clin Chim Acta*, 2000, 297(1-2):217-23.

Weinkove C, "Measurement of Catecholamines and Their Metabolites in Urine," *J Clin Pathol*, 1991, 44(4):269-75.

- ♦ **Cb1** *see* Cobalamin, Serum *on page 150*

- ♦ **CCCT** *see* Follicle Stimulating Hormone, Serum, Plasma, or Urine *on page 175*

- ♦ **CDT** *see* Carbohydrate-Deficient Transferrin, Serum *on page 134*

- ♦ **CEA** *see* Carcinoembryonic Antigen, Serum *on page 135*

- ♦ **CEA, Body Fluid** *see* Body Fluid Chemical Analysis *on page 123*

- ♦ **Central Venous Blood** *see* Blood Gases and pH, Venous *on page 122*

- ♦ **Cephalin Flocculation** *replaced by* Alanine Aminotransferase, Serum *on page 87*

- ♦ **Cephalin Flocculation** *replaced by* Aspartate Aminotransferase, Serum *on page 112*

- ♦ **Cerebrospinal Fluid Angiotensin Converting Enzyme** *see* Angiotensin Converting Enzyme, Serum *on page 105*

Cerebrospinal Fluid Glucose

Related Information

Bacterial Culture, Cerebrospinal Fluid *on page 569*
Body Fluid Glucose *on page 124*
Cerebrospinal Fluid Analysis: Overview *on page 416*
Cerebrospinal Fluid Lactate Dehydrogenase *on page 142*
Cerebrospinal Fluid Lactic Acid *on page 143*
Cerebrospinal Fluid Protein *on page 517*
Cerebrospinal Fluid Protein Electrophoresis *on page 518*

Synonyms CSF Glucose; Glucose, Cerebrospinal Fluid; Spinal Fluid Glucose

Applies to Hypoglycorrhachia; Neuroglycopenia

Abstract For diagnosis of meningitis, culture and Gram staining have priority over all other testing when only a small quantity of cerebrospinal fluid (CSF) is available. Cell count with differential deserve the next priority, followed by glucose and protein.

Patient Preparation Blood (ie, plasma) glucose is needed also. Ideally, it should be drawn 2 hours before the lumbar puncture, the equilibration time.

Specimen Cerebrospinal fluid

Container Clean, sterile CSF tube

Reference Interval 40-70 mg/dL (SI: 2.2-3.9 mmol/L) in fasting patients, should be interpreted with plasma glucose. Values may be somewhat higher in infants and young children, 60-80 mg/dL (SI: 3.4-4.5 mmol/L).[1] CSF glucose should be 60% to 70% of plasma glucose. However, equilibration between plasma and CSF glucose levels may require several hours. In premature and newborn infants, CSF glucose may be 80% or more of plasma glucose, possibly due to greater permeability of the blood-brain barrier and/or increased rate of cerebral blood flow.

Critical Values Less than 40% of simultaneously analyzed serum glucose

Possible Panic Range <40 mg/dL (SI: <2.2 mmol/L), especially with increased cells and/or protein

Use Evaluate viral, bacterial, tuberculous, fungal and other types of meningitis; neoplastic involvement of meninges; other neurological disorders. Diagnose neuroglycopenia, even in the presence of normal plasma glucose. CSF glucose values may be helpful in the distinction of bacterial versus viral meningitis; the CSF glucose values are low (hypoglycorrhachia) in bacterial and tuberculous meningitis. Hypoglycorrhachia may be seen in extensive neoplastic disease of meninges and with subarachnoid hemorrhage. CSF glucose is generally normal in viral disease, but occasionally it may be low with aseptic meningitis.

While the finding of glucose in clear nasal discharge has in past years been considered indicative of CSF rhinorrhea,[2] studies have shown that glucose may be present in non-CSF nasal fluids[3,4] and is therefore not recommended alone for the diagnosis of CSF rhinorrhea. CSF transferrin levels have been used as a marker of CSF leak (see Iron and Total Iron Binding Capacity/Transferrin, Serum *on page 203*). Recommended procedures include CSF protein electrophoresis and use of chloride as well as glucose content and imaging procedures.

Limitations Falsely decreased levels may result from cellular and bacterial utilization of glucose if the test is not performed immediately. Visibly xanthochromic samples may give misleading results. The sensitivity of CSF glucose for bacterial meningitis was only 72% in a series from Minnesota, inferior to the sensitivity of the nucleated blood cell count,[5] but multiple tests are used together. Bloody taps cause falsely increased glucose, since there is more glucose in blood.

Methodology Same procedures as used for blood glucose (eg, glucose oxidase, hexokinase reactions); a reagent strip and a handheld analyzer method have been reported as reliable for use in the bedside determination of CSF glucose.[6]

Additional Information Elevation implies hyperglycemia 2-4 hours earlier. In acute bacterial meningitis, cerebrospinal fluid glucose levels are classically <40 mg/dL (SI: <2.2 mmol/L) in a fasting patient with normal plasma glucose. The frequency of low CSF glucose in bacterial meningitis varies somewhat between series. A major textbook of pediatrics points out that acute viral meningitis is often differentiated from acute bacterial meningitis because the latter is characterized by a CSF glucose <30 mg/dL, a CSF glucose:blood glucose ratio <0.2-0.3 as well as a protein >200 mg/dL, a CSF PMN count >1000/mm^3, and an 80% to 90% likelihood of positive Gram stain in an illness often occurring during the winter in a child younger than 2 years of age.[7] The magnitude of the seasonal curves for viral versus bacterial meningitis (the former more frequent in the summer) is greater than some clinicians appreciate.[8] In 134 Gram stain positive cases, CSF glucose was 14.4/30.6/50.4 mg/dL, 25th percentile/ median/75th percentile.[8] **The gold standard for the diagnosis of bacterial meningitis is the culture,**[5,9] which is fundamental to appropriate diagnosis and treatment.[10] Decreased CSF glucose is characteristically but not invariably found in tuberculous, fungal, and amebic meningitis (*Naegleria*) as well as in bacterial meningitis. Glucose is usually normal in viral meningitis, but in herpes or mumps meningoencephalitis, lymphocytic choriomeningitis, and with enterovirus infection, glucose may be low. Sarcoidosis and neurosyphilis are reported causes of low CSF glucose. Other very uncommon causes of low CSF glucose include meningeal cysticercosis, trichinosis, and with the chemical meningitis which accompanies intrathecal therapy. Low CSF glucose may also occur in subarachnoid hemorrhage and neoplasia (eg, medulloblastoma). Low CSF glucose may be found in CNS leukemia. Decrease has led to the diagnosis of insulinoma presenting with CNS symptoms. Rheumatoid meningitis and lupus myelopathy may cause low CSF glucose.[10] CSF glucose levels ≤20 mg/dL are highly correlated with bacterial meningitis.[11]

Lactic acid may be useful in the diagnosis of bacterial meningitis, but values overlap those found with viral meningitis (aseptic meningitis).[10,12]

Footnotes

1. Painter RC, Cope JY, and Smith JL, "Reference Information for Clinical Laboratory," *Tietz Textbook of Clinical Chemistry*, 3rd ed, Burtis CA and Ashwood ER, eds, Philadelphia, PA: WB Saunders Co, 1999, 1815.
2. Beckhardt RN, Setzen M, and Carras R, "Primary Spontaneous Cerebrospinal Fluid Rhinorrhea," *Otolaryngol Head Neck Surg*, 1991, 104(4):425-32.
3. Hull HF and Morrow G, "Glucorrhea Revisited: Prolonged Promulgation of Another Plastic Pearl," *JAMA*, 1975, 234:1052-3.
4. Steedman DJ and Gordon M, "CSF Rhinorrhea: Significance of the Glucose Oxidase Strip Test," *Injury*, 1987, 18(5):327-8.
5. Rodewald LE, Woodin KA, Szilagyi PG, et al, "Relevance of Common Tests of Cerebrospinal Fluid in Screening for Bacterial Meningitis," *J Pediatr*, 1991, 119(3):363-9.
6. Slovis CM, Negus RA, Amerson SM, et al, "Bedside Cerebrospinal Fluid Glucose Analysis," *Ann Emerg Med*, 1989, 18(9):931-3.
7. Behrman RE, Kliegman RM, and Jenson HB, *Nelson Textbook of Pediatrics*, 16th ed, Philadelphia, PA: WB Saunders Co, 2000, 1793-802.
8. Spanos A, Harrell FE Jr, and Durack DT, "Differential Diagnosis of Acute Meningitis. An Analysis of the Predictive Value of Initial Observations," *JAMA*, 1989, 262(19):2700-7.
9. Smith AL, "Bacterial Meningitis," *Pediatr Rev*, 1993, 14(1):11-8.
10. Fishman RA, *Cerebrospinal Fluid in Diseases of the Nervous System*, 2nd ed, Philadelphia, PA: WB Saunders Co, 1992, 219-21.
11. Greenlee JE, "Approach to Diagnosis of Meningitis - Cerebrospinal Fluid Evaluation," *Infect Dis Clin North Am*, 1990, 4(4):583-98.
12. Leib SL, Boscacci R, Gratzl O, et al, "Predictive Value of Cerebrospinal Fluid (CSF) Lactate Level Versus CSF/Blood Glucose Ratio for the Diagnosis of Bacterial Meningitis Following Neurosurgery," *Clin Infect Dis*, 1999, 29(1):69-74.

References

Avery GM, "Measurement of Glucose in Cerebrospinal Fluid With Reagent Strips and a Reflectance Photometer," *Clin Chem*, 1991, 37(4):590-1.
Bonadio WA and Smith D, "Cerebrospinal Fluid Changes After 48 Hours of Effective Therapy for *Haemophilus influenzae* Type B Meningitis," *Am J Clin Pathol*, 1990, 94(4):426-8.
Givens TG, Paul RI, Bothner JP, et al, "Cerebrospinal Fluid Glucose and Protein in Disposition and Treatment Decisions," *Acad Emerg Med*, 2000, 7(3):298-302.
Gray LD and Fedorko DP, "Laboratory Diagnosis of Bacterial Meningitis," *Clin Microbiol Rev*, 1992, 5(2):130-45.
Olukoga AO, Bolodeoku J, and Donaldson D, "Cerebrospinal Fluid Analysis in Clinical Diagnosis," *J Clin Pathol*, 1997, 50(3):187-92.

Schutte CM and van der Meyden CH, "Prospective Study of Glasgow Coma Scale (GCS), Age, CSF-Neutrophil Count, and CSF-Protein and Glucose Levels as Prognostic Indicators in 100 Adult Patients With Meningitis," *J Infect*, 1998, 37(2):112-5.

Cerebrospinal Fluid Glutamine

Related Information
  Ammonia, Plasma *on page 102*

Synonyms CSF Glutamine; Glutamine, Spinal Fluid

Abstract CSF glutamine is increased in diseases causing hyperammonemia. These include liver disease, urea cycle defects, and certain organic acidurias. Ammonia, toxic to the nervous system, combines with alphaketoglutarate to yield glutamine. Such glutamine formation serves to protect the nervous system.[1]

Specimen Cerebrospinal fluid

Container Clean, sterile CSF tube

Collection Tube should be labeled with the number indicating the sequence in which tubes were obtained.

Storage Instructions With immediate deproteinization CSF samples may be stored for 9 months at -80°C.[2]

Causes for Rejection Samples contaminated with red blood cells

Special Instructions Specimen must be transported **immediately** to the laboratory.

Reference Interval Varies with lab and age. Published ranges include:[2]
  • neonates: 216-1200 µmol/L
  • 3 months to 2 years: 320-676 µmol/L
  • 2-10 years: 299-627 µmol/L
  • adults: 522-658 µmol/L
  See Methodology.

Use Evaluate hepatic encephalopathy and aid in assessment of its severity; evaluate coma; increased in many instances of Reye syndrome (20 of 27 cases); work up hyperammonemic encephalopathies.[3] Levels from 25-95 mg/dL are seen with hepatic coma. Values >35 mg/dL are almost always related to encephalopathy.[1]

Limitations Higher levels are reported with parenteral nutrition, meningitis, and in cerebral hemorrhage. This test is not used extensively.

Methodology Enzymatic, amino acid analyzer, high performance liquid chromatography (HPLC), capillary-isotachophoresis.[4] Glutamine/glutamate levels vary widely with different methods and in particular with specimen handling and preparation prior to analysis. This may be due importantly to *in vitro* hydrolysis of glutamine to glutamate. Immediate deproteinization of CSF may circumvent this problem.

Additional Information Glutamine is the most prominent amino acid in CSF. CSF glutamine levels may be used with plasma ammonia determinations in diagnosis of hepatic encephalopathy. In hepatic encephalopathy, plasma glutamine values correlate better with the clinical course than do values for plasma ammonia.[1] There is evidence that CSF glutamine concentrations are within normal range in a variety of infectious, inflammatory, degenerative and metabolic neurologic disorders.[5] Levels are increased in some cases of meningitis and associated with CSF pleocytosis. Elevated CSF total protein (>40 mg/dL [SI: >0.4 g/L]), in which some examples of loss of integrity of the blood-brain-CSF would be expected, is not accompanied by increase in CSF glutamine unless cell count is also increased. With response of meningitis to therapy (and fall in CSF cell count), CSF glutamine also declines.[5] Increase in CSF glutamine relating to pleocytosis is of a much lesser magnitude than the high levels occurring in cases of hepatic coma. CSF glutamine values are extraordinarily high (75,000 µM) in ornithine transcarbamylase and argininosuccinate lyase deficiency.[3] Increased values are reported in various neurological diseases, including Alzheimer disease and in depression.[6]

Footnotes

1. Fishman RA, *Cerebrospinal Fluid in Diseases of the Nervous System*, 2nd ed, Philadelphia, PA: WB Saunders Co, 1992, 238-9.
2. Painter RC, Cope JY, and Smith JL, "Reference Information for Clinical Laboratory," *Tietz Textbook of Clinical Chemistry*, 3rd ed, Burtis CA and Ashwood ER, eds, 1999, Philadelphia, PA: WB Saunders Co, 1815.
3. Scriver CR, Kaufman S, Eisensmith RC, et al, "Amino Acids," Part 5, *The Metabolic and Molecular Basis of Inherited Disease*, 7th ed, Scriver CR, Beaudet AL, Sly WS, et al, New York, NY: McGraw-Hill Inc, 1995, 1015-368.
4. Tucci S, Pinto C, Goyo J, et al, "Measurement of Glutamine and Glutamate by Capillary Electrophoresis and Laser Induced Fluorescence Detection In Cerebrospinal Fluid of Meningitis Sick Children," *Clin Biochem*, 1998, 31(3):143-50.
5. Hiraoka A, Miura I, Tominaga I, et al, "Capillary-Isotachophoretic Determination of Glutamine in Cerebrospinal Fluid of Various Neurological Disorders," *Clin Biochem*, 1989, 22(4):293-6.
6. Levine J, Panchalingam K, Rapoport A, et al, "Increased Cerebrospinal Fluid Glutamine Levels in Depressed Patients," *Biol Psychiatry 1*, 2000, 47(7):586-93.

References

Mizock BA, Sabelli HC, Dubin A, et al, "Septic Encephalopathy. Evidence for Altered Phenylalanine Metabolism and Comparison With Hepatic Encephalopathy," *Arch Intern Med*, 1990, 150(2):443-9.
Olukoga AO, Bolodeoku J, and Donaldson D, "Cerebrospinal Fluid Analysis in Clinical Diagnosis," *J Clin Pathol*, 1997, 50(3):187-92.
Teerlink T, Hennekes MW, Van Leeuwen PA, et al, "Rapid Determination of Glutamine in Biological Samples by High Performance Liquid Chromatography," *Clin Chim Acta*, 1993, 218(2):159-68.

Cerebrospinal Fluid Glycine

Related Information
Amino Acids, Plasma *on page 100*
Amino Acids, Urine *on page 101*

Synonyms CSF Glycine; Glycine, Cerebrospinal Fluid

Applies to Isovaleric Aciduria; Methylmalonic Aciduria; Nonketotic Hyperglycinemia; Propionic Aciduria

Test Includes Cerebrospinal fluid (CSF) and plasma glycine

Abstract Glycine is a nonessential amino acid. CSF glycine is increased in nonketotic hyperglycinemia (NKH), due to a genetic defect in the glycine cleavage system. Of the four forms of NKH (neonatal, infantile, late onset, and transient), neonatal is the most common type. Patients with NKH develop rapidly progressive neurological symptoms (eg, muscular hypotonia, seizures, apneic attacks and lethargy, and coma). CSF glycine is also increased in certain organic acidurias (eg, methylmalonic, propionic, isovaleric). Increase in CSF:plasma glycine ratio is more diagnostic than absolute CSF or plasma values in the diagnosis of NKH.

Specimen Cerebrospinal fluid; blood sample should also be drawn at the same time for plasma glycine.

Container CSF tube, green top (heparin) tube for blood

Sampling Time Fasting sample is preferred.

Causes for Rejection Traumatic CSF tap (falsely increases glycine values)

Reference Interval
- Plasma: 120-375 μmol/L
- CSF: 3-10 μmol/L
- CSF:plasma ratio: 0.01-0.04

Critical Values The following pathological values have been reported.[1]
Plasma:
- neonatal type: 460-2580 μmol/L
- late-onset type: 340-920 μmol/L
CSF: neonatal type: 33-440 μmol/L
CSF:plasma ratio:
- neonatal type: 0.09-0.25 (diagnostic)
- late-onset type: 0.06-0.10

Use CSF and plasma glycine levels are used in the diagnosis of nonketotic hyperglycinemia.

Limitations WIth traumatic tap, contamination of CSF with blood makes the test invalid.

Methodology Amino acid analyzer (ion-exchange chromatography), high performance liquid chromatography (HPLC)

Additional Information NKH is an autosomal recessive disorder, due to deficiency of the glycine cleavage system. Several mutations have been identified in the glycine cleavage enzyme complex.[2] The disorder is clinically divided into two major types: neonatal and late-onset. Two other forms, infantile and transient, have been described. Most patients have neonatal phenotype. These patients present, in the first few days of life, with lethargy, hypotonia, and myoclonic jerks, generally progressing to apnea and often death. Those who survive such episodes develop intractable seizures and profound mental retardation. A minority of the patients develop symptoms later in life. These patients present with progressive spastic diplegia and optic atrophy. However, they patients do not develop seizures, and their intellectual function remains preserved.[3]

Apnea and hiccuping in NKH is thought to be due to an inhibitory effect of glycine on the spinal cord and brain stem. Intractable seizures and brain damage in NKH are probably due to excitatory effects of glycine on N-methyl-D-aspartate receptor.[3]

The diagnosis of NKH is based on increased CSF:plasma glycine ratio. The confirmatory diagnosis is measurement of activity of glycine cleavage complex in liver tissue. Although no uniformly effective treatment exists, therapies are directed to reduce glycine levels by giving benzoate to the patients and blocking N-methyl-D-aspartate receptor.[4,5,6,7] Benzoate binds to glycine to form hippurate, which is excreted in the urine. Prenatal diagnosis for NKH by enzymatic analysis of chorionic villus samples in 28 families and by DNA analysis in 2 families was recently published.[8]

Footnotes

1. Tada K, "Disorders of Glycine and Imino Acids," *Physician's Guide to the Laboratory Diagnosis of Metabolic Diseases*, Blau N, Duran M, and Blaskovics, eds, London: Chapman & Hall, 1996, 201-8.

2. Toone JR, Applegarth DA, Coulter-Mackie MB, et al, "Biochemical and Molecular Investigations of Patients With Nonketotic Hyperglycinemia," *Mol Genet Metab*, 2000, 70(2):116-21.

3. Hamosh A, Johnston MV, and Valle D, "Nonketotic Hyperglycinemia," *The Metabolic and Molecular Basis of Inherited Disease*, 7th ed, Scriver CR, Beaudet AL, Sly WS, et al, eds, New York, NY: McGraw-Hill Inc, 1995, 1337-48.

4. Neuberger JM, Schweitzer S, Rolland MO, et al, "Effect of Sodium Benzoate in the Treatment of Atypical Nonketotic Hyperglycinaemia," *J Inherit Metab Dis*, 2000, 23(1):22-6.

5. Wiltshire EJ, Poplawski NK, Harrison JR, et al, "Treatment of Late-Onset Nonketotic Hyperglycinaemia: Effectiveness of Imipramine and Benzoate," *J Inherit Metab Dis*, 2000, 23(1):15-21.

6. Hamosh A, Maher JF, Bellus GA, et al, "Long-Term Use of High-Dose Benzoate and Dextromethorphan for the Treatment of Nonketotic Hyperglycinemia," *J Pediatr*, 1998, 132(4):709-13.

7. Deutsch SI, Rosse RB, and Mastropaolo J, "Current Status of NMDA Antagonist Interventions in the Treatment of Nonketotic Hyperglycinemia," *Clin Neuropharmacol*, 1998, 21(2):71-9.

8. Kure S, Rolland MO, Leisti J, et al, "Prenatal Diagnosis of Nonketotic Hyperglycinaemia: Enzymatic Diagnosis in 28 Families and DNA Diagnosis Detecting Prevalent Finnish and Israeli-Arab Mutations," *Prenat Diagn*, 1999, 19(8):717-20.

References

Boneh A, Degani Y, and Harari M, "Prognostic Clues and Outcome of Early Treatment of Nonketotic Hyperglycinemia," *Pediatr Neurol*, 1996, 15(2):137-41.

Kure S, Tada K, and Narisawa K, "Nonketotic Hyperglycinemia: Biochemical, Molecular, and Neurological Aspects," *Jpn J Hum Genet* 1997, 42(1):13-22.

Lu FL, Wang PJ, Hwu WL, et al, "Neonatal Type of Nonketotic Hyperglycinemia," *Pediatr Neurol* 1999, 20(4):295-300.

Maeda T, Inutsuka M, Goto K, et al, "Transient Nonketotic Hyperglycinemia in an asphyxiated Patient With Pyridoxine-Dependent Seizures," *Pediatr Neurol*, 2000, 22(3):225-7.

Steiner RD, Sweetser DA, Rohrbaugh JR, et al, "Nonketotic Hyperglycinemia: Atypical Clinical and Biochemical Manifestations," *J Pediatr*, 1996, 128(2):243-6.

Van Hove JL, Kishnani P, Muenzer J, et al, "Benzoate Therapy and Carnitine Deficiency in Nonketotic Hyperglycinemia," *Am J Med Genet*, 1995, 59(4):444-53.

Cerebrospinal Fluid Lactate Dehydrogenase

Related Information
Body Fluid Lactate Dehydrogenase *on page 125*
Cerebrospinal Fluid Glucose *on page 140*
Cerebrospinal Fluid Lactic Acid *on page 143*
Lactate Dehydrogenase Isoenzymes, Serum *on page 206*
Lactate Dehydrogenase, Serum *on page 207*

Synonyms Cerebrospinal Fluid LD; CSF LD; Lactate Dehydrogenase, Cerebrospinal Fluid; Spinal Fluid LD

Applies to Lactic Acid Dehydrogenase, Fluid

Abstract Lactate dehydrogenase (LD) is a normal component of cerebrospinal fluid (CSF).

Specimen Cerebrospinal fluid

Container Clean, sterile CSF tube

Reference Interval CSF LD (LDH) activity is normally much less than the plasma LD activity. Normal spinal fluid LD levels are about 10% of serum values (<20 units/L). In children, the reference range is 0-23.5 units/L.[1] LD_4 and LD_5 are often not found.

Use Elevated CSF LD, nearly equal to the serum activity, is usually associated with ischemic necrosis, meningitis, leukemia, primary or metastatic CNS cancer, and CNS lymphoma. CSF LD has been used by some to identify bacterial meningitis,[1] but overlapping with results in cases of viral meningitis is recognized.[2] CSF lactate, LD, and LD isoenzymes do not provide definitive data for a diagnosis of bacterial meningitis in childhood.[3]

With CK and AST, cerebrospinal fluid LD has been advocated to distinguish cortical from lacunar stroke. These three enzymes are increased in cases of cortical stroke. While CK and AST are not increased with lacunar stroke, LD is only slightly elevated. CSF LD is increased in patients with severe brain injury but is not useful (as is CK-BB) in assessing the degree of injury or in monitoring outcome.[4] Other monitors of CNS injury include S-100, Serum and Neuron-Specific Enolase, Serum *on page 229*.

Another possible application of LD measurement is the differential diagnosis of intracranial hemorrhage in neonates versus traumatic tap. Lactate dehydrogenase is elevated in proportion to severity of CNS hemorrhage. CSF LDH is higher in stroke than in transient ischemic attack.[5]

Limitations This test has very limited usefulness, due to its nonspecificity.

Methodology Enzymatic

Additional Information A tabulation of CSF enzymes in neurological diseases is available.[2]

Footnotes

1. Knight JA, Dudek SM, and Haymond RE, "Early (Chemical) Diagnosis of Bacterial Meningitis - Cerebrospinal Fluid Glucose, Lactate, and Lactate Dehydrogenase Compared," *Clin Chem*, 1981, 27(8):1431-4.

2. Fishman RA, *Cerebrospinal Fluid in Diseases of the Nervous System*, 2nd ed, Philadelphia, PA: WB Saunders Co, 1992, 215-6.

3. Castro-Gago M, Couce ML, Losada MC, et al, "C-Reactive Protein, Lactate, and LDH Isoenzymes in the Cerebrospinal Fluid in the Diagnosis in Childhood Meningitis," *An Esp Pediatr*, 1988, 28(1):31-3.

4. Paşaoğlu A and Paşaoğlu H, "Enzymatic Changes in the Cerebrospinal Fluid as Indices of Pathological Change," *Acta Neurochir*, 1989, 97(1-2):71-6.

5. Lampl Y, Paniri Y, Eshel Y, et al, "Cerebrospinal Fluid Lactate Dehydrogenase Levels in Early Stroke and Transient Ischemic Attacks," *Stroke*, 1990, 21(6):854-7.

References

Donnan GA, Zapf P, Doyle AE, et al, "CSF Enzymes in Lacunar and Cortical Stroke," *Stroke*, 1983, 14:266-9.

Lampl Y, Paniri Y, Eshel Y, et al, "LDH Isoenzymes in Cerebrospinal Fluid in Various Brain Tumours," *J Neurol Neurosurg Psychiatry*, 1990, 53(8):697-9.

Nolli ML, Picinni P, Polamarasetti T, et al, "Cerebrospinal Fluid Examination as a Possible Predictor of Neurological Outcome in Patients With Acute Liver Failure," *Transplant Proc*, 1993, 25(3):2218-9.

Cerebrospinal Fluid Lactic Acid

Related Information
Cerebrospinal Fluid Glucose *on page 140*
Lactic Acid, Whole Blood or Plasma *on page 208*

Synonyms CSF Lactic Acid; Lactic Acid, Cerebrospinal Fluid; Spinal Fluid Lactic Acid

Abstract Interest in CSF lactic acid is related to increases in bacterial meningitis and partially treated bacterial meningitis, in contrast to the usual finding of normal lactic acid with viral meningitis. However, overlapping concentrations in tuberculous, other bacterial and viral meningitis have limited its diagnostic value.[1,2]

Specimen Cerebrospinal fluid

Container Clean, sterile CSF tube

Storage Instructions Unstable at room temperature[3]

Reference Interval Increased in first 2 weeks of life. Approximate reference range is 4.5-28.8 mg/dL (SI: 0.5-3.2 mmol/L).[4]

Possible Panic Range Lactic acid >30.1 mg/dL (SI: >3.34 mmol/L) is present in essentially all instances of bacterial meningitis, inversely related to CSF glucose. Lower results are reported in partially treated bacterial meningitis.

Use CSF lactic acid has been used in differentiation of bacterial and nonbacterial meningitis. Rutledge et al reported that with equivocal clinical and spinal fluid findings, CSF lactic acid failed to distinguish between bacterial and nonbacterial infections.[5] CSF lactate must not be used in place of the traditional laboratory evaluation of meningitis. CSF lactate was elevated in all patients (group of 21) with culture proven tuberculous meningitis.[6] It was also elevated in cases of biopsy proven Creutzfeldt-Jakob disease (CJD) and has been suggested as a biochemical marker of that disease.[7] CSF lactic acid increase is a characteristic finding of acute infarct of cerebrum. Increased concentrations are found with cerebral hemorrhage, subarachnoid hemorrhage, primary CSF acidosis, malignant hypertension, hepatic encephalopathy, diabetes mellitus, hypoglycemic coma, and in the first 3 days following head injury.[1] An entity of developmental delay with infantile seizures and with depressed CSF glucose and lactate levels is noteworthy, because it responds to a special diet.[1]

Limitations Increases must be interpreted in light of the clinical setting and in concert with conventional parameters of meningitis work-up (glucose, protein, cell count, Gram stain, and culture). Slight increases have been described with craniocerebral trauma, stroke, seizures (up to 81.1 mg/dL (9.0 mmol/L)), and brain tumor. Results from neurosurgical cases must be interpreted cautiously. It is reported as elevated in fungal infections,[1] but concentrations have been reported to be erratic in cryptococcal meningitis. *Staphylococcus epidermidis* meningitis after shunt installation and very early neonatal bacterial meningitis have been described without increased lactic acid levels. Overlapping results limit the value of lactate assays in differential diagnosis between viral meningitis, partially treated bacterial meningitis, and tuberculous meningitis. The assay for lactic acid has not been shown to contribute to accuracy of diagnosis in instances of possible meningitis.[1]

Methodology Enzymatic, gas-liquid chromatography (GLC), amperometric utilizing a lactate-sensitive electrode[3]

Additional Information A linear increase in CSF lactate in relation to lactate producing inflammatory cells with high levels at cell counts >350/mm[3] has been noted.[8] It is implied that increase in CSF lactate results from CSF pleocytosis. Antimicrobial therapy given prior to collection of spinal fluid may decrease reliability of the usual diagnostic tests (Gram stain, cell count, culture, protein, and glucose levels). Equivocal results of tests in some instances of aseptic meningitis may lead to an erroneous diagnosis of bacterial etiology. The Gram stain may be negative in as many as 25% of culture-proven bacterial meningitides. Lactate determination may provide an indicator of the presence or absence of bacterial meningitis. Lactic acid in viral meningitis will occasionally fall between 2.78-3.34 mmol/L. Relapse has been detected by lactic acid assay, which may be of value in calibration of therapeutic response. In early stage of tuberculous meningitis, increased CSF lactate persists even with adequate antituberculous therapy.[8] Spinal fluid lactate levels are said to be independent of plasma levels.

A recent study has shown that following neurosurgery the predictive value of CSF lactate in the diagnosis of bacterial meningitis is higher than a CSF:blood glucose ratio.[9]

Footnotes
1. Fishman RA, *Cerebrospinal Fluid in Diseases of the Nervous System*, 2nd ed, Philadelphia, PA: WB Saunders Co, 1992.
2. Lebel MH, "Meningitis," *Oski's Pediatrics: Principles and Practice*, 3rd ed, McMillan JA, DeAngelis CD, Feigin RD, et al, eds, Philadelphia, PA: JB Lippincott Co, 1999, 413-6.
3. Brook I, "Stability of Lactic Acid in Cerebrospinal Fluid Specimens," *Am J Clin Pathol*, 1982, 77(2):213-6.
4. Cameron PD, Boyce JM, and Ansori BM, "Cerebrospinal Fluid Lactate in Meningitis and Meningocarcinoma," *J Infect*, 1993, 26(3):245-52.
5. Rutledge J, Benjamin D, Hood L, et al, "Is the CSF Lactate Measurement Useful in the Management of Children With Suspected Bacterial Meningitis?" *J Pediatr*, 1981, 98:20-4.
6. Tang LM, "Serial Lactate Determinations in Tuberculous Meningitis," *Scand J Infect Dis*, 1988, 20(1):81-3.
7. Awerbuch G, Peterson P, and Sandyk R, "Elevated Cerebrospinal Fluid Lactic Acid Levels in Creutzfeldt-Jakob Disease," *Int J Neurosci*, 1988, 42(1-2):1-5.
8. Kolmel HW and von Maravic M, "Correlation of Lactic Acid Level, Cell Count and Cytology in Cerebrospinal Fluid of Patients With Bacterial and Nonbacterial Meningitis," *Acta Neurol Scand*, 1988, 78(1):6-9.
9. Leib SL, Boscacci R, Gratzl O, et al, "Predictive Value of Cerebrospinal Fluid (CSF) Lactate Level Versus CSF/Blood Glucose Ratio for the Diagnosis of Bacterial Meningitis Following Neurosurgery," *Clin Infect Dis*, 1999, 29(1):69-74.

References
Gerber J, Tumani M, Kolenda M, et al, "Lumbar and Ventricular CSF Protein, Leukocytes and Lactate in Suspected Bacterial CNS Infections," *Neurology*, 1998, 51:1710-4.
Latcha S and Cunha BA, "*Listeria monocytogenes* Meningoencephalitis: The Diagnostic Importance of CSF Lactic Acid," *Heart Lung*, 1994, 23(2):177-9.
Stacpoole PW, Bunch ST, Neiberger RE, et al, "The Importance of Cerebrospinal Fluid Lactate in the Evaluation of Congenital Lactic Acidosis," *J Pediatr*, 1999, 134(1):99-102.

♦ **Cerebrospinal Fluid LD** *see* Cerebrospinal Fluid Lactate Dehydrogenase *on page 142*

Ceruloplasmin, Serum

Related Information
Copper, Serum *on page 816*
Copper, Urine *on page 818*
Liver Biopsy *on page 65*
Liver Disease: Laboratory Assessment, Overview *on page 216*

Applies to Transcuprein

Abstract Ceruloplasmin, a liver product, is the copper-containing protein of plasma. About 70% to 90% of copper in plasma is bound to this protein. It is decreased in Wilson disease (hepatolenticular degeneration), Menkes syndrome, and nutritional deficiency. It is an acute phase reactant and as such is increased in infections, malignancy, in pregnancy, with estrogens, and in trauma. Wilson disease (WD) is an autosomal recessive abnormality of copper metabolism. Diagnosis of WD can sometimes be made on the basis of hypoceruloplasminemia, hypocupremia, and hypercupruria,[1] with abnormalities in liver-related tests. Liver biopsy is often necessary for diagnosis of WD.

Specimen Serum

Container Red top tube

Collection Draw in chilled tube. Keep specimen on ice. Prolonged storage at room temperature leads to decreased levels. Although serum copper and serum ceruloplasmin are normally parallel one with the other, both are needed in Wilson disease and with acute copper toxicity.

Storage Instructions Separate serum and freeze.

Reference Interval Neonatal levels are lower than adults. Adult concentrations are reached 3-6 months after birth. Adults: 20-40 mg/dL (SI: 1.26-2.52 µmol/L). Ranges depend on methods, but <10 mg/dL (SI: <0.63 µmol/L) is strong evidence for Wilson disease.

Use Serum ceruloplasmin is decreased in most (>75%) patients with Wilson disease (WD). However, interpretive caution is essential because ceruloplasmin is an acute phase reactant; multiple specimens may be required. WD is a devastating disease which can, however, be treated. The diagnosis of WD requires consideration of history, physical findings, multiple laboratory tests, and family studies.[2] In Wilson disease, there is decreased ability to incorporate copper into apoceruloplasmin. As a result, free copper levels in plasma and in tissue, especially liver and brain, are greatly increased.

Ceruloplasmin assay should be considered in cases of central nervous system disease of obscure etiology. Neurological symptoms include problems of coordination.

Ceruloplasmin is **low** in Menkes kinky hair syndrome (in Menkes syndrome the defect is secondary to poor absorption and utilization of dietary copper), and with protein loss such as the nephrotic syndromes, malabsorption, and with some cases of advanced liver disease in which decreases of serum proteins have occurred.

Ceruloplasmin is **high** in a variety of neoplastic and inflammatory states, since it behaves as an acute phase reactant, although levels rise more slowly than do those of other acute phase reactants. Increases are described in carcinomas, leukemias, Hodgkin disease, primary biliary cirrhosis, systemic lupus erythematosus, and rheumatoid arthritis. High levels occur in pregnancy, with estrogens, and with oral contraceptive use when the agent contains estrogen as well as progesterone. Increased in copper intoxication.

Limitations A normal ceruloplasmin result does not rule out Wilson disease, especially in childhood cases. Serum and liver copper should often be measured. Discrepancies occur between immunologic and enzymatic assays in serum of patients with Wilson disease.

Methodology Spectrophotometric, nephelometric, radial immunodiffusion (RID). Multiplying ceruloplasmin level (mg/L) by three gives the contribution of the binding protein to serum copper (µg/L). This may be as great as 90% to 95% of total serum copper. Performing this maneuver allows the clinician to exert a measure of quality control on the laboratory results.

Additional Information Ceruloplasmin is an α_2-globulin containing copper. About 70% of total serum copper is associated with ceruloplasmin, 7% with a high molecular weight protein, transcuprein, 19% with albumin, and 2% with amino acids.[3]
(Continued)

Ceruloplasmin, Serum *(Continued)*

Liver biopsy is usually essential for the diagnosis of Wilson disease. In addition to H&E microscopy, tissue copper concentrations can establish the diagnosis of Wilson disease.[1] Demonstration of failure to incorporate radio-labeled copper into ceruloplasmin is a definitive test for Wilson disease. Liver and CNS manifestations of Wilson disease need not both be present. Kayser-Fleischer rings are extremely helpful findings, but are often absent.

Excessive therapeutic zinc may lead to block of intestinal absorption of copper and a copper deficiency syndrome characterized by hypochromic microcytic anemia with leukopenia/neutropenia and zero level of ceruloplasmin. A prolonged period of time may be required to eliminate the excess zinc, overcome the block of intestinal copper absorption, and obtain increase in serum copper and ceruloplasmin levels.[4]

More information relevant to serum and urine copper, Wilson disease, and other states is provided in the entries Copper, Serum *on page 816* and Copper, Urine *on page 818*. The former monograph includes a table relevant to ceruloplasmin as well as copper.

Footnotes

1. Ludwig J, Moyer TP, and Rakela J, "The Liver Biopsy Diagnosis of Wilson's Disease," *Am J Clin Pathol*, 1994, 102(4):443-6.
2. Gahl WA, "Wilson Disease," *Cecil Textbook of Medicine*, 21st ed, Goldman L and Bennett JC, eds, Philadelphia, PA: WB Saunders Co, 2000, 1130-2.
3. Barrow L and Tanner MS, "Copper Distribution Among Serum Proteins in Pediatric Liver Disorders and Malignancies," *Eur J Clin Invest*, 1988, 18(6):555-60.
4. Hoffman HN II, Phyliky RL, and Fleming CR, "Zinc-Induced Copper Deficiency," *Gastroenterology*, 1988, 94(2):508-12.

References

Cauza E, Maier-Dobersberger T, Polli C, et al, "Screening for Wilson's Disease on Patients With Liver Diseases by Serum Ceruloplasmin," *J Hepatol*, 1997, 27(2):358-62.
Houwen RH, Van Hattum J, and Hoogenraad T, "Wilson's Disease," *Neth J Med*, 1993, 43(1-2):26-37.
Menkes JH, "Kinky Hair Disease: Twenty-Five Years Later," *Brain Dev*, 1988, 10(2):77-9.
Milne DB and Johnson PE, "Assessment of Copper Status: Effect of Age and Gender on Reference Ranges in Healthy Adults," *Clin Chem*, 1993, 39(5):883-7.

♦ **Chloride:Phosphorus Ratio** *see* Calcium, Serum *on page 131*

Chloride, Serum, Plasma, or Blood

Related Information

Anion Gap, Serum, Plasma, or Urine *on page 106*
Bicarbonate, Blood *on page 115*
Carbon Dioxide, Total, Blood *on page 135*
Chloride, Urine *on page 145*
Electrolyte Panel, Serum *on page 168*
Point-of-Care Testing *on page 43*
Sodium, Serum or Plasma *on page 275*

Synonyms Cl, Serum

Applies to Bromism

Abstract Chloride is a negatively charged electrolyte that makes up ~66% of the anions in plasma. Its high extracellular fluid concentration accounts for its major role, along with sodium, in maintaining plasma osmotic homeostasis. Chloride is usually a component of the serum electrolyte panel and is used in the evaluation of a wide variety of hyper-, normo-, and hypochloremic conditions, acid-base balance, and hydration status. Its measurement is required for calculation of the anion gap. The two major extracellular anions are chloride and bicarbonate.

Specimen Serum, plasma, or whole blood

Container Red top tube or green top (heparin) tube

Collection Pediatrics: Blood drawn from heelstick for capillary.

Storage Instructions Refrigerate

Reference Interval Premature: 95-110 mmol/L (SI: 95-110 mmol/L); full-term: 96-106 mmol/L (SI: 96-106 mmol/L); children and adults: 97-107 mmol/L (SI: 97-107 mmol/L)

Possible Panic Range <80 mmol/L (SI: <80 mmol/L), >115 mmol/L (SI: >115 mmol/L)

Use Chloride measurement is used for evaluation of electrolyte status, acid-base balance, water balance, and ketosis. Chloride generally increases and decreases with sodium.

Chloride is **increased** in mineralocorticoid deficiency, with ammonium chloride administration, and the causes of hyperchloremic (nongap) metabolic acidosis: excessive infusion of hyperchloremic (normal) saline, diarrhea/GI losses, renal tubular acidosis, pancreatic fistula, and enterovesical fistula. Chloride is higher in hyperparathyroidism than in some of the other causes of hypercalcemia, but a great deal of overlap exists.

Chloride is **decreased** with overhydration, congestive failure, syndrome of inappropriate secretion of ADH, vomiting, gastric suction, chronic or compensated respiratory acidosis, Addison disease, salt-losing nephritis, burns, metabolic alkalosis, diabetic ketoacidosis, and in some instances of diuretic therapy.

Chloride measurement is useful in the differential diagnosis of acidemias and alkalemias; an important use of chloride is in application of the anion gap. Consult Anion Gap, Serum, Plasma, or Urine *on page 106* for more information.

In differential diagnosis of emesis of uncertain etiology in early infancy, higher bicarbonate and lower chloride (mean 95.7 vs 104 mmol/L) favor pyloric stenosis over gastroesophageal reflux. Serum CL ≤98 mmol signaled the diagnosis of pyloric stenosis with sensitivity of 50%, specificity 99%, positive predictive value 97%.[1]

Limitations Interference from bromide occurs in hospital patients, in some of whom bromide concentrations have been detectable.[2,3] Chloride is not used independently, but only with sodium and commonly with potassium and carbon dioxide. Postprandial specimens have slightly lower serum chloride levels than fasting specimens.

Methodology Coulometric-amperometric titration, spectrophotometry, mercurimetric titration, and ion-selective electrode (ISE) methods

Additional Information Like other electrolytes, chloride cannot be interpreted without clinical knowledge of the patient. A diagnostic approach to the evaluation of hyperchloremic metabolic acidosis includes use of the urinary anion gap in conjunction with measurement of plasma potassium and urinary pH.[4] Direct (no dilution) ISE method is free of the volume displacement error that occurs with specimens with high lipid or protein content.

Superb reviews of acid-base disorders have been published recently.[5,6,7]

The genetic disorders of renal electrolyte transport have recently been reviewed. These include Liddle syndrome, pseudohypoaldosteronism, Bartter syndrome, Gitelman syndrome, Dent disease, familial benign hypercalcemia, and X-linked hypophosphatemic rickets.[8]

Footnotes

1. Smith GA, Mihalov L, and Shields BJ, "Diagnostic Aids in the Differentiation of Pyloric Stenosis From Severe Gastroesophageal Reflux During Early Infancy: the Utility of Serum Bicarbonate and Serum Chloride," *Am J Emerg Med*, 1999, 17(1):28-31.
2. Wenk RE, Lustagarten JA, Pappas NJ, et al, "Serum Chloride Analysis, Bromide Detection, and the Diagnosis of Bromism," *Am J Clin Pathol*, 1976, 65(1):49-57.
3. Rehak NN and Andersen TE, "Evaluation of Gilford Chemistry Control Interference With the Chloride Method in the Beckman Synchron CX3 System Analyzer: Cumulative Effect of Bromide on Chloride Results," *Clin Chem*, 1989, 35(7):1538.
4. Batlle DC, Hizon M, Cohen E, et al, "The Use of the Urinary Anion Gap in the Diagnosis of Hyperchloremic Metabolic Acidosis," *N Engl J Med*, 1988, 318(10):594-9.
5. Adrogué HJ and Madias NE, "Management of Life-Threatening Acid-Base Disorders," First of Two Parts, *N Engl J Med*, 1998, 338(1):26-34, Second of Two Parts, *N Engl J Med*, 1998, 338(2):107-11.
6. Adrogué HJ and Madias NE, "Hypernatremia," *N Engl J Med*, 2000, 342(20):1493-9.
7. Adrogué HJ and Madias NE, "Hyponatremia," *N Engl J Med*, 2000, 342(21):1581-9.
8. Scheinman SJ, Guay-Woodford LM, Thakker RV, et al, "Genetic Disorders of Renal Electrolyte Transport," *N Engl J Med*, 1999, 340(15):1177-87.

References

Koch SM and Taylor RW, "Chloride Ion in Intensive Care Medicine," *Crit Care Med*, 1992, 20(2):227-40.
McCleane GJ, "Urea and Electrolyte Measurement in Preoperative Surgical Patients," *Anaesthesia*, 1988, 43(5):413-5.
Rothenberg DM, Berns AS, Barkin R, et al, "Bromide Intoxication Secondary to Pyridostigmine Bromide Therapy," *JAMA*, 1990, 263(8):1121-2.
Scott MG, Heusel JW, LeGrys VA, et al, "Electrolytes and Blood Gases," *Tietz Textbook of Clinical Chemistry*, 3rd ed, Chapter 31, Burtis CA and Ashwood ER, eds, Philadelphia, PA: WB Saunders Co, 1999, 1056-92.
Wrenn KD, Slovis CM, Minion GE, et al, "The Syndrome of Alcoholic Ketoacidosis," *Am J Med*, 1991, 91(2):119-28.

Chloride, Sweat

Related Information

Cystic Fibrosis DNA Detection *on page 705*
d-Xylose Absorption Test, Serum, Urine *on page 167*

Synonyms Cystic Fibrosis Sweat Test; Iontophoresis; Sweat, Chloride

Applies to Pilocarpine Iontophoresis; *Pseudomonas aeruginosa*, Mucoid; Sodium, Sweat; Trypsin Activity, Stool; Trypsinogen, Immunoreactive

Test Includes Sodium level may also be measured.

Abstract Sweat chloride is used in the diagnostic evaluation of persons, usually infants and small children, with clinical manifestations suggesting possible cystic fibrosis (CF).[1,2] In this test, forearm sweating is induced by pilocarpine iontophoresis, and the resulting sweat is collected on to filter paper, gauze, or a macroduct tube. The sweat is then assayed for chloride. Some authorities have assayed sweat for sodium, but chloride measurements have superior predictive values. Individuals contemplating performing or interpreting sweat chloride tests should study the NCCLS Document 34.A.[3]

Specimen Sweat

Causes for Rejection Not enough sweat collected (<75 mg on 2" x 2" stimulated skin area)

Reference Interval

Children and adults to age 20 years:
- normal: 0-40 mmol/L
- borderline/indeterminate: 41-60 mmol/L
- consistent with cystic fibrosis: >60 mmol/L

Adults older than 20 years: consistent with cystic fibrosis >70 mmol/L

Note: All values should be interpreted with family history and clinical presentations. Sweat chloride values <40 mmol/L have been documented in patients with genetically proven CF; clinical correlation is necessary.

Critical Values Strongly positive and (with characteristic clinical findings or family history) confirmatory: ≥80 mmol/L.[4]

Use Evaluate possible CF in children with family history of CF, frequent and/or foul stools, diarrhea, malnutrition and failure to thrive, depletion of the fat-soluble vitamins, malabsorption, pancreatic insufficiency, history of meconium ileus, neonatal intestinal obstruction, rectal prolapse, infant celiac disease, chronic sinopulmonary and pulmonary disease, asthma, chronic cough, digital clubbing, salt depletion syndromes, chronic metabolic alkalosis, and *Pseudomonas* bronchitis. Evaluation of young adult males for aspermia[3] and for absence of vas deferens.

Limitations Skin involved by inflammation should not be tested. Elevations have been reported in several other diseases; see table. Shwachman and Mahmoodian emphasize that in some of the diseases listed, sweat chloride and sodium elevations lack the constancy that is found in CF.[5] False low results have been described with edema, hypoproteinemia, and excessive sweating. Results are highly variable in adults, especially women in whom sweat chloride levels vary with the menstrual cycle. Sweat chloride levels in adults must be interpreted cautiously: false positives and false negatives may occur.

The differential diagnosis of an elevated sweat chloride includes several disorders other than CF.[6] See table.

Anorexia nervosa
Atopic dermatitis
Autonomic dysfunction
Ecodermal dysplasia
Environmental deprivation
Familial cholestasis
Fucosidosis
Glucose-6-phosphate dehydrogenase deficiency
Glycogen storage disease: type 1
Hypogammaglobulinemia
Klinefelter syndrome
Long-term prostaglandin E1 infusion
Mauriac syndrome
Mucopolysaccharidosis type 1
Nephrogenic diabetes insipidus
Nephrosis
Protein calorie malnutrition
Pseudohypoaldosteronism
Psychosocial failure to thrive
Untreated adrenal insufficiency
Untreated hypothyroidism

Borderline tests must be repeated.[7] Even negative tests should be repeated if the clinical picture suggests cystic fibrosis. Warwick and Hansen are among those who have advocated subsequent confirmation of positives.[8] U.S. Cystic Fibrosis Foundation recommends repeating all positives on a separate occasion. Sweat chloride test does not identify carriers (heterozygotes). Reliability in the first weeks of life is questionable.[9]

A small fraction of CF patients do not have diagnostic sweat chloride patterns.[1,5,9,10] The measurement of sodium and the determination of the Na:Cl ratio may be useful. An application of evolving technology involves isolation of DNA with amplification utilizing the polymerase chain reaction: see Cystic Fibrosis DNA Detection *on page 705*. Molecular recombinant DNA diagnostic techniques may ultimately be the best way to diagnose the disease and the carrier states.

Contraindications Dermatitis. Do not collect sweat from the palm of the hand, or from any site following excessive sweating such as following high temperature or heavy exercise. Improper placement of pad or electrode can cause skin burn.[5]

Methodology Chloride in sweat from the forearm by pilocarpine-ionotophoresis. Coulometric titration by chloridometer. Measurement by an ion-specific electrode (ISE). If gauze or filter paper method of sweat collection is used, at least 75 mg of sweat, on 2" x 2" stimulated skin, must be collected for test validity.[3] Usual collections, using proper equipment producing 1.5-4 mA, range from 100-400 mg of sweat. Laboratory confirmation of the diagnosis of CF requires two or more sweat tests done on separate days with duplicated samples of sweat weighing >75 mg. If microtube tubing is used for sweat collection, minimal volume should be 15 µL.

Additional Information Meconium ileus, very strongly associated with cystic fibrosis, is a separate entity from the meconium plug syndrome.

Other laboratory abnormalities in CF may include culture of mucoid *Pseudomonas aeruginosa*, nonmucoid strains, *Staphylococcus aureus* and *Burkholderia cepacia*; low total protein; prolongation of prothrombin time and liver disease, with abnormalities which may relate to evolving hepatic cirrhosis.

Testing of stool samples for decreased trypsin activity (due to pancreatic exocrine dysfunction) has also been used as a screening test for CF in infants and young children. However, testing for stool trypsin activity is less reliable than the sweat chloride test and should not be used in its place. Assay of immunoreactive trypsinogen on dried blood spots in CF screening programs is improved when combined with DNA analysis, which provides increased sensitivity and specificity.[11,12]

Different clinical facets of CF are recognized. Mutations which cause less severe pancreatic disease are known, and mutations associated with mild lung disease are described.[2,13]

Footnotes

1. Highsmith WE, Burch LH, Zhou Z, et al, "A Novel Mutation in the Cystic Fibrosis Gene in Patients With Pulmonary Disease but Normal Sweat Chloride Concentrations," *N Engl J Med*, 1994, 331(15):974-80.
2. Gan KH, Veeze HJ, van den Ouweland AMW, et al, "A Cystic Fibrosis Mutation Associated With Mild Lung Disease," *N Engl J Med*, 1995, 333(2):95-9.
3. National Committee for Clinical Laboratory Standards (NCCLS), "Sweat Testing: Sample Collection and Quantitative Analysis: Approved Guidelines," *NCCLS Document*, C34-A2, 2000, 20(14):1-40.
4. Stern RC, "The Diagnosis of Cystic Fibrosis," *N Engl J Med*, 1997, 336(7):487-91.
5. Schwachman H and Mahmoodian A, "The Sweat Test and Cystic Fibrosis," *Diagn Med*, 1982, 61-77.
6. LeGrys VA, "Sweat Testing for the Diagnosis of Cystic Fibrosis: Practical Considerations," *J Pediatr*, 1996, 129(6):892-7.
7. Stern RC, Boat TF, Abramowsky CR, et al, "Intermediate-Range Sweat Chloride Concentration and *Pseudomonas* Bronchitis. A Cystic Fibrosis Variant With Preservation of Exocrine Pancreatic Function," *JAMA*, 1978, 239:2676-80.
8. Warwick WJ and Hansen L, "Measurement of Chloride in Sweat With the Chloride-Selective Electrode," *Clin Chem*, 1978, 24(11):2050-3.
9. Behrman RE, Kliegman RM, and Janson HB, *Nelson Textbook of Pediatrics*, 14th ed, Philadelphia, PA: WB Saunders Co, 2000, 1319-22.
10. Stewart B, Zabner J, Shuber AP, et al, "Normal Sweat Chloride Values Do Not Exclude the Diagnosis of Cystic Fibrosis," *Am J Respir Crit Care Med*, 1995, 151(3 Pt 1):899-903.
11. Farrell PM, Kosorok MR, Laxova A, et al, "Nutritional Benefits of Neonatal Screening for Cystic Fibrosis," *N Engl J Med*, 1997, 337(14):963-69.
12. Dankert-Roelse JE and te Meerman GJ, "Screening for Cystic Fibrosis - Time to Change Our Position?" *N Engl J Med*, 1997, 337(14):997-8.
13. Chmiel JF, Drumm ML, Konstan MW, et al, "Pitfall in the Use of Genotype Analysis as the Sole Diagnostic Criterion for Cystic Fibrosis," *Pediatrics*, 1999, 103(4 Pt 1):823-6.

References

Durieu I, Bey-Omar F, Rollet J, et al, "Diagnostic Criteria for Cystic Fibrosis in Men With Congenital Absence of the Vas Deferens," *Medicine*, 1995, 74(1):42-7.
Grody, WW, "Cystic Fibrosis: Molecular Diagnosis, Population Screening, and Public Policy," *Arch Pathol Lab Med*, 1999, 123(11):1041-6.
Hammond KB, Turcios NL, and Gibson LE, "Clinical Evaluation of the Macroduct Sweat Collection System and Conductivity Analyzer in the Diagnosis of Cystic Fibrosis," *J Pediatr*, 1994, 124(2):255-60.
Hanukoglu A, Bistritzer T, Rakover Y, et al, "Pseudohypoaldosteronism With Increased Sweat and Saliva Electrolyte Values and Frequent Lower Respiratory Tract Infections Mimicking Cystic Fibrosis," *J Pediatr*, 1994, 125(5 Pt 1):752-5.
Hillman BC, "Sweat Test vs Genetic Testing for Cystic Fibrosis," *Lab Med*, 1997, 28(7):433-4.
Kirk JM, Keston M, McIntosh I, et al, "Variation of Sweat Sodium and Chloride With Age in Cystic Fibrosis and Normal Populations: Further Investigations in Equivocal Cases," *Ann Clin Biochem*, 1992, 29(Pt 2):145-52.
Larsen J, Campbell S, Faragher EB, et al, "Cystic Fibrosis Screening in Neonates - Measurement of Immunoreactive Trypsin and Direct Genotype Analysis for Delta F508 Mutation," *Eur J Pediatr*, 1994, 153(8):569-73.
LeGrys VA and Burnett RW, "Current Status of Sweat Testing in North America," *Arch Pathol Lab Med*, 1994, 118(9):865-7.
Polack FP, Transue DJ, Belknap WM, et al, "Transient Evaluation of Sweat Chloride Concentration in a Malnourished Girl With the Mauriac Syndrome," *J Pediatr*, 1995, 126(2):261-3.
Ravnik-Glavac M, Glavac D, Chernick M, et al, "Screening for CF Mutations in Adult Cystic Fibrosis Patients With a Directed and Optimized SSCP Strategy," *Hum Mutat*, 1994, 3(3):231-8.
Resnikoff JR and Conrad DJ, "Recent Advances in the Understanding and Treatment of Cystic Fibrosis," *Curr Opin Pulm Med*, 1998, 4(3):130-4.
Rodrigues ME, Melo MC, Reis FJ, et al, "Concentration of Electrolytes in the Sweat of Malnourished Children," *Arch Dis Child*, 1994, 71(2):141-3.
Rosenstein BJ and Cutting GR, "The Diagnosis of Cystic Fibrosis: A Consensus Statement," *J Pediatr*, 1998, 132(4):589-95.
Rosenstein ME and Zeitlin PL, "Cystic Fibrosis," *Lancet*, 1998, 351(9098):277-82.
Waters DL, Dorney SFA, Gaskin KJ, et al, "Pancreatic Function in Infants Identified as Having Cystic Fibrosis in a Neonatal Screening Program," *N Engl J Med*, 1990, 322(5):303-8.

Internet Web Sites
www.nccls.org

Chloride, Urine

Related Information

Anion Gap, Serum, Plasma, or Urine *on page 106*
Blood Gases and pH, Arterial *on page 119*
Chloride, Serum, Plasma, or Blood *on page 144*
Potassium, Urine *on page 259*
Sodium, Urine *on page 278*
Urine Collection, 24-Hour *on page 47*

Synonyms Cl, Urine; Urine Cl

Applies to Alkalosis

(Continued)

Chloride, Urine *(Continued)*

Replaces Electrolytes, Urine

Abstract Urinary chloride is used as an aid in the evaluation of metabolic alkalosis.

Specimen Timed or random urine

Container No preservative

Reference Interval 110-250 mmol/24 hours (SI: 110-250 mmol/day) in adults, lower values in infancy and childhood. Results depend on ingestion of chloride. In older adults, values may be somewhat lower.

Use Urinary chloride is used to evaluate acid-base balance, and particularly to distinguish whether or not a case of metabolic alkalosis is chloride-responsive (salt responsive). Sherman and Eisinger[1,2] discuss bicarbonate excretion, blood volume, potassium depletion, and the differential diagnosis of metabolic alkalosis with loss of gastric juice (emesis, intubation) and after diuretics. Chloride depleted patients excrete urine with low chloride, <10 mmol/L. Such patients are chloride-responsive (ie, they respond to chloride sufficient to return body stores to normal). Metabolic alkalosis with low urine chloride may also be found with villous tumors of the colon.

Endogenous or exogenous corticosteroids produce urine chloride values in excess of 20 mmol/L. Such patients are chloride resistant. The finding of chloride resistant metabolic alkalosis may provide a stimulus to identify an ACTH or aldosterone producing neoplasm (eg, Cushing syndrome or Conn syndrome). A diagrammatic presentation of the differential diagnosis of hypokalemia includes application of urinary chloride (see Potassium, Urine *on page 259*). In Bartter syndrome with metabolic alkalosis, there is usually increased urine chloride. The complex relationships of chronic pulmonary disease with metabolic alkalosis are mentioned by Sherman and Eisinger.

Limitations Halogens other than chloride (bromide), which are also present in urine, may erroneously elevate the chloride result. Isolated urine chloride, without urine sodium or potassium or without serum or plasma electrolytes, can provide misleading information. Discussion of electrolyte balance is beyond the scope of this manual (eg, effect of profound potassium depletion on impairment of chloride reabsorption). Fetal urinary electrolytes are an unreliable guide to evaluate fetal renal function.[3]

Methodology Coulometric titration, ion-selective electrode (ISE)

Additional Information Urine chloride is often ordered with sodium and potassium as a timed urine. The **urinary anion gap** [$Na^+ - (Cl^- + HCO_3^-)$] or [$(Na^+ + K^+) - (Cl^-)$] may be used in the initial evaluation of hyperchloremic metabolic acidosis,[4] and is discussed in the listing Anion Gap, Serum, Plasma, or Urine *on page 106*. In metabolic alkalosis, spot urine chloride in the presence of hypertension can provide important information.[5]

Urinary chloride, sodium, and calcium were shown to be low prenatally in the urine of a mother carrying a fetus with Bartter syndrome and may be useful in prenatal diagnosis.[6]

Footnotes

1. Sherman RA and Eisinger RP, "The Use (and Misuse) of Urinary Sodium and Chloride Measurements," *JAMA*, 1982, 247:3121-4.
2. Sherman RA and Eisinger RP, "Urinary Sodium and Chloride During Renal Salt Retention," *Am J Kidney Dis*, 1983, 3(2):121-3.
3. Elder JS, O'Grady JP, Ashmead G, et al, "Evaluation of Fetal Renal Function: Unreliability of Fetal Urinary Electrolytes," *J Urol*, 1990, 144(2 Pt 2):574-8.
4. Battle DC, Hizon M, Cohen E, et al, "The Use of the Urinary Anion Gap in the Diagnosis of Hyperchloremic Metabolic Acidosis," *N Engl J Med*, 1988, 318(10):594-9.
5. Preuss HG, "Fundamentals of Clinical Acid-Base Evaluation," *Clin Lab Med*, 1993, 13(1):103-16.
6. Matsushita Y, Suzuki Y, Oya N, et al, "Biochemical Examination of Mother's Urine Is Useful for Prenatal Diagnosis of Bartter Syndrome," *Prenat Diagn*, 1999, 19(7):671-3.

References

Guay-Woodford LM, "Bartter Syndrome: Unraveling the Patholphysiologic Enigma," *Am J Med*, 1998, 105(2):151-61.

Harrington JT and Cohen JJ, "Measurement of Urinary Electrolytes - Indications and Limitations," *N Engl J Med*, 1975, 293:1241-3.

Kamel KS, Magner PO, Ethier JH, et al, "Urine Electrolytes in the Assessment of Extracellular Fluid Volume Contraction," *Am J Nephrol*, 1989, 9(4):344-7.

Pan WH, Chen JY, Chen YC, et al, "Diurnal Electrolyte Excretion Pattern Affects Estimates of Electrolyte Status Based on 24-Hour, Half-Day, and Overnight Urine," *Chin J Physiol*, 1994, 37(1):49-53.

♦ **Cholecalciferol** *see* Vitamin D, Serum *on page 300*

♦ **Cholesterol Ester Transfer Protein** *see* High Density Lipoprotein Cholesterol, Serum *on page 192*

♦ **Cholesterol:HDLC Ratio** *see* Cholesterol, Total, Serum or Plasma *on page 146*

♦ **Cholesterol:HDLC Ratio** *see* High Density Lipoprotein Cholesterol, Serum *on page 192*

♦ **Cholesterol, Total** *see* High Density Lipoprotein Cholesterol, Serum *on page 192*

♦ **Cholesterol, Total** *see* Lipids, Overview *on page 213*

Cholesterol, Total, Serum or Plasma

Related Information

Apolipoprotein A-I, Serum *on page 109*

Apolipoprotein B-100, Serum *on page 109*
C-Reactive Protein, Serum *on page 523*
Endomysial Antibodies *on page 525*
High Density Lipoprotein Cholesterol, Serum *on page 192*
Homocyst(e)ine, Plasma *on page 193*
Lipid Panel, Serum *on page 212*
Lipids, Overview *on page 213*
Low Density Lipoprotein Cholesterol *on page 218*
Mevalonic Acid, Urine or Amniotic Fluid *on page 225*
Triglycerides, Serum or Plasma *on page 288*

Applies to Cholesterol:HDLC Ratio

Abstract See Lipids, Overview *on page 213*.

Patient Preparation To support proper interpretation of lipid analysis:

- For optimum patient condition at the time of blood drawing: no change in diet for 3 weeks, stable body weight, and fasting (no food, except water and possibly black coffee without sugar in the morning) for 12 hours. (Fasting is not important for cholesterol analysis but is important when determining other lipids, eg, triglycerides.)
- Posture may be a significant factor: cholesterol values may be 10% to 15% lower after 20 minutes in a recumbent position. From standing to a sitting position values are about 6% lower after 20 minutes.
- Increases of 2% to 5% in cholesterol may be seen if tourniquet is applied for 2 minutes during sampling. Emotional and physical stress may also be factors influencing cholesterol levels.
- Abstinence from alcohol for 72 hours may be desirable, but only inconclusive information is available.

Specimen Serum

Container Red top tube

Storage Instructions At -70°C, a decrease of 2%/year on average takes place.[1]

Reference Interval The National Cholesterol Education Program (NCEP) suggested limit: <200 mg/dL (but age stratification was not provided) (SI: <5.1 mmol/L). Although the relationship between hypercholesterolemia and coronary heart disease is attenuated in elderly individuals,[2] serum total cholesterol remains an important risk factor for acute myocardial infarct beyond age 55 years. In a 1999 paper, hypercholesterolemia was defined as >251 mg/dL for such individuals.[3] See Lipids, Overview *on page 213* and table.

Population Distributions for Total Cholesterol (mg/dL)

Age (y)	5	10	25	50	75	90	95
Male							
0-4	114			155			203
5-9	125	131	141	153	168	183	189
10-14	124	132	144	161	173	191	204
15-19	118	123	135	152	168	183	191
20-24	118	126	142	159	179	197	212
25-29	130	137	154	176	199	223	234
30-34	142	152	161	190	213	237	258
35-39	147	157	176	195	222	248	267
40-44	150	161	179	204	229	251	260
45-49	163	171	188	210	234	255	275
50-54	156	168	189	211	234	262	274
55-59	161	172	188	214	236	260	280
60-64	163	170	191	215	237	262	287
65-69	166	174	192	213	250	275	288
≥70	144	160	185	214	236	253	265
Female							
0-4	112			156			200
5-9	131	135	150	164	177	189	197
10-14	125	131	142	159	171	191	205
15-19	119	126	140	157	176	198	208
20-24	121	132	147	165	186	220	237
25-29	130	142	158	178	198	217	231
30-34	133	141	158	178	197	215	227
35-39	139	149	165	186	209	233	249
40-44	146	156	172	193	220	241	259
45-49	148	162	182	204	213	256	268
50-54	163	171	188	314	240	267	281
55-59	167	182	201	229	251	270	294
60-64	172	186	207	226	251	282	300
65-60	167	179	212	233	259	282	291
≥70	173	181	196	226	249	268	280

To convert to mmol/L, multiply by 0.0259.

Adapted from Lipid Research Clinical Program Epidemiology Committee, "Plasma Lipid Distributions in Selected North American Population: The Lipid Research Clinics Program Prevalence Study," *Circulation*, 1979, 60:427-39 and Lipid Metabolism Branch, Division of Heart, Lung, and Blood Institute: *The Lipid Research Clinics Population Studies Data Book*, Volume I, The Prevalence Study. NIH Publication No. 80-1527, Bethesda, MD: National Institutes of Health, 1980.

Critical Values Borderline high cholesterol: 200-229 mg/dL; high cholesterol:[4,5] ≥240 mg/dL

Use See Lipids, Overview *on page 213.*

Limitations Coronary heart disease is rare without some degree of elevation of low density lipoprotein cholesterol.[5] Thus, for evaluation of coronary atherogenesis, cholesterol is best measured with other risk factors.

In identification of individuals at risk of occlusion after vascular/endovascular surgical therapy, the best predictors of reocclusion or restenosis, in decreasing order, were LDLC, lipoprotein (a), total cholesterol/HDLC, HDLC, and total cholesterol.[6]

Factors additional to cholesterol are relevant to atherosclerosis.[7] A large number of drugs effect cholesterol.[8]

Methodology Enzymatic, ferric chloride-sulfuric acid, Leibermann-Burchardt reaction

Additional Information Markers of cardiovascular risk were recently evaluated. The efficiency of each for prediction of myocardial infarct is shown in the following figure.[9]

Plasma cholesterol values are up to 10% lower than serum values. This difference should be considered when comparing patient values to published reference tables.

Among anemic patients, cholesterol concentrations <156 mg/dL may signal celiac disease.[10]

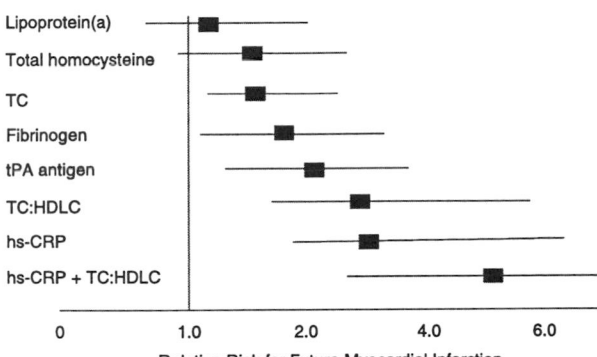

Relative Risk for Future Myocardial Infarction

Relative risk for future myocardial infarction among apparently healthy middle-aged men in the *Physicians' Health Study,* according to baseline levels of lipoprotein(a), total plasma homocysteine, total cholesterol (TC), fibrinogen, tissue-type plasminogen activator (tPA) antigen, the ratio of total cholesterol to high-density lipoprotein cholesterol (HDLC), and high-sensitivity C-reactive protein (hs-CRP). For consistency, risks are computed for men in the top compared with the bottom quartile for each marker.

From Ridker PM, "Evaluating Novel Cardiovascular Risk Factors: Can We Better Predict Heart Attacks?" *Ann Intern Med*, 1999, 130(11):933-7.

Footnotes

1. Shih WJ, Bachorik PS, Haga JA, et al, "Estimating the Long-Term Effects of Storage at -70°C on Cholesterol, Triglyceride, and HDL-Cholesterol Measurements in Stored Sera," *Clin Chem*, 2000, 46(3):351-64.
2. Avins AL and Browner WS, "Improving the Prediction of Coronary Heart Disease to Aid in the Management of High Cholesterol Levels," *JAMA*, 1998, 279(6):445-9.
3. Houterman S, Verschuren WM, Hofman A, et al, "Serum Cholesterol Is a Risk Factor for Myocardial Infarction in Elderly Men and Women: The Rotterdam Study," *J Intern Med*, 1999, 246(1):25-33.
4. Stamler J, Daviglus ML, Garside DB, et al, "Relationship of Baseline Serum Cholesterol Levels in 3 Large Cohorts of Younger Men to Long-Term Coronary, Cardiovascular, and All-Cause Mortality and to Longevity," *JAMA*, 2000, 284(3):311-8.
5. Grundy SM, "Early Detection of High Cholesterol Levels in Young Adults," *JAMA*, 2000, 284(3):365-7.
6. Lippi G, Verald GF, Dorucci V, et al, "Usefulness of Lipids, Lipoproten(a) and Fibrinogen Measurements in Identifying Subjects at Risk of Occlusive Complications Following Vascular and Endovascular Surgery," *Scand J Clin Lab Invest*, 1998, 58:497-504.
7. Ross R, "Atherosclerosis - An Inflammatory Disease," *N Engl J Med*, 1999, 340(2):115-26.
8. Young DS, "Effects of Drugs on Clinical Laboratory Tests," 5th ed, Volume 1: Listing by Test, Washington, DC: AACC Press, American Association of Clinical Chemistry, 2000, Section 3, 182-206.
9. Ridker PM, "Evaluating Novel Cardiovascular Risk Factors: Can We Better Predict Heart Attacks?" *Ann Intern Med*, 1999, 130(11):933-7.
10. Ciacci C, Cirillo M, Giorgetti G, et al, "Low Plasma Cholesterol: A Correlate of Nondiagnosed Celiac Disease in Adults With Hypochromic Anemia," *Am J Gastroenterol*, 1999, 94(7):1888-91.

References

Rifai N, Bachorik PS, and Albers JS, "Lipids, Lipoproteins and Apolipoproteins," *Tietz Textbook of Clinical Chemistry*, 3rd ed, Burtis CA and Ashwood ER, eds, Philadelphia, PA: WB Saunders Co, 1999, 809-61.

◆ **Cholinesterase, Erythrocytic** *see* Acetylcholinesterase, Red Cell *on page 81*

◆ **Cholinesterase I** *see* Acetylcholinesterase, Red Cell *on page 81*

◆ **Cholinesterase II** *see* Pseudocholinesterase, Serum *on page 270*

◆ **Cholinesterase, Serum** *see* Pseudocholinesterase, Serum *on page 270*

◆ **Chorionic Gonadotropin, Beta Subunit** *see* Chorionic Gonadotropin, Human, Serum and Urine *on page 147*

Chorionic Gonadotropin, Human, Serum and Urine

Related Information

Alpha₁-Fetoprotein, Serum *on page 97*
Amniotic Fluid, Chromosome and Genetic Abnormality Analysis *on page 360*
Estriol, Unconjugated, Pregnancy, Serum, Plasma, or Urine *on page 171*
Heterophilic Antibodies *on page 191*
Inhibin A, Serum *on page 199*
Placental Lactogen, Human, Serum *on page 254*
Pregnancy-Associated Protein A, Serum *on page 260*
Pregnancy Test, Serum or Urine *on page 260*
Progesterone, Serum *on page 261*

Synonyms Beta Subunit, hCG; Chorionic Gonadotropin, Beta Subunit; hCG; Human Chorionic Gonadotropin

Applies to GnRH; Pregnancy Testing; Triple Test

Replaces Aschheim-Zondek Test; Friedman's Test; Galli Mainini Test

Abstract A glycoprotein heterodimer, hCG derives from syncytiotrophoblastic cells. Gonadotropin releasing hormone (GnRH) may stimulate its production. Physiologically, it stimulates progesterone secretion by the corpus luteum, which maintains secretory endometrium. In pregnancy, hCG promotes trophoblastic differentiation.

Increased in most nonseminomatous germ cell tumors and less often in subjects with seminoma, it is a marker for trophoblastic tumors, including hydatidiform mole and choriocarcinoma.

Serum markers for screening for Down syndrome include hCG, AFP, uE₃, PAPP-A, inhibin A, and urinary beta-core fragment of hCG, as well as maternal age.

Adverse fetal outcomes are associated with increased second trimester AFP, increased hCG and low uE₃ concentrations. MIC2 is detected by ordinary immunoperoxidase procedures. See table in Alpha₁-Fetoprotein, Serum *on page 97.*

Increased hCG is found with multiparous gestation and with hemolytic disease of the newborn.

Specimen Serum; cerebrospinal fluid to manage intracranial germ cell tumors; urine for beta-core fragment measurement

Container Red top tube

Sampling Time Second trimester screening of maternal serum for Down syndrome (trisomy 21) and Edwards syndrome (trisomy 18) includes sampling at 15-21 weeks gestation when testing also includes AFP and unconjugated estriol.[1] Optimally, collection should be between 16 and 18 weeks.[2]

Storage Instructions Serum is stable 24 hours at 25°C and 4 days at 4°C. Freeze at -20°C for longer storage. If urine is used for beta-core fragment, freezing and prolonged storage should be avoided.

Special Instructions For females, state date of last menstrual period. Length of gestation is relevant for prenatal screening. To monitor patients with testicular tumors, both α-fetoprotein (AFP) and hCG should be measured, and LD as well.

Reference Interval Depends on application and methodology. <5 mIU/mL (SI: <5 IU/L) usually normal (nonpregnant). Mayo Medical Laboratories recently implemented the following for serum:

• male: <0.7 IU/L
• female: premenopausal: <0.8 IU/L, postmenopausal <3.3 IU/L
• cerebrospinal fluid: <1.5 IU/L.[3]

Greater than 300% differences in means of different methods has been documented. Concentration of hCG doubles each 1.5-2.5 days during the first 6 weeks of gestation, peaking at 100,000 IU/L 60-70 days following implantation. Wide individual variation is seen, partly explained by maternal plasma volume increases. The reference range in gestation relates to maternal weight and gestational age; β-hCG >50,000 IU/L supports but does not guarantee the diagnosis of viable intrauterine pregnancy.

Critical Values In subjects with concentration <2000 IU/L, increase of serum hCG <66% in 2 days is suggestive of spontaneous abortion or ruptured ectopic gestation in appropriate clinical setting. Rate of increase diminishes with gestation. After the 14th week, hCG continues its rise in gestational trophoblastic disease but falls in normal pregnancy. Levels of hCG >100,000 IU/L can be found in the sera of patients with choriocarcinoma.

Use Work up and manage **germ cell neoplasms** including choriocarcinoma and embryonal carcinoma. The highest levels are found with **gestational trophoblastic tumors** (hydatidiform mole, partial mole and choriocarcinoma). Increases are found with multiple gestation pregnancy and with erythroblastosis fetalis. Some islet cell tumors may make hCG, as may some carcinomas of lung, stomach, colon, pancreas, liver, and breast. Concentrations of hCG in cerebrospinal fluid may detect CNS involvement; the ratio of plasma levels to CSF values tends to be <60 in the presence of cerebral metastases.[4]

Prenatal screening for trisomy 21 (Down syndrome), trisomy 18 (Edwards syndrome), neural tube defects, and other open fetal abnormalities. Serum

(Continued)

Chorionic Gonadotropin, Human, Serum and Urine
(Continued)

hCG is increased about 100% in trisomy 21, for which it is the best single chemical marker. It is decreased about 64% in trisomy 18.[5] Screening for Down syndrome in the first trimester may be done with measurement in maternal serum of pregnancy-associated protein A with either hCG or its free β-subunits.[6,7,8] In combination with serum unconjugated estriol and serum AFP (triple marker screening), detection of Down syndrome is increased. See Amniotic Fluid, Chromosome and Genetic Abnormality Analysis *on page 360*. Decreases occur in settings in which trophoblastic function is compromised such as **ectopic pregnancy** and **spontaneous abortion**. Extremely high hCG concentrations, at least 4-5 multiples of the median, increase risk of adverse outcome of gestation.[9] Increased hCG concentrations in pregnancy are associated with hypertension, miscarriage, prematurity, and fetal death.

Limitations Normal hCG levels do not rule out germ cell tumor. The same test method may not be suitable for use as a tumor marker and for pregnancy testing. Several reference preparations including World Health Organization sources may be used as standards, but different methods calibrated against different materials, and differences in circulating forms of hCG make interlaboratory comparisons difficult. At least 50 commercial kits for serum have been available in the 1990s. Although overlap exists between inevitable abortion and ectopic pregnancy, the rate of change of hCG and progesterone concentrations distinguish normal intrauterine gestation from pathologic pregnancies (ectopic gestation and inevitable abortion).[10] A single hCG determination falls short in determination of the outcome of a pregnancy.

Heterophilic antibodies, also known as human antimouse antibodies (HAMA), occasionally produce a false-positive **serum** assay for hCG, and such erroneous results have led to needless therapy for gestational trophoblastic neoplasia. See discussion in Heterophilic Antibodies *on page 191*.

Methodology Chemiluminometric sandwich immunoassay is available.[10] Two site immunoradiometric assay (IRMA), radioimmunoassay (RIA); two site enzyme-linked immunosorbent assay (ELISA) methods have been especially successful commercially to assist the diagnosis of early pregnancy.[11,12] Time resolved europium-chelate fluorescence procedures may exceed RIA in sensitivity.[13] Two site fluorescent immunoassay is capable of measurement to the 1 mIU/mL.[14] Assay of hCG by RIA measures the immunologic activities of both hCG and its free β-subunit (sometimes called total beta assays). Total β-hCG may be preferred as a tumor marker.

The multiple hCG-related molecules of serum and urine and the large number of immunoassays available cause interassay discordance. Such variations are especially troublesome in irregular gestations.[15]

Additional Information Human chorionic gonadotropin is normally produced by the developing placenta, and aberrantly produced by some germ cell neoplasms. It is composed of glycopeptide α- and β-subunits. The α-subunit, a 92-amino acid sequence, is essentially identical with that of luteinizing hormone, follicle stimulating hormone, and thyroid stimulating hormone. It is this shared structure which accounts for some false positives in pregnancy tests not based on the β-subunit. The β-subunit, a 145 amino acid sequence, is unique to hCG, and specific assays based on the β-subunit are not subject to hormonal cross reactivity. β-subunit specific assays are now sensitive enough to detect a normal pregnancy 6-14 days after implantation; hCG can be detected as low as 5 mIU/mL (SI: 5 IU/L).

About 10% of hCG molecules in the first trimester are "nicked" by enzymatic cleavage, rendering them inactive and unstable. Nicked molecules reach 20% in the third trimester and contribute to variability between assays. β-core fragments also circulate.

While β-hCG doubles about every 1-3 days in a normal gestation, in most ectopic pregnancies β-hCG doubles more slowly, plateaus, or diminishes. Chorionic gonadotropin assays are sometimes used to support the diagnosis of **ectopic pregnancy**. Ectopic gestations typically secrete decreased amounts of hCG and progesterone compared to intrauterine pregnancies, but it is the slope which must be considered. Abnormally low hCG levels with abnormal rates of change[10] coupled with transvaginal ultrasound detect many ectopic pregnancies prior to rupture.[16] It is helpful to use hCG and progesterone sequentially every other day to detect a lack of rise in the levels. The rate of change of hCG can be calculated.[10] It has been demonstrated that viable and nonviable pregnancy can be distinguished by the ratio of serial hCG values separated by 48 hours. The relationship for various sampling intervals has been plotted on the accompanying chart by Dr LB Baskin,[17] based on prior investigation by Kadar et al and Romero et al. The sampling interval is plotted on the horizontal axis and the ratio of the determined β-hCG values for that interval is plotted on the vertical axis. If the intersection of the lines extending from those two points (the sampling interval and the β-hCG ratio) is above the curve, it is likely a viable intrauterine pregnancy, and if below the line, it is a nonviable pregnancy.

The detection of fetal **trisomy 21 (Down syndrome)** is well established using hCG with other investigation. Mothers carrying fetuses with Down syndrome are more likely to have decreased AFP and unconjugated estriol concentrations with increased hCG at 16 weeks. Although maternal age older than 35 has been a "magic number," in fact, 70% to 80% of children

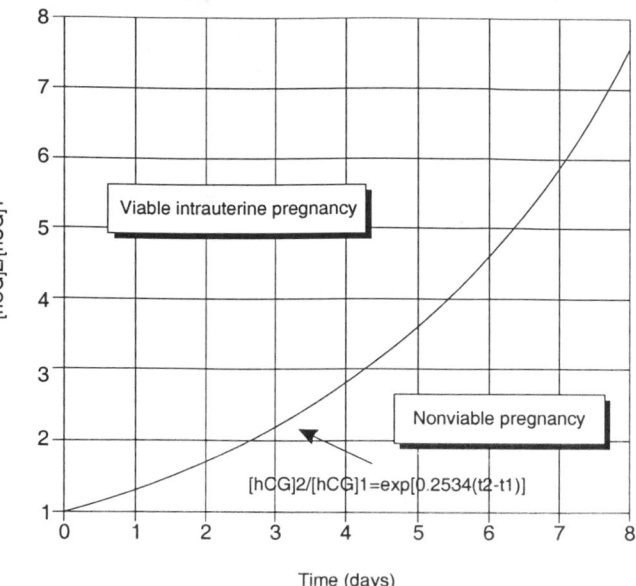

Serum hCG Concentration

$$[hCG]2/[hCG]1 = exp[0.2534(t2-t1)]$$

Time (days)

Minimum increase in viable IUP during 1st trimester:
The ratio of successive serum hCG concentrations during the first trimester of a viable intrauterine pregnancy based on an exponential increase of 66% in 2 days (0.2534 days^{-1} = ln(1.66)/2 days), (sensitivity~90%; specificity~87%).

Courtesy of Leland B. Baskin, MD, assistant professor, the University of Texas Southwestern Medical Center at Dallas, with permission.

From Kadar N, Caldwell BV, and Romero R, "A Method for Screening for Ectopic Pregnancy and Its Indications," *Obstet Gynecol*, 1981, 58:162-5. Romero R, Kadar N, Copel JA, et al, "The Value of Serial Human Chorionic Gonadotropin Testing as a Diagnostic Tool in Ectopic Pregnancy," *Am J Obstet Gynecol*, 1986, 155:392-4.

with Down syndrome are born to mothers younger than age 35.[18] Measurement of the β-subunit offers improved detection.[10] Detection of Down syndrome is enhanced with use of inhibin A.[8]

Decrease in hCG at midtrimester is found with **trisomy 18** (Edwards syndrome).

See table in listing, Alpha$_1$-Fetoprotein, Serum *on page 97*.

Serum hCG levels are extremely useful in following those **germ cell neoplasms** which produce hCG, particularly trophoblastic neoplasms. While hCG concentrations are extremely high with complete molar pregnancy, hCG >100,000 mIU/mL is exceptional in pre-evacuation sera from patients with partial hydatidiform molar pregnancy. Ultrasonography is a sensitive additional technique for support of these diagnoses. Following evacuation of a trophoblastic lesion, serum β-hCG concentrations should return to normal in 9-11 weeks. Following evacuation of a mole, hCG concentrations should be monitored weekly until undetectable for three consecutive weeks, then monthly monitoring until undetectable for six consecutive months.[4] Oral contraceptive use may delay this fall. Any other delay in the fall, or subsequent rise, is an indication for further evaluation. CSF hCG is useful for diagnosis of intracranial germinal neoplasms, germ cell tumors of the pineal gland. Complications of complete molar pregnancy may include hyperthyroidism, even thyroid storm.

In germ cell neoplasms in the male, β-hCG and α-fetoprotein are both useful tumor markers. They can be demonstrated histochemically in tissue to confirm diagnosis and can be followed in serum to evaluate recurrence. Prognostic factors for metastatic testicular germ cell neoplasms include pretreatment evaluation of concentrations of LD, hCG, and AFP.[19] Both AFP and hCG are increased with embryonal carcinoma, AFP is increased with yolk sac tumors and hCG is increased with choriocarcinoma and in about 10% of seminomas. Its presence with seminoma may provide evidence of the presence of coexisting choriocarcinoma. Neither AFP nor hCG are increased with uncomplicated teratoma. AFP and/or hCG is(are) increased in 80% to 90% of subjects with testicular tumors other than seminomas.

Some of the hCG methods available are only intended for pregnancy applications. Such assays do not necessarily detect degraded or more homogenous molecules found in trophoblastic diseases.[20]

The hCG molecule has high carbohydrate content, 30% of its molecular weight is due to sugars, 8% to 9% is the result of sialic acid. Removal of sialic acid residues from the β-subunit decreases biologic activity by 50%. Considerable understanding of the molecular structure and molecular biologic function has developed.

Footnotes

1. Haddow JE and Palomaki GE, "Biochemical Markers of Fetal Disorders in Maternal Serum and Amniotic Fluid," *Medicine of the Fetus and Mother*, 2nd ed, Chapter 40, Reece EA and Hobbins JC, eds, Philadelphia, PA: Lippincott-Raven, 1999, 689-706.
2. Ashwood ER, "Clinical Chemistry of Pregnancy," *Tietz Textbook of Clinical Chemistry*, 3rd ed, Chapter 48, Burtis CA and Ashwood ER, eds, Philadelphia, PA: WB Saunders Co, 1999, 1736-75.
3. Mayo Medical Laboratories, "Method and Reference Value Changes for Chorionic Gonadotropin, Beta-Subunit Tests," *Mayo Communique*, Rochester, MN, 1999, 24(11).
4. Berkowitz RS and Goldstein DF, "Chorionic Tumors," *N Engl J Med*, 1996, 335(23):1740-8.
5. Baskin LB, "Pregnancy and Prenatal Testing," *The Handbook of Clinical Pathology*, 2nd ed, Chapter 21, McKenna RW and Keffer JH, eds, Chicago, IL: ASCP Press, American Society of Clinical Pathologists, 2000.
6. Haddow JE, Palomaki GE, Knight GJ, et al, "Screening of Maternal Serum for Fetal Downs Syndrome in the First Trimester," *N Engl J Med*, 1998, 338(14):955-61.
7. Spencer K, "Screening for Down Syndrome. The Role of Intact hCG and Free Subunit Measurement," *Scand J Clin Lab Invest Suppl*, 1993, 216:79-96.
8. Aitken DA, Wallace EM, Crossley JA, "Dimeric Inhibin A as a Marker for Down Syndrome in Early Pregnancy," *N Engl J Med*, 1996, 334(19):1231-6.
9. Luthy DA, "Maternal Markers and Complications of Pregnancy," *N Engl J Med*, 1999, 341(27):2085-7.
10. Stewart BK, Nazar-Stewart V, and Toivola B, "Biochemical Discrimination of Pathologic Pregnancy From Early, Normal Intrauterine Gestation in Symptomatic Patients," *Am J Clin Pathol*, 1995, 103(4):386-90.
11. Bandi ZL, Schoen I, and DeLara M, "Enzyme-Linked Immunosorbent Urine Pregnancy Tests: Clinical Specificity Studies," *Am J Clin Pathol*, 1987, 87(2):236-42.
12. Braunstein GD, Kelley L, Farber S, et al, "Two Rapid, Sensitive, and Specific Immunoenzymatic Assays of Human Choriogonadotropin in Urine Evaluated," *Clin Chem*, 1986, 32(7):1413-4.
13. Lövgren T, Hemmilä I, Pettersson K, et al, "Time-Resolved Fluorometry in Immunoassays," *Alternative Immunoassays*, Collins WP, ed, New York, NY: John Wiley and Sons, 1985, 203-17.
14. Pettersson K, Siitari H, Hemmilä I, et al, "Time-Resolved Fluoroimmunoassay of Human Choriogonadotropin," *Clin Chem*, 1983, 29(1):60-4.
15. Cole LA, "Immunoassay of Human Chorionic Gonadotropin, Its Free Subunits, and Metabolites," *Clin Chem*, 1997, 43(12):2233-43.
16. Churgay CA and Apgar BS, "Ectopic Pregnancy. An Update on Technologic Advances in Diagnosis and Treatment," *Prim Care*, 1993, 20(3):629-38.
17. Baskin LB, "Ectopic Pregnancy: Laboratory Detection and Monitoring, Contribution of hCG and Progesterone," *3rd Annual Progress in Clinical Pathology*, Dallas, TX: University of Texas Southwestern Medical Center, Sept 28-30, 1995.
18. Pauker SP and Pauker SG, "Prenatal Diagnosis - Why Is 35 a Magic Number?" *N Engl J Med*, 1994, 330(16):51-2 (editorial).
19. Bosl GJ, "Prognostic Factors for Metastatic Testicular Germ Cell Tumours: The Memorial Sloan-Kettering Cancer Model," *Eur Urol*, 1993, 23(1):182-7.
20. Cole LA, Kohorn EI, and Kim GS, "Detecting and Monitoring Trophoblastic Disease. New Perspectives on Measuring Human Chorionic Gonadotropin Levels," *J Reprod Med*, 1994, 39(3):193-200.

References

Bahado-Singh R, Oz U, Rinne K, et al, "Elevated Maternal Urine Level of Beta-Core Fragment of Human Chorionic Gonadotropin Versus Serum Triple Test in the Second-Trimester Detection of Down syndrome," *Am J Obstet Gynecol*, 1999, 181(4):929-33.
Baskin LB and Charles RA, "Detecting Ectopic Pregnancy," *Lab Med*, 1997, 28(2):103-5.
DeCherney AH and Eichhorn JH, "Severe Abdominal Pain During Early Pregnancy in a Woman With Previous Infertility," Case Records of the Massachusetts General Hospital, Case 3-1996, Scully RE, Mark EJ, McNeely WF, et al, eds, *N Engl J Med*, 1996, 334(4):255-60.
Dickerman LH and Redline RW, "Pathologic Findings in Pregnancies With Unexplained Increases in Midtrimester Maternal Serum Human Chorionic Gonadotropin Levels," *Am J Clin Pathol*, 1999, 111(2):209-15.
Goldstein PP and Berkowitz RS, "Current Management of Complete and Partial Molar Pregnancy," *J Reprod Med*, 1994, 39(3):139-46.
Hellemans P, Gerris J, Joostens M, et al, "Serum hCG Decline Following Salpingotomy or Salpingectomy for Extrauterine Pregnancy," *Eur J Obstet Gynecol Reprod Biol*, 1994, 53(1):59-64.
Kantoff PW and Oliva E, "A 27-Year-Old Man With a Painful Retroperitoneal Mass," Case Records of the Massachusetts General Hospital, Case 1-2000, Scully RE, Mark EJ, McNeely WF, et al, eds, *N Engl J Med*, 2000, 342(2):69-144.
Khazaeli MB, Buchina ES, Pattillo RA, et al, "Radioimmunoassay of Free Beta-Subunit of Human Chorionic Gonadotropin in Diagnosis of High-Risk and Low-Risk Gestational Trophoblastic Disease," *Am J Obstet Gynecol*, 1989, 160(2):444-9.
Klee GG, "Human Chorionic Gonadotropin," *Mayo Clin Proc*, 1994, 69(4):391-2.
Kovalevskaya G, Birken S, Kakuma T, et al, "Evaluation of Nicked Human Chorionic Gonadotropin Content in Clinical Specimens by a Specific Immunometric Assay," *Clin Chem*, 1999, 45(1):68-77.
Liu DF, Dickerman LH, and Redline RW, "Pathologic Findings in Pregnancies With Unexplained Increases in Midtrimester Maternal Serum Human Chorionic Gonadotropin Levels," *Am J Clin Pathol*, 1999, 111(2):209-15.
Nomura F, Ohnishi K, and Tanabe Y, "Clinical Features and Prognosis of Hepatocellular Carcinoma With Reference to Serum Alpha-Fetoprotein Levels," *Cancer*, 1989, 64(8):1700-7.
Stenman UH, Unkila-Kallio L, Korhonen J, et al, "Immunoprocedures for Detecting Human Chorionic Gonadotropin: Clinical Aspects and Doping Control," *Clin Chem*, 1997, 43(7):1293-8.
Tyrey L, "Human Chorionic Gonadotropin Assays and Their Uses," *Obstet Gynecol Clin North Am*, 1988, 15(3):457-75.
Udoji WC, Victory DF, Cartwright PS, et al, "Diagnostic Problems With Variant Forms of Human Chorionic Gonadotropin," *Lab Med*, 1998, 29(4):243-8.
Ulbright TM, "Protocol for the Examination of Specimens From Patients With Malignant Germ Cell and Sex Cord-Stromal Tumors of the Testis, Exclusive of Paratesticular Malignancies," *Arch Pathol Lab Med*, 1999, 123(1):14-9.
Wald NJ, George L, Smith D, et al, "Serum Screening for Down's Syndrome Between 8 and 14 Weeks of Pregnancy," *Br J Obstet Gynaecol*, 1996, 103(5):407-12.
Walton DL, Norem CT, Schoen EJ, et al, "Second-Trimester Serum Chorionic Gonadotropin Concentrations and Complications and Outcome of Pregnancy," *N Engl J Med*, 1999, 341(27):2033-8.
Yaron Y, Cherry M, Kramer RL, et al, "Second-Trimester Maternal Serum Marker Screening: Maternal Serum Alpha-Fetoprotein, Beta-Human Chorionic Gonadotropin Estriol, and Their Various Combinations as Predictors of Pregnancy Outcome," *Am J Obstet Gynecol*, 1999, 181(4):968-74.

♦ **Chromogranin A, Plasma** see Catecholamines, Fractionation, Plasma *on page 138*

♦ **Chromogranin A, Plasma** see 5-Hydroxyindoleacetic Acid, Quantitative, Urine *on page 197*

♦ **Chromogronin A, Serum** see Calcitonin, Serum or Plasma *on page 129*

♦ **Chylomicronemia** see Lipids, Overview *on page 213*

♦ **Chylomicrons** see Triglycerides, Serum or Plasma *on page 288*

♦ **Chylous Fluid** see Body Fluid Chemical Analysis *on page 123*

Citrate, Serum, Plasma, or Urine

Related Information
Kidney Stone Analysis *on page 877*
Magnesium, Urine *on page 222*
Oxalate, Urine *on page 238*
Urine Collection, 24-Hour *on page 47*

Abstract Citrate inhibits nephrolithiasis, partly due to binding of calcium in urine. Drug therapy with potassium citrate is useful in prevention of types of stone formation.

Specimen 24-hour urine

Container Plastic container

Collection Some laboratories require preservatives, others do not.

Storage Instructions Refrigerate

Reference Interval Adults: male: 115-921 mg (0.6-4.8 mmol)/24 hours, female: 250-1152 mg (1.3-6.0 mmol)/24 hours;[1] 320-1240 mg (1.7-6.5 mmol)/24 hours[2]

Critical Values Hypocitraturia is defined as <300 mg/24 hours (female) and <250 mg/24 hours (male).[1] (Other sources use other reference intervals.)

Use Hypocitraturia in patients who form kidney stones may be idiopathic, secondary to defective urine acidification, due to small intestinal malabsorption, secondary to hypokalemia or magnesemia, or due to metabolic acidosis. Excessive consumption of protein may stimulate citrate transport in the proximal tubules, leading to hypocitraturia.[3] High sodium diet also causes hypocitraturia. Selected patients at risk for nephrolithiasis may be encouraged to consume more citrus fruits, depending on urinary citrate levels.

Methodology Gas chromatography (GC), ion chromatography, capillary electrophoresis, enzyme-mediated reactions[1]

Additional Information Urinary tests that are sometimes recommended on patients who have had or are likely to develop nephrolithiasis are included in Kidney Stone Analysis *on page 877*. Serum is often assayed for sodium, potassium, chloride, bicarbonate, calcium, phosphorus, alkaline phosphatase, parathyroid hormone, and calcitriol. Analysis of stones is needed; stone composition is the key to preventive therapy.[3]

The pharmacologic treatment of calcium stones requires lowering urinary calcium excretion with thiazides and increasing the inhibitory activity of stone formation by increasing urinary citrate excretion. Potassium citrate is preferred over sodium citrate as sodium increases calcium excretion.[4]

In a recent study on the etiology of idiopathic calcium urolithiasis in children, hypocitraturia was the most important risk factor for stone formation.[5]

Footnotes

1. Newman DJ and Price CP, "Renal Function and Nitrogen Metabolites," *Tietz Textbook of Clinical Chemistry*, 3rd ed, Burtis CA and Ashwood ER, eds, Philadelphia, PA: WB Saunders Co, 1999, 1204-70.
2. Weiss RL, *ARUP Interpretive Data Guide*, ARUP Laboratories Inc, 1999, 178-9.
3. Hruska K, "Renal Calculi (Nephrolithiasis)," *Cecil Textbook of Medicine*, 21st ed, Chapter 114, Goldman L and Bennett JC, eds, Philadelphia, PA: WB Saunders Co, 2000, 622-7.
4. Goldfarb DS and Coe FL, "Prevention of Recurrent Nephrolithiasis," *Am Fam Phys*, 1999, 60(8):2269-76.
5. Tekin A, Tekgul S, Atsu N, et al, "A Study of the Etiology of Idiopathic Calcium Urolithiasis in Children: Hypocitruria Is the Most Important Risk Factor," *J Urol*, 2000, 164(1):162-5.

References

Fuselier HA, Moore K, Lindberg J, "Agglomeration Inhibition Reflected Stone-Forming Activity During Long-Term Potassium Citrate Therapy in Calcium Stone Formers," *Urology*, 1998, 52(6):988-94.
Ganter K, Bongartz D, and Hesse A, "Tamm-Horsfall Protein Excretion and its Relation to Citrate in Urine of Stone-Forming Patients," *Urology*, 1999, 53(3):492-5.
Hoppe B, Kemper MJ, Hvizd MG, et al, "Simultaneous Determination of Oxalate, Citrate and Sulfate in Children's Plasma With Ion Chromatography," *Kidney Int*, 1998, 53(5):1348-52.

(Continued)

Citrate, Serum, Plasma, or Urine *(Continued)*

Hoppe B and Langman CB, "Hypocitraturia in Patients With Urolithiasis," *Arch Dis Child*, 1997, 76(2):174-5.

Melnick JZ, Preisig PA, Haynes S, et al, "Converting Enzyme Inhibition Causes Hypocitraturia Independent of Acidosis or Hypokalemia," *Kidney Int*, 1998, 54(5):1670-4.

Mayo Reference Services Publication, "Supersaturation Profile, Urine," *New Test Announcement*, #82029, Rochester, MN: Mayo Medical Laboratories, May 2000.

♦ **CK** *see* Creatine Kinase, Serum *on page 158*

♦ **CK-2** *see* Creatine Kinase Isoenzymes/Isoforms, Serum *on page 157*

♦ **CK Index** *see* Creatine Kinase Isoenzymes/Isoforms, Serum *on page 157*

♦ **CK Isoenzymes** *see* Creatine Kinase Isoenzymes/Isoforms, Serum *on page 157*

♦ **CK Isoforms** *see* Creatine Kinase Isoenzymes/Isoforms, Serum *on page 157*

♦ **CK-MB and Total CK** *see* Creatine Kinase Isoenzymes/Isoforms, Serum *on page 157*

♦ **Clomid® Test** *see* Clomiphene Test *on page 150*

♦ **Clomiphene Citrate Challenge Test** *see* Follicle Stimulating Hormone, Serum, Plasma, or Urine *on page 175*

Hofmann GE, Danforth DR, and Seifer DB, "Inhibin-B: The Physiologic Basis of the Clomiphene Citrate Challenge Test for Ovarian Reserve Screening," *Fertil Steril*, 1998, 69(3):474-7.

Li TC and Warren MA, "Ovulation Induction for Luteal Phase Defects and Luteal Phase Defects After Ovulation Induction," *Baillieres Clin Obstet Gynaecol*, 1993, 7(2):389-419.

Murakawa H, Hasegawa I, Kurabayashi T, et al, "Polycystic Ovary Syndrome. Insulin Resistance and Ovulatory Responses to Clomiphene Citrate," *J Reprod Med*, 1999, 44(1):23-7.

Scott RT, Leonardi MR, Hoffman GE, et al, "A Prospective Evaluation of Clomiphene Citrate Challenge Test. Screening of the General Infertility Population," *Obstet Gynecol*, 1993, 82(4 Pt 1):539-44.

♦ **Clonidine Suppression Test** *see* Catecholamines, Fractionation, Plasma *on page 138*

♦ **Cl, Serum** *see* Chloride, Serum, Plasma, or Blood *on page 144*

♦ **Cl, Urine** *see* Chloride, Urine *on page 145*

♦ **Clusterin (Apo J)** *see* Apolipoprotein E, Plasma *on page 110*

♦ **CO_2** *see* Bicarbonate, Blood *on page 115*

♦ **CO_2** *see* Carbon Dioxide, Total, Blood *on page 135*

♦ **CO_2 Content** *see* Carbon Dioxide, Total, Blood *on page 135*

Clomiphene Test

Related Information
Follicle Stimulating Hormone, Serum, Plasma, or Urine *on page 175*
Luteinizing Hormone, Blood or Urine *on page 219*

Synonyms Clomid® Test

Test Includes Pre- and post-clomiphene serum FSH and LH analysis

Abstract Clomiphene is a very weak nonsteroidal antiestrogenic agent, a synthetic estrogen analogue, which competes with estradiol at the hypothalamus, thereby blocking the negative feedback of the endogenous gonadal steroids on the hypothalamus. In the presence of an intact hypothalamic-pituitary-gonadal axis, administration of clomiphene leads to increased secretion of LH and FSH, inducing ovulation in many anovulatory patients.

Patient Preparation Four weeks of basal body temperatures are recorded. Ascertain that the patient is not pregnant and that the ovaries are not enlarged. No isotopes administered 24 hours prior to venipuncture. Females initially take 50 mg clomiphene orally daily for 5 days beginning on the fifth day of the induced or spontaneous menstrual cycle.

Specimen Serum

Container Red top tube

Sampling Time Draw pre- and post-clomiphene samples. Because of the pulsatile nature of pituitary gonadotropins, it is recommended that three separate samples, 20 minutes apart, be drawn for baseline and post-clomiphene assays.

Collection Female: draw 5-9 days after last oral dose.

Storage Instructions Refrigerate serum. LH and FSH stable at least 7 days in refrigerated serum.

Special Instructions Provide information if post-clomiphene sample(s).

Reference Interval FSH and LH are expected to peak 5-9 days after completing Clomid®. FSH increase >40% above baseline; LH increase >120% above baseline. Ovulation assessed by basal body temperature or serum progesterone 2 weeks after last clomiphene dose.

Use Clomiphene may be used to evaluate the integrity of the hypothalamic-pituitary-gonadal axis and to enhance fertility in anovulatory patients with normal ovarian function.

Limitations Clomiphene has induced severe hypertriglyceridemia and pancreatitis.[1]

Contraindications In females, observation of hyperstimulation of ovaries but unusual on doses <200 mg, and there is a small risk of multiple pregnancies, about 5%.

Methodology Radioimmunoassay (RIA) or double antibody immunoassay with chemiluminescent read out

Additional Information The structure of clomiphene is similar to that of tamoxifen.

Footnotes
1. Castro MR, Nguyen TT, and O'Brien T, "Clomiphene-Induced Severe Hypertriglyceridemia and Pancreatitis," *Mayo Clin Proc*, 1999, 74(11):1125-8.

References
Blankstein J and Quigley MM, "The Anovulatory Patient. An Orderly Approach to Evaluation and Treatment," *Postgrad Med*, 1988, 83(5):97-102.

Check JH, Chase JS, Nowroozi K, et al, "Empirical Therapy of the Male With Clomiphene in Couples With Unexplained Infertility," *Int J Fertil*, 1989, 34(2):120-2.

Dickey RP and Taylor S, "Future Use of Clomiphene in Ovarian Stimulation," *Hum Reprod*, 1998, 13(9):2358-62.

Dickey RP, Olar TT, Taylor SN, et al, "Relationship of Follicle Number and Other Factors to Fecundability and Multiple Pregnancy in Clomiphene Citrate-Induced Intrauterine Insemination Cycles," *Fertil Steril*, 1992, 57(3):613-9.

Fedele L, Brioschi D, Dorta M, et al, "Prediction and Self-Prediction of Ovulation in Clomiphene Citrate-Treated Patients," *Eur J Obstet Gynecol Reprod Biol*, 1988, 28(4):297-303.

Fujii S, Fukui A, Fukushi Y, et al, "The Effects of Clomiphene Citrate on Normally Ovulatory Women," *Fertil Steril*, 1997, 68(6):997-9.

Cobalamin, Serum

Related Information
Anemia Flowchart *on page 392*
Bone Marrow *on page 410*
Complete Blood Count *on page 419*
Folic Acid, RBC *on page 435*
Folic Acid, Serum *on page 435*
Gastric Analysis *on page 180*
Gastrin, Serum *on page 181*
Helicobacter pylori Biopsy-Based Tests: The Urease Tests, Culture, Cytology, and PCR *on page 620*
Hemoglobin *on page 442*
Homocyst(e)ine, Plasma *on page 193*
Intrinsic Factor Blocking Antibody *on page 537*
Methylmalonic Acid, Serum, Plasma, Urine, or Amniotic Fluid *on page 224*
Parietal Cell Antibody *on page 541*
Pepsinogen I and II, Serum or Plasma *on page 246*
Phlebotomy, Therapeutic *on page 849*
Red Blood Cell Indices *on page 477*
Red Cell Count *on page 478*
Schilling Test *on page 483*
Vitamin B_{12} Unsaturated Binding Capacity *on page 495*
Zidovudine, Serum or Plasma *on page 771*

Synonyms Antipernicious Anemia Factor; B_{12}; Cb1; Cyanocobalamin (Cobalamin) True; Extrinsic Factor of Castle; Vitamin B_{12}

Applies to DIDMOAD Syndrome; Intrinsic Factor; Orotic Aciduria; Transcobalamins; Wolfram Syndrome

Abstract Radioisotopic method replaces *Euglena* microbiological assay for detection of cobalamin deficiency. This assay has lower than desirable positive predictive value for clinical cobalamin deficiency. Serum methylmalonic acid and homocyst(e)ine provide a sensitive indication of early cobalamin deficiency.[1,2] Additional evaluation is important in order to establish the presence of clinical cobalamin (vitamin B_{12}) deficiency. The daily requirement for cobalamin is <2 µg/day. A 4- to 5-year supply is normally stored in the liver. Thus, impaired absorption/transport may be present for several years before deficiency becomes clinically evident. There is recent interest in the ability of serum methylmalonic acid levels to identify the presence of early and/or subclinical cobalamin deficiency (see Methylmalonic Acid, Serum, Plasma, Urine, or Amniotic Fluid *on page 224*).

Patient Preparation A fasting specimen is preferred; draw before transfusions or B_{12} therapy is started.

Specimen Serum

Container Red top tube

Storage Instructions Separate serum and freeze; protect from light. Obtain hematocrit from EDTA tube before freezing the whole blood specimen.

Causes for Rejection Stored specimen, not frozen

Reference Interval The lower reference limit, which is critical to the diagnosis of cobalamin (vitamin B_{12}) deficiency/pernicious anemia, is not clearly established. It is likely in the range of 100-250 pg/mL (SI: 74-185 pmol/L).[3] Values are method and laboratory dependent. Because of overlap in serum levels between cobalamin-deficient and normal individuals, use of an indeterminate range is necessary. The following are interpretive ranges for serum cobalamin:[4]
- normal: 200-900 pg/mL
- indeterminate: 160-200 pg/mL
- low: <160 pg/mL

Clinical correlation and multiple test documentation of the etiology of macrocytic anemia are advised. Occasionally, patients with significant neuropsychiatric abnormalities may have no hematologic abnormalities (absence of anemia or macrocytosis), but vitamin B_{12} level <200 pg/mL (SI: <150 pmol/L), or more commonly between 100 and 200 pg/mL (SI: 75-150 pmol/L).[5] See table for pediatric reference ranges.

Pediatric Serum B_{12} Reference Ranges

Age (y)	Male (pg/mL)		Female (pg/mL)	
	Low	High	Low	High
0-1	216	891	168	1117
2-3	195	897	307	892
4-6	181	795	231	1038
7-9	200	863	182	866
10-12	135	803	145	752
13-18	158	638	134	605

Adapted from Hicks JM, Cook J, Godwin ID, et al, "Vitamin B_{12} and Folate — Pediatric Reference Ranges," *Arch Pathol Lab Med*, 1993, 117:705.

Use Detect cobalamin (Cb1) deficiency in those patients who have hematologic (weakness, anemia, oval macrocytosis, hypersegmented neutrophils, leukopenia/thrombocytopenia) or neurologic (numbness, tingling, loss of vibratory sensation in extremities) findings suggestive of such deficiency. Because of problems associated with verifying the lower limits of "normal," this assay should not be employed as a screening test for functional cobalamin deficiency.[3,5] Evaluate folic acid deficiency; evaluate hypersegmentation of granulocyte nuclei; investigate MCV >98 fL; diagnose macrocytic and megaloblastic anemia; study alcoholism, prenatal care, malabsorption, including jejunoileal bypass patients operated on for massive obesity, and certain neurological disorders.

Limitations Drugs capable of interference with absorption of Cb1 and/or folic acid include chemotherapeutic (methotrexate), antimalarial (pyrimethamine), diuretics (triamterene), protozoacides (pentamidine, isethionate), antibacterials (trimethoprim), anticonvulsants (phenytoin), sedatives (barbiturates), oral contraceptives, antituberculosis agents (cycloserine, paraaminosalicylic acid), antigout (colchicine), oral hypoglycemic, biguanide group (metformin, phenformin). Establishing functional cobalamin (B_{12}) sufficiency in any individual patient may require consideration of intra-individual variation, functional status of the gastric mucosa (in particular in elderly individuals) and transcobalamin II binding.[3] See following discussion of application of serum methylmalonic acid.

Contraindications B_{12}/folate levels should be drawn before performance of Schilling test and before administration of any other radioactivity.

Methodology Radioimmunoassay (RIA) based on competitive protein binding has largely replaced earlier microbiologic assays. Patient's unlabeled endogenous serum B_{12} competes with radiolabeled B_{12} for specific sites on a binding protein (intrinsic factor) and is compared to the behavior of a standard. Most assays measure all forms of B_{12} after conversion to cyanocobalamin. A chemiluminescence receptor assay utilizing intrinsic factor immobilized on magnetic particles (solid phase) has been developed.[6]

Additional Information Vitamin B_{12} (cyanocobalamin) analogues form the base compound in coenzymes having important biologic functions. The vitamin has an intriguing ring structure, a planar tetrapyrrole corrin ring around an asymmetric cobalt atom. The structure is reminiscent of the relation of iron to heme. The corrin system, like porphyrin (heme), is synthesized from delta aminolevulinic acid. The basic compound is named cobalamin. The term vitamin B_{12} refers to hydroxocobalamin or cyanocobalamin and in general use, "B_{12}" applies to all cobalamin forms. The form with attached cyanide group (cyanocobalamin - vitamin B_{12}) was upon original isolation from the liver, actually an artifact generated *in vitro*. Methylcobalamin predominates in the serum, deoxyadenosyl cobalamin in the cytosol. Immunoassays for "B_{12}" measure all forms after conversion to cyanocobalamin. Two metabolically important cobamides (vitamin B_{12} containing coenzymes) are deoxyadenosyl cobamide and methyl cobamide. Cobamides are required for DNA synthesis, methylation, and citric acid cycle reactions.[5]

Cobalamin (Cb1) is not synthesized by humans. In nature, it is supplied only by Cb1-producing microorganisms. It is a requisite dietary component widely available in animal products (meat, fish, eggs, butter, milk, and cheese). The minimum daily requirement (MDR) is 1-5 µg/day, body stores are 2000-5000 µg, and obligatory daily loss is only about 0.1%. B_{12} is absorbed by mucosal epithelial cells (microvilli) of the terminal ileum, a pH and divalent cation dependent process. The vitamin is ingested in food sources nonspecifically bound to protein. Peptic digestion (at low pH in the stomach) is required for release of Cb1 from food protein. Some 25% to 50% of the elderly develop hypochlorhydria or achlorhydria with resultant decrease in proteolysis by pepsin and incomplete release of protein-bound Cb1. This situation can result in Cb1 deficiency but in normal stage I Schilling test (these individuals **can** absorb crystalline CN-[^{57}Co] Cb1 as used in the Schilling Test *on page 483*). Its absorption is dependent upon a gastric glycoprotein, intrinsic factor (IF). Gastric acid splits the B_{12} protein linkage. IF binding is by a benzimidazole nucleotide, which is independent of the analogue chemical form and which protects against digestive enzymes. After the IF-B_{12} complex is absorbed by the ileal mucosa, the vitamin enters the portal circulation where it is bound by a system of carrier proteins, the transcobalamins I, II, and III. See Vitamin B_{12} Unsaturated

Binding Capacity *on page 495* and Schilling Test *on page 483*. Transcobalamins I and III are of leukocyte origin, transcobalamin II is synthesized by the liver and is the plasma carrier protein.

Cobalamin analogues, present in some human plasmas have higher affinity for "R proteins" (R for rapid electrophoretic migrating) than for intrinsic factor, with resultant masking of cobalamin deficiency. Spurious high B_{12} results have been reported in the past relating to anti-intrinsic factor-blocking antibodies and high or low results relating to endogenous B_{12} binding proteins (R proteins).

Conditions associated with decreased serum cobalamin include hypochlorhydria; pernicious anemia (PA) in which cobalamin levels may vary from 0 to overlapping lower limits of patients without PA; dietary deficiency (uncommon); disorders of intestinal absorption; inflammatory bowel disease; bacterial overgrowth, small intestine; *Diphyllobothrium* fish tapeworm, small intestine; prior gastric surgery; intestinal surgery (diminished B_{12} or folate or both are found in 88% of patients with jejunoileal bypass operated for morbid obesity); resection of terminal ileum as for Crohn disease which prevents absorption of B_{12}; oral contraceptives; abnormalities of cobalamin transport or metabolism; Imerslund syndrome;[7,8] and from therapeutic use of gastric H_2 blockers, chronic use of omeprazole, and possibly drug-induced lack of IF secretion.[9] Omeprazole acts by inhibiting a gastric parietal cell proton pump (H^+/K^+ adenosine triphosphatase).[8] **A significant rise in red blood cell mean corpuscular volume (MCV) may be an important early indicator of B_{12} deficiency.** Conditions associated with increased serum cobalamin include chronic granulocytic leukemia (and to a lesser degree leukemoid states); chronic renal failure; severe congestive heart failure; diabetes; obesity; COPD; and cases of liver cell damage (eg, acute hepatitis). Currently, macrocytosis in a hospitalized urban population is most commonly associated with AIDS patients undergoing zidovudine therapy. This may result from AIDS-associated malabsorption and/or a possible DNA-inhibiting effect of zidovudine.[10,11]

DNA Disorders With Macrocytic (Megaloblastic) Anemias Not Due to Cobalamin or Folate Deficiency

Congenital
- Orotic aciduria
- Lesch-Nyhan syndrome
- Congenital dyserythropoietic anemia

Acquired
- Wolfram (DIDMOAD) syndrome: mitochondrial DNA deletion[12]
- Malignancy: erythroleukemia, refractory sideroblastic anemias, antineoplastic chemotherapeutics that inhibit DNA synthesis
- DNA-inhibiting zidovudine and other HIV, other viral antinucleosides
- Toxins, alcohol, others

Elevated serum or urine methylmalonic acid (MMA) level is probably a more definitive indication of early cobalamin (B_{12}) deficiency than the serum cobalamin level. MMA serum level, when increased, reflects decreased tissue cobalamin and is an early indicator of B_{12} deficiency. Cobalamin dependent neurologic disease with normal hematologic parameters and serum B_{12} levels may be associated with significant elevations of serum methylmalonic acid. To avoid dietary influence serum MMA levels have preference over urine studies in nonfasting patients.[13]

Folate deficiency may be a cause of low levels of serum cobalamin. Low serum B_{12} levels may be seen in some individuals deficient only in folate. It is important to note that a normal level of cobalamin in the serum does not always exclude cobalamin deficiency. Individuals with low serum B_{12} require clinical confirmation of deficiency. In pregnancy low serum B_{12} level does not usually indicate deficiency at the biochemical level. Elevation of serum homocyst(e)ine concentrations (in the absence of folate deficiency) may be of value in establishing true B_{12} deficiency. Serum MMA level may be independent of B_{12} status in the pregnant patient.[14]

Footnotes

1. Carmel R, "Current Concepts in Cobalamin Deficiency," *Annu Rev Med*, 2000, 51:357-75.
2. Savage DG, Lindenbaum J, Stabler SP, et al, "Sensitivity of Serum Methylmalonic Acid and Total Homocysteine Determinations for Diagnosing Cobalamin and Folate Deficiencies," *Am J Med*, 1994, 96(3):239-46.
3. Lindstedt G, Lundberg PA, Johansson PM, et al, "High Prevalence of Atrophic Gastritis in the Elderly: Implications for Health-Associated Reference Limits for Cobalamin in Serum," *Clin Chem*, 1989, 35(7):1557-9.
4. Fish MB, "Gastrointestinal Absorption of Cobalamin (Vitamin B_{12})," *Diagnostic Nuclear Medicine*, 3rd ed, Volume 2, Sandler MP, Coleman RE, Wackers FJ, et al, eds, Baltimore, MD: Lippincott Williams & Wilkins, 1996, 840.
5. Lindenbaum J, Healton EB, Savage DG, et al, "Neuropsychiatric Disorders Caused by Cobalamin Deficiency in the Absence of Anemia or Macrocytosis," *N Engl J Med*, 1988, 318(26):1720-8.
6. Leonard H, Klukas C, Williams M, et al, "A Chemiluminescence Receptor Assay for Vitamin B_{12}," *Clin Chem*, 1989, 35:1194.
7. Abdelaal MA and Ahmed AF, "Imerslund-Gräsbeck Syndrome in a Saudi Family," *Acta Paediatr Scand*, 1991, 80(11):1109-12.
8. Russo CL, Hyman PE, and Oseas RS, "Megaloblastic Anemia Characterized by Microcytosis: Imerslund-Gräsbeck Syndrome With Coexistent Alpha-Thalassemia," *Pediatrics*, 1988, 81(6):875-6.
9. Marcuard SP, Albernaz L, and Khazanie PG, "Omeprazole Therapy Causes Malabsorption of Cyanocobalamin," *Ann Intern Med*, 1994, 120(3):211-5.
10. Snower DP and Weil SC, "Changing Etiology of Macrocytosis: Zidovudine as a Frequent Causative Factor," *Am J Clin Pathol*, 1993, 99(1):57-60.

(Continued)

Cobalamin, Serum (Continued)

11. Rule SA, Hooker M, Costello C, et al, "Serum Vitamin B$_{12}$ and Transcobalamin Levels in Early HIV Disease," *Am J Hematol*, 1994, 47(3):167-71.

12. Borgna-Pignatti C, Marradi P, Pinelli L, et al, "Thiamine-Responsive Anemia in DIDMOAD Syndrome," *J Pediatr*, 1989, 114(3):405-10.

13. Rasmussen K, "Studies on Methylmalonic Acid in Humans. I. Concentrations in Serum and Urinary Excretion in Normal Subjects After Feeding and During Fasting and After Loading With Protein, Fat, Sugar, Isoleucine, and Valine," *Clin Chem*, 1989, 38(12):2271-6.

14. Metz J, McGrath K, Bennett M, et al, "Biochemical Indices of Vitamin B$_{12}$ Nutrition in Pregnant Patients With Subnormal Serum Vitamin B$_{12}$ Levels," *Am J Hematol*, 1995, 48:251-5.

References

Antony AC, "Megaloblastic Anemias," *Hematology: Basic Principles and Practice*, 3rd ed, Chapter 28, Hoffman R, Benz EJ Jr, Shattil SJ, et al, eds, Philadelphia, PA: Churchill Livingstone, 2000, 446-85.

Bolann BJ, Solli JD, Schneede J, et al, "Evaluation of Indicators of Cobalamin Deficiency Defined as Cobalamin-Induced Reduction in Increased Serum Methylmalonic Acid," *Clin Chem*, 2000, 46(11):1744-50.

Hicks JM, Cook J, Godwin ID, et al, "Vitamin B$_{12}$ and Folate: Pediatric Reference Ranges," *Arch Pathol Lab Med*, 1993, 117(7):704-6.

Matchar DB, McCrory DC, Millington DS, et al, "Performance of the Serum Cobalamin Assay for Diagnosis of Cobalamin Deficiency," *Am J Med Sci*, 1994, 308(5):276-83.

Oosterhuis WP, Niessen RW, Bossuyt PM, et al, "Diagnostic Value of the Mean Corpuscular Volume in the Detection of Vitamin B$_{12}$ Deficiency," *Scand J Clin Lab Invest*, 2000, 60(1):9-18.

Schilling RF and Williams WJ, "Vitamin B$_{12}$ Deficiency: Underdiagnosed, Overtreated?" *Hosp Pract*, 1995, 30(7):47-54.

Snow CF, "Laboratory Diagnosis of Vitamin B$_{12}$ and Folate Deficiency: A Guide for the Primary Care Physician," *Arch Intern Med*, 1999, 159(12):1289-98.

Wickramasinghe SN, "Newer B$_{12}$ and Folate Assays and Functional Measurements," *Clin Lab Haematol*, 1997, 19:289-320.

♦ **Collagen Cross-Link-Associated C-Telopeptide** *see* Osteocalcin, Serum or Plasma *on page 237*

♦ **Collagen Cross-Link-Associated N-Telopeptide** *see* Osteocalcin, Serum or Plasma *on page 237*

♦ **Collagen Type-1** *see* N-Telopeptides, Urine *on page 233*

♦ **Combined Test** *see* Pregnancy-Associated Protein A, Serum *on page 260*

♦ **Complexed PSA** *see* Prostate Specific Antigen, Free *on page 263*

♦ **Compound F** *see* Cortisol, Serum or Plasma *on page 154*

♦ **Congenital Disorders of Glycosylation** *see* Carbohydrate-Deficient Transferrin, Serum *on page 134*

♦ **Conjugated Hyperbilirubinemia** *see* Bilirubin, Direct, Serum *on page 117*

♦ **Connecting Peptide Insulin** *see* C-Peptide, Serum *on page 156*

♦ **Coproporphyrins** *see* Porphyrins, Quantitative, Urine *on page 255*

♦ **Corticotropin** *see* Adrenocorticotropic Hormone, Plasma *on page 86*

♦ **Corticotropin-Releasing Hormone** *see* Insulin Tolerance Test *on page 202*

Corticotropin-Releasing Hormone Stimulation Test

Related Information
Adrenal Cortex: Laboratory Assessments Overview *on page 84*
Adrenocorticotropic Hormone, Plasma *on page 86*
Corticotropin Stimulation Test (Rapid) *on page 153*
Cortisol, Free, Urine *on page 154*
Cortisol, Serum or Plasma *on page 154*
Insulin Tolerance Test *on page 202*
Metyrapone Stimulation Test, Serum *on page 225*
Urinary Cortisol/Creatinine Increment *on page 296*

Synonyms CRH Stimulation Test

Applies to Dexamethasone-CRH Protocol

Abstract Corticotropin-releasing hormone (CRH) is an ACTH secretagogue which is used in the evaluation of patients with suspected Cushing syndrome (CS).

Patient Preparation

Systemic protocol: The patient fasts for 4 hours and an intravenous line is inserted. After obtaining a baseline blood specimen, ovine CRH, 1 µg/kg body weight,[1] is given intravenously as a bolus. CRH injection may be given at 9 AM or 8 PM.

Inferior petrosal protocol: An intravenous line is placed in a peripheral vein. Catheters are inserted through the femoral veins into the right and left inferior petrosal sinuses.[2] Precise localization is critical; the technique requires a radiologist experienced in this technique.

Dexamethasone-CRH protocol: Investigators at the NIH[3] developed a variation of the CRH stimulation test in which the patient receives pretreatment with 0.5 mg dexamethasone given orally every 6 hours for a total of 8 doses. CRH, 0.1 µg/kg body weight, is given intravenously 2 hours after the last dose of dexamethasone.

Specimen Serum

Container Red top tube

Sampling Time

Systemic protocol: A baseline sample is always obtained 15 minutes before, and then just before, the CRH injection. Subsequent specimens are obtained according to one of these schedules:
- 5, 15, 30, 60, 120, and 180 minutes after CRH[1]
- 5, 10, 15, 30, 45, 60, 90, and 120 minutes after CRH[4]

Samples are assayed for cortisol and/or ACTH, depending on clinical indication.

Inferior petrosal protocol: Specimens are obtained from each inferior petrosal sinus and the peripheral site at the following times: before CRH, and then at 2 and 5 minutes after CRH.[4] Some suggest an additional specimen at 10 minutes after CRH.[1] Specimens may be assayed for ACTH and cortisol, but the diagnostic criteria are based primarily on the ACTH values.

Dexamethasone-CRH protocol: In the original description of this test, specimens for serum cortisol and ACTH were obtained at 15, 10, 5, and 0 minutes before CRH, and then at 5, 15, 30, 45, and 60 minutes after CRH. Since experience with this protocol is limited, the original description should be consulted if its use is contemplated.[3]

Reference Interval

Systemic protocol: The following values are associated with a pituitary source of ACTH in a patient with CS.[1]

ACTH:
- 9:30 AM: 80 ±7 pg/mL (SI:17.6 ±1.5 pmol/L)
- 8:30 PM: 29 ±2.6 pg/mL (SI: 6.38 ±0.57 pmol/L)

Cortisol:
- 10 AM: 13.1 ±1.0 µg/dL (SI: 358.8 ±27.6 nmol/L)
- 9 PM: 17 ±0.7 µg/dL (SI: 470.2 ±19.4 nmol/L)

Inferior petrosal protocol: Following CRH, a central to peripheral serum ACTH ratio >3.0 is strong evidence for a pituitary source of ACTH in an adult patient with CS.[1,4] In children and adolescents, the corresponding cutoff is >2.5.[5]

Dexamethasone-CRH protocol: The following values are from an NIH study of 58 patients, 39 of whom proved to have CS and 19 of whom had pseudo-CS.[3]
- Serum cortisol before CRH: >1.38 µg/dL (SI: >38 nmol/L); sensitivity 90%, specificity 100%
- Serum cortisol 15 minutes after CRH: >1.38 µg/dL (SI: >38 nmol/L); sensitivity/specificity 100%
- Serum ACTH 30 minutes after CRH: >16 pg/mL (SI: >3.5 pmol/L); sensitivity 74%, specificity 100%

Use The CRH test is used to differentiate Cushing disease (ACTH-dependent) vs other causes of Cushing syndrome (eg, adrenal adenoma, ectopic ACTH - see Adrenal Cortex: Laboratory Assessments Overview *on page 84*). The systemic protocol is somewhat less sensitive than the inferior petrosal protocol (see Limitations). The dexamethasone-CRH protocol was developed to differentiate mild cases of Cushing disease from pseudo-Cushing states.

Limitations As many as 8% of patients with Cushing disease will not have the expected increase in ACTH and/or cortisol. Most of these nonresponders will, however, have a central to peripheral ratio ≥3.0 in the inferior petrosal protocol.[4]

Footnotes

1. Demers LM and Whitley RJ, "Function of the Adrenal Cortex," *Tietz Textbook of Clinical Chemistry*, 3rd ed, Burtis CA and Ashwood ER, eds, Philadelphia, PA: WB Saunders Co, 1999, 1544.

2. Oldfield EH, Doppman JL, Nieman LK, et al, "Petrosal Sinus Sampling With and Without Corticotropin-Releasing Hormone for the Differential Diagnosis of Cushing's Syndrome," *N Engl J Med*, 1991, 325:897-905 (published erratum *N Engl J Med*, 1992, 326:1172).

3. Yanovski JA, Cutler GB Jr, Chrousos GP, et al, "Corticotropin-Releasing Hormone Stimulation Following Low-Dose Dexamethasone Administration," *JAMA*, 1993, 269:2232-38.

4. Orth DN and Kovacs WJ, "The Adrenal Cortex," *Williams Textbook of Endocrinology*, 9th ed, Wilson JD, Foster DW, Kronenberg HM, et al, eds, Philadelphia, PA: WB Saunders Co, 1998, 621.

5. Magiakou MA, Mastorakos GM, Oldfield EH, et al, "Cushing's Syndrome in Children and Adolescents," *N Engl J Med*, 1994, 331:629-36.

References

Bornstein SR, Stratakis CA, and Chrousos GP, "Adrenocortical Tumors: Recent Advances in Basic Concepts and Clinical Management," *Ann Intern Med*, 1999, 130(9):759-71.

Orth DN, "Cushing's Syndrome," *N Engl J Med*, 1995, 332:791-803 (published erratum *N Engl J Med* 1995, 332:1527).

Corticotropin Stimulation Test (Rapid)

Related Information

Adrenal Cortex: Laboratory Assessments Overview *on page 84*
Adrenocorticotropic Hormone, Plasma *on page 86*
Corticotropin-Releasing Hormone Stimulation Test *on page 152*
Cortisol, Free, Urine *on page 154*
Cortisol, Serum or Plasma *on page 154*
Insulin Tolerance Test *on page 202*
Metyrapone Stimulation Test, Serum *on page 225*
Thorn Test *on page 490*
Urinary Cortisol/Creatinine Increment *on page 296*

Synonyms Cortrosyn® Test; Cosyntropin Stimulation Test; Rapid (or Short) ACTH Test; Synthetic α 1-24-ACTH Stimulation Test

Replaces ACTH Infusion Test; Bovine ACTH

Abstract Corticotropin, in the context of adrenal testing, refers to a synthetic polypeptide, consisting of the biologically active 1-24 amino acid sequence of human ACTH. This polypeptide stimulates the secretion of cortisol, and other corticosteroids, from the adrenal cortex, and, as a testing agent, is used to evaluate possible adrenocortical insufficiency, and late-onset congenital adrenal hyperplasia (CAH) due to 21-hydroxylase deficiency. It has a very short half-life. In a hospital formulary, this product is often listed under the generic term, cosyntropin; in Europe, the equivalent term is tetracosactrin (see Adrenal Cortex: Laboratory Assessments Overview *on page 84*).

The rapid corticotropin (cosyntropin) stimulation test is performed at two dose levels. The older, more conventional high-dose protocol uses a pharmacologic 250 μg dose (I.V. or I.M.), with blood samples for cortisol obtained just prior to the injection (baseline), and at 30 and 60 minutes postinjection.

The newer low-dose protocol[1,2,3] uses a physiologic 1 μg (or 0.5 μg/m² body surface area). Blood samples for cortisol may be obtained at 30 minutes, or at 30 and 60 minutes postinjection. Some authors include a baseline specimen[1], while others do not[2]. The low-dose test is more sensitive than the high-dose test[4,5] (see Use and Limitations).

Specimen Serum

Container Red top tube

Sampling Time The test is usually performed in the morning, before 10 AM.
- High-dose protocol: Baseline and 60 minutes postinjection (in certain special situations, specimens may also be obtained at 20 and 30 minutes; consult references for guidelines).
- Low-dose protocol: The 30-minutes postinjection value is critical.[2] Some authors also include a baseline and a 60-minute value.[1,6]

Storage Instructions Separate serum and freeze.

Reference Interval

Adrenal insufficiency: Both high-dose and low-dose protocols: Normal adrenal responsiveness is suggested by either:
- a serum cortisol value of 18-20 μg/dL (SI: 500-550 nmol/L) at 30 or 60 minutes, or
- a serum cortisol increment over baseline of 7 μg/dL (SI: 193 nmol/L) at 30 or 60 minutes

However, when using the high-dose protocol, a response that meets one of these criteria of normalcy does not necessarily imply that the patient will have an adequate response to a prolonged stress (such as that associated with surgical procedures, infection, neoplastic disease or trauma).[7]

Congenital adrenal hyperplasia (21-hydroxylase deficiency):
- High-dose protocol: The diagnosis of CAH is confirmed if the 17-hydroxyprogesterone is >1500 ng/dL (SI: >45.0 nmol/L) at 30 or 60 minutes,[8] or if an increase over baseline >1333 ng/dL (SI: >40.0 nmol/L) is seen at 30 or 60 minutes.[9]

Prognosis in septic shock: See Use.

Use Adrenal insufficiency is a potentially life-threatening, but subtle, disorder. The integration of clinical and laboratory information by an experienced clinician is essential in recognizing the possibility of, and diagnosing, adrenal insufficiency (AI). Total reliance on either clinical or laboratory information can have disastrous consequences for the patient. The diagnosis of AI is ruled out if, in an unstressed (not acutely ill) patient, a random serum cortisol result is >20 μg/dL (SI: 550 nmol/L). The diagnosis of AI is confirmed if the basal morning serum cortisol is <3.1 μg/dL (SI: 86 nmol/L). In between these two extremes, and in an acutely ill (stressed) patient, the corticotropin stimulation test is recommended.[6]

Primary adrenal insufficiency (PAI): Included in this category are patients with chronic PAI (Addison disease) due to destruction (by neoplasm, infection, or autoimmune inflammation) of the adrenal, or metabolic adrenal dysfunction (adrenomyeloneuropathy). Classical findings are low serum cortisol, elevated serum ACTH, and hyperpigmentation of the skin.

PAI may also occur as an acute process with an abrupt onset. Causes include acute hemorrhage or necrosis of the adrenal (eg, sepsis, anticoagulant therapy, adrenal vein thrombosis, antiphospholipid antibody syndrome). These patients may have catecholamine-resistant hypotension and hyponatremia. Immediate diagnosis and treatment are essential.

Secondary adrenal insufficiency: This category includes patients with pituitary or hypothalamic dysfunction. In the former category are patients who have received long-term corticosteroid medication (including inhaled corticosteroids). Findings may be similar to primary AI, except that serum ACTH levels are not elevated and hyperpigmentation of the skin is not observed. An abnormal result in the high-dose protocol can be interpreted as definite evidence of AI and signals the need for corticosteroid treatment. However, some patients with secondary or tertiary AI (confirmed by metyrapone and

insulin-tolerance testing) have a normal response to the high-dose protocol.[7] The recognition of these patients led to the development of the low-dose protocol.[1,2,3] The low-dose protocol is a more sensitive test, and therefore is preferred in the setting of secondary AI.

When the result is borderline with the low-dose protocol (eg, 16 μg/dL [SI: 441.6 nmol/L] at 1-hour postinjection), a Metyrapone Stimulation Test, Serum *on page 225* or Insulin Tolerance Test *on page 202* may be useful; caution is warranted, however, since these tests may precipitate acute adrenal crisis in patients with severe AI.

Prognosis in septic shock: A major determinant of survival in septic shock is the functional integrity of the hypothalamic-pituitary-adrenal (HPA) axis. A French study of 189 ICU patients, investigated the Corticotropin Stimulation Test (high-dose protocol) and found that high basal cortisol and small incremental responses to corticotropin indicated a poor prognosis for survival.[10] Further analysis of their data revealed three survival patterns based on the test results. See table.

Corticotropin Stimulation Test in Septic Shock

Basal Cortisol	Delta Max Cortisol	Likelihood of Survival	28-Day Mortality
≤34 μg/dL (SI: <938.4 nmol/L)	>9 μg/dL (SI: >248.4 nmol/L)	High	26%
≤34 μg/dL (SI: 938.4 nmol/L)	<9 μg/dL (SI: <248.4 nmol/L)	Intermediate	67%
≥34 μg/dL	>9 μg/dL (SI: >248.4 nmol/L)	Intermediate	67%
>34 μg/dL (SI: >938.4 nmol/L)	<9 μg/dL (SI: <248.4 nmol/L)	Low	82%

Another French group, investigating a much smaller population of 22 patients and using a different data analysis approach,[11] did not find this test helpful.

Congenital adrenal hyperplasia, 21-hydroxylase deficiency (CAH): CAH is usually diagnosed in infancy or early childhood on the basis of physical findings accompanied by marked elevations of corticosteroid hormones proximal to the enzyme defect.[9] A few patients, however, have an attenuated form of late-onset (nonclassical) CAH, and in these individuals the rapid corticotropin test (high-dose protocol) is useful. Testing in this situation begins with a basal morning 17-hydroxyprogesterone (17-Pr); if the result is <230 ng/dL (SI: <6.9 nmol/L), the diagnosis of CAH is excluded. If 17-Pr is >1500 ng/dL (SI: 45.0 nmol/L), the diagnosis is confirmed. The rapid corticotropin test, **high-dose protocol**, is used for patients whose basal 17aPr results fall between 230 and 1500 ng/dL.[8,12]

For additional information about the less common forms of CAH in children see Levine et al, and in adults see New et al (see References).

Limitations As indicated above (see Use), the **high-dose** protocol can produce a misleadingly normal result, especially in patients with subtle secondary or tertiary AI. A normal result in the **high-dose** protocol does not imply that the cortisol output will be sufficient during a prolonged stress (eg, surgical procedures, infections, trauma, or neoplastic disease).

Methodology Immunoassays (multiple labels)

Additional Information Estrogen medication raises serum cortisol.

Footnotes

1. Tordjman K, Jaffe A, Grazas N, et al, "The Role of the Low Dose (1 μg) Adrenocorticotropin Test in the Evaluation of Patients With Pituitary Diseases," *J Clin Endocrinol Metab*, 1995, 80(4):1301-5.
2. Thaler LM and Blevins LS, "The Low Dose (1 μg) Adrenocorticotropin Stimulation Test in the Evaluation of Patients With Suspected Central Adrenal Insufficiency," *J Clin Endocrinol Metab*, 1998, 83(8):2726-9.
3. Soferman R, Kivity S, Dickstein G, et al, "Low-Dose Adrenocorticotropin Test Reveals Impaired Adrenal Function in Patients Taking Inhaled Corticosteroids," *J Clin Endocrinol Metab*, 1995, 80(4):1243-6.
4. Krasner AS, "Glucocorticoid-Induced Adrenal Insufficiency," *JAMA*, 1999, 282(7):671-6.
5. Amatruda TT, Hollingsworth DR, D'Esopo ND, et al, "A Study of the Mechanism of the Steroid Withdrawal Syndrome: Evidence for Integrity of the Hypothalamic-Pituitary-Adrenal System," *J Clin Endocrinol Metab*, 1960, 20:339-54.
6. Oelkers W, "Adrenal Insufficiency," *N Engl J Med*, 1996, 335(16):1206-12.
7. Streeten DH, Anderson GH Jr, and Bonaventura MM, "The Potential for Serious Consequences From Misinterpreting Normal Responses to the Rapid Adrenocorticotropin Test," *J Clin Endocrinol Metab*, 1996, 81(1):285-90.
8. Gronowski AM and Landau-Levine M, "Reproductive Endocrine Function," *Tietz Textbook of Clinical Chemistry*, 3rd ed, Burtis CA and Ashwood ER, eds, Philadelphia, PA: Saunders Co, 1999, 1619-20.
9. Addison GM, *Biochemical Basis of Pediatric Disease*, Soldin SJ, Rifai N, and Hicks JMB, eds, Washington, DC: AACC Press, American Association of Clinical Chemistry, 1992, 228-9.
10. Annane D, Sebille V, Troche G, et al, "A 3-Level Prognostic Classification in Septic Shock Based on Cortisol Levels and Cortisol Response to Corticotropin," *JAMA*, 2000, 283(8):1038-45.
11. Bouachour G, Roy PM, and Guiraud MP, "The Repetitive Short Corticotropin Stimulation Test in Patients With Septic Shock," *Ann Intern Med*, 1995, 123(12):962-3.
12. Rittmaster RS, "Hirsutism," *Lancet*, 1997, 349(9046):191-5.

References

Levine LS and DiGeorge AM, *Nelson Textbook of Pediatrics*, Behrman RE, Kliegman RM, and Jenson HB, eds, 16th ed, Philadelphia, PA: WB Saunders Co, 2000, 1729-36.

(Continued)

Corticotropin Stimulation Test (Rapid) *(Continued)*

Levy NT, Young WF, Habermann TM, et al, "Adrenal Insufficiency as a Manifestation of Disseminated non-Hodgkin's Lymphoma," *Mayo Clin Proc*, 1997, 72(9):818-22.

Merke DP and Cutler GB, "New Approaches to the Treatment of Congenital Adrenal Hyperplasia," *JAMA*, 1997, 277(3):1073-6.

New MI and Josso N, "Disorders of Sexual Differentiation," *Cecil Textbook of Medicine*, Goldman L and Bennett JC, eds, 21st ed, Philadelphia, PA: WB Saunders Co, 2000, 1300-6.

♦ **Cortisol** *see* Insulin Tolerance Test *on page 202*

♦ **Cortisol-Binding Globulin** *see* Cortisol, Serum or Plasma *on page 154*

♦ **Cortisol-Binding Globulin** *see* Urinary Cortisol/Creatinine Increment *on page 296*

Cortisol, Free, Urine

Related Information

Adrenal Cortex: Laboratory Assessments Overview *on page 84*
Corticotropin-Releasing Hormone Stimulation Test *on page 152*
Cortisol, Serum or Plasma *on page 154*
17-Hydroxycorticosteroids, Urine *on page 196*
Insulin Tolerance Test *on page 202*
Metyrapone Stimulation Test, Serum *on page 225*
Urinary Cortisol/Creatinine Increment *on page 296*
Urine Collection, 24-Hour *on page 47*

Synonyms Urinary Cortisol; Urine Cortisol

Test Includes Creatinine concentration and total volume, to support adequacy of collection

Abstract The diagnosis of Cushing syndrome (CS) requires evidence of cortisol hypersecretion. While serum cortisol levels fluctuate unpredictably and are strongly dependent on concurrent cortisol-binding globulin (CBG) levels, a 24-hour urine specimen integrates the cortisol production for an entire day and is not affected by CBG. Urinary cortisol reflects the portion of serum-free cortisol filtered by the kidney, and correlates well with cortisol secretion rate.

The most common causes of CS are pituitary adenoma (65% to 70%), adrenal tumor (15% to 20%), and the ectopic CS (10% to 15%). (See Adrenal Cortex: Laboratory Assessments Overview *on page 84*.)

Patient Preparation Radioisotopes may interfere if assay method is by radioimmunoassay. Patient should avoid spironolactone or quinacrine. Avoid patient stress.

Specimen 24-hour urine

Container Either 25 mL of 50% acetic acid or 10 g boric acid can be added before collection is started. If no preservative is used, it is necessary to refrigerate during collection.

Sampling Time Two or three 24-hour collections may be needed.

Collection A normal diurnal rhythm exists with highest levels in the morning, but this circadian rhythm is lost in Cushing syndrome.[1]

When assessing the completeness of urine collection, there should be <10% variation in the creatinine concentrations of each 24-hour specimen. A variation >10% suggests incomplete collection. Because cortisol secretion is episodic, the creatinine concentration difference cannot be used to "correct" the cortisol result from an incomplete specimen.

Reference Interval Method dependent; typical ranges (age ranges not exact) include:

HPLC:[1]
- 0-10 years: 2-27 µg/day (SI: 5.52-74.5 nmol/day)
- 11-17 years: 1-55 µg/day (SI: 2.76-151.8 mmol/day)
- adults: 5-55 µg/day (SI: 13.8-151.8 nmol/day)

RIA (extracted):[2]
- 0-10/ years: 2-27 µg/day (SI: 5.52-74.5 nmol/day)
- 11-20 years: 5-55 µg/day (SI: 13.8-151.8 nmol/day)
- adults: 20-90 µg/24 hours (SI: 55.2-248.4 nmol/day)

Use This test is useful in the initial evaluation of patients with suspected Cushing syndrome (CS).[3,4] Patients with CS usually have urine free cortisol >100 µg/24 hours (SI: 276.0 nmol/day), but there is wide variation and no single cutoff can be used safely. If the 24-hour urine free cortisol is elevated, additional testing is indicated to differentiate among pituitary-dependent CS, pituitary-independent CS, and pseudo-Cushing syndrome.[4] (See Adrenal Cortex: Laboratory Assessments Overview *on page 84*.)

Some patients with an elevated 24-hour urine cortisol do not have Cushing syndrome, and are often classified as pseudo-Cushing syndrome. Establishing this diagnosis requires additional testing which includes the low-dose dexamethasone suppression test, the CRH stimulation test, or a protocol that combines them both.[5] (See Adrenal Cortex: Laboratory Assessments Overview *on page 84*.)

The diagnosis of CS requires a meticulous history and physical examination,[4] and these should precede a biochemical evaluation.

Limitations Not useful in the evaluation of adrenal insufficiency (AI). Results in AI overlap with normal ranges. Increased in pregnancy and with oral contraceptives. Increased excretion may be found with pseudo-Cushing syndrome, trauma, or infection.[4] Tetracyclines may cause false elevation of results.

Murphy has challenged the specificity of contemporary immunoassay methods for cortisol.[6,7] He believes that immunoassay cortisol results are falsely elevated because the antibodies cross-react with other corticosteroids.

Methodology Immunoassays (multiple labels) after extraction, high performance liquid chromatography (HPLC), gas chromatography/mass spectrometry (GC/MS)

Footnotes

1. Leavelle DE, ed, *Interpretive Handbook*, Mayo Medical Laboratories, Rochester, MN, 1997, 163-4.
2. Demers LM and Whitley RJ, "Function of the Adrenal Cortex," *Tietz Textbook of Clinical Chemistry*, 3rd ed, Burtis CA and Ashwood ER, eds, Philadelphia, PA: WB Saunders Co, 1997, 1559-60.
3. Watts NB and Keffer JH, "Adrenal Cortex," *Practical Endocrinology*, 4th ed, Philadelphia, PA: Lea & Febiger, 1989, 91-120.
4. Orth DN, "Cushing's Syndrome," *N Engl J Med*, 1995, 332(12):791-803 (published erratum appears in *N Engl J Med*, 1995, 332:1527).
5. Yanovski JA, Cutler GB, Chrousos GP, et al, "Corticotropin-Releasing Hormone Stimulation Following Low-Dose Dexamethasone Administration. A New Test to Distinguish Cushing's Syndrome From Pseudo-Cushing's States," *JAMA*, 1993, 269(17):2232-8.
6. Murphy BEP, "Lack of Specificity of Urinary Free Cortisol Determinations: Why Does it Occur?" *J Clin Endocrinol Metab*, 1999, 84(6):2258-9.
7. Murphy BEP, "How Much UFC Is Really Cortisol?" *Clin Chem*, 2000, 46(6 Pt 1):793-4.

References

Bornstein SR, Stratakis CA, and Chrousos GP, "Adrenocortical Tumors: Recent Advances in Basic Concepts and Clinical Management," *Ann Intern Med*, 1999, 130(9):759-71.

Cortisol, Serum or Plasma

Related Information

Adrenal Cortex: Laboratory Assessments Overview *on page 84*
Adrenocorticotropic Hormone, Plasma *on page 86*
Androstenedione, Serum *on page 104*
Corticotropin-Releasing Hormone Stimulation Test *on page 152*
Corticotropin Stimulation Test (Rapid) *on page 153*
Cortisol, Free, Urine *on page 154*
Estradiol, Serum *on page 170*
17-Hydroxycorticosteroids, Urine *on page 196*
17-Hydroxyprogesterone, Serum or Plasma *on page 197*
Metyrapone Stimulation Test, Serum *on page 225*
Testosterone, Total and Free, Serum or Plasma *on page 280*
Thorn Test *on page 490*
Urinary Cortisol/Creatinine Increment *on page 296*

Synonyms Compound F; Hydrocortisone, Serum

Applies to Cortisol-Binding Globulin; Dexamethasone Suppression Test

Abstract Cortisol, the major adrenal glucocorticoid, is secreted in a circadian pattern, with maximum values, 5-25 µg/dL, in the early morning and minimum values, 3-16 µg/dL, in the late afternoon. Most of the cortisol in the blood is protein-bound to cortisol-binding globulin (CBG) and albumin. Under normal circumstances, cortisol has a half-life in the blood of ~80-100 minutes. The serum concentration of CBG, normally 35-40 ng/L[1] has moderate interindividual variability, and is also influenced by a number of hormones. Of particular importance is the fact that medicinal estrogens can produce a two- to threefold increase in CBG (in both women and men), and CBG is also increased during pregnancy. After metabolic inactivation in the liver, most cortisol metabolites are excreted in the urine. Only ~1% of cortisol is excreted unchanged into urine, but this urine free cortisol is important diagnostically (see Cortisol, Free, Urine *on page 154*). Cortisol secretion fluctuates rapidly in response to a variety of stimuli, including sepsis, surgical procedures, and other stressors. It stimulates catabolism of protein and fat.

Low plasma corticotropin with concurrent increased concentration of serum or plasma cortisol provides indication of autonomous adrenocortical activity.[2]

Patient Preparation

Single sleeping midnight cortisol: In this protocol,[3] which applies to hospitalized patients in a controlled environment, the patient retires ~11 PM and is awakened, as gently as possible, 1 hour later for venipuncture.

Overnight DST: The patient, not necessarily hospitalized, is given dexamethasone 1 mg orally at bedtime (~11 PM) and a blood specimen is drawn the next morning at 8 AM.[4]

Low-dose DST: 24-hour urine specimens are collected on four consecutive days. Beginning at 8 AM on day 2, the patient is given dexamethasone 0.5 mg orally every 6 hours for a total of 8 doses. Blood specimens are obtained at 8 AM and 8 PM on day 1, and again at 8 AM on day 5. The blood specimens are assayed for cortisol. Each urine specimen is assayed for free cortisol and creatinine.[4] (Some clinicians also measure urinary 17-hydroxycorticosteroids.)

High-dose DST: 24-hour urine specimens are collected on four consecutive days. Beginning at 8 AM on day 2, the patient is given dexamethasone 2 mg orally every 6 hours for a total of 8 doses. Blood specimens are obtained at 8 AM and 8 PM on day 1, and again at 8 AM on day 5. The blood specimens are assayed for cortisol. Each urine specimen is assayed for free cortisol and creatinine.[4] (Some clinicians also measure urinary 17-hydroxycorticosteroids.)

Specimen Serum or plasma

Container Red top tube or green top (heparin) tube

Sampling Time See Patient Preparation.

Storage Instructions Stable 7 days at 4°C to 25°C.

Reference Interval See table.

Children[5]		
Age	5-11 AM	5-11 PM
0-24 mo	0.1-3.4 µg/dL (SI: 28-938 nmol/L)	0.1-8.0 µg/dL (SI: 28-828 nmol/L)
2-10 y	0.1-3.3 µg/dL (SI: 28-911 nmol/L)	0.1-2.4 µg/dL (SI: 28-662 nmol/L)
11-18 y	0.1-2.8 µg/dL (SI: 28-773 nmol/L)	0.1-2.2 µg/dL (SI: 10-220 nmol/L)

Adults[4]	
8 AM	5-25 µg/dL (SI: 138-690 nmol/L)
4 PM	3-16 µg/dL (SI: 83-442 nmol/L)
8 PM	50% of 8 AM value
Midnight	<5 µg/dL (SI: 138 nmol/L)

The evening nadir is not found in subjects with Cushing syndrome.

Use Cortisol excess and deficiency are at the center of several major disease processes which require laboratory testing for diagnosis (see Adrenal Cortex: Laboratory Assessments Overview *on page 84*). Random measurements of serum cortisol are often useless. Even in patients with cortisol excess or deficiency, the many factors influencing cortisol can result in cortisol values which overlap the reference range. Diagnostically useful cortisol measurements require standardized testing protocols in which one or more preanalytic variables are held constant.

High cortisol occurs in adrenocortical hypersecretion, adrenal cortical hyperplasia, adenoma, primary pigmented nodular adrenocortical disease,[6] or carcinoma (Cushing syndrome), and with excess pituitary ACTH (Cushing disease) or production of ACTH by a nonpituitary tumor (ectopic corticotropin syndrome, most caused by small cell carcinomas of lung), adrenal cortical adenomas, hyperplasias, and carcinomas (corticotropin-independent Cushing syndrome). When **cortisol excess** (Cushing syndrome - CS) is suspected, the primary tests include one or more of the following: a single sleeping midnight serum cortisol;[3] one of the dexamethasone suppression tests (DST - overnight or low-dose); and measurement of urine free cortisol (see Cortisol, Free, Urine *on page 154*). A midnight sleeping cortisol <1.8 µg/dL (SI: <50 nmol/L) is strong evidence against CS;[3] a higher value may indicate the need for additional testing.

In the **overnight DST**, a serum cortisol at 8 AM <3 µg/dL (SI: 82.8 nmol/L) is strong evidence against CS. Most patients with CS will have an 8 AM serum cortisol >10 µg/dL (SI: 276.0 nmol/L). Patients with results between these two limits may need additional testing.

In the **low-dose DST**, normal persons will have serum cortisol and urine free cortisol values on day 4 that are at least 50% below the baseline (day 1) results. (Some clinicians will also measure urinary 17-hydroxycorticosteroids.)

The **high-dose DST** is one of several procedures intended to differentiate between an adrenal cause of CS, and a cause located in the pituitary, hypothalamus, or an ectopic site. The high-dose test is therefore performed only after the diagnosis of CS has been biochemically confirmed. The high-dose protocol will produce significant suppression of cortisol output in a patient with Cushing disease (a pituitary ACTH-secreting adenoma), but not in a patient with adrenal tumor secreting cortisol or the ectopic corticotropin syndrome. If the patient has Cushing disease, the plasma cortisol will be <10 µg/dL (SI: <27.6 nmol/L) on day 5, and the urine free cortisol (and 17-hydroxycorticosteroids, if obtained) will decrease to at least 50% of baseline by day 4. If the patient has an adrenal tumor secreting cortisol, a lower degree of suppression, or no suppression, will be found.[4] See Adrenal Cortex: Laboratory Assessments Overview *on page 84* for additional information.

Causes of **low cortisol** include pituitary destruction or failure, with resultant loss of ACTH to stimulate the adrenal, and metabolic errors or destruction of the adrenal gland itself (adrenogenital syndromes, primary adrenocortical insufficiency, Addison disease, [idiopathic, tuberculosis, histoplasmosis, other diseases]). When **cortisol deficiency** is suspected, an 8 AM serum cortisol <5 µg/dL (SI: <140 nmol/L) [some authorities prefer <3 µg/dL (SI: <86 nmol/L)] confirms the diagnosis, and a result >20 µg/dL (SI: >550 nmol/L) excludes the diagnosis **in an unstressed patient.** (Stress in this context means a stimulus which approximates the intensity of severe sepsis or a major surgical procedure). Between these extremes, additional testing is required. The next step is often the Corticotropin Stimulation Test (Rapid) *on page 153*. See Adrenal Cortex: Laboratory Assessments Overview *on page 84* for additional information.

Pediatric adrenocortical insufficiency and hypofunction include a variety of congenital and acquired entities which include disorders of the hypothalamus, pituitary, or adrenal cortex. **Congenital adrenal hyperplasia** includes a group of autosomal recessive diseases. Their characteristics include postnatal virilization in boys and girls, prenatal virilization with genital ambiguity in neonatal girls, and adrenocortical insufficiency which may include salt wasting. Cortisol production is impaired, sometimes with impairment of aldosterone production, with ACTH stimulation of the adrenal cortices, and overproduction of androgens and cortisol precursors. Adrenal medullary production of epinephrine and metanephrine are diminished as well.[7] Ninety percent of patients with congenital adrenal hyperplasia have **deficiency of 21-hydroxylase**, for which neonatal screening programs have been developed.[8,9]

Limitations Random serum cortisol may be misleading because of circadian variation in secretion. Method may have a high cross reaction with corticosterone and with 11-deoxycortisol. Falsely abnormal results in both the overnight and low-dose DST tests are associated with a wide variety of concurrent conditions and medications (eg, obesity, depression, diphenylhydantoin, phenobarbital).

Not useful for following dosage of exogenous, synthetic corticosteroids. Cushing syndrome may have normal urinary free cortisol levels, normal cortisol production rates, or normal nocturnal cortisol levels. Cortisol is physiologically increased in patients with hypoglycemia, stress, and in pregnancy. Normal cortisol can be found with partial pituitary deficiency. Aging may suppress both cortisol secretion and the external manifestations of Cushing syndrome.

Contraindications Single samples taken under uncontrolled conditions have no diagnostic value.

Methodology Immunoassays (multiple labels), high performance liquid chromatography (HPLC); measurement by RIA after paper chromatography may more accurately estimate serum cortisol in patients with chronic renal failure.[10]

Additional Information Cortisol represents about 80% of the total 17-hydroxycorticosteroids in blood. Cortisol is the major adrenal glucocorticoid steroid hormone and is normally under feedback control by pituitary ACTH and the hypothalamus. Circadian variation in serum cortisol appears to influence the circadian pattern of serum osteocalcin and urinary calcium excretion, but not markers of bone resorption (N-telopeptide of type I collagen and free deoxypyridinoline).[11]

Footnotes

1. Orth DN and Kovacs WJ, "The Adrenal Cortex," *Williams Textbook of Endocrinology*, 9th ed, Philadelphia, PA: WB Saunders Co, 1998, 517-664.
2. Bornstein SR, Stratakis CA, and Chrousos GP, "Adrenocortical Tumors: Recent Advances in Basic Concepts and Clinical Management," *Ann Intern Med*, 1999, 130(9):759-71.
3. Newell-Price J, Trainer P, Perry L, et al, "A Single Sleeping Midnight Cortisol Has 100% Sensitivity for the Diagnosis of Cushing's Syndrome," *Clin Endocrinol (Oxf)*, 1995, 43(5):545-50.
4. Demers LM and Whitley RJ, "Function of the Adrenal Cortex," *Tietz Textbook of Clinical Chemistry*, 3rd ed, Burtis CA and Ashwood ER, eds, Philadelphia, PA: WB Saunders Co, 1999, 1530-69, 1808.
5. Soldin SJ, Murthy JN, Agarwalla PK, et al, "Pediatric Reference Ranges for Creatine Kinase, CK-MB, Troponin I, Iron and Cortisol," *Clin Biochem*, 1999, 32(1):77-80.
6. Stratakis CA, Sarlis N, Kirschner LS, et al, "Paradoxical Response to Dexamethasone in the Diagnosis of Primary Pigmented Nodular Adrenocortical Disease," *Ann Intern Med*, 1999, 131(8):585-91.
7. Merke DP, Chrousos GP, Eisenhofer G, et al, "Adrenomedullary Dysplasia and Hypofunction in Patients With Classic 21-Hydroxylase Deficiency," *N Engl J Med*, 2000, 343(19):1362-8.
8. Levine LS and DiGeorge AM, "Disorders of the Adrenal Glands," *Nelson Textbook of Pediatrics*, 16th ed, Behrman RE, Kliegman RM, and Jenson HB, eds, Philadelphia, PA: WB Saunders Co, 2000, 1722-43.
9. Merke DP and Cutler GB, "New Approaches to the Treatment of Congenital Adrenal Hyperplasia," *JAMA*, 1997, 277(13):1073-6.
10. Van Herle AJ, Birnbaum JA, Slomowitz LA, et al, "Paper Chromatography Prior to Cortisol RIA Allows for Accurate Use of the Dexamethasone Suppression Test in Chronic Renal Failure," *Nephron*, 1998, 80(1):79-84.
11. Heshmati HM, Riggs BL, Burrit MF, et al, "Effects of the Circadian Variation in Serum Cortisol on Markers of Bone Turnover and Calcium Homeostasis in Normal Postmenopausal Women," *J Clin Endocrinol Metab*, 1998, 83(3):751-6.

References

Aardal-Eriksson E, Karlberg BE, and Holm AC, "Salivary Cortisol - An Alternative to Serum Cortisol Determinations in Dynamic Function Tests," *Clin Chem Lab Med*, 1998, 36(4):215-22.
Al-Saadi N, Diederich S, and Oelkers W, "A Very High Dose Dexamethasone Suppression Test for Differential Diagnosis of Cushing's Syndrome," *Clin Endocrinol*, 1998, 48(1):45-51.
Avgerinos PC, Yanovski JA, Oldfield EH, et al, "The Metyrapone and Dexamethasone Suppression Tests for the Differential Diagnosis of the Adrenocorticotropin-Dependent Cushing Syndrome: A Comparison," *Ann Intern Med*, 1994, 121(5):318-27.
Bergadá I, Verara M, Maglio S, et al, "Functional Adrenal Cortical Tumors in Pediatric Patients: A Clinicopathologic and Immunohistochemical Study of a Long-Term Follow-up Series," *Cancer*, 1996, 77(4):771-7.
Dam H, "Dexamethasone Suppression Test," *Acta Psychiatr Scand Suppl*, 1988, 345:38-44.
Desai SP and Isa-Pratt S, *Clinician's Guide to Laboratory Medicine*, Cleveland, OH: Lexi-Comp, 2000, Chapters 17, 20.
Frothingham R, "Medical Mystery - The Answer Revealed," *N Engl J Med*, 1998, 338(4):266-7.
Georges R, Knappe G, Geri H, et al, "Diagnosis of Cushing's Syndrome: Re-evaluation of Midnight Plasma Cortisol vs Urinary Free Cortisol and Low-Dose Dexamethasone Suppression Test in a Large Patient Group," *J Endocrinol Invest*, 1999, 22(4):241-9.

(Continued)

Cortisol, Serum or Plasma *(Continued)*

Katayama M, Nomura K, Ujihara M, et al, "Age Dependent Decline in Cortisol Levels and Clinical Manifestations in Patients With ACTH-Independent Cushing's Syndrome," *Clin Endocrinol (Oxf)*, 1998, 49(3):311-6.

Kidess AI, Caplan RH, Reynertson RH, et al, "Transient Corticotropin Deficiency in Critical Illness," *Mayo Clin Proc*, 1993, 68(5):435-41.

Lupien SJ, Nair NP, Briere S, et al, "Increased Cortisol Levels and Impaired Cognition in Human Aging: Implication for Depression and Dementia in Later Life," *Rev Neurosci*, 1999, 10(2):117-39.

Magiakou MA, Mastorakos G, Oldfield EH, et al, "Cushing's Syndrome in Children and Adolescents - Presentation, Diagnosis, and Therapy," *N Engl J Med*, 1994, 331(10):629-36.

Nierenberg AA and Feinstein AR, "How to Evaluate a Diagnostic Marker Test. Lessons From the Rise and Fall of Dexamethasone Suppression Test," *JAMA*, 1988, 259(11):1699-702.

Orth DN, "The Cushing Syndrome: Quest for the Holy Grail," *Ann Intern Med*, 1994, 121(5):377-8.

Papanicolaou DA, Yanovski JA, Cutler GB Jr, et al, "A Single Midnight Serum Cortisol Measurement Distinguishes Cushing's Syndrome From Pseudo-Cushing States," *J Clin Endocrinol Metab*, 1998, 83(4):1163-7.

Riordan FA, Thomson AP, Ratcliffe JM, et al, "Admission Cortisol and Adrenocorticotropic Hormone Levels in Children With Meningococcal Disease: Evidence of Adrenal Insufficiency?" *Crit Care Med*, 1999, 27(10):2257-61.

Samuels MH, Brandon DD, Isabelle LM, et al, "Cortisol Production Rates in Subjects With Suspected Cushing's Syndrome: Assessment by Stable Isotope Dilution Methodology and Comparison to Other Diagnostic Methods," *J Clin Endocrinol Metab*, 2000, 85(1):22-8.

Snow K, Jiang NS, and Kao PC, "Biochemical Evaluation of Adrenal Dysfunction: The Laboratory Perspective," *Mayo Clin Proc*, 1992, 67(11):1055-65.

Tantivit P, Subramanian N, Garg M, et al, "Low Serum Cortisol in Term Newborns With Refractory Hypotension," *J Perinatol*, 1999, 19(5):352-7.

"The Dexamethasone Suppression Test: An Overview of its Current Status in Psychiatry," The APA Task Force on Laboratory Tests in Psychiatry, *Am J Psychiatry*, 1987, 144(10):1253-62.

Vance ML, "Hypopituitarism," *N Engl J Med*, 1994, 330(23):1651-62.

Weiner MF, "Age and Cortisol Suppression by Dexamethasone in Normal Subjects," *J Psychiatr Res*, 1989, 23(2):1633-8.

♦ **Cortrosyn® Test** *see* Corticotropin Stimulation Test (Rapid) *on page 153*

♦ **Cosyntropin Stimulation Test** *see* Corticotropin Stimulation Test (Rapid) *on page 153*

♦ **C-Peptide** *see* Insulin, Serum *on page 201*

C-Peptide, Serum

Related Information
Glucose, Fasting, Plasma *on page 183*
Glucose Tolerance Test, Plasma *on page 186*
Insulin Antibody, Serum *on page 200*
Insulin, Serum *on page 201*
Ketone Bodies, Blood *on page 205*

Synonyms Connecting Peptide Insulin; Insulin-Connecting Peptide

Applies to Beta-Cell Peptides; Beta-Hydroxybutyrate; C-Peptide Suppression Test; Insulin; Insulin Antibodies; Proinsulin

Test Includes Simultaneously obtained specimens for glucose, insulin, proinsulin, beta-hydroxybutyrate, and insulin antibodies. C-peptide is rarely obtained as an isolated test. Glucose assay is usually needed at the time a C-peptide specimen is drawn. Refer to the particular testing protocol being used (eg, footnote 1).

Abstract Proinsulin, a polypeptide synthesized in the beta cells of the pancreatic islets of Langerhans, is cleaved into two peptides: C-peptide and insulin in equimolar concentrations. Proinsulin and C-peptide are traditionally believed to be biologically inactive (but see Forst et al 1998, two references, and De La Tour et al 1998). C-peptide is excreted in the urine, disappearing from the plasma with a half-life of about 35 minutes. Insulin has a much shorter half-life, usually 5-10 minutes. These three peptides (proinsulin, insulin, and C-peptide) are often collectively referred to as beta-cell peptides.

Patient Preparation Patients are usually fasting, but refer to the particular testing protocol being used. No recent radioactivity. Drug effects are summarized.[2]

Specimen Serum

Container Red top tube

Collection Date and time must be absolutely correct. Draw in chilled tube. Keep specimen on ice.

Storage Instructions Spin in centrifuge at 4°C. Take off serum. Freeze immediately in a plastic tube.

Reference Interval Varies among laboratories. A typical range for fasting C-peptide in serum is 0.51-2.70 ng/mL (SI: 170-900 pmol/L). After stimulation with glucose or glucagon, values rise to 5.6 ng/mL (SI: 1870 pmol/L).

Use C-peptide measurements are used in five clinical contexts:
- differential diagnosis of hypoglycemia
- classification of diabetes mellitus
- assessment of beta-cell function in diabetes
- forecasting the survival of pancreas transplants
- evaluating the completeness of surgical pancreatectomy

Hypoglycemia: C-peptide is one of a group of analytes used in standardized testing protocols for the differential diagnosis of hypoglycemia. Before embarking on such a protocol, the criteria for Whipple's triad[3] must be satisfied. The triad includes low blood glucose, simultaneous hypoglycemic signs and symptoms, and relief of the signs and symptoms by correcting the low blood glucose. Stated another way, if, during a symptomatic episode, a normal blood glucose value is obtained, a hypoglycemic disorder is thereby excluded and further testing is not indicated.

Patients with insulin-secreting neoplasms have high levels of all three beta-cell peptides (insulin, C-peptide, proinsulin). In contrast, patients with factitious hypoglycemia from surreptitious insulin administration will have low levels of C-peptide and proinsulin in the presence of elevated (exogenous) serum insulin. Ingestion of an insulin secretagogue, such as a sulfonylurea drug, closely mimics insulinoma, because these drugs stimulate the secretion of proinsulin, insulin, and C-peptide. In patients who are evaluated by a standardized, supervised 72-hour fast[1], those with insulinoma or sulfonylurea effect have insulin levels >6.0 µU/mL (SI: >35.7 pmol/L), C-peptide levels >0.61 ng/mL (SI: >0.2 nmol/L), and proinsulin levels >5.0 pmol/L with symptoms of hypoglycemia and blood glucose <45 mg/dL (25 mmol/L). Laboratory differentiation between these two diagnoses requires detection of the sulfonylurea (or other drug) in plasma. Patients with surreptitious insulin administration will have, after the 72-hour supervised fasting protocol, insulin >6.0 µU/mL (often as high as 100 µU/mL or 1000 µU/mL (SI: 694.5 and 6945.0 pmol/L, respectively)), C-peptide <0.61 ng/mL (SI: <0.2 nmol/L), and proinsulin <5.0 pmol/L. **Patients who have noninsulin-mediated hypoglycemia** (eg, secondary to nonislet cell neoplasm) will have, after the supervised 72-hour fast, normal islet cell peptide levels (insulin <6.0 µIU/mL (<35.7 pmol/L), C-peptide <0.61 ng/mL, and proinsulin <5.0 pmol/L). For additional details, see Rizza and Service 2000 and Le Roith.[1,4]

Classification of diabetes mellitus: The classification of diabetes mellitus is usually accomplished by history, physical findings, and blood glucose values. An occasional patient will require additional testing, including serum C-peptide and, even less often, serum insulin. Patients with type 2 diabetes mellitus usually have normal or elevated levels of C-peptide and insulin, and do not have beta-cell autoantibodies. In patients with type 1 diabetes mellitus, serum C-peptide (and serum insulin) are low or, in the late stages, undetectable; 85% to 90% of patients with type 1 diabetes have detectable beta-cell autoantibodies when hyperglycemia is first detected.[5,6]

Beta-cell function in diabetes: C-peptide may also be useful in evaluation of residual beta-cell function in insulin-dependent diabetics, some of whom have antibodies that interfere with insulin assays. Glucagon-stimulated C-peptide concentration has been described as a discriminator between insulin-requiring and noninsulin-requiring diabetic patients.[7,8,9]

Pancreas transplants: A relatively new use for C-peptide levels is in the evaluation of viability and survival of pancreas transplants.[10]

Pancreatectomy: C-peptide should be undetectable following a total pancreatectomy.[11]

Limitations C-peptide levels are increased in renal failure. (C-peptide is normally excreted by the kidneys.) Instances of insulinoma have been described in which proinsulin was increased but insulin and C-peptide were not.

Methodology Immunoassays (multiple labels)

Additional Information C-peptide can be measured in urine, but the test has few, if any, clinical applications.

The C-peptide suppression test depends on suppression of beta cell secretion during hypoglycemia to a lesser degree in patients with insulinoma than in normal individuals.[1]

Footnotes

1. Rizza RA and Service JF, "Hypoglycemic/Pancreatic Islet Cell Disorders," Goldman L and Bennett JC, eds, *Cecil Textbook of Medicine*, Philadelphia, PA: WB Saunders Co, 2000, 1285-92.

2. Young DS, *Effects of Drugs on Clinical Laboratory Tests*, 5th ed, Volume 1: Listing by Test, Washington, DC: AACC Press, American Association of Clinical Chemistry, 2000, Section 3, 232-3.

3. Whipple AO, "The Surgical Therapy of Hyperinsulinism," *J Int Chir*, 1938, 3:237-76.

4. Le Roith D, "Tumor-Induced Hypoglycemia," *N Engl J Med*, 1999, 341(10):757-8.

5. The Expert Committee on the Diagnosis and Classification of Diabetes Mellitus, "Report of the Expert Committee on the Diagnosis and Classification of Diabetes Mellitus," *Diabetes Care*, 1999, 22(Suppl):S5-S19.

6. American Diabetes Association, "Consensus Statement: Type 2 Diabetes in Children and Adolescents," *Diabetes Care*, 2000, 23:381-9.

7. Koskinen PJ, Viikari JS, and Irjala KM, "Glucagon-Stimulated and Postprandial Plasma C-Peptide Values as Measures of Insulin Secretory Capacity," *Diabetes Care*, 1988, 11(4):318-22.

8. Laakso M, Sarlund H, Korhonen T, et al, "Stopping Insulin Treatment in Middle-Aged Diabetic Patients With High Postglucagon Plasma C-Peptide. Effect on Glycaemic Control, Serum Lipids and Lipoproteins," *Acta Med Scand*, 1988, 223(1):61-8.

9. Service FJ, Rizza RA, Zimmerman BR, et al, "The Classification of Diabetes by Clinical and C-Peptide Criteria. A Prospective Population-Based Study," *Diabetes Care*, 1997, 20(2):198-201.

10. Sasaki TM, Gray RS, Ratner RE, et al, "Successful Long-Term Kidney-Pancreas Transplants in Diabetic Patients With High C-Peptide Levels," *Transplantation*, 1998, 65(11):1510-12.

11. Sacks DB, "Carbohydrates," *Tietz Textbook of Clinical Chemistry*, 3rd ed, Burtis CA and Ashwood ER, eds, Philadelphia, PA: WB Saunders Co, 1999, 762.

References

Argoud GW, Schade DS, Eaton RP, et al, "C-Peptide Suppression Test and Recurrent Insulinoma," *Am J Med*, 1989, 86(3):335-7.

Bonora E, Rizzi C, Lesi C, et al, "Insulin and C-Peptide Plasma Levels in Patients With Severe Chronic Pancreatitis and Fasting Normoglycemia," *Dig Dis Sci*, 1988, 33(6):732-6.

De La Tour DD, Raccah D, Jannot MF, et al, "Erythrocyte Na/K ATPase Activity and Diabetes: Relationship With C-Peptide Level," *Diabetologia*, 1998, 41:1080-4.

Forst T, Kunt T, Beyer J, et al, "New Aspects on Biological Activity of C-Peptide in IDDM Patients," *Exp Clin Endocrinol Diabetes*, 1998, 106(4):270-6 (review).

Forst T, Kunt T, Pohlmann T, et al, "Biological Activity of C-Peptide on the Skin Microcirculation in Patients With Insulin-Dependent Diabetes Mellitus," *J Clin Invest*, 1998, 101(10):2036-41.

Karjalainen J, Salmela P, Ilonen J, et al, "A Comparison of Childhood and Adult Type I Diabetes Mellitus," *N Engl J Med*, 1989, 320(14):881-6.

Service FJ, "Hypoglycemic Disorders," *N Engl J Med*, 1995, 332(17):1144-52.

Van Cauter E, Mestrez F, Sturis J, et al, "Estimation of Insulin Secretion Rates From C-Peptide Levels. Comparison of Individual and Standard Kinetic Parameters for C-Peptide Clearance," *Diabetes*, 1992, 41(3):368-77.

◆ **C-Peptide Suppression Test** *see* C-Peptide, Serum *on page 156*

◆ **CPK** *see* Creatine Kinase, Serum *on page 158*

◆ **CPK Isoenzymes** *see* Creatine Kinase Isoenzymes/Isoforms, Serum *on page 157*

Creatine Kinase Isoenzymes/Isoforms, Serum

Related Information

Cardiac Markers: Laboratory Assessment, Overview *on page 137*
Creatine Kinase, Serum *on page 158*
Heterophilic Antibodies *on page 191*
Myoglobin, Blood, Serum, or Plasma *on page 228*
Troponins, Serum *on page 291*

Synonyms CK-2; CK Isoenzymes; CK Isoforms; CK-MB and Total CK; CPK Isoenzymes; Creatine Phosphokinase-MB Isoenzyme and Total Creatine Phosphokinase, Serum

Applies to Cardiac Index; CK Index; Isoform Ratio

Test Includes Separation of enzyme CK into its isoenzymes

Abstract Three isoenzymes may be seen on electrophoresis: CK-MM (CK-3), CK-MB (CK-2), and CK-BB (CK-1). CK-MB is the isoenzyme of most interest because it is present in large quantities in myocardium. Diagnostic elevations of CK-MB isoenzyme typically are seen earlier than 6 hours after the onset of chest pain In Individuals with acute myocardial infarct. Assays for the subforms can support diagnosis earlier. CK-MB, myoglobin, and cardiac specific troponin I (cTnI) appear to be the most valuable current markers of myocardial injury. cTnI continues to hold promise as the ultimate marker of choice because of its cardiospecificity and prolonged activity.[1] CK-MB usually peaks between 15-20 hours after the onset of a myocardial infarct.

Specimen Serum, plasma; ethylenediamine tetraacetic acid (EDTA) for isoforms

Container Red top tube, green top (lithium heparin) tube

Sampling Time CK-MB is most commonly elevated in acute myocardial infarct (AMI), in which it has its greatest usefulness. Collection of specimen at onset of symptoms to establish baseline values is needed. A patient at onset of AMI may have normal results. Some patients reach medical attention at or beyond CK peak, while many seek medical assistance after several hours when serum CK-MB values are still rising. Current recommendations suggest using CK-MB and concurrent cTnI followed by use of the cardiac index (CK index) when CK-MB exceeds the reference range.[1] (The cardiac index is an expression of CK-MB mass as a ratio to total CK. The index is useful when extremely high or low.[1]) Some have suggested sampling times at 0, 3, 6, and 12 hours to detect the rise of CK-MB,[2] others 0, 3, 6, and 9 hours. The same sampling times should be used to assess effective myocardial reperfusion after thrombolytic therapy. In this case, the CK and CK-MB rise very early and very high compared to patients not reperfused.[3] CK-MB may be diagnostic on presentation to the emergency department in 46% of patients and diagnostic in 93% of such patients after 3 hours with specificity of 98%, using the following criteria: elevation in CK-MB and relative index on either the initial or 3-hour sample or an increase in CK-MB by at least a factor of 2, still within normal limits.[4]

When increased CK-MB values have returned to normal, CK isoenzyme determinations are usually no longer required.

Collection Avoid hemolysis.

Storage Instructions Separate serum from red cells and refrigerate.

Turnaround Time Less than 1 hour using CK-MB mass assay

Reference Interval Method dependent. CK-MB normally is <6% of total CK. The most common cause of elevation of MB is AMI. The best reference range is established with an individual patient's own baseline, followed by serial sampling.[1,4] Mass assay of CK-MB gives a reference range of 0-3 µg/mL with a relative index of 0-2.5. **Relative index** or **CK index** is the CK-MB value (in mass units) divided by the total CK (in enzyme units) times 100. The CK index was intended to provide correction for injury to striated muscle, but it can be misleading in situations such as cardiac surgery, in which cardiac and striated muscle damage both exist.[5] An **isoform ratio** (CK-MB2:CK-MB1) >1.5 is indicative of AMI. The reference ratio is near 1.0.

Critical Values CK-MB/total CK index >5%; increasing and decreasing values relevant to time of draws are more relevant than strict adherence to cutoff limits.

Use Diagnosis of AMI. Three fractions may be found, each an isoenzyme.
- MM is present in normal serum. It may originate from both cardiac tissue and skeletal muscle.
- MB is the myocardial fraction associated with AMI. It occurs in certain other states. MB can be used in estimation of infarct size. Despite its specificity for myocardial tissue, MB comprises only 15% to 30% of total CK activity of myocardium.[6]
- BB: *vide infra*

A study using the chemiluminescence mass concentration assay for CK-MB showed that a CK-MB ≥10 ng/mL and CK relative index >3.0 (ng/mL CK-MB per unit CK x 100) gave these results: sensitivity = 1.00; specificity = 0.97; positive predictive value = 1.00; diagnostic efficiency = 0.97.[7] Others have also found that serial CK-MB mass assays resulted in a sensitivity of 1.00 and a specificity of 0.983 with negative predictive value of 1.00 but with positive predictive value of 0.414.[8] Changes of CK-MB isoforms may precede significant elevations of CK-MB by up to 4 hours, potentially providing for earlier diagnosis of AMI.[6] The tissue isoform (CK-MB2) is low in normal serum but increases rapidly after AMI. The CK-MB2:CK-MB1 (isoform) ratio is used as the most sensitive indicator; an increase becoming detectable within 1.5 hours from the onset of chest pain.[6]

Limitations False positives occur (eg, increased CK-MB has been described in marathon runners without MI).[9]

MB increases have been reported with other entities which cause damage to the myocardium, such as myocarditis, some instances of cardiomyopathy, and with extensive rhabdomyolysis, Duchenne muscular dystrophy, malignant hyperthermia, polymyositis, dermatomyositis, mixed connective tissue disease, myoglobinemia, Rocky Mountain spotted fever, Reye's syndrome, and rarely in rheumatoid arthritis with high titer RF.[10] CK-MB does not generally abruptly rise and fall in such nonacute MI settings, as it does in acute myocardial infarct (AMI). Increased CK-MB may occur with hypothyroidism[11] and increases in total CK are even more common, in about 50% of cases.

BB is rarely present. BB has been described as a marker for adenocarcinoma of prostate, breast, ovary, colon, adenocarcinomas of gastrointestinal tract, and for small cell anaplastic carcinoma of lung. BB has been reported with severe shock and/or hypothermia, infarction of bowel,[12] brain injury, stroke, as a genetic marker in some families with malignant pyrexia, and with MB in alcoholic myopathy.

Total CK can be normal early in acute MI, when CK-MB is increased.[13] It is for this reason that the currently accepted standard is to obtain CK-MB first and then obtain a cardiac index if CK-MB is above reference range. Conversely, cases have been reported in which elderly patients have elevated CK-MB without other evidence of myocardial injury.[14] A single CK isoenzyme determination may be misleading, as may any other enzyme or isoenzyme for diagnosis of AMI. **The diagnosis of myocardial injury should be supported by clinical findings, ECG, and often other laboratory parameters.** For non-Q-wave myocardial infarcts, measurement of cTnI for confirmation of elevated CK-MB or index is recommended.[1]

Heterophilic antibodies (eg, human antimurine antibodies) may cause spuriously increased levels of CK-MB when the assay is run by two-site murine antibody-based immunoassay.[15]

Creatine kinase isoforms are elevated slightly earlier than CK-MB following myocardial infarct, but have the same myocardial specificity drawbacks as does CK-MB.[16] Cryoablation of the prostate gland may lead to significant elevations of both total CK and CK-MB.[17] CK is decreased in pregnancy, but may elevate to two fold above the reference range around the time of parturition.[18]

A report of The Ontario Laboratory Proficiency Testing Program has detailed significant variations of results both between different analyzer systems and among identical analyzers.[19] This problem has been explained as being due to lack of suitable reference materials. Use of recently reported recombinant human CK-MB may allow for tighter quality control.[20]

Methodology Measurement of CK-MB by electrophoresis and immunoinhibition methods are relatively insensitive methods that have been supplanted by CK-MB mass concentration assay methods. There is no place for measurement of CK-MB by electrophoretic nor immunoinhibition methods in the 21st century laboratory. Measurement of CK-MB mass concentration by monoclonal anti-CK-MB antibodies is a very sensitive method utilizing microparticulate fluorescence, enhanced luminescence, fluorescence, or chemiluminescence. A very rapid test is that of Hybritech®, which uses the immunocentration format (ICON®). Isoelectric focusing may be used to measure isoforms.

Additional Information CK-MB is found in much higher concentrations in cardiac muscle than in ordinary skeletal muscle although myocardium contains considerable CK-MM isoenzyme, necessitating the use of the relative index when CK-MB mass assay rises above the reference range. **CK-MB is usually not elevated** in exercise (total CK elevated); injections into muscle (total CK elevated); strokes, CVA, and other brain disorders in which total CK may be increased; pericarditis; pneumonias or other lung diseases; pulmonary embolus; seizures (CK may be very high but no great MB increase, if any). Although CK-MB is not usually increased in angina, (Continued)

Creatine Kinase Isoenzymes/Isoforms, Serum
(Continued)

some CK-MB elevations are described in angina patients, depending partly on laboratory methodology and on definitions.

Atypical forms of CK occur. **Macro-CK** migrates between MM and MB and is composed of immunoglobulin complexes of normal isoenzymes. This is found mainly in elderly women and is of no clinical significance. **Mitochondrial-CK** migrates cathodal to MM and is found in seriously ill patients, especially those with metastatic carcinoma. Its presence is a poor prognostic sign.

CK-MM and CK-MB **isoforms** (subforms) are post-translational modifications of the M and B subunits of creatine kinase. There are several isoforms of MM (MM$_1$, MM$_2$, and MM$_3$) and at least three subforms of MB. Only two of these subforms are detectable in human plasma: MB1 and MB2. Increased serum MM$_3$ is a nonspecific marker of muscle damage. An increased CK-MB2:CK-MB1 ratio may be seen in AMI as early as 1-1^1/$_2$ hours after the onset of chest pain.[6] Thus, CK-MB isoforms may have value for early detection of AMI and for assessing myocardial reperfusion following AMI. Several reports have attested to increased sensitivity and specificity of CK-MB isoforms.[21,22,23] A rapid method for measuring CK-MB2 by immuno-chemical extraction followed by automated measurement may replace the previously complex and cumbersome methods.[24] Presently, isoforms of CK have not enjoyed wide acceptance: they are expensive and are reported to lack needed levels of specificity.

The concept of myocardial infarct is still evolving. The current pathophysiological changes of the ischemic myocardium recognizes a continuum from unstable angina through non-Q wave to Q-wave AMI with or without chest pain.[25] Keffer states that microinfarction has confounded many older studies of the biochemical markers based on clinical criteria for distinguishing unstable angina from AMI. The real question is whether there is evidence of active plaque rupture and coronary thrombosis with attendant risk.[1] The sensitivity of troponins for detection of myocardial damage is such that a substantial proportion of patients with unstable angina develop elevations of troponins in the absence of creatine kinase MB increase. Such patients have an increased risk of cardiac events over the short-term and long-term similar to that of patients with definite myocardial infarct.[26] One cost-effective measure proposes to use troponin I as a second-line assay in a subset of higher-risk patients in whom the CK-MB is normal and early exercise testing is not an option.[27]

Use of CK-MB and isoforms may diminish with wider application of myoglobin and troponin I for diagnosis of AMI.

Footnotes

1. Keffer JH, "The Cardiac Profile and Proposed Practice Guidelines for Acute Ischemic Heart Disease," *Am J Clin Pathol*, 1997, 107(4):398-409.
2. Marin MM and Teichman SL, "Use of Rapid Serial Sampling of Creatine Kinase MB for Very Early Detection of Myocardial Infarction in Patients With Acute Chest Pain," *Am Heart J*, 1992, 123(2):354-61.
3. Lott JA and Stang JM, "Differential Diagnosis of Patients With Abnormal Serum Creatine Kinase Isoenzymes," *Clin Lab Med*, 1989, 9(4):627-42.
4. Kontos MC, Anderson FP, Schmidt KA, et al, "Early Diagnosis of Acute Myocardial Infarction in Patients Without ST-Segment Elevation," *Am J Cardiol*, 1999, 83(2):155-8.
5. Schreiber WE, "Laboratory Assessment of Myocardial Damage: Which Test Is Best?" *Am J Clin Pathol*, 1997, 107(4):383-4.
6. Robinson DJ and Christenson RH, "Creatine Kinase and Its CK-MB Isoenzyme: The Conventional Marker for the Diagnosis of Acute Myocardial Infarction," *J Emerg Med*, 1999, 17(1):95-104.
7. Pearson JR and Carrea F, "Evaluation of the Clinical Usefulness of a Chemiluminometric Method for Measuring Creatine Kinase MB," *Clin Chem*, 1990, 36(10):1809-11.
8. Gibler WB, Runyon JP, Levy RC, et al, "A Rapid Diagnostic and Treatment Center for Patients With Chest Pain in the Emergency Department," *Ann Emerg Med*, 1992, 21:504-12.
9. Seigel AJ, Silverman LM, and Evans WJ, "Elevated Skeletal Muscle Creatinine Kinase MB Isoenzyme Levels in Marathon Runners," *JAMA*, 1983, 250(20):2835-7.
10. Wolf PL, "Common Causes of False-Positive CK-MB Test for Acute Myocardial Infarction," *Clin Lab Med*, 1986, 6(3):577-81.
11. Keffer JH, "Assessment of Myocardial Injury," *The Handbook of Clinical Pathology*, 2nd ed, Chapter 17, McKenna RW and Keffer JH, eds, Chicago: ASCP Press, American Society of Clinical Pathologists, 2000, 235-44.
12. Fried MW, Murthy UK, Hassig SR, et al, "Creatine Kinase Isoenzymes in the Diagnosis of Intestinal Infarction," *Dig Dis Sci*, 1991, 36(11):1589-93.
13. Lloyd-Jones DM, Camargo CA Jr, and Giugliano RP, et al, "Characteristics and Prognosis of Patients With Suspected Acute Myocardial Infarction and Elevated MB Relative Index but Normal Total Creatine Kinase," *Am J Cardiol*, 1999, 84(9):957-62.
14. Alterman P, Vigder C, Feldman J, et al, "Creatine Kinase MB Isoenzyme of Noncardiac Origin in Elderly Patients," *Coron Artery Dis*, 1999, 10(7):533-6.
15. Sosolik RC, Hitchcock CL, and Becker WJ, "Heterophilic Antibodies Produce Spuriously Elevated Concentrations of the MB Isoenzyme of Creatine Kinase in a Selected Patient Population," *Am J Clin Pathol*, 1997, 107(5):506-10.
16. Christenson RH, Newby LK, and Ohman EM, "Cardiac Markers in the Assessment of Acute Coronary Syndromes," *Md Med J*, 1997, Suppl:18-24.
17. Long JP, Fallick ML, and Rand W, "Increased Serum Total Creatine Kinase and Creatine Kinase Isoenzyme MB After Cryosurgical Ablation of the Prostate," *J Urol*, 1997, 157(5):1723-6.
18. Shivvers SA, Wians FH Jr, Keffer JH, et al, "Maternal Cardiac Troponin I Levels During Normal Labor and Delivery," *Am J Obstet Gynecol*, 1999, 180(1 Pt 1):122.
19. Henderson AR, Krishnan S, Webb S, et al, "Proficiency Testing of Creatine Kinase and Creatine Kinase-2: The Experience of the Ontario Laboratory Proficiency Testing Program," *Clin Chem*, 1998, 44(1):124-33.
20. Christenson RH, Vaidya H, Landt Y, et al, "Standardization of Creatine Kinase-MB (CK-MB) Mass Assays: The Use of Recombinant CK-MB as a Reference Material," *Clin Chem*, 1999, 45(9):1414-23.
21. Bock, JL, Brogan GX Jr, McCuskey, et al, "Evaluation of CK-MB Isoform Analysis for the Early Diagnosis of Myocardial Infarction," *J Emerg Med*, 1999, 17(1):75-79.
22. Zimmerman, J, Fromm R, Meyer D, et al, "Diagnostic Marker Cooperative Study for the Diagnosis of Myocardial Infarction," *Circulation*, 1999, 99(13):1671-77.
23. Puleo PR, Meyer D, Wathen C, et al, "Use of a Rapid Assay of Subforms of Creatine Kinase MB to Diagnose or Rule Out Acute Myocardial Infarction," *N Engl J Med*, 1994, 331(9):561-6.
24. McBride JH and Schotters SB, "Immunochemical Extraction and Automated Measurement of Plasma Creatine Kinase MB Isoenzyme and Creatine Kinase MB2 Isoform," *J Clin Lab Anal*, 1997, 11(3):163-8.
25. Fuster V, "Elucidation of the Role of Plaque Instability and Rupture in Acute Coronary Events," *Am J Cardiol*, 1995, 76:24c-33c.
26. Galvani M, Ferrini D, Puggioni R, et al, "New Markers for Early Diagnosis of Acute Myocardial Infarction," *Int J Cardiol*, 1998, 65(Suppl 1):S17-22.
27. Polaczyk CA, Kuntz KM, Sacks DB, et al, "Emergency Department Triage Strategies for Acute Chest Pain Using Creatine Kinase-MB and Troponin I Assays: A Cost-Effectiveness Analysis," *Ann Intern Med*, 1999, 131(12):909-18.

References

Adams J, Schechtman K, Landt J, et al, "Comparable Detection of Acute Myocardial Infarction by Creatine Kinase MB Isoenzyme and Cardiac Troponin I," *Clin Chem*, 1994, 40(7 Pt 1):1291-5.

Alexander JH, Sparapani RA, Mahaffey KW, et al, "Association Between Minor Elevations of Creatine Kinase-MB Level and Mortality in Patients With Acute Coronary Syndromes Without ST-Segment Elevation," *JAMA*, 2000, 283(3):347-53.

Bakker AJ, Gorgels JP, Van Vlies B, et al, "Contribution of Creatine Kinase MB Mass Concentration at Admission to Early Diagnosis of Acute Myocardial Infarction," *Br Heart J*, 1994, 72(2):112-8.

Bhayana V, Cohoe S, Leung FY, et al, "Diagnostic Evaluation of Creatine Kinase-2 Mass and Creatine Kinase-3 and -2 Isoform Ratios in Early Diagnosis of Acute Myocardial Infarction," *Clin Chem*, 1993, 39(3):488-95.

Fox, AC and Levin RI, "Ruptured Plaques and Leaking Cells: Cost Effectiveness in the Diagnosis of Acute Coronary Syndromes," *Ann Intern Med*, 1999, 131(12):968-970. (Editorial)

Gensini GF, Fusi C, Conti AA, et al, "Cardiac Troponin I and Q-Wave Perioperative Myocardial Infarction After Coronary Artery Bypass Surgery," *Crit Care Med*, 1998, 26(12):1986-90.

Hamm CW, "New Serum Markers for Acute Myocardial Infarction," *N Engl J Med*, 1994, 331(9):607-8.

Hood D, Van Lente F, and Estes M, "Serum Enzyme Alterations in Chronic Muscle Disease. A Biopsy-Based Diagnostic Assessment," *Am J Clin Pathol*, 1991, 95(3):402-7.

Hossein-Nia M, Kallis P, Brown PA, et al, "Creatine Kinase MB Isoforms: Sensitive Markers of Ischemic Myocardial Damage," *Clin Chem*, 1994, 40(7 Pt 1):1265-71.

Isouard G, "A Quality Management Intervention to Improve Clinical Laboratory Use in Acute Myocardial Infarction," *Med J Aust*, 1999, 170(1):11-4.

Kilpatrick WS, Wasornu D, McGuinness JB, et al, "Early Diagnosis of Acute Myocardial Infarction: CK-MB and Myoglobin Compared," *Ann Clin Biochem*, 1993, 30(Pt 5):435-8.

Lee TH and Goldman L, "Evaluation of the Patient With Acute Chest Pain," *N Engl J Med*, 2000, 342(16):1187-95.

Savonitto S, Ardissino D, Granger CB, et al, "Prognostic Value of the Admission Electrocardiogram in Acute Coronary Syndromes," *JAMA*, 1999, 281(8):707-13.

Smith RM and Neuman TS, "Elevation of Serum Creatine Kinase in Divers With Arterial Gas Embolization," *N Engl J Med*, 1994, 330(1):19-24.

Thygesen K and Alpert JS, "Myocardial Infarction Redefined - A Concensus Document of The Joint European Society of Cardiology/American College of Cardiology Committee for the Redefinition of Myocardial Infarction," The Joint European Society of Cardiology/American College of Cardiology Committee, *J Am Coll Cardiol*, 2000, 36(3):959-69.

Voss EM, Sharkey SW, Gernert AE, et al, "Human and Canine Cardiac Troponin T and Creatine Kinase-MB Distribution in Normal and Diseased Myocardium, Infarct Sizing Using Serum Profiles," *Arch Pathol Lab Med*, 1995, 119(9):799-806.

Zalenski RJ, McCarren M, Roberts R, et al, "An Evaluation of a Chest Pain Diagnostic Protocol to Exclude Acute Cardiac Ischemia in the Emergency Department," *Arch Intern Med*, 1997, 157(10):1085-91.

Creatine Kinase, Serum

Related Information

Synonyms CK; CPK; Creatine Phosphokinase, Total, Serum

Abstract Creatine kinase catalyzes the transfer of inorganic phosphate from creatine phosphate to adenosine diphosphate (ADP), producing adenosine triphosphate (ATP) and creatine. It occurs principally in striated muscle, brain, and heart. Other tissues (eg, kidney) contain much lower levels of activity. Creatine kinase is a sensitive though nonspecific marker for myocardial as well as skeletal muscle injury.

Patient Preparation Avoid exercise before venipuncture. Increased concentrations may be anticipated in the immediate postoperative period following surgical procedures involving incision through muscle.

Specimen Serum, plasma

Container Red top tube, green top (lithium heparin) tube

Storage Instructions Separate serum from red cells. Store in refrigerator. Avoid hemolysis.[1]

Reference Interval Method dependent, but for assays at 37°C (most current assays) usually 50-200 units/L for males. Females have levels 20% to 25% less than males. Infants to 1 year of age may have levels two times adult. On average, African Americans have higher levels. Overnight bedrest may lower CK 10% to 20%.

Use Test for acute myocardial infarct (AMI) and for skeletal muscular disease or damage. Although CK is elevated in some individuals who have malignant hyperthermia syndrome, interval screening is most effective to detect susceptible subjects. Elevated in muscular dystrophy: CK is a marker for Duchenne muscular dystrophy, with elevations of 20-200 times normal.[2] CK is increased in female carriers of this X-linked disease, and in muscular stress, in polymyositis, dermatomyositis, and with muscle trauma. Elevated in myocarditis. Extremely high values are seen in some instances of myositis and in the postictal state of a recent grand mal seizure. CK may be elevated in a number of entities, including the eosinophilia-myalgia syndrome.[3] Marked increases occur with rhabdomyolysis including that with cocaine intoxication.[4] CK is sometimes increased with cerebrovascular accident. Malignancy (advanced) may show increased CK.[5] Cardioversion with multiple shocks may release CK-MB and may result in a false-positive diagnosis of myocardial infarction.[6] Low CK may reflect decreased muscle mass. It has been reported in a number of entities, including metastatic neoplasia, steroid therapy, alcoholic liver disease,[7] connective tissue diseases,[8] ectopic pregnancy (without CK-MB increase), and rheumatoid arthritis.[9]

Limitations CK is a relatively sensitive marker for myocardial infarct, but it lacks myocardial specificity. **Normal at earliest onset of AMI** unless the subject has been exercising or doing physical work; CK is elevated following exercise. Intramuscular injections increase serum CK activity. Elevation of CK following AMI may not be observed until 6 or more hours after onset. CK returns to normal in approximately 48-72 hours after onset of AMI. Total CK can be normal early in AMI when CK-MB may be increased.[10] Conversely, cases have been reported in which elderly patients have elevated CK-MB without other evidence of myocardial injury.[11] Newer tests, especially cardiac troponin I (cTnI) which has greater myocardial specificity, may permit better detection of myocardial injury/infarct than can routine CK and CK-MB measurements. Creatine kinase isoforms are elevated slightly earlier than CK-MB following myocardial infarct, but have the same myocardial specificity drawbacks as does CK-MB.[12] Low serum CK does not rule out myositis in patients with the connective tissue diseases.[7] Cryoablation of the prostate gland may lead to significant elevations of both total CK and CK-MB.[13] CK is decreased in pregnancy but may elevate to twofold above the reference range around the time of parturition.[14] Elevated in some patients with myxedema (hypothyroidism). CK is possibly a marker for ectopic pregnancy.[15]

Methodology Kinetic - UV spectrophotometric

Additional Information High CK is found after trauma, surgery, and exercise without elevation of CK-MB. To distinguish myoglobinuria from hemoglobinuria, serum CK and qualitative urine myoglobin may be helpful. CK is normal with uncomplicated hemolysis and a preparation of an 80% saturated urine solution by ammonium sulfate will precipitate hemoglobin. When myoglobin is released, 40-fold elevation of CK may be anticipated without elevation of troponin I. In rhabdomyolysis, substances which are increased include potassium, myoglobin, LDH and the aminotransferases. CK can reach vast multiples of its upper limit and CK-MB may be increased as well. Cardiac troponin T (cTnT) may be increased.

Footnotes

1. Greenson JK, Farber SJ, and Dubin SB, "The Effect of Hemolysis on Creatine Kinase Determination," Arch Pathol Lab Med, 1989, 113(2):184-5.

2. Rosalki SB, "Serum Enzymes in Disease of Skeletal Muscle," Clin Lab Med, 1989, 9(4):767-81.

3. Kilbourne EM, Swygert LA, Philen RM, et al, "Interim Guidance on the Eosinophilia-Myalgia Syndrome," Ann Intern Med, 1990, 112(2):85-7.

4. Roth D, Alarcón FJ, Fernandez JA, "Acute Rhabdomyolysis Associated With Cocaine Intoxication," N Engl J Med, 1988, 319(11):673-7.

5. Eng C, Skolnick AE, and Come SE, "Elevated Creatine Kinase and Malignancy," Hosp Pract (Off Ed), 1990, 25(12):123, 126, 129-30.

6. O'Neill PG, Faitelson L, Taylor A, et al, "Time Course of Creatine Kinase Release After Termination of Sustained Ventricular Dysrhythmias," Am Heart J, 1991, 122(3 Pt 1):709-14.

7. Nanji AA and Blank D, "Low Serum Creatine Kinase Activity in Patients With Alcoholic Liver Disease," Clin Chem 1981, 27(11):1954.

8. Wei N, Pavlidis N, Tsokos G, et al, "Clinical Significance of Low Creatine Phosphokinase Values in Patients With Connective Tissue Diseases," JAMA, 1981, 246:1921-3.

9. Sanmarti R, Collado A, Gratacos J, et al, "Reduced Activity of Serum Creatine Kinase in Rheumatoid Arthritis: A Phenomenon Linked to the Inflammatory Response," Br J Rheumatol, 1994, 33(3):231-4.

10. Lloyd-Jones DM, Camargo CA Jr, Giugliano RP, et al, "Characteristics and Prognosis of Patients With Suspected Acute Myocardial Infarction and Elevated MB Relative Index but Normal Total Creatine Kinase," Am J Cardiol, 1999, 84(9):957-62.

11. Alterman P, Vigder C, Feldman J, et al, "Creatine Kinase MB Isoenzyme of Noncardiac Origin in Elderly Patients," Coron Artery Dis, 1999, 10(7):533-6.

12. Christenson RH, Newby LK, and Ohman EM, "Cardiac Markers in the Assessment of Acute Coronary Syndromes," Md Med J, 1997, Suppl:18-24.

13. Long JP, Fallick ML, and Rand W, "Increased Serum Total Creatine Kinase and Creatine Kinase Isoenzyme MB After Cryosurgical Ablation of the Prostate," J Urol, 1997, 157(5):1723-6.

14. Shivvers SA, Wians FH Jr, Keffer J, et al, "Maternal Cardiac Troponin I Levels During Normal Labor and Delivery," Am J Obstet Gynecol, 1999, 180(1 Pt 1):122.

15. Saha PK, Gupta I, and Ganguly NK, "Evaluation of Serum Creatine Kinase as a Diagnostic Marker for Tubal Pregnancy," Aust NZ J Obstet Gynecol, 1999, 39(3):366-7.

References

Beek AM, Verheugt FW, and Meyer A, "Usefulness of Electrocardiographic Findings and Creatine Kinase Levels on Admission in Predicting the Accuracy of the Interval Between Onset of Chest Pain of Acute Myocardial Infarction and Initiation of Thrombolytic Therapy," Am J Cardiol, 1991, 68(13):1287-90.

Gambino R, "Creatine Kinase in Tubal Pregnancy," Lab Rep, 1994, 16(11):89-90.

Henderson AR, Krishnan S, Webb S, et al, "Proficiency Testing of Creatine Kinase and Creatine Kinase-2: The Experience of the Ontario Laboratory Proficiency Testing Program," Clin Chem, 1998, 44(1):124-33.

Kini A, Marmur JD, Kini S, et al, "Creatine Kinase-MB Elevation After Coronary Intervention Correlates With Diffuse Atherosclerosis, and Low-to-Medium Level Elevation Has a Benign Clinical Course: Implications for Early Discharge After Coronary Intervention," J Am Coll Cardiol, 1999, 34(3):663-71.

Kong TQ, Davidson CJ, Meyers SN, et al, "Prognostic Implication of Creatine Kinase Elevation Following Elective Coronary Artery Interventions," JAMA, 1997, 277(6):461-6.

Leung FY, Griffith AP, Jablonsky G, et al, "Comparison of the Diagnostic Utility of Timed Serial (Slope) Creatine Kinase Measurements With Conventional Serum Tests in the Early Diagnosis of Myocardial Infarction," Ann Clin Biochem, 1991, 28(Pt 1):78-82.

Ohman EM and Tardiff BE, NC, "Periprocedural Cardiac Marker Elevation After Percutaneous Coronary Artery Revascularization," JAMA, 1997, 277(6):495-6.

Polaczyk CA, Kuntz KM, Sacks DB, et al, "Emergency Department Triage Strategies for Acute Chest Pain Using Creatine Kinase-MB and Troponin I Assays: A Cost-Effectiveness Analysis," Ann Intern Med, 1999, 131(12):909-18.

Robinson DJ and Christenson RH, "Creatine Kinase and its CK-MB Isoenzyme: The Conventional Marker for the Diagnosis of Acute Myocardial Infarction," J Emerg Med, 1999, 17(1):95-104.

Zalenski RJ, McCarren M, Roberts R, et al, "An Evaluation of a Chest Pain Diagnostic Protocol to Exclude Acute Cardiac Ischemia in the Emergency Department," Arch Intern Med, 1997, 157(10):1085-91.

♦ **Creatine Phosphokinase-MB Isoenzyme and Total Creatine Phosphokinase, Serum** see Creatine Kinase Isoenzymes/Isoforms, Serum on page 157

♦ **Creatine Phosphokinase, Total, Serum** see Creatine Kinase, Serum on page 158

Creatinine, 12- or 24-Hour Urine

Related Information
Creatinine Clearance on page 160
Creatinine, Serum or Plasma on page 161
Osmolality, Serum on page 236
Osmolality, Urine on page 236
Sodium, Serum or Plasma on page 275
Sodium, Urine on page 278
Uric Acid, Urine on page 295
Urinalysis on page 887
Urine Collection, 24-Hour on page 47
Vanillylmandelic Acid, Urine on page 297

Synonyms Urine Creatinine

Test Includes Urine creatinine in mg/dL and mg/24 hours or mg/12 hours

Abstract Timed urine collection is a portion of creatinine clearance.

Specimen 12- or 24-hour urine

Container Plastic urine container

Collection If the specimen is a 24-hour collection, instruct the patient to void at 8 AM and discard the specimen. Then collect all urine including the final specimen voided at the end of the 24-hour collection period (ie, 8 AM the next morning). Keep specimen on ice during collection. Container must be labeled with patient's name, date, and time collection started and date and time collection finished.

Storage Instructions Refrigerate

Causes for Rejection Incomplete collection

Reference Interval Children: 2-3 years: 6-22 mg/kg/24 hours (SI: 52.8-193.6 µmol/kg/day), older than 3 years: 12-30 mg/kg/24 hours (SI: 105.0-264.0 µmol/kg/day); adults: male: 1-2 g/24 hours (SI: 8.8-17.7 mmol/day), female: 0.8-1.8 g/24 hours (SI: 7.1-15.9 mmol/day). Creatinine excretion decreases with advanced age as muscle mass diminishes. Normal age-adjusted values for anticipated creatinine excretion stratified for each sex by height are published. These tables assume ideal weight.[1]

Use Urine creatinine provides a portion of a widely used renal function test, when used as part of creatinine clearance. It is also used as a crude marker for completeness of 24-hour urine collections when collected for other *(Continued)*

Creatinine, 12- or 24-Hour Urine *(Continued)*

purposes. It is useful as a renal function test only when done as part of a creatinine clearance. Renal tubular function in acute oliguria may be assessed with measurements of sodium and creatinine concentrations in plasma and urine.[2,3]

Limitations Complete urine collections require vigilance on the part of nursing personnel. Ingestion of meat may increase creatinine values of urine collections as well as serum creatinine values. Application of urine creatinine excretion as a marker for complete collection has been questioned, but is still in widespread use. **Drugs** interfering with tubular creatinine secretion include cimetidine, trimethoprim, and probenecid. Creatinine **reabsorption** occurs with very low urine flow rates. Entities in which reabsorption occurs include severe congestive heart failure, uncontrolled diabetes mellitus, and acute renal failure.[4] Creatinine absorption may also occur physiologically in newborn infants.[5]

Analytical increases are caused by cefoxitin, cephalothin, and other drugs. Physiological increases occur with corticosteroids, including prednisone and with nadrolone.[6]

Methodology Jaffé reaction (alkaline picrate); enzymatic, kinetic or endpoint

Additional Information Urine creatinine is not ordered alone. Creatinine clearance, which requires a serum creatinine, offers useful renal function data. Serum creatinine alone is not an adequate index of glomerular filtration rate.[4] See table to help to ascertain whether acute renal failure is due to prerenal causes or acute tubular injury.

Urinary Indexes in Patients With Acute Renal Failure

Index	Prerenal Causes	Acute Tubular Injury
Urinary sodium concentration (mEq/L)	<20	>40
Fractional excretion of sodium (%)*	<1	>1
Ratio of urine to plasma creatinine	>40	<20
Osmolality (mOsm/kg H_2O) urine	>500	<350

*[Urine (Na) / serum (Na)] + [urine (creatinine) / serum (creatinine)] x 100.

Adapted from Klahr S and Miller SB, "Acute Oliguria," *N Engl J Med*, 1998, 338(10):671-5 and Mitch WE, "Acute Renal Failure," *Cecil Textbook of Medicine*, 21st ed, Chapter 103, Goldman L and Bennett JC, eds, Philadelphia, PA: WB Saunders Co, 2000, 567-71.

Footnotes

1. Walser M, "Creatinine Excretion as a Measure of Protein Nutrition in Adults of Varying Age," *JPEN J Parenter Enteral Nutr*, 1987, 11(5 Suppl):73S-8S.
2. Klahr S and Miller SB, "Acute Oliguria," *N Engl J Med*, 1998, 338(10):671-5.
3. Mitch WE, "Acute Renal Failure," *Cecil Textbook of Medicine*, 21st ed, Chapter 103, Goldman L and Bennett JC, eds, Philadelphia, PA: WB Saunders Co, 2000, 567-71.
4. Levey AS, Perrone RD, and Madias NE, "Serum Creatinine and Renal Function," *Annu Rev Med*, 1988, 39:465-90.
5. Guignard JP and Drukker A, "Why Do Newborn Infants Have a High Plasma Creatinine?" *Pediatrics*, 1999, 103(4):e49.
6. Young DS, *Effects of Drugs on Clinical Laboratory Tests*, 5th ed, Volume 1: Listing by Test, Washington, DC: AACC Press, American Association of Clinical Chemistry, 2000, Section 3, 258.

References

Huang CC, Wang ST, Chang YC, et al, "Measurement of the Urinary Lactate:Creatinine Ratio for the Early Identification of Newborn Infants at Risk for Hypoxic-Ischemic Encephalopathy," *N Engl J Med*, 1999, 341(5):328-35.

Pesola G, Akhaven I, Carlton G, "Urinary Creatinine Excretion in the ICU: Low Excretion Does Not Mean Inadequate Collection," *Am J Crit Care*, 1993, 2(6):462-6.

Schwab SJ, Christensen RL, Dougherty K, et al, "Quantitation of Proteinuria by the Use of Protein-to-Creatinine Ratios in Single Urine Samples," *Arch Intern Med*, 1987, 147(5):943-4.

Creatinine, Amniotic Fluid

Related Information

Body Fluid Chemical Analysis *on page 123*
Lecithin:Sphingomyelin Ratio, Amniotic Fluid *on page 210*
Phosphatidylglycerol, Amniotic Fluid *on page 251*
Pulmonary Surfactant, Amniotic Fluid *on page 271*

Synonyms Amniotic Fluid Creatinine

Abstract Amniotic fluid creatinine is a measure of fetal kidney maturity, which indirectly assesses lung maturity. Much better tests are available for assessing fetal lung maturity (see Lecithin:Sphingomyelin Ratio, Amniotic Fluid *on page 210* and Phosphatidylglycerol, Amniotic Fluid *on page 251*).

Reference Interval See table.

Amniotic Fluid Creatinine*

	mg/dL	μmol/L[1]
Immature fetus	<1.5	<132.6
Equivocal	1.5-2.0	132.6-176.8
Mature fetus	<2.0	>176.8

Use Amniotic fluid creatinine for estimation of fetal maturity is primarily of historical interest.

Limitations Oligohydramnios, related to fetal urinary tract obstruction or to renal agenesis, or polyhydramnios, affect interpretation. Elevation of maternal creatinine may cause increases in the amniotic fluid creatinine level. Complications of amniocentesis may occur.

Methodology Colorimetry, Jaffé reaction

Additional Information Fetal lung and kidney development are related, and normal lung development is dependent on the normal development of the kidneys. Estimation of fetal kidney maturity by measuring amniotic fluid creatinine, therefore, provides an indirect assessment of fetal lung maturity. In addition to creatinine, **amniotic fluid urea nitrogen** has been suggested as a marker for fetal renal maturity and as a predictor of respiratory distress syndrome.[2]

Most laboratories use amniotic fluid phosphatidylglycerol, lecithin:sphingomyelin ratio (see Lecithin:Sphingomyelin Ratio, Amniotic Fluid *on page 210* and Phosphatidylglycerol, Amniotic Fluid *on page 251*), surfactant to albumin ratio, and/or lamellar body count to assess fetal lung maturity.

Footnotes

1. Pitkin RM and Zwirek SJ, "Amniotic Fluid Creatinine," *Am J Obstet Gynecol*, 1967, 98(8):1135-9.
2. Almeida OD and Kitay DZ, "Amniotic Fluid Urea Nitrogen in the Prediction of Respiratory Distress Syndrome," *Am J Obstet Gynecol*, 1988, 159(2):465-8.

References

Darling RE and Zlatnik FJ, "Comparison of Amniotic Fluid Optical Density, L/S Ratio and Creatinine Concentration in Predicting Fetal Pulmonary Maturity," *J Reprod Med*, 1985, 30(6):460-4.

Kjeldsberg CR and Knight JA, "Amniotic Fluid," *Body Fluids: Laboratory Examination of Amniotic, Cerebrospinal, Seminal, Serous & Synovial Fluids*, 3rd ed, Chicago, IL: ASCP Press, American Society of Clinical Pathologists, 1993, 1-63.

Raghav M, Vijay G, Chowdhary DR, et al, "Amniotic Fluid Amino Acids, Urea, Creatinine in Normal and Toxemic Pregnancies," *Indian J Med Sci*, 1985, 39(12):291-3.

Troccoli R, Stella C, Pachi A, et al, "Hydroxyproline and Creatinine Levels in Normal Amniotic Fluid," *Ric Clin Lab*, 1986, 16(1):37-41.

Tyden O, Eriksson U, Agren H, et al, "Estimation of Fetal Maturity by Amniotic Fluid Cytology, Creatinine, Lecithin/Sphingomyelin Ratio and Phosphatidylglycerol," *Gynecol Obstet Invest*, 1983, 16:317-26.

Creatinine Clearance

Related Information

Creatinine, 12- or 24-Hour Urine *on page 159*
Creatinine, Serum or Plasma *on page 161*
Cystatin C, Serum or Plasma *on page 163*
Kidney Biopsy *on page 64*
Kidney Stone Analysis *on page 877*
Protein, Quantitative, Urine *on page 883*
Urea Nitrogen, Serum or Plasma *on page 293*
Uric Acid, Serum *on page 293*
Urine Collection, 24-Hour *on page 47*

Applies to Body Surface Area; Glomerular Filtration Rate

Replaces Urea Clearance; Urea Nitrogen Clearance

Test Includes Serum creatinine, urine creatinine

Abstract The most common test for evaluation of renal function is serum creatinine; the next is creatinine clearance.

Patient Preparation Avoid cephalosporins. If possible, drugs should be stopped beforehand. Have patient drink water before the clearance is begun and continue good hydration throughout the clearance. A meat-free diet has been recommended.[1]

Specimen 24-hour urine and serum; test can be done for shorter periods. The use of two consecutive 2-hour clearances has been advocated.[2]

Container Urine container and red top tube

Collection Instruct the patient to void at 8 AM and discard the specimen. Then collect all urine including the final specimen voided at the end of the 24-hour collection period (ie, 8 AM the next morning). Keep specimen on ice during collection. Bottle must be labeled with patient's name, date and time for a 24-hour collection. Especially for creatinine clearance, accuracy and precision of collection are important. Complete, carefully timed (usually 24-hour) collection is needed; 4- and 12-hour collections are acceptable. Urine flows >2 mL/minute are required for good clearance measurements.

Storage Instructions Refrigerate urine specimen.

Causes for Rejection No blood creatinine ordered, urine specimen not timed

Special Instructions Blood creatinine should be ordered at the same time. Patient's age, height, and weight are needed.

Reference Interval A healthy 70 kg adult excretes about 1 g/day. Clearance for: children: 70-140 mL/minute/1.73 m² (SI: 1.17-2.33 mL/s/1.73 m²); adults: male: 85-125 mL/minute/1.73 m² (SI: 1.42-2.08 mL/s/1.73 m²), female: 75-115 mL/minute/1.73 m² (SI: 1.25-1.92 mL/s/1.73 m²). For each age decades after 40, creatinine clearance decreases 6-7 mL/minute/1.73 m². When used in a series to evaluate completeness of collection for other substances (eg, urinary cortisol), up to about 10% variation is acceptable.

Critical Values Moderate renal impairment (adult): 30-40 mL/minute/1.73 m²

Possible Panic Range Severe renal impairment (adult): <28 mL/minute/1.73 m²

Use Renal function test to estimate GFR; follow possible progression of renal disease; adjust dosages of medications in which renal excretion is pivotal (eg, aminoglycosides, methotrexate, cisplatin). Assay of creatinine is widely used to assess whether or not a 24-hour urine collection for another substance (eg, cortisol) is complete.

Limitations Because of the exponential rise in serum creatinine concentration with decline of GFR, a 25% increase in serum creatinine actually represents a substantial diminution of GFR. As muscle mass and kidney function diminish in parallel with advancing age, an elderly woman with perceived normal creatinine concentration may have a GFR only 30% that of a young adult.[3]

Exercise may cause increased creatinine clearance. The GFR is substantially increased in pregnancy. Ascorbic acid, ketone bodies (acetoacetate), hydantoin, numerous cephalosporins[4,5] and glucose may influence creatinine determinations. Trimethoprim, cimetidine, quinine, quinidine, procainamide reduce creatinine excretion. Icteric samples, lipemia and hemolysis may interfere with determination of creatinine. Since tubular secretion of creatinine is fractionally more important in progressing renal failure, the creatinine clearance overestimates GFR with high serum creatinine levels (ie, as the severity of renal dysfunction increases). Methods for estimating creatinine clearance also become less accurate as the severity of hepatic dysfunction increases.[6] While ingestion of cooked meats may cause some increase in creatinine level, in practice this seems to make a difference only occasionally. Intraindividual variation in creatinine clearance is about 15%. Males excrete more creatinine and have slightly higher clearance than females.

Serum creatinine and creatinine clearance are relatively insensitive indicators for glomerular filtration rate, especially in early stages of renal failure. The estimation can be improved by treating the patient with cimetidine, which blocks tubular excretion of creatinine, before and during the conduction of creatinine clearance.[7,8]

Methodology Jaffé reaction (alkaline picrate) or enzymatic. The calculation for corrected creatinine clearance in mL/minute = [(urine volume per minute x urine creatinine)/serum creatinine] x (1.73/surface area of body in square meters). Body surface area is obtained from nomograms which require height and weight.

Body surface area can be calculated from the following equation:
$$S = M^{0.425} \times H^{0.725} \times 71.84$$

where:
S = body surface in cm^2
M = mass in kg
H = height in cm

Additional Information Glomerular filtration rate is low in newborns and gradually increases towards adult values by age 1-2 years. Glomerular filtration rate declines about 10% per decade after 50 years of age. Some patients with significant impairment of glomerular filtration rate have only slightly elevated serum creatinine.[9] Corrected creatinine clearance is calculated on the basis of the surface area of the patient. Corrected clearance = urine creat (mg/dL) x rate of urine flow (mL/minute) / plasma creat (mg/dL) x 1.73 / patient surface area in square meters. The estimated error of determining creatinine clearance utilizing serum and 24-hour urine collection has been found to be in the range of 10% to 15%. Any test requiring a 24-hour urine collection may also be run on this specimen (eg, protein, quantitative, 24-hour urine, cortisol).

Prediction equations have been proposed to estimate the GFR. One developed from the Modification of Diet in Renal Disease (MDRD) Study was thought to provide more accurate estimation of GFR than did measured creatinine clearance, but has not been validated in subjects without renal disease. It utilizes serum creatinine, urea nitrogen, and albumin concentrations, as well as age, sex, and ethnicity.[10]

Footnotes
1. Gambino R, "Crock-Pot Creatinine Revisited - Measure Creatinine Clearance While Patients Are on a Meat-Free Diet," *Lab Rep*, 1995, 17(2):15.
2. Herget-Rosenthal S, Kribben A, Pietruck F, et al, "Two by Two-Hour Creatinine Clearance - Repeatable and Valid," *Clin Nephrol*, 1999, 51(6):348-54.
3. Turney JH, "Acute Renal Failure - A Dangerous Condition," *JAMA*, 1996, 275(19):1516-7.
4. Swain RR and Briggs SL, "Positive Interference With the Jaffe Reaction by Cephalosporin Antibiotics," *Clin Chem*, 1977, 23(7):1340-2.
5. Levey AS, Perrone RD, and Madias NE, "Serum Creatinine and Renal Function," *Annu Rev Med*, 1988, 39:465-90.
6. Lam NP, Sperelakis R, Kuk J, et al, "Rapid Estimation of Creatinine Clearances in Patients With Liver Dysfunction," *Dig Dis Sci*, 1999, 44(6):1222-7.
7. Hellerstein S, Berenbom M, Alon US, et al, "Creatinine Clearance Following Cimetidine for Estimation of Glomerular Filtration Rate," *Pediatr Nephrol*, 1998, 12(1):49-54.
8. Walser M, "Assessing Renal Function From Creatinine Measurements in Adults With Chronic Renal Failure," *Am J Kidney Dis*, 1998, 32(1):23-31.
9. Klahr S, "The Modifications of Diet in Renal Disease Study," *N Engl J Med*, 1989, 320(13):864-6.
10. Levey AS, Bosch JP, Lewis JB, et al, "A More Accurate Method to Estimate Glomerular Filtration Rate From Serum Creatinine: A New Prediction Equation," Modification of Diet in Renal Disease Study Group, *Ann Intern Med*, 1999, 130(6):461-70.

References
Duarte CG and Preuss HG, " Assessment of Renal Function: Glomerular and Tubular," *Clin Lab Med*, 1993, 13(1):33-52.

Luke DR, Halstenson CE, Opsahl JA, et al, "Validity of Creatinine Clearance Estimates in the Assessment of Renal Function," *Clin Pharmacol Ther*, 1990, 48(5):503-8.
Payne RB, "Biological Variation of Serum and Urine Creatinine and Creatinine Clearance," *Ann Clin Biochem*, 1989, 26(Pt 6):565-6.
Sokoll LJ, Russell RM, Sodowski JA, et al, "Establishment of Creatinine Clearance Reference Values for Older Women," *Clin Chem*, 1994, 40(12):2276-81.
Van Lente F and Suit P, "Assessment of Renal Function by Serum Creatinine and Creatinine Clearance: Glomerular Filtration Rate Estimated by Four Procedures," *Clin Chem*, 1989, 35(12):2326-30.
Young DS, *Effects of Drugs on Clinical Laboratory Tests*, 5th ed, Volume 1: Listing by Test, Washington, DC: AACC Press, American Association of Clinical Chemistry, 2000, Section 3, 258-61.

◆ **Creatinine, Ratio** see *Body Fluid pH* on page 125

Creatinine, Serum or Plasma

Related Information

Applies to Glomerular Filtration Rate

Abstract A primary renal function test. There were 300,000 patients receiving renal replacement therapy in the U.S. in 1998. Of these, 220,000 were on dialysis and the remainder survive with a successful kidney graft. The average age at which renal replacement therapy is presently needed by individuals in renal failure is 60 years. There are about two million subjects in the U.S. who have chronic renal failure. Two entities, diabetes mellitus and primary hypertensive renal disease, cause 66% of cases of end-stage kidney disease.[1]

Patient Preparation Fasting may be desirable. Certain cephalosporins, especially cefoxitin and other drugs, cause misleading high results.[2] High serum bilirubin levels can cause misleading low results with Jaffé reaction method,[3] but not as much by enzymatic methods.

Specimen Serum, plasma

Container Red top tube; gray top (sodium fluoride) tube or green top (heparin) tube can be used if assay is done by Jaffé method.

Collection Pediatrics: Blood drawn from heelstick.

Causes for Rejection Hemolysis

Reference Interval Children: 1-5 years: 0.3-0.5 mg/dL (SI: 27-44 µmol/L), 5-10 years: 0.5-0.8 mg/dL (SI: 44-71 µmol/L); adults: male: up to 1.2 mg/dL (SI: 106 µmol/L), female: up to 1.1 mg/dL (SI: 97 µmol/L).[4] Variation between sources for serum creatinine normal ranges is perhaps greater than for many other important tests. There are slight differences between the sexes with males higher, since the range relates to the amount of muscle mass present. The glomerular filtration rate increases in pregnancy; thus, serum creatinine should be slightly less during that period. In older patients, decrease of muscle mass must be considered in interpretation of results; the elderly have reduced creatinine generation. Similarly, other patients may have creatinine levels in which muscle abnormalities must be considered, including long-term corticosteroid therapy, hyperthyroidism, muscular dystrophy, paralysis, dermatomyositis, and polymyositis.

Critical Values Chronic renal insufficiency is defined by serum creatinine concentration of 1.5-3.0 mg/dL. Chronic renal failure is defined as serum creatinine concentration >3.0 mg/dL.[1] This figure, in children, varies by age.

Use The most common clinical renal function test, providing a rough approximation of glomerular filtration. In children with normal muscle mass, serum creatinine can be used to estimate glomerular filtration rate (GFR) expressed in mL/minute/1.73 m^2 by using the formula:

$$GFR = \delta L / S_{Cr}$$

Where:
L = body length in cm
S_{Cr} = serum creatinine in mg/dL
δ = constant of proportionality (age and sex dependent)

See table on following page.

Causes of high creatinine include renal diseases and insufficiency with decreased glomerular filtration (uremia or azotemia if severe); urinary tract obstruction; reduced renal blood flow including congestive heart failure, shock and dehydration; rhabdomyolysis causes high serum creatinine, which may be elevated out of proportion to BUN, or to the reduction in renal
(Continued)

Creatinine, Serum or Plasma (Continued)

Mean Values and Histograms of δ*

Age	δ (mean)	δ (range)	% Within Range
Low-birth weight infants <1 y	0.33	0.20-0.50	77
Term <1 y	0.45	0.30-0.70	79
Children 2-12 y	0.55	0.40-0.70	83
Male 13-21 y	0.70	0.50-0.90	82
Female 13-21 y	0.55	0.40-0.70	77

*GFR = δL/S_{Cr}

Adapted from Schwartz GJ, Brion LP, and Spitzeer A, "The Use of Plasma Creatinine Concentration for Estimating Glomerular Filtration Rate in Infants, Children, and Adolescents," Pediatr Clin North Am, 1987, 34:571-90.

function. Creatinine >2 mg/dL is among factors for identification of patients with acute necrotizing pancreatitis at risk for adverse outcome.[5] Creatinine with urea nitrogen and electrolytes may be indicated in patients with vomiting, diarrhea, or decreased oral intake.[6] Increased serum creatinine concentrations are found in some patients with hypertension, diabetes mellitus, and cardiovascular disease. Increases in creatinine correlate with age older than 55 years.

Causes of low creatinine include small stature, debilitation, decreased muscle mass, some complex cases of severe hepatic disease. In advanced liver disease, low creatinine may result from decreased hepatic production of creatinine and inadequate dietary protein as well as reduced muscle mass.[2]

Limitations With reduced renal blood flow, creatinine rises less quickly than urea nitrogen. Concentration of creatinine only becomes abnormal when about half or more of the nephrons have stopped functioning in chronic progressive renal disease. Thus, it is not a sensitive indicator of early renal disease. Renal failure is underestimated by serum creatinine and creatinine clearance in patients with hepatic cirrhosis.[7]

Increased serum creatinine results may occur from noncreatinine substances, including meat ingestion, glucose, pyruvate, uric acid, fructose, guanidine, ketonemia (acetoacetate), hydantoin, ascorbic acid, and numerous cephalosporin antibiotics, especially cefoxitin. Cefoxitin levels fall in patients with normal kidney function, such that a sample can be drawn 2 hours after a dose but preferably, 4 hours or more afterwards.[8] With severe renal disease, creatinine is not reliable in the presence of cefoxitin therapy. There is less interference reported from the cephalosporins cephalothin, cephaloridine, cephadrile sodium, and cephaloglycin dihydrate.[9] Cefazolin and cefamandole may cause increased colorimetric values.[10] Cephapirin and moxalactam are described as not causing interference.[11,12] Differences in the interference of such cephalosporins between assay systems are published.[9,11,12] Methyldopa and trimethoprim may increase serum creatinine levels.[13] Cimetidine stops creatinine excretion in the renal tubule, causing a rise in creatinine without reduction in renal function.[14] High creatinine in serum has been reported with methanol intoxication.[15] An antifungal drug, 5-flucytosine, and glucose interfere with the imidohydrolase method.[10] Similarly, lipemia, hemolysis, and bilirubin may interfere.[16,17] Moderate variation of results exists among chemistry analyzer systems. Many drugs cause interference documented with particular assay systems, in small numbers of individuals, or in occasional reports. Others (eg, gentamicin) may cause nephrotoxicity. Overall, a substantial number of drugs may cause pharmacologic/physiologic, analytical, or toxic changes in serum creatinine.[12]

Serum creatinine is only a crude guide to the progress of renal disease.[10] Moderate changes in the glomerular filtration rate (GFR) may not be detected by serum creatinine levels. Levey et al and others emphasize that the serum creatinine does **not** provide an adequate estimate of GFR.[10,18] A fraction of urine creatinine is from tubular secretion. Such tubular secretion increases with declining renal function.

Methodology Alkaline picrate (Jaffé reaction), enzymatic, o-nitrobenzaldehyde (Sakaguchi reaction), imidohydrolase (Ektachem®). Many interference problems are still unresolved in the Jaffé reaction.[19]

Additional Information Serum creatinine level is proportional to lean body muscle mass. It is unaffected by most diet or activity and is freely filtered by the glomerulus. Both BUN and creatinine are often ordered to follow renal problems. Creatinine overall is the more reliable index, but each has pitfalls. As creatinine increases in chronic renal failure, the hematocrit decreases, total carbon dioxide and bicarbonate fall, and serum phosphate and BUN increase. Uric acid increases, usually subsequently. When serum creatinine increases postoperatively, a group of patients may be identified who are at risk for more severe renal failure. Creatinine clearances have a role in such investigations. Serum creatinine has a role in determination of dosages of some drugs (eg, the aminoglycosides and digoxin), especially in elderly subjects.

Patients with diabetes mellitus or hypertension should be monitored with blood pressure measurement, evaluation of urinalysis, serum creatinine and microalbuminuria testing.[20]

Footnotes

1. Luke RG, "Chronic Renal Failure - A Vasculopathic State," N Engl J Med, 1998, 339(12):841-3.
2. Takabatake T, Ohta H, Ishida Y, et al, "Low Serum Creatinine Levels in Severe Hepatic Disease," Arch Intern Med, 1988, 148(6):1313-5.
3. Chadha V, Warady BA, Garg U, et al, "Sieving Coefficient Inaccuracies During Hemodiafiltration in Patients With Hyperbilirubinemia," Pediatr Nephrol, 2000, 15:33-35.
4. Savory DJ, "Reference Ranges for Serum Creatinine in Infants, Children, and Adolescents," Ann Clin Biochem, 1990, 27(Pt 2):99-101.
5. Talamini G, Uomo G, Pezzilli R, et al, "Serum Creatinine and Chest Radiographs in the Early Assessment of Acute Pancreatitis," Am J Surg, 1999, 177(1):7-14.
6. McGee S, Abernethy WB 3rd, and Simel DL, "Is This Patient Hypovolemic?" JAMA, 1999, 281(11):1022-9.
7. Caregaro L, Menon F, Angeli P, et al, "Limitations of Serum Creatinine Level and Creatinine Clearance as Filtration Markers in Cirrhosis," Arch Intern Med, 1994, 154(2):201-5.
8. Durham SR, Bignell AH, and Wise R, "Interference of Cefoxitin in the Creatinine Estimation and its Clinical Relevance," J Clin Pathol, 1979, 32:1148-51.
9. Saah AJ, Koch TR, and Drusano GL, "Cefoxitin Falsely Elevates Creatinine Levels," JAMA, 1982, 247:205-6.
10. Levey AS, Perrone RD, and Madias NE, "Serum Creatinine and Renal Function," Annu Rev Med, 1988, 39:465-90.
11. Kirby MG, Gal P, Baird HW, et al, "Cefoxitin Interference With Serum Creatinine Measurement Varies With the Assay System," Clin Chem, 1982, 28(9):1981.
12. Young DS, Effects of Drugs on Clinical Laboratory Tests, 5th ed, Volume 1: Listing by Test, Washington, DC: AACC Press, American Association of Clinical Chemistry, 2000, Section 3, 240-58.
13. Porter GA and Bennett WM, "Toxic Nephropathies," The Kidney, 2nd ed, Brenner BM and Rector FC Jr, eds, Philadelphia, PA: WB Saunders Co, 1981, 2045-108.
14. Hellerstein S, Berenbom M, Alon US, et al, "Creatinine Clearance Following Cimetidine for Estimation of Glomerular Filtration Rate," Pediatr Nephrol, 1998, 12(1):49-54
15. Wu AH, Stout R, and McComb RB, "Falsely High Serum Creatinine Concentration Associated With Severe Methanol Intoxication," Clin Chem, 1983, 29(1):205-8.
16. Bowers LD and Wong ET, "Kinetic Serum Creatinine Assays. II. A Critical Evaluation and Review," Clin Chem, 1980, 26(5):555-61.
17. Soldin SJ, Henderson L, and Hill JG, "The Effect of Bilirubin and Ketones on Reaction Rate Methods for the Measurement of Creatinine," Clin Biochem, 1978, 11(3):82-6.
18. Walser M, "Assessing Renal Function From Creatinine Measurements in Adults With Chronic Renal Failure," Am J Kidney Dis, 1998, 32(1):23-31.
19. Weber JA and van Zanten AP, "Interferences in Current Methods for Measurements of Creatinine," Clin Chem, 1991, 37(5):695-700.
20. McCarthy JT, "A Practical Approach to the Management of Patients With Chronic Renal Failure," Mayo Clin Proc, 1999, 74(3):269-73.

References

Adrogué HJ and Madias NE, "Medical Progress: Management of Life-Threatening Acid-Base Disorders (First of Two Parts)," N Engl J Med, 1998, 338(1):26-34.

Blijenberg BG, Brouwer HJ, Kuller TJ, et al, "Improvements in Creatinine Methodology: A Critical Assessment," Eur J Clin Chem Clin Biochem, 1994, 32(7):529-37.

Couchoud C, Pozet N, Labeeuw M, et al, "Screening Early Renal Failure: Cutoff Values for Serum Creatinine as an Indicator of Renal Impairment," Kidney Int, 1999, 55(5):1878-84.

Culleton BF, Larson MG, Evans JC, et al, "Prevalence and Correlates of Elevated Serum Creatinine Levels: The Framingham Heart Study," Arch Intern Med, 1999, 159(15):1785-90.

Duarte CG and Preuss HG, "Assessment of Renal Function: Glomerular and Tubular," Clin Lab Med, 1993, 13(1):33-52.

Fink JC, Burdick RA, Kurth SJ, et al, "Significance of Serum Creatinine Values in New End-Stage Renal Disease," Am J Kidney Dis, 1999, 34(4):694-701.

Fossati P, Ponti M, Passoni G, et al, "A Step Forward in Enzymatic Measurement of Creatinine," Clin Chem, 1994, 40(1):130-7.

Hricik DE, Chung-Park M, and Sedor JR, "Glomerulonephritis," N Engl J Med, 1998, 339(13):888-99.

Klahr S and Miller SB, "Acute Oliguria," N Engl J Med, 1998, 338(10):671-5.

Lemann J, Bidani AK, Bain RP, et al, "Use of the Serum Creatinine to Estimate Glomerular Filtration Rate in Health and Early Diabetic Nephropathy. Collaborative Study Group of Angiotensin Converting Enzyme Inhibition in Diabetic Nephropathy," Am J Kidney Dis, 1990, 16(3):236-43.

Cyclic AMP, Plasma

Related Information
Calcium, Ionized, Serum *on page 130*
Parathyroid Hormone, Serum *on page 243*

Synonyms AMP, Cyclic, Plasma; cAMP, Plasma; 3′, 5′-Cyclic Adenosine Monophosphate, Plasma

Abstract Cyclic adenosine monophosphate (cAMP) is an intracellular second messenger which serves as an effector in mediating the action of several peptide hormones. Although once used as an adjunct in the diagnosis of primary hyperparathyroidism, there are now better ways to approach this diagnosis. On rare occasions, urinary cAMP is measured in the evaluation of pseudohypoparathyroidism, and plasma specimens are often a required accompaniment.

References
Logue FC, Fraser WD, Gallacher SJ, et al, "The Loss of Circadian Rhythm for Intact Parathyroid Hormone and Nephrogenous Cyclic AMP in Patients With Primary Hyperparathyroidism," *Clin Endocrinol (Oxf)*, 1990, 32(4):475-83.

Cyclic AMP, Urine

Related Information
Calcium, Ionized, Serum *on page 130*
Calcium, Serum *on page 131*
Parathyroid Hormone, Serum *on page 243*

Synonyms AMP, Cyclic, Urine; cAMP, Urine; Cyclic Adenosine Monophosphate, Urine; 3′, 5′-Cyclic Adenosine Monophosphate, Urine

Abstract Cyclic adenosine monophosphate (cAMP), an intracellular second messenger, serves as an effector in mediating the action of several peptide hormones, including parathyroid hormone (PTH). In normal persons, the infusion of PTH produces a sharp increase in urinary cAMP; this spike is not seen in persons with pseudohypoparathyroidism (the syndrome of target organ resistance to PTH).

Patient Preparation Following an overnight fast, a fluid intake of 400 mL/hour should be maintained for the 2 hours preceding the test until the test is concluded.[1]

Specimen Six consecutive 30-minute urine specimens; a plasma specimen at the midpoint of each 30-minute interval; specimens are assayed for cAMP, phosphorus, and creatinine.[1] Consult your reference laboratory for additional instructions.

Sampling Time See footnote 1, page 114. At the beginning of the fourth urine collection interval, synthetic PTH (teriparatide - a product unavailable at the time of this writing), 3 units/kg to a maximum of 200 units, is given I.V. over a 10-minute period.

Storage Instructions Consult your reference laboratory.

Reference Interval
Random specimen: 1.3-3.7 nmol/dL glomerular filtrate[2]

Stimulation testing with synthetic PTH: A normal response to PTH is a 10-12-fold increase in cAMP excretion, and a 20% decrease in the ratio of the clearance of phosphate relative to the creatinine clearance (TmP/GFR). In states of resistance to PTH, the following are observed:[1]

- Type I pseudohypoparathyroidism: Less than a fivefold increase in urinary cAMP and <10% fall in TmP/GFR.
- Type II pseudohypoparathyroidism: Normal increase in urinary cAMP and <10% fall in TmP/GFR.

Use

Pseudohypoparathyroidism: Pseudohypoparathyroidism names a group of disorders characterized by high or normal serum levels of PTH, end-organ resistance to the action of PTH, and hypocalcemia. These are among the least common causes of hypocalcemia.[1] The biochemical confirmation of pseudohypoparathyroidism involves measuring the urinary cAMP response to intravenous synthetic PTH. The testing protocol described in the reference cited in footnote 1 is based on the original communication cited in footnote 3.

Primary hyperparathyroidism: Test protocols involving the assay of cAMP were once used to diagnose primary hyperparathyroidism in a small number of hypercalcemic patients with otherwise equivocal findings. These tests are no longer necessary since better tests are now available (see Parathyroid Hormone, Serum *on page 243*). In addition, the cAMP-based tests are nonspecific since increased urinary cAMP is found both in primary hyperparathyroidism and in many patients with humoral hypercalcemia of malignancy.[4,5]

Methodology High performance liquid chromatography (HPLC)[2]

Footnotes
1. Cundy T and Reid I, "Calcium, Phosphate and Magnesium," *Clinical Biochemistry*, Marshall WJ and Bangert SK, eds, New York, NY: Churchill Livingstone, 1995, 99-115.
2. Leavelle DE, *Interpretive Handbook*, Mayo Medical Laboratories, Rochester, MN, 1997, 184.
3. Mallette LE, Kirkland JL, Gagel RF, et al, "Synthetic Human Parathyroid Hormone (1-34) for the Study of Pseudohypoparathyroidism," *J Clin Endocrinol Metab*, 1988, 67:964-72.
4. Endres DB and Rude RK, "Mineral and Bone Metabolism," *Tietz Textbook of Clinical Chemistry*, 3rd ed, Burtis CA and Ashwood ER, eds, Philadelphia, PA: Saunders Co, 1999, 1438.

5. Spiegel AM, "The Parathyroid Glands, Hypercalcemia and Hypocalcemia," *Cecil Textbook of Medicine*, 21st ed, Goldman L and Bennett JC, eds, Philadelphia, PA: Saunders Co, 2000, 1403-4.

♦ **Cystathionine** *see* Amino Acids, Urine *on page 101*

Cystatin C, Serum or Plasma

Related Information
Creatinine Clearance *on page 160*
Creatinine, Serum or Plasma *on page 161*

Applies to Glomerular Filtration Rate

Abstract A new marker of glomerular filtration rate (GFR), cystatin C is an endogenous and low molecular weight protein. In children, it is independent of age, height, gender, and body composition. It may prove to be more sensitive and specific for GFR than serum creatinine concentrations.

Patient Preparation This analyte is presently considered independent of diet.

Specimen Serum, plasma (EDTA or heparin)

Storage Instructions Stable for 7 days at 20°C, for 6 months at -80°C.

Reference Interval Children older than 1 year of age to adulthood: 0.63-1.33 mg/L[1]

A cutoff concentration of 1.39 mg/L provided 90% sensitivity and 86% specificity for detection of abnormal GFR.[2]

Use Cystatin C provides estimation of glomerular filtration rate; assessment of allograft function and therapeutic nephrotoxicity. It is independent of muscle mass.

Limitations Greater cost than that of creatinine concentration. Assays are not presently readily available.

Methodology Latex particle enhanced turbidimetric or nephelometric immunoassay; other methods[3,4,5]

Additional Information Cystatin C is freely filtered in the glomeruli and catabolized in the tubules. No extrarenal routes of elimination are known. Most of the studies of this analyte have been provided by European investigators. Its low molecular weight and high pI (9.2) enables it to be freely filtered through the glomerulus. Cystatin C is synthesized by all nucleated cells at a constant rate. Using receiver operator analysis, cystatin C is superior to creatinine in the assessment of GFR.[6,7]

Footnotes
1. Helin I, Axenram M, and Grubb A, "Serum Cystatin C as a Determinant of Glomerular Filtration Rate in Children," *Clin Nephrol*, 1998, 49(4):221-5.
2. Bokenkamp A, Domanetzki M, Zinck R, et al, "Cystatin C - A New Marker of Glomerular Filtration Rate in Children Independent of Age and Height," *Pediatrics*, 1998, 101(5):875-81.
3. Harmoinen AP, Kouri TT, Wirta OR, et al, "Evaluation of Plasma Cystatin C as a Marker for Glomerular Filtration Rate in Patients With Type 2 Diabetes," *Clin Nephrol*, 1999, 52(6):363-70.
4. Erlandsen EJ, Randers E, and Kristensen JH, "Evaluation of the Dade Behring N Latex Cystatin C Assay on the Dade Behring Nephelometer II System," *Scand J Clin Lab Invest*, 1999, 59(1):1-8.
5. Finney H, Newman DJ, Gruber W, et al, "Initial Evaluation of Cystatin C Measurement by Particle-Enhanced Immunonephelometry on the Behring Nephelometer Systems," *Clin Chem*, 1997, 43(6 Pt 1):1016-22.
6. Newman DJ and Price CP, "Renal Function and Nitrogen Metabolites," *Tietz Textbook of Clinical Chemistry*, 3rd ed, Burtis CA and Ashwood ER, eds, Philadelphia, PA: WB Saunders Co, 1999, 1204-70.
7. Stabuc B, Vrhovec L, Stabuc-Silih M, et al, "Improved Prediction of Decreased Creatinine Clearance by Serum Cystatin C: Use in Cancer Patients Before and During Chemotherapy," *Clin Chem*, 2000, 46(2):193-7.

References
Bokenkamp A, Ozden N, Dieterich C, et al, "Cystatin C and Creatinine After Successful Kidney Transplantation in Children," *Clin Nephrol*, 1999, 52(6):371-6.

Bostom AG, Gohh RY, Bausserman L, et al, "Serum Cystatin C as a Determinant of Fasting Total Homocysteine Levels in Renal Transplant Recipients With Normal Serum Creatinine," *J Am Soc Nephrol*, 1999, 10(1):164-6.

Keevil BG, Kilpatrick ES, Nichols SP, et al, "Biological Variation of Cystatin C: Implications for the Assessment of Glomerular Filtration Rate," *Clin Chem*, 1998, 44(7):1535-9.

Le Bricon T, Thervet E, Benlakehal M, et al, "Changes in Plasma Cystatin C After Renal Transplantation and Acute Rejection in Adults," *Clin Chem*, 1999, 45(12):2243-9.

Norlund L, Fex G, Lanke J, et al, "Reference Intervals for the Glomerular Filtration Rate and Cell-Proliferation Markers: Serum Cystatin C and Serum Beta 2-Microglobulin/Cystatin C-Ratio," *Scand J Clin Lab Invest*, 1997, 57(6):463-70.

Randers E, Kristensen JH, Erlandsen EJ, et al, "Serum Cystatin C as a Marker of the Renal Function," *Scand J Clin Lab Invest*, 1998, 58(7):585-92.

Stickle D, Cole B, Hock K, et al, "Correlation of Plasma Concentrations for Cystatin C and Creatinine to Inulin Clearance in a Pediatric Population," *Clin Chem*, 1998, 44(6 Pt 1):1334-8.

♦ **Cysteine, Qualitative** *see* Cystine, Urine *on page 164*

♦ **Cyst Fluid Chemistry** *see* Body Fluid Chemical Analysis *on page 123*

♦ **Cystic Fibrosis Sweat Test** *see* Chloride, Sweat *on page 144*

♦ **Cystine** *see* Amino Acids, Urine *on page 101*

Cystine, Urine

Related Information

Amino Acids, Urine *on page 101*
Kidney Stone Analysis *on page 877*
Urinalysis *on page 887*

Applies to Arginine; Cysteine, Qualitative; Homocyst(e)ine, Qualitative; Lysine; Nitroprusside Screening; Ornithine

Test Includes Homocystine, cysteine

Abstract Cystinuria is an inherited autosomal recessive disease in which excessive dibasic amino acids (lysine, ornithine, arginine, cystine) are excreted in the urine. Cystine is not soluble and causes stones. Patients with cystine stones face recurrent urolithiasis (33% recurrence rate) and repeated urinary tract infections.

Patient Preparation Penicillamine (a chelating agent) can cause false-negative results.

Specimen Random urine

Collection Random urine or 24-hour collection for quantitation

Storage Instructions Acidify to pH 2-3 or freeze specimen at -20°C, or 20 mL toluene can be added to the container prior to the start of a 24-hour collection.

Reference Interval Normal: 40-60 mg cystine/g creatinine; heterozygotes: <300 mg/g; homozygotes: >250 mg/g[1]

Use Detect cystinuria, homocystinuria and other diseases related to the sulfur-containing amino acids. Work up nephrolithiasis.[2,3,4] Cystine stones account for 1% to 3% of renal calculi.[5] Early age at onset, positive family history, and recurrence of urolithiasis are features suggestive of cystine lithiasis.[6]

Limitations Cystinosis, a different entity from **cystinuria,** is not detected by this test. Patients with cystinosis are diagnosed with cystine crystals in biopsies, corneal crystals on slit lamp examination or elevated leukocyte cystine levels.[7]

Methodology Microscopic examination of the sediment of a first morning urine sample can include the hexagonal crystals in samples from homozygotes.[1]

Nitroprusside (cyanide-nitroprusside) screening test is positive with cystine or homocystine. The urine nitroprusside test reacts positively at levels of 75-125 mg cystine/g creatinine,[1] but false positives occur. High performance liquid chromatography (HPLC), ion exchange chromatography are used for quantitation and distinction of cystine from homocyst(e)ine, as well as for confirmation of nitroprusside results.

Additional Information Classical cystinuria is the most common inborn error of amino acid transport. It is due to a transport defect in the third carrier system.[8] A positive screening test should be followed up by a quantitative procedure for cystine. In cystinosis, plasma cystine is usually normal, but increased cystine may be found in tissues. Therapy for cystinuria includes hydration, diet low in protein, urinary alkalinization (pH of urine maintained >7.5), chelation with thiol-containing compounds, surgery, and chemolysis. Cystine stones are radiopaque. They can cause staghorn calculi, can form a nidus of calcium oxalate stones, and appear to be more resistant to lithotripsy than most stones.[5] Percutaneous ultrasonic lithotripsy is described for such patients.[6]

Footnotes

1. Asplin JR, Coe FL, and Favus MJ, "Nephrolithiasis," *Harrison's Principles of Internal Medicine*, 14th ed, Chapter 279, Fauci AS, Braunwald E, Isselbacher KJ, et al, eds, New York, NY: McGraw-Hill Inc, 1998, 1569-74.
2. Wilson DM, "Clinical and Laboratory Approaches for Evaluation of Nephrolithiasis," *J Urol*, 1989, 141(3 Pt 2):770-4.
3. Pak CY, "Etiology and Treatment of Urolithiasis," *Am J Kidney Dis*, 1991, 18(6):624-37.
4. Sakhaee K, Poindexter JR, and Pak CY, "The Spectrum of Metabolic Abnormalities in Patients With Cystine Nephrolithiasis," *J Urol*, 1989, 141(4):819-21.
5. Singh A, Marshall FF, and Chang R, "Cystine Calculi: Clinical Management and *In Vitro* Observations," *Urology*, 1988, 31(3):207-10.
6. Knoll LD, Segura JW, Patterson DE, et al, "Long-Term Follow-up in Patients With Cystine Urinary Calculi Treated by Percutaneous Ultrasonic Lithotripsy," *J Urol*, 1988, 140(2):246-8.
7. Markello TC, Bernardini IM, and Gahl WA, "Improved Renal Function in Children With Cystinosis Treated With Cysteamine," *N Engl J Med*, 1993, 328(16):1157-62.
8. Kinne RK, "Amino Acid Transporters," *Curr Opin Nephrol Hypertens*, 1995, 4(5):412-5.

References

Asplin JR and Coe FL, "Hereditary Tubular Disorders," *Harrison's Principles of Internal Medicine*, 14th ed, Chapter 278, Fauci AS, Braunwald E, Isselbacher KJ, et al, eds, New York, NY: McGraw-Hill Inc, 1998, 1562-9.

Elsas LJ, Longo N, and Rosenberg LE, "Inherited Disorders of Amino Acid Metabolism and Storage," *Harrison's Principles of Internal Medicine*, 14th ed, Chapter 349, Fauci AS, Braunwald E, Isselbacher KJ, et al, eds, New York, NY: McGraw-Hill Inc, 1998, 2194-203.

Ng CS and Streem SB, "Contemporary Management of Cystinuria," *J Endourol*, 1999, 13(9):647-51.

Singer A and Das S, "Cystinuria: A Review of the Pathophysiology and Management," *J Urol*, 1989, 142(3):669-73.

◆ **Dehydroepiandrosterone** *see* 17-Ketosteroids Fractionation, Urine *on page 206*

Dehydroepiandrosterone and Dehydroepiandrosterone Sulfate, Serum or Plasma

Related Information

Adrenocorticotropic Hormone, Plasma *on page 86*
Androstenedione, Serum *on page 104*
Cortisol, Free, Urine *on page 154*
Cortisol, Serum or Plasma *on page 154*
Estradiol, Serum *on page 170*
17-Hydroxyprogesterone, Serum or Plasma *on page 197*
Testosterone, Total and Free, Serum or Plasma *on page 280*

Synonyms DHEA; DHEA-S

Applies to Androstenedione; Dehydroepiandrosterone, Serum; Dehydroepiandrosterone Sulfate, Serum; Epitestosterone; Estradiol; 17-Ketosteroids; Testosterone

Abstract Dehydroepiandrosterone (DHEA) and its conjugated sulfate metabolite, DHEA-S are 19-carbon steroids synthesized in and secreted by the adrenal cortex, under the influence of adrenocorticotropin (ACTH). In the adrenal and in peripheral tissues, DHEA and DHEA-S are interconvertible into each other. In healthy women, the adrenal cortex is the exclusive site of DHEA and DHEA-S synthesis. In men, the adrenal cortex is the principal site of DHEA and DHEA-S synthesis. In addition, ~10% to 25% of DHEA and ~5% of DHEA-S originates in the testes. While both DHEA and DHEA-S are themselves weak androgens, both can be converted, in peripheral tissues, into more potent androgens (eg, androstenedione or testosterone), and into estrogens (eg, estradiol). In normal persons, the serum concentration (molar basis) of DHEA-S is approximately 300-500 times higher than the concentration of DHEA. This concentration difference is, at least in part, due to the much slower metabolic clearance of DHEA-S: the half-life of DHEA-S is 10-20 hours, while the half-life of DHEA is 1-3 hours.[1,2] DHEA exhibits only diurnal variation, while DHEA-S exhibits only very minimal diurnal variation. DHEA and DHEA-S serum levels fall shortly after birth, remain low in early childhood, and then rise from about age 8 years and reach a peak at about 30 years of age. After age 30, there is a gradual decrease in serum levels of both DHEA and DHEA-S. By age 70-80, DHEA and DHEA-S values are ~10% to 25% of their peak values.[2] The significance of this decline is widely studied, but not understood. A cross-sectional analysis of older adults has found that men with DHEA-S levels in the highest quartile are more fit, more lean, and have higher levels of total and free testosterone, than do comparable men with DHEA-S values in the lowest quartile. No comparable correlation was found in women.[3]

Special Instructions Often both tests are ordered at the same time. When only one is obtained, it is usually DHEA-S.

Specimen Serum or plasma

Container Red top tube or lavender top (EDTA) tube

Storage Instructions Separate within 1 hour of collection. Serum or plasma stable 24 hours at 4°C. Freeze for longer storage.

Patient Preparation Avoid recently administered radioisotopes if assay method is RIA.

Causes for Rejection Recently administered radioisotopes if RIA is used for assay

Reference Interval See table.

Reference Intervals for Dehydroepiandrosterone Sulfate and Unconjugated Dehydroepiandrosterone in Serum

Age	Male (μg/dL)	Female (μg/dL)	Male (μmol/L)	Female (μmol/L)
Dehydroepiandrosterone Sulfate				
Children				
1-5 d	12-254	10-248	0.3-6.9	0.3-6.7
1 mo to 5 y	1-41	5-55	0.03-1.1	0.1-1.5
6-9 y	2.5-145	2.5-140	0.07-3.9	0.07-3.8
10-11 y	15-115	15-260	0.4-3.1	0.4-7.0
12-17 y	20-555	20-535	0.5-15.0	0.5-14.4
Pubertal Levels (Tanner Stage)				
1	5-265	5-125	0.1-7.2	0.1-3.4
2	15-380	15-150	0.4-10.3	0.4-4.0
3	60-505	20-535	1.6-13.6	0.5-14.4
4	65-560	35-485	1.8-15.1	0.9-13.1
5	165-500	75-530	4.4-13.5	2.0-14.3
Adults				
18-30 y	125-619	45-380	3.4-16.7	1.2-10.3
31-50 y	59-452	12-379	1.6-12.2	0.8-10.2
51-60 y	20-413		0.5-11.1	
61-83 y	10-285		0.36-7.7	
Postmenopausal female		30-260		0.8-7.0
Dehydroepiandrosterone, Unconjugated				
6-9 y	13-187	18-189	0.45-6.49	0.62-6.55
10-11 y	31-205	112-224	1.07-7.11	3.88-7.77
12-14 y	83-258	98-360	2.88-8.95	3.40-12.5
Adults	180-1250	130-980	6.25-43.4	4.51-34.0

Gronowski AM and Landau-Levine M. "Reproductive Endocrine Function," *Tietz Textbook of Clinical Chemistry*, 3rd ed, Burtis CA and Ashwood ER, eds, Philadelphia, PA: WB Saunders Co, 1999, 1632.

Use

Adrenal hyperfunction. Because of metabolic blockade, DHEA and DHEA-S are elevated in congenital adrenal hyperplasias (CAH) (both the 11-beta hydroxylase and the 21-beta hydroxylase forms). Virilizing adrenal neoplasms are often responsible for elevated DHEA and DHEA-S serum levels. In the clinical context of female hirsutism, elevated basal DHEA-S and testosterone usually point to an adrenal cause. When a woman with hirsutism has normal basal DHEA-S and testosterone values, an adrenal tumor is unlikely.[4]

Virilization in girls. Signs of virilization in pubertal or prepubertal girls are most commonly due to the onset of adrenarche, the adrenal contribution to puberty, a normal physiologic condition involving the onset of adrenal androgen secretion. Less commonly, virilization in girls is due to late-onset congenital adrenal hyperplasia (CAH) or a virilizing adrenal neoplasm. All three conditions are associated with elevated serum DHEA-S. Biochemical differentiation among these requires additional testing.[5]

Adrenal insufficiency. Many patients, especially women, with adrenal insufficiency have low basal DHEA and DHEA-S values. Arlt et al[6] have reported beneficial effects of treating such patients with DHEA in addition to the standard glucocorticoid and mineralocorticoid replacement. Editorial comments on this are published.[7]

Reversing certain effects of aging. The dramatic decrease in serum DHEA and DHEA-S values after age 30 (see Abstract)[2] and research results showing a positive correlation between DHEA and DHEA-S serum levels with markers of good health in older persons[3] have led many to speculate that DHEA dietary supplements, accompanied by laboratory monitoring, might make a beneficial contribution to the physiology of older persons.[2,8,9,10] Others warn, to the contrary, that a randomized prospective clinical trial has not been conducted, and there may be detrimental effects on hormone-sensitive organs (eg, breast and prostate), and the quantity and distribution of body fat may be important in determination of the overall effects of such supplementation.[11]

Methodology Immunoassay (multiple labels and formats) and gas chromatography/mass spectrometry (GC/MS)

Additional Information Extensive compilations of DHEA and DHEA-S levels in a wide range of medical conditions are available: the effects of various activities known to influence endogenous DHEA and DHEA-S levels, the effects of drugs on endogenous DHEA and DHEA-S levels, and DHEA and DHEA-S blood levels associated with the administration of DHEA by various dosages and routes are available.[2]

Thyroid disease. Tagawa et al have reported that serum DHEA and DHEA-S levels are low in patients with hypothyroidism; in hyperthyroidism, DHEA-S was increased, but DHEA was normal.[12]

Athletic performance enhancement. As part of a program to detect the abuse of anabolic steroids, the International Olympic Commission and the U.S. military measure urinary testosterone (T) and its metabolite, epitestosterone (E). These organizations use a T:E ratio >6.0 as an indication of exogenous steroid use. Bowers[13] has reported that higher DHEA doses can be associated with T:E ratios >6.0. In another report, none of 12 men taking 25 mg of DHEA per day had a T:E ratio >6.0.[14] In December 1996, DHEA was added to the list of prohibited compounds by the International Olympic Commission.[13]

Of historical interest is the fact that urinary DHEA and DHEA-S are major constituents of the urine test, "17-ketosteroids," once a mainstay of the laboratory evaluation of adrenal function.

Footnotes

1. Orth DN and Kovacs WJ, "The Adrenal Cortex," *Williams Textbook of Endocrinology,* 9th ed, Wilson JD, Foster DW, Kronenberg HM, et al, eds, Philadelphia, PA: WB Saunders Co, 1998, 517-664.
2. Kroboth PD, Salek FS, Pittenger AL, et al, "DHEA and DHEA-S: A Review," *J Clin Pharmacol,* 1999, 39(4):327-48.
3. Abbasi A, Duthi EH, Sheldahl L, et al, "Association of Dehydroepiandrosterone Sulfate, Body Composition, and Physical Fitness in Independent Community-Dwelling Older Men and Women," *J Am Geriatr Soc,* 1998, 46(3):263-73.
4. Derksen J, Nagesser SK, Meinders AE, et al, "Identification of Virilizing Adrenal Tumors in Hirsute Women," *N Engl J Med,* 1994, 331(15):968-73.
5. Street ME, Weber A, Camacho-Hubner C, et al, "Girls With Virilization in Childhood: A Diagnostic Protocol for Investigation," *J Clin Pathol,* 1997, 50(5):379-83.
6. Arlt W, Callies F, Vlijmen JC, et al, "Dehydroepiandrosterone Replacement in Women With Adrenal Insufficiency," *N Engl J Med,* 1999, 341(14):1013-20.
7. Oelkers W, "Dehydroepiandrosterone for Adrenal Insufficiency," *N Engl J Med,* 1999, 341(14):1073-4.
8. Morales AJ, Nolan JJ, Nelson JC, et al, "Effects of Replacement Dose of Dehydroepiandrosterone in Men and Women of Advancing Age," *J Clin Endocrinol Metab,* 1994, 78(6):1360-7.
9. Casson PR, Andersen RN, Herrod HG, et al, "Oral Dehydroepiandrosterone in Physiologic Doses Modulates Immune Function in Postmenopausal Women," *Am J Obstet Gynecol,* 1993, 169(6):1536-9.
10. Morales AJ, Haubrich RH, Hwang JY, et al, "The Effect of Six Months Treatment With a 100 mg Daily Dose of Dehydroepiandrosterone (DHEA) on Circulating Sex Steroids, Body Composition and Muscle Strength in Age-Advanced Men and Women," *Clin Endocrinol,* 1998, 49(4):421-32.

11. Skolnick AA, "Scientific Verdict Still Out on DHEA," *JAMA,* 1996, 276(17):1365-7.
12. Tagawa N, Tamanaka J, Fujinami A, et al, "Serum Dehydroepiandrosterone, Dehydroepiandrosterone Sulfate, and Pregnenolone Sulfate Concentrations in Patients With Hyperthyroidism and Hypothyroidism," *Clin Chem,* 46(4):523-8.
13. Bowers LD, "Oral Dehydroepiandrosterone Supplementation Can Increase the Testosterone/Epitestosterone Ratio," *Clin Chem,* 1999, 45(2):295-7.
14. Dehnnin L, Ferry M, Lafarge P, et al, "Oral Administration of Dehydroepiandrosterone to Healthy Men: Alteration of the Urinary Androgen Profile and Consequences for the Detection of Abuse in Sport by Gas Chromatography-Mass Spectrometry," *Steroids,* 1998, 63(2):80-7.

References

Arlt W, Haas J, Callies F, et al, "Biotransformation of Oral Dehydroepiandrosterone in Elderly Men: Significant Increase in Circulating Estrogens," *J Clin Endocrinol Metab,* 1999, 84(6):2170-6.

Barnhart KT, Freeman E, Grisso JA, et al, "The Effect of Dehydroepiandrosterone Supplementation to Symptomatic Perimenopausal Women on Serum Endocrine Profiles, Lipid Parameters, and Health-Related Quality of Life," *J Clin Endocrinol Metab,* 1999, 84(11):3896-902.

Ebeling P and Koivisto VA, "Physiological Importance of Dehydroepiandrosterone," *Lancet,* 1994, 343(8911):1479-81.

Flynn MA, Weaver-Osterholtz D, Sharpe-Timms KL, et al, "Dehydroepiandrosterone Replacement in Aging Humans," *J Clin Endocrinol Metab,* 1999, 84(5):1527-33.

Gronowski AM and Landau-Levine M, "Reproductive Endocrine Function," *Tietz Textbook of Clinical Chemistry,* 3rd ed, Burtis CA and Ashwood ER, eds, Philadelphia, PA: WB Saunders Co, 1999, 1632.

Herbert J, "The Age of Dehydroepiandrosterone," *Lancet,* 1995, 345(8959):1193-4.

Mazza E, Maccario M, Ramunni J, et al, "Dehydroepiandrosterone Sulfate Levels in Women. Relationships With Age, Body Mass Index and Insulin Levels," *J Endocrinol Invest,* 1999, 22(9):681-7.

Tilvis RS, Kahonen M, and Harkonen M, "Dehydroepiandrosterone Sulfate, Diseases and Mortality in a General Aged Population," *Aging,* 1999, 11(1):30-4.

♦ **Dehydroepiandrosterone, Serum** *see* Dehydroepiandrosterone and Dehydroepiandrosterone Sulfate, Serum or Plasma *on page 164*

♦ **Dehydroepiandrosterone Sulfate, Serum** *see* Dehydroepiandrosterone and Dehydroepiandrosterone Sulfate, Serum or Plasma *on page 164*

Delta (5)-Aminolevulinic Acid, Urine

Related Information

Lead, Blood *on page 793*
Lead, Urine *on page 795*
Porphobilinogen, Qualitative, Urine *on page 255*
Porphyrins, Quantitative, Urine *on page 255*
Protoporphyrin, Free Erythrocyte *on page 269*
Protoporphyrin, Zinc, Blood *on page 270*

Synonyms ALA; Aminolevulinic Acid; 5-Aminolevulinic Acid; Delta-ALA

Applies to ALA Dehydratase

Abstract Delta (5)-aminolevulinic acid (ALA) is a precursor of the porphyrins (uroporphyrin, coproporphyrin, and protoporphyrin). The acute neurological porphyrias are associated with ALA and porphobilinogen (PBG). Toxins including alcohol, lead and other heavy metals cause increase in ALA by inhibiting porphobilinogen synthase. The other conditions which increase ALA are acute intermittent porphyria, hereditary coproporphyria, porphyria variegata, and some malignancies.[1]

Specimen 24-hour urine

Container Dark urine container, kept on ice

Collection Acidify with acetic acid to pH 3-4.5; some laboratories use 2 g barbituric acid as a preservative. Sodium bicarbonate is appropriate as a preservative also for porphyrins and porphobilinogen.

Storage Instructions Protect from light and freeze.

Reference Interval Normal: 1.3-7.0 mg/24 hours urine (SI: 53 μmol/day), depending on method and laboratory

Possible Panic Range >20 mg/24 hours (SI: 9.9-53.4 μmol/day)

Use Diagnose porphyrias: delta-ALA may be increased in attacks of acute intermittent porphyria, hereditary coproporphyria, and porphyria variegata. Evaluate lead or mercury poisoning, and certain neurological problems with abdominal pain. Urinary delta-ALA is not a sensitive indicator of lead poisoning in children because it does not increase until blood lead concentration is 40 μg/dL, well above the recommended level of <10 μg/dL. ALA is increased also in tyrosinemia.[2] **Porphobilinogen, delta aminolevulinic acid, and uroporphyrinogen-1 synthase are the tests of choice for acute intermittent porphyria.**

Limitations ALA may be normal during latent period of acute intermittent porphyria, hereditary coproporphyria, and porphyria variegata. For the diagnosis of lead poisoning, measurement of blood and urine lead, free erythrocyte protoporphyrin and ALA dehydratase in red cells are available.

Methodology Ion-exchange resin columns, colorimetry. An alternative photometric method for rapid testing has been proposed.[3]

Additional Information ALA is highly soluble in water, and it has low renal threshold. Consequently, it concentrates in the urine and remains at low concentrations in blood. Conversion of ALA to porphobilinogen is inhibited by lead and mercury; thus, **lead poisoning** causes increased urinary delta-ALA as well as increases of coproporphyrin, free erythrocyte protoporphyrin, and inhibition of ALA dehydratase. Molecular lesions have been identified in a severely affected homozygote with delta aminolevulinate dehydratase deficient porphyria.[4] See Lead, Blood *on page 793* and Porphyrins, Quantitative, Urine *on page 255.*
(Continued)

Delta (5)-Aminolevulinic Acid, Urine *(Continued)*

Footnotes

1. Nuttall KL, "Porphyrins and Disorders of Porphyrin Metabolism," *Tietz Textbook of Clinical Chemistry*, 3rd ed, Burtis CA and Ashwood ER, eds, Philadelphia: WB Saunders Co, 1999, 1711-35.
2. "Hereditary Tyrosinemia," *Lancet*, 1990, 335(8704):1500-1.
3. Buttery JE, Stuart S, and Pannall PR, "An Improved Direct Method for the Measurement of Urinary Delta-Aminolevulinic Acid," *Clin Biochem*, 1995, 28(4):477-80.
4. Plewinska M, Thunell S, Holmberg L, et al, "Delta-Aminolevulinate Dehydratase Deficient Porphyria: Identification of the Molecular Lesions in a Severely Affected Homozygote," *Am J Hum Genet*, 1991, 49(1):167-74.

References

Bird TD, Wallace DM, and Labbe RF, "The Porphyria, Plumbism, Pottery Puzzle," *JAMA*, 1982, 247:813-4.

Elder GH, Smith SG, and Smyth SJ, "Laboratory Investigation of the Porphyrias," *Ann Clin Biochem*, 1990, 27(Pt 5):395-412.

Sassa S, "ALAD Porphyria," *Semin Liver Dis*, 1998, 18(1):95-101.

Sassa S, "Hematological Aspects of Porphyrias," *Int J Hematol*, 2000, 71(1):1-17.

Takebayashi T, Omae K, Hosada K, et al, "Evaluation of Delta-Aminolevulinic Acid in Blood of Workers Exposed to Lead," *Br J Ind Med*, 1993, 50(1):49-54.

♦ **Delta-ALA** *see* Delta (5)-Aminolevulinic Acid, Urine *on page 165*

♦ **Delta Aminolevulinic Acid** *see* Porphobilinogen, Qualitative, Urine *on page 255*

♦ **Delta Base** *see* Base Excess, Blood *on page 114*

♦ **Delta Bilirubin** *see* Bilirubin, Direct, Serum *on page 117*

♦ **Deoxycorticosterone** *see* 17-Hydroxyprogesterone, Serum or Plasma *on page 197*

♦ **11-Deoxycortisol** *see* Metyrapone Stimulation Test, Serum *on page 225*

♦ **Deoxypyridinoline** *see* Osteocalcin, Serum or Plasma *on page 237*

♦ **Deoxypyridinoline** *see* Pyridinolines (Pyridinoline and Deoxypyridinoline), Urine *on page 272*

♦ **Deoxypyridoline** *see* N-Telopeptides, Urine *on page 233*

♦ **De Ritis Ratio** *see* Liver Disease: Laboratory Assessment, Overview *on page 216*

♦ **Dermatan Sulfates** *see* Mucopolysaccharides, Urine *on page 226*

♦ **11-Desoxycortisol** *see* 17-Hydroxyprogesterone, Serum or Plasma *on page 197*

♦ **Dexamethasone-CRH Protocol** *see* Corticotropin-Releasing Hormone Stimulation Test *on page 152*

♦ **Dexamethasone Suppression** *see* Adrenocorticotropic Hormone, Plasma *on page 86*

♦ **Dexamethasone Suppression Test** *see* Adrenal Cortex: Laboratory Assessments Overview *on page 84*

♦ **Dexamethasone Suppression Test** *see* Cortisol, Serum or Plasma *on page 154*

♦ **1,4-α-D Glucanohydrolase, Serum** *see* Amylase, Serum *on page 102*

♦ **1,4-α-D Glucanohydrolase, Urine** *see* Amylase, Urine *on page 104*

♦ **DHEA** *see* Dehydroepiandrosterone and Dehydroepiandrosterone Sulfate, Serum or Plasma *on page 164*

♦ **DHEA-S** *see* Dehydroepiandrosterone and Dehydroepiandrosterone Sulfate, Serum or Plasma *on page 164*

♦ **Dialysis** *see* Urea Nitrogen, Serum or Plasma *on page 293*

♦ **Diamond-Blackfan Syndrome** *see* Erythropoietin Receptor *on page 169*

Dibucaine Number, Serum or Plasma

Related Information

Acetylcholinesterase, Red Cell *on page 81*
Organophosphate Pesticides, Urine, Blood, or Serum *on page 804*
Pseudocholinesterase, Serum *on page 270*

Synonyms Pseudocholinesterase Inhibition by Dibucaine

Applies to Dibucaine Toxicity; Fluoride Inhibition of Cholinesterase

Abstract Dibucaine is a substance which inhibits the normal variant of the enzyme cholinesterase. Abnormal variants are less inhibited. Percent inhibition (dibucaine number) is obtained by comparing results from the inhibited reaction with noninhibited reaction.

Specimen Serum or plasma

Container Red top tube or green top (heparin) tube

Collection Do not collect within 24 hours of administration of muscle relaxant.

Storage Instructions Serum cholinesterase (pseudocholinesterase) is stable and may be stored at 0°C to 4°C or at room temperature for 1 year or more and may be frozen/thawed a number of times without changing activity of the enzyme.[1]

Reference Interval Normal individuals have normal (high) amounts of serum cholinesterase (pseudocholinesterase) activity which can be inhibited by dibucaine. Approximately 70% to 86% inhibition is normal; atypical enzyme shows resistance to inhibition, at about the level of only 20%. See reference range of laboratory doing the test.

Possible Panic Range Homozygotes for abnormal cholinesterase activity have low results (low percent inhibition) in assay for serum cholinesterase (pseudocholinesterase). Administration of succinylcholine may pose a risk to patients with abnormal pseudocholinesterase, because there is abnormal persistence of the succinylcholine effect.

Use Assess presence of homozygous or heterozygous "atypical" cholinesterase variant in patients who have normal or low result (low inhibition) of serum cholinesterase assay and may be at risk of apnea when given succinylcholine muscle relaxant. Dibucaine inhibition provides identification of an abnormal allele. Sensitivity of pseudocholinesterase to dibucaine inhibition may distinguish congenital from acquired forms of abnormal pseudocholinesterase activity. About 4% of the population have abnormal inherited forms.[2]

Limitations No single simple test currently exists that can detect all enzyme variants. Traditional tests including dibucaine inhibition are not adequate to identify all variants. Instances of prolonged response to succinylcholine still go without explanation.

Methodology Hydrolysis of propionylthiocholine or butyrylthiocholine with and without dibucaine at 20°C to 40°C; fluoride inhibition at 25°C.[3,4,5]

Additional Information The degree of serum cholinesterase inhibition produced by dibucaine (and fluoride) is under genetic control. Sensitivity to succinylcholine is dependent upon at least four allelic genes. The most widely accepted system of classification (Motulsky) designates E_1 as the first locus for plasma cholinesterase (see table). The $E_1{}^u$ gene codes for the most common form of the plasma enzyme. The $E_1{}^a$ gene is responsible for the atypical enzyme which resists inhibition by dibucaine, $E_1{}^f$ gene for the enzyme that is fluoride resistant, and the $E_1{}^s$ (silent) gene results in an enzyme with little or no activity. An international gene nomenclature conference has proposed a system designating the four alleles as "CHE1·U," "CHE1·A," "CHE1·F," and "CHE1·QO." Single quantitative cholinesterase determinations may not be reliable in detecting sensitivity to succinylcholine, as variant enzymes exhibit qualitative and quantitative differences in substrate specificity. Another common phenotypic designation (of the 15 different phenotypes known) is those at risk, AF; FS and FF (moderate risk); and AA, AS, and SS (severe risk).

Genotype	Phenotype	Previous Term	Dibucaine Number
$E_1{}^u E_1{}^u$	U	Usual	84
$E_1{}^u E_1{}^a$	I	Intermediate	73
$E_1{}^a E_1{}^a$	A	Atypical	32
$E_1{}^u E_1{}^s$	U	Usual	
$E_1{}^s E_1{}^s$	S	Silent	81
$E_1{}^u E_1{}^f$	UF		
$E_1{}^f E_1{}^f$	F		

Dibucaine and fluoride numbers indicate the percent inhibition of enzyme activity by these agents when a serum sample is tested under standard conditions (inhibition expressed as a percent). This approach to screening for presence of serum cholinesterase variants does not entirely avoid the problem of variation in reactivity with some atypical enzymes. Individuals with the genotype $E_1{}^u$, $E_1{}^f$ show resistance to fluoride inhibition (low fluoride number) but do not show resistance to dibucaine inhibition (the normal situation with high dibucaine number). This variant was published almost 30 years ago by Harris and Whittaker.[6] Prolonged apnea following hemodilutional cardiopulmonary bypass has been reported in a patient whose preoperative plasma cholinesterase level was slightly below the normal range.[7]

Accidental dibucaine ingestion in children can be fatal. Toxicity may be manifested by emesis, lethargy, tonic-clonic seizures, and bradycardia, ventricular tachycardia, and dysrhythmia.[8]

Footnotes

1. Huizenga JR, van der Belt K, Gips CH, et al, "The Effect of Storage at Different Temperatures on Cholinesterase Activity in Human Serum," *J Clin Chem Clin Biochem*, 1985, 23(5):283-5.
2. Holownia P, Newman DJ, Bruno C, et al, "Automated Dibucaine Number Measurement With DuPont Dimension® ES and AR Analyzers," *Clin Chem*, 1995, 41(5):664-7.
3. Abernethy MH, George PM, Herron JL, et al, "Plasma Cholinesterase Phenotyping With Use of Visible-Region Spectrophotometry," *Clin Chem*, 1986, 32(1 Pt 1):194-7.
4. Abernethy MH, George PM, and Melton VE, "A New Succinylcholine-Based Assay of Plasma Cholinesterase," *Clin Chem*, 1984, 30(2):192-5.
5. Evans RT and Wroe J, "Is Serum Cholinesterase Activity a Predictor of Succinyl Choline Sensitivity? An Assessment of Four Methods," *Clin Chem*, 1978, 24(10):1762-6.
6. Harris H and Whittaker M, "Differential Inhibition of Human Serum Cholinesterase With Fluoride: Recognition of Two New Phenotypes," *Nature*, 1961, 496-8.
7. Jackson SH, Bailey GW, and Stevens G, "Reduced Plasma Cholinesterase Following Haemodilutional Cardiopulmonary Bypass," *Anaesthesia*, 1982, 37(3):319-20.
8. Dayan PS, Litovitz TL, Crouch BI, et al, "Fatal Accidental Dibucaine Poisoning in Children," *Ann Emerg Med*, 1996, 28(4):442-5.

References

Hosseini J, Firuzian F, and Feely J, "Ethnic Differences in Frequency Distribution of Serum Cholinesterase Activity," *Ir J Med Sci*, 1997, 166(1):10-2.

Kambam JR, Horton B, Parris WC, et al, "Pseudocholinesterase Activity in Human Cerebrospinal Fluid," *Anesth Analg*, 1989, 68(4):486-8.

Marrs TC, "Organophosphate Poisoning," *Pharmacol Ther*, 1993, 58(1):51-66.

Pantuck EJ, "Plasma Cholinesterase: Gene and Variations," *Anesth Analg*, 1993, 77(2):380-6.

♦ **Dibucaine Toxicity** *see* Dibucaine Number, Serum or Plasma *on page 166*

♦ **DIDMOAD Syndrome** *see* Cobalamin, Serum *on page 150*

♦ **Dihydropteridine Reductase** *see* Newborn Screen for Phenylketonuria *on page 229*

♦ **Dihydrotestosterone** *see* Testosterone, Total and Free, Serum or Plasma *on page 280*

Dihydrotestosterone, Serum

Related Information
Testosterone, Total and Free, Serum or Plasma *on page 280*

Abstract Dihydrotestosterone (DHT) is produced from testosterone by the action of 5-alpha reductase, an enzyme found in many androgen-sensitive tissues (eg, skin, prostate, other internal genitalia). Whereas testosterone may be metabolized to DHT or to the estrogen, estradiol, DHT is not converted into estrogen and is much more potent an androgen than is testosterone. Most disorders involving excess or insufficient testicular androgen are well evaluated by measuring Testosterone, Total and Free, Serum or Plasma *on page 280*. In the 46X,Y fetus, the development of the external genitalia depends on the action of DHT.[1]

Specimen Serum

Container Red top tube

Storage Instructions Separate serum and freeze.

Special Instructions No recent radioisotopes

Reference Interval The reference interval is not well defined at present. Below are indicated intervals from two reference laboratories.[2,3]

Male:
- ≤20 years: not established
- 20-39 years: 150-1240 pg/mL[2]
- 20-49 years: 155-553 pg/mL[3]
- >40 years: 150-980 pg/mL[2]
- >50 years: 36-573 pg/mL[3]

Female:
- ≤20 years: not established
- 20-39 years: 50-250 pg/mL[2]
- 15-49 years: 5.5-170 pg/mL[3]
- >40 years: 50-137 pg/mL[2]
- >50 years: 36-573 pg/mL[3]

Use

Drugs which inhibit 5-alpha reductase: Certain drugs (eg, finasteride) used to treat benign prostatic hyperplasia exert their effect by inhibiting 5-alpha reductase, an enzyme in peripheral tissues which converts testosterone to DHT. Therefore, serum DHT may be useful in monitoring treatment with this drug class.

Congenital 5-alpha reductase deficiency: This rare autosomal recessive disorder classically includes a phenotypic male, 46XY infant with hypospadias, a urogenital sinus opening on the perineum, a blind vaginal pouch, and normal appearing testes which may be cryptorchid or in labioscrotal folds.[4] With the onset of puberty, plasma testosterone (total and free) values are normal, but dihydrotestosterone values are very low, reflecting the absence of 5-alpha reductase.[5]

Methodology Radioimmunoassay (RIA)

Additional Information Of all the androgenic hormones, serum DHT is the only one that has been shown to correlate with male sexual functioning.[6]

Footnotes
1. Hughes IA, "A Novel Explanation for Resistance to Androgens," *N Engl J Med*, 2000, 343(12):881-2
2. Mayo Medical Laboratories, *2001 Test Catalogue*, Rochester, MN, 196.
3. ARUP Laboratories, *1999-2000 User's Guide*, 262.
4. New MI and Josso N, "Disorders of Sexual Differentiation," *Cecil Textbook of Medicine*, 21st ed, Chapter 246, Goldman L and Bennett JC, eds, Philadelphia, PA: WB Saunders Co, 2000, 1267-1306.
5. Grumbach MM and Conte FA, *Williams Textbook of Endocrinology*, 9th ed, Wilson JD, Foster DW, Kronenberg HM, et al, eds, Philadelphia, PA: WB Saunders Co, 1998, 1391-4.
6. Mantzoros CS, Georgiadis EI, and Trichopoulos D, "Contribution of Dihydrotestosterone to Male Sexual Behaviour," *BMJ*, 1995, 310(6990):1289-91.

References

Adachi M, Takayanagi R, Tomura A, et al, "Androgen-Insensitivity Syndrome as a Possible Coactivator Disease," *N Engl J Med*, 2000, 343(12):856-62.

♦ **1,25-Dihydroxy Vitamin D₃** *see* Vitamin D, Serum *on page 300*

♦ **2,3-Diphosphoglycerate (2,3-DPG)** *see* Oxygen Saturation, Blood *on page 240*

♦ **Direct Bilirubin** *see* Bilirubin, Direct, Serum *on page 117*

♦ **Disaturated Phosphatidylcholine** *see* Lecithin:Sphingomyelin Ratio, Amniotic Fluid *on page 210*

♦ **D-Lactate** *see* Lactic Acid, Whole Blood or Plasma *on page 208*

♦ **Dopamine** *see* Catecholamines, Fractionation, Plasma *on page 138*

♦ **Dopamine** *see* Vanillylmandelic Acid, Urine *on page 297*

♦ **Dopamine, Urine** *see* Catecholamines, Fractionation, Urine *on page 139*

♦ **Double Test** *see* Pregnancy-Associated Protein A, Serum *on page 260*

♦ **DPD** *see* Osteocalcin, Serum or Plasma *on page 237*

♦ **2,3-DPG** *see* Oxygen Saturation, Blood *on page 240*

♦ **2,3-DPG** *see* P_{50}, Blood *on page 241*

d-Xylose Absorption Test, Serum, Urine

Related Information
Endomysial Antibodies *on page 525*
Gliadin IgG/IgA Antibodies *on page 526*

Synonyms Xylose Absorption Test; Xylose Tolerance Test

Applies to [^{14}C] d-Xylose Breath Test

Abstract d-Xylose is a five-carbon monosaccharide not normally present in significant amounts in the blood. It is passively absorbed unchanged by the normal duodenum and jejunum, and it is excreted unmetabolized by the kidneys. The d-xylose absorption test is used as a screening test for intestinal carbohydrate malabsorption. An oral dose of d-xylose is administered to the fasting patient, and, after a specified period, d-xylose is measured in the patient's timed urine collection and/or serum specimen. Low recoveries in the urine are consistent with intestinal malabsorption syndromes.

Patient Preparation Urea nitrogen, creatinine, and first morning urinalysis should be normal. Patient must fast a minimum of 8 hours prior to administration of d-xylose. Pediatric patients must be fasting for at least 4 hours. Patient must remain in a supine position for duration of the test, except during urine collection. No food is permitted during the test. Since d-xylose is a pentose, the patient should refrain from eating foods containing pentoses. These include fruits, jams, jellies, and pastries. Many medications, including aspirin, indomethacin, other nonsteroidal anti-inflammatory drugs, neomycin, glipizide, or atropine interfere. These and preferably all medications should be discontinued for 24 hours prior to the test. No water restriction is required; in fact, patients should be encouraged to drink during the fasting period and during the test. Start the test in the AM. If a urine collection is to be done, instruct patient to void completely and discard this urine. If a blood determination is to be done and the testing laboratory so requires, draw a fasting blood specimen.

Administer the dose of d-xylose orally (adults, usually 25 g or 5 g, if specified by physician; children younger than 12 years, 5 g or a weight-based dosage equal to 0.5 g/kg body weight up to a maximum of 25 g). The dose should be dissolved in water, making an ~10% (w/v) solution with a maximum of 500 mL. Patient should drink the entire amount. Fill cup with 250 mL of water and have patient drink this as well. Have patient drink another cup with 250 mL of water after 1 hour. Collect urine for 5 hours after administration of d-xylose.

Specimen The specimens usually include, as indicated, a 5-hour, postdose urine collection, (preserved by refrigeration or freezing, according to the instructions of the testing laboratory) and a 1-hour, postdose serum or plasma specimen. (Some protocols call for a 2-hour postdose blood collection rather than a 1-hour, and others call for serial, hourly blood draws up to 5 hours postdose. Check with the testing laboratory beforehand.)

Craig and Atkinson[1] recommended (in a 1988 paper) a 25 g d-xylose absorption test with a 5-hour urine collection and a 1-hour serum specimen for adults with normal renal function and a 1-hour serum specimen only in adult patients with intermediate renal insufficiency. However, Peled et al[2] subsequently showed that the 5-hour urine collection much more accurately reflects abnormal intestinal absorption than the 1-hour serum specimen; therefore, many laboratories recommend that only the 5-hour urine collection be done in adults (12 years or older) with normal renal function.

In children and infants younger than 12 years of age, only a 1-hour serum specimen is recommended. Urine specimens should not be collected due to difficulties with collections in these age groups.

Container Containers include an appropriately labeled urine container, red top tube, green top (heparin) tube, or gray top (sodium fluoride/potassium) tube as required by testing needs and/or testing laboratory.

Reference Interval Reference intervals vary with the protocol used. Reference range for a 5-hour urine collection in adults ≥12 years (25-gram dose) is **≥4 g/5 hours (SI: ≥26.6 mmol/5 hours)**. The table below summarizes the serum ranges recommended by Craig and Atkinson.[1] See following table.

Craig, Atkinson, and others urge that urine tests be abandoned for children younger than 12 years of age[1,3] due to difficulties associated with timed urine collections in these age groups. For accurately performed 5-hour urine collections, however, the pediatric reference interval is 6% to 33% of the dose ingested.

Since a 25-gram dose can cause diarrhea, nausea, and abdominal discomfort in some adult patients, a 5-gram dose is sometimes used. For a 5-gram dose in an adult, a level of serum d-xylose between 20-40 mg/dL (SI: 1.3-
(Continued)

d-Xylose Absorption Test, Serum, Urine (Continued)

2.7 mmol/L) should be reached in 30-60 minutes and maintained for a further 60 minutes; the 5-hour urine collection should yield results >1.2 grams (SI: 8.0 mmol).

1-Hour d-Xylose Absorption Test

Serum	mg/dL	mmol/L (SI)
Adult, 1 h (dose, 25 g)	≥25	≥1.7
Adult with intermediate renal insufficiency, 1 h (dose, 25 g)	≥20	≥1.3
Pediatric <12 y, 1 h (dose, 5 g)	≥20	≥1.3

Use The d-xylose test is used primarily to evaluate the functional integrity of the jejunum in possible enterogenous malabsorption and to distinguish mucosal disease from the malabsorption of chronic pancreatic disease. The differential diagnosis of an abnormal result includes celiac disease, tropical sprue, Crohn disease, surgical bowel resection, AIDS, and other less common small bowel disorders. Craig and Atkinson[1] report that the test (25-gram dose with a 5-hour urine collection and a 1-hour serum specimen) is 91% sensitive and 98% specific for detecting intestinal malabsorption in the absence of renal impairment or bacterial overgrowth.

Limitations d-Xylose absorption is often abnormal in amyloidosis, lymphoma, small bowel ischemia, Whipple disease, eosinophilic gastroenteritis, Zollinger-Ellison syndrome, radiation enteritis, scleroderma, following massive bowel resection, bacterial overgrowth, and with certain parasitic infestations. False-positive results are seen with ascites. Poor renal function, vomiting, decreased or very rapid gastric emptying, hypomotility, intestinal stasis syndromes (eg, surgical blind loops), dehydration/hypovolemia, and certain drugs may cause low urine values **not** secondary to intestinal malabsorption. Renal function may present a problem in geriatric and other patients. Incomplete urine collection causes false-positive results. Results can be normal in the presence of limited disease. The usefulness of the test has been somewhat controversial. Krawitt and Beeken concluded in 1975 that no reason exists to do such d-xylose testing when jejunal biopsies are available.[4] Biopsies of the small intestine provide specific diagnoses in Whipple disease, lymphangiectasia, lymphoma, amyloidosis, celiac disease, many infectious diseases and other entities.

Methodology Methods include enzymatic procedures with colorimetric or fluorometric measurements, gas chromatography, or gas chromatography/mass spectrometry (GC/MS).[5]

Additional Information Normal renal function is necessary if urine values alone are determined. BUN and creatinine serum levels should be measured to exclude patients with renal impairment, resulting in poor xylose excretion and elevated blood xylose levels. Low blood and urine xylose levels indicate malabsorption. Absorption and excretion of d-xylose increase with age. Renal excretion diminishes in patients older than 60 years of age. Therefore, elderly individuals with normal intestinal absorption may have elevated blood xylose levels and decreased urine xylose levels due to mild (subclinical) renal impairment.

The [14C] d-xylose breath test, has been suggested as a useful means for identifying malabsorption due to small intestinal bacterial overgrowth.[1] However, direct culture of gastric and small intestinal aspirates may be the better approach.[6]

Pancreatic enzymes are not required for absorption of d-xylose. The d-xylose test is normal in the chronic nonspecific diarrhea syndrome of infancy. To differentiate patients with pancreatic insufficiency from those with small intestinal malabsorption, the d-xylose absorption test has been paired with the N-benzoyl-L-tyrosyl-p-aminobenzoic acid test (BZ-TY-PABA, PABA test, bentiromide, or BTP test) for pancreatic function.[7]

Footnotes

1. Craig RM and Atkinson AJ Jr, "D-xylose Testing: A Review," *Gastroenterology*, 1988, 95(1):223-31.
2. Peled Y, Doron O, Laufer H, et al, "D-xylose Absorption Test. Urine or Blood?" *Dig Dis Sci*, 1991, 36(2):188-92.
3. Lifschitz CH and Polanco I, "The D-xylose Test in Pediatrics: Is It Useful?" *Gastroenterology*, 1999, 97(1):246-7.
4. Krawitt EL and Beeken WL, "Limitations of the Usefulness of the d-Xylose Absorption Test," *Am J Clin Pathol*, 1975, 63(2):261-3.
5. Deutsch JC, Kolli VR, Santhosh-Kumar CR, et al, "Serum Xylose Analysis by Gas Chromatography/Mass Spectrometry," *Am J Clin Pathol*, 1994, 102(5):595-9.
6. Riordan SM, McIver CJ, Duncombe VM, et al, "Factors Influencing the 1-g 14C-C-Xylose Breath Test for Bacterial Overgrowth," *Am J Gastroenterol*, 1995, 90(9):1455-60.
7. Deutsch JC, Santhosh-Kumar CR, and Kolli VR, "A Noninvasive Stable-Isotope Method to Simultaneously Assess Pancreatic Exocrine Function and Small Bowel Absorption," *Am J Gastroenterol*, 1995, 90(12):2182-5.

References

Casellas F, Chicharro L, and Malagelada JR, "Potential Usefulness of Hydrogen Breath Test With D-Xylose in Clinical Management of Intestinal Malabsorption," *Dig Dis Sci*, 1993, 38(2):321-7.
Casellas F and Malagelada JR, "Clinical Applicability of Shortened D-Xylose Breath Test for Diagnosis of Intestinal Malabsorption," *Dig Dis Sci*, 1994, 39(11):2320-6.

Ehrenpreis ED, Gulino SP, Patterson BK, et al, "Kinetics of D-xylose Absorption in Patients With Human Immunodeficiency Virus Enteropathy," *Clin Pharmacol Ther*, 1991, 49(6):632-40.
Henderson AR and Rinker AD, "Gastric, Pancreatic, and Intestinal Function," *Tietz Textbook of Clinical Chemistry*, 3rd ed, Chapter 36, Burtis CA and Ashwood ER, eds, Philadelphia, PA: WB Saunders Co, 1999, 1271-327.
Hommes FA, ed, *Techniques in Diagnostic Human Biochemical Genetics*, New York, NY: Wiley-Liss, 1991.
Labib M, Gama R, and Marks V, "Predictive Value of D-xylose Absorption Test and Erythrocyte Folate in Adult Coeliac Disease: A Parallel Approach," *Ann Clin Biochem*, 1990, 27(Pt 1):75-7.

♦ **EC 3.1.3.5** *see* 5' Nucleotidase, Serum *on page 234*

♦ **Ecstasy** *see* Liver Disease: Laboratory Assessment, Overview *on page 216*

♦ **Elastase, Serum** *see* Lipase, Serum *on page 212*

♦ **Electrolyte Gap** *see* Anion Gap, Serum, Plasma, or Urine *on page 106*

Electrolyte Panel, Serum

Related Information

Anion Gap, Serum, Plasma, or Urine *on page 106*
Bicarbonate, Blood *on page 115*
Blood Gases and pH, Arterial *on page 119*
Blood Gases and pH, Capillary *on page 121*
Blood Gases and pH, Venous *on page 122*
Carbon Dioxide, Total, Blood *on page 135*
Chloride, Serum, Plasma, or Blood *on page 144*
Drugs of Abuse Testing, Urine *on page 788*
Ibuprofen, Serum *on page 793*
Magnesium, Serum *on page 221*
Osmolality, Calculated, Serum or Plasma *on page 234*
Osmolality, Serum *on page 236*
pCO₂, Blood *on page 246*
pH, Blood *on page 247*
Potassium, Serum or Plasma *on page 258*
Sodium, Serum or Plasma *on page 275*

Synonyms Plasma Electrolytes; Serum Electrolytes

Test Includes The HCFA-defined electrolyte panel includes **sodium, potassium, chloride,** and **carbon dioxide**.[1] **Anion gap** is calculated from the panel results and included on the report from many laboratories.

Abstract The electrolyte panel is used to evaluate electrolyte and acid-base balance in a wide variety of disorders.

Specimen Serum, plasma, or whole blood

Container Red top tube or green top (heparin) tube

Collection Specimen is best collected without a tourniquet if possible. Do **not** allow patient to clench-unclench his/her hand. See Venous Blood Collection *on page 47*. Collect specimen anaerobically and avoid hemolysis during collection. Separate serum or plasma from cells as soon as possible following venipuncture.

Storage Instructions Specimen should be delivered to the laboratory and testing should occur as soon as possible. If delay is inevitable, refrigerate the specimen.

Causes for Rejection Gross hemolysis or lipemia

Use See individual listings for tests involved.

Limitations Hemolysis and prolonged contact of serum with cells produces elevation of potassium. Exposure of specimen to air causes loss of carbon dioxide.

Footnotes

1. *Current Procedural Terminology (CPT™) 2001*, American Medical Association, 2001.

References

Graber M and Corish D, "The Electrolytes in Hyponatremia," *Am J Kidney Dis*, 1991, 18(5):527-45.
Kapsner CO and Tzamaloukas AH, "Understanding Serum Electrolytes. How to Avoid Mistakes," *Postgrad Med*, 1991, 90(8):151-4, 157-8, 161.
Lowe RA, Arst HF, and Ellis BK, "Rational Ordering of Electrolytes in the Emergency Department," *Ann Emerg Med*, 1991, 20(1):16-21.
Scott MG, Heusel JW, LeGrys VA, et al, "Electrolytes and Blood Gases," *Tietz Textbook of Clinical Chemistry*, 3rd ed, Chapter 31, Burtis CA and Ashwood ER, eds, Philadelphia, PA: WB Saunders Co, 1999, 1056-92.
Touitou Y, Touitou C, Bogdan A, et al, "Circadian and Seasonal Variations of Electrolytes," *Clin Chim Acta*, 1989, 180(3):245-54.

♦ **Electrolytes, Urine** *replaced by* Chloride, Urine *on page 145*

♦ **Electrolytes, Urine** *replaced by* Potassium, Urine *on page 259*

♦ **Electrolytes, Urine** *replaced by* Sodium, Urine *on page 278*

♦ **Electrophoresis, Protein, Urine** *see* Protein Electrophoresis, Urine *on page 268*

♦ **Electrophoresis, Serum** *see* Protein Electrophoresis, Serum *on page 267*

♦ **Epinephrine** *see* Metanephrines, Urine or Plasma *on page 223*

♦ **Epinephrine, Norepinephrine, Dopamine** *see* Catecholamines, Fractionation, Plasma *on page 138*

◆ **Epinephrine, Urine** *see* Catecholamines, Fractionation, Urine *on page 139*

◆ **Epitestosterone** *see* Dehydroepiandrosterone and Dehydroepiandrosterone Sulfate, Serum or Plasma *on page 164*

◆ **Epoetin Beta** *see* Erythropoietin, Serum *on page 169*

◆ **Ergocalciferol (Vitamin D₂)** *see* Vitamin D, Serum *on page 300*

◆ **Erythrocyte Cholinesterase** *see* Acetylcholinesterase, Red Cell *on page 81*

◆ **Erythrocyte Porphobilinogen Deaminase** *see* Porphobilinogen Deaminase, Erythrocyte *on page 254*

◆ **Erythrocyte Uroporphyrinogen I Synthase** *see* Porphobilinogen Deaminase, Erythrocyte *on page 254*

Erythropoietin Receptor

Related Information
Apoptosis Assays *on page 402*
Blood Volume *on page 407*
Bone Marrow *on page 410*
Erythropoietin, Serum *on page 169*
Red Cell Mass *on page 478*

Applies to Diamond-Blackfan Syndrome; Idiopathic Erythrocytosis; Primary Familial Polycythemia

Abstract For over a decade, erythropoietin (EPO), the lineage-specific regulator for survival, proliferation, and differentiation of erythroid precursors and the erythropoietin receptor (EPO-R) have been studied as to their role in the development of erythrocytosis (as well as other hematologic disorders). The EPO-R resides on the surface of erythroid precursor cells. There is no evident significant or constant representation of EPO-R in serum, urine, or other body fluid. Thus, direct routine clinical analysis is not currently available. Application of cell culture, genetic and molecular pathologic techniques, however, indicate that secondary erythrocytosis not otherwise explained, may be the result of mutations in the EPO-R gene. Research level laboratory investigation may define the molecular pathophysiology responsible for such cases of "idiopathic erythrocytosis."[1]

Limitations The requirement for culture of erythroid progenitor cells, Southern blot analysis, and nucleotide sequencing of DNA may limit the quest for mutated EPO-R in many clinical situations.

Methodology An affordable readily available direct assay for EPO-R is not currently available due to the cellular site of the target (EPO-R); the soluble form of the EPO-R does not actively bind erythropoietin. Thus, determination of serum soluble EPO-R is not of clinical value.

Additional Information EPO, produced largely in the kidney (with much lesser amounts originating in the liver) is often referred to as the cytokine regulator providing for the survival, proliferation, and differentiation of committed erythroid progenitor cells. EPO is a true hormone, produced at one site (predominantly the kidneys) and transported through the blood to the primary site of its action, the bone marrow. The primary function of EPO appears to be the suppression of apoptosis. The majority of marrow erythroid precursors are destined to succumb (before achieving full functional status) due to genetically programmed cell death (apoptosis). The latter can be seen as a "default program" for normal cells that must be blocked (eg, by EPO) if cell survival is to occur. Erythroid precursors show heterogeneity to EPO sensitivity. EPO increases the level of circulating hemoglobin by early release of maturing normoblasts from the marrow, by increasing the amount of hemoglobin synthesized per red cell, and by expanding the pool of erythroid burst-forming and colony-forming units. EPO functions synergistically with other multilineage growth factors. The usual function of EPO is to stimulate the cell surface EPO-R of erythroid precursor cells.

D'Andrea et al obtained cDNA for the EPO-R in 1989 using a functional expression cloning system.[2] The gene for human EPO-R is on chromosome 19p and encodes a cell surface protein of some 55kDa (multiple forms with molecular weights 64, 66, 70, and 78 kDa, dependent upon the degree of glycosylation, have been identified).[3] The human receptor is formed of 508 amino acids including an extracellular domain, an hydrophobic transmembrane domain, and a cytoplasmic domain. EPO-R belongs to the same superfamily of cytokine receptors which includes receptors for granulocyte-macrophage colony-stimulating factor (GM-CSF). EPO induces homodimerization of the receptor which initiates phosphorylation of protein kinase (JAK[2]) and is followed by phosphorylation of other signal transduction proteins and involvement of tyrosines of the receptor molecule (cytoplasmic domain) as part of a negative regulatory system allowing for down regulation of cell proliferation/differentiation.

Polycythemia vera (PV), a clonal hematopoietic stem cell proliferation, is usually characterized by low serum EPO levels. Structural abnormalities or point mutations of EPO-R have not been identified in PV or in the Diamond-Blackfan syndrome.[1] In idiopathic erythrocytosis (patient does not have PV but has increase in red cell mass without other evident cause of secondary polycythemia), EPO-R mutations have been identified, in particular when there is low serum level of EPO.[1] However, mutations of other genes in the signaling pathway of the EPO-R may be involved.

See Erythropoietin, Serum *on page 169.*

Footnotes
1. McMullin MF and Percy MJ, "Erythropoietin Receptor and Hematological Disease," *Am J Hematol*, 1999, 60(1):55-60.
2. D'Andrea AD, Lodish HF, and Wong GG, "Expression Cloning of the Murine Erythropoietin Receptor," *Cell*, 1989, 57(2):277-85.
3. Kaushansky K, "Hematopoietic Growth Factors and Receptors," *The Molecular Basis of Blood Diseases*, 3rd ed, Philadelphia, PA: WB Saunders Co, 2001, 28-31, 54-5.

References
Gregg XT and Prchal JT, "Erythropoietin Receptor Mutations and Human Disease," *Semin Hematol*, 1997, 34(1):70-6.
Lacombe C and Mayeux P, "Erythropoietin (EPO) Receptor and EPO Mimetics," *Advances in Nephrology*, Volume 29, Chapter 11, 1999, 177-89.
Papayannopoulou T, Abkowitz J, and D'Andrea A, "Biology of Erythropoiesis, Erythroid Differentiation, and Maturation," *Hematology: Basic Principles and Practice*, 3rd ed, Chapter 15, Hoffman R, Benz EJ Jr, Shattil SJ, et al, eds, New York, NY: Churchill Livingstone, 2000, 207-10.
Youssoufian H, Longmore G, Neumann D, et al, "Structure, Function, and Activation of the Erythropoietin Receptor," *Blood*, 1993, 81(9):2223-36.

Erythropoietin, Serum

Related Information
Alkaline Phosphatase, Neutrophil Membrane (mNAP) *on page 402*
Autologous Transfusion, Preoperative Deposit *on page 837*
Blood Volume *on page 407*
Erythropoietin Receptor *on page 169*
Ferritin, Serum *on page 173*
Hemoglobin *on page 442*
Heterophilic Antibodies *on page 191*
Iron and Total Iron Binding Capacity/Transferrin, Serum *on page 203*
Oxygen Saturation, Blood *on page 240*
P_{50}, Blood *on page 241*
Phlebotomy, Therapeutic *on page 849*
Red Cell Count *on page 478*
Red Cell Mass *on page 478*
Thrombopoietin, Serum or Plasma *on page 491*
Viscosity, Blood *on page 494*
Vitamin B_{12} Unsaturated Binding Capacity *on page 495*

Applies to Epoetin Beta

Test Includes Serum iron

Abstract A glycoprotein formed mainly in the kidney, erythropoietin (EPO) has been purified and its gene, found on chromosome 7, has been cloned. EPO is the primary regulatory hormone for red cell production in marrow. Hypoxia increases EPO production; bilateral nephrectomy drastically reduces EPO synthesis and thereby inhibits erythropoiesis.

Polycythemia vera (PV) (primary polycythemia) is a clonal disease in which erythropoiesis is autonomous, independent of EPO. EPO in that disorder is decreased or normal in the presence of polycythemia, involving a negative feedback loop to the kidneys. Other (secondary) types of polycythemia are characterized by increased or normal EPO. Distinction of PV from relative polycythemia and secondary erythrocytosis also includes application of family history, patient history, arterial oxygen saturation, P_{50}, measurement of red cell mass, and plasma volume. PV-related features include the presence of persistent leukocytosis, thrombocytosis, microcytosis, unusual thromboses, splenomegaly, pruritus, and erythromelalgia.

Recombinant EPO (epoetin beta) is now available for treatment of anemia associated with chronic renal failure, HIV infection treated with zidovudine, cancer (including therapy-associated anemia), surgical procedures, and autologous blood donation.[1]

Patient Preparation Recent exposure to radioisotopes may interfere if assay method is RIA.

Specimen Serum

Container Red top tube

Special Instructions Done only by a few laboratories

Reference Interval 5-36 mIU/mL[2] (SI: 5-36 IU/L). EPO increases in pregnancy, in which significantly higher levels are found before the 24th week.[3] Reference values in children from a study of 1122 subjects aged 1-18 years: male: 1.0-21.0 mIU/mL; female: 1.1-20.5 mIU/mL.[4]

Use The test is used to investigate obscure anemias and the anemia of end-stage renal disease. Failure of renal erythropoietin production is the essential cause of the anemia of renal failure. This anemia can be successfully treated with exogenous erythropoietin. The availability of assays for EPO should provide the means to identify patients who will benefit from epoetin beta therapy.[5]

EPO is used to differentiate secondary from primary polycythemia. Low EPO concentrations are fairly specific for PV. EPO is increased with states such as cyanotic heart disease, venous/arterial shunts, hypoxic pulmonary diseases, habitation at high altitudes, and with mutant hemoglobins with high affinity for oxygen. It may be increased in cases of Cushing syndrome, renal artery stenosis, renal cysts, and certain tumors (eg, hemangioblastoma of cerebellum, pheochromocytoma, hepatoma, nephroblastoma, rarely leiomyomas, and renal adenocarcinoma). Some overlap exists between these groups.[6,7]

The physiologic effects of EPO have not escaped the attention of elite athletes seeking preternatural endurance and speed.[8] EPO may have been
(Continued)

Erythropoietin, Serum *(Continued)*

related to the mysterious deaths of 19 cyclists between 1987 and 1990.[9] The International Olympic Committee announced testing for EPO randomly selected participants in the 2000 Olympics, using both a urine test for EPO itself and a blood test which detects an inappropriate proportion of young erythrocytes.[10]

Limitations Serum EPO levels may be increased by phlebotomy, anabolic steroids, androgens, TSH, ACTH, angiotensin, epinephrine, daunorubicin, fenoterol, growth hormone levels, and other drugs. Decreases follow acetazolamide, amphotericin B, cisplatin, enalapril, furosemide, and theophylline.[11] Transfusions and estrogens may lower EPO levels. Normal EPO concentrations do not absolutely rule out PV.

Methodology Radioimmunoassays and immunoradiometric assays (RIA, IRMA),[6,12,13,14] enzyme-linked immunoassays (ELISA), immunoprecipitin assays,[15] and immunochemiluminometric assays are available.

Additional Information Bone marrow examination with cytogenetic evaluation is indicated to establish the diagnosis of PV, recognize the presence of marrow fibrosis or a clonal cytogenetic disorder, or both.

A rare familial EPO receptor mutant disorder occurs with low EPO.

In chronic renal disease, the serum EPO level is generally lower than expected from the magnitude of the anemia. Serum EPO is inappropriately low in adult nephrotic syndrome mostly because of renal/urinary loss of the protein which contributes to the anemia.[16] In chronic iron deficiency, the serum EPO is increased, but the increase may not be as high as expected for the degree of anemia.

EPO response to anemia (excluding renal disease and pregnancy) in older subjects is similar to that of younger subjects.[17]

Epoetin beta has diminished the need for transfusions in very low birthweight infants,[1,18] though such therapy has been associated with vascular thrombosis, neutropenia, thrombocytopenia, infection, and other complications.[18]

Winearls et al[19] report 10 patients with end-stage renal disease, all of whom responded to epoetin beta with increased hemoglobin levels, but complications were recognized. Some similar results were reported by Eschbach.[20]

Epoetin beta has been used to improve the yield of autologous units of blood before orthopedic surgery. It was given twice a week for 21 days, 600 units/kg, intravenously.[21]

Autoantibodies have been demonstrated against EPO in pure red-cell aplasia[22] and against recombinant human EPO in EPO-resistant anemia.[23] A method for detecting antirecombinant human EPO antibodies has been reported.[24]

In contrast to patients with PV, most subjects with apparent polycythemia lack splenomegaly.[25]

See Erythropoietin Receptor *on page 169.*

Footnotes

1. Goodnough LT, Monk TG, and Andriole GL, "Erythropoietin Therapy," *N Engl J Med*, 1997, 336(13):933-8.
2. Goldwasser E and Sherwood JB, "Radioimmunoassay of Erythropoietin," *Br J Haematol*, 1981, 48(3):359-63.
3. Riikonen S, Saijonmaa O, Jarvenpaa AL, et al, "Serum Concentrations of Erythropoietin in Healthy and Anemic Pregnant Women," *Scand J Clin Lab Invest*, 1994, 54(8):653-7.
4. Krafte-Jacobs B, Williams J, and Soldin S, "Plasma Erythropoietin Reference Ranges in Children," *J Pediatr*, 1995, 126(4):601-3.
5. Spivak JL, "The Clinical Physiology of Erythropoietin," *Semin Hematol*, 1993, 30(4 Suppl 6):2-11.
6. Casadevall N, "Determination of Serum Erythropoietin. Its Value in the Differential Diagnosis of Polycythemias," *Nouv Rev Fr Hematol*, 1994, 36(2):173-6.
7. Birgegard G and Wide L, "Serum Erythropoietin in the Diagnosis of Polycythaemia and After Phlebotomy Treatment," *Br J Haematol*, 1992, 81(4):603-6.
8. Barnes J, "The Hardest Test: Drugs and the Tour de France," *The New Yorker*, August 21, 2000, 94-301.
9. Eichner ER, "Better Dead Than Second," *J Lab Clin Med*, 1992, 120(3):359-60.
10. Clarey C, "EPO Tests Approved for Games in Sydney," *NY Times*, August 29, 2000.
11. Young DS, "Effects of Drugs on Clinical Laboratory Tests," 5th ed, Volume 1: Listing by Test, Washington, DC: AACC Press, American Association of Clinical Chemistry, 2000, Section 3, 311-2.
12. Egrie JC, Cotes PM, Lane J, et al, "Development of Radioimmunoassays for Human Erythropoietin Using Recombinant Erythropoietin as Tracer and Immunogen," *J Immunol Methods*, 1987, 99(2):235-41.
13. Mason-Garcia M, Beckman BS, Brookins JW, et al, "Development of a New Radioimmunoassay for Erythropoietin Using Recombinant Erythropoietin," *Kidney Int*, 1990, 38(5):969-75.
14. Schlageter MH, Toubert ME, Podgorniak MP, et al, "Radioimmunoassay of Erythropoietin: Analytical Performance and Clinical Use in Hematology," *Clin Chem*, 1990, 36(10):1731-5.
15. Widness JA, Schmidt RL, Veng-Pedersen P, et al, "A Sensitive and Specific Erythropoietin Immunoprecipitation Assay: Application to Pharmacokinetic Studies," *J Lab Clin Med*, 1992, 119(3):285-94.
16. Vaziri ND, Kaupke CJ, Barton CH, et al, "Plasma Concentration and Urinary Excretion of Erythropoietin in Adult Nephrotic Syndrome," *Am J Med*, 1992, 92(1):35-40.
17. Powers JS, Krantz SB, Collins JC, et al, "Erythropoietin Response to Anemia as a Function of Age," *J Am Geriatr Soc*, 1991, 39(1):30-2.
18. Maier RF, Obladen M, Scigalla P, et al, "The Effect of Epoetin Beta (Recombinant Human Erythropoietin) on the Need for Transfusion in Very-Low-Birth-Weight Infants. European Multicentre Erythropoietin Study Group," *N Engl J Med*, 1994, 330(17):1173-8.
19. Winearls CG, Oliver DO, Pippard MJ, et al, "Effect of Human Erythropoietin Derived From Recombinant DNA on the Anaemia of Patients Maintained by Chronic Haemodialysis," *Lancet*, 1986, 2(8517):1175-8.
20. Eschbach JW, Egrie JC, Downing MR, et al, "Correction of the Anemia of End-Stage Renal Disease With Recombinant Human Erythropoietin. Results of a Combined Phase I and II Clinical Trial," *N Engl J Med*, 1987, 316(2):73-8.
21. Goodnough LT, Rudnick S, Price TH, et al, "Increased Preoperative Collection of Autologous Blood With Recombinant Human Erythropoietin Therapy," *N Engl J Med*, 1989, 321(17):1163-8.
22. Casadevall N, Dupuy E, Molho-Sabatier P, et al, "Brief Report: Autoantibodies Against Erythropoietin in a Patient With Pure Red-Cell Aplasia," *N Engl J Med*, 1996, 334(10):630-3.
23. Peces R, de la Torre M, Alcazar R, et al, "Antibodies Against Recombinant Human Erythropoietin in a Patient With Erythropoietin-Resistant Anemia," *N Engl J Med*, 1996, 335(7):523-4.
24. Urra JM, de la Torre M, Alcazar R, et al, "Rapid Method for Detection of Antirecombinant Human Erythropoietin Antibodies as a New Form of Erythropoietin Resistance," *Clin Chem*, 1997, 43(5):848-9.
25. Carneskog J, Safaj-Kutti S, Suurkuyla M, et al, "The Red Cell Mass, Plasma Erythropoietin and Spleen Size in Apparent Polycythemia," *Eur J Haematol*, 1999, 62(1):43-8.

References

Adamson JW and Eschbach JW, "Erythropoietin for End-Stage Renal Disease," *N Engl J Med*, 1998, 339(9):625-7.

Beguin Y, Clemons GK, Pootrakul P, et al, "Quantitative Assessment of Erythropoiesis and Functional Classification of Anemia Based on Measurements of Serum Transferrin Receptor and Erythropoietin," *Blood*, 1993, 81(4):1067-76.

Greendyke RM, Sharma K, and Gifford FR, "Serum Levels of Erythropoietin and Selected Other Cytokines in Patients With Anemia of Chronic Disease," *Am J Clin Pathol*, 1994, 101(3):338-41.

Ifudu O, Feldman J, and Friedman EA, "The Intensity of Hemodialysis and the Response to Erythropoietin in Patients With End-Stage Renal Disease," *N Engl J Med*, 1995, 334(7):420-5.

Kario K, Matsuo T, and Nakao K, "Serum Erythropoietin Levels in the Elderly," *Gerontology*, 1991, 37(6):345-8.

Nissenson AR, "Erythropoietin Overview - 1993," *Blood Purif*, 1994, 12(1):6-13.

Pressac M, Morgant G, Farnier MA, et al, "Enzyme Immunoassay of Serum Erythropoietin in Healthy Children: Reference Values," *Ann Clin Biochem*, 1991, 28(Pt 4):345-50.

Ridley DM, Dawkins F, and Perlin E, "Erythropoietin: A Review," *J Natl Med Assoc*, 1994, 86(2):129-35.

Tanebe M, Teshima S, Hanyu T, et al, "Rapid and Sensitive Method for Erythropoietin in Serum," *Clin Chem*, 1992, 38(9):1752-5.

Tefferi A, "Diagnosing Polycythemia Vera: A Paradigm Shift," *Mayo Clin Proc*, 1999, 74(2):159-62.

♦ **Estradiol** *see* Dehydroepiandrosterone and Dehydroepiandrosterone Sulfate, Serum or Plasma *on page 164*

♦ **Estradiol** *see* Testosterone, Total and Free, Serum or Plasma *on page 280*

♦ **Estradiol-17β** *see* Estradiol, Serum *on page 170*

Estradiol, Serum

Related Information

Estriol, Unconjugated, Pregnancy, Serum, Plasma, or Urine *on page 171*
Estrogens, Urine *on page 172*
Follicle Stimulating Hormone, Serum, Plasma, or Urine *on page 175*
Heterophilic Antibodies *on page 191*
Luteinizing Hormone, Blood or Urine *on page 219*
Progesterone, Serum *on page 261*

Synonyms 17β-Estradiol; Estradiol-17β

Applies to Estrone

Abstract Estradiol (E2) is the most potent endogenous estrogen. In nonpregnant females, most of the E2 originates in the ovaries, with smaller contributions from the adrenals. The placenta is an additional source in pregnancy. In males, E2 is produced in the testes and adrenals.

Patient Preparation Recent exposure to radioactivity (eg, scan) may interfere if assay method is RIA.

Specimen Serum

Container Red top tube

Sampling Time In females, the phase of the menstrual cycle should be recorded for interpretation. In assisted reproduction protocols, specimens for E2 must be obtained according to a specific schedule.

Storage Instructions Serum specimen is stable if refrigerated for 24 hours or frozen for up to 2 months.

Reference Interval Children 6 months to 10 years: <15 pg/mL (SI: <55 pmol/L); adult male: 10-50 pg/mL (SI: 37-184 pmol/L); female: premenopausal: 30-400 pg/mL (SI: 110-1468 pmol/L) (depending on phase of menstrual cycle); postmenopausal: 0-30 pg/mL (SI: 0-110 pmol/L)

Use

Disorders of ovarian function: E2 is an indicator of overall ovarian function. Values are decreased in ovarian failure (all causes), Turner syndrome, and most hypogonadal states. When ovarian failure is secondary to hypopituitary states, FSH and LH also are decreased. When ovarian failure is primary (ie, due to ovarian disease), FSH and LH are increased. In patients with infertility or irregular menses (including amenorrhea), E2 values, interpreted together with serum FSH, LH, progesterone, other hormones, and menstrual history, are useful in differential diagnosis.

Assisted reproduction: Many assisted reproduction protocols involve the administration of pharmacologic agents (eg, gonadotropins) to induce ovulation. E2 results usually play a key role in such protocols. For example, the magnitude of the E2 increment after the first dose of gonadotropins is a major determinant of the size of the second dose; in like fashion, the E2 increment following the second dose is a determinant of the next dose, etc.[1] Very high serum E2 levels are not detrimental to clinical outcome of *in vitro* fertilization,[2] and change in E2 level following gonadotropin-releasing hormone analogue stimulation has been shown to be an effective predictor of ovarian reserve when accompanied by basal, serum FSH evaluation.[3]

Hormonally active tumors: Rare tumors of the ovary,[4] testis, adrenal, or nonendocrine sites may cause high E2 levels.

Limitations Significant interlaboratory variability is observed,[5] though efforts are underway toward method standardization.[6,7]

In menopausal females, estrone (E_1), rather than E2, is the predominant circulating estrogen; therefore, serum E1 measurements may be indicated in this age group in place of, or in addition to, E2 levels.

E2 increases with hepatic cirrhosis. Oral contraceptives decrease serum levels. E2 levels can be normal in women who have hypogonadism.[8]

Contraindications E2 measurements are not useful in pregnant females or to evaluate fetal well-being, because they do not measure estriol (E3) which comprises >90% of maternal estrogens. However, E2 may be useful in the diagnosis of ectopic pregnancy.[9]

Methodology Routine testing methods include isotopic and nonisotopic immunoassays with and without extraction. The reference/definitive method is isotope-dilution-gas chromatography/mass spectrometry (ID-GC/MS).

Additional Information Elevated serum E2 and testosterone levels have been associated with a high risk of breast cancer,[10] and undetectable E2 levels have been associated with an increased risk of hip and vertebral fracture.[11] E2 levels may become useful in the titration of effective dosages of hormone replacement therapy.[12,13]

Footnotes

1. Gronowski AM and Landau-Levine M, "Reproductive Endocrine Function," *Tietz Textbook of Clinical Chemistry*, 3rd ed, Chapter 45, Burtis CA and Ashwood ER, eds, Philadelphia, PA: WB Saunders Co, 1999, 1601-41.
2. Chenette PE, Sauer MV, and Paulson RJ, "Very High Serum Estradiol Levels Are Not Detrimental to Clinical Outcome of *In Vitro* Fertilization," *Fertil Steril*, 1990, 54(5):858-63.
3. Ranieri DM, Quinn F, Makhlouf A, et al, "Simultaneous Evaluation of Basal Follicle-Stimulating Hormone and 17β-Estradiol Response to Gonadotropin-Releasing Hormone Analogue Stimulation: An Improved Predictor of Ovarian Reserve," *Fertil Steril*, 1998, 70(2):227-33.
4. Young RH and Scully RE, "Sex Cord-Stromal, Steroid Cell, and Other Ovarian Tumors With Endocrine, Parendocrine, and Paraneoplastic Manifestations," *Blaustein's Pathology of the Female Genital Tract*, 4th ed, Kurman RJ, ed, New York, NY: Springer-Verlag, 1994, 783-847.
5. Hershlag A, Lesser M, Montefusco D, et al, "Interinstitutional Variability of Follicle-Stimulating Hormone and Estradiol Levels," *Fertil Steril*, 1992, 58(6):1123-6.
6. Thienpont LM, "Meeting Report: First and Second Estradiol International Workshops," *Clin Chem*, 1996, 42(7):1122-4.
7. Thienpont LM and De Leenheer AP, "Efforts by Industry Toward Standardization of Serum Estradiol-17β Measurements," *Clin Chem*, 1998, 44(3):671-4.
8. Vance ML, "Hypopituitarism," *N Engl J Med*, 1994, 330(23):1651-62.
9. Guillaume J, Benjamin F, Sicuranza BJ, et al, "Serum Estradiol as an Aid in the Diagnosis of Ectopic Pregnancy," *Obstet Gynecol*, 1990, 76(6):1126-9.
10. Cauley JA, Lucas FL, Kuller LH, et al, "Elevated Serum Estradiol and Testosterone Concentrations Are Associated With a High Risk for Breast Cancer," *Ann Intern Med*, 1999, 130(4 Pt 1):270-7.
11. Cummings SR, Browner WS, Bauer D, et al, "Endogenous Hormones and the Risk of Hip and Vertebral Fractures Among Older Women," *N Engl J Med*, 1998, 339(11):733-8.
12. Walsh BW, Spiegelman D, Morrissey M, et al, "Relationship Between Serum Estradiol Levels and the Increases in High-Density Lipoprotein Levels in Postmenopausal Women Treated With Oral Estradiol," *J Clin Endocrinol Metab*, 1999, 84(3):985-9.
13. van de Weijer PH, Barentsen R, De Vries M, et al, "Relationship of Estradiol Levels to Breakthrough Bleeding During Continuous Combined Hormone Replacement Therapy," *Obstet Gynecol*, 1999, 93(4):551-7.

References

Bouve J, De Boever J, Leyseele D, et al, "Direct Enzyme Immunoassay of Estradiol in Serum of Women Enrolled in an *In Vitro* Fertilization and Embryo Transfer Program," *Clin Chem*, 1992, 38(8 Pt 1):1409-13.

Darne J, McGarrigle HH, and Lachelin GC, "Saliva Oestriol, Oestradiol, Oestrone, and Progesterone Levels in Pregnancy: Spontaneous Labour at Term Is Preceded by a Rise in the Saliva Oestriol:Progesterone Ratio," *Br J Obstet Gynaecol*, 1987, 94(3):227-35.

Hayes FJ and Eichhorn JH, "A 60-Year-Old Man With Persistent Gynecomastia After Excision of a Pituitary Adenoma," Case Records of the Massachusetts General Hospital, Case 12-2000, Scully RE, Mark EJ, McNeely WF, et al, eds, *N Engl J Med*, 2000, 342(16):1196-204.

Kiel DP, Baron JA, Plymate SR, et al, "Sex Hormones and Lipoproteins in Men," *Am J Med*, 1989, 87(1):35-9.

Phillips GB, Yano K, and Stemmermann GN, "Decrease in Serum Estradiol Values With Storage," *N Engl J Med*, 1984, 311(25):1635.

Pont A, Goldman ES, Sugar AM, et al, "Ketoconazole-Induced Increase in Estradiol-Testosterone Ratio," *Arch Intern Med*, 1985, 145(8):1429-31.

Potischman N, Falk RT, Laiming VA, et al, "Reproducibility of Laboratory Assays for Steroid Hormones and Sex Hormone-Binding Globulin," *Cancer Res*, 1994, 54(20):5363-7.

Stewart MO, Whittaker PG, Persson B, et al, "A Longitudinal Study of Circulating Progesterone, Oestradiol, hCG and hPL During Pregnancy in Type 1 Diabetic Mothers," *Br J Obstet Gynaecol*, 1989, 96(4):415-23.

Studd J, Savvas M, Waston N, et al, "The Relationship Between Plasma Estradiol and the Increase in Bone Density in Postmenopausal Women After Treatment With Subcutaneous Hormone Implants," *Am J Obstet Gynecol*, 1990, 163(5 Pt 1):1474-9.

Veldhuis JD, Evans WS, and Stumpf PG, "Mechanisms That Subserve Estradiol's Induction of Increased Prolactin Concentrations: Evidence of Amplitude Modulation of Spontaneous Prolactin Secretory Bursts," *Am J Obstet Gynecol*, 1989, 161(5):1149-58.

♦ **Estriol, Free** *see* Estriol, Unconjugated, Pregnancy, Serum, Plasma, or Urine on page 171

Estriol, Unconjugated, Pregnancy, Serum, Plasma, or Urine

Related Information

Alpha₁-Fetoprotein, Serum *on page 97*
Chorionic Gonadotropin, Human, Serum and Urine *on page 147*
Estradiol, Serum *on page 170*
Inhibin A, Serum *on page 199*
Pregnancy-Associated Protein A, Serum *on page 260*
Urine Collection, 24-Hour *on page 47*

Synonyms Estriol, Free; 16-Hydroxyestradiol; uE_3; Unconjugated Estriol, Pregnancy; Unconjugated Estrogen, Serum

Applies to Multiple Marker Screening Test; Triple Test

Abstract Estriol is the major estrogen of pregnancy, but its role in laboratory evaluation has become somewhat controversial. Replacement of uE_3 by inhibin A for identification of Down syndrome, in the multiple marker screening test, is advocated.[1]

Specimen Serum or plasma, 24-hour urine

Container Plain red top tube (not SST™ tube) or (depending on laboratory) green top (heparin) tube for blood; 24-hour urine container

Sampling Time Second trimester screening of maternal serum for Edwards syndrome (trisomy 18) and Down syndrome (trisomy 21) includes sampling at 15-21 weeks gestation when testing also includes AFP and hCG.[2] Optimally, these tests should be drawn between 16 and 18 weeks.[3]

Collection Since circadian rhythms exist, serum estriol should be drawn at the same time of day on each visit.

Storage Instructions 4°C for up to 24 hours; for longer periods freeze at -20°C.

Special Instructions Include maternal birth date, first day of last menstrual period, gestational age by ultrasound and by physical examination, expected date of delivery, maternal weight, race, and diabetic status with request.

Reference Interval Urine concentrations of estriol increase with gestation, from 2 mg/24 hours (SI: 7 nmol/day) at 16 weeks gestation to 10-40 mg/24 hours (SI: 35-139 nmol/day) at term. A wide normal range exists. Reference ranges depend upon maternal weight as well as upon gestational age, like hCG and AFP. **Serum** levels in the table do not represent reference ranges for all laboratories. Different assays lead to wide differences of estriol in the same sample.

Normal Serum or Plasma Unconjugated Estriol Values[4,5,6] (Fetal Well-Being)

Weeks of Gestation	µg/L	SI: nmol/L
25	3.5-10.0	12-35
28	4.0-12.5	14-43
30	4.5-14.0	16-49
32	5.0-16.0	17-55
34	5.5-18.5	19-64
36	7.0-25.0	24-87
37	8.0-28.0	28-97
38	9.0-32.0	31-111
39	10.0-34.0	35-118
40	5.0-40.0	17-139

Note: This table is to be used to monitor fetal well-being.

Possible Panic Range Value of urinary estriol <4 mg/24 hours or 40% below mean of three prior values demands immediate evaluation of fetal well-being.

Use Serial estriol values, depending upon the integrity of the fetal-placental-maternal unit, had been thought to assess fetal well-being, a role no longer in wide use.

(Continued)

Estriol, Unconjugated, Pregnancy, Serum, Plasma, or Urine (Continued)

Estriol may decrease with pregnancy-induced hypertension, small for gestational age pregnancies, fetal growth restriction,[4] molar gestation, chromosomal abnormalities, fetal demise, placental sulfatase deficiency, fetal adrenal aplasia or hypoplasia, and in anencephaly. See table in Alpha$_1$-Fetoprotein, Serum *on page 97*.

Limitations Single values are almost impossible to interpret; trends in a series of measurements are much more important. Other causes of decreased estriol levels include subjects living at high altitudes, on penicillin or related drugs, corticosteroids, dexamethasone, betamethasone, diuretics, Mandelamine®, probenecid, estrogens, phenazopyridine, meprobamate, phenolphthalein, cascara, senna, and glutethimide. It is decreased with anemia and severe liver disease. Estriol may be increased with multiple pregnancy and with oxytocin. It is not reliable in the presence of renal disease. Use of the test has become controversial. It is no longer done in a number of laboratories. Screening for Down syndrome without uE$_3$ is proposed.[5]

Methodology Radioimmunoassay (RIA) or high performance liquid chromatography (HPLC)

Additional Information Estriol, E$_3$, is synthesized in the placenta from 16-α-hydroxydehydroepiandrosterone of fetal origin. Thus, normal production has been thought to serve as a measure of the integrity of the fetoplacental unit. Sequential monitoring of estriol in high risk pregnancy has made early intervention possible. Chronically low estriol values are found in intrauterine growth retardation but also are sometimes seen in normal pregnancy. A decreasing trend is indicative of fetal distress. The sensitivity and specificity of this test for detecting fetal distress are very poor; thus, its use for this purpose has been largely abandoned.

Since estriol comprises ~90% of the estrogen in maternal urine in later pregnancy, many laboratories measure total urinary estrogen levels instead of estriol.

Combined evaluation of unconjugated serum estriol, maternal serum hCG, maternal serum AFP, and maternal age has been used in prediction of risk for fetal chromosomal abnormalities during pregnancy (the **triple screen test** for Down syndrome), but note a paper on unconjugated estriol use by Macri et al.[6] Serum uE$_3$ is low in about 25% of instances of trisomy 21 and in about 55% of cases of trisomy 18.[7] Triple screen testing identifies nearly 60% of pregnancies bearing Down syndrome conceptions. A 5% false-positive rate is accepted for it.

Estriol:creatinine ratios have been advocated for evaluation of urinary estriol excretion.

Footnotes

1. Wenstrom KD, Owen J, Chu DC, et al, "Elevated Second-Trimester Dimeric Inhibin A Levels Identify Down Syndrome Pregnancies," *Am J Obstet Gynecol*, 1997, 177(5):992-6.
2. Haddow JE and Palomaki GE, "Biochemical Markers of Fetal Disorders in Maternal Serum and Amniotic Fluid," *Medicine of the Fetus and Mother*, 2nd ed, Chapter 40, Reece EA and Hobbins JC, eds, Philadelphia, PA: Lippincott-Raven, 1999, 689-706.
3. Ashwood ER, "Clinical Chemistry of Pregnancy," *Tietz Textbook of Clinical Chemistry*, 3rd ed, Burtis CA and Ashwood ER, eds, Chapter 48, Philadelphia, PA: WB Saunders Co, 1999, 1736-75.
4. Kowalczyk TD, Cabaniss ML, and Cusmano L, "Association of Low Unconjugated Estriol in the Second Trimester and Adverse Pregnancy Outcome," *Obstet Gynecol*, 1998, 91(3):396-400.
5. Haddow JE, Palomaki GE, Knight GJ, et al, "Screening of Maternal Serum for Fetal Down's Syndrome in the First Trimester," *N Engl J Med*, 1998, 338(14):955-61.
6. Macri JN, Kasturi RV, Krantz DA, et al, "Maternal Serum Down Syndrome Screening: Unconjugated Estriol Is Not Useful," *Am J Obstet Gynecol*, 1990, 162(3):672-3.
7. Baskin LB, "Pregnancy and Prenatal Testing," *The Handbook of Clinical Pathology*, 2nd ed, Chapter 21, McKenna RW and Keffer JH, eds, Chicago, IL: ASCP Press, American Society of Clinical Pathologists, 2000, 281-92.

References

Bradley LA, Canick JA, Palomaki GE, et al, "Undetectable Maternal Serum Unconjugated Estriol Levels in the Second Trimester: Risk of Perinatal Complications Associated With Placental Sulfatase Deficiency," *Am J Obstet Gynecol*, 1997, 176(3):531-5.

Frishman GN, Canick JA, Hogan JW, et al, "Serum Triple-Marker Screening in *In Vitro* Fertilization and Naturally Conceived Pregnancies," *Obstet Gynecol*, 1997, 90(1):98-101.

Goodwin TM, "A Role for Estriol in Human Labor, Term and Preterm," *Am J Obstet Gynecol*, 1999, 180(1 Pt 3):S208-13.

Haddow JE, "Antenatal Screening for Down's Syndrome: Where Are We and Where Next?" *Lancet*, 1998, 352(9125):336-7.

Jackson M and Dudley DJ, "Endocrine Assays to Predict Preterm Delivery," *Clin Perinatol*, 1998, 25(4):837-57.

Kisbeth RM, Mayo Medical Laboratories, *2000 Test Catalogue*, Rochester, MN.

Macri JN, Kasturi RV, Krantz DA, et al, "Sensitivity and Specificity of Screening for Down Syndrome With Alpha-Fetoprotein, hCG, Unconjugated Estriol, and Maternal Age," *Obstet Gynecol*, 1991, 77(6):63-8.

Ross HL and Elias S, "Maternal Serum Screening for Fetal Genetic Disorders," *Obstet Gynecol Clin North Am*, 1997, 24(1):33-47.

Santolaya-Forgas J, Jessup J, Burd LI, et al, "Pregnancy Outcome in Women With Low Midtrimester Maternal Serum Unconjugated Estriol," *J Reprod Med*, 1996, 41(2):87-90.

Wald NJ, Watt HC, and Hackshaw AK, "Integrated Screening for Down's Syndrome on the Basis of Tests Performed During the First and Second Trimesters," *N Engl J Med*, 1999, 341(7):461-7.

Wyllie JP, Madar RJ, Wright M, et al, "Strategies for Antenatal Detection of Down's Syndrome," *Arch Dis Child Fetal Neonatal Ed*, 1997, 76(1):F26-30.

Yankowitz J, Fulton A, Williamson R, et al, "Prospective Evaluation of Prenatal Maternal Serum Screening for Trisomy 18," *Am J Obstet Gynecol*, 1998, 178(3):446-50.

Yaron Y, Cherry M, Kramer RL, et al, "Second-Trimester Maternal Serum Marker Screening: Maternal Serum Alpha-Fetoprotein, Beta-Human Chorionic Gonadotropin, Estriol, and Their Various Combinations as Predictors of Pregnancy Outcome," *Am J Obstet Gynecol*, 1999, 181(4):968-74.

Zalel Y, Kedar I, Tepper R, et al, "Differential Diagnosis and Management of Very Low Second Trimester Maternal Serum Unconjugated Estriol Levels With Special Emphasis on the Diagnosis of X-Linked Ichthyosis," *Obstet Gynecol Surv*, 1996, 51(3):200-3.

Estrogens, Urine

Related Information
Estradiol, Serum *on page 170*
Estriol, Unconjugated, Pregnancy, Serum, Plasma, or Urine *on page 171*
Follicle Stimulating Hormone, Serum, Plasma, or Urine *on page 175*
Hormonal Evaluation, Cytologic *on page 384*
Luteinizing Hormone, Blood or Urine *on page 219*

Abstract Urinary total estrogens (estradiol, estrone, estriol) have been used to predict ovulation and evaluate numerous hypo- and hyperestrogenic states. Total urinary estrogen testing largely has been replaced by serum Estriol *on page 171*, Estradiol *on page 170*, LH *on page 219*, and FSH *on page 175* measurements.

Use The test is mainly of historic interest.

References
Avioli LV, "Hyperparathyroidism, Estrogens, and Osteoporosis," *Hosp Pract (Off Ed)*, 1991, 26(1):115-22, 127-8, 133-4.

Bartelsmeyer JA and Petrie RH, "Erythema Nodosum, Estrogens, and Pregnancy," *Clin Obstet Gynecol*, 1990, 33(4):777-81.

Goldin BR and Gorbach SL, "Effect of Diet on the Plasma Levels, Metabolism, and Excretion of Estrogens," *Am J Clin Nutr*, 1988, 48(3 Suppl):787-90.

Ishikawa M, Hoshiai H, Tozawa H, et al, "Monitoring Follicular Maturation Through Measurement of Urinary Estrogen Excretion by Latex Agglutination Inhibition Reaction," *Fertil Steril*, 1987, 48(4):688-90.

Katsouyanni K, Boyle P, and Trichopoulos D, "Diet and Urine Estrogens Among Postmenopausal Women," *Oncology*, 1991, 48(6):490-4.

Longcope C, Goldfield SR, Brambilla DJ, et al, "Androgens, Estrogens, and Sex Hormone-Binding Globulin in Middle-Aged Men," *J Clin Endocrinol Metab*, 1990, 71(6):1442-6.

Longcope C, Herbert PN, McKinlay SM, et al, "The Relationship of Total and Free Estrogens and Sex Hormone-Binding Globulin With Lipoproteins in Women," *J Clin Endocrinol Metab*, 1990, 71(1):67-72.

Silberstein SD and Merriam GR, "Estrogens, Progestins, and Headache," *Neurology*, 1991, 41(6):786-93.

Stampfer MJ, "Smoking, Estrogen, and Prevention of Heart Disease in Women," *Mayo Clin Proc*, 1989, 64(12):1553-7.

♦ **Estrone** *see* Estradiol, Serum *on page 170*

♦ **Etiocholanolone** *see* 17-Ketosteroids Fractionation, Urine *on page 206*

♦ **Euthyroid Sick Syndrome** *see* Reverse T$_3$, Serum *on page 274*

♦ **Extrinsic Factor of Castle** *see* Cobalamin, Serum *on page 150*

♦ **Familial Dysalbuminemic Hyperthyroxinemia** *see* Thyroxine Binding Globulin, Serum *on page 284*

♦ **Familial Hypercholesterolemia** *see* Low Density Lipoprotein Cholesterol *on page 218*

♦ **Fast Hemoglobins** *see* Glycated Hemoglobin (Hemoglobin A$_{1c}$), Blood *on page 188*

♦ **Fasting Bilirubin Test** *see* Bilirubin, Total, Serum *on page 118*

♦ **Fasting Blood Sugar** *see* Glucose, Fasting, Plasma *on page 183*

♦ **Fat, Quantitative, 72-Hour Stool Collection** *see* Fecal Fat, Quantitative, 72-Hour Collection *on page 172*

♦ **FBS** *see* Glucose, Fasting, Plasma *on page 183*

♦ **Fe and TIBC** *see* Iron and Total Iron Binding Capacity/Transferrin, Serum *on page 203*

Fecal Fat, Quantitative, 72-Hour Collection

Related Information
Cholesterol, Total, Serum or Plasma *on page 146*
d-Xylose Absorption Test, Serum, Urine *on page 167*
Endomysial Antibodies *on page 525*
Fat, Semiquantitative, Stool, Acid Steatocrit *on page 305*
Fat, Semiquantitative, Stool, Sudan III Stain *on page 306*
Fecal Fat by Near-Infrared Reflectance Analysis *on page 307*
Fecal Pancreatic Elastase 1 *on page 308*
Gliadin IgG/IgA Antibodies *on page 526*

Hemoglobin *on page 442*
Meat Fibers, Stool *on page 313*
Methylene Blue Stain, Stool *on page 313*
pH, Stool *on page 317*
Vitamin D, Serum *on page 300*

Synonyms Fat, Quantitative, 72-Hour Stool Collection; Quantitative Fecal Fat, 72-Hour Collection; Stool Fat, Quantitative

Abstract Test for the investigation of malabsorption and steatorrhea.

Patient Preparation 100-150 g/day fat diet for 3 days before and during 72-hour collection period. Barium interferes.

Specimen 72-hour stool collection, usually in the fourth, fifth, and sixth days of the 100 g/day fat diet

Container Plastic stool container, preweighed

Sampling Time 72 hours; shorter collection periods are not usually acceptable

Collection Specimen should be refrigerated during its collection. A dietary fat intake of 50-150 g/day for **at least** 2 days before and during the collection period.

Storage Instructions Freeze on dry ice if analysis is not to be done promptly.

Causes for Rejection Improper container (ie, paper cartons, coffee cans, plastic bags, etc), foreign matter other than feces inside of container (ie, spoons, tongue depressors, plastic bags, toilet paper, etc), patient not on special diet, not 72-hour collection

Special Instructions Date and time collection started, date and time collection finished are needed.

Reference Interval 2-7 g/24 hours (SI: 2-7 g/day); <20% of total solids

Use Diagnose the presence of steatorrhea, supporting a diagnosis of one of the malabsorption syndromes, including nontropical sprue, Crohn disease, chronic pancreatitis, cystic fibrosis, Whipple disease, or tuberculous enteropathy

Limitations Fecal fat collection does not provide a diagnostic explanation for the presence of steatorrhea. Stool fat collection is an unpleasant experience for the patient as well as others. It may be within normal limits in the presence of advanced loss of pancreatic parenchyma. Fecal fat measurement is regarded as unnecessary for investigation of pancreatic insufficiency.[1]

Contraindications Patient taking mineral oil

Methodology Extraction and titration of long chain fatty acids by sodium hydroxide. Fatty acids represent 60% to 80% of total fecal lipids.

Additional Information Identification of types of stool fat (eg, free fatty acids, triglycerides, neutral fats, phospholipids) is of little value. Fecal fat excretion >7 g/day is abnormal but nonspecific. Small intestinal, pancreatic or hepatobiliary diseases may cause such increased excretion. Increased fecal fat levels do not differentiate between pancreatic (maldigestion) and intestinal (malabsorption) steatorrhea.[2]

Mechanisms in the production of diarrhea include secretory and osmotic diarrhea and motility disorders. A summary of possible laboratory investigation of the first may include stool cultures, gastrin, 5-hydroxyindoleacetic acid, calcitonin, and vasoactive intestinal polypeptide. For the second, lactose tolerance test occasionally may be appropriate. The third category may include sTSH for hyperthyroidism.

If fat malabsorption occurs, the physician may consider the fat soluble vitamins A, D, E, and K. Of these, vitamin D lends itself to investigation not only with serum levels but with utilization of bone density as well.

Footnotes
1. Holmes GK and Hill PG, "Do We Still Need to Measure Faecal Fat?" *Br Med J (Clin Res Ed)*, 1988, 296(6636):1552-3.
2. Bai JC, Andrush A, Matelo G, et al, "Fecal Fat Concentration in the Differential Diagnosis of Steatorrhea," *Am J Gastroenterol*, 1989, 84(1):27-30.

References
Beath S, Willis K, Hooley I, et al, "New Method for Determining Faecal Fat Excretion in Infancy," *Arch Dis Child*, 1993, 69(5):545-7.
Fine KD and Fordtran JS, "The Effect of Diarrhea on Fecal Fat Excretion," *Gastroenterology*, 1992, 102(6):1936-9.
Simko V and Michael S, "Absorptive Capacity for Dietary Fat in Elderly Patients With Debilitating Disorders," *Arch Intern Med*, 1989, 149(3):557-60.

♦ **FENA** *see* Sodium, Urine *on page 278*

♦ **Fenci-Stewart Method** *see* Anion Gap, Serum, Plasma, or Urine *on page 106*

♦ **FEP** *see* Protoporphyrin, Free Erythrocyte *on page 269*

♦ **Ferric Chloride Test** *see* Phenylalanine, Urine *on page 249*

Ferritin, Serum

Related Information
Anemia Flowchart *on page 392*
Bone Marrow *on page 410*
Complete Blood Count *on page 419*
Erythropoietin, Serum *on page 169*
Hereditary Hemochromatosis DNA Test *on page 709*
Iron and Total Iron Binding Capacity/Transferrin, Serum *on page 203*
Iron Stain, Bone Marrow *on page 452*
Lead, Blood *on page 793*

Lead, Urine *on page 795*
Liver Biopsy *on page 65*
Liver Disease: Laboratory Assessment, Overview *on page 216*
Occult Blood, Stool *on page 315*
Phlebotomy, Therapeutic *on page 849*
Protoporphyrin, Free Erythrocyte *on page 269*
Protoporphyrin, Zinc, Blood *on page 270*
Red Cell Count *on page 478*
Transferrin Receptor, Soluble, Serum or Plasma *on page 493*

Applies to Hepatic Iron Index; HLA-A3; Liver Iron Concentration; Transferrin Receptor

Abstract Used as an aid in the distinction of iron deficiency anemias from others. Ferritin serum level is generally proportional to the body's iron store and reflects cellular iron stores. Serum ferritin is the best single test for the diagnosis of iron deficiency. It is also used to support diagnosis and follow therapy of patients with hemochromatosis. Ferritin is an acute phase reactant.

Specimen Serum

Container Red top tube

Storage Instructions Separate serum from clot and refrigerate specimen. Ferritin is stable for 2 days when refrigerated or for longer periods when frozen.

Reference Interval 1 ng/mL of serum ferritin in normal subjects corresponds to ~8 mg of storage iron. Ferritin increases in adulthood in men to about the fifth decade and in women after menopause. Typical reference ranges have been in use:[1]
- newborns: 25-200 ng/mL (SI: 25-200 µg/mL)
- 1 month: 200-600 ng/mL (SI: 200-600 µg/mL)
- 2-5 months: 50-200 ng/mL (SI: 50-200 µg/mL)
- 6 months to 15 years: 7-140 ng/mL (SI: 7-140 µg/mL)
- adult male: 20-250 ng/mL (SI: 20-250 µg/L)
- adult female: younger than 40 years: 12-122 ng/mL (SI: 12-122 µg/L); older than 40 years: 12-250 ng/mL (SI: 12-250 µg/L).[2]

Serious gastrointestinal disease has been reported in subjects whose serum ferritin is ≤50 ng/mL, and endoscopic examination is considered warranted in such patients.[3]

In subjects with hepatic cirrhosis, at concentrations <50 ng/L, iron therapy has been recommended.[4]

Reference ranges of ferritin vary with age and sex.

Critical Values
Iron deficiency: <12 ng/mL (SI: <20 µg/L)
iron overload:[5] male: >325 µg/L, female: >125 µg/L

Use Useful in the differential diagnosis of hypochromic, microcytic anemias. **Decreased** in iron deficiency anemia and **increased** in iron overload. Ferritin levels correlate with and are useful in the evaluation of total body storage iron.

In hemochromatosis, both ferritin and iron saturation are increased. Ferritin levels in hemochromatosis may be >1000 ng/mL (SI: >1000 µg/L), but a normal serum ferritin cannot rule out homozygous hemochromatosis. Screening for hemochromatosis is better done with transferrin saturation. If saturation is consistently >60% in men or >50% in women, serum ferritin should be assayed. If it is high for age and sex, liver biopsy may be considered.[6] Genetic tests have become available in aiding the diagnosis of hemochromatosis (see Hereditary Hemochromatosis DNA Test *on page 709* and the following text). Normal ferritin does not exclude iron deficiency anemia.[7]

Limitations Ferritin escapes from necrotic hepatocytes. It may be increased in alcoholics who are actively abusing alcohol, in individuals with other liver diseases such as autoimmune hepatitis and hepatitis C. A quarter of patients with chronic hepatitis have increased ferritin.[8] In the presence of liver disease, with inflammation such as rheumatoid arthritis, with malignancy or with iron therapy, iron deficiency may not be reflected by low serum ferritin. Increased in inflammatory and infectious disorders. Ferritin, an acute phase reactant, is elevated as well with acute renal failure.[9] Ferritin determinations are not fully reliable when the patient is on iron therapy. Bone marrow aspiration may be needed in some settings, such as low-normal ferritin and low serum iron in the presence of apparent anemia of chronic disease, low-normal ferritin in the presence of liver disease.[2]

The differential diagnosis of transfusional siderosis versus hemochromatosis is largely dependent on clinical history; serum ferritin is less reliable than other diagnostic measures.[10]

Contraindications Ferritin is not of value to evaluate iron stores in alcoholics with liver disease. Ferritin is higher in abusing cirrhotics than in abstaining cirrhotics. Extremely high ferritin may be seen in patients with acute hepatitis.

Ferritin is elevated in hyperthyroidism.[11]

Methodology Enzyme-linked immunosorbent assay (ELISA), fluoroenzymoimmunometric assay, immunoenzymometric,[12] radioimmunometric, radioimmunoassay (RIA)

Additional Information Other than a bone marrow examination, serum ferritin is the most reliable indicator of total body iron stores. When combined with serum iron and percent saturation of iron binding capacity/transferrin, it can usually differentiate the microcytic hypochromic anemias into **iron deficiency anemia** (ferritin low, iron low, saturation low, TIBC
(Continued)

Ferritin, Serum (Continued)

high, transferrin high), the **anemia of chronic disease** (ferritin normal or high, iron low, normal to low transferrin or TIBC), or **thalassemia** (ferritin normal or high). A low serum ferritin level and elevated serum transferrin-receptor indicate iron deficiency anemia, while the ferritin may be normal or raised with low-normal to normal transferrin receptor levels in anemia of chronic disease. (See table in Iron and Total Iron Binding Capacity/Transferrin, Serum *on page 203* and see Anemia Flowchart *on page 392*.) In iron deficiency, the **red cell distribution width** is increased, while it is normal with heterozygous alpha or beta thalassemia trait. The **MCV** is reduced in iron deficiency and alpha or beta thalassemia trait; each is normal with lead poisoning. Ferritin is low with combined iron deficiency and thalassemia. **In adults**, serum ferritin level ≤20 ng/mL indicates iron deficiency.

High serum ferritin may be associated with inflammation, liver disease, megaloblastic anemia, hemolytic anemia, sideroblastic anemia, thalassemia, iron overload (hemochromatosis, hemosiderosis), and malignant diseases. The latter include leukemia and malignant lymphoma. Very high levels usually indicate iron overload. Oral and injected iron increase ferritin levels. Increased serum ferritin is considered a risk factor in primary hepatocellular carcinoma.[6,13]

Primary hemochromatosis is inherited as an autosomal recessive trait, but clinically it is much more common in males. Only homozygotes bear full clinical expression of hemochromatosis. The frequency of homozygosity has been estimated at 3-10 per 1000 in some populations, but the frequency of hemochromatosis when liver biopsy is required for diagnosis is up to 3.7 per 1000. Hemochromatosis can be recognized before disease develops when only homozygosity for the mutant allele is required. The gold standard for diagnosis is liver biopsy with liver iron concentration and calculation of hepatic iron index (ratio of hepatic iron to patient age).[14] Effective therapy (phlebotomies) is available[6] (see Phlebotomy, Therapeutic *on page 849*). **HLA-A3** alloantigen is found in about 70% of subjects who have hemochromatosis.[6] The gene is present on the short arm of chromosome 6. Genetic tests for detection of hemochromatosis mutations (C282Y and H63D) have become available. Homozygosity for C282Y mutation is responsible for up to 90% of hemochromatosis patients. The other mutation, H63D, has been seen in some patients with C282Y mutation, but has reduced penetrance of <2%.[15,16] Inappropriate increase in iron absorption and parenchymal tissue deposition may eventuate in hepatic cirrhosis, diabetes, testicular atrophy, cardiomyopathy, arthropathy, and bronze to slate gray skin pigmentation and very high serum ferritin levels (usually >1000 ng/mL).

Red cell ferritin in conjunction with plasma ferritin may be useful in distinguishing iron deficiency from iron overload in patients who have β-thalassemia.[17]

The decline in serum ferritin occurring during adolescence has been shown to be due to the onset of menarche rather than as a result of the accompanying growth spurt.[18]

Elevated serum ferritin levels in patients with cancer is associated with a poor prognosis which may be due in part to deleterious biological effects of tumor ferritins on lymphocyte and granulocyte function.[19] Data on the nature of isoferritins and their association with and possible utilization in the evaluation of malignant neoplasia is available.[20]

An immunoassay utilizing calibrated mixtures of anti-H and anti-L ferritin subunit monoclonal antibodies has been shown to recognize intermediate isoferritins but was not found to have significant application to tumor monitoring.[21]

Serum transferrin receptor measurements distinguish iron deficiency anemia from the anemia of chronic disease, used with assays of hemoglobin, hematocrit, and ferritin.[7,22,23] See Transferrin Receptor, Soluble, Serum or Plasma *on page 493*.

Footnotes

1. Painter RC, Cope JY, and Smith JL, "Reference Information for Clinical Laboratory," *Tietz Textbook of Clinical Chemistry*, 3rd ed, Burtis CA and Ashwood ER, eds, 1999, Philadelphia, PA: WB Saunders Co, 1813.
2. Sheehan RG, Newton MJ, and Frenkel EP, "Evaluation of a Packaged Kit Assay of Serum Ferritin and Application to Clinical Diagnosis of Selected Anemias," *Am J Clin Pathol*, 1978, 70(1):79-84.
3. Lee JG, Sahagun G, Oehlke MA, et al, "Serious Gastrointestinal Pathology Found in Patients With Serum Ferritin ≤50 ng/mL," *Am J Gastroenterol*, 1998, 93(5):772-6.
4. Intragumtornchai T, Rojnukkarin P, Swasdikul D, et al, "The Role of Serum Ferritin in Diagnosis of Iron Deficiency in Liver Cirrhosis," *J Intern Med*, 1998, 243(2):133-41.
5. Bulaj ZJ, Ajioka RS, Phillips JD, et al, "Disease-Related Conditions in Relatives of Patients With Hemochromatosis," *N Engl J Med*, 2000, 343(21):1529-35.
6. Edwards CQ and Kushner JP, "Screening for Hemochromatosis," *N Engl J Med*, 1993, 328(22):1616-20.
7. Cook JD, "Iron-Deficiency Anemia," *Baillieres Clin Haematol*, 1994, 7(4):787-804.
8. Bell H, Skinningsrud A, Raknerud N, et al, "Serum Ferritin and Transferrin Saturation in Patients With Chronic Alcoholic and Nonalcoholic Liver Diseases," *J Intern Med*, 1994, 236(3):315-22.
9. Mavromatidis K, Fytil C, Kynigopoulou P, et al, "Serum Ferritin Levels Are Increased in Patients With Acute Renal Failure," *Clin Nephrol*, 1998, 49(5):296-8.
10. Andrews NC, "Disorders of Iron Metabolism," *N Engl J Med*, 1999, 341(26):1986-94.
11. Gambino R, "Serum Ferritin Levels Are Elevated in Hyperthyroidism," *Lab Rep*, 1994, 16(10):81.
12. Ramm GA, Duplock LR, Powell LW, et al, "Sensitive and Rapid Colorimetric Immunoenzymometric Assay of Ferritin in Biological Samples," *Clin Chem*, 1990, 36(6):837-40.
13. Hann HW, Kim CY, London WT, et al, "Increased Serum Ferritin in Chronic Liver Disease: A Risk Factor for Primary Hepatocellular Carcinoma," *Int J Cancer*, 1989, 43(3):376-9.
14. "A 25-Year-Old Man With the Recent Onset of Diabetes Mellitus and Congestive Heart Failure," Case Records of the Massachusetts General Hospital, Case 31-1994, Scully RE, Mark EJ, McNeely WF, et al, eds, *N Engl J Med*, 1994, 331(7):460-6.
15. Beutler E, Gelbart T, West C, et al, "Mutation Analysis in Hereditary Hemochromatosis," *Blood Cells Mol Dis*, 1996, 22(2):187-94.
16. Edwards CQ, Griffen LM, Ajioka RS, et al, "Screening for Hemochromatosis: Phenotype Versus Genotype," *Semin Hematol*, 1998, 35(1):72-6.
17. Van Der Weyden MB, Fong H, Hallam LJ, et al, "Red Cell Ferritin and Iron Overload in Heterozygous Beta-Thalassemia," *Am J Hematol*, 1989, 30(4):201-5.
18. Kagamimori S, Fujita T, Naruse Y, et al, "A Longitudinal Study of Serum Ferritin Concentration During the Female Adolescent Growth Spurt," *Ann Hum Biol*, 1988, 15(6):413-9.
19. Hann HW, Stahlhut MW, Lee S, et al, "Effects of Isoferritins on Human Granulocytes," *Cancer*, 1989, 63(12):2492-6.
20. Albertini A, Arosio P, Chiancone E, et al, "Ferritins and Isoferritins as Biochemical Markers," *Proceedings of Advanced Course on Ferritins and Isoferritins as Biochemical Markers*, Amsterdam, Holland: Elsevier/North Holland Biomedical Press, 1984.
21. Cozzi A, Levi S, Bazzigaluppi E, et al, "Development of an Immunoassay for All Human Isoferritins, and Its Application to Serum Ferritin Evaluation," *Clin Chim Acta*, 1989, 184(3):197-206.
22. Testa U, Pelosi E, and Peschle C, "The Transferrin Receptor," *Crit Rev Oncog*, 1993, 4(3):241-76.
23. Cook JD, Skikne BS, and Baynes RD, "Serum Transferrin Receptor," *Annu Rev Med*, 1993, 44:63-74.

References

Beutler E, Felitti V, Gelbart T, et al, "The Effects of HFE Genotypes on Measurements of Iron Overload in Patients Attending a Health Appraisal Clinic," *Ann Intern Med*, 2000, 133(5):329-37.

Brittenham GM, Cohen AR, McLaren CE, et al, "Hepatic Iron Stores and Plasma Ferritin Concentration in Patients With Sickle Cell Anemia and Thalassemia Major," *Am J Hematol*, 1993, 42(1):81-5.

Conrad ME and Umbreit JN, "A Concise Review: Iron Absorption - The Mucin-Mobilferrin-Integrin Pathway. A Competitive Pathway for Metal Absorption," *Am J Hematol*, 1993, 42(1):67-73.

Dawson DW, Fish DI, and Shackleton P, "The Accuracy and Clinical Interpretation of Serum Ferritin Assays," *Clin Lab Haematol*, 1992, 14(1):47-52.

Felitti VJ and Beutler E, "New Developments in Hereditary Hemochromatosis," *Am J Med Sci*, 1999, 318(4):257-68.

Hann HW, Lange B, Stahlhut MW, et al, "Prognostic Importance of Serum Transferrin and Ferritin in Childhood Hodgkin Disease," *Cancer*, 1990, 66(2):313-6.

Holyoake TL, Stott DJ, McKay PJ, et al, "Use of Plasma Ferritin Concentration to Diagnose Iron Deficiency in Elderly Patients," *J Clin Pathol*, 1993, 46(9):857-60.

Looker AC, Dallman PR, Carroll MD, et al, "Prevalence of Iron Deficiency in the United States," *JAMA*, 1997, 277(12):973-6.

Oski FA, "Iron Deficiency in Infancy and Childhood," *N Engl J Med*, 1993, 329(3):190-3.

Powell LW, George DK, McDonnell SM, et al, "Diagnosis of Hemochromatosis," *Ann Intern Med*, 1998, 129(11):925-31.

Tancabelic J, Sheth S, Paik M, et al, "Serum Transferrin Receptor as a Marker of Erythropoietic Suppression in Patients on Chronic Transfusion," *Am J Hematol*, 1999, 60(2):121-5.

♦ **Fetal Fibronectin, Cervicovaginal Secretions** *see* Fibronectin, Fetal, Cervicovaginal Secretions *on page 174*

Fibronectin, Fetal, Cervicovaginal Secretions

Related Information
Bacterial Culture, Genital Specimen *on page 571*
Point-of-Care Testing *on page 43*

Synonyms Fetal Fibronectin, Cervicovaginal Secretions

Abstract Fetal fibronectin (fFN) is a high molecular weight glycoprotein, distinguishable from other fibronectins by a specific epitope (the "oncofetal domain") which is recognized by the FDC-6 monoclonal antibody.[1,2,3] FN is found in malignant tissues and cell lines, fetal connective tissue, amniotic fluid, and placenta.[1] With respect to the latter, fFN is localized to the region at which the placenta and its membranes contact the wall of the uterus, suggesting a possible role for the glycoprotein in the adhesion of the placenta to the uterus during pregnancy.[4] This location permits fFN leakage into the vagina prior to the onset of labor, initiated, perhaps, by mechanical or infectious processes.[4,5] Fetal fibronectin is normally present in cervicovaginal fluid before 21 weeks gestation. However, after 21 weeks, fFN ceases to be present in cervicovaginal secretions until just before delivery at about 37 weeks,[4] its reappearance correlating with cervical ripening.[6,7] **The abnormal presence of fFN in cervicovaginal secretions between 21-37 weeks gestation is associated with preterm delivery.**[4,8,9,10,11,12,13]

Patient Preparation Patients with signs and symptoms of premature labor should be sampled between 24 weeks, 0 days and 34 weeks, and 6 days gestation. Amniotic membranes should be intact, and cervical dilation should be minimal (<3 cm). There should be no cervical cerclage; moderate or gross vaginal bleeding should also be absent.[13,14,15]

Asymptomatic patients should be sampled between 22 weeks, 0 days and 30 weeks, 6 days in order to achieve maximum sensitivity.[11] There should be no cervical cerclage, no placenta previa, and no history of sexual intercourse within the 24 hours prior to specimen collection.[11,15]

The sampling area should be free of lubricants, soaps, disinfectants, or creams. Specimens should be obtained prior to digital cervical examination or vaginal probe ultrasound examination as manipulation of the cervix may cause the release of fFN.[15,16]

Aftercare Fetal fibronectin is said to identify subjects at risk for delivery in the following 7 days.

Specimen Cervicovaginal secretions, swab of vaginal vault

Sampling Time Clinical criteria for testing:[17]
- intact amniotic membranes
- cervical dilatation <2 cm and effacement <80%
- sampling not earlier than 24 weeks and not later than 34 weeks, 6 days gestation

Collection During speculum examination, a Dacron® swab is used to obtain specimen from the posterior vaginal fornix or cervix.[11] The specimen is eluted from the swab into a buffer solution.

Storage Instructions Store for up to 3 days at 2°C to 8°C until analysis.

Turnaround Time ≤2 hours is recommended[17]

Reference Interval Fetal fibronectin is not normally found in the maternal vagina before 37 weeks gestation. Results are reported as negative or positive. Negative results correspond to concentrations <50 ng/mL and are associated with a low likelihood of preterm delivery. Positive results correspond to concentrations ≥50 ng/mL and are indicative of increased risk of preterm labor and delivery.[4]

Use Fetal fibronectin is approved by the United States FDA to assess the risk of preterm delivery in symptomatic and asymptomatic pregnant women. Off-label uses include confirmation of ruptured membranes,[18] prediction of term and post-term delivery,[19,20,21] and prediction of successful labor induction.[21,22,23] With identification of expectant mothers likely to go into early premature labor, intervention can support continued maturation of the fetus with diminution of risk of neonatal respiratory distress syndrome.[17]

Limitations The overall sensitivity of the fFN test in screening for the likelihood of preterm delivery in low risk, asymptomatic patients is poor. However, sensitivity in this group improves somewhat by sampling during the early gestational stages (eg, 22-26 weeks). Specificity and negative predictive value of the fFN test in asymptomatic patients is high.[11]

Methodology Enzyme-linked immunosorbent assay (ELISA) and lateral flow, solid-phase immunosorbent assay. Adeza® rapid assay is in use in a tertiary care center.[17]

Additional Information The presence of fFN in the cervicovaginal secretions of symptomatic patients at risk for preterm delivery is a particularly sensitive and specific indicator of delivery within 7 days, with sensitivities of 90.5% to 93% and negative predictive values of 99% to 99.7%. Sensitivity of the test decreases in predicting longer intervals to delivery, whereas the negative predictive values remain high.[10,13] A recent, prospective study of symptomatic patients showed reduced preterm labor admissions, lengths of stay, and prescriptions for tocolytic agents as a result of testing.[24]

See Bacterial Culture, Genital Specimen *on page 571.*

Footnotes
1. Matsuura H and Hakomori S, "The Oncofetal Domain of Fibronectin Defined by Monoclonal Antibody FDC-6: Its Presence in Fibronectins From Fetal and Tumor Tissues and Its Absence in Those From Adult Tissues and Plasma," *Proc Natl Acad Sci U S A*, 1985, 82:6517-21.
2. Matsuura H, Takio K, Titani K, et al, "The Oncofetal Structure of Human Fibronectin Defined by Monoclonal Antibody FDC-6," *J Biol Chem*, 1988, 263(7):3314-22.
3. Matsuura H, Greene T, and Hakomori S, "An α-N-Acetylgalactosaminylation at the Threonine Residue of a Defined Peptide Sequence Creates the Oncofetal Peptide Epitope in Human Fibronectin," *J Biol Chem*, 1989, 264(18):10472-6.
4. Lockwood CJ, Senyei AE, Dische MR, et al, "Fetal Fibronectin in Cervical and Vaginal Secretions as a Predictor of Preterm Delivery," *N Engl J Med*, 1991, 325(10):669-74.
5. Goldenberg RL, Thom E, Moawad AH, et al, "The Preterm Prediction Study: Fetal Fibronectin, Bacterial Vaginosis, and Peripartum Infection," *Obstet Gynecol*, 1996, 87(5 Pt 1):656-60.
6. Ekman G, Granstrom L, Malmstrom A, et al, "Cervical Fetal Fibronectin Correlates to Cervical Ripening," *Acta Obstet Gynecol Scand*, 1995, 74(9):698-701.
7. Sennstrom MB, Granstrom LM, Lockwood CJ, et al, "Cervical Fetal Fibronectin Correlates to Prostaglandin E₂-Induced Cervical Ripening and Can Be Identified in Cervical Tissue," *Am J Obstet Gynecol*, 1998, 178(3):540-5.
8. Lockwood CJ, Wein R, Lapinski R, et al, "The Presence of Cervical and Vaginal Fetal Fibronectin Predicts Preterm Delivery in an Inner-City Obstetric Population," *Am J Obstet Gynecol*, 1993, 169(4):798-804.
9. Nageotte MP, Casal D, and Senyei AE, "Fetal Fibronectin in Patients at Increased Risk for Premature Birth," *Am J Obstet Gynecol*, 1994, 170(1 Pt 1):20-5.
10. Iams JD, Casal D, McGregor JA, et al, "Fetal Fibronectin Improves the Accuracy of Diagnosis of Preterm Labor," *Am J Obstet Gynecol*, 1995, 173(1):141-5.
11. Goldenberg RL, Mercer BM, Meis PJ, et al, "The Preterm Prediction Study: Fetal Fibronectin Testing and Spontaneous Preterm Birth," *Obstet Gynecol*, 1996, 87(5 Pt 1):643-8.
12. Goldenberg RL, Mercer BM, Iams JD, et al, "The Preterm Prediction Study: Patterns of Cervicovaginal Fetal Fibronectin as Predictors of Spontaneous Preterm Delivery," *Am J Obstet Gynecol*, 1997, 177(1):8-12.
13. Peaceman AM, Andrews WW, Thorp JM, et al, "Fetal Fibronectin as a Predictor of Preterm Birth in Patients With Symptoms: A Multicenter Trial," *Am J Obstet Gynecol*, 1997, 177(1):13-8.

14. "Fetal Fibronectin Preterm Labor Risk Test," ACOG Committee Opinion Number 187, Committee on Obstetric Practice, Washington, DC: The American College of Obstetricians and Gynecologists, September 1997.
15. Lukes AS, Thorp JM Jr, Eucker B, et al, "Predictors of Positivity for Fetal Fibronectin in Patients With Symptoms of Preterm Labor," *Am J Obstet Gynecol*, 1997, 176(3):639-41.
16. McKenna DS, Chung K, and Iams JD, "Effect of Digital Cervical Examination on the Expression of Fetal Fibronectin," *J Reprod Med*, 1999, 44:(9) 796-800.
17. Heise RH and Rommel S, "Fetal Fibronectin: Bedside and In-House Testing for Prediction of Preterm Labor," *Mayo Reference Services Communique*, Rochester, MN, 2000.
18. Eriksen NL, Parisi VM, Daoust S, et al, "Fetal Fibronectin: A Method for Detecting the Presence of Amniotic Fluid," *Obstet Gynecol*, 1992, 80:451-4.
19. Ahner R, Kiss H, Egarter C, et al, "Fetal Fibronectin as a Marker to Predict the Onset of Term Labor and Delivery," *Am J Obstet Gynecol*, 1995, 172(1):134-7.
20. Lockwood CJ, Moscarelli RD, Wein R, et al, "Low Concentrations of Vaginal Fetal Fibronectin as a Predictor of Deliveries Occurring After 41 Weeks," *Am J Obstet Gynecol*, 1994, 171(1):1-4.
21. Blanch G, Olah KS, and Walkinshaw S, "The Presence of Fetal Fibronectin in the Cervicovaginal Secretions of Women at Term - Its Role in the Assessment of Women Before Labor Induction and in the Investigation of the Physiologic Mechanisms of Labor," *Am J Obstet Gynecol*, 1996, 174(Pt 1):262-6.
22. Ahner R, Egarter C, Kiss H, et al, "Fetal Fibronectin as a Selection Criterion for Induction of Term Labor," *Am J Obstet Gynecol*, 1995, 173(5):1513-7.
23. Garite TJ, Casal D, Garcia-Alonso A, et al, "Fetal Fibronectin: A New Tool for the Prediction of Successful Induction of Labor," *Am J Obstet Gynecol*, 1996, 175(6):1516-21.
24. Joffe GM, Jacques D, Bemis-Heys R, et al, "Impact of the Fetal Fibronectin Assay on the Admissions for Preterm Labor," *Am J Obstet Gynecol*, 1999, 180(3 Pt 1):581-6.

References
Ascarelli MH and Morrison JC, "Use of Fetal Fibronectin in Clinical Practice," *Obstet Gynecol Surv*, 1997, 52(4 Suppl):S1-S12.

Chien PF, Khan KS, Ogston S, et al, "The Diagnostic Accuracy of Cervico-Vaginal Fetal Fibronectin in Predicting Preterm Delivery: An Overview," *Br J Obstet Gynaecol*, 1997,104(4):436-44.

Faron G, Boulvain M, Irion O, et al, "Prediction of Preterm Delivery by Fetal Fibronectin: A Meta-Analysis," *Obstet Gynecol*, 1998, 92:153-8.

Leitich H, Egarter C, Kaider A, et al, "Cervicovaginal Fetal Fibronectin as a Marker for Preterm Delivery: A Meta-Analysis," *Am J Obstet Gynecol*, 1999, 180(5):1169-76.

Revah A, Hannah ME, and Sue-A-Quan AK, "Fetal Fibronectin as a Predictor of Preterm Birth: An Overview," *Am J Perinatol*, 1998, 15(11):613-21.

♦ **Finasteride** *see* Prostate Specific Antigen, Serum *on page 263*

♦ **Fluid, Pericardial** *see* Body Fluid Chemical Analysis *on page 123*

♦ **Fluid, Peritoneal** *see* Body Fluid Chemical Analysis *on page 123*

♦ **Fluid, Pleural** *see* Body Fluid Chemical Analysis *on page 123*

♦ **Fluoride Inhibition of Cholinesterase** *see* Dibucaine Number, Serum or Plasma *on page 166*

♦ **Foam Stability Index or Shake Test** *see* Pulmonary Surfactant, Amniotic Fluid *on page 271*

Follicle Stimulating Hormone, Serum, Plasma, or Urine

Related Information
Adrenal Cortex: Laboratory Assessments Overview *on page 84*
Estradiol, Serum *on page 170*
Estrogens, Urine *on page 172*
Heterophilic Antibodies *on page 191*
Luteinizing Hormone, Blood or Urine *on page 219*
Urine Collection, 24-Hour *on page 47*

Synonyms Follitropin; FSH

Applies to CCCT; Clomiphene Citrate Challenge Test; FSH:LH Ratio; Gonadotropic Hormones; Pituitary Gonadotropins

Abstract Follicle stimulating hormone (FSH) and luteinizing hormone (LH) are glycoprotein gonadotropic hormones, produced by the same pituitary cell type. The alpha subunits of LH, FSH, thyroid stimulating hormone (TSH), and human chorionic gonadotropin (hCG) are identical; specificity resides in the beta subunits. In females, FSH promotes the development of ovarian follicles and, together with LH, stimulates secretion of estradiol from the maturing follicles. In males, FSH stimulates spermatogenesis.

Patient Preparation If a radioimmunoassay method is used, avoid recently administered radioisotopes.

Specimen Serum or plasma, timed urine collection

Container Red top tube or green top (heparin) tube; plastic urine container with or without preservative as required by testing laboratory

Collection Refrigerate urine during collection.

Storage Instructions Separate and refrigerate or freeze serum or plasma; avoid hemolysis. Serum FSH is stable 4 hours at 4°C to 25°C, 2 weeks at -20°C, 3 months at -70°C. In urine, FSH is stable 3 months at -20°C.[1,2] Avoid repeated freeze/thaw cycles.

Special Instructions For females, menstrual history is necessary for interpretation.
(Continued)

Follicle Stimulating Hormone, Serum, Plasma, or Urine *(Continued)*

Reference Interval Reference intervals for serum and urine FSH vary among laboratories and are dependent upon the units used and length of urine collection.

Serum:
- prepubertal children: <10 IU/L (SI: <10 IU/L)
- adults: male: <22 IU/L (SI: <22 IU/L)
- adults: female:
  - nonmidcycle: <20 IU/L (SI: <20 IU/L)
  - midcycle surge: <40 IU/L (SI: <40 IU/L) (ovulatory midcycle peak about twice the basal level)
  - postmenopause: 40-160 IU/L (SI: 40-160 IU/L).

Urine:
- male:
  - 0-8 years of age: <5 IU/24 hours (SI: <5 IU/day)
  - older than 9 years: <22 IU/24 hours (SI: <22 IU/day)
- female:
  - 0-8 years: <5 IU/24 hours (SI: <5 IU/day)
  - 9-15 years: <22 IU/24 hours (SI: <22 IU/day)
  - older than 15 years: <30 IU/24 hours (SI: <30 IU/day)
  - postmenopausal: two to three times cycling level.

Results can only interpreted with clinical information. A recent report,[3] which included 3388 women 35-60 years of age, showed that 73% of women having serum FSH levels ≥20 IU/L were postmenopausal. The same study showed that serum FSH levels increase with age and are increased in smokers.

Use Elevated FSH and LH are found in primary hypogonadism, anorchia, gonadal failure,[4] complete testicular feminization syndrome, Klinefelter syndrome, alcoholism, and castration. FSH and LH are pituitary products and are useful in distinguishing primary gonadal failure from secondary (hypothalamic/pituitary) causes of gonadal failure. They are used in investigation of impotence, gynecomastia, and menstrual disturbances including oligomenorrhea and amenorrhea. FSH and LH are useful infertility evaluations of women and men. Both FSH and LH are low in pituitary or hypothalamic (gonadotroph) failure. Timed urinary collections for FSH mitigate the problems of pulsatile, episodic secretion. They are used mainly for women undergoing *in vitro* fertilization and children being worked up for precocious puberty.

Methodology Radioimmunoassay (RIA) and two-site immunometric assay with radioisotope, fluorometric, enzyme, or chemiluminescent detection are used.

Additional Information Secretion of both LH and FSH is pulsatile, in response to the normal intermittent release of gonadotropin releasing hormone (GnRH). In addition, in females both FSH and LH vary over the course of the menstrual cycle, with peaks at time of ovulation. In this patient population it has been suggested that samples should be obtained at 15- to 30-minute intervals and equal volumes of serum should be pooled to decrease the effect of pulsatile excretion. Normal values do not exclude pituitary deficiency.

FSH and LH are under complex regulation by hypothalamic GnRH and by gonadal sex hormones: estrogen and progesterone in females, and testosterone in males. On the simplest level, FSH and LH are high in conditions in which sex hormones cannot be elaborated, and low in conditions of primary pituitary dysfunction. FSH acts on granulosa cells of the ovary and the Sertoli cells of testis. LH acts on Leydig (interstitial) cells of the gonads. Normally FSH increase occurs at an early stage of puberty and it is 2-4 years before LH reaches similar levels.

FSH **is high** in Klinefelter syndrome and in some subjects with precocious puberty. It is decreased with precocious puberty related to adrenal tumors or congenital adrenal hyperplasia. Normal FSH, in an adult nonovulating female, indicates dysfunction at the central nervous system hypothalamic/pituitary level.

High LH:FSH ratio (>1.5) is found in the polycystic ovary syndrome.[5]

FSH is used as a test of ovarian reserve for the purpose of predicting potential fertility in women participating in assisted reproductive technologies. Either a basal serum FSH level alone is done on day 3 of the menstrual cycle or a clomiphene citrate challenge test (CCCT) is done. In the latter, a basal FSH level is done on day 3 of the cycle. Then, on each of days 5-9, 100 mg of oral clomiphene citrate is given. On day 10 another serum FSH level is done. Elevated results on either day 3 or day 10 are consistent with a positive test for infertility. Overall, the CCCT is 26% sensitive and 98% specific with a positive predictive value of 96% and a negative predictive value of 42%.[6]

Low serum FSH levels in women have been reported to be associated with increased risk of ovarian cancer.[7]

Cases of hypogonadism and delayed puberty have been shown to be associated with mutations in the gene for the beta subunit of FSH.[8,9]

Footnotes

1. Kubasik NP, Ricotta M, Hunter T, et al, "Effect of Duration and Temperature of Storage on Serum Analyte Stability: Examination of 14 Selected Radioimmunoassay Procedures," *Clin Chem*, 1982, 28(1):164-5.

2. Livesey JH, Hodgkinson SC, Roud HR, et al, "Effect of Time, Temperature and Freezing on the Stability of Immunoreactive LH, FSH, TSH, Growth Hormone, Prolactin and Insulin in Plasma," *Clin Biochem*, 1980, 13(4):151-5.

3. Backer LC, Rubin CS, Kieszak SM, et al, "Serum Follicle-Stimulating Hormone and Luteinizing Hormone Levels in Women Aged 35-60 in the U.S. Population: The Third National Health and Nutrition Examination Survey (NHANES III, 1988-1994)," *Menopause*, 1999, 6(1):29-35.

4. Layman LC, Wilson JT, Huey LO, et al, "Gonadotropin-Releasing Hormone, Follicle-Stimulating Hormone Beta, Luteinizing Hormone Beta Gene Structure in Idiopathic Hypogonadotropic Hypogonadism," *Fertil Steril*, 1992, 57(1):42-9.

5. Turhan NO, Toppare MF, Seckin NC, et al, "The Predictive Power of Endocrine Tests for the Diagnosis of Polycystic Ovaries in Women With Oligoamenorrhea," *Gynecol Obstet Invest*, 1999, 48(3):183-6.

6. Barnhart K and Osheroff J, "Follicle Stimulating Hormone as a Predictor of Fertility," *Curr Opin Obstet Gynecol*, 1998, 10(3):227-32.

7. Helzlsouer KJ, Alberg AJ, Gordon GB, et al, "Serum Gonadotropins and Steroid Hormones and the Development of Ovarian Cancer," *JAMA*, 1995, 274(24):1926-30.

8. Layman LC, Lee EJ, Peak DB, et al, "Delayed Puberty and Hypogonadism Caused by Mutations in the Follicle-Stimulating Hormone B-Subunit Gene," *N Engl J Med*, 1997, 337(9):607-11.

9. Phillip M, Arbelle JE, Segev Y, et al, "Male Hypogonadism Due to a Mutation in the Gene for the B-Subunit of Follicle-Stimulating Hormone," *N Engl J Med*, 1998, 338(24):1729-32.

References

Bancsi LF, Huijs AM, Den Ouden CT, et al, "Basal Follicle-Stimulating Hormone Levels Are of Limited Value in Predicting Ongoing Pregnancy Rates After *In Vitro* Fertilization," *Fertil Steril*, 2000, 73(3):552-7.

Howanitz JH, "Review of the Influence of Polypeptide Hormone Forms on Immunoassay Results," *Arch Pathol Lab Med*, 1993, 1174(4):369-72.

Jaakkola T, Ding YQ, Kellokumpu-Lehtinen P, et al, "The Ratios of Serum Bioactive/Immunoreactive Luteinizing Hormone and Follicle-Stimulating Hormone in Various Clinical Conditions With Increased and Decreased Gonadotropin Secretion: Reevaluation by a Highly Sensitive Immunometric Assay," *J Clin Endocrinol Metab*, 1990, 70(6):1496-505.

Kim YK, Wasser SK, Fujimoto VY, et al, "Utility of Follicle Stimulating Hormone (FSH), Luteinizing Hormone (LH), Oestradiol and FSH:LH Ratio in Predicting Reproductive Age in Normal Women," *Hum Reprod*, 1997, 12(6):1152-5.

Pandian MR, Odell WD, Carlton E, et al, "Development of Third-Generation Immunochemiluminometric Assays of Follitropin and Lutropin and Clinical Application in Determining Pediatric Reference Ranges," *Clin Chem*, 1993, 39(9):1815-9.

Qiu Q, Kuo A, Todd H, et al, "Enzyme Immunoassay Method for Total Urinary Follicle-Stimulating Hormone (FSH) Beta Subunit and Its Application for Measurement of Total Urinary FSH," *Fertil Steril*, 1998, 69(2):278-85.

Taylor AE, Khoury RH, and Crowley WF Jr, "A Comparison of 13 Different Immunometric Assay Kits for Gonadotropins: Implications for Clinical Investigation," *J Clin Endocrinol Metab*, 1994, 79(1):240-7.

Vance ML, "Hypopituitarism," *N Engl J Med*, 1994, 330(23):1651-62.

♦ **Free Thyroxine Assays** *see* Free Thyroxine Index *on page 177*

Free Thyroxine Index

Related Information
Heterophilic Antibodies *on page 191*
T_3 Uptake, Serum or Plasma *on page 279*
Thyroid Stimulating Hormone, Serum *on page 282*
Thyroperoxidase Autoantibody *on page 545*
Thyroxine Binding Globulin, Serum *on page 284*
Thyroxine, Free, Serum *on page 285*
Thyroxine, Serum *on page 286*
Triiodothyronine, Serum *on page 290*

Synonyms Free Thyroid Index; FT_4I; FT_4 Index; FTI

Applies to Free T_3; Free T_4; Free Thyroxine Assays; Sick Euthyroid Syndrome

Test Includes T_3 uptake and T_4

Abstract The free thyroxine index (FTI) may be calculated as the product of T_3 resin uptake (RT_3U) and total T_4 level; it is usually proportional to actual FT_4. It is an imperfect measure but provides acceptable results with pregnant subjects and in a variety of other settings in which thyroxine binding globulin is altered. In the past, FTI had been widely used, due to unreliability of FT_4 assays. **In recent years, assays for TSH have improved, free thyroxine assays have become more reliable, and use of FTI has decreased.**

With the continuous improvement of the sensitivity of measurements for TSH, free T_4, and free T_3, determination of the free thyroxine index is becoming less relevant. The FTI is no longer considered a useful test.

Patient Preparation No recent administration of radioactive substances (eg, no recent scans) if RIA testing is in place.

Specimen Serum is preferred; plasma may be used.

Container Red top tube; lavender top (EDTA) tube or green top (heparin) tube is acceptable.

Storage Instructions Separate serum or plasma within 48 hours and refrigerate.

Reference Interval 10 years to adult: normal: 5.0-13.0, low: ≤4.8, high: ≥14.0. Normal ranges will differ somewhat between laboratories. The units are similar to total T_4 units.

Use To estimate free thyroxine. Presently, the FTI may be used to monitor therapy for hyperthyroidism and to supplement the sTSH, but its application is becoming progressively only of historic interest.

Limitations The "sick euthyroid syndrome" is an expression used to describe a euthyroid subject whose T_4 and FTI are decreased with severe illness.

The free T_4 index based on T_3 binding to serum proteins (eg, T_3 uptake) is not entirely reliable when decreased serum thyroxine is caused by decreased thyroid hormone binding to thyroxine binding globulin. That is, the value of the free thyroxine index is limited in the differential diagnosis of low total T_4.

See T_3 Uptake, Serum or Plasma *on page 279* for additional limitations.

Methodology Calculation from results of T_3 uptake and T_4.

$$FTI = [\%T_3U \text{ (patient)} / \%T_3U \text{ (reference serum)}] \times T_4$$

Additional Information Calculation includes the T_4 and T_3 uptake values. T_3 uptake and T_4 are influenced by pregnancy, contraceptive pills, abnormalities of serum proteins and other factors, mostly in opposite directions. The free thyroxine index permits interpretation by balancing out most nonthyroidal factors. For example, a pregnant euthyroid patient would have an increased T_4, but the FTI would be normal due to decreased T_3 uptake. An euthyroid patient with nephrotic syndrome may have a decreased T_4 (due to decreased levels by binding proteins), but the FTI would be normal due to increased T_3 uptake.

Drugs that influence thyroid function are tabulated in the listing Thyroxine Binding Globulin, Serum *on page 284*.

References
Attia J, Margetts P and Guyatt G, "Diagnosis of Thyroid Disease in Hospitalized Patients: A Systematic Review," *Arch Intern Med*, 1999, 159(7):658-65.
Dayan CM, "Interpretation of Thyroid Function Tests," *Lancet*, 2001, 357:619-24.
Ercan-Fang S, Schwartz HL, Mariash CN, et al, "Quantitative Assessment of Pituitary Resistance to Thyroid Hormone From Plots of the Logarithm of Thyrotropin Versus Serum Free Thyroxine Index," *J Clin Endocrinol Metab*, 2000, 85(6):2299-303.
Faix JD, Rosen HN, and Velazquez FR, "Indirect Estimation of Thyroid Hormone-Binding Proteins to Calculate Free Thyroxine Index: Comparison of Nonisotopic Methods That Use Labeled Thyroxine ("T-Uptake")," *Clin Chem*, 1995, 41(1):41-7.
Helfand M and Redfern CC, "Clinical Guideline Part 2. Screening for the Thyroid Disease: An Update," American College of Physicians, *Ann Intern Med*, 1998, 129(2):144-58.
Lewis GF, Alessi CA, Imperial JG, et al, "Low Serum Free Thyroxine Index in Ambulating Elderly Is Due to a Resetting of the Threshold of Thyrotropin Feedback Suppression," *J Clin Endocrinol Metab*, 1991, 73(4):843-9.
Mandel SJ, Larsen PR, Seely EW, et al, "Increased Need for Thyroxine During Pregnancy in Women With Primary Hypothyroidism," *N Engl J Med*, 1990, 323(2):91-6.
Mechanick JI, Sacks HS, Cobin RH, et al, "Hypothalamic-Pituitary Axis Dysfunction in Critically Ill Patients With a Low Free Thyroxine Index," *J Endocrinol Invest*, 1997, 20(8):462-70.
Oxley DK, "Screening for Hyperthyroidism," *Arch Pathol Lab Med*, 1991, 1201-2.
Schussler GC, "The Thyroxine-Binding Proteins," *Thyroid*, 2000, 10(2):141-9.
Whitley RJ, "Thyroid Function," *Tietz Textbook of Clinical Chemistry*, 3rd ed, Burtis CA and Ashwood ER, eds, Philadelphia, PA: WB Saunders Co, 1999, 1496-529.

♦ **Free Thyroxine Index, Calculated** *see* Thyroxine Binding Globulin, Serum *on page 284*

♦ **Free-Zone CE** *see* Protein Electrophoresis, Capillary Zone *on page 266*

♦ **Friedewald Equation** *see* Low Density Lipoprotein Cholesterol *on page 218*

♦ **Friedewald Equation** *see* Triglycerides, Serum or Plasma *on page 288*

♦ **Friedman's Test** *replaced by* Chorionic Gonadotropin, Human, Serum and Urine *on page 147*

Fructosamine, Serum

Related Information
Glucose, Fasting, Plasma *on page 183*
Glucose, Noninvasive *on page 185*
Glucose, Whole Blood *on page 188*
Glycated Hemoglobin (Hemoglobin A_{1c}), Blood *on page 188*
Microalbuminuria *on page 879*

Synonyms Glycated Albumin; Glycated Proteins; Ketoamines, Plasma Protein

Abstract A fructosamine is the result of covalently linked glucose with albumin or other proteins, producing a glycated product, a stable ketoamine. It is less expensive than glycated hemoglobin. However, its use is not widely accepted at present. Its application remains under evaluation.

Patient Preparation Patients should not take ascorbic acid for at least 24 hours prior to collection.

Specimen Serum

Container Red top tube

Storage Instructions Refrigerate. Freeze sample if assay is not done within 2 hours.

Reference Interval Normal ranges vary considerably according to method. Ranges in children are slightly lower than those in adults. Nondiabetics: 1.5-2.7 mmol/L; diabetics: ≥2.0-5.0 mmol/L depending on the degree of control. Consult ranges of the particular laboratory providing the assay. The second generation assays are superior and provide much lower reference ranges than did first generation tests.

Use Monitor diabetic control, reflecting diabetic control over a shorter time period (2-3 weeks) than that represented by glycated hemoglobin (hemoglobin A_{1c}) (4-8 weeks). Indicated as an index of longer term control than glucose levels, especially in diabetic subjects with abnormal hemoglobins, patients with gestational diabetes,[1] and in type I diabetes in children.[2] Fructosamine levels may be useful in screening geriatric populations.[3] Glycated albumin, because of its short half-life, lends itself as a test to monitor and control gestational diabetes.[1] Fructosamine may well find a role, especially in subjects with abnormal hemoglobins.

Low concentrations may provide a signal of poor nutrition. Fructosamine may represent a tool to identify women at risk of hip fracture.[4]

Limitations Fructosamine, like Hb A_{1c}, is not useful for diagnosis of diabetes mellitus. Very low albumin concentrations (<3.0 g/dL) may result in falsely low fructosamine values.

Not all proteins are glycated at the same rate. Therefore, altered albumin:globulin ratios will affect results.

Contraindications This test should not be done in the sera of patients with very low albumin concentrations (eg, those with nephrotic syndromes or hepatic cirrhosis), or in those with abnormal serum proteins (eg, monoclonal gammopathies).

Methodology Colorimetry or affinity chromatography. Methods suitable for automated analyzers have been described.[5]

Additional Information Fructosamine is found in the plasma of both normal and diabetic individuals. "Fructosamine" is the term used to describe proteins that have been glycated (ie, are derivatives of the nonenzymatic reaction product of glucose and albumin). It has been advocated as an alternative test to hemoglobin A_{1c} for the monitoring of long-term diabetic control. Fructosamine and hemoglobin A_{1c} do not measure exactly the same thing, since fructosamine has a shorter half-life and probably is somewhat more sensitive to short-term variations in glucose levels. However, this is not necessarily a disadvantage. Much of the development of fructosamine has occurred outside the United States. Although the tests are not identical, probably one or the other is sufficient in routine diabetic patients for assessment of long-term control of hyperglycemia. It is not necessary to order both tests in all patients, although both may be of value in selected problem patients. Fructosamine is clearly superior in patients with abnormal hemoglobins because of the interference of abnormal hemoglobins in the anion-exchange chromatography methods for Hb A_{1c}. An ion-capture immunoassay (Abbott Laboratories) can measure Hb A_{1c} in the presence of abnormal hemoglobins.

Footnotes
1. Narayanan S, "Laboratory Monitoring of Gestational Diabetes," *Ann Clin Lab Sci*, 1991, 21(6):392-401.
2. Cefalu WT, Mejia E, Puente GR, et al, "Correlation of Serum Fructosamine Activity in Type I Diabetic Children," *Am J Med Sci*, 1989, 297(4):244-6.
(Continued)

Fructosamine, Serum *(Continued)*

3. Croxson SC, Absalom S, and Burden AC, "Fructosamine in Diabetes Screening of the Elderly," *Ann Clin Biochem*, 1991, 28(Pt 3):279-82.
4. Jamal SA, Stone K, Browner WS, et al, "Serum Fructosamine Level and the Risk of Hip Fracture in Elderly Women: A Case-Cohort Study Within the Study of Osteoporotic Fractures," *Am J Med*, 1998, 105(6):488-93.
5. Hill RP, Hindle EJ, Howey JE, et al, "Recommendations for Adopting Standard Conditions and Analytical Procedures in the Measurement of Serum Fructosamine Concentration," *Ann Clin Biochem*, 1990, 27(Pt 5):413-24.

References

Allgrove J and Cockrill BL, "Fructosamine or Glycated Haemoglobin as a Measure of Diabetic Control?" *Arch Dis Child*, 1988, 63(4):418-22.

Austin GE, Wheaton R, Nanes MS, et al, "Usefulness of Fructosamine for Monitoring Outpatients With Diabetes," *Am J Med Sci*, 1999, 318(5):316-23.

Browner WS, Pressman AR, Lui LY, et al, "Association Between Serum Fructosamine and Mortality in Elderly Women: The Study of Osteoporitic Fractures," *Am J Epidemiol*, 1999, 149(5):471-5.

Desjarlais F, Comtois R, Beauregard H, et al, "Technical and Clinical Evaluation of Fructosamine Determination in Serum," *Clin Biochem*, 1989, 22(4):329-35.

Furnseth K, Bruusgaard D, Rutle O, et al, "Fructosamine Cannot Replace Hb A$_{1c}$ in the Management of Type 2 Diabetes (NIDDM)," *Scand J Prim Health Care*, 1994, 12(3):219-24.

Gebhart SS, Wheaton RN, Mullins RE, et al, "A Comparison of Home Glucose Monitoring With Determinations of Hemoglobin A$_{1c}$, Total Glycated Hemoglobin, Fructosamine, and Random Serum Glucose in Diabetic Patients," *Arch Intern Med*, 1991, 151(6):1133-7.

Hartland AJ, Smith JM, Clark PM, et al, "Establishing Trimester- and Ethnic Group-related Reference Ranges for Fructosamine and HbA1c in Nondiabetic Pregnant Women," *Ann Clin Biochem*, 1999, 36 (Pt 2):235-7.

Horn F and Ettinger B, "Comparison of Serum Fructosamine vs Glycohemoglobin as Measures of Glycemic Control in a Large Diabetic Population," *Acta Diabetol Lat*, 1998, 35(1):48-51.

Jerntorp P, Sundkvist G, Fex G, et al, "Clinical Utility of Serum Fructosamine in Diabetes Mellitus Compare With Hemoglobin A$_{1c}$," *Clin Chim Acta*, 1988, 175(2):135-42.

Kennedy DM, Johnson AB, and Hill PG, "A Comparison of Automated Fructosamine and HbA1c Methods for Monitoring Diabetes in Pregnancy," *Ann Clin Biochem*, 1998, 35(Pt 2):283-9.

Ko GT, Chan JC, Yeung VT, et al, "Combined Use of a Fasting Plasma Glucose Concentration and HbA1c or Fructosamine Predicts the Likelihood of Having Diabetes in High-Risk Subjects," *Diabetes Care*, 1998, 21(8):1221-5.

Lapolla A, Poli T, Barison A, et al, "Fructosamine Assay: An Index of Medium-Term Metabolic Control Parameters in Diabetic Disease," *Diabetes Res Clin Pract*, 1988, 4(3):231-5.

Miller JC, "Importance of Glycemic Index in Diabetes," *Am J Clin Nutr*, 1994, 59(3 Suppl):747S-52S.

Negoro H, Morley JE, and Rosenthal MJ, "Utility of Serum Fructosamine as a Measure of Glycemia in Young and Old Diabetic and Nondiabetic Subjects," *Am J Med*, 1988, 85(3):360-4.

Roberts AB, Baker JR, James AG, et al, "Fructosamine in the Management of Gestational Diabetes," *Am J Obstet Gynecol*, 1988, 159(1):66-71.

Galactokinase, Blood

Related Information

Galactose-1-Phosphate, Blood *on page 178*
Galactose-1-Phosphate Uridyl Transferase, Blood *on page 179*
Newborn Screening Tests for Galactosemia *on page 232*

Synonyms RBC Galactokinase

Abstract An overview of the galactosemias is offered in Newborn Screening Tests for Galactosemia *on page 232*.

The activity of this enzyme is decreased in galactokinase-deficient galactosemia. This form of galactosemia is milder than the galactosemia due to galactose-1-phosphate uridyl transferase deficiency. Patients with galactokinase deficiency express juvenile cataracts without mental retardation.

Patient Preparation Avoid radioisotope scans or recently administered radioisotopes prior to collection of specimen, if radioactive method for the enzyme assay is being used.

Specimen Whole blood

Container Green top (heparin) tube

Collection Send blood immediately (on ice, not frozen) to the laboratory.

Storage Instructions Red blood cells must be washed repeatedly immediately after receipt in laboratory, therefore, transportation to the laboratory is critical.

Special Instructions Communicate with laboratory, as this test is not usually routinely available and may require referral.

Reference Interval Large interlaboratory differences exist. The following are examples and do not apply to all laboratories:

- children: 0-2 years: 11-150 mU/g Hb (levels in infants are 3-4 times those of adults)
- 2-18 years: 11-54 mU/g Hb
- adults: 12-40 mU/g Hb

Use Establish the diagnosis of galactokinase-deficiency galactosemia. Galactosemia may also be caused by a deficiency of galactose-1-phosphate uridyl transferase and uridine diphosphoglucose 4-epimerase.[1]

Methodology Radioisotopic: RBCs are hemolyzed and the hemolysate is incubated with radiolabeled galactose. The 1-^{14}C-galactose-1-phosphate is quantitated after binding to DEAE chromatography paper. High performance liquid chromatography (HPLC).[2]

Additional Information This condition should enter into the differential diagnosis of any child with cataracts.[3] It is an autosomal recessive inherited enzyme deficiency, 0.2% of the population is heterozygous for the defect. Homozygotes have a form of galactosemia that is associated with cataracts but usually do not suffer mental retardation, liver disease, or problems in the newborn period resulting from galactose exposure (eg, failure to thrive, vomiting, or liver disease/jaundice). Heterozygotes are at risk for the development of cataracts in young adult life. In each of the different forms of galactosemia, an alternative route of galactose metabolism is utilized. Reduction (of galactose) to galactitol and oxidation to galactonate occurs. Galactitol accumulates in the lens, producing osmotic imbalance resulting in cataract formation. An incidence of 6.9% of galactokinase deficiency has been found in a group of idiopathic cataract patients 50 years of age or younger.[4] Heterozygotes have about 50% of the normal enzyme activity. Galactokinase deficiency is in the differential diagnosis of patients with pseudotumor cerebri.[5,6] Therapy, as for transferase deficiency, consists of galactose restriction.

Footnotes

1. Beutler E, "Galactosemia: Screening and Diagnosis," *Clin Biochem*, 1991, 24(4):293-300.
2. Mizoguchi N, Eguchi T, Sakura N, et al, "Erythrocyte Galactokinase Assay With High Performance Liquid Chromatography," *Clin Chim Acta*, 1993, 216(1-2):145-51.
3. Stevens RE, Datiles MB, Srivastava SK, et al, "Idiopathic Presenile Cataract Formation and Galactosaemia," *Br J Ophthalmol*, 1989, 73(1):48-51.
4. Elman MJ, Miller MT, and Matalon R, "Galactokinase Activity in Patients With Idiopathic Cataracts," *Ophthalmology*, 1986, 93(2):210-5.
5. Litman N, Kanter A, and Finberg L, "Galactokinase Deficiency Presenting as Pseudotumor Cerebri," *J Pediatr*, 1975, 86:410-2.
6. Roe T and Ng WG, "Disorders of Carbohydrate and Glycogen Metabolism," *The Physician's Guide to the Laboratory Diagnosis of Metabolic Diseases*, Blau N, Duran M, and Blaskovics ME, eds, New York, NY: Chapman and Hall, 1996, 277-94.

References

Applegarth DA, Dimmick JE, and Toone JR, "Laboratory Detection of Metabolic Disease," *Pediatr Clin North Am*, 1989, 36(1):49-65.

Chung MA, "Galactosemia in Infancy: Diagnosis, Management, and Prognosis," *Pediatr Nurs*, 1997, 23(6):563-9.

Gitzelmann R, "Disorders of Galactose Metabolism," *Inborn Metabolic Diseases: Diagnosis and Treatment*, Fernandes J, Saudubray JM, and Van den Berghe G, eds, 3rd ed, New York, NY: Springer-Verlag, 2000, 103-9.

Holton JB, "Galactosaemia: Pathogenesis and Treatment," *J Inherit Metab Dis*, 1996, 19(1):3-7.

Petry KG and Reichardt JK, "The Fundamental Importance of Human Galactose Metabolism: Lessons From Genetics and Biochemistry," *Trends Genet*, 1998, 14(3):98-102.

Segal S and Berry GT, "Disorders of Galactose Metabolism: Galactokinase Deficiency Galactosemia," *The Metabolic and Molecular Bases of Inherited Disease*, 7th ed, Chapter 25, Scriver CR, Beaudet AL, Sly WS, et al, eds, New York, NY: McGraw-Hill Inc, 1995, 987-9.

♦ **Galactokinase Deficiency** *see* Galactose-1-Phosphate Uridyl Transferase, Blood *on page 179*

Galactose-1-Phosphate, Blood

Related Information

Galactokinase, Blood *on page 178*
Galactose-1-Phosphate Uridyl Transferase, Blood *on page 179*
Newborn Screening Tests for Galactosemia *on page 232*

Abstract See Newborn Screening Tests for Galactosemia *on page 232* for an overview of the galactosemias. Red cell concentration of galactose-1-phosphate is increased in patients with galactosemia due to deficiency of galactose-1-phosphate uridyl transferase or uridine diphosphate galactose-4-epimerase. The concentration of galactose-1-phosphate is the most sensitive index of dietary control in patients with galactosemia.

Specimen Whole blood

Container Green top (heparin) tube

Storage Instructions Store at 4°C.

Causes for Rejection Specimen more than 3 hours old

Reference Interval Normal ranges:[1]

- nongalactosemic: 5-49 μg/g hemoglobin

- galactosemic on galactose restricted diet; 80-125 µg/g hemoglobin
- galactosemic on unrestricted diet: >125 µg/g hemoglobin

Use Monitor galactosemic patients on a galactose-free diet

Limitations Analysis is offered by only a few specialized laboratories. Monitoring of galactose-free diet may be more simply achieved with less cost by using whole blood filter paper spot tests.

Methodology Enzymatic rate reaction (absorbance of NADH). Methods to detect galactose and galactose-1-phosphate from dried blood has been described.[2,3]

Additional Information Galactosemia, the result of an inherited cellular deficiency of galactose-1-phosphate uridyl transferase or uridine diphosphate galactose-4-epimerase, is characterized by galactosuria and increased red cell galactose-1-phosphate. The level of galactose in the blood relates to the dietary intake of lactose (as present in milk but also in foods containing lactose but not so labeled, eg, candy, breads, frankfurters, etc). Patients with congenital galactosemia maintained on a milk-free diet should have level of galactose-1-phosphate <2 mg/100 mL lysed packed red cells. If such patients are ingesting lactose (eg, drinking milk), levels of 9-20 mg/100 mL packed red cell lysate will be obtained.[1] A range of characteristic abnormalities result from galactose toxicity including failure to thrive, vomiting, abnormal liver function with resultant cirrhosis, and mental retardation.[4] Signs and symptoms (including even cataracts) will regress under the influence of a galactose-free diet. An increased frequency of hypergonadotropic hypogonadism in females (ovarian failure with decreased or absent ovarian tissue) has been reported[5] and occurs especially in subjects in whom diet therapy was delayed.

Footnotes

1. Leavelle DE, *Mayo Medical Laboratories: Interpretive Handbook*, Rochester, MN, 1997, 248.
2. Diepenbrock F, Heckler R, Schickling H, et al, "Colorimetric Determination of Galactose and Galactose-1-Phosphate From Dried Blood," *Clin Biochem*, 1992, 25(1):37-9.
3. Rhode H, Elei E, and Taube I, "Newborn Screening for Galactosemia: Ultramicroassay for Galactose-1-Phosphate-Uridyltransferase Activity," *Clin Chim Acta*, 1998, 274(1):71-87.
4. Segal S and Berry GT, "Disorders of Galactose Metabolism," *The Metabolic and Molecular Bases of Inherited Disease*, 7th ed, Chapter 25, Scriver CR, Beaudet AL, Sly WS, et al, eds, New York, NY: McGraw-Hill Inc, 1995, 967-1000.
5. Kaufman FR, Kogut MD, Donnell GN, et al, "Hypergonadotropic Hypogonadism in Female Patients With Galactosemia," *N Engl J Med*, 1981, 304:994-8.

References

Beutler E, "Galactosemia: Screening and Diagnosis," *Clin Biochem*, 1991, 24(4):293-300.

Gitzelmann R, "Disorders of Galactose Metabolism," *Inborn Metabolic Diseases: Diagnosis and Treatment*, Fernandes J, Saudubray JM, and Van den Berghe G, eds, 3rd ed, New York, NY: Springer-Verlag, 2000, 103-9.

Gitzelmann R, "Galactose-1-Phosphate in the Pathophysiology of Galactosemia," *Eur J Pediatr*, 1995, 154(7 Suppl 2):S45-9.

Holton JB, "Galactosaemia: Pathogenesis and Treatment," *J Inherit Metab Dis*, 1996, 19(1):3-7.

Petry KG and Reichardt JK, "The Fundamental Importance of Human Galactose Metabolism: Lessons From Genetics and Biochemistry", *Trends Genet*, 1998, 14(3):98-102.

Reichardt JK, Packman S, and Woo SL, "Molecular Characterization of Two Galactosemia Mutations: Correlation of Mutations With Highly Conserved Domains in Galactose-1-Phosphate Uridyl Transferase," *Am J Hum Genet*, 1991, 49(4):860-7.

Galactose-1-Phosphate Uridyl Transferase, Blood

Related Information

Galactokinase, Blood *on page 178*
Galactose-1-Phosphate, Blood *on page 178*
Newborn Screening Tests for Galactosemia *on page 232*
Reducing Substances, Urine *on page 885*

Applies to Galactokinase Deficiency; UDP Galactose-4-Epimerase Deficiency

Abstract An overview of the galactosemias is provided in Newborn Screening Tests for Galactosemia *on page 232*. Deficiency of this enzyme is the most common cause of galactosemia. Infants with the enzyme deficiency demonstrate failure to thrive, with onset of vomiting and diarrhea within days of milk intake. The urine from these infants will show the presence of **reducing substance** which does not react with glucose oxidase reagents. In untreated patients, the long-term effects include liver damage, cataracts, and mental deterioration.

Patient Preparation Avoid radioisotope scans or recently administered radioisotopes prior to collection of specimen, if a radioactive assay is used.

Specimen Whole blood

Container Green top (heparin) tube, lavender top (EDTA) tube

Storage Instructions Stable 14 days at room temperature, 4 weeks at 4°C; do not freeze.

Reference Interval 17-37 units (µmol/hour/g hemoglobin)

Use Diagnose galactosemia (galactose-1-phosphate uridyl transferase deficiency). Two other enzyme deficiencies that cause galactosemia are galactokinase and UDP galactose-4-epimerase.

Methodology Radioactive with ^{14}C-galactose-1-phosphate as the substrate, fluorometric,[1] colorimetric (dried blood)[2]

Additional Information Galactosemia is an autosomal recessive disorder of galactose metabolism most often caused by a deficiency of galactose-1-

---

phosphate uridyl transferase, rarely by a deficiency of galactokinase or UDP galactose-4-epimerase. Molecular genetic studies have revealed molecular heterogeneity which is related to the variable clinical outcome observed in this disorder.[3] More than 150 different base changes have been found in galactose-1-phosphate uridyl transferase gene; most frequently cited are Q188R, K285N, S135L, and N314D.[4] The resulting accumulation of galactitol and/or galactose-1-phosphate can result in juvenile cataracts, liver failure, failure to thrive, and mental retardation in galactose-1-phosphate uridyl transferase deficiency. Dietary restriction of galactose is a very effective treatment, and liver and lens changes are reversible. Quantitative assays can generally recognize the following genotypes.

- Normal-normal (NN)
- Duarte heterozygote (ND)
- Classical heterozygote (NG)
- Duarte homozygote (DD)
- Duarte galactosemia compound heterozygote (DG)
- Galactosemia-galactosemia (GG)

Cognitive outcome appears to be related to genotype rather than metabolic control. Homozygosity for Q188R has poor outcome.[5]

Blood for galactosemia screening should be obtained as early in life as possible (less than 3-4 days) so that effective therapy can be instituted.

Footnotes

1. Fujimoto A, Okano Y, Miyagi T, et al, "Quantitative Beutler Test for Newborn Mass Screening of Galactosemia Using a Fluorometric Microplate Reader," *Clin Chem*, 2000, 46(6 Pt 1):806-10.
2. Diepenbrock F, Heckler R, Schickling H, et al, "Colorimetric Determination of Galactose and Galactose-1-Phosphate From Dried Blood," *Clin Biochem*, 1992, 25(1):37-9.
3. Reichardt JK, Packman S, and Woo SL, "Molecular Characterization of Two Galactosemia Mutations: Correlation of Mutations With Highly Conserved Domains in Galactose-1-Phosphate Uridyl Transferase," *Am J Hum Genet*, 1991, 49(4):860-7.
4. Tyfield L, Reichardt J, and Fridovich-Keil J, "Classical Galactosemia and Mutations at the Galactose-1-Phosphate Uridyl Transferase (GALT) Gene," *Hum Mutat*, 1999, 13(6):417-30.
5. Shield JP, Wadsworth EJ, MacDonald A, et al, "The Relationship of Genotype to Cognitive Outcome in Galactosaemia," *Arch Dis Child*, 2000, 83(3):248-50.

References

Gitzelmann R, "Disorders of Galactose Metabolism," *Inborn Metabolic Diseases: Diagnosis and Treatment*, Fernandes J, Saudubray JM, and Van den Berghe G, eds, 3rd ed, New York, NY: Springer-Verlag, 2000, 103-9.

Holton JB, "Galactosaemia: Pathogenesis and Treatment," *J Inherit Metab Dis*, 1996, 19(1):3-7.

Kelley RI and Segal S, "Evaluation of Reduced Activity Galactose-1-Phosphate Uridyl Transferase by Combined Radioisotopic Assay and High-Resolution Isoelectric Focusing," *J Lab Clin Med*, 1989, 114(2):152-6.

Lagrou K and Declercq PE, "Simplified Assay of Galactose-1-Phosphate Uridyltransferase," *Clin Chem*, 1991, 37(12):2157-8.

Petry KG and Reichardt JK, "The Fundamental Importance of Human Galactose Metabolism: Lessons From Genetics and Biochemistry," *Trends Genet*, 1998, 14(3):98-102.

◆ **Galactosemia Screening, Filter Paper** *see* Newborn Screening Tests for Galactosemia *on page 232*

◆ **Galactosyl Hydroxylysine** *see* N-Telopeptides, Urine *on page 233*

◆ **Galli Mainini Test** *replaced by* Chorionic Gonadotropin, Human, Serum and Urine *on page 147*

Gamma-Glutamyl Transferase, Serum

Related Information

Alanine Aminotransferase, Serum *on page 87*
Alkaline Phosphatase, Heat Stable, Serum *on page 91*
Alkaline Phosphatase, Serum *on page 93*
Aspartate Aminotransferase, Serum *on page 112*
Bilirubin, Total, Serum *on page 118*
Carbohydrate-Deficient Transferrin, Serum *on page 134*
Leucine Aminopeptidase (LAP), Serum and Urine *on page 211*
Liver Biopsy *on page 65*
Liver Disease: Laboratory Assessment, Overview *on page 216*
5' Nucleotidase, Serum *on page 234*

Synonyms Gamma-Glutamyl Transpeptidase; GGT; GGTP; γ-Glutamyl Transferase; Glutamyl Transpeptidase; GT; GTP

Applies to AST:ALT Ratio; Body Fluid GGT

Replaces BSP

Abstract A biliary excretory enzyme (a peptidase), GGT is especially responsive to obstructive hepatobiliary diseases and is sensitive to ethanol use.

Patient Preparation The patient ideally should fast for 8 hours prior to collection of the specimen. Since elevations may occur with phenytoin or phenobarbital therapy, an alternate test, including alkaline phosphatase, leucine aminopeptidase (LAP) or 5' nucleotidase, is preferable in such patients.

Specimen Serum, ascitic fluid

Container Red top tube

Storage Instructions Hemolysis and prolonged contact with erythrocytes do not interfere. Stable 1 month at 4°C and 1 year at -20°C.
(Continued)

Gamma-Glutamyl Transferase, Serum *(Continued)*

Reference Interval Varies between laboratories. Higher in newborns, in first 3-6 months; male, 6 months and older: 2-30 units/L (SI: 0.03-0.51 µkat/L), female, 6 months and older: 1-24 units/L (SI: 0.02-0.41 µkat/L). Values in adult males are 25% higher than adult females.

Use An enzyme that is especially useful in the diagnosis of obstructive jaundice, intrahepatic cholestasis, and pancreatitis;[1] a major application is in differential diagnosis of patients with increased serum alkaline phosphatase.[2] See diagram in Alkaline Phosphatase, Serum *on page 93*. GGT is more responsive to biliary obstruction than are aspartate aminotransferase (AST) (SGOT) and alanine aminotransferase (ALT) (SGPT). In obstructive disease values as high as 5-50 times upper limit of normal are seen. In infectious hepatitis, values seldom go above 5 times normal.

Increased in hepatoma and carcinoma of pancreas. Useful in diagnosis of metastatic carcinoma in the liver. Increasing levels in carcinoma patients relate to tumor progression and diminishing levels to response to treatment.[3] CEA, alkaline phosphatase, and GGT used together are useful markers for hepatic metastasis from primaries in breast and colon. GGT is elevated in some instances of seminoma.

Useful in diagnosis of chronic alcoholic liver disease, but some heavy drinkers do not have GGT increases. GGT > twice the upper level of reference range with **AST:ALT** ratio >2:1 is strongly suggestive of alcohol abuse.[4] Serial determinations of serum GGT, AST, and ALT levels can distinguish recovering alcoholics who resume drinking from those who remain abstinent.[5,6] Increase in body mass is positively correlated with increased GGT levels.[7] GGT may be a marker for visceral and hepatic fat and an independent risk factor for noninsulin-dependent diabetes mellitus.[8] GGT, postprandial glucose, and triglycerides have some correlation in certain groups of patients, including those with alcoholism and diabetes mellitus. With MCV of red cells and carbohydrate-deficient transferrin, GGT is useful as a screen for alcoholism.[9,10] AST, bilirubin, alkaline phosphatase, and AST:ALT ratio are also helpful.

GGT is the test for cholestasis during or immediately following pregnancy. It is commonly elevated in cirrhosis and hepatitis. The transaminases, AST and ALT rise higher in acute viral hepatitis; these tests with GGT and other assays are best used together in work-up of liver disease.

It is increased in systemic lupus erythematosus.[3] Very high concentrations are common in primary biliary cirrhosis. High GGT is found in infants with biliary atresia. It is increased with hyperthyroidism and decreased in those with hypothyroidism. It was elevated in 93% of cases of adult glycogen storage disease.[11] GGT is comparable in many ways to two other biliary tests, LAP and 5′ nucleotidase. In some cases, several tests (including alkaline phosphatase and bilirubin) are necessary to evaluate the biliary tract. GGT usually is the most sensitive.

In **ascitic fluid**, very high GGT is increased in some, but not all cases of hepatoma, as compared to cirrhosis or liver metastases. As in serum, it is high in the ascitic fluid of those with alcoholic cirrhosis.

Limitations Acetaminophen toxicity has been reported to cause an increase. The combination of high alkaline phosphatase and normal GGT does not rule out liver disease completely. Activity is not significantly increased in sera of patients with lymphoma (unless there is hepatic involvement by the lymphoma). Used alone as a preoperative screening test for metastasis from colorectal carcinoma, GGT is unsatisfactory. As part of a screening battery for carcinoma patients, 19% of GGT results from patients with progressive disease were not abnormal, and 4% of values from patients without evidence of tumor were high.[3] Increases have been reported with diseases of the pancreas, myocardial infarct, renal failure, chronic obstructive pulmonary disease, and diabetes.[4]

Drugs that may cause levels of GGT to **diminish** include azathioprine, clofibrate, conjugated estrogens, methotrexate, and ursodiol. Many agents cause **increased** results, including acetaminophen (poisoning even in some mild cases); aminoglutethimide; anticonvulsants including phenytoin, barbiturates, carbamazepine, and diphenylhydantoin; esterified estrogens; interferon alpha-n3; medroxyprogesterone; oral contraceptives; phenothiazine; streptokinase; and valproic acid.[12]

Methodology Kinetic by photometry. Various substrates have been used. IFCC recommends use of L-γ-glutamyl-2-carboxy-4-nitroanilide as a donor substrate and glycylglycine as the acceptor.[13]

Additional Information GGT provides greater specificity for hepatic disease than does alkaline phosphatase. It is normal in most instances of renal failure. GGT has no origin in bone or placenta, unlike alkaline phosphatase, and age beyond infancy does not influence GGT levels. It is commonly elevated in patients with infectious mononucleosis. When GGT and alkaline phosphatase are both high, but one is disproportionately elevated, suspect the possibility of drug-induced cholestasis (including alcoholism if it is GGT which is much higher).

Treatment of hypertriglyceridemia may also lead to decreased GGT. **GGT is normal** in normal children, adolescents, and in pregnant women. Unlike AST, it is not elevated in skeletal muscle disease. High levels of GGT are present in the prostate, which probably accounts for a higher reference range in males.

High levels have been reported in a family.[2]

Footnotes

1. Stein TA, Burns GP, and Wise L, "Diagnostic Value of Liver Function Tests in Bile Duct Obstruction," *J Surg Res*, 1989, 46(3):226-9.
2. Bibas M, Zampa G, Procopio A, et al, "High Serum Gamma-Glutamyltransferase Concentrations in a Family," *N Engl J Med*, 1994, 330(25):1832-3 (letter).
3. Sahm DF, Murray JL, Munson PL, et al, "Gamma Glutamyltranspeptidase Levels as an Aid in the Management of Human Cancer," *Cancer*, 1983, 52(9):1673-8.
4. Pratt DS and Kaplan MM, "Evaluation of Abnormal Liver-Enzyme Results in Asymptomatic Patients," *N Engl J Med*, 2000, 342(17):1266-71.
5. Irwin M, Baird S, Smith TL, et al, "Use of Laboratory Tests to Monitor Heavy Drinking by Alcoholic Men Discharged From a Treatment Program," *Am J Psychiatry*, 1988, 145(5):595-9.
6. Frimpong NA and Lapp JA, "Effects of Moderate Alcohol Intake in Fixed or Variable Amounts on Concentration of Serum Lipids and Liver Enzymes in Healthy Young Men," *Am J Clin Nutr*, 1989, 50(5):987-91.
7. Robinson D and Whitehead TP, "Effect of Body Mass and Other Factors on Serum Liver Enzyme Levels in Men Attending for Well Population Screening," *Ann Clin Biochem*, 1989, 26(Pt 5):393-400.
8. Perry IJ, Wannamethee SG, and Shaper AG, "Prospective Study of Serum Gamma-Glutamyltransferase and Risk of NIDDM," *Diabetes Care*, 1998, 21(5):732-7.
9. Meerkerk GJ, Njoo KH, Bongers IM, et al, "Comparing the Diagnostic Accuracy of Carbohydrate-Deficient Transferrin, Gamma-Glutamyltransferase, and Mean Cell Volume in a General Practice Population," *Alcohol Clin Exp Res*, 1999, 23(6):1052-9.
10. Anton RF, Stout RL, Roberts JS, et al, "The Effect of Drinking Intensity and Frequency on Serum Carbohydrate-Deficient Transferrin and Gamma-Glutamyltransferase Levels in Outpatient Alcoholics," *Alcohol Clin Exp Res*, 1998, 22(7):1456-62.
11. Talente GM, Coleman RA, Alter C, et al, "Glycogen Storage Disease in Adults," *Ann Intern Med*, 1994, 120(3):218-26.
12. Young DS, *Effects of Drugs on Clinical Laboratory Tests*, 5th ed, Volume 1: Listing by Test, Washington, DC: AACC Press, American Association of Clinical Chemistry, 2000, Section 3, 374-9.
13. Burtis CA and Ashwood ER, *Tietz Textbook of Clinical Chemistry*, 3rd ed, Philadelphia, PA: WB Saunders Co, 1999, 686-89.

References

Bellini M, Tumino E, Giordani R, et al, "Serum Gamma-Glutamyltranspeptidase Isoforms in Alcoholic Liver Disease," *Alcohol Alcohol*, 1997, 32(3):259-66.

Daeppen JB, Smith TL, and Schuckit MA, "Influence of Age and Body Mass Index on Gamma-Glutamyltransferase Activity: A 15-Year Follow-up Evaluation in a Community Sample," *Alcohol Clin Exp Res*, 1998, 22(4):941-4.

Gjerde H, Amundsen A, Skog OJ, et al, "Serum Gamma Glutamyltransferase: An Epidemiological Indicator of Alcohol Consumption?" *Br J Addict*, 1987, 82(9):1027-31.

Hanigan MH, "Gamma-Glutamyl Transpeptidase, a Glutathionase: Its Expression and Function in Carcinogenesis," *Chem Biol Interact*, 1998, 111-112:333-42.

Helander A, Vabo E, Levin K, et al, "Intra- and Interindividual Variability of Carbohydrate-Deficient Transferrin, Gamma-Glutamyltransferase, and Mean Corpuscular Volume in Teetotalers," *Clin Chem*, 1998, 44(10):2120-5.

Mizutani Y, Nakano Y, Yamada S, et al, "A New Assay Method for Gamma-Glutamyltransferase With 4-Aminobenzoate Hydroxylase from *Agaricus bisporus* as a Coupling Enzyme," *Clin Chim Acta*, 1999, 287(1-2):83-97.

Yao DF, Huang ZW, Chen SZ, et al, "Diagnosis of Hepatocellular Carcinoma by Quantitative Detection of Hepatoma-Specific Bands of Serum Gamma-Glutamyltransferase," *Am J Clin Pathol*, 1998, 110(6):743-9.

♦ **Gamma-Glutamyl Transpeptidase** *see* Gamma-Glutamyl Transferase, Serum *on page 179*

♦ **Gap** *see* Anion Gap, Serum, Plasma, or Urine *on page 106*

♦ **Gases, Arterial** *see* Blood Gases and pH, Arterial *on page 119*

♦ **Gastric Acid Stimulation Test** *see* Gastric Analysis *on page 180*

Gastric Analysis

Related Information

Cobalamin, Serum *on page 150*
Gastrin, Serum *on page 181*
Helicobacter pylori Biopsy-Based Tests: The Urease Tests, Culture, Cytology, and PCR *on page 620*
Helicobacter pylori Serology *on page 621*
Intrinsic Factor Blocking Antibody *on page 537*
Methylmalonic Acid, Serum, Plasma, Urine, or Amniotic Fluid *on page 224*
Parietal Cell Antibody *on page 541*
Pepsinogen I and II, Serum or Plasma *on page 246*
Vasoactive Intestinal Polypeptide, Plasma *on page 297*
Vitamin B_{12} Unsaturated Binding Capacity *on page 495*

Synonyms Gastric Acid Stimulation Test; Pentagastrin Stimulation Test; Peptavlon® Stimulation Test

Replaces Gastric Analysis, Nocturnal Acid Output; Histalog™ Stimulation Test; Tubeless Gastric Analysis

Test Includes Basal and four poststimulation specimens for pH, volume, and acid output

Abstract Acid (HCl) output of the stomach is relevant to peptic ulcer. Measurement of acid secretion in evaluation of selected ulcer patients is helpful in particular circumstances, but is not needed for the diagnosis of peptic ulcer. Although fiberoptic endoscopy and availability of gastrin assays have contributed to the decline of gastric analysis, documentation of very high or no output still is clinically relevant in selected cases.

Patient Preparation Antacids and H_2-receptor antagonists should not be given to patient for 24-48 hours prior to testing. Drugs that affect gastric acid secretion, such as tricyclic antidepressants, anticholinergics and reserpine should be discontinued overnight to 72 hours prior to testing. The patient must fast after the evening meal on the day prior to the test day, but may have water up to 1 hour before the test. After pentagastrin has been administered, medical supervision should be maintained since untoward reactions may occur.

Specimen Gastric secretions, four 15-minute basal and four 15-minute post-stimulation collections. Entire volume collected. Longer periods are sometimes used (eg, 24-hour measurement) but are not well standardized and may be dangerous.

Container No preservative

Collection A cold lubricated gastric (Levine) tube is inserted orally or nasally while the patient is in a sitting or reclining position on his/her left side. The tube must have a radiopaque tip. Nasal intubation is used if the patient has a hyperactive gag reflex. It should be positioned in the stomach so that the tip is opposite the angularis or "re-entrant angle" in the most dependent portion of the stomach. In a patient who has had a subtotal gastrectomy, the tube should be placed well within the lumen of the stomach, below the fundus and above the anastomosis. Proper positioning of the tube is confirmed by fluoroscopy or x-ray. Wait 10-15 minutes for the patient to adjust to the tube. The patient should be in a sitting position. Gentle constant suction is needed, except for brief intervals when a small quantity of air can be injected to clear the tube. The first two or three specimens immediately following intubation (the first 15-30 minutes) do not accurately reflect the basal state. Give no liquids to the patient during the test and request that the patient expectorate saliva. The basal specimen is obtained by continuous aspiration of the gastric fluid with a Toomey syringe for 60 minutes as four 15-minute specimens. These are the **BAO (basal acid output)**. After the basal sample has been collected, pentagastrin is injected (see package insert). The collection of the poststimulation specimens must begin immediately. The gastric content is continuously aspirated for the next 60 minutes, during which time the gastric contents obtained from each of four 15-minute periods are collected into separate plastic containers labeled **poststimulation** number 1, 2, 3, and 4 respectively, **the maximal acid output, MAO**. Securely fasten the lids on the containers and send the eight specimens (four basal and four poststimulation) to the laboratory. The containers must identify the order in which the specimens were collected.

Storage Instructions Refrigerate if test delayed more than 4 hours.

Causes for Rejection Contamination of specimens with duodenal contents, indicated by the yellow color of bile

Reference Interval Normal gastric juice may be clear or contain some bile. If red or black, test for blood.

A major disadvantage of gastric analysis is the breadth of values in normal individuals, overlapping results in those with duodenal and gastric ulcer. Normal BAO is up to 10.5 mmol/hour (men) and 5.6 mmol/hour (women). BAO represents gastric acid secretion in the absence of stimulation. It follows circadian rhythm and is highest from 2-11 PM. Brady et al defined basal hypersecretion as basal acid output >11 mmol/hour (men) and 6 mmol/hour (women).[1]

Normal MAO (maximal acid output) is up to 48 mmol/hour (men) and 30 mmol/hour (women). MAO is the sum of four 15-minute collections following pentagastrin.

Normal PAO (peak acid output) is 11-60 mmol/hour (men) and 8-40 mmol/hour (women).

Normal BAO to PAO is <0.29 (men) and <0.23 (women).

BAO and MAO decline with advancing age.

Critical Values More than 90% of patients with Z-E syndrome have BAO >15 mEq/hour if prior gastric surgery has not been done or >5 mEq/L if prior gastric resection or vagotomy had taken place.[2]

Use Evaluate gastric function. Support the diagnosis of pernicious anemia: provision of evidence of gastric mucosal atrophy; evaluation of recurrent peptic ulcer, Zollinger-Ellison (Z-E) syndrome, and Ménétrier disease. **Zollinger-Ellison (Z-E) syndrome** usually includes fulminant peptic ulcer diathesis with massive acid secretion. The Zollinger-Ellison syndrome includes the presence of gastrinoma, neuroendocrine tumors which secrete gastrin, pancreatic or extrapancreatic. The diagnosis of the Zollinger-Ellison syndrome is established by demonstration of gastric acid hypersecretion, basal acid secretion >15 mmol/hour in an unoperated subject with peptic ulcer, with fasting gastrin level >1000 pg/mL (SI: >1000 ng/L). Fasting gastrin >1000 with pH <2.5 provides strong evidence for Z-E syndrome.[2] The Z-E syndrome sometimes does not include peptic ulcer disease, but hyperchlorhydria is characteristic. About 33% of gastrinoma patients have diarrhea and 7% have only diarrhea.

Pernicious anemia: Anacidity is characteristic of PA. High gastrin levels are found, *vide infra.*

Gastritis: Severe gastritis with mucosal atrophy is associated with anacidity. Gastritis produces progressive loss of secretory ability. See Gastritis in the Key Word Index.

Gastric carcinoid tumors are classified into two groups: those that arise in the background of chronic atrophic gastritis and those arising independently.

Ulcer recurrence: The explanation for ulcer recurrence following surgery may be sought with investigation of gastric acid secretion.

Gastric carcinoma: Few if any cases clinically, endoscopically and/or radiologically considered to be carcinoma, presently have gastric analysis. Gastric carcinoma and gastric polyps, classically, have often been associated with decreased-to-absent hydrochloric acid. Of course, carcinoma may occur without anacidity and anacidity occurs without carcinoma. The demonstration of complete anacidity to maximal stimulation (pentagastrin-fast achlorhydria) in the presence of a gastric ulcer strongly supports (but does not prove) a diagnosis of malignancy. Patients with gastric ulcers generally show low to normal basal and maximum acid output.

Limitations Tube not in proper place for aspiration, incomplete volume collection. Losses of gastric juice into the duodenum occur, especially in patients who have had pyloroplasty or gastroenterostomy.

Gastric analysis itself is insufficient for the diagnosis of gastrinoma. Substantial overlap exists between patients with gastrinoma, with common duodenal ulcer and normal subjects in rates of gastric acid output.[3] Gastric analysis is time consuming, uncomfortable for the patient and it is expensive.

Contraindications Gastric intubation is contraindicated for patients with esophageal varices, diverticula, stenosis, malignant neoplasm of the esophagus, aortic aneurysm, severe gastric hemorrhage, and congestive heart failure. It is not necessary for the usual duodenal ulcer patient in whom the Zollinger-Ellison is not suspected.

Patient must not receive medication that influences gastric secretion; such contraindications include antacids, anticholinergic drugs, reserpine, alcohol, adrenergic blocking agents, and adrenocorticosteroids.

Asthma and other severely hyperallergenic problems are thought not to be contraindications when pentagastrin (Pepavlon®) is used as the stimulant (see package insert). It is a pentapeptide consisting of the active carboxy-yterminal tetrapeptide of gastrin with beta-alanine and is the preferred agent. Hypersensitivity or idiosyncrasy to pentagastrin is described.

Methodology Volume measurement, pH measurement by pH meter. Do not use pH paper.[4] **Peak acid output (PAO)** is a calculation, in which the two highest 15-minute MAO specimens are combined and multiplied by 2.

Additional Information "Anacidity" (achlorhydria) is regarded as pH >6 following stimulation, an abnormal finding. If specimens become grossly bloody, physician should be contacted to ascertain if procedure should be continued. Confirm if indicated with a test for hemoglobin.

Basal gastric analysis: Specimens should be collected at 15-minute intervals for 1 hour, labeled basal 1, basal 2, etc, and sent to the laboratory.

Maximal stimulation gastric analysis: This measures the response to maximal stimulation by pentagastrin. This material is administered after collection of the basal specimens. Thirty minutes after administration of pentagastrin, four 15-minute specimens of gastric juice are aspirated as described, labeled "Max 1", "2", etc, and sent to the laboratory. The patient should be observed regularly, preferably by the physician. With proper precautions, side effects are rare.

Availability of assays for gastrin diminish the need for gastric analysis.

Contemporary work-up for pernicious anemia (PA) includes cobalamin (vitamin B_{12})/folate, methylmalonic acid if needed, occasionally the Schilling test, and sometimes, testing for antibodies to intrinsic factor and to parietal cells (see Related Information for specific listings).

In recent years, fiberoptic endoscopy with endoscopic biopsies is replacing gastric analysis as well as radiologic examination.[5]

Footnotes
1. Brady CE 3d, Hadfield TL, Hyatt JR, et al, "Acid Secretion and Serum Gastrin Levels in Individuals With *Campylobacter pylori*," *Gastroenterology*, 1988, 94(4):923-7.
2. Jensen RT and Fraker DL, "Zollinger-Ellison Syndrome - Advances in Treatment of Gastric Hypersecretion and the Gastrinoma," *JAMA*, 1994, 271(18):1429-35.
3. Wolfe MM, "Diagnosis of Gastrinoma: Much Ado About Nothing?" *Ann Intern Med*, 1989, 111(9):697-9.
4. Caballero GA, Ausman RK, Quebbeman EJ, et al, "Gastric Secretion pH Measurement: What You See Is Not What You Get!" *Crit Care Med*, 1990, 18(4):396-9.
5. Rosenfeld L, "Gastric Tubes, Meals, Acid, and Analysis: Rise and Decline," *Clin Chem*, 1997, 43(5):837-42.

References
Fenoglio-Preiser CM, Noffsinger AE, Stemmermann GN, et al, *Gastrointestinal Pathology*, Philadelphia, PA: Lippincott-Raven, 1999.
Iijima K and Ohara S, "A New Endoscopic Method of Gastric Acid Secretory Testing," *Am J Gastroenterol*, 1998, 93(11):2113-8.
Malagelada JR, Davis CS, O'Fallon WM, et al, "Laboratory Diagnosis of Gastrinoma. 1. A Prospective Evaluation of Gastric Analysis and Fasting Serum Gastrin Levels," *Mayo Clin Proc*, 1982, 57:211-8.
Tomassetti P, Migliori M, Caletti GC, et al, "Treatment of Type II Gastric Carcinoid Tumors With Somatostatin Analogues," *N Engl J Med*, 2000, 343(8):551-4.

♦ **Gastric Analysis, Nocturnal Acid Output** *replaced by* Gastric Analysis *on page 180*

Gastrin, Serum

Related Information
Cobalamin, Serum *on page 150*
Gastric Analysis *on page 180*
(Continued)

Gastrin, Serum (Continued)

Helicobacter pylori Biopsy-Based Tests: The Urease Tests, Culture, Cytology, and PCR *on page 620*

Pepsinogen I and II, Serum or Plasma *on page 246*

Schilling Test *on page 483*

Applies to Secretin Test

Abstract Gastrin, a polypeptide hormone secreted by neuroendocrine G cells located in the gastric antrum (and occasionally at other gastrointestinal sites), is known primarily as a gastric acid secretagogue. However, gastrin is also trophic for histamine-secreting enterochromaffin-like (ECL) cells in the gastric mucosa, and, in chronic hypergastrinemia, these cells undergo hyperplasia leading, in extreme cases, to the development of gastric carcinoid tumors. At least three molecular forms of gastrin, all biologically active, circulate in the blood, and clinical assays measure the sum of all these; fractionation is not clinically useful. Gastrin is measured clinically to evaluate the possibility of gastrin-secreting carcinoid tumors (gastrinomas). A common clinical substrate for gastrin-secreting neoplasms is the Zollinger-Ellison syndrome (ZES).[1] Gastric carcinoids occur in association with chronic atrophic gastritis and, on rare occasions, sporadically. Gastrinomas also occur in the duodenum, pancreas, and other locations.

Recent evidence supports the concept that G cells may rarely be found in lymph nodes within the "gastrinoma triangle."[2]

Patient Preparation For **basal** values, a 12-hour overnight fast is required. For dynamic testing (the **secretin challenge** - see below), follow a specific protocol;[3] also summarized in footnotes 4 and 5.

Specimen Serum (plasma is not acceptable)

Container Red top tube

Sampling Time For the **secretin challenge** test, specimens are obtained at 2, 5, 10, 15, 20, and 30 minutes following the bolus injection of porcine secretin, 2 units/kg.[3,4,5]

Collection Transport specimen immediately to the laboratory following collection. Postprandial specimens should be so indicated.

Storage Instructions Separate in a refrigerated centrifuge and freeze immediately. Stable 4 hours at 4°C and 30 days at -20°C. For long-term storage, specimens should be kept at -70°C. Serum specimens loose up to 50% of immunoreactivity during 48 hours at 4°C.

Causes for Rejection Anticoagulated specimen

Reference Interval

Fasting:[5]
- cord blood: 20-290 ng/L
- 0-4 days: 120-183 ng/L
- childhood: <10-125 ng/L
- adults 16-60 years: 25-90 ng/L
- adults older than 60 years: <100 ng/L

Secretin challenge test:[3,4,5] In normal persons, serum gastrin levels decrease, or increase by <200 ng/L in comparison with the preinjection value. An increase >200 ng/L is indicative of gastrinoma.[4]

Use The key to the diagnosis of the Zollinger-Ellison syndrome (ZES) is the combination of high fasting gastrin (often >1000 ng/L) and fasting gastric hyperacidity (often with gastric pH <2.5) in a patient who does not have a retained gastric antrum. When these criteria are fulfilled, in the appropriate clinical context, the diagnosis of gastrinoma is confirmed and further biochemical testing is not needed. Patients whose values do not meet these criteria are candidates for a secretin challenge test. In normal persons, a bolus of secretin decreases serum gastrin (or produces a small increase), but in patients with a gastrinoma there is a paradoxical increase in serum gastrin, >200 ng/L, in response to secretin.

Methodology Radioimmunoassay (RIA). Most assays are specific for C-terminal of gastrin and react equally with G-34, G17, and G-14.

Additional Information There are a number of conditions in which elevated serum gastrin occurs as an appropriate physiological response to the common denominator of low (or absent) gastric acid (atrophic gastritis, Addisonian pernicious anemia, postvagotomy); these patients lack the gastric hyperacidity necessary to diagnose a gastrinoma. Patients receiving proton pump inhibitors will also have elevated gastrin, and should be off this class of medication for at least a week before gastrin testing, either fasting or secretin challenge. Other situations in which patients may have elevated serum gastrin include renal failure, isolated retained antrum, rheumatoid arthritis, cirrhosis, postresection of large portions of the small bowel, and primary gastrin-cell (G cell) hyperplasia of the gastric antrum. The only one of these which causes confusion with ZES is primary gastrin-cell hyperplasia.

Following biochemical confirmation of ZES, the next step is localization of the gastrinoma. Somatostatin-receptor scintigraphy is often successful in localizing these neoplasms, but occasionally other imaging modalities are required. Approximately 90% of gastrinomas are located in the duodenum, pancreas, or a peripancreatic lymph node; the other 10% are widely scattered and may be found in the liver, ovary, heart, stomach, omentum, common bile duct, or small bowel.[4]

Approximately 75% of ZES patients have sporadic gastrinomas, and 25% have the type I multiple endocrine neoplasia syndrome (MEN 1).[4] In a large NIH-based study, patients with sporadic gastrinomas had a better response to operative treatment than those with MEN 1.[4] Following successful surgical therapy for gastrinoma, fasting gastrin levels fall rapidly to normal.

Recurrence is detected by fasting serum gastrin levels and, if needed, the secretin challenge, using the same criteria as used for the initial diagnosis.[6]

Dynamic tests, other than the secretin challenge, have been used to diagnose the ZES. The calcium infusion test has undesirable side effects as well as lower predictive values than the secretin challenge test. The so-called "standard meal" does not have sharply defined cutoff values.[5]

Although there are multiple biochemical forms of gastrin,[5] there is little, if any, clinical usefulness to fractionation studies.

Footnotes

1. Zollinger RM and Ellison EH, "Primary Peptic Ulcerations of the Jejunum Associated With Islet Cell Tumors of the Pancreas," *Ann Surg*, 1955, 142:709-28.
2. Hermann ME, Ciesla MC, Chejfec G, et al, "Primary Nodal Gastrinomas," *Arch Pathol Lab Med*, 2000, 124(6):832-5.
3. Frucht H, Howard JM, Slaff JI, et al, "Secretin and Calcium Provocative Tests in the Zollinger-Ellison Syndrome: A Prospective Study," *Ann Intern Med*, 1989, 111(9):713-22.
4. Norton JA, Fraker DL, Alexander R, et al, "Surgery to Cure the Zollinger-Ellison Syndrome," *N Engl J Med*, 1999, 341(9):635-44.
5. Henderson AR and Rinker AD, "Gastric, Pancreatic, and Intestinal Function," *Tietz Textbook of Clinical Chemistry*, 3rd ed, Burtis CA and Ashwood ER, eds, Philadelphia, PA: Saunders Co, 1999, 1273-8.
6. Fishbeyn VA, Norton JA, Benya RV, et al, "Assessment and Prediction of Long-Term Cure in Patients With the Zollinger-Ellison Syndrome: The Best Approach," *Ann Intern Med*, 1993, 119(3):199-206.

References

Kaplan LM and Graeme-Cook FM, "A 39-Year-Old Woman With Pernicious Anemia and a Gastric Mass," Case Records of the Massachusetts General Hospital, Case 9-1997, Scully RE, Mark EJ, McNeely WE, et al, eds, *N Engl J Med*, 1997, 336(12):861-7.

Stabile BE, Morrow DJ, and Passaro E Jr, "The Gastrinoma Triangle: Operative Implications," *Am J Surg*, 1984, 147(10):25-31.

Tomassetti P, Migliori M, Caletti GC, et al, "Treatment of Type II Gastric Carcinoid Tumors With Somatostatin Analogues," *N Engl J Med*, 2000, 343(8):551-4.

Glucagon, Plasma

Related Information

Adrenocorticotropic Hormone, Plasma *on page 86*

Gastrin, Serum *on page 181*

Glucose, Fasting, Plasma *on page 183*

5-Hydroxyindoleacetic Acid, Quantitative, Urine *on page 197*

Insulin, Serum *on page 201*

Pancreatic Polypeptide, Human, Serum or Plasma *on page 242*

Vasoactive Intestinal Polypeptide, Plasma *on page 297*

Abstract A single chain polypeptide, glucagon provides primary defense against hypoglycemia.[1] Glucagonoma (alpha cell tumor) is an extremely rare neuroendocrine tumor. Most arise in the pancreas. Primary tumors of the duodenum are recognized. Those tumors found in the glucagonoma syndrome usually solitary and very often malignant, but sometimes associated with prolonged survival. (All the neuroendocrine tumors associated with hyperglucagonemia in a 1996 Mayo series were malignant.[2]) Hyperglucagonemia is found in patients with glucagonomas, and some patients with insulinomas, Zollinger-Ellison syndrome, carcinoid syndrome, and multiple endocrine neoplasia (type 1). Polyfunctional hormone production may cause several endocrine syndromes.[2]

Patient Preparation Overnight fasting for basal levels. If diabetic, patient should be in good control before specimen is drawn. Avoid recent radioactive tracer (eg, for radioactive scan).

Specimen Plasma

Container Draw blood into a chilled lavender top (EDTA) tube. Deliver to the laboratory immediately.

Storage Instructions Freeze. Stable 2 months at -20°C.

Special Instructions Mix the blood immediately and centrifuge in a refrigerated centrifuge.

Reference Interval ≤60 pg/mL (SI: ≤60 ng/L) at one laboratory, but other intervals are in use (eg, 20-100 pg/mL)

Critical Values Most patients with glucagonoma have levels >500 pg/mL (SI: >500 ng/L); >1000 pg/mL (SI: >1000 ng/L) is diagnostic.[1] The highest values are found with glucagonoma syndrome and with insulinomas. Fasting hyperglucagonemia has been defined as glucagon concentrations ≥120 pg/mL.[2]

Use Diagnose glucagonoma. The most common clinical presentations of hyperglucagonemia are the Zollinger-Ellison syndrome and the glucagonoma syndrome. Glucagonoma syndromes include a characteristic skin rash (necrolytic migratory erythema), diabetes mellitus (or impaired glucose tolerance), weight loss, abdominal pain, diarrhea, peptic ulcer disease, anemia, and venous thrombosis. This form usually is characterized by very high glucagon levels, >1000 pg/mL (SI: >1000 ng/L). Another presentation is associated with severe diabetes.

Contraindications Recent radioisotopes

Methodology Radioimmunoassay (RIA); ethanol extraction removes "big" glucagon, which is not considered biologically active.

Additional Information Glucagon is normally secreted by α_2-cells of pancreatic islets in response to hypoglycemia. Among the counter-regulatory hormones, it exerts a counterbalancing effect to insulin in regulation of glucose metabolism. It stimulates glycogenolysis, gluconeogenesis, and ketogenesis. Normally inhibited by hypoglycemia, glucagon is increased in diabetes mellitus, even with hyperglycemia.

Glucagon exists in "true" form (3500 daltons - biologically active form) and "big" form (160,000 daltons). This form may represent binding of the 3500-dalton glucagon to plasma protein, and rare families have increased amounts of "big" glucagon circulating. Very high levels of glucagon are seen with glucagonomas, and secondary elevations are also seen in diabetic ketoacidosis, stress, uremia, Cushing syndrome, hepatic cirrhosis, hyperosmolality, acute pancreatitis, burns, trauma, surgery, and hypoglycemia. Decreased values are found in cystic fibrosis, chronic pancreatitis, and in the postpancreatectomy state.

Glucagon can be identified in paraffin sections.

Footnotes
1. Service FJ, "Hypoglycemic Disorders," *N Engl J Med*, 1995, 332(17):1144-52.
2. Wermers RA, Fatourechi V, and Kvols LK, "Clinical Spectrum of Hyperglucagonemia Associated With Malignant Neuroendocrine Tumors," *Mayo Clin Proc*, 1996, 71:1020-8.

References
Boden G, "Glucagonomas and Insulinomas," *Gastroenterol Clin North Am*, 1990, 18(4):831-45.
Diem P, Redmon JB, Abid M, et al, "Glucagon, Catecholamine, and Pancreatic Polypeptide Secretion in Type I Diabetic Recipients of Pancreas Allografts," *J Clin Invest*, 1990, 86(6):2008-13.
Holst JJ, "Glucagon-Like Peptide 1: A Newly Discovered Gastrointestinal Hormone," *Gastroenterology*, 1994, 107(6):1848-55.
Krejs GJ, "Noninsulin-Secreting Tumors of the Gastroenteropancreatic System," *Williams Textbook of Endocrinology*, 9th ed, Wilson JD, Foster DW, Kronenberg HM, et al, eds, Philadelphia, PA: WB Saunders Co, 1998, 1663-6.
Liu D, Moberg E, Kollind M, et al, "A High Concentration of Circulating Insulin Suppresses the Glucagon Response to Hypoglycemia in Normal Man," *J Clin Endocrinol Metab*, 1991, 73(5):1123-8.
Magnusson I, Rothman DL, Gerard DP, et al, "Contribution of Hepatic Glycogenolysis to Glucose Production in Humans in Response to a Physiological Increase in Plasma Glucagon Concentration," *Diabetes*, 1995, 44(2):185-9.
Rosai J, *Ackerman's Surgical Pathology*, 8th ed, St Louis, MO: CV Mosby, 1996.
Rothe AJ, Young JW, Keramati B, et al, "The Value of Glucagon in Routine Barium Investigations of the Gastrointestinal Tract," *Invest Radiol*, 1987, 22(10):786-91.

♦ **Glucose, 2-Hour Postprandial, Plasma** *replaced by* Glucose, Postglucose Load, Plasma *on page 185*

♦ **Glucose, Body Fluid** *see* Body Fluid Glucose *on page 124*

♦ **Glucose, Cerebrospinal Fluid** *see* Cerebrospinal Fluid Glucose *on page 140*

Glucose, Fasting, Plasma

Related Information

Synonyms Blood Sugar, Fasting; Fasting Blood Sugar; FBS; Sugar, Fasting

Applies to Glucose:Insulin Ratio; Tolbutamide Test

Abstract The three tests recommended by the American Diabetes Association (ADA) for the diagnosis of **diabetes mellitus** are fasting plasma glucose, random plasma glucose, and two-hour postglucose load. Testing for **gestational diabetes mellitus** involves a first step screening plasma glucose **1 hour after a 50 g glucose load**, and if this result is abnormal, a **100 g glucose load test**[1] (see Glucose, Postglucose Load, Plasma *on page 185*).

Patient Preparation Patient should be fasting for at least 8 hours before testing. Fasting is defined as no consumption of food or beverage other than water.

Specimen Plasma or serum

Container Gray top (sodium fluoride or iodacetate) tube is preferred; heparin (green top) and red top tubes are acceptable only if specimen is rapidly separated from the red cells and analyzed promptly.

Sampling Time Morning

Collection Venous specimens are recommended from all age groups, except for neonates, whose specimens are most often drawn from heelsticks.

Storage Instructions Glucose will decrease at a rate of 5-10 mg/dL per hour in unseparated, room temperature blood not collected in gray top tubes.

Reference Interval Premature infants: may have glucose values as low as 30 mg/dL (SI:1.6 mmol/L); newborns: 40-60 mg/dL (SI: 2.2-3.3 mmol/L); children: 60-100 mg/dL (SI: 3.3-5.6 mmol/L); adults: 60-109 mg/dL (SI: 3.3-6.0 mmol/L)

ADA Criteria for the Diagnosis of Diabetes Mellitus[1]

Any one of the following findings is diagnostic of diabetes, if confirmed by any one of the following findings on a subsequent day:

- Symptoms of diabetes plus a random plasma glucose level ≥200 mg/dL (11.1 mmol/L). Symptoms include polyuria, polydipsia, and unexplained weight loss.
- Fasting plasma glucose ≥126 mg/dL (7 mmol/L) after a minimum 8-hour fast.
- Two-hour postload glucose ≥200 mg/dL (11.1 mmol/L) during an oral glucose tolerance test conducted as described by the World Health Organization, using glucose load containing the equivalent of 75-g anhydrous glucose dissolved in water

In an unstressed, nonpregnant individual, fasting plasma glucose values between 110-125 mg/dL (SI: 6.1-6.9 mmol/L) are classified as **impaired fasting glucose**, a term intended to convey the presence of a metabolic abnormality between normal and diabetes.[1]

Fasting plasma glucose results in the range of 47-60 mg/dL are consistent with, but not fully diagnostic of, **hypoglycemia**, a diagnosis which has no established biochemical criterion, and which requires careful correlation with clinical features (see table, Clinical Classification of Hypoglycemic Disorders).

Possible Panic Range Infants: <40 mg/dL (SI: <2.2 mmol/L); adults: male: <50 mg/dL (SI: <2.75 mmol/L), female: <40 mg/dL (SI: <2.2 mmol/L); adults: male and female: >400 mg/dL (SI: >22 mmol/L)

Use The test is used to establish the diagnosis of diabetes mellitus and to monitor therapy and support control of diabetes. In addition, fasting glucose measurements are useful in the diagnosis and treatment of certain metabolic disorders (eg, acidosis, ketosis, dehydration, coma).

Causes of **high plasma glucose** other than diabetes include nonfasting specimen, recent or current intravenous infusions of glucose, stress states (eg, myocardial infarct,[2] brain damage, CVA,[3] convulsive episodes, trauma, general anesthesia), Cushing disease, acromegaly, pheochromocytoma, glucagonoma, severe liver disease, pancreatitis, and drugs (thiazide and other diuretics, glucocorticoids, β-blockers, nicotinic acid, estrogen-containing products, and many others).[4]

For the evaluation of hypoglycemia, symptoms must be correlated with plasma glucose. Hypoglycemia has a lengthy, differential diagnosis[5,6] (see following table).

The overnight fasting glucose level is the optimal test, supplemented by additional glucose specimens drawn during symptoms. Outlined below are common diagnostic problems.

- Pancreatic islet cell tumors (insulinomas) - cause hypoglycemia in fasting individuals or after exercise. Measurement of simultaneous glucose, C-peptide, and insulin levels at the time of spontaneous hypoglycemia help to differentiate insulinoma from other conditions. The **glucose:insulin ratio** is useful in the diagnosis of insulinoma as insulin levels are inappropriately increased for plasma glucose (see Insulin, Serum *on page 201*). An intravenous tolbutamide test with plasma glucose and serum insulin determinations may be used for evaluation of insulin-secreting islet cell tumors. The test is positive in ~75% of patients with these tumors.[7] Glucagon and leucine stimulation tests are less frequently utilized.
- Extrapancreatic tumors - rare bulky fibromas, sarcomas, mesotheliomas, and carcinomas, including hepatoma and adrenal tumors
- Adrenal insufficiency (Addison disease), including congenital adrenal hyperplasia
- Hypopituitarism, isolated growth hormone or ACTH deficiency

(Continued)

Glucose, Fasting, Plasma (Continued)

- Starvation, malabsorption - but starvation does not cause hypoglycemia in normal persons. The plasma glucose of normal fasting individuals may drop to <50 mg/dL.[5]
- Hereditary fructose intolerance, galactosemia, leucine sensitivity
- Drugs including insulin (see above), oral hypoglycemic agents, and alcoholism, especially with starvation. Salicylates, quinine, haloperidol, and many other drugs, and conditions[5] can depress glucose levels. Anti-insulin antibodies, spontaneously produced, causing hypoglycemia are reported.[8]
- Liver damage, including fulminant hepatic necrosis (hepatitis, toxicity), and severe congestive failure
- Tumor-induced hypoglycemia appears to be caused by increased production of an insulin-like substance (insulin-like growth factor II) by the tumor. This substance induces increased utilization of glucose by the peripheral tissues and the tumor, and impairs the counterregulatory effect of growth hormone by suppressing growth hormone secretion.[9,10]

Clinical Classification of Hypoglycemic Disorders

Healthy-Appearing Patient
No Coexisting Disease
Cause of predisposing condition
Drugs: ethanol, salicylates, quinine, haloperidol
Insulinoma; nonislet insulin-secreting tumors
Factitious hypoglycemia induced by insulin
Intense exercise
Ketotic hypoglycemia
Coexisting Disease Under Treatment
Diabetes mellitus
Cause of predisposing condition
Drugs: dispensing error, disopyramide, β-adrenergic-blocking agents, drugs containing sulfhydryl or thiol and autoimmune insulin syndrome
Ackee-fruit poisoning and undernutrition
Ill-Appearing Patient
Cause or Predispositing Condition
Drugs
Pentamidine for pneumocystis pneumonia
Trimethoprim-sulfamethoxazole and renal failure
Propoxyphene and renal failure
Quinine for cerebral malaria
Quinidine for malaria
Topical salicylates and renal failure
Illness or condition
Small size for gestational age in infants
Beckwith-Wiedemann syndrome
Erythroblastosis fetalis
Hyperinsulinemia in infants due to maternal diabetes
Glycogen storage disease
Defects in amino acid and fatty acid metabolism
Reye syndrome
Cyanotic congenital heart disease
Hypopituitarism
Isolated growth hormone deficiency
Isolated corticotropin deficiency
Addison disease
Galactosemia
Hereditary fructose intolerance
Carnitine deficiency
Defective type 1 glucose transporter in the brain
Acquired severe liver disease
Large nonbeta-cell tumor
Sepsis
Renal failure
Congestive heart failure
Lactic acidosis
Starvation, malnutrition
Anorexia nervosa
Surgical removal of pheochromocytoma
Insulin-antibody hypoglycemia
Hospitalized Patient
Cause or Predisposing Condition
Hospitalization for a predisposing condition
Total parenteral nutrition and insulin therapy
Interference of cholestyramine with glucocorticoid absorption
Shock

Adapted from Service FH, "Hypoglycemic Disorders," *N Engl J Med*, 1995, 332(17):1144-52.

Infancy and childhood: The causes of neonatal hypoglycemia include delayed first feeding. Rapid glucose measurement is required for infants with tremor, convulsions, and/or respiratory distress, particularly in the presence of maternal diabetes and hemolytic disease of the newborn (erythroblastosis fetalis). Newborns too large or small for gestational age should have a glucose level measured in the first 24 hours of life. A large number of entities cause neonatal hypoglycemia, including glycogen storage diseases,[11] galactosemia, hereditary fructose intolerance, ketotic hypoglycemia of infancy, fructose-1,6-diphosphatase deficiency, carnitine deficiency (a treatable disease presenting as Reye syndrome), and nesidioblastosis (see Insulin, Serum *on page 201*).[12]

Control of diabetes is needed to avoid complications (see Glucose, Whole Blood *on page 188*). Laboratory measures of importance include fasting plasma glucose, urine microalbumin and albumin, creatinine, BUN, glycated hemoglobin or fructosamine, and home measurements of whole blood glucose.[13,14,15,16]

Limitations Measurement of plasma glucose without spinal fluid glucose can miss neuroglycopenia. Fingerstick (whole blood) glucose determination in shock are lower than venous glucose and are dangerously misleading (see Glucose, Whole Blood *on page 188*).[17]

Artifactual hypoglycemia is cause by leukocytosis, hemolysis, glycolysis in specimens overheated or old, and delay in separating serum or heparinized plasma from red cells. Very prompt removal of plasma or serum, followed by prompt glucose analysis, is necessary for accurate results. Hypoglycemia should be confirmed by specimens drawn in gray top tubes. Isolated postchallenge hyperglycemia (IPH) is defined as fasting glucose <126 mg/dL (7.0 mmol/L) and two-hour glucose ≥200 mg/dL (11.1 mmol/L). Reliance placed only on the fasting glucose in diabetes screening must miss significant numbers of individuals with IPH. IPH is a major risk factor for cardiovascular mortality.[18] In another study, high normal concentrations of fasting blood glucose are reported to correlate with increased risk of cardiovascular mortality.[19]

Methodology Specific enzyme-based assays using glucose oxidase or hexokinase

Additional Information Glycosylated hemoglobin, self-monitoring of blood glucose, and urine microalbumin determinations are recommended for monitoring diabetes control and complications.[13]

Etiologic Classification of Diabetes Mellitus[1]

I. Type 1 diabetes (β-cell destruction, usually leading to absolute insulin deficiency)
a. immune-mediated
b. idiopathic
II. Type 2 diabetes (may range from predominantly insulin resistance with relative insulin deficiency to a predominantly secretory defect with insulin resistance)
III. Other specific types
a. genetic defects of β-cell function
b. genetic defects in insulin action
c. diseases of the exocrine pancreas
d. endocrinopathies
e. drug- or chemical-induced
f. infections
g. uncommon forms of immune-mediated diabetes
h. other genetic syndromes sometimes associated with diabetes
IV. Gestational diabetes mellitus (GDM)

Since the 1997 ADA criteria for the diagnosis of diabetes mellitus lowered the fasting glucose threshold, the prevalence of diabetes will probably increase.[20] Some observers have objected to the immediate implementation of these criteria because they are not based on a prospective trial.[21] Others urge quick adoption in order to reduce diabetes-related complications.[22]

Footnotes

1. American Diabetes Association, "Report of the Expert Committee on the Diagnosis and Classification of Diabetes Mellitus," *Diabetes Care*, 1997, 20(7):1183-97.
2. Madsen JK, Haunsoe S, Helquist S, et al, "Prevalence of Hyperglycemia and Undiagnosed Diabetes Mellitus in Patients With Acute Myocardial Infarction," *Acta Med Scand*, 1986, 220(4):329-32.
3. Berger L and Hakim AM, "The Association of Hyperglycemia With Cerebral Edema in Stroke," *Stroke*, 1986, 17(5):865-71.
4. Young DS, *Effects of Drugs on Clinical Laboratory Tests*, 5th ed, Volume 1: Listing by Test, Washington, DC: AACC Press, American Association of Clinical Chemistry, 2000, Section 3, 349-67.
5. Service FJ, "Hypoglycemic Disorders," *N Engl J Med*, 1995, 332(17):1144-52.
6. Le Roith D, "Tumor-Induced Hypoglycemia," *N Engl J Med*, 1999, 341(10):757-8.
7. Field JB, "Hypoglycemia: A Systematic Approach to Specific Diagnosis," *Hosp Pract*, 1986, 21(9):187-94.
8. Polonsky KS, "A Practical Approach to Fasting Hypoglycemia," *N Engl J Med*, 1992, 326(15):994-8.
9. Daughaday WH, Emanuele MA, Brooks MH, et al, "Synthesis and Secretion of Insulin-Like Growth Factor II by a Leiomyosarcoma With Associated Hypoglycemia," *N Engl J Med*, 1988, 319(22):1434-40.
10. Axelrod L and Ron D, "Insulin-Like Growth Factor II and the Riddle of Tumor-Induced Hypoglycemia," *N Engl J Med*, 1988, 319(22):1477-9.
11. Talente GM, Coleman RA, Alter C, et al, "Glycogen Storage Disease in Adults," *Ann Intern Med*, 1994, 120(3):218-26.
12. Stanley CA and Baker L, "The Causes of Neonatal Hypoglycemia," *N Engl J Med*, 1999, 340(15):1200-1.

13. Barbosa J, Steffes MW, Sutherland DER, et al, "Effect of Glycemic Control on Early Diabetic Renal Lesions - A 5-Year Randomized Controlled Clinical Trial of Insulin-Dependent Diabetic Kidney Transplant Recipients," *JAMA*, 1994, 272(8):600-6.

14. Watts NB, "Bedside Monitoring of Blood Glucose in Hospitals. Speed vs Precision and Accuracy," *Arch Pathol Lab Med*, 1993, 117:1078-9.

15. American Diabetes Association, "Standards of Medical Care for Patients With Diabetes Mellitus," *Diabetes Care*, 2000, 23(1 Suppl):S32-S42.

16. Clark CM Jr and Lee DA, "Prevention and Treatment of the Complications of Diabetes Mellitus," *N Engl J Med*, 1995, 332(18):1210-7.

17. Atkin SH, Dasmahapatra A, Jaker MA, et al, "Fingerstick Glucose Determination in Shock," *Ann Intern Med*, 1991, 114:(12)1020-4.

18. Shaw JE, Hodge AM, de Courten M, et al, "Isolated Postchallenge Hyperglycaemia Confirmed as a Risk Factor for Mortality," *Diabetologia*, 1999, 42(9):1050-4.

19. Bjornholt JV, Erikssen G, Aaser E, et al, "Fasting Blood Glucose: An Underestimated Risk Factor for Cardiovascular Death. Results From a 22-Year Follow-up of Healthy Nondiabetic Men," *Diabetes Care*, 1999, 22(1):45-9.

20. American Diabetes Association, "Standards of Medical Care for Patients With Diabetes Mellitus," *Diabetes Care*, 2000, 23(1 Suppl):S32-S42.

21. DECODE Study Group, "Will New Diagnostic Criteria for Diabetes Mellitus Change Phenotype of Patients With Diabetes? Reanalysis of European Epidemiologic Data," *BMJ*, 1998, 317(7155):371-5.

22. Vinicor F, "When Is Diabetes Diabetes?" *JAMA*, 1999, 281(13):1222-4.

References

Aono J, Ueda W, and Manabe M, "Alteration in Glucose Metabolism by Crying in Children," *N Engl J Med*, 1993, 329(15):1129.

Astles JR, Petros WP, Peters WP, et al, "Artifactual Hypoglycemia Associated With Hematopoietic Cytokines," *Arch Pathol Lab Med*, 1995, 119(8):713-6.

Atkinson MA and Maclaren NK, "The Pathogenesis of Insulin-Dependent Diabetes Mellitus," *N Engl J Med*, 1994, 331(21):1428-36.

Desai SP and Isa-Pratt S, *Clinician's Guide to Laboratory Medicine*, Hudson, OH: Lexi-Comp Inc, 2000, Chapter 15.

Fery F, Plat L, van de Borne P, et al, "Impaired Counter-Regulation of Glucose in a Patient With Hypothalamic Sarcoidosis," *N Engl J Med*, 1999, 340(11):852-6.

"Glucose Tolerance and Mortality: Comparison of WHO and American Diabetes Association Diagnostic Criteria. The DECODE Study Group. European Diabetes Epidemiology Group. Diabetes Epidemiology: Collaborative Analysis Of Diagnostic Criteria in Europe," *Lancet*, 1999, 354(9179):617-21.

Magni F, Paroni R, Bonini P, et al, "Determination of Serum Glucose Concentration by a Candidate Definitive Method," *Clin Chem*, 1994, 40(10):1978-80.

Palardy J, Havrankova J, Lepage R, et al, "Blood Glucose Measurements During Symptomatic Episodes in Patients With Suspected Postprandial Hypoglycemia," *N Engl J Med*, 1989, 321(21):1421-5.

Perucchini D, Fischer U, Spinas GA, et al, "Using Fasting Plasma Glucose Concentrations to Screen for Gestational Diabetes Mellitus: Prospective Population Based Study," *BMJ*, 1999, 319(7213):812-5.

Rett K, "The Relationship Between Insulin Resistance and Cardiovascular Complications of the Insulin Resistance Syndrome," *Diabetes Obes Metab*, 1999, 1(Suppl 1):S8-16.

Sacks DB, "Implications of the Revised Criteria for Diagnosis and Classification of Diabetes Mellitus," *Clin Chem*, 1997, 43(12):2230-2.

Seckl MJ, Mulholland PJ, Bishop AE, et al, "Hypoglycemia Due to an Insulin-Secreting Small-Cell Carcinoma of the Cervix," *N Engl J Med*, 1999, 341(10):733-6.

"The Cost-Effectiveness of Screening for Type 2 Diabetes. CDC Diabetes Cost-Effectiveness Study Group, Centers for Disease Control and Prevention," *JAMA*, 1998, 280(20):1757-63.

Thomas S, Gough J, Benson N, et al, "Accuracy of Fingerstick Glucose Determination in Patients Receiving CPR," *South Med J*, 1994, 87(11):1072-5.

Triosi RJ, Cowie CC, and Harris MI, "Diurnal Variation in Fasting Plasma Glucose. Implications for Diagnosis of Diabetes in Patients Examined in the Afternoon," *JAMA*, 2000, 284(24):3157-9.

Yarnell JW, Patterson CC, Thomas HF, et al, "Fasting Plasma Glucose and Subsequent Macrovascular Disease After 10 Years Follow-up: A Collaborative Study on Two Populations," *QJM*, 1999, 92(4):207-10.

♦ **Glucose:Insulin Ratio** *see* Glucose, Fasting, Plasma *on page 183*

Glucose, Noninvasive

Related Information
Glucose, Fasting, Plasma *on page 183*
Glucose, Postglucose Load, Plasma *on page 185*
Glucose, Random, Plasma *on page 186*
Glucose Tolerance Test, Plasma *on page 186*
Glucose, Whole Blood *on page 188*
Point-of-Care Testing *on page 43*

Abstract Self-monitoring of blood glucose by diabetic patients is now commonplace. Traditionally, such monitoring has been accomplished by point-of-care measuring devices requiring a small quantity of whole blood obtained by skin micropuncture; this device provides a continuous recording of glucose in interstitial fluid and does not require a blood sample.[1]

Methodology Reverse iontophoresis.[2] Another approach uses transdermal ultrasound to release interstitial fluid with subsequent assay of glucose (and other analytes).

Footnotes
1. Tamada JA, Garg S, Jovanovic L, et al, "Noninvasive Glucose Monitoring: Comprehensive Clinical Results. Cygnus Research Team," *JAMA*, 1999, 282(19):1839-44.
2. Rao G, Guy RH, Glikfeld P, et al, "Reverse Iontophoresis: Noninvasive Glucose Monitoring *In Vivo* in Humans," *Pharm Res*, 1995, 12(12):1869-73.

Glucose, Postglucose Load, Plasma

Related Information
Fructosamine, Serum *on page 177*
Glucose, Quantitative, Urine *on page 874*
Glucose, Random, Plasma *on page 186*
Glucose, Semiquantitative, Urine *on page 875*
Glucose Tolerance Test, Plasma *on page 186*
Glutamic Acid Decarboxylase (GAD65) Antibody *on page 527*
Glycated Hemoglobin (Hemoglobin A$_{1c}$), Blood *on page 188*
Islet Cell Antibody *on page 538*
Ketones, Urine *on page 877*
Microalbuminuria *on page 879*
Reducing Substances, Urine *on page 885*

Synonyms 2-Hour PP Glucose; Oral Glucose Tolerance Test; Postprandial Glucose; PP, 2-Hour

Replaces Glucose, 2-Hour Postprandial, Plasma

Test Includes Glucose level 2 hours after a meal or after a measured glucose load

Abstract The three tests recommended by the American Diabetes Association (ADA) for the diagnosis of **diabetes mellitus** are fasting plasma glucose, random plasma glucose, and the **2-hour postload** plasma glucose. Testing for **gestational diabetes mellitus** involves a first step screening plasma glucose **1 hour after a 50 g glucose load**, and if this result is abnormal, a **100 g glucose load test** (see below).[1]

Patient Preparation Patient should be fasting (no food or beverage, except for water and prescribed medications) for 8 hours. Testing is best done in the early morning.

- **75 g load:** This test is for diabetes mellitus. Patient should drink the glucose, usually a commercially available product specific for this test, and observe labeling precautions.
- **50 g load:** This is the first stage screen for **gestational diabetes mellitus**. The patient need not be fasting, but fasting is acceptable. Patient should drink the glucose, usually a commercially available product specific for this test, and observe labeling precautions.
- **100 g load:** This is the second stage in the diagnosis of **gestational diabetes mellitus**. The patient should be fasting and drink the glucose, usually a commercially available product specific for this test, and observe the labeling precautions.

Specimen Plasma or serum

Container Gray top (sodium fluoride or iodoacetate) tube; red top tubes are acceptable only if specimen is rapidly separated from the red cells and analyzed promptly.

Sampling Time
- **75 g load:** Draw specimen 2 hours after glucose.
- **50 g load:** Draw specimen 1 hour after glucose
- **100 g load:** Draw specimens fasting (preglucose), 1-hour, 2-hour, and 3-hour postglucose (3-hour OGTT).

Reference Interval

ADA Criteria for the Diagnosis of Diabetes Mellitus[1]

Any one of the following findings is diagnostic of diabetes, if confirmed by any one of the following findings on a subsequent day:

- Symptoms of diabetes plus a random plasma glucose level ≥200 mg/dL (11.1 mmol/L). Symptoms include polyuria, polydipsia, and unexplained weight loss.
- Fasting plasma glucose ≥126 mg/dL (7 mmol/L) after a minimum 8-hour fast.
- Two-hour postload glucose ≥200 mg/dL (11.1 mmol/L) during a 75 g glucose load.

ADA Criteria for the Diagnosis of Gestational Diabetes Mellitus[1]

Step 1. A plasma glucose >140 mg/dL (SI: >7.8 mmol/L) 1 hour after a 50 g load indicates the need for additional testing (Step 2).

Step 2. Gestational diabetes mellitus is diagnosed if two or more values, in the 3-hour OGTT, exceed these criteria:
- Fasting: 105 mg/dL, 5.8 mmol/L
- 1-hour: 190 mg/dL, 10.5 mmol/L
- 2-hour: 165 mg/dL, 9.2 mmol/L
- 3-hour: 145 mg/dL, 8.0 mmol/L

Use Diagnose diabetes mellitus. Isolated postchallenge hyperglycemia (IPH) is defined as fasting glucose <126 mg/dL (7.0 mmol/L) and 2-hour glucose ≥200 mg/dL (11.1 mmol/L). IPH is a major risk factor for mortality from cardiovascular disease.[2]

Methodology Specific enzyme-based assays using glucose oxidase or hexokinase

Additional Information When the fasting plasma glucose is in the range of 110-126 mg/dL (SI: 6.1-7.0 mmol/L), the so-called impaired fasting glucose category, some authorities (eg, the World Health Organization, WHO), but not the American Diabetes Association, recommend a 2-hour oral glucose tolerance test, performed as follows: following an overnight fast, a **75 g** glucose load is taken over a 5-minute period. For children, the dose is 1.75 g glucose/kg body weight. Results are classified as follows.

- Impaired fasting glucose: 0-hour specimen: 110-126 mg/dL (SI: 6.1-7.0 mmol/L); 2-hour specimen: <140 mg/dL (SI: 7.8 mmol/L)

(Continued)

Glucose, Postglucose Load, Plasma *(Continued)*

- Impaired glucose tolerance: 0-hour specimen: <126 mg/dL (SI: <7.0 mmol/L); 2-hour specimen: 140-200 mg/dL (SI: 7.8-11.1 mmol/L)
- Diabetes mellitus: 0-hour specimen: >126 mg/dL (SI: >7.0 mmol/L); 2-hour specimen: >200 mg/dL (SI: >11.1 mmol/L)

Footnotes

1. American Diabetes Association, "Report of the Expert Committee on the Diagnosis and Classification of Diabetes Mellitus," *Diabetes Care*, 1997, 20(7):1183-201.
2. Shaw JE, Hodge AM, de Courten M, et al, "Isolated Postchallenge Hyperglycaemia Confirmed as a Risk Factor for Mortality," *Diabetologia*, 1999, 42(9):1050-4.

References

Hanson RL, Nelson RG, McCance DR, et al, "Comparison of Screening Tests for Noninsulin Dependent Diabetes Mellitus," *Arch Intern Med*, 1993, 153(18):2133-40.

Home P, "The OGTT: Gold That Does Not Shine," *Diabet Med*, 1988, 5(4):313-4.

Jarrett RJ, Keen H, and McCartney P, "The Whitehall Study: Ten Year Follow-up Report on New With Impaired Glucose Tolerance With Reference to Worsening to Diabetics and Predictors of Death," *Diabet Med*, 1984, 1(4):279-83.

McCance DR, Hanson RL, Charles MA, et al, "Comparison of Tests for Glycated Haemoglobin and Fasting and Two-Hour Plasma Glucose Concentrations as Diagnostic Methods for Diabetes," *BMJ*, 1994, 308(6940):1323-8.

Reichelt AJ, Spichler ER, Branchtein L, et al, "Fasting Plasma Glucose Is a Useful Test for the Detection of Gestational Diabetes. Brazilian Study of Gestational Diabetes (EBDG) Working Group," *Diabetes Care*, 1998, 21(8):1246-9.

Shivvers SA and Lucas MJ, "Gestational Diabetes. Is a 50-g Screening Result ≥200 mg/dL Diagnostic?" *J Reprod Med*, 1999, 44(8):685-8.

Glucose, Random, Plasma

Related Information

Related Information
C-Peptide, Serum *on page 156*
Drugs of Abuse Testing, Urine *on page 788*
Glucose, Fasting, Plasma *on page 183*
Glucose, Noninvasive *on page 185*
Glucose, Postglucose Load, Plasma *on page 185*
Glucose Tolerance Test, Plasma *on page 186*
Glucose, Whole Blood *on page 188*
Insulin, Serum *on page 201*
Ketone Bodies, Blood *on page 205*
Ketones, Urine *on page 877*
Microalbuminuria *on page 879*
Point-of-Care Testing *on page 43*
Salicylate, Serum or Plasma *on page 806*

Abstract The three tests recommended by the American Diabetes Association (ADA) for the diagnosis of **diabetes mellitus** are fasting plasma glucose, random plasma glucose, and the two-hour postglucose load. Testing for **gestational diabetes mellitus** involves a first step screening plasma glucose **1 hour after a 50 g glucose load**, and if this result is abnormal, a **100 g glucose load test**[1] (see Glucose, Postglucose Load, Plasma *on page 185*).

Specimen Plasma or serum

Container Gray top (sodium fluoride or iodoacetate) tube is preferred; red top tubes are acceptable only if specimen is rapidly separated from the red cells and analyzed promptly.

Collection Venous specimens are recommended from all age groups, except for neonates, whose specimens are usually obtained from heelsticks. (In postprandial states, a capillary specimen will have a slightly higher glucose concentration than a venous specimen.)

Storage Instructions Glucose will decrease at a rate of 5-10 mg/dL per hour in unseparated, room temperature blood not collected in gray top tubes.

Reference Interval Newborns: <115 mg/dL (SI: <6.4 mmol/L); adults and children: <200 mg/dL (SI: <11.1 mmol/L)

ADA Criteria for the Diagnosis of Diabetes Mellitus[1]

Any one of the following findings is diagnostic of diabetes, if confirmed by any one of the following findings on a subsequent day.

- Symptoms of diabetes plus a random plasma glucose level ≥200 mg/dL (11.1 mmol/L). Symptoms include polyuria, polydipsia, and unexplained weight loss.
- Fasting plasma glucose ≥126 mg/dL (7 mmol/L) after a minimum 8-hour fast.
- Two-hour postload glucose ≥200 mg/dL (11.1 mmol/L) during an oral glucose tolerance test conducted as described by the World Health Organization using glucose load containing the equivalent of 75-g anhydrous glucose dissolved in water.

Random plasma glucose results 47-60 mg/dL are consistent with, but not fully diagnostic of, **hypoglycemia**, a diagnosis which has no established biochemical criterion, and which requires careful correlation with clinical features (see table in Glucose, Fasting, Plasma *on page 183*).

Possible Panic Range Neonates: <40 mg/dL (SI: <2.2 mmol/L); adults: male: <50 mg/dL (SI: <2.8 mmol/L), >400 mg/dL (SI: >22.2 mmol/L); adults female: <40 mg/dL (SI: <2.2 mmol/L), >400 mg/dL (SI: >22.2 mmol/L)

Use The test is used to diagnose diabetes mellitus and to monitor therapy and support control of diabetes. In addition, fasting glucose measurements are useful in the diagnosis and treatment of certain metabolic disorders (eg, acidosis, ketosis, dehydration, coma). **Hypoglycemia** values approximately <45 mg/dL (SI: <2.5 mmol/L) if present, should be investigated with C-

peptide, insulin and proinsulin levels as well (see C-Peptide, Serum *on page 156*).[2] The diagnosis of **insulinoma** is suggested when random glucose <40 mg/dL is found with inappropriate plasma insulin levels following prolonged fasting[3] (see Insulin, Serum *on page 201*). See Glucose, Fasting, Plasma *on page 183* for the differential diagnosis of hypoglycemia. Determination of blood glucose on admission in patients who have had an out-of-hospital cardiac arrest can serve as a predictor of neurologic recovery. Higher levels are indicative of more severe brain ischemia and difficult resuscitation.[4]

Limitations Glucose will decrease in samples left on the clot, and in tubes other than gray top tubes, if not processed and analyzed promptly.

Methodology Specific enzyme-based assays using glucose oxidase or hexokinase

Additional Information Whole blood glucose values are not equivalent to **plasma glucose,** unless the whole blood assay has been calibrated to match plasma values (see Glucose, Whole Blood *on page 188* and Point-of-Care Testing *on page 43*). Small, handheld, whole blood glucose meters are designed for use at the point-of-care and for patient self-monitoring. The wide use of such devices has underscored the need for reliable instrumentation and quality control procedures to ensure valid results from this type of testing (see Glucose, Whole Blood *on page 188*).[5,6,7] Evaluation of glycated hemoglobin, self-monitoring of blood glucose, and use of microalbuminemia testing are ongoing means for monitoring glycemic control in diabetic patients.[8] Noninvasive devices for monitoring glycemic status are being developed.[9,10,11]

In addition to random (casual) plasma glucose levels, fasting plasma glucose levels and 2-hour postload (75-gram, glucose tolerance test in nonpregnant subjects) plasma glucose levels are used to diagnose diabetes mellitus.[1]

If glucose is >400 mg/dL (SI: >22 mmol/L), the possibility of ketonemia should be considered. The incidence of hypoglycemia in hospitalized patients appears to be significant, but may be better controlled if frequent monitoring of glucose levels is employed.[12]

Footnotes

1. American Diabetes Association, "Report of the Expert Committee on the Diagnosis and Classification of Diabetes Mellitus," *Diabetes Care*, 1997, 20(7):1183-97.
2. Axelrod L, "Insulinoma: Cost-Effective Care in Patients With a Rare Disease," *Ann Intern Med*, 1995, 123(4):311-2.
3. Doppman JL, Chang R, Fraker DL, et al, "Localization of Insulinomas to Regions of the Pancreas by Intra-Arterial Stimulation With Calcium," *Ann Intern Med*, 1995, 123(4):269-73.
4. Longstreth WT Jr, Diehr P, Cobb LA, et al, "Neurologic Outcome and Blood Glucose Levels During Out-of-Hospital Cardiopulmonary Resuscitation," *Neurology*, 1986, 36(9):1186-91.
5. Kiechle FL, "Blood Glucose: Measurement in the Point-of-Care Setting," *Lab Med*, 2000, 31(5):276-82.
6. Leroux ML and Desjardins PR, "Establishment and Maintenance of a Hospital Glucose Meter Program," *Lab Med*, 1989, 97-9.
7. Bain OF, Brown KD, Sacher RA, et al, "A Hospital-Wide Blind Control Program for Bedside Glucose Meters," *Arch Pathol Lab Med*, 1999, 113(12):1370-5.
8. Singer DE, Coley CM, Samet JH, et al, "Tests of Glycemia in Diabetes Mellitus - Their Use in Establishing a Diagnosis and in Treatment," *Ann Intern Med*, 1989, 110(2):125-37.
9. Khalil OS, "Spectroscopic and Clinical Aspects of Noninvasive Glucose Measurements," *Clin Chem*, 1999, 45(2):165-77.
10. MacKenzie HA, Ashton HS, Spiers S, et al, "Advances in Photoacoustic Noninvasive Glucose Testing," *Clin Chem*, 1999, 45(9):1587-95.
11. Burmeister JJ and Arnold MA, "Evaluation of Measurement Sites for Noninvasive Blood Glucose Sensing With Near-Infrared Transmission Spectroscopy," *Clin Chem*, 1999, 45(9):1621-7.
12. Fischer KF, Lees JA, and Newman JH, "Hypoglycemia in Hospitalized Patients. Causes and Outcomes," *N Engl J Med*, 1986, 315(20):1245-50.

References

Aono J, Ueda W, and Manabe M, "Alteration in Glucose Metabolism by Crying in Children," *N Engl J Med*, 1993, 329(15):1129.

Bolli GB and Fanelli CG, "Unawareness of Hypoglycemia," *N Engl J Med*, 1995, 333(26):1771-2.

Boyle PJ, Kempers SF, O'Connor AM, et al, "Brain Glucose Uptake and Unawareness of Hypoglucemia in Patients With Insulin-Dependent Diabetes Mellitus," *N Engl J Med*, 1995, 333(26):1726-31.

Brandt KR and Miles JM, "Relationship Between Severity of Hyperglycemia and Metabolic Acidosis in Diabetic Ketoacidosis," *Mayo Clin Proc*, 1988, 63(11):1071-4.

Gill GV, Hardy KJ, Patrick AW, et al, "Random Blood Glucose Estimation in Type 2 Diabetes: Does It Reflect Overall Glycaemic Control?" *Diabet Med*, 1994, 11(7):705-8.

Palardy J, Havrankova J, Lepage R, et al, "Blood Glucose Measurements During Symptomatic Episodes in Patients With Suspected Postprandial Hypoglycemia," *N Engl J Med*, 1989, 321(21):1421-5.

Weiner CP, Faustich M, Burns J, et al, "The Relationship Between Capillary and Venous Glucose Concentration During Pregnancy," *Am J Obstet Gynecol*, 1986, 155(1):61-4.

♦ **Glucose Suppression Test** *see* Growth Hormone, Serum *on page 189*

Glucose Tolerance Test, Plasma

Related Information

Glucose, Fasting, Plasma *on page 183*
Glucose, Postglucose Load, Plasma *on page 185*

Glutamic Acid Decarboxylase (GAD65) Antibody *on page 527*
Islet Cell Antibody *on page 538*

Synonyms GTT; OGTT; Oral Glucose Tolerance Test

Applies to Gestational Diabetes Screening Test

Test Includes Fasting blood glucose followed by glucose levels drawn at timed intervals after administration of a glucose load. Urine is no longer collected or examined for the GTT.

Abstract The oral glucose tolerance test (OGTT) is used for the diagnosis of gestational diabetes mellitus. It has also been used for the diagnosis of types 1 and 2 diabetes mellitus, but is not the optimal test for that purpose.[1]

Patient Preparation Patient should not smoke due to glucose stimulation by nicotine. Patient should be active and have had adequate food intake with adequate carbohydrates (at least 150 g carbohydrate daily) for 3 days, and then fast 12 hours prior to test. Many drugs interfere (eg, steroids, diuretics, antihypertensives, anticonvulsants, psychoactive drugs, antituberculous agents, and anti-inflammatory drugs).[2] Patient should not be stressed.

In **pregnant patients**, a screening test (fasting **not** required) is conducted as follows: A 50-g oral-glucose load is administered, and a blood sample is drawn after 1 hour. The gestational screening test is positive when the postload plasma glucose result is ≥140 mg/dL (SI: ≥7.8 mmol/L).[3,4] Additional testing is then performed as specified in Glucose, Postglucose Load, Plasma *on page 185*.

Specimen Plasma

Container Gray top (sodium fluoride or iodoacetate) tube

Collection Nongestational OGTT: After a fasting blood specimen is obtained, administer the oral glucose solution. (The adult dose is 75 g. Children receive 1.75 g/kg body weight up to 75 g). Collect a blood specimen at 2-hours postglucose administration.

The patient should remain seated and consume nothing but water after the glucose solution is administered. Physical activity should be minimized and some recommend that the patient be kept supine throughout.[5] Vomiting or diarrhea may alter test results.

Causes for Rejection Incorrect or no anticoagulant, time not marked on tubes, nonfasting patient. Stressed patients (eg, following surgery, with infections, on corticosteroids) should not have a OGTT.

Reference Interval

Nongestational OGTT - normal glucose tolerance:
- fasting: <110 mg/dL (SI: <6.1 mmol/L)
- 2-hour: <140 mg/dL (SI: <7.8 mmol/L)

Impaired glucose tolerance:
- fasting: ≥110-<126 mg/dL (SI: ≥6.1-<7.0 mmol/L)
- 2-hour: ≥140-<200 mg/dL (SI: ≥ 7.8 -<11.1 mmol/L)

Diabetes mellitus:
- fasting: ≥126 mg/dL (SI: ≥7.0 mmol/L)
- 2-hour: ≥200 mg/dL (SI: ≥11.1 mmol/L)[1]

Criteria for interpretation for gestational diabetes mellitus: See Glucose, Postglucose Load, Plasma *on page 185*.

Use The OGTT is used for, but is not optimal for, the diagnosis of diabetes mellitus (type 1, type 2) and has been used in the evaluation of unexplained hypertriglyceridemia, neuropathy, impotence, diabetes-like renal diseases, retinopathy, and necrobiosis lipoidica diabeticorum. The gestational OGTT is used in pregnancy to predict perinatal morbidity, risk of fetal abnormality, and perinatal mortality.[6]

Limitations Slight glucose intolerance is seen in patients on oral contraceptives and in postmenopausal women on hormone replacement therapy.[7] Failure to have patient on a 3-day high carbohydrate diet may result in a false-positive OGTT. Impaired glucose tolerance is **not** equivalent to diabetes mellitus. A normal result does not assure that diabetes will not subsequently develop. Criticisms of the OGTT include poor reproducibility, patient inconvenience, and strong propensity for overdiagnosis of diabetes mellitus. The American Diabetes Association (ADA) recommends the fasting plasma glucose determination rather than the OGTT for the diagnosis of type 1 and type 2 diabetes mellitus.

The 5-hour oral glucose tolerance test is discredited.[8] See Glucose, Fasting, Plasma *on page 183*, Insulin, Serum *on page 201*, and C-Peptide, Serum *on page 156* for discussions on the work-up of **hypoglycemia**.

Contraindications The OGTT is contraindicated in the presence of obvious diabetes mellitus. Emesis is often an indication to cancel the remainder of an OGTT for that day; decision is up to the patient's physician.

Methodology Glucose is usually determined by specific, enzyme-based assays using glucose oxidase or hexokinase.

Additional Information Fasting plasma glucose levels ≥126 mg/dL (SI: ≥7.0 mmol/L) and/or symptoms of diabetes plus random plasma glucose levels ≥200 mg/dL (SI: ≥11.1 mmol/L) on two, separate occasions are diagnostic of diabetes mellitus and obviate the need for a OGTT. However, studies of obese[9] and postpartum, gestational diabetic[10] subjects have shown greater diagnostic sensitivity of the OGTT compared to the fasting plasma glucose in these populations.

Glucose intolerance in obese subjects is due to progressive insulin resistance and ultimate decreased insulin secretion.[11] Excessive growth hormone, adrenocortical hormones (eg, Cushing syndrome), thyroid hormones and catecholamines (eg, pheochromocytoma) cause decreased glucose tolerance.

The OGTT lacks specificity and sensitivity for predicting the complications of diabetes mellitus. Approximately 1% to 5% of patients with **impaired glucose tolerance** become overtly diabetic yearly. Patients with impaired glucose tolerance[12] as well as patients with a history of isolated postchallenge hyperglycemia[4] have increased risk for cardiovascular disease.

An increased prevalence of idiopathic hemochromatosis is recognized in the diabetic population.[13]

Pregnant women with an abnormal OGTT are at risk for preeclampsia/eclampsia and delivery of a macrosomic infant.[14,15] Infants of mothers with gestational diabetes are also subject to hypoglycemia, jaundice, respiratory distress syndrome, polycythemia, and hypocalcemia. The complications in labor and delivery of macrosomia are significant.[16]

Nonketotic hyperglycemic syndrome is characterized by glucose levels >600 mg/dL with hyperosmolarity and absence of significant ketonuria.[17]

Footnotes

1. American Diabetes Association, "Report of the Expert Committee on the Diagnosis and Classification of Diabetes Mellitus," *Diabetes Care*, 1997, 20(7):1183-97.
2. Young DS, "Effects of Drugs on Clinical Laboratory Tests," 5th ed, Volume 1, Listing by Test, Washington, DC: AACC Press, American Association of Clinical Chemistry, 2000, Section 3, 349-67.
3. Catalano PM, Vargo KM, Bernstein IM, et al, "Incidence and Risk Factors Associated With Abnormal Postpartum Glucose Tolerance in Women With Gestational Diabetes," *Am J Obstet Gynecol*, 1991, 165(4 Pt 1):914-9.
4. Barrett-Connor E and Ferrara A, "Isolated Postchallenge Hyperglycemia and the Risk of Fatal Cardiovascular Disease in Older Women and Men. The Rancho Bernardo Study," *Diabetes Care*, 1998, 21(8):1236-9.
5. Gambino R, "Is It Time to Abandon the Oral Glucose Tolerance Test?" *Lab Rep*, 1995, 17(10):72.
6. Forest JC, Garrido-Russo M, Lemay A, et al, "Reference Values for the Oral Glucose Tolerance Test at Each Trimester of Pregnancy," *Am J Clin Pathol*, 1983, 80(6):828-31.
7. Espeland MA, Hogan PE, Fineberg SE, et al, "Effect of Postmenopausal Hormone Therapy on Glucose and Insulin Concentrations. PEPI Investigators. Postmenopausal Estrogen/Progestin Interventions," *Diabetes Care*, 1998, 21(10):1589-95.
8. Service FJ, "Hypoglycemic Disorders," *N Engl J Med*, 1995, 332(17):1144-52.
9. Mannucci E, Bardini G, Ognibene A, et al, "Comparison of ADA and WHO Screening Methods for Diabetes Mellitus in Obese Patients. American Diabetes Association," *Diabet Med*, 1999, 16(7):579-85.
10. Conway DL and Langer O, "Effects of New Criteria for Type 2 Diabetes on the Rate of Postpartum Glucose Intolerance in Women With Gestational Diabetes," *Am J Obstet Gynecol*, 1999, 181(3):610-4.
11. Carlsson S, Persson PG, Alvarsson M, et al, "Weight History, Glucose Intolerance, and Insulin Levels in Middle-Aged Swedish Men," *Am J Epidemiol*, 1998, 148(6):539-45.
12. Meigs JB, Nathan DM, Wilson PW, et al, "Metabolic Risk Factors Worsen Continuously Across the Spectrum of Nondiabetic Glucose Tolerance. The Framingham Offspring Study," *Ann Intern Med*, 1998, 128(7):524-33.
13. Phelps G, Chapman I, Hall P, et al, "Prevalence of Genetic Hemochromatosis Among Diabetic Patients," *Lancet*, 1989, 2(8657):233-4.
14. Lindsay MK, Graves W, and Klein L, "The Relationship of One Abnormal Glucose Tolerance Test Value and Pregnancy Complications," *Obstet Gynecol*, 1989, 73(1):103-6.
15. Neiger R and Coustan DR, "The Role of Repeat Glucose Tolerance Tests in the Diagnosis of Gestational Diabetes," *Am J Obstet Gynecol*, 1991, 165(4 Pt 1):787-90.
16. Kjos SL and Buchanan TA, "Gestational Diabetes Mellitus," *N Engl J Med*, 1999, 341(23):1749-56.
17. Rother KI and Schwenk WF 2d, "An Unusual Case of the Nonketotic Hyperglycemic Syndrome During Childhood," *Mayo Clin Proc*, 1995, 70(1):62-5.

References

Astles JR, Petros WP, Peters WP, et al, "Artifactual Hypoglycemia Associated With Hematopoietic Cytokines," *Arch Pathol Lab Med*, 1995, 119(8):713-6.

Atkinson MA and Maclaren NK, "The Pathogenesis of Insulin-Dependent Diabetes Mellitus," *N Engl J Med*, 1994, 331(21):1428-36.

Davies MJ, Muehlbayer S, Garrick P, et al, "Potential Impact of a Change in the Diagnostic Criteria for Diabetes Mellitus on the Prevalence of Abnormal Glucose Tolerance in a Local Community at Risk of Diabetes: Impact of New Diagnostic Criteria for Diabetes Mellitus," *Diabet Med*, 1999, 16(4):343-6.

de Leacy EA and Cowley DM, "Evidence That the Oral Glucose Tolerance Test Does Not Provide a Uniform Stimulus to Pancreatic Islets in Pregnancy," *Clin Chem*, 1989, 35(7):1482-5.

Kritz-Silverstein D, Barrett-Connor E, and Wingard DL, "The Effect of Parity on the Later Development of Noninsulin-Dependent Diabetes Mellitus or Impaired Glucose Tolerance," *N Engl J Med*, 1989, 321(18):1214-9.

Langer O, Brustman L, Anyaegbunam A, et al, "The Significance of One Abnormal Glucose Tolerance Test Value on Adverse Outcome in Pregnancy," *Am J Obstet Gynecol*, 1987, 157(3):758-63.

Neiger R and Coustan DR, "Are the Current ACOG Glucose Tolerance Test Criteria Sensitive Enough?" *Obstet Gynecol*, 1991, 78(6):1117-20.

Nelson RL, "Oral Glucose Tolerance Test: Indications and Limitations," *Mayo Clin Proc*, 1988, 63(3):263-9.

Nolan JJ, Ludvik B, Beersden P, et al, "Improvement in Glucose Tolerance and Insulin Resistance in Obese Subjects Treated With Troglitazone," *N Engl J Med*, 1994, 331(18):1188-93.

Sacks DA, Abu-Fadil S, Karten GJ, et al, "Screening for Gestational Diabetes With the One-Hour 50-g Glucose Test," *Obstet Gynecol*, 1987, 70(1):89-93.

Tallarigo L, Giampietro O, Penno G, et al, "Relation of Glucose Tolerance to Complications of Pregnancy in Nondiabetic Women," *N Engl J Med*, 1986, 315(16):989-92.

Glucose, Whole Blood

Related Information

Glucose, Fasting, Plasma *on page 183*
Glucose, Postglucose Load, Plasma *on page 185*
Glucose, Random, Plasma *on page 186*
Glucose Tolerance Test, Plasma *on page 186*
Glycated Hemoglobin (Hemoglobin A_{1c}), Blood *on page 188*
Ketones, Urine *on page 877*
Microalbuminuria *on page 879*
Point-of-Care Testing *on page 43*
Reducing Substances, Urine *on page 885*

Abstract For most purposes, fasting plasma is the preferred specimen for glucose measurements. Such purposes include the initial diagnosis and classification of diabetes mellitus, and monitoring the metabolic status of diabetic patients and other patients who are seriously ill. There are situations, however, in which whole blood is an appropriate substitute for plasma. Such situations include self-monitoring of diabetes (see also Additional Information), point-of-care (POC) testing in acute and chronic care facilities, and hospitalized patients having arterial blood gas measurements (glucose can be assayed without drawing an additional specimen).

Most of the information in the monograph Glucose, Fasting, Plasma *on page 183* also applies to measurements in whole blood. Described below are important **differences** between whole blood and plasma measurements.

Specimen Whole blood, obtained by venipuncture or skin micropuncture

Container Green top (heparin) tube or none (drop of blood placed directly in/on assay device or on reagent container)

Causes for Rejection Failure to meet instrument criteria, specimen delayed (more than 15 minutes) in reaching testing laboratory

Turnaround Time Within 30 minutes.[1] Most of the POC instruments give whole blood glucose values in <2 minutes.

Special Instructions Must be assayed immediately

Reference Interval Adults: 65-95 mg/dL (SI: 3.5-5.3 mmol/L)[2]

Glucose concentrations in plasma are ~11% higher than in simultaneously obtained whole blood specimen when the hematocrit is normal. To mitigate the potential confusion which can result from the fact that whole blood and plasma glucose concentrations are different, the whole blood instrument can be calibrated using a serum-based reference material. When this is done, the whole blood result is the same as the simultaneously obtained plasma sample. Most of the manufacturers of whole blood glucose instruments have adopted this approach.

Use Whole blood glucose assays are used for monitoring the treatment of patients with an established diagnosis of diabetes mellitus, to determine insulin dose, and for monitoring the metabolic status of seriously ill patients. **The initial diagnosis of diabetes mellitus or gestational diabetes should be made on the basis of glucose assays in fasting venous plasma** (see Glucose, Fasting, Plasma *on page 183*).

Limitations Some devices used in POC testing for blood glucose have larger imprecision and bias characteristics than the analyzers used for plasma glucose measurements in medical laboratories. The National Committee for Clinical Laboratory Standards (NCCLS) has made the following recommendation: For test readings >100 mg/dL (SI: >5.5 mmol/L), the discrepancy between ancillary blood glucose testing (ABGT) concentrations and laboratory concentrations on the same specimen should be <20%; for test readings ≤100 mg/dL, the discrepancy should be no more than 15 mg/dL (SI: 0.83 mmol/L).[3] Mannitol causes interference in trilayer electrochemical biosensor testing.[1] Hematocrit levels are relevant.[4] Drug interference was recently addressed.[5] Lack of bidirectional communication between POC devices and information systems represents a major disadvantage.[6]

The most frequent errors include inadequate instrument cleaning, incorrect quality control, improper technique, and inappropriate match with test strip calibration. Other factors include drug interference, hematocrit extremes, pO_2 (for glucose oxidase methods), and low total protein concentrations in extracorporeal circulation procedures.[7]

Methodology Specific enzyme-based assays using glucose oxidase or hexokinase, trilayer biosensors[1]

Additional Information Because clinical research has demonstrated the advantages of intensive diabetes management, self-monitoring of blood glucose by diabetic patients is now commonplace. Such glucose testing is most frequently performed using POC instruments requiring a small amount of whole blood obtained by skin micropuncture. A new generation of less invasive self-monitoring devices, which are based on the technique of iontophoresis and do not require a blood sample, are becoming available.[8] See Glucose, Noninvasive *on page 185*.

Footnotes

1. Kost GJ, Nguyen TH, and Tang Z, "Whole-Blood Glucose and Lactate. Trilayer Biosensors, Drug Interference, Metabolism, and Practice Guidelines," *Arch Pathol Lab Med*, 2000, 124(8):1128-34.

2. Painter PC, Cope JY, and Smith JL, "Reference Information for the Clinical Laboratory," *Tietz Textbook of Clinical Chemistry*, 3rd ed, Burtis CA and Ashwood ER, eds, Philadelphia, PA: WB Saunders Co, 1999, 1815.

3. National Committee for Clinical Laboratory Standards (NCCLS), "Ancillary (Bedside) Blood Glucose Testing in Acute and Chronic Care Facilities; Approved Guideline," NCCLS document C30-A (ISBN 1-56238-232-2), 1994.

4. Tang Z, Lee JH, Louie RF, et al, "Effects of Different Hematocrit Levels on Glucose Measurements With Handheld Meters for Point-of-Care Testing," *Arch Pathol Lab Med*, 2000, 124(8):1135-40.

5. Tang Z, Du X, Louie RF, et al, "Effects of Drugs on Glucose Measurements With Handheld Glucose Meters and a Portable Glucose Analyzer," *Am J Clin Pathol*, 2000, 113(1):75-86.

6. Kost GJ, "Connectivity. The Millennium Challenge for Point-of-Care Testing," *Arch Pathol Lab Med*, 2000, 124(8):1108-10.

7. Kiechle FL, "Blood Glucose: Measurement in the Point-of-Care Setting," *Lab Med*, 2000, 31(5):276-82.

8. Tamada JA, Garg S, Jovanovic L, et al, "Noninvasive Glucose Monitoring: Comprehensive Clinical Results. Cygnus Research Team," *JAMA*, 1999, 282(19):1839-44.

References

Koch B, "Glucose Monitoring as a Guide to Diabetes Management. Critical Subject Review," *Can Fam Physician*, 1996, 42:1142-6, 1149-52.

Wright J, "Better Data Capture in Glucose Testing's Future," *CAP Today*, September 2000, 47-55.

♦ **Glutamic Oxaloacetic Transaminase, Serum** *see* Aspartate Aminotransferase, Serum *on page 112*

♦ **Glutamic Pyruvate Transaminase** *see* Alanine Aminotransferase, Serum *on page 87*

♦ **Glutamine, Spinal Fluid** *see* Cerebrospinal Fluid Glutamine *on page 141*

♦ **γ-Glutamyl Transferase** *see* Gamma-Glutamyl Transferase, Serum *on page 179*

♦ **Glutamyl Transpeptidase** *see* Gamma-Glutamyl Transferase, Serum *on page 179*

♦ **Glycated Albumin** *see* Fructosamine, Serum *on page 177*

Glycated Hemoglobin (Hemoglobin A_{1c}), Blood

Related Information

Fetal Hemoglobin *on page 431*
Fructosamine, Serum *on page 177*
Glucose, Fasting, Plasma *on page 183*
Glucose, Semiquantitative, Urine *on page 875*
Glucose, Whole Blood *on page 188*
Hemoglobin Electrophoresis *on page 444*
Microalbuminuria *on page 879*
Triglycerides, Serum or Plasma *on page 288*

Synonyms Fast Hemoglobins; GHb; Glycohemoglobin; Hb A_1; Hemoglobin A_{1a}, A_{1b}, A_{1c}

Applies to Protein Glycosylation

Abstract Glycated hemoglobins (GHb), also called glycohemoglobins, comprise a chemically heterogeneous group of substances formed by the reaction between sugars and hemoglobin. The rate at which GHb is formed is proportional to the concentration of blood glucose. Since red blood cells survive an average of 120 days in the circulation, the measurement of GHb provides an index of a person's average blood glucose concentration (glycemia) during a 2- to 4-month period.[1,2]

The various chemical species of GHb have been named with reference to their order of elution when separated by chromatographic techniques (eg, Hb A_0, Hb A_{1a}, Hb A_{1b}, Hb A_{1c}, Hb A_{1d}, Hb A_2, Hb A_3, and so forth). Some assays measure all GHb species in a sample, while other assays measure only one or two species. In an attempt to standardize the clinical measurements, most assays now in use clinically measure Hb A_{1c}, or are calibrated to produce a result equivalent to such a measurement.

The measurement of Hb A_{1c} is important because of evidence showing that tight glycemic control results in a reduced incidence of diabetic nephropathy[3] and other long-term complications of diabetes mellitus.[2]

Specimen Whole blood

Container Lavender top (EDTA) tube; check with the laboratory.

Sampling Time Fasting specimens are not required. Testing at 3-month intervals is recommended for patients with type I diabetes. For patients with type II diabetes, glycated hemoglobins at diagnosis and at 6-month intervals, or as often as required for good control,[2] are desirable.[1]

Storage Instructions Stable 7 days at 4°C.

Reference Interval Method-dependent. For assays that measure **total GHb** (eg, affinity column chromatography) reported reference intervals include 5.3% to 7.5%[4] and 4% to 7%.[5]

With assays that measure Hb A_{1c}, reported reference intervals include 4.5% to 5.7% (HPLC) and 4.5% to 8.5% (column chromatography).[4] For other intervals see Footnotes 6, 7, 8, 9, 10, 11.

Critical Values The risk of microalbuminuria with insulin-dependent diabetes mellitus increases when Hb A_{1c} exceeds 8.1% (equivalent to Hb A_1 >10.1%). This value corresponds with average daily blood glucose levels ~200 mg/dL (SI: ~11.1 mmol/L).[3,12] See Microalbuminuria *on page 879* with graphic.

Use Glycated hemoglobin values are used to assess long-term glucose control in diabetes. The test should be performed at the time of initial diagnosis, and then **at least quarterly** in insulin-dependent diabetes, and

as frequently as needed in noninsulin dependent diabetes.[2] GHb measurements reflect the level of control present over the preceding 60-120 days; more recent levels have greater influence. Continued high levels of blood glucose are reflected in high GHb concentrations.

Singer et al,[1] Gambino,[13] and Peters et al,[14] have suggested a diagnostic approach in which glycated hemoglobin may be substituted for glucose testing and also advocate it as an adjunct in gestational diabetes.[1] Davidson et al advocate application of Hb A_{1c} concentrations to support the diagnosis of diabetes in subjects whose fasting plasma glucose concentrations are <140 mg/dL (7.8 mmol/L) unless excessive glycosylation is demonstrated.[15] Vinicor, however, notes that both false-positive and false-negative diagnoses would result, assuming that a fasting plasma concentration <110 mg/dL (6.1 mmol/L) or >139 mg/dL (7.7 mmol/L) is definitely normal or indicative of diabetes, respectively.[16] Glycated hemoglobin is also useful in evaluation of fetal risk in type II diabetics who become pregnant. Glycated hemoglobin predicts the progression of retinopathy.[17]

Limitations Chronic blood loss, renal failure, and hemolytic anemia result in a misleading decrease in the glycated hemoglobin level. Low values also derive (with use of ion-exchange resin chromatography/cation chromatography) from blood containing hemoglobin S or C, including Hb C trait.[18] Pregnancy may lower glycated hemoglobin. Misleading high levels of glycated hemoglobin are found when testing is done by ion exchange resin columns in patients who have elevated levels of fetal hemoglobin (Hb F) (or beta-thalassemia);[19] high levels of Hb F are found in young children (younger than 2 years of age) and in some hemoglobinopathies. The various analytical methods for glycated hemoglobin are differently affected in the presence of hemoglobinopathies. Increased Hb A_{1c} concentrations in the presence of iron deficiency, should be interpreted cautiously.[20] The multiplicity of methods with varying reference ranges leads to lack of standardization.[21] See also listing Hemoglobin Electrophoresis *on page 444.*

Methodology Immunoassay, high performance liquid chromatography (HPLC), isoelectric focusing, electrospray ionization mass spectrometry, ion-exchange chromatography, boronate affinity with either column chromatographic or ion capture separation, electrophoresis, colorimetry, and spectrophotometry. The American Diabetes Association (ADA)[22,23] recommends that laboratories use only methods certified as traceable to the Diabetes Control and Complications Trial (DCCT) reference method[24,25] and participate in proficiency testing programs that use whole blood specimens with targets set by the National Glycohemoglobin Standardization Program Laboratory Network.

Additional Information This test is essential for optimal management of diabetes mellitus. If a result does not seem consistent with the clinical findings, an assay for abnormal hemoglobins and hemoglobin variants should be performed.

The ADA recommends that the goal of therapy is a GHb <7% in patients with diabetes and that treatment be re-evaluated if values consistently are >8%.[22] These values apply only to DCCT-traceable GHb methods. The ADA does not currently recommend GHb testing for screening or for diagnosis of diabetes.

Diabetes mellitus may be suspected in the presence of glycosuria. Hypertriglyceridemia may provide indication of diabetes.

Footnotes

1. Singer DE, Coley CM, Samet JH, et al, "Tests of Glycemia in Diabetes Mellitus - Their Use in Establishing a Diagnosis and in Treatment," *Ann Intern Med*, 1989, 110(2):125-37.
2. Goldstein DE, Little RR, Lorenz RA, et al, "Tests of Glycemia in Diabetes," *Diabetes Care*, 1995, 18(6):896-906.
3. Krolewski AS, Laffel LMB, Krolewski M, et al, "Glycosylated Hemoglobin and the Risk of Microalbuminuria in Patients With Insulin-Dependent Diabetes Mellitus," *N Engl J Med*, 1995, 332(19):1251-5.
4. Painter PC, Cope JY, and Smith JL, "Reference Information for the Clinical Laboratory," *Tietz Textbook of Clinical Chemistry*, 3rd ed, Philadelphia, PA: WB Saunders Co, 1999, 1816.
5. Mayo Medical Laboratories, *2000 Test Catalogue*, Rochester, MN.
6. Halwachs-Baumann G and Katzensteiner S, "Comparative Evaluation of Three Assay Systems for Automated Determination of Hemoglobin A_{1c}," *Clin Chem*, 1997, 43(3):511-7.
7. Turpeinen U, Karjalainen U, and Stenman UH, "Three Assays for Glycohemoglobin Compared," *Clin Chem*, 1995, 41(2):191-5.
8. Weykamp CW, Penders TJ, Muskiet FA, et al, "Effect of Calibration on Dispersion of Glycohemoglobin Values Determined by 111 Laboratories Using 21 Methods," *Clin Chem*, 1994, 40(1):138-44.
9. Little RR, Wiedmeyer HM, England JD, et al, "Interlaboratory Standardization of Measurements of Glycohemoglobins," *Clin Chem*, 1992, 38(12):2472-8.
10. Bodor GS, Little RR, Garrett N, et al, "Standardization of Glycohemoglobin Determinations in the Clinical Laboratory: Three years of Experience," *Clin Chem*, 1992, 38(12):2414-8.
11. Gillery P, Labbé D, Dumont G, et al, "Glycohemoglobin Assays Evaluated in a Large-Scale Quality-Control Survey," *Clin Chem*, 1995, 41(11):1644-8.
12. Viberti G, "A Glycemic Threshold for Diabetic Complications?" *N Engl J Med*, 1995, 332(19):1293-4.
13. Gambino R, "Is It Time to Abandon the Oral Glucose Tolerance Test?" *Lab Rep*, 1995, 17(10):72.
14. Peters AL, Davidson MB, Schriger DL, et al, "A Clinical Approach for the Diagnosis of Diabetes Mellitus: An Analysis Using Glycosylated Hemoglobin Levels. Meta-analysis Research Group on the Diagnosis of Diabetes Using Glycated Hemoglobin Levels," *JAMA*, 1996, 276(15):1246-52.
15. Davidson MB, Schriger DL, Peters AL, et al, "Relationship Between Fasting Plasma Glucose and Glycosylated Hemoglobin," *JAMA*, 1999, 281(13):1203-10.
16. Vinicor F, "When Is Diabetes Diabetes?" *JAMA*, 1999, 281(13):1222-4.
17. Klein R, Klein BE, Moss SE, et al, "Glycosylated Hemoglobin Predicts the Incidence and Progression of Diabetic Retinopathy," *JAMA*, 1988, 260(19):2864-71.
18. Holt GS, Wofford JL, and Velez R, "Hemoglobinopathies Affect Hemoglobin A_{1c} Measurement," *Ann Intern Med*, 1991, 115(1):68-9.
19. Bergstrom RW, Kelley JR, and Ward WK, "Fetal Hemoglobin Alters Hemoglobin A_{1c} Measurements," *Ann Intern Med*, 1991, 115(8):656.
20. Tarim O, Kucukerdogan A, Gunay U, et al, "Effects of Iron Deficiency on Hemoglobin A_{1c} in Type 1 Diabetes Mellitus," *Pediatr Int*, 1999, 41(4):357-62.
21. Burton L, "Diagnosing and Monitoring Patients With Diabetes," *Lab Med*, 2000, 31(2):84-90.
22. American Diabetes Association, "Standards of Medical Care for Patients With Diabetes Mellitus," Position Statement, *Diabetes Care*, 2000, 23(Suppl 1):S32-S42.
23. American Diabetes Association, "Tests of Glycemia in Diabetes," Position Statement, *Diabetes Care*, 2000, 23(Suppl 1):S80-S82.
24. The DCCT Research Group, "Feasibility of Centralized Measurements of Glycated Hemoglobin in the Diabetes Control and Complications Trial: A Multicenter Study," *Clin Chem*, 1987, 33(12):2267-71.
25. The Diabetes Control and Complications Trial Research Group, "The Effect of Intensive Treatment of Diabetes on the Development and Progression of Long-Term Complications in Insulin-Dependent Diabetes Mellitus," *N Engl J Med*, 1993, 329(14):977-86.

References

Benjamin RJ and Sacks DB, "Glycated Protein Update: Implications of Recent Studies, Including the Diabetes Control and Complications Trial," *Clin Chem*, 1994, 40(5):683-7.

Bouma M, Dekker JH, de Sonnaville JJ, et al, "How Valid Is Fasting Plasma Glucose as a Parameter of Glycemic Control in Noninsulin Using Patients With Type 2 Diabetes?" *Diabetes Care*, 1999, 22(6):904-7.

Cox T, Hess PP, Thompson GD, et al, "Interference With Glycated Hemoglobin by Hemoglobin F May Be Greater Than Is Generally Assumed," *Am J Clin Pathol*, 1993, 99(2):137-41.

Goldstein DE, Little RR, Wiedmeyer HM, et al, "Is Glycohemoglobin Testing Useful in Diabetes Mellitus? Lessons From the Diabetes Control and Complications Trial," *Clin Chem*, 1994, 40(8):1637-40.

Hom F and Ettinger B, "Comparison of Serum Fructosamine vs Glycohemoglobin as Measures of Glycemic Control in a Large Diabetic Population," *Acta Diabetol Lat*, 1998, 35(1):48-51.

Kilpatrick ES, Rumley AG, Dominiczak MH, et al, "Glycated Haemoglobin Values: Problems in Assessing Blood Glucose Control in Diabetes Mellitus," *BMJ*, 1994, 309(6960):983-6.

Kullberg CE and Arnqvist HJ, "Elevated Long-Term Glycated Haemoglobin Precedes Proliferative Retinopathy and Nephropathy in Type 1 (Insulin-Dependent) Diabetic Patients," *Diabetologia*, 1993, 36(10):961-5.

McCance DR, Hanson RL, Charles M, et al, "Comparison of Tests for Glycated Haemoglobin and Fasting and Two Hour Plasma Glucose Concentrations as Diagnostics Method for Diabetes," *BMJ*, 1994, 308(6940):1323-8.

Nuttall FQ, "Comparison of Percent Total GHb With Percent Hb A_{1c} People With and Without Known Diabetes," *Diabetes Care*, 1998, 21(9):1475-8.

Palumbo PJ, "Diabetes Control and Complications Trial: The Continuing Challenge Ahead," *Mayo Clin Proc*, 1993, 68(11):1126-7 (editorial).

♦ **Glycated Proteins** *see* Fructosamine, Serum *on page 177*

♦ **Glycine** *see* Amino Acids, Urine *on page 101*

♦ **Glycine, Cerebrospinal Fluid** *see* Cerebrospinal Fluid Glycine *on page 142*

♦ **Glycohemoglobin** *see* Glycated Hemoglobin (Hemoglobin A_{1c}), Blood *on page 188*

♦ **Glycolic Acid, Urine** *see* Oxalate, Urine *on page 238*

♦ **Glyoxylic Acid, Urine** *see* Oxalate, Urine *on page 238*

♦ **GnRH** *see* Chorionic Gonadotropin, Human, Serum and Urine *on page 147*

♦ **Goiter** *see* Thyroxine, Serum *on page 286*

♦ **Gonadotropic Hormones** *see* Follicle Stimulating Hormone, Serum, Plasma, or Urine *on page 175*

♦ **Gonadotropic Hormones** *see* Luteinizing Hormone, Blood or Urine *on page 219*

♦ **Gonadotropin-Releasing Hormone** *see* Testosterone, Total and Free, Serum or Plasma *on page 280*

♦ **GOT** *see* Aspartate Aminotransferase, Serum *on page 112*

♦ **GPT** *see* Alanine Aminotransferase, Serum *on page 87*

Growth Hormone, Serum

Related Information

Insulin-Like Growth Factor-1 (IGF-1), Serum or Plasma *on page 200*
Insulin-Like Growth Factor Binding Protein 3, Serum *on page 201*
Insulin Tolerance Test *on page 202*
Placental Lactogen, Human, Serum *on page 254*
Prolactin, Serum *on page 262*

Synonyms GH; hGH; Somatotropin
(Continued)

Growth Hormone, Serum (Continued)

Applies to GHRH; GHRH Plus; GHRP-6; GHRP-6 Stimulation Test; Glucose Suppression Test; Insulin-Like Growth Factors; Somatomedin-C; Somatomedins; Somatostatin

Abstract Human growth hormone (GH) is a 191-amino acid polypeptide secreted by the anterior pituitary. GH is structurally similar to prolactin and human placental lactogen. The secretion of GH from the pituitary occurs in the form of multiple short spikes, often secondary to environmental stimuli. Maximum GH secretion occurs after the onset of deep (Stages III and IV) sleep; smaller spikes occur after exercise and after eating. Release of GH from the pituitary is influenced by three hypothalamic factors: GH releasing hormone (GHRH); GH-releasing peptide-6 (GHRP-6); and GH inhibitory hormone (GHIH), also known as somatostatin. Somatostatin is also found in the pancreatic islets and in the gut mucosa.

The half-life of GH in the blood is ~20 minutes. GH is, as suggested by its name, a potent stimulant of growth in children. In adults, GH causes multiple physiologic effects and influences lipolysis, protein synthesis, cardiac function, muscle mass, and red cell mass. GH causes its effects both directly and indirectly, via the action of insulin-like growth factors (IGF), formerly called somatomedins, but renamed because of striking chemical similarities to insulin.[1]

Excessive GH secretion, usually caused by a GH-secreting pituitary adenoma, most commonly produces the clinical syndrome of acromegaly in adults. When this occurs in childhood, the term pituitary gigantism is used. Growth hormone deficiency is one cause of short stature in childhood. GH deficiency in adulthood causes a metabolic disorder with an increase in body fat, decrease in muscle mass, reduced muscle strength, reduced bone density, abnormalities of lipoprotein and carbohydrate dynamics, and altered renal and cardiac function.[2]

Patient Preparation

Glucose suppression test (suspected GH excess). The patient fasts overnight and remains in bed for the test. A baseline blood specimen is obtained, after which the patient drinks a solution containing 100 g of glucose.[1]

Suspected GH deficiency. As specified in the following table (see Use).

GHRH plus GHRP-6 stimulation test. Following an overnight fast, an indwelling catheter is placed in a forearm vein and kept open with slow infusion of 150 mmol/L sodium chloride. GHRH 1 µg/kg body weight plus GHRP-6 1 µg/kg body weight is given as a bolus at time 0.

Specimen Serum

Container Red top tube

Sampling Time

Glucose suppression test: 0, 30, 60 minutes

GHRH plus GHRP-6 stimulation test. A baseline specimen is obtained at -30 min. Poststimulation blood samples are obtained at 30 and 60 minutes.

Other stimulation protocols. As specified in the following table (see Use).

Storage Instructions Label tube with time and date of collection and identifying data. Separate serum and freeze in plastic container. Stable 4 hours at 25°C and 1 year at -20°C.[3]

Reference Interval

Basal or random specimens:[4]
- cord: 8-41 ng/mL
- newborns: 5-53 ng/mL
- infants: 1-12 months: 2-10 ng/mL
- adults: male: 0-4 ng/mL; female: 0-18 ng/mL
- >60 years: male: 1-9 ng/mL; female: 1-16 ng/mL

Glucose suppression testing. The 60-minute or the 120-minute post-glucose specimen GH is <2 ng/mL.

Insulin tolerance test: A normal response is a poststimulation value of at least 10.0 ng/mL. (For complete protocol, see Insulin Tolerance Test *on page 202*.)

Other dynamic tests. A normal response is any poststimulation value of at least 20 ng/mL.

Use

Growth hormone excess. GH secretion is not uniform throughout the day, and the variations are so unpredictable that random serum GH values may be within the reference interval in patients with acromegaly or pituitary gigantism. The key to the diagnosis is to demonstrate that GH is not suppressed normally in response to a standard glucose load. Using the 100 g glucose suppression test (see above, Patient Preparation and Sampling Time) a normal person will have a serum GH <2 ng/mL.

Growth hormone deficiency. Basal and random specimens often fail to discriminate between normals and persons with GH deficiency. Therefore, dynamic testing is usually performed. The traditional gold standard dynamic test is the Insulin Tolerance Test *on page 202*. Since the ITT involves some risk for the patient and requires the presence of a physician, it is rarely used in practice. All the other tests are less sensitive than the ITT; therefore, many authorities recommend using two of the stimulation tests. The stimulation testing protocols which may be used follow.

Dynamic Tests for Growth Hormone Insufficiency

Stimulus	Protocol	Sampling Time
Exercise	Vigorous exercise for 20 minutes	20 minutes after starting to exercise
Sleep	Patient goes to sleep at usual time	1 hour after onset of deep sleep (Stage III or IV), documented by EEG
Arginine	Arginine hydrochloride, 0.5 g/kg body weight intravenously over 30 minutes	60-120 minutes
Glucagon	0.03 mg/kg body weight (not to exceed 1.0 mg), intramuscularly or subcutaneously	120-180 minutes
L-dopa	0.5 g/1.73 m² body surface area, orally with lunch	30-120 minutes
Clonidine	0.15 mg/m² body surface, orally	90 minutes
Diazepam	0.15 mg/kg body weight, orally	60 minutes
Pentagastrin	1.5 mg/kg body weight/hour for 75 minutes	75 minutes

Adapted from Demers L, "Pituitary Function," *Tietz Textbook of Clinical Chemistry*, 3rd ed, Philadelphia, PA: WB Saunders Co, 1999, 1470-95.

GHRH plus GHRP-6 Stimulation Test. A newly described, well documented testing protocol uses two agents, growth hormone releasing hormone (GHRH), 1 µg/kg body weight, plus growth hormone-releasing peptide-6 (GHRP-6), 1 microgram/kg body weight, both given intravenously at time 0. This combination constitutes the most potent stimulation of GH available. Patients with a poststimulation value >20 ng/mL are classified as normal. Patients with both poststimulation values <10 ng/mL are classified as GH-deficient. Values in between constitute an intentional gray zone, indicating the need for additional studies and the exercise of clinical judgment. This protocol was compared with the insulin tolerance test and found to produce higher and more clear cut GH peaks than the ITT.[2]

Limitations Patients with a GH deficiency because of hypothalamic disease may have a normal response to the GHRH plus GHRP-6 stimulation protocol. In patients with suspected hypothalamic disease, the ITT may be more useful than the GHRH plus GHRP-6 test.[5]

Methodology Immunoassays (multiple labels and formats)

Additional Information GH is a substance which can enhance athletic performance.[6] Some athletes surreptitiously inject themselves with recombinant human GH (rhGH) and believe that the recombinant material is chemically undetectable. Physician-investigators in Germany, however, have reported a dual immunoassay system with measurements of both total human GH and a 22 kilodalton isoform of human GH. Persons who inject rhGH have relatively more of the 22kD isoform, and thus the value of their ratio is higher than in persons who do not inject.[7]

Footnotes

1. Demers L, "Pituitary Function," *Tietz Textbook of Clinical Chemistry*, 3rd ed, Burtis CA and Ashwood ER, eds, Philadelphia, PA: WB Saunders Co, 1999, 1470-95.
2. Popovic V, Leal A, Micic D, et al, "GH-Releasing Hormone and GH-Releasing Peptide-6 for Diagnostic Testing in GH-Deficient Adults," *Lancet*, 2000, 356(9236):1137-42.
3. Kubasik NP, Ricotta M, Hunter T, et al, "Effect of Duration and Temperature of Storage on Serum Analyte Stability: Examination of 14 Radioimmunoassay Procedures," *Clin Chem*, 1982, 28(1):164-5.
4. Painter PC, Cope JY, and Smith JL, "Reference Information for the Clinical Laboratory," *Tietz Textbook of Clinical Chemistry*, 3rd ed, Burtis CA and Ashwood ER, eds, Philadelphia, PA: WB Saunders Co, 1999, 1816.
5. Ho KKY, "Diagnosis of Adult GH Deficiency," *Lancet*, 2000, 356(9236):1125-6.
6. Healy ML and Russel-Jones D, "Growth Hormone and Sport: Abuse, Potential Benefits and Difficulties in Detection," *Br J Sports Med*, 1997, 31(4):267-8.
7. Wu Z, Bidlingmaier M, Dall R, et al, "Detection of Doping With Human Growth Hormone," *Lancet*, 1999, 353(9156):895-6.

References
Hoffman DM, O'Sullivan AJ, Baxter RC, et al, "Diagnosis of Growth-Hormone Deficiency in Adults," *Lancet*, 1994, 343(8905):1064-8.

Laron Z, "Short Stature Due to Genetic Defects Affecting Growth Hormone Activity," *N Engl J Med*, 1996, 334(7):463-5.

Takahashi Y, Kaji H, Okimura Y, et al, "Brief Report: Short Stature Caused By a Mutant Growth Hormone," *N Engl J Med*, 1996, 334(7):432-6.

♦ **GT** *see* Gamma-Glutamyl Transferase, Serum *on page 179*

♦ **GTP** *see* Gamma-Glutamyl Transferase, Serum *on page 179*

♦ **GTT** *see* Glucose Tolerance Test, Plasma *on page 186*

♦ **Guanosine Triphosphate Cyclohydrolase 1 Deficiency** *see* Newborn Screen for Phenylketonuria *on page 229*

♦ **Guanosine Triphosphate Cyclohydrolase 1 Deficiency** *see* Phenylalanine, Blood *on page 248*

♦ **Guthrie Test** *see* Phenylalanine, Blood *on page 248*

♦ **Guthrie Test** *see* Phenylalanine, Urine *on page 249*

Haptoglobin, Serum

Related Information

Alpha₁-Acid Glycoprotein, Serum *on page 95*

Anemia Flowchart *on page 392*
C-Reactive Protein, Serum *on page 523*
Hemoglobin, Plasma *on page 446*
Myoglobin, Blood, Serum, or Plasma *on page 228*
Transfusion Reaction Work-up *on page 864*

Abstract Haptoglobin, a serum protein which irreversibly binds hemoglobin, is a tetramer of two alpha chains (with many polymorphisms) and two beta chains (fewer polymorphisms). There are three principal phenotypes, denoted Hp 1-1, Hp 2-2, and Hp 2-1. Haptoglobin is synthesized in the liver (and possibly other sites),[1] migrates electrophoretically in the alpha$_2$ position, and is an acute phase reactant. Some investigators suggest that the "role" of haptoglobin is to modulate the inflammatory reaction.[2]

Specimen Serum

Container Red top tube

Causes for Rejection Hemolysis from traumatic venipuncture

Reference Interval
- Neonates have very low values.
- Children and young adults: 22-164 mg/dL[2]
- Adults: 30-200 mg/dL; decreased values during pregnancy or when estrogen medication is taken[2]

Use

Hemolysis: Episodes of severe hemolysis are usually obvious from routine first- and second-line hematologic studies and, thus, do not require haptoglobin measurements. Haptoglobin is used to detect episodes of more subtle or mild hemolysis, in which situation haptoglobin levels are **decreased.** Haptoglobin is typically absent from serum when the red cell half-life, measured by radioactive chromium-51 labeled autologous red cells, is <17.5 days (normal range by this technique is a half-time of ~26 days).[2,3] It is useful to recall that ineffective erythropoiesis (megaloblastic anemias, hemoglobinopathies), as well as hematomas and soft tissue hemorrhage are conditions with a hemolytic component and are associated with a decrease in haptoglobin. Haptoglobin is decreased by a number of drugs which cause hemolytic anemia.[4] It may be decreased even with extravascular hemolysis.

Forensics and epidemiology: The existence of genetically-determined haptoglobin phenotypes, usually differentiated by electrophoresis, has been used in forensic applications (eg, parentage testing,[2] Patzelt et al 1998) and in epidemiologic studies of genetically influenced disease processes.

Limitations Haptoglobin is an acute phase reactant and the increase which occurs during episodes of **acute inflammation** may mask the decrease produced by concurrent hemolysis. The simultaneous measurement of another acute phase reactant (eg, C-reactive protein or alpha$_1$ acid glycoprotein) can help resolve this interpretive difficulty. **Corticosteroids, androgens,** and **protein-losing states** (eg, nephrotic syndrome, protein-losing enteropathies) produce a similar elevation in haptoglobin, and masking of hemolysis. **Liver disease** and **estrogen** medication produce decreased levels of haptoglobin which can be misinterpreted as evidence of hemolysis. **Rare examples** of genetic absence of haptoglobin and genetic hypohaptoglobinemia have been reported.[2]

Methodology Immunologic methods including radial immunodiffusion (RID), nephelometry, automated immunoprecipitation, hemoglobin binding capacity. In forensic (paternity exclusion) work, starch or acrylamide gel electrophoresis; one-dimensional isoelectric focusing/immunoblotting.[5] Differences in size of various haptoglobin phenotypes renders quantitation by RID inaccurate.

Additional Information Compensatory increases in haptoglobin generation do not take place with hemolysis.

Footnotes
1. Dobryszycka W, "Biological Functions of Haptoglobin - New Pieces to an Old Puzzle," *Euorp J Clin Chem & Clin Biochem*, 1997, 35(9):647-54.
2. Burtis CA and Ashwood ER, eds, *Tietz Textbook of Clinical Chemistry*, 3rd ed, Philadelphia, PA: WB Saunders Co, 1998, 24, 88, 90, 102, 137, 227, 322, 325, 337.
3. Kjeldsberg CR, ed, *Practical Diagnosis of Hematologic Disorders*, Chicago, IL: ASCP Press, 1995, 349-50.
4. Young DS, *Effects of Drugs on Clinical Laboratory Tests*, 5th ed, Volume 1, Listing by Test, Washington, DC: AACC Press, American Association for Clinical Chemistry, 2000, Section 3, 390-1.
5. Teige B, Olaisen B, Pedersen L, et al, "Forensic Aspects of Haptoglobin: Electrophoretic Patterns of Haptoglobin Allotype Products and an Evaluation of Typing Procedure," *Electrophoresis*, 1988, 9(8):384-92.

References
Patzelt D, Geserick G, and Schröder H, "The Genetic Haptoglobin Polymorphism: Relevance of Paternity Assessment," *Electrophoresis*, 1988, 9(8):393-7.

Heterophilic Antibodies

Related Information

Synonyms Human Antianimal Antibodies; Human Antimouse Antibodies

Abstract

Terminology: Heterophilic antibodies refers to circulating human antibodies with specificity for some particular animal protein, most often an animal immunoglobulin. Such antibodies exhibit a high degree of species and class specificity. **Heterophilic antibodies** must be distinguished from heterophil antibodies which have broad species reactivity and are useful in the diagnosis of infectious mononucleosis. (For diagnosis of infectious mononucleosis, see Infectious Mononucleosis Screening Test *on page 643*.) For clarity in communication, **human antianimal antibodies** (HAAA) may be a better term. Because mouse monoclonal antibodies are extensively used in diagnosis and treatment, the vast majority of HAAA are murine; as a result, the term **human antimouse antibodies** (HAMA) is used often in the medical literature.

Clinical issues: HAAA can result from medications (eg, antibody-targeted drugs, antithymocyte globulin), radionuclide imaging agents, blood transfusions, and vaccination. These antibodies can cross the placenta. HAAA can cause interference in any immunoassay. Interferences have been reported in assays for all the analytes listed above (see Related Information). Depending on the assay format, the interference can result in a false increase or decrease in the results. Moreover, such interferences are largely unpredictable. The FDA now recommends that a warning be included in package inserts if a diagnostic test kit employs mouse monoclonal antibodies.[1]

Interference from HAAA is unpredictable, varies among different assays, and usually is identified when a clinician reports that a result appears inexplicably discordant with the clinical situation. The most dramatic of the HAAA errors reported have been in assays for serum human chorionic gonadotropin (hCG). In this situation, HAAA circulating in the patient react with mouse monoclonal IgG used as the capture antibody in the hCG assay. Such patients have had falsely elevated serum hCG results, typically 20-500 IU/L, which have led to erroneous diagnoses of malignant trophoblastic disease, followed by chemotherapy.[2]

Specimen The ideal specimen is the specimen which produced the result that is being questioned. Alternatively, a new specimen can be used; ordinarily it should be collected in the same way as was the original.

Critical Values Whenever an erroneous result due to HAAA is suspected, the clinician(s) should be notified promptly. Often, of course, the clinician will be the source of the information that a result is suspect.

Use

General guidelines: When a clinician reports that an immunoassay result is inconsistent with the clinical situation, or with another assay result, HAAA interference should be suspected. Appropriate preliminary evaluation might include: a) assaying multiple dilutions of the suspected sample; b) assaying for other molecular species that usually accompany the analyte of interest; or c) assaying the analyte of interest by another method, as different assays show highly variable interference effects.[3] Assays for human antimouse antibodies (HAMA), the most common subset of HAAA, can be performed using any one of six commercially available kits, most of which are ELISA formats.[1] These kits will not, however, detect all of the possible HAAA interferents. At the present time, however, most laboratorians will (Continued)

Heterophilic Antibodies (Continued)

submit the specimen in question to the reagent manufacturer for definitive evaluation. Some reference laboratories offer assays for HAAA.

hCG assays: Rotmensch and Cole have recommended that protocols for the diagnosis and treatment of gestational trophoblastic disease include a test for hCG in the urine.[2] Such a requirement would have avoided the problems caused by HAAA cited in their report. In addition, hCG specimens may be referred to the HCG Reference Service, Department of Obstetrics and Gynecology, University of New Mexico, Albuquerque, NM 87131, USA (505-272-6137)[4] Additional information about this reference service is available at the following website: www.hcglab.com.

TSH assays: Patients with heterophil antibodies may have normal thyroid status, but have TSH reported as raised. They may then incorrectly be given thyroxine.[5]

Limitations Undoubtedly, there are erroneous results due to HAAA which will never be detected, a situation which will continue unless and until it becomes feasible to test all patients for HAAA.

Methodology Enzyme-linked immunosorbent assay (ELISA), radioimmuno-assay (RIA)

Footnotes

1. Kricka L, "Human Antianimal Antibody Interferences in Immunological Assays," *Clin Chem*, 1999, 45(7):942-56.
2. Rotmensch S and Cole LA, "False Diagnosis and Needless Therapy of Presumed Malignant Disease in Women With False-Positive Human Chorionic Gonadotropin Concentrations," *Lancet*, 2000, 355(9205):712-5.
3. Kazmierczak SC, Catrou PG, and Briley KP, "Transient Nature of Interference Effects From Heterophil Antibodies: Examples of Interference With Cardiac Marker Measurements," *Clin Chem Lab Med*, 2000, 38(1):33-9.
4. Cole L, personal communication, May 2000.
5. Dayan CM, "Interpretation of Thyroid Function Tests," *Lancet*, 2001, 357:619-24.

References

Bagshawe KD, "Limitations of Tests for Human Chorionic Gonadotropin," *Lancet*, 2000, 355(9205):671.

Internet Web Sites

www.hcglab.com

♦ **Hexosaminidase** *see* Beta-Hexosaminidase, Serum, White Blood Cells *on page 114*

♦ **β-Hexosaminidase, Serum** *see* Beta-Hexosaminidase, Serum, White Blood Cells *on page 114*

♦ **hGH** *see* Growth Hormone, Serum *on page 189*

♦ **5-HIAA, Quantitative, Urine** *see* 5-Hydroxyindoleacetic Acid, Quantitative, Urine *on page 197*

♦ **High Density Lipoprotein Cholesterol (HDLC)** *see* Lipids, Overview *on page 213*

High Density Lipoprotein Cholesterol, Serum

Related Information

Apolipoprotein A-I, Serum *on page 109*
Cholesterol, Total, Serum or Plasma *on page 146*
Lipid Panel, Serum *on page 212*
Lipids, Overview *on page 213*
Lipoprotein (a), Serum *on page 215*
Low Density Lipoprotein Cholesterol *on page 218*
Triglycerides, Serum or Plasma *on page 288*

Synonyms Alpha$_1$ Lipoprotein Cholesterol; HDL; HDLC; HDL Cholesterol

Applies to Apolipoprotein A-I; Cholesterol Ester Transfer Protein; Cholesterol:HDLC Ratio; Cholesterol, Total

Abstract High density lipoprotein cholesterol (HDLC) is a class of heterogeneous particles occurring in serum. These particles contain both lipid and protein in varying ratios, resulting in different densities and sizes. The other clinically relevant lipoproteins are low density (LDL), very low density lipoprotein (VLDL), and chylomicrons. Intermediate density lipoprotein (IDL) and lipoprotein (a) (Lp(a)) are also known. HDLC includes cholesterol esters and free cholesterol, triglycerides, phospholipids, and A, C, and E apolipoproteins. Two subclasses of HDL predominate: HDL$_2$ and smaller, denser HDL$_3$. HDL may function in reverse transport of cholesterol to the liver from peripheral tissues. An independent, strong, inverse relationship of HDL cholesterol and coronary arterial disease (CAD) has been essentially confirmed in the industrial world.[1] Approximately 20% of total serum cholesterol is HDLC.

Patient Preparation Patient ideally should be on a stable diet for 3 weeks and should fast for 9-10 hours prior to collection of specimen. Recent fat intake influences HDL. See Preparation in listing Cholesterol, Total, Serum or Plasma *on page 146*. HDLC is usually done as part of lipid profile.

Specimen Serum

Container Red top tube

Storage Instructions Analysis promptly after sampling is best. The specimen can be refrigerated up to several days at 4°C or frozen for several weeks. For long-term storage use -70°C.[2]

Causes for Rejection Specimen collected in citrate or heparin anticoagulants

Reference Interval See Lipids, Overview *on page 213*, and table.

Population Distributions for High Density Lipoprotein Cholesterol (mg/dL)

Age (y)	Percentile						
	5	10	25	50	75	90	95
Male							
5-9	38	43	49	55	64	70	75
10-14	37	40	46	55	61	71	74
15-19	30	34	39	46	52	59	63
20-24	30	32	38	45	51	57	63
25-29	31	32	37	44	50	58	63
30-34	28	32	38	45	52	59	63
35-39	29	31	36	43	49	58	62
40-44	27	31	36	43	51	60	67
45-49	30	33	38	45	52	60	64
50-54	28	31	36	44	51	58	63
55-59	28	31	38	46	55	64	71
60-64	30	34	41	49	61	69	74
65-69	30	33	39	49	52	74	75
≥70	31	33	40	48	56	70	75
Female							
5-9	36	38	48	52	60	67	73
10-14	37	40	45	52	58	64	70
15-19	35	38	43	51	61	68	74
20-24	33	37	44	51	62	72	79
25-29	37	39	47	55	63	74	83
30-34	36	40	46	55	64	73	77
35-39	34	38	44	53	64	75	82
40-44	34	39	48	56	65	79	88
45-49	34	41	47	58	68	82	87
50-54	37	41	50	62	71	84	92
55-59	37	41	50	60	73	85	91
60-64	38	44	51	61	75	87	92
65-69	35	38	49	62	73	85	96
≥70	33	38	45	60	71	82	92

To convert to mmol/L, multiply by 0.0259.

Adapted from Lipid Research Clinical Program Epidemiology Committee, "Plasma Lipid Distributions in Selected North American Population: The Lipid Research Clinics Program Prevalence Study," *Circulation*, 1979, 60:427-39.

Use Low HDLC is an important predictor of coronary atherosclerosis and coronary heart disease. HDL may act as a protective scavenger molecule (reverse cholesterol transport). The liver is the major site of cholesterol **excretion**. When a slightly increased cholesterol is due to high HDL, therapy is not indicated.[3]

Limitations About 50% of patients treated with etretinate have decreases.[4]

A relationship between variation of the cholesterol ester transfer protein gene locus and progression of coronary arterial atherosclerosis is independent of HDLC.[5]

Methodology The CDC reference method[6] uses ultracentrifugation to isolate HDL and LDL from chylomicrons and VLDL. The LDL in the isolate is selectively precipitated with heparin/MnCl$_2$, and the resulting HDL-containing supernatant is analyzed for cholesterol by a modified Abell-Kendall procedure.[7] This is the method against which modern routine methods ultimately are standardized; however for practical reasons, the Cholesterol Reference Method Laboratory Network has validated and adopted recently a designated comparison method to assist manufacturers in calibrating their products.[8]

Routine methods include first- and second-generation, heterogeneous assays that employ selective precipitation of LDL and VLDL, followed by cholesterol analysis of the HDL-containing supernatant by enzymatic methods. Precipitating agents include heparin/MnCl$_2$, heparin/CaCl$_2$, dextran sulfate/MgCl$_2$, sodium phosphotungstate/MgCl$_2$, and polyethylene glycol. More recently, third-generation, homogeneous (direct) assays have become available that are entirely automated, rapid, and reproducible. These methods employ reagents that sequester LDL and VLDL in stable, soluble complexes, leaving only nonsequestered HDL available for enzymatic cholesterol analysis.[9,10,11,12]

Additional Information Total cholesterol and triglycerides are required as well for determination of lipid risk factors for coronary artery disease. HDLC is especially apt to be low in male subjects who are obese and sedentary, in those who smoke cigarettes, and in those who have diabetes mellitus. Uremia is also associated with lower HDLC. Exercise, appropriate diet, and moderate ethanol intake increase HDLC.

Those **at least risk** for development of CAD have low TC, low triglycerides, and high HDLC. Even in men with moderately low cholesterol, HDLC is protective against CAD.[13] Women have higher serum HDLC than men. This may be explained by hormonal factors.[14]

Thiazides and nonselective beta-adrenergic blocking agents may decrease HDLC.[3]

Apolipoprotein A-I is the major protein of HDL. Apolipoprotein A-I determination may eventually be shown to be superior to HDLC in prediction of coronary disease risk.[1,15] Increased apoprotein A-I is associated with a diminished risk of atherogenesis. It is measured by RIA[16] and by nephelometry.

Factors contributing to decreased HDLC include:
- genetic factors: primary hypoalphalipoproteinemia[17]
- cigarette smoking[18]
- obesity[18]
- hypertriglyceridemia[18]
- lack of exercise[19]
- steroids - androgens, progestogens, anabolic
- thiazides
- beta-adrenergic blockers
- probucol
- neomycin

Many other substances may affect coronary artery disease risk, often by mechanisms not involving serum HDL cholesterol concentrations directly. Such substances include phytosterols, tocotrienols, arginine, and antioxidant vitamins.[20] See Lipids, Overview on page 213.

The rare entity, **Tangier disease**, is characterized by very low HDL, total cholesterol, and low density lipoprotein cholesterol. Cholesterol esters accumulate in tissues. Severe coronary arterial sclerosis with extremely low HDL (1.4 mg/dL) was reported in a subject with Tangier disease.[21]

New information suggests that very active middle-aged men and women have higher plasma lipoprotein concentrations of HDL cholesterol and often moderately low levels of LDL cholesterol.[19] Evidence suggests that fat loss by dieting alone or by exercising alone results in similar elevations of HDL cholesterol.[22]

Chylomicron remnants have been linked to CAD progression. This linkage is not explained by any relationship to the high density lipoprotein system and may indicate a direct atherogenic effect of chylomicron remnants themselves.[23] There is evidence, however, of beneficial effects of aggressive lipoprotein management.[24,25]

The **cholesterol to HDLC ratio** has predictive value. An increase of one unit of this ratio bears association with increased risk of 53% following adjustment for nonlipid risk factors.[26] The best predictor of CAD risk in males younger than 50 years of age was total cholesterol:HDL cholesterol ratio ≥5 in a 1998 paper.[27]

The inverse relationship between moderate alcohol intake and risk of acute infarct of myocardium is thought to be mediated through HDL_2 and HDL_3.[28]

An association is perceived between low HDLC levels and propensity for restenosis following percutaneous transluminal coronary angioplasty.[29]

See Apolipoprotein A-I, Serum on page 109.

Footnotes
1. Gordon DJ and Rifkind BM, "High Density Lipoprotein - The Clinical Implications of Recent Studies," N Engl J Med, 1989, 321(19):1311-6.
2. Nanjee MN and Miller NE, "Evaluation of Long-Term Frozen Storage of Plasma for Measurement of High-Density Lipoprotein and Its Subfractions by Precipitation," Clin Chem, 1990, 36(5):783-8.
3. Betteridge DJ, "High Density Lipoprotein and Coronary Heart Disease," BMJ, 1989, 298(6679):974-5.
4. Young DS, "Effects of Drugs on Clinical Laboratory Tests," 5th ed, Volume 1: Listing by Test, Washington DC: AACC Press, American Association of Clinical Chemistry, 2000, Section 3, 436.
5. Kuivenhoven JA, Jukema JW, Zwinderman AH, et al, "The Role of a Common Variant of the Cholesteryl Ester Transfer Protein Gene in the Progression of Coronary Atherosclerosis," N Engl J Med, 1998, 338(2):86-93.
6. Hainline A, Karon J, and Lippel K, eds, "Manual of Laboratory Operations," Lipid Research Clinics Program, Lipid and Lipoprotein Analysis, 2nd ed, Bethesda, MD: U.S. Department of Health and Human Services, 1982.
7. Abell LL, Levy BB, Brodie BB, et al, "Simplified Methods for the Estimation of Total Cholesterol in Serum and Demonstration of Its Specificity," J Biol Chem, 1951, 195:357-66.
8. Kimberly MM, Leary ET, Cole TD, et al, "Selection, Validation, Standardization, and Performance of a Designated Comparison Method for HDL-Cholesterol for Use in the Cholesterol Reference Method Laboratory Network," Clin Chem, 1999, 45(10):1803-12.
9. Wiebe DA and Warnick GR, "Measurement of High-Density Lipoprotein Cholesterol," Handbook of Lipoprotein Testing, Rifai N, Warnick GR, and Dominiczak MH, eds, Washington, DC: AACC Press, American Association of Clinical Chemistry, 1997, 127-44.
10. Hubbard RS, Hirany SV, Dedvaraj S, et al, "Evaluation of a Rapid Homogeneous Method for Direct Measurement of High-Density Lipoprotein Cholesterol," Am J Clin Pathol, 1998, 110(4):495-502.
11. Halloran P, Roetering H, Pisani T, et al, "Reference Standardization and Analytical Performance of a Liquid Homogeneous High-Density Lipoprotein Cholesterol Method Compared With Chemical Precipitation Method," Arch Pathol Lab Med, 1999, 123(4):317-26.
12. Hoang MP, Hirany SV, Parupia J, et al, "Comparison of 2 Homogeneous High-Density Lipoprotein Cholesterol Assays," Arch Pathol Lab Med, 1998, 122(11):1005-9.
13. Kitamura A, Iso H, Naito Y, et al, "High-Density Lipoprotein Cholesterol and Premature Coronary Heart Disease in Urban Japanese Men," Circulation, 1994, 89(6):2533-9.
14. Kesteloot H and Sasaki S, "On the Relationship Between Nutrition, Sex Hormones and High-Density Lipoproteins in Women," Acta Cardiol, 1993, 48(4):355-63.

15. Miller NE, "Associations of High Density Lipoprotein Subclasses and Apolipoproteins With Ischemic Heart Disease and Coronary Atherosclerosis," Am Heart J, 1987, 113(2 Pt 2):589-97.
16. Maciejko JJ, Holmes DR, Kottke BA, et al, "Apolipoprotein A-1 as a Marker of Angiographically Assessed Coronary Artery Disease," N Engl J Med, 1983, 309:385-9.
17. Grundy SM, Goodman DS, Rifkind BM, et al, "The Place of HDL in Cholesterol Management: A Perspective From the National Cholesterol Education Program," Arch Intern Med, 1989, 149(3):505-10.
18. Frohlich JJ and Pritchard PH, "The Clinical Significance of Serum High Density Lipoproteins," Clin Biochem, 1989, 22(6):417-23.
19. Knight S and Bermingham M, "Regular Nonvigorous Physical Activity and Cholesterol Levels in the Elderly," Gerontology, 1999, 45(4):213-9.
20. Fraser GE, "Diet and Coronary Heart Disease: Beyond Dietary Fats and Low Density Lipoprotein Cholesterol," Am J Clin Nutr, 1994, 59(5 Suppl):1117S-23S.
21. Mautner SL, Sanchez JA, Rader DJ, et al, "The Heart in Tangier Disease. Severe Coronary Atherosclerosis With Near Absence of High-Density Lipoprotein Cholesterol," Am J Clin Pathol, 1992, 98(2):191-8.
22. Wood PD, "Physical Activity, Diet, and Health: Independent and Interactive Effects," Med Sci Sports Exerc, 1994, 26(7):838-43.
23. Hamsten A, "Lipids as a Coronary Risk Factor: Analysis of Hyperlipidaemias," Postgrad Med J, 1993, 69(Suppl 1):S8-11.
24. Superko HR and Krauss RM, "Coronary Artery Disease Regression. Convincing Evidence for the Benefit of Aggressive Lipoprotein Management," Circulation, 1994, 90(2):1056-69.
25. Harper CR and Jacobson TA, "New Perspectives on the Management of Low Levels of High Density Lipoprotein Cholesterol," Arch Intern Med, 1999, 159(10):1049-57.
26. Hostetter AL, "Screening for Dyslipidemia. Practice Parameter," Am J Clin Pathol, 1995, 103(4):380-5.
27. Cubero GI, Reguero JR, Batalla A, et al, "Plasma Lipids, HDL and Apolipoproteins, and Coronary Heart Disease in Men Less Than 50 Years Old," Acta Cardiol, 1998, 53:269-73.
28. Gaziano JM, Buring JE, Breslow JL, et al, "Moderate Alcohol Intake, Increased Levels of High-Density Lipoprotein and its Subfractions, and Decreased Risk of Myocardial Infarction," N Engl J Med, 1993, 329(25):1829-34.
29. Roth A, Eshchar Y, Keren G, et al, "Serum Lipids and Restenosis After Successful Percutaneous Transluminal Coronary Angioplasty. Ichilov Magnesium Study Group," Am J Cardiol, 1994, 73(16):1154-8.

References
Arranz-Pena ML, Tasende-Mata J, and Martin-Gil FJ, "Comparison of Two Homogeneous Assays With a Precipitation Method and an Ultracentrifugation Method for the Measurement of HDL-Cholesterol," Clin Chem, 1998, 44(12):2499-505.

Asayama K, Miyao A, and Kato K, "High-Density Lipoprotein (HDL), HDL2, and HDL3 Cholesterol Concentrations Determined in Serum of Newborns, Infants, Children, Adolescents, and Adults by Use of a Micromethod for Combined Precipitation Ultracentrifugation," Clin Chem, 1990, 36(1):129-31.

Brunner D, Weisbort J, Meshulam N, et al, "Relation of Serum Total Cholesterol and High Density Lipoprotein Cholesterol Percentage to the Incidence of Definite Coronary Events: Twenty Year Follow-up of the Donolo-Tel Aviv Prospective Coronary Artery Disease Study," Am J Cardiol, 1987, 59(15):1271-6.

Burtis CA and Ashwood ER, eds, Tietz Textbook of Clinical Chemistry, 3rd ed, Philadelphia, PA: WB Saunders Co, 1999, 828, 1818.

Gordon DJ, Probstfield JL, Garrison RJ, et al, "High-Density Lipoprotein Cholesterol and Cardiovascular Disease: Four Prospective American Studies," Circulation, 1989, 79(1):8-15.

Kannel WB, "Low High Density Lipoprotein Cholesterol and What to Do About It," Am J Cardiol, 1992, 70(7):810-4.

Pocock SJ, Shaper AG, and Phillips AN, "Concentrations of High Density Lipoprotein Cholesterol, Triglycerides, and Total Cholesterol in Ischaemic Heart Disease," Br Med J (Clin Res Ed), 1989, 298(6679):998-1002.

Rifai N, Bachorik PS, and Albers JS, "Lipids, Lipoproteins and Apolipoproteins," Tietz Textbook of Clinical Chemistry, 3rd ed, Burtis CA and Ashwood ER, eds, Philadelphia, PA: WB Saunders Co, 1999, 809-61.

Rifkind BM, "High-Density Lipoprotein Cholesterol and Coronary Artery Disease: Survey of the Evidence," Am J Cardiol, 1990, 66(6):3A-6A.

Rigotti A and Krieger M, "Getting a Handle on 'Good' Cholesterol With the High-Density Lipoprotein Receptors," N Engl J Med, 1999, 341(2):2011-13.

Rosenson RS, "Low Levels of High Density Lipoprotein Cholesterol (Hypoalphalipoproteinemia). An Approach to Management," Arch Intern Med, 1993, 153(13):1528-38.

Schectmen G and Sasse E, "Variability of Lipid Measurements: Relevance for the Clinician," Clin Chem, 1993, 39(7):1495-503.

Weitzman JB and Vladutiu AO, "Very High Values of Serum High Density Lipoprotein Cholesterol," Arch Pathol Lab Med, 1992, 116(8):831-6.

♦ **Hill Plots** see P_{50}, Blood on page 241

♦ **Histalog™ Stimulation Test** replaced by Gastric Analysis on page 180

♦ **hK3** see Prostate Specific Antigen, Serum on page 263

♦ **HLA-A3** see Ferritin, Serum on page 173

♦ **HMG-CoA Reductase Inhibitor** see Mevalonic Acid, Urine or Amniotic Fluid on page 225

♦ **Hoesch Test** see Porphobilinogen, Qualitative, Urine on page 255

♦ **Homocyst(e)ine** see Amino Acids, Urine on page 101

Homocyst(e)ine, Plasma

Related Information
Anemia Flowchart on page 392
(Continued)

Homocyst(e)ine, Plasma (Continued)

Cholesterol, Total, Serum or Plasma *on page 146*
Cobalamin, Serum *on page 150*
Factor V Leiden *on page 339*
Folic Acid, RBC *on page 435*
Folic Acid, Serum *on page 435*
Hypercoagulation Panel *on page 345*
Intrinsic Factor Blocking Antibody *on page 537*
Lipids, Overview *on page 213*
Methionine Loading Test *on page 224*
Methylmalonic Acid, Serum, Plasma, Urine, or Amniotic Fluid *on page 224*
Schilling Test *on page 483*
Vitamin B_{12} Unsaturated Binding Capacity *on page 495*

Abstract Homocyst(e)ine circulates in plasma in several different forms: 80% to 90% is bound to protein; 5% to 10% is in the oxidized form, homocyst(e)ine; 5% to 10% is combined with cysteine-forming mixed disulfides; and <2% is free.[1,2] Most clinical assays measure the sum of all these entities, and some authors refer to this measurement as **total homocysteine**, although that term is technically incorrect. In this book we follow the practice[3] of using the intentionally ambiguous term homocyst(e)ine (abbreviated Hcy) to refer to the clinical measurement.

Homocyst(e)ine is formed in the metabolism of dietary methionine, an essential amino acid. Once formed, Hcy may undergo **remethylation** to form methionine (a process requiring vitamin B_{12}, folic acid, and riboflavin); **transulfuration** resulting in the synthesis of cysteine and glutathione (a process requiring vitamin B_6 and riboflavin); and **oxidation** to form homocystine and mixed disulfides.[4]

Specimen Fasting plasma is preferred because Hcy increases after the ingestion of protein. Immediate centrifugation mitigates the increase in plasma Hcy due to migration from blood cells. The optimal anticoagulation procedure employs potassium EDTA and requires that the specimen be placed on ice and centrifuged immediately, after which the plasma is immediately frozen. The plasma can then be kept for at least 3 months.[5] Anticoagulation with citrate[6] or heparin/sodium fluoride[7] is also acceptable, and investigation continues into other anticoagulation procedures.[8,9] Unfortunately, there is evidence that different anticoagulants are associated with slightly different reference ranges;[5] therefore, caution is warranted in the selection of an anticoagulant other than EDTA. Serum has also been used (but see Limitations).[1]

Causes for Rejection Plasma not separated from cells within 1 hour

Reference Interval Current information allows only tentative recommendations. Values in adult men are ~25% higher than in premenopausal women. Based on 182 carefully studied individuals, with total plasma Hcy assayed by an isotope dilution method,[10] age- and gender-specific reference ranges have been proposed as follows:

• 0-30 years: 4.6-8.1 μmol/L
• 30-59 years: male: 6.3-11.2 μmol/L; female: 4.5-7.9 μmol/L
• older than 59 years: 5.8-11.9 μmol/L

Based on results from 1437 adult white males, with total plasma Hcy assayed by HPLC methodology,[11] a reference range of 4.9-11.7 μmol/L has been suggested. The point for emphasis is that the medical significance of these ranges remains undefined.

Similar to the situation with cholesterol measurements, the population-based 95th percentile range, approximately 5-15 μmol/L for plasma Hcy,[1] has little relevance to the desirable, or optimal target. Unlike the situation with cholesterol measurements, there has been no large prospective study from which to derive desirable target values. There are also problems resulting from interlaboratory and intermethod precision and bias (see Limitations).

Use Raised blood Hcy is a strong, independent, dose-related risk factor for coronary, aortic, carotid, and peripheral vascular **atherosclerosis**.[12,13,14,15,16] Most of the data on this association were obtained from studies of white subjects. However, a large, cross-sectional study shows that raised Hcy is also a risk factor for myocardial infarction in black and Hispanic subjects.[17] The mechanism(s) linking Hcy and atherosclerosis remains unidentified. One study suggests that copper-dependent interactions may be important.[18]

Raised blood Hcy is a **thrombophilic state** associated with arterial thrombosis and venous thromboembolic disease[19] (although one investigator has challenged this concept and suggests that raised Hcy, in the context of thrombosis, is simply epiphenomenon reflecting ischemic tissue damage and repair).[20]

Raised blood Hcy is a marker for four **dietary vitamin deficiency states** (B_6, B_{12}, folic acid, and riboflavin).[21,22,23] It is used with methylmalonic acid in the investigation of vitamin B_{12} (cobalamin) deficiency states (see Methylmalonic Acid, Serum, Plasma, Urine, or Amniotic Fluid *on page 224*). Elevation of Hcy may be one of the earliest manifestations of vitamin B_{12} deficiency, preceding anemia and macrocytosis. Persons with raised blood Hcy due to a nutritional vitamin deficiency (folic acid, B_6, or B_{12}) will have a normalization of the Hcy when adequate vitamins are supplied.

In pregnancy, raised blood Hcy, reflecting maternal folate deficiency, is associated with an increased incidence of **neural-tube defects**.[24]

Raised blood Hcy is typically present in certain **inborn errors of cobalamin**[12] and **folate metabolism;**[25] it is also found in **homocystinuria**, a rare autosomal recessive metabolic defect resulting from a defect in one of the enzymes involved in homocyst(e)ine metabolism.[26]

Long-term monitoring: Since many persons with raised Hcy will be placed on long-term interventions to reduce their Hcy levels, the long-term, within-person variability is a crucial issue. In one study of healthy volunteers, the biological CV for **fasting** Hcy was 7%, and the critical between-measurement difference (at a 90% probability) was 32% over 4 weeks.[27] In this study, a high reliability coefficient (R=0.94) showed that Hcy concentrations in an individual are relatively constant for at least 1 month. Another study of healthy volunteers found a similar within-person CV of 8.1% over a 5-week period. This variability was, however, significantly increased when blood was collected from subjects in a supine position.[28] However, much greater variability is likely to be encountered when serial measurements are made in different laboratories or by different methods (see Limitations).

Limitations Plasma Hcy is increased when the separation of cells from plasma (or serum) is delayed. Plasma Hcy increases ~10% in 1 hour at room temperature. This process is slowed by placing the specimen on ice.[1]

Clinical interpretation of Hcy values is complicated by inter- and intramethod and inter- and intralaboratory imprecision and bias. The current status is delineated in a recent study of fourteen research level laboratories.[29] Significant intermethod variability has also been shown by a study of three commercially available methods, and one in-house method, at two university laboratories.[30]

At present there is no true **reference method** for Hcy (although GC/MS is often assumed to be a gold standard), and no standard reference material is available. Intermethod and interlaboratory variability is therefore not unexpected. A proficiency testing program for Hcy is available from the College of American Pathologists.[31] The 1998 results from a Scandinavian proficiency testing program are available.[32]

Elevation of Hcy is regularly present in renal insufficiency and hypothyroidism. Certain drugs are associated with marked elevations of Hcy, including corticosteroids, cyclosporine, phenytoin, methotrexate,[33] and trimethoprim.[34] A subset of 52 patients with peripheral arterial disease (ADMIT Trial) who were given niacin (steady state dose 1000 mg daily) to lower their plasma lipids, experienced marked increases in their plasma Hcy values, averaging 55% at 18 weeks.[35]

Methodology Enzyme immunoassay (EIA), fluorescence polarization immunoassay (FPIA), high performance liquid chromatography (HPLC), gas chromatography/mass spectrometry (GC/MS), ion-exchange chromatography, liquid chromatography electrospray tandem mass spectrometry

Additional Information Approximately 5% to 15% of the general population is homozygous for a thermolabile variant of the enzyme 5,10-methylenetetrahydrofolate reductase (MTHFR). These individuals often have raised blood Hcy. Most importantly, they require folic acid intakes that exceed those recommended for the general population.[36]

Individuals with hereditary homocystinuria should probably be tested for factor V Leiden because of the greatly increased risk of thrombosis.[37]

Indian Asians have a 40% higher coronary heart disease mortality than do most European populations, and this increase is not accounted for by cigarette use, hypertension, or raised cholesterol.[38] Of interest in this regard is the recent finding that Indian Asian men residing in the UK have fasting blood Hcy values that are ~6% higher than the values in native Europeans.[39]

In healthy postmenopausal women, estradiol reduces Hcy levels by ~5%, and combined estradiol-progestogen replacement reduces Hcy by an average of 9%, in comparison with a placebo; the largest decreases are experienced by women with the highest baseline Hcy values.[40]

Footnotes

1. Ueland PM, Refsum H, Stabler SP, et al, "Total Homocysteine in Plasma or Serum: Methods and Clinical Applications," *Clin Chem*, 1993, 39(9):1764-79.
2. Jacobsen DW, "Determinants of Hyperhomocysteinemia: A Matter of Nature and Nurture," *Am J Clin Nutr*, 1996, 64(4):641-2.
3. Mudd SH and Levy HL, "Plasma Homocyst(e)ine or Homocysteine?" *N Engl J Med*, 1995, 333(5):325 (letter).
4. Hankey GJ and Eikelboom JW, "Homocysteine and Vascular Disease," *Lancet*, 1999, 354(9176):407-13.
5. Salazar JF, Herbeth B, Siest G, et al, "Stability of Blood Homocysteine and Other Thiols: EDTA or Acidic Citrate?" *Clin Chem*, 1999, 45(11):2016-9.
6. Willems HP, Bos GM, Gerrits WB, et al, "Acidic Citrate Stabilizes Blood Samples for Assay of Total Homocysteine," *Clin Chem*, 1999, 44(2):342-5.
7. Moller J and Rasmussen K, "Homocysteine in Plasma: Stabilization of Blood Samples With Fluoride," *Clin Chem* 1995, 41(5):758-9.
8. Probst R, Brandl R, Blumke M, et al, "Stabilization of Homocysteine in Whole Blood," *Clin Chem*, 1998, 44(7):1567-9.
9. al-Kyhafaji F, Bowron A, Day AP, et al, "Stabilization of Blood Homocysteine by 3-Deazaadenosine," *Ann Clin Biochem*, 1998, 35:780-2.
10. Rasmussen K, Moller J, Lyngbak M, et al, "Age- and Gender-Specific Reference Intervals for Total Homocysteine and Methylmalonic Acid in Plasma Before and After Vitamin Supplementation," *Clin Chem* 1996, 42(2):630-6.
11. Ubbink JB, Becker PJ, Vermaak WJ, et al, "Results of B-Vitamin Supplementation Study Used in a Prediction Model to Define a Reference Range for Plasma Homocysteine," *Clin Chem*, 1995, 41(7):1033-7.

12. Boushey CJ, Beresford SA, Omenn GS, et al, "A Quantitative Assessment of Plasma Homocysteine as a Risk Factor for Vascular Disease: Probable Benefits of Increasing Folic Acid Intakes," *JAMA*, 1995, 274(13):1049-57.

13. Stampfer MJ, Malinow MR, Willett WC, et al, "A Prospective Study of Plasma Homocyst(e)ine and Risk of Myocardial Infarction in U.S. Physicians," *JAMA*, 1992, 268:877-81.

14. Nygard O, Nordrehaug JE, Refsum H, et al, "Plasma Homocysteine Levels and Mortality in Patients With Coronary Artery Disease," *N Engl J Med*, 1997, 337(4):230-6.

15. Whincup PH, Refsum H, Perry IJ, et al, "Serum Total Homocysteine and Coronary Heart Disease: Prospective Study in Middle Aged Men," *Heart*, 1999, 82(4):448-54.

16. Bots ML, Launer LJ, Lindemans J, et al, "Homocysteine and Short-Term Risk of Myocardial Infarction and Stroke in the Elderly," *Arch Intern Med*, 1999, 159(1):38-44.

17. Giles WH, Croft JB, Geenlund KJ, et al, "Association Between Total Homocyst(e)ine and the Likelihood for a History of Acute Myocardial Infarction by Race and Ethnicity: Results From the Third National Health and Nutrition Examination Survey," *Am Heart J*, 2000, 139(3):446-53.

18. Mansoor MA, Bergmark C, Haswell SJ, et al, "Correlation Between Plasma Total Homocysteine and Copper in Patients With Peripheral Vascular Disease," *Clin Chem*, 2000, 46(3):385-91.

19. den Heijer M, Koster T, Blom HJ, et al, "Hyperhomocysteinemia as a Risk Factor for Deep-Vein Thrombosis," *N Engl J Med*, 1996, 334(21):759-62.

20. Dudman NP, "An Alternative View of Homocysteine," *Lancet*, 1999, 354(9195):2072-4.

21. Selhub J, Jacques PF, Wilson PW, et al, "Vitamin Status and Intake as Primary Determinants of Homocysteinemia in an Elderly Population," *JAMA*, 1993, 270(22):2693-8.

22. Fenton WA and Rosenberg LE, "Inherited Disorders of Cobalamin Transport and Metabolism," *The Metabolic and Molecular Bases of Inherited Disease*, 7th ed, Volume 2, Scriver CR, Beaudet AL, Sly WS, et al, eds, New York, NY: McGraw-Hill, 1995, 3133.

23. Hustad S, Ueland PM, Vollset SE, et al, "Riboflavin as a Determinant of Plasma Total Homocysteine: Effect of Modification by the Methylene-Tetrahydrofolate Reductase C677T Polymorphism," *Clin Chem*, 2000, 46(8 Pt 1):1065-71.

24. Mills JL, McPartin JM, Kirke PN, et al, "Homocysteine Metabolism in Pregnancies Complicated by Neural-Tube Defects," *Lancet*, 1995, 345(8943):149-51.

25. Rosenblatt DS, "Inherited Disorders of Folate Transport and Metabolism," *The Metabolic and Molecular Bases of Inherited Disease*, 7th ed, Volume 2, Scriver CR, Beaudet AL, Sly WS, et al, eds, New York, NY: McGraw-Hill, 1995, 3111-49.

26. Mudd SH, Levy HL, and Skovby, "Disorders of Transulfuration," *The Metabolic and Molecular Bases of Inherited Disease*, 7th ed, Volume 2, Scriver CR, Beaudet AL, Sly WS, et al, eds, New York, NY: McGraw-Hill, 1995, 1286-7.

27. Garg UC, Zheng ZJ, Folsom AR, et al, "Short-Term and Long-Term Variability of Plasma Homocysteine Measurement," *Clin Chem*, 1997, 43(1):141-5.

28. Rasmussen K, Moller J, and Lyngbak M, "Within-Person Variation of Plasma Homocysteine and Effects of Posture and Tourniquet Application," *Clin Chem*, 1999, 45(10):1850-5.

29. Pfeiffer CM, Huff DL, Smith SJ, et al, "Comparison of Plasma Total Homocysteine measurements in 14 Laboratories: An International Study," *Clin Chem*, 1999, 45(8 Pt 1):1261-8.

30. Yu HH, Joubrab R, Asmi M, et al, "Agreement Among Four Homocysteine Assays and Results in Patients With Coronary Atherosclerosis and Controls," *Clin Chem*, 2000, 46(2):258-64,

31. Burrs CAP, personal communication, July 2000.

32. Moller J, Rasmussen K, and Christensen L, "External Quality Assessment of Methylmalonic Acid and Total Homocysteine," *Clin Chem*, 1999, 45(9):1536-42.

33. Refsum H, Ueland P, and Kvinnsland S, "Acute and Long-Term Effects of High-Dose Methotrexate Treatment on Homocysteine in Plasma and Urine," *Cancer Res*, 1986, 46(10):5385-91.

34. Smulders YM, de Man AM, Stehouwer CD, et al, "Trimethoprim and Fasting Plasma Homocysteine," *Lancet*, 1998, 352(9143):1827-8.

35. Garg R, Malinow MR, Pettinger M, et al, "Niacin Treatment Increases Plasma Homocyst(e)ine Levels," *Am Heart J*, 1999, 138(6 Pt 1) :1082-7.

36. Molloy AM, Daly S, Mills JL, et al, "Thermolabile Variant of 5,10-Methylenetetrahydrofolate Reductase Associated With Low Red-Cell Folates: Implications for Folate Intake Recommendations," *Lancet*, 1997, 349(9065):1591-3.

37. Mandel H, Brenner B, Berant M, et al, "Coexistence of Hereditary Homocystinuria nd Factor V Leiden - Effect on Thrombosis," *N Engl J Med*, 1996, 334(12):763-8.

38. Balarajan R, "Ethnicity and Variations in Mortality From Coronary Heart Disease," *Health Trends*, 1996, 28:45-51.

39. Chambers JC, Obeid OA, Refsum H, et al, "Plasma Homocysteine Concentrations and Risk of Coronary Heart Disease in UK Indian Asian and European Men," *Lancet*, 2000, 355(9203):523-7.

40. van Baal WM, Smolders RG, van der Mooren MJ, et al, "Hormone Replacement Therapy and Plasma Homocysteine Levels," *Obstet Gynecol*, 1999, 94(4):485-91.

References

Bostom AG, Rosenberg IH, Silbershatz H, et al, "Nonfasting Plasma Total Homocysteine Levels and Stroke Incidence in Elderly Persons: The Framingham Study," *Ann Intern Med*, 1999, 131(5):352-5.

Bostom AG, Silbershatz H, and Rosenberg IH, et al, "Nonfasting Plasma Total Homocysteine Levels and All-Cause and Cardiovascular Disease Mortality in Elderly Framingham Men and Women," *Arch Intern Med*, 1999, 159(10):1077-80.

Chan HH, Douketis JD, and Nowaczyk MJ, "Acute Renal Vein Thrombosis, Oral Contraceptive Use, and Hyperhomocysteinemia," *Mayo Clin Proc*, 2001, 76(2):212-4.

den Heijer M, Koster T, Blom HJ, et al, "Hyperhomocysteinemia as a Risk Factor for Deep-Vein Thrombosis," *N Engl J Med*, 1996, 334(12):759-62.

Eikelboom JW, Lonn E, Genest J J, et al, "Homocyst(e)ine and Cardiovascular Disease: A Critical Review of the Epidemiologic Evidence," *Ann Intern Med*, 1999, 131(5):363-75.

Goldhaber SZ, "Pulmonary Embolism," *N Engl J Med*, 1998, 339(2):93-104.

Graham IM, Daly LE, Refsum HM, et al, "Plasma Homocysteine as a Risk Factor for Vascular Disease," The European Concerted Action Project, *JAMA*, 1997, 277(22):1775-81.

Jacques PF, Selhub J, Bostom AG, et al, "The Effect of Folic Acid Fortification on Plasma Folate and Total Homocysteine Concentrations," *N Engl J Med*, 1999, 340(19):1449-54.

Kark JD, Selhub J, Adler B, et al, "Nonfasting Plasma Total Homocysteine Level and Mortality in Middle-Aged and Elderly Men and Women in Jerusalem," *Ann Intern Med*, 1999, 131(5):321-30.

Kolata G, "New Clue to Heart Disease: A Vitamin Lack," *The New York Times*, July 4, 1995, 19-20.

Malinow MR, Duell PB, Hess DL, et al, "Reduction of Plasma Homocyst(e)ine Levels by Breakfast Cereal Fortified With Folic Acid in Patients With Coronary Heart Disease," *N Engl J Med*, 1998, 338(15):1009-15.

McCully KS, "Homocysteine, Folate, Vitamin B_6, and Cardiovascular Disease," *JAMA*, 1998, 279(5):392-3.

McCully KS, "Vascular Pathology of Homocysteinemia: Implications for the Pathogenesis of Atherosclerosis," *Am J Pathol*, 1969, 56(1):111-28.

Miner SES, Evrovski J, and Cole DE, "Clinical Chemistry and Molecular Biology of Homocysteine Metabolism: An Update," *Clin Biochem*, 1997, 30(3):189-210.

Moat SJ, Bonham JR, Tanner MS, et al, "Recommended Approaches for the Laboratory Measurement of Homocysteine in the Diagnosis and Monitoring of Patients With Hyperhomocysteinaemia," *Ann Clin Biochem*, 1999, 36(Pt 3):372-9.

Mohan IV and Stansby G, "Nutritional Hyperhomocysteinemia," *BMJ*, 1999, 318(7198):1569-70.

Nelen WL, Blom JH, Steegers EA, et al, "Homocysteine and Folate Levels as Risk Factors for Recurrent Early Pregnancy Loss," *Obstet Gynecol*, 2000, 95(4):519-24.

Osganian SK, Stampfer MJ, Spiegelman D, et al, "Distribution of and Factors Associated With Serum Homocysteine Levels in Children," Child and Adolescent Trial for Cardiovascular Health, *JAMA*, 1999, 281(13):1189-96.

Ridker PM, Manson JE, Buring JE, et al, "Homocysteine and Risk of Cardiovascular Disease Among Postmenopausal Women," *JAMA*, 1999, 281(19):1817-21.

Selhub J, Jacques PF, Rosenberg IH, et al, "Serum Total Homocysteine Concentrations in the Third National Health and Nutrition Examination Survey (1991-1994): Population Reference Ranges and Contribution of Vitamin Status to High Serum Concentrations," *Ann Intern Med*, 1999, 131(5):331-9.

Still RA and McDowell IF, "ACP Broadsheet No 152: March 1998. Clinical Implications of Plasma Homocysteine Measurement in Cardiovascular Disease," *J Clin Pathol*, 1998, 51(3):183-8.

Taylor LM, Moneta GL, Sexton GJ, et al, "Prospective Blinded Study of the Relationship Between Plasma Homocysteine and Progression of Symptomatic Peripheral Arterial Disease," *J Vasc Surg*, 1999, 29(1):8-21.

Wald NJ, Watt HC, Law MR, et al, "Homocysteine and Ischemic Heart Disease: Results of a Prospective Study With Implications Regarding Prevention," *Arch Intern Med*, 1998, 158(8):862-7.

Welch GN and Loscalzo J, "Homocysteine and Atherothrombosis," *N Engl J Med*, 1998, 338(15):1042-50.

♦ **Homocyst(e)ine, Qualitative** *see* Cystine, Urine *on page 164*

Homovanillic Acid, Urine

Related Information

Catecholamines, Fractionation, Plasma *on page 138*
Catecholamines, Fractionation, Urine *on page 139*
Metanephrines, Urine or Plasma *on page 223*
Urine Collection, 24-Hour *on page 47*
Vanillylmandelic Acid, Urine *on page 297*

Synonyms HVA

Test Includes Measurement of creatinine excretion as well as HVA

Abstract Homovanillic acid (HVA) is a major terminal metabolite of dopamine. More than three fourths of patients with neuroblastoma excrete increased HVA and/or vanillylmandelic acid (VMA). Increased concentrations of norepinephrine and dopamine are excreted. High VMA:HVA ratio correlates with favorable prognosis.

Patient Preparation Patients should avoid aspirin, disulfiram, reserpine, and pyridoxine, if possible, at least 48 hours prior to collection of the specimen. Levodopa should be avoided for 2 weeks before collection.

Specimen 24-hour urine is preferred. Smaller collections for adults and pediatric patients are acceptable.

Container Plastic urine container

Collection Urine specimen should not contact metal. Depending on laboratory, boric, acetic, or hydrochloric acid must initially be added to the container as a preservative. The specimen should have pH 2.0-4.0. Check with your laboratory for volume and concentration.

Storage Instructions Measure 24-hour urine volume, adjust to pH 2-4 and aliquot 100 mL sample and refrigerate. Stable 7 days at 4°C.

Special Instructions For work-up for neuroblastoma, excretion of VMA should also be measured. Patient's age is needed, as the values are age dependent.

Reference Interval Adult normal range is usually <8.0 mg/24 hours (SI: <44.0 µmol/day). Pediatric values are up to 35.0 µg HVA/mg creatinine (SI: 22.0 mmol HVA/mol creatinine) in infancy. See table on following page.

Use Detect neuroblastoma and ganglioneuroblastoma; follow course of tumor treatment

Limitations Almost all patients with neuroblastoma have elevations of HVA, while only about 80% have elevations of urinary catecholamines. Increased HVA levels, however, are not specific for neuroblastoma.
(Continued)

Homovanillic Acid, Urine *(Continued)*

Homovanillic Acid, Urine

Age	µg HVA/mg creatinine	SI: mmol HVA/mol creatinine
0-1 y	1.2-35.0	0.7-21.7
1-2 y	4.0-23.0	2.5-14.3
2-5 y	0.5-20.0	0.3-12.4
5-10 y	0.5-15.0	0.3-9.3
10-15 y	0.25-12.0	0.2-7.4
Adults	0.25-7.0	0.2-4.4

Adults: <8 mg/24 h.

Methodology High performance liquid chromatography (HPLC), gas chromatography-mass spectroscopy (GC/MS), solvent extraction, colorimetry,[1] and capillary electrophoresis.[2]

Additional Information HVA is the major terminal metabolite of the dopamine pathway. VMA is the major terminal metabolite of the norepinephrine pathway. HVA is often excreted in excess amounts by neuroblastomas, ganglioneuroblastomas, pheochromocytomas, and in Riley-Day syndrome. Excretion may be intermittent. Plasma HVA is increased in schizotypal personality disorders.[3] Approximately 20% of subjects with neuroblastoma do not have increased VMA.

Carcinoembryonic antigen is an additional marker found in many patients with neuroblastoma. Relevant to neuroblastoma are N-*myc* Amplification and Cell Cycle Analysis by Flow Cytometry *on page 53*.

Depressed patients who have attempted suicide have been reported to have decreased urinary HVA compared to patients who have not attempted suicide.[4]

As neuroblastoma is one of the most common malignant tumors in the pediatric population, mass screening for HVA and VMA has been performed.[5,6,7]

Footnotes
1. Davidson DF, "Simultaneous Assay for Urinary 4-Hydroxy-3-Methoxy-Mandelic Acid, 5-Hydroxyindoleacetic Acid and Homovanillic Acid by Isocratic HPLC With Electrochemical Detection," *Ann Clin Biochem*, 1989, 26(Pt 2):137-43.
2. Garcia A, Heinanen M, Jimenez LM, et al, "Direct Measurement of Homovanillic, Vanillylmandelic and 5-Hydroxyindoleacetic Acids in Urine by Capillary Electrophoresis," *J Chromatogr*, A25, 2000, 871(1-2):341-50.
3. Siever LJ, Amin F, Coccaro EF, et al, "Plasma Homovanillic Acid in Schizotypal Personality Disorder," *Am J Psychiatry*, 1991, 148(9):1246-8.
4. Roy A, "Recent Biological Studies on Suicide," *Suicide Life Threat Behav*, 1994, 24(1):10-4.
5. Fauler G, Leis HJ, and Huber E, "Determination of Homovanillic Acid and Vanillylmandelic Acid in Neuroblastoma Screening by Stable Isotope Dilution GC/MS," *J Mass Spectrom*, 1997, 32(5):507-14.
6. Bernstein ML and Woods WG, "Screening for Neuroblastoma," *Cancer Treat Res*, 1996, 86:149-63.
7. Parker L, "Newborn Screening for Neuroblastoma," *Curr Opin Pediatr*, 1997, 9(1):70-3.

References
Fitzgibbon MC and Tormey WP, "Paediatric Reference Ranges for Urinary Catecholamines/Metabolites and Their Relevance in Neuroblastoma Diagnosis," *Ann Clin Biochem*, 1994, 31(Pt 1):1-11.

Javors MA, Bowden CL, and Maas JW, "3-Methoxy-4-Hydroxyphenylglycol, 5-Hydroxyindoleacetic Acid, and Homovanillic Acid in Human Cerebrospinal Fluid. Storage and Measurement by Reversed-Phase High Performance Liquid Chromatography and Coulometric Detection Using 3-Methoxy-4-Hydroxyphenylacetic Acid as an Internal Standard," *J Chromatogr*, 1984, 336(2):259-69.

Rosano TG and Whitley RJ, "Catecholamines and Serotonin," *Tietz Textbook of Clinical Chemistry*, 3rd ed, Burtis CA and Ashwood ER, eds, Philadelphia, PA: WB Saunders Co, 1999, 1570-600.

♦ **2-Hour PP Glucose** *see* Glucose, Postglucose Load, Plasma *on page 185*

♦ **hPL** *see* Placental Lactogen, Human, Serum *on page 254*

♦ **hPP** *see* Pancreatic Polypeptide, Human, Serum or Plasma *on page 242*

♦ **5-HT** *see* Serotonin, Blood, Cerebrospinal Fluid *on page 274*

♦ **Human Antianimal Antibodies** *see* Heterophilic Antibodies *on page 191*

♦ **Human Antimouse Antibodies** *see* Heterophilic Antibodies *on page 191*

♦ **Human Chorionic Gonadotropin** *see* Chorionic Gonadotropin, Human, Serum and Urine *on page 147*

♦ **Human Chorionic Gonadotropin, Urine** *see* Pregnancy Test, Serum or Urine *on page 260*

♦ **Human Chorionic Somatomammotropin** *see* Placental Lactogen, Human, Serum *on page 254*

♦ **Human Kallikrein 3** *see* Prostate Specific Antigen, Serum *on page 263*

♦ **Human Pancreatic Polypeptide** *see* Pancreatic Polypeptide, Human, Serum or Plasma *on page 242*

♦ **Hunter Syndrome** *see* Mucopolysaccharides, Urine *on page 226*

♦ **Hurler Syndrome** *see* Mucopolysaccharides, Urine *on page 226*

♦ **HVA** *see* Homovanillic Acid, Urine *on page 195*

♦ **Hydrocortisone, Serum** *see* Cortisol, Serum or Plasma *on page 154*

♦ **11-Hydroxyandrosterone** *see* 17-Ketosteroids Fractionation, Urine *on page 206*

♦ **β-Hydroxybutyrate** *see* Ketone Bodies, Blood *on page 205*

17-Hydroxycorticosteroids, Urine

Related Information
Adrenal Cortex: Laboratory Assessments Overview *on page 84*
Cortisol, Free, Urine *on page 154*
Cortisol, Serum or Plasma *on page 154*
Metyrapone Stimulation Test, Serum *on page 225*
Urine Collection, 24-Hour *on page 47*

Synonyms 17-OHCS; Porter-Silber Chromogens, Urine

Abstract This test measures the metabolites of cortisol and other adrenal corticosteroids. Two methods are used: Porter-Silber chromogens and 17-ketogenic steroids (Norymberski method). The former measures fewer metabolites.

Patient Preparation Ideally, all drugs should be withheld for several days prior to collection of urine, if possible, without doing harm to the patient. Avoid patient stress.

Specimen 24-hour urine

Container Plastic container with hydrochloric or acetic acid as preservative

Storage Instructions Refrigerate during collection, refrigerate or freeze after collection. Stable 45 days if refrigerated and acidified.

Reference Interval Performed in only a few laboratories. Some variation exists between published ranges and the two different methods that may be used.

17-Hydroxycorticosteroids, Urine

Age	mg/day	µmol/day
0-1 y	0.5-1.0	1.4-2.8
>1 y	1.0-5.6	2.8-15.5
Adults		
male	3.0-10.0	8.2-27.6
female	2.0-8.0	5.5-22.0

Adapted from Painter PC, Cope JY, and Smith JL, "Reference Information for the Clinical Laboratory," *Tietz Textbook of Clinical Chemistry*, 3rd ed, Philadelphia, PA: WB Saunders Co, 1999, 1819.

Use A presently rarely performed adrenal function test which has been done in the evaluation of glucocorticoid production; increased in ectopic ACTH syndrome, Cushing syndrome, and stress; decreased in Addison disease, adrenogenital syndrome, pituitary insufficiency.[1] Urinary metabolites of glucocorticoids can be measured as 17-ketogenic steroids and 17-hydroxycorticosteroids.

Limitations Subject to variability due to unreliable 24-hour urine collections and interferences. Serum or urine cortisol measurements are preferred. **This test has, for the most part, been replaced by the measurement of urinary free cortisol, which is a more sensitive and specific test for hypercortisolism.[2,3]**

17-OHCS (Porter-Silber) does not measure pregnanetriol.

Methodology Porter-Silber color reaction

Additional Information The Porter-Silber color reaction detects steroids with a dihydroxyacetone group at carbon 17, including major glucocorticoid metabolites. By pretreating with a strong reducing agent, one increases the number of metabolites detected (ie, 17-ketogenic steroids). Either 17-hydroxysteroid or 17-ketogenic steroid measurements can be used as an estimate of adrenal steroid production, either as baseline values or in stimulation or suppression tests.

Deoxycorticosterone (DOC), corticosterone (compound B) and aldosterone lack a 17-hydroxyl group and are not detected in 17-KG and 17-OHCS procedures.[3]

Footnotes
1. Zeiger MA, Nieman LK, Cutler GB, et al, "Primary Bilateral Adrenocortical Causes of Cushing's Syndrome," *Surgery*, 1991, 110(6):1106-15.
2. Flack MR, Oldfield EH, Cutler GB Jr, et al, "Urine Free Cortisol in the High-Dose Dexamethasone Suppression Test for the Differential Diagnosis of the Cushing Syndrome," *Ann Intern Med*, 1992, 116(3):211-7.
3. Wilson J and Foster D, *Williams Textbook of Endocrinology*, 9th ed, Philadelphia, PA: WB Saunders Co, 1998, 615.

References
Speroff L, Glass RH, and Kase NG, *Clinical Gynecologic Endocrinology and Infertility*, 4th ed, Baltimore, MD: Lippincott Williams & Wilkins, 1989.

♦ **16-Hydroxyestradiol** *see* Estriol, Unconjugated, Pregnancy, Serum, Plasma, or Urine *on page 171*

♦ **11-Hydroxyetiocholanolone** *see* 17-Ketosteroids Fractionation, Urine *on page 206*

5-Hydroxyindoleacetic Acid, Quantitative, Urine

Related Information
Serotonin, Blood, Cerebrospinal Fluid *on page 274*
Urine Collection, 24-Hour *on page 47*

Synonyms 5-HIAA, Quantitative, Urine

Applies to Chromogranin A, Plasma; Serotonin, Cerebrospinal Fluid; Serotonin, Metabolite

Abstract Carcinoid tumors are neuroendocrine neoplasms which arise in the gastrointestinal and respiratory tracts and in a broad range of additional sites. Most are less aggressive than are usual adenocarcinomas. Indolent versus aggressive characteristics correlate with site of origin, histopathologic characteristics, size, and concentration of 5-HIAA, but survival in large series is difficult to project.[1] 5-HIAA is a serotonin metabolite used as a marker for carcinoid tumors.

Patient Preparation A number of foods are high in serotonin. For a 48-hour period or more prior to and during collection, **avoid** bananas, avocados, chocolate, plums, eggplant, tomatoes, plantain, pineapples, walnuts, acetaminophen, salicylates, phenacetin, cough syrup containing glyceryl guaiacolate, naproxen (Naprosyn®, Anaprox®), mephenesin, methocarbamol, imipramine, isoniazid, MAO inhibitors, methenamine, methyldopa, reserpine, and phenothiazines. Drug interference relates to method;[2] check with laboratory.

Specimen 24-hour urine

Container Check with testing laboratory. Usually, a urine container with no preservative is given to the patient.

Collection Check with testing laboratory. A 24-hour urine specimen is collected, usually without preservative. The specimen should be kept refrigerated during collection. When the specimen is received in the laboratory, its pH may be adjusted to 2-3, depending upon the protocol of the laboratory.

Storage Instructions Stable 14 days if acidified and refrigerated. Acidification is done with hydrochloric or boric acids, depending upon individual laboratory methods. Acetic acid has been shown to decrease recovery of 5-HIAA and is not generally recommended.[3]

Reference Interval Approximately 1-9 mg/24 hours (SI: 5-48 µmol/day); some variation in reference ranges is found.

Critical Values >25 mg/24 hours, without dietary interference, is diagnostic of carcinoid.[4]

Use Urine 5-HIAA measurement is used as an adjunct in the diagnosis of carcinoid tumors, syndrome, and subsequent patient monitoring. Values >25 mg/24 hours (higher if the patient has malabsorption) are strong evidence for carcinoid. Midgut carcinoids are most often associated with the carcinoid syndrome, elevated 5-HIAA excretion, and hepatic metastases.

Limitations Urine 5-HIAA concentrations may be normal with nonmetastatic carcinoid tumor and carcinoid syndrome, particularly in subjects without diarrhea. Some patients with the carcinoid syndrome excrete nonhydroxylated indolic acids, not measured as 5-HIAA. Patients with renal disease may have falsely low urinary 5-HIAA levels. 5-HIAA is increased in untreated patients with malabsorption, who have increased urinary tryptophan metabolites (eg, patients with celiac disease, tropical sprue, Whipple disease, stasis syndrome, and cystic fibrosis), and in those with chronic intestinal obstruction and with some noncarcinoid islet cell tumors. Though used prognostically in carcinoid syndrome,[5] a poor correlation exists between urine 5-HIAA level and clinical severity of disease.

Increased 5-HIAA has been seen with pregnancy, ovulation, and stress as well as those who consume foods rich in serotonin.

Contraindications Falsely elevated results are observed from foods ingested within 2 days prior to specimen collection containing serotonin or drugs producing metabolites that react with nitrosonaphthol, a reagent used in 5-HIAA determinations.

Methodology Spectrophotometry, gas chromatography (GC), high performance liquid chromatography (HPLC),[6] fluorescence polarization immunoassay (FPIA). A carbon fiber electrode technique allows *in vivo* monitoring of 5-HIAA in brain tissue.[7]

Additional Information 5-HIAA is the major urinary metabolite of serotonin (5-hydroxytryptamine) (5-HT), a ubiquitous bioactive amine. Serotonin, and consequently 5-HIAA, are produced in excess by most carcinoid tumors, especially those producing the carcinoid syndrome of flushing, hepatomegaly, diarrhea, bronchospasm, and ultimately right-sided valvular heart disease. Subjects with carcinoid heart disease have higher concentrations of serum serotonin and urine 5-HIAA. Quantitation of urinary 5-HIAA is the best laboratory test for carcinoid, but scrupulous care must be taken that specimen collection and patient preparation have been correct. Carcinoid tumors may cause increased excretion of tryptophan, 5-hydroxytryptophan, histamine, its metabolite N-methylhistamine, and chromogranin A, as well as serotonin. Serum serotonin assay may detect some carcinoids missed by 5-HIAA assay. It may be done by HPLC, RIA, or radioenzymatic assay, but it is not offered by many laboratories. Serotonin measured in blood platelets may be more sensitive than measurement of 5-HIAA or serum serotonin.[8] Of 75 patients with carcinoid tumors, 75% had increased urinary 5-HIAA excretion and 64% had increased serotonin excretion. A few patients with increased urinary serotonin have normal urinary 5-HIAA. Plasma chromogranin A is an independent signal of adverse prognosis.[1]

Increased 5-HIAA concentrations in men with flushing and secondary hypogonadism are found in pseudocarcinoid syndrome with hypogonadism.[9]

An increased urinary ratio of 5-hydroxytryptophol (5-HTOL) divided by 5-HIAA has been reported as a means for detecting recent alcohol consumption.[10,11,12]

Low concentrations of 5-HIAA in cerebrospinal fluid are strongly associated with aggressive behavior.[13]

Footnotes
1. Kulke MH and Mayer RJ, "Carcinoid Tumors," *N Engl J Med*, 1999, 340(11):858-68.
2. Young DS, "Effects of Drugs on Clinical Laboratory Tests," 5th ed, Volume 1: Listing by Test, Washington DC: AACC Press, American Association of Clinical Chemistry, 2000, 3-450-1.
3. Deacon AC and Bartlett WA, "Interference by Acetic Acid in Urinary 5-Hydroxyindoleacetic Acid Determination," *Clin Chem*, 1982, 28(1):250-1.
4. Oates JA, "Multiple-Organ Syndromes: Carcinoid Syndrome," *Cecil Textbook of Medicine*, 21st ed, Chapter 245, Goldman L and Bennett JC, eds, Philadelphia, PA: WB Saunders Co, 2000, 1295-7.
5. Agranovich AL, Anderson GH, Manji M, et al, "Carcinoid Tumour of the Gastrointestinal Tract: Prognostic Factors and Disease Outcome," *J Surg Oncol*, 1991, 47(1):45-52.
6. Stroomer AE, Overmars H, Abeling NG, et al, "Simultaneous Determination of Acidic 3,4-Dihydroxyphenylalanine Metabolites and 5-Hydroxyindole-3-Acetic Acid in Urine by High Performance Liquid Chromatography," *Clin Chem*, 1990, 36(10):1834-7.
7. Suaud-Chagny MF, Cespuglio R, Rivot JP, et al, "High Sensitivity Measurement of Brain Catechols and Indoles In Vivo Using Electrochemically Treated Carbon Fiber Electrodes," *J Neurosci Methods*, 1993, 48(3):241-50.
8. DeVries EG, Kerma IP, Slooff MJ, et al, "Recent Development in Diagnosis and Treatment of Metastatic Carcinoid Tumors," *Scand J Gastroenterol Suppl*, 1993, 200:87-93.
9. Shakir KM, Jasser MZ, Yoshihashi AK, et al, "Pseudocarcinoid Syndrome Associated With Hypogonadism and Response to Testosterone Therapy," *Mayo Clin Proc*, 1996, 71:1145-9.
10. Helander A, Beck O, and Jones AW, "Laboratory Testing for Recent Alcohol Consumption: Comparison of Ethanol, Methanol, and 5-Hydroxytryptophol," *Clin Chem*, 1996, 42(4):618-24.
11. Jones AW and Helander A, "Time Course and Reproducibility of Urinary Excretion Profiles of Ethanol, Methanol, and the Ratio of Serotonin Metabolites After Intravenous Infusion of Ethanol," *Alcohol Clin Exp Res*, 1999, 23(12):1921-6.
12. Helander A, von Wachenfeldt J, Hiltunen A, et al, "Comparison of Urinary 5-Hydroxytryptophol, Breath Ethanol, and Self-Report for Detection of Recent Alcohol Use During Outpatient Treatment: A Study on Methadone Patients," *Drug Alcohol Depend*, 1999, 56(1):33-8.
13. Stanley B, Molcho A, Stanley M, et al, "Association of Aggressive Behavior With Altered Serotonergic Function in Patients Who Are Not Suicidal," *Am J Psychiatry*, 2000, 157(4):609-14.

References
Deacon AC, "The Measurement of 5-Hydroxyindoleacetic Acid in Urine," *Ann Clin Biochem*, 1994, 31(Pt 3):215-32.
Farmer KL, "Additional Tests of Interest to the Dermatologist," *Dermatol Clin*, 1994, 12(1):191-9.
Lechago J, "Neuroendocrine Cells of the Gut and Their Disorders," *Gastrointestinal Pathology*, Goldman H, Appelman HD, and Kaufman N, eds, Baltimore, MD: Lippincott Williams & Wilkins, 1990, 181-219.

♦ **21-Hydroxylase** *see* 17-Hydroxyprogesterone, Serum or Plasma *on page 197*

♦ **Hydroxylysylpyridinoline** *see* Pyridinolines (Pyridinoline and Deoxypyridinoline), Urine *on page 272*

♦ **Hydroxymethylbilane Synthase** *see* Porphobilinogen Deaminase, Erythrocyte *on page 254*

♦ **17α-Hydroxyprogesterone** *see* 17-Hydroxyprogesterone, Serum or Plasma *on page 197*

17-Hydroxyprogesterone, Serum or Plasma

Related Information
Adrenal Cortex: Laboratory Assessments Overview *on page 84*
Adrenocorticotropic Hormone, Plasma *on page 86*
Androstenedione, Serum *on page 104*
Cortisol, Free, Urine *on page 154*
Cortisol, Serum or Plasma *on page 154*
Pregnanetriol, Urine *on page 261*
Progesterone, Serum *on page 261*
Renin Activity, Plasma *on page 273*

Synonyms 17α-Hydroxyprogesterone; 17-OHP

Applies to 11-Beta-Hydroxylase; Deoxycorticosterone; 11-Desoxycortisol; 21-Hydroxylase; 17-OHP, Amniotic Fluid; 17-OHP, Saliva

Replaces Urine 17-Ketogenic Steroids; Urine Pregnanetriol Assay

Abstract A C-21 steroid, 17-hydroxyprogesterone (17-OHP) is produced by adrenal cortices, ovaries, testes, and placenta. It is the metabolic product of progesterone and 17-hydroxypregnenolone. It is a precursor of cortisol, and is markedly elevated in patients with congenital adrenal hyperplasia (CAH). **Congenital adrenal hyperplasia** is the designation for a group of autosomal recessive diseases in which deficiency of cortisol leads to increased ACTH. This then causes adrenal cortical hyperplasia with stimulation to production of other substances. Ninety percent of cases or more are caused by 21-hydroxylase deficiency. Pregnanetriol, cortisol and ACTH assays are relevant as well.
(Continued)

17-Hydroxyprogesterone, Serum or Plasma
(Continued)

A number of states in the U.S. screen for CAH by assaying 17-OHP in blood collected onto filter paper for newborn screening.

Patient Preparation No recent radioactive isotopes, if RIA is used

Specimen Serum or plasma, whole blood

Container Red top tube or lavender top (EDTA) tube; check with laboratory. Whole blood, used for screening neonatal specimen, may be collected and dried onto filter paper. Check with newborn screening laboratory for proper collection details.

Sampling Time Blood levels peak in the morning.

Storage Instructions Separate serum or plasma within 4 hours. Serum or plasma stable for up to 4 days at 4°C and for up to 1 month at -20°C.

Causes for Rejection Incorrect/insufficient filter paper saturation, inadequate specimen labelings

Reference Interval Ranges vary between laboratories. The following are examples.
Prepubertal children: <100 ng/dL (SI: <3.0 nmol/L)
Male: 50-200 ng/dL (SI: 1.5-6.0 nmol/L)
Female:
- follicular: 20-80 ng/dL (SI: 0.6-2.4 nmol/L)
- luteal: 100-300 ng/dL (SI: 3.0-9.0 nmol/L)
- postmenopausal: <50 ng/dL (SI: <1.5 nmol/L)

Allen et al[1] recommended the following birth-weight-dependent thresholds of abnormality for 17-OHP in newborn screening using dried whole blood samples collected onto filter paper. See table.

Newborn Screening for CAH
17-OHP in Dried Whole Blood Specimens

Weight (g)	Possibly Abnormal 17-OHP ng/dL (SI: nmol/L)	Definitely Abnormal 17-OHP ng/dL (SI: nmol/L)
<1299	≥13,500 (≥405)	
1300-1699	11,5000-13,400 (345-402)	≥13,500 (≥405)
1700-2199	6500-8900 (195-267)	≥9000 (≥270)
≥2200	4000-8900 (120-267)	≥9000 (≥270)

Critical Values Low levels of adrenocortical steroids can be life-threatening. Early diagnosis and therapy are indicated.

Use 17-OHP is used
- to diagnose CAH in symptomatic patients and to monitor the effectiveness of cortisol replacement therapy in patients with the disease.
- in newborn screening programs that include testing for CAH.
- to evaluate hirsutism, infertility, and/or hermaphroditism in female patients with possible 21-hydroxylase deficiency.
- to assess certain adrenal or ovarian tumors which may have endocrine activity.

Limitations 17-OHP is elevated, but less so, in the 11-beta-hydroxylase deficiency form of CAH. Measurement of serum 11-desoxycortisol (substance S) and deoxycorticosterone (DOC) differentiates these abnormalities. Because of increased synthesis of mineralocorticoid precursors, hypernatremia and hypertension may develop. Thus, assays for serum sodium and renin activity (suppressed) are desirable.

High false-positive rates are observed from newborn screening analyses of 17-OHP in dried blood on filter paper, leading to unnecessary follow up, especially in preterm, low-birth-weight neonates.[2] Utilization of different decision thresholds for different birth weights improves screening performance.[1] Dried blood cortisol determinations may be used to exclude some infants with falsely increased 17-OHP levels from further testing for CAH, but such differentiation is not sufficiently good to recommend it for routine purposes.[3]

Methodology Radioimmunoassay (RIA), fluoroimmunoassay (FIA), enzyme-linked immunosorbent assay (ELISA), chemiluminescent immunoassay (CIA), high performance liquid chromatography (HPLC), gas chromatography mass spectrometry (GC/MS).

Additional Information 17-OHP is the substrate for subsequent 21- and 11-hydroxylation, in the pathway to cortisol. The two critical enzymes, 21-hydroxylase and 11-beta-hydroxylase, participate in cortisol biosynthesis. If hydroxylation, at either position, cannot take place because of enzyme deficiency, cortisol synthesis decreases, accompanied by increased ACTH. CAH and adrenogenital syndrome result from lack of normal glucocorticoids and build-up of precursors (mostly virilizing). Lack of 21-hydroxylase is the most common cause of adrenogenital syndrome. The syndrome of 21-hydroxylase deficiency is often characterized by androgen excess (virilization) and mineralocorticoid deficiency. Mutations in the gene that encodes 21-hydroxylase have been described,[4] and methods for screening for these mutations are available.[5,6] Over 200 mutations have been described.[7]

CAH caused by 21-hydroxylase deficiency is the most common cause of female hermaphroditism,[8] an autosomal recessive disease. Basal 17-OHP levels can be normal in late-onset 21-hydroxylase deficiency presenting as hirsutism. Such patients are described as having a dramatically increased 17-OHP response to ACTH. Patients with 21-hydroxylase deficiency have increased 17-ketosteroids, urine pregnanetriol, as well as, high 17-OHP.

17-hydroxyprogesterone assay has been used to identify the heterozygous state of 21-hydroxylase deficiency, by testing basal and 30 and 60 minutes after ACTH stimulation. The following figure illustrates basal and stimulated 17-hydroxyprogesterone concentration.[9]

Basal and Stimulated 17-Hydroxyprogesterone

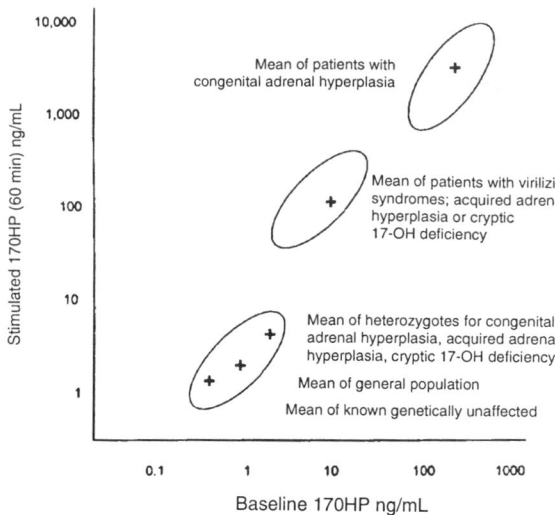

Weiss RL, *ARUP Interpretive Data Guide*, ARUP Laboratories Inc,

Prenatal diagnosis of congenital adrenal hyperplasia is possible by HLA typing, by DNA analysis, or by hormone measurements from amniotic fluid, including 17-OHP.[8]

17-OHP levels in saliva from healthy neonates recently were reported and may become useful alternatives to whole blood determinations in this age group.[10]

Footnotes

1. Allen DB, Hoffman GL, Fitzpatrick P, et al, "Improved Precision of Newborn Screening for Congenital Adrenal Hyperplasia Using Weight-Adjusted Criteria for 17-Hydroxyprogesterone Levels," *J Pediatr*, 1997, 130(1):128-33.
2. al-Saedi SA, Dean H, Dent W, et al, "Screening for Congenital Adrenal Hyperplasia: The DELFIA Screening Test Overestimates Serum 17-Hydroxyprogesterone in Preterm Infants," *Pediatrics*, 1996, 97(1):100-2.
3. Mitchell ML and Hermos RJ, "Cortisol in Dried Blood Screening Specimens From Newborns With Raised 17-Hydroxyprogesterone and Congenital Adrenal Hyperplasia," *Clin Endocrinol*, 1998, 48(6):757-60.
4. White PC, Tasie-Luna MT, New MI, et al, "Mutations in Steroid 21-Hydroxylase (CYP21)," *Hum Mutat*, 1994, 3(4):373-8.
5. Krone N, Rosher AA, Schwarz HP, et al, "Comprehensive Analytical Strategy for Mutation Screening in 21-Hydroxylase Deficiency," *Clin Chem*, 1998, 44(10):2075-82.
6. Killeen AA, Jiddou RR, and Sane KS, "Characterization of Frequent Polymorphisms in Intron 2 of CYP21: Application to Analysis of Segregation of CYP21 Alleles," *Clin Chem*, 1998, 44(12):2410-5.
7. Kapelari K, Ghanaati Z, Wollmann H, et al, "A Rapid Screening for Steroid 21-Hydroxylase Mutations in Patients With Congenital Adrenal Hyperplasia. Mutations in Brief No. 247. Online," *Hum Mutat*, 1999, 13(6):505.
8. Pang S, Pollack MS, Marshall RN, et al, "Prenatal Treatment of Congenital Adrenal Hyperplasia Due to 21-Hydroxylase Deficiency," *N Engl J Med*, 1990, 322(2):111-5.
9. Weiss RL, *ARUP Interpretive Data Guide*, ARUP Laboratories, Inc, 1999, 308.
10. Kiess J, "Cortisol and 17-Hydroxy Progesterone Levels in Saliva of Neonates: Normative Data and Relation to Body Mass Index, Arterial Cord Blood, pH, and Time of Sampling After Birth," *Biol Neonate*, 2000, 78:22-6.

References

Bachega TA, Billerbeck AE, Marcondes JA, et al, "Influence of Different Genotypes on 17-Hydroxyprogesterone Levels in Patients With Nonclassical Congenital Adrenal Hyperplasia due to 21-Hydroxylase Deficiency," *Clin Endocrinol*, 2000, 52(5), 601-7.

Bode HH, Rivkees SA, Cowley DM, et al, "Home Monitoring of 17-Hydroxyprogesterone Levels in Congenital Adrenal Hyperplasia With Filter Paper Blood Samples," *J Pediatr*, 1999, 134(2):185-9.

Check JH, Vaze MM, Epstein R, et al, "17-Hydroxyprogesterone Level as a Marker for Corpus Luteum Function in Aborters Versus Nonaborters," *Int J Fertil*, 1990, 35(2):112-5.

Demers LM and Whitley RJ, "Function of the Adrenal Cortex," *Tietz Textbook of Clinical Chemistry*, Chapter 43, Burtis CA and Ashwood ER, eds, 1999, 1530-69.

Honour JW and Rumsby G, "Problems in Diagnosis and Management of Congenital Adrenal Hyperplasia Due to 21-Hydroxylase Deficiency," *J Steroid Biochem Mol Biol*, 1993, 45(1-3):69-74.

Lee A and Ellis G, "Serum 17-Alpha-Hydroxyprogesterone in Infants and Children as Measured by a Direct Radioimmunoassay Kit," *Clin Biochem*, 1991, 24(6):505-11.

Levine LS and DiGeorge AM, "Disorders of the Adrenal Glands," *Nelson Textbook of Pediatrics*, 16th ed, Bohrman RE, Kliegman RM, and Jenson HB, eds, Philadelphia, PA: WB Saunders Co, 2000, 1722-44.

Summers RH, Herold DA, and Seely BL, "Hormonal and Genetic Analysis of a Patient With Congenital Adrenal Hyperplasia," *Clin Chem*, 1996, 42(9):1483-7.

♦ **Hydroxyproline** *see* Amino Acids, Urine *on page 101*

Hydroxyproline, Total, Urine

Related Information

Alkaline Phosphatase, Heat Stable, Serum on page 91
Alkaline Phosphatase Isoenzymes, Serum on page 92
Alkaline Phosphatase, Serum on page 93
Calcium, Serum on page 131
Calcium, Urine on page 133
N-Telopeptides, Urine on page 233
Osteocalcin, Serum or Plasma on page 237
Osteocalcin (Undercarboxylated), Serum on page 238
Pyridinolines (Pyridinoline and Deoxypyridinoline), Urine on page 272
Urine Collection, 24-Hour on page 47

Abstract Collagen has a very high content of proline and hydroxyproline. Urinary excretion of hydroxyproline reflects bone matrix metabolism/catabolism, and is high in periods of rapid bone turnover (eg, Paget disease of bone). Elevated serum alkaline phosphatase occurs with increased bone formation. Excretion of hydroxyproline and pyridinolines provides an index of bone resorption or destruction. About half of urinary hydroxyproline derives from breakdown of collagen of bone. This assay has been replaced by more specific markers (pyridinolines and N-telopeptides) of bone resorption.

Patient Preparation Avoid foods containing gelatin (cooked collagen) and meat at least 24 hours prior to and during urine collection. These include gelatin desserts (Jello®), ice creams, candies. Patient must avoid aspirin-containing drugs. Hormonal agents affect quantitation.

Specimen 24-hour urine

Collection Add 30 mL of 6N HCl to container before the beginning of collection. Refrigerate during collection. A 2-hour collection after overnight fast may also be used.

Special Instructions Provide patient's age and sex to the laboratory.

Reference Interval Adult male: 15-45 mg/24 hours (1-4 mg/2 hours) (7-20 µg/mg creatinine) (SI: 76-381 µmol/day). Adult female values are about one-half the male ranges. Infants, children, and adolescents variably higher, depending on growth spurts. Normal range is higher in infancy, childhood, and adolescence, especially during growth spurts. **Care must be taken to note the type of diet employed in establishing the reference range of a given laboratory.** Most reference values have been obtained on low-dose gelatin, not gelatin-free diets.

Use Evaluate collagen metabolism of bone, bone resorption, bone destruction. High in Paget disease of bone, healing fracture, primary and secondary hyperparathyroidism. Congenital hydroxyprolinemias are extremely rare. Iminoglycinuria occurs with a frequency of about 1:16,000. A benign autosomal recessive disease, it represents a renal tubular defect. Excessive excretion of glycine, proline, and hydroxyproline occurs. Other hydroxyprolinurias also exist, also without established clinical entities. Measured in osteomalacia when serum alkaline phosphatase is normal, or with coexisting hepatic disease and secondary increase of alkaline phosphatase. It is increased with elevated thyroid function, probably because of increased bone turnover.[1]

Limitations Subject to interference by diet and various diseases, urinary hydroxyproline lacks specificity for bone turnover/resorption. Collagen is found in the diet, in soft tissues, skin and other organs additional to that in bone. A single measurement, subject to high biological variation, provides limited utility.[2]

Biochemical markers of bone turnover provide only limited help in individual osteoporotic patients.[3]

Methodology Extraction/colorimetry, high performance liquid chromatography (HPLC)[4]

Additional Information Increased urinary excretion of hydroxyproline occurs in osteoporosis, osteomalacia, rickets, with prolonged bedrest, pregnancy, and acromegaly. Hydroxyproline may be measured as a marker of metastasis to bone. Multiple myeloma may increase urinary hydroxyproline levels. Urinary hydroxyproline, like serum alkaline phosphatase, may be used in evaluation and response to treatment of Paget disease of bone.

Other markers for the evaluation of bone turnover include assay for pyridinolines, urine N-telopeptides, procollagen I fragments, osteocalcin, and a bone-specific isoenzyme of alkaline phosphatase.[5]

Footnotes

1. Krakauer JC and Kleerekoper M, "Borderline-Low Serum Thyrotropin Level Is Correlated With Increased Fasting Urinary Hydroxyproline Excretion," Arch Intern Med, 1992, 152(2).360-4.
2. Beck-Jensen JE, Kollerup G, Sorensen HA, et al, "A Single Measurement of Biochemical Markers of Bone Turnover Has Limited Utility in the Individual Person," Scand J Clin Lab Invest, 1997, 57(4):351-9.
3. Eastell R and Blumsohn A, "The Value of Biochemical Markers of Bone Turnover in Osteoporosis," J Rheumatol, 1997, 24(6):1215-7.
4. Inoue H and Iguchi H, "Highly Sensitive Determination of N-Terminal Propyl Dipeptides, Proline, and Hydroxyproline in Urine by High Performance Liquid Chromatography Using a New Fluorescent Labeling Reagent," J Chromatogr, 1999, 724(2):221-3.
5. Van Daele PL, Birkenhager JC, and Pols HA, "Biochemical Markers of Bone Turnover: An Update," Neth J Med, 1994, 44(2):65-72.

References

Delmas PD, "Biochemical Markers of Bone Turnover. I: Theoretical Considerations and Clinical Use in Osteoporosis," Am J Med, 1993, 95(5A):11S-6S.

Gilbertson TJ, Branden MN, Gruszczyk SB, et al, "Serum Total Hydroxyproline Assay Effects of Age, Sex, and Paget's Bone Disease," J Clin Chem Clin Biochem, 1983, 21:129-32.

Kim SZ, Varvogli L, Waisbren SE, et al, "Hydroxyprolinemia: Comparison of a Patient and Her Unaffected Twin Sister," J Pediatr, 1997, 130(3):437-41.

Watts NB, "Clinical Utility of Biochemical Markers of Bone Remodeling," Clin Chem, 1999, 45(8B):1359-68.

♦ **5-Hydroxytryptamine, Blood** see Serotonin, Blood, Cerebrospinal Fluid on page 274

♦ **25-Hydroxy Vitamin D₃** see Vitamin D, Serum on page 300

♦ **Hypercapnia** see pCO₂, Blood on page 246

♦ **Hyperphenylalaninemia, Maternal** see Newborn Screen for Phenylketonuria on page 229

♦ **Hyperphenylalaninemia Screen** see Phenylalanine, Blood on page 248

♦ **Hypertonicity** see Sodium, Serum or Plasma on page 275

♦ **Hyperventilation** see pCO₂, Blood on page 246

♦ **Hypoalphalipoproteinemia** see Lipids, Overview on page 213

♦ **Hypoglycorrhachia** see Cerebrospinal Fluid Glucose on page 140

♦ **Hypothalamic-Pituitary-Adrenal Axis** see Insulin Tolerance Test on page 202

♦ **Hypoventilation** see pCO₂, Blood on page 246

♦ **ICSH** see Luteinizing Hormone, Blood or Urine on page 219

♦ **ICTP** see Osteocalcin, Serum or Plasma on page 237

♦ **Idiopathic Erythrocytosis** see Erythropoietin Receptor on page 169

♦ **IGF-1** see Insulin-Like Growth Factor-1 (IGF-1), Serum or Plasma on page 200

♦ **IGFBP-3** see Insulin-Like Growth Factor Binding Protein 3, Serum on page 201

♦ **IGF-I** see Insulin-Like Growth Factor-1 (IGF-1), Serum or Plasma on page 200

♦ **iMg²⁺ₛ (Ionized Serum Magnesium)** see Magnesium, Serum on page 221

♦ **Immunoelectrophoresis** see Protein Electrophoresis, Urine on page 260

♦ **Immunoglobulins** see Protein Electrophoresis, Capillary Zone on page 266

♦ **Immunoglobulins** see Protein Electrophoresis, Serum on page 267

♦ **Immunoreactive Insulin** see Insulin, Serum on page 201

♦ **Immunoreactive PTH** see Parathyroid Hormone, Serum on page 243

♦ **Immunosubtraction Electrophoresis** see Protein Electrophoresis, Capillary Zone on page 266

♦ **Inborn Errors of Metabolism Screen** see Amino Acids, Plasma on page 100

Inhibin A, Serum

Related Information

Alpha₁-Fetoprotein, Serum on page 97
Amniotic Fluid, Chromosome and Genetic Abnormality Analysis on page 360
Chorionic Gonadotropin, Human, Serum and Urine on page 147
Chorionic Villus Sampling, Chromosome and Genetic Abnormality Analysis on page 361
Estriol, Unconjugated, Pregnancy, Serum, Plasma, or Urine on page 171
Pregnancy-Associated Protein A, Serum on page 260
Testosterone, Total and Free, Serum or Plasma on page 280

Applies to Four-Marker Test; Multiple Marker Screening Test; Triple Test

Abstract Inhibin is the major gonadal inhibitory peptide regulating secretion of FSH in both sexes. It is synthesized in the placenta and plateaus during weeks 14-30. The α subunit combines with a β subunit to form inhibin A (Aβ) or inhibin B (Bβ).[1] This test is used with other studies for prediction of Down syndrome. Studies discussed as second trimester tests include AFP, hCG, and inhibin A with[2] or without[3,4] unconjugated estriol (uE₃). Replacement of estriol with inhibin A in the multiple marker screening test has been advocated in screening for Down syndrome.[3] Fetal chromosome analysis provides reliable diagnosis.

Specimen Serum

Sampling Time Measurements of inhibin A are used only after 14 weeks.

Special Instructions Maternal age is needed.

Use In conjunction with other facets, to screen for Down syndrome only after 14 weeks gestation.[5] Dimeric inhibin A is elevated about twofold in the second trimester of Down syndrome gestations. Down syndrome bears association with low maternal AFP and uE₃ and high hCG and inhibin levels. Maternal AFP, dimeric inhibin A with maternal age, as a combination, detect as well autosomal trisomies other than Down syndrome.[6] (Continued)

Inhibin A, Serum (Continued)

Dimeric inhibin A is reported to detect 92% of trisomy 18 and 71% of trisomy 13 afflicted gestations. It is also used for Turner syndrome with AFP, at a 53% detection rate, with a false-positive rate of ~20%.[1] Inhibin levels are not influenced by maternal age.

Limitations Inhibin A is not as pivotal a test as certain other parameters; risk cutoff in the integrated test of 1 in 120 becomes 1 in 190 without serum inhibin A.[7]

Methodology Radioimmunoassay, enzyme-linked immunoassay (ELISA).[8] A two-site enzyme immunoassay, selective for inhibin A (αβ A dimer) is described.

Additional Information The **triple test** (or **triple screen**) testing includes maternal AFP, uE₃, hCG, and age. The **four-marker test** includes also inhibin A.[2] Addition of dimeric inhibin A enhances the rate of detection of Down syndrome gestations to nearly 75% at a 5% false-positive rate.[1]

Maternal age itself is an insensitive marker for Down syndrome; 80% of infants with Down syndrome are born to women younger than age 35.[9]

Threefold increased concentrations of maternal inhibin A in the second trimester predict pre-eclampsia.[1,10,11,12,13]

Footnotes

1. Demers LM, "Dimeric Inhibin A, A Fourth Maternal Serum Screening Marker for Down's Syndrome," *Diagnostic Endocrinology, Immunology, and Metabolism*, 2000, 18(5):131-3.
2. Lambert-Messerlian GM and Canick JA, "Endocrine Analytes in Multiple-Marker Screening," *Clin Perinatol*, 1998, 25(4):963-81, vii.
3. Wenstrom KD, Owen J, Chu DC, et al, "Elevated Second-Trimester Dimetric Inhibin A Levels Identify Down Syndrome Pregnancies," *Am J Obstet Gynecol*, 1997, 177(5):992-6.
4. Aitken DA, Wallace EM, Crossley JA, et al, "Dimeric Inhibin A as a Marker for Down's Syndrome in Early Pregnancy," *N Engl J Med*, 1996, 334(19):1231-6.
5. Wald NJ, George L, Smith D, et al, "Serum Screening for Down's Syndrome Between 8 and 14 Weeks of Pregnancy," *Br J Obstet Gynaecol*, 1996, 103(5):407-12.
6. Wenstrom KD, Chu DC, Owen J, et al, "Maternal Serum Alpha-Fetoprotein and Dimeric Inhibin A Detect Aneuploidies Other Than Down Syndrome," *Am J Obstet Gynecol*, 1998, 179(4):966-70.
7. Wald NJ, Watt HC, and Hackshaw AK, "Integrated Screening for Down Syndrome Based on Tests Performed During the First and Second Trimesters," *N Engl J Med*, 1999, 341(7):461-7.
8. Wallace EM, Crossley JA, Ritoe SC, et al, "Evolution of an Inhibin A ELISA Method: Implications for Down's Syndrome Screening," *Ann Clin Biochem*, 1998, 35(Pt 5):656-64.
9. Copel JA and Bahado-Singh RO, "Prenatal Screening for Down Syndrome - A Search for the Family's Values," *N Engl J Med*, 1999, 341(7):521-2.
10. Aquilina J, Barnett A, Thompson O, et al, "Second-Trimester Maternal Serum Inhibin A Concentration as an Early Marker for Preeclampsia," *Am J Obstet Gynecol*, 1999, 181(1):131-6.
11. Silver HM, Lambert-Messerlian GM, Star JA, et al, "Comparison of Maternal Serum Total Activin A and Inhibin A in Normal, Preeclamptic, and Nonproteinuric Gestationally Hypertensive Pregnancies," *Am J Obstet Gynecol*, 1999, 180(5):1131-7.
12. Cuckle H, Sehmi I, and Jones R, "Maternal Serum Inhibin A Can Predict Preeclampsia," *Br J Obstet Gynaecol*, 1998, 105(10):1101-3.
13. Muttukrishna S, Knight PG, Groome NP, et al, "Activin A and Inhibin A as Possible Endocrine Markers for Preeclampsia," *Lancet*, 1997, 349(9061):1285-8.

References

Haddow JE, Palomaki GE, Knight GJ, et al, "Screening of Maternal Serum for Fetal Down Syndrome in the First Trimester," *N Engl J Med*, 1998, 338(14):955-61.

Hayes FJ, Hall JE, Boepple PA, et al, "Clinical Review 96: Differential Control of Gonadotropin Secretion in the Human: Endocrine Role of Inhibin," *J Clin Endocrinol Metab*, 1998, 83(6):1835-41.

Jackson M and Dudley DJ, "Endocrine Assays to Predict Preterm Delivery," *Clin Perinatol*, 1998, 25(4):837-57, vi.

♦ **Insulin** see C-Peptide, Serum *on page 156*

♦ **Insulin Antibodies** see C-Peptide, Serum *on page 156*

Insulin Antibody, Serum

Related Information
Insulin, Serum *on page 201*

Test Includes Antibodies to both beef and pork insulin

Abstract Essentially all patients treated with beef or pork insulin develop anti-insulin antibodies. Clinically apparent antibody-mediated insulin resistance, however, develops in a very small proportion (0.01%) of treated persons.[1] Patients with insulin antibodies require large doses of insulin. Most anti-insulin antibodies are IgG, but a few are IgE. Assays are performed only in reference laboratories.

Patient Preparation Avoid radioisotopes prior to collection.

Specimen Serum

Container Red top tube

Storage Instructions Serum stable for 7 days at 4°C.

Reference Interval Method dependent. Results may be reported as percent binding of patient's serum to labeled insulin, in which case the reference range is <3%.[2]

Use Determine the presence of antibodies against heterologous insulins. Insulin antibodies may cause misleading results of assays for insulin.

Limitations Anti-insulin antibodies have little clinical significance. Clinical and other biochemical findings are now used to evaluate the syndrome of insulin resistance in patients with type 1 diabetes mellitus.[3]

Methodology Radioimmunoassay (RIA) or enzyme-linked immunosorbent assay (ELISA)

Additional Information Human insulin is less antigenic than are those derived from other species. Insulin antibodies may interfere with insulin assay.

Footnotes

1. Unger RH and Foster DW, "Diabetes Mellitus," *Williams Textbook of Endocrinology*, 9th ed, Wilson JD, Foster DW, Kronenberg HM, et al, eds, Philadelphia, PA: WB Saunders Co, 1998, 1034.
2. Palumbo PJ, Molnar GD, Taylor WF, et al, "Insulin Antibody Binding in Diabetes Mellitus and Facitious Hypoglycemia," *Mayo Clin Proc*, 1969, 44:725-37.
3. Williams KV, Erbey JR, Becker D, et al, "Can Clinical Factors Estimate Insulin Resistance in Type 1 Diabetes?" *Diabetes*, 2000, 49(4):626-32.

References

Despres JP and Marette A, "Relation of Components of Insulin Resistance Syndrome to Coronary Disease Risk," *Curr Opin Lipidol*, 1994, 5(4):274-89.

Greenbaum CJ, Palmer JP, Kuglin B, et al, "Insulin Autoantibodies Measured by Radioimmunoassay Methodology Are More Related to Insulin-Dependent Diabetes Mellitus Than Those Measured by Enzyme-Linked Immunosorbent Assay: Results of the Fourth International Workshop on the Standardization of Insulin Autoantibody Measurement," *J Clin Endocrinol Metab*, 1992, 74(5):1040-4.

Schernthaner G, "Immunogenicity and Allergic Potential of Animal and Human Insulins," *Diabetes Care*, 1993, 16(Suppl 3):155-65.

Taylor SI, Accili D, Haft CR, et al, "Mechanisms of Hormone Resistance: Lessons From Insulin-Resistant Patients," *Acta Paediatr Scand Suppl*, 1994, 399:95-104.

♦ **Insulin-Connecting Peptide** see C-Peptide, Serum *on page 156*

♦ **Insulin-Induced Hypoglycemia Test** see Insulin Tolerance Test *on page 202*

Insulin-Like Growth Factor-1 (IGF-1), Serum or Plasma

Related Information
Growth Hormone, Serum *on page 189*
Insulin-Like Growth Factor Binding Protein 3, Serum *on page 201*
Insulin Tolerance Test *on page 202*

Synonyms IGF-1; IGF-I; Sm-C; Somatomedin-C; Sulfation Factor

Abstract The insulin-like growth factors (IGFs, also called somatomedins) are peptides which are related to the concentration of growth hormone (GH). Two IGFs are of medical interest: IGF-1 (somatomedin C) and IGF-2. The former is used in evaluation of growth disorders,[1] and is generally a better test than is assay for basal- and glucose-suppressed growth hormone. IGF-1 circulates in the body, mostly bound to insulin-like growth factor binding proteins (IGFBPs) mainly IGFBP3 (see Insulin-Like Growth Factor Binding Protein 3, Serum *on page 201*).

Patient Preparation Overnight fast is preferable, no recent administration of radioactivity if assay is to be done by RIA.

Specimen Plasma or serum, depending upon method of assay

Container Lavender top (EDTA) tube (check with the laboratory), red top tube

Storage Instructions Separate plasma immediately by centrifuging at 4°C. Freeze plasma in a plastic tube at -20°C.

Reference Interval GH and IGF-1 are elevated during normal puberty. Values vary with age, sex, and among laboratories. Adults: 130-450 ng/mL. Range is lower in males. It is increased with puberty and pregnancy.[2]

Use An excellent test for acromegaly, in which IGF-1 and GH are increased; evaluate hypopituitarism and hypothalamic lesions in children (diagnosis of dwarfism and response to therapy). IGF-1 is the assay of choice for the diagnosis of acromegaly, since little variation in blood levels is found throughout the day, unlike GH. Used in monitoring growth hormone treatment. Normal IGF-1 results are evidence against growth hormone deficiency, but IGF-1 is not consistently valid to screen for growth hormone deficiency.[2] Low levels occur in undernutrition and Laron dwarfism, an entity in which GH is increased. IGF-1 has been used recently in the treatment of Laron dwarfism.[3] (Laron-type dwarfism is the prototypical syndrome of growth hormone insensitivity.) IGF-1 is used as a measure of effects of growth hormone.[4]

Limitations Malnutrition will cause low IGF-1 levels in spite of normal amounts of circulating growth hormone. The IGF-1 level does not distinguish pituitary dwarfism from constitutional delay of growth and development.[5] Various stimulation tests can distinguish between the two (see Footnote 6 for protocols).

Methodology Radioimmunoassay (RIA) following dissociation from binding protein and chromatography, immunoradiometric assay (IRMA), chemiluminescence immunoassay

Additional Information IGF-1 is a polypeptide hormone produced by the liver and other tissues, with effect on growth promoting activity and glucose metabolism (insulin-like activity). IGF-1 is carried in blood bound to IGF-binding proteins. Its level is, therefore, more constant than that of growth hormones. A single measurement of IGF-1 is considered a true reflection of growth hormone production.

Low values are described with the extremes of age (first 5-6 years and advanced age), hypopituitarism, malnutrition, diabetes mellitus, hypothyroidism, maternal deprivation syndrome, pubertal delay, cirrhosis, hepatoma, Laron dwarfism, and some cases of short stature and normal GH response to pharmacologic tests.[1] Low values may be found with nonfunctioning pituitary tumors, with constitutional delay of growth and development, and with anorexia nervosa.[5]

High values occur with adolescence, true precocious puberty, pregnancy, obesity, pituitary gigantism, **acromegaly**, and diabetic retinopathy.[1]

Since IGF-1 is decreased with malnutrition, its concentration provides a useful index with which to monitor therapy for food deprivation.

Provocative testing is done for assays of growth hormone; IGF-1 provides another approach for evaluation of pituitary GH secretion. Treatment of patients who have acromegaly, with growth-hormone receptor antagonists, results in decrease in IGF-1 and clinical improvement.[6]

Footnotes
1. Jones JI and Clemmons DR, "Insulin-Like Growth Factors and Their Binding Proteins: Biological Actions," *Endocr Rev*, 1995, 16(1):3-34.
2. Vance ML, "Hypopituitarism," *N Engl J Med*, 1994, 330(23):1651-62.
3. Laron Z, "The Essential Role of IGF-1: Lessons From the Long-Term Study and Treatment of Children and Adults With Laron Syndrome," *J Clin Endocrinol Metab*, 1999, 84(12):4397-404.
4. Fazio S, Sabatini D, Capaldo B, et al, "A Preliminary Study of Growth Hormone in the Treatment of Dilated Cardiomyopathy," *N Engl J Med*, 1996, 334(13):809-14.
5. Rosen CJ, "Serum Insulin-like Growth Factors and Insulin-Like Growth Factor-Binding Proteins: Clinical Implications," *Clin Chem*, 1999, 45(8 Pt 2):1384-90.
6. Trainer PJ, Drake WM, Katznelson L, et al, "Treatment of Acromegaly With the Growth Hormone-Receptor Antagonist Pegvisomant," *N Engl J Med*, 2000, 342(16):1171-7.

References
Le Roith D, "Seminars in Medicine of the Beth Israel Deaconess Medical Center. Insulin-Like Growth Factors," *N Engl J Med*, 1997, 336(9):633-40.
Le Roith D and Butler AA, "Insulin-like Growth Factors in Pediatric Health and Disease," *J Clin Endocrinol Metab*, 1999, 84(12):4355-61.
Pintor C, Cella SG, and Baumann G, "Correction and Withdrawal of Conclusion - A Child With Phenotypic Laron Dwarfism and Normal Somatomedin Levels," *N Engl J Med*, 1992, 323(21):1485.
Reiter EO and Rosenfeld RG, "Normal and Aberrant Growth," *Williams Textbook of Endocrinology*, 9th ed, Wilson JD, Foster DW, Kronenberg HM, et al, eds, Philadelphia, PA: WB Saunders Co, 1998, 1470-6.
Rosenfeld RG, "Biochemical Diagnostic Strategies in the Evaluation of Short Stature: The Diagnosis of Insulin-Like Growth Factor Deficiency," *Horm Res*, 1996, 46(4-5):170-3.
Shalet SM, Toogood A, Rahim A, et al, "The Diagnosis of Growth Hormone Deficiency in Children and Adults," *Endocr Rev*, 1998, 19(2):203-23.

Insulin-Like Growth Factor Binding Protein 3, Serum

Related Information
Growth Hormone, Serum *on page 189*
Insulin-Like Growth Factor-1 (IGF-1), Serum or Plasma *on page 200*
Insulin, Serum *on page 201*

Synonyms IGFBP-3; Somatomedins

Abstract Insulin-like growth factors (IGFs), formerly known as somatomedins, circulate in plasma bound to proteins, the insulin-like growth factor binding proteins (IGFBPs), a category which now has 10 members.[1] The serum levels of the IGFs and IGFBPs are, in general, proportional to output of growth hormone (GH). Unlike GH, however, the IGFs and IGFBPs have long serum half-lives and have been investigated as markers of GH secretion. Of all the IGFBPs, IGFBP-3 is the most intensely studied. IGFBP-3 is the most abundant IGFBP in the circulation and binds ~95% of the IGFs in the blood. Originally, it was believed that the major, or only, function of the IGFBPs was to transport the IGFs and modulate their availability to IGF receptors. Recently, however, IGF-independent activities of IGFBP-3 have been identified.[2] In particular, IGFBP-3 is now known to be a potent apoptotic agent, thus inhibiting cell proliferation.

Specimen Serum
Container Red top tube
Reference Interval See table.[3]

Insulin-Like Growth Factor Binding Protein 3, Serum

Age (y)	Male (mg/L)	Female (mg/L)	Age (y)	Male (mg/L)	Female (mg/L)
0-1	0.94-1.79	0.66-2.51	22-23	1.45-4.75	1.45-5.69
2-3	1.12-2.33	0.84-3.77	24-25	1.15-4.27	1.51-4.47
4-5	1.16-3.13	1.32-3.60	26-27	1.24-5.18	1.38-4.70
6-7	1.32-3.38	1.21-4.66	28-29	1.23-4.27	1.19-5.43
8-9	1.35-3.94	1.58-3.99	30-34	1.29-4.06	1.29-4.06
10-11	1.53-5.02	1.93-5.46	35-39	1.50-3.44	1.50-3.44
12-13	1.73-5.11	1.78-6.08	40-44	1.33-3.58	1.33-3.58
14-15	1.90-6.40	2.02-5.44	45-49	1.44-2.75	1.44-2.75
16-17	1.70-6.04	1.88-5.29	50-54	1.31-2.52	1.31-2.52
18-19	1.52-6.01	1.63-6.02	55-59	1.53-2.43	1.53-2.43
20-21	1.79-5.41	1.82-5.35	60-70	1.40-3.22	1.40-3.22

Storage Instructions Refrigerate up to 2 days; freeze thereafter.
Causes for Rejection Recently administered isotopes, if testing is to be done by radioimmunoassay methods; EDTA or heparinized plasma specimen
Use Growth hormone deficiency: Originally proposed as a convenient (because of long half-life) marker of GH activity in the diagnosis of GH deficiency, the clinical accuracy is somewhat less than ideal. For example, Juul et al[4] report the following results, comparing IGFBP-3 against dynamic testing with arginine provocation and clonidine provocation:
- <10 years: 60% sensitivity, 97.9% specificity
- 10-20 years: 56.5% sensitivity, 78.7% specificity

Limitations Poor predictive values (see Use)
Methodology Immunoassays (multiple labels)
Footnotes
1. Rechler MM, "Growth Inhibition by Insulin-Like Growth Factor (IGF) Binding Protein 3 - What's IGF Got to Do With It?" *Endocrinology*, 1997, 138(7):2645-7.
2. Diamandi A, Mistry J, Krishna RG, et al, "Immunoassay of Insulin-Like Growth Factor-Binding Protein-3 (IGFBP-3): New Means to Quantifying IGFBP-3 Proteolysis," *J Clin Endocrinol Metab*, 2000, 85(6):2327-33.
3. ARUP Laboratories, *1999-2000 User's Guide*, 415.
4. Juul A and Skakkebaek NE, "Prediction of the Outcome of Growth Hormone Provocative Testing in Short Children by Measurement of Serum Levels of Insulin-Like Growth Factor 1 and Insulin-Like Growth Factor Binding Protein 3," *J Pediatr*, 1997, 130(2):197-204.

♦ **Insulin-Like Growth Factor-II (IGF-II)** see Insulin, Serum *on page 201*
♦ **Insulin-Like Growth Factors** see Growth Hormone, Serum *on page 189*

Insulin, Serum

Related Information
Ammonia, Plasma *on page 102*
C-Peptide, Serum *on page 156*
Glucose, Fasting, Plasma *on page 183*
Glucose, Random, Plasma *on page 186*
Glucose Tolerance Test, Plasma *on page 186*
Insulin Antibody, Serum *on page 200*
Insulin-Like Growth Factor Binding Protein 3, Serum *on page 201*
Microalbuminuria *on page 879*
Pancreatic Polypeptide, Human, Serum or Plasma *on page 242*

Synonyms Immunoreactive Insulin

Applies to C-Peptide; Insulin-Like Growth Factor-II (IGF-II); Pancreatic Polypeptides; Proinsulin; SUR 1 Mutation

Test Includes Glucose must be drawn simultaneously.

Abstract Within the pancreatic beta cell, the polypeptide, **preproinsulin**, is metabolized via a complex mechanism[1] to three substances which are measured clinically: **proinsulin, insulin,** and **C-peptide,** often collectively referred to as **pancreatic polypeptides**. These analytes are commonly measured in the evaluation of hypoglycemia but are usually not measured in the diagnosis or subsequent management of diabetes mellitus. Observation of onset of symptoms while fasting is relevant as well.[2]

Authoritative opinion[3] holds that disorders variously designated as reactive hypoglycemia, alimentary hypoglycemia, and "early diabetes" hypoglycemia do not exist as scientifically definable entities. Causes of fasting hypoglycemia in both adults and children include islet cell tumor (insulinoma), exogenous insulin or oral hypoglycemic drugs, alcohol use, pituitary or adrenal insufficiency, bulky extrapancreatic tumor, and instances of very severe hepatic disease. In infancy and childhood, there are also familial and sporadic diseases known collectively as persistent hyperinsulinemic hypoglycemia of infancy (PHHI).

Patient Preparation In most instances, patients should be fasting.
Specimen Serum or plasma
Container Red top tube
Storage Instructions Separate serum and freeze until time for assay.
Reference Interval Fasting:[4]
- Infants: 0-12 μIU/mL (SI: 0-90 pmol/L)
- adults: 0-17 μIU/mL (SI: 0-118 pmol/L)

There is moderate interlaboratory variability. Consult with the selected reference laboratory.

Use

Hypoglycemia: Diagnostic criteria for the hypoglycemic disorders (insulinoma, surreptitious insulin administration, and hypoglycemic drug effect) are presented in the discussion of C-peptide. (See C-Peptide, Serum *on page 156*.)

Hypoglycemic disorders of infancy and childhood, in patients who do not have ketosis or acidosis, are usually due to hyperinsulinemia and are collectively referred to as **persistent hyperinsulinemic hypoglycemia of infancy** (PHHI). Clinically subdivided into three forms of varying severity,[5] these disorders share the features of serum glucose <54 mg/dL (SI:<2.9 mmol/L), serum insulin >10 μU/mL (SI: >69.45 pmol/L), and increases in serum C-peptide and proinsulin. The autosomal recessive, clinically most
(Continued)

Insulin, Serum *(Continued)*

severe form, is usually detected within the first few hours of life. An autosomal dominant, less severe form, may be detected anytime in infancy or childhood. A third form, also less severe, is accompanied by hyperammonemia (100-200 µmol N/L). In some children, an additional study involves measuring the glucose response to intravenous glucagon (30 µg/kg[4]) at the time of hypoglycemia; an increase in serum glucose of 40 mg/dL (SI: 2.2 mmol/L) at 10 minutes postinjection[6] is further evidence for PHHI, and also implies that the patient's glycogen stores and glycogenolytic enzymes are intact.[5] Infants with severe PHHI are candidates for pancreatic resection; the decision between partial and near-total resection is guided by intraoperative frozen section of biopsies from the head, body and tail.[7] SUR 1 gene mutations have recently been discussed.[7,8]

Tumor-induced hypoglycemia: Insulinoma (beta-cell tumor) is the most common type of islet cell tumor and is the most common tumor causing hypoglycemia. About 90% are benign. Diagnostic criteria are provided in the listing C-Peptide, Serum *on page 156.* In >85% of cases of insulinoma, proinsulin is >25%; normally it is <25% of total immunoreactive insulin.

Other neoplastic entities causing hypoglycemia include fibrosarcomas, mesotheliomas, leiomyosarcomas, hemangiopericytomas, hepatomas, and carcinomas of stomach, exocrine pancreas, lung, and elsewhere. Most are large. They frequently secrete insulin-like growth factor II (IGF-II). Support for classification as hypoglycemia induced by nonislet cell tumor includes normal to high IGF-II, with low levels of growth hormone, IGF-1, IGF-binding protein 3, and insulin.[2]

A small-cell carcinoma of the uterine cervix, recently reported, was characterized by increased immunoreactive insulin, C-peptide, and proinsulin levels.[9]

Ischemic heart disease: In the Quebec Cardiovascular Study, including 4637 men ages 35-64, high fasting serum insulin levels were identified as an independent risk factor for ischemic heart disease. In this study, subjects who, in 5 years, developed ischemic heart disease had mean fasting serum insulin at entry of 13.3 ±3.9 µIU/L (SI: 92.1 ±27.5 pmol/L); matched controls had a mean fasting serum insulin at entry of 11.26 ±4.1 µIU/mL (SI: 78.2 ±28.8 pmol/L).[10]

Syndrome of insulin resistance: Fasting hyperinsulinemia may be the central defect in a clinical syndrome which includes hypertension, an unfavorable lipid profile, Type II diabetes, obesity, and coronary heart disease. For additional information, see footnotes 11,12,13.

Limitations See Insulin Antibody, Serum *on page 200.*

Methodology Immunoassays (multiple labels)

Additional Information See graphic in listing Microalbuminuria *on page 879* relevant to years of insulin-dependent diabetes and glomerular filtration rate.

Footnotes

1. Sacks DB, *Tietz Textbook of Clinical Chemistry*, 3rd ed, Burtis CA and Ashwood ER, eds, Philadelphia, PA: WB Saunders Co, 1999, 750-808.
2. Le Roith D, "Tumor-Induced Hypoglycemia," *N Engl J Med*, 1999, 341(10):757-8.
3. Service FJ, "Hypoglycemic Disorders," *N Engl J Med*, 1995, 332(17):1144-52.
4. Painter PC, Cope JY, and Smith JL, "Reference Information for the Clinical Laboratory," *Tietz Textbook of Clinical Chemistry*, 3rd ed, Philadelphia, PA: WB Saunders Co, 1999.
5. Sperling MA, "Hypoglycemia," Behrman RE, Kliegman RM, and Jenson HB, eds, *Nelson Textbook of Pediatrics*, 16th ed, Philadelphia, PA: WB Saunders Co, 2000:439-50.
6. Daneman MB, "Disorders of Carbohydrate Metabolism in Infants and Children," *Biochemical Basis of Pediatric Disease*, Soldin SJ, Rifai N, and Hicks JMB, eds, Washington, DC: AACC Press, American Association of Clinical Chemistry, 1992, 261-91.
7. de Lonlay-Debeney P, Poggi-Travert F, Fournet JC, et al, "Clinical Features of 52 Neonates With Hyperinsulinism," *N Engl J Med*, 1999, 340(15):1169-75.
8. Stanley CA and Baker L, "The Causes of Neonatal Hypoglycemia," *N Engl J Med*, 1999, 340(15):1200-1.
9. Seckl MJ, Mulholland PJ, Bishop AE, et al, "Brief Report: Hypoglycemia Due to an Insulin-Secreting Small-Cell Carcinoma of the Cervix," *N Engl J Med*, 1999, 341(10):733-6.
10. Despres JP, Lamarche B, Mauriege P, et al, "Hyperinsulinemia as an Independent Risk Factor for Ischemic Heart Disease," *N Engl J Med*, 1996, 334(15):952-7.
11. Reaven GM, "Pathophysiology of Insulin Resistance in Human Disease," *Physiol Rev*, 1995, 75(3):473-86.
12. Ferrannini E, Haffner SM, Mitchell BD, et al, "Hyperinsulinemia: The Key Feature of a Cardiovascular and Metabolic Syndrome," *Diabetologia*, 1991, 34:416-22.
13. Ferrannini E, "Insulin Resistance, Iron and the Liver," *Lancet*, 2000, 355(9222):2181-2.

References

Dunne MJ, Kane C, Shepherd RM, et al, "Familial Persistent Hyperinsulinemic Hypoglycemia of Infancy and Mutations in the Sulfonylurea Receptor," *N Engl J Med*, 1997, 336(10):703-6.

Glaser B, Kesavan P, Heyman M, et al, "Familial Hyperinsulinism Caused by an Activating Glucokinase Mutation," *N Engl J Med*, 1998, 338(4):226-30.

Insulin Tolerance Test

Related Information

Adrenal Cortex: Laboratory Assessments Overview *on page 84*
Adrenocorticotropic Hormone, Plasma *on page 86*

Corticotropin-Releasing Hormone Stimulation Test *on page 152*
Corticotropin Stimulation Test (Rapid) *on page 153*
Cortisol, Free, Urine *on page 154*
Cortisol, Serum or Plasma *on page 154*
Growth Hormone, Serum *on page 189*
Insulin-Like Growth Factor-1 (IGF-1), Serum or Plasma *on page 200*
Insulin-Like Growth Factor Binding Protein 3, Serum *on page 201*
Insulin, Serum *on page 201*
Metyrapone Stimulation Test, Serum *on page 225*
Urinary Cortisol/Creatinine Increment *on page 296*

Synonyms Insulin-Induced Hypoglycemia Test; ITT

Applies to Corticotropin-Releasing Hormone; Cortisol; Hypothalamic-Pituitary-Adrenal Axis

Abstract The insulin tolerance test (ITT) was introduced into medical practice in 1969 to provide an objective basis for the diagnosis of relative adrenal insufficiency (AI) caused by long-term exogenous corticosteroid medication.[1] The original study included both clinical and biochemical endpoints, and the ITT has become the gold standard for investigation of the hypothalamic-pituitary-adrenal (HPA) axis. Insulin-induced hypoglycemia is a stress which stimulates the release of hypothalamic corticotropin-releasing hormone (CRH). If the HPA axis is intact, hypoglycemia is followed by increases in serum ACTH and cortisol (as well as growth hormone (GH) and prolactin). The ITT is used clinically as a test to evaluate either the functional integrity of the HPA axis or the capacity of the pituitary to release GH.

Patient Preparation The patient must be attended by a physician during this procedure. The patient should fast for at least 8 hours before the test, and remain supine during the procedure. As a precaution, an intravenous preparation of 50% glucose (at least 30 mL) must be available at the bedside, ready for immediate infusion. An intravenous line should be used to inject the insulin (and glucose, if needed) and to obtain blood specimens.

After a baseline blood sample has been obtained, the patient is given regular insulin, 0.1-0.15 units/kg body weight, intravenously. The 0.1 unit/kg dose is preferred for patients with suspected pituitary or adrenal insufficiency. Some authorities recommend increasing the dose to 0.25 units/kg for patients with obesity, "insulin resistance" (see discussion for Insulin, Serum *on page 201*), suspected Cushing syndrome, or suspected acromegaly.[1]

Blood glucose values must be measured stat, ideally at the bedside (see Sampling Time). An adequate hypoglycemic response is variously defined as 40 mg/dL (SI: 2.2 mmol/L)[2] or 35 mg/dL (SI: 1.9 mmol/L).[1] If this degree of hypoglycemia is not achieved, a second dose of insulin is given.

Specimen Serum

Container Red top tube

Sampling Time A baseline sample is always obtained, just before insulin injection. Subsequent specimens are obtained according to one of these schedules: 30 and 45 minutes after insulin;[2] at 30, 60, and 90 minutes after insulin;[3] or 30, 45, 60, and 90 minutes after insulin.[4] Specimens are assayed for glucose (stat), and sent to the laboratory for either cortisol or growth hormone, depending on the purpose of the test.

Reference Interval If the HPA axis is functioning normally, serum cortisol should reach, or exceed, 20 µg/dL (SI: 550 nmol/L).[2,3,4] (The original procedure had the additional criterion of a peak cortisol value which was 5 µg/dL (SI: 138 nmol/L) over baseline.)[1] In normal persons, serum growth hormone should rise to 10 ng/mL.

Use

Adrenal insufficiency (AI): Although the ITT is the gold standard for HPA axis evaluation, in practice the ITT is a tertiary test and, therefore, used only occasionally. For example, if the morning serum cortisol is <5 µg/dL (SI: 140 nmol/L) or if the urine free cortisol (in an adult) is <20 µg/day (SI: 55 nmol/day), the diagnosis of AI is biochemically confirmed and the ITT is not needed. Most patients with AI will be correctly diagnosed with some combination of **primary tests** (see Cortisol, Free, Urine *on page 154*, and Corticotropin Stimulation Test (Rapid) *on page 153*) and **secondary tests** (see Metyrapone Stimulation Test, Serum *on page 225*, Corticotropin-Releasing Hormone Stimulation Test *on page 152*, and Urinary Cortisol/Creatinine Increment *on page 296*).

AI is confirmed if, during the ITT, the cortisol fails to reach 20 µg/dL (SI: 550 nmol/L).

Growth hormone (GH) deficiency: Most patients with GH or insulin-like growth factor (IGF) deficiency are diagnosed using **primary tests** (see Growth Hormone, Serum *on page 189*, Insulin-Like Growth Factor-1 (IGF-1), Serum *on page 200* and Insulin-Like Growth Factor Binding Protein 3, Serum *on page 201*) and **secondary tests** (ie, GH response to various stimuli).[3] Only an occasional patient will require the ITT. **GH deficiency** is confirmed if, during the ITT, serum GH does not reach 10 ng/mL.

Cushing syndrome (CS): The ITT is very rarely indicated in the evaluation of patients with suspected CS. The ITT may be used in a patient to resolve the differential diagnosis of CS vs pseudo-CS. A normal cortisol response to the ITT favors the diagnosis of pseudo-CS (see Adrenal Cortex: Laboratory Assessments Overview *on page 84*).

Contraindications The ITT is contraindicated in persons with seizure disorders, coronary heart disease, and cardiac failure.[3]

Additional Information Burke has published his view that the ITT has no usefulness except in suspected acromegaly.[5]

Footnotes

1. Plumpton FS and Besser GM, "The Adrenocortical Response to Surgery and Insulin-Induced Hypoglycemia in Corticosteroid-Treated and Normal Subjects," *Br J Surg*, 1969, 56(3):216-9.
2. Orth DN and Kovacs WJ, "The Adrenal Cortex," *Williams Textbook of Endocrinology*, 9th ed, Wilson JD, Foster DW, Kronenberg HM, et al, eds, Philadelphia, PA: WB Saunders Co, 1998, 517-664.
3. Demers LM, "Pituitary Function," *Tietz Textbook of Clinical Chemistry*, 3rd ed, Burtis CA and Ashwood ER, eds, Philadelphia, PA: WB Saunders Co, 1999, 1470-95.
4. Thorner MO, Vance ML, Laws ER Jr, et al, "The Anterior Pituitary," *Williams Textbook of Endocrinology*, 9th ed, Wilson JD, Foster DW, Kronenberg HM, et al, eds, Philadelphia, PA: WB Saunders Co, 1998, 249-340.
5. Burke CW, "The Pituitary Megatest: Outdated?" *Clin Endocrinol (Oxf)*, 1992, 36(2):133-4.

References

Cuttler L, Silvers JB, Singh J, et al, "Short Stature and Growth Hormone Therapy," *JAMA*, 1996, 276(7):531-7.
Demers LM and Whitley RJ, "Function of the Adrenal Cortex," *Tietz Textbook of Clinical Chemistry*, 3rd ed, Burtis CA and Ashwood ER, eds, Philadelphia, PA: WB Saunders Co, 1999, 1530-69.
Hoffman DM, O'Sullivan AJ, Baxter RC, et al, "Diagnosis of Growth Hormone Deficiency in Adults," *Lancet*, 1994, 343:1064-8.
Reiter EO and Rosenfeld RG, "Normal and Aberrant Growth," *Williams Textbook of Endocrinology*, 9th ed, Wilson JD, Foster DW, Kronenberg HM, et al, eds, Philadelphia, PA: WB Saunders Co, 1998, 1427-507.
Vance ML and Mauras N, "Growth Hormone Therapy in Adults and Children," *N Engl J Med*, 1999, 341(16):1206-16.

♦ **Integrated Test** see Pregnancy-Associated Protein A, Serum on page 260

♦ **Interleukin-6** see Amylase, Serum on page 102

♦ **Intermediate Density Lipoprotein Cholesterol** see Lipids, Overview on page 213

♦ **Interstitial Cell Stimulating Hormone** see Luteinizing Hormone, Blood or Urine on page 219

♦ **Intramural pH** see pH, Gastric Intramucosal on page 250

♦ **Intrinsic Factor** see Cobalamin, Serum on page 150

♦ **In Vitro Base Excess** see Base Excess, Blood on page 114

♦ **In Vivo Base Excess** see Base Excess, Blood on page 114

♦ **Ion Gap** see Anion Gap, Serum, Plasma, or Urine on page 106

♦ **Ionized Calcium** see Calcium, Ionized, Serum on page 130

♦ **Iontophoresis** see Chloride, Sweat on page 144

Iron and Total Iron Binding Capacity/Transferrin, Serum

Related Information

Anemia Flowchart on page 392
Complete Blood Count on page 419
Copper, Serum on page 816
Deferoxamine Infusion Test on page 819
Erythropoietin, Serum on page 169
Ferritin, Serum on page 173
Hemoglobin on page 442
Hemosiderin Stain, Urine on page 876
Hereditary Hemochromatosis DNA Test on page 709
Iron Stain, Bone Marrow on page 452
Lead, Blood on page 793
Lead, Urine on page 795
Liver Biopsy on page 65
Liver Disease: Laboratory Assessment, Overview on page 216
Occult Blood, Stool on page 315
Phlebotomy, Therapeutic on page 849
Porphyrins, Quantitative, Urine on page 255
Protoporphyrin, Free Erythrocyte on page 269
Protoporphyrin, Zinc, Blood on page 270
Schilling Test on page 483
Transferrin Receptor, Soluble, Serum or Plasma on page 493

Synonyms Fe and TIBC; Iron Binding Capacity; Iron Profile; TIBC; Total Iron Binding Capacity

Applies to Iron Poisoning; Transferrin

Test Includes Serum iron, total iron binding capacity and/or transferrin, percent transferrin saturation

Abstract Diseases of iron homeostasis rank among the most common of human diseases. These include states of **iron deficiency**, including those characterized by **inadequate absorption** (eg, celiac disease, inflammatory bowel disease, bowel resection, dietary causes, bioavailability disorders, and intrinsic red cell defects), and those related to **increased loss**. The latter includes patients with tumors, inflammatory bowel disease, varices, gastritis, ulcer, parasitic infestations, and other gastrointestinal disorders. Genitourinary and other losses are relevant as well.

Diseases of **iron overload** include two major settings. When erythropoiesis is normal but iron exceeds iron binding capacity of transferrin (eg, hemochromatosis), iron is deposited in parenchymal cells of liver and other organs. When catabolism of red cells causes iron overload (eg, transfusional iron overload), Fe is deposited in macrophages of the reticuloendothelial system.[1]

Tests of iron status also include erythrocyte protoporphyrin, serum ferritin, and transferrin saturation, with hemoglobin and other hematologic parameters.

Patient Preparation Specimen should be drawn fasting in the morning (circadian rhythm affects iron; levels are lower in the evening). Sample should be drawn before patient is given therapeutic iron or blood transfusion. Iron determinations on patients who have had blood transfusions should be delayed several days.

Specimen Serum

Container Red top tube

Sampling Time Morning; marked daily variation occurs. Serum iron levels are 30% higher in the morning and blood levels should be determined on fasting AM samples.

Collection Blood should be drawn before other specimens which require anticoagulated tubes. Separate serum from cells as soon as possible.

Storage Instructions Stable 1 week at 4°C

Causes for Rejection Hemolysis

Reference Interval A variety of approaches to the estimation of serum iron, TIBC, and transferrin are in use. Expect normal ranges to vary between laboratories as they are in part method dependent. Iron: 50-160 µg/dL (SI: 9.0-28.8 µmol/L) for adult males; slightly lower (5% to 10%) values for adult females. **Iron binding capacity**: 250-350 µg/dL (SI: 45-63 µmol/L). **Percent saturation (transferrin saturation)**: 20% to 50%, lower in children. **Transferrin**: 200-380 mg/dL (SI: 2.0-3.8 g/L). **TIBC is an approximation of transferrin**. Quantitative assays for transferrin are widely available. A mathematical relationship between TIBC and transferrin can be derived. When transferrin value is known, TIBC can be calculated. TIBC (µg/dL) = transferrin (mg/dL) x 1.25.

Critical Values Transferrin saturation >62% predicts homozygous genotype for hemochromatosis in 92% of cases, but in women, >50% is recommended;[2] vide infra.
• Mild iron toxicity: ≥350 µg/dL (SI: ≥63 µmol/L)
• Serious iron toxicity: 500 µg/dL (SI: 89.5 µmol/L)
• Death from iron toxicity: 1000 µg/dL (SI: 179 µmol/L)

Use Differential diagnosis of anemia, especially with hypochromia and/or low MCV. The **percent saturation** is more helpful than the serum iron to estimate iron stores and iron deficiency anemia. Evaluate thalassemia and possible sideroblastic anemia; work up hemochromatosis, in which iron is increased and iron saturation is high. Decrease in iron level after performance of a Schilling test supports the diagnosis of vitamin B_{12} deficiency, vide infra. Evaluate iron poisoning (toxicity) and overload in renal dialysis patients or patients with transfusion dependent anemias. Use of TIBC in iron toxicity may be less useful than previously believed.[3,4] TIBC or transferrin is a useful index of nutritional status. See table for iron status indicators in various disease states.

Iron Status Indicators in Various Disease States

Disease	Ferritin	Transferrin / TIBC	Serum Iron	Iron Saturation
Uncomplicated iron deficiency	↓	↑	↓	N/↓
Anemia of chronic disease	N/↑	N/↓	↓	N/↓
Sideroblastic anemias	↑	N/↓	N/↑	↑
Hemolytic anemias	↑	N/↓	↑	↑
Hemochromatosis	↑	Slight ↓	↑	↑↑
Protein depletion		N/↓	N/↓	N/↓
Acute liver disease	↑	Var	↑	↑

↑ = increase
↓ = decrease
N = normal
Var = variable

Uncomplicated iron deficiency: Serum transferrin (and TIBC) high, serum iron low, saturation low. Usual causes of depleted iron stores are due to blood loss and inadequate dietary iron. RBCs in moderately severe iron deficiency are hypochromic and microcytic. The red cell distribution width increases and MCV decreases. Stainable marrow iron is absent. Serum ferritin decrease is the earliest indicator of iron deficiency if inflammation is absent.

Anemia of chronic disease: Serum transferrin (and TIBC) low to normal, serum iron low, saturation low or normal, ferritin increased. Transferrin decreases with many inflammatory diseases. With chronic disease there is a block in movement to and utilization of iron by marrow. This leads to low serum iron and decreased erythropoiesis. Examples include acute and chronic infections, malignancy, and renal failure.
(Continued)

Iron and Total Iron Binding Capacity/Transferrin, Serum (Continued)

In inflammatory, infectious, or malignant disease, measurement of usual parameters of iron status may not be sufficient for differentiating iron deficiency anemia from anemia of chronic disease. Bone marrow iron stain is the most definitive assessment of iron status. However, due to complications of bone marrow procedures, a measurement of serum soluble **transferrin receptor (sTfR)** may be useful. Serum soluble transferrin receptor increases in iron deficiency anemia and is usually unaffected in chronic disease; see Transferrin Receptor, Soluble, Serum or Plasma *on page 493*. The transferrin cycle has recently been beautifully diagrammed.[1]

Sideroblastic anemia: Serum transferrin (and TIBC) normal to low, serum iron normal to high, saturation high.

Hemolytic anemias: Serum transferrin (and TIBC) normal to low, serum iron high, saturation high.

Hemochromatosis: Serum transferrin (and TIBC) slightly low, serum iron high, saturation very high. Transferrin saturation >55% with serum ferritin >400 µg/L establishes the diagnosis[2] in the appropriate clinical setting. Liver biopsy can confirm iron overload and represents the gold standard when hepatic iron concentration is measured.[5] **Increased saturation** occurs with HLA-related (classical) hemochromatosis before ferritin is greatly increased, and also with iron overload (eg, cirrhosis and portacaval shunt), in hemolytic anemias, and with iron therapy. Sample contamination and the vagaries of fluctuation in serum iron levels can make percent saturation misleading on occasion. Genetic tests for detecting hemochromatosis mutations (C282Y and H63D) are available. Homozygosity for C282Y mutation is responsible for up to 90% of hemochromatosis patients; see Hereditary Hemochromatosis DNA Test *on page 709*. The H63D mutation has been seen in some patients with heterozygous C282Y mutation, but has reduced penetrance to <2%.[6,7]

Protein depletion: Serum transferrin (and TIBC) may be low, serum iron normal or low (if patient also is iron deficient). This may occur as a result of malnutrition, liver disease, renal disease (eg, nephrosis), or other entities.

Liver disease: Serum transferrin variable; with acute viral hepatitis, high along with serum iron and ferritin. With chronic liver disease (eg, cirrhosis), transferrin may be low. Patients who have cirrhosis and portacaval shunting have saturated TIBC/transferrin as well as high ferritin.

Chronic dialysis for renal failure: Monitor iron levels in patients undergoing dialysis. To follow treatment for iron overload with deferoxamine or with regimen of recombinant human erythropoietin and phlebotomy.[8]

Limitations Except for iron poisoning, a serum iron without TIBC or transferrin is of limited value. Ferritin levels are also useful for iron deficiency. Low iron level may not indicate iron deficiency in acute infection with leukocytosis. Low iron levels may be misleading in chronic infection, inflammation, and malignancy; high ferritin levels occur in many such states. TIBC and transferrin are increased in patients on oral contraceptives, with normal saturation. Transferrin saturation is depressed with acute and chronic inflammation. Gross hemolysis may interfere with serum iron. Some laboratories may have high coefficients of variability, suggesting unacceptable accuracy.[4]

A group of patients exists who have iron-deficiency anemia with normal plasma transferrin concentration.[1]

Deferoxamine, used in therapy of iron toxicity, interferes with TIBC. TIBC may be overestimated in the presence of excessive free iron (ie, iron toxicity), thus, the IBC has only limited value in acute iron overdose.[9] It falsely increases TIBC, and interferes with colorimetric iron methods, causing spuriously low results.[10]

Contraindications Parenteral iron before sample is drawn will cause misleading high iron results. Recent blood transfusion may have only a small positive effect on the serum iron level.

Methodology Ferrozine, bathophenanthroline (iron), nephelometry, turbidimetry (transferrin), $MgCO_3$ column, other methods (TIBC), atomic absorption, anodal stripping, inductively-coupled plasma atomic emission spectroscopy (iron)

Additional Information Serum iron is **increased** in hemosiderosis, hemolytic anemias (especially thalassemia), sideroblastic anemias, hepatitis, acute hepatic necrosis, hemochromatosis, and with inappropriate iron therapy.

Iron may reach high levels with **iron poisoning**, which presents with emesis and severe abdominal pain. Metabolic acidosis with increased anion gap, leukocytosis and hyperglycemia may be found with increased bilirubin, AST, ALT and LD. Pill fragments may be found on abdominal x-ray examination.

Some patients who receive multiple transfusions (eg, some hemolytic anemias, thalassemia, renal dialysis patients) will have increased serum iron levels.

Serum iron is **decreased** with insufficient dietary iron, chronic blood loss (including the hemolytic anemias, paroxysmal nocturnal hemoglobinuria), inadequate absorption of iron, and impaired release of iron stores as in inflammation, infection, and chronic diseases. The combination of low iron, high TIBC and/or transferrin, and low saturation indicates iron deficiency.

Without all of these findings together, iron deficiency is unproven. Low ferritin confirms the diagnosis of iron deficiency. **Detection of iron deficiency may lead to detection of adenocarcinoma of gastrointestinal tract, a point which cannot be overemphasized.**

In recovery from pernicious anemia, especially just after B_{12} dose, iron levels are low. In fact, the **drop in serum iron one to several days after the Schilling test flushing dose** of vitamin B_{12} may be more useful in diagnosis of B_{12} deficiency than the radioactivity of the 24-hour urine collection. Serum iron is reported to drop with acute infarct of myocardium. Changes in TIBC parallel the changes in transferrin.

TIBC is increased in iron-deficiency, use of oral contraceptives, and in pregnancy.

TIBC decreased in hypoproteinemia from many causes, including kwashiorkor, and in a number of inflammatory states.

The serum **ferritin** is usually a more sensitive test than the serum iron or TIBC for iron deficiency and for iron overload. When all these tests are used together, as is often necessary, they usually can distinguish between iron deficiency anemia and the anemia of chronic disease. (See the introduction to Hematology for the Anemia Flowchart *on page 391*.) The best and most reliable evaluation of total body iron stores is by **bone marrow aspiration and biopsy**. The best evaluation of iron deficiency in childhood (unless lead toxicity is suspected) is **free erythrocyte porphyrins**.

With recombinant erythropoietin therapy serum iron, transferrin saturation, and ferritin levels decline due to rapid utilization by stimulated erythropoiesis with resultant decrease in storage iron.[8]

While iron is usually considered in relation to hematopoiesis and oxygen transport functions of red cells, it is also of prime import to the lymphomyeloid systems.[11] The immune response appears to be resistant to alterations in iron status that might impair other systems. It is suggested that cells of the immune system are adapted to have high priority access to iron when supply is low and high level protection against iron related toxicity when supply is in excess.[12]

Footnotes

1. Andrews NC, "Disorders of Iron Metabolism," *N Engl J Med*, 1999, 341(26):1986-94.
2. Edwards CQ and Kushner JP, "Screening for Hemochromatosis," *N Engl J Med*, 1993, 328(22):1616-20.
3. Tenenbein M and Yatscoff RW, "The Total Iron-Binding Capacity in Iron Poisoning. Is It Useful?" *Am J Dis Child*, 1991, 145(4):437-9.
4. Thompson DF, "Reassessment of Measuring Total Iron Binding Capacity in Acute Iron Overdose," *Ann Pharmacother*, 1994, 28(1):63-6.
5. "A 25-Year-Old Man With Congestive Heart Failure and Atrial Fibrillation," Case Records of the Massachusetts General Hospital, Case 1994, Scully RE, Mark EJ, McNeely WF, et al, eds, *N Engl J Med*, 1994, 331(7):460-6.
6. Beutler E, Gelbart T, West C, et al, "Mutation Analysis in Hereditary Hemochromatosis," *Blood Cells Mol Dis*, 1996, 22(2):187-94.
7. Edwards CQ, Griffen LM, Ajioka RS, et al, "Screening for Hemochromatosis: Phenotype Versus Genotype," *Semin Hematol*, 1998, 35(1):72-6.
8. McCarthy JT, Johnson WJ, Nixon DE, et al, "Transfusional Iron Overload in Patients Undergoing Dialysis: Treatment With Erythropoietin and Phlebotomy," *J Lab Clin Med*, 1989, 114(2):193-9.
9. Siff JE, Meldon SW, and Tomassoni AJ, "Usefulness of the Total Iron Binding Capacity in the Evaluation and Treatment of Acute Iron Overdose," *Ann Emerg Med*, 1999, 33(1):73-6.
10. Williams RH and Erickson T, "Evaluating Lead and Iron Intoxication in an Emergency Setting," *Lab Med*, 1998, 29(4):224-31.
11. deSousa M and Brock JH, *Iron in Immunity, Cancer and Inflammation*, New York, NY: John Wiley and Sons, 1989.
12. Kemp JD, "The Role of Iron and Iron Binding Proteins in Lymphocyte Physiology and Pathology," *J Clin Immunol*, 1993, 13(2):81-92.

References

Angelucci E, Brittenham GM, McLaren CD, et al, "Hepatic Iron Concentration and Total Body Iron Stores in Thalassemia Major," *N Engl J Med*, 2000, 343(5):327-31.

Artiss JD, Yang WC, Harake B, et al, "Application of a Sensitive and Specific Reagent for the Determination of Serum Iron to the Bayer DAX48," *Am J Clin Pathol*, 1997, 108(3):269-74.

Beutler E, Felitti V, Gelbart T, et al, "The Effect of HFE Genotypes on Measurements of Iron Overload in Patients Attending a Health Appraisal Clinic," *Ann Intern Med*, 2000, 133(5):329-7.

Brandhagen DJ, Fairbanks VF, Batts KP, et al, "Update on Hereditary Hemochromatosis and the HFE Gene," *Mayo Clin Proc*, 1999, 74(9):917-21.

Brown EB, "Iron Metabolism: A 40 Year Overview," *Am J Med*, 1989, 87(3N):35N-39N.

Bulaj ZJ, Ajioka RS, Phillips JD, et al, "Disease-Related Conditions in Relatives of Patients With Hemochromatosis," *N Engl J Med*, 2000, 343(21):1529-35.

Burns ER, Goldberg SN, Lawrence C, et al, "Clinical Utility of Serum Test for Iron Deficiency in Hospitalized Patients," *Am J Clin Pathol*, 1990, 93(2):240-5.

Feelders RA, Kuiper-Kramer EP, and Van Eijk HG, "Structure, Function, and Clinical Significance of Transferrin Receptors," *Clin Chem Lab Med*, 1999, 37(1):1-10.

Finch CA and Huebers H, "Perspectives in Iron Metabolism," *N Engl J Med*, 1982, 306(25):1520-8.

Fine KD, "The Prevalence of Occult Gastrointestinal Bleeding in Celiac Sprue," *N Engl J Med*, 1996, 334(18):1163-7.

Looker AC, Dallman PR, Carroll MD, et al, "Prevalence of Iron Deficiency in the United States," *JAMA*, 1997, 277(12):973-6.

Oski FA, "Iron Deficiency in Infancy and Childhood," *N Engl J Med*, 1993, 329(3):190-3.

Wharton BA, "Iron Deficiency in Children: Detection and Prevention," *Br J Haematol*, 1999, 106(2):270-80.

♦ **Iron Binding Capacity** *see* Iron and Total Iron Binding Capacity/Transferrin, Serum *on page 203*

♦ **Iron Poisoning** *see* Iron and Total Iron Binding Capacity/Transferrin, Serum *on page 203*

♦ **Iron Profile** *see* Iron and Total Iron Binding Capacity/Transferrin, Serum *on page 203*

♦ **Isocitric Dehydrogenase** *replaced by* Alanine Aminotransferase, Serum *on page 87*

♦ **Isoenzymes of Alkaline Phosphatase** *see* Alkaline Phosphatase Isoenzymes, Serum *on page 92*

♦ **Isoform Ratio** *see* Creatine Kinase Isoenzymes/Isoforms, Serum *on page 157*

♦ **Isoleucine** *see* Amino Acids, Urine *on page 101*

♦ **Isopropyl Alcohol Intoxication** *see* Osmolality, Calculated, Serum or Plasma *on page 234*

♦ **Isovaleric Aciduria** *see* Cerebrospinal Fluid Glycine *on page 142*

♦ **ITT** *see* Insulin Tolerance Test *on page 202*

♦ **Kaliuresis** *see* Potassium, Urine *on page 259*

♦ **Keratan Sulfate** *see* Mucopolysaccharides, Urine *on page 226*

♦ **Ketoamines, Plasma Protein** *see* Fructosamine, Serum *on page 177*

♦ **11-Ketoandrosterone** *see* 17-Ketosteroids Fractionation, Urine *on page 206*

♦ **11-Ketoetiocholanolone** *see* 17-Ketosteroids Fractionation, Urine *on page 206*

17-Ketogenic Steroids, Urine

Synonyms 17-KGS

Abstract 17-KGS, once a mainstay in the work-up of suspected disorders involving the hypothalamic-pituitary-adrenal axis, is now rarely, if ever, needed for this purpose. The test measures the metabolic products of cortisol plus other 21-hydroxysteroids, and this is probably why the results are nonspecific. The test is still available at some reference laboratories; they can be consulted regarding appropriate specimen collection and result interpretation.

Additional Information See Adrenal Cortex: Laboratory Assessments Overview *on page 84*.

Ketone Bodies, Blood

Related Information
Anion Gap, Serum, Plasma, or Urine *on page 106*
Bicarbonate, Blood *on page 115*
Blood Gases and pH, Arterial *on page 119*
Blood Gases and pH, Capillary *on page 121*
Blood Gases and pH, Venous *on page 122*
Glucose, Fasting, Plasma *on page 183*
Glucose, Random, Plasma *on page 186*
Ketones, Urine *on page 877*
Osmolality, Calculated, Serum or Plasma *on page 234*
Osmolality, Serum *on page 236*
pH, Blood *on page 247*
Urea Nitrogen, Serum or Plasma *on page 293*

Synonyms Ketones, Blood; Nitroprusside Reaction, Blood

Applies to Acetoacetate; Acetone; Beta-Hydroxybutyrate; β-Hydroxybutyrate

Abstract Carbohydrate deprivation and increased catabolism of fatty acids leads to increases in the ketone bodies (acetoacetate and acetone). Beta-hydroxybutyrate is also increased and is usually listed with the "ketone" bodies, although it is not a ketone. Blood beta-hydroxybutyrate and acetoacetate are among tests indicated to assess an ill infant or child in whom an inborn error of metabolism is suspected.[1]

Specimen Serum, plasma, or whole blood are acceptable, depending upon assay methodology.

Container Red top tube or green top (heparin) tube

Collection Capillary tubes should be filled as much as possible using technique to avoid air bubbles. Heelsticks should be free flowing. Avoid hemolysis.

Causes for Rejection Hemolysis

Special Instructions Placement of peripheral venous catheter on admission may be useful in selected cases, such as instances of ketoacidosis. Lactic acid, glucose, electrolytes, urea nitrogen, venous or arterial pH should also be measured in possible ketoacidosis, with alcohol level, CBC, and urinalysis if clinically indicated. Serum osmolality is often needed.

Reference Interval Negative in normal nutritional states by semiquantitative/qualitative nitroprusside screening tests (eg, Bayer Acetest® tablets and Bayer Ketostix® reagent strips).

Random quantitative beta-hydroxybutyrate levels in healthy individuals are <0.4 mmol/L;[2] other sources[3] use 0.02-0.27 mmol/L.

Possible Panic Range Positivity of Acetest® in 1:32 dilution indicates severe ketosis; β-hydroxybutyrate level >5.0 mmol/L is consistent with ketoacidosis.

Use Ketone bodies are elevated in metabolic states that lead to lipolysis such as chronic starvation and diabetes mellitus, and are used to assess ketonemia or ketoacidosis resulting from diabetes mellitus, alcoholism, stress, intestinal disorders including emesis, glycogen storage disease (von Gierke's), infantile organic acidemias, and other metabolic disorders. Determination of the presence of ketone bodies is useful when isopropanol ingestion is suspected.

Limitations False negatives or falsely weak reactions may occur. Up to 33% of cases of diabetic ketoacidosis also have lactic acidosis.

The presenting acidosis typical in the ketoacidotic patient shifts the equilibrium away from the ketone bodies (acetoacetate and acetone) and toward formation of beta-hydroxybutyrate. However, beta-hydroxybutyrate is **not** measured by nitroprusside, which reacts only with acetoacetic acid and, to an ~tenfold lesser extent, acetone. **Thus, as the ketoacidosis is treated, a paradoxically more positive positive Acetest® is observed while there is an actual reduction of total plasma ketone body concentration.** Quantitative beta-hydroxybutyrate measurement, therefore, may be preferable to the nitroprusside test,[4,5] though others have concluded otherwise.[6] Ketostix® false positives occur with large amounts of levodopa. Drugs containing free-sulfhydryl groups can give false-positive results in the Acetest®.[7]

Nonketotic coma in diabetes may be caused by hyperosmolarity.

Methodology The nitroprusside reaction with colorimetric endpoint provides the basis of the qualitative/semiquantitative testing that is done using Bayer Acetest® tablets or the qualitative testing done with the Bayer Ketostix® reagent strips. Gas chromatography (GC) and enzymatic methods are used. A rapid, bedside, quantitative beta-hydroxybutyrate test system (GDS STAT-Site®) is available that uses a dry-reagent, enzymatic method. Very recently, a hand-held device for home monitoring has become available that uses an electrochemical sensor for measuring β-hydroxybutyrate.[8]

Additional Information Strongly positive serum acetone without severe acidosis, with normal anion gap, bicarbonate, and plasma glucose suggests the possibility of isopropanol (rubbing alcohol) intoxication. Look for dehydration with ketosis. Ketoacidosis in diabetes usually occurs with decreased plasma pH and bicarbonate, increased glucose and other abnormalities. As ketoacidosis and metabolic acidosis are treated, hypokalemia may become evident. A normal or low potassium on admission of a patient with ketoacidosis may indicate severe potassium depletion. Thus, potassium is especially important among the parameters to follow in treatment of ketoacidosis. Hypophosphatemia may evolve. Acetone may be elevated due to absolute or relative starvation, especially in children. A significant mortality rate exists; in children younger than 10 years of age, diabetic ketoacidosis is reported to account for 70% of diabetes related deaths.[9] Risk factors for cerebral edema in children with diabetic ketoacidosis were recently addressed. They include decreased pCO_2 and increased serum urea nitrogen.[10,11]

A multipoint kinetic method allows determination of acetoacetate, beta-hydroxybutyrate, lactate and pyruvate in a single cuvette.[12]

A recent, large study found the urine ketone dip test (see Ketones, Urine *on page 877*) to have a high sensitivity and a high negative predictive value, respectively, for detecting or excluding diabetic ketoacidosis in hyperglycemic patients.[13]

Footnotes

1. Lindor NM and Karnes PS, "Initial Assessment of Infants and Children With Suspected Inborn Errors of Metabolism," *Mayo Clin Proc*, 1995, 70(10):987-8.
2. Mayo Medical Laboratories, *2000 Test Catalogue*, Rochester, MN.
3. Burtis CA and Ashwood ER, *Tietz Textbook of Clinical Chemistry*, 3rd ed, Philadelphia, PA: WB Saunders Co, 1999.
4. Foreback CC, "β-Hydroxybutyrate and Acetoacetate Levels," *Am J Clin Pathol*, 1997, 108(5):602-4.
5. Umpierrez GE, Watts NB, and Phillips LS, "Clinical Utility of Beta-Hydroxybutyrate Determined by Reflectance Meter in the Management of Diabetic Ketoacidosis," *Diabetes Care*, 1995, 18(1):137-8.
6. Porter WH, Yao HH, and Karounos DG, "Laboratory and Clinical Evaluation of Assays for β-Hydroxybutyrate," *Am J Clin Pathol*, 1997, 107(3):353-8.
7. Csako G and Elin RJ, "Unrecognized False-Positive Ketones From Drugs Containing Free-Sulfhydryl Group(s)," *JAMA*, 1993, 269(13):1634.
8. Byrne HA, Tieszen KL, Hollis S, et al, "Evaluation of an Electrochemical Sensor for Measuring Blood Ketones," *Diabetes Care*, 2000, 23(4):500-3.
9. Bonadio WA, Gutzeit MF, Losek JD, et al, "Outpatient Management of Diabetic Ketoacidosis," *Am J Dis Child*, 1988, 142(4):448-50.
10. Glaser N, Barnett P, McCaslin I, et al, "Risk Factors for Cerebral Edema in Children With Diabetic Ketoacidosis," *N Engl J Med*, 2001, 344(4):264-9.
11. Dunger DB and Edge JA, "Predicting Cerebral Edema During Diabetic Ketoacidosis," *N Engl J Med*, 2001, 344(4):302-3.
12. Nuwayhid NF, Johnson GF, and Feld RD, "Multipoint Kinetic Method for Simultaneously Measuring the Combined Concentrations of Acetoacetate-Beta-Hydroxybutyrate and Lactate-Pyruvate," *Clin Chem*, 1989, 35(7):1526-31.
13. Schwab TM, Hendey GW, and Soliz TC, "Screening for Ketonemia in Patients With Diabetes," *Ann Emerg Med*, 1999, 34(3):342-6.

References

Adrogué HJ and Madias NE, "Management of Life-Threatening Acid-Base Disorders," First of Two Parts, *N Engl J Med*, 1998, 338(1):26-34, Second of Two Parts, *N Engl J Med*, 1998, 338(2):107-11.

(Continued)

Ketone Bodies, Blood *(Continued)*

Hagay ZJ, "Diabetic Ketoacidosis in Pregnancy: Etiology, Pathophysiology, and Management," *Clin Obstet Gynecol*, 1994, 37(1):39-49.

Rosenbloom AL and Hanas R, "Diabetic Ketoacidosis (DKA): Treatment Guidelines," *Clin Pediatr* (Phila), 1996, 35(5):261-6.

Shaffer PA, "Antiketogenesis: Its Mechanism and Significance. 1932 (Classical Article)," *Medicine (Baltimore)*, 1990, 69(5):317-23.

♦ **Ketones, Blood** *see* Ketone Bodies, Blood *on page 205*

♦ **17-Ketosteroids** *see* Dehydroepiandrosterone and Dehydroepiandrosterone Sulfate, Serum or Plasma *on page 164*

17-Ketosteroids Fractionation, Urine

Related Information
Adrenal Cortex: Laboratory Assessments Overview *on page 84*

Synonyms 17-KS Fractionation

Applies to Androsterone; Dehydroepiandrosterone; Etiocholanolone; 11-Hydroxyandrosterone; 11-Hydroxyetiocholanolone; 11-Ketoandrosterone; 11-Ketoetiocholanolone

Test Includes Quantitation of some or all of the following: androsterone, etiocholanolone, and dehydroepiandrosterone (DHEA); these are the three major metabolites of androgens in the urine. Such fractionation may also include 11-ketoandrosterone, 11-ketoetiocholanolone, 11-hydroxyandrosterone, 11-hydroxyetiocholanolone, pregnanediol, pregnanetriol, delta-5-pregnanetriol, and 11-ketopregnanetriol.

Abstract This test is rarely, if ever, needed in the evaluation of endocrine abnormalities. Assays can be obtained from some reference laboratories, which can be consulted regarding appropriate specimen collection and result interpretation.

17-Ketosteroids, Total, Urine

Related Information
Adrenal Cortex: Laboratory Assessments Overview *on page 84*

Dehydroepiandrosterone and Dehydroepiandrosterone Sulfate, Serum or Plasma *on page 164*

Testosterone, Total and Free, Serum or Plasma *on page 280*

Synonyms 17-KS

Abstract Once widely used to investigate endocrine disorders, the test is now rarely, if ever, needed. The assay is available from some reference laboratories, which can be consulted for information relevant to appropriate specimen collection and result interpretation.

♦ **17-KGS** *see* 17-Ketogenic Steroids, Urine *on page 205*

♦ **17-KS** *see* 17-Ketosteroids, Total, Urine *on page 206*

♦ **K⁺, Serum or Plasma** *see* Potassium, Serum or Plasma *on page 258*

♦ **17-KS Fractionation** *see* 17-Ketosteroids Fractionation, Urine *on page 206*

♦ **K⁺, Urine** *see* Potassium, Urine *on page 259*

♦ **Lactate, Blood** *see* Lactic Acid, Whole Blood or Plasma *on page 208*

♦ **Lactate Dehydrogenase, Cerebrospinal Fluid** *see* Cerebrospinal Fluid Lactate Dehydrogenase *on page 142*

Lactate Dehydrogenase Isoenzymes, Serum

Related Information
Anemia Flowchart *on page 392*

Cardiac Markers: Laboratory Assessment, Overview *on page 137*

Cerebrospinal Fluid Lactate Dehydrogenase *on page 142*

Creatine Kinase Isoenzymes/Isoforms, Serum *on page 157*

Infectious Mononucleosis Screening Test *on page 643*

Lactate Dehydrogenase, Serum *on page 207*

Liver Disease: Laboratory Assessment, Overview *on page 216*

Myoglobin, Blood, Serum, or Plasma *on page 228*

Myoglobin, Qualitative, Urine *on page 880*

Troponins, Serum *on page 291*

Synonyms Lactic Acid Dehydrogenase Isoenzymes; LDH Isoenzymes; LD Isoenzymes

Replaces Alpha-Hydroxybutyric Dehydrogenase, Serum

Test Includes Total serum LD (LDH) and electrophoretic quantitation of isoenzymes

Abstract LD is found in all body cells and exists in five molecular forms (isoenzymes). Changes of LD isoenzymes have historically been serially measured following onset of chest pain, to study the relationships of the anodic fractions and to provide information for the differential diagnosis of acute infarct of myocardium (AMI) ("LD_1/LD_2 flip" indicating AMI, peaking after CK and CK-MB). **The troponins are elevated for as long as 4-6 days after myocardial infarct and have essentially eliminated LD isoenzymes for detection of myocardial infarct.** The differential diagnosis of certain other diseases is enhanced with use of LD isoenzymes. LD_5 provides a degree of specificity when liver problems are investigated, and LD_1 is useful in work-up of hemolytic and megaloblastic anemias.

Specimen Serum

Container Red top tube

Sampling Time Cardiac enzymes and isoenzymes are best interpreted as a sequential series, at admission (or initial event) and at subsequent intervals. This applies particularly to CK-MB, troponin I, and myoglobin. LD isoenzymes usually become diagnostic at about 36-55 hours after onset and return to normal 3-14 days after onset. Change in pattern over time is useful to establish diagnosis.

Collection Avoid hemolysis

Causes for Rejection Specimen collected in oxalate, citrate, fluoride, or other anticoagulants

Special Instructions Normal total LD is not necessarily always a contraindication to isoenzymes. $LD_1:LD_2$ flip may be found occasionally in sera in which total LD is within normal range.

Reference Interval Method dependent. Normally LD separates electrophoretically into five bands, each an isoenzyme. One set of normal ranges, based on agarose: LD_1: 22% to 36%, LD_2: 35% to 46%, LD_3: 13% to 26%, LD_4: 3% to 10%, LD_5: 2% to 12%. LD_1 and LD_2 (anodal fractions) are associated with cardiac and RBC origin. LD_5 and LD_4 are associated with hepatic and skeletal muscle origin. LD_2 is greater than LD_1 normally. Thus, the $LD_1:LD_2$ ratio is normally 0.50-0.80. In myocardial damage, such as AMI, there is flip or inversion of $LD_1:LD_2$ (LD_1 becoming greater than LD_2). (Some laboratories use an $LD_1:LD_2$ ratio >0.9 as indicative of a flip. This is method dependent; in other laboratories a moderate fraction of normal employees normally have LD 1:2 of 0.9.) LD_4 is normally less than LD_5, and the normal $LD_5:LD_4$ ratio is up to 0.8.

Possible Panic Range $LD_1:LD_2$ flip in a patient not in a coronary unit, not known to have pernicious anemia or hemolytic anemia.

Use Useful in the differential diagnosis of megaloblastic anemia (folate deficiency, pernicious anemia), hemolytic anemia, and very occasionally renal infarct. These three entities are characterized by LD_1 increases, often with $LD_1:LD_2$ inversion.

The **isomorphic pattern** (total LD significantly high with no significant increase in percentage, of any fraction) is seen with neoplasia, cardiorespiratory diseases, hypothyroidism, infectious mononucleosis, and other inflammatory states, uremia, and necrosis.[1]

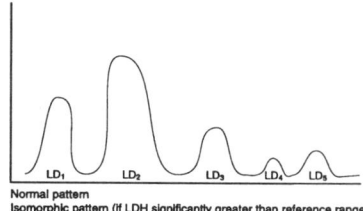

Normal pattern
Isomorphic pattern (if LDH significantly greater than reference range)

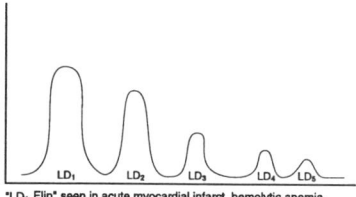

"LD_1 Flip" seen in acute myocardial infarct, hemolytic anemia, megaloblastic anemia, and occasionally in renal injury

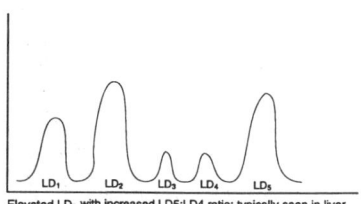

Elevated LD_5 with increased LD5:LD4 ratio; typically seen in liver disease, skeletal muscle injury, and pulmonary edema

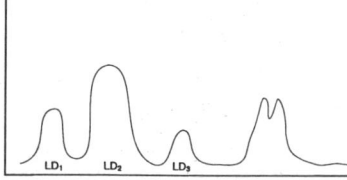

Macroenzyme complex (compare with others)

LD_5 **increases** are seen with striated muscle lesions (eg, trauma) and with liver diseases (eg, hepatic congestion, congestive heart failure, hepatitis, cirrhosis, alcoholism). LD_5 increase is probably more significant when the $LD_5:LD_4$ ratio is increased. LD_5 is considerable more specific for liver disease or injury than are the aminotransferases (AST, ALT), especially when CK is normal.[2] See Liver Disease: Laboratory Assessment, Overview *on page 216*.

In many laboratories, a few percent of normal individuals may have $LD_1:LD_2$ ratios as high as 0.81. A ratio of 0.82-0.99 is suspicious of myocardial injury. A ratio >1.0 is essentially diagnostic of myocardial injury, if other clinical criteria are met, especially in the absence of anemia or increased MCV (ie, without hemolysis or megaloblastic anemia).

Persistent $LD_1:LD_2$ flip following AMI may represent a marker for reinfarction.[3] Especially when AMI is complicated by shock, the isomorphic pattern may be found.[4] $LD_1:LD_2$ inversion commonly appears subsequent to the isomorphic pattern in instances of AMI.[1]

Limitations LDH isoenzymes have been replaced by the troponins for the diagnosis of myocardial infarct. Many laboratories no longer offer this test for the work-up of chest pain.

High-dose allopurinol may diminish activities of LD_1 and LD_2. Tissue-type plasminogen activator may reduce LD_1 activity. Streptokinase may cause broadening of the band between LD_3 and LD_4 and absent LD_5; complex described between LD_3 and IgA. Bismuth subsalicylate increases LD_1 and LD_2. Morphine may increase LD_5, likely due to sphincter spasm.[5]

Methodology Electrophoresis; immunochemical methods have been introduced, including immunoprecipitation.

Additional Information Patterns of LD isoenzymes in acute pulmonary edema include the isomorphic pattern and LD_5 increases.[6] Serum LD increases also in patients with bacterial pneumonia, in whom LD isoenzyme patterns are described.[7]

Macroenzymes, high molecular weight complexes, occur with LD as well as with CK and other enzymes. LD isoenzymes may complex to IgA or IgG. Such LD macroenzymes are characterized by abnormal position of isoenzyme bands, broadening or abnormal motility of a band, and otherwise unexplained increase of total serum LD. Some of these patients have abnormal ANA results and IgG complexes.[8] Some have abnormalities of light chains. Treatment with streptokinase was found to produce a LD-streptokinase complex which was seen as a band at the origin in electrophoresis.[9]

An isoenzyme band cathodal to LD_5 has been called **LD_6**. It is not an immunoglobulin complex. It has occurred in subjects with liver disease and is said to indicate a grave prognosis.[10]

An inverted $LD_5:LD_4$ ratio is not to be confused with $LD_1:LD_2$ ratio. There is evidence that when LD_5 sufficiently exceeds LD_4, liver disease may exist. Such liver disease might be primary or secondary (eg, congestive heart failure). Additional tests which may be useful, if clinically indicated, to work up such possible liver disease or injury might include ALT (SGPT), GGT, serum protein electrophoresis, and prothrombin time. LD_5 is the striated muscle fraction as well as the liver fraction. Although striated muscle problems are usually clinically obvious, occasionally the physician does not get a clinical history of the postictal state or of various withdrawal syndromes. In such situations, serum CK may be helpful.

The association between LD_1 and testicular seminoma has been widely recognized. Its relationship to nonseminomatous testicular tumors as well are described.[11] The ovarian equivalent of seminoma is dysgerminoma, which also may relate to LD_1 increases.[12,13] A variety of malignant tumors are characterized by total LD increases, sometimes with isomorphic patterns[1] or with LD_5 increases.[14] Increase $LD_5:LD_1$ ratio is suggestive of prostatic carcinoma or other cancers.[15]

In a series of 220 patients with carcinoma of breast, LD was the most commonly elevated enzyme. The nonspecificity of single enzyme elevation is well known, but enzymes provide an inexpensive baseline for postoperative follow-up. Enzyme elevation defines a subgroup of patients deserving further evaluation.[16] In malignancy of various types, there is reported an abnormal isoenzyme of LD migrating between albumin and LD_1 on agarose gel electrophoresis.[17]

LD with LD isoenzymes is useful as a tumor marker. Schwartz has outlined applications in adenocarcinoma of lung, colorectal carcinoma, malignant germ cell tumors, and in lymph nodes.[18] LD_3 may be useful in chronic granulocytic leukemia.[19]

Footnotes

1. Jacobs DS, Robinson RA, Clark GM, et al, "Clinical Significance of the Isomorphic Pattern of the Isoenzymes of Serum Lactate Dehydrogenase," *Ann Clin Lab Sci*, 1977, 7(5):411-21.
2. Zimmerman HJ, *Hepatotoxicity: The Adverse Effects of Drugs and Other Chemicals on the Liver*, 2nd ed, Baltimore, MD: Lippincott Williams & Wilkins, 1999, 208-13.
3. Rotenberg Z, Weinberger I, Sagie A, et al, "Lactate Dehydrogenase Isoenzymes in Serum During Recent Acute Myocardial Infarction," *Clin Chem*, 1987, 33(8):1419-20.
4. Rotenberg Z, Weinberger I, Davidson E, et al, "Atypical Patterns of Lactate Dehydrogenase Isoenzymes in Acute Myocardial Infarction," *Clin Chem*, 1988, 34(6):1096-8.
5. Young DS, *Effects of Drugs on Clinical Laboratory Tests*, 5th ed, Volume 1: Listing by Test, Washington, DC: AACC Press, American Association for Clinical Chemistry, 2000, Section 3, 491.
6. Rotenberg Z, Weinberger I, Davidson E, et al, "Patterns of Lactate Dehydrogenase Isoenzymes in Serum of Patients With Acute Pulmonary Edema," *Clin Chem*, 1988, 34(9):1882-4.
7. Rotenberg Z, Weinberger I, Davidson E, et al, "Significance of Isolated Increases in Total Lactate Dehydrogenase and Its Isoenzymes in Serum of Patients With Bacterial Pneumonia," *Clin Chem*, 1988, 34(7):1503-5.
8. Gorus F, Aelbrecht W, and Van Camp B, "Circulating IgG-LD Complex, Dissociable by Addition of NAD+," *Clin Chem*, 1982, 28(1):236-9.

9. Podlasek SJ, DuFour DR, and McPherson RA, "Alterations in Lactate Dehydrogenase Isoenzyme Patterns After Therapy With Streptokinase or Streptococcal Infection," *Clin Chem*, 1989, 35(8):1763-6.
10. Wolf PL, "Lactate Dehydrogenase-6. A Biochemical Sign of Serious Hepatic Circulatory Disturbance," *Arch Intern Med*, 1985, 145(8):1396-7.
11. Law TM, Motzer RJ, Bajorin DF, et al, "The Management of Patients With Advanced Germ Cell Tumors - Seminoma and Nonseminoma," *Urol Clin North Am*, 1994, 21(14):773-83.
12. Schwartz PE and Morris JM, "Serum Lactic Dehydrogenase: A Tumor Marker for Dysgerminoma," *Obstet Gynecol*, 1988, 72(3 Pt 2):511-5.
13. Yoshimura T, Takemori K, Okazaki T, et al, "Serum Lactic Dehydrogenase and Its Isoenzymes in Patients With Ovarian Dysgerminoma," *Int J Gynaecol Obstet*, 1988, 27(3):459-65.
14. Rotenberg Z, Weinberger I, Sagie A, et al, "Total Lactate Dehydrogenase and Its Isoenzymes in Serum of Patients With Non-Small-Cell Lung Cancer," *Clin Chem*, 1988, 34(4):668-70.
15. Manzo V, Sun T, and Lien YY, "Misdiagnosis of Acute Myocardial Infarction," *Ann Clin Lab Sci*, 1990, 20(5):324-8.
16. Clark CP 3d, Foreman ML, Peters GN, et al, "Efficacy of Preoperative Liver Function Tests and Ultrasound in Detecting Hepatic Metastasis in Carcinoma of the Breast," *Surg Gynecol Obstet*, 1988, 167(6):510-4.
17. Giannoulaki EE, Kalpaxis DL, Tentas C, et al, "Lactate Dehydrogenase Isoenzyme Pattern in Sera of Patients With Malignant Diseases," *Clin Chem*, 1989, 35(3):396-9.
18. Schwartz MK, "Lactic Dehydrogenase: An Old Enzyme Reborn as a Cancer Marker?" *Am J Clin Pathol*, 1991, 96(4):441-3.
19. Buchsbaum RM, Liu FJ, and Trujillo JM, "Serum Lactate Dehydrogenase-3 Isoenzyme in Chronic Granulocytic Leukemia," *Am J Clin Pathol*, 1991, 96(4):464-9.

References

Kagawa FT, Kirsch CM, Yenokida GG, et al, "Serum Lactate Dehydrogenase Activity in Patients With AIDS and *Pneumocystis carinii* Pneumonia: An Adjunct to Diagnosis," *Chest*, 1988, 94(5):1031-3.

Wukich DK, Callaghan JJ, Graeber GM, et al, "Operative Treatment of Acute Hip Fractures: Its Effect on Serum Creatine Kinase, Lactate Dehydrogenase and Their Isoenzymes," *J Trauma*, 1989, 29(3):375-9.

Lactate Dehydrogenase, Serum

Related Information

Alanine Aminotransferase, Serum *on page 87*
Anemia Flowchart *on page 392*
Aspartate Aminotransferase, Serum *on page 112*
Body Fluid Lactate Dehydrogenase *on page 125*
Cardiac Markers: Laboratory Assessment, Overview *on page 137*
Creatine Kinase, Serum *on page 158*
Hemosiderin Stain, Urine *on page 876*
Hepatitis B Core Antibody *on page 622*
Hepatitis C Virus RNA Detection and Quantitation *on page 626*
Infectious Mononucleosis Screening Test *on page 643*
Lactate Dehydrogenase Isoenzymes, Serum *on page 206*
Liver Disease: Laboratory Assessment, Overview *on page 216*
Myoglobin, Blood, Serum, or Plasma *on page 228*

Synonyms Lactic Acid Dehydrogenase; LD; LDH

Applies to LDH:AST Ratio

Abstract LD, an enzyme in the glycolytic pathway, catalyzes the interconversion of lactate and pyruvate. Released with cell damage (eg, hypoxia, necrosis), it is increased in a wide variety of neoplastic states and in other disease entities. Some correlation with tumor bulk exists. High serum LDH before treatment is an adverse risk factor for non-Hodgkin lymphoma.

Specimen Serum, body fluid

Container Red top tube, serum separator tube is acceptable. Green top (heparin) tube is also acceptable.

Storage Instructions Stable 2-3 days at room temperature.

Causes for Rejection Hemolysis in collection of sample

Reference Interval Normal ranges for serum LD vary among methods. They are higher in childhood. For adults, in most laboratories, the range is up to ~200 units/L for lactate to pyruvate assays which are by far the most common.

Lactate Dehydrogenase

Age	Units/L
0-2 y	125-275
2-3 y	166-232
3-4 y	112-221
4-5 y	108-206
5-6 y	104-205
6-7 y	100-204
7-8 y	95-203
8-12 y	90-201
12-14 y	90-199
14-16 y	Up to 168
16-17 y	Up to 161
17-43 y	90-156
≥43 y	90-176

(Continued)

Lactate Dehydrogenase, Serum (Continued)

Use Causes of **high LD**: **Neoplastic states** (especially with high alkaline phosphatase, very high total LD, and isomorphic pattern of LD isoenzymes) or with LD_5 increase. High LDH may be found with lymphomas, leukemias, tumors of testis, neuroblastoma, and with a variety of carcinomas, including primaries of lung, breast, pancreas, and gastrointestinal tract. High LDH may be found with **hypoxia; cardiorespiratory diseases**, including cardiac failure and myocarditis (LDH is especially elevated in patients with HIV and *Pneumocystis* pneumonia); **hemolytic anemia,** including that secondary to prosthetic cardiac valves; **megaloblastic anemias**, including pernicious anemia (levels may be >2000 units/L and LD isoenzymes reveal LD_1:LD_2 flip); **infectious mononucleosis; inflammation; hypothyroidism** (some cases); **myocardial infarct**: LD begins to rise about 12 hours after infarct and remains elevated for up to 1-2 weeks after CK and AST have returned to normal; isoenzymes usually most useful 48 hours from onset of infarct to reveal LD_1:$LD_2 \geq 1.0$ ("flip"); **pulmonary infarct** (LD increase is typically present, sometimes with the triad of LD, bilirubin, AST increases); other **lung diseases**.

Diseases of **liver**, including cirrhosis. Total LD in cirrhosis is usually not greatly increased. In acute viral hepatitis, LD is not notably elevated and AST is usually three or more times higher (in relation to the upper limit of normal) than LD; **chronic alcoholism** is usually associated with some combination of elevated MCV (mean corpuscular volume), triglyceride, alkaline phosphatase, AST (SGOT), ALT (SGPT), GGT, and bilirubin with low folate.

Renal infarct - high LD, out of proportion to AST and alkaline phosphatase; **seizures, other CNS diseases**; acute **pancreatitis; collagen diseases**; excessive **destruction of cells; fracture**, other **trauma**, including head trauma, **muscle damage; muscular dystrophy; focal necrosis; shock, hypotension; intestinal obstruction**.

LD isoenzymes may be useful in the diagnosis of a number of the disease states mentioned above including myocardial infarction, neoplastic states, hemolytic anemia, megaloblastic anemias including pernicious anemia, infectious mononucleosis, some cases of hypothyroidism, diseases of the liver, renal infarct, and excessive destruction of cells, especially in hematopoietic neoplasms. See Lactate Dehydrogenase Isoenzymes, Serum *on page 206*.

Other causes of increased LD include specimen tube artifact, such as serum contact with clot or exposure to heat. Test profile with very high LD and no glucose may relate to unseparated serum and cells in a tube at room temperature or higher.

Useful with protein in initial assessment of pleural effusion.[1]

Limitations Artifactual as well as clinical hemolysis elevates LD results. Oxalate inhibits LD. Physiological serum decrease may be seen with anticonvulsants. Analytical serum increases include method-dependent observations relevant to acetaminophen, fluosol-DA, and phenobarbital. Physiological serum increases may be seen with amiodarone, anabolic steroids, dicumarol, gentamicin, isotretinoin, methotrexate, nitrofurantoin, penicillamine, sulfisoxazole, valproic acid, and other drugs.[2]

Methodology Lactate to pyruvate monitored at 340 nm is predominant method but pyruvate to lactate is rarely used. Pyruvate to lactate assay produces values about twice those of the lactate to pyruvate method. The temperature is usually 37°C but 30°C is very seldom used.

Additional Information In **infectious mononucleosis**, LD is usually more elevated than AST, and there is usually an isomorphic pattern of LD isoenzymes. In **viral hepatitis**, by contrast, AST and ALT (the aminotransferases or transaminases) are much more increased than is LD, about three or more times higher than total LD, and LD_5 is high. The differential diagnosis of acute infarct of myocardium includes pericarditis and angina, entities in which enzymes are usually not substantially increased. LD is useful in selected settings as a tumor marker,[3,4,5,6,7] but LD is not helpful as a screening test for cancer. Tumor burden in Hodgkin disease and non-Hodgkin lymphoma is estimated by serum LDH concentration and disease stage.[8] High pretreatment concentrations of serum LDH are an important adverse risk factor in subjects with non-Hodgkin lymphoma and with small cell carcinoma of lung.[9] Increases may be found with dysgerminoma of ovary, seminoma of testis and other germ cell tumors, neuroblastoma, and a wide variety of other neoplastic states. High serum LDH has been described as a marker for drug resistance with high tumor volume in multiple myeloma.[10] (Other applications as a tumor marker are included in the listing Lactate Dehydrogenase Isoenzymes, Serum *on page 206*.)

LDH:AST ratio >18, in patients with biliary pancreatitis, has been proposed as an indicator of pancreatic necrosis.[11]

Footnotes

1. Dev D and Basran GS, "Pleural Effusion: A Clinical Review," *Monaldi Arch Chest Dis*, 1994, 49(1):25-35.
2. Young DS, *Effects of Drugs on Clinical Laboratory Tests*, 5th ed, Volume 1, Listing by Test, Washington, DC: AACC Press, American Association for Clinical Chemistry, 2000, Section 3, 486-91.
3. Barlogie B, Smallwood L, Smith T, et al, "High Serum Levels of Lactate Dehydrogenase Identify a High-Grade Lymphoma-Like Myeloma," *Ann Intern Med*, 1989, 110(7):521-5.
4. Farley FA, Healey JH, Caparros-Sison B, et al, "Lactase Dehydrogenase as a Tumor Marker for Recurrent Disease in Ewing's Sarcoma," *Cancer*, 1987, 59(7):1245-8.

5. Ganz PA, Ma PY, Wang HJ, et al, "Evaluation of Three Biochemical Markers for Serially Monitoring the Therapy of Small-Cell Lung Cancer," *J Clin Oncol*, 1987, 5(3):472-9.
6. Hamrick RM III and Murgo AJ, "Lactate Dehydrogenase Values and Bone Scans as Predictors of Bone Marrow Involvement in Small-Cell Lung Cancer," *Arch Intern Med*, 1987, 147(6):1070-1.
7. Schwartz MK, "Lactic Dehydrogenase: An Old Enzyme Reborn as a Cancer Marker?" *Am J Clin Pathol*, 1991, 96(4):441-3.
8. Sandlund JT, Downing JR, and Crist WM, "Non-Hodgkin Lymphoma in Childhood," *N Engl J Med*, 1996, 334(19):1238-48.
9. Stokkel MP, van Eck-Smit BL, Zwinderman AH, et al, "Pretreatment Serum LDH as Additional Staging Parameter in Small-Cell Lung Carcinoma," *Neth J Med*, 1998, 52(2):65-70.
10. Dimopoulos MA, Barlogie B, Smith TL, et al, "High Serum Lactate Dehydrogenase Level as a Marker for Drug Resistance and Short Survival in Multiple Myeloma," *Ann Intern Med*, 1991, 115(12):931-5.
11. Isogai M, Yamaguchi A, Hori A, et al, "LDH:AST Ratio in Biliary Pancreatitis - a Possible Indicator of Pancreatic Necrosis: Preliminary Results," *Am J Gastroenterol*, 1998, 93(3):363-7.

References

Gulbis B, Unger P, Lenaers A, et al, "Mass Concentration of Creatine Kinase MB Isoenzyme and Lactate Dehydrogenase Isoenzyme 1 in Diagnosis of Perioperative Myocardial Infarction After Coronary Bypass Surgery," *Clin Chem*, 1990, 36(10):1784-8.

Hornykewyez S, Gabriel H, and Huber K, "Biochemical Markers of Myocardial Necrosis in Acute Myocardial Infarction and Thrombolysis," *Ann Hematol*, 1994, 69(4):S59-63.

Kagawa FT, Kirsch CM, Yenokida GG, et al, "Serum Lactate Dehydrogenase Activity in Patients With AIDS and *Pneumocystis carinii* Pneumonia: An Adjunct to Diagnosis," *Chest*, 1988, 94(5):1031-3.

Kantoff PW and Oliva E, "A 27-Year-Old Man With a Painful Retroperitoneal Mass," Case Records of the Massachusetts General Hospital, Case 1-2000, Scully RE, Mark EJ, McNeely WF, et al, eds, *N Engl J Med*, 2000, 342(2):115-22.

Reis GJ, Kaufman HW, Horowitz GL, et al, "Usefulness of Lactate Dehydrogenase and Lactate Dehydrogenase Isoenzymes for Diagnosis of Acute Myocardial Infarction," *Am J Cardiol*, 1988, 61(10):754-8.

Ulbright TM, "Protocol for the Examination of Specimens From Patients With Malignant Germ Cell and Sex Cord-Stromal Tumors of the Testis, Exclusive of Paratesticular Malignancies," *Arch Pathol Lab Med*, 1999, 123(1):14-9.

♦ **Lactic Acid, Body Fluid** *see* Body Fluid Chemical Analysis *on page 123*

♦ **Lactic Acid, Cerebrospinal Fluid** *see* Cerebrospinal Fluid Lactic Acid *on page 143*

♦ **Lactic Acid Dehydrogenase** *see* Lactate Dehydrogenase, Serum *on page 207*

♦ **Lactic Acid Dehydrogenase, Fluid** *see* Cerebrospinal Fluid Lactate Dehydrogenase *on page 142*

♦ **Lactic Acid Dehydrogenase Isoenzymes** *see* Lactate Dehydrogenase Isoenzymes, Serum *on page 206*

Lactic Acid, Whole Blood or Plasma

Related Information

Ammonia, Plasma *on page 102*
Anion Gap, Serum, Plasma, or Urine *on page 106*
Cyanide, Blood *on page 787*
Ethanol, Blood, Urine, and Other Sources *on page 789*
Ibuprofen, Serum *on page 793*
pH, Blood *on page 247*
Salicylate, Serum or Plasma *on page 806*

Synonyms Blood Lactate; Lactate, Blood

Applies to Biotin; D-Lactate; Metformin; Oxygen Transport; Phenformin

Abstract Lactate (lactic acid), an intermediate in carbohydrate metabolism, is formed from pyruvate (pyruvic acid) in the process of glycolysis in skeletal muscle, erythrocytes, brain, skin, and kidney. Strenuous exercise can produce a 10- or 15-fold increase in venous plasma lactate within several seconds. Blood lactate is lowest during fasting and reaches the upper end of the reference range in the postprandial state. **Lactic acidosis**, with elevated blood lactate, occurs in two clinical contexts. **Type A** lactic acidosis is due to hypoxia and is the more common form; **type B** lactic acidosis does not develop from hypoxia and may be due to drugs, inborn errors of metabolism, severe liver disease, or a metabolic myopathy.[1,2]

Patient Preparation Mannitol interference is described for a whole-blood analysis method.[3]

Specimen Whole blood, arterial or venous, or plasma, *vide infra*. Arterial blood is preferred, since contraction of muscles can cause increase in lactate in venous blood.

Container Gray top (sodium fluoride) tube; heparinized syringe, heparin-containing tube, anaerobic draw,[4] depending upon available instrumentation

Collection Avoid hand-clenching, and if possible use of a tourniquet. A tourniquet or a patient clenching and unclenching his/her hand will lead to build-up of potassium and lactic acid from the hand muscles.

Lactic acid is commonly needed with or as stat follow-up to venous or arterial pH. Serial determinations are often valuable.[5] **Send specimen on wet ice.**

Storage Instructions Centrifuge immediately and take off plasma (unless laboratory uses a whole blood method). Keep plasma on ice or at 2°C to 8°C, analyze promptly. A study of blood handling techniques and their effect on lactate concentration has been published.[6]

Causes for Rejection Specimen not received on ice

Turnaround Time Good agreement between whole blood and plasma lactate is reported. Use of whole blood enhances turnaround time.[3,4]

Special Instructions Keep tube on ice until delivered. Tube must be processed within 15 minutes of being drawn.

Reference Interval See table.

Whole Blood Lactate		
	mmol/L*	mg/dL*
Venous		
at rest	0.5-1.3	5-11
in hospital	0.9-1.7	8-15
Arterial		
at rest	0.36-0.75	3-7
in hospital	0.36-1.25	3-11
Plasma Lactate		
	mmol/L†	mg/dL†
Venous	0.5-2.2	4.5-19.8
Arterial	0.5-1.6	4.5-14.4

*Sacks DB, "Carbohydrates," *Tietz Textbook of Clinical Chemistry*, 3rd ed, Burtis CA and Ashwood ER, eds, Philadelphia, PA: WB Saunders Co, 1999, 789.

†Painter PC, Cope JY, and Smith JL, "Reference Information for the Clinical Laboratory," *Tietz Textbook of Clinical Chemistry*, 3rd ed, Burtis CA and Ashwood ER, eds, Philadelphia, PA: WB Saunders Co, 1999, 1822.

Critical Values In general, an inverse relationship between hyperlactatemia and survival exists; high blood lactate serves as a prognostic indicator in critically ill patients. Lactate >36 mg/dL (4 mmol/L) is a strong predictor of need for hospital admission from Emergency Department (ED) as well as predictor of mortality.[4]

Possible Panic Range ≥45.0 mg/dL

Use The differential diagnosis of type A lactic acidosis includes hypoxemia (eg, carbon monoxide, anemia, methemoglobinemia, respiratory failure), hypotension, shock, decreased perfusion, and strenuous exercise.[7] Increased lactate concentrations have a predictive value for acute myocardial infarction with EKG findings. Possible causes of type B lactic acidosis include ethanol, methanol, ethylene glycol, phenformin, cyanide, nitroprusside, salicylate, nalidixic acid, streptozocin, diabetes, liver failure, renal failure, infection, systemic malignancy, and inborn errors of metabolism.[7]

Lactic acid determination is generally indicated if anion gap is >20 mmol/L and if pH is <7.25 and the pCO_2 is not elevated.

Suspect lactic acidosis when unexplained high anion gap metabolic acidosis is encountered, especially if azotemia or ketoacidosis are not present; see Anion Gap, Serum, Plasma, or Urine *on page 106*.

Fetal scalp lactate may have a role in evaluation of intrapartum fetal asphyxia.[8]

Limitations Gross hemolysis depresses results. Intravenous injections or infusions which modify acid-base balance, may cause alterations in lactate levels. Epinephrine and exercise elevate lactate, as may I.V. sodium bicarbonate, glucose, and hyperventilation. False low values with a high LD (LDH) value.

Normal L-lactate occurs with high D-lactate in **D-lactic acidosis**. Metabolic acidosis following jejunoileal bypass for obesity, related to altered gastrointestinal flora, may develop in subjects who develop dysarthria, cerebellar ataxia, and confusion as well, in whom D-lactate is the causative anion. The common laboratory methods do not measure D-lactate. Although jejunoileal bypass is presently rarely performed, a number of individuals have short bowel syndrome secondary to inflammatory bowel disease, vascular disease, and other settings in which a short small intestine is present with an intact colon. Excessive D-lactate production by abnormal flora may develop. Normal D-lactate levels are 0-0.25 mmol/L. Increased anion gap and low bicarbonate are found.[9,10]

The reliability of lactate as an indicator of hypoxia in injury or sepsis has recently been discussed relevant to aerobic glycolysis.[11]

Contraindications Absence of acidosis is **not** a contraindication for this test.

Methodology Enzymatic; other methods include gas chromatography (GC), amperometric, enzymatic, substrate-specific electrode.[4] Whole blood analysis by trilayer-biosensors is available.[3]

Additional Information When lactate is <45 mg/dL (SI: <5.0 mmol/L), suspect carbohydrate infusions, exercise, diabetic ketoacidosis, or ethanol. When lactate is >45 mg/dL, suspect shock, severe anemia, severe congestive failure, or systemic malignancy.

Additional factors which affect lactate levels include glycolysis, catabolism, hepatic metabolism, and pyruvate dehydrogenase. Unlike phenformin (which was removed from the market in the U.S. in 1977, but is available in other countries), metformin is relatively safe. It bears a risk of lactic acidosis of about three cases per 100,000 patient-years, and the risk is found predominantly in subjects whose renal function is impaired. Used in patients without hypoxia or renal impairment, metformin would not be anticipated to cause lactic acidosis.[12,13]

Lactate is increased with mesenteric ischemia, bacterial peritonitis and was found in half of a series of instances of intestinal obstruction.[14]

Lactic acidosis with hepatic steatosis associated with stavudine is reported.[15]

Footnotes

1. Sacks DB, "Carbohydrates," *Tietz Textbook of Clinical Chemistry*, 3rd ed, Burtis CA and Ashwood ER, eds, Philadelphia, PA: WB Saunders Co, 1999, 789.
2. Marshall WJ, "Hydrogen Ion Homeostasis, Tissue Oxygenation and Their Disorders," *Clinical Biochemistry*, Marshall WJ and Bangert SK, eds, New York, NY: Churchill Livingstone, 1995, 61-86.
3. Kost GJ, Nguyen TH, and Tang Z, "Whole-Blood Glucose and Lactate. Trilayer Biosensors, Drug Interference, Metabolism, and Practice Guidelines," *Arch Pathol Lab Med*, 2000, 124(8):1128-34.
4. Aduen J, Bernstein WK, Khastgir T, et al, "The Use and Clinical Importance of a Substrate-Specific Electrode for Rapid Determination of Blood Lactate Concentrations," *JAMA*, 1994, 272(21):1678-85.
5. Artiss JD, Karcher RE, and Cavanaugh KT, "A Liquid-Stable Reagent for Lactic Acid Levels - Application to the Hitachi 911 and Beckman CX7," *Am J Clin Pathol*, 2000, 114(1):139-43.
6. Bishop PA, May M, Smith, JF, et al, "Influence of Blood Handling Techniques on Lactic Acid Concentrations," *Int J Sports Med*, 1992, 13(1):56-9.
7. Desai SP and Isa-Pratt S, *Clinician's Guide to Laboratory Medicine*, Cleveland, OH: Lexi-Comp Inc, 2000, 234-5.
8. Westgren M, Kruger K, Ek S, et al, "Lactate Compared With pH Analysis at Fetal Scalp Blood Sampling: A Prospective Randomised Study," *Br J Obstet Gynaecol*, 1998, 105(1):29-33.
9. Uribarri J, Oh MS, and Carroll HJ, "D-Lactic Acidosis. A Review of Clinical Presentation, Biochemical Features, and Pathophysiologic Mechanisms," *Medicine*, 1998, 77(2):73-82.
10. Vella A and Farrugia G, "D-Lactic Acidosis: Pathologic Consequences of Saprophytism," *Mayo Clin Proc*, 1998, 73(5):451-6.
11. James JH, Luchette FA, McCarter FD, et al, "Lactate Is an Unreliable Indicator of Tissue Hypoxia in Injury or Sepsis," *Lancet*, 1999, 354(9177):505-8.
12. Crofford OB, "Metformin," *N Engl J Med*, 1995, 333(9):588-9.
13. Chan NN, Brain HP, and Feher MD, "Metformin-Associated Lactic Acidosis: a Rare or Very Rare Clinical Entity?" *Diabet Med*, 1999, 16(4):273-81.
14. Lange H and Jäckel R, "Usefulness of Plasma Lactate Concentration in the Diagnosis of Acute Abdominal Disease," *Eur J Surg*, 1994, 160(6-7):381-4.
15. Miller KD, Cameron M, Wood LV, et al, "Lactic Acidosis and Hepatic Steatosis Associated With Use of Stavudine: Report of Four Cases," *Ann Intern Med*, 2000, 133(3):192-6.

References

Adrogue HJ and Madias NE, "Medical Progress: Management of Life-Threatening Acid-Base Disorders (First of Two Parts)," *N Engl J Med*, 1998, 338(1):26-34.

Forsythe SM and Schmidt GA, "Sodium Bicarbonate for the Treatment of Lactic Acidosis," *Chest*, 2000, 117(1):260-7.

Hood VL and Tannen RL, "Protection of Acid-Base Balance by pH Regulation of Acid Production," *N Engl J Med*, 1998, 339(12):819-26.

Prayson RA and Wang N, "Mitochondrial Myopathy, Encephalopathy, Lactic Acidosis, and Strokelike Episodes (MELAS) Syndrome," *Arch Pathol Lab Med*, 1998, 122(11):978-81.

Stacpoole PW, "Lactic Acidosis," *Endocrinol Metab Clin North Am*, 1993, 22(2):221-45.

Stacpoole PW, "Lactic Acidosis and Other Mitochondrial Disorders," *Metabolism*, 1997, 46(3):306-21.

Toffaletti J, "Elevations in Blood Lactate: Overview of Use in Critical Care," *Scand J Clin Lab Invest Suppl*, 1996, 224:107-10.

Toffaletti J, "Physiology and Regulation. Ionized Calcium, Magnesium and Lactate Measurements in Critical Care Settings," *Am J Clin Pathol*, 1995, 104(4 Suppl 1):S88-94.

Lactose Tolerance Test

Related Information
d-Xylose Absorption Test, Serum, Urine *on page 167*
Fat, Semiquantitative, Stool, Sudan III Stain *on page 306*
Fecal Fat by Near-Infrared Reflectance Analysis *on page 307*
Fecal Fat, Quantitative, 72-Hour Collection *on page 172*
pH, Stool *on page 317*
Reducing Substances, Stool *on page 317*

Synonyms Tolerance Test, Lactose

Applies to Breath Hydrogen Analysis

Test Includes Fasting, 30-, 60-, 120-, 180-, and 240-minute glucose measurements after oral lactose challenge

Abstract Lactose intolerance provides an example of osmotic diarrhea from ingestion of solutes not absorbable by a given subject. The lactose tolerance test reflects lactase deficiency of enterocytes, most commonly secondary to decreased synthesis. **Since lactase deficiency can be inferred from effects of ingestion of milk and observation of the effects of a lactose-free diet, the lactose tolerance test is not often needed or done. If available, breath tests are preferable.**

Patient Preparation A trial of withdrawal from lactose-containing food is advocated first. Such a trial may make the test unnecessary. Patient should fast for 8 hours before testing, usually overnight. No smoking or gum chewing allowed during test. Occurrence of any vomiting should be reported to the patient's physician. Patient is encouraged to drink a moderate amount of water during the test, one to two glasses. Patient should remain seated or in bed.

(Continued)

Lactose Tolerance Test (Continued)

Aftercare Test may produce diarrhea and cramps.

Specimen Plasma or 24-hour urine

Container Gray top (sodium fluoride) tube, plastic 24-hour urine container

Collection Draw specimens in gray top tubes fasting and at 30 minutes, 1, 2, 3, and 4 hours after lactose load to be analyzed for glucose. (Samples can be taken fasting, 15 minutes, 30 minutes, 45 minutes, 1 hour, and 2 hours.) Record patient symptoms (especially cramps, nausea, watery diarrhea).

Special Instructions Lactose load: Adults: 50 g/m² body surface or 1 g/kg body weight should be consumed in 5-10 minutes. If severe lactase deficiency is suspected, the dose should be lowered. In infants and young children suspected of severe intolerance, a lower lactose dose should be used to avoid extreme reaction. Ingestion of 15 g lactose in 250 mL of water has been suggested.[1]

Reference Interval An increase in plasma glucose >30 mg/dL (SI: >1.7 mmol/L) is normal. An increase of plasma glucose <20 mg/dL (SI: <1.1 mmol/L) over the fasting level, with symptoms, is considered abnormal and is evidence for lactase deficiency. A flat curve can be defined as an increase <20 mg/dL (SI: <1.1 mmol/L) and is seen in most subjects with lactose deficiency who are not diabetic. Urine reference range: children: <1.5 mg/100 dL; adults: 12-40 mg/dL (SI: 0.7-2.2 mmol/L).

Breath hydrogen increase <10 ppm (0.9×10^{-6} g hydrogen/L air, or 0.45 µmol/L).[1] Less than 10 ppm H_2 gas in the exhaled breath is normal. Lactase deficient subjects usually have ≥50 ppm H_2 in exhaled air. Peak increased hydrogen is anticipated 3-6 hours after ingestion.

Use Work-up for gas, distension, diarrhea and/or cramping after ingestion of milk or dairy products. Diagnose idiopathic lactase deficiency, which is found in a majority of black, native American, and Oriental adults, as well as in 5% to 20% of adult American Caucasians. It is also found in children. Evaluate lactose intolerance, malabsorption syndromes.

Limitations Lactase is an easily injured enteric enzyme and rate limiting for the absorption of lactose. Secondary lactose deficiency is common in infectious enteritis, bacterial overgrowth, immune defects, and inflammatory bowel disease, among other conditions. Up to 20% incidence of false positives and false negatives is reported. Especially since lactase-deficient patients have had normal tolerance curves, this test is of questionable value. It may be abnormal with Crohn disease, small bowel resections, jejunitis, sprue, *Giardia lamblia* infestation, Whipple disease, and in cystic fibrosis of the pancreas.

Methodology Blood specimens are analyzed for glucose after an oral dose of lactose. Hydrogen breath analysis is a better alternate method, if available. It can be done by gas chromatography (GC).

Additional Information Lactose is a disaccharide digested by lactase. It yields glucose and galactose. The latter is converted to glucose by the liver after its absorption. Glucose is measured and it is the increase or lack of increase over the fasting specimen that is used for interpretation.

The breath hydrogen analysis (hydrogen breath test) detects increases in expired H_2 after ingestion of lactose. Increased breath H_2 implies that the lactose is escaping absorption in the small bowel and arrives in the colon. Colonic organisms metabolize lactose and produce hydrogen gas.

The most direct diagnostic test for lactase deficiency is histochemical examination of intestinal epithelium taken by peroral biopsy.

Diabetic patients may have abnormal lactose tolerance curves due to abnormal carbohydrate metabolism and not necessarily due to lactose intolerance. Ethanol can prevent conversion of galactose to glucose by the liver; blood or urine galactose can be measured.

Subjective lactose intolerance is increased in patients with irritable bowel syndrome, despite a lack of increase in the prevalence of lactose maldigestion.[2]

See Reducing Substances, Stool *on page 317*, in which further information is provided.

Footnotes
1. Suarez FL, Savaiano DA, and Levitt MD, "A Comparison of Symptoms After the Consumption of Milk or Lactose-Hydrolyzed Milk by People With Self-Reported Severe Lactose Intolerance," *N Engl J Med*, 1995, 333(1):1-4.
2. Mascolo R and Saltzman JR, "Lactose Intolerance and Irritable Bowel Syndrome," *Nutr Rev*, 1998, 56(10):306-8.

References
Arola H, "Diagnosis of Hypolactasia and Lactose Malabsorption," *Scand J Gastroenterol Suppl*, 1994, 202:26-35.
Brummer RJ, Karibe M, and Stockbrugger RW, "Lactose Malabsorption. Optimalization of Investigational Methods," *Scand J Gastroenterol*, 1993, 200(Suppl):65-9.
Malagelada JR, "Lactose Intolerance," *N Engl J Med*, 1995, 333(1):53-4.
Rings EH, Grand RJ, and Buller HA, "Lactose Intolerance and Lactase Deficiency in Children," *Curr Opin Pediatr*, 1994, 6(5):562-7.
Shaw AD and Davies GJ, "Lactose Intolerance: Problems in Diagnosis and Treatment," *J Clin Gastroenterol*, 1999, 28(3):208-16.

♦ **Ladders Light Chain** *see* Protein Electrophoresis, Urine *on page 268*

♦ **L-Alanine-2-Oxoglutarate Aminotransferase, Serum** *see* Alanine Aminotransferase, Serum *on page 87*

♦ **Lamellar Body Count** *see* Pulmonary Surfactant, Amniotic Fluid *on page 271*

♦ **LAP** *see* Leucine Aminopeptidase (LAP), Serum and Urine *on page 211*

♦ **L-Aspartate-2-Oxoglutarate Aminotransferase** *see* Aspartate Aminotransferase, Serum *on page 112*

♦ **LD** *see* Lactate Dehydrogenase, Serum *on page 207*

♦ **LD, Body Fluid** *see* Body Fluid Chemical Analysis *on page 123*

♦ **LD, Body Fluid** *see* Body Fluid Lactate Dehydrogenase *on page 125*

♦ **LDH** *see* Lactate Dehydrogenase, Serum *on page 207*

♦ **LDH** *replaced by* Troponins, Serum *on page 291*

♦ **LDH:AST Ratio** *see* Lactate Dehydrogenase, Serum *on page 207*

♦ **LDH Isoenzymes** *see* Lactate Dehydrogenase Isoenzymes, Serum *on page 206*

♦ **LDH Isoenzymes** *replaced by* Troponins, Serum *on page 291*

♦ **LD Isoenzymes** *see* Cardiac Markers: Laboratory Assessment, Overview *on page 137*

♦ **LD Isoenzymes** *see* Lactate Dehydrogenase Isoenzymes, Serum *on page 206*

♦ **LDLC** *see* Low Density Lipoprotein Cholesterol *on page 218*

♦ **LDLC:HDLC Ratio** *see* Low Density Lipoprotein Cholesterol *on page 218*

♦ **LDL Cholesterol:HDL Cholesterol** *see* Triglycerides, Serum or Plasma *on page 288*

♦ **Lecithin:Sphingomyelin Ratio** *see* Lecithin:Sphingomyelin Ratio, Amniotic Fluid *on page 210*

Lecithin:Sphingomyelin Ratio, Amniotic Fluid

Related Information
Creatinine, Amniotic Fluid *on page 160*
Lamellar Bodies, Amniotic Fluid *on page 454*
Phosphatidylglycerol, Amniotic Fluid *on page 251*
Pulmonary Surfactant, Amniotic Fluid *on page 271*

Synonyms Amniotic Fluid Lecithin:Sphingomyelin Ratio; Lecithin:Sphingomyelin Ratio; L:S Ratio; Lung Profile, Amniotic Fluid; Phospholipid Profile, Amniotic Fluid

Applies to Disaturated Phosphatidylcholine; Phosphatidylglycerol; Phosphatidylinositol

Test Includes L:S ratio; may include qualitative determination of phosphatidylglycerol (PG) and phosphatidylinositol (PI).

Abstract Amniotic fluid (AF) phospholipid testing assesses fetal lung maturity from which physicians infer the probability of respiratory distress syndrome (RDS) (hyaline membrane disease) in the neonate. The major component of pulmonary surfactant is disaturated lecithin (phosphatidylcholine). Lecithin (L) concentrations in AF increase with advancing gestational age and lung maturation, whereas sphingomyelin (S) concentrations remain relatively stable. The L:S ratio, therefore, is a determination of the relative amount of lecithin, and the ratio increases with increasing fetal lung maturity, rising sharply during the final weeks of gestation.[1]

Aftercare All nonsensitized Rh-negative patients should receive anti-D immunoglobulin after amniocentesis.

Specimen Amniotic fluid

Collection Ultrasound-guided, transabdominal amniocentesis is performed by the physician. Vaginal pool specimens are discouraged.

Storage Instructions The specimen should be centrifuged at low speed in a refrigerated centrifuge. The supernatant may be stored at 4°C for up to 10 days or it may be frozen indefinitely.

Special Instructions Fetal sacs of multiple pregnancies should be sampled and analyzed individually.[2] Send sample(s) to the laboratory **immediately** after collection.

Reference Interval Reference ranges for the L:S ratio vary according to the analytical methods used. The following summarize the L:S reference ranges reported by Kulovich, Hallman, and Gluck.[3]
- Mature: ratio ≥2.0
- Transitional: ratio 1.5-1.9
- Immature, premature: ratio: <1.5

Possible Panic Range An L:S ratio <1.5 predicts RDS on delivery and is associated with a gestational age of 34 weeks or less.

Use Measurement of the L:S ratio in AF is done prior to delivery to assess the likelihood of hyaline membrane disease (RDS) development in the newborn. Results are used to determine the optimal time for obstetrical intervention in cases of possible fetal distress due to maternal diabetes, toxemia, hemolytic disease of the newborn, or postmaturity.

Limitations Conventional testing for the L:S ratio is technically difficult, labor intensive, and not automated. Thin-layer chromatographic patterns are subjective and require experienced interpretation.

Though the predictive value of a mature result is on the order of 95% to 100%, the predictive value of an immature result is only 33% to 50%.[4] False predictions of maturity using the L:S ratio traditionally have been recognized in uncontrolled diabetic gestations, which have been associated with altered or delayed fetal lung maturation. Measurement of PG (see Phosphatidylglycerol, Amniotic Fluid *on page 251*) has been used to improve diagnostic accuracy in these cases. However, studies have shown that in reliably dated, well-controlled, gestational diabetic pregnancies, the L:S and PG correlate with gestational age similarly to nondiabetic control groups without evidence of significant delay in lung maturation[5] or difference in outcome.[6]

Blood contamination of the AF specimen invalidates the L:S result due to the presence of lecithin and sphingomyelin in plasma. Though meconium recently was shown to contain neither lecithin nor sphingomyelin, its presence in AF will cause misleading results.[7] The measurement of PG is unaffected by blood or meconium contamination, and its **accurate** detection in AF is highly predictive of lung maturity.[8]

Methodology One- or two-dimensional, thin-layer chromatography (TLC) is used for the determination of L/S and other AF phospholipids. High performance liquid chromatography (HPLC), also, has been used, albeit less commonly.[9]

Additional Information The incidence of RDS at ≥37 weeks gestation is extremely low in most pregnancies (with the exception of poorly controlled maternal diabetic pregnancies), whereas the incidence of RDS risk becomes significantly high at ≤34 weeks. Consequently, fetal lung maturity testing is most useful in reliably dated, high-risk pregnancies that would benefit from early delivery during the 34-37 week gestational period.[8]

In addition to L:S and PG, assessments of AF phosphatidylinositol (PI) and disaturated (acetone-precipitable) lecithin have been used to enhance interpretation.[3,4] Peak PI concentrations occur at 35-36 weeks, when PG first appears, facilitating further differentiation between transitional and mature patterns. The disaturated form of lecithin is the surface-active lecithin found in pulmonary surfactant; its use in the L:S ratio rather than total lecithin may better reflect fetal lung maturation, though inconsistencies have been reported with the cold acetone precipitation.[8]

With the availability of rapid tests for PG (see Phosphatidylglycerol, Amniotic Fluid *on page 251*) and other rapid tests for assessing fetal lung maturity (see Pulmonary Surfactant, Amniotic Fluid *on page 271*), cascade-testing approaches have been suggested to minimize the cost, time, and effort of performing L:S ratios. It has been recommended that the L:S ratio and PG by TLC be done only by laboratories that have at least fifteen requests per week[10] or be eliminated from the panel of fetal lung maturity testing altogether.[8]

Footnotes

1. Gluck L and Kulovich MV, "Lecithin/Sphingomyelin Ratios in Amniotic Fluid in Normal and Abnormal Pregnancy," *Am J Obstet Gynecol*, 1973, 115(4):539-46.
2. Whitworth NS, Magann EF, and Morrison JC, "Evaluation of Fetal Lung Maturity in Diamniotic Twins," *Am J Obstet Gynecol*, 1999, 180(6 Pt 1):1438-41.
3. Kulovich MV, Hallman MB, and Gluck L, "The Lung Profile. I. Normal Pregnancy," *Am J Obstet Gynecol*, 1979, 135(1):57-63.
4. "ACOG Educational Bulletin, Assessment of Fetal Lung Maturity, Number 230, November 1996," *Int J Gynecol Obstet*, 1997, 56(2):191-8.
5. Berkowitz K, Reyes C, Saadat P, et al, "Fetal Lung Maturation. Comparison of Biochemical Indices in Gestational Diabetic and Nondiabetic Pregnancies," *J Reprod Med*, 1997, 42(12):793-800.
6. Piper JM, Samueloff A, and Langer O, "Outcome of Amniotic Fluid Analysis and Neonatal Respiratory Status in Diabetic and Nondiabetic Pregnancies," *J Reprod Med*, 1995, 40(11):780-4.
7. Longo SA, Towers CV, Strauss A, et al, "Meconium Has No Lecithin or Sphingomyelin But Affects the Lecithin/Sphingomyelin Ratio," *Am J Obstet Gynecol*, 1998, 179(6 Pt 1):1640-42.
8. Dubin SB, "Assessment of Fetal Lung Maturity Practice Parameter," *Am J Clin Pathol*, 1998, 110(6):723-32.
9. Lotze A, Stroud CY, and Soldin SJ, "Serial Lecithin/Sphingomyelin Ratios and Surfactant/Albumin Ratios in Tracheal Aspirates From Term Infants With Respiratory Failure Receiving Extracorporeal Membrane Oxygenation," *Clin Chem*, 1995, 41(8):1182-8.
10. Ashwood ER, "Standards of Laboratory Practice: Evaluation of Fetal Lung Maturity," *Clin Chem*, 1997, 43(1):211-4.

References

Field NT and Gilbert WM, "Current Status of Amniotic Fluid Tests of Fetal Maturity," *Clin Obstet Gynecol*, 1997, 40(2):366-86.
Garite TJ, Freeman RK, and Nageotte MP, "Fetal Maturity Cascade: A Rapid and Cost-Effective Method for Fetal Lung Maturity Testing," *Obstet Gynecol*, 1986, 67(5):619-22.
Gluck L, Kulovich MV, Borer RC, et al, "The Interpretation and Significance of the Lecithin-Sphingomyelin Ratio in Amniotic Fluid," *Am J Obstet Gynecol*, 1974, 120(1):142-55.
Shaver DC, Spinnato JA, Whybrew D, et al, "Comparison of Phospholipids in Vaginal and Amniocentesis Specimens of Patients With Premature Rupture of Membranes," *Am J Obstet Gynecol*, 1987, 156(2):454-7.

Leptin, Serum or Plasma

Applies to Body Mass Index (BMI)

Abstract Leptin, an obesity-related 16kDa serum protein, was discovered in 1994 and has been the subject of hundreds of research papers since then. In humans, leptin is produced only in white adipose tissue. Leptin appears to be a cytokine-like molecule which produces its effect(s) by interacting with receptors in the CNS and peripheral tissues.[1] Increased levels suppress appetite and increase thermogenesis. Leptin gene mutations producing leptin deficiency lead to massive obesity.

Specimen Serum; plasma may be used.

Container Red top tube, green top (heparin) tube

Sampling Time 12-hour fast

Collection If heparin is used, add no more than 10 IU/mL of blood.

Storage Instructions Store at -20°C or lower.

Turnaround Time 1-3 days, depending on how often test is run

Reference Interval Varies with the laboratory performing the test. One RIA procedure uses 7.5 ±9.3 ng/mL in lean subjects, and 31.3 ±24.1 ng/mL in obese subjects.[2,3] Serum leptin is directly proportional to body-mass index (BMI) (see Additional Information). When men and women of equivalent BMI are compared, leptin levels are higher in women. It has been suggested that this is not a true gender difference, but a reflection of the fact that leptin levels are most closely correlated with percentage of body fat and, at any given BMI, women have higher percentage body fat than men.[4] Determining a well-defined reference range is made more difficult by relatively large short-term biologic coefficients of variation (10.9% in lean subjects and 22.5% in obese subjects).[2]

Use Although assays of serum leptin are available from a few reference laboratories, the significance of the results is not yet well understood. Leptin is still both a tool for research into obesity and an object of obesity research. Until its pathophysiology is better understood, serum leptin will probably not have an important role in diagnosis. A possible role in monitoring obesity treatment, however, is easy to envision. Preliminary trials of leptin as a drug have been reported.[5]

Methodology Radioimmunoassay (RIA) (Linco Research, Inc), limit of quantification is 0.2 ng/mL;[6] enzyme-linked immunosorbent assay (ELISA)

Additional Information Many studies of obesity use the body-mass index (BMI) as a measurement of obesity. The BMI is calculated as follows:

$$\text{BMI (kg)} / (\text{m}^2) = \text{body weight (kg)} / \text{height (m}^2)$$

The normal reference interval for the BMI is usually stated as 18.5-24.9 kg/m^2. The interval of 25.0-29.9 kg/m^2 is often called "overweight", while the term "obesity" is reserved for those with values >30 kg/m^2.[7] While the BMI is probably an adequate index of obesity for many individuals, obviously it mistakenly classifies as obese those who have an unusually large muscle mass and very little fat. Another approach to obesity classification measures the distribution of body fat - the ratio of waist circumference to hip circumference. A waist:hip ratio reflecting a "central" distribution of fat (eg, >0.90 in women and >1.0 in men) is correlated with a higher risk for morbidity than a ratio reflecting a "peripheral" distribution of fat (eg, <0.75 in women and <0.85 in men.)[8] Body fat can also be measured by magnetic resonance imaging, but such measurements are not widely available. The ideal index of obesity remains undefined.

Footnotes

1. Auwerx J and Staels B, "Leptin," *Lancet*, 1998, 351(9104):737-42.
2. Ma Z, Gingerich L, Santiago JV, et al, "Radioimmunoassay of Leptin in Human Plasma," *Clin Chem*, 1996, 42(6 Pt 1):942-6.
3. Considine RV, Sinha MK, Heiman ML, et al, "Serum Immunoreactive-Leptin Concentrations in Normal-Weight and Obese Humans," *N Engl J Med*, 1996, 334(5):292-5.
4. Considine RV and Caro JF, "Leptin in Humans: Current Progress and Future Directions," *Clin Chem*, 1996, 42(6 Pt 1):843-4.
5. Heymsfield SB, Greenberg AS, Fujioka K, et al, "Recombinant Leptin for Weight Loss in Obese and Lean Adults," *JAMA*, 1999, 282(16):1568-75.
6. Hicks J and Young D, *Directory of Rare Analyses 97-99*, Washington, DC: AACC Press, American Association of Clinical Chemistry, 1999.
7. Bray GA, "Obesity: A Time Bomb to Be Defused," *Lancet*, 1998, 352(9123):160-1.
8. Rosenbaum M, Leibel RL, and Hirsch J, "Obesity," *N Engl J Med*, 1997, 337(6):396-406.

References

Barash I and Cheung C, "Leptin Is a Metabolic Signal to the Reproductive System," *Endocrinology*, 1996, 137(7):3144-7.
Halaas J and Gajiwala K, "Weight-Reducing Effects of the Plasma Protein Encoded by the Obese (oba0) Gene," *Science*, 1995, 269(5223):543-6.
Imagawa K, Matsumoto Y, Numata Y, et al, "Development of a Sensitive ELISA for Human Leptin, Using Monoclonal Antibodies," *Clin Chem*, 1998, 44(10):2165-71.
Rosenbaum M and Leibel RL, "The Role of Leptin in Human Physiology," *N Engl J Med*, 1999, 341(12):913-5.
Ruige JB and Dekker JM, "Leptin and Variables of Body Weight, Adiposity, Energy, Balance, and Insulin Resistance in a Population-Based Study," *Diabetes Care*, 1999, 22(7):1097-104.

♦ **Leucine** see Amino Acids, Urine *on page 101*

Leucine Aminopeptidase (LAP), Serum and Urine

Related Information

Alkaline Phosphatase, Serum *on page 93*
Bilirubin, Total, Serum *on page 118*
Gamma-Glutamyl Transferase, Serum *on page 179*
Liver Disease: Laboratory Assessment, Overview *on page 216*

Synonyms Arylamidase; Arylamidase Naphthylamidase; LAP

Abstract LAP was used occasionally to determine whether an elevated serum alkaline phosphatase value was due to a process in the liver/biliary tract vs bone or other site; this application has decreased dramatically with the elimination of alkaline phosphatase from most biochemical panels. LAP has been suggested as a tumor marker for neoplasms of the liver and pancreas, but is rarely employed for this purpose. A potential, but as yet unproven, use is the assay for LAP in urine to detect early renal tubular injury in diabetes.[1] Serum LAP levels are elevated in patients with systemic lupus erythematosus (SLE). It has been proposed as a potential activity indicator for SLE.[2]

(Continued)

Leucine Aminopeptidase (LAP), Serum and Urine

(Continued)

Specimen Serum, ascitic fluid

Container Red top tube

Use LAP increases in cholestasis; it is a biliary excretory enzyme which is not increased with bone disease.

Limitations LAP increases in late pregnancy.

Footnotes

1. Bedir A, Ozener IC, and Emerk K, "Urinary Leucine Aminopeptidase Is a More Sensitive Marker of Early Renal Damage in Noninsulin-Dependent Diabetics Than Is Microalbuminuria," *Nephron*, 1996, 74(1):110-3.
2. Inokuma S, Setoguchi K, Ohta T, et al, "Serum Leucine Aminopeptidase as an Activity Indicator in Systemic Lupus Erythematosus: A Study of 46 Consecutive Cases," *Rheumatology (Oxford)* 1999, 38(8):705-8.

♦ **Leydig Cells** *see* Luteinizing Hormone, Blood or Urine *on page 219*

♦ **LFTs** *see* Liver Disease: Laboratory Assessment, Overview *on page 216*

♦ **L-Glyceric Acid, Urine** *see* Oxalate, Urine *on page 238*

♦ **LH** *see* Luteinizing Hormone, Blood or Urine *on page 219*

♦ **Light Chains** *see* Protein Electrophoresis, Serum *on page 267*

♦ **Light Chains, Urine** *see* Protein Electrophoresis, Capillary Zone *on page 266*

♦ **Light Chains, Urine** *see* Protein Electrophoresis, Urine *on page 268*

♦ **Liley Test** *see* Bilirubin, Amniotic Fluid, Delta A450 *on page 116*

Lipase, Serum

Related Information

Amylase, Serum *on page 102*
Amylase, Urine *on page 104*
Bilirubin, Total, Serum *on page 118*
Body Fluid Amylase *on page 122*
Fat, Semiquantitative, Stool, Acid Steatocrit *on page 305*
Fat, Semiquantitative, Stool, Sudan III Stain *on page 306*

Synonyms Triacylglycerol Acylhydrolase

Applies to Body Fluid Lipase; Elastase, Serum

Abstract Lipase, a glycoprotein, is an enzyme which hydrolyzes glycerol esters of long-chain fatty acids. Almost all serum lipase is synthesized in pancreatic acinar cells. **The new lipase methods are superior to total serum amylase in sensitivity and specificity for the diagnosis of acute pancreatitis,**[1] **but both are useful.** Simultaneous determination of both lipase and amylase is widely recommended for patients with abdominal pain.[2] Lipase levels are usually increased in both alcoholic and nonalcoholic forms of pancreatitis.

Specimen Serum; lipase (unlike amylase) is not applicable to urine. Lipase may be measured in pleural or peritoneal fluid.

Container Red top tube

Storage Instructions Stable 1 week at 25°C, 3 weeks at 4°C.

Reference Interval Method dependent but typically <200 units/L (triolein methods by titration or turbidimetry). An enzymatic colorimetric assay utilizing co-lipase and deoxycholate as activators provides reference values of 3-73 units/L.[3]

Critical Values Significant elevation is usually considered three times the upper limit of normal, but patients with small increases of amylase/lipase concentrations on admission may also develop severe pancreatitis.[4]

Use Diagnose acute and chronic pancreatitis. Since amylase levels are apt to return to normal range first, assay of serum lipase is especially helpful in subjects who appear several days after onset.

Limitations EDTA anticoagulant may interfere. Hemoglobin at ≥250 mg/dL may interfere, depending on method. Fifty-five percent of patients with primary biliary cirrhosis had raised serum lipase activity.[5] Lipase is increased in about 50% of the patients with chronic renal failure. About 75% of such patients have increased serum amylase as well.[6] Serum lipase concentrations increase with hemodialysis.[7] This increase is apparently due to heparin-induced lipolytic activity. Therefore, predialysis blood samples are recommended for lipase measurement. Elevated lipase with normal amylase is reported with acute cholecystitis, with hypertriglyceridemia, and with lipolytic enzymes due to malignant tumors as well as with pancreatitis.[2] Serum lipase may be elevated in the absence of acute pancreatitis,[8] an observation published relevant to chronic alcoholics[9] but applicable to others as well.

Drugs may cause increase. Some cause spasm of the sphincter of Oddi (eg, bethanechol, cholinergics, codeine, meperidine, methacholine, narcotics including morphine, pentazocine, secretin). Others may cause pancreatitis (eg, calcitriol, cerivastatin, chlorothiazide, clozapine, diazoxide, didanosine, dideoxyinosine, estropipate, felbamate, hydrocortisone, mercaptopurine, metolazone, metronidazole, minocycline, nitrofurantoin, oral contraceptives, pegaspargase, prednisolone, sulfamethoxazole). Other drugs causing increase include acetaminophen overdose and valproic acid.[10]

An association of intracranial bleeding with increased concentrations of amylase and lipase, in individuals without pancreatitis, is recognized.[11]

Methodology Turbidimetric (using triolein), spectrophotometric, fluorometric, titrimetric, immunoassay

Additional Information Serum lipase is usually normal in those patients with elevated serum amylase, without pancreatitis, who have peptic ulcer, salivary adenitis, inflammatory bowel disease, intestinal obstruction, and macroamylasemia. Lipase activity is usually absent in urine, possibly from inactivation of the enzyme. Coexistence of increased serum amylase with normal lipase may be a helpful clue to the presence of macroamylasemia.[12] Lipase is elevated with amylase in acute pancreatitis, but the elevation of lipase is more prolonged.

Pancreatic isoamylase may be useful in mild elevations of total serum amylase. Electrolytes, serum calcium, glucose, and acetone are also often needed. Serum trypsin is technically more difficult than lipase and probably no better. The serum lipase:amylase ratio is no longer considered useful to distinguish alcoholic from nonalcoholic acute pancreatitis.[13,14]

The most common obstructive etiology of acute pancreatitis is gallstone disease. The most common toxin causing acute pancreatitis is ethyl alcohol, and over 85 drugs have been implicated. Additional causes include hypertriglyceridemia, hypercalcemia, and other entities.[15]

Laboratory and other factors useful to project severity of pancreatitis include C-reactive protein.[15] Important concepts in recognition and management of clinically **severe acute pancreatitis** were recently tabulated. They include age older than 55 years, WBC >16,000/mm^3, glucose >200 mg/dL, LDH >350 IU/L, AST >250 IU/L, decreased Hct >10%, increased BUN >5 mg/dL, serum calcium <8 mg/dL, arterial PaO$_2$ <60 mm Hg, base deficit >4 mmol/L, and fluid sequestration >6 L.[16] Amylase and lipase may be normal or minimally increased in **chronic pancreatitis**. Bilirubin and alkaline phosphatase may be abnormal. Fecal fat excretion may be increased if malabsorption develops.[17]

Footnotes

1. Chase CW, Barker DE, Russell WL, et al, "Serum Amylase and Lipase in the Evaluation of Acute Abdominal Pain," *Am J Surg*, 1996, 62(12):1028-33.
2. Frank B and Gottlieb K, "Amylase Normal, Lipase Elevated: Is it Pancreatitis? A Case Series and Review of the Literature," *Am J Gastroenterol*, 1999, 94(2):463-9.
3. Mayo Medical Laboratories, "Method and Reference Value Change for Lipase, Serum," *Mayo Communique*, Rochester, MN, 1999, 24(11).
4. Lankisch PG, Burchard-Reckert S, and Lehnick D, "Underestimation of Acute Pancreatitis: Patients With Only a Small Increase in Amylase/Lipase Levels Can Also Have or Develop Severe Acute Pancreatitis," *Gut*, 1999, 44(4):542-4.
5. Fonseca V, Epstein O, Katrak A, et al, "Serum Immunoreactive Trypsin and Pancreatic Lipase in Primary Biliary Cirrhosis," *J Clin Pathol*, 1986, 39(6):638-40.
6. Royse VL, Jensen DM, and Corwin HL, "Pancreatic Enzymes in Chronic Renal Failure," *Arch Intern Med*, 1987, 147(3):537-9.
7. Vaziri ND, Chang D, Malekpour A, et al, "Pancreatic Enzymes in Patients With End-Stage Renal Disease Maintained on Hemodialysis," *Am J Gastroenterol*, 1988, 83(4):410-2.
8. Orebaugh SL, "Normal Amylase Levels in the Presentation of Acute Pancreatitis," *Am J Emerg Med*, 1994, 12:21-4.
9. Gumaste VV, Sereny G, Dave P, et al, "Serum Lipase Levels in Chronic Alcoholics," *J Clin Gastroenterol*, 1991, 13(4):407-10.
10. Young DS, *Effects of Drugs on Clinical Laboratory Tests*, 5th ed, Volume 1: Listing by Test, Washington, DC: AACC Press, American Association for Clinical Chemistry, 2000, Section 3, 526-8.
11. Justice AD, Di Benedetto RJ, and Stanford E, "Significance of Elevated Pancreatic Enzymes in Intracranial Bleeding," *South Med J*, 1994, 87(9):889-93.
12. Andrews PA and Thomas PA, "Macroamylasaemia as a Cause of Persistently Raised Serum Amylase," *Br J Surg*, 1988, 75(10):1035.
13. Pezzilli R, Billi P, Barakat B, et al, "Lipase-Amylase Ratio Does Not Determine the Etiology Acute Pancreatitis. Another Myth Bites the Dust," *J Clin Gastroenterol*, 1998, 26(1):34-8.
14. Ansari E, Talenti DA, Scopelliti JA, et al, "Serum Lipase and Amylase Ratio in Acute Alcoholic and Nonalcoholic Pancreatitis by Using Dupont ACA Discrete Clinical Analyzer," *Dig Dis Sci*, 1996, 41(9):1823-7.
15. Steinberg W and Tenner S, "Acute Pancreatitis," *N Engl J Med*, 1994, 330(17):1198-210.
16. Baron TH and Morgan DE, "Acute Necrotizing Pancreatitis," *N Engl J Med*, 1999, 340(18):1412-17 (review paper).
17. Steer ML, Waxman I, and Freedman S, "Chronic Pancreatitis," *N Engl J Med*, 1995, 332(22):1482-90 (review paper).

Lipid Panel, Serum

Related Information

Apolipoprotein A-I, Serum *on page 109*
Apolipoprotein B-100, Serum *on page 109*
Cholesterol, Total, Serum or Plasma *on page 146*
High Density Lipoprotein Cholesterol, Serum *on page 192*
Lipids, Overview *on page 213*
Low Density Lipoprotein Cholesterol *on page 218*
Triglycerides, Serum or Plasma *on page 288*

Test Includes This is a HCFA-defined panel which must include these three measurements:[1]

* Cholesterol (total), serum
* High density lipoprotein cholesterol, serum
* Triglycerides, serum

In addition, many laboratories will calculate a low density lipoprotein cholesterol value based on these measurements, using the Friedewald equation, *vide infra*.

Patient Preparation An early morning specimen after a 14-hour fast is ideal.

Specimen Serum

Container Red top tube

Storage Instructions If testing is not performed the same day the specimen is drawn, store at 4°C.

Reference Interval See tables in Lipids, Overview *on page 213*.

Use See Lipids, Overview *on page 213*.

Methodology See discussions in monographs on the individual analytes (Related Information). The Friedewald equation produces a calculated value for LDL cholesterol:

LDLC (mg/dL) = cholesterol, total (mg/dL) - HDLC (mg/dL) - [triglycerides (mg/dL) / 5]

The formula is valid for samples having a fasting triglyceride concentration up to 400 mg/dL. Specimens with fasting triglycerides >400 mg/dL require a direct measurement of LDLC or may be referred to a specialized lipid laboratory for ultracentrifugal analysis.

Footnotes

1. *Current Procedural Terminology (CPT™) 2001*, American Medical Association, 2001.

Lipids, Overview

Related Information

Apolipoprotein A-I, Serum *on page 109*
Apolipoprotein B-100, Serum *on page 109*
Cholesterol, Total, Serum or Plasma *on page 146*
C-Reactive Protein, Serum *on page 523*
High Density Lipoprotein Cholesterol, Serum *on page 192*
Homocyst(e)ine, Plasma *on page 193*
Lipid Panel, Serum *on page 212*
Lipoprotein (a), Serum *on page 215*
Low Density Lipoprotein Cholesterol *on page 218*
Mevalonic Acid, Urine or Amniotic Fluid *on page 225*
Triglycerides, Serum or Plasma *on page 288*

Applies to Apo-A-I; Apo B-100; Cholesterol, Total; Chylomicronemia; High Density Lipoprotein Cholesterol (HDLC); Hypoalphalipoproteinemia; Intermediate Density Lipoprotein Cholesterol; Lipoprotein-Associated Phospholipase A$_2$; Low Density Lipoprotein Cholesterol (LDLC); Triglycerides; Very Low Density Lipoprotein Cholesterol

Abstract The assessment of coronary artery disease (CAD) risk requires simultaneous consideration of multiple risk factors, of which the most important include smoking status, systolic blood pressure, presence of diabetes mellitus, obesity, left ventricular hypertrophy, EKG abnormalities, aging, family history, physical activity/inactivity, and serum lipids. The serum lipid risk "factor" actually consists of at least four separate biochemical fractions: total cholesterol (TC), low density lipoprotein cholesterol (LDLC), high density lipoprotein cholesterol (HDLC), and serum triglycerides (TG), which often serves as a surrogate for very low density lipoprotein cholesterol (VLDLC). TC includes HDLC, LDLC, and VLDLC. These fractions lack sharp boundaries, except when testing is done by ultracentrifugation. For example, the LDLC fraction, and to a lesser extent the VLDLC fraction, also contain intermediate density lipoprotein cholesterol (IDLC).

Some physicians believe that if an individual's TC is sufficiently low (*vide infra*), the other lipid fractions need not be measured. However, since physicians often recommend interventions which decrease one fraction, LDLC, and increase another, HDLC, measuring each fraction separately is required to monitor the effectiveness of such interventions. Some experts recommend measuring these fractions as cholesterol fractions, but others believe that more accurate risk information is provided by measuring the apoproteins themselves (eg, apo-A-I instead of HDLC, and apo B-100 instead of LDLC).

Patient Preparation Patient should be on stable diet ideally for 2-3 weeks prior to collection of blood and should fast for at least 10 hours before collection of the specimen. There is inconclusive evidence for 72 hours of abstinence from alcohol before sampling for lipid profile. See Preparation in the listing Cholesterol, Total, Serum or Plasma *on page 146*.

Specimen Serum

Container Red top tube

Collection Lipid concentrations fluctuate rapidly and unpredictably following an acute coronary event. Lipid testing should be deferred until 3 months after such an illness.

Storage Instructions Lipoproteins are labile. Even stored at 4°C, analysis should not be delayed more than a few days.

Reference Interval A reference interval, usually the central 95% of a population distribution,[1] is not relevant to cholesterol measurements. This is because, at least in the U.S., CAD is so prevalent, and has such a long symptom-free latent period, that it is not possible to define a reference population free of the disease. There is, however, a rich database from the Lipid Research Clinics (LRC) and the Framingham Study which link fasting serum cholesterol values to CAD risk.[2,3] Such risk estimates, stratified by gender and age, go far beyond the dichotomous classification, normal vs abnormal, and provide for each individual a quantitative assessment of CAD risk. Similar risk estimates are also available for the cholesterol fractions: Low Density Lipoprotein Cholesterol *on page 218*, High Density

Lipoprotein Cholesterol, Serum *on page 192*, and Triglycerides, Serum or Plasma *on page 288*. See tables 1-8.

Table 1. Selected Reference Values for Plasma Total Cholesterol in White Male Subjects (mg/dL)

Age (y)	No.	Mean	Percentile			
			5	75	90	95
0-19	5749	155	115	170	185	200
20-24	882	165	125	185	205	220
25-29	2042	180	135	200	225	245
30-34	2444	190	140	215	240	255
35-39	2320	200	145	225	250	270
40-44	2428	205	150	230	250	270
45-69	7710	215	160	235	260	275
70+	850	205	150	230	250	270

Table 2. Selected Reference Values for Plasma Total Cholesterol in White Female Subjects (mg/dL)

Age (y)	No.	Mean	Percentile			
			5	75	90	95
0-19	5470	160	120	175	190	200
20-24	1566	170	125	190	215	230
25-34	4340	175	130	195	220	235
35-39	2012	185	140	205	230	245
40-44	2050	195	145	215	235	255
45-49	2149	205	150	225	250	270
50-54	1992	220	165	240	265	285
55+	4478	230	170	250	275	295

Table 3. Selected Reference Values for Plasma Low-Density Lipoprotein Cholesterol in White Male Subjects (mg/dL)

Age (y)	No.	Mean	Percentile			
			5	75	90	95
5-19	713	95	65	105	120	130
20-24	118	105	65	120	140	145
25-29	253	115	70	140	155	165
30-34	403	125	80	145	165	185
35-39	371	135	80	155	175	190
40-44	385	135	85	155	175	185
45-69	1162	145	90	165	190	205
70+	119	145	90	165	180	185

Table 4. Selected Reference Values for Plasma Low-Density Lipoprotein Cholesterol in White Female Subjects (mg/dL)

Age (y)	No.	Mean	Percentile			
			5	75	90	95
5-19	652	100	65	110	125	140
20-24	199	105	55	120	140	160
25-34	646	110	70	125	145	160
35-39	299	120	75	140	160	170
40-44	318	125	75	145	165	175
45-49	326	130	80	150	175	185
50-54	256	140	90	160	185	200
55+	668	150	95	170	195	215

Table 5. Selected Reference Values for Plasma High-Density Lipoprotein Cholesterol in White Male Subjects (mg/dL)

Age (y)	No.	Mean	Percentile		
			5	10	95
5-14	438	55	35	40	75
15-19	299	45	30	35	65
20-24	118	45	30	30	65
25-29	253	45	30	30	65
30-34	403	45	30	30	65
35-39	371	45	30	30	60
40-44	383	45	25	30	65
45-69	1162	50	30	30	70
70+	119	50	30	35	75

(Continued)

Lipids, Overview (Continued)

Table 6. Selected Reference Values for Plasma High-Density Lipoprotein Cholesterol in White Female Subjects (mg/dL)

Age (y)	No.	Mean	Percentile 5	Percentile 10	Percentile 95
5-19	666	55	35	40	70
20-24	199	55	35	35	80
25-34	649	55	35	40	80
35-39	298	55	35	40	80
40-44	318	60	35	40	90
45-49	328	60	35	40	85
50-54	256	60	35	40	90
55+	668	60	35	40	95

Table 7. Selected Reference Values for Plasma Triglycerides in White Male Subjects (mg/dL)

Age (y)	No.	Mean	Percentile 5	Percentile 90	Percentile 95
0-9	1491	55	30	85	100
10-14	2278	65	30	100	125
15-19	1980	80	35	120	150
20-24	882	100	45	165	200
25-29	2042	115	45	200	250
30-34	2444	130	50	215	265
35-39	2320	145	55	250	320
40-54	6862	150	55	250	320
55-64	2526	140	60	235	290
65+	1600	135	55	210	260

Table 8. Selected Reference Values for Plasma Triglycerides (mg/dL) in White Female Subjects

Age	No.	Mean	Percentile 5	Percentile 90	Percentile 95
0-9 y	1304	60	35	95	110
10-19 y	4166	75	40	115	130
20-34 y	5906	90	40	145	170
35-39 y	2012	95	40	160	195
40-44 y	2050	105	45	170	210
45-49 y	2149	110	45	185	230
50-54 y	1992	120	55	190	240
55-64 y	2768	125	55	200	250
65+ y	1710	130	60	205	240

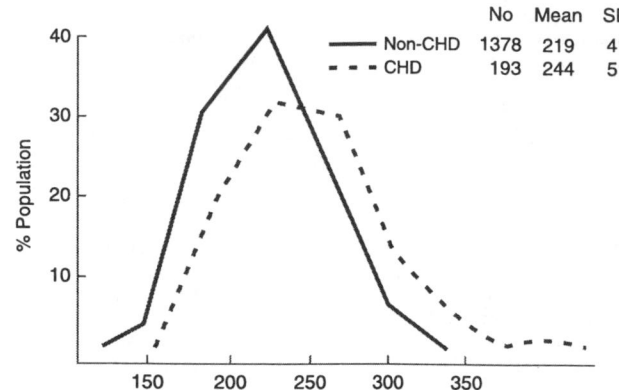

Serum cholesterol in subjects free of coronary heart disease versus those in whom coronary heart disease developed within 16 years.

Adapted from Castelli WP, "Epidemiology of Coronary Heart Disease: The Framingham Study," *Am J Med*, 1984, 76:4-12.

Use

CAD RISK

In CAD, total cholesterol (TC) is a risk factor, **not** a diagnostic test. This important distinction is illustrated in the figure taken from the original Framingham Study cohort.[3] Simple inspection of the figure reveals that TC is not a diagnostic test for CAD risk, since the degree of overlap between diseased and nondiseased is much too great. However, we know from many studies, including Framingham, that TC is a measurement which has a continuous and graded relationship to CAD; the higher the TC, the greater the risk. Use of the LRC data (see tables) allows a relatively precise estimation of CAD risk, an estimate that provides more information than any single target or cutoff.[4] For example, a total cholesterol (TC) value of 200 mg/dL (SI: 5.17 mmol/L) implies a relatively high risk (75th percentile) for a 34-year old woman, but a much lower risk (30th percentile) for a 65-year old man.

Since an individual will have many cholesterol measurements over a lifetime, **biologic variability** is important and should be kept in mind by clinicians advising patients. The mean intraindividual biologic coefficient of variation (CVb) for TC ranges from 5% to 10%.[5,6] The CVb is higher in individuals with very high cholesterol values. Cooper and colleagues (CDC) have recommended that intraindividual CVb can be minimized by measuring two or more TC values and calculating a relative range (RR); the RR is "...the difference between the lowest and highest concentration values observed for a person, divided by the mean of all the observed values."[7] See Footnote 7 citation for more information.

Equally important for multiple measurements over the long-term is **intermethod variability.** Historically, this has been a major obstacle to useful cholesterol results. The Laboratory Standardization Panel (LSP), created by the National Cholesterol Education Program (NCEP), recommended in 1988 that laboratories achieve a bias not exceeding ±3%, and, in addition, precision sufficient that the analytic coefficient of variation (CVa) also not exceed ±3%.[8] An additional recommendation was that all clinical cholesterol methods be traceable to the CDC reference method (a modified Abell-Kendall technique) or to the National Institute for Standards and Technology (NIST) definitive method (isotope-dilution mass spectrometry).[9]

More recently, analytical goals have been developed by the NCEP for LDLC and HDLC. For LDLC, the total analytic error should not exceed 12%; this criterion can be met in a laboratory in which the bias does not exceed ±4%, and the analytical imprecision (CVa) also does not exceed ±4%.[10] For HDLC the total analytical error should not exceed 13%; this can be achieved if the bias is ±5%, and the analytical imprecision (CVa) is <4%.[11] After an individual's lipid fractions have been measured, they should be placed into the context of **overall CAD risk,** which includes assessment of blood pressure, diabetes, smoking history, and family history.

Quite a different approach to cholesterol testing, recommended by some British scientists, involves assessing individuals for blood pressure, smoking, diabetes, and left ventricular enlargement risk factors. Cholesterol testing is provided only for those individuals who have, based on these other risk factors, a >3% estimated likelihood of a coronary event in the present year.[12] While we do not endorse this practice, we present it for completeness. Interested readers should consult the citation in Footnote 12.

PRIMARY LIPID DISORDERS[13]

Patients with **familial hypercholesterolemia** (an autosomal dominant disease) have elevated TC as a result of deficient or defective LDL receptors. Heterozygotes (1 in 500 persons) have TC values ~400-500 mg/dL, and, if untreated, often experience their first coronary event and signs of peripheral vascular disease in their fourth or fifth decade. Homozygotes (much rarer) have TC ~1000 mg/dL, premature vascular disease, and often have tendon xanthomas. **Familial defective apolipoprotein B** (also autosomal dominant) has a very similar biochemical phenotype, but is due to defective ligand binding with markedly delayed clearance of LDL cholesterol. Patients with **familial hyperalphalipoproteinemia** have elevated TC, but fractionation reveals that the major increase is in HDL cholesterol, not LDL cholesterol. Such individuals have a decreased incidence of CAD.

Lipoprotein lipase deficiency and **apoprotein C II deficiency** present with markedly elevated triglycerides (see Triglycerides, Serum or Plasma *on page 288*); TC may be normal or slightly elevated.

Familial chylomicronemia is a rare, autosomal recessive disorder characterized by very high serum TG. Either lipoprotein lipase or apo-C II is defective or deficient. In **familial dysbetalipoproteinemia,** also autosomal recessive, serum TG is also very high, and identifying the defective apoE phenotype requires referral to a specialized lipid laboratory.

Familial hypoalphalipoproteinemia (low HDLC) is probably a heterogeneous group of individuals having the common denominator of low serum HDLC. Within this group are marked differences in premature CAD, xanthomas, and many other features.

Polygenic hypercholesterolemia is the name given to individuals with high LDLC, but whose findings do not support a diagnosis of FH or any other of the foregoing diagnostic categories. Since this is a default category, it is almost certain that the individuals assigned thereto are a heterogeneous grouping, and one that will be altered on the basis of additional research.

SECONDARY HYPERLIPIDEMIAS[13]

Numerous drugs and certain diseases produce changes in blood lipids. Of most concern are those which produce elevations of TC (eg, high fat diet, hypothyroidism, Cushing syndrome, oral contraceptives, chronic liver disease) and TG (high carbohydrate diet, excessive ethanol, Cushing syndrome, hypothyroidism, pregnancy, obesity, pancreatitis, diabetes mellitus, diuretics, estrogen use, beta blocker therapy).

An association exists between hypothyroidism and increased cholesterol, triglycerides, HDLC, apolipoprotein A-1 and B-100, and Lp(a). Thyroid replacement therapy leads to improvement.[14]

Methodology See individual listings.

Additional Information Other markers of coronary risk exist as well, including C-reactive protein, fibrinogen concentrations, and white cell count. They have recently been summarized in an important editorial.[15]

Lipoprotein-associated phospholipase A_2 is proposed as a potential risk factor.[16]

Footnotes

1. Solberg HE, "Establishment and Use of Reference Values," *Tietz Textbook of Clinical Chemistry*, 3rd ed, Philadelphia, PA: WB Saunders Co, 1999, 336-56.
2. Gotto AM, Bierman EL, Connor WE, et al, "Recommendations for Treatment of Hyperlipidemia in Adults. A Joint Statement of the Nutrition Committee and the Council on Arteriosclerosis," *Circulation*, 1984, 69(5):1067A-90A.
3. Castelli WP, "Epidemiology of Coronary Heart Disease: The Framingham Study," *Am J Med*, 1984, 76(2A):4-12.
4. Oxley DK, "Cholesterol Measurements: Quality Assurance and Medical Usefulness Interrelationships," *Arch Pathol Lab Med*, 1988, 112(4):387-91.
5. Hegsted DM and Nicolosi RJ, "Individual Variation in Serum Cholesterol Levels," *Proc Natl Acad Sci U S A*, 1987, 84(17):6259-61.
6. Statland BE and Winkel P, "Effects of Preanalytical Factors on the Intra-Individual Variations of Analyses in the Blood of Healthy Subjects," *CRC Crit Rev Clin Lab Sci*, 1977, 8(2):105-44.
7. Cooper GR, Smith SJ, Myers GL, et al, "Estimating and Minimizing Effects of Biologic Sources of Variation by Relative Range When Measuring the Mean of Serum Lipids and Lipoproteins," *Clin Chem*, 1994, 40(2):227-32.
8. "Current Status of Blood Cholesterol Measurement in Clinical Laboratories in the U.S.: A Report From the Laboratory Standardization Panel of the National Cholesterol Education Program," *Clin Chem*, 1988, 34(1):193-201.
9. Myers GL, Cooper GR, Henderson LO, et al, "Standardization of Lipid and Lipoprotein Measurements," *Handbook of Lipoprotein Testing*, Rifai N, Warnick GR, and Dominiczak MH, eds, Washington, DC: AACC Press, American Association of Clinical Chemistry, 1997, 223-50.
10. Bachorik P, "Measurement of Low-Density Lipoprotein Cholesterol," *Handbook of Lipoprotein Testing*, Rifai N, Warnick GR, and Dominiczak MH, eds, Washington, DC: AACC Press, American Association of Clinical Chemistry, 1997, 145-60..
11. Wiebe DA and Warnick GR, "Measurement of High Density Lipoprotein Cholesterol," *Handbook of Lipoprotein Testing*, Rifai N, Warnick GR, and Dominiczak MH, eds, Washington, DC: AACC Press, American Association of Clinical Chemistry, 1997, 127-44.
12. Ramsay LE, Haq IU, Jackson PR, et al, "Targeting Lipid-Lowering Drug Therapy for Primary Prevention of Coronary Disease: An Updated Sheffield Table," *Lancet*, 1996, 348(9024):387-8.
13. Jones PH, Grundy SM, and Gotto AM, "Assessment and Management of Lipid Abnormalities," *Hurst's The Heart*, Alexander RW, Schlant RC, Fuster V, et al, eds, New York, NY: McGraw-Hill, 1998, 1553-81.
14. Martínez-Triguero ML, Hernández-Mijares A, Nguyen TT, et al, "Effect of Thyroid Hormone Replacement on Lipoprotein(a), Lipids, and Apolipoproteins in Subjects With Hypothyroidism," *Mayo Clin Proc*, 1998, 73(9):837-41.
15. Rader DJ, "Inflammatory Markers of Coronary Risk," *N Engl J Med*, 2000, 343(16):1179-82.
16. Packard CJ, O'Reilly DS, Caslake MJ, et al, "Lipoprotein-Associated Phospholipase A_2 as an Independent Predictor of Coronary Heart Disease," *N Engl J Med*, 2000, 343(16):1148-55.

References

Austin GE, Hollman J, Lynn MJ, et al, "Serum Lipoprotein Levels Fail to Predict Postangioplasty Recurrent Coronary Artery Stenosis," *Cleve Clin J Med*, 1989, 56(5):509-14.

Brown WV, "Lipoprotein Disorders in Diabetes Mellitus," *Med Clin North Am*, 1994, 78(1):143-61.

Fraser GE, "Diet and Coronary Heart Disease: Beyond Dietary Fats and Low-Density-Lipoprotein Cholesterol," *Am J Clin Nutr*, 1994, 59(5 Suppl):1117S-23S.

Gaziano JM, Buring JE, Breslow JL, et al, "Moderate Alcohol Intake, Increased Levels of High-Density Lipoprotein and Its Subfractions, and Decreased Risk of Myocardial Infarction," *N Engl J Med*, 1993, 329(25):1829-34.

Lichtenstein AH, Ausman LM, Jalbert SM, et al, "Effects of Different Forms of Dietary Hydrogenated Fats on Serum Lipoprotein Cholesterol Levels," *N Engl J Med*, 1999, 340(25):1933-40.

Ozturk IC and Killeen AA, "An Overview of Genetic Factors Influencing Plasma Lipid Levels and Coronary Artery Disease Risk," *Arch Pathol Lab Med*, 1999, 123:1219-22.

Rosenson RS, "Low Levels of High Density Lipoprotein Cholesterol (Hypoalphalipoproteinemia). An Approach to Management," *Arch Intern Med*, 1993, 153(13):1528-38.

Schectman G and Sasse E, "Variability of Lipid Measurements: Relevance for the Clinician," *Clin Chem*, 1993, 39(7):1495-503.

Segrest JP and Anantharamaiah GM, "Pathogenesis of Atherosclerosis," *Curr Opin Cardiol*, 1994, 9(4):404-10.

Slyper AH, "Low-Density Lipoprotein Density and Atherosclerosis. Unraveling the Connection," *JAMA*, 1994, 272(4):305-8.

Stern MP, Patterson JK, Haffner SM, "Lack of Awareness and Treatment of Hyperlipidemia in Type II Diabetes in a Community Survey," *JAMA*, 1989, 262(3):360-4.

Witztum JL and Steinberg D, "The Hyperlipoproteinemias," *Cecil Textbook of Medicine*, 21st ed, Chapter 328, Goldman L and Bennett JC, eds, Philadelphia, PA: WB Saunders Co, 2000, 1090-100.

Lipoprotein (a), Serum

Related Information

Apolipoprotein A-I, Serum *on page 109*
Apolipoprotein B-100, Serum *on page 109*
Apolipoprotein E, Plasma *on page 110*
Lipid Panel, Serum *on page 212*
Lipids, Overview *on page 213*
Low Density Lipoprotein Cholesterol *on page 218*

Synonyms Lp(a)

Applies to Lp(a)-C

Abstract "Lipoprotein-little a" [Lp(a)], a cholesterol- and kringle-containing plasma lipoprotein with a lipid composition very similar to low-density lipoprotein (LDL), has two apoprotein constituents: apo B-100 (the major structural protein of LDL and VLDL) and apo(a), which is unique to Lp(a) and is, because of structural heterogeneity, a source of difficulty in assay development. Lp(a) is thought to be a risk factor for coronary heart disease (CHD) and cerebrovascular disease. Lp(a) can be measured using a variety of methods, but there is a high degree of intermethod variability in results. At present, two approaches are widely used: immunochemical mass assays [reported as Lp(a)] and cholesterol-based mass assays [reported as Lp(a)-C]. The immunochemical assays suffer from variations in antibody specificity resulting from the structural heterogeneity of apo(a). This has made it difficult to develop assay calibrators that are representative of patient specimens.[1,2] Presently, three assay formats are used:

1. an ELISA format with monoclonal antibodies against unique apo(a) epitopes
2. a sandwich ELISA with an antiapo(a) capture antibody and an antiapoB signal antibody
3. a cholesterol-based assay which requires a relatively complex separation of lipoproteins prior to the cholesterol measurement

Lp(a) levels are genetically determined and show extremely wide intrapopulation and interpopulation variabllity. Across all human populations studied to date, the naturally occurring values of Lp(a) vary by more than 1000-fold.[3] Values in whites have a skewed distribution while values in blacks have a gaussian distribution. The median value in blacks is three times higher than the median in whites. The fact that CHD is equally prevalent in the black and white populations implies that the significance of a particular value is not the same in whites as it is in blacks. Therefore, the reference intervals, and the risk-factor cutoff values, should be ethnically based.

Many case-control studies have shown a positive correlation between serum Lp(a) values and prevalent coronary heart disease.[4,5,6] While at least seven prospective studies (one of which included only postmenopausal women)[7] have shown that Lp(a) is a risk factor for CHD;[7,8,9,10,11] at least three studies have failed to confirm such a relationship (see footnote 3).

Specimen Serum

Container Red top tube

Storage Instructions Serum is stable at 4°C for 1 week and frozen for months.

Reference Interval There are no well documented reference values based on large populations, and there is no large database establishing risk percentiles. Traditionally, Lp(a) mass values >30 mg/dL (SI: 1.05 mmol/L) have been classified as reflecting a high risk. Other authorities prefer a cutoff >25 mg/dL (SI: 0.88 mmol/L).

A report from the Framingham Offspring Study,[12] including 3332 white subjects, and using a cholesterol-based assay, found the following reference intervals, based on the central 90% of values: Lp(a)-cholesterol:

- male: 1.35-19.62 mg/dL (SI: 0.035-0.508 mmol/L)
- female: 1.24-20.06 mg/dL (SI: 0.032-0.519 mmol/L)

Lp(a) mass assays performed on a subset of 1000 of these subjects showed that, although the Lp(a) mass result was always higher than the corresponding Lp(a)-C result, the results were strongly correlated.[12]

Use Because of uncertainty about the significance of particular values, Lp(a) measurements are not recommended for general screening.[3] Some investigators do, however, recommend Lp(a) measurements in persons who have a family history of CHD, stroke or "elevated lipid values". **To be useful in practice, Lp(a) results should be reported with ethnically-specific, and gender-specific, population based reference values; moreover, the result should be accompanied by an interpretive statement indicating which reference population percentile corresponds to the patient result.** Results that exceed the 80th percentile are often interpreted as indicative of high risk.

Limitations See Abstract and Use.

(Continued)

Lipoprotein (a), Serum (Continued)

Methodology
- Lp(a) mass: Enzyme-linked immunosorbent assay (ELISA), radial immunodiffusion, radioimmunoassay, latex immunoassay, immunonephelometry, electroimmunodiffusion, immunoturbidimetric, fluorescence assay[2]
- Lp(a) cholesterol: Ultracentrifugation followed by spectrophotometry[3]
- Apo(a) phenotypes: Immunoblotting[13]

Additional Information

Apo(a) phenotypes. A recent case-controlled study[13] demonstrates a strong correlation between apo(a) phenotype and the age at onset of CHD. Thirty different phenotypes were identified among the 705 subjects.

Correlates of high Lp(a) values include a wide array of pathologic conditions, including preeclampsia,[14] recurrent fetal loss,[15] early renal insufficiency,[16] left atrial thrombus,[17] childhood thromboembolism,[18] and children without growth hormone deficiency who are treated with growth hormone.[19]

Risk factor modification. Niacin reduces Lp(a) levels.[3] In a large study (n=2759) of postmenopausal women, treatment with estrogen and progesterone was associated with a lowering of Lp(a) values; this effect was most pronounced in women with the highest baseline Lp(a) values.[7] Other drugs which may lower Lp(a) levels include tamoxifen[20] and anabolic steroids.[21] Exercise may not favorably modify one's Lp(a).[22]

Footnotes
1. Albers JJ, Marcovina SM, and Lodge MS, "The Unique Lipoprotein(a): Properties and Immunochemical Measurement," *Clin Chem*, 1990, 36(12):2019-26.
2. Marcovina SM and Koschinsky ML, "Lipoprotein(a): Structure, Measurement and Clinical Significance," *Handbook of Lipoprotein Testing*, Rifai N, Warnick GR, and Dominiczak MH, eds, Washington, DC: AACC Press, American Association of Clinical Chemistry, 1997, 283-301.
3. Marcovina SM and Koschinsky ML, "Lipoprotein(a) as a Risk Factor for Coronary Artery Disease," *Am J Cardiol*, 1998, 82(12A):57U-66U.
4. Dahlen G and Ramberg UB, "Prebeta-1 Lipoprotein and Early Detection of Risk Factors for Coronary Heart Disease," *Acta Med Scand*, 1974, 195(5):341-4.
5. Dahlen G, Frick MH, Berg K, et al, "Further Studies on Lp(a) Lipoprotein/Prebeta-1-Lipoprotein in Patients With Coronary Heart Disease," *Clin Genet*, 1975, 8(3):183-9.
6. Genest JJ, Martin-Murley SS, McNamara JR, et al, "Familial Lipoprotein Disorders in Patients With Premature Coronary Artery Disease," *Circulation*, 1992, 85(6):2025-33.
7. Shlipak MG, Simon JA, Vittinghoff E, et al, "Estrogen and Progestin, Lipoprotein(a), and the Risk of Recurrent Coronary Heart Disease Events After Menopause," *JAMA*, 2000, 283(14):1845-52.
8. Bostom AG, Gagnon DR, Cupples LA, et al, "A Prospective Investigation of Elevated Lipoprotein(a) Detected by Electrophoresis and Cardiovascular Disease in Women: The Framingham Heart Study," *Circulation*, 1994, 90(45):1688-95.
9. Bostom AG, Cupples LA, Jenner JL, et al, "Elevated Plasma Lipoprotein(a) and Premature Coronary Heart Disease in Framingham Men: A Prospective Study," *JAMA*, 1996, 276(7):544-8.
10. Schaefer EJ, Lamon-Fava S, Jenner JL, et al, "Lipoprotein(a) Levels and Risk of Coronary Artery Disease in Men: The Lipid Research Clinics Coronary Primary Prevention Trial," *JAMA*, 1994, 271:999-1003.
11. Wald NJ, Law M, Watt HC, et al, "Apolipoproteins and Ischaemic Heart Disease: Implications for Screening," *Lancet*, 1994, 343:75-9.
12. Seman LJ, DeLuca C, Jenner JL, et al, "Lipoprotein(a) Cholesterol and Coronary Heart Disease in the Framingham Heart Study," *Clin Chem*, 1999, 45(7):1039-46.
13. Gazzaruso C, Garzaniti A, Buscaglia P, et al, "Association Between Apolipoprotein(a) Phenotypes and Coronary Heart Disease at Young Age," *J Am Coll Cardiol*, 1999, 33(1):157-63.
14. Wang J, Mimuro S, Lahoud R, et al, "Elevated Levels of Lipoprotein(a) in Women With Preeclampsia," *Am J Obstet Gynecol*, 1998, 178(1 Pt 1):146-9.
15. Szczepanski M, Bauer A, Gardas A, et al, "Antiphospholipid Antibodies and Lipoprotein(a) in Women With Recurrent Fetal Loss," *Int J Gynecol Obstet*, 1998, 61(1):39-44.
16. Sechi LA, Zingaro L, DeCarli S, et al, "Increased Serum Lipoprotein(a) Levels in Patients With Early Renal Failure," *Ann Intern Med*, 1998, 129(6):457-61.
17. Igarashi Y, Yamaura M, Ito M, et al, "Elevated Serum Lipoprotein(a) Is a Risk Factor for Left Atrial Thrombus in Patients With Chronic Atrial Fibrillation: A Transesophageal Echocardiographic Study," *Am Heart J*, 1998, 136(6):965-71.
18. Nowak-Gottl U, Debus O, Findeisen M, et al, "Lipoprotein(a): Its Role in Childhood Thromboembolism," *Pediatrics*, 1997, 99(6):E11.
19. Hershkovitz E, Belotserkovsky O, Limony Y, et al, "Increase of Serum Lipoprotein(a) Levels During Growth Hormone Therapy in Normal Short Children," *Eur J Pediatr*, 1998, 157(1):4-7.
20. Elisaf M, Bairaktari E, Nicolaides C, et al, "The Beneficial Effect of Tamoxifen on Serum Lipoprotein-A Levels: An Additional Antiatherogenic Property," *Anticancer Res*, 1996, 16(5A):2725-8.
21. Crook D, Sidhu M, Seed M, et al, "Lipoprotein Lp(a) Levels Are Reduced by Danazol, an Anabolic Steroid," *Atherosclerosis*, 1992, 92(1):41-7.
22. Mackinnon LT and Hubinger LM, "Effects of Exercise on Lipoprotein(a)," *Sports Med*, 1999, 28 (1):11-24.

References
Cantin B, Gagnon F, Moorjani S, et al, "Is Lipoprotein(a) an Independent Risk Factor for Ischemic Heart Disease in Men?" *J Am Coll Cardiol*, 1998, 31:519-25.
Jialal I, "Evolving Lipoprotein Risk Factors: Lipoprotein(a) and Oxidized Low-Density Lipoprotein," *Clin Chem*, 1998, 44(8B):1827-32.
Milionis HJ, Winder AF, and Mikhailidis DP, "Lipoprotein (a) and Stroke," *J Clin Pathol*, 2000, 53:487-96.

♦ **Lipoprotein-Associated Phospholipase A$_2$** see Lipids, Overview on page 213

Lipoprotein Electrophoresis

Related Information
Lipids, Overview on page 213

Synonyms Lipoprotein Phenotyping

Abstract Electrophoresis is no longer the optimal technique for the separation of lipoproteins. The technique is presently of historic interest.

♦ **Lipoprotein Phenotyping** see Lipoprotein Electrophoresis on page 216

♦ **Liver Battery** see Liver Disease: Laboratory Assessment, Overview on page 216

Liver Disease: Laboratory Assessment, Overview

Related Information
Acetaminophen, Serum on page 778
Alanine Aminotransferase, Serum on page 87
Albumin, Serum on page 88
Alkaline Phosphatase, Serum on page 93
Alpha$_1$-Antitrypsin Phenotyping on page 95
Alpha$_1$-Antitrypsin, Serum on page 96
Amiodarone, Serum on page 735
Antimitochondral Antibody on page 505
Aspartate Aminotransferase, Serum on page 112
Bilirubin, Total, Serum on page 118
Bilirubin, Urine on page 870
Body Fluid Chemical Analysis on page 123
Carbohydrate-Deficient Transferrin, Serum on page 134
Carcinoembryonic Antigen, Serum on page 135
Ceruloplasmin, Serum on page 143
Copper, Serum on page 816
Copper, Urine on page 818
Echinococcosis Serological Test on page 602
Ethanol, Blood, Urine, and Other Sources on page 789
Ferritin, Serum on page 173
Gamma-Glutamyl Transferase, Serum on page 179
Hepatitis B Core Antibody on page 622
Hepatitis B DNA Detection on page 623
Hepatitis B$_e$ Antibody on page 624
Hepatitis B$_e$ Antigen on page 624
Hepatitis B Surface Antibody on page 625
Hepatitis B Surface Antigen on page 625
Hepatitis C Virus RNA Detection and Quantitation on page 626
Hepatitis C Virus Serology on page 627
Hepatitis D Serology on page 627
Hepatitis E Serology on page 628
Hepatitis: Laboratory Assessment, Overview on page 629
Iron and Total Iron Binding Capacity/Transferrin, Serum on page 203
Isoniazid, Serum or Plasma on page 753
Lactate Dehydrogenase, Serum on page 207
Leucine Aminopeptidase (LAP), Serum and Urine on page 211
Liver Biopsy on page 65
Liver/Kidney Microsomal Type 1 Antibodies on page 539
5′ Nucleotidase, Serum on page 234
Protein Electrophoresis, Serum on page 267
Prothrombin Time on page 354
Smooth Muscle Antibody on page 543
Yellow Fever on page 697

Synonyms Liver Battery; Liver Panel; Liver Profile

Applies to Acetaminophen; ALT:AST Ratio; AST:ALT Ratio; De Ritis Ratio; Ecstasy; LFTs; Liver Function Tests, So-Called

Test Includes The differential diagnosis of liver disease often requires albumin; bilirubin, total; bilirubin, direct; alkaline phosphatase; aspartate aminotransferase (AST/SGOT); alanine aminotransferase (ALT/SGPT); protein, total; and often GGT (GGTP). It may also include serum protein electrophoresis, prothrombin time, and hepatitis serological tests when indicated. Alpha$_1$-antitrypsin phenotype and quantitation on occasion explains cases otherwise difficult to classify but is rarely, if ever, included in liver profiles. Other tests which may be helpful in evaluation of liver disease include immunoglobulins IgG, IgA, IgM; ANA; antimitochondrial antibody; smooth muscle antibody; liver/kidney microsomal type 1 antibodies, alphafetoprotein, and 2-hour urine urobilinogen. Ammonia is useful in selected cases, **(eg, Reye syndrome, urea cycle disorders**, and certain **organic acidurias)**. Lactate dehydrogenase and LD isoenzymes may be useful in the differential diagnosis of icterus.

Abstract Characterization of liver disease requires correlation of the medical history, physical examination, laboratory test results, and, when indicated, the liver biopsy. Classification of liver disease includes hepatocellular, cholestatic (intra- or extrahepatic) and infiltrative states. Clinical assessment includes patient history and physical examination. Family history is especially relevant in cases of hemolytic anemia, Gilbert syndrome, Dubin-Johnson syndrome, Wilson disease, hemochromatosis, and α_1-antitrypsin deficiency.[1]

Storage Instructions Protect specimens for bilirubin from light.

Causes for Rejection Hemolysis interferes with certain tests (see individual listings).

Special Instructions Note listings for individual tests. The specimens should be handled with extra precaution, especially if there is a greater than usual possibility of viral hepatitis.

Use Evaluate hepatobiliary disease, hepatoma, autoimmune hepatitis and cirrhosis, including biliary cirrhosis; investigate otherwise unexplained increases in such tests as AST, ALT, alkaline phosphatase, or prolongation of prothrombin time; work up possible alcoholism.

A number of useful tests include those to work up **pancreatitis**, such as serum and urine amylase and serum lipase.

The two most common causes of persistent abnormalities of liver function in Western countries are hepatitis C and heavy alcohol consumption.[2] Use of blood alcohol determinations for investigation of liver disease has been advocated, because the test is cheap and simple. Other tests useful in alcoholism include carbohydrate deficient transferrin, MCV, albumin, and folate levels, triglycerides, GGT, and bilirubin. AST increment is greater than that of ALT in alcoholic hepatitis; the **AST:ALT ratio** is >2.0 and AST is not increased more than 250 units/L.[1] Prothrombin time is often helpful. An estimated 15-20 million Americans are alcoholics. Alcoholism causes malnutrition including deficiencies of vitamins, including thiamine and vitamin A as well as folate. It leads to hyperlacticacidemia, hyperuricemia, ketosis, and hyperlipidemia. Alcoholics are vulnerable to a wide variety of substances, solvents, and medications including acetaminophen. Alcoholism may lead to a variety of complications including cirrhosis, gastritis, malnutrition, pancreatitis, and cardiomyopathy.[3]

Cholestasis and biliary tract: alkaline phosphatase, GGT, total bilirubin, conjugated bilirubin, eosinophil count, urine bile (as part of urinalysis) are used. In **extrahepatic biliary obstruction** the serum alkaline phosphatase is increased two to three times or more while AST remains <300 units/L. Very high alkaline phosphatase levels may be found with intrahepatic cholestasis, such that alkaline phosphatase which is high out of proportion to the severity of jaundice, may indicate an intrahepatic disease. Viral, alcoholic, or drug-related cholestatic hepatitis may give rise to chemistry tests indistinguishable from those of extrahepatic obstruction. Primary biliary cirrhosis, primary sclerosing cholangitis, overlap syndrome, and autoimmune cholangiopathy sometimes represent difficult differential diagnosis.[4]

Liver excretory function: urine urobilinogen, total bilirubin, conjugated bilirubin.

In **viral hepatitis**, ALT is greater than AST, but in chronic liver diseases the **AST:ALT ratio** is less useful. In cirrhosis caused by hepatitis B and other agents, the AST:ALT ratio may be >1.0.[1] In acute viral hepatitis, AST is usually three to five times or more higher (as multiples of the upper limit of normal) than LD; in cases which clinically resemble hepatitis, but in which LD equals or exceeds AST, LD isoenzymes may be useful. LD_4 and LD_5 are the hepatic fractions. An isomorphic pattern, if detected, may suggest infectious mononucleosis, CMV infection, neoplasm, or cirrhosis/alcoholism, depending on clinical setting. Transaminases increase in viral and drug-induced hepatitis and peak within 7-14 days, usually in the low thousands range, returning to normal in about 6 weeks in uncomplicated viral hepatitis.[1] At onset they are generally more than 10 times the upper limit of reference range. Alkaline phosphatase is only moderately elevated. Acute viral hepatitis includes at least five separate disease entities. See Hepatitis: Laboratory Assessment, Overview *on page 629.*

Appropriate positive serological tests support a diagnosis of viral hepatitis, while negative ones provide support for other disorders including drug-induced hepatitis. Resolution of liver disease with removal of the offending agent enhances the latter diagnosis. Excellent reviews of **drug-induced hepatotoxicity** have been published.[5,6] Ecstasy, a synthetic amphetamine, may cause hepatic damage resembling acute viral hepatitis.[7]

Table 2 in the listing Liver Biopsy *on page 65,* summarizes histopathologic findings with AST and ALT in toxic hepatic injury.

Chronic hepatitis includes chronic hepatitis B, C, and D and autoimmune hepatitis. It clinically may resemble alcoholic and nonalcoholic steatohepatitis. A review of its classification, criteria, and grading is available.[8] **Nonalcoholic steatohepatitis (NASH)**, a common cause of liver disease in Western countries, is associated with type 2 diabetes, hyperlipidemia, jejunoileal bypass, and drugs including amiodarone and perhexilene. The only clinical manifestation of hepatic steatosis and NASH may be moderate increases of aminotransferase concentrations. The ratio of **ALT to AST** (**ALT:AST ratio** or De Ritis ratio) is >1, but <1.0 in alcoholic liver disease (it is normally <1). Liver biopsy is needed.[2]

Immunologic stimulation: Protein electrophoresis: features suggestive of cirrhosis but not always present in that disease include low albumin, low alpha$_2$, polyclonal or oligoclonal gammopathy, and beta/gamma bridging. Oligoclonal gammopathy is found in <50% of cases of autoimmune hepatitis. HLA phenotypes may be relevant.

Autoimmune hepatitis, found predominantly in young to middle-aged women, is recognized by the presence of increased immunoglobulins and the presence of autoantibodies. More than 80% have hypergammaglobulinemia. Two other major groups of autoimmune liver diseases are recognized, primary biliary cirrhosis and primary sclerosing cholangitis. The distinction between autoimmune hepatitis and chronic viral hepatitis with hyperglobulinemia and/or autoantibodies is sometimes blurred. Wilson

disease also enters this differential diagnosis. In autoimmune hepatitis, classical laboratory features include elevation of serum aminotransferases, bilirubin and alkaline phosphatase, and increased gamma globulins, especially IgG with autoantibodies (ANA and antismooth muscle antibodies in autoimmune hepatitis type 1). In type 2 autoimmune hepatitis, anti-liver-kidney-microsomal 1 antibodies are detected. Soluble liver antigen and smooth muscle antibody are anticipated in type 3. See discussion and table in Smooth Muscle Antibody *on page 543.* Liver biopsy is needed for disease confirmation.

In **ischemic hepatitis**, as develops in instances of cardiac failure and hypotension, the transaminases may be >10,000 IU/L, and vast increases of LDH may be found. Such increased transaminase concentrations may be seen as well with **acetaminophen overdose** and with **herpes simplex hepatitis.**[1]

In the presence of liver disease with hemolysis, **Wilson disease** must be considered. With hypoceruloplasminemia, hypocupremia, and hypercupruria, a diagnosis of Wilson disease is expedited, but liver biopsy for microscopy including rhodamine and orcein stains and tissue copper analysis are worthwhile.[9] See Copper, Urine *on page 818* and Copper, Serum *on page 816.*

Hemochromatosis: Mild abnormalities in liver profile tests (AST, ALT, ALP) may occur in hemochromatosis.[10] Iron, IBC, transferrin, ferritin, and molecular testing are available. Liver biopsy is considered essential for confirmation of the diagnoses of Wilson disease and of hemochromatosis, save that biopsy may be unnecessary in patients younger than age 40 with normal results. See Hereditary Hemochromatosis DNA Test *on page 709* and Hemochromatosis in the Key Word Index.

Liver disease related to **alpha$_1$-antitrypsin deficiency** is associated with periodic acid-Schiff positive diastase-resistant globules[11] and an abnormal α_1-antitrypsin phenotype, PiZZ homozygotes, and several other alleles. (The MM phenotype (PiMM) is normal.) See Alpha$_1$-Antitrypsin Deficiency in the Key Word Index.

Hepatic functional reserve: Both albumin and prothrombin time are useful in evaluation of the liver, but they are nonspecific. Albumin reflects hepatic synthesis and nutritional status but is lost in a variety of gastrointestinal and renal diseases.

Liver metabolic function: Serum ammonia may increase in liver necrosis and cirrhosis as well as in Reye syndrome.

Hepatoma (carcinoma, liver) and other tumors: Useful assays include alkaline phosphatase, GGT, total LD, CEA, HB$_s$Ag (hepatitis B surface antigen). Alpha$_1$-fetoprotein may increase moderately in nonmalignant liver diseases; rising or high levels may indicate hepatoma. Such clinical laboratory tests do not prove tumor without imaging and biopsy. Other primary tumors of liver, benign and malignant, are found.

Metastatic tumors are the most common malignant neoplasms of the liver. The most frequent primaries include carcinoma of the stomach, colon, pancreas, esophagus, lung, and breast. The liver is a site of spread of malignant lymphomas.

Limitations Some types of hepatic injury may not be accompanied by very much increase in enzymes (eg, injury from ethionine or phosphorus).[6]

More specialized tests are often necessary to establish an etiologic diagnosis. Liver biopsy is often needed to provide precise diagnosis in subjects with subacute to chronic abnormalities.[1] See table.

Groups of Serum Enzymes According to Their Sensitivities

Enzyme	Cholestasis*	Hepatocellular Necrosis	Chronic Injury	Injury of Other Organs†
Group I Cholestasis > Hepatic Injury				
ALP, GGT	↑↑↑	↑	↑	+
Group II Hepatic Injury > Cholestasis				
A - Extrahepatic and Hepatic Disease				
AST, LDH	↑	↑↑↑	↑	↑
B - More Specificity for the Liver				
ALT	↑	↑↑↑	↑	↑
C - Still Greater Specificity for Hepatic Injury/Disease				
LDH$_5$	↑	↑↑↑	↑	
Group III Insensitivity to Liver Injury				
CK	Normal	Normal	Normal	↑

5'N = 5'-nucleotidase; ALP = alkaline phosphatase; ALT = alanine aminotransferase; AST = aspartate aminotransferase; CK = creatine kinase; LAP = leucine aminopeptidase; LDH$_5$ = least anodic isoenzyme of lactic dehydrogenase; LDH = lactase dehydrogenase; ↑ = increased; ↑↑↑ = markedly increased; ± = little change.

*Obstructive jaundice or intrahepatic cholestasis.

†Cardiac or skeletal muscle, brain, or kidney.

Modified from Zimmerman HJ, *Hepatotoxicity: The Adverse Effects of Drugs and Other Chemicals on the Liver,* 2nd ed, Philadelphia, PA: Lippincott Williams and Wilkins, 1999.

Many physicians prefer to order tests individually, as clinically indicated. Tests appropriate for specific clinical indications may not be included among tests predefined as laboratory profiles. Few physicians recall accurately the content of a liver profile offered by a specific clinical laboratory. However, the concept of a battery of tests designated "Liver Profile" has expedited order transmission. The enzymes which are often called "LFTs"

(Continued)

Liver Disease: Laboratory Assessment, Overview
(Continued)

("liver function tests") often lack specificity for the liver when used alone, and reflect injury or disease of other organs as well. Use of LDH isoenzymes supports specificity: LDH$_5$ reflects disease of liver or of striated muscle, and CK arises from injury to the latter.

Additional Information Relevant topics in the Key Word Index include Acetaminophen, Biliary Function Tests, Carcinoma (Liver), Cirrhosis, Cirrhosis (Primary Biliary), Hemochromatosis, Hepatic Necrosis/Failure, Hepatitis, Hepatitis (Autoimmune), Jaundice, and Wilson Disease.

Footnotes
1. Kamath PS, "Clinical Approach to the Patient With Abnormal Liver Test Results," *Mayo Clin Proc*, 1996, 71:1089-95.
2. James O and Day C, "Non-alcoholic Steatohepatitis; Another Disease of Affluence," *Lancet*, 1999, 353(9165):1634-6.
3. Lieber CS, "Medical Disorders of Alcoholism," *N Engl J Med*, 1995, 333(16):1058-65.
4. Krawitt EL, "Autoimmune Hepatitis," *N Engl J Med*, 1996, 334(14):897-903.
5. Lee WM, "Drug-Induced Hepatotoxicity," *N Engl J Med*, 1995, 333(17):1118-27.
6. Zimmerman HJ, *Hepatotoxicity: The Adverse Effects of Drugs and Other Chemicals on the Liver*, 2nd ed, Baltimore, MD: Lippincott Williams & Wilkins, 1999.
7. Andrew V, Mao A, Bruguera M, et al, "Ecstasy: A Common Cause of Severe Acute Hepatotoxicity," *J Hepatol*, 1998, 29(3):394-7.
8. Batts KP and Ludwig J, "Chronic Hepatitis: An Update on Terminology and Reporting," *Am J Surg Pathol*, 1995, 19(12):1409-17.
9. Ludwig J, Moyer TP, and Rakela J, "The Liver Biopsy Diagnosis of Wilson's Disease. Methods in Pathology," *Am J Clin Pathol*, 1994, 102(4):443-6.
10. Lin E and Adams PC, "Biochemical Liver Profile in Hemochromatosis. A Survey of 100 Patients," *J Clin Gastroenterol*, 1991, 13(3):316-20.
11. Iezzoni JC, Gaffey MJ, Stacy EK, et al, "Hepatocytic Globules in End-Stage Hepatic Disease: Relationship to Alpha$_1$-Antitrypsin Phenotype," *Am J Clin Pathol*, 1997, 107(6):692-7.

References
Berg CL and Graeme-Cook FM, "A 68-Year Old Woman With Hepatic Encephalopathy," Case Records of the Massachusetts General Hospital, Case 10-1997, Scully RE, Mark EJ, McNeely WF, et al, eds, *N Engl J Med*, 1997, 336(13):939-47.

Kamath PS, Jalihal A, and Chakraborty A, "Differentiation of Typhoid Fever From Fulminant Hepatic Failure in Patients Presenting With Jaundice and Encephalopathy," *Mayo Clin Proc*, 2000, 75(5):462-6.

Lee WM, "Acute Liver Failure," *N Engl J Med*, 1993, 329(25):1862-72.

Pratt DS and Kaplan MM, "Evaluation of Abnormal Liver-Enzyme Results in Asymptomatic Patients," *N Engl J Med*, 2000, 342(17):1266-71.

Schiff ER, "Update in Hepatology," *Ann Intern Med*, 1999, 130(1):52-7.

Schiff ER, "Update in Hepatology," *Ann Intern Med*, 2000, 132(6):460-6.

Tilg H and Diehl AM, "Cytokines in Alcoholic and Nonalcoholic Steatohepatitis," *N Engl J Med*, 2000, 343(20):1467-76.

♦ **Liver Function Tests, So-Called** *see* Liver Disease: Laboratory Assessment, Overview *on page 216*

♦ **Liver Iron Concentration** *see* Ferritin, Serum *on page 173*

♦ **Liver Panel** *see* Liver Disease: Laboratory Assessment, Overview *on page 216*

♦ **Liver Profile** *see* Liver Disease: Laboratory Assessment, Overview *on page 216*

♦ **Loperamide Inhibition Test** *see* Adrenal Cortex: Laboratory Assessments Overview *on page 84*

♦ **Lovastatin** *see* Mevalonic Acid, Urine or Amniotic Fluid *on page 225*

Low Density Lipoprotein Cholesterol

Related Information
Apolipoprotein A-I, Serum *on page 109*
Apolipoprotein B-100, Serum *on page 109*
Cholesterol, Total, Serum or Plasma *on page 146*
High Density Lipoprotein Cholesterol, Serum *on page 192*
Lipid Panel, Serum *on page 212*
Lipids, Overview *on page 213*
Triglycerides, Serum or Plasma *on page 288*

Synonyms Beta Lipoproteins; LDLC

Applies to Familial Hypercholesterolemia; Friedewald Equation; LDLC:HDLC Ratio

Abstract The concentration of cholesterol in this lipoprotein is positively correlated with coronary heart disease risk (see table). It is also a risk factor for dementia with stroke. For additional information, see Lipids, Overview on page 213.

Patient Preparation See Preparation in the listing Cholesterol, Total, Serum or Plasma *on page 146*.

Specimen Serum

Container Red top tube

Sampling Time 12- to 14-hour fast before drawing

Reference Interval See Lipids, Overview *on page 213* and following table.

Population Distributions
for Low Density Lipoprotein Cholesterol (mg/dL)

Age (y)	Percentile						
	Male						
	5	10	25	50	75	90	95
5-9	63	69	80	90	103	117	129
10-14	64	73	82	94	109	123	133
15-19	62	68	80	93	109	123	130
20-24	66	73	85	101	118	138	147
25-29	70	75	96	116	138	157	165
30-34	78	88	107	124	144	166	185
35-39	81	92	110	131	154	176	189
40-44	87	98	115	135	157	173	186
45-49	97	106	120	140	163	185	202
50-54	89	102	118	143	162	185	197
55-59	88	103	123	145	168	191	203
60-64	83	107	121	143	165	188	210
65-69	98	104	125	146	170	199	210
≥70	88	100	119	142	164	182	186
	Female						
5-9	68	73	88	98	115	125	140
10-14	68	73	81	94	110	126	136
15-19	59	73	78	93	110	129	137
20-24	57	65	82	102	118	141	159
25-29	71	75	90	108	126	148	164
30-34	70	77	91	109	129	146	156
35-39	75	81	96	116	139	161	172
40-44	74	84	104	122	146	165	174
45-49	79	89	105	127	150	173	186
50-54	88	94	111	134	160	186	201
55-59	89	97	120	145	168	199	210
60-64	100	105	126	149	168	191	224
65-69	92	99	125	151	184	205	221
≥70	96	108	126	147	170	189	206

To convert to mmol/L, multiply by 0.0259.

Adapted from Lipid Research Clinical Program Epidemiology Committee, "Plasma Lipid Distributions in Selected North American Population: The Lipid Research Clinics Program Prevalence Study," *Circulation*, 1979, 60:427-39.

Critical Values >160 mg/dL (4.14 mmol/L). A goal of LDLC <130 mg/dL (3.36 mmol/L) is desirable in subjects with diabetes mellitus, with triglycerides <200 mg/dL (2.26 mmol/L).[1] The National Cholesterol Education Program recommends diminution of LDLC ≤100 mg/dL (2.59 mmol/L) in patients with established coronary heart disease. The National Committee for Quality Assurance (NCQA), as part of the Health Plan Employer and Data Information Set (HEDIS) endorses achievement of concentrations <130 mg/dL (3.36 mmol/L) 60-365 days following discharge for major coronary heart disease events, a performance measure.[2,3]

Possible Panic Range In subjects homozygous for familial hypercholesterolemia, LDLC reaches 700-1200 mg/dL (18.1-31.0 mmol/L).[4] These are extremely high figures.

Use See Lipids, Overview *on page 213* and table.
Aggressively lowering LDLC to <100 mg/dL diminishes progression of atherosclerosis in saphenous vein coronary bypass grafts.[5]

The heterozygous form of familial hypercholesterolemia affects about 1 in 500 individuals; thus, it is among the more common genetic diseases. In its presence, the risk of a first coronary heart event is 51% by age 50 years among men. Among women, the risk is 58% by age 60 years.[6]

Limitations If triglyceride is >400 mg/dL, LDL cannot be calculated accurately by the Friedewald equation. See notes in methodology. For reliable LDLC levels by calculation, accurate HDLC, cholesterol, and triglyceride methods are necessary.

A large number of drugs affect LDLC.[7]

Methodology Though a true reference method for LDLC does not exist, β-quantification methods similar to those used in large-scale clinical and epidemiological studies are the generally accepted gold standards of measurement. These methods employ ultracentrifugation and polyanion precipitation steps.[8]

The Friedewald equation[9] produces a calculated value for LDLC and is the method currently recommended by the National Cholesterol Education Program (NCEP) for routine use by clinical laboratories.[10]

LDLC (mg/dL) = cholesterol, total (mg/dL) - HDLC (mg/dL) - [triglycerides (mg/dL) / 5]

The equation is valid for samples having a fasting triglyceride concentration up to 400 mg/dL. Specimens with fasting triglycerides >400 mg/dL require a direct measurement of LDLC or may be referred to a specialized lipid laboratory for ultracentrifugal analysis.

Methods for direct measurement of LDLC include heterogeneous immunochemical[11] as well as fully-automatable, detergent-based homogeneous[12,13] assays. These methods are precise, do not require fasting specimens, and generally show satisfactory agreement with the Friedewald and β-quantification methods. Inaccuracy of calculated LDLC increases when triglyceride is >200 mg/dL.[14]

Additional Information Human low density lipoproteins are the major transport proteins for cholesterol and comprise a spectrum of particles that have been characterized by size, chemical composition, metabolic behavior, and atherogenicity. LDL has been subfractionated into three fractions: buoyant, intermediate, and small dense (LDL1-LDL3).[15] There is speculation that oxidized LDL is taken up by macrophages forming the foam cells of atherosclerotic plaques.[16,17] Tissue factor pathway inhibitor (TFPI), a potent inhibitor of extrinsic coagulation is associated with and regulated by LDL.[18] Phenolic substances in red wine inhibit LDL oxidation,[19] possibly explaining why red wine appears to be protective against atherosclerosis in epidemiologic studies in France. Recent studies suggest that white wines contain oxidation inhibitors. Interestingly, at least one study has shown that LDL proteins from diabetics have *in vivo* modifications in protein and lipid moiety, that are able to induce massive cholesterol accumulation in cultured aortic intimal cells.[20]

The importance of physical activity in management of LDLC is emphasized.[21]

LDLC is an independent risk factor for development of dementia with stroke.[22]

Footnotes

1. O'Brian T, Nguyen TT, and Zimmerman BR, "Hyperlipidemia and Diabetes Mellitus," *Mayo Clin Proc*, 1998, 73, 969-76.
2. Lee TH, Cleeman JI, Grundy SM, et al, "Clinical Goals and Performance Measures for Cholesterol Management in Secondary Prevention of Coronary Heart Disease," *JAMA*, 2000, 283(1):94-8.
3. Allison TG, Squires RW, Johnson BD, et al, "Achieving National Cholesterol Education Program Goals for Low-Density Lipoprotein Cholesterol in Cardiac Patients: Importance of Diet, Exercise, Weight Control, and Drug Therapy," *Mayo Clin Proc*, 1999, 74:466-73.
4. Steinberg D and Gotta AM Jr, "Preventing Coronary Artery Disease by Lowering Cholesterol Levels - Fifty Years From Bench to Bedside," *JAMA*, 1999, 282(21):2043-50.
5. "The Effect of Aggressive Lowering of Low-Density Lipoprotein Cholesterol Levels and Low-Dose Anticoagulation on Obstructive Changes in Saphenous-Vein Coronary-Artery Bypass Grafts," Postcoronary Artery Bypass Graft Trial Investigators, *N Engl J Med*, 1997, 336(3):153-62.
6. Rifkind BM, Schucker B, and Gordon DJ, "When Should Patients With Heterozygous Familial Hypercholesterolemia Be Treated?" *JAMA*, 1999, 281(2):180-1.
7. Young DS, "Effects of Drugs on Clinical Laboratory Tests," 5th ed, Volume 1: Listing by Test, Washington DC: AACC Press, American Association of Clinical Chemistry, 2000, Section 3, 495-507.
8. Bachorik PS, "Measurement of Low-Density Lipoprotein Cholesterol," *Handbook of Lipoprotein Testing*, Rifai N, Warnick GR, and Dominiczak MH, eds, Washington, DC: AACC Press, American Association of Clinical Chemistry, 1997, 145-60.
9. Friedewald WT, Levy RI, and Fredrickson DS, "Estimation of the Concentration of Low-Density Lipoprotein Cholesterol in Plasma, Without Use of the Preparative Ultracentrifuge," *Clin Chem*, 1972, 18(6):499-502.
10. Bachorik PS and Ross JW, "National Cholesterol Education Program Recommendations for Measurements of Low-Density Lipoprotein Cholesterol: Executive Summary. National Cholesterol Education Program Working Group on Lipoprotein Measurements," *Clin Chem*, 1995, 41(10):1414-20.
11. Jialal I, Hirany SV, Devaraj S, et al, "Comparison of an Immunoprecipitation Method for Direct Measurement of LDL-Cholesterol With Beta-Quantification (Ultracentrifugation)," *Am J Clin Pathol*, 1995, 104(1):76-81.
12. Nauck M, Graziani MS, Bruton D, et al, "Analytical and Clinical Performance of a Detergent-Based Homogeneous LDL-Cholesterol Assay: A Multicenter Evaluation," *Clin Chem*, 2000, 46(4):506-14.
13. Rifai N, Iannotti E, DeAngelis K, et al, "Analytical and Clinical Performance of a Homogeneous Enzymatic LDL-Cholesterol Assay Compared With the Ultracentrifugation-Dextran Sulfate-Mg^{2+} Method," *Clin Chem*, 1998, 44(6):1242-50.
14. Branchi A, Rovellini A, Torri A, et al, "Accuracy of Calculated Serum Low-Density Lipoprotein Cholesterol for the Assessment of Coronary Heart Disease Risk in NIDDM Patients," *Diabetes Care*, 1998, 21(9):1397-1402.
15. Watson TD, Caslake MJ, Freeman DJ, et al, "Determinants of LDL Subfraction Distribution and Concentrations in Young Normolipemic Subjects," *Arterioscler Thromb*, 1994, 14(6):902-10.
16. Young SG and Parthasarathy S, "Why Are Low-Density Lipoproteins Atherogenic?" *West J Med*, 1994, 160(2):153-64.
17. Kanazawa T, Osanai T, Uemura T, et al, "Evaluation of Oxidized Low-Density Lipoprotein and Large Molecular Size Low-Density Lipoproteins in Atherosclerosis," *Pathobiology*, 1993, 61(3-4):200-10.
18. Hansen JB, Huseby NE, Sandset PM, et al, "Tissue-Factor Pathway Inhibitor and Lipoproteins. Evidence for Association With and Regulation by LDL in Human Plasma," *Arterioscler Thromb*, 1994, 14(2):223-9.
19. "Inhibition of LDL Oxidation by Phenolic Substances in Red Wine: A Clue to the French Paradox," *Nutr Rev*, 1993, 51(6):185-7.
20. Solenin IA, Tehton VV, and Ohekhov AN, "Characterization of Chemical Composition of Native and Modified Low Density Lipoprotein Occurring in the Blood of Diabetic Patients," *Int Angiol*, 1994, 13(1):78-83.
21. Stefanick ML, Mackey S, Sheehan M, et al, "Effects of Diet and Exercise in Men and Postmenopausal Women With Low Levels of HDL Cholesterol and High Levels of LDL Cholesterol," *N Engl J Med*, 1998, 339(1):12-20.
22. Moroney JT, Tang MX, Berglund L, et al, "Low-Density Lipoprotein Cholesterol and the Risk of Dementia With Stoke," *JAMA*, 1999, 282(3):254-60.

References

Austin MA, Breslow JL, Hennekens CH, et al, "Low-Density Lipoprotein Subclass Patterns and Risk of Myocardial Infarction," *JAMA*, 1988, 260(13):1917-21.

Goodman DS, Hulley SB, Clark LT, et al, "Report of the National Cholesterol Education Program Expert Panel on Detection, Evaluation, and Treatment of High Blood Cholesterol in Adults," *Arch Intern Med*, 1988, 148(1):36-69.

Hostetter AL, "Screening for Dyslipidemia, Practice Parameter," *Am J Clin Pathol*, 1995, 103(4):380-5.

"National Cholesterol Education Program, Adult Treatment Panel Report 1987," National Cholesterol Education Program, National Heart, Lung, and Blood Institute, National Institutes of Health, 1987, C-200, Bethesda, MD.

Pitt B, Waters D, Brown WV, et al, "Aggressive Lipid-Lowering Therapy Compared With Angioplasty in Stable Coronary Artery Disease," *N Engl J Med*, 1999, 341(2):70-6.

Rifai N, Bachorik PS, and Albers JS, "Lipids, Lipoproteins and Apolipoproteins," *Tietz Textbook of Clinical Chemistry*, 3rd ed, Burtis CA and Ashwood ER, eds, Philadelphia, PA: WB Saunders Co, 1999, 809-61.

Rifai N, Warnick GR, McNamara JR, et al, "Measurement of Low Density Lipoprotein Cholesterol in Serum: A Status Report," *Clin Chem*, 1992, 38(1):150-60.

Steinberg D, Parthasarathy S, Carew TE, et al, "Beyond Cholesterol. Modifications of Low-Density Lipoprotein That Increase Its Atherogenicity," *N Engl J Med*, 1989, 320(14):915-24.

Warnick GR, Knopp RH, Fitzpatrick V, et al, "Estimating Low Density Lipoprotein Cholesterol by the Friedewald Equation Is Adequate for Classifying Patients on the Basis of Nationally Recommended Cutpoints," *Clin Chem*, 1990, 36(1):15-9.

♦ **Low Density Lipoprotein Cholesterol (LDLC)** see Lipids, Overview on *page 213*

♦ **Lp(a)** see Lipoprotein (a), Serum on *page 215*

♦ **Lp(a)-C** see Lipoprotein (a), Serum on *page 215*

♦ **L:S Ratio** see Lecithin:Sphingomyelin Ratio, Amniotic Fluid on *page 210*

♦ **Lung Profile, Amniotic Fluid** see Lecithin:Sphingomyelin Ratio, Amniotic Fluid on *page 210*

♦ **Luteinizing Hormone** see Testosterone, Total and Free, Serum or Plasma on *page 280*

Luteinizing Hormone, Blood or Urine

Related Information

Adrenal Cortex: Laboratory Assessments Overview on *page 84*
Clomiphene Test on *page 150*
Estradiol, Serum on *page 170*
Estrogens, Urine on *page 172*
Follicle Stimulating Hormone, Serum, Plasma, or Urine on *page 175*
Growth Hormone, Serum on *page 189*
Heterophilic Antibodies on *page 191*
Progesterone, Serum on *page 201*
Prolactin, Serum on *page 262*
Testosterone, Total and Free, Serum or Plasma on *page 280*
Urine Collection, 24-Hour on *page 47*

Synonyms Follitropin; ICSH; Interstitial Cell Stimulating Hormone; LH

Applies to Gonadotropic Hormones; Leydig Cells; Pituitary Gonadotropins

Test Includes Usually measured with FSH

Abstract Luteinizing hormone (LH) and follicle stimulating hormone (FSH) are glycoprotein gonadotropic hormones produced by the same pituitary cell type. The alpha subunits of LH, FSH, thyroid stimulating hormone (TSH), and human gonadotropin (hCG) are identical; specificity resides in the beta subunits.

LH and FSH are under complex regulation by hypothalamic gonadotropin releasing hormone (GnRH) and by the gonadal sex hormones: estrogen and progesterone in females, and testosterone in males. FSH and LH, respectively, stimulate spermatogenesis and production of testosterone by the Leydig cells of the testes.

Levels of LH and FSH are used to assess anterior pituitary gonadotropic function, sexual differentiation, fertility, and pseudohermaphroditism. In general, FSH and LH are elevated in conditions in which sex hormones cannot be elaborated and are decreased in conditions of primary pituitary dysfunction.

Patient Preparation Avoid radioisotope administration to patient prior to collection of specimen if RIA is used for assay.

Specimen Serum or 24-hour urine

Container Red top tube; plastic urine container containing boric acid

Storage Instructions Separate serum from cells. Stable 14 days at 4°C to 25°C.

Special Instructions In females, date of last menstrual period should be supplied. It is important to measure both FSH and LH.

Reference Interval Check with the testing laboratory as there is considerable variation among laboratories. Results can only be interpreted with clinical information. Some representative ranges are as follows.[1]

Serum:
- prepubertal children: <1.0 IU/L
- adults, male: 1.0-9.0 IU/L
- adults, female:
  - follicular: 1.0-18.0 IU/L
  - midcycle: 20.0-80.0 IU/L
  - luteal: 0.5-18.0 IU/L
  - postmenopausal: 12.0-55.0 IU/L

Urine:
- prepubertal children: <0.2 IU/24 hours
- adults, male: 0.2-5.0 IU/24 hours

(Continued)

Luteinizing Hormone, Blood or Urine (Continued)

- adults, female:
  - nonmidcycle: <5.0 IU/24 hours
  - postmenopausal: >5.0 IU/24 hours

Use Excessive FSH and LH production occurs in anorchia, gonadal failure, complete testicular feminization syndrome, and menopause. FSH and LH are pituitary products, useful for distinguishing primary gonadal failure from secondary (hypothalamic/pituitary) causes of gonadal failure, menstrual disturbances, and amenorrhea. Both FSH and LH are low with primary pituitary or hypothalamic failure. When one is high and the other low, a gonadotropin-producing pituitary tumor is likely.

FSH and LH are useful in infertility evaluation of women and testicular dysfunction in men. Elevated basal LH with high LH:FSH ratio (>2), accompanied by an increase of ovarian androgen in an essentially nonovulatory adult female, is presumptive evidence of Stein-Leventhal syndrome in the appropriate clinical setting. High concentrations of LH (during the follicular phase) in patients with polycystic ovary syndrome interfere with conception and may contribute to early pregnancy loss in these patients.[2]

LH acts upon and is used to assess Leydig cell function in males. It regulates male sexual differentiation, androgenization, and sexual function.[3] In males, LH has been called interstitial cell stimulating hormone (ICSH) because of its effect on testosterone production by Leydig cells, necessary for normal maturation of spermatozoa.

Urinary LH and FSH are used in children who have precocious puberty, in many of whom serum FSH and LH levels overlap the normal range. An advantage of 24-hour urine collections is that they overcome problems of pulsatile secretion spikes.

FSH, LH and testosterone are low in Kallmann syndrome. Isolated LH deficiency is a variant of Kallmann syndrome. Patients who have growth hormone deficiency have FSH and/or LH deficiency as well.

Limitations Secretion of both LH and FSH are pulsatile, in response to the normal intermittent release of gonadotropin releasing hormone (GnRH). Problems of secretion spikes are minimized with 24-hour urine collections. While both are pulsatile, LH exhibits a circadian rhythm while FSH does not.[4] In addition, in females both FSH and LH vary over the course of the menstrual cycle, with peaks at time of ovulation. Thus, interpretation of a single determination may be difficult. Only 75% of patients with polycystic ovary syndrome have increased LH. Increased LH with normal or low FSH may occur with obesity, hyperthyroidism, and in liver disease. Normal LH and FSH (RIA) levels can occur in hypoestrogenic patients. The glycoprotein hormones can be heterogeneous inactive molecules which may circulate and cross react with reagent antibodies in the radioimmunoassay to give a false value. FSH and LH within normal range can occur with CNS/pituitary failure.

Gonadal resistance to LH caused by mutations to the LH receptor gene are described.[3]

Methodology Radioimmunoassay (RIA), immunoradiometric assay (IRMA), radioreceptor assay,[5] dissociation enhanced lanthanide fluoroimmunoassay (DELFIA),[6] chemiluminescence immunoassay (CIA),[7] immunofluorometric assay

Additional Information A retrospective study of 100 patients with gonadotroph pituitary adenomas found that hypersecretion of LH or FSH is unusual in these patients.[8] Another study did not find useful serum LH or FSH measurements for the diagnosis of prepubertal monorchism.[9]

A combination of serum LH and FSH measurements on day 1 of the menstrual cycle has been shown to be a good indicator of ovarian reserve (reproductive age) in normally cycling women.[10] The LH/FSH ratio has been reported to be a predictor of ovarian hyperstimulation syndrome, an iatrogenic complication of gonadotropin therapy.[11] However, serum LH, unlike serum FSH and serum estradiol, was not shown to be a good predictor of ovarian response to stimulation with highly purified FSH after pituitary down-regulation with leuprolide acetate.[12]

LH increases in urine after the pituitary's LH surge that precedes ovulation by 24-36 hours. Home use test kits for qualitative urine LH are available for predicting when ovulation is likely to occur and have been reported to be effective for this use.[13]

Footnotes

1. Mayo Medical Laboratories, *2000 Test Catalogue*, Rochester, MN.
2. Homburg R, Armar NA, Eshel A, et al, "Influence of Serum Luteinizing Hormone Concentrations on Ovulation, Conception, and Early Pregnancy Loss in Polycystic Ovary Syndrome," *Br Med J*, 1988, 297(6655):1024-6.
3. Latronico AC, Anasti J, Arnhold IJ, et al, "Brief Report: Testicular and Ovarian Resistance to Luteinizing Hormone Caused by Inactivating Mutations of the Luteinizing Hormone-Receptor Gene," *N Engl J Med*, 1996, 334(8):507-12.
4. Dunkel L, Alfthan H, Stenman UH, et al, "Developmental Changes in 24-Hour Profiles of Luteinizing Hormone and Follicle-Stimulating Hormone From Prepuberty to Midstages of Puberty in Boys," *J Clin Endocrinol Metab*, 1992, 74(4):890-7.
5. Whitcomb RW and Schneyer AL, "Development and Validation of a Radioligand Receptor Assay for Measurement of Luteinizing Hormone in Human Serum," *J Clin Endocrinol Metab*, 1990, 71(3):591-5.
6. Menjivar M, Ortiz G, Cardenas M, et al, "Comparison of the DELFIA and RIA Methods for Measuring Luteinizing and Follicle Stimulating Hormones in Serum," *Rev Invest Clin*, 1993, 45(6):579-84.

7. Rojanasakul A, Udomsubpayakul U, and Chinsomboom S, "Chemiluminescence Immunoassay Versus Radioimmunoassay for the Measurement of Reproductive Hormones," *Int J Gynaecol Obstet*, 1994, 45(2):141-6.
8. Young WF, Scheithauer BW, Kovacs KT, et al, "Gonadotroph Adenoma of the Pituitary Gland: A Clinicopathologic Analysis of 100 Cases," *Mayo Clin Proc*, 1996, 71(7):649-56.
9. Palmer LS, Gill B, and Kogan SJ, "Endocrine Analysis of Childhood Monorchism," *J Urol*, 1997, 158(2):594-6.
10. Kim YK, Wasser SK, Fujimoto VY, et al, "Utility of Follicle Stimulating Hormone (FSH), Luteinizing Hormone (LH), Oestradiol and FSH:LH Ratio in Predicting Reproductive Age in Normal Women," *Hum Reprod*, 1997, 12(6):1152-5.
11. Bodis J, Torok A, and Tinneberg HR, "LH/FSH Ratio as a Predictor of Ovarian Hyperstimulation Syndrome," *Hum Reprod*, 1997, 12(4):869-70.
12. Develioglu OH, Cox B, Toner JP, et al, "The Value of Basal Serum Follicle Stimulating Hormone, Luteinizing Hormone and Oestradiol Concentrations Following Pituitary Down-Regulation in Predicting Ovarian Response to Stimulation With Highly Purified Follicle Stimulating Hormone," *Hum Reprod*, 1999, 14(5):1168-74.
13. Miller PB and Soules MR, "The Usefulness of a Urinary LH Kit for Ovulation Prediction During Menstrual Cycles of Normal Women," *Obstet Gynecol*, 1996, 87(1):13-7.

References

Apter D, Cacciatore B, Alfthan H, et al, "Serum Luteinizing Hormone Concentrations Increase 100-Fold in Females From 7 Years to Adulthood, as Measured by Time-Resolved Immunofluorometric Assay," *J Clin Endocrinol Metab*, 1989, 68(1):53-7.

Backer LC, Rubin CS, Marcus M, et al, "Serum Follicle-Stimulating Hormone and Luteinizing Hormone in Levels in Women Aged 35-60 in the U.S. Population: The Third National Health and Nutrition Examination Survey (NHANES III, 1988-1994)," *Menopause*, 1999, 6(1):29-35.

Demers LM, "Pituitary Function," *Tietz Textbook of Clinical Chemistry*, 3rd ed, Chapter 41, Burtis CA and Ashwood ER, eds, Philadelphia, PA: WB Saunders Co, 1999, 1470-95.

Franks S, "Polycystic Ovary Syndrome," *N Engl J Med*, 1995, 333(13):853-61.

Kossoy LR, Hill GA, Parker RA, et al, "Luteinizing Hormone and Ovulation Timing in a Therapeutic Donor Insemination Program Using Frozen Semen," *Am J Obstet Gynecol*, 1989, 160(5 Pt 1):1169-72.

Liu G, Duranteau L, Carel JC, et al, "Leydig-Cell Tumors Caused by an Activating Mutation of the Gene Encoding the Luteinizing Hormone Receptor," *N Engl J Med*, 1999, 341(23):1731-6.

Nippoldt TB, Reame NE, Kelch RP, et al, "The Roles of Estradiol and Progesterone in Decreasing Luteinizing Hormone Pulse Frequency in the Luteal Phase of the Menstrual Cycle," *J Clin Endocrinol Metab*, 1989, 69(1):67-76.

Turhan NO, Toppare MF, Seckin NC, et al, "THe Predictive Power of Endocrine Tests for the Diagnosis of Polycystic Ovaries in Women With Oligoamenorrhea," *Gynecol Obstet Invest*, 1999, 48(3):183-6.

Vance ML, "Hypopituitarism," *N Engl J Med*, 1994, 330(23):1651-62.

- **Lymphocyte, Vacuolated** *see* Mucopolysaccharides, Urine *on page 226*

- **Lysine** *see* Cystine, Urine *on page 164*

Lysophosphatidic Acid, Plasma

Synonyms Ovarian Cancer Activating Factor

Abstract Lysophosphatidic acid (LPA), a heterogeneous substance originally purified from the ascites fluid of patients with ovarian carcinoma, has undergone preliminary evaluation at the Cleveland Clinic as a biomarker for ovarian and other gynecologic cancers.[1]

Specimen Plasma

Container Lavender top (EDTA) tube

Sampling Time Not determined

Collection Whole blood is centrifuged at 580 g for 5 minutes; supernatant is transferred to microcentrifuge and centrifuged at 8000 g for 5 minutes (to remove remaining platelets).

Storage Instructions Store plasma at -70°C.

Reference Interval <1.3 μmol/L[1]

Critical Values Not established

Use Not yet established. In a sample of patients with various gynecologic cancers and healthy controls, and a cutoff value of 1.3 μmol/L, the overall sensitivity for gynecologic cancer was 95% and the specificity was 98%. Eight of 9 patients (89%) with FIGO Stage I ovarian cancer had elevated LPA, as compared with 2 of 9 (22%) who had elevated CA 125 (>35 kU/L). All of 24 patients with FIGO Stages II, III, and IV ovarian cancer had elevated LPA results, as did all of 14 patients with recurrent ovarian cancer.

Limitations Since LPA is released by platelets during the coagulation process, specimen collection and handling must be optimal to avoid erroneous values.

Methodology Research assay (Cleveland Clinic) includes thin layer chromatographic (TLC) separation followed by gas chromatography (GC).

Footnotes

1. Xu Y, Shen Z, Wiper DW, et al, "Lysophosphatidic Acid as a Potential Biomarker for Ovarian and Other Gynecologic Cancers," *JAMA*, 1998, 280(8):719-23.

- **Lysylpyridinoline** *see* Pyridinolines (Pyridinoline and Deoxypyridinoline), Urine *on page 272*

- **Magnesium:Creatinine Ratio, Urine** *see* Magnesium, Urine *on page 222*

- **Magnesium-Loading Test** *see* Magnesium, Urine *on page 222*

- **Magnesium Retention Test** *see* Magnesium, Urine *on page 222*

Magnesium, Serum

Related Information

Aminoglycosides, Serum *on page 734*
Calcium, Serum *on page 131*
Digoxin, Serum *on page 746*
Magnesium, Urine *on page 222*
Potassium, Urine *on page 259*

Synonyms

Mg, Serum

Applies to

iMg^{2+}_s (Ionized Serum Magnesium); tMg_s (Total Magnesium, Serum); tMg (Total Magnesium)

Abstract

Magnesium (Mg) is one of the major inorganic cations; the others are sodium, potassium, and calcium. It is the second most abundant cation within the cell, after potassium and the most important intracellular divalent cation. Intracellular Mg concentrations are much higher than extracellular (serum) values, but measurement of serum Mg is still relevant. Most intracellular Mg is complexed. The clinical importance of hypomagnesemia in the critically ill is still being developed. It is a cofactor for multiple enzyme systems. Up to 40% of hypokalemic patients are also hypomagnesemic.[1] Urinary Mg declines before serum magnesium. Cardiovascular benefits of doses of Mg following myocardial infarct may need further study. Changes may occur with administration of blood components.

Patient Preparation

Smoking negatively interferes with NOVA Mg ion-specific electrode.[2]

Specimen

Serum. Mg can also be measured in erythrocytes and in mononuclear blood cells.

Container

Red top tube

Collection

Draw without venous stasis, separate serum from red cells as soon as possible.

Storage Instructions

Refrigerate. Serum separated from cells is stable at 2°C to 6°C for several days.

Causes for Rejection

Hemolysis

Reference Interval

tMg_s: 1.5-2.3 mg/dL (SI: 0.62-0.95 mmol/L or 1.2-1.9 mEq/L), although slightly different ranges are reported by different laboratories.[3] Four sets of units are in use to express concentration of Mg: 1.0 mEq/L = 1.22 mg/dL = 0.5 mmol/L = 12.2 mg/L. Mg, like calcium, is partly protein bound. Slightly low values in the presence of hypoalbuminemia or hypoproteinemia should not, therefore, be of major concern. A 1996 paper provides a range of 1.8-2.2 mg/dL.[3]

iMg^{2+}_s: 1.1-1.6 mg/dL (SI: 0.47-0.65 mmol/L)[4]

Possible Panic Range

Symptoms appear at <1.2 mg/dL (SI: <0.5 mmol/L); serum concentrations at <1.2 mg/dL are regarded as severe depletion. Slightly low levels should be repeated on a new specimen. Hospital diet often improves Mg levels, especially in those who have not been on a normal diet. Toxic symptoms appear >4.9 mg/dL (SI: >2.0 mmol/L). Possible death from respiratory failure >14.6 mg/dL (SI: >6.0 mmol/L).

Hypomagnesemia iMg^{2+}_s <1.1 mg/dL (<0.46 mmol/L).[4]

Use

Magnesium deficiency produces neuromuscular spasm, fasciculations, hyperactivity and may cause weakness, dizziness, tremors, tetany, and convulsions. Coronary arterial spasm, hypertension and development of kidney stones may relate to hypomagnesemia. Magnesium deficiency may be associated with and may cause cardiac arrhythmias, especially in the presence of hypokalemia. An association with acute infarct and sudden death exists. Magnesium depletion induces vitamin D resistance.[3] Usually of nutritional origin, hypomagnesemia is associated with hypocalcemia; hypokalemia; phosphate deficiency; long-term hyperalimentation; intravenous therapy; diabetes mellitus, especially during treatment of ketoacidosis; acidosis/alkalosis; alcoholism and other types of malnutrition; pancreatitis; short bowel syndrome; malabsorption and chronic diarrhea; hyperparathyroidism; dialysis; pregnancy; glomerulonephritis; and hyperaldosteronism. Renal loss of magnesium occurs, including that with cisplatin therapy and in those taking mercurial diuretics or ammonium chloride. Alfrey also adds amphotericin toxicity to the causes of hypomagnesemia. Significantly decreased tMg was found in chronic alcoholics.[5] See Summary of Indications.

Increased magnesium levels relate mostly to patients in renal failure. Marked increases may be found in such patients who take magnesium salts (eg, as antacids which contain magnesium). Increased serum magnesium is also found with Addison disease, and in pregnant patients with severe preeclampsia or eclampsia who are receiving magnesium sulfate as an anticonvulsant. Hypermagnesemia may occur in patients using magnesium-containing cathartics.[6] Increased Mg concentrations may occur with dehydration and diabetic acidosis. High magnesium levels are manifested by decreased reflexes, somnolence, and heart block.

Indications for measurement of serum magnesium include the presence of unexplained hypocalcemia, instances in which hypokalemia is unresponsive to potassium supplementation, and in patients who have cardiac disorders in which hypomagnesemia may be especially hazardous such as congestive failure, myocardial infarct, ventricular ectopy, digitalis use, or left ventricular hypertrophy. Serum magnesium is indicated only selectively in patients on diuretics: those on high dose thiazides, loop diuretics (eg, furosemide), or hydrochlorothiazide in doses >50 mg/day.

Because an association between aminoglycoside therapy and severe hypomagnesemia is described, a recommendation is published to measure serum magnesium in subjects receiving aminoglycosides. Recommendations also exist to measure it in patients on cyclosporine[7] or cisplatin.

Summary of Indications

for the measurement of serum magnesium concentration:[1,8]

- myocardial infarct
- refractory cardiac arrhythmia
- alcoholism
- refractory hypokalemia, hypocalcemia, hyponatremia
- diuretic therapy, particularly with multiple agents
- digoxin toxicity
- aminoglycoside therapy
- amphotericin B therapy
- parenteral nutrition
- severe or chronic diarrhea
- unexplained electrolyte disturbance
- unexplained neuromuscular irritability, particularly in the absence of hypocalcemia
- treatment with nephrotoxic or cytotoxic agents
- neurological abnormalities in the neonate
- preeclampsia or eclampsia

Limitations

Hemolysis will yield elevated results as levels in erythrocytes are two to three times higher than serum. Bilirubin may cause falsely low values by methylthymol blue photometric assays. Although measured low levels of Mg provide evidence of Mg deficiency, serum Mg concentrations may not adequately reflect magnesium status. Serum magnesium constitutes only a small fraction of total body stores and may not predict magnesium status correctly.[3,4,9] **Magnesium deficiency sufficiently severe to lead to hypocalcemia and cardiac arrhythmias may exist in the presence of normal levels of serum magnesium.**[3] Declining before serum Mg, urinary Mg is reported as an earlier and more reliable signal of evolving Mg deficiency.[3] Huijgen et al found that about 70% of patients hypomagnesemic by tMg_s are no longer so when iMg^{2+} is measured.[4]

Methodology

Spectrophotometry using calmagite dye, methylthymol blue; fluorometry; enzymatic methods; atomic absorption spectrophotometry (AAS).[1,4] These methods were found to correlate, although a slight bias to higher values was reported with the Du Pont aca®, for levels >2.4 mg/dL (SI: >1.0 mmol/L). Inductively-coupled plasma emission spectroscopy is in use.[3] Measurement of intracellular Mg would be desirable but is not routinely available.

The application of ion-selective electrodes is under active investigation.[1,4,5,10,11,12] About 50% to 60% of plasma Mg exists in a free ionized form. Mg by ion-selective electrode is independent of protein binding.[4]

Additional Information

Magnesium is the second most abundant intracellular ion. Ionized magnesium (Mg^{2+}) is the physiologically active form with the protein bound and chelated magnesium forming a pool. Approximately 50% of the total body magnesium is present in soft tissues with the other half stored in bone. Less than 1% of the total body magnesium is present in serum.[13]

Only about 1% of intracellular magnesium is present in the free ionized form (Mg^{2+}) (iMg^{2+}_s). Free Mg^{2+} levels are carefully controlled within the cell. Total cellular magnesium is maintained at the expense of extracellular and bone magnesium.[14] The most important binding protein in blood of Mg is albumin. A negative correlation exists between serum albumin and iMg^{2+}_s. Decreased tMg was more common than diminished iMg^{2+}_s in a series examining critically ill patients.[4]

Parathormone enhances tubular reabsorption of magnesium. Measure magnesium in patients with hypocalcemia, of whom 23%, without renal failure, were found in one study to have hypomagnesemia. Magnesium-containing drugs can cause toxic levels in patients with impaired renal function. A causal relation between decreased Mg^{2+} content of cardiac muscle/coronary arteries and nonocclusive sudden-death ischemic heart disease has been proposed. Magnesium acts as a metallic cofactor in over 300 enzymatic reactions.[15] A positive correlation between normomagnesemia and successful resuscitation is reported. Serum magnesium has prognostic importance in congestive heart failure.[16] Magnesium-depleted ICU patients have higher mortality rates than magnesium-repleted patients.[17] There is an association between development of type 2 diabetes and low serum magnesium, although a relation with low dietary intake has not been established.[18]

Footnotes

1. Ryan MF and Barbour H, "Magnesium Measurement in Routine Clinical Practice," *Ann Clin Biochem*, 1998, 35(Pt 4):449-59.
2. Niemela JE, Cecco SA, Rehak NN, et al, "The Effect of Smoking on the Serum Ionized Magnesium Concentration Is Method Dependent," *Arch Pathol Lab Med*, 1997, 121(10):1087-92.
3. Fleming CR, George L, Stoner GL, et al, "The Importance of Urinary Magnesium Values in Patients With Gut Failure," *Mayo Clin Proc*, 1996, 71(1):21-4.
4. Huijgen HJ, Soesan M, Sanders R, et al, "Magnesium Levels in Critically Ill Patients. What Should We Measure?" *Am J Clin Pathol*, 2000, 114(5):688-95.
5. Hristova EN, Rehak NN, Cecco S, et al, "Serum Ionized Magnesium in Chronic Alcoholism: Is It Really Decreased?" *Clin Chem*, 1997, 43(2):394-9.
6. Gerard SK, Hernandez C, and Khayam-Bashi H, "Extreme Hypermagnesemia Caused by an Overdose of Magnesium-Containing Cathartics," *Ann Emerg Med*, 1988, 17(7):728-31.

(Continued)

Magnesium, Serum *(Continued)*

7. Chernow B, Bamberger S, Stoiko M, et al, "Hypomagnesemia in Patients in Postoperative Intensive Care," *Chest*, 1989, 95(2):391-7.
8. Ryan MF, "The Role of Magnesium in Clinical Biochemistry: An Overview," *Ann Clin Biochem*, 1991, 28(Pt 1):19-26.
9. Elin RJ, "Assessment of Magnesium Status," *Clin Chem*, 1987, 33(11):1965-70.
10. Foley C and Zaritsky A, "Should We Measure Ionized Magnesium?" *Crit Care Med*, 1998, 26(12):1949-50.
11. Fiser RT, Torres A, Butch AW, et al, "Ionized Magnesium Concentrations in Critically Ill Children," *Crit Care Med*, 1998, 26(12):2048-52.
12. Wu C and Kenny MA, "Circulating Total and Ionized Magnesium After Ethanol Ingestion," *Clin Chem*, 1996, 42(4):625-9.
13. Elin RJ, "Magnesium: The Fifth But Forgotten Electrolyte," *Am J Clin Pathol*, 1994, 102(5):616-22.
14. Quamme GA, "Magnesium Homeostasis and Renal Magnesium Handling," *Miner Electrolyte Metab*, 1993, 19(4-5):218-25.
15. Reinhart RA, "Clinical Correlates of the Molecular and Cellular Actions of Magnesium on the Cardiovascular System," *Am Heart J*, 1991, 121(5):1513-21.
16. Gottlieb SS, Baruch L, Kukin ML, et al, "Prognostic Importance of the Serum Magnesium Concentration in Patients With Congestive Heart Failure," *J Am Coll Cardiol*, 1990, 16(4):827-31.
17. Olerich MA and Rude RK, "Should We Supplement Magnesium in Critically Ill Patients?" *New Horiz*, 1994, 2(2):186-92.
18. Kao W, Folsom AR, Nieto FJ, et al, "Serum and Dietary Magnesium and the Risk for Type 2 Diabetes Mellitus," *Arch Intern Med*, 1999, 159(18):2151-9.

References

Castelbaum AR, Donofrio PD, Walker FO, et al, "Laxative Abuse Causing Hypermagnesemia, Quadriparesis, and Neuromuscular Junction Defect," *Neurology*, 1989, 39(5):746-7.

Gottlieb SS, "Importance of Magnesium in Congestive Heart Failure," *Am J Cardiol*, 1989, 63(14):39G-42G.

Gren J and Woolf A, "Hypermagnesemia Associated With Catharsis in a Salicylate-Intoxicated Patient With Anorexia Nervosa," *Ann Emerg Med*, 1989, 18(2):200-3.

Lum G, "Hypomagnesemia in Acute and Chronic Care Patient Populations," *Am J Clin Pathol*, 1992, 97(6):827-30.

Quamme GA, "Laboratory Evaluation of Magnesium Status: Renal Function and Free Intracellular Magnesium Concentration," *Clin Lab Med*, 1993, 13(1):209-23.

Rubenowitz E, Axelsson G, and Rylander R, "Magnesium and Calcium in Drinking Water and Death From Acute Myocardial Infarction in Women," *Epidemiology*, 1999, 10(1):31-6.

Siddiqui MN, Zafar H, Alvi R, et al, "Hypomagnesemia in Postoperative Patients: An Important Contributing Factor in Postoperative Mortality," *Int J Clin Pract*, 1998, 52(4):265-7.

Toffaletti J, "Physiology and Regulation. Ionized Calcium, Magnesium, and Lactate Measurements in Critical Care Settings," *Am J Clin Pathol*, 1995, 104(4 Suppl 1):S88-94.

Weber CA and Santiago RM, "Hypermagnesemia. A Potential Complication During Treatment of Theophylline Intoxication With Oral Activated Charcoal and Magnesium-Containing Cathartics," *Chest*, 1989, 95(1):56-9.

Magnesium, Urine

Related Information

Aminoglycosides, Serum *on page 734*
Amphotericin B, Serum *on page 737*
Calcium, Serum *on page 131*
Calcium, Urine *on page 133*
Citrate, Serum, Plasma, or Urine *on page 149*
Cyclosporine, Blood *on page 744*
Digoxin, Serum *on page 746*
Ketone Bodies, Blood *on page 205*
Kidney Stone Analysis *on page 877*
Magnesium, Serum *on page 221*
Oxalate, Urine *on page 238*
Potassium, Serum or Plasma *on page 258*
Urine Collection, 24-Hour *on page 47*
Vitamin D, Serum *on page 300*

Synonyms Mg, Urine

Applies to Magnesium:Creatinine Ratio, Urine; Magnesium-Loading Test; Magnesium Retention Test

Abstract Hypomagnesemia is manifested by neuromuscular abnormalities, including fasciculation and tremor; see Magnesium, Serum *on page 221*. The kidneys provide the major excretory path for magnesium. Urine magnesium collections may be used to evaluate urine magnesium loss and balance; magnesium balance is controlled by magnesium excretion. Urinary magnesium may diminish before serum magnesium does and may provide earlier indication of evolving deficiency. Magnesium deficiency sufficiently severe to lead to hypocalcemia and cardiac arrhythmias can exist in the presence of normal serum magnesium concentrations.[1]

Patient Preparation Patient should be instructed to use a plastic bedpan; *vide infra.*

Specimen 24-hour urine is preferred[2]

Container Plastic acid-washed urine container; addition of an acidifying agent such as hydrochloric acid as preservative is desirable; check with laboratory. Acidification to pH 1.0 is recommended.[2]

Collection Since a circadian rhythm exists for magnesium excretion, 24-hour collections are indicated. In children, in whom a timed collection may not be feasible, **urine magnesium:creatinine ratio** can be used.[3] See graphic.

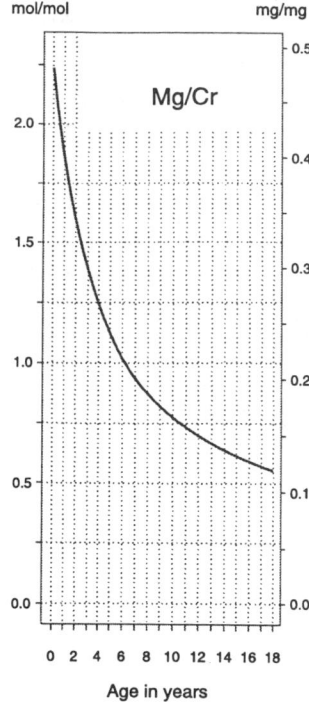

Estimated 95th percentiles for urinary
Mg/Cr ratios in relation to age.

Storage Instructions Refrigerate

Causes for Rejection Specimen allowed to contact metal.

Reference Interval 6.0-10.0 mEq/day (SI: 3-5 mmol/day). Some laboratories report in mg/24 hours: 120-160 mg/day. The mean in control subjects was 127 mg/24 hours in a 1996 paper. See information regarding units in the listing Magnesium, Serum *on page 221*. Values are slightly higher in males.

Use Urinary collection is valuable to detect magnesium deficiency due to gastrointestinal causes (eg, gut failure or Crohn disease).[1,4] Replacement of Mg in patients with gut failure should be directed at normalization of urinary Mg. The propensity to form calcium oxalate kidney stones is related to urine concentrations of oxalate and calcium, and inversely to those of citrate and Mg.[1]

Urinary excretion is not diminished if depletion is caused by a renal leak.[5] Magnesium urinary excretion is enhanced by increasing blood alcohol levels, diuretics, Bartter syndrome, Gitelman syndrome, corticosteroids, cis-platinum therapy, and aldosterone. Renal magnesium wasting occurs in renal transplant recipients who are on cyclosporine and prednisone. Other drugs which may lead to magnesium depletion include aminoglycosides, cyclosporine, pentamidine, and foscarnet.[5] Renal conservation of magnesium is diminished by hypercalciuria, salt-losing conditions, and the syndrome of inappropriate secretion of antidiuretic hormone. Urinary magnesium analyses have been advocated before and after therapeutic magnesium administration to further investigate the significance of an apparent low serum concentration.[6] Significantly diminished urinary magnesium concentration is found in some subjects whose serum magnesium is within normal limits.[1]

Limitations A lack of uniformity exists among references regarding boundaries of reference range for urine magnesium. Lack of consistent normal ranges for serum magnesium between published papers, laboratories, and geographic areas is also evident. High urinary concentrations of Mg can lead to errors by calmagite photometric assays if such specimens are not appropriately diluted.[2]

Methodology Atomic absorption (AA), inductively-coupled plasma emission spectroscopy, enzymatic methods, photometric assays. Methods have been compared and tabulated.[2]

Additional Information Regulation of magnesium balance is via intestinal absorption (dietary source) and renal excretion. Magnesium is filtered at the glomerulus and reabsorbed along various tubular segments. The loop of Henle plays the major role in orchestration of magnesium resorption and urinary magnesium excretion.[7]

Hypercalcemia, hypophosphatemia, and acidosis, including diabetic ketoacidosis, are among inhibitors of tubular reabsorption of magnesium. A magnesium retention test is described to assess magnesium deficit in bone, but problems exist.[4] A criterion used to ascertain the magnitude of magnesium deficiency is the magnesium-loading test.[1]

Gitelman and Bartter syndromes have been recently reviewed.[8]

Footnotes

1. Fleming CR, George L, Stoner GL, et al, "The Importance of Urinary Magnesium Values in Patients With Gut Failure," *Mayo Clin Proc*, 1996, 71(1):21-4.
2. Ryan MF and Barbour H, "Magnesium Measurement in Routine Clinical Practice," *Ann Clin Biochem*, 1998, 35(Pt 4):449-59.
3. Matos V, Van Melle G, Boulat O, et al, "Urinary Phosphate/Creatinine, Calcium/Creatinine and Magnesium/Creatinine Ratios in a Healthy Pediatric Population," *J Pediatr*, 1997, 131(2):252-7.
4. Elin RJ, "Magnesium: The Fifth but Forgotten Electrolyte," *Am J Clin Pathol*, 1994, 102(5):616-22.
5. Alfrey AC, "Disorders of Magnesium Metabolism," *Cecil Textbook of Medicine*, Chapter 223, 21st ed, Goldman L and Bennett JC, eds, Philadelphia, PA: WB Saunders Co, 2000, 1137-9.
6. Chernow B, Bamberger S, Stoiko M, et al, "Hypomagnesemia in Patients in Postoperative Intensive Care," *Chest*, 1989, 95(2):391-7.
7. Quamme GA, "Magnesium Homeostasis and Renal Magnesium Handling," *Miner Electrolyte Metab*, 1993, 19(4-5):218-25.
8. Scheinman SJ, Guay-Woodford LM, Thakker RV, et al, "Genetic Disorders of Renal Electrolyte Transport," *N Engl J Med*, 1999, 340(15):1177-87.

References

Dorup I, "Magnesium and Potassium Deficiency. Its Diagnosis, Occurrence and Treatment in Diuretic Therapy and Its Consequences for Growth, Protein Synthesis and Growth Factors," *Acta Physiol Scand*, 1994, 618(Suppl):1-55.

Nicoll GW, Struthers AD, and Fraser CG, "Biological Variation of Urinary Magnesium," *Clin Chem*, 1991, 37(10 Pt 1):1794-5.

Roelofsen JM, Berkel GM, Uttendorfsky OT, et al, "Urinary Excretion Rates of Calcium and Magnesium in Normal and Complicated Pregnancies," *Eur J Obstet Gynecol Reprod Biol*, 1988, 27(3):227-36.

Metanephrines, Urine or Plasma

Related Information

Catecholamines, Fractionation, Plasma *on page 138*
Catecholamines, Fractionation, Urine *on page 139*
Homovanillic Acid, Urine *on page 195*
Multiple Endocrine Neoplasia/Familial Medullary Thyroid Carcinoma *on page 727*
Urine Collection, 24-Hour *on page 47*
Vanillylmandelic Acid, Urine *on page 297*

Synonyms Metanephrine; Normetanephrine; Total Metanephrines

Applies to Catecholamines; Epinephrine; Metanephrine:Creatinine Ratio, Urine; Norepinephrine

Test Includes Metanephrine and normetanephrine

Abstract The collective term "metanephrines" includes metanephrine and normetanephrine, the *O*-methylated metabolites of the catecholamines, epinephrine, and norepinephrine, respectively. Clinical interest in the metanephrines is focused on the catecholamine-secreting neoplasms predominantly arising from the adrenal medulla: pheochromocytomas, paragangliomas and neuroblastomas. Measurement of metanephrines is highly sensitive for the diagnosis of pheochromocytoma, and the urine **metanephrine:creatinine ratio** may be even better; its published sensitivity of 100% and negative predictive value of 100% seem impressive.[1,2]

Patient Preparation Methylxanthine-containing food products and smoking should be avoided after midnight.[3] A number of drugs may interfere with testing. They include buspirone, labetalol, sotalol, levodopa, acetaminophen, methyldopa, oxprenolol, oxytetracycline, phenylephrine, hydrazine derivatives, monoamine oxidase inhibitors and prochlorperazine.[4] Other drugs reported to cause interference have included antihypertensive drugs, bromocriptine, phenothiazines, tricyclic antidepressants, and propranolol.[5] Check with testing laboratory for specific instructions (see Limitations).

Emotional and physical stress should be minimized prior to and during specimen collection. Patient should be at rest during urine collections and should rest prior to blood collections (see Collection).

Specimen 24-hour urine, plasma

Container Plastic urine container; green top (heparin) tube or lavender top (EDTA) tube, check with the laboratory.

Collection

Urine: Specimens for catecholamines, VMA, and metanephrines should be obtained while the patient is resting, not on medications, and without recent exposure to imaging contrast materials.[6] The likelihood of detection of pheochromocytoma is enhanced if the collection period is initiated by or includes a hypertensive crisis. Acidify urine to pH 2-4 after collection is complete. Check with laboratory for instructions.

Blood: Collection of blood specimens should be done from an indwelling catheter in an antecubital vein after the patient has rested supine for at least 20 minutes; arterial blood can be used.[3] Collect blood into precooled tubes containing appropriate anticoagulant; centrifuge within 30 minutes.[3]

Overnight collections for urinary catecholamines and metanephrines have been advocated for diagnosis of pheochromocytoma.[7]

Storage Instructions Keep urine collection cold. Freeze plasma until assay.

Reference Interval Reference ranges vary among laboratories. Urinary metanephrine levels are slightly higher among men.[2]

Urine:

- metanephrines, total: <1.4 mg/24 hours (SI: <7 μmol/day)[6] or ≤1.2 μg/mg creatinine (SI: ≤0.69 mmol/mol creatinine).[8]
- normetanephrine (free plus conjugated): <0.4 mg/24hours (SI: <2.0 μmol/day)[6]
- metanephrine (free plus conjugated): <0.3 mg/24hours (SI: <1.5 μmol/day)[6]
- urinary metanephrine:creatinine ratios:
  men: 0.152 ±0.074
  women: 0.181 ±0.090
  upper limit of normal: 0.354[2]

Plasma:

- normetanephrine (free): ≤0.66 nmol/L[3]
- metanephrine (free): ≤0.30 nmol/L[3]

Use Measurement of metanephrines in urine or plasma is one of the most effective biochemical approaches to the diagnosis of a catecholamine-secreting neoplasm. Chemical testing is indicated for postoperative follow-up.

Limitations Urine: Overestimation or underestimation of time of collection of a urine specimen remain problematic. False-negative **urinary** results occur (eg, interference by methylglucamine in x-ray contrast medium).[5] False-positive **urinary** results occur; results should be confirmed by repeat testing, imaging or other means, such as urine catecholamines and VMA. False positives can be caused by stress and drugs. Interfering substances partly depend on analytical methods. Drugs causing interference are addressed above. New immunoassays are reported to provide advantages from drug interference.[9]

Blood: A few patients with stroke, respiratory or cardiac failure or other severe diseases have increased plasma metanephrines. False-positive plasma assays may occur in patients with hypertension or chronic renal disease.

Methodology Photometry, fluorometry, gas chromatography (GC), high performance liquid chromatography (HPLC), radioenzymatic methods, and immunoassay. HPLC with electrochemical detection is the most commonly used method, and is superior to colorimetric assays. Héron, et al, used HPLC with electrochemical detection in their study, which included urinary metanephrine to creatinine ratio. Measurement of urinary metanephrines by liquid chromatography almost eliminates false positives from food or drugs.[2]

Additional Information Because the secretion from a pheochromocytoma is usually episodic, plasma catecholamine levels drawn during asymptomatic periods may be normal, while total urinary metanephrines collected over 24 hours are likely to be abnormal. On the other hand, a tumor could be intermittently active, but secrete over a full 24-hour period total metanephrines that are within reference ranges. Analyses of 24-hour urine specimens are preferable to spot (random) urine samples for catecholamines, VMA, and metanephrines.

Assay of urinary total urinary metanephrines has provided the highest number of true positive results for pheochromocytoma. It has become the first choice as a screening test. Recent reports, however, have suggested that measurement of metanephrine and norepinephrine in plasma is even more sensitive and specific than measurement of urine metanephrines in the diagnosis of pheochromocytoma.[3,10] Although normal plasma metanephrine concentrations are reported to rule out pheochromocytoma, normal urine metanephrine and normal plasma catecholamine concentrations do not.[3]

Most pheochromocytomas are sporadic, but some are familial. Pheochromocytoma may be a manifestation of von Hippel-Lindau disease or multiple endocrine neoplasia (MEN) 2A or 2B. Tumors of kidney, pancreas and epididymus, cerebellar hermangioblastoma and retinal angiomas occur in von Hippel-Lindau disease. Such patients in a 1999 series had especially high plasma levels of normetanephrine.[10] Bilaterality is suggestive of von Hippel-Lindau disease, or MEN 2A, in which medullary carcinoma of thyroid and hyperparathyroidism also are found.[11] Familial pheochromocytoma also is found in von Recklinghausen disease, neurofibromatosis type 1.

When only a spot urine sample is available or the 24-hour urine collection is incomplete, simultaneous measurement of urine creatinine permits expression of the metanephrine:creatinine ratio. Reference intervals for 24-hour urinary metanephrines in hypertensives are available.[12] Pheochromocytomas cause hypertension that is classically paroxysmal. They may cause sudden headache, pallor, perspiration, and palpitation. Rarely, hypotension presents as the initial manifestation.[7]

Other tests for neuroblastoma include HVA, VMA, and CEA.

Footnotes

1. Bravo EL, "Plasma or Urinary Metanephrines for the Diagnosis of Pheochromocytoma? That Is the Question," *Ann Intern Med*, 1996, 125(4):331-2.
(Continued)

Metanephrines, Urine or Plasma (Continued)

2. Héron E, Chatellier G, Billaud E, et al, "The Urinary Metanephrine-to-Creatinine Ratio for the Diagnosis of Pheochromocytoma," Ann Intern Med, 1996, 125(4):300-3.

3. Lenders JW, Keiser HR, Goldstein DS, et al, "Plasma Metanephrines in the Diagnosis of Pheochromocytoma," Ann Intern Med, 1995, 123(2):101-9.

4. Young DS, Effects of Drugs on Clinical Laboratory Tests, 5th ed, Volume 1: Listing by Test, Washington, DC: AACC Press, 2000, 3:551-2.

5. Sheps SG, Jiang NS, Klee GG, et al, "Recent Developments in the Diagnosis and Treatment of Pheochromocytoma," Mayo Clin Proc, 1990, 65(1):88-95.

6. Pisano JJ, "A Simple Analysis of Normetanephrine and Metanephrine in Urine," Clin Chim Acta, 1960, 5:406-14.

7. Peaston RT, Lennard TW, and Lai LC, "Overnight Excretion of Urinary Catecholamines and Metabolites in the Detection of Pheochromocytoma," J Clin Endocrinol Metab, 1996, 81(4):1378-84.

8. Rosano TG and Whitley RJ, "Catecholamines and Serotonin," Tietz Textbook of Clinical Chemistry, 3rd ed, Chapter 14, Burtis CA and Ashwood ER, eds, Philadelphia, PA: WB Saunders Co, 1999, 1570-600.

9. Wassell J, Reed P, Kane J, et al, "Freedom From Drug Interference in New Immunoassays for Urinary Catecholamines and Metanephrines," Clin Chem, 1999, 45(12):2216-23.

10. Eisenhofer G, Lenders JWM, Linehan WM, et al, "Plasma Normetanephrine and Metanephrine for Detecting Pheochromocytoma in Von Hippel-Lindau Disease and Multiple Endocrine Neoplasia Type 2," N Engl J Med, 1999, 340(24):1872-9.

11. Pomares FJ, Canas R, Rodriguez JM, et al, "Differences Between Sporadic and Multiple Endocrine Neoplasia Type 2A Phaeochromocytoma," Clin Endocrinol, 1998, 48(2):195-200.

12. Kairisto V, Koskinen P, Mattila K, et al, "Reference Intervals for 24-Hour Urinary Normetanephrine, Metanephrine, and 3-Methoxy-4-Hydroxymandelic Acid in Hypertensive Patients," Clin Chem, 1992, 38(3):416-20.

References

Eisenhofer G, Keiser H, Friberg P, et al, "Plasma Metanephrines Are Markers of Pheochromocytoma Produced by Catechol-O-Methyltransferase Within Tumors," J Clin Endocrinol Metab, 1998, 83(6):2175-85.

Fonseca V and Bouloux PM, "Pheochromocytoma and Paraganglioma," Baillieres Clin Endocrinol Metab, 1993, 7(2):509-44.

Jessurun CR, Adam K, Moise KJ Jr, et al, "Pheochromocytoma-Induced Myocardial Infarction in Pregnancy. A Case Report and Literature Review," Tex Heart Inst J, 1993, 20(2):120-2.

Klingler PJ, Fox TP, Menke DM, et al, "Pheochromocytoma in an Incidentally Discovered Asymptomatic Cystic Adrenal Mass," Mayo Clin Proc, 2000, 75(5):517-20.

Krakoff LR, "Searching for Pheochromocytoma: A New and Better Test?" Ann Intern Med, 1995, 123(2):150-1.

Lenders JW, Eisenhofer G, Armando I, et al, "Determination of Metanephrines in Plasma by Liquid Chromatography With Electrochemical Detection," Clin Chem, 1993, 39(1):97-103.

Lucon A, Pereira M, Mendonca B, et al, "Pheochromocytoma: Study of 50 Cases," J Urol, 1997, 157:1208-12.

Pacak K, Linehan WM, Eisenhofer G, et al, "Recent Advances in Genetics, Diagnosis, Localization, and Treatment of Pheochromocytoma," Ann Intern Med, 2001, 134(4):315-29.

Rosano TG, Swift TA, and Hayes LW, "Advances in Catecholamine and Metabolite Measurements for Diagnosis of Pheochromocytoma," Clin Chem, 1991, 37(10 Pt 2):1854-67.

Witteles RM, Kaplan EL, and Roizen MF, "Sensitivity of Diagnostic and Localization Tests for Pheochromocytoma in Clinical Practice," Arch Intern Med, 2000, 160(16):2521-4.

♦ **Metformin** see Lactic Acid, Whole Blood or Plasma on page 208

♦ **Methanol** see Osmolality, Calculated, Serum or Plasma on page 234

♦ **Methionine** see Amino Acids, Urine on page 101

Methionine Loading Test

Related Information

Cobalamin, Serum on page 150
Folic Acid, RBC on page 435
Folic Acid, Serum on page 435
Homocyst(e)ine, Plasma on page 193
Vitamin B_6, Plasma or Serum on page 299

Abstract This test includes the measurement of plasma homocyst(e)ine (Hcy - see Homocyst(e)ine, Plasma on page 193) at certain intervals (eg, 2, 4, or most commonly, 6 hours) following an oral dose of methionine (100 mg L-methionine/kg body weight).[1]

Reference Interval Not well defined. Increased risk of atherogenesis is correlated with 6-hour postmethionine plasma homocyst(e)ine values >40 µmol/L.

Use This test is used in three different clinical situations:

1. Detection of mild (heterozygous) cases of homocystinuria, by stressing the transulfuration pathway of methionine metabolism.[1]
2. Assessment of vitamin (B_6, B_{12}, and folate) status[2]
3. More recently, to identify individuals at increased risk for thrombotic events despite normal fasting Hcy levels[3] (see Homocyst(e)ine, Plasma on page 193)

Limitations For all applications, the appropriate reference ranges are uncertain. Testing results appear to be much less specific than was anticipated by theoretical consideration.[1]

Additional Information For examples of how this test is used in clinical research studies, see the references by Chambers et al and Vermeulen et al.

Footnotes

1. Still RA and McDowell IFW, "Clinical Implications of Plasma Homocysteine Measurement in Cardiovascular Disease," J Clin Pathol, 1998, 51:183-8.

2. McCormick DB and Greene HL, "Vitamins," Tietz Textbook of Clinical Chemistry, 3rd ed, Burtis CA and Ashwood ER, eds, Philadelphia, PA: WB Saunders Co, 1999, 1018.

3. Mayo Medical Laboratories, "New Test Available - Methionine Load, Plasma," Rochester, MN, October 1998.

References

Chambers JC, Obeid OA, Refsum H, et al, "Plasma Homocysteine Concentrations and Risk of Coronary Heart Disease in UK Asian and European Men," Lancet, 2000, 355(9203):523-7.

Domagala TB, Libura M, and Szczeklik A, "Hyperhomocysteinemia Following Oral Methionine Load Is Associated With Increased Lipid Peroxidation," Thrombosis Research, 1997, 87(4):411-6.

Vermeulen EG, Stehouwer CD, Twisk JW, et al, "Effect of Homocysteine-Lowering Treatment With Folic Acid Plus Vitamin B_6 on Progression of Subclinical Atherosclerosis: A Randomized, Placebo-Controlled Trial," Lancet, 2000, 355(9203):517-22.

♦ **3-Methoxy-4-Hydroxymandelic Acid** see Vanillylmandelic Acid, Urine on page 297

Methylmalonic Acid, Serum, Plasma, Urine, or Amniotic Fluid

Related Information

Anemia Flowchart on page 392
Cobalamin, Serum on page 150
Folic Acid, RBC on page 435
Folic Acid, Serum on page 435
Gastric Analysis on page 180
Helicobacter pylori Biopsy-Based Tests: The Urease Tests, Culture, Cytology, and PCR on page 620
Homocyst(e)ine, Plasma on page 193
Schilling Test on page 483

Abstract The predominant cause of cobalamin deficiency is pernicious anemia. Recommended initial testing in macrocytic/megaloblastic anemia includes serum levels of cobalamin with serum and red cell folate, utilizing methylmalonic acid (MMA) and homocyst(e)ine concentrations as follow-up evaluation when necessary.[1] Recently, a more important role, as initial test modalities, that can detect early and subclinical functional cobalamin deficiency has been pursued for these metabolites[2,3,4,5,6,7] (with some detractors).[8] Since cobalamin is required for conversion of methylmalonic acid to succinic acid, subjects with cobalamin deficiency have increased serum and urine concentrations of methylmalonic acid which decrease following cobalamin administration.

MMA is also a diagnostic marker for methylmalonic acidemias and acidurias, a group of some eight inherited disorders, inborn errors of organic acid metabolism.

Patient Preparation Broad spectrum antibiotics can cause decreased to normal levels in patients who have cobalamin deficiency by inhibition of gut flora, but such drugs do not change increased homocyst(e)ine concentrations.

Specimen Serum, plasma (EDTA), urine; amniocentesis obtained between 16-19 weeks gestational age.[9]

Reference Interval 70-270 nmol/L; the median concentration in cases of cobalamin deficiency is about 3500 nmol/L, but values as great as 2,000,000 nmol/L are described. In cobalamin responsive methylmalonic aciduria, following initiation of treatment, concentrations return to normal in 5-10 days.

Use Confirm cobalamin deficiency; detect early/subclinical cobalamin deficiency; distinction between cobalamin and folate deficiency; methylmalonic acid is increased in >95% of subjects who have cobalamin deficiency. Methylmalonic acid concentrations are not increased with folate deficiency. (Serum homocyst(e)ine concentrations are increased in both). Folate therapy in cobalamin-deficient individuals does not cause a decrease of methylmalonic acid concentrations. Cobalamin deficiency, prevalent following gastric surgery,[10] occurs following resection of distal small intestine (eg, as with Crohn disease) as well as in Addisonian pernicious anemia.

Limitations Renal failure and volume depletion may increase levels of both methylmalonic acid and homocyst(e)ine. In a study of patients who had undergone gastric surgery and had cobalamin deficiency, 20% had only elevation of serum total homocyst(e)ine levels without abnormal methylmalonic acid concentrations.[10]

Methodology Gas chromatography-mass spectrometry (GC/MS); other method. Recently, liquid chromatography-electrospray tandem mass spectrometry (LC-MS/MS) methods have been developed for the routine determination of total homocyst(e)ine[11] and of methylmalonic acid[12] with apparent advantages (analytic time per test of 3 minutes and lower cost).[12]

Additional Information Homocyst(e)ine accumulates with deficiency of either vitamin B_{12} or folate. Conversion of methylmalonyl coenzyme A to succinyl coenzyme A is impaired by deficiency of vitamin B_{12}, leading to accumulation of methylmalonic acid. Methylmalonic acid and homo-cyst(e)ine concentrations provide strong evidence of deficiency. They have a high level of sensitivity to early and subclinical cobalamin deficiency, greater than that of the traditional cobalamin level and Schilling test studies.[2,3,4,5,6,7] They provide confirmation of diagnosis when confirmation is needed.

Isolated methylmalonyl CoA mutase deficiency is associated with clinical neonatal or infantile metabolic ketoacidosis. There may be absence of mutase (mut[0]) or structurally altered mutase (mut·) in affected cells. Affected children have methylmalonic acidemia and methylmalonic aciduria that do not respond to cobalamin treatment, but may be treated by protein restriction.[13] In infants with methylmalonic acidurias, cobalamin deficiency must be excluded, particularly in infants who are breast-fed by a mother who is either a strict vegetarian or who has subclinical pernicious anemia.[14]

Footnotes

1. Allen RH, "Megaloblastic Anemias," *Cecil Textbook of Medicine*, 21st ed, Goldman L and Bennett JC, eds, Philadelphia, PA: WB Saunders Co, 2000, 859-67.
2. Savage DG, Lindenbaum J, Stabler SP, et al, "Sensitivity of Serum Methylmalonic Acid and Total Homocysteine Determinations for Diagnosing Cobalamin and Folate Deficiencies," *Am J Med*, 1994, 96(3):239-46.
3. Green R, "New Assays of Folate and Vitamin B$_{12}$ Metabolism," *Clin Lab Haematol*, 1997, 19:289-320.
4. Björkregren K and Svärdsudd K, "Elevated Serum Levels of Methylmalonic Acid and Homocysteine in Elderly People. A Population-Based Intervention Study," *J Intern Med*, 1999, 246(6):317-24.
5. Carmel R, "Current Concepts in Cobalamin Deficiency," *Annu Rev Med*, 2000, 51:357-75.
6. Klee GG, "Cobalamin and Folate Evaluation: Measurement of Methylmalonic Acid and Homocysteine vs Vitamin B$_{12}$ and Folate," *Clin Chem*, 2000, 46(8 Pt 2):1277-83.
7. Zittoun J and Zittoun R, "Modern Clinical Testing Strategies in Cobalamin and Folate Deficiency," *Semin Hematol*, 1999, 36(1):35-46.
8. Chanarin I and Metz J, "Diagnosis of Cobalamin Deficiency: The Old and the New," *Br J Haematol*, 1997, 97(4):695-700.
9. Mayo Reference Services Publication, "Methylmalonic Acid (MMA), Amniotic Fluid," *New Test Announcement*, #81921, Rochester, MN: Mayo Medical Laboratories, September 2000.
10. Sumner AE, Chin MM, Abraham JL, et al, "Elevated Methylmalonic Acid and Total Homocysteine Levels Show High Prevalence of Vitamin B$_{12}$ Deficiency After Gastric Surgery," *Ann Intern Med*, 1996, 124(5):469-76.
11. Magera MJ, Lacey JM, Casetta B, et al, "Method for the Determination of Total Homocysteine in Plasma and Urine by Stable Isotope Dilution and Electrospray Tandem Mass Spectrometry," *Clin Chem*, 1999, 45(9):1517-22.
12. Magera MJ, Helgeson JK, Matern D, et al, "Methylmalonic Acid Measured in Plasma and Urine by Stable-Isotope Dilution and Electrospray Tandem Mass Spectrometry," *Clin Chem*, 2000, 46(11):1804-10.
13. Fenton WA and Rosenberg LE, "Disorders of Propionate and Methylmalonate Metabolism," *The Metabolic and Molecular Bases of Inherited Disease*, 7th ed, Volume 1, Chapter 41, Scriver CR, Beaudet AL, Sly WS, et al, eds, New York, NY: McGraw-Hill Inc, 1995, 1425-49.
14. deBaulny HO and Saudubray JM, "Branched-Chain Organic Acidurias," *Inborn Metabolic Diseases: Diagnosis and Treatment*, Fernandes J, Saudubray JM, and Van den Berghe G, eds, New York, NY: Springer-Verlag, 2000, 195-212.

References

Holleland G, Schneede J, Ueland PM, et al, "Cobalamin Deficiency in General Practice: Assessment of the Diagnostic Utility and Cost-Benefit Analysis of Methylmalonic Acid Determination in Relation to Current Diagnostic Strategies," *Clin Chem*, 1999, 45(2):189-98.

Koehler KM, Romero LJ, Stauber PM, et al, "Vitamin Supplementation and Other Variables Affecting Serum Homocysteine and Methylmalonic Acid Concentrations in Elderly Men and Women," *J Am Coll Nutr*, 1996, 15(4):364-76.

Lindgren A, Swolin B, Nilsson O, et al, "Serum Methylmalonic Acid and Total Homocysteine in Patients With Suspected Cobalamin Deficiency: A Clinical Study Based on Gastrointestinal Histopathological Findings," *Am J Hematol*, 1997, 56(4):230-8.

Nicolaides P, Leonard J, and Surtees R, "Neurological Outcome of Methylmalonic Acidaemia," *Arch Dis Child*, 1998, 78(6):508-12.

Norman EJ, "Urinary Methylmalonic Acid/Creatinine Ratio: A Gold Standard Test for Tissue Vitamin B$_{12}$ Deficiency," *J Am Geriatr Soc*, 1999, 47(9):1158-9.

Norman EJ, "Urinary Methylmalonic Acid/Creatinine Ratio Defines True Tissue Cobalamin Deficiency," *Br J Haematol*, 1998, 100(3):614-5.

Pettersson T, Friman C, Abrahamsson L, et al, "Serum Homocysteine and Methylmalonic Acid in Patients With Rheumatoid Arthritis and Cobalaminopenia," *J Rheumatol*, 1998, 25(5):859-63.

Pfeiffer CM, Smith SJ, Miller DT, et al, "Comparison of Serum and Plasma Methylmalonic Acid Measurements in 13 Laboratories: An International Study," *Clin Chem*, 1999, 45(12):2236-42.

Rasmussen K, Moller J, Lyngba M, et al, "Age- and Gender-Specific Reference Intervals for Total Homocysteine and Methylmalonic Acid in Plasma Before and After Vitamin Supplementation," *Clin Chem*, 1996, 42(4):630-6.

Rifai N, Hagen T, Bradley L, et al, "Determination of Serum Physiological Concentration of Methylmalonic Acid by Gas Chromatography-Mass Spectrometry With Selected Ion Monitoring," *Ann Clin Biochem*, 1998, 35(Pt 5):633-6.

Sniderman LC, Lambert M, Giguere R, et al, "Outcome of Individuals With Low-moderate Methylmalonic Aciduria Detected Through a Neonatal Screening Program," *J Pediatr*, 1999, 134(6):675-80.

Snow CF, "Laboratory Diagnosis of Vitamin B$_{12}$ and Folate Deficiency," *Arch Intern Med*, 1999, 159(12):1289-98.

Stabler SP, Lindenbaum J, and Allen RH, "Vitamin B$_{12}$ Deficiency in the Elderly: Current Dilemmas," *Am J Clin Nutr*, 1997, 66(4):741-9.

♦ **Methylmalonic Aciduria** *see Cerebrospinal Fluid Glycine on page 142*

Metyrapone Stimulation Test, Serum

Related Information

Adrenal Cortex: Laboratory Assessments Overview *on page 84*
Adrenocorticotropic Hormone, Plasma *on page 86*
Cortisol, Free, Urine *on page 154*
Cortisol, Serum or Plasma *on page 154*
17-Hydroxycorticosteroids, Urine *on page 196*

Applies to 11-Deoxycortisol

Test Includes Oral metyrapone at midnight, followed at 8 AM by serum levels of cortisol, 11-deoxycortisol, and ACTH

Abstract The metyrapone stimulation test (MST) is a secondary test of adrenal function which is used in the setting of suspected adrenal insufficiency (AI) or Cushing syndrome (CS) (see Adrenal Cortex: Laboratory Assessments Overview *on page 84*). There are three MST protocols: overnight, 2-day, and 3-day.[1] In this book, we deal only with the overnight protocol, the one most commonly used. MST tests the functional integrity of the hypothalamic-pituitary-adrenal (HPA) axis. Metyrapone inhibits the conversion of 11-deoxycortisol to cortisol and thereby produces a marked decrease in serum cortisol which, when sensed by the pituitary, results in an increase in pituitary output, and serum level, of ACTH. The endpoints of the overnight MST are the serum levels of cortisol, 11-deoxycortisol, and ACTH, drawn at 8 AM the morning after a midnight dose of metyrapone.

Patient Preparation At midnight, the patient is given metyrapone by mouth (with milk or a snack) on a weight-adjusted scale: <70 kg receives 2 grams; 70-90 kg receives 2.5 grams; >90 kg receives 3 grams. Since metyrapone is metabolized by enzymes that are induced by drugs that enhance steroid metabolism (eg, phenytoin, rifampin, phenobarbital, mitotane, and corticosteroids), these drugs should be discontinued before conducting the MST.[1]

Specimen Serum

Container Red top tube

Sampling Time 8 AM on the morning after oral metyrapone

Storage Instructions Freeze serum if assay is not performed within 24 hours.

Reference Interval The 8 AM serum cortisol should be <3 µg/dL (SI: <83 nmol/L). Failure to achieve this level makes the other values uninterpretable. Possible causes of a serum cortisol above this level include failure to take the metyrapone and rapid metyrapone clearance (see Patient Preparation) and 4% of otherwise normal persons also exhibit this phenomenon.[1] When the HPA is intact, the following thresholds are met or exceeded in the 8 AM specimen:[1]
- serum 11-deoxycortisol: >7 µg/dL (SI: >210 nmol/L)
- serum ACTH: >75 pg/mL (SI: >17 pmol/L)

Use

Adrenal insufficiency (AI): The MST is useful in patients being evaluated for secondary AI (pituitary- or hypothalamic-based AI). Patients with secondary AI will have serum 11-deoxycortisol and ACTH values less than the criteria indicated above, indicating pituitary or hypothalamic dysfunction. The MST is not used in the diagnosis of primary AI (see Adrenal Cortex: Laboratory Assessments Overview *on page 84*).

Cushing syndrome: The MST is useful in distinguishing pituitary-based CS from adrenal-based CS (see Adrenal Cortex: Laboratory Assessments Overview). When a patient with CS has MST results which meet or exceed the criteria indicated above, the diagnosis is usually pituitary-based CS (Cushing disease). In CS patients whose MST results do not meet these criteria, the differential diagnosis includes adrenal tumor vs the ectopic corticotropin syndrome (ECS). Patients with adrenal tumor typically have very low, or undetectable, serum ACTH, while those with ECS have normal or elevated (sometimes markedly elevated) serum ACTH level

Methodology See individual analytes.

Footnotes

1. Orth DN and Kovacs WJ, "The Adrenal Cortex," *Williams Textbook of Endocrinology*, 9th ed, Wilson JD, Foster DW, Kronenberg HM, et al, eds, Philadelphia, PA: WB Saunders Co, 1998, 620-1.

References

Avgerinos PC, Yanovski JA, Oldfield EH, et al, "The Metyrapone and Dexamethasone Suppression Tests for the Differential Diagnosis of the Adrenocorticotropin-Dependent Cushing Syndrome: A Comparison," *Ann Intern Med*, 1994, 121(5):318-27.

Orth DN, "Cushing's Syndrome," *N Engl J Med*, 1995, 332(12):791-803.

Mevalonic Acid, Urine or Amniotic Fluid

Related Information

Amino Acids, Plasma *on page 100*
Amino Acids, Urine *on page 101*
Immunoglobulin D *on page 532*
Inherited Diseases of Metabolism and Cell Structure *on page 449*
Lipids, Overview *on page 213*
Urine Collection, 24-Hour *on page 47*

Synonyms Urinary MVA

Applies to HMG-CoA Reductase Inhibitor; Lovastatin; Pravastatin

Abstract Urinary mevalonic acid (MVA) is considered as a marker of cholesterol biosynthesis *in vivo*.[1] Decrease in urinary MVA reflects the effect of "statin" therapy on *in vivo* cholesterol metabolism. Mevalonic aciduria (a (Continued)

Mevalonic Acid, Urine or Amniotic Fluid (Continued)

rare form of organic aciduria) is the result of an inherited deficiency of mevalonate kinase (see the following diagram for biochemical pathway and metabolic relationships).[2]

The Branched Pathway of Cholesterol and Nonsterol Isoprene Biosynthesis

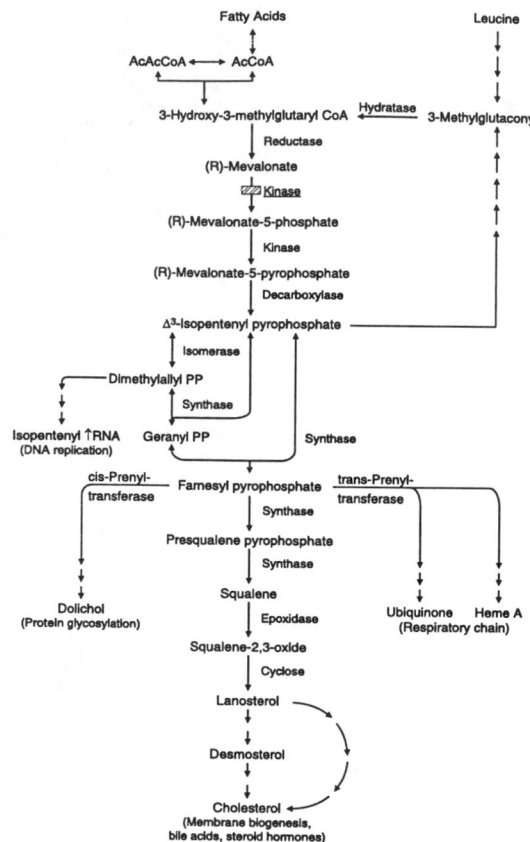

Mevalonic acid is the first committed intermediate of the pathway. The position of the defective enzyme in mevalonic aciduria is indicated by the hatched rectangle. PP denotes pyrophosphate.

Adapted from Hoffmann G, Gibson KM, Brandt IK, et al, "Mevalonic Aciduria - An Inborn Error of Cholesterol and Nonsterol Isoprene Biosynthesis," *N Engl J Med*, 1986, 314(25):1610-4.

Specimen Urine, amniotic fluid

Reference Interval See table.

Subject	Age	MVA µmol/day mean ±SD (range)
Male	21-58	2.32 ±0.82 (0.70-4.76)
Female	19-58	1.85 ±0.47 (0.73-3.19)
Male (before pravastatin)	25-50	2.32 ±0.65 (1.50-3.58)
Male (after prevastatin)	25-50	1.47 ±0.49 (1.03-2.38)

Adapted from Hiramatus M, Hayashi A, Hidaka H, et al, "Enzyme Immunoassay of Urinary Mevalonic Acid and Its Clinical Application," *Clin Chem*, 1998, 44(10):2152-7.

Limitations The presence of time-related variation in cholesterol synthesis and simultaneous increase in plasma and urinary MVA (with peak at midnight) has been noted with earlier methods, but was not observed with enzyme immunoassay.[1]

Methodology Enzyme immunoassay[1,3] (with intra-assay coefficient of variation, 3.4%[1] and interassay valuation (VC) of 6.9%); radioimmunoenzyme assay;[4] liquid partition chromatography with subsequent gas chromatography and gas chromatography-mass spectrometry of the trimethylsilyl and methylester trimethylsilyl ether derivatives[3]

Additional Information Plasma mevalonate is a measure of cholesterol synthesis in man. Mevalonic acid (MVA) level in plasma correlates with whole body cholesterol synthesis. MVA is a metabolic precursor of cholesterol and nonsterol isoprenes, including heme A, ubiquinone, dolichol, and isopentyl adenine. MVA can be considered as an indicator of the *in vivo* rate of cholesterol biosynthesis. MVA, which is hydrophilic, is excreted in urine in proportion to its concentration in plasma. Thus, urinary MVA provides a window on cholesterol biosynthesis. After being given pravastatin, 3-hydroxy-3-methylglutaryl-coenzyme A (HMG-CoA) reductase, urinary MVA was decreased (sample size of only 9 men).[1]

A young male child who suffered severe failure to thrive, developmental delay, anemia, and hepatomegaly with central cataracts and dysmorphic features was found to excrete very large amounts of mevalonic acid (46,000-56,200 mmol/mol of creatinine vs 0.2-0.3 mmol/mol in normal children).[2] Mevalonate kinase was significantly deficient in extracts of cultured patient's fibroblasts and lymphocytes. Parents had intermediate levels of activity. Mevalonic aciduria is an autosomal recessive disorder. The gene is present on chromosome 12. As of 1995, some 11 patients have been identified. Prenatal diagnosis is supported by the finding of increased MVA in amniotic fluid and confirmed by the assay of cultured amniocytes.[2]

Footnotes

1. Hiramatsu M, Hayashi A, Hidaka H, et al, "Enzyme Immunoassay of Urinary Mevalonic Acid and its Clinical Application," *Clin Chem*, 1998, 44(10):2152-7.
2. Hoffmann G, Gibson KM, Brandt IK, et al, "Mevalonic Aciduria - an Inborn Error of Cholesterol and Nonsterol Isoprene Biosynthesis," *N Engl J Med*, 1986, 314(25):1610-4.
3. Hiramatsu M, Hayashi A, Hamanaka N, et al, "Enzyme Immunoassay of Human Urinary Mevalonic Acid Using Highly Specific Monoclonal Antibody," *Rinsyo Kagaku*, 1995, 24(1):94-100.
4. Pappu AS, Illingworth DR, and Bacon S, "Reduction in Plasma Low-Density Lipoprotein Cholesterol and Urinary Mevalonic Acid by Lovastatin in Patients With Heterozygous Familial Hypercholesterolemia," *Metabolism*, 1989, 38(6):542-9.

References

Naoumova RP, Marais AD, Mountney J, et al, "Plasma Mevalonic Acid, an Index of Cholesterol Synthesis *In Vivo*, and Responsiveness to HMG-CoA Reductase Inhibitors in Familial Hypercholesterolaemia," *Atherosclerosis*, 1996, 119(2):203-13.

Sweetman L and Williams JC, "Branched Chain Organic Acidurias," *The Metabolic and Molecular Bases of Inherited Disease*, 7th ed, Volume 1, Chapter 40, Scriver CR, Beaudet AL, Sly WS, et al, eds, New York, NY: McGraw-Hill Inc, 1995, 1387-8, 1402-5.

♦ **Mg, Serum** see Magnesium, Serum *on page 221*

♦ **Mg, Urine** see Magnesium, Urine *on page 222*

♦ **Microbilirubin** see Bilirubin, Neonatal, Serum *on page 117*

♦ **Midnight to Morning Urinary Cortisol Increment** see Urinary Cortisol/Creatinine Increment *on page 296*

♦ **Monoclonal Gammopathy** see Protein Electrophoresis, Capillary Zone *on page 266*

♦ **Monoclonal Gammopathy** see Protein Electrophoresis, Serum *on page 267*

♦ **Monoclonal Gammopathy** see Protein Electrophoresis, Urine *on page 268*

♦ **Monoclonal Light Chains** see Protein Electrophoresis, Urine *on page 268*

♦ **M-Proteins** see Protein Electrophoresis, Capillary Zone *on page 266*

♦ **M-Proteins** see Protein Electrophoresis, Serum *on page 267*

♦ **MUC1** see CA 15-3, Serum *on page 127*

♦ **MUC1 Gene** see CA 27.29, Serum *on page 128*

Mucopolysaccharides, Urine

Related Information

Amniotic Fluid, Chromosome and Genetic Abnormality Analysis *on page 360*

Chorionic Villus Sampling, Chromosome and Genetic Abnormality Analysis *on page 361*

Inherited Diseases of Metabolism and Cell Structure *on page 449*

Muscle Biopsy *on page 69*

Peripheral Blood: Differential Leukocyte Count *on page 464*

Urinalysis *on page 887*

Urine Collection, 24-Hour *on page 47*

Applies to Dermatan Sulfates; Heparan; Hunter Syndrome; Hurler Syndrome; Keratan Sulfate; Lymphocyte, Vacuolated; Sulfatase

Abstract Increased excretion of urinary mucopolysaccharides (dermatan and/or heparan sulfates) occurs in the mucopolysaccharidoses (forms of lysosomal storage diseases). The mucopolysaccharides are currently referred to as glycosaminoglycans (GAGs). "Mucopolysaccharidosis" is still generally used in the medical literature. Glycosaminoglycans (with the exception of hyaluronic acid) have a protein core "backbone" and are thus referred to as proteoglycans. Degradation of the latter occurs in lysosomes by the action of proteases and the sequential action of lysosomal hydrolases. Inherited deficiency or absence of these enzymes results in a number of clinical pathologic entities, the mucopolysaccharidoses.

Specimen 24-hour urine collection is preferred due to circadian variation of GAG excretion.[1]

Container Plastic urine container

Storage Instructions Freeze

Special Instructions Do not collect specimen while patient is receiving intravenous heparin.

Reference Interval

- Younger than 1 year: 20-40 mg/mmol creatinine
- 1-5 years: 10-15 mg/mmol creatinine
- 5 years and older: 3-8 mg/mmol creatinine

Consult laboratory performing the test.

Use Screen for the presence of mucopolysaccharidose

Limitations "Spot" tests may be associated with a 20% to 30% incidence of false-positive or false-negative results.[1,2]

Methodology Spectrophotometry (quantitative) based on a colorimetric reaction with 1,9-dimethylmethylene blue;[2,3] electrophoretic separation of glycosaminoglycans (GAG)

Additional Information Glycosaminoglycans (GAGs) consist of repetitive sulfated and/or carboxylated disaccharide units of 7 types: hyaluronic acid, chondroitin 4-sulfate, chondroitin 6-sulfate, dermatan sulfate, keratin sulfate, heparin and heparan sulfate. Linked to proteins (to form proteoglycans) they are major components of the ground substance of connective tissue. If an enzyme or enzyme activity is missing in the stepwise degradation of a GAG, undegraded molecules gradually accumulate in the lysosome, the underlying basis for 7 (over 10 if variants are included) forms of mucopolysaccharidosis, MPS I-VII. See table.

These disorders, often clinically apparent, can be detected by the identification of specific GAG segments in the urine and verified by assay of the specific hydrolases in leukocytes or fibroblasts. As an example, Hunter syndrome (MPS II-XR) is due to loss of iduronate sulfate sulfatase activity with excess dermatan and heparan sulfate accumulation in the urine. To assist with the diagnosis, assays for defective enzyme activity can be applied to serum, cultured fibroblasts, amniotic fluid, cultured amniotic cells and/or chorionic villi.[4] Inheritance is autosomal recessive with the exception of MPS II (Hunter) which is X-linked. The involved genes for most of the mucopolysaccharidoses have been identified and cloned. Some of the phenotypes, as with Hurler syndrome, include early onset, growth retardation, mental retardation, severe dementia, seizures, and early death, a pediatric neurologic constellation. Other phenotypes (eg, MPS II-XR and MPS IV-B) have less severe involvement with survival into adulthood. The Hurler phenotype may include cytoplasmic inclusions, seen in lymphocytes on study of peripheral blood smears.[4] A number of lysosomal storage diseases may be associated with vacuolated lymphocytes:[1]

- aspartylglucosaminuria
- fucosidosis
- galactosialidosis
- alpha-mannosidosis
- mucolipidosis I-III
- Salla disease
- Pompe disease - all patients
- Wolman disease

Up to 5% of lymphocytes with vacuoles may be considered normal and such cells may occur with sepsis.

Elevation of G_{M2} and G_{M3} gangliosides in central nervous system tissue of MPS IIIA patients has been identified by tandem mass spectrometry.[5]

Sophisticated analytic procedures have been developed for the analysis of GAGs, in particular, the structure of the oligosaccharide components. Recently, surface noncovalent affinity mass spectrometry (SNA-MS) and matrix-assisted laser desorption ionization mass spectrometry (MALDI-MS) have been described.[6]

Bone marrow transplantation has been performed in some cases (eg, children with Hurler syndrome) with occasional documented therapeutic effect.[7,8] Gene therapy is under development.[9,10] Ten patients with mucopolysaccharidosis I (including examples of Hurler-Scheie, Hurler, and Scheie syndrome) have been treated with recombinant-human α-L-iduronidase administered intravenously. A dose of 125,000 units/kg of body weight once/week was given for 52 weeks. This therapy produced significant decrease in hepatosplenomegaly, normalization of liver size for patient weight and age, decrease in urinary glycosaminoglycan excretion, and improvement in many impaired musculoskeletal and cardiorespiratory functional characteristics.[11]

Footnotes

1. Ullrich K, "Screening for Lysosomal Disorders," *Eur J Pediatr*, 1994, 153(Suppl 1):S38-S43.

2. de Jong JGN, Wevers RA, Laarakkers C, et al, "Dimethylmethylene Blue-Based Spectrophotometry of Glycosaminoglycans in Untreated Urine: A Rapid Screening Procedure for Mucopolysaccharidoses," *Clin Chem*, 1989, 35(7):1472-7.

3. van de Lest CHA, Versteeg EMM, Veerkamp JH, et al, "A Spectrophotometric Method for the Determination of Heparan Sulfate," *Biochim Biophys Acta*, 1994, 1201(2):305-11.

4. Spranger J, "Mucopolysaccharidoses," *Emery and Rimoin's Principles and Practice of Medical Genetics*, 3rd ed, Volume 11, Rimoin DL, Connor MJ, and Pyeritz RE, eds, New York, NY: Churchill Livingstone, 1997, 2071-9.

5. Whitfield PD, Sharp P, Meikle PJ, et al, "Characterization of Ganglioside Storage in Mucopolysaccharidosis IIIA by Tandem Mass Spectrometry," *J Inherit Metab Dis*, 2000, 23(Suppl 1):237.

6. Keiser N, Venkataraman G, Shriver Z, et al, "Direct Isolation and Sequencing of Specific Protein-Binding Glycosaminoglycans," *Nat Med*, 2001, 7(1):123-8.

7. Tanaka A, Toshiyuki S, Kono K, et al, "MR Images in 23 Patients With Mucopolysaccharidoses and the Effect of Bone Marrow Transplantation," *J Inherit Metab Dis*, 2000, 23(Suppl 1):235.

8. Venditti LN, Lee SJ, Venditti CP, et al, "Cost-Effectiveness of Bone Marrow Transplantation for Children With Hurler Syndrome," *J Inherit Metab Dis*, 2000, 23(Suppl 1):234.

9. Winchester B, Burton S, Estruch E, et al, "Gene Therapy for Mucopolysaccharidoses Types I, IIIA, and IIIB: Herpes Simplex Virus-Mediated Gene Transfer and Expression," *J Inherit Metab Dis*, 2000, 23(Suppl 1):237.

10. Stronock DF, Hubel A, Shankar SR, et al, "Retroviral Transduction and Expansion of Peripheral Blood Lymphocytes for the Treatment of Mucopolysaccharidosis Type II, Hunter's Syndrome," *Transfusion*, 1999, 39(4):343-50.

11. Kakkis ED, Muenzer J, Tiller GE, et al, "Enzyme-Replacement Therapy in Mucopolysaccharidosis I," *N Engl J Med*, 2001, 344(3):182-8.

Disorder	Clinical Feature	Enzyme Defect	Assay*
MPS I-H Hurler syndrome	Mental retardation, progressive, beginning at age 1; corneal opacities; coarse facies; stiff joints; dwarfing; organomegaly; death, usually by age 14	α-L-iduronidase	L, F, Ac, CV
MPS I-S Scheie syndrome	Mild form of I-H; stiff joints; corneal opacity; mild-to-absent mental retardation; aortic stenosis; survive to adult	α-L-iduronidase	L, F, Ac, CV
MPS I-H/S Hurler/Scheie syndrome	Intermediate phenotype between I-H and I-S; some are Hurler-Scheie double heterozygotes	α-L-iduronidase	L, F, Ac, CV
MPS II-XR Hunter syndrome	Similar to MPS I-H but with clear cornea; may be deafness; later onset and longer survival (to adulthood)	Iduronate sulfate sulfatase	S, F, Af, Ac, CV
MPS III-A MPS III-B	Most common of the MPS with behaviorial problems, progressive dementia, seizures, intrafamilial variability, hirsute with coarse hair; survival to 2nd or 3rd decade of life	Heparan N-sulfatase α-N-acetylglucosaminidase	L, F, Ac, CV
MPS III-C MPS III-D Sanfilippo A-D syndromes		α-glucosaminide-N-acetyltransferase N-acetylglucosamine-6-sulfate sulfatase	F, Ac
MPS IV-A Morquio A syndrome	Short trunk dwarfism; fine corneal opacities; short neck; odontoid anomalies; normal intellect	Galactosamine-6-sulfate sulfatase	L, F, Ac
MPS IV-B Morquio B syndrome	Mild form of IV-A	β-galactosidase	L, F, Ac, CV
MPS V	Formerly Scheie disease		
MPS VI Maroteaux-Lamy syndrome	Hurler phenotype with severe-to-mild dysostosis multiplex; gross corneal opacity; growth retardation; normal intellect	Arylsulfatase B	L, F, Ac
MPS VII Glucuronidase deficiency Sly syndrome	Highly variable with mild mental retardation; tendency to coarse facies; gingivitis; organomegaly; inclusions in granulocytes	β-glucuronidase	S, F, Ac

*With the exception of MPS IV-B and MPS VII, the above mucopolysaccharidoses are characterized by the presence of excess urinary mucopolysaccharides, dermatan and/or heparan sulfates. Keratan sulfate is present in urine from cases of MPS IV-A. Quantitative enzyme assay is applicable to each of the above conditions.

L = leukocytes, S = serum, F = cultured fibroblasts, Ac = cultured amniotic cells, Af = amniotic fluid, CV = chorionic villi

Adapted from O'Brien J, "Lysosomal Storage Disease," *Tietz Textbook of Clinical Chemistry*, 3rd ed, Chapter 49, Burtis CA and Ashwood ER, eds, Philadelphia, PA: WB Saunders Co, 1999, 1777-80 and from Spranger J, "Mucopolysaccharidoses," *Emery and Rimoin's Principles and Practice of Medical Genetics*, 3rd ed, Chapter 96, Rimoin DL, Connor JM, and Pyeritz RE, eds, New York, NY: Churchill Livingstone, 1997, 2073.

(Continued)

Mucopolysaccharides, Urine *(Continued)*

References

Baynes J and Dominiczak MH, "The Extracellular Matrix," *Medical Biochemistry*, Chapter 26, London, England: Mosby, 1999, 333-43.

Berry HK, "Mucopolysaccharides," *Methods in Clinical Chemistry*, Pesce AJ and Kaplan LA, eds, St Louis, MO: CV Mosby Co, 1987, 189-99.

Bower L and Warren C, "Human Serum and Urine Glycosaminoglycans in Health and in Patients With Chronic Renal Failure," *Ann Clin Biochem*, 1992, 29(2):190-5.

Brunngraber EG, "Neuropathology," *Neurochemistry of Amniosugars: Neurochemistry and Neuropathology of the Complex Carbohydrates*, Chapter XIV, Springfield, IL: Charles C Thomas, 1979, 579-93.

Busoni P and Fognani G, "Failure of the Laryngeal Mask to Secure the Airway in a Patient With Hunter's Syndrome (Mucopolysaccharidosis Type II)," *Paediatr Anaesth*, 1999, 9(2):153-5.

Dawson G and Hancock LW, "Inborn Errors of Complex Carbohydrate Catabolism," *Neurobiology of Glycoconjugates*, Chapter 15, Margolis RU and Margolis RK, eds, New York, NY: Plenum Press, 1989, 421-45.

de la Cruz-Amoros V, Cortes-Castell E, and Moya M, "Urinary Excretion of Mucopolysaccharides in Pediatric and Adolescent Patients," *An Esp Pediatr*, 1999, 50(4):361-6.

Kelly TE, revised by Rucknagel DL, "Diseases of Genetic Origin," *Clinical Chemistry: Theory, Analysis, and Correlation*, 3rd ed, Chapter 47, Kaplan LA, Pesce AJ, and Kazmierczak SC, eds, St Louis, MO: Mosby, 1996, 947-51.

O'Brien JF, "Lysosomal Storage Disease," *Tietz Textbook of Clinical Chemistry*, 3rd ed, Chapter 49, Burtis CA and Ashwood ER, eds, Philadelphia, PA: WB Saunders Co, 1999, 1776-9.

Orliaguet O, Pepin JL, Veale D, et al, "Hunter's Syndrome and Associated Sleep Apnea Cured by CPAP and Surgery," *Eur Respir J*, 1999, 13(5):1195-7.

Su PH, Hwu WL, Chiang SC, et al, "Mucopolysaccharidosis Type II (Hunter's Syndrome) in Taiwan," *J Formos Med Assoc*, 1998, 97(3):186-90.

♦ **Multiple Endocrine Neoplasia (MEN) Type 1** *see* Parathyroid Hormone, Serum *on page 243*

♦ **Multiple Marker Screening Test** *see* Estriol, Unconjugated, Pregnancy, Serum, Plasma, or Urine *on page 171*

♦ **Multiple Marker Screening Test** *see* Inhibin A, Serum *on page 199*

♦ **Murphy-Pattee** *replaced by* Thyroxine, Serum *on page 286*

♦ **Myocardial Infarct Panel** *see* Cardiac Markers: Laboratory Assessment, Overview *on page 137*

Myoglobin, Blood, Serum, or Plasma

Related Information

Carboxyhemoglobin, Blood *on page 784*
Cardiac Markers: Laboratory Assessment, Overview *on page 137*
Creatine Kinase Isoenzymes/Isoforms, Serum *on page 157*
Creatine Kinase, Serum *on page 158*
Haptoglobin, Serum *on page 190*
Lactate Dehydrogenase, Serum *on page 207*
Muscle Biopsy *on page 69*
Myoglobin, Qualitative, Urine *on page 880*
Troponins, Serum *on page 291*

Applies to CA-III; Carbonic Anhydrase III

Abstract Myoglobin is an oxygen-binding low molecular weight (17,800 d) cytoplasmic heme protein which is found in cardiac and striated muscle. A rapid increase in its concentration (rate of expression) is a useful marker for very early detection of recent myocardial infarct, but only a narrow window, at presentation, is available for assay. Its best use is in combination with other markers in a serial mode,[1] usually CK-MB and/or troponins.[2] It is useful to rule out acute damage to myocardium. Myoglobin must be supplanted by other markers to confirm the diagnosis of acute myocardial infarct (AMI), usually CK, CK-MB, and/or troponin I (TnI).

Other applications for myoglobin are applied to urinary myoglobins (see Myoglobin, Qualitative, Urine *on page 880*).

Specimen Serum, plasma

Container Red top tube, green top (lithium heparin) tube

Sampling Time Myoglobin presents 1-3 hours following damage to cardiac or skeletal muscle. Use of two to three samples at 1- to 2-hour intervals has been advocated at presentation of AMI.[3,4] Myoglobin is best measured in patients whose chest pain began less than 6 hours before evaluation.[5]

Storage Instructions Serum may be stored at 4°C for 2 years or frozen at -20°C.[4]

Turnaround Time 2 minutes to 4 hours, analytical TUT, depending upon methods. Methods <16 minutes include latex agglutination, nephelometry, turbidimetric immunoassay, fluorometric enzyme immunoassay, fluorometric radial partition enzyme immunoassay, and indirect chemiluminescence immunoassay.[2]

Reference Interval Approximate range: 5-70 µg/L (immunonephelometric assay). Varies with method. Level may be up to 25% higher in men.

Critical Values Increase >40 µg/L between T_o and 2-hour specimens is indicative of an acute episode.

Use Myoglobin is used to rule out AMI or skeletal muscle injury.

Serum myoglobin is detectable earlier than CK or CK-MB increase in patients with AMI.[3,4] Increased serum myoglobin has been found also in 50% of patients with acute coronary insufficiency. Myoglobin concentrations correlate with size of infarct.[3] Serum myoglobin levels have their greatest utility as an early negative indicator, especially when used with CK-MB. Myoglobin is useful as well in combination with TnI; increases are seen very early in AMI when TnI is still within normal limits. Myoglobin is useful for the evaluation of reperfusion.

Urinary as well as serum myoglobin are used in the diagnosis of rhabdomyolysis. It is found with trauma, malignant hyperthermia, ischemia, dermatomyositis, polymyositis, and muscular dystrophy.

Limitations False positives limit the role of myoglobin for evaluation of chest pain. Increased myoglobin levels occur after intramuscular injections, other muscle injury and shock. Increased myoglobin has been reported after high voltage electrical accident. Many laboratories prefer CK isoenzymes (CK-MB does not rise after intramuscular injection) and others use CK-MB with myoglobin levels. Better specificity is seen with CK-MB[4] and with troponin I. As an index of AMI, myoglobin returns rapidly to baseline levels. **Rising serum myoglobin concentrations may be missed if there is patient delay in seeking medical attention following the onset of chest pain.** Therefore, its role in the diagnosis of AMI may be limited in populations in which there is a delay in patients seeking treatment for acute chest pain. Myoglobin is released following open heart surgery and false positives occur with renal failure and following strenuous exercise. It is not tightly bound to protein and is rapidly excreted.[6] In patients with massive myoglobinemia, blood myoglobin may rapidly fall independent of renal function or therapeutic manipulation.[6]

Methodology Fluorometric immunoassay, immunoturbidimetry, dual-label time-resolved fluoroimmunoassay, nephelometry, two-site sandwich monoclonal assay, indirect chemiluminescence assay, electrochemical immunosensor.[2] Radioimmunoassay (RIA) is presently considered too slow (see Turnaround Time).

Additional Information Serum myoglobin is rapidly cleared by the kidneys. Elevated levels may be associated with cocaine use.[7] It is increased in cardiac surgery, and thrombolytic therapy,[8,9] as well as myocardial infarction. Its **main advantage** is as a sensitive (99% to 100%) marker for **early myocardial injury** because it is released earlier from necrotic cells than CK, allowing for earlier detection of myocardial infarction. Levels rise as early as 1 hour after infarct and peak within 4-12 hours. Repeat myoglobin that has doubled within 1-2 hours after presentation, even if still within the normal range, may signify an acute myocardial infarct.[10]

Because myoglobin is not specific to myocardial muscle, the issue of specificity arises in cases of acute myocardial injury associated with muscle trauma, a situation in which a distinction cannot be made as to the origin of myoglobin. If one measures **carbonic anhydrase III (CA-III)**, an 18,000-d cytoplasmic protein present in skeletal muscle but **not** in cardiac muscle, such separation can be made;[6] the myoglobin:CA-III ratio provides appreciable sensitivity, but turnaround time for CA-III has been prolonged.[2] Simultaneous assay of both proteins shows that in skeletal muscle injury the ratio of myoglobin to carbonic anhydrase III is constant; while in patients with AMI, the ratio shows a temporal pattern similar to myoglobin alone. Serum troponin I concentration presents significant advantages (see Troponins *on page 291*) because of high specificity.

Footnotes

1. Kost GJ, Kirk JD, and Omand K, "A Strategy for the Use of Cardiac Injury Markers (Troponin I and T, Creatine Kinase-MB Mass and Isoforms, and Myoglobin) in the Diagnosis of Acute Myocardial Infarction," *Arch Pathol Lab Med*, 1998, 122(3):245-51.

2. Plebani M and Zaninotto M, "Diagnostic Strategies Using Myoglobin Measurement in Myocardial Infarction," *Clin Chim Acta*, 1998, 272(1):69-77.

3. Woo J, Lacbawan FL, Sunheimer R, et al, "Is Myoglobin Useful in the Diagnosis of Acute Myocardial Infarction in the Emergency Department Setting?" *Am J Clin Pathol*, 1995, 103(6):725-9.

4. Montague C and Kircher T, "Myoglobin in the Early Evaluation of Acute Chest Pain," *Am J Clin Pathol*, 1995, 104(4):472-6.

5. Chang CC, Ip MP, Hsu RM, et al, "Evaluation of a Proposed Panel of Cardiac Markers for the Diagnosis of Acute Myocardial Infarction in Patients With Atraumatic Chest Pain," *Arch Pathol Lab Med*, 1998, 122(4):320-4.

6. Wakabayashi Y and Kikuno T, Ohwada T, et al, "Rapid Fall in Blood Myoglobin in Massive Rhabdomyolysis and Acute Renal Failure," *Intensive Care Med*, 1994, 20(2):109-12.

7. Pogue VA and Nurse HM, "Cocaine-Associated Acute Myoglobinuric Renal Failure," *Am J Med*, 1989, 86(2):183-6.

8. McCullough DA, Harrison PG, Forshall JM, et al, "Serum Myoglobin and Creatine Kinase Enzymes in Acute Myocardial Infarction Treated With Anistreplase," *J Clin Pathol*, 1992, 45(5):405-7.

9. Laperche T, Steg PG, Benessiano J, et al, "Patterns of Myoglobin and MM Creatine Kinase Isoforms Release Early After Intravenous Thrombolysis of Direct Percutaneous Transluminal Coronary Angioplasty for Acute Myocardial Infarction, and Implications for the Early Noninvasive Diagnosis of Reperfusion," *Am J Cardiol*, 1992, 70(13):1129-34.

10. Tucker JF, Collins RA, Anderson AJ, et al, "Value of Serial Myoglobin Levels in the Early Diagnosis of Patients Admitted for Acute Myocardial Infarction," *Ann Emerg Med*, 1994, 24(4):704-8.

References

Delanghe J, Chapelle JP, el Allaf M, et al, "Quantitative Turbidimetric Assay for Determining Myoglobin Evaluated," *Ann Clin Biochem*, 1991, 28(Pt 5):474-9.

Lee HS, Cross SJ, Garthwaite P, et al, "Comparison of the Value of Novel Rapid Measurement of Myoglobin, Creatine Kinase, and Creatine Kinase-MB With the Electrocardiogram for the Diagnosis of Acute Myocardial Infarction," *Br Heart J*, 1994, 71(4):311-5.

Miyata M, Abe S, Arima S, et al, "Rapid Diagnosis of Coronary Reperfusion by Measurement of Myoglobin Level Every 15 Min in Acute Myocardial Infarction," *J Am Coll Cardiol*, 1994, 23(5):1009-15.

♦ **Na⁺** *see* Sodium, Serum or Plasma *on page 275*

♦ **N-Acetyl-β-Hexosaminidase A** *see* Beta-Hexosaminidase, Serum, White Blood Cells *on page 114*

♦ **NAG** *see* Beta-Hexosaminidase, Serum, White Blood Cells *on page 114*

♦ **β-NAG A** *see* Beta-Hexosaminidase, Serum, White Blood Cells *on page 114*

♦ **Nagao Isoenzyme** *see* Alkaline Phosphatase, Heat Stable, Serum *on page 91*

♦ **Nagao Isoenzyme** *see* Alkaline Phosphatase Isoenzymes, Serum *on page 92*

♦ **Naloxone Stimulation Test** *see* Adrenal Cortex: Laboratory Assessments Overview *on page 84*

♦ **Naproxen** *see* Porphyrins, Quantitative, Urine *on page 255*

♦ **Na, Urine** *see* Sodium, Urine *on page 278*

♦ **Neurofibrillary Tangles** *see* Apolipoprotein E, Plasma *on page 110*

♦ **Neuroglycopenia** *see* Cerebrospinal Fluid Glucose *on page 140*

♦ **Neuronal Thread Proteins** *see* AD7c Neural Thread Protein, CSF or Urine *on page 83*

Neuron-Specific Enolase, Serum

Synonyms NSE; Phosphopyruvate Hydratase

Applies to S-100, Serum

Abstract Neuron-specific enolase (NSE), a glycolytic enzyme found in neurons, neuroendocrine cells, erythrocytes, and platelets, has been proposed, and is undergoing evaluation, as a serum marker for neuroendocrine neoplasms and for cerebral tissue injury.[1,2]

Specimen Serum

Container Red top tube

Collection Must avoid hemolysis. Place blood on ice immediately after collecting.

Storage Instructions Centrifuge within 30-45 minutes. Maintain at 4°C and analyze same day or freeze at -70°C until assayed.

Causes for Rejection Specimen with hemolysis (RBCs contain γ-enolase). Hemolysis will cause false-positive results.

Turnaround Time Approximately 1 week, as this analysis will usually be performed by a reference laboratory.

Reference Interval Not well established. Check with reference laboratory.
Serum:
- 0-30 ng/mL[3]
- 0-12.5 ng/mL[4]
- 7.1 ±3.6 ng/mL[5]

CSF: 0-13 years: 0-4.8 ng/mL[6]; values may be age- and sex-dependent[5]

Use

Tumor marker: NSE has no established role in screening for, or early detection of, neoplastic disease. Some investigators have found that, in patients with small cell lung carcinoma, NSE measured after the first cycle of chemotherapy is useful as an early and independent predictor of complete response and survival.[7] In a study of 770 patients with small cell lung carcinoma treated in 9 centers, NSE has been used, together with disease stage and performance status, in a formula to calculate a prognostic index.[8] Investigators from the National Cancer Institute in Milan have found serum NSE useful as in treatment monitoring and prognosis assessment in patients with neuroblastoma.[9]

Brain injury and dysfunction: Serum NSE is elevated in patients with traumatic brain injury and can be used to predict outcome.[10] Likewise, serum NSE (S-NSE) is elevated in patients with stroke, but S-100, serum (a related protein) appears to correlate better with infarct size and outcome.[2] In elderly patients undergoing coronary artery bypass grafting, the S-NSE at 24 hours correlates well with neuropsychologically measured cognitive function.[11] In patients resuscitated after cardiac arrest, a S-NSE >33 ng/mL predicts coma.[12] The NSE level in CSF correlates with the duration and outcome of status epilepticus.[13] The NSE level in amniotic fluid is reported to be a potentially useful marker of brain injury in neonates.[14]

Methodology Immunoassays (multiple labels)

Footnotes

1. Chan DW and Sell S, "Tumor Markers," *Tietz Textbook of Clinical Chemistry*, 3rd ed, Burtis CA and Ashwood ER, eds, Philadelphia, PA: WB Saunders Co, 1999, 728-9.
2. Missler U, Weismann M, Friedrich C, et al, "S-100 Protein and Neuron-Specific Enolase Concentrations in Blood as Indicators of Infarction Volume and Prognosis in Acute Ischemic Stroke," *Stroke*, 1998, 28:1956-60.
3. Mayo Medical Laboratories, *Test Catalogue*, Rochester, MN, 1999, 394.
4. Ashwood ER, personal communication. July 2000.
5. Nygaard O, Langbakk B, and Romner B, "Neuron-Specific Enolase Concentrations in Serum and Cerebrospinal Fluid in Patients With no Previous History of Neurological Disease," *Scand J Clin Lab Invest*, 1998, 58(3):183-6.

6. Rodriguez-Nunez A, Cid E, Eiris J, et al, "Neuron-Specific Enolase Levels in the Cerebrospinal Fluid of Neurologically Healthy Children," *Brain and Development*, 1999, 21(1):16-9.
7. Fizazi K, Cojean I, Pignon JP, et al, "Normal Serum Neuron Specific Enolase After the First Cycle of Chemotherapy: An Early Predictor of Complete Response and Survival in Patients With Small Cell Lung Carcinoma," *Cancer*, 1998, 82(3):1049-55.
8. Jorgensen LG, Osterlind K, Gomm J, et al, "Serum Neuron Specific Enolase (S-NSE) and the Prognosis in Small Cell Lung Cancer (SCLS): A Combined Multivariable Analysis on Data From Nine Centers," *Br J Cancer*, 1996, 74:(4)463-7 (published erratum *Br J Cancer*, 1996, 74:2043).
9. Massaron S, Seregni E, Luksch R, et al, "Neuron Specific Enolase Evaluation in Patients With Neuroblastoma," *Tumor Biology*, 1998, 19:261-8.
10. McKeating EG, Andrews PJ, and Mascia L, "Relationship of Neuron Specific Enolase and Protein S-100 Concentrations in Systemic and Jugular Venous Serum to Injury Severity and Outcome After Traumatic Brain Injury," *Acta Neurochirurgica*, 1998, 71(Suppl):117-9.
11. Rasmussen LS, Christiansen M, Hansen PB, et al, "Do Blood Levels of Neuron-Specific Enolase and S-100 Protein Reflect Cognitive Dysfunction After Coronary Artery Bypass?" *Acta Anaesthesiologica Scand*, 1999, 43(5):495-500.
12. Fogel W, Krieger D, Veith M, et al, "Serum Neuron Specific Enolase as Early Predictor of Outcome After Cardiac Arrest," *Crit Care Med*, 1997, 25(5):1133-8.
13. Correale J, Rabinowicz AL, Heck CN, et al, "Status Epilepticus Increases CSF Levels of Neuron-Specific Enolase and Alerts the Blood-Brain Barrier," *Neurology*, 1998, 50(4 Pt 1):1388-91.
14. Elimian A, Figueroa R, Verma U, et al, "Amniotic Fluid Neuron-Specific Enolase: A Role in Predicting Neonatal Neuronal Injury?" *Obstet Gynecol*, 1998, 92(4 Pt 1):546-50.

Newborn Screen for Phenylketonuria

Related Information
Amino Acids, Plasma *on page 100*
Newborn Screen for T_4, Filter Paper *on page 230*
Newborn Screen for TSH, Filter Paper *on page 231*
Phenylalanine, Blood *on page 248*

Synonyms Phenylketonuria, Newborn Screen; PKU, Neonatal

Applies to BH_4 Cofactor Deficiencies; Dihydropteridine Reductase; Guanosine Triphosphate Cyclohydrolase 1 Deficiency; Hyperphenylalaninemia, Maternal; Phenylalanine Hydroxylase Activity; Pyruvoyl Tetrahydropterin Synthase Deficiency; Tetrahydrobiopterin Pathway

Test Includes Phenylalanine screen using filter paper collection. Samples for newborn screens for congenital hypothyroidism and galactosemia are usually obtained at the same time.

Abstract Autosomal recessive aminoacidopathy due to phenylalanine hydroxylase (≥97% cases) or biopterin (folic acid constituent) cofactor deficiencies. Detection by low cost dried blood spot screening can result in early treatment, intended to prevent mental retardation.

Patient Preparation Newborns should have milk (protein) feeding ideally for 48 hours before testing; sample should be taken as late as possible prior to discharge from hospital. Blood should be obtained 2-4 days after birth. Collection is recommended at 4-10 days for low birth weight infants.

Specimen Whole blood, serum or plasma

Container Newborns: PKU test card; screening: filter paper sheet. Pediatrics: Small red top tube, gray top (sodium fluoride) tube or green top (heparin) tube; check with the laboratory.

Sampling Time Just before infant is discharged from the nursery

Collection Test card must be labeled with patient's name, date, time, date of birth, and time of first milk feeding. In order to obtain accurate test results for PKU, blood collection should preferably be made when the infant is 48-120 hours of age and has been on a protein feeding for at least 24 hours. Do not oversaturate filter paper. Do not fill circles on one side and then fill circles on reverse side. Do not collect blood with a capillary tube to apply to filter paper. Include information regarding blood transfusions and antibiotics or other medications administered to the infant, which may influence screening test results.

Storage Instructions Newborns: Air dry specimens at room temperature in a horizontal position for at least 2 hours. Do not use hermetically sealed envelopes. Pediatrics: Separate serum and transfer to a plastic vial containing 10 mg NaF. (Check with the laboratory for other possible specimen requirements.) Separate within 4 hours of collection. Serum or plasma is stable 5 days at 4°C. Care in handling the filter paper specimens is essential, because exposure to extreme heat or light or touching the filter paper portion of the form can cause erroneous test results. Specimens containing contaminants, such as alcohol or other liquids, or antibiotics may not be satisfactory for testing. (See following discussion.) The phenylalanine in filter paper dried blood spots is stable for years when not exposed to environmental extremes.

Causes for Rejection Filter paper not thoroughly saturated, inadequate specimen identification, specimens which are respotted (several drops of blood applied to the same circle), specimens which are QNS (quantity not sufficient). **Cord blood cannot be used because phenylalanine is not significantly increased at birth.** Blood should **not** be drawn before milk diet of at least 24 hours prior to sampling, but need to sample before discharge from the nursery may take priority if outpatient sampling is not assured.

Reference Interval Phenylalanine: ≤2 mg/dL (SI: ≤121 µmol/L) by Guthrie bacterial inhibition assay; <4 mg/dL (SI: <242 µmol/L) by fluorometry in some laboratories.
(Continued)

Newborn Screen for Phenylketonuria (Continued)

Possible Panic Range Phenylalanine: ≥4 mg/dL (SI: ≥242 μmol/L) by Guthrie bacterial inhibition assay. Specific diagnosis after identification of a candidate case (by screening program) requires that plasma levels of phenylalanine be >2 mg/dL (SI: >121 μmol/L) on 2 consecutive days.

Use Screen for PKU in newborns (mandatory in the U.S. and many other parts of the world); prevent mental retardation by early diagnosis. Siblings of children with PKU, PHP (persistent hyperphenylalaninemias) deserve special priority.[1]

Limitations When a baby is discharged early (before 72 hours of age), many states, hospitals, and physicians prefer to take a sample early, rather than risk no sample at all.[1] Early sampling for **PKU** risks some false-negative results. Essentially all phenylketonurics may be positive within the first 24 hours if a cutoff of 2 mg/dL is used.[2] Subclassification of phenylalanine hydroxylase deficiency can be made based on blood phenylalanine levels.[3] Identification of non-PKU forms of hyperphenylalaninemia (see following information) requires additional testing for tetrahydrobiopterin pathway enzyme defects. **Not all individuals with increased blood phenylalanine have phenylketonuria.** When an infant is tested for PKU before 24 hours of age, there is a 16% chance of missing a positive case. When screened between 24 and 72 hours of age, there is a 4% chance of missing a positive.[2] If screening (PKU) occurs before 24 hours of life, rescreening should be done. Sick and/or premature infants should be screened (PKU) by age 7 days independent of feeding history or antibiotic therapy.[1]

Any inadequate specimen must be repeated.

Screening must be integrated with follow-up, confirmation of diagnosis, and treatment. Problems have included failure to screen all neonates and imperfect compliance with follow-up screening.

Methodology Guthrie bacterial inhibition method is widely used for neonatal PKU testing. Phenylalanine can also be quantitated by fluorometry. False-positive PKU tests due to antibiotic usage, in particular ampicillin, have been noted and methods for their avoidance (use of penicillinase in test agar or fixing with formic acid vapors) have been reported.[4,5,6]

Additional Information Successful detection of phenylketonuria by screening newborns for hyperphenylalaninemia has as its goal the identification of infants subject to central nervous system damage (in particular mental retardation) due to excessive levels of phenylalanine. Cofactor variants must be correctly diagnosed to provide appropriate therapy. Once identified, harmful CNS effects can be largely avoided by dietary measures, notably a semisynthetic diet low in phenylalanine in the usual cases. In young PKU patients, the tolerance for dietary phenylalanine (to maintain nontoxic plasma levels) is about 250-550 mg/day. Widespread institution of PKU screening programs, worldwide, is an outstanding public health triumph of the 20th century. Incidence is 1:10,000 to 1:15,000 in the United States. For African-Americans in Maryland, the reported incidence is 1:50,000.

Scriver and Clow indicate that an adequate sample is obtained from a term neonate at least 24 hours after milk feeding is started and as close to hospital discharge as possible. For the premature infant, they define an adequate sample as one obtained between the fifth and seventh days of life.[7]

The standard is established that all infants be tested for PKU and congenital hypothyroidism (see Newborn Screen for T$_4$, Filter Paper *on page 230*) **prior to discharge.**

Presence of hyperphenylalaninemia implies a disorder of phenylalanine hydroxylation (to tyrosine). PKU due to phenylalanine hydroxylase (PAH) deficiency is the common example. However, in addition to PAH, hydroxylation requires oxygen and tetrahydrobiopterin (BH$_4$) as a cofactor. A defect in the metabolism of BH$_4$ that results in BH$_4$ deficiency will impair hydroxylation and result in increased plasma phenylalanine concentrations. In the past 15 years, three types of inborn errors of BH$_4$ metabolism ("atypical PKU") have been identified. Defects in BH$_4$ synthesis are guanosine triphosphate cyclohydrolase I deficiency and pyruvoyl tetrahydropterin synthase deficiency. The third type of defect involves the regeneration of BH$_4$ catalyzed by the enzyme dihydropteridine reductase. Experience with treatment of PKU over the past 25 years has shown that some 3% (variable between different populations) fail to respond. These are largely cases of BH$_4$ cofactor deficiency. There are important differences in therapy between classical PKU and the various BH$_4$ cofactor deficiencies. "PKU-positive" cases (identified as the result of phenylalanine screening tests) should be additionally tested for BH$_4$ deficiency.

To maintain intellectual function, the importance of long-term (eg, beyond 10 years) dietary control of the blood phenylalanine level has been recently re-emphasized. Significant phenylalanine hydroxylation *in vivo* in PKU homozygotes has been demonstrated. Such findings suggest significant alternative pathway activity such as tyrosine hydroxylase. Promotion of such latent hydroxylating capabilities may eventually lead to therapies which will complement phenylalanine restriction.

Spuriously high blood phenylalanine levels (false positives) may occur with Guthrie test screening due to uninterpretable "clear zone" effect, the result of antibiotics (usually ampicillin). Because of an increase in the number of cases and amounts of the awards in litigation involving PKU screening (usually false-negative cases), vagaries of PKU testing, while uncommon, are of considerable import and generate comment and innovation.

Intrauterine fetal injury results from exposure of the developing fetus to increased intrapartum maternal plasma phenylalanine levels. There is a high incidence of resultant fetal damage including microcephaly, intrauterine growth retardation, mental retardation, and congenital heart disease, as a result of **maternal hyperphenylalaninemia.** Dietary management of mothers identified by newborn screening programs has as its goal the maintenance of near normal maternal phenylalanine levels throughout pregnancy. In order to retain the achievements of over three decades of early detection and treatment of PKU, increasing attention is being turned to control of maternal hyperphenylalaninemia. The risk of maternal phenylketonuria and hyperphenylalaninemia syndrome is increasing. There is a nearly 100% risk of recurrence if treatment is not given. A number of suggestions have been made to deal with the growing problem of maternal PKU including use of genetic registers. A recent study determined whether dietary treatment during pregnancy of women with PKU affects development outcome of offspring. Scores on the McCarthy General Cognitive Index decreased as weeks to metabolic control increased. Offspring of women who had metabolic control prior to pregnancy had a mean score of 99. Forty-seven percent of offspring whose mothers did not have metabolic control by 20 weeks gestation have a General Cognitive Index score 2 SDs below the norm. Overall, 30% of children born to mothers with PKU had social and behavioral problems. The data suggest that delayed development in offspring of women with PKU is associated with lack of maternal metabolic control prior to or early in pregnancy. Treatment at any time during pregnancy may reduce the severity of delay.[8]

High performance liquid chromatography and polymerase chain reaction based tests have been suggested to screen for carriers of PKU.[9,10,11]

Footnotes

1. American Academy of Pediatrics, Committee on Genetics, "Newborn Screening Fact Sheets: Congenital Hypothyroidism and Phenylketonuria," *Pediatrics*, 1989, 83(3):454-6, 461-2.
2. Doherty LB, Rohr FJ, and Levy HL, "Detection of Phenylketonuria in the Very Early Newborn Blood Specimen," *Pediatrics*, 1991, 87(2):240-4.
3. Matalon R and Michals K, "Phenylketonuria: Screening, Treatment, and Maternal PKU," *Clin Biochem*, 1991, 24(4):337-42.
4. Mabry CC, Reid MC, and Kuhn RJ, "A Source of Error in Phenylketonuria Screening," *Am J Clin Pathol*, 1988, 90(3):279-83.
5. Wilcken B, Brown AR, Liu A, et al, "Eliminating Some Possible Errors in Phenylketonuria Screening," *Am J Clin Pathol*, 1989, 92(3):396.
6. Kremensky I and Kalaydjieva L, "Avoiding Sources of Error in PKU Screening," *Am J Clin Pathol*, 1989, 92(3):396-7.
7. Scriver CR and Clow CL, "Phenylketonuria: Epitome of Human Biochemical Genetics," *N Engl J Med*, 1989, 303:1336-42, 1394-400.
8. Waisbren SE, Hanley W, and Levy HL, "Outcome at Age 4 Years in Offspring of Women With Maternal Phenylketonuria: The Maternal PKU Collaborative Study," *JAMA*, 2000, 283(6):756-62.
9. Hilton MA, Sharpe JN, Hicks LG, et al, "A Simple Method for Detection of Heterozygous Carriers of the Gene for Classic Phenylketonuria," *J Pediatr*, 1986, 109(4):601-4.
10. Eisnesmith RC, Goltsov AA, and Woo SLC, "A Simple, Rapid, and Highly Informative PCR-Based Procedure for Prenatal Diagnosis and Carrier Screening of Phenylketonuria," *Prenat Diagn*, 1994, 14:1113-8.
11. Enns GM, Martinez DR, Kuzmin AI, et al, "Molecular Correlations in Phenylketonuria: Mutation Patterns and Corresponding Biochemical and Clinical Phenotypes in a Heterogeneous California Population," *Pediatr Res*, 1999, 46(5):594-602.

References

Koch R, Levy HL, Matalon R, et al, "The North American Collaborative Study of Maternal Phenylketonuria. Status Report 1993," *Am J Dis Child*, 1993, 147(11):1224-30.

Levy HL, "Phenylketonuria: Old Disease, New Approach to Treatment," *Proc Natl Acad Sci U S A*, 1999, 96(5):1811-3.

Levy HL, Lobbregt D, Sansaricq C, et al, "Comparison of Phenylketonuric and Nonphenylketonuric Sibs From Untreated Pregnancies in a Mother With Phenylketonuria," *Am J Med Genet*, 1992, 44(4):439-42.

Mabry CC, "Phenylketonuria: Contemporary Screening and Diagnosis," *Ann Clin Lab Sci*, 1990, 20(6):393-7.

Michals K, Azen C, Acosta P, et al, "Blood Phenylalanine Levels and Intelligence of 10-Year-Old Children With PKU in the National Collaborative Study," *J Am Diet Assoc*, 1988, 88(10):1226-9.

Scriver CR, "Whatever Happened to PKU?" *Clin Biochem*, 1995, 28(2):137-44.

Scriver CR and Waters PJ, "Monogenic Traits Are Not Simple: Lessons From Phenylketonuria," *Trends Genet*, 1999, 15(7):267-72.

Waisbren SE, Mahon BE, Schnell RR, et al, "Predictors of Intelligence Quotient and Intelligence Quotient Change in Persons Treated for Phenylketonuria Early in Life," *Pediatrics*, 1987, 79(3):351-5.

Newborn Screen for T$_4$, Filter Paper

Related Information

Newborn Screen for Phenylketonuria *on page 229*
Newborn Screen for TSH, Filter Paper *on page 231*
Newborn Screening Tests for Galactosemia *on page 232*
Phenylalanine, Blood *on page 248*
Thyroxine, Free, Serum *on page 285*
Thyroxine, Serum *on page 286*

Synonyms T$_4$ Neonatal; Thyroid Screen for Newborns

Abstract Untreated newborns with congenital hypothyroidism suffer from irreversible mental retardation and physical deformities. Very successful outcome from early treatment makes this disorder an excellent candidate for newborn screening. Screening for congenital hypothyroidism now occurs in all 50 states of the U.S., in most of Europe, and in many other parts of the world.

Specimen Whole blood collected on newborn screening filter paper

Container Special filter paper collection card

Sampling Time Just before infant is discharged from the nursery

Collection Obtain heelstick whole blood sample and thoroughly saturate circles on the filter paper. Label the card with the patient's name, age, and physician. Prompt collection and processing of infants' blood samples is crucial to early detection of these disorders. Steps for collection: Warm the foot and/or massage the leg. Clean the puncture site with an alcohol swab, then dry with a sterile sponge to remove alcohol. Puncture the infant's heel with a sterile lancet <2.5 mm. Wipe away the first drop of blood. Touch the filter paper to the drops and allow them to flow onto the filter paper and diffuse through the circles. Apply a sterile covering to the puncture site.

Causes for Rejection Filter paper not thoroughly saturated, radioactive tracer given to baby before the sample is obtained, exposure of card to extreme heat or light. Touching the filter paper portion, where the blood is spotted, can cause erroneous test results.

Special Instructions The T_4 specimen is usually collected at the same time the PKU specimen is obtained. Optimal collection time is 3-7 days after birth, 4-10 days after birth is recommended for low birth weight infants. With early release (less than 24 hours postdelivery), babies must be brought back to the physician's office for thyroid screening.

Reference Interval T_4 results in infancy are higher than adult ranges. Thyroxine levels are lower in prematures. Peak occurs at about 24 hours; then T_4 decreases. Newborns that have a low T_4 are tested for TSH. For infants 1-2 weeks old: 10-17 µg/dL.

Possible Panic Range Low result for T_4; high TSH. Abnormal value for infants 7 days old or younger: T_4 ≤6.5 µg/dL (SI: ≤84 nmol/L); for infants 8 days old and older: T_4 ≤5.0 µg/dL (SI: ≤64 nmol/L). See report of individual laboratory.

Use Screen for congenital hypothyroidism

Limitations Congenital thyroxine binding globulin deficiency, an X-linked trait, will result in low total T_4 values even though the patient is euthyroid. These patients have normal free thyroxine and TSH. Severe acute illnesses (respiratory distress syndrome, sepsis) cause false-positive results.

Methodology Radioimmunoassay (RIA), enzyme immunoassay (EIA), fluorescent immunoassay

Additional Information Congenital hypothyroidism is a common preventable cause of mental retardation. The overall incidence is approximately 1 in 4000 in the Caucasian population; females are affected about twice as often as males. Persons from African descent have a lower rate of incidence (1 in 32,000). There is evidence that growth becomes thyroid hormone dependent immediately after birth. Decreased growth rate, short stature, and abnormal epiphyseal maturation are clinical features of thyroid deficiency. While height may be normal at birth, growth velocity is decreased during the first weeks of life, increasing after the start of therapy.[1] Patients who are not detected and who do not receive early therapy will develop mental retardation, variable growth failure, metabolic changes of hypothyroidism, deafness and neurologic abnormalities. There is a higher incidence of detection from screening programs than from clinical surveillance since clinical signs in the great majority of cases are minimal at birth. Timing of sampling, retesting, and hazards of screening are important considerations.[2] Transient hypothyroxinemia and transient hyperthyroxinemia occur.[3]

If low values are obtained, the patient must have confirmatory tests run: T_4, TSH, sometimes T_3 uptake, and possibly TBG assessment. For rescreening, combined T_4 and TSH is recommended, when the initial T_4 is low.[2] Thyroid scintigraphy, using ^{99m}Tc or ^{123}I, is the most accurate diagnostic test to detect thyroid dysgenesis or one of the inborn errors of T_4 synthesis.[4]

Newborn screening protocols for congenital hypothyroidism vary from state to state.[5] Some states test for both T_4 and TSH, whereas other states first screen by T_4 or TSH followed by the other test on recognition of abnormal results. Use of receiver operator curves (ROC) has shown that primary TSH screening is more effective for mass screening in reducing false-positive and false-negative cases, than primary thyroxine (T_4) with secondary TSH screening.[6]

Excessive quantities of TBG result in increased T_4, while deficiency in TBG has the opposite effect. Extrathyroidal conditions resulting in depressed T_4 levels include low birth weight (LBW), respiratory distress syndrome, and sepsis. In normal as well as LBW infants, the T_4 will be lower, between 5 and 9 days, compared to 3-5 days after birth. In a Netherlands study, the incidence of total organification defect (an autosomal process) was about 1 in 60,000 neonates.[7] **Seven million newborns are screened annually for hypothyroidism. Three hundred and sixty are spared delayed growth and severe mental retardation while 1200 more babies avoid subnormal intelligence with early diagnosis.[8]**

Although early treatment of congenital hypothyroidism avoids major abnormalities, a brief period of thyroid hormone deficiency results in decline in IQ, poorer visuomotor and visuospatial abilities, delayed speech and language development, selective neuromotor deficiencies, and poorer attention and memory skills.[9,10] Furthermore, recently it has been shown that hypothyroidism in pregnant women may adversely affect their fetuses, and therefore screening for thyroid deficiency during pregnancy may be warranted.[11]

Footnotes

1. Leger J and Czernichow P, "Congenital Hypothyroidism: Decreased Growth Velocity in the First Week of Life," *Biol Neonate*, 1989, 55(4-5):218-23.
2. "Newborn Screening Fact Sheets," American Academy of Pediatrics. Committee on Genetics, *Pediatrics*, 1996, 98(3 Pt 1):473-501.
3. Catlin EA and Lee MM, "Neonatal Endocrinology," *Oski's Pediatrics: Principles and Practice*, 3rd ed, McMillan JA, DeAngelis CD, Feigin RD, et al, eds, eds, Philadelphia, PA: JB Lippincott Co, 1999, 345-56.
4. La Franchi S, "Congenital Hypothyroidism: Etiologies, Diagnosis, and Management," *Thyroid*, 1999, 9(7):735-40.
5. Stoddard JJ and Farrell PM, "State-to-State Variations in Newborn Screening Policies," *Arch Pediatr Adolesc Med*, 1997, 151(6):561-4.
6. Wang ST, Pizzolato S, and Demshar HP, "Diagnostic Effectiveness of TSH Screening and of T_4 With Secondary TSH Screening for Newborn Congenital Hypothyroidism," *Clin Chim Acta*, 1998, 274(2):151-8.
7. Vulsma T, Gons MH, and de Vijlder JJM, "Maternal-Fetal Transfer of Thyroxine in Congenital Hypothyroidism Due to a Total Organification Defect or Thyroid Agenesis," *N Engl J Med*, 1989, 321(1):13-6.
8. Willi SM and Moshang T Jr, "Diagnostic Dilemmas. Results of Screening Tests for Congenital Hypothyroidism," *Pediatr Clin North Am*, 1991, 38(3):555-66.
9. Rovet JF, "Congenital Hypothyroidism: Long-Term Outcome," *Thyroid*, 1999, 9(7):741-8.
10. Simons WF, Fuggle PW, Grant DB, et al, "Educational Progress, Behaviour, and Motor Skills at 10 Years in Early Treated Congenital Hypothyroidism," *Arch Dis Child*, 1997, 77(3):219-22.
11. Dugbartey AT, "Neurocognitive Aspects of Hypothyroidism," *Arch Intern Med*, 1998, 158(13):1413-8. 12. Haddow JE, Palomaki GE, Allan WC, et al, "Maternal Thyroid Deficiency During Pregnancy and Subsequent Neuropsychological Development of the Child," *N Engl J Med*, 1999, 341(8):549-55.

References

Burrow GN, Fisher DA, and Larsen PR, "Maternal and Fetal Thyroid Function," *N Engl J Med*, 1994, 331(16):1072-8.

Delange F, "Neonatal Screening for Congenital Hypothyroidism: Results and Perspectives," *Horm Res*, 1997, 48(2):51-61.

Gruters A, "Congenital Hypothyroidism," *Pediatr Ann*, 1992, 21(1):15, 18-21, 24-8.

Helfand M and Redfern CC, "Screening for Thyroid Disease: An Update," *Ann Intern Med*, 1998, 129(2):144-58.

La Franchi SH, Hanna CE, Krainz PL, et al, "Screening for Congenital Hypothyroidism With Specimen Collection at Two Time Periods: Results of the Northwest Regional Screening Program," *Pediatrics*, 1985, 76(5):734-40.

Morreale de Escobar G and Escobar del Rey F, "Maternal Thyroid Deficiency During Pregnancy and Subsequent Neuropsychological Development of the Child," *N Engl J Med*, 1999, 341(26):2015-6.

Van Vliet G, "Neonatal Hypothyroidism: Treatment and Outcome," *Thyroid*, 1999, 9(1):79-84.

Woeber KA, "The Year in Review: The Thyroid," *Ann Intern Med*, 1999, 131(12):959-62.

Newborn Screen for TSH, Filter Paper

Related Information

Newborn Screen for Phenylketonuria *on page 229*
Newborn Screen for T_4, Filter Paper *on page 230*
Newborn Screening Tests for Galactosemia *on page 232*
Phenylalanine, Blood *on page 248*
Thyroxine, Free, Serum *on page 285*
Thyroxine, Serum *on page 286*

Synonyms Thyroid Stimulating Hormone Screen, Filter Paper; TSH, Filter Paper

Applies to Thyroid Screen for Newborns

Abstract Untreated newborns with congenital hypothyroidism suffer from irreversible mental retardation and physical deformities. The importance of newborn screening for case detection and early initiation of treatment has led to filter paper screening programs of T_4 and/or TSH in many countries of the world. If hypothyroidism is undetected, growth and mental retardation occur, and in rare instances, death.

Patient Preparation After cleansing infant's heel, puncture to obtain free-flowing blood for spotting on collection card. Spot blood directly on card, using no pipets or blood collection equipment. Avoid radioisotope administration before collection of specimen if RIA is used for assay.

Specimen Whole blood, soaked through special (newborn screening) collection paper

Container Special filter paper collection card

Sampling Time Test newborn at 7-10 days. Generally, the sample is collected before the infant leaves the hospital.

Collection Cord blood can be used, or sample can be collected at 3-5 days after birth. Using a large drop of blood, soak through the special collection paper at a minimum of one spot.

Causes for Rejection Blood not soaked through collection card, recently administered radioisotope if RIA is used for assay

Reference Interval TSH peaks just after birth, then declines.[1] "Normal" after immediate postpartum period is <7 mIU/L. Adult levels are reached by 10 days of age. Adults: 0.4-4.2 mIU/L.

Possible Panic Range Elevated TSH with low T_4, or high TSH with normal T_4

Use Newborn screening for congenital hypothyroidism

Limitations Although an elevated TSH level is a better indicator of hypothyroidism than a decreased level of T_4, the TSH surge at birth can cause false-positive results if the sample is collected too early.[1] When TSH is used (Continued)

Newborn Screen for TSH, Filter Paper (Continued)

as the primary screen, cases of secondary or tertiary hypothyroidism are not detected.

Methodology Enzyme immunoassay (EIA), radioimmunoassay (RIA), fluorescent immunoassay, chemiluminescent immunoassay

Additional Information The incidence of congenital hypothyroidism in the United States (on the basis of screening programs) is from 1 in 3600 to 1 in 5000; females are affected about twice as often as males. The incidence is significantly less in black populations (1 in 32,000). Without screening the diagnosis is likely to be missed because signs are usually minimal just after birth. Without detection and treatment mental and physical disability results, including retardation, poor growth, low metabolic rate, constipation, bradycardia, and myxedema. Screening for congenital hypothyroidism is now performed by all states of the USA. Newborn screening protocols for congenital hypothyroidism vary from state to state.[2] Some states test for both T_4 and TSH, whereas other states first screen by T_4 or TSH followed by the other test on abnormal results from the first. Use of receiver operator curves (ROC) has shown that primary TSH screening is more effective for mass screening in reducing false-positive and false-negative cases, than is primary thyroxine (T_4) with secondary TSH screening.[3] Neonatal TSH screening can also find newborns with congenital hyperthyroidism.[4]

Although early treatment of congenital hypothyroidism avoids major abnormalities, deficiencies in IQ, visuomotor and visuospatial abilities, speech and language development, and attention and memory skills exist.[5,6,7]

Footnotes

1. Hannon WH and Therrell BL Jr, "Laboratory Methods for Detecting Congenital Hypothyroidism," *Laboratory Methods for Neonatal Screening*, Therrell BL Jr, ed, Washington, DC: American Public Health Association, 1993, 139-54.
2. Stoddard JJ and Farrell PM, "State-to-State Variations in Newborn Screening Policies," *Arch Pediatr Adolesc Med*, 1997, 151(6):561-4.
3. Wang ST, Pizzolato S, and Demshar HP, "Diagnostic Effectiveness of TSH Screening and of T_4 With Secondary TSH Screening for Newborn Congenital Hypothyroidism," *Clin Chim Acta*, 1998, 274(2):151-8.
4. Kopp P, van Sande J, Parma J, et al, "Brief Report: Congenital Hyperthyroidism Caused by a Mutation in the Thyrotropin-Receptor Gene," *N Engl J Med*, 1995, 332(3):150-4.
5. Rovet JF, "Congenital Hypothyroidism: Long-Term Outcome," *Thyroid*, 1999, 9(7):741-8.
6. Simons WF, Fuggle PW, Grant DB, et al, "Educational Progress, Behaviour, and Motor Skills at 10 Years in Early Treated Congenital Hypothyroidism," *Arch Dis Child*, 1997, 77(3):219-22.
7. Dugbartey AT, "Neurocognitive Aspects of Hypothyroidism," *Arch Intern Med*, 1998, 158(13):1413-8.

References

Burrow GN, Fisher DA, and Larsen PR, "Maternal and Fetal Thyroid Function," *N Engl J Med*, 1994, 331(16):1072-8.

Delange F, "Neonatal Screening for Congenital Hypothyroidism: Results and Perspectives," *Horm Res*, 1997, 48(2):51-61.

Morreale de Escobar G and Escobar del Rey F, "Maternal Thyroid Deficiency During Pregnancy and Subsequent Neuropsychological Development of the Child," *N Engl J Med*, 1999, 341(26):2015-6.

"Newborn Screening Fact Sheets," American Academy of Pediatrics, Committee on Genetics, *Pediatrics*, 1996, 98(3 Pt 1):473-501.

Van Vliet G, "Neonatal Hypothyroidism: Treatment and Outcome," *Thyroid*, 1999, 9(1):79-84.

Newborn Screening Tests for Galactosemia

Related Information

Amino Acids, Urine *on page 101*
Galactokinase, Blood *on page 178*
Galactose-1-Phosphate, Blood *on page 178*
Galactose-1-Phosphate Uridyl Transferase, Blood *on page 179*
Newborn Screen for T_4, Filter Paper *on page 230*
Reducing Substances, Urine *on page 885*

Synonyms Beutler-Baluda Test; Beutler Test; Blood Spot Screen for Galactose/Galactose-1-Phosphate; Galactosemia Screening, Filter Paper; Paigen Test (*E. coli* Bacteriophage Resistance to Lysis Assay)

Test Includes Combinations of screening tests for red cell galactose/galactose-1-phosphate (increase) and red cell galactose-1-phosphate uridyl transferase (absence or low activity)

Abstract Galactosemia may occur with any of three metabolic abnormalities but is usually the result of an inherited **deficiency of galactose-1-phosphate uridyl transferase** activity. This condition, if undetected and untreated, is characterized clinically by failure to thrive, vomiting, cataracts, mental retardation, liver disease, amino aciduria, hypoglycemia, and death. Incidence, generally is about 1:60,000 but estimates worldwide have ranged from 1:18,000 to 1:180,000. A number of variants have been defined with gel electrophoresis, of which the Duarte and Los Angeles types are the most common.[1] The Duarte variant is characterized by intermediate levels of transferase (higher than those of the classical deficiency) and by an electrophoretically distinctive enzyme. Duarte form appears clinically benign. The Indiana variant is an unstable electrophoretically distinct enzyme. Individuals with Los Angeles variant do not have abnormal galactose metabolism.

Deficiency of cellular galactokinase results in a galactose toxicity that is usually milder and limited to development of cataracts.

The third cause of galactosemia, **uridine diphosphate galactose-4-epimerase deficiency**, occurs in two forms. One involves only red and white blood cells and is benign. The second form is unusual and requires care in dietary management. It manifests as does transferase deficiency with hypotonia and nerve deafness. It responds to dietary restriction of galactose. A low level of galactose must be maintained in the diet, however, since epimerase is involved in supplying UDP-galactose for complex carbohydrate, galactolipid and galactoprotein synthesis. While estimates of incidence of galactokinase and epimerase deficiencies have been in the 1:20,000 to 1:40,000 range, very few clinically deficient cases have been reported as compared to cases of transferase deficiency.

The enzyme deficiencies responsible for galactosemia have an autosomal recessive mode of inheritance.

Screening for galactose-1-phosphate uridyl transferase deficiency is the most common method for galactosemia screening. Some states also screen for total galactose.

Specimen Whole blood, dried as a spot on filter paper; may use heparinized whole blood

Sampling Time Screening should be performed within the first 3 days of life after the milk feeding has begun; may be method/diet dependent.

Collection Drop of whole blood soaked into provided filter paper. See Phenylalanine, Blood *on page 248* for collection details.

Storage Instructions Avoid exposure to high temperature during transit to the laboratory (eg, especially during heat of summer) (applies primarily to Beutler test).[2,3]

Causes for Rejection Insufficient or improper application of blood to filter paper spot, excessive exposure to heat, specimen paper without proper label/identification, blood collected in acid-citrate-dextrose or EDTA in some cases[3]

Reference Interval Normal neonates: blood galactose <1 mg/dL (SI: <0.06 mmol/L) in 88%, 1-5 mg/dL (SI: 0.06-0.28 mmol/L) in 12% of cases. Galactosemic infants usually have blood galactose >20 mg/dL (SI: >1.11 mmol/L) (Paigen test).[4]

Use Detect galactosemia; monitor dietary therapy of galactosemia

Limitations Antibiotics present in the sample apparently do not cause a false-negative result in the Paigen test (*E. coli* bacteriophage resistance to lysis), see following information. The Beutler-Baluda test will detect transferase deficient cases of galactosemia only (galactose kinase and epimerase deficiencies although uncommon, would be missed). The Paigen screen for increased RBC galactose/galactose-1-phosphate, if positive, should be followed by a transferase screen (eg, Beutler test) which, if negative, would indicate a different cause for the galactosemia (eg, galactose kinase or epimerase deficiency, see following information). A galactose screening test that is not sensitive also to galactose-1-phosphate will require that the newborn have ingested milk prior to testing or a false-positive result may be obtained. **Transfusion may result in a false-negative Beutler-Baluda test for as long as 2-3 months.**

Methodology Urine can be screened for galactosuria by reagents usually commonly available in the Urinalysis and/or Chemistry sections of most clinical laboratories. Specimen is first tested for reducing substances by a cupric ion reduction method (eg, Benedict's Test, Clinitest® tablets). If positive, a glucose oxidase specific method is applied. If the specific test for glucose is negative, but a reducing substance is present, there is presumptive evidence for one of the three forms of galactosemia.

Screening programs for galactosemia have been established by most states in the United States and many countries of the world. Ease of specimen transport to high volume reference laboratories favors dried blood spot over urine testing. A variety of applicable tests utilizing whole blood samples spotted on filter paper have been described.[5]

The Beutler test has a fluorescent end point, tests for deficiency of galactose-1-phosphate uridyl transferase, and can be performed rapidly. A recently described fluorescent method can distinguish patients with galactose-1-phosphate uridyl transferase deficiency from healthy subjects and heterozygote carriers.[3]

The Paigen assay screens for increase in galactose and galactose-1-phosphate. It is the most effective **single** test available for all forms of galactosemia.[5] The procedure uses a strain of *E. coli* that resists C21 bacteriophage lysis in the presence of galactose. Thus, bacterial growth occurs around filter paper blood spots in cases of galactosemia. In the absence of galactose (normal nongalactosemic newborn), no growth occurs as the bacteria are killed by the phage. The diameter of the growth zone is proportional to the concentration of galactose.[4]

An enzymatic centrifugal analyzer chemical method has been developed. Galactose is determined by measuring the change in absorbance of reduced NADH at 340 nm after addition of galactose dehydrogenase.[6] A presumptive positive is defined as a blood galactose plus galactose-1-phosphate level >0.30 mmol/L. Each presumptive positive is also screened with a Beutler spot test to assess transferase activity. This method for galactosemia screening is rapid, sensitive and may be the method of choice for mass screening.[6] A microplate fluorometric method based on the GADH-NAD+/NADH system has similar advantages to the Manitoba system noted above, is rapid, reliable, and applicable to routine screening of newborns.[7]

Third generation cephalosporin antibiotics may cause false-positive results in *E. coli* W5 based tests (in which presence of galactose inhibits bacterial growth).[8] Presence of galactosemia, however, is not excluded, until another sample is appropriately tested by a different method.

Additional Information Urine from normal newborns may have levels of galactose as high as 60 mg/dL (SI: 3.33 mmol/L) (physiologic melituria); in premature infants this may occur over the first 2 weeks of life.[9] High level of milk intake may also produce galactosuria.[10] In cases of galactosemia, galactosuria may be intermittent (partly relating to the intake of milk) and may be missed if urine is very dilute. A screening program based on a copper reduction test, then, may result in false negatives. Early identification and treatment of the infant with galactosemia is critical as cataracts, mental retardation, liver disease with hepatosplenomegaly, and death due to septicemia (in particular, *E. coli* septicemia) may occur in the untreated individual. Specific enzyme assays should be employed to define abnormalities detected by screening tests.

While dietary measures (galactose-restricted diets) control the acute life-threatening disorder, long-term outcome may be unfavorable. Developmental delay, learning disability, impaired motor function and balances, speech disorder, gonadal failure, and personality disorders occur in later years.[11]

Galactosemia screening programs also detect **transient galactosemia**, prognosis of which is almost always favorable. Patients with transient galactosemia should be followed for at least 1 year.[12]

Footnotes

1. Segal S and Berry GT, "Disorders of Galactose Metabolism," *The Metabolic and Molecular Bases of Inherited Disease*, 7th ed, Chapter 25, Scriver CR, Beaudet AL, Sly WS, et al, eds, New York, NY: McGraw-Hill Inc, 1995, 967-1000.
2. "American Academy of Pediatrics, Committee on Genetics, Newborn Screening Fact Sheets," *Pediatrics*, 1989, 83(3):458-60.
3. Fujimoto A, Okano Y, Miyagi T, et al, "Quantitative Beutler Test for Newborn Mass Screening of Galactosemia Using a Fluorometric Microplate Reader," *Clin Chem*, 2000, 46(6 Pt 1):806-10.
4. Paigen K, Pacholec F, and Levy HL, "A New Method of Screening for Inherited Disorders of Galactose Metabolism," *J Lab Clin Med*, 1982, 88:895-907.
5. Beutler E, "Galactosemia: Screening and Diagnosis," *Clin Biochem*, 1991, 24(4):293-300.
6. Greenberg CR, Dilling LA, Thompson R, et al, "Newborn Screening for Galactosemia: A New Method Used in Manitoba," *Pediatrics*, 1989, 84(2):331-5.
7. Yamaguchi A, Fukushi M, Mizushima Y, et al, "Microassay for Screening Newborns for Galactosemia With Use of a Fluorometric Microplate Reader," *Clin Chem*, 1989, 35(9):1962-4.
8. Schunk JP, Bradley JS, Buist NR, et al, "Interference by Third Generation Cephalosporins With Neonatal Screening for Galactosemia," *J Pediatr*, 1988, 112(5):842.
9. Dahlquist A and Svenningsen NW, "Galactose in the Urine of Newborn Infants," *J Pediatr*, 1969, 75:454.
10. Holl WK, Cravey CE, Chen PT, et al, "An Evaluation of Galactosuria," *J Pediatr*, 1970, 77:625.
11. Holton JB and Leonard JV, "Clouds Still Gathering Over Galactosaemia," *Lancet*, 1994, 344(8932):1242-3.
12. Ono H, Mawatari H, Mizoguchi N, et al, "Transient Galactosemia Detected by Neonatal Mass Screening," *Pediatr Int*, 1999, 41(3):281-4.

References

Applegarth DA, Dimmick JE, and Toone JR, "Laboratory Detection of Metabolic Disease," *Pediatr Clin North Am*, 1989, 36(1):49-65.

Berry HK and Croft CC, "Reagent That Restores Galactose-1-Phosphate Uridyltransferase Activity in Dry Blood Spots," *Clin Chem*, 1987, 33(8):1471-2.

Gitzelmann R, "Disorders of Galactose Metabolism," *Inborn Metabolic Diseases: Diagnosis and Treatment*, Fernandes J, Saudubray JM, and Van den Berghe G, eds, 3rd ed, New York, NY: Springer-Verlag, 2000, 103-9.

Gitzelmann R and Steinmann B, "Galactosemia," *Eur J Pediatr*, 1995, 154(7 Suppl 2):S2-S105.

Holton JB, "Galactosaemia: Pathogenesis and Treatment," *J Inherit Metab Dis*, 1996, 19(1):3-7.

Kwon C and Farrell PM, "The Magnitude and Challenge of False-Positive Newborn Screening Test Results," *Arch Pediatr Adolesc Med*, 2000, 154(7):714-8.

Petry KG and Reichardt JK, "The Fundamental Importance of Human Galactose Metabolism: Lessons From Genetics and Biochemistry," *Trends Genet*, 1998, 14(3):98-102.

Sokol RJ, McCabe ER, Kotzer AM, et al, "Pitfalls in Diagnosing Galactosemia: False-Negative Newborn Screening Following Red Blood Cell Transfusion," *J Pediatr Gastroenterol Nutr*, 1989, 8(2):266-8.

♦ **NH₃, Blood** *see* Ammonia, Plasma *on page 102*

♦ **Nitroprusside Reaction, Blood** *see* Ketone Bodies, Blood *on page 205*

♦ **Nitroprusside Screening** *see* Cystine, Urine *on page 164*

♦ **Nonketotic Hyperglycinemia** *see* Cerebrospinal Fluid Glycine *on page 142*

♦ **Nonthyroidal Illness** *see* Reverse T₃, Serum *on page 274*

♦ **Norepinephrine** *see* Metanephrines, Urine or Plasma *on page 223*

♦ **Norepinephrine, Urine** *see* Catecholamines, Fractionation, Urine *on page 139*

♦ **Normetanephrine** *see* Metanephrines, Urine or Plasma *on page 223*

♦ **NSE** *see* Neuron-Specific Enolase, Serum *on page 229*

♦ **5'NT** *see* 5' Nucleotidase, Serum *on page 234*

♦ **N-Telopeptides of Type-1 Collagen** *see* N-Telopeptides, Urine *on page 233*

N-Telopeptides, Urine

Related Information

Alkaline Phosphatase, Heat Stable, Serum *on page 91*
Alkaline Phosphatase Isoenzymes, Serum *on page 92*
Alkaline Phosphatase, Serum *on page 93*
Calcium, Serum *on page 131*
Calcium, Urine *on page 133*
Hydroxyproline, Total, Urine *on page 199*
Osteocalcin, Serum or Plasma *on page 237*
Parathyroid Hormone, Serum *on page 243*
Phosphorus, Serum *on page 251*
Phosphorus, Urine *on page 253*
Pyridinolines (Pyridinoline and Deoxypyridinoline), Urine *on page 272*
Urine Collection, 24-Hour *on page 47*

Synonyms N-Telopeptides of Type-1 Collagen; NTx

Applies to Collagen Type-1; C-Telopeptide; Deoxypyridoline; Galactosyl Hydroxylysine; Pyridinoline; Telopeptides

Abstract Bone remodeling is a constant process, through osteoclast-mediated resorption and osteoblast-mediated osteogenesis. N-telopeptide (NTx) is a specific marker of bone resorption. When bone is resorbed, NTx is released from bone and excreted in urine. The rate of NTx excretion in urine is used as an index of bone resorption.

Sampling Time Second morning void or 24-hour urine. Due to diurnal variation, 24-hour urine sample is preferred. NTx excretion is higher at night. Following baseline assay(s), repeat assay about 3 months following beginning of antiresorptive treatment, repeat at 12 months, then annually if medically necessary.[1]

Collection Refrigerate during collection

Storage Instructions Refrigerate. Freeze for longer storage (>2 days).

Reference Interval NTx levels are higher in children. In the literature, there is a wide variation in reference ranges, even with the same methodology, particularly in children.[2,3,4,5] Approximate adult reference ranges for 24-hour urine are:

- male : <65 pmol/μmol creatinine
- female: premenopausal: <65 pmol/μmol creatinine; postmenopausal: <131 pmol/μmol creatinine

Use The major roles of biochemical markers of bone remodeling are as monitors of response to therapy.[6] These markers are also used to evaluate bone resorption and to identify patients at high risk for fractures. NTx is used to predict bone response to hormonal replacement in postmenopausal women, and antiresorptive treatment in osteoporosis and Paget disease of bone.

The Negotiated Rulemaking Committee of HCFA has listed the following indications for collagen cross-link assays (any method):

- Identifying individuals with elevated bone resorption, who have osteoporosis, in whom response to treatment is being monitored
- Predict response (as assessed by bone mass measurements) to FDA-approved antiresorptive therapy in postmenopausal women
- Assess effectiveness of osteoporosis treatment including FDA-approved antiresorptive therapies in postmenopausal women, individuals with osteoporosis, Paget disease of bone and antiestrogen or selective estrogen therapies.[1]

Limitations Substantial variability between methods and specimens is recognized. Therefore, a second baseline assay is not inappropriate. NTx is affected by renal clearance.

Methodology Enzyme-linked immunosorbent assay (ELISA), competitive immunoassay, radioimmunoassay (RIA)

Additional Information Type 1 collagen makes up ~90% of organic matrix of bone. It is cross-linked at N- and C-terminals by amino acids, predominantly deoxypyridinoline and pyridinoline. Urinary deoxypyridinoline, pyridinoline, galactosyl hydroxylysine, and N- and C-telopeptides are used as markers of bone resorption. These bone resorption markers are released from bone with osteoclast activity.[7]

NTx levels are increased in osteoporosis, Paget disease, metastatic bone disease, primary and secondary hyperparathyroidism, hyperthyroidism, and other diseases with increased bone resorption. NTx levels are increased in aging individuals, predominantly postmenopausal women, as compared to premenopausal controls.

Diseases, conditions, and drugs that cause increased or unbalanced levels of bone turnover markers include:[8,9]

- postmenopausal estrogen deficiency
- osteoporosis
- hypercortisolism, hypogonadism, hyperparathyroidism, and hyperthyroidism
- Paget disease of bone
- renal insufficiency or renal failure
- gastrointestinal diseases related to nutrition and mineral metabolism, osteomalacia
- rheumatoid arthritis, polymyalgia rheumatica, and other connective tissue disorders

(Continued)

N-Telopeptides, Urine (Continued)

- osteogenesis imperfecta, acromegaly, growth hormone/receptor deficiency, and other growth disorders
- multiple myeloma, hypercalcemia of malignancy, and metastatic neoplasms
- chronic immobilization
- alcoholism and tobacco use
- recent fracture
- chronic therapy with anticonvulsants, corticosteroids (glucocorticoids), excess thyroid hormone, gonadotropin-releasing hormone agonists, or heparin

Treatment of osteoporotics and postmenopausal women with biphosphonates and/or estrogen replacement therapy and other means decreases bone resorption markers. As compared to pyridinolines, NTx responds better to antiresorptive therapy. A typical response to antiresorptive therapy may be seen as a decrease of 30% to 40% from baseline after 3 months of treatment. An adequate therapeutic response is signaled by a ≥50% reduction in the resorption marker.[1,6]

Footnotes

1. Mayo Reference Services Publication, "NTx Telopeptide, Urine," *New Test Announcement*, Rochester, MN: Mayo Medical Laboratories, 2000.
2. Bollen AM and Eyre DR, "Bone Resorption Rates in Children Monitored by the Urinary Assay of Collagen Type I Cross-Linked Peptides," *Bone*, 1994, 15(1):31-4.
3. Zanze M, Souberbielle JC, Kindermans C, et al, "Procollagen Propeptide and Pyridinium Cross-Links as Markers of Type I Collagen Turnover: Sex- and Age-Related Changes in Healthy Children," *J Clin Endocrinol Metab*, 1997, 82(9):2971-7.
4. Mora S, Prinster C, Bellini A, et al, "Bone Turnover in Neonates: Changes of Urinary Excretion Rate of Collagen Type I Cross-Linked Peptides During the First Days of Life and Influence of Gestational Age," *Bone*, 1997, 20(6):563-6.
5. Mora S, Prinster C, Proverbio MC, et al, "Urinary Markers of Bone Turnover in Healthy Children and Adolescents: Age-Related Changes and Effect of Puberty," *Calcif Tissue Int*, 1998, 63(5):369-74.
6. Hurley DL and Khosla S, "Update on Primary Osteoporosis," *Mayo Clin Proc*, 1997, 72(10):943-9.
7. Christenson RH, "Biochemical Markers of Bone Metabolism: An Overview," *Clin Biochem*, 1997, 30(8):573-93.
8. Miller PD, Baran DT, Bilezikian JP, et al, "Practical Clinical Application of Biochemical Markers of Bone Turnover: Consensus of an Expert Panel," *J Clin Densitom*, 1999, 2(3):323-42.
9. Delmas PD, "Biochemical Markers of Bone Turnover in Paget's Disease of Bone," *J Bone Miner Res*, 1999, 14(Suppl 2):66-9.

References

Beck-Jensen JE, Kollerup G, Sorensen HA, et al, "A Single Measurement of Biochemical Markers of Bone Turnover Has Limited Utility in the Individual Person," *Scand J Clin Lab Invest*, 1997, 57(4):351-9.

Knott L and Bailey AJ, "Collagen Cross-Links in Mineralizing Tissues: A Review of Their Chemistry, Function, and Clinical Relevance," *Bone*, 1998, 22(3):181-7.

Lane JM and Nydick M, "Osteoporosis: Current Modes of Prevention and Treatment," *J Am Acad Orthop Surg*, 1999, 7(1):19-31.

Papapoulos SE and Frolich M, "Prediction of the Outcome of Treatment of Paget's Disease of Bone With Bisphosphonates From Short-Term Changes in the Rate of Bone Resorption," *J Clin Endocrinol Metab*, 1996, 81(11):3993-7.

Seibel MJ and Woitge HW, "Basic Principles and Clinical Applications of Biochemical Markers of Bone Metabolism: Biochemical and Technical Aspects," *J Clin Densitom*, 1999, 2(3):299-321.

Souberbielle JC, Cormier C, and Kindermans C, "Bone Markers in Clinical Practice," *Curr Opin Rheumatol*, 1999, 11(4):312-9.

Urena P and De Vernejoul MC, "Circulating Biochemical Markers of Bone Remodeling in Uremic Patients," *Kidney Int*, 1999, 55(6):2141-56.

Watts NB, "Clinical Utility of Biochemical Markers of Bone Remodeling," *Clin Chem*, 1999, 45(8 Pt 2):1359-68.

- ♦ **NTP** see AD7c Neural Thread Protein, CSF or Urine *on page 83*
- ♦ **NTx** see N-Telopeptides, Urine *on page 233*
- ♦ **NTX** see Osteocalcin, Serum or Plasma *on page 237*

5′ Nucleotidase, Serum

Related Information

Alkaline Phosphatase, Serum *on page 93*
Gamma-Glutamyl Transferase, Serum *on page 179*
Liver Disease: Laboratory Assessment, Overview *on page 216*

Synonyms EC 3.1.3.5; 5′NT; 5′-Ribonucleotide Phosphohydrolase: NTP

Abstract A plasma membrane enzyme relevant to the biliary tract. The test is not widely available.

Patient Preparation A fasting specimen is preferred.

Specimen Serum

Container Red top tube

Storage Instructions Stable 4 days at 4°C or 3 months at -20°C. Unstable at room temperature.

Reference Interval Varies with laboratory. Adults: 2-17 units/L.[1]

Use 5′NT is used in the differential diagnosis of diseases involving the liver and the porta hepatic area. Marked increases (4-6 times the upper limit of normal) are found in hepatobiliary diseases (eg, obstruction of common duct, biliary cirrhosis, intrahepatic cholestasis). Normal values, or very small increases, are found in parenchymal liver disease (eg, hepatitis) and skeletal diseases. In the past, 5′NT was among the tests used to evaluate

persons with an elevated alkaline phosphatase result on a biochemical screen, but this application is decreasing.

Methodology Kinetic with spectrophotometric detection

Additional Information The diseases identified by elevations of 5′NT parallel closely those identified by Gamma-Glutamyl Transferase, Serum *on page 179*, and there does not appear to be a need for two tests providing the same information. In patients receiving antiepileptic drugs, the frequency of enzyme elevation was similar to that of alkaline phosphatase but lower than that of GGT.[2]

It has recently been reported that a ratio of GGT:5′NT is significantly lower in patients with intrahepatic cholestasis as compared to extrahepatic cholestasis. A threshold of GGT:5′NT <1.9 had a sensitivity of 40% and specificity of 100% for diagnosis of intrahepatic cholestasis.[3]

Footnotes

1. Moss DW and Henderson AR, "Clinical Enzymology," *Tietz Textbook of Clinical Chemistry*, 3rd ed, Burtis CA and Ashwood ER, eds, Philadelphia, PA: WB Saunders Co, 1999, 617-21.
2. Fortman CS and Witte DL, "Serum 5′ Nucleotidase in Patients Receiving Antiepileptic Drugs," *Am J Clin Pathol*, 1985, 84(2):197-201.
3. Sapey T, Mendler MH, Guyader D, et al, "Respective Value of Alkaline Phosphatase, Gamma-Glutamyl Transpeptidase and 5′-Nucleotidase Serum Activity in the Diagnosis of Cholestasis: A Prospective Study of 80 Patients," *J Clin Gastroenterol*, 2000, 30(3):259-63.

- ♦ **O₂ Binding Capacity (BO₂)** see Oxygen Saturation, Blood *on page 240*
- ♦ **O₂ Content (ctO₂)** see Oxygen Saturation, Blood *on page 240*
- ♦ **OD 450 Method** see Bilirubin, Amniotic Fluid, Delta A450 *on page 116*
- ♦ **OGTT** see Glucose Tolerance Test, Plasma *on page 186*
- ♦ **1,25-(OH)₂ D₃** see Vitamin D, Serum *on page 300*
- ♦ **17-OHCS** see 17-Hydroxycorticosteroids, Urine *on page 196*
- ♦ **25-(OH) D₃** see Vitamin D, Serum *on page 300*
- ♦ **17-OHP** see 17-Hydroxyprogesterone, Serum or Plasma *on page 197*
- ♦ **17-OHP, Amniotic Fluid** see 17-Hydroxyprogesterone, Serum or Plasma *on page 197*
- ♦ **17-OHP, Saliva** see 17-Hydroxyprogesterone, Serum or Plasma *on page 197*
- ♦ **o-Phosphoric-Monoester Phosphohydrolase** see Acid Phosphatase, Plasma *on page 82*
- ♦ **Optical Density at 650 nm** see Pulmonary Surfactant, Amniotic Fluid *on page 271*
- ♦ **Oral Glucose Tolerance Test** see Glucose, Postglucose Load, Plasma *on page 185*
- ♦ **Oral Glucose Tolerance Test** see Glucose Tolerance Test, Plasma *on page 186*
- ♦ **Organic Acids** see Amino Acids, Plasma *on page 100*
- ♦ **Organic Acids** see Amino Acids, Urine *on page 101*
- ♦ **Organophosphate Toxicity** see Acetylcholinesterase, Red Cell *on page 81*
- ♦ **Ornithine** see Amino Acids, Urine *on page 101*
- ♦ **Ornithine** see Cystine, Urine *on page 164*
- ♦ **Orosomucoid** see Alpha₁-Acid Glycoprotein, Serum *on page 95*
- ♦ **Orotic Aciduria** see Cobalamin, Serum *on page 150*
- ♦ **Osmolal Gap** see Osmolality, Calculated, Serum or Plasma *on page 234*
- ♦ **Osmolal Gap** see Osmolality, Serum *on page 236*
- ♦ **Osmolal Gap** see Sodium, Serum or Plasma *on page 275*
- ♦ **Osmolal Gap, Urine** see Osmolality, Urine *on page 236*

Osmolality, Calculated, Serum or Plasma

Related Information

Anion Gap, Serum, Plasma, or Urine *on page 106*
Antidiuretic Hormone, Plasma *on page 107*
Bicarbonate, Blood *on page 115*
Electrolyte Panel, Serum *on page 168*
Ethanol, Blood, Urine, and Other Sources *on page 789*
Ethylene Glycol, Serum or Plasma *on page 790*
Ketone Bodies, Blood *on page 205*
Osmolality, Serum *on page 236*
Osmolality, Urine *on page 236*
pH, Blood *on page 247*
Sodium, Serum or Plasma *on page 275*
Sodium, Urine *on page 278*
Volatile Screen, Blood or Urine *on page 809*

Applies to Isopropyl Alcohol Intoxication; Methanol; Osmolal Gap

Test Includes Sodium, urea nitrogen (BUN), glucose

Abstract Serum osmolality may be directly measured, or predicted, using one of several equations based on the concentrations of serum sodium, glucose, and urea. Each equation has its own set of advantages and disadvantages. The purpose of each equation is the necessity, now unique to the U.S., of converting the conventionally reported glucose and urea results into molar (or SI) units. A formula widely used by clinicians, to calculate osmolality in mOsm/kg H_2O, is:

Calculated osmolality = 2[Na] + BUN / 2.8 + GLU / 18

in which BUN is the serum urea nitrogen in mg/dL; and GLU is the plasma or serum glucose in mg/dL. Dividing the BUN by 2.8 converts the measurement from mg/dL to mmol/L. The same is true for dividing the glucose by 18. Multiplying the sodium, already in mmol/L, by 2 is done to account for the osmotically active anions (mostly chloride and bicarbonate) associated with the sodium. Osterloh et al support application of this formula.[1] (Other formulas may be found in the reference by Dr Weisberg and in textbooks of clinical chemistry.) The **osmal gap** is the arithmetic difference between the measured osmolality and the calculated osmolality.

The **sodium** value used in the equation should be one measured without dilution by a sodium-selective ion electrode. This avoids using the erroneous value (euphemistically called pseudohyponatremia) which results from a sodium measurement made after dilution by flame photometry on a specimen with an increased concentration of lipid or protein.

Patient Preparation Patient ideally should be fasting for 8 hours, a setting not usually possible when the need for investigation of osmolality arises.

Specimen Serum or plasma

Container Red top tube, green top (heparin) tube

Collection Keep one green top tube on ice, should a pH be needed.

Causes for Rejection Gross hemolysis

Reference Interval
- Calculated osmolality: 290 mOsm/kg H_2O
- Measured osmolality: up to age 60 years: 275-295 mOsm/kg H_2O, older than 60 years: 280-301 mOsm/kg H_2O
- Osmolal gap: 9.0 (±6.4) mOsm/kg H_2O

Possible Panic Range A gap >20 mOsm/kg H_2O (SI: >20 mmol/kg H_2O)

Use Hyponatremia is a laboratory finding which raises the possibility of an osmolal disturbance and prompts additional laboratory studies. Since some, but by no means all, patients with hyponatremia are at risk for acute cerebral edema, prompt diagnosis is essential. The following table details typical findings in various clinical conditions having hyponatremia as a common denominator. See Sodium, Serum or Plasma on page 275.

The differential diagnosis of an **increased osmolal gap** associated with a high anion gap metabolic acidosis includes chronic renal failure, diabetic ketoacidosis, methanol intoxication, ethylene glycol intoxication, and lactic acidosis.[2] An increased osmolal gap with normal blood pH and ketosis occurs in ethanol and isopropyl alcohol intoxication (see Anion Gap, Serum, Plasma, or Urine on page 106). See table.

Limitations Considerable variability occurs in the normal osmolal gap.[1]

Methodology The tests above can be done on a variety of instruments, that have in common the items necessary to calculate osmolality and to follow many of the patients seen in hospital practice, with other tests ordered, as clinically indicated. See individual listings for sodium, BUN, and glucose.

Additional Information Look for crystalluria in the urinary sediment to further investigate ethylene glycol toxicity. Calcium oxalate and/or hippurate crystals would support this impression, as would the documentation of severe high anion gap metabolic acidosis.[3]

Footnotes
1. Osterloh JD, Kelly TJ, Khayam-Bashi H, et al, "Discrepancies in Osmolal Gaps and Calculated Alcohol Concentrations," *Arch Pathol Lab Med*, 1996, 120(7):637-41.
2. Desai SP and Isa-Pratt S, *Clinician's Guide to Laboratory Medicine*, Cleveland, OH: Lexi-Comp Inc, 2000, 228-35.
3. Terlinsky AS, Grochowski J, Geoly KL, et al, "Identification of Atypical Calcium Oxalate Crystalluria Following Ethylene Glycol Ingestion," *Am J Clin Pathol*, 1981, 76(2):223-6.

References
Baker RJ, "Biochemical Gaps: Osmolal and Anion," *Curr Surg*, 1987, 44(5):378-81.
Eder AF, McGrath CM, Dowdy YG, et al, "Ethylene Glycol Poisoning: Toxokinetic and Analytical Factors Affecting Laboratory Diagnosis," *Clin Chem*, 1998, 44(1):168-77.
Emmett M and Narins RG, "Clinical Use of the Anion Gap," *Medicine (Baltimore)*, 1977, 56:38-54.
Halperin ML, Margolis BL, Robinson LA, et al, "The Urine Osmal Gap: A Clue to Estimate Urine Ammonium in "Hybrid" Types of Metabolic Acidosis," *Clin Invest Med*, 1988, 11(3):198-202.

Causes of Increased Osmolal Gap, Overview

Exogenous Causes
- Acetone
- Methanol
- Ethanol
- Isopropanol
- Ethylene glycol
- Propylene glycol
- Ethyl ether
- Dimethyl sulfoxide*
- Glycine*
- Mannitol*
- Osmotic contrast dyes

Diseases
- Chronic renal failure
- Lactate acidosis?
- Alcoholic ketoacidosis
- Diabetic ketoacidosis
- Hyperlipidemia,† hyperglobulinemia†

Artifactual
- Lavender top (EDTA‡) tube 15 mOsm/L§
- Gray top (sodium fluoride - potassium oxalate) tube 150 mOsm/L§
- Blue top (citrate) tube 10 mOsm/L§
- Green top (lithium heparin) tube 6 mOsm/L§

*These agents are given by intravenous infusion.
†Sodium was measured by flame emission spectrophotometry.
‡EDTA indicates ethylenediaminetetraacetic acid.
§Values are reported as calculated contributions.
Adapted from Osterloh JD, Kelly TJ, Khayam-Bashi H, et al, "Discrepancies in Osmolal Gaps and Calculated Alcohol Concentrations.," *Arch Pathol Lab Med*, 1996, 120(7):637-41.

Typical Serum Sodium, Osmolality, and Effective Osmolality (Tonicity) in Different Clinical States*

Condition	Serum Sodium mmol/L	Blood Glucose mmol/L (mg/dL)	Serum Urea Nitrogen mmol/L (mg/dL)	Mannitol or Ethanol mmol/L	Osm$_c$ mmol/kg H_2O	Osm$_m$ mmol/kg H_2O	Osmolal Gap mmol/kg H_2O	Effective Osmolality mmol/kg H_2O†	Risk of Cerebral Edema‡
Normal	140	5 (90)	5 (14)	0	290	290	0	285 (normal)	None
Hyponatremia (without abnormal amounts of other solutes)	120	5 (90)	5 (14)	0	250	250	0	245 (low)	Increased
Pseudohyponatremia (eg, from extreme hypertriglyceridemia)	120	5 (90)	5 (14)	0	250	290	40	285 (normal)	Unchanged
Hyponatremia caused by severe hyperglycemia	120	75 (1350)	5 (14)	0	320	320	0	315 (high)	Variable**
Hyponatremia caused by retention of mannitol	120	5 (90)	5 (14)	75§	250	325	75	320 (high)	Decreased
Hyponatremia together with high serum urea nitrogen¶	120	5 (90)	45 (126)	0	290	290	0	245 (low)	Increased
Hyponatremia together with high blood ethanol level¶	120	5 (90)	5 (14)	40#	250	290	40	245 (low)	Increased
Hypernatremia	160	5 (90)	5 (14)	0	330	330	0	325 (high)	Decreased

*Osm$_c$ indicates calculated osmolality (calculated as 2[Na] + SUN / 2.8 + GLU / 18, where SUN indicates serum urea nitrogen, and GLU glucose); Osm$_m$ indicates measured osmolality (assume that normal osmal gap is zero). Osmal gap is Osm$_m$ - Osm$_c$.
†Effective osmolality (tonicity) is that portion of osmolality inducing transmembrane water movement; the cited values for effective osmolality were calculated by subtracting the contributions of urea and ethanol (if present) from the measured osmolality.
‡Immediate risk of the osmotic type of cerebral edema before treatment (the more acute the hyponatremia, the greater the risk, since osmotic adaptation is less advanced).
**Effect on intracellular fluid volume depends on clinical circumstances.
§Neglecting the correction factor for serum water content. 75 mmol of mannitol per liter corresponds to approximately 1365 mg/dL.
¶Substances (eg, urea and ethanol) that easily cross cell membranes contribute to measured osmolality, but not to tonicity.
#Neglecting the correction factor for serum water content. 40 mmol of ethanol per liter corresponds to approximately 184 mg/dL.
Adapted from Oster JR and Singer I, "Hyponatremia, Hypo-osmolality, and Hypotonicity," *Arch Intern Med*, 1999, 159(4):333-6.

(Continued)

Hertford JA, McKenna JP, and Chamovitz BN, "Metabolic Acidosis With an Elevated Anion Gap," *Am Fam Phys*, 1989, 39(4):159-68.

Hirasawa H, Odaka M, Sugai T, et al, "Prognostic Value of Serum Osmolality Gap in Patients With Multiple Organ Failure Treated With Hemopurification," *Artif Organs*, 1988, 12(5):382-7.

Norris SH, "Quiz of the Month. Severe Acidosis and an Osmolar Gap in an Alcoholic," *Am J Nephrol*, 1989, 9(2):144, 175-6.

Oster JR, Perez GO, and Materson BJ, "Use of the Anion Gap in Clinical Medicine," *South Med J*, 1988, 81(2):229-37.

Sklar AH and Linas SL, "The Osmolal Gap in Renal Failure," *Ann Intern Med*, 1983, 98:481-2.

Sweeney TE and Beuchat CA, "Limitations of Methods of Osmometry: Measuring the Osmolality of Biological Fluids," *Am J Physiol*, 1993, 264(3 Pt 2):R469-80.

Weisberg HF, "Unraveling the Laboratory Model of a Syndrome: The Osmolality Model," *Clinician and Chemist. The Relationship of the Laboratory to the Physician*, Young DS, Hicks J, Nipper H, et al, eds, Washington, DC: AACC Press, American Association of Clinical Chemistry, 1979, 200-43.

Osmolality, Serum

Related Information

Anion Gap, Serum, Plasma, or Urine *on page 106*
Antidiuretic Hormone, Plasma *on page 107*
Carbohydrate-Deficient Transferrin, Serum *on page 134*
Drugs of Abuse Testing, Urine *on page 788*
Electrolyte Panel, Serum *on page 168*
Ethanol, Blood, Urine, and Other Sources *on page 789*
Ethylene Glycol, Serum or Plasma *on page 790*
Ketone Bodies, Blood *on page 205*
Osmolality, Calculated, Serum or Plasma *on page 234*
Osmolality, Urine *on page 236*
pH, Blood *on page 247*
Sodium, Serum or Plasma *on page 275*
Specific Gravity, Urine *on page 886*
Urea Nitrogen:Creatinine Ratio *on page 292*

Synonyms Serum Osmolality

Applies to Osmolal Gap; Osmolality:Serum Ratio; Sodium, Serum:Osmolality, Serum Ratio; Urine:Serum Osmolality Ratio

Replaces Osmolarity

Abstract The osmolality of a solution is the number of particles (molecules or ions) in a liter of solution. Osmolality is independent of particle size or charge. Nonpolar solutions yield one molecule (eg, glucose) while polar solutions yield multiples of the number of ions solubilized (eg, sodium chloride yields two ions while magnesium chloride yields three ions).

Ethanol ingestion is the most common cause of increased osmolality and is responsible for most osmolal gaps.[1]

Specimen Serum

Container Red top tube

Collection Pediatrics: Blood drawn from heelstick

Storage Instructions Refrigerate or freeze serum if not run within 4 hours.

Reference Interval 275-295 mOsm/kg H_2O (SI: 275-295 mmol/kg H_2O)

• Urine:serum osmolality ratio: 1.0-3.0 with fluid restriction: 3.0-4.7
• Sodium, serum:osmolality:serum ratio:[2] 0.43-0.50

Possible Panic Range <265 mOsm/kg H_2O (SI: <265 mmol/kg H_2O), >320 mOsm/kg H_2O (SI: >320 mmol/kg H_2O). Result of 385 mOsm/kg H_2O (SI: 385 mmol/kg H_2O) may reflect stupor in hyperglycemia. Values 400-420 mOsm/kg H_2O (SI: 400-420 mmol/kg H_2O) may reflect grand mal seizures. Values >420 mOsm/kg H_2O (SI: >420 mmol/kg H_2O) may be lethal.

Use Serum osmolality is used to evaluate electrolyte and water balance, hyperosmolar status, hydration/dehydration status, acid-base balance, seizures, antidiuretic hormone function, liver disease, and hyperosmolar coma. Osmolality is proportional to the concentration of particles in solution.

Freezing point depression serum osmolality with calculated osmolal gap is useful in screening for and approximating the serum concentrations of certain low molecular weight toxins, such as ethanol, ethylene glycol, isopropanol, and methanol,[3,4] especially as a rapid approximation for emergent situations. See Limitations.

High serum osmolality may result from hypernatremia, dehydration, hypovolemia, hyperglycemia, mannitol therapy, azotemia, and ingestion of ethanol, methanol, or ethylene glycol. Thus, osmolality has a role in toxicology and in coma evaluation. Very low birth weight infants may have elevated serum osmolality for the first week of life.[5]

Low serum osmolality may be secondary to overhydration, hyponatremia, and the syndrome of inappropriate antidiuretic hormone secretion (SIADH).

Serum osmolality measurements do not measure the fraction of serum that is water. Osmolality measurement by freezing point depression is also indifferent to permeability of solutes to cell membranes.[6]

Limitations When vapor pressure osmometry is used, volatile solutes (eg, alcohols and glycols) may remain in the vapor phase and not be detected.[3]

Methodology Freezing point depression (more often used) or vapor pressure elevation

Additional Information Measured osmolality usually exceeds the calculated osmolality. If measured osmolality is >15 mOsm/kg H_2O (SI: >15 mmol/kg H_2O) greater than calculated, the differential diagnosis includes: methanol, ethylene glycol, ethanol, or other toxicity; shock and trauma. Elevated serum osmolality with normal sodium suggests hyperglycemia, uremia, or alcoholism.[7] Both serum and urine values and calculated osmolality (see Osmolality, Calculated, Serum or Plasma *on page 234*) are sometimes required for accurate diagnosis. Although lactic acidosis theoretically should not contribute to the osmolal gap, increases in the osmolal gap in lactic acidosis have been reported.[8] Drugs including thiazide diuretics, steroids, cimetidine, and others have been implicated in the development of hyperosmolar hyperglycemic nonketotic coma.[9] Elevations of endogenous glycerol, acetone, and acetone metabolite levels are reported to cause an increased osmolal gap in alcoholics.[10] Slight elevation of serum osmolality over expected values have been reported in the elderly.[11,12]

After overnight dehydration, **urine:serum osmolality ratio** is usually ≥3.[7] Even with fluid restriction, the ratio is 0.2-0.7 in diabetes insipidus. It is usually normal in neurogenic polyuria without fluid restriction and is increased with fluid restriction.[2]

The expression "urinary:plasma ratio" is also used. See Osmolality, Urine *on page 236*. Laboratory criteria for hypovolemia include elevation of urea nitrogen:creatinine ratio >25 and/or increased serum osmolality and sodium concentration.[13] Serum sodium and osmolality increase in dehydration; the **serum sodium:serum osmolality ratio** remains within normal limits.

Footnotes

1. Osterloh JD, Kelly TJ, Khayam-Bashi H, et al, "Discrepancies in Osmolal Gaps and Calculated Alcohol Concentration," *Arch Pathol Lab Med*, 1996, 120(7):637-41.
2. Newman DJ and Price CP, "Renal Function and Nitrogen Metabolites," *Tietz Textbook of Clinical Chemistry*, 3rd ed, Chapter 35, Burtis CA and Ashwood ER, eds, Philadelphia, PA: WB Saunders Co, 1999, 1204-70.
3. Eisen TF, Lacouture PG, and Woolf A, "Serum Osmolality in Alcohol Ingestions: Differences in Availability Among Laboratories of Teaching Hospital, Nonteaching Hospital, and Commercial Facilities," *Am J Emerg Med*, 1989, 7(3):256-9.
4. DuFour DR, "Laboratory Recognition and Testing in Acid-Base Disorders," *Lab Med*, 1999, 30(12):776-82.
5. Giacoia GP, Miranda R, and West KI, "Measured vs Calculated Plasma Osmolality in Infants With Very Low Birth Weights," *Am J Dis Child*, 1992, 146(6):712-7.
6. Gennari FJ, "Current Concepts, Serum Osmolality, Uses and Limitations," *N Engl J Med*, 1984, 310(2):102-5.
7. Weisberg HF, "Unraveling the Laboratory Model of a Syndrome: The Osmolality Model," *Clinician and Chemist. The Relationship of the Laboratory to the Physician*, Young DS, Hicks J, Nipper H, et al, eds, Washington, DC: AACC Press, American Association of Clinical Chemistry, 1979, 200-43.
8. Schelling JR, Howard RL, Winter SD, et al, "Increased Osmolal Gap in Alcoholic Ketoacidosis and Lactic Acidosis," *Ann Intern Med*, 1990, 113(8):580-2.
9. Pope DW and Dansky D, "Hyperosmolar Hyperglycemic Nonketotic Coma," *Emerg Med Clin North Am*, 1989, 7(4):849-57.
10. Braden GL, Strayhorn CH, Germain MJ, et al, "Increased Osmolal Gap in Alcoholic Acidosis," *Arch Intern Med*, 1993, 153(20):2377-80.
11. McLean KA, O'Neill PA, Davies I, et al, "Influence of Age on Plasma Osmolality: A Community Study," *Age Ageing*, 1992, 21(1):56-60.
12. O'Neill PA, Faragher EB, Davies I, et al, "Reduced Survival With Increasing Plasma Osmolality in Elderly Continuing-Care Patients," *Age Ageing*, 1990, 19(1):68-71.
13. McGee S, Abernethy WB 3rd, and Simel DL, "Is This Patient Hypovolemic?" *JAMA*, 1999, 281(11):1022.

References

Aabakken L, Johansen KS, Rydningen EB, et al, "Osmolal and Anion Gaps in Patients Admitted to an Emergency Medical Department," *Hum Exp Toxicol*, 1994, 13(2):131-4.

Baker RJ, "Biochemical Gaps: Osmolal and Anion," *Curr Surg*, 1987, 44(5):378-81.

Demedts P, Theunis L, Wauters A, et al, "Excess Serum Osmolality Gap After Ingestion of Methanol: A Methodology-Associated Phenomenon?" *Clin Chem*, 1994, 40(8):1587-90.

Fraser CL and Arieff AI, "Fatal Central Diabetes Mellitus and Insipidus Resulting From Untreated Hyponatremia: A New Syndrome," *Ann Intern Med*, 1990, 112(2):113-9.

Galvan LA and Watts MT, "Generation of an Osmolality Gap-Ethanol Nomogram From Routine Laboratory Data," *Ann Emerg Med*, 1992, 21(11):1343-8.

Maffly RH, "Renal Function and Disorders of Water, Sodium, and Potassium Balance," *Scientific American Medicine*, Section 10, Chapter 1, Rubenstein E and Federman DD, eds, New York, NY: Scientific American Inc, 1990, 2-34.

Roberts WL and Paulson WD, "Method-Specific Reference Intervals for Serum Anion Gap and Osmolality," *Clin Chem*, 1998, 44(7):1582.

Snyder H, Williams D, Zink B, et al, "Accuracy of Blood Ethanol Determination Using Serum Osmolality," *J Emerg Med*, 1992, 10(2):129-33.

Sweeny TE and Beuchat CA, "Limitations of Methods of Osmometry: Measuring the Osmolality of Biological Fluids," *Am J Physiol*, 1993, 264(3 Pt 2):R469-80.

Worthley LI, Guerin M, and Pain RW, "For Calculating Osmolality, the Simplest Formula Is the Best," *Anaesth Intensive Care*, 1987, 15(2):199-202.

♦ **Osmolality:Serum Ratio** *see* Osmolality, Serum *on page 236*

Osmolality, Urine

Related Information

Antidiuretic Hormone, Plasma *on page 107*
Osmolality, Calculated, Serum or Plasma *on page 234*
Osmolality, Serum *on page 236*
Sodium, Serum or Plasma *on page 275*
Specific Gravity, Urine *on page 886*

Synonyms Urine Osmolality

Applies to Osmolal Gap, Urine; U:P Ratio; Urine Osmolar Gap; Urine:Serum Osmolality Ratio

Abstract Osmolality is a definitive measure of urine concentration.

Specimen Random or timed urine (1 mL minimum)

Storage Instructions Refrigerate

Reference Interval Random urine: neonates: 75-300 mOsm/kg H_2O (SI: 75-300 mmol/kg H_2O); children and adults: 250-900 mOsm/kg H_2O (SI: 250-900 mmol/kg H_2O). Normal range of serum sodium (mmol/L) to osmolality (mOsm/kg) ratio is 0.43-0.50.[1] Patients with normal renal function after 14-hour restriction of fluids should be able to concentrate to >800 mOsm/kg H_2O (SI: >800 mmol/kg H_2O).

Critical Values <400 mOsm/kg H_2O (SI: <400 mmol/kg H_2O) is interpreted by Weisberg as severe renal impairment.[2] Prolonged dehydration may be dangerous for some patients.

Possible Panic Range <100 mOsm/kg H_2O (SI: <100 mmol/kg H_2O) in overhydration, >800 mOsm/kg H_2O (SI: >800 mmol/kg H_2O) in dehydration

Use Urine osmolality is use to evaluate the concentrating ability of the kidneys (eg, in acute and chronic renal failure), electrolyte and water balance, renal disease, syndrome of inappropriate antidiuretic hormone secretion (SIADH), diabetes insipidus, dehydration, and amyloidosis. It is sometimes used in addition to urinalysis when the patient has been administered radiopaque substances or has glycosuria or proteinuria.[2] Estimation of urinary ammonium concentration and detection of increased osmolarity due to unusual molecules are possible using the urine osmolal gap.[3] Osmolality is desirable in examination of neonatal urine when protein or glucose are present.[4]

Limitations Serum osmolality is often needed to interpret urine osmolality.

Methodology Freezing point depression

Additional Information Osmolality is a better measurement of urine concentration than specific gravity and is a measure of renal tubular concentration, depending on the state of hydration. Simultaneous determination of urine and serum osmolalities facilitates interpretation of results. High **urinary:plasma ratio** (U:P) is seen in concentrated urine. Normal ranges for the U:P ratio are given by Dr Weisberg as approximately 0.2-4.7, and >3.0 with overnight dehydration.[2] With poor concentrating ability the ratio is low but still ≥1.0. In SIADH urine sodium and urine osmolality are high for plasma osmolality.[5] The ability of the kidney to produce a concentrated urine decreases with age.[6] (The expression urine:serum osmolality ratio is also used, see Osmolality, Serum *on page 236*.)

Specifically derived regression equations are advocated in neonates to predict urine osmolality from specific gravity measurements.[4] Low birthweight infants have been reported to have increased serum osmolality with normal urine osmolality.[7]

The urine osmolal gap is described as the sum of urinary concentrations of sodium, potassium, bicarbonate, chloride, glucose, and urea compared to measured urine osmolality. The gap is normally 80-100 mOsm/kg H_2O (SI: 80-100 mmol/kg H_2O) greater for measured than for calculated. Determination of the urine osmolal gap is used to characterize metabolic acidosis. High urine osmolal gap can be used semiquantitatively.[8]

Footnotes

1. Pincus MR, Preuss HG, and Henry JB, "Evaluation of Renal Function, Water, Electrolytes, Acid-Base Balance, and Blood Gases" *Clinical Diagnosis and Management by Laboratory Methods*, 19th ed, Henry JB, ed, Philadelphia, PA: WB Saunders Co, 1996, 139-61.
2. Weisberg HF, "Unraveling the Laboratory Model of a Syndrome: The Osmolality Model," *Clinician and Chemist. The Relationship of the Laboratory to the Physician*, Young DS, Hicks J, Nipper H, et al, eds, Washington, DC: AACC Press, American Association of Clinical Chemistry, 1979, 200-43.
3. Kamel KS, Ethier JH, Richardson RM, et al, "Urine Electrolytes and Osmolality: When and How to Use Them," *Am J Nephrol*, 1990, 10(2):89-102.
4. Leech S and Penney MD, "Correlation of Specific Gravity and Osmolality of Urine in Neonates and Adults," *Arch Dis Child*, 1987, 62(7):671-3.
5. Kovacs L and Robertson GL, "Syndrome of Inappropriate Antidiuretics," *Endocrinol Metab Clin North Am*, 1992, 21(4):859-75.
6. O'Neill PA and McLean KA, "Water Homeostasis and Aging," *Med Lab Sci*, 1992, 49:291-8.
7. Giacoia GP, Miranda R, and West KI, "Measured vs Calculated Plasma Osmolality in Infants With Very Low Birth Weights," *Am J Dis Child*, 1992, 146(6):712-7.
8. Halperin ML, Margolis BL, Robinson LA, et al, "The Urine Osmolal Gap: A Clue to Estimate Urine Ammonium in 'Hybrid' Types of Metabolic Acidosis," *Clin Invest Med*, 1988, 11(3):198-202.

References

Davis BB and Zenser TV, "Evaluation of Renal Concentrating and Diluting Ability," *Clin Lab Med*, 1993, 13(1):131-4.

Fraser CL and Arieff AI, "Fatal Central Diabetes Mellitus and Insipidus Resulting From Untreated Hyponatremia: A New Syndrome," *Ann Intern Med*, 1990, 112(2):113-9.

♦ **Osmolarity** *replaced by* Osmolality, Serum *on page 236*

Osteocalcin, Serum or Plasma

Related Information

Alkaline Phosphatase Isoenzymes, Serum *on page 92*
Alkaline Phosphatase, Serum *on page 93*
Aluminum, Bone and Bone Biopsy *on page 813*
Calcium, Serum *on page 131*

Calcium, Urine *on page 133*
Hydroxyproline, Total, Urine *on page 199*
N-Telopeptides, Urine *on page 233*
Osteocalcin (Undercarboxylated), Serum *on page 238*
Parathyroid Hormone, Serum *on page 243*
Pyridinolines (Pyridinoline and Deoxypyridinoline), Urine *on page 272*
Vitamin D, Serum *on page 300*

Synonyms BGP; Bone GLA Protein

Applies to Bone Formation; Bone Resorption; Collagen Cross-Link-Associated C-Telopeptide; Collagen Cross-Link-Associated N-Telopeptide; Deoxypyridinoline; DPD; ICTP; NTX; PYD; Pyridinoline

Abstract Osteocalcin (OC), the major noncollagen calcium-binding protein of bone matrix, is synthesized by osteoblasts and has a high affinity for hydroxyapatite. The serum concentration of OC is believed to be directly proportional to concurrent bone formation. OC synthesis is vitamin D dependent. The osteogenic activity of OC requires post-translational carboxylation, a process which is vitamin K dependent, and is biochemically analogous to the carboxylation of the vitamin K-dependent coagulation factors. OC serum levels are high during childhood, and peak levels occur in early puberty.[1] A second peak occurs in females at menopause.[2]

The important markers of bone formation include OC and bone-specific alkaline phosphatase (BAP). The markers of bone resorption are urinary hydroxyproline, urinary pyridinoline (PYD), urinary deoxypyridinoline (DPD), urinary collagen cross-link-associated N-telopeptide (NTX), and serum collagen cross-link-associated C-telopeptide (IGTP).[3] Urinary calcium lacks sensitivity and specificity for assessment of bone remodeling.

As bone is undergoing remodeling, use of a bone formation marker with a resorption marker may provide better information than use of a single test.[4]

Decrease in bone mass with microarchitectural deterioration of the skeleton, with bone fragility and propensity for fracture, is designated osteoporosis.[4]

Specimen Serum or plasma; because there are method-dependent decreases in immunoreactivity with some antibodies, collect on ice, and separate serum immediately. Keep frozen until ready to assay.

Container Red top tube

Sampling Time Circadian rhythm: peak in late afternoon-evening; nadir in early morning. A morning specimen is usually preferred.

Storage Instructions Proteolytic enzymes degrade OC. Separate from red cells quickly. Stable frozen.

Reference Interval Tentative guidelines are indicated as follows.[5] Interpretive caution is necessary since results are method-dependent.[6]

Male:
- 0-1 years: not established
- 2-10 years: 10-43 ng/mL
- 11-19 years: not established
- 20-50 years: 2-15 ng/mL
- 51-70 years: 2-10 ng/mL

Female:
- 0-1 years: not established
- 2-10 years: 10-43 ng/mL
- 11-19 years: not established
- 20-50 years: 2-15 ng/mL
- 51-80 years: 6-22 ng/mL

Use Results are **not** diagnostic of osteoporosis.[7] Results may be helpful in:
- **monitoring drug, exercise and/or hormone treatment of osteoporosis**; decreasing serum levels of osteocalcin are interpreted as evidence of a favorable response to treatment
- monitoring bone metabolic changes secondary to Cushing syndrome,[8,9] primary hyperparathyroidism,[10] malabsorption syndromes,[11] including inflammatory bowel disease[12] and plasma cell myeloma[13]
- monitoring bone metabolic changes occurring as a result of resistance exercise training[14]
- selecting the most appropriate treatment for patients with hypercalciuria[15]

Limitations Most assays measure total OC. Interpretation of total OC results is confounded when patients are on treatment with a vitamin K antagonist such as warfarin, or are consuming a diet deficient in vitamin K. In such situations, a significant fraction of the osteocalcin is undercarboxylated and, therefore lacks osteogenic functionality. These patients may have a normal or high total OC serum level which does not reflect osteogenic activity. One approach to resolve such interpretive ambiguity is to use an ELISA test with specificity for undercarboxylated osteocalcin;[16] an assay is not widely available at this time. (See Osteocalcin (Undercarboxylated), Serum *on page 238*.)

Bone marker assays must be used in concert with other biochemical tests, bone mineral densitometry, and imaging studies. Bone mineral densitometry is the gold standard for the evaluation of osteoporosis.

OC is reduced in lipemic serum. Assays lack standardization.

Bone remodeling is characterized by diurnal rhythm and is subject to phases of the menstrual cycle, seasons of the year, bedrest, exercise, diet, and variation over time. Day to day variation for bone formation markers is ~10%. Bone markers increase as much as 60% following fracture.

False-negative and false-positive results are estimated for bone markers in 20% to 30% of patients.[3]

(Continued)

Osteocalcin, Serum or Plasma (Continued)

Methodology Immunoassays (multiple labels), hydroxyapatite binding

Additional Information Results are higher in summer than winter (see References, Woitge et al). Much about the physiology of OC remains to be explored. Mice missing OC gene have denser and stronger bones than their normal littermates.[17]

Footnotes

1. Mora S, Pitukcheewanont P, Kaufman FR, et al, "Biochemical Markers of Bone Turnover and the Volume and the Density of Bone in Children at Different Stages of Sexual Development," *J Bone Miner Res*, 1999, 14(10):1664-71.

2. Peris P, Alvarez L, Monegal A, et al, "Biochemical Markers of Bone Turnover After Surgical Menopause and Hormone Replacement Therapy," *Bone*, 1999, 25(3):349-53.

3. Watts NB, "Clinical Utility of Biochemical Markers of Bone Remodeling," *Clin Chem*, 1999, 45(8B):1359-68.

4. Hurley DL and Khosla S, "Update on Primary Osteoporosis," *Mayo Clin Proc*, 1997, 72(10):943-9.

5. Leavelle DE, *Mayo Medical Laboratories Interpretive Handbook*, Rochester, MN: Mayo Medical Laboratories, 1997, 406-7.

6. Diaz Diego ED, Guerrero R, and de la Piedra C, "Six Osteocalcin Assays Compared," *Clin Chem*, 1994, 40(11):2071-7.

7. Finkelstein JS, "Osteoporosis," *Cecil Textbook of Medicine*, 21st ed, Goldman L and Bennett JC, eds, Philadelphia, PA: WB Saunders Co, 2000, 1368-70.

8. Sartorio A, Conti A, Ferraro S, et al, "Serum Bone G1a Protein and Carboxy-Terminal Cross-Linked Telopeptide of Type I Collagen in Patients With Cushing's Syndrome," *Postgrad Med J*, 1996, 72(849):419-22.

9. Sartorio A, Conti A, Ferrero S, et al, "Evaluation of Markers of Bone and Collagen Turnover in Patients With Active and Preclinical Cushing's Syndrome and in Patients With Adrenal Incidentaloma," *Eur J Endocrinol*, 1998, 138(2):146-52.

10. Thorsen K, Kristoffersson AO, and Lorentzon RP, "Changes in Bone Mass and Serum Markers of Bone Metabolism After Parathyroidectomy," *Surgery*, 1997, 122(5):882-7.

11. Pratico G, Caltabiano L, Bottaro G, et al, "Serum Levels of Osteocalcin and Type I Procollagen in Children With Celiac Disease," *J Pediatr Gastroenterol Nutr*, 1997, 24(2):170-3.

12. Bjarnason I, MacPherson A, Mackintosh C, et al, "Reduced Bone Density in Patients With Inflammatory Bowel Disease," *Gut*, 1997, 40(2):228-33.

13. Abildgaard N, Bentzen SM, Nielsen JL, et al, "Serum Markers of Bone Metabolism in Multiple Myeloma: Prognostic Value of the Carboxy-Terminal Telopeptide of Type I Collagen (ICTP). Nordic Myeloma Study Group (NMSG)," *Br J Haematol*, 1997, 96(1):103-10.

14. Fujimura R, Ashizawa N, Watanabe M, et al, "Effect of Resistance Exercise Training on Bone Formation and Resorption in Young Male Subjects Assessed by Biomarkers of Bone Metabolism," *J Bone Miner Res*, 1997, 12:656-62.

15. Strohmaier WL, Schlee-Giehl K, and Bichler KH, "Osteocalcin Response to Calcium-Restricted Diet: A Helpful Tool for the Workup of Hypercalciuria," *European Urology*, 1996, 103:103-7.

16. Vergnaud P, Garnero P, Meunier OJ, et al, "Undercarboxylated Osteocalcin Measured With a Specific Immunoassay Predicts Hip Fracture in Elderly Women: The EPIDOS Study," *J Clin Endocrinol Metab*, 1997, 82(3):719-24.

17. Ducy P, Desbois C, Boyce B, et al, "Increased Bone Formation in Osteocalcin-Deficient Mice," *Nature*, 1996, 382(6590):448-52.

References

Craciun AM, Vermeer C, Eisenwiener HG, et al, "Evaluation of a Bead-Based Enzyme Immunoassay for the Rapid Detection of Osteocalcin in Human Serum," *Clin Chem*, 2000, 46(2):252-7 (new method).

Eyre DR, "Bone Biomarkers as Tools in Osteoporosis Management," *Spine*, 1997, 22(24 Suppl):17S-24S.

Griesmacher A, Peichl P, Pointinger P, et al, "Biochemical Markers in Menopausal Women," *Scand J Clin Lab Invest Suppl*, 1997, 227:64-72.

Kakonen SM, Hellman J, Karp M, et al, "Development and Evaluation of Three Immunofluorometric Assays That Measure Different Forms of Osteocalcin in Serum," *Clin Chem*, 2000, 46(3):332-7 (biochemical heterogeneity).

Minisola S, Rosso R, Romagnoli E, et al, "Serum Osteocalcin and Bone Mineral Density at Various Skeletal Sites: A Study Performed With Three Different Assays," *Clin Lab Med*, 1997, 129(4):422-9.

Ravn P, Bidstrup M, Wasnich RD, et al, "Alendronate and Estrogen-Progestin in the Long-Term Prevention of Bone Loss: Four-Year Results From the Early Postmenopausal Intervention Cohort Study," *Ann Intern Med*, 1999, 131(12):935-42.

Urena P and De Vernejoul MC, "Circulating Biochemical Markers of Bone Remodeling in Uremic Patients," *Kidney Int*, 1999, 55(6):2141-56.

Woitge HW, Scheidt-Nave C, Kissling C, et al, "Seasonal Variation of Biochemical Indexes of Bone Turnover: Results of a Population-Based Study," *J Clin Endocrinol Metab*, 1998, 83(1):68-75.

Osteocalcin (Undercarboxylated), Serum

Related Information

Alkaline Phosphatase Isoenzymes, Serum *on page 92*
Alkaline Phosphatase, Serum *on page 93*
Aluminum, Bone and Bone Biopsy *on page 813*
Calcium, Serum *on page 131*
Calcium, Urine *on page 133*
Hydroxyproline, Total, Urine *on page 199*
N-Telopeptides, Urine *on page 233*
Osteocalcin, Serum or Plasma *on page 237*
Parathyroid Hormone, Serum *on page 243*
Prothrombin Time *on page 354*
Pyridinolines (Pyridinoline and Deoxypyridinoline), Urine *on page 272*
Vitamin D, Serum *on page 300*

Abstract Osteocalcin (OC) is a bone-specific protein, which is dependent on both vitamin D and vitamin K (see Osteocalcin, Serum or Plasma *on page 237*). Under ordinary circumstances, total serum OC is assumed to be a reflection of concurrent bone formation. However, this assumption does not hold for persons taking a vitamin K antagonist (warfarin) or persons consuming a diet deficient in vitamin K. Total serum OC in such individuals will contain a substantial proportion of undercarboxylated OC (uOC), a peptide which lacks osteoblastic functionality.

Specimen Serum; because there are method-dependent decreases in immunoreactivity with some antibodies, collect on ice, and separate serum immediately. Keep frozen until ready to assay.

Container Red top tube

Sampling Time Circadian rhythm: peak in late afternoon-evening; nadir in early morning. A morning specimen is usually preferred.

Reference Interval Interpretive caution is essential, since methods are only now being validated. One source,[1] using an in-house enzyme-linked immunoassay (ELISA) method and a hydroxyapatite-binding (HAP) method, report following from a study of elderly French women:

ELISA: uOC: 5.8 (±4.1) ng/mL (±1 SD)
HAP: uOC: 4.4 (±3.3) ng/mL (±1 SD)

Be certain to verify the reference range of the laboratory doing the analysis.

Use Results are **not** diagnostic of osteoporosis.

Clinical investigators have studied the role of uOC in prediction of the risk of femoral fracture in elderly persons.[1,2,3] In these evaluations, the serum uOC in considered together with bone mineral density in arriving at a predictive metric.

Another potential application for serum uOC is in the evaluation of vitamin K nutritional status. Sokoll et al[4] have reported that serum uOC is much more sensitive than the prothrombin time in detecting subtle vitamin K deficiency. Other sensitive markers of dietary vitamin K deficiency were plasma phylloquinone and urinary gamma-carboxylgutamic acid.

Limitations Bone marker assays must be used in concert with bone mineral densitometry, other biochemical markers, and various imaging studies. Bone mineral densitometry is the gold standard for the diagnosis of osteoporosis.

Methodology immunoassays (various labels), hydroxyapatite binding

Footnotes

1. Vergnaud P, Garnero PJ, Meunier PJ, et al, "Undercarboxylated Osteocalcin Measured With a Specific Immunoassay Predicts Hip Fracture in Elderly Women: The EPIDOS Study," *J Clin Endocrinol Metab*, 1997, 82(3):719-24.

2. Seibel MJ, Robins SP, and Bilezikian JP, "Serum Undercarboxylated Osteocalcin and the Risk of Hip Fracture," *J Clin Endocrinol Metab*, 1997, 82(3):7171-8.

3. Szulc P, Chapuy MC, Meunier PJ, et al, "Serum Undercarboxylated Osteocalcin Is a Marker of the Risk of Hip Fracture: A Three Year Follow-up Study," *Bone*, 1996, 18(50):487-8.

4. Sokoll LJ, Booth SL, O'Brien ME, et al, "Changes in Serum Osteocalcin, Plasma Phylloquinone, and Urinary Gamma-Carboxyglutamic Acid in Response to Altered Intakes of Dietary Phylloquinone in Human Subjects," *Am J Clin Nutr*, 1997, 65(3):779-84.

♦ **Ovarian Cancer Activating Factor** *see* Lysophosphatidic Acid, Plasma *on page 220*

Oxalate, Urine

Related Information

Ascorbic Acid, Serum or Plasma *on page 112*
Citrate, Plasma, Serum, or Urine *on page 149*
Ethylene Glycol, Serum or Plasma *on page 790*
Kidney Stone Analysis *on page 877*
Magnesium, Serum *on page 221*
Magnesium, Urine *on page 222*
Urinalysis *on page 887*
Urine Collection, 24-Hour *on page 47*

Synonyms Calcium Oxalate, Urine; Urine Oxalate

Applies to Glycolic Acid, Urine; Glyoxylic Acid, Urine; L-Glyceric Acid, Urine; Vitamin C

Abstract Calcium oxalate stones are common in the urinary tract. Oxalate excretion is a predictor of oxalate nephrolithiasis; hyperoxaluria can be detected in up to 33% of patients with calcium oxalate stones.[1]

Patient Preparation Avoid vitamin C for 24 hours before collection. Pyridoxine is said to diminish oxaluria. The patient should be ambulatory, preferably at home, on usual fluid and food intake, to best interpret risk factors for nephrolithiasis.

Specimen 24-hour urine; first morning urine may give oxalate concentrations similar to 24-hour collections.[2] Total amount of oxalate excreted might be estimated using first morning urinary oxalate concentration and an estimate of daily urine output. Oxalate can also be measured in plasma,[3] but such testing is not widely available at the present time.

Container Acid-washed plastic container with 20 mL of 6N HCl added prior to collection (depending upon laboratory). Acid prevents oxalate crystallization and conversion of ascorbate to oxalate. No metal cap.

Collection Urine creatinine is often determined. In children, second morning urine specimen can be used to determine oxalate/creatinine ratio. Between ages 0-6 years, the ratio is inversely related to age. The ratio plateaus at age 6 years.[4] See graphic.

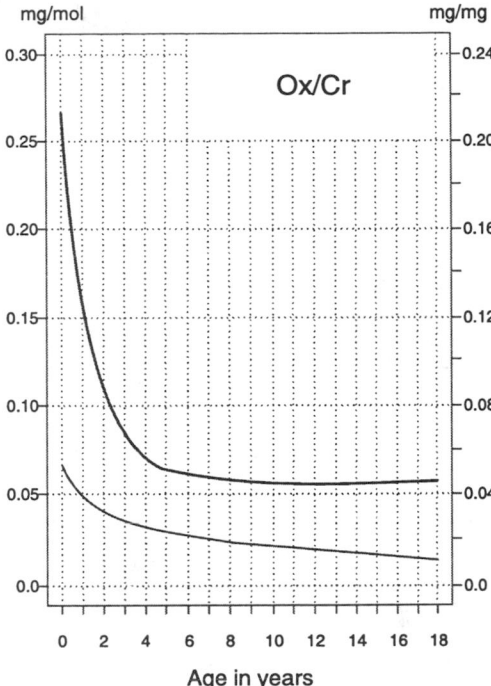

Estimated 95th and 5th percentiles for oxalate (Ox) to creatinine (Cr) ratios related to age.

Reference Interval 20-60 mg/24 hours (SI: 0.23-0.68 mmol/day)[5] in those whose diets include oxalate-rich foods; *vide infra*. Without excess of such foods, normal men excrete up to 45 mg (500 µmol) and women up to 40 mg (444 µmol).[6] Greater excretion of oxalic acid in men is recognized in healthy subjects as well as in stone formers. The differences were unexplained on the basis of body surface. A relationship with age was not found.[7]

Use Calcium oxalate renal stones are common. Patients who form calcium oxalate kidney stones appear to absorb and excrete a higher fraction of dietary oxalate in urine than do normals. Hyperoxaluria is not uncommon in subjects with malabsorption, including fat malabsorption. Twenty-four hour urine collections for oxalate are indicated in patients with surgical loss of distal small intestine, especially those with Crohn disease. The incidence of nephrolithiasis in patients who have inflammatory bowel disease is 2.6% to 10%.[8]

Oxaluria is characteristic of ethylene glycol intoxication.

Hyperoxaluria is regularly present after jejunoileal bypass for morbid obesity; such patients may develop nephrolithiasis and oxalate nephrosis.[9]

Limitations Interference by ascorbate is a major impediment in developing a simple assay. Urine specimens containing significant amounts of ascorbic acid (10-325 µg/dL) experience interference in two forms. First, ascorbic acid is converted nonenzymatically to oxalate at alkaline pH or if urine is not acidified after bicarbonate administration.[10] Second, ascorbate inhibits oxalate oxidase (enzymatic method) and markedly decreases recovery of oxalates.[11,12] Methods to eliminate ascorbate meet with varied success depending upon the urine ascorbate concentration.[12]

Methodology Colorimetry following anion exchange resin; atomic absorption (AA) after precipitation with calcium; enzymatic, oxalate oxidase; high performance liquid chromatography (HPLC). Methods for routine clinical urinary oxalate have been reported.[13,14]

Additional Information Oxalic acid excretion is increased with methoxyflurane.

Hyperoxaluria may occur with high intake of gelatin, strawberries, pepper, rhubarb, beans, beets, spinach, tomatoes, chocolate, cocoa, tea, pecans, peanuts, okra, and lime peel.[6,15] Hyperoxaluria is described with pyridoxine deficiency. Urinary oxalate derives from the metabolism of glycine and ascorbic acid more than from dietary ingestion. Oxalate excretion was increased in vegetarians, despite low animal protein ingestion.[16] Calcium taken orally with oxalate loads decreases urinary oxalate excretion in patients with ileal disease. Calcium supplements taken with meals are less likely to lead to nephrolithiasis.[17]

Vitamin C increases oxalate excretion and may be a risk factor for calcium oxalate nephrolithiasis in individuals consuming "megadose" vitamin C. Such ingestion can usually be determined by history. If a vitamin C using stone former is found to have high urine oxalate excretion, the habit should be stopped. If oxalate excretion drops to normal, additional therapy to prevent stones may not be required.

Hyperoxaluria can result from intestinal hyperabsorption related to low calcium intake or high calcium enteric binding to compounds such as phytates. Conversely, increased dietary calcium may reduce the absorption of oxalate in patients with recurrent oxalate kidney stones.[15] Unabsorbed fat can bind calcium. Increased urinary uric acid excretion is frequently found in subjects who have calcium oxalate nephrolithiasis. Calcium nephrolithiasis in patients with hyperuricosuria has been related to urate-induced crystallization of calcium oxalate.[18] Urinary oxalate concentrations have been found to be increased in very low birth weight infants receiving parenteral amino acid solutions.[19]

Rare genetic disorders which increase endogenous oxalate production; there are two types of primary hyperoxaluria. They are characterized by elevated urinary oxalate excretion and recurrent oxalate nephrocalcinosis. In type I, an autosomal recessive, a defect in glyoxalate metabolism is found, leading to increased oxalate synthesis.[20] Excessive quantities of urinary glyoxylic and glycolic acid excretion occur. Type II is rare; it is characterized by excessive urinary excretion of oxalic and L-glyceric acids with normal excretion of glycolic acid.[21] type I causes renal failure and systemic oxalosis, but type II rarely does so.[22] Urinary oxalate excretion in both forms is >135-270 mg (SI: >1523-3000 µmol) daily.[6]

Glycine irrigation during transurethral prostatic resections does not raise the urinary oxalate level during the postoperative period. This suggests that post-transurethral forced diuresis may not be indicated solely for bladder irrigation with glycine.[23]

The importance of magnesium supplements to prevent calcium oxalate nephrolithiasis in subjects with gastrointestinal disease has been recently addressed.[24] See Magnesium, Serum *on page 221* and Magnesium, Urine *on page 222.*

Footnotes

1. Hesse A, Schneeberger W, Engfeld S, et al, "Intestinal Hyperabsorption of Oxalate in Calcium Oxalate Stone Formers: Application of a New Test With [13C2]Oxlate," J Am Soc Nephrol, 1999, 10(Suppl 14):S329-33.
2. Balchin ZEC, Moss PA, and Fraser CG, "Biological Variation of Urinary Oxalate in Different Specimens Types," Ann Clin Biochem, 1991, 28(Pt 6):622-3.
3. Hoppe B, Kemper MJ, Hvizd MG, et al, "Simultaneous Determination of Oxalate, Citrate and Sulfate in Children's Plasma With Ion Chromatography," Kidney Int, 1998, 53(5):1348-52.
4. Matos V, Van Melle G, Werner D, et al, "Urinary Oxalate and Urate to Creatinine Ratios in Healthy Pediatric Population," Am J Kidney Dis, 1999, 34(2):6E.
5. Wilson DM and Liedtke RR, "Modified Enzyme-Based Colorimetric Assay of Urinary and Plasma Oxalate With Improved Sensitivity and No Ascorbate Interference: Reference Values and Sample Handling Procedures," Clin Chem, 1991, 37(7):1229-35.
6. Hruska K, "Renal Calculi (Nephrolithiases)," Cecil Textbook of Medicine, 21st ed, Chapter 114, Goldman L and Bennett JC, eds, Philadelphia, PA: WB Saunders Co, 2000, 622-7.
7. Hesse A, Klocke K, Classen A, et al, "Age and Sex as Factors in Oxalic Acid Excretion in Healthy Persons and Calcium Oxalate Stone Patients," Contrib Nephrol, 1987, 58:16-20.
8. Earnest DL, "Enteric Hyperoxaluria," Adv Intern Med, 1979, 24:407-27.
9. Hicks K, Evans GB, Rogerson ME, et al, "Jejuno-Ileal Bypass, Enteric Hyperoxaluria, and Oxalate Nephrosis: A Role for Polarised Light in the Renal Biopsy," J Clin Pathol, 1998, 51(9):700-2.
10. Lemann J Jr, Hornick LJ, Pleuss JA, et al, "Oxalate Is Overestimated in Alkaline Urines Collected During Administration of Bicarbonate With No Specimen pH Adjustment," Clin Chem, 1989, 35(10):2107-10.
11. Li MG and Madappally MM, "Rapid Enzymatic Determination of Urinary Oxalate," Clin Chem, 1989, 35(12):2330-3.
12. Inamdar KV, Raghavan KG, and Pradhan DS, "Five Treatment Procedures Evaluated for the Elimination of Ascorbate Interference in the Enzymatic Determination of Urinary Oxalate," Clin Chem, 1991, 37(6):864-8.
13. Mazzuchin A, Michelutti L, and Falter H, "Modifications to Commercial Oxalate Oxidase Based Determination of Urinary Oxalate: A Method Suitable for Routine Clinical Analysis," Clin Biochem, 1990, 23(2):173-7.
14. Sriboonlue P, Suwantrai S, and Prasongwatana V, "An Indirect Method for Urinary Oxalate Estimation," Clin Chim Acta, 1998, 273(1):59-68.
15. Massey LK, Roman-Smith H, and Sutton RA, "Effect of Dietary Oxalate and Calcium on Urinary Oxalate and Risk of Formation of Calcium Oxalate Kidney Stones," J Am Diet Assoc, 1993, 93(8):901-6.
16. Marangella M, Bianco I, Martini C, et al, "Effect of Animal and Vegetable Protein Intake on Oxalate Excretion in Idiopathic Calcium Stone Disease," Br J Urol, 1989, 63(4):348-51.
17. Curhan GC, Willett WC, Rimm EB, et al, "A Prospective Study of Dietary Calcium and Other Nutrients and the Risk of Symptomatic Kidney Stones," N Engl J Med, 1993, 328(12):833-8.
18. Pak CY and Peterson R, "Successful Treatment of Hyperuricosuric Calcium Oxalate Nephrolithiasis With Potassium Citrate," Arch Intern Med, 1986, 146(5):863-7.
19. Campfield T and Braden G, "Urinary Oxalate Excretion by Very Low Birth Weight Infants Receiving Parenteral Nutrition," Pediatrics, 1989, 84(5):860-3.
20. Bastani B and Nahass G, Images in Clinical Medicine, "Type I Primary Hyperoxaluria," N Engl J Med, 1999, 341(26):1979.
21. Yendt ER and Cohanim M, "Response to Physiologic Dose of Pyridoxine in Type 1 Primary Hyperoxaluria," N Engl J Med, 1985, 312(15):953-7.
22. Marangella M, Petrarulo M, Cosseddu D, et al, "End-Stage Renal Failure in Primary Hyperoxaluria Type 2," N Engl J Med, 1994, 330(23):1690.
23. Hahn RG, "Glycine Irrigation and Urinary Oxalate Excretion," Br J Urol, 1989, 64(3):287-9.
24. Fleming CR, George L, Stoner GL, et al, "The Importance of Urinary Magnesium Values in Patients With Gut Failure," Mayo Clin Proc, 1996, 71(1):21-4.

(Continued)

Oxalate, Urine (Continued)

References

Allen LC, Kadijevic L, and Romaschin AD, "An Enzymatic Method for Oxalate Automated With the Cobas Fara Centrifugal Analyzer," *Clin Chem*, 1989, 35(10):2098-100.

Barratt TM, Kasidas GP, Murdoch I, et al, "Urinary Oxalate and Glycolate Excretion and Plasma Oxalate Concentration," *Arch Dis Child*, 1991, 66(4):501-3.

Cowley DM, McWhinney BC, Brown JM, et al, "Effect of Citrate on the Urinary Excretion of Calcium and Oxalate: Relevance to Calcium Oxalate Nephrolithiasis," *Clin Chem*, 1989, 35(1):23-8.

Goldfarb S, "Diet and Nephrolithiasis," *Annu Rev Med*, 1994, 45:235-43.

Holmes RP and Assimos DG, "Glyoxylate Synthesis, and its Modulation and Influence on Oxalate Synthesis," *J Urol*, 1998, 160(5):1617-24.

Levine M, Rumsey SC, Daruwala R, et al, "Criteria and Recommendations for Vitamin C Intake," *JAMA*, 1999, 281(15):1415-23.

Messa P, Marangella M, Paganin L, et al, "Different Dietary Calcium Intake and Relative Supersaturation of Calcium Oxalate in the Urine of Patients Forming Renal Stones," *Clin Sci*, 1997, 93(3):257-63.

Milliner DS, Eickholt JT, Bergstralh EJ, et al, "Results of Long-Term Treatment With Orthophosphate and Pyridoxine in Patients With Primary Hyperoxaluria," *N Engl J Med*, 1994, 331(23):1553-8.

Petrarulo M, Marangella M, Bianco O, et al, "Preventing Ascorbate Interference in Ion-Chromatographic Determinations of Urinary Oxalate: Four Methods Compared," *Clin Chem*, 1990, 36(9):1642-5.

Ruml LA, Pearle MS, and Pak CY, "Medical Therapy, Calcium Oxalate Urolithiasis," *Urol Clin North Am*, 1997, 24(1):117-33.

Sharma S, Nath R, and Thind SK, "Recent Advances in Measurement of Oxalate in Biological Materials," *Scanning Microsc*, 1993, 7(1):431-41.

♦ **Oximeters, Pulse** see Carbon Dioxide, Total, Blood on page 135

♦ **Oximetry, Pulse** see Oxygen Saturation, Blood on page 240

♦ **Oxygen-Hemoglobin Dissociation Curve (ODC)** see Oxygen Saturation, Blood on page 240

♦ **Oxygen-Hemoglobin Dissociation Curve (ODC)** see P₅₀, Blood on page 241

♦ **Oxygen Radical Absorbance Capacity** see Antioxidant Concentrations, Plasma on page 108

♦ **Oxygen Saturation** see Blood Gases and pH, Arterial on page 119

Oxygen Saturation, Blood

Related Information

Arterial Blood Collection on page 40
Blood Gases and pH, Arterial on page 119
P₅₀, Blood on page 241
pH, Blood on page 247
Point-of-Care Testing on page 43
Red Blood Cells on page 857
Uncrossmatched Blood, Emergency on page 865
Whole Blood on page 866

Synonyms SaO₂; SO₂; sO₂

Applies to 2,3-Diphosphoglycerate (2,3-DPG); 2,3-DPG; Fractional Oxyhemoglobin (FO_2Hb); O₂ Binding Capacity (BO_2); O₂ Content (ctO_2); Oximetry, Pulse; Oxygen-Hemoglobin Dissociation Curve (ODC); Pulse Oximetry, Transcutaneous

Test Includes A complete O₂ status evaluation includes concentration of total hemoglobin ($ctHb$), hematocrit (Hct), O₂ content (ctO_2), O₂ binding capacity (BO_2), partial pressure of O₂ or O₂ tension (pO_2), partial pressure of O₂ at which SO₂ is 50% (p50), SO₂, fractional oxyhemoglobin (FO_2Hb), fractional carboxyhemoglobin ($FCOHb$), fractional methemoglobin ($FMetHb$), and fractional deoxyhemoglobin ($FHHb$). pH and pCO₂ are often included. Electrolytes and other analytes are relevant.

Abstract Hemoglobin oxygen saturation (SO₂) is the percentage or fraction of functional hemoglobin (ie, hemoglobin able to bind oxygen) that is oxygenated. It is determined by the following equation:

$$SO_2\ (\%) = [cO_2Hb\ /\ (cO_2Hb + cHHb)] \times 100$$

where cO_2Hb is the concentration of oxyhemoglobin and $cHHb$ is the concentration of deoxyhemoglobin.

Specimen Whole blood, arterial

Container Heparinized syringe, capillary tubes, or green top (heparin) tube

Collection Draw specimen anaerobically into heparinized syringe, avoid air bubbles, and stopper tightly. Place heparinized specimen on ice. Take to the laboratory immediately.

Causes for Rejection Specimens received with clots or air bubbles in the syringe, specimens not on ice, specimens not tightly stoppered

Special Instructions If capillary tubes are used to collect the specimen, warm skin 10-15 minutes prior to puncture to obtain free flow of blood with a sufficiently deep puncture ("arterialized capillary blood"). Fill heparinized capillary tubes completely full, cap the tubes, and mix well.

Reference Interval Newborns: 85% to 90% (SI: 0.85-0.90); thereafter: 95% to 99% (SI: 0.95-0.99)

Possible Panic Range Arterial pO₂ of 20 mm Hg and SO₂ of 35% (SI: 0.35) are critically low, life-endangering levels; the same values from mixed venous blood indicate tissue hypoxia. Arterial pO₂ of 40 mm Hg and SO₂ of 75% (SI: 0.75) are panic values that correlate with cyanosis, but these values are normal for mixed venous blood.

Use SO₂ (together with pO₂, $FHbO_2$, ctO_2, $FMetHb$, and $FCOHb$) is used to assess the extent of oxygenation of hemoglobin and adequacy of tissue oxygenation in the evaluation of hypoxia (due to lung and/or cardiac disease or dysfunction, cyanosis, or toxic exposure) and monitor respiratory function during mechanical ventilation.[1] It allows for the evaluation of oxygenation and oxyhemoglobin dissociation of blood with use of the oxygen dissociation curve (ODC).

Limitations Accuracy and precision may be affected by the presence of other pigments in the blood (eg, other heme derivatives, carotene, bilirubin, diagnostic dyes), low hemoglobin concentrations, plasma turbidity (eg, lipemia), and presence of cell fragments. Interpretation is more meaningful if the nature of patient's inspired gas is recorded (ie, room air or mixture of gases with a controlled oxygen content).

Though reference intervals are virtually identical, SO₂ **should not** be used interchangeably with fractional oxyhemoglobin (FO_2Hb) or estimated oxygen saturation (abbreviated by NCCLS[2] as "O₂Sat") as these can have substantially different values in critically ill patients or patients with abnormal hemoglobins. SO₂, by definition, is not affected by dyshemoglobinemia or hemoglobin variants, whereas FO_2Hb, which is the concentration of oxyhemoglobin (cO_2Hb) divided by the concentration of total hemoglobin ($ctHb$), is decreased under these circumstances. Consequently, the NCCLS[2] recommends that SO₂ results be reported together with FO_2Hb results or only after ruling out dyshemoglobinemia. Simple oximeters (eg, pulse oximeters, indwelling fiber optic oximeters) that use only two wavelengths of light measure only O₂Hb and HHb and report only a result for SO_2; these instruments are incapable of determining FO_2Hb or detecting the presence of dyshemoglobins and should be used with caution and preferably only after dyshemoglobinemia is ruled out.

Estimated oxygen saturation (O₂Sat) is calculated empirically from the results of pH, pO₂, and hemoglobin measurements. Errors result from the fact that the equations assume normal O₂ affinity for hemoglobin, normal erythrocyte 2,3-diphosphoglycerate (2,3-DPG) concentration, and absence of dyshemoglobinemia. Values obtained by these equations may vary significantly from SO₂ and should not be used in further calculations (eg, shunt fraction) or assumed to be equivalent to FO_2Hb.[2]

Contraindications Contraindications of arterial puncture

Methodology Spectrophotometric analysis of hemolysate is performed using oximetry instrumentation that directly measures the fractions of O₂Hb and HHb and, using the results of these measurements, automatically calculates the SO₂. At minimum, blood is analyzed at two wavelengths, one with a large difference in absorbance between oxygenated and deoxygenated hemoglobin, the other at the isobestic point (molar absorbance identical for the oxygenated and deoxygenated forms). Modern oximetry, however, employs multiple wavelengths for detection of not only these functional hemoglobins, but for detection of common, interfering dyshemoglobins (eg, carboxyhemoglobin, methemoglobin, sulfhemoglobin) as well. Transcutaneous pulse oximetry measures the absorption of different wavelengths of light passed through living tissue. See following discussion and footnotes.

Additional Information The terms, "O₂ content (ctO_2)," "O₂ binding capacity (BO_2)," and "SO₂", refer to various definitions of the amount of O₂ carried in the blood. ctO_2 is the **total** amount of O₂ present (bound to hemoglobin and dissolved in plasma) in the blood. BO_2 is the maximum amount of O₂ that can be carried by hemoglobin if **all** the hemoglobin capable of binding O₂ were oxygenated. SO₂ is defined in the Abstract (see above).

The binding of O₂ by hemoglobin is dependent upon (primarily) pH (and thereby CO₂ parameters that contribute to the control of pH), temperature, the concentration of 2,3-DPG, and the molecular species of hemoglobin. When graphed, the relationship results in a sigmoid (S-shaped) O₂-hemoglobin dissociation curve (ODC). The SO₂ (in %) is represented on the Y axis, the pO₂ (in mm Hg) on the X axis with the curve shifted to the right or left (isobars) by changes in pH or other parameters. This is a biochemically fixed relation such that if any two of the three determinants, pH, pO₂, or SO₂ are known, the other may roughly be predicted. With the ODC in hand one can assess whether the three reported values are consistent with each other as defined by the ODC (assuming normal molecular species of hemoglobin, concentration of 2,3-DPG, and constant temperature).

Red cell 2,3-DPG concentration plays an important role in regulation of hemoglobin's affinity for O₂. 2,3-DPG binds to the beta chains of O₂Hb and results in displacement of O₂ by the following equation:[3]

$$Hb\ O_2 + 2,3\text{-}DPG = Hb\text{-}2,3\text{-}DPG + O_2$$

An increase in 2,3-DPG will cause a shift of the reaction to the right. Greater affinity of fetal hemoglobin (Hb F) for O₂ has been ascribed to the poor binding of 2,3-DPG by the gamma chains of Hb F. Increased erythrocyte 2,3-DPG concentrations decrease intracellular pH resulting in a further reduction in O₂ affinity. 2,3-DPG is increased with hypoxia.

Red cells of newborns contain ~80% Hb F. Hb F has a slightly higher O₂ affinity compared to hemoglobin A (normal adult hemoglobin) and binds 2,3-DPG less strongly than hemoglobin A. Following birth, O₂ affinity decreases as red cell 2,3-DPG concentrations rise (20% during the first week of life). At 1-4 weeks, healthy prematures have p50 values approaching those of normal adults.[4]

Decreased SO_2 relates to impaired cardiorespiratory function at the macro-organ level of heart and/or lungs (due to a variety of diseases) or at the intracellular chemical respiratory level. The four mechanisms of abnormal gas exchange are hypoventilation, ventilation-perfusion disturbance, diffusion defect, and venous admixture. The hypoxemia accompanying right-to-left shunting in cardiac diseases (venous admixture) is preferentially evaluated with SO_2, which provides a more direct indication of the size of the shunt than pO_2.[5] Decreased central venous SO_2 was found to correlate better with estimated blood loss volumes in 26 trauma patients than vital signs including heart rate, blood pressure, central venous pressure, pulse pressure, and urine output. In this series of trauma patients, all had normal vital signs upon admission and a significant percentage of these patients had serious injuries and ongoing blood loss that required immediate attention.[6]

Arterial oxygen desaturation occurs after sedation for peritoneoscopy with resultant hypoxemia, hypercarbia, and acidosis.[7]

There is widespread use of **transcutaneous pulse oximetry** to determine SO_2, particularly in premature and in critically ill newborns and children. This noninvasive technique avoids the rigor and hazard of arterial puncture and necessity of subsequent proper sample handling, and provides continual monitoring. It is reliable and useful in monitoring adequacy of oxygenation, effectiveness of resuscitative efforts, detection of development of prolonged periods of decreased SO_2 in neonates, and monitoring preterm infant's response to physical therapy.[1,8,9,10,11,12] Pulse oximetry has also been applied to detection of hyperoxemia in newborns but has low specificity.[13] Limitations of pulse oximetry have included overestimation of SO_2 at values 65% and less,[11,14] and variation from in vitro determined SO_2 in samples with >50% Hb F as compared with samples having <25% Hb F.[10] A study of pulse oximeter determined SO_2 in pregnant patients and their newborns has found that SO_2 in neonates is commonly ≤90% within 10 minutes after birth and may not always be indicative of pathologic hypoxia.[15] Specialized devices (eg, balloon-tipped, thermodilution, fiberoptic, pulmonary arterial catheter) have been developed for the intraoperative monitoring of mixed venous oxygen saturation.[16]

Pulse oximetry may be unreliable as a measure of adequacy of ventilation.[17]

See P₅₀, Blood on page 241.

Footnotes

1. Shannon DC, "Rational Monitoring of Respiratory Function During Mechanical Ventilation of Infants and Children," *Intensive Care Med*, 1989, 15(Suppl 1):S13-6.
2. "National Committee for Clinical Laboratory Standards: Fractional Oxyhemoglobin, Oxygen Content and Saturation, and Related Quantities in Blood: Terminology, Measurement, and Reporting," Approved Guideline, C25-A, Wayne, PA: National Committee for Clinical Laboratory Standards, 1997.
3. Ganong WF, *Review of Medical Physiology*, 15th ed, Norwalk, CT: Appleton & Lange, 1991, 616-22.
4. Bunn HF and Forget BG, "Oxygen and Carbon Dioxide Transport," *Hemoglobin: Molecular, Genetic and Clinical Aspects*, Chapter 5, Philadelphia, PA: WB Saunders Co, 1986, 91-125.
5. Siggaard-Andersen O, "Hydrogen Ions and Blood Gases," *Chemical Diagnosis of Disease*, Brown SS, Mitchell FL, and Young DS, eds, New York, NY: Elsevier/North Holland Biomedical Press, 1979, 219-38.
6. Scalea TM, Hartnett RW, Duncan AO, et al, "Central Venous Oxygen Saturation: A Useful Clinical Tool in Trauma Patients," *J Trauma*, 1990, 30(12):1539-43.
7. Brady CE III, Harkleroad LE, and Pierson WP, "Alterations in Oxygen Saturation and Ventilation After Intravenous Sedation for Peritoneoscopy," *Arch Intern Med*, 1989, 149(5):1029-32.
8. Deckardt R, Schneider KT, and Graeff H, "Monitoring Arterial Oxygen Saturation in the Neonate," *J Perinat Med*, 1987, 15(4):357-60.
9. House JT, Schultetus RR, and Gravenstein N, "Continuous Neonatal Evaluation in the Delivery Room by Pulse Oximetry," *J Clin Monit*, 1987, 3(2):96-100.
10. Jennis MS and Peabody JL, "Pulse Oximetry: An Alternative Method for the Assessment of Oxygenation in Newborn Infants," *Pediatrics*, 1987, 79(4):524-8.
11. Lewallen PK, Mammel MC, Coleman JM, et al, "Neonatal Transcutaneous Arterial Oxygen Saturation Monitoring," *J Perinatol*, 1987, 7(1):8-10.
12. Kelly MK, Palisano RJ, and Wolfson MR, "Effects of a Developmental Physical Therapy Program on Oxygen Saturation and Heart Rate in Preterm Infants," *Phys Ther*, 1989, 69(6):467-74.
13. Bucher HU, Fanconi S, Baeckert P, et al, "Hyperoxemia in Newborn Infants: Detection by Pulse Oximetry," *Pediatrics*, 1989, 84(2):226-30.
14. Fanconi S, "Pulse Oximetry and Transcutaneous Oxygen Tension for Detection of Hypoxemia in Critically Ill Infants and Children," *Adv Exp Med Biol*, 1987, 220:159-64.
15. Porter KB, Goldhamer R, Mankad A, et al, "Evaluation of Arterial Oxygen Saturation in Pregnant Patients and Their Newborns," *Obstet Gynecol*, 1988, 71(3 Pt 1):354-7.
16. Thys DM, Cohen E, and Eisenkraft JB, "Mixed Venous Oxygen Saturation During Thoracic Anesthesia," *Anesthesiology*, 1988, 69(6):1005-9.
17. Ayas N, Bergstrom LR, Schwab TR, et al, "Unrecognized Severe Postoperative Hypercapnia: A Case of Apneic Oxygenation," *Mayo Clin Proc*, 1998, 73:51-4.

References

Grebstad JA, Svendsen L, and Gulsvik A, "Precision of Arterial Blood Gases and Cutaneous Oxygen Saturation in Healthy Nonsmokers," *Scand J Clin Lab Invest*, 1989, 49(3):265-8.
Hsia CCW, "Respiratory Function of Hemoglobin," *N Engl J Med*, 1998, 338(4):239-46.
Mendelson Y, "Pulse Oximetry: Theory and Applications for Noninvasive Monitoring," *Clin Chem*, 1992, 38(9):1601-7.

Scott MG, Heusel JW, LeGrys VA, et al, "Electrolytes and Blood Gases," *Tietz Textbook of Clinical Chemistry*, 3rd ed, Chapter 31, Burtis CA and Ashwood ER, eds, Philadelphia, PA: WB Saunders Co, 1999, 1078-9.
Zijlstra WG, Buursma A, and Meeuwsen-van der Roest WP, "Absorption Spectra of Human Fetal and Adult Oxyhemoglobin, De-Oxyhemoglobin, Carboxyhemoglobin, and Methemoglobin," *Clin Chem*, 1991, 37(9):1633-8.

♦ **Oxygen Transport** see Lactic Acid, Whole Blood or Plasma on page 208

♦ **P-5'-P** see Vitamin B₆, Plasma or Serum on page 299

P₅₀, Blood

Related Information

Blood Volume on page 407
Carboxyhemoglobin, Blood on page 784
Erythropoietin, Serum on page 169
Fetal Hemoglobin on page 431
Methemoglobin, Whole Blood on page 800
Oxygen Saturation, Blood on page 240

Synonyms Blood Gas P-50; pO₂ (0.5); pO₂ at Half Saturation

Applies to 2,3-DPG; Hill Plots; Oxygen-Hemoglobin Dissociation Curve (ODC)

Abstract P₅₀ is that pO₂ (partial pressure of oxygen) at which hemoglobin is 50% saturated with oxygen (O₂). It is affected by pH, temperature, pCO₂ (partial pressure of carbon dioxide), concentration of 2,3-diphosphoglycerate (2,3-DPG), and the presence of fetal hemoglobin, variant hemoglobins, or dyshemoglobins (eg, carboxyhemoglobin and methemoglobin). P₅₀ is inversely related to the binding affinity of hemoglobin for oxygen.[1] The affinity of hemoglobin for O₂ is graphically illustrated with a sigmoid O₂ dissociation curve (ODC), which is a plot of O₂ saturation (SO_2) versus pO_2. See figure.

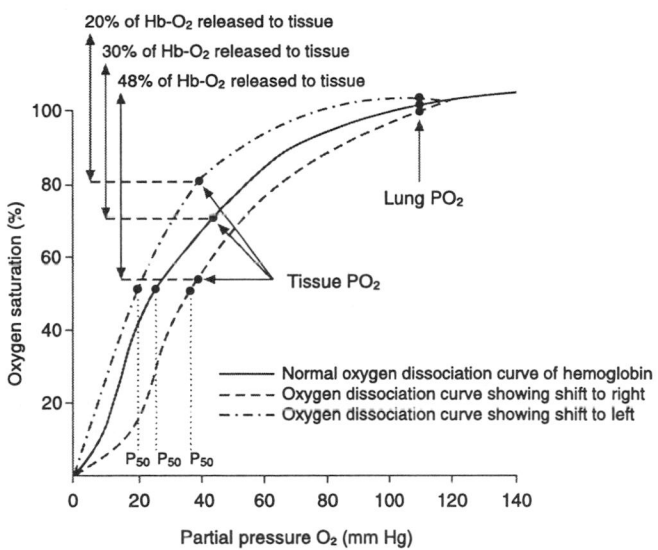

Oxygen dissociation curves under different conditions.

Adapted from *Technical Manual*, 13th ed, Chapter 8, Bethesda, MD: American Association of Blood Banks, 1999, 165.

Shifts in the curves to the left and right reflect, respectively, increased and decreased affinity of hemoglobin for O₂. Determination of P₅₀ value assumes that a tightly maintained physiologic relation between pO_2 and oxygen saturation exists and by implication that hemoglobin function is normal. This assumption does not necessarily apply to all hemoglobin types.

Specimen Arterial or venous whole blood

Container Heparinized syringe

Collection Avoid contact with air, insert needle into cork or hard rubber block, place on ice, and deliver to the laboratory immediately.

Causes for Rejection Specimen clotted, air bubbles in syringe, needle not tightly capped

Reference Interval Newborns: 18-24 mm Hg (because Hb F is present); adults: 25-29 mm Hg (corrected to pH 7.4, measured at 37°C); 26.3 mm Hg at sea level

Use The P₅₀ is used to assess affinity of hemoglobin for O₂ (ie, in detection of abnormalities in the affinity of hemoglobin for oxygen from diseases or from hemoglobin variants).[1] Decreased affinities (ie, **increased P₅₀** values with curve shifts to the right) result from acidemia, hypercapnia, hyperthermia, conditions associated with increased 2,3-DPG, and some hemoglobinopathies (eg, hemoglobin Seattle). See figure. Increased affinities (ie, **decreased P₅₀** values with curve shifts to the left) are observed in alkalemia, hypocapnia, conditions associated with decreased 2,3-DPG, (Continued)

P₅₀, Blood (Continued)

dyshemoglobinemias, and some hemoglobinopathies. Thus, P_{50} is an indirect measure of 2,3-DPG. Change in 2,3-DPG concentration is the most common cause of change in P_{50}. Other causes of altered P_{50} include carboxyhemoglobin, methemoglobin, or increased hemoglobin F.

Individuals with hemoglobin variants which have high affinity for oxygen may have secondary erythrocytosis but are usually asymptomatic; thus, the differential diagnosis would include possible polycythemia vera.

Limitations In vivo P_{50} changes with body temperature, CO_2T, and pH.

Methodology The P_{50} is most accurately determined by construction of the O_2 dissociation curve. A wide variety of "discontinuous" and "continuous" methods have been described to accomplish this, and these are well reviewed in the introduction to a paper by Zwart et al.[2] In each of these methods, either pO_2 or SO_2 or both are measured with additional measurement or control of pH and/or pCO_2. These methods are cumbersome and not routinely available in most clinical laboratories. With the availability of blood gas analyzer/multi-wavelength oximeter combinations, single point calculation methods for determining P_{50} have been described.[3,4] These methods are suitable for detection of clinically significant abnormalities in O_2 affinity such as those that occur in patients with abnormal hemoglobins and carbon monoxide poisoning, but do not provide truly accurate P_{50} and Hill values and are unable to discriminate between high and low values for P_{50} within the reference range.[3]

Additional Information The characteristic sigmoid configuration of the ODC curve relates to the interaction of the components of the hemoglobin tetramer ("heme-heme interaction") and to the acceptance by the tetramer of 2,3-DPG as O_2 is progressively bound or released. In effect, conformational changes occur at the molecular level with actual physical changes in the globin chain configuration and chain-to-chain positions with oxygenation/deoxygenation. When 2,3-DPG is decreased and the P_{50} is increased (and ODC shifts to the right), less O_2 is attached to hemoglobin and more released to the tissues at any given pO_2. When 2,3-DPG is increased, the P_{50} is decreased (and ODC shifts to the left), more O_2 is attached to hemoglobin and less released to the tissues at any given pO_2. The following is a summary:

$$\uparrow\ \substack{RBC\\2,3\text{-DPG}} \rightarrow\ \uparrow P\text{-}50 \begin{cases} \uparrow pO_2 \text{ necessary to} \rightarrow 50\% \text{ saturation Hgb with } O_2 \\ \downarrow O_2 \text{ affinity, } \uparrow \text{ tissue availability} \end{cases}$$

$$\downarrow\ \substack{RBC\\2,3\text{-DPG}} \rightarrow\ \downarrow P\text{-}50 \begin{cases} \downarrow pO_2 \text{ necessary to} \rightarrow 50\% \text{ saturation Hgb with } O_2 \\ \uparrow O_2 \text{ affinity, } \downarrow \text{ tissue availability} \end{cases}$$

Some hemoglobinopathies are characterized by altered affinity for O_2. A variety of molecular bases for large numbers of different hemoglobins with high and low O_2 affinities are recognized. Of multiple α-chain and β-chain hemoglobin variants with increased O_2 affinity, not all have polycythemia or cyanosis. A number of α-chain and β-chain variants have decreased O_2 affinity, some with cyanosis, and/or hemolysis and/or "anemia." The "anemia" may reflect a condition defined by a laboratory result rather than a physiologic deficiency, as the lowered affinity should allow a decreased mass of circulating hemoglobin to deliver a sufficient amount of O_2. Hemoglobin Seattle, among many others, appears to be such an example. A laboratory study of the ODC is important in cases of suspect hemoglobinopathy as some (eg, Hemoglobin Malmo[5]) have normal electrophoretic patterns using routine techniques. P_{50} has been found to decrease with use of some radiologic contrast agents.[6] Slight decrease in P_{50} has also been reported in the critically ill.[7] Phosphates may increase the P_{50}.[8]

Footnotes

1. Hsia CCW, "Respiratory Function of Hemoglobin," N Engl J Med, 1998, 338(4):239-46.
2. Zwart A, Kwant G, Oeseburg B, et al, "Oxygen Dissociation Curves for Whole Blood, Recorded With an Instrument That Continuously Measures pO_2 and SO_2 Independently at Constant t, pCO_2, and pH," Clin Chem, 1982, 28(6):1287-92.
3. Kwant G, Oeseburg B, and Zijistra WG, "Reliability of the Determination of Whole-Blood Oxygen Affinity by Means of Blood-Gas Analyzers and Multiwavelength Oximeters," Clin Chem, 1989, 35(5):773-7.
4. Scott MG, Heusel JW, LeGrys VA, et al, "Electrolytes and Blood Gases," Tietz Textbook of Clinical Chemistry, 3rd ed, Chapter 31, Burtis CA and Ashwood ER, eds, Philadelphia, PA: WB Saunders Co, 1999, 1056-92
5. Fairbanks VF, Maldonado JE, Charache S, et al, "Familial Erythrocytosis Due to Electrophoretically Undetectable Hemoglobin With Impaired Oxygen Dissociation (Hemoglobin Malmo $\alpha_2 \beta_2^{97gln}$)," Mayo Clin Proc, 1971, 46:721-7.
6. Kim SJ, Salem MR, Joseph NJ, et al, "Contrast Media Adversely Affect Oxyhemoglobin Dissociation," Anesth Analg, 1990, 71(1):73-6.
7. Myburgh JA, Webb RK, and Worthley LIG, "The P50 Is Reduced in Critically Ill Patients," Intensive Care Med, 1991, 17(6):355-8.
8. Clerbaux T, Reynaert M, Willems E, et al, "Effect of Phosphate on Oxygen-Hemoglobin Affinity, Diphosphoglycerate and Blood Gases During Recovery From Diabetic Ketoacidosis," Intensive Care Med, 1989, 15(8):495-8.

References

Dodson SR, Hensley FA Jr, Martin DE, et al, "Continuous Oxygen Saturation Monitoring During Cardiac Catheterization in Adults," Chest, 1988, 94(1):28-31.

Konzuki H, Enoki Y, Sakata S, et al, "A Simple Microtonometric Method for Whole Blood Oxygen Dissociation Curve and a Critical Evaluation of the Single Point Procedure for Blood P_{50}," Jpn J Physiol, 1983, 33:987-94.

Lichtman MA, Murphy MS, and Adamson JW, "Detection of Mutant Hemoglobins With Altered Affinity for Oxygen. A Simplified Technique," Ann Intern Med, 1976, 84(5):517-20.

Samaja M, Melotti D, Rovida E, et al, "Effect of Temperature on the P_{50} Value for Human Blood," Clin Chem, 1983, 29(1):110-4.

♦ **Paigen Test (E. coli Bacteriophage Resistance to Lysis Assay)** see Newborn Screening Tests for Galactosemia on page 232

Pancreatic Polypeptide, Human, Serum or Plasma

Related Information

Glucagon, Plasma on page 182
Insulin, Serum on page 201
Multiple Endocrine Neoplasia/Familial Medullary Thyroid Carcinoma on page 727
Vasoactive Intestinal Polypeptide, Plasma on page 297

Synonyms hPP; Human Pancreatic Polypeptide

Abstract Human pancreatic polypeptide (hPP) is a 36-amino acid, peptide hormone produced primarily by the endocrine type F cells of the pancreatic islets. Plasma levels rise in a biphasic manner after a meal, regulated initially by vagal cholinergic stimulation and later by cholecystokinin release. The exact physiologic role of hPP is unknown, but it appears to be involved in the modulation of gastrointestinal functions. It influences gastric secretion, inhibits pancreatic secretion, decreases gallbladder activity, and slows gastric and upper intestinal motilities. Plasma levels of hPP are increased in some patients with pancreatic islet cell neoplasms, multiple endocrine neoplasia (MEN), and pancreatic endocrine tumors. Patients with pancreatic exocrine failure have reduced levels of hPP.

Patient Preparation Patient must fast overnight for basal evaluations. Avoid recent radioactive scan. Antacid medications or medications that affect insulin levels should be discontinued, if possible, for at least 48 hours prior to sample collection.

Specimen Serum or plasma

Container Red top tube or lavender top (EDTA) tube; check with reference laboratory for specific instructions.

Storage Instructions Process blood promptly in a refrigerated centrifuge. Serum or plasma should be frozen until analysis.

Reference Interval There is considerable variation among laboratories and literature reports. A study of basal serum levels from 623 fasting, adult subjects gave the following age- and gender-specific reference intervals.[1]

Male (pg/mL = pmol/L x 4.1817):
- 20-29 years: 3-47 pmol/L; 13-197 pg/mL
- 30-39 years: 4-74 pmol/L; 17-309 pg/mL
- 40-49 years: 5-102 pmol/L; 21-427 pg/mL
- 50-59 years: 7-156 pmol/L; 29-652 pg/mL
- 60-69 years: 5-146 pmol/L; 21-611 pg/mL

Female (pg/mL = pmol/L x 4.1817):
- 20-29 years: 2-48 pmol/L; 8-201 pg/mL
- 30-39 years: 2-71 pmol/L; 8-297 pg/mL
- 40-49 years: 3-84 pmol/L; 13-351 pg/mL
- 50-59 years: 5-121 pmol/L; 21-506 pg/mL
- 60-69 years: 10-76 pmol/L; 42-318 pg/mL

Basal hPP levels of 233 ±147 pg/mL were reported from a study of 45 healthy, pediatric patients ranging in age from 0-15 years.[2]

Use Human pancreatic polypeptide is used as a pancreatic endocrine tumor marker (pancreatic islet cell neoplasms, including insulinomas, glucagonomas, VIPomas); a marker for multiple endocrine neoplasia (MEN-1), and as an indicator of vagal function (after a meal or sham feeding).

Limitations Low diagnostic sensitivity has been reported for the prediction of pancreatic endocrine tumors[3,4] and the subset of pancreatic islet cells neoplasms.[5] With respect to the latter, however, a study of 202 patients with multiple endocrine neoplasia type 1 showed that markedly elevated (>3 times normal), basal, plasma hPP levels were 95% sensitive and 88% specific for the presence of radiographically detectable pancreatic islet cell tumors.[6]

Methodology Radioimmunoassay (RIA)

Additional Information An atropine suppression test is used to distinguish tumor-related secretion of hPP from normal. Release of hPP from normal cells is under cholinergic control, inhibited by atropine, while autonomous secretion from a tumor is anticipated.[3] Pancreatic endocrine tumors often secrete more than a single peptide. Peptides associated with such tumors include hPP, vasoactive intestinal polypeptide, gastrin, glucagon, somatostatin, and neurotensin.[3] Though a distinct clinical syndrome due to excessive secretion of hPP has not been established, a recent case report suggests that hPP hyperplasia may cause a watery diarrhea syndrome.[7] Most hPP-secreting neuroendocrine tumors originate from the pancreas; however, there was a recent case reported of a pure, hPP-secreting neuroendocrine carcinoma of the gallbladder in a patient whose high levels of hPP may have contributed to presenting symptoms of cholestasis and cholelithiasis.[8] Insulin-dependent diabetic patients predisposed to development of autonomic neuropathy may demonstrate decreased hPP (and epinephrine) levels in response to insulin-induced hypoglycemia.[9] Blunted hPP responses after meal ingestion in type 1 diabetics may be due to vagal neuropathy or islet cell dysfunction.[10] Human pancreatic polypeptide may be a glucoregulatory hormone.[11,12] Its release appears to be dependent upon intraluminal starch digestion.[13] Measurement of hPP has been used as an indicator or pancreatic endocrine function post-transplantation.[14,15]

Footnotes

1. Brimnes Damholt M, Rasmussen BK, Hilsted L, et al, "Basal Serum Pancreatic Polypeptide Is Dependent on Age and Gender in an Adult Population," *Scand J Clin Lab Invest*, 1997, 57(8):695-702.
2. Hanukoglu A, Chalew S, and Kowarski AA, "Human Pancreatic Polypeptide in Children and Young Adults," *Horm Metabol Res*, 1990, 22:41-3.
3. Adrian TE, Uttenthal LO, Williams SJ, et al, "Secretion of Pancreatic Polypeptide in Patients With Pancreatic Endocrine Tumors," *N Engl J Med*, 1986, 315(5):287-91.
4. Chiang H-CV, O'Dorisio TM, Huang SC, et al, "Multiple Hormone Elevations in Zollinger-Ellison Syndrome - Prospective Study of Clinical Significance and of the Development of a Second Symptomatic Pancreatic Endocrine Tumor Syndrome," *Gastroenterology*, 1990, 99(6):1565-75.
5. Langstein HN, Norton JA, Chiang H-CV, et al, "The Utility of Circulating Levels of Human Pancreatic Polypeptide as a Marker for Islet Cell Tumors," *Surgery*, 1990, 108(6):1109-16.
6. Mutch MG, Frisella MM, DeBenedetti MK, et al, "Pancreatic Polypeptide Is a Useful Plasma Marker for Radiographically Evident Pancreatic Islet Cell Tumors in Patients With Multiple Endocrine Neoplasia Type 1," *Surgery*, 1997, 122(6):1012-20.
7. Pasieka JL and Hershfield N, "Pancreatic Polypeptide Hyperplasia Causing Watery Diarrhea Syndrome: A Case Report," *Can J Surg*, 1999, 42(1):55-8.
8. Marrano NN, Blevins LS, Gal AA, et al, "Pancreatic Polypeptide Hypersecretion Associated With a Neuroendocrine Carcinoma of the Gallbladder," *Am J Med Sci*, 1999, 317(1):55-8.
9. Kennedy FP, Go VL, Cryer PE, et al, "Subnormal Pancreatic Polypeptide and Epinephrine Responses to Insulin-Induced Hypoglycemia Identify Patients With Insulin-Dependent Diabetes Mellitus Predisposed to Develop Overt Autonomic Neuropathy," *Ann Intern Med*, 1988, 108(1):54-8.
10. Rasmussen MH, Carstensen H, List S, et al, "Impaired Pancreatic Polypeptide Response to a Meal in Type 1 Diabetic Patients: Vagal Neuropathy or Islet Cell Dysfunction?" *Acta Endocrinol*, 1993, 128:221-4.
11. Seymour NE, Brunicardi FC, Chaiken RL, et al, "Reversal of Abnormal Glucose Production After Pancreatic Resection by Pancreatic Polypeptide Administration in Man," *Surgery*, 1988, 104(2):119-29.
12. Brunicardi FC, Chaiken RL, Ryan AS, et al, "Pancreatic Polypeptide Administration Improves Abnormal Glucose Metabolism in Patients With Chronic Pancreatitis," *J Clin Endocrinol Metab*, 1996, 81(10):3566-72.
13. Layer P, Go VL, and DiMagno EP, "Carbohydrate Digestion and Release of Pancreatic Polypeptide in Health and Diabetes Mellitus," *Gut*, 1989, 30(9):1279-84.
14. Diem P, Redmon JB, Abid M, et al, "Glucagon, Catecholamine, and Pancreatic Polypeptide Secretion in Type 1 Diabetic Recipients of Pancreas Allografts," *J Clin Invest*, 1990, 86:2008-13.
15. Pyzdrowski KL, Kendall DN, Halter JB, et al, "Preserved Insulin Secretion and Insulin Independence on Recipients of Islet Autografts," *N Engl J Med*, 1992, 327(4):220-6.

References

Gehlert DR, "Multiple Receptors for the Pancreatic Polypeptide (PP-Fold) Family: Physiological Implications," *Proc Soc Exp Biol Med*, 1998, 218(1):7-22.

Gelston AL, Delisle MB, and Patel YC, "Multiple Endocrine Adenomatosis Type I. Occurrence in Octogenarian With High Levels of Circulating Pancreatic Polypeptide," *JAMA*, 1982, 247:665-6.

Hazelwood RL, "The Pancreatic Polypeptide (PP-Fold) Family: Gastrointestinal, Vascular, and Feeding Behavioral Implications," *Proc Soc Exp Biol Med*, 1993, 202(1):44-63.

Meier R, Hildebrand P, Thumshirn M, et al, "Effect of Loxiglumide, a Cholecystokinin Antagonist, on Pancreatic Polypeptide Release in Humans," *Gastroenterology*, 1990, 99(6):1757-62.

♦ **Pancreatic Polypeptides** *see* Insulin, Serum *on page 201*

♦ **PAP** *see* Acid Phosphatase, Plasma *on page 82*

♦ **PAPP-A** *see* Pregnancy-Associated Protein A, Serum *on page 260*

♦ **Paracentesis Fluid Analysis** *see* Body Fluid Chemical Analysis *on page 123*

♦ **Parathormone** *see* Parathyroid Hormone, Serum *on page 243*

♦ **Parathormone** *see* Vitamin D, Serum *on page 300*

♦ **Parathyroid Hormone, C-Terminal** *see* Parathyroid Hormone, Serum *on page 243*

♦ **Parathyroid Hormone, Intact** *see* Parathyroid Hormone, Serum *on page 243*

♦ **Parathyroid Hormone, N-Terminal** *see* Parathyroid Hormone, Serum *on page 243*

♦ **Parathyroid Hormone (PTH), Whole Molecule** *see* Parathyroid Hormone, Serum *on page 243*

♦ **Parathyroid Hormone-Related Protein** *see* Calcium, Serum *on page 131*

Parathyroid Hormone-Related Protein, Serum

Related Information

Calcium, Ionized, Serum *on page 130*
Calcium, Serum *on page 131*
Calcium, Urine *on page 133*

Parathyroid Hormone, Serum *on page 243*

Synonyms PTHrP

Abstract The association of cancer with hypercalcemia has been observed for many decades, but the fact that this hypercalcemia may result from tumor production of parathyroid hormone-related protein (PTHrP) is a relatively recent discovery. PTHrP, the major factor causing humoral hypercemia of malignancy, may be made by tumor cells without bone metastases. Squamous cell carcinomas account for about 50% of cases. Primaries in breast, kidney, ovary, bladder, and hematologic neoplasms account for most of the remainder.[1]

PTHrP and parathyroid hormone (PTH) share many important biological effects, including the production of hypercalcemia, activation of osteoclasts and increasing bone resorption, enhanced renal conservation of calcium and excretion of phosphate, and increased absorption of calcium from the gut (via stimulation of 1,25OH vitamin D synthesis). Chemically, PTHrP is the name of three proteins, all of which show close homology to parathyroid hormone (PTH) in their first 13 amino acids. Unlike PTH, which consists of 84 peptides, PTHrP occurs in three forms with 139, 141, and 173 peptides, respectively.

Hypersecretion of PTH by nonparathyroid tumors is extremely rare.[2]

Specimen EDTA plasma (check with reference laboratory for additional preservatives)

Container Lavender top (EDTA) tube

Collection Centrifuge promptly and freeze immediately (check with reference laboratory)

Reference Interval 0-1.5 pmol/L[3]

Possible Panic Range Hypercalcemia in cancer patients appears abruptly and carries a poor prognosis; median survival is only ~6 weeks.[4]

Use A large proportion (33% to 50%) of patients presenting with hypercalcemia have malignancy associated hypercalcemia (MAH) as the cause. Of patients with malignancy associated hypercalcemia, many have bone metastases. At least 80% of patients with solid tumors and hypercalcemia have increased PTHrP.[4] Most of the other patients have primary hyperparathyroidism (PHPT). Therefore the PTHrP assay is highly useful in the differential diagnosis of hypercalcemia. Most patients with PHPT have normal or undetectable PTHrP.

Limitations This assay is not yet widely available. In addition to patients with MAH, PTHrP is also elevated in women who are lactating and correlates with the associated decrement in bone density.[5]

Methodology Immunoradiometric assay (IRMA)

Additional Information PTHrP production by benign tumors rarely occurs. It is called humoral hypercalcemia of benignancy.[6]

PTHrP has been demonstrated immunohistochemically in a tumor causing humoral hypercalcemia of malignancy.[1]

Footnotes

1. Crespo M, Sopena B, Orloff JJ, et al, "Immunohistochemical Detection of Parathyroid Hormone-Related Protein in a Cutaneous Squamous Cell Carcinoma Causing Humoral Hypercalcemia of Malignancy," *Arch Pathol Lab Med*, 1999, 123(8):725-30.
2. Marx SJ, "Hyperparathyroid and Hypoparathyroid Disorders," *N Engl J Med*, 2000, 343(25):1863-75.
3. Associated Regional and University Pathologists, Inc (ARUP), 1999-2000 User's Guide, 524. ARUP Laboratories phone: 801-583-2787.
4. Strewler GJ, "Mechanisms of Disease. The Physiology of Parathyroid Hormone-Related Protein," *N Engl J Med*, 2000, 342(3):177-85.
5. Sowers MF, Hollis BW, Shapiro B, et al, "Elevated Parathyroid Hormone-Related Peptide Associated With Lactation and Bone Density Loss," *JAMA*, 1996, 276(7):549-54.
6. Knecht TP, Behling CA, Burton DW, et al, "The Humoral Hypercalcemia of Benignancy. A Newly Appreciated Syndrome," *Am J Clin Pathol*, 1996, 105(4):487-92.

References

Bilezikian JP, "Clinical Utility of Assays for Parathyroid Hormone-Related Protein," *Clin Chem*, 1992, 38:179-81.

Burtis WJ, "Parathyroid Hormone-Related Protein: Structure, Function, and Measurement," *Clin Chem*, 1992, 38:2171-83.

Guise TA, "Parathyroid Hormone-Related Protein and Bone Metastases," *Cancer*, 1997, 80:1572-80.

Pandian MR, Morgan CH, Carlton E, et al, "Modified Immunoradiometric Assay of Parathyroid Hormone-Related Protein: Clinical Application in the Differential Diagnosis of Hypercalcemia," *Clin Chem*, 1992, 38(2):282-8.

Rankin W, Grill V, and Martin TJ, "Parathyroid Hormone-Related Protein and Hypercalcemia," *Cancer*, 1997, 80(8 Suppl):1564-71.

Seymour JF, "Malignancy-Associated Hypercalcemia," *Scientific American Science and Medicine*, 1995, 48-57.

Stewart AF and Broadus AE, "Humoral Hypercalcemia of Malignancy," *Advances in Endocrinology and Metabolism*, 1990, 1:1-21.

Internet Web Sites

www.arup-lab.com

Parathyroid Hormone, Serum

Related Information

Aluminum, Bone and Bone Biopsy *on page 813*
Calcium, Ionized, Serum *on page 130*
Calcium, Serum *on page 131*
Calcium, Urine *on page 133*
Creatinine, Serum or Plasma *on page 161*
Cyclic AMP, Plasma *on page 163*
(Continued)

Parathyroid Hormone, Serum *(Continued)*

Cyclic AMP, Urine *on page 163*
Kidney Stone Analysis *on page 877*
Multiple Endocrine Neoplasia/Familial Medullary Thyroid Carcinoma *on page 727*
Osteocalcin, Serum or Plasma *on page 237*
Parathyroid Hormone-Related Protein, Serum *on page 243*
Phosphorus, Serum *on page 251*
Phosphorus, Urine *on page 253*
Vitamin D, Serum *on page 300*

Synonyms Immunoreactive PTH; Parathormone; PTH

Applies to Multiple Endocrine Neoplasia (MEN) Type 1; Parathyroid Hormone, C-Terminal; Parathyroid Hormone, Intact; Parathyroid Hormone, N-Terminal; Parathyroid Hormone (PTH), Whole Molecule

Test Includes Concomitant serum calcium is required for interpretation. Age, sex, serum phosphorus and creatinine are also important (*vide infra*, see Use).

Abstract The parathyroid glands regulate concentrations of plasma calcium and metabolism of bone, through secretion of PTH.

Hyperparathyroidism causes nephrolithiasis (in ~20%) and osteopenia/osteoporosis (osteopenia occurs in ~25%), and rarely presently, osteitis fibrosa cystica. Many contemporary American cases present with few symptoms or seem asymptomatic. Eighty-five percent to 90% of cases are caused by solitary parathyroid adenomas, and <1% are caused by parathyroid carcinoma.

Hypersecretion of PTH causes hypercalcemia. When hypercalcemia is found, unless its cause is obvious (eg, use of large doses of vitamin D or cancer) the next steps include assay of PTH.

Parathyroid hormone (PTH), a single-chain polypeptide containing 84 amino acid residues, is synthesized and stored in the parathyroid glands, from which it is secreted at a rate inversely proportional to ambient concentration of ionized serum calcium. The **half-life** of PTH in the plasma is 2-5 minutes. The overall biochemical effects of PTH, increasing the serum concentrations of both ionized and total calcium and decreasing the serum concentration of phosphorus, are mediated by actions in bone, kidney, and gut. PTH mobilizes calcium from bone (by activating osteoclasts), increases reabsorption of calcium from tubular urine, decreases reabsorption of phosphorus from tubular urine, and increases gastrointestinal absorption of calcium (by stimulating the formation of $1,25(OH)_2$ vitamin D).

Of historical interest are assays for the amino-terminal (N-terminal) fragment of PTH and other assays for the carboxy-terminal (C-terminal) fragment of PTH. Now that reliable assays are available for **whole molecule PTH** (also called intact PTH), there are few, if any, indications for N-terminal and C-terminal assays.

Patient Preparation Patient should be fasting. Lithium and thiazides may alter PTH secretion and calcium concentration. (About 5% of subjects on long-term lithium treatment develop mild hyperparathyroidism.)

Specimen Serum; plasma is acceptable in some protocols.

Container Red top tube for serum; check with reference laboratory for preferred anticoagulant if plasma is to be used.

Sampling Time Because a circadian rhythm is present, specimen collection times should be standardized to reduce biologic variation. Draw in early morning, before 10 AM.

Collection Centrifuge promptly. Freeze immediately. Consult reference laboratory for specific instructions regarding exact PTH moiety being analyzed.

Reference Interval The reference intervals vary with the method, patient age, and gender (in children).

Pediatrics:[1] See table.

Serum Intact PTH

Age (y)	n	Median (ng/L)	2.5th-97.5th Percentiles (ng/L)
2.1-4	M: 48 F: 42	M: 12.46 F: 12.80	M: 5.7-34.2 F: 3.6-32.0
4.1-6	M: 46 F: 39	M: 9.65 F: 8.71	M: 4.4-15.6 F: 1.0-13.0
6.1-8	M: 48 F: 54	M: 9.93 F: 10.91	M: 2.5-27.3 F: 2.7-24.6
8.1-10	M: 60 F: 66	M: 13.11 F: 12.88	M: 4.6-33.8 F: 2.0-30.2
10.1-12	M: 57 F: 67	M: 13.02 F: 16.53	M: 2.5-25.4 F: 4.3-33.9
12.1-14	M: 54 F: 65	M: 12.84 F: 15.62	M: 1.4-25.5 F: 1.6-36.5
14.1-16	M: 72 F: 76	M: 13.57 F: 13.98	M: 4.5-35.8 F: 1.2-39.0

Adapted from Cioffi M, Corradino M, Gazzerro P, et al, "Serum Concentrations of Intact Parathyroid Hormone in Healthy Children," *Clin Chem*, 2000 46(6):863.

Adults:
- whole molecule, immunochemiluminometric assay (ICMA):[2] 1.0-5.2 pmol/L

- whole molecule, radioimmunoassay (RIA):[3] 10.0-65.0 pg/mL
- whole molecule, immunoradiometric, double antibody (IRMA):[4] 1.0-6.0 pmol/L

In normal persons serum calcium and serum PTH are in a negative feedback loop such that the higher the serum calcium, the lower the serum PTH. This relationship is disturbed in some diseases.

A few reference laboratories still perform N-terminal PTH and C-terminal PTH assays, and they should be consulted regarding their reference intervals.

Use

Differential diagnosis of hypercalcemia: The most common causes of hypercalcemia are primary hyperparathyroidism (**PHP**) and malignancy-associated hypercalcemia (**MAH**). These two diagnoses account for >90% of patients with hypercalcemia.[4] Less common causes include familial hypocalcuric hypercalcemia (**FHH**), granulomatous diseases, certain lymphomas, thyrotoxicosis, and vitamin D intoxication.[4] Rare causes of hypercalcemia include lithium medication, thiazide therapy, Addison disease, hypothyroidism, milk-alkali syndrome, immobilization, PTH receptor defects, recovery from renal failure and following renal transplant.[4]

PHP and FHH: If the serum PTH is elevated, PHP is the most likely diagnosis. A family history will help identify the small number of patients with FHH, an autosomal dominant genetic disease caused by a mutation in the calcium-sensing receptor.[5] Patients with FHH have low urine calcium, and the **urinary calcium:creatinine ratio** is usually <0.01. Interpretation of the PTH result is not optimal without simultaneous measurements of serum calcium, creatinine and phosphorus. A homeostatic relationship exists between serum calcium and PTH (see Abstract) and this relationship is disturbed in PHP and FHH.

MAH: If the serum PTH is appropriate for the concurrent calcium (this relationship is often recorded in the laboratory results), then MAH is the most likely diagnosis. MAH occurs by two mechanisms, and both mechanisms can be operative in the same patient.
- Many tumors secrete parathyroid hormone-related protein (**PTHrP**) which shares many biologic properties with PTH. PTHrP mobilized calcium from bone (by osteoclast activation), produces renal conservation of calcium, and stimulates the formation of $1,25(OH)_2$ vitamin D (calcitriol).[6]
- Tumors in bone release cytokines which activate osteoclasts and produce hypercalcemia by this mechanism, sometimes called **local osteolytic hypercalcemia** (LOH).

The LOH mechanism is particularly prominent in plasma cell myeloma. For most patients with MAH, the diagnosis of MAH can be made with a PTH assay (including serum calcium, phosphorus, and creatinine) **in addition to** a thorough work-up for malignancy. Only rarely is it necessary to obtain a PTHrP assay. In some patients with cancer and hypercalcemia, the cause is attributed to "ectopic" PTH production, but this presently is considered very rare, if it exists at all.

Endogenous vitamin D intoxication: In normal individuals, 25 hydroxy vitamin D (25OH vitamin D) is converted in the kidney to 1,25 dihydroxy vitamin D [$1,25(OH)_2$ vitamin D]. In some patients with granulomatous diseases (and a few with lymphomas not involving bone), lesional (non-neoplastic) macrophages also have the ability to affect this conversion, which then leads to hypercalcemia.

When PHP, MAH, FHH, and endogenous vitamin D intoxication have been ruled out, the search for a diagnosis focuses on the rare conditions listed above (Differential Diagnosis).

Intraoperative Monitoring of PTH: The surgical treatment of primary hyperparathyroidism requires an intraoperative decision about whether the disease involves just one gland (adenoma) or multiple glands (hyperplasia or multiple adenomas). Pathologic evaluation by frozen section sometimes may be an imperfect tool for this purpose.[7] Investigators at the Mayo Clinic[8] originally reported a modification of their immunochemiluminometric (ICMA) whole molecule PTH assay, which required only 15 minutes of assay time and therefore allowed the assay results to be reported quickly enough for intraoperative monitoring. These investigators also found that when a parathyroid gland(s) is hyperfunctioning, the other (normal) glands are suppressed and do not regain function for up to 130 minutes after resection; therefore, intraoperative PTH levels are not affected by the function of previously suppressed parathyroid tissue. Improvements in assay technique now provide a 10 minute assay, and actual experience with that assay indicates that a decrease of 50% or more from the baseline PTH predicts operative success with an overall accuracy of 97%.[9] When the PTH decrement is <50% of baseline, further exploration to find additional hyperfunctioning tissue is indicated.[10] Intraoperative PTH assays, combined with differential venous sampling assists in the localization of difficult-to-find parathyroid glands.[11,12,13]

Differential diagnosis of hypocalcemia: Causes include hypoparathyroidism (including familial hypocalcemia due to a mutation in the calcium-sensing receptor),[14] rickets, low serum albumin, acute pancreatitis, sepsis, medication effect, hungry bone syndrome, tumor lysis syndrome, rhabdomyolysis, chronic renal insufficiency, and magnesium deficiency.[15]

Hypocalcemia from hypoparathyroidism is a recognized risk following thyroid surgery.[16] Hypoparathyroidism may be due to organ destruction (iron overload or autoimmunity, granulomatous disease, metastatic neoplasm), and failure to develop (DiGeorge syndrome). These patients have low serum calcium with inappropriately low serum PTH. Rickets is most often due to dietary Vitamin D deficiency (but may also be caused by an inborn error of vitamin D metabolism). Dietary deficiency is usually confirmed by the serum 25OH vitamin D assay (see Vitamin D, Serum *on page 300*); such patients are expected to have elevated serum PTH due to the negative feedback loop described above (see Abstract). An inborn error of metabolism responsive to high doses of Vitamin D may be due to a mutation in the 25OH vitamin D 1-alpha-hydroxylase gene.[17] Dietary calcium deficiency is less common than vitamin D deficiency. Some hypocalcemic patients have malabsorption of vitamin D, calcium, or both; gluten-sensitive enteropathy and postsurgical bowel are leading causes. When serum albumin is low, the total serum calcium can be corrected using the following formula:

Corrected calcium = measured calcium [mg/dL] + 0.8 (4 - patient albumin [g/dL])[15]

When acute pancreatitis or sepsis cause hypocalcemia, the basic underlying disease is usually obvious. Following surgical removal of hyperfunctioning parathyroid tissue, patients with bone disease secondary to hyperparathyroidism often experience transient hypocalcemia as calcium is taken up by bone. Tumor lysis syndrome occurs in cancer patients, typically (but not exclusively) a patient on chemotherapy; the laboratory profile also includes elevations of uric acid, phosphate, and potassium. In rhabdomyolysis, other findings include elevation of creatine kinase, potassium, phosphate, and myoglobin in urine and blood.

Drugs causing hypocalcemia include calcitonin, mithramycin, biphosphonates, phosphates, phenytoin plus phenobarbital, and foscarnet.

Pseudohypoparathyroidism refers to conditions in which there is end organ unresponsiveness to PTH. Typical biochemical findings are hypocalcemia, accompanied by elevated serum phosphate and PTH.

Limitations Not all patients with PHP have elevated serum PTH. Both serum calcium and PTH may be intermittently elevated. In an evaluation of 60 patients with surgically proven primary hyperparathyroidism (PHP), 59 (98.3%) patients had elevated ionized calcium and 49 (82%) had elevated serum PTH. Therefore, clinical judgment is important in evaluation of such patients, and special testing (eg, renal handling of calcium and phosphate) may occasionally be needed.[18]

Methodology Immunochemiluminometric assay (ICMA), two-site immunoradiometric assay

Additional Information Patients who seem asymptomatic with hyperparathyroidism are not necessarily unharmed. Many have diminished bone density and therefore increased risk of fracture.[19]

About 85% of individuals with **Multiple endocrine neoplasia (MEN) type 1** by age 40 have hyperparathyroidism. Primary hyperparathyroidism occurs in **MEN type 2A** (in which medullary thyroid carcinoma and pheochromocytoma are found).

Parathyroid carcinoma should be considered when a patient presents with features of hyperparathyroidism, a palpable neck mass, both bone disease and nephrolithiasis, and marked increases of both serum calcium and PTH levels.[20,21]

When a nonparathyroid tumor is associated with hypercalcemia, decreased serum phosphorus and increased concentrations of parathyroid hormone-related peptide, the neoplasm is most often squamous cell bronchogenic carcinoma (other primaries include squamous carcinomas of head and

neck, and carcinomas of breast and kidney). This clinical syndrome, recently called **ectopic hyperparathyroidism**, is now named **humoral hypercalcemia of malignancy.**[22] Parathyroid hormone-related peptide is now considered to be the major mediator of humoral hypercalcemia of malignancy.[23] See Parathyroid Hormone-Related Protein, Serum *on page 243.*

Neonatal severe primary hyperparathyroidism is rare. There are very high PTH and calcium concentrations.

The interrelationships between serum PTH and calcium in three common clinical situations and in normals are illustrated in the figure.[2]

SUMMARY: The two most important tests for primary hyperparathyroidism are PTH and serum ionized calcium.

Footnotes

1. Cioffi M, Corradino M, Gazzerro P, et al, "Serum Concentrations of Intact Parathyroid Hormone in Healthy Children," *Clin Chem*, 2000, 46(6 Pt 1):863-4.
2. Mayo Medical Laboratories, *2000 Test Catalogue*, Rochester, MN, 403.
3. Painter PC, Cope JY, and Smith JL, "Reference Information for the Clinical Laboratory," *Tietz Textbook of Clinical Chemistry*, Burtis CA and Ashwood ER, eds, Philadelphia, PA: WB Saunders Co, 1999, 1788-1846.
4. Selby PL and Adams PH, "The Investigation of Hypercalcemia," *J Clin Pathol*, 1994, 47:579-84.
5. Pearce SH and Brown EM, "The Genetic Basis of Endocrine Disease: Disorders of Calcium Ion Sensing," *J Clin Endocrinol Metab*, 1996, 81:2030-5.
6. Burtis WJ, "Parathyroid Hormone-Related Protein: Structure, Function, and Measurement," *Clin Chem*, 1992, 38(11):2171-83.
7. LiVolsi VA and Hamilton R, "Intraoperative Assessment of Parathyroid Gland Pathology," *Am J Clin Pathol*, 1994, 102(3):365-73.
8. Kao P, Van Heerden JA, and Taylor RL, "Intraoperative Monitoring of Parathyroid Procedures by a 15-minute Parathyroid Hormone Immunochemiluminometric Assay," *Mayo Clin Proc*, 1994, 69:532-7.
9. Irvin GL and Carneiro DM, "Rapid Parathyroid Hormone Assay Guided Exploration," *Operative Tech Gen Surg*, 1999, 1:18-27.
10. Irvin GL and Carneiro DM, "Management Changes in Primary Hyperparathyroidism," *JAMA*, 2000, 284(8):934-6.
11. Irvin GL, Molinari AS, Figueroa C, et al, "Improved Success Rate in Reoperative Parathyroidectomy With Intraoperative PTH Assay," *Ann Surg*, 1999, 229(6):874-8.
12. Wenk RE and Efron G, "Central Laboratory Analyses of Intact PTH Using Intraoperative Samples," *Lab Med*, 2000, 31(3):158-61.
13. Wians FH Jr, Balko JA, Hsu RM, et al, "Intraoperative vs Central Laboratory PTH Testing During Parathyroidectomy Surgery," *Lab Med*, 2000, 31(11):616-21.
14. Pearce SH, Williamson C, Kifor O, et al, "A Familial Syndrome of Hypocalcemia With Hypercalciuria Due to Mutations in the Calcium-Sensing Receptor," *N Engl J Med*, 1996, 335:1115-22.
15. Desai SP and Isa-Pratt S, *Clinician's Guide to Laboratory Medicine*, Hudson, OH: Lexi-Comp, 2000, 201-20.
16. Pattou F, Combemale F, Fabre S, et al, "Hypocalcemia Following Thyroid Surgery: Incidence and Prediction of Outcome," *World J Surg*, 1998, 22(7):718-24.
17. Kitanaka S, Takeyama K, Murayama A, et al, "Inactivating Mutations in the 25-Hydroxyvitamin D_3 Alpha-Hydroxylase Gene in Patients With Pseudovitamin D-Deficiency Rickets," *N Engl J Med*, 1998, 338:653-61.
18. Glendenning P, Gutteridge DH, Retallack RW, et al, "High Prevalence of Normal Total Calcium and Intact PTH in 60 Patients With Proven Primary Hyperparathyroidism: A Challenge to Current Diagnostic Criteria," *Aust N Z J Med*, 1998, 28(2):173-8.
19. Utiger RD, "Treatment of Primary Hyperparathyroidism," *N Engl J Med*, 1999, 341(17):1301-2.
20. Wynne AG, van Heerden J, Carney JA, et al, "Parathyroid Carcinoma: Clinical and Pathologic Features in 43 Patients," *Medicine (Baltimore)*, 1992, 71(4):197-205.
21. Jaffey P, Kahky M, and Ackerman E, "Pathologic Quiz Case: Recurrent Hypercalcemia," *Arch Pathol Lab Med*, 2000, 124(7):1087-8.
22. Wysolmerski JJ and Broadus AE, "Hypercalcemia of Malignancy: The Central Role of Parathyroid Hormone-Related Protein," *Annu Rev Med*, 1994, 45:189-200.
23. Law F, Ferrari S, Rizzoli R, et al, "Parathyroid Hormone-Related Protein and Calcium Phosphate Metabolism," *Pediatr Nephrol*, 1993, 7(6):827-33.

References

DeLellis RA, "Tumors of the Parathyroid Gland," *Atlas of Tumor Pathology*, Third Series, Fascicle 6, Bethesda, MD: Armed Forces Institute of Pathology under the Auspices of Universities Associated for Research and Education in Pathology, Inc, 1993.
Glendenning P, Gutteridge DH, Retallack RW, et al, "High Prevalence of Normal Total Calcium and Intact PTH in 60 Patients With Proven Primary Hyperparathyroidism: A Challenge to Current Diagnostic Criteria," *Aust N Z J Med*, 1998, 28(2):173-8.
Jorde R, Bonaa KH, and Sundsfjord J, "Population Based Study on Serum Ionised Calcium, Serum Parathyroid Hormone, and Blood Pressure," *Eur J Endocrinol*, 1999, 141(4):350-7.
Kinnaert P, Tielemans C, Dhaene M, et al, "Evaluation of Surgical Treatment of Renal Hyperparathyroidism by Measuring Intact Parathormone Blood Levels on First Postoperative Day," *World J Surg*, 1998, 22(7):695-9.
Malberti F, Farina M, and Imbasciati E, "The PTH-Calcium Curve and the Set Point of Calcium in Primary and Secondary Hyperparathyroidism," *Nephrol Dial Transplant*, 1999, 14(10):2398-406.
Michelangeli VP, Heyma P, Colman PG, et al, "Evaluation of a New, Rapid and Automated Immunochemiluminometric Assay for the Measurement of Serum Intact Parathyroid Hormone," *Ann Clin Biochem*, 1997, 34(Pt 1):97-103.
Silverberg SJ, Shane E, Jacobs TP, et al, "A 10-Year Prospective Study of Primary Hyperparathyroidism With or Without Parathyroid Surgery," *N Engl J Med*, 1999, 341(17):1249-55.
Utiger RD, "Treatment of Primary Hyperparathyroidism," *N Engl J Med*, 1999, 341:1301-2.
(Continued)

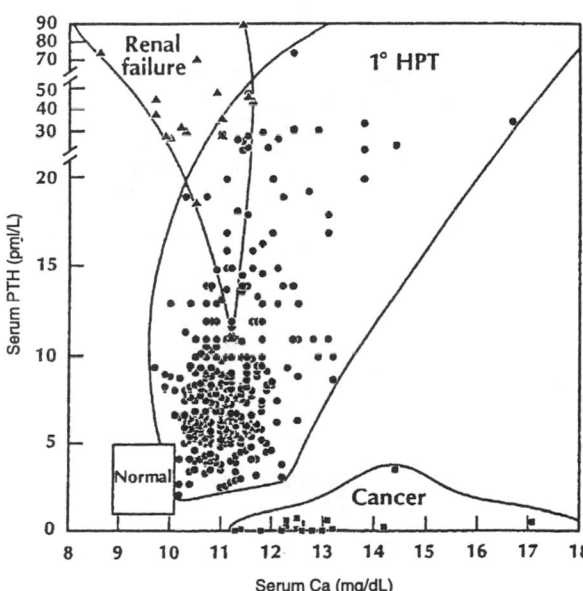

Overlapping domains are seen, especially early in the course of the disorders shown.

Parathyroid Hormone, Serum *(Continued)*

Young DS, *Effects of Drugs on Clinical Laboratory Tests*, 5th ed, Volume 1: Listing by Test, Washington, DC: AACC Press, American Association of Clinical Chemistry, 2000, Section 3, 599-601.

Zahrani AA and Levine MA, "Primary Hyperparathyroidism," *Lancet*, 1997, 349:1233-38.

♦ **Pbg-D** *see* Porphobilinogen Deaminase, Erythrocyte *on page 254*

♦ **PBI** *replaced by* Thyroxine, Serum *on page 286*

♦ **PChE** *see* Pseudocholinesterase, Serum *on page 270*

♦ **pCO₂** *see* Blood Gases and pH, Arterial *on page 119*

pCO₂, Blood

Related Information
Arterial Blood Collection *on page 40*
Bicarbonate, Blood *on page 115*
Blood Gases and pH, Arterial *on page 119*
Blood Gases and pH, Capillary *on page 121*
Blood Gases and pH, Venous *on page 122*
Carbon Dioxide, Total, Blood *on page 135*
pH, Blood *on page 247*
Point-of-Care Testing *on page 43*

Applies to Acid-Base Status; Hypercapnia; Hyperventilation; Hypoventilation; Respiratory Acidosis; Respiratory Alkalosis

Test Includes Test is part of blood gas panels and often, electrolyte panels

Abstract pCO₂ is the partial pressure of dissolved carbon dioxide in blood and is useful in evaluating acid-base status. Disturbances of respiration primarily affect pCO₂, while metabolic disturbances are reflected by bicarbonate levels.

Specimen Whole blood (arterial, venous, or capillary)

Collection Specimen should be collected anaerobically. See Arterial Blood Collection *on page 40*, Venous Blood Collection *on page 47*, and Skin Puncture Blood Collection *on page 45*. Deliver specimen immediately to the laboratory. When pCO₂ is drawn as a venous specimen, avoid a tourniquet if possible. Especially, **avoid fist clenching**.

Storage Instructions Specimen should be analyzed immediately. However, if delay in analysis is unavoidable, the specimen should be placed in a slurry of ice chips and water. Analysis should not be delayed beyond 1 hour. *In vitro* pCO₂ will increase by about 0.5 mm Hg/hour at 4°C.[1]

Causes for Rejection Specimen with clots, air bubbles, or not received on ice; needle not tightly stoppered

Turnaround Time Usually 30 minutes or less

Reference Interval
- Newborns, infants, and children up to ~2 years of age, with **arterialized capillary blood** (heel, fingertip, big toe) or arterial blood: 27-40 mm Hg
- Children older than 2 years of age (arterial) 27-41 mm Hg
- Adults, arterial: male: 35-48 mm Hg, female: 32-45 mm Hg
- Adults, venous: 40-45 mm Hg

Critical Values Partial pressure of arterial carbon dioxide (PaCO₂) >45 mm Hg may be a risk factor for pulmonary complications. In limited numbers of reviewed cases, such patients had significant airway obstruction on spirometry.[2]

Possible Panic Range <20 mm Hg, >70 mm Hg

Use Alveolar ventilation varies inversely as arterial pCO₂; therefore, pCO₂ is an indication of adequacy of CO₂ elimination by the lungs. **Respiratory alkalosis** (hyperventilation) results in low pCO₂ with elevated pH. **Respiratory acidosis** (hypoventilation) results in high pCO₂ with lowered pH.

Limitations Venous and arterial values are sensitive to sampling technique.

Methodology Analysis is done with blood gas instrumentation equipped with a pCO₂ electrode. This is a modified pH electrode which is present in a carbonate-bicarbonate buffer system. A plastic membrane (permeable to CO₂) is positioned between the blood sample and the electrode's surrounding buffer. CO₂ from the sample diffuses into the buffer; any pH change is detected by the electrode, and the resultant voltage change is read as pCO₂.

Additional Information Respiratory compensation for metabolic acidosis and alkalosis involves adjustment of the pCO₂ level by hypoventilation (as in cases of metabolic alkalosis with resultant rise in pCO₂) or by hyperventilation (as in cases of metabolic acidosis with decreasing pCO₂). As CO₂ is highly soluble, there is a quickly attained equilibrium between arterial carbon dioxide tension **(PaCO₂)** and alveolar carbon dioxide tension. Therefore, the arterial CO₂ measurement also determines the status of ventilation. PaCO₂ has a reverse relationship to alveolar ventilation.[1]

The expression "**hypercapnia**" indicates the presence of excessive carbon dioxide in the blood. Disorders associated with hypercapnia include central respiratory depression, abnormal neuromuscular function, chest wall abnormality, upper or lower respiratory tract disease, or hypercapnia secondary to cardiac disease.[3] Arterial pCO₂ may be an indicator of systemic perfusion during cardiopulmonary resuscitation.[4] Increased venous-arterial pCO₂ gradients do not appear to be a reliable indicator of inadequate tissue perfusion during cardiopulmonary bypass.[5] Transcutaneous measurements of pCO₂ may be a convenient means of monitoring the neonate in intensive care units. Acidosis does affect the ability to correlate transcutaneous and arterial pCO₂ values.[6]

Regulation of cerebral blood flow and volume appears to rely heavily upon changes in arterial pCO₂.[7]

Footnotes
1. Scott MG, Heusel JW, LeGrys VA, et al, "Electrolytes and Blood Gases," *Tietz Textbook of Clinical Chemistry*, 3rd ed, Chapter 31, Burtis CA and Ashwood ER, eds, Philadelphia, PA: WB Saunders Co, 1999, 1056-92.
2. Smetana GW, "Preoperative Pulmonary Evaluation," *N Engl J Med*, 1999, 340(12):937-53.
3. Weinberger SE, Schwartzstein RM, and Weiss JW, "Hypercapnia," *N Engl J Med*, 1989, 321(18):1223-31.
4. Gazmuri RJ, von Planta M, Weil MH, et al, "Arterial pCO₂ as an Indicator of Systemic Perfusion During Cardiopulmonary Resuscitation," *Crit Care Med*, 1989, 17(3):237-40.
5. Ariza M, Gothard JW, Macnaughton P, et al, "Blood Lactate and Mixed Venous-Arterial pCO₂ Gradient as Indices of Poor Peripheral Perfusion Following Cardiopulmonary Bypass Surgery," *Intensive Care Med*, 1991, 17(6):320-4.
6. Hand IL, Shepard EK, Krauss AN, et al, "Discrepancies Between Transcutaneous and End-Tidal Carbon Dioxide Monitoring in the Critically Ill Neonate With Respiratory Distress Syndrome," *Crit Care Med*, 1989, 17(6):556-9.
7. Madden JA, "The Effect of Carbon Dioxide on Cerebral Arteries," *Pharmacol Ther*, 1993, 59(2):229-50.

References
Burnett RW and Itano M, "An Interlaboratory Study of Blood-Gas Analysis: Dependence of pO₂ and pCO₂ Results on Atmospheric Pressure," *Clin Chem*, 1989, 35(8):1779-81.

Gay PC and Edmonds LC, "Severe Hypercapnia After Low-Flow Oxygen Therapy in Patients With Neuromuscular Disease and Diaphragmatic Dysfunction," *Mayo Clin Proc*, 1995, 70(4):327-30.

Hansen JE, Casaburi R, Crapo RO, et al, "Assessing Precision and Accuracy in Blood Gas Proficiency Testing," *Am Rev Respir Dis*, 1990, 141(5 Pt 1):1190-3.

Meyerhoff ME, "New *In Vitro* Analytical Approaches for Clinical Chemistry Measurements in Critical Care," *Clin Chem*, 1990, 36(8 Pt 2):1567-72.

Narins RG and Emmett M, "Simple and Mixed Acid-Base Disorders: A Practical Approach," *Medicine (Baltimore)*, 1980, 59:161-87.

Preuss HG, "Fundamentals of Clinical Acid-Base Evaluation," *Clin Lab Med*, 1993, 13(1):103-16.

Tobin MJ and Jubran A, "Oxygen Takes the Breath Away: Old Sting, New Setting," *Mayo Clin Proc*, 1995, 70(4):403-4.

♦ **Pentagastrin Stimulation Test** *see* Calcitonin, Serum or Plasma *on page 129*

♦ **Pentagastrin Stimulation Test** *see* Gastric Analysis *on page 180*

♦ **Pepsinogen A** *see* Pepsinogen I and II, Serum or Plasma *on page 246*

♦ **Pepsinogen A:C Ratio** *see* Pepsinogen I and II, Serum or Plasma *on page 246*

♦ **Pepsinogen C** *see* Pepsinogen I and II, Serum or Plasma *on page 246*

Pepsinogen I and II, Serum or Plasma

Related Information
Cobalamin, Serum *on page 150*
Gastric Analysis *on page 180*
Gastrin, Serum *on page 181*
Helicobacter pylori Antigen Detection by EIA *on page 619*
Helicobacter pylori Biopsy-Based Tests: The Urease Tests, Culture, Cytology, and PCR *on page 620*
Helicobacter pylori Serology *on page 621*

Synonyms Pepsinogen A; Pepsinogen C; PG I; PG II

Applies to Pepsinogen A:C Ratio; Pepsinogen I:II Ratio; PG I:PG II Ratio

Abstract Pepsinogen I (PG I) and pepsinogen II (PG II) are groups of gastric mucosal proenzymes of pepsins, aspartate proteinases involved in protein digestion. PG I and PG II differ electrophoretically and immunologically, and their serum concentrations reflect the morphological and functional status of the gastric mucosa.[1] Both PG I and PG II are secreted by chief cells and mucous neck cells of the gastric fundus and corpus; PG-II is also secreted by the pyloric glands of the antrum and Brunner's glands of the proximal duodenum. In general, acute or mild chronic gastric inflammation causes increased secretion of both PG I and PG II; atrophy causes decreased secretion. However, corpus atrophy results in chief cells being replaced by pyloric glands, resulting in decreased serum levels of PG I with no change or increase in PG II and decreased PG I:PG II ratios.

Patient Preparation Patient should fast for 10-12 hours and discontinue antacids or other medications affecting stomach acidity or gastrointestinal mobility for at least 48 hours prior to collection.

Specimen Serum, plasma

Container Red top tube, lavender top (EDTA) tube

Storage Instructions Freeze specimen immediately after centrifugation and transport to referral laboratory on dry ice.

Reference Interval PG I: 20-107 µg/L; PG II: 3-19 µg/L; PG I:PG II ratio: 5-6

Use Ratios are decreased in patients with atrophic gastritis, gastric cancer, and gastric body ulcer. Ratios are increased in duodenal ulcer patients and in patients with achlorhydria (eg, pernicious anemia).

Limitations The test is not widely available, even among the large referral laboratories. Considerable overlap in values is found between healthy individuals and those with abnormality.

Methodology Radioimmunoassay (RIA), fluorometric immunoassay, enzyme-linked immunosorbent assay (ELISA)

Additional Information The combination of a PG I level <70 μg/L and a PG I:PG II ratio <3.0 was 84.6% sensitive and 73.5% specific for detecting gastric cancer in one large study of 5113 subjects who also underwent endoscopy.[2] The combined detection of *H. pylori* antibodies and decreased serum PG I[3,4,5] is associated with an increased risk of gastric cancer. Increased levels of PG II are associated with *H. pylori* infection;[6,7] however, recent studies vary with regard to whether its measurement or that of the ratio are sufficiently reliable indicators for monitoring success of *H. pylori* treatment.[8,9]

Footnotes

1. Konishi N, Matsumoto K, Hiasa Y, et al, "Tissue and Serum Pepsinogen I and II in Gastric Cancer Identified Using Immunohistochemistry and Rapid ELISA," *J Clin Pathol*, 1995, 48(4):364-7.
2. Kitahara F, Kobayashi K, Sato T, et al, "Accuracy of Screening for Gastric Cancer Using Serum Pepsinogen Concentrations," *Gut*, 1999, 44(5):693-7.
3. Aromaa A, Kosunen TU, Knekt P, et al, "Circulating Anti-*Helicobacter pylori* Immunoglobulin A Antibodies and Low Serum Pepsinogen I Level Are Associated With Increased Risk of Gastric Cancer," *Am J Epidemiol*, 1996, 144(2):142-9.
4. Webb PM, Hengels KJ, Moller H, et al, "The Epidemiology of Low Serum Pepsinogen A Levels and an International Association With Gastric Cancer Rates," *Gastroenterology*, 1994, 107:1335-44.
5. Knight T, Wyatt J, Wilson A, et al, "*Helicobacter pylori* Gastritis and Serum Pepsinogen Levels in a Healthy Population: Development of a Biomarker Strategy for Gastric Atrophy in High-Risk Groups," *Br J Cancer*, 1996, 73(6):819-24.
6. Sarker SA, Mahalanabis D, Hildebrand P, et al, "*Helicobacter pylori*: Prevalence, Transmission, and Serum Pepsinogen II Concentrations in Children of a Poor Periurban Community in Bangladesh," *Clin Infect Dis*, 1997, 25:(5)990-5.
7. Matsumoto K, Konishi N, Ohshima M, et al, "Association Between *Helicobacter pylori* Infection and Serum Pepsinogen Concentrations in Gastroduodenal Disease," *J Clin Pathol*, 1996, 49:1005-8.
8. Al-Assi MT, Miki K, Walsh JH, et al, "Noninvasive Evaluation of *Helicobacter pylori* Therapy: Role of Fasting or Postprandial Gastrin, Pepsinogen I, Pepsinogen II, or Serum IgG Antibodies," *Am J Gastroenterol*, 1999, 94(9):2367-72.
9. Gisbert JP, Boixeda D, Al-Mostafa A, et al, "Basal and Stimulated Gastrin and Pepsinogen Levels After Eradication of *Helicobacter pylori*: A 1-Year Follow-up Study," *Eur J Gastroenterol Hepatol*, 1999, 11(2):189-200.

References

Diamandis EP, Nadkarni S, Bhaumik B, et al, "Immunofluorometric Assay of Pepsinogen C and Preliminary Clinical Applications," *Clin Chem*, 1997, 43(8):1365-71.

Henderson RA and Rinker AD, "Gastric, Pancreatic, and Intestinal Function," *Tietz Textbook of Clinical Chemistry*, 3rd ed, Chapter 36, Burtis CA and Ashwood ER, eds, Philadelphia, PA: WB Saunders Co, 1999, 1271-327.

Kokkola A, Haapiainen R, Laxen F, et al, "Risk of Gastric Carcinoma in Patients With Mucosal Dysplasia Associated With Atrophic Gastritis: A Follow Up Study," *J Clin Pathol*, 1996, 49:979-84.

pH, Blood

Related Information

Synonyms Blood pH

Abstract Blood pH is used to indicate the presence of acidemia or alkalemia.

Specimen Whole blood (arterial, venous, or capillary)

Container Green top (heparin) tube or heparinized syringe

Collection See Arterial Blood Collection *on page 40*, Venous Blood Collection *on page 47*, and Skin Puncture Blood Collection *on page 45*. For a venous sample, it is best to collect without a tourniquet if possible. **Do not allow the patient to clench/unclench his/her hand**, an activity which builds up lactic acid. Draw the specimen into an air-free heparinized syringe with needle quickly stoppered, making sure that no air bubbles remain. Capillary tubes should be filled as much as possible, metal flea inserted, capped, and mixed well with a magnet. All specimens should be on ice and brought to the laboratory immediately. For capillary collection, the skin area to be punctured should be warmed 10-15 minutes. The puncture should be deep enough to allow a free flow of blood.

Storage Instructions Specimen should be analyzed immediately. However, if delay in analysis is unavoidable, the specimen should be placed in a slurry of ice chips and water. Analysis should not be delayed beyond 1 hour. *In vitro* pH will decrease by <0.01 pH unit/hour at 4°C.[1]

Causes for Rejection Specimen with clots, air bubbles, and not properly iced; needle not tightly stoppered

Turnaround Time Usually reported in less than 30 minutes.

Reference Interval Newborns (<2 months), with **arterialized capillary blood** (heel, fingertip, big toe) or arterial blood: 7.32-7.49; 2 months to 2 years, arterialized capillary or arterial blood: 7.34-7.46; children (>2 years) and adults: **arterial:** 7.35-7.45, **venous:** 7.32-7.43. Blood pH can be measured from either arterial or venous blood samples, usually with only very small differences.

Possible Panic Range <7.20, >7.60. Occasionally, patients with acidosis as severe as pH 6.80 survive. Many of these present with diabetic ketoacidosis, for which effective therapy is available.

Use The measurement of pH is used to diagnose acidosis (eg, ketoacidosis) and alkalosis (eg, emesis with loss of gastric juice), and to evaluate acid-base balance; to assess significance of serum or plasma potassium levels (eg, in hypokalemia); and in interpretation of oxyhemoglobin dissociation curves. It may be useful for assessment of birth asphyxia in the depressed newborn.

Blood pH is **increased** with uncompensated metabolic and respiratory alkalosis and **decreased** with uncompensated metabolic and respiratory acidosis.

Limitations pH values are sensitive to sampling technique.

Methodology Glass pH electrode

Additional Information pH should be judged in relation to other measurements such as pCO_2, HCO_3, Na^+, K^+, Cl^-, glucose, ketone bodies, phosphorus, lactic acid, BUN, creatinine, and osmolality of serum and urine. The osmolal gap is addressed in the listing Osmolality, Calculated, Serum or Plasma *on page 234*.

Causes of metabolic acidosis with normal and with increased anion gap are published[2] and are addressed in Anion Gap, Serum, Plasma, or Urine *on page 106*. See Blood Gases and pH, Arterial *on page 119*, and the Key Word Index.

Methanol, ethylene glycol, paraldehyde, salicylate toxicity, diabetic ketoacidosis, alcoholic ketoacidosis, lactic acidosis, renal failure, and starvation are causes of **high anion gap metabolic acidosis**.

Additional to electrolytes and other tests listed above, relevant laboratory findings in acidemia may also include ketones, ethanol concentration, uric acid, albumin, CBC, urinalysis with examination for oxalate crystals, and salicylate concentration.

Hypoproteinemia causes a metabolic alkalosis.[3]

Umbilical artery pH may be useful in the assessment of birth asphyxia[4,5] of the depressed neonate. Others contend that infants must be severely depressed with Apgar scores ≤3 at 1 and 5 minutes to be reflected in a decreased serum pH.[6] Blood may be obtained from a clamped umbilical segment up to 1 hour after delivery.[7] See Blood Gases and pH, Umbilical Cord *on page 121*.

In hypotensive patients, tissue hypoxia may be assessed by measurements of arterial pH, mixed venous pH, and bicarbonate concentrations.[8] Such measurements do not appear to reliably assess tissue hypoxia in patients with fulminant hepatic failure.[9] For such patients, oxygen flux (the difference between arterial and venous oxygen) remains the best way to detect the presence of covert tissue hypoxia.

Footnotes

1. Scott MG, Heusel JW, LeGrys VA, et al, "Electrolytes and Blood Gases," *Tietz Textbook of Clinical Chemistry*, 3rd ed, Chapter 31, Burtis CA and Ashwood ER, eds, Philadelphia, PA: WB Saunders Co, 1999, 1056-92.
2. Narins RG and Emmett M, "Simple and Mixed Acid-Base Disorders: A Practical Approach," *Medicine*, 1980, 59:161-87.
3. McAuliffe JJ, Lind LJ, Leith DE, et al, "Hypoproteinemic Alkalosis," *Am J Med*, 1986, 81(1):86-90.
4. Goldaber KG and Gilstrap LC 3d, "Correlations Between Obstetric Clinical Events and Umbilical Cord Blood Acid-Base and Blood Gas Values," *Clin Obstet Gynecol*, 1993, 36(1):47-59.
5. Blackstone J and Young BK, "Umbilical Cord Blood Acid-Base Values and Other Descriptors of Fetal Condition," *Clin Obstet Gynecol*, 1993, 36(1):33-46.
6. Gilstrap LC 3d, Leveno KJ, Burris J, et al, "Diagnosis of Birth Asphyxia on the Basis of Fetal pH, Apgar Score, and Newborn Cerebral Dysfunction," *Am J Obstet Gynecol*, 1989, 161(3):825-30.

(Continued)

pH, Blood *(Continued)*

7. Duerbeck NB, Chaffin DG, and Seeds JW, "A Practical Approach to Umbilical Artery pH and Blood Gas Determinations," *Obstet Gynecol*, 1992, 79(6):959-62.
8. Adrogué HJ, Rashad MN, Gorin AB, et al, "Assessing Acid-Base Status in Circulatory Failure: Differences Between Arterial and Central Venous Blood," *N Engl J Med*, 1989, 320(20):1312-6.
9. Wendon JA, Harrison PM, Keays R, et al, "Arterial-Venous pH Differences and Tissue Hypoxia in Patients With Fulminant Hepatic Failure," *Crit Care Med*, 1991, 19:(11)1362-4.

References
Adrogué HJ and Madias NE, "Management of Life-Threatening Acid-Base Disorders," First of Two Parts, *N Engl J Med*, 1998, 338(1):26-34, Second of Two Parts, *N Engl J Med*, 1998, 338(2):107-11.
Adrogué HJ, Wilson H, Boyd AE III, et al, "Plasma Acid-Base Patterns in Diabetic Ketoacidosis," *N Engl J Med*, 1982, 307:1603-10.
Brandenburg MA and Dire DJ, "Comparison of Arterial and Venous Blood Gas Values in the Initial Emergency Department Evaluation of Patients With Diabetic Ketoacidosis," *Ann Emerg Med*, 1998, 31(4):459-65.
Hood VL and Tannen RL, "Protection of Acid-Base Balance by pH Regulation of Acid Production," *N Engl J Med*, 1998, 339(12):819-26.
Nicolaides KH, Economides DL, and Soothill PW, "Blood Gases, pH, and Lactate in Appropriate- and Small-for-Gestational-Age Fetuses," *Am J Obstet Gynecol*, 1989, 161(4):996-1001.
Preuss HG, "Fundamentals of Clinical Acid-Base Evaluation," *Clin Lab Med*, 1993, 13(1):103-16.
Scheinman SJ, Guay-Woodford LM, Thakker RV, et al, "Genetic Disorders of Renal Electrolyte Transport," *N Engl J Med*, 1999, 340(15):1177-87.
Shapiro BA, "pH and Blood Gas Measurements: Discerning Innovation From Sophistication," *Crit Care Med*, 1989, 17(9):966.
Shapiro BA, Cane RD, Chomka CM, et al, "Preliminary Evaluation of an Intra-Arterial Blood Gas System in Dogs and Humans," *Crit Care Med*, 1989, 17(5):455-60.
Thorp JA, Sampson JE, Parisi VM, et al, "Routine Umbilical Cord Blood Gas Determinations?" *Am J Obstet Gynecol*, 1989, 161(3):600-5.
Wang F, Butler T, Rabbani GH, et al, "The Acidosis of Cholera: Contributions of Hyperproteinemia, Lactic Acidemia, and Hyperphosphatemia to an Increased Serum Anion Gap," *N Engl J Med*, 1986, 315(25):1591-5.

♦ **pH Body Fluid** *see Body Fluid pH on page 125*

♦ **Phenformin** *see Lactic Acid, Whole Blood or Plasma on page 208*

♦ **Phenistix®** *see Phenylalanine, Urine on page 249*

♦ **Phenylalanine** *see Amino Acids, Urine on page 101*

Phenylalanine, Blood

Related Information
Amino Acids, Plasma *on page 100*
Amino Acids, Urine *on page 101*
Newborn Screen for Phenylketonuria *on page 229*
Newborn Screen for T₄, Filter Paper *on page 230*
Newborn Screen for TSH, Filter Paper *on page 231*
Phenylalanine, Urine *on page 249*

Synonyms Guthrie Test; Hyperphenylalaninemia Screen; Phenylalanine Screening Test, Blood; Phenylketonuria Test; PKU Test

Applies to Biopterin Cofactor Deficiency; Guanosine Triphosphate Cyclohydrolase 1 Deficiency; Pyruvoyl Tetrahydropterin Synthase Deficiency; Tetrahydrobiopterin Cofactor Deficiency

Abstract Autosomal recessive aminoacidopathy due to phenylalanine hydroxylase or biopterin (folic acid constituent) cofactor deficiencies. Detection by low cost dried blood spot screening can result in early treatment, intended to prevent mental retardation. Clinical diversity relates to genetic heterogeneity.

Patient Preparation Newborn should have milk (protein) feeding ideally for 48 hours before testing; sample as late as possible prior to discharge from hospital. Collection is recommended at 4-10 days for low birth weight infants. Antibiotics interfere with the Guthrie test.

Specimen Whole blood, serum or plasma

Container Newborns: PKU test card; screening: filter paper sheet. Pediatrics: Small red top tube, gray top (sodium fluoride) tube or green top (heparin) tube; check with laboratory

Sampling Time With newborn, just before infant is discharged from the nursery

Collection Test card must be labeled with patient's name, date, time, date of birth and time of first milk feeding. In order to obtain accurate tests results for PKU, blood collection should preferably be made when the infant is 48-120 hours of age and has been on a protein feeding for at least 24 hours. Do not oversaturate filter paper. Do not fill circles on one side and then fill circles on reverse side. Do not collect blood with a capillary tube to apply to filter paper. Include information regarding blood transfusions and antibiotics or other medications administered to the infant, which may influence screening test results.

Storage Instructions Newborns: Air dry specimens at room temperature in a horizontal position for at least 2 hours. Do not use hermetically sealed envelopes. Pediatrics: Separate serum and transfer to plastic vial containing 10 mg NaF. (Check with laboratory for other possible specimen requirements.) Separate within 4 hours of collection. Serum or plasma is stable 5 days at 4°C. Care in handling the filter paper specimens is essential, because exposure to extreme heat or light or touching the filter paper portion of the form can cause erroneous test results. Specimens containing contaminants, such as alcohol or other liquids, or antibiotics may not be satisfactory for testing. (See following discussion.) The phenylalanine in filter paper dried blood spots is stable for years when not exposed to environmental extremes.

Causes for Rejection Filter paper not thoroughly saturated, inadequate specimen identification, specimens which are respotted (several drops of blood applied to the same circle), specimens which are QNS (quantity not sufficient). **Cord blood cannot be used. Phenylalanine is not significantly increased at birth.** Blood should not be drawn before milk diet of at least 24 hours prior to sampling, but need to sample before discharge from the nursery may take priority if outpatient sampling is not assured.

Reference Interval ≤2 mg/dL (SI: ≤121 μmol/L) by Guthrie bacterial-inhibition assay; <4 mg/dL (SI: <242 μmol/L) by fluorometry in some laboratories. Positive tests by Guthrie assay should be confirmed by a chemical method (fluorometry or chromatography).

Possible Panic Range ≥4 mg/dL (SI: ≥242 μmol/L) by Guthrie bacterial-inhibition assay. Specific diagnosis after identification of a candidate case (by screening program) requires that plasma levels of phenylalanine be >2 mg/dL (SI: >121 μmol/L) on 2 consecutive days.

Use Evaluate patients for phenylketonuria, monitor therapy with phenylalanine restricted diet

Limitations Cases have been missed because blood phenylalanine was not increased, even after the third day of life.[1] Identification of non-PKU forms of hyperphenylalaninemia (see following information) requires additional testing for tetrahydrobiopterin pathway enzyme defects. **Not all individuals with increased blood phenylalanine have phenylketonuria.** When the infant is tested for PKU before 24 hours of age, there is a 16% chance of missing a positive case. When screened between 24 and 48 hours of birth, there is a 2.2% chance of missing a positive, between 48 and 72 hours, 0.3% chance.

Methodology Guthrie testing (microbiologic inhibition assay) (semiquantitative), gas chromatography-mass spectrometry (GC/MS), high performance liquid chromatography (HPLC), fluorometry, enzymatic, polymerase chain reaction (PCR) for mutation analysis. Because antibiotics interfere with the Guthrie test, many neonatal screening laboratories have switched to fluorometric techniques.

Additional Information Successful detection of phenylketonuria by screening newborns for hyperphenylalaninemia has as its goal the identification of infants subject to central nervous system damage (in particular mental retardation) due to excessive levels of phenylalanine. Once identified, harmful CNS effects can be largely avoided by dietary measures, notably a semisynthetic diet low in phenylalanine. In young PKU patients, the tolerance for dietary phenylalanine (to maintain nontoxic plasma levels) is about 250-550 mg/day. Widespread institution of PKU screening programs, worldwide, is an outstanding public health triumph of the 20th century. Incidence is 1:10,000 to 1:15,000 in the United States, highest in Caucasians. For blacks in Maryland the reported incidence is 1:50,000.[2]

State laws require PKU testing of infants within 28 days or less; in some states, prior to hospital discharge regardless of age. Disease caused by lack of phenylalanine hydroxylase leads to mental retardation if not treated. A second screening should be considered but is not universally mandated in infants whose first test occurred within the first 24 hours of life. Screening generally includes testing for hypothyroidism and in some areas for galactosemia and maple syrup disease. Every effort must be made to assure that immediate diagnosis and treatment is provided for infants with abnormal results.

Presence of hyperphenylalaninemia implies a disorder of phenylalanine hydroxylation (to tyrosine). PKU due to phenylalanine hydroxylase (PAH) deficiency is the common example. However, in addition to PAH, hydroxylation requires oxygen and tetrahydrobiopterin (BH₄) as a cofactor. A defect in the metabolism of BH₄ that results in BH₄ deficiency will impair hydroxylation and result in increased plasma phenylalanine concentrations. In the past 15 years three types of inborn errors of BH₄ metabolism ("atypical PKU") have been identified. Defects in BH₄ synthesis are guanosine triphosphate cyclohydrolase I deficiency and pyruvoyl tetrahydropterin synthase deficiency. The third type of defect involves the regeneration of BH₄ catalyzed by the enzyme dihydropteridine reductase. Experience with treatment of PKU over the past 25 years has shown that some 3% (variable between different populations) fail to respond.[3] These are largely cases of BH₄ cofactor deficiency. There are important differences in therapy between classical PKU and the various BH₄ cofactor deficiencies. "PKU positive" cases (identified as the result of phenylalanine screening tests) should be additionally tested for BH₄ deficiency. Clinical features; urine, blood, and enzyme analyses; prenatal diagnosis; and therapy of BH₄ deficiencies have been reviewed.[3]

Classical PKU is an autosomal recessive disorder. Relatives (eg, siblings) of a PKU homozygote or heterozygote have a 50% to 66.7% probability of being heterozygous for PKU. High performance liquid chromatography and PCR-based methods have been proposed as screening tests for PKU heterozygotes.[4]

To maintain intellectual function, the importance of long-term (eg, beyond 10 years) dietary control of the blood phenylalanine level has been recently re-emphasized.[5,6] Significant phenylalanine hydroxylation *in vivo* in PKU homozygotes has been demonstrated.[7] Such findings suggest significant alternative pathway activity such as tyrosine hydroxylase. Promotion of such latent hydroxylating pathways may eventually lead to therapies which will complement phenylalanine restriction.

Spuriously high blood phenylalanine levels (false positives) may occur with Guthrie test screening due to uninterpretable "clear zone" effect, the result of antibiotics (usually ampicillin). Because of an increase in the number of cases and amounts of the awards in litigation involving PKU screening (usually false-negative cases), vagaries of PKU testing, while uncommon, are of considerable importance and generate comment and innovation.[8,9,10]

Due to interference of antibiotics in the Guthrie test, a number of newborn screening laboratories are using fluorometric techniques. Continuous flow and microplate (Isolab, Inc, Akron, OH) fluorometric methods are available. Performance of Guthrie, microplate, and an enzymatic method was compared and all methods were found to be suitable for newborn PKU screening.[11]

Consult references (below) by Scriver et al and by Güttler et al for review of the genetic/molecular biology of the hyperphenylalaninemias. Clinical heterogeneity of PKU relates to the existence of multiple different mutations in the PAH gene and to combinations of mutations. Such genetic considerations have important implications for therapy and its outcome.

Intrauterine fetal injury results from exposure of the developing fetus to increased intrapartum maternal plasma phenylalanine levels. There is a high incidence of resultant fetal damage including microcephaly, intrauterine growth retardation, mental retardation, and congenital heart disease, as a result of **maternal hyperphenylalaninemia**.[12] Dietary management of mothers identified by newborn screening programs has as its goal the maintenance of near normal maternal phenylalanine levels throughout pregnancy. Treatment at anytime during pregnancy reduces the risk of severity of PKU.[13] In order to retain the achievements of over three decades of early detection and treatment of PKU, increasing attention is being turned to control of maternal hyperphenylalaninemia. The risk of maternal phenylketonuria and hyperphenylalaninemia syndrome is increasing. There is a nearly 100% risk of recurrence if treatment is not given. A number of suggestions have been made to deal with the growing problem of maternal PKU including use of genetic registers.[14]

Gas chromatography-mass spectrometry (GC/MS) and MS/MS have recently become available for newborn screening. These analytical techniques allow rapid and simultaneous screening of more than 30 constituents with high specificity and sensitivity. Due to complexity of these techniques, currently they are not widely used in newborn screening.[15,16,17]

Footnotes

1. Committee on Genetics. American Academy of Pediatrics, "New Issues in Newborn Screening for Phenylketonuria and Congenital Hypothyroidism," *Pediatrics*, 1982, 69:104-6.

2. Hofman KJ, Steel G, Kazazian HH, et al, "Phenylketonuria in U.S. Blacks: Molecular Analysis of the Phenylalanine Hydroxylase Gene," *Am J Hum Genet*, 1991, 48(4):791-8.

3. Matalon R, Michals K, Blau N, et al, "Hyperphenylalaninemia Due to Inherited Deficiencies of Tetrahydrobiopterin," *Advanced Pediatrics*, eds, Barness LA, DeViro DC, Morrow G, et al, Chicago, IL: Year Book Medical Publishers, 1989, 36:67-89.

4. Eisensmith RC, Goltsov AA, and Woo SLC, "A Simple, Rapid, and Highly Informative PCR-Based Procedure for Prenatal Diagnosis and Carrier Screening of Phenylketonuria," *Prenat Diagn*, 1994, 14(12):1113-8.

5. Waisbren SE, Mahon BE, Schnell RR, et al, "Predictors of Intelligence Quotient and Intelligence Quotient Change in Persons Treated for Phenylketonuria Early in Life," *Pediatrics*, 1987, 79(3):351-5.

6. Michals K, Azen C, Acosta P, et al, "Blood Phenylalanine Levels and Intelligence of 10-Year-Old Children With PKU in the National Collaborative Study," *J Am Diet Assoc*, 1988, 88(10):1226-9.

7. Thompson GN and Halliday D, "Significant Phenylalanine Hydroxylation *In Vivo* in Patients With Classical Phenylketonuria," *J Clin Invest*, 1990, 86(1):317-22.

8. Mabry CC, Reid MC, and Kuhn RJ, "A Source of Error in Phenylketonuria Screening," *Am J Clin Pathol*, 1988, 90(3):279-83.

9. Clemens PC and Plettner C, "Phenylketonuria Screening: Avoiding a Source of Error by Simplifying the Procedure," *Am J Clin Pathol*, 1989, 91(6):747.

10. Wilcken B, Brown AR, Liu A, et al, "Eliminating Some Possible Errors in Phenylketonuria Screening," *Am J Clin Pathol*, 1989, 92(3):396.

11. Wang ST, Pizzolato S, and Demshar HP, "Receiver Operating Characteristic Plots to Evaluate Guthrie, Wallac, and Isolab Phenylalanine Kit Performance for Newborn Phenylketonuria Screening," *Clin Chem*, 1997, 43(10):1838-42.

12. Brenton DP, "Cardiac Defects in the Children of Mothers With High Concentrations of Plasma Phenylalanine," *Br Heart J*, 1990, 63(3):143-4.

13. Waisbren SE, Hamley W, and Levy HL, "Outcome at Age 4 Years in Offspring of Women With Maternal Phenylketonuria: The Maternal PKU Collaborative Study," *JAMA*, 2000, 283(6):756-62.

14. Luder AS and Greene CL, "Maternal Phenylketonuria and Hyperphenylalaninemia: Implications for Medical Practice in the United States," *Am J Obstet Gynecol*, 1989, 161(5):1102-5.

15. Chace DH, DiPerna JC, and Naylor EW, "Laboratory Integration and Utilization of Tandem Mass Spectrometry in Neonatal Screening: A Model for Clinical Mass Spectrometry in the Next Millennium," *Acta Paediatr Suppl*, 1999, 88(432):45-7.

16. Levy HL, "Newborn Screening by Tandem Mass Spectrometry: A New Era," *Clin Chem*, 1998, 44(12):2401-2.

17. Sweetman L, "Newborn Screening by Tandem Mass Spectrometry (MS-MS)," *Clin Chem*, 1996, 42(3):345-6.

References

"American Academy of Pediatrics, Committee on Genetics, Newborn Screening Fact Sheets: Phenylketonuria," *Pediatrics*, 1989, 83(3):461-2.

Atherton ND, "HPLC Measurement of Phenylalanine by Direct Injection of Plasma Onto an Internal-Surface Reverse-Phase Silica Support," *Clin Chem*, 1989, 35(6):975-8.

de Freitas O, Izumi C, Lara MG, et al, "New Approaches to the Treatment of Phenylketonuria," *Nutr Rev*, 1999, 57(3):65-70.

Gerasimova NS, Steklova IV, and Tuuminen T, "Fluorometric Method for Phenylalanine Microplate Assay Adapted for Phenylketonuria Screening," *Clin Chem*, 1989, 35(10):2112-5.

Güttler F and Guldberg P, "Mutations in the Phenylalanine Hydroxylase Gene: Genetic Determinants for the Phenotypic Variability of Hyperphenylalaninemia," *Acta Paediatr Suppl*, 1994, 407:49-56.

Koch RK, "Issues in Newborn Screening for Phenylketonuria," *Am Fam Phys*, 1999, 60(5):1462-6.

"Phenylketonuria - Past, Present, Future," Proceedings of a Symposium Held in Elsinore, Denmark, May 23-25, 1994, *Acta Paediatr Scand Suppl*, 407:1-129.

Scriver CR, "Whatever Happened to PKU?" *Clin Biochem*, 1995, 28(2):137-44.

Scriver CR, Kaufman S, Eisensmith RC, et al, "The Hyperphenylalaninemias," *The Metabolic and Molecular Bases of Inherited Disease*, 7th ed, Volume 1, Chapter 27, Scriver CR, Beaudet AL, Sly WS, et al, eds, New York, NY: McGraw-Hill Inc, 1995, 1015-75.

Tessari P, Inchiostro S, Vettore M, et al, "A Fast High Performance Liquid Chromatographic Method for the Measurement of Plasma Concentration and Specific Activity of Phenylalanine," *Clin Biochem*, 1991, 24(5):425-8.

♦ **Phenylalanine Hydroxylase Activity** *see* Newborn Screen for Phenylketonuria *on page 229*

♦ **Phenylalanine Screening Test, Blood** *see* Phenylalanine, Blood *on page 248*

Phenylalanine, Urine

Related Information
Newborn Screen for Phenylketonuria *on page 229*
Phenylalanine, Blood *on page 248*

Synonyms Phenylpyruvic Acid, Urine; PKU, Urine Test

Applies to Ferric Chloride Test; Guthrie Test; Phenistix®; Tyrosyluria

Abstract Hyperphenylalaninemia is a disorder of phenylalanine catabolism, primarily due to deficiency of phenylalanine hydroxylase. Phenylalanine inhibits synthesis of catecholamines and serotonin, resulting in neurological deterioration.

Specimen Freshly voided random urine

Collection Transport specimen to the laboratory within 1 hour of collection. Container must state date and time of collection.

Reference Interval Negative (level of detection with Phenistix® is 5-10 mg/100 mL)

Use Assist in the detection of hyperphenylalaninemia, including phenylalanine hydroxylase deficiency (phenylketonuria, PKU and non-PKU hyperphenylalaninemia), and tetrahydrobiopterin cofactor deficiency.[1] **Urine is not used as an initial screening test for PKU.** See Phenylalanine, Blood *on page 248*. **After birth, 2-6 weeks may pass before phenylpyruvic acid is excreted in the urine.**[2] After the diagnosis of PKU has been established, a urine screening test may be employed to follow adequacy of dietary control, including monitoring of dietary intake of pregnant women who lack phenylalanine hydroxylase.

Limitations Diluted urine may cause false negatives. The urine screening tests may miss a significant number of cases due to interferences and insensitivity. Tyrosyluria, the result of transitory tyrosinemia in prematures due to immaturity of hepatic metabolism, may result in a positive ferric chloride test.

Contraindications The ferric chloride method should not be used to screen newborns for PKU. Its primary use is to monitor dietary adherence in known cases. The level of phenylalanine in the blood is correlated with urine phenylpyruvic acid in older children.

Methodology Screening tests:
- Ferric chloride method - green color
- Phenistix® urine reagent strips (a ferric chloride method) - a persistent blue-gray to gray-green color is produced with phenylpyruvic acid. (Salicylates or phenothiazine derivatives give pink to purple colors.) Tyrosyluria in the premature or newborn due to liver disease will produce a fading green color with ferric chloride screening tests.[2]

Confirmatory tests may be done by one of several methods:
- High voltage electrophoresis followed by chromatography
- Cation exchange column chromatography for plasma and urine phenylalanine quantitation
- More sensitive and specific methods, detecting phenylpyruvic acid in the urine by chemiluminescent or fluorometric techniques.[3] High performance liquid chromatography with fluorescent detection is also used, and can detect the low levels of phenylpyruvic acid in normal adults or newborns.
- Phenylpyruvic acid can be detected by gas chromatography-mass spectrometry during organic acids analysis.

Additional Information The incidence of classic PKU varies considerably in different countries. Mental retardation is the main clinical finding. There are over 200 known mutations at loci of chromosomes that encode components of the phenylalanine hydroxylation reaction.[1] This is the genetic basis for the heterogeneous phenotype of hyperphenylalaninemia. Many mutations result in only transient or variable elevations in blood phenylalanine (Continued)

Phenylalanine, Urine (Continued)

and presence of urine phenylalanine, tyrosine metabolites, or other amino acids. Some are associated with non-PKU hyperphenylalaninemia. Phenylalanine hydroxylase deficient PKU (phenylketonuria) is characterized by impaired postnatal mental and physical development. A blood level of 10-20 mg/dL of phenylpyruvic acid (phenylalanine metabolite) is required to produce a urine level ≥8 mg/dL, which is the approximate threshold of the screening tests. **The Guthrie bacterial inhibition test performed on blood is more sensitive and is the preferred and accepted screening procedure.** Positive results of screening tests should be confirmed by a fluorometric method. **The test should be performed after the newborn has had 24 hours of milk feeding.** A metabolite of acetaminophen, has been reported to interfere with chromatographic analyses identifying phenylalanine.[4]

Monitoring of urinary excretion of phenylalanine metabolites (by gas chromatography/mass spectrometry) to avoid neurotoxic effects in children with PKU has been undertaken with the goal of identifying a range of blood phenylalanine that is associated with normal levels of excretion of such products.[5] The importance of controlling blood phenylalanine levels by diet during pregnancy in women with hyperphenylalaninemia (including those with diagnosed and undiagnosed phenylketonuria) has been emphasized in order to decrease the risk of maternal phenylketonuria syndrome.[6] Treatment at anytime during pregnancy reduces the risk of severity of PKU.[7]

Footnotes

1. Erlandsen H and Stevens RC, "The Structural Basis of Phenylketonuria," *Mol Genet Metab*, 1999, 68(2):103-25.
2. Strasinger SK, *Urinalysis and Body Fluids: A Self Instructional Text*, Philadelphia, PA: FA Davis Co, 1985, 116-9.
3. Sano A, Ogawa M, and Takitani S, "Fluorometric Determination of Phenylpyruvic Acid With 1,4-Dimethyl-3-Carbamoylpyridinium Chloride," *Chem Pharm Bull (Tokyo)*, 1987, 35(9):3746-9.
4. Shih VE, Nikiforov V, and Carney MM, "Acetaminophen Metabolite Interferes in Analysis for Amino Acids," *Clin Chem*, 1985, 31(1):148.
5. Michals K, Lopus M, and Matalon R, "Phenylalanine Metabolites as Indicators of Dietary Compliance in Children With Phenylketonuria," *Biochem Med Metab Biol*, 1988, 39(1):18-23.
6. Luder AS and Greene CL, "Maternal Phenylketonuria and Hyperphenylalaninemia: Implications for Medical Practice in the United States," *Am J Obstet Gynecol*, 1989, 161(5):1102-5.
7. Waisbren SE, Hanley W, Levy HL, et al, "Outcome at Age 4 Years in Offspring of Women With Maternal Phenylketonuria: The Maternal PKU Collaborative Study," *JAMA*, 2000, 283(6):756-62.

References

de Freitas O, Izumi C, Lara MG, et al, "New Approaches to the Treatment of Phenylketonuria," *Nutr Rev*, 1999, 57(3):65-70.

Scriver CR, Kaufman S, and Eisensmith RC, "The Hyperphenylalaninemias," *The Metabolic and Molecular Basis of Inherited Disease*, 7th ed, Chapter 27, Scriver CK, Beaudet AL, Sly WS, et al, eds, New York, NY: McGraw-Hill Inc, 1995, 1015-75.

♦ **Phenylketonuria, Newborn Screen** *see* Newborn Screen for Phenylketonuria *on page 229*

♦ **Phenylketonuria Test** *see* Phenylalanine, Blood *on page 248*

♦ **Phenylpyruvic Acid, Urine** *see* Phenylalanine, Urine *on page 249*

---

pH, Gastric Intramucosal

Related Information

Bicarbonate, Blood *on page 115*
Blood Gases and pH, Arterial *on page 119*
Lactic Acid, Whole Blood or Plasma *on page 208*
pCO₂, Blood *on page 246*
pH, Blood *on page 247*

Synonyms Intramural pH; pH$_i$

Abstract Successful management of critically ill patients often relies upon the detection and treatment of tissue hypoperfusion. Gastric intramucosal pH (pH$_i$) is an indirect indicator of splanchnic hypoxia and is used as an index of therapeutic tissue oxygenation and a predictor of multiorgan dysfunction syndrome. Decreased levels are associated with increased morbidity and mortality in critically ill patients.

Patient Preparation A nasogastric tonometer consisting of a balloon-tip catheter is inserted into the stomach and its position is confirmed radiographically. It is recommended by some that a histamine-2-receptor antagonist be administered and enteral feedings be stopped for the duration of the testing.[1,2] Once inserted the tonometer is filled with 2.5 mL of normal saline solution. The silicone balloon is permeable only to gases and, after proper placement and filling, is allowed to equilibrate for 60 to ≥90 minutes, permitting carbon dioxide (CO_2) produced by the gastric mucosal cells to diffuse across the balloon wall and dissolve in the saline solution.

Specimen After the equilibration period the saline is aspirated anaerobically and submitted to the laboratory for pCO_2 measurement. A concurrent arterial blood specimen is drawn for bicarbonate (HCO_3^-) determination (see Arterial Blood Collection *on page 40*, Blood Gases and pH, Arterial *on page 119*, and Bicarbonate, Blood *on page 115*).

Container Glass or plastic syringe with no anticoagulant for the saline specimen; glass or plastic heparinized blood gas syringe for the arterial blood specimen

Sampling Time The equilibration time should be recorded.

Collection Collection of saline and arterial blood specimens should be done anaerobically. Expel air from syringe tip and seal securely.

Storage Instructions Analysis should be done immediately. However, if delay in analysis of more than 10-15 minutes is unavoidable or otherwise anticipated, place specimens in a slurry of ice chips and water. Delay of analysis should not exceed 1 hour.

Causes for Rejection Air bubbles in syringes, unsealed/open syringes, specimen incorrectly iced

Special Instructions The equilibration time should be noted on the requisition as it affects the calculation of pH$_i$.

Reference Interval pH$_i$ ≥7.32

Critical Values A pH$_i$ result <7.32 has been shown to have a sensitivity of 89% and a specificity of 77% for predicting early mortality in critically ill adult patients.[3] This threshold also predicts mortality in children ages 1 month to 16 years of age.[4]

Use The test is used as an assessment of the adequacy of systemic tissue oxygenation, which is an indicator of prognosis in critically ill patients.[3,5] Monitoring pH$_i$ is useful for guiding treatment to increase systemic O_2 transport or to reduce O_2 demand when the pH$_i$ drops into the critical range.[6]

Limitations Since standard blood gas instrumentation is designed for analyses of whole blood specimens, pCO_2 measurements in a matrix of saline may be unreliable.[7,8,9] Takala et al[7] showed that saline pCO_2 measurement can be an important source of error in pH$_i$ measurement, depending upon the blood gas instrument in use and the pCO_2 level, and that only changes in pH$_i$ ≥0.06 are clinically meaningful given the accuracy and precision observed from their study. Some blood gas instruments significantly underestimate the pCO_2 in the saline specimen and should not be used.

The pH$_i$ reflects not only mucosal perfusion but also metabolic abnormalities and is, therefore, affected unpredictably by therapy with vasoactive drugs[10] and should not be used to guide resuscitation efforts.[11]

The assumption that the arterial HCO_3^- accurately reflects the mucosal HCO_3^- has recently been brought into question, and its use has been shown to cause underestimations of pH$_i$.[12]

Methodology The pH$_i$ is monitored by gas tonometry. The tonometer consists of a balloon-tip catheter positioned in the stomach and inflated with saline solution. Carbon dioxide (CO_2) produced by the mucosal cells of the stomach diffuses through the balloon wall, dissolving in the saline solution. After an equilibration period, the saline is aspirated, and the pCO_2 of the saline specimen is measured. The measured pCO_2 is adjusted to a steady-state value, using a correction factor derived from the equilibration interval. The pH$_i$ is calculated, using the arterial blood bicarbonate (HCO_3^-) concentration and the Henderson-Hasselbalch equation. Continuous monitoring with capnometric recirculating gas tonometric devices[13] and fiberoptic CO_2 sensors[14] have been described.

Additional Information Other methods for assessing adequate tissue perfusion include hemodynamic monitors, systemic indicators of oxygen transport, capillary filling time, central-peripheral temperature difference, urine output, arterial pH, and lactic acid measurements.

Footnotes

1. Marik PE and Lorenzana A, "Effect of Tube Feedings on the Measurement of Gastric Intramucosal pH," *Crit Care Med*, 1996, 24(9):1498-1500.
2. Heard SO, Helsmoortel CM, Kent JC, et al, "Gastric Tonometry in Healthy Volunteers: Effect of Ranitidine on Calculated Intramural pH," *Crit Care Med*, 1991, 19(2):271-4.
3. Gutierrez G, Bismar H, Dantzker DR, et al, "Comparison of Gastric Intramucosal pH With Measures of Oxygen Transport and Consumption in Critically Ill Patients," *Crit Care Med*, 1992, 20(4):451-7.
4. Casado-Flores J, Mora E, Perez-Corral F, et al, "Prognostic Value of Gastric Intramucosal pH in Critically Ill Children," *Crit Care Med*, 1998, 26(6):1123-7.
5. Marik PE, "Gastric Intramucosal pH. A Better Predictor of Multiorgan Dysfunction Syndrome and Death Than Oxygen-Derived Variables in Patients With Sepsis," *Chest*, 1993, 104(1):225-9.
6. Gutierrez G, Palizas F, Doglio G, et al, "Gastric Intramucosal pH as a Therapeutic Index of Tissue Oxygenation in Critically Ill Patients," *Lancet*, 1992, 339(8787):195-9.
7. Takala J, Parviainen I, Siloaho M, et al, "Saline pCO_2 Is an Important Source of Error in the Assessment of Gastric Intramucosal pH," *Crit Care Med*, 1994, 22(11):1877-9.
8. Riddington D, Venkatesh B, Clutton-Brock T, et al, "Potential Hazards in Estimation of Gastric Intramucosal pH," *Lancet*, 1992, 340(8818):547.
9. Guzman JA, Sobek SB, and Kruse JA, "Accuracy and Precision of Saline pCO_2 Assay Using Blood Gas Analyzers: Implications for Clinical Assessment of Gastric Intramucosal pH by Tonometry," *Crit Care Med*, 1996, 24(1 Suppl):A59.
10. Silva E, DeBacker D, Creteur J, et al, "Effects of Vasoactive Drugs on Gastric Intramucosal pH," *Crit Care Med*, 1998, 26(10):1749-58.
11. Gomersall CD, Joynt GM, Freebairn RC, et al, "Resuscitation of Critically Ill Patients Based on the Results of Gastric Tonometry: A Prospective, Randomized, Controlled Trial," *Crit Care Med*, 2000, 28(3):607-14.
12. Morgan TJ, Venkatesh B, and Endre ZH, "Accuracy of Intramucosal pH Calculated From Arterial Bicarbonate and the Henderson-Hasselbalch Equation: Assessment Using Simulated Ischemia," *Crit Care Med*, 1999, 27(11):2495-9.
13. Guzman JA and Kruse JA, "Continuous Assessment of Gastric Intramucosal pCO_2 and pH in Hemorrhagic Shock Using Capnometric Recirculating Gas Tonometry," *Crit Care Med*, 1997, 25(3):533-7.
14. Knichwitz G, Rotker J, Mollhoff T, et al, "Continuous Intramucosal pCO_2 Measurement Allows the Early Detection of Intestinal Malperfusion," *Crit Care Med*, 1998, 26(9):1550-7.

References

Carcillo JA, "Can Gastric Intramucosal pH Measurement Be Useful in Pediatric Critical Illness?" *Crit Care Med*, 1998, 26(6):999-1000.

Chang MC, Cheatham ML, Nelson LD, et al, "Gastric Tonometry Supplements Information Provided by Systemic Indicators of Oxygen Transport," *J Trauma*, 1994, 37(3):488-94.

Elizalde JI, Hernandez C, Llach J, et al, "Gastric Intramucosal Acidosis in Mechanically Ventilated Patients: Role of Mucosal Blood Flow," *Crit Care Med*, 1998, 26(5):827-32.

Gys T, Hubens A, Neels H, et al, "Prognostic Value of Gastric Intramural pH in Surgical Intensive Care Patients," *Crit Care Med*, 1988, 16(12):1222-4.

Maynard N, Bihari D, Beale R, et al, "Assessment of Splanchnic Oxygenation by Gastric Tonometry in Patients With Acute Circulatory Failure," *JAMA*, 1993, 270(10):1203-10.

Perez A, Schnitzler EJ, and Minces PG, "The Value of Gastric Intramucosal pH in the Postoperative Period of Cardiac Surgery in Pediatric Patients," *Crit Care Med*, 2000, 28(5):1585-9.

♦ **pH$_i$** *see* pH, Gastric Intramucosal *on page 250*

♦ **Phosphatase, Acid** *see* Acid Phosphatase, Plasma *on page 82*

♦ **Phosphatase, Alkaline** *see* Alkaline Phosphatase, Serum *on page 93*

♦ **Phosphate, Blood** *see* Phosphorus, Serum *on page 251*

♦ **Phosphatidylglycerol** *see* Lecithin:Sphingomyelin Ratio, Amniotic Fluid *on page 210*

Phosphatidylglycerol, Amniotic Fluid

Related Information
Creatinine, Amniotic Fluid *on page 160*
Lamellar Bodies, Amniotic Fluid *on page 454*
Lecithin:Sphingomyelin Ratio, Amniotic Fluid *on page 210*
Pulmonary Surfactant, Amniotic Fluid *on page 271*

Synonyms Amniotic Fluid Phosphatidylglycerol

Abstract Amniotic fluid (AF) phospholipid testing assesses fetal lung maturity from which physicians infer the probability of respiratory distress syndrome (RDS)/hyaline membrane disease in the neonate. Phosphatidylglycerol (PG), a component of pulmonary surfactant, first appears in the AF at 35-36 weeks gestation. The **accurate** determination of its presence in AF is highly predictive of fetal lung maturity.[1,2] The most important facet of management of hyaline membrane disease is prevention of prematurity. AF testing supports avoidance, when possible, of suboptimal timing of caesarean section.

Aftercare All nonsensitized Rh-negative patients should receive anti-D immunoglobulin after amniocentesis.

Specimen Amniotic fluid; the detection of PG is unaffected by blood or meconium contamination.[2]

Collection Ultrasound-guided, transabdominal amniocentesis is performed by the physician. Vaginal pool specimens are discouraged.

Storage Instructions The specimen should be centrifuged at low speed in a refrigerated centrifuge. The supernatant may be stored at 4°C for up to 10 days or it may be frozen indefinitely.

Special Instructions Fetal sacs of multiple pregnancies should be sampled and analyzed individually.[3] Send sample(s) to the laboratory **immediately** after collection.

Reference Interval
• Mature: PG present
• Immature: PG absent

The predictive value of a mature result is virtually 100%, whereas the predictive value of an immature result ranges from 30% to 50%.[2,4]

Use Determination of the presence or absence of PG in AF is done prior to delivery to assess the likelihood of hyaline membrane disease (RDS) development in the newborn. Results are used to determine the optimal time for obstetrical intervention in cases of possible fetal distress due to maternal diabetes, preeclampsia/toxemia, hemolytic disease of the newborn, or postmaturity.

Limitations Thin-layer chromatographic (TLC) methods are technically difficult, labor intensive, not automated, and require experienced interpretation. In addition, comigrating substances in TLC methods can interfere with accurate PG identification. Immunoagglutination testing improves analytical specificity and turnaround time. However, false-positive PG results due to normal vaginal flora may occur in vaginal pool specimens regardless of analytical method.[5,6]

Methodology PG can be detected by rapid immunologic agglutination and enzymatic assays,[7] as well as by more time-consuming and technically-demanding TLC methods.[1]

Additional Information The incidence of RDS at ≥37 weeks gestation is extremely low in most pregnancies (with the exception of poorly controlled maternal diabetic pregnancies), whereas the incidence of RDS risk becomes significantly high at ≤34 weeks. Consequently, fetal lung maturity testing is most useful in reliably dated, high-risk pregnancies that would benefit from early delivery during the 34-37 week gestational period.[2]

The measurement of PG has been used to enhance the diagnostic accuracy of the L:S ratio (see Lecithin:Sphingomyelin Ratio, Amniotic Fluid *on page 210*), especially in uncontrolled diabetic gestations.

With the availability of rapid tests for PG and other rapid tests for assessing fetal lung maturity (see Pulmonary Surfactant, Amniotic Fluid *on page 271*), cascade-testing approaches have been suggested to minimize the cost, time, and effort of performing L:S ratios.[2,8]

Footnotes

1. Kulovich MV, Hallman MB, and Gluck L, "The Lung Profile. I. Normal Pregnancy," *Am J Obstet Gynecol*, 1979, 135(1):57-63.

2. Dubin SB, "Assessment of Fetal Lung Maturity Practice Parameter," *Am J Clin Pathol*, 1998, 110(6):723-32.

3. Whitworth NS, Magann EF, and Morrison JC, "Evaluation of Fetal Lung Maturity in Diamniotic Twins," *Am J Obstet Gynecol*, 1999, 180(6 Pt 1):1438-41.

4. "ACOG Educational Bulletin, Assessment of Fetal Lung Maturity, Number 230, November 1996," *Int J Gynecol Obstet*, 1997, 56(2):191-8.

5. Lambers DS, Brady K, Leist PA, et al, "Ability of Normal Vaginal Flora to Produce Detectable Phosphatidylglycerol in Amniotic Fluid *In Vitro*," *Obstet Gynecol*, 1995, 85(5):651-5.

6. Pastorek JG, Letellier RL, and Gebbia K, "Production of Phosphatidylglycerol-Like Substance by Genital Flora Bacteria," *Am J Obstet Gynecol*, 1988, 159(1):199-202.

7. Eisenbrey AB, Epstein E, Zak B, et al, "Phosphatidylglycerol in Amniotic Fluid. Comparison of an "Ultrasensitive" Immunologic Assay With TLC and Enzymatic Assay," *Am J Clin Pathol*, 1989, 91(3):293-7.

8. Ashwood ER, "Standards of Laboratory Practice: Evaluation of Fetal Lung Maturity," *Clin Chem*, 1997, 43(1):211-4.

References

Berkowitz K, Reyes C, Saadat P, et al, "Fetal Lung Maturation. Comparison of Biochemical Indices in Gestational Diabetic and Nondiabetic Pregnancies," *J Reprod Med*, 1997, 42(12):793-800.

Field NT and Gilbert WM, "Current Status of Amniotic Fluid Tests of Fetal Maturity," *Clin Obstet Gynecol*, 1997, 40(2):366-86.

Garite TJ, Freeman RK, and Nageotte MP, "Fetal Maturity Cascade: A Rapid and Cost-Effective Method for Fetal Lung Maturity Testing," *Obstet Gynecol*, 1986, 67(5):619-22.

Piper JM, Samueloff A, and Langer O, "Outcome of Amniotic Fluid Analysis and Neonatal Respiratory Status in Diabetic and Nondiabetic Pregnancies," *J Reprod Med*, 1995, 40(11):780-4.

Saad SA, Fadel HE, Fahmy K, et al, "The Reliability and Clinical Use of a Rapid Phosphatidylglycerol Assay in Normal and Diabetic Pregnancies," *Am J Obstet Gynecol*, 1987, 157(6):1516-20.

Shaver DC, Spinnato JA, Whybrew D, et al, "Comparison of Phospholipids in Vaginal and Amniocentesis Specimens of Patients With Premature Rupture of Membranes," *Am J Obstet Gynecol*, 1987, 156(2):454-7.

Stoll BJ and Kliegman RM, "The Fetus and the Neonatal Infant," Part XI, Section 1, "Hyaline Membrane Disease," *Nelson Textbook of Pediatrics*, 16th ed, Behrman RE, Kliegman RM, and Jenson HB, eds, Philadelphia, PA: WB Saunders Co, 2000, 498-505.

Strassner HT Jr, Golde SH, Mosley GH, et al, "Effect of Blood in Amniotic Fluid on the Detection of Phosphatidylglycerol," *Am J Obstet Gynecol*, 1980, 138(6):697-702.

Teng SH, Andrews AG, and Horacek I, "Rapid Enzyme Analysis of Amniotic Fluid Phospholipids Containing Choline: A Comparison With the Lecithin to Sphingomyelin Ratio in Prenatal Assessment of Fetal Lung Maturity," *J Clin Pathol*, 1985, 38(11):1304-8.

Towers CV and Garite TJ, "Evaluation of the New Amniostat-FLM Test for the Detection of Phosphatidylglycerol in Contaminated Fluids," *Am J Obstet Gynecol*, 1989, 160(2):298-303.

♦ **Phosphatidylinositol** *see* Lecithin:Sphingomyelin Ratio, Amniotic Fluid *on page 210*

♦ **Phospholipid Profile, Amniotic Fluid** *see* Lecithin:Sphingomyelin Ratio, Amniotic Fluid *on page 210*

♦ **Phosphopyruvate Hydratase** *see* Neuron-Specific Enolase, Serum *on page 229*

Phosphorus, Serum

Related Information
Amino Acids, Urine *on page 101*
Anion Gap, Serum, Plasma, or Urine *on page 106*
Calcium, Serum *on page 131*
Ethanol, Blood, Urine, and Other Sources *on page 789*
Ketone Bodies, Blood *on page 205*
Kidney Stone Analysis *on page 877*
Lactic Acid, Whole Blood or Plasma *on page 208*
Parathyroid Hormone, Serum *on page 243*
Vitamin D, Serum *on page 300*

Synonyms Phosphate, Blood

Abstract Of total body phosphate, <1% exists in plasma. Most is in bone, then in striated muscle. Phosphorus plays a pivotal role in cell physiology. Its metabolism is regulated principally by the renal tubules. With exclusion of factitious types of hyperphosphatemia, causes of increased phosphate include diminished glomerular filtration, increased absorption in the renal tubules, and/or increased exogenous or endogenous phosphate loads. Hypophosphatemia and its complications are outlined. The expression, "phosphate depletion", indicates diminution of total body phosphates, secondary to impaired absorption or urinary wasting.

Patient Preparation Ideally, patient should be fasting. Phosphate levels may fluctuate following meals.

Specimen Serum

Container Red top tube

(Continued)

Phosphorus, Serum (Continued)

Sampling Time A mean diurnal variation 0.6 ±0.1 mg/dL nadirs about 11 AM, plateaus about 4 PM, and peaks at 12:30 AM.[1]

Collection Pediatrics: Blood drawn from heelstick for capillary

Storage Instructions Serum should be promptly separated from the clot to avoid false elevations. Avoid overheating.

Causes for Rejection Observable hemolysis

Reference Interval Both low and high ends of the normal range are higher in children than in adults. Infants: 4.5-7.5 mg/dL (SI: 1.45-2.42 mmol/L). Children: ~4.0-6.0 mg/dL (SI: 1.29-1.94 mmol/L). Adults: 2.5-4.5 mg/dL (SI: 0.81-1.45 mmol/L). Some variation in reference interval exists among authorities.

Possible Panic Range <1.0 mg/dL is critical; <1.5 mg/dL indicates severe hypophosphatemia.

Use Serum phosphorus is commonly analyzed, because abnormalities in phosphate concentration can jeopardize life.

Causes of **high phosphorus:** Youth; exercise; dehydration and hypovolemia; high phosphorus content enema; acromegaly; hypoparathyroidism; pseudohypoparathyroidism; bone metastases; hypervitaminosis D; sarcoidosis; milk-alkali syndrome; liver disease, such as portal cirrhosis; catastrophic events such as cardiac resuscitation, pulmonary embolism, renal failure; diabetes mellitus with ketosis; serum artifact - sample not refrigerated; overheated, hemolyzed sample, or serum allowed to remain too long on the clot. Thrombocytosis causes elevated serum concentrations, but plasma phosphate remains unaltered.[2]

Although phosphate accumulation occurs as renal disease progresses, hyperphosphatemia is not a feature of early renal failure; it does not usually develop before renal function has diminished to about 25% of normal.[3] Osteitis fibrosa in uremic subjects, from excessive bone turnover, relates to hyperparathyroidism.

Causes of **low phosphorus:** Hypophosphatemia may occur with or without phosphate depletion, but clinically relevant hypophosphatemia is usually found in subjects with phosphate depletion. (Starvation is among the exceptions to this generalization.[1]) Serum levels vary as much as 2.0 mg/dL (SI: 0.65 mmol/L) during the day.

Antacids (especially those containing aluminum), diuretics, and long-term steroids are among common agents bearing a relationship to severe hypophosphatemia.[4] Recent carbohydrate ingestion decreases phosphorus, as does intravenous glucose administration; cases of hypophosphatemia relate to I.V. carbohydrate,[4] dialysis, hyperalimentation, prolonged intravenous administration of phosphate-free fluids, metabolic states involving glucose, potassium, and pH. The hypophosphatemic refeeding syndrome includes situations, such as prolonged intravenous hydration, in which patients are provided large quantities with inadequate amounts of phosphate.[1] Depletion of phosphate occurs in diabetic ketoacidosis. Like potassium, phosphorus returns to the cell with therapy of diabetic ketoacidosis, and serum levels may diminish significantly during treatment. Osmotic diuresis induced by glycosuria in poorly controlled diabetes may lead to urinary phosphate losses with negative phosphorus balance. Phosphate levels may prove useful in initiation of insulin therapy, in diabetic ketoacidosis and other situations of insulin lack; with hyperglucagonemia, corticosteroid and epinephrine use, and in respiratory alkalosis. Association of hypophosphatemia with impaired glucose metabolism is recognized. Alcoholism and other hepatic disorders are found very frequently among patients with low phosphate. Alcoholic ketosis and alcohol withdrawal are among causes of hypophosphatemia. There is a slight decrease in serum phosphorus in the last trimester of pregnancy.

Primary hyperparathyroidism and other causes of calcium elevation, including humoral hypercalcemia of malignancy.

Tumoral calcinosis, a form of soft tissue calcification, may be found with severe hyperparathyroidism.

Patients with sepsis, including Legionnaires' disease and other respiratory infections. Twenty-two percent of instances of respiratory infections had serum phosphorous ≤2.4 mg/dL. Halevy and Bulvik report gram-negative septicemia as a common cause of severe hypophosphatemia among 55,000 chemistry profiles of hospitalized patients they studied.[4] (Hypophosphatemia impairs bactericidal activity).

Vitamin D deficiency; osteomalacia, inherited and sporadic forms of hypophosphatemic rickets. In work-up for osteomalacia, look for decreased calcium and phosphorus and increased alkaline phosphatase. Biopsy, however, can be abnormal even when these biochemical parameters are within normal limits.

Renal tubular disorders (Fanconi syndrome, renal tubular acidosis); use of antacids that bind phosphorus (look for hypercalciuria, low urinary phosphorus, high alkaline phosphatase); dialysis; vomiting; saline or lactate I.V.; steatorrhea, malabsorption, severe diarrhea, nasogastric suction; hypokalemia; negative nitrogen balance, including starvation (very severely malnourished subjects may have low phosphate levels, but even in starvation, phosphorus levels usually are normal); other considerations include decreased dietary phosphate intake; recovery from severe burn injury; salicylate poisoning; acute gout; tumor-related: described as including hemangiopericytomas (uncommon pathologic entities) and neurofibromatosis; transfusion of blood; arteriography.

Low serum phosphate may be found in postoperative patients. It can be observed after renal transplantation due to hyperactive parathyroid glands or renal phosphate leak.

Hypophosphatemia can be caused by respiratory alkalosis.

The signs and symptoms of phosphate depletion may include neuromuscular, neuropsychiatric, gastrointestinal, skeletal, and cardiopulmonary systems. Manifestations usually are accompanied by serum levels <1.0 mg/dL (SI: <0.32 mmol/L).

Tumor-induced osteomalacia (oncogenic osteomalacia) is a rare entity in which hypophosphatemia, hyperphosphaturia, low 1,25-dihydroxy-vitamin D and rickets or osteomalacia are reversed with removal of the tumor.[5]

Severe hypophosphatemia is most common in elderly patients and is often found in postoperative subjects.[4]

Complications of hypophosphatemia: Effect on RBC 2,3-diphosphoglycerate and oxygen dissociation. Depression of myocardial function (contractibility), decreased cardiac output; respiratory failure and respiratory muscle weakness; increased incidence of sepsis, impairment of bactericidal activities.[6] CNS consequences: polyradiculopathy, paresthesias, tremor, ataxia, weakness, slurred speech, stupor, coma, seizure; joint stiffness; myopathy; renal stones, hypercalciuria secondary to renal phosphate leak; insulin resistance, glucose intolerance. Rhabdomyolysis may complicate marked hypophosphatemia. A mortality rate of 20% is described in patients whose phosphorus concentration was 1.1-1.5 mg/dL (SI: 0.36-0.48 mmol/L).[4]

Manifestations of Hypophosphatemia[1]

- Musculoskeletal: chronic myopathy, rhabdomyolysis, osteopenia, osteomalacia
- Cardiovascular: cardiomyopathy, arrhythmias
- Pulmonary: respiratory failure, failure of weaning ventilator support
- Neurologic: delirium, seizures, encephalopathy, hallucinations, peripheral neuropathy
- Hematologic: impaired oxygen release, hemolysis, leukocyte dysfunction
- Metabolic: metabolic acidosis, glucose intolerance

Limitations Ninety-seven percent of hyperparathyroid subjects with normal renal function have <3.3 mg/dL serum phosphate, 80% <3.0 mg/dL and 40% <2.5 mg/dL. Collection of multiple data points throughout the day may help to establish the diagnosis of primary hyperparathyroidism in patients with borderline serum biochemistries.[7] Thus, some hyperparathyroid patients have serum phosphorus levels within normal limits. Hemolysis, glassware contaminated with detergents, hyperbilirubinemia, or dysproteinemia may cause increased results. Spurious hyperphosphatemia may be due to increased serum triglycerides. Phosphorus measurement on the Du Pont aca® was reported to be low with I.V. mannitol administration. Falsely elevated serum phosphate concentrations have been reported in patients with multiple myeloma using a molybdate colorimetric assay on the Hitachi® 717.[8] Other **drug effects**, including analytical and physiologic/pharmacologic effects, have been summarized. They include acetazolamide, albuterol, alendronate, aluminum hydroxide and salts, anabolic steroids, anesthetic agents, anticonvulsants, azathioprine, ascorbic acid, aldatense, cefotaxime, cidofovir, cisplatin, ergocalciferol, etidronate, etretinate, fluosol-DA, foscarnet, fosphenytoin, furosemide, gallium nitrate, hydrochlorothiazide, 1-α-hydroxy vitamin D, insulin, isoniazid, lithium, mannitol, medroxyprogesterone, methyltestosterone, mestranol, nafarelin, niacin, nicardipine, oral contraceptives, pamidronate, phenothiazine, Phospho®-Soda, primidone, promethazine, and tacrolimus.[9]

Contraindications Sampling not long after a phosphorus-containing enema can provide startlingly high phosphate levels.

Methodology Phosphomolybdate - colorimetric; modified molybdate - enzymatic, colorimetric[8]

Additional Information Increasing dietary intake of potassium has been reported to increase serum phosphate concentrations apparently by decreasing renal excretion of phosphate.[10] During the last trimester of pregnancy, there is a sixfold increase in calcium and phosphorus accumulation as the fetus triples its weight. Plasma phosphorus concentrations may provide a useful means to assess response to phosphate supplements in the premature infant.[11] Control of serum phosphorus in dialysis patients is a complex topic which includes nutritional needs with protein intake.[12]

Footnotes

1. Subramanian R and Khardori R, "Severe Hypophosphatemia: Pathophysiologic Implications, Clinical Presentations, and Treatment," *Medicine*, 2000, 79(1):1-8.
2. Lutomski DM and Bower RH, "The Effect of Thrombocytosis on Serum Potassium and Phosphorus Concentrations," *Am J Med Sci*, 1994, 307(4):255-8.
3. Coburn JW and Salusky IB, "Control of Serum Phosphorus in Uremia," *N Engl J Med*, 1989, 320(17):1140-2.
4. Halevy J and Bulvik S, "Severe Hypophosphatemia in Hospitalized Patients," *Arch Intern Med*, 1988, 148(1):153-5.
5. Cai Q, Hodgson SF, Kao PC, et al, "Brief Report: Inhibition of Renal Phosphate Transport by a Tumor Product in a Patient With Oncogenic Osteomalacia," *N Engl J Med*, 1994, 330(23):1645-9.
6. Knochel JP, "The Pathophysiology and Clinical Characteristics of Severe Hypophosphatemia," *Arch Intern Med*, 1977, 137(2):203-20.
7. Lobaugh B, Neelon FA, Oyama H, et al, "Circadian Rhythms for Calcium, Inorganic Phosphorus, and Parathyroid Hormone in Primary Hyperparathyroidism: Functional and Practical Considerations," *Surgery*, 1989, 106(6):1009-16.

8. Bakker AJ, Bosma H, and Christen PJ, "Influence of Monoclonal Immunoglobulins in Three Different Methods for Inorganic Phosphorus," *Ann Clin Biochem*, 1990, 27(Pt 3):227-31.

9. Young DS, *Effects of Drugs on Clinical Laboratory Tests*, 5th ed, Volume 1: Listing by Test, Washington, DC: AACC Press, American Association of Clinical Chemistry, 2000, Section 3, 616-21.

10. Sebastian A, Hernandez RE, Portale AA, et al, "Dietary Potassium Influences Kidney Maintenance of Serum Phosphorus Concentration," *Kidney Int*, 1990, 37(5):1341-9.

11. Mayne PD and Kovar IZ, "Calcium and Phosphorus Metabolism in the Premature Infant," *Ann Clin Biochem*, 1991, 28(Pt 2):131-42.

12. Delmez JA and Slatopolsky E, "Hyperphosphatemia: Its Consequences and Treatment in Patients With Chronic Renal Disease," *Am J Kidney Dis*, 1992, 19(4):303-17.

References

Alon US and Chan JCM, *Phosphate in Pediatric Health and Disease*, Boca Raton: CRC Press, 1993.

Bourke E and Yanagawa M, "Assessment of Hyperphosphatemia and Hypophosphatemia," *Clin Lab Med*, 1993, 13(1):183-207.

DeVizia B and Mansi A, "Calcium and Phosphorus Metabolism in Full-Term Infants," *Monatsschr Kinderheilkd*, 1992, 140(9 Suppl 1):S8-12.

Econs MJ and Drezner MK, "Tumor-Induced Osteomalacia - Unveiling a New Hormone," *N Engl J Med*, 1994, 330(23):1679-81 (editorial).

Hodgson SF and Hurley DL, "Acquired Hypophosphatemia," *Endocrinol Metab Clin North Am*, 1993, 22(2):397-409.

Laaban JP, Waked M, Laromiguiere M, et al, "Hypophosphatemia Complicating Management of Acute Severe Asthma," *Ann Intern Med*, 1990, 112(1):68-9.

Loghman-Adham M, "Role of Phosphate Retention in the Progression of Renal Failure," *J Lab Clin Med*, 1993, 122(1):16-26.

Root AW and Diamond FB Jr, "Disorders of Calcium and Phosphorus Metabolism in Adolescents," *Endocrinol Metab Clin North Am*, 1993, 22(3):573-92.

Phosphorus, Urine

Related Information

Calcitonin, Serum or Plasma *on page 129*
Calcium, Serum *on page 131*
Calcium, Urine *on page 133*
Growth Hormone, Serum *on page 189*
Kidney Stone Analysis *on page 877*
Parathyroid Hormone, Serum *on page 243*
Parietal Cell Antibody *on page 541*
Urine Collection, 24-Hour *on page 47*

Synonyms Urine Phosphorus

Test Includes Phosphorus on random or timed urine specimen

Abstract Urinary phosphorus helps in evaluation of calcium/phosphorus balance.

Specimen Timed or random urine. Diurnal variation exists.

Storage Instructions Refrigerate. Laboratory adjusts final pH of urine aliquot to 6.

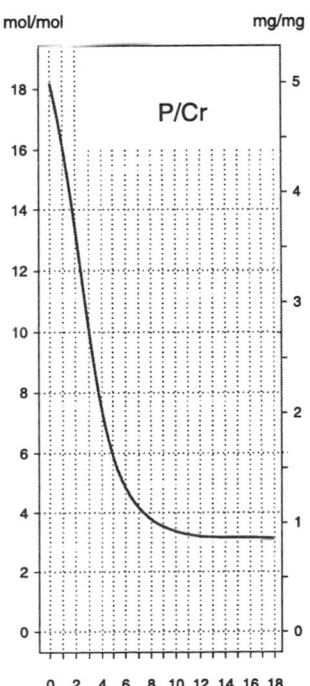

Estimated 95th percentiles for urinary P/Cr ratios in relation to age.

Reference Interval Adults: 0.9-1.3 g/24 hours (SI: 29-42 mmol/day), dependent on dietary intake. In children, between the ages of 0-6 years, an inverse correlation exists between urine phosphate:creatinine ratio and age. The upper limit of normal then stabilizes around the value of 1.0.[1] See graphic.

Use Evaluate calcium/phosphorus balance. **High** urinary phosphorus (ie, increased renal losses) occurs in primary hyperparathyroidism, vitamin D deficiency, renal tubular acidosis, diuretic use. Phosphates are among the substances which may be lost in the Fanconi syndrome and other proximal tubular abnormalities. Renal loss of phosphate may lead to rickets or osteomalacia. **Low** in malnutrition, hypoparathyroidism, pseudohypoparathyroidism, and vitamin D intoxication.

Effects on Phosphorus Transport

Atrial natriuretic peptide	↓
Calcitonin	↓
Glucocorticoid	↑
Growth hormone	↑
Insulin-like growth factor-I	↑
Metabolic acidosis (chronic)	↓
Metabolic alkalosis	↑
Parathyroid hormone	↓
Parathyroid hormone-related peptide (HHM factor)	↓
Phosphorus supply	↑ or ↓
Vasopressin	↓
Vitamin D	↑
Volume expansion	↓

Adapted from Hruska KA, "Phosphate Balance and Metabolism," *The Principles and Practice of Nephrology*, Chapter 19, Jacobson HR, Striker GE, and Klahr S, eds, Philadelphia, PA: Mosby-Year Book Inc, 1991, 122.

Evaluate nephrolithiasis. Hypophosphatemia with normal serum calcium, high alkaline phosphatase, hypercalciuria, low urinary phosphorus occurs with osteomalacia from excessive antacid ingestion. Observations of renal phosphate excretion have led to the classical theory of a maximal transport capacity (T_m). By this model, phosphate is reabsorbed to a maximum rate after which phosphate appears in the urine once the T_m is exceeded. The T_m can be calculated by simultaneously measuring random urine and serum phosphate and creatinine. Mechanisms and effectors of tubular phosphate reabsorption are described.[2] The table lists some important effectors of phosphate transport in the proximal nephron. Largely, however, urine phosphate simply reflects phosphate intake in patients not on phosphate-binding medications.

Limitations A number of drugs and chemicals alter phosphate excretion, including aluminum salts, diltiazem, phloridzin, acetazolamide, asparaginase, aspirin, bicarbonate, calcitonin, corticosteroids, dihydrotachysterol, hydrochlorothiazide, mercurial diuretics, metolazone, and orthophosphate.[3]

Methodology Enzymatic, colorimetric[4]

Additional Information Children with thalassemia may have normal phosphorus absorption but high renal phosphaturia, leading to a deficiency of phosphorus. Increasing dietary intake of potassium has been reported to increase serum phosphate concentrations apparently by decreasing renal excretion of phosphate.[5] During the last trimester of pregnancy, there is a sixfold increase in calcium and phosphorus accumulation as the fetus triples its weight. Plasma phosphorus concentrations and increased urinary phosphate may provide a useful means to assess response to phosphate supplements in the premature infant.[6]

Tumor-induced osteomalacia (oncogenic osteomalacia) is a rare entity in which hypophosphatemia, hyperphosphaturia, low 1,25-dihydroxy vitamin D, and rickets or osteomalacia can be reversed with removal of the tumor.[7]

Footnotes

1. Matos V, Van Melle G, Boulat O, et al, "Urinary Phosphate/Creatinine, Calcium/Creatinine, and Magnesium/Creatinine Ratios in a Healthy Pediatric Population," *J Pediatr*, 1997, 131(2):252-7.

2. Hruska KA, "Phosphate Balance and Metabolism," *The Principles and Practice of Nephrology*, Chapter 19, Jacobson HR, Striker GE, and Klahr S, eds, Philadelphia, PA: BC Decker Inc, 1991, 122.

3. Young DS, *Effects of Drugs on Clinical Laboratory Tests*, 5th ed, Volume 1: Listing by Test, Washington, DC: AACC Press, American Association of Clinical Chemistry, 2000, Section 3, 621-2.

4. Berti G, Fossati P, Tarenghi G, et al, "Enzymatic Colorimetric Method for the Determination of Inorganic Phosphorus in Serum and Urine," *J Clin Chem Clin Biochem*, 1988, 26(6):399-404.

5. Sebastian A, Hernandez RE, Portale AA, et al, "Dietary Potassium Influences Kidney Maintenance of Serum Phosphorus Concentration," *Kidney Int*, 1990, 37(5):1341-9.

6. Mayne PD and Kovar IZ, "Calcium and Phosphorus Metabolism in the Premature Infant," *Ann Clin Biochem*, 1991, 28(Pt 2):131-42.

7. Cai Q, Hodgson SF, Kai PC, et al, "Brief Report: Inhibition of Renal Phosphate Transport by a Tumor Product in a Patient With Oncogenic Osteomalacia," *N Engl J Med*, 1994, 330(23):1645-9.

References

Alon US and Chan JCM, *Phosphate in Pediatric Health and Disease*, Boca Raton: CRC Press, 1993.

(Continued)

Phosphorus, Urine (Continued)

Bakker AJ, Bosma H, and Christen PJ, "Influence of Monoclonal Immunoglobulins in Three Different Methods for Inorganic Phosphorus," *Ann Clin Biochem*, 1990, 27(Pt 3):227-31.

Somell A and Alveryd A, "Diurnal Variations in the Urinary Excretion of Calcium and Phosphate in Hyperparathyroidism," *Acta Chir Scand*, 1976, 142(5):357-9.

Subramanian R and Khardori R, "Severe Hypophosphatemia: Pathophysiologic Implications, Clinical Presentations, and Treatment," *Medicine*, 2000, 79(1):1-8.

Weintraub Z, Iancu TC, Sheinfeld M, et al, "Urinary and Blood Levels of Adenosine 3′, 5′-Monophosphate, Phosphorus, and Calcium in Infants," *Biol Neonate*, 1989, 55(4-5):233-7.

◆ **pH, Umbilical Venous Blood Gases (pCO$_2$ and pO$_2$)** see Blood Gases and pH, Umbilical Cord *on page 121*

◆ **Pilocarpine Iontophoresis** see Chloride, Sweat *on page 144*

◆ **Pituitary Gonadotropins** see Follicle Stimulating Hormone, Serum, Plasma, or Urine *on page 175*

◆ **Pituitary Gonadotropins** see Luteinizing Hormone, Blood or Urine *on page 219*

◆ **PKU, Neonatal** see Newborn Screen for Phenylketonuria *on page 229*

◆ **PKU Test** see Phenylalanine, Blood *on page 248*

◆ **PKU, Urine Test** see Phenylalanine, Urine *on page 249*

Placental Lactogen, Human, Serum

Related Information
Chorionic Gonadotropin, Human, Serum and Urine *on page 147*

Synonyms hCS; hPL; Human Chorionic Somatomammotropin

Abstract Human placental lactogen (hPL) is a hormone secreted by trophoblastic cells, both placental and extravillous.[1] Serum levels are proportional to placental size and fetal birth weight. Very low levels of hPL can be detected in both male and female adults.[2]

Patient Preparation As specified by research laboratory.

Specimen Serum or plasma

Container As specified by research laboratory.

Storage Instructions As specified by research laboratory.

Reference Interval Varies with duration of gestation. Levels rise with advancing gestation to plateau at about 37 weeks. May reach a maximum of 11 µg/mL (SI: 509 nmol/L).

Use Biochemical assays and immunohistochemical preparations are used in research projects studying various aspects of fetal and placental growth and metabolism. Increased serum levels of hPL are seen in preeclampsia;[3] decreased levels are seen in chorioamnionitis[4] and during the first trimester of diabetic pregnancies. However, the predictive values of all these relationships are too low to be of clinical usefulness.[5]

Limitations No clinical application has yet been established for this serum test.

Methodology Immunoassays (multiple labels)

Additional Information Human placental lactogen is used as an immunohistochemical reaction in surgical pathology.

Footnotes
1. Rhoton-Vlasak A, Wagner JM, Rutgers JL, et al, "Placental Site Trophoblastic Tumor: Human Placental Lactogen and Pregnancy-Associated Major Basic Protein as Immunohistologic Markers," *Hum Pathol*, 1998, 29(3):280-8.

2. Madersbacher S, Untergasser G, Gerth R, et al, "Reassessment of the Role of Human Placental Lactogen in Physiological Nonpregnant and Pathological Conditions," *Experimental and Clinical Endocrinology and Diabetes*, 1998, 106(1):61-7.

3. Murai JT, Muzykanskiy E, and Taylor RN, "Maternal and Fetal Modulators of Lipid Metabolism Correlate With the Development or Preeclampsia," *Metabolism*, 1997, 46(8):963-7.

4. Okada H, Matsuzaki N, Sawai K, et al, "Chorioamnionitis Reduces Placental Endocrine Functions: The Role of Bacterial Lipopolysaccharide and Superoxide Anion," *J Endocrinol*, 1997, 155(3):401-10.

5. Markestad T, Bergsjo P, Aakvaag A, et al, "Prediction of Fetal Growth Based on Maternal Serum Concentrations of Human Chorionic Gonadotropin, Human Placental Lactogen and Estriol," *Acta Obstetrica et Gynecologica Scandinavia*, 1997, 165(Suppl):50-5.

References
Ashwood ER, "Clinical Chemistry of Pregnancy," *Tietz Textbook of Clinical Chemistry*, 3rd ed, Burtis CA and Ashwood ER, eds, Philadelphia, PA: WB Saunders Co, 1999, 1738-9.

◆ **Plasma Cholinesterase** see Pseudocholinesterase, Serum *on page 270*

◆ **Plasma Electrolytes** see Electrolyte Panel, Serum *on page 168*

◆ **Pleural Fluid Analysis** see Body Fluid Chemical Analysis *on page 123*

◆ **Pleural Fluid pH** see Body Fluid pH *on page 125*

◆ **pO$_2$** see Blood Gases and pH, Arterial *on page 119*

◆ **pO$_2$ (0.5)** see P$_{50}$, Blood *on page 241*

◆ **pO$_2$ at Half Saturation** see P$_{50}$, Blood *on page 241*

◆ **Polymorphic Epithelial Mucin** see CA 15-3, Serum *on page 127*

◆ **Porphobilinogen** see Porphyrins, Quantitative, Urine *on page 255*

Porphobilinogen Deaminase, Erythrocyte

Related Information
Porphobilinogen, Qualitative, Urine *on page 255*
Porphyrins, Quantitative, Urine *on page 255*
Uroporphyrinogen III Synthase, Erythrocyte *on page 296*

Synonyms Erythrocyte Porphobilinogen Deaminase; Erythrocyte Uroporphyrinogen I Synthase; Hydroxymethylbilane Synthase; Pbg-D; Uroporphyrinogen-Cosynthetase; Uroporphyrinogen I Synthase

Abstract The enzymatic defect of acute intermittent porphyria (AIP) is a partial deficiency of uroporphyrin I synthase in erythrocytes and other cells.[1,2] Inheritance of AIP is autosomal dominant with low penetrance. The incidence of AIP is estimated to be 5-10 persons per 100,000. This assay is described as the most reliable test for diagnosis of AIP.

Patient Preparation Patient should fast for 12-14 hours, abstain from alcohol and ideally be off medications for 2 weeks.

Specimen Whole blood (done on erythrocytes)

Container Green top (heparin) tube, lavender top (EDTA) tube

Storage Instructions If test can be done promptly, a red cell hemolysate is prepared directly from whole blood. The whole blood sample can be stored for 1 week at 4°C. If there will be a delay of over a week, centrifuge heparinized specimen. After plasma and buffy layer are removed, wash red cells three times with cold isotonic saline. Pack by centrifugation. Freeze in dry ice-acetone.[1] Store at -20°C. There is loss of activity at 4°C, more at room temperature as red cells age. The test is done on a red cell hemolysate.

Turnaround Time Usually sent to reference laboratory with turnaround time of approximately 7 days

Special Instructions Hemoglobin and reticulocyte count should also be ordered.

Reference Interval ≥7.0 nmol/second/L red cells; ELISA assay: >110 µg/g hemoglobin

Varies among methods and among laboratories. Patients with acute intermittent porphyria have levels about half normal; *vide infra*. Hemoglobin determination is done on the hemolysate for calculation of activity on a per gram of hemoglobin basis.

Critical Values Indeterminate: 3.5-3.9 nmol/second/L; diminished: <3.5 nmol/second/L

Use Evaluate subjects with episodes of abdominal pain, especially when such episodes are recurrent, and with tachycardia. Uroporphyrin-1-synthase is low in the latent or carrier state of acute intermittent porphyria, normal in the other hereditary porphyrias. It is thought to provide support in the differential diagnosis of acute intermittent porphyria from other neurological porphyrias,[1] following the first steps of PBG and ALA.

Limitations Only a minority of carriers of the defective enzyme will experience clinical AIP.[2] A small overlap with normals exists. Repeat assay at a later time is indicated to confirm carrier status. Qualitative and quantitative urinary porphobilinogen and family studies are also useful. Indeterminate or normal values for this enzyme may occur in some patients with acute intermittent porphyria. Interpretation is difficult at the low end of the normal range. Red cell uroporphyrin-1-synthase activity varies with cell age. Younger red cells (newborn subjects) or other settings in which younger red cells are found, with reticulocytosis ≥5%, may lead to increased activity of this assay, which therefore may be high in various anemias, and may also mask the diagnosis of acute intermittent porphyria. Measurement of porphobilinogen deaminase activity is of limited use in assessing patients with latent acute intermittent porphyria.

Methodology Fluorometric assay, ELISA assay, electrophoresis for molecular analysis;[3] method at Mayo Medical Laboratories is published.[4]

Additional Information See tables in Porphyrins, Quantitative, Urine *on page 255*. More than 130 mutations causing AIP are described.[3] This is the enzyme which converts porphobilinogen to uroporphyrinogen I. Uroporphyrin I synthase is a method of detection of asymptomatic carriers of acute intermittent porphyria. Another is quantitation of urine porphobilinogen. Both are recommended. Uroporphyrin-1-synthase is normal or increased with lead poisoning, because of anemia in plumbism.[5] In acute intermittent porphyria excessive excretion of porphobilinogen and delta aminolevulinic acid occurs during acute attacks, but excretion may be normal between them. Red blood cell porphobilinogen deaminase (uroporphyrinogen I synthase) activity, measured by a spectrofluorometric assay on erythrocytes, defines most patients with acute intermittent porphyria, while 55 of 56 subjects with other porphyrias were reported as having normal activity. This assay identified a number of latent carriers but not all patients with assumed acute intermittent porphyria.[6] Either Pbg-D or ALA-D (aminolevulinic acid dehydratase) in red cells is expected to be decreased in subjects with AIP.[4]

More than 90% of the individuals who carry a defective gene never experience an episode of the disease. An acute attack is mostly caused by endogenous hormonal factors and through exposure to various chemicals or drugs.[2]

Footnotes
1. Forman DT, "Erythrocyte Uroporphyrinogen I Synthase Activity as an Indicator of Acute Porphyria," *Ann Clin Lab Sci*, 1989, 19(2):128-32.

2. Nuttall KL, "Porphyrins and Disorders of Porphyrin Metabolism," *Tietz Textbook of Clinical Chemistry*, 3rd ed, Burtis CA and Ashwood ER, eds, Philadelphia, PA: WB Saunders Co, 1999, 1711-35.

3. Tchernitchko D, Lamoril J, Puy H, et al, "Evaluation of Mutation Screening by Heteroduplex Analysis in Acute Intermittent Porphyria: Comparison With Denaturing Gradient Gel Electrophoresis," *Clin Chim Acta*, 1999, 279(1-2):133-43.
4. Leavelle DE, *Mayo Medical Laboratories Interpretive Handbook*, Rochester, MN: Mayo Medical Laboratories, 1997.
5. Bird TD, Wallace DM, and Labbe RF, "The Porphyria, Plumbism, Pottery Puzzle," *JAMA*, 1982, 247:813-4.
6. Pierach CA, Weimer MK, Cardinal RA, et al, "Red Blood Cell Porphobilinogen Deaminase in the Evaluation of Acute Intermittent Porphyria," *JAMA*, 1987, 257(1):60-1.

References

Hindmarsh JT, Oliveras L, and Greenway DC, "Biochemical Differentiation of the Porphyrias," *Clin Biochem*, 1999, 32(8):609-19.
Kushner JP, "Laboratory Diagnosis of the Porphyrias," *N Engl J Med*, 1991, 324(20):1432-4.
Sassa S and Kappas A, "Molecular Aspects of the Inherited Porphyrias," *J Intern Med*, 2000, 247(2):169-78.

Porphobilinogen, Qualitative, Urine

Related Information

Delta (5)-Aminolevulinic Acid, Urine *on page 165*
Lead, Blood *on page 793*
Porphobilinogen Deaminase, Erythrocyte *on page 254*
Porphyrins, Quantitative, Urine *on page 255*
Protoporphyrin, Free Erythrocyte *on page 269*
Uroporphyrinogen III Synthase, Erythrocyte *on page 296*

Synonyms Watson-Schwartz Test

Applies to Delta Aminolevulinic Acid; Hoesch Test; Porphyrins, Fecal; Uroporphyrinogen Synthase

Test Includes Qualitative screen for urobilinogen and porphobilinogen

Abstract Porphobilinogen (PBG) and delta aminolevulinic acid (ALA) are early porphyrin precursors, which are excreted. Acute intermittent porphyria (AIP) can be fatal. Urine delta ALA and/or PBG is/are increased in acute neurological porphyrias during attacks. These include acute intermittent porphyria, hereditary coproporphyria, and variegate porphyria. Most porphyrias are transmitted as autosomal dominant disorders.

Specimen Random urine

Container Any clean dark container, no preservative

Sampling Time PBG levels in the urine should be measured during acute attacks of abdominal pain, extremity pain or paresthesias, tachycardia, hypertension, nausea and vomiting, neurologic abnormalities, and in the investigation of dark urine.

Collection Keep refrigerated during collection and thereafter. Prevent exposure to light. Some authorities suggest collecting in a dark bottle with 5 g sodium bicarbonate, as well as keeping under refrigeration.

Storage Instructions Specimen may be stored for a brief period in refrigerator, but must be analyzed promptly. Adjust to pH 6-7 with sodium bicarbonate. Stabilized specimen is stable 12 hours at 25°C and 7 days at 4°C.

Reference Interval Negative

Use PBG is a screen for **acute intermittent porphyria (AIP)**, which is characterized by urinary excretion of PBG and delta ALA during acute attacks. The Watson-Schwartz test may detect some patients in latent periods who have AIP. Increased urinary excretion of PBG may also be caused by acute attacks of **variegate porphyria** or of **hereditary coproporphyria**, and rarely in lead poisoning. In lead poisoning, urinary ALA measurement is more useful.

Limitations False negatives may occur. The major drawback of the Watson-Schwartz and Hoesch tests is the need for subjective interpretation of the visual endpoint.[1] Schreiber et al have described an anion-exchange resin. Columns were prepared by packing polybenzimidazole resin.[1] Positive results must be confirmed by other methods, including quantitative tests for PBG and for ALA. A quantitative method using a condensation reaction with *p*-dimethylaminobenzaldehyde, with spectrophotometric analysis, is widely used. (Normal 0.0-2.0 mg/day or 0.0-8.8 mmol/day.)

May be negative in the patient with asymptomatic (latent) phase of AIP, in whom uroporphyrinogen I synthase may detect the presence of AIP; see Porphobilinogen Deaminase, Erythrocyte *on page 254* for this assay.

The intoxication porphyrinurias (including lead poisoning) are better detected by delta aminolevulinic acid and other tests.

Fecal porphyrins are elevated with the neurocutaneous porphyrias. Fecal porphyrins are useful in hereditary coproporphyria and variegate porphyria and to distinguish these from AIP. In variegate porphyria and erythropoietic protoporphyria, increased fecal protoporphyrins are anticipated.

Methodology Watson-Schwartz test, Ehrlich's reagent. A variant of the Watson-Schwartz test, the newer **Hoesch test** does not react with urobilinogen, an advantage. In both tests, there is a chemical interference (decrease in results) if indolic compounds (indole, indican, 5-HIAA) are present in large amounts.

Polybenzimidazole (PBI) resin columns:[1] A Dowex 2 resin is used to adsorb alkaline PBG, then acid elution of the PBG, followed by reaction with Ehrlich's reagent, and reading by spectrophotometry. The sensitivity is greatly increased.[2] Others have quantified the eluate by HPLC.[3]

Recently, a commercial semiquantitative kit (Trace, Miami, FL) for urinary porphobilinogen (PBG), in which urine is pretreated with ion-exchange resin

and the color of the Ehrlich-PBG adduct matched against a set of surrogate standards, has been described. The method was compared with qualitative screening methods (Watson-Schwartz) in common use. For 129 urine samples with raised PBG, 95% samples were positive with Trace kit as compared to only 38% positive by qualitative tests. Sixteen out of 91 results for pigmented urine samples with normal PBG were reported as positive using qualitative screening tests, but only one using the Trace kit. Therefore, the Trace method seems far more sensitive and specific than the qualitative screening tests. The study recommended that Watson-Schwartz-type screening tests should be abandoned and, ideally, all urine samples analyzed by quantitative methods. However, the Trace method is a convenient alternative which is adequate for the initial screening of symptomatic patients.[4]

Additional Information Acute attacks of AIP are precipitated by drugs, including barbiturates, sulfa drugs, heavy metals, hydantoins, hormones, infection, and diet. The most common symptom of AIP is abdominal pain. The most common sign is tachycardia. Such autonomic attacks include emesis, fever, leukocytosis, and neurologic findings. Subjects with the porphyrias may pass urine the color of port wine. The term porphyria derives from the Greek "porphyria," an expression for the color purple.

Quantitative urine PBG will pick up many but not all patients with acute intermittent porphyria in the latent period.

The Watson-Schwartz test is negative with porphyria cutanea tarda and in Günther's disease, congenital erythropoietic porphyria.

Footnotes

1. Schreiber WE, Jamani A, and Pudek MR, "Screening Tests for Porphobilinogen Are Insensitive. The Problem and Its Solution," *Am J Clin Pathol*, 1989, 92(5):644-9.
2. Buttery JE, Chamberlain BR, and Beng CG, "A Sensitive Method of Screening for Urinary Porphobilinogen," *Clin Chem*, 1989, 35(12):2311-2.
3. Jamani A, Pudek M, and Schreiber WE, "Liquid-Chromatographic Assay of Urinary Porphobilinogen," *Clin Chem*, 1989, 35(3):471-5.
4. Deacon AC and Peters TJ, "Identification of Acute Porphyria: Evaluation of a Commercial Screening Test for Urinary Porphobilinogen," *Ann Clin Biochem*, 1998, 35(Pt 6):726-32

References

Buttery JE, Carrera AM, and Pannall PR, "Analytical Sensitivity and Specificity of Two Screening Methods for Urinary Porphobilinogen," *Ann Clin Biochem*, 1990, 27(Pt 2):165-6.
Buttery JE and Stuart S, "Measurement of Porphobilinogen in Urine by a Simple Resin Method With Use of A Surrogate Standard," *Clin Chem*, 1991, 37(12):2133-6.
Desnick RJ, "The Porphyrias," *Harrison's Principles of Internal Medicine*, 14th ed, Chapter 343, Fauci AS, Braunwald E, Isselbacher KJ, et al, eds, New York, NY: McGraw-Hill Inc, 1998, 2152-8.
Hindmarsh JT, "Variable Phenotypic Expression of Genotypic Abnormalities in the Porphyrias," *Clin Chim Acta*, 1993, 217(1):29-38.
Hindmarsh JT, Oliveras L, and Greenway DC, "Biochemical Differentiation of the Porphyrias," *Clin Biochem*, 1999, 32(8):609-19
Lip GY, McColl KE, and Moore MR, "The Acute Porphyrias," *Br J Clin Pract*, 1993, 47(1):38-43.
Meola T and Lim HW, "The Porphyrias," *Dermatol Clin*, 1993, 11(3):583-96.
Moore MR, "Biochemistry of Porphyria," *Int J Biochem*, 1993, 25(10):1353-68.
Nuttall KL, "Porphyrins and Disorders of Porphyrin Metabolism," *Tietz Textbook of Clinical Chemistry*, 3rd ed, Burtis CA and Ashwood ER, eds, Philadelphia, PA: WB Saunders Co, 1999, 1711-35.
Tefferi A, Colgan JP, and Solberg LA Jr, "Acute Porphyrias: Diagnosis and Management," *Mayo Clin Proc*, 1994, 69(10):991-5.
Tefferi A, Solberg LA Jr, and Ellefson, "Porphyrias: Clinical Evaluation and Interpretation of Laboratory Tests," *Mayo Clin Proc*, 1994, 69(3):289-90.

♦ **Porphyrins, Erythrocytes** *see* Porphyrins, Quantitative, Urine *on page 255*

♦ **Porphyrins, Fecal** *see* Porphobilinogen, Qualitative, Urine *on page 255*

♦ **Porphyrins, Fecal** *see* Porphyrins, Quantitative, Urine *on page 255*

♦ **Porphyrins, Plasma** *see* Porphyrins, Quantitative, Urine *on page 255*

Porphyrins, Quantitative, Urine

Related Information

Delta (5)-Aminolevulinic Acid, Urine *on page 165*
Iron and Total Iron Binding Capacity/Transferrin, Serum *on page 203*
Lead, Blood *on page 793*
Lead, Urine *on page 795*
Liver Biopsy *on page 65*
Phlebotomy, Therapeutic *on page 849*
Porphobilinogen Deaminase, Erythrocyte *on page 254*
Porphobilinogen, Qualitative, Urine *on page 255*
Protoporphyrin, Free Erythrocyte *on page 269*
Urine Collection, 24-Hour *on page 47*
Uroporphyrinogen III Synthase, Erythrocyte *on page 296*

Synonyms Coproporphyrins; Porphobilinogen; Uroporphyrins

Applies to Naproxen; Porphyrins, Erythrocytes; Porphyrins, Fecal; Porphyrins, Plasma; Uroporphyrinogen Decarboxylase

Test Includes Uroporphyrins (octacarboxylporphyrins), heptacarboxylporphyrins, hexacarboxylporphyrins, pentacarboxylporphyrins, coproporphyrins (tetracarboxylporphyrins)[1]

Abstract Porphyrins are byproducts of porphyrinogens. Accumulations of either cause porphyrias, which are hereditary enzyme disorders. They *(Continued)*

Porphyrins, Quantitative, Urine *(Continued)*

affect the heme biosynthetic pathway and are characterized by increased excretion of porphyrins, porphyrinogens, or their precursors. Such precursors include delta aminolevulinic acid (ALA) and porphobilinogen (PBG). These are water soluble and appear in the urine, in common with coproporphyrin and uroporphyrin. The disease entities relate to specific enzyme defects. Most are inherited as autosomal dominant with low disease penetrance.

There is also a group of acquired porphyrias which most commonly result from either lead poisoning or hereditary tyrosinemia. In lead poisoning there is increased excretion of ALA due to inhibition of PBG synthase. In hereditary tyrosinemia the increase in ALA excretion is due to inhibition of PBG synthase by succinylacetone.

Patient Preparation Avoid alcohol and excessive fluid intake during collection. Phenothiazines may cause misleading porphobilinogen results.

Specimen 24-hour urine

Container Clean, dark container. Must be kept covered.

Collection Check with laboratory; 5 g sodium bicarbonate is usually added to container before collection. Specimen should be kept cool during collection. Transport specimen immediately to the laboratory upon completion of collection. Adjust to pH 6-7 with sodium bicarbonate.

Storage Instructions Refrigerate during collection. **Protect specimen from light.**

Causes for Rejection Sodium phosphate is undesirable as a preservative.

Reference Interval Total porphyrins: <320 nmol/L; see also literature from individual laboratory.

Use There are a number of clinical situations in which patients are investigated for porphyrias. The most common clinical presentations and tests selection are summarized in the following table.[2]

Selection of Laboratory Tests in Common Clinical Presentations

Clinical Presentation	Primary Test	Supplemental Test
Acute neuropsychiatric porphyria	Random urine PBG	Second urine PBG Urine ALA
Chronic neuropsychiatric porphyria	Urine PBG	Fecal porphyrins
Differentiating among the neurological porphyrias	Fecal porphyrins	Serum and urine porphyrins Enzyme and gene-based tests
Latent neurological porphyria	None	Urine PBG and porphyrins Fecal and serum porphyrins Enzyme and gene-based tests
Acute photosensitivity	Serum or fecal porphyrins	Liver function tests Urine porphyrins
Bullous skin lesions	Urine porphyrins	Serum and fecal porphyrins Urine PBG
Following porphyria cutanea tarda	Urine porphyrins	Serum porphyrins
Elevated coproporphyrin	None	Evaluation of diet Liver function tests
Identification of iron disorders	Zinc protoporphyrin	Serum ferritin Other iron studies
Lead exposure	Whole blood lead	Zinc protoporphyrin

In **congenital erythropoietic porphyria**, a decrease of red cell uroporphyrinogen III synthase of red cells occurs. Severe hemolysis and photosensitivity are found; see Uroporphyrinogen III Synthase, Erythrocyte *on page 296.*

In **acute intermittent porphyria**, porphobilinogen and delta aminolevulinic acid are elevated in acute attacks, and mild increases of urinary uroporphyrin and coproporphyrin may be found. Porphobilinogen is increased in many but not all patients with acute intermittent porphyria in latent periods. Quantitative porphobilinogen is a better test than delta aminolevulinic acid overall for acute intermittent porphyria, but both are used (as well as the Watson-Schwartz test).[3] Porphobilinogen deaminase activity can be measured; see Porphobilinogen Deaminase, Erythrocyte *on page 254.*

Coproporphyrin and porphobilinogen excretion in urine are markedly increased during acute attacks of **hereditary coproporphyria**, increase of urinary uroporphyrin may be found, and increased fecal coproporphyrin III is described. Urinary ALA and PBG are increased with acute attacks.

In **variegate porphyria (VP)** in acute attacks, results are similar to those of acute intermittent porphyria. Porphobilinogen and ALA are increased with acute attacks but are prone to become normal between attacks. Urine coproporphyrin exceeds uroporphyrin excretion during acute attacks. Plasma can be used to identify **porphyria cutanea tarda** (PCT)[4] and distinguish it from VP.[5]

Chemical porphyrias occur. Porphyrinogenic chemicals include certain halogenated hydrocarbons which cause the excretion of increased uroporphyrin. A number of drugs, infections, heavy metals, hormones, and chemicals cause porphyrias.[6]

In **lead poisoning** elevation of delta aminolevulinic acid greater than that of porbobilinogen occurs and porphobilinogen may be normal. Urinary coproporphyrin characteristically is increased. Free erythrocyte protoporphyrin and zinc protoporphyrin (ZPP) are increased. (See Lead, Blood *on page 793.*) Toxins such as lead interfere with heme synthesis and cause porphyrinuria.

Increased urine excretion of uroporphyrinogen, uroporphyrin, and coproporphyrin occurs in **porphyria cutanea tarda (PCT)**. Uroporphyrinogen decarboxylase is decreased. It is done on red cells; whole blood is collected. It is normal in acquired PCT and in some inherited cases.[1] It is found in middle-aged men who like ethanol, young women on oral contraceptives, in selective hydrocarbon exposure, in subjects on dialysis. These patients do not excrete increased porphobilinogen, but may have slight elevations of delta aminolevulinic acid. Iron overload is found with the acquired form, for which treatment includes repeated phlebotomies.

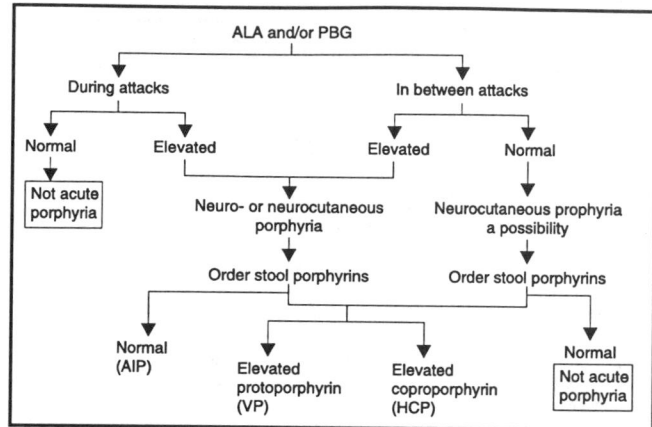

Interpretation of urine studies, as the cause of symptoms, during evaluation of acute porphyria. AIP = acute intermittent porphyria; ALA = Δ- aminolevulinic acid; HCP = hereditary coproporphyria; PBG = porphobilinogen; VP = variegate porphyria. From Tefferi A, Solberg LA, and Ellefson RD, "Porphyrias: Clinical Evaluation and Interpretation of Laboratory Tests," *Mayo Clin Proc,* 1994, 69:289-90 with permission.

Limitations Increased porphobilinogen may occur in patients on oral contraceptives. This test and delta aminolevulinic acid will not detect protoporphyria. Coproporphyrinuria alone lacks specificity and sensitivity for lead screening. Erythrocyte uroporphyrinogen I synthase is decreased in latent acute intermittent porphyria, and is needed in patients with possible latent acute intermittent porphyria. Quantitative porphobilinogen is of value in active and in many cases of latent acute intermittent porphyria, but will miss some of the latter when compared to red cell uroporphyrinogen I synthase.

Increased urine porphyrin excretion may be secondary to other diseases (eg, hepatobiliary diseases), especially coproporphyrin excretion. These are secondary porphyrinurias. They lack increased urinary porphobilinogen or ALA, with the important exception of lead poisoning.[6]

Methodology High performance liquid chromatography (HPLC) is the method of choice; spectrophotometry and fluorometry are also used.

Additional Information Heme is a component not only of hemoglobin, but of enzymes such as the cytochrome P-450 system. It includes a tetrapyrole ring (protoporphyrin IX) and iron.

The table provides an abbreviated overview of the porphyrias. Porphyrin fractionation of plasma can be done. Increases of urine porphyrins are found with congenital erythropoietic porphyria, acute intermittent porphyria, hereditary coproporphyria, variegate porphyria, and porphyria cutanea tarda.

Fecal porphyrin examination for hereditary coproporphyria, variegate porphyria, and protoporphyria can be used for adult patients. Stool examination for coproporphyrin and protoporphyrin is recommended for diagnosis of variegate porphyria.[7]

Neurologic dysfunction occurs in the **hepatic porphyrias**, the types of porphyria in which acute attacks develop: acute intermittent porphyria, variegate porphyria, hereditary coproporphyria, and ALA dehydrase deficiency. Abdominal pain, caused by autonomic neuropathy, occurs with acute attacks (eg, acute intermittent porphyria). It is the most common symptom of acute intermittent porphyria.[6]

The acute porphyrias include acute intermittent porphyria (AIP), variegate porphyria, and hereditary coproporphyria. Attacks may be life-threatening.[8] Symptoms may include colicky abdominal pain, fever, vomiting, neuritis, and psychosis.

The nonacute porphyrias include cutaneous hepatic porphyria, erythropoietic protoporphyria, and congenital porphyria. Dermatological symptoms are caused by circulating porphyrins which cause photosensitivity.[8]

Hepatic complications are found with **porphyria cutanea tarda** and **protoporphyria**. Fluorescence is demonstrable in liver biopsies from patients with the former, as well as siderosis. Crystalline deposits may be found in

Porphyrias: Overview

Disorder	Inheritance	Age of Clinical Onset	Primary Organ Involvement	Useful Tests	Primary Signs and Symptoms

Congenital erythropoietic porphyria
 	
(Günther disease)
	Autosomal recessive
	
	Rare
		Birth – 5 y	Erythroid cells	Urinary porphyrins
				Fecal porphyrins
				Uroporphyrinogen III synthase, erythrocytes
				
				Fluorescence of a diaper under Wood's light
					Severe photosensitivity
					
					Red urine
					  Stains diapers
					  Hemolytic anemia
					  Splenomegaly

Acute intermittent porphyria Precipitating causes include barbiturates, hydantoins, sulfonamides	Autosomal dominant Most common acute hepatic porphyria in U.S.	Adults	Hepatic, probably erythroid cells	Urine porphobilinogen Porphobilinogen deaminase, erythrocyte Urine porphyrins Urinary delta aminolevulinic acid Erythrocyte uroporphyrinogen 1 synthase Fecal porphyrins	Mild to severe neurologic/visceral (autonomic) symptoms Acute attacks
Hereditary coproporphyria	Autosomal dominant	Adults	Hepatic, possibly erythroid cells	Urine PBG and ALA in acute attacks Urine porphyrins including coproporphyrin Fecal porphyrins Plasma porphyrins	Similar to variegate porphyria Acute attacks
Variegate porphyria	Autosomal dominant	Adults	Hepatic, possibly erythroid cells	Urine PBG and ALA in acute attacks Urine porphyrins Fecal porphyrins Plasma porphyrins Erythrocyte uroporphyrinogen-1-synthase	Mild to severe photosensitivity and neurologic-visceral symptoms Acute attacks
Porphyria cutanea tarda	Autosomal dominant, type II (inherited type); sporadic type also known Most common porphyria in U.S.	Adults	Hepatic, possibly erythroid cells; photosensitivity	Urine porphyrins Plasma porphyrins Uroporphyrinogen decarboxylase, type II (RBCs)	Similar to variegate porphyria Photosensitization Liver damage
Protoporphyria	Autosomal dominant	Usually childhood	Erythroid cells, probably liver	Protoporphyrin, free erythrocyte	Photosensitization Liver damage
Acquired (intoxication) porphyria	Acquired	Children and adults	Hepatic, erythroid cells	Erythrocyte porphyrins Urinary delta aminolevulinic acid Urine porphobilinogen Urine porphyrins Fecal porphyrins	Mild photosensitivity

protoporphyria.[6] The amount of porphobilinogen excreted in acute intermittent porphyria is usually greater than the excretion of ALA. When there is more ALA, another diagnosis should be considered, including lead poisoning, another type of porphyria, or hereditary tyrosinemia.[6] See Protoporphyrin, Free Erythrocyte *on page 269*, which pertains to lead poisoning, and erythropoietic protoporphyria. The differential diagnosis of lead poisoning is relevant,[9] *vide supra*. Drugs can cause confusion. Naproxen is reported to cause a reaction clinically and histopathologically similar to porphyria cutanea tarda.[10]

This is a complex group of diseases, of which most are uncommon. Some are extremely rare (eg, hepatoerythropoietic porphyria). Larger sources are recommended for more comprehensive review.[11,12,13,14]

The pathogenesis of most inherited porphyrias has now been defined at the molecular level, and it is clear that there is a great deal of genetic heterogeneity in each porphyria. Currently, molecular testing for porphyria is done only in research laboratories. With advances in methodology, it may eventually become possible to perform molecular testing for porphyria in clinical laboratories in a cost-effective manner.[15,16,17]

Footnotes

1. Leavelle DE, *Mayo Medical Laboratories Interpretive Handbook*, Rochester, MN: Mayo Medical Laboratories, 1997.
2. Nuttall KL, "Porphyrins and Disorders of Porphyrin Metabolism," *Tietz Textbook of Clinical Chemistry*, 3rd ed. Burtis CA and Ashwood ER, eds, Philadelphia, PA: WB Saunders Co, 1999, 1711-35.
3. Tschudy DP, "Porphyrins," *Chemical Diagnosis of Disease*, Brown SS, Mitchell FL, and Young DS, eds, Amsterdam, Holland: Elsevier/North Holland Biomedical Press, 1979, 1039-58.
4. Hindmarsh JT, Oliveras L, and Greenway DC, "Plasma Porphyrins in the Porphyrias," *Clin Chem*, 1999, 45(7):932-3.
5. Desnick RJ, "The Porphyrias," *Harrison's Principles of Internal Medicine*, 14th ed, Chapter 343, Fauci AS, Braunwald E, Isselbacher KJ, et al, eds, New York, NY: McGraw-Hill Inc, 1998, 2152-8.
6. Downey DC, "Porphyria and Chemicals," *Med Hypotheses*, 1999, 53(2):166-71.
7. Bloomer JR and Bonkovsky HL, "The Porphyrias," *Dis Mon*, 1989, 35(1):1-54.
8. Muhlbauer JE, Pathak MA, Tishler PV, et al, "Variegate Porphyria in New England," *JAMA*, 1982, 247:3095-102.
9. Moore MR, "Biochemistry of Porphyria," *Int J Biochem*, 1993, 25(10):1353-68.
10. Bird TD, Wallace DM, and Labbe RF, "The Porphyria, Plumbism, Pottery Puzzle," *JAMA*, 1982, 247:813-4.
11. Fitzpatrick JE, "New Histopathologic Findings in Drug Eruptions," *Dermatol Clin*, 1992, 10(1):19-36.
12. Bickers DR, "Photosensitivity and Other Reactions to Light," *Harrison's Principles of Internal Medicine*, 14th ed, Chapter 58, Fauci AS, Braunwald E, Isselbacher KJ, et al, eds, New York, NY: McGraw-Hill Inc, 1998, 328-34.
13. Tefferi A, Colgan JP, and Solberg LA, "Acute Porphyrias: Diagnosis and Management," *Mayo Clin Proc*, 1994, 69(10):991-5.

14. Tefferi A, Solberg LA Jr, and Ellefson RD, "Porphyrias: Clinical Evaluation and Interpretation of Laboratory Tests," *Mayo Clin Proc*, 1994, 69(3):289-90.
15. Sassa S and Kappas A, "Molecular Aspects of the Inherited Porphyrias," *J Intern Med*, 2000, 247(2):169-78.
16. Schreiber WE, "A Molecular View of the Neurologic Porphyrias," *Clin Lab Med*, 1997, 17(1):73-83.
17. Elder GH, "Genetic Defects in the Porphyrias: Types and Significance," *Clin Dermatol*, 1998, 16(2):225-33.

References

"A 29-Year-Old Woman With Abdominal Pain, Myalgia, and Muscle Weakness," Case Records of the Massachusetts General Hospital, Case 39-1984, Scully RE, Mark EJ, McNeely WF, et al, eds, *N Engl J Med*, 1984, 311(13):839-47.

Ayala F and Santoianni P, "Drug-Induced Cutaneous Porphyria," *Clin Dermatol*, 1993, 11(4):535-9.

Edwards CQ, Griffen LM, Goldgar DE, et al, "HLA-Linked Hemochromatosis Alleles in Sporadic Porphyria Cutanea Tarda," *Gastroenterology*, 1989, 97(4):972-81.

Elder GH, Urquhart AJ, De Salamanca RE, et al, "Immunoreactive Uroporphyrinogen Decarboxylase in the Liver in Porphyria Cutanea Tarda," *Lancet*, 1985, 2(8449):229-33.

Hift RJ, Meissner PN, Todd G, et al, "Homozygous Variegate Porphyria: An Evolving Clinical Syndrome," *Postgrad Med J*, 1993, 69(816):781-6.

Hindmarsh JT, "Variable Phenotypic Expression of Genotypic Abnormalities in the Porphyrias," *Clin Chim Acta*, 1993, 217(1):29-38.

Hindmarsh JT, Oliveras L, and Greenway DC, "Biochemical Differentiation of the Porphyrias," *Clin Biochem*, 1999, 32(8):609-19.

Lip GY, McColl KE, and Moore MR, "The Acute Porphyrias," *Br J Clin Pract*, 1993, 47(1):38-43.

Martinelli AL, Villanova MG, Roselino AM, et al, "Abnormal Uroporphyrin Levels in Chronic Hepatitis C Virus Infection," *J Clin Gastroenterol*, 1999, 29(4):327-31.

Meola T and Lim HW, "The Porphyrias," *Dermatol Clin*, 1993, 11(3):583-96.

Pierach CA and Ippen H, "A Porphyrin-Soaked Diaper," *N Engl J Med*, 1994, 330(23):1690.

Scarlett YV and Brenner DA, "Porphyrias," *J Clin Gastroenterol*, 1998, 27(3):192-8.

Todd DJ, "Erythropoietic Protoporphyria," *Br J Dermatol*, 1994, 131(6):751-66.

Westerlund J, Pudek M, and Schreiber WE, "A Rapid and Accurate Spectrofluorometric Method for Quantification and Screening of Urinary Porphyrins," *Clin Chem*, 1988, 34(2):345-51.

Internet Web Sites

www.enterprise.net/apf/

♦ **Porter-Silber Chromogens, Urine** *see* 17-Hydroxycorticosteroids, Urine *on page 196*

♦ **Postprandial Glucose** *see* Glucose, Postglucose Load, Plasma *on page 185*

♦ **Potassium, Arterial** *see* Potassium, Serum or Plasma *on page 258*

Potassium, Serum or Plasma

Related Information

Synonyms K[+], Serum or Plasma

Applies to Potassium, Arterial

Abstract
The major intracellular cation, K[+] is very commonly measured as one of the serum/plasma or urine electrolytes.

Specimen Serum, plasma

Container Red top tube or green top (heparin) tube

Collection
Avoid very small needles if possible. Avoid stasis, use of tourniquet if possible and **avoid hand clenching.** Fist clenching increases K[+]. If a tourniquet must be used, sample blood 1-2 minutes after the hand is relaxed and the tourniquet removed. Avoid potassium-containing tubes such as potassium oxalate. Potassium can be reported from arterial as well as from venous blood. If arterial puncture is done for pO_2, plasma can be tested for Na[+], K[+], and Cl[-] so long as lithium and not potassium heparinate anticoagulant is used, sparing the patient a venipuncture.

Storage Instructions
Remove plasma or serum from red cells within 4 hours before specimen is refrigerated. Storage of unspun blood at 4°C causes serum and plasma K[+] to increase.

Causes for Rejection
Hemolyzed specimen, serum specimen not removed from clot in patient with high platelet count. Such specimens may be analyzed but the likelihood of a falsely high potassium level must be recognized and stated in report.

Reference Interval
Plasma: 3.5-5.0 mmol/L. Add **approximately** 0.1 to normal ranges if serum is sampled rather than plasma. Pediatric ranges are sometimes reported as slightly higher than adult levels. Differences may partially relate to the amount of hemolysis in specimens used to establish normal ranges. In daily practice some degree of hemolysis may occur in neonatal and pediatric specimens. Although grossly hemolyzed specimens are usually rejected, the acceptability of samples with slight hemolysis is debatable. Even slight hemolysis can dramatically increase K[+] results; red cells have an intracellular K[+] concentration of 100-120 mmol/L or more.

Possible Panic Range
Newborns: <2.5 mmol/L (SI: <2.5 mmol/L), >7.0 mmol/L (SI: >7.0 mmol/L); adults: <2.5 mmol/L (SI: <2.5 mmol/L), >6.5 mmol/L (SI: >6.5 mmol/L). With unanticipated high or low K[+], EKG may be indicated. If potassium is high and serum was used, examine peripheral blood smear for thrombocytosis and/or leukocytosis; obtain platelet and white count if indicated, *vide infra.*

Use
Evaluate electrolyte balance; K[+] level should be followed especially in elderly patients, those on intravenous hyperalimentation, in patients on diuretic therapy and in cases of renal disease, particularly patients with acute renal failure and those on hemodialysis. As one of the major electrolytes, serum K[+] concentrations are a part of regular assessment of acid-base balance, management of intravenous therapy, and evaluation of patients with hypertension.

Evaluate muscular weakness and irritability, mental confusion, weakness; manage leukemia, diseases of gastrointestinal tract including laxative abuse, hepatic encephalopathy, fistulas and tube drainage; evaluate and prevent cardiac arrhythmias;[1,2] evaluate alcoholism with delirium tremens; detect, diagnose, and manage mineralocorticoid excess or deficiency, renal tubular abnormalities, heat stroke, licorice ingestion mineralocorticoid effect.

Hypokalemia[3] **(low potassium)** has been found in 80% to 90% of hypertensive patients with primary aldosteronism.[4] This uncommon entity is a curable cause of hypertension (see Adrenal Cortex: Laboratory Assessments Overview *on page 84*). Hypokalemia can be observed in patients with secondary hyperaldosteronism as in those with renal artery stenosis. Low K[+] occurs with endogenous or exogenous increase in other corticosteroids, including that in Cushing syndrome as well as with dietary or parenteral deprivation of K[+] (eg, parenteral therapy without adequate K[+] replacement). Hypokalemia occurs with vomiting, diuretics, β₂-adrenergic agonist medications, burns, excessive perspiration, alkalosis, Bartter syndrome, Gitelman syndrome, malnutrition, ureterosigmoidostomy, alcoholism, theophylline overdose, toluene inhalation, anabolic states, insulin overdose, folic acid deficiency, and renal tubular disorders.

Other drugs causing hypokalemia include bronchodilators; tocolytic agents; caffeine; verapamil intoxication; chloroquine intoxication; diuretics; mineralocorticoids and substances such as licorice; high-dose glucocorticoids; high-dose penicillin; nafcillin, ampicillin, and carbenicillin; aminoglycosides; cisplatin; foscarnet; amphotericin B; phenolphthalein; and sodium polystyrene sulfonate.[5]

Causes of K[+] loss in stools include laxatives, diarrhea, tumors (eg, VIPoma, colorectal villous tumor, and Zollinger-Ellison syndrome), jejunoileal bypass, enteric fistulas, malabsorption, chemotherapy, radiation enteropathy, and other entities[5] (see Potassium, Urine *on page 259*).

Hyperkalemia (high potassium) reflects generally inadequate renal excretion, mobilization of potassium from the tissues, or excessive intake or administration. Hyperkalemia occurs with trauma,[6] with administration of K[+] salts of some drugs, ACE inhibitors, Addison disease, acidosis including ketoacidosis as in diabetes mellitus, insulin lack, with increased osmolality (eg, glucose, mannitol), and in other entities as well as in renal diseases with azotemia, with malignant hyperthermia, and with renal tubular acidosis. Increased K[+] can occur with potassium-sparing diuretics, nonsteroidal anti-inflammatory drugs, especially in the presence of renal disease. Systemic heparin therapy can suppress aldosterone release and increase K[+], especially in the presence of other factors. Hyperkalemia is reported with high-dose trimethoprim-sulfamethoxazole therapy.[7] Other factors which may cause hyperkalemia include dehydration, exercise, pregnancy, standing posture, and hyperventilation.[8] Hyperkalemia can be caused by ingestion of large quantities of water from a potassium-based water softener in subjects in renal failure.[9] **Artifact causing hyperkalemia includes hemolysis from collection, storage, or processing.**

Limitations Drug effects are summarized.[10] Inadequate sodium intake may mask the hypokalemia of aldosteronism; sodium loading in that setting may make hypokalemia recognizable. Heparinized plasma is probably the specimen of choice for K[+], because clotting causes cytolysis and may elevate serum values, usually but not always only slightly. Artifactual hyperkalemia may be found in serum (but not plasma) in patients with essential thrombocythemia.[11]

Be wary of potentially falsely high K[+] concentrations in blood samples that have sat unattended for several hours. Such samples may have falsely elevated K[+] in the absence of visible hemolysis ("pocket syndrome"). If doubt exists, repeat measurements on a fresh specimen.

While acute hypokalemia is reflected largely by serum/plasma K[+] concentration, chronic hypokalemia is more apt to be accompanied by reduction of total body stores, as well as serum/plasma concentrations.

Methodology Ion-selective electrode (ISE) in most laboratories

Additional Information Patients scheduled for cardiac surgery may benefit from preoperative serum/plasma potassium measurement and repletion therapy.[12] Low K[+] is much more significant with a low pH than with a high pH. When pH increases by 0.1, K[+] decreases ~0.6 mmol/L. With low pH, as in ketoacidosis, as therapeutic adjustment towards normal pH is made, plasma/serum K[+] concentrations will decrease. Phosphorus concentrations tend to follow potassium downwards during therapy of diabetic ketoacidosis; both are largely intracellular. With insulin therapy (and increased utilization of carbohydrate), potassium moves into cells and serum/plasma concentrations fall. Hyperalimentation may have a similar effect. Hypokalemia has been reported in slightly >50% of a series of 32 patients with acute myelogenous leukemia, but thrombocytosis can increase serum K[+] levels, *vide supra.*

Consider magnesium status in patients who have hypokalemia.[13]

Since platelets release K[+] during coagulation, samples from patients who have thrombocytosis (eg, some cases of polycythemia vera and other myeloproliferative diseases) yield spuriously elevated K[+] concentrations. This "pseudohyperkalemia" may also occur in cases of leukemia with high WBC count (notably chronic myelogenous leukemia) as potassium is released from WBCs and platelets during clot formation. For such patients it is best to assay K[+] on a heparinized sample. Pseudohyperkalemia in serum specimens may be due to increased platelets.[14] Serum potassium increases with the platelet count in normal subjects and in those with thrombocytosis and spherocytosis, and such pseudohyperkalemia increment is an artifact.[15] Plasma concentrations are not affected.

A discussion of the relation between lactic acidosis, ketoacidosis, and elevated serum K[+] levels is provided in a paper by Fulop.[16]

Footnotes

1. Clausen TG, Brocks K, and Ibsen H, "Hypokalemia and Ventricular Arrhythmias in Acute Myocardial Infarction," *Acta Med Scand,* 1988, 224(6):531-7.
2. Weiner ID and Wingo CS, "Hyperkalemia: A Potential Silent Killer," *J Am Soc Nephrol,* 1998, 9(8):1535-43.
3. Weiner ID and Wingo CS, "Hypokalemia - Consequences, Causes and Correction," *J Am Soc Nephrol,* 1997, 8(7):179-88.
4. Blumenfeld JD, Sealey JE, Schlussel Y, et al, "Diagnosis and Treatment of Primary Hyperaldosteronism," *Ann Intern Med,* 1994, 121(11):877-85.
5. Gennari FJ, "Hypokalemia," *N Engl J Med,* 1998, 339:451-58.
6. Vanek VW, Seballos RM, Chong D, et al, "Serum Potassium Concentrations in Trauma Patients," *South Med J,* 1994, 87(1):41-6.
7. Greenberg S, Reiser IW, and Chou SY, "Hyperkalemia With High-Dose Trimethoprim-Sulfamethoxazole Therapy," *Am J Kidney Dis,* 1993, 22(4):603-6.
8. Gambino R, "Nondisease Factors That Affect Potassium Levels," *Lab Rep,* 1995, 17(10):69-71.

9. Graves JW, "Hyperkalemia Due to a Potassium-Based Water Softener," *N Engl J Med*, 1998, 339(24):1790-1.

10. Young DS, "Effects of Drugs on Clinical Laboratory Tests," 5th ed, Volume 1: Listing by Test, Washington, DC: AACC Press, American Association of Clinical Chemistry, 2000, Section 3, 644-54.

11. Howard MR, Ashwell S, Bond LR, et al, "Artifactual Serum Hyperkalaemia and Hypercalcaemia in Essential Thrombocythaemia," *J Clin Pathol*, 2000, 53(2):105-9.

12. Wahr JA, Parks R, Boisvert D, et al, "Preoperative Serum Potassium Levels and Perioperative Outcomes in Cardiac Surgery Patients," *JAMA*, 1999, 281(23):2203.

13. Ryan MP, "Interrelationships of Magnesium and Potassium Homeostasis," *Miner Electrolyte Metab*, 1993, 19(4-5):290-5.

14. Colussi G and Cipriani D, "Pseudohyperkalemia in Extreme Leukocytosis," *Am J Nephrol*, 1995, 15(5):450-2.

15. Alani FS, Dyer T, Hindle E, et al, "Pseudohyperkalaemia Associated With Hereditary Spherocytosis in Four Members of a Family," *Postgrad Med J*, 1994, 70(828):749-51.

16. Fulop M, "Hyperkalemia in Diabetic Ketoacidosis," *Am J Med Sci*, 1990, 299(3):164-9.

References

Agarwal R, Afzalpurkar R, and Fordtran JS, "Pathophysiology of Potassium Absorption and Secretion by the Human Intestine," *Gastroenterology*, 1994, 107(2):548-71.

Alpern RJ and Toto RD, "Hypokalemic Nephropathy - A Clue to Cystogenesis?" *N Engl J Med*, 1990, 322(6):398-9.

Brem AS, "Disorders of Potassium Homeostasis," *Pediatr Clin North Am*, 1990, 37(2):419-27.

Corr LA, Grounds RM, Beacham JL, et al, "Effects of Circulating Endogenous Catecholamines on Plasma Glucose, Potassium, and Magnesium," *Clin Sci*, 1990, 78(2):185-91.

Desai SP and Isa-Pratt S, "Adrenal Cortical Function Tests," *Clinician's Guide to Laboratory Medicine*, Cleveland, OH: Lexi-Comp, 2000, 181-200.

Faria SH, "Assessing Laboratory Values: Serum Na+, K+, and Ca+," *Home Care Provid*, 1998, 3(2):73-6.

Gambino R, "Hypokalemia and Heat Stress - Men vs Women. A Closer Look at the Untold Medical Story Behind the Headlines of the Citadel Incident," *Lab Med*, 1995, 17(9):61-4.

Gitelman HJ, "Unresolved Issues in the Pathogenesis of Bartter's Syndrome and Its Variants," *Curr Opin Nephrol Hypertens*, 1994, 3(4):471-4.

Halperin ML and Kamel KS, "Potassium," *Lancet*, 1998, 352(9122):135-40.

Higham PD, Adams PC, Murray A, et al, "Plasma Potassium, Serum Magnesium, and Ventricular Fibrillation: A Prospective Study," *Q J Med*, 1993, 86(9):609-17.

Krishna GG, "Role of Potassium in the Pathogenesis of Hypertension," *Am J Med Sci*, 1994, 307(Suppl 1):S21-5.

Latta K, Hisano S, and Chan JC, "Perturbations in Potassium Balance," *Clin Lab Med*, 1993, 13(1):149-56.

Phillips SL and Polzin DJ, "Clinical Disorders of Potassium Homeostasis. Hyperkalemia and Hypokalemia," *Vet Clin North Am Small Anim Pract*, 1998, 28(3):545-64.

Shaffer SG, Kilbride HW, Hayen LK, et al, "Hyperkalemia in Very Low Birth Weight Infants," *J Pediatr*, 1992, 121(2):275-9.

Solomon R, Weinberg MS, and Dubey A, "The Diurnal Rhythm of Plasma Potassium: Relationship to Diuretic Therapy," *J Cardiovasc Pharmacol*, 1991, 17(5):854-9.

Torres VE, Young WF Jr, Offord KP, et al, "Association of Hypokalemia, Aldosteronism, and Renal Cysts," *N Engl J Med*, 1990, 322(6):345-51.

Wong KC, Schafer PG, and Schultz JR, "Hypokalemia and Anesthetic Implications," *Anesth Analg*, 1993, 77(6):1238-60.

Potassium, Urine

Related Information

Synonyms K+, Urine; Urine K+

Applies to Kaliuresis

Replaces Electrolytes, Urine

Abstract Urine potassium studies provide explanation for disturbances of serum or plasma values. Urinary potassium losses may reflect primary hyperaldosteronism (adrenocortical adenoma or carcinoma, bilateral adrenocortical hyperplasia); congenital adrenal hyperplasia (22-β-hydroxylase deficiency, 17-α-hydroxylase deficiency); renin-secreting tumors, ectopic corticotropin syndrome, Cushing syndrome (pituitary or adrenocortical disease); glucocorticoid-responsive aldosteronism, renovascular hypertension, malignant hypertension, vasculitis; Liddle syndrome; 11-β-hydroxysteroid dehydrogenase deficiency; Bartter syndrome and Gitelman syndrome.[1]

Specimen Random or timed urine (ie, 8-, 12-, or 24-hour)

Container No preservative

Storage Instructions Refrigerate

Reference Interval 26-123 mmol/24 hours, markedly intake dependent. If significantly decreased serum or plasma K+ has existed for days or more, urine K+ excretion should be low: ≤15 mmol/L (SI: ≤15 mmol/L), or ≤30 mmol/24 hours (SI: ≤30 mmol/day). There is significant diurnal variation, output greater at night.[2]

Use Evaluate electrolyte balance, acid-base balance; evaluate hypokalemia; Carroll and Oh point out that urinary loss of 40 mmol/24 hours (SI: 40 mmol/

day) in the presence of hypokalemia <3 mmol/L is excessive.[3] In the presence of such hypokalemia, urine excretion is helpful to separate renal from nonrenal losses. Excretion <20 mmol/24 hours (SI: <20 mmol/day) is evidence that hypokalemia is not from renal loss.[2] Causes include vomiting, nasogastric tube suctioning, villous tumor, VIPoma, laxative abuse, and hyperhidrosis. Renal loss >50 mmol/L in a hypokalemic, hypertensive patient not on a diuretic may indicate primary or secondary hyperaldosteronism/hyper-reninemia. The kidneys do not respond quickly to potassium deprivation. There is renal wastage of K+ in secondary aldosteronism. Glucocorticoids, including endogenous steroids in Cushing syndrome, are among the causes of kaliuresis. A 24-hour urine collection for potassium represents an appropriate screening test for hyperaldosteronism, preferably following K+ repletion to achieve serum level >3 mmol/L.[4] Urine sodium:potassium ratio helps in the evaluation of children with hypercalciuria.[5]

Limitations A number of agents cause alterations in urinary K+ excretion.[6]

Methodology Ion-selective electrode (ISE) in most laboratories

Additional Information Urinary K+ may be elevated with dietary (food and/or medicinal) increase, hyperaldosteronism, renal tubular acidosis, onset of alkalosis, and with other disorders. Characteristics of primary aldosteronism include hypertension, hypokalemia, decreased plasma renin and increased plasma aldosterone concentrations. Such patients have inappropriate kaliuresis, 24-hour urinary K+ >30 mmol, in the presence of hypokalemia (serum K+ <3.0 mmol/L).[7]

Time relationships are important in interpretation. K+ will decrease in Addison disease and in renal disease with decreased urine flow (nephrosclerosis, pyelonephritis, glomerulonephritis).

An algorithm for the differential diagnosis of hypokalemia is given in the flowchart.[8] See Chloride, Urine *on page 145*.

Differential Diagnosis of Hypokalemia

Diuretic therapy is the most common cause of hypokalemia (see Gennari footnote).

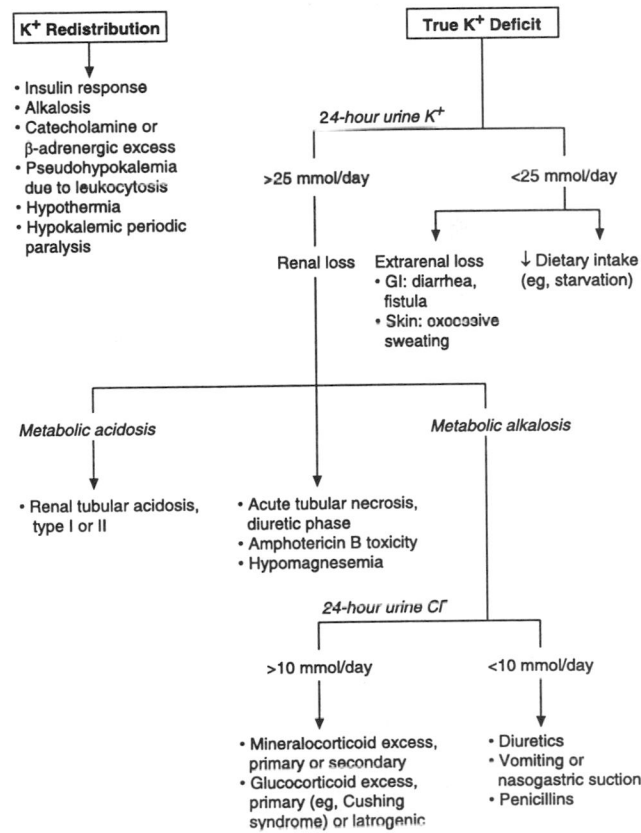

Adapted from Heusel JW, Siggard-Anderson O, and Scott MG, "Physiology and Disorders of Water, Electrolyte and Acid-Base Metabolism," *Tietz Textbook of Clinical Chemistry*, 3rd ed, Burtis CA and Ashwood ER, eds, Philadelphia, PA: WB Saunders Co, 1999, 1095-124.

Footnotes

1. Gennari FJ, "Hypokalemia," *N Engl J Med*, 1998, 339(7):451-8.

2. Moore-Ede MC, Czeisler CA, and Richardson GS, "Circadian Timekeeping in Health and Disease, Part 2. Clinical Implications of Circadian Rhythmicity," *N Engl J Med*, 1983, 309:530-6.

3. Carroll HJ and Oh MS, *Water Electrolyte and Acid-Base Metabolism: Diagnosis and Management*, Philadelphia, PA: JB Lippincott Co, 1978.

(Continued)

Potassium, Urine (Continued)

4. "A 52-Year-Old Man With Hypertension, Hypokalemia, and an Adrenal Mass," Case Records of the Massachusetts General Hospital, Case 24-1992, Scully RE, Mark EJ, McNeely WF, et al, eds, *N Engl J Med*, 1992, 326(24):1617-23.
5. Osorio AV and Alon US, "The Relationship Between Urinary Calcium, Sodium and Potassium Excretion and the Role of Potassium in Treating Idiopathic Hypercalciuria," *Pediatrics*, 1997, 100(4):675-81.
6. Young DS, "Effects of Drugs on Clinical Laboratory Tests," 5th ed, Volume 1: Listing by Test, Washington, DC: AACC Press, American Association of Clinical Chemistry, 2000, Section 3, 654-5.
7. Ghose RP, Hall PM, and Bravo EL, "Medical Management of Aldosterone-Producing Adenomas," *Ann Intern Med*, 1999, 131(2):105-8.
8. Heusel JW, Siggaard-Andersen O, and Scott MG, "Physiology and Disorders of Water, Electrolyte and Acid-Base Metabolism," *Tietz Textbook of Clinical Chemistry*, 3rd ed, Burtis CA and Ashwood ER, eds, Philadelphia, PA: WB Saunders Co, 1999, 1095-124.

References

Giebisch G, "Renal Potassium Transport: Mechanisms and Regulation," *Am J Physiol*, 1998, 274(5 Pt 2):F817-33.

Tannen RL, "Potassium Disorders," *Fluids and Electrolytes*, 2nd ed, Kokko JA and Tannen RL, eds, Philadelphia, PA: WB Saunders Co, 1990, 195-300.

White PC, "Disorders of Aldosterone Biosynthesis and Action," *N Engl J Med*, 1994, 331(4):250-8.

♦ **PP, 2-Hour** *see* Glucose, Postglucose Load, Plasma *on page 185*

♦ **Pravastatin** *see* Mevalonic Acid, Urine or Amniotic Fluid *on page 225*

♦ **Prealbumin** *see* Transthyretin, Serum *on page 287*

Pregnancy-Associated Protein A, Serum

Related Information

Alpha$_1$-Fetoprotein, Serum *on page 97*

Amniotic Fluid, Chromosome and Genetic Abnormality Analysis *on page 360*

Chorionic Gonadotropin, Human, Serum and Urine *on page 147*

Chorionic Villus Sampling, Chromosome and Genetic Abnormality Analysis *on page 361*

Estriol, Unconjugated, Pregnancy, Serum, Plasma, or Urine *on page 171*

Inhibin A, Serum *on page 199*

Synonyms PAPP-A

Applies to Combined Test; Double Test; Integrated Test; Triple Test

Abstract In the first trimester of pregnancy, Down syndrome is associated with high concentrations of maternal free β-hCG or hCG, low concentrations of pregnancy-associated plasma protein A, and equivocally, high values for fetal nuchal translucency, the last measured by ultrasonography. Application of such testing has reached sensitivity levels of first trimester screening up to as much as 80%.[1]

Specimen Serum

Sampling Time Measure maternal serum pregnancy-associated plasma protein A and hCG or its free beta subunit at 10-14 weeks gestation. Measurements of PAPP-A are used only before 14 weeks of gestation.

Storage Instructions Separate serum and refrigerate.

Special Instructions Maternal age is needed.

Reference Interval PAPP-A values are low in affected pregnancies throughout the 8- to 14-week period, more at 8-11 weeks than at 12-14 weeks.[2]

Use Screening for Down syndrome in the first trimester with PAPP-A and either hCG or its free β-subunit in maternal serum is feasible. Indications for such screening include advanced maternal age, family history of Down syndrome, family history of another chromosomal abnormality or of another genetic disorder. Risk according to maternal age can be estimated with an equation.[3]

Limitations At 8-14 weeks gestation, the detection rate is 62% for a 5% false-positive rate.[2]

Methodology Two-site immunometric assay,[2] enzyme-linked immunosorbent assay (ELISA)[3]

Additional Information The markers, PAPP-A and β-hCG at 10 weeks of pregnancy, are combined with maternal age to estimate risk of Down syndrome. These three indices were better than the **double test** (α-fetoprotein and hCG and maternal age) and similar to the **triple test** (α-fetoprotein, unconjugated estriol and hCG with maternal age) at 15-22 weeks.[2] **The combined test** proposes application of PAPP-A, free β subunit of hCG, and nuchal translucency by ultrasonography at 10-13 weeks (first trimester).

Rates of detection of Down syndrome were 42% for PAPP-A, 29% for free hCG, 25% for free β-subunit of hCG, 17% for α-fetoprotein, and 4% for unconjugated estriol at 5% false-positive rates. In combination with maternal age and PAPP-A, the detection rate of hCG was 63% while 60% was the rate for free β-subunit hCG.[3]

Screening for Down syndrome is an effective means to select patients for chorionic villus sampling or amniocentesis.[4]

The **integrated test** integrates measurements of first and second trimester markers including PAPP-A and nuchal translucency in the first trimester. Second trimester serum markers are low maternal α-fetoprotein and unconjugated estriol with high hCG and inhibin A concentrations. The integrated test achieves low false-positive rates.[4] However, in the U.S., the practice is to provide patients with timely results.[1]

Footnotes

1. Copel JA and Bahado-Singh RO, "Prenatal Screening for Down's Syndrome - A Search for the Family's Values," *N Engl J Med*, 1999, 341(7):521-2.
2. Wald NJ, George L, Smith D, et al, "Serum Screening for Down's Syndrome Between 8 and 14 Weeks of Pregnancy," *Br J Obstet Gynaecol*, 1996, 103(5):407-12.
3. Haddow JE, Palomaki GE, Knight GJ, et al, "Screening of Maternal Serum for Fetal Down's Syndrome in the First Trimester," *N Engl J Med*, 1998, 338(14):955-61.
4. Wald NJ, Watt HC, and Hackshaw AK, "Integrated Screening for Down's Syndrome Based on Tests Performed During the First and Second Trimesters," *N Engl J Med*, 1999, 341(7):461-7.

♦ **Pregnancy Testing** *see* Chorionic Gonadotropin, Human, Serum and Urine *on page 147*

Pregnancy Test, Serum or Urine

Related Information

Chorionic Gonadotropin, Human, Serum and Urine *on page 147*

Progesterone, Serum *on page 261*

Synonyms Beta Subunit Human Chorionic Gonadotropin, Urine or Serum; hCG, Slide Test, Stat; hCG, Urine; Human Chorionic Gonadotropin, Urine

Abstract Amenorrhea, morning sickness, breast symptoms, and enlarged uterus with soft cervix are among clinical indicators of pregnancy. Urinary human chorionic gonadotropin (β-hCG) is used as an indication of pregnancy or of hCG-producing tumors. The gold standard is a urine or serum hCG test.[1]

Specimen Serum or urine; first voided morning specimen is preferred if urine is tested (to obtain most concentrated specimen).

Container Red top tube or urine container

Storage Instructions Serum should be frozen at -20°C if not run within 48 hours. Urine is stable 4 hours at 25°C and 3 days at 4°C.

Causes for Rejection Urine specimen grossly contaminated, low urinary specific gravity, proteinuria (applicable to certain tests), gross lipemia or turbidity

Turnaround Time 1 hour (in laboratory ~15 minutes)

Special Instructions Centrifuge turbid urine specimens prior to testing.

Reference Interval Normal male/nonpregnant female: negative; normal pregnant female: positive. Sensitivity and specificity of β-subunit two point RIA or EIA tests may allow early diagnosis of pregnancy, within 6 days after conception. Presently, qualitative tests are positive when intact hCG exceeds 25 IU/L (International Reference Preparation, IRP (also called Third International Standard, 3rd IS), from World Health Organization).[2,3] Concentration of hCG in urine is parallel to that of serum, with about equal quantities in 1 L of serum and in a 24-hour urine collection.[4]

Use Establish diagnosis of pregnancy; screen for women at risk of being pregnant prior to performance of x-ray, sterilization, menstrual regulation, and curettage procedures and/or prior to the initiation of gestation/embryo/fetal potentially injurious medication (eg, to avoid teratogenic drugs), evaluation of abdominal pain; detection and/or evaluation of incomplete/complete abortion; detection of ectopic gestation. A sensitive and quantitative test for the presence of hCG is preferable to rule out or follow gestational trophoblastic neoplasia or ectopic hCG-producing tumor.

False negative pregnancy tests lead to delay in prenatal care and possible continuation of teratogenic exposures.

Limitations Results may be negative in early pregnancy or with low specific gravity urine. In early pregnancy, incomplete abortion, recent complete abortion, ectopic pregnancy (in which hCG level is low), slide test endpoints may be difficult to interpret. Methods using covalent bonded latex particles and tests producing macroagglutination are more reliably interpreted. Reliability of serum and urine tests are comparable.[1]

Methodology Slide or tube agglutination-inhibition tests (urine) are largely replaced by enzyme immunoassay (EIA); β-subunit hCG by radioimmunoassay (RIA) (serum or urine); immunoradiometric (IRMA) (eg, Tandem® hCG which incorporates two monoclonal antibodies, each with immunospecificity for different sites on the hCG molecule, one coated on a plastic bead on which the solid phase develops). Enzyme immunoassay, including sensitive (to 5-40 mIU/mL level of hCG, SI: 5-40 IU/L) two-point urine or serum qualitative/quantitative membrane based tests of which Tandem® ICON® is most well known.

Additional Information Pregnancy testing may be performed on serum or urine. It is based on detection of human chorionic gonadotropin (hCG). Concentrations of hCG in the urine approach those seen in serum. In normal pregnancy, hCG levels rise at implantation and peak at 8-12 weeks. Although newer urine pregnancy tests are quite sensitive, false negatives can occur early in gestation. In such cases, if ectopic pregnancy is suspected, serial serum hCG and progesterone assays may be of value; see these listings.

Early in the first trimester of pregnancy (1-2 weeks) serum hCG concentrations are from 50-500 mIU/mL (SI: 50-500 IU/L). Current generation sensitive tests can detect pregnancy shortly (2-3 days) after implantation of the ovum. By 3-4 weeks of gestation, hCG is at the 500-10,000 mIU/mL level (SI: 500-10,000 IU/L). Serum hCG level peaks during the second to third month of gestation (30,000-100,000 mIU/mL) (SI: 30,000-100,000 IU/L).

Use of serum for pregnancy testing may provide greater sensitivity, of special value in cases of early pregnancy, and is of greater value in serial testing for follow-up of an abnormal gestation (eg, ectopic pregnancy or a gestational trophoblastic neoplasm). If serum (or urine) hCG concentrations do not appear to correlate with the anticipated clinical situation, periodic repeat hCG and progesterone determinations may be helpful.[5,6,7] If there is demise of the developing embryo/fetus (eg, ectopic pregnancy), hCG and progesterone concentrations will fall. Because of slow clearance from the serum, hCG may be detected in serum/urine for as long as 4 weeks following abortion.

Currently, the tests most commonly used to screen for pregnancy are two-point EIA "concentration" methods. A variety of different forms are commercially available. An antibody (frequently monoclonal) is immobilized on a membrane or other solid phase and the sample hCG is "concentrated" in a small central area of the surface (a membrane, bead, paddle, tube, or dipstick). Color development occurs within minutes of addition of enzyme tagged monoclonal anti-β-hCG. These tests are sensitive, specific, and fast. They have largely supplanted slide/tube screening procedures.

A study of specificity (six commercially available ELISA urine pregnancy tests) utilizing specimens from men and postmenopausal females found variable performance by the different methods, not explained by review of the medical records. Variations in results may be explained by the large number of antibody specificities available.[3,8,9,10] Test systems with provision for a negative reference area gave fewer false-positive results (had greater specificity).[11] Correlation was found between mucous content of the postmenopausal female group's urine samples and the incidence of false-positive hCG results.

One year of routine use of Tandem® ICON® system for urine pregnancy testing (University of Texas Southwestern) did not result in a report of known false-positive results. Stability of color development after addition of color reagents and presence or absence of a built in positive control could influence choice of a test system for routine use.

Serum progesterone levels used with β-hCG levels may assist in differentiating normal intrauterine from abnormal intrauterine or **ectopic pregnancy** (cutoff: 15 ng/mL) (SI: 48 nmol/L). β-hCG and progesterone levels are lower in abnormal pregnancies. Less overlap occurs, however, between progesterone (as compared to β-hCG) values in normal versus ectopic and abnormal pregnancies.[5,6,7,12] When a positive pregnancy test is obtained, differential considerations should include the possibility of simultaneous intrauterine and extrauterine gestations[13] (albeit unlikely) and the possibility of passively acquired hCG as in an individual recently transfused with fresh frozen plasma prepared from pregnant donors[14] (also unlikely). When a gestation is large enough to produce in excess of 1600 IU/L hCG (3rd IS) (at about 5 weeks gestation) one may anticipate that in normal gestation the sac should be visible on transvaginal ultrasonography, **depending upon methods**.[9]

A number of commercially successful home pregnancy tests have been available since their introduction in 1976. They have been found to vary widely in performance, particularly in accuracy, sensitivity, specificity, and human factor usability.[15]

Footnotes
1. Bastion LA and Piscitelli JT, "Is This Patient Pregnant? Can You Reliably Rule In or Rule Out Early Pregnancy by Clinical Examination?" *JAMA*, 1997, 278(7):586-91.
2. Hussa RO, *The Clinical Marker hCG*, New York, NY: Praeger Publishers, 1987.
3. Smikle CB, Sorem KA, Wians FH, et al, "Measuring Quantitative Serum Human Chorionic Gonadotropin: Variations in Levels Between Kits," *J Repro Med*, 1995, 40(6):439-42
4. Baskin LB and Charles RA, "Detecting Ectopic Pregnancy," *Lab Med*, 1997, 28(2):103-5.
5. Stewart BK, Nazar-Stewart V, and Toivola B, "Biochemical Discrimination of Pathologic Pregnancy From Early, Normal Intrauterine Gestation in Symptomatic Patients," *Am J Clin Pathol*, 1995, 103(4):386-90.
6. Stovall TG, Kellerman AL, Ling FW, et al, "Emergency Department Diagnosis of Ectopic Pregnancy," *Ann Emerg Med*, 1990, 19(10):1098-103.
7. Al-Sebai MA, Kingsland CR, Diver M, et al, "The Role of a Single Progesterone Measurement in the Diagnosis of Early Pregnancy Failure and the Prognosis of Fetal Viability," *Br J Obstet Gynaecol* 1995, 102(5):364-9.
8. Cole LA, "Human Choriogonadotropin and Related Molecules," *AACC Endo*, 1994, 12:207-24.
9. Klee GG, "Human Chorionic Gonadotropin," *Mayo Clin Proc*, 1994, 69(4):391-2.
10. Mishalani SH, Seliktar J, and Braunstein GD, "Four Rapid Serum-Urine Combination Assays of Choriogonadotropin (hCG) Compared and Assessed for Their Utility in Quantitative Determination of hCG," *Clin Chem*, 1994, 40(10):1944-9.
11. Bandi ZL, Schoen I, and DeLara M, "Enzyme-Linked Immunosorbent Urine Pregnancy Tests: Clinical Specificity Studies," *Am J Clin Pathol*, 1987, 87(2):236-42.
12. Riss PA, Radivojevic K, and Bieglmayer C, "Serum Progesterone and Human Chorionic Gonadotropin in Very Early Pregnancy: Implications for Clinical Management," *Eur J Obstet Gynecol Reprod Biol*, 1989, 32(2):71-7.
13. Boutiette LA and Anderson GV Jr, "Heterotopic Pregnancy," *J Emerg Med*, 1989, 7(1):33-5.
14. Kruskall MS, Owings DV, Donovan LM et al, "Passive Transfusion of Human Chorionic Gonadotropin From Plasma Donated During Pregnancy," *Vox Sang*, 1989, 56(2):71-4.
15. Bastian LA, Nanda K, Hasselblad V, et al, "Diagnostic Efficiency of Home Pregnancy Test Kits: A Meta-analysis," *Arch Fam Med*, 1998, 7(5):465-9.

References
Norman RJ, Gilmore TA, and McLoughlin JW, "Simple Quantitative Measurement of Serum Choriogonadotropin Compared With Immunoradiometric, Immunoenzymometric, and Chemiluminescent Assays," *Clin Chem*, 1992, 38(1):144-7.
Taylor CA Jr, Overstreet JW, Samuels SJ, et al, "Prospective Assessment of Early Fetal Loss Using An Immunoenzymometric Screening Assay for Detection of Urinary Human Chorionic Gonadotropin," *Fertil Steril*, 1992, 57(6):1220-4.
Wyte CD, "Diagnostic Modalities in the Pregnant Patient," *Emerg Med Clin North Am*, 1994, 12(1):9-43.

Pregnanetriol, Urine

Related Information
17-Hydroxyprogesterone, Serum or Plasma *on page 197*

Abstract Pregnanetriol is a metabolite of 17-hydroxyprogesterone. Increased urinary excretion is observed when the serum level of 17-hydroxyprogesterone is elevated.

Patient Preparation Avoid exercise before and during collection.

Specimen 24-hour urine

Collection Preserve with boric acid.

Reference Interval Varies with laboratory.[1]
- 0-5 years: <0.1 mg/day (SI: <0.3 μmol/day)
- 6-9 years: <0.3 mg/day (SI: <0.9 μmol/day)
- adult male: 0.4-2.5 mg/day (SI: 1.2-7.5 μmol/day)
- adult female: follicular: 0.1-0.8 mg/day (SI: 0.3-5.3 μmol/day); luteal: 0.9-2.2 mg/day (SI: 2.7-6.5 μmol/day)

Use Urinary pregnanetriol is increased in congenital adrenal hyperplasia (21-hydroxylase type), but this test is not usually required in the diagnostic evaluation for this disorder.

Limitations The expected elevation in urinary pregnanetriol is not observed in infants.[2] Muscular exercise may increase urinary pregnanetriol.

Methodology Gas-liquid chromatography (GLC)

Footnotes
1. Painter PC, Cope JY, and Smith JL, "Reference Information for the Clinical Laboratory," *Tietz Textbook of Clinical Chemistry*, 3rd ed, Burtis CA and Ashwood ER, eds, Philadelphia, PA: WB Saunders Co, 1999,1831.
2. Grumbach MM and Conte FA, "Disorders of Sex Differentiation," *Williams Textbook of Endocrinology*, 9th ed, Wilson JD, Foster DW, Kronenberg HM, et al, eds, Philadelphia, PA: WB Saunders Co, 1998, 1303-425.

References
Shackleton CH, Irias J, McDonald C, et al, "Late-Onset 21-Hydroxylase Deficiency: Reliable Diagnosis by Steroid Analysis of Random Urine Collections," *Steroids*, 1986, 48(3-4):239-50.

♦ **Pressor Amines** see Catecholamines, Fractionation, Plasma *on page 138*

♦ **Primary Familial Polycythemia** see Erythropoietin Receptor *on page 169*

Progesterone, Serum

Related Information
Chorionic Gonadotropin, Human, Serum and Urine *on page 147*
Estradiol, Serum *on page 170*
Estrogens, Urine *on page 172*
Heterophilic Antibodies *on page 191*
17-Hydroxyprogesterone, Serum or Plasma *on page 197*
Pregnancy Test, Serum or Urine *on page 260*

Abstract A C-21 steroid, progesterone is made by the corpus luteum. It promotes development of the secretory phase of endometrium. Its major source in pregnancy, by 40-50 days after implantation, is the placenta. The serum level of progesterone rises during the luteal (secretory) phase of the endometrial cycle (indicating ovulation) and increases dramatically from the end of the first trimester to term. Progesterone is required for maintenance of pregnancy. Lower values occur with ectopic gestation or miscarriage.[1]

Specimen Serum, saliva

Container Red top tube

Storage Instructions Serum stable 4 days at 4°C and 3 months at -20°C.

Special Instructions Patient's LMP (last menstrual period) and trimester of pregnancy are relevant.

Reference Interval
Serum:[2]
- prepubertal: 7-52 ng/dL (SI: 0.2-1.7 nmol/L)
- adult male: 13-97 ng/dL (SI: 0.4-3.1 nmol/L)
- female: follicular: 15-70 ng/dL (SI: 0.5-2.2 nmol/L); luteal 200-2500 ng/dL (SI: 6.4-79.5 nmol/L)
- pregnancy: 1st trimester: 725-4400 ng/dL (SI: 23.0-140.0 nmol/L); 2nd trimester: 1950-8250 ng/dL (SI: 62.0-262.4 nmol/L); 3rd trimester: 6500-22,900 ng/dL (SI: 206.7-728.2 nmol/L)

Saliva: Assays not widely available. Check with your reference laboratory. One publication indicates:[3]
- follicular: 0.5-4.0 ng/dL (SI: 0.016-0.127 nmol/L)
- luteal: 6.0-12.0 ng/dL (SI: 0.19-0.38 nmol/L)

Critical Values In a pregnant patient with first trimester bleeding, a serum progesterone >250 ng/dL (SI: >7.95 nmol/L) predicts a normal intrauterine pregnancy, while a value <150 ng/dL (SI: <4.77 nmol/L) predicts an
(Continued)

Progesterone, Serum (Continued)

abnormal gestation. The serum progesterone cannot, however, distinguish between an ectopic pregnancy and an abnormal intrauterine pregnancy.[4]

Use

Disorders of the first trimester: Serum progesterone levels are occasionally used in a patient with bleeding to evaluate the possibility of miscarriage or of an ectopic gestation. The usual combination of tests includes serial serum hCG levels and progesterone concentration combined with ultrasound.

Evaluation of infertility: Midluteal luteinizing hormone and progesterone on day 21: progesterone concentration ≥10 µg/mL usually indicates adequate luteinization. Endometrial biopsy between days 24 and 26 provides assessment of secretory phase endometrium.[5]

Assisted reproduction: The test is useful for monitoring patients having ovulation during induction with hCG, hMG, FSH/LHRH, or clomiphene.

Screening for Down syndrome: Serum progesterone levels do not have an established role in this application. At the research level, Kratzer et al have used the serum progesterone level, together with the total serum hCG and free beta-hCG to calculate an "aneuploidy index".[4] See Chorionic Gonadotropin, Human, Serum and Urine on page 147.

Limitations High concentrations of 17-hydroxyprogesterone falsely increase progesterone levels in a number of assays.

Methodology Immunoassays (multiple labels)

Footnotes

1. Baskin LB, "Pregnancy and Prenatal Testing," The Handbook of Clinical Pathology, 2nd ed, McKenna RW and Keffer JH, eds, Chicago, IL: ASCP Press, American Society of Clinical Pathologists, 2000, 281-92.
2. Gronowski AM and Landau-Levine M, "Reproductive Endocrine Function," Tietz Textbook of Clinical Chemistry, 3rd ed, Burtis CA and Ashwood ER, eds, Philadelphia, PA: WB Saunders Co, 1999, 1601-41.
3. Rosevear S, "Bleeding in Early Pregnancy," High Risk Pregnancy, James DK, Steer PJ, Weiner CP, et al, eds, Philadelphia, PA: WB Saunders Co, 1999, 61-89.
4. Kratzer PG, Golbus S, Monroe SE, et al, "First Trimester Aneuploidy Screening Using Serum Human Chorionic Gonadotropin (hCG), Free hCG, and Progesterone," Prenat Diagn, 1991, 11:751-65.
5. Byrd EW Jr, "Andrology and Fertility Assessment," The Handbook of Clinical Pathology, 2nd ed, McKenna RW and Keffer JH, eds, Chicago, IL: ASCP Press, American Society of Clinical Pathologists, 2000, 537-48.

References

Baskin LB and Charles RA, "Clinical Pathology Rounds-Detecting Ectopic Pregnancy," Lab Med, 1997, 28(2):103-5.

Daily CA, Laurent SL, and Nunley WC, "The Prognostic Value of Serum Progesterone and Quantitative Beta-Human Chorionic Gonadotropin in Early Human Pregnancy," Am J Obstet Gynecol, 1994, 171(2):380-4.

Darne J, McGarrigle HH, and Lachelin GC, "Saliva Oestriol, Oestradiol, Oestrone and Progesterone Levels in Pregnancy: Spontaneous Labour at Term Is Preceded by a Rise in the Saliva Oestriol:Progesterone Ratio," Br J Obstet Gynaecol, 1987, 94(3):227-35.

Daya S, "Optimal Time in the Menstrual Cycle for Serum Progesterone Measurement to Diagnose Luteal Phase Defects," Am J Obstet Gynecol, 1989, 161(4):1009-11.

Finn MM, Gosling JP, Tallon DF, et al, "Normal Salivary Progesterone Levels Throughout the Ovarian Cycle as Determined by a Direct Enzyme Immunoassay," Fertil Steril, 1988, 50(6):882-7.

Tay JT, Moore J, and Walker JJ, "Ectopic Pregnancy," BMJ, 2000, 320(7239):916-9.

♦ **Proinsulin** see C-Peptide, Serum on page 156

♦ **Proinsulin** see Insulin, Serum on page 201

Prolactin, Serum

Related Information

Amoxapine, Serum or Plasma on page 736

Dehydroepiandrosterone and Dehydroepiandrosterone Sulfate, Serum or Plasma on page 164

Estradiol, Serum on page 170

Follicle Stimulating Hormone, Serum, Plasma, or Urine on page 175

Heterophilic Antibodies on page 191

Abstract Prolactin (PRL), so named because it initiates and maintains lactation, is one of the anterior pituitary hormones. The hypothalamic secretion of dopamine inhibits the release of PRL from the pituitary. Hormones that stimulate the release of PRL are not well understood, and **may** include thyrotropin-releasing hormone (TRH), vasoactive intestinal polypeptide, and other peptides. PRL is secreted in pulses which are superimposed on a circadian rhythm. A number of physiologic stimuli (eg, sleep, exercise, and hyperglycemia) cause short-term increases in serum PRL.

The most common type of pituitary adenoma (25% to 40%) is the prolactin cell adenoma (prolactinoma). It may or may not be symptomatic. Over 80% are minoadenomas (<10 mm) in reproductive age women.[1] Amenorrhea, irregular menses, and in infertility, galactorrhea provide sensitive signals in reproductive age women; males and older females, lacking most of these indicators, appear later, often with invasion and mass effect.

Patient Preparation Fasting specimen is preferred. In both males and females, the most common cause of elevated PRL is a drug side effect.[2]

Specimen Serum

Container Red top tube

Collection Venipuncture itself can occasionally elevate prolactin level. Draw between 8 AM and 10 AM. Draw in chilled tube. Keep specimen on ice.

Storage Instructions Separate serum in refrigerated centrifuge and freeze. Stable 3 months at -20°C.

Special Instructions When used as a tumor marker, some laboratories can perform prolactin assay on tumor tissue and various body fluids.

Reference Interval Reference ranges are method-dependent. The normal range has little medical importance.

Male:[3]
- 0-1 month: 0-90 ng/mL
- 2-11 months: 0-30 ng/mL
- 1-18 years: 1-15 ng/mL
- >19 years: 4-23 ng/mL

Female:[3]
- 0-1 month: 0-90 ng/mL
- 2-11 months: 0-30 ng/mL
- 1-18 years: 1-15 ng/mL
- >19 years: 4-30 ng/mL

Critical Values In macroadenomas (>10 mm), prolactin concentrations are usually >250 ng/mL, and essentially all are characterized by concentrations >100 ng/mL.

Biochemical cure: Permanent postoperative diminution in prolactin levels to <18 ng/mL in males and <23 ng/mL in females.

Biochemical persistence: Continued postoperative hyperprolactinemia

Biochemical recurrence: Increased prolactin, above normal range after initial postoperative normalization.[1]

Use Features of hyperprolactinemia in women include ovulatory/menstrual dysfunction including amenorrhea, hypoestrogenism, galactorrhea, and infertility.

In males, hyperprolactinemia causes diminished libido, impotence and hypogonadism with suppressed LH and FSH and decreased testosterone concentrations.[1,4] In men and older individuals, the tumors are often macroprolactinomas, which may cause hypopituitarism or visual effects.

Elevated serum PRL usually accompanies galactorrhea.

The differential diagnosis of **hyperprolactinemia** includes drug side effect, PRL-secreting pituitary adenoma, and other diseases of the hypothalamic-pituitary stalk region. Rare causes include renal disease, primary hypothyroidism, and endogenous estrogen overproduction.

Pituitary tumors: The principal clinical use for PRL levels is in the diagnosis of PRL-secreting pituitary adenomas. In this clinical setting, PRL values **must** be interpreted together with imaging studies.

A single PRL value >200 ng/mL is consistent with prolactinoma in a patient with concordant imaging findings. Some patients will require multiple specimens before this criterion is met.[5]

Preoperative Serum Prolactin Levels Stratified by Various Factors

Group	No. of Patients	Serum Prolactin (ng/mL)	
		Median	Range
Young females	38	188	43-3300
Older females	12	370	55-42,000
Males	18	1152	105-6688
Microadenoma	29	179	43-2900
Macroadenoma	39	1000	55-42,000
Noninvasive adenoma	31	141	43-4600
Invasive adenoma	37	705	60-42,000
No mitoses	48	220	43-6400
Mitoses present	20	2062	83-42,000

Adapted from Calle-Rodrigue RD, Giannini C, Scheithauer BW, et al, "Prolactinomas in Male and Female Patients: A Comparative Clinicopathologic Study," Mayo Clin Proc, 1998, 73:1046-52.

In a patient with imaging evidence of a pituitary abnormality and multiple PRL values falling short of these size-referenced criteria, consider the diagnosis of a non-PRL-secreting pituitary tumor (or other similarly located disease process) causing hyperprolactinemia by mechanical compression of the pituitary stalk, thus, interfering with the physiologic inhibition of PRL by dopamine.[5] Some investigators refer to such tumors as "pseudoprolactinomas."

Male Infertility: Some physicians include PRL measurements in their evaluation of subfertile males. When elevated PRL levels are found in this setting, treatment with bromocriptine may be effective in carefully selected patients.[6] Men with **gynecomastia** usually have normal prolactin.[7]

Limitations Many drugs produce increased PRL as a side effect. Estrogens cause prolactin cell hyperplasia and may promote growth of prolactinomas. Other drugs include antipsychotic drugs (especially dopamine receptor antagonists), tricyclic antidepressants, opiates, cimetidine, reserpine, phenothiazines, verapamil, methyldopa, metoclopramide, amphetamines, and fluoxetine.[8] We recommend checking with an authoritative source of drug information before excluding drug side effect as a cause of hyperpro-lactinemia.[2]

Methodology Immunoassay (multiple labels)

Additional Information Estrogens from any source will increase PRL levels. Therefore, patients (male and female) with endogenous hyper-estrogenism, such as occurs in estrogen-secreting neoplasms, will have elevated serum PRL. Estrogen and progesterone receptors are found in prolactinomas.

Approximately 25% to 30% of pituitary adenomas appear not to be hormon-ally active. Of the remainder, PRL is the most commonly secreted hormone.

Footnotes

1. Calle-Rodrigue RD, Giannini C, Scheithauer BW, et al, "Prolactinomas in Male and Female Patients: A Comparative Clinicopathologic Study," *Mayo Clin Proc*, 1998, 73:1046-52.
2. Young DS, "Effects of Drugs on Clinical Laboratory Tests," 5th ed, Volume 1: Listing by Test, Washington, DC: AACC Press, American Association of Clinical Chemistry, 2000, Section 3, 662.
3. Mayo Medical Laboratories, *2000 Mayo Test Catalogue*, Rochester, MN, 423.
4. Molitch ME, "Anterior Pituitary," *Cecil Textbook of Medicine*, 21st ed, Chapter 237, Goldman L and Bennett JC, eds, Philadelphia, PA: WB Saunders Co, 2000, 1208-25.
5. Demers LM, "Pituitary Function," *Tietz Textbook of Clinical Chemistry*, 3rd ed, Burtis CA and Ashwood ER, eds, Philadelphia, PA: WB Saunders, 1999, 1478-80.
6. Vandekerckhove P, Lilford R, Vail A, et al, "Bromocriptine for Idiopathic Oligo-/Asthenospermia (Cochrane Review)," *The Cochrane Library*, Issue 3, 1999, Oxford: Update Software.
7. Frantz AG and Wilson JD, "Endocrine Disorders of the Breast," *Williams Textbook of Endocrinology*, 9th ed, Wilson J, Foster DW, Kronenberg HM, et al, eds, Philadelphia, PA: WB Saunders Co, 1998, 891-2.
8. Peterson MC, "Reversible Galactorrhea and Prolactin Elevation Related to Fluoxetine Use," *Mayo Clin Proc*, 2001:76(2):215-6.

References

Freeman ME, Kanyicska B, Lerant A, et al, "Prolactin: Structure, Function, and Regulation of Secretion," *Physiol Rev*, 2000, 80(4):1523-631.
Schulster D, Gaines-Das RE, and Jeffcoate SL, "International Standards for Human Prolactin: Calibration by International Collaborative Study," *J Endocrinol*, 1989, 121(1):157-66.
Zikel OM, Atkinson JL, and Hurby DL, "Prolactinoma Manifesting With Symptomatic Hydrocephalus," *Mayo Clin Proc*, 1999, 74(5):475-7.

♦ **Proline** see Amino Acids, Urine *on page 101*

♦ **Propionic Aciduria** see Cerebrospinal Fluid Glycine *on page 142*

Prostate Specific Antigen, Free

Related Information
Prostate Specific Antigen, Serum *on page 263*

Synonyms fPSA; Free PSA

Applies to Complexed PSA; Free PSA:Total PSA Ratio

Abstract Upon release into the blood, most PSA is enzymatically active, but is rapidly inactivated by protease inhibitors, the two principal ones being alpha₁ antichymotrypsin and alpha₂ macroglobulin. In normal individuals, most PSA (~80% to 90%) is bound to alpha₁ antichymotrypsin with lesser quantities bound to alpha₂ macroglobulin and other proteins. In patients with adenocarcinoma of the prostate, a higher proportion of PSA is bound (>90%). The unbound fraction is called "free PSA" while the bound fraction is called "complexed PSA". The measurement of both free and complexed fractions may be useful in screening men with other equivocal findings. Goals include reduction of the number of unnecessary biopsies in men with total PSA concentrations between 4 and 10 ng/mL, the gray zone. It is not helpful when total PSA is <2.5 or 3.0[1] or 4.0.[2] Free PSA increases specificity with only slight loss of sensitivity, providing stratification of cancer risk in the gray zone. Low levels of fPSA are associated with adverse characteristics.[3]

Patient Preparation Fasting specimen is preferred. The practice of sampling at least 4 weeks following digital rectal examination and needle biopsy is published;[4] *vide infra*. Avoid recent exposure to radioactivity if RIA is used.

Specimen Serum

Container Red top tube

Sampling Time Recent prostatic manipulation probably should be avoided; *vide supra*. PSA has little diurnal variation[5]. Although it is often sampled together with prostatic acid phosphatase (PAP), the latter has fallen into disrepute.

Collection Rectal examination within 48 hours of specimen collection may cause elevation of results.

Storage Instructions PSA is stable in serum for 48 hours if refrigerated. For longer periods, store at -20°C or colder.[5] No special treatment of serum is required. Ship to a reference laboratory in a plastic vial on dry ice.

Special Instructions Individuals should be followed with the same assays consistently.

Reference Interval Method dependent. Median free PSA % is lower in subjects with prostatic carcinoma. Free PSA/total PSA is typically >25% in normal men and <25% in men with prostatic adenocarcinoma. It has been recommended that men with mildly elevated total PSA (4-10 ng/mL) and a free PSA/total PSA <20% to 30% be evaluated further. Use of percentage free PSA cutoff of 25% detected 98% of carcinomas at ages 50-59 years,

94% at 60-69 years, 90% at 70-75 years, and in men 50-75 years of age with a palpably benign prostate and total PSA of 4-10 ng/mL.[6]

Use The free PSA:total PSA ratio is a useful screening test for identifying men with equivocal laboratory or physical findings who may benefit from prostate biopsy. This group includes those with mildly elevated total PSA (4-10 ng/mL)[6] or those with enlarged prostate volumes detected by ultrasound.

A high risk of carcinoma exists when the percentage of free PSA is very low, cancer occurring in 55% of individuals with levels of 0% to 10%. Cancer risk was 5% to 9% when concentrations were >25%.[6] Its use in monitoring and determining prognosis of men with prostate carcinoma has not been established.[7] A role in prostatic intraepithelial neoplasia is described.[8]

Limitations As with other immunoassays, it is important to use the same method when following a patient or at least to be aware of the relationship between the operational characteristics of different immunoassay methods. This is even more important when using a ratio such as the free PSA:total PSA. Although using different manufacturers' assays for the two measurements is acceptable, it is highly recommended that they be used consistently.

Methodology Two-site immunometric assay. Typically, the capture antibody recognizes an epitope that is present on both free and complexed forms while the signal antibody recognizes an epitope that is blocked by alpha₁ antichymotrypsin in the complexed form. The effect of other bound proteins may be variable, since some molecules such as alpha₂ macroglobulin may block the immunoreactivity of PSA.

Additional Information Assays for complexed PSA are also available. These may recognize either PSA complexed to alpha₁ antichymotrypsin or to alpha₂ macroglobulin.

Footnotes

1. Vashi AR and Oesterling JE, "Percent Free Prostate-Specific Antigen: Entering a New Era in the Detection of Prostate Cancer," *Mayo Clin Proc*, 1997, 72(4):337-44.
2. Carlson GD, Calvanese CB, and Childs SJ, "The Appropriate Lower Limit for the Percent Free Prostate-Specific Antigen Reflex Range," *Urology*, 1998, 52(3):450-4.
3. Horninger W, Rogatsch H, Reissigl A, et al, "Correlation Between Preoperative Predictors and Pathologic Features in Radical Prostatectomy Specimens in PSA-Based Screening," *Prostate*, 1999, 40(1):56-61.
4. Lechevallier E, Echazarian C, Ortega JC, et al, "Kinetics of Postbiopsy Levels of Serum Free Prostate-Specific Antigen and Percent Free Prostate-Specific Antigen," *Urology*, 1999, 53(4):731-5.
5. Schifman RB, Ahmann FR, Elvick A, et al, "Analytical and Physiological Characteristics of Prostate-Specific Antigen and Prostatic Acid Phosphatase in Serum Compared," *Clin Chem*, 1987, 33(11):2086-8.
6. Catalona WJ, Partin AW, Slawin KM, et al, "Use of the Percentage of Free Prostate-Specific Antigen to Enhance Differentiation of Prostate Cancer From Benign Prostatic Disease: A Prospective Multicenter Clinical Trial," *JAMA*, 1998, 279(19):1542-7.
7. Sokoll LJ and Chan DW, "Clinical Applications of the Molecular Forms of Prostate-Specific Antigen," *Diag Endo Metab*, 1998, 16:133-48.
8. Kilic S, Kukul E, Danisman A, et al, "Ratio of Free to Total Prostate-Specific Antigen in Patients With Prostatic Intraepithelial Neoplasia," *Eur Urol*, 1998, 34(3):176-80.

References

Allard WJ, Zhou Z, and Yeung KK, "Novel Immunoassay for the Measurement of Complexed Prostate-Specific Antigen in Serum," *Clin Chem*, 1998, 44(6 Pt 1):1216-23.
Black MH, Giai M, Ponzone R, et al, "Serum Total and Free Prostate-Specific Antigen for Breast Cancer Diagnosis in Women," *Clin Cancer Res*, 2000, 6(2):467-73.
Bostwick DG, Grignon DJ, Hammond MEH, et al, "Prognostic Factors in Prostate Cancer: College of American Pathologists Consensus Statement 1999," *Arch Pathol Lab Med*, 2000, 124(7):995-1000.
Gion M, Mione R, Barioli P, et al, "Percent Free Prostate-Specific Antigen in Assessing the Probability of Prostate Cancer Under Optimal Analytical Conditions," *Clin Chem*, 1998, 44(12):2462-70.
Henricks WH, England BG, Giacherio DA, et al, "Serum Percent-Free PSA Does Not Predict Extraprostatic Spread of Prostate Cancer," *Am J Clin Pathol*, 1998,109(5):533-9.
Jacobsen SJ, Katusic SK, Bergstralh EJ, et al, "Incidence of Prostate Cancer Diagnosis In the Eras Before and After Serum Prostate-Specific Antigen Testing," *JAMA*, 1995, 274(18):1445-9.
Kuriyama M, Kawada Y, Arai Y, et al, "Significance of Free to Total PSA Ratio in Men With Slightly Elevated Serum PSA Levels: A Cooperative Study," *Jpn J Clin Oncol*, 1998, 28(11):661-5.
Leung HY, Lai LC, Day J, et al, "Serum Free Prostate-Specific Antigen in the Diagnosis of Prostate Cancer," *Br J Urol*, 1997, 80(2):256-9.
Roehrborn CG, Gregory A, McConnell JD, et al, "Comparison of Three Assays for Total Serum Prostate-Specific Antigen and Percentage of Free Prostate-Specific Antigen in Predicting Prostate Histology," *Urology*, 1996, 48(6A Suppl):23-32.
Ruckle HC, Klee GG, and Oesterling JE, "Prostate-Specific Antigen: Critical Issues for the Practicing Physician," *Mayo Clin Proc*, 1994, 69(1):59-68.
Stenman UH, Leinonen J, Zhang WM, et al, "Prostate-Specific Antigen," *Sem Cancer Biol*, 1999, 9(2):83-93.
The Internal Medicine Clinic Research Consortium, "Effect of Digital Rectal Examination on Serum Prostate-Specific Antigen in a Primary Care Setting," *Arch Intern Med*, 1995, 155(4):389-92.
Wians FH Jr, "The Role of Prostate-Specific Antigen (PSA) Testing in the Diagnosis, Treatment and Follow-up of Patients With Adenocarcinoma of the Prostate," *ASCP Check Sample*, 1997, 37:77-103.

Prostate Specific Antigen, Serum

Related Information
Acid Phosphatase, Plasma *on page 82*
(Continued)

Prostate Specific Antigen, Serum *(Continued)*

Immunoperoxidase Procedures *on page 60*
Prostate Specific Antigen, Free *on page 263*

Synonyms hK3; Human Kallikrein 3; PSA

Applies to Finasteride; PSA Density; PSA Velocity

Abstract The best, most accurate and the most useful marker for adenocarcinoma of the prostate, PSA is increased in most men with clinically significant prostate cancer, but it is sometimes increased in benign entities and may fall within normal range even with advanced prostatic adenocarcinoma. It increases rates of **detection** of prostatic adenocarcinoma, but some of the carcinomas it detects are biologically insignificant.[1] It is best when the blood sample is collected prior to digital rectal examination,[2] to which it is complementary. Serially measured, PSA is extremely useful in monitoring presurgical, as well as postsurgical patients. PSA level, PSA density, ratio of free to total PSA, and needle biopsy histopathologic observations represent predictors of extent of tumor. PSA density, PSA velocity and fractions of bound or free PSA are called "PSA derivatives" and a consensus does not yet exist about their precise utility.[3] Ultimately, it is clinical outcome which is most important. Category I of the College of American Pathologists rankings, factors proven to be of prognostic importance and useful in clinical patient management, include preoperative serum PSA, TNM stage, Gleason score, and surgical margin status.[3] (Other important factors associated with progression of prostatic carcinoma include positive lymph nodes, intraprostatic vascular invasion, and seminal vesicle invasion). PSA has become an indispensable predictor for recurrent adenocarcinoma in postsurgical patients and those treated with radiation therapy.[4,5,6,7] Stamey et al define biochemical failure as a PSA concentration of at least 0.07 ng/mL, and rising in subsequent samples, using the equimolar automated Tosoh A1A-600 assay. A single sample, confirmed by a second serum specimen >0.07 was also considered an acceptable indication of failure.[8] Pound et al use a detectable serum PSA of at least 0.2 ng/mL as evidence of biochemical failure. They used Hybritech® Tandem R and E and Tosoh PSA assays (Hybritech/Beckman). They use prostate-specific antigen doubling time, timing of the initial PSA increase, and Gleason score as well to predict development of metastatic carcinoma.[9] PSA doubling time is not a useful predictor when the time to PSA recurrence is known.[10]

Patient Preparation Fasting specimen is preferred. The practice of sampling at least 4 weeks following digital rectal examination and needle biopsy is published;[1] *vide infra*. Avoid recent exposure to radioactivity if a radioisotopic method is used.

Specimen Serum

Container Red top tube

Sampling Time Recent prostatic manipulation should be avoided. PSA has little diurnal variation.[11] Although it has often been sampled together with prostatic acid phosphatase (PAP), the latter has fallen into disrepute.

Collection Digital rectal examination within 48 hours of specimen collection may cause elevation of results.[12]

Storage Instructions PSA is stable in serum for 48 hours if refrigerated. For longer periods, store at -20°C or colder.[11] No special treatment of serum is required. Ship to a reference laboratory in a plastic vial on dry ice.

Turnaround Time 1 hour in laboratory

Special Instructions Individual patients should be followed with the same assay consistently. When a decision is made to follow patients without immediate therapy, serial assays are recommended to ascertain rate of change of PSA. This is called **PSA velocity**,[1] defined as change in PSA at 1-year intervals.[13]

Reference Interval Male: <4 ng/mL; female <0.5 ng/mL (immunoassay method); *vide infra*. Age adjusted reference ranges have been advocated; PSA results increase moderately with age; *vide infra*. Use of upper limit of 4.5 ng/mL for men 60-69 years of age and 6.5 ng/mL for those 70 years and older would decrease sensitivity from 86% to 77% but would enhance specificity from 56% to 67%. It would decrease the numbers of biopsies.[14]

For most PSA assays, sensitivity = ~73% to 84%; specificity = ~59% to 93%.[13]

Use Prostate specific antigen, human kallikrein-3 (hK3), is a serine protease that is produced almost exclusively by epithelial cells of prostatic tissue. It is present at high concentrations in seminal fluid and functions in the liquefaction of seminal coagulum.[15] Preoperative PSA serum levels correlate (but imperfectly) with extent of disease in patients with prostate cancer. **PSA density** is obtained by division of serum PSA result by prostatic weight utilizing transrectal ultrasound **(TRUS)** volumetric measurements:

PSA density = [PSA] / total prostate volume; units = ng/mL/cc[13]

Results of PSA density are not definitive; it is increased with prostatitis[16] but may be useful in patient selection for radical prostatectomy.[17] With PSA assay and histopathologic interpretation from prostate needle biopsy, correlation of **extent of tumor** can be improved. (Of these, TRUS has not consistently been found to predict tumor extent.)[1] PSA is useful in detection of residual tumor and disease progression in postoperative stage of prostate cancer. When PSA rises in patients who have previously had prostatectomy and who have no detectable disease, metastases are likely, in spite of inability to detect them.[10]

PSA has several advantages over prostatic acid phosphatase (PAP). It is more stable and does not have a significant diurnal variation. It has been shown to be elevated in 95% of newly diagnosed cases of prostatic carcinoma (vs 60% for PAP) and in 97% of recurrent cases (PAP 66%).[18]

PSA relates to increasing Gleason score and outcome. (Unfortunately, Gleason scores are themselves sometimes problematical.) PSA is successfully widely used in screening selected populations of patients with or without symptoms indicative of prostate cancer and has led to increased detection of prostate cancer. It detects incidental, as well as, aggressive neoplasms. Some of the former are biologically indolent, posing no threat to the life of the patient.[1] Sensitivity for aggressive carcinoma of prostate was 87% for tumors occurring within the first 4 years.[19,20] PSA lacks sufficient sensitivity and specificity to be used alone as a screening test for prostatic carcinoma in the present screening format. In conjunction with digital rectal examination and TRUS, PSA greatly increases prostatic carcinoma detection rates.[21] A strategy which begins at an earlier age but screens biennially rather than annually has been suggested.[22]

A significant shift to lower stage carcinomas, fewer nondiploid, more frequently organ-confined tumors at initial assessment has been recognized since the advent of PSA testing at a large referral center.[23] A new clinical stage category, stage T1c, has evolved following experience with PSA; it is nonpalpable carcinoma detected by increased serum concentration of PSA and diagnosed by examination of needle biopsies. The number of men with metastatic cancer at initial assessment has diminished. Application of PSA has led to diagnosis of lower stage and smaller volume carcinomas. Migration to tumors with more favorable prognostic characteristic, with use of PSA, is described.[24]

A PSA assay is indicated prior to initiation of finasteride therapy for benign hyperplasia of prostate, since this drug causes an ~50% decrease in serum PSA concentration.

Limitations Approximately 25% to 46% of men with benign prostatic hyperplasia have an elevated serum PSA concentration. One-third of men with PSA >4 ng/mL will have carcinoma on prostate biopsy but two-thirds will not.[3] Between 20% and 40% of patients with organ-confined prostatic carcinoma have serum PSA concentrations within the reference range.[13] PSA is not acceptable used alone for staging[23] and alone should not be used to select candidates for radical prostatectomy. Physiologic fluctuation ≤30% is described. PSA is not specific for prostatic adenocarcinoma, but serum levels are specific for prostatic tissue. Elevations may also be associated with digital rectal examination, prostatic massage, urethral instrumentation, prostatitis, TUR, prostatic needle biopsy, urinary retention, or prostatic ischemia or infarct. PSA occasionally has been associated with sources other than prostate.[25,26,27,28] Used in preoperative patients, PSA does not sharply distinguish intracapsular from extracapsular carcinoma. Despite wide availability of screening tests to detect prostatic carcinoma, trials have not shown conclusively overall prolongation of survival.[29] A lack of specificity is recognized between 4-10 ng/mL.[30]

PSA values in the gray zone, between 4 and 10 ng/mL, include some carcinomas. Of men whose PSA values fall in this range and whose digital rectal examination is negative, 75% do not have carcinoma in the initial biopsy.

It is now known that 50% to 90% of serum PSA is bound to an inhibitor called α_1-antichymotrypsin. (See Prostate Specific Antigen, Free *on page 263*.) The antibodies used in assays have different affinities for bound and free PSA. An effort has been made to provide a calibration with 90% bound and 10% free PSA, which should be appropriate for the vast majority of men. When following patient values, it is most important to continue use of the same assay.[31]

Methodology Radioimmunoassay (RIA), enzymetric immunoassay, immunofluorometric assay,[32] monoclonal two-site immunoradiometric assay (IRMA).[33] An ultrasensitive RIA has been developed.[34] Over 30 different assay are available.[3]

Additional Information The PSA-alpha$_1$-antichymotrypsin (PSA-ACT) complex is the predominant molecular form of serum PSA with the free noncomplexed form of serum PSA constituting the remainder.[35] It has been suggested that assays measuring the PSA-ACT complex only may improve the differentiation between prostatic carcinoma and benign prostatic hyperplasia.[36] The ratio of free to complexed PSA can be determined and may be relevant. A lower proportion of free PSA is found in patients with prostate carcinoma (<10% free suggests carcinoma). (See Prostate Specific Antigen, Free *on page 263*.)

Three to 6 months after radical prostatectomy, PSA is reported to provide a sensitive indicator of persistent disease. Six months following introduction of antiandrogen therapy, PSA is reported as capable of distinguishing patients with favorable response from those in whom limited response is anticipated.[37]

Following prostatectomy for carcinoma, persistent increase in PSA signals residual disease, but undetectable results do not assure cure. Increasing PSA concentrations can be seen months or even years before other evidence of progression. Clinical objectives in management of rising postoperative PSA include prevention of possible symptoms, metastases, or death from prostate carcinoma. "Advanced" prostatic carcinoma indicates PSA increase only; "lethal" indicates detection of metastases on imaging.

Use of age-specific reference ranges may make PSA density superfluous.[38] Use of age-specific reference ranges for PSA has been claimed to provide greater sensitivity in patients younger than the age of 60 and greater specificity in older patients.[38,39]

PSA velocity is an expression used to indicate rate of change of PSA. It may provide an index capable of earlier detection of adenocarcinoma of prostate with distinction from benign hyperplasia and normal and may support clinical decisions following radical prostatectomy.[40] PSA increase of 0.8 ng/mL/year in a man whose PSA is within reference range, with a minimum of three assays, is described as an indication for further investigation.[38] Such measurements should be based on two-year intervals.[41]

Prostatic specific antigen is a reliable immunocytochemical marker for primary and metastatic adenocarcinoma of prostate, reacting with at least some cells in almost all adequate biopsies.

Footnotes

1. Epstein JI, Walsh PC, Carmichael M, et al, "Pathologic and Clinical Findings to Predict Tumor Extent of Nonpalpable (Stage T1c) Prostate Cancer," *JAMA*, 1994, 271(5):368-74.
2. Woolf SH, "Screening for Prostate Cancer With Prostate-Specific Antigen. An Examination of the Evidence," *N Engl J Med*, 1995, 333(21):1401-5.
3. Bostwick DG, Grignon DJ, Hammond MEH, et al, "Prognostic Factors in Prostate Cancer: College of American Pathologists Consensus Statement 1999," *Arch Pathol Lab Med*, 2000, 124(7):995-1000.
4. Chauvet B, Félix-Faure C, Lupsascka N, et al, "Prostate-Specific Antigen Decline: A Major Prognostic Factor for Prostate Cancer Treated With Radiation Therapy," *J Clin Oncol*, 1994, 12(7):1402-7.
5. Ruckle HC, Klee GG, and Oesterling JE, "Prostate-Specific Antigen: Concepts for Staging Prostate Cancer and Monitoring Response to Therapy," *Mayo Clin Proc*, 1994, 69(1):69-79.
6. Fowler JE Jr, Pandey P, Braswell NT, et al, "Prostate Specific Antigen Progression Rates After Radical Prostatectomy or Radiation Therapy for Localized Prostate Cancer," *Surgery*, 1994, 116(2):302-6.
7. Epstein JI, "Pathologic Features That Predict Progression of Disease Following Radical Prostatectomy," *Pathology of the Prostate*, Foster CS and Bostwick DG, eds, Philadelphia, PA: WB Saunders Co, 1998, 228-42.
8. Stamey TA, McNeal JE, Yemoto CM, et al, "Biological Determinants of Cancer Progression in Men With Prostate Cancer," *JAMA*, 1999, 281(15):1395-400.
9. Pound CR, Partin AW, Eisenberger MA, et al, "Natural History of Progression After PSA Elevation Following Radical Prostatectomy," *JAMA*, 1999, 281(17):1591-7.
10. Scher HI, "Management of Prostate Cancer After Prostatectomy: Treating the Patient, Not the PSA," *JAMA*, 1999, 281(17):1642-5.
11. Schifman RB, Ahmann FR, Elvick A, et al, "Analytical and Physiological Characteristics of Prostate-Specific Antigen and Prostatic Acid Phosphatase in Serum Compared," *Clin Chem*, 1987, 33(11):2086-8.
12. Lechevallier E, Eghazarian C, Ortega JC, et al, "Effect of Digital Rectal Examination on Serum Complexed and Free Prostate-Specific Antigen and Percentage of Free Prostate-Specific Antigen," *Urology*, 1999, 54(5):857-61.
13. Wians FH Jr, "PSA Today," *6th Annual Progress in Clinical Pathology*, Dallas, Texas: University of Texas Southern Medical Center, 1999.
14. Oesterling JE, Jacobsen SJ, and Cooner WH, "The Use of Age-Specific Reference Ranges for Serum Prostate-Specific Antigen in Men 60 Years Old or Older," *J Urol*, 1995, 153(4):1160-3.
15. Oesterling JE, "Prostate-Specific Antigen and Diagnosing Early Malignancies of the Prostate," *J Cell Biochem Suppl*, 1992, 16H:31-43.
16. Bare R, Hart L, and McCullough DL, "Correlation of Prostate-Specific Antigen and Prostate-Specific Antigen Density With Outcome of Prostate Biopsy," *Urology*, 1994, 43(2):191-6.
17. Seaman EK, Whang IS, Cooner W, et al, "Predictive Value of Prostate-Specific Antigen Density for the Presence of Micrometastatic Carcinoma of the Prostate," *Urology*, 1994, 43(5):645-8.
18. Rainwater LM, Morgan WR, Klee GG, et al, "Prostate-Specific Antigen Testing in Untreated and Treated Prostatic Adenocarcinoma," *Mayo Clin Proc*, 1990, 65(8):1118-26.
19. Krahn MD, Mahoney JE, Eckman MH, et al, "Screening for Prostate Cancer. A Decision Analytic View," *JAMA*, 1994, 272(10):773-80.
20. Lange PH, "New Information About Prostate-Specific Antigen and the Paradoxes of Prostate Cancer," *JAMA*, 1995, 273(4):336-7.
21. Crawford ED and De Antoni EP, "PSA as a Screening Test for Prostate Cancer," *Urol Clin North Am*, 1993, 20(4):637-46.
22. Ross KS, Carter HB, Pearson JD, et al, "Comparative Efficiency of Prostate-Specific Antigen Screening Strategies for Prostate Cancer Detection," *JAMA*, 2000, 284(11):1399-405.
23. Amling CL, Blute ML, Lerner SE, et al, "Influence of Prostate-Specific Antigen Testing on the Spectrum of Patients With Prostate Cancer Undergoing Radical Prostatectomy at a Large Referral Practice," *Mayo Clin Proc*, 1998, 73(5):401-6.
24. Humphrey PA, "Prostate Cancer in the Serum Prostate-Specific Antigen Era," *Mayo Clin Proc*, 1998, 73(5):489-90.
25. Yu H and Diamandis EP, "Prostate-Specific Antigen in Milk of Lactating Women," *Clin Chem*, 1995, 41(1):54-8.
26. James GK, Pudek M, Berean KW, et al, "Salivary Duct Carcinoma Secreting Prostate-Specific Antigen," *Am J Clin Pathol*, 1996, 106(2):242-7.
27. Zarghami N, Levesque M, D'Costa M, et al, "Frequency of Expression of Prostate-Specific Antigen mRNA in Lung Tumors," *Am J Clin Pathol*, 1997, 108(2):184-90.
28. Mannello F, Malatesta M, Luchetti F, et al, "Immunoreactivity, Ultrastructural Localization, and Transcript Expression of Prostate-Specific Antigen in Human Neuroblastoma Cell Lines," *Clin Chem*, 1999, 45(1):78-84.
29. Small EJ, "Prostate Cancer: Who to Screen and What the Results Mean," *Geriatrics*, 1993, 48(12):28-30, 35-8.
30. Catalona WJ, Partin AW, Slawin KM, et al, "Use of the Percentage of Free Prostate-Specific Antigen to Enhance Differentiation of Prostate Cancer From Benign Prostatic Disease: A Prospective Multicenter Clinical Trial," *JAMA*, 1998, 279(19):1542-7.
31. Catalona WJ, Smith DS, Wolfert RL, et al, "Evaluation of Percentage of Free Serum Prostate Specific Antigen to Improve Specificity of Prostate Cancer Screening," *JAMA*, 1995, 274(15):1214-20.
32. Jacobsen SJ, Klee GG, Lilja H, et al, "Stability of Serum Prostate-Specific Antigen Determination Across Laboratory, Assay, and Storage Time," *Urology*, 1995, 45(3):447-53.
33. Lindstedt G, Jacobsson A, Lundberg PA, et al, "Determination of Prostate-Specific Antigen in Serum by Immunoradiometric Assay," *Clin Chem*, 1990, 36(1):53-8.
34. Graves HC, Wehner N, and Stamey TA, "Ultrasensitive Radioimmunoassay of Prostate-Specific Antigen," *Clin Chem*, 1992, 38(5):735-42.
35. Lilja H, "Significance of Different Molecular Forms of Serum PSA. The Free, Noncomplexed Form of PSA Versus That Complexed to Alpha$_1$-Antichymotrypsin," *Urol Clin North Am*, 1993, 20(4):681-6.
36. Wu JT, "Assay for Prostate Specific Antigen (PSA): Problems and Possible Solutions," *J Clin Lab Anal*, 1994, 8(1):51-62.
37. Zietman AL, Shipley WU, and Willett CG, "Residual Disease After Radical Surgery or Radiation Therapy for Prostate Cancer. Clinical Significance and Therapeutic Implications," *Cancer*, 1993, 71(3 Suppl):959-69.
38. Ruckle HC, Klee GG, and Oesterling JE, "Prostate-Specific Antigen: Critical Issues for the Practicing Physician," *Mayo Clin Proc*, 1994, 69(1):59-68.
39. Cooner WH, "Prostate-Specific Antigen and Transrectal Ultrasound of the Prostate in Detection of Prostate Cancer," *Clin Invest Med*, 1993, 16(6):471-4.
40. Partin AW, Pearson JD, Landis PK, et al, "Evaluation of Serum Prostate-Specific Antigen Velocity After Radical Prostatectomy to Distinguish Local Recurrence From Distant Metastases," *Urology*, 1994, 43(5):649-59.
41. Carter HB, Pearson JD, Waclawiw Z, et al, "Prostate-Specific Antigen Variability in Men Without Prostate Cancer: Effect of Sampling Interval on Prostate-Specific Antigen Velocity," *Urology*, 1995, 45(14):591-6.

References

Allard WJ, Zhou Z, and Yeung KK, "Novel Immunoassay for the Measurement of Complexed Prostate-Specific Antigen in Serum," *Clin Chem*, 1998, 44(6 Pt 1):1216-23.

Andriole GL, Guess HA, Epstein JI, et al, "Treatment With Finasteride Preserves Usefulness of Prostate-Specific Antigen in the Detection of Prostate Cancer: Results of a Randomized, Double-Blind, Placebo-Controlled Clinical Trial," PLESS Study Group. Proscar Long-Term Efficacy and Safety Study, *Urology*, 1998, 52(2):195-201-2.

Babaian RJ, Mettlin C, Kane R, et al, "The Relationship of Prostate-Specific Antigen to Digital Rectal Examination and Transrectal Ultrasonography," Findings of the American Cancer Society National Prostate Cancer Detection Project, *Cancer*, 1992, 69(5):1195-200.

Benson MC, Whang IS, Olsson CA, et al, "The Use of Prostate Specific Antigen Density to Enhance the Predictive Value of Intermediate Levels of Serum Prostate Specific Antigen," *J Urol*, 1992, 147(3 Pt 2):817-21.

Catalona WJ, "Management of Cancer of the Prostate," *N Engl J Med*, 1994, 331(15):996-1004

Clinton JJ, "From the Agency for Health Care Policy and Research," *JAMA*, 1994, 271(15):1151.

Cohen RJ, Haffejee Z, Steele GS, et al, "Advanced Prostate Cancer With Normal Serum Prostate-Specific Antigen Values," *Arch Pathol Lab Med*, 1994, 118(11):1123-6.

Critz FA, Levinson AK, Williams WH, et al, "Prostate Specific Antigen Nadir Achieved by Men Apparently Cured of Prostate Cancer by Radiotherapy," *J Urol*, 1999, 161(4):1199-203-5.

Crook JM, Choan E, Perry GA, et al, "Serum Prostate-Specific Antigen Profile Following Radiotherapy for Prostate Cancer: Implications for Patterns of Failure and Definition of Cure," *Urology*, 1998, 51(4):566-72

D'Amico AV, Schultz D, Loffredo M, et al, "Biochemical Outcome Following External Beam Radiation Therapy With or Without Androgen Suppression Therapy for Clinically Localized Prostate Cancer," *JAMA*, 2000, 284(10):1280-3.

Drago JR and York JP, "Prostate-Specific Antigen, Digital Rectal Examination, and Transrectal Ultrasound in Predicting the Probability of Cancer," *J Surg Oncol*, 1992, 49(3):172-5.

"Effect of Digital Rectal Examination on Serum Prostate-Specific Antigen in a Primary Care Setting, the Internal Medicine Clinic Research Consortium, " *Arch Intern Med*, 1995, 155(4):389-92.

Epstein JL, "Prostate Biopsy Interpretation," 1989, NY: Raven Press.

Gann PH, Hennekens CH, and Stampfer MJ, "A Prospective Evaluation of Plasma Prostate-Specific Antigen for Detection of Prostate Cancer," *JAMA*, 1995, 273(4):289-94.

Gillenwater JY, "Digital Rectal Examination-Associated Alterations in Serum Prostate-Specific Antigen," *Am J Clin Pathol*, 1992, 97(4):466-7.

Glenski WJ, Malek RS, Myrtle JF, et al, "Sustained, Substantially Increased Concentration of Prostate-Specific Antigen in the Absence of Prostatic Malignant Disease: An Unusual Clinical Scenario," *Mayo Clin Proc*, 1992, 67(3):249-52.

Grignon DJ and Hammond EH, "College of American Pathologists Conference XXVI on Clinical Relevance of Prognostic Markers in Solid Tumors. Report of the Prostate Cancer Working Group," *Arch Pathol Lab Med*, 1995, 119(12):1122-6.

Howanitz JH, "Immunoassay for Measuring Prostate-Specific Antigen," *Lab Med*, 1996, 27(4):255-8.

Jacobsen SJ, Katusic SK, Bergstralh EJ, et al, "Incidence of Prostate Cancer Diagnosis in the Eras Before and After Serum Prostate-Specific Antigen Testing," *JAMA*, 1995, 274(18):1445-9.

Kestin LL, Vicini FA, Ziaja EL, et al, "Defining Biochemical Cure for Prostate Carcinoma Patients Treated With External Beam Radiation Therapy," *Cancer*, 1999, 86(8):1557-66.

Leibman BD, Dillioglugil O, Wheeler TM, et al, "Distant Metastasis After Radical Prostatectomy in Patients Without an Elevated Serum Prostate Specific Antigen Level," *Cancer*, 1995, 76:2530-4.

Oesterling JE, Roy J, Agha A, et al, "Biologic Variability of Prostate-Specific Antigen and its Usefulness as a Marker for Prostate Cancer: Effects of Finasteride," Finasteride PSA Study Group, *Urology*, 1998, 51(4A Suppl):58-63.

Pollack A, Zagars GK, and Kavadi VS, "Prostate Specific Antigen Doubling Time and Disease Relapse After Radiotherapy for Prostate Cancer," *Cancer*, 1994, 74(2):670-8.

(Continued)

Prostate Specific Antigen, Serum (Continued)

Porter JR, and Brawer MK, "Prostatic Intraepithelial Neoplasia and Prostate-Specific Antigen," *World J Urol*, 1993, 11(4):196-200.

Poteat HT, Ho GT, Lee ML, et al, "The Utility of Patient Age in Evaluating Prostate Cancer," *Am J Clin Pathol*, 1997, 107(3):337-44.

"Prostate Disease and PSA Testing," *Mayo Communique*, Mayo Reference Service Publication, January, 2001.

Renshaw AA, Richie JP, Loughlin KR, et al, "Maximum Diameter of Prostatic Carcinoma Is a Simple, Inexpensive, and Independent Predictor of Prostate-Specific Antigen Failure in Radical Prostatectomy Specimens. Validation in a Cohort of 434 Patients," *Am J Clin Pathol*, 1999, 111(5):641-4.

Roehrborn CG, Boyle P, Gould AL, et al, "Serum Prostate-Specific Antigen as a Predictor of Prostate Volume in Men With Benign Prostatic Hyperplasia," *Urology*, 1999, 53(3):581-9.

Roehrborn CG, Gregory A, McConnell JD, et al, "Comparison of Three Assays for Total Serum Prostate-Specific Antigen and Percentage of Free Prostate-Specific Antigen in Predicting Prostate Histology," *Urology*, 1996, 48(6A Suppl):23-32.

Sershon PD, Barry MJ, and Oesterling JE, "Serum Prostate-Specific Antigen Discriminates Weakly Between Men With Benign Prostatic Hyperplasia and Patients With Organ-Confined Prostate Cancer," *Eur Urol*, 1994, 25(4):281-7.

Slovacek KJ, Riggs MW, Spiekerman AM, et al, "Use of Age-Specific Normal Ranges for Serum Prostate-Specific Antigen," *Arch Pathol Lab Med*, 1998, 122(4):330-2.

Smith DC, Dunn RL, Strawderman MS, et al, "Change in Serum Prostate-Specific Antigen as a Marker of Response to Cytotoxic Therapy for Hormone-Refractory Prostate Cancer," *J Clin Oncol*, 1998, 16(5):1835-43.

Sokoll LJ and Chan DW, "Clinical Applications of the Molecular Forms of Prostate-Specific Antigen," *Diag Endo Metab*, 1998, 16:133-48.

Srigley JR, Amin MB, Bostwick DG, et al, "Updated Protocol for the Examination of Specimens From Patients With Carcinoma of the Prostate Gland. A Basis for Checklists," *Arch Pathol Lab Med*, 2000, 124(7):1034-9.

Stenman UH, Leinonen J, Zhang WM, et al, "Prostate-Specific Antigen," *Sem Cancer Biol*, 1999, 9(2):83-93.

Thomson RD and Clejan S, "Digital Rectal Examination-Associated Alterations in Serum Prostate-Specific Antigen," *Am J Clin Pathol*, 1992, 97(4):528-34.

Vashi AR and Oesterling JE, "Percent Free Prostate-Specific Antigen: Entering a New Era in the Detection of Prostate Cancer," *Mayo Clin Proc*, 1997, 72(4):337-44.

Wians FH Jr, "The Role of Prostate-Specific Antigen (PSA) Testing in the Diagnosis, Treatment and Follow-up of Patients With Adenocarcinoma of the Prostate," *ASCP Check Sample*, 1997, 37:77-103.

Young RH, Srigley JR, Amin MB, et al, "Tumors of the Prostate Gland, Seminal Vesicles, Male Urethra, and Penis," *Atlas of Tumor Pathology*, Washington, DC: Armed Forces Institute of Pathology under the Auspices of Universities Associated for Research and Education in Pathology, Inc, Bethesda, MD, 2000.

Internet Web Sites

www.niddk.nih.gov/health/urolog/pubs/prostate/index.htm

♦ **Prostatic Acid Phosphatase** *see* Acid Phosphatase, Plasma *on page 82*

♦ **Protease Inhibitors** *see* Alpha₁-Antitrypsin Phenotyping *on page 95*

♦ **Protease Inhibitors** *see* Alpha₁-Antitrypsin, Serum *on page 96*

♦ **Protein, Body Fluids** *see* Body Fluid Chemical Analysis *on page 123*

Protein Electrophoresis, Capillary Zone

Related Information

Immunofixation Electrophoresis, Serum or Urine *on page 530*
Immunoglobulin G *on page 535*
Immunoglobulin M *on page 537*
Protein Electrophoresis, Serum *on page 267*
Protein Electrophoresis, Urine *on page 268*

Synonyms Capillary Electrophoresis; Free-Solution CE; Free-Zone CE

Applies to Bisalbuminemia; Immunoglobulins; Immunosubtraction Electrophoresis; Light Chains, Urine; Monoclonal Gammopathy; M-Proteins; Serum and Urine Protein Electrophoresis

Abstract Advances in capillary technology have permitted their use in electrophoresis systems. Capillary zone electrophoresis (CZE) may be used to analyze proteins for reasons analogous to other electrophoretic methods. Monoclonal gammopathy includes monoclonal immunoglobulin heavy chain (gamma, alpha, mu, delta, epsilon) and/or light chain (kappa or lambda). During long-term follow-up of asymptomatic subjects with a small monoclonal gammopathy (monoclonal gammopathy of undetermined significance), up to 25% develop multiple myeloma, macroglobulinemia of Waldenström, or amyloidosis.[1] Monoclonal proteins are a tumor marker in subjects with myeloma and Waldenström macroglobulinemia.

Specimen Serum, urine

Container Red top tube

Storage Instructions Refrigerate

Reference Interval
- Albumin: 3.7-5.2 g/dL
- Alpha₁: 0.2-0.57 g/dL
- Alpha₂: 0.3-0.76 g/dL
- Beta: 0.5-1.1 g/dL
- Gamma: 0.6-1.48 g/dL
- A:G ratio: 1.62 (1.09-2.16)

From Katzmann et al.[1]

Use As with protein electrophoresis, the primary applications are to detect and to monitor monoclonal gammopathies (paraproteins). It is more sensitive for small monoclonal protein abnormalities, especially IgA paraproteins, which can hide in the beta area in agarose gel separations.[2] It has also been reported to be useful for therapeutic drug monitoring, hemoglobin, and amino acid quantitation.[3,4,5,6] It provides better resolution with separation of the beta region into transferrin and C3 components, and offers advantages in cost and sensitivity (eg, in detection of bisalbuminemia).[2,7,8]

Limitations Of 13 instances of free monoclonal light chains in the Katzmann paper, 9 had abnormality by capillary electrophoresis and 6 by agarose gel electrophoresis. Monoclonal IgA was not detected in three cases by agarose gel or capillary electrophoresis.[1]

Methodology Capillary electrophoresis (CE) uses high voltage applied across a buffer-filled fused-silica small bore capillary (20-100 microns diameter x ~100 cm long) to cause differential migration of the sample components. Typically, analytes are detected by passage of a light beam near one end of the capillary. Using CE, one can rapidly achieve high-resolution separation of molecules ranging in size from small ions to nucleotides and even to whole cells using small samples. Separation may be determined by analyte size, charge, hydrophobicity, ligand-binding, and chirality. The advantages of CE accrue from the small bore that allows for 1) small sample variation, 2) high length to diameter ratio, 3) high surface area to volume ratio that allows for rapid dispersion of heat and, thus, high voltage and 4) electro-osmotic flow (EOF).[5,6,9,10]

Capillary zone electrophoresis (CZE, also called free-zone CE or free-solution CE) is the simplest form of CE performed under alkaline conditions. It uses EOF extensively to separate proteins and smaller molecules.[5,6,9] Its primary use has been to identify and quantitate monoclonal paraproteins. A method called **"immunosubtraction"** has been introduced in which the serum or urine is incubated with specific antibodies that are immobilized. This removes the specific protein, and the resultant electropherogram can then be compared to one performed without incubation. Comparison of the two electropherograms allows quantitation of the specific protein.[10]

Additional Information The primary advantages of CZE over agarose gel electrophoresis include better quantitation, small sample size, simple operation, rapid output, and low cost. It is more sensitive than agarose gel electrophoresis in detection of low concentrations of monoclonal proteins.[2] The disadvantages include decreased sensitivity due to short light path, inability to separate uncharged molecules, and potential protein adsorption to capillary wall.[5,6,10]

Immunosubtraction electrophoresis is reported to be less accurate than immunofixation electrophoresis in determination of the immunotype of a monoclonal protein. Its patterns may be difficult to interpret. Its detection of only 60% to 75% of immunotyping of monoclonal proteins has been described as unacceptable.[2]

CZE may be more sensitive for detection of bisalbuminemia than agarose gel electrophoresis.[8] Bisalbuminemia, a double band of albumin, can be inherited or acquired. Familial bisalbuminemia is clinically inconsequential. Acquired (and transitory) bisalbuminemia may be associated with antibiotic overdose, ascites, or pancreatic pseudocyst.

Footnotes

1. Katzmann JA, Clark R, Sanders E, et al, "Prospective Study of Serum Protein Capillary Zone Electrophoresis and Immunotyping of Monoclonal Proteins by Immunosubtraction," *Am J Clin Pathol*, 1998, 110(4):503-9.
2. Litwin CM, Anderson SK, Philipps G, et al, "Comparison of Capillary Zone and Immunosubtraction With Agarose Gel and Immunofixation Electrophoresis for Detecting and Identifying Monoclonal Gammopathies," *Am J Clin Pathol*, 1999, 112(3):411-7.
3. Chen FT, Liu CM, Hsieh YZ, et al, "Capillary Electrophoresis: A New Clinical Tool," *Clin Chem*, 1991, 37(1):14-9.
4. Chen FT, "High-Resolution Protein Analysis by Automated Capillary Electrophoresis," *Clin Chem*, 1992, 38:1651-3.
5. Landers JP, "Clinical Capillary Electrophoresis," *Clin Chem*, 1995, 41(4):495-509.
6. Shihabi ZK, "Applications of Capillary Electrophoresis in the Clinical Laboratory," *ASCP Check Sample*, 1993, CC93-4 (CC-242):1-8.
7. Smalley DL, Mayer R, and Gardner C, "Evaluation of Capillary Zone Electrophoresis Assessment of Beta Proteins," *Clin Lab Science*, 1999, 12(5):262-5.
8. Jaeggi-Groisman SE, Byland C, and Gerber H, "Improved Sensitivity of Capillary Electrophoresis for Detection of Bisalbuminemia," *Clin Chem*, 2000, 46(6):880-1.
9. Keren DF, "Capillary Zone Electrophoresis in the Evaluation of Serum Protein Abnormalities," *Am J Clin Pathol*, 1998, 110(2):248-52.
10. Palfrey SM, ed, *Clinical Applications of Capillary Electrophoresis*, Totawa, NJ: Human Press, 1999.

References

Altria KD, "Overview of Capillary Electrophoresis and Capillary Electrochromatography," *J Chromatogr A*, 1999, 856(1-2):443-63.

Bossuyt X, Bogaerts A, Schiettekatte G, et al, "Detection and Classification of Paraproteins by Capillary Immunofixation/Subtraction," *Clin Chem*, 1998, 44(4):760-4.

Bossuyt X, Schiettekatte G, Bogaerts A, et al, "Serum Protein Electrophoresis by CZE 2000 Clinical Capillary Electrophoresis System," *Clin Chem*, 1998, 44(4):749-59.

Dong M, Ding XQ, Pinon DI, et al, "Structurally Related Peptide Agonist, Partial Agonist, and Antagonist Occupy a Similar Binding Pocket Within the Colecystokinin Receptor," *J Biol Chem*, 1999, 274(8):4778-85.

Jenkins MA and Guerin MD, "Quantification of Serum Proteins Using Capillary Electrophoresis," *Ann Clin Biochem*, 1995, 32(Pt 5):493-7.

Jorgenson JW and Lukacs KD, "Capillary Zone Electrophoresis," *Science*, 1983, 222:266-72.

Perrett D, "Capillary Electrophoresis in Clinical Chemistry," *Ann Clin Biochem*, 1999, 36(Pt 2):133-50.

Rosenzweig IB, "Capillary Electrophoresis: A New Methodology for Therapeutic Drug Monitoring and Drugs-of-Abuse Confirmation," *Ther Drug Monitor Toxicol*, 1996, 17:143-60.

Wan QH and Le XC, "Fluorescence Polarization Studies of Affinity Interactions in Capillary Electrophoresis," *Anal Chem*, 1999, 71(19):4183-9.

Wijnen PA and van Dieijen-Visser MP, "Capillary Electrophoresis of Serum Proteins. Reproducibility, Comparison With Agarose Gel Electrophoresis and a Review of the Literature," *Eur J Clin Chem Clin Biochem*, 1997, 35(5):393-4.

Xian J, Harrington MG, and Davidson EH, "DNA-Protein Binding Assays From a Single Sea Urchin Egg: A High-Sensitivity Capillary Electrophoresis Method," *Proc Natl Acad Sci U S A*, 1996, 93(1):86-90.

Internet Web Sites

www.ceandcec.com

Protein Electrophoresis, Serum

Related Information

Albumin, Serum *on page 88*
Alpha₁-Antitrypsin Phenotyping *on page 95*
Alpha₁-Antitrypsin, Serum *on page 96*
Cerebrospinal Fluid Protein Electrophoresis *on page 518*
Immunofixation Electrophoresis, Serum or Urine *on page 530*
Immunoglobulin A *on page 532*
Immunoglobulin G *on page 535*
Immunoglobulin M *on page 537*
Liver Disease: Laboratory Assessment, Overview *on page 216*
Protein Electrophoresis, Capillary Zone *on page 266*
Protein Electrophoresis, Urine *on page 268*
Protein, Total, Serum *on page 269*
Smooth Muscle Antibody *on page 543*
Viscosity, Serum or Plasma *on page 495*

Synonyms Electrophoresis, Serum; Serum Protein Electrophoresis; Zone Electrophoresis

Applies to Beta-Gamma Bridging; Globulin, Serum; Immunoglobulins; Light Chains; Monoclonal Gammopathy; M-Proteins

Test Includes Serum electrophoresis for quantitation of albumin, alpha₁, alpha₂, beta, and gamma globulins. A total protein value is needed, since the fractions are otherwise available only as percentages. Used with total protein, the fractions can be expressed as absolute quantities.

Abstract Serum proteins have different net charges and can be separated by electrophoresis into several distinct bands: albumin, alpha 1-globulin (α_1G), alpha 2-globulin (α_2G), beta globulin (βG), and gamma globulins (γG). Protein concentrations are altered as results of different disease states.

Serum and urine protein electrophoresis are among pivotal studies in the diagnosis and differential diagnosis of multiple myeloma, Waldenström macroglobulinemia, amyloidosis, and monoclonal gammopathy of undetermined significance (MGUS). The latter is the most common form of monoclonal gammopathy.

Specimen Serum

Container Red top tube or SST™ tube

Storage Instructions Refrigerate separated serum.

Reference Interval Values in the table are representative, but variation between methods and laboratories exists. The figures in the table are based on an agarose system. Values in infancy and early childhood are not identical to adult reference ranges.

Table 1. Protein Electrophoresis, Serum

Component	Relative (%) Normal Range	Absolute (g/dL) Normal Range
Total protein		5.90-8.00
Albumin	58.0-74.0	4.00-5.50
Alpha₁	2.0-3.5	0.15-0.25
Alpha₂	5.4-10.6	0.43-0.75
Beta	7.0-14.0	0.50-1.00
Gamma	8.0-18.0	0.60-1.30
A/G ratio		1.4-2.6

Critical Values Monoclonal globulin levels >3.0 g/dL indicate a malignant disease, IgG or IgA myeloma, or IgM of Waldenström macroglobulinemia.[1]

Use Serum protein electrophoresis is a part of evaluation of patients when multiple myeloma, macroglobulinemia of Waldenström or primary amyloidosis is considered. Interpretation of serum protein electrophoresis patterns is helpful in screening for or evaluation of the diagnosis of disease states such as acute phase reaction, chronic inflammation, autoimmune hepatitis, cirrhosis, humoral immunodeficiency, α_1-antitrypsin abnormalities, and monoclonal, oligoclonal, and polyclonal gammopathies.

Narrow, intensely stained bands appearing as tall, narrow peaks in densitometric tracings are **monoclonal gammopathies** (paraproteins, monoclonal immunoglobulins, M-proteins), found in multiple myeloma, macroglobulinemia of Waldenström, amyloidosis, lymphoproliferative diseases, and in heavy-chain diseases. They occur also in 11% of patients with hepatitis C.[2]

Monoclonal gammopathy of undetermined significance (MGUS) is characterized by the presence of monoclonal IgG or IgA without evidence of multiple myeloma. Hematologic malignancy ultimately developed in 64% of patients with MGUS on 31-year follow-up in a small New Zealand series.[3] Special efforts to establish diagnosis are indicated in the presence of bone lesions, hypercalcemia, or anemia, which have prognostic relevance in cases of myeloma. Serum protein electrophoresis should be repeated in 1 year for asymptomatic patients with a monoclonal protein <1.5 g/dL who have normal values of hemoglobin, calcium, and creatinine. Electrophoresis should be repeated in 2-3 months if the monoclonal protein is between 1.5 and 2.5 g/dL. Patients being treated for multiple myeloma, Waldenström macroglobulinemia or amyloidosis should be monitored at 1- to 2-month intervals.

Smoldering myeloma is a designation applied to cases with monoclonal gammopathy, with atypical marrow plasma cells, without anemia, bone lesions, or renal failure.

Indications for Protein Electrophoresis

- Consideration of multiple myeloma, macroglobulinemia of Waldenström, or primary amyloidosis
- Back pain, especially in subjects >50 years old
- Osteoporosis
- Osteolytic lesions by imaging
- Hypercalcemia
- Presence of Bence Jones protein (monoclonal light chains) in urine
- Increasing serum creatinine
- Recurrent infections
- Unexplained peripheral neuropathy
- Congestive heart failure refractory to usual therapy
- Nephrotic syndrome
- Malabsorption in subjects >50 years old
- Unexplained hepatomegaly and/or splenomegaly and/or anemia
- Initial screening for α_1-antitrypsin deficiency (most of α_1 globulin is α_1-antitrypsin)
- Evaluation of chronic liver disease: decreased albumin, polyclonal gammopathy, β- and γ-bridging are prototypical findings of hepatic cirrhosis; the γ increase is IgM in primary biliary cirrhosis
- Increased ESR[4]

Limitations Serum protein electrophoresis may be normal in some patients with plasma cell dyscrasia. Such individuals may have monoclonal light chains (Bence Jones protein) in urine. See Protein Electrophoresis, Urine and Immunofixation Electrophoresis.[1] Capillary zone electrophoresis is more sensitive than agarose gel in detection of low levels of monoclonal proteins; agarose methodology failed to detect three of 14 IgA monoclonal proteins which were found with capillary zone technology in one series. However, such IgA abnormalities can be missed with capillary zone electrophoresis as well.[5] While agarose gel electrophoresis provided sensitivity and specificity of 91% and 99%, respectively, capillary zone electrophoresis provided 95% and 99%.[6]

Methodology Cellulose acetate and agarose electrophoresis are widely used methods, quantitated by densitometry. Stains include Ponceau S and Coomassie brilliant blue. Capillary zone and immunosubtraction electrophoretic methods are gaining acceptance (see Protein Electrophoresis, Capillary Zone *on page 266*).

Additional Information The most commonly recognized electrophoresis patterns are summarized in the following table.

The most common presentations of myeloma include osteolytic lesions, anemia, renal insufficiency, and recurrent bacterial infections. The diagnosis is supported by the presence of a monoclonal immunoglobulin in serum or urinary light chains.[7] Immunofixation is needed to characterize monoclonal gammopathies.[8]

Most patients with immunoglobulin amyloidosis have monoclonal immunoglobulin in serum, urine, or both.[9]

Footnotes

1. Alexanian R, Weber D, and Liu F, "Differential Diagnosis of Monoclonal Gammopathies," *Arch Pathol Lab Med*, 1999, 123(2):108-13.
2. Andreone P, Zignego AL, Cursaro C, et al, "Prevalence of Monoclonal Gammopathies in Patients With Hepatitis C Virus Infection," *Ann Intern Med*, 1998, 129(4):294-8.
3. Colls BM, "Monoclonal Gammopathy of Undetermined Significance (MGUS): 31-Year Follow up of a Community Study," *Aust N Z J Med*, 1999, 29(4):500-4.
4. Mayo Medical Laboratories, "Improved Procedures for Investigation of Monoclonal Proteins," *Mayo Communique*, Rochester, MN, June 1998, 23(3).
5. Litwin CM, Anderson SK, Philipps G, et al, "Comparison of Capillary Zone and Immunosubtraction With Agarose Gel and Immunofixation Electrophoresis for Detecting and Identifying Monoclonal Gammopathies," *Am J Clin Pathol*, 1999, 112(3):411-7.
6. Katzmann JA, Clark R, Sanders E, et al, "Prospective Study of Serum Protein Capillary Zone Electrophoresis and Immunotyping of Monoclonal Proteins by Immunosubtraction," *Am J Clin Pathol*, 1998, 110(4):503-9.
7. Bataille R and Harousseau JL, "Multiple Myeloma," *N Engl J Med*, 1997, 336(23):1657-64.
8. Kyle RA, "Sequence of Testing for Monoclonal Gammopathies," *Arch Pathol Lab Med*, 1999, 123(2):114-8.
9. Benson MD, "Aging, Amyloid, and Cardiomyopathy," *N Engl J Med*, 1997, 336(7):502-4.

(Continued)

Protein Electrophoresis, Serum *(Continued)*

Table 2.

Pattern	Protein Changes	Frequently Associated Diseases
Acute inflammation	Normal or ↓ albumin ↑ α_1G and/or α_2G	Acute infection and inflammatory disorders (acute phase reaction)
Chronic inflammation	Normal or ↓ albumin ↑ α_1G and/or α_2G ↑ γG	Autoimmune diseases, chronic liver disease including chronic autoimmune hepatitis, primary biliary cirrhosis, chronic infection, cancer
Hypoalbuminemia	↓ albumin	Metastatic cancer, CHF, malnutrition, protein-losing disorders
Hypogammaglobulinemia	Normal or ↓ albumin ↓ γG	Lymphoproliferative disorders, inflammatory bowel disease, congenital immunodeficiencies
Polyclonal gammopathy	↑ γG	Autoimmune disease, chronic infections, infestations such as visceral leishmaniasis, liver disease including autoimmune hepatitis and cirrhosis
Cirrhosis	Often ↓ albumin ↑ γG, Beta-gamma bridging	Cirrhosis Autoimmune hepatitis
Protein-losing disorder	↓ albumin ↑ α_2G ↓ γG	Nephrotic syndrome, exudative skin disorders, gastroenteropathies
Monoclonal gammopathy	Normal or ↓ albumin ↑ γG	Myeloma, macroglobulinemia, MGUS, CLL, lymphoma, amyloidosis, Gaucher disease (25% or patients), AIDS (15% of patients)
Antitrypsin deficiency	Absent or low α_1G	Alpha-1 antitrypsin deficiency
Hyperbetaglobulinemia	Normal or ↓ albumin ↑ βG	Hyperlipidemia, diabetes mellitus, iron deficiency anemia
Immune deficiency	↓ or absent γG	Congenital or acquired immunodeficiency states

α_1G = alpha-1 globulin; α_2G = alpha-2 globulin; βG = beta globulin; γG = gamma globulin

References

Gerard SK, Chen KH, and Khayam-Bashi H, "Immunofixation Compared With Immunoelectrophoresis for the Routine Characterization of Paraprotein Disorders," *Am J Clin Pathol*, 1987, 88(2):198-203.

Goeken JA and Keren DF, "Introduction to the Report of the Consensus Conference on Monoclonal Gammopathies," *Arch Pathol Lab Med*, 1999, 123(2):104-5.

Keren DF, "Capillary Zone Electrophoresis in the Evaluation of Serum Protein Abnormalities," *Am J Clin Pathol*, 1998, 110(2):248-52.

Keren DF, "Clinical Indications for Electrophoresis and Immunofixation," Section A, Immunological Methods, Nakamura RM, volume ed, *Manual of Clinical Laboratory Immunology*, Rose NR, deMacario EC, Folds JD, et al, eds, 5th ed, Chapter 9, Washington, DC: ASM Press, American Society of Microbiology, 1997, 65-74.

Keren DF, "Procedures for the Evaluation of Monoclonal Immunoglobulins," *Arch Pathol Lab Med*, 1999, 123(2):126-32.

Keren DF, Alexanian R, Goeken JA, et al, "Guidelines for Clinical and Laboratory Evaluation of Patients With Monoclonal Gammopathies," *Arch Pathol Lab Med*, 1999, 123:106-7.

Tsianos EV, Di Bisceglie AM, Papadopoulos NM, et al, "Oligoclonal Immunoglobulin Bands in Serum in Association With Chronic Viral Hepatitis," *Am J Gastroenterol*, 1990, 85(8):1005-8.

Winkelmann RK, Litzow MR, Umbert IJ, et al, "Giant Cell Granulomatous Pulmonary and Myocardial Lesions in Necrobiotic Xanthogranuloma With Paraproteinemia," *Mayo Clin Proc*, 1997, 72(11):1028-33.

Protein Electrophoresis, Urine

Related Information

Immunofixation Electrophoresis, Serum or Urine *on page 530*
Immunoglobulin G *on page 535*
Microalbuminuria *on page 879*
Protein Electrophoresis, Serum *on page 267*
Protein, Quantitative, Urine *on page 883*
Protein, Semiquantitative, Urine *on page 885*
Urine Collection, 24-Hour *on page 47*
Viscosity, Serum or Plasma *on page 495*

Synonyms Electrophoresis, Protein, Urine; Globulins, Urine; Urine Electrophoresis; Urine Protein Electrophoresis

Applies to Immunoelectrophoresis; Ladders Light Chain; Light Chains, Urine; Monoclonal Gammopathy; Monoclonal Light Chains; Pseudo-oligoclonal Bands

Replaces Bence Jones Protein

Test Includes Quantitative total urine protein, urine albumin, urine $alpha_1$, urine $alpha_2$, urine beta, and urine gamma globulin fractions

Abstract Normal glomerular and tubular function results in excretion <150 mg of protein/day. Two thirds of the filtered protein is comprised of albumin, transferrin, low molecular weight proteins, and some immunoglobulins. Renal injury may result in proteinuria. Urine protein electrophoresis separates proteins according to charge and allows classification of the type of renal injury. Protein patterns are interpreted by a clinical pathologist and reported as glomerular, tubular, or mixed patterns.

Excretion of monoclonal light chains >50 mg/day is evidence against the benign character of monoclonal gammopathy.

Specimen 24-urine (preferred)

Container Container, no preservative

Storage Instructions Refrigerate during and after the collection

Causes for Rejection Total protein too low to measure or to yield usable electrophoretic pattern

Reference Interval A normal urine protein pattern consists of albumin and occasionally faint alpha-1 and beta bands.
- Total protein: <150 mg/24-hour specimen
- Albumin: <50% of total
- Total globulin: 60% to 67% of total

Use Classify type of renal injury

Limitations May not detect pathologic light chains due to insufficient sensitivity of this method; immunofixation electrophoresis is the next step.

Contraindications Reagent strips, sulfosalicylic acid, and acidified heat precipitation are unsuitable for characterization of monoclonal free light chains.[1]

Methodology Electrophoresis, cellulose acetate, and agarose gel are most commonly used. Evaluation of monoclonal free light chains is best accomplished with quantitation of 24-hour urinary protein excretion, densimetry, and immunofixation.[1]

Additional Information Glomerular filtration produces fluid containing very little protein with molecular weights >40,000 daltons. Proteins with molecular weights <15,000 daltons pass freely through the glomerulus but are then almost completely reabsorbed in the proximal tubules. Normal glomerular and tubular function results in excretion <150 mg of protein per day. Two thirds of the filtered protein is comprised of albumin, transferrin, low molecular weight proteins, and some immunoglobulins. The remainder, such as Tamm-Horsfall glycoprotein, is derived from the urinary tract itself.

Glomerular proteinuria occurs when the glomerulus begins to lose its ability to retain large proteins in the plasma. The most common causes are minimal change disease, glomerulonephritis, and diabetic nephropathy. Heavy glomerular proteinuria is often associated with the nephrotic syndrome. The urine contains increased levels of albumin and other proteins of similar size such as $alpha_1$-antitrypsin, $alpha_1$-acid glycoprotein, and transferrin. The electrophoretic pattern shows increased albumin, $alpha_1$- and $beta_1$-globulin bands.

Tubular proteinuria occurs when the renal tubules cannot reabsorb low molecular weight proteins. Tubular proteinuria is associated with drug toxicity (aminoglycosides, cephalosporins, and cyclosporine), pyelonephritis, renal vascular disease, and transplant rejection. This protein pattern reveals a small amount of albumin, two protein bands in the $alpha_2$ region ($alpha_1$-microglobulin, retinol binding protein), and one band in the $beta_2$ region ($beta_2$-microglobulin).

Mixed glomerular/tubular proteinuria occurs when both glomerular and tubular functions are compromised. This pattern is typically seen in chronic renal failure. The urine protein pattern often resembles serum with increased amounts of both large proteins (albumin, transferrin, $alpha_1$-antitrypsin) and low molecular weight proteins (retinol binding protein and $beta_2$-microglobulin). Albumin, $alpha_1$-, $alpha_2$-, and beta-globulin bands are increased.

Multiple evenly spaced bands (usually 3-5 in number) have been referred to as "the ladder light chain pattern" (upon urine immunofixation electrophoresis).[2] The original report concluded (on the basis of two dimensional electrophoresis and silver staining) that this pattern could be attributed to polyclonal light chain. A recent report, however, found over 15 equidistant narrow bands in the β- and γ-globulin regions and clinical pathologic features of multiple myeloma, light chain type (all narrow bands were of a light chain type), including kidney biopsy showing "myeloma kidney" pattern.[3]

Monoclonal gammopathy (M-protein) is found with myeloma, Waldenström macroglobulinemia, lymphoproliferative diseases including chronic lymphocytic leukemia, and primary systemic amyloidosis. A more common entity, monoclonal gammopathy of undetermined significance (MGUS), is an important consideration in differential diagnosis. Bence Jones protein (monoclonal light chains) in MGUS is absent or <50 mg/day. In asymptomatic multiple myeloma, Bence Jones proteinuria >50 mg/day is associated with earlier progression.[4]

Footnotes

1. Keren DF, Alexanian R, Goeken JA, et al, "Guidelines for Clinical and Laboratory Evaluation of Patients With Monoclonal Gammopathies," *Arch Pathol Lab Med*, 1999, 123(2):106-7.
2. Harrison HH, "The "Ladders Light-Chain" or Pseudo-oligoclonal Pattern in Urinary Immunofixation Electrophoresis (IEF) Studies: A Distinct IFE Pattern and an Explanatory Hypothesis Relating it to Free Polyclonal Light Chains," *Clin Chem*, 1991, 37(9):1559-64.
3. Roach BM, Meinke JS, Sridhar N, et al, "Multiple Narrow Bands in Urine Protein Electrophoresis," *Clin Chem*, 1999, 45(5):716-8.
4. Alexanian R, Weber D, and Liu F, "Differential Diagnosis of Monoclonal Gammopathies," *Arch Pathol Lab Med*, 1999, 123(2):108-13.

References

Baskin LB and Hsu RM, "Laboratory Evaluation of Proteinuria," *MLO*, 1999, 30-6.

Deegan MJ, Abraham JP, Sawdyk M, et al, "High Incidence of Monoclonal Proteins in the Serum and Urine of Chronic Lymphocytic Leukemia Patients," *Blood*, 1984, 64(6):1207-11.

Larson TS, "Evaluation of Proteinuria," *Mayo Clin Proc*, 1994, 69:1154-8.

♦ **Protein Glycosylation** *see* Glycated Hemoglobin (Hemoglobin A₁c), Blood *on page 188*

Protein, Total, Serum

Related Information
Albumin:Globulin Ratio, Serum *on page 88*
Albumin, Serum *on page 88*
Cerebrospinal Fluid Protein Electrophoresis *on page 518*
Immunofixation Electrophoresis, Serum or Urine *on page 530*
Immunoglobulin A *on page 532*
Immunoglobulin G *on page 535*
Immunoglobulin G Subclasses *on page 536*
Immunoglobulin M *on page 537*
Protein Electrophoresis, Capillary Zone *on page 266*
Protein Electrophoresis, Serum *on page 267*
Protein, Quantitative, Urine *on page 883*

Synonyms Total Protein, Serum

Applies to Globulin, Serum

Abstract Used to evaluate protein nutritional status and protein altering diseases

Specimen Serum or plasma

Container Red top tube, green top (heparin) tube

Collection Pediatrics: Blood drawn from heelstick for capillary.

Storage Instructions Separate serum from cells. Refrigerate at 2°C to 8°C.

Reference Interval 6.0-8.0 g/dL (SI: 60-80 g/L) in later childhood and adults. Lower ranges occur in early childhood. Ambulatory values are slightly higher than are those found in recumbency. If normal ranges are set for inpatients, then many outpatients appear to be a little above the upper limit. Because plasma contains fibrinogen, the plasma protein concentration may be up to 0.4 g/dL higher than serum protein concentration.

Use Evaluate nutritional status; investigate edema.

In the entities which follow, the diseases listed are sometimes increased or decreased as indicated, but are not always so.

Causes of **high total protein:** dehydration; some cases of chronic liver disease, including autoimmune hepatitis and cirrhosis; neoplasms, especially myeloma; macroglobulinemia of Waldenström; tropical diseases (eg, kala-azar, leprosy, and others); granulomatous diseases, such as sarcoidosis; diseases in which total protein is sometimes high include collagen disease (eg, lupus erythematosus (SLE), and other instances of acute or chronic infection/inflammation).

Causes of **low total protein:** pregnancy; intravenous fluids; cirrhosis or other liver disease, including chronic alcoholism; prolonged immobilization; heart failure; nephrotic syndromes; glomerulonephritis; neoplasia; protein losing enteropathies; Crohn disease and chronic ulcerative colitis; starvation, malabsorption, or malnutrition; hyperthyroidism; burns; severe skin disease; and other chronic diseases.

Very low total protein (<4.0 g/dL (SI: <40 g/L)) and low albumin cause edema (eg, nephrotic syndromes).

Limitations Venous stasis during venipuncture can lead to increased values. Hemolysis can falsely elevate total protein. Clinical interpretation is greatly enhanced by examination of the fractions composing total protein, when such separation is clinically indicated (ie, serum protein electrophoresis, methods for IgG, IgA, IgM, immunofixation).

Methodology Biuret for total protein, refractometry, BCG for albumin[1,2]

Additional Information Total protein and albumin normally decrease by 5% to 10% upon recumbency, as in hospitalization. "Globulin" may be provided as a calculation, total protein - albumin = globulin. Such a result is a screening test, much less definitive than other methods. Total protein and albumin are commonly measured on chemistry profiling instruments.

Following an acute phase stimulus such as infection or trauma, many liver derived plasma proteins increase in concentration ("acute phase reactants"), while albumin decreases. Thus, while the total serum protein concentration may remain the same in acute phase reactions, the composition of the serum proteins is altered.[3]

Drug effects are summarized. **Increases** related to analytical methods include fluosol-DA, phenazopyradine, radiographic agents and sulfasalazine. Pharmacological increases include effects of anabolic steroids, angiotensin, bumetanide, corticosteroids, digitalis, furosemide, insulin isoretinoin, oral contraceptives, progesterone, and other drugs. **Decreases** are related to carvedilol, hetastarch, laxatives (with continued use), tacrolimus, and other drugs.[4]

Footnotes
1. Dawnay AB, Hirst AD, Perry DE, et al, "A Critical Assessment of Current Analytical Methods for the Routine Assay of Serum Total Protein and Recommendations for Their Improvement," *Ann Clin Biochem*, 1991, 28(Pt 6):556-67.
2. Camara PD, Wright C, Dextraze P, et al, "Comparison of a Commercial Method for Total Protein With a Candidate Reference Method," *Ann Clin Lab Sci*, 1991, 21(5):335-9.
3. Steel DM and Whitehead AS, "The Major Acute Phase Reactants: C-Reactive Protein, Serum Amyloid P Component and Serum Amyloid A Protein," *Immunol Today*, 1994, 15(2):81-8.

4. Young DS, *Effects of Drugs on Clinical Laboratory Tests*, 5th ed, Volume 1: Listing by Test, Washington, DC: AACC Press, American Association of Clinical Chemistry, 2000, Section 3, 672, 677.

References
Johnson AM, Rohlfs EM, and Silverman LM, "Proteins," *Tietz Textbook of Clinical Chemistry*, 3rd ed, Chapter 20, Burtis CA and Ashwood ER, eds, Philadelphia, PA: WB Saunders Co, 1999; 477-540.

Protoporphyrin, Free Erythrocyte

Related Information
Delta (5)-Aminolevulinic Acid, Urine *on page 165*
Ferritin, Serum *on page 173*
Iron and Total Iron Binding Capacity/Transferrin, Serum *on page 203*
Lead, Blood *on page 793*
Lead, Urine *on page 795*
Porphobilinogen, Qualitative, Urine *on page 255*
Porphyrins, Quantitative, Urine *on page 255*
Protoporphyrin, Zinc, Blood *on page 270*
Transferrin Receptor, Soluble, Serum or Plasma *on page 493*

Synonyms FEP; Free Erythrocyte Protoporphyrin; Protoporphyrins, Fractionation, Erythrocytes; RBC Protoporphyrin

Abstract Free erythrocyte protoporphyrin expresses the amount of nonheme protoporphyrin in red cells. Unless lead toxicity is suspected, it is useful for evaluation of iron deficiency in childhood and its differential diagnosis; molecules accumulate with slowing of hemoglobin synthesis with iron deficiency. Erythropoietic protoporphyria is an erythropoietic porphyria for which red cell protoporphyrin is tested. It is due to deficiency of ferrochelatase.

Specimen Whole blood (test done on washed erythrocytes)

Container Lavender top (EDTA) tube (preferred) or green top (heparin) tube

Collection Pediatrics: Blood drawn from heelstick for capillary.

Storage Instructions Stable 3 weeks at 4°C. Do not freeze.

Special Instructions Current hematocrit must be measured or specified.

Reference Interval Depends on method; ascertain ranges for individual testing laboratory. The FEP is considered unreliable in infants younger than 6 months of age.[1] Pediatric upper limit is 50 µg/dL (SI: 0.89 µmol/L) RBC. Higher levels prevail through infancy. Adults: male: <30 µg/dL (SI: <0.53 µmol/L), female: <40 µg/dL (SI: <0.71 µmol/L) by hematofluorometer; 11-45 µg/dL (SI: 0.20-0.80 µmol/L) for adult men and 19-52 µg/dL (SI: 0.34-0.92 µmol/L) for adult women by Piomelli. FEP is expressed as µg/dL blood.[2]

A recent decline in free erythrocyte protoporphyrin concentrations has been paralleled by a decrease in lead levels.[3]

Possible Panic Range >190 µg/dL (SI: >3.38 µmol/L)

Use Differential diagnosis of disorders of heme production versus diseases of globin synthesis.[4] FEP is increased in lead poisoning, erythropoietic protoporphyria, in iron deficiency,[5,6,7,8] as well as in anemia of chronic disease and with some sideroblastic anemias.[4] With lead poisoning and iron deficiency, photosensitivity is not found. FEP levels are also increased in entities characterized by marked increase in erythropoiesis, such as severe hemolytic anemias. Thus, FEP is useful in work-up of the microcytic anemias. FEP is not increased in acute intermittent porphyria.[9,10,11] FEP is reported normal with presumed alpha thalassemia trait, hemoglobin H, beta thalassemia trait, and hemoglobin E.

Limitations Fluorescent substances in plasma may interfere with hematofluorometer results. Elevated FEPs should be verified by retesting washed RBCs or by microextraction. Skin contamination may lead to false elevations. Both this test and blood lead are needed for full evaluation.

Methodology Hematofluorometer, extraction method, and high performance liquid chromatography (HPLC). The hematofluorometer measures porphyrins unbound in erythrocytes. With iron deficiency and diminished heme synthesis, free porphyrin accumulates in the red blood cell. A definitive fluorometric method has been published by the National Committee for Clinical Laboratory Standards (NCCLS).[12]

Additional Information "Free" protoporphyrin is not complexed, nonheme protoporphyrin. **Lead poisoning** is characterized by elevated plasma and urine delta aminolevulinic acid and increased urinary coproporphyrin as well as increased blood lead. Urinary porphobilinogen and uroporphyrin are normal to slightly increased. Free erythrocyte protoporphyrin is a sensitive test for lead toxicity or chronic exposure,[11] **although, a careful study based on receiver operator curves showed that erythrocyte protoporphyrin levels should not be used as a screening test for lead poisoning in children.** It is insensitive to blood lead levels ≤35 µg/dL. The diagnosis of lead exposure or poisoning includes consideration of environmental exposure, as well as symptoms and abnormal erythrocyte protoporphyrin. FEP is given as 92-288 µg/dL (SI: 1.63-5.12 µmol/L) RBC in level II increased lead absorption, with higher FEP results in level III. Increased lead absorption is reported in the presence of iron deficiency.[13] Increased erythrocyte protoporphyrin exists as free protoporphyrin in protoporphyria, not as a zinc chelate, in contrast to lead poisoning and iron deficiency.[14] Zinc protoporphyrin and metal-free protoporphyrin can be distinguished from each other by spectrophotofluorometry.

Ferrochelatase activity can be assayed using red blood cells and fibroblasts.

(Continued)

Protoporphyrin, Free Erythrocyte *(Continued)*

Footnotes

1. Benjamin JT, Dickens MD, Ford RF, et al, "Normative Data of Hemoglobin Concentration and Free Erythrocyte Protoporphyrin in a Private Pediatric Practice," *Clin Pediatr (Phila)*, 1986, 25(4):206-8.
2. Marsh WL Jr, Nelson DP, and Koenig HM, "Free Erythrocyte Protoporphyrin (FEP) I. Normal Values for Adults and Evaluation of the Hematofluorometer," *Am J Clin Pathol*, 1983, 79(6):655-60.
3. Looker AC, Dallman PR, Carroll MD, et al, "Prevalence of Iron Deficiency in the United States," *JAMA*, 1997, 277(12):973-6.
4. Marsh WL Jr, Nelson DP, and Koenig HM, "Free Erythrocyte Protoporphyrin (FEP) II. The FEP Test Is Clinically Useful in Classifying Microcytic RBC Disorders in Adults," *Am J Clin Pathol*, 1983, 79(6):661-6.
5. Benjamin JT, Dickens MD, Ford RF, et al, "Normative Data of Hemoglobin Concentration and Free Erythrocyte Protoporphyrin in A Private Pediatric Practice: A 1990 Update," *Clin Pediatr (Phila)*, 1991, 30(2):74-6.
6. Parsons PJ, Stanton NV, Gunter EW, et al, "An Interlaboratory Comparison of Control Materials for Use With Hematofluorometers," *Clin Chem*, 1989, 35(10):2059-65.
7. Brown RG, "Determining the Cause of Anemia. General Approach, With Emphasis on Microcytic Hypochromic Anemias," *Postgrad Med*, 1991, 89(6):161-4, 167-70.
8. Beaton GH, Corey PN, and Steele C, "Conceptual and Methodological Issues Regarding the Epidemiology of Iron Deficiency and Their Implications for Studies of the Functional Consequences of Iron Deficiency," *Am J Clin Nutr*, 1989, 50(3 Suppl):575-88.
9. Turk DS, Schonfeld DJ, Cullen M, et al, "Sensitivity of Erythrocyte Protoporphyrin as a Screening Test for Lead Poisoning," *N Engl J Med*, 1992, 326(2):137-8.
10. McElvaine MD, Orbach HG, Binder S, et al, "Evaluation of the Erythrocyte Protoporphyrin Test as a Screen for Elevated Blood Lead Levels," *J Pediatr*, 1991, 119(4):548-50.
11. DeBaun MR and Sox HC Jr, "Setting the Optimal Erythrocyte Protoporphyrin Screening Decision Threshold for Lead Poisoning: A Decision Analytic Approach," *Pediatrics*, 1991, 88(1):121-31.
12. National Committee for Clinical Laboratory Standards, "Erythrocyte Protoporphyrin Testing: Approved Guidelines," *NCCLS Document*, C42-A, Wayne, PA: NCCLS, 1996.
13. Carraccio CL, Bergman GE, and Daley BP, "Combined Iron Deficiency and Lead Poisoning in Children. Effect on FEP Levels," *Clin Pediatr (Phila)*, 1987, 26(12):644-7.
14. Thadani H, Deacon A, and Peters T, "Diagnosis and Management of Porphyria," *BMJ*, 2000, 320(7250):1647-51.

References

Bird TD, Wallace DM, and Labbe RF, "The Porphyria, Plumbism, Pottery Puzzle," *JAMA*, 1982, 247:813-4.

Downey DC, "Porphyria and Chemicals," *Med Hypotheses*, 1999, 53(2):166-71.

Hindmarsh JT, Oliveras L, and Greenway DC, "Biochemical Differentiation of the Porphyrias," *Clin Biochem*, 1999, 32(8):609-19.

McCabe ER, "The Metabolic Encephalopathies," *Oski's Pediatrics: Principles and Practice*, 3rd ed, McMillan JA, De Angelis CD, Feigin RD, et al, eds, Philadelphia, PA: JB Lippincott Co, 1999, 1996-2004.

Zanella A, Gridelli L, Berzuini A, et al, "Sensitivity and Predictive Value of Serum Ferritin and Free Erythrocyte Protoporphyrin for Iron Deficiency," *J Lab Clin Med*, 1989, 113(1):73-8.

- ◆ **Protoporphyrins, Fractionation, Erythrocytes** *see* Protoporphyrin, Free Erythrocyte *on page 269*

Protoporphyrin, Zinc, Blood

Related Information

Delta (5)-Aminolevulinic Acid, Urine *on page 165*
Ferritin, Serum *on page 173*
Iron and Total Iron Binding Capacity/Transferrin, Serum *on page 203*
Lead, Blood *on page 793*
Protoporphyrin, Free Erythrocyte *on page 269*

Synonyms Protoporphyrin, Zinc, Erythrocyte; Zinc Protoporphyrin; ZPP

Abstract Zinc protoporphyrin measurement may in some cases, be a useful adjunct in the diagnosis of nonanemic iron deficiency[1] but is not useful in screening programs for lead intoxication.[2] It may also be increased in erythropoietic protoporphyria, however erythrocyte protoporphyrin concentrations are much higher as compared to zinc protoporphyrin.

Specimen Whole blood

Container Lavender top (EDTA) tube, green top (heparin) tube

Collection Routine venipuncture

Storage Instructions Do not centrifuge. Refrigerate and protect from light. Stable 1 week at 4°C.

Causes for Rejection Hemolysis, icterus

Reference Interval 20-80 µg/dL whole blood (SI: 0.27-1.23 µmol/L). Results may be obtained as ZPP:heme ratio; reference range: 30-80 µmol/mol heme. It is moderately increased with pregnancy.

Critical Values >100 µg/dL (SI: >1.6 µmol/L)

Use Evaluate reduction of body iron storage, especially in nonanemic iron deficiency. ZPP is superior to hemoglobin in identifying female blood donors with nonanemic iron deficiency.[1]

Limitations Zinc protoporphyrin is increased in lead poisoning but not with thalassemia. ZPP alone should **not** be used to screen or diagnose lead poisoning.[2,3] High concentrations of aluminum in subjects on hemodialysis can cause increased levels. It may be increased with the anemia of chronic disease, including cases of lymphoma, sideroblastic and hemolytic anemia, and secondary polycythemia.

Methodology Hematofluorometry (front-face); if washed erythrocytes are used, the assay becomes more specific and sensitive.[4]

Additional Information Zinc protoporphyrin (ZPP) levels increase as blood lead levels increase. Various authorities caution using ZPP as a screening test for lead poisoning. The Centers for Disease Control has lowered the cutoff level for lead intoxication in children younger than 6 years of age to **10 µg/dL (SI: 0.48 µmol/L)**, and this level is so low that **ZPP is not useful** in this context because it is insensitive to such a lead level, and is increased only when blood lead levels are >25 µg/dL. Therefore, it is mandatory to measure lead levels in any screening program, rather than ZPP. ZPP appears only in new RBCs and remains for the life of the RBC; therefore, ZPP does not increase until several weeks after the onset of lead exposure and remains high long after exposure to lead. It is a reasonable indicator of total body burden of lead and remains a useful adjunct to the diagnosis of iron deficiency, particularly in nonanemic or questionably anemic patients. It reflects iron depletion in the bone marrow. However, in uremic patients, use of ZPP as a first-line diagnostic marker is questionable.[5]

Footnotes

1. Jensen BM, Sando SH, Grandjean P, et al, "Protoporphyrin for Iron Deficiency in Nonanemic Female Blood Donors," *Clin Chem*, 1990, 36(6):846-8.
2. Turk DS, Schonfeld DJ, Cullen M, et al, "Sensitivity of Erythrocyte Protoporphyrin as a Screening Test for Lead Poisoning," *N Engl J Med*, 1992, 326(2):137-8.
3. Rolfe PB, Marcinak JF, Nice AJ, et al, "Use of Zinc Protoporphyrin Measured by the Protofluor-Z Hematofluorometer in Screening Children for Elevated Blood Lead Levels," *Am J Dis Child*, 1993, 147(1):66-8.
4. Hastka J, Lasserre JJ, Schwarzbeck A, et al, "Washing Erythrocytes to Remove Interferents in Measurement of Zinc Protoporphyrin by Front-Face Hematofluorometry," *Clin Chem*, 1992, 38(11):2184-9.
5. Canavese C, Grill A, Decostanzi E, et al, "Limited Value of Zinc Protoporphyrin as a Marker of Iron Status in Chronic Hemodialysis Patients," *Clin Nephrol*, 2000, 53(1):42-7.

References

Cone DC, "Lead Screening and Follow-up in an Urban Pediatric Clinic," *N Y State J Med*, 1992, 92(8):338-42.

Hastka J, Lasserre JJ, Schwarzbeck A, et al, "Zinc Protoporphyrin in Anemia of Chronic Disorders," *Blood*, 1993, 81(5):1200-4.

Labbe RF, "Clinical Utility of Zinc Protoporphyrin," *Clin Chem*, 1992, 38(11):2167-8.

Labbe RF, Vreman HJ, and Stevenson DK, "Zinc Protoporphyrin: A Metabolite With a Mission," *Clin Chem*, 1999, 45(12):2060-72.

McCabe ER, "The Metabolic Encephalopathies," *Oski's Pediatrics: Principles and Practice*, 3rd ed, McMillan JA, DeAngelis CD, Feigin RD, et al, eds, Philadelphia, PA: JB Lippincott Co, 1999, 1996-2004.

Zwennis WC, Franssen AC, and Wijnans MJ, "Use of Zinc Protoporphyrin in Screening Individuals for Exposure to Lead," *Clin Chem*, 1990, 36(8 Pt 1):1456-9.

- ◆ **Protoporphyrin, Zinc, Erythrocyte** *see* Protoporphyrin, Zinc, Blood *on page 270*
- ◆ **PSA** *see* Prostate Specific Antigen, Serum *on page 263*
- ◆ **PSA Density** *see* Prostate Specific Antigen, Serum *on page 263*
- ◆ **PSA Velocity** *see* Prostate Specific Antigen, Serum *on page 263*
- ◆ **Pseudocholinesterase Inhibition by Dibucaine** *see* Dibucaine Number, Serum or Plasma *on page 166*

Pseudocholinesterase, Serum

Related Information

Acetylcholinesterase, Red Cell *on page 81*
Dibucaine Number, Serum or Plasma *on page 166*
Organophosphate Pesticides, Urine, Blood, or Serum *on page 804*

Synonyms Acylcholine Acylhydrolase; Benzoyl Cholinesterase; Cholinesterase II; Cholinesterase, Serum; PChE; Plasma Cholinesterase

Abstract Two types of cholinesterase are found in blood: **"true" cholinesterase (acetylcholinesterase)** in red cells, lung, and brain, while **"pseudocholinesterase"** (acylcholine acylhydrolase) (PChE) is found in serum (plasma). PChE, a sialated glycoprotein, is synthesized in the liver. Organophosphorus-containing insecticides inhibit RBC cholinesterase and depress serum pseudocholinesterase. Serum pseudocholinesterase is more sensitive than the red cell enzyme to organophosphate compounds. See Acetylcholinesterase, Red Cell *on page 81*.

Specimen Serum

Container Red top tube

Storage Instructions Stable at room temperature for 6 hours, 1 week at 4°C, and 6 months at -70°C. Avoid repeat freezing and thawing.

Causes for Rejection Gross hemolysis

Reference Interval Low in infancy, then increasing to adult levels by the second month.[1] Ranges vary between methods and laboratories. Typical values[2] are 5-12 units/mL (with propionyl thiocholine); 7-19 units/mL (with butylthiocholine). Intermediate levels are found in heterozygotes.

Possible Panic Range Serious neuromuscular symptoms occur at decreases of ~80%.

Use Screen preoperative patients for inherited succinylcholine (suxamethonium) anesthetic sensitivity, genetic or secondary to insecticide exposure, in appropriate circumstances. The diagnosis of the cholinergic syndrome is based on clinical findings as well as PChE activity. Prevent or evaluate prolonged anesthetic effect, prolonged apnea, after surgery. Very small amounts (0.04-0.06 mg/kg) of succinylcholine are needed to obtain 90% of neuromuscular blockade in patients with an abnormal allele who have low levels of plasma cholinesterase activity.

Monitor and diagnose organophosphorous exposure and poisoning, in which pseudocholinesterase level is decreased; establish patient's baseline value before exposure. Cholinesterase activity is inhibited by organic insecticides including parathion, sarin, and tetraethyl pyrophosphate. Indications include pesticide exposure for patients with miosis, blurred vision, muscle weakness, twitching, and fasciculation, bradycardia, nausea, diarrhea, vomiting, salivation, sweating, respiratory failure, pulmonary edema, ventricular arrhythmias, and convulsions. The value of assessment of risk status in persons exposed to organophosphate insecticides on the basis of plasma cholinesterase levels alone has been called into question. See Organophosphate Pesticides, Urine, Blood, or Serum *on page 804*.

Family studies may be done when an individual with a genetically abnormal type is documented by serum pseudocholinesterase deficiency and, ideally, confirmed by phenotyping. See Dibucaine Number, Serum or Plasma *on page 166*.

Limitations Serum pseudocholinesterase may be decreased in patients on estrogens and oral contraceptives. Fluoride interferes. Pseudocholinesterase is also low in some instances of liver disease, including decompensated cirrhosis, hepatitis, metastatic carcinoma, CHF, and in malnutrition, but not sufficiently consistently enough to be a useful clinical test for such disorders. Decreases up to 70% are found in some cases of advanced hepatic disease. Genetic atypical enzyme does not explain every instance of prolonged postsurgical apnea (ie, normal serum PChE does not entirely assure lack of sensitivity to succinylcholine). Red cell cholinesterase is more useful for chronic insecticide exposure. Carbamate-poisoned persons can appear to have near normal or normal levels of pseudocholinesterase. PChE is elevated in obese and diabetic individuals.[3]

Contraindications Not useful to screen for toxicity from chlorinated insecticides.

Methodology Colorimetry, kinetic enzyme utilizing different substrates, fluorometry[1,4]

Additional Information Low serum cholinesterase activity may relate to exposure to insecticides or to one of a number of variant genotypes. Dibucaine and fluoride numbers are useful to phenotype such homozygous and heterozygous individuals, who are genetically sensitive to succinylcholine. A case of inherited pseudocholinesterase deficiency has been reported.[5]

One patient in 1500 is susceptible to succinyldicholine anesthetic mishap.

Plasmapheresis has been noted to decrease the level of plasma cholinesterase. Patients with abnormally low cholinesterase activity after transfusion of blood or plasma will experience temporary augmentation of enzyme level. In estimating the duration of this enhanced activity, measures of plasma cholinesterase half-life have been utilized. The true half-life value is, however, uncertain. A half-life value determined by measuring the rate of disappearance after intravenous injection of human cholinesterase has provided an average value of 11 days.[6]

A low level of activity of pseudocholinesterase has been demonstrated in cerebrospinal fluid, at about 1/20 to 1/100 the activity present in the corresponding plasma. With clinical conditions characterized by bleeding into the CSF, pseudocholinesterase activity increases 25% to 50% that of plasma.

Increase in acetylcholinesterase activity by histochemistry, without ganglion cells, in rectal biopsy (not as measured in serum) has provided discriminatory diagnostic value in some cases of Hirschsprung disease.

Some patients with high pseudocholinesterase activities show marked difficulty in intubation.[7]

Footnotes
1. Moss DW and Henderson AR, "Clinical Enzymology," *Tietz Textbook of Clinical Chemistry*, 3rd ed, Chapter 22, Burtis CA and Ashwood ER, eds, Philadelphia, PA: WB Saunders Co, 1999, 617-721.
2. Painter PC, Cope JY, and Smith JL, "Reference Information for the Clinical Laboratory," *Tietz Textbook of Clinical Chemistry*, 3rd ed, Burtis CA and Ashwood ER, eds, Philadelphia, PA: WB Saunders Co, 1999, 1807.
3. Kutty KM and Payne RH, "Serum Pseudocholinesterase and Very-Low-Density Lipoprotein Metabolism," *J Clin Lab Anal*, 1994, 8(4):247-50.
4. Kusu F, Tsuneta T, and Takamura K, "Fluorometric Determination of Pseudocholinesterase Activity in Postmortem Blood Samples," *J Forensic Sci*, 1990, 35(6):1330-4.
5. Ho VW and Osiovich H, "A Case of Pseudocholinesterase Deficiency in the Neonate," *Am J Perinatol*, 1999, 16(7):351-3.
6. Ostergaard D, Viby-Mogensen J, Hanel HK, et al, "Half-Life of Plasma Cholinesterase," *Acta Anaesthesiol Scand*, 1988, 32(3):266-9.
7. Yao FS and Savarese JJ, "Pseudocholinesterase Hyperactivity With Succinylcholine Resistance: An Unusual Case of Difficult Intubation," *J Clin Anesth*, 1997, 9(4):328-30.

References
Bardin PG, van Eeden SF, Moolman JA, et al, "Organophosphate and Carbamate Poisoning," *Arch Intern Med*, 1994, 154(13):1433-41.
Burgess JL, Bernstein JN, and Hurlbut K, "Aldicarb Poisoning. A Case Report With Prolonged Cholinesterase Inhibition and Improvement After Pralidoxime Therapy," *Arch Intern Med*, 1994, 154(2):221-4.
Hoffman RS, Henry GC, Howland MA, et al, "Association Between Life-Threatening Cocaine Toxicity and Plasma Cholinesterase Activity," *Ann Emerg Med*, 1992, 21(3):247-53.

Jokanovic M and Maksimovic M, "Abnormal Cholinesterase Activity: Understanding and Interpretation," *Eur J Clin Chem Clin Biochem*, 1997, 35(1):11-6.
Lessenger JE and Reese BE, "Rational Use of Cholinesterase Activity Testing in Pesticide Poisoning," *J Am Board Fam Pract*, 1999, 12(4):307-14.
Marrs TC, "Organophosphate Poisoning," *Pharmacol Ther*, 1993, 58(1):51-66.
Pantuck EJ, "Plasma Cholinesterase: Gene and Variations," *Anesth Analg*, 1993, 77(2):380-6.

♦ **Pseudomonas aeruginosa, Mucoid** *see* Chloride, Sweat *on page 144*

♦ **Pseudo-oligoclonal Bands** *see* Protein Electrophoresis, Urine *on page 268*

♦ **PTH** *see* Parathyroid Hormone, Serum *on page 243*

♦ **PTHrP** *see* Parathyroid Hormone-Related Protein, Serum *on page 243*

Pulmonary Surfactant, Amniotic Fluid

Related Information
Lamellar Bodies, Amniotic Fluid *on page 454*
Lecithin:Sphingomyelin Ratio, Amniotic Fluid *on page 210*
Phosphatidylglycerol, Amniotic Fluid *on page 251*

Synonyms Amniotic Fluid Pulmonary Surfactant

Applies to Foam Stability Index or Shake Test; Lamellar Body Count; Optical Density at 650 nm; Surfactant:Albumin Ratio

Abstract As the fetal lungs mature with increasing gestational age, fetal pulmonary surfactant is secreted into the amniotic fluid. Analyses of amniotic fluid pulmonary surfactant assess fetal lung maturity and the probability of hyaline membrane disease (respiratory distress syndrome - RDS). This section addresses commonly used amniotic fluid pulmonary surfactant tests other than the L:S ratio and PG.

Aftercare All nonsensitized Rh-negative patients should receive anti-D immunoglobulin after amniocentesis.

Specimen Amniotic fluid; specimen volume required varies with analytical method (1 mL minimum).

Container The use of siliconized collection tubes will interfere with the shake test and should not be used.[1]

Collection Ultrasound-guided amniocentesis is performed by the physician. Vaginal pool specimens are discouraged.

Reference Interval The following table summarizes the reference ranges[1,2] for the various pulmonary surfactant tests.

Amniotic Fluid Pulmonary Surfactant

Pulmonary Surfactant Test	Maturity Threshold
Surfactant:albumin ratio (S/A)	>55 mg/g
Lamellar body count (LB)	>50,000/μL
Foam stability index (FSI)	≥47
Optical density at 650 nm (OD_{650})	≥0.15

Use The analysis of amniotic fluid pulmonary surfactant is done prenatally in high-risk pregnancies to evaluate fetal lung maturity and the newborn's risk for developing RDS/hyaline membrane disease.

Limitations Contamination of specimen with blood, meconium, or vaginal mucus and debris may falsely affect results by all methods. One study showed that blood contamination tends to yield falsely immature or borderline values in truly mature specimens by the automated S/A assay, but mature results from blood contaminated specimens are valid.[3] Another study concluded that all bloody specimens with S/A results <90 mg/g be tested for PG by the rapid immunoagglutination method for confirmation.[4]

There is considerable variation in diagnostic thresholds for lamellar body (LB) counts due to variation in centrifugation speeds and times and commercial hematology counters. Neither bilirubin nor meconium interferes with this test, but red cells decrease results.[2] Consistent centrifugation conditions are necessary for both LB counts and OD_{650} determinations.[2]

Though the predictive value of mature results are close to 100% for any of the pulmonary surfactant tests, the predictive value of immature results range from 30% to 50%.[2] Sequential (cascade) testing procedures are sometimes used, employing combinations of these procedures and/or L/S or PG determinations to further characterize initial, "immature" results.

Methodology Fluorescence polarization (S/A), platelet channel counting (LB), light scattering (LB, OD_{650}), ethanol dilution (FSI, Shake Test)

Additional Information The original reagent formulation for the automated fluorescence polarization determination of S/A had a maturity threshold >70 mg/g and should be kept in mind while reviewing the earlier literature on this method. This higher threshold has been shown to be valid in diabetic pregnancies.[5,6] Fetal lung maturity testing by fluorescence polarization in preterm labor has been shown to be most cost-effective between 34 and 36 weeks gestation[7] and to have diagnostic power equivalent to or better than the L:S ratio.[8]

Lamellar bodies are surfactant-containing structures that are secreted from type II pneumocytes. Because of their size (1-5 μm), estimations of lamellar body counts in amniotic fluid may be made using the platelet counting chamber of standard cell counters. See Lamellar Bodies, Amniotic Fluid *on page 454*.
(Continued)

Pulmonary Surfactant, Amniotic Fluid *(Continued)*

Theoretically, chronic oligohydramnios/polyhydramnios has a minimal effect on surfactant concentration measurement in amniotic fluid. However, acute oligohydramnios/polyhydramnios may significantly affect the amniotic fluid surfactant measurement if the acute change in volume is due to decreased/increased volume of inflow.[9] Fluorescence polarization S/A results are unaffected by amniotic fluid volume changes.

Footnotes

1. "ACOG Educational Bulletin. Assessment of Fetal Lung Maturity. Number 230, November 1996," *Int J Gynaecol Obstet*, 1997, 56(2):191-8.
2. Dubin SB, "Assessment of Fetal Lung Maturity Practice Parameter," *Am J Clin Pathol*, 1998, 110(6):723-32.
3. Carlan SJ, Gearity D, and O'Brien WF, "The Effect of Maternal Blood Contamination on the TDx-FLM II Assay," *Am J Perinatol*, 1997, 14(8):491-4.
4. Wong SS, Schenkel O, and Qutishat A, "Strategic Utilization of Fetal Lung Maturity Tests," *Scand J Clin Lab Invest*, 1996, 56(6):525-32.
5. Livingston EG, Herbert WN, Hage ML, et al, "Use of the TDx-FLM Assay in Evaluating Fetal Lung Maturity in an Insulin-Dependent Diabetic Population," *Obstet Gynecol*, 1995, 86(5):826-9.
6. Del Valle GO, Adair CD, Ramos EE, et al, "Interpretation of the TDx-FLM Fluorescence Polarization Assay in Pregnancies Complicated by Diabetes Mellitus," *Am J Perinatol*, 1997, 14(5):241-4.
7. Myers ER, Alvarez JG, Richardson DK, et al, "Cost-Effectiveness of Fetal Lung Maturity Testing in Preterm Labor," *Obstet Gynecol*, 1997, 90(5):824-9.
8. Bender TM, Stone LR, and Amenta JS, "Diagnostic Power of Lecithin/Sphingomyelin Ratio and Fluorescence Polarization Assays for Respiratory Distress Syndrome Compared by Relative Operating Characteristic Curves," *Clin Chem*, 1994, 40(4):541-5.
9. Nelson GH and Nelson SJ, "Theoretical Effects of Amniotic Fluid Volume Changes on Surfactant Concentration Measurements," *Am J Obstet Gynecol*, 1985, 152(7 Pt 1):870-8.

References

Bonebrake RG, Towers CV, Rumney PJ, et al, "Is Fluorescence Polarization Reliable and Cost Efficient in a Fetal Lung Maturity Cascade?" *Am J Obstet Gynecol*, 1997, 177(4):835-41.

Dalence CR, Bowie LJ, Dohnal JC, et al, "Amniotic Fluid Lamellar Body Count: A Rapid and Reliable Fetal Lung Maturity Test," *Obstet Gynecol*, 1995, 86(2):235-9.

Greenspoon JS, Rosen DJ, Roll K, et al, "Evaluation of Lamellar Body Number Density as the Initial Assessment in Fetal Lung Maturity Test Cascade," *J Reprod Med*, 1995, 40(4):260-6.

Lee IS, Cho YK, Ahm K, et al, "Lamellar Body Count in Amniotic Fluid as a Rapid Screening Test for Fetal Lung Maturity," *J Perinatol*, 1996, 16(3 Pt 1):176-80.

Lewis PS, Lauria MR, Dzieczkowski J, et al, "Amniotic Fluid Lamellar Body Count: Cost-Effective Screening for Fetal Lung Maturity," *Obstet Gynecol*, 1999, 93(3):387-91.

Nakamura Y, Yamamoto I, Funatsu Y, et al, "Decreased Surfactant Level in the Lung With Oligohydramnios: A Morphometric and Biochemical Study," *J Pediatr*, 1988, 112(3):471-4.

Sher G, Statland B, and Freer DE, "Clinical Evaluation of the Quantitative Foam Stability Index Test," *Obstet Gynecol*, 1980, 55:617-20.

Statland BE and Sher G, "Reliability of Amniotic Fluid Surfactant Measurements," *Am J Clin Pathol*, 1985, 83(3):382-4.

♦ **Pulse Oximetry, Transcutaneous** *see* Oxygen Saturation, Blood *on page 240*

♦ **PYD** *see* Osteocalcin, Serum or Plasma *on page 237*

♦ **Pyridinium Collagen Cross-Links** *see* Pyridinolines (Pyridinoline and Deoxypyridinoline), Urine *on page 272*

♦ **Pyridinoline** *see* N-Telopeptides, Urine *on page 233*

♦ **Pyridinoline** *see* Osteocalcin, Serum or Plasma *on page 237*

Pyridinolines (Pyridinoline and Deoxypyridinoline), Urine

Related Information

Alkaline Phosphatase Isoenzymes, Serum *on page 92*
Alkaline Phosphatase, Serum *on page 93*
Calcium, Serum *on page 131*
Calcium, Urine *on page 133*
Hydroxyproline, Total, Urine *on page 199*
N-Telopeptides, Urine *on page 233*
Osteocalcin, Serum or Plasma *on page 237*
Parathyroid Hormone, Serum *on page 243*
Phosphorus, Serum *on page 251*
Phosphorus, Urine *on page 253*
Urine Collection, 24-Hour *on page 47*
Vitamin D, Serum *on page 300*

Synonyms Deoxypyridinoline; Hydroxylysylpyridinoline; Lysylpyridinoline; Pyridinium Collagen Cross-Links

Test Includes Pyridinoline and deoxypyridinoline

Abstract The cross-links of the helical structure of type 1 collagen are the pyridinolines and deoxypyridinolines. Pyridinolines are, like hydroxyproline, markers of bone resorption, of osteoclast activity. During bone resorption, pyridinolines are released and excreted in the urine. The rate of excretion of pyridinolines in urine is used as an index of bone matrix degradation and resorption.

Specimen Urine

Sampling Time Due to diurnal variation, 24-hour urine collection is preferred. However, for deoxypyridinoline the variation is less as compared to N-telopeptide.[1] Excretion of deoxypyridinoline is greater at night.

Resorption markers fall faster than formation markers when a change in rate of remodeling occurs: 2-12 weeks for resorption markers, 3-6 months for formation markers.

Storage Instructions Refrigerate. Freeze for longer storage (>2 days).

Special Instructions Avoid exposure to light.

Reference Interval Pyridinoline levels are higher in children as compared to adults. There is considerable variation in reference ranges from different laboratories. The following are the reference ranges (**pmol/mmol creatinine**), in relation to pubertal stages, from a recent publication.[2]

Pubertal Stage	Pyridinoline (pmol/mmol creatinine)		Deoxypyridinoline (pmol/mmol creatinine)	
	Boys	Girls	Boys	Girls
1	383 ±16	440 ±35	66 ±3	75 ±7
2	369 ±31	511 ±42	59 ±6	82 ±7
3	407 ±54	357 ±67	58 ±9	57 ±13
4	404 ±61	250 ±43	63 ±9	39 ±7
5	126 ±15	151 ±21	20 ±3	21 ±3
Adults	83 ±5	88 ±5	17 ±1	15 ±1

Values are mean ±SEM.

Use The major roles of biochemical markers of bone remodeling are as monitors of response to therapy. These markers can also be used to evaluate bone metabolism, bone resorption (eg, in osteopenia, osteoporosis[3]); identify patients at high risk of fracture; assess patients with carcinoma as markers of bone metastasis as well as indicators of response to therapy.[4,5,6,7]

Limitations Day-to-day variation is ~20% for bone resorption markers.[8] Pyridinium cross-links are affected by renal clearance.

Methodology High performance liquid chromatography (HPLC), enzyme-linked immunosorbent assay (ELISA), chemiluminescence immunoassay, radioimmunoassay

Additional Information Bone biopsy and bone density scans are used to assess bone mass. However, with these methods, 6-12 months are needed to measure a true change in bone mass. Biochemical markers of bone formation and resorption are very sensitive to bone mass changes. Collagen fibers are linked together by pyridinium cross-links (pyridinoline and deoxypyridinoline). During bone resorption, both pyridinoline and deoxypyridinoline are released, approximately in a ratio of 3:1. Deoxypyridinoline is a more specific marker of bone resorption as compared to pyridinoline because it is formed during collagen maturation, not biosynthesis and originates only as a degradation product of the mature bone matrix. It does not appear to be metabolized prior to excretion in the urine. Bone is a major source of deoxypyridinoline and it is not absorbed from the diet.[9]

Pyridinolines are increased in osteoporosis, Paget disease, metastatic bone disease,[10] primary and secondary hyperparathyroidism, hyperthyroidism, and other diseases with increased bone resorption.[11,12,13,14,15] Urinary excretion of pyridinium cross-links is diminished in hypothyroidism.[16]

In normal individuals, ~40% of pyridinolines are released as free and 60% bound to protein. However, in health and disease the ratio of total to free pyridinolines varies considerably.[8] Total deoxypyridinoline increases more than free deoxypyridinoline in postmenopausal women and in patients with osteoporosis, Paget disease, and hyperthyroidism. Treatment of Paget disease and osteoporotic patients with biphosphanates decreases total but not free deoxypyridinoline, whereas both are decreased during estrogen therapy of postmenopausal women.[11,17] In patients with Paget disease treated with biphosphanates, N-telopeptides are suppressed more than deoxypyridinoline and best predict the outcome of therapy.[11,17,18] Pyridinolines are increased in breast cancer and prostate cancer patients with bone metastases. These markers are more sensitive than CA 15-3 tumor markers for breast cancer in assessing response to treatment in women with bone metastases.

In differential diagnosis of osteoporosis, CBC, serum calcium, phosphorus, creatinine, alkaline phosphatase, protein electrophoresis, urinary calcium, TSH, parathormone, and vitamin D may be useful, as well as pyridinolines, N-telopeptides, and osteocalcin.

Bone density remains the major marker for osteoporosis/osteopenia.

Footnotes

1. Ju HS, Leung S, Brown B, et al, "Comparison of Analytical Performance and Biological Variability of Three Bone Resorption Assays," *Clin Chem*, 1997, 43(9):1570-6.
2. Mora S, Prinster C, Proverbio MC, et al, "Urinary Markers of Bone Turnover in Healthy Children and Adolescents: Age-Related Changes and Effect of Puberty," *Calcif Tissue Int*, 1998, 63(5):369-74.
3. Hurley DL and Khosla S, "Subspecialty Clinics: Endocrinology, Metabolism, and Nutrition. Update on Primary Osteoporosis," *Mayo Clin Proc*, 1997, 72(10):943-9.
4. Walls J, Assiri A, Howell A, et al, "Measurement of Urinary Collagen Cross-Links Indicate Response to Therapy in Patients With Breast Cancer and Bone Metastases," *Br J Cancer*, 1999, 80(8):1265-70.
5. Maeda H, Koizumi M, Yoshimura K, et al, "Correlation Between Bone Metabolic Markers and Bone Scan in Prostatic Cancer," *J Urol*, 1997, 157(2):539-43.

6. Nemoto R, Nakamura I, Nishijima Y, et al, "Serum Pyridinoline Crosslinks as Markers of Tumour-Induced Bone Resorption," *Br J Urol*, 1997, 80(2):274-80.

7. Ikeda I, Miura T, and Kondo I, "Pyridinium Cross-Links as Urinary Markers of Bone Metastases in Patients With Prostate Cancer," *Br J Urol*, 1996, 77(1):102-6.

8. Watts NB, "Clinical Utility of Biochemical Markers of Bone Remodeling," *Clin Chem*, 1999, 45(8 Pt 2):1359-68.

9. Colwell A, Russell RG, and Eastell R, "Factors Affecting the Assay of Urinary 3-Hydroxy Pyridinium Cross-Links of Collagen as Markers of Bone Resorption," *Eur J Clin Invest*, 1993, 23(6):341-9.

10. Takeuchi S, Arai K, Saitoh H, et al, "Urinary Pyridinoline and Deoxypyridinoline as Potential Markers of Bone Metastasis in Patients With Prostate Cancer," *J Urol*, 1996, 156(5):1691-5.

11. Alvarez L, Guanabens N, Peris P, et al, "Discriminative Value of Biochemical Markers of Bone Turnover in Assessing the Activity of Paget's Disease," *J Bone Miner Res*, 1995, 10(3):458-65.

12. Urena P and De Vernejoul MC, "Circulating Biochemical Markers of Bone Remodeling in Uremic Patients," *Kidney Int*, 1999, 55(6):2141-56.

13. Engler H, Oettli RE, and Riesen WF, "Biochemical Markers of Bone Turnover in Patients With Thyroid Dysfunctions and in Euthyroid Controls: A Cross-Sectional Study," *Clin Chim Acta*, 1999, 289(1-2):159-72.

14. Walls J, Assiri A, Howell A, et al, "Measurement of Urinary Collagen Cross-Links Indicate Response to Therapy in Patients With Breast Cancer and Bone Metastases," *Br J Cancer*, 1999, 80(8):1265-70.

15. Langdahl BL, Loft AG, Eriksen EF, et al, "Bone Mass, Bone Turnover and Body Composition in Former Hypothyroid Patients Receiving Replacement Therapy," *Eur J Endocrinol*, 1996, 134(6):702-9.

16. Nakamura H, Mori T, Genma R, et al, "Urinary Excretion of Pyridinoline and Deoxypyridinoline Measured by Immunoassay in Hypothyroidism," *Clin Endocrinol (Oxf)*, 1996, 44(4):447-51.

17. Garnero P, Gineyts E, Arbault P, et al, "Different Effects of Bisphosphonate and Estrogen Therapy on Free and Peptide-Bound Bone Cross-Links Excretion," *J Bone Miner Res*, 1995, 10(4):641-9.

18. Blumsohn A, Naylor KE, Assiri AM, et al, "Different Responses of Biochemical Markers of Bone Resorption to Bisphosphonate Therapy in Paget Disease," *Clin Chem*, 1995, 41(11):1592-8.

References

Body JJ, Dumon JC, Gineyts E, et al, "Comparative Evaluation of Markers of Bone Resorption in Patients With Breast Cancer-Induced Osteolysis Before and After Bisphosphonate Therapy," *J Bone J Cancer*, 1997, 75(3):408-12.

Endres DB and Rude RK, "Mineral and Bone Metabolism," *Tietz Textbook of Clinical Chemistry*, 3rd ed, Burtis CA and Ashwood ER, eds, 1999, Philadelphia, PA: WB Saunders Co, 1395-1457.

Garnero P and Delmas PD, "Biochemical Markers of Bone Turnover: Applications for Osteoporosis," *Endocrinol Metab Clin North Am*, 1998, 27(2):303-23.

Robins SP, Duncan A, Wilson N, et al, "Standardization of Pyridinium Crosslinks, Pyridinoline and Deoxypyridinoline, for Use as Biochemical Markers of Collagen Degradation," *Clin Chem*, 1996, 42(10):1621-6.

Stewart A, Black A, Robins SP, et al, "Bone Density and Bone Turnover in Patients With Osteoarthritis and Osteoporosis," *J Rheumatol*, 1999, 26(3):622-6.

Wolinsky-Friedland M, "Drug-Induced Metabolic Bone Disease," *Endocrinol Metab Clin North Am*, 1995, 24(2):395-420.

♦ **Pyridoxal-5-Phosphate** *see* Vitamin B₆, Plasma or Serum *on page 299*

♦ **Pyridoxine** *see* Vitamin B₆, Plasma or Serum *on page 299*

♦ **Pyruvoyl Tetrahydropterin Synthase Deficiency** *see* Newborn Screen for Phenylketonuria *on page 229*

♦ **Pyruvoyl Tetrahydropterin Synthase Deficiency** *see* Phenylalanine, Blood *on page 248*

♦ **Quantitative Fecal Fat, 72-Hour Collection** *see* Fecal Fat, Quantitative, 72-Hour Collection *on page 172*

♦ **Rapid (or Short) ACTH Test** *see* Corticotropin Stimulation Test (Rapid) *on page 153*

♦ **RBC Galactokinase** *see* Galactokinase, Blood *on page 178*

♦ **RBC Protoporphyrin** *see* Protoporphyrin, Free Erythrocyte *on page 269*

♦ **[¹⁴C] d-Xylose Breath Test** *see* d-Xylose Absorption Test, Serum, Urine *on page 167*

♦ **Regan Isoenzyme** *see* Alkaline Phosphatase, Heat Stable, Serum *on page 91*

♦ **Regan Isoenzyme** *see* Alkaline Phosphatase Isoenzymes, Serum *on page 92*

♦ **Renin** *see* Aldosterone, Serum or Plasma *on page 90*

♦ **Renin** *see* Aldosterone, Urine *on page 91*

Renin Activity, Plasma

Related Information
Adrenal Cortex: Laboratory Assessments Overview *on page 84*
Aldosterone, Serum or Plasma *on page 90*
Aldosterone, Urine *on page 91*
Electrolyte Panel, Serum *on page 168*
Potassium, Serum or Plasma *on page 258*
Potassium, Urine *on page 259*
Sodium, Serum or Plasma *on page 275*

Applies to Angiotensin; Captopril Test

Test Includes Fasting supine or upright specimens, catheterization studies

Abstract Renin, secreted by the juxtaglomerular cells adjacent to renal afferent arterioles, converts angiotensinogen to angiotensin I. The latter is, in turn, converted to angiotensin II, a biologically active peptide, which both 1) stimulates adrenocortical secretion of aldosterone, and 2) has direct vasopressor activity. Clinical interest in measuring plasma renin (PR) centers on patients who have aldosterone excess. There are two types of aldosterone excess: 1) **primary hyperaldosteronism** (Conn syndrome) in which the aldosterone excess is autonomously produced by an adrenal adenoma or hyperplasia, and 2) **secondary hyperaldosteronism** in which the increased aldosterone is a physiological response to a disease process such as cardiac failure, cirrhosis, renovascular hypertension, a renin-secreting tumor (Bartter syndrome), diuretic medication, or protracted vomiting. In primary hyperaldosteronism PR is characteristically low, while in secondary hyperaldosteronism PR is characteristically high. Interpretation of a PR result is difficult because 1) some assays are indirect and therefore nonspecific, 2) many preanalytic variables affect renin production (sodium balance, posture, medications), and 3) the circadian variation in renin production (maximum in early morning, minimum in late afternoon). Renin secretion is stimulated by upright posture, low sodium intake, and diuretic medication. (See also Aldosterone, Serum or Plasma *on page 90*.) Renin and aldosterone concentrations with other studies, including especially serum/plasma potassium, are needed to evaluate the renin-angiotensin-aldosterone system; *vide infra*.

Patient Preparation Preanalytic variables which must be controlled are sodium balance, posture, blood pressure medications, and time of day. Specific protocols are available.[1] Samples for PR are commonly drawn at the end of a 24-hour collection of urine for sodium and creatinine and after several days of stable sodium intake controlled by the physician. Check with the laboratory for particular patient preparation instructions.

Specimen Plasma, peripheral venous blood, bilateral renal vein samples

Container Lavender top (EDTA) tube

Sampling Time Timing of sampling (morning) and the posture of the patient before sampling (upright) require standardization.[2] Maximum activity is found early in the morning, during sleep. Minimum renin activity occurs in the late afternoon.[3]

Collection Draw specimen into a prechilled syringe. Place in chilled lavender top tubes (with the rubber stopper off). Recap, mix, and immediately place on ice and deliver to the laboratory. **Posture of the patient must be recorded.**

Storage Instructions Place in an ice-water bath. After the specimen is well cooled, centrifuge at 4°C. Separate plasma immediately and freeze in a plastic container. Avoid freeze-thaw cycles.

Causes for Rejection Clotted sample, patient preparation incorrect for the analysis needed; hemolysis

Reference Interval Method dependent, with large interlaboratory variation.

Indirect assay of angiotensin I:[4]
Sodium replete:
- 18-39 years: <0.6-4.3 ng/mL/hour
- >40 years: <0.6-3.0 ng/mL/hour
Sodium depleted:
- 18-39 years: 2.9-24.0 ng/mL/hour
- >40 years: 2.9-10.8 ng/mL/hour

Direct immunoassay of active renin: see table on following page.

Critical Values Ratio of plasma aldosterone to renin >30-50. A ratio >30 deserves further evaluation.[2]

Use

Primary hyperaldosteronism: Basal PR is low and does not increase in response to normal physiologic stimuli (ie, volume depletion, hyponatremia, and upright posture). This can be tested for by:
1. Placing the patient on a low sodium diet for 5-7 days and measuring basal (8 AM) PR 2 hours after the patient has been upright and walking.
2. Same as above plus a diuretic (such as furosemide). This constitutes a maximum stimulation. Some patients with Conn syndrome may show a misleading increase in PR.[1]
3. Failure of an elevated aldosterone value to be suppressed by a saline infusion.[1]

When primary hyperaldosteronism is suspected, PR **must** be interpreted with concurrent serum aldosterone values and information relevant to sodium balance, medications, and posture. Serum/plasma electrolytes, including potassium, are needed. Inappropriate kaliuresis (urine potassium >30 mmol) in the presence of hypokalemia (potassium <3.0 mmol/l) is found in primary hyperaldosteronism.

Secondary hyperaldosteronism: Basal PR is high, reflecting a normal physiologic response to volume depletion or decreased effective renal blood flow. Concentrations of plasma renin and aldosterone are high in patients with congestive heart failure.[5]

Other hypertensive patients: Although it was once popular to classify all hypertensive patients into high-renin, normal-renin, or low-renin categories, this is rarely done today **except** when there is clinical suspicion of primary hyperaldosteronism as the cause.

Limitations Nonspecificity is a problem since many reference laboratories use an indirect assay, measuring the generation of angiotensin I, rather than renin itself. Since preanalytic variables are difficult to control, reference intervals are wide.
(Continued)

Renin Activity, Plasma *(Continued)*

Renin: Direct Immunoassay

Reference Values for Healthy Adults

Range of Active Renin (ng/L)	Upright			Supine		
	Number of Persons	Frequency	Cumulative Frequency	Number of Persons	Frequency	Cumulative Frequency
<10	20	0.20	0.20	48	0.48	0.48
10-14	22	0.42	0.42	30	0.30	0.78
15-19	16	0.58	0.58	14	0.14	0.92
20-24	14	0.72	0.72	8	0.08	1.00
25-29	16	0.88	0.88			
30-34	4	0.92	0.92			
35-39	4	0.96	0.96			
>40	4	1.00	1.00			

Adapted from Simon D, Hartman DJ, Badouaille G, et al, "Two-site Direct Immunoassay Specific for Active Renin," *Clin Chem*, 1992, 38:1959-62.

Methodology Immunoassay (various labels); an immunoradiometric assay specific for active renin utilizes two monoclonal antibodies.[1]

Additional Information The captopril protocol for aldosteronism has fallen short of expectations.[2]

In patients with renal artery stenosis, bilateral renal vein sampling can provide PR ratio (affected/nonaffected side) to predict blood pressure response to revascularization,[6] but newer imaging studies may render this obsolete. Correlation with urine sodium excretion is relevant to evaluation for renal arterial stenosis.[1]

Footnotes

1. Demers LM and Whitley RJ, "Function of the Adrenal Cortex," *Tietz Textbook of Clinical Chemistry*, 3rd ed, Burtis CA and Ashwood ER, eds, Philadelphia, PA: WB Saunders, 1999, 1530-69.
2. Ganguly A, "Primary Aldosteronism," *N Engl J Med*, 1998, 339(25):1828-34.
3. Young DS and Bermes EW, "Specimen Collection and Processing: Sources of Biological Variation," *Tietz Textbook of Clinical Chemistry*, 3rd ed, Chapter 2, Burtis CA and Ashwood ER, eds, Philadelphia, PA: WB Saunders Co, 1999, 42-72.
4. Mayo Medical Laboratories, *2000 Test Catalogue*, Rochester, MN, 436.
5. Schrier RW and Abraham WT, "Hormones and Hemodynamics in Heart Failure," *N Engl J Med*, 1999, 341(8):577-84.
6. Canzanello VJ and Textor SC, "Noninvasive Diagnosis of Renovascular Disease," *Mayo Clin Proc*, 1994, 69(12):1172-81.

References

Simon D, Hartmann DJ, Badouaille G, et al, "Two-Site Direct Immunoassay Specific for Active Renin," *Clin Chem*, 1992, 38:1959-62.

♦ **Resin Triiodothyronine Uptake** *see* T₃ Uptake, Serum or Plasma *on page 279*

♦ **Resin Uptake Ratio** *see* T₃ Uptake, Serum or Plasma *on page 279*

♦ **Respiratory Acidosis** *see* pCO₂, Blood *on page 246*

♦ **Respiratory Alkalosis** *see* pCO₂, Blood *on page 246*

♦ **Retinoids** *see* Vitamin A, Serum or Plasma *on page 298*

♦ **Retinol, Serum** *see* Vitamin A, Serum or Plasma *on page 298*

Reverse T₃, Serum

Related Information

Free Thyroxine Index *on page 177*
Thyroid Stimulating Hormone, Serum *on page 282*
Thyroxine, Free, Serum *on page 285*
Thyroxine, Serum *on page 286*

Synonyms rT₃; Triiodothyronine Reverse

Applies to Euthyroid Sick Syndrome; Nonthyroidal Illness

Abstract Reverse T₃ (rT₃), which differs from T₃ by the site of iodination of an aromatic ring, is biologically inactive and may be a waste product. Small amounts are secreted by the thyroid gland.

Patient Preparation Avoid radioisotope administration prior to collection of specimen if testing is by RIA.

Specimen Serum

Container Red top tube

Storage Instructions Separate serum and store at 4°C if the test is done within 24 hours. Freeze for longer periods of storage. Frozen samples are stable for at least 1 month.

Reference Interval Values are higher in cord blood and newborns. Ranges are as follows:[1]
- cord blood: 130-300 ng/dL (SI: 2.00-4.62 nmol/L)
- 1 day: 83-194 ng/dL (SI: 1.28-2.99 nmol/L)
- 2 days: 107-209 ng/dL (SI: 1.65-3.22 nmol/L)
- 3 days: 102-166 ng/dL (SI: 1.57-2.56 nmol/L)
- 1 month to 20 years: 10-35 ng/dL (SI: 0.15-0.54 nmol/L)
- adults: 10-28 ng/dL (SI: 0.17-0.51 nmol/L)

Use Evaluation of euthyroid sick patients with low T₃ levels

Limitations The rT₃ test is generally not necessary. It is not to be confused with T₃.

Methodology Radioimmunoassay (RIA)

Additional Information In peripheral tissues of healthy individuals, approximately 40% of T₄ is converted to T₃ (3,5,3'-L-triiodothyronine), and about 45% of T₄ is converted to reverse T₃ (rT₃, 3,3',5'-L-triiodothyronine).[1,2] rT₃ is biologically inactive. In normal individuals levels of T₄ and rT₃ tend to change in the same direction. T₄ and rT₃ are low in hypothyroidism and high in hyperthyroidism. However, in patients with metabolic abnormalities involving energy (eg, starvation, anorexia nervosa, severe trauma, hemorrhagic shock, hepatic dysfunction, postoperative state, severe infection, and burns), conversion of T₄ to T₃ is decreased and to rT₃ is increased. Such patients, with nonthyroidal illness, are generally euthyroid, and measurement of rT₃ in this so-called "sick euthyroid" syndrome may be useful.[3,4]

In neonates with low T₄ and normal T₃ uptake and TSH, reverse T₃ has been used to distinguish euthyroid sick syndrome from central hypothyroidism. Low reverse T₃ levels can help to distinguish infants with central hypothyroidism from sick and well infants who tend to have relatively elevated reverse T₃ levels.[5]

Footnotes

1. Whitley RJ, "Thyroid Function," *Tietz Textbook of Clinical Chemistry*, 3rd ed, Burtis CA and Ashwood ER, eds, Philadelphia, PA: WB Saunders Co, 1999, 1496-529.
2. Visser TJ, "Pathways of Thyroid Hormone Metabolism," *Acta Med Austriaca*, 1996, 23(1-2):10-6.
3. McIver B and Gorman CA, "Euthyroid Sick Syndrome: An Overview," *Thyroid*, 1997, 7(1):125-32.
4. Stockigt JR, "Guidelines for Diagnosis and Monitoring of Thyroid Disease: Nonthyroidal Illness," *Clin Chem*, 1996, 42(1):188-92.
5. Faase EM, Meacham LR, Novack CM, et al, "Decreased Reverse T₃ Levels in Neonates With Central Hypothyroidism," *J Perinatol*, 1997, 17(1):15-7.

References

Camacho PM and Dwarkanathan AA, "Sick Euthyroid Syndrome. What to Do When Thyroid Function Tests Are Abnormal in Critically Ill Patients," *Postgrad Med*, 1999, 105(4):215-9.

Chopra IJ, "Clinical Review 86: Euthyroid Sick Syndrome: Is It a Misnomer?" *J Clin Endocrinol Metab*, 1997, 82(2):329-34.

Kaplan MM, "Clinical Perspectives in the Diagnosis of Thyroid Disease," *Clin Chem*, 1999, 45(8 Pt 2):1377-83.

Klee GG and Hay ID, "Biochemical Testing of Thyroid Function," *Endocrinol Metab Clin North Am*, 1997, 26(4):763-75.

Lamb EJ and Martin J, "Thyroid Function Tests: Often Justified in the Acutely Ill," *Ann Clin Biochem*, 2000, 37(Pt 2):158-64.

♦ **Rheumatoid Effusion** *see* Body Fluid pH *on page 125*

♦ **Rheumatoid Factor, Body Fluid** *see* Body Fluid Chemical Analysis *on page 123*

♦ **5'-Ribonucleotide Phosphohydrolase: NTP** *see* 5' Nucleotidase, Serum *on page 234*

♦ **rT₃** *see* Reverse T₃, Serum *on page 274*

♦ **S-100, Serum** *see* Neuron-Specific Enolase, Serum *on page 229*

♦ **SaO₂** *see* Oxygen Saturation, Blood *on page 240*

♦ **Sarin Exposure** *see* Acetylcholinesterase, Red Cell *on page 81*

♦ **Secretin Test** *see* Gastrin, Serum *on page 181*

Serotonin, Blood, Cerebrospinal Fluid

Related Information

5-Hydroxyindoleacetic Acid, Quantitative, Urine *on page 197*

Synonyms 5-HT; 5-Hydroxytryptamine, Blood

Applies to Serotonin, Cerebrospinal Fluid

Abstract Serotonin (5-hydroxytryptamine [5-HT]) is synthesized from tryptophan in the intestinal chromaffin cells or in central and peripheral neurons. The major metabolite of serotonin, 5-HIAA, is measured more commonly than 5-HT (parent compound). The latter test is rarely utilized.

Patient Preparation Monoamine oxidase inhibitor drugs should be discontinued for at least 1 week prior to sampling, since they tend to increase the level of serotonin. Avoid application of radioisotopes (eg, scans) before collection of specimen if RIA is used for assay. Some methods require a low indole diet for several days. Avoid eggplant, avocado, bananas, tomatoes, pineapple, walnuts, and red plums.

Specimen Whole blood, cerebrospinal fluid

Container Tube with EDTA, sometimes with ascorbic acid. Check with laboratory if the assay is available at all.

Collection Draw in chilled tubes. Keep on ice.

Storage Instructions Place whole blood in plastic bottle containing 10 mg EDTA and 75 mg ascorbic acid. Freeze within 4 hours of collection. Stable 7 days at -20°C.

Reference Interval 10-30 µg/dL (SI: 570-1700 nmol/L). Values vary among laboratories and are method dependent. In serum, serotonin (5-hydroxytryptamine) levels in females are about 1.3-fold that of males. By RIA, a study provided ranges: male: 7-12 µg/dL (SI: 380-680 nmol/L), female: 9-16 µg/dL (SI: 520-900 nmol/L).[1]

Use This assay is used in the diagnosis of carcinoid syndrome only in unusual circumstances. The classical syndrome includes flushing and vasomotor instability, diarrhea, hepatomegaly, and endocardial lesions. Ectopic production may occur from oat cell carcinomas of lung, islet cell tumors of pancreas, and medullary carcinoma of thyroid. Carcinoid tumors occur in multiple endocrine neoplasia, types I or II. Clinically, serotonin plays a role in depression.

Limitations Serotonin assays are not widely available and only rarely used. It may be useful to measure serotonin when normal or borderline increases of 5-HIAA are seen in a patient with clinical evidence of carcinoid syndrome. **Urinary 5-HIAA is more sensitive and specific for diagnosis of carcinoid tumors.** Engbaek and Voldby indicate that 5-methoxytryptamine and tryptamine cross react with their RIA method.[1]

Methodology Spectrophotometry, fluorometry, radioimmunoassay (RIA), gas chromatography (GC), high performance liquid chromatography (HPLC) with electrochemical detection, radioenzymatic assay. For sensitive and specific determination, HPLC is preferred.

Additional Information Serotonin is produced by cells of the APUD system, including the enterochromaffin (Kulchitsky) cells distributed through the mucosa of the gastrointestinal tract. Most serotonin in blood is usually concentrated in platelets, which release it during platelet aggregation. Serotonin may be measured to confirm the diagnosis of carcinoid syndrome if a problem emerges with conventional investigation. The carcinoid syndrome usually originates with primary carcinoids of the ileum, occasionally with primary carcinoids of the stomach. Other organs give rise to carcinoids, including pancreas, duodenum, bronchus, thymus, thyroid, testis, and ovary. Hepatic metastases are most common from small bowel primaries. The common carcinoids of appendix rarely metastasize, and those from the large intestine almost never cause endocrine effects. A role of serotonin in psychiatric disorders has been suggested.[2] A urinary serotonin assay is described but also is not widely available.[3]

In humans, serotonin has been implicated in a variety of behavioral patterns including sleep, perception of pain, social behavior, schizophrenia, and mental depression. In depressed-serotonin-deficient patients, treatment with antidepressant drugs, which inhibit serotonin uptake by presynaptic neurons, gives favorable clinical response.[4,5]

Footnotes

1. Engbaek F and Voldby B, "Radioimmunoassay of Serotonin (5-Hydroxytryptamine) in Cerebrospinal Fluid, Plasma, and Serum," *Clin Chem*, 1982, 28(4 Pt 1):624-8.
2. Meltzer HY, "The Role of Serotonin in Schizophrenia and the Place of Serotonin-Dopamine Antagonist Antipsychotics," *J Clin Psychopharmacol*, 1995, 15(1 Suppl 1):2S-3S.
3. Feldman JM, "Urinary Serotonin in the Diagnosis of Carcinoid Tumors," *Clin Chem*, 1986, 32(5):840-4.
4. Abi-Dargham A, Laruelle M, Aghajanian GK, et al, "The Role of Serotonin in the Pathophysiology and Treatment of Schizophrenia," *J Neuropsychiatry Clin Neurosci*, 1997, 9(1):1-17.
5. Kent JM, "SNaRIs, NaSSAs, and NaRIs: New Agents for the Treatment of Depression," *Lancet*, 2000, 355(9207):911-8.

References

Rosano TG and Whitley RJ, "Catecholamines and Serotonin," *Tietz Textbook of Clinical Chemistry*, 3rd ed, Burtis CA and Ashwood ER, eds, Philadelphia, PA: WB Saunders Co, 1999, 1570-600.
Williams JW Jr, Mulrow CD, Chiquette E, et al, "A Systematic Review of Newer Pharmacotherapies for Depression in Adults: Evidence Report Summary," *Ann Intern Med*, 2000, 132(9):743-56.

Sodium, Serum or Plasma

Related Information

Synonyms Na+

Applies to Hypertonicity; Osmolal Gap; Sodium, Arterial Blood; Sodium, Corrected

Abstract Sodium with its accompanying anions is the most important extracellular osmotically active solute.[1] The major cation of extracellular fluid, Na+ is extremely important in maintenance of water and osmotic pressure equilibrium in the extracellular compartment.

Specimen Serum or plasma

Container Red top tube or green top (lithium heparin, not sodium heparin) tube

Collection Pediatrics: Blood drawn from heelstick for capillary sample. Na+, with K+ and Cl-, can be reported from arterial or venous blood. If an arterial puncture is done for pO$_2$, lithium heparin anticoagulant must be used.

Reference Interval

Infants:[2]
- 0-7 days: 133-146 mmol/L
- 7-31 days: 134-144 mmol/L
- 1-6 months: 134-142 mmol/L
- 6 months to 1 year: 133-142 mmol/L
- older than 1 year: 134-143 mmol/L

Adults: 136-145 mmol/L

Possible Panic Range <125 mmol/L, >150 mmol/L

Use Evaluation of electrolytes, acid-base balance, water balance, water intoxication, dehydration

Hypernatremia occurs from loss of water or from Na+ retention.[1] It is found in dehydration and with diuretic use. Increased insensible water loss with fever, burns, hyperpnea, sweating, and ambient temperature causes hypernatremia (see Figure 1). Nasogastric protein feeding with insufficient fluids may cause hypernatremia, as can vomiting and diarrhea. Hypernatremia without obvious cause may relate to Cushing syndrome, central or nephrogenic diabetes insipidus with insufficient fluids, adipsia, primary aldosteronism, and other diseases. Often, patients who have primary aldosteronism have mild hypernatremia.[1] Severe hypernatremia may be associated with volume contraction, lactic acidosis, and azotemia. Increased hematocrit may provide evidence of dehydration. The corrected serum Na+ is often high in nonketotic hyperosmolar coma. (A corrected Na+ is calculated by increasing Na+ by 1.3-1.6 mmol/L for each 100 mg/dL increment in serum or plasma glucose). The corrected serum Na+ level should be calculated in nonketotic hyperosmolar coma. **Apparent mild hyponatremia with very high glucose may actually mean hypernatremia.**[3] Infusion of hypertonic saline or sodium bicarbonate or ingestion of Na+ may cause sodium retention. The pathophysiology of hypernatremia is (Continued) reviewed by Adrogué et al; its differential diagnosis is presented in Table 1 from that source.[4] Hypernatremia denotes hypertonicity.

Hyponatremia (serum Na$^+$ <136 mmol/L) can be found with low, normal, or high tonicity. The most common type is dilutional, from retention of water. Hyponatremia occurs with nephrotic syndrome, cachexia, hypoproteinemia, intravenous glucose (salt-free) infusion, congestive heart failure, mineralocorticoid deficiency, and cystic fibrosis. Mineralocorticoid deficiency leads to hyponatremia, hypovolemia, and hyperkalemia through inadequate Na$^+$ and water resorption and diminished potassium excretion.[5] Serum sodium is a factor predictive of cardiovascular mortality in patients with severe congestive heart failure.[3] Hyponatremia without congestive heart failure or dehydration may occur with hypothyroidism, the syndrome of inappropriate secretion of antidiuretic hormone (SIADH), renal failure, or renal sodium loss. See Table 2.[6]

The evaluation of hyponatremia includes Addison disease, hypopituitarism, liver disease including cirrhosis, hypertriglyceridemia, and psychogenic polydipsia. Diuretics and other drugs may cause hyponatremia. Sodium decreasing to levels <120 mmol/L can lead to significant neurological dysfunction with cerebral edema, increased intracranial pressure and uncal herniation, a life-threatening complication.[7] See Osmolality, Calculated, Serum or Plasma *on page 234.*

The differential diagnosis of hyponatremia includes determination of urine sodium and osmolality and serum urea nitrogen (BUN). BUN is often normal or decreased in SIADH, but is increased in states in which hyponatremia is related to volume depletion. (Extracellular volume is normal or increased in SIADH.) Hyperlipidemia, hyperproteinemia, and hyperglycemia must be considered; *vide infra.*

Table 1. Causes of Hypernatremia

Net Water Loss

Pure water

  Unreplaced insensible losses (dermal and respiratory)

  Hypodipsia

  Neurogenic diabetes insipidus

    Post-traumatic

    Tumors, cysts, histiocytosis, tuberculosis, sarcoidosis

    Idiopathic

    Aneurysms, meningitis, encephalitis, Guillain-Barré syndrome

    Ethanol ingestion (transient)

  Congenital nephrogenic diabetes insipidus

  Acquired nephrogenic diabetes insipidus

    Renal disease (eg, medullary cystic disease)

    Hypercalcemia or hypokalemia

    Drugs (lithium, demeclocycline, foscarnet, methoxyflurane, amphotericin B, vasopressin V$_2$-receptor antagonists)

Hypotonic fluid

  Renal

    Loop diuretics

    Osmotic diuresis (glucose, urea, mannitol)

    Postobstructive diuresis

    Polyuric phase of acute tubular necrosis

    Intrinsic renal disease

  Gastrointestinal

    Vomiting

    Nasogastric drainage

    Enterocutaneous fistula

    Diarrhea (most common cause in infancy)

    Use of osmotic cathartic agents (eg, lactulose)

  Cutaneous

    Burns

    Excessive sweating

Hypertonic Sodium Gain

Hypertonic sodium bicarbonate infusion (eg, resuscitation)

Hypertonic feeding preparation

Ingestion of sodium chloride

Ingestion of sea water

Sodium chloride-rich emetics

Hypertonic saline enemas

Intrauterine injection of hypertonic saline

Hypertonic sodium chloride infusion

Hypertonic dialysis

Primary hyperaldosteronism

Cushing syndrome

Adapted from Adrogué HJ and Madias NE, "Hypernatremia," *N Engl J Med*, 2000, 342(20):1493-9.

Table 2. Causes of Hypotonic Hyponatremia

Impaired Capacity of Renal Water Excretion
Decreased Volume of Extracellular Fluid

Renal sodium loss

  Diuretic agents

  Osmotic diuresis (glucose, urea, mannitol)

  Adrenocortical insufficiency

  Salt-wasting nephropathy

  Bicarbonaturia (renal tubular acidosis, disequilibrium stage of vomiting)

  Ketonuria

Extrarenal sodium loss

  Diarrhea

  Vomiting

  Blood loss

  Excessive sweating (eg, in marathon runners)

  Fluid sequestration in "third space"

    Bowel obstruction

    Peritonitis

    Pancreatitis

    Muscle trauma

    Burns

Increased volume of extracellular fluid

Congestive heart failure

Cirrhosis

Nephrotic syndrome

Renal failure (acute or chronic)

Pregnancy

Essentially normal volume of extracellular fluid

Thiazide diuretics*

Hypothyroidism

Adrenocortical insufficiency

Syndrome of inappropriate secretion of antidiuretic hormone

  Cancer

    Pulmonary neoplasms

    Mediastinal neoplasms

    Extrathoracic neoplasms

  Central nervous system disorders

    Acute psychosis

    Mass lesions

    Inflammatory and demyelinating diseases

    Stroke

    Hemorrhage

    Trauma

  Drugs

    Desmopressin

    Oxytocin

    Prostaglandin-synthesis inhibitors

    Nicotine

    Phenothiazines

    Tricyclics

    Serotonin-reuptake inhibitors

    Opiate derivatives

    Chlorpropamide

    Clofibrate

    Carbamazepine

    Cyclophosphamide

    Vincristine

  Pulmonary conditions

    Infections

    Acute respiratory failure

    Positive-pressure ventilation

  Miscellaneous

    Postoperative state

    Pain

    Severe nausea

    Infection with the human immunodeficiency virus

Decreased intake of solutes

  Beer potomania

  Tea-and-toast diet

Excessive Water Intake

Primary polydipsia†

Dilute infant formula

Sodium-free irrigant solutions (used in hysteroscopy, laparoscopy, or transurethral resection of the prostate)‡

Accidental intake of large amounts of water (eg, during swimming lessons)

Multiple tap-water enemas

*Sodium depletion, potassium depletion, stimulation of thirst, and impaired urinary dilution are implicated

†Often a mild reduction in the capacity for water excretion is also present.

‡Hyponatremia is not always present.

Adapted from Androgueé HJ and Madias NE, "Hyponatremia," *N Engl J Med*, 2000, 342(21):1581-9.

Figure 1.
Extracellular-Fluid and Intracellular-Fluid Compartments Under Normal Conditions and During States of Hypernatremia

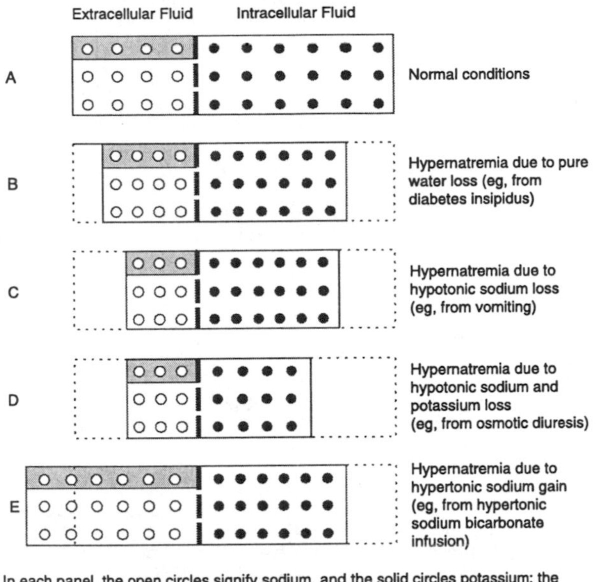

In each panel, the open circles signify sodium, and the solid circles potassium; the broken line between the two compartments represents the cell membrane, and the shading indicates the intravascular volume.

The extracellular-fluid and intracellular-fluid compartments normally account for 40% and 60% of total body water, respectively (Panel A). Pure water loss reduces the size of each compartment proportionally (Panel B). The volume of extracellular fluid in this setting is reduced, not normal, although the reduction is often not clinically evident. The sodium content of extracellular fluid remains unaltered, yet 1 of each 2.5 liters of water that is lost is from the extracellular-fluid compartment. Hypotonic sodium loss causes a relatively larger loss of volume in the extracellular-fluid compartment than in the intracellular-fluid compartment (Panel C). Potassium loss in addition to hypotonic sodium loss further reduces the intracellular-fluid compartment (Panel D). Hypertonic sodium gain results in an increase in extracellular fluid but a decrease in intracellular fluid (Panel E).

Adapted from Adrogué HJ and Madias NE, "Hypernatremia," *N Engl J Med*, 2000, 342(20):1493-9.

Figure 2.
Extracellular-Fluid and Intracellular-Fluid Compartments Under Normal Conditions and During States of Hyponatremia

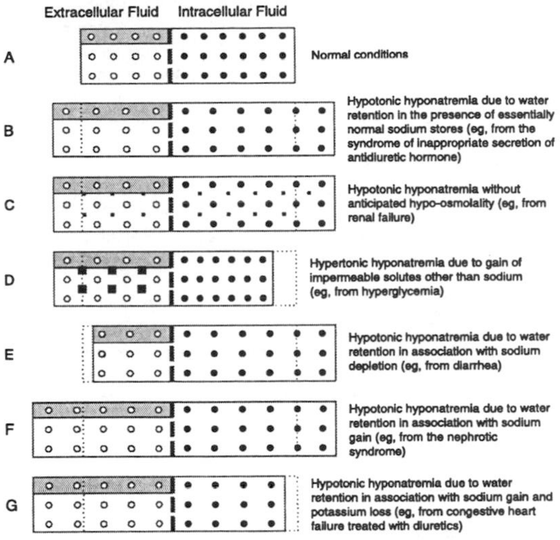

In each panel, open circles signify sodium, solid circles potassium, large squares impermeable solutes other than sodium, and small squares permeable solutes; the broken line between the two compartments represents the cell membrane, and the shading indicates the intravascular volume.

The extracellular-fluid and intracellular-fluid compartments normally make up 40% and 60% of total body water, respectively (Panel A). With the syndrome of inappropriate secretion of antidiuretic hormone, the volumes of extracellular fluid and intracellular fluid expand (although a small element of sodium and potassium loss, not shown, occurs during inception of the syndrome) (Panel B). Water retention can lead to hypotonic hyponatremia without the anticipated hypo-osmolality in patients who have accumulated ineffective osmoles, such as urea (Panel C). A shift of water from the intracellular-fluid compartment to the extracellular-fluid compartment, driven by solutes confined in the extracellular fluid, results in hypertonic (translocational) hyponatremia (Panel D). Sodium depletion (and secondary water retention) usually contracts the volume of extracellular fluid but expands the intracellular-fluid compartment. At times, water retention can be sufficient to restore the volume of extracellular fluid to normal or even above-normal levels (Panel E). Hypotonic hyponatremia in sodium-retentive states involves expansion of both compartments, but predominantly the extracellular-fluid compartment (Panel F). Gain of sodium and loss of potassium in association with a defect of water excretion, as they occur in congestive heart failure treated with diuretics, lead to expansion of the extracellular-fluid compartment but contraction of the intracellular-fluid compartment (Panel G).

Adapted from Adrogué HJ and Madias NE, "Hyponatremia," *N Engl J Med*, 2000, 342(21):1581-9.

Limitations Care should be taken that one is not dealing with "pseudohyponatremia;" *vide infra*.

Blood collection in inappropriate tubes can lead to a preanalytic error, (eg, sodium fluoride - gray, sodium citrate - light blue or black, EDTA - lavender, sodium heparin - green).

Sodium contamination of specimens in the laboratory or office can derive from bleach (sodium hypochlorite), baking soda cleanser (sodium bicarbonate), and liquid soap.[8]

Methodology Ion-selective electrode (ISE), flame emission photometry

Additional Information The ratio of serum sodium to osmolality is normally 0.43-0.50; a decreased ratio is found in uremia and other states in which there are increased substances with osmotic activity (see Osmolality, Calculated, Serum or Plasma *on page 234* and Osmolality, Serum *on page 236*).

See Urea Nitrogen, Serum or Plasma *on page 293* regarding hyponatremia with sodium <128 mmol/L, hypo-osmolality, low BUN, and the syndrome of inappropriate secretion of antidiuretic hormone.

A number of situations result in "pseudohyponatremia." In these circumstances, treatment may be undesirable. With pseudohyponatremia serum sodium is decreased but the serum is not hypotonic (serum osmolality is normal or even increased). This may occur as the result of other molecules replacing water in relation to sodium. The water content is effectively lowered - sodium is "diluted." In severe hypertriglyceridemia or paraprotein-related marked increase in protein, the concentration of sodium in relation to water is normal but the analytic result is determined as mmol/L of serum. Osmolality in this situation is determined as the amount of particles per kg of water and will be normal. Analysis by ion-selective electrode of the direct potentiometric type (requires no dilution) is not artifactually low in patients with hyperlipidemia.[9] If large amounts of solute, such as glucose or mannitol, are present, movement of intracellular water into the extracellular space may produce dilutional hyponatremia. In this case, sodium concentration in relation to water is actually low. "Osmolal gap" however exists between measured and calculated serum osmolality. Other substances capable of increasing serum osmolality (eg, ethanol) may also cause increase in the osmolal gap.

Another cause of pseudohyponatremia is increased serum viscosity due to increased globulin proteins, occurring particularly in Waldenström's macroglobulinemia. Analyzers may aspirate too little sample when viscosity is so high, leading to a factitious low sodium concentration.

Studying a geriatric group, hyponatremia on admission to hospital bears association with poor prognosis.[10]

Drug effects are summarized.[11]

Footnotes

1. Gregoire JR, "Adjustment of the Osmostat in Primary Aldosteronism," *Mayo Clin Proc*, 1994, 69(11):1108-10.
2. Soldin SJ and Hicks JM, eds, "Pediatric Reference Ranges," Washington, DC: AACC Press, American Association of Clinical Chemistry, 1995, 122.
3. Daugirdas JT, Kronfol NO, Tzamaloukas AH, et al, "Hyperosmolar Coma: Cellular Dehydration and the Serum Sodium Concentration," *Ann Intern Med*, 1989, 110(11):855-7.
4. Adrogué HJ and Madias NE, "Hypernatremia," *N Engl J Med*, 2000, 342(20):1493-9.
5. White PC, "Disorders of Aldosterone Biosynthesis and Action," *N Engl J Med*, 1994, 331(4):250-8.
6. Adrogué HJ and Madias NE, "Hyponatremia," *N Engl J Med*, 2000, 342(21):1581-9.
7. Knochel JP, "Hypoxia Is the Cause of Brain Damage in Hyponatremia," *JAMA*, 1999, 281(24):2342-3.
8. Klosinski DD, "Troubleshooting Elevated Sodium Levels," *Lab Med*, 1997, 28(6):369.
9. Aw TC and Kiechle FL, "Pseudohyponatremia," *Am J Emerg Med*, 1985, 3(3):236-9.
10. Terzian C, Frye EB, and Piotrowski ZH, "Admission Hyponatremia in the Elderly: Factors Influencing Prognosis," *J Gen Intern Med*, 1994, 9(2):89-91.
11. Young DS, "Effects of Drugs on Clinical Laboratory Tests," 5th ed, Volume 1: Listing by Test, Washington, DC: AACC Press, American Association of Clinical Chemistry, 2000, Section 3, 714-20.

References

Ayus JC and Arieff AI, "Chronic Hyponatremic Encephalopathy in Postmenopausal Women - Association of Therapies With Morbidity and Mortality," *JAMA*, 1999, 281(24):2299-304.

Ayus JC, Varon J, and Arieff AI, "Hyponatremia, Cerebral Edema, and Norcardiogenic Pulmonary Edema in Marathon Runners," *Ann Intern Med*, 2000, 132(9):711-14.

Briggs JP, Sawaya BE, and Schnermann J, "Disorders of Salt Balance," *Fluids and Electrolytes*, 2nd ed, Kokko JP and Tannen RL, eds, Philadelphia, PA: WB Saunders Co, 1990, 70-138.

DeVita MV and Michelis MF, "Perturbations in Sodium Balance: Hyponatremia and Hypernatremia," *Clin Lab Med*, 1993, 13(1):135-48.

(Continued)

Sodium, Serum or Plasma (Continued)

Faria SH, "Assessing Laboratory Values: Serum Na⁺, K⁺, and Ca⁺," *Home Care Provid*, 1998, 3(2):73-6.

Kumar S and Berl T, "Sodium," *Lancet*, 1998, 352(9134):1146-7.

Leehey DJ, Daugirdas JT, Manahan FJ, et al, "Prolonged Hypernatremia Associated With Azotemia and Hyponatruria," *Am J Med*, 1989, 86(4):494-6.

Maffly RH, "Renal Function and Disorders of Water, Sodium, and Potassium Balance," *Scientific American Medicine*, Section 10, Chapter 1, Rubenstein E and Federman DD, eds, New York, NY: Scientific American Inc, 1990, 2-34.

Oh MS and Carroll HJ, "Disorders of Sodium Metabolism: Hypernatremia and Hyponatremia," *Crit Care Med*, 1992, 20(1):94-103.

Polderman KH, Schreuder WO, van Schijndel R, et al, "Hypernatremia in the Intensive Care Unit: An Indicator of Quality Care?" *Crit Care Med*, 1999, 27:1105-8.

Votey SR, Peters AL, and Hoffman JR, "Disorders of Water Metabolism: Hyponatremia and Hypernatremia," *Emerg Med Clin North Am*, 1989, 7(4):749-69.

♦ **Sodium, Serum:Osmolality, Serum Ratio** *see* Osmolality, Serum *on page 236*

♦ **Sodium, Sweat** *see* Chloride, Sweat *on page 144*

Sodium, Urine

Related Information

Aldosterone, Serum or Plasma *on page 90*
Anion Gap, Serum, Plasma, or Urine *on page 106*
Chloride, Urine *on page 145*
Creatinine, 12- or 24-Hour Urine *on page 159*
Electrolyte Panel, Serum *on page 168*
Kidney Stone Analysis *on page 877*
Osmolality, Calculated, Serum or Plasma *on page 234*
Osmolality, Serum *on page 236*
Osmolality, Urine *on page 236*
Potassium, Urine *on page 259*
Sodium, Serum or Plasma *on page 275*
Urine Collection, 24-Hour *on page 47*

Synonyms Na, Urine; Urine Na

Applies to FENA; Fractional Excretion of Sodium

Replaces Electrolytes, Urine

Abstract Urinary sodium excretion normally relates to intake. Body sodium stores are based upon intake and renal excretion.

Specimen Timed or random urine

Container Plain urine container

Reference Interval 24-hour urine: 27-287 mmol/day, varies markedly with dietary intake of sodium. There is diurnal variation (output is lower at night). A European study provides average sodium excretion: male: 162 mmol/day, range: 143-208 mmol/day; female: 134 mmol/day, range: 119-165 mmol/day; within person CV: male: 30%, female: 34%.[1]

Use Work up volume depletion, acute renal failure, acute oliguria, and differential diagnosis of hyponatremia.[2] See tables on following page.

Limitations It is often advantageous to request urine potassium and always necessary to obtain urine creatinine along with sodium measurement. High urine sodium does not necessarily indicate that total body sodium is increased (eg, salt-losing nephropathy). This area is complex; the reader is referred to the footnotes and references.

Methodology Ion-selective electrode (ISE), flame emission photometry.

Fractional excretion of sodium (FENa) is calculated as follows:

FENa = (urine Na⁺ / urine Cr) x (serum Cr / serum Na⁺) x 100

Additional Information In cases of hyponatremia, random urine Na⁺ <10 mmol/L or FENa <1% commonly indicates extrarenal depletion: dehydration (gastrointestinal or sweat loss), congestive heart failure, liver disease or nephrotic syndrome. With renal or adrenal diseases, urinary Na⁺ concentration is usually >20 mmol/L.

Random urine Na⁺ >10 mmol/L may indicate diuretics, emesis, intrinsic renal diseases, Addison disease, hypothyroidism, or syndrome of inappropriate antidiuretic hormone (SIADH).[3] In hypothyroidism and in SIADH, Na⁺ and Cl⁻ may be >40 mmol/L.[4] (Depending on intake, such results also can be found in normal individuals.)

In SIADH, random urinary sodium usually is >20 mmol/L. SIADH has been found in 7% of patients with small cell lung cancer.[5] Medications, CNS disease, and other pulmonary diseases are additional causes of SIADH. Such patients have hyponatremia, often severe, with hypo-osmolar serum, absence of clinical evidence of volume depletion, high urinary sodium excretion with urine osmolality greater than that of serum. Urine may not be maximally concentrated in some patients but it should not have osmolarity less than that of serum.

The classification as presented here is overly abbreviated for clinical application. Pitfalls exist (eg, increase of Na⁺ necessary to balance excretion of penicillin).[4]

Urine Na⁺ >40 mmol/L in oliguria is found in acute tubular necrosis.[4,6] However, a better indicator is the fractional excretion of Na⁺ based on simultaneously obtained random urine and blood Na⁺ and creatinine.[7] (See Methodology above.)

Low Na⁺ excretion may be found with early obstructive uropathy and with the oliguria of acute glomerulonephritis[4] and in some patients with x-ray contrast acute renal failure.

It is important to know the urinary sodium concentration in patients with unexplained hyperchloremic metabolic acidosis when the diagnosis of distal renal tubular acidosis is being considered.[8]

The urinary anion gap is discussed in the listing, Anion Gap, Serum, Plasma, or Urine *on page 106*.

An autosomal recessive disorder, pseudohypoaldosteronism type I, is characterized by renal salt wasting and high concentrations of sodium in stool, sweat, and saliva; hypokalemia; increased renin activity; and aldosterone levels.[9]

Footnotes

1. Knuiman JT, Hautvast JG, van der Heijden L, et al, "A Multicentre Study on Within-Person Variability in the Urinary Excretion of Sodium, Potassium, Calcium, Magnesium, and Creatinine in 8 European Centers," *Hum Nutr Clin Nutr*, 1986, 40(5):343-8.

2. Harrington JT and Cohen JJ, "Measurement of Urinary Electrolytes - Indications and Limitations," *N Engl J Med*, 1975, 293:1241-3.

3. DeVita MV and Michelis MF, "Perturbations in Sodium Balance: Hyponatremia and Hypernatremia," *Clin Lab Med*, 1993, 13(1):135-48.

4. Sherman RA and Eisinger RP, "The Use (and Misuse) of Urinary Sodium and Chloride Measurements," *JAMA*, 1982, 247:3121-4.

5. Hainsworth JD, Workman R, and Greco FA, "Management of the Syndrome of Inappropriate Antidiuretic Hormone Secretion in Small Cell Lung Cancer," *Cancer*, 1983, 51(1):161-5.

6. Schrier RW, "Acute Renal Failure," *JAMA*, 1982, 247:2518-22, 2524.

7. Kaloynides GJ, "Acute Renal Failure," *Therapy of Renal Diseases*, 3rd ed, Suki WN and Massri SG, eds, Boston, MA: Kluwer Academic Publishers, 1997, 359-86.

8. Battle DC, von Riotte A, and Schlueter W, "Urinary Sodium in the Evaluation of Hyperchloremic Metabolic Acidosis," *N Engl J Med*, 1987, 316(3):140-4.

9. Scheinman SJ, Guay-Woodford LM, Thakker RV, et al, "Genetic Disorders of Renal Electrolyte Transport," *N Engl J Med*, 1999, 340(15):1177-87.

References

Andreoli TE, "An Overview of Salt Absorption by the Nephron," *J Nephrol*, 1999, 12(Suppl 2):S3-15.

Ayus JC and Arieff AI, "Pathogenesis and Treatment of Hypoosmolar and Hyperosmolar States," *Therapy of Renal Diseases*, 3rd ed, Suki WN and Massri SG, eds, Boston, MA: Kluwer Academic Publishers, 1997, 1-20.

Kamel KS, Ethier JH, Richardson RM, et al, "Urine Electrolytes and Osmolality: When and How to Use Them," *Am J Nephrol*, 1990, 10(2):89-102.

Robillard JE, Smith FG, and Segai JL, et al, "Mechanisms Regulating Renal Sodium Excretion During Development," *Pediatr Nephrol*, 1992, 6(2):205-13.

♦ **Somatomedin-C** *see* Growth Hormone, Serum *on page 189*

♦ **Somatomedin-C** *see* Insulin-Like Growth Factor-1 (IGF-1), Serum or Plasma *on page 200*

♦ **Somatomedins** *see* Growth Hormone, Serum *on page 189*

♦ **Somatomedins** *see* Insulin-Like Growth Factor Binding Protein 3, Serum *on page 201*

♦ **Somatostatin** *see* Growth Hormone, Serum *on page 189*

♦ **Somatotropin** *see* Growth Hormone, Serum *on page 189*

♦ **Spinal Fluid Glucose** *see* Cerebrospinal Fluid Glucose *on page 140*

♦ **Spinal Fluid Lactic Acid** *see* Cerebrospinal Fluid Lactic Acid *on page 143*

♦ **Spinal Fluid LD** *see* Cerebrospinal Fluid Lactate Dehydrogenase *on page 142*

♦ **Standard Base Excess** *see* Base Excess, Blood *on page 114*

♦ **Stool Fat, Quantitative** *see* Fecal Fat, Quantitative, 72-Hour Collection *on page 172*

♦ **sTSH** *see* Thyroid Stimulating Hormone, Serum *on page 282*

♦ **Succinylcholine Sensitivity** *see* Acetylcholinesterase, Red Cell *on page 81*

♦ **Sugar, Fasting** *see* Glucose, Fasting, Plasma *on page 183*

♦ **Sulfatase** *see* Mucopolysaccharides, Urine *on page 226*

♦ **Sulfation Factor** *see* Insulin-Like Growth Factor-1 (IGF-1), Serum or Plasma *on page 200*

♦ **SUR 1 Mutation** *see* Insulin, Serum *on page 201*

♦ **Surfactant:Albumin Ratio** *see* Pulmonary Surfactant, Amniotic Fluid *on page 271*

♦ **Sweat, Chloride** *see* Chloride, Sweat *on page 144*

♦ **Synthetic α 1-24-ACTH Stimulation Test** *see* Corticotropin Stimulation Test (Rapid) *on page 153*

♦ **T₃ Resin Uptake** *see* T₃ Uptake, Serum or Plasma *on page 279*

♦ **T₃RU** *see* T₃ Uptake, Serum or Plasma *on page 279*

♦ **T₃, Total** *see* Triiodothyronine, Serum *on page 290*

♦ **T₃U** *see* T₃ Uptake, Serum or Plasma *on page 279*

Evaluation and Treatment of **Hyponatremic** Patient

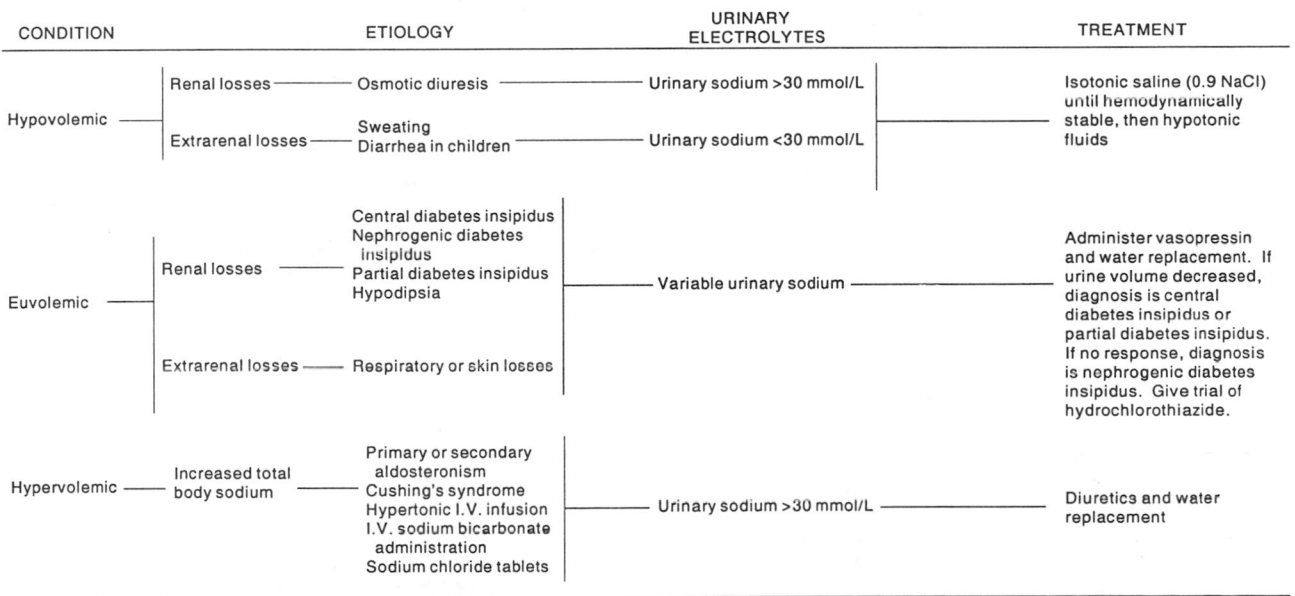

CONDITION	CLINICAL PRESENTATION	URINARY ELECTROLYTES	ETIOLOGY	TREATMENT
Hypovolemic	Orthostatic hypotension Tachycardia Azotemia	Urinary sodium >30 mmol/L	Diuretics, RTA, mineralocorticoid deficiency, salt-wasting nephritis	0.9 NaCl I.V.
		Urinary sodium <30 mmol/L	Extrarenal losses: vomiting, diarrhea, burns, sequestration	
Euvolemic	No evidence of volume depletion or overload. Subclinical increase in total body water may be present.	Urinary sodium >20 mmol/L	Hypothyroidism	Thyroid replacement
			Glucocorticoid deficiency	I.V. glucocorticoids
			SIADH, drugs, acute water intoxication	Fluid restriction
Hypervolemic	Volume excess Edema	Urinary sodium >30 mmol/L	Acute and chronic renal failure	Fluid restriction; treat renal failure
		Urinary sodium <10 mmol/L	Cirrhosis Cardiac failure Nephrotic syndrome	Fluid restriction; sodium restriction; treat underlying disorders

From Devita MV and Michelis MF, "Perturbations in Sodium Balance: Hyponatremia and Hypernatremia," *Clinics in Laboratory Medicine*, Vol 13, Preuss HG, ed, Philadelphia, PA: WB Saunders Co, 1993, 135-48, with permission.

Evaluation and Treatment of the **Hypernatremic** Patient

CONDITION	ETIOLOGY		URINARY ELECTROLYTES	TREATMENT
Hypovolemic	Renal losses	Osmotic diuresis	Urinary sodium >30 mmol/L	Isotonic saline (0.9 NaCl) until hemodynamically stable, then hypotonic fluids
	Extrarenal losses	Sweating Diarrhea in children	Urinary sodium <30 mmol/L	
Euvolemic	Renal losses	Central diabetes insipidus Nephrogenic diabetes insipidus Partial diabetes insipidus Hypodipsia	Variable urinary sodium	Administer vasopressin and water replacement. If urine volume decreased, diagnosis is central diabetes insipidus or partial diabetes insipidus. If no response, diagnosis is nephrogenic diabetes insipidus. Give trial of hydrochlorothiazide.
	Extrarenal losses	Respiratory or skin losses		
Hypervolemic	Increased total body sodium	Primary or secondary aldosteronism Cushing's syndrome Hypertonic I.V. infusion I.V. sodium bicarbonate administration Sodium chloride tablets	Urinary sodium >30 mmol/L	Diuretics and water replacement

From Devita MV and Michelis MF, "Perturbations in Sodium Balance: Hyponatremia and Hypernatremia", *Clinics in Laboratory Medicine*, Vol 13, Preuss HG, ed, Philadelphia, PA: WB Saunders Co, 1993, 135-48, with permission.

T₃ Uptake, Serum or Plasma

Related Information
Free Thyroxine Index *on page 177*
Thyroid Stimulating Hormone, Serum *on page 282*
Thyroxine Binding Globulin, Serum *on page 284*
Thyroxine, Serum *on page 286*

Synonyms Resin Triiodothyronine Uptake; Resin Uptake Ratio; T₃ Resin Uptake; T₃RU; T₃U

Applies to Free T₄ Index (FT₄I); FTI; T₇; T₁₂; Thyroid Hormone Binding Ratio; Thyroxine Ratio

Test Includes The thyroid profile has been done very widely by most laboratories. It includes T₃ uptake with T₄ or equivalent.

Abstract T₃U is an indirect measure of unsaturated binding sites on thyroid binding globulin (TBG). T₃ uptake does **not** measure serum T₃ levels. The first T₃ uptake assay was described using red blood cells. Radioactive T₃ was used in preference to T₄ because of lesser affinity of TBG for T₃ compared to T₄. Such red cells were subsequently replaced by resins. The use of T₃ uptake is limited to testing with T₄ (thyroxine) to calculate the free thyroxine index (FTI), which provides the indirect estimate of free thyroxine. **In recent years, free thyroxine assays have become more reliable and use of T₃ uptake has decreased.** However, according to year 2000 College of American Pathologist surveys, there remain still over 900 laboratories performing this test. If free thyroxine and/or sTSH assays are available, use of T₃ uptake should be discouraged.

Patient Preparation Avoid recent isotope scan before collection of specimen if a radioactive method is used.

Specimen Serum is preferred, plasma may also be acceptable.
(Continued)

T_3 Uptake, Serum or Plasma *(Continued)*

Container Red top tube; lavender top (EDTA) tube or green top (heparin) tube is also acceptable.

Storage Instructions Separate within 48 hours. Store at 2°C to 8°C.

Reference Interval Varies with different laboratories. A range of 24% to 34% is frequently used. The T_3 uptake can be expressed in several ways. The Committee on Nomenclature of the American Thyroid Association recommends that raw uptake results be normalized by dividing the raw T_3 uptake by the T_3 uptake of normal pooled serum, to form the **thyroid hormone binding ratio (THBR)**. The THBR in all laboratories will have a reference range centered on 1.00 and is usually given as 0.90-1.10. See also table in Thyroxine Binding Globulin, Serum *on page 284*.

Use A thyroid function test for the diagnosis of hypothyroidism or hyperthyroidism, T_3U is used with T_4 or equivalent to provide free thyroxine index (free T_4 index, FT_4I). An indirect measure of binding protein, the T_3 uptake reflects available binding sites (ie, reflects TBG) and estimation of free thyroxine concentration. T_3 uptake is **not** a measurement of serum T_3. It should never be used alone; rather, its usual application is in conjunction with total T_4 measurement. THBR is preferred and should be used instead of T_3U. Better assays for sTSH, selectively with tests for free T_3 and/or free T_4, are presently recommended for initial thyroid evaluation.[1] See table for typical examples of use.

Diagnostic Utility of T_3U and FT_4I

Clinical Condition	T_4	T_3U	FT_4I
Normal	Normal	Normal	Normal
Hyperthyroid	Increased	Increased	Increased
Hypothyroid	Decreased	Decreased	Decreased
Increased TBG (eg, pregnancy)	Increased	Decreased	Normal
Decreased TBG (eg, nephrotic syndrome)	Decreased	Increased	Normal

Limitations An **increase** in T_3U occurs in hyperthyroidism; in situations in which drugs displace T_4 from TBG (eg, high doses of salicylates, phenytoin, phenylbutazone, etc); and in cases in which the TBG concentration decreases (eg, nephrotic syndrome, malnutrition, active acromegaly). Nicotinic acid increases T_3 resin uptake ratios. A **decrease** in T_3U occurs in hypothyroidism and in cases in which an increase in TBG occurs, such as estrogen administration (as contraceptive, during menopause, or treatment of osteoporosis), during pregnancy, and in conjunction with perphenazine.

Alterations in binding capacity of TBG are described with major illness and with high doses of salicylates and corticosteroids, and with use of heroin, methadone, phenytoin, and perphenazine. Alterations occur with malnutrition, such as in metastatic malignancy, and are found in patients with abnormal serum protein patterns (eg, nephrotic syndromes, cirrhosis). Other states in which changes in TBG occur include infancy, acromegaly, molar and ordinary pregnancy, oral contraceptives, and with exogenous hormones including androgens, anabolic steroids, and estrogens. Hereditary increase and decrease of TBG occurs. **Most authorities have abandoned this test in favor of more specific, sensitive tests such as FT_4, sTSH, and FT_3.**

Contraindications This test should not be ordered alone; it is only useful with T_4 type tests.

Methodology Resin sponge uptake, charcoal bead uptake, related methods, based on *in vitro* competition for thyroid hormone between thyroid binding globulin and the added inert receptor. For THBR, divide patient's T_3U by T_3U for normal or reference serum.

Additional Information Free thyroxine index is calculated as:

$$FT_4I = [\% \ T_3U \ (patient) \ / \ \% \ T_3U \ (reference \ serum)] \times T_4$$

The FT_4I range usually approximates the range for total T_4. In the presence of thyroid binding globulin abnormalities, the free thyroxine index is a useful laboratory parameter regarding clinical thyroid status. A number of pseudonyms, including thyroxine ratio, T_7, and T_{12}, for FT_4I are used in the literature. Use of these terms should be discouraged.

Footnotes
1. Dayan CM, "Interpretation of Thyroid Function Tests," *Lancet*, 2001, 357:619-24.

References
Attia J, Margetts P, and Guyatt G, "Diagnosis of Thyroid Disease in Hospitalized Patients: A Systematic Review," *Arch Intern Med*, 1999, 159(7):658-65.

Christofides ND, Wilkinson E, Stoddart M, et al, "Assessment of Serum Thyroxine Binding Capacity-Dependent Biases in Free Thyroxine Assays," *Clin Chem*, 1999, 45(4):520-5.

Faix JD, Rosen HN, and Velazquez FR, "Indirect Estimation of Thyroid Hormone-Binding Proteins to Calculate Free Thyroxine Index: Comparison of Nonisotopic Methods That Use Labeled Thyroxine ("T-Uptake")," *Clin Chem*, 1995, 41(1):41-7.

Feldkamp CS and Carey JL, "An Algorithmic Approach to Thyroid Function Testing in a Managed Care Setting. 3-Year Experience," *Am J Clin Pathol*, 1996, 105(1):11-6.

Franklyn JA, "The Management of Hyperthyroidism," *N Engl J Med*, 1994, 330(24):1731-8.

Oxley DK, "Screening for Hyperthyroidism," *Arch Pathol Lab Med*, 1991, 1201-2.

Whitley RJ, "Thyroid Function," *Tietz Textbook of Clinical Chemistry*, 3rd ed, Burtis CA and Ashwood ER, eds, Philadelphia, PA: WB Saunders Co, 1999, 1496-529.

♦ **T_4** *see* Thyroxine, Serum *on page 286*

♦ **T_4-Binding Globulin** *see* Thyroxine Binding Globulin, Serum *on page 284*

♦ **T_4 CPB** *replaced by* Thyroxine, Serum *on page 286*

♦ **T_4, Free** *see* Thyroxine, Free, Serum *on page 285*

♦ **T_4 Neonatal** *see* Newborn Screen for T_4, Filter Paper *on page 230*

♦ **T_7** *see* T_3 Uptake, Serum or Plasma *on page 279*

♦ **T_{12}** *see* T_3 Uptake, Serum or Plasma *on page 279*

♦ **TAG-72** *see* CA 19-9, Serum *on page 128*

♦ **Tartrate-Resistant Acid Phosphatase** *see* Acid Phosphatase, Plasma *on page 82*

♦ **Tau Protein** *see* Apolipoprotein E, Plasma *on page 110*

♦ **TBG** *see* Thyroxine Binding Globulin, Serum *on page 284*

♦ **TBG** *see* Thyroxine, Serum *on page 286*

♦ **TCO_2** *see* Bicarbonate, Blood *on page 115*

♦ **TCO_2** *see* Blood Gases and pH, Arterial *on page 119*

♦ **TCO_2** *see* Carbon Dioxide, Total, Blood *on page 135*

♦ **Telopeptides** *see* N-Telopeptides, Urine *on page 233*

♦ **Testosterone** *see* Dehydroepiandrosterone and Dehydroepiandrosterone Sulfate, Serum or Plasma *on page 164*

Testosterone, Total and Free, Serum or Plasma

Related Information
Adrenal Cortex: Laboratory Assessments Overview *on page 84*
Adrenocorticotropic Hormone, Plasma *on page 86*
Androstenedione, Serum *on page 104*
Cortisol, Serum or Plasma *on page 154*
Dehydroepiandrosterone and Dehydroepiandrosterone Sulfate, Serum or Plasma *on page 164*
Dihydrotestosterone, Serum *on page 167*
Follicle Stimulating Hormone, Serum, Plasma, or Urine *on page 175*
Infertility Screen *on page 310*
Inhibin A, Serum *on page 199*
17-Ketosteroids, Total, Urine *on page 206*
Luteinizing Hormone, Blood or Urine *on page 219*
Semen Analysis, Advanced *on page 318*
Semen Analysis, Basic *on page 319*
Sperm Mucus Penetration Test (Human or Bovine Cervical Mucus) *on page 320*
Sperm Penetration Assay (Zona-Free Hamster Egg Penetration Test) *on page 321*
Swim Up/Swim Down Procedures (Spermatozoa) *on page 323*

Applies to Dihydrotestosterone; Estradiol; Free Testosterone; Gonadotropin-Releasing Hormone; Luteinizing Hormone; Sex-Hormone Binding Globulin

Abstract Testosterone (T) is the most abundant androgen secreted by the testicular Leydig cells. T is both an androgen itself, and a prohormone which can be converted into an even more potent androgen, dihydrotestosterone (DHT), and an estrogenic hormone, estradiol (E2). The conversion into DHT occurs in tissues containing the enzyme, 5-alpha reductase (skin, prostate, other internal genitalia), while the conversion into E2 occurs in tissues containing the enzyme, aromatase (fat tissue, breast). Secretion of T is primarily dependent on stimulation of the testicular Leydig cells by pituitary luteinizing hormone (LH), which is, in turn, dependent on stimulation of pituitary gonadotrophic cells by hypothalamic gonadotropin-releasing hormone (GnRH). T is part of a classical negative feedback mechanism: increased serum levels of T suppress serum levels of LH, while decreased T leads to marked increases in serum LH. T has a diurnal variation, with peak serum levels at 0400-0800 and minimum levels at 1600-2000. T circulates in the plasma ~65% bound to sex-hormone binding globulin (SHBG) and ~30% to 32% bound to albumin; ~1% to 4% of T in plasma is free (not bound to protein).[1]

Patient Preparation Avoid recent administration of radioactive isotopes if assay is to be done by RIA.

Specimen Serum or plasma

Container Red top tube, green top (heparin) tube, or lavender top (EDTA) tube

Storage Instructions Separate serum or plasma and freeze.

Use

Total vs free T. For most clinical purposes, when an assessment of T is needed, measurement of total T provides all of the needed diagnostic information. Measurement of free (unbound) T is rarely needed but may be useful in obese patients who sometimes have low SHBG concentrations, which make total T levels seem inappropriately low.[2]

Polycystic ovary syndrome (PCOS). PCOS is a highly prevalent disorder characterized by signs of androgen excess (anovulation accompanied by hirsutism, acne, and male-pattern baldness). Most patients with PCOS have elevated serum T; other biochemical features include elevated serum androstenedione and LH. The differential diagnosis includes late-onset congenital adrenal hyperplasia, a diagnosis which is usually excluded if the patient has a normal response in 17-alpha hydroxyprogesterone to synthetic corticotropin (ACTH). Other elements in the differential diagnosis are acromegaly, hyperprolactinemia, and androgen-secreting tumors of the ovary or adrenal.[3]

Female hirsutism. The differential diagnosis of hirsutism in an adult female includes;

- a) PCOS (see discussion above and Key Word Index)
- b) late-onset congenital adrenal hyperplasia (CAH)
- c) Cushing syndrome
- d) hormone-secreting tumors of the adrenal or ovary
- e) idiopathic hirsutism

See Adrenal Cortex: Laboratory Assessments Overview *on page 84* for a discussion of possibilities (b) and (c), and see Dehydroepiandrosterone and Dehydroepiandrosterone Sulfate, Serum or Plasma *on page 164* for possibility (d). Idiopathic hirsutism is usually a diagnosis of exclusion; such patients typically have normal serum T. Fiet et al recommend using a coordinated set of immunoassays for eight hormones in the differential diagnosis of hirsutism and acne in women.[4]

Male hypogonadism. Primary testicular insufficiency or failure is characterized by low serum T and elevated serum LH and FSH. Primary hypogonadism must be differentiated from secondary hypogonadism (low serum T and with LH and FSH near lower end of reference interval) because patients with secondary hypogonadism are potentially fertile, while patients with primary hypogonadism are not.[2]

Androgen insensitivity syndrome. In the fetus with a 46X,Y genotype, T and DHT combine with the nuclear androgen receptor to mediate the development of male internal and external genitalia. When, because of a genetic mutation, the nuclear androgen receptor is absent or inactive, the individual with a 46X,Y (male) genotype will have a female phenotype (ie, female external genitalia, breast development, and a female habitus) - a disorder historically referred to as the testicular feminization syndrome, but now renamed the androgen-insensitivity syndrome. Such patients have a vagina, no uterus, and bilaterally cryptorchid testes.[5] Androgen insensitivity is also a possible diagnosis when a phenotypically female infant has inguinal hernias and a mass in the inguinal area or labia.[6]

Anabolic steroid abuse. Some athletes take androgenic hormones in an attempt to increase muscle mass; the effects, if any, on serum T and DHT are unpredictable since the exogenous hormone suppresses endogenous hormone production. In a randomized controlled trial, androstenedione supplementation did **not** increase serum T (nor did it improve adaptation to resistance training).[7]

Reference Interval See table.

Testosterone, Total and Free

Total Testosterone			
Male			
Age (y)	ng/dL	nmol/L	% Free
<1	Not established		
1-9	<40	<1.39	
10-11	<200	<6.94	
12-13	<800	<27.76	
14	<1200	<41.64	
15-16	100-1200	3.47-41.64	
17-18	300-1200	10.41-41.64	
19-40	300-950	10.41-32.97	
>40	240-950	8.32-32.97	
Female			
<1	Not established		
1-9	<40	<1.39	
10-11	<75	<2.60	
12-16	<120	<4.16	
17-18	20-120	0.69-4.16	
>18	20-80	0.69-2.77	
Free Testosterone			
Male	9-30	0.31-1.04	2.0-4.8
Female	0.3-1.9	0.01-0.07	0.9-3.8

Adapted from Mayo Medical Laboratories, *2000 Test Catalog*, Rochester, MN, 2000, 470.

Limitations Total serum testosterone may be normal in women with hirsutism, who may have abnormal free testosterone. Plasma testosterone level may be elevated in patients using cimetidine. In **Klinefelter syndrome**, testosterone can be at the low end of the reference range or lower. Even when it is almost normal, LH levels are increased.

Methodology Radioimmunoassay (RIA), chemiluminescent immunoassay (CIA). Free testosterone is generally done by RIA or CIA after ultrafiltration or equilibrium dialysis.

Additional Information Cresswell et al have emphasized that there are at least two common, but distinct, forms of PCOS: one profile comprises

normal body weight and elevated serum LH; the other comprises obesity, signs of androgen excess (especially hirsutism), and elevated serum LH and T. These investigators present evidence suggesting that these two forms of PCOS are due to different patterns of intrauterine development.[8,2]

Patients with the androgen-insensitivity syndrome (see above) often consult a gynecologist because of their failure to initiate menses. It is important that the cryptorchid testes in such individuals not be misinterpreted as Sertoli-Leydig cell neoplasms.[5]

Footnotes

1. Gronowski AM and Landau-Levine M, "Reproductive Endocrine Function," *Tietz Textbook of Clinical Chemistry*, 3rd ed, Burtis CA and Ashwood ER, eds, Philadelphia, PA: WB Saunders Co, 1999, 1601-43.
2. Bagatell CJ and Bremner WJ, "Androgens in Men - Uses and Abuses," *N Engl J Med*, 1996, 334(11):707-14.
3. Franks S, "Polycystic Ovary Syndrome," *N Engl J Med*, 1995, 333(13):853-61.
4. Fiet J, Gosling JP, Soliman H, et al, "Hirsutism and Acne in Women: Coordinated Radioimmunoassays for Eight Relevant Plasma Steroids," *Clin Chem*, 1994, 40(12):2296-305.
5. Rosai J, *Ackerman's Surgical Pathology*, 8th ed, St. Louis, MO: Mosby-Year Book Inc., 1996, 1463-4.
6. Grumbach MM and Conte FA, "Disorders of Sex Differentiation," *Williams Textbook of Endocrinology*, 9th ed, Wilson JD, Foster DW, Kronenberg HM, et al, eds, Philadelphia, PA: WB Saunders Co, 1998, 1385-6.
7. King DS, Sharp RL, Vukovich MD, et al, "Effect of Oral Androstenedione on Serum Testosterone and Adaptations to Resistance Training in Young Men: A Randomized Controlled Trial," *JAMA*, 1999, 281(21):2020-8.
8. Creswell JL, Barker DJP, Osmond C, et al, "Fetal Growth, Length of Gestation, and Polycystic Ovaries in Adult Life," *Lancet*, 1997, 350(9085):1131-5.

References

Adachi M, Takayanagi R, Tomura A, et al, "Androgen Insensitivity Syndrome as a Possible Coactivator Disease," *N Engl J Med*, 2000, 343(12):856-62.
Street ME, Weber A, Camacho-Hubner C, "Girls With Virilization in Childhood: A Diagnostic Protocol for Investigation," *J Clin Pathol*, 1997, 50(5):379-83.

Thyroglobulin, Serum

Abstract Thyroglobulin is a secretory product of thyroid follicular epithelium, a high molecular weight (660,000 daltons) iodinated glycoprotein. Its only origin is the thyroid gland. It is the storage form of the thyroid hormones, T_4, and T_3. Its major clinical use is as a tumor marker, in the management (not diagnosis) of differentiated thyroid carcinomas. It is increased in papillary carcinoma, follicular carcinoma, and mixed papillary follicular carcinoma. It is not increased in medullary carcinoma of thyroid.

Patient Preparation Avoid scans and other recent prior administration of radioisotopes before collection of specimen if RIA is used for assay. Do not draw a specimen for this test soon after needle biopsy, thyroid surgery, or radioiodine therapy. The test is most sensitive for detection of thyroid cancer when the patient is off thyroxine replacement long enough to have increased TSH. This may take as long as 6 weeks.

Specimen Serum

Container Red top tube

Storage Instructions Freeze serum.

Special Instructions This is **not** thyroxine binding globulin (TBG).

Reference Interval Approximately 3-42 ng/mL. Detectable in most healthy adults; moderately elevated (several fold) in the last trimester of gestation and in neonates. In athyroidic patient, <5 ng/mL. Levels >15 ng/mL are significant when the patient has not been on thyroid hormone replacement therapy after thyroidectomy.

Critical Values Thyroglobulin levels >50.0 ng/mL are associated with tumor recurrence in patients who lack thyroid tissue.

Use Thyroglobulin is elevated in several thyroid disorders: endemic goiter, untreated Graves disease, thyroiditis, and differentiated thyroid carcinomas (papillary and follicular). It is also useful in the investigation of cases of self-induced hyperthyroidism due to exogenous intake of thyroxine.

Those thyroid cancer patients who have no remaining thyroid tissue, following surgery and/or irradiation, would not be expected to have a source of thyroglobulin. Thyroglobulin then is **a tumor marker useful to assess the presence of residual papillary-follicular carcinoma of thyroid**,[1,2] (Continued)

Thyroglobulin, Serum (Continued)

following resection, including tumors which fail to concentrate radioiodine. High values are found with many instances of tumor dissemination. Thus, thyroglobulin assays are used to monitor postoperative thyroid carcinoma patients. Such assays are best used in concert with total body scans. Possibly it will be useful in patients with bone metastases in whom the primary site is unknown.

Thyroglobulin is elevated in patients with thyroiditis and thyrotoxicosis. Low or undetectable levels are a clue to thyrotoxicosis factitia (surreptitious use of thyroid hormone). The assay may be used to support a diagnosis of subacute thyroiditis and may be used to monitor response to treatment of nodular or diffuse nontoxic goiter. The absence of thyroglobulin from the serum of neonates suggests congenital athyreosis.[3] Circulating thyroglobulin is also absent when TSH receptor function is lost.[4]

Limitations Thyroglobulin is useful in the management but not diagnosis of differentiated thyroid carcinomas. Thyroglobulin is not valid as a tumor marker for anaplastic or medullary carcinoma of thyroid or for thyroid lymphoma. High values are reported with surgery or irradiation to the thyroid, with thyroiditis, T_4 binding globulin deficiency, with administration of TRH, TSH, iodine, and of anticancer drugs. High levels of thyroglobulin occur in goiter and in many types of hyperthyroidism. Normal levels are found in patients with small thyroid carcinomas. Low values occur with thyroid hormone administration. This is not a screening test for thyroid cancer. RIA methods are subject to interference in serums containing autoantibodies (eg, most patients with Hashimoto thyroiditis). Newer methods, using IRMA are less prone to interference from autoantibodies.[5] There is wide variation in thyroglobulin levels measured by different assays.[6,7] Thyroglobulin is decreased with fasting.[8]

Methodology Radioimmunoassay (RIA), immunoradiometric assay (IRMA), sandwich enzyme immunoassay (EIA), immunochemiluminometric assays (ICMA)

Additional Information Although functioning metastatic thyroid carcinoma causing hyperthyroidism is extremely uncommon, serial thyroglobulin assays provide a means of following such patients.[1] Serial thyroglobulin determinations may be helpful for detection of metastases which do not accumulate radioiodine.[9] Patients with small thyroidal remnants demonstrable by ^{131}I scan may not have elevated thyroglobulin. Therefore, thyroglobulin should be used as an adjunct, not a replacement to ^{131}I scanning.

Footnotes

1. Black EG and Sheppard MC, "Serum Thyroglobulin Measurements in Thyroid Cancer: Evaluation of "False"-Positive Results," *Clin Endocrinol (Oxf)*, 1991, 35(6):519-20.
2. Utiger RD, "Follow-up of Patients With Thyroid Carcinoma," *N Engl J Med* 1997, 337(13):928-30.
3. LaFranchi S, "Disorders of Thyroid Gland," *Nelson Textbook of Pediatrics*, 16th ed, Behrman RE, Kliegman RM, and Jenson HB, eds, Philadelphia, PA: WB Saunders Co, 2000, 1696-714.
4. Tonacchera M, Agretti P, Pinchera A, et al, "Congenital Hypothyroidism With Impaired Thyroid Response to Thyrotropin (TSH) and Absent Circulating Thyroglobulin: Evidence for a New Inactivating Mutation of the TSH Receptor Gene," *J Clin Endocrinol Metab*, 2000, 85(3):1001-8.
5. Marquet PY, Daver A, Sapin R, et al, "Highly Sensitive Immunoradiometric Assay for Serum Thyroglobulin With Minimal Interference From Autoantibodies," *Clin Chem*, 1996, 42(2):258-62.
6. Spencer CA, Takeuchi M, and Kazarosyan M, "Current Status and Performance Goals for Serum Thyroglobulin Assays," *Clin Chem*, 1997, 43(2):413-5.
7. Spencer CA and Wang CC, "Thyroglobulin Measurement. Techniques, Clinical Benefits, and Pitfalls," *Endocrinol Metab Clin North Am*, 1995, 24(4):841-63.
8. Unger J, "Fasting Induces a Decrease in Serum Thyroglobulin in Normal Subjects," *J Clin Endocrinol Metab*, 1988, 67(6):1309-11.
9. Botsch H, Glatz J, Shulz E, et al, "Long-Term Follow-up Using Serial Serum Thyroglobulin Determinations in Patients With Differentiated Thyroid Carcinoma," *Cancer*, 1983, 52(10):1856-9.

References

Hay ID and Klee GG, "Thyroid Cancer Diagnosis and Management," *Clin Lab Med*, 1993, 13(3):725-34.
Ng DC, Sundram FX, and Sin AE, "[99]mTc-Sestamibi and [131]I Whole-Body Scintigraphy and Initial Serum Thyroglobulin in the Management of Differentiated Thyroid Carcinoma," *J Nucl Med*, 2000, 41(4):631-5.
Schlumberger MJ, "Papillary and Follicular Thyroid Carcinoma," *N Engl J Med*, 1998, 338(5):297-306.
Schlumberger MJ and Baudin E, "Serum Thyroglobulin Determination in the Follow-up of Patients With Differentiated Thyroid Carcinoma," *Eur J Endocrinol*, 1998, 138(3):249-52.
Schlumberger MJ, Mancusi F, Baudin E, et al, "[131]I Therapy for Elevated Thyroglobulin Levels," *Thyroid*, 1997, 7(2):273-6.

♦ **Thyroid Hormone Binding Ratio** see T_3 Uptake, Serum or Plasma *on page 279*

♦ **Thyroid Screen for Newborns** see Newborn Screen for T_4, Filter Paper *on page 230*

♦ **Thyroid Screen for Newborns** see Newborn Screen for TSH, Filter Paper *on page 231*

♦ **Thyroid Stimulating Hormone Screen, Filter Paper** see Newborn Screen for TSH, Filter Paper *on page 231*

Thyroid Stimulating Hormone, Serum

Related Information

Cholesterol, Total, Serum or Plasma *on page 146*
Fine Needle Aspiration, Deep Masses *on page 381*
Free Thyroxine Index *on page 177*
Heterophilic Antibodies *on page 191*
Lithium, Serum *on page 754*
T_3 Uptake, Serum or Plasma *on page 279*
Thyroperoxidase Autoantibody *on page 545*
Thyrotropin Receptor Antibody, Serum *on page 545*
Thyroxine, Free, Serum *on page 285*
Thyroxine, Serum *on page 286*
Triglycerides, Serum or Plasma *on page 288*
Triiodothyronine, Serum *on page 290*

Synonyms Fourth Generation TSH; sTSH; Third Generation TSH; Thyrotropin; TSH; Ultrasensitive TSH

Applies to TRH Stimulation Test

Abstract Produced by the anterior pituitary gland, thyroid stimulating hormone (TSH) stimulates secretion of T_4 (thyroxine) and T_3 (triiodothyronine). TSH secretion is physiologically regulated by T_4 and T_3 (feedback inhibition) and is stimulated by TRH (thyrotropin releasing hormone) from the hypothalamus. TSH assay was originally used to diagnose or confirm primary hypothyroidism. The new sensitive assays (sTSH) permit recognition of **hyperthyroidism**, including Graves disease, multinodular goiter or toxic nodule (sTSH undectable or low). Thus, with the availability of sTSH assays, diagnostic thyroid testing strategies have been altered.[1,2] Sensitive TSH has become the best single test for thyroid function screening.[3,4] Not bound to carrier proteins, TSH is not plagued with problems of estrogen and androgen administration, or hepatic or renal disorders which influence other important thyroid tests. TSH measurement is also used to distinguish primary from secondary **hypothyroidism**. Thyroid tests are interpreted in clinical context, including history, physical examination, additionally with free T_4 and free T_3 concentrations and other tests as needed.

A normal TSH concentration, or result of any other serum test, does not necessarily assure that an individual patient's thyroid gland is well (eg, a patient with a thyroid nodule requires further investigation).

Patient Preparation Avoid radioisotope administration before collection of specimen if RIA is used for assay.

Specimen Serum

Container Red top tube

Sampling Time A diurnal rhythm exists. Peak levels occur at about 11 PM. TSH release is pulsatile.

Storage Instructions Separate serum within 4 hours and refrigerate. Stable 4 days at 4°C.

Reference Interval Reference ranges are age dependent and somewhat method dependent. For prematures and during the first week of life, TSH values are significantly higher. Approximate values using third generation TSH assay are as follows:[5]

- prematures, 28-36 weeks: 0.7-27.0 mIU/L
- birth to 4 days: 1.0-39.0 mIU/L
- 2-20 weeks: 1.7-9.1 mIU/L
- 21 weeks to 20 years: 0.7-6.4 mIU/L
- 21-54 years: 0.4-4.2 mIU/L
- 55-87 years: 0.5-8.9 mIU/L

Critical Values <0.1 mIU/L provides indication of primary hyperthyroidism or exogenous thyrotoxicosis. Risk exists for atrial fibrillation at TSH levels <0.1 mIU/L, but the degree of risk is controversial.

Use Hypothyroidism implies a deficiency in thyroxine (T_4) output relative to physiological requirements. T_4 production is regulated by the pituitary-thyroid feedback loop: when there is inadequate T_4 in the periphery, increased TSH is secreted from the pituitary. **Primary hypothyroidism** (ie, due to disease in the thyroid itself) is usually identified by finding an elevated serum TSH. The dynamics of the pituitary-thyroid feedback loop are such that an elevation of TSH precedes a recognizably decreased T_4 (total or free). Patients with **central hypothyroidism** (ie, due to pituitary failure, and also called **secondary hypothyroidism**), by contrast, usually have a TSH value that is low in relation to the simultaneously obtained T_4, but TSH may be within, at, or above, the adult reference interval. In such patients, the pituitary cannot fully respond to the low T_4 in the periphery.[6] When a patient has a low T_4 (total or free) and a normal TSH, the clinician will probably investigate further; however, when only the TSH has been obtained (the practice in many clinics) and is normal, there is a danger of overlooking the diagnosis of central hypothyroidism. Such a scenario can be further complicated if the patient has a surgical procedure or intercurrent illness and thereby develops, in addition to the unrecognized central hypothyroidism, the **euthyroid sick syndrome** in which there is a transient, additional decrement in TSH; Waise et al have described six such examples.[7] An additional problem is recognizing patients who have **resistance to thyroid hormone** (RTH), a familial disease first described in 1967.[8] In such patients, the pituitary and most other organs and tissues are relatively insensitive to thyroid hormone, and the characteristic biochemical profile includes elevated T_4 (free and total), elevated T_3 (free and total), and an inappropriately "normal" (or elevated) TSH.[9] Testing for RTH may include a challenge dose of L-T_4 (eg, 2 mg by mouth), or T_3 (eg, 3000 mcg of

Cytomel®), and observing that the normal suppression of TSH (to <10% of baseline) does not occur.[10] This challenge test is also useful in the diagnosis of rare TSH-secreting pituitary neoplasms.[10] An important hazard for persons with RTH is receiving the erroneous diagnosis, and treatment, for hyperthyroidism. Such a scenario is most likely to arise when a physician looks only at the laboratory results and fails to correlate them with the clinical findings.[10] The treatment of patients with RTH is controversial.[11]

An increasingly common practice, but still controversial, involves diagnosing and treating **subclinical hypothyroidism**, understood as individuals who appear eumetabolic by clinical criteria, have normal serum T_4 (total and free) and elevated TSH.[12,13] Its usual causes include thyroiditis and inadequate treatment of hypothyroidism.[14]

A novel, and presumably rare, form of hypothyroidism in children appears to be due to **pituitary-thyroid feedback hypersensitivity**. The patient reported in 2000[15] was a 17-year-old male with hypothyroid facies, tiredness, growth delay, and poor academic progress. The free T_4, total T_4, and free T_3 were low and the total T_3 was at the lower limit of the reference interval; the TSH was inappropriately normal and the TSH response to thyrotropin-release-hormone stimulation was low for the concurrent T_4 and T_3 levels.

TSH has become the primary thyroid function test for stable ambulatory subjects who lack pituitary or neuropsychiatric illness.[1,3,4] An sTSH result within the accepted reference range provides strong evidence for euthyroidism. A simple algorithm for thyroid testing can be found in the following chart, modified from that at the Mayo Clinic Laboratory.[16]

The Mayo Medical Laboratories Thyroid Function Cascade (modified)

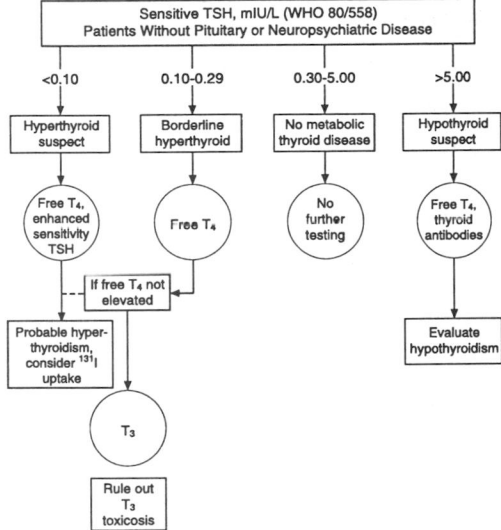

Subclinical hyperthyroidism is defined as suppression of sTSH concentrations with normal levels of serum thyroxine and triiodothyronine. This disorder may lead to diminution of bone mineral density, and increases risk of atrial fibrillation in patients older than 60 years of age. The most common cause of subclinical hyperthyroidism is excessive thyroid hormone treatment.[14]

Limitations TSH is decreased by glucocorticoids, levodopa, dopamine, and may be affected by stress and by severe nonthyroidal illness, and these remain limitations even for the new, sensitive TSH assays. Acute illness reduces the specificity of sTSH tests for thyroid disease. The positive likelihood ratio associated with an abnormal sTSH test result in ill inpatients is about 10 compared with about 100 in outpatients.[17] Causes of transient increase in TSH include lithium, methimazole, propylthiouracil, valproate, and in certain patients, iodine, amiodarone, and radiologic contrast media. Effects of drugs upon thyroid testing and physiology have recently been reviewed.[18] Normal TSH levels in the presence of hypothyroidism have been reported with head injury. TSH is not elevated in secondary hypothyroidism (that due to hypopituitarism) nor in hypothalamic hypothyroidism.

Probably no single test, even the sensitive immunoassays, can be expected to adequately reflect thyroid status under all circumstances. Among possible problems are the recovery phase of nonthyroidal illness, states of resistance to thyroid hormone, thyrotropin-producing tumors, thyroid masses, thyroid status in acute psychiatric illness, early thyrotoxicosis and subacute thyroiditis. Heterophilic antibodies remain a problem[19] (see Heterophilic Antibodies *on page 191*).

Common errors in interpretation by thyroid function tests are described in the following table.[20]

Malabsorption of prescribed thyroxine from small intestinal disease, cholestyramine or iron therapy can lead to TSH increase.

Common Errors in Interpretation of Thyroid Function Tests

Thyroid Function Test Results	Circumstance	Wrong Interpretation	Correct Interpretation
Low TSH, low FT_3 or FT_4	Post-treatment for thyrotoxicosis	Persistent hyperthyroidism	Profoundly hypothyroid
Low TSH, high FT_3 or FT_4	Short history of neck pain	Established thyrotoxicosis	Possible self-resolving thyroiditis
Low or normal TSH, low or normal FT_3 or FT_4	Patient systemically ill	Hypothyroid	Nonthyroidal illness
Normal TSH (FT_3 or FT_4 not tested)	Pituitary disease	Euthyroid	Possibly hypothyroid - check FT_3 or FT_4
High TSH, normal FT_3 or FT_4	TSH fails to fall with T_4	Noncompliance with T_4	Possible interfering heterophil or an antibody

FT_3 = free T_3; FT_4 = free T_4.

Adapted from Dayan CM, "Interpretation of Thyroid Function Tests," *Lancet*, 2001, 357:619-24.

When thyroid function tests are discrepant with the clinical appearance of the patient, or with one another, further investigation may well be desirable. This is especially so when there is history of childhood thyroid abnormality or of familial disease.[20]

Methodology Immunoassays including radioimmunoassay (RIA), immunochemiluminometric assays (ICMA), sandwich immunoradiometric assays (IRMA), fluorometric enzyme immunoassay with use of monoclonal antibodies, microparticle enzyme immunoassay (MEIA) on IMx and AxSym (Abbott Laboratories). Most assays presently in use are beyond the first generation of tests.

Additional Information TSH is the single most sensitive test for primary hypothyroidism. With the availability of ultrasensitive TSH assay, the diagnostic capability of the assay has expanded to the detection of hyperthyroidism. Elevated TSH in apparently euthyroid individuals can be followed by third generation FT_4 and assay for thyroperoxidase antibodies. If positive for thyroperoxidase antibodies, such patients are at risk for subsequent evolution of hypothyroidism, especially if FT_4 is marginally decreased. Such risk is between 5% and 26% annually. It has been suggested that tests for antibodies be done when TSH levels are increased.[1] If there is clear evidence for hypothyroidism and the TSH is not elevated, secondary or tertiary hypothyroidism should be considered. In these situations, the TRH stimulation test may be useful, but is often not necessary.

When TSH is used to monitor thyroxine therapy, generally 6-8 weeks are required to achieve normal TSH levels. Likewise, TSH levels lag behind the return of thyroxine concentration to normal after thyroid replacement therapy, thyroid ablation, or antithyroid medication for hyperthyroidism. The most common cause of low TSH among outpatients is excessive replacement of thyroid hormone.

TSH levels have been **elevated** in some patients with thyrotropin-secreting pituitary adenomas (thyrotroph adenomas). TSH-secreting pituitary adenoma (TSH-oma), can be detected by computed tomographic (CT) scan or magnetic resonance imaging (MRI). Surgical, radiotherapy or octreotide treatment may be assessed by TSH levels. Undetectable TSH, 1 week postsurgery, suggests cure.[21]

As the prevalence of hypothyroidism is very high (up to 14%) in the elderly population, screening for hypothyroidism in this population is justified, and TSH is used as a primary screening test. Subclinical hypothyroidism, as defined by elevated TSH and normal FT_4, is an independent risk factor for atherosclerosis and myocardial infarction in the elderly population.[22] Recently, a filter paper method for screening for hypothyroidism in an elderly population has been tried. Although the method was adequate when TSH levels were >10 mIU/L, it was not sensitive for screening for subclinical hypothyroidism.[23]

Different strategies have been proposed for the laboratory investigation of thyroid function.[1] The American Association of Clinical Endocrinologists, the American Thyroid Association, and many others endorse sensitive TSH measurements as "the single best screening test" for thyroid disease.[1,3,4,24] The National Academy of Clinical Biochemistry recommends use of sensitive TSH as "the initial step in the diagnosis" of hypothyroidism.[25] The Royal College of Physicians of London recommends use of TSH and T_4 or FT_4.[26]

See table in Thyroxine Binding Globulin, Serum *on page 284* for effects of some drugs on thyroid function tests.

An outstanding recent review of Graves disease includes clinical photographs, outlines of pathogenesis, genetic factors, environmental and endogenous facets, clinical manifestations and review of diagnostic studies.[27]

Subclinical hypothyroidism and subclinical hyperthyroidism are addressed in the listing, Thyroxine, Free, Serum *on page 285*.

Hypothyroidism leads to increase in total cholesterol, triglycerides, HDLC, apolipoprotein A-1 and B-100, and Lp(a). Thyroid hormone replacement leads to less atherogenic lipid studies.[28]

Fetuses may be adversely affected by undiagnosed hypothyroidism in pregnant women. Screening for hypothyroidism during pregnancy may be needed.[29,30]

(Continued)

Thyroid Stimulating Hormone, Serum (Continued)

Among those age 60 and older, low TSH (<0.1 mIU/L) is a risk factor for atrial fibrillation.[31,32]

Footnotes

1. Klee GG and Hay ID, "Biochemical Testing of Thyroid Function," *Endocrinol Metab Clin North Am*, 1997, 26(4):763-5.
2. Utiger RD, "Subclinical Hyperthyroidism - Just a Low Serum Thyrotropin Concentration, or Something More?" *N Engl J Med*, 1994, 331(19):1302-3.
3. Garcia M, Baskin HJ, Feld S, et al, "AACE Clinical Practice Guidelines for the Evaluation and Treatment of Hyperthyroidism and Hypothyroidism," *Endocr Pract*, 1995, 1:56-62.
4. Ladenson PW, Singer PA, Ain K, et al, "American Thyroid Association Guidelines for Detection of Thyroid Dysfunction," *Arch Intern Med*, 2000, 160(11):1573-5.
5. Whitley RJ, "Thyroid Function," *Tietz Textbook of Clinical Chemistry*, 3rd ed, Burtis CA and Ashwood ER, eds, Philadelphia: WB Saunders Co, 1999, 1496-529.
6. Spencer CA, Takeuchi M, and Kazarosyan M, "Current Status and Performance Goals for Serum Thyrotropin (TSH) Assays," *Clin Chem*, 1996, 42(1):140-5.
7. Waise A and Belchetz PE, "Lesson of the Week: Unsuspected Central Hypothyroidism," *BMJ*, 2000, 321(7271):1275-7.
8. Refetoff S, DeWind LT, and DeGroot LJ, "Familial Syndrome Combining Deaf-Mutism, Stuppled Epiphyses, Goiter and Abnormally High PBI: Possible Target Organ Refractoriness to Thyroid Hormone," *J Clin Endocrinol Metab*, 1967, 27(2):279-94.
9. Brucker-Davis F, Skarulis MC, Grace MB, et al, "Genetic and Clinical Features of 42 Kindreds With Resistance to Thyroid Hormone," The National Institutes of Health Prospective Study, *Ann Intern Med*, 1995, 123(8):572-83.
10. Gladwin MT and Duell PB, "Inappropriate Thyroid Gland Ablation in Patients With Generalized Resistance to Thyroid Hormone. A Common Sequela of a Rare Disorder," *Arch Intern Med*, 1996, 156(1):106-9.
11. Weiss RE and Refetoff S, "Treatment of Resistance to Thyroid Hormone - primum non nocere," *J Clin Endocrinol Metab*, 1999, 84(2):401-4.
12. Weetman AP, "Hypothyroidism: Screening and Subclinical Disease," *BMJ*, 1997, 314(7088):1175-8.
13. O'Reilly DS, "Thyroid Function Tests - Time for a Reassessment," *BMJ*, 2000, 320(7245):1332-4.
14. Fatourechi V, "Subclinical Thyroid Disease," *Mayo Clin Proc*, 2001, 76(5):413-7.
15. Frankton S, Karmali R, Mirkine N, et al, "Pituitary-Thyroid Feedback Hypersensitivity as a Novel Cause of Hypothyroidism in Children," *Lancet*, 2000, 356(9237):1238-40.
16. Leavelle DE, *Mayo Medical Laboratories Interpretive Handbook*, Rochester, MN: Mayo Medical Laboratories, 1997, 502-3.
17. Attia J, Margetts P, and Guyatt G, "Diagnosis of Thyroid Disease in Hospitalized Patients: A Systematic Review," *Arch Intern Med*, 1999, 159(7):658-65.
18. Young DS, *Effects of Drugs on Clinical Laboratory Tests*, 5th ed, Volume 1: Listing by Test, Washington, DC: AACC Press, American Association of Clinical Chemistry, 2000, Section 3, 753-7.
19. Ward G, McKinnon L, Badrick T, et al, "Heterophilic Antibodies Remain a Problem for the Immunoassay Laboratory," *Am J Clin Pathol*, 1997, 108(4):417-21.
20. Dayan CM, "Interpretation of Thyroid Function Tests," *Lancet*, 2001, 357:619-24.
21. Beck-Peccoz P, Persani L, Mantovani S, et al, "Thyrotropin-Secreting Pituitary Adenomas," *Metabolism*, 1996, 45(8 Suppl 1):75-9.
22. Hak AE, Pols HA, Visser TJ, et al, "Subclinical Hypothyroidism Is an Independent Risk Factor for Atherosclerosis and Myocardial Infarction in Elderly Women: The Rotterdam Study," *Ann Intern Med*, 2000, 132(4):270-8.
23. Takats IK, Peter F, Rimanoczi E, et al, "The Blood Spot Thyrotropin Method Is Not Adequate to Screen for Hypothyroidism in the Elderly Living in Abundant-Iodine Intake Areas: Comparison to Sensitive Thyrotropin Measurements," *Thyroid*, 2000, 10(1):79-85.
24. Feldkamp CS and Carey JL, "An Algorithmic Approach to Thyroid Function Testing in a Managed Care Setting. 3-Year Experience," *Am J Clin Pathol*, 1996, 105(1):11-6.
25. Kaplan LA and Sawin CT, eds, "Standard of Laboratory Practice: Laboratory Support for the Diagnosis and Monitoring of Thyroid Disease," Washington, DC: National Academy of Clinical Biochemistry, 1996, 1-55.
26. Vanderpump MP, Ahlquist JA, Franklyn JA, et al, "Consensus Statement for Good Practice and Audit Measures in the Management of Hypothyroidism and Hyperthyroidism," *BMJ*, 1996, 313(7056): 539-44.
27. Weetman AP, "Graves' Disease," *N Engl J Med*, 2000, 343(17):1236-48.
28. Martínez-Triguero ML, Hernández-Mijares A, Nguyen TT, et al, "Effect of Thyroid Hormone Replacement on Lipoprotein(a), Lipids, and Apolipoproteins in Subjects With Hypothyroidism," *Mayo Clin Proc*, 1998, 73(9):837-41.
29. Haddow JE, Palomaki GE, Allan WC, et al, "Maternal Thyroid Deficiency During Pregnancy and Subsequent Neuropsychological Development of the Child," *N Engl J Med*, 1999, 341(8):549-55.
30. Utiger RD, "Maternal Hypothyroidism and Fetal Development," *N Engl J Med*, 1999, 341(8):601-2.
31. Sawin CT, Geller A, Wolf PA, et al, "Low Serum Thyrotropin Concentrations as a Risk Factor for Atrial Fibrillation in Older Patients," *N Engl J Med*, 1994, 331(19):1249-52.
32. Gangemi D, Ponzetto M, Scarafiotti C, et al, "Atrial Fibrillation and Thyroid Function in Elderly Hospitalized Subjects," *J Endocrinol Invest*, 1999, 22(10 Suppl):43.

References

Bahn RS and Heufelder AE, "Pathogenesis of Graves' Ophthalmopathy," *N Engl J Med*, 1993, 329(20):1468-75.

Beck-Peccoz P, Brucker-Davis F, Persani L, et al, "Thyrotropin-Secreting Pituitary Tumors," *Endocr Rev*, 1996, 17(6):610-38.

Greenspan SL and Greenspan FS, "The Effect of Thyroid Hormone on Skeletal Integrity," *Ann Intern Med*, 1999, 130(9):750-8.

Helfand M, "More on Screening for Mild Thyroid Failure," *JAMA*, 1997, 277(6):458-9.

Helfand M and Redfern CC, "Screening for Thyroid Disease: An Update," *Ann Intern Med*, 1998, 129:144-58.

Howanitz JH, "Review of the Influence of Polypeptide Hormone Forms on Immunoassay Results," *Arch Pathol Lab Med*, 1993, 117(4):369-72.

Kaplan MM, "Clinical Perspectives in the Diagnosis of Thyroid Disease," *Clin Chem*, 1999, 45(8 Pt 2):1377-83.

Lindsay RS and Toft AD, "Hypothyroidism," *Lancet*, 1997, 349:413-7.

Madsen JR and Karluk D, "A 71-Year-Old Woman With an Enlarging Pituitary Mass," Case Records of the Massachusetts General Hospital, Case 34-2000, Scully RE, Mark EJ, McNeely WF, et al, eds, *N Engl J Med*, 2000, 343(19):1399-406.

Martinez M, Derksen D, and Kapsner P, "Making Sense of Hypothyroidism. An Approach to Testing and Treatment," *Postgrad Med*, 1993, 93(6):135-8, 141-5.

Masters PA and Simons RJ, "Clinical Use of Sensitive Assays for Thyroid-Stimulating Hormone," *J Gen Intern Med*, 1996, 11(2):115-27.

McDermott MT and Ridgway EC, "Thyroid Hormone Resistance Syndromes," *Am J Med*, 1993, 94(4):424-32.

Smallridge RC, "Disclosing Subclinical Thyroid Disease. An Approach to Mild Laboratory Abnormalities and Vague or Absent Symptoms," *Postgrad Med*, 2000, 107(1):143-6, 149-52.

Woeber KA, "The Year in Review: The Thyroid," *Ann Intern Med*, 1999, 131(12):959-62.

♦ **Thyrotropin** see Thyroid Stimulating Hormone, Serum on page 282

Thyroxine Binding Globulin, Serum

Related Information

Free Thyroxine Index on page 177
T$_3$ Uptake, Serum or Plasma on page 279
Thyroxine, Free, Serum on page 285
Thyroxine, Serum on page 286

Synonyms T$_4$-Binding Globulin; TBG

Applies to Familial Dysalbuminemic Hyperthyroxinemia; Free Thyroxine Index, Calculated; Transthyretin

Abstract Serum thyroid binding proteins include albumin, transthyretin (thyroid binding prealbumin), and, most important, thyroxine binding globulin (TBG). As >75% of T$_3$ and T$_4$ are bound to TBG, any change, either genetic or acquired, in TBG concentration affects total T$_3$ and T$_4$ values. Abnormal total but normal free T$_3$ and T$_4$, in an euthyroid individual, suggests TBG deficiency or excess. In such circumstances, measurement of TBG may help to explain confusing results. TBG is a glycoprotein. Its abnormalities are not clinical diseases (ie, they do not themselves require treatment). **This test should not be confused with thyroglobulin.**

Patient Preparation No recent administration of radioactive isotopes or *in vivo* uptakes if method is by RIA.

Specimen Serum

Container Red top tube

Reference Interval The reference ranges are higher in children as compared to adults.

- 0-1 week: 3-8 mg/dL
- 1-12 months: 3-6 mg/dL
- 2-10 years: 2-5 mg/dL
- Adults: 1.2-2.5 mg/dL; adult levels are reached about age 14.

Use TBG is used to clarify thyroid function status in euthyroid individuals with increased binding by TBG, who have increased T$_4$ and normal levels of free hormones. It provides documentation of cases of hereditary deficiency or increase of TBG. In work-up of thyroid disease, in patients with low T$_4$, high T$_3$ uptake or the reverse, who clinically seem eumetabolic and have normal free T$_4$ or FTI, measurement of TBG is only occasionally needed. Some such patients may have hereditary anomalies of TBG. The most common explanation for increased TBG is increased endogenous or exogenous estrogens.[1] TBG is also increased by tamoxifen, pregnancy, perphenazine, and in some cases of liver disease, including infectious or chronic active hepatitis. Neonates and patients with acute intermittent porphyria have increased TBG. TBG is increased in about 50% of individuals who have prolonged history of heroin use or who are treated with methadone.[1] Increased TBG is found in certain genetically determined states, with a prevalence of 1 in 25,000.[2]

Decreased TBG is found with some instances of chronic liver disease, nephrotic syndrome, and systemic disease, and with large amounts of glucocorticoids and in acromegaly. Individuals on androgens or anabolic steroids remain euthyroid in spite of decreased TBG and T$_4$ concentrations.[1] Decreased TBG is also seen in cases of severe acidosis, large doses of aspirin, elevated testosterone, severe illness or certain inherited disorders. The reported prevalence of familial TBG deficiency is 1 in 5000.[3] Although alterations of TBG are usually resolved by the thyroid profile, TBG must occasionally be directly measured.

A number of drugs have been shown to effect thyroid function tests. Some of the common drugs which effect thyroid functions are listed in the following table.[4,5] Other references, on the effects of drugs on thyroid function, are also available.[1,6]

Kindreds are described with elevated TBG and hyperthyroxinemia as a harmless genetic abnormality. They have normal levels of TSH and free T$_4$ and decreased T$_3$ uptake. Structural variants of TBG are inherited as X-chromosome linked traits; most inherited structural abnormalities in TBG cause decreased affinity for thyroid hormone.[1] A number of families have been described with complete TBG deficiency. Although, in most of these individuals, TBG deficiency does not cause any thyroid dysfunction, TBG deficiency has been associated with hypothyroidism in a recent report.[7]

Effects of Some Drugs on Tests of Thyroid Function

Cause	Drug	Effect
Inhibit TSH secretion	Dopamine L-dopa Glucocorticoids Somatostatin	$\downarrow T_4$; $\downarrow T_3$; $\downarrow$TSH
Inhibit thyroid hormone synthesis or release	Iodine Lithium	$\downarrow T_4$; $\downarrow T_3$; $\uparrow$TSH
Inhibit conversion of T_4 to T_3	Amiodarone Glucocorticoids Propranolol Propylthiouracil Radiographic contrast agents	$\downarrow T_3$; $\uparrow$rT_3; $\downarrow$, $\longleftrightarrow$, $\uparrow T_4$ and FT_4; $\longleftrightarrow$, $\uparrow$TSH
Inhibit binding of T_4/T_3 to serum proteins	Salicylates Phenytoin Carbamazepine Furosemide Nonsteroidal anti-inflammatory agents Heparin (in vitro effect)	$\downarrow T_4$; $\downarrow T_3$; $\downarrow FT_4E$; $\longleftrightarrow$, $\uparrow FT_4$; $\longleftrightarrow$TSH
Stimulate metabolism of iodothyronines	Phenobarbital Phenytoin Carbamazepine Rifampicin	$\downarrow T_4$; $\downarrow FT_4$; $\longleftrightarrow$TSH
Inhibit absorption of ingested T_4	Aluminum hydroxide Ferrous sulfate Cholesytramine Colestipol Iron sucralfate Soybean preparations Kayexalate	$\downarrow T_4$; $\downarrow FT_4$; $\uparrow$TSH
Increase in concentration of T_4 binding proteins	Estrogen Clofibrate Opiates (heroin, methadone) 5-Fluouracil Perphenazine	$\uparrow T_4$; $\uparrow T_3$; $\longleftrightarrow FT_4$; $\longleftrightarrow$TSH
Decrease in concentration of T_4 binding proteins	Androgens Glucocorticoids	$\downarrow T_4$; $\downarrow T_3$; $\longleftrightarrow FT_4$; $\longleftrightarrow$TSH

$\downarrow$, reduced serum level; $\uparrow$, increased serum level; $\longleftrightarrow$, no change

Limitations TBG is normal in **familial dysalbuminemic hyperthyroxinemia**, an entity which can be incorrectly identified as thyrotoxicosis.[8] Low T_3 uptake and normal free T_4 or free T_4 index or thyroxine binding ratio often make measurement of TBG unnecessary.

Methodology Double antibody precipitation, radioimmunoassay (RIA)

Additional Information The usual thyroid function studies (eg, free T_4 and TSH) should be performed before considering this test. The major indication for TBG testing is in diagnosis of **hereditary deficiency of TBG**. Complete deficiency of thyroxine-binding globulin (TBG-CD) is defined as undetectable TBG in the serum of affected hemizygous subjects. Five distinct mutations have been identified in the TBG gene that cause this phenotype.[9] Most of these subjects with TBG deficiency can be expected to have low T_4 but normal TSH.[1] However, TBG deficiency can cause hypothyroidism.[7]

See Thyroxine, Serum on page 286.

Footnotes

1. Surks MI and Sievert R, "Drugs and Thyroid Function," N Engl J Med, 1995, 333(25):1688-94.
2. Komatsu M, Hanamura N, Seki T, et al, "A Family With Hereditary High Serum Thyroxine-Binding Globulin," Endocr J, 1994, 41(4):467-70.
3. Tojo K, Miura Y, Mori Y, et al, "Familial Thyroxine-Binding Globulin Deficiency Associated With Hyperthyroldism," Intern Med, 1995, 34(5):413-7.
4. Stockigt JR, "Thyroid Hormone Changes in Critical Illness: The Sick Euthyroid Syndrome," Diag Endo Metab, 1997, 15:39-46.
5. Whitley RJ, "Thyroid Function," Tietz Textbook of Clinical Chemistry, 3rd ed, Burtis CA and Ashwood ER, eds, Philadelphia, PA: WB Saunders Co, 1999, 1496-529.
6. Young DS, Effects of Drugs on Clinical Laboratory Tests, 5th ed, Volume 1: Listing by Test, Washington, DC: AACC Press, American Association of Clinical Chemistry, 2000, Section 3, 753-67.
7. Carrel AL and Allen DB, "Persistent Infantile Hypothyroidism Attributable to Thyroxine-Binding Globulin Deficiency," Pediatrics, 1999, 104(2 Pt 1):312-4.
8. Ruiz M, Rajatanavin R, Young RA, et al, "Familial Dysalbuminemic Hyperthyroxinemia: A Syndrome That Can Be Confused With Thyrotoxicosis," N Engl J Med, 1982, 306:635-9.
9. Carvalho GA, Weiss RE, Valdutiu AO, et al, "Complete Deficiency of Thyroxine-Binding Globulin (TBG-CD Buffalo) Caused by a New Nonsense Mutation in the Thyroxine-Binding Globulin Gene," Thyroid, 1998, 8(2):161-5.

References

Bartalena L, Bogazzi F, Brogioni S, et al, "Measurement of Serum Free Thyroid Hormone Concentrations: An Essential Tool for the Diagnosis of Thyroid Dysfunction," Horm Res, 1996, 45(3-5):142-7.

Langsteger W, Stockigt JR, Docter R, et al, "Familial Dysalbuminaemic Hyperthyroxinaemia and Inherited Partial TBG Deficiency: First Report," Clin Endocrinol (Oxf), 1994, 40(6):751-8.

Refetoff S, "Inherited Thyroxine-Binding Globulin Abnormalities in Man," Endocr Rev, 1989, 10(3):275-93.

Schussler GC, "The Thyroxine-Binding Proteins," Thyroid, 2000, 10(2):141-9.

♦ **Thyroxine-Binding Prealbumin** see Transthyretin, Serum on page 287

♦ **Thyroxine-Binding Protein Electrophoresis** see Thyroxine, Serum on page 286

♦ **Thyroxine by RIA** see Thyroxine, Serum on page 286

Thyroxine, Free, Serum

Related Information

Free Thyroxine Index on page 177
Newborn Screen for TSH, Filter Paper on page 231
Thyroid Stimulating Hormone, Serum on page 282
Thyrotropin Receptor Antibody, Serum on page 545
Thyroxine Binding Globulin, Serum on page 284
Thyroxine, Serum on page 286
Triiodothyronine, Serum on page 290

Synonyms Free T_4; Free Thyroxine; FT_4; T_4, Free; Unbound T_4

Applies to FTI

Abstract Free T_4 (FT_4) is a very small fraction of total thyroxine (0.03% to 0.04%); it is the metabolically active fraction and is precursor of T_3. Measurement of free T_4 is very helpful in patients who are suspected of having binding proteins changes, such as those in pregnancy and sex steroid therapy. It is less sensitive to changes in the serum binding proteins.[1]

Patient Preparation Recent injection of radioisotope may interfere, depending on assay system in use.

Specimen Serum

Container Red top tube

Storage Instructions Separate serum within 48 hours. Stable 2 weeks at 4°C.

Reference Interval Newborns: 2.6-6.3 ng/dL (SI: 33.5-81.3 pmol/L); adults: 0.8-2.7 ng/dL (10.3-35 pmol/L)

Use A sensitive test for thyroid function, free T_4 is increased with hyperthyroidism and decreased in hypothyroidism. It is a better indicator of thyroid function than total T_4 because it is not affected by changes in thryoxine-binding proteins. Free T_4 is indicated when binding globulin (TBG) problems are perceived, or when conventional test results are borderline or seem inconsistent with clinical observations. Free thyroxine is normal in subjects with high thyroxine binding globulin hormone binding who are euthyroid (ie, free thyroxine should be normal in nonthyroidal diseases). It should be normal in familial dysalbuminemic hyperthyroxinemia. FT_4 is used to assess the severity of hyperthyroidism (eg, when sTSH is suppressed). FT_4 or thyroxine clarifies patient status in situations such as secondary hypothyroidism related to pituitary damage. When sTSH, used as the primary screening test is suppressed and FT_4 is normal, measurement of serum T_3 is indicated.[2] The combination of low TSH with normal free T_3 or free T_4 occurs with ingestion of thyroxine as well as with subclinical hyperthyroidism.[3] A diagnostic strategy for diagnostic work up of thyroid disease using TSH and FT_4 can be found in Thyroid Stimulating Hormone, Serum on page 282.

Limitations As FT_4 is only a small fraction of total T_4, direct measurement of FT_4 in serum presents a considerable technical challenge. Most reliable methods (eg, equilibrium dialysis and ultrafiltration), which physically separate FT_4 from protein bound hormone, are too cumbersome for use in routine clinical laboratory. The results are misleading in the presence of antithyroxine autoantibodies and rheumatoid factor,[4] and with low molecular weight heparin treatment.[5] FT_4 is increased in familial dysalbuminemic hyperthyroxinemia, amiodarone treatment, states of resistance to thyroid hormone, and acute psychiatric illness.[3] Free T_4 will not detect T_3 thyrotoxicosis. Increased free T_4 levels may occur in subjects with nonthyroid diseases. Such elevations are described as transient.[6] Low values are reported in patients with nonthyroidal illness. Discrepancies in free T_4 levels between methods are recognized,[7,8] and discrepant results are still seen with extreme changes in binding proteins, nonthyroidal disorders, anticonvulsants, and some other drugs.[3] Concentrations of sTSH become abnormal before FT_4 levels do so, early in primary hypo- and hyperthyroidism.

Methodology Equilibrium dialysis is the reference method. Routinely used methods are radioimmunoassay (RIA), fluorescent immunoassay, and chemiluminescent immunoassay.

Additional Information Estimation of FT_4 and FTI has decreased over time, due to availability of more reliable free T_4 assays, but they still are in widespread use. Generally, the FTI and the free T_4 provide comparable information. Using a combination of thyrotropin and FTI as a gold standard for defining thyroid status, the Technicon Immuno-1 FT_4 method had a sensitivity of 100% and specificity of 98.3% for hyperthyroidism, versus 93.8% and 99.3%, respectively, for hypothyroidism.[9]

Subclinical hypothyroidism (normal FT_4 and elevated TSH or low FT_4 and normal TSH) is an independent risk factor for atherosclerosis and myocardial infarction,[10,11] and progression to overt hypothyroidism.[12]

In **subclinical hyperthyroidism** (TSH <0.3-0.4 µU/L with normal concentrations of free thyroxine and free triiodothyronine), there is increased risk for atrial fibrillation, osteoporosis, and progression to overt hyperthyroidism.[12]

Footnotes

1. Schussler GC, "The Thyroxine-Binding Proteins," Thyroid, 2000, 10(2):141-9.
(Continued)

Thyroxine, Free, Serum *(Continued)*

2. Klee GG and Hay ID, "Biochemical Thyroid Function Testing," *Mayo Clin Proc*, 1994, 69(5):469-70.

3. Dayan CM, "Interpretation of Thyroid Function Tests," *Lancet*, 2001, 357:619-24.

4. Norden AG, Jackson RA, Norden LE, et al, "Misleading Results From Immunoassays of Serum Free Thyroxine in the Presence of Rheumatoid Factor," *Clin Chem*, 1997, 43(6 Pt 1):957-62.

5. Stevenson HP, Archbold GP, Johnston P, et al, "Misleading Serum Free Thyroxine Results During Low Molecular Weight Heparin Treatment," *Clin Chem*, 1998, 44(5):1002-7.

6. Cooke RR and Pratt R, "Thyroid Function Tests in Acutely Ill Patients. Comparison of Analogue Based Free Thyroid Hormone Assays With Free Thyroxine Index," *Pathology*, 1986, 18(1):94-7.

7. Christofides ND, Wilkinson E, Stoddart M, et al, "Assessment of Serum Thyroxine Binding Capacity-Dependent Biases in Free Thyroxine Assays," *Clin Chem*, 1999, 45(4):520-5.

8. Wang R, Nelson JC, Weiss RM, et al, "Accuracy of Free Thyroxine Measurements Across Natural Ranges of Thyroxine Binding to Serum Proteins," *Thyroid*, 2000, 10(1):31-9.

9. Bock JL, Morris D, Cheng J, et al, "Evaluation of the Technicon Immuno 1 Free Thyroxine Assay," *Am J Clin Pathol*, 1996, 105(5):583-8.

10. Bruckert E, Giral P, and Chadarevian R, "Low Free-Thyroxine Levels Are a Risk Factor for Subclinical Atherosclerosis in Euthyroid Hyperlipidemic Patients," *J Cardiovasc Risk*, 1999, 6(5):327-31.

11. Hak AE, Pols HA, Visser TJ, et al, "Subclinical Hypothyroidism Is an Independent Risk Factor for Atherosclerosis and Myocardial Infarction in Elderly Women: The Rotterdam Study," *Ann Intern Med*, 2000, 132(4):270-8.

12. Woeber KA, "The Year in Review: The Thyroid," *Ann Intern Med*, 1999, 131(12):959-62.

References

Attia J, Margetts P, and Guyatt G, "Diagnosis of Thyroid Disease in Hospitalized Patients: A Systematic Review," *Arch Intern Med*, 1999, 159(7):658-65.

Bartalena L, Bogazzi F, Brogioni S, et al, "Measurement of Serum Free Thyroid Hormone Concentrations: An Essential Tool for the Diagnosis of Thyroid Dysfunction," *Horm Res*, 1996, 45(3-5):142-7.

Helfand M and Redfern CC, "Clinical Guideline Part 2. Screening for Thyroid Disease: An Update," *Ann Intern Med*, 1998, 129(2):144-58.

Kaptein EM, "Clinical Application of Free Thyroxine Determinations," *Clin Lab Med*, 1993, 13(3):653-72.

Surks MI and Sievert R, "Drugs and Thyroid Function," *N Engl J Med*, 1995, 333(25):1688-94.

Utiger RD, "Subclinical Hyperthyroidism - Just a Low Serum Thyrotropin Concentration, or Something More?" *N Engl J Med*, 1994, 331(19):1302-3

Internet Web Sites

www.thyroid.org/

♦ **Thyroxine Ratio** *see* T$_3$ Uptake, Serum or Plasma *on page 279*

Thyroxine, Serum

Related Information

Free Thyroxine Index *on page 177*
Heterophilic Antibodies *on page 191*
Lithium, Serum *on page 754*
Newborn Screen for TSH, Filter Paper *on page 231*
T$_3$ Uptake, Serum or Plasma *on page 279*
Thyroid Stimulating Hormone, Serum *on page 282*
Thyroperoxidase Autoantibody *on page 545*
Thyroxine Binding Globulin, Serum *on page 284*
Thyroxine, Free, Serum *on page 285*
Triiodothyronine, Serum *on page 290*

Synonyms T$_4$; Tetraiodothyronine; Thyroxine by RIA

Applies to Free Thyroid Index; FT$_4$I; Goiter; TBG; Thyroxine-Binding Protein Electrophoresis

Replaces T$_4$ CPB; Murphy-Pattee; PBI

Abstract Thyroxine (T$_4$) and triiodothyronine (T$_3$) are the major secretory products of the thyroid gland. T$_4$ is carried through the blood bound (in equilibrium) to thyroxine binding globulin (TBG), prealbumin, and albumin (>99.9%). T$_4$ secretion is stimulated by thyrotropin (thyroid stimulating hormone) (TSH). In peripheral tissues, thyroxine is converted to triiodothyronine (T$_3$), the active hormone.

Although very commonly used in assessing thyroid function, popularity of serum total T$_4$ as a laboratory test has waned, because it has been recognized that abnormal T$_4$ results occur in euthyroid individuals having altered thyroxine binding protein. Free T$_4$ and sTSH are recommended in preference to total T$_4$. Sensitive TSH assays are replacing T$_4$ as screening tests for evaluation of thyroid function.[1]

Thyroid hormones are required for growth and development.

Patient Preparation Avoid radioisotope administration prior to collection of specimen if testing is by RIA.

Specimen Serum

Container Red top tube

Storage Instructions Separate serum within 48 hours and refrigerate. Separated serum stable 1 week at 25°C.

Reference Interval Reference ranges may vary somewhat between laboratories. Values are much higher in the first few weeks of life and fall with age. Approximate ranges are found in the following table.[2]

Age	μg/dL	SI: nmol/L
1-3 d	11.8-22.6	152-292
1-2 wk	9.8-16.6	126-214
1-4 mo	7.2-14.4	93-186
4-12 mo	7.8-16.5	101-213
1-5 y	7.3-15.0	94-194
5-10 y	6.4-13.3	83-172
10-15 y	5.6-11.7	72-151
≥15 y	5.0-11.0	65-138

Normal range is increased in women on birth control pills, owing to increased TBG. Free thyroxine index and free T$_4$ will still be within the normal range. Normal range in pregnancy: approximately 5.5-16.0 mcg/dL (SI: 71-206 nmol/L).

Possible Panic Range At values <2.0 μg/dL (SI: <26 nmol/L), myxedema coma is possible. At values >20 μg/dL (SI: >257 nmol/L), thyroid storm is possible.

Use Following detection of abnormality of sTSH, laboratory testing may include T$_4$ or FT$_4$. As methods for FT$_4$ have improved in recent years, measurement of FT$_4$ over T$_4$ is preferred.[1] In lieu of FT$_4$, some laboratories perform **free thyroxine index**. If FT$_4$ assay is available, free thyroxine index measurement should be discouraged. See Free Thyroxine Index *on page 177.*

Those most likely to benefit from thyroid testing include the elderly, women in the postpartum state 4-8 weeks following delivery, patients with autoimmune disorders, and those with family history of thyroid disease.[3] **Decreased** in hypothyroidism, in genetically or acquired disorders (eg, nephrotic syndrome, chronic liver disease, GI protein loss), decreased thyroxine binding globulin (TBG), decreased thyroxine-binding prealbumin, drugs (phenytoin, carbamazepine), and in the third stage of (painful) subacute thyroiditis; **increased** with hyperthyroidism, peripheral resistance to thyroid hormone, drugs (amiodarone, amphetamines), with subacute thyroiditis in its first stage, with thyrotoxicosis due to Graves disease, with increased TBG (pregnancy, genetically increased TBG, acute intermittent porphyria, primary biliary cirrhosis), thyrotoxicosis factitia, and occasionally in euthyroid patients with familial dysalbuminemic hyperthyroxinemia. Used to diagnose T$_4$ thyrotoxicosis.

Primary hypothyroidism (hypometabolism) is caused by Hashimoto thyroiditis, idiopathic myxedema, prior radioactive iodine therapy for hyperthyroidism, prior thyroid surgery, endemic goiter, use of lithium carbonate, and other entities. Congenital causes include enzyme blocks and agenesis. Causes of **secondary hypothyroidism** include primary pituitary disease [eg, postpartum pituitary necrosis (Sheehan syndrome) and pituitary tumors]. The expression "myxedema" indicates advanced clinical hypothyroidism, with dermal mucopolysaccharide deposits. A diagnosis of primary hypothyroidism should be confirmed by sTSH assay.

Graves disease is classical thyrotoxicosis (hypermetabolism), an immune or autoimmune disorder. Other causes of **hyperthyroidism** include toxic multinodular or uninodular goiter, phases of thyroiditis, and a number of uncommon to rare entities which cause increased T$_4$.

T$_4$, sTSH, FT$_4$, and other tests are used to investigate **goiter**, an expression for thyroid enlargement, which may be found with hypothyroidism, euthyroidism, or hyperthyroidism.

Limitations T$_4$ may be increased with excess intake of iodine or with surreptitious use of thyroxine. T$_4$ levels may be abnormal in the presence of systemic nonthyroidal disease. Alterations in binding capacity or quantity of TBG may increase or decrease total thyroxine without causing symptoms. A cause of elevated T$_4$ in nonthyroidal disease is said to be liver disease.

Serum thyroxine is increased in **familial dysalbuminemic hyperthyroxinemia**, a euthyroid syndrome in which an abnormal binding site has affinity for thyroxine. The T$_3$ is usually normal in this entity, as is T$_3$ uptake. **Thyroxine-binding protein electrophoresis** on polyacrylamide gel can be used to characterize such proteins.[3]

T$_4$ is less sensitive than sTSH in the diagnosis of early primary hypothyroidism or hyperthyroidism.[1]

Euthyroid hyperthyroxinemia is an expression used as a collective term for nonthyroidal diseases and states which increase thyroxine levels with normal thyroid tissue and metabolism. In addition to congenital or acquired thyroid hormone binding globulin changes (excessive thyroid binding globulin, familial dysalbuminemic hyperthyroxinemia, and others[3]) and drug-related phenomena, peripheral resistance to thyroid hormones and increases related to medical and acute psychiatric illness are described. Hyperemesis gravidarum and hyponatremia may cause euthyroid hyperthyroxinemia.

Anti-T$_4$ antibodies may exist, interfering with T$_4$ and free T$_4$ determinations.

Contraindications T$_4$ alone as an initial screen is not advised.[4]

Methodology Radioimmunoassay (RIA), enzyme-linked immunosorbent assay (ELISA), fluorescence polarization immunoassay (FPIA), chemiluminescence immunoassay (CIA)

Additional Information The combination of the serum T$_4$ and free T$_4$ or T$_3$ uptake (an estimate of FT$_4$I) as an assessment of TBG, helps to determine whether an abnormal T$_4$ value is due to alterations in serum thyroxine binding globulin or to changes of thyroid hormone levels. The **free thyroid index** is T_4 x T_3 uptake. It is used as spinoff (reflex testing) to evaluate selected results from sTSH screening.[5] Deviations of both tests in the same direction usually indicate that an abnormal T_4 is due to abnormalities in thyroid hormone. Deviations of the two tests in opposite directions provide evidence that an abnormal T_4 may relate to alterations in TBG. Free T_4 assays are preferred over free thyroxine index. See Free Thyroxine Index *on page 177*.

Thyroid Tests With Disease and Varying TBG

Diagnosis	T_4	FT_4 (or FT_4I)	TSH
Normal	Normal	Normal	Normal
Hyperthyroidism	Increased	Increased	Decreased
Hypothyroidism	Decreased	Decreased	Increased
Increased TBG	Increased	Normal	Normal
Decreased TBG	Decreased	Normal	Normal

Causes of increased TBG binding include neonatal state, molar and conventional pregnancy, estrogens, oral contraceptives, heroin, methadone, 5-fluorouracil, clofibrate, infectious hepatitis, autoimmune hepatitis and primary biliary cirrhosis, acute intermittent porphyria, lymphoma, and hereditary TBG increase.

Causes of decreased TBG binding include abnormal protein states. These include nephrotic syndrome, androgens, anabolic steroids, prednisone, acromegaly, liver or other systemic illness, severe stress, and hereditary TBG deficiency. Salicylates, T_3, and diphenylhydantoin may lower T_4 significantly, and nicotinic acid appears to do so.[6] Amiodarone may cause increased thyroxine levels and can cause hypothyroidism or hyperthyroidism.

Lithium carbonate may cause goiter with or without hypothyroidism.

Carbamazepine (Tegretol®) and phenytoin are reported to cause decreased values of total thyroxine by displacing thyroxine from its binding proteins.[7,8]

This brief review must point out that clinical interpretation of patients' signs and symptoms has primary significance. Definitive treatment based on insufficient laboratory investigation is condemned.

Different strategies have been proposed for laboratory testing of thyroid function.[1] The American Association of Clinical Endocrinologists, the American Thyroid Association, and many others endorse sensitive TSH measurements as "the single best screening test" for thyroid disease.[1,5,9,10] The National Academy of Clinical Biochemistry recommends use of sensitive TSH as "the initial step in the diagnosis" of hypothyroidism.[11] The Royal College of Physicians of London recommends use of TSH and T_4 or FT_4.[12]

Relationships of drugs to thyroid testing and physiology have recently been updated.[7,8] See table in Thyroxine Binding Globulin, Serum *on page 284*.

Footnotes

1. Klee GG and Hay ID, "Biochemical Testing of Thyroid Function," *Endocrinol Metab Clin North Am*, 1997, 26(4):763-75.
2. Whitley RJ, "Thyroid Function," *Tietz Textbook of Clinical Chemistry*, 3rd ed, Burtis CA and Ashwood ER, eds, Philadelphia, PA: WB Saunders Co, 1999, 1496-529.
3. Smith SA, "Commonly Asked Questions About Thyroid Function," *Mayo Clin Proc*, 1995, 70(6):573-7.
4. Dayan CM, "Interpretation of Thyroid Function Tests," *Lancet*, 2001, 357:619-24.
5. Feldkamp CS and Carey JL, "An Algorithmic Approach to Thyroid Function Testing in a Managed Care Setting. 3-Year Experience," *Am J Clin Pathol*, 1996, 105(1):11-6.
6. Shakir KM, Kroll S, Aprill BS, et al, "Nicotinic Acid Decreases Serum Thyroid Hormone Levels While Maintaining a Euthyroid State," *Mayo Clin Proc*, 1995, 70(6):556-8.
7. Young DS, *Effects of Drugs on Clinical Laboratory Tests*, 5th ed, Volume 1: Listing by Test, Washington, DC: AACC Press, American Association of Clinical Chemistry, 2000, Section 3, 760-1.
8. Surks MI and Sievert R, "Drugs and Thyroid Function," *N Engl J Med*, 1995, 333(25):1688-94.
9. Garcia M, Baskin HJ, Feld S, et al, "AACE Clinical Practice Guidelines for the Evaluation and Treatment of Hyperthyroidism and Hypothyroidism," *Endocrin Pract*, 1995, 1:56-62.
10. Ladenson PW, Singer PA, Ain K, et al, "American Thyroid Association Guidelines for Detection of Thyroid Dysfunction," *Arch Intern Med*, 2000, 160(11):1573-5.
11. Kaplan LA and Sawin CT, eds, *Standard of Laboratory Practice: Laboratory Support for the Diagnosis and Monitoring of Thyroid Disease*, Washington, DC: National Academy of Clinical Biochemistry, 1996, 1-55.
12. Vanderpump MP, Ahlquist JA, Franklyn JA, et al, "Consensus Statement for Good Practice and audit Measures in the Management of Hypothyroidism and Hyperthyroidism," *BMJ*, 1996, 313(7056):539-44.

References

Brent GA, "The Molecular Basis of Thyroid Hormone Action," *N Engl J Med*, 1994, 331(13):847-53.

Dabon-Almirante CL and Surks MI, "Clinical and Laboratory Diagnosis of Thyrotoxicosis," *Endocrinol Metab Clin North Am*, 1998, 27(1):25-35.

Drake WM and Wood DF, "Thyroid Disease in Pregnancy," *Postgrad Med J*, 1998, 74(876):583-6.

Franklyn JA, "The Management of Hyperthyroidism," *N Engl J Med*, 1994, 330(24):1731-8.

Kaplan MM, "Clinical Perspectives in the Diagnosis of Thyroid Disease," *Clin Chem*, 1999, 45(8 Pt 2), 1377-83.

Rallison ML, Dobyns BM, Meikle AW, et al, "Natural History of Thyroid Abnormalities: Prevalence, Incidence, and Regression of Thyroid Diseases in Adolescents and Young Adults," *Am J Med*, 1991, 91(4):363-70.

Ruiz M, Rajatanavin R, Young RA, et al, "Familial Dysalbuminemic Hyperthyroxinemia: A Syndrome That Can Be Confused With Thyrotoxicosis," *N Engl J Med*, 1982, 306:635-9.

Staub JJ, Althaus BU, Engler H, et al, "Spectrum of Subclinical and Overt Hypothyroidism: Effect on Thyrotropin, Prolactin, and Thyroid Reserve, and Metabolic Impact on Peripheral Target Tissues," *Am J Med*, 1992, 92(6):631-42.

Surks MI and Ocampo E, "Subclinical Thyroid Disease," *Am J Med*, 1996, 100(2):217-23.

Toft AD, "Thyroxine Therapy," *N Engl J Med*, 1994, 331(3):174-80.

Tomer Y and Davies TF, "Infection, Thyroid Disease, and Autoimmunity," *Endocr Rev*, 1993, 14(1):107-20.

Wheetman AD, "Medical Progress: Grave's Disease," *N Engl J Med*, 2000, 343(17):1236-48.

Woeber KA, "The Year in Review: The Thyroid," *Ann Intern Med*, 1999, 131(12):959-62.

Wolf PG and Meek JC, "Practical Approach to the Treatment of Hypothyroidism," *Am Fam Phys*, 1992, 45(2):722-31.

Transthyretin, Serum

Related Information
C-Reactive Protein, Serum *on page 523*

Synonyms Prealbumin; Thyroxine-Binding Prealbumin

Abstract Transthyretin is a tryptophan-rich, tetrameric protein (54,000 daltons) synthesized primarily in the liver and, to a lesser extent, in the choroid plexus of the CNS. It migrates electrophoretically ahead of albumin, which is the reason for the term, **prealbumin**. Transthyretin has a relatively short half-life of ~48 hours. It functions as a serum transport protein for thyroxine, triiodothyronine, and the vitamin A/retinol binding complex, and it is a negative acute phase reactant. Transthyretin in plasma decreases in rapid response to diminished protein-calorie intake, being significantly decreased in a matter of 3-4 days. Levels return quickly to normal once adequate nutrition status is restored. Decreased serum levels also occur as a result of inflammation, malignancy, liver disease, kidney disease, or (Continued)

Transthyretin, Serum *(Continued)*

malnutrition. Increased levels may occur as a result of decreased renal function, transthyretin-producing tumor, or Hodgkin disease.

Patient Preparation Adults should fast overnight prior to specimen collection.

Specimen Serum or plasma may be used depending upon assay methodology.

Storage Instructions Specimen may be stored at 4°C for up to 72 hours, at -20°C for up to 6 months, and indefinitely at -70°C.

Causes for Rejection Lipemia or hemolysis depending upon assay methodology

Reference Interval Ranges reported in healthy adults generally span from 12-50 mg/dL (SI: 120-500 mg/L) with individual reference ranges dependent upon study populations and analytical methods.[1] The range in infants is approximately 4-19 mg/dL (SI: 40-190 mg/L)[2] with a gradual rise thereafter into childhood and puberty.[3] A cord blood range of 8.1-18.7 mg/dL (SI: 81-187 mg/L) has been reported, which was similar to the newborn (1-3 days old) range reported in the same study.[4]

Critical Values Concentrations in adults <11 mg/dL (SI: 110 mg/L) are considered high risk, requiring major nutritional intervention.[1] Moderate risk includes concentrations in the range of 11-17 mg/dL (SI: 110-170 mg/L), and little to no risk is associated with values >17 mg/dL (SI: >170 mg/L).

Use Transthyretin is used primarily as an indicator of nutritional status in adults, children, and newborns. Of the several circulating proteins sometimes used for this purpose (eg, albumin, transferrin, fibronectin, retinol-binding protein), transthyretin appears to be one of the best in terms of diagnostic sensitivity and specificity, largely due to its intermediate half-life and relative rapid response to changes in protein/energy homeostasis.[1,5,6,7,8,9,10,11]

Limitations Transthyretin has been shown in some studies to be insufficiently sensitive or of no additional value to standard methods for the assessment or monitoring of protein-calorie malnutrition.[12,13,14,15] Its plasma concentration is affected by conditions that alter its rate of synthesis, utilization, and excretion. Thus, decreased serum levels occur as a result of inflammation, malignancy, liver disease, and kidney disease, and increased levels may occur as a result of compromised renal function. The measurement of C-reactive protein together with transthyretin is sometimes used to rule in or out the presence of concomitant inflammation.

Methodology Rate immunonephelometry, particle-enhanced turbidimetric immunoassay, turbidimetric immunoassay, enzyme immunoassay (EIA), electroimmunoassay, and radial immunodiffusion (RID)

Additional Information There is no single, ideal marker for evaluation of the short-term response to nutritional therapy. A combination of assessments, in addition to plasma protein levels, is often required, including anthropometric measurements and determination of nitrogen balance. Transthyretin levels appear to reflect protein intake more than total energy intake,[16] possibly due to its relatively high essential-to-nonessential amino acid composition.

Footnotes

1. Bernstein LH, Leukhardt-Fairfield CJ, Pleban W, et al, "Usefulness of Data on Albumin and Prealbumin Concentrations in Determining Effectiveness of Nutritional Support," *Clin Chem*, 1989, 35(2):271-4.
2. Lee C, Berrett PG, and Richmond SA, "Determination of Serum Prealbumin (Transthyretin) by Competitive Enzyme Immunoassay," *Lab Med*, 1992, 23(7):473-6.
3. Malvy DJM, Poveda JD, Debruyne M, et al, "Laser Immunonephelometry Reference Intervals for Eight Serum Proteins in Healthy Children," *Clin Chem*, 1992, 38(3):394-9.
4. Raubenstine DA, Ballantine TVN, Greecher CP, et al, "Neonatal Serum Protein Levels as Indicators of Nutritional Status: Normal Values and Correlation With Anthropometric Data," *J Pediatr Gastroenterol Nutr*, 1990, 10(1):53-61.
5. Chwals WJ, Fernandez ME, Charles BJ, et al, "Serum Visceral Protein Levels Reflect Protein-Calorie Repletion in Neonates Recovering From Major Surgery," *J Pediatr Surg*, 1992, 27(3):317-21.
6. Winkler MF, Gerrior SA, Pomp A, et al, "Use of Retinol-Binding Protein and Prealbumin as Indicators of the Response to Nutrition Therapy," *J Am Diet Assoc*, 1989, 89(5):684-7.
7. Elhasid R, Laor A, Lischinsky S, et al, "Nutritional Status of Children With Solid Tumors," *Cancer*, 1999, 86(1):119-25.
8. Yoder MC, Anderson DC, Gopalakrishna GS, et al, "Comparison of Serum Fibronectin, Prealbumin, and Albumin Concentrations During Nutritional Repletion in Protein-Calorie Malnourished Infants," *J Pediatr Gastroenterol Nutr*, 1987, 6(1):84-8.
9. Bourry J, Milano G, Caldani C, et al, "Assessment of Nutritional Proteins During the Parenteral Nutrition of Cancer Patients," *Ann Clin Lab Sci*, 1982, 12(3):158-162.
10. Moskowitz SR, Pereira G, Spitzer A, et al, "Prealbumin as a Biochemical Marker of Nutritional Adequacy in Premature Infants," *J Pediatr*, 1983, 102(5):749-53.
11. Smith FR, Suskind R, Thanangkul O, et al, "Plasma Vitamin A, Retinol-Binding Protein and Prealbumin Concentrations in Protein-Calorie Malnutrition. III. Response to Varying Dietary Treatments," *Am J Clin Nutr*, 1975, 28:732-8.
12. Nadeau L, Forest JC, Masson M, et al, "Biochemical Markers in the Assessment of Protein-Calorie Malnutrition in Premature Neonates," *Clin Chem*, 1986, 32(7):1269-73.
13. Rettmer RL, Williamson JC, Labbe RF, et al, "Laboratory Monitoring of Nutritional Status in Burn Patients," *Clin Chem*, 1992, 38(3):334-7.
14. Elmore MF, Wagner DR, Knoll DM, et al, "Developing an Effective Adult Nutrition Screening Tool for a Community Hospital," *J Am Diet Assoc*, 1994, 94(10):1113-8, 1121.
15. Ferguson RP, O'Connor P, Crabtree B, et al, "Serum Albumin and Prealbumin as Predictors of Clinical Outcomes of Hospitalized Elderly Nursing Home Residents," *J Am Geriatr Soc*, 1993, 41(5):545-9.
16. Polberger SKT, Fex GA, Axelsson IE, et al, "Eleven Plasma Proteins as Indicators of Protein Nutritional Status in Very Low Birth Weight Infants," *Pediatrics*, 1990, 86(6):916-21.

References

Benjamin DR, "Laboratory Tests and Nutritional Assessment," *Pediatr Clin North Am*, 1989, 36(1):139-61.
Holownia P, Newman DJ, Thakkar H, et al, "Development and Validation of an Automated Latex-Enhanced Immunoassay for Prealbumin," *Clin Chem*, 1998, 44(6 Pt 1):1316-24.
Spiekerman AM, "Proteins Used in Nutritional Assessment," *Clin Lab Med*, 1993, 13(2):353-69.
Ulicny KS and Hiratzka LF, "Nutrition and the Cardiac Surgical Patient," *Chest*, 1992, 101(3):836-42.

- ◆ **TRH Stimulation Test** *see* Thyroid Stimulating Hormone, Serum *on page 282*
- ◆ **Triacylglycerol Acylhydrolase** *see* Lipase, Serum *on page 212*
- ◆ **Triacylglycerols** *see* Triglycerides, Serum or Plasma *on page 288*
- ◆ **Triglycerides** *see* Lipids, Overview *on page 213*

Triglycerides, Serum or Plasma

Related Information

Apolipoprotein A-I, Serum *on page 109*
Apolipoprotein B-100, Serum *on page 109*
Cholesterol, Total, Serum or Plasma *on page 146*
Glycated Hemoglobin (Hemoglobin A$_{1c}$), Blood *on page 188*
High Density Lipoprotein Cholesterol, Serum *on page 192*
Lipid Panel, Serum *on page 212*
Lipids, Overview *on page 213*
Low Density Lipoprotein Cholesterol *on page 218*

Synonyms Triacylglycerols

Applies to Chylomicrons; Friedewald Equation; HDL:LDL Cholesterol; LDL Cholesterol:HDL Cholesterol; VLDL

Test Includes In efforts to identify individuals at risk for coronary heart disease (CHD), triglycerides are included in the lipid profiles (lipoprotein analyses) of most laboratories.

Abstract Triglycerides (TG) are a family of complex lipids composed of glycerol esterified with three fatty acids (saturated or unsaturated) of the same or different lengths. Triglycerides are not soluble in blood and are therefore transported as chylomicrons (TG from exogenous source) or as VLDL (TG from endogenous source). Triglycerides constitute 95% of tissue storage fat. See Lipids, Overview *on page 213*.

Patient Preparation The patient should be fasting for 10-14 hours and should be on a stable diet 3 weeks prior to collection of blood. Alcohol should be avoided for 3 days and strenuous exercise for at least 24 hours prior to collection of blood. See Preparation in Cholesterol, Total, Serum or Plasma *on page 146*.

Specimen Serum or plasma

Container Red top tube; lavender top (EDTA) tube is used by some outstanding laboratories.

Storage Instructions 4°C; long-term at -70°C, a 2.8% decrease/year takes place.[1]

Causes for Rejection Specimen collected in a glycerinated tube, nonfasting specimen

Reference Interval Although fasting TG levels of 100-200 mg/dL (SI: 1.13-2.26 mmol/L) have been considered normal by the National Cholesterol Education Program, such levels indicate increased risk for CHD. New coronary arterial events are increased in patients whose triglyceride concentrations are 100-199 mg/dL (SI: 1.13-2.25 mmol/L).[2,3] Although a cutoff >100 mg/dL (SI: >1.13 mmol/L) has been proposed,[2,3] generally that level is lower than widely accepted reference ranges.

The following tables are based on plasma triglycerides. Triglyceride values increase with aging. With cholesterol values within normal ranges, triglyceride levels <250 mg/dL (SI: <2.82 mmol/L) (90th percentile) were not thought to be related to risk.

Reference Values for Plasma Triglycerides for White Males* (mg/L)

Age (y)	Percentile			
	5	50	90	95
0-9	300	550	850	1000
10-14	300	650	1000	1250
15-19	350	800	1200	1500
20-24	450	1000	1650	2000
25-29	450	1150	2000	2500
30-34	500	1300	2150	2650
35-39	550	1450	2500	3200
40-54	550	1500	2500	3200
55-64	600	1400	2350	2900
65+	550	1350	2100	2600

*Adapted from the LRC Prevalence Study (North America).

Reference Values for Plasma Triglycerides for White Females* (mg/L)

Age (y)	Percentile			
	5	50	90	95
0-9	350	600	950	1100
10-19	400	750	1150	1300
20-34	400	900	1450	1700
35-39	400	950	1600	1950
40-44	450	1050	1700	2100
45-49	450	1100	1850	2300
50-54	550	1200	1900	2400
55-64	550	1250	2000	2500
65+	600	1300	2050	2400

*Adapted from the LRC Prevalence Study (North America).

Reference Values for Plasma Triglycerides for Black Males* (mg/L)

Age (y)	Percentile†			
	5	50	90	95
0-9	310	470	750	880
10-19	310	530	880	1020
20-29	–	710	1250	–
30-39	420	910	1660	2240
40-49	520	970	2150	2940
50-59	–	1050	–	–
60+	–	960	–	–

†5th and 95th percentiles not given if n <100; 90th percentile not given if n <75.

*Adapted from the LRC Prevalence Study (North America).

Reference Values for Plasma Triglycerides for Black Females* (mg/L)

Age (y)	Percentile†			
	5	50	90	95
0-9	330	500	830	940
10-19	360	600	950	1100
20-29	380	680	1180	1370
30-39	380	740	1290	1500
40-49	430	840	1530	1880
50-59	–	940	1760	–
60+	–	1060	–	–

†5th and 95th percentiles not given if n <100; 90th percentile not given if n <75.

*Adapted from the LRC Prevalence Study (North America).

The Copenhagen Male Study found an increase in the relative risk for ischemic heart disease of 1.0 for each increase in TG concentration >89 mg/dL (1 mmol/L).[4]

A 40% increase in TG, cholesterol, phospholipids, and free fatty acids is found in pregnancy.

Critical Values A goal of TG <200 mg/dL (SI: <2.26 mmol/L) is recommended for patients with diabetes mellitus.[5] Baseline TG concentrations are higher in subjects with multivessel stenosis.[3]

Use Evaluate turbid samples of blood, plasma, and serum; work-up of chylomicronemia; evaluate hyperlipidemia; occasional cases of diabetes mellitus and/or pancreatitis are detected by hypertriglyceridemia. High levels may occur with hypothyroidism, nephrotic syndromes (cholesterol alone or cholesterol and TG),[6] carbohydrate-sensitive hypertriglyceridemia, glycogen storage disease, and in hyperlipoproteinemias. Some alcoholics have hypertriglyceridemia which disappears with abstinence. Extremely high triglyceride levels may occur with alcohol abuse. Disturbances in triglyceride metabolism relate to diabetes and are an interactive risk factor for atherosclerotic disease.[7] Although the role of hypertriglyceridemia as a risk factor for coronary arterial disease has been somewhat controversial, men and women with low serum HDL cholesterol and high serum triglyceride concentrations have a higher relative risk of coronary artery disease (vide infra). The combination of low HDL and high TG is important to project outcome following coronary bypass.[8] In familial combined hyperlipidemia, hypertriglyceridemia may be found before hypercholesterolemia. Many knowledgeable authorities favor screening with lipid profiles, including triglycerides, for reasons discussed elsewhere in this listing and in other listings. In exogenous hypertriglyceridemia, chylomicrons float as a layer in the tube of refrigerated, stored serum. Triglyceride determination is needed with cholesterol and HDLC to calculate LDLC. The Friedewald estimation is addressed in Low Density Lipoprotein Cholesterol on page 218. This formula is valid when TG levels are <400 mg/dL (<10.4 mmol/L) without chylomicrons or floating beta VLDL, type III dyslipidemia.

Limitations If triglyceride is >400 mg/dL, LDL cannot be calculated accurately by the Friedewald equation, but direct methods to calculate LDL may be employed up to a triglyceride value of 1000 mg/dL; above this, beta quantification should be used.[9] Correction for free serum glycerol in critically ill patients or patients on hyperalimentation with glycerol-based solutions may be necessary in some enzymatic methods.[10] The most common cause of triglyceride increase is inadequate patient fasting, which is a cause for rejection of the specimen.

Methodology Enzymatic, colorimetric. A method for direct measurement of LDLC is available. In this procedure, HDL and VLDL are separated from LDL by a filter which traps antibody-coated latex beads. Several commercially available methods exist for direct measurement of LDLC.

Additional Information Classic research from the Framingham studies in the 1970s identified major risk factors for coronary artery disease as hypertension, high serum cholesterol concentrations, and cigarette smoking. Subsequent analyses from the Framingham heart study demonstrated that men and women with high serum triglyceride concentrations (>151 mg/dL, SI: >1.7 mmol/L) and low serum HDL concentrations have a significantly higher rate of coronary artery disease. This high risk group (high serum triglycerides, low serum HDL) appears independent of the major risk factors including low serum HDL concentrations.[11] The Helsinki Heart Study reported a 5 year randomized coronary prevention trial among dyslipemic, middle-aged men. This study found a relative risk of 3.8 for those men with an LDL cholesterol:HDL cholesterol ratio >5 and serum triglycerides >203 mg/dL (>2.3 mmol/L), compared with men with LDL cholesterol:HDL cholesterol ratios ≤5 and serum triglyceride concentrations ≤2.3 mmol/L. In individuals with TG >2.3 mmol/L and LDLC:HDLC ratio ≤5, relative risk was 1.2.[12] A similar European study[13] reported similar findings. Clearly, serum triglyceride concentration is a factor interacting with effects of cholesterol and HDL cholesterol. Variations in apolipoprotein A-I and triglyceride concentrations account for 66% of the population variance in serum HDL cholesterol concentrations.[14] Fundamental relationships observed between HDL cholesterol, apolipoprotein A-I, and triglyceride were unaltered by levels of factors under personal volition such as obesity, physical activity/inactivity, and smoking.[14] Triglycerides commonly increase with obesity and may increase with chronic renal or liver disease. A positive association exists between diabetes mellitus and hypertriglyceridemia. Extremely high triglyceride levels suggest the possibility of pancreatitis. **Chylomicronemia**, although associated with pancreatitis, is not accompanied by increased atherogenesis. Chylomicrons are not seen in normal fasting serum, but are found in the sera of normal subjects following a fatty meal as exogenous triglycerides. Left refrigerated, chylomicrons float to the surface of a sample overnight; VLDL remains in suspension. Triglyceride physiologically is carried mostly as very low density lipoproteins (VLDL). The triglyceride in VLDL is endogenous from hepatic synthesis.

When turbidity of blood, serum, or plasma is seen, triglyceride is often >350 mg/dL. **Fasting chylomicronemia** occurs with, but is not limited to, deficiency of apo-CII (apolipoprotein work-up). It occurs also with deficiency of **lipoprotein lipase.**

Healthy first-degree male relatives of subjects with type 2 diabetes mellitus exhibited postprandial lipid intolerance with fasting TG concentrations within normal limits. Their postprandial hypertriglyceridemia was substantial.[15]

Increased TG concentrations are found in women with the polycystic ovary syndrome.[16]

A positive association exists between gout and hypertriglyceridemia.

Hypertriglyceridemia is found in glycogen storage disease Ia with other abnormalities.[17]

Hypertriglyceridemia can result from the state which has been designated Type V dyslipoproteinemia, which occurs in adults and presents with fasting chylomicronemia and elevated VLDL levels. In these patients, a secondary factor such as alcohol, diabetes, drugs, obesity, or renal failure usually increased triglyceride values.

Drug effects have been recently extensively reviewed.[18] Some women on estrogens and high estrogen oral contraceptives have an increase of triglyceride. Increases occur with pregnancy, similar to those with oral contraceptives. Hypertriglyceridemia is associated with use of steroids, thiazide diuretics, and beta-adrenergic blocking agents. Rarely, tamoxifen has been associated with severe hypertriglyceridemia. Clomiphene has recently been reported to induce hypertriglyceridemia and pancreatitis.[19]

Footnotes

1. Shih WJ, Bachorik PS, and Haga JA, "Estimating the Long-Term Effects of Storage at -70°C on Cholesterol, Triglyceride, and HDL-Cholesterol Measurements in Stored Sera," *Clin Chem*, 2000, 46(3):351-64.
2. Miller M, Seidler A, Moalemi A, et al, "Normal Triglyceride Levels and Coronary Artery Disease Events: The Baltimore Coronary Long-Term Study," *J Am Coll Cardiol*, 1998, 31(6):1252-7.
3. Miller M, "Is Hypertriglyceridemia an Independent Risk Factor for Coronary Heart Disease? The Epidemiological Evidence," *Eur Soc Cardiol*, 1998, 19(Suppl H):H18-H22.

(Continued)

Triglycerides, Serum or Plasma (Continued)

4. Jeppesen J, Hein HO, Suadicani P, et al, "Triglyceride Concentration and Ischemic Heart Disease: An Eight-Year Follow-up in the Copenhagen Male Study," *Circulation*, 1998, 97(11):1029-36.
5. O'Brien T, Nguyen TT, and Zimmerman BR, "Hyperlipidemia and Diabetes Mellitus," *Mayo Clin Proc*, 1998, 73(10):969-76.
6. Orth SR and Ritz E, "The Nephrotic Syndrome," *N Engl J Med*, 1998, 338(17):1202-11.
7. Rifkind BM and Segal P, "Lipid Research Clinics Program Reference Values for Hyperlipidemia and Hypolipidemia," *JAMA*, 1983, 250:1869-72.
8. Lindén T, Bondjers G, Karlsson T, et al, "Serum Triglycerides and HDL Cholesterol - Major Predictors of Long-Term Survival After Coronary Surgery," *Eur Heart J*, 1994, 15(6):747-52.
9. Friedewald WT, Levy RI, and Fredrickson DS, "Estimation of the Concentration of Low-Density Lipoprotein Cholesterol in Plasma, Without Use of the Preparative Ultracentrifuge," *Clin Chem*, 1972, 18(6):499-502.
10. Jessen RH, Dass CJ, and Eckfeldt JH, "Do Enzymatic Analyses of Serum Triglycerides Really Need Blanking for Free Glycerol?" *Clin Chem*, 1990, 36(7):1372-5.
11. Castelli WP, "Epidemiology of Triglycerides: A View From Framingham," *Am J Cardiol*, 1992, 70(19):3H-9H.
12. Manninen V, Tenkanen L, Koskinen P, et al, "Joint Effects of Serum Triglyceride and LDL Cholesterol and HDL Cholesterol Concentrations on Coronary Heart Disease Risk in the Helsinki Heart Study - Implications for Treatment," *Circulation*, 1992, 85(1):37-45.
13. Assmann G and Schulte H, "Role of Triglycerides in Coronary Artery Disease: Lessons From the Prospective Cardiovascular Münster Study," *Am J Cardiol*, 1992, 70(19):10H-13H.
14. Patsch W, Sharrett AR, Sorlie PD, et al, "The Relation of High Density Lipoprotein Cholesterol and Its Subfractions to Apolipoprotein A-I and Fasting Triglycerides: The Role of Environmental Factors - The Atherosclerosis Risk in Communities (ARIC) Study," *Am J Epidemiol*, 1992, 136(5):546-57.
15. Axelsen M, Smith U, Eriksson JW, et al, "Postprandial Hypertriglyceridemia and Insulin Resistance in Normoglycemic First-Degree Relatives of Patients With Type 2 Diabetes," *Ann Intern Med*, 1999, 131(1):27-31.
16. Lobo RA and Carmina E, "The Importance of Diagnosing the Polycystic Ovary Syndrome," *Ann Intern Med*, 2000, 132(12):989-93.
17. Talente GM, Coleman RA, Alter C, et al, "Glycogen Storage Disease in Adults," *Ann Intern Med*, 1994, 120(3):218-26.
18. Young DS, *Effects of Drugs on Clinical Laboratory Tests*, 5th ed, Volume 1: Listing by Test, Washington, DC: AACC Press, American Association of Clinical Chemistry, 2000, Section 3, 781-801.
19. Castro MR, Nguyen TT, and O'Brien T, et al, "Clomiphene-Induced Severe Hypertriglyceridemia and Pancreatitis," *Mayo Clin Proc*, 1999, 74(11):1125-8.

References

Criqui MH, Heiss G, Cohn R, et al, "Plasma Triglyceride Level and Mortality From Coronary Heart Disease," *N Engl J Med*, 1993, 328(17):1220-5.

Hostetter AL, "Screening for Dyslipidemia, Practice Parameter" *Am J Clin Pathol*, 1995, 103(4):380-5.

Kihara S, Matsuzawa Y, Kubo M, et al, "Autoimmune Hyperchylomicronemia," *N Engl J Med*, 1989, 320(19):1255-9.

Maeda I, Hayashi S, Fushimi R, et al, "Error Detection of High Concentrations of Endogenous Free Glycerol in Determination of Serum Triglyceride With the TBA-80S Automated Discrete Analyzer," *Clin Chem*, 1992, 38(7):1376-7.

McQueen MJ, Henderson AR, Patten RL, et al, "Results of a Province-Wide Quality Assurance Program Assessing the Accuracy of Cholesterol, Triglycerides, and High-Density Lipoprotein Cholesterol Measurements and Calculated Low-Density Lipoprotein Cholesterol in Ontario, Using Fresh Human Serum," *Arch Pathol Lab Med*, 1991, 115(12):1217-22.

O'Meara NM, Lewis GF, Cabana VG, et al, "Role of Basal Triglyceride and High Density Lipoprotein in Determination of Postprandial Lipid and Lipoprotein Responses," *J Clin Endocrinol Metab*, 1992, 75(2):465-71.

Peterson CM, Jovanovic-Peterson L, Mills JL, et al, "The Diabetes in Early Pregnancy Study: Changes in Cholesterol, Triglycerides, Body Weight, and Blood Pressure," *Am J Obstet Gynecol*, 1992, 166(2):513-8.

Sady SP, Thompson PD, Cullinane EM, et al, "Prolonged Exercise Augments Plasma Triglyceride Clearance," *JAMA*, 1986, 256(18):2552-5.

Uiterwaal CS, Grobbee DE, Witteman JC, et al, "Postprandial Triglyceride Response in Young Adult Men and Familial Risk for Coronary Atherosclerosis," *Ann Intern Med*, 1994, 121(8):576-83.

Yeshurun D and Gotto AM Jr, "Hyperlipidemia: Perspectives in Diagnosis and Treatment," *South Med J*, 1995, 88(4):379-91.

♦ **Triiodothyronine Reverse** see Reverse T3, Serum *on page 274*

Triiodothyronine, Serum

Related Information

Free Thyroxine Index *on page 177*
Heterophilic Antibodies *on page 191*
Thyroglobulin, Serum *on page 281*
Thyroid Stimulating Hormone, Serum *on page 282*
Thyrotropin Receptor Antibody, Serum *on page 545*
Thyroxine, Free, Serum *on page 285*
Thyroxine, Serum *on page 286*

Synonyms T_3, Total; Total T_3; Triiodothyronine, Total

Applies to Free T_3; Free T_4

Abstract T_3 (triiodothyronine) is a thyroid hormone produced mainly (80%) from peripheral conversion of T_4 (a prohormone). T_3 has greater biological activity than T_4 and binds to thyroid binding globulin (TBG) less tightly than T_4. Only 0.3% exists in free form. When total or free thyroxine (T_4 or FT_4) are normal and TSH is low, high T_3 confirms triiodothyronine toxicosis.

Patient Preparation Avoid radioisotope administration prior to collection of specimen if RIA is used for assay.

Specimen Serum

Container Red top tube

Storage Instructions Separate serum within 48 hours. Stable up to 7 days at 25°C. Refrigeration is preferred. Stable for at least 30 days at -20°C.

Reference Interval Values in infancy and childhood are higher than in adults. Reference ranges also vary between different methods and populations. Published expected values are found in the following table.[1]

Age	ng/dL	SI: nmol/L
1-3 d	100-740	1.54-11.40
1-11 mo	105-245	1.62-3.77
1-5 y	105-269	1.62-4.14
6-10 y	94-241	1.45-3.71
11-15 y	82-213	1.26-3.28
16-20 y	80-210	1.23-3.23
20-50 y	70-204	1.08-3.14
50-90 y	40-181	0.62-2.79

Use This thyroid function test is indicated in patients with decreased sTSH and normal free thyroxine and/or total thyroxine levels. Useful in evaluation of hyperthyroid states, particularly in the diagnosis of T_3 thyrotoxicosis, in which T_3 is increased and T_4 is within normal limits. (See a diagnostic diagram in Thyroid Stimulating Hormone, Serum *on page 282*.) T_3 toxicosis is occasionally found in Graves disease. It occurs with a single toxic nodule, multinodular thyrotoxicosis, and following treatment with T_3 (Cytomel®).[2] It is increased in and helpful for confirmation of the diagnosis of conventional hyperthyroidism, in which commonly both serum T_3 and T_4 concentrations are increased. It is normal to slightly increased with familial dysalbuminemic hyperthyroxinemia. Recommended for patients with supraventricular tachycardia, for patients with fatigue and weight loss not otherwise explained, or for those with proximal myopathy, in whom T_4 concentrations are not elevated. It is also helpful in monitoring T_4 replacement therapy.

Limitations T_3 is decreased with nonthyroidal chronic diseases and influenced by the state of nutrition. It may be normal with thyrotoxicosis (thyroxine thyrotoxicosis).[3,4] Variations in TBG and other binding proteins can affect T_3. In these situations, free T_3 should be measured, as free T_3 is not altered with changes in TBG. It is decreased with nicotinic acid.[5] Increases may be found with use of oral contraceptives, pregnancy, and other binding protein abnormalities outlined in Thyroxine, Serum *on page 286*.

Contraindications T_3 **is not reliable for evaluation of hypothyroidism**, since T_3 typically remains normal in mild and moderate thyroid gland failure.

Methodology Radioimmunoassay (RIA), immunochemiluminometric assay, fluorescence polarization immunoassay (FPIA), fluorometric immunoassay

Additional Information Thyroid hormones exist in human plasma as free and bound forms (ie, free T_3 and free T_4, as well as bound T_3 and bound T_4). Less than 1% of total serum T_3 is in the free form. Serum concentrations of the free forms of T_3 and T_4 are regulated by feedback systems and appear to parallel rates of cellular uptake. Thus, the free hormone fraction determines the thyroid status of the individual. Essentially, bound fractions are unavailable to exert metabolic effects. Proteins that bind T_3 include thyroxine binding globulin, transthyretin, and albumin. As the serum concentrations of the binding proteins rise so does the total T_3, while the free T_3 fraction may be unchanged. Examples include pregnancy and estrogen therapy. Reduced total T_3 levels occur in drug therapy with androgens, prednisone, dexamethasone, and glucocorticoids. T_3 levels are also reduced in iodine deficiency, nonthyroidal illness, and anorexia nervosa.[2,3] T_3 has a higher metabolic potency relative to T_4. As ~33% of T_4 is converted to T_3, T_4 appears to have little intrinsic metabolic activity in humans. See table for comparison of T_3 with T_4.

Comparison of T_3 and T_4 in Humans

	T_3	T_4
Serum concentration		
total (µg/dL)	0.14	8.0
free (ng/dL)	0.4	1.6
Fraction of total serum hormone that is in the free form (%)	0.3	0.02
Distribution volume (L)	35	10
Fraction intracellular (%)	64	10-20
Half-life (days)	1	7
Production rate (µg/day)	33	80
Fraction directly from thyroid (%)	20	100
Relative metabolic potency	1	0.3

From Larsen PR, "The Thyroid," *Cecil Textbook of Medicine*, Vol 2, Wyngarden JB, Smith LH, and Bennett JC, eds, Philadelphia, PA: WB Saunders Co, 1992, 1250, with permission.

Increased T_3 often occurs in hyperthyroidism, but in ~5% of cases only T_3 is elevated, "T_3 toxicosis." Do not confuse T_3 with T_3 uptake; these are two different tests. The latter has been done very commonly as part of the usual thyroid profile.

Patients with hypothyroidism are usually treated with thyroxine (levothyroxine) only, but the studies have shown that in patients with hypothyroidism, partial substitution of triiodothyronine for thyroxine may improve mood and neuropsychological function.[6]

Footnotes

1. Whitley RJ, "Thyroid Function," *Tietz Textbook of Clinical Chemistry*, 3rd ed, Burtis CA and Ashwood ER, eds, Philadelphia, PA: WB Saunders Co, 1999, 1496-529.
2. Kaplan MM, "Clinical Perspectives in the Diagnosis of Thyroid Disease," *Clin Chem*, 1999, 45(8 Pt 2):1377-83.
3. Dabon-Almirante CL and Surks MI, "Clinical and Laboratory Diagnosis of Thyrotoxicosis," *Endocrinol Metab Clin North Am*, 1998, 27(1):25-35.
4. Woeber KA, "Thyrotoxicosis and the Heart," *N Engl J Med*, 1992, 327(2):94-8.
5. Shakir KM, Kroll S, Aprill BS, et al, "Nicotinic Acid Decreases Serum Thyroid Hormone Levels While Maintaining a Euthyroid State," *Mayo Clin Proc*, 1995, 70(6):556-8.
6. Bunevicius R, Kazanavicius G, Zalinkevicius R, et al, "Effects of Thyroxine as Compared With Thyroxine Plus Triiodothyronine in Patients With Hypothyroidism," *N Engl J Med*, 1999, 340(6):424-9.

References

Attia J, Margetts P, and Guyatt G, "Diagnosis of Thyroid Disease in Hospitalized Patients: A Systematic Review," *Arch Intern Med*, 1999, 159(7):658-65.

Dayan CM, "Interpretation of Thyroid Function Tests," *Lancet*, 2001, 357:619-24.

Franklyn JA, "The Management of Hyperthyroidism," *N Engl J Med*, 1994, 330(24):1731-8.

Helfand M and Redfern CC, "Screening for Thyroid Disease: An Update," *Ann Intern Med*, 1998, 129:144-58.

Klee GG, "Clinical Usage Recommendations and Analytic Performance Goals for Total and Free Triiodothyronine Measurements," *Clin Chem*, 1996, 42(1):155-9.

Motomura K and Brent GA, "Mechanisms of Thyroid Hormone Action. Implications for the Clinical Manifestation of Thyrotoxicosis," *Endocrinol Metab Clin North Am*, 1998, 27(1):1-23.

Runnels BL, Garry PJ, Hunt WC, et al, "Thyroid Function in a Healthy Elderly Population: Implications for Clinical Evaluation," *J Gerontol*, 1991, 46(1):B39-44.

Utiger RD, "Altered Thyroid Function in Nonthyroidal Illness and Surgery. To Treat or Not to Treat?" *N Engl J Med*, 1995, 333(23):1562-3.

Woeber KA, "The Year in Review: The Thyroid," *Ann Intern Med*, 1999, 131(12):959-62.

Troponins, Serum

Related Information

Cardiac Markers: Laboratory Assessment, Overview *on page 137*
Creatine Kinase Isoenzymes/Isoforms, Serum *on page 157*
Creatine Kinase, Serum *on page 158*
Heterophilic Antibodies *on page 191*
Myoglobin, Blood, Serum, or Plasma *on page 228*

Synonyms Cardiac Troponin; TnI (Troponin I); TnT (Troponin T)

Applies to Troponin C; Troponin I; Troponin T

Replaces LDH; LDH Isoenzymes

Abstract The first test for immediate recognition of chest pain is the electrocardiogram, a tool which has limitations in sensitivity. Cardiac **troponin I (TnI)**, superior to **troponin T (TnT)**, is very useful in the diagnosis of acute myocardial injury because it provides a high degree of cardiac specificity and provides better sensitivity than CK-MB or myoglobin.[1] TnT may be increased in patients with chronic renal failure, acute trauma involving muscle, rhabdomyolysis, polymyositis, or dermatomyositis. This nonspecificity is not shared by TnI. Cardiac TnI is alone among markers for myocardial injury which is not expressed in a regenerative phase of striated (skeletal) muscle. Thus, troponin I is the laboratory marker of choice for assessment of acute coronary syndromes. The presence of any level provides evidence of necrosis of myocardial tissue.[2] Use of troponin I provides simpler, more cost-effective care than routine application of echocardiography for diagnosis of acute myocardial infarct.[3] The need for serial measurements of cardiac enzymes and isoenzymes is stressed.

Noncardiac diseases must be considered in those with chest pain and normal concentrations of troponins.

Specimen Serum, plasma

Container Red top tube, green top (lithium heparin) tube

Sampling Time Serial sampling, tracking sequential increases and decreases in analyte concentration is optimal for troponin I as it is for CK, CK-MB, myoglobin, and LDH and LDH isoenzymes to document or rule out acute myocardial infarct (AMI). Baseline, 3-, 6-, and 12-hour testing has

been advocated for myoglobin, CK-MB, and TnI. New episodes of pain cause the clock to start again.[2] TnI rise is similar to that of CK-MB but its more prolonged elevation (of several days) provides a desirable kinetic feature. It sometimes may be detected even before CK-MB.

Storage Instructions Serum stable 4 days at 4°C.

Causes for Rejection Specimen hemolyzed

Turnaround Time Use of plasma decreases turnaround time.[4]

Reference Interval Depends on method; undetectable[2]

Critical Values TnI: >1.5 ng/mL. Timing and results of the rise and fall in serial sampling are more important than cutoff values.

Possible Panic Range Any elevation of troponin concentration is considered abnormal.

Use Diagnose AMI and minor myocardial cell damage from a few hours after onset of symptoms to as long as 5-7 days. CK-MB may be more sensitive in some cases during the first 4 hours after onset of chest pain. Troponin remains increased longer than CK-MB and is more cardiac specific. Its superior specificity over CK-MB in detection of perioperative myocardial injury or AMI is documented. Troponin I may be warranted following even minor trauma when the differential diagnosis includes AMI. Combined with myoglobin, troponin I provides satisfactory analytical turnaround time.[5] TnI is used as a sensitive risk stratification marker in subjects with unstable angina. TnI provides a sensitive indicator of unstable angina when it is slightly increased without positive results for any other cardiac marker.[6,7]

Limitations Chemical markers do not signal an infarct beginning to take place at the moment of sampling. A single determination may be misleading. A bedside assay for cardiac troponin T is qualitative. For instance, it may not detect reinfarction.[8] Fibrin strands in serum may cause unanticipated fluctuations,[9] a problem which can be avoided by the use of plasma.[4] Heterotopic antibodies have caused problems.

TnT may be increased in patients with renal failure, muscle injury, disease or rhabdomyolysis. This nonspecificity is not shared by TnI. Troponin T provides no advantage over that of troponin I.

Troponin I provides cardiospecificity but may be detected in patients with causes of myocardial necrosis other than AMI (eg, myocarditis, trauma, scleroderma).

The troponins are not helpful in detection of repeated episodes of injury of myocardium.

Methodology Enzyme immunoassay (EIA), one-step;[10] double monoclonal sandwich enzyme immunoassay (EIA); fluorescent immunoassay

Additional Information The contractile proteins of the myofibril include the regulatory protein, troponin. Troponin is a complex of three proteins, **troponin C** (the calcium-binding subunit, molecular weight 18 kD), **troponin I** (the actomyosin-adenosine triphosphatase-inhibiting subunit, molecular weight 26.5 kD), and **troponin T** (the tropomysin-binding subunit, molecular weight 39 kD). The distribution of these isoforms varies between cardiac muscle and slow- and fast-twitch skeletal muscle. Their importance lies in the fact that some isoforms show a high degree of cardiac specificity. The measurement of troponin I has become the most important addition to the clinical laboratory assessment of myocardial injury.

Antman et al evaluated cardiac troponin T as a bedside assay for AMI. They found it rapid and sensitive.[8] However, they did not compare it to quantitative laboratory assay for troponin I or several other useful markers.[11]

Troponin I assays have excellent diagnostic accuracy of AMI following noncardiac surgery. The assay avoids many of the false positives seen with use of CK-MB.[3] Troponin I assays may be performed rapidly to provide suitable emergency room application. Wide application of TnI, CK-MB, and myoglobin is taking place.

Increased risk is recognized for patients who lack other criteria for AMI but have elevation of troponin concentrations. Increased TnI in subjects with unstable angina is a predictor of adverse prognosis.

A study advocating cost-effectiveness has recommended use of troponin I in a subset of higher risk patients, in whom CK-MB is normal and early exercise testing is not an option.[12]

Footnotes

1. Feng YJ, Chen C, Fallon JT, et al, "Comparison of Cardiac Troponin I, Creatine Kinase-MB, and Myoglobin for Detection of Acute Ischemic Myocardial Injury in a Swine Model," *Am J Clin Pathol*, 1998, 110(1):70-7.
2. Keffer JH, "Assessment of Myocardial Injury," *The Handbook of Clinical Pathology*, 2nd ed, Chapter 17, McKenna RW and Keffer JH, eds, Chicago, IL: ASCP Press, American Society of Clinical Pathologists, 2000, 235-44.
3. Adams JE 3rd, Sicard GA, Allen BT, et al, "Diagnosis of Perioperative Myocardial Infarction With Measurement of Cardiac Troponin I," *N Engl J Med*, 1994, 330(10):670-4.
4. Plebani M and Zaninotto M, "Diagnostic Strategies Using Myoglobin Measurement in Myocardial Infarction," *Clin Chim Acta*, 1998, 272(1):69-77.
5. Plebani M and Zaninotto M, "The Author's Reply," *Am J Clin Pathol*, 2000, 113(4):593.
6. Caragher TE, Fernandez BB, and Barr LA, "Long-Term Experience With an Accelerated Protocol for Diagnosis of Chest Pain," *Arch Pathol Lab Med*, 2000, 124(10):1434-9.
7. Sobel BE and LeWinter MM, "Ingenuous Interpretation of Elevated Blood Levels of Macromolecular Markers of Myocardial Injury: A Recipe for Confusion," *J Am Coll Cardiol*, 2000, 35(5):1355-8.
8. Antman EM, Grudzien C, and Sacks DB, "Evaluation of a Rapid Bedside Assay for Detection of Serum Cardiac Troponin T," *JAMA*, 1995, 273(16):1279-82.

(Continued)

Troponins, Serum (Continued)

9. Burdick CO, "Suspected Myocardial Infarction," *Am J Clin Pathol*, 2000, 113(4):592-3.
10. Katus HA, Looser S, Hallermayer K, et al, "Development and *In Vitro* Characterization of A New Immunoassay of Cardiac Troponin T," *Clin Chem*, 1992, 38(3):386-93.
11. Borzak S, "Bedside Serum Cardiac Troponin T Analysis Was Sensitive for Myocardial Infarction," *ACP J Club*, 1995, 123(3):72.
12. Polaczyk CA, Kuntz KM, Sacks DB, et al, "Emergency Department Triage Strategies for Acute Chest Pain Using Creatine Kinase-MB and Troponin I Assays: A Cost-Effectiveness Analysis," *Ann Intern Med*, 1999, 131(12):909-18.

References

Carrier M, Pelletier LC, Martineau R, et al, "In Elective Coronary Artery Bypass Grafting, Preoperative Troponin T Level Predicts the Risk of Myocardial Infarction," *J Thorac Cardiovasc Surg*, 1998, 115(6):1328-34.

del Rey JM, Madrid AH, Valino JM, et al, "Cardiac Troponin I and Minor Cardiac Damage: Biochemical Markers in a Clinical Model of Myocardial Lesions," *Clin Chem*, 1998, 44(11):2270-6.

De Paulis R, Colagrande L, Seddio F, et al, "Levels of Troponin I and Cardiac Enzymes After Reinfusion of Shed Blood in Coronary Operations," *Ann Thorac Surg*, 1998, 65(6):1617-20.

Edouard AR, Mimoz O, Sami K, et al, "Circulating Cardiac Troponin I in Trauma Patients Without Cardiac Contusion," *Intensive Care Med*, 1998, 24(6):569-73.

Fulda GJ, Giberson F, Hailstone D, et al, "An Evaluation of Serum Troponin T and Signal-Averaged Electrocardiography in Predicting Electrocardiographic Abnormalities After Blunt Chest Trauma," *J Trauma*, 1997, 43(2):304-10.

Gensini GF, Fusi C, Conti AA, et al, "Cardiac Troponin I and Q-Wave Perioperative Myocardial Infarction After Coronary Artery Bypass Surgery," *Crit Care Med*, 1998, 26(12):1986-90.

Keffer JH, "Myocardial Markers of Injury. Evolution and Insights," *Am J Clin Pathol*, 1996, 105(3):305-20.

Khan I, Tun A, Wattanasauwan N, et al, "Elevation of Serum Cardiac Troponin I in Noncardiac and Cardiac Diseases Other Than Acute Coronary Syndromes," *Am J Emerg Med*, 1999, 17(3):225-9.

Lee TH and Goldman L, "Evaluation of the Patient With Acute Chest Pain," *N Engl J Med*, 2000, 342(16):1187-95.

Martins JT, Li DJ, Baskin LB, et al, "Comparison of Cardiac Troponin I and Lactate Dehydrogenase Isoenzymes for the Late Diagnosis of Myocardial Injury," *Am J Clin Pathol*, 1996, 106(6):705-8.

Missov E and Mair J, "A Novel Biochemical Approach to Congestive Heart Failure: Cardiac Troponin T," *Am Heart J*, 1999, 138(1 Pt 1):95-8.

Newby LK, Christenson RH, Ohman EM, et al, "Value of Serial Troponin T Measurements for Early and Late Risk Stratification in Patients With Acute Coronary Syndromes," *Circulation*, 1998, 98(18):1853-9.

Olatidoye AG, Wu AH, Feng Y, et al, "Prognostic Role of Troponin T Versus Troponin I in Unstable Angina Pectoris for Cardiac Events With Meta-Analysis Comparing Published Studies," *Am J Cardiol*, 1998, 81(12):1405-10.

Ooi DS and House AA, "Cardiac Troponin T in Hemodialysis Patients," *Clin Chem*, 1998, 44(7):1410-6.

Porter GA, Norton T, and Bennett WB, "Troponin T, a Predictor of Death in Chronic Hemodialysis Patients," *Eur Heart J*, 1998, 19(Suppl N):N34-N37.

Rao AC, Collinson PO, Canepa-Anson R, et al, "Troponin T Measurement After Myocardial Infarction Can Identify Left Ventricular Ejection of Less Than 40 Percent," *Heart*, 1998, 80(3):223-5.

Roppolo LP, Fitzgerald R, Dillow J, et al, "A Comparison of Troponin T and Troponin I as Predictors of Cardiac Events in Patients Undergoing Chronic Dialysis at a Veteran's Hospital: A Pilot Study," *J Am Coll Cardiol*, 1999, 34(2):448-54.

Shivvers SA, Wians FH, Keffer JH, et al, "Maternal Cardiac Troponin I Levels During Normal Labor and Delivery," *Am J Obstet Gynecol*, 1999, 180(1 Pt 1):122-7.

Shyu K, Kuan P, Cheng J, et al, "Cardiac Troponin T, Creatine Kinase, and its Isoform Release After Successful Percutaneous Transluminal Coronary Angioplasty With or Without Stenting," *Am Heart J*, 1998, 135(5 Pt 1):862-7.

Stromme JH, Johansen O, Brekke M, et al, "Markers of Myocardial Injury in Blood Following PTCA: A Comparison of CK-MB, Cardiospecific Troponin T and Troponin I," *Scand J Clin Lab Invest*, 1998, 58(8):693-9.

Thygesen K and Alpert JS, "Myocardial Infarction Redefined - A Concensus Document of The Joint European Society of Cardiology/American College of Cardiology Committee for the Redefinition of Myocardial Infarction," The Joint European Society of Cardiology/American College of Cardiology Committee, *J Am Coll Cardiol*, 2000, 36(3):959-69.

Zaninotto M, Altinier S, Lachin M, et al, "Strategies for the Early Diagnosis of Acute Myocardial Infarction Using Biochemical Markers," *Am J Clin Pathol*, 1999, 111(3):399-405.

♦ **Troponin T** *see* Troponins, Serum *on page 291*

♦ **True Cholinesterase** *see* Acetylcholinesterase, Red Cell *on page 81*

♦ **Trypsin Activity, Stool** *see* Chloride, Sweat *on page 144*

♦ **Trypsin, Immunoreactive** *see* Amylase, Urine *on page 104*

♦ **Trypsinogen Activation Peptide** *see* Amylase, Serum *on page 102*

♦ **Trypsinogen, Immunoreactive** *see* Chloride, Sweat *on page 144*

♦ **Tryptophan** *see* Amino Acids, Urine *on page 101*

♦ **TSH** *see* Thyroid Stimulating Hormone, Serum *on page 282*

♦ **TSH, Filter Paper** *see* Newborn Screen for TSH, Filter Paper *on page 231*

♦ **Tubeless Gastric Analysis** *replaced by* Gastric Analysis *on page 180*

♦ **Tyrosine** *see* Amino Acids, Urine *on page 101*

♦ **Tyrosyluria** *see* Phenylalanine, Urine *on page 249*

♦ **UDP Galactose-4-Epimerase Deficiency** *see* Galactose-1-Phosphate Uridyl Transferase, Blood *on page 179*

♦ **uE₃** *see* Estriol, Unconjugated, Pregnancy, Serum, Plasma, or Urine *on page 171*

♦ **U-III-S** *see* Uroporphyrinogen III Synthase, Erythrocyte *on page 296*

♦ **Ultrasensitive TSH** *see* Thyroid Stimulating Hormone, Serum *on page 282*

♦ **Umbilical Arterial Blood Gases (pCO₂ and pO₂)** *see* Blood Gases and pH, Umbilical Cord *on page 121*

♦ **Unbound T₄** *see* Thyroxine, Free, Serum *on page 285*

♦ **Unconjugated Estriol, Pregnancy** *see* Estriol, Unconjugated, Pregnancy, Serum, Plasma, or Urine *on page 171*

♦ **Unconjugated Estrogen, Serum** *see* Estriol, Unconjugated, Pregnancy, Serum, Plasma, or Urine *on page 171*

♦ **U:P Ratio** *see* Osmolality, Urine *on page 236*

♦ **Urate** *see* Uric Acid, Serum *on page 293*

♦ **Urate, Urine** *see* Uric Acid, Urine *on page 295*

♦ **Urea Clearance** *replaced by* Creatinine Clearance *on page 160*

♦ **Urea Nitrogen Clearance** *replaced by* Creatinine Clearance *on page 160*

Urea Nitrogen:Creatinine Ratio

Related Information

Creatinine, Serum or Plasma *on page 161*
Osmolality, Serum *on page 236*
Urea Nitrogen, Serum or Plasma *on page 293*

Synonyms BUN:Creatinine Ratio

Test Includes Serum creatinine and urea nitrogen

Abstract The urea nitrogen:creatinine ratio is used with other investigation to attempt to distinguish between prerenal failure, intrinsic failure, and obstruction.

Increased ratio occurs with prerenal and postrenal disorders, while the ratio is normal in renal disease states. It is also relevant to transit of blood through the gastrointestinal tract.

Specimen Serum

Reference Interval 10-20 (up to 30 in infants); about 14 for a person on a normal diet. The ratio is usually normal with intrinsic renal failure.

Critical Values Ratio is generally >20:1 in prerenal failure (decreased renal blood flow, decreased perfusion), gastrointestinal bleeding, or in urinary tract obstruction

Use High BUN:creatinine ratio is found in overproduction or lowered excretion of urea nitrogen.[1] High ratios occur with prerenal azotemia[2] (eg, congestive heart failure), decreased renal perfusion, shock, volume depletion/hypovolemia, hypotension, and dehydration. High ratio with normal creatinine concentration may be found in catabolic states. Often the BUN:creatinine ratio is greatly elevated in gastrointestinal bleeding and with swallowed blood from the upper airway. A BUN:creatinine ratio >36 suggests upper gastrointestinal bleeding, whereas a ratio <36 is not helpful in locating the source of bleeding.[3] Correlation exists between upper GI bleeding, male gender, and age younger than 50 years. With consideration of age and gender, a ratio of 36 or more provided sensitivity about 90%, specificity 27%, positive predictive value 79%, and negative predictive value 57%.[4]

The ratio may be increased with high protein diet, with ileal conduit, and with urinary tract obstruction.[5] It may also be increased with tetracyclines or steroids. These conditions frequently occur with normal serum creatinine levels. In postrenal obstruction and in prerenal azotemia superimposed on renal disease a high BUN:creatinine ratio is present with elevated serum creatinine.

Low BUN:creatinine ratio may be found in low protein diet, malnutrition, pregnancy, severe liver disease, rhabdomyolysis, prolonged I.V. fluid therapy, ketosis (acetoacetic acid interferes with and falsely elevates creatinine), repeated hemodialysis, inappropriate secretion of antidiuretic hormone, with drugs which increase creatinine but not urea nitrogen (eg, cimetidine, trimethoprim), and with tetracycline use (antianabolic effect).[6]

Limitations Patients' variability in protein intake and mass of voluntary muscle can cause this ratio to be misleading.[2] It is only a preliminary guide.

Additional Information In hypovolemia, increased serum osmolality and sodium concentrations may be anticipated, as well as increased urea nitrogen:creatinine ratio.[7] See Osmolality, Serum *on page 236*, in which the urine:serum osmolality ratio and the sodium, serum:osmolality ratio are addressed.

Footnotes

1. Maher JF, "Disparity in BUN and Plasma Creatinine Test Results in Patient," *JAMA*, 1977, 237:2535.
2. Beck LH, "Hypouricemia in the Syndrome of Inappropriate Secretion of Antidiuretic Hormone," *N Engl J Med*, 1979, 301:528-30.

3. Richards RJ, Donica MB, and Grayer D, "Can the Blood Urea Nitrogen/Creatinine Ratio Distinguish Upper From Lower Gastrointestinal Bleeding?" *J Clin Gastroenterol*, 1990, 12(5):500-4.

4. Ernst AA, Haynes ML, Nick TG, et al, "Usefulness of the Blood Urea Nitrogen/Creatinine Ratio in Gastrointestinal Bleeding," *Am J Emerg Med*, 1999, 17(1):70-2.

5. Dossetor JB, "Creatininemia Versus Uremia: The Relative Significance of Blood Urea Nitrogen and Serum Creatinine Concentrations in Azotemia," *Ann Intern Med*, 1966, 65(6):1287-99.

6. Jurado R and Mattix H, "The Decreased Serum Urea Nitrogen-Creatinine Ratio," *Arch Intern Med*, 1998, 158(22):2509-11.

7. McGee S, Abernethy WB 3rd, and Simel DL, et al, "Is This Patient Hypovolemic?" *JAMA*, 1999, 281(11):1022-9.

References

Lindeman RD, "Assessment of Renal Function in the Old: Special Considerations," *Clin Lab Med*, 1993, 13(1):269-77.

Olsen LH and Andreassen KH, "Stools Containing Altered Blood-Plasma Urea: Creatinine Ratio as a Simple Test for the Source of Bleeding," *Br J Surg*, 1991, 78(1):71-3.

Urea Nitrogen, Serum or Plasma

Related Information

Bicarbonate, Blood *on page 115*
Creatinine Clearance *on page 160*
Creatinine, Serum or Plasma *on page 161*
Cystatin C, Serum or Plasma *on page 163*
Kidney Biopsy *on page 64*
Kidney Stone Analysis *on page 877*
Osmolality, Calculated, Serum or Plasma *on page 234*
Sodium, Serum or Plasma *on page 275*
Urea Nitrogen:Creatinine Ratio *on page 292*

Synonyms Blood Urea Nitrogen; BUN

Applies to Dialysis; Urea Reduction Ratio

Abstract The end product of protein metabolism, urea is synthesized by the liver. Easily filtered by renal glomeruli and highly diffusible, urea nitrogen reflects the ratio between urea **production** and **clearance**. Increased urea nitrogen may be due to increased production or decreased excretion. Although many use the expression "BUN," (for blood urea nitrogen), most laboratories use serum, occasionally plasma, but never whole blood.

Specimen Serum, plasma

Container Red top tube. Avoid fluoride and sodium citrate tubes if urease reaction is used and ammonium heparin tubes when conductimetric method is used. EDTA is suitable as well as lithium heparin for young children.

Collection Pediatrics: Blood drawn from heelstick for capillary (lithium heparin tube)

Storage Instructions Stable 1 day at room temperature, 3 days at 4°C to 8°C, and 3 months at -20°C.

Reference Interval 1 week: 3-25 mg/dL (SI: 1.07-8.9 mmol/L);[1] 1 year: 4-16 mg/dL (SI: 1.4-5.7 mmol/L); 1-40 years: 5-20 mg/dL (SI: 1.8-7.1 mmol/L); gradual slight increase subsequently occurs over 40 years of age. It is 8-23 mg/dL in subjects older than 60 years of age. It is decreased in pregnancy.

Possible Panic Range BUN >100 mg/dL (SI: >35.7 mmol/L) has been used in the definition of uremia.[2]

Use Useful to assess renal function, especially with serum creatinine. **High BUN** occurs in acute and chronic renal diseases. BUN is useful to follow hemodialysis and other therapy. (A highly diffusible molecule, urea falls rapidly with dialysis.) "Uremia" was defined by Luke as an expression of a constellation of signs and symptoms in patients with severe azotemia secondary to acute or chronic renal failure.[2] Other causes of increased BUN include severe congestive heart failure, increased protein catabolism, tetracyclines, diuretic use, hyperalimentation, ketoacidosis, shock, and dehydration. Even moderate dehydration can cause BUN to increase up to about 24 mg/dL, usually with normal creatinine concentrations.[1] It is dependent on renal blood flow and urine flow rates. Corticosteroids tend to increase BUN by causing increased protein catabolism. Bleeding from the gastrointestinal tract is an important cause of high urea nitrogen, commonly accompanied by disproportionate increase in BUN relative to creatinine (see Urea Nitrogen:Creatinine Ratio *on page 292*). Nephrotoxic drugs must be considered.

Borderline high values may occur after recent ingestion of high protein meal and with muscle wasting.

Low BUN occurs in late normal pregnancy, decreased protein intake, with intravenous fluids, with some antibiotics, and in severe liver damage. BUN has a role in assessment of nutritional support.

The BUN is especially important when creatinine values are misleading (eg, with certain cephalosporins). The BUN is superior to creatinine in assessing the function of the filter in hyperbilirubinemic patients undergoing hemodiafiltration for renal failure.[3]

In the syndrome of inappropriate secretion of antidiuretic hormone (SIADH), findings include hyponatremia with serum or plasma Na+ ≤128 mmol/L, serum hypo-osmolality, <260 mOsm/kg, with urine osmolality >300 mOsm/kg (SI: >300 mmol/kg) with low BUN. Such observations occur in situations in which patients are overhydrated. Clinical findings included absence of edema or evidence of heart, liver, thyroid, renal or adrenal disease.[4] Hypouricemia, with uric acid levels in 16 of 17 patients <4 mg/dL (SI: <238 µmol/L), is reported with the syndrome of inappropriate secretion of antidiuretic

hormone.[5] (SIADH can be seen with higher serum sodiums and higher osmolalities. Urine osmolality is greater than serum osmolality in SIADH.)[5,6]

BUN is needed to assess calculated osmolality. Osmolality (mOsm/kg H_2O) may be calculated as follows:

Osmolality = [Na+ (mmol/L) x 2] + urea N (mg/dL)/2.8 + glucose (mg/dL)/18

Limitations Creatinine is usually more specific for glomerular function but may be less sensitive to some types of early renal disease. Uremia and other types of renal dysfunction are best evaluated with creatinine as well as urea nitrogen. In both prerenal and postrenal azotemia, BUN is apt to be increased somewhat more than is creatinine. However, in a series of dehydrated children with gastroenteritis who had metabolic acidosis and increased anion gap, 88% had BUN concentration ≤18 mg/dL (SI: ≤6.4 mmol/L). The authors found bicarbonate and anion gap more sensitive indices in this setting.[7] In chronic progressive renal disease, about 75% of renal parenchyma must be damaged or destroyed before azotemia develops. BUN lacks sensitivity and specificity, but still remains a useful test. It is insensitive to early diminution of glomerular filtration rate.

Methodology Diacetyl monoxime; urease, Berthelot reaction; rate conductivity

Additional Information Although creatinine is generally considered a more specific test to evaluate renal function, BUN and creatinine are commonly used together. Luke points out that clinical renal failure is variable between individual patients.[2]

BUN before and following dialysis and between dialysis treatments is among the determinants of patients so treated. The **urea reduction ratio** (percent reduction in concentration of BUN during a dialysis treatment) is not as powerful as serum albumin as a predictor of death. Its calculation: $100 \times (1-[C_t/C_o])$; C_t is the BUN 5 minutes following the end of dialysis, C_o is predialysis BUN. This ratio bears relationship to blood clearance by dialysis, length of dialysis, and volume of distribution of urea in the patient. The ratio represents quantitation of an individual's urea clearance during a single dialysis.[8]

BUN concentrations are used to evaluate patients with lymphoma at risk for tumor lysis after chemotherapy.[9]

Drug effects have been summarized. A large number of substances and drugs affect the concentration of urea nitrogen by pharmacologic/physiologic or by analytic means, including those causing nephrotoxicity, dehydration, and volume depletion.[10]

Other tests are relevant to the differential diagnosis of renal failure. Hypercalcemia with hyperuricemia may indicate a neoplastic state. High CK may point to rhabdomyolysis. Abnormalities in serum and/or urine proteins may indicate myeloma. Allergic interstitial nephritis may be signaled by eosinophilia. An osmolal gap and oxalate crystalluria may point to ethylene glycol toxicity. Glomerular basement membrane antibody, ANA, ANCA, and other immunologic studies may be helpful.

Footnotes

1. Neuman DJ and Price CP, "Renal Function and Nitrogen Metabolites," *Tietz Textbook of Clinical Chemistry*, 3rd ed, Burtis CA and Ashwood ER, eds, Philadelphia, PA: WB Saunders Co, 1999, 1204-70.
2. Luke RG, "Uremia and the BUN," *N Engl J Med*, 1981, 305:1213-5.
3. Chadha V, Warady BA, Garg U, et al, "Inaccuracies During Hemodiafiltration in Patients With Hyperbilirubinemia," *Pediatr Nephrol* (in press).
4. Decaux G, Genette F, and Mockel J, "Hypouremia in the Syndrome of Inappropriate Secretion of Antidiuretic Hormone," *Ann Intern Med*, 1980, 93(5):716-7.
5. Beck LH, "Hypouricemia in the Syndrome of Inappropriate Secretion of Antidiuretic Hormone," *N Engl J Med*, 1979, 301:528-30.
6. Decaux G, Unger J, Brimioulle S, et al, "Hyponatremia in the Syndrome of Inappropriate Secretion of Antidiuretic Hormone. Rapid Correction With Urea, Sodium Chloride, and Water Restriction Therapy," *JAMA*, 1982, 247:471-4.
7. Bonadio WA, Hennes HH, Machi J, et al, "Efficacy of Measuring BUN in Assessing Children With Dehydration Due to Gastroenteritis," *Ann Emerg Med*, 1989, 18(7):755-7.
8. Owen WF Jr, Lew NL, Liu Y, et al, "The Urea Reduction Ratio and Serum Albumin Concentration as Predictors of Mortality in Patients Undergoing Hemodialysis," *N Engl J Med*, 1993, 329(14):1001-6.
9. Hande KR and Garrow GC, "Acute Tumor Lysis Syndrome in Patients With High-Grade Non-Hodgkin Lymphoma," *Am J Med*, 1993, 94(2):133-9.
10. Young DS, *Effects of Drugs on Clinical Laboratory Tests*, 5th ed, Volume 1: Listing by Test, Washington, DC: AACC Press, American Association of Clinical Chemistry, 2000, Section 3, 806-17.

References

Seifter JL and Nickeleit V, "A 67-Year-Old Woman With Vomiting, Bloody Diarrhea, and Azotemia," *Case Records of the Massachusetts General Hospital, Case 17-1997*, Scully RE, Mark EJ, McNeely WF, et al, eds, *N Engl J Med*, 1997, 336(22):1587-94.

Thadhani R, Pascual M, and Bonventre JV, "Acute Renal Failure," *N Engl J Med*, 1996, 334(22):1448-60.

◆ **Urea Reduction Ratio** *see* Urea Nitrogen, Serum or Plasma *on page 293*

◆ **Uric Acid/Creatinine Ratio, Urine** *see* Uric Acid, Urine *on page 295*

Uric Acid, Serum

Related Information

Ammonia, Plasma *on page 102*
(Continued)

Uric Acid, Serum (Continued)

Complete Blood Count on page 419
Creatinine Clearance on page 160
Creatinine, Serum or Plasma on page 161
Ethanol, Blood, Urine, and Other Sources on page 789
Kidney Stone Analysis on page 877
Lead, Blood on page 793
Molybdenum, Blood on page 821
Sodium, Serum or Plasma on page 275
Sputum Cytology on page 387
Synovial Fluid Analysis on page 323
Uric Acid, Urine on page 295

Synonyms Urate

Abstract Classic gouty podagra ("foot seizure") causes onset of a painful, swollen great toe in an upperclass man, especially depicted in 18th century Britain as a badge of the landed gentry. Antoni van Leeuwenhoek described crystals from a gouty tophus in the mid-17th century.[1] Such sodium urate crystals in synovial fluid are diagnostic. Gout, a clinical entity, is caused by deposition of monosodium urate monohydrate (urate) crystals. In most cases, the onset of acute monoarticular arthritis in a peripheral joint in a lower extremity is followed by remission, then by a series of recurrences, ultimately followed by tophi in some subjects. Factors which contribute to hyperuricemia include obesity, high purine diet, regular use of ethanol, and diuretic therapy. At physiologic pH, 99% of the molecules are in the form of urate.[2] Uric acid, the end product of catabolism of purines, is increased in a variety of clinicopathologic entities in addition to gout. Hyperuricemia can be caused by **increased formation** or **decreased excretion**. Primary causes of **increased formation** include increased purine synthesis or inherited metabolic disorder. Secondary causes of increased formation include excessive dietary purine intake and altered ATP metabolism. **Decreased excretion** can be primary or secondary to chronic renal failure or increased renal reabsorption.[3]

Patient Preparation Ideally, patient should be fasting. Diurnal variations occur. Uric acid concentration is usually higher in the morning and lower in the evening.

Specimen Serum

Container Red top tube

Collection Separate serum. Do not collect in lavender top (EDTA) tube or gray top (sodium fluoride) tube for urease method.

Storage Instructions Urate is stable in serum for 3 days at 25°C, 3-7 days at 4°C, and 6-12 months at -20°C.

Special Instructions Alcoholic beverages are best avoided before collection.

Reference Interval An increase occurs during childhood. Adults: male: 3.4-7.0 mg/dL (SI: 202-416 μmol/L), female: 2.4-6.0 mg/dL (SI: 143-357 μmol/L), if specific laboratory methods are used. Values >7.0 mg/dL (SI: >416 μmol/L) are sometimes arbitrarily regarded as hyperuricemia, but there is no sharp line between normals on the one hand, and the serum uric acid of those with clinical gout. Normal ranges cannot be adjusted for purine ingestion, but high purine diet increases uric acid. Uric acid may be increased with body size, exercise, and stress.

Possible Panic Range "Severe hyperuricemia" has been classified as uric acid >12.0 mg/dL (SI: >714 μmol/L).

Use An increased uric acid level does not necessarily translate to a diagnosis of gout; only about 10% to 15% of instances of hyperuricemia are manifested by gout. The extensive overlap in serum uric acid levels between those with and without gout is shown in a study in which the lowest level in a gouty subject was 6 mg/dL (SI: 357 μmol/L), while the highest uric acid in a nongouty person was 9.5 mg/dL (SI: 565 μmol/L).[4] Among subjects with serum urate concentrations of 9.0 mg/dL (SI:535.5 μmol/L), the incidence of acute gout is about 5% per year. Gouty tophi form in cooler portions of the body because uric acid solubility varies directly with the temperature.

Elevations of uric acid occur in renal diseases with renal failure[5] and prerenal azotemia (eg, dehydration) as well as gout. Three types of kidney disease are caused by precipitation: acute uric acid nephropathy, nephrolithiasis, and chronic urate nephropathy.[6]

Asymptomatic hyperuricemia is found in the population at large, especially in family members of subjects with gout.

Hereditary gout: Lesch-Nyhan syndrome (X-linked) with choreoathetosis, spasticity, self-mutilation, hyperuricemia, hyperuricaciduria, increased urate:creatinine ratio, and marked decrease in the conversion of hypoxanthine to inosine monophosphate and guanine to guanine monophosphate (urine acid "salvage") due to decreased activity of hypoxanthine-guanine phosphoribosyl transferase (HGPRT).[3]

Other causes of increased uric acid concentration include increased 5-phosphoribosyl-1-pyrophosphate synthetase, glycogen storage disease type 1a,[7] and glucose-6-phosphatase deficiency.

Lead poisoning (saturnine gout) from paint, batteries, and moonshine is a secondary type of decreased excretion. A causal relationship between plumbism and gout was recognized before 1876. Gout as a common complication of subclinical lead poisoning is described among the Roman aristocracy.[8]

Another secondary cause of decreased excretion is acidosis: Lactic acidosis, diabetic ketoacidosis, recent and/or prolonged alcohol ingestion,

alcoholic ketosis. Increased uric acid concentrations in subjects with cirrhosis are related to renal function, particularly renal plasma flow.[9] Shock and hypoxia relate to hyperuricemia. Attention has been directed at the cause of hyperuricemia in the intensive care unit; severely increased uric acid levels in acutely ill patients is explained by degradation of ATP with degradation of accumulated nucleotides to purine metabolites, uric acid among them. Such ATP degradation may occur with strenuous exercise and the adult respiratory distress syndrome. With metabolism of ethanol to acetyl CoA, the degradation of ATP explains the hyperuricemia of alcohol use. Hyperuricemia becomes then a marker for cell injury crisis.[7] Hypouricemia is found as well in the ICU; vide infra.

Preeclampsia, diet, weight loss, fasting, or starvation.

Excessive cell destruction (increased formation, secondary): Neoplasia, even before as well as following chemotherapy and radiation therapy, especially lymphoma and leukemia; hemolytic anemia, resolving pneumonia and other inflammation; psoriasis; polycythemia, myeloma, pernicious anemia, infectious mononucleosis, congestive heart failure, large myocardial infarct.

Triglyceride increase bears an association with hyperuricemia, as do diabetes mellitus and obesity. Hyperuricemia bears an association with hypertension and statistical association with myocardial infarct (vide infra). Hyperuricemia in early essential hypertension correlates with renal vascular resistance and inversely with renal blood flow. Increased serum uric acid may indicate renal involvement.[10,11]

Serum uric acid concentration can provide information on the severity of primary pulmonary hypertension and has been recommended to assess the effects of therapy.[12]

Drugs: A large number of drugs cause analytical and pharmacologic **elevations** in serum uric acid concentrations. These include, but are not limited to, acetaminophen, acetazolamide, aldatense, aldesleukin, aluminum nicotinate, aminothiadiazole, ampicillin, anabolic steroids, angiotensin I.V., antineoplastic agents, aspirin (low doses), atenolol, azathioprine, azathymine, azauridine, basiliximab, bendroflumethiazide, bisoprolol, bumetanide, busulfan, calcitriol, capreomycin, chlorambucil, chloroform, cisplatin, cyclosporine, cyclosporine A, cytarabine, defibrotide I.V., diapamide, diazoxide, dichlorphenamide, didanosine, dideoxyinosine, diltiazem, doxorubicin, ethacrynic acid, ethambutol, etoposide, furosemide, hydroxyurea, ibuprofen, indapamide, levodopa, mechlorethamine, mercaptopurine, mercurial diuretics, methchlorethamine (especially in subjects with lymphoma), methicillin, methyldopa, metolazone, mitomycin, niacin, niacinamide, nicotinic acid (large doses), oxytetracycline, p-aminophenol, pentostatin, phenylbutazone (low doses), propranolol, propylthiouracil, pyrazinamide, rifampin, sulfanilamide, tetracycline, theophylline, thiazides including benzthiazide and chlorothiazide, thioneine, thiotepa, thiouric acid, threonine, triamterene, vincristine, warfarin, and zidovudine.[13]

Low Uric Acid

Poor dietary intake of purines and protein; tea, coffee.

Renal tubular defects, Fanconi syndrome, late in Wilson disease, outdated tetracycline, cystinosis, galactosemia, heavy metal poisoning, malignant neoplasms, hypereosinophilic syndrome.

Xanthinuria (deficiency of xanthine oxidase).

Hypouricemia is reported with acute intermittent porphyria, severe liver disease (especially obstructive biliary disease), and as an isolated defect in the tubular transport of uric acid.

With increased renal clearance of urate, hypercalciuria, and decreased bone density, diabetes,[14] and in SIADH.

With hyponatremia, serum hypo-osmolarity: Beck has described low uric acid with the syndrome of inappropriate secretion of antidiuretic hormone (SIADH): 16 of 17 patients with this syndrome were hypouricemic, with serum urate ≤4.0 mg/dL (SI: ≤238 μmol/L). All 13 patients with other causes of hyponatremia had serum urate ≥5.0 mg/dL (SI: ≥297 μmol/L).[15] Volume expansion, as with SIADH, causes decreased uric acid. The combination of low uric and low Na+ may also be found in instances of liver disease and was anticipated with ticrynafen.

In hospital patients, hypouricemia was most common in patients in intensive care. Hypouricemia was found in oncology patients, especially with hematologic malignant disease, with diabetics on insulin therapy, and with SIADH.[16]

Idiopathic hypouricemia commonly is transient. Familial hypouricemia has been described.

Drugs: A substantial number of drugs may cause analytical and/or pharmacologic **decreases** in serum uric acid concentrations. These include, but are not limited to, allopurinol, aspirin (high doses), azlocillin, cefotaxime, corticosteroids, corticotropin, massive doses of vitamin C and ascorbic acid are uricosuric. Others include albuterol, azathioprine, benzbromarone, benziodarone, canola oil, chlorothiazide, chlorpromazine, chlorprothixene, clofibrate, dicumarol, dipyrone, dobutamine, griseofulvin, indomethacin, levodopa, methotrexate, methyldopa, oxyphenbutazone, phenylbutazone (high doses), prednisolone, probenecid, radiographic agents, spironolactone, and verapamil.[13]

Limitations Uncommonly, gout may occur without hyperuricemia,[17] and the presence of hyperuricemia in a patient with arthritis does not necessarily establish the diagnosis of gout.[2]

Hyperuricosuria rather than hyperuricemia may be the only clue to the diagnosis of purine overproduction in children who have enzymatic defects or who develop hyperuricemia in the course of treatment of malignancies, due to a high uric acid clearance which occurs prior to puberty.[18]

Methodology Phosphotungstate (PTA), uricase, high performance liquid chromatography (HPLC). Uricase methods are more specific and have replaced PTA methods in most of the current instruments.

Additional Information Increased concentrations of uric acid are recently reported to bear independent and significant association with cardiovascular mortality risk.[19]

When gouty tophi are biopsied, their histopathologic appearance is often diagnostic in H&E. Alcohol fixation is highly desirable for such biopsies. Staining methods are available.[20]

The differential diagnosis between gout and calcium pyrophosphate deposition disease is tabulated and discussed in Synovial Fluid Analysis *on page 323.*

Footnotes

1. McCarty DJ (book review), Porter R, and Rousseau GS, *Gout: The Patrician Malady, N Engl J Med,* 1999, 340(11):898.
2. Emmerson BT, "The Management of Gout," *N Engl J Med,* 1996, 334(7):445-51.
3. Newman DJ and Price CP, "Renal Function and Nitrogen Metabolites," *Tietz Textbook of Clinical Chemistry,* 3rd ed, Chapter 35, Burtis CA and Ashwood ER, eds, Philadelphia, PA: WB Saunders Co, 1999, 1204-70.
4. Seegmiller JE, Laster L, and Howell RR, "Biochemistry of Uric Acid and Its Relation to Gout," *N Engl J Med,* 1983, 268:712-6.
5. Langford HG, Blaufox MD, Borhani NO, et al, "Is Thiazide-Produced Uric Acid Elevation Harmful?" *Arch Intern Med,* 1987, 147(4):645-9.
6. Dykman D and Simon EE, "Hyperuricemia and Uric Acid Nephropathy," *Arch Intern Med,* 1987, 147(7):1341-5.
7. Talente GM, Coleman RA, Alter C, et al, "Glycogen Storage Disease in Adults," *Ann Intern Med,* 1994, 120(3):218-26.
8. Nriagu JO, "Saturnine Gout Among Roman Aristocrats," *N Engl J Med,* 1983, 308:660-3.
9. Lee WC, Lin HC, Hou MC, et al, "Serum Uric Acid Levels in Patients With Cirrhosis: A Reevaluation," *J Clin Gastroenterol,* 1999, 29(3):261-5.
10. Larson AW and Strong CG, "Initial Assessment of the Patient With Hypertension," *Mayo Clin Proc,* 1989, 64(12):1533-42.
11. Nunez BD, Frohlich ED, Garavaglia GE, et al, "Serum Uric Acid in Renovascular Hypertension: Reduction Following Surgical Correction," *Am J Med Sci,* 1987, 294(6):419-22.
12. Nagaya N, Uematsu M, Satoh T, et al, "Serum Uric Acid Levels Increase in Proportion to Severity of Primary Pulmonary Hypertension," *Am J Respir Crit Care Med,* 1999, 160(2):487-92.
13. Young DS, *Effects of Drugs on Clinical Laboratory Tests,* 5th ed, Volume 1: Listing by Test, Washington, DC: AACC Press, American Association of Clinical Chemistry, 2000, Section 3, 817-30.
14. Shichiri M, Iwamoto H, and Shiigai T, "Diabetic Renal Hypouricemia," *Arch Intern Med,* 1987, 147(2):225-8.
15. Beck LH, "Hypouricemia in the Syndrome of Inappropriate Secretion of Antidiuretic Hormone," *N Engl J Med,* 1979, 301:528-30.
16. Crook M, "Hypouricaemia in a Hospital Population," *Scand J Clin Lab Invest,* 1993, 53(8):883-5.
17. McCarty DJ, "Gout Without Hyperuricemia," *JAMA,* 1994, 271(4):302-3.
18. Pascual E, "Hyperuricemia and Gout," *Curr Opin Rheumatol,* 1994, 6(4):454-8.
19. Fang J and Alderman MH, "Serum Uric Acid and Cardiovascular Mortality - The NHANES I Epidemiologic Follow-up Study, 1971-1992," *JAMA,* 2000, 283(18):2404-10.
20. Shidham V and Shidham G, "Staining Method to Demonstrate Urate Crystals in Formalin-Fixed, Paraffin-Embedded Tissue Sections," *Arch Pathol Lab Med,* 2000, 124(5):774-6.

References

Conger JD, "Acute Uric Acid Nephropathy," *Med Clin North Am,* 1990, 74(4):859-71.
Devgun MS and Dhillon HS, "Importance of Diurnal Variations on Clinical Value and Interpretation of Serum Urate Measurements," *J Clin Pathol,* 1992, 45(2):110-3.
Hande KR and Garrow GC, "Acute Tumor Lysis Syndrome in Patients With High-Grade Non-Hodgkin Lymphoma," *Am J Med,* 1993, 94(2):133-9.
Harris MD, Siegel LB and Alloway JA, "Gout and Hyperuricemia," *Am Fam Physician,* 1999, 59(4):925-34.
Joseph J and McGrath H, "Gout or Pseudogout: How to Differentiate Crystal-Induced Arthropathies," *Geriatrics,* 1995, 50(4):33-9.
Lieber CS, "Medical Disorders of Alcoholism," *N Engl J Med,* 1995, 333(16):1058-65.
Lin HY, Rocher LL, McQuillan MA, et al, "Cyclosporine-Induced Hyperuricemia and Gout," *N Engl J Med,* 1989, 321(5):287-92.
Lindor NM and Karnes PS, "Initial Assessment of Infants and Children With Suspected Inborn Errors of Metabolism," *Mayo Clin Proc,* 1995, 70(10):987-8.
Low RK and Stoller ML, "Uric Acid-Related Nephrolithiasis," *Urol Clin North Am,* 1997, 24(1):135-48.
Mejias E, Navas J, Lluberes R, et al, "Hyperuricemia, Gout, and Autosomal Dominant Polycystic Kidney Disease," *Am J Med Sci,* 1989, 297(3):145-8.

Uric Acid, Urine

Related Information

Synonyms Urate, Urine

Applies to Uric Acid/Creatinine Ratio, Urine

Abstract Uric acid concentration is the product of *de novo* synthesis and dietary sources. Seventy-five percent of urate is eliminated through the kidney and 25% through the intestine. Renal excretion of urate involves reabsorption by the proximal tubules, secretion by the distal portion of the proximal tubules, and further reabsorption by the distal tubules.

Patient Preparation Twenty-four hour uric acid excretion is most often measured in patients with nephrolithiasis, in whom it is desirable to know the excretion of uric acid and other substances while the patient is on a **usual** diet. Ethanol causes reduced excretion of uric acid. Alcoholic beverages should be excluded during this urine collection.

In children, the upper limit of normal of second morning urine specimen uric acid to creatinine ratio has been established.[1] See graphic.

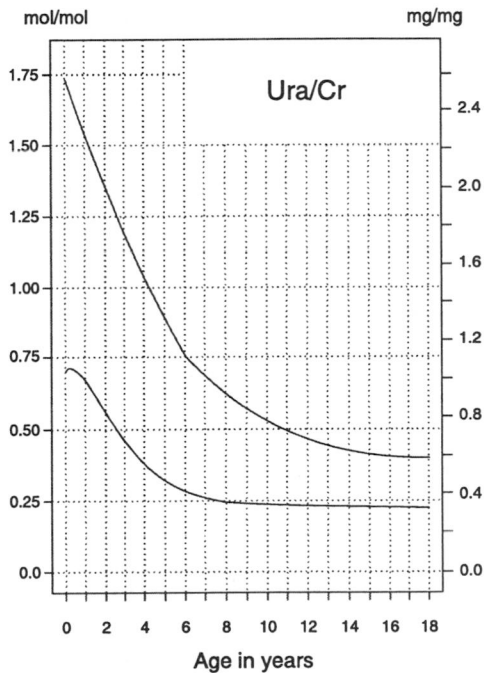

Estimated 95th and 5th percentiles for urate (Ura) to creatinine (Cr) ratios related to age.

A number of drugs affect uric acid excretion including aspirin, other anti-inflammatory preparations, x-ray contrast agents, vitamin C, and warfarin. Diuretics decrease uric acid excretion.

Specimen 24-hour urine, random urine with creatinine determination

Container To prevent precipitation in acid urine, add 10 mL of sodium hydroxide solution (12.5 M) to specimen container prior to collection.

Storage Instructions Do not refrigerate. Stable about 3 days.

Reference Interval Approximately 250-750 mg/24 hours (SI: 1.5-4.5 mmol/day) for women. Range for men may extend to 800 mg/24 hours (SI: 4.8 mmol/day) on ordinary diet. Increases on purine-rich diet. Of those with idiopathic gout, about 10% have overexcretion of uric acid.

Use Hyperuricosuria, as well as hyperuricemia, is associated with renal calculus formation. Identify overexcretors to determine risk of stone formation; identify genetic defects, Influence of overexcretion on therapy of gout. Uric acid nephrolithiasis occurs in primary gout or in secondary hyperuricemia (eg, malignant diseases). Uric acid nephrolithiasis may complicate ulcerative colitis, Crohn disease, and surgical jejunoileal bypass. Most subjects with uric acid stones do not have gout. Evaluate uric acid metabolism in gout.

Methodology Phosphotungstate, uricase, high performance liquid chromatography (HPLC). The uricase method is more specific and is in wide use in modern chemistry analyzers.

Additional Information Even mild renal failure decreases uric acid excretion. Uric acid excretion is decreased with hypertension.

A young patient with acute gouty arthritis, uric acid stones, and any patient who excretes >1000 mg uric acid/24 hours (SI: >5.9 mmol/day), should be screened for hypoxanthine-guanine phosphoribosyltransferase (HPRT) deficiency.[2] The uric acid:creatinine ratio has been used as a screen for Lesch-Nyhan syndrome (HPRTase deficiency). Normal control patients 0.21-0.59; partial enzyme deficient group 0.62-2.00; complete enzyme deficiency 1.98-5.35. Determinations of serum uric acid, as well as of urine uric acid:creatinine ratio, are of value in initiation of investigation of purine-related metabolic diseases.[3]

(Continued)

Uric Acid, Urine *(Continued)*

The ratio of uric acid to creatinine concentration on a random urine specimen has also been shown to be >1.0 in patients with acute renal failure secondary to acute uric acid nephropathy, but <1.0 in patients with acute renal failure resulting from other causes.

Risk for uric acid stone formation correlates with the degree of uric acid supersaturation in the urine, depending upon the degree of uric acid concentration and urinary pH.[4] Patients may develop uric acid urolithiasis in the face of normal uric acid excretion if the urine is persistently very acidic. Protection against uric acid nephropathy includes urine alkalinization.

A supersaturation profile for urine is available from a major reference laboratory. Its concept involves the balance between levels of supersaturation and of inhibitor activity. The analytes subject to such evaluation include potassium, calcium, phosphorus, oxalate, uric acid, citrate, magnesium, sodium, chloride, sulfate, and pH.[5] Urine volume, not usually regarded as an analyte, is relevant. Its goal is management of nephrolithiasis.

Footnotes
1. Matos V, Van Melle G, Werner D, et al, "Urinary Oxalate and Urate to Creatinine Ratios in a Healthy Pediatric Population," *Am J Kidney Dis*, 1999, 34(2):6E.
2. Wilson JM, Young AB, and Kelley WN, "Hypoxanthine-Guanine Phosphoribosyltransferase Deficiency. The Molecular Basis of the Clinical Syndromes," *N Engl J Med*, 1983, 309:900-10.
3. Valik D and Jones JD, "Hereditary Disorders of Purine and Pyrimidine Metabolism: Identification of Their Biochemical Phenotypes in the Clinical Laboratory," *Mayo Clin Proc*, 1997, 72(8):719-25.
4. Halabe A and Sperling O, "Uric Acid Nephrolithiasis," *Miner Electrolyte Metab*, 1994, 20(6):424-31.
5. Mayo Reference Services Publication, "Supersaturation Profile, Urine," *New Test Announcement*, Rochester, MN: Mayo Medical Laboratories, 2000.

References
Dykman D and Simon EE, "Hyperuricemia and Uric Acid Nephropathy," *Arch Intern Med*, 1987, 147(7):1341-5.

Preminger GM, "Renal Calculi: Pathogenesis, Diagnosis, and Medical Therapy," *Semin Nephrol*, 1992, 12(2):200-16.

♦ **Urinary Cortisol** *see* Cortisol, Free, Urine *on page 154*

Urinary Cortisol/Creatinine Increment

Related Information
Adrenal Cortex: Laboratory Assessments Overview *on page 84*
Adrenocorticotropic Hormone, Plasma *on page 86*
Corticotropin-Releasing Hormone Stimulation Test *on page 152*
Corticotropin Stimulation Test (Rapid) *on page 153*
Cortisol, Free, Urine *on page 154*
Cortisol, Serum or Plasma *on page 154*
Creatinine, 12- or 24-Hour Urine *on page 159*
Insulin Tolerance Test *on page 202*
Metyrapone Stimulation Test, Serum *on page 225*

Synonyms Midnight to Morning Urinary Cortisol Increment; Urinary Cortisol Increment

Applies to Cortisol-Binding Globulin

Abstract This test for adrenal insufficiency (AI) uses **sleep** as a stimulus for ACTH release. The endpoints of the test are cortisol measurements in two urine specimens collected under standardized conditions. A double voiding technique is used to assure that the cortisol measured corresponds to the cortisol secretion at the time of urine collection, and the cortisol measurement is normalized to the concurrent creatinine to allow for interindividual differences in urinary flow rate. The urine free cortisol (see Cortisol, Free, Urine *on page 154*) in a 1-hour collection, beginning immediately after a postawakening void, is compared with the cortisol in a baseline 1-hour urine specimen collected from 11 PM to midnight the night before. The cortisol results are divided by the concurrent urinary creatinine, resulting in a ratio. The midnight ratio is subtracted from the morning ratio to obtain the urinary cortisol/creatinine increment (UCCI).[1]

Sampling Time The specimens are usually collected at home. The patient is instructed to collect urine samples (5-20 mL) at bedtime and on awakening, and to place them in prelabeled containers. A double-voiding technique is used: the patient empties the bladder at 11 PM and collects a urine sample for testing 1 hour later; the patient next empties the bladder on awakening and collects the second sample for testing 1 hour later.

Storage Instructions Check with reference laboratory or use a preservative appropriate for free cortisol.[2]

Reference Interval In persons with a normal hypothalamic-pituitary axis, the UCCI is >9.[1]

Use This is a noninvasive test for **adrenal insufficiency** (AI), and is useful when the results of primary testing (see Cortisol, Serum or Plasma *on page 154*, Cortisol, Free, Urine *on page 154*, and Adrenocorticotropic Hormone, Plasma *on page 86*), are equivocal. The use of urine cortisol overcomes some of the limitations of serum cortisol measurements, such as unpredictable short-term fluctuations and dependence on normal levels of cortisol-binding globulin (CBG). The positive predictive value of the test (in a population of 40 patients with AI and 40 controls), using the Insulin Tolerance Test *on page 202* as the gold standard, was 95%; in this study, patients who had a normal UCCI and an abnormal ITT also had low serum CBG, which may have masked a truly normal adrenal response.

Limitations This is a relatively new test. While it seems very promising, it is not possible to predict what the results of larger studies will be.

Footnotes
1. Kong WM, Alaghband-Zadeh J, Jones J, et al, "The Midnight to Morning Urinary Cortisol Increment Is an Accurate, Noninvasive Method for Assessment of the Hypothalamic-Pituitary-Adrenal Axis," *J Clin Endocrinol Metab*, 1999, 84(9):3093-8.
2. Mayo Medical Laboratories, *1999 Test Handbook*, Rochester, MN, 611.

♦ **Urinary Cortisol Increment** *see* Urinary Cortisol/Creatinine Increment *on page 296*

♦ **Urinary MVA** *see* Mevalonic Acid, Urine or Amniotic Fluid *on page 225*

♦ **Urine 17-Ketogenic Steroids** *replaced by* 17-Hydroxyprogesterone, Serum or Plasma *on page 197*

♦ **Urine Cl** *see* Chloride, Urine *on page 145*

♦ **Urine Cortisol** *see* Cortisol, Free, Urine *on page 154*

♦ **Urine Creatinine** *see* Creatinine, 12- or 24-Hour Urine *on page 159*

♦ **Urine Electrophoresis** *see* Protein Electrophoresis, Urine *on page 268*

♦ **Urine K⁺** *see* Potassium, Urine *on page 259*

♦ **Urine Na** *see* Sodium, Urine *on page 278*

♦ **Urine Osmolality** *see* Osmolality, Urine *on page 236*

♦ **Urine Osmolar Gap** *see* Osmolality, Urine *on page 236*

♦ **Urine Oxalate** *see* Oxalate, Urine *on page 238*

♦ **Urine Phosphorus** *see* Phosphorus, Urine *on page 253*

♦ **Urine Pregnanetriol Assay** *replaced by* 17-Hydroxyprogesterone, Serum or Plasma *on page 197*

♦ **Urine Protein Electrophoresis** *see* Protein Electrophoresis, Urine *on page 268*

♦ **Urine:Serum Osmolality Ratio** *see* Osmolality, Serum *on page 236*

♦ **Urine:Serum Osmolality Ratio** *see* Osmolality, Urine *on page 236*

♦ **Uroporphyrinogen-Cosynthetase** *see* Porphobilinogen Deaminase, Erythrocyte *on page 254*

♦ **Uroporphyrinogen Decarboxylase** *see* Porphyrins, Quantitative, Urine *on page 255*

♦ **Uroporphyrinogen III Co-synthase** *see* Uroporphyrinogen III Synthase, Erythrocyte *on page 296*

Uroporphyrinogen III Synthase, Erythrocyte

Related Information
Porphyrins, Quantitative, Urine *on page 255*

Synonyms U-III-S; Uroporphyrinogen III Co-synthase

Abstract Congenital erythropoietic porphyria (Günther's disease) is caused by an autosomal recessive trait. Decreased enzyme activity is found in red blood cells. This enzyme catalyzes conversion of hydroxymethylbilane to uroporphyrinogen and produces the type III isomer.[1] This disorder is rarely a diagnostic dilemma because the presentation is very specific: severe photosensitivity and red-to-dark urine.

Patient Preparation Avoid medications for 1 week before test; fasting state for 12 hours before test; abstinence from ethanol for 24 hours before test.[2]

Specimen Blood

Container Green top (heparin) tube

Collection Place on wet ice immediately.[2] See instructions of reference laboratory.

Storage Instructions Maintain low temperatures; follow recommendations of laboratory which will perform the test.

Reference Interval ≥40 relative units

Critical Values ≤10 relative units (congenital erythropoietic porphyria)[3]

Use Diagnose congenital erythropoietic porphyria (erythropoietic uroporphyria); investigate dark red urine, red to brown stained diapers, hemolytic anemia, splenomegaly, photosensitivity, mostly in neonates; investigate stained teeth, hirsutism, scarring of sun-exposed skin

Methodology Incubation of washed red cells[3]

Additional Information Teeth and fluid from vesicles are recognized by red fluorescence with ultraviolet light. The high porphyrin content of urine has been observed to cause characteristic reddish fluorescence on a diaper examined under Wood's light (320-420 nm).[4] Long-term biochemical and clinical effectiveness of allogenic bone marrow transplantation seems to be promising.[5]

Footnotes
1. Nuttall KL, "Porphyrins and Disorders of Porphyrin Metabolism," *Tietz Textbook of Clinical Chemistry*, 3rd ed, Burtis CA and Ashwood ER, Philadelphia, PA: WB Saunders Co, 1999, 1711-35.
2. Kisabeth RM, Mayo Medical Laboratories, *2000 Test Catalogue*, Rochester, MN.
3. Leavelle DE, *Mayo Medical Laboratories Interpretive Handbook*, Rochester, MN: Mayo Medical Laboratories, 1997.
4. Pollock SS and Rosenthal MS, Images in Clinical Medicine, "Diaper Diagnosis of Porphyria," *N Engl J Med*, 1994, 330:114.
5. Tezcan I, Xu W, Gurgey A, et al, "Congenital Erythropoietic Porphyria Successfully Treated by Allogeneic Bone Marrow Transplantation," *Blood*, 1998, 92(11):4053-8.

References

Desnick RJ, "The Porphyrias," *Harrison's Principles of Internal Medicine*, 14th ed, Chapter 343, Fauci AS, Braunwald E, Isselbacher KJ, et al, New York, NY: McGraw-Hill Inc, 1998, 2152-8.

Fritsch C, Bolsen K, Ruzicka T, et al, "Congenital Erythropoietic Porphyria," *J Am Acad Dermatol*, 1997, 36(4):594-610.

Hindmarsh JT, Oliveras L, and Greenway DC, "Biochemical Differentiation of the Porphyrias," *Clin Biochem*, 1999, 32(8):609-19.

Kushner JP, "Laboratory Diagnosis of the Porphyrias," *N Engl J Med*, 1991, 324(20):1432-4.

◆ **Uroporphyrinogen I Synthase** *see* Porphobilinogen Deaminase, Erythrocyte *on page 254*

◆ **Uroporphyrinogen Synthase** *see* Porphobilinogen, Qualitative, Urine *on page 255*

◆ **Uroporphyrins** *see* Porphyrins, Quantitative, Urine *on page 255*

◆ **Valine** *see* Amino Acids, Urine *on page 101*

Vanillylmandelic Acid, Urine

Related Information
Catecholamines, Fractionation, Plasma *on page 138*
Catecholamines, Fractionation, Urine *on page 139*
Creatinine, 12- or 24-Hour Urine *on page 159*
Homovanillic Acid, Urine *on page 195*
Metanephrines, Urine or Plasma *on page 223*
Urine Collection, 24-Hour *on page 47*

Synonyms 3-Methoxy-4-Hydroxymandelic Acid; VMA

Applies to Dopamine

Abstract Vanillylmandelic acid (VMA) tests for neuroblastoma/pheochromocytoma with other tests, homovanillic acid, and metanephrines. VMA is a major metabolite of both epinephrine and norepinephrine, the result of the actions of both carboxy-o-methyl transferase and monoamine oxidase. It may be significantly elevated in conditions in which overproduction of catecholamines occurs. VMA is less sensitive than metanephrines in evaluation for pheochromocytoma.[1,2] Evaluating a number of urinary tests for pheochromocytoma, Lucon et al found sensitivity of VMA second to that of metanephrines and comparable to that of norepinephrine. Its sensitivity exceeded that of epinephrine and dopamine.[3] Witteles et al found VMA slightly less sensitive than plasma total catecholamines and urine total metanephrines.[4]

Patient Preparation Interfering substances relate to methodology. Drug and diet recommendations from the laboratory used are desirable. Many laboratories restrict foods, such as coffee, tea, bananas, and other foods. Some ask for no drug use (except for digitalis) for 2 weeks before the test. Aspirin, pyridoxine, levodopa, amoxicillin, carbidopa, reserpine, and disulfiram commonly interfere. Monoamine oxidase inhibitors decrease VMA excretion. See Limitations.

Specimen A small urine collection for pediatrics, up to 24-hour urine for adults

Container Plastic container with hydrochloric or acetic acid preservative added before collection, according to the protocol of the laboratory which will perform the test. Adjust to pH 2-4 after collection, according to procedures of the laboratory doing the analysis.

Collection Patient should be at rest during the collection, if possible taking no medication and without recent exposure to radiographic materials.

Creatinine is measured concomitantly in a random or 24-hour urine specimen to ensure adequate collection and to calculate the excretion ratio of VMA/creatinine and metanephrine/creatinine (see table). Twenty-four hour urine is preferred due to diurnal variation, the zenith occurring in the morning and nadir at night.[5]

Storage Instructions Refrigerate. Stable up to 2 weeks when the sample is acidified.

Vanillylmandelic Acid, Urine

24-Hour Collection	mg/24 h	SI: μmol/d
0-1 y	≤1.8	≤ 9
1-4 y	≤3	≤15
4-15 y	≤4	<20
15 y to adult	7-9	35-45
24- or 12-Hour Collection	**μg/mg Creatinine**	
<1 y	15-27	
1-5 y	11-13	
6-15 y	≤7	
15 y - adult	≤4.5	
Adults	≤7	
24-Hour Collection	**μg/kg Body Weight/24 h**	
<1 mo	≤180	
1 mo - 2 y	≤230	
>2 y	≤150	

Special Instructions For neuroblastoma, both HVA (homovanillic acid) and VMA should be collected. Metanephrines are recommended as a first test for pheochromocytoma.[2,3,6]

Reference Interval Adult normal range is usually up to approximately 7-9 mg/24 hours (SI: 35-45 μmol/day). See table.

Use VMA is used for diagnosis and follow-up of neuroblastoma, ganglioneuroma, and ganglioneuroblastoma. Most neuroblastoma patients excrete excess HVA in 24-hour collections. If VMA and HVA are both used in work-up, up to 80% of cases will be detected.

VMA is also used in the diagnosis of pheochromocytoma with metanephrines, imaging, and other tests.

Limitations MAO inhibitors may produce misleading results. Coffee, vanilla, and chocolate should be omitted before testing. VMA in a random specimen may yield a false-negative value; 24-hour collections are preferred for adults. Carbidopa causes false positives. Propranolol interferes. Normal VMA values are reported in patients with pheochromocytoma whose tumors secrete only epinephrine. VMA lacks diagnostic sensitivity.[7] Its specificity is limited as well for pheochromocytoma; urinary VMA falls somewhat short.[8] Some neuroblastoma patients are positive for urinary homovanillic acid abnormality but do not excrete increased VMA.[9] Twenty percent to 32% of patients with neuroblastoma do **not** have elevation of VMA. Many will have other laboratory abnormalities such as increased metanephrines, homovanillic acid (HVA), or dopamine. Serum and urine metanephrines provide the best diagnostic sensitivity and specificity overall for pheochromocytoma.

Methodology High performance liquid chromatography (HPLC), spectrophotometric following extraction, gas chromatography/mass spectrometry (GC/MS)

Additional Information Ninety-five percent of patients with neuroblastoma have an increase in VMA or HVA, or both. Interpretation of all results should be tempered by knowledge of influences causing false negatives and false positives (eg, stress, drugs, compounds that interfere with the assays).[6,10] The status of a mass screening program in Japan is reported. Virtually all 387 cases detected were at an early stage and 97% are expected to be cured.[11]

Footnotes

1. Lenders JW, Keiser HR, Goldstein DS, et al, "Plasma Metanephrines in the Diagnosis of Pheochromocytoma," *Ann Intern Med*, 1995, 123:101-9.
2. Héron E, Chatellier G, Billaud E, et al, "The Urinary Metanephrine-to-Creatinine Ratio for the Diagnosis of Pheochromocytoma," *Ann Intern Med*, 1996, 125(4):300-3.
3. Lucon AM, Pereira MA, Mendonca BB, et al, "Pheochromocytoma: Study of 50 Cases," *J Urol*, 1997, 157:1208-12.
4. Witteles RM, Kaplan EL, and Roizen MF, "Sensitivity of Diagnostic and Localization Tests for Pheochromocytoma in Clinical Practice," *Arch Intern Med*, 2000, 160(16):2521-4.
5. Rosano TG and Whitley RJ, "Catecholamines and Serotonin," *Tietz Textbook of Clinical Chemistry*, 3rd ed, Burtis CA and Ashwood ER, eds, Philadelphia, PA: WB Saunders Co, 1999, 1570-600.
6. Sheps SG, Jiang NS, Klee GG, et al, "Recent Developments in the Diagnosis and Treatment of Pheochromocytoma," *Mayo Clin Proc*, 1990, 65(1):88-95.
7. Gerlo EA and Sevens C, "Urinary and Plasma Catecholamines and Urinary Catecholamine Metabolites in Pheochromocytoma: Diagnostic Value in 19 Cases," *Clin Chem*, 1994, 40(2):250-6.
8. Krakoff LR, "Searching for Pheochromocytoma: A New and Better Test?" *Ann Intern Med*, 1995, 123(2):150-1.
9. Rothstein A, "Determination of Urinary Homovanillic Acid Using the Nitrosonaphthol Reaction," *Am J Clin Pathol*, 1987, 87(5):644-8.
10. Young DS, *Effects of Drugs on Clinical Laboratory Tests*, 5th ed, Volume One: Listing by Test, Washington, DC: AACC Press, 2000, 3:835-6.
11. Sawada T, Sugimoto T, Kawakatsu H, et al, "Mass Screening for Neuroblastoma in Japan," *Pediatr Hematol Oncol*, 1991, 8(2):93-109.

References

Bell S, Parker L, Craft AW, et al, "False Positive Results in a Neuroblastoma Screening Programme," *Med Pediatr Oncol*, 1994, 22(3):181-6.
Young WF Jr, "Pheochromocytoma and Primary Aldosteronism: Diagnostic Approaches," *Endocrinol Metab Clin North Am*, 1997, 26(4):801-27.

◆ **Vascular Endothelial Growth Factor** *see* Body Fluid Chemical Analysis *on page 123*

Vasoactive Intestinal Polypeptide, Plasma

Related Information
Gastric Analysis *on page 180*
Glucagon, Plasma *on page 182*
Pancreatic Polypeptide, Human, Serum or Plasma *on page 242*

Synonyms VIP

Abstract Vasoactive intestinal polypeptide (VIP), a nonadrenergic noncholinergic neurotransmitter, is found widely distributed in cells of the central and peripheral nervous systems. The highest concentrations are in the brain, spinal cord, and peripheral nerves of the gastrointestinal tract. Under normal circumstances, VIP has an extremely short half-life in the circulation (~1 minute). Clinical interest in VIP centers on tumors which secrete VIP (so-called **VIPomas**) and thereby cause a high-volume secretory diarrhea much like cholera. Long-term elevations of VIP may inhibit gastric acid secretion, resulting in achlorhydria. The term **pancreatic cholera** has been applied since, in adults, most VIPomas are in the tail of the pancreas. A clinically identical syndrome of secretory diarrhea, also due (Continued)

Vasoactive Intestinal Polypeptide, Plasma
(Continued)

to VIP, occurs in children, but the tumors are most commonly in the adrenal (see Use).

Patient Preparation Avoid recent administration of radioactive isotopes. Patient must be completely fasting for 10-12 hours. Not even water may be taken. No antacids for 24 hours prior to collection. All medications should be discontinued for 24-48 hours prior to collection.

Specimen Plasma

Sampling Time 6 AM to 8 AM

Collection Collect specimen in lavender top (EDTA) tube and centrifuge immediately. Freeze plasma in plastic vial.

Storage Instructions Transport frozen on dry ice.

Reference Interval Method-dependent, with wide interlaboratory variation. One publication states <50 pg/mL,[1] and another <75 pg/mL.[2]

Use In the appropriate clinical context, increased VIP levels support a diagnosis of VIPoma, but provide no information about the location of the tumor(s). The most common location in adults is the tail of the pancreas. In a review of 18 adult patients, the preoperative VIP levels ranged from 15.0-5975.0 pg/mL; only one patient had a value below their laboratory cutoff of 75 pg/mL.[3]

In children, most VIPomas are ganglioneuromas or ganglioneuroblastomas. Reported locations include the adrenal, gastrointestinal tract, lung, and paravertebral soft tissue. A recent report of six cases indicated elevated plasma VIP (~4-5 times the upper limit of normal) in the four children who had the measurement.[4]

Limitations Not all patients with a syndrome of pancreatic cholera have increased VIP. Increased VIP can be found in healthy controls and in laxative abusers.[5]

Methodology Radioimmunoassay (RIA)

Additional Information Other features of some cases of VIPoma have included hypercalcemia, flushing, and glucose intolerance.[5] A study of islet cell tumors in patients with multiple endocrine neoplasia (MEN) included vasoactive intestinal polypeptide tumor (VIPoma) as well as Zollinger-Ellison syndrome and insulinoma.[6] A VIP-producing tumor causing the pancreatic cholera syndrome was a well-differentiated mucinous adenocarcinoma.[7]

Footnotes
1. Henderson AR and Rinker AD, "Gastric, Pancreatic, and Intestinal Function," *Tietz Textbook of Clinical Chemistry*, 3rd ed, Burtis CA and Ashwood ER, eds, Philadelphia, PA: WB Saunders, 1999, 1279-80.
2. Mayo Medical Laboratories, *2000 Test Catalogue*, Rochester, MN, 495.
3. Smith SL, Branton SA, Avino AJ, et al, "Vasoactive Intestinal Polypeptide Secreting Islet Cell Tumors: A 15-Year Experience and Review of the Literature," *Surgery*, 1998, 124(6):1050-5.
4. Murphy MS, Sibal A, and Mann JR, "Persistent Diarrhea and Occult VIPomas in Children," *BMJ*, 2000, 320(7248):1524-6.
5. Krejs GJ, "Noninsulin-Secreting Tumors of the Pancreatic Islets," *Williams Textbook of Endocrinology*, 9th ed, Wilson JD, Foster DW, Kronenberg HM, et al, eds, Philadelphia, PA: WB Saunders, 1998, 1667.
6. Sheppard BC, Norton JA, Doppman JL, et al, "Management of Islet Cell Tumors in Patients With Multiple Endocrine Neoplasia: A Prospective Study," *Surgery*, 1989, 106(6):1108-18.
7. Rood RP, DeLellis RA, Dayal Y, et al, "Pancreatic Cholera Syndrome Due to a Vasoactive Intestinal Polypeptide-Producing Tumor: Further Insights Into the Pathophysiology," *Gastroenterology*, 1988, 94(3):813-8.

References
Delcore R and Friesen SR, "Gastrointestinal Neuroendocrine Tumors," *J Am Coll Surg*, 1994, 178(2):187-211.
Grier JF, "WDHA (Watery Diarrhea, Hypokalemia, Achlorhydria) Syndrome: Clinical Features, Diagnosis, and Treatment," *South Med J*, 1995, 88(1):22-4.

♦ **Vasopressin** *see* Antidiuretic Hormone, Plasma *on page 107*

♦ **Venous Blood Gases** *see* Blood Gases and pH, Venous *on page 122*

♦ **Very Low Density Lipoprotein Cholesterol** *see* Lipids, Overview *on page 213*

♦ **VIP** *see* Vasoactive Intestinal Polypeptide, Plasma *on page 297*

Vitamin A, Serum or Plasma

Related Information
Antioxidant Concentrations, Plasma *on page 108*
Vitamin E, Serum or Plasma *on page 301*
Zinc, Serum *on page 824*
Zinc, Urine *on page 825*

Applies to Carotene; Retinoids; Retinol, Serum

Test Includes Vitamin A and beta-carotene determination

Abstract Dietary vitamin A is derived from animal sources as well as supplements. Carotenoids including beta-carotene are synthesized from plants and are partly converted to retinol. The present recommended daily allowance for women is 800 retinol equivalents (about 2700 IU vitamin A) daily. The expression "vitamin A" refers to retinoids which have the biologic activity of retinol.[1] Vitamin A is a fat-soluble essential vitamin which is necessary for the integrity of epithelial cells. It also plays an important role in the visual cycle and is required for normal growth, development, and

reproduction. With vitamins D, E, and K, vitamin A is fat soluble. Its two natural forms are **retinol** (vitamin A_1) and **3-dehydro-retinol** (vitamin A_2). Vitamin A_1 is predominant. β-**carotene** is the most common provitamin A of the 50-60 known compounds and represents ~25% of the total of serum carotenoids. Antioxidant properties are not uniform among the different carotenoids.[2]

Patient Preparation Patient must fast a minimum of 8 hours.

Specimen Serum or plasma

Container Red top tube, green top (heparin) tube

Collection Draw in chilled tube. Protect from light. Keep specimen on ice.

Storage Instructions Separate serum or plasma in a 4°C centrifuge and freeze in a plastic vial immediately. Stable 2 years frozen. Stable 4 weeks at 4°C, although freezing is preferred. Protect from light.

Reference Interval
- Vitamin A: adults: 30-120 µg/dL (SI: 1.05-4.20 µmol/L). Normal range is less in childhood. Concentrations in males are about 20% greater than those in females.
- Beta-carotene: 10-85 µg/dL (SI: 0.19-1.58 µmol/L)

Critical Values Vitamin A levels <10 µg/dL (SI: <0.35 µmol/L) may provide evidence of marked deficiency; >140 µg/dL (SI: >4.89 µmol/L) signals toxicity.

Use Differential diagnosis of hypervitaminosis A, which may include toxicity; *vide infra.*

A combination of a low serum carotene level and a low vitamin A suggests inadequate vitamin A nutrition. Individuals with fat malabsorption are especially likely to develop vitamin A deficiency.

Limitations Serum levels do not correlate well with liver stores because of homeostatic control exerted by the liver. Increased in patients on oral contraceptives. β-carotene may be increased with hypothyroidism and with hyperlipidemia of diabetes mellitus.

Probucol (Lorelco®) may interfere.

Methodology Fluorescence or UV/VIS spectroscopy and other methods; presently, the method of choice is high performance liquid chromatography (HPLC), which permits simultaneous determination of vitamins A and E.

Additional Information **Decreased levels** of vitamin A are commonly due to dietary deficiency,[3] or may occur in conditions of deficient pancreatic digestive enzymes (eg, cystic fibrosis), impaired intestinal absorption and zinc deficiency resulting in decreased retinol-binding protein (RBP) levels, or deficient bile. Vitamin A deficiency is found most commonly in children younger than 5 years of age and is usually due to insufficient dietary intake. Vitamin A deficiency is found with prolonged ethanol consumption.[4] Hypovitaminosis A may lead to impaired skeletal growth, blindness, xerophthalmia, increased susceptibility to respiratory infections, and keratomalacia. Other less specific deficiency symptoms include increased susceptibility to infection, loss of appetite, and keratinization of the epithelial cells of the respiratory tract and other organs. Night blindness is the most common result.

Hypervitaminosis A may be due to increased intake, or conditions causing impaired disposal such as myxedema, diabetes mellitus, or renal disease. The toxic effects of increased vitamin A include elevation of intracranial pressure, skin desquamation, hair loss, joint pain, headache, nausea, fever, vertigo, and visual disorientation. Chronic hypervitaminosis A may cause anorexia, dry skin, alopecia, hepatomegaly, and fatigue. Toxicity is best assessed by measuring retinyl esters which normally comprise 5% of total vitamin A, but may comprise >30% of total vitamin A in toxicity (taking >50,000 IU/day). Toxicity appears when vitamin A levels exceed the capacity of retinol-binding protein (RBP) to bind to it.

Retinoids can be teratogenic.[1]

Vitamin A deficiency may occur when diseases or conditions impair the conversion of carotene to vitamin A or reduce the levels of RBP. Children with hypovitaminosis A have increased morbidity with measles.[5,6] Depressed immune response to tetanus in children with vitamin A deficiency is recognized.[7] Serum vitamin A levels may be decreased during periods of infection.[8,9]

In one 1996 paper, 12 years of supplementation with beta carotene led to no harm or benefit relevant to cancer risk or risks of cardiovascular disease or death from all causes.[10] In another study, following 4 years of supplementation, beta carotene and vitamin A provided no benefit, and may have had an adverse effect, on lung carcinoma incidence and/or risk of death from carcinoma of lung, cardiovascular disease, and any cause in smokers and individuals exposed to asbestos.[11] These papers led to an editorial observation that the tens of millions of dollars spent annually on beta carotene supplements should be diverted to more useful purposes.[12]

Attention has recently been directed at the antioxidants, including beta carotene and vitamin E. Efficacy of these substances has not been proven at present to prevent colorectal tumors[13] or lung carcinoma in smokers.[14] A possible decreased risk of age-related macular degeneration by consumption of certain carotenoid-containing foods requires further study.[15]

Footnotes
1. Rothman KJ, Moore LL, Singer MR, et al, "Teratogenicity of High Vitamin A Intake," *N Engl J Med*, 1995, 333(21):1369-73.
2. Kritchevsky SK, "Beta-Carotene, Carotenoids, and Prevention of Coronary Heart Disease," *J Nutr*, 1999, 129:5-8.
3. Usha N, Sankaranarayanan A, Walia BN, et al, "Early Detection of Vitamin A Deficiency in Children With Persistent Diarrhoea," *Lancet*, 1990, 335(8686):422.

4. Lieber CS, "Medical Disorders of Alcoholism," *N Engl J Med*, 1995, 333(16):1058-65.
5. Division of Field Epidemiology, Centers for Disease Control, "Vitamin A Levels and Severity of Measles. New York City," *Am J Dis Child*, 1992, 146(2):182-6.
6. Hussey GD and Klein M, "A Randomized, Controlled Trial of Vitamin A in Children With Severe Measles," *N Engl J Med*, 1990, 323(3):160-4.
7. Semba RD, Muhilal S, Scott AL, et al, "Depressed Immune Response to Tetanus in Children With Vitamin A Deficiency," *J Nutr*, 1992, 122(1):101-7.
8. Velasquez-Melendez G, Okani ET, Kiertsman B, et al, "Plasma Levels of Vitamin A, Carotenoids, and Retinol Binding Protein in Children With Acute Respiratory Infections and Diarrheal Diseases," *Rev Saude Publica*, 1994, 28(5):357-64.
9. Velasquez-Melendez G, Okani ET, Kiertsman B, et al, "Vitamin A Status in Children With Pneumonia," *Eur J Clin Nutr*, 1995, 49(5):379-84.
10. Hennekens CH, Buring JE, Manson JE, et al, "Lack of Effect of Long-Term Supplementation With Beta Carotene on the Incidence of Malignant Neoplasms and Cardiovascular Disease," *N Engl J Med*, 1996, 334(18):1145-9.
11. Omenn GS, Goodman GE, Thornquist MD, et al, "Effects of a Combination of Beta Carotene and Vitamin A on Lung Cancer and Cardiovascular Disease," *N Engl J Med*, 1996, 334(18):1150-5.
12. Greenberg ER and Sporn MB, "Antioxidant Vitamins, Cancer, and Cardiovascular Disease," *N Engl J Med*, 1996, 334(18):1189-90.
13. Greenberg ER, Baron JA, Tosteson TD, et al, "A Clinical Trial of Antioxidant Vitamins to Prevent Colorectal Adenoma," *N Engl J Med*, 1994, 331(3):141-7.
14. "The Effect of Vitamin E and Beta Carotene on the Incidence of Lung Cancer and Other Cancers in Male Smokers. The Alpha-Tocopherol, Beta Carotene Cancer Prevention Study Group," *N Engl J Med*, 1994, 330(15):1029-35.
15. Seddon JM, Ajani UA, Sperduto RD, et al, "Dietary Carotenoids, Vitamins A, C, and E, and Advanced Age-Related Macular Degeneration," *JAMA*, 1994, 272(18):1413-20.

References
Bloem MW, Wedel M, Egger RJ, et al, "Mild Vitamin A Deficiency and Risk of Respiratory Tract Diseases and Diarrhea in Preschool and School Children in Northeastern Thailand," *Am J Epidemiol*, 1990, 131(2):332-9.
"Detecting Vitamin A Deficiency Early," *Lancet*, 1992, 339(8808):1514-5.
Jakob E and Elmadfa I, "Rapid HPLC Assay for the Assessment of Vitamin K₁, A, E, and Beta-Carotene Status in Children (7-19 Years)," *Int J for Vitamin & Nutrition Research*, 1995, 65(1):31-5.
McCormick DB and Greene HL, "Vitamins," *Tietz Textbook of Clinical Chemistry*, 3rd ed, Chapter 29, Burtis CA and Ashwood ER, eds, Philadelphia, PA: WB Saunders Co, 1999, 999-1028.
Oakley GP Jr and Erickson JD, "Vitamin A and Birth Defects - Continuing Caution Is Needed," *N Engl J Med*, 1995, 333(21):1414-5.
Russell RM, "The Vitamin A Spectrum: From Deficiency to Toxicity," *Am J Clin Nutr*, 2000, 71(4):878-84.
Suan EP, Bedrossian EH Jr, Eagle RC Jr, et al, "Corneal Perforation in Patients With Vitamin A Deficiency in the United States," *Arch Ophthalmol*, 1990, 108(3):350-3.
Werler MM, Lammer EJ, and Mitchell AA, "Teratogenicity of High Vitamin A Intake," *N Engl J Med*, 1996, 334(18):1195-7.

Vitamin B₆, Plasma or Serum

Related Information
Homocyst(e)ine, Plasma *on page 193*
Synonyms P 5' P; Pyridoxal-5-Phosphate; Pyridoxine
Abstract Vitamin B₆, a water soluble vitamin, acts as a coenzyme (pyridoxal-5-phosphate) in protein, carbohydrate, and lipid metabolism, as well as in heme synthesis.
Patient Preparation Avoid radioisotope scan prior to collection of specimen if RIA is used for assay.
Specimen Serum or plasma
Container Red top tube, lavender top (EDTA) tube
Collection Transport specimen **immediately** to the laboratory following collection. Avoid exposing specimen to light.
Storage Instructions Separate plasma or serum and freeze **immediately**. Avoid exposure to light. Stable 10 days at -80°C; 50% loss in 7 days at -20°C.
Causes for Rejection Specimen more than 30 minutes in transit to the laboratory.
Special Instructions Communicate with laboratory before this test is ordered; it is not always routinely available. Scheduling and/or use of a reference laboratory may be required.
Reference Interval 5-30 ng/mL (SI: 20-121 nmol/L) (varies considerably with method).
Critical Values <5 ng/mL (SI: <20 nmol/L) indicates deficiency
Use Detect vitamin B₆ deficiency (eg, subjects with xanthurenic aciduria, primary cystathioninuria, homocystinuria, and hyperhomocystinemia). B₆ deficiency may lead to dermatitis with cheilitis and glossitis.[1]

Penicillamine (eg, those treated for Wilson disease), levodopa, disulfiram, oral contraceptive agents, theophylline, phenelzine,[2] and the antituberculous drugs isoniazid, cycloserine, and pyrazinoic acid may cause B₆ depletion in some cases with apparently associated sideroblastic anemia. B₆ supplements may be necessary.

B₆ may be decreased with pregnancy, lactation, alcoholism, diabetes mellitus, and in an uncommon B₆ dependency state, vitamin B₆ responsive neonatal convulsions. The effects of megadose vitamin B₆ consumption are controversial. There is evidence of significant neurotoxicity associated with pyridoxine megavitaminosis; tingling, numbness, clumsiness, gait disturbances, pseudoathetosis, with doses >2 g/day.[3]

Vitamin B₆ deficiency impairs immune function by inhibiting interleukin-2 production and lymphocyte proliferation.[4]
Limitations Evaluation is complicated by an unusually high requirement for vitamin B₆ in some individuals.
Methodology Enzyme assay, high performance liquid chromatography (HPLC) with fluorometric detection, immunoradiometric assay (IRMA). Vitamin B₆ nutriture is best assessed by a combination of three assessment methods, including plasma pyridoxal phosphate levels, urinary excretion of 4-phosphatidic acid, and the response of urinary metabolites to a 2 g tryptophan load.
Additional Information The family of "vitamin B₆" compounds includes pyridoxine as well as B₆ activity contributed by aldehyde (pyridoxal) and amine (pyridoxamine) derivatives, pyridoxine being the alcohol form of the 3-hydroxy-2-methylpyridine basic structure. In biologic material the B₆ compounds exist largely as phosphorylated derivatives. The vitamin is synthesized by plants and many microorganisms but not by the higher animals. It is widely available in natural diets, being present in fish, chicken, some fruits and vegetables, and wheat germ. It is partially destroyed by cooking and food processing. Vitamin B₆ is water soluble and is absorbed largely from the jejunum. A series of phosphorylase, oxidase, and kinase enzymes provide for extensive *in vivo* interconversion of pyridoxine and its derivatives.

Most B₆-dependent enzymes utilize pyridoxal-5-phosphate (the aldehyde form) in a coenzyme role. Critical amino acid/protein metabolic pathways (eg, transamination and decarboxylation reactions) are dependent upon B₆ enzymes. Glycogen phosphorylase requires B₆ as does delta aminolevulinic acid synthetase, and pyridoxal phosphate is required for DNA synthesis. With dietary deficiency, conservation of pyridoxal phosphate-dependent enzymes occurs with redistribution of available coenzyme and maintenance of more essential functions, thus rendering some clinical deficiency states difficult to define.

Deficiency of this vitamin has been implicated in a wide variety of clinical conditions. Vitamin B₆ deficiency rarely occurs alone and is most commonly seen in people who are deficient in several B-complex vitamins. As protein intake increases, onset of deficiency becomes more rapid. (This relationship of protein intake and vitamin B₆ is believed to reflect the major role of pyridoxal phosphate in amino acid metabolism.) Important in neonatology is the syndrome of jittery characteristics, colic, irritability, easy startling and seizures due to B₆ deficiency following ingestion of formula rendered B₆ depleted by excessive heating. B₆ may be decreased with malabsorption and inflammatory disease of the small bowel and in some cases of jejunoileal bypass.

Pyridoxine is required for heme synthesis. With deficiency, a hypochromic form of sideroblastic anemia may occur, characterized by the presence of ring sideroblasts (iron positive granules deposited about the nuclei of red cell precursors). Occasionally, the anemia may have megaloblastic characteristics. Most cases are the result of a block in the conversion of pyridoxine to pyridoxal phosphate, which inhibits the production of delta aminolevulinic acid and thus the production of heme. This form of sideroblastic anemia responds to large doses (>2 g) of pyridoxal phosphate per day. Inherited abnormalities of apoenzymes that bind with pyridoxal phosphate are responsible for newborn conditions characterized by mental retardation, skeletal deformities, thrombotic conditions, osteoporosis, and visual defects. Some are associated with increased urinary amino acids (eg, hyperhomocyst(e)inemia, homocystinuria, hypermethioninemia, cystathioninuria). If the alterations in these amino acids is due to deficiency of cystathionine-beta-synthase, in some patients, it can be controlled with large doses of vitamin B₆.

In adults, elevated serum homocyst(e)ine levels due to vitamin B₆ deficiency may promote atherogenesis with resultant arteriosclerotic and thromboembolic cerebral, coronary, and/or peripheral vascular events.[5] With B₆ deficiency the activity of cystathionine β-synthase (which functions in amino acid metabolism) is inhibited. Pyridoxal-5'-phosphate is a cofactor for this enzyme. The influence of B₆ on serum cholesterol levels and platelet aggregation is controversial. Decreased plasma pyridoxal phosphate levels have been found in patients with acute myocardial infarct.[6] Therapy with vitamin B₆ and folic acid apparently normalizes homocyst(e)ine metabolism in essentially all patients with cardiovascular disease and mild hyperhomocyst(e)inemia.[7] Metabolic evidence of B₆, as well as B₁₂/folate deficiency, in the presence of normal serum levels may be common in the elderly.[8] There is evidence against increased need for vitamin B₆ by athletes.[9]

Pais et al report that children with leukemia had lower pyridoxal-5 phosphate levels than age-matched control children.[10]

Acute toxicity of vitamin B₆ is low. However, high levels can cause ataxia and a severe sensory neuropathy and symptoms disappear within 6 months of discontinuing the source of vitamin B₆.

Footnotes
1. McCormick DB and Greene HL, "Vitamins," *Tietz Textbook of Clinical Chemistry*, Burtis CA and Ashwood ER, eds, 3rd ed, Chapter 29, Philadelphia, PA: WB Saunders Co, 1999, 999-1028.
2. Malcolm DE, Yu PH, Bowen RC, et al, "Phenelzine Reduces Plasma Vitamin B₆," *J Psychiatr Neurosci*, 1994, 19(5):332-4.
3. Schaumburg H, Kaplan J, Windebank A, et al, "Sensory Neuropathy From Pyridoxine Abuse," *N Engl J Med*, 1983, 309:445-8.
4. Rosenburg, IH, "Vitamin B₆ and Immune Function in the Elderly and HIV-Seropositive Subjects," *Nutr Rev*, 1992, 50(5):145-7.
(Continued)

Vitamin B₆, Plasma or Serum (Continued)

5. Robinson K, Mayer E, and Jacobsen DW, "Homocysteine and Coronary Artery Disease," *Cleve Clin J Med*, 1994, 61(6):438-50

6. Kok FJ, Schrijver J, Hofman A, et al, "Low Vitamin B₆ Status in Patients With Acute Myocardial Infarction," *Am J Cardiol*, 1989, 63(9):513-6.

7. van den Berg M, Franken DG, Boers GH, et al, "Combined Vitamin B₆ Plus Folic Acid Therapy in Young Patients With Arteriosclerosis and Hyperhomocysteinemia," *J Vasc Surg*, 1994, 20(6):933-40.

8. Naurath HJ, Joosten E, Riezler R, et al, "Effects of Vitamin B₁₂, Folate, and Vitamin B₆ Supplements in Elderly People With Normal Serum Vitamin Concentrations," *Lancet*, 1995, 346(8967):85-9.

9. Dreon DM and Butterfield GE, "Vitamin B₆ Utilization in Active and Inactive Young Men," *Am J Clin Nutr*, 1986, 43(5):816-24.

10. Pais RC, Vanous E, Hollins B, et al, "Abnormal Vitamin B₆ Status in Childhood Leukemia," *Cancer*, 1990, 66(11):2421-8.

References

Bender DA, "Novel Functions of Vitamin B₆," *Proc Nutr Soc*, 1994, 53:625-30.

Borschel MW, Kirksey A, and Hannemann RE, "Effects of Vitamin B₆ Intake on Nurture and Growth of Young Infants," *Am J Clin Nutr*, 1986, 43(1):7-15.

♦ **Vitamin B₁₂** *see* Cobalamin, Serum *on page 150*

♦ **Vitamin C** *see* Ascorbic Acid, Serum or Plasma *on page 112*

♦ **Vitamin C** *see* Oxalate, Urine *on page 238*

♦ **Vitamin D₁** *see* Vitamin D, Serum *on page 300*

Vitamin D, Serum

Related Information

Aluminum, Bone and Bone Biopsy *on page 813*
Amino Acids, Urine *on page 101*
Calcium, Serum *on page 131*
Calcium, Urine *on page 133*
Fecal Fat, Quantitative, 72-Hour Collection *on page 172*
Kidney Stone Analysis *on page 877*
Magnesium, Serum *on page 221*
Magnesium, Urine *on page 222*
Osteocalcin, Serum or Plasma *on page 237*
Parathyroid Hormone, Serum *on page 243*
Phosphorus, Serum *on page 251*

Synonyms Cholecalciferol

Applies to Calcitonin; Calcitriol; 1,25-Dihydroxy Vitamin D₃; Ergocalciferol (Vitamin D₂); 25-Hydroxy Vitamin D₃; 1,25-(OH)₂ D₃; 25-(OH) D₃; Parathormone; Vitamin D₁

Test Includes Assays are available for the precursor substance, vitamin D, and two vitamin D metabolites: 25-hydroxy vitamin D and 1,25-dihydroxy vitamin D (*vide infra*).

Abstract The term, vitamin D, is generic and includes several metabolically interrelated sterol substances that have hormonal activity. In the skin, 7-dehydrocholesterol is converted by ultraviolet light to vitamin D₃ (cholecalciferol); both of these sterols are biologically inactive in humans. Vitamin D₃ is converted in the liver to 25-hydroxy vitamin D [25OH-vitamin D], and the latter is converted in the kidney to 1,25-dihydroxy vitamin D [1,25-OH vitamin D]. Vitamin D₂ is usually acquired from the diet and undergoes an analogous series of biochemical reactions to a (25OH) form and a (1,25OH) form. In this monograph, "25OH vitamin D" refers to the (25OH) metabolite of both vitamins D₃ and D₂; likewise, "1,25OH vitamin D" refers to the (1,25OH) metabolite of both vitamins D₃ and D₂. Of these metabolites, 1,25OH vitamin D is the major biologically active fraction and has a plasma half-life of 4-6 hours. 25OH vitamin D, with a plasma half-life of 2-3 weeks, is the substance usually measured to assess vitamin D deficiency or excess.[1]

In the medical literature, **calcitriol**, is a synonym for the biologically active metabolite, 1,25OH vitamin D.

Acting in conjunction with parathormone and calcitonin, 1,25OH vitamin D regulates calcium homeostasis. In the alimentary tract, 1,25 OH vitamin D stimulates calcium absorption. In bone, 1,25OH vitamin D stimulates both osteoblastic and osteoclastic activity.

Patient Preparation Avoid radioisotope administration if RIA is used as the assay.

Specimen Serum, plasma

Container Red top tube, green top (heparin) tube

Storage Instructions Stable 3 days at 4°C to 25°C. Processed serum stable for months at -20°C, tolerates freeze-thaw cycles.[2]

Causes for Rejection Administration of radioisotopes if RIA is used for assay

Reference Interval Varies with method and environmental conditions (eg, recent sunlight exposure and diet). Following is a sampling of reference ranges:

Vitamin D (precursor): <0.2-20 ng/mL (SI: <0.5-52 nmol/L)[1]
25OH vitamin D: 10-50 ng/mL (SI: 25-125 nmol/L)[1]
• winter: 14-42 ng/mL (high performance liquid chromatography)[3]
• summer: 15-80 ng/mL (high performance liquid chromatography)[3]
1,25OH vitamin D: 15-60 ng/mL (SI: 36-144 nmol/L)[1]
• 15-60 ng/mL (high performance liquid chromatography)[3]

Use 25OH vitamin D is the preferred measurement to assess nutritional adequacy. Decreased values are associated with dietary vitamin D insufficiency, liver disease, malabsorption, inadequate sun exposure, and nephrotic syndrome. Increased values of 25OH vitamin D are associated with vitamin D intoxication.

1,25OH vitamin D is particularly useful in evaluating patients with hypercalcemia due to extrarenal conversion of 25OH vitamin D to 1,25OH vitamin D (calcitriol). Such a situation occurs in sarcoidosis,[4] cat-scratch disease,[5] and certain lymphomas.[6] These patients have **increased** levels of 1,25OH vitamin D. The underlying biochemical abnormality is the 1-alpha hydroxylation of 25OH vitamin D (a process normally restricted to kidney) in lesional histiocytes which accompany these disease processes.[6] This endogenous form of vitamin D intoxication is, in many series, the third most common cause of hypercalcemia, following primary hyperparathyroidism and malignancy.

1,25OH vitamin D is also **increased** in primary hyperparathyroidism, dietary vitamin D intoxication, and type II vitamin D-dependent rickets, a disease characterized by end-organ unresponsiveness to 1,25OH vitamin D.[1]

1,25OH vitamin D is **decreased** in hypoparathyroidism, pseudohypoparathyroidism, hypercalcemia of malignancy, renal failure, hyperphosphatemia, hypomagnesemia, and vitamin D-dependent rickets (type 1).[1]

Methodology Competitive binding assay, radioimmunoassay (RIA), radioreceptor assay (RRA), high performance liquid chromatography (HPLC)

Additional Information Chronic vitamin D deficiency leads to osteopathy (low serum 25OH vitamin D and elevated serum parathormone) and ultimately to osteomalacia. There is evidence that hypovitaminosis D-associated osteopathy is underdiagnosed in certain populations.[7]

Magnesium depletion leads to vitamin D resistance syndrome in which skeletal tissue is unresponsive to 1,25OH vitamin D.[8]

Tumor-induced (oncogenic) osteomalacia is a rare entity characterized by hypophosphatemia, hyperphosphaturia, low 1,25OH vitamin D levels, and osteomalacia. Tumor removal leads resolution of such abnormalities.[9] The following table lists vitamin D levels in hypocalcemic and hypercalcemic disorders.[10]

Anticipated Vitamin D Levels in Hypocalcemic and Hypercalcemic Disorders

Clinical Disorder	Hypocalcemia	
	25(OH)D*	1,25(OH)₂D*
Vitamin D deficiency	D	D,N,I
Severe hepatocellular disease	D	D,N
Nephrotic syndrome	D	D,N
Renal failure	N	D
Hyperphosphatemia	N	D
Hypoparathyroidism	N	D,N
Pseudohypoparathyroidism	N	D,N
Hypomagnesemia	N	D,N
Vitamin D-dependent rickets, type I (pseudovitamin D deficiency rickets)	N,I	D
Vitamin D-dependent rickets, type II (pseudovitamin D resistant rickets)	N,I	D
	Hypercalcemia	
Vitamin D, 25(OH)D intoxication	I	D,N
1,25(OH)₂D intoxication	N	I
Granulomatous diseases	N	N,I
Lymphoma	N	N,I
Hypercalcemia of malignancy	N	D,N
Hyperparathyroidism	N	N,I
Idiopathic hypercalciuria	N	N,I

Adapted from Weiss RL, "ARUP Interpretive Data Guide," ARUP Labs, 1999, 509-10.

*D = decreased, N = normal, I = increased

Footnotes

1. Endres DB and Rude RK, "Mineral and Bone Metabolism," *Tietz Textbook of Clinical Chemistry*, 3rd ed, Burtis CA and Ashwood ER, eds, Philadelphia, PA: WB Saunders Co, 1999, 1395-457.

2. Lissner D, Mason RS, and Posen S, "Stability of Vitamin D Metabolites in Human Blood Serum and Plasma," *Clin Chem*, 1981, 27(5):773-4.

3. Mayo Medical Laboratories, *2000 Test Catalogue*, Rochester, MN, 500-1.

4. Young C, Burrows R, Katz J, et al, "Hypercalcaemia in Sarcoidosis," *Lancet*, 1999, 353(9150):374.

5. Bosch X, "Hypercalcemia Due to Endogenous Overproduction of Active Vitamin D in Identical Twins With Cat-Scratch Disease," *JAMA*, 1998, 279(7):532-4.

6. Seymour JF, Gagel RF, Hagemeister FB, et al, "Calcitriol Production in Hypercalcemic and Normocalcemic Patients With non-Hodgkin Lymphoma," *Ann Intern Med*, 1994, 121(9):633-40.

7. Nellen JF, Smulders YM, Frissen PH, et al, "Hypovitaminosis D in Immigrant Women: Slow to Be Diagnosed," *BMJ*, 1996, 312(7030):570-2.

8. Fleming CR, George L, Stoner GL, et al, "The Importance of Urinary Magnesium Values in Patients With Gut Failure," *Mayo Clin Proc*, 1996, 71(1):21-4.

9. Cai Q, Hodgson SF, Kao PC, et al, "Brief Report: Inhibition of Renal Phosphate Transport by a Tumor Product in a Patient With Oncogenic Osteomalacia," *N Engl J Med*, 1994, 330(23):1645-9.

10. Weiss RL, "ARUP Interpretive Data Guide," ARUP Labs, 1999, 509-10.

References

Bosch X, López-Soto A, Morelló A, et al, "Vitamin D Metabolite-Mediated Hypercalcemia in Wegener's Granulomatosis," *Mayo Clin Proc*, 1997, 72(5):440-4.

Fraser DR, "Vitamin D," *Lancet*, 1995, 345(8942):104-7.

van der Wielen RP, Löwik MR, van den Berg H, et al, "Serum Vitamin D Concentrations Among Elderly People in Europe," *Lancet*, 1995, 346(8969):207-10.

Vitamin E, Serum or Plasma

Related Information

Antioxidant Concentrations, Plasma *on page 108*

Cholesterol, Total, Serum or Plasma *on page 146*

Vitamin A, Serum or Plasma *on page 298*

Synonyms Alpha Tocopherol; Tocopherol; α-Tocopherol

Abstract Vitamin E is a lipid soluble vitamin that acts as antioxidant, preventing damage to membranes by free radicals. Naturally occurring structures with vitamin E activity include four tocopherols and four tocotrienols (alpha, beta, gamma, delta). Tocotrienols differ from tocopherols in that they have an unsaturated side chain. Tocopherols that occur naturally have the RRR stereochemistry. The most active form is d-α-tocopherol.

Specimen Serum, plasma

Container Red top tube, green top (heparin) tube

Sampling Time Oral vitamin E may circulate for 1-2 days.

Storage Instructions Separate serum or plasma within 2 hours. Protect from light. Serum or plasma is stable 2 weeks at 25°C, 14 days at 4°C, and 1 year at -20°C.

Reference Interval 0.5-1.8 mg/dL (SI: 12-42 μmol/L) for adults.[1] Reference ranges vary with method and age (ranges for premature babies, neonates, children, and adults can be stratified.)

Critical Values Values <0.2 mg/dL indicate need for supplementation.

Possible Panic Range Although vitamin E toxicity has not been clearly established, values >4 mg/dL indicate significant excess.

Use Evaluate vitamin E deficiency in hemolytic disease in premature infants and neuromuscular disease in infants (and adults) with chronic biliary disease/chronic cholestasis including biliary atresia; evaluate patients on long-term parenteral nutrition and those on long-term dialysis; evaluate patients with malignancy or malabsorption (eg, patients with cystic fibrosis, cases of intestinal bypass surgery); investigate brown-bowel syndrome; investigate weakness in subjects who may be vitamin E deficient. Patients with malabsorption can develop myopathy and neuropathy.

Isolated vitamin E deficiency, a hereditary entity, resembles Friedrich ataxia.[2]

Vitamin E deficiency may occur with acanthocytosis (abetalipoproteinemia).

Methodology High performance liquid chromatography (HPLC) is recommended.[1] Other methods include fluorometry after solvent extraction, colorimetry, thin layer chromatography (TLC). Vitamin E concentrations assessed by HPLC are more accurate than those measured by spectrophotometric methods or TLC. If HPLC is used, vitamin A can be measured simultaneously.

Additional Information Vitamin E (α-tocopherol) is an antioxidant so widely distributed in foodstuffs that deficiency rarely occurs in normal adults from diet. However, vitamin E is fat soluble, and malabsorption and deficiency may develop in cases of chronic intraluminal intestinal bile deficiency. This has been particularly noted in premature infants and children with biliary atresia or cystic fibrosis (chronic intrahepatic cholestasis).[3] Clinically, this may lead to a hemolytic anemia, due to increased erythrocyte fragility, or to a slowly progressive neurologic disorder characterized by ataxia, areflexia, gaze disturbances, and loss of proprioception and vibratory sensation. A similar syndrome has been reported in adults with malabsorption. The syndrome may respond to treatment with parenteral vitamin E.

Early treatment with vitamin E may delay or prevent the neuropathy with ataxia that develops during the course of abetalipoproteinuria. Vitamin E therapy, in some cases, may have a favorable effect on moderate and severe cases of the retinopathy of prematurity[4] and the retinopathy of abetalipoproteinemia. While lipid malabsorption syndrome (with steatorrhea and malabsorption of vitamin E) may be etiologically related to ataxic spinocerebellar neurologic degenerative disease, there are reports of familial and sporadic vitamin E deficiency with neurologic impairment in the absence of fat malabsorption or demonstrated plasma lipoprotein level abnormality.[5,6,7]

Vitamin E is transported into plasma lipoproteins. Hepatic tocopherol binding or transfer protein (TBP or TTP) appears to be deficient in some individuals who are vitamin E deficient.[7] The importance of not overlooking a treatable cause of neurologic degenerative disease has been emphasized.[8]

As an antioxidant, vitamin E assists the prevention of peroxidation of unsaturated fatty acids. Deficiency may result in accumulation of oxidized lipids which may polymerize with polysaccharides to form ceroid/lipofuscin pigment. This PAS positive material deposits in tissue as intracytoplasmic pigment granules. In three patients with "brown-bowel syndrome," vitamin E levels were found to be "extremely low" (0.1-0.2 mg/dL (SI: 2-5 μmol/L)).[9]

Furthermore, low vitamin E intakes have been thought to be associated with increased cardiovascular disease, while increased intakes were considered cardioprotective. Several lines of evidence have accumulated pointing to an intracellular antiatherogenic role for alpha-tocopherol, the most potent member of the vitamin E family.

There continues to be interest in correlating plasma vitamin E levels with a variety of plasma constituents, with some positive and some negative results. Significance and/or validity of some associations is uncertain. Notably, abnormal serum levels of vitamin E have not been shown to relate significantly to clinical patency of ductus arteriosus,[10] sickle cell anemia,[11] moderate freshwater fish consumption,[12] insulin-dependent diabetics,[13] and risk of cancer.[14,15,16] Plasma vitamin E level, in one study, showed a positive correlation with serum cholesterol, non-HDL cholesterol, triglycerides, and apolipoprotein B.[17] Vitamin E has been reported to reduce the risk of coronary heart disease in men[18] and women.[19] However, question remained about the efficacy of supplemental doses of vitamin E.[20,21] Recently, a study of patients at high risk for cardiovascular events concluded that vitamin E had no apparent effect on cardiovascular outcomes in individuals 55 years of age or older.[22]

See Antioxidant Concentrations, Plasma *on page 108*; some desirable effects of antioxidants are discussed.

Vitamin E antagonizes functions of other fat-soluble vitamins at high doses and can lead to diminished bone mineralization, decreased storage of vitamin A, problems in coagulation, and impaired immune response.[23] It enhances certain T-cell mediated functions in healthy elderly subjects.[24] It has been proposed that nutritional indices such as vitamin E/phospholipids and vitamin E/total lipids are better indicators of vitamin E status than single plasma or serum vitamin concentrations.[25] While evaluating the vitamin E status of an individual, plasma lipid levels should be taken into account because all plasma vitamin E is transported in plasma lipoproteins.

Footnotes

1. McCormick DB and Greene HL, "Vitamins," *Tietz Textbook of Clinical Chemistry*, Burtis CA and Ashwood ER, 3rd ed, Chapter 29, Philadelphia, PA: WB Saunders Co, 1999, 999-1028.

2. Brust JCM, "Nutritional Disorders of the Nervous System," *Cecil Textbook of Medicine*, 21st ed, Chapter 489, Goldman L and Bennett JC, eds, Philadelphia, PA: WB Saunders Co, 2000, 2175-8.

3. Issa S, Rotthauwe HW, and Burmeister W, "25-Hydroxyvitamin D and Vitamin E Absorption in Healthy Children and Children With Chronic Intrahepatic Cholestasis," *Eur J Pediatr*, 1989, 148(7):605-9.

4. Johnson L, Quinn GE, Abbasi S, et al, "Effect of Sustained Pharmacologic Vitamin E Levels on Incidence and Severity of Retinopathy of Prematurity: A Controlled Clinical Trial," *J Pediatr*, 1989, 114(5):827-38.

5. Harding AE, Matthews S, Jones S, et al, "Spinocerebellar Degeneration Associated With a Selective Defect of Vitamin E Absorption," *N Engl J Med*, 1985, 313(1):32-5.

6. Sokol RJ, Kayden HJ, Bettis DB, et al, "Isolated Vitamin E Deficiency in the Absence of Fat Malabsorption - Familial and Sporadic Cases: Characterization and Investigation of Causes," *J Lab Clin Med*, 1988, 111(5):548-59.

7. Traber MG, "Determinants of Plasma Vitamin E Concentrations," *Free Radic Biol Med*, 1994, 16(2):229-39.

8. Harding AE, Macevilly CJ, and Muller DPR, "Serum Vitamin E Concentrations in Degenerative Ataxias," *J Neurol Neurosurg Psychiatry*, 1989, 52(1):132.

9. Michowitz M, Noy S, Chayen D, et al, "Brown-Bowel Syndrome," *Am J Surg*, 1989, 55(9):566-9.

10. Rudolph N, Schiller MS, and Wong SL, "Vitamin E and Selenium in Preterm Infants: Lack of Effect on Clinical Patency of Ductus Arteriosus," *Int J Vitam Nutr Res*, 1989, 59(2):140-6.

11. Broxson EH Jr, Sokol RJ, and Githens JH, "Normal Vitamin E Status in Sickle Hemoglobinopathies in Colorado," *Am J Clin Nutr*, 1989, 50(3):497-503.

12. Haglund O, Agren JJ, Laitinen MV, et al, "Dose-Response Relationships in Blood Lipids During Moderate Freshwater Fish Diet," *Ann Med*, 1989, 21:203-7.

13. Basu TK, Tze WJ, and Leichter J, "Serum Vitamin A and Retinol-Binding Protein in Patients With Insulin-Dependent Diabetes Mellitus," *Am J Clin Nutr*, 1989, 50(2):329-31.

14. Connett JE, Kuller LH, Kjelsberg MO, et al, "Relationship Between Carotenoids and Cancer. The Multiple Risk Factor Intervention Trial (MRFIT) Study," *Cancer*, 1989, 64(1):126-34.

15. "The Effect of Vitamin E and Beta Carotene on the Incidence of Lung Cancer and Other Cancers in Male Smokers. The Alpha-Tocopherol, Beta Carotene Cancer Prevention Study Group," *N Engl J Med*, 1994, 330(15):1029-35.

16. Greenberg ER, Baron JA, Tosteson TD, et al, "A Clinical Trial of Antioxidant Vitamins to Prevent Colorectal Adenoma," *N Engl J Med*, 1994, 331(3):141-7.

17. Rubba P, Mancini M, Fidanza F, et al, "Plasma Vitamin E, Apolipoprotein B and HDL Cholesterol in Middle-Aged Men From Southern Italy," *Atherosclerosis*, 1989, 77(1):25-9.

18. Rimm EB, Stampfer MJ, Ascherio A, et al, "Vitamin E Consumption and the Risk of Coronary Heart Disease in Men," *N Engl J Med*, 1993, 328(20):1450-6.

19. Stampfer MJ, Hennekens CH, Manson JE, et al, "Vitamin E Consumption and the Risk of Coronary Disease in Women," *N Engl J Med*, 1993, 328(20):1444-9.

20. Kushi LH, Folsom AR, Prineas RJ, et al, "Dietary Antioxidant Vitamins and Death From Coronary Heart Disease in Postmenopausal Women," *N Engl J Med*, 1996, 334(18):1156-62.

21. Greenberg ER and Sporn MB, "Antioxidant Vitamins, Cancer, and Cardiovascular Disease," *N Engl J Med*, 1996, 334(18):1189-90.

22. Yusuf S, Dagenais G, Pogue J, et al, "Vitamin E Supplementation and Cardiovascular Events in High-Risk Patients. The Heart Outcomes Prevention Evaluation Study Investigators," *N Engl J Med*, 2000, 342(3):154-60.

23. Chandra RK, "Graying of the Immune System. Can Nutrient Supplements Improve Immunity in the Elderly?" *JAMA*, 1997, 277(17):1398-9.

(Continued)

Vitamin E, Serum or Plasma *(Continued)*

24. Meydani SN, Meydani M, Blumberg JB, et al, "Vitamin E Supplementation and *In Vivo* Immune Response in Healthy Elderly Subjects," A Randomized Controlled Trial, *JAMA*, 1997, 277(17):1380-6.
25. Gomez Vida JM, Bayes Garcia R, and Molina Font JA, "Materno-Fetal Nutritional Status Related to Vitamin E," *An Esp Pediatr*, 1992, 36(3):197-200.

References

Anderson R, "Assessment of the Roles of Vitamin C, Vitamin E, and Beta-Carotene in the Modulation of Oxidant Stress Mediated by Cigarette Smoke-Activated Phagocytes," *Am J Clin Nutr*, 1991, 53(1 Suppl):358S-61S.

Kelleher J, Miller MG, Littlewood JM, et al, "The Clinical Effect of Correction of Vitamin E Depletion in Cystic Fibrosis," *Int J Vitam Nutr Res*, 1987, 57(3):253-9.

Munoz SJ, Heubi JE, Balistreri WF, et al, "Vitamin E Deficiency in Primary Biliary Cirrhosis: Gastrointestinal Malabsorption, Frequency and Relationship to Other Lipid-Soluble Vitamins," *Hepatology*, 1989, 9(4):525-31.

Seddon JM, Ajani UA, Sperduto RD, et al, "Dietary Carotenoids, Vitamins A, C, and E, and Advanced Age-Related Macular Degeneration. Eye Disease Case-Control Study Group," *JAMA*, 1994, 272(18):1413-20.

CLINICAL MICROSCOPY

Wayne R. DeMott, MD

David S. Jacobs, MD

Use of the microscope to study all manner of materials (in particular body fluids and tissues) of human/animal origin is one of the oldest disciplines of medical/patient investigation. The microscope has played, and continues to play, a central role in the evolution of medical science. This edition of the *Laboratory Test Handbook* finds a shortened Clinical Microscopy section due to separate chapter status of Urinalysis. Some expansion of the residual Clinical Microscopy material is the result of new listings being placed with their older, more established counterparts, as is true in particular (and by design) with fecal analysis.

◆ **Acid Steatocrit** *see* Fat, Semiquantitative, Stool, Acid Steatocrit *on page 305*

◆ **Acid Steatocrit** *see* Fat, Semiquantitative, Stool, Sudan III Stain *on page 306*

◆ **Advanced Semen Analysis** *see* Semen Analysis, Advanced *on page 318*

◆ **Andrology** *see* Infertility Screen *on page 310*

◆ **Antispermatozoal Antibody Test** *see* Infertility Screen *on page 310*

◆ **Arthrocentesis** *see* Synovial Fluid Analysis *on page 323*

Bile Fluid Examination

Related Information
Ova and Parasites, Stool *on page 666*

Synonyms Biliary Drainage Examination; Biliary Sludge Examination; Crystal Examination; Duodenal Drainage Examination

Abstract A variety of bile/duodenal content specimens obtained by tube aspiration, endoscopic retrograde cholangiopancreatography, or direct gallbladder puncture are studied for the presence of cholesterol, calcium bilirubinate, calcium carbonate crystals, bilirubin crystals, or parasites (predominantly *Giardia lamblia*). Crystals may support diagnoses of gallbladder and/or pancreatic disease. **Biliary sludge** is a suspension of precipitates of cholesterol monohydrate crystals or calcium bilirubinate granules in bile,[1] but other calcium salts including calcium carbonate microspheroliths may be relevant as well.[2] Such material may be embedded in strands of mucin.

Sludge in most persons resolves without treatment, but other outcomes include correlation with cholecystolithiasis, biliary colic, acute pancreatitis, and acute cholecystitis.[3]

Patient Preparation Specimen is obtained by use of a gastroduodenal endoscopy study, either by direct aspiration or into a trap. Patient must take nothing by mouth after midnight before the test.

Specimen Bile fluid, duodenal drainage specimen (gallbladder bile is preferred over hepatic bile)

Collection The collection may be divided into multiple containers, usually three: "A" bile (yellow - common duct origin), "B" bile (viscous and green or green-brown - gallbladder bile), and "C" bile (lighter color - hepatic bile duct origin). Many physicians send only one specimen, either a "pool" or a collection of largely "B" bile. Such "B" bile (gallbladder origin) may have a volume of 30-50 mL.

Storage Instructions Cholesterol that does not redissolve may crystallize with freezing. Centrifuge the specimen if it cannot be examined immediately; such sediment can be safely frozen. Refrigeration of whole bile samples may be followed by bacterial proliferation.[3]

Reference Interval Gallbladder bile is normally clear and brown. Normal bile should not include any significant number of cholesterol crystals, calcium bilirubinate or bilirubin crystals, parasites, or inflammatory cells. Ko et al regard two crystals/100x field or >4 crystals/sample as positive.[3] Ceftriaxone may be an important component.

Use Evaluate cholelithiasis, cholecystitis, and biliary colic in cases in which a high index of suspicion exists, but in which primary tests are negative. Direct microscopy of gallbladder content is more sensitive for detection of sludge than is ultrasonography.[3] To evaluate results of litholytic therapy, cholesterol crystals in bile can identify most cholesterol calculi and calcium bilirubinate granules can be used to identify pigment stones.[4] Bile fluid examination may be used to detect occult microlithiasis in cases of "idiopathic" acute pancreatitis.[5] Biliary sludge has been described with pregnancy, rapid weight loss, prolonged fasting, prolonged parenteral nutrition, ceftriaxone or octreotide use, and with transplantation.[3]

Such fluid may be used to establish the presence of giardiasis. See also Ova and Parasites, Stool *on page 666*.

Limitations Specimen pH <4.5 may produce a false-positive bilirubin precipitate which may be confused with calcium bilirubinate.

This diagnostic approach for identification of crystals and diagnosis of cholelithiasis is not widely used and is not found in all major textbooks. It is less clinically applicable than ultrasonography. The sensitivity of transabdominal ultrasonography for sludge is only ~55% while sensitivity of endoscopic ultrasonography is ~96%.[3]

Gallstones are formed only in a minority of subjects with sludge.[3]

Methodology Sludge can be diagnosed by ultrasonography or by bile microscopy. Transabdominal ultrasonography should be the initial test.[3]

Variation in processing of duodenal bile specimens prior to microscopic examination has contributed to difficulty in comparison of results of published series. For patients undergoing endoscopy, Ko et al recommend aspiration of duodenal content following cholecystokinin infusion, 0.05-0.1 mg/kg of body weight intravenously over 10 minutes. Sampling for 10-20 minutes after infusion usually provides 5-15 mL of duodenal content which includes gallbladder bile.

For patients not undergoing endoscopic examination, a nasogastric tube is placed in the duodenum with fluoroscopic guidance. Cholecystokinin infusion is begun with intermittent mild negative suction (-5 to -10 mm Hg) for 20 minutes, yielding 5-15 mL of duodenal fluid containing gallbladder bile.

The specimen is centrifuged at 3000 g for 15 minutes. The sediment is placed on a slide with a drop of distilled water and examined.[3] Both light and polarizing microscopy are recommended. The appearance of the crystals is described and illustrated.[3]

Other approaches are described.[6,7]

Neoptolemos et al[8] examined a second sediment obtained by recentrifuging the supernatant after incubation at 37°C for 24 hours. Ramond et al,[9] studying gallbladder bile obtained by direct puncture at cholecystectomy, found sensitivity was increased by a second microscopic examination at 24 hours. They kept the bile samples at 37°C for at least 1 hour, centrifuged it at 12,000 rpm for 5 minutes, and examined the bile sample and pellet for crystals initially and after a 24-hour incubation at 37°C. Need for temperature control at 37°C is debatable.[3]

Stones can be classified by quantitative infrared spectroscopy.

Additional Information Microscopy of duodenal drainage bile may be useful in the investigation of cholelithiasis, "idiopathic" pancreatitis, and parasitism.[6,7,8,9,10] Analysis of aspirated stimulated "duodenal bile" can provide presumptive evidence of calculous biliary tract disease in patients with suggestive symptoms but negative gallbladder radiologic and ultrasonic studies.

In studies of gallbladder bile (obtained at cholecystectomy), presence of rhomboid, birefringent cholesterol crystals as an indication of cholesterol gallstones has a sensitivity approaching 90% and a specificity of nearly 100%.[9] Reddish brown bilirubinate crystals alone as predictors of pigment stones have a lower level of sensitivity (about 70%) and specificity (slightly >90%).[9] Ramond et al found cholesterol crystals (in the absence of stones) in 4 of 11 patients with biliary stenosis, raising the possibility that bile stasis induces the formation of cholesterol crystals. As duodenal bile is diluted with variable amounts of gastric and small intestinal content, sensitivity of microscopy for crystals is likely somewhat decreased. Van Erpecum et al found the sensitivity (84%) of cholesterol crystals in fresh bile only slightly reduced in dilute gallbladder bile. They note "...examination of fresh bile for cholesterol crystals is a specific and reasonably sensitive test for cholesterol gallstone disease."[10]

Almost 70% of cases of acute pancreatitis are caused by gallstones or alcohol abuse.[1] Duodenal bile crystal analysis has been found useful in the investigation of "idiopathic" pancreatitis.[8] Microscopic examination of centrifuged duodenal bile in patients recovering from an episode of acute pancreatitis found cholesterol, bilirubinate, or calcium carbonate microspheroliths in 67% of cases while bile from postalcoholic pancreatitis patients was negative for crystals.[5] Study of gallbladder bile obtained at cholecystectomy (and/or serial GB ultrasonography) found biliary sludge or microlithiasis in 73% of patients.[5]

Bile cholesterol supersaturation with nearly all patients having cholesterol crystals in their bile has been reported in postcolectomy ulcerative colitis patients.[11] Cholesterol monohydrate predominates in pregnancy, with weight loss, and with octreotide therapy.[3]

Calcium bilirubinate sludge is found in patients receiving total parenteral nutrition and following bone marrow transplantation.[3]

A sensitivity of 83% and specificity of 100% for recognition of cholelithiasis has been reported on the basis of microscopic examination of bile samples obtained at endoscopic retrograde cholangiography.[12]

Dahan et al report different figures for sensitivity and specificity but conclude that when ultrasonography and microscopic examination of duodenal bile are negative, the risk of underdiagnosis of cholecystolithiasis is negligible.[13]

When endoscopic drainage is utilized for initial control of severe acute cholangitis caused by choledocholithiasis, the drainage material may be cultured.[14]

While a variety of protozoan, trematode and nematode parasites have been found in duodenal specimens, *Giardia lamblia* is most frequently encountered.[6] In patients clinically suspected of opisthorchiasis, in whom stool specimens are negative for ova, bile microscopy may be of special importance in establishing the diagnosis.[15]

Footnotes

1. Lee SP, Nicholls JF, and Park HZ, "Biliary Sludge as a Cause of Acute Pancreatitis," *N Engl J Med*, 1992, 326(9):589-93.
2. Steinberg WM, "Acute Pancreatitis - Never Leave a Stone Unturned," *N Engl J Med*, 1992, 326(9):635-7.
3. Ko CW, Sekijima JH, and Lee SP, "Biliary Sludge," *Ann Intern Med*, 1999, 130(4 Pt 1):301-11.
4. Agarwal DK, Choudhuri G, Saraswat VA, et al, "Utility of Biliary Microcrystal Analysis in Predicting Composition of Common Bile Duct Stones," *Scand J Gastroenterol*, 1994, 29(4):352-4.
5. Ros E, Navarro S, Bru C, et al, "Occult Microlithiasis in 'Idiopathic' Acute Pancreatitis: Prevention of Relapses by Cholecystectomy or Ursodeoxycholic Acid Therapy," *Gastroenterology*, 1991, 101(6):1701-9.
6. Juniper K and Burson EN Jr, "Biliary Tract Studies: II. The Significance of Biliary Crystals," *Gastroenterology*, 1957, 32:175-211.
7. Burnstein MJ, Vassal KP, and Strasberg SM, "Results of Combined Biliary Drainage and Cholecystokinin Cholecystography in 81 Patients With Normal Oral Cholecystograms," *Ann Surg*, 1982, 196(6):627-32.

8. Neoptolemos JP, Davidson BR, Winder AF, et al, "Role of Duodenal Bile Crystal Analysis in the Investigation of "Idiopathic" Pancreatitis," *Br J Surg*, 1988, 75(5):450-3.

9. Ramond MJ, Dumont M, Belghiti J, et al, "Sensitivity and Specificity of Microscopic Examination of Gallbladder Bile for Gallstone Recognition and Identification," *Gastroenterology*, 1988, 95(5):1339-43.

10. van Erpecum KJ, van Berge Henegouwen GP, Stoelwinder B, et al, "Cholesterol and Pigment Gallstone Disease: Comparison of the Reliability of Three Bile Tests for Differentiation Between the Two Stone Types," *Scand J Gastroenterol*, 1988, 23(8):948-54.

11. Harvey PR, McLeod RS, Cohen Z, et al, "Effect of Colectomy on Bile Composition, Cholesterol Crystal Formation, and Gallstones in Patients With Ulcerative Colitis," *Ann Surg*, 1991, 214(4):396-401.

12. Buscail L, Escourrou J, Delvaux M, et al, "Microscopic Examination of Bile Directly Collected During Endoscopic Cannulation of the Papilla - Utility in Patients With Suspected Microlithiasis," *Dig Dis Sci*, 1992, 37(1):116-20.

13. Dahan P, Andant C, Levy P, et al, "Prospective Evaluation of Endoscopic Ultrasonography and Microscopic Examination of Duodenal Bile in the Diagnosis of Cholecystolithiasis in 45 Patients With Normal Conventional Ultrasonography," *Gut*, 1996, 38(2):277-81.

14. Lai EC, Mok FP, Tan ES, et al, "Endoscopic Biliary Drainage for Severe Acute Cholangitis," *N Engl J Med*, 1992, 326(24):1582-6.

15. Dao AH, Barnwell SF, and Adkins RB Jr, "A Case of Opisthorchiasis Diagnosed by Cholangiography and Bile Examination," *Am J Surg*, 1991, 57(4):206-9.

References

Bockus HL, Shay H, Willard JH, et al, "Comparison of Biliary Drainage and Cholecystography in Gallstone Diagnosis: With Especial Reference to Bile Microscopy," *JAMA*, 1931, 96:311-17.

Janowitz P, Swobodnik W, Wechsler JG, et al, "Comparison of Gallbladder Bile and Endoscopically Obtained Duodenal Bile," *Gut*, 1990, 31(12):1407-10.

Magnuson TH, Lillemoe KD, Scheeres DE, et al, "Altered Bile Composition During Cholesterol Gallstone Formation: Cause or Effect?" *J Surg Res*, 1990, 48(6):584-9.

Marks JW, Broomfield P, Bonorris GG, et al, "Factors Affecting the Measurement of Cholesterol Nucleation in Human Gallbladder and Duodenal Bile," *Gastroenterology*, 1991, 101(1):214-9.

Paumgartner G and Sauerbruch T, "Secretions, Composition, and Flow of Bile," *Clin Gastroenterol*, 1983, 12(1):3-23.

Sahlin S, Ahlberg J, Angelin B, et al, "Nucleation Time of Gallbladder Bile in Gallstone Patients: Influence of Bile Acid Treatment," *Gut*, 1991, 32(12):1554-7.

♦ **Biliary Drainage Examination** *see* Bile Fluid Examination *on page 304*

♦ **Biliary Sludge Examination** *see* Bile Fluid Examination *on page 304*

♦ **Blood, Occult, Stool** *see* Occult Blood, Stool *on page 315*

♦ **Bovine Cervical Mucus Penetration Test** *see* Sperm Mucus Penetration Test (Human or Bovine Cervical Mucus) *on page 320*

♦ **Breath Hydrogen Analysis** *see* Reducing Substances, Stool *on page 317*

♦ **Calcium Pyrophosphate Dihydrate Crystals** *see* Synovial Fluid Analysis *on page 323*

♦ **CASA** *see* Infertility Screen *on page 310*

♦ **CASA** *see* Semen Analysis, Basic *on page 319*

♦ **CASA** *see* Sperm Penetration Assay (Zona-Free Hamster Egg Penetration Test) *on page 321*

♦ **Cervical Mucus Interaction, Cross Hostility Tests** *see* Sperm Mucus Penetration Test (Human or Bovine Cervical Mucus) *on page 320*

♦ **Chloridorrhea, Congenital** *see* pH, Stool *on page 317*

♦ **Cholesterol-Binding Pancreatic Proteinase** *see* Fecal Pancreatic Elastase 1 *on page 308*

♦ **CMPT** *see* Sperm Mucus Penetration Test (Human or Bovine Cervical Mucus) *on page 320*

♦ **$^{13}CO_2$ Breath Test** *see* Reducing Substances, Stool *on page 317*

♦ **Computer-Assisted Semen Analysis** *see* Infertility Screen *on page 310*

♦ **Computer-Assisted Semen Analysis** *see* Sperm Penetration Assay (Zona-Free Hamster Egg Penetration Test) *on page 321*

♦ **Computer-Assisted Sperm Analysis** *see* Semen Analysis, Basic *on page 319*

♦ **Crystal Examination** *see* Bile Fluid Examination *on page 304*

♦ **Duodenal Drainage Examination** *see* Bile Fluid Examination *on page 304*

♦ **Elastase, Fecal Pancreatic** *see* Fecal Pancreatic Elastase 1 *on page 308*

Fat, Semiquantitative, Stool, Acid Steatocrit

Related Information

d-Xylose Absorption Test, Serum, Urine *on page 167*
Fat, Semiquantitative, Stool, Sudan III Stain *on page 306*
Fecal Fat by Near-Infrared Reflectance Analysis *on page 307*
Fecal Fat, Quantitative, 72-Hour Collection *on page 172*
Fecal Pancreatic Elastase 1 *on page 308*

Meat Fibers, Stool *on page 313*
Methylene Blue Stain, Stool *on page 313*
pH, Stool *on page 317*

Synonyms Acid Steatocrit

Applies to Steatocrit

Abstract The steatocrit and its improved version, the acid steatocrit, are simple, low cost methods for the estimation of fecal fat. Routine glass hematocrit tubes and a standard hematocrit centrifuge (readily available laboratory equipment) are used in performance of these tests. Results are used to assess the presence of steatorrhea and to study malabsorptive/maldigestive processes, including exocrine pancreatic function in cystic fibrosis and chronic pancreatitis.

Patient Preparation To provide for adequate sensitivity in testing stool for fat, test subjects must be maintained on a high fat diet. An adult patient should be ingesting about 100-150 g of dietary fat (60 g/m² body surface area) per day for about 1 week before and during the test. High fiber content diet should be avoided for a few days prior to the test.

Specimen Random spot stool specimen; a 72-hour sample provides better correlation with 72-hour quantitative fecal fat.[1]

Container Glass or plastic tube or specimen container

Storage Instructions Store at -20°C if there is a delay in analysis.[1]

Turnaround Time 12-24 hours

Reference Interval

Steatocrit:

- small for gestational age premature infants: 29% ±1%
- appropriate for gestational age premature infants: 17% ±1%[2]
- children 3-12 years of age (mean ±SE) 1.1% ±0.4%

Acid steatocrit:

- premature and many formula-fed term infants to 6 months of age (but clinically well, thus "physiologic steatorrhea"): >60%. **Note:** Human milk-fed infants have steatocrit and acid steatocrit values lower than those of formula-fed babies.[3]
- children: 6 months to 3 years: <10%[3]; 3-12 years (mean ±SEM): 3.8% ±1%
- adults (median with interquartile range): 14.5(8-23)%[1]

Use Confirm the presence of steatorrhea; assist with the diagnostic study of malabsorption and/or maldigestion (as with exocrine pancreatic failure in some cases of cystic fibrosis, chronic pancreatitis, and pancreatectomy); monitor results of therapy (use in clinical follow-up) in patients with chronic diarrhea and in patients receiving exogenous enzyme therapy

Limitations There may be concern for safety of laboratory personnel (handling of stool specimens in breakable hematocrit tubes, aerosol production by hematocrit centrifuge). Plastic hematocrit tubes are available. The effect of olestra (a nonabsorbable fat substitute consisting of 6-8 fatty acids esterified to a sucrose molecule) on the results of this test has not yet been described. One should consider the possibility of false-positive test results (see Limitations in listing Fat, Semiquantitative, Stool, Sudan III Stain *on page 306*).

Methodology

Steatocrit: An aliquot of stool (at least 0.5 g) is diluted 1:3 with deionized water (a drop of 1% w/w Sudan III solution can be added to increase accuracy of measurement), followed by homogenization, and subsequently sampled into a 75 µL glass hematocrit tube. Using a standard hematocrit centrifuge, the tube is spun (horizontally) at 13,000 rpm for 15 minutes. The steatocrit is defined by dividing the upper (fatty) layer length (using a graduated magnifying lens) by the sum of the upper (fatty) and lower (solid) layer lengths.[4]

Acid steatocrit: Same as above steatocrit method with the exception that prior to filling the capillary tube, the homogenate is acidified with 5 N perchloric acid (using $\frac{1}{5}$ of the volume of the homogenate) and mixed for 1 minute (Vortex mixer).[4]

Additional Information Candidates for alternatives to the only clinically proven quantitative measurement for fecal fat (the 72-hour chemical titrimetric method of van de Kamer et al[5]) have recently been developed. The acid steatocrit appears to provide a practical, low-cost alternative that requires no special equipment. The 72-hour fecal fat test of van de Kamer (the gold standard) requires a 6-day high-fat diet and a 3-day collection of stool, logistically and aesthetically difficult for patients and medical personnel. The steatocrit, proposed some 20 years ago as a simple method to estimate stool fat content in newborn infants,[6,7] considered unreliable by some[8], has been improved recently by fecal acidification.[4] At low pH values, all fatty acids are protonated, fat extraction is improved, and boundaries between layers in the hematocrit tubes are sharpened, improving accuracy of reading.[4] A **spot stool acid steatocrit** has been considered to estimate the quantitative fecal fat (g/24 hours) by the equation:

fecal fat = -0.43 + [0.45 x (acid steatocrit %)][1]

The upper limit of normal fecal fat excretion in adults is 7 g/day (on a diet of 100 g/fat daily).[1,9,10]

The acid steatocrit (performed on random spot stools) has been reported to have a sensitivity of 100%, specificity of 95%, and a positive predictive value of 90% in the detection of steatorrhea (mixed population of subjects from normal to those with severe steatorrhea).[1] In a study of children (ages 6.5 months to 18 years), 50% with and 50% without malabsorption acid steatocrit values correlate with fecal fat excretion and concentration. Sensitivity for malabsorption was 90% with specificity at 100%.[11] On the basis of

(Continued)

Fat, Semiquantitative, Stool, Acid Steatocrit
(Continued)

statistical considerations, it has been suggested that "acid steatocrit not be used for clinical diagnosis," a matter of some controversy.[12]

Footnotes

1. Amann S, Josephson SA, and Toskes PP, "Acid Steatocrit: A Simple, Rapid Gravimetric Method to Determine Steatorrhea," *Am J Gastroenterol*, 1997, 92(12):2280-4.
2. Böhler T, Krämer T, Janecke AR, et al, "Increased Energy Expenditure and Fecal Fat Excretion Do Not Impair Weight Gain in Small-for-Gestational-Age Preterm Infants," *Early Hum Dev*, 1993, 54(3):223-34.
3. Van den Neucker A, Forget P, Veneberg JA, et al, "Acid Steatocrit During Infancy," *Acta Paediatr*, 1996, 85(10):1153-5.
4. Tran M, Forget P, van den Neucker A, et al, "The Acid Steatocrit: A Much Improved Method," *J Pediatr Gastroenterol Nutr*, 1994, 19(3):299-303.
5. Van de Kamer JH, ten Bokkel Huinink H, and Weyers HA, "Rapid Method for the Determination of Fat in Feces," *J Biol Chem*, 1949, 177(1):349-55.
6. Phuapradit P, Narang A, Mendonca P, et al, "The Steatocrit: A Simple Method for Estimating Stool Fat Content in Newborn Infants," *Arch Dis Child*, 1981, 56(9):725-7.
7. Iacono G, Carroccio A, Cavataio F, et al, "Steatocrit Test: Normal Range and Physiological Variations in Infants," *J Pediatr Gastroenterol Nutr*, 1990, 11(1):53-7.
8. Walters MP, Kelleher J, Gilbert J, et al, "Clinical Monitoring of Steatorrhea in Cystic Fibrosis," *Arch Dis Child*, 1990, 65(1):99-102.
9. Bai JC, Andrush A, Matelo G, et al, "Fecal Fat Concentration in the Differential Diagnosis of Steatorrhea," *Am J Gastroenterol*, 1989, 84(1):27-30.
10. Van den Neucker A, Pestel N, Tran TD, et al, "Clinical Use of Acid Steatocrit," *Acta Paediatr*, 1997, 86(5):466-9.
11. Addison GM, "Acid Steatocrit," *J Pediatr Gastroenterol Nutr*, 1996, 22(3):227 (letter).
12. Tran M, Forget P, and Van den Neucker A, "Author's Reply to Acid Steatocrit," *J Pediatr Gastroenterol Nutr*, 1997, 24(3):365 (letter).

References

Riley SA and Marsh MN, "Maldigestion and Malabsorption," *Sleisenger and Fordtran's Gastrointestinal and Liver Disease*, 6th ed, Chapter 88, Feldman M, Scharschmidt BF, and Sleisenger MH, eds, Philadelphia, PA: WB Saunders Co, 1998, 1501-22.

Steer ML, Waxman I, and Freedman S, "Chronic Pancreatitis," *N Engl J Med*, 1995, 332(22):1482-90.

Tran M, Forget P, Van den Neucker A, et al, "Improved Steatocrit Results Obtained by Acidification of Fecal Homogenates Are Due to Improved Fat Extraction," *J Pediatr Gastroenterol Nutr*, 1996, 22(2):157-60.

Tran TD, Van den Neucker A, Hendriks JE, et al, "Effects of a Proton-Pump Inhibitor in Cystic Fibrosis," *Acta Paediatr*, 1998, 87(5):553-8.

Fat, Semiquantitative, Stool, Sudan III Stain

Related Information
d-Xylose Absorption Test, Serum, Urine *on page 167*
Fat, Semiquantitative, Stool, Acid Steatocrit *on page 305*
Fecal Fat by Near-Infrared Reflectance Analysis *on page 307*
Fecal Fat, Quantitative, 72-Hour Collection *on page 172*
Fecal Lactoferrin *on page 308*
Fecal Pancreatic Elastase 1 *on page 308*
Meat Fibers, Stool *on page 313*
Methylene Blue Stain, Stool *on page 313*
pH, Stool *on page 317*

Synonyms Fatty Acid, Stool; Fecal Fat Stain, Sudan III Stain, Stool; Neutral Fat, Stool; Stool Fat, Semiquantitative

Applies to Acid Steatocrit; Fecal Fat Analysis, 72-Hour; Fecal Fat by Infrared Reflectance Analysis; Infrared Reflectance Analysis; Steatocrit

Abstract In this simple and low cost procedure, fecal fat is stained with Sudan III. The test is used as a screen for the presence of fecal neutral fat and fatty acids and may assist in the determination of the cause of steatorrhea. More recently developed tests for the semiquantitative assessment of fecal fat include the steatocrit, acid steatocrit, fecal elastase 1, and near-infrared reflectance spectroscopy as well as a Sudan III "quantitative" fecal fat microscopy method.[1] The diagnosis of steatorrhea, however, should still be defined by results of a quantitative 72-hour fecal fat determination.

Patient Preparation An adult patient should be on a diet containing about 100-150 g of dietary fat (60 g/m² body surface area) per day for about 1 week before and during the test and should avoid high fiber for a few days prior to the test. The patient should not use suppositories or mineral oil before the specimen is collected. Oily material (eg, creams, lubricants, etc) should be avoided prior to collection of the specimen.

Specimen Fresh random stool or, preferably, aliquot of homogenized 72-hour fecal collection. Some methods are claimed to provide useful test results without use of the ideal 3-day stool specimen.

Storage Instructions Maintain specimen at 4°C until analysis. For prolonged storage, keep at -20°C.

Causes for Rejection Contamination with water or urine; absence of proper labeling, including patient identification and duration of collection

Reference Interval Neutral fat: <50 fat globules/hpf, reported as normal. Fatty acids: <100 fat globules/hpf is considered normal.

Use Confirm the presence of steatorrhea; assist with the diagnostic study of malabsorption and/or maldigestion (as with exocrine pancreatic failure in some cases of cystic fibrosis); monitor results of therapy (use in clinical follow-up) in patients with chronic diarrhea and in patients receiving exogenous enzyme therapy

Limitations Castor oil or mineral oil droplets can mimic neutral fat. Ingestion of the fat substitute olestra (a nonabsorbable substance consisting of 6-8 fatty acids esterified to a sucrose molecule) may cause false-positive results with resultant erroneous diagnosis.[2]

This is not a definitive test; ***vide infra.***

Contraindications Administration of barium, bismuth, Metamucil®, castor oil, or mineral oil within 1 week prior to collection of the specimen

Methodology A small amount of stool sample is mixed with two drops of water, two drops of 95% ethanol, and three to four drops of Sudan III stain. Increased yellow-orange refractile fat globules (direct Sudan III stain) identifies neutral fats. Fatty acids and fat soaps are detected after hydrolysis by mixing stool sample with two to three drops each of Sudan III and glacial acetic acid, followed by heating before microscopic examination.

A recently described quantitative fecal fat microscopy method uses a small drop of homogenized stool placed on a glass slide followed by 36% acetic acid and 1% Sudan III stain followed by heat x3. A calibrated ocular micrometer is used to count and assign stained fat droplets into six groups by size from which a "fecal fat droplet total size-number product" is derived.[1]

Additional Information The test consists of determination of the presence of neutral fats and of total fats representing fatty acids. The results are reported semiquantitatively. Results of Sudan stain for fecal fat lack sensitivity and may be misleading with some dietary fatty acids or with constipation.[3] In a comparison of screening tests for enteropathy in children, results of lactose breath hydrogen, 1-hour d-xylose absorption, and 72-hour fecal fat tests were compared with the results of jejunal biopsy. Only the d-xylose and fecal fat tests correlated significantly with biopsy results.[4] See Meat Fibers, Stool *on page 313*. The new quantitative fecal fat microscopy test (see above) has not yet undergone extensive comparison studies. On the basis of evaluation of 180 patients with chronic diarrhea, however, there was significant linear correlation with chemically measured fecal fat output. The quantitative method had a sensitivity of 94% and specificity of 95% vs 76% and 99%, respectively, for the traditional method. The quantitative test performed on spot specimens was considered capable of excluding clinically significant steatorrhea (when negative results were obtained on each of two randomly collected stool specimens).[1]

Presence of steatorrhea can be established by the results of a 72-hour fecal fat analysis. Maldigestion or malabsorption may cause steatorrhea. Some patients with maldigestion may excrete excess triglyceride while patients with malabsorption excrete excess fatty acid. The 72-hour fecal fat determination involves saponification and does not usually provide for selective quantitation of triglyceride and fatty acid. The two-step Sudan III staining procedure (see Methodology) has been considered capable of distinguishing triglyceride from fatty acid (and thereby, theoretically, maldigestion from malabsorption). However, there is evidence that in adults with pancreatic insufficiency, the fecal triglyceride content may be normal. At least, the fecal triglyceride expressed in mg/g of fecal weight is not increased in all cases of pancreatic insufficiency.[5] One may not be able to differentiate maldigestion from malabsorption (pancreatic vs intestinal steatorrhea) by comparing fecal triglyceride/fatty acid or fecal fat concentration.[6,7,8] The influence of extrapancreatic lipase (eg, gastric lipase) must be considered.[9] The steatocrit, a semiquantitative method for detection of steatorrhea, has been reported to correlate with chemical methods.[10] See Fat, Semiquantitative, Stool, Acid Steatocrit *on page 305*. Fecal acidification enhances the sensitivity of the Sudan fecal staining method.[5] Acidification of the fecal homogenate (with 5N $HClO_4$) improves the steatocrit method (significantly higher correlation with chemically determined fecal fat content).[11,12] See Fat, Semiquantitative, Stool, Acid Steatocrit *on page 305*. There is controversy as to whether the acid steatocrit should be used for diagnostic purposes.[13,14]

Recently introduced infrared reflectance spectroscopy methods are direct, easy to perform, and provide results comparable with the standard 72-hour chemical method but require use of an infrared spectrophotometer. "InfraAlyzer" (Technicon Instrument Corporation) is available (see Fecal Fat by Near-Infrared Reflectance Analysis *on page 307*).

A linear relationship exists between the amount of long chain fatty acids consumed and the quantity in the stools.[15]

Footnotes

1. Fine KD and Ogunji F, "A New Method of Quantitative Fecal Fat Microscopy and Its Correlation With Chemically Measured Fecal Fat Output," *Am J Clin Pathol*, 2000, 113(4):528-34.
2. Balasekaran R, Porter JL, Santa Ana CA, et al, "Positive Results on Tests for Steatorrhea in Persons Consuming Olestra Potato Chips," *Ann Intern Med*, 2000, 132(4):279-82.
3. Riley SA and Marsh MN, "Maldigestion and Malabsorption," *Sleisenger and Fordtran's Gastrointestinal and Liver Disease*, 6th ed, Chapter 88, Feldman M, Scharschmidt BF, and Sleisenger MH, eds, Philadelphia, PA: WB Saunders Co, 1998, 1505-6.
4. Levine JJ, Seidman E, and Walker WA, "Screening Tests for Enteropathy in Children," *Am J Dis Child*, 1987, 141(4):435-8.
5. Bernstein LH, "Old Insight Into a New Insight Into an Old Test," *Gastroenterology*, 1989, 97(2):552-3.
6. Khouri MR, Ng SN, Huang G, et al, "Fecal Triglyceride Excretion Is Not Excessive in Pancreatic Insufficiency," *Gastroenterology*, 1989, 96(3):848-52.
7. Lembcke B, Grimm K, and Lankisch PG, "Raised Fecal Fat Concentration Is Not a Valid Indicator of Pancreatic Steatorrhea," *Am J Gastroenterol*, 1987, 82(6):526-31.
8. Kaunitz JD, "Dietary Fat Intake, 72-Hour Excretion, and Sudan Stain for Fecal Fat," *Gastroenterology*, 1989, 97(2):550-1.

9. Moreau H, Laugier R, Gargouri Y, et al, "Human Preduodenal Lipase Is Entirely of Gastric Fundic Origin," *Gastroenterology*, 1988, 95(5):1221-6.

10. Sugai E, Srur G, Vazquez H, et al, "Steatocrit: A Reliable Semiquantitative Method for Detection of Steatorrhea," *J Clin Gastroenterol*, 1994, 19(3):206-9.

11. Tran M, Forget P, Van den Neucker A, et al, "The Acid Steatocrit: A Much Improved Method," *J Pediatr Gastroenterol Nutr*, 1994, 19(3):299-303.

12. Van den Neucker A, Pestel N, Tran TD, et al, "Clinical Use of Acid Steatocrit," *Acta Paediatr*, 1997, 86(5):466-9.

13. Addison GM, "Acid Steatocrit," *J Pediatr Gastroenterol Nutr*, 1996, 22(2):227 (letter).

14. Tran M, Forget P, and Van den Neucker A, "Authors' Reply to Acid Steatocrit," *J Pediatr Gastroenterol Nutr*, 1996, 24(3):365.

15. Donowitz M, Kokke FT, and Saidi R, "Evaluation of Patients With Chronic Diarrhea," *N Engl J Med*, 1995, 332(11):725-9.

References

Ahnen DJ, "Nutrient Assimilation," *Textbook of Internal Medicine*, 3rd ed, Chapter 116, Kelley WN, editor-in-chief, Philadelphia, PA: Lippincott-Raven Publishers, 1997, 719-20.

Vuoristo M, Väänänen H, and Miettinen TA, "Cholesterol Malabsorption in Pancreatic Insufficiency: Effects of Enzyme Substitution," *Gastroenterology*, 1992, 102(2):647-55.

♦ **Fatty Acid, Stool** *see* Fat, Semiquantitative, Stool, Sudan III Stain *on page 306*

♦ **Fecal Elastase 1** *see* Fecal Pancreatic Elastase 1 *on page 308*

♦ **Fecal Fat Analysis, 72-Hour** *see* Fat, Semiquantitative, Stool, Sudan III Stain *on page 306*

♦ **Fecal Fat by Infrared Reflectance Analysis** *see* Fat, Semiquantitative, Stool, Sudan III Stain *on page 306*

Fecal Fat by Near-Infrared Reflectance Analysis

Related Information

d-Xylose Absorption Test, Serum, Urine *on page 167*
Fat, Semiquantitative, Stool, Acid Steatocrit *on page 305*
Fat, Semiquantitative, Stool, Sudan III Stain *on page 306*
Fecal Fat, Quantitative, 72-Hour Collection *on page 172*
Fecal Pancreatic Elastase 1 *on page 308*
Meat Fibers, Stool *on page 313*
Methylene Blue Stain, Stool *on page 313*
pH, Stool *on page 317*

Synonyms Fecal Fat by Near-Infrared Reflectance Spectrometry

Applies to Fecalogram

Abstract Stool fat, nitrogen, and water can be assayed simultaneously by near-infrared reflectance spectroscopy.[1,2,3,4] After homogenization of the stool specimen, a sample is placed in a cup, covered by a glass slide or placed on other appropriate surface, and loaded into the infrared (IR) analyzer. The method is simple, rapid, and reproducible but requires IR equipment. Results are applicable to the study of steatorrhea/malabsorption/maldigestion.

Patient Preparation Diet should contain 80-100 g fat/day for 3-5 days prior to and during sample collection.

Specimen Stool

Container Preweighed plastic container

Sampling Time 72 hours (preferred)

Collection 72-hour stool collection will provide results most comparable to classic chemical methods for fecal fat. Refrigerate during collection. For the study of patients with chronic diarrhea (fecal output in adult celiac disease), 24-hour stool specimens are preferred (decreases risk of false-negative results).[5]

Storage Instructions Fecal fat level is stable for weeks (at least 8 weeks) at -24°C.[4] Nitrogen and water content may change, however, water due to evaporation, nitrogen in relation to bacterial activity. Thus, samples for combined analysis should be processed promptly or stored for only a few days.[3]

Causes for Rejection Improper patient identification or preparation, specimen contaminated (eg, urine or other material)

Turnaround Time 1 hour; less under favorable circumstances

Special Instructions Include date and time collection started and finished.

Reference Interval Same as chemical reference methods (procedure is standardized on these methods), 2-7 g/24 hours (SI: 2-7 g/day)

Use Diagnosis, evaluation, and quantitative surveillance of steatorrhea as in cases of chronic pancreatic insufficiency and a number of intestinal diseases characterized by malabsorption

Limitations Requires availability of infrared (IR) analyzer. The effect of olestra (a nonabsorbable fat substitute) on results of this test has not been described. The possibility of a false-positive test result for steatorrhea malabsorption should be considered. (See Limitations in listing Fat, Semiquantitative, Stool, Sudan III Stain *on page 306*.)

Methodology Fecal near-infrared reflectance analysis (NIRA) depends on the measurement and computer processing of signal data from matrix and substrate-specific relationships involving reflectance of IR-specific wave lengths diffused by the fecal surface relative to the composition of the sample.[4] Reflectance readings from multiple discrete wave lengths are applied to multiple fecal samples correlated with computer assistance to obtain "reflectance scaling factors" (F values). F values are determined for each of the wave lengths at which NIRA measurement is being made. Thus, sample results are calculated from calibration derived from known samples whose IR characteristics are evaluated relative to specific components determined by a reference method (eg, fat by titrimetric method of van de Kamer[6] - the gold standard).

Fecal components of interest have functional groups (eg, CH, NH, OH) that have specific absorption bands in the near IR range. The near-infrared portion of the electromagnetic spectrum is within the wave length range of 780-2526 nm, between the visible 400-780 nm and the basic IR regions (2526-150,000 nm).[7] Currently, the most commonly employed instruments are the 450 InfraAlyzer (Technicon Instruments) and Fenir 8820 (Esetek Instruments). With the former, analytic parameters, including calibration curves, are fixed by the manufacturer. Optimal wave length combinations, however, have been found to vary possibly due to a change in stool matrix (the result of different eating habits) or change in detector characteristic curves between different analyzers. Thus, it has been recommended that each laboratory calibrate their own InfraAlyzer with a sufficient number of samples.[3]

The analyzer itself is operationally simple. A sample of the homogenized stool is placed in a cup and covered with a flat surface (eg, glass slide). The cup is placed on a sample drawer, pushed into the machine (ie, InfraAlyzer), and the wave length program is initiated.[1] Each analyte is determined and results displayed in under 1 minute.

Additional Information Reflectance infrared analysis is not widely applied in medically-oriented (clinical) laboratories. Infrared spectroscopy is used in clinical chemistry for analysis of urinary calculi and methods have been developed for a few constituents (eg, cholesterol, glucose, others) in serum/plasma/blood.[8]

Both near and medium IR spectroscopic methods have been described.[7,8] The methods are operationally simple, requiring no reagents after homogenization of the sample and only minimal manipulation of the stool. They are, however, secondary methods and require IR analytic instruments not available in many clinical laboratories. Calibration is recommended (see Methodology). Linear regression analyses show excellent correlation with the results of standard chemical methods.[1,2,3,4,7,8,9] Coefficients of variation are low, in the 1% to 3% range. Quantitative recoveries have been reported as between 95% and 105%.[2] NIRA was found to be 94.9% as sensitive and 98.2% as specific for the diagnosis of steatorrhea as the gas-liquid chromatography (GLC) method of Lapage and 87.5% as sensitive and 90.0% as specific as the van de Kamer method.[10] The NIRA method was inaccurate, however, in the determination of neutral sterols, bile acids, and short-chain fatty acids (as compared to results of conventional methods).[10]

A "fecalogram" (including fecal dry weight, total nitrogen, total fat, and hydrolyzed fat) has been developed using simultaneous determinations by NIRA for detection of steatorrhea and its identification as of pancreatic (maldigestive) or intestinal (malabsorptive) origin.[1] Using NIRA, the high value of fecal fat, nitrogen, and water in celiac disease has been found to be the result of fecal weight. The percentage composition of stool was not found to be of additional diagnostic value.[5]

The accuracy, rapidity, simplicity, and cost-effectiveness make NIRA practical for serial analyses in the clinical monitoring of patients with malabsorption/maldigestion syndromes,[2] including congenital exocrine pancreatic insufficiency (EPI) most commonly the result of cystic fibrosis. The second most common cause of inherited EPI, Shwachman syndrome (SS), has apparently not been reported as studied or monitored using NIRA. Shwachman syndrome (estimated incidence of 1:100,000 to 1:200,000 live births) is characterized by EPI and, in many cases, by short stature, bone dysplasia, bone marrow dysfunction (with anemia, neutropenia, thrombocytopenia), increase in Hb F, impaired glucose tolerance, and other abnormalities.[11,12]

Footnotes

1. Peuchant E, Salles C, and Jensen R, "Value of a Spectroscopic "Fecalogram" in Determining the Etiology of Steatorrhea," *Clin Chem*, 1988, 34(1):5-8.

2. Picarelli A, Greco M, Di Giovambattista F, et al, "Quantitative Determination of Faecal Fat, Nitrogen and Water by Means of a Spectrophotometric Technique: Near Infrared Reflectance Analysis (NIRA). Assessment of its Accuracy and Reproducibility Compared With Chemical Methods," *Clin Chim Acta*, 1995, 234(1-2):147-56.

3. Neumeister V, Henker J, Kaltenborn G, et al, "Simultaneous Determination of Fecal Fat, Nitrogen and Water by Near-Infrared Reflectance Spectroscopy," *J Pediatr Gastroenterol Nutr*, 1997, 25(4), 388-93.

4. Stein J, Purschian B, Bieniek U, et al, "Near-Infrared Reflectance Analysis: A New Dimension in the Investigation of Malabsorption Syndromes," *Eur J Gastroenterol Hepatol*, 1994, 6(10):889-94.

5. Picarelli A, Di Giovambattista F, Cedrone C, et al, "Quantitative Analysis of Stool Losses in Adult Celiac Disease: Use of Near-Infrared Analysis Reconsidered," *Scand J Gastroenterol*, 1998, 33(10):1052-6.

6. van de Kamer JH, ten Bokkel Huinink H, and Weyers HA, "Rapid Method for the Determination of Fat in Feces," *J Biol Chem*, 1949, 177(1):347-87.

7. Koumantakis G and Radcliff FJ, "Estimating Fat in Feces by Near-Infrared Reflectance Spectroscopy," *Clin Chem*, 1987, 33(4):502-6.

8. Franck P, Sallerin JL, Schroeder H, et al, "Rapid Determination of Fecal Fat by Fourier Transform Infrared Analysis (FTIR) With Partial Least-Squares Regression and an Attenuated Total Reflectance Accessory," *Clin Chem*, 1996, 42(12):2015-20.

9. Benini L, Caliari S, Guidi GC, et al, "Near Infrared Spectrometry for Faecal Fat Measurement: Comparison With Conventional Gravimetric and Titrimetric Methods," *Gut*, 1989, 30(10):1344-7.

(Continued)

Fecal Fat by Near-Infrared Reflectance Analysis
(Continued)

10. Nakamura T, Takeuchi T, Terada A, et al, "Near-Infrared Spectrometry Analysis of Fat, Neutral Sterols, Bile Acids, and Short-Chain Fatty Acids in the Feces of Patients With Pancreatic Maldigestion and Malabsorption," *Int J Pancreatol*, 1998, 23(2):137-43.

11. Cipolli M, D'Orazio C, Delmarco A, et al, "Shwachman's Syndrome: Pathomorphosis and Long-Term Outcome," *J Pediatr Gastroenterol Nutr*, 1999, 29(3):265-72.

12. Mack DR, Forstner GG, Wilschanski M, et al, "Shwachman Syndrome: Exocrine Pancreatic Dysfunction and Variable Phenotypic Expression," *Gastroenterology*, 1996, 111(6):1593-1602.

♦ **Fecal Fat by Near-Infrared Reflectance Spectrometry** *see* Fecal Fat by Near-Infrared Reflectance Analysis *on page 307*

♦ **Fecal Fat Stain, Sudan III Stain, Stool** *see* Fat, Semiquantitative, Stool, Sudan III Stain *on page 306*

Fecal Lactoferrin

Related Information
Bacterial Culture, Stool *on page 575*
Clostridium difficile Toxin Assay and Culture *on page 592*
Cryptosporidium Direct Staining Procedures *on page 596*
d-Xylose Absorption Test, Serum, Urine *on page 167*
Entamoeba histolytica Serology *on page 605*
Fat, Semiquantitative, Stool, Acid Steatocrit *on page 305*
Fat, Semiquantitative, Stool, Sudan III Stain *on page 306*
Fungal Culture, Stool *on page 614*
Meat Fibers, Stool *on page 313*
Methylene Blue Stain, Stool *on page 313*
Occult Blood, Stool *on page 315*
Ova and Parasites, Stool *on page 666*

Synonyms Lactoferrin, Fecal; Leukotest®, Stool

Abstract Lactoferrin, an iron-binding glycoprotein present in the cytoplasmic granules of polymorphonuclear white blood cells (PMNs), can be used as a marker for fecal leukocytes.[1,2] A commercially available (Leukotest®) latex agglutination procedure has undergone evaluation as a screening test for inflammatory bacterial diarrhea including, *Clostridium difficile* colitis.[3,4,5,6]

Specimen Stool

Container Plastic specimen container or rayon tipped swab[1]

Storage Instructions Specimen may be stored refrigerated (4°C) for up to 6 days[1]

Reference Interval
- Pediatrics: titer up to 1:200 in children without diarrhea
- Adults: fecal lactoferrin titer ≤1:50

Titers from 1:50-1:200 may relate to mild inflammation (eg, enteric parasites) or protein malabsorption (including subclinical malabsorption of milk). Sensitivity of detection (*in vitro* suspension, not in clinical stool specimens) is <1 ng (0.31 ng/μL) of purified lactoferrin per μL (equivalent to 60 PMNs per mm^3).[1]

Use Marker for the presence of fecal leukocytes; useful in detection of and screening for inflammatory bacterial diarrhea

Limitations Breast-fed infants (stools with lactoferrin containing human milk) may produce false positives even when high titers of fecal lactoferrin are detected.[2]

Methodology Antihuman lactoferrin antibody-coated latex bead agglutination[1]

Additional Information Lactoferrin, an iron-binding glycoprotein, is present as one of the components of polymorphonuclear white blood cell (neutrophil) granules. By chelating iron, lactoferrin inhibits the growth of microorganisms. For the diagnosis of inflammatory diarrhea, detection of a constituent of PMNs (eg, lactoferrin) can serve as an alternative to microscopic study of stool for leukocytes with some inherent advantages.[1] The latex agglutination test, utilizing antilactoferrin antibody, has been shown to be sensitive (in stool specimens, with definite 1+ to 2+ agglutination) to 120-280 PMNs per μL.[1] Sensitivity is maintained after refrigeration of specimens for up to 6 days. Swab specimens do not show the loss of sensitivity that characterizes microscopic examination for fecal PMNs.[1]

False-positive reactions in breast-fed infants relate to characteristics of the reagent antibody. Infectious diarrheal illness in the pediatric age group, however, is uncommon before children are weaned.[2]

When used as a screen for inflammatory bacterial enteritis, the lactoferrin assay was found to have a negative predictive value of 98.4%.[3] When used to screen stool specimens for those likely to be positive for enteric pathogens on culture, the negative predictive value was 99.4%.[3] While the lactoferrin stool test may be more sensitive than microscopic identification of PMNs and a cost-effective approach in the choice of patients for culture studies,[3,4,5] some authorities note that neither stool PMNs or lactoferrin studies are sufficiently sensitive to serve as screening tests for *Campylobacter*, *Salmonella*, *Shigella*, or *Clostridium difficile* pathogens.[5,6,7]

Footnotes

1. Guerrant RL, Araujo V, Soares E, et al, "Measurement of Fecal Lactoferrin as a Marker of Fecal Leukocytes," *J Clin Microbiol*, 1992, 30(5):1238-42.

2. Quiroga T, Garcia P, Goycoolea M, et al, "Fecal Lactoferrin as a Marker of Fecal Leukocytes," *J Clin Microbiol*, 1994, 32(10):2629-30.

3. Silletti, RP, Lee G, and Ailey E, "Role of Stool Screening Tests in Diagnosis of Inflammatory Bacterial Enteritis and in Selection of Specimens Likely to Yield Invasive Enteric Pathogens," *J Clin Microbiol*, 1996, 34(5):1161-5.

4. Choi SW, Park CH, Silva TMJ, et al, "To Culture or Not to Culture: Fecal Lactoferrin Screening for Inflammatory Bacterial Diarrhea," *J Clin Microbiol*, 1996, 34(4):928-32.

5. Yong WH, Mattia AR, and Ferraro MJ, "Comparison of Fecal Lactoferrin Latex Agglutination Assay and Methylene Blue Microscopy for Detection of Fecal Leukocytes in *Clostridium difficile*-Associated Disease," *J Clin Microbiol*, 1994, 32(5):1360-1.

6. Ruiz-Peláez JG and Mattar S, "Accuracy of Fecal Lactoferrin and Other Stool Tests for Diagnosis of Invasive Diarrhea at a Colombian Pediatric Hospital," *Pediatr Infect Dis J*, 1999, 18(4):342-6.

7. Nachamkin I, "Fecal Lactoferrin Screening Assay for Inflammatory Bacterial Diarrhea," *J Clin Microbiol*, 1996, 34(9):2337-8

References

Dowdy LM, "Infectious Diarrhea," *Clinical Practice of Gastroenterology*, Chapter 60, Brandt LJ, ed, Philadelphia, PA: Current Medicine, Inc, 1999, 529-30.

Huicho L, Campos M, Rivera J, et al, "Fecal Screening Tests in the Approach to Acute Infectious Diarrhea: A Scientific Overview," *Pediatr Infect Dis J*, 1996, 15(6):486-94.

Manabe YC, Vinetz JM, Moore RD, et al, "*Clostridium difficile* Colitis: An Efficient Clinical Approach to Diagnosis," *Ann Intern Med*, 1995, 123(11):835-40.

Miller JR, Barrett LJ, Kotloff K, et al, "A Rapid Test for Infectious and Inflammatory Enteritis," *Arch Intern Med*, 1994, 154(23):2660-4.

♦ **Fecal Leukocyte Stain** *see* Methylene Blue Stain, Stool *on page 313*

♦ **Fecal Occult Blood Test** *see* Occult Blood, Stool *on page 315*

♦ **Fecalogram** *see* Fecal Fat by Near-Infrared Reflectance Analysis *on page 307*

Fecal Pancreatic Elastase 1

Related Information
Fat, Semiquantitative, Stool, Acid Steatocrit *on page 305*
Fat, Semiquantitative, Stool, Sudan III Stain *on page 306*
Fecal Fat by Near-Infrared Reflectance Analysis *on page 307*
Fecal Fat, Quantitative, 72-Hour Collection *on page 172*

Synonyms Cholesterol-Binding Pancreatic Proteinase; Elastase, Fecal Pancreatic; Fecal Elastase 1

Abstract Pancreatic elastase 1, an endoprotease and sterol-binding protein, is present in pancreatic secretions and feces and is not degraded during intestinal transit. It can serve as a noninvasive tubeless test of pancreatic function.

Specimen Small sample of stool, aliquot of an homogenized 24-hour stool collection is preferred.

Storage Instructions Stable up to at least 3 days at room temperature (24°C). May be frozen at -20°C for up to 30 days (possibly longer) prior to analysis.[1] Enzyme is stable for months at 4°C.[2]

Reference Interval Normal value is considered as >200 μg elastase/g stool (cutoff value). Control population has shown a range of 200-1500 μg/g (95% of all values - spot stool samples).[3] Values rise during the first month after birth to 586 μg/g ±65 μg/g and are generally >500 μg/g during childhood.[4]

Use Noninvasive (tubeless) test for the evaluation of pancreatic function; evaluate severity of chronic pancreatitis; assist in the differentiation of maldigestion from malabsorption in cases of steatorrhea.

Limitations Reproducibility of fecal elastase 1 test (FET) results may relate to variable dilution of the enzyme in stool and variable dietary pancreatic stimulation. A significant correlation has been shown, however, between the results of FET and the secretin and pancreozymin test (SPT).[3,5]

Methodology Enzyme-linked immunosorbent assay (ELISA), a "sandwich"-type enzyme immunoassay available commercially in kit form (ScheBo-Tech Diagnostica GmbH, Wettenberg, Germany). This ELISA test incorporates two monoclonal antibodies with specificity against two different epitopes of human pancreatic elastase.

Additional Information Human pancreatic elastase 1 (E1) is a sterol-binding proteinase produced by the exocrine pancreas. It combines with bile acids and neutral sterols to transport cholesterol and derived metabolites along the intestinal lumen. As described by Sziegoleit in 1984[6] it is secreted in pancreatic juice and found intact in stool in concentrations five to six times those in pancreatic secretions.[7] The amino acid sequence of E1 has been determined.[8] E1 survives intestinal passage and its presence in stool is considered to reflect exocrine pancreatic function.[9] ELISA assay has been developed for serum[10] and is available commercially as a FET.[1] The assay has acceptable precision with intra-assay coefficient of variation (CV) of 3.3% to 6.3% (mean 4.8%) and interassay CV of 4.1% to 10.2% (mean 7.7%).[1] While the secretin and pancreozymin test may still be considered as the gold standard for evaluating pancreatic function, it is invasive (requiring injection/intubation), costly, time consuming, subject to technical error, and not commonly available. Alternative indirect tubeless pancreatic function tests include the fecal chymotrypsin test (FCT). While the FCT is procedurally simple, it has low sensitivity and the enzyme undergoes variable inactivation during intestinal transit. In addition, enzyme interference requires cessation of enzyme therapy 72 or more hours prior to obtaining the stool specimen. Elastase passes intact along the intestinal lumen and is measured as human-specific elastase. Thus, the FET is not subject to the problems noted to occur with the FCT. A number of recent studies have found the FET to be a simple and accurate, although indirect, test for chronic pancreatitis and to provide significant correlation with the gold standard.[1,5,11,12,13] The FET has been applied to the assessment of exocrine pancreatic insufficiency in children with cystic fibrosis. High levels of sensitivity and specificity (90% to 100%) have been reported.[13,14,15] When the FET was studied in relation to graded severity of exocrine pancreatic insufficiency (ie, mild, moderate, severe), the test was found to lack sensitivity for mild-to-moderate forms of the disease, which are the more frequent and difficult clinical problems.[15,16,17] It is disturbing that one study[17] found decreased fecal elastase 1 in 5 of 7 patients with malabsorption of nonpancreatic origin; evidence that the FET lacks specificity. The study sample size (7), however, was quite small. Studies utilizing FET in both adults[18] and children[19] indicate that fat malabsorption in immunodeficient, virus-infected patients may be due to exocrine pancreatic insufficiency in conjunction with intestinal malabsorption, although the decrease in pancreatic function may not be a major contributor to the malabsorption.[18,19] A significant negative correlation was found between fecal elastase 1 level and steatocrit.[19]

Footnotes

1. Stein J, Jung M, Sziegoleit A, et al, "Immunoreactive Elastase 1: Clinical Evaluation of a New Noninvasive Test of Pancreatic Function," *Clin Chem*, 1996, 42(2):222-6.
2. Sziegoleit A, "Purification and Characterization of a Cholesterol-Binding Protein From Human Pancreas," *Biochem J*, 1982, 207(3):573-82.
3. Stein J, Jung M, Zeuzem S, et al, "Fecal Elastase 1: A New Tubeless Test in the Diagnosis of Pancreatic Insufficiency," *Gastroenterology*, 1994, 106(4 Suppl):A325.
4. Terbrack HG, Gürtler KH, Klör HU, et al, "Human Pancreatic Elastase 1 Concentration in Faeces of Healthy Children and Children With Cystic Fibrosis," *Gut*, 1995, 37(Suppl 2):A253.
5. Löser C, Mölgaard A, and Fölsch UR, "Elastase 1 in Faeces: A Novel Sensitive and Specific Pancreatic Function Test for Easy and Inexpensive Routine Application," *Digestion*, 1995, 56(4):301.
6. Sziegoleit A, "A Novel Proteinase From Human Pancreas," *Biochem J* 1984, 219(3):735-42.
7. Sziegoleit A, Linder D, Schlüter M, et al, "Studies on the Specificity of the Cholesterol-Binding Pancreatic Proteinase and Identification as Human Pancreatic Elastase 1," *Eur J Biochem*, 1985, 151(3):595-9.
8. Shen W, Fletcher TS, and Largman C, "Primary Structure of Human Pancreatic Protease E Determined by Sequence Analysis of the Cloned mRNA," *Biochemistry*, 1987, 26(12):3447-52.
9. Sziegoleit A, Krause E, Klör HU, et al, "Elastase 1 and Chymotrypsin B in Pancreatic Juice and Feces," *Clin Biochem*, 1989, 22(2):85-9.
10. Sziegoleit A, Knäpler H, and Peters B, "ELISA for Human Pancreatic Elastase 1," *Clin Biochem*, 1989, 22(2):79-83.
11. Dominquez-Munoz JE, Hieronymus C, Sauerbruch T, et al, "Fecal Elastase Test: Evaluation of a New Noninvasive Pancreatic Function Test," *Am J Gastroenterol*, 1995, 90(10):1834-7.
12. Löser C, Möllgaard A, and Fölsch UR, "Faecal Elastase 1: A Novel, Highly Sensitive, and Specific Tubeless Pancreatic Function Test," *Gut*, 1996, 39(4):580-6.
13. Soldan W, Henker J, and Sprössig C, "Sensitivity and Specificity of Quantitative Determination of Pancreatic Elastase 1 in Feces of Children," *J Pediatr Gastroenterol Nutr*, 1997, 24(1):53-5.
14. Gullo L, Graziano L, Babbini S, et al, "Faecal Elastase 1 in Children With Cystic Fibrosis," *Eur J Pediatr* 1997, 156(10):770-2.
15. Walkowiak J, Cichy WK, and Herzig KH, "Comparison of Fecal Elastase-1 Determination With the Secretin-Cholecystokinin Test in Patients With Cystic Fibrosis," *Scand J Gastroenterol*, 1999, 34(2):202-7.
16. Lankisch PG, Schmidt I, König H, et al, "Faecal Elastase 1: Not Helpful in Diagnosing Chronic Pancreatitis Associated With Mild to Moderate Exocrine Pancreatic Insufficiency," *Gut*, 1998, 42(4):551-4.
17. Amann ST, Bishop M, Curington C, et al, "Fecal Pancreatic Elastase 1 Is Inaccurate in the Diagnosis of Chronic Pancreatitis," *Pancreas*, 1996, 13(3):226-30.
18. Carroccio A, Di Prima L, Di Grigoli, et al, "Exocrine Pancreatic Function and Fat Malabsorption in Human Immunodeficiency Virus-Infected Patients," *Scand J Gastroenterol*, 1999, 34(7):729-34.
19. Carroccio A, Fontana M, Spagnuolo MI, et al, "Pancreatic Dysfunction and its Association With Fat Malabsorption in HIV Infected Children," *Gut*, 1998, 43(4):558-63.

References

Mariani A, Mezzi G, Masci E, et al, "Accuracy of the Plasma Amino-Acid-Consumption Test in Detecting Pancreatic Diseases Is Due to Different Methods," *Pancreas*, 1999, 18(2):203-11.

♦ **Fecal pH** *see* pH, Stool *on page 317*

♦ **First Order Red Compensator** *see* Synovial Fluid Analysis *on page 323*

♦ **FOBT** *see* Occult Blood, Stool *on page 315*

♦ **Franklin-Dukes Test** *see* Infertility Screen *on page 310*

♦ **Gram Stain, Stool** *see* Methylene Blue Stain, Stool *on page 313*

♦ **Guaiac, Stool** *see* Occult Blood, Stool *on page 315*

♦ **Hamster Egg Penetration Test** *see* Sperm Penetration Assay (Zona-Free Hamster Egg Penetration Test) *on page 321*

♦ **Hamster Oocyte Penetration Assay** *see* Sperm Penetration Assay (Zona-Free Hamster Egg Penetration Test) *on page 321*

♦ **Hamster Test** *see* Sperm Penetration Assay (Zona-Free Hamster Egg Penetration Test) *on page 321*

♦ **Hamster Zona-Free Ovum Test** *see* Sperm Penetration Assay (Zona-Free Hamster Egg Penetration Test) *on page 321*

♦ **Hemizona Binding Assay** *see* Infertility Screen *on page 310*

♦ **Herbal Effects, Sperm Function** *see* Sperm Penetration Assay (Zona-Free Hamster Egg Penetration Test) *on page 321*

♦ **Heterologous Ovum Penetration Test** *see* Sperm Penetration Assay (Zona-Free Hamster Egg Penetration Test) *on page 321*

♦ **Humster (Human + Hamster) Test** *see* Sperm Penetration Assay (Zona-Free Hamster Egg Penetration Test) *on page 321*

♦ **Hyaluronate Concentration, Synovial Fluid** *see* Mucin Clot Test *on page 314*

Hypo-osmotic Swelling Test (Spermatozoa)

Related Information
Infertility Screen *on page 310*
Semen Analysis, Basic *on page 319*
Sperm Mucus Penetration Test (Human or Bovine Cervical Mucus) *on page 320*
Sperm Penetration Assay (Zona-Free Hamster Egg Penetration Test) *on page 321*

Applies to Sperm Penetration Assay

Abstract The HOS test evaluates the functional integrity of the sperm tail membrane. Results are correlated with the *in vitro* fertilizing ability of spermatozoa (ie, hamster egg sperm penetration assay, sperm motility and morphology).[1]

Specimen Semen

Container Clean, dry, wide-mouth glass or plastic bottle maintained warm and free of detergent or other toxic compounds

Collection Physician usually provides instruction for collection. Specimen quality is enhanced when collected in physician's office or laboratory, obviating delay in testing and exposure to extremes of temperature occasioned by transportation. Alternately, specimen may be obtained at patient's house by coitus interruptus or masturbation and delivered to the laboratory as soon as possible.[2] Collection of semen during intercourse using a seminal collection device may yield a specimen of higher quality.[3,4] Use of such a Silastic condom-type seminal pouch (with a small pencil lead-size perforation) to obtain a specimen for analysis in overcoming human infertility is acceptable to and falls within the principles of the Catholic Church.[5]

Storage Instructions Patient should be instructed to bring specimen to the laboratory within 30-60 minutes after collection maintaining warmth (37°C) during transport. Patient should be instructed to transport specimen in a pocket close to the skin. Low temperature during transport may decrease motility of sperm.

Causes for Rejection Specimen older than 60 minutes; semen specimen should be tested within 60 minutes after complete liquefaction

Turnaround Time 1-2 hours

Special Instructions Requisition should specify infertility study or postvasectomy study. Semen, as with all blood, urine, and body fluid specimens, because of the risk of AIDS, should be received and handled with attention to universal precautions. Gloves must be worn during the handling and manipulation of sperm/semen containing fluids. Persons with sores/open wounds of the skin must avoid contact with semen.

Reference Interval The test result is normal if >60% of spermatozoa undergo tail swelling. The semen specimen is abnormal if <50% of spermatozoa show tail swelling.

Use This test measures the functional integrity of the sperm membrane. Change in the properties of the sperm membrane is a requirement of successful spermatocyte/oocyte interaction (ie, sperm capacitation, acrosome reaction, and binding of spermatozoa to the surface of the ovum). As such, the hypo-osmotic swelling test result is an indicator of the fertilizing ability of spermatozoa. The test is a relatively simple low cost addition to standard semen analysis.

Limitations Rarely, a semen specimen may contain >5% swollen spermatozoa or coiled tails (swollen spermatozoa may be seen occasionally in untreated semen, usually in the range of 3% to 5%), or require more than 30-60 minutes for complete liquefaction. Test results in these circumstances may lack significance. The test protocol should include examination of the ejaculate before its addition to the HOS solution. The percent of spermatozoa with curled tails subtracted from the percentage obtained after treatment may provide a useful "true percentage" of sperm that reacted in the test.

Methodology Whole semen (0.1 mL) and hypo-osmotic solution (1 mL of equal parts of fructose and sodium citrate, each 150 mOsm, with resultant calculated ionic strength of 0.15) are mixed and incubated at 37°C for at least 30 minutes but for no longer than 120 minutes. After the mixture is allowed to stand for at least 1 minute, spermatozoa are examined using phase contrast microscopy for presence of changes in shape of the tail (see graphic following page). The number of swollen spermatozoa (as a result of a 200 cell count in duplicate) is used to calculate the mean percentage of sperm showing tail abnormalities indicative of swelling.

Additional Information Successful fertilization of a human ovum involves penetration of that ovum and subsequent fusion activities by a normally functioning spermatozoon. This process depends importantly upon the functional integrity of the sperm membrane. The hypo-osmotic swelling test (HOS Test) was developed to provide a simple assessment of the overall
(Continued)

Hypo-osmotic Swelling Test (Spermatozoa)
(Continued)

functional characteristics of the sperm membrane.[1] The test involves microscopic detection and percent quantification of morphologic swollen spermatozoa resulting from exposure to a hypotonic sugar/salt solution (half and half each 150 mOsm fructose and sodium citrate). If there is swelling under hypo-osmotic conditions intact membrane function is implied (in as much as the membrane allows passage of water to establish fluid equilibrium between intracellular and external environments). HOS test results have shown good correlation (r=0.90) with the hamster oocyte penetration test, even though the latter test has not shown good correlation with sperm morphology/motility parameters.[6] Sperm swelling relates poorly to sperm morphology (r=0.30) but somewhat better to sperm motility (r=0.61).

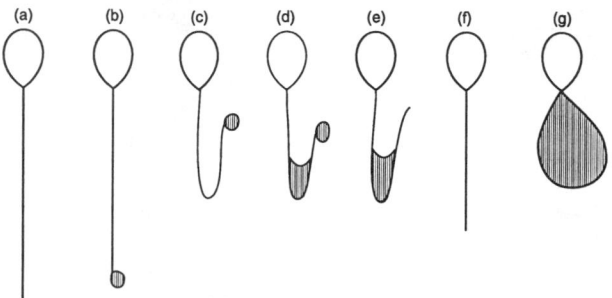

Schematic representation of typical morphological changes of human spermatozoa subjected to hypo-osmotic stress: a = no change; b-g = various types of tail changes. Tail region showing swelling is indicated by the hatched area.

Adapted from Jeyendran RS, Van der Ven HH, Perez-Pelaez M, et al, "Development of an Assay to Assess the Functional Integrity of the Human Sperm Membrane and Its Relationship to Other Semen Characteristics," *J Reprod Fertil*, 1984, 70(1):219-28.

Footnotes
1. Jeyendran RS, Van der Ven HH, Perez-Pelaez M, et al, "Development of an Assay to Assess the Functional Integrity of the Human Sperm Membrane and Its Relationship to Other Semen Characteristics," *J Reprod Fertil*, 1984, 70(1):219-28.
2. Sarkar S and Henry JB, "Semen Analysis," *Todd-Sanford-Davidsohn Clinical Diagnosis and Management by Laboratory Methods*, 19th ed, Henry JB, ed, Philadelphia, PA: WB Saunders Co, 1996, 510-11.
3. Zavos PM, "Seminal Parameters of Ejaculates Collected From Oligospermic and Normospermic Patients Via Masturbation and at Intercourse With the Use of a Silastic Seminal Fluid Collection Device," *Fertil Steril*, 1985, 44(4):517-20.
4. Zavos PM and Goodpasture JC, "Clinical Improvements of Specific Seminal Deficiencies Via Intercourse With a Seminal Collection Device Versus Masturbation," *Fertil Steril*, 1989, 51(1):190-3.
5. Griese ON, Rev Msgr, *Catholic Identity in Healthcare: Principles and Practice*, The Pope John Center, 1987, 51-3.
6. World Health Organization, *WHO Laboratory Manual for the Examination of Human Semen and Sperm-Cervical Mucus Interaction*, 4th ed, Cambridge, UK: Cambridge University Press, 1999, 4-11, 60-1.

References
Esteves SC, Sharma RK, Thomas AJ Jr, et al, "Sperm Viability Assays - A Matter of Life and Death," *Fertil Steril*, 1999, 72(1):184-5.
World Health Organization Laboratory Manual for the Examination of Human Semen and Sperm-Cervical Mucus Interaction, 4th ed, Cambridge, UK: Cambridge University Press, 1999, 29, 69-70.

Infertility Screen

Related Information

Applies to Andrology; Antispermatozoal Antibody Test; CASA; Computer-Assisted Semen Analysis; Franklin-Dukes Test; Hemizona Binding Assay; Leukocytospermia; MH61; Prosaposin; rSMP-B; Semen, Brown Colored; Sperm Agglutination and Inhibition; Sperm Antibodies; Sperm-Oolemma Binding Test

Test Includes Semen analysis. Specialized infertility/andrology laboratories perform infertility testing, but there is not a standardized test menu.

Abstract Extensive and sophisticated methodology for the evaluation of spermatozoa has been developed during the last decade. Expanding capabilities related to continuing growth in *in vitro* fertilization (IVF)/artificial insemination/intracytoplasmic sperm-spermatid injection has provided impetus for the study of sperm function, in particular by specialized andrology laboratories. The following is an overview of infertility evaluation, emphasis largely on the "male factor". It is hoped that the accompanying footnotes and references will provide entry to additional study and to the details of test methodology.

Patient Preparation Follow physician's instructions. Ejaculation should be avoided for 2-3 days prior to collection of the specimen. The entire ejaculate must be collected (initial portion may contain the majority of spermatozoa).[1]

Specimen Serum (both partners) and semen

Container Blood: red top tube; semen: clean, dry, wide-mouth glass or plastic container known to be free of detergent or other toxic agents. Storage in a plastic container may reduce motility of the spermatozoa. Examination should be conducted immediately upon liquefaction (or specimen placed in a glass container) if collection has been made initially in plastic.[1]

Collection Semen: Postcoital or masturbation using condom-like Silastic seminal fluid collection device (see Semen Analysis, Basic *on page 319*). There is evidence that some seminal deficiency test parameters are improved by semen collection via intercourse using a seminal collection device as opposed to masturbation.[2]

Storage Instructions Tests should be started as soon as possible after collection of semen at least within 2-3 hours, preferably within 1 hour or immediately after liquefaction.

Causes for Rejection Semen specimen more than 2 hours old, unlabeled specimen, specimen subjected to extremes of temperature or toxic material

Turnaround Time Test dependent, usually 1-2 days

Special Instructions Semen, as with all blood, urine, and body fluid specimens, because of the risk of AIDS, should be received and handled with care to avoid contamination of laboratory personnel. Gloves must be worn during the handling and manipulation of sperm/semen-containing fluids. Persons with sores/open wounds of the skin must avoid contact with semen. Infertility screen testing is not offered by many routine clinical laboratories. Specialized infertility/andrology laboratories perform infertility testing.

Reference Interval Individual test and laboratory dependent

Use Evaluate infertility; guide application of assisted reproductive techniques. The possibility that a couple is infertile can be considered when there is failure to conceive after about 1 year of unimpaired intercourse.

Limitations While the existence of sperm antibodies relating to infertility seems firmly established, methodology of some early testing procedures has not proven to be highly technically reliable. Tests utilizing methanol-fixed spermatozoa may give unpredictable and nonreproducible results.[2]

Computer-assisted semen analysis results have been found to be unreliable if sperm count is <20 million/mL. Sperm motility may be underestimated by computer-assisted analysis on post-thaw (after freezing) specimens.[3]

Methodology Routine semen analysis protocols, semen function tests, computer-assisted sperm morphology/motility studies, Kibrick agglutination assay with or without the use of gelatin, method of Franklin and Dukes,[4] microagglutination tests, sperm immobilization/cytotoxicity tests (eg, Isojima assay), mixed antiglobulin reaction assay (MAR), enzyme-linked immunosorbent assay (ELISA) using as antigen glutaraldehyde-fixed spermatozoa, Immunobead™ binding assay,[5] antisperm antibodies by indirect fluorescence using flow cytometry,[6] fluorescence *in situ* hybridization,[7] human sperm activation assay[8]

Additional Information Approximately 95% of normal couples should conceive within 13-15 months.[9] Many factors may be responsible for infertility. These may be divided into **"female factors"** and **"male factors"**. Common causes of female infertility include endometriosis, tubal factors (often pelvic inflammatory disease), ovulation and cervical/uterine factors. A "male factor" is responsible in some 20% of cases.[9] Basic evaluation (American Fertility Society) includes history and examination of the female, postcoital test, evaluation of tubal patency (hysterosalpingogram), evaluation of hormonal factors, history and examination of the male, and semen analyses.[10] To overcome the effect of transient variables, multiple and/or periodic study of spermatozoa may be necessary. Most cases of male infertility are classified as **idiopathic oligospermia** and **asthenospermia**, defined as <50 million/ejaculate and <50% motility respectively. Immunologic factors are a potential important cause of infertility. It has been estimated that 7% to 14% of men attending a fertility clinic have sperm-bound antibodies (as compared to an incidence of 1% to 2% in fertile men without history of vasovasostomy).[11]

This text deals largely with tests that identify "male factor" causes of infertility. The past 20 years have seen continuing interest in the evaluation of spermatozoa, reflecting increased understanding of sperm physiology with accompanying new test development. Thus, the growing number and capability of fertility/andrology laboratories, usually in support of assisted reproduction programs. The latter include such procedures as *in vitro* fertilization and embryonic transfer (IVF-ET), gamete-intrafallopian tube transfer (GIFT), and intracytoplasmic sperm injection (ICSI). The American Fertility Society has published guidelines for human andrology laboratories including recognition of the National Committee for Clinical Laboratory Standards (NCCLS) specified format.[12] An example of a quality control and quality assurance program has been published.[13] An excellent review presents an array of tests of human sperm function including:[14]

- resistance of sperm to decondensation in sodium dodecyl sulfate
- acidic aniline blue stain for immature sperm nuclei
- acridine orange stain for abnormal nuclear chromatin

- trypan blue or eosin Y membrane dye exclusion test
- follicular fluid induction of acrosome reaction
- calcium ionophore A23187 induction of acrosome reaction
- acrosome assessment by *Pisum sativum* agglutinin fluorescein stain
- measurement of acrosomal proteinase activity
- assessment of hyaluronidase activity
- sperm-oolemma binding test
- hypo-osmotic swelling test
- hemizona binding assay
- variety of tests for determination of antisperm antibodies (see below)

Presence of **antisperm antibodies** has not been clearly associated with disease states but bears association with diminished fertility. When clumping of sperm or sperm with poor motility is found, antibodies should be considered.[15] Such antibodies may be found in the circulation, free or as immune complexes, in seminal plasma, and/or attached to the sperm surface. In semen, sperm antibodies are usually immunoglobulin class IgA or IgG with the former, generally, of greater clinical significance. IgM antibodies, possibly relating to their larger size, are not usually present in semen.[16] Tests that measure immunoglobulin on the sperm surface have greater sensitivity than assays of serum antisperm antibodies. Some males may have blood negative for sperm antibodies but have demonstrable antibody on the surface of spermatozoa. Sperm-bound antibody measured by ELISA has been found present in a greater percentage of infertile men with varicoceles than infertile men without varicoceles.[17] Results of a modification of the Seminobead™ test (in which the beads are coated with MH61, a monoclonal antibody specific for acrosome-reacted sperm) have been shown to correlate with outcomes of sperm penetration assays (SPA) and *in vitro* fertilization (IVF).[18]

Antibodies are found in some males with testicular disease. They are also seen in some cases of autoimmune aspermatogenesis experimentally induced by immunization with semen, spermatozoa, or testicular homogenates. There may be a cause and effect relationship between spermatozoal antibodies in serum of females and unexplained infertility. Both members of the couple should have their serum tested. The use of a single type of test may not be adequate. Studies indicate that each test has a different incidence of positive results in an infertile population. Repeat of a test procedure will, at times, give different results for a particular serum sample. A number of immunologic-based methods for detection of antisperm antibodies (ASA) have been developed. The Immunobead™ test and the mixed antiglobulin reaction (MAR) IgG and IgA tests are the most commonly used screening tests.[16] Antisperm antibody tests are critiqued in the text by Glover et al and include immunofluorescence (IF); gelatin agglutination test (GAT), Kibrick method; tube-slide agglutination test (TSAT), Franklin Dukes method; tray agglutination test (TAT); slide agglutination test (SAT); modified slide agglutination test (MSAT); sperm immobilization test (SIT); mixed antiglobulin reaction (MAR); Immunobead™ test (IBT); and enzyme-linked immunosorbent assay (ELISA).[19]

Serious shortcomings of currently used ASA tests (both qualitative and quantitative) are detailed by Helmerhorst et al with the conclusion "...it is difficult to consider the routinely used ASA tests as an essential procedure in the fertility work-up. It is even more difficult to justify a treatment on the basis of such tests." Bronson, on the other hand, concludes that current tests have practical clinical value even as future generations of more specific tests that detect ASA directed against defined fertilization-related antigens are being developed.[20] Such development involves application of modern procedural tools, including immunoblotting, affinity chromatography, and flow cytometry. rSMP-B, a sperm protein localized to the surface of the tail and midpiece region of human sperm, has been proposed as the target antigen of sperm - immobilizing antibodies and measured using an enzyme-linked immunosorbent assay with synthetic peptide segment rSMP-230 as substrate (corresponds with the hydrophilic domain of rSMP-B).[21] Immunologic mechanisms may, theoretically, interfere with the sperm-egg binding protein, prosaposin, and/or its sperm receptors.[22]

Electro-optical and computer-assisted devices and systems are available for the semiautomated/automated study of sperm morphology and motility, that is, computer-assisted semen analysis (CASA). These are utilized by a growing number of andrology laboratories. Some aspects of their evaluation and application are detailed.[23,24,25] Early opinion cautioned against clinical use of CASA results in prediction of *in vivo* fertility. However, with emphasis on proper sample characteristics and preparation, technical competence with adherence to instrument manufacturer's operating instructions, and careful quality assurance procedures, a role is evolving for use of CASA by routine andrology laboratories.[26,27,28,29]

Sperm concentration, motility and concentration of progressively motile cells, along with CASA determined simple sperm morphometry characteristics appear to relate to time to conception.[26,27] Sperm concentration determination by CASA is improved by use of fluorescent DNA stains.[30] A recently developed automated system allows for the measurement of numerous (some 30 plus) sperm morphometric characteristics.[31] A standard terminology is applied to sperm movement characteristics (eg, ALH - amplitude of lateral head displacement).[26,29] An intralaboratory and interlaboratory comparison of sperm morphology (strict criteria) found good correlation between manual analysis of liquefied samples as compared with washed samples with both Diff-Quik™ and Papanicoulau-stained slides with intraclass coefficient (ICC) of 0.93 and 0.83. Intralaboratory correlation of within-computer readings (washed samples) was high (ICC of 0.93). Interlaboratory computer comparisons (study limited to just two centers, each on different continents) showed moderate correlation (ICC of 0.72). However, a low level of agreement (ICC of 0.57) was noted with interlaboratory manual comparison.[32] Computerized morphology has been applied to the identification of mature spermatozoa (midpiece and tail dimensions varied between mature and decreased maturity sperm fractions).[33]

Analysis of sperm donor's specimens, none azoospermic, by manual standard methods (WHO standards) and the Sperm Quality Analyzer IIB (SQA IIB) have been compared with unfavorable results.[34]

The finding of apparent decline of sperm counts in fertile men over the past 50 years is disputed by recent studies.[35,36,37]

Exposure to aromatic solvents appears to be associated with reduced sperm quality (low sperm count, low % motility, and low % normal forms).[38]

Infertility may be the first clinical sign of male genitourinary tuberculosis.[39] Semen/sperm parameters are usually normal with the exception of leukocytospermia (pyospermia), which occasionally may be massive. Results of a morning urine culture can establish the diagnosis.

The cellular and molecular basis for infertility in spinal cord injury is the subject of a recent review.[40] Brown-colored semen has been noted in 27% (on at least one ejaculation) of men with spinal cord injury.[40] This finding could not be attributed to the presence of RBCs (in 50% of specimens) or to the presence of heme pigment (in 33% of specimens). The brown color may relate to seminal-vesicle dysfunction involving phagocytosis, degradation, and processing of sperm by macrophages with generation of lipofusion-like pigment.[41]

Andrology research has resulted in numerous proposed tests or approaches to testing that may have clinical applicability. Included are cell imaging and manipulative techniques (eg, electron microscopy,[42,43] atomic force microscopy,[44] and flow cytometry[45,46,47]), biochemical analyses (eg, calcium,[48] trace metals,[49,50] reactive oxygen species[51,52,53]), and multiantigen/enzyme studies[54] (with the finding that decreased prostaglandin D synthase may be a new marker of post-testicular obstruction). Glycerophosphorylcholine:choline ratio (determined by magnetic resonance spectroscopy) may be able to differentiate different forms of azoospermia (eg, different forms of spermatogenic failure and obstructive azoospermia).[55]

With the advent of treatment of male factor infertility by intracytoplasmic sperm injection (ICSI) - the intracytoplasmic injection of a single spermatozoon directly into an oocyte - concern has arisen about possible transmission of genetic (DNA) abnormalities, in particular, aneuploid chromosome number.[56,57,58,59,60,61]

A minimum level of extracellular ionized calcium is necessary to the maintenance of normal sperm motility. Spermatozoa appear to be dependent on intracellular translocation of calcium ions rather than on the extracellular concentration of ionized calcium.[62]

Evaluation of spermatozoal function has been approached by measuring surrogate cervical mucus penetration (see also Sperm Mucus Penetration Test (Human or Bovine Cervical Mucus) *on page 320*) and the determination of sperm capacitation index, based on the degree of polyspermy in penetration of zona-free, pellucida-free hamster ova.[63] See also Sperm Penetration Assay (Zona-Free Hamster Egg Penetration Test) *on page 321.*

Heavy smoking appears to be associated with detrimental effects on sperm viability and morphology.[64,65,66] This effect may be mediated by smoker's seminal plasma, replacement of which, by physiological media, may possibly enhance the fertilizing capability of involved spermatozoa in assisted reproductive procedures.[66] The use of cocaine has been associated with low sperm concentration, low sperm motility, and presence of abnormal morphology.[67]

Increased frequency of chromosomal as well as numerical abnormalities has been found in sperm from infertile males.[7]

Hypogonadotropic hypogonadism is an uncommon explanation for male infertility, for which therapy is available.[15]

Clinical features of cystic fibrosis (CF) include male infertility. Over 95% of men with CF are azoospermic due to a variety of regressive abnormalities of the mesonephric duct (Wolffian duct-derived anomalies) of which congenital bilateral absence of the vas deferens (CBAVD) is most common. Over 60% of patients with CBAVD have one or more mutations of the cystic fibrosis transmembrane conductance regulator (CFTR) gene. CBAVD patients may carry the most common (ΔF508) mutation but may also harbor rare mutations (ie, R117H). The CFTR gene abnormalities associated with obstructive azoospermia anomalies are found uncommonly in the classic CF population. As routine testing for CFTR mutations may miss the unusual abnormalities and as epididymal/testicular aspiration and intracytoplasmic sperm injection are now available, it has been recommended that genetic analyses and counselling be pursued due to the possibility of iatrogenic transmission of CFTR mutations.[68,69]

Footnotes

1. McBride LJ, "Seminal Fluid Analysis," *Textbook of Urinalysis and Body Fluids: A Clinical Approach,* Chapter 12, Philadelphia, PA: Lippincott-Raven Publishers, 1998, 219-22.

(Continued)

Infertility Screen (Continued)

2. Zavos PM and Goodpasture JC, "Clinical Improvements of Specific Seminal Deficiencies Via Intercourse With a Seminal Collection Device Versus Masturbation," Fertil Steril, 1989, 51(1):190-3.

3. Sidhu RS, Sharma RK, Lee JC, et al, "Accuracy of Computer-Assisted Semen Analysis in Prefreeze and Post-thaw Specimens With High and Low Sperm Counts and Motility," Urology, 1998, 51(2):306-12.

4. Franklin RR and Dukes CD, "Further Studies on Sperm-Agglutinating Antibody and Unexplained Infertility," JAMA, 1964, 190:682.

5. Clarke GN, Elliott PJ, and Smaila C, "Detection of Sperm Antibodies in Semen Using the Immunobead™ Test: A Survey of 813 Consecutive Patients," Am J Reprod Immunol Microbiol, 1985, 7(3):118-23.

6. Sinton EB, Riemann DC, and Ashton ME, "Antisperm Antibody Detection Using Concurrent Cytofluorometry and Indirect Immunofluorescence Microscopy," Am J Clin Pathol, 1991, 95(2):242-6.

7. Moosani N, Pattinson HA, Carter MD, et al, "Chromosomal Analysis of Sperm From Men With Idiopathic Infertility Using Sperm Karyotyping and Fluorescence iIn Situ Hybridization," Fertil Steril, 1995, 64(4):811-7.

8. Brown DB, Hayes EJ, Uchida T, et al, "Some Cases of Human Male Infertility Are Explained by Abnormal In Vitro Human Sperm Activation," Fertil Steril, 1995, 64(3):612-22.

9. Talbert LM, "Overview of the Diagnostic Evaluation," Infertility - A Practical Guide for the Physician, 3rd ed, Hammond MG and Talbert LM, eds, Boston, MA: Blackwell Scientific Publications, 1992, 1-10.

10. Taymor ML, Infertility - A Clinician's Guide to Diagnosis and Treatment, New York, NY: Plenum Medical Book Company, 1990, 12-3.

11. Glover TD, Barratt CL, Tyler JP, et al, "Seeking Possible Causes of Dysfunction," Human Male Fertility and Semen Analysis, San Diego, CA: Academic Press, 1990, 109.

12. Byrd W, Boldt JP, and Wolf DP, Guidelines for Human Andrology Laboratories, Birmingham, AL: The American Fertility Society, Fertil Steril, 1992, 58(4 Suppl 1):11S-16S.

13. Muller CH, "The Andrology Laboratory in an Assisted Reproductive Technologies Program - Quality Assurance and Laboratory Methodology," J Androl, 1992, 13(5):349-60.

14. Liu DY and Baker HWG, "Tests of Human Sperm Function and Fertilization In Vitro," Fertil Steril, 1992, 58(3):465-83.

15. Howards SS, "Treatment of Male Infertility," N Engl J Med, 1995, 332(5):312-7.

16. World Health Organization Laboratory Manual for the Examination of Human Semen and Sperm-Cervical Mucus Interaction, 4th ed, Cambridge, UK: Cambridge University Press, 1999, 23-7 and 77-80.

17. Gilbert BR, Witkin SS, and Goldstein M, "Correlation of Sperm-Bound Immunoglobulins With Impaired Semen Analysis in Infertile Men With Varicoceles," Fertil Steril, 1989, 52(3):469-73.

18. Ohashi K, Saji F, Kato M, et al, "Evaluation of Acrosomal Status Using MH61-Beads Test and Its Clinical Application," Fertil Steril, 1992, 58(4):803-8.

19. Glover TD, Barratt CL, Tyler JP, et al, Human Male Fertility and Semen Analysis, San Diego, CA: Academic Press, 1990, 137-42.

20. Helmerhorst FM, Finken MJ, and Erwich JJ, "Detection Assays for Antisperm Antibodies: What Do They Test?" Bronson R, "Detection of Antisperm Antibodies: An Argument Against Therapeutic Nihilism," Debate: Antisperm Antibodies, Hum Reprod, 1999, 14(7):1669-73.

21. Kamada M, Yamamoto S, Takikawa M, et al, "Identification of the Human Sperm Protein That Interacts With Sperm-Immobilizing Antibodies in the Sera of Infertile Women," Fertil Steril, 1999, 72(4):691-5.

22. Amann R, Shabanowitz RB, Huszar G, et al, "Increased In Vitro Binding of Fresh and Frozen-Thawed Human Sperm Exposed to a Synthetic Peptide," J Androl, 1999, 20(5):655-9.

23. Wang C, Leung A, Tsoi WL, et al, "Computer-Assisted Assessment of Human Sperm Morphology: Comparison With Visual Assessment," Fertil Steril, 1991, 55(5):983-8.

24. Kruger TF, DuToit TC, Franken DR, et al, "A New Computerized Method of Reading Sperm Morphology (Strict Criteria) Is as Efficient as Technician Reading," Fertil Steril, 1993, 59(1):202-9.

25. Davis RO and Gravance CG, "Standardization of Specimen Preparation, Staining, and Sampling Methods Improves Automated Sperm-Head Morphometry Analysis," Fertil Steril, 1993, 59(2):412-7.

26. Irvine DS, Macleod IC, Templeton AA, et al, "A Prospective Clinical Study of the Relationship Between the Computer-Assisted Assessment of Human Semen Quality and the Achievement of Pregnancy In Vivo," Hum Reprod, 1994, 9(12):2324-34.

27. Mortimer D and Frasser L, "Consensus Workshop on Advanced Diagnostic Andrology Techniques," ESHRE (European Society of Human Reproduction and Embryology) Andrology Special Interest Group, Hum Reprod, 1996, 11(7):1463-79.

28. "Guidelines on the Application of CASA Technology in the Analysis of Spermatozoa," ESHRE Andrology Special Interest Group, Hum Reprod, 1998, 13(1):142-5.

29. World Health Organization, WHO Laboratory Manual for the Examination of Human Semen and Sperm-Cervical Mucus Interaction, 4th ed, Cambridge, UK: Cambridge University Press, 1999, 30-1, 33, 90-3.

30. Zinaman MJ, Uhler ML, Vertuno E, et al, "Evaluation of Computer-assisted Semen Analysis (CASA) With IDENT Stain to Determine Sperm Concentration," J Androl, 1996, 17(3):288-92.

31. Garrett C and Baker HW, "A New Fully Automated System for the Morphometric Analysis of Human Sperm Heads," Fertil Steril, 1995, 63(6):1306-17.

32. Barroso G, Mercan R, Ozgur K, et al, "Intra- and Interlaboratory Variability in the Assessment of Sperm Morphology by Strict Criteria: Impact of Semen Preparation, Staining Techniques, and Manual Versus Computerized Analysis," Hum Reprod, 1999, 14(8):2036-40.

33. Gergely A, Kovanci E, Senturk L, et al, "Morphometric Assessment of Mature and Diminished-Maturity Human Spermatozoa: Sperm Regions That Reflect Differences in Maturity," Hum Reprod, 1999, 14(8):2007-14.

34. Makler A, Shiram E, Geva H, et al, "Evaluation of the SQA IIB: A New Version of a Sperm Quality Analyzer," Fertil Steril, 1999, 71(4):761-4.

35. Fisch H, Goluboff ET, Olson JH, et al, "Semen Analysis in 1283 Men From the United States Over a 25-Year Period: No Decline in Quality," Fertil Steril, 1996, 65(5):1009-14.

36. Emanuel ER, Goluboff ET, and Fisch H, "Macleod Revisited: Sperm Count Distribution in 374 Fertile Men From 1971 to 1994," Urol 1998, 51(1):86-8.

37. Paulsen CV, Berman NG, and Wang C, "Data From Men in Greater Seattle Area Reveals no Downward Trend in Semen Quality: Further Evidence That Deterioration of Semen Quality Is Not Geographically Uniform," Fertil Steril, 1996, 65(5):1015-20.

38. Tielemans E, Burdorf A, te Velde ER, et al, "Occupationally Related Exposures and Reduced Semen Quality: A Case-Control Study," Fertil Steril, 1997, 71(4):690-6.

39. Lübbe J, Ruef C, Spirig W, et al, "Infertility as the First Symptom of Male Genitourinary Tuberculosis," Urol Int, 1996, 56(3):204-6.

40. Rajasekaran M and Monga M, "Cellular and Molecular Causes of Male Infertility in Spinal Cord Injury," J Androl, 1999, 20(3):326-30.

41. Wieder JA, Lynne CM, Ferrell SM, et al, "Brown-Colored Semen in Men With Spinal Cord Injury," J Androl, 1999, 20(5):594-600.

42. Carbone DJ Jr, McMahon JT, Levin HS, et al, "Role of Electron Microscopy of Sperm in the Evaluation of Male Infertility During the Era of Assisted Reproduction," Urology, 1998, 52(2):301-5.

43. Nogueira D, Bourgain C, Verheyen G, et al, "Light and Electron Microscopic Analysis of Human Testicular Spermatozoa and Spermatids From Frozen and Thawed Testicular Biopsies," Hum Reprod , 1999, 14(8):2041-9.

44. Mai A, Rattanachaiyanont M, Lender A, et al, "Atomic Force Microscopy of Human Sperm: A New Approach to Human Sperm Morphology Analysis," Fertil Steril, 1998, 70(3 Suppl 1):S95-S96.

45. Cooper TG and Yeung CH, "A Flow Cytometric Technique Using Peanut Agglutinin for Evaluating Acrosomal Loss From Human Spermatozoa," J Androl, 1998, 19(5):542-50.

46. Carver-Ward JA, Jaroudi KA, Hollanders JM, et al, "High Fertilization Prediction by Flow Cytometric Analysis of the CD46 Antigen on the Inner Acrosomal Membrane of Spermatozoa," Hum Reprod, 1996, 11(9):1923-8.

47. Ziyyat A, Lassalle B, Testart J, et al, "Flow Cytometry Isolation and Reverse Transcriptase-Polymerase Chain Reaction Characterization of Human Round Spermatids in Infertile Patients," Hum Reprod, 1999, 14(2):379-87.

48. Kilic S, Sarica K, Yaman O, et al, "Effect of Total and Ionized Calcium Levels of Seminal Fluid on Sperm Motility," Urol Int, 1996, 56(4):215-8.

49. Carpino A, Siciliano L, Petrone MF, et al, "Low Seminal Zinc Bound to High Molecular Weight Proteins in Asthenozoospermic Patients: Evidence of Increased Sperm Zinc Content in Oligoasthenozoospermic Patients," Hum Reprod, 1998, 13(1):111-4.

50. Hovatta O, Venäläinen ER, Kuusimäki L, et al, "Aluminum, Lead, and Cadmium Concentrations in Seminal Plasma and Spermatozoa, and Semen Quality in Finnish Men," Hum Reprod, 1998, 13(1):115-9.

51. World Health Organization, WHO Laboratory Manual for the Examination of Human Semen and Sperm-Cervical Mucus Interaction, 4th ed, World Health Organization, Cambridge, UK: Cambridge University Press, 1999, 31-2, appendix XVI, 99-101.

52. Donnelly ET, McClure N, and Lewis SM, "Antioxidant Supplementation In Vitro Does Not Improve Human Sperm Motility," Fertil Steril, 1999, 72(3):484-95.

53. Zini A, O'Bryan MK, Israel L, et al, "Human Sperm NADH and NADPH Diaphorase Cytochemistry: Correlation With Sperm Motility," Urology, 1998, 51(3):464-8.

54. Diamandis PE, Arnett WP, Foussias G, et al, "Seminal Plasma Biochemical Markers and Their Association With Semen Analysis Findings," Urology, 1999, 53(3):596-603.

55. Hamamah S, Seguin F, Bujan L, et al, "Quantification by Magnetic Resonance Spectroscopy of Metabolites in Seminal Plasma Able to Differentiate Different Forms of Azoospermia," Hum Reprod, 1998, 13(1):132-5.

56. Pfeffer J, Pang MG, Hoegerman SF, et al, "Aneuploidy Frequencies in Semen Fractions From Ten Oligoasthenoteratozoospermic Patients Donating Sperm for Intracytoplasmic Sperm Injection," Fertil Steril, 1999, 72(3):472-8.

57. Lim AS, Fong Y, and Yu SL, "Analysis of the Sex Chromosome Constitution of Sperm in Men With a 47,XYY Mosaic Karyotype by Fluorescence In Situ Hybridization," Fertil Steril, 1999, 72(1):121-3.

58. Carrell DT, Emery BR, and Liu L, "Characterization of Aneuploidy Rates, Protamine Levels, Ultrastructure, and Functional Ability of Round-Headed Sperm From Two Siblings and Implications for Intracytoplasmic Sperm Injection," Fertil Steril, 1999, 71(3):511-6.

59. Colombero CT, Hariprashad JJ, Tsai MC, et al, "Incidence of Sperm Aneuploidy in Relation to Semen Characteristics and Assisted Reproductive Outcome," Fertil Steril, 1999, 72(1):90-6.

60. Lee JD, Kamiguchi Y, and Yanagimachi R, "Analysis of Chromosome Constitution of Human Spermatozoa With Normal and Aberrant Head Morphologies After Injection Into Mouse Ooxytes," Hum Reprod, 1996, 11(9):1942-6.

61. Zini A, Mak V, Phang D, et al, "Potential Adverse Effect of Semen Processing on Human Sperm Deoxyribonucleic Acid Integrity," Fertil Steril, 1999, 72(3):496-9.

62. Aaberg RA, Sauer MV, Sikka S, et al, "Effects of Extracellular Ionized Calcium, Diltiazem and cAMP on Motility of Human Spermatozoa," J Urol, 1989, 141(5):1221-4.

63. Smith RG, Johnson A, Lamb D, et al, "Functional Tests of Spermatozoa. Sperm Penetration Assay," Urol Clin North Am, 1987, 14(3):451-8.

64. Sofikitis N, Miyagawa I, Dimitriadis D, et al, "Effects of Smoking on Testicular Function, Semen Quality and Sperm Fertilizing Capacity," J Urol, 1995, 154(3):1030-4.

65. Zavos PM, Correa JR, Karagounis CS, et al, "An Electron Microscopic Study of the Axonemal Ultrastructure in Human Spermatozoa From Male Smokers and Nonsmokers," Fertil Steril, 1998, 69(3):430-4.

66. Zavos PM, Correa JR, Antypas S, et al, "Effects of Seminal Plasma From Cigarette Smokers on Sperm Viability and Longevity," Fertil Steril, 1998, 69(3):425-9.

67. Bracken MB, Eskenazi B, Sachse K, et al, "Association of Cocaine Use With Sperm Concentration, Motility, and Morphology," Fertil Steril, 1990, 53(2):315-22.

68. Dohle CR, Veeze HJ, Overbeek SE, et al, "The Complex Relationship Between Cystic Fibrosis and Congenital Bilateral Absence of the Vas Deferens: Clinical, Electrophysiological, and Genetic Data," Hum Reprod, 1999, 14(2):371-4.

69. Mak V, Zielenski J, Tsui LC, et al, "Proportion of Cystic Fibrosis Gene Mutations Not Detected by Routine Testing in Men With Obstructive Azoospermia," *JAMA*, 1999, 281(23):2217-24.

References

Adelman MM and Cahill EM, *Atlas of Sperm Morphology*, Chicago, IL: American Society of Clinical Pathologists, 1989.

Auger J, Kunstmann JM, Czyglik F, et al, "Decline in Semen Quality Among Fertile Men in Paris During the Past 20 Years," *N Engl J Med*, 1995, 332(5):281-5.

Baker DJ and Witmyer J, "Semen Analysis Training Tool," *Reproduction Educational Resources*, Lexington, KY, 1998. Review, Adelman MM, "Media Reviews," *Lab Med*, 1999, 30(10):687-8.

Bohring C and Krause W, "The Intra- and Inter-Assay Variation of the Indirect Mixed Antiglobulin Reaction Test: Is a Quality Control Suitable?" *Hum Reprod*, 1999, 14(7):1802-5.

College of American Pathologists Conference XX, "New Developments in Reproductive Biology: August 21-23, 1991," *Arch Pathol Lab Med*, 1992, 116(4):323-43.

Comhaire FH, "Sperm Antibodies - Gold Standard?" *Fertil Steril*, 1993, 59(1):242-3.

Damjanov I, "Clinical Evaluation of the Infertile Couple," *Pathology of Infertility*, Chapter 2, St Louis, MO: CV Mosby Co, 1993, 7-42.

De Jonge C, "Attributes of Fertile Spermatozoa: An Update," Andrology Lab Corner, *J Androl*, 1999, 20(4):463-73.

Downie SE, Flaherty SP, and Matthews CD, "Detection of Chromosomes and Estimation of Aneuploidy in Human Spermatozoa Using Fluorescence *In Situ* Hybridization," *Mol Hum Reprod*, 1997, 3(7):585-98.

Glover TD and Barratt CR, *Male Infertility and Infertility*, Cambridge, UK: Cambridge University Press, 1999.

Gwatkin RBL, Collins JA, Jarrell JF, et al, "The Value of Semen Analysis and Sperm Function Assays in Predicting Pregnancy Among Infertile Couples," *Fertil Steril*, 1990, 53(4):693-9.

Hurowitz EH, Leung A, and Wang C, "Evaluation of the CellTrak Computer-Assisted Sperm Analysis in Comparison to the Cellsoft System to Measure Human Sperm Hyperactivation," *Fertil Steril*, 1995, 64(2):427-32.

Jeremias J and Witkin SS, "Molecular Approaches to the Diagnosis of Male Infertility," *Mol Hum Reprod*, 1996, 2(3):195-202.

Kjeldsberg CR and Knight JA, *Body Fluids - Laboratory Examination of Amniotic, Cerebrospinal, Seminal, Serous, and Synovial Fluids*, 3rd ed, Chicago, IL: ASCP Press, American Society of Clinical Pathologists, 1993, 255-64, 344-66.

Lähteenmäki A, "*In Vitro* Fertilization in the Presence of Antisperm Antibodies Detected by the Mixed Antiglobulin Reaction (MAR) and the Tray Agglutination Test (TAT)," *Hum Reprod*, 1993, 8(1):84-8.

Liu DY and Baker HWG, "Morphology of Spermatozoa Bound to the Zona Pellucida of Human Oocytes That Failed to Fertilize *In Vitro*," *J Reprod Fertil*, 1992, 94(1):71-84.

Mackenna A, Barratt CLR, Kessopoulou E, et al, "The Contribution of a Hidden Male Factor to Unexplained Infertility," *Fertil Steril*, 1993, 59(2):405-11.

McLendon WW, "The American Fertility Society - College of American Pathologists Collaborative Program for Accreditation of *In Vitro* Fertilization Laboratories: Building Bridges to Enhance Patient Care," *Arch Pathol Lab Med*, 1992, 116(4):317-8.

Mortimer ST, "A Critical Review of the Physiological Importance and Analysis of Sperm Movement in Mammals," *Hum Reprod Update*, 1997, 3(5):403-29.

Nasseri A and Grifo JA, "Barriers to Success in Assisted Reproduction," *Curr Probl Obstet Gynecol Fertil*, 1998, 21(5):132-41.

Shen HM, Chia SE, Ni ZY, et al, "Detection of Oxidative DNA Damage in Human Sperm and the Association With Cigarette Smoking," *Reprod Toxicol*, 1997, 11(5):675-80.

Sherins RJ, "Are Semen Quality and Male Fertility Changing?" *N Engl J Med*, 1995, 332(5):327-8.

Takihara H, "The Treatment of Obstructive Azoospermia in Male Fertility - Past, Present, and Future," *Urology*, 1998, 51(Suppl 5A):150-5.

Turek PJ and Lipshultz LI, "Immunologic Infertility," *Urol Clin North Am*, 1994, 21(3):447-68.

Yablonsky T, "Male Fertility Testing. New Tests Yield More Predictive Power: But Are They Useful?" *Lab Med*, 1996, 27(6):378-80.

♦ **Infrared Reflectance Analysis** *see* Fat, Semiquantitative, Stool, Sudan III Stain *on page 306*

♦ **Intestinal Converted Fraction** *see* Occult Blood, Stool *on page 315*

♦ **In Vivo Cervical Mucus Penetration (Postcoital) Test** *see* Sperm Mucus Penetration Test (Human or Bovine Cervical Mucus) *on page 320*

♦ **Joint Fluid Analysis** *see* Synovial Fluid Analysis *on page 323*

♦ **Kremer Sperm Penetration Test** *see* Sperm Mucus Penetration Test (Human or Bovine Cervical Mucus) *on page 320*

♦ **Lactoferrin, Fecal** *see* Fecal Lactoferrin *on page 308*

♦ **Leukocytospermia** *see* Infertility Screen *on page 310*

♦ **Leukotest® (Fecal Lactoferrin)** *see* Methylene Blue Stain, Stool *on page 313*

♦ **Leukotest®, Stool** *see* Fecal Lactoferrin *on page 308*

Meat Fibers, Stool

Related Information

d-Xylose Absorption Test, Serum, Urine *on page 167*
Fat, Semiquantitative, Stool, Sudan III Stain *on page 306*
Fecal Fat by Near-Infrared Reflectance Analysis *on page 307*
Fecal Fat, Quantitative, 72-Hour Collection *on page 172*
Fecal Lactoferrin *on page 308*
Fecal Pancreatic Elastase 1 *on page 308*
Methylene Blue Stain, Stool *on page 313*

pH, Stool *on page 317*
Reducing Substances, Stool *on page 317*

Synonyms Muscle Fiber, Stool; Stool Meat Fibers

Abstract Stool is examined microscopically for the presence of striated muscle fibers as an indicator of malabsorption/pancreatic insufficiency. While simple and inexpensive, this test is largely ignored (due to lack of sensitivity and in particular, lack of specificity) in favor of more specific screening tests for malabsorption (eg, d-xylose and vitamin D absorption tests) and fecal fat determination.[1,2]

Patient Preparation Patient is required to eat adequate amounts of red meat for 24-72 hours before testing. Specimens may be obtained with warm saline or Fleet Phospho®-Soda enema. Specimens obtained with mineral oil, bismuth, or magnesium compounds are unsatisfactory. Barium procedures or laxatives should be avoided for 1 week prior to collection of the specimen.

Specimen Stool

Causes for Rejection Purgatives other than saline or Fleet® Phospho®-Soda

Reference Interval Negative for muscle fibers

Use Initial evaluation of malabsorption syndromes, pancreatic exocrine dysfunction, or gastrocolic (fecal) fistula

Methodology Stool is mixed with a 10% solution of eosin in ethanol, stained on a slide for 3 minutes, and coverslipped. Only rectangular-shaped fibers with identifiable cross striations are counted.

Additional Information The presence of fecal undigested muscle fibers implies impaired intraluminal digestion. There is good correlation with stool fat determinations. Study of stool for muscle fibers when a high meat intake has been maintained is an inexpensive but necessarily nonspecific test for malabsorption. The presence of fecal muscle fibers cannot differentiate pancreatic insufficiency from other causes of malabsorption.[3] More sophisticated tests of pancreatic exocrine function (secreting ability) include the pancreozymin secretin test, cerulein secretin test, NBT-PABA test, and pancreatic dual-label Schilling test.[4] Muscle fibers reported as present in urine are suggestive of fecal contamination of the specimen (eg, fecal fistula).[5]

Footnotes

1. Kalser MH, "Malabsorption Syndromes," *Bockus Gastroenterology*, 5th ed, Chapter 58, Haubrich WS, Schaffner F, and Berk JE, eds, Philadelphia, PA: WB Saunders Co, 1995, 996-8.
2. Powell DW, "Approach to the Patient With Diarrhea," *Textbook of Gastroenterology*, 2nd ed, Chapter 38, Yamada T, ed, Philadelphia, PA: JB Lippincott Co, 1995, 813.
3. Moore JG, Englert E Jr, Bigler AH, et al, "Simple Fecal Tests of Absorption - A Prospective Study and Critique," *Am J Dig Dis*, 1971, 16(2):97-105.
4. Chen WL, Morishita R, Eguchi T, et al, "Clinical Usefulness of Dual-Label Schilling Test for Pancreatic Exocrine Function," *Gastroenterology*, 1989, 96(5 Pt 1):1337-45.
5. Birch DF, Fairley KF, Becker GJ, et al, *A Color Atlas of Urine Microscopy*, London: Chapman and Hall Medical, 1994, 8, 11.

References

Fischbach FT, *A Manual of Laboratory and Diagnostic Testing*, 5th ed, Philadelphia, PA: JB Lippincott Co, 1996, 269.

Kao YS, Liu FJ, and Alexander DR, "Laboratory Diagnosis of Gastrointestinal Tract and Exocrine Pancreatic Disorders," *Clinical Diagnosis and Management by Laboratory Methods*, 19th ed, Chapter 23, Henry JB, ed, Philadelphia, PA: WB Saunders Co, 1996, 538.

Strasinger SK, "Fecal Analysis," *Urinalysis and Body Fluids*, 3rd ed, Chapter 10, Philadelphia, PA: FA Davis Co, 1994, 201.

Methylene Blue Stain, Stool

Related Information

Bacterial Culture, Stool *on page 575*
Clostridium difficile Toxin Assay and Culture *on page 592*
Cryptosporidium Direct Staining Procedures *on page 596*
d-Xylose Absorption Test, Serum, Urine *on page 167*
Entamoeba histolytica Antigen Detection *on page 604*
Entamoeba histolytica Serology *on page 605*
Fat, Semiquantitative, Stool, Sudan III Stain *on page 306*
Fecal Fat by Near-Infrared Reflectance Analysis *on page 307*
Fecal Fat, Quantitative, 72-Hour Collection *on page 172*
Fecal Lactoferrin *on page 308*
Fungal Culture, Stool *on page 614*
Meat Fibers, Stool *on page 313*
Occult Blood, Stool *on page 315*
Ova and Parasites, Stool *on page 666*
pH, Stool *on page 317*

Synonyms Fecal Leukocyte Stain; Stool, Methylene Blue Stain

Applies to Gram Stain, Stool; Leukotest® (Fecal Lactoferrin); Wright Stain, Stool

Test Includes Methylene blue, Gram, or Wright stain of stool smear

Abstract Evaluation for fecal leukocytes is a part of the initial evaluation of chronic diarrhea.[1] In general, the presence of fecal leukocytes provides indication for stool culture. Absence of fecal leukocytes, however, does not exclude bacterial diarrhea or the need for stool collection.

Patient Preparation Collect specimen prior to barium procedures if possible.

Specimen Fresh random stool, rectal swab

(Continued)

Methylene Blue Stain, Stool *(Continued)*

Container Cup specimen is more sensitive than swab specimen in detection of fecal leukocytes.

Storage Instructions Refrigerate

Reference Interval No predominance of yeast, cocci in clusters, or leukocytes

Use Examine fecal specimens for the presence of leukocytes as an indicator of inflammatory diarrhea (eg, invasive enteric infection). Diarrhea for more than 4 weeks is an indication for evaluation.[1] The presence of blood (occult or gross) with leukocytes in the stool is a characteristic feature of inflammatory diarrhea.

Limitations Ten percent to 15% of stools which yield an invasive bacterial pathogen on culture have an absence of fecal leukocytes. Fecal leukocytes are present in idiopathic inflammatory bowel disease.

Methodology Smear of stool (preferably mucus) with one drop methylene blue, coverslip, and observe the presence of leukocytes.

Additional Information Conditions associated with marked fecal leukocytes, blood, and mucus include predominantly bacterial infections including invasive *E. coli*, shigellosis, salmonellosis, *Helicobacter*, *Yersinia* infection, ulcerative colitis, and cases of antibiotic-associated colitis and pseudomembranous colitis. *Salmonella typhi* may evoke a monocyte response. Conditions associated with modest numbers of fecal leukocytes include early shigellosis involving small bowel, and cases of antibiotic-associated colitis. In amebiasis, stool leukocytes are variable. Diarrhea can be watery or bloody.[1] See *Entamoeba histolytica* Serology *on page 605*. Conditions associated with an absence of fecal leukocytes include toxigenic bacterial infection including *Vibrio cholerae*, giardiasis, and viral infections. The methylene blue stain for polymorphonuclear leukocytes has a high sensitivity (85%) and specificity (88%) for bacterial diarrhea (*Shigella*, *Salmonella*, *Helicobacter*). Positive predictive value is 59%. Negative predictive value is 97%. Combined with a history of abrupt onset, more than four stools per day, and no vomiting before the onset of diarrhea, the stool methylene blue stain for fecal polymorphonuclear leukocytes is a very effective presumptive diagnostic test for bacterial diarrhea.[2] A positive occult blood test may also be suggestive of acute bacterial diarrhea being more sensitive (79% vs 42%) than the fecal leukocyte test (in detection of invasive bacteria in pediatric patients). The occult blood test in this setting, however, lacks specificity and has been found to have a positive predictive value of only 24%.[3] Occult blood negative samples (adult and pediatric) correlate reliably with absence of invasive bacteria (negative predictive value of 87% for adults, 96% for pediatrics).[3] Culture results were used as the criterion for bacterial detection. The processing for enteropathogens included testing for enterotoxigenic *E. coli*, some strains of which (eg, *E. coli* O157:H7) are not identified by routine stool culture.[4]

Neither absence of fecal occult blood and/or leukocytes should pre-empt the use of culture.[5] When both tests were positive, there was a sensitivity of 81% and specificity of 74% for bacterial diarrhea.[6]

A retrospective review of 172 patients with a diagnosis of collagenous colitis at Mayo Clinic found that 55% had fecal leukocytes (64 of 116 patients). This finding was considered to confirm the inflammatory basis of collagenous colitis.[7]

A commercially available latex agglutination screening test (Leukotest®) for the leukocyte marker lactoferrin has several advantages over the microscopic-based detection of fecal leukocytes.[8,9] Both tests, however, are insufficiently sensitive to be used as screening tests for such pathogens as *Campylobacter*, *Salmonella*, or *Shigella* spp.[10,11] See Fecal Lactoferrin *on page 308*.

Footnotes

1. Donowitz M, Kokke FT, and Saidi R, "Evaluation of Patients With Chronic Diarrhea," *N Engl J Med*, 1995, 332(11):725-9.
2. DeWitt TG, Humphrey KF, and McCarthy P, "Clinical Predictors of Acute Bacterial Diarrhea in Young Children," *Pediatrics*, 1985, 76(4):551-6.
3. McNeely WS, Dupont HL, Mathewson JJ, et al, "Occult Blood Versus Fecal Leukocytes in the Diagnosis of Bacterial Diarrhea: A Study of U.S. Travelers to Mexico and Mexican Children," *Am J Trop Med Hyg*, 1996, 55(4):430-3.
4. Slutsker L, Ries AA, Greene KD, et al, "*Escherichia coli* O157:H7 Diarrhea in the United States: Clinical and Epidemiologic Features," *Ann Intern Med*, 1997, 126(7):505-13.
5. Huicho L, Sanchez D, Contreras M, et al, "Occult Blood and Fecal Leukocytes as Screening Tests in Childhood Infectious Diarrhea: An Old Problem Revisited," *Pediatr Infect Dis J*, 1993, 12(6):474-7.
6. Siegel D, Cohen PT, Neighbor M, et al, "Predictive Value of Stool Examination in Acute Diarrhea," *Arch Pathol Lab Med*, 1987, 111(8):715-8.
7. Zins BJ, Tremaine WJ, and Carpenter HA, "Collagenous Colitis: Mucosal Biopsies and Association With Fecal Leukocytes," *Mayo Clin Proc*, 1995, 70(5):430-3.
8. Choi SW, Park CH, Silva TM, et al, "To Culture or Not to Culture: Fecal Lactoferrin Screening for Inflammatory Bacterial Diarrhea," *J Clin Microbiol*, 1996, 34(4):928-32.
9. Silleti RP, Lee G, and Ailey E, "Role of Stool Screening Tests in Diagnosis of Inflammatory Bacterial Enteritis and in Selection of Specimens Likely to Yield Invasive Enteric Pathogens," *J Clin Microbiol*, 1996, 34(5):1161-5.
10. Nachamkin I, "Fecal Lactoferrin Screening Assay for Inflammatory Bacterial Diarrhea," *J Clin Microbiol*, 1996, 34(9):2337-8 (letter).
11. Ruiz-Peláez JG and Mattar S, "Accuracy of Fecal Lactoferrin and Other Stool Tests for Diagnosis of Invasive Diarrhea at a Colombian Pediatric Hospital," *Pediatr Infect Dis*, 1999, 18(4):342-6.

References

Dowdy LM, "Infectious Diarrhea," *Clinical Practice of Gastroenterology*, Chapter 60, Brandt LJ, ed, Philadelphia, PA: Current Medicine Inc, 1999, 529-30.

Gilligan PH, Janda JM, Karmali MA, et al, "Laboratory Diagnosis of Bacterial Diarrhea," *Cumitech 12A*, Nolte FS, ed, Washington, DC: American Society for Microbiology, 1992.

Kao YS, Liu FJ, and Alexander DR, "Laboratory Diagnosis of Gastrointestinal Tract and Exocrine Pancreatic Disorders," *Clinical Diagnosis and Management by Laboratory Methods*, 19th ed, Chapter 23, Henry JB, ed, Philadelphia, PA: WB Saunders Co, 1996, 538.

◆ **MH61** *see* Infertility Screen *on page 310*

◆ **Monosodium Urate Crystals** *see* Synovial Fluid Analysis *on page 323*

Mucin Clot Test

Related Information
Synovial Fluid Analysis *on page 323*

Synonyms Synovial Fluid Mucin Clot Test; Synovial Fluid Ropes Test; Synovial Fluid Viscosity

Applies to Hyaluronate Concentration, Synovial Fluid; Synovial Fluid Hyaluronate Concentration

Abstract Qualitative test for the nature of hyaluronic acid in synovial fluid. In rheumatoid arthritis, clot is friable. This test lacks specificity, but bears correlation with the presence of inflammation.[1] It is considered by some to be only of historical interest,[2] but is still in use as a simple, rapid, and practical measure of inflammatory change in joint fluid. The test estimates the degree of polymerization of hyaluronate such that clots can be categorized as to their quality (eg, good, fair, or poor).

Specimen Synovial fluid

Container Sterile tube or lavender top (EDTA) tube; avoid oxalate anticoagulants.

Storage Instructions Refrigerate if there is delay in analysis.

Reference Interval Mucin clot - positive (firm clot)

Use Differential diagnosis of joint disease. Findings are somewhat nonspecific and alone are not diagnostic of a single pathologic entity.

Limitations Results should be assessed with other cellular, chemical, and microscopic joint fluid characteristics, as the mucin clot test lacks specificity (ie, it is not indicative of a single entity). Sibley et al[3] have argued that the mucin clot test should be excluded from the 11 criteria of rheumatoid arthritis by American Rheumatism Association. They felt that the low specificity (49%) and positive predictive value (52%) make the test of little value. Others find the mucin clot test to be of questionable value and state that it may be omitted from the "routine" synovial fluid analysis.[4] Similar information may be obtained from measurement of synovial fluid viscosity.

Methodology Evaluate clot formed on reaction of synovial fluid with acetic acid. Equal amounts of fluid and 5% acetic acid are mixed on a glass slide. Quality of the clot may be graded as "good", "fair", or "poor". This test reflects the physical chemical status of hyaluronic acid in a qualitative manner. Inflammation degrades the quality of the mucin clot. Viscosity relates to mucin hyaluronate content and also can be evaluated by the quality of the string produced. Normal (noninflammatory) fluids produce long strings. Inflammatory fluids (low viscosity) produce short strings. Synovial fluid hyaluronate concentration and degree of polymerization as determined by a high performance liquid chromatography (HPLC) procedure has been found to correlate with quality of the mucin clot.[5] It was considered that rheumatology units with HPLC analytic capability could use the more reproducible HPLC determinations to replace older mucin clot test/synovial fluid viscosity studies.

Additional Information In osteoarthritis the clot is firm and the surrounding fluid remains clear even after agitation. In rheumatoid arthritis the clot is friable and the surrounding fluid is turbid. In acute rheumatic fever the clot is firm, and in lupus erythematosus the clot is firm (ie, normal).

Footnotes

1. Bentz JS and Adams B, "Laboratory Examination of Synovial Fluid," *Clin Lab Sci*, 1994, 7(2):90-4.
2. Baker DG, "Chemistry, Serology, and Immunology," *A Practical Handbook of Joint Fluid Analysis*, 2nd ed, Gatter RA and Schumacher HR, eds, Philadelphia, PA: Lea & Febiger, 1991, 70.
3. Sibley JT, Harth M, and Burns DE, "The Mucin Clot Test and the Synovial Fluid Rheumatoid Factor as Diagnostic Criteria in Rheumatoid Arthritis," *J Rheumatol*, 1983, 10(6):889-93.
4. Smith GP and Kjeldsberg CR, "Cerebrospinal, Synovial, and Serous Body Fluids," *Clinical Diagnosis and Management by Laboratory Methods*, 19th ed, Chapter 19, Henry JB, ed, Philadelphia, PA: WB Saunders Co, 1996, 470.
5. Saari H and Konttinen YT, "Determination of Synovial Fluid Hyaluronate Concentration and Polymerization by High Performance Liquid Chromatography," *Ann Rheum Dis*, 1989, 48(7):565-70.

References

McCarty DJ, "Synovial Fluid," *Arthritis and Allied Conditions: A Textbook of Rheumatology*, Koopman WJ, ed, 13th ed, Chapter 4, Philadelphia, PA: Lea & Febiger, 1997, 84-5.

Sack U, Kinne RW, Marx T, et al, "Interleukin-6 in Synovial Fluid Is Closely Associated With Chronic Synovitis in Rheumatoid Arthritis," *Rheumatol Int*, 1993, 13(2):45-51.

van Leeuwen MA, Westra J, Limburg PC, et al, "Interleukin-6 in Relation to Other Proinflammatory Cytokines, Chemotactic Activity, and Neutrophil Activation in Rheumatoid Synovial Fluid," *Ann Rheum Dis*, 1995, 54(1):33-8.

- ◆ **Mucin Test for Hyaluronic Acid** *see* Synovial Fluid Analysis *on page 323*

- ◆ **Muscle Fiber, Stool** *see* Meat Fibers, Stool *on page 313*

- ◆ **Neutral Fat, Stool** *see* Fat, Semiquantitative, Stool, Sudan III Stain *on page 306*

Occult Blood, Stool

Related Information
Carcinoembryonic Antigen, Serum *on page 135*
Colon Cancer, Hereditary Nonpolyposis Type *on page 724*
[51]Cr Red Cell Survival *on page 422*
Fecal Lactoferrin *on page 308*
Ferritin, Serum *on page 173*
Iron and Total Iron Binding Capacity/Transferrin, Serum *on page 203*
Methylene Blue Stain, Stool *on page 313*

Synonyms Blood, Occult, Stool; Fecal Occult Blood Test; FOBT

Applies to Guaiac, Stool; Intestinal Converted Fraction; Stool Guaiac

Abstract Occult bleeding can be defined as the presence of blood in stool for which detection requires chemical testing (ie, which is not apparent to the patient). It may present as iron deficiency anemia. The most common global cause is hookworm infestation, but in industrialized countries, the most important cause is colorectal adenocarcinoma. Colorectal carcinoma is the second leading cause of death from cancer in the U.S. Fecal occult blood testing (FOBT) is applied both to screening and to case detection. It is relatively insensitive as a screen for colorectal neoplasia and is even less sensitive for detection of polyps. Efficacy is poor. Less than 30% of carcinomas and larger polyps bleed sufficiently to be detected by occult blood screening. Detection of small adenomas by FOBT is unlikely. False positives as well as false negatives occur. In spite of its shortcomings, annual fecal occult blood testing does diminish deaths from colorectal carcinomas, especially when used in concert with episodic colonoscopy and sigmoidoscopy. Successful detection and therapy of even a fraction of the ~150,000 new U.S. cases annually is meaningful. However, technical and other serious flaws work against implementation of broad-based population surveillance at this time.[1] Positive FOBT may derive from the upper gastrointestinal tract or small intestine as well as from colorectal disease.

Patient Preparation Patient should not receive vitamin C (ascorbic acid) for 5 days prior to occult blood testing by guaiac. 250 mg vitamin C intake leads to false-negative FOBT based on guaiac methods. Vitamin C does not affect the HemoQuant® test. A high bulk, red meat free diet with restriction of peroxidase-rich vegetables (turnips, horseradish, artichokes, mushrooms, radishes, broccoli, bean sprouts, cauliflower, apples, oranges, bananas, cantaloupes and other melons, grapes) has been recommended for 3-5 days prior to guaiac testing and during testing, to decrease the incidence of false positives. Ingestion of red meat or use of aspirin or other nonsteroidal anti-inflammatory drugs for 3 days before or during the collection may affect results for guaiac tests or HemoQuant®,[2] but low-dose aspirin, in doses used for cardiovascular prophylaxis, probably should not be stopped.[3] Alcohol and aspirin, especially together, and other gastric irritants should also be avoided. Social use of ethanol alone is unlikely to cause false-positive HemoQuant® results but therapeutic doses of aspirin may do so.[4] Halogens and cimetidine can cause reactions with guaiac tests. Oral iron is reported to not cause positive guaiac[5,6,7] or HemoQuant® stool assay results.[8] Positive stool reactions from subjects on therapeutic doses of oral iron should not be dismissed as false positives.[8]

Specimen Guaiac tests: Follow manufacturer's instructions. HemoQuant®: 1 g feces from a single defecation, collected with a sampler provided with the kit.

Container For HemoQuant®, the sampler is inserted in a screw-capped tube.

Collection Stool collection is offensive, unwieldy, and awkward under the best of circumstances. Mostly left to their own inspiration, some patients are unwilling or unable to comply. Up to 75% of blood leaches from the fecal surface into surrounding toilet water in 4-12 minutes. Many toilet sanitizers generate chlorine and are reported to cause false-positive reactions to guaiac tests. False positives can be traced to toilet bowl water containing blood from menstruation or urine. A collection device has been described.[9] Toilet sanitizers and detergents exert marked reductions in hemoglobin concentration or antigenicity of immunologic tests.[10]

Storage Instructions Delay in examination can adversely affect Hemoccult® results and also affects HemoQuant® results. Refrigerated HemoQuant® specimen must arrive at reference laboratory within 24 hours of collection, or be sent frozen on dry ice.

Special Instructions Tests for stool occult blood are not appropriately applied to detection of blood in gastric juice by virtue of possible ingestion of drugs and the pH of gastric juice.

Reference Interval Normal blood loss into the gastrointestinal tract is 0.5-1.5 mL/day, a quantity not detected by FOBT.

Guaiac: negative. (A positive report has much more significance than does a negative). No consistent fecal hemoglobin level exists above which guaiac tests are reliably positive or below which they are not.[7,11] HemoQuant®: <2 mg total hemoglobin/g of feces is considered normal, 2-3 mg total hemoglobin/g of feces is marginal, >3 mg total hemoglobin/g of feces is elevated.[2]

Use Detection of gastrointestinal bleeding, especially that from large bowel adenocarcinoma. FOBT is applied to case finding as well as to population screening. The importance of fecal blood and leukocytes as markers for the inflammatory diarrheas is discussed in Methylene Blue Stain, Stool *on page 313*.

Disease of the **upper** gastrointestinal tract may first be recognized by FOBT.[12,13] Even gastritis associated with *H. pylori*, as well as gastric cancer, can cause positive FOBT.[14,15] Bleeding from the upper gastrointestinal tract is best detected by hemeporphyrin FOBT; guaiac-based FOBT are not as sensitive, and immunochemical tests are insensitive to this source.[7] Celiac disease is also a cause of occult bleeding.[16] Other causes of positive FOBT in the small intestine include tumors, Meckel's diverticulum, and vascular ectasias.[7,17] However, both upper gastrointestinal diseases and colorectal carcinoma are common; identification of the former should not necessarily exclude colonoscopy.

Limitations Most methods lack sensitivity to small amounts of blood and might fail to detect slow rates of blood loss. Many adenomas and carcinomas do not bleed. When occult GI bleeding is suspected, at least three samples, preferably of separate bowel movements, should be submitted. Many substances and conditions interfere with guaiac tests. Vitamin C (ascorbic acid) and antacids may cause false negatives to guaiac tests. False-positive results may be caused by excessive dietary intake of vegetable peroxidases, especially horseradish. Drugs shown to be associated with gastrointestinal blood loss in normal subjects include salicylates (aspirin), steroids, rauwolfia derivatives, all nonsteroidal anti-inflammatory drugs, and colchicine. The sensitivity of the slides is increased by rehydration prior to development. Such increment in sensitivity provided by rehydration can be a useful adjunct,[18] but decreases its specificity; *vide infra*. Other means to increase sensitivity include testing on three consecutive days or use of more sensitive tests.

Ahlquist and Bakken quote Sherlock Holmes' observation[19] that the old guaiacum test is clumsy and uncertain, and they quote his lament of the lack of a reliable test ("A Study in Scarlet"). They describe the still current truth of Arthur Conan Doyle's criticism of guaiac false positives and negatives,[20] which are outlined in the table. Guaiac tests present a number of additional problems. Acid pH, heat, and dry stools lead to some false negatives, while watery stools are more apt to test positive. **Intestinal converted fraction** is an expression which describes the fraction of heme converted to porphyrins and iron during fecal transit, a phenomenon which is not detected by guaiac-based tests, but is detected by heme-porphyrin assay.[20,21,22]

Colorectal adenomas and carcinomas cause a minority of positive guaiac tests;[11] 70% of carcinomas and 80% of adenomas larger than 2 cm are missed.[23] The sensitivity of Hemoccult® for detection of intraluminal cancer recurrence, all new primary carcinomas, and Dukes A and B carcinomas was respectively only 21%, 33%, and 29%, and sensitivity for detection of polyps ≥2.0 cm was 20% for Hemoccult® and HemoQuant®.[24] A 1993 *JAMA* editorial concludes that the real limit to occult blood stool testing is likely to be that many asymptomatic carcinomas do not lead to abnormal blood loss.[25] The high incidence of positivity of fecal screening for occult blood, using rehydrated Hemoccult® slides, about 10%, occurs for entities and reasons other than carcinoma or polyp.[26] Ransohoff and Lang express their opinion that sensitivity below about 95% (false-positive rates >5%) is unacceptable, because of the effort and expense of investigation. Hemoccult® II with rehydration yields false-positive rates ≥10%.

Patients with unexplained iron deficiency anemia or with evidence or symptoms of gastrointestinal disease must be investigated, whether or not their FOBTs are positive.

FOBT are not sufficiently sensitive to replace endoscopy in high-risk situations such as familial colorectal carcinoma.[27]

Methodology Guaiac is a leuko-dye. Guaiac tests are inexpensive but nonspecific, with substantial problems of specificity and sensitivity. Commercially generated tests based on it include Colo-Screen® (Helena Laboratories), Colo-Rect® (Roche Diagnostics), Hema-Chek® (Miles Laboratories), Quick-Cult® (Laboratory Diagnostics), Hemoccult® II (SmithKline) and Hemoccult® II Sensa. The peroxidase-like activity of hemoglobin or nonspecific oxidants catalyze the reaction of peroxide and the chromogen ortho-toluidine to form blue oxidized orthotolidine.

New methodology, based on heme-derived porphyrin fluorescence, is more expensive (**HemoQuant®**). It detects peroxidase-negative heme-derived porphyrins, peroxidase-positive hemoglobin, and free heme spectrofluorometrically.[7,28] HemoQuant® has been described as more expensive and cumbersome. An author expressed his opinion that there is no place for HemoQuant®.[29]

Immunologic tests have been developed,[29] but enteric degradation of hemoglobin interferes with immunologic as well as guaiac tests. Immunologic tests do not react with drugs, red meats, or nonhemoglobin peroxidase compounds. They utilize antibodies against human globin epitopes. Sensitivity compared favorably with that of a guaiac test.[30] See following table.

When paper slides impregnated with guaiac are not promptly processed, drying occurs, which may diminish sensitivity. Such slides may be rehydrated with a drop of deionized water, as was done in a major study.[31] Rehydration increased the number of positives but caused diminution of specificity,[31,32] increasing positivity rates from 2% to 3% to 8% to 16% with (Continued)

Occult Blood, Stool (Continued)

Occult Blood, Stool

	Guaiac	Heme-Derived Porphyrin Fluorescence	Immunoassays
Cost	Low	High	Intermediate
Reliability	False-positives, false-negatives; best at detection of large, distal lesions; questions about accuracy	Little better	Intermediate; loss of globin antigenicity at room temperature
Specificity	Poor	Measures both heme and porphyrins, but a high false-positive rate limits application of this test	Improved over guaiac
Availability	Almost anywhere	Specimens must be sent to a reference laboratory, Mayo Medical Laboratories, Rochester, MN.	Limited availability
Recognition of porphyrin derived from heme	No	Yes	N/A
Recognition of bleeding from right colon (intestinal converted fraction)	Like immunologic tests, especially insensitive-enteric heme degradation	Sensitive	Similar to guaiac
Sensitivity deteriorates with time, fecal storage (eg, mailed in specimens)*	Yes (Hemoccult II Sensa® more sensitive than Hemoccult II®)	No	Similar to guaiac
Such reducing substances as ascorbic acid cause false-negatives*	Yes	No	No
Antacids cause false-negatives*	Yes	No	No
Dietary (red meats) hemoglobin†	Yes	Yes	No
Vegetable peroxidases†	False-positives	Not affected	Not affected
Rehydration†	Yes Raises sensitivity but reduces specificity	No	No
Iron, dietary	No	No	No
Ease of test performance	Not difficult	Complex	Complex - an enzyme immunoassay is available and counter immunoelectrophoresis is described.
Commonly used tests	Hemoccult II® Hemoccult II Sensa®	HemoQuant®	Heme-Select® FlexSure OBT®

*Causes of false-negative results.

†Causes of false-positive results.

Table partially based on 1999 review article (see Rockey footnote).

average positivity about 10%. Rehydration is recommended but important criticisms are published.[26,33,34]

Additional Information Methods for guaiac tests of stool for occult blood utilize peroxidation of a chromogen by stool peroxidases. Hemoglobin acts as a peroxidase, but stool may also contain meat, bacterial and plant peroxidases. Hemoccult® begins to turn positive at about 5 mg hemoglobin/g feces, which is considered to be the upper limit of normal stool peroxidase activity. This method is capable of detection of 6 mg of added hemoglobin/g feces in 90% of observations, but will fail 80% of the time to detect up to 1.5 mg/g feces. After ingestion of 8 oz of cooked red meat per day, reactions remain negative 95% of the time. Hemoccult® II Sensa is more sensitive in detection of polyps and carcinomas than Hemoccult® II but its specificity has been reported to be poor.[35] The heme-derived porphyrin based method (HemoQuant®) has been shown to correlate closely with ^{51}Cr-labeled RBC radioisotope measurements of short-term (12 day) quantitation of fecal blood loss.[36]

Stool obtained by digital rectal examination did not increase the number of false positives in asymptomatic patients at average risk.[37] New lesions have been identified by this means.[7]

Recommendations for screening are published.[38]

Approximately 56,000 deaths occur in the U.S. annually from colorectal cancer.[31,34] 150,000 new cases a year are anticipated. Family history is also relevant when it has been found in first degree relatives.[34]

Alternatives include colonoscopy, which is an expensive gold standard,[34] and serum ferritin.[39]

Footnotes

1. Simon JB, "Should All People Over the Age of 50 Have Regular Fecal Occult-Blood Tests?" *N Engl J Med*, 1998, 338(16):1151-2.
2. Kisabeth RM, Mayo Medical Laboratories, *2000 Test Catalogue*, Rochester, MN.
3. Greenberg PD, Cello JP, and Rockey DC, "Relationship of Low-Dose Aspirin to GI Injury and Occult Bleeding: A Pilot Study," *Gastrointest Endosc*, 1999, 50(5):618-22.
4. Fleming JL, Ahlquist DA, McGill DB, et al, "Influence of Aspirin and Ethanol on Fecal Blood Levels as Determined by Using the HemoQuant® Assay," *Mayo Clin Proc*, 1987, 62(3):159-63.
5. McDonnell WM, Ryan JA, Seeger DM, et al, "Effect of Iron on the Guaiac Reaction," *Gastroenterology*, 1989, 96(1):74-8.
6. Anderson GD, Yuellig TR, and Krone RE Jr, "An Investigation Into the Effects of Oral Iron Supplementation on *In Vivo* Hemoccult® Stool Testing," *Am J Gastroenterol*, 1990, 85(5):558-61.
7. Rockey DC, "Occult Gastrointestinal Bleeding," *N Engl J Med*, 1999, 341(1):38-46.
8. Coles EF and Starnes EC, "Use of HemoQuant® Assays to Assess the Effect of Oral Iron Preparations on Stool Hemoccult® Tests," *Am J Gastroenterol*, 1991, 86(10):1442-4.
9. Ahlquist DA, Schwartz S, Isaacson J, et al, "A Stool Collection Device: The First Step in Occult Blood Testing," *Ann Intern Med*, 1988, 108(4):609-12.
10. Imafuku Y, Nagai T, and Yoshida H, "The Effect of Toilet Sanitizers and Detergents on Immunological Occult Blood Tests," *Clin Chim Acta*, 1996, 253(1-2):51-9.

11. Ahlquist DA, "Fecal Blood Testing: Demystifying the Occult," Annual Clinical Conference on Cancer, 30:Gastrointestinal Cancer: Current Approaches to Diagnosis and Treatment, University of Texas System Cancer Center, 1988.
12. Bini EJ, Rajapaksa RC, Valdes MT, et al, "Is Upper Gastrointestinal Endoscopy Indicated in Asymptomatic Patients With a Positive Fecal Occult Blood Test and Negative Colonoscopy?" *Am J Med*, 1999, 106(6):613-8.
13. Rockey DC, Auslander A, and Greenberg PD, "Detection of Upper Gastrointestinal Blood With Fecal Occult Blood Tests," *Am J Gastroenterol*, 1999, 94(2):344-50.
14. Yip R, Limburg PJ, Ahlquist DA, et al, "Pervasive Occult Gastrointestinal Bleeding in an Alaska Native Population With Prevalent Iron Deficiency," *JAMA*, 1997, 277(14):1135-9.
15. Wood H and Feldman M, "*Helicobacter pylori* and Iron Deficiency," *JAMA*, 1997, 277(14):1166-7 (editorial).
16. Fine KD, "The Prevalence of Occult Gastrointestinal Bleeding in Celiac Sprue," *N Engl J Med*, 1996, 334(18):1163-7.
17. Morris AJ, "Small-Bowel Investigation in Occult Gastrointestinal Bleeding," *Semin Gastrointest Dis*, 1999, 10(2):65-70.
18. Macrae FA, St John DJ, Caligiore P, et al, "Optimal Dietary Conditions for Hemoccult® Testing," *Gastroenterology*, 1982, 82(5 Pt 1):899-903.
19. Ahlquist DA and Bakken CL, "Fecal Blood Tests," *ASCP Check Sample*, Chicago, IL: American Society of Clinical Pathologists, 1988.
20. Doyle AC, *A Study in Scarlet*, Philadelphia, PA: JB Lippincott Co, 1902.
21. Ahlquist DA, McGill DB, Schwartz S, et al, "HemoQuant®, A New Quantitative Assay for Fecal Hemoglobin," *Ann Intern Med*, 1984, 101(3):297-302.
22. Ahlquist DA, McGill DB, Schwartz S, et al, "Fecal Blood Levels in Health and Disease. A Study Using HemoQuant®" *N Engl J Med*, 1985, 312(22):1422-8.
23. Sandler RS, "Fecal Occult Blood Screening for Colorectal Neoplasia," *ACP J Club*, 1993, 119(Suppl 1):25.
24. Ahlquist DA, Wieand HS, Moertel CG, et al, "Accuracy of Fecal Occult Blood Screening for Colorectal Neoplasia - A Prospective Study Using Hemoccult® and HemoQuant® Tests," *JAMA*, 1993, 269(10):1262-7.
25. Selby JV, "How Should We Screen for Colorectal Cancer?" *JAMA*, 1993, 269(10):1294-6 (editorial).
26. Lang CA and Ransohoff DF, "Fecal Occult Blood Screening for Colorectal Cancer - Is Mortality Reduced by Chance Selection for Screening Colonoscopy?" *JAMA*, 1994, 271(13):1011-3.
27. Hunt LM, Rooney PS, Bostock K, et al, "Chemical and Immunological Testing for Faecal Occult Blood in Screening Subjects at Risk of Familial Colorectal Cancer," *Gut*, 1997, 40(1):110-2.
28. Selby JV, Friedman GD, Quesenberry CP Jr, et al, "Effect of Fecal Occult Blood Testing on Mortality From Colorectal Cancer," *Ann Intern Med*, 1993, 118(1):1-6.
29. Nakama H, Kamijo N, Fujimori K, et al, "Relationship Between Fecal Sampling Times and Sensitivity and Specificity of Immunochemical Fecal Occult Blood Tests for Colorectal Cancer: A Comparative Study," *Dis Colon Rectum*, 1997, 40(7):781-4.
30. Robinson MH, Marks CG, Farrands PA, et al, "Screening for Colorectal Cancer With an Immunological Faecal Occult Blood Test: 2-year Follow-up," *Br J Surg*, 1996, 83(4):500-1.
31. Mandel JS, Bond JH, Church TR, et al, "Reducing Mortality From Colorectal Cancer by Screening for Fecal Occult Blood," *N Engl J Med*, 1993, 328(19):1365-71.
32. Winawer SJ, "Colorectal Cancer Screening Comes of Age," *N Engl J Med*, 1993, 328(9):1416-7.

33. Ahlquist DA, Moertel CG, and McGill DB, "Screening for Colorectal Cancer," *N Engl J Med*, 1993, 329(18):1351.

34. Toribara NW and Sleisenger MH, "Screening for Colorectal Cancer," *N Engl J Med*, 1995, 332(13):861-7.

35. Allison JE, Tekawa IS, Ransom LJ, et al, "A Comparison of Fecal Occult-Blood Tests for Colorectal-Cancer Screening," *N Engl J Med*, 1996, 334(3):155-9.

36. Leahy MB, Pippard MJ, Salzmann MB, et al, "Quantitative Measurement of Faecal Blood Loss: Comparison of Radioisotopic and Chemical Analyses," *J Clin Pathol*, 1991, 44(5):391-4.

37. Bini EJ, Rajapaksa RC, and Weinshel EH, "The Findings and Impact of Nonrehydrated Guaiac Examination of the Rectum (FINGER) Study: A Comparison of 2 Methods of Screening for Colorectal Cancer in Asymptomatic Average-Risk Patients," *Arch Intern Med*, 1999, 159(17):2022-6.

38. Levin B, "Colorectal Cancer Screening," *Cancer*, 1993, 72(3 Suppl):1056-60.

39. Nelson RL, "Elevation of Serum Ferritin Is Superior to Fecal Occult Blood Testing as a Screening Test for Colonic Adenoma... and Not Only Because Patients Do Not Have to Handle Their Own Stool," *Dis Colon Rectum*, 1996, 39(12):1441-2.

References

Blebea J and McPherson RA, "False-Positive Guaiac Testing With Iodine," *Arch Pathol Lab Med*, 1985, 109(5):437-40.

Bond JH, "Fecal Occult Blood Tests in Occult Gastrointestinal Bleeding," *Semin Gastrointest Dis*, 1999, 10(2):48-52.

Bouvier V, Launoy G, Herbert C, et al, "Colorectal Cancer After a Negative Haemoccult II Test and Programme Sensitivity After a First Round of Screening: The Experience of the Department of Calvados (France)," *Br J Cancer*, 1999, 81(2):305-9.

Frazier AL, Colditz GA, Fuchs CS, et al, "Cost-Effectiveness of Screening for Colorectal Cancer in the General Population," *JAMA*, 2000, 284(15):1954-61.

Klos SE, Drinka P, and Goodwin JS, "The Utilization of Fecal Occult Blood Testing in the Institutionalized Elderly," *J Am Geriatr Soc*, 1991, 39(12):1169-73.

Losek JD and Fiete RL, "Intussusception and the Diagnostic Value of Testing Stool for Occult Blood," *Am J Emerg Med*, 1991, 9(1):1-3.

Mandel JS, Church TR, Bond JH, et al, "The Effect of Fecal Occult-Blood Screening on the Incidence of Colorectal Cancer," *N Engl J Med*, 2000, 343(22):1603-7.

Palmer KR, Hayes PC, and Forrest JA, "Gastrointestinal Bleeding," *Diseases of the Gastrointestinal Tract*, 3rd ed, Shearman DJC, Finlayson N, Camilleri M, et al, eds, New York, NY: Churchill Livingstone, 1997, 497-8.

Pye G, Jackson J, Thomas WM, et al, "Comparison of ColoScreen Self-Test and Haemoccult Faecal Occult Blood Tests in the Detection of Colorectal Cancer in Symptomatic Patients," *Br J Surg*, 1990, 77(6):630-1.

Ransohoff DF and Lang CA, "Improving the Fecal Occult-Blood Test," *N Engl J Med*, 1996, 334(3):189-90.

Rozen P, Knaani J, and Samuel Z, "Performance Characteristics and Comparison of Two Immunochemical and Two Guaiac Fecal Occult Blood Screening Tests for Colorectal Neoplasia," *Dig Dis Sci*, 1997, 42(10):2064-71.

Schrock TR, "Colon and Rectum: Diagnostic Techniques," *Shakelford's Surgery of the Alimentary Tract*, 4th ed, Volume IV, Zuidema GD, ed, Philadelphia, PA: WB Saunders Co, 1996, 24-5.

Sinatra MA, St John DJ, and Young GP, "Interference of Plant Peroxidases With Guaiac-Based Fecal Occult Blood Tests Is Avoidable," *Clin Chem*, 1999, 45(1):123-6.

Solomon MJ and McLeod RS, "Periodic Health Examination, 1994 Update: Screening Strategies for Colorectal Cancer. Canadian Task Force on the Periodic Health Examination," *Can Med Assoc J*, 1994, 150(12):1961-70.

St-John DJB, Young GP, McHutchison JG, et al, "Comparison of the Specificity and Sensitivity of Hemoccult® and HemoQuant® in Screening for Colorectal Neoplasia," *Ann Intern Med*, 1992, 117(5):376-82.

Winawer SJ, Zauber AG, Gerdes H, et al, "Risk of Colorectal Cancer in the Families of Patients With Adenomatous Polyps," *N Engl J Med*, 1996, 334(2):82-7.

Woolf SH, "The Best Screening Test for Colorectal Cancer - A Personal Choice," *N Engl J Med*, 2000, 343(22):1641-3.

♦ **Osteoarthritis** see Synovial Fluid Analysis on page 323

---

pH, Stool

Related Information
Clostridium difficile Toxin Assay and Culture on page 592
Fat, Semiquantitative, Stool, Sudan III Stain on page 306
Fecal Fat by Near-Infrared Reflectance Analysis on page 307
Fecal Fat, Quantitative, 72-Hour Collection on page 172
Meat Fibers, Stool on page 313
Methylene Blue Stain, Stool on page 313
Reducing Substances, Stool on page 317

Synonyms Fecal pH; Stool pH

Applies to Chloridorrhea, Congenital

Abstract Evaluation for diarrhea depends first on history and physical examination. Nocturnal diarrhea, weight loss >5 kg, increased ESR, and/or decreased Hb/Hct favor presence of organic disease. Investigation of chronic diarrhea may include examination for fecal leukocytes, ova and parasites, *C. difficile* toxin assay, stool pH, stool for reducing substances; CBC and differential, ESR, electrolytes, BUN/creatinine, TSH, T_4, gastrin; vasoactive intestinal polypeptide if hypokalemia is present and diarrhea volume >1 liter/day; assay for *Giardia* antigen and other studies, including imaging and endoscopy.[1]

Patient Preparation Barium procedures and laxatives should be avoided for 1 week prior to collection of the specimen.

Specimen Fresh random stool

Storage Instructions Refrigerate

Causes for Rejection Specimen contaminated with urine

Reference Interval Diet dependent; normal: neutral to slightly alkaline or acid. Stool pH is usually slightly acidic at a pH of ~6. pH is increased with protein breakdown, decreased with carbohydrate or fat malabsorption. Breast-fed infants have slightly acid stools, bottle-fed infants, neutral or slightly alkaline. Acid stool is formed with fat malabsorption. In a South African population of control subjects, the mean stool pH of rural African-Americans was significantly lower (pH 6.14) than that in urban African-American individuals (pH 6.77) and in patients with chronic pancreatitis (pH 6.61).[2]

Critical Values Stool pH <5.3 is diagnostic of carbohydrate intolerance; stool pH >6.8 is evidence of cholerheic enteropathy.[1]

Use Screen for carbohydrate and fat malabsorption; evaluate small intestinal disaccharidase deficiencies

Limitations Limited value due to dependence on stool volume and transit time. The diagnosis of steatorrhea requires 72-hour specimen with diet of 75-100 g fat/24 hours; see Fecal Fat, Quantitative, 72-Hour Collection on page 172.

Methodology Aqueous stool suspension measured with pH paper

Additional Information Stool pH is dependent in part on fermentation of sugars. Colonic fermentation of normal amounts of carbohydrate sugars and production of fatty acids accounts for the normally slightly acidic pH. If disaccharide intolerance is suspect, simple screening tests may be performed. Slightly alkaline pH may occur in cases of secretory diarrhea without food intake, colitis, villous tumor, and possibly with antibiotic usage (with resultant impaired colonic fermentation). A stool pH <6 (measured by pH paper) is suggestive evidence of sugar malabsorption and is more likely to be associated with osmotic than with secretory diarrhea.[3] Children and some adults notice that their stools have a sickly sweet smell as the result of volatile fatty acids and the presence of undigested lactose. Low stool pH also contributes to excoriation of perianal skin which frequently accompanies diarrhea.[4]

Intestinal resections may cause postprandial bile acid diarrhea, cholerheic enteropathy, with stool pH >6.8. It responds to cholestyramine.[5]

Osmotic diarrhea is due to an excess of nonabsorbable solutes, while secretory diarrhea is the result of intestinal mucosal secretory activity exceeding absorptive capacity.

Congenital chloridorrhea or defect in jejunal brush border Na^+-H^+ exchange is rarely the underlying cause of life-long watery diarrhea and dehydration. Stool pH in chloridorrhea is slightly acidic (about 6) and the sum of stool water sodium and potassium levels is less than the chloride level. Change in daily stool weight (between a period of normal intake and a 48-hour fast) is more reliable than determination of osmolarity and osmolar gap. Unchanged stool weight with fast indicates secretory diarrhea.[5]

Determination of fecal reducing substances is a more reliable screening test for disaccharidase deficiency. See Reducing Substances, Stool on page 317 and Fat, Semiquantitative, Stool, Sudan III Stain on page 306.

High fecal pH may be a risk factor for colorectal cancer.[6,7] Intake of oat bran (75-100 g/day over a 14-day period) has been shown capable of reducing fecal pH by 0.4 units.[6] There is evidence, however, that high fecal pH may be secondarily rather than primarily related to cancer risk.[8]

Footnotes

1. Donowitz M, Kokke FT, and Saidi R, "Evaluation of Patients With Chronic Diarrhea," *N Engl J Med*, 1995, 332(11):725-9.

2. Riedel L, Walker ARP, Segal I, et al, "Limitations of Faecal Chymotrypsin as a Screening Test for Chronic Pancreatitis," *Gut*, 1991, 32(3):321-4.

3. Castro-Rodriguez JA, Salazar-Lindo E, and León-Barúa R, "Differentiation of Osmotic and Secretory Diarrhoea by Stool Carbohydrate and Osmolar Gap Measurements," *Arch Dis Child*, 1997, 77(3):201-5.

4. Cooper BT, "Lactase Deficiency and Lactose Malabsorption," *Dig Dis*, 1986, 4(2):72-82.

5. Ammon HV, "Diarrhea and Constipation," *Bockus Gastroenterology*, 5th ed, Volume 1, Chapter 8, Haubrich WS, Schaffner F, and Berk JE, eds, Philadelphia, PA: WB Saunders Co, 1995, 97.

6. Kashtan H, Stern HS, Jenkins DJ, et al, "Manipulation of Fecal pH by Dietary Means," *Prev Med*, 1990, 19(6):607-13.

7. Kashtan H, Gregoire RC, Bruce WR, et al, "Effects of Sodium Sulfate on Fecal pH and Proliferation of Colonic Mucosa in Patients at High Risk for Colon Cancer," *J Natl Cancer Inst*, 1990, 82(11):950-2.

8. Walker AR, Walker BF, and Walker AJ, "Faecal pH, Dietary Fibre Intake, and Proneness to Colon Cancer in Four South African Populations," *Br J Cancer*, 1986, 53(4):489-95.

References

Branski D, Lerner A, and Lebenthal E, "Chronic Diarrhea and Malabsorption," *Pediatr Clin North Am*, 1996, 43(2):307-31.

Read NW, "Diarrhea, Chronic," *Difficult Diagnosis*, Taylor RB, ed, Philadelphia, PA: WB Saunders Co, 1985, 109-10.

♦ **Prosaposin** see Infertility Screen on page 310

♦ **Psoriatic Arthritis** see Synovial Fluid Analysis on page 323

♦ **RA Cells** see Synovial Fluid Analysis on page 323

Reducing Substances, Stool

Related Information
d-Xylose Absorption Test, Serum, Urine on page 167
(Continued)

Reducing Substances, Stool *(Continued)*

Lactose Tolerance Test *on page 209*
Meat Fibers, Stool *on page 313*
pH, Stool *on page 317*

Synonyms Stool Reducing Substances

Applies to Breath Hydrogen Analysis; $^{13}CO_2$ Breath Test

Test Includes Stool weight, stool pH, and total reducing substances

Abstract Screening test for fecal reducing substance (eg, sugars) as an indication of disaccharidase (sucrase, lactase) deficiency and to assist in the differentiation of osmotic from secretory diarrhea

Specimen Fresh random stool

Collection Transport the specimen to the laboratory as soon as possible; delay may cause falsely low results.

Storage Instructions Freeze specimen if testing is delayed.

Causes for Rejection Specimen collected in a diaper or other absorbent surface

Reference Interval Normal: <2 mg/g stool; borderline: between 2-5 mg/g stool; abnormal: >5 mg/g stool. Even though premature infants have relative lactase deficiency and pancreatic insufficiency, there is evidence that older (32 weeks gestation) prematures have insignificant fecal loss of intact carbohydrate. Comparison of fecal carbohydrate excretion in infants fed formulas of 50% lactose vs 50% lactose plus 50% glucose polymers found no significant difference. Mean excretion was <0.2 g/day (<1% of carbohydrate intake).[1]

Use Detect deficiency of intestinal border enzymes, primarily sucrase and lactase (disaccharidases) due to congenital deficiency or nonspecific mucosal injury

Limitations Bacterial fermentation may give falsely low results if specimen is not analyzed within 1 hour. In the neonatal period, high Clinitest® results may be observed.

Methodology Clinitest® performed on a 1:3 dilution of supernatant from a diarrheal stool.[2] A result >200-250 mg/dL of stool may be considered abnormal (normal is <2 mg/g of stool).

Additional Information Sugars should be rapidly absorbed in the upper small intestine. If not, however, they remain in the intestine and cause osmotic diarrhea by the osmotic pressure of the unabsorbed sugar in the intestine, drawing fluid and electrolytes into the gut. Carbohydrate malabsorption is a major cause of the watery diarrhea and electrolyte imbalance seen in patients with the short bowel syndrome. As a result of bacterial fermentation, the stools become acid with a high concentration of lactic acid. The pH measurement reflects this process. The unabsorbed sugars are measured as reducing substances. Although sucrose is not a reducing sugar, it is subjected to acid hydrolysis in the gut, and thus, is also measured as a reducing substance. The presence of excess fecal reducing substances in infants and children admitted with watery diarrhea is reported as a sensitive and specific indicator favoring osmotic over secretory diarrhea.[3]

Idiopathic lactase deficiency is common, occurring in 70% to 75% of Southern European Greeks and Italians, 70% of black adults, >90% of Oriental adults, and 5% to 20% of white American adults. Lactase activity declines with age in humans and is controlled genetically. It is influenced in its phenotypic expression as lactase malabsorption by several nongenetic factors (eg, adaption to nutritional intake of dairy products, biological (circadian) rhythm of enzyme activity, hormones and hormonal changes of the body and the brain, gastrointestinal functions such as motility and the nutritional components of digested food).[4] On the other hand, a strong correlation has been noted between a genetic polymorphism in the apolipoprotein A-IV gene (apo A-IV-2) and lactase persistence polymorphisms (that determine the prevalence of adult lactase persistence). Noting that the Apo-IV-2 allele frequently was highest in Iceland, it is proposed that the allele was disseminated by conferring a nutritional advantage to a population with high milkfat intake and that subsequently spread South and East by Viking migrations.[5]

The **breath hydrogen analysis** test may provide more definitive information.[6,7] A positive breath hydrogen result (as with lactose intolerance) will exceed 20 parts (hydrogen) per million.[6] The $^{13}CO_2$ **breath test** is reportedly more sensitive and specific than the H_2 test in the detection of low jejunal lactase activity.[8] A ^{13}C-lactose digestion test has shown (on the basis of increase in the plasma ^{13}C-glucose concentration after consumption of ^{13}C-lactose) a higher prevalence of lactose maldigestion (Caucasian population) than indicated by the H_2 breath test. It appears that the hydrogen breath test does not provide as accurate a measure of small intestinal lactose digestive capacity as does the ^{13}C-lactose digestive test.[9] There is considerable variation in lactose tolerance between lactase deficient subjects. A 50 g lactose load has been reported to cause symptoms in 75% of lactase deficient adults whereas 10 g causes symptoms in only 50%.[10] A glass of milk has ~12 g of lactose. Classically, stools from patients with disaccharidase deficiency are liquid, acid, and frothy in appearance. The use of mucosal disaccharidase enzyme activity as an isolated diagnostic criterion may have limited value.[11]

Footnotes

1. Ameen VZ and Powell GK, "Quantitative Fecal Carbohydrate Excretion in Premature Infants," *Am J Clin Nutr*, 1989, 49(6):1238-42.
2. Kerry KR and Anderson CM, "A Ward Test for Sugars in Feces," *Lancet*, 1964, 1(7340):981.
3. Castro-Rodriguez JA, Salazar-Lindo E, and León-Barúa R, "Differentiation of Osmotic and Secretory Diarrhoea by Stool Carbohydrate and Osmolar gap Measurements," *Arch Dis Child*, 1997, 77(3):201-5.
4. Enck P and Whitehead WE, "Lactase Deficiency and Lactose Malabsorption. A Review," *Z Gastroenterol*, 1986, 24(3):125-34.
5. Weinberg RB, "Apolipoprotein A-IV-2 Allele: Association of its Worldwide Distribution With Adult Persistence of Lactase and Speculation on its Function and Origin," *Genet Epidemiol*, 1999, 17(4):285-97.
6. Matthews SB and Campbell AK, "When Sugar Is Not So Sweet," *Lancet*, 2000, 355(9212):1330.
7. Ostrander CR, Cohen RS, Hopper AO, et al, "Breath Hydrogen Analysis: A Review of the Methodologies and Clinical Applications," *J Pediatr Gastroenterol Nutr*, 1983, 2(3):525-33.
8. Hiele M, Ghoos Y, Rutgeerts P, et al, "$^{13}CO_2$ Breath Test Using Naturally ^{13}C-Enriched Lactose for Detection of Lactase Deficiency in Patients With Gastrointestinal Symptoms," *J Lab Clin Med*, 1988, 112(2):193-200.
9. Vonk RJ, Lin Y, Koetse HA, et al, "Lactose (mal)Digestion Evaluated by the ^{13}C-Lactose Digestion Test," *Eur J Clin Invest*, 2000, 30(2):140-6.
10. Cooper BT, "Lactase Deficiency and Lactose Malabsorption," *Dig Dis*, 1986, 4(2):72-82.
11. Calvin RT, Klish WJ, and Nichols BL, "Disaccharidase Activities, Jejunal Morphology, and Carbohydrate Tolerance in Children With Chronic Diarrhea," *J Pediatr Gastroenterol Nutr*, 1985, 4(6):949-53.

References

Ameen VZ, Powell GK, and Jones LA, "Quantitation of Fecal Carbohydrate Excretion in Patients With Short Bowel Syndrome," *Gastroenterology*, 1987, 92(2):493-500.

Brunzel NA, "Fecal Analysis," *Fundamentals of Urine and Body Fluid Analysis*, Philadelphia, PA: WB Saunders Co, 1994, 324.

Goldstein R, Braverman D, and Stankiewicz H, "Carbohydrate Malabsorption and the Effect of Dietary Restriction on Symptoms of Irritable Bowel Syndrome and Functional Bowel Complaints," *Isr Med Assoc J*, 2000, 2(8):583-7.

Hammer HF, Fine KD, Santa Ana CA, et al, "Carbohydrate Malabsorption. Its Measurement and Its Contribution to Diarrhea," *J Clin Invest*, 1990, 86(6):1936-44.

Koetse HA, Stellaard F, Bijleveld CM, et al, "Noninvasive Detection of Low-Intestinal Lactase Activity in Children by Use of a Combined 13CO₂/H₂ Breath Test," *Scand J Gastroenterol*, 1999, 34(1):35-40.

Lloyd ML and Olsen WA, "A Study of the Molecular Pathology of Sucrase-Isomaltase Deficiency. A Defect in the Intracellular Processing of the Enzyme," *N Engl J Med*, 1987, 316(8):438-42.

Szajewska H, Kantecki M, Albrecht P, et al, "Carbohydrate Intolerance After Acute Gastroenteritis - A Disappearing Problem in Polish Children," *Acta Paediatr*, 1997, 86(4):347-50.

Udall JN, "Secretory Diarrhea in Children: Newly Recognized Toxins and Hormone-Secreting Tumors," *Pediatr Clin North Am*, 1996, 43(2):333.

♦ **rSMP-B** *see* Infertility Screen *on page 310*

Semen Analysis, Advanced

Related Information

Infertility Screen *on page 310*
Semen Analysis, Basic *on page 319*
Sperm Mucus Penetration Test (Human or Bovine Cervical Mucus) *on page 320*
Sperm Penetration Assay (Zona-Free Hamster Egg Penetration Test) *on page 321*
Testosterone, Total and Free, Serum or Plasma *on page 280*

Synonyms Advanced Semen Analysis

Test Includes Semen Analysis, Basic plus sperm processing through a density gradient preparation plus sperm survival after 24-hour incubation

Abstract The recently described "Advanced Semen Analysis" is a set of simple procedures, results of which are useful in predicting the success of intrauterine insemination (IUI). The analysis includes basic semen analysis, assessment of total motile sperm available for insemination, and 24-hour survival of spermatozoa.

Specimen Semen specimen from a subject who has abstained from ejaculation for 2-5 days; semen from ejaculate specimen

Container Sterile specimen container; clean, dry, wide mouth glass or plastic bottle maintained warm and known to be free of detergent or other toxic compounds

Collection See Semen Analysis, Basic *on page 319*.

Causes for Rejection Specimen more than 1 hour old, exposed to cold, contaminated, or not liquefied

Turnaround Time 1-2 days

Special Instructions Semen, as with all blood, urine, and body fluid specimens, because of the risk of AIDS, should be received and handled with attention to universal precautions. Gloves must be worn during the handling and manipulation of sperm/semen containing fluids. Persons with sores/open wounds of the skin must avoid contact with semen.

Reference Interval

- Processed (through Percoll or other gradient) total motile sperm count: lower limit of 5×10^6, optimum level of $\geq 10 \times 10^6$
- Sperm survival test: >70% correlates with high pregnancy rate as a result of IUI

Use Prediction of success of intrauterine insemination

Methodology Analysis includes basic studies (ie, semen volume, sperm concentration, motility, sperm morphology, and seminal leukocytes). Total mobile sperm count is determined after processing through a density gradient preparation (discontinuous two-layered Percoll gradient, 40% to

80%), with two centrifugation and wash cycles. Percoll has been withdrawn from use in human clinical applications, alternative products may be used (eg, PureSperm or Isolate as described in the WHO manual, 4th edition).[1] After sperm count and assessment of motility, specimen is adjusted to a maximum concentration of 10×10^6 motile sperm/mL of medium and incubated at 37°C in 5% CO_2. After 24 hours, the percentage of sperm motility is again determined.

Additional Information The parameters of basic semen analysis (ie, semen volume, sperm concentration, motility, sperm morphology, and seminal leukocytes) correlate poorly with the success of intrauterine insemination. A recently developed and described "Advanced Semen Analysis" includes, in addition to the basic studies, a processed (after density gradient sperm separation) motile sperm fraction determination and a 24-hour incubation study (to assess sperm survival). In the initial report of "Advanced Semen Analysis," the basic semen analysis findings again showed no significant correlation with pregnancy rate resulting from IUI. Processed total motile sperm count <5 x 10⁶ was associated with unsuccessful IUI (ie, no pregnancies). Sperm survival test was highly predictive of successful IUI. With survival >70%, 89% (162 of 182) of couples became pregnant as the result of IUI with a 21.4% per cycle pregnancy rate. In 23% of men with normal basic semen analysis parameters, but abnormally low 24-hour motility or processed total motile sperm results, the per cycle pregnancy rate was only 1.8%. Thus, findings suggest that Advanced Semen Analysis may predict results of intrauterine insemination (IUI) independent of the basic semen analysis. The procedure may also be used to screen for couples that may require intracytoplasmic sperm injection.[2]

Footnotes

1. *World Health Organization Laboratory Manual for the Examination of Human Semen and Sperm-Cervical Mucus Interaction*, 4th ed, Cambridge, UK: Cambridge University Press, 1999, 105-6.
2. Correa-Pérez JR, "Advanced Sperm Analysis - A Step in the Right Direction?" *Fertil Steril*, 1999, 72(6):1150-1.

References

Branigan EF, Estes MA, and Muller CH, "Advanced Semen Analysis: A Simple Screening Test to Predict Intrauterine Insemination Success," *Fertil Steril*, 1999, 71(3):547-51.

Semen Analysis, Basic

Related Information

Synonyms Seminal Cytology; Sperm Count; Sperm Examination; Sperm Morphology Study

Applies to CASA; Computer-Assisted Sperm Analysis; Semen, Brown Colored; Semen, Yellow Colored; Spermatids, Round

Test Includes A variety of parameters may be included in a "standard" or "basic" semen analysis, generally an assessment of number, motility, and morphology of the spermatozoa. More specifically, volume of the semen specimen, concentration of sperm, total count, liquefaction status, viscosity, color, odor, assessment of motility, determination of viability, and detection of abnormal morphologic forms. Direct microscopy of wet preparations and/or a modified Papanicolaou method may be utilized.

Abstract Analysis usually consists of a number of measurements including physical characteristics (eg, volume, color, odor, consistency, etc) of the semen and the morphologic characteristics/functional ability of its constituent spermatozoa. Computer-assisted assessment of sperm morphology and motility can enrich the basic study by providing analysis of individual spermatozoon motility characteristics (sperm kinematics).

Patient Preparation Ejaculation should be avoided for 2-3 days (but not more than 7 days) prior to collection.

Specimen Semen from ejaculate specimen

Container Clean, dry, wide mouth glass or plastic bottle maintained warm (20°C to 40°C) and known to be free of detergent or other toxic compounds

Sampling Time Because of apparent diurnal variation in semen quality (see below), late afternoon seminal fluid collection is preferable.[1]

Collection Physician usually provides instruction for collection. Specimen quality is enhanced when collected in physician's office or laboratory, obviating delay in testing and exposure to extremes of temperature occasioned by transportation. Alternately, specimen may be obtained at patient's home by masturbation and delivered to the laboratory within 1 hour.[1] Collection of semen during intercourse using a seminal collection device may yield a

specimen of higher quality.[2] Use of such a Silastic condom-type seminal pouch (with a small pencil lead-size perforation) to obtain a specimen for analysis in overcoming human infertility is acceptable to and falls within the principles of the Catholic Church.[3] Ordinary latex condoms may interfere with the viability of spermatozoa and should not be used. Because of sample contamination (eg, bacteria, cells, and pH effects of vaginal fluid) and loss of the first portion of the ejaculate, coitus interruptus should not be used.[4] The first portion of the ejaculate usually contains the most spermatozoa. The semen specimen should be complete.

Storage Instructions Patient should be instructed to bring specimen to the laboratory within 30-60 minutes after collection maintaining warmth (37°C) during transport. Patient should be instructed to transport specimen in a pocket close to the skin. Low temperature during transport may decrease motility of sperm.

Causes for Rejection Specimen more than 2 hours old, improper collection, specimen unlabeled

Turnaround Time Dependent upon component tests of analysis, minimum of 2-3 days

Special Instructions Requisition should specify infertility study or postvasectomy study. Semen, as with all blood, urine, and body fluid specimens, because of the risk of AIDS, should be received and handled with attention to universal precautions. Gloves must be worn during the handling and manipulation of sperm/semen containing fluids. Persons with sores/open wounds of the skin must avoid contact with semen.

Because semen/sperm parameters may vary significantly from day to day in any one individual, two samples should be collected and studied at initial evaluation. The sample interval should be from 7-21 days apart.

Reference Interval

- Volume: 2-5 mL
- Appearance: white to gray, opalescent, viscid, opaque
- Clotting and liquefaction: complete in 20-30 minutes, rarely over 60 minutes
- pH: 7.2-8.0
- Sperm count: ≥20 million/mL
- Total sperm count: ≥40 million/ejaculate
- Motility: at least 50% motile
- Morphology: about 70% normal oval-headed forms (<15% normal forms is usually associated with decreased *in vitro* fertilization rate)
- Leukocytes (largely neutrophils): <1 million/mL[4]

A diurnal rhythm in sperm quality has been reported.[5] Afternoon specimens showed higher number and concentration of spermatozoa as compared to morning specimens.

Use Infertility studies, postvasectomy studies; diagnose azoospermia, oligospermia

Limitations Lack of standardization of many test parameters

Methodology Macroscopic and microscopic analysis; direct observation, enumeration, and description, preferentially using the "stricter criteria" of Menkveld et al.[6] Morphologic "stricter criteria" (for normal spermatozoon) include the following.

- Head; smooth oval configuration with a well-defined acrosome comprising ~40% to 70% of the sperm head.
- Acrosome should cover more than $1/3$ of the head surface.
- Head length 3 and 5 μm, width between 2 and 3 μm.
- Head width between $3/5$ and $2/3$ of the head length.
- "Borderline normal" head forms and/or spermatozoa with nearly oval heads with no gross abnormalities are considered to be abnormal.
- No neck, midpiece, or tail defects allowed.
- Midpiece slender, axially attached, ≤1 μm in width and about 1½ times the head length.
- Cytoplasmic droplets less than $1/2$ the size of the sperm can be present.
- Tail - uniform, slightly thinner than midpiece, uncoiled, and ~45 μm long.

Systems for computer-assisted study of morphology and motility (CASA) are increasingly employed. A progressive spurious increase in sperm concentration occurs with ever longer delay in applying the cover glass (Makler Counting Chamber) when sperm are suspended in seminal plasma or in culture medium.[7] The improved Neubauer hemocytometer has been considered as the standard for sperm counting.[8]

Additional Information The semen sample may be red-brown if red blood cells or heme pigments are present or in cases of spinal cord injury (see Infertility Screen *on page 310*). Increase in leukocytes seen in semen of men with spinal cord injury appear to be the result of urinary tract infection.[9] Semen may be yellow in some cases of pyospermia, in jaundiced patients, and in some individuals taking certain vitamins.[4] If pH is <7 and there is azoospermia, obstruction of the ejaculatory ducts or bilateral congenital absence of the vas deferens may be present.[4] Sperm counts may be reduced in patients taking cimetidine and possibly other histamine-receptor blockers. Other drugs that may be responsible for decrease in sperm count include sulfasalazine, nitrofurantoin, cyclophosphamide, nitrogen mustard, procarbazine, vincristine, methotrexate, and possibly other chemotherapeutics. Estrogens and methyltestosterone may suppress spermatogenesis. Orchitis, testicular atrophy (as after mumps), varicocele, testicular failure, obstruction of vas deferens (as after vasectomy), and hyperpyrexia may be associated with hypospermia or azoospermia and/or morphologically aberrant forms of spermatozoa. The motility of spermatozoa is dependent upon the level of ionized calcium, in particular the intracellular translocation of

(Continued)

Semen Analysis, Basic *(Continued)*

calcium ions.[10] Cigarette smoking is associated with decrease in volume of semen; coffee drinking with increase in sperm density and percentage of abnormal forms.[11] Alcohol consumption may not affect sperm function at least as measured at semen analysis.[11] Use of cocaine may be associated with low sperm concentration, low sperm motility, and presence of abnormal morphology.[12] Other illicit drugs which may interfere with spermatogenesis include marijuana; anabolic steroids, lead, and arsenic also do so.[13]

In some cases of infertility, cytologically abnormal spermatocytes or spermatogonia may be seen. A number of associations and known etiologies not withstanding, the cause of oligospermia in most infertile men remains unknown. Fertility correlates most closely with the parameters of sperm motility and morphology. A role for image analysis in selected settings such as oligozoospermia is published.[14]

Testicular biopsy and fine needle biopsy are in use,[15] and other types of investigation are available as well.

Recent studies appear to refute previous findings indicating a decline in the quality of sperm from men living in industrialized countries.[16,17,18]

There is considerable research activity in andrology and related laboratory testing. A small sampling is included in the footnotes below. These recent articles have been chosen and loosely grouped to allow perusal of categories with potential clinical application such as: cytokines, receptors, hormones,[19,20,21,22,23,24] round spermatids,[25] hyperactivated spermatozoa,[26,27] prediction of fertilization *in vitro*,[28,29] chromosomal considerations,[30,31] and nutritional considerations.[32]

Footnotes

1. Sarkar S and Henry JB, "Semen Analysis," *Todd-Sanford-Davidsohn Clinical Diagnosis and Management by Laboratory Methods*, 19th ed, Henry JB, ed, Philadelphia, PA: WB Saunders Co, 1996, 510-11.
2. Zavos PM and Goodpasture JC, "Clinical Improvements of Specific Seminal Deficiencies Via Intercourse With a Seminal Collection Device Versus Masturbation," *Fertil Steril*, 1989, 51(1):190-3.
3. Griese ON, Rev Msgr, *Catholic Identity in Healthcare: Principles and Practice*, The Pope John Center, 1987, 51-3.
4. World Health Organization, *WHO Laboratory Manual for the Examination of Human Semen and Sperm-Cervical Mucus Interaction*, 4th ed, Cambridge, UK: Cambridge University Press, 1999, 4-11, 60-1.
5. Cagnacci A, Maxia N, and Volpe A, "Diurnal Variation of Semen Quality in Human Males," *Hum Reprod*, 1999, 14(1):106-9.
6. Menkveld R, Stander FS, Kotze TJ, et al, "The Evaluation of Morphological Characteristics of Human Spermatozoa According to Stricter Criteria," *Hum Reprod*, 1990, 5(5):586-92.
7. Matson P, Irving J, Zuvela E, et al, "Delay in the Application of the Cover Glass Is a Potential Source of Error With the Makler Counting Chamber," *Fertil Steril*, 1999, 72(3):559-61.
8. Mahmoud AM, Depoorter B, Peins N, et al, "The Performance of 10 Different Methods for the Estimation of Sperm Concentration," *Fertil Steril*, 1997, 68(2):340-5.
9. Aird IA, Vince GS, Bates MD, et al, "Leukocytes in Semen From Men With Spinal Cord Injuries," *Fertil Steril*, 1999, 72(1):97-103.
10. Aaberg RA, Sauer MV, Sikka S, et al, "Effects of Extracellular Ionized Calcium, Diltiazem, and cAMP on Motility of Human Spermatozoa," *J Urol*, 1989, 141(5):1221-4.
11. Marshburn PB, Sloan CS, and Hammond MG, "Semen Quality and Association With Coffee Drinking, Cigarette Smoking, and Ethanol Consumption," *Fertil Steril*, 1989, 52(1):162-5.
12. Bracken MB, Eskenazi B, Sachse K, et al, "Association of Cocaine Use With Sperm Concentration, Motility, and Morphology," *Fertil Steril*, 1990, 53(2):315-22.
13. Howards SS, "Treatment of Male Infertility," *N Engl J Med*, 1995, 332(5):312-7.
14. Mazzilli F, Rossi T, Sabatini L, et al, "Superimposed Image Analysis System (SIAS) Software: A New Approach to Sperm Motility Assessment," *Fertil Steril*, 1995, 64(3):653-6.
15. Gottschalk-Sabag S, Weiss DB, Folb-Zacharow N, et al, "Is One Testicular Specimen Sufficient for Quantitative Evaluation of Spermatogenesis?" *Fertil Steril*, 1995, 64(2):399-402.
16. Fisch H, Goluboff ET, Olson JH, et al, "Semen Analyses in 1,283 Men From the United States Over a 25-Year Period: No Decline in Quality," *Fertil Steril*, 1996, 65(5):1009-14.
17. Acacio BD, Gottfried T, Israel R, et al, "Evaluation of a Large Cohort of Men Presenting for a Screening Semen Analysis," *Fertil Steril*, 2000, 73(3):595-7.
18. Becker S and Berhane K, "A Meta-analysis of 61 Sperm Count Studies Revisited," *Fertil Steril*, 1997, 67(6):1103-8.
19. Loras B, Vételé F, Malki AE, et al, "Seminal Transforming Growth Factor-β in Normal and Infertile Men," *Hum Reprod*, 1999, 14(6):1534-9.
20. Blume-Jensen P, Jiang G, Hyman R, et al, "Kit/Stem Cell Factor Receptor-Induced Activation of Phosphatidylinositol 3′-Kinase Is Essential for Male Fertility," *Nat Genet*, 2000, 24(2):157-2.
21. Siow Y, Fallat ME, Amin FA, et al, "Müllerian Inhibiting Substance Improves Longevity of Motility and Viability of Fresh and Cryopreserved Sperm," *J Androl*, 1998, 19(5):568-72.
22. Gupta S, Li H, and Sampson NS, "Characterization of Fertilin Beta-Disintegrin Binding Specificity in Sperm-Egg Adhesion," *Bioorg Med Chem*, 2000, 8(4):723-9.
23. Tapanainen JS, Aittomäki K, Min J, et al, "Men Homozygous for an Inactivating Mutation of the Follicle-Stimulating Hormone (FSH) Receptor Gene Present Variable Suppression of Spermatogenesis and Fertility," *Nat Genet*, 1997, 15(4):205-6.
24. Mulryan K, Gitterman DP, Lewis CJ, et al, "Reduced Vas Deferens Contraction and Male Infertility in Mice Lacking P2X₁ Receptors," *Nature*, 2000, 403(6765):86-9.
25. Hendin BN, Patel B, Levin HS, et al, "Identification of Spermatozoa and Round Spermatids in the Ejaculates of Men With Spermatogenic Failure," *Urology*, 1998, 51(5):816-9.
26. Green S and Fishel S, "Morphology Comparison of Individually Selected Hyperactivated and Nonhyperactivated Human Spermatozoa," *Hum Reprod*, 1999, 14(1):123-30.
27. Green S, Fishel S, and Rowe P, "The Incidence of Spontaneous Acrosome Reaction in Homogeneous Populations of Hyperactivated Human Spermatozoa," *Hum Reprod*, 1999, 14(7):1819-22.
28. Duran EH, Gürgan T, Günalp S, et al, "A Logistic Regression Model Including DNA Status and Morphology of Spermatozoa for Prediction of Fertilization *In Vitro*," *Hum Reprod*, 1998, 13(5):1235-9.
29. Kruger TF, Acosta AA, Simmons KF, et al, "Predictive Value of Abnormal Sperm Morphology in *In Vitro* Fertilization," *Fertil Steril*, 1988, 49(1):112-7.
30. Chemes HE, Puigdomenech ET, Carizza C, et al, "Acephalic Spermatozoa and Abnormal Development of the Head-Neck Attachment: A Human Syndrome of Genetic Origin," *Hum Reprod*, 1999, 14(7):1811-8.
31. Spano M, Bonde JP, Hjollund HI, et al, "Sperm Chromatin Damage Impairs Human Fertility," *Fertil Steril*, 2000, 73(1):43-50.
32. Wong WY, Thomas CM, Merkus JM, et al, "Male Factor Subfertility: Possible Causes and the Impact of Nutritional Factors," *Fertil Steril*, 2000, 73(3):435-42.

References

Adelman MM and Cahill EM, *Atlas of Sperm Morphology*, Chicago, IL: ASCP Press, American Society of Clinical Pathologists, 1989.

Auger J, Kunstmann JM, Czyglik F, et al, "Decline in Semen Quality Among Fertile Men in Paris During the Past 20 Years," *N Engl J Med*, 1995, 332(5):281-5

Ginsburg KA, Sacco AG, Ager JW, et al, "Variation of Movement Characteristics With Washing and Capacitation of Spermatozoa. II. Multivariate Statistical Analysis and Prediction of Sperm Penetrating Ability," *Fertil Steril*, 1990, 53(4):704-8.

Glover TD, Barratt CL, Tyler JP, et al, *Human Male Fertility and Semen Analysis*, San Diego, CA: Academic Press Inc, 1990, 123-45.

Gottschalk-Sabag S, Weiss DB, and Sherman Y, "Assessment of Spermatogenic Process by Deoxyribonucleic Acid Image Analysis," *Fertil Steril*, 1995, 64(2):403-7.

Hanson MA and Dumesic DA, "Initial Evaluation and Treatment of Infertility in a Primary-Care Setting," *Mayo Clin Proc*, 1998, 73(7):681-5.

Irvine DS and Aitken RJ, "Seminal Fluid Analysis and Sperm Function Testing," *Endocrinol Metab Clin North Am*, 1994, 23(4):725-48.

Kiessling AA, Lamparelli N, Yin HZ, et al, "Semen Leukocytes: Friends or Foes?" *Fertil Steril*, 1995, 64(1):196-8.

Kjeldsberg CR and Knight JA, *Body Fluids - Laboratory Examination of Amniotic, Cerebrospinal, Seminal, Serous, and Synovial Fluids: A Textbook Atlas*, 3rd ed, Chicago, IL: American Society of Clinical Pathologists, 1993, 255-64, 349-66.

Mansour RT, Aboulghar MA, Serour GI, et al, "The Effect of Sperm Parameters on the Outcome of Intracytoplasmic Sperm Injection," *Fertil Steril*, 1995, 64(5):982-6.

McElreavey K, "The Genetic Basis of Male Infertility," Book Review, *Hum Genet*, 2000, 106(5):572.

Sheriff DS, "Analysis of Semen in a Constantly Changing Social Context of Medicine," *Arch Androl*, 1995, 34(3):125-32.

Sherins RJ, "Are Semen Quality and Male Fertility Changing?" *N Engl J Med*, 1995, 332(5):327-8.

Sokol RZ, Shulman P, and Paulson RJ, "Comparison of Two Methods for the Measurement of Sperm Concentration," *Fertil Steril*, 2000, 73(3):591-4.

Van Thiel DH, Gavaler JS, Smith WI, et al, "Hypothalamic-Pituitary-Gonadal Dysfunction in Men Using Cimetidine," *N Engl J Med*, 1979, 300(18):1012-5.

World Health Organization, *WHO Laboratory Manual for the Examination of Human Semen and Sperm-Cervical Mucus Interaction*, 4th ed, Cambridge, UK: Cambridge University Press, 1999.

Yablonsky T, "Male Fertility Testing. New Tests Yield More Predictive Power: But Are They Useful?" *Lab Med*, 1996, 27(6):378-80.

Zamboni L, "Clinical Relevance of Evaluation of Sperm and Ova," *Pathology of Reproductive Failure*, Kraus FT, Damjanov I, and Kaufman N, eds, Baltimore, MD: Lippincott Williams & Wilkins, 1991, 10-31.

Sperm Mucus Penetration Test (Human or Bovine Cervical Mucus)

Related Information

Testosterone, Total and Free, Serum or Plasma *on page 280*

Synonyms Bovine Cervical Mucus Penetration Test; CMPT; Kremer Sperm Penetration Test; Sperm-Cervical Mucus Interaction: The Capillary Tube Test

Applies to Cervical Mucus Interaction, Cross Hostility Tests; *In Vivo* Cervical Mucus Penetration (Postcoital) Test

Test Includes Migration distance, penetration density, migration reduction (decrease in penetration density at 4.5 cm cf at lcm), and duration of progressive movements in cervical mucus in hours

Patient Preparation Follow physician's instructions. Ejaculation should be avoided for 2-3 days prior to collection.

Specimen Liquefied semen. Normal seminal fluid should be liquefied by about 30 minutes after collection (at 37°C). Test should be started within 1 hour after collection of the sample.

Container Clean, dry, wide mouth glass or plastic bottle known to be free of detergent or substances toxic to spermatozoa

Collection Postcoital or masturbation using condom-like Silastic seminal fluid collection device (see Semen Analysis, Basic *on page 319*) or directly into sterile glass jar.

Storage Instructions Samples should be tested as soon as possible after collection. Time between ejaculation and start of test should not be over 2-3 hours, preferably 1 hour. Human cervical mucus (obtained during time of ovulation) may be stored for some hours at 4°C in the refrigerator.

Causes for Rejection Specimen more than 2 hours old

Turnaround Time 2 days

Special Instructions Semen, as with all blood, urine, and body fluid specimens, because of the risk of AIDS, should be received and handled with close attention to cleanliness. Gloves must be worn during the handling and manipulation of sperm/semen containing fluids. Persons with sores/open wounds of the skin must avoid contact with semen.

Reference Interval ≥30 mm penetration by the "vanguard sperm" (Penetrak™ test)

Use Evaluate interaction between spermatozoa and cervical mucus

Limitations Test provides information additional to other semen tests (sperm count, motility, morphology; see Semen Analysis, Basic *on page 319*). It is not intended for use without other evaluation.

Methodology Miller and Kurzrok, in 1932, developed and made clinical application of a semen-mucus phase boundary test. A 3 mm-sized fragment of cervical mucus and a similar sized drop of semen were placed 3 mm from each other on a glass slide. A coverslip was applied with minimal motion and the events occurring at the semen-mucus interface were studied by microscopy.[1] In 1965 Kremer described the construction of a "sperm penetration meter" and its use in a cervical mucus sperm penetration test.[2] In the commercially available "Penetrak™" test, bovine cervical mucus is kept frozen in flat sealed capillary tubes. Using a standardized technique, sperm migration through the mucus over a 90-minute period is measured. The distance traveled by the sperm the furthest down the tube (the "vanguard sperm") is measured and reported. The average of duplicate values is reported. If values differ by more than 15 mm, it is recommended that the test be repeated on a different specimen.

Additional Information In a study published in 1981, the bovine CMPT identified a group of individuals with inadequate penetration (<15 mm) who had mean sperm density of 53.8 ±6.8 x 10^6/mL (sperm counts within normal limits).[3] Significant numbers of individuals (5%, 10%, and 15% of different groups) had inadequate penetration, but adequate to high sperm counts or levels of motility. Results of *in vitro* tests of sperm penetration have been found to correlate with fertility (pregnancy). Cervical mucus penetration testing has been found of value in assessment of fertility prognosis, in particular when modified to produce a crossmatching penetrability test. The latter study compares results of penetration using cervical mucus of the patient's wife by subject's spermatozoa and additionally with use of semen from fertile donors.[4] The use of hormonally standardized human cervical mucus from female partners has been considered superior to bovine cervical mucus as a penetration medium and as to ability to provide information about sperm function.[5] There are data to suggest that the ability of cervical mucus to accept spermatozoa is dependent upon the carbohydrate composition of mucus glycoproteins.[6]

Footnotes

1. Miller EG Jr and Kurzrock R, "Biochemical Studies of Human Semen. III. Factors Affecting Migration of Sperm Through the Cervix," *Am J Obstet Gynecol*, 1932, 24:19-26.
2. Kremer J, "A Simple Sperm Penetration Test," *Int J Fertil*, 1965, 10:209-15.
3. Alexander NJ, "Evaluation of Male Infertility With an *In Vitro* Cervical Mucus Penetration Test," *Fertil Steril*, 1981, 36:201-8.
4. Eggert-Kruse W, Gerhard I, Tilgen W, et al, "Clinical Significance of Crossed *In Vitro* Sperm-Cervical Mucus Penetration Test in Infertility Investigation," *Fertil Steril*, 1989, 52(6):1032-40.
5. Eggert-Kruse W, Leinhos G, Gerhard I, et al, "Prognostic Value of *In Vitro* Sperm Penetration Into Hormonally Standardized Human Cervical Mucus," *Fertil Steril*, 1989, 51(2):317-23.
6. Morales P, Roco M, and Vigil P, "Human Cervical Mucus: Relationship Between Biochemical Characteristics and Ability to Allow Migration of Spermatozoa," *Hum Reprod*, 1993, 8(1):78-83.

References

Adelman MM and Cahill EM, *Atlas of Sperm Morphology*, Chicago, IL: American Society of Clinical Pathologists, 1989, 99.

World Health Organization Laboratory Manual for the Examination of Human Semen and Sperm-Cervical Mucus Interaction, 4th ed, Cambridge, UK: Cambridge University Press, 1999, 51-8 and 110-13.

♦ **Sperm-Oolemma Binding Test** *see Infertility Screen on page 310*

♦ **Sperm Penetration Assay** *see Hypo-osmotic Swelling Test (Spermatozoa) on page 309*

Sperm Penetration Assay (Zona-Free Hamster Egg Penetration Test)

Related Information

Hypo-osmotic Swelling Test (Spermatozoa) *on page 309*
Infertility Screen *on page 310*
Semen Analysis, Advanced *on page 318*
Semen Analysis, Basic *on page 319*
Sperm Mucus Penetration Test (Human or Bovine Cervical Mucus) *on page 320*
Testosterone, Total and Free, Serum or Plasma *on page 280*

Synonyms Hamster Egg Penetration Test; Hamster Oocyte Penetration Assay; Hamster Test; Hamster Zona-Free Ovum Test; Heterologous Ovum Penetration Test; Humster (Human + Hamster) Test

Applies to CASA; Computer-Assisted Semen Analysis; Herbal Effects, Sperm Function; St John's Wort, Mutagenesis, Sperm Cells

Abstract The sperm penetration assay (SPA) is an *in vitro* test that can provide a measure of the fertilizing capacity of human spermatozoa. The test measures the ability of human sperm to penetrate zona-free hamster oocytes. The test thus reflects the ability of sperm to capacitate, acrosome react, fuse with the oolemma, and to undergo nuclear decondensation (within zona-free hamster oocytes). It is not a global test for male infertility.

Patient Preparation Abstinence for a period of at least 48 hours prior to test; less than 48 hours (12 or 24 hours) is associated with reduced penetration potential even though sperm count or motility may not be decreased.[1]

Specimen Semen

Container Clean, wide-mouth glass or plastic container; condom-like device (Silastic seminal fluid collection device - available commercially) placed in a clean jar. Containers should be known free of detergent or other toxic compounds.

Collection Proper collection and handling of the semen specimen is critically necessary to obtain representative results. Semen collection by masturbation in a special room within or adjacent to the laboratory performing the analysis is ideal for some patients. This allows for direct transfer to the laboratory of a fresh specimen without risking degradation of spermatozoa by aging or temperature extremes incurred during transportation.[2] Patient preference, however, may dictate the use of a coital specimen (collected during intercourse) using a Silastic seminal fluid collection device. Commercial sources for such devices include (but may not be limited to) Male-Factor Pak manufactured by Apex Medical Technologies Inc, available from Fertility Technologies Inc, Natick, Massachusetts; HDC Corporation, Mountain View, California. There is evidence that semen quality is improved when collected during intercourse using such a device.[3,4] Specimen must be delivered to the laboratory within 30-60 minutes after collection. Avoid exposure to extremes of heat or cold during transport (patient should be instructed to carry specimen in a pocket close to the skin).

Storage Instructions Specimen is maintained in the laboratory at room temperature, allowed to liquefy (usually occurs within 30 minutes, abnormal if not liquefied by 60 minutes), standard semen analysis is commonly initiated, and specimen is buffered (see below) and incubated at 4°C for 18 hours or longer.

Causes for Rejection Question concerning authenticity of specimen identification (label, content), exposure to extreme of temperature, specimen more than 1 hour old (sperm should not stay in contact with seminal fluid for more than 1-2 hours prior to processing)

Turnaround Time Results usually available within 36 hours (dependent upon preincubation time which in current procedures may be as long as 18-22 hours).

Special Instructions Semen, as with all blood, urine, and body fluid specimens, because of the risk of AIDS, should be received and handled with close attention to cleanliness. Gloves must be worn during the handling and manipulation of sperm-/semen-containing fluids. Persons with sores/open wounds of the skin must avoid contact with semen specimens.

Reference Interval Penetration of 21% to 100% - ("good category");[5] penetration index of over 0.2. The terms "penetration index,"[5] "fertilization index," and "sperm capacitation index,"[6] are a measure of polyspermy (the average number of penetrations per ovum).

Use Evaluate fertilizing capability of human spermatozoa;[6] application to the study of effect that environmental factors have on male fertility; a clinical test of sperm function in conjunction with semen analysis and other studies as a screen for *in vitro* fertilization. The SPA measures components of sperm penetration including capacitation (see below), acrosome reaction, chromatin decondensation, and ability to fuse with oolemma. SPA-failed spermatozoa may still be functional in intracytoplasmic sperm injection (ICSI), as the injection procedure bypasses the need for independent sperm oocyte penetration.
(Continued)

Sperm Penetration Assay (Zona-Free Hamster Egg Penetration Test) *(Continued)*

Limitations SPA does not assess all functions of human spermatozoa. The test does not measure the ability of sperm to penetrate human ova with granulosa cells and zona pellucida intact. Ability of spermatozoa to bind the zona pellucida is species specific. Thus, semen with a positive SPA result may not necessarily have sperm with normal penetrating ability (false-positive result). Patients with low scores on SPA may subsequently initiate pregnancy (false-negative result). The test suffers from lack of standardization and is relatively expensive. Cumulus and zona-free hamster oocytes are not true physiologic models. Extensive experience with the SPA used in conjunction with *in vitro* fertilization indicates that in most individuals, sperm capable of penetrating zona-free hamster ova can also penetrate intact human eggs.[7]

Methodology The original method of Yanagimachi et al utilized a modified Krebs-Ringer's culture medium developed by Biggers, Whitten, and Whittingham (BWW medium) supplemented with human serum albumin.[8] Ova were obtained from superovulated hamsters and prepared by treatment with bovine testicular hyaluronidase (divests the surrounding cumulus cells). The zona pellucida was removed by treatment with bovine pancreatic trypsin. A drop of filtered, washed human semen (sperm suspension) was placed with ova in BWW medium and examined (phase contrast microscopy) for evidence of sperm penetration. Evidence of penetration (fertilization) was presence of swollen sperm heads within the cytoplasm of an oocyte.

The assay has undergone continuing improvement and simplification. Cryopreserved hamster ova have become commercially available, simplifying the SPA procedure. Use of these ova provides a baseline for use in quality control procedures. The frozen ova were found to be statistically equivalent (% penetration and penetration index) to unfrozen ova in a study of the SPA using 547 frozen hamster ova.[9]

A modification of the SPA uses 10 μL wells of Teraski tissue typing plates allowing the study of very small numbers of spermatozoa as they interact with single hamster ova. This modification may be of value clinically in cases of severe abnormality when few motile spermatozoa can be recovered.[10] Frozen semen is recommended for quality control.[11]

Additional Information There is a lack of consensus and a surprisingly wide variety of opinion concerning the value of the sperm penetration assay in the study of fertility. The 1992 review by Liu and Baker[6] noted that "the clinical significance of the SPA in predicting male fertility is still disputed" but that "the SPA has been widely used as a clinical test of sperm function." Correlation with the results of *in vitro* fertilization (IVF) has been variable.[5] Lack of standardized test parameters, small sample size, and/or variable, often poorly defined parameters of the patient test population characterize many studies. Comparisons and conclusions are problematic.

There is unanimity of opinion that the SPA does assess sperm capacitation, acrosome reaction, ability to fuse with oolemma, and chromatin decondensation with head swelling in cytoplasm of the ovum.[5,6] These are major physiologic events necessary to fertilization. With the acrosome reaction there is fusion and vesiculation of membranes, formation of pores, and eventual loss of sperm, and outer acrosomal membranous envelope anterior to the equator of the sperm head. The acrosome reaction must occur before the sperm can penetrate the zona pellucida. Round headed spermatozoa (without acrosomes) are thus not capable of fertilization. Before ejaculated spermatozoa are functional, they require a period of time (within the female tract or *in vitro*) before they can fertilize. This process is termed "capacitation" and is followed by an influx of calcium ions and cytoplasmic alkalinization[12] leading to the acrosome reaction. These calcium and pH changes can be achieved artificially by use of the divalent cation ionophore, A23187. Capacitation is not associated with a recognizable morphologic change, thus, the important role of functional based assays such as the SPA.

A large study (241 couples) published in 1992 compared the results of SPA under conditions that enhance sperm capacitation (use of TES and TRIS - yolk-extender buffer system and cool incubation) with outcome of *in vitro* fertilization.[5] A significant correlation was found between SPA penetration category (poor: 0% to 20%; good: 21% to 100%), and pregnancy rate after IVF. No pregnancy occurred (among eight embryo transfers) in the 31 cases falling into the "poor SPA" category. On the other hand there were 73 pregnancies (34.8%) in the 210 cases falling into the "good SPA" category. Sperm quality (count, motility, and morphology) were all significantly higher in "good SPA" versus the "poor SPA" categories. The authors concluded that the SPA "is a useful screening assay before IVF together with sperm morphology."[5]

Findings from computer-assisted semen analysis have been compared with SPA penetration rates. Total motile oval count (TMO), defined as the product of total count, percent motility, and percent normal (oval) forms in the semen specimen, was a greater risk factor than percent sperm with oval morphology in relation to the outcome of SPA.[13] Below 20% penetration in the SPA assay, both TMO and percent oval sperm were comparable predictive factors.

Acceptance of SPA for clinical assessment of fertility is hampered by interlaboratory variation, cost, and presence of false-negative results. (Spermatozoa fail the SPA test but are able to fertilize human oocytes *in vitro* or *in vivo*.) Perhaps of limited use in a routine infertility practice, SPA may be useful in predicting results of *in vitro* fertilization and need for ICSI although even recent studies do not provide unanimity of opinion on this matter.[14,15] The test continues to find application at the scientific/research level as a model for the study of sperm-oocyte fusion, including environmental and pharmaceutical effects upon this important process. A study of herbal effects on the penetration of zona-free hamster oocytes suggested that high concentrations of St John's wort, ginkgo, and Echinacea damage reproductive cells and that St John's wort may be mutagenic to sperm cells (results of denaturing gradient gel electrophoresis).[16]

Footnotes

1. Rogers BJ, Perreault SD, Bentwood BJ, et al, "Variability in the Human-Hamster *In Vitro* Assay for Fertility Evaluation," *Fertil Steril*, 1983, 39(2):204-11.
2. Overstreet JW and Katz DF, "Semen Analysis," *Urol Clin North Am*, 1987, 14(3):441-9.
3. Zavos PM, "Seminal Parameters of Ejaculates Collected From Oligospermic and Normospermic Patients Via Masturbation and at Intercourse With the Use of a Silastic Seminal Fluid Collection Device," *Fertil Steril*, 1985, 44(4):517-20.
4. Zavros PM, "Characteristics of Human Ejaculates Collected Via Masturbation and a New Silastic Seminal Fluid Collection Device," *Fertil Steril*, 1985, 43(3):491-2.
5. Soffer Y, Golan A, Herman A, et al, "Prediction of *In Vitro* Fertilization Outcome by Sperm Penetration Assay With TEST-Yolk Buffer Preincubation," *Fertil Steril*, 1992, 58(3):556-62.
6. Liu DY and Baker HW, "Tests of Human Sperm Function and Fertilization *In Vitro*," *Fertil Steril*, 1992, 58(3):465-83.
7. Smith RG, Johnson A, Lamb D, et al, "Functional Tests of Spermatozoa. Sperm Penetration Assay," *Urol Clin North Am*, 1987, 14(3):451-8.
8. Yanagimachi R, Yanagimachi H, and Rogers BJ, "The Use of Zona-Free Animal Ova as a Test-System for the Assessment of the Fertilizing Capacity of Human Spermatozoa," *Biol Reprod*, 1976, 15(4):471-6.
9. Leibo SP, Giambernardi TA, Meyer TK, et al, "The Efficacy of Cryopreserved Hamster Ova in the Sperm Penetration Assay," *Fertil Steril*, 1990, 53(5):906-12.
10. Bronson RA, Oula L, and Bronson SK, "A Microwell Sperm Penetration Assay," *Fertil Steril*, 1992, 58(5):1078-80.
11. Johnson A, Bassham B, Lipshultz LI, et al, "A Quality Control System for the Optimized Sperm Penetration Assay," *Fertil Steril*, 1995, 64(4):832-7.
12. Aitken J, "On the Future of the Hamster Oocyte Penetration Assay," *Fertil Steril*, 1994, 62(1):17-9.
13. Brandeis VT, "Importance of Total Motile Oval Count in Interpreting the Hamster Ovum Sperm Penetration Assay," *J Androl*, 1993, 14(1):53-9.
14. Shibahara H, Mitsuo M, Inoue M, et al, "Relationship Between Human *In Vitro* Fertilization and Intracytoplasmic Sperm Injection and the Zona-Free Hamster Egg Penetration Test," *Hum Reprod*, 1998, 13(7):1928-32.
15. Zainul Rashid MZ, Fishel SB, Thornton S, et al, "The Predictive Value of the Zona-Free Hamster Egg Penetration Test in Relation to *In Vitro* Fertilization at Various Insemination Concentrations," *Hum Reprod*, 1998, 13(3):624-9.
16. Ondrizek RR, Chan PJ, Patton WC, et al, "An Alternative Medicine Study of Herbal Effects on the Penetration of Zona-Free Hamster Oocytes and the Integrity of Sperm Deoxyribonucleic Acid," *Fertil Steril*, 1999, 71(3):517-22.

References

Auger J, Kunstmann JM, Czyglik F, et al, "Decline in Semen Quality Among Fertile Men in Paris During the Past 20 Years," *N Engl J Med*, 1995, 332(5):281-5.

Bar-Chama N and Lamb DJ, "Evaluation of Sperm Function: What Is Available in the Modern Andrology Laboratory?" *Urol Clin North Am*, 1994, 21(3):433-46.

British Andrology Society Guidelines for the Screening of Semen Donors for Donor Insemination (1999), *Hum Reprod*, 1999, 14(7):1823-6.

Chuang AT and Howards SS, "Male Infertility: Evaluation and Nonsurgical Therapy," *Urol Clin North Am*, 1998, 25(4):703-13.

Fraser L, Barratt CL, Canale D, et al, "Consensus Workshop on Advanced Diagnostic Andrology Techniques," *ESHRE Andrology Special Interst Group, Hum Reprod*, 1997, 12(4):873.

Fraser L, Barratt CL, Canale D, et al, "Consensus Workshop on Advanced Diagnostic Andrology Techniques," *ESHRE Andrology Special Interest Group, Hum Reprod*, 1997, 12(4):873.

Howards SS, "Treatment of Male Infertility," *N Engl J Med*, 1995, 332(5):312-7.

Mortimer D and Frasser L, "Consensus Workshop on Advanced Diagnostic Andrology Techniques," *ESHRE (European Society of Human Reproduction and Embryology) Andrology Special Interest Group, Hum Reprod*, 1996, 11(7):1463-79.

World Health Organization Laboratory Manual for the Examination of Human Semen and Sperm-Cervical Mucus Interaction, 4th ed, Cambridge, UK: Cambridge University Press, 1999, 31, 94-8.

Yablonsky T, "Male Fertility Testing. New Tests Yield More Predictive Power: But Are They Useful?" *Lab Med*, 1996, 27(6):378-80.

Swim Up/Swim Down Procedures (Spermatozoa)

Related Information
Infertility Screen *on page 310*
Semen Analysis, Basic *on page 319*
Testosterone, Total and Free, Serum or Plasma *on page 280*

Applies to Sex Selection, Swim Up Procedure

Abstract Preparatory techniques used to obtain spermatozoa from seminal plasma for use in a variety of diagnostic and therapeutic procedures. The harvested sperm are largely morphologically normal and highly motile. Nonmotile/dead spermatozoa, white blood cells, and debris are eliminated. The resultant preparations can be used for intrauterine insemination (IUI) and for attempted gender preselection utilizing IUI.

Specimen Semen

Container Sterile specimen container; clean, dry, wide mouth glass or plastic bottle maintained warm and known to be free of detergent or other toxic compounds

Collection Physician usually provides instruction for collection. Specimen quality is enhanced when collected in physician's office or laboratory, obviating delay in testing and exposure to extremes of temperature occasioned by transportation. Alternately, specimen may be obtained at patient's house by coitus interruptus or masturbation and delivered to the laboratory as soon as possible. Collection of semen during intercourse using a seminal collection device may yield a specimen of higher quality. Use of such a Silastic condom-type seminal pouch (with a small pencil lead-size perforation) to obtain a specimen for analysis in overcoming human infertility is acceptable to and falls within the principles of the Catholic Church.

Storage Instructions Patient should be instructed to bring specimen to the laboratory within 30-60 minutes after collection, maintaining warmth (37°C) during transport. Patient should be instructed to transport specimen in a pocket close to the skin. Low temperature during transport may decrease motility of sperm. Procedures should be performed just after liquefaction of the specimen (within 1 hour of collection of the ejaculate).

Turnaround Time 1-2 hours

Special Instructions Specimens for use in assisted reproduction procedures such as *in vitro* fertilization/intrauterine insemination (IVF)/IUI, if obtained with diluents having human serum albumin as a constituent, must use highly purified albumin that is free from viral, bacterial, and prior contamination. Requisition should specify infertility study or postvasectomy study. Semen, as with all blood, urine, and body fluid specimens, because of the risk of HIV, should be received and handled with attention to universal precautions. Gloves must be worn during the handling and manipulation of sperm/semen containing fluids. Persons with sores/open wounds of the skin must avoid contact with semen.

Use Separation of spermatozoa from semen for use in some therapeutic/diagnostic procedures in clinical andrology. The resultant preparations are enriched by morphologically normal and motile spermatozoa.

Methodology

Swim up: A variety of methods have been used.[1,2,3,4] Basically, a preovulatory human tubal fluid-like diluent is placed over the liquefied semen specimen and spermatozoa are allowed to migrate into the diluent. The WHO Laboratory Manual, 1999,[3] recommends use of a supplemented Earle's medium which includes pyruvate and lactate and either patient's heat inactivated serum or human serum albumin (see Special Instructions). Sperm are collected for 30-60 minutes in absence of light at 37°C. A 5% CO_2 environment may be utilized. The upper 1 mL of diluent (contains the motile spermatozoa) is removed, gently centrifuged, and resuspended in diluent. Aliquots are used to determine sperm concentration, morphology, function, and/or for insemination.

Swim down: In this procedure, an aliquot of a centrifuged, resuspended serum sample is layered on top of 10% bovine serum albumin and incubated at 37°C for 45-60 minutes. Sperm in the bottom two-thirds of the albumin layer are then analyzed for concentration, morphology, and motility. The bottom layer may also be washed, resuspended, and used for insemination.

Gradient centrifugation: Preparation of spermatozoa by passage through Percoll gradients, or Sephadex and Ficoll columns has also been used.[3,5] Percoll, however, has been withdrawn from use in clinical situations (may only be used for nonclinical research studies). Alternative products (for human clinical applications) include PureSperm (NidaCon Labs, Gothenburg, Sweden) and Isolate (Irvine Scientific, NidaCon, Santa Ana, CA, USA).

Stimulation techniques: Sperm can also be prepared by incubation with stimulants in order to increase motility and/or capacitation. These include pentoxifylline (phosphodiesterase inhibitor) and calcium ionophore A23187 (calcium transport modulator). Sperm refrigeration in high-albumin solutions and sperm incubation with heparin may also stimulate sperm capacitation.[5]

Additional Information Sperm preparation by washing (and diluting) with culture media and with multiple cycles of centrifugation serves to remove inactive, fragmented and dead spermatozoa, white blood cells, and seminal debris as well as capacitation inhibitors and prostaglandins. Cyclic centrifugation and compaction of the sample, however, is traumatic and usually results in significant loss (or absence) of sperm motility. Functional spermatozoa which are more motile and have higher density can be harvested by the relatively more gentle swim-up, swim-down, or discontinuous density gradient procedures.

Direct swim-up procedures are preferred for the separation of motile spermatozoa. Centrifugation of sperm prior to swim-up may produce reactive oxygen species/cell membrane damage and should be avoided. Swim-up is easily performed. It consists of layering a human tubal fluid-like cell culture medium on top of the liquefied semen sample and allowing motile spermatozoa to migrate ("swim-up") into the medium.[3] The motility of such migrated sperm has been reported in the range of 80% to 100%.[1,2,4] Significant increase in the number of sperm recovered has been reported by minimizing the effects of gravity during swim-up. In this modification, sperm were exposed to an antigravitational force during swim-up.[6] No significant differences in percent motile sperm or in progressive motile sperm recovery between swim-up with or without "antigravitational" centrifugation was noted.

The results of five sperm preparation techniques on pregnancy rates (PR) following artificial insemination with husband semen has concluded that swim-up and Percoll gradient preparations result in higher PRs than the wash, swim-down and refrigeration/heparin methods.[5]

X and Y bearing sperm have been relatively "separated" using a discontinuous Percoll density gradient (Y-bearing sperm present in the fraction lighter than 1.06 g/mL was 73.1% ±3.3%; fraction >1.11g/mL contained 27.4% ±3.4% Y-bearing sperm - result of a 1983 study).[7] While there has been controversy as to whether the swim-up method can enrich samples with either X- or Y-bearing spermatozoa, a 1998 study (6 year clinical experience) using male spouse semen specimens and a modified swim-up method resulted in a 86.7% success rate in conceiving a female child and 89.2% success rate in conceiving a male child (as compared to control groups).[8]

Evaluation of the "swim-up" technique using fluorescent *in situ* hybridization (FISH) with DNA probes, however, has shown that the ratio of male- to female-producing sperm does not change.[9] Spermatozoa can be sorted (as to their X or Y chromosome) by flow cytometry.[10,11]

Footnotes
1. Lopata A, Patullo MJ, Chang A, et al, "A Method for Collecting Motile Spermatozoa From Human Semen," *Fertil Steril,* 1976, 27(6):677-84.
2. Urry RL, Middleton RG, McNamara L, et al, "The Effect of Single-Density Bovine Serum Albumin Columns on Sperm Concentration, Motility, and Morphology," *Fertil Steril,* 1983, 40(5):666-9.
3. *World Health Organization Laboratory Manual for the Examination of Human Semen and Sperm-Cervical Mucus Interaction,* 3rd ed, Cambridge, UK: Cambridge University Press, 1992, 40, 99-100.
4. Harris SJ, Milligan MP, Masson GM, et al, "Improved Separation of Motile Sperm in Asthenospermia and Its Application to Artificial Insemination Homologous (AIH)," *Fertil Steril,* 1981, 36(2):219-21.
5. Carrell DT, Kuneck PH, Peterson CM, et al, "A Randomized, Prospective Analysis of Five Sperm Preparation Techniques Before Intrauterine Insemination of Husband Sperm," *Fertil Steril,* 1998, 69(1):122-6.
6. Babbo CJ, Hecht BR, and Jeyendran RS, "Increased Recovery of Swim-Up Spermatozoa by Application of Antigravitational Centrifugation," *Fertil Steril,* 1999, 72(3):556-8.
7. Kaneko S, Yamaguchi J, Kobayashi T, et al, "Separation of Human X- and Y-Bearing Sperm Using Percoll Density Gradient Centrifugation," *Fertil Steril,* 1983, 40(5):661-5.
8. Khatamee MA, Horn SR, Weseley A, et al, "A Controlled Study for Gender Selection Using Swim-Up Separation," *Gynecol Obstet Invest,* 1999, 48(1):7-13.
9. De Jonge CJ, Flaherty SP, Barnes AM, et al, "Failure of Multitube Sperm Swim-Up for Sex Preselection," *Fertil Steril,* 1997, 67(6):1109-14.
10. Vidal F, Fugger EF, Blanco J, et al, "Efficacy of Microsort Flow Cytometry for Producing Sperm Populations Enriched in X- or Y-Chromosome Haplotypes: A Blind Trial Assessed by Double and Triple Colour Fluorescent *In Situ* Hybridization," *Hum Reprod,* 1998, 13(2):308-12.
11. Mastroianni L Jr, "Swimming Upstream: Views on the Ethics of Preconception Gender Selection," *J Androl,* 1999, 20(3):332-5.

References
World Health Organization Laboratory Manual for the Examination of Human Semen and Sperm-Cervical Mucus Interaction, 4th ed, Cambridge, UK: Cambridge University Press, 1999, 34-5, 104-6.

Synovial Fluid Analysis

Related Information
Antinuclear Antibody *on page 507*
Bacterial Culture, Biopsy or Body Fluid *on page 565*
Body Cavity Fluid Cytology *on page 372*
Body Fluid Analysis, Cell Count *on page 408*
Body Fluid Glucose *on page 124*
Body Fluid Lactate Dehydrogenase *on page 125*
Chlamydia trachomatis Culture *on page 590*
Chlamydia trachomatis Direct Antigen Test *on page 590*
Chlamydia trachomatis Nucleic Acid Detection *on page 591*
Fungal Culture, Biopsy or Body Fluid *on page 610*
Gram Stain *on page 617*
Lyme Disease DNA Detection *on page 649*
Lyme Disease Serology *on page 650*
Mucin Clot Test *on page 314*
Mycobacterial Culture, Biopsy or Body Fluid *on page 655*
(Continued)

Synovial Fluid Analysis (Continued)

Neisseria gonorrhoeae Culture and Smear *on page 662*
Rheumatoid Factor, Serum or Body Fluid *on page 541*
Uric Acid, Serum *on page 293*

Synonyms Joint Fluid Analysis

Applies to Arthrocentesis; Calcium Pyrophosphate Dihydrate Crystals; First Order Red Compensator; Monosodium Urate Crystals; Mucin Test for Hyaluronic Acid; Osteoarthritis; Psoriatic Arthritis; RA Cells; Whipple Disease

Test Includes May vary between laboratories but should include cell count and differential, cultures and Gram stain for pathogens and polarizing microscopic examination for crystals. Other tests, depending on the clinical situation, may be of value including viscosity, clot lysis, uric acid, rheumatoid factor, cytokines, and cytology.

Abstract Analysis of joint fluid usually includes multiple studies (eg, cell count, microscopic exam, culture) to determine if joint disease is present and to assess its nature and severity. Analyses are particularly helpful in differentiating traumatic arthritis from the immune-based and crystal-induced arthritides.

Patient Preparation As per physician's usual aseptic aspiration technique

Specimen Joint fluid; simultaneously drawn venous blood in red top tube often helpful, especially with order for serum chemistry profile

Container Capped syringe or three sterile tubes, one with sodium heparin (or liquid EDTA) and two red top tubes for joint fluid;[1] one to two red top tubes of venous blood desirable; Thayer-Martin agar is best inoculated with joint fluid at bedside if gonococcal (GC) infection is suspected. Avoid anticoagulants composed of crystalline EDTA, or oxalate or lithium heparin.

Collection An experienced physician, using sterile technique, obtains the specimen (arthrocentesis). Media appropriate for culture of *N. gonorrhoeae*, *M. tuberculosis*, and other organisms should be available if indicated.

Storage Instructions Testing should be initiated, in most cases, shortly after receipt of the specimen. It may be prudent to save a portion of the specimen for possible additional analyses (eg, bacterial and crystal-induced diseases) if such testing is not performed initially. An average 42% decrease in white blood cell count has been noted during the first 6 hours after obtaining the specimen.[1] Calcium pyrophosphate crystals decrease in a few days, while monosodium urate (MSU) crystals maintain their number, size, and birefringence over the first days but decrease over a few weeks.[2]

Causes for Rejection Some constituent tests of the analysis may not be performed if gross contamination has occurred.

Turnaround Time From hours to days (eg, culture results)

Comparison of Gout and CPPD Crystal Deposition Disease*

Feature	Gout	CPPD Crystal Deposition Disease
Male-female ratio	7:1	1.5:1
Age-group affected	Middle-aged men, postmenopausal women	Elderly
Hereditary forms?	Yes	Yes
Hyperuricemia present?	Yes	No
Clinical picture	Asymptomatic phase, acute and chronic arthritis, tophi, renal disease	Asymptomatic phase, acute and chronic arthritis, tophus-like collections only rarely
Typical joint localization	First MTP joints, midfoot, ankles, knees, wrists	Knees, wrists, MCP joints, elbows, shoulders
Radiologic findings	Erosions with overlying edge of displaced bone	Chondrocalcinosis
Findings on synovial fluid analysis	Evidence of inflammation, MSU crystals	Evidence of inflammation, CPPD crystals
Birefringence of synovial fluid crystals	Strong with negative elongation	Weak with positive elongation
Symptomatic treatment	NSAID, colchicine, corticosteroid (intra-articular or systemic)	NSAID, colchicine (occasionally), corticosteroid (intra-articular)
Definitive treatment	Allopurinol (Zyloprim®) or probenecid (Benemid®) to decrease serum uric acid level	None
Possible underlying disease	Diabetes, obesity, hypertension, hyperlipidemia	Hyperparathyroidism, hemochromatosis, hypomagnesemia, hypophosphatasia, severe hypothyroidism

*Formerly called pseudogout.

CPPD = calcium pyrophosphate dihydrate; MCP = metacarpophalangeal; MSU = monosodium urate; MTP = metatarsophalangeal; NSAID = nonsteroidal anti-inflammatory drugs

Adapted from Beutler A and Schumacher HR Jr, "Gout and Pseudogout: When Are Arthritic Symptoms Caused by Crystal Deposition?" *Postgrad Med*, 1994, 95(2):103-16.

Special Instructions Specimens should be delivered immediately to the laboratory and placed in the hands of a medical technologist. **Physician should indicate clinical impression and indicate tests he/she feels are necessary.** If presence of monosodium urate (MSU) crystals (as are present with gout) is a consideration, alcohol-based fixatives and stains must be used. MSU crystals are water soluble.

Reference Interval When synovial fluid can be aspirated, abnormality is probably evident. Normal synovial fluid does not clot spontaneously, because it lacks fibrinogen. Clotting bears an implication of inflammation. There should be <200 WBCs/mm³, 0% to 25% neutrophils, protein should be ≤3.0 g/dL (SI: ≤30 g/L) and uric acid should be <8.0 mg/dL (SI: <476 μmol/L) and fluid LD (LDH) should be the same or less than that of the patient's serum drawn at the same time. Glucose is significantly abnormal in the nonfasting subject when it is <40 mg/dL (SI: <2.2 mmol/L). There should be a long string produced normally when synovial fluid is poured from a container and the mucin clot test is normally positive (ie, a firm mucin clot is formed in the presence of acetic acid).

Use Aid the diagnosis of rheumatic disease and diseases which cause joint symptoms, pain, increase in joint fluid or destruction of joint space, including rheumatoid arthritis, joint infection, gout, and pseudogout. In cases with appropriate clinical presentation (see table), synovial fluid analysis using polarized light should be done to confirm presence of a crystal-induced arthropathy. When infection is **not** in question, routine synovial fluid analysis has a low diagnostic yield and does not contribute significantly to the management of cases with previously established rheumatic disease.[3]

Limitations Appropriate work-up may not be accomplished unless there is discussion between physician and analyst. Oxalate anticoagulants may lead to problems in crystal identification. The anticoagulants sodium EDTA, ammonium oxalate, and lithium heparin can form crystals in joint fluid.[1] If a laboratory is unaware of a possibility of gonococcal arthritis, it may not inoculate specimen on Thayer-Martin medium. If GC infection is in the differential consideration, the physician, ideally, should plate out the Thayer-Martin medium at the bedside at time of aspiration. Limited sensitivity and specificity exist overall for synovial fluid analysis.

Methodology Includes polarizing and phase as well as conventional microscopy. Laboratory notes volume, clarity, color, and presence of clot in centrifuged specimen. Cultures are made from centrifuged sediment and media inoculated for acid-fast bacteria, fungus, routine culture, and Gram stain smear. Rheumatoid factor titer is desirable in suspected cases of rheumatoid arthritis. Other testing methodologies may be applied as indicated or ordered. The use of Testsimplet™ supravital staining (glass slide precoated with methylene blue and crystal violet) has been found advantageous in microscopy of synovial fluid.[4]

The contribution of the laboratory to diagnosis of joint disease depends importantly on its ability to identify crystals present in the patient's synovial fluid. The two most common crystals are monosodium urate (needle-shaped and found in an intracellular situation in neutrophils/monocytes in 90% of cases of acute gout) and calcium pyrophosphate dihydrate (often rhomboid and the cause of "pseudogout," for which the preferred term is now, calcium pyrophosphate deposition disease). Both MSU and CPPD crystals are birefringent. The physician should verify that laboratory personnel are experienced in the use of birefringence in crystal analysis. A polarizing microscope and first-order red compensator must be available to determine the sign of birefringence of the crystal. An excellent discussion of this subject with clear and helpful illustrations has been provided by Judkins and Cornbleet.[1]

A recent study, with the goal of estimating operating characteristics of synovial fluid examination for crystals found only sparse data about the accuracy of crystal identification. Literature review (four studies identified) concluded that rates of interobserver agreement were low and false-negative rates in identification of calcium pyrophosphate crystals were high. Recommendations for interpretation of crystal analysis, use of likelihood ratios, and the foundation of a quality assurance approach for crystal analysis were provided.[5,6]

Additional Information Normal fluid is rarely obtained because of its small volume; therefore, any fluid which is aspirated is potentially a diagnostic specimen. When results of analyses are combined with the clinical impression of the physician, a high rate of accurate diagnosis is obtained. Some diagnoses cannot be made without such analysis. Detection of synovial fluid monosodium urate crystals is important in establishing a diagnosis of gout. A heparinized tube is needed for cell count and differential. A red cell count is not necessary, but if grossly bloody, a hematocrit should be ordered. Joint fluid uric acid significantly higher than serum uric acid may be diagnostic of gout. Other chemistries are usually of little value with the occasional exception of protein, LD (LDH), and glucose. Decreased fluid glucose indicates inflammation, but the result should be compared to that of serum or plasma. High synovial LD but normal serum LD suggests RA, infectious arthritis, or gout. Synovial LD is normal in degenerative joint disease.

Sediment or fluid may be examined in the cytology laboratory for presence of cartilage. Presence of cartilage cells supports a diagnosis of traumatic arthritis or osteoarthritis. While involvement of joints by malignancy is uncommon, both primary and metastatic tumors should be included in differential consideration.[7] Cytologic examination may support diagnosis of pigmented villonodular synovitis or Reiter's syndrome. While rhomboid cholesterol crystals have been reported in chronic joint effusions of rheumatoid arthritis and osteoarthritis, birefringent lipid bodies (lipid microspherules, liposomes, smectic mesophases, lipid liquid crystals), intra- and extracellular, at least partly formed of cholesterol ester, have been found in fluids from acute and chronic arthritis, traumatic arthritis, and pigmented villonodular synovitis.[8,9]

Phase microscopy is used to look for intracellular inclusions in pus cells. These are "RA cells" only if the rheumatoid titer is positive. Synovial fluid in pseudogout, traumatic arthritis and osteoarthritis rarely also may contain intraleukocytic cytoplasmic inclusions. Polarizing microscopy is done to identify crystals of urate and pyrophosphate, the causes, respectively, of gout and pseudogout. Calcium pyrophosphate dihydrate (CPPD) crystal deposition disease does not equate exclusively with a diagnosis of pseudogout (chondrocalcinosis). It is important to recognize that CPPD disease encompasses an array of disorders occurring largely in the aged.[10] These include asymptomatic chondrocalcinosis, acute pseudogout, and chronic pyrophosphate arthropathy. As an example, asymptomatic chondrocalcinosis occurs in 10% to 15% in those 65-75 years of age and in 30% to 60% of those older than 80 years of age.[10] Cases of CPPD disease may be sporadic, familial, or secondary to degenerative or metabolic disease. Hyperparathyroidism and hemochromatosis may be associated with CPPD deposition. Cholesterol crystals occur occasionally, indicating RA. Steroid crystals after therapeutic injection may be found. LE cells may be noted in synovial fluid aspirate.

Test for viscosity and mucin test for hyaluronic acid measure the physical character of the synovial fluid. Abnormality in either of these tests indicates dilution or inflammation. Viscosity can be evaluated by the quality of stringing; inflammatory fluids of low viscosity produce very short strings, but normal or noninflammatory fluids produce long strings. Viscosity is generally equivalent to mucin hyaluronate content.

In some large urban areas, gonococcal infection is the most common cause of infectious arthritis. While peripheral blood white cell counts may not be helpful, synovial fluid white cell levels average some 50,000 cells/µL with Gram stains positive in about 25% of cases.[11] In cases with tenosynovitis following migratory arthralgia, some 40% of patients have positive blood cultures. Nongonococcal acute bacterial arthritis, usually occurring in immune impaired or traumatized patients, is most commonly the result of Staphylococcus aureus infection. Group A/B streptococci, E. coli, and Pseudomonas aeruginosa should also be considered. When the white cell count in the synovial fluid is >100,000/µL, largely neutrophils, blood culture is positive in some 50% of patients.[11]

More than 2% eosinophils in synovial fluid may be a clue to presence of Lyme disease. Rheumatoid factor negative patients with oligoarthritis of unknown etiology were tested for Chlamydia trachomatis utilizing antigen specific synovial T-cell response and detection of bacterial antigen. Antigen specific lymphocyte proliferation was found in the synovial fluid of 34% of such patients. C. trachomatis was the most frequent single agent detected. Only chlamydial antigen was found in synovial fluid cells by monoclonal antibody technique.[12]

The finding of amyloid in synovial fluid (using Congo red stained sections of 10% formol saline fixed, paraffin-embedded, centrifuged sediment) has been considered a sufficient finding to establish a diagnosis of amyloid arthropathy.[13]

A variety of cytokines have been found in synovial fluid. Some (IL-6 and IL-8) are increased in cases of inflammatory arthritis (RA) as compared with cases of osteoarthritis.[14]

Individual laboratories may not be proficient in the identification of crystals present in synovial fluid. Artifacts and unexplained birefringent materials may be present. Patients with hemarthrosis may develop solid and angular birefringent crystals of two different types. Rectangular hemoglobin- like crystals within red cells are weakly birefringent. Golden brown rhomboid crystals (likely hematoidin) are intensely birefringent with positive or negative elongation. These red cell-derived crystals may be confused with pathogenic crystals.[15]

Advantages have been found in the use of atomic force microscopy (AFM) in the detection of synovial fluid crystals, in particular small crystals and octacalcium phosphate. Small sample size (only a few microliters are required), minimal sample preparation, and in some cases greater sensitivity (AFM vs polarized light microscopy) have been reported.[16]

Synovial fluid analysis has found some application in the evaluation of articulating surfaces in surgical hip replacement procedures.[17]

Arthritis is one of the characteristic features of Whipple disease (WD). The arthritis, episodic and migratory, is the presenting symptom (oligoarthritis or polyarthritis) in 60% of patients with WD. Synovial fluid from the hip joint of a patient with a clinical course consistent with WD contained 7500 neutrophils/mm³ and bacterial DNA of Tropheryma whippelii (most likely causative agent of WD) was identified by polymerase chain reaction.[18]

Various aspects of psoriatic arthritis have been studied, including measurement of synovial fluid levels of IL-1β and IL-6.[19] IL-1β may play a role in psoriasis as suggested by the finding that psoriatic fibroblasts produce increased IL-1β.[20] Increased levels of IL-6 have been reported in synovial fluid from post-traumatic psoriatic arthritis patients.[21] Synovial fluid level IL-1β may be useful in predicting the evolution of monoarticular psoriatic

arthritis to polyarthritis.[22] Higher concentrations of IL-1β and of IL-6 are found in synovial fluid of elderly onset than of younger onset psoriatic arthritis, possibly relating to the more severe onset and destructive course of psoriatic arthritis in elderly patients.[23]

Footnotes

1. Judkins SW and Cornbleet PJ, "Synovial Fluid Crystal Analysis," Lab Med, 1997, 28(12):774-9.
2. Kerolus G, Clayburne G, and Schumacher HR Jr, "Is it Mandatory to Examine Synovial Fluids Promptly After Arthrocentesis?" Arthritis Rheum, 1989, 32(3):271-8.
3. Pal B, Nash J, Oppenheim B, et al, "Is Routine Synovial Fluid Analysis Necessary? Lessons and Recommendations From an Audit," Rheumatol Int, 1999, 18(5-6):181-2.
4. Reginato AJ, Maldonado I, Reginato AM, et al, "Supravital Staining of Synovial Fluid With Testsimplets," Diagn Cytopathol, 1992, 8(2):147-52.
5. Segal JB and Albert D, "Diagnosis of Crystal-Induced Arthritis by Synovial Fluid Examination for Crystals: Lessons From an Imperfect Test," Arthritis Care Res, 1999, 12(6):376-80.
6. Dieppe P, Swan A, and Amer Hanya, "The Diagnosis of Crystal-Induced Arthritis: Comment on the Article by Segal and Albert," Arthritis Care Res, 2000, 13(4):246.
7. Chakravarty KK and Webley M, "Monarthritis: An Unusual Presentation of Renal Cell Carcinoma," Ann Rheum Dis, 1992, 51(5):681-2.
8. Ugai K, Kurosaka M, and Hirohata K, "Lipid Microspherules in Synovial Fluid of Patients With Pigmented Villonodular Synovitis," Arthritis Rheum, 1988, 31(11):1442-6.
9. Baer AN and Wright EP, "Lipid Laden Macrophages in Synovial Fluid: A Late Finding in Traumatic Arthritis," J Rheumatol, 1987, 14(4):848-51.
10. Bonafede RP, "Evaluating CPPD Crystal Deposition, An Important Disease of Aging," Geriatrics, 1988, 43(11):59-68.
11. Lowery CL, "Sudden Joint and Extremity Pain in Pregnancy," Obstet Gynecol Clin North Am, 1995, 22(1):173-90.
12. Sieper J, Braun J, Brandt J, et al, "Pathogenetic Role of Chlamydia, Yersinia, and Borrelia in Undifferentiated Oligoarthritis," J Rheumatol, 1992, 19(8):1236-42.
13. Muñoz-Gómez J, Gómez-Pérez R, Solé-Arques M, et al, "Synovial Fluid Examination for the Diagnosis of Synovial Amyloidosis in Patients With Chronic Renal Failure Undergoing Haemodialysis," Ann Rheum Dis, 1987, 46(4):324-6.
14. Remick DG, DeForge LE, Sullivan JF, et al, "Profile of Cytokines in Synovial Fluid Specimens From Patients With Arthritis - Interleukin 8 (IL-8) and IL-6 Correlate With Inflammatory Arthritides," Immunol Invest, 1992, 21(4):321-7.
15. Tate GA, Schumacher HR Jr, Reginato AJ, et al, "Synovial Fluid Crystals Derived From Erythrocyte Degradation Products," J Rheumatol, 1992, 19(7):1111-4.
16. Blair JM, Sorensen LB, Arnsdorf MF, et al, "The Application of Atomic Force Microscopy for the Detection of Microcrystals in Synovial Fluid From Patients With Recurrent Synovitis," Semin Arthritis Rheum, 1995, 24(5):359-69.
17. Dorr LD, Hilton KR, Wan Z, et al, "Modern Metal on Metal Articulation for Total Hip Replacements," Clin Orthop, 1996, (333):108-17.
18. Lange U and Teichmann J, "Diagnosis of Whipple's Disease by Molecular Analysis of Synovial Fluid," concise communications, Arthritis Rheum, 1999, 42(8):1777-8.
19. Debets R, Hegmans JP, Deleuran M, et al, "Expression of Cytokines and Their Receptors by Psoriatic Fibroblasts. I. Altered IL-6 Synthesis," Cytokine, 1996, 8(1):70-9.
20. Espinoza LR, Espinoza CG, Cuellar ML, et al, "Fibroblast Function in Psoriatic Arthritis. II. Increased Expression of Beta Platelet Derived Growth Factor Receptors and Increased Production of Growth Factor and Cytokines," J Rheumatol, 1994, 21(8):1507-14.
21. Punzi L, Pianon M, Bertazzolo N, et al, "Clinical, Laboratory and Immunogenetic Aspects of Post-traumatic Psoriatic Arthritis: A Study of 25 Patients," Clin Exp Rheumatol, 1998, 16(3):277-81.
22. Punzi L, Bertazzolo N, Pianon M, et al, "Value of Synovial Fluid Interleukin-1β Determination in Predicting the Outcome of Psoriatic Monoarthritis," Ann Rheum Dis, 1996, 55(9):642-4.
23. Punzi L, Pianon M, Rossini P, et al, "Clinical and Laboratory Manifestations of Elderly Onset Psoriatic Arthritis: A Comparison With Younger Onset Disease," Ann Rheum Dis, 1999, 58(4):226-9.

References

Beutler A and Schumacher HR Jr, "Gout and Pseudogout: When Are Arthritic Symptoms Caused by Crystal Deposition?" Postgrad Med, 1994, 95(2):103-6, 109, 113-6.
Dieppe P and Swan A, "Identification of Crystals in Synovial Fluid," Ann Rheum Dis, 1999, 58(5):261-3.
Ivorra J, Rosas J, and Pascual E, "Most Calcium Pyrophosphate Crystals Appear as Nonbirefringent," Ann Rheum Dis, 1999, 58(9):582-4.
Johnson KD, "Synovial Fluid," Body Fluids - Laboratory Examination of Amniotic, Cerebrospinal, Seminal, Serous, and Synovial Fluids, 3rd ed, Chapter 6, Kjeldsberg CR and Knight JA, eds, Chicago, IL: ASCP Press, American Society of Clinical Pathologists, 1993, 265-301.
Lazarevic MB, Skosey JL, Vitic J, et al, "Cholesterol Crystals in Synovial and Bursal Fluid," Semin Arthritis Rheum, 1993, 23(2):99-103.
Lossos IS, Yossepowitch O, Kandel L, et al, "Septic Arthritis of the Glenohumoral Joint. A Report of 11 Cases and Review of the Literature," Medicine (Baltimore), 1998, 77(3):177-87.
Luukkainen R, Hakala M, Sajanti E, et al, "Predictive Value of Synovial Fluid Analysis in Estimating the Efficacy of Intra-articular Corticosteroid Injections in Patients With Rheumatoid Arthritis," Ann Rheum Dis, 1992, 51(7):874-6.
Myers SL, "Synovial Fluid Markers in Osteoarthritis," Rheum Dis Clin North Am, 1999, 25(2):433-49.
O'Connell JX, "Pathology of the Synovium," Am J Clin Pathol, 2000, 114(5):773-84.
Shmerling RH, "Synovial Fluid Analysis. A Critical Reappraisal," Rheum Dis Clin North Am, 1994, 20(2):503-12.
Wollheim FA, "Serum Markers of Articular Cartilage Damage and Repair," Rheum Dis Clin North Am, 1999, 25(2):417-32.

♦ **Synovial Fluid Hyaluronate Concentration** see Mucin Clot Test on page 314

- **Synovial Fluid Mucin Clot Test** *see* Mucin Clot Test *on page 314*
- **Synovial Fluid Ropes Test** *see* Mucin Clot Test *on page 314*
- **Synovial Fluid Viscosity** *see* Mucin Clot Test *on page 314*

- **Whipple Disease** *see* Synovial Fluid Analysis *on page 323*
- **Wright Stain, Stool** *see* Methylene Blue Stain, Stool *on page 313*

COAGULATION

Elizabeth M. Van Cott, MD

Michael Laposata, MD, PhD

Hemostasis requires a balance between procoagulant and anticoagulant pathways. Normal hemostasis involves the formation of blood clots to stop bleeding from injured vessels, with natural anticoagulant and fibrinolytic systems that limit clot formation to sites of injury to prevent excessive clot formation. Fibrinolysis (degradation of clots) also helps restore normal blood flow by removing the clot once it is no longer needed. An imbalance between the procoagulant and anticoagulant systems can result in disorders of hemostasis, which may be hereditary or acquired. Defects in clot formation, due to insufficient quantity or function of platelets or coagulation factors, can lead to bleeding disorders. Excessive fibrinolysis can also lead to bleeding disorders (eg, in rare hereditary disorders). Defects in the natural anticoagulant systems or, less commonly defective fibrinolysis, lead to hypercoagulability. New evidence suggests that elevated levels of coagulation factors may also be associated with hypercoagulability. A growing menu of laboratory tests can be used to provide a specific diagnosis in affected patients. Several new therapeutic anticoagulants are also commonly in use, in particular danaparoid, hirudin, and argatroban. The Coagulation Laboratory can offer new tests to monitor these anticoagulants.

♦ **Aα Fragment** *see* Hypercoagulation Panel *on page 345*

♦ **Ac-Globulin (Factor V)** *see* Coagulation Factor Assays *on page 335*

♦ **ACT** *see* Activated Clotting Time *on page 328*

♦ **ACT** *see* Heparin Neutralization *on page 344*

Activated Clotting Time

Related Information
Activated Partial Thromboplastin Time *on page 328*
Heparin Antifactor Xa Assay *on page 342*
Heparin Neutralization *on page 344*
Platelet Count *on page 468*
Point-of-Care Testing *on page 43*

Synonyms ACT; Activated Coagulation Time

Applies to Heparin

Abstract The ACT is a bedside clotting test that is most useful for monitoring high-dose heparin anticoagulation.

Specimen Whole blood

Container One tube containing an activator of coagulation, such as celite (diatomaceous earth), kaolin, or glass particles. For methods that use cartridges rather than tubes, whole blood may be collected into a plastic syringe or tube and then immediately transferred into the cartridge.

Collection Routine venipuncture. Do not collect from a line that contains heparin. Some tubes require approximately 10 vigorous shakes to disperse the activator; other tubes require gentle mixing. Perform test immediately.

Storage Instructions Specimen cannot be stored; test is performed immediately after collection.

Turnaround Time Minutes

Reference Interval Reference range varies considerably depending on the method; it usually falls somewhere within 70-180 seconds. With cardiopulmonary bypass heparinization, the goal is to exceed 400-500 seconds (commonly >480 seconds), depending on the method, representing a mean heparin level of approximately 4-5 units/mL.[1,2] For other indications, the ACT goal is typically lower than it is for cardiopulmonary bypass. The ACT goal can also vary depending on the test method. For example, Hemochron® ACT measurements tend to be higher than HemoTec® ACT measurements, although this is not always the case. A HemoTec® ACT >275-300 seconds or a Hemochron® ACT >350 seconds has been recommended for coronary angioplasty.[2,3]

Use Monitor high-dose heparin anticoagulation, such as during cardiopulmonary bypass surgery. May also be used when an immediate measure of heparin anticoagulation is required at the bedside, such as with extracorporeal membrane oxygenation (ECMO), hemodialysis, cardiac catheterization, and vascular surgery.

Limitations The ACT is less precise than the PTT, and lacks high correlation with the PTT or with heparin antifactor Xa levels. The ACT is influenced by a number of variables, including platelet count, platelet function, lupus anticoagulants, factor deficiencies, ambient temperature, hypothermia, and hemodilution. The various methods are not standardized, and therefore, results from different methods are not interchangeable. Aprotinin prolongs celite-based ACTs but generally not kaolin-based ACTs. Thus, celite-based ACTs may overestimate the amount of heparin anticoagulation when aprotinin is present. However, very high doses of aprotinin, such as following a large initial bolus, may prolong kaolin-based ACTs.

Methodology Whole blood is collected into a tube containing an activator of coagulation, such as celite (diatomaceous earth), kaolin, or glass particles.[4] These activate the intrinsic pathway of coagulation, causing the blood to clot. The tubes are placed into a specialized coagulation analyzer (eg, Hemochron®, International Technidyne; Actalyke®, Helena Laboratories), which measures the time it takes for the blood to clot. Clot formation can be detected by the mobility of a magnet inside the blood test tube. As the instrument rolls the test tube, the magnet rolls along the bottom. When the clot forms, the clot pulls the magnet away from a magnetic detector. With other methods, whole blood is placed into a specialized cartridge that contains an activator of coagulation, such as celite, kaolin or silica, and the clotting time is measured (eg, HemoTec®, Medtronics Inc; i-STAT, i-STAT Corp; GEM PCL, Instrumentation Laboratories). The Medtronics instrument detects clotting by a plunger that moves through the blood sample. When a clot forms, the clot resists the plunger. With the i-STAT instrument, clotting is detected indirectly by the presence of a substrate for thrombin in the cartridge. The substrate resembles the site on fibrinogen that thrombin normally cleaves to form fibrin clot. Thrombin is generated as coagulation is activated, and it cleaves the substrate, releasing an electroactive compound that is detected amperometrically. With GEM PCL cartridges, clot formation is monitored as the instrument draws the blood back and forth across a light detection window. Once the blood clots, the blood no longer flows across the window.

Additional Information With high doses of heparin, the PTT cannot be used to monitor heparin therapy because the PTT is unclottable. The ACT or heparin antifactor Xa levels are used instead of the PTT in such situations. Rarely, ACTs are collected in anticoagulated tubes and the test is performed in a central laboratory.[1]

Footnotes
1. Olson JD, Arkin CF, Brandt JT, et al, "College of American Pathologists Conference XXXI on Laboratory Monitoring of Anticoagulant Therapy. Laboratory Monitoring of Unfractionated Heparin Therapy," *Arch Pathol Lab Med*, 1998, 122(9):782-98.
2. Hirsh J, Warkentin TE, Raschke R, et al, "Heparin and Low-Molecular Weight Heparin. Mechanisms of Action, Pharmacokinetics, Dosing Considerations, Monitoring, Efficacy, and Safety," *Chest*, 1998, 114(5 Suppl):489-510.
3. Ferguson JJ, "Conventional Antithrombotic Approaches," *Am Heart J*, 1995, 130(3 Pt 2):651-7.
4. Hattersley PG, "Activated Coagulation Time of Whole Blood," *J Am Med Assoc*, 1966, 196(5):436-40.

References
Despotis GJ, Joist JH, Hogue CW, et al, "More Effective Suppression of Hemostatic System Activation in Patients Undergoing Cardiac Surgery by Heparin Dosing Based on Heparin Blood Concentrations Rather Than ACT," *Thromb Haemost*, 1996, 76(6):902-8.

♦ **Activated Coagulation Time** *see* Activated Clotting Time *on page 328*

Activated Partial Thromboplastin Time

Related Information
Activated Clotting Time *on page 328*
Activated Protein C Resistance and the Factor V Leiden Mutation *on page 330*
Antiphospholipid Antibody (Lupus Anticoagulant and/or Anticardiolipin Antibody) *on page 331*
Coagulation Factor Assays *on page 335*
Cryoprecipitate *on page 838*
Disseminated Intravascular Coagulation Screen *on page 338*
Factor Inhibitors *on page 340*
Factor IX Concentrate *on page 841*
Factor VIII Concentrate *on page 841*
Fibrinogen *on page 341*
Heparin Antifactor Xa Assay *on page 342*
Heparin Neutralization *on page 344*
High-Molecular Weight Kininogen *on page 344*
Mixing Studies *on page 346*
Plasma, Fresh Frozen *on page 851*
Platelet Count *on page 468*
Point-of-Care Testing *on page 43*
Prekallikrein *on page 350*
Prothrombin Time *on page 354*
Reptilase® Time *on page 355*
Thrombin Time *on page 356*
Warfarin *on page 770*

Synonyms APTT; aPTT; Partial Thromboplastin Time; PTT

Applies to Argatroban; Common Pathway; Extrinsic Pathway; Heparin; Heparin Resistance; Hirudin; Intrinsic Pathway

Abstract The activated partial thromboplastin time (PTT) measures the clotting time from the activation of factor XII, through the formation of fibrin clot (see figure). This measures the integrity of the intrinsic and common pathways of coagulation, whereas the prothrombin time (PT) measures the integrity of the extrinsic and common pathways of coagulation. PTT prolongations are caused by either factor deficiencies (especially of factors VIII, IX, XI, and/or XII), or inhibitors (most commonly, lupus anticoagulants, or therapeutic anticoagulants such as heparin, hirudin, or argatroban).

Specimen Plasma

Container One blue top (citrate) tube; 3.2% citrate tubes are now recommended instead of 3.8% citrate tubes.[1]

Sampling Time See Additional Information for sampling times with the various anticoagulant therapies.

Collection Routine venipuncture. If multiple tests are being drawn, draw blue top tubes after any red top tubes but before any lavender top (EDTA), green top (heparin), or gray top (oxalate/fluoride) tubes. Recent data suggest that an initial discard tube is not necessary.[2] Immediately invert tube gently at least 4 times to mix. Tubes must be appropriately filled. Deliver tubes immediately to the laboratory, otherwise factor VIII may degrade thereby falsely raising the PTT, or falsely low values may occur in heparinized samples as platelets release platelet factor 4 (PF4) which neutralizes heparin.

Specimens drawn from a heparinized line are easily contaminated with heparin, even when the initial volume drawn is discarded. Therefore, coagulation tests are best drawn directly from a peripheral vein, avoiding the arm in which heparin, hirudin, or argatroban is being infused (if relevant).

Storage Instructions Separate plasma from cells as soon as possible, preferably within 1 hour if the PTT is used to monitor heparin, otherwise, PF4 released from platelets neutralizes heparin and can falsely lower the PTT value. To minimize the amount of PF4 in specimens, laboratories should ensure that the plasma contains <10 x 10^9/L platelets. With or without heparin, plasma may be stored on ice for up to 4 hours, otherwise, store frozen.

Causes for Rejection Specimen received more than 4 hours after collection, tubes not filled, clotted specimens, visible hemolysis

Turnaround Time Less than 1 day; often less than 1 hour if requested stat. The PT and PTT are the most readily available coagulation tests.

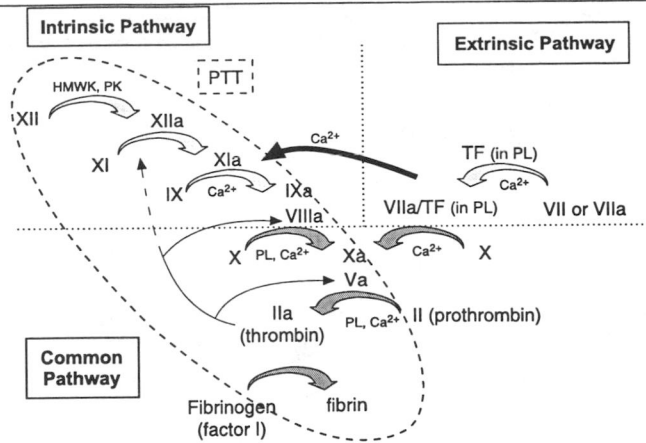

Intrinsic Pathway

Extrinsic Pathway

Common Pathway

The PTT measures the clotting time from factor XII through fibrin formation (intrinsic and common pathways of coagulation). The PT measures the clotting time from factor VII through fibrin formation (extrinsic and common pathways of coagulation). The intrinsic pathway is activated when factor XII binds to a negatively charged "foreign" surface exposed to the blood, with sequential activation of factor XI, then IX, then X, followed by II, and finally fibrinogen is converted to fibrin. Factors V and VIII and phospholipid serve as cofactors. Many steps also require calcium. It is now believed that *in vivo*, coagulation is primarily initiated through the extrinsic pathway, upon exposure of blood to tissue factor (TF) at sites of tissue injury. In this model of coagulation, the ability to activate factor IX (by TF/VIIa) and factor XI (by thrombin) without factor XII indicates that factor XII, prekallikrein, and HMWK of the intrinsic pathway are not needed in normal procoagulant pathways. This is consistent with the observation that deficiencies of the latter three factors are not associated with bleeding symptoms, whereas, deficiencies of the other factors may cause a bleeding tendency.

Key:
TF = tissue factor (a transmembrane protein; thus, it is associated with phospholipid *in vivo*).
PK = prekallikrein.
HMWK = high molecular weight kininogen.
PL = phospholipid.
Ca^{2+} = calcium.

Adapted from Van Cott EM and Laposata M, "Coagulation, Fibrinolysis and Hypercoagulation," *Clinical Diagnosis and Management by Laboratory Methods*, 20th ed, Henry JG, ed, Philadelphia, PA: WB Saunders Co, in press.

Reference Interval Varies significantly among different reagent-instrument combinations. The approximate lower limit of normal is 20-25 seconds; the approximate upper limit of normal is 32-39 seconds. Newborns normally have prolonged PTTs in comparison with adults. The PTT is up to 55 seconds at birth, and the PTT gradually decreases into the adult normal range by the age of 6 months.[3] However, newborns and infants do not normally experience bleeding, because a balance between procoagulants and natural anticoagulants is maintained.

Critical Values >100-150 seconds (varies depending on reagent-instrument combination and laboratory policies)

Use To screen the integrity of the intrinsic pathway of coagulation (factors VIII, IX, XI, and XII) and to a lesser extent the common pathway (fibrinogen and factors II, V, and X). May detect lupus anticoagulants, but the PTT should not be used to screen for lupus anticoagulants because the PTT may or may not be prolonged (depending on the reagents). Also used to monitor therapeutic heparin, hirudin, or argatroban anticoagulation.

Limitations With single factor deficiencies, the deficient factor has to be below 15% to 45% before the PTT becomes prolonged, depending on the reagent and the deficient factor. The PTT is more sensitive to intrinsic pathway factor deficiencies than to common pathway factor deficiencies. With multiple factor deficiencies, the PTT becomes prolonged with less severe decreases in factor levels.[4] Factor VIII elevations shorten the PTT. Factor VIII elevations are common because they occur during acute phase reactions.

Factors VII and XIII do not affect the PTT. The PT can screen for factor VII (and common pathway factor) deficiencies and a specific factor XIII assay can screen for factor XIII deficiencies.

Lupus anticoagulants and deficiencies of certain factors (eg, factor XII) may prolong the baseline PTT and/or accentuate the prolongation of the PTT when heparin is added. Therefore, in these situations, an alternative assay, such as the Heparin Antifactor Xa Assay *on page 342*, should be used rather than the PTT to monitor heparin. If the heparin anti-Xa assay demonstrates that the heparinized PTT is not affected by the lupus anticoagulant, cautious use of the PTT may be considered in that patient.

With very high doses of heparin, as used in cardiac bypass surgery, the PTT is unclottable (>150 seconds) and therefore not useful. The activated coagulation time (ACT) is typically used instead in such situations.

Methodology PTT reagent (phospholipid with an intrinsic pathway activator such as silica, celite, kaolin, ellagic acid) and calcium are added to patient plasma, and the time until clot formation is measured in seconds. Phospholipid in the PTT assay is called "partial thromboplastin" because tissue factor is not present. Tissue factor is present with phospholipid in (complete) thromboplastin reagents that are used for PT assays. Tissue factor activates the extrinsic pathway of coagulation, which is not measured in PTT assays. Phospholipid and calcium are required cofactors in the coagulation cascade. Citrate in the blue top tube prevents clotting by chelating calcium. When the PTT test is ready to be performed, excess calcium is added to overcome citrate.

More recently point-of-care PTT test methods have become available which use a single drop of whole blood, and these methods are undergoing evaluation.[5]

Additional Information To determine the etiology of an unexplained PTT prolongation, the first step is usually to determine if heparin contamination is the cause (see Heparin Neutralization *on page 344*). If this demonstrates that heparin is not present, a mixing study is usually the next step (see Mixing Studies *on page 346*). Mixing studies can predict whether the cause of the PTT prolongation is a factor deficiency or an inhibitor.

Factor deficiencies that prolong PTT: The PTT is more sensitive to deficiencies of the intrinsic pathway (factors VIII, IX, XI, XII, prekallikrein, HMWK) than it is to deficiencies of the common pathway (fibrinogen, and factors II, V, and X). If a mixing study suggests a factor deficiency, assays for factors VIII, IX, XI, and XII can be performed. If the PT is also prolonged, assays for fibrinogen and factors II, V, VII, and X can also be performed. Prekallikrein and HMWK are often not assayed because deficiencies of these two factors are rare and do not cause bleeding, despite causing a prolonged PTT. Factor XII deficiencies also do not cause bleeding, but factor XII deficiencies are relatively common. If the factor assays are all normal, lupus anticoagulant tests can be considered, because occasionally the mixing study will not detect the presence of a lupus anticoagulant.

The effects of hereditary or acquired factor deficiencies on PT and PTT are shown in Tables 1 and 2 in Coagulation Factor Assays *on page 335*.

Inhibitors that prolong PTT: Inhibitors are usually antibodies (lupus anticoagulants or specific factor inhibitors) or anticoagulants such as heparin, hirudin, or argatroban. Lupus anticoagulants bind to phospholipid and interfere with phospholipid's role as an essential cofactor in the coagulation cascade, thereby prolonging various clotting times such as the PTT. Despite the PTT prolongation, lupus anticoagulants are associated with thrombosis rather than bleeding. Specific factor inhibitors are antibodies directed against a specific coagulation factor, such as a factor VIII inhibitor. PTT mixing studies have a characteristic pattern when a factor VIII inhibitor is present. In such cases, factor VIII inhibitor tests should be performed (see Mixing Studies *on page 346* and Factor Inhibitors *on page 340*). When a PTT mixing study suggests an inhibitor other than a factor VIII inhibitor is present, lupus anticoagulant tests may be performed, as lupus anticoagulants are by far the most common inhibitor. If the lupus anticoagulant tests are negative, factor assays may be performed as described above. If one factor is significantly decreased, specific factor inhibitor assays may be performed to determine if there is an inhibitor against that factor (see Factor Inhibitors). Specific factor inhibitors are rare.

Acquired causes of PTT prolongations are much more common than hereditary causes, especially among inpatients (see following list). The liver synthesizes all of the coagulation factors. Therefore, with liver disease, multiple factor deficiencies can develop which prolong the PT earlier and more than the PTT. Coumadin® or vitamin K deficiency impairs the function of factors II, VII, IX, and X, leading to PT and eventually PTT prolongations. In disseminated intravascular coagulation (DIC), multiple factor deficiencies may arise due to activation and consumption of factors, prolonging the PT more often than the PTT.[6] Heparin inhibits activated factors II, X, IX, XI, XII, and kallikrein by enhancing antithrombin activity. Hirudin and argatroban inhibit only activated factor II (thrombin).

Causes of PTT Prolongations
Hereditary:
- Deficiency of factor VIII, IX, XI, XII, prekallikrein, or HMWK *(PT is normal)*
- Deficiency of fibrinogen or factor II, V, or X *(PT is also prolonged)*

Acquired:
- Lupus anticoagulants *(PT usually normal)*
- Heparin *(PT less affected than PTT, PT may be normal)*
- Hirudin or argatroban *(PT usually also prolonged)*
- Liver dysfunction *(PT affected earlier and more than PTT)*
- Vitamin K deficiency *(PT affected earlier and more than PTT)*
- Coumadin® *(PT affected earlier and more than PTT)*
- Disseminated intravascular coagulation (DIC) *(PT affected earlier and more than PTT)*
- Specific factor inhibitors *(PT normal except in the rare cases of an inhibitor against fibrinogen, factor II, V, or X)*

Monitoring heparin: Low-dose, subcutaneous, prophylactic unfractionated heparin (eg, 5000 units two or three times daily) is typically not monitored with coagulation tests. Platelet counts should be followed to ensure that if heparin-induced thrombocytopenia develops, the diagnosis will be made promptly. These low levels of unfractionated heparin usually do not affect the PTT. Full-dose, therapeutic levels of unfractionated heparin should be monitored, and the platelet count also followed. The PTT is the most commonly used assay for unfractionated heparin monitoring because it is inexpensive, automated, and usually available 24 hours a day. The therapeutic range is the PTT range that corresponds to an antifactor Xa level of
(Continued)

Activated Partial Thromboplastin Time (Continued)

0.3-0.7 units/mL. Each laboratory determines its own therapeutic range, but it is often a PTT range that is about 1.5-2.5 times the mean of normal PTT. Therapeutic levels of heparin are most often administered as an initial intravenous bolus followed by a continuous intravenous infusion. The PTT is measured every 6 hours during the first day of unfractionated heparin therapy and 6 hours after any dosage change. If the PTT is therapeutic, it can be checked once daily while patients are on heparin. A less common approach is to administer therapeutic unfractionated heparin doses subcutaneously twice daily, drawing the PTT 6 hours after injection.[7,8] Peak levels are reached 2-4 hours after subcutaneous injection, although this is variable. If patients on unfractionated heparin are started on Coumadin,® heparin is continued until the INR is therapeutic for 2 days. With some PT reagents, heparin can prolong the PT (and therefore the INR) to some extent. Conversely, the PTT can be prolonged somewhat by Coumadin.® Low-molecular weight heparin (LMWH) usually does not significantly prolong the PTT, therefore, the PTT is not used to monitor LMWH. Antifactor Xa assays can be used to monitor LMWH, when indicated.

Heparin resistance is a condition in which the PTT does not prolong as much as expected despite high doses of heparin. This is commonly due to an acute phase reaction, because many acute phase reactant proteins bind and neutralize heparin. Additionally, factor VIII becomes elevated during acute phase reactions, which shorten the PTT. Rarely, heparin resistance is due to antithrombin deficiency. Mild decreases of antithrombin commonly occur as a result of heparin therapy, but mild decreases do not cause significant heparin resistance. Thus, if a patient has heparin resistance, indices of an acute phase reaction may be ordered (eg, fibrinogen, factor VIII), and a heparin assay (antifactor Xa assay) may be helpful.

Monitoring hirudin (lepirudin, Refludan™): Hirudin is a direct thrombin inhibitor that is commonly used as an anticoagulant for the treatment of thrombosis in patients with heparin-induced thrombocytopenia. Hirudin treatment should be monitored with the PTT. The usual therapeutic dose of hirudin in patients with normal kidney function is 0.4 mg/kg intravenous bolus followed by 0.15 mg/kg/hour continuous intravenous infusion. The dose has to be significantly reduced when the creatinine is >1.6 mg/dL. The PTT is performed 4 hours after starting hirudin and 4 hours after any dosage change. If the PTT is in the desired therapeutic range (1.5-2.5 times mean of normal PTT), the PTT can be checked once daily while on hirudin.
Note: See Coagulation Factor Assays on page 335 for the use of chromogenic factor X assays to monitor Coumadin® in patients receiving hirudin or argatroban.

Footnotes

1. National Committee for Clinical Laboratory Standards (NCCLS), "Collection, Transport, and Processing of Blood Specimens for Coagulation Testing and General Performance of Coagulation Assays: Approved Guideline 3rd edition," NCCLS document H21-A3, NCCLS, 940 West Valley Road, Wayne, Pennsylvania 19087, USA, 1998.

2. Gottfried EL and Adachi MM, "Prothrombin Time and Activated Partial Thromboplastin Time Can Be Performed on the First Tube," *Am J Clin Pathol*, 1997, 107(6):681-3.

3. Andrew M, Paes B, and Johnston M, "Development of the Hemostatic System in the Neonate and Young Infant," *Am J Pediatr Hematol Oncol*, 1990, 12(1)95-104.

4. Burns ER, Goldberg SN, and Wenz B, "Paradoxic Effect of Multiple Mild Coagulation Factor Deficiencies on the Prothrombin Time and Activated Partial Thromboplastin Time," *Am J Clin Pathol*, 1993, 100(2):94-8.

5. Solomon HM, Mullins RE, Lyden P, et al, "The Diagnostic Accuracy of Bedside and Laboratory Coagulation: Procedures Used to Monitor the Anticoagulation Status of Patients Treated With Heparin," *Am J Clin Pathol*, 1998, 109(4):371-8.

6. Spero JA, Lewis JH, and Hasiba U, "Disseminated Intravascular Coagulation: Findings in 346 Patients," *Thromb Haemost*, 1980, 43(1):28-33.

7. Prandoni P, Bagatella P, Bernardi E, et al, "Use of an Algorithm for Administering Subcutaneous Heparin in the Treatment of Deep Venous Thrombosis," *Ann Intern Med*, 1998, 129(4):299-302.

8. Kearon C, Harrison L, Crowther M, et al, "Optimal Dosing of Subcutaneous Unfractionated Heparin for the Treatment of Deep Vein Thrombosis," *Thromb Res*, 2000, 97(6):395-403.

References

Bajaj SP and Joist JH, "New Insights Into How Blood Clots: Implications for the Use of APTT and PT as Coagulation Screening Tests and in Monitoring of Anticoagulant Therapy," *Semin Thromb Hemost*, 1999, 25(4):407-18.

Hyers TM, Agnelli G, Hull RD, et al, "Antithrombotic Therapy for Venous Thrombotic Disease," *Chest*, 1998, 114(5 Suppl):561S-78S.

Laposata M, Green D, Van Cott EM et al, "College of American Pathologists Conference XXXI on Laboratory Monitoring of Anticoagulant Therapy: The Clinical Use and Laboratory Monitoring of Low-Molecular Weight Heparin, Danaparoid, Hirudin and Related Compounds, and Argatroban," *Arch Pathol Lab Med*, 1998, 122(9):799-807.

Olson JD, Arkin CF, Brandt JT, et al, "College of American Pathologists Conference XXXI on Laboratory Monitoring of Anticoagulant Therapy: Laboratory Monitoring of Unfractionated Heparin Therapy," *Arch Pathol Lab Med*, 1998, 122(9):782-98.

♦ **Activated Protein C Resistance** see Activated Protein C Resistance and the Factor V Leiden Mutation on page 330

♦ **Activated Protein C Resistance** see Hypercoagulation Panel on page 345

Activated Protein C Resistance and the Factor V Leiden Mutation

Related Information

Activated Partial Thromboplastin Time on page 328
Antithrombin on page 333
Hypercoagulation Panel on page 345
Polymerase Chain Reaction on page 713
Protein C on page 351
Protein S on page 352

Synonyms Activated Protein C Resistance; APC; Protein C Resistance, Activated

Abstract Resistance to activated protein C (APC) is a condition which leads to a hypercoagulable state with an increased risk for venous thrombosis. The effect of exogenous APC on patient's clotting time (usually activated partial thromboplastin time (PTT)) is used to detect presence of resistance to APC (as occurs in individuals with the factor V Leiden mutation). A few laboratories might use clotting times other than the PTT. DNA-based assays can be used to directly detect the presence of the factor V Leiden mutation.

Specimen Plasma (for clotting time-based screening assay) and whole blood (for DNA-based confirmatory assay)

Container Blue top (sodium citrate) tube for screening assay. Container varies with laboratory for DNA-based assay (blue top, yellow top, or lavender top).

Collection Routine venipuncture. If multiple tests are being drawn, draw blue top tubes after any red top tubes but before any lavender top (EDTA), green top (heparin), or gray top (oxalate/fluoride) tubes. Immediately invert tube gently at least 4 times to mix. Tubes must be appropriately filled. Deliver tubes immediately to the laboratory.

Storage Instructions Clotting-time based assay: Store plasma at 4°C or room temperature if testing is performed within 4 hours; otherwise, store frozen until testing. According to one manufacturer, storage up to 24 hours without freezing is acceptable (Coatest APC Resistance V by Chromogenix). **DNA-based assay:** Store whole blood at 4°C or at room temperature.

Causes for Rejection Tube not full, specimen clotted, specimen received more than 4-24 hours after collection

Turnaround Time Clotting-time based assay: usually less than 1 day. DNA-based assay: several days (depending on how often test batches are performed).

Special Instructions Do not centrifuge or freeze whole blood specimen for DNA-based assay.

Reference Interval APC prolongs the PTT usually more than twofold in controls (normal persons) and less than twofold in affected individuals.

Some laboratories report the result as a normalized ratio, which is the result of the activated protein C resistance assay for the patient, divided by the result for normal pooled plasma.

Use The clotting-time assay identifies individuals who have resistance to APC. The DNA test identifies factor V Leiden as the cause of the APC resistance. Activated protein C resistance is the most prevalent hereditary predisposition to venous thrombosis. It is present in 5% of the general Caucasian population and is less common or rare in other ethnic groups.[1,2,3] It accounts for 20% of unselected patients with a first deep vein thrombosis and 50% of familial cases of thrombosis.[4,5,6] The vast majority of cases are due to the factor V Leiden mutation, which renders factor V resistant to degradation by activated protein C, resulting in an increased risk for venous thrombosis.[7,8]

Limitations Lupus anticoagulants, hirudin, or argatroban may cause inaccurate results in the commonly used PTT clotting-time based assay but do not affect DNA-based tests. Various alternative assays are not affected by lupus anticoagulants.[9,10,11,12]

Methodology Clotting time (usually PTT)-based. Test provides a measure of the APC-dependent prolongation of the clotting time (PTT), in essence, of the ability of APC to act as an anticoagulant. The specimen is first diluted 1:5 in factor V deficient plasma. An activated partial thromboplastin time (PTT) is performed on the diluted specimen, in the presence and absence of exogenously supplied activated protein C.[4,13] Exogenous activated protein C degrades the patient's factors Va and VIIIa, thereby prolonging the PTT. The ratio of the PTT with activated protein C divided by the baseline PTT is calculated. Normal individuals usually have a ratio >2.0, whereas individuals with factor V Leiden usually have a ratio <2.0 because their mutated factor Va resists activated protein C degradation (each laboratory determines its own reference range). If the result is abnormal, a DNA-based assay (eg, polymerase chain reaction (PCR)-based assay) should be performed to determine if the patient has the factor V Leiden mutation, which confers activated protein C resistance. DNA-based methods allow precise determination of heterozygosity and homozygosity for the mutation.

The sensitivity and specificity of the PTT-based assay for detection of factor V Leiden mutation approach 100%.[14] Some laboratories do not include the dilution into factor V deficient plasma described above, in which case the sensitivity is reduced to 50% to 86% and the specificity is reduced to 75% to 98% for detecting the factor V Leiden mutation.[15,16,17] In addition, patients with an abnormal baseline PTT (usually including patients receiving Coumadin® or heparin) cannot be tested without the dilution step. Whether or not the test without the dilution step provides information regarding hypercoagulability is currently under investigation.[18]

Additional Information The anticoagulant action of activated protein C normally involves degradation of activated factors V and VIII by proteolytic cleavage at specific arginine residues, thereby inhibiting coagulation. Individuals with factor V Leiden have a mutation at one of the arginine cleavage sites in factor V, such that factor V resists degradation by activated protein C. The factor V Leiden mutation is a point mutation in which the guanine at nucleotide position 1691 is replaced by an adenine, resulting in substitution of arginine with glutamine at amino acid residue 506. One, and possibly two, additional factor V mutations at another arginine cleavage site are a very rare cause of activated protein C resistance,[19,20] and other factor V mutations are also under investigation.[21] Mutations in the factor VIII gene causing resistance to activated protein C are theoretically possible but have not yet been described. Using the normalized ratio reduces intra- and interlaboratory variability in the assay. However, it has not improved the ability of the assay to distinguish activated protein C resistance from normal.[8,22,23]

See Hypercoagulation Panel *on page 345*.

Footnotes

1. Hooper WC, Dilley A, Ribeiro MJA, et al, "A Racial Difference in the Prevalence of the Arg506 → Gln Mutation," *Thromb Res*, 1996, 81(5):577-81.

2. Rees DC, Cox M, and Clegg JB, "World Distribution of Factor V Leiden," *Lancet*, 1995, 346(8983):1133-4.

3. Ridker PM, Miletich JP, Hennekens CH, et al, "Ethnic Distribution of Factor V Leiden in 4047 Men and Women," *J Am Med Assoc*, 1997, 277(16):1305-7.

4. Svensson PJ and Dahlbäck B, "Resistance to Activated Protein C as a Basis for Venous Thrombosis," *N Engl J Med*, 1994, 330(8):517-22.

5. Griffin JH, Evatt B, Wideman C, et al, "Anticoagulant Protein C Pathway Defective in Majority of Thrombophilic Patients," *Blood*, 1993, 82(7):1989-93.

6. Koster T, Rosendaal FR, de Ronde H, et al, "Venous Thrombosis Due to Poor Anticoagulant Response to Activated Protein C: Leiden Thrombophilia Study," *Lancet*, 1993, 342(8886-7):1503-6.

7. Bertina RM, Koeleman BPC, Koster T, et al, "Mutation in Blood Coagulation Factor V Associated With Resistance to Activated Protein C," *Nature*, 1994, 369(6475):64-7.

8. Voelkerding KV, Wu L, Williams EC, et al, "Factor V R506Q Gene Mutation Analysis by PCR-RFLP: Optimization, Comparison With Functional Testing for Resistance to Activated Protein C, and Establishment of Cell Line Controls," *Am J Clin Pathol*, 1996, 106(1):100-6.

9. Akhtar MS, Blair AJ, King TC, et al, "Whole Blood Screening Test for Factor V Leiden Using a Russell Viper Venom Time-Based Assay," *Am J Clin Pathol*, 1998, 109(4):387-91.

10. Le DT, Griffin JH, Greengard JS, et al, "Use of a Generally Applicable Tissue-Factor-Dependent Factor V Assay to Detect Activated Protein C-Resistant Factor Va in Patients Receiving Warfarin and in Patients With a Lupus Anticoagulant," *Blood*, 1995, 85(7):1704-11.

11. Martorell JR, Munoz-Castillo A, and Gil JL, "False-Positive Activated Protein C Resistance Test Due to Antiphospholipid Antibodies Is Corrected by Platelet Extract," *Thromb Haemost*, 1995, 74(2):796-7.

12. van Oerle R, van Pampus L, Tans G, et al, "The Clinical Application of a New Specific Functional Assay to Detect the Factor V (Leiden) Mutation Associated With Activated Protein C Resistance," *Am J Clin Pathol*, 1997, 107(5):521-6.

13. Dahlbäck B, Carlsson M, and Svensson PJ, "Familial Thrombophilia Due to a Previously Unrecognized Mechanism Characterized by Poor Anticoagulant Response to Activated Protein C: Prediction of a Cofactor to Activated Protein C," *Proc Natl Acad Sci U S A*, 1993, 90(3):1004-8.

14. Jorquera JI, Montoro JM, Fernandez MA, et al, "Modified Test for Activated Protein C Resistance," *Lancet*, 1994, 344:1162-3.

15. Strobl FJ, Hoffman S, Huber S, et al, "Activated Protein C Resistance Assay Performance: Improvement by Sample Dilution With Factor V-Deficient Plasma," *Arch Pathol Lab Med*, 1998, 122(5):430-3.

16. Sweeney JD, Blair AJ, and King TC, "Comparison of an Activated Partial Thromboplastin Time With a Russell Viper Venom Time Test in Screening for Factor V (Leiden) (FVR506Q)," *Am J Clin Pathol*, 1997, 108(1):74-7.

17. Zehnder JL and Benson RC, "Sensitivity and Specificity of the APC Resistance Assay in Detection of Individuals With Factor V Leiden," *Am J Clin Pathol*, 1996, 106(1):107-11.

18. de Visser MC, Rosendaal FR, and Bertina RM, "A Reduced Sensitivity for Activated Protein C in the Absence of Factor V Leiden Increases the Risk of Venous Thrombosis," *Blood*, 1999, 93(4):1271-6.

19. Chan WP, Lee CK, Kwong YL, et al, "A Novel Mutation of Arg 306 of Factor V Gene in Hong Kong Chinese," *Blood*, 1998, 91(4):1135-9.

20. Williamson D, Brown K, Luddington R, et al, "Factor V Cambridge: A New Mutation (Arg306 → Thr) Associated With Resistance to Activated Protein C," *Blood*, 1998, 91(4):1140-4.

21. Faioni EM, "Factor V HR2: An Ancient Haplotype Out of Africa - Reasons for Being Interested," *Thromb Haemost*, 2000, 83(3):358-9.

22. Brandt G, Gruppo R, Gluek CJ, et al, "Sensitivity, Specificity, and Predictive Value of Modified Assays for Activated Protein C Resistance in Children," *Thromb Haemost*, 1998, 79(3):567-70.

23. Tripodi A, Chantarangkul V, Negri B, et al, "Standardization of the APC Resistance Test: Effects of Normalization of Results by Means of Pooled Normal Plasma," *Thromb Haemost*, 1998, 79(3):564-6.

References

Dahlbäck B, "Molecular Genetics of Thrombophilia: Factor V Gene Mutation Causing Resistance to Activated Protein C as a Basis of the Hypercoagulable State," *J Lab Clin Med*, 1995, 125(5):566-71.

De Stefano V, Finazzi G, and Mannucci PM, "Inherited Thrombophilia: Pathogenesis, Clinical Syndromes, and Management," *Blood*, 1996, 87(9):3531-44.

- ♦ **Acute Phase Reactants** *see* Fibrinogen *on page 341*
- ♦ **Acute Phase Reactants** *see* Plasminogen *on page 347*
- ♦ **Acute Phase Reactants** *see* Plasminogen Activator Inhibitor 1 *on page 347*
- ♦ **Acute Phase Reactants** *see* von Willebrand Factor *on page 357*
- ♦ **Afibrinogenemia** *see* Fibrinogen *on page 341*
- ♦ **Aggregometer Test** *see* Platelet Aggregation *on page 348*
- ♦ **Alpha$_2$-Antiplasmin** *see* Antiplasmin *on page 332*
- ♦ **Antifactor Xa Assay** *see* Heparin Antifactor Xa Assay *on page 342*
- ♦ **Antihemophilic Factor (Factor VIII)** *see* Coagulation Factor Assays *on page 335*
- ♦ **Antiphosphatidylserine Antibodies** *see* Antiphospholipid Antibody (Lupus Anticoagulant and/or Anticardiolipin Antibody) *on page 331*

Antiphospholipid Antibody (Lupus Anticoagulant and/or Anticardiolipin Antibody)

Related Information

Activated Partial Thromboplastin Time *on page 328*
Anticardiolipin Antibody *on page 503*
Antinuclear Antibody *on page 507*
Chlorpromazine, Serum *on page 743*
Factor Inhibitors *on page 340*
HIV-1/HIV-2 Antibody Screen and Western Blot *on page 636*
Hypercoagulation Panel *on page 345*
Platelet Count *on page 468*
RPR *on page 677*
VDRL, Serum *on page 688*

Synonyms Lupus Inhibitor

Applies to Antiphosphatidylserine Antibodies; Beta-2-Glycoprotein I; Circulating Anticoagulant; Lupus Anticoagulant; PTT

Abstract Antiphospholipid antibodies are associated with an increased risk of thrombosis, thrombocytopenia, and recurrent fetal loss.

Specimen Lupus anticoagulant: plasma; anticardiolipin antibody: serum

Container Lupus anticoagulant: blue top (sodium citrate) tube; anticardiolipin antibody: red top tube

Collection Routine venipuncture. If multiple tests are being drawn, draw blue top tubes after any red top tubes but before any lavender top (EDTA), green top (heparin), or gray top (oxalate/fluoride) tubes. Immediately invert gently at least 4 times, mixing thoroughly. Blue top tubes must be appropriately filled. Deliver immediately to the laboratory.

Storage Instructions Separate plasma (or serum) from cells as soon as possible. Plasma (or serum) may be stored on ice for up to 4 hours; otherwise, store frozen. Platelet count must be <10 x 10^9/L in plasma prior to freezing, or false-negative lupus anticoagulant results may occur.

Causes for Rejection Blue top specimen received more than 4 hours after collection; clotted specimen; blue top not filled; patient on hirudin, danaparoid, or argatroban anticoagulation

Turnaround Time Lupus anticoagulant: less than 1 day if negative, longer if positive because confirmatory assays need to be performed; anticardiolipin: often several days because testing is batched.

Special Instructions Notify laboratory if patient is on heparin, including subcutaneous low-dose heparin or low-molecular weight heparin. In some assays, heparin may cause false-positive lupus anticoagulant results. Therefore, heparin must first be removed from the specimen by the laboratory. Other assays contain a heparin neutralizer that tolerates specimens containing up to 1 unit/mL heparin. Results can be interpreted correctly in patients on Coumadin®. Hirudin, danaparoid, or argatroban anticoagulation may cause false-positive results in some assays.

Reference Interval Negative for lupus anticoagulant; <15 units of anticardiolipin antibody

Use If an antiphospholipid antibody is suspected, assays for both lupus anticoagulant and anticardiolipin antibody should be performed. Used to evaluate hypercoagulable states, recurrent miscarriage, thrombocytopenia, or prolonged PTT. Lupus anticoagulants may or may not prolong the PTT.

Limitations Factor VIII inhibitors can cause false positive lupus anticoagulant[1] tests (a factor VIII assay showing normal factor VIII levels rules out this possibility). The transient presence of antiphospholipid antibodies may accompany infections or drugs; *vide infra*.

Methodology

Anticardiolipin antibody: Enzyme-linked immunosorbent assay (ELISA) using cardiolipin, a phospholipid, as the antigen. Newer ELISA assays are available that test for anti-β_2-glycoprotein I antibodies or antiphosphatidylserine antibodies.

Lupus anticoagulant: To improve sensitivity, two screening tests are suggested.[2] These tests are clotting-time based assays, such as the Russell viper venom time, PTT-based assays, kaolin clotting time, or dilute prothrombin time (tissue thromboplastin inhibition test). Lupus anticoagulants prolong various clotting times in the laboratory because they bind to phospholipid and thereby interfere with the ability of phospholipid to serve

(Continued)

Antiphospholipid Antibody (Lupus Anticoagulant and/or Anticardiolipin Antibody) *(Continued)*

its essential cofactor function in the coagulation cascade. Lupus anticoagulant screening assays usually have a low concentration of phospholipid to enhance sensitivity. Any abnormal (prolonged) screening result is repeated after a 1:1 mixture of patient plasma with normal plasma to demonstrate that the clotting time remains prolonged upon mixing. Confirmatory assays are performed if the screening assay remains abnormal after the 1:1 mixture. Confirmatory assays typically demonstrate that upon addition of excess phospholipid, the clotting time shortens toward normal. The "platelet neutralization procedure" is a confirmatory assay in which the source of the excess phospholipid is freeze-thawed platelets. **Note:** The routine PTT may or may not be prolonged, depending on the amount of phospholipid in the reagent. In addition, elevated factor VIII can normalize an otherwise prolonged PTT. PTT-based lupus anticoagulant screening assays have a low concentration of phospholipid to enhance sensitivity. When the PTT is prolonged, a PTT mixing study may be a useful first test. **When lupus anticoagulants are present, the PTT remains prolonged upon mixing with an equal volume of normal plasma.**

Additional Information The two principal types of antiphospholipid antibodies are lupus anticoagulants and anticardiolipin antibodies. They are present in 0% to 5% of the general population and in 12% or more of patients with thrombosis.[3,4] Antiphospholipid antibodies are acquired autoantibodies directed against phospholipid-protein complexes. These antibodies are associated with an increased risk for arterial or venous thrombosis,[3,5] thrombocytopenia,[6] and fetal loss.[7] Associations with cardiac valve disease, livedo reticularis, and other features are also recognized.[8] The mechanism of thrombosis is not entirely clear, although a number of mechanisms have been proposed. In a recent prospective study involving individuals with antiphospholipid antibodies, the **incidence of thrombosis** per year was 1% in individuals with no history of thrombosis, 4% in patients with systemic lupus erythematosus, 5.5% in patients with a history of thrombosis, and 6% in individuals with high titer IgG anticardiolipin antibody (>40 units).[9]

The diagnosis of **antiphospholipid antibody syndrome** requires a positive test in the antiphospholipid antibody panel (lupus anticoagulant and/or anticardiolipin antibody) on two separate occasions, at least 6 weeks apart, in the setting of thrombosis, thrombocytopenia, or recurrent miscarriage.[10]

Anticardiolipin antibodies recognize cardiolipin bound to β_2-glycoprotein I. Most lupus anticoagulants recognize phospholipid bound to prothrombin, but others recognize phospholipid bound to β_2-glycoprotein I or other proteins. Rarely, prothrombin levels become decreased as a result of a lupus anticoagulant, and an increased risk for bleeding may develop.[11] As cardiolipin is the antigen used for syphilis screening tests (VDRL, Venereal Disease Research Laboratories; and RPR, rapid plasma reagin), false-positive syphilis tests may occur in patients with anticardiolipin antibodies. Conversely, true syphilis infections can cause positive anticardiolipin antibody test results.

Despite the prolonged clotting times, bleeding is not a typical feature associated with these antibodies. Thrombocytopenia, if present, is usually mild. Patients may have either a lupus anticoagulant or an anticardiolipin antibody or they may have both antibodies. A high percentage of patients with systemic lupus erythematosus (SLE) or related autoimmune diseases have these antibodies. These antibodies may also develop in patients without an underlying disorder. The antibodies can appear transiently in association with certain medications (eg, hydralazine, phenytoin) or infections. The human immunodeficiency virus (HIV) is commonly associated with positive tests for antiphospholipid antibodies.[12] Infection-associated antibodies may not be associated with clinical symptoms of antiphospholipid antibody syndrome, and they tend to recognize phospholipid rather than the phospholipid-protein complexes described above.[13]

Heparin treatment in patients with lupus anticoagulants can be complicated by the fact that lupus anticoagulants may prolong the baseline PTT and/or accentuate the PTT prolongation when heparin is added. As such, heparin may be monitored with antifactor Xa assays. If the antifactor Xa assay demonstrates that the heparinized PTT is not affected by the lupus anticoagulant, cautious use of the PTT may be considered for that patient.

Footnotes

1. Goudemand J, Caron C, De Prost D, et al, "Evaluation of Sensitivity and Specificity of a Standardized Procedure Using Different Reagents for the Detection of Lupus Anticoagulants," *Thromb Haemost*, 1997, 77(2):336-42.

2. Brandt JT, Triplett DA, Alving B, et al, "Criteria for the Diagnosis of Lupus Anticoagulants: An Update," *Thromb Haemost*, 1995, 74(4):1185-90.

3. Ginsburg KS, Liang MH, Newcomer L, et al, "Anticardiolipin Antibodies and the Risk for Ischemic Stroke and Venous Thrombosis," *Ann Intern Med*, 1992, 117(12):997-1002.

4. Doig RG, O'Malley CJ, Dauer R, et al, "An Evaluation of 200 Consecutive Patients With Spontaneous or Recurrent Thrombosis for Primary Hypercoagulable States," *Am J Clin Pathol*, 1994, 102(6):797-801.

5. Vaarala O, Manttari M, Manninen V, et al, "Anticardiolipin Antibodies and Risk of Myocardial Infarction in a Prospective Cohort of Middle-aged Men," *Circulation*, 1995, 91(1):23-7.

6. Galli M, Finazzi G and Barbui T, "Thrombocytopenia in the Antiphospholipid Syndrome," *Br J Haematol*, 1996, 93(1):1-5.

7. Yasuda M, Takakuwa K, Tokunaga A, et al, "Prospective Studies of the Association Between Anticardiolipin Antibody and Outcome of Pregnancy," *Obstet Gynecol*, 1995, 86(4 Pt 1):555-9.

8. Hogan WJ, McBane RD, Santrach PJ, et al, "Antiphospholipid Syndrome and Perioperative Hemostatic Management of Cardiac Valvular Surgery," *Mayo Clin Proc*, 2000, 75(9):971-6.

9. Finazzi G, Brancaccio V, Moia M, et al, "Natural History and Risk Factors for Thrombosis in 360 Patients With Antiphospholipid Antibodies: A Four-Year Prospective Study From the Italian Registry," *Am J Med*, 1996, 100(5):530-6.

10. Wilson WA, Gharavi AE, Koike T, et al, "International Consensus Statement on Preliminary Classification Criteria for Definite Antiphospholipid Syndrome," *Arthritis Rheum*, 1999, 42(7):1309-11.

11. Bajaj SP, Rapaport SI, Fierer DS, et al, "A Mechanism for the Hypoprothrombinemia of the Acquired Hypoprothrombinemia-Lupus Anticoagulant Syndrome," *Blood*, 1983, 61(4):684-92.

12. de Larranaga GF, Forastiero RR, Carreras LO, et al, "Different Types of Antiphospholipid Antibodies in AIDS: A Comparison With Syphilis and the Antiphospholipid Syndrome," *Thromb Res*, 1999, 96(1):19-25.

13. McNally T, Purdy G, Mackie IJ, et al, "The Use of an Antibeta-2-Glycoprotein-I Assay for Discrimination Between Anticardiolipin Antibodies Associated With Infection and Increased Risk of Thrombosis," *Br J Haematol*, 1995, 91(2):471-3.

References

Galli M and Barbui T, "Antiprothrombin Antibodies: Detection and Clinical Significance in the Antiphospholipid Syndrome," *Blood*, 1999, 93(7):2149-57.

Galli M, Finazzi G and Barbui T, "Antiphospholipid Antibodies: Predictive Value of Laboratory Tests," *Thromb Haemost*, 1997, 78(1):75-8.

Roubey RAS, "Antiphospholipid Antibody Syndrome," *Arthritis and Allied Condition*, Koopman WJ, ed, Baltimore, MD: Lippincott Wilkins & Wilkins, 1997, 1393-406.

Triplett DA, "Protean Clinical Presentation of Antiphospholipid-Protein Antibodies (APA)," *Thromb Haemost*, 1995, 74(1):329-37.

Antiplasmin

Related Information

Hypercoagulation Panel *on page 345*
Plasminogen *on page 347*
Plasminogen Activator Inhibitor 1 *on page 347*

Synonyms Alpha$_2$-Antiplasmin; α_2-Antiplasmin; Plasmin Inhibitor

Abstract Antiplasmin is a major inhibitor of plasmin. Hereditary antiplasmin deficiency is a rare familial bleeding disorder due to excessive fibrinolysis.

Specimen Plasma

Container Blue top (sodium citrate) tube

Collection Routine venipuncture. If multiple tests are being drawn, draw blue top tubes after any red top tubes but before any lavender top (EDTA), green top (heparin), or gray top (oxalate/fluoride) tubes. Immediately invert tube gently at least 4 times to mix. Tubes must be appropriately filled. Deliver tubes immediately to the laboratory.

Storage Instructions Separate plasma from cells as soon as possible; plasma may be stored on ice for up to 4 hours; otherwise store frozen.

Causes for Rejection Specimen received more than 4 hours after collection, tube not filled, clotted specimen

Turnaround Time Several days, because test is often sent out

Special Instructions Specimens for functional assays should not contain fibrinolysis inhibitors (eg, epsilon-aminocaproic acid, aprotinin) or heparin. Elevated α_2-macroglobulin levels >200% may slightly interfere with functional assays.

Reference Interval Approximately 80% to 130% functional; approximately 48-80 mg/dL antigen. Antiplasmin levels (measured by antigen assay) are slightly lower during the first 5 days of life.[1]

Use Not a commonly performed clinical assay. May be considered in patients with strong evidence for a familial bleeding disorder and normal test results for more common bleeding disorders, such as von Willebrand disease.

Methodology

Functional (activity) assays: Excess plasmin is added to patient plasma. Antiplasmin in the patient plasma binds to and inhibits plasmin, forming a plasmin-antiplasmin complex. Residual plasmin then cleaves a chromogenic substrate, releasing a colored compound that can be detected spectrophotometrically. The amount of plasmin detected is inversely proportional to the concentration of antiplasmin in the patient specimen.

Antigen (immunologic) assay by radial immunodiffusion: Plasma is placed in a cylindrical well of an agarose gel. The agarose gel contains an antibody monospecific for antiplasmin. Antiplasmin in the specimen diffuses from the well into the gel where it forms a complex with the antibody, creating a precipitin ring. The size of the ring is proportional to the amount of antiplasmin in the plasma.

Additional Information Plasmin mediates fibrinolysis, and antiplasmin inhibits plasmin. Activated factor XIII cross-links antiplasmin to fibrin, and antiplasmin protects fibrin from plasmin-mediated fibrinolysis. Antiplasmin also binds to plasminogen and may inhibit plasminogen binding to fibrin. Antiplasmin is synthesized in the liver. Acquired causes of decreased antiplasmin include liver disease, thrombolytic therapy, and disseminated intravascular coagulation (DIC). Hereditary deficiencies of antiplasmin are either type I or type II. Type I deficiencies are quantitative, in which both functional and antigen levels are reduced. Type II deficiencies are qualitative, with decreased functional levels but normal or near normal antigen levels.

Footnotes

1. Andrew M, Paes B, Milner R, et al, "Development of the Human Coagulation System in the Full-Term Infant," *Blood*, 1987, 70(1):165-72.

References

Lijnen HR, Okada K, Matsuo O, et al, "α2-Antiplasmin Gene Deficiency in Mice Is Associated With Enhanced Fibrinolytic Potential Without Overt Bleeding," *Blood*, 1999, 93(7):2274-81.

Yoshinaga H, Hirosawa S, Chung DH, et al, "A Novel Point Mutation of the Splicing Donor Site in the Intron 2 of the Plasmin Inhibitor Gene," *Thromb Haemost*, 2000, 84(2):307-11.

♦ **α₂-Antiplasmin** see Antiplasmin on page 332

Antithrombin

Related Information

Activated Protein C Resistance and the Factor V Leiden Mutation on page 330
Heparin Antifactor Xa Assay on page 342
Hypercoagulation Panel on page 345
Protein C on page 351
Protein S on page 352

Applies to Heparin; Heparin Cofactor II; Heparin Resistance

Replaces Antithrombin III Assay

Abstract A deficiency of antithrombin, a natural anticoagulant protein, leads to a hypercoagulable state with an increased risk for venous thrombosis. Acquired antithrombin deficiencies are more common than hereditary deficiencies.

Specimen Plasma

Container One blue top (sodium citrate) tube

Collection Routine venipuncture. If multiple tests are being drawn, draw blue top tubes after any red top tubes but before any lavender top (EDTA), green top (heparin), or gray top (oxalate/fluoride) tubes. Immediately invert tube gently at least 4 times to mix. Tubes must be appropriately filled. Deliver tubes immediately to the laboratory.

Storage Instructions Separate plasma from cells as soon as possible. Plasma may be stored on ice for up to 4 hours, otherwise, store frozen.

Causes for Rejection Specimen received more than 4 hours after collection, tubes not filled, clotted specimens

Turnaround Time 2-4 hours; longer if testing is batched

Reference Interval Results are often reported as a percent of the amount expected in normal plasma. By definition, the mean value in normal plasma is 100%. The reference range is approximately 80% to 130%.

Results may also be reported in mg/dL; reference range is approximately 17-39 mg/dL (SI: 170-390 mg/L).

At birth, antithrombin levels average 63% (range 39% to 87%) of adult levels. Antithrombin increases to adult values within 6 months.[1] Spontaneous thromboses do not develop in normal infants because a balance between procoagulants and inhibitors is maintained.

Use A functional assay should be performed first, because both type I and type II hereditary antithrombin deficiencies will be detected. If the result of the functional assay is decreased, the antigenic assay is needed to differentiate between type I and type II deficiencies. If the antigen assay is performed without the functional assay, type II deficiencies will not be detected (see Additional Information).

Antithrombin Levels

Increased With	Decreased With
Coumadin® (possibly)	Heparin
	Liver disease
	Thrombosis (eg, pulmonary embolism, acute myocardial infarction, thrombophlebitis)
	Disseminated intravascular coagulation (DIC)
	Surgery
	Nephrotic syndrome
	Oral contraceptives, pregnancy (possibly)

Limitations

Chromogenic (functional) assays: Heparin cofactor II, another natural thrombin inhibitor, produces falsely elevated levels of antithrombin in some thrombin-based assays.[2] One commercially available kit uses heparin that has been treated with a bacterial enzyme (chondroitinase) such that the heparin no longer enhances heparin cofactor II activity, and heparin cofactor II interference is thus essentially eliminated.[3] In factor Xa-based assays, high levels of heparin cofactor II will not lead to an overestimate of antithrombin, because heparin cofactor II does not inhibit factor Xa.

Hirudin or argatroban anticoagulation can interfere with thrombin-based assays.

Antigenic assays: If used without the functional assay, type II antithrombin deficiencies will not be detected. An antigenic test is usually performed only if the functional test result is decreased, to determine if the patient has type I or type II deficiency (see Additional Information).

Methodology Functional (activity) and antigenic (immunologic) tests are available. Functional assays are usually chromogenic. To perform the chromogenic test, heparin and thrombin are added to the patient's plasma. Antithrombin in the patient's plasma will bind and inhibit thrombin. A chromogenic substrate that resembles thrombin's natural substrate is then added. Any unbound thrombin will cleave the substrate, liberating a chromogenic substance that can be measured spectrophotometrically. The amount detected is inversely proportional to the amount of antithrombin in the patient.[4] Factor Xa-based methods are also available; these are similar in principle to the thrombin-based assays described above, except that factor Xa is used instead of thrombin.[2] Antigenic (immunologic) assay: A commonly used automated method involves latex particles coated with antibodies directed against antithrombin. In the presence of antithrombin, the latex particles form aggregates that absorb light passing through the specimen. The amount of light absorbance is directly related to the amount of antithrombin in the specimen.[5]

Additional Information Antithrombin is a natural inhibitor of thrombin as well as factors Xa, IXa, XIa, XIIa, and kallikrein. The activity of antithrombin is greatly accelerated by interaction with the glycosaminoglycans, heparan sulfate or heparin. Heparan sulfate is naturally located in vivo on the endothelial cell surface. Antithrombin deficiency is present in 0.17% of the general population.[6] It accounts for 1.1% of unselected patients with venous thrombosis and up to 5% of patients younger than age 70 years with thrombosis.[7,8] Over 127 mutations in the antithrombin gene are known to cause hereditary antithrombin deficiency.[9] Individuals heterozygous for antithrombin deficiency have a fivefold increased risk for venous thrombosis.[10] Homozygous deficiencies are incompatible with life, except for patients with type II deficiency due to heparin-binding mutations. Heterozygotes generally have antithrombin levels between 45% to 75%,[11] although levels as high as 78% have been observed. The risk for thrombosis is further increased in the presence of a second risk factor.[12] The age at onset of thrombosis is usually between 10-50 years (peak 15-35 years) in heterozygous individuals. The risk of arterial thrombosis remains uncertain, but 2% of individuals developed arterial thrombosis in one study.[13]

Decreased antithrombin also arises from acquired conditions, such as:

- decreased hepatic synthesis from liver disease or L-asparaginase treatment
- consumption from thrombosis, DIC (disseminated intravascular coagulation) or surgery
- increased clearance from full-dose heparin use[14]
- proteinuria

Mild decreases occasionally result from elevated estrogen levels (eg, pregnancy or oral contraceptive use). Colitis has been associated with low antithrombin levels. If a patient with low antithrombin has any of the conditions listed above, the test should be repeated once the condition is no longer present, if possible. Confirmation of a hereditary antithrombin deficiency may require documenting antithrombin deficiency in a relative. In contrast to protein C and protein S, which are decreased by Coumadin®, antithrombin levels may increase while on Coumadin®. Antithrombin levels in premenopausal women may be somewhat lower than in men, but postmenopausal women have higher levels than men.[15]

Antithrombin deficiencies are quantitative (type I) or qualitative (type II).[11] In type I deficiencies, normal antithrombin molecules are made, but in reduced quantity. In type II deficiencies, normal amounts of antithrombin are made, but the antithrombin is defective. Accordingly, type I deficiencies have decreased antithrombin in both functional and antigenic assays. Type II deficiencies have normal (or near normal) antigenic antithrombin levels, with decreased functional antithrombin. Thus, if only antigenic assays are performed, type II deficiencies will not be detected. Therefore, a functional assay should be used as the initial screening assay. If the result is decreased, an antigenic assay should be performed to determine if the deficiency is type I or type II. According to one study, 0.02% of the general population have type I antithrombin deficiency and 0.15% have type II.[6] The heparin-binding variant, which is one of the mutations that causes type II deficiency, has a low risk of thrombosis in comparison to the other mutations, and it is present in at least 0.01% of the general population.[6] For patients with test results suggesting type II deficiency, a method has been described that tests for the heparin-binding mutation.[16]

Patients with marked decreases in antithrombin may demonstrate heparin resistance, in which very high doses of heparin are required to obtain a therapeutic PTT prolongation. Antithrombin concentrates are available for the treatment of hereditary antithrombin deficiency. The use of antithrombin concentrates for certain acquired antithrombin deficiencies, such as DIC, is under investigation.[17]

See Hypercoagulation Panel on page 345.

Footnotes

1. Andrew M, Paes B, Milner R, et al, "Development of the Human Coagulation System in the Full-Term Infant," *Blood*, 1987, 70(1):165-72.
2. Demers C, Henderson P, Blajchman MA, et al, "An Antithrombin III Assay Based on Factor Xa Inhibition Provides a More Reliable Test to Identify Congenital Antithrombin III Deficiency Than an Assay Based on Thrombin Inhibition," *Thromb Haemost*, 1993, 69:231-5.
3. Triscott MX and Eggerding VC, "Improved Differentiation Between Normal and Abnormal Antithrombin Levels Using a Thrombin Based Chromogenic Assay," *Thromb Haemost*, 1999, (Suppl):379.

(Continued)

Antithrombin (Continued)

4. Odegard O, Lie M, and Ablidgaard U, "Heparin Cofactor II Activity Measured With an Amidolytic Method," *Thromb Res*, 1975, 6:287-94.
5. Laroche P, Plassart V, and Amiral J, "Rapid Quantitative Latex Immunoassays for Diagnosis of Thrombotic Disorders," *Thromb Haemost*, 1989, 62:379.
6. Tait RC, Walker ID, Perry DJ, et al, "Prevalence of Antithrombin Deficiency in the Healthy Population," *Br J Haematol*, 1994, 87(1):106-12.
7. Rodeghiero F and Tosetto A, "The Epidemiology of Inherited Thrombophilia: The VITA Project," *Thromb Haemost*, 1997, 78(1):636-40.
8. Melissari E, Monte G, Lindo VS, et al, "Congenital Thrombophilia Among Patients With Venous Thromboembolism," *Blood Coagul Fibrinolysis*, 1992, 3(6):749-58.
9. Bayston TA and Lane DA, "Antithrombin: Molecular Basis of Deficiency," *Thromb Haemost*, 1997, 78(1):339-43.
10. van der Meer FJM, Koster T, Vandenbroucke JP, et al, "The Leiden Thrombophilia Study (LETS)," *Thromb Haemost*, 1997, 78(5):631-5.
11. Lane DA, Bayston T, Olds RJ, et al, "Antithrombin Mutation Database: 2nd (1997) Update," *Thromb Haemost*, 1997, 77(1):197-211.
12. van Boven HH, Vandenbroucke JP, Briet E, et al, "Gene-Gene and Gene-Environment Interactions Determine Risk of Thrombosis in Families With Inherited Antithrombin Deficiency," *Blood*, 1999, 94:2590-4.
13. Demers C, Ginsberg JS, Hirsh J, et al, "Thrombosis in Antithrombin III-Deficient Persons: Report of a Large Kindred and Literature Review," *Ann Intern Med*, 1992, 116(9):754-61.
14. Rao AK, Niewiarowski S, Guzzo J, et al, "Antithrombin III Levels During Heparin Therapy," *Thromb Res*, 1981, 24:181-6.
15. Meade TW, Dyer S, Howarth DJ, et al, "Antithrombin III and Procoagulant Activity: Sex Differences and Effects of the Menopause," *Br J Haematol*, 1990, 74(1):77-81.
16. Sas G, Pepper DS, and Cash JD, "Further Investigations on Antithrombin III in the Plasmas of Patients With the Abnormality of Antithrombin III Budapest," *Thromb Diath Haemorrh*, 1975, 33:564-72.
17. Eisele B and Lamy M. "Clinical Experience With Antithrombin III Concentrates in Critically Ill Patients With Sepsis and Multiple Organ Failure," *Semin Thromb Hemost*, 1998, 24:(1)71-80.

References
Blajchman MA, Austin RC, Fernandez-Rachubinski F, et al, "Molecular Basis of Inherited Human Antithrombin Deficiency," *Blood*, 1992, 80(9):2159-71.
De Stefano V, Finazzi G, and Mannucci PM, "Inherited Thrombophilia: Pathogenesis, Clinical Syndromes, and Management," *Blood*, 1996, 87(9):3531-44.

Bleeding Time

Related Information
Platelet Aggregation on page 348
Platelet Count on page 468
Platelet Transfusion on page 854
von Willebrand Factor on page 357

Applies to Bleeding Time, Duke; Bleeding Time, Ivy; Bleeding Time, Mielke

Abstract The bleeding time is intended to measure platelet function, but it is neither a sensitive nor a specific test. For this reason, its use is declining and at some institutions this test has been eliminated.

Patient Preparation Aspirin prolongs the bleeding time, and therefore, patients should not have taken aspirin or related compounds for at least 1 week prior to testing.

Clinicians may wish to inform the patient that a scar might form as a result of a bleeding time test, particularly if the patient has a history of keloids.

Aftercare A butterfly bandage is placed over the incision and kept in place for 24 hours.

Specimen None - performed at bedside by a coagulation technologist or other trained healthcare professional.

Turnaround Time 30 minutes or less after the coagulation technologist arrives at the bedside

Reference Interval Approximately 1.5-9.5 minutes (shorter in newborns)[1]

Use Its intended use is as a measure of platelet function, but due to its inaccuracies, it is generally not useful.

Limitations Lacks sensitivity and specificity. Platelet counts <100,000/μL, low hematocrit, aspirin, other platelet inhibitory drugs, and certain other medications can prolong the bleeding time. Many variables influence the result, including skin thickness, temperature, blood vessel characteristics, the blade, orientation of the incision (horizontal vs vertical), location of the incision, handedness, and other features.

Methodology A trained healthcare professional makes a small incision on the patient's arm, and every 30 seconds gently blots the blood with filter paper to see if the bleeding has stopped. The filter paper must not touch the wound. Prior to making the cut, a blood pressure cuff is placed on the patient's arm at 40 mm Hg.

Additional Information The bleeding time can be prolonged in von Willebrand disease and other hereditary platelet function disorders, uremia, macroglobulinemia, and a variety of other conditions. However, it is not a reliable test for diagnosis or for predicting bleeding risk. In 1990, an analysis of 862 publications on the bleeding time concluded that the bleeding time is not a useful test, particularly as a preoperative screening test in a patient with a negative bleeding history.[2] More recent publications continue to support this concept.[3,4,5,6,7]

Historically, the Duke bleeding time was used, in which the earlobe or fingertip was pierced with a lancet. This was later replaced with the Ivy bleeding time, in which a blood pressure cuff was placed on the arm at 40 mm Hg and the forearm was cut with a lancet. This approach was later modified into the template bleeding time (Mielke bleeding time), which attempted to standardize the size and depth of the cut by placing a template on the skin. A spring-loaded blade within the template device creates a cut through a slit in the template. Two such template devices are Surgicutt® (International Technidyne Corp) and Simplate® (Organon Teknika Corp).

Footnotes
1. Andrew M, Paes B, Bowker J, et al, "Evaluation of an Automated Bleeding Time Device in the Newborn," *Am J Hematol*, 1990, 35(4):275-7.
2. Rodgers RP and Levin J, "A Critical Reappraisal of the Bleeding Time," *Semin Thromb Hemost*, 1990, 16(1):1-20.
3. Basili S, Ferro D, Leo R, et al, "Bleeding Time Does Not Predict Gastrointestinal Bleeding in Patients With Cirrhosis," *J Hepatol*, 1996, 24(5):574-80.
4. de Rossi SS and Glick MG, "Bleeding Time: An Unreliable Predictor of Clinical Hemostasis," *J Oral Maxillofac Surg*, 1996, 54(9):1119-20.
5. Gewirtz AS, Miller ML, and Keys TF, "The Clinical Usefulness of the Preoperative Bleeding Time," *Arch Pathol Lab Med*, 1996, 120(4):353-6.
6. Munro J, Booth A, and Nicholl J, "Routine Preoperative Testing: A Systematic Review of the Evidence," *Health Technol Assess*, 1997, 1(12):1-62.
7. Peterson P, Hayes TE, Arkin CF, et al, "The Preoperative Bleeding Time Test Lacks Clinical Benefit," *Arch Surg*, 1998, 133(2):134-9.

References
Brown BA, *Hematology: Principles and Procedures*, 6th ed, Philadelphia, PA: Lea and Febiger, 1993, 267-70.

Clot Retraction

Related Information
Fibrinogen on page 341
Platelet Aggregation on page 348
Platelet Count on page 468

Test Includes Test may include description of clot retraction, clot size and firmness, RBC fallout, serum "drip-out".

Abstract This test has been replaced by newer tests for platelet function and for Glanzmann thrombasthenia in most coagulation laboratories.

Specimen Whole blood

Container Red top tube

Collection Routine venipuncture; transport specimen to the laboratory immediately. (Note: Contact the laboratory prior to collecting the specimen, as the laboratory may not offer the test.)

Turnaround Time 24 hours

Reference Interval Clot retraction occurs within 4 hours.[1]

Optional considerations:[2] With normal clots and normal hematocrits, the clot in a red top tube occupies 40% to 60% of the original volume. The remaining 40% to 60% consists of serum as well as red cells that fall out of the clot and settle to the bottom of the tube ("red cell fall-out"). Red cell fall-out is usually <5% of the original blood sample volume (centrifuged, after removing the clot). When normal clots are removed from the tube, serum drips from the clot at a rate of two drops or less in 2 minutes.

Use Currently, it is an infrequently used clinical test. In the past, it was a test for Glanzmann thrombasthenia and platelet function.

Limitations Platelet counts <100,000/μL, aspirin and related medications, monoclonal gammopathy (paraproteinemia), and polycythemia reduce the amount of clot retraction. Anemia increases clot retraction. With polycythemia, the increased number of red blood cells within the clot limits the extent to which the clot can retract.

Methodology The red top tube is kept at 37°C and the clot is examined at 1, 2, 4, and 24 hours for clot retraction. When the clot retracts, it pulls away from the walls of the tube. Normally, a few red blood cells fall out of the clot, and they can be seen at the bottom of the tube.

Optional approach:[2] The initial blood specimen can be placed in a graduated tube such that volumes can be approximated. A wooden stick can be placed in the tube prior to clot formation, so that the clot can be removed from the tube for examination. A normal clot is firm and tightly attached to the stick.

Additional Information During clot formation, platelets aggregate as fibrinogen binds to platelet glycoprotein IIb/IIIa, linking platelets to each other. Normally, clot retraction occurs subsequently, as platelets within the clot contract. Glycoprotein IIb/IIIa is necessary for platelet aggregation as well as for clot retraction. In Glanzmann thrombasthenia, clot retraction and platelet aggregation are reduced because glycoprotein IIb/IIIa is deficient. With dysfibrinogenemia, hypofibrinogenemia, or disseminated intravascular coagulation (DIC), the clot can be small and an increased number of red blood cells fall out of the clot.

Footnotes

1. Brown BA, *Hematology: Principles and Procedures*, 6th ed, Philadelphia, PA: Lea and Febiger, 1993, 271.
2. Sirridge MS and Shannon R, *Laboratory Evaluation of Hemostasis and Thrombosis*, 3rd ed, Philadelphia, PA: Lea and Febiger, 1983, 83-90.

References

Hantgan RR and Mousa SA, "Inhibition of Platelet-Mediated Clot Retraction by Integrin Antagonists," *Thromb Res*, 1998, 89(6):271-9.

Rooney MM, Farrell DH, van Hemel BM, et al, "The Contribution of the Three Hypothesized Integrin-Binding Sites in Fibrinogen to Platelet-Mediated Clot Retraction," *Blood*, 1998, 92(7):2374-81.

Coagulation Factor Assays

Related Information

Activated Partial Thromboplastin Time *on page 328*
Antiphospholipid Antibody (Lupus Anticoagulant and/or Anticardiolipin Antibody) *on page 331*
Factor Inhibitors *on page 340*
Factor IX Concentrate *on page 841*
Factor VIII Concentrate *on page 841*
Factor XIII *on page 339*
Fibrinogen *on page 341*
High-Molecular Weight Kininogen *on page 344*
Mixing Studies *on page 346*
Occult Blood, Stool *on page 315*
Prekallikrein *on page 350*
Prothrombin Time *on page 354*
von Willebrand Factor *on page 357*
Warfarin *on page 770*

Synonyms Ac-Globulin (Factor V); Antihemophilic Factor (Factor VIII); Autoprothrombin I (Factor VII); Autoprothrombin II (Factor IX); Christmas Disease Factor (Factor IX); Hageman Factor (Factor XII); Labile Factor (Factor V); Plasma Thromboplastin Antecedent (Factor XI); Plasma Thromboplastin Component (Factor IX); Proaccelerin (Factor V); Proconvertin (Factor VII); Prothrombin (Factor II); Stable Factor (Factor VII); Stuart Factor (Factor X); Stuart-Prower Factor (Factor X)

Applies to DDAVP; Desmopressin; Factor(s) II, V, VII, VIII, IX, X, XI, XII; Factor VIII:von Willebrand Factor Ratio; Hemophilia A (Factor VIII Deficiency); Hemophilia B (Factor IX Deficiency); INR; International Normalized Ratio

Abstract Isolated factor deficiencies can be hereditary, but this is much more rare than multiple, acquired factor deficiencies produced by liver disease, disseminated intravascular coagulation, warfarin, or the inhibitory effects in factor assays from lupus anticoagulants, heparin, or other anticoagulants.

Specimen Plasma

Container Three blue top (sodium citrate) tubes if all factor assays are requested

Collection Routine venipuncture. If multiple tests are being drawn, draw blue top tubes after any red top tubes but before any lavender top (EDTA), green top (heparin), or gray top (oxalate/fluoride) tubes. Immediately invert tube gently at least 4 times to mix. Tubes must be appropriately filled. Deliver tubes immediately to the laboratory.

Avoid heparin contamination during specimen collection. Heparin, hirudin, or argatroban anticoagulation can interfere with factor assays by acting as an "inhibitor", resulting in falsely decreased factor levels. Heparin, if present, must be removed from specimens by the laboratory. Warfarin decreases factors II, VII, IX, and X.

Storage Instructions Separate plasma from cells as soon as possible. Store plasma at room temperature for up to 2 hours, at 2°C to 8°C for up to 4 hours, or store frozen. Factor VIII, and to a lesser extent factor V, degrade if specimens are kept unfrozen for prolonged periods.

Causes for Rejection Specimen received more than 4 hours after collection, tubes not filled, clotted specimen

Turnaround Time Less than 1 day, unless test has to be sent out to a reference laboratory

Reference Interval Factor levels are expressed as percent of normal plasma concentrations. By definition, normal plasma contains 100% (1 unit/mL) of each factor. The reference range is approximately 60% to 140%. Factor VIII levels are not decreased at birth or throughout childhood. The other factor levels are below adult reference range at birth, ranging approximately from 10% to 100%. The levels increase toward the adult reference range by age 6 months, although they may remain mildly below adult normal range throughout childhood.[1,2] However, newborns and children do not normally experience bleeding, because a balance between coagulation factors and natural coagulation inhibitors is maintained throughout development. Factor XI can decrease during pregnancy, whereas fibrinogen and factor VIII increase.

Use To determine the etiology of a prolonged PT or PTT. Usually performed after a mixing study has been completed (see Mixing Studies *on page 346*), to identify specific factor deficiencies or inhibitors. Assays for factors VIII, IX, XI, and XII are performed to evaluate a prolonged PTT (with normal PT). Assays for fibrinogen, factors II, V, VII, and X are performed to evaluate a prolonged PT (with normal PTT). If PT and PTT are both prolonged, all eight factors and fibrinogen may be performed to establish the cause for the prolongations. Because acquired causes of factor deficiencies are generally more common than hereditary causes, a patient found to have a factor deficiency should be evaluated for possible acquired etiologies, especially if multiple factor deficiencies are present (see Tables 1 and 2). If a hereditary etiology for the decrease appears likely, the diagnosis can be confirmed by measuring the factor in relatives.

Table 1. Effects of Hereditary or Acquired Factor Deficiencies on PT and PTT

PTT Prolonged, PT Normal
Deficiencies of factor(s) VIII, IX, XI, and/or XII (intrinsic pathway)
PT Prolonged, PTT Normal
Deficiency of factor VII (extrinsic pathway)
Occasionally, mild-to-moderate deficiencies of factor(s) II, V, X, and/or fibrinogen (common pathway)
Both PT and PTT Prolonged
Deficiencies of factor(s) II, V, X, and/or fibrinogen (common pathway)
Multiple factor deficiencies

Table 2. Acquired Causes of Factor Deficiencies

Acquired Conditions Affecting PT Sooner and More Significantly Than PTT	
Warfarin or vitamin K deficiency	Decreased function of factors II, VII, IX, and X
Liver dysfunction	Decreases hepatic synthesis of coagulation factors. All factors may be decreased except for factor VIII. Factor VII has the shortest half-life and therefore is often the earliest and most severely decreased factor. Factors XI and XII have the longest half-lives and therefore are often the last to be affected.
Disseminated intravascular coagulation (DIC)	All factors can be variably decreased, including factor VIII, due to factor activation and consumption.
Amyloidosis	Factor X, and occasionally other factors, can be decreased, due to binding of factor(s) to amyloid.
Acquired Conditions Affecting PTT Sooner and More Significantly Than PT	
Prolonged specimen transit to laboratory	Degradation of factors V and VIII
Proteinuria	Occasionally, decreased factors XI and XII. PT usually normal.
Acquired Conditions That Can Interfere With Factor Assays	
Heparin	Inhibits activated factors II, X, IX, XI, and XII, prolonging the PTT earlier and more than PT, and interfering in PTT-based factor assays more than PT-based factor assays, without causing a true decrease in factor levels.
Lupus anticoagulants	Inhibits the phospholipid cofactor function in coagulation, often prolonging the PTT. PT is usually normal. Can interfere in PTT-based factor assays, without causing a true decrease in factor levels. Rarely, a lupus anticoagulant can bind to factor II and cause a true decrease in factor II, prolonging the PT.
Hirudin and argatroban	Inhibit activated factor II (thrombin), prolonging both the PT and PTT, and interfering in PT- or PTT-based factor assays without causing a true decrease in factor levels.
Factor inhibitors	

(Continued)

Coagulation Factor Assays (Continued)

Chromogenic factor X assays are useful for monitoring warfarin in the presence of a lupus anticoagulant, hirudin, or argatroban. Lupus anticoagulants, hirudin or argatroban can prolong the PT and therefore the international normalized ratio (INR).[3] In these situations, the INR can overestimate the amount of warfarin anticoagulation and lead to inappropriate reductions in warfarin dose. Warfarin decreases factor X (as well as factors II, VII, and IX), and a chromogenic assay is available for factor X which has no interference from lupus anticoagulants, hirudin or argatroban. When the INR is 2-3, the chromogenic factor X level is approximately 20% to 40%. Each laboratory should determine its own chromogenic factor X therapeutic range.

Relatives of patients with a known hereditary factor deficiency may chose to have PT, PTT, and/or factor assay(s) performed to determine if they also have the deficiency or if they are a carrier.

Factor VIII assays are part of a von Willebrand disease evaluation. Factor VIII assays, together with von Willebrand factor assays, can also assess for hemophilia A carrier status in females. In hemophilia A carriers, the factor VIII:von Willebrand factor ratio is approximately 0.5.

An increased risk for thrombosis has been reported with elevated levels of certain coagulation factors (eg, fibrinogen, factor VII, factor VIII, factor XI).[4,5,6,7] In addition, factor VII levels may be affected by dietary lipids, and factor VII levels correlate with triglyceride and cholesterol levels.[8] However, factor assays have not yet been added to most hypercoagulation panels.

Methodology Factor assays are PT- or PTT-based reactions. These assays are performed by mixing patient plasma with plasma that is deficient in the factor that is being measured. Based on the resulting PT or PTT of this mixture, the amount of factor can be determined by comparing the PT or PTT clotting time to a standard curve that plots known factor levels against clotting times. Factor VIII, IX, XI, and XII assays are PTT-based. Factor II, VII, and X assays are PT-based. PT- and PTT-based assays are both available for factor V.

The presence of an inhibitor, such as a lupus anticoagulant, can cause artifactual decreases in the *in vitro* factor level. Therefore, laboratories should perform factor assays at multiple dilutions. At higher dilutions, the inhibitor interference will decrease due to dilution of the inhibitor.

Chromogenic factor assays and immunoassays (antigen assays) are commercially available for some of the coagulation factors. For example, chromogenic assays are commercially available for factors II, VII, VIII, and X; antigen assays are commercially available for factors VII, VIII, IX, and X. Therapeutic anticoagulants, lupus anticoagulants, and other inhibitors do not interfere with these assays (except in some instances when the inhibitor or anticoagulant is directed specifically against the factor being assayed or against another factor that participates in the assay).

Additional Information Factor deficiencies can be quantitative or qualitative. In quantitative disorders, the factor level determined by routine PT- or PTT-based methods (functional activity assays) is similar to the result obtained by immunological (antigen) assays. In qualitative disorders, the PT- or PTT-based (functional) assay result is decreased, but the antigen level is normal or significantly higher than the functional level, indicating the presence of a dysfunctional protein. Antigen assays are not available for some factors.

Hereditary Deficiencies of Factor VIII (Hemophilia A) or Factor IX (Hemophilia B)

Hemophilia A (factor VIII deficiency) is the most common severe hereditary bleeding disorder, affecting 1 in 5000-10,000 males.[9,10] Hemophilia B (factor IX deficiency) is also a severe hereditary bleeding disorder, affecting 1 in 25,000-30,000 males. Hemophilia A and B are X-linked recessive disorders, because the factor VIII and factor IX genes are located on the X chromosome. Therefore, typically only males are affected. Females carrying the hemophilia mutation on one of their two X chromosomes are carriers. Female carriers with factor VIII levels <50% and bleeding symptoms have been reported.

The clinical severity of hemophilia A or B depends on the factor level. In hemophilia, <1% factor VIII or IX produces severe hemophilia with spontaneous bleeding, 1% to 5% produces moderate bleeding, and >5% is considered mild hemophilia in which bleeding occurs primarily with trauma or surgery rather than spontaneously. The baseline factor level remains relatively constant within an individual and within a kindred. Bleeding manifestations include hemarthrosis, soft tissue hematomas including bleeding into muscles, easy bruising, excessive bleeding with surgery, trauma, dental extractions, and circumcision, bleeding in the gastrointestinal or genitourinary tract, epistaxis, poor wound healing, and uncommonly, umbilical stump bleeding. Intracranial hemorrhages can occur, particularly following trauma.

Hemophilia testing is suggested for male patients with unexplained bleeding, especially if the PTT is prolonged with a normal PT and platelet count. Decreases in factor VIII or IX to <20% to 30% can cause PTT prolongations, depending on the PTT reagent and instrument. Since up to 30% of hemophilia A or B cases arise from new mutations, a positive family history will not always be present. If a family history is present, the inheritance pattern is X-linked recessive. The initial tests for hemophilia are the

factor VIII and factor IX assays. A von Willebrand test panel is usually also performed. In von Willebrand disease, factor VIII levels are decreased secondary to a decrease in von Willebrand factor. Thus, the tests for von Willebrand factor assess whether a decrease in factor VIII represents von Willebrand disease or hemophilia A. The von Willebrand panel is also useful in predicting hemophilia A carrier status in females. In hemophilia A carrier females, the ratio of factor VIII to von Willebrand factor is approximately 0.5:1. In normal persons, the ratio is approximately 1:1, since factor VIII circulates in the plasma with von Willebrand factor. Confirmation of carrier status often requires family or genetic studies (see below). Both factor VIII and von Willebrand factor can be elevated during acute phase reactions, including pregnancy. Therefore, if a patient is determined to have elevated acute phase reactants, testing should be repeated at a time when the acute phase reaction has subsided. Lastly, factor VIII is labile at room temperature. Consequently, a mild to moderate decrease in factor VIII may be seen in specimens that have not been processed and stored appropriately.

The factor VIII gene is quite large, and numerous mutations causing hemophilia A have been identified. Therefore, genetic testing can be difficult. An inversion mutation of Intron® 22 has been shown to cause up to 40% of severe hemophilia A in Caucasians, which simplifies genetic testing in these families.[11] Restriction fragment length polymorphism (RFLP) studies or methods that directly identify the mutation may be useful in families without the Intron® 22 inversion.

Numerous mutations causing hemophilia B have also been identified. Like hemophilia A, genetic testing for female carrier status or prenatal detection can often be achieved with restriction fragment length polymorphism (RFLP) analysis or methods that directly demonstrate the mutation.

Many patients with hemophilia became infected with human immunodeficiency virus (HIV) as a result of treatment with factor concentrates prior to the availability of HIV testing of blood donors. Currently, factor VIII and IX concentrates are treated to destroy HIV and other viruses, and blood donors are screened for HIV. Desmopressin (DDAVP) elevates factor VIII (and von Willebrand factor) levels approximately two- to threefold over baseline for 6-12 hours. Therefore, it is often used to treat bleeding episodes in patients with mild hemophilia.

Hereditary Deficiencies of Other Coagulation Factors (Factors II, V, VII, X, XI, XII)

Unlike factor VIII and IX deficiencies, which have X-linked recessive inheritance, hereditary deficiencies of the other coagulation factors have autosomal inheritance. Hereditary deficiencies of factors II, V, VII, and X are rare. Factor XI deficiency is common among individuals of Ashkenazi Jewish descent. Factor XII deficiency is relatively common, but it is not associated with any bleeding risk. With the other factor deficiencies, bleeding symptoms may include easy bruising, epistaxis, menorrhagia, bleeding with surgery, trauma, dental extractions, postpartum, or circumcision, umbilical stump bleeding (especially with factor XIII deficiency or afibrinogenemia, described separately) and bleeding in the gastrointestinal or genitourinary tract. Intracranial hemorrhage has been reported with severe deficiencies of factor II, V, VII, or X. Hemarthrosis and bleeding into muscles, characteristic of factor VIII and IX deficiencies, are less common but can occur in other factor deficiencies.[12,13,14,15,16] Factor deficiencies may prolong the PT and/or PTT, depending on the factor and the severity of the decrease in factor level (see Table 1 on previous page).

In general, with hereditary factor deficiencies, heterozygous deficient individuals have approximately 50% (most commonly within 30% to 60%) of the normal value for the affected factor. Homozygous deficient individuals have a more severe decrease in the affected factor. As previously mentioned, heterozygous or homozygous deficiencies of factor XII do not cause bleeding.[17] Heterozygous deficiencies of the other factors are usually either asymptomatic or have a milder bleeding tendency than homozygous deficiencies (see Table 3). Factor XI deficient heterozygotes may have bleeding symptoms.[16] Factor II or factor X deficient heterozygotes sometimes have mild bleeding symptoms. With rare exceptions, heterozygous factor V or VII deficiencies are asymptomatic. In contrast, homozygous deficiencies of these factors (II, V, VII, X, XI) do have an increased incidence of bleeding symptoms. However, factor V, VII, or XI levels do not always correlate with severity of symptoms. In general, factor VIII and IX deficiencies tend to be the most severe, while deficiencies of factors II, V, or XI tend to be milder than factor VIII or IX deficiencies. Severe deficiencies of factor VII or X can have a clinical presentation as severe as hemophilia A or B.

Hereditary Combined Coagulation Factor Deficiencies

Combined factor deficiencies are very rare. A combined deficiency of factors V and VIII is an autosomal recessive disorder arising, in most families studied so far, from a mutation in an endoplasmic reticulum-Golgi intermediate compartment gene on chromosome 18 which appears to decrease intracellular transportation of factors V and VIII.[18] A combined deficiency of the vitamin K-dependent factors II, VII, IX, and X has been described which, in at least some families, is due to a mutation in the gamma-glutamyl carboxylase gene.[19] The gene codes for an enzyme that carboxylates glutamate residues in the vitamin K dependent coagulation factors, a reaction that is necessary for normal function of these vitamin K-dependent factors.

Table 3. Coagulation Factor Deficiencies and Factor Half-Lives

Factor Deficiency	Level Required for Surgical Hemostasis	Bleeding Risk in Homozygous Deficiency?	Bleeding Risk in Heterozygous Deficiency?	Biologic Half-life of Factor
Fibrinogen (factor I)	100 mg/dL	Yes	Sometimes	72-120 h
Prothrombin (factor II)	10%-40%	Yes	Sometimes	72 h (48-120 h)
Factor V	10%-30%	Yes*	No (rare exceptions)	12-36 h
Factor VII	10%-25%	Yes*	No (rare exceptions)	4-7 h
Factor VIII	Major surgery or major bleeding: 80%-100% / Postoperative: 30%-50% / Minor bleeding: 30%-50%	Yes (X-linked recessive)	No (rare exceptions; heterozygotes are carrier females)	8-12 h
Factor IX	Major surgery or major bleeding: 50%-80% / Postoperative: 40% / Minor bleeding: 30%-50%	Yes (X-linked recessive)	No (rare exceptions; heterozygotes are carrier females)	18-24 h
Factor X	10%-40%	Yes	Sometimes	24-48 h
Factor XI	15%-50%	Sometimes*	Sometimes	40-84 h
Factor XII	0%	No	No	48-52 h
Factor XIII	>5%-50%†	Yes	Sometimes	9-12 d

*Factor V, VII, or XI levels do not always correlate well with severity of bleeding.

†Factor XIII levels >1%-5% have traditionally been considered asymptomatic; however, recent evidence suggests heterozygous deficiencies with levels up to 50% can be associated with excess bleeding.

Adapted from Van Cott EM and Laposata M, "Coagulation, Fibrinolysis, and Hypercoagulation," *Clinical Diagnosis and Management by Laboratory Methods*, 20th ed, Henry JB, ed, New York, NY: WB Saunders Co, in press.

References:

Menitove 1995, Edmunds 1994, Laposata 1989, Roberts 1995, Roberts 1994, and see text for references regarding bleeding risk with heterozygous and homozygous deficiencies.

Footnotes

1. Andrew M, Vegh P, Johnston M, et al, "Maturation of the Hemostatic System During Childhood," *Blood*, 1992, 80(8):1998-2005.
2. Andrew M, Paes B, and Johnston M, "Development of the Hemostatic System in the Neonate and Young Infant," *Am J Pediatr Hematol Oncol*, 1990, 12(1):95-104.
3. Moll S and Ortel TL, "Monitoring Warfarin Therapy in Patients With Lupus Anticoagulants," *Ann Intern Med*, 1997, 127(3):177-85.
4. Iacoviello L, Di Castelnuovo A, de Knijff P, et al, "Polymorphisms in the Coagulation Factor VII Gene and the Risk of Myocardial Infarction," *N Engl J Med*, 1998, 338(2):79-85.
5. Ma J, Hennekens CH, Ridker PM, et al, "A Prospective Study of Fibrinogen and Risk of Myocardial Infarction in the Physician's Health Survey," *J Am Coll Cardiol*, 1999, 33(5):1347-52.
6. van der Meer FJ, Koster T, Vandenbroucke JP, et al, "The Leiden Thrombophilia Study (LETS)," *Thromb Haemost*, 1997, 78(1):631-5.
7. Meijers JC, Tekelenburg WLH, Bouma BN, et al, "High Levels of Coagulation Factor XI as a Risk Factor for Venous Thrombosis," *N Engl J Med*, 2000, 342(10):696-701.
8. Mennen LI, Schouten EG, Grobbee DE, et al, "Coagulation Factor VII, Dietary Fat and Blood Lipids: A Review," *Thromb Haemost*, 1996, 76(4):492-9.
9. Hoyer LW, "Hemophilia A," *N Engl J Med*, 1994, 330(1):38-47.
10. Ljung R, Petrini P, and Nilsson M, "Diagnostic Symptoms of Severe and Moderate Haemophilia A and B. A Survey of 140 Cases," *Acta Paediatr Scand*, 1990, 79(2):196-200.
11. Naylor JA, Green PM, Rizza CR, et al, "Factor VIII Gene Explains All Cases of Haemophilia A," *Lancet*, 1992, 340(8827):1066-7.
12. Giangrande PLF, "Other Inherited Disorders of Blood Coagulation," Rizza C and Lowe G, eds, *Haemophilia and Other Inherited Bleeding Disorders*, London, WB Saunders Co, 1997, 291-307.
13. Kane WH and Davie EW, "Blood Coagulation Factors V and VIII: Structural and Functional Similarities and Their Relationship to Hemorrhagic and Thrombotic Disorders," *Blood*, 1988, 71(3):539-55.
14. Cooper DN, Millar DS, Wacey A, et al, "Inherited Factor VII Deficiency: Molecular Genetics and Pathophysiology," *Thromb Haemost*, 1997, 78(1):151-60.
15. Cooper DN, Millar DS, Wacey A, et al, "Inherited Factor X Deficiency: Molecular Genetics and Pathophysiology," *Thromb Haemost*, 1997, 78(1):161-72.
16. Modi GJ and Musclow CE, "Factor XI: A Piece of the Coagulation Puzzle," *Lab Med*, 1993, 24:353-6.
17. Halbmayer WM, Haushofer A, Schon R, et al, "The Prevalence of Moderate and Severe FXII (Hageman Factor) Deficiency Among the Normal Population: Evaluation of the Incidence of FXII Deficiency Among 300 Healthy Blood Donors," *Thromb Haemost*, 1994, 71(1):68-72.
18. Nichols WC, Seligsohn U, Zivelin A, et al, "Mutations in the ER-Golgi Intermediate Compartment Protein ERGIC-53 Cause Combined Deficiency of Coagulation Factors V and VIII," *Cell*, 1998, 93(1):61-70.
19. Brenner B, Sanchez-Vega B, Wu SM, et al, "A Missense Mutation in Gamma-Glutamyl Carboxylase Gene causes Combined Deficiency of all Vitamin K-Dependent Blood Coagulation Factors," *Blood*, 1998, 92(12):4554-9.

References

Edmunds LH and Salzman EW, "Hemostatic Problems, Transfusion Therapy, and Cardiopulmonary Bypass in Surgical Patients," *Hemostasis and Thrombosis: Basic Principles and Clinical Practice*, 3rd ed, Colman RW, Hirsh J, Marder VJ, et al, eds, Philadelphia, PA: Churchill Livingstone, 1994, 958.

Laposata M, Connor AM, Hicks DG, et al, *The Clinical Hemostasis Handbook*, Chicago, IL: Yearbook Medical Publishers, Inc, 1989.

Menitove JE, Gill JC, and Montgomery RR, "Preparation and Clinical Use of Plasma and Plasma Fractions," *William's Hematology*, 5th ed, Beutler E, Lichtman MA, Coller BS, et al, eds. New York, NY: McGraw-Hill, 1995, 1657.

Roberts HR and Hoffman M, "Hemophilia and Related Conditions - Inherited Deficiencies of Prothrombin (Factor II), Factor V, and Factors VII to XII," *William's Hematology*, 5th ed, Beutler E, Lichtman MA, Coller BS, et al, eds, New York, NY: McGraw-Hill, 1995, 1413-39.

Roberts HR and Lefkowitz JB, "Inherited Disorders of Prothrombin Conversion," *Hemostasis and Thrombosis: Basic Principles and Clinical Practice*, 3rd ed, Colman RW, Hirsh J, Marder VJ, et al, eds, Philadelphia, PA: Churchill Livingstone, 1994, 200-18.

♦ **Common Pathway** *see* Activated Partial Thromboplastin Time *on page 328*

♦ **Common Pathway** *see* Prothrombin Time *on page 354*

♦ **Conjunctivitis, Ligneous** *see* Plasminogen *on page 347*

♦ **Consumptive Coagulopathy Screen** *see* Disseminated Intravascular Coagulation Screen *on page 338*

♦ **Coumadin®** *see* Heparin-Induced Thrombocytopenia *on page 343*

♦ **Coumadin®** *see* Prothrombin Time *on page 354*

♦ **Cryocrit** *see* Cryofibrinogen *on page 337*

Cryofibrinogen

Related Information

Cold Agglutinin Titer *on page 594*

Cryoglobulin, Qualitative, Serum and Plasma *on page 524*

Applies to Cryocrit

Abstract Cryofibrinogen precipitates at cold temperatures, causing predominantly cutaneous symptoms on cold-exposed areas. It is also commonly asymptomatic.

Specimen Plasma

Container Two blue top (sodium citrate) tubes or EDTA tubes; also one red top tube for cryoglobulin. Tubes may be prewarmed to 37°C if necessary.

Collection Immediately place specimens in warm water and transport to laboratory.

Causes for Rejection Improper tube, specimen more than 2 hours in transit to the laboratory, specimen not warm upon arrival to laboratory

Turnaround Time 24-72 hours

Reference Interval Negative: no cryofibrinogen detected

Use Consider a cryofibrinogen assay for patients with unexplained cutaneous ulcers, ischemia or necrosis on cold-exposed areas. Occasionally, routine blood samples are noted to form a gel during or soon after blood drawing.

Contraindications Specimens containing heparin should not be used, because heparin nonspecifically precipitates fibrinogen in this assay.

Methodology Plasma is obtained by centrifuging the warm specimen at 37°C. The plasma is then refrigerated overnight, usually in a tube that can measure "cryocrit", such as a Wintrobe tube. To determine if fibrinogen precipitate has formed, the tube is centrifuged at 4°C. Each millimeter of visible precipitate represents 1% of "cryocrit" (in this case, cryofibrinogen). The cryocrit is the volume percent of the precipitate compared with the total volume of test plasma. Also, if cryofibrinogen is present, plasma fibrinogen levels are lower after refrigeration compared with fibrinogen measurements performed on the warm specimen prior to refrigeration.[1] A cryoglobulin test is simultaneously performed, to ensure that the plasma precipitate is not cryoglobulin. Cryoglobulin precipitates in plasma or serum at cold temperatures, whereas cryofibrinogen precipitates in cold plasma but not serum (because fibrinogen is not present in serum). Cryoglobulin and cryofibrinogen disappear upon rewarming the specimen. See Cryoglobulin, Qualitative, Serum and Plasma *on page 524*.

Additional Information Cryofibrinogen consists of fibrinogen and other substances that precipitate at cold temperatures. Cryoglobulins are immunoglobulins that precipitate at cold temperatures. Cryofibrinogenemia or cryoglobulinemia both can produce cold-induced skin symptoms in the extremities, ears or nose. Such symptoms include purpura, ulceration, necrosis, gangrene, bleeding, cold urticaria, bullae, livedo reticularis, and Raynaud syndrome. In one study, 13% of cryofibrinogenemia patients had venous and/or arterial thrombosis.[2] Cryofibrinogenemia can be a primary (essential) condition or it may arise in association with an underlying condition, such as malignancy, infection, inflammation, diabetes, pregnancy, scleroderma, or oral contraceptives. A few familial cases have been reported. Skin biopsies may show leukocytoclastic vasculitis.

Footnotes

1. Gluek HI and Herrman LG, "Cold-Precipitable Fibrinogen, Cryofibrinogen," *Arch Intern Med*, 1964, 113:748-57.
2. Blain H, Cacoub P, Musset L, et al, "Cryofibrinogenaemia: A Study of 49 Patients," *Clin Exp Immunol*, 2000, 120(2):253-60.

(Continued)

Cryofibrinogen *(Continued)*

References
Kallemuchikkal U and Gorevic PD, "Evaluation of Cryoglobulins," *Arch Pathol Lab Med*, 1999, 123(2):119-25.

Klein AD and Kerdel FA, "Purpura and Recurrent Ulcers on the Lower Extremities. Essential Cryofibrinogenemia," *Arch Dermatol*, 1991, 127(1):113-8.

♦ **Danaparoid** *see* Heparin Antifactor Xa Assay *on page 342*

♦ **Danaparoid** *see* Heparin-Induced Thrombocytopenia *on page 343*

♦ **Danaparoid** *see* Mixing Studies *on page 346*

♦ **DDAVP** *see* Coagulation Factor Assays *on page 335*

♦ **DDAVP** *see* von Willebrand Factor *on page 357*

♦ **D-Dimers** *see* D-Dimers and Fibrin Degradation Products *on page 338*

♦ **D-Dimers** *see* Hypercoagulation Panel *on page 345*

D-Dimers and Fibrin Degradation Products

Related Information
Disseminated Intravascular Coagulation Screen *on page 338*
Hypercoagulation Panel *on page 345*

Synonyms D-Dimers; FBP; FDP; Fibrin Breakdown Products; Fibrin Split Products; FSP

Applies to Fibrinolysis; Plasmin; Thrombin; Thrombolysis

Abstract Fibrinolysis is mediated by plasmin, which degrades fibrin clots into D-dimers and fibrin degradation products (FDP). Plasmin can also degrade intact fibrinogen, generating fibrinogen degradation products (FDP) that are detected in FDP assays.

Specimen Plasma (some FDP assays require serum; the SimpliRed® D-dimer assay uses whole blood)

Container One blue top (citrate) tube (some FDP serum assays require special tubes that contain thrombin to clot the blood, and a fibrinolysis inhibitor to prevent FDP formation in the test tube)

Collection Routine venipuncture. If multiple tests are being drawn, draw blue top tubes after any red top tubes but before any lavender top (EDTA), green top (heparin), or gray top (oxalate/fluoride) tubes. Immediately invert tube gently at least 4 times to mix. Tubes must be appropriately filled. Deliver tubes immediately to the laboratory.

Storage Instructions Separate plasma from cells as soon as possible. Store plasma at room temperature for up to 8 hours, on ice for up to 24 hours, or store frozen. (Serum: Once serum is obtained, it may be refrigerated for up to 1 week, or it may be stored frozen.)

Causes for Rejection Clotted specimens are unsuitable for plasma-based tests.

Turnaround Time Less than 1 day (latex agglutination methods take less than 1 hour; standard ELISA methods take 5 hours; rapid ELISA methods have been developed)

Reference Interval D-dimer: approximately <0.5 µg/mL; FDP: approximately <5 µg/mL

Use D-dimers or FDP are part of a panel of tests required for diagnosing DIC. In DIC, both thrombin and plasmin are generated, causing an elevation in D-dimers and FDP. See Disseminated Intravascular Coagulation Screen *on page 338*.

D-dimers assist with the diagnosis of deep venous thrombosis (DVT) and pulmonary embolism (PE), but only if a very sensitive method is used. If the test is positive in a patient suspected to have DVT or PE, clinicians proceed with further diagnostic tests for DVT or PE. If the test is negative, depending on the clinical situation and the sensitivity of the D-dimer assay, DVT or PE is considered unlikely and further diagnostic tests for DVT or PE might not be pursued.[1,2]

Monitoring thrombolytic therapy is not routinely required. However, if monitoring is desired, D-dimers or FDP are one of several tests that can be performed to confirm that thrombolysis (fibrinolysis) is occurring. D-dimers and FDP should become increased with thrombolytic therapy.

Limitations D-dimers and FDP can become elevated whenever the coagulation and fibrinolytic systems are activated. This occurs in a variety of conditions, and therefore the tests are not specific for any one diagnosis.

Manual latex agglutination and certain other methods are not sufficiently sensitive to exclude the diagnosis of DVT or PE when the test result is negative. Even with the most sensitive methods (eg, ELISA assays), a patient with PE or DVT may test negative for D-dimers.

High rheumatoid factor (RF) levels may cause false-positive results with some assays.

Methodology Assays are semiquantitative or quantitative immunoassays.

Latex agglutination: Patient plasma is mixed with latex particles which are coated with monoclonal anti-FDP antibodies.[3] If FDP are present in the patient plasma, the latex particles agglutinate as FDP bind to the antibodies on the particles. These large agglutinated clumps are detected visually by the technologist. Various dilutions of patient plasma can be tested to provide an estimation of the FDP titer (semiquantitative result). Latex agglutination assays are also available for D-dimers. Automated, quantitative versions of this assay are commercially available for D-dimers (MDA® D-

dimer, Organon Teknika; STA Liatest®, Diagnostica Stago), in which the agglutination is detected turbidimetrically by a coagulation analyzer rather than visually by a technologist.[4,5]

Enzyme-linked immunosorbent (ELISA) assays: Quantitative ELISA assays are available for FDP, D-dimers, or fibrinogen degradation products. An automated, rapid ELISA assay for D-dimers is available (VIDAS®, bioMerieux Inc).[1,2,6]

Other methods: SimpliRed® D-dimer (American Diagnostica) is a semiquantitative red blood cell agglutination assay that can be performed on whole blood. Other methods have been developed that are not yet available in the United States.

Additional Information A D-dimer is a specific FDP that is formed only by plasmin degradation of fibrin, and not by plasmin degradation of intact fibrinogen. Thus, the presence of D-dimers indicates that fibrin has been formed and degraded. In contrast, a positive FDP assay indicates that fibrin and/or fibrinogen is being degraded by plasmin, because the FDP assay detects fibrin degradation products, including D-dimers, and fibrinogen degradation products. D-dimers and FDP can be positive with DIC or thrombosis, including DVT, PE and myocardial infarction. They also may be positive in liver disease due to decreased hepatic clearance. They can become elevated postoperatively, and with significant bleeding, hemodialysis, eclampsia, sickle cell crisis, and other conditions. Cancer patients often have positive D-dimers and FDP, usually representing low-grade, chronic DIC. D-dimers and FDP mildly increase in pregnancy.

In the past, FDP had to be performed on serum samples, because the polyspecific antibodies cross-react with fibrinogen in plasma. Fibrinogen is not present in serum because it has been converted into fibrin clot, centrifuged, and discarded. Currently, monoclonal antibodies specific for FDP, without cross-reactivity against fibrinogen, allow the test to be performed in plasma. There is some evidence that the older, serum-based assays are not as reliable as the newer, plasma-based assays, because serum-based FDP may give low values due to trapping of FDP in the clot, or high values due to generation of FDP during clot formation.[7]

Footnotes
1. van der Graaf F, van den Borne H, van der Kolk M, et al, "Exclusion of Deep Venous Thrombosis With D-Dimer testing. Comparison of 13 D-Dimer Methods in 99 Outpatients Suspected of Deep Venous Thrombosis Using Venography as Reference Standard," *Thromb Haemost*, 2000, 83(2):191-8.
2. Perrier A, Desmarais S, Miron MJ, et al, "Noninvasive Diagnosis of Venous Thromboembolism in Outpatients," *Lancet*, 1999, 353(9148):190-5.
3. Mirshahi M, Soria J, Soria C, et al, "A Latex Immunoassay of Fibrin/Fibrinogen Degradation Products in Plasma Using a Monoclonal Antibody," *Thromb Res*, 1986, 44(6):715-28.
4. Escoffre-Barbe M, Oger E, Leroyer C, et al, "Evaluation of a New Rapid D-Dimer Assay for Clinically Suspected Deep Venous Thrombosis (Liatest® D-Dimer)," *Am J Clin Pathol*, 1998, 109(6):748-53.
5. Bates SM, Grand'Maison A, Johnston M, et al, "A Latex D-Dimer Reliably Excludes Venous Thromboembolism," *Thromb Haemost*, 1999, 82(Suppl):258.
6. Pittet JL, de Moerloose P, Reber G, et al, "VIDAS® D-Dimer: Fast Quantitative ELISA for Measuring D-Dimer in Plasma," *Clin Chem*, 1996, 42(3):410-15.
7. Gaffney PJ and Perry MJ, "Unreliability of Current Serum Fibrin Degradation Product (FDP) Assays," *Thromb Haemost*, 1985, 53(3):301-302.

References
Freyburger G, Trillaud H, and Labrouche S, "D-Dimer Strategy in Thrombosis Exclusion. A Gold Standard Study in 100 Patients Suspected of Deep Venous Thrombosis or Pulmonary Embolism: 8 DD Methods Compared," *Thromb Haemost*, 1998, 79(1):32-7.

♦ **Desmopressin** *see* Coagulation Factor Assays *on page 335*

♦ **Desmopressin** *see* von Willebrand Factor *on page 357*

♦ **DIC Screen** *see* Disseminated Intravascular Coagulation Screen *on page 338*

Disseminated Intravascular Coagulation Screen

Related Information
Activated Partial Thromboplastin Time *on page 328*
Anemia Flowchart *on page 392*
D-Dimers and Fibrin Degradation Products *on page 338*
Fibrinogen *on page 341*
Platelet Count *on page 468*
Prothrombin Time *on page 354*

Synonyms Consumptive Coagulopathy Screen; DIC Screen; Screen for Disseminated Intravascular Coagulation

Applies to Fibrinolysis; Schistocytes

Abstract The most useful panel of tests to screen for disseminated intravascular coagulation (DIC) includes D-dimer or fibrin degradation products (FDP), prothrombin time (PT), activated partial thromboplastin time (PTT), platelet count, and fibrinogen. **These tests are not, however, specific for DIC.**

Specimen Plasma (and whole blood for platelet count and peripheral blood smear)

Container Blue top (sodium citrate) tube; lavender top (EDTA) tube for platelet count and peripheral blood smear

Collection Routine venipuncture. Draw blue top before lavender top (EDTA) tube. If a red top is drawn, draw red top tube before blue top tube. Immediately invert tube gently at least 4 times to mix. Blue top tubes must be appropriately filled. Deliver tubes immediately to the laboratory.

Storage Instructions Blue top tube: separate plasma from cells as soon as possible; plasma may be stored on ice for up to 4 hours; otherwise store frozen

Causes for Rejection Blue top tube received more than 4 hours after collection, blue top tube not filled, clotted specimens

Turnaround Time 1-2 hours (often less than 1 hour if requested stat)

Reference Interval See individual tests.

Use Diagnose DIC in patients with an underlying disorder known to cause DIC and/or with clinical suspicion of DIC

Limitations D-dimer and FDP are positive with physiologic clot formation and lysis, and they may be positive in liver disease because they are normally cleared by the liver. Therefore, DIC can be difficult to diagnose in the presence of liver disease in some cases. Results should be reviewed in relation to the clinical situation.

Methodology See individual tests.

Additional Information DIC is a common acquired coagulation disorder resulting from excessive activation of the coagulation system, usually due to massive tissue injury, sepsis, or certain pregnancy complications. The normal anticoagulant and fibrinolytic systems are overwhelmed and cannot contain the coagulation activation, which becomes systemic, resulting in disseminated microvascular thrombi. Thrombosis consumes platelets, coagulation factors, and the natural anticoagulants, which consequently become depleted. The decrease in coagulation factors causes PT and PTT prolongations, and may lead to bleeding. Depletion of platelets also contributes to the bleeding risk. The fibrinolytic system is activated to dissolve the fibrin thrombi, resulting in consumption of plasminogen as it is converted into plasmin, and the formation of fibrin degradation products (FDP) including D-dimers as plasmin degrades fibrin clots. FDP can contribute to bleeding, because they impair fibrin clot formation and interfere with platelet function. In acute DIC, the most obvious clinical symptom is bleeding, although the insidious underlying disseminated microvascular thrombosis may lead to tissue ischemia and consequently multiorgan failure. **The key laboratory findings** are elevated D-dimers or FDP, prolonged PT and/or PTT, and decreased or decreasing platelets and fibrinogen. Repeat testing may be needed to show that fibrinogen and/or platelets are decreasing over time. Fibrinogen is decreased in ~50% of acute DIC cases; the PT is prolonged in ~70%; and the PTT is prolonged in ~50% of acute DIC cases. **Thus, it is important to note that these tests can be normal in a substantial percentage of DIC cases.**[1,2] D-dimer or FDP should be positive in DIC. See D-Dimers and Fibrin Degradation Products *on page 338.*

Chronic DIC may develop when the activation of the coagulation system is low-grade and prolonged, as occurs with malignancy, retained dead fetus, aneurysm,[3] or hemangioma. The clinical features and laboratory findings in chronic DIC can be much more subtle than with acute DIC. Fibrinogen and platelet levels are commonly elevated, because they can increase during acute phase reactions in response to illness (including malignancy), injury, or other conditions. The PT and PTT may actually be short, possibly due to increased circulating activated coagulation factors. Large-vessel thrombosis can occur in chronic DIC of malignancy. The main laboratory abnormality for acute or chronic DIC is positive D-dimers or FDP, neither of which are specific for DIC.

Schistocytes are present on the peripheral blood smear in 50% or more of acute DIC cases.[4,5] Schistocytes are generated by microangiopathic hemolysis of red blood cells severed by flowing through fibrin strands. A large number of other coagulation tests may be abnormal in acute or chronic DIC, but their clinical utility for DIC diagnosis remains uncertain. These include decreases in the natural anticoagulant proteins antithrombin, protein C, and protein S; prolonged thrombin time; elevated markers of coagulation activation (eg, prothrombin fragment 1.2, fibrinopeptide A, fibrinopeptide B, fibrin monomers,[6] thrombin-antithrombin complexes[6]), and the appearance of markers of fibrinolysis (plasmin-antiplasmin complexes,[6] decreased plasminogen, and antiplasmin) (see Hypercoagulation Panel *on page 345*). The thrombin time is often prolonged because of decreased fibrinogen and/or elevated FDP. Elevated FDP interfere with fibrin polymerization, prolonging the thrombin time. Plasma markers of platelet activation, such as platelet factor 4 and beta-thromboglobulin, may also be detected. None of these markers are specific for DIC.

Treatment of the underlying condition is the primary treatment of DIC, along with supportive care including transfusions if needed for bleeding. Heparin use is controversial. New strategies, such as antithrombin concentrates or recombinant activated protein C, are under investigation.[7]

Footnotes

1. Spero JA, Lewis JH, and Hasiba U, "Disseminated Intravascular Coagulation: Findings in 346 Patients," *Thromb Haemost*, 1980, 43:28-33.
2. Siegal T, Seligsohn U, Aghai E, et al, "Clinical and Laboratory Aspects of Disseminated Intravascular Coagulation (DIC): A Study of 118 Cases," *Thromb Haemost*, 1978, 39(1):122-34.
3. Sakakibara Y, Takeda T, Hori M, et al, "Disseminated Intravascular Coagulation in Aortic Aneurysms: Assessment of Consumption Site Using Labeled-Platelet Scintigraphy," *Thorac Cardiovasc Surg*, 1999, 47(3):162-5.
4. Chuansumrit A, Hotrakitya S, Sirinavin S, et al, "Disseminated Intravascular Coagulation Findings in 100 Patients," *J Med Assoc Thai*, 1999, 82(Suppl 1):S63-8.
5. Gilbert JA and Scalzi RP, "Disseminated Intravascular Coagulation," *Emerg Med Clin North Am*, 1993, 11(2):465-80.
6. Wada H, Sakuragawa N, Mori Y, et al, "Hemostatic Molecular Markers Before the Onset of Disseminated Intravascular Coagulation," *Am J Hematol*, 1999, 60(4):273-8.
7. Eisele B and Lamy M, "Clinical Experience With Antithrombin III Concentrates in Critically Ill Patients With Sepsis and Multiple Organ Failure," *Semin Thromb Hemost*, 1998, 24(1):71-80.

References

Baglin T, "Disseminated Intravascular Coagulation: Diagnosis and Treatment," *BMJ*, 1996, 312(7032):683-7.
Levi M and ten Cate H, "Disseminated Intravascular Coagulation," *N Engl J Med*, 1999, 341(8):586-92.
Marder VJ, Feinstein DI, Francis CW, et al, "Consumptive Thrombohemorrhagic Disorders," *Hemostasis and Thrombosis: Basic Principles and Clinical Practice*, 3rd ed, Chapter 52, Colman RW, Hirsh J, Marder VJ, et al, eds, Philadelphia, PA: Churchill Livingstone, 1994, 1023-63.

♦ **Dysfibrinogenemia** *see* Fibrinogen *on page 341*

♦ **Dysfibrinogenemia** *see* Hypercoagulation Panel *on page 345*

♦ **Extrinsic Pathway** *see* Activated Partial Thromboplastin Time *on page 328*

♦ **Extrinsic Pathway** *see* Prothrombin Time *on page 354*

Factor V Leiden

Related Information

Activated Protein C Resistance and the Factor V Leiden Mutation *on page 330*

Coagulation Factor Assays *on page 335*

Homocyst(e)ine, Plasma *on page 193*

Abstract See Activated Protein C Resistance and Factor V Leiden Mutation *on page 330.* The term "factor V Leiden" is often used interchangeably with activated protein C resistance, although they are not true synonyms. The factor V Leiden mutation causes the vast majority of cases of activated protein C resistance. Whether or not additional mutations other than factor V Leiden can cause clinically-significant activated protein C resistance is under continued investigation.

Factor XIII

Related Information

Coagulation Factor Assays *on page 335*

Cryoprecipitate *on page 838*

Plasma, Fresh Frozen *on page 851*

Synonyms Fibrin Stabilizing Factor; Fibrinoligase; Laki-Lorand Factor

Abstract Activated factor XIII stabilizes fibrin clots by cross-linking fibrin strands. Factor XIII deficiency can cause a hereditary bleeding disorder with features including delayed bleeding, umbilical stump bleeding, and miscarriages.

Specimen Plasma

Container One blue top (sodium citrate) tube

Collection Routine venipuncture. If multiple tests are being drawn, draw blue top tubes after any red top tubes but before any lavender top (EDTA), green top (heparin), or gray top (oxalate/fluoride) tubes. Immediately invert tube gently at least 4 times to mix. Tubes must be appropriately filled. Deliver tubes immediately to the laboratory.

Storage Instructions Separate plasma from cells as soon as possible. Plasma may be stored on ice for up to 4 hours; otherwise, store frozen.

Causes for Rejection Specimen received more than 4 hours after collection, tubes not filled, clotted specimens

Turnaround Time Screening assay: 24 hours after incubation begins; quantitative assay: several days (typically it is a send-out test)

Reference Interval Screening assay: Clot stable in 5 M urea for at least 24 hours. If factor XIII deficiency is present, clot will usually dissolve in 1-2 hours. Quantitative assay: 70% to 140% of normal (some newborns have lower levels than adults).[1]

Use Consider this test in patients with evidence for a familial bleeding disorder and a normal PT, PTT, and von Willebrand panel (because factor XIII deficiencies do not prolong the PT or PTT, and von Willebrand disease is a much more common disorder than factor XIII deficiency).

Factor XIII deficiency is rare. It causes delayed bleeding because although fibrin clots can form initially, they are weak and subsequently lyse. Factor XIII consists of two catalytic A subunits and two noncatalytic B subunits. Most mutations causing factor XIII deficiency have so far been found in the A subunit. The PT and PTT are normal in factor XIII deficiency because factor XIII stabilizes the clot after a fibrin clot has formed, whereas the PT and PTT measure the clotting time through initial fibrin formation. Inheritance is autosomal. Formerly, it was believed that heterozygotes are asymptomatic, but more recent evidence suggests they can have bleeding symptoms.[2] Symptoms include poor wound healing, umbilical stump bleeding, miscarriage, prolonged bleeding from superficial wounds, and intracranial hemorrhage, in addition to a number of other bleeding symptoms.

(Continued)

Factor XIII *(Continued)*

Limitations Screening assay: will not detect heterozygotes; quantitative assay: expensive, not readily available, and high ammonia levels may falsely decrease the result

Methodology A qualitative factor XIII assay evaluates clot stability in 5 M urea. The patient sample is clotted by adding calcium, and then after 30 minutes at 37°C the clot is placed in 5 M urea for 24 hours at room temperature. Clots formed by normal individuals remain stable in 5 M urea, while clots from factor XIII deficient patients dissolve in urea. This assay detects only the most severely affected homozygous patients with 1% to 2% factor XIII activity or less. A quantitative assay can detect heterozygous deficiencies (with values of ~50%), but this test is not yet readily available in most U.S. laboratories. In the quantitative assay, factor XIII is activated by thrombin. Activated factor XIII then attaches glycine ethyl ester to a specific peptide substrate, releasing ammonia. The released ammonia generates a subsequent reaction that is detected by a photometer.

Additional Information When fibrin initially forms, fibrin monomers are held together by weak noncovalent hydrogen bonds. Factor XIII is a transglutaminase that stabilizes fibrin clot by cross-linking fibrin monomers with covalent bonds. Calcium is required for its activation by thrombin as well as its activity. It also cross-links antiplasmin to fibrin, which protects the clot from fibrinolysis by plasmin.

A factor XIII polymorphism (Val34Leu), present in nearly half of the population, is suspected to protect against deep venous thrombosis and is somewhat more frequent in patients with intracranial hemorrhage.[3,4] Factor XIII has a long half-life of 10-12 days. Therefore, treatment of factor XIII deficiency can be successful with infrequent doses of cryoprecipitate, fresh frozen plasma, or if available, factor XIII concentrates. Acquired decreases in factor XIII can arise in liver disease (decreased hepatic synthesis), disseminated intravascular coagulation (DIC), certain inflammatory diseases (Crohn, ulcerative colitis, Henoch-Schönlein purpura), leukemia, myelodysplasia, and myeloproliferative disorders. Over 25 cases of inhibitors (antibodies) against factor XIII have been reported.[5,6]

Footnotes

1. Andrew M, Paes B, and Johnston M, "Development of the Hemostatic System in the Neonate and Young Infant," *Am J Pediatr Hematol Oncol*, 1990,12(1):95-104.
2. Seitz R, Duckert F, Lopaciuk S, et al, "ETRO Working Party on Factor XIII Questionnaire on Congenital Factor XIII Deficiency in Europe: Status and Perspectives," *Semin Thromb Hemost*, 1996, 22(5):415-8.
3. Catto AJ, Kohler HP, Coore J, et al, "Association of a Common Polymorphism in the Factor XIII Gene With Venous Thrombosis," *Blood*, 1999; 93(3):906-8.
4. Catto AJ, Kohler HP, Bannan S, et al, "Factor XIII Val 34 Leu: A Novel Association With Primary Intracerebral Hemorrhage," *Stroke*, 1998, 29(4):813-6.
5. Standen G, Birchall J, Morse C, et al, "A Large Bruise," *Lancet*, 1999, 353(9168):1934.
6. Lorand L, Velasco PT, Murthy P, et al, "Autoimmune Antibody in a Hemorrhagic Patient Interacts With Thrombin-Activated Factor XIII in a Unique Manner," *Blood*, 1999, 93(3):909-17.

References

Egbring R, Kroniger A, and Seitz R, "Factor XIII Deficiency: Pathogenic Mechanisms and Clinical Significance," *Semin Thromb Hemost*, 1996, 22(5):419-25.
Mikkola H and Palotie A, "Gene Defects in Congenital Factor XIII Deficiency," *Semin Thromb Hemost*, 1996, 22(5):393-8.

♦ **Factor Assays** *see* Mixing Studies *on page 346*

♦ **Factor I** *see* Fibrinogen *on page 341*

Factor Inhibitors

Related Information

Anticardiolipin Antibody *on page 503*
Antinuclear Antibody *on page 507*
Antiphospholipid Antibody (Lupus Anticoagulant and/or Anticardiolipin Antibody) *on page 331*
Coagulation Factor Assays *on page 335*
Cryoprecipitate *on page 838*
Factor IX Concentrate *on page 841*
Factor VIII Concentrate *on page 841*
Mixing Studies *on page 346*

Synonyms Bethesda Assay; Circulating Anticoagulant; Modified Bethesda Assay

Abstract Specific factor inhibitors are antibodies that inhibit the activity of a specific coagulation factor. A severe acquired bleeding disorder may develop.

Specimen Plasma

Container Three blue top (sodium citrate) tubes

Collection Routine venipuncture. If multiple tests are being drawn, draw blue top tubes after any red top tubes but before any lavender top (EDTA), green top (heparin), or gray top (oxalate/fluoride) tubes. Immediately invert tube gently at least 4 times to mix. Tubes must be appropriately filled. Deliver tubes immediately to the laboratory. Avoid heparin contamination of specimens during specimen collection.

Storage Instructions Separate plasma from cells as soon as possible. Plasma may be stored on ice for up to 4 hours; otherwise, store frozen.

Causes for Rejection Specimen received more than 4 hours after collection, tubes not filled, clotted specimens

Turnaround Time 1 full day or longer (usually performed in a specialized laboratory)

Special Instructions Specific factor inhibitors, such as factor VIII inhibitors, can cause a severe bleeding disorder and treatment can be difficult. Therefore, the specimen should be sent to a laboratory that can perform the assay promptly.

Reference Interval The inhibitor is quantitated in Bethesda units (BU). Each Bethesda unit of inhibitor decreases the factor concentration in the assay by 50%. For example, one unit of factor VIII inhibitor decreases factor VIII from 100% (normal) to 50%, two units decrease it to 25%, three units decrease it to 12.5%, and so on.

Use Performed when mixing studies and factor assays suggest the presence of a specific factor inhibitor, and the findings are not due to a lupus anticoagulant, heparin, or other anticoagulants (see Mixing Studies *on page 346*). For example, if a mixing study shows the characteristic pattern for a factor VIII inhibitor, and factor VIII is the only markedly decreased factor (usually <1% to 10%; mean normal value is 100%), a Bethesda assay should be performed to identify and titer the factor VIII inhibitor.

Methodology Bethesda assay for factor VIII inhibitor:[1] Serial patient plasma dilutions in citrated saline are prepared, from 1:1 up to 1:160 (or higher if necessary for high-titer factor inhibitors). The purpose of these dilutions is to dilute out the inhibitor. The patient plasma dilutions are then mixed with an equal volume of normal plasma containing a normal amount of coagulation factors. The mixed dilutions are usually incubated for up to 2 hours, because certain inhibitors show an inhibitory effect only after prolonged incubation (particularly factor V and factor VIII inhibitors). Factor VIII assays are then performed on each mixed dilution. The dilution that inhibits 50% of factor VIII in the assay defines the titer of the inhibitor. For example, if the 1:40 dilution inhibits 50% of the factor VIII in the assay, the patient is reported to have a titer of 40 BU of factor VIII inhibitor.

Porcine factor VIII can be substituted for normal plasma (which contains human factor VIII) in the Bethesda assay to determine if the factor VIII inhibitor cross-reacts with porcine factor VIII. If there is little or no cross-reactivity, porcine factor VIII is often used to treat bleeding due to a factor VIII inhibitor.

The Bethesda assay can be modified to identify and titer other specific factor inhibitors. For example, if a factor V inhibitor is suspected, factor V assays are performed on the mixed dilutions instead of factor VIII assays.

Additional Information Antibodies that inhibit the activity of a specific coagulation factor can develop spontaneously or in association with certain medications, autoimmune diseases, or other conditions. These antibodies may also arise when a patient with a hereditary factor deficiency is transfused with a product containing the factor, such as a factor concentrate or fresh frozen plasma. The immune system in the patient with the deficiency views the transfused factor as foreign, and forms an antibody against the transfused factor. This complication makes treatment of bleeding episodes difficult in such patients. The most common clinically significant factor inhibitor is a factor VIII inhibitor. Factor VIII inhibitors develop in approximately 10% to 20% of patients with severe hemophilia A and less commonly with mild or moderate hemophilia A, following the infusion of factor VIII-containing products. Rarely, factor VIII inhibitors can also arise spontaneously in persons without hereditary hemophilia. Factor VIII inhibitors cause decreased factor VIII activity and consequently a prolonged PTT. Factor VIII inhibitors exhibit a characteristic pattern in the PTT mixing study where the mixed plasma PTT is initially normal (or significantly more normal than the patient plasma's PTT) but becomes prolonged (typically by increasing at least 8-10 seconds) over the course of a 1- to 2-hour incubation.

Factor IX inhibitors develop in approximately 2% to 12% of patients with severe hemophilia B, and less commonly with mild or moderate hemophilia B, following transfusion of factor IX-containing products.[2] Very rarely, factor IX inhibitors can also arise spontaneously in persons without hereditary hemophilia B. Factor IX inhibitors cause decreased factor IX activity and consequently a prolonged PTT. The prolonged PTT caused by a factor IX inhibitor is immediately prolonged in the PTT mixing study.

Other factor inhibitors arise occasionally following exposure to "fibrin glue" preparations, which are administered topically and intraoperatively to help achieve hemostasis. Fibrin glue is prepared by adding bovine thrombin to human fibrinogen, in the form of cryoprecipitate. The affected patient's immune system views the bovine thrombin as foreign, and forms an antibody against it. Frequently, traces of bovine factors V, VII, or X are also present and antibodies can be generated against these factors as well. The antibodies to bovine coagulation factors sometimes cross-react against the corresponding human coagulation factor, which can lead to bleeding. In one series, 1.7% of patients exposed to bovine thrombin preparations developed a clinically significant inhibitor with bleeding.[3]

Other specific factor inhibitors have also been observed, but most are exceedingly rare. These include inhibitors to factors I (fibrinogen), II, V, VII, X, XI, XII, XIII, and prekallikrein.

Factor V inhibitors may behave like factor VIII inhibitors in the mixing study, with increasing PTT (or PT) prolongation over a 1- to 2-hour incubation.[4] Other factor inhibitors most likely behave like factor IX inhibitors in mixing studies, with immediate prolongation of the PTT (or PT) in the mixed plasma.

Note: Factor inhibitors can cause artifactual decreases in the *in vitro* factor level of other coagulation factors. Therefore, laboratories should perform factor assays at multiple dilutions. At higher dilutions, the inhibitor interference will decrease due to dilution of the inhibitor. For example, a factor VIII inhibitor sometimes causes false decreases in factor IX, XI, or XII assays. Typically, the false decreases, if any, are mild to moderate, whereas the decrease in the truly inhibited factor is typically severe.

Rarely, nonspecific factor inhibition is found with monoclonal gammopathy (paraproteinemia) which can appear to nonspecifically inhibit clotting reactions in the laboratory without targeting any particular coagulation factor. The PT and PTT may be prolonged, and multiple factor assays are nonspecifically inhibited.

Footnotes

1. Brown BA, *Hematology: Principles and Procedures*, 6th ed, Philadelphia, PA: Lea & Febiger, 1993, 256-8.
2. Shapiro SS and Hultin M, "Acquired Inhibitors to the Blood Coagulation Factors," *Semin Thromb Hemost*, 1975, 336-85.
3. Dorion RP, Hamati HF, Landis B, et al, "Risk and Clinical Significance of Developing Antibodies Induced by Topical Thrombin Preparations," *Arch Pathol Lab Med*, 1998, 122(10):887-94.
4. Crowell EB, "Observations on a Factor-V Inhibitor," *Br J Haematol*, 1975, 29(3):397-404.

References

Sahud MA, "Laboratory Diagnosis of Inhibitors," *Semin Thromb Hemost*, 2000, 26(2):195-203.

- ◆ **Factor(s) II, V, VII, VIII, IX, X, XI, XII** *see* Coagulation Factor Assays *on page 335*

- ◆ **Factor VIII:von WIllebrand Factor Ratio** *see* Coagulation Factor Assays *on page 335*

- ◆ **Factor VIII:von Willebrand Factor Ratio** *see* von Willebrand Factor *on page 357*

- ◆ **FBP** *see* D-Dimers and Fibrin Degradation Products *on page 338*

- ◆ **FDP** *see* D-Dimers and Fibrin Degradation Products *on page 338*

- ◆ **FDP** *see* Hypercoagulation Panel *on page 345*

- ◆ **Fibrin Breakdown Products** *see* D-Dimers and Fibrin Degradation Products *on page 338*

- ◆ **Fibrin Monomer** *see* Hypercoagulation Panel *on page 345*

Fibrinogen

Related Information

Activated Partial Thromboplastin Time *on page 328*
Clot Retraction *on page 334*
Coagulation Factor Assays *on page 335*
Cryoprecipitate *on page 838*
D-Dimers and Fibrin Degradation Products *on page 338*
Disseminated Intravascular Coagulation Screen *on page 338*
Factor XIII *on page 339*
Hypercoagulation Panel *on page 345*
Mixing Studies *on page 346*
Plasma, Fresh Frozen *on page 851*
Prothrombin Time *on page 354*
Sedimentation Rate, Erythrocyte *on page 484*
Thrombin Time *on page 356*
Zeta Sedimentation Ratio *on page 500*

Synonyms Factor I

Applies to Acute Phase Reactants; Afibrinogenemia; Dysfibrinogenemia; Plasmin; Sedimentation Rate; Thrombin

Abstract Fibrinogen is converted into fibrin clot by thrombin. Fibrinogen levels <100 mg/dL can be associated with bleeding. Acquired decreases in fibrinogen (eg, with liver dysfunction or DIC) are much more common than hereditary deficiencies.

Specimen Plasma

Container Blue top (sodium citrate) tube

Collection Routine venipuncture. If multiple tests are being drawn, draw blue top tubes after any red top tubes but before any lavender top (EDTA), green top (heparin), or gray top (oxalate/fluoride) tubes. Immediately invert tube gently at least 4 times to mix. Tubes must be appropriately filled. Deliver tubes immediately to the laboratory.

Storage Instructions Separate plasma from cells as soon as possible. Store plasma at room temperature for up to 2 hours, at 2°C to 8°C for up to 4 hours, or store frozen.

Causes for Rejection Specimen received more than 4 hours after collection, tubes not filled, clotted specimen

Turnaround Time Less than 1 day

Reference Interval Approximately 150-400 mg/dL

Use One of several tests performed in a DIC panel, a prolonged PT or PTT evaluation, and an evaluation of a patient with an unexplained bleeding history

Limitations Heparin concentrations >0.6 units/mL can falsely decrease the result with the Clauss method (described below). Usual therapeutic doses of heparin do not significantly affect PT-based methods. The Ellis method is more sensitive to heparin than the Clauss method. Some reagents contain hexadimethrine bromide (Polybrene) to neutralize heparin, allowing fibrinogen to be measured in specimens containing heparin. Fibrin degradation products (FDP) >30-100 µg/mL may decrease fibrinogen values with the Clauss method. Hirudin or argatroban anticoagulation may falsely decrease fibrinogen levels levels with the Clauss and Ellis method, and possibly the PT-based method

Methodology

Functional (activity) assays: The majority of clinical laboratories use the **Clauss**[1] method, which is essentially a dilute thrombin time. A high concentration of thrombin is added to dilute patient plasma, which converts fibrinogen into fibrin clot. The clotting time is inversely proportional to the amount of fibrinogen in the sample. In the **Ellis**[2] method, a lower amount of thrombin is added to undiluted patient plasma and change in turbidity is measured in a spectrophotometer. In the **PT-based method**,[3,4] thromboplastin (tissue factor with phospholipid) is added to undiluted patient plasma to generate endogenous thrombin, and light scatter or turbidity is measured. The measured optical change (before and after fibrin clot formation) is proportional to the amount of fibrinogen in the sample.

Antigen assays (immunoassays) for fibrinogen measure the quantity of fibrinogen without assessing fibrinogen function. This method is not routinely indicated and is usually a send-out test (see Additional Information for its use in dysfibrinogenemia evaluations).

Additional Information Fibrinogen decreases with liver disease, due to decreased hepatic synthesis. However, fibrinogen may be normal or even elevated until late stages of hepatic disease. Fibrinogen decreases in DIC due to excessive thrombin generation, which converts fibrinogen into fibrin. Fibrinogen also decreases with thrombolytic therapy and fibrinolysis because plasmin breaks down fibrinogen in addition to fibrin.

Fibrinogen becomes elevated during acute phase reactions and during pregnancy. As with certain other acute phase reactants (eg, C-reactive protein), elevated fibrinogen has been associated with an increased risk of myocardial infarction.[5]

Hereditary deficiencies of fibrinogen are rare. The PT and PTT may be prolonged. Bleeding symptoms may include bruising, epistaxis, menorrhagia, bleeding with surgery, trauma, dental extractions, and postpartum, and bleeding in the gastrointestinal or genitourinary tract. Miscarriage and poor wound healing are also complications of fibrinogen deficiency. Umbilical stump bleeding and bleeding with circumcision may be noted in newborns with afibrinogenemia. Intracranial hemorrhage has been reported with afibrinogenemia.[6,7,8] In general, deficiencies of fibrinogen tend to be milder than factor VIII or IX deficiencies (hemophilia).

There are three major types of fibrinogen deficiency. The homozygous quantitative form, called afibrinogenemia, results in a severe quantitative deficiency of fibrinogen and an increased risk for bleeding. The heterozygous form of this deficiency is hypofibrinogenemia, with less severe reductions in the fibrinogen level and little or no bleeding.[7] Fibrinogen consists of two copies of each of three polypeptide chains called α, β, and γ. Among the afibrinogenemia mutations that have been characterized thus far, most have been found in the α-fibrinogen chain gene.[9]

Dysfibrinogenemia is a qualitative fibrinogen deficiency, characterized by the production of dysfunctional fibrinogen.[6,8,10] Many different mutations are known to cause hereditary dysfibrinogenemia. Most patients with hereditary dysfibrinogenemia are heterozygous. Rare homozygous cases have been reported. Dysfibrinogenemia patients are usually asymptomatic or have mild bleeding, but severe bleeding has been reported. Interestingly, some dysfibrinogenemia cases are associated with thrombosis, with or without bleeding. Dysfibrinogenemia has an estimated prevalence of 0.8% in patients with venous thrombosis.[6] Arterial thrombosis is less frequent than venous thrombosis in these patients. Acquired forms of dysfibrinogenemia, of uncertain clinical significance, can be seen with liver disease or acute phase reactions with generation of high levels of fibrinogen (Galanakis D, personal communication 1999). The thrombin time and Reptilase® time, which measure the clotting time during the conversion of fibrinogen into fibrin, are often prolonged in dysfibrinogenemia. The PT and PTT may also be prolonged. In dysfibrinogenemia, assays that measure fibrinogen function show lower levels than assays that measure fibrinogen quantity (immunological or "antigen" assays), because fibrinogen function is impaired but fibrinogen quantity is not. This potentially diagnostic disparity between functional and antigen levels may be less pronounced with PT-based functional fibrinogen assays than with Clauss-based functional assays.[3] See Table 3 in Coagulation Factor Assays *on page 335*.

See Thrombin Time *on page 356*.

Footnotes

1. Clauss A, "Rapid Physiological Coagulation Method for the Determination of Fibrinogen [German]," *Acta Haematol*, 1957, 17:237-46.
2. Ellis BC and Stransky A, "A Quick and Accurate Method for the Determination of Fibrinogen in Plasma," *J Lab Clin Med*, 1961, 58:477-88.
3. Rossi E, Mondonico P, Lombardi A, et al, "Method for the Determination of Functional (Clottable) Fibrinogen by the New Family of ACL Coagulometers," *Thromb Res*, 1988, 52(5):453-68.
4. Tan V, Doyle CJ, and Budzynski AZ, "Comparison of the Kinetic Fibrinogen Assay With the von Clauss Method and the Clot Recovery Method in Plasma of Patients With Conditions Affecting Fibrinogen Coagulability," *Am J Clin Pathol*, 1995, 104(4):455-62.

(Continued)

Fibrinogen (Continued)

5. Ma J, Hennekens CH, Ridker PM, et al, "A Prospective Study of Fibrinogen and Risk of Myocardial Infarction in the Physician's Health Survey," *J Am Coll Cardiol*, 1999, 33(5):1347-52.

6. Haverkate F and Samama M, "Familial Dysfibrinogenemia and Thrombophilia. Report on a Study of the SSC Subcommittee on Fibrinogen," *Thromb Haemost*, 1995, 73(1):151-61.

7. Al-Mondhiry H and Ehmann WC, "Congenital Afibrinogenemia," *Am J Hematol*, 1994, 46(4):343-7.

8. Galanakis DK, "Fibrinogen Anomalies and Disease. A Clinical Update," *Hematol Oncol Clin North Am*, 1992, 6(5):1171-87.

9. Neerman-Arbez M, de Moerloose P, Bridel C, et al, "Mutations in the Fibrinogen Aα Gene Account for the Majority of Cases of Congenital Afibrinogenemia," *Blood*, 2000, 96(1):149-52.

10. Cote HC, Lord ST, and Pratt KP, "γ-Chain Dysfibrinogenemias: Molecular Structure-Function Relationships of Naturally Occurring Mutations in the γ Chain of Human Fibrinogen," *Blood*, 1998, 92(7):2195-212.

References

Giangrande PLF, "Other Inherited Disorders of Blood Coagulation," *Haemophilia and Other Inherited Bleeding Disorders*, Rizza C and Lowe G, eds, London: WB Saunders Co, 1997, 291-307.

Heparin Antifactor Xa Assay

Related Information

Synonyms Antifactor Xa Assay; Anti-Xa Assay; Heparin Assay

Applies to Danaparoid; Heparin; LMWH; Low-Molecular Weight Heparin; Orgaran®; PF4; Platelet Factor 4; PTT

Abstract Two relatively new anticoagulants, low-molecular weight heparin (LMWH) and danaparoid (Orgaran®), when present at therapeutic levels, usually do not significantly prolong the activated partial thromboplastin time (PTT). Therefore, when laboratory tests are used to monitor therapeutic anticoagulant levels of LMWH or danaparoid, antifactor Xa assays are necessary. In addition, in some instances the PTT cannot be used to monitor unfractionated heparin. For example, lupus anticoagulants* or certain factor deficiencies (eg, factor XII deficiencies) may prolong the baseline PTT and/or accentuate the PTT prolongation when heparin is added. In these cases, unfractionated heparin may be monitored with antifactor Xa assays (*Note: if the antifactor Xa assay demonstrates that the heparinized PTT is not affected by the lupus anticoagulant, cautious use of the PTT may be tried in that patient).

Specimen Plasma

Container One blue top (sodium citrate) tube

Sampling Time Draw specimen 4 hours after subcutaneous injection of LMWH or 6 hours after subcutaneous injection of danaparoid, otherwise, falsely low values may occur. The therapeutic antifactor Xa ranges with subcutaneous LMWH and danaparoid are defined for the peak levels.

Collection Routine venipuncture. Deliver tube to laboratory immediately, otherwise falsely low values may occur (because platelets release platelet factor 4 (PF4) which can neutralize heparin, LMWH, or danaparoid). If multiple tests are being drawn, draw blue top tubes after any red top tubes but before any lavender top (EDTA), green top (heparin), or gray top (oxalate/fluoride) tubes. Immediately invert tube gently at least 4 times to mix. Tubes must be appropriately filled.

Storage Instructions Separate plasma from cells as soon as possible, ideally within 1 hour of specimen collection. Otherwise, falsely low values may occur (because platelets release PF4, which can neutralize heparin, LMWH, or danaparoid). Plasma can be stored for 2 hours at room temperature or on ice; otherwise, store frozen.

Turnaround Time 1 day, unless testing is batched less frequently

Special Instructions Notify the laboratory specifically as to which drug should be measured (heparin, LMWH, or danaparoid), because the laboratory must construct a standard curve using the same drug that the patient is receiving.

Reference Interval

Patients not on anticoagulants: 0 units/mL

Therapeutic range for **treatment** of existing deep venous thrombosis (DVT):
- heparin 0.3-0.7 units/mL
- LMWH: 0.4-1.1 units/mL for twice daily subcutaneous dosing. For once daily subcutaneous LMWH dosing, the therapeutic range is less certain but is approximately 1-2 units/mL.
- danaparoid: 0.5-0.8 units/mL

Target range for deep vein thrombosis (DVT) prophylaxis (prevention): There is no defined target range for **prophylaxis** of deep vein thrombosis (DVT) because such anticoagulation is not usually monitored. When anti-Xa levels have been measured, mean values have been <0.45 units/mL.

Use Determine if the patient is at the desired level of anticoagulation with therapeutic doses of heparin, LMWH, or danaparoid

Limitations More expensive and less readily available than the PTT for heparin monitoring

Methodology Chromogenic.[1] Patient plasma is added to a known amount of excess factor Xa with excess antithrombin. If heparin (or LMWH or danaparoid) is present in the patient plasma, it will bind to antithrombin and inhibit factor Xa. The amount of residual factor Xa is inversely proportional to the amount of heparin in the plasma. The amount of residual factor Xa is detected by adding a chromogenic substrate that resembles the natural substrate of factor Xa. Factor Xa cleaves the chromogenic substrate, releasing a colored compound that can be detected by a spectrophotometer. Results are reported as anticoagulant concentration in antifactor Xa units/mL, such that high antifactor Xa values indicate high levels of anticoagulation and low antifactor Xa values indicate low levels of anticoagulation. Deficiencies of antithrombin in the patient do not affect the assay, because excess antithrombin is provided in the reaction.

Additional Information Therapeutic doses of unfractionated heparin require intense laboratory monitoring, because the amount of *in vivo* anticoagulation for a given dose is variable. That is, the dose-response for heparin is unpredictable. In contrast, LMWH and danaparoid do have a predictable dose-response, therefore, laboratory monitoring is usually not essential. In fact, if a LMWH or danaparoid antifactor Xa level is subtherapeutic, the most common causes are drawing the specimen at the wrong time (see below) or specimen transportation was longer than 2 hours. Most of the time, LMWH and danaparoid antifactor Xa levels are in the appropriate range when specimens are drawn correctly. Occasions in which periodic monitoring of LMWH might be considered include renal failure, pregnancy (increased dosage requirement in the third trimester), pediatric patients (increased dosage requirement in newborns), obesity, underweight patients, prolonged use, or patients at high risk for bleeding or thrombosis. It is probably also advisable to periodically monitor danaparoid in these same conditions.

The dose-response for unfractionated heparin is unpredictable because many of the heparin chains are long. The long chains can bind nonspecifically to a variety of proteins and cells, and the amounts of these heparin-binding proteins in particular vary considerably among patients, and even vary within the same patient at different times. In contrast, LMWH and danaparoid consist of shorter chains (ie, low-molecular weight) that have much less nonspecific binding.

Causes of subtherapeutic antifactor Xa level:
- specimen drawn at incorrect time (correction times are 4 hours after injection of LMWH, 6 hours after injection of danaparoid)
- specimen transportation longer than 2 hours
- patient receiving prophylactic dose, therefore, therapeutic range is not applicable and anti-Xa level is actually appropriate for dose
- higher dose needed (uncommon with LMWH or danaparoid, more common with heparin, eg, an acute phase state often increases the heparin dose requirement)

Causes of supratherapeutic antifactor Xa level:
- renal failure (with LMWH or danaparoid) (decreased renal clearance)

- heparin contamination, if specimen was drawn from a line
- lower dose needed (uncommon with LMWH or danaparoid, more common with heparin)

Footnotes

1. Teien AN and Lie M, "Evaluation of an Amidolytic Heparin Assay Method: Increased Sensitivity by Adding Purified Antithrombin III," *Thromb Res*, 1977, 10:399-410.

References

Hirsh J, Warkentin TE, Raschke R, et al, "Heparin and Low-Molecular Weight Heparin. Mechanisms of Action, Pharmacokinetics, Dosing Considerations, Monitoring, Efficacy and Safety," *Chest*, 1998, 114(5 Suppl):489-510.

Laposata M, Green D, Van Cott EM, et al, "College of American Pathologists Conference XXXI on Laboratory Monitoring of Anticoagulant Therapy. The Clinical Use and Laboratory Monitoring of Low-Molecular Weight Heparin, Danaparoid, Hirudin and Related Compounds, and Argatroban," *Arch Pathol Lab Med*, 1998, 122(9):799-807.

Olson JD, Arkin CF, Brandt JT, et al, "College of American Pathologists Conference XXXI on Laboratory Monitoring of Anticoagulant Therapy. Laboratory Monitoring of Unfractionated Heparin Therapy," *Arch Pathol Lab Med*, 1998, 122(9):782-98.

♦ **Heparinase** *see* Heparin Neutralization *on page 344*

♦ **Heparin Assay** *see* Heparin Antifactor Xa Assay *on page 342*

♦ **Heparin Cofactor II** *see* Antithrombin *on page 333*

♦ **Heparin Cofactor II** *see* Hypercoagulation Panel *on page 345*

Heparin-Induced Thrombocytopenia

Related Information

Platelet Count *on page 468*
Platelet Transfusion *on page 854*
Warfarin *on page 770*

Synonyms HIT

Applies to Argatroban; Coumadin®; Danaparoid; Heparin; Hirudin; PF4; Platelet Factor 4; Serotonin Release Assays

Abstract Heparin-induced thrombocytopenia (HIT) is a common, serious complication of heparin therapy, with a high risk of potentially catastrophic venous or arterial thrombosis and high mortality.

Specimen Plasma (some laboratories may use serum)

Container Blue top (sodium citrate) tube for plasma (or red top tube if serum is requested); one tube suffices for ELISA or platelet aggregation, more tubes may be required for serotonin release assay.

Collection Routine venipuncture

Storage Instructions Plasma (or serum) can be stored for 24 hours at room temperature; otherwise, store frozen.

Turnaround Time 1 day, unless testing is batched less frequently

Special Instructions For serotonin release or platelet aggregation assays, notify laboratory if patient is receiving heparin. Such specimens should ideally not contain heparin. If heparin is present, it may be removed (adsorbed) by the laboratory prior to testing.

Reference Interval Negative for HIT antibody (HIT antibody not present)

Use Determine if thrombocytopenia or thrombosis in a patient exposed to heparin is due to heparin-induced thrombocytopenia

Limitations The antibody disappears after heparin is discontinued, usually within weeks to months but occasionally longer. Therefore, testing should be performed in the acute setting when HIT is presently suspected.

Methodology Three methods are commonly in use. Enzyme-linked immunosorbent assays (ELISA) use heparin complexed to platelet factor 4 (PF4) as the antigen. In platelet aggregation assays, patient plasma (or serum) is added to normal donor platelets and heparin. If the HIT antibody is present, it stimulates the platelets to aggregate. In serotonin release assays, patient plasma (or serum) and heparin are added to normal platelets that contain radiolabeled serotonin. If the HIT antibody is present, it activates the platelets which then release their serotonin. The released radiolabeled serotonin can then be detected.

Additional Information Thrombocytopenia and thrombosis are the predominant clinical features of HIT. Despite the thrombocytopenia, bleeding complications are uncommon.[1] Up to 8% of heparinized patients develop the antibody that causes HIT without becoming thrombocytopenic.[2,3] Another 1% to 5% of patients on heparin progress further to HIT with thrombocytopenia,[3,4,5,6] and of those, at least 33% develop venous and/or arterial thrombosis.[3,5,6,7,8,9] Thrombosis usually occurs only in HIT patients who are thrombocytopenic. However, thrombosis has been reported in HIT patients with normal platelet counts.[10] Thrombosis in HIT is associated with a mortality of approximately 20% to 30%, with an equal number becoming permanently disabled by amputation, stroke, or other causes.[1,7,8,11] HIT can develop from even small amounts of heparin, such as line flushes or heparin-coated catheters.

In patients receiving heparin for the first time, the platelet count begins to decrease in HIT 4-20 days after initiation of heparin exposure, most commonly between days 5 and 12, with the median on day 10.[1,12] In patients who were sensitized to heparin in the past, platelet counts may decrease within the first 3 days or even hours after re-exposure to heparin.[1,13] A progressive decline in platelet count >50% from baseline or to <100,000/µL is typical of HIT. The median nadir is 50,000/µL (range 20,000-150,000/µL). In patients developing HIT for the first time, the nadir is reached about 5 days after the onset of the decline, although this is variable. In previously sensitized patients, the nadir can be reached as soon as

the first day or two after heparin re-exposure. After discontinuing heparin, the platelet count starts to rise after 2-3 days and usually returns to normal within 4-10 days. However, occasionally the recovery requires up to 25 days.[1,13]

HIT is due to an antibody that recognizes heparin bound to platelet factor 4 (PF4) on the platelet surface. The antibody binds to the heparin-PF4 complex, which then allows the antibody to bind the Fc receptor on the platelet.[14] Interaction with the Fc receptor activates the platelet, resulting in platelet loss (thrombocytopenia) and platelet aggregation (thrombosis). A minority of cases of HIT may involve an antigen other than the PF4-heparin complex.[15]

Among the HIT tests, the ELISA is the most sensitive and platelet aggregation the least sensitive.[16,17,18] The sensitivity of serotonin release or ELISA is ≥90%. Thus, a negative test for HIT does not rule out the diagnosis with complete certainty if HIT is suspected clinically. All three tests have high specificity. However, the significance of a positive ELISA in the absence of thrombocytopenia or thrombosis is uncertain. There is at least one case reported in which the antibody was detected by ELISA 5 days prior to the onset of thrombocytopenia.[18]

Heparin should be permanently discontinued in HIT patients (special arrangements are made for patients who require bypass surgery). Platelet transfusions should be avoided. Patients with HIT are often treated with danaparoid, hirudin, or argatroban. Low-molecular weight heparin (LMWH) has a lower incidence of HIT than unfractionated heparin.[3] However, the cross-reactivity of the HIT antibody against LMWH is high enough that LMWH is also contraindicated for HIT patients, now that the newer alternatives mentioned above are available. Coumadin® should not be used alone in the setting of acute HIT, because it may precipitate venous limb gangrene.[19] If Coumadin® is used, an immediate-acting alternative anticoagulant (eg, hirudin, danaparoid, argatroban) should be used with it until Coumadin® is therapeutic.

Footnotes

1. Greinacher A, "Antigen Generation in Heparin-Associated Thrombocytopenia: The Nonimmunologic Type and the Immunologic Type Are Closely Linked in Their Pathogenesis," *Semin Thromb Hemost*, 1995, 21(1):106-16.
2. Kappers-Klunne MC, Boon DMS, Hop WC, et al, "Heparin-Induced Thrombocytopenia and Thrombosis: A Prospective Analysis of the Incidence in Patients With Heart and Cerebrovascular Diseases," *Br J Haematol*, 1997, 96(3):442-6.
3. Warkentin TE, Levine MN, Hirsch J, et al, "Heparin-Induced Thrombocytopenia in Patients Treated With Low-Molecular Weight Heparin or Unfractionated Heparin," *N Engl J Med*, 1995, 332(20):1330-5.
4. Schmitt BP and Adelman B, "Heparin-Associated Thrombocytopenia: A Critical Review and Pooled Analysis," *Am J Med Sci*, 1993, 305(4):208-15.
5. Warkentin TE and Kelton JG, "Interaction of Heparin With Platelets, Including Heparin-Induced Thrombocytopenia," *Low-Molecular Weight Heparins in Prophylaxis and Therapy of Thromboembolic Diseases*, Bounameaux H, ed, New York, NY: Marcel Dekker Inc, 1994, 75-127.
6. Baglin TP, "Heparin-Induced Thrombocytopenia/Thrombosis Syndrome (HIT): Diagnosis and Treatment," *Platelets*, 1997, 8:72-4.
7. Demasi R, Bode AP, Knupp C, et al, "Heparin-Induced Thrombocytopenia," *Am J Surg*, 1994, 60(1):26-9.
8. Nand S, Wong W, Yuen B, et al, "Heparin-Induced Thrombocytopenia With Thrombosis: Incidence, Analysis of Risk Factors, and Clinical Outcomes in 108 Consecutive Patients Treated at a Single Institution," *Am J Hematol*, 1997, 56(1):12-6.
9. Warkentin TE and Kelton JG, "A 14-Year Study of Heparin-Induced Thrombocytopenia," *Am J Med*, 1996, 101(5):502-7.
10. Hach-Wunderle V, Kainer K, Salzmann G, et al, "Heparin-Related Thrombosis Despite Normal Platelet Counts in Vascular Surgery," *Am J Surg*, 1997, 173(2):117-9.
11. Magnani HN, "Heparin-Induced Thrombocytopenia (HIT): An Overview of 230 Patients Treated With Orgaran (Org 10172)," *Thromb Haemost*, 1993, 70(4):554-61.
12. King DJ and Kelton JG, "Heparin-Associated Thrombocytopenia," *Ann Intern Med*, 1984, 100(4):535-40.
13. Miller ML, "Heparin-Induced Thrombocytopenia," *Cleve Clin J Med*, 1989, 56(5):483-90.
14. Newman PM and Chong BH, "Heparin-Induced Thrombocytopenia: New Evidence for the Dynamic Binding of Purified Anti-PF4-Heparin Antibodies to Platelets and the Resultant Platelet Activation," *Blood*, 2000, 96(1)182-7.
15. Amiral J, Wolf M, Marfaing-Koka A, et al, "Characteristics of Antibodies to PF4, IL-8, and NAP-2 Complexed to Heparin in Patients With Heparin-Induced Thrombocytopenia. A study of 187 cases," *Thromb Haemost* , 1997, (Suppl):449.
16. Chong BH, Burgess J, and Ismail F, "The Clinical Usefulness of the Platelet Aggregation Test for the Diagnosis of Heparin-Induced Thrombocytopenia," *Thromb Haemost*, 1995, 69:344-50.
17. Arepally G, Reynolds C, Tomaski A, et al, "Comparison of PF4/Heparin ELISA Assay With the 14C-Serotonin Release Assay in the Diagnosis of Heparin-Induced Thrombocytopenia," *Am J Clin Pathol*, 1995, 104(6):648-54.
18. Amiral J, Bridey F, Wolf M, et al, "Antibodies to Macromolecular Platelet Factor 4-Heparin Complexes in Heparin-Induced Thrombocytopenia: A Study of 44 Cases," *Thromb Haemost*, 1995, 73(1):21-8.
19. Warkentin TE, "Heparin-Induced Thrombocytopenia: IgG-Mediated Platelet Activation, Platelet Microparticle Generation, and Altered Procoagulant/Anticoagulant Balance in the Pathogenesis of Thrombosis and Venous Limb Gangrene Complicating Heparin-Induced Thrombocytopenia," *Transfus Med Rev*, 1996, 10(4):249-58.

References

Warkentin TE, Chong BH, and Greinacher A, "Heparin-Induced Thrombocytopenia: Toward Consensus," *Thromb Haemost*, 1998, 79(1):1-7.

Heparin Neutralization

Related Information
Activated Clotting Time *on page 328*
Activated Partial Thromboplastin Time *on page 328*
Heparin Antifactor Xa Assay *on page 342*

Synonyms
Heparinase; Hepzyme®

Applies to
ACT; Heparin; PTT

Abstract
Heparin contamination of specimens is a common cause of an unexpected PTT prolongation. Heparinase (Hepzyme®) can be used to determine if the PTT prolongation is due to heparin. In addition, while patients are receiving heparin, it is sometimes necessary to perform coagulation tests that are affected by heparin. In such cases, heparinase can be used to remove heparin from the specimen so that coagulation tests can be performed without heparin interference.

Specimen
Plasma

Container
Blue top (sodium citrate) tube

Collection
Routine venipuncture. If multiple tests are being drawn, draw blue top tubes after any red top tubes but before any lavender top (EDTA), green top (heparin), or gray top (oxalate/fluoride) tubes. Immediately invert tube gently at least 4 times to mix. Tubes must be appropriately filled. Deliver tubes immediately to the laboratory.

Storage Instructions
Separate plasma from cells as soon as possible, ideally within 1 hour of collection. Store plasma according to the guidelines for the individual postheparinase coagulation tests that will be performed.

Causes for Rejection
Specimen received more than 4 hours after collection, tube not full, specimen clotted

Turnaround Time
1 day, unless testing is batched less frequently

Reference Interval
If heparin is the explanation for the prolonged PTT, the PTT will become normal after treatment of the specimen with heparinase.

Use
Determine if an unexpected PTT prolongation is due to heparin contamination; remove known heparin from a specimen so that coagulation tests can be performed without heparin interference

Methodology
To determine if a prolonged PTT is due to heparin, measure the PTT before and after heparinase treatment. 1 mL of patient plasma is added to one vial of heparinase and kept at room temperature for 15 minutes. Heparinase is an enzyme that degrades unfractionated heparin (and low-molecular weight heparin) by cleaving it at multiple sites including within the pentasaccharide sequence. The pentasaccharide sequence is the antithrombin binding site and therefore is required for heparin anticoagulation. Heparinase degradation yields small fragments of about 1000 daltons that lack anticoagulant activity.[1] Heparinase is produced by the bacterium *Flavobacterium heparinum.* Up to 2 units/mL heparin can be degraded. As an alternative to heparinase, heparin-binding cellulose can be used to remove heparin from specimens. The cellulose material is added to the specimen, where it binds to heparin. The specimen is then centrifuged, bringing cellulose and heparin into the pellet. The supernatant plasma is then free of heparin.

Additional Information
Some laboratories use thrombin time to detect heparin. The thrombin time is very sensitive to heparin, therefore, if the thrombin time is normal, heparin cannot account for a PTT prolongation.

In one study, heparin contamination accounted for 39% of unexpected PTT prolongations in patients who were not receiving heparin or Coumadin® treatments.[2] Heparin contamination may account for an unexplained PTT prolongation even when a heparinized line is carefully flushed to remove heparin prior to specimen collection.

If the PTT shortens significantly but remains prolonged after heparinase, a coagulation abnormality may be present in addition to heparin contamination. If a markedly prolonged PTT (eg, >150 seconds) shortens significantly but remains slightly prolonged after heparinase, a small amount of residual heparin is a possible explanation, because the initial amount of heparin contamination was very high. If a second heparinase treatment of the specimen produces a normal PTT, heparin is the confirmed explanation.

Footnotes
1. Lindhardt R, Grant A, Cooney CL, et al, "Differential Anticoagulant Activity of Heparin Fragments Prepared Using Microbial Heparinase," *J Biol Chem,* 1982, 257:7310-3.
2. Newman RS and Fagin AR, "Heparin Contamination in Coagulation Testing and a Protocol to Avoid It and the Risk of Inappropriate FFP Transfusion," *Am J Clin Pathol,* 1995, 104(4):447-9.

References
Ameer GA, Barabino G, Sasisekharan R, et al, "*Ex Vivo* Evaluation of a Taylor-Couette Flow, Immobilized Heparinase I Device for Clinical Application," *Proc Natl Acad Sci U S A,* 1999, 96(5):2350-5.

Hutt ED and Kingdon HS, "Use of Heparinase to Eliminate Heparin Inhibition in Routine Coagulation Assays," *J Lab Clin Med,* 1972, 79(6):1027-34.

Michelsen LG, Kikura M, Levy JH, et al, "Heparinase I (Neutralase) Reversal of Systemic Anticoagulation," *Anesthesiology,* 1996, 85(2):339-46.

◆ **Heparin Resistance** *see* Activated Partial Thromboplastin Time *on page 328*

◆ **Heparin Resistance** *see* Antithrombin *on page 333*

◆ **Hepzyme®** *see* Heparin Neutralization *on page 344*

High-Molecular Weight Kininogen

Related Information
Activated Partial Thromboplastin Time *on page 328*
Coagulation Factor Assays *on page 335*
Mixing Studies *on page 346*
Prekallikrein *on page 350*

Synonyms
HMWK, Fitzgerald Factor; HMW Kininogen; Williams-Fitzgerald-Flaujeac Factor

Abstract
High molecular weight kininogen (HMWK) is a coagulation protein involved in the early stages of intrinsic pathway activation. HMWK deficiency can cause a marked prolongation of the PTT, but it does not cause bleeding. The same is true for factor XII deficiency and prekallikrein deficiency.

Specimen
Plasma

Container
One blue top (sodium citrate) tube

Collection
Routine venipuncture. If multiple tests are being drawn, draw blue top tubes after any red top tubes but before any lavender top (EDTA), green top (heparin), or gray top (oxalate/fluoride) tubes. Immediately invert tube gently at least 4 times to mix. Tubes must be appropriately filled. Deliver tubes immediately to the laboratory.

Storage Instructions
Separate plasma from cells as soon as possible. If test is not performed within 4 hours, freeze plasma.

Causes for Rejection
Specimen received more than 4 hours after collection, tubes not filled, clotted specimens

Turnaround Time
Less than 1 day (longer if test is a send-out)

Special Instructions
Patients cannot be on hirudin or argatroban anticoagulation, which can interfere with mixing studies and HMWK assays. Danaparoid may also interfere with these assays. If heparin is present, notify the laboratory because heparin must be removed prior to testing.

Reference Interval
60% to 140% of normal. Newborns have lower levels than adults; the values increase to near adult normal range by age 6 months.[1]

Use
May be performed when a routine prolonged PTT evaluation finds no explanation for the prolongation (see Mixing Studies *on page 346*). The assay for HMWK (and prekallikrein) can be considered when the following findings are present: the PTT is normal in the mixing study; factors VIII, IX, XI, and XII are normal; the PT and fibrinogen are normal; and lupus anticoagulant assays are negative.

Methodology
A factor assay for HMWK can be performed which is similar to other coagulation factor assays. Patient plasma is mixed with HMWK-deficient plasma and a PTT is performed on the mixture. The amount of HMWK in the patient plasma is determined from a standard curve that plots known amounts of HMWK against PTT values.

Additional Information
HMWK is one of the contact factors that participates in the activation of the intrinsic pathway of coagulation when blood is exposed to a negatively charged foreign surface. With contact activation, activated factor XII (XIIa) converts prekallikrein into kallikrein. Kallikrein then activates more factor XII. HMWK acts as a cofactor in both of these reactions. HMWK also acts as a cofactor in the activation of factor XI by factor XIIa. Kallikrein releases bradykinin from HMWK, which has vasoactive activities. Fibrinolysis is also activated by contact activation. Recent evidence suggests that, *in vivo*, activation of prekallikrein occurs before activation of factor XII.

HMWK deficiency is rare and does not cause bleeding, despite PTT prolongations. The lack of bleeding is presumably because the extrinsic pathway of coagulation, via factor VII and tissue factor, remains intact, and factor XI can be activated by thrombin generated from the extrinsic pathway.[2,3] Thus, factor XI can be activated without the need for HMWK, prekallikrein, or factor XII. This is consistent with the observation that deficiencies of the latter three factors are not associated with bleeding. Acquired, usually mild-to-moderate decreases in HMWK may be found in liver disease or disseminated intravascular coagulation (DIC).

Footnotes
1. Andrew M, Paes B, and Johnston M, "Development of the Hemostatic System in the Neonate and Young Infant," *Am J Pediatr Hematol Oncol,* 1990,12(1):95-104.
2. Gailani D and Broze GJ, "Factor XI Activation in a Revised Model of Blood Coagulation," *Science,* 1991, 253(5022):909-12.
3. Naito K and Fujikawa K, "Activation of Human Blood Coagulation Factor XI Independent of Factor XII. Factor XIa Is Activated by Thrombin and Factor XIa in the Presence of Negatively Charged Surfaces," *J Biol Chem,* 1991, 266(12):7353-8.

References
Schmaier AH, Rojkjaer R, and Shariat-Madar Z, "Activation of the Plasma Kallikrein/Kinin System on Cells: A Revised Hypothesis," *Thromb Haemost,* 1999, 82(2):226-33.

◆ **Hirudin** *see* Activated Partial Thromboplastin Time *on page 328*

◆ **Hirudin** *see* Heparin-Induced Thrombocytopenia *on page 343*

◆ **Hirudin** *see* Mixing Studies *on page 346*

◆ **Hirudin** *see* Prothrombin Time *on page 354*

◆ **HIT** *see* Heparin-Induced Thrombocytopenia *on page 343*

◆ **HMWK, Fitzgerald Factor** *see* High-Molecular Weight Kininogen *on page 344*

♦ **HMW Kininogen** *see* High-Molecular Weight Kininogen *on page 344*

♦ **Hypercoagulable State, Platelet Aggregation** *see* Platelet Hyperaggregation *on page 350*

Hypercoagulation Panel

Related Information
Activated Protein C Resistance and the Factor V Leiden Mutation *on page 330*
Anticardiolipin Antibody *on page 503*
Antiphospholipid Antibody (Lupus Anticoagulant and/or Anticardiolipin Antibody) *on page 331*
Antiplasmin *on page 332*
Antithrombin *on page 333*
C-Reactive Protein, Serum *on page 523*
Heparin Neutralization *on page 344*
Homocyst(e)ine, Plasma *on page 193*
Lipoprotein (a), Serum *on page 215*
Plasminogen *on page 347*
Plasminogen Activator Inhibitor 1 *on page 347*
Platelet Hyperaggregation *on page 350*
Protein C *on page 351*
Protein S *on page 352*
Prothrombin G20210A Mutation *on page 353*
Reptilase® Time *on page 355*
Thrombin Time *on page 356*

Synonyms Screen for Hypercoagulation; Thrombophilia Panel; Thrombotic Disease Screen

Applies to Aα Fragment; Activated Protein C Resistance; Antithrombin Deficiency; Bβ 1-42 Fragment; Beta-Thromboglobulin; D-Dimers; Dysfibrinogenemia; FDP; Fibrin Monomer; Fibrinopeptide A; Fibrinopeptide B; Heparin Cofactor II; Hyperhomocyst(e)inemia; PAI-1; PAP; PF4; Plasmin-Antiplasmin Complexes; Platelet Factor 4; Protein C Deficiency; Protein S Deficiency; Prothrombin Fragment 1.2; Thrombin-Antithrombin Complexes; Tissue Plasminogen Activator; tPA

Abstract Testing is often performed in panels, because the presence of more than one predisposition to thrombosis further increases the risk for thrombosis.[1,2]

Specimen Plasma (and serum if including anticardiolipin antibody and whole blood if including DNA tests)

Container Three blue top (sodium citrate) tubes (and one red top tube if including anticardiolipin antibody)

Collection Routine venipuncture. If a red top tube is being drawn, draw blue top tubes after red top tube. Immediately invert tubes gently at least 4 times to mix. Blue top tubes must be appropriately filled. Deliver tubes immediately to the laboratory.

Storage Instructions Separate plasma from cells as soon as possible. Plasma may be stored on ice for up to 4 hours; otherwise, store frozen.

Causes for Rejection Specimen received more than 4 hours after collection, blue top tubes not filled, blue top tubes clotted

Turnaround Time Several days

Special Instructions Notify laboratory if patient is on any anticoagulant (eg, heparin, warfarin, danaparoid, hirudin, or argatroban). Heparin should be removed from the specimen by the laboratory, and not all tests can be performed when other anticoagulants are present.

Reference Interval See individual tests.

Use Evaluate hypercoagulable states (eg, a young person with spontaneous or recurrent deep venous thrombosis, or a family with multiple members affected by deep venous thrombosis)

Methodology See individual tests.

Venous Thrombosis: Acquired Predisposing Conditions

Advanced age
Collagen/vascular disorders
Heparin-induced thrombocytopenia
Hyperhomocyst(e)inemia
Estrogen (oral contraceptives, pregnancy, and estrogen replacement therapy)
Hyperviscosity
Immobilization
Trauma
Inflammatory bowel disease
Antiphospholipid antibodies
Neoplastic disease and chronic disseminated intravascular coagulation (DIC)
Nephrotic syndrome
Myeloproliferative disorders
Paroxysmal nocturnal hemoglobinuria
Postoperative status
Previous episode of thromboembolism
Indwelling catheter
Obesity

Venous Thrombosis: Hereditary Predisposing Conditions

Disorder	Prevalence in General Population (%)	Prevalence in Venous Thrombosis (%)
Antithrombin deficiency	0.17	1-5
Protein C deficiency	0.14-0.50	3-9
Protein S deficiency	0.7	2-8
Prothrombin G20210A mutation	2	6
Hyperhomocyst(e)inemia (hereditary or acquired)	5-10	10-25
Activated protein C resistance	5 (Caucasians)	20-50

Van Cott EM and Laposata M, "Laboratory Evaluation of Hypercoagulable States," *Hematol Oncol Clin North Am*, 1998, 12(6):1141-66.

Additional Information Venous thromboembolism affects 0.1% of the general population in the United States annually, resulting in over 50,000 deaths every year. Hereditary and acquired predisposing conditions are listed in the tables.

A test panel to evaluate a patient with familial venous thrombosis typically includes assays for activated protein C resistance, protein S, and antithrombin (see table). Activated protein C resistance, discovered in 1993, is the most common known hereditary predisposition to thrombosis. Discovered in 1996, the prothrombin G20210A mutation assay is becoming increasingly included in the test panel as this mutation is one of the most common hereditary predispositions to thrombosis. Assays for antiphospholipid antibodies (lupus anticoagulant and anticardiolipin antibodies) are also recommended, although they are not familial conditions. Homocyst(e)ine is often included, as elevated homocyst(e)ine can be a hereditary or acquired predisposition to venous thrombosis.[3,4,5] Elevated homocyst(e)ine is unique among the hypercoagulable states in that it may be treated with vitamins B_{12}, B_6 and folate. If all these initial tests are normal and the suspicion for a hereditary hypercoagulable state remains high, assays for plasminogen, dysfibrinogenemia, heparin cofactor II, or platelet hyperaggregability may be considered. These latter four conditions are rare and/or not well characterized. Dysfibrinogenemia test results are characterized by prolonged thrombin time and/or Reptilase® time, and fibrinogen levels higher by antigen assay than by functional assay.

If a patient is undergoing an evaluation for arterial thrombosis, the panel of tests may be different. Antiphospholipid antibodies should be included, as these are associated with arterial and/or venous thrombosis. Homocyst(e)ine levels can also be considered, as the evidence linking hyperhomocyst(e)inemia with arterial thrombosis (particularly coronary artery disease) is even more extensive than it is for venous thrombosis. When arterial thrombosis occurs in the setting of atherosclerosis (eg, coronary artery disease/myocardial infarction, stroke), lipoprotein (a) may be considered in addition to the routine cholesterol panel and clinical cardiovascular risk factors (family history, diabetes, hypertension, smoking).[6] Other cardiovascular risk markers are under investigation, including C-reactive protein (or other markers of inflammation) and LDL subclasses (small, dense LDL).[7,8] The other tests described above for evaluation of venous thrombosis (eg, activated protein C resistance) have an uncertain association with arterial thrombosis. It is possible that the markers of venous thrombosis increase the risk for arterial thrombosis only when a second risk factor for arterial thrombosis is present, such as smoking, hypertension, or hypercholesterolemia.[9]

Just as deficiencies of certain coagulation factors may cause bleeding, elevated levels of certain coagulation factors have been implicated in thrombotic risk. For example, high levels of fibrinogen and factor VII have been associated with an increased risk of myocardial infarction, and high levels of factor VIII or XI have been implicated in venous thrombosis.[10,11,12,13] Coagulation factor levels have not yet been added to many hypercoagulation panels, at least partly because the levels are difficult to interpret in individual patient cases.

Markers of coagulation activation are also commercially available, mostly on a research basis. These tests, when elevated, indicate on-going coagulation activation, as may occur in the setting of thrombosis or disseminated intravascular coagulation (DIC). Such tests, not routinely used clinically, include prothrombin fragment 1.2, fibrinopeptide A, fibrinopeptide B, fibrin monomers, thrombin-antithrombin complexes (TAT), platelet factor 4 (PF4) and beta-thromboglobulin. As prothrombin is converted into thrombin, a peptide is released from prothrombin, called prothrombin fragment 1.2. As fibrinogen is converted into fibrin, two peptides called fibrinopeptide A and fibrinopeptide B are released from fibrinogen. The remaining portion of fibrinogen is called a fibrin monomer. Fibrin monomers then polymerize to form fibrin clot. As thrombin is formed, antithrombin binds to thrombin, forming a thrombin-antithrombin complex (TAT), thereby inhibiting thrombin to prevent excessive clotting. Platelet consumption (thrombocytopenia) and platelet activation markers (eg, platelet factor 4 and beta-thromboglobulin) may also be present. Fibrinogen and antithrombin may be consumed, as well as protein C and protein S.

Markers of fibrinolysis are also present in patients with thrombosis or DIC. Tests for these markers are commercially available but, except for the D-dimer and FDP, they are not commonly used clinically. Such tests include: (Continued)

Hypercoagulation Panel (Continued)

plasminogen, antiplasmin, plasmin-antiplasmin complexes (PAP), tissue plasminogen activator (tPA), plasminogen activator inhibitor (PAI-1), Bβ 1-42 fragment and Aα fragment. When fibrinolysis is activated, plasminogen levels may decrease as plasminogen is converted into plasmin. As plasmin degrades fibrin, two peptide fragments, called the Bβ 1-42 fragment and Aα fragment, are released, and FDP and D-dimers are formed. As plasmin is formed, antiplasmin binds to plasmin, forming a plasmin-antiplasmin complex (PAP), thereby inhibiting plasmin to prevent excessive fibrinolysis. Antiplasmin and tPA activity can become decreased, and PAI-1 can increase.

Footnotes

1. Ridker PM, Hennekens CH, Selhub J, et al, "Interrelation of Hyperhomocyst(e)inemia, Factor V Leiden, and Risk of Future Venous Thromboembolism," *Circulation*, 1997, 95(7):1777-82.
2. Koeleman BPC, van Rumpt D, Hamulyak K, et al, "Factor V Leiden: An Additional Risk Factor for Thrombosis in Protein S Deficient Families?" *Thromb Haemost*, 1995, 74(2):580-3.
3. den Heijer M, Blom HJ, Gerrits WBJ, et al, "Is Hyperhomocysteinaemia a Risk Factor for Recurrent Venous Thrombosis?" *Lancet*, 1995, 345(8954):882-5.
4. den Heijer M, Koster T, Blom HK, et al, "Hyperhomocysteinemia as a Risk Factor for Deep-Vein Thrombosis," *N Engl J Med*, 1996, 334(12):759-62.
5. Simioni P, Prandoni P, Burlina A, et al, "Hyperhomocysteinemia and Deep-Vein Thrombosis. A Case Control Study," *Thromb Haemost*, 1996, 76(6):883-6.
6. Schlipak MG, Simon JA, Vittinghoff E, et al, "Estrogen and Progestin, Lipoprotein (a), and the Risk of Recurrent Coronary Heart Disease Events After Menopause," *J Am Med Assoc*, 2000, 283(14):1845-52.
7. Ridker PM, Hennekens CH, Buring JE, et al, "C-Reactive Protein and Other Markers of Inflammation in the Prediction of Cardiovascular Disease in Women," *N Engl J Med*, 2000, 342(12):836-43.
8. Lamarche B, Tchernof A, Moorjani S, et al, "Small, Dense Low-Density Lipoprotein Particles as a Predictor of the Risk of Ischemic Heart Disease in Men. Prospective Results From the Quebec Cardiovascular Study," *Circulation*, 1997, 95(1):69-75.
9. Inbal A, Freimark D, Modan B, et al, "Synergistic Effects of Prothrombotic Polymorphisms and Atherogenic Factors on the Risk of Myocardial Infarction in Young Males," *Blood*, 1999, 93(7):2186-90.
10. Iacoviello L, Di Castelnuovo A, de Knijff P, et al, "Polymorphisms in the Coagulation Factor VII Gene and the Risk of Myocardial Infarction," *N Engl J Med*, 1998, 338(2):79-85.
11. Ma J, Hennekens CH, Ridker PM, et al, "A Prospective Study of Fibrinogen and Risk of Myocardial Infarction in the Physician's Health Study," *J Am Coll Cardiol*, 1999, 33(5):1347-52.
12. van der Meer FJM, Koster T, Vandenbroucke JP, et al, "The Leiden Thrombophilia Study (LETS)," *Thromb Haemost*, 1997, 78(1):631-5.
13. Meijers JC, Tekelenburg WL, Bouma BN, et al, "High Levels of Coagulation Factor XI as a Risk Factor for Venous Thrombosis," *N Engl J Med*, 2000, 342(10):696-701.

References

De Stefano V, Finazzi G, and Mannucci PM, "Inherited Thrombophilia: Pathogenesis, Clinical Syndromes, and Management," *Blood*, 1996, 87(9):3531-44.

Simioni P, Sanson BJ, Prandoni P, et al, "Incidence of Venous Thromboembolism in Families With Inherited Thrombophilia," *Thromb Haemost*, 1999, 81(2):198-202.

Tripodi A and Mannucci PM, "Markers of Activated Coagulation and Their Usefulness in the Clinical Laboratory," *Clin Chem*, 1996, 42(5):664-9.

Van Cott EM and Laposata M, "Laboratory Evaluation of Hypercoagulable States," *Hematol Oncol Clin North Am*, 1998, 12(6):1141-66.

Mixing Studies

Related Information

Synonyms Circulating Anticoagulant Screen; Inhibitor Screen

Applies to Argatroban; Danaparoid; Factor Assays; Heparin; Hirudin

Abstract Mixing studies can be performed when the PT or PTT is prolonged, to determine if the etiology of the prolongation is a factor deficiency or an inhibitor.

Specimen Plasma

Container Blue top (sodium citrate) tubes

Collection Routine venipuncture. If multiple tests are being drawn, draw blue top tubes after any red top tubes but before any lavender top (EDTA), green top (heparin), or gray top (oxalate/fluoride) tubes. Immediately invert tube gently at least 4 times to mix. Tubes must be appropriately filled. Deliver tubes immediately to the laboratory.

Storage Instructions Separate plasma from cells as soon as possible. Plasma may be stored on ice for up to 4 hours; otherwise, store frozen.

Causes for Rejection Specimen received more than 4 hours after collection, tubes not filled, clotted specimen

Turnaround Time Several hours; longer if additional follow-up tests are indicated

Special Instructions Notify the laboratory if patient is on heparin (including low-molecular-weight heparin), hirudin, danaparoid, or argatroban anticoagulation, any of which can prolong PTT and/or PT.

Reference Interval There are three types of results in the PTT mixing study:

1. If the PTT of the mixture is normal, and remains normal after prolonged (2-hour) incubation, the results indicate the presence of factor deficiency(ies). The PTT is normal in such mixtures because the normal plasma supplies the factor that is deficient in the patient plasma. There may be one or more deficient factors. Assays for factors VIII, IX, XI, and XII should then be performed to identify the specific factor deficiency(ies). If the PT is also prolonged, common pathway factor assays can also be considered.

2. If the PTT of the mixture remains prolonged, the results suggest the presence of an inhibitor, most commonly, a lupus anticoagulant. Therefore, lupus anticoagulant assays should then be performed. Heparin, hirudin, argatroban, or high-dose danaparoid, if present, will also show this type of result in a mixing study. Specific factor inhibitors against a particular coagulation factor (eg, factor IX, XI, or XII), are very rare possibilities.

3. If the PTT of the mixture is initially normal (or significantly shorter than the patient plasma's PTT) but becomes prolonged after a 1- or 2-hour incubation, the results are characteristic of a factor VIII inhibitor (factor VIII inhibitors show an inhibitory effect only after prolonged incubation). A factor VIII assay should then be performed and, if decreased (usually to <10%), a factor VIII inhibitor assay (Bethesda assay) should be performed.

When the PT is prolonged and the PTT is normal, a PT mixing study may also be useful in determining if the etiology is a factor deficiency or a factor inhibitor, similar to that described for the PTT. However, factor inhibitors that affect only the PT and not the PTT are rare. The results of PT mixing studies in patients on warfarin are consistent with factor deficiencies, because warfarin acts as an anticoagulant by decreasing the activity of factors II, VII, IX, and X.

Methodology When the PTT is prolonged, the laboratory should first determine if the prolongation is due to heparin by treating the specimen to remove heparin (see Heparin Neutralization *on page 344*). Alternatively, some laboratories perform the thrombin time, which is prolonged when even a small amount of heparin is in the sample. If a prolonged PTT is not due to heparin, patient plasma is then mixed with an equal volume of normal plasma, and the PTT is repeated. The resulting PTT of this mixture indicates whether the prolongation is due to a factor deficiency or an inhibitor. Inhibitors are substances that inhibit clotting reactions. They are usually antibodies (eg, lupus anticoagulants or specific factor inhibitors) or anticoagulants such as heparin, hirudin, or argatroban. Based on the mixing study results, factor assays, lupus anticoagulant tests, or tests for factor inhibitors may be indicated. PT mixing studies can be similarly performed to evaluate PT prolongations.

References

Clyne LP, Yen Y, Kriz NS, et al, "The Lupus Anticoagulant. High Incidence of Negative Mixing Studies in a Human Immunodeficiency Virus-Positive Population," *Arch Pathol Lab Med*, 1993, 117(6):595-601.

Kaczor DA, Bickford NN, and Triplett DA, "Evaluation of Different Mixing Study Reagents and Dilution Effect in Lupus Anticoagulant Testing," *Am J Clin Pathol*, 1991, 95(3):408-11.

Van Cott EM and Laposata M, "Coagulation, Fibrinolysis and Hypercoagulation," *Clinical Diagnosis and Management by Laboratory Methods*, 20th ed, Henry JB, ed, New York, NY: WB Saunders Co, in press.

- ♦ **Modified Bethesda Assay** *see* Factor Inhibitors *on page 340*
- ♦ **Multimer Assay** *see* von Willebrand Factor *on page 357*
- ♦ **NAIT** *see* Platelet Antibodies *on page 349*
- ♦ **Neonatal Alloimmune Thrombocytopenia** *see* Platelet Antibodies *on page 349*
- ♦ **Organan®** *see* Heparin Antifactor Xa Assay *on page 342*
- ♦ **PAI-1** *see* Hypercoagulation Panel *on page 345*
- ♦ **PAI-1** *see* Plasminogen Activator Inhibitor 1 *on page 347*
- ♦ **PAP** *see* Hypercoagulation Panel *on page 345*
- ♦ **Partial Thromboplastin Time** *see* Activated Partial Thromboplastin Time *on page 328*
- ♦ **PF4** *see* Heparin Antifactor Xa Assay *on page 342*
- ♦ **PF4** *see* Heparin-Induced Thrombocytopenia *on page 343*
- ♦ **PF4** *see* Hypercoagulation Panel *on page 345*
- ♦ **Plasma Thromboplastin Antecedent (Factor XI)** *see* Coagulation Factor Assays *on page 335*
- ♦ **Plasma Thromboplastin Component (Factor IX)** *see* Coagulation Factor Assays *on page 335*
- ♦ **Plasmin** *see* D-Dimers and Fibrin Degradation Products *on page 338*
- ♦ **Plasmin** *see* Fibrinogen *on page 341*
- ♦ **Plasmin-Antiplasmin Complexes** *see* Hypercoagulation Panel *on page 345*
- ♦ **Plasmin Inhibitor** *see* Antiplasmin *on page 332*

Plasminogen

Related Information
Disseminated Intravascular Coagulation Screen *on page 338*
Hypercoagulation Panel *on page 345*
Plasminogen Activator Inhibitor 1 *on page 347*

Applies to Acute Phase Reactants; Conjunctivitis, Ligneous; Fibrinogenolysis; Fibrinolysis; Tissue Plasminogen Activator; tPA; uPA; Urokinase-Type Plasminogen Activator

Abstract Plasminogen is the precursor of plasmin, which lyses fibrin clots. Hereditary plasminogen deficiency is rare, and it may predispose to venous thrombosis.

Specimen Plasma

Container Blue top (sodium citrate) tube

Collection Routine venipuncture. If multiple tests are being drawn, draw blue top tubes after any red top tubes but before any lavender top (EDTA), green top (heparin), or gray top (oxalate/fluoride) tubes. Immediately invert tube gently at least 4 times to mix. Tubes must be appropriately filled. Deliver tubes immediately to the laboratory.

Storage Instructions Separate plasma from cells as soon as possible. Store plasma on ice for up to 4 hours, or store frozen.

Causes for Rejection Specimen received more than 4 hours after collection, tubes not filled, clotted specimens

Turnaround Time 1 day or longer, depending on how often testing is batched

Reference Interval Functional results are reported as a percent of the amount expected in normal plasma. By definition, the mean value in normal plasma is 100%. The reference range is approximately 75% to 130%. Antigen results may be reported in mg/dL, with a reference range of approximately 6-14 mg/dL. Plasminogen levels can increase during pregnancy. Newborn levels are about 60% of adult values. Newborn levels increase to near adult values by age 6 months.[1]

Use May be considered in patients with familial venous thrombosis and no evidence for more common hypercoagulable states. Occasionally, if monitoring of thrombolytic therapy is desired, plasminogen levels are followed. Plasminogen decreases during thrombolytic therapy. Consider testing plasminogen in patients with ligneous conjunctivitis, a condition that is associated with severe plasminogen deficiency.

Limitations Plasminogen may become elevated during pregnancy and during acute phase reactions. Antigen assays will not detect qualitative (dysfunctional) deficiencies.

Methodology
Functional (activity) assays: Chromogenic assays for plasminogen are available. Streptokinase is added to patient plasma, which binds to plasminogen. The streptokinase-plasminogen complex has plasmin-like activity[2] which cleaves a chromogenic substrate, releasing a colored compound. The amount of color detected spectrophotometrically is proportional to the amount of plasminogen in the sample.

Antigen (immunologic) assays: Radial immunodiffusion methods are commercially available.

Additional Information Plasminogen is converted into plasmin by tissue plasminogen activator (tPA) or urokinase-type plasminogen activator (uPA). Plasmin degrades fibrin clots (fibrinolysis) as well as intact fibrinogen (fibrinogenolysis). Plasmin also inactivates factors Va and VIIIa. Plasminogen can be decreased during thrombolytic therapy, liver disease, disseminated intravascular coagulation (DIC), and rarely, with a hereditary plasminogen deficiency. The incidence of plasminogen deficiency is 0.29% to 0.73% in healthy individuals, up to 1.4% to 2.2% among patients with venous thrombosis, and 1.4% among patients with arterial thrombosis.[3,4,5] In one study, 2.5% of a general population with plasminogen deficiency had a history of thrombosis.[5] Hereditary deficiencies of plasminogen could result in decreased fibrinolysis. However, the association with thrombosis is somewhat uncertain. In some studies, plasminogen-deficient relatives of affected individuals have similar rates of thrombosis as nondeficient relatives,[4] whereas in other studies they do have a higher rate of thrombosis.[6] Severe hereditary plasminogen deficiency is associated with ligneous conjunctivitis, a rare chronic pseudomembranous conjunctivitis characterized histologically by massive deposits of fibrin in the affected tissues.[7,8] Apparently, the fibrin depositions result from decreased or absent clearance of fibrin by plasminogen.

Footnotes
1. Andrew M, Paes B, Milner R, et al, "Development of the Human Coagulation System in the Full-Term Infant," *Blood*, 1987, 70(1):165-72.
2. Reddy KN and Markus G, "Mechanism of Activation of Human Plasminogen by Streptokinase: Presence of Active Center in Streptokinase-Plasminogen Complex," *J Biol Chem*, 1972, 247(6):1683-91.
3. Heijboer H, Brandjes DP, Buller HR, et al, "Deficiencies of Coagulation-Inhibiting and Fibrinolytic Proteins in Outpatients With Deep-Vein Thrombosis," *N Engl J Med*, 1990, 323(22):1512-6.
4. Biasiutti FD, Sulzer I, and Stucki B, "Is Plasminogen Deficiency a Thrombotic Risk Factor? A study on 23 Thrombophilic Patients and Their Family Members," *Thromb Haemost*, 1998, 80:167-70.
5. Tait RC, Walker ID, Conkie JA, et al, "Isolated Familial Plasminogen Deficiency May Not Be a Risk Factor for Thrombosis," *Thromb Haemost*, 1996, 76(6):1004-8.
6. Girolami A, Sartori MT, Saggiorato G, et al, "Symptomatic Versus Asymptomatic Patients in Congenital Hypoplasminogenemia: A Statistical Analysis," *Haematologia (Budap)*, 1994, 26(2):59-65.
7. Schuster V, Seidenspinner S, Zeitler P, et al, "Compound-Heterozygous Mutations in the Plasminogen Gene Predispose to the Development of Ligneous Conjunctivitis," *Blood*, 1999, 93(10):3457-66.
8. De Cock R, Ficker LA, Dart JG, et al, "Topical Heparin in the Treatment of Ligneous Conjunctivitis," *Ophthalmology*, 1995, 102(11):1654-9.

Plasminogen Activator Inhibitor 1

Related Information
Antiplasmin *on page 332*
Plasminogen *on page 347*

Synonyms PAI-1

Applies to Acute Phase Reactants; Tissue Plasminogen Activator; tPA

Abstract PAI-1 inhibits tissue plasminogen activator (tPA). High levels of PAI-1 may be associated with an increased risk of arterial thrombosis due to inhibition of fibrinolysis, and low levels of PAI-1 characterize a rare familial bleeding disorder due to excessive fibrinolysis.[1,2] A causal effect of high levels of PAI-1 on arterial thrombosis has not yet been established.

Specimen Plasma

Container Blue top (sodium citrate) tube. Specialized tubes containing platelet inhibitors (to prevent platelet release of PAI-1) or acid (to prevent PAI-1 from forming a complex with tPA) have been recommended, but are not necessary if specimens are handled appropriately.[3]

Sampling Time PAI-1 has a circadian rhythm: its plasma concentration is highest in the morning, and lowest in the afternoon and evening. In one study, the mean level was 23 ng/mL at 9 AM and 10 ng/mL at 4 PM.[3]

Collection Collect blood from a steadily flowing venipuncture. Discard the first 3-5 mL if PAI-1 is the only test being drawn. If multiple tests are being drawn, draw blue top tubes after any red top tubes but before any lavender top (EDTA), green top (heparin), or gray top (oxalate/fluoride) tubes. Immediately invert tube gently at least 4 times to mix. Tubes must be appropriately filled. Deliver tubes immediately to the laboratory.

Storage Instructions Separate plasma from cells as soon as possible. Laboratories should avoid platelet contamination of plasma because platelets contain PAI-1. Centrifugation at 2000-3000 g for 15 minutes helps ensure platelet-free plasma.[3] Store plasma on ice for up to 2 hours, or store frozen.

Causes for Rejection Specimen received more than 2 hours after collection; tubes not filled; clotted specimens; antifibrinolytic agent present in specimen, such as aprotinin or epsilon-aminocaproic acid, which interfere with functional PAI-1 assays

Turnaround Time Usually at least several days, as testing is often batched

Reference Interval Approximately 4-40 ng/mL in antigen assay[4] and 0-12 units/mL in functional assay (see Sampling Time for note regarding circadian rhythm)

Use Not a commonly performed clinical assay. May be considered in patients with strong evidence for a familial bleeding disorder and normal test results for more common bleeding disorders (eg, von Willebrand disease). May be considered in patients with unexplained premature myocardial infarction. (Continued)

Plasminogen Activator Inhibitor 1 *(Continued)*

Limitations PAI-1 is an acute phase reactant.[5] Therefore, it becomes elevated following a thrombotic event and it should not be measured in the acute setting following thrombosis. A related inhibitor, PAI-2, is normally not present in plasma. However, it becomes elevated in pregnant women and can cause overestimations of PAI-1 during pregnancy. PAI-1 also becomes elevated during pregnancy. Antigen assays will not detect qualitative deficiencies.

Methodology

Functional (activity) assays:[6] Patient plasma is added to a known amount of urokinase; PAI-1 in the patient plasma binds and inhibits the urokinase. The amount of residual urokinase is detected by adding plasminogen, which is converted to plasmin by urokinase. Plasmin cleaves a chromogenic synthetic substrate, releasing a colored compound which can be detected spectrophotometrically. The amount of released color is inversely proportional to the amount of PAI-1 in the sample. This assay contains an inhibitor of antiplasmin and other plasmin inhibitors to prevent these other inhibitors from interfering with the assay. Another version of this assay uses tPA instead of urokinase, and an acidification step to destroy antiplasmin and other plasmin inhibitors.

Antigen (enzyme-linked immunosorbent) assays are also available.[4]

Additional Information PAI-1 is produced by the endothelium and liver and is also present in platelets. PAI-1 inhibits both tPA and urokinase-type plasminogen activator (uPA). PAI-1 may be active, inactive, or complexed with tPA.

The relationship between elevated PAI-1 and coronary artery disease may be at least partly due to its association with established cardiovascular risk factors, namely, the syndrome of insulin resistance. Elevated PAI-1 is associated with an increased incidence of myocardial infarction in prospective studies, but the association has not always remained significant after adjusting for other factors such as insulin resistance.[7] The synthesis of PAI-1 is increased by high glucose or insulin levels. PAI-1 levels are elevated in insulin resistance, which is associated with a constellation of lipid and other abnormalities and an increased risk of coronary artery disease. Weight loss, which may reduce insulin resistance, also reduces PAI-1.[8] Studies are conflicting regarding an association between a PAI-1 polymorphism, higher PAI-1 levels, and myocardial infarction.[9]

Footnotes

1. Fay WP, Shapiro AD, Shih JL, et al, "Brief Report: Complete Deficiency of Plasminogen-Activator Inhibitor Type 1 Due to a Frame-Shift Mutation," *N Engl J Med*, 1992, 327(24):1729-33.
2. Takahashi Y, Tanaka T, Minowa H, et al, "Hereditary Partial Deficiency of Plasminogen Activator Inhibitor-1 Associated With a Life-Long Bleeding Tendency," *Int J Hematol*, 1996, 64(1):61-8.
3. Macy EM, Meilahn EN, Declerck PJ, et al, "Sample Preparation for Plasma Measurement of Plasminogen Activator Inhibitor-1 Antigen in Large Population Studies," *Arch Pathol Lab Med*, 1993, 117(1):67-70.
4. Declerck PJ, Alessi MC, Verstreken M, et al, "Measurement of Plasminogen Activator Inhibitor 1 in Biologic Fluids With a Murine Monoclonal Antibody-Based Enzyme-Linked Immunosorbent Assay," *Blood*, 1988, 71(1):220-5.
5. Jansson JH, Norberg B, and Nilsson TK, "Impact of Acute Phase on Concentrations of Tissue Plasminogen Activator and Plasminogen Activator Inhibitor in Plasma After Deep Vein Thrombosis or Open Heart Surgery," *Clin Chem*, 1989, 35(7):1544-5.
6. Contant G, Nicham F, and Martinoli JL, "Determination of Plasminogen Activator Inhibitor (PAI) by a New Venom-Based Assay," *Fibrinolysis*, 1992, 6(Suppl 3):85-6.
7. Juhan-Vague I, Pyke SD, Alessi MC, et al, "Fibrinolytic Factors and the Risk of Myocardial Infarction or Sudden Death in Patients With Angina Pectoris. ECAT Study Group. European Concerted Action on Thrombosis and Disabilities," *Circulation*, 1996, 94(9):2057-63.
8. Svendsen OL, Hassager C, Christiansen C, et al, "Plasminogen Activator Inhibitor-1, Tissue-Type Plasminogen Activator, and Fibrinogen. Effect of Dieting With or Without Exercise in Overweight Postmenopausal Women," *Arterioscler Thromb Vasc Biol*, 1996, 16(3):381-5.
9. Mikkelsson J, Perola M, Wartiovaara U, et al, "Plasminogen Activator Inhibitor-1 (PAI-1) 4G/5G Polymorphism, Coronary Thrombosis, and Myocardial Infarction in Middle-Aged Finnish Men Who Died Suddenly," *Thromb Haemost*, 2000, 84(1):78-82.

References

Kohler HP and Grant PJ, "Plasminogen-Activator Inhibitor Type I and Coronary Artery Disease," *N Engl J Med*, 2000, 342(24):1792-801.

Lane DA and Grant PJ, "Role of Hemostatic Gene Polymorphisms in Venous and Arterial Thrombotic Disease," *Blood*, 2000, 95(5):1517-32.

Platelet Aggregation

Related Information

Activated Partial Thromboplastin Time *on page 328*
Platelet Count *on page 468*
Platelet Hyperaggregation *on page 350*
Prothrombin Time *on page 354*
von Willebrand Factor *on page 357*

Synonyms Aggregometer Test; Platelet Function Studies

Applies to ATP:ADP Ratio; Beta-Thromboglobulin

Test Includes Response to adenosine diphosphate (ADP), epinephrine, collagen, ristocetin, and arachidonic acid

Abstract Platelet aggregation tests are used to assess platelet function.

Patient Preparation Patients should not have aspirin (or any medication containing aspirin) for at least 7 days prior to testing. Nonsteroidal anti-inflammatory drugs or other platelet-inhibiting agents should also be avoided.

Specimen Platelet-rich plasma

Container Three blue top or plastic (sodium citrate) tubes

Collection Routine venipuncture. Immediately invert tubes gently at least 4 times to mix. Deliver tubes immediately to the laboratory at room temperature (platelets are activated at cold temperatures).

Storage Instructions Keep specimen at room temperature and perform test immediately (or within 2 hours, if transportation to a reference laboratory is required). Do not refrigerate or freeze specimen.

Causes for Rejection Specimen received more than 2 hours after collection, specimen clotted, specimen received on ice.

Turnaround Time Less than 1 day

Special Instructions Usually must be scheduled in advance with the laboratory.

Reference Interval >60% of platelets aggregate with each agonist tested. Normally no significant spontaneous aggregation. Normal newborns can have decreased aggregation compared to adults.[1]

Use Assess platelet function. When a familial bleeding disorder is suspected, this test is usually not performed unless routine tests are normal (PT, PTT, and platelet count) and von Willebrand tests are normal, because von Willebrand disease is much more common than hereditary platelet dysfunction.

Methodology Citrated plasma is centrifuged at a gentle speed, to draw red and white blood cells into a pellet, leaving platelets suspended in the plasma. Various platelet aggregating agents (agonists) are added to aliquots of the platelet-rich plasma, and the resulting platelet aggregation is measured in an aggregometer.[2] The aggregometer measures platelet aggregation by monitoring optical density. As platelets aggregate, more light can pass through the specimen. The platelet agonists commonly include arachidonate, ADP, collagen, epinephrine, and ristocetin. One aliquot usually has no platelet agonist added, to assess for spontaneous platelet aggregation.

A rapid, whole blood point-of-care device has been compared to platelet aggregation in monitoring platelet function during antiplatelet therapy.[3] Another rapid whole blood platelet function analyzer has been studied in small numbers of patients with various platelet function abnormalities.[4]

Additional Information The most common cause of platelet dysfunction detected in this assay is medications. With aspirin and related compounds, arachidonate aggregation is markedly decreased or absent, and other aggregation tracings may be variably impaired. A variety of other platelet-inhibiting agents, such as ticlopidine, clopidogrel, and abciximab, are known to impair platelet aggregation. A vast number of other medications have been implicated in impaired *in vitro* platelet aggregation, and the clinical significance, if any, is usually uncertain. If a patient is found to have impaired platelet aggregation in this assay, a careful review of prescribed, as well as over-the-counter medications, is indicated. An on-line literature search for each medication is often informative. Other acquired causes of impaired platelet aggregation include uremia and paraproteinemia (monoclonal gammopathy). Myeloproliferative disorders can impair platelet aggregation, by epinephrine in particular. Hyperaggregation has also been reported with myeloproliferative disorders.

Hereditary platelet dysfunction is far less common than acquired dysfunction. A hereditary disorder may be considered in patients with bleeding histories and no obvious acquired etiology to account for an abnormal platelet aggregation study. Ideally, the aggregation study is repeated on a fresh specimen to determine if the abnormality is reproducible. The presence of the same abnormality in family members supports the diagnosis of a hereditary defect. Platelet storage pool disorders may variably decrease responses to epinephrine, ADP, and occasionally other agonists. Platelet storage pool disorders are characterized by deficiencies in alpha or dense platelet granules. Alpha granules normally store platelet factor 4 (PF4), beta-thromboglobulin, and other substances. Dense granules normally contain ADP, serotonin, and other compounds. Alpha granule deficiency is a rare disorder called "gray platelet syndrome," because platelets appear gray with light microscopy due to a lack of alpha granules. Alpha granules give normal platelets their purple granular appearance. In gray platelet syndrome, platelets are large; thrombocytopenia may be present; and beta-thromboglobulin (a research test) is decreased in platelets but may be elevated in plasma. A research test for dense granule deficiency is the platelet ATP:ADP ratio, which is increased with dense granule deficiency. Uncommonly, patients are deficient in both alpha and dense granules. Rare genetic disorders may underlie some cases of storage pool deficiency, including Hermansky-Pudlak syndrome (dense granule granule deficiency with pulmonary fibrosis and albinism), Chédiak-Higashi syndrome, Wiskott-Aldrich syndrome, or thrombocytopenia with absent radius syndrome.

Glanzmann thrombasthenia is a rare inherited condition in which platelet glycoprotein IIb/IIIa (GPIIb/IIIa) is deficient. GPIIb/IIIa mediates platelet aggregation using fibrinogen to link platelets to each other. Therefore, in Glanzmann thrombasthenia, aggregation is decreased with all agonists (ADP, collagen, epinephrine, arachidonate) except ristocetin. Ristocetin agglutinates platelets using von Willebrand factor and platelet glycoprotein Ib (GPIb). Bernard-Soulier disease is a rare inherited disorder characterized by GPIb deficiency and therefore decreased ristocetin-induced aggregation.

Giant platelets and often thrombocytopenia are also present. With severe von Willebrand disease, ristocetin aggregation can be decreased, but most cases of von Willebrand disease are mild and ristocetin aggregation is most often normal. For that reason, platelet aggregation is not used to screen for von Willebrand disease.

Note: The term "agglutination" is often used to describe ristocetin-induced platelet aggregation, because true platelet aggregation links platelets through fibrinogen and GPIIb/IIIa, whereas ristocetin links platelets through von Willebrand factor and GPIb.

Footnotes

1. Michelson AD, "Platelet Function in the Newborn," *Semin Thromb Hemost*, 1998, 24(6):507-12.
2. Brown BA, *Hematology: Principles and Procedures*, 6th ed, Philadelphia, PA: Lea & Febiger, 1993, 271-4.
3. Kereiakes DJ, Broderick TM, Roth EM, et al, "Time Course, Magnitude, and Consistency of Platelet Inhibition by Abciximab, Tirofiban, or Eptifibatide in Patients With Unstable Angina Pectoris Undergoing Percutaneous Coronary Intervention," *Am J Cardiol*, 1999, 84(4):391-5.
4. Fressinaud E, Veyradier A, Truchaud F, et al, "Screening for von Willebrand Disease With a New Analyzer Using High Shear Stress: A Study of 60 Cases," *Blood*, 1998, 91(4):1325-31.

References

Gahl WA, Brantly M, Kaiser-Kupfer MI, et al, "Genetic Defects and Clinical Characteristics of Patients With a Form of Oculocutaneous Albinism (Hermansky-Pudlak syndrome)," *N Engl J Med*, 1998, 338(18):1258-64.

Nurden AT, "Inherited Abnormalities of Platelets," *Thromb Haemost*, 1999, 82(2):468-80.

♦ **Platelet Aggregation, Hypercoagulable State** *see* Platelet Hyperaggregation *on page 350*

Platelet Antibodies

Related Information

Heparin-Induced Thrombocytopenia *on page 343*
Platelet Antibody, Immunohematologic *on page 852*
Platelet Count *on page 468*
Platelets, Apheresis, Donation *on page 853*
Platelet Transfusion *on page 854*
Quinidine, Serum *on page 764*
Transfusion Reaction Work-up *on page 864*

Applies to Idiopathic Thrombocytopenic Purpura; ITP; Lymphocytotoxicity Assay; NAIT; Neonatal Alloimmune Thrombocytopenia; Platelet Transfusion Refractoriness; Post-transfusion Purpura; PTP

Abstract Platelet antibodies can be autoimmune (as found in idiopathic thrombocytopenic purpura (ITP)), drug-induced, or alloimmune (as found in neonatal alloimmune thrombocytopenia (NAIT), post-transfusion purpura (PTP), platelet transfusion refractoriness). Heparin-induced thrombocytopenia (HIT), the most common drug-induced immune thrombocytopenia, occurs by a unique mechanism. Therefore, HIT is discussed separately.

Specimen Varies depending on method. Whole blood for direct antibody tests (measuring antibody attached to platelets) or for identifying platelet antigens; serum or plasma for indirect antibody tests (measuring antiplatelet antibody not bound to platelets). DNA testing requires whole blood or other source of DNA.

Container Varies depending on method. Commonly requires lavender top (EDTA - whole blood or plasma) tube and/or red top (serum) tube. Some methods require 6-8 tubes of blood; other methods need only one tube. Specimens should be transported to the laboratory immediately.

Collection Routine venipuncture

Storage Instructions Varies depending on method. Some methods require whole blood at room temperature; others recommend refrigerated whole blood, or refrigerated or frozen serum or plasma.

Turnaround Time Usually several days, because these assays are often send-out tests.

Use Confirm drug-induced thrombocytopenia, NAIT, PTP, or platelet transfusion refractoriness. The tests are not considered necessary for diagnosing ITP, according to an expert panel.[1] For ITP, the tests may lack adequate sensitivity (particularly certain newer methods) or specificity (particularly certain older methods).

Methodology A variety of methods exist. Older methods that measure antibody associated with platelets are generally sensitive but not specific.[2] For example, the use of **radiolabeled antibodies** that bind to other antibodies are used in some specialized coagulation laboratories as either a direct or indirect antiplatelet antibody assay. More recently, a number of enzyme-linked immunosorbent (**ELISA**) assays are available to test for specific antiplatelet antibodies in serum or plasma. The platelet antigen of interest, such as an HLA antigen or glycoprotein Ib/IX, is bound to the surface of a microtiter plate. The patient sample is added and if antibody is present, it will bind to the antigen. In **antigen capture immunoassays**, monoclonal antibodies directed against platelet antigens are used to individually capture various known platelet antigens onto a solid phase. Patient serum is added. If the corresponding antibody is present in the patient serum, it will bind. For example, if an antibody in the patient serum binds in the assay containing the PI^{A1} antigen, then the patient is found to have an anti-PI^{A1} antibody. **Flow cytometry** is also used in some laboratories to detect platelet-associated antibodies.

NAIT: The diagnosis of NAIT often involves typing (identifying) platelet antigens in the mother and father (and newborn), to demonstrate that the mother lacks a platelet antigen that is present on the platelets of the father (and newborn). It can also be demonstrated that there is an antibody in the mother's serum that is directed against a platelet antigen in the father (and newborn). Testing the newborn directly is typically not necessary, if the father can be tested.

PTP: The diagnosis of PTP often involves typing platelet antigens in the patient, and demonstrating that a platelet antibody in the patient's serum is directed against an antigen that is absent on the patient's platelets. Methods for detecting platelet antibodies in serum have been described above. Some of the current methods used for typing platelet antigens are described below.

Platelet antigen typing by antigen-capture immunoassays: Monoclonal antibodies are used to immobilize the patient's platelet antigens onto a solid phase. Various antibodies of known antigen specificity are added. If an antibody binds, the patient's platelets have that particular antigen. For example, if an anti-PI^{A1} antibody binds to the patient's platelet antigens in this assay, then the patient is found to carry the PI^{A1} antigen. If the PI^{A1} antibody does not bind, then the patient's platelets lack the PI^{A1} antigen. Alternatively, polymerase chain reaction (**PCR**) assays can be used to identify the patient's platelet antigens. The platelet-specific antigens that cause platelet antibody formation are polymorphisms of platelet glycoproteins. Many of the alterations in DNA sequence that account for these polymorphisms are known and can be identified by PCR.

Drug-induced thrombocytopenia: The serotonin release assay, flow cytometry or other methods can be used to diagnose drug-induced thrombocytopenia. These tests are not routinely available. In serotonin release assays, patient plasma (or serum) and the suspected drug are added to normal platelets that contain radiolabeled serotonin. If antibodies against the drug are present, they stimulate the platelets to release their serotonin. The released radiolabeled serotonin can then be detected.

A **lymphocytotoxicity assay** (percent reactive antibody, PRA) can be used to detect HLA antibodies in patients who are refractory to platelet transfusions.

Additional Information

ITP: ITP is an isolated thrombocytopenia due to an autoantibody against platelets. The platelet antibodies are most commonly directed against components of platelet glycoprotein IIb/IIIa or to a lesser extent glycoprotein Ib/IX. In children, it is most often an acute disorder that resolves spontaneously. In adults, it is most often a chronic condition. Typically, the only abnormality on a peripheral blood smear is thrombocytopenia with normal to large platelets. Because ITP is a diagnosis of exclusion, laboratory tests recommended by a consensus panel to exclude other disorders include a peripheral blood smear, complete blood count (CBC), HIV testing in individuals with HIV risk factors, thyroid function tests in adults considering splenectomy, liver function tests in pregnant women to exclude HELLP syndrome, and bone marrow biopsy in persons older than age 60, adults considering splenectomy, or chronic cases in children that do not respond to IVIg.[1]

Neonatal alloimmune thrombocytopenia (NAIT) occurs when fetal platelets have an antigen from the father that is absent in the mother, and the mother forms antibodies that cross the placenta and destroy fetal platelets. Newborn platelet counts are often <100,000/μL at birth, returning to normal within 2 weeks after birth. The antigens are usually components of platelet glycoprotein IIb/IIIa, most commonly, an antigen called PI^{A1}. The incidence of NAIT is approximately one case per 1000-5000 live births. See Platelet Transfusion *on page 854*.

Post-transfusion purpura (PTP) is a rare condition that occurs when a patient is transfused with platelets that express an antigen that is absent in the patient. The patient forms antibodies against the donor platelets. For unclear reasons in PTP, these antibodies also destroy the patient's own platelets, even though they lack the offending antigen. As with NAIT, the antigens are usually components of platelet glycoprotein IIb/IIIa, most commonly PI^{A1}. PTP is characterized by the sudden onset of thrombocytopenia 5-12 days after transfusion of a platelet-containing product. The thrombocytopenia is typically severe (<10,000/μL), and it usually begins to resolve within 14 days after the transfusion.

Drug-induced immune thrombocytopenia: A vast number of drugs have been implicated in drug-induced thrombocytopenia, but a cause-effect relationship has not been proven for most drugs. Some of the drugs that cause immune thrombocytopenia include quinidine, quinine, sulfonamides, sulfonylureas, gold salts, and salicylates. Some drugs cause thrombocytopenia through nonimmune mechanisms, including marrow suppression (eg, ethanol, thiazide, procarbazine) or nonimmune destruction (eg, ristocetin, bleomycin, protamine). In the nonimmune cases, there is no antibody and therefore no need for platelet antibody tests. With immune drug-induced thrombocytopenia, platelet counts are often severely decreased (<10,000/μL). Platelet counts typically return to normal within 7 days after discontinuing the drug.

Platelet refractoriness is a condition that occurs in thrombocytopenic patients who have received multiple platelet transfusions. The transfusions expose the patient to a variety of foreign HLA and other platelet antigens, against which the patient forms antibodies. These antibodies destroy (Continued)

Platelet Antibodies (Continued)

subsequently transfused platelets, and, the patient is said to be refractory to platelet transfusion. Platelet refractoriness is most often due to antibodies against HLA-A or HLA-B antigens; less common causes include antibodies against ABO blood group antigens or platelet glycoproteins.

Footnotes

1. George JN, Woolf SH, Raskob GE, et al, "Idiopathic Thrombocytopenic Purpura: A Practice Guideline Developed by Explicit Methods for the American Society of Hematology," *Blood*, 1996, 88(1):3-40.
2. Warner M and Kelton JG, "Laboratory Investigation of Immune Thrombocytopenia," *J Clin Pathol*, 1997, 50(1):5-12.

References

Berchtold P, Muller D, Beardsley D, et al, "International Study to Compare Antigen-Specific Methods Used for the Measurement of Antiplatelet Autoantibodies," *Br J Haematol*, 1997, 96(3):477-83.

Brighton TA, Evans S, Castaldi PA, et al, "Prospective Evaluation of the Clinical Usefulness of an Antigen-Specific Assay (MAIPA) in Idiopathic Thrombocytopenic Purpura and Other Immune Thrombocytopenias," *Blood*, 1996, 88(1):194-201.

Bussel JB, Zabusky MR, Berkowitz RL, et al, "Fetal Alloimmune Thrombocytopenia," *N Engl J Med*, 1997, 337(1):22-6.

Moore SB and DeGoey SR, "Serum Platelet Antibody Testing. Evaluation of Solid-Phase Enzyme Immunoassay and Comparison With Indirect Immunofluorescence," *Am J Clin Pathol*, 1998, 109(2):190-5.

Taaning E and Svejgaard A, "Post-transfusion Purpura: A Survey of 12 Danish Cases With Special Reference to Immunoglobulin G Subclasses of the Platelet Antibodies," *Transfus Med*, 1994, 4(1):1-8

♦ **Platelet Autoaggregation** *see* Platelet Hyperaggregation *on page 350*

♦ **Platelet Factor 4** *see* Heparin Antifactor Xa Assay *on page 342*

♦ **Platelet Factor 4** *see* Heparin-Induced Thrombocytopenia *on page 343*

♦ **Platelet Factor 4** *see* Hypercoagulation Panel *on page 345*

♦ **Platelet Function Studies** *see* Platelet Aggregation *on page 348*

Platelet Hyperaggregation

Related Information

Antithrombin *on page 333*
Hypercoagulation Panel *on page 345*
Platelet Aggregation *on page 348*

Synonyms Hypercoagulable State, Platelet Aggregation; Platelet Aggregation, Hypercoagulable State; Platelet Autoaggregation

Test Includes Evaluation for spontaneous aggregation, and aggregation in response to low concentrations of adenosine diphosphate (ADP), epinephrine, arachidonate, and collagen

Abstract Platelet hyperaggregation in response to platelet agonists, and/or spontaneous platelet aggregation (aggregation without a platelet agonist) has been described in association with hypercoagulability, including strokes, myocardial infarction, and less commonly venous thrombosis.

Patient Preparation Patients should not have aspirin (or any medication containing aspirin) for at least 7 days prior to testing. Nonsteroidal anti-inflammatory drugs or other platelet-inhibiting agents should also be avoided.

Specimen Platelet-rich plasma

Container Four to six blue top or plastic (sodium citrate) tubes

Collection Routine venipuncture. Immediately invert tubes gently at least 4 times to mix. Deliver tubes immediately to the laboratory at room temperature (platelets are activated at cold temperatures).

Storage Instructions Keep specimen at room temperature and perform test within 2 hours of collection. Do not refrigerate or freeze specimen.

Causes for Rejection Specimen received more than 2 hours after collection, specimen clotted, specimen received on ice

Turnaround Time Less than 1 day

Special Instructions Test usually must be scheduled in advance with the laboratory.

Reference Interval No spontaneous platelet aggregation and no hyperaggregation compared to a normal control. Normal newborns can have decreased aggregation compared to adults.[1]

Use Evaluation for excessive platelet aggregation may be useful in patients with evidence of unexplained hypercoagulability and normal values in the routine hypercoagulation test panel.

Limitations Subjective. Results are compared to a normal control. Variable results among patients and controls. Platelet-inhibiting medications interfere. Labor-intensive for the laboratory, therefore, not suitable for high volume clinical testing.

Methodology As described for platelet aggregation, except each platelet agonist is tested at multiple lower-than-usual concentrations. For example, instead of testing epinephrine only at 10 µM, it is tested at 10 µM, 5 µM, 1 µM, and 0.5 µM. No agonist is added to one aliquot to assess for spontaneous aggregation.

Additional Information Various medications can cause increased *in vitro* platelet aggregation. If a patient is found to have increased platelet aggregation in this assay, a careful review of prescribed, as well as over-the-counter medications, is indicated. An on-line literature search for each medication is often informative. Hyperaggregation has also been reported

with myeloproliferative disorders. Hereditary hyperaggregation as a cause of hypercoagulability is not well characterized.

Footnotes

1. Michelson AD, "Platelet Function in the Newborn," *Semin Thromb Hemost*, 1998, 24(6):507-12.

References

Mammen EF, "Sticky Platelet Syndrome," *Semin Thromb Hemost*, 1999, 25(4):361-5.

Landolfi R, Marchioli R, and Patrono C, "Mechanisms of Bleeding and Thrombosis in Myeloproliferative Disorders," *Thromb Haemost*, 1997, 78(1):617-21.

♦ **Platelet Transfusion Refractoriness** *see* Platelet Antibodies *on page 349*

♦ **Post-transfusion Purpura** *see* Platelet Antibodies *on page 349*

Prekallikrein

Related Information

Activated Partial Thromboplastin Time *on page 328*
Coagulation Factor Assays *on page 335*
High-Molecular Weight Kininogen *on page 344*

Synonyms Fletcher Factor

Applies to Kallikrein

Abstract Prekallikrein is a coagulation protein involved in the early stages of intrinsic pathway activation. Prekallikrein deficiency can cause a marked prolongation of the PTT, but it does not cause bleeding. The same is true for factor XII deficiency and high-molecular weight kininogen (HMWK) deficiency.

Patient Preparation Patients cannot be on hirudin or argatroban anticoagulation, which can interfere with mixing studies and PTT-based prekallikrein assays. Danaparoid may also interfere with these assays. If heparin is present, notify the laboratory because heparin must be removed prior to testing.

Specimen Plasma

Container One blue top (sodium citrate) tube

Collection Routine venipuncture. If multiple tests are being drawn, draw blue top tubes after any red top tubes but before any lavender top (EDTA), green top (heparin), or gray top (oxalate/fluoride) tubes. Immediately invert tube gently at least 4 times to mix. Tubes must be appropriately filled. Deliver tubes immediately to the laboratory.

Storage Instructions Separate plasma from cells as soon as possible. If assay is not performed within 4 hours, freeze plasma specimen.

Causes for Rejection Specimen received more than 4 hours after collection, tubes not filled, clotted specimens

Turnaround Time Less than 1 day (longer if test is a send-out)

Reference Interval 60% to 140% of normal. Newborns have lower levels than adults; the values increase to near adult normal range by age 6 months.[1]

Use May be performed when a routine prolonged PTT evaluation finds no explanation for the prolongation (see Mixing Studies *on page 346*). The PTT is normal in the mixing study; factors VIII, IX, XI, and XII are normal; the PT and fibrinogen are normal; and lupus anticoagulant assays are negative. If prekallikrein assays are normal, HMWK assays may be considered.

Methodology

Screening assay: Preincubate a PTT test sample for 10 minutes prior to adding calcium. A prolonged PTT that shortens after the 10-minute incubation is suspicious for a prekallikrein deficiency. In addition, if a PTT is performed with ellagic acid as the intrinsic pathway activator, the PTT will usually be normal in prekallikrein deficiencies.

Specific factor assay for prekallikrein: Can be performed similar to other coagulation factor assays. Patient plasma is mixed with prekallikrein-deficient plasma and a PTT is performed on the mixture. The amount of prekallikrein in the patient plasma is determined from a standard curve that plots known amounts of prekallikrein against PTT values. **Note:** PTT tests are normally incubated for 3 minutes prior to adding calcium. When using the PTT in a prekallikrein factor assay, the incubation period is shortened to 1 minute.[2] A chromogenic prekallikrein assay is also available.

Additional Information Prekallikrein is one of the contact factors that participates in the activation of the intrinsic pathway of coagulation when blood is exposed to a negatively charged foreign surface. With contact activation, activated factor XII (XIIa) converts prekallikrein into kallikrein. Kallikrein then activates more factor XII. HMWK acts as a cofactor in both of these reactions. HMWK also acts as a cofactor in the activation of factor XI by factor XIIa. Kallikrein releases bradykinin from HMWK, which has vasoactive activities. Fibrinolysis is also activated by contact activation. Recent evidence suggests that, *in vivo*, activation of prekallikrein occurs before activation of factor XII.

Prekallikrein deficiency is rare and does not cause bleeding, despite prolongation of the PTT. The lack of bleeding is presumably because the extrinsic pathway of coagulation, via factor VII and tissue factor, remains intact, and factor XI can be activated by thrombin generated from the extrinsic pathway.[3,4] Thus, factor XI can be activated without the need for prekallikrein, HMWK, or factor XII. This is consistent with the observation that deficiencies of the latter three factors are not associated with bleeding.

Acquired, usually mild-to-moderate decreases in prekallikrein may be found in liver disease or disseminated intravascular coagulation (DIC). Rarely, a prekallikrein inhibitor (antibody) has been reported.[5]

Footnotes

1. Andrew M, Paes B, and Johnston M, "Development of the Hemostatic System in the Neonate and Young Infant," *Am J Pediatr Hematol Oncol*, 1990,12(1):95-104.
2. Sibley C and Evatt BL, "Laboratory Suggestions: Improving the Sensitivity of the Fletcher Factor Assay," *Am J Clin Pathol*, 1979, 71(5):570-3.
3. Naito K and Fujikawa K, "Activation of Human Blood Coagulation Factor XI Independent of Factor XII. Factor XIa Is Activated by Thrombin and Factor XIa in the Presence of Negatively Charged Surfaces," *J Biol Chem*, 1991, 266(12):7353-8.
4. Gailani D and Broze GJ, "Factor XI Activation in a Revised Model of Blood Coagulation," *Science*, 1991, 253(5022):909-12.
5. Page JD, DeLa Cadena RA, Humphries JE, et al, "An Autoantibody to Human Plasma Prekallikrein Blocks Activation of the Contact System," *Br J Haematol*, 1994, 87(1):81-6.

References

Sanfelippo MJ, Carafo AJ, and Hollister WN, "APTT Prolonged by Prekallikrein Deficiency," *Lab Med*, 1998, 29(5):274-6.

Schmaier AH, Rojkjaer R, and Shariat-Madar Z, "Activation of the Plasma Kallikrein/Kinin System on Cells: A Revised Hypothesis," *Thromb Haemost*, 1999, 82(2):226-33.

♦ **Proaccelerin (Factor V)** *see* Coagulation Factor Assays *on page 335*

♦ **Proconvertin (Factor VII)** *see* Coagulation Factor Assays *on page 335*

Protein C

Related Information

Activated Protein C Resistance and the Factor V Leiden Mutation *on page 330*
Antithrombin *on page 333*
Hypercoagulation Panel *on page 345*
Protein S *on page 352*
Warfarin *on page 770*

Abstract Protein C, with protein S as a cofactor, is a natural anticoagulant protein. A hereditary deficiency of protein C leads to a hypercoagulable state with an increased risk for venous thrombosis. Type I deficiency is a quantitative deficiency of protein C. Type II deficiencies result from qualitatively abnormal (but often quantitatively normal) protein C.

Patient Preparation Determine if patient is on oral anticoagulants. Protein C levels are decreased by warfarin (Coumadin®).

Specimen Plasma

Container One blue top (sodium citrate) tube

Sampling Time Testing should be deferred until patients have not received Coumadin® for at least 10 days, because Coumadin® decreases protein C levels.

Collection Routine venipuncture. If multiple tests are being drawn, draw blue top tubes after any red top tubes but before any lavender top (EDTA), green top (heparin), or gray top (oxalate/fluoride) tubes. Immediately invert tube gently at least 4 times to mix. Tubes must be appropriately filled. Deliver tubes immediately to the laboratory.

Storage Instructions Separate plasma from cells as soon as possible. Plasma may be stored on ice for up to 4 hours; otherwise, store frozen.

Causes for Rejection Specimen received more than 4 hours after collection, tubes not filled, clotted specimens

Turnaround Time Several hours to several days, depending on how often test batches are performed

Reference Interval Results are reported as a percent of the amount expected in normal plasma. By definition, the mean value in normal plasma is 100%. The reference range is approximately 70% to 140%.[1] At birth, protein C levels are only 35% (range 17% to 53%) of adult normal values.[2] Mean protein C levels rise to above 50% of adult normal values by age 6 months, but may remain below adult normal range until the age of 10-16 years.[3]

Use A functional assay should be performed first, because both type I and type II protein C deficiencies will be detected. The antigen assay is needed only if the functional assay is decreased, in order to determine if the deficiency is type I or type II. If the antigen assay is performed without the functional assay, type II deficiencies will not be detected (see Additional Information).

Limitations Acquired protein C deficiencies are more common than hereditary deficiencies (see Additional Information).

Chromogenic (functional) assays: Certain type II protein C deficiencies may not be detected in the chromogenic assay but will be detected by clot-based assays.[4,5] Assays are usually designed to tolerate up to 1 unit/mL heparin. The advantage of this assay is that it is not affected by lupus anticoagulants, factor VIII levels, factor V Leiden, or other coagulation abnormalities that can interfere with clot-based protein C assays.

Clot-based (functional) assays: Commonly encountered coagulation conditions can interfere. For example, lupus anticoagulants can artifactually increase the protein C test result. Elevations in factor VIII (>200%) can artifactually decrease the result; factor VIII elevations occur in patients with an acute phase reaction. Falsely low values have been reported in patients with the factor V Leiden mutation.[6,7] The advantage of this assay is that all known type I and type II variants should be detected.[4,5] Assays that tolerate

up to 1 unit/mL heparin are available. Cannot be performed in patients on hirudin or argatroban anticoagulation.

Antigen (immunologic) assays: If not used in conjunction with a functional assay, type II deficiencies will not be detected (see Additional Information).

Methodology Assays are functional (chromogenic or clot-based) or antigenic.

Chromogenic assays: Protein C in the patient plasma sample is activated, usually by a specific snake venom. The activated protein C cleaves a synthetic substrate that resembles the natural substrate of protein C, liberating a chromogenic substance that can be measured spectrophotometrically.[8]

Clot-based assays: Protein C in the patient plasma sample is activated, usually by a specific snake venom. The activated protein C then degrades factors Va and VIIIa, thereby prolonging a PTT-based clotting time.

Antigenic (immunoassay): Enzyme-linked immunosorbent assay (ELISA)[9]

Additional Information Protein C, a vitamin K dependent zymogen of a serine protease (activated protein C), has a molecular weight of 62,000 daltons. Protein C functions as an anticoagulant by using protein S as a cofactor to degrade activated factors V and VIII. Protein C must first be converted into activated protein C by interacting with a thrombin-thrombomodulin complex on the surface of endothelial cells. Protein C also indirectly promotes fibrinolysis.[10]

Hereditary protein C deficiency is present in 0.14% to 0.50% of the general population.[11,12] It accounts for 3% of unselected patients with venous thrombosis and up to 9% of patients younger than 70 years of age with thrombosis.[13,14] Over 160 mutations in the protein C gene are known to cause hereditary protein C deficiency.[15,16] Individuals heterozygous for protein C deficiency have a sevenfold increased risk for venous thrombosis.[13] Heterozygotes generally have protein C levels between 35% and 65%, although levels as high as 68% have been reported.[17] The risk for thrombosis is further increased in the presence of a second risk factor.[18] The age at onset of thrombosis is usually between 10-50 years in heterozygous individuals. **Coumadin®-induced skin necrosis** may occur if protein C deficient patients are treated with Coumadin® without the addition of an immediate-acting anticoagulant (eg, heparin) until the Coumadin® levels are therapeutic. Homozygous deficiencies are rare, and are fatal if untreated. They present in the newborn period with severely decreased protein C, **purpura fulminans**, and disseminated intravascular coagulation (DIC).

Decreased protein C can also arise from acquired conditions, such as:
- decreased hepatic synthesis from liver disease or L-asparaginase treatment
- synthesis of a dysfunctional protein due to vitamin K deficiency or warfarin (Coumadin®) use
- consumption from thrombosis, DIC, or surgery

A case of an acquired inhibitor (autoantibody) to protein C has been reported.[19] If a patient with low protein C has any of the conditions listed above, the test should be repeated once the condition is no longer present. Confirmation of a hereditary protein C deficiency may require documenting protein C deficiency in a relative. In nephrotic syndrome, protein C may increase, decrease, or remain unchanged. Malm et al. reported that protein C can increase with oral contraceptives and pregnancy,[20] whereas Kjellberg et al reported no significant increase in protein C during pregnancy.[21] Women may have slightly decreased protein C levels in comparison to men, and premenopausal women may have slightly lower levels than postmenopausal women.[22]

Protein C has a relatively short half-life of 6-8 hours; therefore, it is one of the first hepatic coagulation proteins to decrease with liver dysfunction as well as with Coumadin® initiation.

Protein C deficiencies are quantitative (type I) or qualitative (type II). In type I deficiencies, normal protein C molecules are made, but in reduced quantity. In type II deficiencies, normal amounts of protein C are made, but the protein C is defective. Functional assays measure protein C function (activity). Antigenic assays are immunoassays that measure the quantity of protein C, regardless of the quality of its function. Accordingly, type I deficiencies have decreased protein C in both functional and antigenic assays. Type II deficiencies have normal antigenic protein C levels, with decreased functional protein C. Thus, if only antigenic assays are performed, type II deficiencies will not be detected. Therefore, a functional assay should be used as the initial screening assay. If the result is decreased, an antigenic assay may be performed to determine if the deficiency is type I or type II.

Footnotes

1. Allaart CF, Poort SR, Rosendaal FR, et al, "Increased Risk of Venous Thrombosis in Carriers of Hereditary Protein C Deficiency Defect," *Lancet*, 1993, 341:134-8.
2. Andrew M, Paes B, Milner R, et al, "Development of the Human Coagulation System in the Full-Term Infant," *Blood*, 1987, 70(1):165-72.
3. Andrew M, Vegh P, Johnston M, et al, "Maturation of the Hemostatic System During Childhood," *Blood*, 1992, 80(8):1998-2005.
4. Vasse M, Borg JY, and Monconduit M, "Protein C: Rouen, a New Hereditary Protein C Abnormality With Low Anticoagulant but Normal Amidolytic Activities," *Thromb Res*, 1989, 56:387-98.
5. Wojcik EGC, Simioni P, Berg MVD, et al, "Mutations Which Introduce Free Cysteine Residues in the Gla-domain of Vitamin K Dependent Proteins Result in the Formation of Complexes With α1-microglobulin," *Thromb Haemost*, 1996, 75(1):70-5.
(Continued)

Protein C (Continued)

6. Ireland H, Bayston T, Thompson E, et al, "Apparent Heterozygous Type II Protein C Deficiency Caused by the Factor V 506 Arg to Gln Mutation," *Thromb Haemost*, 1995, 73(4):731-2.

7. Jennings I, Kitchen S, Cooper PC et al, "Further Evidence That Activated Protein C Resistance Affects Protein C Coagulant Activity Assays," *Thromb Haemost*, 2000, 83(1):171-2.

8. Francis RB Jr and Seyfert U, "Rapid Amidolytic Assay of Protein C in Whole Plasma Using an Activator From the Venom of Agkistrodon Contortrix," *Am J Clin Pathol*, 1987, 87(5):619-25.

9. Boyer C, Rothschild C, Wolf M, et al, "A New Method for the Estimation of Protein C by ELISA,"*Thromb Res*, 1984, 36:579-89.

10. Nesheim M, Wang W, Boffa M, et al, "Thrombin, Thrombomodulin and TAFI in the Molecular Link Between Coagulation and Fibrinolysis," *Thromb Haemost*, 1997, 78(1):386-91.

11. Miletich J, Sherman L, and Broze G Jr, "Absence of Thrombosis in Subjects With Heterozygous Protein C Deficiency," *N Engl J Med*, 1987, 317:991-6.

12. Tait RC, Walker ID, Reitsma PH, et al, "Prevalence of Protein C Deficiency in the Healthy Population," *Thromb Haemost*, 1995, 73(1):87-93.

13. van der Meer FJ, Koster T, Vandenbroucke JP, et al, "The Leiden Thrombophilia Study (LETS)," *Thromb Haemost*, 1997, 78(1):631-5.

14. Melissari E, Monte G, Lindo VS et al, "Congenital Thrombophilia Among Patients With Venous Thromboembolism," *Blood Coagul Fibrinolysis*, 1992, 3(6):749-58.

15. Reitsma PH, Bernardi F, Doig RG, et al, "Protein C Deficiency: A Database of Mutations, 1995 Update," *Thromb Haemost*, 1995, 73:876-89.

16. Reitsma PH, "Protein C Deficiency: From Gene Defects to Disease," *Thromb Haemost*, 1997, 78(1):344-50.

17. Finazzi G and Barbui T, "Different Incidence of Venous Thrombosis in Patients With Inherited Deficiencies of Antithrombin III, Protein C and Protein S," *Thromb Haemost*, 1994, 71:15-8.

18. Simioni P, Sanson BJ, Prandoni P, et al, "Incidence of Venous Thromboembolism in Families With Inherited Thrombophilia," *Thromb Haemost*, 1999, 81(2):198-202.

19. Mitchell CA, Rowell JA, Hau L, et al, "A Fatal Thrombotic Disorder Associated With an Acquired Inhibitor of Protein C," *N Engl J Med*, 1987, 317:1638-42.

20. Malm J, Laurell M, and Dahlbäck B, "Changes in the Plasma Levels of Vitamin K-Dependent Proteins C and S and of C4b-Binding Protein During Pregnancy and Oral Contraception," *Br J Haematol*, 1988, 68(4):437-43.

21. Kjellberg U, Andersson NE, Rosen S, et al, "APC Resistance and Other Haemostatic Variables During Pregnancy and Puerperium," *Thromb Haemost*, 1999, 81(4):527-31.

22. Henkens CM, Bom VJ, van der Schaaf W et, al, "Plasma Levels of Protein S, Protein C and Factor X: Effects of Sex, Hormonal State and Age," *Thromb Haemost*, 1995, 74(5):1271-5.

References

Alhenc-Gelas M, Gandrille S, Aubry ML, et al, "Thirty-three Novel Mutations in the Protein C Gene," *Thromb Haemost*, 2000, 83:86-92.

De Stefano V, Finazzi G, and Mannucci PM, "Inherited Thrombophilia: Pathogenesis, Clinical Syndromes, and Management," *Blood*, 1996, 87(9):3531-44.

Gandrille S and Aiach M, "Identification of Mutations in 90 of 121 Consecutive Symptomatic French Patients With a Type I Protein C Deficiency. The French INSERM Network on Molecular Abnormalities Responsible for Protein C and Protein S Deficiencies," *Blood*, 1995, 86(7):2598-605.

Sanson BJ, Simioni P, Tormene D et al, "The Incidence of Venous Thromboembolism in Asymptomatic Carriers of a Deficiency of Antithrombin, Protein C, or Protein S: A Prospective Cohort Study," *Blood*, 1999, 94(11):3702-6.

Schofield KP, Thomson JM, and Poller L, "Protein C Response to Induction and Withdrawal of Oral Anticoagulant Treatment," *Clin Lab Haematol*, 1987, 9(3):255-62.

♦ **Protein C Deficiency** see Hypercoagulation Panel on page 345

♦ **Protein C Resistance, Activated** see Activated Protein C Resistance and the Factor V Leiden Mutation on page 330

Protein S

Related Information

Activated Protein C Resistance and the Factor V Leiden Mutation on page 330

Antithrombin on page 333

Hypercoagulation Panel on page 345

Protein C on page 351

Warfarin on page 770

Abstract Protein S is a required cofactor for the anticoagulant activity of protein C. A hereditary deficiency of protein S leads to a hypercoagulable state with an increased risk for venous thrombosis. Protein S deficiencies are quantitative (type I) or qualitative (type II).

Patient Preparation Determine if patient is on oral anticoagulants or estrogen (eg, oral contraceptives, estrogen replacement) or if the patient is pregnant. Protein S levels are decreased by estrogen, pregnancy, and warfarin (Coumadin®).

Specimen Plasma

Container Blue top (sodium citrate) tube

Sampling Time Testing should be deferred until patients have not received Coumadin® for at least 10 days, because Coumadin® decreases protein S levels.

Collection Routine venipuncture. If multiple tests are being drawn, draw blue top tubes after any red top tubes but before any lavender top (EDTA), green top (heparin), or gray top (oxalate/fluoride) tubes. Immediately invert tube gently at least 4 times to mix. Tubes must be appropriately filled. Deliver tubes immediately to the laboratory.

Storage Instructions Separate plasma from cells as soon as possible. Plasma may be stored on ice for up to 4 hours; otherwise, store frozen.

Causes for Rejection Specimen received more than 4 hours after collection, tubes not filled, clotted specimens

Turnaround Time Several days (because testing is usually batched)

Special Instructions Elevated factor VIII (>200%) is a common cause of artifactually decreased protein S in PTT-based functional assays. It is recommended to measure factor VIII on the same specimen when the functional protein S is decreased by PTT-based methods, to determine if the decrease is due to elevated factor VIII.

Reference Interval Results are reported as a percent of the amount expected in normal plasma. By definition, the mean value in normal plasma is 100%. The reference range is approximately 70% to 140%; lower for women than for men.[1,2] At birth, protein S (total antigen) levels are only 36% (range 12% to 60%) of adult normal values.[3] Protein S rises into the adult reference range by age 6 months.

Use A functional assay should be performed first, because all subtypes of protein S deficiencies will be detected. The free antigen assay is needed only if the functional assay is decreased, and the total antigen assay is needed only if the free antigen is decreased, in order to determine the deficiency subtype. If the antigen assays are performed without the functional assay, patients with certain subtypes will not be detected (see Additional Information and the table).

Limitations Acquired protein S deficiencies are more common than hereditary deficiencies (see Additional Information).

Functional assays: Commonly encountered coagulation conditions interfere. For example, lupus anticoagulants can falsely increase the protein S test result. Elevations in factor VIII (>200%) can artifactually decrease PTT-based results; factor VIII elevations occur in patients with an acute phase reaction. In some assays, falsely low values have been reported in patients with the factor V Leiden.[4,5] Assays that tolerate up to 1-2 units/mL heparin are available. The functional assay cannot be performed in patients on hirudin or argatroban anticoagulation.

Antigen assays: If not used in conjunction with a functional assay, patients with some subtypes will not be detected (see Additional Information and table).

Methodology

Functional (activity) assays: Protein S is measured by its ability to serve as a cofactor required for activated protein C-mediated degradation of activated factors V and VIII, thereby prolonging a PTT- or PT-based clotting time.

Free antigen (immunoassay): Monoclonal antibodies specific for free (unbound) protein S are used in an enzyme-linked immunosorbent assay (ELISA). In an older assay, free protein S was determined by first treating specimens with polyethylene glycol (PEG), which precipitates bound protein S and leaves free protein S in the supernatant. In the new ELISA using monoclonal antibodies specific for free protein S, the PEG step is no longer necessary. Elimination of the PEG-precipitation step has significantly improved the accuracy of the test result.[6]

Total antigen (immunoassay): Measures total (free and bound) protein S by ELISA. An alternative method uses latex particles coated with antibodies directed against protein S. In the presence of protein S, the latex particles form aggregates that absorb light passing through the specimen. The amount of light absorbance is directly related to the amount of protein S in the specimen.[7] A third method, rocket immunoelectrophoresis, is an older method that is still in use in some laboratories.[8]

Additional Information Protein S is a vitamin K dependent protein that is a required cofactor for activated protein C. Activated protein C, with protein S as a cofactor, acts as an anticoagulant by degrading activated factors V and VIII. Sixty percent of total protein S is bound to C4b-binding protein and is inactive. The remainder, called free protein S, is the functionally active form.

Hereditary protein S deficiency is present in 0.7% of the general population.[9] It accounts for 2% of unselected patients with venous thrombosis and up to 7.6% of patients younger than 70 years of age with thrombosis.[10,11] Many different mutations in the protein S gene are known to cause hereditary protein S deficiency.[12] Individuals heterozygous for protein S deficiency have an increased risk for venous thrombosis, and the risk is further increased in the presence of a second risk factor.[13] Heterozygotes generally have protein S levels between 20% to 65%.[6,14] The age at onset of thrombosis is usually between 10-50 years in heterozygous individuals. **Coumadin®-induced skin necrosis** has been reported in protein S deficient patients who are started on Coumadin® without the addition of an immediate-acting anticoagulant (eg, heparin) until the Coumadin® levels are therapeutic. Homozygous deficiencies are rare, and are fatal if untreated. They present in the newborn period with severely decreased protein S, purpura fulminans, and disseminated intravascular coagulation (DIC).[15]

Decreased protein S can also arise from acquired conditions, such as:
- decreased hepatic synthesis from liver disease or L-asparaginase treatment
- synthesis of a dysfunctional protein due to vitamin K deficiency or warfarin (Coumadin®) use
- consumption from thrombosis, DIC or invasive procedures

- estrogen, including oral contraceptives, estrogen replacement therapy, or pregnancy (decreased protein S may persist for up to 2 months after delivery or estrogen discontinuation)
- acute phase reactions (due to elevated C4b-binding protein, which decreases free and consequently functional protein S)

May also become decreased in nephrotic syndrome, varicella infection[16,17,18] or HIV infection.[19] Acquired inhibitors (autoantibodies) to protein S have been reported,[20] some of which arose in association with varicella infections. If an acquired cause is present, the test should be repeated once the condition is no longer present, if possible. Confirmation of a hereditary protein S deficiency may require documenting protein S deficiency in a relative.

In liver disease, protein S is occasionally normal despite decreased protein C and antithrombin (all three proteins are synthesized in the liver). It is speculated that this is because protein S is synthesized in endothelial cells and megakaryocytes in addition to the liver, whereas protein C and antithrombin are synthesized predominantly or exclusively in the liver.

Protein S deficiencies are quantitative (type I) or qualitative (type II). In type I deficiencies, normal protein S molecules are made, but in reduced quantity. In type II deficiencies, normal amounts of protein S are made, but the protein S is defective. Functional assays measure protein S function. The total antigen assay is an immunoassay that measures the total quantity of protein S, regardless of the quality of its function. Free antigen assays are immunoassays that measure only unbound (free) protein S, regardless of the quality of its function. Only free (unbound) protein S is active; protein S that is bound to its binding protein (C4b-binding protein) is inactive. Accordingly, type I deficiencies have decreased protein S in both functional and antigenic assays. Type II deficiencies have normal total antigen levels, with decreased functional protein S. A further type II subtype (known as type IIa or type III) is characterized by decreased functional and free antigen levels with normal total antigen levels (see table). This subtype may be due to mutations causing increased binding of protein S to C4b-binding protein. In summary, if only antigenic assays are performed, type II deficiencies will not be detected. Therefore, a functional assay should be used as the initial screening assay. If the result is decreased, a free antigen assay should be performed to determine the deficiency subtype. If the free antigen is decreased, a total antigen assay may be performed to further determine the deficiency subtype (see table).

Classification of Hereditary Protein S Deficiencies

Type	Functional Protein S	Free Protein S (Free Antigen Assay)	Total Protein S (Total Antigen Assay)
I	Low	Low	Low
II (also called IIb)	Low	Normal	Normal
III (also called IIa)	Low	Low	Normal

Footnotes

1. Leroy-Matheron C, Duchemin J, Levent M, et al, "Influence of the nt 2148 A to G Substitution (Pro 626 Dimorphism) in the PROS1 Gene on Circulation Free Protein S Levels in Healthy Volunteers - Reappraisal of Protein S Normal Ranges," *Thromb Haemost*, 2000, 83(5):798-9.
2. Henkens CM, Bom VJ, van der Schaaf W, et al, "Plasma Levels of Protein S, Protein C and Factor X: Effects of Sex, Hormonal State and Age," *Thromb Haemost*, 1995, 74(5):1271-5.
3. Andrew M, Paes B, Milner R, et al, "Development of the Human Coagulation System in the Full-Term Infant," *Blood*, 1987, 70(1):165-72.
4. D'Angelo SV, Mazzola G, Valle PD, et al, "Variable Interference of Activated Protein C Resistance in the Measurement of Protein S Activity by Commercial Assays," *Thromb Res*, 1995, 77(4):375-8.
5. Faioni EM, Boyer-Neumann C, Franchi F, et al, "Another Protein S Functional Assay Is Sensitive to Resistance to Activated Protein C," *Thromb Haemost*, 1994, 72:648.
6. Aillaud MF, Pouymayou K, Brunet D, et al, "New Direct Assay of Free Protein S Antigen Applied to Diagnosis of Protein S Deficiency," *Thromb Haemost*, 1996, 75(2):283-5.
7. Laroche P, Plassart V, and Amiral J, "Rapid Quantitative Latex Immunoassays for Diagnosis of Thrombotic Disorders," *Thromb Haemost*, 1989, 62:379.
8. Edson JR, Vogt JM, and Huesman DA, "Laboratory Diagnosis of Inherited Protein S Deficiency," *Am J Clin Pathol*, 1990, 94(2):176-86.
9. Rodeghiero F and Tosetto A, "The Epidemiology of Inherited Thrombophilia: The VITA Project," *Thromb Haemost*, 1997, 78(1):636-40.
10. Heijboer H, Brandjes DPM, Buller HR, et al, "Deficiencies of Coagulation-Inhibiting and Fibrinolytic Proteins in Outpatients With Deep-Vein Thrombosis," *N Engl J Med*, 1990, 323:1512-6.
11. Melissari E, Monte G, Lindo VS, et al, "Congenital Thrombophilia Among Patients With Venous Thromboembolism," *Blood Coagul Fibrinolysis*, 1992, 3(6):749-58.
12. Borgel D, Grandrille S, and Aiach M, "Protein S Deficiency," *Thromb Haemost*, 1997, 78(1):351-6.
13. Simioni P, Sanson BJ, Prandoni P, et al, "Incidence of Venous Thromboembolism in Families With Inherited Thrombophilia," *Thromb Haemost*, 1999, 81(2):198-202.
14. Finazzi G and Barbui T, "Different Incidence of Venous Thrombosis in Patients With Inherited Deficiencies of Antithrombin III, Protein C and Protein S," *Thromb Haemost*, 1994, 71:15-8.
15. Pegelow CH, Ledford M, Young J, et al, "Severe Protein S Deficiency in a Newborn," *Pediatrics*, 1992, 89:674-6.
16. Nguyen P, Reynaud J, Pouzol P, et al, "Varicella and Thrombotic Complications Associated With Transient Protein C and Protein S Deficiencies in Children," *Eur J Pediatr*, 1994, 153:646-9.
17. Manco-Johnson MJ, Nuss R, Key N, et al, "Lupus Anticoagulant and Protein S Deficiency in Children With Postvaricella Purpura Fulminans or Thrombosis," *J Pediatr*, 1996, 128(3):319-23.
18. Peyvandi F, Faioni E, Alessandro Moroni G, et al, "Autoimmune Protein S Deficiency and Deep Vein Thrombosis After Chickenpox," *Thromb Haemost*, 1996, 75(1):212-3.
19. Stahl CP, Wideman CS, Spira TJ, et al, "Protein S Deficiency in Men With Long-Term Human Immunodeficiency Virus Infection," *Blood*, 1993, 81(7):1801-7.
20. Sorice M, Arcieri P, Griggi T, et al, "Inhibition of Protein S by Autoantibodies in Patients With Acquired Protein S Deficiency," *Thromb Haemost*, 1996, 75(4):555-9.

References

Makris M, Leach M, Beauchamp NJ, et al, "Genetic Analysis, Phenotypic Diagnosis, and Risk of Venous Thrombosis in Families With Inherited Deficiencies of Protein S," *Blood*, 2000, 95(6):1935-41.

Van Cott EM and Laposata M, "Laboratory Evaluation of Hypercoagulable States," *Hematol Oncol Clin North Am*, 1998, 12(6):1141-66.

♦ **Protein S Deficiency** see Hypercoagulation Panel *on page 345*

♦ **Prothrombin (Factor II)** see Coagulation Factor Assays *on page 335*

♦ **Prothrombin Fragment 1.2** see Hypercoagulation Panel *on page 345*

Prothrombin G20210A Mutation

Related Information

Hypercoagulation Panel *on page 345*
Polymerase Chain Reaction *on page 713*

Abstract This mutation is a common hereditary predisposition to venous thrombosis. DNA-based methods, such as the polymerase chain reaction (PCR)-based assay, are used to determine the presence of a specific mutation at nucleotide position 20210 in the prothrombin gene.

Specimen Whole blood

Container Varies with laboratory

Collection Routine venipuncture

Storage Instructions Do not centrifuge or freeze specimen. Store at 4°C or room temperature.

Turnaround Time Several days or longer (depending on how often test batches are performed)

Reference Interval Normal: prothrombin G20210A mutation not present

Use The test identifies individuals who have the prothrombin G20210A mutation. The results indicate whether an affected individual is heterozygous or homozygous for the mutation. The heterozygous form of the mutation is present in 2.3% of the general population and 6.2% of patients with venous thrombosis.[1] It is present in 18% of cases of familial venous thrombosis.[2]

Methodology Commonly, polymerase chain reaction (PCR). The prothrombin G20210A mutation is a point mutation in which the guanine at nucleotide position 20210 is replaced by an adenine. The nucleotide change also allows the introduction of a new Hind III restriction site during PCR.[2] To perform the test, DNA is isolated from whole blood and the mutation site is amplified by PCR. The PCR product is digested with Hind III and then subjected to agarose gel electrophoresis to separate the DNA bands based on size. The presence of a Hind III site at position 20210 can be determined by the pattern of DNA bands detected on the gel. The presence of a Hind III site at position 20210 indicates the presence of the prothrombin G20210A mutation. Heterozygotes and homozygotes can be specifically identified.

Additional Information The mutation involves a guanine to adenine transition at nucleotide position 20210 in an untranslated region of the gene. It is associated with elevated prothrombin levels and an increased risk for **venous** thrombosis.[2,3,4] Individuals heterozygous for the prothrombin G20210A mutation have a two- to threefold increased risk for venous thrombosis.[1] Homozygous individuals likely have an even higher risk for venous thrombosis. The risk for **venous** thrombosis is further increased in the presence of a second risk factor.[5,6] Some studies have shown an increased risk for **arterial** thrombosis[7] while other studies have not.[8] It is possible that an increased risk for **arterial** thrombosis exists only when additional risk factors for arterial thrombosis are also present.[9]

Footnotes

1. van der Meer FJ, Koster T, Vandenbroucke JP, et al, "The Leiden Thrombophilia Study (LETS)," *Thromb Haemost*, 1997, 78(5):631-5.
2. Poort SR, Rosendaal FR, Reitsma PH, et al, "A Common Genetic Variation in the 3'-Untranslated Region of the Prothrombin Gene Is Associated With Elevated Plasma Prothrombin Levels and an Increase in Venous Thrombosis," *Blood*, 1996, 88(10):3698-703.
3. Soria JM, Almasy L, Souto JC, et al, "Linkage Analysis Demonstrates That the Prothrombin G20210A Mutation Jointly Influences Plasma Prothrombin Levels and Risk of Thrombosis," *Blood*, 2000, 95(9):2780-5.
4. Cattaneo M, Chantarangkul V, Taioli E, et al, "The G20210A Mutation of the Prothrombin Gene in Patients With Previous First Episodes of Deep-Vein Thrombosis: Prevalence and Association With Factor V G1691A, Methylenetetrahydrofolate Reductase C677T and Plasma Prothrombin Levels," *Thromb Res*, 1999; 93(1):1-8
5. Martinelli I, Taioli E, Bucciarelli P, et al, "Interaction Between the G20210A Mutation of the Prothrombin Gene and Oral Contraceptive Use in Deep Vein Thrombosis," *Arterioscler Thromb Vasc Biol*, 1999, 19(3):700-3.

(Continued)

Prothrombin G20210A Mutation *(Continued)*

6. Martinelli I, Sacchi E, Landi G, et al, "High Risk of Cerebral-Vein Thrombosis in Carriers of a Prothrombin Gene Mutation and in Users of Oral Contraceptives," *N Engl J Med*, 1998, 338(25):1793-7.
7. Franco RF, Trip MD, ten Cate H, et al, "The 20210 G/A Mutation in the 3′-Untranslated Region of the Prothrombin Gene and the Risk for Arterial Thrombotic Disease," *Br J Haematol*, 1999, 104(1):50-4.
8. Ridker PM, Hennekens CH, and Miletich JP, "G20210A Mutation in Prothrombin Gene and Risk of Myocardial Infarction, Stroke, and Venous Thrombosis in a Large Cohort of U.S. Men," *Circulation*, 1999, 99(8):999-1004.
9. Inbal A, Freimark D, Modan B, et al, "Synergistic Effects of Prothrombotic Polymorphisms and Atherogenic Factors on the Risk of Myocardial Infarction in Young Males," *Blood*, 1999, 93(7):2186-90.

References

De Stefano V, Chiusolo P, Paciaroni K, et al, "Prothrombin G20210A Mutant Genotype Is a Risk Factor for Cerebrovascular Ischemic Disease in Young Patients," *Blood*, 1998, 91(10) :3562-3565.

Eikelboom JW, Baker RI, Parsons R, et al, "No Association Between the 20210 G/A Prothrombin Gene Mutation and Premature Coronary Artery Disease," *Thromb Haemost*, 1998, 80(6):878-880.

Prothrombin Time

Related Information

Activated Partial Thromboplastin Time *on page 328*
Bilirubin, Total, Serum *on page 118*
Blood, Urine *on page 870*
Coagulation Factor Assays *on page 335*
Cryoprecipitate *on page 838*
Disseminated Intravascular Coagulation Screen *on page 338*
Factor Inhibitors *on page 340*
Fibrinogen *on page 341*
Hepatitis B Core Antibody *on page 622*
Hepatitis C Virus RNA Detection and Quantitation *on page 626*
Liver Disease: Laboratory Assessment, Overview *on page 216*
Mixing Studies *on page 346*
Plasma, Fresh Frozen *on page 851*
Point-of-Care Testing *on page 43*
Protein C *on page 351*
Protein S *on page 352*
Reptilase® Time *on page 355*
Thrombin Time *on page 356*
Warfarin *on page 770*

Synonyms Protime; PT

Applies to Argatroban; Common Pathway; Coumadin®; Extrinsic Pathway; Heparin; Hirudin; INR; International Normalized Ratio; Intrinsic Pathway; Thromboplastin; Vitamin K

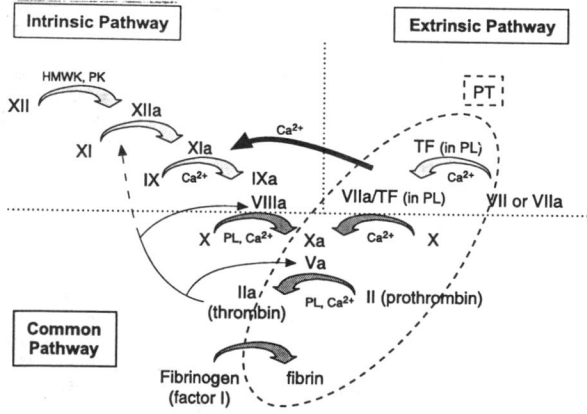

The PTT measures the clotting time from factor XII through fibrin formation (intrinsic and common pathways of coagulation). The PT measures the clotting time from factor VII through fibrin formation (extrinsic and common pathways of coagulation). The intrinsic pathway is activated when factor XII binds to a negatively charged "foreign" surface exposed to the blood, with sequential activation of factor XI, then IX, then X, followed by II, and finally fibrinogen is converted to fibrin. Factors V and VIII and phospholipid serve as cofactors. Many steps also require calcium. It is now believed that *in vivo*, coagulation is primarily initiated through the extrinsic pathway, upon exposure of blood to tissue factor (TF) at sites of tissue injury. In this model of coagulation, the ability to activate factor IX (by TF/VIIa) and factor XI (by thrombin) without factor XII indicates that factor XII, prekallikrein, and HMWK of the intrinsic pathway are not needed in normal procoagulant pathways. This is consistent with the observation that deficiencies of the latter three factors are not associated with bleeding symptoms, whereas, deficiencies of the other factors may cause a bleeding tendency.

Key:
TF = tissue factor (a transmembrane protein; thus, it is associated with phospholipid *in vivo*).
PK = prekallikrein.
HMWK = high molecular weight kininogen.
PL = phospholipid.
Ca²⁺ = calcium.

Adapted from Van Cott EM and Laposata M, "Coagulation, Fibrinolysis and Hypercoagulation," Clinical Diagnosis and Management by Laboratory Methods, 20th ed, Henry JG, ed, Philadelphia, PA: WB Saunders Co, in press.

Abstract The prothrombin time (PT) measures the clotting time from the activation of factor VII, through the formation of fibrin clot (see figure). This test measures the integrity of the extrinsic and common pathways of coagulation, whereas the activated partial thromboplastin time (PTT) measures the integrity of the intrinsic and common pathways of coagulation. PT prolongations are most commonly caused by factor deficiencies involving fibrinogen or factors II, V, VII, or X. Less commonly, PT prolongations are due to an inhibitor, such as therapeutic anticoagulants including heparin, hirudin, or argatroban. Rarely, PT prolongations are caused by lupus anticoagulants or by specific factor inhibitors against fibrinogen or factor II, V, VII, or X.

Specimen Plasma

Container Blue top (sodium citrate) tube; 3.2% citrate tubes are now recommended instead of 3.8% citrate tubes.[1]

Collection Routine venipuncture. If multiple tests are being drawn, draw blue top tubes after any red top tubes but before any lavender top (EDTA), green top (heparin), or gray top (oxalate/fluoride) tubes. Recent data suggest that an initial discard tube is not necessary.[2] Immediately invert tube gently at least 4 times to mix. Tubes must be appropriately filled. Deliver tubes immediately to the laboratory.

Specimens drawn from a heparinized line are easily contaminated with heparin, even when the initial volume drawn is discarded. Although heparin prolongs the PTT, it can also prolong the PT to a lesser extent. Hirudin and argatroban prolong the PT and PTT. Therefore, coagulation tests are best drawn directly from a peripheral vein, avoiding the arm in which heparin, hirudin or argatroban is being infused (if relevant).

Storage Instructions Separate plasma from cells as soon as possible. Plasma (or uncentrifuged specimen) may be stored at room temperature or on ice for up to 24 hours, otherwise store frozen.[1]

Causes for Rejection Specimen received more than 24 hours after collection, tube not filled, clotted specimen, visible hemolysis

Turnaround Time Less than 1 day; often less than 1 hour if requested stat. The PT and PTT are the most readily available coagulation tests.

Reference Interval Varies significantly among different reagent-instrument combinations. The approximate lower limit of normal is 10-12 seconds; the approximate upper limit of normal is 12-14 seconds. Newborns normally have prolonged PTs in comparison with adults. The PT is up to approximately 16 seconds at birth, and the PT gradually shortens into the adult normal range by the age of 6 months.[3] However, newborns and infants do not normally experience bleeding, because a balance between procoagulants and natural anticoagulants is maintained.

Critical Values Longer than 30 seconds is the most commonly used PT panic value in specialized coagulation laboratories according to the College of American Pathologists 1999 Survey CG2-C, but the value varies depending on the reagent-instrument combination and individual laboratory policies.

Use Screen the integrity of the extrinsic (factor VII) and common (fibrinogen and factors II, V, and X) pathways of coagulation; monitor warfarin (Coumadin®) anticoagulation

Limitations With single factor deficiencies, the deficient factor has to be below 15% to 45% before the PT becomes prolonged, depending on the reagent. With multiple factor deficiencies, the PT becomes prolonged with less severe decreases in factor levels.[4]

Deficiencies of factors VIII, IX XI, XII, prekallikrein, or high-molecular weight kininogen do not affect the PT, but do affect the PTT. Factor XIII does not affect the PT nor PTT. A specific factor XIII assay can screen for factor XIII deficiencies.

Heparin can prolong the PT, depending on the reagent. Some reagents contain a heparin neutralizer to reduce or eliminate heparin interference.

Lupus anticoagulants uncommonly prolong the baseline PT. Most PT reagents contain excess phospholipid such that lupus anticoagulants (which are antiphospholipid antibodies) do not prolong the PT. However, with some PT reagents, lupus anticoagulants can accentuate the prolongation of the PT when patients are on warfarin.[5] In these situations, an alternative assay such as a chromogenic factor X assay can be used rather than (or in addition to) the PT to monitor warfarin (see Additional Information).

Methodology PT reagent is called thromboplastin (phospholipid with tissue factor and calcium). It is added to patient plasma, and the time until clot formation is measured in seconds. Tissue factor activates the extrinsic pathway of coagulation. Phospholipid and calcium are required cofactors in the coagulation cascade. Citrate in the blue top tube prevents clotting by chelating calcium. PT reagents contain excess calcium to overcome the citrate. More recently, point-of-care PT test methods have become available which use a single drop of whole blood, and these methods are undergoing evaluation.[6]

Additional Information If indicated, a vitamin K trial may be performed in a patient with an unexplained PT prolongation. If the PT prolongation is due to vitamin K deficiency, the PT becomes normal or significantly shorter within 12-24 hours after vitamin K administration.

To determine the etiology of an unexplained PT prolongation, a mixing study is usually the first step (if the PTT is also prolonged, the presence of heparin or related anticoagulants must first be excluded - see Mixing Studies *on page 346*). Mixing studies can predict whether the cause of the

PT prolongation is a factor deficiency or an inhibitor. The majority of PT prolongations are due to factor deficiencies. If the PT mixing study suggests a factor deficiency, assays for fibrinogen and factors II, V, VII, and X can be performed to identify the deficient factor(s). Inhibitors that prolong the PT are rare. Factor VII inhibitors prolong the PT but not the PTT. Factor II, V, or X inhibitors typically prolong the PTT as well as the PT (see Coagulation Factor Assays *on page 335* for more information). As mentioned above, lupus anticoagulants are inhibitors that commonly prolong the PTT, but uncommonly prolong the PT.

In patients with both a lupus anticoagulant and a prolonged PT, a factor II assay could be considered, because occasionally lupus anticoagulants cause decreased factor II due to increased clearance.

Acquired causes of PT prolongations are much more common than hereditary causes, especially among inpatients (see list below). The liver synthesizes all of the coagulation factors. Therefore, with liver disease, multiple factor deficiencies can develop which prolong the PT earlier and more than the PTT. Coumadin® or vitamin K deficiency impair the function of factors II, VII, IX, and X, leading to PT and eventually PTT prolongations. In disseminated intravascular coagulation (DIC), multiple factor deficiencies may arise due to activation and consumption of factors, prolonging the PT more often than the PTT.[7] Heparin inhibits activated factors II, X, IX, XI, XII, and kallikrein by enhancing antithrombin activity, prolonging the PTT more than the PT. Hirudin and argatroban inhibit only activated factor II (thrombin), prolonging the PT and PTT.

CAUSES OF PT PROLONGATIONS:

Hereditary:
- Deficiency of factor VII *(PTT is normal)*
- Deficiency of fibrinogen or factors II, V, or X *(PTT may also be prolonged)*

Acquired:
- Liver dysfunction *(PT affected earlier and more than PTT)*
- Vitamin K deficiency *(PT affected earlier and more than PTT)*
- Warfarin *(PT affected earlier and more than PTT)*
- Disseminated intravascular coagulation (DIC) *(PT affected earlier and more than PTT)*
- Lupus anticoagulants *(may or may not prolong the PTT; PT is rarely prolonged)*
- Heparin *(PT less affected than PTT, PT may be normal)*
- Hirudin or argatroban *(PTT also prolonged)*
- Specific factor inhibitors *(PTT also prolonged except in the rare case of an inhibitor against factor VII)*

The effects of hereditary or acquired factor deficiencies on PT and PTT are shown in Tables 1 and 2 in Coagulation Factor Assays *on page 335.* Factor half-lives are summarized in Table 3 in that listing.

Monitoring warfarin: Warfarin is monitored by the international normalized ratio (INR). The usual therapeutic goal is an INR of 2-3. The INR is calculated from the PT and is intended to allow valid comparisons of results regardless of the type of PT reagent used among different laboratories:

INR = [patient PT / mean normal PT]^{ISI}

The international sensitivity index (ISI) is a measure of the sensitivity of a particular PT reagent. Different PT reagents have different sensitivities to factor deficiencies. For example, with an insensitive reagent, the PT will not become prolonged until the factor levels are very decreased, whereas with a sensitive reagent, the PT will become prolonged with milder factor deficiencies. Insensitive reagents have higher ISI values, up to about 3.0. Sensitive reagents have lower ISI values, down to about 1.0. The ISI for each reagent is determined by the manufacturer.

During warfarin initiation, the PT/INR is typically checked daily or at least 4-5 times per week until the dose and INR are therapeutic and stable.[8] The interval between PT/INR tests can then be gradually decreased to as infrequently as every 4 weeks, depending on the stability of the dose and the PT/INR result.[8,9] It takes 4-5 days for warfarin's antithrombotic action to take effect, because the half-lives of factors II and X are relatively long. For this reason, patients who need immediate anticoagulation are treated with an immediate-acting anticoagulant (eg, heparin) while waiting for warfarin to become therapeutic. Heparin is typically continued until the INR is in the desired range for two consecutive days.[9]

To treat warfarin overdose (bleeding), vitamin K or fresh frozen plasma can be administered.[9] If the INR is >5 without bleeding, vitamin K administration can be considered. If large doses of vitamin K are administered, patients can become temporarily warfarin resistant.

Warfarin (Coumadin®) and vitamin K deficiency share the same molecular basis for their effects. Warfarin is used as a therapeutic anticoagulant because it impairs the regeneration of active vitamin K, thereby decreasing the amount of active vitamin K. Vitamin K in its active form is a cofactor in a reaction which carboxylates glutamic acid residues to form gamma carboxyglutamic acid residues on factors II, VII, IX, and X as well as protein C and protein S. This carboxylation step is necessary for normal activity of these proteins. As a result, vitamin K deficiency or warfarin therapy decreases the activity of these proteins and prolongs the PT. Patients with mild vitamin K deficiency or low levels of warfarin anticoagulation can have a normal PTT.

In certain situations (eg, lupus anticoagulants or the concomitant use of hirudin or argatroban with warfarin) alternative assays may be used to monitor warfarin because the PT/INR will be elevated by hirudin, argatroban, and occasionally by lupus anticoagulants.[5] Alternative assays (eg, chromogenic factor X assays) are not affected by these interferences. However, alternative assays have not yet been well studied in these settings. An INR of 2-3 corresponds approximately to a chromogenic factor X of 20% to 40%.

Changes in dietary vitamin K (see website reference below) and many medications (many of which are listed in reference 9) can alter the warfarin dose requirement. Hyperthyroidism, liver failure, cancer, fever, or vitamin K deficiency (from malabsorption, steatorrhea, poor nutrition, certain antibiotics etc) tend to decrease the dose required to increase the PT. Hypothyroidism or certain genetic polymorphisms tend to increase the dose requirement.[10] Some patients have hereditary warfarin resistance, an uncommon condition in which very high doses of warfarin are needed to maintain a therapeutic INR.

Warfarin should not be used alone in the acute setting of heparin-induced thrombocytopenia, because paradoxical thrombosis can occur. If warfarin is used in this setting, a rapid-acting anticoagulant (eg, hirudin, danaparoid, or argatroban) must also be used until the INR is therapeutic.[11] A similar approach is used for patients with hereditary protein C or protein S deficiency, to prevent Coumadin®-induced skin necrosis.

Footnotes

1. NCCLS, "Collection, Transport, and Processing of Blood Specimens for Coagulation Testing and General Performance of Coagulation Assays: Approved Guideline 3rd edition," NCCLS Document H21-A3, NCCLS, 940 West Valley Road, Wayne, Pennsylvania 19087, USA 1998.
2. Gottfried EL and Adachi MM, "Prothrombin Time and Activated Partial Thromboplastin Time Can Be Performed on the First Tube," *Am J Clin Pathol*, 1997, 107(6):681-3.
3. Andrew M, Paes B, and Johnston M, "Development of the Hemostatic System in the Neonate and Young Infant," *Am J Pediatr Hematol Oncol*, 1990, 12(1):95-104.
4. Burns ER, Goldberg SN, and Wenz B, "Paradox Effect of Multiple Mild Coagulation Factor Deficiencies on the Prothrombin Time and Activated Partial Thromboplastin Time," *Am J Clin Pathol*, 1993, 100(2):94-8.
5. Moll S and Ortel TL, "Monitoring Warfarin Therapy in Patients With Lupus Anticoagulants," *Ann Intern Med*, 1997, 127(3):177-85.
6. Sawicki PT, Working Group for the Study of Patient Self-Management of Oral Anticoagulation, "A Structured Teaching and Self-Management Program for Patients Receiving Oral Anticoagulation," *J Am Med Assoc*, 1999, 281(2):145-50.
7. Spero JA, Lewis JH, and Hasiba U, "Disseminated Intravascular Coagulation: Findings in 346 Patients," *Thromb Haemost*, 1980, 43(1):28-33.
8. Fairweather RB, Ansell J, van den Besselaar AM, et al, "College of American Pathologists Conference XXXI on Laboratory Monitoring of Anticoagulant Therapy. Laboratory Monitoring of Oral Anticoagulant Therapy," *Arch Pathol Lab Med*, 1998, 122(9):768-81.
9. Hirsh J, Dalen JE, Anderson DR, et al, "Oral Anticoagulants. Mechanism of Action, Clinical Effectiveness, and Optimal Therapeutic Range," *Chest*, 1998, 114(5):445-69S.
10. Taube J, Halsall D, and Baglin T, "Influence of Cytochrome P-450 CYP2C9 Polymorphisms on Warfarin Sensitivity and Risk of Over-Anticoagulation in Patients on Long-Term Treatment," *Blood*, 2000, 96(5):1816-9.
11. Warkentin TE, "Heparin-Induced Thrombocytopenia: IgG-Mediated Platelet Activation, Platelet Microparticle Generation, and Altered Procoagulant/Anticoagulant Balance in the Pathogenesis of Thrombosis and Venous Limb Gangrene Complicating Heparin-Induced Thrombocytopenia," *Transfus Med Rev*, 1996, X:249-58.

References

Bajaj SP and Joist JH, "New Insights Into How Blood Clots: Implications for the Use of APTT and PT as Coagulation Screening Tests and in Monitoring of Anticoagulant Therapy," *Semin Thromb Hemost*, 1999, 25(4):407-18.
Hyers TM, Agnelli G, Hull RD, et al, "Antithrombotic Therapy for Venous Thrombotic Disease," *Chest*, 1998, 114(5):561-578S.

Internet Web Sites
www.nal.usda.gov (foods with vitamin K)

- **Protime** *see* Prothrombin Time *on page 354*
- **PT** *see* Prothrombin Time *on page 354*
- **PTP** *see* Platelet Antibodies *on page 349*
- **PTT** *see* Activated Partial Thromboplastin Time *on page 328*
- **PTT** *see* Antiphospholipid Antibody (Lupus Anticoagulant and/or Anticardiolipin Antibody) *on page 331*
- **PTT** *see* Heparin Antifactor Xa Assay *on page 342*
- **PTT** *see* Heparin Neutralization *on page 344*

Reptilase® Time

Related Information
D-Dimers and Fibrin Degradation Products *on page 338*
Fibrinogen *on page 341*
Hypercoagulation Panel *on page 345*
Thrombin Time *on page 356*

Abstract Clotting time similar to thrombin time except that a snake venom (Reptilase®) is used instead of thrombin. The Reptilase® time is prolonged by decreased or dysfunctional fibrinogen, or high levels of fibrin degradation products (FDP). Dysfibrinogenemia is an uncommon hereditary or acquired condition characterized by dysfunctional fibrinogen.

Specimen Plasma
(Continued)

Reptilase® Time *(Continued)*

Container One blue top (sodium citrate) tube

Collection Routine venipuncture. If multiple tests are being drawn, draw blue top tubes after any red top tubes but before any lavender top (EDTA), green top (heparin), or gray top (oxalate/fluoride) tubes. Immediately invert tube gently at least 4 times to mix. Tubes must be appropriately filled. Deliver tubes immediately to the laboratory.

Storage Instructions Separate plasma from cells as soon as possible. Plasma may be stored at room temperature or on ice for up to 8 hours; otherwise, store frozen.

Causes for Rejection Specimen received more than 4 hours after collection, tube not filled, clotted specimens

Turnaround Time Less than 1 day

Reference Interval 16-24 seconds

Use Performed with thrombin time to diagnose dysfibrinogenemia in patients undergoing evaluation for hypercoagulability and/or a bleeding tendency. Often performed only if an initial panel of tests excludes more common disorders, as dysfibrinogenemia is uncommon. Unlike the thrombin time, Reptilase® time is not prolonged by heparin or hirudin.

Methodology Reptilase® is added to patient plasma and the clotting time is measured in seconds. Reptilase® cleaves fibrinogen, releasing fibrinopeptide A from fibrinogen and converting fibrinogen into fibrin clot. In contrast, when thrombin cleaves fibrinogen, fibrinopeptide A and fibrinopeptide B are both released from fibrinogen.

Additional Information Many different mutations are known to cause hereditary dysfibrinogenemia. Dysfibrinogenemia mutations can cause bleeding, thrombosis, or both, or they may be clinically asymptomatic. If bleeding is present, it is usually mild, but severe bleeding has been reported. Dysfibrinogenemia has an estimated prevalence of 0.8% in patients with venous thrombosis.[1] Arterial thrombosis is less frequent than venous thrombosis in these patients. Most patients with hereditary dysfibrinogenemia are heterozygous. Rare homozygous cases have been reported. The Reptilase® time and thrombin time, which measure the clotting time during the conversion of fibrinogen into fibrin, are often prolonged in dysfibrinogenemia because fibrinogen is dysfunctional. Assays that measure fibrinogen function show lower levels than assays that measure fibrinogen quantity (immunological or "antigen" assays), because fibrinogen function is impaired but fibrinogen quantity is not. The PT and PTT may be prolonged in dysfibrinogenemia.[1,2,3] Causes of acquired dysfibrinogenemia include liver disease, hepatoma,[3] or acute phase reactions with generation of high levels of fibrinogen.[4] The bleeding and thrombosis risk with acquired dysfibrinogenemia is uncertain. Prolongation of the thrombin time and Reptilase® time has been commonly observed with amyloidosis due to inhibition of fibrinogen conversion to fibrin.[5]

Footnotes

1. Haverkate F and Samama M, "Familial Dysfibrinogenemia and Thrombophilia. Report on a Study of the SSC Subcommittee on Fibrinogen," *Thromb Haemost*, 1995, 73(1):151-61.
2. Cote HC, Lord ST, and Pratt KP, "γ-Chain Dysfibrinogenemias: Molecular Structure-Function Relationships of Naturally Occurring Mutations in the γ Chain of Human Fibrinogen," *Blood*, 1998, 92(7):2195-212.
3. Galanakis DK, "Fibrinogen Anomalies and Disease. A Clinical Update," *Hematol Oncol Clin North Am*, 1992, 6(5):1171-87.
4. Galanakis DK, personal communication, 1999.
5. Gastineau DA, Gertz MA, Daniels TM, et al, "Inhibitor of the Thrombin Time in Systemic Amyloidosis: A Common Coagulation Abnormality," *Blood*, 1991, 77(12):2637-40.

♦ **Ristocetin Cofactor** *see* von Willebrand Factor *on page 357*

♦ **Ristocetin-Induced Platelet Aggregation Assay** *see* von Willebrand Factor *on page 357*

♦ **Schistocytes** *see* Disseminated Intravascular Coagulation Screen *on page 338*

♦ **Screen for Disseminated Intravascular Coagulation** *see* Disseminated Intravascular Coagulation Screen *on page 338*

♦ **Screen for Hypercoagulation** *see* Hypercoagulation Panel *on page 345*

♦ **Sedimentation Rate** *see* Fibrinogen *on page 341*

♦ **Serotonin Release Assays** *see* Heparin-Induced Thrombocytopenia *on page 343*

♦ **Stable Factor (Factor VII)** *see* Coagulation Factor Assays *on page 335*

♦ **Stuart Factor (Factor X)** *see* Coagulation Factor Assays *on page 335*

♦ **Stuart-Prower Factor (Factor X)** *see* Coagulation Factor Assays *on page 335*

♦ **Thrombin** *see* D-Dimers and Fibrin Degradation Products *on page 338*

♦ **Thrombin** *see* Fibrinogen *on page 341*

♦ **Thrombin-Antithrombin Complexes** *see* Hypercoagulation Panel *on page 345*

Thrombin Time

Related Information

Activated Partial Thromboplastin Time *on page 328*

D-Dimers and Fibrin Degradation Products *on page 338*
Factor Inhibitors *on page 340*
Fibrinogen *on page 341*
Heparin Antifactor Xa Assay *on page 342*
Heparin Neutralization *on page 344*
Hypercoagulation Panel *on page 345*
Reptilase® Time *on page 355*

Applies to Fibrinopeptide A; Fibrinopeptide B

Abstract Measures clotting time of the last step in the coagulation cascade, which is the conversion of fibrinogen into fibrin by thrombin. Useful for diagnosis of dysfibrinogenemia. Very sensitive to low amounts of heparin, hirudin, or argatroban anticoagulants.

Specimen Plasma

Container One blue top (sodium citrate) tube

Collection Routine venipuncture. If multiple tests are being drawn, draw blue top tubes after any red top tubes but before any lavender top (EDTA), green top (heparin), or gray top (oxalate/fluoride) tubes. Immediately invert tube gently at least 4 times to mix. Tubes must be appropriately filled. Deliver tubes immediately to the laboratory, on ice.

Storage Instructions Separate plasma from cells as soon as possible. Plasma may be stored on ice for up to 4 hours; otherwise, store frozen.

Causes for Rejection Specimen received more than 4 hours after collection, tube not filled, clotted specimens

Turnaround Time Less than 1 day

Reference Interval Approximately 10-13 seconds or 16-24 seconds, depending on thrombin concentration and ionic strength of the reaction conditions

Use Performed together with Reptilase® time to diagnose dysfibrinogenemia in patients undergoing evaluation for hypercoagulability and/or a bleeding tendency. Often performed only if an initial panel of tests excludes more common disorders, because dysfibrinogenemia is uncommon. The thrombin time is an older method for detecting heparin contamination in specimens; direct heparin neutralizing methods are now available for this purpose. The thrombin time has occasionally been used to monitor heparin therapy in patients for whom the PTT could not be used,[1] but now antifactor Xa assays are available for such situations. The thrombin time is often too sensitive to monitor heparin anticoagulation, and the assay is not standardized for this purpose.

Methodology Thrombin is added to patient plasma and the clotting time is measured in seconds. Thrombin cleaves fibrinogen, releasing fibrinopeptide A and fibrinopeptide B from fibrinogen and converting fibrinogen into fibrin clot. Assays use bovine or human thrombin.

Some laboratories use the thrombin time to detect unexpected heparin contamination in specimens. Even small amounts of heparin prolong the thrombin time, because heparin inhibits thrombin. If the thrombin time is prolonged, patient plasma can be mixed with an equal volume of normal plasma. The thrombin time of the mixture remains prolonged if the prolongation is due to heparin, fibrin degradation products (FDP), hirudin, argatroban, or other thrombin inhibitors. If the thrombin time of the mixture is normal, then the etiology of the prolongation is decreased fibrinogen or dysfibrinogenemia. The Reptilase® time is not prolonged by heparin. Many laboratories now use direct heparin neutralizing methods to detect heparin contamination rather than the thrombin time (see Heparin Neutralization *on page 344*).

Additional Information The thrombin time is prolonged when fibrinogen is decreased or dysfunctional, or when a thrombin inhibitor is present. **Dysfibrinogenemia** is an uncommon hereditary or acquired condition characterized by dysfunctional fibrinogen. Many different mutations are known to cause hereditary dysfibrinogenemia. Dysfibrinogenemia mutations can cause bleeding, thrombosis, or both, or they may be clinically asymptomatic. If bleeding is present it is usually mild, but severe bleeding has been reported. Dysfibrinogenemia has an estimated prevalence of 0.8% in patients with venous thrombosis.[2] Arterial thrombosis is less frequent than venous thrombosis in these patients. Most patients with hereditary dysfibrinogenemia are heterozygous. Rare homozygous cases have been reported. The thrombin time and Reptilase® time, which measure the clotting time during the conversion of fibrinogen into fibrin, are often prolonged in dysfibrinogenemia because fibrinogen is dysfunctional. Assays that measure fibrinogen function show lower levels than assays that measure fibrinogen quantity (immunological or "antigen" assays), because fibrinogen function is impaired but fibrinogen quantity is not. The PT and PTT may be prolonged in dysfibrinogenemia.[2,3,4] Causes of acquired dysfibrinogenemia include liver disease, hepatoma,[4] or or acute phase reactions with generation of high levels of fibrinogen.[5] The bleeding and thrombosis risk with acquired dysfibrinogenemia is uncertain. See Fibrinogen *on page 341*.

The thrombin time can be prolonged in disseminated intravascular coagulation (DIC) or thrombolytic therapy due to high levels of FDP and decreased fibrinogen. However, the thrombin time is not a necessary test for DIC diagnosis because fibrinogen and FDP can be measured directly. Prolongation of the thrombin time and Reptilase® time has been commonly observed with amyloidosis due to inhibition of fibrinogen conversion to fibrin.[6] Patients exposed to bovine thrombin may develop thrombin inhibitors that prolong bovine-based thrombin times, and if the antibody cross-reacts against human thrombin, human-based thrombin times can also be prolonged (see Factor Inhibitors *on page 340*). The Reptilase® time is normal with these inhibitors. Rarely, heparin-like anticoagulants have been reported in

COAGULATION: VON WILLEBRAND FACTOR

patients with malignancies or other disorders, with prolonged thrombin times and normal Reptilase® times.

Footnotes

1. Ray MJ, Perrin EJ, Smith IR, et al, "A Proposed Model to Monitor Heparin Therapy Using the Concentrated Thrombin Time Which Allows Standardization of Reagents and Improved Estimation of Heparin Concentrations," *Blood Coagul Fibrinolysis*, 1996, 7(5):515-21.
2. Haverkate F and Samama M, "Familial Dysfibrinogenemia and Thrombophilia. Report on a Study of the SSC Subcommittee on Fibrinogen," *Thromb Haemost*, 1995, 73(1):151-61.
3. Cote HC, Lord ST, and Pratt KP, "γ-Chain Dysfibrinogenemias: Molecular Structure-Function Relationships of Naturally Occurring Mutations in the γ Chain of Human Fibrinogen," *Blood*, 1998, 92(7):2195-212.
4. Galanakis DK, "Fibrinogen Anomalies and Disease. A Clinical Update," *Hematol Oncol Clin North Am*, 1992; 6(5):1171-87.
5. Galanakis D, personal communication, 1999.
6. Gastineau DA, Gertz MA, Daniels TM, et al, "Inhibitor of the Thrombin Time in Systemic Amyloidosis: A Common Coagulation Abnormality," *Blood*, 1991, 77(12):2637-40.

References

Olson JD, Arkin CF, Brandt JT, et al, "College of American Pathologists Conference XXXI on Laboratory Monitoring of Anticoagulant Therapy. Laboratory Monitoring of Unfractionated Heparin Therapy," *Arch Pathol Lab Med*, 1998, 122:782-98.

♦ **Thrombolysis** *see* D-Dimers and Fibrin Degradation Products *on page 338*

♦ **Thrombophilia Panel** *see* Hypercoagulation Panel *on page 345*

♦ **Thromboplastin** *see* Prothrombin Time *on page 354*

♦ **Thrombotic Disease Screen** *see* Hypercoagulation Panel *on page 345*

♦ **Tissue Plasminogen Activator** *see* Hypercoagulation Panel *on page 345*

♦ **Tissue Plasminogen Activator** *see* Plasminogen *on page 347*

♦ **Tissue Plasminogen Activator** *see* Plasminogen Activator Inhibitor 1 *on page 347*

♦ **tPA** *see* Hypercoagulation Panel *on page 345*

♦ **tPA** *see* Plasminogen *on page 347*

♦ **tPA** *see* Plasminogen Activator Inhibitor 1 *on page 347*

♦ **uPA** *see* Plasminogen *on page 347*

♦ **Urokinase-Type Plasminogen Activator** *see* Plasminogen *on page 347*

♦ **Vitamin K** *see* Prothrombin Time *on page 354*

---

von Willebrand Factor

Related Information

Coagulation Factor Assays *on page 335*
Factor VIII Concentrate *on page 841*

Synonyms Multimer Assay; Ristocetin Cofactor; Ristocetin-Induced Platelet Aggregation Assay; von Willebrand Factor Antigen; von Willebrand Factor Assay; von Willebrand Factor Collagen-Binding Assay; von Willebrand Factor Multimer Assay

Applies to Acute Phase Reactants; DDAVP; Desmopressin; Factor VIII:von Willebrand Factor Ratio

Test Includes Assays for von Willebrand factor (vWF) activity (ristocetin cofactor), vWF antigen, and factor VIII should be ordered. If indicated by these results, a vWF multimer analysis and/or low-dose ristocetin aggregation assay can be ordered.

Abstract von Willebrand factor (vWF) mediates platelet adhesion to injured endothelium, the first step in hemostasis. It also helps maintain factor VIII levels. When vWF is deficient, patients have a bleeding disorder called von Willebrand disease (vWD). vWD is the most common hereditary bleeding disorder, of which several subtypes are recognized (see below).

Specimen Plasma

Container Three blue top (sodium citrate) tubes

Collection Routine venipuncture. Deliver tubes to laboratory immediately, otherwise falsely low factor VIII values may occur (factor VIII is labile). If multiple tests are being drawn, draw blue top tubes after any red top tubes but before any lavender top (EDTA), green top (heparin), or gray top (oxalate/fluoride) tubes. Immediately invert tubes gently at least 4 times to mix. Tubes must be appropriately filled.

Storage Instructions Separate plasma from cells as soon as possible. Plasma can be stored for 2 hours on ice, otherwise store frozen. For vWF antigen only, plasma can be stored for 8 hours at room temperature or 24 hours on ice, otherwise store frozen.

Causes for Rejection Specimen received more than 4 hours after collection, tubes not filled, clotted specimens

Turnaround Time Several days (longer if follow-up testing is needed, such as multimer analysis)

Reference Interval Varies with blood type through an unknown mechanism. Results are reported as a percent of the amount expected in normal plasma. By definition, the mean value in pooled normal plasma is 100%. In a large study of normal persons, the mean vWF level was 75% in blood type

O, 106% in type A, 117% in type B, and 123% in type AB individuals. The overall mean vWF level was 100%.[1] Newborns have higher vWF levels than do adults. Values for vWF gradually decrease into the adult normal range by age 6 months.[2]

Use Determine if a patient with a personal or family history of bleeding has von Willebrand disease (vWD); assist in determining hemophilia A carrier status in females

Methodology

Initial tests:

The **ristocetin cofactor assay** assesses vWF function by measuring ristocetin-mediated binding of vWF to platelet GPIb, which leads to platelet agglutination.[3] The ristocetin cofactor assay is performed by mixing patient plasma with ristocetin and formalin-fixed normal platelets and measuring the amount of platelet agglutination in an aggregometer. **Note:** The term "agglutination" is often used to describe ristocetin-induced platelet aggregation, because true platelet aggregation links platelets through fibrinogen and GPIIb/IIIa, whereas ristocetin links platelets through von Willebrand factor and GPIb. The **von Willebrand factor antigen** assay is an enzyme-linked immunosorbent assay (ELISA), which measures the quantity of vWF, independent of vWF function. An alternative automated assay involves latex particles coated with antibodies directed against vWF. In the presence of vWF, the latex particles form aggregates that absorb light passing through the specimen. The amount of light absorbance is directly related to the amount of vWF in the specimen. Rocket immunoelectrophoresis is an older antigen assay that is still in use in some laboratories. The **factor VIII assay** is a PTT-based clotting assay which measures factor VIII activity.

More recently, alternative immunoassays have been designed to assess vWF function.[4] The collagen-binding assay is an ELISA in which collagen is the antigen. If vWF is functional, it binds to collagen and is subsequently detected. Another vWF "functional" ELISA uses monoclonal antibodies that recognize a functional epitope on vWF, but there is conflicting evidence whether this test correlates better with ristocetin cofactor or with vWF antigen. These newer functional assays are not yet as established as the ristocetin cofactor assay.

Interpretation of von Willebrand Factor Assays

RCoF + vWF Ag + FVIII + Fibrinogen (or other acute phase reaction marker):
• Normal:* vWD unlikely if no acute phase reaction, pregnancy, estrogen use, newborn
• Normal* but fibrinogen (or factor VIII) elevated: repeat vWF assays when fibrinogen and factor VIII are normal
• RCoF, vWF Ag, FVIII reduced to a similar extent: **type 1** vWD likely
• RCoF, vWF Ag, FVIII severely reduced (<10%) or undetectable: **type 3** vWD likely
• RCoF reduced more severely than vWF Ag and FVIII:† consider **type 2** vWD (2A, 2B, or 2M); perform multimer analysis and low-dose ristocetin cofactor to determine subtype:
– Multimer analysis normal: type 2M likely (subtle abnormalities in some variants)
– Multimer analysis missing high molecular weight multimers: type 2A likely
– Multimer analysis missing high and intermediate molecular weight multimers: type 2B or platelet type likely
– Increased low-dose ristocetin aggregation: type 2B or platelet type‡
– Normal or decreased low-dose ristocetin aggregation: not type 2B or platelet type
• FVIII reduced (5% to 40%), RCoF and vWF Ag normal:† consider **type 2N** vWD; or in males, mild hemophilia A. In female hemophilia A carriers, factor VIII is approximately 50% with large variability. Consider also factor VIII degradation if prolonged specimen transportation.

*Consider blood type when determining if values are normal.

†Mean RCoF:vWF Ag ratio is 0.3 for type 2A, 0.6 for type 2B, and uncertain (<1) for type 2M. Mean FVIII:vWF Ag ratio is 0.28 for type 2N (see Footnote 13).

‡Thrombocytopenia may occur with type 2B or platelet-type (and rare type 2A variants).
RCoF = ristocetin cofactor assay; vWF Ag = von Willebrand factor antigen assay; FVIII = factor VIII assay

Follow-up tests (performed if indicated, see table):

Multimer analysis is performed when type 2 vWD is suspected.[5] A plasma sample is electrophoresed on a gel to separate the multimers by size. The multimers are then visualized using ^{125}I-labeled anti-vWF antibody or other techniques. **Low-dose ristocetin platelet aggregation assay** is performed when type 2B vWD is suspected.[6] This test is similar to the ristocetin cofactor assay, except that the patient's own platelets are used instead of normal platelets, and lower doses of ristocetin are used. The patient's own platelets and plasma are mixed with ristocetin, and platelet aggregation is measured in an aggregometer. This assay is less sensitive than the ristocetin cofactor assay for diagnosing vWD, but it is useful for confirming a diagnosis of type 2B vWD. Type 2B patients' platelets become abnormally coated with vWF *in vivo*, due to increased affinity of the mutant vWF for platelet GPIb. As a result, the patient's platelets show increased aggregation in this assay. Platelet-type vWD also shows increased aggregation in this assay, due to a mutation on platelet GPIb which increases its affinity for vWF. In contrast, other types of vWD may show decreased ristocetin-induced platelet aggregation due to decreased vWF quantity and/or function. Further specialized coagulation testing can be performed to distinguish type 2B from platelet-type vWD.

Additional Information von Willebrand disease (vWD) is the most common hereditary bleeding disorder, occurring in up to 1% of the general population.[7,8] Many cases remain undiagnosed because of the mild nature
(Continued)

von Willebrand Factor (Continued)

of bleeding in many patients and the fact that acute phase reactions can mask the diagnosis. vWF is a polypeptide synthesized in endothelial cells and megakaryocytes, which polymerizes to form multimers containing up to 100 subunits. Bleeding symptoms resemble those of a platelet function defect, since platelet adhesion is impaired. Thus, the most common symptoms are epistaxis, easy bruising, bleeding with dental extractions, and menorrhagia.

Laboratory testing for vWD is summarized in the table. Repeat testing is often required, because both vWF and factor VIII become elevated above baseline during acute phase reactions (including even minor illnesses, injury, or stress), pregnancy, estrogen use, or in newborns. **An elevation of a low or borderline value for vWF into the normal range during any of these conditions often masks the diagnosis of vWD.** Measurement of an acute phase reactant such as fibrinogen is helpful in assessing the likelihood that a patient is in an acute phase reaction at the time of testing.

vWF serves as the carrier protein for factor VIII, and levels of factor VIII are often decreased when vWF is decreased. When vWF is markedly decreased, the factor VIII level can also become very low, which prolongs the PTT. In most vWD patients, the disease is mild or moderate and the PTT is therefore normal.

Many variants of vWD have been described, but the classification scheme has recently been simplified into three types (see table).[9] Type 1 is by far the most common form, accounting for the majority of cases. Type 1 vWD is characterized by a partial quantitative deficiency of vWF. Although the quantity of vWF is reduced, the function of the individual vWF molecules which are synthesized is normal.

Type 2 vWD is characterized by qualitative (functional) deficiencies of vWF. Often the quantity of vWF is also reduced. Type 2 vWD is further subdivided into four categories (see table). Type 2A and type 2B are characterized by a loss of high molecular weight multimers of vWF. The highest molecular weight multimers have more hemostatic function than the lower molecular weight multimers. Therefore, in these disorders, the overall function relative to the quantity of vWF molecules is reduced. Thus, the functional assay (ristocetin cofactor) result is reduced more than the quantitative assay (von Willebrand factor antigen). In type 2A, the loss of high molecular weight multimers is due to defective multimer assembly and secretion or increased proteolysis of multimers.[10,11]

Type 2B vWD mutations lead to increased binding of vWF to GPIb, the platelet vWF receptor.[6] Platelets coated with vWF are cleared from the bloodstream at an increased rate, leading to loss of high molecular weight multimers as well as thrombocytopenia.

Platelet-type or pseudo-vWD is a rare disorder in which a mutation in the platelet GPIb gene (not the vWF gene) leads to increased binding of vWF to GPIb, resulting in the same findings described above for type 2B vWD.[12]

Types 2M and 2N vWD are rare subtypes of type 2 vWD. Type 2M vWF mutations cause decreased function despite the presence of normal-sized multimers, often because the mutation impairs the ability of vWF to bind to platelet GPIb.[9,13] In type 2N (Normandy) vWD, the factor VIII-binding ability of vWF is impaired, and the half-life of factor VIII is consequently shortened. Thus, vWF is normal in quantity (normal antigen assay) and has normal platelet-adhesion function (normal ristocetin cofactor assay), but factor VIII levels are decreased. **As a result, type 2N patients are frequently misdiagnosed as having hemophilia A.**[14] The family history may be useful in distinguishing type 2N vWD from hemophilia A. Type 2N vWD is inherited autosomally (males and females are affected), whereas hemophilia A is an X-linked recessive disorder (males are affected and females are carriers). An assay which measures the ability of vWF to bind factor VIII is available in a limited number of specialized laboratories. Type 2N patients show decreased binding of factor VIII in this assay.

Type 3 vWD is a rare, severe bleeding disorder characterized by a severe quantitative deficiency of vWF such that vWF is typically undetectable.

The bleeding time is often prolonged in vWD. However, it is neither a necessary nor a reliable test for diagnosis.

In hemophilia A carriers (who are females only), the factor VIII:vWF ratio is ~0.5, instead of the normal ratio of 1. Definitive determination of carrier status may require DNA-based testing for mutations that cause hemophilia A.

Bleeding episodes, in most patients, can be treated with DDAVP (desmopressin) if needed, as DDAVP temporarily increases the levels of vWF and factor VIII two- to threefold. As a small percentage of patients do not respond to DDAVP, patients are usually given a trial dose of DDAVP while asymptomatic, with measurement of their vWF level before and after DDAVP, to ensure that their vWF levels do increase with DDAVP. Bleeding patients who do not respond to DDAVP or patients with severe vWD can be treated with vWF-containing factor VIII concentrates (eg, Humate-P®, Alphanate®, Koāte®). Some consider DDAVP contraindicated in type 2B because it can cause thrombocytopenia. However, others report DDAVP is a beneficial treatment for type 2B patients.

Acquired vWD is a rare condition that can occur spontaneously or in association with a variety of underlying disorders, such as hematologic neoplasms or autoimmune diseases. Thrombotic thrombocytopenic purpura (TTP) is due to a deficiency of a vWF-cleaving protease, usually due to an autoantibody against the protease.[15,16] This could account for the microvascular platelet-rich thrombi and thrombocytopenia that are characteristic of TTP. Unusually large vWF multimers may also be seen in TTP.

Footnotes

1. Gill JC, Endres-Brooks J, Bauer PJ, et al, "The Effect of ABO Blood Group on the Diagnosis of von Willebrand's Disease," *Blood*, 1987, 69(6):1691-5.
2. Andrew M, Paes B, and Johnston M, "Development of the Hemostatic System in the Neonate and Young Infant," *Am J Pediatr Hematol Oncol*, 1990,12(1):95-104.
3. Weiss HJ, Hoyer LW, Rickles FR, et al, "Quantitative Assay of a Plasma Factor Deficient in von Willebrand's Disease That Is Necessary for Platelet Aggregation. Relationship to Factor VIII Procoagulant Activity and Antigen Content," *J Clin Invest*, 1973, 52:2708-16.
4. Favaloro EJ, "Collagen Binding Assay for von Willebrand Factor (VWF:CBA): Detection of von Willebrand's Disease (VWD), and Discrimination of VWD Subtypes, Depends on Collagen Source," *Thromb Haemost*, 2000, 83(1):127-35.
5. Ruggeri ZM and Zimmerman TS, "Variant von Willebrand's Disease: Characterization of Two Subtypes by Analysis of Multimeric Composition of Factor VIII/von Willebrand Factor in Plasma and Platelets," *Blood*, 1980, 65(6):1318-25.
6. Ruggeri ZM, Pareti FI, Mannucci PM, et al, "Heightened Interaction Between Platelets and Factor VIII/von Willebrand Factor in a New Subtype of von Willebrand's Disease," *N Engl J Med*, 1980, 302:1047-51.
7. Rodeghiero F, Castaman G, and Dini E, "Epidemiological Investigation of The Prevalence of von Willebrand's Disease," *Blood*, 1987, 69(2):454-9.
8. Werner EJ, Broxson EH, Tucker EL, et al, "Prevalence of von Willebrand Disease in Children: A Multiethnic Study," *J Pediatr*, 1993, 123:893-8.
9. Sadler JE, "A Revised Classification of von Willebrand Diseases," *Thromb Haemost*, 1994, 71:520-5.
10. Lyons SE, Bruck ME, Bowie EJ, et al, "Impaired Intracellular Transport Produced by a Subset of Type IIA von Willebrand Disease Mutations," *J Biol Chem*, 1992, 267:4424-30.
11. Nichols WC, Seligsohn U, Zivelin A, et al, "Mutations in the ER-Golgi Intermediate Compartment Protein ERGIC-53 Cause Combined Deficiency of Coagulation Factors V and VIII," *Cell*, 1998, 93(1):61-70.
12. Miller JL, "Platelet-Type von Willebrand's Disease," *Thromb Haemost*, 1996, 75(6):865-9.
13. Meyer D, Fressinaud E, Gaucher C, et al, "Gene Defects in 150 Unrelated French Cases With Type 2 von Willebrand's Disease: From the Patient to the Gene," *Thromb Haemost*, 1997, 78(1):451-6.
14. Mazurier C, "von Willebrand's Disease Masquerading as Haemophilia A," *Thromb Haemost*, 1992, 67:391-6.
15. Furlan M, Robles R, Galbusera M, et al, "von Willebrand Factor-Cleaving Protease in Thrombotic Thrombocytopenic Purpura and the Hemolytic-Uremia Syndrome," *N Engl J Med*, 1998, 339(22):1578-84.
16. Tsai HM and Lian EC, "Antibodies to von Willebrand Factor-Cleaving Protease in Acute Thrombotic Thrombocytopenic Purpura," *N Engl J Med*, 1998, 339(22):1585-94.

References

Ewenstein BM, "von Willebrand's Disease," *Annu Rev Med*, 1997, 48:525-42.

Ginsberg D and Sadler JE, "von Willebrand's Disease: A Database of Point Mutations, Insertions and Deletions," *Thromb Haemost*, 1993, 69:177-84.

Internet Web Sites

mmg2.im.med.umich.edu/vwf (database of vWF mutations)

♦ **von Willebrand Factor Antigen** *see* von Willebrand Factor *on page 357*

♦ **von Willebrand Factor Assay** *see* von Willebrand Factor *on page 357*

♦ **von Willebrand Factor Collagen-Binding Assay** *see* von Willebrand Factor *on page 357*

♦ **von Willebrand Factor Multimer Assay** *see* von Willebrand Factor *on page 357*

♦ **Williams-Fitzgerald-Flaujeac Factor** *see* High-Molecular Weight Kininogen *on page 344*

CYTOGENETICS

Diane L. Persons, MD

Contributor: Wayne R. DeMott, MD

Chromosomes, as they appear in a metaphase spread, consist of tightly coiled DNA and protein. A karyotype is the somatic chromosomal complement of an individual or species. For the human, a normal karyotype consists of 46 chromosomes including 22 pairs of autosomes, identical in males and females, and one pair of sex chromosomes, XX in the female and XY in the male. The primary constriction of a chromosome, the centromere, divides the chromosome into an upper (short) arm and lower (long) arm designated "p" (petite) and "q", respectively. The chromosomes are aligned in a standard sequence on the basis of size, centromere location, and banding pattern. The karyotype is one of the basic tools of the cytogeneticist.

Chromosomal abnormalities are defined according to a uniform system, The International System for Cytogenetic Nomenclature. An example of the abbreviations provided in this system include the use of a plus sign to signify gain of a chromosome: +21 is interpreted as gain of one copy of chromosome 21. A translocation is designated by "t" and is defined as the exchange of chromosomal material between two or more nonhomologous chromosomes. A list of some of the most commonly utilized terms is provided in the following table.

Partial Listing of Symbols and Abbreviated Terms

del	Deletion
der	Derivative chromosome
dmin	Double minute
hsr	Homogeneously staining region
i	Isochromosome
ins	Insertion
inv	Inversion
mar	Marker chromosome
mat	Maternal origin
minus (-)	Loss of
p	Short arm
pat	Paternal origin
plus (+)	Gain of
q	Long arm
r	Ring chromosome
t	Translocation

From Mitelman F, *An International System of Human Cytogenetic Nomenclature*, 1995.

The greatest advance in the field of cytogenetics over the last decade has been the development of molecular cytogenetic techniques. Traditionally, cytogenetic data have been obtained through the direct microscopic analysis of chromosomes displaying characteristic bands with Giemsa, quinacrine, or other staining methods from cells arrested in metaphase. Progress in the study of the organization and function of nucleic acid sequences has made it possible to gain information about the chromosomes in an interphase or terminally differentiated cell by means of specially developed chromosome-specific probes and fluorescence *in situ* hybridization (FISH). These probes are labeled with fluorescent dyes, either directly or indirectly. Different combinations of haptenated probes (eg, labeled with biotin, digoxigenin, or dinitrophenol) and different fluorophores [green (fluorescein), red (rhodamine or Texas Red), and blue (AMCA or Cascade Blue)] allows visualization of three or more separate chromosomal DNA sequences concurrently. Specific DNA target sequences in individual cells in tissue sections, single-cell, or chromosome preparations can be detected with FISH. With this approach, DNA sequences can be mapped on specific chromosomes; repositioning of sequences between chromosomes or within a particular chromosome, as a result of a chromosomal rearrangement, can be determined; small rearrangements, not detectable with standard karyotypic analysis, can be uncovered; breakpoints using probes for defined DNA sequences can be detected and characterized; and numerical chromosomal abnormalities can be ascertained in interphase and/or metaphase cells. With respect to the latter, cell culture can be omitted, resulting in an expedited diagnosis. The newly developed techniques of spectral karyotyping and multicolor FISH identify all 24 human chromosomes simultaneously, greatly facilitating recognition of chromosome aberrations.

Another central area of diagnostic testing that has profited from advances in cytogenetic technology is cancer genetics. Cancer is an acquired genetic disorder resulting from loss of normal regulation of cell growth. This loss is manifested in a number of different ways, including alteration of the normal chromosomal complement. Cytogenetic analysis of both benign and malignant neoplasms has resulted in the definition of characteristic chromosomal anomalies which serve as important, if not essential, diagnostic aids. Identification of the aberrant chromosomal bands has provided a basis for molecular approaches in establishing the definitive genes affected and the associated consequences of these gene alterations. Moreover, many of these abnormalities are important prognostically.

Dr Julia Bridge is acknowledged with appreciation for her significant contributions to this chapter in the previous edition.

Amniotic Fluid, Chromosome and Genetic Abnormality Analysis

Related Information

Alpha₁-Fetoprotein, Amniotic Fluid on page 96
Alpha₁-Fetoprotein, Serum on page 97
Autosomal Dominant Polycystic Kidney Disease DNA Detection on page 704
Beta-Hexosaminidase, Serum, White Blood Cells on page 114
Bilirubin, Amniotic Fluid, Delta A450 on page 116
Chorionic Gonadotropin, Human, Serum and Urine on page 147
Chorionic Villus Sampling, Chromosome and Genetic Abnormality Analysis on page 361
Chromosome Analysis, Blood on page 361
Chromosome Analysis, Products of Conception on page 365
Creatinine, Amniotic Fluid on page 160
Cystic Fibrosis DNA Detection on page 705
Duchenne/Becker Muscular Dystrophy DNA Detection on page 706
Fluorescence In Situ Hybridization on page 367
Fragile X Syndrome DNA Test on page 708
Inherited Diseases of Metabolism and Cell Structure on page 449
Inhibin A, Serum on page 199
Lecithin:Sphingomyelin Ratio, Amniotic Fluid on page 210
Mucopolysaccharides, Urine on page 226
Phosphatidylglycerol, Amniotic Fluid on page 251
Polymerase Chain Reaction on page 713
Pregnancy-Associated Protein A, Serum on page 260
Pulmonary Surfactant, Amniotic Fluid on page 271

Synonyms Chromosome Studies, Amniotic Fluid; Karyotype, Amniotic Fluid

Applies to Enzyme Deficiency Analyses; Molecular Genetic Disorders

Test Includes Chromosomal complement of fetal cells in amniotic fluid are examined for determination of abnormalities.

Abstract A karyotype is the somatic chromosomal complement of an individual or species. For the human, a normal karyotype consists of 46 chromosomes aligned in a standard sequence on the basis of size, centromere location, and banding pattern. Amniocentesis is performed to obtain cells of fetal origin in the amniotic fluid for culturing and chromosomal analysis. Examination of the chromosomes by banding techniques can reveal numerical and/or structural abnormalities.

Patient Preparation The patient should be placed on her abdomen for ~20 minutes prior to the amniocentesis. Traditional amniocentesis is performed around 15-16 weeks gestation and early amniocentesis may be performed before 15 weeks (11-14 weeks). Ultrasound studies (to verify fetal life, detect multiple gestation, confirm fetal age, localize placenta, and detect fetal/uterine/adnexal abnormality) are usually carried out.

The Related Information field includes relevant tests in Chemistry and other chapters.

Specimen Amniotic fluid

Container Sterile container

Sampling Time At or after 16 weeks gestation

Collection An optimum quantity of 20 mL should be obtained by amniocentesis, using strict aseptic technique. Pertinent medical findings should accompany the request, including maternal age, gestational age by sonography, reason for study, relevant history, medication history, transfusion history, note of any viral infection, number of pregnancies and miscarriages, and suspected diagnosis. In the case of twins or triplets, amniotic fluid must be collected separately from each amniotic sac.

Storage Instructions Specimen should be transported to the laboratory at room temperature and under sterile conditions as quickly as possible.

Causes for Rejection Specimen frozen or clotted (due to excess contamination with blood)

Turnaround Time 1-2.5 weeks may be needed.

Reference Interval Forty-six chromosomes to include 22 sets of normal autosomal chromosomes and one set of normal sex chromosomes (XX for female; XY for male). Interpretative information is usually included.

Use Prenatal detection of chromosomal abnormalities, especially Down syndrome, in groups of pregnant women at risk. Such groups include women age 35 years or older, previous child with a chromosomal abnormality or multiple congenital abnormalities, three or more previous spontaneous abortions, familial history of a chromosomal abnormality, or known carrier of an X-linked disorder. At the same time that amniotic fluid is collected for chromosomal analysis, additional sample can be obtained for testing of inherited metabolic disorders (enzyme deficiency analyses on cultured cells), molecular genetic disorders, or neural tube defects (alpha₁-fetoprotein).

Limitations Failure of cells to grow in culture and/or contamination precludes complete analysis (fluorescence in situ hybridization may be of use if this occurs). Overall culture success rate has been reported as 97% with a fetal loss (within 4 weeks of the amniocentesis) of 1.2%. Higher fetal loss and increased incidence of musculoskeletal foot deformities have been described in early amniocentesis (11-12 weeks) compared to midtrimester (14-16 weeks) amniocentesis.[1]

Contraindications Environment lacking capability in ultrasonography, genetic counseling, amniocentesis, amniotic fluid culturing, and chromosomal analysis techniques

Methodology Cell culturing of fetal cells, subsequent harvesting, and chromosome analysis with Giemsa or quinacrine banding techniques

Additional Information At least 0.5% of newborns are born with a chromosomal abnormality. Among these, the most common is trisomy 21 or Down syndrome. It affects approximately 1 in 800 newborns and is a major cause of mental retardation. The incidence is higher in children born to mothers 35 years of age and older. For example, the incidence is 1 in 25 liveborn children of mothers older than 45 years of age. The risk of obstetric complications for amniocentesis is <0.5%. Because the risk of having a child with a chromosomal abnormality for a mother older than 35 years of age is greater than the risk of the procedure for amniocentesis or chorionic villus sampling, maternal age is an indication for prenatal testing. Rapid detection (24 hours) of the most common chromosome abnormalities (trisomy 21, 18, and 13 and sex chromosome aneusomy) can also be accomplished using fluorescence in situ hybridization (FISH) on interphase nuclei of uncultured amniocytes. See Fluorescence In Situ Hybridization on page 367.[2] In addition to numeric chromosome abnormalities, structural chromosome rearrangements are also detected by cytogenetic analysis.[3]

Birth defects and genetic disorders are encountered in ~3% of liveborn infants (less than 1/3 of which are the result of a chromosomal abnormality). Prenatal diagnosis is possible for more than 1000 inherited diseases, including inborn errors of metabolism. See the table for some of the most common metabolic, chromosome, and molecular genetic disorders that can be diagnosed prenatally.

Methods for Prenatal Diagnosis of Genetic Disorders	
Biochemical Analysis	
Adenosine deaminase deficiency	Lesch-Nyhan disease
Argininosuccinic aciduria	Mannosidosis
Batten disease	Maple syrup urine disease
Citrullinemia	Menkes disease
Cystinosis	Methylmalonic aciduria
Fabry disease	Mucopolysaccharidosis (I, II, III, VI, VII)
Farber disease	Niemann-Pick
Fucosidosis	Orotic aciduria
Galactosemia	Pyruvate decarboxylate deficiency
Gaucher disease	Refsum disease
Generalized gangliosidosis	Sandhoff disease
Glycogen storage disease (II, III, IV)	Steroid sulfatase deficiency
Homocystinuria	Tay-Sachs disease
I-cell disease	Wolman disease
Krabbe disease	
Cytogenetic Analysis	
Cri Du Chat syndrome (deletion 5)	**Chromosome Instability**
Down syndrome (trisomy 21)	Ataxia telangiectasia
Edwards syndrome (trisomy 18)	Bloom's syndrome
Klinefelter syndrome (XXY)	Fanconi anemia
Miller-Dieker syndrome (deletion 17)	
Patau syndrome (trisomy 13)	
Prader-Willi syndrome (deletion 15)	
Retinoblastoma (deletion 13)	
Unbalanced translocation	
Velocardiofacial/DiGeorge syndrome (deletion 22)	
Wiedemann-Beckwith syndrome (deletion 11)	
Wilms tumor (deletion 11)	
XXX syndrome (XXX)	
Molecular Genetic Analysis	
Adult polycystic kidney disease	Lesch-Nyhan syndrome
Alpha₁-antitrypsin deficiency	Multiple endocrine neoplasia (types 1 and 2a)
Alpha-thalassemia	Myotonic muscular dystrophy
Beta-thalassemia	Neurofibromatosis I
Carbamyl phosphate synthetase I deficiency	Norrie disease
Congenital adrenal hyperplasia	Ornithine transcarbamylase deficiency
Cystic fibrosis	Osteogenesis imperfecta
Duchenne/Becker muscular dystrophy	Phenylketonuria
Ehlers-Danlos syndrome	Retinoblastoma
Familial amyloidosis	Sickle cell disease
Fragile X syndrome	Tay-Sachs disease
Friedrich ataxia	Wiskott-Aldrich syndrome
Hemophilias A and B	X-linked lymphoproliferative disease
Huntington disease	

Footnotes

1. Delisle MF and Wilson RD, "First Trimester Prenatal Diagnosis: Amniocentesis," Semin Perinatol, 1999, 23(5):414-23.
2. Pergament E, Chen PX, Thangvelu M, et al, "The Clinical Application of Interphase FISH in Prenatal Diagnosis," Prenat Diagn, 2000, 20(3):215-20.

3. Warburton D, "*De novo* Balanced Chromosome Rearrangements and Extra Marker Chromosomes Identified at Prenatal Diagnosis: Clinical Significance and Distribution of Breakpoints," *Am J Hum Genet*, 1991, 49(5):995-1013.

References

Beaudet AL, Scriver CR, Sly WS, et al, "Genetics, Biochemistry, and Molecular Basis of Variant Human Phenotypes," *The Metabolic Basis of Inherited Disease*, 7th ed, Chapter 1, Scriver CR, Beaudet AL, Sly WS, et al, eds, New York, NY: McGraw-Hill Inc, 1995, 53-228.

Bridge JA and Sandberg AA, "Cytogenetics," *Anderson's Textbook of Pathology*, 10th ed, Damjanov I and Linder J, eds, 1996, 223-57.

DiLiberti JH, Greenstein MA, and Rosengren SS, "Prenatal Diagnosis," *Pediatr Rev*, 1992, 13(9):334-42.

- ♦ **Aneuploidy** *see* Chromosome Analysis, Bone Marrow *on page 362*

- ♦ **Aneusomy** *see* Chromosome Analysis, Bone Marrow *on page 362*

- ♦ **Aneusomy** *see* Fluorescence *In Situ* Hybridization *on page 367*

- ♦ **Bloom Syndrome** *see* Fanconi Anemia, Chromosome Breakage Study *on page 365*

- ♦ **Bone Marrow Chromosome Analysis** *see* Chromosome Analysis, Bone Marrow *on page 362*

Chorionic Villus Sampling, Chromosome and Genetic Abnormality Analysis

Related Information

Alpha$_1$-Fetoprotein, Amniotic Fluid *on page 96*
Alpha$_1$-Fetoprotein, Serum *on page 97*
Amniotic Fluid, Chromosome and Genetic Abnormality Analysis *on page 360*
Chorionic Gonadotropin, Human, Serum and Urine *on page 147*
Chromosome Analysis, Blood *on page 361*
Chromosome Analysis, Products of Conception *on page 365*
Cystic Fibrosis DNA Detection *on page 705*
Duchenne/Becker Muscular Dystrophy DNA Detection *on page 706*
Fluorescence *In Situ* Hybridization *on page 367*
Fragile X Syndrome DNA Test *on page 708*
Inherited Diseases of Metabolism and Cell Structure *on page 449*
Inhibin A, Serum *on page 199*
Mucopolysaccharides, Urine *on page 226*
Polymerase Chain Reaction *on page 713*
Pregnancy-Associated Protein A, Serum *on page 260*

Synonyms Chromosome Karyotype, Chorionic Villus Sampling; Chromosome Studies, Chorionic Villus Sampling; CVS, Chromosome and Genetic Abnormality Analysis

Test Includes Chromosomal complement of fetal trophoblast cells are examined for determination of abnormalities

Specimen Chorionic villi

Container Sterile container

Sampling Time 8-12 weeks gestation

Collection Fetal trophoblast tissue is aspirated from placental chorionic villi transcervically or transabdominally with ultrasound guidance as early as the 8th week of gestation, usually performed at 9-12 weeks of gestation.

Vascularized and budding villi of the chorion frondosum are collected transcervically or transabdominally by aseptic technique with ultrasound guidance between the 8th and 12th weeks of gestation. Maternally derived tissue such as maternal blood, decidua, and cervical mucus is carefully separated from other tissues under a dissecting microscope to prevent maternal cell contamination.

Pertinent medical findings should accompany the request, including maternal age, gestational age by sonography, reason for study, relevant history, medication history, transfusion history, note of viral infection, number of pregnancies and miscarriages, and suspected diagnosis.

Storage Instructions Specimen should be transported to the laboratory at room temperature and under sterile conditions as quickly as possible.

Causes for Rejection Specimen frozen or lacking in viable chorionic villi

Turnaround Time 1-2.5 weeks may be needed.

Reference Interval Forty-six chromosomes to include 22 sets of normal autosomal chromosomes and one set of normal sex chromosomes (XX for female; XY for male). Interpretative information is usually included.

Use Prenatal detection of chromosomal abnormalities, especially Down syndrome, in groups of pregnant women at risk. Such groups include women age 35 years or older, previous child with a chromosomal abnormality or multiple congenital abnormalities, three or more previous spontaneous abortions, familial history of a chromosomal abnormality, or known carrier of an X-linked disorder. At the same time that chorionic villi are collected for chromosomal analysis, additional sample can be obtained for testing of inherited metabolic disorders.

Limitations Failure of cells to grow in culture and/or contamination precludes complete analysis (fluorescence *in situ* hybridization may be of use if this occurs). The overall success rate of chromosome analysis is slightly lower than with amniocentesis. The rate of fetal loss due to CVS, when the fetus is viable at 8-12 weeks gestation, is approximately 1% to 3.5%.[1] Chromosome aberrations observed in the CVS specimen but not in the fetus (confined placental mosaicism) occur in ~1% of cases.[2] Additional invasive testing may be required in these cases.

Contraindications Environment lacking capability in ultrasonography, genetic counseling, CVS, chorionic villi culturing, and chromosomal analysis techniques

Methodology Cell culturing of fetal trophoblast, subsequent harvesting, and chromosome analysis with Giemsa or quinacrine banding techniques

Additional Information CVS is still a limited service in many centers. A distinct advantage of CVS is the earlier gestational age in which the specimen may be collected, thus reducing the period of uncertainty and allowing termination, if elected, to be performed on an outpatient basis, in the first trimester. Additionally, there is a rapid technique to visualize spontaneous metaphases in the cytotrophoblast layer yielding results in 1-3 days if desired. A disadvantage is that amniotic fluid alpha-fetoprotein (AFAFP) measurement cannot be performed at this stage; it must be done later.

Footnotes

1. Kim SK, Cho DJ, Kim JW, et al, "Adverse Pregnancy Outcome Following Postchorionic Villus Sampling Amniocentesis Compared to Chorionic Villus Sampling," *J Obstet Gynaecol Res*, 2000, 26(3):209-13.
2. Farra C, Giudicelli B, Pellissier MC, et al, "Fetoplacental Chromosomal Discrepancy," *Prenat Diagn*, 2000, 20(3):190-3.

References

Goldberg JD and Golbus MS, "Chorionic Villus Sampling," *Adv Hum Genet*, 1988, 17:1-25.

Jenkins TM and Wapner RJ, "First Trimester Prenatal Diagnosis: Chorionic Villus Sampling," *Semin Perinatol*, 1999, 23(5):403-13.

Chromosome Analysis, Blood

Related Information

Amniotic Fluid, Chromosome and Genetic Abnormality Analysis *on page 360*
Bone Marrow *on page 410*
Breakpoint Cluster Region Rearrangement in CML *on page 721*
Chorionic Villus Sampling, Chromosome and Genetic Abnormality Analysis *on page 361*
Chromosome Analysis, High-Resolution *on page 363*
Chromosome Analysis, Lymph Node and Solid Tumor *on page 364*
Chromosome Analysis, Products of Conception *on page 365*
Fluorescence *In Situ* Hybridization *on page 367*
Fragile X Syndrome DNA Test *on page 708*
Lymph Node Biopsy *on page 67*

Synonyms Chromosome Karyotype, Blood; Chromosome Studies, Blood; Cytogenetics, Blood; Karyotype, Blood

Abstract The constitutional karyotype (chromosome complement) of each individual is determined during fertilization or during the first few cell divisions. If the karyotype is abnormal, development may be altered. In general, chromosome abnormalities with gains or losses of large amounts of chromatin will manifest early in development and often result in spontaneous abortion. Examples of such abnormalities include trisomies, monosomy X, triploids, and large unbalanced structural rearrangements. Approximately 1 in 156 live births have a major chromosome abnormality. Congenital anomalies and/or mental retardation or phenotypic abnormalities which appear later on in life are observed in about half of these cases. Some chromosome abnormalities go undetected during prenatal and perinatal periods. Physical and mental developmental delays first noted during childhood may be associated with small unbalanced rearrangements, small interstitial deletions (microdeletions), and mosaic trisomies. Sex chromosome abnormalities may not be clinically evident until puberty when inappropriate secondary sexual development occurs or when infertility is recognized later in life. Finally, normal individuals who are carriers of balanced rearrangements may remain unrecognized until adulthood, at which time they can present with multiple miscarriages or abnormal offspring.

Specimen Whole blood

Container Green top (sodium heparin) tube. **Note:** Specimens in lavender top (EDTA) tubes, blue top (sodium citrate) tubes, or green top (lithium heparin) tubes are not acceptable.

Storage Instructions Specimen should be delivered to the laboratory immediately; do not freeze.

Causes for Rejection Clotted or hemolyzed specimen, use of improper anticoagulant, improper storage

Reference Interval Forty-six chromosomes including 22 sets of normal autosomal chromosomes and one set of normal sex chromosomes (XX for female, XY for male). Interpretive information should be included.

Use Evaluate congenital anomaly (birth defect), developmental delay, ambiguous genitalia, mental retardation, cryptorchidism, hypogonadism, primary amenorrhea, infertility, multiple miscarriages, or the carrier status in relatives of patients with known chromosome abnormalities.

Limitations Failure to obtain metaphases occurs infrequently and may be due to collection in inappropriate anticoagulant or improper specimen storage (eg, frozen specimen).

Methodology Accessibility of peripheral blood along with the success of mitogen stimulation has made lymphocyte culture the test of choice in studying constitutional chromosomes. At times, other tissues, such as skin biopsy, may be used for studying the mosaic status of an abnormality or for detection of tissue-specific abnormalities. The method for lymphocyte analysis involves phytohemagglutinin stimulation during lymphocyte culture, (Continued)

Chromosome Analysis, Blood (Continued)

colchicine arrest of cells in metaphase, methanol:acetic acid fixation, spread preparation using hypotonic solution, banding of chromosomes, microscopic chromosome analysis, and preparation of karyotypes by photography or computerized image analysis. Conventional banding techniques employ trypsin treatment of chromosomes followed by staining with Giemsa (or a similar stain). Alternative banding techniques and special stains for identification of specific chromosome regions include quinacrine banding, reverse banding, C-banding (constitutive heterochromatin banding), DAPI technique, Ag-Nor technique (silver stain), and fluorescence *in situ* hybridization.

Additional Information The highest proportion of chromosome abnormalities occurs in early spontaneous abortions (50%) (see Chromosome Analysis, Products of Conception *on page 365*). Approximately 7% of stillbirths and perinatal deaths are chromosomally abnormal, and 0.65% of newborns have a major chromosome abnormality. Trisomy 21 (Down syndrome) is the most frequent chromosome anomaly, with an incidence of 1 in 700-850 births. Sex chromosome aneusomies are the next most common. One XXY and one XYY is present in every 1000 male births, and one XXX is seen in every 1000 female births. Structural balanced rearrangements have a frequency of about 1 in 500 live births. Carriers of such balanced rearrangements are phenotypically normal but have an increased risk for having abnormal offspring and multiple miscarriages.

Chromosome abnormalities are present in about 10% of mentally retarded children. When mentally retarded children are examined who also have multiple birth defects or low birth weights, the incidence of chromosome abnormalities increases to 23%, half of which are Down syndrome. In addition, 3% to 6% of males and 3% to 4% of females with mental retardation will have the fragile X syndrome. (See Fragile X Syndrome DNA Test *on page 708*.)

No single phenotype is exclusive to any chromosome syndrome. The combination of phenotypic abnormalities, however, allows certain syndromes to be recognized (see table). In general, complex organ systems are often adversely affected by a great variety of chromosomal abnormalities. The heart, brain (mental retardation), head, eyes, genitourinary system, hands, and feet frequently are abnormal when an autosomal chromosome anomaly is present. In contrast, sex chromosome anomalies usually have less severe phenotypic abnormalities, with the reproductive organs most commonly involved, and mental retardation being only rarely

Common Chromosomal Syndromes

Autosome Syndromes		
Syndrome	Chromosome Abnormality	Features
Down syndrome	Trisomy 21	Epicanthal folds, simian crease of palm, flat nasal bridge, congenital heart disease, mental retardation
Patau syndrome	Trisomy 13	Microcephaly, cleft lip/palate, congenital heart disease, polydactaly, mental retardation
Edward syndrome	Trisomy 18	Micrognathia, congenital heart disease, mental retardation, clenched 3rd/4th fingers/overlapped fifth, rocker-bottom feet
Wolf-Hirschhorn syndrome	Deletion 4p	Microcephaly, growth retardation, mental retardation, carp mouth
Cri-du-chat syndrome	Deletion 5p	Cat-like cry, microcephaly, hypertelorism, retrognathia, mental retardation
Warkam syndrome	Mosaic trisomy 8	Malformed ears, bulbous nose, deep palmar creases, absent or hypoplastic patellae
Beckwith-Weidemann syndrome	Duplication 11p15	Macroglossia, omphalocele, ear lobe creases
Pallister-Killian syndrome	Trisomy 12p	Psychomotor delay, sparse anterior scalp hair, micrognathia, hypotonia
Cat's eye syndrome	Trisomy 22q11-pter	Anal atresia, coloboma
Sex Chromosome Syndromes		
Syndrome	Chromosome Abnormality	Features
Klinefelter syndrome	47,XXY	Hypogonadism, infertility, underdeveloped secondary sexual characteristics, learning disabilities
XYY syndrome	47,XYY	Tall stature, increased risk of behavior problems
Triple X syndrome	47,XXX	Increased risk of infertility and learning disabilities
Turner-Ullrich syndrome	45,X (and other structural abnormalities of X)	Short stature, gonadal dysgenesis, webbed neck, broad chest, low posterior hairline, renal and cardiovascular anomalies

observed. In addition to the classic chromosome syndromes listed in the table, syndromes associated with minute deletions (microdeletion syndromes) are detected using special high-resolution chromosome analysis (see Chromosome Analysis, High-Resolution *on page 363* and Fluorescence *In Situ* Hybridization *on page 367*).

References

Gosden CM, Davidson C, and Robertson M, "Lymphocyte Culture," *Human Cytogenetics: A Practical Approach*, 3rd ed, Rooney DE and Czepulkowski BH, eds, New York, NY: Oxford University Press, 2001.

Robinson A and Linden M, *Clinical Genetics Handbook*, 2nd ed, Boston, MA: Blackwell Scientific Publications, 1993.

Miller OJ and Thurman E, *Human Chromosomes*, 4th ed, New York, NY: Springer-Verlag, 2001.

Van Dyke DL and Wiktor A, "Clinical Cytogenetics," *Clinical Laboratory Medicine*, 2nd ed, McClatchey KD, ed, Baltimore, MD: Lippincott Williams & Wilkins, 2001.

Internet Web Sites

www.ncbi.nlm.nih.gov/omim/ onlinemendelianinheritanceinman

Chromosome Analysis, Bone Marrow

Related Information

Bone Marrow *on page 410*
Breakpoint Cluster Region Rearrangement in CML *on page 721*
Chromosomal Translocations, Molecular Detection *on page 723*
Chromosome Analysis, Lymph Node and Solid Tumor *on page 364*
Fluorescence *In Situ* Hybridization *on page 367*
Lymph Node Biopsy *on page 67*
White Blood Cell Count *on page 496*

Synonyms Bone Marrow Chromosome Analysis; Cytogenetics, Bone Marrow; Karyotype, Bone Marrow

Applies to Aneuploidy; Aneusomy; FAB Types; Karyotypic Abnormalities; Monosomy; Philadelphia Chromosome; Retinoic Acid Receptor Alpha; Translocation; Trisomy

Abstract Cytogenetic analysis is often needed in the diagnostic study of patients with or suspected of having, a hematologic disorder. Numerous consistently occurring primary chromosome abnormalities have been well established in both acute and chronic hematologic diseases. Select abnormalities have specific associations with morphologic subtypes of disorders, and are therefore useful in establishing specific diagnoses. Cytogenetic findings at diagnosis have also been shown to be an independent prognostic factor associated with complete remission, duration of remission, and ultimate survival in many hematologic disorders. Chromosome analysis is also used for monitoring patients following standard treatment or bone marrow transplantation.

Specimen Bone marrow aspirate

Container 1-3 mL bone marrow should be transported in a sterile container containing preservative-free sodium heparin; specimens in EDTA, citrate, or heparin anticoagulants are not acceptable.

Storage Instructions Maintain the specimen at room temperature and transport **immediately** to the Cytogenetics Laboratory.

Causes for Rejection Clotted or hemolyzed specimen

Use Chromosome analysis of bone marrow aids in diagnosis of hematologic disorders, supplies prognostic information, and is used to monitor patients following therapy or bone marrow transplantation.

Limitations Neoplastic cells may fail to grow in culture. Since normal bone marrow stem cells can divide *in vitro*, a normal cytogenetic result may reflect either a diploid neoplastic population or the analysis of normal cells. Sensitivity may be limited in detecting minimal residual disease since only 20-30 metaphases are routinely analyzed. Fluorescence *in situ* hybridization may be used to aid in diagnosis of a genetic abnormality in all of the above stated limitations.

Methodology Bone marrow aspirates are the specimen of choice for cytogenetic analysis of hematologic disorders. In cases of lymphoma, lymph node biopsies or aspirates are more appropriate. At times, unstimulated peripheral blood cultures may be useful, for example, in chronic lymphocytic leukemia, or following a dry bone marrow tap. A combination of two to three methods for obtaining metaphases is normally employed for bone marrow specimens. A "direct harvest" technique may be used to analyze cells undergoing spontaneous division. One or more short-term cultures (24- and/or 48-hour) are usually performed. Short-term cultures, in contrast to the direct technique, may be necessary for consistent detection of certain abnormalities including t(8;21) and t(15;17). Culturing of cells in chronic lymphocytic diseases may be enhanced with the use of B- or T-cell mitogens. Colchicine arrest of cells in metaphase, followed by routine harvesting of metaphases is performed prior to banding and microscopic analysis of chromosomes.

Additional Information Acute myelogenous leukemia: More than 30 different structural chromosome abnormalities have been implicated as primary rearrangements in AML (see table 1). Several abnormalities are specifically associated with FAB (French-American-British) subclasses. For example, t(8;21) typically occurs in FAB group M2, t(15;17) in M3, inv(16)/del(16) in M4 with eosinophilia, and t(9;11) in M5. High complete remission rates have been noted in patients with t(8;21), while patients with hyperdiploid karyotypes or combined abnormalities of chromosome 5 and 7 have low remission rates. Although a significant loss of patients with M3 may occur early in the disease because of hemorrhagic complications, the t(15;17) subgroup of AML patients go into remission readily. The duration of complete remission has been shown to be long for patients with t(8;21), t(15;17), and inv(16). However, a subset of patients with t(8;21) has a high incidence of relapse. Short durations of complete remission have been associated with abnormalities of chromosomes 5 or 7. Abnormalities of chromosomes 5 and 7, +8, and 11q23 rearrangements generally are associated with a short mean disease-free survival. In adult patients, inv(16) has been associated with relatively long survival, while in children, a more intermediate survival has been observed. In general, patients with abnormalities of chromosome 5 have a poor prognosis, while those with inv(16), t(8;21), or t(15;17) have a good prognosis. Secondary AML (therapy-related or environmental mutagen-related) usually has a larger number of chromosome abnormalities than *de novo* AML. Hypodiploidy, -7, del(5q), der(11q), del(7q), and der(1;7) are among the characteristic chromosome abnormalities observed in secondary AML.

Table 1. Common Chromosome Abnormalities in Acute Myeloid Leukemia

FAB Correlation	Karyotypic Abnormality	Comments
M1	t(9;22)(q34;q11.2)	Also seen in M2
	inv(3)(q21q26), ins(3;3)(q26;q21q26), t(3;3)9q21;q26)	Platelet and megakaryocytic abnormalities, also seen in M7 and MDS
M2	t(8;21)(q22;q22)	Auer rod positive
	t(6;9)(p23;q34)	Basophilia, also seen in M1, M4, and MDS
M3	t(15;17)(q22;q12)	
M4	trans 11q23 with 1q21, 2p21, 6q27, 10p11-15, 17q25, 19p13	
	del(11)(q23)	
	inv(16)(p13q22) del(16)(q22)	M4Eo, with eosinophilia
	+4	Also seen in M2
M5	t(9;11)(p22;q23)	Mostly M5a
ALL classes	+8	Also seen in MDS, MPD
Therapy-related AML	-5/del(5q)	Also seen in MDS
	-7/del(7q)	Also seen in MDS
	t(1;7)(p10;q10)	Also seen in MDS

FAB = French-American-British

Chronic myeloproliferative disorders: The first chromosome abnormality found to be consistently associated with a neoplastic process, was a small marker chromosome, referred to as the Philadelphia chromosome (Ph). Greater than 90% of patients with chronic myelogenous leukemia (CML) were found to be Ph-positive. It was later shown that the Ph originated from a balanced translocation, t(9;22)(q34;q11.2). Complex-variant translocations are found in 5% to 10% of CML patients and have the same molecular rearrangement as the classic t(9;22). Actual Ph-negative CML may be quite rare. Many of the cases thought to be Ph-negative in the past have been reclassified into disorders other than CML or have been shown, by molecular methods, to have a submicroscopic *bcr/abl* rearrangement. Since the Ph-positive clone persists following most modes of standard chemotherapy, the use of cytogenetics in monitoring such patients is of limited value. However, the detection of additional cytogenetic abnormalities (most commonly +Ph, +8, iso(17q), +19) can be helpful in predicting the accelerated phase or impending blast crisis. Secondary cytogenetic abnormalities often precede clinical blast crisis by several months. Although no karyotypic abnormality is specific for the other myeloproliferative disorders (polycythemia vera, idiopathic myelofibrosis, and essential thrombocythemia), the most frequently observed chromosome changes include rearrangements of the long arm of chromosome 1, -7, del(7q), del(5q), +8, +9, del(13q), and del(20q).

Myelodysplastic syndrome: Chromosome abnormalities are detected in approximately one-third to one-half of all *de novo* myelodysplastic syndromes (MDS), varying in frequency among the FAB subgroups. Among the most common recurring, nonrandom chromosome aberrations are del(5q), -7, +8, del(20q), del(7q), and del(13q). Although these abnormalities do not aid in subclassification of the FAB subgroups and can also be seen in other disorders, the detection of an acquired clonal abnormality within bone marrow cells establishes the diagnosis of a neoplastic disorder. This is especially helpful in cases of refractory anemia in which morphological changes may be subtle. Deletion of 5q is the most common chromosome abnormality in MDS (~30% of abnormal cases). 5q can be observed in any subgroup of MDS and in some other hematologic disorders. A subgroup of patients with del(5q) as the sole abnormality have specific clinicohematologic characteristics referred to as the "5q- syndrome". These patients characteristically are elderly women with refractory macrocytic anemia, elevated or normal platelet counts, and hypolobulated megakaryocytes. The clinical course is generally mild with only rare transformation to AML. A poorer prognosis is associated with del(5q) when accompanied by additional chromosome abnormalities. In addition to the prognostic significance associated with del(5q), the presence of monosomy 7 or complex

karyotypes has been associated with a poor prognosis of MDS. The frequency of chromosome abnormalities is generally higher in secondary MDS. Deletions or monosomy of chromosomes 5 and/or chromosome 7 are often observed especially following exposure to alkylating agents. Likewise, rearrangements involving 11q23 have been associated with exposure to drugs targeted against topoisomerase II.

Acute lymphocytic leukemia: Approximately two-thirds of all acute lymphocytic leukemias (ALL) have abnormal karyotypes. Table 2 illustrates some of the most common abnormalities and the FAB subgroups and cell types with which they are associated. Loci involved in normal development of lymphocytes are often part of a chromosome rearrangement observed in both acute and chronic lymphocytic disorders. These loci include immunoglobulin genes; the heavy-chain locus (IGH) at 14q32, the kappa light-chain locus (IGK) at 2p12, the lambda light-chain locus (IGL) at 22q11, and T-cell receptor molecules; the α-chain locus (TCRA) at 14q11, the β-chain locus (TCRB) at 7q34-36, and the γ-chain locus (TCRG) at 7p13. The karyotype has been shown to be an important independent prognostic factor in ALL. Patients with a modal chromosome number >50 (hyperdiploid) have the most favorable cytogenetic prognosis. When, however, structural abnormalities coexist within the hyperdiploid karyotype, the prognosis is no longer favorable. Hypodiploidy is associated with a poor prognosis, as are specific translocations such as t(1;19), t(4;11), t(9;22) and t(8;14). A normal karyotype appears to have an intermediate prognosis. The t(12;21), observed primarily in children, has been associated with a good prognosis.

Table 2. Common Chromosome Abnormalities in Acute Lymphocytic Leukemia

Karyotypic Abnormality	FAB Type	Cell Type
t(8;14)(q24;q32)	L3	B
t(8;22)(q24;q11)	L3	B
t(2;8)(p12q24)	L3	B
t(12;21)(p12;q22)	L1, L2	B
t(1;19)(q23;p13)	L1, L2	Pre-B
t(8;14)(q24;q11)	L1, L2	T
t(11;14)(p13;q11)	L1, L2	T
del(9p)	L1, L2	T
del(6)(q21q25)	L1, L2	CALLA and early pre-B
t(9;22)(q34;q11)	L1, L2	Pre-B
t(4;11)(q21;q23)	L1, L2	Mixed lineage

FAB = French-American-British

Chronic lymphoproliferative disorders: As in acute lymphocytic leukemias, immunoglobulin gene and T-cell receptor gene loci are often involved in clonal chromosome rearrangements. Other characteristic cytogenetic findings include trisomy 12 and del(13q) in chronic lymphocytic leukemia, del(6q) in numerous B- and T-cell derived chronic disorders, and 2p rearrangements in Sézary syndrome.

References

Dewald GW, Morris MA, and Lilla VC, "Chromosome Studies in Neoplastic Hematologic Disorders," *Clinical Laboratory Medicine*, 2nd ed, McClatchey KD, ed, Baltimore, MD: Lippincott Williams & Wilkins, 2001.

Heim S and Metelman F, *Cancer Cytogenetics: Chromosomal and Molecular Genetic Aberrations of Tumor Cells*, 2nd ed, New York, NY: Wiley-Liss, 1995.

Rooney DE and Czepulkowski BH, *Human Cytogenetics: Malignancy and Acquired Abnormalities*, 3rd ed, Volume II, New York, NY: Oxford University Press, 2001.

Internet Web Sites

www.infobiogen.fr/services/chromcancer/index.html

Chromosome Analysis, High-Resolution

Related Information

Chromosome Analysis, Blood *on page 361*
Fluorescence *In Situ* Hybridization *on page 367*

Synonyms Microdeletion Study; Prometaphase Study; Prophase Study

Applies to Microdeletion Syndrome

Abstract Standard blood culture and chromosome-staining techniques result in metaphase chromosomes with 400 to 500 total bands per haploid set of chromosomes. The recognition of various chromosome abnormalities resulting from subtle gains or losses of genetic material consisting of single bands or even smaller portions of chromosomes, has resulted in the development of techniques for detection of these minute abnormalities. High-resolution techniques arrest cells in prophase or prometaphase, resulting in elongated chromosomes with identifiable bands in the 550 to 1200 band stage. Such techniques are used when microdeletions or other subtle chromosome abnormalities are suspected.

Specimen Whole blood

Container Green top (sodium heparin) tube. **Note:** Specimens in lavender top (EDTA) tubes, blue top (sodium citrate) tubes, or green top (lithium heparin) tubes are not acceptable.

Storage Instructions Specimen should be delivered to the laboratory immediately; do not freeze.

(Continued)

Chromosome Analysis, High-Resolution (Continued)

Causes for Rejection Clotted or hemolyzed specimen, use of improper anticoagulant, improper storage (frozen specimen)

Reference Interval Forty-six chromosomes including 22 sets of normal autosomal chromosomes and one set of normal sex chromosomes (XX for female, XY for male). Interpretive information is usually included.

Use Detect small chromosomal deletions, duplications, or rearrangements

Limitations Failure to obtain metaphases occurs infrequently and may be due to collection in inappropriate anticoagulant or improper specimen storage (eg, frozen specimen). The detection limit is a function of the resolution of the microscope; therefore, submicroscopic abnormalities (deletions, duplications, or rearrangements) may remain undetected by these methods. Fluorescence *in situ* hybridization is a useful adjunct in detecting microdeletions (see Chromosome Analysis, Bone Marrow *on page 362*).

Methodology High-resolution chromosomes can be obtained by synchronizing cells in particular stages of prophase or prometaphase. Antimetabolites, such as methotrexate, can be used to arrest cells in S-phase, followed by release with thymidine resulting in synchronization. Alternatively, addition of substances such as actinomycin D or ethidium bromide will interfere with condensation, resulting in elongated chromosomes.

Additional Information High-resolution chromosome analysis is useful in situations in which a small chromosome deletion, duplication, or rearrangement may be clinically suspected. A number of disorders have been shown to be associated with minute deletions or duplications of chromatin. Examples of the major microdeletion/duplication syndromes and their clinical characteristics are shown in the table. These disorders are often referred to as "contiguous gene syndromes". It is thought that each of several contiguous genes involved in the abnormality is responsible for a portion of the clinical manifestations associated with the disorder. Therefore, clinical manifestations can be variable depending on the extent of material deleted or duplicated. Some individuals with these syndromes have no chromosome abnormality, and others may have abnormalities too small (submicroscopic) to be detected even by high-resolution cytogenetic methods. DNA probes for select microdeletion syndromes are now commercially available. They are used in conjunction with high-resolution chromosome analysis for confirmation of microdeletions within metaphases using fluorescence *in situ* hybridization (FISH). In some cases, FISH may confirm the presence of a submicroscopic deletion that is beyond the resolution of high-resolution cytogenetic analysis.

Major Microdeletion Syndromes

Syndrome	Deletion	Features
Williams	7q11.23	Congenital heart disease, intermittent hypercalcemia, dysmorphic facial features, mental retardation
Langer-Giedion	8q24.11-q24.13	Multiple exostoses, mental retardation, sparse hair, bulbous nose
Anirida/Wilms tumor (WAGR)	11p13	Wilms' tumor with aniridia, gonodoblastoma, and retardation
Retinoblastoma	13q14	Retinoblastoma, osteosarcoma, bossed head
Angelman	15q11-q13	Hypotonia, ataxia, seizures, mental retardation, excessive laughter
Prader-Willi	15q11-q13	Neonatal hypotonia, hypogonadism, obesity, small hands and feet, mental retardation
Smith-Magenis	17p11.2	Hyperactive, self-destructive behavior, facial dysmorphism, mental retardation
Miller-Dieker	17p13.3	Lissencephaly, facial dysmorphism, mental retardation
DiGeorge/ Velocardiofacial	22q11.2	Hypoplasia of parathyroid and thymus, facial anomalies, congenital heart disease
Steroid sulfatase	Xp22.3	X-linked disorder, ichthyosis
Kallmann	Xp22.3	X-linked disorder, deafness, renal and cardiac anomalies

References

Gosden CM, Davidson C, and Robertson M, "Lymphocyte Culture," *Human Cytogenetics: A Practical Approach*, 3rd ed, Rooney DE and Czepulkowski BH, eds, New York, NY: Oxford University Press, 2001.

Thompson MW, McInnes RR, and Willard HF, *Genetics in Medicine*, 5th ed, Philadelphia, PA: WB Saunders Co, 1991.

Van Dyke DL and Wiktor A, "Clinical Cytogenetics," *Clinical Laboratory Medicine*, 2nd ed, McClatchey KD, ed, Baltimore, MD: Lippincott Williams & Wilkins, 2001.

Internet Web Sites

www.ncbi.nlm.nih.gov/omim/ onlinemendelianinheritanceinman

Chromosome Analysis, Lymph Node and Solid Tumor

Related Information

Cell Cycle Analysis by Flow Cytometry *on page 53*
Chromosome Analysis, Blood *on page 361*
Chromosome Analysis, Bone Marrow *on page 362*
Colon Cancer, Hereditary Nonpolyposis Type *on page 724*
Fluorescence *In Situ* Hybridization *on page 367*
Gene Rearrangement for Leukemia and Lymphoma *on page 725*
Histopathology *on page 59*
Immunophenotypic Analysis of Tissues by Flow Cytometry *on page 62*
Lymph Node Biopsy *on page 67*

Synonyms Chromosome Studies, Lymph Node and Solid Tumor; Karyotype, Lymph Node and Solid Tumor

Test Includes Lymph nodal or solid tumor tissue is examined cytogenetically for clonal chromosomal abnormalities

Abstract Cytogenetic analyses of both benign and malignant solid tumors and lymphoma have revealed abnormalities in the number and/or structure of chromosomes. Many such changes are specific for a particular tumor type and thus, play a direct, potentially decisive role in examination and therapy of these lesions. In addition to adding a new dimension to the formulation of diagnosis, the cytogenetic findings provide prognostic information and resolution of cellular origin. Identification of aberrant chromosomal bands has served as a basis of molecular approaches to establish the definitive genes affected and the associated consequences of these gene alterations. In some instances, recognition of the cytogenetic abnormality is the first clue that a mutated gene resides at a particular locus.

Specimen Lymph node or solid tumor

Container Sterile container

Collection A portion of lymph node or tumor specimen surgically removed for histopathologic diagnosis is submitted fresh and aseptically for cytogenetic analysis. The sample should represent the neoplastic process, and adjacent normal tissue should be discarded.

Common Chromosomal Abnormalities in Lymphoma and Solid Tumors

Diagnosis	Chromosomal Abnormality
B-Cell non-Hodgkin Lymphoma	
(Burkitt) small noncleaved cell	t(8;14) (q24;q32)
(Burkitt) small noncleaved cell	t(2;8) (p12;q24)
(Burkitt) small noncleaved cell	t(8;22); (q24;q11)
Small lymphocytic or diffuse large cell	+12
Diffuse large cell	t(3;14) (q27;q32)
Diffuse large cell	t(3;22) (q27;q11)
Centrocytic (variable zone) with CD5-positive cells	t(11;14) (q13;q32)
Mixed, small cleaved and large cell follicular	t(14;18) (q32;q21)
T-Cell Lymphoma	t(11;14) (p13;q11)
	inv(14) (q11;?)
	t(14;?) (q11;?)
Anaplastic large cell (Ki-1)	t(2;5) (p23;q35)
Solid Tumors	
Clear cell sarcoma/malignant melanoma of soft parts	t(12;22) (q13;q12)
Desmoplastic small round cell tumor	t(11;22) (p13;q12)
Ewing sarcoma/peripheral neuroectodermal tumor	t(11;22) (q24;q12)
	t(21;22) (q22;q12)
	t(7;22) p22;q12)
Extraskeletal myxoid chondrosarcoma	t(9;22) (q22;q12)
	t(9;17) (q22;q11)
Glioma	double minutes
	+7
	-10
Germ-cell tumors	i(12) (p10)
Leiomyoma	t(12;14) (q14;q23)
Lipoma	t(12;?) (q14;?)
Medulloblastoma	i(17) (q10)
Meningioma	-22/del(22)(q12)
Myxoid liposarcoma	t(12;16) (q13;p11)
	t(12;22) (q13;q12)
Neuroblastoma	double minutes
	homogeneously staining regions
	del(1) (p31-32)
Pleomorphic adenoma	t(3;8) (p21;q12)
Renal cell carcinoma	del(3p)
Retinoblastoma	del(13) (q14)
Rhabdomyosarcoma (alveolar)	t(2;13) (q37;q14)
	t(1;13) (p36;q14)
Small cell lung carcinoma	del(3) (p14;p23)
Synovial sarcoma	t(X;18) (p11.2;q11.2)

A 1-2 cm³ sample (approximately 0.5-1 g) should be provided for analysis, preferably as part of the specimen submitted for surgical pathology. Pertinent medical findings such as age and sex of the patient, location of the lesion, indication, relevant history, note of any viral infection, and suspected diagnosis should be submitted.

Storage Instructions Specimen should be submitted to the laboratory as soon as possible. If overnight storage is necessary, the sample can be refrigerated in sterile isotonic saline or culture media containing serum.

Causes for Rejection Specimen frozen

Turnaround Time 2-14 days

Reference Interval Normal lymph node and solid tissue cells contain 46 chromosomes with 22 pairs of autosomal chromosomes and one set of sex chromosomes (XX for female; XY for male). Clonal numerical and/or structural chromosomal abnormalities are detected in neoplastic tissue. An abnormal clone is defined as two or more cells exhibiting a gain of the same chromosome or structural alteration, or three or more cells exhibiting loss of the same chromosome. Many of the characteristic or tumor-specific chromosomal abnormalities are listed (see table on previous page).

Use Cytogenetic analysis of lymphoma and solid tumors (in particular sarcomas), is a useful and sometimes, essential diagnostic adjunct. Cytogenetic analysis also provides prognostic information for some malignancies.

Limitations Failure of cells to grow in culture, overgrowth of normal supporting stromal cells (fibroblasts) and/or contamination precludes complete analysis (fluorescence *in situ* hybridization may be of use if this occurs).

Methodology Cell culturing of neoplastic cells, subsequent harvesting, and chromosome analysis with Giemsa or quinacrine banding techniques

Additional Information In some cases, molecular methods are subsequently used to further define chromosomal abnormalities.

References
Bridge JA, "Cytogenetic and Molecular Cytogenetic Techniques in Orthopedic Surgery," *J Bone Joint Surg*, 1993, 75(4):606-14.
Heim S and Metelman F, *Cancer Cytogenetics: Chromosomal and Molecular Genetic Aberration of Tumor Cells*, 2nd ed, New York, NY: Wiley-Liss, 1995.
Sandberg AA and Bridge JA, *The Cytogenetics of Bone and Soft Tissue Tumors*, Austin, TX: RG Landes Co, 1994.

Internet Web Sites
www.infobiogen.fr/services/chromcancer/index.html

Chromosome Analysis, Products of Conception

Related Information
Amniotic Fluid, Chromosome and Genetic Abnormality Analysis *on page 360*
Chorionic Villus Sampling, Chromosome and Genetic Abnormality Analysis *on page 361*
Chromosome Analysis, Blood *on page 361*
Endometrial Cytology *on page 380*
Fluorescence *In Situ* Hybridization *on page 367*

Synonyms Chromosome Karyotype, Products of Conception, Spontaneous Miscarriage or Abortion; Chromosome Studies, Products of Conception, Spontaneous Miscarriage or Abortion

Test Includes Chromosomal complement of products of conception are examined for determination of abnormalities

Abstract The overall incidence of chromosomal abnormalities in spontaneous abortions approaches 50%. Trisomy has been identified for all the human autosomes except chromosome 1. Generally, trisomies result in spontaneous abortions. Appreciable numbers of live births occur only for trisomies 13, 18, and 21, and these children are always abnormal. Chromosomal abnormalities most commonly seen in spontaneous abortions include trisomy (62.1%), triploidy (12.4%), monosomy X (10.5%), tetraploidy (9.2%), and structural chromosome anomalies (4.7%).[1]

Specimen Products of conception

Container Sterile container

Collection Products of conception are the evacuated contents of the uterus after termination of an early pregnancy or the spontaneously aborted material collected after early miscarriage. The latter specimen generally consists of variably recognizable fetal parts and remnants of the sac and placenta. Although some fetal specimens may be severely autolyzed (depending on the time elapsed between death and specimen collection), it is important not to be dissuaded from attempting culture because the placenta will have recently been attached to the maternal circulation and may still contain viable cells.

Causes for Rejection Specimen frozen or lacking in viable fetal cells

Turnaround Time 1-3 weeks

Reference Interval Forty-six chromosomes to include 22 sets of normal autosomal chromosomes and one set of normal sex chromosomes (XX for female; XY for male). Interpretative information is usually included.

Use Detection of chromosomal abnormality in a spontaneously aborted fetus is important for genetic counseling and to assess risks for future abnormal pregnancies. For example, young women (younger than 35 years of age) who have previously given birth to a trisomic infant or who have had a trisomic fetus detected prenatally are at high risk for having a second trisomic abortion.

Limitations Failure of cells to grow in culture and/or contamination precludes complete analysis (fluorescence *in situ* hybridization may be of use if this occurs).

Contraindications Environment lacking capability in genetic counseling, products of conception culture, and chromosomal analysis techniques

Methodology Cell culture most commonly of fetal fibroblasts, subsequent harvesting, and chromosome analysis with Giemsa or quinacrine banding techniques

Footnotes
1. Eiben B, Bartels I, Bahr-Porsch S, et al, "Cytogenetic Analysis of 750 Spontaneous Abortions With the Direct-Preparation Method of Chorionic Villi and its Implications for Studying Genetic Causes of Pregnancy Wastage," *Am J Hum Genet*, 1990, 47(4):656-63.

References
Griffin DK, Millie EA, Redline RW, et al, "Cytogenetic Analysis of Spontaneous Abortions: Comparison of Techniques and Assessment of the Incidence of Confined Placental Mosaicism," *Am J Med Genet*, 1997, 72(3):297-301.
Qumsiyeh MB, "Chromosome Abnormalities in the Placenta and Spontaneous Abortions," *J Matern Fetal Med*, 1998, 7(4):210-2.
Warburton D, Kline J, Stein Z, et al, "Does the Karyotype of a Spontaneous Abortion Predict the Karyotype of a Subsequent Abortion? Evidence From 273 Women With Two Karyotyped Spontaneous Abortions?" *Am J Hum Genet*, 1987, 41(3):465-83.

♦ **Chromosome Breakage Syndrome, Fanconi Anemia** *see* Fanconi Anemia, Chromosome Breakage Study *on page 365*

♦ **Chromosome Instability Test** *see* Fanconi Anemia, Chromosome Breakage Study *on page 365*

♦ **Chromosome Karyotype, Blood** *see* Chromosome Analysis, Blood *on page 361*

♦ **Chromosome Karyotype, Chorionic Villus Sampling** *see* Chorionic Villus Sampling, Chromosome and Genetic Abnormality Analysis *on page 361*

♦ **Chromosome Karyotype, Products of Conception, Spontaneous Miscarriage or Abortion** *see* Chromosome Analysis, Products of Conception *on page 365*

♦ **Chromosome Stress Test** *see* Fanconi Anemia, Chromosome Breakage Study *on page 365*

♦ **Chromosome Studies, Amniotic Fluid** *see* Amniotic Fluid, Chromosome and Genetic Abnormality Analysis *on page 360*

♦ **Chromosome Studies, Blood** *see* Chromosome Analysis, Blood *on page 361*

♦ **Chromosome Studies, Chorionic Villus Sampling** *see* Chorionic Villus Sampling, Chromosome and Genetic Abnormality Analysis *on page 361*

♦ **Chromosome Studies, Lymph Node and Solid Tumor** *see* Chromosome Analysis, Lymph Node and Solid Tumor *on page 364*

♦ **Chromosome Studies, Products of Conception, Spontaneous Miscarriage or Abortion** *see* Chromosome Analysis, Products of Conception *on page 365*

♦ **Comparative Genomic Hybridization** *see* Fluorescence *In Situ* Hybridization *on page 367*

♦ **CVS, Chromosome and Genetic Abnormality Analysis** *see* Chorionic Villus Sampling, Chromosome and Genetic Abnormality Analysis *on page 361*

♦ **Cytogenetics, Blood** *see* Chromosome Analysis, Blood *on page 361*

♦ **Cytogenetics, Bone Marrow** *see* Chromosome Analysis, Bone Marrow *on page 362*

♦ **Diepoxybutane** *see* Fanconi Anemia, Chromosome Breakage Study *on page 365*

♦ **Diepoxybutane Stress Test** *see* Fanconi Anemia, Chromosome Breakage Study *on page 365*

♦ **Enzyme Deficiency Analyses** *see* Amniotic Fluid, Chromosome and Genetic Abnormality Analysis *on page 360*

♦ **FAB Types** *see* Chromosome Analysis, Bone Marrow *on page 362*

Fanconi Anemia, Chromosome Breakage Study

Related Information
Alpha₁-Fetoprotein, Serum *on page 97*
Bone Marrow *on page 410*
Complete Blood Count *on page 419*
Fluorescence *In Situ* Hybridization *on page 367*
Lymphocyte Transformation Test *on page 539*
Platelet Count *on page 468*

Synonyms Chromosome Breakage Syndrome, Fanconi Anemia; Chromosome Instability Test; Chromosome Stress Test; Diepoxybutane Stress Test; Mitomycin C Stress Test

Applies to Bloom Syndrome; Diepoxybutane; TRACE

Test Includes Detection of increased spontaneous and chemically-induced chromosome breakage in the patient's lymphocytes compared to control lymphocytes
(Continued)

Fanconi Anemia, Chromosome Breakage Study
(Continued)

Abstract Fanconi anemia (FA) is an autosomal recessive disorder affecting approximately 1 in 360,000 people. In FA there is cytogenetic hypersensitivity to bifunctional alkylating agents, suggestive of a defect in the repair of DNA interstrand cross-links. Clinically, there is bone marrow failure, predisposition to the development of malignancy, and presence of multiple congenital anomalies. With marrow failure there is involvement of all marrow elements resulting in anemia, leukopenia, and thrombocytopenia. FA is associated with increased risk of malignancy (especially acute myeloid leukemia which occurs in ~9% of patients) but cancers may also develop in skin, gastrointestinal, and gynecologic systems. Frequent congenital malformations include radial ray defects, microcephaly, renal malformations, and mental retardation. Some 33% of FA patients lack congenital malformation.

Clinical findings (variable) of Fanconi anemia:
- growth retardation
- short stature
- microcephaly
- micro-ophthalmia
- microstomia
- mental retardation
- bone marrow failure
- skeletal abnormalities: face (elf-like), upper limb (absent radii of thumb, wrist, forearm)
- skin pigment abnormalities
- genitourinary
- risk of malignancy (especially acute myeloid leukemia)

FA cells manifest spontaneous chromosome breakage and display enhanced chromosome breakage upon exposure to bifunctional DNA cross-linking agents including mitomycin C, diepoxybutane (DEB), and nitrogen mustard.

Specimen Whole blood; antenatal diagnosis may utilize chorionic villus cells or fetal blood sample.

Container Green top (sodium heparin) tube. **Note:** Specimens in lavender top (EDTA) tubes, blue top (sodium citrate) tubes, or green top (lithium heparin) tubes are not acceptable.

Storage Instructions Specimen should be delivered to the laboratory immediately.

Causes for Rejection Clotted or hemolyzed specimen, specimen more than 24 hours old, use of improper anticoagulant

Special Instructions Call laboratory so that test can be arranged and scheduled.

Reference Interval An increased frequency of chromosomal damage is observed compared to control specimens for both spontaneous breakage and chemically-induced chromosome breakage following exposure to DEB or mitomycin C. Interpretation is usually provided with report. Presence or absence of monosomy 7 is of especial interest, as it is a frequent cytogenetic finding in the bone marrow of patients with FA and acute myeloid leukemia.[1]

Use Increased levels of chromosome instability provide an important aid to the clinical diagnosis of Fanconi anemia (FA)

Limitations Discrepancies exist between the clinical classification of some patients and the diagnosis suggested by *in vitro* cytogenetic findings. Therefore, the definitive diagnosis should not be based solely on cytogenetic results.

Methodology Peripheral T cells from PHA-stimulated blood cultures of the patient and a control are exposed to a bifunctional DNA cross-linking agent such as mitomycin C or diepoxybutane (DEB). In addition, spontaneous breakage is evaluated from untreated specimens from both the patient and control. Cells are harvested in a routine fashion and either banded or unbanded chromosomes are evaluated for chromosome breakage and rearrangements. The chromosomal instability in FA is primarily characterized by breaks and gaps and nonhomologous multiradials.

Additional Information Seven complementation groups (different genetic defects with the ability to correct for one another) have been identified in FA on the basis of results from somatic cell fusion studies.[2] The number of FA genes implicated on the basis of complementation studies has grown rapidly over the past few years from 4 to 8. Recently, FA-H (represented by a single patient) has been reassigned to group A[2] (see table).

Complementation Groups of Fanconi Anemia

Group	Estimated % of FA patients	Chromosome Location
A	66	16q24.3
B	4	
C	12	9q22.3
D	4	3p25.3
E	12	
F	Rare	
G	Rare	9p13

Four of the groups (A, C, D, and G) have been mapped to discreet chromosomal loci, respectively, 16q24.3, 9q22.3, 3p22-26 and 9p13. Thus, FA is genetically heterogeneous in contrast to ataxia telangiectasia and Bloom syndrome (which are chromosomal breakage syndromes arising from single gene mutations). FA genes A, C, and G have been cloned and encode "orphan" proteins (no similar proteins in the GenBank).

FA cells, in addition to DNA cross-linking sensitivity, also show defects in cell cycle regulation and apoptosis. The cells are hypersensitive to interferon gamma and tumor necrosis factor α likely with pathogenic significance to the development of aplastic anemia in FA patients.[3,4] Mutational analyses performed on FA genes FANCC, FANCA, and FANCG, and study of the encoded FA proteins are providing an understanding of the molecular basis of FA.[5] FANCA and FANCC (gene products) bind and form an intranuclear protein complex. Cytoplasmic FANCA and FANCC proteins are hypothesized to undergo phosphorylation after appropriate (?) cellular stimulus, binding occurs, and the complex is translocated to the cell nucleus where a nuclear function (ie, DNA repair or chromosome stabilization) is mediated. Defects (including mutated involved proteins) may result in chromosome instability.[5] With the availability of the FA genes, mutations can be identified at the molecular level providing an adjunctive procedure to the diepoxybutane test.

Carriers (heterozygotes) have an increased risk of cancer, although no excess of any specific cancer type has been noted. The study of chromosome breakage by use of DEB and mitomycin C is usually a reliable technique for identification of homozygotes. However, cytogenetic analysis is not dependable for identification of FA heterozygotes.

The hematologic manifestations in FA (bone marrow dependent) undergo variable progression. Macrocytosis and pancytopenia develop during the first decade of life. Platelet and red cell deficiencies usually antedate white cell abnormalities. Patients demonstrate progressively impaired erythropoiesis with fetal-like characteristics (increased i antigen and hemoglobin F). Serum erythropoietin levels may be increased. There is variable progression to pancytopenia.

Currently, treatment of FA is supportive (transfusion for marrow failure). Bone marrow transplant (allogeneic, using a histocompatible sibling donor or, potentially, umbilical cord blood stem cells for patients without appropriate donors) results in restoration of hematopoiesis in some 80% of cases. Siblings, heterozygous for FA, may be suitable donors. Marrow transplantation does not ameliorate the risk of malignancy.

On the basis of morphmetric analyses of red blood cells (RBCs) (with cell shrinkage and bleb formation) cytoskeletal changes, attributed to changes in spectrin, have been described.[6] These changes were frequent and occurred in both homozygous and heterozygous individuals raising the possibility (if substantiated) that abnormalities in RBCs might assist in the identification of FA heterozygotes or minimally symptomatic homozygotes.[6]

Median survival is about 25% (in untreated individuals) with FA. Some 20% of patients with FA develop malignancy. About 10% of patients develop acute myeloblastic leukemia (at an average age of 15 years). Leukemia is the presenting feature in some 25% of these affected FA patients. Cancer usually develops in older FA patients (mean age of 23 years). Squamous cell carcinoma is especially common, occurring in about 5% of patients. The oropharynx and gastrointestinal/genitourinary tracts are most commonly involved.[7]

Elevated serum alpha-fetoprotein (AFP) has been noted in FA patients.[8] AFP assay (fluoroimmunoassay based on TRACE technology) reportedly had a sensitivity of 93% and a specificity of 100% (61 FA patients/27 controls), elevations not apparently related to liver disease. Allogeneic marrow transplantation did not modify AFP levels; heterozygotes had normal levels.

Footnotes

1. Thurston VC, Ceperich TM, Vance GH, et al, "Detection of Monosomy 7 in Bone Marrow by Fluorescence *In Situ* Hybridization. A Study of Fanconi Anemia Patients and Review of the Literature," *Cancer Genet Cytogenet*, 1999, 109(2):154-60.
2. Joenje H, Levitus M, Waisfisz Q, et al, "Complementation Analysis in Fanconi Anemia: Assignment of the Reference FA-H Patient to Group A," *Am J Hum Genet*, 2000, 67(3):759-62.
3. Rathbun RK, Faulkner GR, Ostroski MH, et al, "Inactivation of the Fanconi Anemia Group C Gene Augments Interferon-Gamma-Induced Apoptotic Responses in Hematopoietic Cells," *Blood*, 1997, 90(3):974-85.
4. Whitney MA, Royle G, Low MJ, et al, "Germ Cell Defects and Hematopoietic Hypersensitivity to Gamma-Interferon in Mice With a Targeted Disruption of the Fanconi Anemia C Gene," *Blood*, 1996, 88(1):49-58.
5. Garcia-Higuera I, Kuang Y, and D'Andrea AD, "The Molecular and Cellular Biology of Fanconi Anemia," *Curr Opin Hematol*, 1999, 6(2):83-8.
6. Straface E, Masella R, Principe DD, et al, "Spectrin Changes Occur in Erythrocytes From Patients With Fanconi's Anemia and Their Parents," *Biochem Biophys Res Commun*, 2000, 273(3):899-901.
7. Shinton NK, *CRC Desk Reference for Hematology*, Boca Raton, FL: CRC Press, 1998, 219-21.
8. Cassinat B, Guardiola P, Chevret S, et al, "Constitutive Elevation of Serum Alpha-Fetoprotein in Fanconi Anemia," *Blood*, 2000, 96(3):859-63.

References

Alter BP, "Bone Marrow Failure Syndromes" *Clin Lab Med*, 1999, 19(1):113-33.
Auerbach AD, Rogatko A, and Schroeder-Kurth TM, "International Fanconi's Anemia Registry: Relation of Clinical Symptoms to Diepoxybutane Sensitivity," *Blood*, 1989, 73(2):391-6.

Ayas M and Mustafa MM, "Results of Allogeneic BMT in 16 Patients With Fanconi's Anemia," *Bone Marrow Transplant*, 2000, 25(12):1321-2.

Berger R, Le Coniat M, and Gendron MC, "Fanconi Anemia. Chromosome Breakage and Cell Cycle Studies," *Cancer Genet Cytogenet*, 1993, 69(1):13-6.

D'Andrea AD and Grompe M, "Molecular Biology of Fanconi Anemia: Implications for Diagnosis and Therapy," *Blood*, 1997, 90(5):1725-36.

de Winter JP, Rooimans MA, van der Weel L, et al, "The Fanconi Anaemia Gene FANCF Encodes a Novel Protein With Homology to ROM," *Nat Genet*, 2000, 24(1):15-6.

Freedman MH, "Inherited Forms of Bone Marrow Failure," 3rd ed, Chapter 18, *Hematology: Basic Principles and Practice*, Hoffman R, Benz EJ Jr, Shattil SJ, et al, eds, Philadelphia, PA: Churchill Livingstone, 2000.

Giampietro PF, Verlander PC, Davis JG, et al, "Diagnosis of Fanconi Anemia in Patients Without Congenital Malformations: An International Fanconi Anemia Registry Study," *Am J Med Genet*, 1997, 68(1):58-61.

Hejna JA, Timmers CD, Reifsteck C, et al, "Localization of the Fanconi Anemia Complementation Group D Gene to a 200-kb Region on Chromosome 3p25.3," *Am J Hum Genet*, 2000, 66(5):1540-51.

Kaushansky K, "Hematopoietic Growth Factors and Receptors," *The Molecular Basis of Blood Diseases*, 3rd ed, Chapter 2, Stamatoyannopoulos G, Majerus PW, Perlmutter RM, et al, eds, Philadelphia, PA: WB Saunders Co, 2001.

McKusick VA, *Mendelian Inheritance in Man: A Catalog of Human Genes and Genetic Disorders*, 12th ed, Volume 3, Baltimore, MD: Johns Hopkins University Press, 1998, 2211-18.

Pang Q, Fagerlie S, Christianson TA, et al, "The Fanconi Anemia Protein FANCC Binds to and Facilitates the Activation of Stat1 by Gamma Interferon and Hematopoietic Growth Factors," *Mol Cell Biol*, 2000, 20(13):4724-35.

Waisfisz Q, Morgan NV, Savino M, et al, "Spontaneous Functional Correction of Homozygous Fanconi Anaemia Alleles Reveals Novel Mechanistic Basis for Reverse Mosaicism," *Nat Genet*, 1999, 22(4):379-83.

♦ **FISH** *see* Fluorescence *In Situ* Hybridization *on page 367*

Fluorescence *In Situ* Hybridization

Related Information

Synonyms FISH; *In Situ* Chromosome Hybridization; Molecular Cytogenetics

Applies to Aneusomy; Comparative Genomic Hybridization; Microdeletions; Spectral Karyotyping

Abstract Fluorescence *in situ* hybridization (FISH) is a technique in which specific nucleic acid sequences can be visualized, utilizing fluorescent-labeled probes in individual metaphase or interphase cells from fresh or aged samples such as blood smears, touch and cytospin preparations, or paraffin-embedded tissue. FISH, a powerful technique which has revolutionized the field of cytogenetics, has numerous applications. The three main areas of clinical use are diagnosis of individuals with birth defects and mental retardation, prenatal diagnosis and screening, and identification and monitoring of acquired chromosome abnormalities in leukemia/cancer. Importantly, analysis with FISH is not contingent on dividing or mitosing cells and provides cellular localization of DNA sequences in a heterogeneous cell population.

Several different types of chromosomal probes are commercially available. Those most commonly used include probes to chromosome-specific repeated sequences (such as alpha satellite and satellite III DNA, regions around the chromosomal centromere); sequence or loci-specific probes such as those which are unique for the different chromosomal regions of deletion in the microdeletion syndromes (see table in Chromosome Analysis, High-Resolution *on page 363*); or translocation breakpoint flanking or spanning probes or amplified regions of DNA; telomere-specific probes;[1] and whole chromosome "painting" probes. The latter are composed of a mixture of sequences that will bind to the entire length of a particular chromosome and are useful for resolving structural rearrangements. In addition to chromosome-specific and region-specific probes, FISH techniques are also available for detection of alterations on a genome-wide scale. Comparative genomic hybridization (CGH) is a technique that permits the detection of chromosome gains or losses throughout the entire genome.[2] Spectral karyotyping (SKY) and multicolor FISH (MFISH) are techniques that provide distinct identification of all 24 human chromosomes, thereby greatly facilitating the recognition of chromosome aberrations.[3,4,5]

Specimen The specimen required will depend on the reason the test is requested; it may include blood, peripheral blood lymphocytes, bone marrow, amniotic fluid, chorionic villus sample, products of conception, lymph nodes, or solid tumors. All specimens should be sent fresh if standard cytogenetic studies will also be performed. Frozen, fixed, or paraffin-embedded samples are acceptable for detection of numerical abnormalities and some translocations and deletions, but are not suitable for all types of structural rearrangements.

Container Blood should be collected in a green top (sodium heparin) tube, 5 mL minimum; bone marrow should be collected in a heparinized syringe (20-25 units heparin), 1-2 mL minimum; amniotic fluid, chorionic villi, products of conception, lymph node and solid tumor tissue should be submitted in a sterile container. See Amniotic Fluid, Chromosome and Genetic Abnormality Analysis *on page 360*; Chorionic Villus Sampling, Chromosome and Genetic Abnormality Analysis *on page 361*; Chromosome Analysis, Blood *on page 361*; Chromosome Analysis, Bone Marrow *on page 362*; Chromosome Analysis, Lymph Node and Solid Tumor *on page 364*; Chromosome Analysis, Products of Conception *on page 365* for further collection information.

Storage Instructions All fresh specimens must be sent to the laboratory immediately after collection. Maintain at room temperature.

Causes for Rejection Specimen more than 48 hours old, specimen clotted or hemolyzed due to the use of improper anticoagulant will yield suboptimal results.

Turnaround Time 24-72 hours

Reference Interval Normal chromosome number and structure. Interpretation is usually provided with the report.

Table 1. Common FISH-Based Tests for Microdeletions

Abnormality	Microdeletion Syndrome
del(4)(p15)	Wolf-Hirschorn
del(5)(p15)	Cri-du-chat
del (7)(q11.2q11.2)	Williams
del(15)(q11.2q11.2)	Prader-Willi
del(15)(q11.2q11.2)	Angelman
del(17)(p11.2p11.2)	Smith-Magenis
del(17)(p13.3p13.3)	Miller-Dieker
del(22)(q11.2q11.2)	DiGeorge/velocardiofacial

Table 2. Common FISH-Based Tests for Acquired Abnormalities

Abnormality	Related Disorder
Leukemia/Lymphoma	
t(2;5)(p23;q35)	NHL (Ki-1)
del(5)(q12-31q31-35)/monosomy 5	MDS, MPD, AML
del(7)(q11-34q31-35)/monosomy 7	MDS, MPD, AML
trisomy 8	CML, AML, MPD, MDS
t(8;14)(q24;q32)	Burkitt lymphoma/leukemia
t(8;21)(q22;q22)	AML(M2)
t(9;22)(q34;q11.2)	CML, ALL, AML
t(11;14)(q13;q32)	NHL (mantle cell), CLL, MM
11q23 rearrangements	AML, ALL, MDS
trisomy 12	CLL, CLD
t(12;21)(p13;q22)	ALL
del(13)(q14.3)	CLL, MM, NHL
IgH rearrangements (14q32)	B-cell disorders
t(14;18)(q32;q21)	NHL (follicular, diffuse large cell)
t(15;17)(q22;q12)	AML(M3)
inv(16)(p13q22)	AML(M4-EO), MDS
p53 deletion (17p13.1)	CLL
del(20)(q11-13)	MPD, MDS, AML
Solid Tumors	
Abnormality	**Related Solid Tumor***
N-*myc* amplification (2p24.1)	Neuroblastoma
c-*myc* amplification (8q24.12-q24.13)	Breast, prostate, gastric, colorectal cancer
p16 deletion (9p21)	Bladder, breast, prostate, colorectal cancer
Cyclin D1 amplification (11q13)	Breast, esophageal, bladder cancer
RB-1 deletion (13q14.3)	Retinoblastoma, colon cancer, osteosarcoma
p53 deletion (17p13.1)	Bladder, cervical, colorectal, breast cancer
HER-2/*neu* amplification (17q11.2-q12)	Breast, ovarian cancer
Topoisomerase II-α amplification (17q11.2-q12)	Breast cancer
20q13.2 amplification	Breast cancer
Androgen receptor gene (Xq12)	Prostate cancer

*Not meant to be inclusive; many abnormalities listed may be associated with several additional hematologic disorders or solid tumors.

ALL = acute lymphoblastic leukemia; AML = acute myelogenous leukemia; CLD = chronic lymphocytic disorder; CLL = chronic lymphocytic leukemia; CML = chronic myelogenous leukemia; MDS = myelodysplastic syndrome; MM = multiple myeloma; MPD = myeloproliferative disorder; NHL = non-Hodgkin lymphoma.

(Continued)

Fluorescence *In Situ* Hybridization *(Continued)*

Use Numerous applications of FISH exist. Prenatal screening for detection of aneusomy (loss or gain of one or more chromosomes) such as Turner syndrome (45,X), trisomy 21 (Down syndrome), or other autosomal or sex chromosomal disorders such as Klinefelter syndrome, trisomy 13, and trisomy 18 is becoming increasingly common.[6,7] An advantage of FISH is that mitosing cells are not required and results for a suspected disorder can be obtained within 24 hours if necessary.[8] FISH can uncover small rearrangements that are not detectable with standard karyotypic analysis. For instance, the presence of a microdeletion (see table in Chromosome Analysis, High-Resolution *on page 363* and Table 1 which follows) can be detected by the absence of signal on one of a homologous chromosome pair.

FISH is also useful in the evaluation of neoplasia (see Table 2 on previous page). For example, the 9;22 translocation characteristic of CML can be detected quickly in interphase cells with high sensitivity and may be seen in the absence of the translocation visible cytogenetically (cryptic rearrangement). FISH can be used to determine bone marrow transplant engraftment in sex-mismatched donors and recipients using sex chromosome-specific probes. FISH is often used to characterize chromosomal abnormalities that are difficult to define with traditional cytogenetic analysis, such as marker and supernumerary chromosomes using specific FISH probes or the SKY or MFISH techniques. The utility of FISH continues to rapidly expand as evidenced by its recent application for detection of HER-2/*neu* amplification in breast cancer[9] and detection of recurrent bladder cancer[10] using multicolor FISH probe mixtures.

Limitations FISH can only provide information with respect to the specific probe being utilized. For example, using an X chromosome-specific probe to rule out Turner syndrome will not disclose chromosomal abnormalities involving other chromosomes such as trisomy 21, 18, or 13.

Methodology Cells from the specimen are first immobilized on a microscope slide and fixed with a methanol:acetic acid fixative. FISH is performed using probes selected for specific chromosomes or chromosomal regions. DNA sequences in the target and probe (which are complementary) are denatured and then mixed together so that the probe binds to the chromosomal regions in which it has high homology. The bound probe is detected using a series of fluorescent-labeled reagents and fluorescence microscopy.

Additional Information FISH is utilized for detection of aneusomy (loss or gain of one or more chromosomes) or structural rearrangements (most commonly deletions and translocations) in metaphase or interphase cells in a wide variety of specimens.

Footnotes

1. Knight SJ and Flint J, "Perfect Endings: A Review of Subtelomeric Probes and Their Use in Clinical Diagnosis," *J Med Genet*, 2000, 37(6):401-9.

2. Weiss MM, Hermsen MA, Meijer GA, et al, "Comparative Genomic Hybridization," *Mol Pathol*, 1999, 52(5):243-51.

3. Rothmann C, Bar-Am I, and Malik Z, "Spectral Imaging for Quantitative Histology and Cytogenetics," *Histol Histopathol*, 1998, 13(3):921-6.

4. Fleischman EW, Reshmi S, Sokova OI, et al, "Increased Karyotype Precision Using Fluorescence *In Situ* Hybridization and Spectral Karyotyping in Patients With Myeloid Malignancies," *Cancer Genet Cytogenet*, 1999, 108(2):166-70.

5. Mohr B, Bornhauser M, Thiede C, et al, "Comparison of Spectral Karyotyping and Conventional Cytogenetics in 39 Patients With Acute Myeloid Leukemia and Myelodysplastic Syndrome," *Leukemia*, 2000, 14(6):1031-8.

6. Thilaganathan B, Sairam S, Ballard T, et al, "Effectiveness of Prenatal Chromosomal Analysis Using Multicolor Fluorescent *In Situ* Hybridization," *Br J Obstet Gynaecol*, 2000, 107(2):262-6.

7. Lewin J, Kleinfinger P, Bazin A, et al, "Defining the Efficiency of Fluorescence *In Situ* Hybridization on Uncultured Amniocytes on a Retrospective Cohort of 27,407 Prenatal Diagnosis," *Prenat Diagn*, 2000, 20(1):1-6.

8. Pergament E, Chen PX, Thangavelu M, et al, "The Clinical Application of Interphase FISH in Prenatal Diagnosis," *Prenat Diagn*, 2000, 20(3):215-20.

9. Pauletti G, Dandekar S, Rong H, et al, "Assessment of Methods for Tissue-Based Detection of the HER-2/*neu* Alteration in Human Breast Cancer: A Direct Comparison of Fluorescence *In Situ* Hybridization and Immunohistochemistry," *J Clin Oncol*, 2000, 18(21):3651-64.

10. Sokolova IA, Halling KC, Jenkins RB, et al, "The Development of a Multitarget, Multicolor Fluorescence *In Situ* Hybridization Assay for Detection of Urothelial Carcinoma in Urine," *J Mol Diagn*, 2000, 2(3):166-23.

References

De Lellis RA, "*In Situ* Hybridization Techniques for the Analysis of Gene Expression: Applications in Tumor Pathology," *Hum Pathol*, 1994, 25(6):580-5.

Gozzetti A and Le Beau MM, "Fluorescence *In Situ* Hybridization: Uses and Limitations," *Semin Hematol*, 2000, 37(4):320-33.

Haddad BR, Schrock E, Meck J, et al, "Identification of *de novo* Chromosomal Markers and Derivatives by Spectral Karyotyping," *Hum Genet*, 1998, 103(5):619-25.

Luke S and Shepelsky M, "FISH: Recent Advances and Diagnostic Aspects," *Cell Vis*, 1998, 5(1):49-53.

Patel AS, Hawkins AL, and Griffin CA, "Cytogenetics and Cancer," *Curr Opin Oncol*, 2000, 12(1):62-7.

Tkachuk DC, Westbrook CA, Andreeff M, et al, "Detection of *bcr-abl* Fusion in Chronic Myelogenous Leukemia by *In Situ* Hybridization," *Science*, 1990, 250(4980):559-62.

Watson MS, Buchanan PD, Cohen MM, et al, Test and Technology Transfer Committee, American College of Medical Genetics, "Technical and Clinical Assessment of Fluorescence *In Situ* Hybridization: An ACMG/ASHG Position Statement. I. Technical Considerations," *Genet Med*, 2000, 2(6):356-60.

Wolman SR, "Fluorescence *In Situ* Hybridization: A New Tool for the Pathologist," *Hum Pathol*, 1994, 25(6):586-90.

CYTOPATHOLOGY

Celeste N. Powers, MD, PhD

Christopher D. Ackley, MD, PhD

Jennifer A. Brainard, MD

Leigh Ann Cahill, BS, CT (ASCP), CMIAC

Mary Ann Pedigo, BS, CT (ASCP), CMIAC

David S. Jacobs, MD

Cytopathology is the study of alterations within individual cells reflective of changes within their environment. Examination of such alterations at the cellular, as well as molecular level, allows the diagnosis of a wide range of benign, preneoplastic and malignant conditions. Like all morphologic studies, clinical and radiologic findings are of inestimable value in the accurate diagnosis of cytologic specimens. In addition, proper specimen procurement is absolutely essential for reliable interpretation.

Cytopathology can be divided into two major areas: exfoliative and aspiration cytopathology. The most well known and widely used cytopathology test is the Pap smear. Developed by Dr George Papanicolaou in the 1940s, the implementation of the Pap smear as a screening technique for cervical cancer has resulted in the dramatic decline of cervical cancer over the past 50 years. Current advances include The Bethesda System, a classification scheme developed by gynecologists, pathologists, and oncologists; development of better sampling and preparatory devices; and computer-assisted screening of Pap smears.

Screening techniques have also been developed for other body sites such as lung (sputum), bladder (urine), effusions, and cerebrospinal fluids and have established the utility of the Cytopathology Laboratory in the interpretation of nongynecologic specimens. Advances in endoscopic procedures have allowed more extensive evaluations of the respiratory, gastrointestinal, and urinary tracts by cytologic methods. The advent of fine needle aspiration (FNA) techniques utilized for both superficial or palpable masses and deep lesions requiring radiologic guidance has brought the Cytopathology Laboratory into the forefront of diagnostic pathology. FNA is rapid, safe, and cost-effective, and, in experienced hands, has a diagnostic accuracy approaching that of surgical biopsy.

In addition to light microscopy, numerous ancillary techniques can be used to evaluate cellular material. While electron microscopy, immunocytochemistry, and flow/laser cytometry are proven methods, newer molecular diagnostic techniques are being evaluated for diagnostic and prognostic reliability.

Excellence in patient care is always the goal of the Cytopathology Laboratory; however, its ability to provide accurate and timely results is directly linked to the clinician's ability to provide appropriate clinical information and satisfactory specimens. This chapter is designed to provide clinicians and their assistants with the necessary information to accomplish this goal.

ABSOLUTELY ESSENTIAL INFORMATION

To facilitate the correct processing of a specimen for interpretation by cytopathologists, certain necessary documentation must accompany the sample. Such documentation includes patient demographics, relevant history, clinical impression and prior abnormal pathology results, as well as referring physician information for report distribution. In addition, the submitting physician must designate an ICD-9-CM (International Classification of Disease, 9th revision, Clinical Modification) code or diagnostic narrative for each specimen. ICD-9 codes are extremely important for all types of samples and absolutely necessary to differentiate between screening and diagnostic Pap smears, as currently required by Medicare and other payers. Since Medicare may not pay for a particular test, such as annual screening Pap smear, patients need to sign an ABN (Advanced Beneficiary Notice) which documents their agreement to pay for a test if it is denied.

ICD-9 codes designated by the ordering physician are required to identify the reason (signs/symptoms/history) the test is performed. The CPT (Current Procedural Terminology) coding is used by the laboratory for reporting medical services performed, with each specimen being assigned one or more of these codes. CPT codes indicate the method of slide evaluations (manual, computer assisted, automated screening, etc) as well as the type of preparation of the sample (monolayer, smear, cytospin, etc) The list of CPT codes is maintained by the AMA for annual review/revision.

Cytology laboratories are inspected by a variety of enforcing agencies and must comply with the government mandated CLIA '88 (Clinical Laboratory Improvement Amendments of 1988) Final Rules. CLIA '88 sets standards for laboratory personnel, quality assurance, and controls workload limits. Proficiency testing of all individuals screening or interpreting gynecologic cytology is proposed. In an attempt to detect errors and improve performance, CLIA '88 requires that each cytology laboratory must: 1) review at least 10% of gynecologic cases interpreted as negative; 2) compare all malignant and premalignant gynecologic reports with corresponding histopathology reports to determine the cause of any discrepancies; 3) and for each patient with a current diagnosis of a high grade lesion or above, the laboratory must perform a retrospective review of all negative Pap smears within the previous 5 years. If any significant discrepancies are found that would affect current patient care, the laboratory must issue an amended report to the patient's physician.

In an attempt to standardize reporting terminology and better communicate with clinicians, the Bethesda System (TBS) for reporting cervical/vaginal cytology was developed at the National Cancer Institute in 1988 and further modified in 1991. The format of TBS includes a statement of specimen adequacy, a classification of the Pap smear based of the worst type of cellular change present, and a descriptive diagnosis. This method of reporting, though designed to simplify and group diagnoses according to prognostic outcomes, has not been adopted by all laboratories and applies only to gynecologic cytology at this time.

References

American Medical Association, *Current Procedural Terminology (CPT) 2001*, Standard Edition.
CLIA '88 Final Rules, Northfield, IL: College of American Pathologists, February, 1992.
Kurman and Solomon, *The Bethesda System for Reporting Cervical/Vaginal Cytologic Diagnosis*, New York, NY: Springer-Verlag, 1994.
Procedural Coding Crosswalk: Cross-Reference ICD-9 CM Volume 3 Codes to CPT Codes, Washington, DC: St Anthony Publishing, 1999.

- ◆ **Abdominal Mass Aspiration** *see* Fine Needle Aspiration, Deep Masses *on page 381*

- ◆ **Adrenal Mass Aspiration** *see* Fine Needle Aspiration, Deep Masses *on page 381*

Asbestos, Lung or Sputum

Related Information
Body Cavity Fluid Cytology *on page 372*
Bronchoalveolar Lavage (BAL) *on page 375*

Synonyms Asbestos Preparation; Ferruginous Body Count

Test Includes Cytologic evaluation of slides after processing (membrane filtration procedure, preferably nucleopore). Number of filtration preparations varies according to quantity of ferruginous bodies present. Precise weight of lung required - 5 grams is the standard sample. Lung tissue or sputum will be digested which may take 24 hours before preparation can be started. Results will be an exact count of ferruginous bodies (partial and complete) in the entire sample.

Abstract Asbestiform minerals include chrysotile, crocidolite, amosite, tremolite, anthophyllite, and actinolite. The risk of development of diffuse malignant mesothelioma (DMM) is greatest with exposure to crocidolite, but amosite is more often associated with DMM than is crocidolite in North America. They are equally represented in the UK.[1]

Ferruginous bodies are baton-shaped refractile rods onto which iron salts have precipitated. They are strongly associated with asbestosis.

This method provides a quantitative analysis of ferruginous bodies, particularly for patients suspected of long-term exposure to asbestos, fiberglass, carbon, or other minerals. Iron stain may be helpful in detection.[2]

Patient Preparation Informed consent for thoracotomy or endoscopy is needed if lung biopsy is obtained as part of an intraoperative procedure, tissue specimen most often from autopsy. If sputum sample is collected, advise patient not to remove fixative from container.

Specimen Fresh tissue, tissue fixed in appropriate fixative for lung biopsy, single or continuous multiple expectorated sputum samples

Container Wide-neck jar with appropriate fixative for lung biopsy. If fresh tissue is obtained, submit in sterile gauze premoistened with saline, enclosed in a plastic bag. Wide-mouth jar with Saccomanno fixative used for expectorated sputa sample. Each specimen container must be labeled with patient's name.

Collection Lung biopsies collected during procedures should be placed directly into fixative or wrapped in moistened gauze. Sputa samples can be collected at the patient's bedside or a container with fixative can be sent home with the patient for collection.

Storage Instructions Specimen should be delivered to the Cytology Laboratory as soon as possible. Unfixed tissue should be either refrigerated or processed immediately. Appropriate documentation (see Absolutely Essential Information *on page 369*) needs to accompany the specimen.

Use It was recognized in 1960 that many subjects with mesothelioma had asbestos exposure.[1]

Asbestos is considered responsible for 4000-6000 annual deaths from carcinoma of lung, including all histopathologic subtypes. A synergistic and multiplicative effect is postulated for smoking and exposure to asbestos.[3]

Limitations Acceptable range of ferruginous bodies is not clearly established. Random sampling may yield results that do not substantiate clinical suspicions. Cases are often the subject of legal proceedings.

Footnotes
1. Battifora H and McCaughey WT, "Tumors of the Serosal Membranes," *Atlas of Tumor Pathology*, Third Series, Fascicle 15, Washington, DC: Armed Forces Institute of Pathology, 1995.
2. DeMay R, *The Art and Science of Cytopathology-Exfoliative Cytology*, Chicago, IL: ASCP Press, American Society of Clinical Pathologists, 1996.
3. Colby TV, Koss MN, and Travis WD, "Tumors of the Lower Respiratory Tract," *Atlas of Tumor Pathology*, Third Series, Fascicle 13, Washington, DC: Armed Forces Institute of Pathology, American Registry of Pathology, 1995.

References
Guzman y Rotaeche J and Costabel U, "Bronchoalveolar Lavage in Diagnostic Cytology," *Compendium on Diagnostic Cytology*, 8th ed, Wied GL, Bibbo M, Keebler CM, et al, eds, Chicago, IL: Tutorials of Cytology, 1997, 233-47.
Hammar SP, "Pleural Diseases," *Pulmonary Pathology Tumors*, Chapter 5, Dar DH, Hammar SP, and Colby TV, eds, New York, NY: Springer-Verlag, 1995, 405-522.
Medical College of Virginia Hospitals, *Cytopathology Procedure Manual*, Richmond, VA: Virginia Commonwealth University, 1998, 165-71.

- ◆ **Asbestos Preparation** *see* Asbestos, Lung or Sputum *on page 371*

- ◆ **Ascitic Fluid Cytology** *see* Body Cavity Fluid Cytology *on page 372*

- ◆ **AutoCyte Prep** *see* Automation in Cytology, Preparation *on page 371*

- ◆ **AutoCyte Prep** *see* Automation in Cytology, Screening *on page 371*

Automation in Cytology, Preparation

Related Information
Automation in Cytology, Screening *on page 371*
Body Cavity Fluid Cytology *on page 372*
Bronchial Brushings Cytology *on page 373*

Bronchial Washings Cytology *on page 374*
Cerebrospinal Fluid Cytology *on page 376*
Cervical/Vaginal Cytology *on page 377*
Fine Needle Aspiration Culture *on page 609*
Sputum Cytology *on page 387*
Urinary Tract Cytology *on page 389*

Synonyms AutoCyte Prep; Monolayer Preparations; Thin-Layer Preparations; Thin Prep

Applies to Bladder Washings; Body Cavity Fluids Cytology; Esophageal Brushings/Washings Cytology; Esophageal Cytology; Fine Needle Aspiration Biopsy Cytology; Gastrointestinal Tract Brushings/Washings; Gastrointestinal Tract Cytology; Respiratory Tract Cytology; Urinary Cytology

Test Includes Automated preparations of slides from cells collected in a fluid suspension[1]

Abstract There are two new methods of sample collection and slide preparation designed to significantly improve screening and diagnostic accuracy especially in gynecologic cytology.[1] These methods can also be used in the preparation of nongynecologic specimens. The new technologies are Thin Prep by Cytyc Corporation and AutoCyte PREP by TriPath Imaging, Inc.

Patient Preparation The patient should be informed concerning the particular technology that the Cytology Laboratory is utilizing and sign a consent form especially for gynecologic specimens where the patient may be responsible for any charges not covered by the insurance company.

Container Use the vial of preservative material which is usually a buffered alcohol or alcohol-based solution (PreserveCyt® for Thin Prep and CytoRich® for AutoCyte PREP).

Collection Use the desired collection device for gynecologic samples (ie, Ayre spatula, cytobrush, cervix broom). Collect the specimen and rinse the collection device in the vial of preservative. For nongynecologic specimens, collect the specimen in accordance with instructions for the specific specimen. The Cytology Laboratory will add the appropriate preservative upon receipt of the specimen. Nongynecologic specimens can be collected directly into the preservative vial if deemed necessary by the Cytology Laboratory.

Storage Instructions Gynecologic samples collected in the vial of preservative do not need to be refrigerated. Any specimens (nongynecologic) not collected in the preservative must be refrigerated until the preservative is added.

Causes for Rejection Specimen not properly labeled, specimen not collected in correct preservative, specimen not refrigerated with correct preservative added

Special Instructions Provide all the pertinent patient information including clinical history, radiologic findings, history of cancer, insurance information, etc.

Use Liquid-based monolayer technologies have been developed as an alternative and/or replacement for the conventional Pap smear in an effort to improve diagnostic accuracy.[2,3] Studies have shown an overall increased detection rate of epithelial cell abnormalities for both liquid-based systems.[3] Multiple slide preparations can be made from a single vial which may prove useful for laboratory quality control.[1] The residual material in the vial may be used for test modalities such as DNA hybridization.

Limitations Allowing the collection device to air dry prior to rinsing it in the vial of preservative will yield drying artifacts and degeneration. Specimen may need to be recollected.

Footnotes
1. Zahniser D and Sullivan PJ, "CYTYC Corporation," *Acta Cytol*, 1996, 40(1):37-44.
2. Vassilakos P, Saurel J, and Rondez R, "Direct-To-Vial Use of the AutoCyte PREP Liquid-Based Preparation for Cervical-Vaginal Specimens in Three European Laboratories," *Acta Cytol*, 1999, 43(1):65-8.
3. Austin RM and Ramzy I, "Increased Detection of Epithelial Cell Abnormalities by Liquid-Based Gynecologic Preparations: A Review of Accumulated Data," *Acta Cytol*, 1998, 42(1):178-84.

References
Bishop JW, Bigner SH, Colgan TJ, et al, "Multicenter Masked Evaluation of AutoCyte PREP Thin Layers With Matched Conventional Smears: Including Initial Biopsy Results," *Acta Cytol*, 1998, 42(1):189-97.
Bolick DR and Hellman DJ, "Laboratory Implementation and Efficacy Assessment of the ThinPrep Cervical Cancer Screening System," f*Acta Cytol*, 1998, 42(1):209-13.
Papillo JL, Zarka MA, and St, John TL, "Evaluation of the ThinPrep Pap Test in Clinical Practice: A Seven Month, 16314-Case Experience in Northern Vermont," *Acta Cytol*, 1998, 42(1):203-8.

Automation in Cytology, Screening

Related Information
Automation in Cytology, Preparation *on page 371*
Cervical/Vaginal Cytology *on page 377*

Synonyms AutoCyte Prep; Monolayer Preparations; Thin-Layer Preparations; Thin Prep

Test Includes Automated screening of Pap smears by new technologies using the principles of image analysis algorithms or neural network processing

Abstract New technologies for automating the screening of Pap smears have been developed in order to improve consistency and reduce the number of false-negative cases.[1] The AutoPap 300 System by TriPath Imaging, Inc is FDA approved for primary screening of conventional smears and is undergoing FDA approval for screening of monolayer slides prepared (Continued)

Automation in Cytology, Screening (Continued)

with the AutoCyte Prep System. The AutoCyte Interactive System is undergoing FDA approval for screening of monolayer cervical smears.[2]

Patient Preparation The patient should be informed that her Pap smear will be screened/rescreened by the particular technology utilized by the laboratory and that a consent must be signed that the patient will pay any charges not covered by her insurance company, if applicable.

Container Refer to container methods for Cervical/Vaginal Cytology *on page 377* and Automation in Cytology, Preparation *on page 371*.

Collection Refer to collection methods for Cervical/Vaginal Cytology *on page 377* and Automation in Cytology, Preparation *on page 371*.

Storage Instructions Gynecologic samples collected in the vial of preservative do not need to be refrigerated. Any specimens (nongynecologic) not collected in the preservative must be refrigerated until the preservative is added.

Causes for Rejection Each automated device with have set protocols for rejection (eg, excessive bubbles, receding mounting medium, limited cells, thickness of the conventional smear, etc).

Special Instructions Provide all the pertinent patient information including clinical history, radiologic findings, history of cancer, abnormal Pap smears, and so forth.

Use These technologies have been developed for use as either a primary screening system or for quality control rescreening.

Limitations The AutoPap 300 System from TriPath Imaging, Inc. has been FDA approved for primary screening allowing for up to 25% of Pap smears to be "archived" without human review.[1]

Footnotes

1. Schofield K, "Cervical Cancer Detection Improvements," *Advance*, April, 2000, 66-9.
2. Icho N, "The Automation Trend in Cytology," *Lab Med*, 2000, 31(4):218-21.

References

Godfrey SE, "The Pap Smear, Automated Rescreening, and Negligent Nondisclosure," *Am J Clin Pathol*, 1999, 111(1):14-7.

Knesel EA, "Roche Image Analysis Systems, Inc," *Acta Cytol*, 1996, 40(1):60-6.

Lee JS, Kuan L, Oh S, et al, "A Feasibility Study of the AutoPap System Location-Guided Screening." *Acta Cytol*, 1998, 42(1):221-6.

Patten SF Jr, Lee JS, and Nelson AC, "NeoPath, Inc: NeoPath AutoPap 300 Automatic Pap Screener System," *Acta Cytol*, 1996, 40(1):45-52.

Takahashi M, Kimura M, Akagi A, et al, "AutoCyte SCREEN Interactive Automated Primary Cytology Screening System: A Preliminary Evaluation," *Acta Cytol*, 1998, 42(1):185-8.

Wilbur DC, Prey MU, Miller WM, et al, "The AutoPap System for Primary Screening in Cervical Cytology: Comparing the Results of a Prospective, Intended-Use Study With Routine Manual Practice," *Acta Cytol*, 1998, 42(1):214-20.

♦ **BAL Cytology** *see* Bronchoalveolar Lavage (BAL) *on page 375*

♦ **Barr Bodies** *see* Buccal Smear for Sex Chromatin Evaluation *on page 376*

♦ **Bladder, Ureteral, and Pelvicocalyceal Barbotage Specimens** *see* Urinary Tract Cytology *on page 389*

♦ **Bladder Washings** *see* Automation in Cytology, Preparation *on page 371*

♦ **Bladder Washings Cytology** *see* Urinary Tract Cytology *on page 389*

Body Cavity Fluid Cytology

Related Information

Asbestos, Lung or Sputum *on page 371*
Bacterial Culture, Aerobes *on page 563*
Bacterial Culture, Biopsy or Body Fluid *on page 565*
Body Fluid Amylase *on page 122*
Body Fluid Analysis, Cell Count *on page 408*
Body Fluid Chemical Analysis *on page 123*
Body Fluid Glucose *on page 124*
Body Fluid Lactate Dehydrogenase *on page 125*
Body Fluid pH *on page 125*
Bronchoalveolar Lavage (BAL) *on page 375*
CA 27.29, Serum *on page 128*
CA 125, Serum *on page 126*
Carcinoembryonic Antigen, Serum *on page 135*
Cell Cycle Analysis by Flow Cytometry *on page 53*
Cyst Fluid Cytology *on page 379*
Fine Needle Aspiration, Deep Masses *on page 381*
Flow Cytometry, Overview *on page 432*
Fungal Culture, Biopsy or Body Fluid *on page 610*
Gene Rearrangement for Leukemia and Lymphoma *on page 725*
Gram Stain *on page 617*
Herpesvirus 8 *on page 634*
Immunoperoxidase Procedures *on page 60*
Immunophenotypic Analysis of Tissues by Flow Cytometry *on page 62*
Mycobacterial Culture, Biopsy or Body Fluid *on page 655*
Polymerase Chain Reaction *on page 713*
Synovial Fluid Analysis *on page 323*
Viral Culture *on page 689*
Viral Culture, Body Fluid *on page 691*
Washing Cytology *on page 390*

Synonyms Body Fluid Cytology; Effusion Cytology; Fluids Cytology; Serous Effusion Cytology; Serous Fluid Cytology

Applies to Ascitic Fluid Cytology; Culdocentesis; Paracentesis Fluid Cytology; Pericardial Fluid Cytology; Peritoneal Fluid Cytology; Pleural Fluid Cytology; Synovial Fluid Cytology; Thoracentesis Fluid Cytology

Test Includes Cytologic evaluation of smears, cytocentrifuge preparations, filter preparations, and cell block preparations when indicated

Abstract The major coelomic cavities are the pleural spaces, the pericardial sac, and the peritoneum. The tunica vaginalis testis exists in males. Cytologic evaluation of body fluids, in conjunction with chemical analysis and clinical profile, can render and/or enhance diagnosis of a variety of benign and malignant conditions. Fluid may be obtained during staging surgical procedures (see Washing Cytology *on page 390*) or by puncture. The most common cause of fluid accumulations in the body spaces is congestive heart failure. The second most common cause is neoplastic disease.[1]

Patient Preparation Patient should sign informed consent prior to procedure. Puncture site should be carefully cleaned and prepared as for any tap. In cases of suspected malignancy, the smallest gauge needle (22 g) should be used, as tract seeding has been reported post-thoracentesis with large bore needles.

Specimen Fresh body fluid

The volume, clarity or opalescence, color, malodor, or viscosity may be relevant. For example, the epithelial type of diffuse malignant mesothelioma frequently gives rise to hyaluronic acid, which increases viscosity.

Container Use clear container to which anticoagulant can be added prior to collection. The optimal amount of fluid for cytology is 200-500 mL. The practice of salvaging large amounts (in excess of 500 mL) of fluid for cytologic examination is not recommended. The best diagnostic aliquot is the last portion that is drawn off, not the first. See Special Instructions.

Collection Gently agitate the container as fluid is collected in order to mix the heparin with the fluid; fluid may also be collected fresh without anticoagulant and sent to the laboratory in the fresh state immediately. Other tests are usually needed as well; see Related Information above. **Venous blood** drawn at the same time may be helpful; comparisons between serum and body fluid protein, LD, glucose, and other tests are often useful. See Body Fluid Analysis, Cell Count *on page 408*, Body Fluid Chemical Analysis *on page 123*, and related monographs. When pleural fluid is sampled, a **pleural biopsy** may provide diagnosis, especially of granulomatous diseases as well as carcinoma.

Storage Instructions Fluid with or without anticoagulant may be stored at 4°C; cells in the fluid can be preserved at this temperature for up to 1 week, without appreciable deterioration of cellular detail. With special techniques, specimens may be kept frozen at -70°C for 1 year without serious loss of cellular details.[2]

Causes for Rejection Added fixation of any type, unless previously discussed with Cytology Laboratory personnel; prolonged period (over 2 hours) at room temperature; improper container (thoracentesis and paracentesis drainage bags and large syringes are not acceptable containers)

Special Instructions Add 1 mL of heparin per 100 mL of fluid anticipated (each mL of heparin contains 1000 units). The common anticoagulants that can be used are heparin, 5-10 units per mL of fluid to be placed in the collecting vessel; or 3.8% sodium citrate, 1 mL per 10 mL of fluid; or EDTA, 1 mg per 1 mL of fluid. The cells in these fluids do not deteriorate rapidly if refrigerated, and no fixative need be added if the **fluid is refrigerated** within 30 minutes of collection. Fixation precludes the use of certain stains which may be useful for particular diagnoses. Include pertinent clinical information on requisition including previous malignancy, drugs, radiation therapy, or history of alcohol abuse.

Use Establish the presence of primary or metastatic neoplasms including gastric and gynecologic primaries. Aid in the diagnosis of rheumatoid pleuritis; systemic lupus erythematosus; myeloproliferative and lymphoproliferative disorders; viral, fungal, and parasitic infestation;[3] and fistulas involving serous cavities. Examination of effusion fluid is more sensitive and specific than blind pleural biopsy in the diagnosis of malignant pleural disease. The presence of malignant neoplastic cells in body fluid usually indicates that the patient has widespread metastases, with the exception of patients with primary pulmonary lesions. Positive peritoneal cytology is associated with advanced disease and is a strong predictor of unresectability of adenocarcinoma of pancreas.[4] Effusion fluid may be submitted for flow cytometric analysis in those cases suspected of myeloproliferative or lymphoproliferative disorder, and gene rearrangement analysis can be useful as well. The pleura is involved in 6% to 19% of patients with non-Hodgkin lymphoma. Pleural biopsy is advocated when >50% of cells in a pleural effusion are lymphocytes. In that situation, the likelihood of neoplastic disease or of tuberculosis is 95%.[5] In addition to lymphoma and TB, sarcoidosis is a cause of pleural fluid lymphocytosis.[1]

Examination of **synovial fluid** from a joint effusion may aid in the diagnosis of metabolic arthritis (gout or pseudogout), rheumatoid arthritis, or traumatic arthritis as well as septic arthritis (gonococcal arthritis). See Synovial Fluid Analysis *on page 323*. Occasional neoplasms may be detected.

Limitations Allowing fluid to stand for prolonged period before processing may cause deterioration and artifacts. In such fluids a second tap may be required after the reaccumulation of fluid for optimal cytologic interpretation. Clots may contain diagnostic cells which are available for recovery by preparation of a cell block while routine smears may fail to reveal such cells. Malignant cells cannot be recovered from all fluids from all subjects with malignant disease. Very well differentiated carcinomas may be difficult to distinguish from reactive states.

Ascitic fluid from patients with cirrhosis may contain markedly atypical cells which may be derived from mesothelial cells.[6]

Contraindications Relative contraindications include documented bleeding diathesis and full anticoagulated state.

Methodology Cholesterol crystals are dissolved in conventional processing. A wet-film technique can expose them.[3]

Additional Information Fluids should be submitted **fresh, unfixed**, and **heparinized** with anticoagulant added before collection to provide well-preserved, representative, diagnostic material. Exfoliated cells deteriorate rapidly in effusions, both in and out of the body. The amount of anticoagulant recommended is minimal but adequate to prevent clotting of body cavity fluids and to act as a preservative; excess amounts will not alter cytologic detail. Cytologic evaluation may classify the type of neoplasm and suggest its site of origin. Fixatives, such as formalin and alcohol, or other types of fixatives must not be used since they prevent adherence of the cells to the slides, do not allow cells to flatten out for optimal presentation of cellular details, and hinder quality staining by the Papanicolaou method. Alcohol also causes precipitation of protein which may interfere with cell analysis. If feasible, cell blocks can be prepared from the fluid sediment.[7] Cell blocks may be especially helpful in evaluation of clotted specimens, and for ultrastructural examination, special staining, and immunocytochemistry. Naylor considers cell blocks indispensable.[3]

Mucinous or mucinous-like fluids can be caused by pseudomyxoma peritonei primary in ovary or appendix, or colloid carcinomas of stomach, breast, ovary, or colorectum. Mesotheliomas produce hyaluronic acid.[1]

Tumor markers support discrimination between benign and malignant effusions. **Carcinoembryonic antigen** (CEA) is used both as an immunocytochemical marker and as a test available for serum and other body fluids. As a fluid marker, it is significantly increased with many carcinomas of lung, especially adenocarcinomas,[8] while mesotheliomas do not cause significant elevations of fluid CEA. Other primary sites likely to cause CEA elevations include breast and gastrointestinal tract. Some increase may be encountered in the presence of empyema, pancreatitis, tuberculosis, and cirrhosis. See Carcinoembryonic Antigen, Serum *on page 135*. The differential diagnosis between mesothelioma and adenocarcinoma of lung may be difficult in tissue sections as well as in cytologic material. Electron microscopy and/or immunocytochemistry are not infrequently needed.[9,10] Since initial presentation of most pleural mesotheliomas is effusion, study of aspiration fluid provides opportunity for early diagnosis. Reliable diagnosis is possible in as many as 80% of cases in experienced hands.[10]

CA 125 elevation with negative CEA assay occurs with serous and endometrioid carcinomas of ovary and adenocarcinoma of endometrium and fallopian tube.[11,12] By contrast, increased fluid CEA with negative CA 125 results are found with mucinous adenocarcinomas of ovary, lungs, gastrointestinal tract (including pancreas), or breast.[12] Both antigens are within normal range with lymphoma, melanoma, and with benign effusions. See CA 125, Serum *on page 126*.

Lymphoblastic lymphoma classically presents as a mediastinal mass, with which pleural effusion is often found.[13]

Molecular detection of pathogens can be applied (eg, body cavity-based lymphoma and human herpesvirus 8).[14,15]

Other techniques may also supplement classical cytologic methods (eg, chemistry). See Body Fluid Chemical Analysis *on page 123* and Flow Cytometry, Overview *on page 432*.[16]

When fluids are examined in the clinical microscopy laboratory, detection of neoplastic cells cannot be expected to compare with the capabilities of the cytopathology laboratory.[17]

See also Washing Cytology *on page 390*.

Footnotes

1. DeMay RM, "Fluids," *The Art and Science of Cytopathology*, Chapter 8, Chicago, IL: ASCP Press, American Society of Clinical Pathologists, 1996, 257-325.
2. McCorriston J, "New Method for Preserving Cytology Specimens," *J Clin Pathol*, 1989, 42(10):1101-3.
3. Naylor B, "Pleural, Peritoneal and Pericardial Fluids," *Comprehensive Cytopathology*, 2nd ed, Chapter 24, Bibbo M, ed, Philadelphia, PA: WB Saunders Co, 1997, 551-621.
4. Merchant NB, Conlon KC, Saigo P, et al, "Positive Peritoneal Cytology Predicts Unresectability of Pancreatic Adenocarcinoma," *J Am Coll Surg*, 1999, 188(4):421-6.
5. Mansoor A, Wagner RP, and DePalma L, "Waldenström Macroglobulinemia Presenting as a Pleural Effusion," *Arch Pathol Lab Med*, 2000, 124(6):891-3.
6. Guzman J, Bross KJ, Schölmerich J, et al, "Immunocytochemical Analysis of Ascitic Fluid Due to Cirrhosis - A Contribution to Understanding the Origin of Markedly Atypical Cells," *Acta Cytol*, 1992, 36(2):236-40.
7. Nathan NA, Narayan E, Smith MM, et al, "Cell Block Cytology. Improved Preparation and its Efficacy in Diagnostic Cytology," *Am J Clin Pathol*, 2000, 114(4):599-606.
8. Kjeldsberg CR and Knight JA, *Body Fluids - Laboratory Examination of Amniotic, Cerebrospinal, Seminal, Serous, and Synovial Fluids*, 3rd ed, Chicago, IL: American Society of Clinical Pathologists, 1993, 159-254.
9. Carella R, Deleonardi G, D'Errico A, et al, "Immunohistochemical Panels for Differentiating Epithelial Malignant Mesothelioma From Lung Adenocarcinoma: A Study With Logistic Regression Analysis," *Am J Surg Pathol*, 2001, 25(1):43-50.

10. Battifora H and McCaughey WT, "Tumors of the Serosal Membranes," *Atlas of Tumor Pathology*, Third Series, Fascicle 15, Washington, DC: Armed Forces Institute of Pathology, 1995.
11. Pinto MM, Bernstein LH, Brogan DA, et al, "Immunoradiometric Assay of CA 125 in Effusions. Comparison With Carcinoembryonic Antigen," *Cancer*, 1987, 59(2):218-22.
12. Rudolph RA, Pinto MM, and Bernstein LH, "Measuring Decision Values for CEA and CA 125 in Effusions," *Lab Med*, 1990, 21(9):574-8.
13. Sandlund JT, Downing JR, and Crist WM, "Non-Hodgkin Lymphoma in Childhood," *N Engl J Med*, 1996, 334(19):1238-48.
14. Alkan S, Eltoum IA, Tabbara S, et al, "Usefulness of Molecular Detection of Human Herpesvirus-8 in the Diagnosis of Kaposi Sarcoma by Fine-Needle Aspiration," *Am J Clin Pathol*, 1999, 111(1):91-6.
15. Mullaney BP, Ng VL, Herndier BG, et al, "Comparative Genomic Analyses of Primary Effusion Lymphoma," *Arch Pathol Lab Med*, 2000, 124(6):824-6.
16. Horn KD and Penchansky L, "Chylous Pleural Effusions Simulating Leukemic Infiltrate Associated With Thoracoabdominal Disease and Surgery in Infants," *Am J Clin Pathol*, 1999, 111(1):99-104.
17. Ben-Ezra J, Stastny JF, Harris AC, et al, "Comparison of the Clinical Microscopy Laboratory With the Cytopathology Laboratory in the Detection of Malignant Cells in Body Fluids," *Am J Clin Pathol*, 1994, 102(4):439-42.

References

Brandstetter RD, Velazquez V, Viejo C, et al, "Postural Changes in Pleural Fluid Constituents," *Chest*, 1994, 105(5):1458-61.

Covell JL, Lowry EH, and Feldman PS, "Cytologic Diagnosis of Blastomycosis in Pleural Fluid," *Acta Cytol*, 1982, 26(6):833-6.

Drew PA and Krauss JS, "Identification of *Giardia lamblia* in Peritoneal Fluid of Trauma Patients," *Acta Cytol*, 1989, 33(2):283-4.

Fam AG, Voorneveld C, Robinson JB, et al, "Synovial Fluid Immunocytology in the Diagnosis of Leukemic Synovitis," *J Rheumatol*, 1991, 18(2):293-6.

Hallman JR and Geisinger KR, "Cytology of Fluids From Pleural, Peritoneal and Pericardial Cavities in Children. A Comprehensive Survey," *Acta Cytol*, 1994, 38(2):209-17.

Hammar SP, "Pleural Diseases," *Pulmonary Pathology Tumors*, Chapter 5, Dail DH, Hammar SP, and Colby TV, eds, New York, NY: Springer-Verlag, 1995, 405-522.

Hira PR, Lindberg LG, Ryd W, et al, "Cytologic Diagnosis of Bancroftian Filariasis in a Nonendemic Area," *Acta Cytol*, 1988, 32(2):267-9.

Koss LG, "Examination of Effusions - Pleural, Ascitic, and Pericardial Fluids," *Compendium on Diagnostic Cytology*, 8th ed, Wied GL, Bibbo M, Keebler CM, et al, eds, Chicago, IL: Tutorials of Cytology, 1997, 292-4.

Lidang Jensen M and Johansen P, "Immunocytochemical Staining of Serous Effusions: An Additional Method in the Routine Cytology Practice?" *Cytopathology*, 1994, 5(2):93-103.

Mezger J, Stötzer O, Schilli G, et al, "Identification of Carcinoma Cells in Ascitic and Pleural Fluid - Comparison of Four Panepithelial Antigens With Carcinoembryonic Antigen," *Acta Cytol*, 1992, 36(1):75-81.

Naylor B, "Cytological Aspects of Pleural, Peritoneal, and Pericardial Fluids From in Patients With Systemic Lupus Erythematosus," *Cytopathology*, 1992, 3(1):1-8.

Naylor B, "The Pathognomonic Cytologic Picture of Rheumatoid Pleuritis," *Acta Cytol*, 1990, 34(4):465-73.

Okuyama T, Imai S, and Tsuburu Y, "Egg of *Schistosoma japonicum* in Ascitic Fluid," *Acta Cytol*, 1985, 29(4):651-2.

Raab SS, "Significance of Atypical Cells in Cytologic Serous Fluid Specimens," *Am J Clin Pathol*, 1999, 111(1):11-3.

Weaver KM, Novak PM, and Naylor B, "Vegetable Cell Contaminants in Cytologic Specimens. Their Resemblance to Cells Associated With Various Normal and Pathologic States," *Acta Cytol*, 1981, 25(3):210-4.

Wilbur DC, "Body Cavity Fluid Cytology - An Approach to Evaluation and Differential Diagnosis," *Compendium on Diagnostic Cytology*, 8th ed, Wied GL, Bibbo M, Keebler CM, et al, eds, Chicago, IL: Tutorials of Cytology, 1997, 295-301.

Wojno KJ, Olson JL, and Sherman ME, "Cytopathology of Pleural Effusions After Radiotherapy," *Acta Cytol*, 1994, 38(1):1-8.

Bronchial Brushings Cytology

Related Information

(Continued)

Bronchial Brushings Cytology (Continued)

Synonyms Bronchial Brush Cytology

Test Includes Cytologic evaluation of direct smears, cytocentrifuge (cytospin) preparations, and/or monolayer preparations most commonly; membrane filtration preparations and cell blocks are less often used.

Abstract Bronchial brushings are generally used with bronchial washings for diagnosis of potential pulmonary neoplasms in patients with abnormal imaging findings or persistent respiratory symptoms. Bronchial cytology is useful in the evaluation of patients with abnormal sputum cytology.[1,2] Visualization of tumor results in excellent diagnostic yield.

Specimen Direct smears may be prepared by rolling the brush onto a frosted or plain glass slide and immediately fixing in 95% ethanol. Alternatively, the brush end may be placed in physiologic saline and sent to the Cytology Laboratory for processing. The brush is rolled between two glass slides which are then fixed and stained with a Papanicolaou stain. Cytospins, monolayer preparations, and/or cell blocks may be prepared after the brush is placed in physiologic saline and vortexed.

Collection Brushings are obtained using a circular, stiff-bristled brush in an area of bronchoscopic abnormality.

Storage Instructions If a delay in processing must occur, the brushing specimen should be refrigerated.

Causes for Rejection Prolonged period (more than 1 hour) at room temperature

Special Instructions Indicate the type of specimen submitted as well as all pertinent clinical information (ie, age, clinical impression, history of malignancy, prior chemotherapy or radiation, radiographic findings). Provision of clinical history supports diagnostic accuracy.[3] Specify need for special stains for microorganisms.

Use Bronchial cytology is generally used to evaluate patients with the clinical symptoms of prolonged cough, localized wheezing, hemoptysis, or bronchial obstruction, structural deformity, extrinsic compression,[4] as well as those with radiographic abnormalities including a new solitary pulmonary nodule, atelectasis or persistent pulmonary infiltrates.[1,2] The various types of diagnostic respiratory cytology are complementary to one another. Bronchial cytology is useful in the diagnosis of both central and peripheral pulmonary lesions. Pleural based lesions or those in the extreme periphery of the pulmonary parenchyma may not be accessible to the bronchoscope. Bronchial brushing is most sensitive for the diagnosis of squamous cell carcinoma and most specific in identifying small cell carcinoma and adenocarcinoma.[1] Bronchial brushing should be used in combination with bronchial washing to maximize diagnostic yield. The combination of cytology with biopsy provides specific diagnosis more often than either alone.[5] Repeat specimens may be helpful in the setting of an initial negative result in the presence of a high degree of clinical suspicion. An unequivocal diagnosis of cancer can be made by cytologic means in ~50% of sputum specimens, and in ~65% of bronchial brushings or bronchoalveolar lavage samples. With computed tomography guidance, the sensitivity of FNA is ~90%.[5]

Respiratory infections may also be diagnosed using this technique, though bronchoalveolar lavage (BAL) is generally more useful.

Limitations To be considered adequate, the specimen should contain large numbers of well-preserved bronchial epithelial cells and pulmonary macrophages.[2] Sparsely cellular samples or specimens composed predominantly of oral squamous cells are unsatisfactory for evaluation. Obscuring inflammation, blood, or extensive air-drying artifact may also render a specimen unsatisfactory. A specimen is considered less than optimal for evaluation if there is a lack of accompanying clinical information.

Limited extent of sampling is provided by bronchial brushings.

Additional Information Useful comparisons between sputum, bronchial brush cytology, and FNA biopsy have recently been tabulated.[6]

Cytologic observations with increased antineutrophil cytoplasmic antibody (C-ANCA) concentrations and negative cultures, may support the diagnosis of Wegener granulomatosis.[7]

Footnotes

1. DeMay RM, The Art and Science of Cytopathology, Chicago, IL: ASCP Press, American Society of Clinical Pathologists, 1996, 207-56.
2. Papanicolaou Society Task Force on Standards of Practice, "Guidelines of the Papanicolaou Society of Cytopathology for the Examination of Cytologic Specimens Obtained From the Respiratory Tract," Diagn Cytopathol, 1999, 21(1):61-9.
3. Rabb SS, Oweity T, Hughes JH, et al, "Effect of Clinical History on Diagnostic Accuracy in the Cytologic Interpretation of Bronchial Brush Specimens," Am J Clin Pathol, 2000, 114(1):78-83.
4. Barker AL, "Bronchiectasis and Localized Airway/Parenchymal Disorders," Cecil Textbook of Medicine, 21st ed, Chapter 77, Goldman L and Bennett JC, eds, Philadelphia, PA: WB Saunders Co, 2000, 405-9.
5. Linder J, "Lung Cancer Cytology - Something Old, Something New," Am J Clin Pathol, 2000, 114(2):169-71.
6. Johnston WW, "Cytopathology of the Lung: Diagnostic Applications of Sputum, Bronchial Brushings, and Fine Needle Aspiration Biopsy Specimens," Compendium on Diagnostic Cytology, 8th ed, Wied GL, Bibbo M, Keebler CM, et al, eds, Chicago, IL: Tutorials of Cytology, 1997, 216-29.

7. Michael CW and Flint A, "The Cytologic Features of Wegener's Granulomatosis," Am J Clin Pathol, 1998, 110(1):10-5.

References

Bibbo M, "Bronchial Brushing," Compendium on Diagnostic Cytology, 8th ed, Wied GL, Bibbo M, Keebler CM, et al, eds, Chicago, IL: Tutorials of Cytology, 1997, 231-2.
Johnston WW and Elson CE, "Respiratory Tract," Comprehensive Cytopathology, 2nd ed, Chapter 16, Bibbo M, ed, Philadelphia PA: WB Saunders Co, 1997, 325-401.
Popp W, Merkle M, Schreiber B, et al, "How Much Brushing Is Enough for the Diagnosis of Lung Tumors?" Cancer, 1992, 70:2278-80.
Powers CN, "Respiratory Cytopathology," Atlas of Difficult Diagnoses in Cytopathology, Chapter 3, Atkinson BF and Silverman JF, eds, Philadelphia, PA: WB Saunders Co, 1998, 113-44.

◆ **Bronchial Wash Cytology** see Bronchial Washings Cytology on page 374

Bronchial Washings Cytology

Related Information

Synonyms Bronchial Wash Cytology; Tracheal Aspiration Cytology; Tracheal Washings

Test Includes Cytologic evaluation of cytocentrifuge (cytospin) preparations and/or monolayer preparations most commonly; membrane filtration preparations and cell blocks are less often used.

Abstract Bronchial washings are generally used with bronchial brushings for diagnosis of potential pulmonary neoplasms in patients with abnormal imaging findings or persistent respiratory symptoms. Bronchial cytology is useful in the evaluation of patients with abnormal sputum cytology.[1,2]

Specimen The freshly aspirated washing specimen should be immediately sent to the Cytopathology Laboratory without fixative for processing.

Collection Washings are obtained by repetitive instillation of 3-5 mL of sterile physiologic saline through the bronchoscope in the area of clinical suspicion followed by reaspiration of the fluid. Blind sampling in the absence of bronchoscopic abnormality has little or no utility.

Storage Instructions If a delay in processing must occur, the washing specimen should be refrigerated.

Causes for Rejection Prolonged period (more than 1 hour) at room temperature

Special Instructions Indicate the type of specimen submitted as well as all pertinent clinical information (ie, age, clinical impression, history of malignancy, prior chemotherapy or radiation, radiographic findings). Specify need for special stains for microorganisms.

Use Bronchial cytology is generally used to evaluate patients with the clinical symptoms of prolonged cough, localized wheezing, hemoptysis, or bronchial obstruction as well as those with radiographic abnormalities including a new solitary pulmonary nodule, atelectasis, or persistent pulmonary infiltrates.[1,2] The various types of diagnostic respiratory cytology are complementary to one another. Bronchial cytology is useful in the diagnosis of both central and peripheral pulmonary lesions. Pleural based lesions or those in the extreme periphery of the pulmonary parenchyma may not be accessible to the bronchoscope. Bronchial washing is most sensitive for the diagnosis of squamous cell carcinoma and most specific in identifying squamous cell carcinoma and small cell carcinoma.[1] It is as sensitive in the diagnosis of adenocarcinoma as bronchial brushing and sputum cytology. Bronchial washing should be used in combination with bronchial brushing to maximize diagnostic yield. Repeat specimens may be helpful in the setting of an initial negative result and a high degree of clinical suspicion. Respiratory infections may also be diagnosed using this technique, though bronchoalveolar lavage (BAL) is generally more useful. Special stains for microorganisms may be performed on the washing material.

Limitations To be considered adequate, the specimen should contain large numbers of well-preserved bronchial epithelial cells and pulmonary macrophages.[2] Sparsely cellular samples or specimens composed predominantly of oral squamous cells are unsatisfactory for evaluation. Obscuring inflammation, blood, or extensive air drying artifact may also render a specimen unsatisfactory. A specimen is considered less than optimal for evaluation if there is a lack of accompanying clinical information.

Footnotes

1. DeMay RM, "The Art and Science of Cytopathology: Exfoliative Cytology," Respiratory Cytology, Chapter 7, Chicago, IL: ASCP Press, 1996, 207-56.
2. Papanicolaou Society Task Force on Standards of Practice, "Guidelines of the Papanicolaou Society of Cytopathology for the Examination of Cytologic Specimens Obtained From the Respiratory Tract," Diagn Cytopathol, 1999, 21(1):61-9.

References

Johnston WW and Elson CE, "Respiratory Tract," Comprehensive Cytopathology, 2nd ed, Chapter 16, Bibbo M, ed, Philadelphia PA: WB Saunders Co, 1997, 325-401.
Powers CN, "Respiratory Cytopathology," Atlas of Difficult Diagnoses in Cytopathology, Chapter 3, Atkinson BF and Silverman JF, eds, Philadelphia, PA: WB Saunders Co, 1998, 113-44.

Sturgis CD, Nassar DL, D'Antonio JA, et al, "Cytologic Features Useful for Distinguishing Small Cell From Nonsmall Cell Carcinoma in Bronchial Brush and Wash Specimens," *Am J Clin Pathol*, 2000, 114(2):197-202.

Bronchoalveolar Lavage (BAL)

Related Information

Synonyms BAL Cytology

Test Includes Cytologic evaluation of slides after processing. Special stains for microorganisms and/or cell count with differential. Identification of hemosiderin-laden macrophages. Combined use of cytocentrifugation, liquid-based monolayer techniques, direct smears, and filter membrane techniques may be beneficial in some circumstances.[1]

Abstract Useful in the diagnosis of cancer, opportunistic infections in immunocompromised patients, culture in those with aspiration pneumonia, pneumonia secondary to chronic disease or to complications (eg, the postoperative state), interstitial lung disease, granulomatous disease (including sarcoid), hypersensitivity pneumonia, drug-induced pulmonary toxicity, asbestosis, pulmonary hemorrhage, and evaluation of transplant rejection.[2]

Patient Preparation Informed consent for procedure. Premedication is often given. Topical anesthesia of the pharynx and upper respiratory tract is necessary. Sedation is useful but often precluded by patient's clinical status.

Aftercare Transient fever, chills, and myalgias have been reported to occur in up to 50% of cases. Antipyretic analgesics may be indicated.

Specimen Lavage fluid

Container Sterile, leakproof disposable container

Collection More than 80% of pulmonologists use the right middle lobe as the sampling site due to increased volume recovered and higher cell count. The bronchoscope is wedged in a subsegmental bronchus. 100-300 mL of warm, pyrogen-free, isotonic, sterile solution is infused with recovery of 40% to 60%. Fixative should not be used.[2,3]

Storage Instructions Specimen should be delivered to the Cytology Laboratory as soon as possible. Refrigeration of the specimen is essential if there is a delay in delivering to the laboratory or delay in specimen processing. Detection of *Pneumocystis carinii* is not compromised by delayed processing; however, it is more difficult to identify in patients who are already receiving treatment for this organism.

Special Instructions Specify need for special stains for microorganisms or cell count. Routine processing in many cytology laboratories includes only Papanicolaou stained smears.

Use Bronchoalveolar lavage (BAL) is useful in the diagnosis of infections of the lung and is now commonly used as the preliminary diagnostic procedure in severe diffuse lung infections in both normal and immunocompromised patients, including pneumonia caused by gram-negative bacilli,[4] and particularly opportunistic infectious organisms such as cytomegalovirus, *P. carinii*, herpes simplex virus (HSV), and atypical mycobacteria and fungi. BAL is also useful in the diagnosis and management of sarcoid; fibrosing alveolitis; bronchiolitis obliterans organizing pneumonia; eosinophilic pneumonia; pneumoconioses including silica particles, asbestosis, titaneum, tantalum, nickel, and chromium lung disease; chronic beryllium disease; alveolar proteinosis;[5] idiopathic pulmonary hemosiderosis; and interstitial lung disease.[6] The presence of foamy cytoplasm in alveolar macrophages results from accumulation of phospholipids in amiodarone toxicity.[7] With electron microscopy, a diagnosis of Langerhans cell (eosinophilic) granulomatosis can be established. Various neoplastic processes are diagnosed by this method including primary bronchogenic carcinoma, bronchoalveolar carcinoma, metastatic tumors including lymphangitic carcinomatosis, leukemias, and lymphomas.[3]

Atypical type II pneumocytes in the lavage fluid due to toxic injury may indicate progression of damage. BAL is useful in evaluation of response to therapy and follow up (eg, allergic alveolitis).[3]

Limitations Wide variability in cell type and numbers recovered, particularly in smokers. Standardized volumes and concentrations not yet established.

Contraindications Severe hypoxemia with impending respiratory failure

Methodology Liquid-based monolayer techniques, cytocentrifugation and membrane filter techniques, and fractionated analysis; Papanicolaou, May-Grünwald-Giemsa staining. Immunofluorescence, immunoperoxidase, PAS, PAS diastase, alcian blue PAS, iron stains, silver methenamine; laser scanning cytometry, flow cytometry.

Additional Information BAL can help to separate inflammatory processes in which lymphocytes predominate (ie, sarcoid, hypersensitivity pneumonia including drug reaction, berylliosis) from those in which neutrophils or macrophages predominate (ie, idiopathic pulmonary fibrosis, cytotoxic drug reaction, Langerhans histiocytosis).[2]

A Diff-Quik™ stained cytospin preparation of BAL is an excellent rapid screening procedure for pathogens, especially in immunocompromised patients including *P. carinii*, CMV, HSV, *Cryptococcus neoformans*, *Candida* spp, *Blastomyces dermatitidis*, and *Aspergillus* spp as well as *Nocardia* spp and *Actinomyces* spp. The presence of bacteria phagocytosed by >7% of lavaged cells is thought to bear predictive relevance and may be useful to direct antimicrobial treatment before the results of cultures become available.[8] Detection of lipid-laden macrophages in increased numbers (>40% of cells) correlates well with chronic aspiration pneumonia.

Footnotes

1. Thompson AB, Robbins RA, Ghafouri MA, et al, "Bronchoalveolar Lavage Fluid Processing - Effect of Membrane Filtration Preparation on Neutrophil Recovery," *Acta Cytol*, 1989, 33(4):544-9.
2. DeMay RM, *The Art and Science of Cytopathology*, Chicago, IL: ASCP Press, American Society of Clinical Pathologists, 1996, 212.
3. Taskinen EI, Tukiainen PS, Alitalo RL, et al, "Bronchoalveolar Lavage: Cytological Techniques and Interpretation of the Cellular Profiles," *Pathol Annu*, Rosen PP and Fechner RE, eds Norwalk, CT: Appleton & Lange, 1994, 29(2):121-54.
4. Johnson WG, "Pneumonia Caused by Aerobic Gram-Negative Bacilli," *Cecil Textbook of Medicine*, 21st ed, Chapter 321, Goldman L and Bennett JC, eds, Philadelphia, PA: WB Saunders Co, 2000, 1612-15.
5. Burkhalter A, Silverman JF, Hopkins MB, et al, "Bronchoalveolar Lavage Cytology in Pulmonary Alveolar Proteinosis," *Am J Clin Pathol*, 1996, 106(4):504-10.
6. Guzman y Rotaeche J and Costabel U, "Bronchoalveolar Lavage in Diagnostic Cytology," *Compendium on Diagnostic Cytology*, 8th ed, Wied GL, Bibbo M, Keebler CM, et al, eds, Chicago, IL: Tutorials of Cytology, 1997, 233-47.
7. Faling LJ and Marke J, "A 65-Year-Old woman With a Dry Cough and Pulmonary Nodules," Case Records of the Massachusetts General Hospital, Case 35-1997, Scully RE, Mark EJ, McNeely WF, et al, eds, *N Engl J Med*, 1997, 337(20):1449-58.
8. Johanson WG, "Pneumonia Caused by Aerobic Gram-Negative Bacilli," *Cecil Textbook of Medicine*, 21st ed, Chapter 321, Goldman L and Bennett JC, eds, Philadelphia PA: WB Sanders Co, 2000, 1612-15.

References

Allen JN, Davis WB, and Pacht ER, "Diagnostic Significance of Increased Bronchoalveolar Lavage Fluid Eosinophils," *Am Rev Respir Dis*, 1990, 142(3):642-7.
Baughman RP, Dohn MN, Loudon RG, et al, "Bronchoscopy With Bronchoalveolar Lavage in Tuberculosis and Fungal Infections," *Chest*, 1991, 99(1):92-7.
Buhl R, Stahl E, and Meier-Sydow J, "*In Vivo* Assessment of Pulmonary Oxidant Damage: The Role of Bronchoalveolar Lavage," *Monaldi Arch Chest Dis*, 1994, 49(3 Suppl 1):1-8.
Konstan MW, Hilliard KA, Norvell TM, et al, "Bronchoalveolar Lavage Findings in Cystic Fibrosis Patients With Stable, Clinically Mild Lung Disease Suggest Ongoing Infection and Inflammation," *Am J Respir Crit Care Med*, 1994, 150(2):448-54.
Martin WJ 2d, "Diagnostic Bronchoalveolar Lavage in Immunosuppressed Patients With New Pulmonary Infiltrates," *Mayo Clin Proc*, 1992, 67(3):296-8.
Meduri GU, Stover DE, Greeno RA, et al, "Bilateral Bronchoalveolar Lavage in the Diagnosis of Opportunistic Pulmonary Infections," *Chest*, 1991, 100(5):1272-6.
Moumouni H, Garaud P, Diot P, et al, "Quantification of Cell Loss During Bronchoalveolar Lavage Fluid Processing. Effects of Fixation and Staining Methods," *Am J Respir Crit Care Med*, 1994, 149(3 Pt 1):636-40.
Pisani RJ, Witzig TE, Li CY, et al, "Confirmation of Lymphomatous Pulmonary Involvement by Immunophenotypic and Gene Rearrangement Analysis of Bronchoalveolar Lavage Fluid," *Mayo Clin Proc*, 1990, 65(5):651-6.
Popp W, Ritschka L, Scherak O, et al, "Bronchoalveolar Lavage in Rheumatoid Arthritis and Secondary Sjögren's Syndrome," *Lung*, 1990, 168(4):221-31.
Radio SJ, Rennard SI, Kessinger A, et al, "Breast Carcinoma in Bronchoalveolar Lavage. A Cytologic and Immunochemical Study," *Arch Pathol Lab Med*, 1989, 113(4):333-6.
Rennard SI, "Bronchoalveolar Lavage in the Diagnosis of Cancer," *Lung*, 1990, 168(Suppl):1035-40.
Rennard SI, "Future Directions for Bronchoalveolar Lavage," *Lung*, 1990, 168(Suppl):1050-6.
Roggli VL, Piantadosi CA, and Bell DY, "Asbestos Bodies in Bronchoalveolar Lavage Fluid: A Study of 20 Asbestos-Exposed Individuals and Comparison to Patients With Other Chronic Interstitial Lung Disease," *Acta Cytol*, 1986, 30(5):470-6.
Schumann GB and Swensen JJ, "Comparison of Papanicolaou's Stain With the Gomori Methenamine Silver (GMS) Stain for the Cytodiagnosis of *Pneumocystis carinii* in Bronchoalveolar Lavage (BAL) Fluid," *Am J Clin Pathol*, 1991, 95(4):583-6.
Silverman JF, Turner RC, West RL, et al, "Bronchoalveolar Lavage in the Diagnosis of Lipoid Pneumonia," *Diagn Cytopathol*, 1989, 5(1):3-8.
Stanley MW, Henry-Stanley MJ, and Iber C, "Bronchoalveolar Lavage," *Cytology and Clinical Application*, New York, NY: Igaku-Shoin, 1991.
Woods GL, Thompson AB, Rennard SL, et al, "Detection of Cytomegalovirus in Bronchoalveolar Lavage Specimens. Spin Amplification and Staining With a Monoclonal Antibody to the Early Nuclear Antigen for Diagnosis of Cytomegalovirus Pneumonia," *Chest*, 1990, 98(3):568-75.

♦ **Bronchopulmonary Lavage for** *Pneumocystis* see *Pneumocystis carinii* Preparation *on page 386*

Brushings Cytology

Related Information
Bronchial Brushings Cytology *on page 373*
Sputum Cytology *on page 387*

Abstract Brushing of epithelial lined surfaces in diagnostic cytopathology has greatly advanced with the use of flexible fiberoptic devices. Cytologic specimens using endoscopy and the brushing technique can be obtained from the respiratory and gastrointestinal tracts. Additionally, the endoscope has also provided a means of obtaining small tissue biopsies for histologic examination. The general principle in this type of cytology is that the lesion is visible endoscopically and must primarily involve the tissue surface.

In the respiratory tract, specimens obtained by bronchial brushing have a higher yield (more sensitive) than those obtained by either bronchial washings or sputum examination. Interestingly, tumor type affects the diagnostic sensitivity of brushing cytology, with metastatic carcinomas having the highest sensitivity and squamous cell carcinomas the lowest. Additionally, bronchial brushing cytology can be used for diagnosis of granulomatous and infectious processes involving the lung.

Gastrointestinal tract cytology specimens are obtained almost exclusively by endoscopy in symptomatic or high-risk patients. Cytologic examination of gastrointestinal lesion(s) can lead to a diagnostic yield of 80% to 85%. Application of endoscopic retrograde cholangiopancreatography (ERCP) has provided increasing numbers of brush specimens from the biliary tract and pancreatic ducts.[1,2] Like respiratory tract tumors, the specific nature of the tumor influences the diagnostic yield (exophytic greater than endophytic). Cytologic brushing samples can also be beneficial in the diagnosis of infectious disease involving the GI tract, inflammatory lesions as well as neoplastic lesions, but again the process must involve the surface to be sampled by brushing techniques.

Use In addition to the differential diagnosis of neoplastic and tumor-like lesions, infectious agents are encountered. These include histoplasmosis, candidiasis, herpes infections, CMV, mycobacterial and *H. pylori* infections, infestation by giardiasis, cryptosporidiosis, and microsporidiosis.

Footnotes
1. Ducatman BS and Wang HH, "Gastrointestinal Cytology," *Atlas of Difficult Diagnoses in Cytopathology*, Chapter 6, Atkinson BF and Silverman JF, eds, Philadelphia, PA: WB Saunders Co, 1998, 201-29.
2. Renshaw AA, Madge R, Jiroutek M, et al, "Bile Duct Brushing Cytology: Statistical Analysis of Proposed Diagnostic Criteria," *Am J Clin Pathol*, 1998, 110(5):635-40.

References
Geisinger KR, "Alimentary Tract (Esophagus, Stomach, Small Intestine, Colon, Rectum, Anus, Biliary Tract)," *Comprehensive Cytopathology*, 2nd ed, Bibbo M, ed, Philadelphia, PA: WB Saunders, 1997, 413-44.

Geisinger KR, Teot LA, and Richter JE, "A Comparative Cytopathologic and Histologic Study of Atypia, Dysplasia, and Adenocarcinoma in Barrett's Esophagus," *Cancer*, 1992, 69(1):8-16.

Johnston WW, "Cytopathology of the Lung: Diagnostic Applications of Sputum, Bronchial Brushings and Fine Needle Aspiration Biopsy Specimens," *Compendium on Diagnostic Cytology*, 8th ed, Wied GL, Bibbo M, Keebler CM, et al, eds, Chicago, IL: Tutorials of Cytology, 1997, 216-29.

Johnston WW and Elson CE, "Respiratory Tract," *Comprehensive Cytopathology*, 2nd ed, Bibbo M, ed, Philadelphia, PA: WB Saunders, 1997, 325-401.

Rumalla A, Baron TH, Leontovich O, et al, "Improved Diagnostic Yield of Endoscopic Biliary Brush Cytology by Digital Image Analysis," *Mayo Clin Proc*, 2001, 76(1):29-33.

Stanley MW, "False-Positive Diagnoses in Exfoliative Cytology," *Am J Clin Pathol*, 1995, 104(2):117-9.

♦ **Buccal Smear for Barr-Body Study** see Oral Cavity Cytology *on page 386*

Buccal Smear for Sex Chromatin Evaluation

Related Information
Oral Cavity Cytology *on page 386*

Synonyms Barr Bodies; Sex Chromatin

Test Includes Cell count of Barr bodies under oil immersion; fluorescent Y chromosome examination

Abstract The Barr body is the heterophilic X chromosome found adjacent to the interphase nuclear membrane.[1]

Patient Preparation Rinse mouth prior to obtaining specimens for adults. In infants, collection should be performed between feedings.

Aftercare Usually not needed but saline rinses may be used.

Specimen Scrape of buccal mucosa (right and left sides submitted separately)

Collection Scrape buccal mucosa with tongue depressor and **discard**. Then firmly scrape again with **clean** tongue depressor and spread evenly on frosted side of glass slides; fix immediately in 95% ethanol. Label frosted slide with patient's name. Label bottle.

Causes for Rejection Improper fixation, air drying

Special Instructions Provide age, phenotype, sex, and pertinent clinical information including tentative diagnosis to the laboratory.

Reference Interval For practical purposes, the presence of ≥4% cells in which clear sex chromatin bodies are found is diagnostic of XX chromosomal constitution.[2]

Use Confirm the presence or absence of sex chromatin and the presence or absence of fluorescent portion of the "Y" chromosome

Limitations Chromatin testing of newborn infants should be deferred for 1 week. The incidence of chromatin-positive cells may fall in both the mother and in a normal female infant; thus, the buccal smear of an infant female may be erroneously interpreted as chromatin negative in the first few days of life. The incidence of chromatin-positive nuclei rises slowly to reach normal ranges within 3-4 days. **This is a screening test only.** It is subject to marked technical variability in interpretation. It is also unable to detect chimeric states reliably. For complete sex chromatin evaluation, a formal karyotype is needed.

This is not a contemporary procedure.

Contraindications Mouth lesions, bleeding abnormalities

Additional Information In a phenotypic mature female, vaginal wall scrapings are suitable and possibly more accurate than buccal scrapings.

Footnotes
1. Silverman S Jr, "Oral Cavity," *Comprehensive Cytopathology*, 2nd ed, Bibbo M, ed, Philadelphia, PA: WB Saunders Co, 1997, 403-12.
2. Koss LG, ed, *Diagnostic Cytology and its Histopathologic Bases*, 4th ed, Philadelphia, PA: JB Lippincott Co, 1992, 867.

♦ **Catheterized Urine Cytology** see Urinary Tract Cytology *on page 389*

Cerebrospinal Fluid Cytology

Related Information
Bacterial Culture, Cerebrospinal Fluid *on page 569*
Beta₂-Microglobulin, Serum or Urine *on page 509*
Cell Cycle Analysis by Flow Cytometry *on page 53*
Cerebrospinal Fluid Analysis: Overview *on page 416*
Cerebrospinal Fluid Lactate Dehydrogenase *on page 142*
Cerebrospinal Fluid Protein Electrophoresis *on page 518*
Cryptococcal Antigen Titer *on page 595*
Flow Cytometry, Overview *on page 432*
Fungal Culture, Cerebrospinal Fluid *on page 611*
Immunoperoxidase Procedures *on page 60*
Immunophenotypic Analysis of Tissues by Flow Cytometry *on page 62*
Mycobacterial Culture, Cerebrospinal Fluid *on page 656*
Polymerase Chain Reaction *on page 713*
Viral Culture, Central Nervous System Symptoms *on page 692*

Synonyms CSF Cytology; Spinal Fluid Cytology

Test Includes Cytologic evaluation of cytocentrifuge (cytospin) preparations, monolayer preparations, or membrane filtration preparations. Direct smears are generally inadequate for evaluation secondary to low cellular yield. Depending on the clinical setting, immunohistochemistry, flow cytometry, and other ancillary tests can be performed on cerebrospinal fluid (CSF) specimens.

Abstract Cytologic examination of CSF fluid is generally used as a diagnostic test in patients with clinical or radiologic evidence of central nervous system abnormality. Once a diagnosis has been established, serial evaluations of CSF specimens may be used to monitor therapy.

Specimen Cerebrospinal fluid specimens should be collected in sterile, leak-proof, plastic containers and sent immediately to the Cytopathology Laboratory for processing. The second or third tube collected is usually preferred for cytologic evaluation. The volume of CSF sent to cytopathology is usually 1-3 mL. If a malignancy is suspected, at least 3 mL should be submitted if possible. Sample volumes less than 1 mL are suboptimal.

Collection A cerebrospinal fluid specimen is most commonly obtained by lumbar puncture, which involves inserting a 23-gauge spinal needle through the L1-L2 interspinous space and dura mater into the subarachnoid space. Alternatively, CSF may be collected from cysternum, ventricle, parenchymal cyst, ventricular shunt, or reservoir.

Storage Instructions If a delay in processing must occur, the CSF specimen must be promptly refrigerated. Without immediate processing, degeneration of cells in the spinal fluid begins within 20 minutes at room temperature.

Causes for Rejection Prolonged periods (more than 1 hour) at room temperature

Special Instructions It is imperative to indicate the type of CSF specimen obtained (lumbar puncture versus shunt/reservoir or other source) as well as all pertinent clinical information including age, working diagnosis, history of malignancy, prior chemotherapy, radiation or surgery, imaging findings, and tumor location.

Use Cytologic examination of the CSF is generally used in the diagnostic work-up of patients with neurologic symptoms. Cerebrospinal fluid cytology may aid in the diagnosis of neoplasm, infection, trauma, vascular disorders or demyelinating disease. Depending on the clinical impression, CSF cytology may be used in conjunction with microbiologic studies and hematologic evaluation to maximize diagnostic yield. In the appropriate clinical context, these examinations are complementary. Secondary malignancies, including lymphoma/leukemia and metastases, are much more commonly diagnosed in the CSF than primary brain tumors. It has been estimated that of positive CSF specimens from adult patients, 60% represent metastases,

30% are from lymphoma/leukemia, and 10% derive from primary brain tumors. Common sites of origin of tumors metastatic to the brain include lung, breast, stomach, kidney, bladder, prostate, ovary, and pancreas. CNS metastases are also frequently seen with melanoma and choriocarcinoma. In general, most primary brain tumors are deeply situated in the brain parenchyma and not amenable to diagnosis by exfoliative cytology. Medulloblastoma is the primary brain tumor most commonly diagnosed in the CSF. Cerebrospinal fluid cytology also may aid in the diagnosis of meningitis. In some cases, a specific infectious agent can be identified morphologically (ie, *Cryptococcus*, CMV). In other cases, the types of cells present provide clues to the infectious agent. Examination of the CSF in AIDS patients is helpful in identification of opportunistic pathogens as well as in the diagnosis of primary CNS lymphoma. Once a diagnosis of malignancy or infection has been established, serial CSF examinations may be used to monitor response to therapy.

Limitations Only processes that exfoliate cells and involve the leptomeninges or are located adjacent to the ventricles can be diagnosed with cerebrospinal fluid cytology. Thus, a negative CSF cytology does not exclude malignancy. Repeat evaluations of CSF may be helpful to maximize diagnostic yield in cases of suspected malignancy. Certain diagnostic procedures including lumbar puncture and myelography as well as chemotherapy and radiation may produce striking reactive changes that may be mistaken for malignancy. A specimen is considered less than optimal for evaluation if there is a lack of accompanying clinical information.

Methodology A variety of methods are available, including filtration procedures and the cytocentrifuge. The latter is considered optimal by some authorities.[1,2,3] Wright, Giemsa, Diff-Quik®, and Papanicolaou staining are used.[3]

Additional Information Additional studies which may be helpful include CEA and other serum tumor markers. Similarly, immunohistochemical studies (eg, epithelial membrane antigen, PSA, AFP, and others) may be extremely useful.[1]

Tachyzoites of *Toxoplasma gondii* were identified in ventricular rather than lumbar puncture specimens in a series of two cases of 6090 CSF specimens. Each of the patients was immunocompromised.[4]

Footnotes

1. Rosenthal DL, "Cytopathology of the Central Nervous System," *Compendium on Diagnostic Cytology*, 8th ed, Wied GL, Bibbo M, Keebler CM, et al, eds, Chicago, IL: Tutorials of Cytology, 1997, 303-9.
2. Stanton C and Stanley MW, "Cytopathology of Cerebrospinal Fluid and Brain," *Atlas of Difficult Diagnoses in Cytopathology*, Chapter 8, Atkinson BF and Silverman JF, eds, Philadelphia, PA: WB Saunders Co, 1998, 259-98.
3. DeMay RM, "Cerebrospinal FLuid," *The Art and Science of Cytopathology - Exfoliative Cytology*, Chapter 11, Chicago, IL: ASCP Press, American Society of Clinical Pathologists, 1996, 427-62.
4. Brogi E and Cibas ES, "Cytologic Detection of *Toxoplasma gondii* Tachyzoites in Cerebrospinal Fluid," *Am J Clin Pathol*, 2000, 114(6):951-5.

♦ **Cervical Smear** *see* Cervical/Vaginal Cytology *on page 377*

Cervical/Vaginal Cytology

Related Information

Synonyms Cervical Smear; Gynecologic Cytology, Liquid-Based Thin-Layer or Monolayer Prep; Pap Smear; Vaginal Cytology

Applies to Herpes Smear; Human Papillomaviruses (HPV); Koilocytosis; The Bethesda System; Vira Pap®; Vira Type®; Vulvar Cytology

Test Includes Fast smear, cervical scraping smear, vaginal pool smear, lateral vaginal wall smear, direct scraping smear, cytobrush, or monolayer preparation

Abstract The spectrum of abnormality of cervical epithelium includes benign inflammatory processes (often due to bacterial, fungal, parasitic, or viral infections), low-grade squamous intraepithelial lesions (**LSIL**, mild dysplasia, **CIN 1**), high-grade squamous intraepithelial lesions (**HSIL**, moderate and severe dysplasia, **CIS, CIN 2-3**), and carcinoma. About 80% of carcinomas of the uterine cervix are squamous. Most of the remainder are adenocarcinomas and mixed adenosquamous carcinomas. Other entities which may be detected include adenocarcinoma of endometrium, sarcomas, carcinoids, endocrine carcinomas, and other rare epithelial tumors and metastatic cancers.

A notable reduction in mortality from cervical cancer followed implementation of Pap smear screening, but problems in sampling, specimen adequacy, microscopic screening, and interpretation remain. Even with strict federal guidelines, compliance requirements, and inspection by

approved agencies, false negatives can occur in the best cytopathology laboratory.

Presently, >80% of those women dying of carcinoma of the cervix have either never had a Pap smear or have not had one in the prior 5 years.[1]

Patient Preparation Patients are advised to avoid douches 48-72 hours prior to examination; however, this should not preclude taking of the smear. Provide relevant information including age, last menstrual period (LMP), and pertinent clinical history.

Specimen Cervical scrape and endocervical brush samples are recommended in all cases. The optimal sample for hormonal evaluation is a lateral vaginal wall scrape, but aspiration of posterior vaginal fornix fluid (vaginal pool) may be used. Endometrial aspirations are not advised for routine use. For lesions of the vagina or vulva, scrapings made directly from the lesion are most diagnostic.

Container Bottle filled with 95% ethanol, cardboard mailer or plastic slide holder if slides are spray-fixed. **Hair spray should never be used to fix Pap smear slides.** Appropriate vials with collection fluid are used for liquid-based preparations.

Collection Using a graphite pencil, write the patient's name on the frosted end of the glass slide. It is possible to label nonfrosted slides with a diamond point pen. Collection vials for liquid-based preparations should be labeled according to the directions. The speculum must be introduced **without** lubricant; in certain cases, running the speculum through warm saline will prove helpful prior to insertion into atrophic, stenotic, or small introitus.

Sampling:

Endocervix: Gentle scrape or brush of endocervical canal
- Scrape - Rotate narrow end of spatula in the cervical os and gently smear onto labeled glass slide and fix immediately.
- Brush - Use a synthetic fiber brush to sample endocervical cells; remove mucous plug if present, before sampling the endocervical canal. Do not rub onto the slide; rather, lightly roll brush over the slide surface.

Ectocervical scrape: With spatula thoroughly scrape the entire ectocervix with emphasis on the squamocolumnar junction (transformation zone). Spread material evenly onto labeled glass slide and fix immediately. Immediate fixation is imperative.

Lateral vaginal wall smear: Scraping from upper lateral one-third of vaginal mucosa. Used for cytohormonal evaluations.

Direct scraping smear: Direct scrape of grossly visible lesion, smeared and fixed as previously described.

Liquid-based preparations require a brush instrument for sample collection. The brush may be disconnected or cut and submerged in the collection fluid provided. The vial is then submitted to the laboratory for processing.

Special Instructions Include pertinent clinical history such as age, LMP, parity, postmenopausal status, surgery, exogenous hormones, history of carcinoma, radiation, chemotherapy, abnormal vaginal bleeding, and history of previous abnormal Pap smears.

Use Diagnose primary or metastatic neoplasms; diagnose cervical dysplasia (cervical intraepithelial neoplasia (CIN)); diagnose genital infections with herpes, *Candida* species, *Trichomonas vaginalis*, cytomegalovirus and *Actinomyces*; aid in the diagnosis of vaginal adenosis, cervicovaginal endometriosis, condyloma, human papillomavirus infection, lymphogranuloma venereum; aid in evaluation of hormonal status.

Presently, the primary concerns should be consistent availability and use of the Pap test for screening with adequate follow-up.[2]

Limitations In spite of its great success, the Pap smear (gynecologic cytology) should still be considered a screening test.[3] And the interpretation of Pap smears, even though based on well-documented criteria, is a subjective evaluation. Higher areas of disease prevalence are related to higher levels of sensitivity.[4] There are guidelines that establish the adequacy of gynecologic samples. Each report should contain a statement of adequacy.

"Satisfactory for evaluation" indicates that the specimen has all of the following:
- appropriate labeling and identifying information
- relevant clinical information
- adequate numbers of well-preserved and well-visualized squamous epithelial cells
- an adequate endocervical/transformation zone component (from those patients who have a cervix)[5]

A specimen is **"satisfactory for evaluation but limited by..."** if:
- lack of pertinent clinical patient information (age, date of last menstrual period as a minimum; additional information as appropriate)
- partially obscuring blood, inflammation, thick areas, poor fixation, air-drying artifact, contaminant, etc, that precludes interpretation of approximately 50% to 70% of the epithelial cells.
- absence of an endocervical/transformation zone component as defined above

The above implies that a diagnosis can be made, however interpretation might be compromised due to the above.[5]

A specimen is **"unsatisfactory for evaluation..."** if any of the following apply:
- lack of patient identification on the specimen and/or requisition form
- a slide that is broken and cannot be repaired

(Continued)

Cervical/Vaginal Cytology (Continued)

- scant squamous epithelial component (well preserved and well visualized squamous epithelial cells covering <10% of the slide surface)
- obscuring blood, inflammation, thick areas, poor fixation, air-drying artifact, contaminant, etc, that precludes interpretation of ~75% or more of the epithelial cells.[5]

The "unsatisfactory" designation indicates that the specimen is unreliable for detection of cervical epithelial abnormalities. A diagnosis should not be made.

About two-thirds of false negatives result from sampling error, the remaining third from detection error.[4]

Interobserver agreement in classification of AGUS lesions (atypical glandular cells of undetermined significance) remains a problem.[6] HPV DNA testing has been proposed for identification of high-risk cases for referral for colposcopy.[7]

The greatest obstacle to prevention of carcinoma of the cervix in the U.S. is failure to be tested.[8] An Agency for Health Care Policy and

Cervical/Vaginal Cytology

Bethesda System
ADEQUACY OF THE SPECIMEN
Satisfactory for evaluation
Satisfactory for evaluation but limited by...(specify reason)
Unsatisfactory for evaluation...(specify reason)
GENERAL CATEGORIZATION (optional)
Within normal limits
Benign cellular changes: see Descriptive Diagnoses.
Epithelial cell abnormality: see Descriptive Diagnoses.
DESCRIPTIVE DIAGNOSES
Benign Cellular Changes
Infection
Trichomonas vaginalis
Fungal organisms morphologically consistent with *Candida* sp
Predominance of coccobacilli consistent with shift in vaginal flora
Bacteria morphologically consistent with *Actinomyces* sp
Cellular changes associated with herpes simplex virus
Other*
Reactive Changes
Reactive cellular changes associated with:
Inflammation (includes typical repair)
Atrophy with inflammation ("atrophic vaginitis")
Radiation
Intrauterine contraceptive device (IUD)
Other
Epithelial Cell Abnormalities
Squamous Cell
Atypical squamous cells of undetermined significance (**ASCUS**): qualify†
Low grade squamous intraepithelial lesion (**LSIL**) encompassing:
HPV* mild dysplasia/**CIN 1**
High grade squamous intraepithelial lesion (**HSIL**) encompassing: moderate and severe dysplasia, **CIS/CIN 2**, and **CIN 3**
Squamous cell carcinoma (**SCC**)
Glandular Cell
Endometrial cells, cytologically benign in a postmenopausal woman
Atypical glandular cells of undetermined significance (**AGUS**): qualify†
Endocervical adenocarcinoma
Endometrial adenocarcinoma
Extrauterine adenocarcinoma
Adenocarcinoma, NOS
Other Malignant Neoplasms: Specify
Hormonal Evaluation (applies to vaginal smears only)
Hormonal pattern compatible with age and history
Hormonal pattern incompatible with age and history: specify
Hormonal evaluation not possible due to: specify

*Cellular changes of human papillomavirus (**HPV**) — previously termed **koilocytosis, koilocytotic atypia,** and **condylomatous atypia** — are included in the category of LSIL.

†Atypical squamous or glandular cells of undetermined significance should be further qualified, if possible, as to whether a reactive or premalignant/malignant process is favored.

Research Evidence Report/Technology Assessment recognized that "...a large proportion of cervical cancer occurs in women with very limited or no screening" but the assessment "...did not examine programs or policies designed to improve screening compliance."[4]

Pap smears are presently underused.[2]

Contraindications Air drying of smears prior to fixation must not be permitted.

Additional Information The earliest identified event in the etiology of carcinogenesis of the uterine cervix is infection with types of human papillomavirus (HPV). HPV infections may lead to low grade squamous intraepithelial lesion (LSIL) (mild dysplasia) (CIN 1 on biopsy), which can be expressed as koilocytotic condylomatous atypia. Such infections are common, and ultimately tend to resolve even at the molecular level. Less commonly, these infections persist and may progress to higher grade lesions. Infrequently, biopsy of patients with smear results of LSIL reveal CIN 2 or 3. Risk factors include HPV type but other steps, factors, or cofactors exist as well,[9] including patient age.[10] Important pitfalls exist with analysis for human papillomavirus (HPV) infection in cervix and its correlation with smears and biopsies.[11] Detection of genital human papillomavirus (HPV) can be done by polymerase chain reaction,[12] Southern blot hybridization, dot blot hybridization, and Hybrid capture liquid hybridization kit. Although most of the ±440,000 global cases of cervical cancer are attributed to HPV infection, carcinoma of the cervix is uncommon when compared to lifetime cumulative incidence of HPV infection of the cervix. Cytologic diagnosis of LSIL represents only up to about 30% of HPV infection which can be detected by DNA technology.[9] See Human Papillomavirus DNA Probe Test *on page 641.*

Discrepancies occur between cervicovaginal smears and subsequent biopsies, even when done by quality laboratories. The most common cause for such discrepancy at the University of Kentucky was colposcopic biopsy sampling. Other causes included problems in cytologic interpretation, cytologic sampling, histotechnical processing, and cytologic screening.[13] Sampling problems making smears inadequate are reported in 12.3% of cases. SIL may be underestimated in 17.5% of cases. About 15% to 25% of individuals with SIL are reported to have normal cervical/vaginal cytology.[14]

The practitioner and patients should insist on case evaluation by licensed cytotechnologists and board certified pathologists and should be cautious about simply seeking the lowest price. The present Pap smear liability crisis is primarily a threat to women and the public health.[3] Analysis and interpretation of the Pap smear is a sophisticated professional consultation which should be selected with the same care utilized in selection of surgeons or other specialists.[15]

Conferences of leading cytopathologists and gynecologists, held at Bethesda in 1988 and 1991, formulated recommendations for uniform diagnostic terminology for cervical/vaginal cytology. Such recommendations eliminated reporting by classes. These conferences, sponsored by the National Cancer Institute, led to a new classification, the Bethesda System (TBS). See table. TBS provides a means to support communication of cervical/vaginal cytologic diagnoses in a format which is concise, reproducible, and easily understood.[16]

Footnotes

1. Frable WJ, "Toward a Process Standard in Cytopathology," *Cancer*, 1998, 84(3):127-9.
2. Cain JM and Howett MK, "Preventing Cervical Cancer," *Science*, 2000, 288(5472):1753-4.
3. Godfrey SE, "The Pap Smear, Automated Rescreening, and Negligent Nondisclosure," *Am J Clin Pathol*, 1999, 111(1):14-7.
4. Agency for Health Care Policy and Research, Evidence Report/Technology Assessment No. 5, "Evaluation of Cervical Cytology," *AHCPR*, No. 99-E009, January, 1999.
5. Solomon D and Kurman RJ, *The Bethesda System for Reporting Cervical/Vaginal Cytologic Diagnoses*, New York, NY: Springer-Verlag, 1994, 6-8.
6. Raab SS, Geisinger KR, Silverman JF, et al, "Interobserver Variability of a Papanicolaou Smear. Diagnosis of Atypical Glandular Cells of Undetermined Significance," *Am J Clin Pathol*, 1998, 110(5):653-9.
7. Manos MM, Kinney WK, Hurley LB, et al, "Identifying Women With Cervical Neoplasia. Using Human Papillomavirus DNA Testing for Equivocal Papanicolaou Results," *JAMA*, 1999, 281(17):1605-10.
8. Garber AM, "Making the Most of Pap Testing," *JAMA*, 1998, 279(3):240-1.
9. Schiffman MH and Brinton LA, "The Epidemiology of Cervical Carcinogenesis," *Cancer*, 1995, 76(10 Suppl):1888-901.
10. Cox JT, "Evaluating the Role of HPV Testing for Women With Equivocal Papanicolaou Test Findings," *JAMA*, 1999, 281(17):1645-6.
11. Herrington CS, Evans MF, Gray W, et al, "Morphological Correlation of Human Papillomavirus Infection of Matched Cervical Smears and Biopsies From Patients With Persistent Mild Cervical Cytological Abnormalities," *Hum Pathol*, 1995, 26(9):951-5.
12. Mayelo V, Garaud P, Renjard L, et al, "Cell Abnormalities Associated With Human Papillomavirus-Induced Squamous Intraepithelial Cervical Lesions. Multivariate Data Analysis," *Am J Clin Pathol*, 1994, 101(1):13-8.
13. Tritz DM, Weeks JA, Spires SE, et al, "Etiologies for Noncorrelating Cervical Cytologies and Biopsies," *Am J Clin Pathol*, 1995, 103(5):594-7.
14. Cannistra SA and Niloff JM, "Cancer of the Uterine Cervix," *N Engl J Med*, 1996, 334(16):1030-8.
15. Austin RM and McLendon WW, "The Papanicolaou Smear: Medicine's Most Successful Cancer Screening Procedure Is Threatened," *JAMA*, 1997, 277(9):754-5.
16. Wildes JW, "The ABCs of TBS - A Novice's Guide to the Bethesda System," *Lab Med*, 1998, 29(9):546-52.

References

Abdul-Karim FW and Al-Kaisi N, "Gynecologic Cytopathology," *Atlas of Difficult Diagnoses in Cytopathology*, Chapter 2, Atkinson BF and Silverman JF, eds, Philadelphia, PA: WB Saunders Co, 1998, 29-112.

Betsill WL Jr and Clark AH, "Early Endocervical Glandular Neoplasia," *Acta Cytol*, 1986, 30(2):115-26.

Bibbo M, *Comprehensive Cytopathology*, 2nd ed, Philadelphia, PA: WB Saunders Co, 1997.

Bibbo M and Wied GL, "Inflammation Reaction and Microbiology of the Female Productive Tract," *Compendium on Diagnostic Cytology*, Wied GL, Bibbo M, Keebler CM, et al, eds, Chicago, IL: Tutorials of Cytology, 1992, 63-8.

Brown AD and Garber AM, "The Cost-Effectiveness of 3 Methods to Enhance the Sensitivity of Papanicolaou Testing," *JAMA*, 1999, 281(4):347-53.

Buntinx F, Knottnerus JA, Andre J, et al, "The Effect of Different Sampling Devices on the Presence of Endocervical Cells in Cervical Smears. A Systematic Literature Review," *Eur J Cancer Prev*, 1994, 3(1):23-30.

Chakrabarti S, Guijon FB, and Paraskevas M, "Brush vs Spatula for Cervical Smears. Histologic Correlation With Concurrent Biopsies," *Acta Cytol*, 1994, 38(3):315-8.

Chua KL and Hjerpe A, "Persistence of Human Papillomavirus (HPV) Infections Preceding Cervical Carcinoma," *Cancer*, 1996, 77(1):121-7.

Crum CP, "Papillomavirus-Related Changes and Premalignant and Malignant Squamous Lesions of the Uterine Cervix," *Tumors and Tumor-Like Lesions of the Uterine Corpus and Cervix*, Volume 19, Clement PB and Young RH, eds, New York, NY: Churchill Livingstone, 1993, 51-83.

Davey DD, Nielsen MI, Rosenstock W, et al, "Terminology and Specimen Adequacy in Cervicovaginal Cytology: The College of American Pathologists' Interlaboratory Comparison Experience," *Arch Pathol Lab Med*, 1992, 116(9):903-7.

Davila RM, "Cervicovaginal Smear, True or False?" *Am J Clin Pathol*, 1994, 101(1):1-2.

DeMay RM, "The Pap Smear," *The Art and Science of Cytopathology - Exfoliative Cytology*, Chapter 6, Chicago, IL: ASCP Press, American Society of Clinical Pathologists, 1996, 61-205.

Ellerbrock TV, Chiasson MA, Bush TJ, et al, "Incidence of Cervical Squamous Intraepithelial Lesions in HIV-Infected Women," *JAMA*, 2000, 283(8):1031-7.

Gay JD, Donaldson LD, and Goellner JR, "False-Negative Results in Cervical Cytologic Studies," *Acta Cytol*, 1985, 29(6):1043-6.

Genest DR, Stein L, Cibas E, et al, "A Binary (Bethesda) System for Classifying Cervical Cancer Precursors: Criteria, Reproducibility, and Viral Correlates," *Hum Pathol*, 1993, 24(7):730-6.

Granter SR and Lee KR, "Cytologic Findings in Minimal Deviation Adenocarcinoma (Adenoma Malignum) of the Cervix: A Report of Seven Cases," *Am J Clin Pathol*, 1996, 105(3):327-33.

Grenko RT, Abendroth CS, Frauenhoffer EE, et al, "Variance in the Interpretation of Cervical Biopsy Specimens Obtained for Atypical Squamous Cells of Undetermined Significance," *Am J Clin Pathol*, 2000, 114(5):735-40.

Ho GYF, Bierman R, Beardsley L, et al, "Natural History of Cervicovaginal Papillomavirus Infection in Young Women," *N Engl J Med*, 1998, 338(7):423-8.

Holowaty P, Miller AB, Rohan T, et al, "Natural History of Dysplasia of the Uterine Cervix," *J National Cancer Institute*, 1999, 91(3):252-8.

Ibrahim SN, Krigman HR, Coogan AC, et al, "Prospective Correlation of Cervicovaginal Cytologic and Histologic Specimens," *Am J Clin Pathol*, 1996, 106(3):319-24.

Jones BA, "Rescreening in Gynecologic Cytology, Rescreening of 3762 Previous Cases for Current High-Grade Squamous Intraepithelial Lesions and Carcinoma - A College of American Pathologists Q-Probes Study of 312 Institutions," *Arch Pathol Lab Med*, 1995, 119(12):1097-103.

Jones HW 3d, "Impact of the Bethesda System," *Cancer*, 1995, 76(10):1914-8.

Korn AP, Judson PL, and Zaloudek CJ, "Importance of Atypical Glandular Cells of Uncertain Significance in Cervical Cytologic Smears," *J Reprod Med*, 1998, 43(9):774-8.

Levine AJ, Harper J, Hilborne L, et al, "HPV DNA and the Risk of Squamous Intraepithelial Lesions of the Uterine Cervix in Young Women," *Am J Clin Pathol*, 1993, 100(1):6-11.

Luff RD, "The Bethesda System for Reporting Cervical/Vaginal Cytologic Diagnoses. Report of 1991 Bethesda Workshop," *JAMA*, 1992, 98(2):152-4.

Meyer MP, Carbonell RI, Mauser NA, et al, "Detection of Human Papillomavirus in Cervical Swab Samples by ViraPap® and in Cervical Biopsy Specimens by *In Situ* Hybridization," *Am J Clin Pathol*, 1993, 100(1):12-7.

National Cancer Institute Workshop, "The 1988 Bethesda System for Reporting Cervical/Vaginal Cytologic Diagnoses," *JAMA*, 1989, 262(7):931-4.

Nielsen ML, Davey DD, and Kline TS, "Specimen Adequacy Evaluation in Gynecologic Cytopathology: Current Laboratory Practice in the College of American Pathologists Interlaboratory Comparison Program and Tentative Guidelines for Future Practice," *Diagn Cytopathol*, 1993, 9(4):394-403.

Raab SS, Bishop NS, and Zaleski MS, "Cost Effectiveness of Rescreening Cervicovaginal Smears," *Am J Clin Pathol*, 1999, 111(5):601-9.

Raab SS, Bishop NS, and Zaleski MS, "Long-Term Outcome and Relative Risk in Women With Atypical Squamous Cells of Undetermined Significance," *Am J Clin Pathol*, 1999, 112(1):57-62.

Raab SS, Snider TE, Potts SA, et al, "Atypical Glandular Cells of Undetermined Significance: Diagnostic Accuracy and Interobserver Variability Using Select Cytologic Criteria," *Am J Clin Pathol*, 1997, 107(3):299-307.

Renshaw AA and Granter SR, "Appropriate Follow-up Interval for Biopsy Confirmation of Squamous Intraepithelial Lesions Diagnosed by Cervical Smear Cytology," *Am J Clin Pathol*, 1997, 108(3):275-9.

Renshaw AA, Friedman MM, Rahemtulla A, et al, "Accuracy and Reproducibility of Estimating the Adequacy of the Squamous Component of Cervicovaginal Smears," *Am J Clin Pathol*, 1999, 111(1):38-42.

Schumann JL, O'Connor DM, Covell JL, et al, "Pap Smear Collection Devices: Technical, Clinical, Diagnostic, and Legal Considerations Associated With Their Use," *Diagn Cytopathol*, 1992, 8(5):492-503.

Shroyer KR, Brookes CG, Markham NE, et al, "Detection of Human Papillomavirus in Anorectal Squamous Cell Carcinoma: Correlation With Basaloid Pattern of Differentiation," *Am J Clin Pathol*, 1995, 104(3):299-305.

Wied GL, Bibbo M, Keebler CM, et al, *Compendium on Diagnostic Cytology*, 8th ed, Chicago, IL: Tutorials of Cytology, 1997.

Wright TC, Denny L, Kuhn L, et al, "HPV DNA Testing of Self-Collected Vaginal Samples Compared With Cytologic Screening to Detect Cervical Cancer," *JAMA*, 2000, 283(1):81-6.

Cyst Fluid Cytology

Related Information
Body Cavity Fluid Cytology *on page 372*
Body Fluid Amylase *on page 122*
Body Fluid Chemical Analysis *on page 123*
Breast Biopsy *on page 51*
Fine Needle Aspiration, Deep Masses *on page 381*
Fine Needle Aspiration, Superficial Masses (Palpable) *on page 382*
Washing Cytology *on page 390*

Applies to Brain Cyst Fluid Cytology; Breast Cyst Fluid Cytology; Hepatic Cyst fluid Cytology; Hydrocele Fluid Cytology; Ovarian Cyst Fluid Cytology; Pancreatic Cyst Fluid Cytology; Renal Cyst Fluid Cytology; Thyroid Cyst Fluid Cytology

Test Includes Cytologic evaluation of direct smears, cytocentrifuge (cytospin) preparations and/or monolayer preparations most commonly; membrane filter preparations and cell blocks are less routinely used.

Abstract Fine needle aspiration is a safe and reliable way of diagnosing non-neoplastic cysts as well as benign and malignant cystic neoplasms. Cyst aspiration may be both diagnostic and therapeutic.

Specimen Freshly aspirated cyst fluid should be collected in a leakproof plastic container and transported to the Cytopathology Laboratory for processing. A small amount of cyst fluid may be directly smeared onto a glass slide and either air-dried for Diff-Quik™ staining or immediately fixed in alcohol for Papanicolaou staining.

Collection Cyst fluid should be obtained using the techniques described for fine needle aspiration of superficial or deep masses depending on location (see Fine Needle Aspiration, Deep Masses *on page 381* and Fine Needle Aspiration, Superficial Masses (Palpable) *on page 382*). The cyst should be drained as completely as possible. Importantly, any palpable residual mass present following cyst drainage should be aspirated.

Storage Instructions If a delay in processing must occur, the cyst fluid specimen should be refrigerated.

Use Fine needle aspiration cytology is useful in establishing the nature of cystic lesions. The majority of cysts are non-neoplastic and aspiration may be therapeutic as well as diagnostic. However, cystic neoplasms and malignancies with a cystic component do occur and represent a common source of false-negative cytologic diagnoses. It cannot be overemphasized that any residual mass following cyst drainage must be reaspirated to ensure that the lesion has been adequately sampled. Most benign cysts yield clear or light yellow fluid and contain few cells, which are predominantly histiocytes. Malignant cystic lesions are more likely than benign cysts to be bloody, but a bloody aspirate is not in itself indicative of malignancy. Malignant cyst aspirates are in, in general, highly cellular. A variety of cystic neoplasms yield mucoid fluid.

Aspirates of hydatid hepatic cysts contain scoleces. Hooklets remain in old cysts. The two major types of hepatic abscess are pyogenic and amebic, entities which can be diagnosed by cytologic means.[1]

Limitations False-negative diagnoses may occur due to failure to sample malignant cells, even with appropriate aspiration technique. Always keeping in mind the possibility of a neoplastic cyst improves diagnostic accuracy.

Fluids may contain degenerated material. Distinction of histiocytes from epithelial cells can be difficult by light microscopy. Sometimes, in such circumstances, electron microscopy may prove useful.[2]

Methodology See Fine Needle Aspiration, Deep Masses *on page 381*.

Footnotes
1. Tao LC, "Liver and Pancreas," *Comprehensive Cytopathology*, 2nd ed, Chapter 32, Bibbo M, ed, Philadelphia, PA: WB Saunders Co, 1997, 827-63.
2. Frias-Hidvegi D, Gurley AM, Cajulis RS, et al, "Electron Microscopy," *Comprehensive Cytopathology*, 2nd ed, Chapter 36, Bibbo M, ed, Philadelphia, PA: WB Saunders Co, 1997, 929-50.

(Continued)

Cyst Fluid Cytology *(Continued)*

References

Bardales RH, "Fine Needle Aspiration Cytology of Papillary Neoplasms," *Clinics in Laboratory Medicine: Fine Needle Aspiration*, Volume 18, No 3, Stanley MW, ed, Philadelphia, PA: WB Saunders Co, 1998, 373-99.

Centeno BA, "Fine Needle Aspiration of the Pancreas," *Clinics in Laboratory Medicine: Fine Needle Aspiration*, Volume 18, No 3, Stanley MW, ed, Philadelphia, PA: WB Saunders Co, 1998, 401-27.

Gaetje R and Popp LW, "Is Differentiation of Benign and Malignant Cystic Adnexal Masses Possible by Evaluation of Cysts Fluids With Respect to Color, Cytology, Steroid Hormones, and Tumor Markers?" *Acta Obstet Gynecol Scand*, 1994, 73(6):502-7.

Ingram EA and Helikson MA, "Echinococcosis (Hydatid Disease) in Missouri: Diagnosis by Fine Needle Aspiration of a Lung Cyst," *Diagn Cytopathol*, 1991, 7(5):527-31.

Katz LB and Ehya H, "Aspiration Cytology of Papillary Cystic Neoplasm of the Pancreas," *Am J Clin Pathol*, 1990, 94(3):328-33.

Lewandrowski KB, Southern JF, Pins MR, et al, "Cyst Fluid Analysis in the Differential Diagnosis of Pancreatic Cysts. A Comparison of Pseudocysts, Serous Cystadenoma, Mucinous Cystic Neoplasm, and Mucinous Cystadenocarcinoma," *Ann Surg*, 1993, 217(1):41-7.

Löwhagen T, Tani EM, and Skoog L, "Salivary Glands and Rare Head and Neck Lesions," *Comprehensive Cytopathology*, 2nd ed, Chapter 27, Bibbo M, ed, Philadelphia, PA: WB Saunders Co, 1997, 649-71.

Orell SR, Sterrett GF, Walters MN, et al, *Manual and Atlas of Fine Needle Aspiration Cytology*, New York, NY: Churchill Livingstone, 1992.

Patel KR and Boon AP, "Metastatic Breast Cancer Presenting as an Ovarian Cyst: Diagnosis by Fine Needle Aspiration Cytology," *Cytopathology*, 1992, 3(3):191-5.

Pinto MM, Bernstein LH, Brogan DA, et al, "Measurement of CA 125, Carcinoembryonic Antigen, and Alpha-Fetoprotein in Ovarian Cyst Fluid: Diagnostic Adjunct to Cytology," *Diagn Cytopathol*, 1990, 6(3):160-3.

Rogers LR and Barnett G, "Percutaneous Aspiration of Brain Tumor Cysts Via the Ommaya Reservoir System," *Neurology*, 1991, 41(2 Pt 1):279-82.

Sherman ME, "Cytopathology," *Blaustein's Pathology of the Female Genital Tract*, 4th ed, Chapter 25, Kurman RJ, ed, New York, NY: Springer-Verlag, 1994, 1097-130.

Stanley MW, Horwitz CA, and Frable WJ, "Cellular Follicular Cyst of the Ovary: Fluid Cytology Mimicking Malignancy," *Diagn Cytopathol*, 1991, 7(1):48-52.

♦ **Cytology, Sputum** *see* Sputum Cytology *on page 387*

♦ **Cytomegalic Inclusion Bodies** *see* Cytomegalovirus Cytology *on page 380*

♦ **Cytomegalic Inclusion Disease Cytology** *see* Cytomegalovirus Cytology *on page 380*

Cytomegalovirus Cytology

Related Information

Bacterial Culture, Bronchoscopy/Bronchial Brush/Bronchoalveolar Lavage Specimen *on page 568*
Bronchoalveolar Lavage (BAL) *on page 375*
Brushings Cytology *on page 376*
Cytomegalovirus Antigen Detection *on page 598*
Cytomegalovirus Culture *on page 598*
Cytomegalovirus Nucleic Acid Detection *on page 599*
Cytomegalovirus Serology *on page 600*
Urinary Tract Cytology *on page 389*
Viral Culture, Urine *on page 695*

Synonyms CMV Smear; Cytomegalic Inclusion Bodies; Cytomegalic Inclusion Disease Cytology; Viral Study

Test Includes Filter or cytocentrifuge preparations for identification of nuclear and/or cytoplasmic viral inclusion bodies

Abstract Cytomegalovirus (CMV) maybe a potentially fatal infection in infants and immunocompromised patients, but it may also be present in asymptomatic adult carriers who are otherwise healthy. CMV is a member of the herpesvirus family. Infections are characterized by both intranuclear and cytoplasmic inclusions. The definitive diagnosis of CMV is seldom made solely on the basis of a cytologic specimen, due to the paucity of infected cells. However, cytology, when positive, can provide a rapid diagnosis. CMV viral inclusions may be identified in specimens obtained from the genitourinary tract, gastrointestinal tract, and respiratory tract as well as serous fluids and cerebrospinal fluid.

Specimen Bronchoalveolar lavage fluid, fresh urine, washing fluid, alcohol-fixed brushing specimen, cervical secretions

Sampling Time Several fresh specimens are indicated when urine is to be evaluated, since shedding is intermittent but cell disintegration is rapid.

Causes for Rejection Nonfixed specimen not processed within 1 hour

Special Instructions History is needed, especially relevant to immunosuppression, radiation, and/or chemotherapy.

Use Establish the presence of cytomegalovirus infection, especially in immunosuppressed patients, including those with bone marrow and other transplantation procedures and AIDS. A presumptive diagnosis of CMV can be provided in 25% to 50% of instances of symptomatic congenital infection by cytologic techniques.[1]

Limitations Viral culture is often described as the method of choice for definitive diagnosis of CMV, but cytology can provide more rapid information. Cytology is often described as less sensitive than culture for CMV, even when immunohistochemical staining is employed. Solans et al have reported biopsy to be more helpful in lung transplant recipients who are clinically symptomatic.[2] A negative cytologic examination for CMV does not exclude the possibility of this etiology, and culture results are usually needed. Separation between CMV as a cause of clinical disease versus its presence as an incidental finding in a given patient remains a source of interpretive error.[3]

Methodology Conventional cytologic methods, immunofluorescence microscopy

Additional Information Immunohistochemistry, applying monoclonal antibodies to immediate-early and early CMV nuclear antigens, is reported to provide evidence of evolution of CMV pneumonitis prior to development of cytopathic biopsy changes.[2]

More than 10 PMNs/hpf in CSF in patients with AIDS, in whom an infectious agent is not found, may signal CMV radiculopathy in spite of lack of viral cytopathic inclusions.[4]

See information about this topic in the Infectious Disease chapter.

Footnotes

1. Hodinka RL, "Human Cytomegalovirus," *Manual of Clinical Microbiology*, 7th ed, Chapter 66, Murray PR, Baron EJ, Pfaller MA, et al, eds, Washington, DC: ASM Press, American Society for Microbiology, 1999, 888-99.
2. Solans EP, Garrity ER Jr, McCabe M, et al, "Early Diagnosis of Cytomegalovirus Pneumonitis in Lung Transplant Patients," *Arch Pathol Lab Med*, 1995, 119(1):33-5.
3. Martin WJ II, "Diagnostic Bronchoalveolar Lavage in Immunosuppressed Patients With New Pulmonary Infiltrates," *Mayo Clin Proc*, 1992, 67(3):296-8.
4. Granter SR, Doolittle MH, and Renshaw AA, "Predominance of Neutrophils in the Cerebrospinal Fluid of AIDS Patients With Cytomegalovirus Radiculopathy," *Am J Clin Pathol*, 1996, 105(3):364-6.

References

Crawford SW, Bowden RA, Hackman RC, et al, "Rapid Detection of Cytomegalovirus Pulmonary Infection by Bronchoalveolar Lavage and Centrifugation Culture," *Ann Intern Med*, 1988, 108(2):180-5.

Emanuel D, Peppard J, Stover D, et al, "Rapid Immunodiagnosis of Cytomegalovirus Pneumonia by Bronchoalveolar Lavage Using Human and Murine Monoclonal Antibodies," *Ann Intern Med*, 1986, 104(4):476-81.

Gupta PK, "Microbiology, Inflammation, and Viral Infections," *Comprehensive Cytopathology*, 2nd ed, Bibbo M, ed, Philadelphia, PA: WB Saunders Co, 1997, 125-60.

Rimsza LM, Vela EE, Yvette MS, et al, "Rapid Automated Combined *In Situ* Hybridization and Immunohistochemistry for Sensitive Detection of Cytomegalovirus in Paraffin-Embedded Tissue Biopsies," *Am J Clin Pathol*, 1996, 106(4):544-8.

Rosenthal DL, "Cytologic Diagnosis of Infectious Diseases of the Lung," *Compendium on Diagnostic Cytology*, 8th ed, Wied GL, Bibbo M, Keebler CM, et al, eds, Chicago, IL: Tutorials of Cytology, 1997, 208-15.

Rotaeche JG and Costabel U, "Bronchoalveolar Lavage in Diagnostic Cytology," *Compendium on Diagnostic Cytology*, 8th ed, Wied GL, Bibbo M, Keebler CM, et al, eds, Chicago, IL: Tutorials of Cytology, 1997.

Teot LA, Ductman BS, and Geisinger KR, "Cytologic Diagnosis of Cytomegaloviral Esophagitis: A Report of Three Acquired Immunodeficiency Syndrome-Related Cases," *Acta Cytol*, 1993, 37(1):93-6.

♦ **Effusion Cytology** *see* Body Cavity Fluid Cytology *on page 372*

Endometrial Cytology

Related Information

Bacterial Culture, Genital Specimen *on page 571*
Cervical/Vaginal Cytology *on page 377*
Chromosome Analysis, Products of Conception *on page 365*

Synonyms Endo-Pap®; Gravlee Jet® Wash; Isaac's Aspirator®; Medhosa Cannula®; Mi-Mark® Procedure; Tao Brush; Vakutage®

Test Includes Smears, filter, cytocentrifuge, and cell block preparations

Abstract The frequency of endometrial carcinoma has increased during the last several decades. The Pap smear, proven so very successful as a screening test for cervical cancer, is not a reliable source for the diagnosis of endometrial neoplasia, although the diagnosis is rendered from time to time. Nonetheless, cytology can provide a means of diagnosis of endometrial cancer, if a direct and optimal sample is obtained. Widespread use of the office endometrial biopsy has diminished the need for endometrial cytology.

Specimen Endometrial scrape, wash, or aspiration

Collection Smear cellular material from collecting instrument thinly and evenly on a clean glass slide. Immediately spray or wet fix. Any remaining cellular material is deposited in a formalin bottle for cell block preparation. Slides and specimen bottle are labeled with patient's name and identification number. Aspirated fluid must be brought to the laboratory at once. Fluid specimens may be processed either by cytocentrifuge or cell block method.

Special Instructions Include all relevant clinical data on requisition including LMP, age, prior diagnoses, history of bleeding, hypertension, diabetes, parity, as well as hormone use.

Use Evaluate possible endometrial carcinoma or hyperplasia

Limitations Hypocellular specimen, poorly fixed specimen limits interpretation. Alterations and pitfalls accompany pregnancy.[1]

Contraindications Cervical or vaginal infections, cervical stenosis

Methodology Smears and cytocentrifuged specimens are examined microscopically; cell blocks and tissue fragments are processed as surgical tissue specimens for histopathologic examination. Differences between adenocarcinomas of endometrial and endocervical origin are recognized.[2,3]

Additional Information This procedure may be useful in women who are at high risk of developing endometrial carcinoma or in women on whose routine cervical Pap smear endometrial cells were identified. Evidence supporting screening for endometrial carcinoma is scanty. Moreover, patients may be screened with a well performed combined Fast smear. The presence of noncyclic endometrial cells in a routine Pap smear may be abnormal, depending upon clinical history and cellular appearance.

A series utilizing the Tao Brush has recently been reported. It has been approved by the U.S. Food and Drug Administration. Its application for detection of endometrial carcinoma and atypical hyperplasia is described.[4]

The diagnosis of extrauterine cancer in specimens from the endometrial cavity, cervical canal, or posterior vaginal fornix may include primaries from the ovary, gastrointestinal tract, fallopian tube, pancreas, urethra, breast, peritoneum, and other organs.[5]

In addition to several clinicopathologic types of adenocarcinomas primary in the endometrium, a variety of primary sarcomas of the uterus are known.[6]

Footnotes

1. DeMay RM, "Cytology of the Glandular Epithelium," *The Art and Science of Cytopathology*, Chapter 6, Chicago, IL: ASCP Press, American Society of Clinical Pathologists, 1996, 120-35.
2. Ng ABP, "Endometrial Hyperplasia and Carcinoma and Extrauterine Cancer," *Comprehensive Cytopathology*, 2nd ed, Chapter 12, Bibbo M, ed, Philadelphia, PA: WB Saunders Co, 1997, 251-77.
3. Ng ABP and Reagan JW, "Pathology and Cytopathology of Adenocarcinoma of the Uterus," *Compendium on Diagnostic Cytology*, 8th ed, Wied GL, Bibbo M, Keebler CM, et al, eds, Chicago, IL: Tutorials of Cytology, 1997, 157-72.
4. Wu HHJ, Harshbarger KE, Berner HW, et al, "Endometrial Brush Biopsy (Tao Brush): Histologic Diagnosis of 200 Cases With Complementary Cytology - an Accurate Sampling Technique for the Detection of Endometrial Abnormalities," *Am J Clin Pathol*, 2000, 114(3):412-18.
5. Ng ABP and Reagan JW, "Diagnosis of Extrauterine Cancer," *Compendium on Diagnostic Cytology*, 8th ed, Wied GL, Bibbo M, Keebler CM, et al, eds, Chicago, IL: Tutorials of Cytology, 1997, 173-5.
6. Patten SF and Patten FW, "Cytopathology of Uterine Sarcomas and Their Differential Diagnosis," *Compendium on Diagnostic Cytology*, 8th ed, Wied GL, Bibbo M, Keebler CM, et al, eds, Chicago, IL: Tutorials of Cytology, 1997, 176-9.

References

Byrne AJ, "Endocyte Endometrial Smears in the Cytodiagnosis of Endometrial Carcinoma," *Acta Cytol*, 1990, 34(3):373-81.

Koss LG, Schreiber K, Oberlander SG, et al, "Detection of Endometrial Carcinoma and Hyperplasia in Asymptomatic Women," *Obstet Gynecol*, 1984, 64(1):1-11.

Osmers RG and Kuhn W, "Endometrial Cancer Screening," *Curr Opin Obstet Gynecol*, 1994, 6(1):75-9.

Tao LC, *Cytopathology of the Endometrium*, Chicago, IL: ASCP Press, 1993.

♦ **Endo-Pap®** *see* Endometrial Cytology *on page 380*

♦ **Eosinophilic Index** *replaced by* Hormonal Evaluation, Cytologic *on page 384*

♦ **Esophageal Brushings/Washings Cytology** *see* Automation in Cytology, Preparation *on page 371*

♦ **Esophageal Cytology** *see* Automation in Cytology, Preparation *on page 371*

♦ **Esophageal Washings Cytology** *see* Washing Cytology *on page 390*

♦ **Estrogen Effect** *see* Hormonal Evaluation, Cytologic *on page 384*

♦ **Eye Smear for Cytology** *see* Ocular Cytology *on page 385*

♦ **Ferruginous Body Count** *see* Asbestos, Lung or Sputum *on page 371*

♦ **Fine Needle Aspiration Biopsy Cytology** *see* Automation in Cytology, Preparation *on page 371*

♦ **Fine Needle Aspiration Biopsy Cytology** *see* Fine Needle Aspiration, Superficial Masses (Palpable) *on page 382*

Fine Needle Aspiration, Deep Masses

Related Information

Bacterial Culture, Abscess *on page 562*
Bacterial Culture, Biopsy or Body Fluid *on page 565*
CA 15-3, Serum *on page 127*
CA 19-9, Serum *on page 128*
CA 125, Serum *on page 126*
Carcinoembryonic Antigen, Serum *on page 135*
Cyst Fluid Cytology *on page 370*
Electron Microscopy *on page 54*
Fine Needle Aspiration Culture *on page 609*
Fine Needle Aspiration, Superficial Masses (Palpable) *on page 382*
Flow Cytometry, Overview *on page 432*
Fluorescence *In Situ* Hybridization *on page 367*
Fungal Culture, Biopsy or Body Fluid *on page 610*
Image Analysis *on page 59*
Immunoperoxidase Procedures *on page 60*
Immunophenotypic Analysis of Tissues by Flow Cytometry *on page 62*
Mycobacterial Culture, Biopsy or Body Fluid *on page 655*
Polymerase Chain Reaction *on page 713*
Thyroid Stimulating Hormone, Serum *on page 282*
Transbronchial Fine Needle Aspiration *on page 388*

Synonyms CT-Guided FNA; FNA; FNAB; FNA, Deep Masses; Ultrasound Guided FNA

Applies to Abdominal Mass Aspiration; Adrenal Mass Aspiration; Bone Needle Aspiration Cytology; Brain Needle Aspiration; Liver Needle Aspiration Cytology; Lung Needle Aspiration Cytology; Lymph Node Aspiration Cytology; Mediastinal Mass Aspiration; Neck Mass Aspiration; Needle Biopsy Cytology; Pancreas Needle Aspiration Cytology; Renal Mass Aspiration; Retroperitoneal Mass Aspiration; Thyroid Needle Aspiration Cytology

Test Includes Examination of air-dried, Diff-Quik™ stained, and/or ethanol-fixed, Papanicolaou-stained direct smears, cytospin or cell block preparations. Useful adjuncts include microbiological cultures, special stains, flow cytometry, laser scanning cytometry, and immunohistochemistry.

Abstract Techniques for imaging deep organs have led to a reliable means of sampling, using fine needle aspiration biopsy. Successful cytologic diagnosis is dependent upon adequate sampling and correct slide preparation. As sample size is small, aspirated material can only be accurately interpreted when cytologic findings are placed in a clinical context.

Patient Preparation Signed informed consent from the patient is required. The patient is prepped surgically to produce a sterile field. One percent lidocaine is used for local anesthesia of skin and overlying subcutaneous tissue. Sedation and/or analgesics may be needed. The suite in which the biopsies are done should be equipped for the handling of complications, such as pneumothorax (chest tube trays, etc).

Aftercare Patient should be advised of possible discomfort, local pain, and bleeding. A postpulmonary biopsy routine chest x-ray is obtained, as are routine cuts of liver, and/or other sites; post-CT biopsy, to exclude hematoma. Occasionally, antibiotics may be required, depending upon clinical circumstances.[1]

Collection Aspiration equipment includes a 15 cm graduated 22-gauge sterile Chiba needle with stylet and attached 20 mL plastic syringe. The aspiration is usually performed by the radiologist, surgeon, or pathologist in the CT or ultrasound suite. Most important is the accurate localization of the needle tip within the mass. Scans should be performed to confirm appropriate needle placement prior to performing FNA. Smears and needle rinses are usually prepared by a cytotechnologist or cytopathologist present at the procedure. Immediate evaluation of air-dried Diff-Quik™ stained smears is possible, and rapidly determines the adequacy of the specimen, and ensures appropriate specimen triage. Material for culture may be obtained by this method.

Storage Instructions All material should be immediately brought to the Cytology Laboratory. The needle rinse, if immediate delivery to the laboratory is not possible, should be refrigerated at 4°C.

Special Instructions The cytopathologist often needs the insight of adequate clinical information.

Use With advances in radiologic imaging, a variety of deeply situated masses became accessible to fine needle aspiration. FNA may rapidly and safely obtain diagnostic material that would otherwise have to be obtained by thoracotomy or laparotomy. FNA is most often used to diagnose neoplasms and may be particularly helpful in identifying metastasis and tumor recurrence as well as in staging. Its applications include head and neck cancer, especially when carcinoma is suspected, no primary site is identified, and a neck mass is found.[2] FNA is useful in evaluation of selected thyroid nodules, in which adequate tissue is obtained in ~90% of patients. Correct diagnosis can be established by aspiration of thyroid nodules in <90%, with ~4% false negatives and ~1% false positives.[3] Differential diagnostic considerations include cystic lesions, goiter, thyroiditis, benign neoplasms, papillary/follicular carcinoma, medullary carcinoma, anaplastic carcinoma and lymphoma, as well as other entities.[4,5] Fine needle aspiration of soft tissue lesions may be challenging.[6] FNA may also assist in the diagnosis of infectious and inflammatory processes (eg, human herpesvirus 8).[7]

Limitations Sampling error, particularly with small (1 cm or less) pulmonary nodules; lesions completely surrounded by bone; or when the procedure must be terminated due to complications or patient discomfort.

Excisional biopsy of lymph nodes for lymphoma provides evaluation of lymph node architecture. Flow cytometry with cytomorphology enhances FNA diagnoses, but false-negative diagnosis remains possible: Hodgkin disease, for instance, yielded a false-negative diagnosis in a recent series.[8]

Needlestick risks for healthcare personnel include infections (eg, hepatitis and AIDS).[9]

Contraindications Severe chronic obstructive pulmonary disease is a contraindication to pulmonary aspiration, which has a 15% to 30% risk of pneumothorax; coagulopathy; adrenal or extra-adrenal mass in which the diagnosis of pheochromocytoma is being considered.

Methodology Procedures have recently been reviewed.[4,10,11,12,13,14] Immunocytochemistry is described as the backbone of the Cytopathology Section of the Laboratory of Pathology of the National Institutes of Health. Fluorescence *in situ* hybridization (FISH) lends to cytopathology. The polymerase chain reaction is utilized.[12]

Additional Information The smallest gauge needle should be used, routinely a 22-gauge needle is used. Needle tracking of malignancy has been reported in the literature but occurs only rarely. Although the majority of such cases were 18-gauge or greater needles, incidents of tracking with 22- and 23-gauge needles, especially of high-grade pancreatic carcinoma, have been reported. Other significant complications include pneumothorax, empyema, hemorrhage, nerve damage, and sudden death due to aspiration or to pheochromocytoma. Most deep-seated FNA biopsies proceed (Continued)

Fine Needle Aspiration, Deep Masses (Continued)

uneventfully. Good communication among radiologist, cytopathologist, and clinician maximizes the usefulness of this procedure.

Cell blocks may contribute to diagnosis.[15]

See Tumor Markers in the Key Word Index.

Footnotes

1. Ulich TR and Layfield LJ, "Fatal Septic Shock After Fine Needle Aspiration of a Pancreatic Pseudocyst," *Acta Cytol*, 1985, 29(5):879-81.
2. Concus AP and Singer MI, "Head and Neck Cancer," *Cecil Textbook of Medicine*, 21st ed, Chapter 518, Goldman L and Bennett JC, eds, Philadelphia, PA: WB Saunders Co, 2000, 2257-62.
3. Dillmann WH, "The Thyroid," *Cecil Textbook of Medicine*, 21st ed, Chapter 239, Goldman L and Bennett JC, eds, Philadelphia, PA: WB Saunders Co, 2000, 1231-50.
4. Gutman PD and Henry M, "Fine Needle Aspiration Cytology of the Thyroid," *Clin Lab Med*, 1998, 18(3):461-82.
5. Schlinkert RT, van Heerden JA, Goellner JR, et al, "Factors That Predict Malignant Thyroid Lesions When Fine-Needle Aspiration Is Suspicious for Follicular Neoplasm," *Mayo Clin Proc*, 1997, 72(10):913-6.
6. Abdul-Karim FW and Rader AE, "Fine Needle Aspiration of Soft Tissue Lesions," *Clin Lab Med*, 1998, 18(3):507-40.
7. Alkan S, Eltoum IA, Tabbara S, et al, "Usefulness of Molecular Detection of Human Herpesvirus 8 in the Diagnosis of Kaposi Sarcoma by Fine Needle Aspiration," *Am J Clin Pathol*, 1999, 11(1):91-6.
8. Nicol TL, Silberman M, Rosenthal DL, et al, "The Accuracy of Combined Cytopathologic and Flow Cytometric Analysis of Fine-Needle Aspirates of Lymph Nodes," *Am J Clin Pathol*, 2000, 114(1):18-28.
9. DeMay RM, "The Art and Science of Cytopathology - Aspiration Cytology," Chicago, IL: ASCP Press, American Society of Clinical Pathologists, 1996.
10. Dabbs DJ, "The Surgical Pathologist's Approach to Fine Needle Aspiration," *Clin Lab Med*, 1998, 18(3):357-72.
11. Pitman MB, "Fine Needle Aspiration Biopsy of the Liver: Principle Diagnostic Challenges," *Clin Lab Med*, 1998, 18(3):483-506.
12. Abati A, Fetsch P, and Filie A, "If Cells Could Talk: The Application of New Techniques to Cytopathology," *Clin Lab Med*, 1998, 18(3):561-83.
13. Keebler CM, "Cytopreparatory Techniques," *Comprehensive Cytopathology*, 2nd ed, Chapter 34, Bibbo M, ed, Philadelphia, PA: WB Saunders Co, 1997, 889-917.
14. Frable WJ, "Fine Needle Aspiration Biopsy Techniques," *Comprehensive Cytopathology*, 2nd ed, Chapter 25, Bibbo M, ed, Philadelphia, PA: WB Saunders Co, 1997, 623-42.
15. Nathan NA, Narayan R, Smith MM, et al, "Cell Block Cytology. Improved Preparation and its Efficacy in Diagnostic Cytology," *Am J Clin Pathol*, 2000, 114(4):599-606.

References

Austin JH and Cohen MB, "Value of Having a Cytopathologist Present During Percutaneous Fine-Needle Aspiration Biopsy of Lung: Report of 55 Cancer Patients and Meta-analysis of the Literature," *AJR Am J Roentgenol*, 1993, 160(1):175-7.

Bardales RH, "Fine Needle Aspiration Cytology of Papillary Neoplasms," *Clin Lab Med*, 1998, 18(3):373-99.

Centeno BA, "Fine Needle Aspiration Biopsy of the Pancreas," *Clin Lab Med*, 1998, 18(3):401-27.

DeMay RM, "Medicolegal Issues and Fine Needle Aspiration of the Breast: What You Can Do to Decrease Your Risk of Being Sued," *Clin Lab Med*, 1998, 18(3):599-605.

Galera-Davidson H and González-Cámpora R, "Thyroid," *Comprehensive Cytopathology*, 2nd ed, Chapter 28, Bibbo M, ed, Philadelphia, PA: WB Saunders Co, 1997, 673-701.

Katz RL, "Kidneys, Adrenals, and Retroperitoneum," *Comprehensive Cytopathology*, 2nd ed, Chapter 31, Bibbo M, ed, Philadelphia, PA: WB Saunders Co, 1997, 781-826.

Kurtycz DF, "Electronic Imaging in Cytopathology," *Clin Lab Med*, 1998, 18(3):585-98.

Löwhagen T, Tani EM, and Skoog L, "Salivary Glands and Rare Head and Neck Lesions," *Comprehensive Cytopathology*, 2nd ed, Chapter 27, Bibbo M, ed, Philadelphia, PA: WB Saunders Co, 1997, 649-71.

Nguyen GK and Akin MR, "Fine Needle Aspiration Cytology of the Kidney, Renal Pelvis, and Adrenal," *Clin Lab Med*, 1998, 18(3):429-59.

Silverman JF, "Breast," 2nd ed, Chapter 30, Bibbo M, ed, *Comprehensive Cytopathology*, Philadelphia, PA: WB Saunders Co, 1997, 731-80.

Silverman JF and Gay RM, "Fine-Needle Aspiration and Surgical Pathology of Infectious Lesions: Morphologic Features and the Role of the Clinical Microbiology Laboratory for Rapid Diagnosis," *Clin Lab Med*, 1995, 15(2):251-78.

Stanley MW and Löwenhagen T, *Fine Needle Aspiration of Palpable Masses*, Stoneham, MA: Butterworth-Heinemann, 1993.

Tao LC, "Liver and Pancreas," *Comprehensive Cytopathology*, 2nd ed, Chapter 32, Bibbo M, ed, Philadelphia, PA: WB Saunders Co, 1997, 827-63.

Wakely PE, "Fine Needle Aspiration Cytopathology of Malignant Lymphoma," *Clin Lab Med*, 1998, 18(3):541-59.

Yungbluth M, "The Laboratory Diagnosis of Pneumonia. The Role of the Community Hospital Pathologist," *Clin Lab Med*, 1995, 15(2):209-34.

♦ **Fine Needle Aspiration of Lung** see Transbronchial Fine Needle Aspiration on page 388

Fine Needle Aspiration, Superficial Masses (Palpable)

Related Information

Synonyms Fine Needle Aspiration Biopsy Cytology; FNA; FNAB; FNA, Superficial Masses (Palpable); Skinny or Thin Needle Aspiration

Applies to Breast Aspiration Cytology; Cyst Aspiration Cytology; Intraoral Needle Aspiration; Lymph Node Needle Aspiration; Neck Mass Needle Aspiration; Needle Biopsy Cytology; Prostate Needle Aspiration; Salivary Gland Needle Aspiration; Soft Tissue Mass Aspiration; Thyroid Needle Aspiration

Test Includes Examination of both air-dried Diff-Quik™ and 95% ethanol-fixed Papanicolaou stained smears, with needle rinse material submitted for cytospins or cell block preparation. Useful adjuncts include microbiological cultures, special stains for organisms, and flow and laser scanning cytometric immunophenotyping for cell surface markers (RPMI media used for needle rinse).

Abstract In the hands of an experienced operator, fine needle aspiration biopsy is a safe and reliable method of obtaining diagnostic material. It can be performed rapidly with minimal patient discomfort in an outpatient setting. As sample size is small, aspirated material can only be accurately interpreted when cytologic findings are placed in a clinical context.

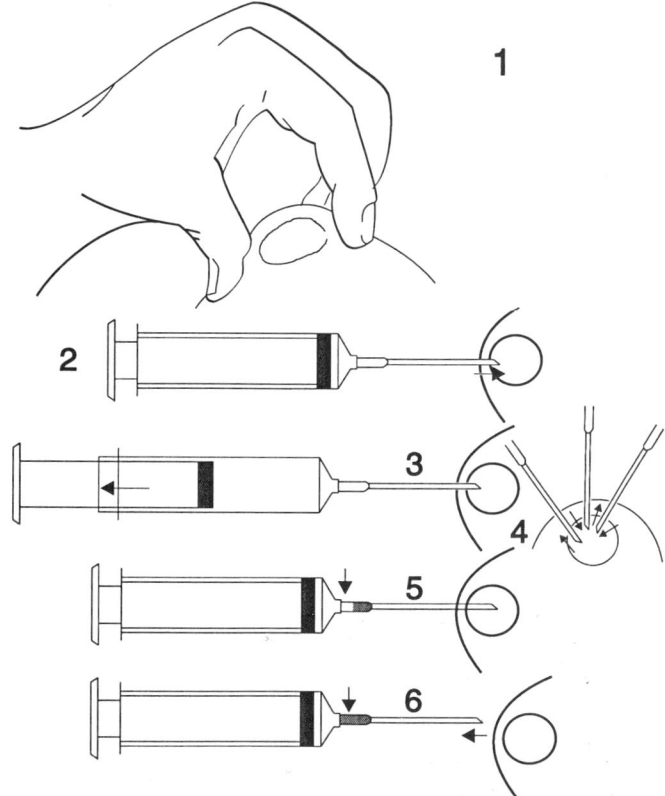

Aspiration Procedure Steps	Suction Applied
Locate, palpate, and stabilize the target lesion (Figure 1).	No
Pass the needle through the skin and into the lesion (Figure 2).	No
Apply suction by pulling back on the syringe plunger (Figure 3).	Yes
Move the tip of the needle with quick tiny movements through the mass along the same needle tract. Multiple passes are generally necessary to adequately sample the mass (Figure 4).	Yes
Release suction by releasing the plunger, **do not pull back or push forward – simply release it** (Figure 5).	No
Remove the needle from the mass (Figure 6).	No
Slides are prepared as follows:	
Detach the needle from the syringe and fill the syringe with air.	
Replace the needle onto the syringe.	
Touch the needle to a glass slide and express a drop of specimen.	
Gently spread drop using care to avoid mechanical distortion.	
Alternate slides are air-dried and alcohol-fixed.	
Rinse needle and syringe with saline or RPMI and collect for processing.	

Patient Preparation A signed informed consent should be obtained. The patient should be comfortably seated or supine in a position which maximizes exposure of and access to the area to be biopsied. The overlying skin should be cleansed with an alcohol or Betadine® wipe and allowed to dry. Local anesthesia with 1% lidocaine is used only in rare cases (eg, possible traumatic neuroma). Intraoral lesions should be sprayed with topical anesthetic spray. Assistance of an otolaryngologist is recommended for biopsies of the posterior mouth and pharynx.

Aftercare Adequate pressure is essential to prevent significant deep hematoma, especially in hyperplastic lymph nodes, thyroid gland, and salivary gland aspirates. If the patient regularly takes aspirin, longer pressure with an ice pack may be required, as in patients on anticoagulants. Mild analgesics may be needed by the patients for 24-48 hours postbiopsy if the area is painful.

Collection Aspiration equipment includes a 1" to 1.5" long 23- to 25-gauge sterile needle with a **clear hub** and an attached 20 mL syringe. The clear-hubbed needle allows the aspirated material to be seen easily. Commercially available syringe holders ("guns") are available. Extensive experience is necessary to become proficient in fine needle aspiration technique. This table outlines the steps of fine needle aspiration. See table and graphics.

As noted in Cyst Fluid Cytology, if a cystic lesion is drained, the area should be re-examined for residual mass, and if present the residual mass should be aspirated. If an infectious process is suspected, appropriate cultures should be appropriately inoculated and immediately sent to the Microbiology Laboratory.

Storage Instructions All materials should be forwarded immediately to the Cytology Laboratory. If the needle rinse cannot be immediately brought to the laboratory, it should be kept refrigerated at 4°C.

Special Instructions Fine needle aspirates are ideally interpreted by the physician who examines the patient and procures the specimen. Close communication between the clinician and cytopathologist is imperative for accurate diagnosis, especially if the cytopathologist does not perform the aspiration. Knowledge of the exact site of the aspirate, texture of the mass, as well as all pertinent clinical history (ie, age, clinical impression, history of malignancy, prior chemotherapy or radiation, radiographic findings, and so forth) is essential. The anticipated need for ancillary studies should be noted beforehand.

Use Fine needle aspiration is a biopsy procedure and should be viewed in the same context as surgical biopsy. It should not be used as a screening test. Virtually any superficially situated palpable mass may be diagnosed by FNA. FNA may be used to diagnose primary benign and malignant neoplasms and is particularly helpful in identifying metastases and tumor recurrence as well as in staging. FNA may assist in the diagnosis of infections, inflammatory processes (ie, sarcoidosis), and amyloidosis. The rapidity of the biopsy procedure allows immediate assessment of specimen adequacy and appropriate specimen triage for ancillary studies. It facilitates early diagnosis and therapeutic planning and may relieve patient anxiety. The procedure is generally convenient and well tolerated by patients. Complications when using fine needles are rare. The diagnostic utility as well as the limitations of FNA are in part site-dependent and knowledge of the uses of FNA in particular locations are important to maximize diagnostic yield. Good communication between clinician and cytopathologist maximizes the usefulness of this procedure. FNA has a high degree of accuracy when in the hands of experienced physicians and cytopathologists. Its use has been steadily increasing in the United States as a consequence of its low morbidity, rapid turnaround time, and high accuracy. FNA of the prostate gland has essentially been replaced by use of the "biopty" gun method.

Fine needle aspiration is used for culture (see Fine Needle Aspiration Culture on page 609) and for molecular detection of pathogens (eg, herpesvirus 8).[1]

Limitations Needle aspiration is subject to sampling error (1% to 10%). Intraepidermal lesions, small, mobile subcutaneous lesions, extensively necrotic lesions, and diffuse plaque-like lesions may cause most of the sampling errors. The limitations of FNA are largely site dependent. For example, aspirations of thyroid follicular lesions cannot reliably indicate if the lesion is an adenoma or carcinoma; histopathologic examination is needed. Also, when an aspiration primary diagnosis of lymphoma is made, an excisional biopsy is sometimes preferable for definitive classification of the lymphoma.

Contraindications Coagulopathy. Patients on anticoagulants may be biopsied, however, extensive and lengthy postbiopsy pressure and application of ice are advised. Such a case should be discussed with the cytopathologist beforehand.

Methodology See Fine Needle Aspiration, Deep Masses on page 381. See Tumor Markers in the Key Word Index.

Additional Information Routinely, FNA of palpable masses is a procedure causing only minor discomfort with local bruising and 24-48 hours of tenderness in the area biopsied. However, some situations **must** be considered if doing FNA, including the following. A neck mass in an elderly patient may represent a calcified atherosclerotic carotid; ultrasound prior to biopsy may be needed to exclude this possibility, as FNA may induce embolization of atheromatous plaque. Thyroid laceration with extensive bleeding may occur if the patient moves during thyroid aspiration. Pneumothorax can be induced by aspiration of a mass in the supraclavicular fossa, most frequently in a markedly cachectic patient. Infarction of a nodule due to FNA and, rarely, infection of aspiration site or nerve damage may occur.

Footnotes
1. Alkan S, Eltoum IA, Tabbara S, et al, "Usefulness of Molecular Detection of Human Herpesvirus-8 in the Diagnosis of Kaposi Sarcoma by Fine Needle Aspiration," *Am J Clin Pathol*, 1999, 111(1):91-6.

References
Abele JS and Miller TR, "Implementation of an Outpatient Needle Aspiration Biopsy Service and Clinic," *Personal Perspective Cytopathology Annual*, Baltimore, MD: Lippincott Williams & Wilkins, 1993, 113-7.
Abele JS, Miller TR, King EB, et al, "Smearing Techniques for the Concentration of Particles From Fine Needle Aspiration Biopsy," *Diagn Cytopathol*, 1985, 1(1):59-65.
DeMay RM, "The Art and Science of Cytopathology - Aspiration Cytology," Chicago, IL: ASCP Press American Society of Clinical Pathologists, 1996.
Frable WJ, "Fine Needle Aspiration Biopsy Techniques," *Comprehensive Cytopathology*, 2nd ed, Chapter 25, Bibbo M, ed, Philadelphia, PA: WB Saunders Co, 1997, 623-42.
Koss LG, Wayke S, and Olsewski W, *Aspiration Biopsy: Cytologic Interpretation and Histologic Bases*, 2nd ed, New York, NY: Igaku-Shoin, 1992.
Orell SR, Sterrett GF, Walters MN, et al, *Manual and Atlas of Fine Needle Aspiration Cytology*, New York, NY: Churchill Livingstone, 1992.
Silverman JF and Gay RM, "Fine-Needle Aspiration and Surgical Pathology of Infectious Lesions - Morphologic Features and the Role of the Clinical Microbiology Laboratory for Rapid Diagnosis," *Clin Lab Med*, 1995, 15(2):251-78.
Stanley MW and Löwhagen T, *Fine Needle Aspiration of Palpable Masses*, Boston, MA: Butterworth-Heinemann, 1993.

Herpesvirus Cytology

Related Information
Herpes Simplex Antibody on page 630
Herpes Simplex Virus Antigen Detection on page 630
Herpes Simplex Virus Culture on page 631
Herpes Simplex Virus DNA Detection on page 632
Oral Cavity Cytology on page 386
Polymerase Chain Reaction on page 713
Skin Biopsy on page 71
Varicella-Zoster Virus Serology on page 687
Viral Culture on page 689
Viral Culture, Dermatological Symptoms on page 693

Synonyms Herpetic Inclusion Bodies; HSV Cytology; Inclusion Body Cytology; Tzanck Smear

Applies to Tzanck Smears; VZV

Test Includes Preparation of cytological smears, both air-dried and Diff-Quik™ stained, as well as alcohol-fixed Papanicolaou stained, with microscopic examination for cellular features of herpesvirus infection

Abstract Herpes simplex virus (HSV) infection may be asymptomatic or lead to ulcerated painful lesions of epithelial lined surfaces. Infected epithelial cells demonstrate characteristic nuclear changes including multinucleation, molding, and chromatin margination. In the Tzanck preparation, cells obtained from herpesvirus-induced vesicles are cytologically examined. This test may lead to a rapid diagnosis, but is only positive in ~50% of
(Continued)

Herpesvirus Cytology (Continued)

cases. Cytologic examination of gastrointestinal tract and genitourinary tract specimens can be used for diagnosis, but tissue biopsy is complimentary to these studies. Herpes simplex virus can also be detected in urine and CSF fluid. Genital herpes simplex virus infection can be associated with neonatal morbidity and mortality and therefore, its diagnosis in pregnant patients is important. Life-threatening herpesvirus infections include those in neonates and encephalitis.

Specimen Scrape of lesion. If a blister is present, the smear should be taken at the edge of the lesion after the blister has been "deroofed". A direct scrape of the area under the blister will be useless, and will reveal only neutrophils.

Collection Firmly scrape the edge of the lesion, preferably a bullous lesion after removal of the bulla. The edge of normal skin and ulcer is to be scraped. In sites other than skin, a direct scrape is done. The scrape may be done with a wooden spatula or tongue blade. Use of cotton swab or Culturette® will recover fewer cells. If a nonblistering lesion is to be scraped, it may be moistened first with sterile saline before scraping. Label slides with patient's name.

Causes for Rejection Hypocellular smears or smears composed only of neutrophilic exudate

Use Establish the presence of herpesvirus infection in genitourinary and gastrointestinal tracts and other sites. The most common cause of viral esophagitis is herpes simplex virus, which causes multiple shallow ulcers.[1]

Limitations Tzanck smears cannot provide distinction between HSV-1 and HSV-2, and treatment is not the same for each. Neonatal herpes is most often due to type 2 infection. Herpes inclusions may not be seen in 50% of active lesions, however, peripheral margination of nuclear chromatin, multinucleated giant cells, and other cellular changes suggestive of herpes infection may point to the correct diagnosis. Interpretation can be difficult. **Viral culture is the definitive diagnostic method.** Polymerase chain reaction has been utilized successfully in detection of HSV and VZV DNA sequences and has been reported as equivalent or superior to viral culture. Biopsy is also useful.

Methodology Air-dried, Diff-Quik™ stained or alcohol-fixed, Pap-stained smear. Both types of smears may be submitted for immunoperoxidase stain for herpes viral antigen. Giemsa or Wright stain may also be used.

Additional Information Diagnostic yield is increased by immunoperoxidase or immunofluorescent procedures, which become positive before characteristic viral cytopathic changes develop. Smears with a heavy inflammatory exudate may be especially difficult to interpret because of nonspecific staining. Smears must be done with and without the primary antibody, and positive and negative controls must be run concurrently.

Additional information relevant to HSV is included in the Infectious Disease chapter.

Footnotes
1. Geisinger KR, "Alimentary Tract (Esophagus, Stomach, Small Intestine, Colon, Rectum, Anus, Biliary Tract)," *Comprehensive Cytopathology*, 2nd ed, Chapter 18, Bibbo M ed, Philadelphia, PA: WB Saunders Co, 1997, 413-44.

References
Arvin AM and Prober CG, "Herpes Simplex Virus," *Manual of Clinical Microbiology*, 7th ed, Murray PR, Baron EJ, Pfaller MA, et al, eds, Washington, DC: ASM Press, American Society for Microbiology, 1999, 878-87.

Atkinson BF and Silverman JF, eds, *Atlas of Difficult Diagnoses in Cytopathology*, Philadelphia, PA: WB Saunders Co, 1998.

Corey L and Handsfield HH, "Genital Herpes and Public Health. Addressing a Global Problem," *JAMA*, 2000, 283(6):791-4.

Gupta PK, "Microbiology, Inflammation, and Viral Infections," *Comprehensive Cytopathology*, 2nd ed, Chapter 9, Bibbo M, ed, Philadelphia, PA: WB Saunders Co, 1997, 125-60.

Nahass GT, Goldstein BA, Zhu WY, et al, "Comparison of Tzanck Smear, Viral Culture, and DNA Diagnostic Methods in Detection of Herpes Simplex and Varicella-Zoster Infection," *JAMA*, 1992, 268(18):2541-4.

♦ **Herpetic Inclusion Bodies** *see* Herpesvirus Cytology *on page 383*

Hormonal Evaluation, Cytologic

Related Information
Cervical/Vaginal Cytology *on page 377*
Estrogens, Urine *on page 172*
Follicle Stimulating Hormone, Serum, Plasma, or Urine *on page 175*
Luteinizing Hormone, Blood or Urine *on page 219*

Synonyms Estrogen Effect; Maturation Index

Replaces Cornification Count; Eosinophilic Index; Karyopyknotic Index

Test Includes Count of at least 100 squamous cells, with assessment of maturation as to parabasal, intermediate, or superficial, with 25% of the count performed in each quadrant of the smeared specimen. The results will be reported as a ratio or percentage of the three cell types to equal 100: P:I:S = 100. The maturation index may also be expressed as an estimated percentage (estimogram) of the overall cell pattern of the entire sample.[1]

Abstract Cytologic smear, if done properly, can provide a simple and inexpensive method for a general impression of hormonal status. Due to the responsiveness of vaginal epithelium to multihormonal substances, hormonal cytology can be useful to suggest a need for hormonal therapy, monitor the effects of hormonal therapy, suggest the estimated time of ovulation, and draw attention to cases in whom the hormonal pattern is not compatible with the patient's age or clinical history.

Patient Preparation Douches should be avoided for 24 hours prior to obtaining the smear.

Specimen The preferred specimen is a scrape of the distal third of the lateral vaginal wall.

Container Bottle filled with 95% ethanol or cardboard mailer if specimen is spray-fixed.

Collection Using a graphite pencil, write the patient's name and vaginal wall on the frosted end of the glass slide. Smear recently shed exfoliated cells from the lateral vaginal wall across the glass slide and fix immediately. 95% ethanol is a suitable fixative.[2] Include patient's age and menstrual status and any indications of hormonal therapy with the patient's history.

Use Establish hormonal status; evaluate ovarian function; institute evaluation for hormone-producing tumors which can alter estrogen effect in children and postmenopausal women[3]

Limitations The presence of infectious organisms or inflammation greatly diminishes the accuracy of the maturation index. The presence of endocervical cells or metaplastic cells in the sample suggests that the specimen was not correctly collected (ie, not from the vaginal wall). The maturation index is of limited value as an isolated procedure, and hormonal assays prove much more sensitive and indicative of hormonal function.

Methodology See published procedures.[2]

Additional Information Estrogens, androgens, and progestogens influence the appearance of vaginal epithelial cells.

Footnotes
1. Keebler K and Somrak T, *The Manual of Cytotechnology*, 7th ed, Chicago IL: ASCP Press, American Society of Clinical Pathologists, 1993, 69.
2. Wied GL and Bibbo M, "Hormonal Cytology," *Comprehensive Cytopathology*, 2nd ed, Chapter 8, Bibbo M, ed, Philadelphia, PA: WB Saunders Co, 1997, 101-24.
3. Weid GL, Bibbo M, and Keebler CM, "Evaluation of the Endocrinologic Condition of the Female Genital Tract by Exfoliative Cytology," *Compendium on Diagnostic Cytology*, 8th ed, Weid GL, Bibbo M, Keebler CM, et al, eds, Chicago, IL: Tutorials of Cytology, 1997, 55-64.

♦ **HSV Cytology** *see* Herpesvirus Cytology *on page 383*

♦ **Human Papillomaviruses (HPV)** *see* Cervical/Vaginal Cytology *on page 377*

♦ **Hydrocele Fluid Cytology** *see* Cyst Fluid Cytology *on page 379*

♦ **Inclusion Body Cytology** *see* Herpesvirus Cytology *on page 383*

♦ **Inclusion Conjunctivitis** *see* Ocular Cytology *on page 385*

♦ **Induced Sputum Technique** *see* Pneumocystis carinii Preparation *on page 386*

♦ **Intraoral Needle Aspiration** *see* Fine Needle Aspiration, Superficial Masses (Palpable) *on page 382*

♦ **Isaac's Aspirator®** *see* Endometrial Cytology *on page 380*

♦ **Karyopyknotic Index** *replaced by* Hormonal Evaluation, Cytologic *on page 384*

♦ **Koilocytosis** *see* Cervical/Vaginal Cytology *on page 377*

♦ **Lavage Cytology** *see* Washing Cytology *on page 390*

♦ **Liver Needle Aspiration Cytology** *see* Fine Needle Aspiration, Deep Masses *on page 381*

♦ **Lung Needle Aspiration Cytology** *see* Fine Needle Aspiration, Deep Masses *on page 381*

♦ **Lymph Node Aspiration Cytology** *see* Fine Needle Aspiration, Deep Masses *on page 381*

♦ **Lymph Node Needle Aspiration** *see* Fine Needle Aspiration, Superficial Masses (Palpable) *on page 382*

♦ **Maturation Index** *see* Hormonal Evaluation, Cytologic *on page 384*

♦ **Medhosa Cannula®** *see* Endometrial Cytology *on page 380*

♦ **Mediastinal Mass Aspiration** *see* Fine Needle Aspiration, Deep Masses *on page 381*

♦ **Mi-Mark® Procedure** *see* Endometrial Cytology *on page 380*

♦ **Monolayer Preparations** *see* Automation in Cytology, Preparation *on page 371*

♦ **Monolayer Preparations** *see* Automation in Cytology, Screening *on page 371*

♦ **Neck Mass Aspiration** *see* Fine Needle Aspiration, Deep Masses *on page 381*

♦ **Neck Mass Needle Aspiration** *see* Fine Needle Aspiration, Superficial Masses (Palpable) *on page 382*

♦ **Needle Biopsy Cytology** *see* Fine Needle Aspiration, Deep Masses *on page 381*

♦ **Needle Biopsy Cytology** *see* Fine Needle Aspiration, Superficial Masses (Palpable) *on page 382*

Nipple Discharge Cytology

Related Information
Breast Biopsy *on page 51*
Fine Needle Aspiration, Superficial Masses (Palpable) *on page 382*
Prolactin, Serum *on page 262*

Synonyms Breast Discharge Cytology

Test Includes Cytologic evaluation of direct smears

Abstract Nipple discharge cytology may be useful in evaluation of patients with abnormal nipple discharge. It is a simple and cost-effective procedure that can facilitate diagnosis of neoplastic or inflammatory lesions and may further direct therapy.

Specimen Prepared smears may be air dried for Diff-Quik™ staining or immediately fixed in 95% ethanol for Papanicolaou staining.

Collection Clean nipple and areola with warm saline then gently grip subareolar area and nipple with thumb and forefinger. Using a milking action, when liquid appears, allow a pea-sized drop to accumulate on the nipple apex. Place a glass slide upon the nipple and slide across quickly. Prepare smears and air dry or immediately fix in alcohol. See diagram.

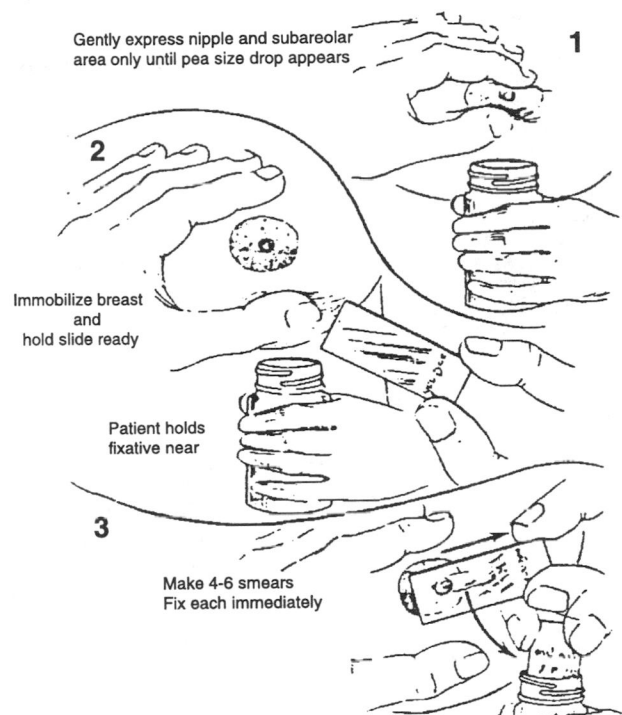

Gently express nipple and subareolar area only until pea size drop appears **1**

2

Immobilize breast and hold slide ready

Patient holds fixative near

3

Make 4-6 smears
Fix each immediately

Special Instructions Indicate type of specimen submitted and all pertinent clinical information (physical examination findings, mammographic and/or ductographic data, medications, clinical history, etc).

Use Abnormal nipple discharge is a common and significant clinical problem requiring thorough investigation. It may be either physiologic or pathologic and may occur in the absence of a palpable or mammographically detectable mass. Abnormal discharges caused by physiologic mechanisms (eg, drugs, elevated prolactin levels) are usually bilateral, arise from multiple ducts, and are milky or serous in character. Nipple discharges caused by intraductal lesions are generally unilateral, arise from a single duct, are persistent, and may be bloody. Most breast lesions associated with a nipple discharge are benign and include papillomas and fibrocystic changes most commonly. Nipple discharge cytology also occasionally picks up cases of breast carcinoma. Nipple discharges in males are more likely to be associated with malignancy than those occurring in females.

Limitations The majority of nipple discharge specimens are acellular. Thus, nipple discharge cytology lacks sensitivity and false-negative diagnoses are common. A negative result does not exclude malignancy.

Rosai considers nipple secretion aspiration cytology of very little value. He notes frequency of false positives, and observes that negative results can cause a false sense of security and delay recognition of carcinoma.[1]

Footnotes
1. Rosai J, *Ackerman's Surgical Pathology*, 8th ed, Volume 2, St Louis, MO: CV Mosby, 1996, 1592.

References
Fung A, Rayter Z, Fisher C, et al, "Preoperative Cytology and Mammography in Patients With Single-Duct Nipple Discharge Treated by Surgery," *Br J Surg*, 1990, 77(11):1211-2.
Johnson TL and Kini SR, "Cytologic and Clinicopathologic Features of Abnormal Nipple Secretions: 225 Cases," *Diagn Cytopathol*, 1991, 7(1):17-22.

Lee MM, Petrakis NL, Wrensch MR, et al, "Association of Abnormal Nipple Aspirate Cytology and Mammographic Pattern and Density," *Cancer Epidemiol Biomarkers Prev*, 1994, 3(1):33-6.
Takeda T, Matsui A, Sato Y, et al, "Nipple Discharge Cytology in Mass Screening for Breast Cancer," *Acta Cytol*, 1990, 34(2):161-4.

Ocular Cytology

Related Information
Bacterial Culture, Conjunctiva *on page 570*
Chlamydia trachomatis Direct Antigen Test *on page 590*
Herpes Simplex Virus Antigen Detection *on page 630*
Herpes Simplex Virus Culture *on page 631*
Viral Culture, Eye or Ocular Symptoms *on page 693*

Synonyms *Chlamydia* Smears Cytology; Conjunctival Smear Cytology; Corneal Cytology; Eye Smear for Cytology; Vitreous Fluid

Applies to Inclusion Conjunctivitis

Test Includes Smears fixed in 95% ethanol and stained with Papanicolaou stain; or air-dried smears stained with Giemsa or Diff-Quik™ stain

Abstract Useful for diagnosis of infections, inflammatory conditions, and primary as well as metastatic malignancies

Specimen Direct smear (scraping, washing) of ocular lesion or fine needle aspiration specimen[1,2,3]

Container Sterile, disposable leakproof container

Collection Swab lesion with cotton-tipped applicator or scrape with sterile ophthalmic spatula and smear on two clean, glass slides, **immediately** spray-fix one slide, let other air dry. Label frosted end of slide with patient's identification. FNA is performed in standard manner. (See Fine Needle Aspiration, Superficial Masses (Palpable) *on page 382*.) Aspirated fluid can be submitted to the laboratory.

Storage Instructions Keep specimen refrigerated until it can be delivered to the laboratory.

Use Diagnose trachoma-inclusion conjunctivitis and evaluate possible dysplastic or malignant conjunctival lesions; evaluation of certain intraocular and/or orbital tumors. Cytologic examination of material aspirated from the aqueous or vitreous has proven useful for large cell lymphoma, retinoblastoma, and phacolytic glaucoma.[4]

Additional Information Diagnosis of viral and chlamydial infections is considerably improved by immunofluorescent and immunoperoxidase stains for organisms. A beautifully illustrated, recent clinical review paper is recommended.[5] A study of 292 palpable orbital and eyelid tumors reported a false-positive rate for malignancy of 1.6% and a false-negative rate of 1.8%.[6] Experience with intraocular fine needle aspirations is limited, but published reports exist.[3]

Footnotes
1. Scroggs MW, Johnston WW, and Klintworth GK, "Intraocular Tumors: A Cytopathologic Study," *Acta Cytol*, 1990, 34(3):401-8.
2. Arora R, Rewari R, and Betharia SM, "Fine Needle Aspiration Cytology of Orbital and Adnexal Masses," *Acta Cytol*, 1992, 36(4):483-91.
3. O'Hara BJ, Ehya H, Shields JA, et al, "Fine Needle Aspiration Biopsy in Pediatric Ophthalmic Tumors and Pseudotumors," *Acta Cytol*, 1993, 37(2):125-30.
4. Rosai J, "Eye and Ocular Adnexa," *Ackerman's Surgical Pathology*, 8th ed, Volume 2, Chapter 30, St Louis, MO: CV Mosby, 1996, 2249-508.
5. Leibowitz HM, "The Red Eye," *N Engl J Med*, 2000, 343(5):345-51.
6. Zajdela A, Vielh P, Schlienger P, et al, "Fine Needle Cytology of 292 Palpable Orbital and Eyelid Tumors," *Am J Clin Pathol*, 1990, 93(1):100-4.

References
Arora R, Rewari R, and Betharia SM, "Fine Needle Aspiration Cytology of Eyelid Tumors," *Acta Cytol*, 1990, 34(2):227-32.
Carlier C, Coste J, Etchepare M, et al, "Conjunctival Impression Cytology With Transfer as a Field-Applicable Indicator of vitamin A Status for Mass Screening," *Int J Epidemiol*, 1992, 21(2):373-80.
Char DH and Miller T, "Orbital Pseudotumor. Fine-Needle Aspiration Biopsy and Response to Therapy," *Ophthalmology*, 1993, 100(11):1702-10.
Char DH, Kroll SM, Stoloff A, et al, "Cytomorphometry of Uveal Melanoma. Comparison of Fine Needle Aspiration Biopsy Samples With Histologic Sections," *Anal Quant Cytol Histol*, 1991, 13(4):293-9.
Connor CG, Campbell JB, Tirey WW, et al, "Modification of Impression Cytology for In-Office Use," *J Am Optom Assoc*, 1991, 62(12):898-901.
Cristallini EG, Bolis GB, and Ottaviano P, "Fine Needle Aspiration Biopsy of Orbital Meningioma - Report of a Case," *Acta Cytol*, 1990, 34(2):236-8.
de Rojas MV, Rodriguez MT, Ces Blanco JA, et al, "Impression Cytology in Patients With Keratoconjunctivitis Sicca," *Cytopathology*, 1993, 4(6):347-55.
Dewan S, Mittal S, D'Souza A, et al, "Cytological Evaluation of Conjunctival Scrape Smears in Cases of Conjunctivitis," *Indian J Pathol Microbiol*, 1992, 35(2):118-24.
Fuchs GJ, Ausayakhun S, Ruckphaopunt S, et al, "Relationship Between Vitamin A Deficiency, Malnutrition, and Conjunctival Impression Cytology," *Am J Clin Nutr*, 1994, 60(2):293-8.
Fuller DG, "Cytology in Anterior Segment Disease," *Optom Clin*, 1992, 2(1):27-40.
Gadkari SS, Adrianwala SD, Prayag AS, et al, "Conjunctival Impression Cytology - A Study of Normal Conjunctiva," *J Postgrad Med*, 1992, 38(1):21-3.
Glasgow BJ and Foos RY, *Ocular Cytopathology*, Boston, MA: Butterworth Heinemen, 1993.
Knop E and Brewitt H, "Conjunctival Cytology in Asymptomatic Wearers of Soft Contact Lenses," *Graefes Arch Clin Exp Ophthalmol*, 1992, 230(4):340-7.
Kobayashi TK, Tsubota K, Ugajin Y, et al, "Presence of Bar-Shaped Nuclear Chromatin in Cell Samples From the Conjunctiva," *Acta Cytol*, 1992, 36(2):163-6.
Paridaens AD, McCartney AC, Curling OM, et al, "Impression Cytology of Conjunctival Melanosis and Melanoma," *Br J Ophthalmol*, 1992, 76(4):198-201.

(Continued)

Ocular Cytology *(Continued)*

Resnikoff S, Luzeau R, Filliard G, et al, "Impression Cytology With Transfer in Xerophthalmia and Conjunctival Diseases," *Int Ophthalmol*, 1992, 16(6):445-51.

Rivas L, Oroza MA, Perez-Esteban A, et al, "Morphological Changes in Ocular Surface in Dry Eyes and Other Disorders by Impression Cytology," *Graefes Arch Clin Exp Ophthalmol*, 1992, 230(4):329-34.

Rivas L, Rodriguez JJ, Alvarez MI, et al, "Correlation Between Impression Cytology and Tear Function Parameters in Sjögren's Syndrome," *Acta Ophthalmol*, 1993, 71(3):353-9.

Schwartz D, Sobottka I, Leitch GJ, et al, "Pathology of Microsporidiosis: Emerging Parasitic Infections in Patients With Acquired Immunodeficiency Syndrome," *Arch Pathol Lab Med*, 1996, 120(2):173-88.

Tsubota K, Kajiwara K, Ugajin S, et al, "Conjunctival Brush Cytology," *Acta Cytol*, 1990, 34(2):233-5.

Tsubota K, Takamura E, Hasegawa T, et al, "Detection by Brush Cytology of Mast Cells and Eosinophils in Allergic and Vernal Conjunctivitis," *Cornea*, 1991, 10(6):525-31.

Tsubota K, Yamada M, Kajiwara K, et al, "Cytologic Evaluation of Conjunctival Epithelium After Cataract Surgery," *Cornea*, 1992, 11(5):418-26.

Vadrevu VL and Fullard RJ, "Enhancements to the Conjunctival Impression Cytology Technique and Examples of Applications in a Clinico-Biochemical Study of Dry Eye," *CLAO J*, 1994, 20(1):59-63.

Oral Cavity Cytology

Related Information

Buccal Smear for Sex Chromatin Evaluation *on page 376*
Herpes Simplex Virus Antigen Detection *on page 630*
Herpes Simplex Virus Culture *on page 631*
Herpesvirus Cytology *on page 383*
Skin Biopsy *on page 71*
Skin Biopsy, Immunofluorescence *on page 72*

Synonyms Buccal Smear for Barr-Body Study; Oral Direct Smear; Oral Scraping Cytology; Pemphigus Smear

Test Includes Evaluation of alcohol-fixed Papanicolaou-stained smears, or alcohol-fixed Aceto-Orcein-stained smears; smears may also be used for immunofluorescent studies screening for monosomies or trisomies.

Abstract This test is used to diagnose infectious, reactive, malignant and premalignant lesions within the oral cavity. Additional stains may assist in screening for some genetic conditions.

Patient Preparation Patient should rinse mouth vigorously several times before scrape is done.

Specimen A direct scrape of a visible lesion may be done with a tongue blade or wooden spatula. All oral lesions should be sampled cytologically since it is impractical to biopsy every visible lesion.[1]

Container Bottle filled with 95% ethanol or cardboard mailer if slide is spray-fixed

Collection Scrape visible lesions with spatula or tongue blade, fix **immediately** in alcohol or spray fix. For genetic assessments, a scraping is taken from the lateral buccal mucosa avoiding the dentate line. Each sample should be submitted to the laboratory with appropriate documentation.

Special Instructions Documentation of patient history needs to include age, physical findings, history of smoking or heavy drinking, presence of dentures, prior diagnosis of cancer or subsequent treatment, and any suspected genetic abnormalities. The periphery of a lesion should be sampled if pemphigus is suspected, or if there is central ulceration.

Use Diagnose dysplastic and malignant disease of the oral cavity, oral pemphigus, oral herpes, and *Candida* spp

Limitations An adequate diagnosis cannot be rendered on poorly fixed or hypocellular specimens. Pitfalls include the presence of a pseudomembrane, very thick saliva, lack of moisture, or excessive bleeding.[2] Overlying leukoplakia in some oral lesions make them better suited for biopsy. Buccal smears for sex chromatin evaluation have become almost obsolete; newer methodology provides more diagnostic genetic information.

Methodology A wooden spatula or a clean, cotton-tipped applicator is suggested.[2] A fairly sharp nonabsorbent instrument (eg, an amalgam spatula) is recommended for scraping leukoplakic lesions.[1]

Additional Information Diseases which occur in the mouth include a variety of hyperkeratotic/parakeratotic lesions, of which some are atypical. Carcinoma and other malignant tumors occur. Inflammatory atypias and features of regeneration and reaction are commonplace. Herpes, pemphigus vulgaris, Darier disease, and other entities occur in the oral mucosa.

Footnotes

1. DeMay R, *The Art and Science of Cytopathology - Exfoliative Cytology*, Chicago, IL: ASCP Press, American Society of Clinical Pathologists, 1996.
2. Silverman S Jr, "Oral Cavity," *Comprehensive Cytopathology*, 2nd ed, Bibbo M, ed, Philadelphia, PA: WB Saunders Co, 1997, 403-12.

References

Das DK, Gulati A, Bhatt NC, et al, "Fine Needle Aspiration Cytology of Oral and Pharyngeal Lesions - A Study of 45 Cases," *Acta Cytol*, 1993, 37(3):333-42.

Günhan O, Doğan N, Celasun B, et al, "Fine Needle Aspiration Cytology of Oral Cavity and Jaw Bone Lesions - A Report of 102 Cases," *Acta Cytol*, 1993, 37(2):135-41.

Medak H and Burlakow P, "Cytology of Pemphigus Vulgaris," *ASCP Check Sample*®, Chicago, IL: American Society of Clinical Pathologists, 1981.

♦ **Oral Direct Smear** *see* Oral Cavity Cytology *on page 386*

♦ **Oral Scraping Cytology** *see* Oral Cavity Cytology *on page 386*

♦ **Ovarian Cyst Fluid Cytology** *see* Cyst Fluid Cytology *on page 379*

♦ **Pancreas Needle Aspiration Cytology** *see* Fine Needle Aspiration, Deep Masses *on page 381*

♦ **Pancreatic Cyst Fluid Cytology** *see* Cyst Fluid Cytology *on page 379*

♦ **Pap Smear** *see* Cervical/Vaginal Cytology *on page 377*

♦ **Paracentesis Fluid Cytology** *see* Body Cavity Fluid Cytology *on page 372*

♦ **Pemphigus Smear** *see* Oral Cavity Cytology *on page 386*

♦ **Pericardial Fluid Cytology** *see* Body Cavity Fluid Cytology *on page 372*

♦ **Peritoneal Fluid Cytology** *see* Body Cavity Fluid Cytology *on page 372*

♦ **Peritoneal Washings Cytology** *see* Washing Cytology *on page 390*

♦ **Pleural Fluid Cytology** *see* Body Cavity Fluid Cytology *on page 372*

Pneumocystis carinii Preparation

Related Information

Automation in Cytology, Preparation *on page 371*
Bacterial Culture, Bronchoscopy/Bronchial Brush/Bronchoalveolar Lavage Specimen *on page 568*
Bronchoalveolar Lavage (BAL) *on page 375*
Pneumocystis Immunofluorescence *on page 671*
Polymerase Chain Reaction *on page 713*
Sputum Cytology *on page 387*
Viral Culture, Respiratory Symptoms *on page 694*

Applies to Bronchial Aspiration for *Pneumocystis*; Bronchopulmonary Lavage for *Pneumocystis*; Induced Sputum Technique; Transbronchial Aspiration Biopsy for *Pneumocystis*; Transthoracic Needle Aspiration for *Pneumocystis*

Test Includes Papanicolaou, Diff-Quik™, Giemsa, methenamine silver stains, or monoclonal antibodies to *Pneumocystis*

Abstract *Pneumocystis carinii* pneumonia is essentially an alveolar disease.[1] The cornerstone of diagnosis is bronchoalveolar lavage (BAL). Diagnosis of *P. pneumonia* in any immunocompromised subject, including individuals with AIDS, postorgan transplant patients, those with hematologic malignant diseases, inflammatory disorders, and those receiving chemotherapeutic regimens. Corticosteroids had been given to most of the patients without AIDS in the month prior to onset.[2]

Patient Preparation Additional to BAL, specimens may be obtained by induced sputum, bronchoscopic lung biopsy, or other means. These procedures have generally replaced open lung biopsy for this disease.

Induced sputum technique: A common method used consists of using a heated (37°C) solution of 15% NaCl and 20% propylene glycol, the vapors of which the patient inhales for 15-20 minutes. Subsequent to this inhalation, the patient usually will produce a large amount of satisfactory sputum. Induced sputum provides a rapid, inexpensive first-line diagnosis for individuals at high risk, especially for patients with HIV infection.[1]

Specimen Lung biopsy, transthoracic needle aspirate, bronchoalveolar lavage fluid, or induced sputum. **Routine sputum is not acceptable** for identification of *Pneumocystis*.

Container Sterile jar, clean glass slides

Collection For **bronchoalveolar lavage**, see Bronchoalveolar Lavage (BAL) *on page 375*. Stager et al used Saccomanno fixative.[3] The addition of bronchoscopic lung biopsy to BAL leads to diagnosis in a few subjects in whom *Pneumocystis* was not identified by BAL.[1] For **tissue lung biopsy**, touch preparations are made from the fresh surgical specimen by lightly touching the fresh tissue in rapid succession along the length of three to four slides. Induced sputum is sent to the laboratory fresh, and prepared in the laboratory.

Use Identify *Pneumocystis carinii* organisms, predominantly in immunocompromised patients

Limitations *Pneumocystis* preparations applied to spontaneously expectorated sputum have an extremely low yield. In about 40% of individuals with AIDS and symptomatic pneumonia caused by other agents, one may anticipate *P. carinii* in bronchoalveolar lavage fluid, unless the patient is receiving treatment for this organism prophylactically. *P. carinii* was correctly identified in 94% of adequate transbronchial biopsies, 95% of bronchoalveolar lavage cell block specimens, 88% of bronchoalveolar smears, and 79% of brushings in a series of 36 autopsy-proven cases.[4] Although a 1985 paper from the city of New York indicated that *Pneumocystis* can be reliably identified in smears of bronchial washes,[5] many presently recommend lavage cytologic procedures.[6,7,8] Martin explains that although sputum analysis remains useful for the diagnosis of *P. carinii* pneumonia in subjects who have AIDS, its utility for diagnosis of *P. carinii* in immunosuppressed patients who do not have AIDS is limited.[7] A 1988 paper recommended the induced sputum technique and provided details of methods.[9]

Methodology In the hands of an experienced cytopathologist, *P. carinii* can be identified with Pap, Giemsa, Diff-Quik™, and methenamine silver stains. Immunofluorescent (IF) staining may be optimal in terms of sensitivity and specificity, but some believe that differences between IF and silver staining are slight.[8] Diagnostic yields were significantly higher for direct immunofluorescence monoclonal antibody-stained bronchoalveolar lavage specimens than for application of Grocott methenamine-silver nitrate in bronchoscopic lung biopsies in a 1996 study.[10] See *Pneumocystis* Immunofluorescence *on page 671*. PCR detection of *P. carinii* is more sensitive than cytology or immunofluorescence.[11]

Additional Information Impaired cellular immunity is the major predisposing background for *Pneumocystis carinii* infection: AIDS, malnutrition, prematurity, immunodeficiency disease entities, and use of immunosuppressive drugs and/or corticosteroids. In subjects with AIDS, the risk of *P. carinii* correlates with the number of CD4 lymphocytes.[12]

This entity is found in patients with clinical diffuse interstitial pneumonitis. Immunocompromised patients have a high incidence of *Pneumocystis carinii* infection (as high as 44% in some series). *Pneumocystis carinii* pneumonia may be, but is not always, rapidly progressive. It may be life-threatening, so that rapid diagnosis is important to allow prompt institution of therapy. *Pneumocystis carinii* is the most frequent cause of death in children with ALL in remission, such that some institutions routinely give prophylactic trimethoprim-sulfamethoxazole to their leukemic children undergoing antineoplastic therapy. *P. carinii* is also the most common infection and most common cause of death in patients with AIDS. If a patient has been receiving prophylactic therapy for *P. carinii* and presents with pneumonitis, the cytopathologist must be notified, because if organisms are present, they will have destroyed or partially destroyed cyst walls, and examination must be extremely meticulous to identify the organisms. Under circumstances of prophylactic therapy for *Pneumocystis*, such organisms are best identified through use of an immunohistochemical or immunofluorescent method.

P. carinii occasionally causes extrapulmonary infections in patients with or without AIDS, usually in patients with advanced HIV infection.[1] It involves liver and spleen, eyes, ears, lymph nodes, thymus, skin, ascitic fluid, portions of the gastrointestinal tract, kidneys, bone marrow, pancreas, adrenals and other tissues. Some of the sites can be diagnosed by aspiration.[13]

Serum carcinoembryonic antigen has been proposed but not proven as prognostic in HIV-related *P. carinii* pneumonia.[14]

Footnotes

1. Limper AH, "Diagnosis of *Pneumocystis carinii* Pneumonia: Does Use of Only Bronchoalveolar Lavage Suffice?" *Mayo Clin Proc*, 1996, 71(11):1121-3.
2. Yale SH and Limper AH, "*Pneumocystis carinii* Pneumonia in Patients Without Acquired Immunodeficiency Syndrome: Associated Illness and Prior Corticosteroid Therapy," *Mayo Clin Proc*, 1996, 71(1):5-13.
3. Stager CE, Fraire AE, Kim HS, et al, "Modification of the Fungi-Fluor and the Genetic Systems Fluorescent Antibody Methods for Detection of *Pneumocystis carinii* in Bronchoalveolar Lavage Specimens," *Arch Pathol Lab Med*, 1995, 119(2):142-7.
4. Gal AA, Klatt EC, Koss MN, et al, "The Effectiveness of Bronchoscopy in the Diagnosis of *Pneumocystis carinii* and Cytomegalovirus Pulmonary Infections in Acquired Immunodeficiency Syndrome," *Arch Pathol Lab Med*, 1987, 111(3):238-41.
5. Rorat E, Garcia RL, and Skolom J, "Diagnosis of *Pneumocystis carinii* Pneumonia by Cytologic Examination of Bronchial Washings," *JAMA*, 1985, 254(14):1950-1.
6. DeFine LA, Saleba KP, Gibson BB, et al, "Cytologic Evaluation of Bronchoalveolar Lavage Specimens in Immunosuppressed Patients With Suspected Opportunistic Infections," *Acta Cytol*, 1987, 31(3):235-42.
7. Martin WJ 2nd, "Diagnostic Bronchoalveolar Lavage in Immunosuppressed Patients With New Pulmonary Infiltrates," *Mayo Clin Proc*, 1992, 67(3):296-8.
8. Zimmerman RL, "Testing for *Pneumocystis carinii* Pneumonia," *Lab Med*, 2000, 31(9):477-8.
9. Masur H, Gill VJ, Ognibene FP, et al, "Diagnosis of *Pneumocystis* Pneumonia by Induced Sputum Technique in Patients Without the Acquired Immunodeficiency Syndrome," *Ann Intern Med*, 1988, 109(9):755-6.
10. Fraser JL, Lilly C, Israel E, et al, "Diagnostic Yield of Bronchoalveolar Lavage and Bronchoscopic Lung Biopsy for Detection of *Pneumocystis carinii*," *Mayo Clin Proc*, 1996, 71(11):1025-9.
11. Leibovitz E, Pollack H, Moore T, et al, "Comparison of PCR and Standard Cytological Staining for Detection of *Pneumocystis carinii* From Respiratory Specimens From Patients With or at High Risk for Infection by Human Immunodeficiency Virus," *J Clin Microbiol*, 1995, 33(11):3004-7.
12. Walzer PD, "*Pneumocystis carinii* - New Clinical Spectrum?" *N Engl J Med*, 1991, 324(4):263-5.
13. "A 29-Year-Old Man With AIDS and Multiple Splenic Abscesses," Case Records of the Massachusetts General Hospital, Case 3-1995, Scully RE, Mark EJ, McNeely WF, et al, eds, *N Engl J Med*, 1995, 332(4):249-57.
14. Bedos JP, Hignette C, Lucet JC, et al, "Serum Carcinoembryonic Antigen: A Prognostic Marker in HIV-Related *Pneumocystis carinii* Pneumonia," *Scand J Infect Dis*, 1992, 24(3):309-15.

References

"A 44-Month-Old Girl With Fever of Unknown Origin After Repair of Tetralogy of Fallot," Case Records of the Massachusetts General Hospital, Case 8-1987, Scully RE, Mark EJ, McNeely WF, et al, eds, *N Engl J Med*, 1987, 316(8):466-75.
Bibbo M, *Comprehensive Cytopathology*, 2nd ed, Philadelphia, PA: WB Saunders Co, 1997.
Koss LG, *Diagnostic Cytology and its Histopathologic Bases*, 4th ed, Philadelphia, PA: JB Lippincott Co, 1992, 741-2.
Rotaeche JG and Costabel U, "Bronchoalveolar Lavage in Diagnostic Cytology," *Compendium on Diagnostic Cytology*, 8th ed, Wied GL, Bibbo M, Keebler CM, et al, eds, Chicago, IL: Tutorials of Cytology, 1997.

Sputum Cytology

Related Information

Synonyms Cytology, Sputum; Pulmonary Cytology Series

Test Includes Three to five consecutive first morning deep cough specimens

Abstract Five major techniques are available for the cytologic diagnosis of carcinoma of lung. Sputum cytology is the most fundamental, beginning with the first major series in 1919. The three bronchoscopic methods are bronchial washing, bronchial brushing, and bronchoalveolar lavage. FNA techniques are performed with imaging guidance or transbronchoscopically.[1] Cytopathological examination of sputum aids in the evaluation of respiratory infections or neoplasms. In suspected carcinoma of lung, sputum cytology as the first test is likely to be cost-effective without adverse effect on patient outcome.[2] About 172,000 U.S. patients are presently diagnosed annually with cancer of lung. It is the most common fatal malignant disease in both sexes in the U.S. Five-year survival is only ≤15%.[3]

The least invasive means to establish pathologic diagnosis, sputum cytology is up to 70% sensitive for central tumors, but provides much lower sensitivity for peripheral neoplasms.

Patient Preparation It should be explained to the patient that the contents of the collection container (fixative material) should not be consumed by the patient.

Specimen Expectorated sputum, **not saliva or nasal aspirates**

Container 50 mL screw-top plastic container; for sputum series it will contain cytologic fixative (ie, Saccomanno fixative, Carbowax®). An antibiotic to prevent bacterial overgrowth is sometimes used.

Collection Upon arising the patient rinses his mouth with water and expectorates a deep cough into the container. The **first** cough specimen is the most rewarding.

Storage Instructions Specimens not delivered during laboratory hours should be placed in a refrigerator (but not allowed to freeze) and delivered as soon as possible. If it is not possible to bring unfixed material to the laboratory, a prefixed specimen (using Carbowax® or 70% ethanol) may be substituted.

Causes for Rejection Specimen consisting of saliva or nasal secretions

Special Instructions Include admitting diagnosis and pertinent clinical history on requisition (ie, age, clinical diagnosis, exposure to carcinogens, radiographic findings, and history of radiation or chemotherapy). (Continued)

Sputum Cytology (Continued)

Use Establish the presence of neoplasm; aid in the diagnosis of respiratory infections with herpesvirus, cytomegalovirus, fungal diseases, *Strongyloides*, *Echinococcus*, and *Paragonimus*; aid in the diagnosis of lipoid pneumonitis, allergic processes, hemosiderosis, Goodpasture syndrome, asbestosis, and alveolar proteinosis.

Limitations If no carbon bearing histiocytes are identified in the specimen, it is considered to be an unsatisfactory specimen (not a deep cough specimen). A 2.1% false-positive rate (97.9% specificity) is recognized.[4] Sputum can be difficult to obtain from some patients. Other means are needed to localize the lesion. It is not optimal for peripheral neoplasms.[5]

Mechanical blending decreases sensitivity for small cell undifferentiated carcinoma by disruption, and that for adenocarcinoma by shearing mucin-containing vacuoles.[1]

Methodology Sputa may be collected fresh, without fixative; make direct smears from white flecks and blood-tinged areas; fix smears immediately in 95% ethanol. Sputa may be collected in Carbowax® if the Saccomanno technique is used.[6] Saccomanno technique involves the collection of sputum material in a mixture of 50% ethanol and 2% polyethylene glycol. If the patient cannot produce sputum spontaneously by deep coughing, it should be induced as described in *Pneumocystis carinii* Preparation *on page 386*. Sputa may be processed by the liquid-based monolayer techniques (see Automation in Cytology, Preparation *on page 371*).

Additional Information Special stains are sometimes needed. When a pulmonary lesion is suspected, a complete sputum series should be examined. The complete sputum series consists of a fresh, early morning, deep cough specimen each day for 3-5 days. A postbronchoscopy sputum should be included in the series. The complete sputum series increases the detection of primary bronchogenic carcinoma from 45% (one specimen) to 86% (three specimens). A 12- to 24-hour specimen is collected in Carbowax® in patients with scanty sputum, when a previous single sputum contains rare malignant cells, or cells highly suspicious for malignancy are present. Sputum cytology can distinguish between undifferentiated carcinoma, small cell type and other (nonsmall cell) bronchogenic carcinomas. Small cell carcinoma nuclei appear larger and more vesicular in specimens from brushings or FNA compared to those from sputum.[1] In cases in which infectious agents are identified by cytology, confirmation with culture is advised. Although some institutions report high accuracy of diagnosis of *P. carinii* with induced sputa, our laboratory has not been able to duplicate these results.

Automated image cytometry can detect a substantial proportion of squamous cell carcinoma cases.[7]

Footnotes

1. Linder J, "Lung Cancer Cytology: Something Old, Something New," *Am J Clin Pathol*, 2000, 114(2):169-71.
2. Raab SS, Hornberger J, and Raffin T, "The Importance of Sputum Cytology in the Diagnosis of Lung Cancer: A Cost-Effectiveness Analysis," *Chest*, 1997, 112(4):937-45.
3. Petty TL, "Screening Strategies for Early Detection of Lung Cancer - The Time Is Now," *JAMA*, 2000, 284(15):1977-80.
4. Tockman MS and Mulshine JL, "Sputum Screening by Quantitative Microscopy: A New Dawn for Detection of Lung Cancer?" *Mayo Clin Proc*, 1997, 72(8):788-90.
5. DeMay RM, "The Art and Science of Cytopathology - Exfoliative Cytology," *Respiratory Cytology*, Chapter 7, Chicago, IL: ASCP Press, 1996, 207-56.
6. Saccomanno G, Saunders RP, Ellis H, et al, "Concentration of Carcinoma or Atypical Cells in Sputum," *Acta Cytol*, 1963, 7:305-10.
7. Payne PW, Sebo TJ, Doudkine A, et al, "Sputum Screening by Quantitative Microscopy: A Reexamination of a Portion of the National Cancer Institute Cooperative Early Lung Cancer Study," *Mayo Clin Proc*, 1997, 72(8):697-704.

References

Blumenfeld W and Griffiss JM, "*Pneumocystis carinii* in Sputum," *Arch Pathol Lab Med*, 1988, 112(8):816-20.

Colby TV, Koss MN, and Travis WD, "Tumors of the Lower Respiratory Tract," *Atlas of Tumor Pathology*, Third Series, Fascicle 13, Washington, DC: Armed Forces Institute of Pathology, 1995.

Dao AH, "*Entamoeba gingivalis* in Sputum Smears," *Acta Cytol*, 1985, 29(4):632-3.

Fontana RS, Sanderson DR, Woolner LB, et al, "Screening for Lung Cancer. A Critique of the Mayo Lung Project," *Cancer*, 1991, 67(4 Suppl):1155-64.

Gupta RK, "Diagnosis of Unsuspected Pulmonary Cryptococcosis With Sputum Cytology," *Acta Cytol*, 1985, 29(2):154-6.

Johnston WW, "Role of Cytopathology in the Diagnosis of Opportunistic Infections of the Respiratory Tract and Other Nongynecologic Sites," *Compendium on Diagnostic Cytology*, 8th ed, Wied GL, Bibbo M, Keebler CM, et al, eds, Chicago, IL: Tutorials of Cytology, 1997, 197-207.

Midgley J, Parsons PA, Shanson DC, et al, "Monoclonal Immunofluorescence Compared With Silver Stain for Investigating *Pneumocystis carinii* Pneumonia," *J Clin Pathol*, 1991, 44(1):75-6.

Powers C, "Respiratory Cytopathology," *Atlas of Difficult Diagnoses in Cytopathology*, Chapter 3, Atkinson BF and Silverman JF, ed, Philadelphia, PA: WB Saunders Co, 1998, 113-44.

Rosenthal DL, "Cytologic Diagnosis of Infectious Diseases of the Lung," *Compendium on Diagnostic Cytology*, 8th ed, Wied GL, Bibbo M, Keebler CM, et al, eds, Chicago, IL: Tutorials of Cytology, 1997, 208-15.

Schwartz D, Sobottka I, Leitch GJ, et al, "Pathology of Microsporidiosis: Emerging Parasitic Infections in Patients With Acquired Immunodeficiency Syndrome," *Arch Pathol Lab Med*, 1996, 120(2):173-88.

◆ **Synovial Fluid Cytology** *see* Body Cavity Fluid Cytology *on page 372*

◆ **Tao Brush** *see* Endometrial Cytology *on page 380*

◆ **The Bethesda System** *see* Cervical/Vaginal Cytology *on page 377*

◆ **Thin-Layer Preparations** *see* Automation in Cytology, Preparation *on page 371*

◆ **Thin-Layer Preparations** *see* Automation in Cytology, Screening *on page 371*

◆ **Thin Prep** *see* Automation in Cytology, Preparation *on page 371*

◆ **Thin Prep** *see* Automation in Cytology, Screening *on page 371*

◆ **Thoracentesis Fluid Cytology** *see* Body Cavity Fluid Cytology *on page 372*

◆ **Thyroid Cyst Fluid Cytology** *see* Cyst Fluid Cytology *on page 379*

◆ **Thyroid Needle Aspiration** *see* Fine Needle Aspiration, Superficial Masses (Palpable) *on page 382*

◆ **Thyroid Needle Aspiration Cytology** *see* Fine Needle Aspiration, Deep Masses *on page 381*

◆ **Tracheal Aspiration Cytology** *see* Bronchial Washings Cytology *on page 374*

◆ **Tracheal Washings** *see* Bronchial Washings Cytology *on page 374*

◆ **Transbronchial Aspiration Biopsy for *Pneumocystis*** *see* Pneumocystis carinii Preparation *on page 386*

Transbronchial Fine Needle Aspiration

Related Information

Bacterial Culture, Bronchoscopy/Bronchial Brush/Bronchoalveolar Lavage Specimen *on page 568*
Bronchial Brushings Cytology *on page 373*
Bronchial Washings Cytology *on page 374*
Bronchoalveolar Lavage (BAL) *on page 375*
Fine Needle Aspiration Culture *on page 609*
Fine Needle Aspiration, Deep Masses *on page 381*

Synonyms Fine Needle Aspiration of Lung; Wang Needle Biopsy

Test Includes Cytologic evaluation of direct smears, cytocentrifuge preparations, and/or monolayer preparations and cell blocks

Abstract Transbronchial fine needle aspiration is useful in the evaluation of patients with pulmonary nodules that involve or are adjacent to major bronchi, as well as in sampling hilar and mediastinal lymph nodes in staging of bronchogenic carcinoma.

Specimen Prepared smears may be air-dried or immediately fixed in 95% ethanol. The needle should be rinsed in a balanced salt solution or formalin for processing by cytocentrifugation or cell block preparation.

Collection The specimen is obtained through a fiberoptic bronchoscope using a long flexible tube with an attached needle and following the techniques for fine needle aspiration. (See Fine Needle Aspiration, Deep Masses *on page 381* and Fine Needle Aspiration, Superficial Masses (Palpable) *on page 382*). Transbronchial FNA should be performed prior to bronchial brushings, washings, or grasp biopsy to minimize contamination by blood and tracheobronchial secretions.

Storage Instructions If a delay in processing must occur, the needle rinse material should be refrigerated.

Special Instructions Indicate the type of specimen submitted as well as all pertinent clinical information (ie, age, clinical impression, history of malignancy, prior chemotherapy or radiation, radiographic findings, etc).

Use Transbronchial fine needle aspiration is a relatively low-risk procedure used as an adjunct to bronchoscopy, in the evaluation of patients with localized pulmonary disease. Though most useful in establishing a diagnosis of lung carcinoma, this technique may also facilitate the identification of infection (eg, TB,[1] histoplasmosis) and inflammatory processes (eg, sarcoidosis). Transbronchial FNA has the greatest diagnostic yield when a submucosal mass is present or when there is extrinsic compression of the bronchi. Lesions which ulcerate the bronchial mucosa may be more accessible to direct forceps tissue biopsy or bronchial brushing. The combination of transbronchial FNA, and bronchial brushing and washing cytology has a diagnostic accuracy approaching 100% for tumors involving the large bronchi. This technique may also be used to sample mediastinal and hilar lymph nodes in the staging of bronchogenic carcinoma.

Limitations In the absence of neoplastic cells, no well-accepted criteria for specimen adequacy with this technique has been established, with the possible exception of the identification of a specific infectious process. Thus, a negative result does not exclude malignancy. False-negative results are usually secondary to sampling error. False-positive results may be due to contaminating bronchial secretions from distal airways or sampling a parenchymal tumor instead of a lymph node. Specimens consisting only of respiratory cells and mucus as well as purported lymph node samples lacking lymphocytes should be considered nondiagnostic.

Contraindications Abnormal coagulation profile, severe hypoxemia, pulmonary hypertension, intrapulmonary vascular lesions, echinococcal cysts.[2]

Methodology Published procedures include those by Johnston.[2]

Footnotes

1. Das DK, "Fine-Needle Aspiration Cytology in the Diagnosis of Tuberculous Lesions," *Lab Med*, 2000, 31(11):625-32.
2. Johnston WW, "Cytopathology of the Lung: Diagnostic Applications of Sputum, Bronchial Brushings, and Fine Needle Aspiration Biopsy Specimens," *Compendium on Diagnostic Cytology*, 8th ed, Wied GL, Bibbo M, Keebler CM, et al, eds, Chicago, IL: Tutorials of Cytology, 1997, 216-29.

References

Colby TV, Koss MN, and Travis WD, "Tumors of the Lower Respiratory Tract," *Atlas of Tumor Pathology*, Third Series, Fascicle 13, Washington, DC: Armed Forces Institute of Pathology, 1995.
Hammar SP, "Pleural Diseases," *Pulmonary Pathology Tumors*, Chapter 5, Dail DH, Hammar SP, and Colby TV, eds, New York, NY: Springer-Verlag, 1995, 405-522.
Johnston WW and Elson CE, "Respiratory Tract," *Comprehensive Cytopathology*, 2nd ed, Chapter 16, Bibbo M, ed, Philadelphia, PA: WB Saunders Co, 1997, 325-401.

♦ **Transthoracic Needle Aspiration for *Pneumocystis*** *see Pneumocystis carinii Preparation on page 386*

♦ **Tzanck Smear** *see Herpesvirus Cytology on page 383*

♦ **Tzanck Smears** *see Herpesvirus Cytology on page 383*

♦ **Ultrasound Guided FNA** *see Fine Needle Aspiration, Deep Masses on page 381*

♦ **Ureteral Washings Cytology** *see Urinary Tract Cytology on page 389*

♦ **Urinary Cytology** *see Automation in Cytology, Preparation on page 371*

Urinary Tract Cytology

Related Information

Applies to Bladder, Ureteral, and Pelvicocalyceal Barbotage Specimens; Bladder Washings Cytology; Catheterized Urine Cytology; Renal Pelvic Washings Cytology; Ureteral Washings Cytology; Voided Urine Cytology

Test Includes Smears, cytocentrifuge preparations, millipore filter preparations, flow cytometry, immunocytochemistry

Abstract Urine cytology may be useful in the evaluation of inflammatory and neoplastic conditions in the urinary system. History is important, including irradiation therapy and drug use.

Patient Preparation Hydrate patient (give several glasses of water) 30 minutes to 1 hour prior to collection. Patient should **not** have had mineral oil cathartics. Inform patient to discard first early morning voided urine. Taking 1 g vitamin C at bedtime the night before the examination can help to improve cell preservation.

Specimen Voided or catheterized urine; intraoperative washings of urinary bladder, ureters, or renal pelvis; ileal conduit urine

Container 100 mL plastic, leakproof, screw-top container; specimen should be submitted in the fresh state as soon as possible to the Cytology Laboratory. If a delay of more than 1 hour is anticipated, addition of Saccomanno or other suitable fixative (1:1 specimen to fixative) is recommended.

Sampling Time Ideally, the specimen should be as fresh as possible. Urine which has been in the bladder for prolonged periods shows extensive cellular degeneration. Specimens sitting out fresh at room temperature demonstrate cellular degeneration within 1 hour.

Collection For detection of upper urinary tract lesions: Catheterize ureters to pelvis for suspected renal or pelvic lesions. Repeat procedure using either ureter for control. For ureteral lesion, catheterize ureter to a point just below the level of the suspected lesion. Catheterize other ureter for control. Collect urine for 30 minutes. Label appropriately, right and left ureteral or right and left pelvic specimen. Hydration over 2-3 hours after initial morning voiding is recommended.[1] Bring specimen immediately to the Cytology Laboratory.

Storage Instructions If the specimen cannot be brought immediately to the Cytology Laboratory, it must be refrigerated at 4°C and fixed with a suitable fixative.

Causes for Rejection 24-hour collection, prolonged period at room temperature with extensive degeneration of cellular detail

Special Instructions First morning voided specimen is unsatisfactory, due to cellular degeneration. Bladder washings should not be collected in a hypotonic solution. Voided urine is the specimen of choice for male patients, and catheterized urine is the specimen of choice for female patients (to avoid vaginal-vulvar squamous contamination). If cytomegalovirus infection is suspected, this concern should be noted. The type of collection must be made known to the cytology service, as the cellular presentation varies with the collection method. Failure to do so, could possibly result in a false-positive diagnosis.

Use Recognition of primary benign or malignant as well as metastatic disease; routine surveillance for recurrent transitional cell carcinoma; follow-up patients receiving intravesicular therapy for transitional cell carcinoma; aid in diagnoses of infections with herpesvirus, polymovirus, cytomegalovirus, fungal diseases, and *Schistosoma*; detect malacoplakia, renal hemosiderosis, hemolytic anemia, cerebral metachromatic leukodystrophy, and endometriosis of the urinary tract

Limitations Low grade (grade 1) papillary transitional cell carcinoma cannot be diagnosed reliably by cytology alone. Polyoma virus infections may sometimes be confused with high grade transitional cell carcinoma.[2] Recent instrumentation and calculi may produce atypical changes in urothelial cells simulating malignancy. History of instrumentation of the bladder must be provided. Numerous chemotherapeutic agents including cyclophosphamide (Cytoxan®), busulfan (Myleran®), thiotepa, and BCG may produce cell changes almost indistinguishable from true dysplasia or neoplasia. For these reasons, complete clinical history is of utmost importance. Urine cytology has a very low sensitivity for detection of primary renal and prostate neoplasms. Diagnostic accuracy of urine cytology appears closely related to the grade of bladder tumors, pretreatment and post-treatment status, and minimally to the type of therapy (radiation, chemotherapy, surgery).[3]

Contraindications 24-hour urine collections are **not** recommended.[1]

Methodology Two preparatory methods to evaluate urine cytology have been compared.[4]

Additional Information Voided urine is much preferred over a catheterized sample due to atypical cell changes induced by trauma of the catheter itself. Barbotage (instilled saline insufflated with air in tiny bubbles to gently exfoliate the urothelium) cytology has the highest sensitivity for detection of transitional cell carcinoma. Although poorly-differentiated carcinomas are diagnosed with relative ease, well-differentiated (low grade) carcinomas may not be diagnosed by usual cytologic methods. DNA flow cytometry (DNA analysis) may detect the presence of an aneuploid population of cells with or without an increased S phase. It is a sensitive indicator for recurrent transitional neoplasia but is of no use in cases in which the primary transitional cell carcinoma is diploid. Maximum sensitivity is obtained using both cell morphology and DNA analysis. Renal tubular cells may be found in the urine secondary to acute tubular injury.[5] Lymphomas may rarely be diagnosed in urine cytology.[6]

Footnotes

1. Rosenthal DL and Mandell DB, "Cytologic Detection of Urothelial Lesions," *Compendium on Diagnostic Cytology*, 8th ed, Wied GL, Bibbo M, Keebler CM, et al, eds, Chicago, IL: Tutorials of Cytology, 1997, 268-75.
2. Boon ME, van Keep JP, and Kok I P, "Polyomavirus Infection Versus High-Grade Bladder Carcinoma - The Importance of Cytologic and Comparative Morphometric Studies of Plastic-Embedded Voided Urine Sediments," *Acta Cytol*, 1989, 33(6):887-93.
3. Wiener HG, Vooijs GP, Van't Hof-Grootenboer B, "Accuracy of Urinary Cytology in the Diagnosis of Primary and Recurrent Bladder Cancer," *Acta Cytol*, 1993, 37(2):163-9.
4. Dhundee J and Rigby HS, "Comparison of Two Preparatory Techniques for Urine Cytology," *J Clin Pathol*, 1990, 43(12):1034-5.
5. Racusen LC and Solez K, "Ideas in Pathology. Exfoliation of Renal Tubular Cells," *Mod Pathol*, 1991, 4(3):368-70.
6. Tanaka T, Yoshimi N, Sawada K, et al, "Ki-1-Positive Large Cell Anaplastic Lymphoma Diagnosed by Urinary Cytology - A Case Report," *Acta Cytol*, 1993, 37(4):520-4.

References

Betz SA, See WA, and Cohen MB, "Granulomatous Inflammation in Bladder Wash Specimens After Intravesical Bacillus Calmette-Guérin Therapy for Transitional Cell Carcinoma of the Bladder," *Am J Clin Pathol*, 1993, 99(3):244-8.
Crosby JH, Allsbrook WC Jr, Koss LG, et al, "Cytologic Detection of Urothelial Cancer and Other Abnormalities in a Cohort of Workers Exposed to Aromatic Amines," *Acta Cytol*, 1991, 35(3):263.
Farrow GM, "Urine Cytology of Transitional Cell Carcinoma: Diagnostic Efficacy," *Compendium on Diagnostic Cytology*, 8th ed, Wied GL, Bibbo M, Keebler CM, et al, eds, Chicago, IL: Tutorials of Cytology, 1997, 280-4.
Koss LG, "Urinary Tract Cytology," *Compendium on Diagnostic Cytology*, 8th ed, Wied GL, Bibbo M, Keebler CM, et al, eds, Chicago, IL: Tutorials of Cytology, 1997, 276-9.
Koss LG, Czerniak B, Herz F, et al, "Flow Cytometric Measurements of DNA and Other Cell Components in Human Tumors: A Critical Appraisal," *Hum Pathol*, 1989, 20(6):528-48.
Matzkin H, Moinuddin SM, and Soloway MS, "Value of Urine Cytology Versus Bladder Washing in Bladder Cancer," *Urology*, 1992, 39(3):201-3.
Murphy WM, "Current Status of Urinary Cytology in the Evaluation of Bladder Neoplasms," *Hum Pathol*, 1990, 21(9):886-96.
Murphy WM, Beckwith JB, and Farrow GM, "Tumors of the Kidney, Bladder, and Related Urinary Structures," *Atlas of Tumor Pathology*, Third Series Fascicle, Washington, DC: Armed Forces Institute of Pathology, 1993.
Radio SJ, Stratta RJ, Linder J, et al, "Histologic Confirmation of Acute Rejection Detected by Urine Cytology in Pancreas Transplant Recipients," *Transplant Proc*, 1994, 26(2):529-30.
Schwartz D, Sobottka I, Leitch GJ, et al, "Pathology of Microsporidiosis: Emerging Parasitic Infections in Patients With Acquired Immunodeficiency Syndrome," *Arch Pathol Lab Med*, 1996, 120(2):173-88.
Schwinn CP and Harris MJ, "Exfoliative Cytology of the Urinary Irrigation System," *Compendium on Diagnostic Cytology*, 8th ed, Wied GL, Bibbo M, Keebler CM, et al, eds, Chicago, IL: Tutorials of Cytology, 1997, 285-91.

♦ **Vaginal Cytology** *see Cervical/Vaginal Cytology on page 377*

♦ **Vakutage®** *see Endometrial Cytology on page 380*

- ♦ **Viral Study** *see* Cytomegalovirus Cytology *on page 380*

- ♦ **Vira Pap®** *see* Cervical/Vaginal Cytology *on page 377*

- ♦ **Vira Type®** *see* Cervical/Vaginal Cytology *on page 377*

- ♦ **Vitreous Fluid** *see* Ocular Cytology *on page 385*

- ♦ **Voided Urine Cytology** *see* Urinary Tract Cytology *on page 389*

- ♦ **Vulvar Cytology** *see* Cervical/Vaginal Cytology *on page 377*

- ♦ **VZV** *see* Herpesvirus Cytology *on page 383*

- ♦ **Wang Needle Biopsy** *see* Transbronchial Fine Needle Aspiration *on page 388*

Washing Cytology

Related Information

Asbestos, Lung or Sputum *on page 371*
Bacterial Culture, Biopsy or Body Fluid *on page 565*
Body Cavity Fluid Cytology *on page 372*
Body Fluid Amylase *on page 122*
Body Fluid Chemical Analysis *on page 123*
Body Fluid Glucose *on page 124*
Body Fluid pH *on page 125*
Fine Needle Aspiration, Deep Masses *on page 381*
Flow Cytometry, Overview *on page 432*
Fungal Culture, Biopsy or Body Fluid *on page 610*
Mycobacterial Culture, Biopsy or Body Fluid *on page 655*
Transbronchial Fine Needle Aspiration *on page 388*

Synonyms Lavage Cytology

Applies to Colon Washings Cytology; Esophageal Washings Cytology; Gastric Washings Cytology; Peritoneal Washings Cytology

Test Includes Smears, cytocentrifuge preparations, filter preparations, cell block

Abstract Used to establish the presence of inflammatory or neoplastic lesions in various body sites. Peritoneal washings provide an inexpensive, effective tool in evaluation and management of neoplastic disease. Serous cavity involvement by neoplastic processes can be undetectable by unaided visual inspection.

Patient Preparation For gastric or esophageal washings, patient must be fasting at least 12 hours prior to procedure. Soft supper the night before, water *ad lib* 1 hour before. For intubation patient should be sitting upright. Dentures, if worn, should be removed. Colon washings specimens should be collected prior to barium examination. If this is not possible, wait at least 24 hours after the barium exam before attempting a cytologic study.

Specimen Gastric washings, colon washings, esophageal washings, peritoneal washings in a fresh unfixed state

Container Plastic, screw-top container, 50 mL; may contain 50% ethanol; **packed in ice**

Collection Gastric washing: Evaluation for neoplasm: Collect resting gastric contents and discard. Then instill 300 mL of a balanced salt solution through the gastric tube. Have patient then sit, lie on back, lie on stomach, lie on right side, and lie on left side. Aspirate as much of injected saline as possible and place in container packed in ice. Label with patient name, identification number, and date. Deliver immediately on ice to the Cytology Laboratory.

Peritoneal washings: Wash peritoneal site vigorously with several hundred mL of a balanced salt solution. Retrieve as much as possible and submit as above, labeled by anatomic site (eg, "subdiaphragm", "cul-de-sac", "left gutter wash", "right gutter wash").

Storage Instructions Due to rapid degeneration of cellular material, storage, even at 4°C for any extended length of time, is not recommended.

Special Instructions Provide pertinent clinical history (eg, suspicion for neoplasm, history of peptic ulcer, endoscopic findings).

Use Establish the presence of primary or metastatic neoplasms. Washing cytology in laparotomies provides detection of occult neoplasms, recognition of tumor persistence and likelihood of recurrence as well as staging.[1] Postive cytologic examinations in peritoneal washings, especially for patients with ovarian and endometrial primaries, are apt to lead to alterations in patient management. Ducatman and Soisson have provided some thoughtful insights into the significance of such washings.[2] Washing cytology also supports recognition of reactive processes and infectious diseases and aids especially in staging of gynecologic and gastrointestinal neoplasms. Peritoneal washings are commonly done with gynecologic surgical procedures. In some cases, recognition of malignant cells in washings changes postoperative staging, greatly influencing therapy and prognosis.[1] Cytopathology may provide the only evidence of extraovarian spread of primary ovarian tumors in approximately 3% to 10% of patients.

Limitations Nondiagnostic if epithelium is not present or poorly preserved; if specimen is grossly contaminated with food or barium sulfate; if no mesothelial cells are identified in peritoneal washings, the specimen is unsatisfactory; may be of limited value in intestinal cases in which the lesion is submucosal; a Wang transmucosal needle aspirate may be helpful (see Transbronchial Fine Needle Aspiration *on page 388*). Difficulties in cytologic interpretation, including false positives, may derive from the presence of reactive mesothelial cells, endosalpingiosis, endometriosis, hemorrhage, and pelvic inflammatory disease, and from effects of chemotherapy and irradiation therapy.[1]

False negatives remain a serious problem.[3]

Contraindications Collection of specimen at a time when it cannot be immediately processed.

Additional Information Lavage is not as sensitive or specific as endoscopically directed brushings or biopsy (aspiration biopsy or tissue forceps biopsy). However, a complete set of peritoneal, pelvic, and diaphragmatic washings are an essential part of the staging of gynecologic, particularly ovarian carcinomas.

Footnotes

1. Mathew S and Erozan YS, "Significance of Peritoneal Washings in Gynecologic Oncology: The Experience With 901 Intraoperative Washings at an Academic Medical Center," *Arch Pathol Lab Med*, 1997, 121(6):604-6.

2. Ducatman BS and Soisson AP, "Peritoneal Washing Cytology. How Significant?" *Arch Pathol Lab Med*, 1997, 121(9):923-4.

3. DeMay RM, "Fluids," *The Art and Science of Cytopathology*, Chapter 8, Chicago, IL: ASCP Press, American Society of Clinical Pathologists, 1996, 257-325.

References

Bibbo M, van Hoeven KH, and Fitzpatrick BJ, "Peritoneal Washings and Ovary," *Comprehensive Cytopathology*, 2nd ed, Bibbo M, ed, Philadelphia, PA: WB Saunders Co, 1997, 315-23.

Drake M, "Esophageal and Gastric Cytology," *Compendium on Diagnostic Cytology*, 8th ed, Wied GL, Bibbo M, Keebler CM, et al, eds, Chicago, IL: Tutorials of Cytology, 1997, 248-56.

Layfield LJ, Reichman A, and Weinstein WM, "Endoscopically Directed Fine Needle Aspiration Biopsy of Gastric and Esophageal Lesions," *Acta Cytol*, 1992, 36(1):69-74.

Sherman ME, "Cytopathology," *Blaustein's Pathology of the Female Genital Tract*, 4th ed, Chapter 25, Kurman RJ, ed, New York, NY: Springer-Verlag, 1994, 1097-130.

Wang HH, Jonasson JG, and Ducatman BS, "Brushing Cytology of the Upper Gastrointestinal Tract: Obsolete or Not?" *Acta Cytol*, 1991, 35(2):195-8.

HEMATOLOGY

Wayne R. DeMott, MD

Barry S. Skikne, MD

Hematology involves the study of blood, bone marrow, and components of the reticuloendothelial system as found in a number of discreet and diffuse organs and systems including liver, spleen, gastrointestinal tract, and lymph nodes. Physiologic and biochemical processes that affect the quantity, quality, and function of the cellular components of blood (erythrocytes, leukocytes, and platelets) are an integral part of this discipline of medicine.

While hematology has deep roots in morphology, there has been significant progress in unraveling and establishing the genetic and molecular biologic bases of hematologic disorders. Understanding of the hemoglobinopathies (including the thalassemias), red cell enzyme deficiencies, and red cell membrane/structural protein abnormalities, continues to expand. Paroxysmal nocturnal hemoglobinuria (PNH), relates to the complement system through glycosyl-phosphatidyl-inositol (GPI) anchored proteins and to the gene PIG-A (for phosphatidylinositol glycan-class A) which is present on the short arm of the X chromosome (Xp 22.1). While uncommon clinically, it is a mighty well head for the understanding of molecular mechanisms of disease. Still only partially unravelled is the association of PNH with bone marrow failure syndromes (eg, myelodysplasia and aplastic anemia).[1] A new generation of analytic techniques is being applied to the analysis of molecular biologic and cell-based mechanisms of hematologic disease. These new methods complement and, in many cases, supplant the earlier generation of morphologic-based observations and concepts. Dissection of lymphocyte function and pathology at the molecular level is of particular importance to a variety of human afflictions that have abnormalities of cell structure, immunology, and/or neoplasia as their basis. Older analytic techniques such as electrophoresis of nucleic acid fragments with Southern (DNA) or Northern (RNA) hybridization, restriction fragment length polymorphism (RFLP) analyses, and cell in situ hybridization are now often pre-empted by more efficient and ever more commonly employed, fluorescence in situ hybridization (FISH),[2,3] polymerase chain reaction (PCR)[4,5] and variants, and flow cytometry[6,7] with its many variations. We are on a fast train, next stop, gene array based testing. With continuing budgetary restraints, the ratio of cost to patient benefit remains an area of serious concern.

Table of Unit Equivalency

Procedure	Conventional Unit	SI Equivalent
Red blood cell count	$10^6/\mu L$ ($10^6/mm^3$)	$10^{12}/L$
White blood cell count	$10^3/\mu L$ ($10^3/mm^3$)	$10^9/L$
Platelet count	$10^3/\mu L$ ($10^3/mm^3$)	$10^9/L$
Reticulocyte count	% (or .../mm³)	% (or ... x $10^9/L$)
Hemoglobin	g/dL	g/L
Mean cell volume	fL	fL
Mean cell hemoglobin	pg	pg
Mean cell hemoglobin concentration	g/dL	g/L
Mean cell diameter	μm	μm
Plasma hemoglobin	mg/dL	mg/L
Vitamin B_{12}, Serum	pg/mL	pmol/L
Folate, serum	ng/mL	nmol/L

Footnotes

1. Bessler M and Atkinson JP, "Paroxysmal Nocturnal Hemoglobinuria," *The Molecular Basis of Blood Diseases*, 3rd ed, Part III, Chapter 17, Stamatoyanno-poulos G, Majerus PW, Perlmutter RM, et al, eds, Philadelphia PA: WB Saunders Company, 2001, 564-77.

2. Le Beau MM and Larson RA, "Cytogenetics and Neoplasia," *Hematology: Basic Principles and Practice*, 3rd ed, Chapter 48, Hoffman R, Benz EJ, Shattil SJ, et al, eds, New York, NY: Churchill Livingstone, 2000, 848-70.

3. Mark HF, Jenkins R, and Miller WA, "Current Applications of Molecular Cytogenetic Technologies," *Ann Clin Lab Sci* 1997, 27(1):47-56.

4. Berliner N, "Use of Molecular Techniques in the Analysis of Hematologic Diseases," *Hematology: Basic Principles and Practice*, 3rd ed, Chapter 160, Hoffman R, Benz EJ, Shattil SJ, et al, eds, New York, NY: Churchill Livingstone, 2000, 2511-9.

5. Abdel-Reheim FA, Edwards E, and Arber DA, "Utility of a Rapid Polymerase Chain Reaction Panel for the Detection of Molecular Changes in B-Cell Lymphomas," *Arch Pathol Lab Med*, 1996, 120(4):357-63.

6. Paraskevas F, "Clinical Flow Cytometry," *Wintrobe's Clinical Hematology*, 10th ed, Chapter 4, Lee RG, Foerster J, Lukens, J, et al, eds, Baltimore, MD: Williams & Wilkins, 1999, 56-71.

7. McCoy JP Jr, Johnson E, Catalano E, et al, "Detection and Monitoring of a Concomitant Atypical Myeloproliferative Disorder and Chronic Lymphocytic Leukemia by Flow-Cytometric Immunophenotyping," *Arch Pathol Lab Med*, 1995, 119(1):1038-43.

HEMATOLOGY — ANEMIA FLOWCHART

The flowchart that follows is intended as an aid in diagnosis of anemia and is a supplement to this chapter to demonstrate how the entries might be placed in a logical order. The flowchart is not meant to replace a standard history and physical for diagnosis. Instead, it is intended as a teaching tool to develop patterns for test ordering in the work-up of anemia. Cost-effectiveness is made a prime concern. Initial evaluation is based on the CBC results typically produced by most modern automated blood counters. This output includes red blood cell count, MCV, and RDW (see Complete Blood Count *on page 419*and the tables in that listing). The method of Bessman has been adapted for this beginning classification. In real life, some conditions may not fit the flowchart precisely, but the majority of cases do. Much of the flowchart centers around the reticulocyte count (section C) and the reticulocyte production index (RPI). See Reticulocyte Count *on page 481* entry for more information.

It will soon become apparent that the flowchart often ends with the diagnosis of iron deficiency anemia. This should not be surprising since iron deficiency anemia is the most common cause of decreased hemoglobin, especially in the outpatient setting. Normal values for many tests will vary between laboratories. Use reference ranges (normal values) from your own laboratory when appropriate. This flowchart is not intended to cover every hematologic possibility. There may not be a direct flow from one category to another in all possible circumstances. In order to follow the pathway of testing in an individual patient, follow the alphabetical designations.

References

Bessman JD, Gilmer PR Jr, and Gardner FH, "Improved Classification of Anemias by MCV and RDW," *Am J Clin Pathol*, 1983, 80(3):322-6.
Geaghan SM, "Hematologic Values and Appearances in the Healthy Fetus, Neonate, and Child," *Clin Lab Med*, 1999, 19(1):1-37.
Goodnough LT, Skikne B, and Brugnara C, "Erythropoietin, Iron, and Erythropoiesis," *Blood*, 2000, 96(3):823-33.

Is the patient anemic?

MCV <80 RDW ≤15	MCV <80 RDW >15	≥80 MCV ≤98 RDW ≤15	≥80 MCV ≤98 RDW >15	MCV >98 RDW ≤15	MCV >98 RDW >15
A	B	C	D	E	F

Patient probably has iron deficiency anemia.

Confirm with ferritin. The value should be:
male <20 µg/L
female <12 µg/L

If ferritin is not decreased, obtain transferrin receptor level. If raised, patient probably has iron deficiency anemia.

Patient may have liver disease, hypothyroidism, or myelodysplastic disorder.

*Although helpful in a number of instances, the RDW is not sufficiently sensitive/specific to make clear decisions in these evaluations.

Note: Hb levels may be higher at elevated altitudes.

A
What is the RBC?

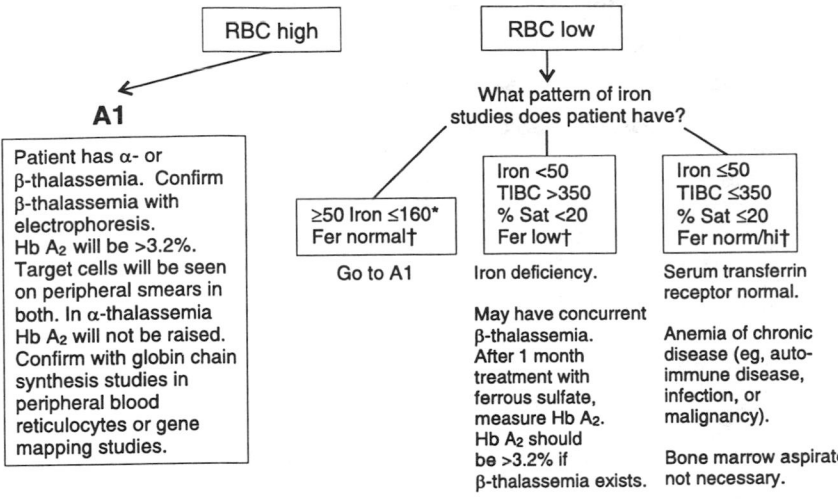

RBC high ⟶ **A1**

RBC low

A1

Patient has α- or β-thalassemia. Confirm β-thalassemia with electrophoresis. Hb A$_2$ will be >3.2%. Target cells will be seen on peripheral smears in both. In α-thalassemia Hb A$_2$ will not be raised. Confirm with globin chain synthesis studies in peripheral blood reticulocytes or gene mapping studies.

What pattern of iron studies does patient have?

≥50 Iron ≤160* Fer normal†	Iron <50 TIBC >350 % Sat <20 Fer low†	Iron ≤50 TIBC ≤350 % Sat ≤20 Fer norm/hi†
Go to A1	Iron deficiency.	Serum transferrin receptor normal.

May have concurrent β-thalassemia. After 1 month treatment with ferrous sulfate, measure Hb A$_2$. Hb A$_2$ should be >3.2% if β-thalassemia exists.

Anemia of chronic disease (eg, auto-immune disease, infection, or malignancy).

Bone marrow aspirate not necessary.

Reference range: mean ± 1 SD

RBC x 10^6/mm^3	Male	Female
15-17 y	5.0 ±0.4	4.5 ±0.3
18-64 y	5.0 ±0.4	4.4 ±0.4
65-74 y	4.8 ±0.5	4.5 ±0.4

*Adult males, values are slightly (5% to 10%) lower for adult females.
†Ferritin, reference range:
   adult male 20-250 ng/mL
   adult female
     <40 y 12-122 ng/mL
     >40 y 12-250 ng/mL

B

Does red cell morphology demonstrate schistocytes?

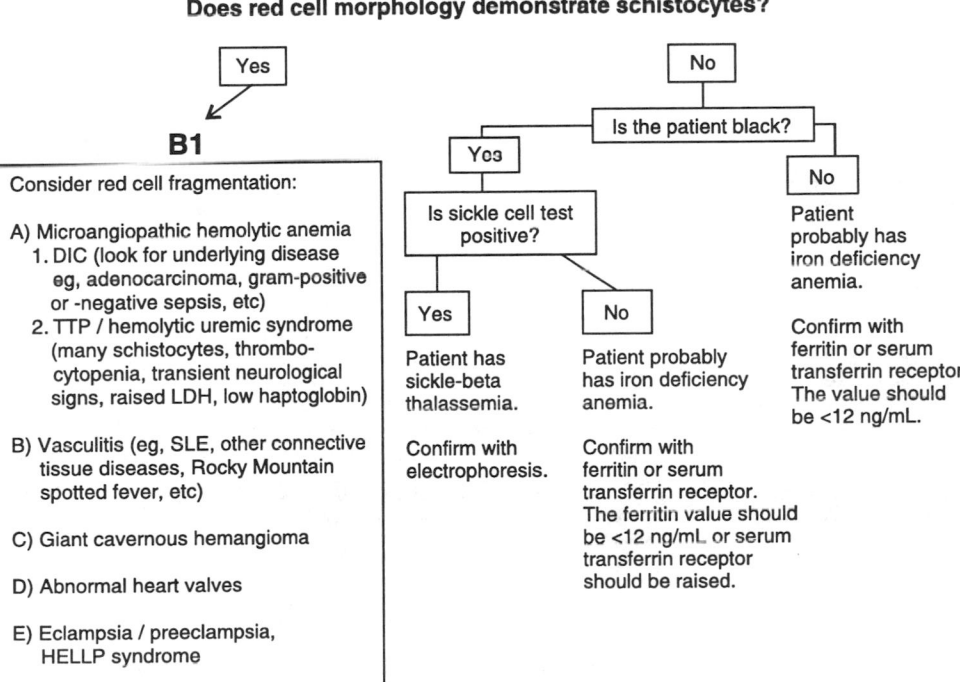

Yes ⟶ **B1**

B1

Consider red cell fragmentation:

A) Microangiopathic hemolytic anemia
  1. DIC (look for underlying disease eg, adenocarcinoma, gram-positive or -negative sepsis, etc)
  2. TTP / hemolytic uremic syndrome (many schistocytes, thrombocytopenia, transient neurological signs, raised LDH, low haptoglobin)

B) Vasculitis (eg, SLE, other connective tissue diseases, Rocky Mountain spotted fever, etc)

C) Giant cavernous hemangioma

D) Abnormal heart valves

E) Eclampsia / preeclampsia, HELLP syndrome

F) March hemoglobinuria

G) Severe burns

H) Others

No

Is the patient black?

Yes

Is sickle cell test positive?

Yes: Patient has sickle-beta thalassemia.

Confirm with electrophoresis.

No: Patient probably has iron deficiency anemia.

Confirm with ferritin or serum transferrin receptor. The ferritin value should be <12 ng/mL or serum transferrin receptor should be raised.

No: Patient probably has iron deficiency anemia.

Confirm with ferritin or serum transferrin receptor. The value should be <12 ng/mL.

C

What is the uncorrected reticulocyte count?

Obtain single correction reticulocyte count (reticulocyte index) (S)

S = reticulocyte count x (patient's hematocrit / 0.45)

Double correction reticulocyte count or reticulocyte production index (RPI) is calculated by dividing the single correction reticulocyte count(s) by the maturation index (T).

Hct	T
0.40 - 0.50	1
0.30 - 0.40	1.5
0.20 - 0.30	2.0
0.10 - 0.20	2.5

Reticulocyte production index = U

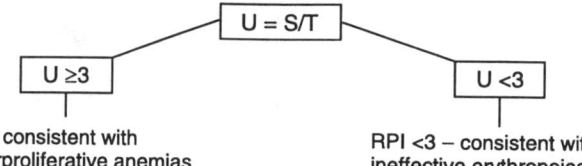

U = S/T

U ≥3

U <3

RPI >3 – consistent with the hyperproliferative anemias (acute hemorrhage or hemolysis, response to hematinics).

Go to C1

RPI <3 – consistent with ineffective erythropoiesis or hypoproliferative anemias.

Go to C100

C1

Raised RPI ≥3

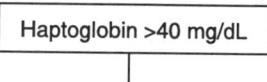

Examine peripheral blood smear for abnormal morphology.

Obtain:
Bilirubin
LDH
Serum free hemoglobin
Urine hemoglobin
Urine hemosiderin
Haptoglobin

Haptoglobin >40 mg/dL

Haptoglobin <30 mg/dL*

Patient probably has/had an acute hemorrhage or is responding to hematinic.

Patient should be evaluated for external or internal bleeding. Stools checked for occult blood.

Probably has hemolytic anemia. Bilirubin is usually between 1.0 and 5.0 mg/dL. Most should be indirect bilirubin. Serum LDH is raised. The LDH isoezymes will show a flipped 1:2 pattern similar to that of an acute myocardial infarction.

If intravascular hemolysis is present, hemoglobinemia, hemoglobinuria, and hemosiderinuria may be present. A bone marrow aspirate (usually not indicated) will reveal erythroid hyperplasia with fairly normal maturation.

*Haptoglobin levels are decreased during pregnancy and with estrogen medication. With acute inflammation, haptoglobin, as an acute phase reactant may increase, masking a decrease relating to concurrent hemolysis (see also Haptoglobin, Serum in Chemistry chapter).

C2

Does the patient have any of the following morphological abnormalities?

C3) Sickle cells
C4) Hb C crystals
C5) Target cells
C6) Spherocytes
C7) Elliptocytes
C8) Acanthocytes
C9) Stomatocytes
C10) Schistocytes
C11) Malaria / *Babesia*
C12) None of the above

C3	C4	C5
Do hemoglobin electro-phoresis. The patient has sickle cell disease (SS) or is doubly heterozygous (SC, SD, SO, S-thal, etc).	The patient probably has homozygous Hb C disease. Confirm with electro-phoresis.	Four possibilities: 1) Liver disease...elevated enzymes, (AST, ALT, LDH, GGT, Alk Phos), decreased albumin, increased PT, etc. 2) Hemoglobin C trait or disease, confirm by electrophoresis. 3) Thalassemia, confirm with elevated A2 (>3.2%) by electrophoresis. 4) Postsplenectomy

C6

Is the antiglobulin test, direct (Coombs test, direct) positive?

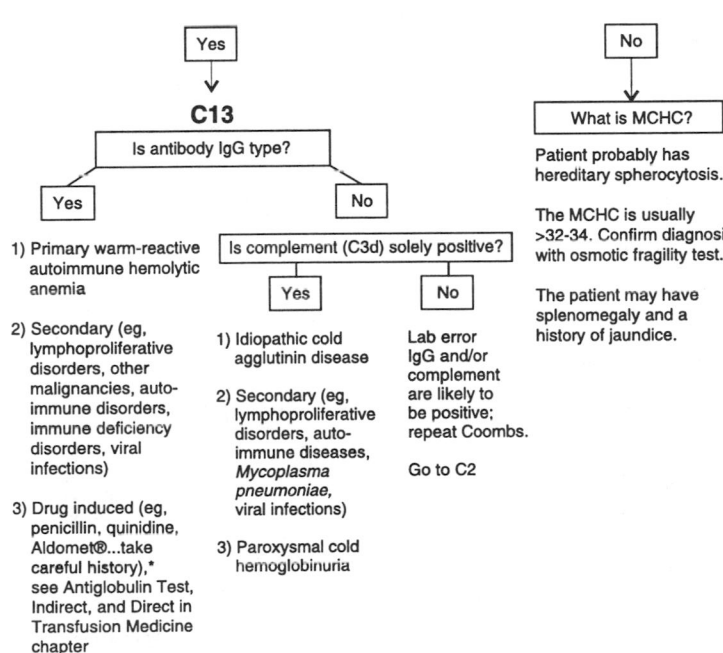

C13

Is antibody IgG type?

Yes

1) Primary warm-reactive autoimmune hemolytic anemia

2) Secondary (eg, lymphoproliferative disorders, other malignancies, auto-immune disorders, immune deficiency disorders, viral infections)

3) Drug induced (eg, penicillin, quinidine, Aldomet®...take careful history),* see Antiglobulin Test, Indirect, and Direct in Transfusion Medicine chapter

No

Is complement (C3d) solely positive?

Yes

1) Idiopathic cold agglutinin disease

2) Secondary (eg, lymphoproliferative disorders, auto-immune diseases, *Mycoplasma pneumoniae*, viral infections)

3) Paroxysmal cold hemoglobinuria

No

Lab error IgG and/or complement are likely to be positive; repeat Coombs.

Go to C2

No

What is MCHC?

Patient probably has hereditary spherocytosis.

The MCHC is usually >32-34. Confirm diagnosis with osmotic fragility test.

The patient may have splenomegaly and a history of jaundice.

*Young DS, *Effects of Drugs on Clinical Laboratory Tests*, 5th ed, Volume One: Listing by Test, Washington, DC: AACC Press, 2000, Section 3, 220-1.

C7

Repeat peripheral smear on another occasion (ensure that results are repeatable). Assure that the result is not an artifact.

If results are repeatable then the diagnosis is hereditary elliptocytosis (very rarely of clinical significance).

C8

Due to:

1) Severe liver disease.
   See Liver Disease: Laboratory Assessment, Overview

2) Congenital abetalipoproteinemia

3) Postsplenectomy

C9

Patient has hereditary stomatocytosis, or changes may be an artifact.

C10

Causes of red cell fragmentation:

A) Microangiopathic hemolytic anemia.

1) DIC* (look for underlying disease eg, adenocarcinoma, gram-positive or -negative sepsis, etc)

2) TTP* (many schistocytes, thrombocytopenia, renal changes, transient neurological signs)

3) Hemolytic uremic syndrome*

B) Vasculitis (eg, SLE, other connective tissue diseases,* Rocky Mountain spotted fever, etc)

C) Prosthetic / abnormal heart valves

D) Eclampsia / preeclampsia, HELLP syndrome*

E) Malignant hypertension

F) March hemoglobinuria*

G) Severe burns

*See listing in Key Word Index.

C12

Do antiglobulin test, direct (Coombs test). Are the results of direct Coombs test positive?

Yes — Go to C13

No — Possible hemoglobinopathy. Do hemoglobin electrophoresis

Are the results positive?

Yes — 8% of American blacks have sickle trait (AS). 0.15% of American blacks have sickle cell disease (SS). Hemoglobin C is 10 times less likely than hemoglobin S. Numerous hemoglobin variants exist, most of them quite rare.

No — Go to C14

C11

The patient has red blood cell inclusions (eg, malaria, *Babesia,* ehrlichiosis). Confirm with thick smear, serological tests.

C14

Do pyruvate kinase (PK) and G-6-PD enzyme screens.

Is PK present?

Is G-6-PD present?

PK (Yes) G-6-PD (No)	PK (No) G-6-PD (Yes)	PK (Yes) G-6-PD (Yes)
The patient has G-6-PD deficiency. False-negatives can occur if measured at time of a high reticulocyte count associated with a hemolytic episode.	Patient has PK deficiency	Other enzyme deficiencies could be the cause of the hemolysis. Send sample of blood to a reference lab for screening. The chance of such deficiency is 1 in 300,000.

C15

Repeat history and physical, examine for splenomegaly.

C25

What are vitamin B_{12}, folate, and RBC folate levels?

B_{12} >250 pg/mL Folate <2 RBC folate <200	B_{12} <250 pg/mL Folate >2 RBC folate >200	B_{12} <250 pg/mL Folate <2 RBC folate <200	Any other combination?
Patient has folate deficiency. Homocysteine level raised, methylmalonic acid level normal. The bone marrow aspirate will show hyperplastic, megaloblastic changes.	The patient has B_{12} deficiency. Homocysteine and methylmalonic acid levels raised. Obtain parietal cell antibody, intrinsic factor blocking antibodies. Schilling test, parts 1 & 2 may distinguish gastric from ileal problem. The bone marrow aspirate will show hyperplastic, megaloblastic changes.	The patient has combined B_{12} and folate deficiencies. The bone marrow aspirate will show hyperplastic, megaloblastic changes.	Do bone marrow aspirate and biopsy and evaluate microscopically. A) Myelophthisic state - this shows replacement of the normal hematopoietic elements of the bone marrow by leukemia, metastic carcinoma, TB, fibrosis, etc. B) Hypoplasia/aplasia - bone marrow shows decreased erythrocytic precursors only (pure red cell aplasia) or panhypoplasia of marrow elements. C) Endocrinopathy - slight hypoplasia due to Hashimoto thyroiditis, Addison disease, etc. Do appropriate endocrine tests; see Key Word Index. D) Normal marrow - obtain heme consult.

C100

What pattern of iron studies does patient have?

Iron <50 TIBC >350 % Sat <20 Fer low	Iron <50 TIBC ≤250 % Sat ≤20 Fer norm/hi	Iron >160 TIBC <250 % Sat >20 Fer norm/hi	≥50 Iron ≤160 Fer norm/hi	Any other combination

The patient has iron deficiency, raised serum transferrin receptor level.

A bone marrow is not necessary, but would show absence of stainable iron.

Anemia of chronic disease (inflammatory disease, infection or malignancy, RE iron block).

Normal serum transferrin receptor level; inappropriately reduced erythropoietin level.

Bone marrow would show the presence of iron stores.

The patient has sideroblastic anemia, either congenital, or acquired (lead poisoning, alcohol, isoniazid, myelodysplasia, etc).

Bone marrow may show normal/increased erythroid precursors, ringed sideroblasts on doing iron stain.

Note: Obtain cytogenetic studies on the bone marrow sample.

A1
Patient has beta thalassemia.

Confirm with electrophoresis.

Hb A will be >3.2%.

Target cells will be seen on peripheral smear.

What is patient's serum creatinine?

Creatinine ≤1.8	Creatinine >2.0

Go to C25

Chronic renal failure

Obtain erythropoietin level.

Bone marrow may show mild hypoplasia due to lack of erythropoietin. Bone marrow is not usually required.

D

Normocytic, heterogeneous anemia is present.

Possible early iron deficiency, sideroblastic or megaloblastic anemia or mixed deficiency is present.

What are ferritin and RBC folate / vitamin B_{12} values?

Ferritin low RBC folate <200 Vitamin B_{12} <250	Ferritin normal RBC folate <200 Vitamin B_{12} <250	Ferritin normal RBC folate >200 Vitamin B_{12} >250

Mixed iron and megaloblastic anemia are present.

Obtain serum transferrin receptor, homocysteine, and methylmalonic acid levels if necessary.

Megaloblastic anemia is present.

Obtain homocysteine and methylmalonic acid levels if necessary.

Sideroblastic anemia may be present. Confirm with observation of ringed sideroblasts in bone marrow.

or

If patient is black, also consider hemoglobinopathy (eg, SS or SC hemoglobinopathy).

or

Myeloproliferative disorder may be present.
A leukoerythroblastic reaction should be present (nucleated RBCs and immature myeloid series). Diagnosis confirmed on bone marrow examination.

F

Do antiglobulin test, direct (Coombs test, direct).
Are results of direct Coombs test positive?

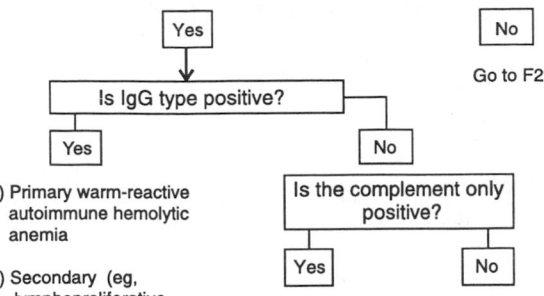

| Yes | No |

Go to F2

Is IgG type positive?

Yes

1) Primary warm-reactive autoimmune hemolytic anemia

2) Secondary (eg, lymphoproliferative disorders, malignancies, autoimmune disorders, immune deficiency disorders, viral infections)

3) Drug induced (eg, penicillin, quinidine, Aldomet®... take careful history)

No

Is the complement only positive?

Yes

1) Idiopathic cold agglutinin disease

2) Secondary (eg, lymphoproliferative disorders, autoimmune disease, *Mycoplasma*, pneumonia, viral infections

3) Paroxysmal cold hemoglobinuria

No

Lab error; IgG and/or complement should be positive: repeat Coombs.

Go to F2

F2

Macrocytic, heterogeneous anemia

What pattern of folate / vitamin B_{12} studies does patient have?

>250 B_{12} <1000 Folate <2 RBC folate <200	B_{12} <250 Folate >2 RBC folate >200	B_{12} <250 RBC folate <200	Normal B_{12} >250 Folate >2 RBC folate >200
The patient has folate deficiency.*	The patient has B_{12} deficiency.*	The patient has both B_{12} and folate deficiencies.*	Ensure no liver disease, alcoholism, raised reticulocyte count (accelerated erythropoiesis), hypothyroidism.
Measure homocysteine and methylmalonic acid, LDH, indirect bilirubin.	Measure homocysteine and methylmalonic acid, LDH, indirect bilirubin.	Measure homocysteine and methylmalonic acid, LDH, indirect bilirubin.	Do bone marrow aspirate with chromosomes and biopsy.
Homocysteine raised confirmed folate deficiency.	Both raised - confirmed vitamin B_{12} deficiency.	Both raised - confirmed vitamin B_{12} deficiency or mixed vitamin B_{12} deficiency and folate deficiency.	If the diagnosis is not apparent (eg, myelodysplastic syndrome) then repeat CBC and begin work-up again.
Bone marrow may not be required.	Obtain intrinsic factor and parietal cell antibody studies to help confirm/exclude pernicious anemia. A Shilling test part 1 and 2 may help to confirm the presence of pernicious anemia.	Obtain intrinsic factor and parietal cell antibody studies to help confirm/exclude pernicious anemia. A Shilling test part 1 and 2 may help to confirm the presence of pernicious anemia.	
	Bone marrow may not be required.	Bone marrow may not be required.	

*A deficiency state may be present in a patient, but this may not necessarily be the cause of the anemia. Confirmatory studies are thus required.

CLUSTER OF DIFFERENTIATION (CD) ANTIGENS

Human Leukocyte Cell Surface (Membrane) Markers

CD #	Synonyms	Cell Type	Identity	Molecular Size of Antigen	Function/Clinical Application
1	T6; Leu-6; OKT6		HLA class I-like molecule	45-kDa	Expressed as complex with β-2 microglobulin on cortical immature thymocytes and on Langerhans' cells
2	T11; Leu-6; OKT11	Pan-T cells	Sheep red blood cell receptor	50-kDa	Involved in T-cell activation; a single chain glycoprotein member of Ig superfamily that transduces signal to T cells
3	T3; Leu-4; OKT3	Pan-T cells	Multicomponent; five polypeptides	16-28 kDa each	Associated with T-cell receptor, T-lymphocyte activation
4	T4; Leu-3a; OKT4	Helper T cells; monocytes; macrophages		59-kDa	A single chain glycoprotein member of Ig superfamily involved in T-cell activation; receptor for HLA class II; receptor for HIV
7	3AI; Leu-9			40-kDa	Member of Ig superfamily; present on T cells, NK cells
8	T8; Leu-2a; OKT8	Suppressor T cells; some monocytes; macrophages	Homo-or heterodimer with α and β chains	32-kDa	Receptor for HLA class I antigens; member of Ig superfamily; involved in T-cell activation
10	T5; CALLA (common acute lymphoblastic leukemia antigen)	Early B and T cells; germinal center cells; neutrophils	Integrin glycoprotein	100-kDa	Single chain glycoprotein; peptide cleavage (endopeptidase)
11a	LFA-1		α-integrin glycoprotein complexed with β-integrin CD18	180-kDa	Receptor for ICAM-1, -2, and -3 adherence molecules
11b	Mac-1; OKM-1; CR3; Leu-15	Monocytes; neutrophils; NK cells	α-integrin glycoprotein complexed with β-integrin CD18	165-kDa	Receptor for ICAM-1 and fibrinogen complement 3b receptor
11c	CR4; Leu-M5; BLY6	Monocytes; activated lymphs; granulocytes	α-integrin glycoprotein complexed with β-integrin CD18	150-kDa	Receptor for ICAM-1 and fibrinogen complement 3b receptor
14	Mo2; MY4; Leu-M3	Monocytes; immature granulocytes	Glycoprotein linked to phosphatidyl-inositol	55-kDa	Lipopolysaccharide receptor
16	FcrRIII	NK cells; macrophages; granulocytes	Glycoprotein	60-kDa	IgG receptor, low affinity antibody-dependent cellular toxicity
18	LFA-1; Mac-1	Leukocytes	β integrin glycoprotein complexed with α-integrins CD 11a, b, or c	95-kDa	
19	B4; Leu-12	B cells; follicular dentritic cells	Single chain glycoprotein	95-kDa	B-lymphocyte activation
20	B1; Bp35; Leu-16; L26	B cells	Single chain protein	35-kDa	Modulates B-cell activation (Ca++ channel involved)
21	CR2	B cells	Single chain complement regulatory protein	145-kDa	B-lymphocyte activation; complement 3 receptor; Epstein-Barr virus receptor; amplified signal from B-cell receptor
22	FCeRII; Bgp135; Leu-14	B cells	Ig superfamily		B-cell activation receptor for IgE
23	FCeRII; B6; Leu-20	Activated B cells; follicular dentritic cells; eosinophils; platelets	Lectin like	45-kDa	Receptor for IgE
25	TAC antigen; IL-2R α-chain	Activated T and B cells; macrophages	Glycoprotein	55-kDa	Low affinity receptor for IL-2
28	TP44	T-cell subset activated B cells	Ig superfamily	44-kD; homodimer	Costimulatory for CD80 binding results in T-cell activation receptor for B7
29	VLA	Numerous	β-integrin complexed with α-integrin chains	130-kDa	
32	FcγRII	Numerous	Single chain protein	40-kDa	IgG receptor
34	MY10	T cells; stem cells	Single chain glycoprotein	110-kDa	?adhesion molecule; ?marker for HSC
35	CRI; C36 receptor	B cells; NK cells; PMNs; monocytes; red blood cells			Binds immune complexes
38	OKT10; T10; CR1; Leu-17	Activated lymphocytes; immature B cells	Single chain glycoprotein	190-250-kDa	Complement 3b receptor
40	gp50	B cells; macrophages; follicular dendritic cells	Single chain polypeptide homologue of tumor necrosis factor receptor, Fas	48-kDa	Growth factor receptor; B-cell activation; involved in B cell apoptosis
43	Leukosialin; leukophorin	Lymphocytes NK; cells monocytes	Glycoprotein	95-135-kDa	Leukocyte activation; cell surface mucin
44	Pgp-1; Hermes receptor type III	Lymphocytes; NK cells; monocytes; red blood cells	Single chain glycoprotein	80-95-kDa	Leukocyte homing; cell migration; adhesion to hyalutonic acid with implication to tumor cell metastasis
45	Leukocyte common antigen; T200 isoforms: CD45RA, CD45RB, CD45RO	Leukocytes	Single chain glycoprotein with differentially expressed isoforms	Multiple isoforms; 180-220-kDa; 220-kDa form; 220, 205, 190-kDa forms; 180-kDa form	B cells; monocytes CD8 SP; T cells; naive T cells; B cells; monocytes; macrophages; subsets of memory T cells; monocytes; thymocytes; activated T cells; memory T cells
46	MCP	Numerous	Dimeric glycoprotein	60-kDa	Cofactor, cleavage of complement 36 and 46
50	ICAM-3	Leukocytes	Single chain glycoprotein; Ig superfamily adhesion molecule	120-kDa	Adhesion molecule binds CD11/CD18
54	ICAM-1	Activated lymphocytes; endothelial cells	Ig superfamily adhesion molecule	90-kDa	Binds CD11/CD18; ligand for LFA-1, rhinoviruses
55	DAF	Many	Single chain glycoprotein	70-kDa	Inactivates complement factors C3 and C5
56	Leu-19	NK cells	Single chain glycoprotein	140-200-kDa	Adhesion molecule
59	Protectin	Many	Glycoprotein	20-kDa	Inhibits production of membrane attack complex of complement
62 E, L, P	Selectins E, L, P; ELAM-1; LAM-1	E: activated endothelium; L: neutrophils/monocytes and NK cells	Single chain glycoprotein	E: 110-kDa L: 76-kDa P: 140-kDa	Adhesion; P-selectin mediates adhesion of platelets
64	FcγRI	Monocytes/macrophages	Single chain glycoprotein	75-kDa	High affinity IgG receptor mediates phagocytosis; ab-dependent cell cytotoxicity; cytokine release
71	Transferrin receptor	Most activated cells	Homodimeric glycoprotein	95-kDa	Receptor for iron uptake protein
73	Ecto 5'-nucleotidase	Lymphocyte subsets			Regulates uptake of nucleotides
74	HLA class II		Single chain glycoprotein	35-kDa	Antigen presentation

Human Leukocyte Cell Surface (Membrane) Markers (continued)

CD #	Synonyms	Cell Type	Identity	Molecular Size of Antigen	Function/Clinical Application
79 a and b	Igα; Igβ	B cells			Part of B-cell antigen receptor
80	B7-1	Activated B cells; monocytes; macrophages; dendritic cells	Ig superfamily	60-kDa	Ligand for CD28
86	B7-2	Activated lymphocytes; monocytes; macrophages; dendritic cells	Ig superfamily		Ligand for CD152
87	Urokinase/plasminogen receptor (uPA-R)	Activated T cells; neutrophils; macrophages	Phosphatidyl-inositol linked single chain glycoprotein anchored by GPI linkage	60-kDa	uPA-R and receptors for plasminogen focus plasmin on surface of tumor (or inflammatory cells) to assist metastatic invasion (and aid diapedesis at inflammatory sites)
95	APO-1; Fas	Activated T and B cells; NK cells	Glycoprotein; member of TNF receptor family	45-kDa	Mediates apoptosis; delivers apoptotic signal on binding Fas ligand; sequence of 65 aas (intracytoplasmic) form the "death domain" (promotes the death signal)
115	M-CSF receptor; c-fms product	Macrophages	Single chain glycoprotein	150-kDa	Growth factor receptor
115w	GM CSF	Myeloid precursors	Single chain glycoprotein	80-kDa	Growth factor receptor
117	c-kit, stem cell factor receptor	Hemopoietic cells	Single chain glycoprotein	145-kDa	Growth factor receptor
117w	IFN-γ receptor	Many	Single chain glycoprotein	90-kDa	Growth factor receptor
120a	Tumor necrosis; factor receptor I; TNFR I	Many	Member NGFR/TNFR superfamily	50-kDa	Cytokine receptor; involved in septic shock
120b	Tumor necrosis; factor receptor II; TNFR II	Many	Member NGFR/TNFR superfamily	75-kDa	Cytokine receptor; induces nitric oxide (NO); activates neutrophils
121a	IL-1 receptor type 1	Activated T and B cells; macrophages	Glycoproteins		Cytokine receptor
121b	IL-1 receptor type 2	Activated T and B cells; macrophages	Glycoproteins		Cytokine receptor
122	IL-2 receptor	B cells; activated macrophages	Glycoproteins	75-kDa	IL-2 receptor, β-chain
123	IL-3 receptor	B cells; hematopoietic stem cells			Binds IL-3; affects early hemopoietic (pluripotential stem cell stage) cell differentiation
124	IL-4 receptor	Many, including B cells, T cells, hemopoietic precursors, marrow stroma, fibroblasts, mast cells, others			IL-4 binding; high affinity switch factor for IgE
125-129	IL-5-9 receptor	Widespread distribution			Multiple cytokine stimulatory functions; signal transduction functions
152	CTLA-4; Ly 56	Activated T cells	Ig superfamily		Negative signals; immune response
154	CD40 ligand, gp39	Activated T cells			Receptor for CD40

131-166 — new CD antigens from the 6th International Workshop on Human Leukocyte Differentiation Antigens

♦ **Abciximab** *see* Platelet Count *on page 468*

♦ **ABC Proteins** *see* Inherited Diseases of Metabolism and Cell Structure *on page 449*

♦ **Absence of Phosphorylation-Induced Gelation of Red Cell Membrane Skeletons** *see* Gelation Assay *on page 437*

♦ **Absolute Eosinophil Count** *see* Eosinophil Count *on page 424*

♦ **Acanthocytes** *see* Peripheral Blood: Differential Leukocyte Count *on page 464*

♦ **Acatalasemia** *see* Red Blood Cell Enzyme Deficiency, Quantitative *on page 475*

♦ **Acid β-Galactosidase** *see* Inherited Diseases of Metabolism and Cell Structure *on page 449*

♦ **Acid Elution for Fetal Hemoglobin** *see* Kleihauer-Betke *on page 453*

♦ **Acid-Fast, Ziehl-Neelsen, Stain for Intracellular Pigment** *see* Leukocyte Cytochemistry *on page 456*

♦ **Acidified Glycerol Lysis Test** *see* Glycerol Lysis Test, Acidified, Modified *on page 439*

♦ **Acidified Serum Test** *see* Ham Test *on page 439*

♦ **Acid Phosphatase Stain With and Without Tartrate** *see* Leukocyte Cytochemistry *on page 456*

♦ **Acid Phosphatase, Tartrate Resistant, Leukocytes** *see* Tartrate Resistant Leukocyte Acid Phosphatase *on page 488*

♦ **Acid Serum Test** *see* Ham Test *on page 439*

♦ **Acid Serum Test for PNH** *see* Ham Test *on page 439*

♦ **Acute Chest Syndrome** *see* Sickle Cell Tests *on page 486*

♦ **Adenosine Deaminase Overproduction** *see* Red Blood Cell Enzyme Deficiency, Quantitative *on page 475*

♦ **Adenylate Kinase Deficiency** *see* Red Blood Cell Enzyme Deficiency, Quantitative *on page 475*

♦ **Adenylate Kinase Deficiency** *see* Red Blood Cell Enzyme Deficiency Screen *on page 476*

♦ **Adrenal Function Eosinophil Count** *see* Thorn Test *on page 490*

♦ **Adrenoleukodystrophy** *see* Inherited Diseases of Metabolism and Cell Structure *on page 449*

♦ **AGLT** *see* Glycerol Lysis Test, Acidified, Modified *on page 439*

♦ **Alder-Rielly Anomaly** *see* Peripheral Blood: Differential Leukocyte Count *on page 464*

Alkaline Phosphatase, Neutrophil Membrane (mNAP)

Related Information
Erythropoietin, Serum *on page 169*
Flow Cytometry, Overview *on page 432*
Ham Test *on page 439*
Leukocyte Alkaline Phosphatase *on page 455*
Leukocyte Cytochemistry *on page 456*
Lysozyme, Blood and Urine *on page 457*
PNH Test (GPI-Anchored Proteins) by Flow Cytometry *on page 472*

Synonyms Membrane Leukocyte Alkaline Phosphatase; mNAP

Abstract Fluorescence intensity of neutrophil surface membrane alkaline phosphatase (mNAP) and the number of neutrophils positive for mNAP is measured with immunofluorescence methodology, using monoclonal antibody and flow cytometer technology. Application to the diagnosis of hematologic disorders, notably myeloproliferative disease, is similar to the measure of intracytoplasmic neutrophil alkaline phosphatase (ALP). (See Leukocyte Alkaline Phosphatase *on page 455*.) The mNAP procedure is said to avoid the vicissitudes of fixation and staining of the slide-based cytochemical method, and in particular the subjective evaluation involved in interpretation and grading of the ALP stained slides.

Specimen Whole blood

Container Blue top (sodium citrate) tube

Storage Instructions Store samples at 4°C and run within 24 hours of collection. After staining and fixation, sample can be stored at 4°C for at least 4 days without significant degradation of fluorescent intensity.

Reference Interval % mNAP + cells = 17% to 89%; mean fluorescence intensity (MFI) = 5.7-40.9

Use Differential diagnosis of chronic myelogenous leukemia (CML), paroxysmal nocturnal hemoglobinuria (PNH), inflammatory leukocytosis, polycythemia vera (PV), and aplastic anemia (AA)

Limitations Methodology requires availability of flow cytometer

Methodology Binding of anti-ALP monoclonal antibody detected by indirect immunofluorescence procedures utilizing a fluorescence-activated cell sorter (FACS)

Additional Information Good correlation has been reported between mNAP and the cytochemical detection of intracytoplasmic neutrophil alkaline phosphatase (NAP) by Tomonaga's[1] rather than Kaplow's[2] method. Patients with inflammatory leukocytosis, PV and AA were found to have mNAP levels that were significantly higher than normal. Patients with PNH and CML had lower levels of mNAP than normal. Reference to "mNAP level" includes both %mNAP and MFI. In patients with PNH, 50% of cases had normal mNAP levels. The fluorescence distribution curves formed two peaks, apparently corresponding to mNAP negative cells (PNH clone) and mNAP positive cells (as shown by 2-color immunofluorescence analysis using anti-CD16 reacting with an independent membrane protein). Patients with myelodysplastic syndrome showed low or high mNAP levels.[3] Membrane leukocyte alkaline phosphatase is one of some 18 glycosyl phosphatidylinositol-anchored proteins that are deficient in paroxysmal nocturnal hemoglobinuria.

Footnotes
1. Shibata A, Bennett JM, Castoldi GL, et al, "Recommended Methods for Cytological Procedures in Haematology. International Committee for Standardization in Haematology (ICSH)," *Clin Lab Haematol*, 1985, 7(1):55-74.
2. Kaplow LS, "A Histochemical Procedure for Localizing and Evaluating Leukocyte Alkaline Phosphatase Activity in Smears of Blood and Marrow," *Blood*, 1955, 10(10):1023-9.
3. Shibano M, Machii T, Nishimori Y, et al, "Assessment of Alkaline Phosphatase on the Surface Membrane of Neutrophils by Immunofluorescence," *Am J Haematol*, 1999, 60(1):12-8.

References
Rambaldi A, Masuhara K, Borleri GM, et al "Flow Cytometry of Leukocyte Alkaline Phosphatase in Normal and Pathologic Leukocytes," *Br J Haematol*, 1997, 96(4):815-22.

♦ **Allele-Specific Oligonucleotide Hybridization for Thalassemia** *see* DNA-Probe Assay for Thalassemia (BeTha Gene Test) *on page 423*

♦ **Alpha-Naphthyl Esterase Stain With and Without Fluoride** *see* Leukocyte Cytochemistry *on page 456*

♦ **Amino Acid Screen, Plasma** *see* Inherited Diseases of Metabolism and Cell Structure *on page 449*

♦ **Amino Acid Screen Qualitative, Urine** *see* Inherited Diseases of Metabolism and Cell Structure *on page 449*

♦ **Amniotic Fluid Lamellar Bodies** *see* Lamellar Bodies, Amniotic Fluid *on page 454*

♦ **Amyloid** *see* Leukocyte Cytochemistry *on page 456*

♦ **Annexin V** *see* Apoptosis Assays *on page 402*

♦ **APL® Cell Test** *see* Promyelocytic Leukemia Assay *on page 474*

Apoptosis Assays

Related Information
bcl-2 Gene Rearrangement *on page 720*
Flow Cytometry, Overview *on page 432*
p53, Functional Assay/Sequencing *on page 728*
Retinoblastoma Gene DNA Detection *on page 729*
White Blood Cell Count *on page 496*

Applies to Annexin V; Caspase Enzymes; CD95; FAS Receptor; Hyaline Globules; Propidium Iodide; Survivin; Thanatosomes; TUNEL Assay

Abstract Apoptosis (a Greek derived term meaning "falling of leaves from the tree") refers to a mechanism of cell death distinct from necrosis. Apoptosis has specific morphologic characteristics, partially defined molecular mechanisms including an endogenous endonuclease (caspase) cascade, and is under genetic control leading to the concept of "programmed cell death".[1] Apoptosis has broad implications for biology and medicine. The process is of critical import to embryogenesis, lymphocyte development, and thus, immunity, and to autoimmunity, inflammation, neoplasia, and the cellular response to toxins (eg, chemotherapeutic drugs and ionizing radiation). Numerous approaches are available to test for apoptosis and its resultant biologic effects, including morphologic observation, flow cytometry, and molecular analysis including electrophoretic-based techniques.[2]

Specimen Specimen requirements are method dependent (see Methodology).

Special Instructions Consult your local laboratory and with laboratory consultants concerning appropriate application and availability of different assays for apoptosis. These procedures have been recently developed and may be performed largely on a research basis but may be offered currently or in the near future by some reference laboratories.

Use Cell, tissue, and molecular-based assays to estimate the presence and/or characteristics of apoptosis in a broad range of pathologic or developmental processes. Assays for apoptosis can be applied to monitor the results of therapy for malignant disease, to assess the presence of apoptotic change in neural cells (as may occur in neurodegenerative disorders), to provide evaluation of transplant rejection, and to evaluate apoptotic change in fibroblast activity in the regulation of tissue repair (ie, as in the control of scar formation). Monitor the results of therapy involving the regulation of apoptosis (eg, in the modulation of disorders of immunodeficiency such as AIDS). Use of these assays is not limited to these examples.

Limitations Methods used to evaluate apoptosis must be well controlled (and may not have been in some, if not many, instances) in order to avoid producing the process (apoptosis) that one is attempting to study (see references by Zhang and Jerome).

Methodology Apoptosis is a multifaceted sequential process (see Additional Information) which has allowed the development and application of a surprising number of laboratory assays, each usually targeting a specific stage and/or event of programmed cell death. Distinct morphologic changes include condensation of nuclear chromatin, shrinkage of cytoplasm, membrane bleb formation, and formation of apoptotic bodies. Some assays respond to early changes while others measure events that occur in later stages. A recent article that deals with mechanisms of HIV-associated lymphocyte apoptosis includes a table of assays commonly applied to the detection and study of apoptosis.[3]

Morphologic observation, Annexin V binding, and TUNEL (terminal dUTP nick end labeling) are especially commonly employed.

Apoptosis - identification by morphologic features: In cultured cells there is loss of adhesion to substrate with cell rounding, surface bleb formation, cell shrinkage with cessation of blebbing, membrane deterioration, nuclear matrix degeneration with chromatin condensation, and formation of condensed apoptotic cell bodies.[4] Phase contrast microscopy showing blebs, spikes, and blisters, as well as a table of cellular changes, as they relate to apoptosis assays is presented in a recent publication.[5]

Criteria for detection of apoptotic leukocytes in peripheral blood smears:[6]

- cell shrinkage
- peripheral condensation of chromatin along the nuclear membrane, nuclear fragmentation, formation of cytoplasmic blebs, membrane-bound apoptotic bodies, and cytoplasmic vacuoles
- persistence of specific granules and plasma membrane

Annexin V (multiple commercial sources for reagents/kits including: R and D Systems, Minneapolis, MN; Immunotech, Boehringer, Mannheim, Germany; Coulter, Hialeah, Florida): Annexin V is a 35 kDA Ca^{2+}-dependent phospholipid-binding anticoagulant protein. It can bind to phosphatidyl serine. The latter is usually situated in a protected position along the inner surface of the plasma membrane but is externally exposed with apoptosis. Annexin V is then able to bind and can be detected by flow cytometry. In its exposed situation, phosphatidyl serine serves as a recognition signal for macrophages that can eliminate apoptotic cells. See diagram.

TUNEL assay (commercial kits for the detection of apoptosis by TUNEL are available from Pharmingen, San Diego, CA and by INSEL, Apoptag kit, Oncor, Gaithersburg, MD). The TUNEL (*in situ* terminal deoxynucleotidyl transferase d uridine triphosphate nick end labeling) and the INSEL (*in situ* DNA end labeling) methods are based on the detection of DNA fragmentation. Both techniques reflect endonuclease dependent cleavage of DNA by labeling nick end DNA with a specific complex conjugated to a chromogen or fluorogen.

Leukocyte viability by light scatter: A rapid and simple method for quantifying apoptosis using the Abbott CD4000 hematology analyzer has been proposed.[7] Based on cellular light scatter properties with the demonstration of membrane fragility (as occurs with apoptosis) this method has been reported to correlate well with TUNEL (slide based) and Annexin V (by flow cytometry). In addition to multiangle cellular light scatter data the Cell-Dyn 4000 measures red fluorescence emitted by cells that have been labeled with propidium iodide, with generation of a leukocyte viability index.

Quantitative Assessment of Apoptosis Using Flow Cytometry

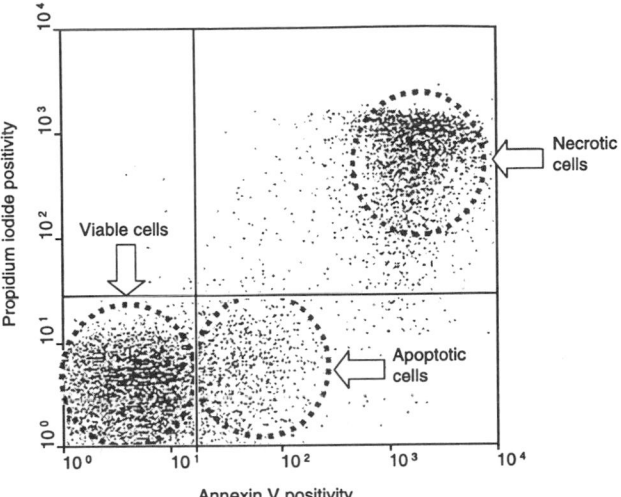

The illustration reflects activated peripheral blood lymphocytes that have been stained with propidium iodide (PI) or annexin V and subjected to fluorescence activated cell sorting. Each dot represents an individual cell. Viable cells stain with neither PI nor annexin V. Apoptotic cells stain with annexin V only, whereas necrotic cells stain with both.
Adapted from Afford S and Randhawa S, "Apoptosis," *Mol Pathol*, 2000, 53(2):55-63.

Additional Information Apoptosis, a term first used in 1972, refers to the process of programmed cell death.[8] It is a critical component, the end stage, of cellular homeostasis and is necessarily closely and highly regulated.[2] It is a coordinated mechanism of cellular death under genetic control, a genetically regulated form of cell suicide morphologically distinct from necrosis.[1] Malignancy, autoimmunity and immunodeficiency may evolve in relation to abnormalities in the regulation of apoptosis.

Assays of Apoptosis Related to Events of Apoptosis

Event	Assays	Detection
Changes in nuclear morphology: Chromatin condensation, segmentation, and formation of apoptotic bodies	DNA stains (DAPI)	Microscopy
Changes in membrane permeability	Vital dyes (PI) Permeable DNA stains: (DAPI, Hoechst 33258)	Microscopy Flow cytometry with simultaneous size determination
Changes in membrane composition: Externalization of phosphatidylserine	Annexin V binding	Flow cytometry Confocal and epifluorescence microscopy
Cleavage of nuclear proteins	Poly ADP ribose polymerase	Western blot

Mitochondrial function and integrity
  Changes in permeability transition ($\Delta\Psi$)
  Accessibility to mitochondrial antigens
  Release of cytochrome C
  Production of free radicals
	Vital dyes ($DiOC_6$, JC-1)
	Apo 2,7 antibody
	Anticytochrome C antibody
	DPPP/dihydroethidium
		Flow cytometry
		Flow cytometry
		Flow cytometry, Western blot
		Flow cytometry

Caspase activation
  Detection of caspase cleavage product
  Detection of active caspase
  Detection of caspase activity
	Known caspase substrates; PARP, caspase 3, caspase 8, DNA-PK, PK-C
	Antiactivated caspase 3 antibody
	Cleavage of fluorescent or colorimetric substrate(s)
		Western blot
		Western blot
		Fluorometer, plate reader

DNA degradation Large fragments	DNA stains (EtBr, SYBR green) DNA stains (EtBr) Radioactivity (C^{14})	Pulse-field gel electrophoresis Comet Detection of radio-labeled DNA by filter binding
Small fragments	DNA stains (EtBr) Radioactivity (C^{14})	Agarose gel electrophoresis (DNA ladder) Detection of radio-labeled DNA by filter binding
Sub-G1 peak detection	DNA stains (PI, Hoechst)	Flow cytometry
Detection of DNA strand breaks	Terminal dUTP nick end labeling (TUNEL) Ligation-mediated polymerase chain reaction	*in situ* hybridization Flow cytometry Agarose or polyacrylamide gel electrophoresis

Adapted from Badley AD, Pilon AA, Landay A, "Mechanisms of HIV-Associated Lymphocyte Apoptosis," *Blood*, 2000, 96(9):2951-6.
(Continued)

Apoptosis Assays (Continued)

Operationally, apoptosis, while continuing to grow in complexity as its mechanisms are dissected, can be conveniently divided into four steps:

- initiation
- monitoring and decision
- execution
- removal

Initially, there is interaction between the cell surface and its environment, mediated importantly by the FAS receptor (CD95). FAS may then activate the second phase of apoptosis, involving the intracellular proteins of the Bcl-2 family. Within this family are molecules that block (Bcl-2, Bcl-x1) and some that promote (BAX, Bcl-xs and BAD) apoptosis. These proteins are situated on the outer mitochondrial surface, act as pore forming units and share protein dimerization sequences. The balance of Bcl-2 family proteins on the mitochondrial surface represents the decision mechanism and controls the fate of the cell (survival or death).[1] A positive suicide decision results in the release of cytochrome C and other factors from mitochondria into the cell cytoplasm. In the third step (execution), cytochrome C activates the caspase family of cysteine proteinase enzymes that lead to a broad range of intracellular events resulting in the dismantling of the cell. The importance of the caspase family of enzymes was developed by Yuan and Horvitz who showed that the protein Ced-3 (from the Nematode Caenorhabditis elegans) was essential for the execution of apoptosis.[9] Ced-3 came to be known as a member of the caspase family. Mutations of Ced-3 that prevented its catalytic activity also prevented apoptosis.[10] Caspase-1, a cytoplasmic protease, activates interleukin-1B, a proinflammatory cytokine, and was originally identified as interleukin-1B converting enzyme (ICE). At present there are 14 known caspase family members in the cascade that modulates apoptosis. In addition, transcription factors, modulate the expression of genes that regulate the production of proapoptotic and antiapoptotic molecules including Bcl-2 (mitochondrial family of proteins), cytochrome C, and the tumor suppressor genes p53 and p21/WAF1 (death promoters).[11] DNA is "cut" by the caspases resulting in a characteristic "laddering" pattern of DNA fragments on electrophoretic study, one of the laboratory modalities for investigation of apoptosis. In the final step, phagocytic macrophages, as a result of signaling (by capsases) at the cell surface are attracted and remove the apoptotic dead cell body, completing the "death" process without inciting a true inflammatory reaction. Recently, noncaspases such as cathepsins, calpains, granzymes, and the proteasome complex (the ubiquitin-proteasome system)[12,13] have been considered to participate in the mediation and promotion of apoptotic cell death.[14]

Many inter-relationships have been described between molecules involved in apoptosis, a limited number are mentioned above. Among others, survivin, an inhibitor of apoptosis (IAP) is a member of a family of such proteins. The survivin gene encodes a protein formed of 142 amino acids that includes a Cys/His-based zinc finger, repeated two to three times and essential for survivin function (the inhibition of apoptosis). Survivin is expressed in several preneoplastic lesions, may appear early during malignant transformation and participates in the emergence of a more aggressive phenotype.[15] Survivin positivity (within tumor) appears to be a significant independent risk factor for progression of colorectal cancer.[16]

The characteristics of hyaline globules, present in a wide variety of benign and malignant conditions, have been considered for their relation to apoptosis.[17] On the basis of changes occurring in 80 malignant tumors, the term "thanatosomes" has been proposed and considered to apply to the entire spectrum of hyaline globules (HG) with emphasis on their relation to cell death. While not specific to any tumor, "thanatosomes" are considered to have evolved from apoptotic degenerative processes, common to all cell types, benign or malignant.[17] In support of this concept it was noted that HG on light microscopy were present in areas of increased apoptosis and often contained apoptotic nuclear fragments. Cytoplasmic blebbing and presence of a variety of plasma proteins on immunohistochemical analysis of cells containing HG were seen as indicative of increased plasma membrane permeability. Double stains for apoptosis and plasma proteins provided results also indicative of increased plasma membrane permeability to proteins of apoptotic cells. Ultrastructural changes were associated with intense cytoplasmic bleb formation. These and other findings led to the conclusion that HG reflect stages of cell injury relating in most cases to apoptotic cell death.[17]

The concept of apoptosis is not without detractors/skeptics, but they are few.[18]

Footnotes

1. Cotran RS, Kumar V, and Collins TC, et al, eds, "Cellular Pathology I: Cell Injury and Cell Death," *Robbins Pathologic Basis of Disease*, 6th ed, Chapter 1, Philadelphia, PA: WB Saunders Company, 1999, 18-25.
2. Cotter FE, "Laboratory Assessment of Apoptosis," *Clin Lab Haematol*, 1997, 19(4):289-320.
3. Badley AD, Pilon AA, Landay A, et al, "Mechanisms of HIV-associated Lymphocyte Apoptosis," *Blood*, 2000, 96(9):2951-64.
4. McKenney CA, Romzek MR, and Ziemba SE, "Apoptosis - When Cells Die," *Lab Med*, 1999, 30(12):791.
5. Willingham MC, "Cytochemical Methods for the Detection of Apoptosis," *J Histochem Cytochem*, 1999, 47(9):1101-10.
6. Shidham VB and Swami VK, "Evaluation of Apoptotic Leukocytes in Peripheral Blood Smears," *Arch Pathol Lab Med*, 2000, 124(9):1291-4.
7. Mentz F, Baudet S, Maloum K, et al, "Quantification of Apoptosis by the Abbott CD4000 Hematology Analyzer," *Hematol Cell Ther*, 1998, 40(5):183-8.
8. Kerr JF, Wyllie AH, and Currie AR, "Apoptosis: A Basic Biological Phenomenon With Wide-Ranging Implications in Tissue Kinetics," *Br J Cancer*, 1972, 26(4):239-57.
9. Yuan JY and Horvitz HR, "The Caenorhabditis Elegans Genes ced-3 and ced-4 Act Cell Autonomously to Cause Programmed Cell Death," *Dev Biol*, 1990, 138(1):33-41.
10. Yuan JY, Shaham S, Ledoux S, et al, "The C. Elegans Cell Death Gene ced-3 Encodes a Protein Similar to Mammalian Interleukin-1 Beta-Converting Enzyme," *Cell*, 1993, 75(4):641-52.
11. Afford S and Randhawa S, "Apoptosis," *Mol Pathol*, 2000, 53(2):55-63.
12. Pickart CM, "Ubiquitin in Chains," *Trends Biochem Sci*, 2000, 25(11):544-8.
13. Goldberg AL, Elledge SJ, and Harper JW, "The Cellular Chamber of Doom," *Sci Am*, 2001, 284(1):68-73.
14. Johnson DE, "Noncaspase Proteases in Apoptosis," *Leukemia*, 2000, 14(9):1695-703.
15. Altieri DC, Marchisio PC, and Marchisio C, "Survivin Apoptosis: An Interloper Between Cell Death and Cell Proliferation in Cancer," *Lab Invest*, 1999, 79(11):1327-33.
16. Kawasaki H, Altieri DC, Lu CD, et al, "Inhibition of Apoptosis by Survivin Predicts Shorter Survival Rates in Colorectal Cancer," *Cancer Res*, 1998, 58(22):5071-4.
17. Papadimitriou JC, Drachenberg CB, Brenner DS, et al, "Thanatosomes: A Unifying Morphogenetic Concept for Tumor Hyaline Globules Related to Apoptosis," *Hum Pathol*, 2000, 31(12):1455-65.
18. Marcella M and Ackerman AB, *A Critical Review of Apoptosis in Historical Perspective*, 1999, Philadelphia, PA: Ardor Scribendi.

References

Akasaka Y, Ishikawa Y, Ono I, et al, "Enhanced Expression of Caspase-3 in Hypertrophic Scars and Keloid: Induction of Caspase-3 and Apoptosis in Keloid Fibroblasts In Vitro," *Lab Invest*, 2000, 80(3):345-57.

Aprikyan AA, Liles WC, and Dale DC, "Emerging Role of Apoptosis in the Pathogenesis of Severe Neutropenia," *Curr Opin Hematol*, 2000, 7(3):131-2.

Aubry JP, Blaecke A, Lecoanet-Henchoz S, et al, "Annexin V Used for Measuring Apoptosis in the Early Events of Cellular Cytotoxicity," *Cytometry*, 1999, 37(3):197-204.

Bandorowicz-Pikula J, Buchet R, and Pikula S, "Annexins as Nucleotide-Binding Proteins: Facts and Speculations," *Bioessays*, 2001, 23(2):170-8.

Bardales RH, Xie SS, and Hsu SM, "In Situ DNA Fragmentation Assay for Detection of Apoptosis in Paraffin-Embedded Tissue Sections. Technical Considerations," *Am J Clin Pathol*, 1997, 107(3):332-6.

Blagosklonny MV, "The Dilemma of Apoptosis in Myelodysplasia and Leukemia: A New Promise of Therapeutic Intervention?," *Leukemia*, 2000, 14(12):2017-8.

Boudard D, Sordet O, Vasselon C, et al, "Expression and Activity of Caspases 1 and 3 in Myelodysplastic Syndromes," *Leukemia*, 2000, 14(12):2045-51.

De Maria R, Testa U, Luchetti L, et al, "Apoptotic Role of Fas/Fas Ligand System in the Regulation of Erythropoiesis," *Blood*, 1999, 93(3):796-803.

Domen J, Cheshier SH, and Weissman IL, "The Role of Apoptosis in the Regulation of Hematopoietic Stem Cells: Overexpression of Bcl-2 Increases Both Their Number and Repopulation Potential," *J Exp Med*, 2000, 191(2):253-64.

Ferri KF and Kroemer G, "Mitochondria - The Suicide Organelles," *Bioessays*, 2001, 23(2):111-5.

Fisher MS, Guerra CG, Hickman JR, et al, "Peripheral Blood Lymphocyte Apoptosis. A Clue to the Diagnosis of Acute Infectious Mononucleosis," *Arch Pathol Lab Med*, 1996, 120(10):951-5.

Gupta S, "Molecular Steps of Cell Suicide: An Insight into Immune Senescence," *J Clin Immunol*, 2000, 20(4):229-39.

Jerome KR and Chen Z, "Apoptosis in HL-60 Cells and Topoisomerase I In Vivo," *Arch Pathol Lab Med*, 2000, 124(6):802-5.

Kindzelskii AL and Petty HR, "Ultrasensitive Detection of Hydrogen Peroxide-Mediated DNA Damage After Alkaline Single Cell Gel Electrophoresis Using Occultation Microscopy and TUNEL Labeling," *Mutat Res*, 1999, 426(1):11-22.

Kolb JP, "Mechanisms Involved in the Pro- and Antiapoptotic Role of NO in Human Leukemia," *Leukemia*, 2000, 14(9):1685-94.

Kumari SR, Mendoza-Alvarez H, and Alvarez-Gonzalez R, "Functional Interactions of p53 With Poly(ADP-Ribose) Polymerase (PARP) During Apoptosis Following DNA Damage: Covalent Poly(ADP-Ribosyl)ation of p53 by Exogenous PARP and Noncovalent Binding of p53 to the M(r) 85,000 Proteolytic Fragment," *Cancer Res*, 1998, 58(22):5075-8.

Miller LJ and Marx J, "Apoptosis," *Science*, 1998, 281(5381):1301-26.

Miller DK, "Activation of Apoptosis and Its Inhibition," *Ann N Y Acad Sci*, 1999, 886:132-57.

Mitra D, Kim J, and MacLow C, et al, "Role of Caspases 1 and 3 and Bcl-2-Related Molecules in Endothelial Cell Apoptosis Associated With Thrombotic Microangiopathies," *Am J Hematol*, 1998, 59(4):279-87.

Piro FR, di Gioia CR, Gallo P, et al, "Is Apoptosis a Diagnostic Marker of Acute Myocardial Infarction?," *Arch Pathol Lab Med*, 2000, 124(6):827-31.

Reed JC, "Caspases and Cytokines: Roles in Inflammation and Autoimmunity," *Advances in Immunology*, Volume 73, Dixon FJ, ed, San Diego, CA: Academic Press, 1999, 265-99.

Solary E, Droin N, Bettaieb A, et al, "Positive and Negative Regulation of Apoptotic Pathways by Cytotoxic Agents in Hematological Malignancies," *Leukemia*, 2000, 14(10):1833-49.

Thatte U and Dahanukar S, "Apoptosis: Clinical Relevance and Pharmacological Manipulation," *Drugs*, 1997, 54(4):511-32.

van Wijk IJ, de Hoon AC, Jurhawan R, et al, "Detection of Apoptotic Fetal Cells in Plasma of Pregnant Women," *Clin Chem*, 2000, 46(5):729-31.

Villa P, Kaufmann SH, and Earnshaw WC, "Caspases and Caspase Inhibitors," *Trends Biochem Sci*, 1997, 22(10):388-93.

Winkler JD, ed, "Introduction - Apoptosis in Inflammatory Cells and Diseases," *Apoptosis and Inflammation. Progress in Inflammation Research*, Basal, Switzerland: Birkhäuser Verlag, 1999, 1-6.

Zhang X, Chen J, Davis B, et al, "Hoechst 33342 Induces Apoptosis in HL-60 Cells and Inhibits Topoisomerase I In Vivo," *Arch Pathol Lab Med*, 1999, 123(10):921-7.

♦ **Apoptosis bcl-x** see White Blood Cell Count on page 496

Apt-Downey Test

Related Information
Fetal Hemoglobin on page 431

Synonyms Fetal Hemoglobin Test in Newborn

Abstract The Apt-Downey test (Apt test) uses alkali denaturation of fetal hemoglobin to determine if blood present in the stool of a newborn is the result of swallowing maternal blood or is due to perinatal/neonatal GI hemorrhage.

Specimen Blood stained diaper, grossly bloody (red) stool, or bloody vomitus or mucus

Container Use clean uncontaminated glass or plastic container for specimen or send blood stained diaper.

Causes for Rejection Specimen is not grossly bloody or there is evidence of melena/coffee ground aspirate (vide infra).

Turnaround Time 1-2 hours

Reference Interval Report will provide indication if blood is of maternal or infant origin (adult or fetal hemoglobin).

Use Diagnose swallowed blood syndrome and differentiate this condition from gastrointestinal hemorrhage in the newborn

Limitations The specimen must be grossly bloody, red, not tarry. Test performed in cases of melena or with coffee ground material (denatured blood) may produce a false-positive result as oxyhemoglobin has been converted to hematin and may be falsely read as adult Hb.[1] Visual judgment of color produced by test procedure may lead to error if only a small amount of blood is present. Bilirubin containing meconium and possibly other substances may cause stool color interference. Use of a spectrophotometric-based or high performance liquid chromatography (HPLC) procedure may avoid these problems.[2,3]

Methodology Dissolved blood (one volume of bloody stool or vomitus mixed with five volumes of water) is treated with 1% NaOH, 1-4 mL of hemolysate (alkali denaturation test). The mixture is then centrifuged at 2000 rpm for 1-2 minutes. Fetal hemoglobin is alkali resistant, and the solution will remain pink. Maternal blood will be converted to alkaline hematin in 1-2 minutes, and the solution becomes yellow to dark green-brown. Thus, if the supernatant remains pink (indicative of fetal blood), additional clinical investigation must be pursued.[4] The newborn's blood should be tested concurrently as a control to exclude the possibility of adult Hb in the test infant. Spectrophotometric, as well as, HPLC methods are available offering improved sensitivity/specificity.[2,3]

Additional Information In the swallowed blood syndrome, blood or bloody stools are passed usually on the second or third day of life. The blood may be swallowed during delivery or may be from a fissure of the mother's nipple. This condition must be differentiated from gastrointestinal hemorrhage of the newborn. With early discharge of newborns from the hospital nursery, the problem may present at the emergency department.[5] The test is based on the fact that the infant's blood contains >60% fetal hemoglobin that is alkali resistant. Swallowed blood of maternal origin contains adult hemoglobin which is converted to brownish alkaline hematin on the addition of alkali. A sensitive and accurate spectrophotometric-based procedure has been developed.[2] It should be of special value when the sample is small and/or only a small amount of blood is present in the sample. The ratio of absorbance of oxyhemoglobin before and after the addition of sodium hydroxide is determined spectrophotometrically at 576 nm. This ratio has been found to be linearly proportional to the percentage of Hb F in the specimen.[2] A modified Apt test has been applied to the evaluation of blood obtained at cordocentesis. The test can discriminate fetal from maternal blood in cordocentesis samples. The test has been described as practical, quick, and inexpensive.[6] If mixed fetal/adult blood in the sample is suspect (possible maternal contamination), a greater number (at least 30) metaphases can be counted to assess possible presence of fetal and maternal chromosomes.[6]

Footnotes
1. Apt L and Downey WS, "Melena Neonatorum: The Swallowed Blood Syndrome. A Simple Test for the Differentiation of Adult and Fetal Hemoglobin in Bloody Stools," J Pediatr, 1955, 47(1):6-12.
2. Liu N, Wu AH, and Wong SS, "Improved Quantitative Apt Test for Detecting Fetal Hemoglobin in Bloody Stools of Newborns," Clin Chem, 1993, 39(11 Pt 1):2326-9.
3. Chen D, Wilhite TR, Smith CH, et al, "HPLC Detection of Fetal Blood in Meconium: Improved Sensitivity Compared With Qualitative Methods," Clin Chem, 1998, 44(11):2277-80.
4. Glader BE, "Recognition of Anemia and Red Blood Cell Disorders During Infancy," Perinatal Hematology, Volume 21, Chapter 6, Alter BD, ed, New York, NY: Churchill Livingstone, 1989, 158-9.
5. Guritzky RP and Rudnitsky G, "Bloody Neonatal Diaper," Ann Emerg Med, 1996, 27(5):662-4.
6. Ogur G, Gül D, Özen S, et al, "Application of the Apt Test in Prenatal Diagnosis to Evaluate the Fetal Origin of Blood Obtained by Cordocentesis: Results of 30 Pregnancies," Prenat Diagn, 1997, 17(9):879-82.

References
Apt L, "Melena Neonatorum: An Experimental Study of the Effect of the Oral Administration of Blood on the Stools," J Pediatr, 1955, 47(1):1-5.
Berry R and Perrault J, "Gastrointestinal Bleeding," Pediatric Gastrointestinal Disease: Pathophysiology-Diagnosis-Management, Volume 1, Chapter 21, Walker WA, Durie PR, Hamilton JR, et al, eds, St Louis, MO: CV Mosby Co, 1996, 329.
Lehman CM and Baron B, "Apt Testing," Q & A, Lab Med, 2000, 31(7):365-6.

Squires RH Jr, "Gastrointestinal Bleeding," Pediatr Rev, 1999, 20(3):95-101.

♦ **Ascitic Fluid Analysis** see Body Fluid Analysis, Cell Count on page 408

♦ **ASD Chloroacetate Esterase Stain** see Leukocyte Cytochemistry on page 456

♦ **Atopic Cough** see Eosinophil Smear on page 428

♦ **Auer Rods** see Peripheral Blood: Differential Leukocyte Count on page 464

♦ **Auramine O** see Reticulated Platelet Count on page 480

Autohemolysis Test

Related Information
Anemia Flowchart on page 392
Glucose-6-Phosphate Dehydrogenase, Quantitative, Blood on page 437
Glucose-6-Phosphate Dehydrogenase Screen, Blood on page 438
Glycerol Lysis Test, Acidified, Modified on page 439
Hemosiderin Stain, Urine on page 876
Hypertonic Cryohemolysis Test on page 448
Osmotic Fragility on page 462
Osmotic Fragility, Incubated on page 463
Peripheral Blood: Red Blood Cell Morphology on page 467
Pyruvate Kinase Assay, Erythrocytes on page 474
Red Blood Cell Enzyme Deficiency, Quantitative on page 475

Applies to Pyropoikilocytosis, Hereditary

Abstract Autohemolysis test measures the degree to which patient's red cells lyse without additives, with glucose, and with ATP. Sterile conditions are required. The test has some application to diagnosis of hereditary spherocytosis (HS) and RBC enzyme deficiencies but is tedious to perform and is of limited value. A recently proposed hypertonic cryohemolysis test may be more sensitive, easier, and rapidly performed than the osmotic fragility and autohemolysis tests.[1,2] (See Hypertonic Cryohemolysis Test on page 448.)

Specimen Defibrinated sterile blood

Container Sterile syringe

Collection Using sterile technique, 25 mL of blood is drawn and immediately defibrinated by swirling in a bottle which contains glass beads.

Storage Instructions Specimen is immediately taken to the laboratory, blood defibrinated, and tubes prepared for incubation.

Causes for Rejection Specimen hemolyzed, specimen clotted, specimen more than 5 minutes in transit, specimen contaminated with bacteria (as from a patient with septicemia)

Special Instructions Defibrinated blood must usually be obtained by laboratory personnel.

Reference Interval Percent of red cell lysis at 48 hours: blood alone: 0.2-2.0; blood and 10% glucose: 0-0.9; blood and 0.4M ATP: 0.5-2.5

Use Diagnosis of **hereditary spherocytosis** (HS); detect conditions producing spontaneous hemolysis, particularly hereditary spherocytosis; categorize RBC enzyme deficiencies; evaluate hemolytic anemia

Limitations Large sample of blood required and must be obtained by a trauma-free venipuncture. Test lacks sensitivity and specificity. While this test may still find application in the diagnosis of hereditary spherocytosis, it has largely been supplanted by specific enzyme spot assays for the diagnosis of nonspherocytic congenital hemolytic anemia.

Contraindications Bacteremic patients

Methodology Defibrinated blood from patient and from a control are incubated without additives, with glucose, and with ATP. Subsequently absorbance determinations are used to calculate the percent hemolysis. Procedure is technically laborious. Sterile glassware must be used.

Additional Information The test must always be run with and compared to a control. Test should be run in duplicate to possibly allow detection of reagent inactivity or bacterial contamination of specimen or reagent. It is difficult to maintain sterility but also full activity of ATP. Normal red cells hemolyze minimally when incubated. **G6PD deficient** RBCs (Dacie type I hemolytic anemia) have increased autohemolysis which corrects significantly with glucose or ATP. **Pyruvate kinase deficiency** (Dacie type II hemolytic anemia) has increased autohemolysis which does not correct and may be aggravated with glucose but does correct toward normal with ATP. **Triosephosphate isomerase** deficiency corrects completely with glucose or ATP. **Hereditary spherocytosis** is a type I hemolytic anemia; the addition of glucose usually, but not always, decreases the rate of autohemolysis to about the same proportion as normal blood. Autohemolysis is normal in **hereditary elliptocytosis** but shows increased RBC hemolysis that is not corrected by adding glucose in cases of hereditary pyropoikilocytosis (HPP).[3]

Glucose by itself can induce hemolysis in the autohemolysis test in patients with HS.[4] This may be the result of a direct effect of glucose on already swollen red cells. The problem can be ameliorated by adding NaCl to isotonic conditions.[4] With autoimmune hemolytic anemia, autohemolysis may be increased, but the effect of adding glucose is unpredictable. Autohemolysis is usually normal in cases of paroxysmal nocturnal hemoglobinuria. Hemolytic anemia due to oxidant drugs is usually associated with increased autohemolysis. Generally, failure of glucose to decrease autohemolysis indicates presence of a glycolytic block. Schröter et al have found (Continued)

Autohemolysis Test *(Continued)*

the autohemolysis test, along with the fresh osmotic fragility test, to be highly diagnostic for HS in the newborn.[5] This is especially important since the MCHC may not be elevated in HS in the newborn and because spherocytes are not uncommon in newborns without HS. See table.

Autohemolysis Test

Condition	Incubation at 37°C for 48 Hours	Incubation + 10% Glucose	Incubation + ATP
Normal	0.2%-2.0%	0.0%-0.9%	0.5%-2.5%
G6PD deficiency	3.0%-5.0%	Normal	Normal
Pyruvate kinase deficiency	12%-16%	12%-16%	Normal
Hereditary spherocytosis	12.0%-15.0%	3.0%-5.0%	3.0%-5.0%

The acidified glycerol lysis test, a modification called the "pink test," and the other autohemolysis tests have also been applied to the diagnosis of HS. Histogram of MCHCs, as provided by some automated hematology analyzers, is a sensitive, accurate, and an inexpensive test for establishing the diagnosis in a patient known to have a relative with HS. This approach lends itself to screening other family members if desired.[6]

Footnotes

1. Streichman S, Gescheidt Y, and Tatarsky I, "Hypertonic Cryohemolysis: A Diagnostic Test for Hereditary Spherocytosis," *Am J Hematol*, 1990, 35(2):104-9.
2. Streichman S and Gescheidt Y, "Cryohemolysis for the Detection of Hereditary Spherocytosis: Correlation Studies With Osmotic Fragility and Autohemolysis," *Am J Hematol*, 1998, 58(3):206-12.
3. Cochran DL and Burnside LK, "Detecting and Identifying Hereditary Pyropoikilocytosis," Clinical Pathology Rounds, *Lab Med*, 1999, 30(1):26-9.
4. Streichman S, Cohen S, and Tatarsky J, "Glucose-Induced Hemolysis of Spheric Red Blood Cells in Hereditary Spherocytosis: New Aspects of the Autohemolysis Test," *Am J Clin Pathol*, 1984, 81(1):122-7.
5. Schröter W and Kahsnitz E, "Diagnosis of Hereditary Spherocytosis in Newborn Infants," *J Pediatr*, 1983, 103:460-3.
6. Gallagher PG, Forget BC, and Lux SE, "Disorders of the Erythrocyte Membrane," *Hematology of Infancy and Childhood*, 5th ed, Chapter 16, Nathan DG and Orkin SH, eds, Philadelphia, PA: WB Saunders Co, 1998, 594-6.

References

Dacie JV and Lewis SM, *Practical Haematology*, 8th ed, New York, NY: Churchill Livingstone, 1995, 222-5.

Grimes AJ, Leets I, and Dacie JV, "The Autohemolysis Test: Appraisal of the Method for the Diagnosis of Pyruvate Kinase Deficiency and the Effect of pH and Additives," *Br J Haematol*, 1968, 14:309-22.

♦ **Automated Differential** *see* Peripheral Blood: Differential Leukocyte Count on page 464

Bacteremia Detection, Buffy Coat Micromethod

Related Information

Acid-Fast Stain *on page 550*
Bacterial Antigens, Rapid Detection Methods *on page 562*
Bacterial Culture, Blood *on page 566*
Bacterial Culture, Intravascular Device *on page 572*
Bacterial Culture, Wounds, Bites *on page 579*
Buffy Coat Smear Study of Peripheral Blood *on page 412*
Gram Stain *on page 617*
Histoplasmosis Antibody *on page 635*
Malaria Smear and Tests *on page 458*
Microfilariae, Peripheral Blood Preparation *on page 460*
Peripheral Blood: Differential Leukocyte Count *on page 464*

Synonyms Buffy Coat Method for Detection of Bacteremia; Microbuffy Coat Method for Detection of Bacteremia; Septicemia Detection, Buffy Coat Micromethod

Applies to *Capnocytophaga canimorsus*; QBC Tube (Quantitative Buffy Coat)

Abstract Glass slide smears of buffy coat of blood (relatively concentrated white cells) are stained for microorganisms. The procedure is a simple, quick, cost-efficient method that can assist in establishing the presence of bacteremia but lacks sensitivity and to some extent, specificity. In select populations (eg, premature infants), careful examination of a routine peripheral blood smear may disclose bacteria within neutrophils without preparation of buffy coat smears.[1,2] Meningococci may be found in meningococcemia. *Histoplasma* organisms may be present on smears from patients with acquired immune deficiency syndrome.

Specimen Blood

Container Heparinized capillary tubes

Collection Transport immediately to the laboratory for processing. Blood should be cultured concurrently.

Turnaround Time 1-2 hours

Reference Interval Negative

Possible Panic Range Positive

Use An infrequently used aid in the diagnosis of acute bacterial blood infection, bacteremia; can provide rapid, prompt diagnosis of septicemia in preterm infants;[1] assist in the detection and identification of rarely encountered microorganisms that may cause potentially fatal septicemia.[2]

Limitations There have been conflicting reports on the usefulness of this technique. Occurrence of false-positive and false-negative results may complicate interpretation.

Methodology Gram stain is applied to smear of buffy coat. Wright stain of buffy coat can show histoplasmosis; Ziehl-Neelsen stain can show mycobacteria.

Additional Information A variety of unusual organisms, sites of infection and clinical circumstances may produce septicemia. Attempts to stain buffy coat of blood samples obtained from children with suspected bacteremia using acridine orange (a DNA-intercalating agent) has proven to be of low diagnostic efficiency.[3] The QBC tube (quantitative buffy coat, utilizing tubes precoated with acridine orange) has been considered to have value in the rapid detection of *Wuchereria bancrofti* microfilarial organisms[4] but had low sensitivity and was frequently (40% of specimens) unable to provide species identification when utilized for malaria case identification in the field.[5] The ability to detect and diagnose *Mycobacterium avium-intracellulare* and *Cryptococcus neoformans* using both a stain of the buffy coat and culture of the buffy coat from AIDS patients has been studied. The results showed that culture of buffy coat was much more effective in early diagnosis of those organisms than examining the stained buffy coat smear microscopically.[6] Another group found that use of the buffy coat smear was rapid and specific for detection of *Mycobacterium avium* complex infection in AIDS patients, although lacking in sensitivity (positive predictive value of 100%, negative predictive value of 22%).[7] Buffy coat smears have been employed in the diagnosis of histoplasmosis in AIDS patients[8] and in the detection of *Malassezia* species deep-line catheter-associated sepsis.[9] In select populations (eg, immunosuppressed patients, hyposplenism, presence of indwelling catheters, especially in premature neonates with signs of illness), intracellular bacteria may be identified on study of routine peripheral blood smears without preparation of buffy coat slides.[1,2]

An unusual but clinically significant microbial cause of septicemia is *Capnocytophaga canimorsus*. Septicemia followed by fatal Waterhouse-Friderichsen syndrome may progress rapidly following inoculation by animal bite (especially dog bite). While occurring in immune-impaired patients, apparently healthy individuals are also at risk. The mortality rate may be as high as 28%. The organism is a fastidious, microaerophilic, gram-negative rod and is susceptible to antibiotics, including penicillin.[2]

Study of buffy coat smears may provide detection of organisms prior to development of clinical signs of infection.[1,6]

Footnotes

1. Howard MR and Smith RA, "Early Diagnosis of Septicaemia in Preterm Infants From Examination of Peripheral Blood Films," *Clin Lab Haematol*, 1999, 21(5):365-8.
2. Mirza I, Wolk J, Toth L, et al, "Waterhouse-Fredericksen Syndrome Secondary to *Capnocytophaga canimorsus* Septicemia and Demonstration of Bacteremia by Peripheral Blood Smear: A Case Report and Review of the Literature," *Arch Pathol Lab Med*, 2000, 124(6):859-63.
3. Henrickson KJ, Powell KR, and Ryan DH, "Evaluation of Acridine Orange Stained Buffy Coat Smears for Identification of Bacteremia in Children," *J Pediatr*, 1988, 112(1):65-6.
4. Freedman DO and Berry RS, "Rapid Diagnosis of Bancroftian Filariasis by Acridine Orange Staining of Centrifuged Parasites," *Am J Trop Med Hyg*, 1992, 47(6):787-93.
5. Mak JW, Normaznah Y, and Chiang GL, "Comparison of the Quantitative Buffy Coat Technique With the Conventional Thick Blood Film Technique for Malaria Case Detection in the Field," *Singapore Med J*, 1992, 33(5):452-4.
6. Damsker B and Bottone EJ, "Mycobacteria and Cryptococci Cultured From the Buffy Coat of AIDS Patients Prior to Symptomatology: A Rationale for Early Therapy," *AIDS Res*, 1986, 2(4):343-8.
7. Nussbaum JM, Dealist C, Lewis W, et al, "Rapid Diagnosis by Buffy Coat Smear of Disseminated *Mycobacterium avium* Complex Infection in Patients With Acquired Immunodeficiency Syndrome," *J Clin Microbiol*, 1990, 28(3):631-2.
8. Kurtin PJ, McKinsey DS, Gupta MR, et al, "Histoplasmosis in Patients With Acquired Immunodeficiency Syndrome," *Am J Clin Pathol*, 1990, 93(3):367-72.
9. Marcon MJ and Powell DA, "Human Infections Due to *Malassezia* spp," *Clin Microbiol Rev*, 1992, 5(2):101-19.

References

Fife A, Hill D, Barton C, et al, "Gram Negative Septicaemia Diagnosed on Peripheral Blood Smear Appearances," *J Clin Pathol*, 1994, 47(1):82-4.

Fowlie PW and Schmidt B, "Diagnostic Tests for Bacterial Infection From Birth to 90 Days - A Systematic Review," *Arch Dis Child Fetal Neonatal Ed*, 1998, 78(2):F92-8.

Gomez R and Buescher ES, Images in Clinical Medicine, "Meningococcemia," *N Engl J Med*, 1997, 336(10):707.

Kostiala AA, Jormalainen S, and Kosunen TU, "Detection of Experimental Bacteremia and Fungemia by Examination of Buffy Coat Prepared by a Micromethod," *Am J Clin Pathol*, 1979, 72(3):437-43.

♦ **Band 3 (Anion Transport Protein)** *see* Osmotic Fragility on page 462

Band 4.2, Red Cell Membrane

Related Information

Autohemolysis Test *on page 405*
Osmotic Fragility *on page 462*

Synonyms Pallidin; Protein 4.2

Applies to Ovalocytes; Protein 4.2[Lisboa]; Stomatocytes

Abstract Complete or partial deficiency of band 4.2, a red cell membrane protein, may be responsible for uncompensated hemolysis and in some cases modest anemia.

Specimen Whole blood (to obtain red blood cells)

Container Lavender top (EDTA) tube

Special Instructions This test is likely to be available only on a research/referral basis.

Use Evaluate hemolytic states; assist in determining cause of red cell stomatocytosis, ovalostomatocytosis

Methodology 1% sodium dodecylsulfate (SDS) polyacrylamide gel electrophoresis (PAGE) with Coomassie blue staining, immunoblotting with anti-band 4.2 antibody

Additional Information Band 4.2 is one of a number of red cell membrane proteins involved in some forms of hereditary spherocytosis (HS). It has a molecular weight of 72 kDa (on SDS-PAGE) and accounts for about 5% of total membrane protein. Chromosome location is at 15q15.[1] Isoforms are largely P4.2L (721 amino acids) and P4.2S (691 amino acids). In healthy Japanese, P4.2S has an incidence of about 97%. Congenital band 4.2 abnormalities are of three types: complete deficiency, partial deficiency, and band 4.2 variants (doublet cases). "Complete" deficiency of band 4.2 is responsible for uncompensated hemolysis and in some cases normochromic anemia. Red cell membrane anion transport activity has been reported as increased in HS due to partial deficiency or absence of band 4.2.[2] In HS, the result of spectrin and ankyrin deficiency anion transport was normal, while with HS due to band 3 deficiency anion transport was decreased.[2] Osmotic fragility is increased into the range seen with hereditary spherocytosis but peripheral blood smear shows ovalostomatocytosis with few or absent spherocytes. Protein 4.2[Lisboa], a mutant that results in complete absence of normal protein 4.2 has clinical characteristics of typical HS.[3] Band 4.2 variant cases are associated with stomatocytosis. The red cell morphologic abnormalities persist after splenectomy.

This condition is uncommon, clinically, and apparently largely isolated to the Japanese (estimated incidence of 1% of all red cell membrane disorders in Japan). Acquired band 4.2 deficiency has been reported with biliary obstruction.[4]

A study (electrophoretic pattern of red cell membrane proteins) of centenarians (mean age 103 years) found a significant increase in the integral protein band 4.2 and in the skeletal protein actin.[4] The possibility is raised that extreme longevity is associated with "substantial integrity" of the red blood cell membrane including improved membrane fluidity and a structurally strengthened cell membrane.[5]

Footnotes
1. Najfeld V, Ballard SG, Menninger J, et al, "The Gene for Human Erythrocyte Protein 4.2 Maps to Chromosome 15q15," *Am J Hum Genet*, 1992, 50(1):71-5.
2. De Franceschi L, Olivieri O, Miraglia del Giudice E, et al, "Membrane Cation and Anion Transport Activities in Erythrocytes of Hereditary Spherocytosis: Effects of Different Membrane Protein Defects," *Am J Hematol*, 1997, 55(3):121-8.
3. Hayette S, Dhermy D, dos Santos ME, et al, "A Deletional Frameshift Mutation in Protein 4.2 Gene (Allele 4.2 Lisboa) Associated With Hereditary Hemolytic Anemia," *Blood*, 1995, 85(1):250-6.
4. Iida H, Hasegawa I, and Nozawa Y, "Biochemical Studies on Abnormal Erythrocyte Membranes. Protein Abnormality of Erythrocyte Membrane in Biliary Obstruction," *Biochim Biophys Acta*, 1976, 443(3):394-401.
5. Caprari P, Scuteri A, Salvati AM, et al, "Aging and Red Blood Cell Membrane: A Study of Centenarians," *Exp Gerontol*, 1999, 34(1):47-57.

References
Cohen CM, Dotimas E, and Korsgren C, "Human Erythrocyte Membrane Protein Band 4.2 (Pallidin)," *Semin Hematol*, 1993, 30(2):119-37.

Gallagher PG and Benz EJ JR, "The Erythrocyte Membrane and Cytoskeleton: Structure, Function, and Disorders," *The Molecular Basis of Blood Diseases*, 3rd ed, Chapter 8, Stamatoyannopoulos G, Majerus PW, Perlmutter RM, et al, eds, Philadelphia, PA: WB Saunders Co, 2001, 291, 304.

Gallagher PG and Jarolin P, "Red Cell Membrane Disorders," *Hematology: Basic Principles and Practice*, 3rd ed, Chapter 33, Hoffman R, Benz EJ, Jr, Shattil SJ, et al, eds, Philadelphia, PA: Churchill Livingstone, 2000, 576-610.

Yawata Y, "Band 4.2 Abnormalities in Human Red Cells," *Am J Med Sci*, 1994, 307(3):190-203.

- ◆ **Beckwith-Wiedemann Syndrome** see Viscosity, Blood on page 494

- ◆ **Ber-EP₄** see Flow Cytometry, Overview on page 432

- ◆ **Bernard-Soulier Syndrome** see Platelet Count on page 468

- ◆ **Berry Spot Test** see Inherited Diseases of Metabolism and Cell Structure on page 449

- ◆ **Beta-Glucuronidase Stain** see Leukocyte Cytochemistry on page 456

- ◆ **BeTha Gene 1 Kit** see DNA-Probe Assay for Thalassemia (BeTha Gene Test) on page 423

- ◆ **Biotin-Labeled Red Cell Survival** see ⁵¹Cr Red Cell Survival on page 422

- ◆ **Bleomycin-Induced Pulmonary Fibrosis** see TGF-β, Serum on page 490

- ◆ **Blood Cell Profile** see Complete Blood Count on page 419

- ◆ **Blood Count** see Complete Blood Count on page 419

- ◆ **Blood Smear for Malarial Parasites** see Malaria Smear and Tests on page 458

- ◆ **Blood Smear Morphology** see Peripheral Blood: Red Blood Cell Morphology on page 467

- ◆ **Blood Viscosity** see Viscosity, Blood on page 494

Blood Volume

Related Information
⁵¹Cr Red Cell Survival on page 422
Erythropoietin, Serum on page 169
Hematocrit on page 441
Peripheral Blood: Red Blood Cell Morphology on page 467
Phlebotomy, Therapeutic on page 849
Red Blood Cell Indices on page 477
Red Cell Mass on page 478

Synonyms Blood Volume, Total; Plasma/Blood Volume

Applies to Plasma Volume Measurement; Red Cell Volume

Test Includes Total blood volume, red cell mass, and plasma volume, measured or derived and with measured values reported with predicted values for comparison

Abstract This procedure measures the patient's total circulating volume of blood and/or fractions (eg, red cell mass) of the blood volume. A component of the blood (eg, albumin) is labeled with a dye (colored) or radioisotope. The dilution of the label is inversely proportional to the size (volume) of the compartment in which it has been diluted. Recently developed modifications of nonradioactive label methods employ carbon monoxide (CO), hydroxyethyl starch, or indocyanine green dye (ICG). These procedures may prove useful in bedside, critical care, or intraoperative situations.[1,2,3] Blood volume study may be an invaluable contribution to some clinical situations (eg, polycythemia, acute blood loss) in which determination of Hb, a concentration, or Hct, a fraction, could be misleading.

Patient Preparation Patient should have all RIA blood work performed, at least drawn, prior to injection of any radioactive material. Technologist will administer injected dose to patient and withdraw blood samples after the appropriate interval (usually 10 minutes). Patient must be available, since timing is important.

Specimen Whole blood; the "seminoninvasive" CO and ICG methods do not require collection of postlabeling blood samples.

Container Method dependent. For ⁵¹Cr-labeled red cell methods, ACD-NIH or Strumia's ACD solution, ratio of one part ACD to five parts blood. EDTA anticoagulated blood may be used, but excess EDTA must be avoided. EDTA causes shrinkage of red cells. The resultant red cell volume is too low unless EDTA is used in a concentration of 1.5 ±0.25 mg/mL of blood. Samples of blood for ¹²⁵I- or ¹³¹I-labeled albumin plasma volume methods may be collected in heparinized syringe.

Sampling Time The laboratory will need to obtain postdose blood samples at specific times. The patient will need to be available for such sampling (critical to successful completion of the test).

Causes for Rejection Patient with recent radioisotope administration (consult laboratory), patient not available for postdose blood sampling

Turnaround Time Procedure/method dependent, varying from 10 minutes to 12 hours; most isotope dilution methods will require 2-6 hours for earliest availability of results, unsatisfactory for many critical care applications.

Reference Interval Normal values are method dependent. Blood volume varies with body habitus, age, sex, weight, and height. There is special correlation with body surface area. As the amount of blood in fat is about 2/35 that of lean tissue, the normal value for an obese individual is less than that for a lean person of same weight. See Red Cell Mass on page 478 for application of biologic impedance measuring devices to normalizing total RBC volume in relation to body fat content. Careful clinical assessment as to degree of obesity, edema, etc, must be a part of the determination of "normal." Difficulties with determination of predicted (calculated) blood volume parameters (using weight, height, and in particular, body surface area) have limited use of these studies in some, especially acute situations.

Estimated Blood Volumes

Age	Plasma Volume (mL/kg) (PV)	Red Cell Mass (mL/kg) (RCM)	Total Blood Volume (mL/kg)	
			From PV	From RCM
Newborns	41.3	43.1	82.1	86.1
	46		78	84.7
1-7 d	51-54	37.9	82-86	77.8
1-12 mo	46.1	25.5	78.1	72.8
1-3 y	44.4	24.9	73.8	69.1
	47.2		81.8	
4-6 y	48.5	25.5	80.0	67.5
	49.6		85.6	
7-9 y	52.2	24.3	87.6	67.5
	49.0		86.1	
10-12 y	51.9	26.3	87.6	67.4
	46.2		83.2	
13-15 y	51.2		88.3	
16-18 y	50.1		90.2	
Adults	39-44	25-30	68-88	55-75

Adapted from Price DC and Ries C, *Nuclear Medicine in Clinical Pediatrics*, Handmaker H and Lowenstein JM, eds, New York, NY: Society of Nuclear Medicine, 1975, 279.

(Continued)

Blood Volume *(Continued)*

Use Differentiate relative from absolute **polycythemia**. Polycythemia may be defined as increased red cells and, in a sense, is the opposite of anemia. Polycythemia is usually considered when hemoglobin is 18 g/dL, hematocrit is 52%, and RBC count is 6 million/mm³. These values do not tell whether the red cell mass is increased or the plasma volume is decreased. Relative polycythemias are caused by decreased plasma volumes such as in burns, severe sweating, shock, dehydration, or any other cause of hemoconcentration. Absolute polycythemia occurs when red cell mass is increased. This can be because of increased erythropoietin in secondary polycythemia (appropriate or inappropriate) or occurs spontaneously as in polycythemia vera, one of the myeloproliferative syndromes in which splenomegaly is usually present.

Limitations Any *in vivo* isotope test may affect radioisotope determined blood volume (eg, bone scans, liver scans, brain scans). Check with the laboratory to see if blood volume determination would be valid. Cost of radioisotope label has increased substantially in recent years. A decline in orders for blood volume determination has occurred over the past two decades relating to technical variations, accuracy concerns, cumulative radiation exposure, and in part to FDA related-withdrawal of some partially automated analytic systems. A dependable, accurate, "double tag" procedure (simultaneous use of ¹²⁵I albumin and ⁵¹Cr-labeled RBCs) is the preferred method but is technically rigorous and time consuming compared to other clinical laboratory procedures. Methods in which the red cell volume or plasma volume are measured and total blood volume is calculated using the packed cell volume are subject to error.

Contraindications Patient actively bleeding, combative, or with situations leading to loss of capillary vascular integrity or "third space" effects

Methodology General concept of dilution technique using ¹²⁵I- or ¹³¹I-tagged albumin, Evans blue, or indocyanine green dye and/or ⁵¹Cr-tagged red blood cells. Technetium (Tc-99m) or indium (¹¹³ᵐIn or ¹¹¹In) labeled red cells have also been used for red cell volume measurements. The isotope based methods, if carefully performed, are most likely to provide reliable and clinically useful results. These methods, however, are technically demanding, time consuming, and require specifically trained personnel. They are costly, with expensive reagents and equipment. They may not be repeatable at frequent intervals because of concerns over the cumulative effects of radiation exposure. These concerns have stimulated interest in the development of rapid and reliable procedures for blood volume determination, in particular in emergency/critical care environments in which hypovolemia (resulting from post-traumatic hemorrhage, intraoperative blood loss, or internal bleeding) may be life threatening.

A number of methods have recently been described and recommended for use, they generally represent significant modifications of, or improvements in, older procedures. The carbon monoxide (CO) method was first suggested in the late 1800s. More recently, the CO method used with an improved delivery system, was studied in both critically ill humans as well as in pigs (for repeatability). It was concluded that the test was of potential bedside use for estimating blood volume and circulating hemoglobin mass.[1] The use of hydroxyethyl starch has been studied. This technique requires hemolysis of starch by acid and heat (boiling water bath).[2] Of particular interest, indocyanine green (ICG) dye measured with pulse-spectrophotometry[3,4] (pulse dye densitometry[5]) may find application in critical care monitoring.[6] The method is noninvasive (after the injection of ICG dye) and uses a device that detects pulsatile changes of tissue optical density of a nostril or finger scanned by a probe that emits infrared wavelengths at 805 and 890 nm. A near-infrared spectroscopy-based method has been used to determine cerebral blood volume in preterm infants in the neonatal intensive care setting.[7] These new blood volume methods have quite limited availability. They are generally of research status and study sample sizes are small.

Additional Information Hb, Hct, or RBC count determinations are concentration expressed parameters and may be misleading when the clinical situation requires assessment of the absolute volume of blood or one of its components. Acute shift in body fluids between the intravascular and extravascular spaces as may occur with heart failure, shock, and third space pooling are examples of such misleading circumstances.

There is an increase in plasma volume in the second to last trimester of pregnancy, toxemia of pregnancy, and in uremia. As red cell volume shows proportionally less rise (or may decrease), there is an element of dilutional anemia. On the basis of independent measure of red cells using ⁵³Cr, a stable, nonradioactive isotope and Evans blue determination of plasma volume ("double tag" study), blood volume was decreased in patients with pre-eclampsia (as compared with normotensive subjects) but was normal in patients with gestational hypertension.[8]

The plasma volume is decreased by some 2 mL/kg as the result of positive/prolonged bedrest. Blood volume may be as much as 16% higher in the evening than in the morning. Blood volume is decreased in cases of subarachnoid hemorrhage.[9] There is evidence that total blood volume (TBV) decreases with age in healthy men of comparable size and levels of physical activity.[10] In postmenopausal women, TBV is decreased in healthy but sedentary subjects but maintained in physically active females.[11] Hormone replacement therapy (in postmenopausal women) had no effect on TBV.[11]

See Red Cell Mass *on page 478*.

See references for further information and tables of predicted normal blood volumes.

Footnotes

1. Dingley J, Foex BA, Swartz M, et al, "Blood Volume Determination by the Carbon Monoxide Method Using a New Delivery System: Accuracy in Critically Ill Humans and Precision in an Animal Model," *Crit Care Med*, 1999, 27(11):2435-41.
2. Tschaikowsky K, Meisner M, Durst R, et al, "Blood Volume Determination Using Hydroxyethyl Starch: A Rapid and Simple Intravenous Injection Method," *Crit Care Med*, 1997, 25(4):599-606.
3. He YL, Tanigami H, Ueyama H, et al, "Measurement of Blood Volume Using Indocyanine Green Measured With Pulse-Spectrophotometry: Its Reproducibility and Reliability," *Crit Care Med*, 1998, 26(8):1446-51.
4. Haruna M, Kumon K, Yahagi N, et al, "Blood Volume Measurement at the Bedside Using ICG Pulse Spectrophotometry," *Anesthesiology*, 1998, 89(6):1322-8.
5. Iijima T, Iwao Y, and Sankawa H, "Circulating Blood Volume Measured by Pulse Dye-Densitometry: Comparison With (131)I-HSA Analysis," *Anesthesiology*, 1998, 89(6):1329-35.
6. Barker SJ, "Blood Volume Measurement: The Next Intraoperative Monitor?" *Anesthesiology*, 1998, 89(6):1310-2.
7. Adcock LM, Wafelman LS, Hegemier S, et al, "Neonatal Intensive Care Applications of Near-Infrared Spectroscopy," *Clin Perinatol*, 1999, 26(4):893-903.
8. Silver HM, Seebeck M, and Carlson R, "Comparison of Total Blood Volume in Normal, Pre-eclamptic, and Nonproteinuric Gestational Hypertensive Pregnancy by Simultaneous Measurement of Red Blood Cell and Plasma Volumes," *Am J Obstet Gynecol*, 1998, 179(1):87-93.
9. Sato K, Karibe H, and Yoshimoto T, "Circulating Blood Volume in Patients With Subarachnoid Hemorrhage," *Acta Neurochir*, 1999, 141(10):1069-73.
10. Davy KP and Seals DR, "Total Blood Volume in Healthy Young and Older Men," *J Appl Physiol*, 1994, 76(5):2059-62.
11. Jones PP, Davy KP, DeSouza CA, et al, "Absence of Age-Related Decline in Total Blood Volume in Physically Active Females," *Am J Physiol*, 1997, 272(6 Pt 2):H2534-40.

References

Berlin NI and Lewis SM, "Measurement of Total RBC Volume Relative to Lean Body Mass for Diagnosis of Polycythemia," *Am J Clin Pathol*, 2000, 114(6):922-6.
Dacie JV and Lewis SM, "Blood Volume," *Practical Haematology*, 8th ed, Chapter 21, New York, NY: Churchill Livingstone, 1995, 391-7.
Kisch H, Leucht S, Lichtwarck-Aschoff M, et al, "Accuracy and Reproducibility of the Measurement of Actively Circulating Blood Volume With an Integrated Fiberoptic Monitoring System," *Crit Care Med*, 1995, 23(5):885-93.
Manaloor EJ, Neiman RS, Heilman DK, et al, "Immunohistochemistry Can Be Used to Subtype Acute Myeloid Leukemia in Routinely Processed Bone Marrow Biopsy Specimens. Comparison With Flow Cytometry," *Am J Clin Pathol*, 2000, 113(6):814-22.
Pollycove M and Tono M, "Blood Volume," *Diagnostic Nuclear Medicine*, 3rd ed, Volume 2, Chapter 42, Sandler MP, Coleman RE, Wackers FJT, et al, eds, Baltimore, MD: Lippincott Williams & Wilkins, 1996, 827-34.
"Recommended Methods for Measurement of Red-Cell and Plasma Volume: International Committee for Standardization in Haematology," *J Nucl Med*, 1980, 21(8):793-800.
Thompson JK, Fogi-Anderson N, Bulow K, et al, "Blood and Plasma Volumes Determined by Carbon Monoxide Gas, ⁹⁹ᵐTc-Labeled Erythrocytes, ¹²⁵I-Albumin and the T 1824 Technique," *Scand J Clin Lab Invest*, 1999, 51(2):185-90.

♦ **Blood Volume, Total** *see* Blood Volume *on page 407*

Body Fluid Analysis, Cell Count

Related Information

Applies to Ascitic Fluid Analysis; Cell Count Ratio; Cyst Fluid Analysis; Joint Fluid Analysis; Paracentesis Fluid Analysis; Pericardial Fluid Analysis; Peritoneal Fluid Analysis; Peritoneal Lavage, Diagnostic; Pleural Fluid Analysis; Serous Fluid Analysis; Thoracentesis Fluid Analysis

Test Includes Total WBC count and differential; total RBC count; multiple additional tests (eg, protein, sugar, LD, amylase) are commonly done on body fluids.

Abstract Benign and/or malignant cells, crystals, bacteria, and various forms of particulate material can be analyzed by cell counting techniques (manual/automated) and by microscopic study of stained slides bearing smears from unprocessed fluid or centrifuged sediment from fluid. Cytocentrifuge preparations, as available from the laboratory, are strongly recommended (in particular for cerebrospinal fluid) in order to obtain the best preservation of cell morphology.

Patient Preparation Aseptic preparation for aspiration

Specimen Body fluid (ie, pleural fluid, synovial fluid, cyst fluid, paracentesis fluid, pericardial fluid, lavage fluid, etc)

Container Glass test tube or large glass container

Collection Add heparin to specimen.

Storage Instructions Specimen should be brought directly to the laboratory after collection. Cell studies should be done within 1 hour of collection. If complement level is measured (synovial fluid), test immediately or freeze specimen at -70°C.

Causes for Rejection Clotted specimen, inadequate volume of specimen for the procedures requested

Special Instructions Requisition must state site of origin. Commonly cytologic, microbiologic and chemical examinations are also helpful.

Reference Interval See table. Glucose and amylase levels in fluids approximate whole blood levels. A pleural fluid LD to serum LD ratio >0.6 suggests exudate. In pleural fluids, total protein >3.0 g/dL indicates exudate, protein <3.0 g/dL indicates transudate. For peritoneal fluid, the cutoff point is lower, 2.0-2.5. Pericardial fluids have no established cutoff point in differentiating transudates from exudates.

Expected Normal Findings – Body Fluids

Type of Fluid	Appearance	Amount (mL)	Cells	Glucose	Total Protein
Pleural	Clear, colorless to pale yellow	1-10	<1000/mm³ <25% polys 0 RBC	Approximates WB glucose	
Peritoneal	Clear, colorless to pale yellow	<100	<500/mm³ <25% polys <100,000 RBC/mm³		
Pericardial	Clear, colorless to pale yellow	20-25	<500 WBC/mm³ <25% polys 0 RBC		
Synovial	No crystals	<4	<200 WBC/mm³ <25% polys	Blood/synovial difference <10 mg/dL	1.0-3.0 g/dL

Use Evaluate body fluids; differential diagnosis of exudate, transudate

Methodology Cells are usually counted/studied using manual methods (hemocytometer). Automated (electronic) methods may be used rarely, under certain conditions, if the fluid specimen is grossly purulent or bloody. Specimen should be observed macroscopically and on initial smear for presence of fibrin clots, cell aggregates, crystals, etc, that might occlude apertures of automated counters. Stained smears of fluid are prepared and/or sediment is obtained from centrifuged fluid. A variety of stains can be applied, including Wright/Giemsa type stains for study of white cell morphology/parasites, Papanicolaou-stained smears for identification and study of tumor cells, Gram stain for bacterial microorganisms, acid-fast stain for mycobacterial organisms, Gomori methenamine silver (GMS), periodic acid Schiff (PAS), and other stains for fungal microorganisms.

Optimal processing is achieved with cytocentrifuge concentration and slide preparation, in particular, for cell studies of cerebrospinal fluid.[1]

For best results, fresh unfixed specimens should be specially processed as indicated including washing cells of serous fluids, liquefaction of synovial fluids with hyaluronidase, agitation of clots (to free up cells for study), and use of albumin.[1] Use of a standardized dilution protocol and a "reagent blank" (to detect bacterial contamination of supposedly sterile reagents) is also recommended.

Additional Information Cultures, cytology, and chemical studies usually must be requested separately and should have a separate specimen if possible. See Body Fluid Chemical Analysis on page 123; Body Fluid Glucose on page 124; Body Fluid Amylase on page 122; Body Fluid pH on page 125; and Body Cavity Fluid Cytology on page 372. Elevated lymphocytes can be associated with congestive heart failure (pleural fluid), tuberculosis, tumors, lymphomas, lymphatic leukemia, rheumatoid arthritis, and postpneumonic effusions. Elevated polymorphonuclear leukocytes are associated with acute infectious processes (ie, bacterial inflammation, eg, bacterial peritonitis). The difference between uninfected ascitic fluid and that of bacterial peritonitis is reported, for example, as WBC count of 122/mm³ vs 2686/mm³. PMN count provides the highest sensitivity; its reliability is enhanced with pH (low with peritonitis, <7.35).[2] Elevated eosinophils are associated with tumors, infarcts, SLE, rheumatoid arthritis, rheumatic fever, parasites, postpneumonic effusions, pneumothorax, or may have no clinical significance. The level of eosinophil granule proteins can be determined in body fluids and may serve as a marker for previously lysed eosinophils (see Eosinophil Granule Proteins on page 426). Elevated plasma cells can be associated with lymphoma, especially Hodgkin disease or with chronic inflammation. Sometimes atypical plasma cells are seen in the presence of multiple myeloma. A low glucose level supports diagnosis of rheumatoid effusion. Creatinine level distinguishes ascitic collection from tap of an overdistended bladder.

Small pleural effusions occur in the immediate postoperative period in some 50% of coronary artery bypass graft (CABG) patients.[3] These usually resolve spontaneously without incident. A small number (<1%) of patients, however, develop moderate to large, occasionally symptomatic effusions, that may not reach maximum size for weeks or months.[4] While such large effusions may be the result of congestive heart failure, pericarditis, or pulmonary embolus, >50% of such fluid accumulations are unexplained. They are usually left-sided and ~50% are bloody, and as might be expected, are associated with higher lactic acid dehydrogenase levels than are nonbloody fluids.[4]

Diagnostic peritoneal lavage (DPL) was introduced in 1965.[5] Classic criteria for a positive DPL have been considered as >100,000 red blood cells (RBC)/mm³, >500 white blood cells (WBC)/mm³, serum amylase >175 IU, or particulate material in the lavage return (with use of 1000 mL of lactated Ringer's solution as lavage fluid). DPL has been considered negative if there are <50,000 RBC/mm³, <100 WBC/mm³, and amylase activity is <75 IU.[6] With positive findings, laparotomy was usually performed. With the advent of noninvasive imaging (eg, computed tomography, ultrasonography) the role (and use) of DPL has been reduced. When imaging is unavailable or results are inconclusive, DPL studies with new diagnostic criteria may assist in determination of the need for laparotomy. In a series of 429 DPLs performed for the question of peritoneal penetration as a result of gunshot wound to the abdomen with threshold criterion of 10,000 red blood cells/mm³, DPL was sensitive (99%), specific (98%), and accurate (98%).[7] In a study of 250 patients with blunt abdominal trauma, classic criteria were used with addition of WBC ≥ RBC/150 (when DPL was positive for hemoperitoneum) for determination of intestinal injury. Diagnostic sensitivity was 97% with specificity of 99% when DPL was performed within the time frame of 3-18 hours after trauma.[8] A **"cell count ratio"** defined as the ratio between WBC count and RBC count of lavage fluid divided by the ratio of the same counts (WBC/RBC) in peripheral blood was applied to 212 patients who had a positive DPL (by classic criteria). A cell count ratio ≥1 predicted hollow organ perforation with a specificity of 97% and sensitivity of 100%.[6] A low (<1) cell count ratio can contribute to more confident nonoperative management. See graphic.

Management of Blunt Abdominal Injury

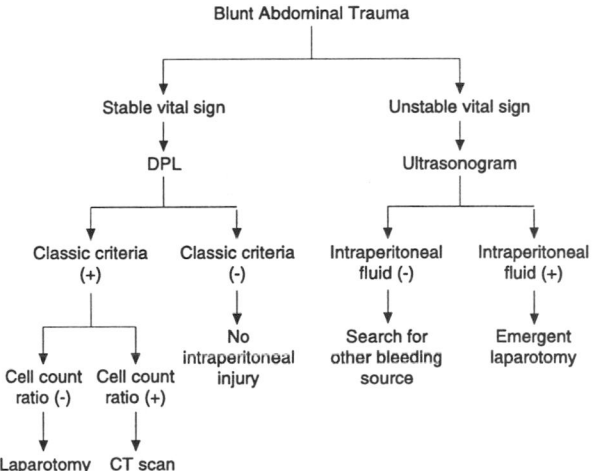

Adapted from Fang JF, Chen RJ, and Lin BC, "Cell Count Ratio: New Criterion of Diagnostic Peritoneal Lavage for Detection of Hollow Organ Perforation," J Trauma, 1998, 45(3):540-4.

A rare cause of ascites and pleural effusion is extramedullary hematopoiesis. A recent report of this condition in a 33-year old woman who had myelofibrosis (agnogenic myeloid metaplasia) for 14 years serves as a reminder that myelofibrosis with extramedullary hematopoiesis can occur at a relatively young age. Examination of peritoneal fluid revealed megakaryocytes, normoblasts, and immature granulocytes.[9]

An unfortunately not so rare cause of serous and/or bloody effusions is malignancy, usually malignant lymphoma or metastatic carcinoma, or less commonly sarcoma or malignant mesothelioma. The malignancy may be an unexpected discovery on study of stained smears of body cavity fluid. Initially or subsequently, cytocentrifuge slide preparations with Wright-Giemsa stain, provide an excellent basis for study and identification of the malignant cell population.[1,10] See table on following page for Wright-Giemsa differential cytodiagnostic features (benign vs malignant conditions) and original article[10] for an excellent set of color photomicrographs illustrating each of these cytologic characteristics.

A cost-efficient management of body fluid clinical laboratory testing is recommended by Albright et al with the description of "transport and rapid accessioning for additional procedures," a two-tiered analytic system.[11] Physician understanding and logistic considerations for standardized (Continued)

Body Fluid Analysis, Cell Count *(Continued)*

handling are involved. Storage of and access to body fluid samples for subsequent testing after limited initial study are the cornerstone of this concept. Cell count, however, must be performed as soon as possible to avoid distortions produced by storage. Microbiologic study and cytology must also receive timely consideration: see Related Information, *vide supra*.

Benign vs Malignant Cell Characteristics
Wright-Giemsa Stained Slides
(cytocentrifuge preparations preferred)

	Malignant (generally epithelial)	Mesothelial Cells – Benign	Ependymal Lining Cells
General Characteristics			
Site of origin	Variable	Lining of body cavities (pleural, pericardial, peritoneal)	Ependymal lining of ventricular spaces
Size	Variable, usually large	Large, small if cells are unstimulated	
Cell groupings	Clusters with morula-like or 3-D appearance, cell overlap, outer border continuous	May occur in loose clusters with "windows" between cells	Choroid cells – single or in clusters
Nuclear Characteristics			
Shape	Irregular	Oval to bean shape	Round to oval
Size	Large	Less than 1/2 to 2/3 of size of cell	
Contour	Irregular	Regular	Regular
Membrane	Indistinct, jagged	Prominent, distinct	Prominent, distinct
Chromatin	Uncondensed, uneven/clumped, parachromatin, spaces prominent	Uniform, smooth, parachromatin, spaces minimal may be fine, uncondensed	
Molding	Important feature of malignancy when present	Rare to absent	
Nuclear:cytoplasmic ratio (N:C ratio)	High	Small to moderate	Moderate
Multinuclearity	May be present, nuclei dissimilar	May be present, nuclei similar in size and shape	Very rare
Mitosis	May be numerous irregular shapes, displaced chromosomes and fragments	Occasional, circumscribed, symmetric	Uncommon
Nucleoli	Common, large, angulated	Small to medium if present	
General	Degenerative changes with peripheral blebs		
Cytoplasmic Characteristics			
Color			Amphophilic (pink-blue)
Granules	Bizarre granules, inclusions may be present	Absent	
Vacuoles	May be large, smooth well-defined border, may coalesce, common with adenocarcinoma, may produce "signet" cells	Small, ground glass-like, cluster in perinuclear location, medium size, seen at periphery, "pseudovacuoles"	
Microvilli	Usually absent	Absent	Present on choroid cells

Adapted from Cornbleet PJ, "Wright-Giemsa Cytology of Body Fluids: Criteria for Identification of Malignant Cells," *Lab Medicine*, 1998, 29(1):26-31.

Footnotes

1. Jones CD and Cornbleet PJ, "Wright-Giemsa Cytology of Body Fluids," *Lab Med*, 1997, 28(11):713-6.
2. Garcia-Tsao G, Conn HO, and Lerner E, "The Diagnosis of Bacterial Peritonitis: Comparison of pH, Lactate Concentration and Leukocyte Count," *Hepatology*, 1985, 5(1):91-6.
3. Daganou M, Dimopoulou I, Michalopoulos N, et al, "Respiratory Complications After Coronary Artery Bypass Surgery With Unilateral or Bilateral Internal Mammary Artery Grafting," *Chest*, 1998, 113(5):1285-9.
4. Light RW, Rogers JT, Cheng DS, et al, "Large Pleural Effusions Occurring After Coronary Artery Bypass Grafting," *Ann Intern Med*, 1999, 130(11):891-6.
5. Root HD, Hauser CW, McKinley CR, et al, "Diagnostic Peritoneal Lavage," *Surgery*, 1965, 57(5):633-7.
6. Fang JF, Chen RJ, and Lin BC, "Cell Count Ratio: New Criterion of Diagnostic Peritoneal Lavage for Detection of Hollow Organ Perforation," *J Trauma*, 1998, 45(3):540-4.

7. Nagy KK, Krosner SM, Joseph KT, et al, "A Method of Determining Peritoneal Penetration in Gunshot Wounds to the Abdomen," *J Trauma*, 1997, 43(2):242-6.
8. Otomo Y, Henmi H, Mashiko K, et al, "New Diagnostic Peritoneal Lavage Criteria for Diagnosis of Intestinal Injury," *J Trauma*, 1998, 44(6):991-9.
9. Oren I, Goldman A, Haddad N, et al, "Ascites and Pleural Effusion Secondary to Extramedullary Hematopoiesis," *Am J Med Sci*, 1999, 318(4):286-8.
10. Cornbleet PJ, "Wright-Giemsa Cytology of Body Fluids: Criteria for Identification of Malignant Cells," *Lab Med*, 1998, 29(1):26-31.
11. Albright RE Jr, Christenson RH, Habig RL, et al, "Cerebrospinal Fluid (CSF) TRAP: A Method to Improve CSF Laboratory Efficiency," *Am J Clin Pathol*, 1988, 90(6):707-10.

References

Albright RE Jr, "Management of Cerebrospinal Fluid and Other Body Fluids," *Practical Laboratory Hematology*, Chapter 13, Koepke JA, ed, New York, NY: Churchill Livingstone, 1991, 295-310.

Gall JJ, "Laboratory Evaluation of Body Fluids," *Clinical Hematology: Principles, Procedures, Correlations*, 2nd ed, Chapter 30, Stiene-Martin EA, Lotspeich-Steininger CA, and Koepke JA, eds, Philadelphia, PA: Lippincott-Raven, 1998, 400-14.

Judkins SW and Cornbleet PJ, "Synovial Fluid Crystal Analysis," *Lab Med*, 1997, 28(12):774-9.

Kjeldsberg CR and Knight JA, *Body Fluids - Laboratory Examination of Amniotic, Cerebrospinal, Seminal, Serous, and Synovial Fluids*, 3rd ed, Chicago, IL: ASCP Press, American Society of Clinical Pathologists, 1993, 159-253, 265-301.

Bone Marrow

Related Information

Anemia Flowchart *on page 392*
Bacterial Culture, Biopsy or Body Fluid *on page 565*
Breakpoint Cluster Region Rearrangement in CML *on page 721*
Buffy Coat Smear Study of Peripheral Blood *on page 412*
Cerebrospinal Fluid Cytology *on page 376*
Chorionic Villus Sampling, Chromosome and Genetic Abnormality Analysis *on page 361*
Chromosomal Translocations, Molecular Detection *on page 723*
Chromosome Analysis, Blood *on page 361*
Chromosome Analysis, Bone Marrow *on page 362*
Cobalamin, Serum *on page 150*
Complete Blood Count *on page 419*
Erythropoietin Receptor *on page 169*
Fanconi Anemia, Chromosome Breakage Study *on page 365*
Flow Cytometry, Overview *on page 432*
Fluorescence *In Situ* Hybridization *on page 367*
Fungal Culture, Biopsy or Body Fluid *on page 610*
Gene Rearrangement for Leukemia and Lymphoma *on page 725*
Immunofixation Electrophoresis, Serum or Urine *on page 530*
Immunoperoxidase Procedures *on page 60*
Immunophenotypic Analysis of Tissues by Flow Cytometry *on page 62*
Iron Stain, Bone Marrow *on page 452*
Leishmaniasis Serology *on page 647*
Leukocyte Alkaline Phosphatase *on page 455*
Leukocyte Cytochemistry *on page 456*
Lymph Node Biopsy *on page 67*
Mycobacterial Culture, Biopsy or Body Fluid *on page 655*
Parvovirus B19 Serology *on page 669*
Peripheral Blood: Differential Leukocyte Count *on page 464*
Polymerase Chain Reaction *on page 713*
Promyelocytic Leukemia Assay *on page 474*
Q Fever Serology *on page 673*
Schilling Test *on page 483*
Siderocyte Stain *on page 487*
Terminal Deoxynucleotidyl Transferase *on page 489*
Viral Culture *on page 689*
Viral Culture, Tissue *on page 695*
White Blood Cell Count *on page 496*

Test Includes H&E stain, Wright or Wright/Giemsa stain, iron stain, cytochemistry, special histochemistry, and immunohistochemistry stains as indicated for the particular disorders/indications under investigation. Always consider obtaining samples for flow cytometry, gene rearrangement studies, and cytogenetics when obtaining a bone marrow. If these are not initially obtained, it is often necessary to do a repeat bone marrow to obtain these additional studies to better clarify diagnoses. In many situations, bone marrow samples in liquid phase (heparinized test tube) can be held prior to sending them for these special studies, and a decision can be made to submit for specific studies after an initial inspection of a stained aspirate slide is made. Bone marrow studies are done in concert with obtaining/examining the peripheral blood smear and obtaining a bone marrow clot section from the aspirated bone marrow material.

Abstract Use a 20 cc plastic syringe for the **bone marrow aspiration**. A number of disposable bone marrow aspiration kits are now available. Sample is obtained from the bone marrow cavity using a bone marrow aspiration needle. A needle guard is used when obtaining sample from the sternum. **Bone marrow biopsy** is obtained using a specialized needle (eg, Jamshidi needle). There are a number of different types of disposable biopsy needles available. Samples are obtained to examine the cellularity of the various normal marrow constituents, for morphological changes in the normal populations of bone marrow cells, to identify and study malignant infiltrates, and to determine the presence of infections, cytogenetic abnormalities, and status of iron stores. There are many other applications.

Patient Preparation Explain procedure and pain potential to the patient. Obtain informed consent from the patient or the patient's guardian. Use local anesthetic, 1% lidocaine. Systemic control of pain (conscious sedation) may be required (eg, Demerol® 25-50 mg I.V. or oral and Valium® 5-10 mg oral or Versed®). If systemic pain control is administered, provide for monitoring of vital signs, oxygen saturation, and facilities to administer oxygen. The procedure is performed using aseptic technique, typically from the posterior superior iliac crest or the sternum. **Note:** Marrow biopsy is never attempted from the sternum.

Aftercare Apply septic barrier/cover to the needle entry site for 24 hours. Instruct the patient not to bathe for 24 hours. If conscious sedation is utilized, ensure that the patient's condition is fully stable prior to releasing patient from the facility where bone marrow was obtained.

Specimen Bone marrow aspirate obtained for making coverslip or glass slide preparations. The smearing technique and rapid handling of the aspirated marrow material is crucial to obtain quality preparations, in view of the tendency of the marrow to clot rapidly. Only 1 mL of aspirated marrow is required for the production of slide preparations. Additional aspirated marrow samples may be obtained for flow cytometry, cytogenetic studies, or for obtaining bacterial, fungal, virology cultures (~5 mL in heparinized test tube). Obtain a 1 mL sample for making slides prior to obtaining larger aspiration volumes for the cytogenetic, flow cytometry, and culture samples.

Container Glass coverslips or slides, pipette for handling/transferring sample to glass coverslip or slide, petri dish for distribution of aspirated material, heparinized tubes for additional studies as noted above; microbiology Isolator™ tubes for culture studies; tubes containing Zenker solution or formalin for clot sections and biopsy samples.

Special Instructions Generally, marrow procedures require advanced planning/scheduling in order to obtain/coordinate other special studies (eg, flow cytometric studies, cytogenetics, gene rearrangement studies, and *in situ* hybridization studies).

Reference Interval Normal ranges for infants and adults have been determined.[1,2]

Use Evaluation of cellularity, morphology of erythroid, myeloid, lymphoid monocytic/macrophage precursors and megakaryocytes; maturation of the precursors of each of these cell lines; and erythroid:myeloid ratio. Establish decrease or increase in any of these cell lines. Abnormal representation/infiltration of the bone marrow by any of these cell lines or cells foreign to the bone marrow. Access presence of abnormal reticulin or myelofibrosis. Quantify iron status by Perl's stain and establish presence/absence of ring sideroblasts. Examine for the presence of infectious organisms in the bone marrow (eg, histoplasmosis, various mycobacteria species, cytomegalovirus, parvovirus inclusions involving erythroid precursors). In general, a bone marrow examination can be omitted in uncomplicated iron deficiency anemia when serum ferritin levels are reduced below 20 µg/L, serum transferrin receptor levels are raised above normal, or the transferrin level/TIBC is raised along with concomitant reduction in the fasting serum iron level <55 mg/dL and resultant transferrin saturation is reduced to <18%. (See the Anemia Flowchart in the Introduction to this chapter.) Repetitive bone marrow examinations are valuable for assessment of response to therapy in cases of hematological malignancies (eg, acute leukemias, lymphomas, multiple myeloma, as well as nonhematological malignancies, eg, Ewing sarcoma, carcinoma).[3] Evaluation of response to therapy may include examination of cytogenetic abnormalities and quantification of abnormal metaphases (eg, chronic myeloid leukemia). The number of Philadelphia-positive metaphases or the number of *bcr-abl* transcripts noted on performing FISH or PCR are invaluable markers of response to therapy.[4] Similarly, FISH and PCR are invaluable in determining minimal disease in acute progranulocytic leukemia.

Limitations Bone marrow involvement may be spotty in certain disorders (eg, multiple myeloma, carcinoma) thus rendering identification of marrow infiltration less sensitive. Therefore, it is necessary to perform bilateral bone marrow biopsies when evaluating possible marrow involvement in Hodgkin lymphoma as well as the non-Hodgkin lymphomas. In certain conditions in which the bone marrow is heavily infiltrated by malignant cells or in which there is underlying myelofibrosis, a "dry tap" is not unusual as a result of attempting to obtain a bone marrow aspirate. Under such circumstances when a cellular aspirate cannot be obtained, touch imprints of the bone marrow biopsy should be performed on a glass coverslip or slide.[5] This may render the diagnosis and provide a clear view of the morphological characteristics of the involved marrow cells. In certain circumstances when a "dry tap" is encountered, it may be possible to obtain a single cell suspension from a bone marrow biopsy sample[6] for flow cytometry or other special studies. It may be difficult to determine the significance of lymphoid aggregates in the bone marrow, even after performing immunocytochemistry. PCR study may be helpful in such cases.[7] Potentially, repeated biopsies from the same site may result in fibrosis which could be misinterpreted and result in false diagnosis of myelofibrosis.[8]

Contraindications Avoid doing a bone marrow from the sternum in any patient with multiple myeloma, or in a patient with a large thoracic aortic aneurysm. Great care should be taken, especially in elderly patients with osteoporosis. **Note:** It is not necessary to correct a low platelet count or coagulopathy prior to performing a bone marrow aspirate/biopsy. Significant bleeding is unusual, even in the presence of a reduced platelet count or

coagulopathy. A pressure dressing and compression over the site is usually all that is required.

Methodology A variety of disposable bone marrow aspirate needles and biopsy needles are currently available. Biopsy needles are based on the Jamshidi needle. In general, bone marrow **aspirates** are obtained from the sternum or the posterior or anterior iliac crests. Bone marrow **biopsies** are obtained from the posterior or anterior iliac crests. In infants, the anterior tibia is usually the preferred site.

Additional Information The French American British classification has generally been used for the classification of acute myeloid leukemia, acute lymphoid leukemia, and the myelodysplastic syndromes. Recently, the WHO classification has been proposed and is likely to be universally accepted as an all encompassing classification of the myeloid and lymphoid malignancies.

WHO CLASSIFICATION (PROPOSED) OF ACUTE MYELOID LEUKEMIAS:

Acute Myeloid Leukemias With Cytogenetic Translocations

AML with t(8;21)(q22;q22)

The morphological features are similar to that seen in AML with maturation. This leukemia was previously classified as an FAB M2 subtype, and accounts for ~50% of FAB M2. Maturation beyond the blast stage to promyelocytes and metamyelocytes may be seen. Auer rods may be present.

Acute Promyelocytic Leukemia; AML with t(15;17) (q22;q11-12), (FAB M3)

This leukemia was classified as FAB M3. Two morphological variants occur:

1. Hypergranular promyelocytic leukemia - Auer rods are frequently present. These may occur in bundles. The WBC count is frequently <10,000/µL at diagnosis.
2. Microgranular promyelocytic variant - granules are not visible on standard microscopy. Granules are numerous on electron microscopy. The nuclei of this subtype are monocytoid in shape. The WBC count may be raised to 15,000/µL at diagnosis.

Both morphological variants stain heavily with the peroxidase stain/Sudan black stain. DIC is classically associated with this subtype. HLA DR negative. CD13, CD33 positive.

AML with abnormal bone marrow eosinophils (inv 16)(p13q22) or t(16;16)(p13;q11).

This subtype is typically an FAB M4 - myelomonocytic leukemia. The bone marrow contains >30% eosinophils and/or eosinophil precursors.

AML with 11q abnormalities - these leukemias frequently occur secondary to treatment with topoisomerase II inhibitors (epipodophyllotoxin and doxorubicin). Dysplastic changes may be present in the bone marrow precursors.

Acute Myeloid Leukemias With Multilineage Dysplasia

AML with prior myelodysplastic syndrome
AML without prior myelodysplastic syndrome

Acute Myeloid Leukemia and Myelodysplastic Syndrome, Therapy Related

Alkylating agent-related
Epipodophyllotoxin and doxorubicin related (topoisomerase II inhibitors)
Other types

Acute Myeloid Leukemia not Otherwise Categorized

AML with minimal differentiation (FAB M0)

May be difficult to differentiate from ALL. Lacks primary granules and Auer rods. Peroxidase positive in <3% blasts. May be CD13, CD33 positive, lymphoid markers negative except for CD7. Tdt positive in ~50%.

AML without maturation (FAB M1)

Primary granules and Auer rods rare/absent. Have <10% maturing granulocyte precursors beyond the blast stage. Peroxidase positive. May express T-cell antigen CD7.

AML with maturation (FAB M2)

Maturation to and beyond the promyelocyte - >10% maturing myeloid cells. Monocytic cells <20% of nonerythroid cells in the bone marrow. Blasts may contain Auer rods and have primary granules. Peroxidase positive and chloroacetate esterase positive.

Acute myelomonocytic leukemia (FAB M4)

Monocytic cell line >20% peripheral blood or bone marrow precursors. Peroxidase, chloroacetate esterase, and butyrate esterase/α-naphthol acetate-esterase positive. The inv(16)(p13,q22) has these morphological characteristics.

Acute monocytic leukemia (FAB M5)

Monocytic cells comprise >80% of the nonerythroid bone marrow cells. Two morphological subtypes may be present:

1. monoblasts without differentiation
2. monoblasts with differentiation to promonocytes and monocytes

Butyrate esterase and/or α-naphthol acetate-esterase positive

Acute erythroid leukemia (FAB M6)

Erythroid precursors >50% of the bone marrow cellularity and myeloblasts >30% of the nonerythroid marrow precursors. Glycophorin positive on flow cytometry in immature erythroid precursors. Myeloid markers are present on the myeloblasts.

(Continued)

Bone Marrow (Continued)

Acute megakaryocytic leukemia (FAB M7)
Myelofibrosis is often prominent. This leads to a dry bone marrow tap. May be CD33, CD34+, CD41+, and von Willebrand factor positive.[9]
Acute basophilic leukemia
Acute panmyelosis with myelofibrosis
This subtype is usually associated with the megakaryocytic leukemias noted above. A subset of patients may not have demonstrable megakaryocytes.

Acute Biphenotypic Leukemias

There are two main subtypes:
Biphenotypic - individual leukemic cells have features of more than one cell type (eg, myeloblasts and erythroid cell lines).
Biclonal - more than one leukemic cell type are present concurrently.

Note: FAB Classification is included in parentheses.

WHO Classification (Proposed) of Acute Lymphoid Leukemias:

Note: These are categorized in part according to the presence or absence of cytogenetic abnormalities, and whether the leukemic cells are of precursor B-cell or precursor T-cell origin. The L1, L2, and L3 subtypes used with the FAB classification have been discarded in view of the fact that the L1 and L2 subtypes do not significantly differ in clinical behavior, genetic abnormalities present, or immunophenotypic features. The L3 subtype is classically of Burkitt-cell origin and is classified as Burkitt-cell leukemia.

Precursor B-cell acute lymphoblastic leukemia

Cytogenetic subgroups:
t(9;22)(q34;q11); *bcr/abl*
t(v;11q23)
t(1;19)(q23;p13)
t(12;21)(p12;q22)

Precursor T-cell acute lymphoblastic leukemia

Burkitt-cell leukemia
Cytogenetic abnormalities
t(8;14); t(8;22); t(2;8)

The WHO classification Has Proposed Significant Changes Related to the Myelodysplastic Syndromes as Follows:

Refractory anemia
Without ringed sideroblasts: Cellularity is normal to increased. Erythroid precursor cells are typically increased, have megaloblastic changes, as well as dyserythropoiesis. Dysplastic changes may also be seen in the myeloid and megakaryocyte series. Blasts account for <5% of the bone marrow nucleated cells.
With ringed sideroblasts: Ringed sideroblasts occur in >15% of the normoblasts on Perl's stain. A dimorphic red blood cell pattern is seen on the peripheral blood smear, one population with normal hemoglobinization and one with hypochromic red blood cells. There is significant erythroid hyperplasia of the bone marrow and significant dyserythropoiesis is classically seen. Blasts are <5% of the nucleated bone marrow elements.
Refractory cytopenia with multilineage dysplasia: All cell lines show significant dysplastic changes. Dyserythropoiesis, dysmyelopoiesis with giant metamyelocytes, and megaloblastic myelopoiesis with left-shifted myelopoiesis are seen. Hypolobated megakaryocytes, micromegakaryocytes are seen. Blasts <5% of the nucleated bone marrow precursors.
Refractory anemia with excess blasts: The changes noted above with refractory cytopenia and multilineage dysplasia occur, but the blast count is between 5% to 20%. A blast count >20% indicates acute leukemia. This replaces the prior FAB category - refractory anemia with excess blasts in transformation.
5q-syndrome: This subtype usually has macrocytic anemia plus normal to increased platelet counts. The bone marrow is normocellular to hypercellular due to erythroid hyperplasia. The megakaryocytes are normal to increased in number and in addition they may be immature with hypolobated nuclei. There may be increased micromegakaryocytes.
Myelodysplastic syndrome, unclassifiable

Note: The previous FAB category, refractory anemia with excess blasts in transformation, has been omitted in the WHO classification. The opinion of the authors of the WHO classification was that a blast count >20% represents acute leukemia and should be treated as such. Chronic myelomonocytic leukemia, previously classified as a myelodysplastic syndrome, is now classified in the myelodysplastic/myeloproliferative syndrome category noted below. Flow cytometric analysis of marrow CD10+ granulocytes may assist in confirming a diagnosis of myelodysplastic syndrome.[10]

WHO Classification of the Myeloproliferative Syndromes

Chronic myelogenous leukemia, Philadelphia chromosome positive t(9;22)(q34;q11); *bcr/abl*
Chronic neutrophilic leukemia
Chronic eosinophilic leukemia/hypereosinophilic syndrome
Chronic idiopathic myelofibrosis
Polycythemia vera
Essential thrombocythemia
Myeloproliferative disease, unclassified

WHO Classification of Myelodysplastic/Myeloproliferative Diseases

Chronic myelomonocytic leukemia
Atypical chronic myelogenous leukemia
Juvenile myelomonocytic leukemia

Footnotes

1. Bain BJ, Clark DM, and Lampert IA, "The Normal Bone Marrow," *Bone Marrow Pathology*, Chapter 1, Cambridge, MA: Blackwell Scientific Publications, 1996, 24-30.
2. Geaghan SM, "Hematologic Values and Appearances in the Healthy Fetus, Neonate, and Child," *Clinics in Laboratory Medicine: Diagnostic Pediatric Hematology*, Volume 19, Philadelphia, PA: WB Saunders, 1999, 1-37.
3. Braun S, Pantel K, Müller P, et al, "Cytokeratin-Positive Cells in the Bone Marrow and Survival of Patients With Stage I, II, or III Breast Cancer," *N Engl J Med*, 2000, 342(8):525-33.
4. Tefferi A, Litzow MR, Noel P, et al, "Chronic Granulocytic Leukemia: Recent Information on Pathogenesis, Diagnosis, and Disease Monitoring," *Mayo Clin Proc*, 1997, 72(5):445-52.
5. Aboul-Nasr R, Estey EH, Kantarjian HM, et al, "Comparison of Touch Imprints With Aspirate Smears for Evaluating Bone Marrow Specimens," *Am J Clin Pathol*, 1999, 111(6):753-8.
6. Dunphy CH, Dunphy FR, and Visconti JL, "Flow Cytometric Immunophenotyping of Bone Marrow Core Biopsies: Report of 8 Patients With Previously Undiagnosed Hematologic Malignancy and Failed Bone Marrow Aspiration," *Arch Pathol Lab Med*, 1999, 123(3):206-12.
7. Ben-Ezra J, Hazelgrove K, Ferreira-Gonzalez A, et al, "Can Polymerase Chain Reaction Help Distinguish Benign From Malignant Lymphoid Aggregates in Bone Marrow Aspirates?" *Arch Pathol Lab Med*, 2000, 124(4):511-5.
8. Salgado C, Feliu E, Blade J, et al, "A Second Bone Marrow Biopsy as a Cause of a False Diagnosis of Myelofibrosis," *Br J Haematol*, 1992, 80(3):407-9.
9. Chuang SS, Yung YC, and Li CY, "von Willebrand Factor Is the Most Reliable Immunohistochemical Marker for Megakaryocytes of Myelodysplastic Syndrome and Chronic Myeloproliferative Disorders," *Am J Clin Pathol*, 2000, 113(4):506-11.
10. Chang CC and Cleveland RP, "Decreased CD10-positive Mature Granulocytes in Bone Marrow From Patients With Myelodysplastic Syndrome," *Arch Pathol Lab Med*, 2000, 124(8):1152-6.

References

Bueno MJ and Herráez J, Images in Clinical Medicine, "Visceral Leishmaniasis," *N Engl J Med*, 1996, 335(14):1034.
Foucar K, *Bone Marrow Pathology*, Chicago, IL: ASCP Press, 1995.
Harris NL, Jaffé ES, Diebold J, et al, "World Health Organization Classification of Neoplastic Diseases of the Hematopoietic and Lymphoid Tissues. Report of the Clinical Advisory Committee Meeting, Airlie House, Virginia, November, 1997," *J Clin Oncol*, 1999, 17(12):3835-49.
Jaffe ES, "Hematopathology: Integration of Morphologic Features and Biologic Markers for Diagnosis," *Mod Pathol*, 1999, 12(2):109-15.
Kröber SM, Greschniok A, Kaiserling E, et al, "Acute Lymphoblastic Leukaemia: Correlation Between Morphological/Immunohistochemical and Molecular Biological Findings in Bone Marrow Biopsy Specimens," *J Clin Pathol Mol Pathol*, 2000, 53(2):83-7.
Shpall EJ, Gee AP, Hogan C, et al, "Bone Marrow Metastases," *Hematol Oncol Clin North Am*, 1996, 10(2):321-43.
Tegg EM, Tuck DM, Lowenthal RM, et al, "The Effect of G-CSF on the Composition of Human Bone Marrow," *Clin Lab Haematol*, 1999, 21(4):265-70.
Young NS and Maciejewski J, "The Pathophysiology of Acquired Aplastic Anemia," *N Engl J Med*, 1997, 336(19):1365-72.

♦ **Bone Marrow Iron Stain** *see* Iron Stain, Bone Marrow *on page 452*

♦ **Buffy Coat Method for Detection of Bacteremia** *see* Bacteremia Detection, Buffy Coat Micromethod *on page 406*

Buffy Coat Smear Study of Peripheral Blood

Related Information

Bacteremia Detection, Buffy Coat Micromethod *on page 406*
Bacterial Culture, Blood *on page 566*
Bone Marrow *on page 410*
Chagas' Disease Serological Test *on page 588*
Ehrlichiosis Serology *on page 603*
Lymph Node Biopsy *on page 67*
Malaria Smear and Tests *on page 458*
Peripheral Blood: Differential Leukocyte Count *on page 464*
Polymerase Chain Reaction *on page 713*
Toxoplasmosis Serology *on page 684*

Applies to *Capnocytophaga canimorsus; Legionella dumoffii*

Abstract The detection of some microorganisms potentially present in peripheral blood can be enhanced by preparing (by centrifugation) and staining the concentrated white cell fraction ("buffy coat") of blood. The buff or pale tan colored layer contains the nucleated blood cells, while the off-white colored top layer usually corresponds to platelets. PCR assays for detecting bacteria, viruses, and parasites have been developed for use on buffy coat white cells.

Specimen Blood

Container Lavender top (EDTA) tube

Storage Instructions Cannot be stored. Specimen is processed and smears are prepared and studied 1-2 hours after blood is obtained, after which stained smears can be archived.

Use Low cost maneuver to detect uncommon cells or pathogenic/parasitic organisms in blood. Can be used for detection of abnormal, immature, blast, or malignant white blood cells or other nucleated cell forms. Used to detect leukemic cells, circulating malignant cells, or immature blood cells in cases of myelofibrosis or other marrow myelophthisic processes; may be used in histochemical evaluation of leukemias when a "dry tap" of the marrow occurs. May assist in the search for circulating plasma cells (as in cases of multiple myeloma) and in the evaluation of megaloblastic anemia (identification of megaloblastic nucleated red cells and hypersegmented neutrophils).

Limitations Preparation of buffy coat smears may distort cells; artifact affects especially fragile cells. When used to detect microorganisms, a variable incidence of false-negative results is anticipated.

Methodology Wright/Giemsa type stained smear of buffy coat developed in centrifuged tube or capillary of anticoagulated whole blood. The cytocentrifuge can be utilized with a WBC rich layer suspended in normal saline to which bovine albumin is added. Some morphologic distortion may be introduced (see description of methods in references below).

Additional Information In some cases, erroneous results from buffy coat study result from an uneven distribution of cells in the buffy coat layer. Removal and mixing of the entire buffy coat layer prior to making smears prevents uneven distribution of the leukocytes and may assist in avoiding artifactual distortion of WBC morphology. Unusual microorganisms, tumor cells, and cells with inclusions (eg, *Strongyloides stercoralis* hyperinfection in an immune-suppressed individual, microfilaria[1], *Borrelia* species spirochetes [cause of relapsing fever], AIDS, Howell-Jolly body-like inclusions,[2] RBC-associated bacillus *Tropheryma whippelii* [causative agent of Whipple disease, which has recently been grown in a human fibroblast cell line (HEL)[3] and can be identified by polymerase chain reaction[4]], *Ehrlichia* neutrophil inclusions in human ehrlichiosis,[5] myeloma[6], and other circulating malignant cells) may be more readily detected by buffy coat study. Spirochetes of relapsing fever may be detected with the help of wet preparations of blood (small numbers of such organisms are revealed by occasional slight agitation of loosely grouped red blood cells). Darkfield microscopy (see Darkfield Examination, Leptospirosis *on page 601*), Wright-Giemsa, or acridine orange-stained thin or dehemoglobinized thick smears of peripheral blood may also be helpful in demonstration of these organisms.[7]

Currently, buffy coat specimens are also obtained to harvest hemopoietic progenitors (stem cells)[8,9] and for performance of polymerase chain reaction (PCR) analyses. PCR detection methods have been applied to a broad spectrum of microbial pathogens including herpesvirus 6 and 7,[10] cytomegalovirus,[11] *Trypanosoma cruzi* (causative agent of Chagas' disease),[12] *Plasmodium falciparum*,[13,14] *Burkholderia pseudo-mallei* (cause of melioidosis, including in particular, septicemic melioidosis),[15] *Coxiella burnetii* (cause of Q fever),[16] *Trypanosoma brucei* (African trypanosomiasis),[17] *Neisseria meningitidis* (cause of meningococcal meningitis),[18] and *Legionella dumoffii*.[19]

Buffy coat smears prepared from peripheral blood and/or bone marrow and stained for specific organisms are still of value. They are technically simple and offer a direct, rapid, and low cost approach to some difficult diagnostic situations (eg, sputum-negative cases of pulmonary tuberculosis and tuberculosis of inaccessible extrapulmonary sites).[20] Evaluation of septicemia due to unusual microorganisms such as *Capnocytophaga canimorsus*, which is rapidly progressive and potentially fatal.[21]

Footnotes

1. Freedman DO and Berry NS, "Rapid Diagnosis of Bancroftian Filariasis by Acridine Orange Staining of Centrifuged Parasites," *Am J Trop Med Hyg*, 1992, 47(6):787-93.
2. Slagel DD, Lager DJ, and Dick FR, "Howell-Jolly Body-Like Inclusions in the Neutrophils of Patients With Acquired Immunodeficiency Syndrome," *Am J Clin Pathol*, 1994, 101(4):429-31.
3. Raoult D, Birg ML, La Scola B, et al, "Cultivation of the Bacillus of Whipple's Disease," *N Engl J Med*, 2000, 342(9):620-5.
4. Lowsky R, Archer GL, Fyles G, et al, "Brief Report: Diagnosis of Whipple's Disease by Molecular Analysis of Peripheral Blood," *N Engl J Med*, 1994, 331(20):1343-6.
5. Rynkiewicz DL and Liu LX, "Human Ehrlichiosis in New England," *N Engl J Med*, 1994, 330(4):292-3.
6. Witzig TE, "Detection of Malignant Gels in the Peripheral Blood of Patients With Multiple Myeloma. Clinical Implications and Research Applications," *Mayo Clin Proc*, 1994, 69(9):903-7.
7. "*Borrelia* (Relapsing Fever)," *2000 Red Book: Report of the Committee on Infectious Diseases*, Pickering LK, Peter G, Baker CJ, et al, eds, 25th ed, Section 3: Summaries of Infectious Diseases, Elk Grove Village, IL: American Academy of Pediatrics, 2000, 190-2.
8. Ghielmini M, Pfister U, Zucca E, et al, "Distribution of Mobilized Progenitor Cells in the Buffy Coat of the Haemonetics MCS3p Cell Separator: A Study to Optimize the Collection of Progenitors by Leukapheresis," *J Hematother*, 1998, 7(3):251-6.
9. Sousa T, de Sousa ME, Godinho MI, et al, "Umbilical Cord Blood Processing: Volume Reduction and Recovery of CD34+ Cells," *Bone Marrow Transplant*, 1997, 19(4):311-3.
10. Moschettini D, De Milito A, Catucci M, et al, "Detection of Human Herpesviruses 6 and 7 in Heart Transplant Recipients by a Multiplex Polymerase Chain Reaction Method," *Eur J Clin Microbiol Infect Dis*, 1998, 17(2):117-9.
11. Evans P, Gray J, and Wreghitt T, "Comparison of Three PCR Techniques for Detecting Cytomegalovirus (CMV) DNA in Serum, Detection of Early Antigen Fluorescent Foci and Culture for the Diagnosis of CMV Infection," *J Med Microbiol*, 1999, 48(11):1029-35.
12. Herwaldt B, Grijalva M, and Newsome A, "Use of Polymerase Chain Reaction to Diagnose the Fifth Reported U.S. Case of Autochthonous Transmission of *Trypanosoma cruzi*, in Tennessee, 1998" *J Infect Dis*, 2000, 181(1):395-9.
13. Craig MH and Sharp BL, "Comparative Evaluation of Four Techniques for the Diagnosis of *Plasmodium falciparum* Infections," *Trans R Soc Trop Med Hyg*, 1997, 91(3):279-82.
14. Carrasquilla G, Banguero M, Sanchez P, et al, "Epidemiologic Tools for Malaria Surveillance in an Urban Setting of Low Endemicity Along the Colombian Pacific Coast," *Am J Trop Med Hyg*, 2000, 62(1):132-7.
15. Dharakul T, Songsivilai S, Viriyachitra S, et al, "Detection of *Burkholderia pseudomallei* DNA in Patients With Septicemic Melioidosis," *J Clin Microbiol*, 1996, 34(3):609-14.
16. Spyridaki I, Gikas A, Kofteridis D, et al, "Q Fever in the Greek Island of Crete: Detection, Isolation, and Molecular Identification of Eight Strains of *Coxiella burnetii* From Clinical Samples," *J Clin Microbiol*, 1998, 36(7):2063-7.
17. Harris E, Detmer J, Dungan J, et al, "Detection of *Trypanosoma brucei* spp. in Human Blood by a Nonradioactive Branched DNA-based Technique," *J Clin Microbiol*, 1996, 34(10):2401-7.
18. Newcombe J, Cartwright K, Palmer WH, et al, "PCR of Peripheral Blood for Diagnosis of Meningococcal Disease," *J Clin Microbiol*, 1996, 34(7):1637-40.
19. Murdoch D and Chambers S, "Detection of *Legionella* DNA in Peripheral Leukocytes, Serum, and Urine From a Patient With Pneumonia Caused by *Legionella dumoffii*," *Clin Infect Dis*, 2000, 30(2):382-3.
20. Sen R, Singh S, Singh HP, et al, "Demonstration of Acid-Fast Bacilli in Buffy Coat and Bone Marrow Smear - a Diagnostic Tool in Pulmonary Tuberculosis," *J Indian Med Assoc*, 1996, 94(10):379-80, 390.
21. Mirza I, Wolk J, Toth L, et al, "Waterhouse-Fredericksen Syndrome Secondary to *Capnocytophaga carnimorsus* Septicemia and Demonstration of Bacteremia by Peripheral Blood Smear: A Case Report and Review of the Literature," *Arch Pathol Lab Med*, 2000, 124(6):859-63.

References

Cooper RI and Neuhauser T, Images in Clinical Medicine, "Borreliosis," *N Engl J Med*, 1998, 338(4):231.

Pan AA and Winkler MA, "The Threat of Chagas' Disease in Transfusion Medicine. The Presence of Antibodies to *Trypanosoma cruzi* in the U.S. Blood Supply," *Lab Med*, 1997, 28(4):269-74.

Shafer JA, "Preparation of Blood Films for Examination," *Clinical Hematology: Principles, Procedures, and Correlations*, 2nd ed, Chapter 3, Stiene-Martin EA, Lotspeich-Steininger CA, and Koepke JA, eds, Philadelphia, PA: Lippincott Raven Publishers, 1998, 26-7.

Walker DH and Dumler JS, "Human Monocytic and Granulocytic Ehrlichioses. Discovery and Diagnosis of Emerging Tick-Borne Infections and the Critical Role of the Pathologist," *Arch Pathol Lab Med*, 1997, 121:785-91.

Westenfeld FW, "Relapsing Fever in a Recent Visitor to Africa," *Lab Med*, 1997, 28(7):436-8.

Wyrick-Glatzel J and Hughes V, "Routine Hematology Methods," *Clinical Hematology and Fundamentals of Hemostasis*, 3rd ed, Chapter 31, Harmening DM, ed, Philadelphia, PA: FA Davis Company, 1997, 609.

♦ **Burr Cells** *see* Peripheral Blood: Differential Leukocyte Count *on page 464*

♦ **Cabot Rings** *see* Peripheral Blood: Differential Leukocyte Count *on page 464*

♦ **Capillary Isoelectric Focusing** *see* Hemoglobin A$_2$ *on page 443*

♦ **Capnocytophaga canimorsus** *see* Bacteremia Detection, Buffy Coat Micromethod *on page 406*

♦ **Capnocytophaga canimorsus** *see* Buffy Coat Smear Study of Peripheral Blood *on page 412*

♦ **Capnocytophaga canimorsus** *see* Peripheral Blood: Differential Leukocyte Count *on page 464*

♦ **Carboxyhemoglobin** *see* Hemoglobin, Unstable, Heat Labile Test *on page 447*

♦ **Carboxyhemoglobin** *see* Hemoglobin, Unstable - Isopropanol Precipitation Test *on page 448*

♦ **Cardiopulmonary Bypass** *see* Hemoglobin, Plasma *on page 446*

♦ **Caspase Enzymes** *see* Apoptosis Assays *on page 402*

♦ **CBC** *see* Complete Blood Count *on page 419*

♦ **CD** *see* Flow Cytometry, Overview *on page 432*

♦ **CD4 Lymphocytes** *see* Flow Cytometry, Overview *on page 432*

♦ **CD8 Lymphocytes** *see* Flow Cytometry, Overview *on page 432*

♦ **CD14** *see* PNH Test (GPI-Anchored Proteins) by Flow Cytometry *on page 472*

♦ **CD16** *see* PNH Test (GPI-Anchored Proteins) by Flow Cytometry *on page 472*

♦ **CD24** *see* PNH Test (GPI-Anchored Proteins) by Flow Cytometry *on page 472*

CD34+ Hematopoietic Stem Cells by Flow Cytometry

Related Information

Flow Cytometry, Overview *on page 432*
Hematopoietic Progenitor Cells, Cord Blood/Placental Blood *on page 843*
Hematopoietic Progenitor Cells, Marrow *on page 844*
Hematopoietic Progenitor Cells, Peripheral Blood *on page 845*
Thrombopoietin, Serum or Plasma *on page 491*
(Continued)

CD34+ Hematopoietic Stem Cells by Flow Cytometry (Continued)

Applies to CD45; Hematopoietic Stem Cells; Integrins; Peripheral Blood Stem Cells; Peripheral Blood Stem Cell Transplantation; Selectin; Umbilical Cord Blood Transplantation; VLA-4; VLA-5

Abstract The CD34 membrane antigen is a heavily glycosylated mucin-like structure which is present on the surface of some 3% of bone marrow hematopoietic precursors or "stem-like" cells and can also be recovered from peripheral blood. These cells constitute only 0.01% to 0.05% of nucleated cells in the peripheral blood of normal individuals but mobilization treatment (ie, administration of hematopoietic growth factors) increases circulating (CD34+) stem cells in patients and in healthy donors, such that peripheral blood stem cells (PBSC) have largely replaced bone marrow as the source for stem cells in marrow transplantation.[1]

Specimen Peripheral whole blood

Container Lavender top (EDTA) tube

Collection Proper identification of the sample is of critical importance. Working Party Guideline[1] recommends that samples be labeled with patient's full name, a numeric patient identifier (eg, hospital number), date of birth, patient location, and date and time of collection.

Storage Instructions Total WBC count must be obtained within 6 hours of sample collection. Specimen should be stored at 4°C and processing completed within 12 hours.

Causes for Rejection Presence of blood clots, hemolysis, receipt after 12 hours of sampling

Special Instructions Timing of stem cell harvesting is dependent on the CD34+ cell count. Harvesting requires a peripheral blood CD34 count >10 cells/μL (with the goal of obtaining ≥2 x 10^6 CD34+ cells).

Use To assess stem cell (hematopoietic progenitor cell) numbers in peripheral blood, cord blood, and apheresis specimens for potential use in PBSC transplantation

Limitations Hematology analyzer white blood cell determinations (used to obtain absolute CD34+ counts) must be properly corrected for presence of nucleated red blood cells, and reverse pipetting used to avoid error from the introduction of bubbles

Methodology *In vitro* assay of colony-forming units (CFU-GM) to assess hematopoietic potential (numbers of clonogenic-committed granulocytic-monocytic progenitor cells grown *in vitro*). Single or dual platform flow cytometry,[1] preferably a whole blood, lyse-no-wash, technique using fixative-free NH₄CL-based red cell lysing reagents.[2] Proprietary kits using a fixative-based reagent must follow the manufacturer's recommendations, as the CD34 antigen may be affected by fixatives used with specific labeling methods. Samples should be analyzed immediately post red blood cell lysis (or kept on melting ice until analysis)[3] and analyses must be completed within 1 hour following lysis. The Working Party Guideline recommends that the fluorochrome phycoerythrin (PE) conjugated to a class II antibody (or class III antibody - any conjugate) be used with an argon laser for enumeration of CD34+ stem cells.[1] Because of interference with class II antibody-binding properties, fluorescein isothiocyanate (FITC) conjugated class II antibodies "must not be used." The Guideline also specifies reagents for detection of the CD45 antigen (the CD34 receptor), and emphasizes that a sufficient number of events must be analyzed to obtain a statistically valid result (an intra-assay coefficient of variation of 10% requires that a minimum of 100 CD34+ events must be collected).[4] A major factor in variability of results between laboratories involves gating strategy. The International Society for Hematotherapy and Graft Engineering (ISHAGE) protocol gives the most reproducible results.[4,5] Four sequential gating steps are used, CD45 monoclonal antibody serves as a "counterstain" and assists in resolving leukocytes from irrelevant cells.[4,5,6] Recently developed CD34+ hematopoietic analysis systems include the STELLer assay which uses the IMAGN 2000 microvolume fluorimeter and Cy5-conjugated anti-CD34,[1,7] and the Sysmex SE-9000 system which is based on phospholipid content.[8]

Additional Information CD34+ hematopoietic precursor blast-like cells were originally described in 1984.[9] Human KG-1a undifferentiated leukemia cells were used as an immunogen to produce monoclonal antibodies against potential cell-surface antigens of blast cells. After screening and winnowing, anti-My-10 was found to have narrow cellular specificity. Thus, the My-10 antigen (CD34) was discovered and found to represent a protein of about 115 kD. The earliest marrow progenitor cells are CD34- with subsequent switch of this resting stem cell from CD34- to CD34+. With external stimulation, prior dormant CD34- cells respond by upregulation of multiple surface receptors (see diagram) and become CD34+ cells. They may then become susceptible to DNA damage and development of leukemia. Currently, there is interest (with therapeutic application) in identifying (and potentially separating) a population of benign (vs malignant) hematopoietic progenitors at this early stage of maturation.[10]

With the exception of a tiny population of very immature hematopoietic progenitor cells (HPC) that are CD34-, the CD34 molecule is unique in that it is expressed at various levels on essentially all HPC.[11] There are <1% of CD34+ cells in all HPC preparations and the expression of CD34+ varies within the HPC population. A number of different glycosylated CD34+ epitopes exist with resultant antigenic diversity.

The CD34 molecule has adhesion properties, the gene resides at chromosome 1q32, a region that encodes adhesion molecules. The extracellular

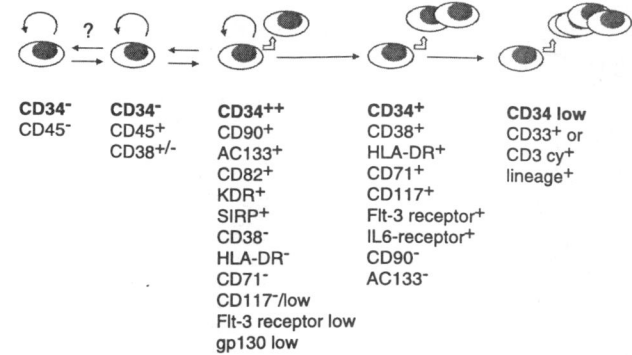

CD34+ Hematopoietic Stem-Cells by Flow Cytometry

CD34-	CD34-	CD34++	CD34+	CD34 low
CD45-	CD45+	CD90+	CD38+	CD33+ or
	CD38+/-	AC133+	HLA-DR+	CD3 cy+
		CD82+	CD71+	lineage+
		KDR+	CD117+	
		SIRP+	Flt-3 receptor+	
		CD38-	IL6-receptor+	
		HLA-DR-	CD90-	
		CD71-	AC133-	
		CD117-/low		
		Flt-3 receptor low		
		gp130 low		

⤺ Self-renewal

⤶ Differentiation capacity

Summarization of recent hypotheses of human stem-cell development. Model of CD34 expression in the human bone marrow during maturation progress. The earliest stem-cell is probably not tissue-determined, quiescent and with self-renewing capacity. Possibly through cell matrix interaction it can acquire a tissue specific phenotype and function. This early hematopoietic progenitor cell with ability for self-renewal seems to be CD34- CD45+ exhibiting variable expresion of CD38. On activation this cell can acquire a CD34+ phenotype and give rise to differentiated progeny. It displays a strong CD34 expression which is reversible if an activation equilibrium occurs. The activated CD34+ cell is partially capable of self-renewal and long-term engraftment, especially if it has a certain pattern of coexpressed antigens indicating an immature developmental stage like CD90+, DR-. As maturation proceeds, the coantigen expression pattern changes and the clonogenic potential improves while self-renewal capacity persists. It should be emphasized that maturation in reality is a continuing process unlike this diagram, which suggests a stepwise maturation with defined stages. Antigen expression is probably a gradually increasing or decreasing process reflecting the fluent maturation progress.

Adapted from Brendel C and Neubauer A, "Characteristics and Analysis of Normal and Leukemic Stem Cells: Current Concepts and Future Directions," *Leukemia*, 2000, 14(10):1711-7.

portion of CD34 has features in common with leukosialin (CD43) and other adhesion molecules. L-selectin (CD62L), an adhesion molecule, binds CD34.[11] The adhesion molecule complement of CD34+ stem cells appears to play a role in mobilization of HPC and in their relation to the marrow microenvironment. The integrins (in particular those of the β₁-subfamily) direct cell-cell and cell-matrix interactions. CD34+ stem cells bind to bone marrow stroma or to extracellular matrix proteins of the marrow microenvironment through the β₁-integrins, in particular VLA-4 and VLA-5. A number of other adhesion molecule/receptor families are involved.[12,13,14,15]

For marrow transplantation and retrovirally-mediated gene transfer, *in vitro* and *in vivo* expansion of hemopoietic stem cell (HSC) populations is of importance. The use of stromal elements, growth factors (in particular thrombopoietin), and culture constituents and characteristics are being defined.[16]

Factors influencing the recovery of CD34+ cells during collection and the significance of rapidity of clearance of CD34+ cells from peripheral blood after HSC infusion have been studied.[17,18] Optimal timing of stem cell collection can be based on rising WBC and platelet counts which provides increased numbers of CD34+ cells in leukapheresis as compared with collection on a fixed day following initiation of the mobilization protocol.[17] The rapidity of clearance of CD34+ from peripheral blood (following infusion of relatively lower doses) is an independent indicator of hematologic recovery.[18]

The use of CD34+ subsets (eg, CD34-38-, CD34+33-, CD34+33+, CD34+41+, CD34+CD61+, CD34+CD105+) in predicting the engraftment success and quality of marrow transplantation and in following early maturation is under investigation.[19,20,21,22]

The bone marrow transplantation treatment modality has been expanded by the discovery that umbilical cord blood (UCB) could be used as an alternate source for HSC.[23,24,25,26] Reconstitution of hemopoiesis after engraftment of UCB cells, however, is slower compared to the use of bone marrow or CD34+ peripheral blood stem cells. Currently, research interest is targeting the nature of the UCB CD34+ cell population and improvement in the rate of post-UCB cell infusion hematologic recovery.[27,28,29,30,31]

Footnotes

1. Barnett D, Janossy G, Lubenko A, et al, "Guideline for the Flow Cytometric Enumeration of CD34+ Haematopoietic Stem Cells. Prepared by the CD34+ Haematopoietic Stem Cell Working Party," General Haematology Task Force of the British Committee for Standards in Haematology, *Clin Lab Haematol*, 1999, 21(5):301-8.

2. Menéndez P, Redondo O, Rodriguez A, et al, "Comparison Between a Lyse-and-Then-Wash Method and a Lyse-non-Wash Technique for the Enumeration of CD34+ Haematopoietic Progenitor Cells," *Cytometry*, 1998, 34(6):264-71.

3. Serke S, van Lessen A, Pardo I, et al, "Selective Susceptibility of CD34-Expressing Cells to Acquire Flow Cytometric Features of Apoptosis/Necrosis on Exposure to an Ammonium Chloride-Based Red Blood Cell Lysing Reagent," *J Hematother*, 1998, 7(4):315-8.

4. Sutherland DR, Anderson L, Keeney M, et al, "The ISHAGE Guidelines for CD34+ Cell Determination by Flow Cytometry. International Society of Hematotherapy and Graft Engineering," *J Hematother*, 1996, 5(3):213-26.

5. Gratama JW, Orfao A, Barnett D, et al, "Flow Cytometric Enumeration of CD34+ Hematopoietic Stem and Progenitor Cells," European Working Group on Clinical Cell Analysis, *Cytometry*, 1998, 34(3):128-42.

6. Serke S, Beyer J, Rick O, et al, "Analysis of CD34-Expressing Cells in Clinical Practice," *Vox Sang*, 1998, 74(Suppl 2):469-75.

7. Dietz LJ, Dubrow RS, Manian BS, et al, "Volumetric Capillary Cytometry: A New Method for Absolute Cell Enumeration," *Cytometry*, 1996, 23(3):177-86.

8. Takekawa K, Yamane T, Suzuki K, et al, "Identification of Hematopoietic Stem Cells by the SE-9000 Automated Hematology Analyzer in Peripheral Blood Stem Cell Harvest Samples," *Acta Haematol*, 1997, 98(1):54-5.

9. Civin I, Strauss LC, Brovall C, et al, "Antigenic Analysis of Hematopoiesis: I. Hematopoietic Progenitor Cell Surface Antigen Defined by a Monoclonal Antibody Raised Against KG-1a Cells," *Blood*, 1984, 133(1):157-65.

10. Brendel C and Neubauer A, "Characteristics and Analysis of Normal and Leukemic Stem Cells: Current Concepts and Future Directions," *Leukemia*, 2000, 14(10):1711-7.

11. Egeland T, "The CD34 Molecule and Hematopoietic Progenitor Cell Studies - A Challenge in Clinical Medicine," *Vox Sang*, 1998, 74(Suppl 2):467-8.

12. DiPersio JF, "Introduction: The Biologic Basis of Stem-Cell Therapy," *Semin Hematol*, 2000, 37(1 Suppl 2):1-2.

13. Cacciola RR, Stagno F, Impera S, et al, "Beta-1-Integrin Expression in Adult Acute Lymphoblastic Leukemia: Possible Relationship With the Stem Cell Antigen CD34," *Acta Haematol*, 1997, 97(1-2):63-6.

14. Liesveld JL, "Expression and Function of Adhesion Receptors in Acute Myelogenous Leukemia: Parallels With Normal Erythroid and Myeloid Progenitors," *Acta Haematol*, 1997, 97(1-2):53-62.

15. Lichterfeld M, Martin S, Burkly I, et al, "Mobilization of CD34+ Haematopoietic Stem Cells Is Associated With a Functional Inactivation of the Integrin Very Late Antigen 4," *Br J Haematol*, 2000, 110(1):71-81.

16. Wagemaker G, "*In Vitro* and *In Vivo* Expansion of Stem Cell Populations," *Vox Sang*, 1998, 74(Suppl 2):463-6.

17. Krieger MS, Schiller G, Berenson JR, et al, "Collection of Peripheral Blood Progenitor Cells (PBPC) Based on a Rising WBC and Platelet Count Significantly Increases the Number of CD34+ Cells," *Bone Marrow Transplant*, 1999, 24(1):25-8.

18. D'Hondt L, Wuu J, André M, et al, "Clearance Kinetics of CD34+ Cells From Peripheral Blood: An Independent Predictor of Hematologic Recovery After High-Dose Chemotherapy and Hematopoietic Stem Cell Transplantation," *Bone Marrow Transplant*, 1999, 24(5):483-9.

19. Stewart DA, Guo D, Luider J, et al, "Factors Predicting Engraftment of Autologous Blood Stem Cells: CD34+ Subsets Inferior to the Total CD34+ Cell Dose," *Bone Marrow Transplant*, 1999, 23(12):1237-43.

20. Johnsen HE, Rasmussen T, and Knudsen LM, "CD34+ Subset and Tumor Cell Quantitation by Flow Cytometry - Step Toward Quality Assessment of Autografts in B Cell Malignancies," *Vox Sang*, 1998, 74(Suppl 2):477-82.

21. Pierelli L, Scambia G, Bonanno G, et al, "CD34+/CD105+ Cells Are Enriched in Primitive Circulating Progenitors Residing in the G0 Phase of the Cell Cycle and Contain All Bone Marrow and Cord Blood CD34+/CD38low/- Precursors," *Br J Haematol*, 2000, 108(3):610-20.

22. Robin C, Bennaceur-Griscelli A, Louache F, et al, "Identification of Human T-lymphoid Progenitor Cells in CD34+ CD38low and CD34+ CD38+ Subsets of Human Cord Blood and Bone Marrow Cells Using NOD-SCID Fetal Thymus Organ Cultures," *Br J Haematol*, 1999, 104(4):809-19.

23. Wagner JE, Kernan NA, Steinbuch M, et al, "Allogeneic Sibling Umbilical-Cord-Blood Transplantation in Children With Malignant and Nonmalignant Disease," *Lancet*, 1995, 346(8969):214-9.

24. Laporte JP, Gorin NC, Rubinstein P, et al, "Cord-Blood Transplantation From an Unrelated Donor in an Adult With Chronic Myelogenous Leukemia," *N Engl J Med*, 1996, 335(3):167-70.

25. Wagner JE, Rosenthal J, Sweetman R, et al, "Successful Transplantation of HLA-matched and HLA-mismatched Umbilical Cord Blood From Unrelated Donors: Analysis of Engraftment and Acute Graft-Versus-Host Disease," *Blood*, 1996, 88(3):795-802.

26. Gluckman E, Rocha V, Boyer-Chammard A, et al, " Outcome of Cord-Blood Transplantation From Related and Unrelated Donors. Eurocord Transplant Group and the European Blood and Marrow Transplantation Group," *N Engl J Med*, 1997, 337(6):373-81.

27. Lucotti C, Malabarba L, Rosti V, et al, "Cell Cycle Distribution of Cord Blood-Derived Haematopoietic Progenitor Cells and Their Recruitment into the S-phase of the Cell Cycle," *Br J Haematol*, 2000, 108(3):621-8.

28. Kusadasi N, van Soest PL, Mayen AE, et al, "Successful Short-Term *Ex Vivo* Expansion of NOD/SCID Repopulating Ability and CAFC Week 6 From Umbilical Cord Blood," *Leukemia*, 2000, 14(11):1944-53.

29. Sousa T, de Sousa ME, Godinho MI, et al, "Umbilical Cord Blood Processing: Volume Reduction and Recovery of CD34+ Cells," *Bone Marrow Transplant*, 1997, 19(4):311-3.

30. Hübl W, Iturraspe J, Martinez GA, et al, "Measurement of Absolute Concentration and Viability of CD34+ Cells in Cord Blood and Cord Blood Products Using Fluorescent Beads and Cyanine Nucleic Acid Dyes," *Cytometry*, 1998, 34(3):121-7.

31. Qiu L, Meagher R, Welhausen S, et al, "*Ex Vivo* Expansion of CD34+ Umbilical Cord Blood Cells in a Defined Serum-Free Medium (QBSF-60) With Early Effect Cytokines," *J Hematother Stem Cell Res*, 1999, 8(6):609-18.

References

Barrett J and Treleaven JG, eds, *The Clinical Practice of Stem-Cell Transplantation*, Volumes 1 and 2, Oxford, UK: Isis Medical Media, 1998.

Belvedere O, Feruglio C, Malangone W, et al, "Phenotypic Characterization of Immunomagnetically Purified Umbilical Cord Blood CD34+ Cells," *Blood Cells Mol Dis*, 1999, 25(3-4):141-6.

Champseix C, Marechal V, Khazaal I, et al, "A Cell Surface Marker Gene Transferred With a Retroviral Vector Into CD34+ Cord Blood Cells Is Expressed by Their T-cell Progeny in the SCID-hu Thymus," *Blood*, 1996, 88(1):107-13.

de Fabritiis P, Gonzalez M, Meloni G, et al, "Monitoring of CD34+ Cells During Leukapheresis Allows a Single, Successful Collection of Hemopoietic Progenitors in Patients With Low Numbers of Circulating Stem Cells," *Bone Marrow Transplant*, 1999, 23(12):1229-36.

Dunbar CE, "Gene Transfer to Hematopoietic Stem Cells: Implications for Gene Therapy of Human Disease," *Annu Rev Med*, 1996, 47:11-20.

Dürig J, Rosenthal C, Elmaagacli A, et al, "Biological Effects of Stroma-Derived Factor-1 Alpha on Normal and CML CD34+ Haemopoietic Cells," *Leukemia*, 2000, 14(9):1652-60.

Gowans ID, Hepburn MD, Clark DM, et al, "The Role of the Sysmex SE-9000 Immature Myeloid Index and Sysmex R-2000 Reticulocyte Parameters in Optimizing the Timing of Peripheral Blood Stem Cell Harvesting in Patients With Lymphoma and Myeloma," *Clin Lab Haematol*, 1999, 21(5):331-6.

Gratama JW, Braakman E, Kraan J, et al, "Comparison of Single and Dual-Platform Assay Formats for CD34+ Haematopoietic Progenitor Cell Enumeration," *Clin Lab Haematol*, 1999, 21(5):337-46.

"Guidelines for Preventing Opportunistic Infections Among Hematopoietic Stem Cell Transplant Recipients," *MMWR Morb Mortal Wkly Rep*, 2000, 49(RR-10):1-125.

Hildebrandt M, Serke S, Meyer O, et al, "Immunomagnetic Selection of CD34+ Cells: Factors Influencing Component Purity and Yield," *Transfusion*, 2000, 40(5):507-12.

Hughes VC, "Cord Blood Transplantation: Hallmarks of the 20th Century," *Lab Med*, 2000, 31(12):672.

Jiang Y, Prosper F, and Verfaillie CM, "Opposing Effects of Engagement of Integrins and Stimulation of Cytokine Receptors on Cell Cycle Progression of Normal Human Hematopoietic Progenitors," *Blood*, 2000, 95(3):846-54.

Kim HJ, Tisdale JF, Wu T, et al, "Many Multipotential Gene-Marked Progenitor or Stem Cell Clones Contribute to Hematopoiesis in Nonhuman Primates," *Blood*, 2000, 96(1):1-8.

Kline RM, "Whose Blood Is It, Anyway?" *Scientific American*, 2001, 284(4):42-9.

Martin-Henao GA, Picón M, Amill B, et al, "Isolation of CD34+ Progenitor Cells From Peripheral Blood by Use of an Automated Immunomagnetic Selection System: Factors Affecting the Results," *Transfusion*, 2000, 40(1):35-43.

Michallet M, Thiebaut A, Dreger P, et al, "Peripheral Blood Stem Cell (PBSC) Mobilization and Transplantation After Fludarabine Therapy in Chronic Lymphocytic Leukaemia (CLL): A Report of the European Blood and Marrow Transplantation (EBMT) CLL Subcommittee on Behalf of the EBMT Chronic Leukaemias Working Party (CLWP)," *Br J Haematol*, 2000, 108(3):595-601.

Paloczi K, "Immunophenotypic and Functional Characterization of Human Umbilical Cord Blood Mononuclear Cells," *Leukemia*, 1999, 13(Suppl 1):S87-9.

Reiser M, Josting A, Draube A, et al, "Successful Peripheral Blood Stem Cell Mobilization With Etoposide (VP-16) in Patients With Relapsed or Resistant Lymphoma Who Failed Cyclophosphamide Mobilization," *Bone Marrow Transplant*, 1999, 23(12):1223-8.

Simnett SJ, Stewart LA, Sweetenham J, et al, "Autologous Stem Cell Transplantation for Malignancy: A Systematic Review of the Literature," *Clin Lab Haematol*, 2000, 22(2):61-72.

Spangrudo GJ and Cooper DD, "Paradigm Shifts In Stem-Cell Biology," *Semin Hematol*, 2000, 37(1 Suppl 2):3-10.

Vaisman B, Konijn AM, and Fibach E, "Isolation of Large and Pure Samples of Human Erythroid Precursors at Different Stages of Maturation Using Immunomagnetic Separation of Cells From Liquid Cultures," *Acta Haematol*, 1999, 101(3):135-9.

Wagner JE, "Umbilical Cord Transplantation," *Leukemia*, 1998, 12(Suppl 1):S30-2

♦ **CD45** *see* CD34+ Hematopoietic Stem Cells by Flow Cytometry *on page 413*

♦ **CD55 by Flow Cytometry** *see* PNH Test (GPI-Anchored Proteins) by Flow Cytometry *on page 472*

♦ **CD55 (Decay Accelerating Factor - DAF)** *see* PNH Test (GPI-Anchored Proteins) by Flow Cytometry *on page 472*

♦ **CD59 by Flow Cytometry** *see* PNH Test (GPI-Anchored Proteins) by Flow Cytometry *on page 472*

♦ **CD59 (Membrane Inhibitor of Reactive Lysis - MIRL)** *see* PNH Test (GPI-Anchored Proteins) by Flow Cytometry *on page 472*

♦ **CD61** *see* Platelet Count *on page 468*

♦ **CD61 Per CP** *see* Reticulated Platelet Count *on page 480*

♦ **CD62P** *see* Platelet Count *on page 468*

♦ **CD66b** *see* PNH Test (GPI-Anchored Proteins) by Flow Cytometry *on page 472*

♦ **CD95** *see* Apoptosis Assays *on page 402*

♦ **Cell Count, CSF** *see* Cerebrospinal Fluid Analysis: Overview *on page 416*

♦ **Cell Count Ratio** *see* Body Fluid Analysis, Cell Count *on page 408*

♦ **Ceramidase** *see* Inherited Diseases of Metabolism and Cell Structure *on page 449*

♦ **Ceramidetrihexoside α-Galactosidase** *see* Inherited Diseases of Metabolism and Cell Structure *on page 449*

Cerebrospinal Fluid Analysis: Overview

Related Information

Synonyms Cell Count, CSF; CSF Analysis; Spinal Fluid Analysis

Applies to CSF Leukocyte Aggregation Score; Lumbar Puncture

Test Includes Color of supernatant, volume, turbidity, WBC/mm³, polys/mm³, lymphs/mm³, RBC/mm³, percent of crenated RBC, protein and glucose, VDRL, and other tests as clinically indicated in selected cases. India ink preparation and cryptococcal antigen titer are best not forgotten.

Abstract Bacterial meningitis is a medical emergency and requires immediate evaluation and treatment[1] (ie, with cerebrospinal fluid (CSF) analysis, and other studies). Examination of CSF also contributes to diagnosis and sometimes management of other disease entities of the central nervous system including encephalitis, encephalopathy, instances of vasculitis, demyelinating diseases, certain tumors, paraneoplastic entities, polyneuritis, cases of seizure disorders, and confusional states.[2] For diagnosis of meningitis, culture and then Gram stain study over all other testing, when only a small quantity of CSF is available. Cell count with differential deserves the next priority, followed by glucose and protein.

Table 1. Differential Diagnosis of Initial Cerebrospinal Fluid Findings in Suppurative Diseases of the Central Nervous System and Meninges

Condition	Pressure (mm H₂O)	Leukocytes/mm³	Protein (mg/dL)	Sugar (mg/dL)	Specific Findings
Acute bacterial meningitis	Usually elevated	Several hundred to >60,000; usually a few thousand; occasionally <100 (especially meningococcal or early in disease); PMNs* predominate	Usually 100-500, occasionally >1000	<40 in >50% of cases (normal glucose does not rule out bacterial meningitis)	Organism usually seen on smear or culture in >90% of cases
Subdural empyema†	Usually elevated; average, 300	<100 to a few thousand; PMNs predominate	Usually 100-500	Normal	No organisms seen on smear or culture unless concurrent meningitis
Brain abscess†	Usually elevated	Usually 10-200; fluid is rarely acellular; lymphocytes predominate	Usually 75-400	Normal	No organisms seen on smear or culture
Ventricular empyema (rupture of brain abscess)†	Considerably elevated	Several thousand to 100,000; usually >90% PMNs	Usually several hundred	Usually <40	Organism may be seen on smear or culture
Cerebral epidural abscess†	Slightly to modestly elevated	Few to several hundred or more cells; lymphocytes predominate	Usually 50-200	Normal	No organisms seen on smear or culture
Spinal epidural abscess†	Usually reduced with spinal block	Usually 10-100; lymphocytes predominate	Usually several hundred	Normal	No organisms seen on smear or culture
Thrombophlebitis (often associated with subdural empyema)	Often elevated	Few to several hundred; PMNs and lymphocytes	Slightly to moderately elevated	Normal	No organisms seen on smear or culture
Bacterial endocarditis (with embolism)	Normal or slightly elevated	Few to <100; lymphocytes and PMNs; pleocytosis in 70%	Elevated, sometimes slightly	Normal to low	No organisms seen on smear or culture. Lymphocytic to PMN predominence; sometimes resembles CSF in purulent meningitis
Acute viral encephalitis	Usually elevated	Few to >1000; PMNs early, followed by mononuclear cells	Moderately elevated	Normal to slightly reduced	No organisms seen on smear or culture; oligoclonal bands may be found
Aseptic meningitis	Slightly increased	10 to >3000 (avg 50-500); neutrophils early, quickly replaced by mononuclear cells	Normal to slightly elevated, usually <100 mg/dL	Normal to <40 mg/dL	Enteroviruses cause >80% of cases
Herpetic meningitis		Mononuclear pleocytosis	Slightly elevated	Normal to slightly low	Etiology HSV-2 by viral culture or PCR
Tuberculous infection	Usually elevated; may be low with dynamic block in advanced stages	Usually 25-100, rarely more than 500; lymphocytes predominate, except in early stages when PMNs may account for 80% of the cells	Nearly always elevated, usually 100-200; may be much higher if dynamic block	Usually reduced; <50 in 75% of cases	Acid-fast organisms may be seen on smear of protein coagulum (pellicle) or recovered from inoculated guinea pig or by culture
Cryptococcal infection	Usually elevated; average, 225	Average, 50 (0-800); lymphocytic pleocytosis; diminished or absent inflammatory response may be found in subjects with and without AIDS	Average, 100; usually 20-500	Reduced in >50% the cases; average 30; often higher in patients with concomitant diabetes mellitus	Organisms may be seen in India ink preparation and on culture (Sabouraud's medium); will usually grow on blood agar; may produce alcohol in cerebrospinal fluid from fermentation of glucose; culture is imperative; large volumes of CSF are recommended for culture (5-10 mL)
Syphilis (acute)	Usually elevated	Average, 500; usually lymphocytes; rare PMNs	Average, 100; - globulin often high, with abnormal colloidal gold curve	Normal (rarely reduced)	Positive results of reagin test for syphilis; spirochetes not demonstrable by usual techniques of smear or culture
Sarcoidosis	Normal to considerably elevated	0 to <100 mononuclear cells	Slight to moderate elevation	Normal	Cultures Negative
Neurocysticercosis		Lymphocytic and eosinophilic pleocytosis (5-500)	Elevated	Decreased	Enzyme-linked immunosorbent assay, Western blot for IgM and IgG antibodies
CMV polyradiculopathy			Marked increase		CMV inclusions on cytology examination

*Polymorphonuclear leukocytes

†Spinal tap may be contraindicated in these conditions

Modified from Feigin RD and Cherry JD, eds, *Textbook of Pediatric Infectious Diseases*, Vol 1, Philadelphia, PA: WB Saunders, 1992, 410.

Patient Preparation Aseptic preparation for aspiration

Specimen Cerebrospinal fluid. A sample of peripheral blood for serum should be obtained concurrently if CSF is being studied for presence of oligoclonal bands (eg, as in demyelinating diseases, in particular multiple sclerosis) or when glucose levels are needed as in cases of possible infection (eg, meningitis or encephalitis). Blood culture and plasma glucose should be drawn as well as CBC and differential in cases of possible meningitis.

Container Sterile test tubes from lumbar puncture (LP) tray

Collection Specimens of spinal fluid and blood for culture should be obtained prior to initiation of antibiotic treatment of meningitis. Tubes must be labeled with patient's name, date, and labeled with number indicating sequence in which tubes were obtained. Specimen must be delivered to the laboratory **promptly**.

Storage Instructions Do **not** store; place in the hands of a laboratory technologist. The laboratory should not discard such specimens for several days; need for additional testing may be subsequently recognized.

Special Instructions When a diagnosis of meningitis is considered, culture of other materials as well as culture of CSF may be helpful. Most children with bacterial meningitis are initially bacteremic, and blood cultures are of value. In neonates and small children, urine culture may be positive. Culture and Gram stain of petechiae may provide immediate diagnosis.

Reference Interval
- Premature neonate: <29 cells/mm³
- Younger than 1 month: <32 cells/mm³
- 1 month to 1 year: <10 cells/mm³
- 1-4 years: <8 cells/mm³
- 5 years to puberty: <5 cells/mm³
- Adults: 0-5 cells/mm³, all lymphocytes and monocytes; 0 red blood cells; protein: lumbar: 15-50 mg/dL, cisternal: 15-25 mg/dL, ventricular: 6-15 mg/dL; glucose: 50-80 mg/dL

Possible Panic Range Increased number of cells

Use Evaluate bacterial or viral encephalitis, meningitis, meningoencephalitis, mycobacterial or fungal infection, parasitic infestations, primary or secondary malignancy, leukemia/malignant lymphoma of CNS, trauma, vascular occlusive disease, vasculitis, heredofamilial and/or degenerative processes. **Table 1** outlines findings, including those with subdural empyema, brain abscess, ventricular empyema, cerebral epidural abscess, spinal epidural abscess, tuberculosis, syphilis, sarcoidosis, and other entities.[2]

The nucleated blood cell count in the cerebrospinal fluid is described as superior to any combination of the other CSF tests for bacterial meningitis. In patients who have not received antimicrobial agents the ultimate diagnosis of bacterial meningitis is based on results of culture.[3] The cell count and differential count are mandatory, and a Gram stain must be examined promptly in work-up of possible meningitis. Glucose and protein are necessary in the work-up for possible meningitis. In a study of aseptic versus bacterial meningitis, the mean CSF cell counts in aseptic and bacterial meningitis were respectively 228 cells/mm³ (range 6-2650) and 4035 cells/mm³ (range 16-17,650).[4] **Early viral infection** as well as **bacterial meningitis** can elicit neutrophil leukocytosis in blood and CSF. In viral meningitis, a shift to mononuclear predominance often occurs subsequently.[5,6,7] In 205 cases of acute **viral** meningitis, the 25th percentile, median, and 75th percentile leukocyte counts (10⁶/L) were 37/100/250, with 3%, 33%, and 75%, respectively PMNs. In 217 cases of acute **bacterial** meningitis, leukocyte counts (10⁶/L) were 330/1195/4400 with 70%, 86%, and 97% PMNs, respectively.[8] Seasonal curves for viral and bacterial infection go in opposite directions; viral meningitis is a disease of midsummer, while bacterial meningitis is relatively more common in the winter.[8]

Table 2. Features of Four Similar Syndromes of Ascending Paralysis

Feature	Tick Paralysis	Guillain-Barré Syndrome	Spinal Cord Lesion	Poliomyelitis
Rate of progression	Hours to days	Days to weeks	Gradual or abrupt	Days to weeks
Babinski sign	Absent	Absent	Present	Absent
Sensory loss	None	Mild	Present	None
Meningeal signs	Absent	Rare	Absent	Present
Fever	Absent	Rare	Absent	Present
Cerebrospinal fluid findings:				
Protein level	Normal	High	Normal or high	High
White cell count/mm³	<10	<10	Variable	>10
Time to recovery	<24h after tick removal	Weeks to months	Variable, depending on cause	Months to years or no recovery (permanent paresis)

Modified from Felz MW, Smith CD, and Swift TR, "Brief Report: A Six-Year-Old Girl With Tick Paralysis," *N Engl J Med*, 2000, 342(2):90-4.

The differential diagnosis of a number of entities requires clinical and laboratory correlation. Botulism is characterized by descending paralysis, but both botulism and tick paralysis can mimic the Guillain-Barré syndrome.[9] Guillain-Barré syndrome progresses to peak neurologic impairment within 4 weeks; in tick paralysis, CSF is normal and progression to peak paralysis requires only hours to a few days.[10] See **Table 2**.

Signals of possible meningeal infection in the newborn: Leukocyte count >30 cells/mm³ with more than 60% PMNs, CSF protein >100 mg/dL, CSF glucose lower than 40% of the level in blood are findings in bacterial meningitis.[11] CSF WBC >10 cells/mm³ in very young infants, and 5 cells/mm³ in older infants and children with >1 PMN/mm³ is abnormal.

Limitations A traumatic (bloody) tap may make interpretation difficult. Normal CSF may be found early in meningitis.

Contraindications Lumbar puncture (LP) is generally considered unsafe and contraindicated in cases of brain abscess proven by neuroimaging. LP may cause tentorial herniation and death. In cases of suspected or possible abscess, neuroimaging, usually with contrast, should be done to exclude brain abscess prior to LP. CSF findings with brain abscess may be normal, or resemble those of bacterial meningitis.

Methodology Manual cell count using hemacytometer. Electronic cell counters lack precision and validity when used to analyze most CSF specimens (background is high relative to total white cell count). Differential cell study using manually prepared smears or cytocentrifuge methods. Bovine albumin, 22%, mixed with spinal fluid specimen is helpful in maintaining the morphologic integrity of smeared cells. For chemical, microbiologic, and other analyses, see appropriate entries.

Additional Information More extensive testing: Cytology, conventional cultures and cultures for mycobacteria, fungi, and viruses, additional chemistry and serologic determinations must usually be ordered separately. Gram stain of punch biopsy or needle aspiration of hemorrhagic skin lesions in meningococcemia can provide rapid diagnosis.

Correction for traumatic tap: If cell counts and protein determinations are performed on CSF and blood obtained at the same time, correction for "bloody tap" can be calculated. All CSF measurements should be made from the same tube. The ratio of RBC count CSF to RBC count blood provides a factor which when multiplied by the blood WBC count or blood protein level indicates the expected level of contribution of these parameters from the blood to the spinal fluid. These contributed WBC or protein values can then be subtracted from the respective values measured in the spinal fluid. For example:

1. RBCs (CSF)/RBCs (blood) x WBCs (blood) or x protein (blood).
2. WBCs (CSF) or protein (CSF) - product calculated In 1 = true CSF WBC or true CSF protein.

If the peripheral blood is normal and traumatic tap occurs, about 1 WBC is added to the CSF for each 700 RBCs that have been transferred into the CSF. RBC contamination from a traumatic tap does not adversely affect the laboratory diagnosis of bacterial meningitis. Prompt centrifugation and analysis of xanthochromic fluid can help to differentiate a traumatic tap from bloody CSF. Clearing of RBCs from tubes 1-4 suggests traumatic tap.

When only a small amount of CSF can be obtained, Gram stain and culture must always have priority over antigen detection testing.[12] Antigen detection methods cannot replace culture and Gram stain. Gram stain of spun sediment is positive in 60% to 80% of cases of bacterial meningitis. A bacterial culture is the first test to be performed on cerebrospinal fluid for meningitis. It is the gold standard for diagnosis.[13] A requirement for 50 or more leukocytes per µL of CSF has been proposed as justification for bacterial antigen testing.[12] Another group found a CSF nucleated blood cell count <6/mm³ provided a criterion for an abbreviated CSF evaluation.[3] Correlation exists between bacterial concentration in CSF and the numbers of PMNs found.[14]

There is substantial mortality and morbidity in subjects with bacterial meningitis. Neurologic sequelae are found in as many as 33% of all survivors in one study.[15] Sequelae occur especially in newborns and children.[12] Particularly when bacterial meningitis follows an insidious pattern, diagnostic delay may be unavoidable.[16] Eight of 21 survivors of neonatal meningitis were normal, eight had mild sequelae, and five had moderate to severe sequelae in a culture-proven series.[17] Despite early diagnosis and the use of appropriate therapy, both complications of meningitis and death may occur. As many as 50% of survivors of meningitis have some sequelae, as summarized by the Task Force on Diagnosis and Management of Meningitis.[18]

A "CSF leukocyte aggregation score" (LAS) has been developed and applied to the rapid differentiation of bacterial (potentially fatal) meningitis from viral meningitis (usually benign). The CSF LAS (ratio of cell clusters of more than 3 cells to individual cells in CSF smears) was standardized and showed <5% intra- and interobserver variability. The mean LAS was significantly higher in bacterial meningitis (32.1% with range of 0% to 84%) than in viral meningitis (0% with range of 0% to 16.6%). In children with meningitis of undefined etiology, the mean LAS score was 0% with a range of 0% to 20.7%. Compared with 11 other laboratory tests, the LAS was the best predictor of bacterial meningitis (odds ratio of 1.6:3.7 in a logistic regression model).[19]

(Continued)

Cerebrospinal Fluid Analysis: Overview (Continued)

White cell pleocytosis is found in only 33% of patients with multiple sclerosis (MS). The white count rarely exceeds 50 cells/mm^3.[20] Most patients with MS (66%) have normal total protein. In contrast, patients with Guillain-Barré syndrome usually have no excess white cells but show elevated CSF protein >40 mg/dL.[10]

A number of the complications of HIV-1 infections are provided in the Key Word Index under Acquired Immunodeficiency Syndrome. Many of these may involve the central nervous system.

Nonsteroidal anti-inflammatory drugs, antibiotics, intravenous immunoglobulins, and monoclonal antibodies against the T$_3$ receptor are the most common causes of drug-induced aseptic meningitis. Neutrophilic pleocytosis with the remainder of clinical and CSF findings obscures distinction from infectious meningitis but resolution takes place several days after discontinuation of the drug.[21]

Footnotes

1. Swartz MN, *Bacterial Meningitis, Cecil Textbook of Medicine*, 21st ed, Chapter 328, Goldman L and Bennett JC, eds, Philadelphia, PA: WB Saunders Co, 2000, 1645-54.
2. Felgin RD and Cherry JD, *Textbook of Pediatric Infectious Diseases*, Philadelphia, PA: WB Saunders Co, 1987, 488.
3. Rodewald LE, Woodin KA, Szilagyi PG, et al, "Relevance of Common Tests of Cerebrospinal Fluid in Screening for Bacterial Meningitis," *J Pediatr*, 1991, 119(3):363-9.
4. Walsh-Kelly C, Nelson DB, Smith DS, et al, "Clinical Predictors of Bacterial Versus Aseptic Meningitis in Childhood," *Ann Emerg Med*, 1992, 21(8):910-4.
5. Connolly KJ and Hammer SM, "The Acute Aseptic Meningitis Syndrome," *Infect Dis Clin North Am*, 1990, 4(4):599-622.
6. Hammer SM and Connolly KJ, "Viral Aseptic Meningitis in the United States: Clinical Features, Viral Etiologies, and Differential Diagnosis," *Curr Clin Top Infect Dis*, 1992, 12:1-25.
7. Amir J, Harel L, Frydman M, et al, "Shift of Cerebrospinal Polymorphonuclear Cell Percentage in the Early Stage of Aseptic Meningitis," *J Pediatr*, 1991, 119(6):938-41.
8. Spanos A, Harrell FE Jr, and Durack DT, "Differential Diagnosis of Acute Meningitis: An Analysis of the Predictive Value of Initial Observations," *JAMA*, 1989, 262(19):2700-7.
9. Schaumburg HH and Herskovitz S, "The Weak Child - A Cautionary Tale," *N Engl J Med*, 2000, 342(2):127-9.
10. Felz MW, Smith CD, and Swift TR, "Brief Report: A Six-Year-Old Girl With Tick Paralysis," *N Engl J Med*, 2000, 342(2):90-4.
11. McCracken GH Jr, "Current Management of Bacterial Meningitis in Infants and Children," *Pediatr Infect Dis J*, 1992, 11(2):169-74.
12. Gray LD and Fedorko DP, "Laboratory Diagnosis of Bacterial Meningitis," *Clin Microbiol Rev*, 1992, 5(2):130-45.
13. Smith AL, "Bacterial Meningitis," *Pediatr Rev*, 1993, 14(1):11-8.
14. La Scolea LJ Jr and Dryja D, "Quantitation of Bacteria in Cerebrospinal Fluid and Blood of Children With Meningitis and Its Diagnostic Significance," *J Clin Microbiol*, 1984, 19(2):187-90.
15. Sáez-Llorens X, Ramilo O, Mustafa MM, et al, "Molecular Pathophysiology of Bacterial Meningitis: Current Concepts and Therapeutic Implications," *J Pediatr*, 1990, 116(5):671-84.
16. Kilpi T, Anttila M, Kallio MJ, et al, "Severity of Childhood Bacterial Meningitis and Duration of Illness Before Diagnosis," *Lancet*, 1991, 338(8764):406-9.
17. Franco SM, Cornelius VE, and Andrews BF, "Long-Term Outcome of Neonatal Meningitis," *Am J Dis Child*, 1992, 146(6):567-71.
18. Klein JO, Feigin RD, and McCracken GH Jr, "Report of the Task Force on Diagnosis and Management of Meningitis," *Pediatrics*, 1986, 78(5):959-82.
19. Michelow IC, Nicol M, Tiemessen C, et al, "Value of Cerebrospinal Fluid Leukocyte Aggregation in Distinguishing the Causes of Meningitis in Children," *Pediatr Infect Dis J*, 2000, 19(1):66-72.
20. Rudick RA, "Multiple Sclerosis and Related Conditions," *Cecil Textbook of Medicine*, 21st ed, Chapter 482, Goldman L and Bennett JC, eds, Philadelphia, PA: WB Saunders Co, 2000, 2141-9.
21. Moris G and Garcia-Monco JC, "The Challenge of Drug-Induced Aseptic Meningitis," *Arch Intern Med*, 1999, 159(11):1185-94.

References

Attia J, Hatala R, Cook DJ, et al, "Does This Adult Patient Have Acute Meningitis?" *JAMA*, 1999, 282(2):175-81.

Bonadio WA, Smith DS, Goddard S, et al, "Distinguishing Cerebrospinal Fluid Abnormalities in Children With Bacterial Meningitis and Traumatic Lumbar Puncture," *J Infect Dis*, 1990, 162(1):251-4.

Feigin RD, McCracken GH Jr, and Klein JO, "Diagnosis and Management of Meningitis," *Pediatr Infect Dis J*, 1992, 11:785-814.

Levy M, Wong E, and Fried D, "Diseases That Mimic Meningitis. Analysis of 650 Lumbar Punctures," *Clin Pediatr (Phila)*, 1990, 29(5):258-61.

Norris CM, Danis PG, and Gardner TD, "Aseptic Meningitis in the Newborn and Young Infant," *Am Fam Phys*, 1999, 59(10):2761-70.

Travlos A, Anton HA, and Wing PC, "Cerebrospinal Fluid Cell Count Following Spinal Cord Injury," *Arch Phys Med Rehabil*, 1994, 75(3):293-6.

Yurdakok M and Kocabas CN, "CSF Erythrocyte Volume Analysis: A Simple Method for the Diagnosis of Traumatic Tap in Newborn Infants," *Pediatr Neurosurg*, 1991-92, 17(4):199.

♦ **Chédiak-Higashi Anomaly** *see* Peripheral Blood: Differential Leukocyte Count *on page 464*

♦ **Chromium-51 Tagged RBC Survival Test** *see* ^{51}Cr Red Cell Survival *on page 422*

♦ **Chronic Idiopathic Neutropenia** *see* TGF-β, Serum *on page 490*

♦ **Circulating Transferrin Receptor** *see* Transferrin Receptor, Soluble, Serum or Plasma *on page 493*

♦ **Clusters of Differentiation** *see* Flow Cytometry, Overview *on page 432*

♦ ***c-mpl*-Ligand (ligand for the receptor encoded by the *c-mpl* proto-oncogene)** *see* Thrombopoietin, Serum or Plasma *on page 491*

♦ **Cobalophilin** *see* Vitamin B$_{12}$ Unsaturated Binding Capacity *on page 495*

Cold Hemolysin Test

Related Information

Cold Agglutinin Titer *on page 594*
Cryofibrinogen *on page 337*
Cryoglobulin, Qualitative, Serum and Plasma *on page 524*
Hemosiderin Stain, Urine *on page 876*
Infectious Mononucleosis Screening Test *on page 643*
Parvovirus B19 DNA *on page 669*
Parvovirus B19 Serology *on page 669*
VDRL, Serum *on page 688*

Synonyms Donath-Landsteiner Test; Paroxysmal Cold Hemoglobinuria Test

Applies to Parvovirus B19

Abstract Test for paroxysmal cold hemoglobinuria (PCH), a condition caused by sensitization of red blood cells (at temperatures less than 30°C) by a complement binding IgG biphasic hemolysin. Warming to 37°C causes hemolysis of patient's RBCs. Patients may develop fever, back/leg pain, abdominal cramps, and shaking chills with hemoglobinemia/hemoglobinuria.

Specimen Blood

Container Red top tube

Collection Obtain 7 mL of blood by routine venipuncture from patient in previously warmed (37°C) red top tube and another 7 mL of blood in previously cooled (3°C to 4°C) red top tube in an ice water bath. Collect similar samples from a normal individual for a negative control. Deliver to hematology laboratory immediately.

Special Instructions Consult laboratory; scheduling will likely be necessary.

Reference Interval Negative

Use Diagnosis of the uncommon disorder, paroxysmal cold hemoglobinuria. PCH may occur with syphilis, infectious mononucleosis, influenza, measles, mumps, chickenpox, parvovirus B19, and other viral illnesses.

Methodology Observation of red cell lysis by patient's cold activated serum. Sample of patient's whole blood is kept at 4°C for 30 minutes and then at 37°C for 30 minutes. A second sample is kept only at 37°C. Both samples are observed for hemolysis after being centrifuged. A positive test is the presence of hemolysis in the 4°C exposed sample. The second (control) specimen should show no hemolysis. (Donath-Landsteiner test for PCH.)

Additional Information There are two types of cold autoantibodies, the cold autoagglutinins/hemolysins (as found in cold-antibody autoimmune hemolytic anemia) and the biphasic hemolysins. These antibodies are characterized by optimal reaction at temperatures less than 30°C. The cold autoagglutinins are usually monoclonal or polyclonal IgM antibodies with anti-H, anti-IH, or anti-i immunospecificity. Anti-Pr is the second most commonly associated antibody. Classic paroxysmal cold hemoglobinuria is caused by an IgG complement binding biphasic hemolysin,[1] an autoantibody that attaches to the RBC membrane at 4°C to 20°C. The antibody causes only weak agglutination of red cells in saline. When the temperature rises to 37°C, hemolysis occurs. The immunohematologic specificity of the Donath-Landsteiner type PCH antibody is usually anti-P.[2] While PCH was the first hemolytic anemia to be recognized, it has become the least common type of autoimmune hemolytic anemia. Previously associated with syphilis, it is now more commonly seen in viral-like illness, largely in children.[3] Parvovirus 19 infection may cause a reticulocytopenic postinfectious hemolytic anemia in children.[4] The red cell P antigen has specificity for the D-L antibody and is also the parvovirus receptor on red cell precursors. The re-emergence of syphilis associated with AIDS may cause a resurgence of PCH.

PCH and D-L type antibodies have been associated with non-Hodgkin's lymphoma,[5,6,7] leading one group of authors to emphasize that "unexplained hemolytic anemia in the elderly should raise the suspicion of an underlying lymphoproliferative disorder."[7]

Footnotes

1. Engelfriet CP, Overbeeke MA, and von dem Borne AE, "Autoimmune Hemolytic Anemia," *Semin Hematol*, 1992, 29(1):3-12.
2. Judd WJ, Wilkinson SL, Issitt PD, et al, "Donath-Landsteiner Hemolytic Anemia Due to an Anti-Pr-Like Biphasic Hemolysin," *Transfusion*, 1986, 26(5):423-5.
3. Nordhagen R, Stensvold A, Winses A, et al, "Paroxysmal Cold Hemoglobinuria. The Most Frequent Acute Autoimmune Haemolytic Anaemia in Children?" *Acta Paediatr Scand*, 1984, 73(2):258-62.
4. Chambers LA and Rauck AM, "Acute Transient Hemolytic Anemia With a Positive Donath-Landsteiner Test Following Parvovirus B19 Infection," *J Pediatr Hematol Oncol*, 1996, 18(2):178-81.
5. Sivakumaran M, Murphy PT, Booker DJ, et al, "Paroxysmal Cold Haemoglobinuria Caused by non-Hodgkin's Lymphoma," *Br J Haematol*, 1999, 105(1):278-9.

6. Ramos RR, Curtis BR, Eby CS, et al, "Fatal Outcome in a Patient With Autoimmune Hemolytic Anemia Associated With an IgM Bithermic Anti-ITP," *Transfusion*, 1994, 34(5):427-31.
7. Sharar AI, Hillsley RE, Wax TD, et al, "Paroxysmal Cold Hemoglobinuria Associated With non-Hodgkin's Lymphoma," *South Med J*, 1994, 87(3):397-9.

References
Dacie JV and Lewis SM, *Practical Haematology*, 8th ed, New York, NY: Churchill Livingstone, 1995, 520-4.

Lycholm LJ and Edmond MB, Images in Clinical Medicine, "Seasonal Hemolysis Due to Cold-Agglutinin Syndrome," *N Engl J Med*, 1996, 334(7):437.

Sherry C, "Acquired Immune Anemias of Increased Destruction," *Clinical Hematology: Principles, Procedures, Correlations*, 2nd ed, Chapter 19, Stiene-Martin EA, Lotspeich-Steininger CA, and Koepke JA, eds, Philadelphia, PA: Lippincott-Raven Publishers, 1998, 286-7.

Sokol RJ, Booker DJ, and Stamps R, "Investigation of Patients With Autoimmune Haemolytic Anemia and Provision of Blood for Transfusion," *J Clin Pathol*, 1995, 48(7):602-10.

Sthoeger ZM, Sthoeger D, Shtalrid M, et al, "Mechanism of Autoimmune Hemolytic Anemia in Chronic Lymphocytic Leukemia," *Am J Hematol*, 1993, 43(4):259-64.

Complete Blood Count

Related Information

Synonyms Blood Cell Profile; Blood Count; CBC; Hematology Profile; Hemogram

Test Includes WBC count, differential count, Hct, Hb, RBC count, WBC and RBC morphology, RBC indices, platelet estimate, platelet count, RDW, and histograms. Although hemoglobin concentration (of individual RBCs), RBC, WBC, and platelet histograms are not usually available on patient charts, they are helpful to the technologist in detecting problems with patients and quality control. Even though the histograms are not on the chart, they can be viewed in the laboratory along with a stained blood smear. Also provided are automated 5-part white cell differentials: granulocytes, monocytes, lymphocytes, eosinophils, basophils, and additional RBC and platelet indices. In addition, current analyzers have reticulocyte capability including determination of a set of reticulocyte indices.

Abstract The CBC is a profile of tests rather than a single test. It is the standard, broadly inclusive, usually automated test for evaluation of RBC, WBC, and platelets. The majority of CBC results are generated by highly automated electronic and pneumatic multichannel analyzers based on aperture-impedance and/or laser beam cell sizing and counting.

Specimen Whole blood

Container Lavender top (EDTA) tube. International Council for Standardization in Hematology recommendation is for use of K_2-EDTA, 1.5-2.2 mg/mL of blood as anticoagulant for blood cell counting and sizing.[1]

Collection Mix specimen 10 times by gentle inversion. If specimen is not brought to the laboratory immediately refrigeration is required. If the anticipated delay in arrival is more than 4 hours, two blood smears should be prepared immediately after the venipuncture and submitted with the blood specimen.

Storage Instructions EDTA-anticoagulated sample should be analyzed within 6 hours at room temperature and within 24 hours when stored at 4°C. Studies using the Cell-Dyn 3500 (Abbott Diagnostics, Mountain View, CA) found blood cell parameters stable for up to 24-48 hours (differential stable for 24 hours) at 4°C.[2,3]

Causes for Rejection Improper tube, clotted specimen, hemolyzed specimen, dilution of blood with I.V. fluid

Turnaround Time If the analyzer is operational, a stat result may be available within 5-10 minutes.

Special Instructions Blood specimen and diluent may require prewarming to obtain meaningful results if cold agglutinins are present.

Reference Interval Accompanying tables summarize differences in red cell parameter normal ranges, note especially important age and sex variances.

Refer to tables. See White Blood Cell Count *on page 496* for review of origin of reference values used by many current texts.

Mean Hematologic Values for Low-Birth-Weight Infants*

Weight and Gestational Age at Birth	Age at Testing	Hemoglobin (g/dL)	Hematocrit (%)	Reticulocytes (%)
<1500 g, 28-32 wk	3 d	17.5 ±1.5	54 ±5	8.0 ±3.5
	1 wk	15.5 ±1.5	48 ±5	3.0 ±1.0
	2 wk	13.5 ±1.1	42 ±4	3.0 ±1.0
	3 wk	11.5 ±1.0	35 ±4	—
	4 wk	10.0 ±0.9	30 ±3	6.0 ±2.0
	6 wk	8.5 ±0.5	25 ±2	11.0 ±3.5
	8 wk	8.5 ±0.5	25 ±2	8.5 ±3.5
	10 wk	9.0 ±0.5	28 ±3	7.0 ±3.0
1500-2000 g, 32-36 wk	3 d	19.0 ±2.0	59 ±6	6.0 ±2.0
	1 wk	16.5 ±1.5	51 ±5	3.0 ±1.0
	2 wk	14.5 ±1.1	44 ±5	2.5 ±1.0
	3 wk	13.0 ±1.1	39 ±4	—
	4 wk	12.0 ±1.0	36 ±4	3.0 ±1.0
	6 wk	9.5 ±0.8	28 ±3	6.0 ±2.0
	8 wk	9.5 ±0.5	28 ±3	5.0 ±1.5
	10 wk	9.5 ±0.5	29 ±3	4.5 ±1.5
2000-2500 g, 36-40 wk	3 d	19.0 ±2.0	59 ±6	4.0 ±1.0
	1 wk	16.5 ±1.5	51 ±5	3.0 ±1.0
	2 wk	15.0 ±1.5	45 ±5	2.5 ±1.0
	3 wk	14.0 ±1.1	43 ±4	—
	4 wk	12.5 ±1.0	37 ±4	2.0 ±1.0
	6 wk	10.5 ±0.9	31 ±3	3.0 ±1.0
	8 wk	10.5 ±0.9	31 ±3	3.0 ±1.0
	10 wk	11.0 ±1.0	33 ±3	3.0 ±1.0

Adapted from Johnson TR, "How Growing Up Can Alter Lab Values in Pediatric Laboratory Medicine," *Diag Med* (special issue), 1982, 5:13-8.

*Mean ±1 SD.

Proposed Classification of Anemic Disorders Based on Red Cell Mean (MCV) and Heterogeneity (RDW)

MCV Low RDW Normal (microcytic homogeneous)	MCV Low RDW High (microcytic heterogeneous)	MCV Normal RDW Normal (normocytic homogeneous)	MCV Normal RDW High (normocytic heterogeneous)	MCV High RDW Normal (macrocytic homogeneous)	MCV High RDW High (macrocytic heterogeneous)
Heterozygous thalassemia*	Iron deficiency*	Normal	Mixed deficiency*	Aplastic anemia	Folate deficiency*
Chronic disease*	S/β -thalassemia	Chronic disease* chronic liver disease*†	Early iron or folate deficiency*	Preleukemia†	Vitamin B_{12} deficiency
	Hemoglobin H	Nonanemic hemoglobinopathy (eg, AS, AC)	Anemic hemoglobinopathy (eg, SS, SC)*		Immune hemolytic anemia
	Red cell fragmentation	Transfusion†	Myelofibrosis		Cold agglutinins
		Chemotherapy	Sideroblastic*		Chronic lymphocytic leukemia, high count
		Chronic lymphocytic leukemia			
		Chronic myelocytic leukemia†			
		Hemorrhage			
		Hereditary spherocytosis			

Adapted from Bessman JD Jr, Gilmer PR, and Gardner FH, "Improved Classification of Anemias by MCV and RDW," *Am J Clin Pathol*, 1983, 80:324. The data for sensitivity of RDW and MCV in each disease category can be obtained from the authors.

*MCV alone <90% sensitive.   †RDW alone <90% sensitive.

(Continued)

Complete Blood Count *(Continued)*

Red Cell Values on First Postnatal Day*

Gestational Age (wk)	24-25	26-27	28-29	30-31	32-33	34-35	36-37	Term
RBC (x 10⁶/mm³)	4.65 ±0.43	4.73 ±0.45	4.62 ±0.75	4.79 ±0.74	5.0 ±0.76	5.09 ±0.5	5.27 ±0.68	5.14 ±0.7
Hb (g/dL)	19.4 ±1.5	19.0 ±2.5	19.3 ±1.8	19.1 ±2.2	18.5 ±2.0	19.6 ±2.1	19.2 ±1.7	19.3 ±2.2
Hct (%)	63 ±4	62 ±8	60 ±7	60 ±8	60 ±8	61 ±7	64 ±7	61 ±7.4
MCV (fL)	135 ±0.2	132 ±14.4	131 ±13.5	127 ±12.7	123 ±15.7	122 ±10.0	121 ±12.5	119 ±9.4
Retic (%)	6.0 ±0.5	9.6 ±3.2	7.5 ±2.5	5.8 ±2.0	5.0 ±1.9	3.9 ±1.6	4.2 ±1.8	3.2 ±1.4

Adapted from Zaizov R and Matoth Y, "Red Cell Values on the First Postnatal Day During the Last 16 Weeks of Gestation," *Amer J Hematol*, 1976, 1:2, 275-8.

*Mean values ±1 SD.

Mean (±1 SD) Reference Ranges for Hematologic Values

Age	Hb (g/dL)	Hct (%)	RBC (x 10⁶/mm³) (x 10¹²/L)	MCV (fL)	MCH (pg)	MCHC (g/dL)	WBC (x 10³/mm³) (x 10⁹/L)
Birth (cord blood)	17.1 ±1.8	52 ±5	4.64 ±0.5	113 ±6	37 ±2	33 ±1	
1 d	19.4 ±2.1	58 ±7	5.30 ±0.5	110 ±6	37 ±2	33 ±1	
2-6 d	19.8 ±2.4	66 ±8	5.40 ±0.7	122 ±14	37 ±4	30 ±3	
14-23 d	15.7 ±1.5	52 ±5	4.92 ±0.6	106 ±11	32 ±3	30 ±2	
24-37 d	14.1 ±1.9	45 ±7	4.35 ±0.6	104 ±11	32 ±3	31 ±3	
40-50 d	12.8 ±1.9	42 ±6	4.10 ±0.5	103 ±11	31 ±3	30 ±2	
2-3.5 mo	11.3 ±1.0	37 ±4	3.81 ±0.5	98 ±9	30 ±3	30 ±2	
5-10 mo	11.6 ±0.7	38 ±3	4.28 ±0.5	91 ±8	27 ±3	30 ±2	
1-3 y	11.9 ±0.6	39 ±2	4.45 ±0.4	87 ±7	27 ±2	30 ±2	
3-5 y	12.3 ±0.8	36 ±3	4.4 ±0.3	81 ±5	28 ±2	34 ±1	7.7 ±2.2
6-8 y	12.7 ±0.9	37 ±2	4.5 ±0.3	83 ±5	28 ±2	34 ±1	7.5 ±2.0
9-11 y	13.1 ±0.9	38 ±2	4.6 ±0.4	83 ±5	28 ±2	34 ±1	7.0 ±1.8
12-14 y							
male	13.8 ±1.0	40 ±3	4.8 ±0.4	84 ±5	29 ±2	34 ±1	7.0 ±1.8
female	13.2 ±1.0	39 ±2	4.5 ±0.3	86 ±5	29 ±2	34 ±1	7.1 ±2.1
15-17 y							
male	14.7 ±1.0	43 ±3	5.0 ±0.4	87 ±5	30 ±2	34 ±1	7.2 ±2.0
female	13.3 ±1.0	39 ±3	4.5 ±0.3	88 ±5	30 ±2	34 ±1	7.7 ±2.1
18-64 y							
male	15.2 ±1.1	44 ±3	5.0 ±0.4	89 ±5	31 ±2	34 ±1	7.4 ±2.1
female	13.5 ±1.1	40.5 ±3	4.4 ±0.4	90 ±6	30 ±2	34 ±1	7.2 ±2.1
65-74 y							
male	14.8 ±1.4	44 ±4	4.8 ±0.5	91 ±6	31 ±2	34 ±1	7.1 ±2.0
female	13.7 ±1.2	40.5 ±3	4.5 ±0.4	90 ±6	31 ±2	34 ±1	6.8 ±2.4

Adapted from Johnson TR, "How Growing Up Can Alter Lab Values in Pediatric Laboratory Medicine," *Diag Med* (special issue), 1982, 5:13-8; and Second National Health and Nutrition Examination Survey (NHANES), "Hematological and National Biochemistry Reference Data for Persons 6 Months - 74 Years of Age," *DHHS Publication No (PHS) 83-1682*, Hyattsville, MD: Public Health Service, Dec 1982.

Above values are reference ranges for the population defined in NHANES II (1976-1980, see above). These ranges are not necessarily identical to "normal ranges" for local populations, but are sufficiently broad such that mean ±2 SD should include most (at least 95%) of normal subjects. NHANES III data (from a 6-year study, 1988-1994) is avaiblabe, in part, as it pertains to iron deficiency. See Looker AC, Dallman PR, Carroll MD, et al, "Prevalence of Iron Deficiency in the United States," *JAMA*, 1997, 277(12):973-6. NHANES III Hb cutoff values were calculated as the mean Hb of the reference group minus 1.645 SD (corresponds to the 5th percentile value for a variable such as Hb that has a gaussian distribution). Thus, adult males (ages 20-49) had Hb level of 15.30 ±0.97 with a cutoff value <13.7/100 mL. Adult females (20-49 years) had Hb level of 13.48 ±0.91 with a cutoff value <12.0 g/100 mL.

Critical Values Critical values: Hematocrit: <18% or >54%; hemoglobin: <6.0 g/dL or >18.0 g/dL; WBC on admission: <2500/mm³ or >30,000/mm³; platelets: <20,000/mm³ or >1,000,000/mm³

Use Evaluate anemia, leukemia, reaction to inflammation and infections, peripheral blood cellular characteristics, state of hydration and dehydration, polycythemia, hemolytic disease of the newborn; manage chemotherapy decisions

Limitations Hemoglobin (and thus the derived MCH and MCHC) may be falsely high if the plasma is lipemic or if the white count is >50,000 cells/mm³. "Spun" (manual centrifuged) microhematocrits are ~3% higher (due to plasma trapping) compared to automated hematocrit levels. The increase is especially pronounced in cases of polycythemia (increased Hct levels) and when the cells are hypochromic and microcytic. The spun Hct level (as compared to automated instruments' calculated level) may be 12% higher at Hct levels of 70% and MCV of 48 fL with decrease in change to 3% higher at Hct levels of 70% with MCV of 100 fL. Cold agglutinins (high titer) may cause spurious macrocytosis and low RBC count. This results when RBC couplets are "seen" and processed as single cells by the detection circuitry. Keeping the blood warm and warming the diluent prior to and during counting can correct this problem. See also Hematocrit *on page 441.* Cryoproteinemia (cryoglobulinemia) may cause pseudoleukocytosis or pseudothrombocytosis.[4] Malaria may be a cause of pseudoreticulocytosis.[5]

Methodology Varies considerably between institutions. Most laboratories have high capacity multichannel instruments in place (available from multiple commercial sources). The majority measure RBC and WBC parameters on the basis of changes in electrical impedance as cells and platelets are pulled through a tiny aperture. These are highly automated devices with extensive computer processing of the electrical signals after analog/digital conversion. Accuracy (with proper standardization) and precision (usually in the 0.5% to 2% range) is significantly improved over older manual and semiautomated methods. Some instruments count light impulses that are generated as cells flow across a laser beam. Proper calibration is a prime requisite. Excellent correlation for all parameters (except basophils) was shown between Cell Dyn 3500, and Coulter STK-S and between CD 3500 and manual methods.[2] The Bayer® H*2 automated counter has been used to count white and red blood cells in cerebrospinal fluid. Reliable results were reported down to the level of 5 x 10⁶ white cells/L and 5 x 10⁸ red cells/L. It was not necessary to change thresholds or sample volumes.[6]

Additional Information Presence of one or more of the following may be indications for further investigation: hemoglobin <10 g/dL, hemoglobin >18 g/dL, MCV >100 fL, MCV <80 fL, MCHC >37%, WBC >20,000/mm³, WBC <2000/mm³, presence of sickle cells, significant spherocytosis, basophilic stippling, stomatocytes, significant schistocytosis, oval macrocytes, tear drop red blood cells, eosinophilia (>10%) monocytosis (>15%), nucleated red blood cells in other than the newborn, malarial organisms or the possibility of malarial organisms, hypersegmented (five or more nuclear segments) PMNs, agranular PMNs, Pelger-Huët anomaly, Auer rods, Döhle bodies, marked toxic granulation, mononuclears in which apparent nucleoli are prominent (blast type cells), presence of metamyelocytes, myelocytes, promyelocytes, neutropenia, presence of plasma cells, peculiar atypical lymphocytes, significant increase or decrease in platelets. Some quantitative elements of the CBC are related to each other, normally, such that examination of the results of any individual analysis allow for the application of a simple but effective case individualized quality control maneuver. The RBC count, hemoglobin, and hematocrit may be analyzed by applying a "rule of three." If red cells are normochromic/normocytic, the RBC count times three should approximately equal the hemoglobin and the hemoglobin multiplied by three should approximate the hematocrit. If there is significant deviation from this relation, one should check for supporting abnormalities in RBC indices and in the peripheral blood smear. The indices themselves offer a quick quality control check of the CBC. If patient transfusion can be excluded, then RBC indices should vary little consecutively from day to day.

Histograms of red cell, white cell, platelet, and hemoglobin distributions have important application to quality assurance, analyzer trouble shooting, and patient diagnosis. Such histograms are usually not charted in patients' medical records but are available for review in the clinical laboratory. See reference by Gulati and Hyun for review of the "Value of Histograms."

Some red cell based parameters (Hb, Hct, but not RBC count) show seasonal variation - lower in summer than winter.[7] Changes in nonsmokers vs smokers were compared. In nonsmokers, Hb concentration and Hct values were lower in summer than in winter. Smokers showed no seasonal differences in Hb level but Hct increased in the summer. Nonsmokers had increases (about 6%) in summertime plasma volume, such increase did not occur in the cigarette smoking group.[7]

Anemias have been classified on the basis of their MCV and RDW (RBC heterogeneity). This classification has been especially helpful in the separation of iron deficiency from thalassemia. Heterozygous thalassemia (thalassemia minor) when associated with normal hemoglobin has a normal RDW (13.4 ±1.2%) while RDW is high with iron deficiency (16.3 ±1.8%).[8] RDW will be increased slightly in cases of thalassemia with slight anemia.[8] Some studies have found that the RDW does not reliably separate iron deficiency from thalassemia minor unless, possibly, a higher cutoff value of 17.0% is utilized.[9] A study evaluating four indices used to discriminate between thalassemic and nonthalassemic microcytosis found that MCV alone was as effective or superior to the mathematically derived values in selecting cases for thalassemia testing.[10] A recently proposed algorithm uses ethnic background and MCV to provide a "high index of suspicion" for detection of thalassemia trait when dealing with multicultural populations.[11] See also Ferritin, Serum *on page 173* and article by Jiménez and by Erler BS et al concerning, respectively, discriminant analysis and neural networks using elements of the CBC in differentiating thalassemia trait from iron deficiency.[12]

In patients who do not have disorders known to result in anisocytosis (eg, liver disease, alcoholism, combined nutritional deficiency) and who have not received a recent blood transfusion, it has been claimed RDW may be helpful in separating the anemia of chronic disease (RDW in normal range) from iron deficiency (RDW increased) thereby reducing the need for marrow study to determine iron stores.[13] It has also been reported, however, on the basis of serum ferritin levels in relatively undefined patient populations that RDW is not clinically useful in distinguishing the anemia of chronic disease from iron deficiency.[14] In some 30% to 50% of patients with anemia of chronic disease, red cells are hypochromic and microcytic, often with decreased serum iron, iron binding capacity and transferrin saturation even with demonstrably adequate iron stores.[15]

Bessman claims that the RDW is increased before the MCV decreases in iron deficiency.[16] Although this is somewhat controversial,[17] it serves as an inexpensive screen for the common iron deficiency anemia. See tables. Histogram of MCHC is of value in the diagnosis of hereditary spherocytosis[18] and the differentiation of α- from β-thalassemic red cells.[19]

As might be anticipated, the RDW is an insensitive parameter for the diagnosis of vitamin B_{12} deficiency, as well as for the diagnosis of folate deficiency, and the RDW has no value in separating alcohol-related macrocytosis from B_{12}/folate deficiency.[20] It has been found that in a hospitalized urban patient population, zidovudine treatment of AIDS is the most common cause of macrocytosis (44%) and B_{12}/folate deficiency are relatively decreased (3% and 4%, respectively).[21]

A study of RDW in healthy pregnant women at 16 and 34 weeks gestation, intrapartum, and 3 and 7 days postpartum found a significant and unexpected rise in RDW during the last 4-6 weeks before onset of labor.[22] The change was interpreted as suggestive of increased bone marrow activity and as a possibly useful indicator of impending parturition.

Most recent generation automated hematology analyzers include leukocyte differential determination and a system of "flags" to indicate presence of abnormal, atypical, and possible immature granulocytes and/or blasts. Numerous studies evaluating performance of flagging systems are now available; only a sample is included in the footnotes below.[23,24,25,26,27] Performance of analyzers in this WBC discriminate function is important in detection and characterization of leukemia.[26,27] Earlier instruments were prone to generation of inappropriate flags, in particular in the presence of atypical lymphocytes/mononuclears.[23] Automated hematology analysis has also been applied to enumeration of bone marrow cells.[28]

Currently, a variety of automated hematology analyzers are available allowing capability to be matched to specific requirements (in particular throughput needs) of the situation. Smaller instruments can be used in clinic situations and as back-up for larger machines but lack cap-piercing and bar code capability, must be hand fed, and require safety precautions (eg, use of shields and biohazard wipes). Large analyzers with the capacity to run thousands of tests per day usually interface with laboratory information systems, have networking capability, and may include "expert" systems that automate the application of complex rule-based review criteria. The test menu continues to expand with enhanced flow cytometry and with ability to perform reticulocyte counts, nucleated red blood cell determinations, CD4:CD8, CD64, immature granulocyte, and variant lymphocyte counts.[29,30] A flow cytometric analysis of platelets, "ImmunoPlt" assay is based in part on CD61 monoclonal antibody labeling (implemented on the Cell-Dyn 4000). It is especially suited for analysis of thrombocytopenic specimens (interference by nonplatelet particles is decreased).[31]

Detailed comparison and/or descriptions of available multiparameter instruments have recently become available.[32,33] Capabilities of instruments (including multiple models and versions) from the following manufacturers are detailed, including interface potential, service features, and price range.

- Abbott Diagnostics (Cell-Dyn 3200, 3700, and 4000)
- ABX Diagnostics Inc (Pentra 60[c+], 120 Retic Hematology Analyzer)
- Bayer® Diagnostics (Advia 120 Hematology System)
- Beckman Coulter, Inc (Coulter GEN-S, HmX, STK-S with Reticulocytes, MAXM with Reticulocytes)
- Roche Diagnostics Corp (Sysmex SF-3000/SF-Alpha, 9500/SE-Alpha II, SE-9500R/SE-Alpha IIR/HST, XE 2100/XE Alpha II/HST)

For consideration of the differential leukocyte count, see Peripheral Blood: Differential Leukocyte Count *on page 464* and also reference by Krause JR.

See White Blood Cell Count *on page 496* for text concerning reference range and data/comments under Additional Information which apply to the white cell count component of the CBC. Text, footnotes, and references may apply also to other components of the CBC or to the CBC in general.

Footnotes

1. "Recommendations of the International Council for Standardization in Haematology for Ethylenediaminetetraacetic Acid Anticoagulation of Blood for Blood Cell Counting and Sizing," *Am J Clin Pathol*, 1993, 100(4):371-2.
2. al-Ismail SA, Bond K, Carter AB, et al, "Two-Centre Evaluation of the Abbott CD3500 Blood Counter," *Clin Lab Haematol*, 1995, 17(1):11-21.
3. Wood BL, Andrews J, Miller S, et al, "Refrigerated Storage Improves the Stability of the Complete Blood Cell Count and Automated Differential," *Am J Clin Pathol*, 1999, 112(5):687-95.
4. Maitra A, Ward PC, Kroft SH, et al, "Cytoplasmic Inclusions in Leukocytes. An Unusual Manifestation of Cryoglobulinemia," *Am J Clin Pathol*, 2000, 113(1):107-12.
5. Hoffman JJ and Pennings JM, "Pseudoreticulocytosis as a Result of Malaria Parasites," *Clin Lab Haematol*, 1999, 21(4):257-60.
6. Aune MW and Sandberg S, "Automated Counting of White and Red Blood Cells in the Cerebrospinal Fluid," *Clin Lab Haematol*, 2000, 22(4):203-10.
7. Kristal-Boneh E, Froom P, Harari G, et al, "Seasonal Differences in Blood Cell Parameters and the Association With Cigarette Smoking," *Clin Lab Haematol*, 1997, 19(3):177-81.
8. Bessman JD, Gilmer PR, and Gardner FH, "Improved Classification of Anemias by MCV and RDW," *Am J Clin Pathol*, 1983, 80(3):322-6.
9. van Zeben D, Bieger R, van Wermeskerken RK, et al, "Evaluation of Microcytosis Using Serum Ferritin and Red Blood Cell Distribution Width," *Eur J Haematol*, 1990, 44(2):106-9.
10. Lafferty JD, Crowther MA, Ali MA, et al, "The Evaluation of Various Mathematical RBC Indices and Their Efficacy in Discriminating Between Thalassemic and Nonthalassemic Microcytosis," *Am J Clin Pathol*, 1996, 106(2):201-5.
11. Kiss TL, Ali MA, Levin M, et al, "An Algorithm to Aid in the Investigation of Thalassemia Trait in Multicultural Populations," *Arch Pathol Lab Med*, 2000, 124(9):1320-3.
12. Jiménez CV, "Iron-Deficiency Anemia and Thalassemia Trait Differentiated by Simple Hematological Tests and Serum Iron Concentrations," *Clin Chem*, 1993, 39(11):2271-5.
13. Kaye FJ and Alter BP, "Red-Cell Size Distribution Analysis: An Evaluation of Microcytic Anemia in Chronically Ill Patients," *Mt Sinai J Med*, 1985, 52(5):319-23.
14. Rice LE, Saleem A, Dunn K, et al, "RDW Fails to Distinguish Iron Deficiency From Anemia of Chronic Disease," *Blood*, 1987, 70(5 Suppl 1):55a.
15. Krantz SB, "Pathogenesis and Treatment of the Anemia of Chronic Disease," *Am J Med Sci*, 1994, 307(5):353-9.
16. McClure S, Custer E, and Bessman JD, "Improved Detection of Early Iron Deficiency in Nonanemic Subjects," *JAMA*, 1985, 253(7):1021-3.
17. Flynn MM, Reppun TS, and Bhagavan NV, "Limitations of Red Cell Distribution Width (RDW) in Evaluation of Microcytosis," *Am J Clin Pathol*, 1986, 85(4):445-9.
18. Lux SE and Palek J, "Disorders of the Red Cell Membrane," *Blood: Principles and Practice of Hematology*, Chapter 54, Handin RI, Lux SE, and Stossel TP, eds, Philadelphia, PA: JB Lippincott Co, 1995, 1701.
19. Bunyaratvej A, Fucharoen S, Greenbaum A, et al, "Hydration of Red Cells in Alpha and Beta Thalassemias Differs. A Useful Approach to Distinguish Between These Red Cell Phenotypes," *Am J Clin Pathol*, 1994, 102(2):217-22.
20. Zuiable A and Wickramasinghe SN, "RDW in Vitamin B_{12} and Folate Deficiency and in Patients With Alcohol-Related Macrocytosis," *Clin Lab Haematol*, 1992, 14(2):164-6.
21. Snower DP and Weil SC, "Changing Etiology of Macrocytosis: Zidovudine as a Frequent Causative Factor," *Am J Clin Pathol*, 1993, 99(1):57-60.
22. Shehata HA, Ali MM, Evans-Jones JC, et al, "Red Cell Distribution Width (RDW) Changes in Pregnancy," *Int J Gynaecol Obstet*, 1998, 62(1):43-6.
23. Bartels PC, Schoorl M, and Willekens FL, "Evaluation of Sysmex SF-3000 Performance Concerning Interpretive Morphology Flagging of the Leukocyte Differential Count," *Clin Lab Haematol*, 1997, 19(3):187-90.
24. Iles-Mann J and Henniker J, "An Evaluation of the Differential From the Abbott CD3500 in a Population of Patients With Haematological Abnormalities," *Clin Lab Haematol*, 1997, 19(3):191-6.

(Continued)

Complete Blood Count (Continued)

25. Corberand JX, Segonds C, Fontanilles AM, et al, "Evaluation of the Vega Haematology Analyzer in a University Hospital Setting," Clin Lab Haematol, 1999, 21(1):3-10.
26. van der Meer W, Swinkels DW, and Willems HL, " The Characterization of Leukaemias With the Sysmex NE-8000," Acta Haematol, 1997, 98(4):195-8.
27. Hoedemakers RM, Pennings JM, and Hoffmann JJ, "Performance Characteristics of Blast Flagging on the Cell Dyn 4000 Haematology Analyzer," Clin Lab Haematol, 1999, 21(5):347-51.
28. Sakamoto C, Yamane T, Ohta K, et al, "Automated Enumeration of Cellular Composition in Bone Marrow Aspirate With the CELL-DYN 4000 Automated Hematology Analyzer," Acta Haematol, 1999, 101(3):130-4.
29. Chapman M, "Hematology Analyzers Offer New Technology and User-Friendliness," Lab Med, 2000, 31(3):146-50.
30. Grimaldi E and Scopacasa F, "Evaluation of the Abbott CELL-DYN 4000 Hematology Analyzer," Am J Clin Pathol, 2000, 113(4):497-505.
31. Gill JE, Davis KA, Cowart WJ, et al, "A Rapid and Accurate Closed-Tube Immunoassay for Platelets on an Automated Hematology Analyzer," Am J Clin Pathol, 2000, 114(1):47-56.
32. Aller RD and Pierre RV, "Getting Better All the Time," CAP Today, 2000, 14(12):27, 28, 30, 32-4.
33. Davis BH and Bigelow NC, "Performance Evaluation of a Hematology Blood Counter With Five-Part Leukocyte Differential Capability," Am Clin Lab, 1999, 18(10):8-9.

References

Dot D, Miró J, and Fuentes-Arderiu X, "Within-Subject Biological Variation of Hematological Quantities and Analytical Goals," Arch Pathol Lab Med, 1992, 116(8):825-6.

Erler BS, Vitagliano P, and Lee S, "Superiority of Neural Networks Over Discriminant Functions for Thalassemia Minor Screening of Red Blood Cell Microcytosis," Arch Pathol Lab Med, 1995, 119(4):350-4.

Fraser CG, Wilkinson SP, Neville RG, et al, "Biologic Variation of Common Hematologic Laboratory Quantities in the Elderly," Am J Clin Pathol, 1989, 92(4):465-70.

Fulwood R, Johnson CL, Bryner JD, et al, "Hematological and Nutritional Biochemistry Reference Data for Persons 6 Months - 74 Years of Age: United States 1976-1980," Vital and Health Statistics, Series 11, No. 232, DHHS Publication No (PHS) 83-1682, 1982.

Gulati GL and Hyun BH, "An Unusual WBC Scattergram and Its Possible Causes," Lab Med, 1996, 27(6):398-9.

Gulati GL and Hyun BH, "The Automated CBC: A Current Perspective," Hematol Oncol Clin North Am, 1994, 8(4):593-603.

Hoyer JD, "Leukocyte Differential," Mayo Clin Proc, 1993, 68(10):1027-8.

Hübl W, Hauptlorenz S, Tlustos L, et al, "Precision and Accuracy of Monocyte Counting: Comparison of Two Hematology Analyzers, the Manual Differential and Flow Cytometry," Am J Clin Pathol, 1995, 103(2):167-70.

Jones RG, Faust AM, and Matthews RA, "Quality Team Approach in Evaluating Three Automated Hematology Analyzers With Five-Part Differential Capability," Am J Clin Pathol, 1995, 103(2):159-66.

Koepke J, "Quantitative Blood Cell Counting," Practical Laboratory Hematology, Chapter 3, Koepke JA, ed, New York, NY: Churchill Livingstone, 1991, 43-60.

Krause JR, "The Automated White Blood Cell Differential: A Current Perspective," Hematol Oncol Clin North Am, 1994, 8(4):605-16.

Lacombe F, Lacoste L, Vial JP, et al, "Automated Reticulocyte Counting and Immature Reticulocyte Fraction Measurement. Comparison of ABX PENTRA 120 Retic, Sysmex R-2000, Flow Cytometry, and Manual Counts," Am J Clin Pathol, 1999, 112(5):677-86.

Lee GR, "Anemia: A Diagnostic Strategy," Wintrobe's Clinical Hematology, 10th ed, Volume 1, Chapter 30, Lee GR, Foerster J, Lukens J, et al, eds, Philadelphia, PA: Lea & Febiger, 1999, 908-40.

Looker AC, Dallman PR, Carroll MD, et al, "Prevalence of Iron Deficiency in the United States," JAMA, 1997, 277(12):973-6.

Picard F, Gicquel C, Marnet L, et al, "Preliminary Evaluation of the New Hematology Analyzer Coulter GEN-S in a University Hospital," Clin Chem Lab Med, 1999, 37(6):681-6.

Second National Health and Nutrition Examination Survey, "Hematological and Nutritional Biochemistry Reference Data for Persons 6 Months-74 Years of Age: United States, 1976-80," Vital and Health Statistics, DHHS Publication No (PHS) 83-1682, 1982.

Sheridan BL, Lollo M, Howe S, et al, "Evaluation of the Roche Cobas Argos 5Diff Automated Haematology Analyzer With Comparison to a Coulter STK-S," Clin Lab Haematol, 1994, 16(2):117-30.

Tsuji T, Sakata T, Hamaguchi Y, et al, "New Rapid Flow Cytometric Method for the Enumeration of Nucleated Red Blood Cells," Cytometry, 1999, 37(4):291-301.

van Duijnhoven HL and Treskes M, "Marked Interference of Hyperglycemia in Measurements of Mean (Red) Cell Volume by Technicon® H Analyzers," Clin Chem, 1996, 42(1):76-80.

♦ **Congenital Neutropenia** see White Blood Cell Count on page 496

♦ **Cordocentesis** see Kleihauer-Betke on page 453

♦ **Cough Variant Asthma** see Eosinophil Smear on page 428

♦ **Crash Syndrome** see Inherited Diseases of Metabolism and Cell Structure on page 449

♦ **Cripps Method (for plasma hemoglobin)** see Hemoglobin, Plasma on page 446

♦ **^{51}Cr-Labeled Red Cell Volume** see Red Cell Mass on page 478

^{51}Cr Red Cell Survival

Related Information

Blood Volume on page 407

Occult Blood, Stool on page 315

Reticulocyte Count on page 481

Synonyms Chromium-51 Tagged RBC Survival Test; Erythrocyte Survival; Red Cell Survival; Survival of Red Blood Cells

Applies to Biotin-Labeled Red Cell Survival

Patient Preparation Obtain signed procedure permit for "^{51}Cr red cell survival." Patient's own ^{51}Cr-labeled red cells are infused. Patient should be provided a schedule for serial blood samples to be drawn.

Specimen Whole blood is drawn, processed (tagged with ^{51}Cr), and reinfused into the patient.

Container Lavender top (EDTA) tube

Collection Scheduled periodic blood samples are drawn for determination of residual radioactivity.

Causes for Rejection Previous isotope procedure with significant radioactivity remaining in patient's blood, significant transfused blood, intermittent bleeding episodes

Turnaround Time Time required for procedure depends on half-time of disappearance of labeled cells and averages 3 weeks.

Special Instructions At least 21 days should be allowed for this study. When selective splenic sequestration as cause of hemolysis is suspected, liver and spleen readings may be performed in conjunction with ^{51}Cr RBC Survival Test.

Reference Interval Presence of half of ^{51}Cr label remaining at 25-35 days (red cell survival half-life of 25-35 days).[1] Given an isotope label that would act as a "perfect" tracer (no loss through elution), one would expect half of the label to disappear at about 55-60 days, half of the average red cell life span of 110-120 days (see discussion that follows). The ratio of spleen to liver counts is usually 1:1 in normal individuals.

Use Provide proof of hemolytic process (ie, determine if patient's RBCs have decreased survival); determine red cell survival in cases of increased red cell destruction (ie, immune hemolytic anemia;[2] spherocytosis, red cell enzyme deficiency, and hemoglobinopathies); evaluate occult blood loss, especially subdural hematomas,[3] and splenic sequestration. In the spleen:liver (S:L) ratio, the average patient with splenomegaly ratio is 1:1; hemolytic anemias show 3:1 or 4:1.

Limitations This test cannot discriminate between red cell loss due to intravascular hemolysis and red cell loss due to bleeding that results in blood loss from the intravascular compartment. Test is expensive.

Methodology Patient's own RBCs incubated with ^{51}Cr under sterile conditions are injected back into the patient's vascular system and periodic blood samples are obtained for measurement of residual radioactivity over a 2- to 3-week period. Activity (counts/minute/mL of RBCs) obtained at 24 hours is usually taken as the starting point (is given a value of 100%). A plot is constructed (should include hematocrit correction)[4] and the ^{51}Cr half-life is determined. A flow cytometry-based method has been found to lack sensitivity and accuracy as compared to conventional ^{51}Cr labeled in vivo red cell survival (when the proportion of transfused cells in the recipient is some 0.2% or less).[5]

Additional Information The ^{51}Cr red cell survival does not equate numerically with one-half of the physiologic RBC lifespan (110-120 days). This is due to elution of the ^{51}Cr label from red cells during the procedure. As a result, the ^{51}Cr survival time does not relate in a simple or direct manner to the red cell lifespan and is best viewed as a semiquantitative index of survival. Given a "perfect" label, half of the activity would be lost at 55-60 days. Di-isopropylfluorophosphate (DFP) ^{14}C, ^{32}P, or tritium labels act, essentially, as a perfect label but are not in common routine clinical use as, lacking gamma emission, imaging or organ uptake studies cannot be performed. In patients with hemolysis, the RBC survival curve results from the rate of elution of the label combined with the rate of random hemolysis. In addition to DFP, red cells may be labeled for survival studies with ^{14}C cyanate, ^{75}Se selenomethionine, ^{14}C or ^{15}N glycine or ^{55}Fe or ^{59}Fe iron. Because of the penetration capability of gamma emitting ^{51}Cr, patients with ^{51}Cr-labeled RBCs can undergo in vivo count rate measurements over the spleen and liver during red cell survival study. See reference by Landaw for clinical significance of spleen:liver ratio, RBC sequestration index, and RBC survival.

A nonradioactive, nontoxic alternative for red cell survival studies has been developed using a canine animal model. Red cells were labeled with Bx NHS (a biotin compound soluble in dimethylformamide) and detected by flow cytometry (FITC-labeled avidin and excitation wavelength of 488 nm).[6] Biotinylated autologous red blood cells have also been used in humans to determine red cell survival.[7]

Footnotes

1. International Committee for Standardization in Haematology, "Recommended Method for Radioisotope Red-Cell Survival Studies," Br J Haematol, 1980, 45:659-66.
2. Levy GJ, Selset G, McQuiston D, et al, "Clinical Significance of Anti-Yt^b. Report of a Case Using ^{51}Chromium Red Cell Survival Study," Transfusion, 1988, 28(3):265-7.
3. Ito H, Yamamoto S, Saito K, et al, "Quantitative Estimation of Hemorrhage in Chronic Subdural Hematoma Using the ^{51}Cr Erythrocyte Labeling Method," J Neurosurg, 1987, 66(6):862-4.
4. Milam JD, Samuels MS, Hidalgo JU, et al, "Use of Hematocrit Values in Evaluation of Red Cell Survival With Chromium-51," Am J Clin Pathol, 1966, 45:56-60.
5. Kumpel BM, Austin EB, Lee D, et al, "Comparison of Flow Cytometric Assays With Isotopic Assays of ^{51}Chromium-Labeled Cells for Estimation of Red Cell Clearance or Survival In Vivo," Transfusion, 2000, 40(2):228-39.

6. Hoffmann-Fezer G, Trastl C, Beisker W, et al, "Preclinical Evaluation of Biotin Labeling for Red Cell Survival Testing," *Ann Hematol*, 1997, 74(5):231-8.

7. Mock DM, Lankford GL, Widness JA, et al, "Measurement of Red Cell Survival Using Biotin-Labeled Red Cells: Validation Against ^{51}Cr-Labeled Red Cells," *Transfusion*, 1999, 39(2):156-62.

References

Brucer M, "How Long Will Red Cells Last?" "Development of the Red Cell Survival Test," *Vignettes in Nuclear Medicine*, St Louis, MO: Mallinckrodt Chemical Works, 1973, 55.

Elghetany MT and Davey FR, "Erythrocytic Disorders," *Clinical Diagnosis and Management by Laboratory Methods*, 19th ed, Chapter 26, Henry JB, ed, Philadelphia, PA: WB Saunders Co, 1996, 604, 632.

Landaw SA, "Hemostasis, Survival, and Red Cell Kinetics: Measurement and Imaging of Red Cell Production," *Hematology: Basic Principles and Practice*, 2nd ed, Chapter 34, Hoffman R, Benz EJ Jr, Shattil SJ, et al, eds, Philadelphia, PA: Churchill Livingstone, 1995, 448-58.

Langan JK, Scheffel U, and McIntyre PA, "The Hematopoietic System," *Nuclear Medicine Technology and Techniques*, Chapter 18, Bernier DR, Christian PE, Langan JK, et al, eds, St Louis, MO: CV Mosby Co, 1989, 493-5.

DNA-Probe Assay for Thalassemia (BeTha Gene Test)

Related Information

Synonyms Allele-Specific Oligonucleotide Hybridization for Thalassemia; BeTha Gene 1 Kit

Test Includes Multiplex polymerase chain reaction (PCR), β-globin gene amplification, allele-specific oligonucleotide hybridization, and enzyme-linked immunosorbent assay (ELISA) visualization/detection

Abstract This assay (as available commercially in kit form) provides for the qualitative detection of eight (includes the most common) Mediterranean β-thalassemia mutations. The thalassemias are a spectrum of disease states characterized by an imbalance of globin chain synthesis. There is a reduced rate of synthesis by one or more globin chain genes. Dependent upon the underlying molecular mechanism, a variety of clinical conditions may result, including some that are fatal. Thalassemia is an important cause of hypochromic microcytic anemia which must be differentiated from other causes of hypochromia/microcytosis (eg, iron deficiency and sideroblastic anemia). A variety of DNA-based analytic techniques are applicable to the diagnosis of thalassemia but are not usually required to establish the diagnosis.

Specimen Whole blood

Container Lavender top (EDTA) tube

Storage Instructions There is evidence that samples are stable at room temperature for 2 days, at 2°C to 8°C for 6 days, and at -20°C for 28 days.[1]

Turnaround Time 2-3 hours (with use of Instagene™ chelex resin kit, Bio-Rad Laboratories, a DNA preparation procedure for provision of PCR-ready DNA)

Special Instructions This procedure may be used for fetal diagnosis using fetal DNA prepared from chorionic villi obtained during amniocentesis. Villus samples must be free of maternal tissue and transported in tissue culture medium. Amniotic fluid (15-20 mL) must be received by the laboratory within 24 hours of collection. If the specimen is to be transported, consult the laboratory performing the analysis to obtain any recommended special buffer for chorionic villus samples or tissue culture medium for transport of amniocytes.

Reference Interval Positive hybridization signal with normal allele-specific oligonucleotides (in the case of BeTha Gene 1 kit, an ELISA soluble yellow product with absorption maximum at 450 nm)

Use Screen for individuals heterozygous for mutations that may cause β-thalassemia. Molecular diagnostic techniques such as DNA probe assays can be used to confirm the diagnosis of β-thalassemia and is especially valuable in prenatal diagnosis which can identify situations in which genetic counseling may be applicable. While therapy of the severe forms of thalassemia is currently largely supportive, advances in bone marrow/stem cell transplantation and developments in genetic engineering will require identification of specific genotypes.

Limitations Availability of DNA analysis for thalassemia is likely to be dependent on geography. Different groups of mutations that cause β-thalassemia are associated with different geographic sites. Each area of the world in which thalassemia is prevalent has a few common mutations and many uncommon or rare varieties. The allele-specific nucleotides incorporated in a particular DNA probe assay will usually target only the common local forms of thalassemia; the test will not detect all forms (ie, the uncommon types) of the condition.

Methodology The BeTha Gene 1 kit provides a four-step procedure utilizing the principle of allele-specific oligonucleotide hybridization.[1] See diagrams.

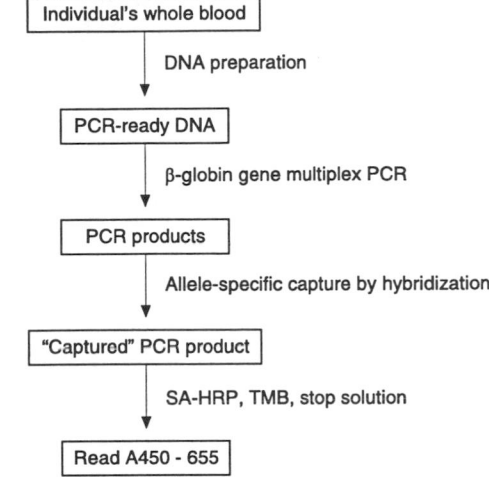

Overview of the steps involved in the determination of the Mediterranean β-thalassemia genotypes with the BeTha Gene 1. SA-HRP is streptavidin-horseradish peroxidase conjugate, and TMB is 3,3'-5,5' tetramethylbenzidine.

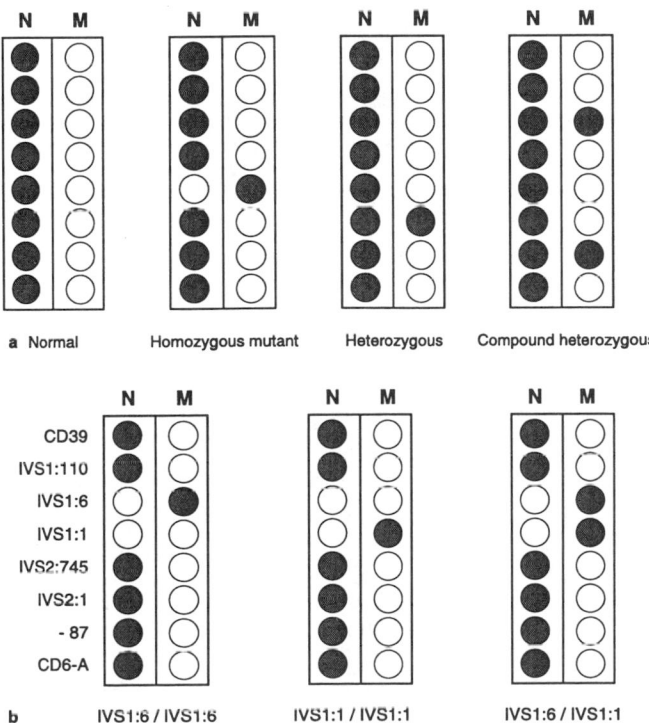

a: Overview of the four possible outcomes for the analysis of the β-thalassemia mutations. N are the eight normal ASO probes, and M are the eight mutant ASO probes. **b:** Example of mutations in close proximity: IVS1:6 and IVS1:1.

Genomic DNA is prepared using the Instagene™ matrix, a chelex resin, part of the Instagene™ whole blood kit (Bio-Rad Laboratories, Hercules, California), which allows the preparation of PCR-ready DNA in 30-45 minutes. The second step consists of *in vitro* DNA amplification by PCR. The β-globin gene is amplified in a multiplex PCR reaction containing four 5' biotinylated oligonucleotide primers. In a third step, a sample of the PCR reaction (Continued)

DNA-Probe Assay for Thalassemia (BeTha Gene Test) *(Continued)*

mixture is chemically denatured and "capture" is achieved in a 96-well ELISA plate by hybridization to an immobilized allele-specific oligonucleotide (ASO) probe. A sample of each denatured product is aliquoted to one strip (of the ELISA plate) containing ASO (immobilized) for normal alleles and one strip with ASO for the mutant alleles (each strip is color coded). After hybridization, visualization is achieved by an ELISA reaction utilizing steptavidin-horseradish peroxidase conjugate, tetramethylbenzidine reagent, and a stop-solution reagent followed by measurement of the difference in absorbance at 450 nm versus 655 nm (difference determined for each well of the ELISA plate).

Additional Information Multiple (over 180) molecular defects in the β-globin genes are responsible for the reduced synthesis of the gene product; the β-globin gene with resultant excess accumulation of α-globin chains. This underlying mechanism (globin chain imbalance) leads to formation of insoluble α-globin tetramers that precipitate within red blood cells. Intrasplenic sequestration and destruction of red cells occurs with reduced size (microcytosis) and fragmentation of red cells and with an increase in hemoglobin A2 levels. There is geographic clustering of the gene abnormalities which, while numerous and diverse, include only a few common forms. Thus, detection of the majority of clinically significant cases of β-thalassemia is possible using allele-specific oligonucleotides tailored to the geographic site. In the Mediterranean area, eight mutations account for >90% of cases of β-thalassemia. These mutations are targeted/detected by the BeTha Gene 1 kit.[1]

Homozygous β-thalassemia patients (β-thalassemia major) have a severe hemolytic disease process requiring transfusion therapy. While a few patients have been treated successfully with bone marrow transplantation techniques,[2] and gene therapy is being developed,[3] most require supportive care. Thus, screening for heterozygous/prenatal diagnosis and genetic counseling as desired may be utilized even though most individuals heterozygous for β-thalassemia are clinically asymptomatic (and have minimal hematologic abnormality).

Footnotes

1. Ugozzoli LA, Lowery JD, Reyes AA, et al, "Evaluation of the BeTha Gene 1 Kit for the Qualitative Detection of the Eight Most Common Mediterranean β-Thalassemia Mutations," *Am J Hematol*, 1998, 59(3):214-22.
2. Giardini C and Lucarelli G, "Bone Marrow Transplantation for Beta-Thalassemia," *Hematol Oncol Clin North Am*, 1999, 13(5):1059-64.
3. May C, Rivella S, Callegari J, et al, "Therapeutic Haemoglobin Synthesis in β-Thalassaemic Mice Expressing Lentivirus-Encoded Human β-Globin," *Nature*, 2000, 406(6791):82-6.

References

Bowie LJ, Reddy PL, Nagabhushan M, et al, "Detection of α-Thalassemias by Multiplex Polymerase Chain Reaction," *Clin Chem*, 1994, 40(12):2260-6.

Maggio A, Giambona A, Cai SP, et al, "Rapid and Simultaneous Typing of Hemoglobin S, Hemoglobin C, and Seven Mediterranean β-Thalassemia Mutations by Covalent Reverse Dot-Blot Analysis: Application to Prenatal Diagnosis in Sicily," *Blood*, 1993, 81(1):239-42.

Olivieri NF, "The Beta-Thalassemias," *N Engl J Med*, 1999, 341(2):99-109.

Saiki RK, Chang CA, Levenson CH, et al, "Diagnosis of Sickle Cell Anemia and Beta-Thalassemia With Enzymatically Amplified DNA and Nonradioactive Allele-Specific Oligonucleotide Probes," *N Engl J Med*, 1998, 319(9):537-41.

Schiliro G, Di Gregorio F, Samperi P, et al, "Genetic Heterogeneity of β-Thalassemia in Southeast Sicily," *Am J Hematol*, 1995, 48(1):5-11.

Weatherall DJ and Provan AB, "Red Cells I: Inherited Anaemias," *Lancet*, 2000, 355(9210):1169-75.

◆ **Döhle Bodies** *see* Peripheral Blood: Differential Leukocyte Count *on page 464*

◆ **Donath-Landsteiner Test** *see* Cold Hemolysin Test *on page 418*

◆ **Elliptocytes** *see* Osmotic Fragility *on page 462*

◆ **Elliptocytes** *see* Peripheral Blood: Differential Leukocyte Count *on page 464*

◆ **Eosinophil Cationic Protein** *see* Eosinophil Granule Proteins *on page 426*

◆ **Eosinophil Catonic Protein** *see* Eosinophil Count *on page 424*

Eosinophil Count

Related Information

Complete Blood Count *on page 419*
Eosinophil Granule Proteins *on page 426*
Eosinophil Smear *on page 428*
Eotaxin, Serum, Plasma, or Urine *on page 429*
Immunoglobulin E *on page 533*
Lysozyme, Blood and Urine *on page 457*
Ova and Parasites, Stool *on page 666*
Ova and Parasites, Urine *on page 667*
Peripheral Blood: Differential Leukocyte Count *on page 464*
Thorn Test *on page 490*

Synonyms Absolute Eosinophil Count; Eosinophil Count, Total

Applies to Eosinophil Catonic Protein; Eosinophilic Pneumonia; Eosinophil-Myalgia Syndrome; Granulocyte/Macrophage Colony Stimulating Factor; Interleukin 3; Interleukin 5

Abstract Eosinophils are granulocytic type white blood cells distinguished by prominent reddish-orange cytoplasmic granules on Wright-Giemsa (Romanowsky-type) stains, frequently with bilobed nuclei, and with both circulating and tissue forms. Manual (using phloxine stain) or automated absolute eosinophil count is requested in certain clinical situations because of expected greater precision/accuracy than is usually obtained using the relative number of eosinophils from the manual differential count. Eosinophil count is increased in a wide variety of conditions including especially, allergy, drug reaction, parasitism, collagen vascular disease, and some malignant states. Eosinophils are decreased with hyperadrenalism.

Specimen Whole blood

Container Lavender top (EDTA) tube

Causes for Rejection Clotted specimen, specimen more than 4 hours old

Reference Interval 15-650/mm³ (0.015 to 0.65 x 10⁹/L).[1] There is diurnal variation with lowest levels in the morning. There may be within-day physiologic variation >40%.[2]

Use Aid in the diagnosis of allergy, drug reaction, parasitic infestations, collagen disease, Hodgkin disease, and myeloproliferative diseases. Increased also in a broad range of less common conditions including sarcoidosis,[3] the acute hypereosinophilic syndrome, angioneurotic edema, acute renal allograft rejection, eosinophilic nonallergic rhinitis, anisakiasis,[4] eosinophilic gastroenteritis,[5] eosinophilia-myalgia syndrome,[6] and others. Decrease in eosinophils (eosinopenia) occurs in Cushing disease (hyperadrenalism) and is seen with a variety of infections, correlating with severity of the infectious process. Absence of eosinophils has unfavorable prognostic implications in cases of infection.

Limitations Manual method is subject to an inherent error of 20% to 30%.[7]

Methodology Manual, using Fuchs-Rosenthal or Speirs-Levy special large volume hemocytometer and eosinophil stain diluent (eg, Pilot's solution or phloxine B solution as used in the Unopette™ Brand System, Becton Dickinson, Rutherford, NJ). Automated method (eg, Bayer® (Technicon®), Coulter, Sysmex) should provide greater precision/accuracy and is recommended for obtaining an absolute eosinophil count.[7]

Additional Information The major cause of eosinophilia is allergy (atopy) which is clinically common and frequently asymptomatic or minimally symptomatic. An important cause of eosinophilia is parasitic infection. Eosinophilia is seen especially with tissue invasion by parasites as occurs with trichinosis, schistosomiasis, filariasis, echinococcal disease, spirochetal infection, liver infestation (as with *Clonorchis sinensis*, *Fasciola hepatica*, *Capillaria hepatica*) and many other parasitic organisms. Occult neoplasm is in the differential consideration but most tumor-associated eosinophilia occurs in cases with widespread metastases.[8] Classification of eosinophilia by degree of severity may be helpful in differential diagnosis.[8] See table.

Likely and Less Likely Causes of Eosinophilia on the Basis of Severity (absolute eosinophil count)

Likely Causes	Less Likely Causes
Mild (0.7-1.5 x 10⁹/L)	
Allergic rhinitis	Neoplasm
Hay fever or atopy	Gastrointestinal disease
Extrinsic asthma	Skin disease
Drug reaction	Certain infectious diseases
Parasitic disease	Long-term dialysis
Occupational lung disease	Radiation therapy
	Immunodeficiency state
Moderate (1.5-5 x 10⁹/L)	
Parasitic disease	Polyarteritis nodosa
Intrinsic asthma	Other connective tissue disorders
Drug reaction	Neoplasm
Pulmonary eosinophilia syndrome	Hypereosinophilic syndrome
Marked (>5 x 10⁹/L)	
Parasitic diseases	Disorder usually associated with moderate eosinophilia
Visceral larva migrans associated with *Toxocara canis* or *Toxocara cati* infestation	Trichinosis, hookworm infection, ascariasis, strongyloidiasis, neoplasm, polyarteritis nodosa
Tissue migration during larval stage (eg, *Ascaris*, *Trichinella*, hookworm, *Strongyloides* sp)	Neoplasm
Hypereosinophilic syndrome	Polyarteritis nodosa
Eosinophilic leukemia	Drug reaction

Adapted from Brigden ML, "A Practical Work-up for Eosinophilia: You Can Investigate the Most Likely Causes Right in Your Office," *Postgrad Med*, 1999, 105(3); 193-210.

Toxocaral disease (visceral larva migrans) is a typical parasitic disease in which eosinophil counts (eosinophils >30% on differential) are usually markedly elevated. However, ~25% of children with toxocariasis have normal eosinophil counts. Thus, normal eosinophil counts do not rule out toxocaral disease or other parasitic infestations.

The T-cell produced cytokines interleukin-3, granulocyte/macrophage colony stimulating factor, and interleukin-5 (IL-5) stimulate eosinophil production in vitro. IL-5 appears to be the prime mediator of eosinophilia in patients with certain parasitic diseases.[9,10] Type 2 helper T cells (CD4+,CD3-), which can produce interleukin-4 (stimulates IgE antibody production) and interleukin-5 (promotes the differentiation and activation of eosinophils) may be involved in causing the hypereosinophilic syndrome (see below).[11] Clonal populations of aberrant T cells produce large amounts of IL-5 in some cases of "idiopathic" eosinophilia.[12] Interleukin-2 and interleukin-15, which stimulate the proliferation of T cells and natural killer cells (CD16 and CD56+), may also be involved.[13]

There is recent interest in the clinical applicability of eosinophil granule protein levels. In some situations, eosinophil proteins may serve as markers for previous eosinophil reaction. The four principal eosinophil granule proteins can be considered as "proinflammatory" and consist of major basic protein (MBP), eosinophil cationic protein (ECP), eosinophil-derived neurotoxin (EDN), and eosinophil peroxidase (EPO). ECP and EDN are potent ribonuclease neurotoxins each with genes localized to the q24-q31 region of chromosome 14. The role of eosinophil granule proteins in pulmonary (in particular, asthma) and in gastrointestinal (in particular, inflammatory bowel disease) pathology is under active investigation (see Eosinophil Cationic Protein).[14,15,16] The possibility that ECP and EDN are also synthesized and/or localized to neutrophil granules may temper enthusiasm for use of these proteins as markers of eosinophil-associated inflammation.[17]

An eosinophil specific chemokine (an eosinophil chemoattractant) has recently been identified, purified and named eotaxin.[18,19] Originally studied in guinea pigs, the gene and cDNA of human eotaxin have been isolated with gene mapping to chromosome 17.[20] Specificity of eotaxin owes to its specific receptor, CCR-3, which is present only on eosinophils. Eotaxin stimulates production and release of bone marrow eosinophils, mediates tissue eosinophilia, and is itself induced by IL-13/IL-4 in fibroblasts.[21] See Eotaxin, Serum, Plasma, or Urine on page 429.

Infiltrative lung diseases, in which peripheral blood eosinophils may be increased, include eosinophilic pneumonia, Löffler's syndrome (often related to Ascaris infestation), and tropical eosinophilia (usually related to filariasis).[22] See following flowchart.

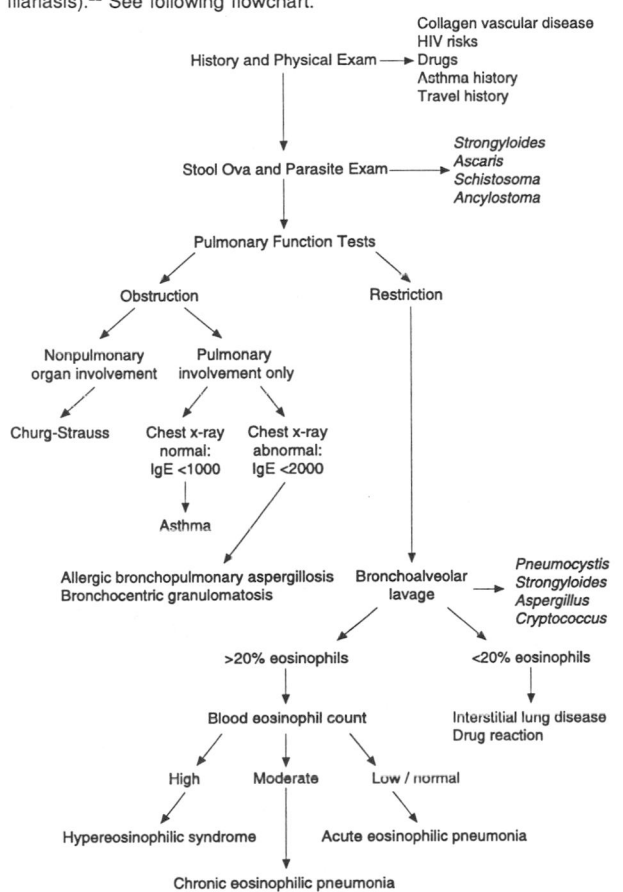

Adapted from Rochester CL, "The Eosinophilic Pneumonias," Fishman's Pulmonary Diseases and Disorders, 3rd ed, Chapter 74, Fishman AP, Elias JA, Fishman JA, et al, eds, New York, NY: McGraw-Hill, Health Professions Division, 1998, 1:113-50.

An important although rare cause of increased eosinophils in the peripheral blood is the acute hypereosinophilic syndrome (HES). Reported mortality

ranges from 81% to 95% in 1-3 years. The HES syndrome includes high peripheral WBC count, circulating early eosinophil forms without blast cells, mental confusion, delusions, near coma, and severe cardiac symptoms. If the absolute eosinophil count is >1.5 x 10^9/L and persists for over 6 months, HES must be considered.[8] Consistently associated with a poor prognosis are WBC count ≥90,000/mm³, blast forms in blood, heart failure, and severe CNS symptoms (confusion, organic psychosis and coma). This condition may not be a true leukemic myeloproliferative disease, although concepts of HES are controversial.

Idiopathic chronic eosinophilic pneumonia is of rare occurrence and unknown cause. There may be no blood eosinophilia but lung biopsy is characterized by interstitial tissue eosinophil infiltrate.[23]

Eosinophilic gastroenteritis may occur with blood eosinophilia.[5]

Eosinophilia-myalgia syndrome (EMS), characterized by an eosinophil count ≥1000 cells/mm³, severe often incapacitating myalgia, fatigue, cough, shortness of breath, rash and headache was associated with ingestion of large amounts of one form of L-tryptophan.[4] Sarcoidosis, granulomatous myositis, collagen vascular diseases, neoplastic myositis, and other entities are in the differential consideration. An EMS-like syndrome has been considered to result from several factors including ingestion of tryptophan, inactivation of indoleamine-2,3-dioxygenase, and possible impairment of the hypothalamic-pituitary-adrenal axis.[24] EMS is potentially fatal (Guillain-Barré like ascending polyneuropathy) with a clinical course resembling the toxic oil syndrome that was epidemic in Spain in 1981 and affected over 20,000 individuals resulting in 277 deaths.[25]

The population of patients with "idiopathic" (and persistent) eosinophilia may harbor subclinical, low grade or frank evolving Sézary syndrome, or other T-cell lymphomas (including those caused by HTLV-I infection).[13,26,27] Thus, it has been suggested that patients with "idiopathic" eosinophilia should be closely observed for lymphoproliferative disorders.

Footnotes

1. Krause JR and Boggs DR, "Search for Eosinophilia in Hospitalized Patients With Normal Blood Leukocyte Concentration," Am J Hematol, 1987, 24(1):55-63.
2. Winkel P, Statland BE, Saunders AM, et al, "Within-Day Physiologic Variation of Leukocyte Types in Healthy Subjects as Assayed by Two Automated Leukocyte Differential Analyzers," Am J Clin Pathol, 1981, 75(5):693-700.
3. Renston JP, Goldman ES, Hsu RM, et al, "Peripheral Blood Eosinophilia in Association With Sarcoidosis," Mayo Clin Proc, 2000, 75(6):586-90.
4. del Pozo V, Arrieta I, Tunon T, et al, "Immunopathogenesis of Human Gastrointestinal Infection by Anisakis simplex," J Allergy Clin Immunol, 1999, 104(3 Pt 1):637-43.
5. Kelly KJ, "Eosinophilic Gastroenteritis," J Pediatr Gastroenterol Nutr, 2000, 30:Suppl:S28-35.
6. Kamb ML, Murphy JJ, Jones JL, et al, "Eosinophilia-Myalgia Syndrome in L-Tryptophan-Exposed Patients," JAMA, 1992, 267(1):77-82.
7. Terrell JC, "Laboratory Evaluation of Leukocytes: Absolute Eosinophil Counting Procedure," Clinical Hematology: Principles, Procedures, Correlations, 2nd ed, Chapter 24, Stiene-Martin EA, Lotspeich-Steininger CA, and Koepke JA, eds, Philadelphia, PA: JB Lippincott Co, 1998, 342-3.
8. Brigden ML, "A Practical Work-up for Eosinophilia: You Can Investigate the Most Likely Causes Right in Your Office," Postgrad Med, 1999, 105(3):193-210.
9. Limaye AP, Abrams JS, Silver JE, et al, "Regulation of Parasitic Induced Eosinophilia: Selectively Increased Interleukin-5 Production in Helminth-Infected Patients," J Exp Med, 1990, 172(1):399-402.
10. Limaye AP, Abrams JS, Silver JE, et al, "Interleukin-5 and the Post-treatment Eosinophilia in Patients With Onchocerciasis," J Clin Invest, 1991, 88(4):1418-21.
11. Cogan E, Schandené L, Crusiaux A, et al, "Brief Report: Clonal Proliferation of Type 2 Helper T Cells in a Man With the Hypereosinophilic Syndrome," N Engl J Med, 1994, 330(8):535-8.
12. Simon HU, Plotz SG, Dummer R, et al, "Abnormal Clones of T Cells Producing Interleukin-5 in Idiopathic Eosinophilia," N Engl J Med, 1999, 341(15):1112-20.
13. Means-Markwell M, Burgess T, deKeratry D, et al, "Eosinophilia With Aberrant T Cells and Elevated Serum Levels of Interleukin-2 and Interleukin-15," N Engl J Med, 2000, 342(21):1568-71.
14. Venge P, Byström J, Carlson M, et al, "Eosinophil Cationic Protein (ECP): Molecular and Biological Properties and the Use of ECP as a Marker of Eosinophil Activation in Disease," Clin Exp Allergy, 1999, 29(9):1172-86.
15. Shields MD, Brown V, Stevenson C, et al, "Serum Eosinophilic Cationic Protein and Blood Eosinophil Counts for the Prediction of the Presence of Airways Inflammation in Children With Wheezing," Clin Exp Allergy, 1999, 29(10):1382-9.
16. Levy AM, Gleich GJ, Sandborn WJ, et al, "Increased Eosinophil Granule Proteins in Gut Lavage Fluid From Patients With Inflammatory Bowel Disease," Mayo Clin Proc, 1997, 72(2):117-23.
17. Sur S, Glitz DG, Kita H, et al, "Localization of Eosinophil-Derived Neurotoxin and Eosinophil Cationic Protein in Neutrophilic Leukocytes," J Leukoc Biol, 1998, 63(6):715-22.
18. Jose PG, Griffiths-Johnson DA, Collins PD, et al, "Eotaxin: A Potent Eosinophil Chemoattractant Cytokine Detected in a Guinea Pig Model of Allergic Airways Inflammation," J Exp Med, 1994, 179(3):881-6.
19. Jose PJ, Adcock IM, Griffiths-Johnson DA, et al, "Eotaxin: Cloning of an Eosinophil Chemoattractant Cytokine and Increased mRNA Expression Allergen-Challenged Guinea Pig Lungs," Biochem Biophy Res Commun, 1994, 205(1):788-94.
20. Kitaura M, Nakajima T, Imai T, et al, "Molecular Cloning of Human Eotaxin, an Eosinophil-Selective CC Chemokine, and Identification of a Specific Eosinophil Eotaxin Receptor, CC Chemokine Receptor 3," J Biol Chem, 1996, 271(13):7725-30.
21. Terada N, Hamano N, Nomura T, et al, "Interleukin-13 and Tumour Necrosis Factor-α Synergistically Induce Eotaxin Production in Human Nasal Fibroblasts," Clin Exp Allergy, 2000, 30(3):348-55.

(Continued)

Eosinophil Count (Continued)

22. Rochester CL, "The Eosinophilic Pneumonias," *Fishman's Pulmonary Diseases and Disorders*, 3rd ed, Chapter 74, Fishman AP, Elias JA, Fishman JA, et al, eds, New York, NY: McGraw Hill, Health Professions Division, 1998, 1, 113-50.

23. Marchand E, Reynaud-Gaubert M, Lauque D, et al, "Idiopathic Chronic Eosinophilic Pneumonia: A Clinical and Follow-up Study of 62 Cases," *Medicine*, 1998, 77(5):299-312.

24. Silver RM, Heyes MP, Maize JC, et al, "Scleroderma, Fasciitis, and Eosinophilia Associated With the Ingestion of Tryptophan," *N Engl J Med*, 1990, 322(13):874-81.

25. Rigau-Pérez JG, Pérez-Alvarez L, Duenas-Castro S, et al, "Epidemiologic Investigation of an Oil-Associated Pneumonic, Paralytic Eosinophilic Syndrome in Spain," *Am J Epidemiol*, 1984, 119(2):250-60.

26. Guitart J, "Idiopathic Eosinophilia," *N Engl J Med*, 2000, 342(9):659-60.

27. Suzuki R, Seto M, and Nakaura S, "Idiopathic Eosinophilia," *N Engl J Med*, 2000, 342(9):660-1.

References

Ackerman SJ and Butterfield JH, "Eosinophilia, Eosinophil-Associated Diseases, and the Hypereosinophilic Syndrome," *Hematology: Basic Principles and Practice*, 3rd ed, Chapter 40, Hoffman R, Benz EJ, Shattil SJ, et al, eds, Philadelphia, PA: Churchill Livingstone, 2000, 702-20.

Bain BJ, "Hypereosinophilia," *Curr Opin Hematol*, 2000, 7(1):21-5.

Carulli G, Sbrana S, Azzara A, et al, "Detection of Eosinophils in Whole Blood Samples by Flow Cytometry," *Cytometry*, 1998, 34(6):272-9.

Duffy J, "Eosinophilia-Myalgia Syndrome," *Mayo Clin Proc*, 1992, 67(12):1201-2.

Katzenstein AL, "Diagnostic Features and Differential Diagnosis of Churg-Strauss Syndrome in the Lung," *Am J Clin Pathol*, 2000, 114(5):767-72.

Kikly KK, Bochner BS, Freeman SD, et al, "Identification of SAF-2, a Novel Siglec Expressed on Eosinophils, Mast Cells, and Basophils," *J Allergy Clin Immunol*, 2000, 105(6 Pt 1):1093-100.

Marone G, "Human Eosinophils," *Chemical Immunology*, Volume 76, Adorini L, Arai K, Berek C, et al, eds, Switzerland: Karger, 2000.

Mayeno AN, Belongia EA, Lin F, et al, "3-(Phenylamino)alanine, a Novel Aniline-Derived Amino Acid Associated With the Eosinophilia-Myalgia Syndrome: A Link to the Toxic Oil Syndrome?" *Mayo Clin Proc*, 1992, 67(12):1134-9.

Moqbel R and Becker AB, "The Human Eosinophil," *Wintrobe's Clinical Hematology*, 10th ed, Chapter 14, Lee GR, Foerster J, Lukens J, et al, eds, Baltimore, MD: Lippincott Williams & Wilkins, 1999, 351-61.

Ramakrishna G, Connolly HM, Tazelaar HD, et al, "Churg-Strauss Syndrome Complicated by Eosinophilic Endomyocarditis," *Mayo Clin Proc*, 2000, 75(6):631-5.

Randolph TG, "Differentiation and Enumeration of Eosinophils in the Counting Chamber With a Glycol Stain; A Valuable Technique in Appraising ACTH Dosage," *J Lab Clin Med*, 1949, 34:1696-1701.

Rothenberg ME, "Eosinophilia," *N Engl J Med*, 1998, 338(22):1592-600.

Smith H and Cook RM, *Immunopharmacology of Eosinophils, The Handbook of Immunopharmacology*, San Diego, CA: Academic Press, 1993, 1-250.

Walsh GM, "Human Eosinophils: Their Accumulation, Activation, and Fate," *Br J Haematol*, 1997, 97(4):701-9.

♦ **Eosinophil Count, Total** *see* Eosinophil Count *on page 424*

♦ **Eosinophil Derived Neurotoxin (EDN) (eosinophil protein X is a synonym for EDN)** *see* Eosinophil Granule Proteins *on page 426*

Eosinophil Granule Proteins

Related Information

Eosinophil Count *on page 424*
Eosinophil Smear *on page 428*
Eotaxin, Serum, Plasma, or Urine *on page 429*
Immunoglobulin E *on page 533*
Pregnancy-Associated Protein A, Serum *on page 260*

Applies to Eosinophil Cationic Protein; Eosinophil Derived Neurotoxin (EDN) (eosinophil protein X is a synonym for EDN); Eosinophilic Cellulitis; Eosinophil Major Basic Protein; Eosinophil Peroxidase; EPX; EPX/EDN; Giant Papillary Conjunctivitis; Idiopathic Pulmonary Fibrosis; Pneumonia, Chronic Eosinophilic; Wells Syndrome

Test Includes ECP and/or EDN and/or others

Abstract Eosinophils (eosinophilic granulocytes) play an important role in the inflammatory process. They are of primary importance in the immune response to parasites and in allergic reactions, especially asthma. The intracytoplasmic eosinophil secondary granules consist largely of four basic proteins. **Major basic protein (MBP)** forms the crystalloid core while **eosinophil cationic protein (ECP)**, **eosinophil-derived neurotoxin (EDN)**, and **eosinophil peroxidase (EPO)** are present in the granule matrix (by electron microscopy).[1,2] Together they comprise 90% of the granule protein. In addition to this potent arsenal of cytoplasmic cytotoxic proteins (see Figures 1 and 2), an array of surface molecules (see Figure 3) indicates broad participation in inflammation, including utilization of chemokines, cytokines, and adhesion molecules.[3,4] An excellent detailed review of the molecular pathophysiology of eosinophils is available and is highly recommended.[5]

Specimen ECP and EDN are the granule proteins of greater clinical interest. These proteins can be measured in a variety of clinical specimens. In particular, urine and feces are appropriate specimens for the determination of EDN. Circadian variation in EDN levels introduces a variable that must be interpreted if such levels are measured in urine. The use of urine is advantageous in the pediatric population as specimen procurement is noninvasive.[6] Variation in eosinophil activation, circadian and otherwise must be considered. Such concerns may extend to use of feces as the specimen.

One is advised to consult with those performing the test as to what specimens may be acceptable and as to specimen handling. Test results are importantly dependent upon viability and lysis of eosinophils and eosinophil granules contained in the specimen.[7] The following indicates the variety of specimens that may be of interest:

- bronchoalveolar lavage fluid, sputum[8]
- nasal lavage fluid[8]
- tears (from patient with vernal keratoconjunctivitis, allergic conjunctivitis, and giant papillary conjunctivitis)[9]
- jejunal perfusion fluids (for evaluation of inflammatory bowel disease)
- fecal samples (study of infants with atopic eczema and food allergy and patients with inflammatory bowel disease)
- urine samples (especially useful in pediatric patients being monitored during respiratory therapy)[7]
- serum/plasma (EDTA or citrate), serum is preferred[8]

Storage Instructions Serum, 24-hour storage at 4°C, following a 1-hour clotting period at 20°C to 22°C (specimens from healthy controls or allergic patients).[10] Freeze serum at -20°C if not analyzed within 1 day of collection. Freeze spot urine samples (for EPX/EDN determination) at -70°C. Simultaneous determination of urine creatinine is necessary to allow evaluation of the extent of dilution of urine.[7]

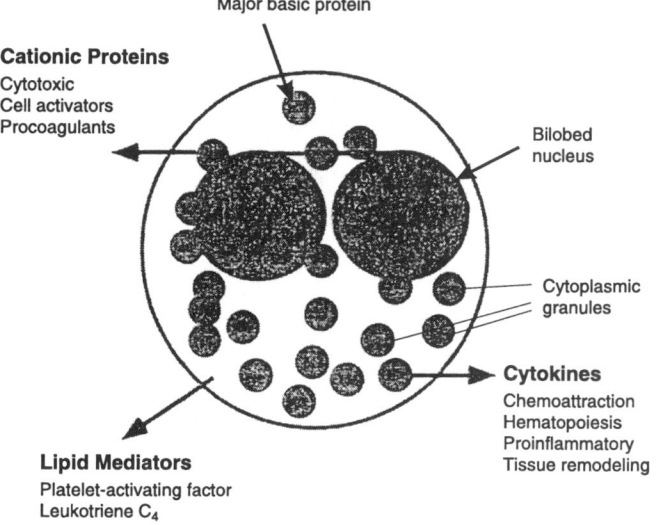

Figure 1. Schematic diagram of the human eosinophil.

Adapted from Thomas LL and Page SM, "Inflammatory Cell Activation by Eosinophil Granule Proteins," *Human Eosinophils, Biological and Clinical Aspects*, Volume 76, Marone G, ed, Basel, Switzerland: Karger, 2000, 99-117.

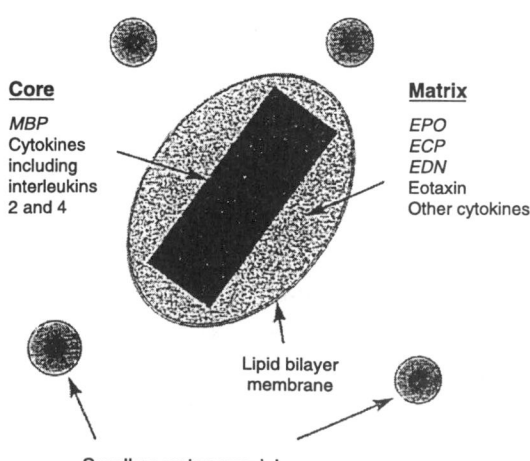

Figure 2. The crystalloid granule contains two internal compartments, the core, and the matrix.

Adapted from Lacy P and Moqbel R, "Eosinophil Cytokines," *Human Eosinophils, Biological and Clinical Aspects*, Volume 76, Marone G, ed, Basel, Switzerland: Karger, 2000, 134-55.

Figure 3

Adhesion Molecules	
CD11a	CD29
CD11b	CD44
CD11c	CD49d
αd	CD49f
CD15	CD62L
CD15s	CD162
CD18	
β7	

Apoptosis, Signaling, and Others	
CD9	CD82
CD17	CD92
CD24	CD95
CD37	CD97
CD39	CD98
CD43	CD99
CD52	CD139
CD53	CD148
CD63	CD149
CD65	CD151
CD69*	CD161
CD76	CD165
CD81	

Chemokine, Complement and Other Chemotactic Factor Receptors

CD35	LTD₄R
CD88	LTE₄R
C3aR	fMLPR
PAFR	CCR1
LTB₄R	CCR3

Immunoglobulin Receptors and Other Members of the Immunoglobulin Superfamily

CD4	CD66
CD16*	CD89
CD31†	CD100
CD47	CD101
CD48	HLA class I
CD50†	HLA-DR*
CD54*†	FCεRI‡
CD58	

Enzymes

CD13	
CD45	
CD45RB	
CD45RO	
CD46	
CD55	
CD59	
CD87	

Cytokines

CD25	CD124
CD116	CD125
CD117	CD129
CD119	CD131
CD120	IL-13R
CD123	TGFβR

Figure 3. Cell surface molecules found on human eosinophils. Many have been identified by flow cytometry, some are inferred based on cellular responsiveness to specific stimuli.

*Activated eosinopils.
†Also considered to be adhesion molecules.
‡Expression, if present, is extremely low.
R = receptor.

Adapted from Tachimoto H and Bochner BS, "The Surface Phenotype of Human Eosinophils," *Human Eosinophils, Biological and Clinical Aspects*, Volume 76, Marone G, ed, Basel, Switzerland: Karger, 2000, 45-62.

Reference Interval Children (nonatopic): 6.5 μg/L (95th percentile, 19 μg/L).[11] Higher levels of ECP are found in serum than in EDTA plasma due to continued release of granule proteins from eosinophils in blood without additives whereas with EDTA the cells are inactivated and do not release granule proteins.[8] There is circadian (diurnal variation in serum ECP with highest levels in the early morning).[6]

Adults: 6.0 μg/L (geometric mean), range (95%) of 2.3-15.9 μg ECP/L[12]

Use Evaluation of allergic/asthmatic, upper/lower respiratory conditions with opportunity to correlate serum, urine, sputum, and bronchial lavage specimens for diagnostic and/or monitoring purposes. Evaluation and monitoring of response to therapy in cases of inflammatory bowel disease (ulcerative colitis and Crohn disease) measure clinical activity of Wells syndrome (eosinophilic cellulitis). Potential use as a maternal serum marker for Down syndrome (eosinophil MBP complexed with pregnancy-associated plasma protein-A).

Limitations Variables that may influence test results include choice of anticoagulant, time allowed for coagulation, ambient temperature and other factors relating to sample handling that may affect the extracellular release of eosinophil proteins.

Methodology Radioimmunoassay[8,11,12] (commercially available, Pharmacia Upjohn, Diagnostics, Milton Keynes, UK); fluoroimmunoassay (Kabi Pharmacia, Pharmacia Diagnostics AB, Uppsala, Sweden); enzyme-linked immunosorbent assay (ELISA), biotin/avidin amplified, for use with serum, urine, and other body fluids[13]

Additional Information Eosinophil cationic protein was isolated some 30 years ago from granules of the myeloid cells of chronic myelogenous leukemia. Subsequently, the protein was localized to the matrix of the larger specific eosinophil cytoplasmic granule. ECP is a zinc-containing protein (a zinc metalloenzyme) with a molecular weight of 16-22 kDa. Variation in the degree of glycosylation accounts for some variation in molecular weight. ECP is a member of the bovine pancreatic ribonuclease A (RNaseA) family which also includes the more active enzyme, eosinophil-derived neurotoxin (EDN). The isoelectric point of ECP is 10.8 (the result of a high arginine content, consistent with the protein's "sticky" nature and tendency to bind to negatively charged molecules as are present on cell membranes). The gene for ECP, located on chromosome 14 (q24-31) is close to a sister protein, EPX/EDN with which it has nearly 70% amino acid sequence homology.

The release of eosinophil granule proteins reflect the activation of eosinophils. ECP has a variety of functions including cytotoxic effects (eg, destruction of parasites and tumor cells, neurotoxicity, cardiovascular and respiratory injury, and antibacterial/antiviral activity). Nontoxic effects include inhibition of T-cell proliferation, release of histamine from basophils, stimulation of secretion of airway mucus, effects on coagulation and anticoagulants (eg, heparin), and interaction with the complement system and adhesion molecules. Cell-killing action likely relates to ECP's ability to make pores (about 50 A°C wide) in cell membranes, with resultant cytotoxic cell death by osmotic lysis. The 6 molecular forms of ECP allow for functional heterogeneity.[1] The half life of ECP in circulation is about 65 minutes.[12]

With some caveats, serum ECP (and blood eosinophil counts when obtained) bears a positive correlation with the severity of asthma and levels show post-therapy decline,[14,15] but do not accurately reflect functional indices of asthma severity in chronic stable patients.[16] While sputum ECP level in sputum (induced) may be helpful in the diagnosis of bronchial asthma,[17] serum ECP may not serve to differentiate asthmatics from nonasthmatics.[18] In children, serum eosinophil count and serum ECP may be able to differentiate patients with asthma from those without the disease but has not been reliably correlated with the intensity of bronchial (mucosal) inflammation.[19] On the other hand, urinary EPX/EDN levels have been considered to have value in the monitoring of bronchial inflammation in asthmatic children.[6] Levels of ECP (and of eosinophils) in bronchoalveolar lavage fluid have been reported to correlate with the severity of asthma but increased with adult respiratory distress syndrome, idiopathic pulmonary fibrosis, chronic eosinophilic pneumonia and postlung transplantation (in association with acute rejection).[8]

ECP and EPX/EDN radioimmunoassays have been applied to the analysis of feces in inflammatory bowel disease (IBD). Fecal ECP and EPX/EDN were increased in both active ulcerative colitis (UC) and active Crohn disease (CD) as compared to their inactive counterparts. Patients with inactive CD who relapsed within 3 months also had increased fecal ECP and EPX/EDN with the latter having more stability in feces than ECP.[20] Eosinophil granule proteins were increased in gut lavage fluid from patients with IBD as compared to control subjects, while differences were not found between patients with UC and those with CD.[21] Fecal ECP and EPX/EDN have also been suggested as a noninvasive method for monitoring allergic intestinal inflammation and disease activity in infants with atopic eczema and food allergy.[22]

Wells syndrome (eosinophilic cellulitis with dermal edema and eosinophil infiltrate) is associated with increase in ECP and interleukin-5 (IL-5) in peripheral blood, levels of which bear a close correlation with clinical activity.[23] IL-5 apparently plays an important role in the pathogenesis of this condition.

The precursor of eosinophil MBP (proMBP) is synthesized by the placenta and secreted into the maternal circulation where it forms a complex with pregnancy-associated plasma protein-A (PAPP-A).[24,25] It may serve as a maternal serum marker for Down syndrome.[24] A significant challenge has been raised as to the specificity of ECP and EPX/EDN for eosinophil granules with the finding (utilizing anti-ECP and anti-EDN-based indirect immunofluorescent and electron microscopic methods) that these apparent eosinophil markers are demonstrable also in neutrophils. Eosinophil MBP was not detected.[26]

Footnotes

1. Thomas LL and Page SM, "Inflammatory Cell Activation by Eosinophil Granule Proteins," *Chem Immunol*, 2000, 76:99-117.
2. Abu-Ghazaleh RI, Dunnette SL, Loegering DA, et al, "Eosinophil Granule Proteins in Peripheral Blood Granulocytes," *J Leukoc Biol*, 1992, 52(6):611-8.
3. Lacy P and Moqbel R, "Eosinophil Cytokines," *Chem Immunol*, 2000, 76:134-55
4. Tachimoto H and Bochner BS, "The Surface Phenotype of Human Eosinophils," *Chem Immunol*, 2000, 76:45-62.
5. Marone G, "Human Eosinophils: Biological and Clinical Aspects," *Chem Immunol*, 2000, 76.
6. O'Sullivan S and Kumlin M, "Eosinophil Markers in Childhood Asthma," *Clin Exp Allergy*, 1999, 29(11):1454-6.
7. Van's Gravesande KS, Mattes J, Grüntjens T, et al, "Circadian Variation of Urinary Eosinophil Protein X in Asthmatic and Healthy Children," *Clin Exp Allergy*, 1999, 29(11):1497-501.
8. Venge P, Byström J, Carlson M, et al, "Eosinophil Cationic Protein (ECP): Molecular and Biological Properties and the Use of ECP as a Marker of Eosinophil Activation in Disease," *Clin Exp Allergy*, 1999, 29(9):1172-86.
9. Montan PG and van Hage-Hamsten M, "Eosinophil Cationic Protein in Tears in Allergic Conjunctivitis," *Br J Ophthalmol*, 1996, 80(6):556-60.
10. Hallden G, Nopp A, Ihre E, et al, "Conditions in Blood Sampling Procedures That Extend the *Ex Vivo* Stability of Eosinophil Activity Markers in Peripheral Blood From Allergic Patients and Healthy Controls," *Ann Allergy Asthma Immunol*, 1999, 83(5):413-21.
11. Fitch PS, Brown V, Schock BC, et al, "Serum Eosinophil Cationic Protein (ECP): Reference Values in Healthy Nonatopic Children," *Allergy*, 1999, 54(11):1199-203.
12. Peterson CG, Enander I, Nystrand J, et al, "Radioimmunoassay of Human Eosinophil Cationic Protein (ECP) by an Improved Method. Establishment of Normal Levels in Serum and Turnover In Vivo," *Clin Exp Allergy*, 1991, 21(5):561-7.
13. Reimert CM, Minuva U, Kharazmi A, et al, "Eosinophil Protein X/Eosinophil Derived Neurotoxin (EPX/EDN). Detection by Enzyme-Linked Immunosorbent Assay and Purification From Normal Human Urine," *J Immunol Methods*, 1991, 141(1):97-104.
14. Dal Negro R, Micheletto C, Tognella S, et al, "Effect of Inhaled Beclomethasone Dipropionate and Budesonide Dry Powder on Pulmonary Function and Serum Eosinophil Cationic Protein in Adult Asthmatics," *J Investig Allergol Clin Immunol*, 1999, 9(4):241-7.
15. Sin A, Terzioglu E, Kokuludag A, et al, "Serum Eosinophil Cationic Protein (ECP) Levels in Patients With Seasonal Allergic Rhinitis and Allergic Asthma," *Allergy Asthma Proc*, 1998, 19(2):69-73.
16. Ronchi MC, Piragino C, Rosi E, et al, "Do Sputum Eosinophils and ECP Relate to the Severity of Asthma?" *Eur Respir J*, 1997, 10(8):1809-13.
17. Park JW, Whang YW, Kim CW, et al, "Eosinophil Count and Eosinophil Cationic Protein Concentration of Induced Sputum in the Diagnosis and Assessment of Airway Inflammation in Bronchial Asthma," *Allergy Asthma Proc*, 1998, 19(2):61-7.

(Continued)

Eosinophil Granule Proteins (Continued)

18. Perfetti L, Galdi E, Brame B, et al, "Serum Eosinophil Cationic Protein (sECP) in Subjects With a History of Asthma Symptoms With or Without Rhinitis," *Allergy*, 1999, 54(9):962-7.

19. Vila-Indurain B, Munoz-Lopez F, and Martin-Mateos M, "Evaluation of Blood Eosinophilia and the Eosinophil Cationic Protein (ECP) in the Serum of Asthmatic Children With Varying Degree of Severity," *Allergol Immunopathol (Madr)*, 1999, 27(6):304-8.

20. Saitoh O, Kojima K, Sugi K, et al, "Fecal Eosinophil Granule-Derived Proteins Reflect Disease Activity in Inflammatory Bowel Disease," *Am J Gastroenterol*, 1999, 94(12):3513-20.

21. Levy AM, Gleich GJ, Sandborn WJ, et al, "Increased Eosinophil Granule Proteins in Gut Lavage Fluid From Patients With Inflammatory Bowel Disease," *Mayo Clin Proc*, 1997, 72(2):117-23.

22. Majamaa H, Laine S, and Miettinen A, "Eosinophil Protein X and Eosinophil Cationic Protein as Indicators of Intestinal Inflammation in Infants With Atopic Eczema and Food Allergy," *Clin Exp Allergy*, 1999, 29(11):1502-6.

23. Espana A, Sanz ML, Sola J, et al, "Wells' Syndrome (Eosinophilic Cellulitis): Correlation Between Clinical Activity, Eosinophil Levels, Eosinophil Cation Protein and Interleukin-5," *Br J Dermatol*, 1999, 140(1):127-30.

24. Christiansen M, Oxvig C, Wagner JM, et al, "The Proform of Eosinophil Major Basic Protein: A New Maternal Serum Marker for Down Syndrome," *Prenat Diagn*, 1999, 19(10):905-10.

25. Overgaard MT, Oxvig C, Christiansen M, et al, "Messenger Ribonucleic Acid Levels of Pregnancy-Associated Plasma Protein-A and the Proform of Eosinophil Major Basic Protein: Expression in Human Reproductive and Nonreproductive Tissues," *Biol Reprod*, 1999, 61(4):1083-9.

26. Sur S, Glitz DG, Kita H, et al, "Localization of Eosinophil-Derived Neurotoxin and Eosinophil Cationic Protein in Neutrophilic Leukocytes," *J Leukoc Biol*, 1998, 63(6):715-22.

References

Bischoff SC, Mayer J, Nguyen QT, et al, "Immunohistological Assessment of Intestinal Eosinophil Activation in Patients With Eosinophilic Gastroenteritis and Inflammatory Bowel Disease," *Am J Gastroenterol*, 1999, 94(12):3521-9.

Boix E, Leonidas DD, Nikolovski Z, et al, "Crystal Structure of Eosinophil Cationic Protein at 2.4 A Resolution," *Biochemistry*, 1999, 38(51):16794-801.

Koller DY, Halmerbauer G, Muller J, et al, "Major Basic Protein, but Not Eosinophil Cationic Protein or Eosinophil Protein X, Is Related to Atopy in Cystic Fibrosis," *Allergy*, 1999, 54(10):1094-9.

Krug N, Napp U, Enander I, et al, "Intracellular Expression and Serum Levels of Eosinophil Peroxidase (EPO) and Eosinophil Cationic Protein in Asthmatic Children," *Clin Exp Allergy*, 1999, 29(11):1507-15.

Leonardi A, Borghesan F, Faggian D, et al, "Tear and Serum Soluble Leukocyte Activation Markers in Conjunctival Allergic Diseases," *Am J Ophthalmol*, 2000, 129(2):151-8.

Morioka J, Kurosawa M, Inamura H, et al, "Development of a Novel Enzyme-Linked Immunosorbent Assay for Blood and Urinary Eosinophil-Derived Neurotoxin: A Preliminary Study in Patients With Bronchial Asthma," *Int Arch Allergy Immunol*, 2000, 122(1):49-57.

Pronk-Admiraal CJ, Bartels PC, and Mulder K, "Eosinophil Cationic Protein in Serum From Nonatopic and Asymptomatic Atopic Individuals After Standardized Blood Clotting at 37°C," *Ann Clin Biochem*, 1999, 36(Pt 3):353-8.

Rothenberg ME, "Eosinophilia," *N Engl J Med*, 1998, 338(22):1592-600.

Xu X and Håkansson L, "Regulation of the Release of Eosinophil Cationic Protein by Eosinophil Adhesion," *Clin Exp Allergy*, 2000, 30(6):794-806.

♦ **Eosinophilic Bronchitis** see Eosinophil Smear on page 428

♦ **Eosinophilic Cellulitis** see Eosinophil Granule Proteins on page 426

♦ **Eosinophilic Pneumonia** see Eosinophil Count on page 424

♦ **Eosinophil Major Basic Protein** see Eosinophil Granule Proteins on page 426

♦ **Eosinophil-Myalgia Syndrome** see Eosinophil Count on page 424

♦ **Eosinophil Peroxidase** see Eosinophil Granule Proteins on page 426

Eosinophil Smear

Related Information

Eosinophil Count on page 424
Eosinophil Granule Proteins on page 426
Eotaxin, Serum, Plasma, or Urine on page 429

Synonyms Fecal Smear for Eosinophils; Nasal Smear for Eosinophils; Sputum Smear for Eosinophils

Applies to Atopic Cough; Cough Variant Asthma; Eosinophilic Bronchitis

Abstract The eosinophil is a major effector in allergic processes. Study of appropriately stained smears of clinical material may help to define the role of the eosinophil in any particular patient's reactive process.

Specimen Two slides of nasal secretion; smear or swab of feces; sputum or induced (with saline) sputum.[1,2,3,4] No fixation is required for slides. Nasal secretions may be submitted on wax paper or plastic wrap.

Container Slides of smeared specimen or nasal secretions on wax paper

Causes for Rejection Slides received in cytology fixative, no specimen on slide, smear, or swab

Special Instructions Requisition must state site of specimen.

Reference Interval No eosinophils identified

Use Investigate allergy, asthmatic disorders, and parasitic infestations

Methodology Wright or May-Grünwald-Giemsa stain and microscopic examination of smear. Gram-stained smears of microbiology specimens will not stain eosinophils.

Additional Information Eosinophils are often increased in the blood and sputum of patients with asthma, usually in relation to the severity of the process.[5] There is no percentage of eosinophils in sputum diagnostic of asthma, but levels >80% (related to proportion of neutrophils) are very suggestive of asthma or of chronic bronchitis with wheezing. There is evidence of an inverse correlation between the numbers of eosinophils in the circulation and/or sputum and pulmonary function (eg, airway flow rates).[6]

Chronic cough is a common clinical problem. Determination of the nature of airway inflammation is assisted by the study of induced sputum.[1,2,3,4] The concept of eosinophilic bronchitis/atopic cough (see table) has evolved with the observation that eosinophilic inflammation, as seen with asthma, can occur in patients with isolated chronic cough but without evidence of variable airflow obstruction and airway hyper-responsiveness (as occur with asthma).[7]

Sputum eosinophilia (>3%) is present.[8] Atopic cough may be responsible for up to 15% of cases with chronic cough. Gastroesophageal reflux-associated cough, postnasal drip-induced cough, angiotensin-converting enzyme inhibitor-induced cough, and cough variant asthma are in the differential diagnosis of nonproductive cough. Establishing a diagnosis of eosinophilic bronchitis has clinical significance as the cough responds to inhaled corticosteroids with accompanying significant decline in follow-up sputum eosinophil count (from 16.8% to 1.6%).[8]

Patients who are smokers and who have chronic airflow limitation (severe obstructive bronchitis) may benefit from sputum eosinophil study. Sputum eosinophilia ≥3% predicted a beneficial response to prednisone.[9] Effort dyspnea, quality of life, and forced expiratory volume$_1$ were improved. There was accompanying decline in median sputum eosinophil percentage from 9.7% to 0.5%

Sputum eosinophil count and eosinophil cationic protein level may not reflect the severity of asthma in cases of chronic stable asthma.[10] There is evidence that change in sputum eosinophils may be useful in predicting loss of asthma control as reflected by loss of airway function.[11]

In cases of idiopathic hypereosinophilic syndrome (sustained hypereosinophilia with organ involvement and with inapparent etiology), see Eosinophil Count on page 424. Eosinophils may show morphologic abnormalities including hypersegmented nuclei and cytoplasmic hypogranularity.[12]

Footnotes

1. Pin I, Gibson PG, Kolendowicz R, et al, "Use of Induced Sputum Cell Counts to Investigate Airway Inflammation in Asthma," *Thorax*, 1992, 47(1):25-9.

2. Fujimura M, Songür N, Kamio Y, et al, "Detection of Eosinophils in Hypertonic Saline-Induced Sputum in Patients With Chronic Nonproductive Cough," *J Asthma*, 1997, 34(2):119-26.

3. Pizzichini E, Pizzichini MMM, Efthimiadis A, et al, "Indices of Airway Inflammation in Induced Sputum: Reproducibility and Validity of Cell and Fluid-Phase Measurements," *Am J Respir Crit Care Med*, 1996, 154(Pt 1 of 2):308-17.

The Characteristics of Cough Variant Asthma, Eosinophilic Bronchitis, and Atopic Cough

	Asthma	Cough Variant Asthma	Eosinophilic Bronchitis Without Asthma	Atopic Cough
Symptoms	Dyspnea, cough, wheeze	Isolated cough	Cough and often associated upper airway symptoms	Isolate cough
Atopy	Common	Common	Same as general population	Common
Variable airflow obstruction	Present	Present	Absent	Absent
Airway hyper-responsiveness	Present	Present	Absent	Absent
Cough reflex hypersensitivity	Normal or increased	Normal or increased	Increased	Increased
Sputum eosinophilia	Usually	Usually	Always at diagnosis	Invariably at diagnosis
Bronchial biopsy eosinophilic infiltration	Yes	Yes	Unknown	Yes
Bronchoalveolar lavage eosinophilia	Yes	Yes	Yes	No

Adapted from Brightling CE and Pavord ID, "Eosinophilic Bronchitis - What Is It and Why Is It Important?" *Clin Exp Allergy*, 2000, 30(1):4-6.

4. Pavord ID, Pizzichini MM, Pizzichini E, et al, "The Use of Induced Sputum to Investigate Airway Inflammation," *Thorax*, 1997, 52(6):498-501.
5. Busse WW and Sedgwick JB, "Eosinophils in Asthma," *Ann Allergy*, 1992, 68(3):286-90.
6. Griffin E, Håkansson L, Formgren H, et al, "Blood Eosinophil Number and Activity in Relation to Lung Function in Patients With Asthma and With Eosinophilia," *J Allergy Clin Immunol*, 1991, 87(2):548-57.
7. Fujimura M, Ogawa H, Yasui M, et al, "Eosinophilic Tracheobronchitis and Airway Cough Hypersensitivity in Chronic Nonproductive Cough," *Clin Exp Allergy*, 2000, 30(1):41-7.
8. Brightling CE, Ward R, Goh KL, et al, "Eosinophilic Bronchitis Is an Important Cause of Chronic Cough," *Am J Respir Crit Care Med*, 1999, 160(2):406-10.
9. Pizzichini E, Pizzichini MM, Gibson P, et al, "Sputum Eosinophilia Predicts Benefit From Prednisone in Smokers With Chronic Obstructive Bronchitis," *Am J Respir Crit Care Med*, 1998, 158(5 Pt 1):1511-7.
10. Ronchi MC, Piragino C, Rosi E, et al, "Do Sputum Eosinophils and ECP Relate to the Severity of Asthma?" *Eur Respir J*, 1997, 10(8):1809-13.
11. Jatakanon A, Lim S, and Barnes PJ, "Changes in Sputum Eosinophils Predict Loss of Asthma Control," *Am J Respir Crit Care Med*, 2000, 161(1):64-72.
12. Kim HJ, Lee YJ, Lee DS, et al, "A Case of Idiopathic Hypereosinophilic Syndrome With Hypersegmented and Hypogranular Eosinophils," *Clin Lab Haematol*, 1999, 21(6):428-30.

References

Bain BJ, "Hypereosinophilia," *Curr Opin Hematol*, 2000, 7(1):21-5

Brightling CE and Pavord ID, "Eosinophilic Bronchitis - What Is It and Why Is It Important?" *Clin Exp Allergy*, 2000, 30(1):4-6.

Mattes J, Storm van's Gravesande K, Reining U, et al, "NO in Exhaled Air Is Correlated With Markers of Eosinophilic Airway Inflammation in Corticosteroid-Dependent Childhood Asthma," *Eur Respir J*, 1999, 13(6):1391-5.

Middleton E Jr, "Chronic Rhinitis in Adults," *J Allergy Clin Immunol*, 1988, 81(5 Pt 2):971-5.

Rothenberg ME, "Eosinophilia," *N Engl J Med*, 1998, 338(22):1592-600.

Eotaxin, Serum, Plasma, or Urine

Related Information

Eosinophil Count *on page 424*
Eosinophil Smear *on page 428*
Immunoglobulin E *on page 533*

Abstract Eotaxin is an eosinophil specific chemoattractant. Eotaxin is a CC (double cysteine) chemokine with a specific receptor, CCR-3, which is present only on eosinophils.[1] In addition, the chemokine stimulates the growth and development of myeloid precursors in the bone marrow and induces rapid release of eosinophils from the marrow.[2] As one of a number of ligands for the CCR-3 receptor, eotaxin plays a role in the pathogenesis of asthma. Plasma eotaxin levels are elevated in patients with acute asthma.[3]

Specimen Serum or plasma (plasma preferred); serum has been considered unsuitable.

Container Lavender top (EDTA) tube or red top tube

Storage Instructions Separate plasma from cells within 2 hours. May store at -20°C until time of assay.

Special Instructions Serum eotaxin levels increase by some 50% to 100% (as compared with plasma levels) over a 2-hour period if the serum is not immediately harvested after obtaining the specimen. The eotaxin is apparently released from red blood cells during clotting.[4] Eotaxin values in EDTA plasma do not change even after incubation at 25°C for 6 hours.[4]

Reference Interval 287 pg/mL, range of 200-378 pg/mL (plasma)

Use Assist with diagnosis of asthma; evaluate lung function in patients with asthma;[5] study the pathogenesis of asthma;[6] assist in the diagnosis of nephritis with tissue eosinophilia (see Additional Information)

Limitations ELISA tests for eotaxin have only recently been developed. Testing will initially be available only from research and/or a few reference laboratories. Multiple cytokines stimulate eosinophils such that the role of eotaxin may be difficult to assess.

Methodology Enzyme-linked immunosorbent assay (ELISA). One method has sensitivity of 30 pg/mL and coefficient of variation (CV) of 10%.[5,6] Recent sensitive sandwich assay (using two monoclonal antibodies and purified recombinant eotaxin as standard) has reported minimal detectable concentration of 1.5 pg/mL with CVs <10%.[6] There was no significant cross-reactivity of other CC chemokines with eosinophil CCR-3 receptors.[4]

Additional Information Eotaxin is a chemotactic cytokine (chemokine) that attracts eosinophils by activating the CCR-3 chemokine receptor. The latter is present on a number of cell types associated with asthma (eg, eosinophils, basophils, and T lymphocytes).[3] While there are many eosinophil-active chemoattractants, eotaxin is unique in that it specifically attracts eosinophils, due to its specific receptor, CCR-3 (expressed only on eosinophils).[6] Chemokines act as chemoattractants for leukocytes. There are four subfamilies, CXC, CC, C, and CX_3C dependent on the nature of the cysteine residues in their primary structures.[7] Human eotaxin is a 74 amino acid residue from the C-C (double cysteine) branch of the platelet factor 4 superfamily of chemotactic cytokines. Eotaxin stimulates myeloid development and release from the bone marrow[2], attracts eosinophils (eg, in inflammatory reactions, reactions to parasites, etc) and mediates tissue eosinophilia. Eotaxin is apparently produced by epithelial cells, endothelial cells, and activated leukocytes (including eosinophils). See figure.

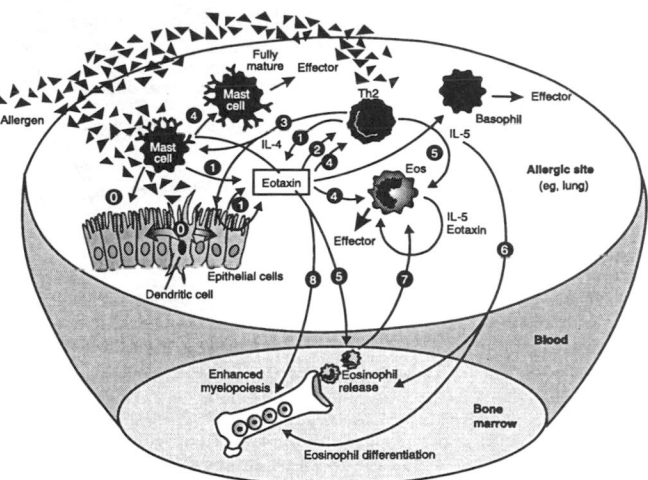

Eotaxin is mainly produced by epithelial cells (1), but in some conditions it is also produced by other cell types, such as mast cells and alveolar macrophages. Signals that trigger the production of eotaxin by epithelial cell (0) come from lymphocytes, but possibly also mast cells and dendritic cells. Eotaxin recruits Th2 cell (2) that in turn produce IL-4 and IL-5 (3) and amplify all the effects on epithelial cells and mast cells, resulting in the production of more eotaxin. Significant levels of eotaxin result (4) in eosinophil recruitment and degranulation, further Th2 recruitment, basophil degranulation and mast cell migration and differentiation. Eotaxin acting on the bone marrow pool of eosinophils induces their rapid mobilization to the blood (5), making them available for recruitment at the inflammatory site (7). IL-5, acting as a chemokinetic factor for eosinophils, synergizes with eotaxin in promoting the fast mobilization of the eosinophil pool from the bone marrow. In the context of a chronic allergic inflammatory response, eotaxin's colony-stimulating factor activity will probably result in enhanced myelopoiesis (8) that, in combination with high levels of IL-5, will result in increased eosinophilopoiesis.
Abbreviations: Eos = eosinophil; IL-4 = interleukin 4; IL-5 = interleukin 5; Th2 = T-helper type 2 cell.

Adapted from Gutierrez-Ramos JC, Lloyd C, and Gonzalo JA, "Eotaxin: From an Eosinophilic Chemokine to a Major Regulator of Allergic Reactions." *Immunol Today*, 1999, 20(11): 500-4.

In at least some situations, fibroblasts (eg, nasal mucosa) stimulated by IL-13 and/or IL-4 are the major source of eotaxin.[8] Fibroblasts in Hodgkin disease tissue express eotaxin with resultant recruitment of eosinophils and T lymphocytes.[9]

Initially detected (in bronchoalveolar lavage fluid),[1] described, studied, and cloned in guinea pigs,[10,11,12] eotaxin has been cloned in humans.[13,14] The gene is present on chromosome 17.

Plasma eotaxin levels have been applied to a number of clinical and pathogenic aspects of asthma. Eotaxin levels were elevated in a series of patients with acute asthma symptoms and airflow obstruction.[3] Increasing eotaxin level correlates with increased risk for asthma and inversely with lung function independent of age, sex, race, and smoking habits.[5] Demonstration of eotaxin in urine may assist in the diagnosis of diffuse interstitial nephritis (with tissue eosinophils).[15]

Footnotes

1. Kitaura M, Nakajima T, Imai T, et al, "Molecular Cloning of Human Eotaxin, an Eosinophil-Selective CC Chemokine, and Identification of a Specific Eosinophil Eotaxin Receptor, CC Chemokine Receptor 3," *J Biol Chem*, 1996, 271(13):7725-30.
2. Palframan RT, Collins PD, Williams TJ, et al, "Eotaxin Induces a Rapid Release of Eosinophils and Their Progenitors From the Bone Marrow," *Blood*, 1998, 91(7):2240-8.
3. Lilly CM, Woodruff PG, Camargo CA Jr, et al, "Elevated Plasma Eotaxin Levels in Patients With Acute Asthma," *J Allergy Clin Immunol*, 1999, 104(No 4, Pt 1):786-90.
4. Morita A, Shimosako K, Kikuoka S, et al, "Development of a Sensitive Enzyme-Linked Immunosorbent Assay for Eotaxin and Measurement of it Levels in Human Blood," *J Immunol Methods*, 1999, 226(1-2):159-67.
5. Nakamura H, Weiss, ST, Israel E, et al, "Eotaxin and Impaired Lung Function in Asthma," *Am J Respir Crit Care Med*, 1999, 160(6):1952-6.
6. Lilly CM, Nakamura H, Kesselman K, et al, "Expression of Eotaxin by Human Lung Epithelial Cells: Induction by Cytokines and Inhibition by Glucocorticoids," *J Clin Invest*, 1997, 99(7):1767-73.
7. Bazan JF, Bacon KB, and Hardiman G, "A New Class of Membrane-Bound Chemokine With a CX_3C Motif," *Nature*, 1997, 385(6617):640-5.
8. Terada N, Hamano N, Nomura T, et al, "Interleukin-13 and Tumour Necrosis Factor-α Synergistically Induce Eotaxin Production in Human Nasal Fibroblasts," *Clin Exp Allergy*, 2000, 30(3):348-55.
9. Jundt F, Anagnostopoulos I, Bommert K, et al, "Hodgkin/Reed Sternberg Cells Induce Fibroblasts to Secrete Eotaxin, A Potent Chemoattractant for T Cells and Eosinophils," *Blood*, 1999, 94(6):2065-71.
10. Griffiths-Johnson DA, Collins PD, Rossi AG, et al, "The Chemokine, Eotaxin, Activates Guinea Pig Eosinophils In Vitro and Causes Their Accumulation into the Lung In Vivo," *Biochem Biophys Res Commun*, 1993, 197(3):1167-72.
11. Jose PJ, Griffiths-Johnson DA, Collins PD, et al, "Eotaxin: A Potent Eosinophil Chemoattractant Cytokine Detected in a Guinea Pig Model of Allergic Airways Inflammation," *J Exp Med*, 1994, 179(3):881-7.
12. Jose PJ, Griffiths-Johnson DA, Berkman N, et al, "Eotaxin: Cloning of an Eosinophil Chemoattractant Cytokine and Increased mRNA Expression in Allergen-Challenged Guinea Pig Lungs," *Biochem Biophys Res Commun*, 1994, 205(1):788-94.
13. Ponath PD, Qin S, Ringler DJ, et al, "Cloning of the Human Eosinophil Chemoattractant, Eotaxin," *J Clin Invest*, 1996, 97(13):604-12.

(Continued)

Eotaxin, Serum, Plasma, or Urine (Continued)

14. Kitaura M, Nakajima T, Imai T, et al, "Molecular Cloning of Human Eotaxin, an Eosinophil-Selective CC Chemokine, and Identification of a Specific Eosinophil Eotaxin Receptor, CC Chemokine Receptor 3," *J Biol Chem*, 1996, 271(13):7725-30.

15. Wada T, Furuichi K, Sakai N, et al, "Eotaxin Contributes to Renal Interstitial Eosinophilia," *Nephrol Dial Transplant*, 1999, 14(1):76-80.

References

Corrigan CJ, "Eotaxin and Asthma: Some Answers, More Questions," *Clin Exp Immunol*, 1999, 116(1):1-3.

Gutierrez-Ramos JC, Lloyd C, and Gonzalo JA, "Eotaxin: From an Eosinophilic Chemokine to a Major Regulator of Allergic Reactions," *Immunol Today*, 1999, 20(11):500-4.

Luster AD, "Chemokines - Chemotactic Cytokines That Mediate Inflammation," *N Engl J Med*, 1998, 338(7):436-45.

Minshall EM and Hamid QA, "Fibroblasts: A Cell Type Central to Eosinophil Recruitment?" *Clin Exp Allergy*, 2000, 30(3):301-3.

Nagase H, Yamaguchi M, Jibiki S, et al, "Eosinophil Chemotaxis by Chemokines: A Study by a Simple Photometric Assay," *Allergy*, 1999, 54(9):994-50.

Worthen GS and Nick JA, "Leukocyte Accumulation in the Lung," *Fishman's Pulmonary Diseases and Disorders*, Fishman AP, Elias MA, Fishman JA, et al, eds, New York, NY: McGraw-Hill Health Professions Division, 1998, 331-2.

Fetal Cell Detection by Flow Cytometry

Related Information

Applies to F Cells; Hb F; Kleihauer Test; Rosetting Test for FMH

Abstract Fluorescent-tagged antibody to an epitope of fetal red blood cells is used to detect and measure (by flow cytometry) occurrence of fetomaternal hemorrhage (FMH). Estimate of volume of FMH serves to guide therapeutic dose of Rh(D) immune globulin (human). See Rh$_o$(D) Immune Globulin (Human) *on page 860*.

This test is also relevant to certain of the hemolytic anemias.

Specimen 5 mL maternal whole blood (red blood cells from EDTA, heparin, or citrate anticoagulated tubes or red cells freed from clotted specimens can be analyzed)

Container Lavender top (EDTA) tube

Storage Instructions Transport specimen to the laboratory promptly for testing or transfer to local/regional center for imminent batch testing. Washed, fixed erythrocytes suspended in phosphate-buffered saline/2% albumin can be stored at -70°C.[1]

Causes for Rejection Gross hemolysis

Turnaround Time 2-3 hours

Reference Interval Normal adults (includes subjects without hemoglobinopathy): Hb F cells <0.01%; full-term newborns: Hb F cells >90%

Use Test of maternal blood for evidence of fetomaternal hemorrhage and to assess magnitude of such hemorrhage, to assist in calculation of dosage of Rh(D) immune globulin (eg, RhoGAM™); aid in the diagnosis of some hemoglobinopathies. See Kleihauer-Betke *on page 453*.

Limitations Effect of transfusion prior to obtaining specimen for analysis must be considered in interpretation of results. Flow cytometer and associated support personnel are required for analysis.

Methodology Flow cytometry (FC); antibodies to different antigens have been used to detect fetal cells admixed within the maternal cell population. These include anti-D antigen, anti-CD71 (transferrin receptor), and antihemoglobin F (anti-Hb F). The latter uses a monoclonal antibody with activity against an epitope of the gamma (γ) chain of Hb F[2,3] or a polyclonal antibody against Hb F.[4] Early methods relied upon the detection of D antigen and showed greater sensitivity and precision than manual methods (Kleihauer-Betke). These tests are applicable only to cases with D incompatibility, admittedly the common form of hemolytic disease of the newborn (HDN) and cannot be used as a test for all cases of suspected FMH.

The antigen CD71 is expressed only on maternal nucleated RBCs and immature reticulocytes. Methods based on this antigen find application in genetic testing. Detection of fetal cells based on antibodies to Hb F has a number of advantages most significant of which is allowance of a broad global approach to fetal cell detection (not restricted to Rh-negative women). In addition, the method can identify different forms of Hb F containing cells (eg, true fetal cells with Hb F as the major form of hemoglobin vs adult cells with only a small proportion of Hb F). As Hb F is intracellular, permeabilization is necessary to allow antibody access.

The Hb F procedure involves fixation of whole blood in glutaraldehyde, subsequent wash steps followed by suspension of cells in a nonionic detergent (Triton X-100, which affects permeabilization), and additional wash steps prior to staining with fluorescein isothiocyanate-labeled Hb F antibody with use of appropriate buffers and environmental conditions.

Additional Information Documentation of fetomaternal hemorrhage (FMH) is the most common application of methods that measure presence of fetal cells. For over 40 years, most clinical laboratories have used the Kleihauer-Betke (K-B) procedure (slide-based microscopic detection and counting of the results of acid elution treated erythrocytes) for the evaluation of FMH. While relatively rapid, simple, and logistically practical, the K-B method suffers from imprecision. The test requires no special or expensive equipment and no mechanical technical expertise, but performance (in particular interpretation of the slide reaction) can be quite variable among technologists, as shown by the results of proficiency tests (eg, College of American Pathologists) with coefficient of variation in the 40% to 60% range (specimens with a fetal cell frequency of 0.2% to 1%).[5] Other methods for determination of FMH include the rosetting test,[6] enzyme-linked antiglobulin test (ELAT),[7] gel agglutination technique,[8] and flow cytometry.[2,3,4] Flow cytometric-based methods appear to offer a simple, reliable, and more precise alternative to the K-B manual method. Many clinical laboratories do not have access, however, to flow cytometry and the required technical expertise.

Flow cytometry is uniquely suited for F-cell quantitation in the study of hemoglobinopathies, in particular, sickle cell disease (SCD) and its variants.[1] The percent of Hb F in whole blood (measured by alkali denaturation or comparable method) is one of many determinants of clinical severity in SCD. With higher levels of Hb F, clinical severity is decreased. Presence of Hb F dilutes intracellular Hb S in addition to which Hb F and its γ-globin chains impair polymerization of Hb S. Clinical severity of SCD is also dependent upon differences in total Hb concentration, mean corpuscular hemoglobin concentration, red cell rheology, percentage of adhesive cells,[9] the proportion of dense cells, concurrent presence or absence of thalassemia and/or the β-globin haplotype.[10] The percent of Hb F, however, is likely the most important laboratory determinant of clinical severity and predictor of early mortality in patients with SCD.[11] At some 10% to 20% or higher level of Hb F there are fewer deleterious clinical events in cases of SCD.[12]

Hb F is not present in all red cells. It is located in a subset of erythrocytes referred to as Hb F containing cells ("F cells"). An exception is hereditary persistence of hemoglobin F in which all red cells are F cells. In normal adults, the percentage of F cells is from 0.5% to 7%. The percentage of F cells (which survive preferentially in the blood of SCD patients) must be considered as well as the absolute amount of Hb F when considering the effect on clinical severity of sickle hemoglobinopathy. A recent study found a logarithmic correlation between the percentage of F cells and the percentage of Hb F in children with SCD with implications for pharmacologic therapy to increase Hb F.[1] Thus, a growing application of flow cytometry may be to monitor the effect of chemical (drug) therapy of SCD on the F-cell population. A reliable and complicated method for the identification of F reticulocytes by fluorescence image cytometry may also be used to monitor the response of SCD patients being treated with drugs such as hydroxyurea and butyrate.[13]

The use of hydroxyurea and butyrate as drugs to increase the level of Hb F in cases of sickle disease and β-thalassemia has led to amelioration of the disease process and interest in assessment of the efficacy of treatment programs (eg, determination of F reticulocytes).[10]

Footnotes

1. Marcus SJ, Kinney TR, Schultz WH, et al, "Quantitative Analysis of Erythrocytes Containing Fetal Hemoglobin (F Cells) in Children With Sickle Cell Disease," *Am J Hematol*, 1997, 54(1):40-6.

2. Davis BH, Olsen S, Bigelow NC, et al, "Detection of Fetal Red Cells in Fetomaternal Hemorrhage Using a Fetal Hemoglobin Monoclonal Antibody by Flow Cytometry," *Transfusion*, 1998, 38(8):749-56.

3. Navenot JM, Merghoub T, Ducrocq R, et al, "New Method for Quantitative Determination of Fetal Hemoglobin-Containing Red Blood Cells by Flow Cytometry: Application to Sickle-Cell Disease," *Cytometry*, 1998, 32(3):186-90.

4. Nelson M, Zarkos K, Popp H, et al, "A Flow-Cytometric Equivalent of the Kleihauer Test," *Vox Sang*, 1998, 75(3):234-41.

5. Davis BH, "Is There an Alternative to the Kleihauer-Betke Method for Quantitation of Fetal-Maternal Hemorrhage?" Q and A, *Lab Med*, 1999, 30(5):307-8.

6. Sebring ES and Polesky HF, "Detection of Fetal Maternal Hemorrhage in Rh Immune Globulin Candidates: A Rosetting Technique Using Enzyme-Treated Rh₂Rh₂ Indicator Erythrocytes," *Transfusion*, 1982, 22(6):468-71.

7. Riley JZ, Ness PM, Taddie SJ, et al, "Detection and Quantitation of Fetal Maternal Hemorrhage Utilizing an Enzyme-Linked Antiglobulin Test," *Transfusion*, 1982, 22(6):472-4.

8. Salama A, Wittmann MDG, Stelzer A, et al, "Use of the Gel Agglutination Technique for Determination of Fetomaternal Hemorrhage," *Transfusion*, 1998, 38(2):177-80.

9. Hebbel RP, "Blockade of Adhesion of Sickle Cells to Endothelium by Monoclonal Antibodies: Clinical Implications of Basic Research," *N Engl J Med*, 2000, 342(25):1910-11.

10. Powars DR, "Sickle Cell Anemia: β^s-Gene-Cluster Haplotypes as Prognostic Indicators of Vital Organ Failure," *Semin Hematol*, 1991, 28(3):202-8.

11. Platt OS, Brambilla DJ, Rosse WF, et al, "Mortality in Sickle Cell Disease: Life Expectancy and Risk Factors for Early Death," *N Engl J Med*, 1994, 330(23):1639-44.

12. Powars DR, Weiss JN, Chan LS, et al, "Is There a Threshold Level of Fetal Hemoglobin That Ameliorates Morbidity in Sickle Cell Anemia?" *Blood*, 1984, 63(4):921-6.

13. Osterhout ML, Ohene-Frempong K, and Horiuchi K, "Identification of F-Reticulocytes by Two-Stage Fluorescence Image Cytometry," *J Histochem Cytochem*, 1996, 44(4):393-7.

References

Horiuchi K, Osterhout ML, Kamma H, et al, "Estimation of Fetal Hemoglobin Levels in Individual Red Cells via Fluorescence Image Cytometry," *Cytometry*, 1995, 20(3):261-7.

Fetal Hemoglobin

Related Information

Apt-Downey Test *on page 405*
Fetal Cell Detection by Flow Cytometry *on page 430*
Glycated Hemoglobin (Hemoglobin A₁c), Blood *on page 188*
Hemoglobin Electrophoresis *on page 444*
Kleihauer-Betke *on page 453*
Sickle Cell Tests *on page 486*

Synonyms Hb F; Hemoglobin, Fetal

Applies to SIDS; Sudden Infant Death Syndrome

Specimen Whole blood

Container Lavender top (EDTA) tube for venipuncture specimen; lavender top Microtainer™ tube for capillary specimen

Reference Interval 6 months to adult: up to 2% of the total hemoglobin; 0-6 months: up to 75% (alkali denaturation method). Term newborn with high performance liquid chromatography (HPLC) method (Diamat, Bio-Rad, Hercules, CA), 61% to 77%.[1]

Use Evaluate hemoglobinopathies, hemolytic anemia; diagnose hereditary persistence of fetal hemoglobin, thalassemia; evaluate sickling hemoglobins; monitor Hb F levels in sickle cell patients receiving hydroxyurea to increase Hb F production.[2]

Limitations Carboxyhemoglobin A is also resistant to alkali denaturation. Assay for Hb F should initially convert carboxyhemoglobin to cyanmethemoglobin or false-positive elevations of Hb F may be obtained.

Methodology Alkali denaturation, high resolution hemoglobin electrophoresis (some methods), acid elution (Kleihauer-Betke), radial immunodiffusion (RID), isoelectric focusing, high performance liquid chromatography (HPLC),[2] enzyme immunoassay (EIA), capillary electrophoresis,[3] capillary isoelectric focusing[4]

Additional Information Fetal hemoglobin is formed of two α-chains and two γ-chains. It is the major hemoglobin during fetal life. Hb F levels decrease after birth by about 3% to 4% per week. In 2-3 weeks fetal hemoglobin is about 65%. By 6 months of age fetal hemoglobin is <2% of the total hemoglobin. See graph. The oxygen dissociation curve of Hb F is shifted to the left as compared with normal Hb A, which may be due to decreased binding of 2,3-DPG by Hb F (γ-chains). This facilitates placental oxygen transfer. With erythroblastosis fetalis and anoxic states of the newborn, however, Hb F is proportionally lower than in a normal newborn. Over 15 inherited abnormalities of γ-chain structure have been described,[5] but most are without clinical significance (fetal Hb normally forms <2% of total hemoglobin). An exception is Hb F Poole which has been reported as a cause of hemolytic disease of the newborn.[6]

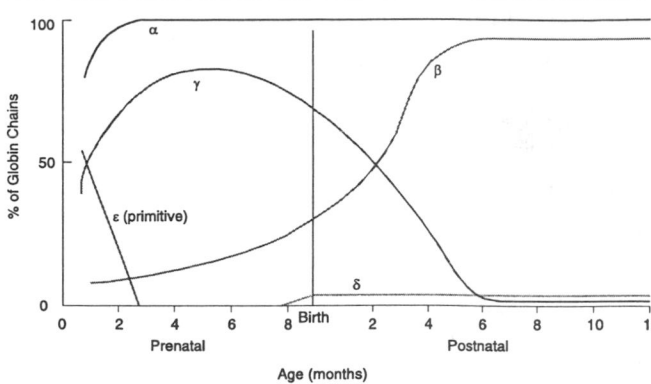

Relative amounts of the several globin chains (ε, α, γ, β, and δ) present during fetal development and the first year of life.

Nonmalignant Conditions Associated With Increased Proportions of Hb F

Condition	Hb F Value (%)
Anemias	
Aplastic anemia (both congenital and acquired)	5-25
Pernicious anemia	2-6
Hereditary spherocytosis	2-5
Hereditary elliptocytosis	2-5
Congenital nonspherocytic hemolytic anemia	3-4
Anemia of chronic infection	2-3
Anemia of blood loss	2-8
Erythropoietic porphyria	2-10
Paroxysmal nocturnal hemoglobinuria	2-25
Hemoglobinopathies	
Unstable hemoglobins	<10
Homozygous Hb S disease	<20
Hb Lepore trait	<5
Hb Kenya trait	6-13
Thalassemias	
β-thalassemia minor	<5
δβ-thalassemia minor	5-20
β-thalassemia major	30-95
α-thalassemia minor	~ 1
Hb H disease	5-15
Hemoglobinopathy-thalassemia interactions	
S/β-thalassemia	10-30
E/β-thalassemia	10-50
C/β-thalassemia	10-30
Hereditary persistence of fetal hemoglobin (HPFH)	
African-type	
heterozygous	15-40
homozygous	100
Greek-type	
heterozygous	10-20
Swiss-type	
heterozygous	1-3

In the adult, hereditary persistence of fetal hemoglobin (HPFH) of multiple varieties, is associated with varying elevations of Hb F. The homozygous form of HPFH is found only in African-Americans. In the heterozygous state, the Hb F level is 15% to 35% in the black type, and 5% to 20% in the Greek type. Homozygous β-thalassemia is associated with Hb F levels >10% to <90%. About 50% of heterozygotes for β-thalassemia have elevated levels around 2%, rarely >5%. The remainder have normal Hb F. Using elements of the CBC, discriminant analysis[7] and use of neural networks have been applied to the differentiation of heterozygous thalassemia from iron deficiency anemia.[8] Heterozygous S/β thalassemia may have Hb F in the 5% to 20% range. With homozygous Hb S disease the level of Hb F varies from 1% to 30%.[9] Hb F inhibits the polymerization of sickle hemoglobin, exerting an ameliorating effect on the sickle disease process. Thus, there is interest in the development and use of drugs that stimulate the production of Hb F (enhance expression of the γ-globin gene in erythroid precursors). Hydroxyurea stimulates Hb F production and has significant clinical benefit in sickle disease.[10] Analogues of butyrate and other short-chain fatty acid derivatives also increase Hb F and may be useful in sickle disease therapy.[10] Gene therapy is under development.[11]

Other conditions associated with elevated Hb F include various anemias (spherocytosis, Fanconi, acquired aplastic, hemolytic, hypoplastic, myelophthisic, megaloblastic including untreated pernicious anemia, paroxysmal nocturnal hemoglobinuria, Blackfan-Diamond anemia); all types of leukemia (especially erythroleukemia and juvenile chronic myelogenous leukemia). (Continued)

Fetal Hemoglobin (Continued)

multiple myeloma and lymphomas, metastatic disease of the bone marrow; bone marrow transplantation; pregnancy; miscellaneous disorders reported include infants small for gestational age, infants with chronic intrauterine anoxia with developmental anomalies; during anticonvulsant drug therapy; diabetes; hyper- and hypothyroidism; and macroglobulinemia. Elevation of Hb F should, then, raise the question of possible underlying disease. Even after exclusion of this variety of disease states, some apparently normal individuals will have elevated Hb F in the 1.5% to 4.0% range. A majority of these result from mutations involving the gamma (γ) chain of Hb F, in particular a cytosine to threonine change at the amino acid 158 position [C $\rightarrow$ T at -158 ($^{G}\gamma$)].[12] Human Hb F consists of two α and two γ chains ($\alpha_2 \gamma_2$). Synthesis of the γ chain has a glycine residue at position 136, $^{A}\gamma$ has alanine at that location. Mutations and the effect of the β globin gene cluster on the expression of γ-globin genes are important participants in regulation of the level of Hb F and thus the clinical severity of sickle disease.

The oxyhemoglobin dissociation curve for Hb F compared to Hb A shows a "left shift" (greater affinity of Hb F c.f. Hb A). Mutant Hb F with decreased oxygen affinity is in the differential diagnosis of newborns presenting with cyanosis of unknown cause.[13] Hb F also causes interference with the laboratory measurement of percent saturation with O_2 and with measurement of fraction of oxygenated hemoglobin. There are a variety of approaches to correction for the effect of Hb F.[14] Modern CO-Oximeter™ instruments nearly eliminate interference by Hb F through appropriate selection of light wavelengths. Neither Hb F nor bilirubin in blood causes clinically significant interference with COHb measurement such that COHb could be used to assist in the diagnosis of hemolysis in the newborn.[15]

Hemoglobin F levels have been studied in relation to risk factors for sudden infant death syndrome (SIDS).[1] Higher levels of Hb F occurred in newborns with shorter gestations and lower birth weights. Newborns older than 38 weeks, whose mothers smoked, had higher Hb F levels than newborns of nonsmoking mothers. Factors associated with high risk for SIDS were found similar to factors leading to higher Hb F levels. The goal is to determine if Hb F levels can identify infants at high risk for SIDS.[1]

Footnotes

1. Cochran DL, Conrad ME, and Matney J, "Hemoglobin F and Risk Factors for Sudden Infant Death Syndrome," *Lab Med*, 1997, 28(1):53-7.
2. Tan GB, Aw TC, Dunstan RA, et al, "Evaluation of High Performance Liquid Chromatography for Routine Estimation of Haemoglobins A₂ and F," *J Clin Pathol*, 1993, 46(9):852-6.
3. Cotton F, Lin C, Fontaine B, et al, "Evaluation of a Capillary Electrophoresis Method for Routine Determination of Hemoglobins A₂ and F," *Clin Chem*, 1999, 45(2):237-43.
4. Conti M, Gelfi C, and Righetti PG, "Screening of Umbilical Cord Blood Hemoglobins by Isoelectric Focusing in Capillaries," *Electrophoresis*, 1995, 16(8):1485-91.
5. Weatherall DJ, Clegg JB, Higgs DR, et al, "The Hemoglobinopathies," *The Metabolic and Molecular Basis of Inherited Disease*, 7th ed, Volume 111, Scriver CR, Beaudet AL, Sly WS, et al, eds, New York, NY: McGraw-Hill Inc, 1995, 3417-84.
6. Lee-Potter JP, Deacon-Smith RA, Simpkiss MJ, et al, "A New Cause of Hemolytic Anemia in the Newborn. A Description of an Unstable Fetal Hemoglobin: F. Poole, $\alpha_2\gamma_2$ 130 Tryptophan Yields Glycine," *J Clin Pathol*, 1975, 28:317-20.
7. Jiménez CV, "Iron-Deficiency Anemia and Thalassemia Trait Differentiated by Simple Hematological Tests and Serum Iron Concentrations," *Clin Chem*, 1993, 39(11 Pt 1):2271-5.
8. Erler BS, Vitagliano P, and Lee S, "Superiority of Neural Networks Over Discriminant Functions for Thalassemia Minor Screening of Red Blood Cell Microcytosis," *Arch Pathol Lab Med*, 1995, 119(4):350-4.
9. Weatherall DJ, Clegg JB, Higgs DR, et al, "The Hemoglobinopathies," *The Metabolic and Molecular Bases of Inherited Disease*, 7th ed, Chapter 113, Scriver CR, Beaudet AK, Sly WS, et al, eds, New York, NY: McGraw Hill Inc, 1995, 3437.
10. Bunn HF, "Pathogenesis and Treatment of Sickle Cell Disease," *N Engl J Med*, 1997, 337(11):762-9.
11. May C, Rivella S, Callegari J, et al, "Therapeutic Haemoglobin Synthesis in β-Thalassaemic Mice Expressing Lentivirus-Encoded Human β-Globin," *Nature*, 2000, 406(6791):82-6.
12. Leonova JY, Kazanetz EG, Smetanina NS, et al, "Variability in the Fetal Hemoglobin Level of the Normal Adult," *Am J Hematol*, 1996, 53(2):59-65.
13. Kohli-Kumar M, Zwerdling T, and Rucknagel DL, "Hemoglobin F-Cincinnati, $\alpha_2{}^G\gamma_2$ 41 (C7) Phe $\rightarrow$ Ser in a Newborn With Cyanosis," *Am J Hematol*, 1995, 49(1):43-7.
14. Moran RF, "Hemoglobin F and Measurement of Oxygen Saturation and Fractional Oxyhemoglobin," *Clin Lab Sci*, 1994, 7(3):162-4.
15. Vreman HJ and Stevenson DK, "Carboxyhemoglobin Determined in Neonatal Blood With a CO-Oximeter™ Unaffected by Fetal Oxyhemoglobin," *Clin Chem*, 1994, 40(8):1522-7.

References

Adekile AD and Huisman THJ, "Hb F in Sickle Cell Anemia," *Experientia*, 1993, 49(1):16-27.

Bowie LJ, Reddy PL, Nagabhushan M, et al, "Detection of α-Thalassemias by Multiplex Polymerase Chain Reaction," *Clin Chem*, 1994, 40(12):2260-6.

Egberts J, Huisman M, van Leeuwen A, et al, "Improved Method for Determining Fetal Hemoglobin (Hb F) by Alkali Denaturation," *Clin Chem*, 1995, 41(12):1778-80.

Kaufman RE, "Analysis of Abnormal Hemoglobins," *Practical Laboratory Hematology*, Koepke JA, ed, New York, NY: Churchill Livingstone, 1991, 251-94.

Papadea C and Cate JC 4th, "Identification and Quantification of Hemoglobins A, F, S, and C by Automated Chromatography," *Clin Chem*, 1996, 42(1):57-63.

Prehu C, Ducrocq R, Godart C, et al, "Determination of Hb F Levels: The Routine Methods," *Hemoglobin*, 1998, 22(5&6):459-67.

Steinberg MH, "Sickle Cell Anemia and Fetal Hemoglobin," *Am J Med Sci*, 1994, 308(5):259-65.

◆ **Fetal Hemoglobin Test in Newborn** see Apt-Downey Test on page 405

◆ **Filarial Infestation** see Microfilariae, Peripheral Blood Preparation on page 460

◆ **Filariasis, Peripheral Blood Preparation** see Microfilariae, Peripheral Blood Preparation on page 460

◆ **Flippase** see Sickle Cell Tests on page 486

◆ **Floppase** see Sickle Cell Tests on page 486

◆ **Flow Cytofluorometry** see Flow Cytometry, Overview on page 432

◆ **Flow Cytometric Analysis for Paroxysmal Nocturnal Hemoglobinuria (PNH)** see PNH Test (GPI-Anchored Proteins) by Flow Cytometry on page 472

◆ **Flow Cytometric Test for GPI-Anchored Protein Deficient Cells** see PNH Test (GPI-Anchored Proteins) by Flow Cytometry on page 472

Flow Cytometry, Overview

Related Information

Alkaline Phosphatase, Neutrophil Membrane (mNAP) on page 402
Apoptosis Assays on page 402
Body Cavity Fluid Cytology on page 372
Body Fluid Chemical Analysis on page 123
Bone Marrow on page 410
CD4/CD8 Enumeration on page 511
CD34⁺ Hematopoietic Stem Cells by Flow Cytometry on page 413
Cell Cycle Analysis by Flow Cytometry on page 53
Complete Blood Count on page 419
Cytomegalovirus Antigen Detection on page 598
Fetal Cell Detection by Flow Cytometry on page 430
Fetal Hemoglobin on page 431
Fine Needle Aspiration Culture on page 609
Fine Needle Aspiration, Deep Masses on page 381
Fine Needle Aspiration, Superficial Masses (Palpable) on page 382
Immunophenotypic Analysis of Tissues by Flow Cytometry on page 62
Infertility Screen on page 310
Kleihauer-Betke on page 453
Leukocyte Cytochemistry on page 456
Lymphocyte Transformation Test on page 539
Mixed Lymphocyte Culture on page 540
Nitroblue Tetrazolium Test on page 461
Platelet Antibodies on page 349
Platelet Count on page 468
Platelet Sizing on page 471
PNH Test (GPI-Anchored Proteins) by Flow Cytometry on page 472
Polymerase Chain Reaction on page 713
Reticulated Platelet Count on page 480
Reticulocyte Count on page 481
Reticulocyte Hemoglobin Content on page 482
Tissue Typing on page 546

Synonyms FACS; FC; FCM; Flow Cytofluorometry; Flow Microfluorometry; Fluorescence Activated Cell Sorter

Applies to Ber-EP₄; CD; CD4 Lymphocytes; CD8 Lymphocytes; Clusters of Differentiation; Mesothelial Cells; Permeabilization; Prion Protein; Suspension Array Technology

Abstract Flow cytometry (FCM) is a technique for the identification, enumeration, and/or separation of particles (including cells) on the basis of light-scattering and/or fluorescence characteristics. Operationally, a column (shaped and contained by a "sheathing" fluid) of particles flows single file past the flow cell analysis point of the cytometer. Important established and expanding uses include immunophenotyping for classification of leukemia/lymphoma, tumor ploidy and S-phase determination, diagnosis of immune deficiency disorders including acquired immunodeficiency syndrome (AIDS), stem cell enumeration, diagnosis of paroxysmal nocturnal hemoglobinuria (PNH), detection of minimal residual disease following therapy of malignancy, enumeration of reticulocyte and platelet parameters, semen analysis, and an evergrowing number of clinical as well as research applications. Multicolor flow cytometry-based suspension array technology (SAT) can perform rapid simultaneous multianalyte immunoassay.

Specimen Whole blood, heparinized. EDTA-anticoagulated blood may be used for many applications.[1] A variety of other clinical specimens can be analyzed (eg, bone marrow, cerebrospinal fluid,[2] serous body fluids/peritoneal washings).[3] Cells must be viable and present as a suspension of single cellular elements. Tissue must be dissociated mechanically and/or by enzyme treatment into an individual cell suspension.

Special Instructions Cell fixation and permeabilization are required for analysis of intracellular targets, see Fetal Hemoglobin on page 431.

Reference Interval Application dependent

Use Broad applications for the unique capabilities of flow cytometric analysis have been, and continue to be, developed in many scientific/analytic disciplines, but are of especial value in clinical hematology and immunology.

Hematology

- Diagnosis/classification of **leukemia** (myeloid, lymphoid, erythroid)
- Diagnosis/classification of lymphoproliferative disorders (**malignant lymphoma** and leukemia)
- Detection of clonality and minimal residual disease
- DNA content and cell cycle analysis
- Reticulocyte count, levels of maturation and indices (reticulocyte mean volume, hemoglobin concentration, and hemoglobin content), see Reticulocyte Count *on page 481* and Hemoglobin *on page 442*
- Granulocyte function and antineutrophil antibody studies
- Assay for leukocyte alkaline phosphatase[4] (a "PIG" protein - see PNH Test (GPI-Anchored Proteins) by Flow Cytometry *on page 472*)
- Platelet count, maturation, and antiplatelet antibody studies
- Diagnosis of PNH by flow cytometry, see PNH Test (GPI-Anchored Proteins) by Flow Cytometry *on page 472*
- F-cell analysis by flow cytometry, see Fetal Cell Detection by Flow Cytometry *on page 430*

Immunology

Identification and enumeration of cell populations identified by surface antigens classified as "clusters of differentiation" (CD) and including numerous members of immunoglobulin, receptor or other "superfamilies" (eg, CD34, member of a family of adhesion molecules-sialomucins and present on hemopoietic stem cells). See CD34+ Hematopoietic Stem Cells by Flow Cytometry *on page 413* and Cluster of Differentiation Antigens Table *on page 400* in the Hematology Introduction.

Limitations Eosinophils may bind unconjugated fluorescein isothiocyanate (trace amounts of which may contaminate reagent kits) and act as a potential source of analytic error.[5] Sensitivity of immunophenotyping is dependent upon characteristics of the monoclonal antibody (eg, specificity, affinity, and properties of the fluorochrome label). Background fluorescence must be minimized. Nonspecific binding of antibody (mediated through the Fc fragment and nonspecies specific) must be decreased by pretreatment with human plasma. FCM may be less than ideally sensitive in detection of T-cell lymphoid malignancy. If malignant cells are few and present admixed with many benign/reactive hematopoietic cells (as occurs with most forms of Hodgkin disease and with T-cell rich B-cell lymphoma) malignancy may not be detected.

Methodology Flow cytometry (FCM) (applied to human cells) is a multiple parameter process involving cell preparation, cell analysis, and data processing/presentation. A variety of scientific disciplines are involved, including antigen/antibody reactions, fluorescence labeling and detection, fluid flow parameters (fluidics), light scattering and detection, and computer/electronic control and analysis techniques.

Study of white blood cells is usually performed after lysis of the red cell population. A method for differentiation of red cells and white cells using dilute whole blood has been described that obviates lysis of red cells or staining of white cells.[6] In the process of flow cytometry, cells are made to pass singly in a fluid stream through a beam of light - the flow cell analysis point (see diagram).

Diagram of Flow Chamber of Cytometer

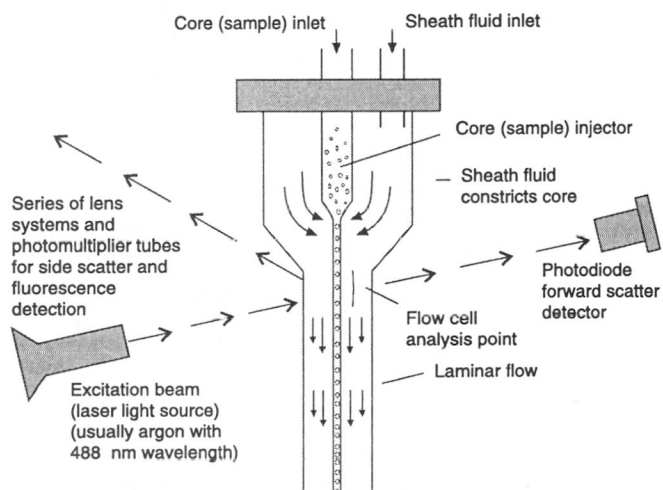

Please refer to Howard Shapiro's clever and entertainingly written informative classic *Practical Flow Cytometry* (3rd ed, John Wiley and Sons, 1995), for a truly revealing color diagram of a FC optical system and for color histograms (between pages 378 and 379), and for Shapiro's *Laws of Flow Cytometry*. If stolen from your local library, it is worthy of purchase for your very own.

As the cells pass through the beam of light (usually a laser light source), photons are emitted and scattered (light scattering). Light scattered along the axis of the beam, forward angle scatter (FS), and light scattered at right angles, 90°C or side scatter (SS), is transmitted optically, and collected by detectors for electronic/computer analysis. The light signal is converted to a

digital signal by photomultiplier tubes (PMT). A PMT produces a signal proportional to the amount of light detected. FS is proportional to the size of the cell; SS corresponds to nuclear complexity and cytoplasmic granularity.

Fluorochrome-conjugated antibodies reacting with cell membrane surface antigens (and/or with intracellular targets after application of cell fixation and "permeabilization" techniques) allow dissection of cell structure and composition. The fluorochromes (eg, fluorescein isothiocyanate - FITC, and phycoerythrin - PE, are commonly used) and have distinctive excitation and emission spectra. The argon laser is of common use in clinical hematology and produces a 488 nm excitation wavelength, capable of exciting many different fluorochromes. Each fluorochrome has a specific and distinct emission wavelength (or spectrum). Two additional fluorochromes (ie, Texas red and cyanine), conjugated with PE, allow argon laser excitation at 488 nm with light emission at three different wavelengths. Thus, "three color" flow cytometry, in which three separate fluorochrome/monoclonal antibody combinations allow for detection of three antigens (total of five parameters) by a single flow cell. Flow cytometers are now available that utilize two lasers and a corresponding greater number of detectors that allow "four-color" (total of six parameters) cytometry with a single flow cell.[7,8]

Propidium iodide (PI) is excited at the same wavelength (488 nm) as FITC and PE. PI stains DNA and can be used in nuclear S-phase and ploidy studies utilizing an argon laser (as with FTIC- and PE-based analyses).

Complex light scattering and fluorescence excitation/emission events, as partially detailed above, occur at the "flow cell analysis point" and depend importantly upon the system fluidics to deliver cells in a uniform single column from a monodisperse suspension. This is accomplished by forcing isotonic fluid under pressure through tubing to the flow cell. Within the flow cell, "sheath fluid" is generated that has laminar flow and a high flow rate (10 m/sec) (see diagram). The sample to be analyzed is fed into the center of the sheath fluid by a computer-driven syringe. Thus, a coaxial stream within a stream is created without mixing of sample and sheath streams. Individual cells must be properly oriented as they pass, single file, past the analysis point. Orientation is assisted by the shape of the tip of the sample insertion needle and by hydrodynamic alignment of cells by pressure of the sheath stream. As the cells pass single file through the flow cell and across the analysis point, they produce light scattering, are excited by the laser light beam, and emit fluorescent light.

Flow cytometry, a near miraculous technical achievement is not without expense and requirements for dedicated space and knowledgeable operating personnel.[9] For additional insight into methodology see Additional Information and consult the outstanding references listed below.

Flow Cytometer Systems for Clinical Application[9]

Cytometer	Manufacturer
FACS Calibur	Becton Dickinson San Jose, CA
XL	Beckman-Coulter Miami, FL
PAS	Partec Munster, Germany
Bryte HS	BioRad Hercules, CA
IMAGN 2000	Biometric Imaging and Becton Dickinson San Jose, CA
Laser Scanning Cytometer	Compucyte Cambridge, MA
Cell Dyn 4000	Abbott Laboratories North Chicago, IL

Additional Information Data gathered from photomultiplier tubes of the flow cytometer (see Methodology) is digitized and can be stored in digital format (computer memory) where it is subject to manipulation by software. The data is commonly displayed as a "dot plot." On the basis of light scatter characteristics, the weak analog signals are amplified (linear or logarithmic) and converted to digital signals, a reflection of which can be represented as a dot on a display device. The example below shows white blood cells identified and displayed on the basis of size (y-axis, ordinate) representing forward light scatter (FS) and on the basis of granularity (x-axis, abscissa) representing side (90°C) light scatter (SS).

The cell populations can be further delineated on the basis of fluorescence from fluorochrome conjugated antibody to specific cell surface (membrane) markers, and in some cases, intracellular targets after cell fixation and permeabilization. The degree of cell membrane electropermeabilization can be monitored by use of a nonpermeant cytotoxic agent (bleomycin).[10] Cell components (eg, G protein-coupled receptors) have also been detected by FCM after solubilization and binding to a fluorescent ligand particle.[11] FCM can detect and measure antigens which are catalogued by "CD" designation.[12] CD refers to cluster designation, "clusters of differentiation", meaning a cluster of antibodies binding to a known antigen.[13]

(Continued)

Flow Cytometry, Overview *(Continued)*

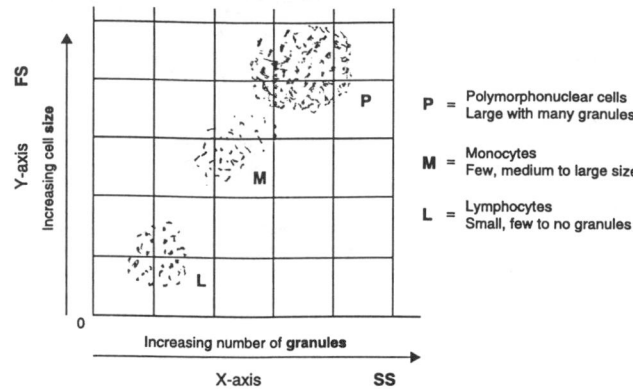

P = Polymorphonuclear cells
Large with many granules

M = Monocytes
Few, medium to large size

L = Lymphocytes
Small, few to no granules

Prognostic Value of Antigen Expression (Composite of Eight Reports)[14]

Prognostic Influence	ALL*		AML†	MM‡
	Childhood	Adults		
Favorable	CD34	CD58	CD58	CD11a
	CD2		CD95	CD56
	CD9			
	CD54			
Adverse	CD45	CD34	CD34	CD20
			CD11b	sIg
			CD7	CD13/CD33
			CD9	CD28
			CD44v6	CD44
			CD56	
			MDRI§	
			LRP¶	

*Acute lymphocytic leukemia.

†Acute myelogenous leukemia.

‡Multiple myeloma.

§MDRI, multidrug-resistant protein.

¶LRP, lung-resistant protein, only in childhood AML.

Perhaps the most valuable and widely used application of FCM is immunophenotyping of hematologic malignancy. Immunophenotyping is important in lineage determination (eg, myeloid, lymphoid), differentiation of acute B-cell from acute T-cell leukemia, establishing presence of mixed lineage

leukemia, assisting in the determination of prognosis and in detection of minimal residual disease. Of 30 or so B-lymphoid cell markers, some 12 have value in analysis of hematologic malignancy. Of 26 T-lymphoid cell markers, 9 are useful in lymphoid malignancy. Of 23 myeloid/monocytic markers, some 9 are useful in hematologic malignancy. See table.

Immunophenotype Markers (Lineage Associations) Useful in Study of Hematologic Malignancy

B-Cell Markers	T-Cell Markers	Myeloid/Monocytic Markers
CD5	CD1-CD5	CD10
CD10	CD7	CD13-CD16
CD19	CD8	CD24
CD20-CD25	CD25	CD33
CD40	CD28	CD34
CD79	CD40L	CD117 (c-kit)
CD103		

CD = Clusters of differentiation, see text and references.

Unfortunately, determination that there is expression of a rare cell marker on a majority of cells may not occur in all cases or may be misleading in some cases of leukemia, thus, the composite phenotype should be utilized (see Leukocyte Cytochemistry *on page 456* for examples of immunophenotypic characteristics of some leukemias).

As hematopoietic (including lymphoid) cells evolve/mature, their cell antigens (in particular, surface membrane antigens) also evolve (change). This process of differentiation may relate to or be mimicked by leukemias/lymphomas, although anomalous development is also common in these malignancies. These anomalies may provide opportunity to monitor disease progression, including detection of residual disease.

Types of abnormal antigen expression include:

1. Lineage infidelity; myeloid antigens are expressed on lymphoid cells or lymphoid antigens are seen on myeloid cells
2. Asynchronous antigen expression; immature and mature antigens are coexpressed
3. Antigen absence; antigens, normally seen together are not both expressed on cells of a tumorous process
4. Intensity of antigen expression is altered (up or down)

A recent broad literature review found that the utility of flow cytometric immunophenotyping of hematologic malignancy (for diagnosis, classification, prognosis, and post-therapeutic monitoring) was rather minimally utilized in routine practice.[14] The following table, indicating the prognostic value of antigen expression on leukemic cells in some cases, is taken with slight modification from this review.[14]

Sensitive methods are required to detect minimal residual disease in cases of acute leukemia. Even though in "clinical" remission, acute leukemia may have up to 10^10 residual malignant cells. FCM can detect one leukemic cell among 10,000 normal bone marrow cells. Because of their sensitivity, FCM and PCR find application in detection of these submicroscopic levels of leukemia.[15]

A system has been introduced for the CD4 and CD8 lymphocyte immunophenotype determination that does not require a high degree of technical sophistication (IMAGN 2000; Becton Dickinson, San Jose, CA).[16] This instrument automatically sets discrimination gates, takes into account volume and sample dilution factors, and has a number of internal quality control features. It directly reports CD4 and CD8 cells per µL of whole blood.[16]

Disorders of granulocyte function (eg, phagocytosis, adhesion defects, production of oxygen radicals in chronic granulomatous disease - CGD) can be assessed by FCM-based methods. The Nitroblue Tetrazolium Test *on page 461*, for diagnosis of CGD, has been largely replaced by FCM-based procedures.[17]

Blood can be analyzed by FCM to determine the percentage of F cells. A method using an isothiocyanate conjugated monoclonal antibody against Hb F has been developed.[18] Washed blood is fixed in formaldehyde and glutaraldehyde and then "permeabilized" in a Triton x-100/PBS solution so that the antibody can gain access to the intracellular Hb F. FCM analysis is then used to determine the percentage of F cells.

FCM may be of value in study of serous effusions harboring malignant cells. Use of Ber-EP₄ (monoclonal antibody directed against two glycopeptides on human epithelial cells) has, in some studies, shown specificity and sensitivity in differentiating between malignant epithelial cells and mesothelial cells.[3]

Multicolor flow cytometer-based suspension array technology (SAT) is ideal for cytokine panel quantitation. Microparticle-based multiplexed immunoassays, affinity assays, and DNA hybridization assays utilizing low-cost miniaturized laser systems have led to commercial FCM dedicated to SAT with the potential to replace most ELISA (enzyme-linked immunoassay) based methods.[19]

FCM's ability to detect and follow cell differentiation has been applied in an evergrowing number of research investigations. An example is elucidation of prion protein's role in the genesis of the transmissible spongiform encephalopathies (TSE) which includes Creutzfeldt-Jakob disease (CJD) in humans.[20] Prion protein is etiologically related to TSE. An isoform of prion protein (PrP^Sc), which accumulates in CJD, is formed as the result of a post-translational process with conformational changes from the **normal** cellular isoform of the prion protein (PrP^c). PrP^Sc apparently replicates by converting PrP^c into PrP^Sc by a process of autocatalysis. FCM studies have shown that PrP^c plays an important role in function and development of some lymphoid hematopoietic cells.[20] Recently, it has been shown that plasminogen selectively binds PrP^Sc. This finding has neuropathogenetic significance and may open avenues for prion removal from blood-derived biological products and to the development of diagnostic procedures.[21] Previously there were no immunoreagents available for clinical use that could reliably differentiate between PrP^Sc and PrP^c. There is interest (especially in Europe) in the development and application of a screening test to detect individuals infected with variant CJD.[22]

Footnotes

1. Stelzer GT, Marti G, Hurley A, et al, "U.S.-Canadian Consensus Recommendations on the Immunophenotypic Analysis of Hematologic Neoplasia by Flow Cytometry: Standardization and Validation of Laboratory Procedures," *Cytometry*, 1997, 30(5):214-30.
2. Finn WG, Peterson LC, James C, et al, "Enhanced Detection of Malignant Lymphoma in Cerebrospinal Fluid by Multiparameter Flow Cytometry," *Am J Clin Pathol*, 1998, 110(3):341-6.
3. Risberg B, Davidson B, Dong HP, et al, "Flow Cytometric Immunophenotyping of Serous Effusions and Peritoneal Washings: Comparison With Immunocytochemistry and Morphological Findings," *J Clin Pathol*, 2000, 53(7):513-7.
4. Rambaldi A, Masuhara K, Borleri GM, et al, "Flow Cytometry of Leukocyte Alkaline Phosphatase in Normal and Pathologic Leukocytes," *Br J Haematol*, 1997, 96(4):815-22.
5. Bedner E, Halicka HD, Cheng W, et al, "High Affinity Binding of Fluorescein Isothiocyanate to Eosinophils Detected by Laser Scanning Cytometry: A Potential Source of Error in Analysis of Blood Samples Utilizing Fluorescein-Conjugated Reagents in Flow Cytometry," *Cytometry*, 1999, 36(1):77-82.
6. Ost V, Neukammer J, and Rinneberg H, "Flow Cytometric Differentiation of Erythrocytes and Leukocytes in Dilute Whole Blood by Light Scattering," *Cytometry*, 1998, 32(3):191-7.
7. Kroft SH, "Q & A Flow Cytometry," *Lab Med*, 2000 31(10):535-6.

8. Stewart CC and Stewart SJ, "Compensation Requirements for Four-Color Immunophenotyping," *Cytometry*, 1999, 38(4):161-75.

9. Bakke AC, "Clinical Applications of Flow Cytometry," *Lab Med*, 2000, 31(2):97-102.

10. Kotnik T, Macek-Lebar A, Miklavcic D, et al, "Evaluation of Cell Membrane Electropermeabilization by Means of a Nonpermeant Cytotoxic Agent," *BioTechniques*, 2000, 28(5):921-6.

11. Sklar LA, Vilven J, Lynam E, et al, "Solubilization and Display of G Protein-Coupled Receptors on Beads for Real-Time Fluorescence and Flow Cytometric Analysis," *BioTechniques*, 2000, 28(5):976-85.

12. Fleisher TA and Tomar RH, "Introduction to Diagnostic Laboratory Immunology," *JAMA*, 1997, 278(22):1823-4.

13. Glassman AB, Hopwood VL, and Schwartz DJ, "Improving Diagnosis of Hematologic Neoplasms," *ADVANCE for Administrators of the Laboratory*, 2000, 9(1):58-61.

14. Orfao A, Schmitz G, Brando B, et al, "Clinically Useful Information Provided by the Flow Cytometric Immunophenotyping of Hematological Malignancies: Current Status and Future Directions," *Clin Chem*, 1999, 45(10):1708-17.

15. Campana D and Coustan-Smith E, "Detection of Minimal Residual Disease in Acute Leukemia by Flow Cytometry," *Cytometry*, 1999, 38(4):139-52.

16. Glencross D, Scott L, Aggett H, et al, "Microvolume Fluorometry for the Determination of Absolute CD4 and CD8 Lymphocyte Counts in Patients With HIV: A Comparative Evaluation," *Clin Lab Haematol*, 1999, 21(6):391-5.

17. Lun A, Schmitt M, and Renz H, "Phagocytosis and Oxidative Burst: Reference Values for Flow Cytometric Assays Independent of Age," *Clin Chem*, 2000, 46(11):1836-9.

18. Campbell TA, Ware RE, and Mason M, "Detection of Hemoglobin Variants in Erythrocytes by Flow Cytometry," *Cytometry*, 1999, 35(3):242-8.

19. Mandy F and Minkus T, "New Applications for Flow Cytometry," *ADVANCE for Administrators of the Laboratory*, 2000, 9(6):80-8.

20. Dürig J, Giese A, Schulz-Schaeffer W, et al, "Differential Constitutive and Activation-Dependent Expression of Prion Protein in Human Peripheral Blood Leukocytes," *Br J Haematol*, 2000, 108(3):488-95.

21. Fischer MB, Roeckl C, Parizek P, et al, "Binding of Disease-Associated Prion Protein to Plasminogen," *Nature*, 2000, 408(6811):479-83.

22. Brown P, Cervenáková L, and Diringer H, "Blood Infectivity and the Prospects for a Diagnostic Screening Test in Creutzfeldt-Jakob Disease," *J Lab Clin Med*, 2001, 137(1):5-13.

References

Alvarez-Barrientos A, Arroyo J, Canton R, et al, "Applications of Flow Cytometry to Clinical Microbiology," *Clin Microbiol Rev*, 2000, 13(2):167-95.

Bakke AC, "The Principles of Flow Cytometry," *Lab Med*, 2001, 32(4):207-11.

Bonanno E, Mauriello A, Partenzi A, et al, "Flow Cytometry Analysis of Atherosclerotic Plaque Cells From Human Carotids: A Validation Study," *Cytometry*, 2000, 39(2):158-65.

Brown M and Wittwer C, "Flow Cytometry: Principles and Clinical Applications in Hematology," *Clin Chem*, 2000, 46(8):1221-9.

Carulli G, Sbrana S, Azzara A, et al, "Detection of Eosinophils in Whole Blood Samples by Flow Cytometry," *Cytometry*, 1998, 34(6):272-9.

Chu PG, Chang KL, Arber DA, et al, "Immunophenotyping of Hematopoietic Neoplasms," *Semin Diagn Pathol*, 2000, 17(3):236-56.

Crucian B, Norman J, Brentz J, et al, "Laboratory Outreach: Student Assessment of Flow Cytometer Fluidics in Zero Gravity," *Lab Med*, 2000, 31(10):569-73.

Fleisher TA, "Flow Cytometry," *Semin Hematol*, 2001, 38(2).

Frizzera G, Wu CD, and Inghirami G, "The Usefulness of Immunophenotypic and Genotypic Studies in the Diagnosis and Classification of Hematopoietic and Lymphoid Neoplasms," *Am J Clin Pathol*, 111(Suppl 1):S13-S39.

Fukushima PI, Khanh Thi Nguyen P, O'Grady P, et al, "Flow Cytometric Analysis of Kappa and Lambda Light Chain Expression in Evaluation of Specimens for B-Cell Neoplasia," *Cytometry*, 1996, 26(4):243-52.

Gratama JW, Bolhuis RL, and Van T Veer MB, "Quality Control of Flow Cytometric Immunophenotyping of Haematological Malignancies," *Clin Lab Haematol*, 1999, 21(5):155-60.

Heiden T, Castanos-Vélez E, Andersson LC, et al, "Combined Analysis of DNA Ploidy, Proliferation, and Apoptosis in Paraffin-Embedded Cell Material by Flow Cytometry," *Lab Invest*, 2000, 80(8).1207-13.

Kjeldsberg CR, Elenitoba-Johnson KS, Foucar K, et al, "Special Techniques: Flow Cytometry, Molecular Diagnostics, Fluorescent *In Situ* Hybridization and Cytogenetics," *Practical Diagnosis of Hematologic Disorders*, 3rd ed, Kjeldsberg CR, ed, Chicago, IL: ASCP Press: American Society of Clinical Pathologists, 2000, 861.

Maccy MG, McCarthy DA, Milne T, et al, "Comparative Study of Five Commercial Reagents for Preparing Normal and Leukaemic Lymphocytes for Immunophenotypic Analysis by Flow Cytometry," *Cytometry*, 1999, 38(4):153-60.

Paraskevas F, "Clinical Flow Cytometry" *Wintrobe's Clinical Hematology*, 10th ed, Chapter 4, Lee GR, Foerster J, Lukens J, et al, eds, Baltimore, MD: Lippincott Williams & Wilkins, 1999, 56-71.

Shapiro HM, "How Flow Cytometers Work," *Practical Flow Cytometry*, 3rd ed, Chapter 4, New York, NY: Wiley-Liss, 1995, 75-178.

Siebert JD, Weeks LM, List LW, et al, "Utility of Flow Cytometry Immunophenotyping for the Diagnosis and Classification of Lymphoma in Community Hospital Clinical Needle Aspiration/Biopsies," *Arch Pathol Lab Med*, 2000, 124(12):1792-9.

Tarapchak P, "Turning the Light on Disease Diagnosis," *ADVANCE for Administrators of the Laboratory*, 1999, 8:34-6.

Willmann K and Dunne JF, "A Flow Cytometric Immune Function Assay for Human Peripheral Blood Dendritic Cells," *J Leukoc Biol*, 2000, 67(4):536-44.

♦ **Flow Microfluorometry**   see Flow Cytometry, Overview on page 432

♦ **Fluorescence Activated Cell Sorter**   see Flow Cytometry, Overview on page 432

♦ **Folate Level**   see Folic Acid, Serum on page 435

Folic Acid, RBC

Related Information

Anemia Flowchart on page 392
Cobalamin, Serum on page 150
Complete Blood Count on page 419
d-Xylose Absorption Test, Serum, Urine on page 167
Folic Acid, Serum on page 435
Hemoglobin on page 442
Homocyst(e)ine, Plasma on page 193
Methylmalonic Acid, Serum, Plasma, Urine, or Amniotic Fluid on page 224
Parietal Cell Antibody on page 541
Phenobarbital, Serum or Plasma on page 760
Primidone, Serum or Plasma on page 762
Schilling Test on page 483
Vitamin B_{12} Unsaturated Binding Capacity on page 495

Synonyms RBC Folate; Red Cell Folate

Patient Preparation Avoid radioisotope scan prior to collection of specimen if RIA is used for assay.

Specimen Erythrocytes

Container Lavender top (EDTA) tube. Green top (heparin) tube may also be used for folate assay, but heparin interferes with serum cobalamin determinations, which are often performed simultaneously.

Sampling Time Fasting specimen is preferred.

Storage Instructions Red cells (or hemolysate) can be stored at 4°C or frozen until assay.

Reference Interval 125-600 ng/mL (SI: 283-1360 nmol/L). The megaloblastic anemia of folate deficiency is usually associated with red cell folate levels <100 ng/mL (SI: <227 nmol/L) RBCs.

Use Detect folate deficiency

Limitations Unfortunately, there is evidence that red cell folate testing methods may be unreliable. In a study of 130 samples from patients with severe folate deficiency, falsely normal red cell folate levels were found in 16% to 40% of cases (different kits). Folate deficiency in these cases was documented on the basis of microbiologic assay of plasma and red cell folate (low levels documented), bone marrow morphologic abnormalities, abnormal dU suppression test, and/or an appropriate response to therapy.[1]

Methodology Radioimmunoassay (RIA), competitive protein binding

Additional Information Since serum folate values fluctuate significantly with diet, measurement of red cell folate is a better measure of tissue folate stores. Elderly patients with decreased serum cobalamin and/or folate (serum and RBC levels) but without hematologic signs of megaloblastosis (MCV <100 FL) likely reflect an uncertain upper limit of normal for the MCV and/or presence of subclinical megaloblastic anemia.[2] Attention to clinical setting is important since a normal red cell folate level can be found in a rapidly developing folic acid deficiency such as the stress of pregnancy. There is evidence that when RBC folate and D-xylose absorption tests, used as a noninvasive screen, are both normal, the predictive accuracy for absence of celiac disease is 100%. When used together, these tests were found ideal for selecting patients for jejunal biopsy from an otherwise unmanageable number with symptoms suggestive of celiac disease.[3]

Footnotes

1. Zittoun J and Zittoun R, "Modern Clinical Testing Strategies in Cobalamin and Folate Deficiency," *Semin Hematol*, 1999, 36(1):35-46.

2. Chanarin I and Metz J, "Diagnosis of Cobalamin Deficiency: The Old and the New," *Br J Haematol*, 1997, 97(4):695-700.

3. Labib M, Gama R, and Marks V, "Predictive Value of D-Xylose Absorption Test and Erythrocyte Folate in Adult Coeliac Disease: A Parallel Approach," *Ann Clin Biochem*, 1990, 27(Pt 1):75-7.

References

Luong KV and Nguyen LT, "Folate and Vitamin B_{12}-Deficiency Anemias in Vietnamese Immigrants Living in Southern California," *South Med J*, 2000, 93(1):53-7.

Miller SM, "Old and New Rationales for Serum B_{12} and Folate Determinations," *Clin Lab Sci*, 1993, 6(5):272-4.

Snow CF, "Laboratory Diagnosis of Vitamin B_{12} and Folate Deficiency: A Guide for the Primary Care Physician," *Arch Intern Med*, 1999, 159(12):1289-98.

Wickramasinghe SN, "Newer B_{12} and Folate Assays and Functional Measurements," *Clin Lab Haematol*, 1997, 19(4):302-3.

Folic Acid, Serum

Related Information

Anemia Flowchart on page 392
Cobalamin, Serum on page 150
Complete Blood Count on page 419
Folic Acid, RBC on page 435
Hemoglobin on page 442
Homocyst(e)ine, Plasma on page 193
Intrinsic Factor Blocking Antibody on page 537
Methylmalonic Acid, Serum, Plasma, Urine, or Amniotic Fluid on page 224
Parietal Cell Antibody on page 541
Phenobarbital, Serum or Plasma on page 760
Primidone, Serum or Plasma on page 762
Schilling Test on page 483
(Continued)

Folic Acid, Serum (Continued)

Vitamin B$_{12}$ Unsaturated Binding Capacity *on page 495*

Synonyms Folate Level; Serum Folate

Abstract Folic acid (pteroylglutamic acid) exists in dihydro- and tetrahydro forms. Reduction occurs by ascorbic acid or by enzyme-folate reductases. Biologic activity in tissue metabolism involves one-carbon transfer of the tetrahydro form (dihydrofolate reductase required). Folate coenzymes are involved in oxidation-reduction and single carbon transfer reactions. Folates are coenzymes involved in many metabolic pathways with one-carbon unit transfers including purine and pyrimidine synthesis and amino acid conversions. The latter is of special importance in the conversion of homocyst(e)ine to methionine (cobalamin also required as a coenzyme). A methyl group is transferred from methyl tetrahydrofolate to cobalamin (forms methyl cobalamin followed by transfer of the methyl group to homocyst(e)ine to form methionine). Elevated homocyst(e)ine levels have important implications for the development of vascular disease (see Homocyst(e)ine, Plasma *on page 193*). Folate deficiency by interfering with nucleoside biosynthesis (includes DNA synthesis) is an important cause of megaloblastic anemia. Folate deficiency/inhibition is common in pregnancy and in those who take alcohol and/or a number of drugs (including methotrexate).

Patient Preparation Patient should be fasting overnight. Collect prior to transfusion or initiation of folate therapy.

Specimen Serum

Container Red top tube

Collection Avoid hemolysis. Transport specimen to the laboratory promptly after collection. Avoid exposure to light. Significant (12% to 19%) loss of folate occurs over 24 hours in specimens kept at room temperature and exposed to light. Specimens exposed to light for more than 8 hours should be redrawn.[1]

Storage Instructions Stable 24 hours at 4°C or store frozen early in hospital stay (feeding malnourished patient may rapidly elevate folate level to normal). Protect from light.

Causes for Rejection Hemolyzed specimen, stored specimen not frozen or protected from light, patient having had isotope scan or Schilling's test prior to collection of specimen

Reference Interval >2 ng/mL (SI: >5 nmol/L). See table for pediatric reference ranges. Hemolysis may result in markedly elevated serum folate levels.

Pediatric Serum Folate Reference Chart

Age	Male (nmol/L)		Female (nmol/L)	
	Low	High	Low	High
0-1 y	16.3	50.8	14.3	51.5
2-3 y	5.7	34.0	3.9	35.6
4-6 y	1.1	29.4	6.1	31.9
7-9 y	5.2	27.0	5.4	30.4
10-12 y	3.4	24.5	2.3	23.1
13-18 y	2.7	19.9	2.7	16.3

Adapted from Hicks JM, Cook J, Godwin ID, et al, "Vitamin B$_{12}$ and Folate – Pediatric Reference Ranges," *Arch Pathol Lab Med*, 1993, 117:705.

B$_{12}$/Folate Levels in Megaloblastic Anemia

Deficiency	Serum B$_{12}$	Serum/RBC Folate
Vitamin B$_{12}$	↓	normal or ↑/↓
Folate	normal or slight ↓	↓/↓
B$_{12}$ and folate	↓	↓/↓

Use Detect folate deficiency; monitor therapy with folate; evaluate megaloblastic and macrocytic anemia; evaluate alcoholic patients and those with prior jejunoileal bypass for morbid obesity or those with intestinal blind-loop syndrome; evaluate cause of increase in serum homocyst(e)ine level

Limitations May be falsely elevated with RBC hemolysis. May be decreased in patients on oral contraceptives. Folate will deteriorate on exposure to light. Usually measured with red cell folate and vitamin B$_{12}$ levels. Significant fluctuation with diet occurs and can result in a false-normal serum folate in a patient with folate deficiency. Concurrent severe iron deficiency may mask presence of folate deficiency. Serum methylmalonic acid, increased in some early cases of B$_{12}$ deficiency, is usually normal with folate deficiency.

Methodology Competitive protein binding radioimmunoassay. Patient's endogenous unlabeled serum folate competes with radiolabeled folate for specific sites on a binding protein (eg, as derived from milk) and is compared to a standard curve. Serum contains multiple forms of folate. Methyltetrahydrofolate is the major serum form of folate. Most immunoassays measure a composite of serum folates.[2] Chemiluminescence receptor assays have been developed in which the serum specimen is combined with a solid substrate (or polyamine solution) that contains a folate-binding protein. After conjugation and binding with a fluorescent substrate, product is measured. Fluorescence is proportional to the concentration of test folate. It employs an acridinium-ester-coupled folate molecule as tracer and folate binding protein on magnetic particles as the solid phase.[3] An ion capture assay (Abbott IMx analyzer) has been developed.[4]

Additional Information Naturally occurring folates are present widely in plant and animal foods taken in the diet and absorbed in the small intestine. Folic acid (pteroylglutamic acid) has a number of biologically active forms (largely conjugates of glutamic acid, eg, N-5-methyltetrahydrofolic acid and N-5-formyltetrahydrofolic acid - folinic acid) that function as coenzymes. Lack of folic acid inhibits DNA synthesis in rapidly dividing cells, thus producing megaloblastic anemia. While a specific folate-binding protein is present in the serum, some 90% of folate is unbound. The binding protein increases with folate deficiency and returns to normal with treatment.

Serum levels are affected by present dietary intake. Drugs that are folate antagonists, such as methotrexate and pentamidine, may induce a deficiency state. Some drugs, such as oral contraceptives, phenytoin, and ethanol impair absorption of folate. In the pH range of physiologic significance, folate binds to aluminum hydroxide. Chronic use of antacids or H$_2$-receptor antagonists by patients with diets marginal in folate may be a cause of folic acid deficiency. Folate levels are commonly high in patients with B$_{12}$ deficiency since this vitamin is needed to allow incorporation of folate into tissue cells. Increased serum homocyst(e)ine level may occur with deficiency of either vitamin B$_{12}$ or folate. Folate (folic acid) deficiency is present in some 33% of pregnant women, many alcoholics, patients with a wide variety of malabsorption syndromes including celiac disease, sprue, Crohn disease, and jejunal/ileal bypass procedure.

Some Drugs With Potential to Cause Megaloblastosis by Effect on Folate Metabolism

- Methotrexate and other antineoplastics
- Anticonvulsants
- Oral contraceptives
- Sulfasalazine
- Trimethoprim
- Pyrimethamine
- Alcohol abuse (most common cause of folate deficiency in U.S.)

Measurement of serum and, in some cases, red cell folate levels constitutes a reliable means of determining the existence of folate deficiency. These tests should be considered in patients who have megaloblastic anemia, as well as for patients who have anemia, hypersegmentation of granulocyte nuclei, and coincident evidence of iron deficiency. The finding of a low serum folate means that the patient's recent diet has been subnormal in folate content and/or that recent absorption of folate has been subnormal, but does not prove that the patient either has or will develop tissue folate depletion requiring folate therapy. Therefore, serum folate assays have a very poor predictive value in diagnosis and should be interpreted with caution. A low red cell folate can mean either that there is tissue folate depletion due to folate deficiency requiring folate therapy, or alternatively, that the patient has primary vitamin B$_{12}$ deficiency blocking the ability of cells to take up folate. In the latter case, the proper therapy would be with vitamin B$_{12}$ rather than with folic acid. For these reasons, it has been considered advisable in the past to determine red cell folate in addition to serum folate, to establish a diagnosis of folate deficiency for which the proper treatment is folic acid. Currently however, analytic limitations of red cell folate assays are cautioned. Additionally, decreases in RBC folate lack specificity for folate deficiency as they also occur in cobalamin deficiency. For thoroughness, serum level should also be determined. In some geographic areas (hospitalized urban patient populations), zidovudine, used in the treatment of acquired immune deficiency syndrome, has been the most common condition associated with macrocytosis.[5]

Folate deficient diets have been proposed for methotrexate responsive malignancy. It has also been suggested that plasma folate concentrations in patients who do and do not respond to folate deprivation/antagonism be compared and ratioed to methotrexate levels as part of tumor therapy regimes.[6] The levels of serum and RBC folate may be significantly increased in hyperthyroidism.[7]

In 1997, the U.S. government mandated fortification of grain products with folic acid.[8,9] The intent was to increase dietary folate to about 100 μg/person/day (diet dependent) in order to decrease the incidence of neural tube defects. The attempt was to set the amount of supplement so as to reduce the incidence of neural tube defects without masking occult cobalamin deficiency. The result was an increase in mean serum folate level from 4.6-10.0 μg/L. The mean serum homocyst(e)ine concentration fell from 10.1 to 9.4 μmol/L.[9] These changes will likely effect "normal" reference ranges for folate and homocyst(e)ine as well as possibly decreasing the number of laboratory folate tests (at least in those without hematologic abnormality) with resultant cost savings.[10]

Footnotes

1. Mastropaolo W and Wilson MA, "Effect of Light on Serum B$_{12}$ and Folate Stability," *Clin Chem*, 1993, 39(5):913.
2. Lucock MD, Daskalakis I, Schorah CJ, et al, "Folate-Homocysteine Interrelations: Potential New Markers of Folate Status," *Mol Genet Metab*, 1999, 67(1):23-35.
3. Klukas C, Comerci C, Campbell J, et al, "A Chemiluminescence Receptor Assay for Folate," *Clin Chem*, 1993, 39(5):913.
4. Wilson DH, Herrmann R, Hsu S, et al, "Ion Capture Assay for Folate With the Abbott IMx Analyzer," *Clin Chem*, 1995, 41(12 Pt 1):1780-1.
5. Snower DP and Weil SC, "Changing Etiology of Macrocytosis: Zidovudine as a Frequent Causative Factor," *Am J Clin Pathol*, 1993, 99(1):57-60.

6. Cohen P and Dix D, "On the Role of Folate Deficiency in Cancer Therapy," *Clin Chem*, 1988, 34(9):1945-6.

7. Ford HC, Carter JM, and Rendle MA, "Serum and Red Cell Folate and Serum Vitamin B$_{12}$ Levels in Hyperthyroidism," *Am J Hematol*, 1989, 31(4):233-6.

8. Malinow MR, Duell PB, Hess DL, et al, "Reduction of Plasma Homocyst(e)ine Levels by Breakfast Cereal Fortified With Folic Acid in Patients With Coronary Heart Disease," *N Engl J Med*, 1998, 338(15):1009-15.

9. Jacques PF, Selhub J, Bostom AG, et al, "The Effect of Folic Acid Fortification on Plasma Folate and Total Homocysteine Concentrations," *N Engl J Med*, 1999, 340(19):1449-54.

10. Cembrowski GS, Zhang MM, Prosser CI, et al, "Folate Is Not What it Is Cracked up to Be," *Arch Intern Med*, 1999, 159(22):2747-8.

References

Allen RH, "Megaloblastic Anemias," *Cecil Textbook of Medicine*, 21st ed, Goldman L and Bennett JC, eds, Philadelphia, PA: WB Saunders, 2000, 859-67.

Antony AC, "Megaloblastic Anemias," *Hematology: Basic Principles and Practice*, Hoffman R, Benz EJ, Shattil SJ, et al, eds, Philadelphia, PA: Churchill Livingstone, 2000, 446-85.

Carmel R, "Current Concepts in Cobalamin Deficiency," *Annu Rev Med*, 2000, 51:357-75.

Hicks JM, Cook J, Godwin ID, et al, "Vitamin B$_{12}$ and Folate: Pediatric Reference Ranges," *Arch Pathol Lab Med*, 1993, 117(7):704-6.

Klee GG, "Cobalamin and Folate Evaluation: Measurement of Methylmalonic Acid and Homocysteine vs Vitamin B$_{12}$ and Folate," *Clin Chem*, 2000, 46(8 Pt 2):1277-83.

Rothenberg SP, "Increasing the Dietary Intake of Folate: Pros and Cons," *Semin Hematol*, 1999, 36(1):65-74.

Zittoun J and Zittoun R, "Modern Clinical Testing Strategies in Cobalamin and Folate Deficiency," *Semin Hematol*, 1999, 36(1):35-46.

♦ **Free Hemoglobin** see Hemoglobin, Plasma on page 446

♦ **Friedreich Ataxia** see Inherited Diseases of Metabolism and Cell Structure on page 449

♦ α-**Fucosidase** see Inherited Diseases of Metabolism and Cell Structure on page 449

♦ **G6PD, Qualitative** see Glucose-6-Phosphate Dehydrogenase Screen, Blood on page 438

♦ **G6PD, Quantitative, Blood** see Glucose-6-Phosphate Dehydrogenase, Quantitative, Blood on page 437

♦ **G6PD Screen, Blood** see Glucose-6-Phosphate Dehydrogenase Screen, Blood on page 438

♦ **Gaisbock Syndrome** see Red Cell Mass on page 478

♦ **Galactocerebroside** see Inherited Diseases of Metabolism and Cell Structure on page 449

♦ β-**Galactosidase** see Inherited Diseases of Metabolism and Cell Structure on page 449

♦ **Gametocytes** see Malaria Smear and Tests on page 458

Gelation Assay

Related Information
Glycerol Lysis Test, Acidified, Modified on page 439
Osmotic Fragility on page 462
Osmotic Fragility, Incubated on page 463

Synonyms Absence of Phosphorylation-Induced Gelation of Red Cell Membrane Skeletons; Erythrocyte Membrane Skeleton Gelation Assay; Gelation Failing Test

Abstract This test, initially reported to be specific for the diagnosis of hereditary spherocytosis (HS), has not gained proponents for its clinical use.

Specimen Whole blood

Container Green top (heparin) tube

Storage Instructions Blood is collected and processed within the same day. cAMP-independent protein kinase may be stored at -20°C.

Reference Interval Normal individuals and patients with a variety of hemolytic anemias show gelation after 30-50 minutes. Patients with hereditary spherocytosis show absence of gelation of erythrocyte membranes including after incubation for 12 hours (positive test is absence of gelation).

Use Diagnosis of hereditary spherocytosis

Limitations Assay is of limited availability. Preparation requires considerable laboratory manual processing. Documentation of sensitivity and specificity is based on small patient samples.

Methodology Red cell membrane (ghosts) and partially purified cAMP-independent kinase are prepared, mixed under standardized conditions in a pipette, and observation for gelation is conducted by visual inspection.

Additional Information This test, based on a visually detectable change in the behavior of erythrocyte membrane ghosts, was developed and investigated as a possibly specific test for hereditary spherocytosis. The gelation assay is based on the observation that upon phosphorylation with cAMP-independent protein kinase, normal red cell membrane ("ghost") preparations set to a gelatinous mass (negative reaction) while those from spherocytosis red cells do not gel (positive reaction). Negative reactions have been observed in cases of hereditary elliptocytosis, hereditary stomatocytosis, β-thalassemia, pyruvate kinase deficiency, glucose phosphate isomerase deficiency, and glucose-6-phosphate dehydrogenase deficiency as well as in normal individuals. The gelation test is technically more involved

and time consuming than the modified acidified glycerol lysis or osmotic fragility screening tests.

References
Armbrust R, Eber SW, and Schröter W, "Absence of Phosphorylation-Induced Gelation of Erythrocyte Membrane Skeletons: A Diagnostic Tool for Hereditary Spherocytosis," *Ann Hematol*, 1992, 64(2):93-6.

♦ **Gelation Failing Test** see Gelation Assay on page 437

♦ **Genetic Chronic Thrombocytopenia** see Platelet Count on page 468

♦ **Giant Papillary Conjunctivitis** see Eosinophil Granule Proteins on page 426

♦ **Glucocerebroside** see Inherited Diseases of Metabolism and Cell Structure on page 449

Glucose-6-Phosphate Dehydrogenase, Quantitative, Blood

Related Information
Autohemolysis Test on page 405
Glucose-6-Phosphate Dehydrogenase Screen, Blood on page 438
Heinz Body Stain on page 440
Hemosiderin Stain, Urine on page 876
Red Blood Cell Enzyme Deficiency, Quantitative on page 475
Red Blood Cell Enzyme Deficiency Screen on page 476

Synonyms G6PD, Quantitative, Blood

Applies to Heinz Bodies

Abstract See Glucose-6-Phosphate Dehydrogenase Screen, Blood on page 438.

Specimen Erythrocytes

Container Lavender top (EDTA) tube, green top (heparin) tube, or acid-citrate-dextrose (ACD) solution

Storage Instructions In above anticoagulants, RBC enzymes stable at 4°C for at least 6 days and stable at 25°C for at least 24 hours.

Special Instructions If sample must be sent to a referral laboratory, ship on wet ice, do not freeze.

Reference Interval 8.34 ±1.59 IU/g hemoglobin, adults measured at 30°C. "Normal" levels in newborns and prematures are apparently higher (these subjects have largely newly formed red cells).

Use Evaluate G6PD deficiency; determine the cause of drug-induced hemolysis or hemolysis secondary to acute bacterial or viral infection or metabolic disorder such as acidosis

Limitations False normal results after hemolysis may occur; *vide infra*.

Contraindications Normal G6PD screen, marked reticulocytosis

Methodology Using hemolysate, measurement of formation of NADPH by following change in absorbance at 340 nm at 37°C

Additional Information The active G6PD enzyme exists as a dimer, each monomer consisting of 515 amino acids. Aggregation of monomers into active forms (largely dimers) is NADP dependent. G6PD catalyzes the first step in the hexose monophosphate pathway which acts to remove peroxide, thus protecting the red cell from oxidative damage. The enzyme provides reducing power in the form of NADPH which with glutathione is requisite for detoxification of H_2O_2. Over 440 G6PD mutations have been described of which some 60 mutations or combination of mutations have been documented in G6PD deficiency. Total deficiency is thought to be incompatible with life.

A G6PD screen is recommended before G6PD quantitative is requested (see Glucose-6-Phosphate Dehydrogenase Screen, Blood on page 438). G6PD hemolysis is associated with formation of Heinz bodies in peripheral red blood cells. It is the older erythrocytes which are most G6PD deficient in affected individuals. These cells are first eliminated in a hemolytic crisis. The younger cells and reticulocytes contain more G6PD. For these reasons after a hemolytic crisis, when only younger erythrocytes and reticulocytes are present, the G6PD values may be spuriously normal. Quantitative assay of G6PD may be helpful in establishing the diagnosis in female patients (who have two RBC populations) or in males with mild G6PD deficiency who have had recent hemolysis. In such cases, assay of the reticulocyte-poor bottom fraction of a centrifuged blood sample may be useful.[1] Mutations responsible for the G6PD deficient state have been identified by use of molecular biologic techniques, in particular, PCR based methods.[2,3,4]

Footnotes
1. Beutler E, "Glucose-6-Phosphate Dehydrogenase Deficiency," *N Engl J Med*, 1991, 324(3):169-74.

2. Huang CS, Tang CJ, Huang MJ, et al, "Diagnosis of Glucose-6-Phosphate Dehydrogenase (G6PD) Mutations by DNA Amplification and Allele-Specific Oligonucleotide Probes," *Acta Haematol*, 1992, 88(2-3):92-5.

3. Liese AM, Siddiqi MQ, and Spolastics Z, "Rapid Detection of Glucose-6-Phosphate Dehydrogenase Type A-Deficiency by Allele-Specific Polymerase Chain Reaction," *Am J Hematol*, 2000, 63(3):159-62.

4. Beutler E, Kuhl W, Vives-Corrons JL, et al, "Molecular Heterogeneity of Glucose-6-Phosphate Dehydrogenase A," *Blood*, 1989, 74(7):2550-5.

References
Beutler E, "G6PD Deficiency," *Blood*, 1994, 84(11):3613-36.

Glader BE and Lukens JN, "Glucose-6-Phosphate Dehydrogenase Deficiency and Related Disorders of Hexose Monophosphate Shunt and Glutathione Metabolism,"
(Continued)

Glucose-6-Phosphate Dehydrogenase, Quantitative, Blood *(Continued)*

Wintrobe's Clinical Hematology, 10th ed, Chapter 43, Lee GR, Foerster J, Lukens J, et al, eds, Baltimore, MD: Lippincott Williams & Wilkins, 1999, 1176-90.

Luzzatto L and Roper D, "Investigation of the Hereditary Haemolytic Anaemias: Membrane and Enzyme Abnormalities," *Practical Haematology*, 8th ed, Chapter 13, Dacie JV and Lewis SM, eds, New York, NY: Churchill Livingstone, 1995, 215-47.

Glucose-6-Phosphate Dehydrogenase Screen, Blood

Related Information

Autohemolysis Test *on page 405*
Glucose-6-Phosphate Dehydrogenase, Quantitative, Blood *on page 437*
Heinz Body Stain *on page 440*
Red Blood Cell Enzyme Deficiency, Quantitative *on page 475*
Red Blood Cell Enzyme Deficiency Screen *on page 476*

Synonyms G6PD, Qualitative; G6PD Screen, Blood

Applies to Fava Beans

Abstract Glucose-6-phosphate dehydrogenase (G6PD) is a red cell enzyme with an X-linked mode of inheritance that is important in maintaining RBC proteins in the reduced state. There are over 440 different mutations recorded,[1] of which 60 by themselves or in combination with other mutations result in premature hemolysis of red cells when the mutant enzyme is stressed. G6PD quantitation may be useful if a deficiency is detected in the screening test.

Specimen Erythrocytes

Container Lavender top (EDTA) tube

Reference Interval G6PD enzyme activity detected

Use Detect drug sensitive populations of red cells due to G6PD deficiency; determine the cause of hemolysis. G6PD deficient hemolysis may also be secondary to acute bacterial or viral infection and metabolic disorder such as acidosis. G6PD quantitation may be useful if a deficiency is detected in the screening test.

Limitations A blood enzyme screen, performed after a hemolytic episode often will not detect G6PD deficiency even if present because the most deficient cells have been destroyed (young G6PD-deficient red cells just released from the bone marrow have relatively high enzyme activity). This procedure can only differentiate between normal and grossly deficient samples. **Test may need to be repeated (if initial result is normal) after the patient recovers from an undiagnosed episode of anemia.** Alternatively, family studies can be performed. Recently developed tests based on allele-specific polymerase chain reaction (AS-PCR) avoid this disadvantage.[2]

Contraindications Marked reticulocytosis

Methodology Fluorescent NADPH spot test. Fluorescence is due to reduced nicotine adenine dinucleotide phosphate (NADPH) formed from NADP in the presence of G6PD. Recently developed polymerase chain reaction based methods can identify G6PD-deficient individuals even after blood loss or acute hemolytic activity which can produce false-negative results with the older generation of enzyme activity based tests.[2] AS-PCR-based G6PD deficiency tests, however, will not screen for all variants of G6PD, and are usually designed to detect one or a few mutant forms common to a particular geographic area.

Additional Information G6PD has been considered a "housekeeping enzyme", protecting the red cells from oxidation damage.[3] G6PD catalyzes the first step in the hexose monophosphate assay. Generation (reduction) of NADPH from NADP represents reducing power which with glutathione removes hydrogen peroxide, protecting the cell against oxidative damage. G6PD deficiency is the most common red cell defect associated with hemolysis and as such is the most common metabolic disorder of red blood cells. Some 400 million people are affected world-wide. There are many genetic variants of G6PD, some causing marked clinical manifestations, others none. Over 440 G6PD enzyme variants (many, on molecular analysis, are identical) have been subclassified by the World Health Organization, largely on the basis of clinical severity.

- Class I: Severe enzyme deficiency with chronic hemolytic anemia (<10% of normal enzyme activity)
- Class II: Severe enzyme deficiency with intermittent hemolysis
- Class III: Moderate enzyme deficiency with intermittent hemolysis usually associated with infection or drugs (10% to 60% of normal enzyme activity)
- Class IV: No enzyme deficiency or hemolysis

G6PD[A-] (Class III) and G6PD[A+] (Class IV) are high frequency G6PD-deficient variants (each found in 10% to 15% of African-Americans). The G6PD[A-] variant is associated with acute intermittent hemolysis and primaquine sensitivity. G6PD[A+], although a common and well-studied isoenzyme variant, has no evident associated hematological phenotype. The common variant G6PD[Mediterranean] (Class II) is found in Caucasians of Mediterranean/Far East ethnic origin. In children, when in steady state, most cases of G6PD deficiency are not anemic. Chronic nonspherocytic hemolytic anemia occurs only in Class I variants which are rare. Class II may be severe with rapid decline of Hb to near fatal levels. Ingestion of fava beans may be associated with severe hemolysis. Class III variants may experience hemolysis that is usually mild and self-limited.[4] Rare sporadic cases, occurring anywhere in the world, may present as nonspherocytic hemolytic anemia.[5]

G6PD deficiency had no adverse effect on the course and fatality rates of a spectrum of diseases (including those with thrombotic associations).[6] While usually mild in black children G6PD deficiency may be severe and life-threatening with oxidative stress, especially that relating to infection (viral in particular), fava bean ingestion, and less often relating to naphthalene exposure. A number of commonly used drugs/chemicals can induce hemolysis in individuals with G6PD deficiency (see table), while evidence has accumulated that some occasionally suspect drugs can be given in therapeutic doses without inducing hemolysis.[7] While G6PD screens may be normal after hemolytic episodes significant reticulocytosis (usually >7%) will reflect presence of the deficiency. Infection rather than use of ASA appears to precipitate hemolytic episodes in cases of G6PD deficiency. If deficiency is severe, impaired granulocyte function occurs with increased susceptibility to infection (G6PD *Barcelona*). Molecular heterogeneity, as reflected by the numerous mutant isoenzymes, is accompanied by biochemical functional diversity including decreased catalytic effectiveness, impaired substrate and cofactor kinetics, variable reactivity with substrate analogues, and variations in electrophoretic migration rates and pH optima. Cloning of the G6PD gene has been accomplished, and there is ongoing activity in cDNA sequencing of G6PD variants.[7,8,9,10]

Drugs and Chemicals That Should Be Avoided by Persons With G6PD Deficiency

Acetanilid	Phenylhydrazine
Acetylsalicylic acid (aspirin)	Primaquine
Chloromycetin	Quinidine
Doxorubicin	Quinine
Furazolidone (Furoxone®)	Sulfacetamide
Isobutyl nitrite	Sulfamethoxazole (Gantanol®)
Methylene blue	Sulfanilamide
Nalidixic acid (NegGram®)	Sulfapyridine
Naphthalene	Sulfisoxazole
Niridazole (Ambilhar®)	Thiazolesulfone
Nitrofurantoin (Furadantin®)	Toluidine blue
Para-aminosalicylic acid	Trinitrotoluene (TNT)
Pentaquine	Urate oxidase
Phenazopyridine (Pyridium®)	

Footnotes

1. Beutler E, "G6PD Deficiency," *Blood*, 1994, 84(11):3613-36.

2. Liese AM, Siddiqi MQ, and Spolarics Z, "Rapid Detection of Glucose-6-Phosphate Dehydrogenase Type A[-202A/376G] Deficiency by Allele-Specific Polymerase Chain Reaction," *Am J Hematol*, 2000, 63(3):159-62.

3. Pandolfi PP, Sonati F, Rivi R, et al, "Targeted Disruption of the Housekeeping Gene Encoding Glucose 6-Phosphate Dehydrogenase (G6PD): G6PD Is Dispensable for Pentose Synthesis but Essential for Defense Against Oxidative Stress," *EMBO J*, 1995, 14(21):5209-15.

4. Glader BE, "Hemolytic Anemia in Children," *Clin Lab Med*, Volume 19, Geaghan SM, ed, Philadelphia, PA: WB Saunders Co, 1999, 87-111.

5. Mason PJ, Sonati MF, MacDonald D, et al, "New Glucose-6-Phosphate Dehydrogenase Mutations Associated With Chronic Anemia," *Blood*, 1995, 85(5):1377-80.

6. Heller P, Best WR, Nelson RB, et al, "Clinical Implications of Sickle Cell Trait and Glucose-6-Phosphate Dehydrogenase Deficiency in Hospitalized Black Male Patients," *N Engl J Med*, 1979, 300:1001-5.

7. Beutler E, "Glucose-6-Phosphate Dehydrogenase Deficiency," *N Engl J Med*, 1991, 324(3):169-74.

8. Martini G, Toniolo D, Vulliamy T, et al, "Structural Analysis of the X-Linked Gene Encoding Human Glucose-6-Phosphate Dehydrogenase," *EMBO J*, 1986, 5(8):1849-55.

9. Chiu DT, Zuo L, Chao L, et al, "Molecular Characterization of Glucose-6-Phosphate Dehydrogenase (G6PD) Deficiency in Patients of Chinese Descent and Identification of New Base Substitutions in the Human G6PD Gene," *Blood*, 1993, 81(8):2150-4.

10. Calabro V, Mason PJ, Filosa S, et al, "Genetic Heterogeneity of Glucose-6-Phosphate Dehydrogenase Deficiency Revealed by Single-Strand Conformation and Sequence Analysis," *Am J Hum Genet*, 1993, 52(3):527-36.

References

Beutler E, "Study of Glucose-6-Phosphate Dehydrogenase: History and Molecular Biology," *Am J Hematol*, 1993, 42(1):53-8.

Luzzatto L, "Glucose-6-Phosphate Dehydrogenase Deficiency and Hemolytic Anemia," *Hematology of Infancy and Childhood*, 5th ed, Chapter 18, Nathan DG and Orkin SH, eds, Philadelphia, PA: WB Saunders Co, 1998, 704-26.

Luzzatto L and Roper D, "Investigation of the Hereditary Haemolytic Anaemias: Membrane and Enzyme Abnormalities," *Practical Haematology*, 8th ed, Chapter 13, Davie JV and Lewis SM, eds, New York, NY: Churchill Livingstone, 1995, 215-47.

Miwa S and Fujii H, "Molecular Basis of Erythroenzymopathies Associated With Hereditary Hemolytic Anemia: Tabulation of Mutant Enzymes," *Am J Hematol*, 1996, 51(2):122-32.

Naylor CE, Rowland P, Basak AK, et al, "Glucose-6 Phosphate Dehydrogenase Mutations Causing Enzyme Deficiency in a Model of the Tertiary Structure of the Human Enzyme," *Blood*, 1996, 87(7):2974-82.

Prchal JT and Gregg XT, "Red Cell Enzymopathies," *Hematology: Basic Principles and Practice*, 3rd ed, Chapter 32, Hoffman R, Benz EJ, Jr, Shattil SJ, et al, eds, Philadelphia, PA: Churchill Livingstone, 2000, 561-76.

♦ **β-Glucosidase** *see* Inherited Diseases of Metabolism and Cell Structure *on page 449*

♦ **Glutamine, Plasma** *see* Malaria Smear and Tests *on page 458*

♦ **γ-Glutamylcysteine Synthetase** *see* Red Blood Cell Enzyme Deficiency, Quantitative *on page 475*

♦ **γ-Glutamylcysteine Synthetase** *see* Red Blood Cell Enzyme Deficiency Screen *on page 476*

♦ **Glutathione Reductase** *see* Red Blood Cell Enzyme Deficiency Screen *on page 476*

♦ **Glutathione Reductase Deficiency, RBC** *see* Red Blood Cell Enzyme Deficiency, Quantitative *on page 475*

♦ **Glycerol Lysis Test** *see* Glycerol Lysis Test, Acidified, Modified *on page 439*

Glycerol Lysis Test, Acidified, Modified

Related Information
Autohemolysis Test *on page 405*
Gelation Assay *on page 437*
Hypertonic Cryohemolysis Test *on page 448*
Osmotic Fragility *on page 462*
Osmotic Fragility, Incubated *on page 463*

Synonyms Acidified Glycerol Lysis Test; AGLT; Glycerol Lysis Test; Pink Test

Applies to Volumetric Glycerol Lysis Test

Abstract A sensitive, specific, simple, inexpensive test applicable to population screening and provisional diagnosis of hereditary spherocytosis (HS). The test is a measure of the property of glycerol to retard osmotic swelling of red blood cells (glycerol in hypotonic saline slows the rate of entry of water into red blood cells, prolonging the time taken for lysis).

Specimen EDTA anticoagulated whole blood; test is performed on less than 100 µL of blood, amenable to finger puncture collection

Container Lavender top (EDTA) tube, microsample container, or buffer containing tube

Collection Whole blood collected by venipuncture or by finger puncture

Storage Instructions Test is usually started by placing skin puncture obtained whole blood into appropriate buffer solution immediately upon collection, but whole blood collected within 24 hours and kept at room temperature can be used.

Turnaround Time 1-2 hours

Reference Interval Half-life for AGLT lysis: normal is over 30 minutes; result is less than 5 minutes in cases of hereditary spherocytosis (major portion of HS cases have half-life between 1 and 2 minutes).[1]

Use Screening test for diagnosis of hereditary spherocytosis

Limitations While 100% specificity is claimed, some 7% of apparent normals may give results of between 5 and 30 minutes ("possibly pathologic"). In the series of 1464 healthy blood donors of Eber et al, these individuals were hematologically normal and did not have increased osmotic fragility. Test is not entirely specific, with a short AGLT found in some cases of chronic renal failure, chronic leukemia, autoimmune hemolytic anemia, and some cases of pregnancy. This test, while not difficult to perform, is offered by only a few laboratories.

Methodology The glycerol lysis time is the time taken for 50% hemolysis of red cells in a blood sample placed in buffered hypotonic saline/glycerol. In the acidified modification,[2] a sample (20 µL) of EDTA anticoagulated whole blood is diluted in buffered saline (0.0093 M sodium phosphate, pH 6.90) and 1 part added to 2 parts of a buffered 0.3 M glycerol solution. Temperature must be controlled at 25°C. Fall in absorbance (625 nm) is measured as the turbidity of the solution decreases due to hemolysis of red cells. Results are given as the half-time for AGLT lysis.

Additional Information Development of a screening test for HS might be considered unfeasible due to the heterogeneous nature of the disease process. Clinically, the hemolytic anemia of HS ranges from mild, asymptomatic fully compensated forms to those with severe hemolysis requiring transfusion. There is not a single underlying molecular red cell structural defect (dependent upon one's definition of "hereditary spherocytosis"). HS or HS like clinical picture occurs with primary structural defects of spectrin, ankyrin, band 3, and protein 4.2 (pallidin) red cell proteins. It is thus somewhat surprising that after a series of modifications over the past 20 years (see reference) following Gottfried and Robertson's original procedure[3] (and the subsequent modification-acidification of Zanella et al),[2] that the current AGLT has been found to be 100% sensitive and nearly 100% specific!

The glycerol lysis test has also been applied to the differential diagnosis of thalassemia and iron deficiency using a Continuous MCV Analyzer (Sysmex-TOA). A small sample (2 µL) of whole blood is placed in buffer/glycerol mixture and after stirring for 3 seconds the MCV is measured every 2 seconds. The change in MCV is plotted as a continuous glycerol hemolysis curve, the procedure is referred to as the "volumetric glycerol lysis test".[4] Thalassemic red cells gradually increase in cell volume while normal red cells rapidly increase in volume followed by lysis.

Footnotes
1. Eber SW, Pekrun A, Neufeldt A, et al, "Prevalence of Increased Osmotic Fragility of Erythrocytes in German Blood Donors: Screening Using a Modified Glycerol Lysis Test," *Ann Hematol*, 1992, 64(2):88-92.
2. Zanella A, Izzo C, Rebulla P, et al, "Acidified Glycerol Lysis Test: A Screening Test for Spherocytosis," *Br J Haematol*, 1980, 45(3):481-6.
3. Gottfried EL and Robertson NA, "Glycerol Lysis Time as a Screening Test for Erythrocyte Disorders," *J Lab Clin Med*, 1974, 83(2):323-33.
4. Wada Y, Tatsumi N, and Fessas P, "Volumetric Glycerol Lysis Test Using Blood Cell Counter for Thalassemia Screening," *Birth Defects Original Article Series*, 1987, 23(5A):181-6.

References
Bucx MJ, Breed WP, and Hoffmann JJ, "Comparison of Acidified Glycerol Lysis Test, Pink Test and Osmotic Fragility Test in Hereditary Spherocytosis: Effect of Incubation," *Eur J Haematol*, 1988, 40(3):227-31.
Gallagher PG and Jarolim P, "Red Cell Membrane Disorders," *Hematology: Basic Principles and Practice*, 3rd ed, Chapter 33, Hoffman R, Benz EJ Jr, Shattil SJ, et al, eds, Philadelphia, PA: Churchill Livingstone, 2000, 588.

♦ **Glycogen Storage Diseases** *see* Inherited Diseases of Metabolism and Cell Structure *on page 449*

♦ **Glycophorin A** *see* PNH Test (GPI-Anchored Proteins) by Flow Cytometry *on page 472*

♦ **Glycophorin C Deficiency** *see* Osmotic Fragility *on page 462*

♦ **GPI-Anchored Proteins** *see* Ham Test *on page 439*

♦ **GPI-Anchored Proteins** *see* PNH Test (GPI-Anchored Proteins) by Flow Cytometry *on page 472*

♦ **Granulocyte/Macrophage Colony Stimulating Factor** *see* Eosinophil Count *on page 424*

♦ **Gray Platelet Syndrome** *see* Platelet Count *on page 468*

♦ **Hairy Cell Leukemia** *see* Tartrate Resistant Leukocyte Acid Phosphatase *on page 488*

♦ **Hairy Cell Leukemia Test** *see* Tartrate Resistant Leukocyte Acid Phosphatase *on page 488*

Ham Test

Related Information
Hemosiderin Stain, Urine *on page 876*
Peripheral Blood: Red Blood Cell Morphology *on page 467*
PNH Test (GPI-Anchored Proteins) by Flow Cytometry *on page 472*
Red Blood Cells, Washed *on page 859*
Sugar Water Test Screen *on page 488*

Synonyms Acid Serum Test; Acid Serum Test for PNH; Acidified Serum Test; Paroxysmal Nocturnal Hemoglobinuria Test; PNH Test; Serum Lysis

Applies to GPI-Anchored Proteins

Abstract A positive Ham test (lysis of patient red cells in acidified serum) may be used as a screening test for paroxysmal nocturnal hemoglobinuria (PNH) and indicates unusual sensitivity of such red cells to the action of complement. PNH is characterized clinically by nocturnal hemoglobinuria, chronic hemolytic anemia, hypoplastic or aplastic hematopoiesis, and tendency to venous thrombosis. It is the result of an acquired defect of hematopoietic stem cells. Affected cells have lost the glycosyl-phosphatidyl-inositol (GPI) anchor to the outer cell membrane. GPI acts to anchor proteins (CD55 and CD59) which protect red blood cells from the action of complement. These changes are the result of an acquired somatic cell mutation that inactivates a gene (PIG-A) that codes for an enzyme needed for GPI biosynthesis.[1]

Specimen Erythrocytes from EDTA anticoagulated whole blood

Container Lavender top (EDTA) tube

Causes for Rejection Specimen hemolyzed

Reference Interval A positive result shows lysis of red cells in acidified serum samples with patient's cells (not with normal cells).

Use Evaluate patients with suspected PNH (paroxysmal nocturnal hemoglobinuria) or suspected congenital dyserythropoietic anemia, type II (HEMPAS); evaluate hemolytic anemia, especially with hemosiderinuria, pancytopenia, decreased RBC acetylcholinesterase, decreased leukocyte alkaline phosphatase, negative direct Coombs' test, and/or apparent marrow failure. Positive in PNH: 10% to 50% lysis in acidified noninactivated serum. Can be as low as 5% or as much as 80%. Low or negative after transfusion. With PNH, suspect patient's red cells have a high sensitivity to complement mediated hemolysis.

Limitations False-positive results may occur in other hematologic diseases: hereditary and acquired spherocytosis, hereditary dyserythropoietic anemia (CDA type II, HEMPAS, *vide infra*), aged red cells (as with old transfused blood), aplastic anemia, leukemia, and myeloproliferative syndromes. In these conditions hemolysis will also occur in the acidified inactivated serum. The latter is negative in PNH since hemolysis is complement dependent. Flow cytometry (see PNH Test (GPI-Anchored Proteins) by Flow Cytometry *on page 472*) is much more sensitive than the Ham test. In populations of bone marrow failure syndromes (in particular myelodysplasia), PNH cells as detected by flow cytometry are relatively common. In patients who have received massive red cell transfusion (most of the patients RBCs are of
(Continued)

Ham Test (Continued)

donor origin), flow cytometry allows study of and identification of PNH neutrophils.[2]

Contraindications Transfusion

Methodology Acidified serum test of Ham. PNH suspect RBCs will lyse in acidified normal and acidified patient's serum (acidified to a pH of 6.2). The normal serum used must be fresh and ABO blood group compatible with test RBCs. Sensitivity is maximized by optimizing pH and serum concentration (see reference by Rosse). Alternatives to acidification of the testing serum are the addition of bovine thrombin, cobra venom factor, insulin, heating, or use of specific antibodies to activate complement. Probably, these tests do not offer advantages over the Ham test and false-negative results may occur if the PNH patient's serum (which may have low serum complement activity) is used.

Additional Information PNH red cells are unusually susceptible to lysis by complement. The Ham (acidified serum) and sucrose hemolysis test can demonstrate this lysis *in vitro*. In PNH, 10% to 50% of lysis (measured as liberated hemoglobin) is usually obtained but lysis may be as great as 80% or as little as 5%.

In some cases, three populations of cells exist in patients with PNH. One is markedly hypersensitive to complement (type III cells), one has a midlevel of sensitivity (type II cells), and the third population has normal sensitivity (type I cells). Type III cells are variably present, are the population which undergoes lysis in the Ham test and relate to the severity of illness.[3] The young PNH cells (reticulocyte-rich) are more susceptible to lysis than the older red cells. PNH RBCs will undergo lysis in acidified normal serum and in the patient's acidified serum.[3]

The membrane defect involves a protein, the membrane inhibitor of reactive lysis (MIRL, "protectin", CD59). It is one of some 18 proteins anchored to the external cell surface by a GPI moiety consisting of phosphatidylinositol, glucosamine, and three mannose molecules.[1,4] This protein regulates the assembly of polymerized C9 in the membrane attack complex, the effector and final stage of the complement activation sequence. MIRL (protectin or CD59) is an 18,000-20,000 MW complement lysis restricting factor that inhibits C5b-8 catalyzed insertion of C9 into lipid bilayers. The protein is also expressed in granulocytes, monocytes, and on platelets; its absence plays a role in the hypercoagulable state present in PNH. The underlying gene defect (in the gene PIG-A) is located on the short arm of the X chromosome and is acquired (present only in somatic hematopoietic cells). As of 1995, 84 PIG-A mutations in 72 patients had been reported; 53 of the 84 were deletion or insertion mutations.[5,6] See PNH Test (GPI-Anchored Proteins) by Flow Cytometry *on page 472*.

The only other disorder which may give a positive Ham test is one of the congenital dyserythropoietic anemias. In CDA type II (HEMPAS - hereditary erythroblastic multinuclearity with positive acidified serum test) the red cells undergo lysis in only a proportion (about 30%) of normal sera, and these RBCs do not undergo lysis in the patient's own acidified serum. The sucrose lysis test and PNH test by flow cytometry are negative in cases of HEMPAS. Heating at 56°C, which destroys the complement in serum, inactivates the lytic system so that if lysis occurs with inactivated serum this cannot be considered positive.

Another type of cell that may lyse in inactivated serum is the spherocyte. Spherocytes may lyse in acidified serum possibly due to the lowered pH.[1,4]

The relationship between aplastic anemia and PNH has been considered for over two decades.[7] A 55% to 65% incidence of PNH occurs in primary myelofibrosis and myeloid metaplasia.

PNH is a disease not only of increased complement sensitivity of red cell membranes, but also granulocytes and platelet membranes, the latter predisposing to venous thrombosis at unusual sites including abdomen and liver. A diagnostic test using flow cytometry and monoclonal antibodies was developed in the early 1990s and is now the preferred method for establishing a diagnosis of PNH.[8] This technique detects missing proteins from granulocytes (GPI-anchored proteins) in patients with PNH. The method has significant advantages over the Ham test for abnormal red cells. See PNH Test (GPI-Anchored Proteins) by Flow Cytometry *on page 472*. Genetic instability may underlie the development of PIG-A mutations that lead to clinical PNH.[9]

Footnotes

1. Kinoshita T, Inoue N, and Takeda J, "Role of Phosphatidylinositol-Linked Proteins in Paroxysmal Nocturnal Hemoglobinuria Pathogenesis," *Annu Rev Med*, 1996, 47:1-10.
2. Dunn DE, Tanawattanacharoen P, Boccuni P, et al, "Paroxysmal Nocturnal Hemoglobinuria Cells in Patients With Bone Marrow Failure Syndromes," *Ann Intern Med*, 1999, 131(6):401-8.
3. Luzzato L and Hillmen P, "Laboratory Methods Used in the Investigation of Paroxysmal Nocturnal Hemoglobinuria (PNH)," *Practical Laboratory Haematology*, Dacie JV and Lewis SM, eds, 8th ed, Chapter 15, New York, NY: Churchill Livingstone, 1995, 287-96.
4. Parker CJ, "Molecular Basis of Paroxysmal Nocturnal Hemoglobinuria," *Stem Cells*, 1996, 14(4):396-411.
5. Rosse WF and Ware RE, "The Molecular Basis of Paroxysmal Nocturnal Hemoglobinuria," *Blood*, 1995, 86(9):3277-86.
6. Miyata T, Yamada N, Iida Y, et al, "Abnormalities of PIG-A Transcripts in Granulocytes From Patients With Paroxysmal Nocturnal Hemoglobinuria," *N Engl J Med*, 1994, 330(4):249-55.

7. Young NS, "The Problem of Clonality in Aplastic Anemia: Dr Dameshek's Riddle, Restated," *Blood*, 1992, 79(6):1385-92.
8. van der Schoot CE, Huizinga TW, van't Veer Korthof ET, et al, "Deficiency of Glycosyl-Phosphatidylinositol-Linked Membrane Glycoproteins of Leukocytes in Paroxysmal Nocturnal Hemoglobinuria, Description of a New Diagnostic Cytofluorometric Assay," *Blood*, 1990, 76(7):1853-9.
9. Purow DB, Howard TA, Marcus SJ, et al, "Genetic Instability and the Etiology of Somatic PIG-A Mutations in Paroxysmal Nocturnal Hemoglobinuria," *Blood Cells Mol Dis*, 1999, 25(5):81-91.

References

Beutler E and Luzzatto L, "Hemolytic Anemia," *Semin Hematol*, 1999, 36(4 Suppl 7):38-47.

Hillmen P and Richards SJ, "Implications of Recent Insights Into the Pathophysiology of Paroxysmal Nocturnal Hemoglobinuria," *Br J Haematol*, 2000, 108(3):470-9.

Marks PW and Mitus AJ, "Congenital Dyserythropoietic Anemias," *Am J Hematol*, 1996, 51(1):55-63.

McMullin MF, "The Molecular Basis of Disorders of the Red Cell Membrane," *J Clin Pathol*, 1999, 52(4):245-8.

Parker CJ and Lee GR, "Paroxysmal Nocturnal Hemoglobinuria," *Wintrobe's Clinical Hematology*, 10th ed, Chapter 47, Lee GR, Foerster J, Lukens J, et al, eds, Baltimore, MD: Lippincott Williams & Wilkins, 1999, 1264-88.

Rosse WF, "Paroxysmal Nocturnal Hemoglobinuria," *Hematology: Basic Principle and Practice*, 3rd ed, Chapter 20, Hoffman R, Benz EJ Jr, Shattil SJ, et al, eds, Philadelphia, PA: Churchill Livingstone, 2000, 331-42.

Wickramasinghe SN, "Congenital Dyserythropoietic Anaemias: Clinical Features, Haematological Morphology and New Biochemical Data," *Blood Reviews*, 1998, 12(3):178-200.

Heinz Body Stain

Related Information
Glucose-6-Phosphate Dehydrogenase, Quantitative, Blood *on page 437*
Hemoglobin, Unstable, Heat Labile Test *on page 447*
Hemoglobin, Unstable - Isopropanol Precipitation Test *on page 448*
n-Butanol Stability Test *on page 460*
Peripheral Blood: Red Blood Cell Morphology *on page 467*
Red Blood Cell Enzyme Deficiency, Quantitative *on page 475*
Red Blood Cell Enzyme Deficiency Screen *on page 476*
Reticulocyte Count *on page 481*

Synonyms Methyl Violet Stain for Heinz Bodies

Applies to Fava Beans; Heinz Bodies; Homoglobinopathies, Unstable

Abstract Heinz bodies (HBs) are microscopically visible intraerythrocyte insoluble aggregates of oxidized denatured hemoglobin that attach to the internal surface of the red blood cell (RBC) membrane. They reflect the presence of a metabolic derangement of or abnormality in the secondary structure of hemoglobin. The afflicted red cell has shortened survival due to injury and/or removal from the circulation by the spleen. Demonstration of HBs in a patient's RBCs indicates the presence of a red cell biochemical defect, commonly glucose-6-phosphate dehydrogenase (G6PD) deficiency, thalassemia, or unstable hemoglobin. Drug-induced oxidative stress may lead to Heinz body (HB) formation.

Specimen Whole blood

Container Lavender top (EDTA) tube, green top (heparin) tube

Collection Obtain a tube of normal control blood at the time patient sample is drawn.

Storage Instructions Refrigerate

Causes for Rejection Clotted specimen, hemolyzed specimen

Reference Interval No Heinz bodies (or only rare HBs) identified. Using blood incubated with acetylphenylhydrazine, normal control may have one to a few (under five) HBs in about one-third of the RBCs. A positive result (indicative of a defective reducing system) will find five or more HBs in about one-third or more of the RBCs. The definition of "abnormal" may vary somewhat between different laboratories.

Use Test for hemolytic disorders associated with Heinz body formation (eg, G6PD deficiency, thalassemia, unstable hemoglobin)

Methodology Supravital stain (methyl violet, new methylene blue, crystal violet, or brilliant cresyl blue) using blood incubated (60 minutes or more) at room temperature with acetylphenylhydrazine or sterile blood incubated 24 and 48 hours at 37°C. Heinz bodies are intraerythrocytic, purple, vary in shape (round, oval, serrated), 1-3 μm across, single or multiple, and close to the cell membrane. They are not usually visible on study of routinely stained (Romanowsky Wright/Giemsa type) blood smears. Rhodanile blue staining offers advantages as a stain for permanent storage.[1,2]

Additional Information Heinz bodies (HBs) are uncommon except with G6PD deficiency immediately following hemolysis, postsplenectomy, and in patients with unstable hemoglobin variants. They are present characteristically in the congenital Heinz body hemolytic anemias (CHBHA - the unstable hemoglobinopathies). There are now some 200 different identified molecular variants of hemoglobin underlying CHBHA. Less than one-half of these are of clinical significance.[1] The three major causes for HB formation and increased hemolysis are exposure to certain chemicals and drugs, deficiency of one of the reducing systems of blood, and presence of an unstable hemoglobin. Oxidative denaturation of the hemoglobin molecule leads to HB formation with the first two situations and is probably the mechanism for the precipitation of unstable hemoglobin.

Heinz bodies are usually removed by the spleen; postsplenectomy they increase in the peripheral blood. While absent in the blood of normal individuals presplenectomy, they occur in sulfonamide-induced hemolytic crisis in cases of Hb Zurich and in cases of Hb Shepherd's Bush, Hb Gun Hill, and Hb Philly. Postsplenectomy, HBs occur in >50% of cells in blood stained supravitally, especially with methyl violet. They can be generated in red cells of unsplenectomized patients by 60 minutes or more incubation with acetylphenylhydrazine or by incubation of sterile blood for 24-48 hours at 37°C. Ability to demonstrate the bodies relates to the degree of instability of the hemoglobin. Cells of Hb Köln require up to 48 hours incubation and the HBs are small. Degradation of HB Köln to a fluorescent yellow pigment (dipyrroles) is associated with green fluorescence seen in the cytoplasm and HBs of Köln red blood cells.[3] With Hb Seattle and Hb Shepherd's Bush the bodies are seen readily after 24 hours incubation.

Heinz bodies are efficiently extracted ("pitted") from red blood cells during their transit through the splenic microvasculature. Study of peripheral blood smears from susceptible individuals may show only morphologic residua or suggestion of HB formation such as presence of "bite" cells (degmacytes). These are RBCs with a semicircular bite-like defect along the edge, resultant from "pitting" or extrusion of HBs with irregular contraction of the remaining RBC. Routinely stained peripheral blood smears showing small protrusions from red cell surfaces are suspicious for HBs and should be confirmed by study of HB stains (as per recent photomicrograph illustrating HB hemolytic anemia in Wilson disease - copper from hepatocytes leading to oxidant-induced hemolytic anemia).[4]

HBs may be found after the administration of sulfonamides, nitrofurans, Dilantin®, streptomycin, fava beans, chlorates, phenylhydrazine, primaquine (in sensitive individuals), and other compounds; omeprazole (in a case of renal failure) has been incriminated.[5] See table.

Footnotes

1. Lukens JN and Lee R, "Unstable Hemoglobin Disease," *Wintrobes' Clinical Hematology*, 10th ed, Part IV, Disorders of Red Cells, Chapter 52, Lee GR, Foerster J. Lukens J, et al, eds, Baltimore, MD: Lippincott Williams & Wilkins, 1999, 1398-1404.

2. Dacie JV and Lewis SM, "Red Cell Cytochemistry," *Practical Haematology*, 8th ed, Chapter 8, Dacie JV and Lewis SM, eds, New York, NY: Churchill Livingstone, 1995, 134-6.

3. Eisinger J, Flores J, Tyson JA, et al, "Fluorescent Cytoplasm and Heinz Bodies of Hemoglobin Köln Erythrocytes: Evidence for Intracellular Heme Catabolism," *Blood*, 1985, 65(4):886-93.

4. Bain BJ, "Heinz Body Haemolytic Anaemia in Wilson's Disease: Images in Haematology," *Br J Haematol*, 1999, 104(4):647.

5. Davidson S, Seldon M, and Jones B, "Omeprazole and Heinz-Body Haemolytic Anaemia," *Aust N Z J Med*, 1997, 27(4):441.

References

Beutler E, "Heinz Body Staining," *Williams Hematology*, 5th ed, Chapter 5, Beutler E, Lichtman MA, Coller BS, et al, eds, New York, NY: McGraw-Hill Inc, 1995, 356 and L26.

Robertson JE, Christopher MM, and Rogers QR, "Heinz Body Formation in Cats Fed Baby Food Containing Onion Powder," *J Am Vet Med Assoc*, 1998, 212(8):1260-6.

♦ **Helmet Cells** *see* Peripheral Blood: Differential Leukocyte Count *on page 464*

♦ **Helminths, Blood** *see* Microfilariae, Peripheral Blood Preparation *on page 460*

Possible Causes of Heinz Body Formation

Intrinsic (Intraerythrocyte Molecular) Abnormalities
Glucose-6-phosphate dehydrogenase deficiency (G6PD)
Unstable hemoglobinopathies (eg, Hb Köln)
Intrinsic Plus Extrinsic (Drug or Chemical) Abnormalities
Unstable hemoglobinopathies (eg, Hb Zurich = sulphonamides)
G6PD deficiency and oxidant stress-producing drugs (eg, acetanilid, dapsone, methylene blue, nalidixic acid, nitrofurantoin, pamaquine, pentaquine, sulphonamides*, thiazolesulfone).
Chemical Exposure
Arsine (arsenic hydride)
Benzene derivatives
Heavy metals (lead, mercury, copper, arsenic)
Potassium chlorate
Naphthalene
Toluidine blue
Trinitrotoluene
Drug Exposure (see also Intrinsic Plus Extrinsic)
Daunorubicin
Diaminodiphenyl sulfone
Niradazole
Omeprazole
Pamaquine
Pentaquine
Quinidine
Sulphonamides*

*Sulphonamides including sulfacetamide, sulfamethoxazole (Gantanol®), sulfapyridine, and sulfanilamide.

Hematocrit

Related Information

Anemia Flowchart *on page 392*
Blood Volume *on page 407*
Complete Blood Count *on page 419*
Hemoglobin *on page 442*
Peripheral Blood: Red Blood Cell Morphology *on page 467*
Red Blood Cell Indices *on page 477*
Red Blood Cells *on page 857*
Red Cell Count *on page 478*
Red Cell Mass *on page 478*
Reticulocyte Count *on page 481*
Uncrossmatched Blood, Emergency *on page 865*

Synonyms Hct; Microhematocrit; Packed Cell Volume; PCV

Applies to H and H

Abstract Percent of whole blood that is red blood cells. A determination that is of importance in the detection and follow-up of anemia and polycythemia. The hematocrit value is used in the calculation of the MCV and MCHC.

Specimen Whole blood

Container Lavender top (EDTA) tube

Collection Routine venipuncture. Invert tube gently to mix. For capillary puncture, establish free flow of blood to minimize dilution with tissue fluid.

Storage Instructions If specimen is not brought to the laboratory within 4 hours, refrigeration should be provided. Perform manual Hct within 6 hours after collection of blood.

Causes for Rejection Clotted or hemolyzed specimen

Reference Interval Male: 2 years of age: 35% to 43%, 6 years of age: 33% to 42%, adults: 42% to 52%; female: 2 years of age: 35% to 43%, 6 years of age: 33% to 42%, adults: 35% to 47%. In general, spun hematocrits are 2% to 3% higher than automated hematocrits, due to plasma trapping. There is evidence that Hct shows slight seasonal variation, lower in summer in nonsmokers but increased in smokers. Mean values for the two groups (summer vs winter) were, however, within the reference range of normal.[1] See tables.

Hematocrit Values – First Postnatal Day[2]

Gestational Age (wk)	Hct (%)
24-25	63
26-27	62
28-29	60
30-31	60
32-33	60
34-35	61
36-37	64
Term	61

(Continued)

Hematocrit (Continued)

**Normal Hematocrit Values –
Newborn**

Age	Hct (%)
Birth - 2 d	54-68
2-3 d	54-66
3-4 d	52-71
4-5 d	39-55
5-6 d	50-64
6-7 d	47-61
7-8 d	47-64
1-2 wk	50-62
2-3 wk	39-53
3-4 wk	37-49

Use Evaluate anemia, blood loss, hemolytic anemia, polycythemia, and other conditions

Limitations During centrifugation, plasma is not completely extruded from the red cell column, plasma trapping amongst red blood cells (RBCs) which may increase the PCV of normal blood by nearly 2%. Plasma trapping is increased if abnormal RBCs (such as microcytes, macrocytes, spherocytes, thalassemic or sickled cells) are present (cells with increased rigidity). When dealing with results of automated instruments falsely high results may occur with cryoproteins, significant leukocytosis, giant platelets; false low results may be seen with microcytosis, in vitro hemolysis or in presence of autoagglutinins.

Methodology Manual microhematocrit centrifugation using disposable 75 mm long capillary tubes of 1 mm bore filled with EDTA anticoagulated whole blood and centrifuged at 10,000-12,000 g for 5 minutes (analyst must wear gloves and observe precautions). The Hct is included (by calculation) in the menu of test results provided by a variety of multiparameter hematology analyzers including different models from Coulter, Sysmex, Abbott/Cell Dyne, Bayer®/Technicon, ABX Diagnostics/Pentra, and Cobas-Helios (see Complete Blood Count on page 419). The Hct is derived by electronic calculation considering that Hct = RBC x MCV / 10 (latter two are directly measured).

Additional Information The degree of plasma trapping is increased in disease with less deformable RBCs (eg, sickle cell disease, hereditary spherocytosis, and iron deficiency).

A large study (17,274 children in apparent good health and residing in the Washington, DC, metropolitan area) found that the lower mean Hct and Hb value in African-American children (as compared to white children) was the result not only of α- and β-thalassemia but also of the presence of Hb AS and Hb AC. The mean Hct of children with Hb AC and Hb AS was 1.5 and 1.0 point lower, respectively, than that of subjects with Hb AA.[3]

Hct levels in the highest quintile have been associated with increased morbidity and mortality from cardiovascular disease.[4] High Hct (≥34%) on arrival in the ICU postcoronary artery bypass grafting was associated with twice the risk for Q-wave myocardial infarction.[5] Elevated Hct (51 or higher) has been noted to increase the risk of stroke.[6] Relatively high Hct (median 45.0% on admission) in patients with necrotizing pancreatitis may reflect early hemoconcentration and can serve as a decision point for hospital admission.[7]

Rapid, near patient (point-of-care) devices have been and are being developed. THe Spuncrit™ is portable (battery operated), consists of an infra-red analyzer with centrifuge, and can provide Hct and hemoglobin values within 90 seconds.[8] Comparison with results obtained by use of a Sysmex NE 1500 (TOA Medical) and Ciba Corning 288 showed good agreement for Hct (2 SD of Spuncrit™ results between -5.66 and +4.42%). The Spuncrit™ estimates the hemoglobin concentration by dividing the measured Hct by a factor of 2.82. For hemoglobin concentration, 2 SD of Spuncrit™ estimates were between 1.6 g/dL below to 1.92 g/dL above the comparison methods. Software for the Spuncrit™ has been modified to improve accuracy of the hemoglobin estimate.[8]

In a renal dialysis population, Hb vs Hct comparison studies, found Hct levels high (by 3% but possibly due to plasma trapping) with adverse effect on patient welfare as the result of inappropriate (low) erythropoietin dosage.[9] Comparison of centrifuged microhematocrit with calculated packed cell volume using different automated hematology analyzers at four Swedish university hospitals found the average difference between the means amounting to 1.9% (centrifuged microhematocrit vs calculated PCV - due to trapped plasma in the former). It was concluded that the therapeutic goal should be to maintain calculated PCV <43 (rather than 45, the goal in the past based on use of centrifuged microhematocrit).[10]

A study of 1000 Israeli airmen over a 15-year period with average number of annual Hct of 13.2 per person (Wintrobe's microhematocrit method) found that variations of up to 3% in Hct over time can be considered within normal in young males.[11]

The red cell indices, MCV and MCHC, depend on the Hct for their derivation and are of use in the evaluation of anemia. See discussion in Complete Blood Count on page 419.

A six parameter (includes Hct) point-of-care handheld portable analyzer that requires just 2 minutes for analyses is available (i-STAT).[12,13]

Footnotes

1. Kristal-Boneh E, Froom P, Harari G, et al, "Seasonal Differences in Blood Cell Parameters and the Association With Cigarette Smoking," Clin Lab Haematol, 1997, 19(3):177-81.
2. Zaizov R and Matoth Y, "Red Cell Values on the First Postnatal Day During the Last 16 Weeks of Gestation," Am J Hematol, 1976, 1(2):275-8.
3. Rana SR, Sekhsaria S, and Castro OL, "Hemoglobin S and C Traits: Contributing Causes for Decreased Mean Hematocrit in African-American Children," Pediatrics, 1993, 91(4):800-2.
4. Gagnon DR, Zhang TJ, Brand FN, et al, "Hematocrit and the Risk of Cardiovascular Disease - The Framingham Study: A 34-Year Follow-up," Am Heart J, 1994, 127(3):674-82.
5. Spiess BD, Ley C, Body SC, et al, "Hematocrit Value on Intensive Care Unit Entry Influences the Frequency of Q-Wave Myocardial Infarction After Coronary Artery Bypass Grafting," J Thorac Cardiovasc Surg, 1998, 116(3):460-7.
6. Wannamethee G, Perry IJ, and Shaper AG, "Haematocrit, Hypertension and Risk of Stroke," J Intern Med, 1994, 235(2):163-8.
7. Baillaregeon JD, Orav J, Ramagopal V, et al, "Hemoconcentration as an Early Risk Factor for Necrotizing Pancreatitis," Am J Gastroenterol, 1998, 93(11):2130-4.
8. Weatherall MS and Sherry KM, "An Evaluation of the Spuncrit™ Infra-red Analyzer for Measurement of Haematocrit," Clin Lab Haematol, 1997, 19(3):183-6.
9. Marooney M, "Comparative Analysis Between Centrifuged Hematocrit and Point-of-Care Hemoglobin: Impact on Erythropoietin Dosing," ANNA J, 1998, 25(5):479-81.
10. Andréasson B, Wahlstrom E, Jacobsson S, et al, "The Measurement of Venous Haematocrit in Patients With Polycythaemia Vera," J Intern Med, 1999, 246(3):293-7.
11. Froom P, Benbassat J, Kiwelowicz A, et al, "Significance of Low Hematocrit Levels in Asymptomatic Young Adults: Results of 15 Years Follow-up," Aviat Space Environ Med, 1999, 70(10):983-6.
12. Woo J, McCabe JB, Chauncey D, et al, "The Evaluation of a Portable Clinical Analyzer in the Emergency Department," Am J Clin Pathol, 1993, 100(6):599-605.
13. Bingham D, Kendall J, and Clancy M, "The Portable Laboratory: An Evaluation of the Accuracy and Reproductibility of i-STAT," Ann Clin Biochem, 1999, 36(Pt 1):66-71.

References

Brown BA, Hematology: Principles and Procedures, 6th ed, Philadelphia, PA: Lea & Febiger, 1993, 85-7, 345-79.
Morris MW and Davey FR, "Basic Examination of Blood," Clinical Diagnosis and Management by Laboratory Methods, 19th ed, Chapter 24, Henry JB, ed, Philadelphia, PA: WB Saunders Co, 1996, 553-6.
Riedinger TM and Rodak BF, "Quantitative Laboratory Evaluation of Erythrocytes," Clinical Hematology: Principles, Procedures, Correlations, 2nd ed, Chapter 9, Stiene-Martin EA, Lotspeich-Steininger CA, and Koepke JA, eds, Philadelphia, PA: Lippincott-Raven Publishers, 1998, 106-24.
Second National Health and Nutrition Examination Survey, "Hematological and Nutritional Biochemistry Reference Data for Persons 6 Months - 74 Years of Age: United States, 1976-80," Vital and Health Statistics, DHHS Publication No (PHS), 83-1682, 1982.

◆ **Hematology Profile** see Complete Blood Count on page 419

◆ **Hematopoietic Stem Cells** see CD34+ Hematopoietic Stem Cells by Flow Cytometry on page 413

◆ **Hemoflagellates** see Microfilariae, Peripheral Blood Preparation on page 460

Hemoglobin

Related Information
Anemia Flowchart on page 392
Cobalamin, Serum on page 150
Complete Blood Count on page 419
Cyanide, Blood on page 787
Erythropoietin, Serum on page 169
Ferritin, Serum on page 173
Folic Acid, RBC on page 435
Folic Acid, Serum on page 435
Hematocrit on page 441
Hemoglobin A_2 on page 443
Hemoglobin, Plasma on page 446
Iron and Total Iron Binding Capacity/Transferrin, Serum on page 203
Methemoglobin, Whole Blood on page 800
Oxygen Saturation, Blood on page 240
P_{50}, Blood on page 241
Protoporphyrin, Free Erythrocyte on page 269
Red Blood Cell Indices on page 477
Red Blood Cells on page 857
Red Cell Count on page 478
Red Cell Mass on page 478
Reticulocyte Count on page 481
Reticulocyte Hemoglobin Content on page 482
Sickle Cell Tests on page 486
Uncrossmatched Blood, Emergency on page 865

Synonyms Hb; Hgb

Applies to H and H

Abstract This procedure determines the concentration of hemoglobin (Hb) in whole blood. Hemoglobin is the major component of the red cell and functions to transport oxygen. It also acts to buffer carbon dioxide formed during metabolic activity. The Hb level is important in the detection and follow up of anemia and polycythemia. The Hb value is used in the calculation of the mean corpuscular hemoglobin (MCH) and mean corpuscular hemoglobin concentration (MCHC).

Specimen Whole blood

Container Lavender top (EDTA) tube

Collection Routine venipuncture. Invert tube gently to mix.

Causes for Rejection Clotted or hemolyzed specimen

Reference Interval See tables in Complete Blood Count *on page 419.*

Use Evaluate anemia, blood loss, hemolysis, polycythemia, and other conditions

Limitations Hyperlipemic plasma (especially if chylomicronemia is present) or white count >50,000/mm³ may falsely elevate the hemoglobin result with corresponding increase in the MCH and MCHC. A method correcting for lipemia has been suggested. Increased turbidity (with resultant interference in sample absorbance) may also be due to presence of a paraprotein or of an abnormal hemoglobin (S or C). A variety of corrective procedures are available[1] (see also reference by Brown).

Methodology While oxyhemoglobin and other chemical approaches to hemoglobinometry exist, nearly all current procedures involve a one or two step procedure in which RBC lysis/dilution occurs with the formation of a cyanmethemoglobin compound. Dilutions are read by spectrophotometer at 540 nm. The majority of routine hematology laboratories obtain the hemoglobin level as one of a number of parameters from an automated multichannel instrument.

Additional Information The hemoglobin determination is one of the best standardized and accurate of available clinical laboratory analyses. The results of current College of American Pathologists (CAP) surveys show good interlaboratory performance for the Hb procedure with low standard deviation and coefficient of variation values. The clinical utility of subject-specific reference values has been delineated and emphasized.[2]

In cyanide poisoned individuals treated with methemoglobin-forming agents (to protect cytochrome oxidase) oxygen carrying capacity is decreased in direct proportion to the amount of methemoglobin (nonoxygen carrying) that is formed. A multiwavelength spectrophotometric method has been developed which allows monitoring of hemoglobin derivatives present in the blood of treated cyanide poisoned patients.[3]

The red cell indices, MCH and MCHC, depend on the Hb for their derivation and are of use in the evaluation of anemia. A report of multiple myeloma (with an IgA-K paraprotein) found MCH and MCHC elevated values that failed Coulter STK-S machine internal limits.[4] The analyzer gave a plasma hemoglobin concentration (in the absence of visible hemolysis) with elevated overall blood Hb value. It was considered that only some one-third of the Hb measurement was caused by the monoclonal protein's apparent plasma contribution, the rest of the error resulting from some "unique property of the paraprotein". Technicon® H*IE and Sysmex NE 8000 were minimally affected by the abnormal protein. The latter likely due to the use of a greater dilution of whole blood, the H*IE likely due to the solubilizing effect, alkaline pH and a zwitterionic surfactant (in high concentration).[4]

Red cell parameters have been noted to undergo seasonal changes probably relating to increase in plasma volume in the summer with corresponding lower levels of Hb and Hct. In smokers, however, the increase in plasma volume did not occur and Hct increased while Hb levels did not change. Thus, smokers did not show the expected summer changes seen with nonsmokers.[5] See also the discussion under Complete Blood Count *on page 419.*

As the red cell ages hemoglobin is gradually lost (see comments in Hemoglobin A₂ *on page 443*). The effects of glycation, carbamylation, and loss of RBC water and Hb (with age) result in changes in the RBC indices and must be taken into consideration in assessment of the expected recovery following blood transfusion.[6]

Footnotes

1. Linz LJ, "Elevation of Hemoglobin, MCH, and MCHC by Paraprotein: How to Recognize and Correct the Interference," *Clin Lab Sci*, 1994, 7(4):211-2.
2. Fraser CG, Wilkinson SP, Neville RG, et al, "Biologic Variation of Common Hematologic Laboratory Quantities in the Elderly," *Am J Clin Pathol*, 1989, 92(4):465-70.
3. Zijlstra WG and Buursma A, "Rapid Multicomponent Analysis of Hemoglobin Derivatives for Controlled Antidotal Use of Methemoglobin-Forming Agents in Cyanide Poisoning," *Clin Chem*, 1993, 39(8):1685-9.
4. Roberts WL, Fontenot JD, and Lehman CM, "Overestimation of Hemoglobin in a Patient With an IgA-K Monoclonal Gammopathy," *Arch Pathol Lab Med*, 2000, 124(4):616-18.
5. Kristal-Boneh E, Froom P, Harari G, et al, "Seasonal Differences in Blood Cell Parameters and the Association With Cigarette Smoking," *Clin Lab Haematol*, 1997, 19(3):177-81.
6. Willekens FL, Bosch FH, Roerdinkholder-Stoelwinder B, et al, "Quantification of Loss of Haemoglobin Components From the Circulating Red Blood Cell *In Vivo*," *Eur J Haematol*, 1997, 58(4):246-50.

References

Brown BA, *Hematology: Principles and Procedures*, 6th ed, Philadelphia, PA: Lea & Febiger, 1993, 83-5, 345-79.

Counter SA, Buchanan LH, Ortega F, et al, "Blood Lead and Hemoglobin Levels in Andean Children With Chronic Lead Intoxication," *Neurotoxicology*, 2000, 21(3):301-8.

Morris MW and Davey FR, "Basic Examination of Blood," *Clinical Diagnosis and Management by Laboratory Methods*, 19th ed, Henry JB, ed, Philadelphia, PA: WB Saunders Co, 1996, 549-53, 587-9, 600-3.

Second National Health and Nutrition Examination Survey, "Hematological and Nutritional Biochemistry Reference Data for Persons 6 Months-74 Years of Age: United States, 1976-80," *Vital and Health Statistics*, DHHS Publication No (PHS) 83-1682, 1982.

Zwart A, "Spectrophotometry of Hemoglobin: Various Perspectives," *Clin Chem*, 1993, 39(8):1570-2.

Hemoglobin A₂

Related Information

Anemia Flowchart *on page 392*
DNA-Probe Assay for Thalassemia (BeTha Gene Test) *on page 423*
Hemoglobin Electrophoresis *on page 444*
Peripheral Blood: Red Blood Cell Morphology *on page 467*
Red Blood Cell Indices *on page 477*

Synonyms Hb A₂

Applies to Capillary Isoelectric Focusing

Abstract Hemoglobin A₂ (Hb A₂) is a tetramer of α- and δ-globulin chains ($α_2 δ_2$). Concentration fluctuates in the thalassemia syndromes and some acquired diseases.

Specimen Whole blood

Container Lavender top (EDTA) tube

Causes for Rejection Specimen clotted

Reference Interval The stable adult Hb A₂ level is 2.0% to 3.2% of total hemoglobin; ≤5 months: 0% to 2.5%; 6 months to 1 year: 1.5% to 2.9%. See table.

Alterations in Hb A₂ in Various Disorders

	Elevated	Reduced
Congenital	β-thalassemia trait	α-thalassemia
	Unstable hemoglobin variants	δβ-thalassemia
	Sickle trait (AS)	δ-thalassemia
	SS with α-thalassemia	HPFH
Acquired	Megaloblastic anemias	Iron deficiency
	Hyperthyroidism	Sideroblastic anemias

Adapted from Bunn HF and Forget BG, *Hemoglobin: Molecular, Genetic, and Clinical Aspects*, Philadelphia, PA: WB Saunders Co, 1986, 61-7

Use Investigate microcytic anemia, for hemoglobinopathies, especially thalassemia, particularly beta-thalassemia trait

Limitations Blood transfusion prior to hemoglobin electrophoresis may make interpretation inconsistent. High levels of hemoglobin F usually are accompanied by lower levels of A₂. Sickle cell trait range is from 1.7% to 4.5% hemoglobin A₂. Presence of Hb S or Hb C will interfere with column chromatographic method.[1] Presence of Hb C interferes with routine electrophoretic method. Quantitation of Hb A₂ by densitometric scanning of electrophoretic pattern may result in misleading (high) results as this method is not uniformly reliable.

Contraindications Recent blood transfusion

Methodology Electrophoresis, DEAE cellulose chromatography, high performance cation-exchange liquid chromatography (HPLC); radial immunodiffusion (RID) has also been used. Capillary electrophoresis[2] and capillary isoelectric focusing have been developed[3,4,5] and found to be rapid (under 15 minutes), precise (coefficient of variation <2% to 6%), sensitive, and high resolution automated methods for determination of Hb variants, comparable to the use of HPLC but with lower cost.[4] Hb A₂ by capillary electrophoresis was not affected by presence of Hb S[5] or Hb D[6] as has been reported to occur with use of HPLC-variant β-thalassemia short program.[1] A recent study has concluded that the use of capillary zone electrophoresis at alkaline pH with "dynamic coating" (which increases negative charge on the capillary surface with resultant high electro-osmotic flow and shortens analysis time) could replace HPLC for the screening of hemoglobinopathies.[7] Due to these partly method-based interpretive difficulties, each laboratory should have and utilize an alternate procedure, the application and performance of which is understood.[6]

Additional Information This test is done in many laboratories as part of the hemoglobin electrophoresis. Hemoglobin A₂ levels have special application to the diagnosis of beta-thalassemia trait, which may be present even though peripheral blood smear is normal. This reflects the underlying genetic spectrum of beta-thalassemia which in reality is a complex of multiple distinct (and some less distinct) conditions, the result of over 180 different mutations.[8] The microcytosis and other morphologic changes of beta-thalassemia trait must be differentiated from iron deficiency. Low MCV may include the majority of beta-thalassemia trait patients but does not differentiate iron deficient individuals. Low Hb A₂ levels occur in untreated iron deficiency. If iron deficiency occurs with beta-thalassemia, the Hb A₂ level may fall to within the normal range.[9]

The most definitive evidence for presence of beta-thalassemia trait is genetic (family study). A well documented report, however, indicates the occurrence of beta-thalassemia minor as a result of a spontaneous initiation codon mutation.[10] Offspring of a person with thalassemia major will have beta-thalassemia trait. Apart from such family/genetic studies (which are (Continued)

Hemoglobin A₂ (Continued)

subject to practical difficulties) gene probes are the most definitive method for identifying beta-thalassemia trait. This method identifies "silent" carriers. See DNA-Probe Assay for Thalassemia (BeTha Gene Test) *on page 423.* Elevated percent Hb A₂ is the next best evidence for the diagnosis of beta-thalassemia trait. Sufficient criteria for the diagnosis of thalassemia trait are an elevated Hb A₂ percentage by a reliable method (Hb electrophoresis with elution and quantitation by spectrophotometry) or column chromatography (assuming Hb S, C, or an unstable hemoglobin are not present).

Hb A₂ may be increased in megaloblastic anemia and may be decreased in sideroblastic anemia, Hb H disease, and erythroleukemia. Approximately 33% of zidovudine (AZT) treated human immunodeficiency virus-1 positive individuals have elevated Hb A₂ levels.[11]

Hemoglobin is gradually lost from the red blood cell during its lifespan. During the first half of the red cell lifespan Hb A and Hb A₂ decrease by glycation and carbamylation. During the second half of the lifespan, additional Hb and chemically altered forms are lost, overall total loss of 20%.[12] Red cells lose water and Hb with age producing changes in the red cell indices (decrease of 30% in MCV, increase of 15% in MCHC).[13] In addition to changes in red cell indices, these considerations have clinical application to the efficacy (expected improvement in Hb/Hct level) of red cell transfusions.[12]

In a study of over 600 β-thalassemia heterozygotes (with multiple different underlying genetic mechanisms including 32 different base changes or frame shifts) severe cases (β°-thalassemia or β⁺-thalassemia) had Hb A₂ levels of 4.5% to 5.5%, mild β⁺-thalassemia had levels of 3.6% to 4.2%, while silent mutations had lower values. Homozygotes often had Hb A₂ levels of 10% or more but many cases had received transfusions such that A₂ values were not representative.[14]

Footnotes

1. Shokrani M, Terrell F, Turner EA, et al, "Chromatographic Measurements of Hemoglobin A₂ in Blood Samples That Contain Sickle Hemoglobin," *Ann Clin Lab Sci,* 2000, 30(2):191-4.
2. Jenkins MA, Hendy J, Smith IL, "Evaluation of Hemoglobin A₂ Quantitation Assay and Hemoglobin Variant Screening by Capillary Electrophoresis," *J Capillary Electrophor,* 1997, 4(3):137-43.
3. Mario N, Baudin B, Aussel C, et al, "Capillary Isoelectric Focusing and High-Performance Cation-Exchange Chromatography Compared for Qualitative and Quantitative Analysis of Hemoglobin Variants," *Clin Chem,* 1997, 43(11):2137-42.
4. Craver RD, Abermanis JG, Warrier RP, et al, "Hemoglobin A₂ Levels in Healthy Persons, Sickle Cell Disease, Sickle Cell Trait, and β-Thalassemia by Capillary-Isoelectric Focusing," *Am J Clin Pathol,* 1997, 107(1):88-91.
5. Cotton F, Lin C, Fontaine B, et al, "Evaluation of a Capillary Electrophoresis Method for Routine Determination of Hemoglobins A₂ and F," *Clin Chem,* 1999, 45(2):237-43.
6. Cotton F, Gulbis B, Hansen V, et al, "Interference of Hemoglobin D in Hemoglobin A₂ Measurement by Cation-Exchange HPLC," *Clin Chem,* 1999, 45(8 Pt 1):1317-8.
7. Mario N, Baudin B, Bruneel A, et al, "Capillary Zone Electrophoresis for the Diagnosis of Congenital Hemoglobinopathies," *Clin Chem,* 1999, 45(2):285-8.
8. Weatherall DJ, "The Thalassemias," *The Molecular Basis of Blood Diseases,* 3rd ed, Chapter 6, Stamatoyannopoulos G, Majerus PW, Perlmutter RM, et al, eds, Philadelphia, PA: WB Saunders Co, 2001, 183-226.
9. Wasi P, Disthasongchan P, and Na-Nakorn S, "The Effect of Iron Deficiency on the Levels of Hemoglobins A₂ and E," *J Lab Clin Med,* 1968, 71:85-91.
10. Beris P, Darbellay R, Speiser D, et al, "De Novo Initiation Codon Mutation (ATG → ACG) of the β-Globin Gene Causing β-Thalassemia in a Swiss Family," *Am J Hematol,* 1993, 42(3):248-53.
11. Routy JP, Monte M, Beaulieu R, et al, "Increase of Hemoglobin A₂ in Human Immunodeficiency Virus-1-Infected Patients Treated With Zidovudine," *Am J Hematol,* 1993, 43(2):86-90.
12. Willekens FL, Bosch FH, Roerdinkholder-Stoelwinder B, et al, "Quantification of Loss of Haemoglobin Components From the Circulating Red Blood Cell *In Vivo,*" *Eur J Haematol,* 1997, 58(4):246-50.
13. Bosch FH, Werre JM, Roerdinkholder-Stoelwinder B, et al, "Characteristics of Red Cell Populations Fractionated With a Combination of Counterflow Centrifugation and Percoll Separation," *Blood,* 1992, 79(1):254-60.
14. Huisman TH, "Levels of Hb A₂ in Heterozygotes and Homozygotes for Beta-Thalassemia Mutations: Influence of Mutations in the CACCC and ATAAA Motifs of the Beta-Globin Gene Promoter," *Acta Haematol,* 1997, 98(4):187-94.

References

Lukens JN, "The Thalassemias and Related Disorders: Quantitative Disorders of Hemoglobin Synthesis," *Wintrobe's Clinical Hematology,* 10th ed, Volume 1, Chapter 53, Lee GR, Foerster J, Lukens J, et al, eds, Baltimore, MD: Lippincott Williams & Wilkins, 1999, 1405-48.

Steinberg MH and Adams JG 3d, "Hemoglobin A₂: Origin, Evolution, and Aftermath," *Blood,* 1991, 78(9):2165-77.

Thonglairoam V, Winichagoon P, Fucharoen S, et al, "Hemoglobin Constant Spring in Bangkok: Molecular Screening by Selective Enzymatic Amplification of the α₂-Globin Gene," *Am J Hematol,* 1991, 38(4):277-80.

Hemoglobin Electrophoresis

Related Information

DNA-Probe Assay for Thalassemia (BeTha Gene Test) *on page 423*
Fetal Hemoglobin *on page 431*
Fructosamine, Serum *on page 177*
Glycated Hemoglobin (Hemoglobin A₁c), Blood *on page 188*
Hemoglobin A₂ *on page 443*
Hemosiderin Stain, Urine *on page 876*
Methemoglobin, Whole Blood *on page 800*
P₅₀, Blood *on page 241*
Peripheral Blood: Red Blood Cell Morphology *on page 467*
Reticulocyte Count *on page 481*
Sickle Cell Tests *on page 486*

Applies to Hb G_Philadelphia

Test Includes Electrophoresis for separation and distribution of hemoglobins, fetal hemoglobin (Hb F) and hemoglobin A₂ (Hb A₂) often by other methods, in particular column or high performance liquid chromatography.

Abstract In this procedure, hemoglobins are caused to separate and migrate. A variety of techniques are utilized. Most commonly hemoglobins are separated as discrete bands as they move through a substrate in a buffer solution across an electric field with subsequent visualization by fixation and staining (hemoglobin electrophoresis). Clinical applications include detection and identification of hemoglobin variants and the investigation of some hemolytic anemias resulting from red cell intracorpuscular defects.

Specimen Whole blood

Container Lavender top (EDTA) tube for venipuncture specimen; lavender top Microtainer™ tube for capillary specimen

Causes for Rejection Specimen clotted

Turnaround Time Method dependent, usually 1-2 days

Reference Interval Hemoglobin A: 95% to 98%; hemoglobin A₂: 1.5% to 3.5%; hemoglobin F: 0% to 2%; hemoglobin C: absent; hemoglobin S: absent

Use Diagnose hemoglobinopathies; evaluate hemolytic anemia; diagnose thalassemia; evaluate sickling hemoglobins, hemoglobin C; with other and specialized techniques, evaluate unstable, low and high oxygen affinity hemoglobinopathies (the latter representing one cause of polycythemia)

Limitations Blood transfusion prior to hemoglobin electrophoresis may make interpretations inconsistent.[1,2] Many abnormal hemoglobins do not separate from normal adult Hb A during application of routine electrophoretic techniques. Rarely, there may be lack of specificity for Hb (eg, as may occur when a monoclonal immunoglobulin is present).[3]

Methodology Electrophoresis using cellulose acetate, agarose gel, citrate agar gel, or starch gel substrates; isoelectric focusing using polyacrylamide or agarose gel substrates; alkali denaturation for fetal hemoglobin; anion exchange resin chromatography for hemoglobin A₂ quantitation; globin chain electrophoresis; capillary electrophoresis; capillary isoelectric focusing; high performance cation-exchange liquid chromatography (HPLC); high performance anion-exchange liquid chromatography (HPLC). Multiple methods may be needed to establish the nature of some complex hemoglobinopathies (ie, Hb SS and SG_Philadelphia associated with α-thalassemia-2), Hb G_Philadelphia is an alpha-chain variant.[4]

Additional Information In this procedure, hemoglobin (Hb), released from lysed red blood cells, is caused to migrate through a substrate in a buffer by application of an electric current. Different types of hemoglobin are separated into specific bands that are subsequently visualized by application of one of a variety of staining procedures. Migration of hemoglobin is defined by interaction of a specific hemoglobin molecule with substrate structure, buffer pH, ionic strength, and other characteristics. By referring to the accompanying table of patterns for cellulose acetate (alkaline pH), one can determine that Hb A, in the allotted time period, migrates relatively far towards the anode (+ charged pole). It is thus "faster" in migration than most other hemoglobins. Even more anodal migrating are the "fast" Hbs H,[5] I, and Bart's. Intermediate migrating Hbs are D, G, S, and Lepore while "slow" Hb include C, E, A₂, and O. The test is of central importance in establishing the presence of common hemoglobinopathies (Hb S, C, D, and E) and in the evaluation of some cases of hemolytic anemia.

Hemoglobin Electrophoresis Pattern

Sample Identity	Cellulose Acetate Alkaline, pH 8.4-8.6							Citrate Agar Gel Acid, pH 6.0-6.2			
	Origin	Carbonic Anhydrase	A₂, C, E, O	S, D, G	F	A₁	Ratio of S/A	C	S	A₁, A₂, D, G, E	F
Control	I	I	■	■	■	■	-	■	■	■	■
Normal (A₁, A₂)	I	I	■			■			■	■	
Cord Blood	I	I			■	■				■	■
Sickle Cell Disease (SCD)	I	I	■	■*			100/0		■		■*
Sickle Cell Trait (SA₁A₂)	I	I	■	■		■	40/60		■	■	
SC Disease	I	I	■	■			-	■	■	■	
SE Disease	I	I	■	■					■	■	
S/B⁺ Thalassemia	I	I	■	■		■	60/40		■	■	
S/Bᵒ Thalassemia	I	I	■	■			100/0		■	■	
CC	I	I	†■					■			
C Trait	I	I	†■			■		■		■	
C_Harlem Trait	I	I	†■	■		■		■	■	■	
D Trait	I	I		■		■				■	

*Amount varies   †A₂ may be slightly separate

Study of peripheral blood smear RBC morphology can assist in the decision to order hemoglobin electrophoresis. Hemoglobin electrophoresis (including determination of Hb F) is indicated if a positive sickle screening test has been obtained. Hb F and Hb A₂ quantitation (often included as part of hemoglobin evaluation) are important in establishing the presence of thalassemia. In some cases, additional study will be needed. Depending upon the abnormality encountered this might include reticulocyte count, haptoglobin level, citrate agar gel electrophoresis at acidic pH, globin chain electrophoresis, mRNA studies, and family studies.

Complete characterization of an abnormal hemoglobin may require sophisticated laboratory studies usually available only in a research setting (eg, as with some of the thalassemia syndromes). Amino acid globin chain sequencing may be used to establish the presence of a hemoglobinopathy.

Hemoglobin electrophoresis of umbilical cord blood can detect α-chain variants Hb F/G and Hb G as well as S and C gene products. Results have been reported as consistent with the predicted frequency (1 in 625) of sickle anemia at birth. Techniques of analysis, such as globin chain electrophoresis, isoelectric focusing, high performance liquid chromatography,[6,7,8] amino acid sequencing, restriction endonuclease studies, and polymerase chain reaction[9] are additional methods, focused at the genetic level, allowing the laboratory to detect and identify hemoglobin variants. A multiplex polymerase chain reaction for detection of α-thalassemia (caused by α-globin gene deletion - the most common genetic abnormality in the world) is said to be applicable to routine performance by clinical laboratories.[10] (See also DNA-Probe Assay for Thalassemia (BeTha Gene Test) *on page 423*.)

Sequential Application of Procedures for Identification of an Abnormal Hemoglobin

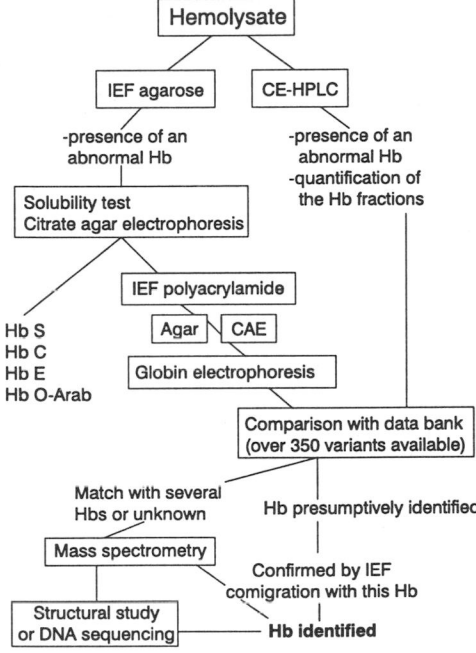

Flow diagram showing procedures applicable to identification of a hemoglobin variant.

When the electrophoretic data match for several Hbs, additional tests (eg, reversed-phase HPLC, measurement of functional properties) may be performed before a structural determination is made.

Adapted from Riou J, Godart C, Hurtrel D, et al, "Cation-Exchange HPLC Evaluated for Presumptive Identification of Hemoglobin Variants," *Clin Chem*, 1997, 43(1):34-9.

Some alkaline gel electrophoretic systems may offer advantages in glycohemoglobin quantitation because of their ability to discriminate Hb F and to simultaneously detect common hemoglobinopathies.[11] Cation exchange HPLC has delineated over 10 minor hemoglobins including Hb A₁c and Hb A₁d₃ with evidence that the latter is useful for assessment of the uremic state.[12] It has been shown that capillary electrophoresis can separate hemoglobin variants within 10 minutes.[13]

Screening of the general population for sickle cell and other hemoglobinopathies had vocal proponents in the late 1960s and early 1970s. Interest waned, largely the result of possible socioeconomic implications of case detection. Since 1986, when the effectiveness of oral penicillin in reducing SCD-related morbidity and mortality in children became established,[14] there has been growing activity in (and state support of) newborn screening for the S gene and for other hemoglobinopathies. Currently, most states screen newborns for SCD.[15,16] Problem areas include false-negative results (associated with the use of dried blood filter paper samples) and maternal contamination of cord blood.[17] Molecular genetic analysis-based screening

programs have been proposed[18,19] in some cases in consideration of the lifetime cost of treatment (eg, in cases of β-thalassemia major).[20] The California Department of Health Services, Genetic Disease Laboratory has determined the distribution of Hb F, A, S, C, E, and D quantities in 4 million dried blood spot newborn screening specimens using an automated 2-minute cation-gradient HPLC method.[21]

A number of interactions between pathologic hemoglobin and glycated hemoglobin (Hb A₁c), the latter used as a measure of long-term blood glucose control in diabetic patients, have been described. A comparison of Hb A₁c results using cation exchange chromatography (Bio-Rad Variant) vs a method based on an immunological reaction (Bayer® DCA 2000) found close agreement of Hb A₁c results on specimens from individuals with Hb S, C, D, and E trait.[22] A mathematical correction, required for correlation of Hb A₁c Bio-Rad Variant results in individuals with D trait has required application of a new correction calculation or use of an immune-based methodology (eg, Bayer® DCA 2000)[23] or use of fructosamine measurement as an alternate to diabetes control (when Hb D or Hb D$_{Los Angeles}$) causes diagnostic confusion as a result of falsely low or high Hb A₁c.[24] A recently available fully automated HPLC assay for Hb A₁c (Tosoh A₁c 2.2 Plus Glycohemoglobin Analyzer, Tosoh Medics, Foster City, California) identifies Hb variants and does not generate an Hb A₁c value if Hb A is significantly decreased.[25]

New Hb variants continue to be described, some, such as hemoglobin Old Dominion/Burton-Upon-Trent (reported in four unrelated persons of Irish or Scots-Irish ancestry) may cause spurious increase in glycated Hb A₁c (with use of ion-exchange chromatography methods).[26] The amino acid substitution is β-143 (H21) His→Tyr which affects a 2,3-diphosphoglycerate binding site with minimal increase in oxygen affinity but without clinical erythrocytosis.[26] On alkaline gel Hb electrophoresis, the variant migrated with Hb A, on acid agar get it was 3.5 mm from Hb A. Characterization of Hb Old Dominion/Burton-Upon-Trent was by electrospray ionization mass spectrometry and peptide analysis.[26] The report by Elder et al (as of April 1998) provides a table (with references) of 26 hemoglobin variants and Hb F that interfere with glycated Hb measurements by ion-exchange chromatography.[26] The following variants were listed.

Andrew-Minneapolis	Hope	Okayama
Bart's	I	Olomouc
Deer Lodge	J	Osler
F	K	Raleigh
Fannin-Lubbock	Le Lamentin	Sherwood Forest
Fukuyama	Lisbon	South Florida
Graz	Marseille/Long Island	Tacoma
H	Malmö	Tatras
Hijiyama	N	

Hb A₁c, a minor Hb variant, is formed *in vivo*, a post-translational modification by glucose with glycated N-terminal β-chains. A recent sophisticated analysis using electrospray ionization mass spectrometry affirmed a curvilinear relationship of patient glucose with Hb A₁c.[27] Multiple species of glycated Hb, however, cochromatographed with Hb A₁c on cation exchange. As glycation increased, β:α-chain ratio glycation increased, and the number of β-chain glycation sites increased. Glycated and nonglycated, both α- and β-chain varieties including some multiply glycated β-chains, were encountered, complicating the standardization of glycohemoglobin clinical assays.[27]

Footnotes

1. Ahmad E and Sykes E, "Clinical Pathology Rounds: Low Levels of Hemoglobin S in a White Woman," *Lab Med*, 1999, 30(9):572.
2. Veillon DM, Kaltenbach JE, Hall CG, et al, "Assays for Hemoglobin S," *Lab Med*, 2000, 31(2):68-9.
3. Sughayer MA and Arkin CF, "Unusual Band on Hemoglobin Electrophoresis Produced by a Monoclonal Immunoglobulin in Serum," *Clin Chem*, 1989, 35(8):1794.
4. Kirk CM, Papadea CN, and Lazarchick J, "Laboratory Recognition of a Rare Hemoglobinopathy: Hemoglobins SS and SG$_{Philadelphia}$ Associated With α-Thalassemia-2," *Arch Pathol Lab Med*, 1999, 123(10):963-6.
5. Chen FE, Ooi C, Ha SY, et al, "Genetic and Clinical Features of Hemoglobin H Disease in Chinese Patients," *N Engl J Med*, 2000, 343(8):544-50.
6. Riou J, Godart C, Hurtrel D, et al, "Cation-Exchange HPLC Evaluated for Presumptive Identification of Hemoglobin Variants," *Clin Chem*, 1997, 43(1):34-9.
7. Papadea C and Cate JC 4th, "Identification and Quantification of Hemoglobins A, F, S, and C by Automated Chromatography," *Clin Chem*, 1996, 42(1):57-63.
8. Wild BJ and Stephens AD, "The Use of Automated HPLC to Detect and Quantitate Haemoglobins," *Clin Lab Haematol*, 1997, 19(3):171-6.
9. Arcasoy MO and Gallagher PG, "Molecular Diagnosis of Hemoglobinopathies and Other Red Blood Cell Disorders," *Semin Hematol*, 1999, 36(4):328-39.
10. Bowie LJ, Reddy PL, and Nagabhushan M, et al, "Detection of α-Thalassemias by Multiplex Polymerase Chain Reaction," *Clin Chem*, 1994, 40(12):2260-6.
11. Bayliss KM, Kopinski WS, and Kueck BD, "Glycohemoglobin Quantitation by Alkaline Gel Electrophoresis. A Reliable Technique With Practical Clinical Advantages," *Am J Clin Pathol*, 1989, 91(5):570-4.
12. Bissé E, Huaman-Guillen P, and Wieland H, "Chromatographic Evaluation of Minor Hemoglobins: Clinical Significance of Hemoglobin A₁d, Comparison With Hemoglobin, A₁c, and Possible Interferences," *Clin Chem*, 1995, 41(5):658-63.
13. Chen FT, Liu CM, Hsieh YZ, et al, "Capillary Electrophoresis - A New Clinical Tool," *Clin Chem*, 1991, 37(1):14-9.

(Continued)

Hemoglobin Electrophoresis (Continued)

14. Gaston MH, Verter JI, Woods G, et al, "Prophylaxis With Oral Penicillin in Children With Sickle Cell Anemia. A Randomized Trial," *N Engl J Med*, 1986, 314(25):1593-9.

15. Pass K and Harris K, "Update: Newborn Screening for Sickle Cell Disease - California, Illinois, and New York, 1998," *JAMA*, 2000, 284(11):1373.

16. "Newborn Screening Task Force. Serving the Family From Birth to the Medical Home," *Pediatrics*, 2000, 106(Part 2 of 3):389-427.

17. Githens JH, Lane PA, McCurdy RS, et al, "Newborn Screening for Hemoglobinopathies in Colorado. The First 10 Years," *Am J Dis Child*, 1990, 144(4):466-70.

18. McCabe ER and McCabe LL, "State-of-the-Art for DNA Technology in Newborn Screening," *Acta Paediatr Suppl*, 1999, 88(432):58-60.

19. Dobrowolski SF, Banas RA, Naylor EW, et al, "DNA Microarray Technology for Neonatal Screening," *Acta Paediatr Suppl*, 1999, 88(432):61-4.

20. Karnon J, Zeuner D, Brown J, et al, "Lifetime Treatment Costs of β-Thalassaemia Major," *Clin Lab Haematol*, 1999, 21(6):377-85.

21. Eastman JW, Lorey F, Arnopp J, et al, "Distribution of Hemoglobin F, A, S, C, E, and D Quantities in 4 Million Newborn Screening Specimens," *Clin Chem*, 1999, 45(5):683-4.

22. Blakney GB, Higgins TN, and Holmes DJ, "Comparison of Hemoglobin A₁c Results by Two Different Methods on Patients With Structural Hemoglobin Variants," *Clin Biochem*, 1998, 31(8):619-26.

23. Blakney GB and Higgins TN, "More on the Measurement of Glycohemoglobin in Patients With Hemoglobin D," *Clin Biochem*, 2000, 33(2):143-5.

24. Schnedl WJ, Lipp RW, and Trinker M, "Hemoglobin D [β121 (GH4) Glu→Gln] Causing Falsely Low and High Hb A₁c Values in HPLC," *Clin Chem*, 1998, 44(9):1999-2000.

25. Khuu HM, Robinson CA, Goolsby K, et al, "Evaluation of a Fully Automated High-Performance Liquid Chromatography Assay for Hemoglobin A₁c," *Arch Pathol Lab Med*, 1999, 123(9):763-7.

26. Elder GE, Lappin TR, Horne AB, et al, "Hemoglobin Old Dominion/Burton-Upon-Trent, β143 (H21) His→Tyr, Codon 143 CAC→TAC - A Variant With Altered Oxygen Affinity That Compromises Measurement of Glycated Hemoglobin in Diabetes Mellitus: Structure, Function, and DNA Sequence," *Mayo Clin Proc*, 1998, 73(4):321-8.

27. Peterson KP, Pavlovich JG, Goldstein D, et al, "What Is Hemoglobin A₁c? An Analysis of Glycated Hemoglobins by Electrospray Ionization Mass Spectrometry," *Clin Chem*, 1998, 44(9):1951-8.

References

Bunn HF, "Human Hemoglobins: Sickle Hemoglobin and Other Mutants," *The Molecular Basis of Blood Diseases*, 3rd ed, Chapter 7, Stamatoyannopoulos G, Majerus PW, Perlmutter RM, et al, eds, Philadelphia, PA: WB Saunders Co, 2001, 227-73.

Cronin EK, Normand C, Henthorn JS, et al, "Organization and Cost-Effectiveness of Antenatal Haemoglobinopathy Screening and Follow-up in a Community-Based Programme," *BJOG*, 2000, 107(4):486-91.

Donaldson A, Old J, Fisher C, et al, "Jamaican Sβ⁺-Thalassaemia: Mutations and Haematology," *Br J Haematol*, 2000, 108(2):290-4.

Fucharoen S and Winichagoon P, "Clinical and Hematologic Aspects of Hemoglobin E β-Thalassemia," *Curr Opin Hematol*, 2000, 7(2):106-12.

Gelehrter TD, Collins FS, and Ginsburg D, "Molecular Genetics of Human Disease: Hemoglobinopathies," *Principles of Medical Genetics*, 2nd ed, Chapter 6, Baltimore, MD: Lippincott Williams & Wilkins, 1998, 91-116.

Sandhaus LM and Harvey FG, "Laboratory Methods for the Detection of Hemoglobinopathies in the Community Hospital," *Clin Lab Med*, 1993, 13(4):801-16.

Shokrani M, Terrell F, Turner EA, et al, "Chromatographic Measurements of Hemoglobin A₂ in Blood Samples That Contain Sickle Hemoglobin," *Ann Clin Lab Sci*, 2000, 30(2):191-4.

Simsek M, Daar S, Ojeli H, et al, "Improved Diagnosis of Sickle Cell Mutation by a Robust Amplification Refractory Polymerase Chain Reaction," *Clin Biochem*, 1999, 32(8):677-80.

Stamatoyannopoulos G, Nienhuis AW, Majerus PW, et al, eds, *The Molecular Basis of Blood Diseases*, 2nd ed, Chapters 4-6, Philadelphia, PA: WB Saunders Co, 1994, 107-256.

Streetly A, "A National Screening Policy for sickle Cell Disease and Thalassaemia Major for the United Kingdom. Questions Are Left After Two Evidence Based Reports," *BMJ*, 2000, 320(7246):1353-4.

Thonglairoam V, Winichagoon P, Fucharoen S, et al, "Hemoglobin Constant Spring in Bangkok: Molecular Screening by Selective Enzymatic Amplification of the α₂-Globin Gene," *Am J Hematol*, 1991, 38(4):277-80.

Weatherall DJ and Clegg JB, "Genetic Disorders of Hemoglobin," *Semin Hematol*, 1999, 36(4 Suppl 7):24-37.

Wenning MR, Kimura EM, Jorge SB, et al, "Molecular Characterization of Hemoglobins Kurosaki [α7 Lys→Glu], G-Pest [α74 Asp→Asn], Stanleyville-II [α78 Asn→Lys] and J-Rovigo [α53 Ala→Asp]," *Acta Haematol*, 1999, 102(4):203-5.

♦ **Hemoglobin, Fetal** *see* Fetal Hemoglobin *on page 431*

♦ **Hemoglobin, Free** *see* Hemoglobin, Plasma *on page 446*

♦ **Hemoglobin Munchausen** *see* Sickle Cell Tests *on page 486*

Hemoglobin, Plasma

Related Information

Haptoglobin, Serum *on page 190*
Hemoglobin *on page 442*
Hemoglobin, Qualitative, Urine *on page 875*
Transfusion Reaction Work-up *on page 864*

Synonyms Free Hemoglobin; Hemoglobin, Free; Plasma Free Hemoglobin

Applies to Cardiopulmonary Bypass; Cripps Method (for plasma hemoglobin); Erythrocyte Adenylate Kinase, Isoenzyme; Human Polymerized Hemoglobin; Poly SFH-P; Soloni Method (for plasma hemoglobin)

Abstract Test used to detect intravascular hemolysis. Increase of hemoglobin in the plasma is a reliable sign of intravascular hemolysis only if lysis of red blood cells during and after obtaining the sample (ie, traumatic puncture) can be definitely excluded.[1] Plasma hemoglobin levels are used to assess damage to blood cells (erythrocytes) caused by a variety of medical devices.

Patient Preparation Special precautions and patient preparation are usually required to draw the specimen. Laboratory should be contacted directly.

Aftercare A pressure bandage should be applied to the site of 18-gauge needle puncture (following the puncture) to stop residual bleeding.

Specimen Plasma

Container Lavender top (EDTA) tube

Collection Recommended procedure for collecting sample without inducing hemolysis: Use 18-gauge needle with attached infusion tubing. Observing HIV precautions, place tourniquet lightly around the upper arm. Puncture antecubital vein with as little trauma as possible. Release tourniquet and clamp tubing off as soon as blood return is seen. Collect 3 mL of blood first in a red top tube with the rubber stopper off. Follow by a 5 mL collection in a green top (heparin) tube with the stopper off. Clamp tubing, withdraw needle, and apply pressure to the site until residual bleeding is stopped. Cap green top tube and gently mix three to five times. Use this specimen for the plasma hemoglobin determination.

Storage Instructions Separate and freeze plasma as soon as possible if test is not run immediately.

Causes for Rejection Traumatic venipuncture causing hemolysis

Reference Interval Under optimal conditions (with absence of hemolysis due to collection of blood) <0.6 mg/dL (<6 mg/L).[1] Practically (allowing for minimal hemolysis during collection), a plasma (or serum) level of hemoglobin >20 mg/dL (200 mg/L) is likely indicative of a pathologic hemolytic process.[2]

Use Evaluate hemolytic anemia, especially intravascular hemolysis; evaluate red cell lysis caused by medical devices (cardiopulmonary bypass machines, left ventricular assist devices, pumps, pulsatile assist devices); evaluate use of human hemoglobin-derived blood substitutes

Limitations Plasma hemoglobin is increased with intravascular hemolysis, in particular as occurs with paroxysmal nocturnal hemoglobinuria, paroxysmal cold hemoglobinuria, the cold-hemagglutinin syndrome, and "blackwater fever" but also as occurs with ABO incompatible transfusion, traumatic hemolysis, falciparum malaria, burns, and march hemoglobinuria. Increase may occur in some cases of extravascular hemolysis, delayed transfusion reaction, with slight increase in sickle cell anemia, and β-thalassemia. In hereditary spherocytosis (hemolysis occurs largely in the spleen), plasma hemoglobin levels are normal or only slightly increased.[1] High bilirubin, turbidity, methemalbuminemia (method measures methemalbumin and hemoglobin together), lipemic plasma, and hemolysis during or after venipuncture may cause falsely elevated values in the plasma hemoglobin test (method based on peroxide oxidation of benzidine). Method based on the fractional absorbance of oxyhemoglobin at 578 nm is proportional even in the presence of those interfering substances. Use of benzidine has been restricted because of reports that it is carcinogenic. An alternative is the use of tetramethylbenzidine which is more readily available but which should also be handled with care.

Methodology An established method utilizes fractional absorbance of oxyhemoglobin at 578 nm. A method utilizing first-derivative spectroscopy (procedure of Soloni et al) has undergone evaluation. It is rapid and not affected by bilirubin, myoglobin, lipemia, or turbidity. It is sensitive down to a level of 1 mg/dL.[3]

Additional Information High bilirubin (up to 36 mg/dL), turbidity of the specimen, or a fair amount of methemalbumin will not affect the method based on fractional absorbance of oxyhemoglobin at 578 nm or the method of Soloni et al.[4] Hemoglobinemia can be detected by gross examination of centrifuged blood. Plasma will have a pink tinge when hemoglobin is present in a concentration ≥200 mg/L.[1]

A variety of pump-based heart/lung machines and associated devices have been and continue to be developed for a growing number of cardiopulmonary (cardiovascular operative procedures, eg, centrifugal pumps, pumps for extracorporeal membrane oxygenation, percutaneous cardiopulmonary support, pulsatile assist devices, etc). Plasma free hemoglobin measurements are important in assessment of trauma to the circulating cells of peripheral blood (assessment of traumatic hemolysis).[5,6] The U.S. Food and Drug Administration (FDA) must review submissions for use of such medical devices but found that there was no standard or widely accepted method for determination of plasma hemoglobin concentration. They found over 20 different assays in clinical use for measurement of plasma hemoglobin. They assessed nine currently used plasma hemoglobin assays for accuracy, reproducibility, sensitivity, interference effects and ease of use.[7] Results were graded on a scale of 1 (worst) to 9 (best). See table. The older direct optical techniques (eg, Cripps method from 1968) had overall good performance while "added chemical" methods (eg, cyanmethemoglobin method) were less satisfactory. The Soloni et al procedure noted above was included, adapted, and is method "A" in the table. It is a "first-derivative absorbance" method and was equivalent to the Cripps procedure.

Plasma hemoglobin monitoring has been used in the evaluation of Poly SFH-P, a polymerized hemoglobin under evaluation as a blood substitute after acute trauma and emergency surgery.[8]

Comparison of Plasma Hemoglobin Assays
Scale of 1 (worst) to 9 (best)

Method (media)	Absolute Accuracy (plasma)	Relative Accuracy (plasma)	Bilirubin Interference (PBS)	Lipid Interference (PBS)	Absolute Accuracy (PBS/ water)	Precision (PBS/ water)	Sensitivity (PBS/ water)	Ease of Use	Time for 20 Samples	Instrumentation (band width)	Overall Use	Convert Abs to mg/dL
Cripps	9	9	9	8	8	9	6	9	9 (10 min)	7 (2 nm)	9	Self calibration
Kahn	2*	2*	8	8	3*	9	6	9	9 (10 min)	7 (2 nm)	4	Equation given
Porter	4†	8	8	4†	9	9	8	9	9 (10 min)	7 (2 nm)	6	Self calibration
Shinowara	5*	6*	8	5*	8	9	4	9	9 (10 min)	7 (2 nm)	5	Self calibration
A'	9	9	9	9	8	8		8	8 (15 min)	6 (2 nm)	8	Self calibration
Harboe	9	9	5*	9	8	8	6	8	8 (17 min)	8 (4 nm)	8	Equation given
Fairbanks	8	9	1‡	9	8	7	6	8	8 (17 min)	8 (4 nm)	7	Equation given
HiCN	1†	8	1¶	1¶	9	8	3	7	7 (19 min)	9 (6 nm)	5	Self calibration
TMB	3*	3*	8	8	3‡	4	9	2	1 (80 min)	9	3	Kit standards

*Negatively interferes with the assay.

†Positively interferes with the assay.

‡Greatly negatively interferes with the assay.

¶Greatly positively interferes with the assay.

Note: The scores (from 1-9) presented in the table are based on relative comparisons between the accuracy, precision, or utility of the methods under each respective column heading as evaluated over the hemoglobin concentration range of 1-200 mg/dL.

Note: Relative accuracy refers to analytical recovery evaluated by subtracting the baseline concentration obtained by each method from the concentration measured by that method when a known amount of hemoglobin was added.

Note: In last column "abs" refers to the measured absorbance quantity and its conversion to a hemoglobin concentration (mg/dL) using a calibration coefficient.

Adapted from Malinauskas RZ, "Plasma Hemoglobin Measurement Techniques for the *in vitro* Evaluation of Blood Damage Caused by Medical Devices," *Artif Organs*, 1997, 21(12):1255-67.

The plasma hemoglobin level along with haptoglobin, indirect bilirubin, LD isoenzymes, reticulocyte count, and perhaps other clinical laboratory studies can be applied to evaluate parts of the spectrum of clinical hemolytic processes. A recently suggested additional marker for hemolysis is erythrocyte adenylate kinase isoenzyme activity.[9]

Footnotes

1. Dacie JV and Lewis SM, "Laboratory Methods Used in the Investigation of the Haemolytic Anaemias," *Practical Haematology*, 8th ed, Chapter 12, Dacie JV and Lewis SM, eds, New York, NY: Churchill Livingstone, 1995, 199-201.
2. Copeland BE, Dyer PJ, and Pesce AJ, "Hemoglobin by First Derivative Spectrophotometry: Extent of Hemolysis in Plasma and Serum Collected in Vacuum Container Devices," *Ann Clin Lab Sci*, 1989, 19(5):383-8.
3. Copeland BE, Dyer PJ, and Pesce AJ, "Hemoglobin Determination in Plasma or Serum by First-Derivative Recording Spectrophotometry," *Am J Clin Pathol*, 1989, 92(5):619-24.
4. Soloni FG, Cunningham MT, and Amazon K, "Plasma Hemoglobin Determination by Recording Derivative Spectrophotometry," *Am J Clin Pathol*, 1986, 85(3):342-7.
5. Kawahito K and Nosé Y, "Hemolysis in Different Centrifugal Pumps," *Artif Organs*, 1997, 21(4):323-6.
6. Iwaya F, Igari T, Hoshino S, et al, "Evaluation of Hemolysis in a Pulsatile Assist Device for Centrifugal Pump," *Artif Organs*, 1997, 21(7):700-3.
7. Malinauskas RA, "Plasma Hemoglobin Measurement Techniques for the *In Vitro* Evaluation of Blood Damage Caused by Medical Devices," *Artif Organs*, 1997, 21(12):1255-67.
8. Gould SA, Moore EE, Moore FA, et al, "Clinical Utility of Human Polymerized Hemoglobin as a Blood Substitute After Acute Trauma and Urgent Surgery," *J Trauma*, 1997, 43(2):325-32.
9. Thomas G and Murthy VV, "Erythrocyte Adenylate Kinase Isoenzyme as a Marker for Hemolysis," *J Clin Lab Anal*, 1997, 11(6):351-6.

References

Fairbanks VF, Ziesmer SC, and O'Brien PC, "Methods for Measuring Plasma Hemoglobin in Micromolar Concentration Compared," *Clin Chem*, 1992, 38(1):132-40.

Lee GR, "The Hemolytic Disorders: General Considerations," *Wintrobe's Clinical Hematology*, 10th ed, Volume 1, Chapter 40, Lee GR, Foerster J, Lukens J, et al, eds, Philadelphia, PA: Lippincott Williams & Wilkins, 1999, 1109-31.

Hemoglobin, Unstable, Heat Labile Test

Related Information
Heinz Body Stain *on page 440*
Hemoglobin, Unstable - Isopropanol Precipitation Test *on page 448*
Hemosiderin Stain, Urine *on page 876*
n-Butanol Stability Test *on page 460*

Synonyms Heat Denaturation; Test for Congenital Heinz Body Hemolytic Anemia; Unstable Hemoglobins

Applies to Carboxyhemoglobin; Hb Köln; Hb Zurich; Heinz Bodies

Abstract A simple, low cost test for detection of unstable hemoglobins. A variety of mutations (>75% involve the β-chain) are responsible for this inherited condition (some, however, are the result of spontaneous mutations). The resultant "unstable" hemoglobins impair hemoglobin solubility or increase susceptibility to oxidation of amino acids forming the involved globin chains. Dependent upon the specific mutation, globin chain folding abnormality, α-β-interaction, and/or globin to heme destabilization occurs with formation of Heinz bodies (precipitates of α- and β-globin chains, globin fragments, and heme). Most of such variant hemoglobin will not separate from Hb A on routine electrophoresis.

Specimen Whole blood

Container Lavender top (EDTA) tube

Causes for Rejection Specimen more than 4 hours old

Reference Interval Less than 1% unstable hemoglobin (quantitation by hemoglobinometry of centrifuged lysate). Normally, test should result in little or no precipitate. A positive result (denatured hemoglobin present) is the presence of turbidity and/or fine flocculation, a readily visible precipitate.

Use Determine the presence of unstable hemoglobins, most of which will not be identified by routine hemoglobin electrophoresis

Limitations False-negative results may occur if only a small amount of abnormal hemoglobin is present. The visual end point in this test may be difficult to interpret. Test should be run along with a normal control. Some degree of slight precipitation may occur in an erratic manner in normals. Quantitation of % unstable hemoglobin (by hemoglobinometry) is desirable. Result can be compared to the isopropanol precipitation test for unstable hemoglobin (see Hemoglobin, Unstable - Isopropanol Precipitation Test *on page 448*).

Methodology Washed cells lysed, acidified, lysate heated at 50°C for 1 hour and examined for turbidity/flocculation (compared to control). Percent unstable hemoglobin may be reported.

Additional Information Another approach to detection of unstable hemoglobins is to search for Heinz bodies. Heinz body test is less specific than heat instability study. Hemolysates containing unstable hemoglobin may precipitate spontaneously on standing a few days in the refrigerator. Some unstable hemoglobins are associated with hemolytic anemia and an appropriate clinical picture including intermittent jaundice and usually splenomegaly. If hypersplenism is present there may be thrombocytopenia. There have been many different unstable hemoglobins reported after the identification of Hb Köln as a cause of "congenital Heinz body anemia".[1] Lukens and Lee in the 10th edition (1999) of *Wintrobe's Clinical Hematology* indicate that some 200 different unstable hemoglobin mutants have been identified.[2] The most common unstable Hb variant is Hb Köln which has wide geographic distribution. Hb Köln is the result of replacement of the amino acid valine by methionine at position 98 of the β-chain (a β98 val → met substitution). A number of unstable hemoglobins have altered oxygen affinity, with Hb Köln, affinity is increased. Such patients have impaired delivery of oxygen to tissues (as compared with normal hemoglobin), the tissue hypoxia results in compensatory increase in erythropoietin production and thus, marrow erythropoiesis. This accounts for higher Hct levels than expected on the basis of severity of hemolysis. Splenectomy (performed in some cases of unstable hemoglobin disease to ameliorate number and severity of hemolytic episodes) may (if the hemoglobin also has high oxygen affinity) result in postsplenectomy polycythemia and thrombotic vascular complications.[3] Hb Zurich (a β63 His → Arg substitution), is an unstable hemoglobin with drug-induced (usually sulfonamide) hemolytic anemia that is ameliorated by smoking. Hb Zurich has a markedly increased

(Continued)

Hemoglobin, Unstable, Heat Labile Test *(Continued)*

affinity for carbon monoxide which stabilizes the molecule against oxidant stresses of drug sensitization. Most unstable hemoglobins have been demonstrated only in single individuals or families. Nearly all unstable hemoglobin diseases have an autosomal dominant mode of inheritance; most patients are heterozygotes.

Footnotes

1. Carrell RW and Lehmann H, "Haemoglobin Köln (β-98 Valine → Methionine): An Unstable Protein Causing Inclusion-Body Anaemia," *Nature*, 1966, 210(5039):915-6.
2. Lukens J and Lee GR, "Unstable Hemoglobin Disease," *Wintrobe's Clinical Hematology*, Lee GR, Foerster J, Lukens J, et al, eds, 10th ed, Volume 1, Chapter 52, Baltimore, MD: Lippincott Williams & Wilkins, 1999, 1398-404.
3. Thuret I, Bardakdjian J, Badens C, et al, "Priapism Following Splenectomy in an Unstable Hemoglobin: Hemoglobin Olmsted β141 (H19) Leu→Arg," *Am J Hematol*, 1996, 51(2):133-6.

References

Bunn HF, "Human Hemoglobins: Sickle Hemoglobin and Other Mutants," *The Molecular Basis of Blood Diseases*, 3rd ed, Chapter 7, Stamatoyannopoulos G, Majerus PW, Perlmutter RM, et al, eds, Philadelphia, PA: WB Saunders Co, 2001, 227-73.

Safko R, "Anemias of Abnormal Globin Development - Hemoglobinopathies," *Clinical Hematology: Principles, Procedures, Correlation*, 2nd ed, Chapter 14, Stiene-Martin EA, Lotspeich-Steininger CA, and Koepke JA, eds, Philadelphia, PA: Lippincott-Raven Publishers, 1998, 209-12.

Williamson D, "The Unstable Haemoglobins," *Blood Rev*, 1993, 7(3):146-63.

Zinkham WH and Winslow RM, "Unstable Hemoglobins: Influence of Environment on Phenotypic Expression of a Genetic Disorder," *Medicine (Baltimore)*, 1989, 68(5):309-20.

Hemoglobin, Unstable - Isopropanol Precipitation Test

Related Information

Heinz Body Stain *on page 440*
Hemoglobin, Unstable, Heat Labile Test *on page 447*
n-Butanol Stability Test *on page 460*

Synonyms Unstable Hemoglobins

Applies to Carboxyhemoglobin; Hb Zurich; Heinz Bodies

Abstract A simple, low cost test for unstable hemoglobins. Most of such variant hemoglobins will not be detected by routine hemoglobin electrophoresis as they migrate with Hb A.

Specimen Whole blood

Container Lavender top (EDTA) tube

Storage Instructions Fresh blood should be used. Sample must be no more than 1 week old.[1]

Reference Interval Absence of a precipitate in buffered isopropanol. Solution should remain clear for 30-40 minutes.

Use Differential diagnosis of hemolytic anemias; detect unstable hemoglobins many of which will not be identified (separated from Hb A) by standard electrophoretic techniques

Limitations Hemoglobin F begins to precipitate about halfway through the incubation period - about the time that one expects unstable Hb to appear. If the patient's Hb F is increased (>4%), a false-positive result for unstable Hb may result.[1] Unstable Hb Zurich has increased affinity for carbon monoxide which stabilizes the molecule against denaturing effect of isopropanol. The rate of isopropanol-induced precipitation varies inversely with carboxyhemoglobin levels in patients with Hb Zurich.[2]

Methodology Mix 2 mL of 17% (unit/unit) isopropanol with 0.2 mL of hemolysate. Incubate at 37°C; check for precipitate at 20 minutes.

Additional Information Heat lability, n-butanol, and Heinz body tests are also applicable to the detection and study of unstable hemoglobins. While simple to perform, interpretation may be difficult. A multitest approach has merit.

Footnotes

1. Brozovic M and Henthorn J (revised by), "Investigation of Abnormal Haemoglobins and Thalassemia," *Practical Haematology*, 8th ed, Chapter 14, Dacie JV and Lewis SM, eds, New York, NY: Churchill Livingstone, 1995, 268-70.
2. Lukens JN and Lee GR, "Unstable Hemoglobin Disease," *Wintrobe's Clinical Hematology*, 10th ed, Volume 1, Chapter 52, Lee GR, Foerster J, Lukens J, et al, Philadelphia, PA: Lippincott Williams & Wilkins, 1999, 1401.

References

Beutler E, Lichtman MA, Coller BS, et al, *Williams Hematology*, 5th ed, Chapters 57 and L34, New York, NY: McGraw-Hill Inc, 1995, 650-4 and L34.

Carrell RW and Kay R, "A Simple Method for the Detection of Unstable Hemoglobins," *Br J Haematol*, 1972, 23:615-9.

Zinkham WH and Winslow RM, "Unstable Hemoglobins: Influence of Environment on Phenotypic Expression of a Genetic Disorder," *Medicine (Baltimore)*, 1989, 68(5):309-20.

♦ **Hemogram** *see* Complete Blood Count *on page 419*

♦ **Hemosiderin Stain** *see* Iron Stain, Bone Marrow *on page 452*

♦ **Hemosiderin Stain** *see* Siderocyte Stain *on page 487*

♦ **Hereditary Macrothrombocytopenia** *see* Platelet Count *on page 468*

♦ **Hereditary Thrombocythemia** *see* Thrombopoietin, Serum or Plasma *on page 491*

♦ **Hexosaminidase A** *see* Inherited Diseases of Metabolism and Cell Structure *on page 449*

♦ **Hexosaminidase B** *see* Inherited Diseases of Metabolism and Cell Structure *on page 449*

♦ **Hgb** *see* Hemoglobin *on page 442*

♦ **Highly Fluorescent Reticulocytes** *see* Reticulocyte Count *on page 481*

♦ **Histidine-Rich Protein (HRP-2)** *see* Malaria Smear and Tests *on page 458*

♦ **Homoglobinopathies, Unstable** *see* Heinz Body Stain *on page 440*

♦ **Howell-Jolly Bodies** *see* Peripheral Blood: Differential Leukocyte Count *on page 464*

♦ **Human Genome Project** *see* Inherited Diseases of Metabolism and Cell Structure *on page 449*

♦ **Human Polymerized Hemoglobin** *see* Hemoglobin, Plasma *on page 446*

♦ **Hyaline Globules** *see* Apoptosis Assays *on page 402*

♦ **Hydroxyurea** *see* Sickle Cell Tests *on page 486*

Hypertonic Cryohemolysis Test

Related Information

Autohemolysis Test *on page 405*
Glucose-6-Phosphate Dehydrogenase, Quantitative, Blood *on page 437*
Glucose-6-Phosphate Dehydrogenase Screen, Blood *on page 438*
Osmotic Fragility *on page 462*
Osmotic Fragility, Incubated *on page 463*
Peripheral Blood: Red Blood Cell Morphology *on page 467*
Pyruvate Kinase Assay, Erythrocytes *on page 474*
Red Blood Cell Enzyme Deficiency, Quantitative *on page 475*

Synonyms Cryohemolysis Test

Abstract Red blood cells from patients with hereditary spherocytosis (HS) are susceptible to hemolysis when suspended in hypertonic solution, incubated at 37°C, and then kept at 0°C. This hypertonic cryohemolysis test is said to be sensitive to essentially all cases of HS including asymptomatic carriers. Specificity of the test is <100% and is not fully established.[1]

Specimen Fresh whole blood, at least 3 mL

Container Lavender top (EDTA) tube

Storage Instructions Do not store sample over one day.

Causes for Rejection Anticoagulated blood, hemolysis

Reference Interval 3% to 5% (hemolysis of red cells)[2]

Limitations Specificity of this test for HS is not yet fully defined.

Methodology Red cells washed in cold saline are placed in warm (37°C) buffered 0.7 M sucrose, incubated for 10 minutes, placed in an ice cold bath for 10 minutes, vortexed, and centrifuged. Absorbance of the supernatant is read at 540 nm and % cryohemolysis is calculated as a ratio of 100% hemolysis (determined as a result of red cells placed in deionized water).

Additional Information Red blood cells in a hypertonic environment undergo significant hemolysis when cooled rapidly from 37°C to 0°C.[2] This may relate to the lipid bilayer of the cell membrane changing from a fluid to a gel. Erythrocytes of hereditary spherocytosis are especially susceptible to hypertonic cryohemolysis.[2] This sensitivity of HS red cells has been confirmed[3] and forms the basis of a new test (subject of this listing) for hereditary spherocytosis.[4] Increased cryohemolysis is also seen in some forms of hereditary elliptocytosis[3] and in some cases of HEMPAS (hereditary erythroblast multinuclearity with positive acidified serum test) - a form of congenital dyserythropoietic anemia (CDA Type II).[4] See Ham Test *on page 439*. The heterogeneous nature of HS relates to a variety of underlying inherited molecular defects in red cell structural proteins including spectrin, ankyrin, band 3, and protein 4.2.[5,6] The cryohemolysis test identifies mild forms and asymptomatic carriers of HS and in this regard is more sensitive than the osmotic fragility and autohemolysis tests. This sensitivity may relate to the mechanism of cryohemolysis which appears to relate to structural protein defects rather than to the surface area to volume ratio (which may not be sufficiently decreased to be detected by osmotic fragility studies).[2]

Footnotes

1. Gallagher PG, Forget BC, and Lux SE, "Disorders of the Erythrocyte Membrane," *Hematology of Infancy and Childhood*, 5th ed, Chapter 16, Nathan DG and Oski SH, eds, Philadelphia, PA: WB Saunders Co, 1998, 594-6.
2. Streichman S and Gesheidt Y, "Cryohemolysis for the Detection of Hereditary Spherocytosis: Correlation Studies With Osmotic Fragility and Autohemolysis," *Am J Hematol*, 1998, 58(3):206-12.
3. Melrose WD, "An Evaluation of the Hypertonic Cryohemolysis Test as a Diagnostic Test for Hereditary Spherocytosis," *Austral J Med Sci*, 1992, 13(1):22.
4. Streichman S, Gesheidt Y, and Tatarsky I, "Hypertonic Cryohemolysis: A Diagnostic Test for Hereditary Spherocytosis," *Am J Hematol*, 1990, 35(2):104-9.
5. Hassoun H, Vassiliadis JN, Murray J, et al, "Characterization of the Underlying Molecular Defect in Hereditary Spherocytosis Associated With Spectrin Deficiency," *Blood*, 1997, 90(1):398-406.
6. Liu SC, Zhai S, Palek J, et al, "Molecular Defect of the Band 3 Protein in Southeast Asian Ovalocytosis," *N Engl J Med*, 1990, 323(22):1530-8.

References

Streichman S, Kahana E, and Tatarsky I, "Hypertonic Cryohemolysis of Pathologic Red Blood Cells," *Am J Hematol*, 1985, 20(4):373-81.

Inherited Diseases of Metabolism and Cell Structure

Related Information

Amniotic Fluid, Chromosome and Genetic Abnormality Analysis *on page 360*

Beta-Hexosaminidase, Serum, White Blood Cells *on page 114*

Chorionic Villus Sampling, Chromosome and Genetic Abnormality Analysis *on page 361*

Methylmalonic Acid, Serum, Plasma, Urine, or Amniotic Fluid *on page 224*

Mevalonic Acid, Urine or Amniotic Fluid *on page 225*

Mucopolysaccharides, Urine *on page 226*

Muscle Biopsy *on page 69*

Urinalysis *on page 887*

Synonyms Glycogen Storage Diseases; Inborn Errors of Metabolism; Large Molecule Diseases; Lipidoses; Lysosomal Storage Diseases; Mucolipidoses; Mucopolysaccharidoses; Small Molecule Diseases; Sphingolipidoses; Storage Disorders; Tests for Uncommon Inherited Diseases of Metabolism and Cell Structure

Applies to ABC Proteins; Acid β-Galactosidase; Adrenoleukodystrophy; Amino Acid Screen, Plasma; Amino Acid Screen Qualitative, Urine; Berry Spot Test; Ceramidase; Ceramidetrihexoside α-Galactosidase; Crash Syndrome; Farber Disease; Friedreich Ataxia; α-Fucosidase; Galactocerebroside; β-Galactosidase; Glucocerebroside; β-Glucosidase; Hexosaminidase A; Hexosaminidase B; Human Genome Project; Krabbe Disease; Leigh Syndrome; Merosin; Metachromatic Leukodystrophy; Neutral β-Galactosidase; Peroxisomes; Persistent Hyperinsulinemic Hypoglycemia of Infancy; Sandhoff Disease; Shindler Disease; Sphingomyelinase; Steroid Sulfatase Deficiency; Sulfatidase; Sulfonylurea Receptor; Zellweger Syndrome

Test Includes Under this heading recognition is given to an ever growing number of genetically determined disorders having a biochemical/metabolic defect (usually an enzyme deficiency or abnormality). The limitations of space allow only brief mention. Most of these disorders can be categorized as to biochemical type (eg, sphingolipidoses, mucopolysaccharidoses, lysosomal storage diseases, glycogen storage diseases, mitochondrial disorders) with overlap between these concepts and with some independent entities.

Of some 500 diseases with a defined biochemical basis, a majority involve abnormalities in enzymes, receptors, and/or structural proteins. The 7th (1995) edition of the monumental text, *The Metabolic and Molecular Bases of Inherited Disease* (with 302 authors) has descriptions of inborn errors of metabolism that include some 900 entities tabulated over 4605 pages. They are grouped by biochemical type (eg, carbohydrate, amino acid, lipoprotein/lipid, purine/pyrimidine, acid lipase), tissue/function type (eg, blood and blood forming organs, transport, peroxisome, immune, etc) and include some 70 **disorders of lysosomal enzymes**, with which this listing will be largely concerned. Clinical features (eg, age at onset, severity, signs and symptoms) may show considerable variation within diagnostic groups. Over 54 specific mutations responsible for the G_{M2} gangliosidoses (includes Tay-Sachs disease and Sandhoff disease) have been characterized. The 12th edition of McKusick's *Mendelian Inheritance in Man (MIM)* lists 8587 (including 2082 new entries) human genes and their disorders as of early June 1997 with 56,163 journal reference citations and including 1644 clinical disorders that have been mapped to specific chromosomal sites. This synopsis of the map of the human genome is updated nearly daily in a computer accessible on line database (catalog) available from the William H Welch Medical Library (Johns Hopkins University School of Medicine). OMIM™ (Online Mendelian Inheritance in Man), an online version of MIM (which is continuously updated), is available on the World Wide Web (Internet) from the National Center for Biotechnology Information (NCBI) at the National Library of Medicine, Bethesda, Maryland. Access is provided by NCBI at http://www.nlm.nih.gov/omim/. Questions about OMIM™ access may be directed to NCBI at (301) 496-2475. The OMIM™ database can be searched by an author's name, a word, or combination of words. A CD-Rom version of OMIM™ (MIM-CD™) is available from the Johns Hopkins University Press, Hampden Station, Baltimore, MD, #21211, or http://www.press.jhu.edu/home.html.

Abstract Inherited diseases of metabolism/cell structure include a very large array of clinical disorders with a variety of underlying genetic bases. Many represent a specific enzyme deficiency with resultant excessive accumulation of substances (substrates) usually present in only small amounts. The disorders range from acute life-threatening crises to episodic conditions with prolonged asymptomatic periods or with developmental delay. Presentation in the pediatric age group is common and as indicated in the reference by Lindor and Karnes, rapid diagnosis and institution of therapy may be lifesaving or may be important to optimizing long-term outcome.

Patient Preparation Appropriate preliminary studies may be critically important to allow narrowing the range of diagnostic testing possibilities. Such investigation might include eye examination (cherry red macula occurs in some gangliosidoses; corneal opacities in Fabry disease; optic atrophy in metachromatic leukodystrophy and Krabbe disease); blood/urine screening tests (Berry spot test positive in G_{M1} gangliosidosis; anemia; vacuolated lymphocytes in fucosidosis and other lysosomal storage diseases - see Mucopolysaccharides, Urine *on page 226*); x-ray studies (for developmental changes in bone as with mucopolysaccharidoses; EEG, nerve conduction time, and bone marrow in search of inclusion bearing or foamy histocytes, eg, as with Gaucher cells). A variety of dietary, pharmacologic, microbiologic, and environmental, as well as analytic factors, may complicate urine testing for organic acidurias (see table).[1]

Nonorganinc Acid Origins of Organic Acidurias

Diagnostic Organic Acid	Associated Organic Acidurias*	Nonorganic Acid Origins
2-oxoglutaric acid	Dihydrolipolyl dehydrogenase (E3) deficiency	Krebs cycle and acid-base alterations
3-OH isovaleric acid	3-methylcrotonyl CoA carboxylase deficiency, 3-methylglutaconyl-CoA hydratase deficiency, 3-OH 3-methylglutaric aciduria, biotinidase deficiency, holocarboxylase synthetase deficiency	Severe ketosis
3-OH propionic acid	Biotinidase deficiency, holocarboxylase synthetase deficiency, methylmalonicaciduria, propionic acidemia	Bacterial origin
4-OH phenylacetic acid	Tyrosinemia	Bacterial origin
5-oxoproline	5-oxoprolinuria, hawkinsinuria	Drug depletion of glutathione
Acetyl-L-tyrosine	Tyrosinemia	Amino acid solution therapy
Adipic acid	Medium-chain acyl-CoA dehydrogenase deficiency, glutaric aciduria type II	Dietary: gelatin and MCT feedings
Azelaic and pimelic acids	Short-chain acyl-CoA dehydrogenase deficiency	Plastic container storage
Dicarboxylic aciduria	Short-chain acyl-CoA dehydrogenase deficiency	MCT feedings; container storage
Lactic acid	Biotinidase deficiency, holocarboxylase synthetase deficiency, lactic acidosis	Bacterial origin and artifactual isomers
Fumaric acid	Fumarase deficiency	Krebs cycle and acid-base alterations
Glycerol	Glyceroluria	Pharmaceutical preparations and ointments
Glycolic acid	Hyperoxaluria type I	Ethylene glycol poisoning
Long-chain organic acids	Lysosomal storage disorders	Equipment conditions

*Sweetman L, "Organic Acid Analysis," *Techniques in Diagnostic Human Biochemical Genetics: A Laboratory Manual*, Hommes FA, ed. New York, NY: Wiley-Liss, 1991, 165-71.

MCT = medium-chain triglyceride containing diet.

Adapted from Joseph F and Russo TM, "Origins of Spurious Organic Acidurias," *Clin Chem*, 2000, 31(11):622.

It has been recommended that urine specimens submitted for organic acid testing be accompanied by a completed query form indicating patient's diet, medication and specimen handling information (eg, when was specimen frozen).[1]

Specimen The majority of tests in this area involve lysosomal enzymes, present in body tissues and fluids. Blood (serum, plasma, or white cells), urine, and tears are the most easily obtained samples for analysis. Solid tissue may be biopsied (eg, skin, liver, muscle). Most commonly used are serum, leukocytes,[2] and cultured fibroblasts (from tissue biopsy).[2] Heparin anticoagulated whole blood, usually at least 5 mL is needed, along with the serum. Specimen preference may be disease dependent (eg, the α-glucosidase deficiency of Pompe disease is best detected by using cultured skin fibroblasts or skeletal muscle). Leukocytes provide a favorable substrate for sphingolipidosis testing but for detection of heterozygotes of Niemann-Pick or Krabbe disease DNA mutation analysis may be required. Use of cultured fibroblasts (with analysis of fatty acid oxidation intermediates) may be preferable for the diagnosis of mitochondrial oxidation disorders.[3] Referral of a leukocyte pellet or biopsy in culture media or even a growing culture of fibroblasts may be required. Molecular analysis for identification of a specific gene defect may be applicable usually with more readily obtained specimen (eg, whole blood).

Turnaround Time Approximately 1 week

Special Instructions For a number of reasons (a sampling follows), the reference laboratory should be contacted before specimens are sent. Details of the preliminary findings can be reviewed, appropriate tests (Continued)

Inherited Diseases of Metabolism and Cell Structure (Continued)

recommended, the preferred samples obtained, need for a clinical photograph established, mode of transport decided, and any other special requirement arranged.

Use Assist in the diagnosis of sphingolipid and mucopolysaccharide lysosomal storage diseases by demonstrating presence of a partial or complete enzyme deficiency. Major symptoms, lipids accumulating, and enzymes involved in the sphingolipidoses are given in the table.

Sphingolipid Storage Diseases (Sphingolipidoses)

Disease	Signs and Symptoms	Enzyme Defect
Fabry disease	Reddish-purple skin rash, kidney failure, pain in lower extremities	Ceramidetrihexoside-α-galactosidase
Farber disease	Hoarseness, dermatitis, skeletal deformation, mental retardation	Ceramidase
Fucosidosis	Cerebral degeneration, muscle spasticity, thick skin	α-fucosidase
Gaucher disease	Spleen and liver enlargement, erosion of long bones and pelvis, mental retardation only in infantile form	Glucocerebroside-β-glucosidase
Generalized gangliosidosis	Mental retardation, liver enlargement, skeletal deformities, about 50% with red spot in retina	β-galactosidase
Krabbe disease (globoid leukodystrophy)	Mental retardation, almost total absence of myelin, globoid bodies in white matter of brain	Galactocerebroside-β-galactosidase
Niemann-Pick disease type I, II and subtypes	Liver and spleen enlargement, mental retardation, about 30% with red spot in retina	Sphingomyelinase
Metachromatic leukodystrophy	Mental retardation, psychological disturbances in adult form, nerves stain yellow-brown with cresyl violet dye	Sulfatidase
Sandhoff disease	Same as Tay-Sachs disease but progressing more rapidly	Hexosaminidase A and B
Shindler disease	Neurodegeneration, psychomotor retardation, cortical blindness, myoclonic seizures	α-N-acetyl-galactosaminidase
Tay-Sachs disease	Mental retardation, red spot in retina, blindness, muscular weakness	Hexosaminidase A

Adapted from Brady RO and Kolodny EH, "The Sphingolipid Storage Disorders: Diagnosis and Detection," *Lab Management*, 1982, 20:28.

Methodology Tests for enzyme deficiency utilizing synthetic substrates (eg, monosaccharide derivatives of 4-methylumbelliferone) have found growing application in this group of diseases.[2,4] In addition to serum or plasma assays, tests utilizing pelleted leukocytes and fibroblast cultures are used. Molecular analyses for identification of a specific gene defect utilizing specific restriction fragment length polymorphism (RFLP), polymerase chain reaction (PCR), synthetic oligonucleotide probes, DNA sequencing, and/or study of linked chromosomal anomalous DNA sequences may be used.[2,5] They may be particularly helpful for identification of heterozygosity.

In the past few years, electrospray tandem mass spectrometry (MS/MS) has been applied to the quantification of amino acids and acylcarnitines in blood spots to screen for metabolic disorders (in particular aminoacidopathies and organic acidurias) of the neonate.[6,7] MS/MS provides an automated, high throughout and broad spectrum screening method (that can replace bacterial inhibition assays) and requires just 2 minutes of analytic time per specimen.

Additional Information The phrase "inborn errors of metabolism" is relatively nonspecific. With continually evolving insight, as provided at the level of molecular biology, the terms "inborn" and "errors of metabolism" are likely overly inclusive. In general usage, "inborn errors of metabolism" refers to numerous disorders that have a genetic basis and are characterized by accumulation of a metabolite that cannot be degraded, usually the result of an enzyme deficiency (absence, partial absence, or functional absence of specific enzyme molecules). The lysosomal storage diseases are the primary examples of such "inborn errors," resulting from an intralysosomal accumulation of metabolites that would normally be degraded by a lysosomal enzyme.[2]

One group of lysosomal storage diseases, the mucopolysaccharidoses are due to genetic defects in enzymes that degrade connective tissue glycosaminoglycan. The table relates the type of mucopolysaccharidosis to the enzyme defect. Urine screening tests are available for initial diagnosis of these diseases (see Mucopolysaccharides, Urine *on page 226*).

A table of glycogen storage diseases follows. Most of these disorders of carbohydrate metabolism are not lysosomal storage diseases. They are all autosomal recessive except one form of liver phosphorylase kinase deficiency in which only males are affected and the inheritance is X-linked.[8]

Mucopolysaccharidoses

Type	Eponymic Designation	Lysosomal Enzyme Defect
I	Three allelic disorders Hurler-Scheie	α-L-iduronidase
II	Hunter severe, mild	Iduronate sulfatase
III (A-D)	Four nonallelic disorders Sanfilippo syndromes A-D	IIIA Heparan N-sulfatase IIIB N-acetyl-α-D-glucosaminidase IIIC Acetyl-CoA: α-glucosaminide N-acetyl transferase IIID N-acetyl-α-D-glucosaminide 6-sulfate sulfatase
IV (A,B)	Two nonallelic disorders Morquio syndromes A,B	IVA Galactosamine 6-sulfate sulfatase IVB β-galactosidase
VI	Several allelic types Maroteaux-Lamy syndrome	Arylsulfatase B
VII	Sly syndrome	β-glucuronidase

Glycogen Storage Diseases

I	von Gierke Ia, Ib	Glucose-6-phosphatase
II	Pompe infantile, adult form	Lysosomal α-1,4-glucosidase
III	Cori Forbe	Amylo-1,6-glucosidase (debrancher enzyme)
IV	Andersen	Amylo-(1,4:1,6)-transglucosidase (brancher enzyme)
V	McArdle	Muscle phosphorylase
VI	Hers, glycogenoses	Hepatic phosphorylase X-linked phosphorylase-β-kinase Autosomal phosphorylase-β-kinase
VII	Tarui	Muscle phosphofructokinase

Disease severity and symptoms vary widely with type and organ site of the defective enzyme activity.

The recognized spectrum of inherited abnormalities of metabolism and structure is continually enlarging. The majority are uncommon to rare, so that resources of equipment and experienced personnel for testing are justifiably limited to the specialized laboratory. Even so there are enough laboratories performing these assays so as to raise the question if any **one** can develop necessary case experience. Dialogue between the referring physician and the specialty laboratory is essential (discussed above in relation to technical considerations) in particular because of the biochemical heterogeneity frequently seen in these conditions. Clinical expression may be variable and unpredictable.

Each of the sphingolipidoses represents not one but several diseases differing in clinical signs and/or enzyme activity. They are characterized by differing age of onset, site of pathology, and amount of residual enzyme activity (total or partial deficiency). As in Tay-Sachs disease more than one form of the involved enzyme may be present. Two lysosomal glycoproteins (hexosaminidase A and G_{M2} activator protein) account for the enzymatic hydrolysis of glycolipids (largely ganglioside G_{M2}). With defective lysosomal degradation, glycolipid accumulates in neurones. Hexosaminidase A is formed of subunits α and β, each under different chromosome control. Hexosaminidase, the enzyme involved exists as two isoenzymes, A and B. In Tay-Sachs disease, hexosaminidase A is decreased or absent while hexosaminidase B is increased. In Sandhoff's disease, a variant form of Tay-Sachs, there is deficiency of both hexosaminidase A and B due to hexosaminidase β-subunit defect (encoded on chromosome 5).[9] In addition, the usual sources of variance may affect enzyme deficiency testing. The activity of β-N-acetyl hexosaminidases in Tay-Sachs is affected by pregnancy, chronic diseases of liver, heart, joints, endocrine system, skin and medications including oral contraceptives, some steroids, thyroid, and Butazolidin®. These factors do not affect the result of hexosaminidase assays performed on leukocytes, fibroblasts, or tears.

Sphingolipid storage diseases involve most cells of the body and thus are expressed as multisystem diseases. Gaucher disease is the most common and may show hepatosplenomegaly, thrombocytopenia, erosion of bone with tendency to pathologic fracture and in a few cases, CNS involvement. All of the lipid storage diseases show autosomal recessive inheritance with the exception of Fabry disease (which is transmitted as X-linked).

The advent of treatment strategies (eg, enzyme infusion,[10] use of recombinant enzymes, and gene therapy) may add further impetus to establishing the diagnosis, detection of carriers, and monitoring of pregnancies at risk (through amniocentesis and culturing of epithelial cells in the amniotic fluid). Macrophage-targeted natural and recombinant glucocerebrosidase is now available for the treatment of Gaucher disease.[10] Imiglucerase (recombinant acid β-glucosidase), replacing the human placental-derived aglucerase, is still associated with hypersensitivity reactions, usually mild to moderate. A severe near-anaphylactic response to imiglucerase, however, has been observed.[11]

Steroid sulfatase deficiency, characterized clinically by low maternal estrogen excretion with normal fetal growth/development, is important to recognize by antenatal diagnosis so that it can be differentiated from more serious fetal defects that are associated with low estrogen levels.[12]

Peroxisomes, cellular organelles involved in oxidative functions are deficient in cases of Zellweger syndrome. There is accumulation of long chain fatty acids, phytanic acid, pipecolic acid, bile acid intermediates, and lack of plasmalogen biosynthesis. Other diseases in this group include adrenoleukodystrophy and a form of chondrodysplasia punctata.[13]

Increased understanding of the molecular pathophysiology responsible for conditions previously catalogued as peroxisomal, mitochondrial, or other (site) disorders has led to the development of classifications (of inborn errors), and in some cases, cross-classifications that are focused upon basic structural biochemical mechanisms. Such clinically diverse conditions as adrenoleukodystrophy (ALD), the cerebro-hepato-renal syndrome of Zellweger, persistent hyperinsulinemic hypoglycemia of infancy (PHHI), a rare disease due to a mutation of the gene for the sulfonylurea receptor (SUR1), and cystic fibrosis (CF) can be considered to be the result of mutated human ABC proteins.[14]

ABC (ATP binding cassette) proteins are one of the largest protein families. Their rapid identification relates to progress of the Human Genome Project and other mass sequencing projects. Over half of human ABC proteins have been discovered in the past few years. Some 30 ABC proteins have been fully sequenced. ABC proteins are formed of transmembrane domains (TMDs) and nucleotide binding domains (NBDs or ATP-binding cassettes) and are defined by presence of the "ABC unit." The latter is a 200-250 amino acid "mini" protein that includes two conserved peptide sequences (Walker A and Walker B). These are involved in ATP binding and are present in other ATP-utilizing proteins. An "ABC signature" protein, also diagnostic to the ABC unit, is present between Walker A and B.[14] ABC proteins serve largely as membrane transporters (translocate a variety of substrates to various compartments) accounting for a wide spectrum of functions. These proteins are further defined structurally by the characteristics of their TMDs and ABCs.

Members of the ABC protein family can be grouped into eight subfamilies:[14]

- **MDR/TAP**: Includes multidrug resistance transporters.
- **ALD**: Members of this adrenoleukodystrophy (ALD) protein are localized to the peroxisomal membrane, mutant forms are involved in peroxisomal disorders (PD) including the most frequent PD, ALD, a severe x-linked neurodegenerative disorder that affects some 1/20,000 males.
- **MRP/CFTR**: The human multidrug resistance-associated protein (hMRP1) confers a drug resistant phenotype to tumor cells. SUR1 interacts with the sulfonylurea receptor and inhibits the conductance of ATP-dependent potassium channels. CFTR forms a cAMP activated chloride channel and is involved in the pathogenesis of CF, one of the most common inherited diseases (prevalence 1:2500 births).
- **ABC1**: Includes hABCR, human retinal ABC transporter
- **White**: ABC8/h white, involved in mitoxantrone and breast cancer resistance and possibly in neurodegenerative disorders
- **OABP**: RNAse L inhibitor
- **ANSA**: ars A and ars B gene products complex and transport arsenite and antimonite out of bacteria
- **GCN20**: ABC50 protein, may not be a transporter

See the references by Applegarth et al, Burlina et al,[6] Shih VE, and the text by Scriver et al for investigation of small molecule diseases; organic acid, urea cycle, and peroxisomal disorders.

Disorders considered to be mitochondrial based include defects in fatty acid oxidation, pyruvate metabolism, and the respiratory chain (due to abnormal enzyme structure/function) and are of especial importance in neonates relating in part to their high energy requirements. Mitochondrial-based disorders may result from defects in mitochondrial DNA (mtDNA) or in nuclear DNA (nDNA). Mitochondria contain their own genetic material, 16,569 base pairs long and encoding 13 respiratory chain proteins, 2 ribosomal proteins, and tRNAs required for assembly of these proteins.[15] Mitochondrial function is thus under dual genetic control (from both mtDNA and nDNA). Over 100 different rearrangements and 50 different point mutations involving mtDNA have been associated with human disease.

HUMAN MITOCHONDRIAL DISORDERS[16]

Mitochondrial DNA Defects
Rearrangements (deletions and duplications, >100 identified)
Chronic progressive external ophthalmoplegia (CPEO)
Kearns-Sayre syndrome
Diabetes and deafness

Point mutations (mtDNA nucleotide positions are on the L-chain) (currently >50 identified)
Protein-encoding genes

Leber hereditary optic neuropathy (G11778A, T14484C, G3460A)
Leber hereditary optic neuropathy/dystonia (G14459A, T14569A)
Neurogenic weakness, ataxia, and retinitis pigmentosa (T8993G/C)
Leigh syndrome (T8993G/C)
tRNA genes
Mitochondrial encephalopathy with lactic acidosis and stroke-like episodes (A3243G, T3271C, A3251G)
Myoclonic epilepsy with ragged-red fibers (A8344G, T8356C)
CPEO (A3243G, T4274C)
Myopathy (T14709C, A12320G)
Cardiomyopathy (A3243G, A4269G)
Diabetes and deafness (A3243G, C12258A)
Encephalomyopathy (G1606A, T10010C)
Leigh syndrome (G1644T)
tRNA genes
Nonsyndromic sensorineural deafness (A7445G)
Aminoglycoside-induced nonsyndromic deafness (A15556)

Nuclear DNA Defects
Nuclear genetic disorders with a mitochondrial basis
Friedreich ataxia (frataxin)
Autosomal-recessive hereditary spastic paraplegia (paraplegin)
Wilson disease (P-type ATPase)

Nuclear genetic disorders of the mitochondrial respiratory chain
Leigh syndrome (complex I deficiency - mutations in AQDQ subunit on chromosome 5)
Optic atrophy and ataxia (complex II deficiency - mutations in Fp subunit of SDH on chromosome 3)
Leigh syndrome (complex IV deficiency - mutations in SURF I gene on chromosome 9q1)

Nuclear genetic disorders associated with multiple mtDNA deletions
Autosomal dominant external ophthalmoplegia (chromosome 10q23.3-q24.3; 3p14.1-21.2)
Mitochondrial neurogastrointestinal encephalomyopathy (thymidine phosphorylase deficiency) - mutations in thymidine phosphorylase gene on chromosome 22q13.32-qter

Mutated and wild type (normal) mtDNA may exist in cells together (heteroplasmy) complicating the analysis and clinical expression of mtDNA and its genetic variants.[17] The mutated mtDNA must reach threshold levels before cellular expression can occur. It may be difficult to document the presence of mtDNA disease. Careful consideration and assimilation of clinical and laboratory data is necessary. In some cases, analysis of skeletal muscle may be required (eg, histochemical study that may reveal subsarcolemmal accumulation of mitochondria ("ragged-red fibers") or mosaic deficiency of cytochrome c oxidase - absence of these findings does not exclude the diagnosis). Analysis of DNA extracted from muscle may be necessary for diagnosis.[16]

The neonate with a mitochondrial-based metabolic disorder may present clinically with hypotonia, lethargy, feeding and respiratory difficulties, failure to thrive, psychomotor delay, seizures, and/or vomiting. Laboratory results that may lead to a diagnosis include abnormal levels of lactate, pyruvate, lactate:pyruvate ratio, glucose, and ketone bodies.[15]

Inborn errors of metabolism may have broad and devastating effects on the development and function of the nervous system. A recent compilation of inherited metabolic disorders having neurologic involvement and with adult onset includes nearly 40 entities (exclusive of subtypes). Included are lysosomal storage diseases, amino acid disorders, organic acid disorders, peroxisomal disorders, lactic acidaemias, disorders of the glycogenolytic and glycolytic pathway and a number of miscellaneous conditions.[18] The adhesion molecules merosin (laminin-2), Po, and L₁, and their associated clinical conditions, congenital muscular dystrophy, peripheral neuropathies, and crash syndrome, respectively, are detailed in a recent review.[19] Another recent review summarizes diseases that result from glycoprotein oligosaccharide structural alteration and are dependent on the identification of glycoprotein glycoforms that are defined by variation in O- or N-linked oligosaccharides (the latter being covalently linked to proteins through oxygen or nitrogen). There is microheterogeneity of these glycans, wild type glycoproteins consisting of mixtures of glycosylated variants (glycoforms). Inherited diseases involving glycan chemistry and associated enzymes include I-cell disease, congenital disorders of glycosylation, leukocyte adhesion deficiency type II, hereditary erythroblastic multinuclearity with a positive acidified serum test, and Wiskott-Aldrich syndrome.[20]

Footnotes

1. Joseph F and Russo TM, "Origins of Spurious Organic Acidurias," *Lab Med*, 2000, 31(11):622.
2. O'Brien JF, "Lysosomal Storage Disease: Method for the Preparation of Leukocytes," *Tietz Textbook of Clinical Chemistry*, 3rd ed, Chapter 49, Burtis CA and Ashwood ER, eds, Philadelphia, PA: WB Saunders Co, 1999, 1776-84.
3. Pourfarzam M, Schaefer J, Turnbull DM, et al, "Analysis of Fatty Acid Oxidation Intermediates in Cultured Fibroblasts to Detect Mitochondrial Oxidation Disorders," *Clin Chem*, 1994, 40(12):2267-75.
4. Brady RO and Kolodny EH, "The Sphingolipid Storage Disorders: Diagnosis and Detection," *Lab Management*, 1982, 20:7, 30-2.
5. Unger ER and Piper MA, "Nucleic Acid Biochemistry and Diagnostic Applications," *Tietz Textbook of Clinical Chemistry*, 3rd ed, Chapter 18, Burtis CA and Ashwood ER, eds, Philadelphia, PA: WB Saunders Co, 1999, 421-43.
(Continued)

Inherited Diseases of Metabolism and Cell Structure *(Continued)*

6. Burlina AB, Bonafé L, and Zacchello F, "Clinical and Biochemical Approach to the Neonate With a Suspected Inborn Error of Amino Acid and Organic Metabolism," *Semin Perinatol*, 1999, 23(2):162-73.
7. Rashed MS, Rahbeeni Z, and Ozand PT, "Application of Electrospray Tandem Mass Spectrometry to Neonatal Screening," *Semin Perinatol*, 1999, 23(2):183-93.
8. Chen YT and Burchell A, "Glycogen Storage Diseases," *The Metabolic Basis of Inherited Disease*, 7th ed, Chapter 24, Scriver CR, Beaudet AL, Sly WS, et al, eds, New York, NY: McGraw-Hill Inc, 1995, 935-65.
9. Gravel RA, Clarke JT, and Kabuck MM, "The GM2 Gangliosidoses," *The Metabolic Basis of Inherited Disease*, 7th ed, Chapter 92, Scriver CR, Beaudet AL, Sly WS, et al, eds, New York, NY: McGraw-Hill Inc, 1995, 2839-79.
10. Duursma SA, guest ed, "Gaucher Disease, Hematologic, Skeletal, Visceral, and Biochemical Effects: Current Understanding, Recent Advances, and Future Directions," *Semin Hematol*, 1995, 32(3 Suppl 1):1-52.
11. Aviner S, Levy Y, Yaniv I, et al, "Anaphylactoid Reaction to Imiglucerase, but Not to Alglucerase, in a Type I Gaucher Patient," *Blood Cells Mol Dis*, 1999, 25(5):92-4.
12. Sherwood RA and Rocks BF, "Antenatal Diagnosis of Steroid Sulfatase Deficiency: Case Report and Literature Survey," *J Clin Pathol*, 1982, 35(11):1236-9.
13. Moser HW, "Peroxisomal Disorders," *Clin Biochem*, 1991, 24(4):343-51.
14. Klein I, Sarkadi B, and Váradi A, "An Inventory of the Human ABC Proteins," *Biochim Biophys Acta*, 1999, 1461(2):237-62.
15. Sue CM, Hirano M, DiMauro S, et al, "Neonatal Presentations of Mitochondrial Metabolic Disorders," *Semin Perinatol*, 1999, 23(2):113-24.
16. Chinnery PF and Turnbull DM, "Mitochondrial DNA and Disease," *Lancet*, 1999, 354(Suppl 1):SI17-SI21.
17. Lightowlers RN, Chinnery PF, Turnbull DM, et al, "Mammalian Mitochondrial Genetics: Heredity, Heteroplasmy and Disease," *Trends Genet*, 1997, 13(11):450-5.
18. Gray RGF, Preece MA, Green SH, et al, "Inborn Errors of Metabolism as a Cause of Neurological Disease in Adults: An Approach to Investigation," *J Neurol Neurosurg Psychiatry*, 2000 69(1):5-12.
19. Kamiguchi H, Hlavin ML, Yamasaki M, et al, "Adhesion Molecules and Inherited Diseases of the Human Nervous System," *Annu Rev Neurosci*, 1998, 21:97-125.
20. Durand G and Seta N, "Protein Glycosylation and Diseases: Blood and Urinary Oligosaccharides as Markers for Diagnosis and Therapeutic Monitoring," *Clin Chem*, 2000, 46(6 Pt 1):795-805.

References

Applegarth DA, Dimmick JE, and Toone JR, "Laboratory Detection of Metabolic Disease," *Pediatr Clin North Am*, 1989, 36(1):49-65.
Beutler E, Demina A, Laubscher K, et al, "The Clinical Course of Treated and Untreated Gaucher Disease. A Study of 45 Patients," *Blood Cells Mol Dis*, 1995, 21(2):73-85.
Beyer EM, Karpova EA, Udalova OV, et al, "The Multiple Cases of Fabry Disease in a Russian Family Caused by an E341K Amino Acid Substitution in the α-Galactosidase A," *Clin Chim Acta*, 1999, 280(1-2):81-9.
Charrow J, Andersson HC, Kaplan P, et al, "The Gaucher Registry: Demographics and Disease Characteristics of 1698 Patients With Gaucher Disease," *Arch Intern Med*, 2000, 160(18):2835-43.
Charrow J, Esplin JA, Gribble TJ, et al, "Gaucher Disease: Recommendations on Diagnosis, Evaluation, and Monitoring," *Arch Intern Med*, 1998, 158(16):1754-60.
Cochat P, Koch Nogueira PC, Mahmoud MA, et al, "Primary Hyperoxaluria in Infants: Medical, Ethical, and Economic Issues," *J Pediatr*, 1999, 135(6):746-50.
Czartoryska B, Tylki-Szymanska A, and Lugowska A, "Changes in Serum Chitotriosidase Activity With Cessation of Replacement Enzyme (Cerebrosidase) Administration in Gaucher Disease," *Clin Biochem*, 2000, 33(2):147-9.
Dowton SB and Slaugh RA, "Diagnosis of Human Heritable Diseases - Laboratory Approaches and Outcomes," *Clin Chem*, 1995, 41(5):785-94.
Frattini A, Orchard PJ, Sobacchi C, et al, "Defects in TCIRG1 Subunit of the Vacuolar Proton Pump Are Responsible for a Subset of Human Autosomal Recessive Osteopetrosis," *Nat Genet*, 2000, 25(3):343-6.
Hyland K, "Presentation, Diagnosis, and Treatment of the Disorders of Monoamine Neurotransmitter Metabolism," *Semin Perinatol*, 1999, 23(2):194-203.
Jansen SM, Groener JE, and Poorthuis BJ, "Lysosomal Phospholipase Activity Is Decreased in Mucolipidosis II and III Fibroblasts," *Biochim Biophys Acta*, 1999, 1436(3):363-9.
Jansen GA, Mihalik SJ, Watkins PA, et al, "Characterization of Phytanoyl-Coenzyme A Hydroxylase in Human Liver and Activity Measurements in Patients With Peroxisomal Disorders," *Clin Chim Acta*, 1998, 271(2):203-11.
Johnson DW, "A Rapid Screening Procedure for the Diagnosis of Peroxisomal Disorders: Quantification of Very Long-Chain Fatty Acids, as Dimethylaminoethyl Esters, in Plasma and Blood Spots, by Electrospray Tandem Mass Spectrometry," *J Inherit Metab Dis*, 2000, 23(5):475-86.
Kolodny EH, "Niemann-Pick Disease," *Curr Opin Hematol*, 2000, 7(1):48-52.
Lindor NM and Karnes PS, "Initial Assessment of Infants and Children With Suspected Inborn Errors of Metabolism," *Mayo Clin Proc*, 1995, 70(10):987-8.
McKusick VA, *Mendelian Inheritance in Man: A Catalog of Human Genes and Genetic Disorders*, 12th ed, Baltimore, MD: John Hopkins University Press, 1998.
Meikle PJ, Hopwood JJ, Clague AE, et al, "Prevalence of Lysosomal Storage Disorders," *JAMA*, 1999, 281(3):249-54.
Rhead WJ, "Inborn Errors of Fatty Acid Oxidation in Man," *Clin Biochem*, 1991, 24(4):319-29.
Rinaldo P, "Inherited Metabolic Disorders in the Neonate," *Semin Perinatol*, 1999, 23(2):99-204.
Rogers DP and Bankaitis VA, "Phospholipid Transfer Proteins and Physiological Functions," *Int Rev Cytol*, 2000, 197:35-81.
Sacks DB, "Carbohydrates: Glycogen Storage Disease," *Tietz Textbook of Clinical Chemistry*, 3rd ed, Chapter 24, Burtis CA and Ashwood ER, eds, 1999, 750-804.
Scriver CR, Beaudet Al, Sly WS, et al, eds, Part 12, "Lysosomal Enzymes," Volume II, *The Metabolic and Molecular Bases of Inherited Disease*, 7th ed, New York, NY: McGraw-Hill Inc, 1995, 2427-879.

Shih VE, "Detection of Hereditary Metabolic Disorders Involving Amino Acids and Organic Acids," *Clin Biochem*, 1991, 24(4):301-9.
Sopelsa AMI, Severini MHA, Da Silva CMD, et al, "Characterization of β-Galactosidase in Leukocytes and Fibroblasts of GM1 Gangliosidosis Heterozygotes Compared to Normal Subjects," *Clin Biochem*, 2000, 33(2):125-9.
Surtees R, "Inborn Errors of Neurotransmitter Receptors," *J Inherit Metab Dis*, 1999, 22(4):374-80.
Zeviani M, Tiranti V, and Piantadosi C, "Reviews in Molecular Medicine: Mitochondrial Disorders," *Medicine*, 1998, 77(1):59-72.

Internet Web Sites
www.nlm.nih.gov/omim/
www.press.jhu.edu/home.html

♦ **Integrins** see CD34⁺ Hematopoietic Stem Cells by Flow Cytometry on page 413

♦ **Interleukin 3** see Eosinophil Count on page 424

♦ **Interleukin 3** see Thrombopoietin, Serum or Plasma on page 491

♦ **Interleukin 5** see Eosinophil Count on page 424

♦ **Interleukin 6** see Thrombopoietin, Serum or Plasma on page 491

♦ **Interleukin 11** see Thrombopoietin, Serum or Plasma on page 491

♦ **Intrinsic Factor** see Schilling Test on page 483

♦ **Iron Stain** see Siderocyte Stain on page 487

Iron Stain, Bone Marrow

Related Information
Bone Marrow on page 410
Ferritin, Serum on page 173
Hereditary Hemochromatosis DNA Test on page 709
Iron and Total Iron Binding Capacity/Transferrin, Serum on page 203
Liver Biopsy on page 65
Reticulocyte Hemoglobin Content on page 482
Siderocyte Stain on page 487
Transferrin Receptor, Soluble, Serum or Plasma on page 493

Synonyms Bone Marrow Iron Stain; Hemosiderin Stain; Marrow Iron Stores; Perls' Test; Prussian Blue Stain; Sideroblast Stain

Applies to Perls' Reaction; Prussian Blue Reaction; Ringed Sideroblasts; Sideroblasts; X-Linked Pyridoxine-Responsive Sideroblastic Anemia; Zinc Protoporphyrin:Heme Ratio

Test Includes Iron stain on sections of marrow aspirate clot and/or bone marrow biopsy and iron stain marrow cover slip smears

Abstract A stain (the Prussian blue reaction) applied to smears of bone marrow particles for iron containing blue to blue-green granular precipitates in macrophages/histiocytes. Seen also in a proportion of red cell precursors in the bone marrow (sideroblasts), in some peripheral red blood cells (siderocytes), and in some marrow immature red cells with impaired iron utilization ("ringed sideroblasts").

Specimen Bone marrow glass coverslip or slide smears, marrow aspirate, or biopsy

Container Coverslips or glass microslides are prepared at the bedside. Biopsy and clot fixed in formalin or other fixative (eg, B5 or Zenker's solution).

Collection Physician obtains bone marrow aspirate specimen by aseptic aspiration technique. Phlebotomist simultaneously obtains blood specimen for the preparation of peripheral blood smears.

Causes for Rejection No marrow obtained ("dry tap") or no bone marrow particles on smears

Special Instructions Requisition should include a brief clinical history.

Reference Interval Results should be interpreted in light of clinical background. Peripheral blood: no stainable iron is usually present (ie, no siderocytes are normally found). Bone marrow: stainable iron present as extracellular granules/globules and/or intracellular in cytoplasm of histiocytes - cells of the reticuloendothelial (RE) system. About one-third of the rubricytes in the marrow may be iron-positive sideroblasts (but not "ringed sideroblasts").

Use Semiquantitation of bone marrow iron stores; sensitive test for the evaluation of iron reserve; aid in the diagnosis of iron deficiency and its differentiation from another hypochromic/microcytic condition, thalassemia, in which iron stores are often increased; aid in the diagnosis of hemosiderosis/hemochromatosis; aid in the diagnosis of sideroblastic anemia (including refractory anemia with ringed sideroblasts) and in the detection of hemophagocytosis

Limitations Specimen should include sufficiently large spicules of marrow. True stainable marrow iron must be differentiated from iron positive artifacts.

Methodology Ferrocyanide ion reacts in acid with ferric ion to form a dark blue-green precipitate called Prussian blue. Presence of this pigment is reported semiquantitatively (and subjectively) as absent, decreased, normal, or increased (or on a scale of 0 to 4+). Some (20% to 40%) of red cell precursors will also have some iron-positive granules. These cells are called sideroblasts. In the common condition, "anemia of chronic disease," iron stores are normal or increased, but sideroblasts are absent. A silver stain has been proposed as a sensitive alternative for the demonstration of ringed sideroblasts.[1]

Additional Information It would appear that when a bone biopsy specimen is decalcified for over 2 hours, "leaching" of iron may occur so that a bone biopsy may be negative for iron while aspirate smear is positive. Krause et al, however, found that in only 35% of 270 cases with iron negative aspirate smears were there also iron negative biopsies (65% iron positive biopsies with iron negative smears).[2] Therefore, without evaluation of both types of specimens a significant overdiagnosis of iron deficiency may occur. Hemochromatosis, hemolytic anemias, and those with ineffective erythropoiesis (eg, thalassemia, megaloblastic and sideroblastic anemias) and anemias of chronic disease (especially inflammation) are characterized by increase in iron stores. The usual sideroblast has small iron positive granules without pattern in the cytoplasm. Ringed sideroblasts are rubricytes with tiny particles of iron located in mitochondria forming a ring around at least two-thirds of the nucleus. These pathologic sideroblasts occur in cases of normoblastic refractory anemia, B_6 responsive anemia including inherited (X-linked) pyridoxine-responsive sideroblastic anemia due to mutant erythroid 5-aminolevulinate synthase,[3] thalassemia, a variety of sideroblastic anemias, in some cases of B_{12}/folic acid deficiency, and in chloramphenicol toxicity.

Review of iron-stained marrow preparations also finds application in the identification of hemophagocytic histiocytosis (evidence of erythrophagocytosis and/or leukophagocytosis).[4]

A proposed silver stain for ringed sideroblasts may have as its chemical basis the demonstration of insoluble phosphates and/or carbonates of iron or other metals. Thus, when marrow iron is decreased (eg, sideroblastic anemia with iron deficiency due to GI bleeding), silver staining may be used to demonstrate ringed sideroblasts that would not be seen with Perls' reaction. Decalcified bone biopsy specimens, however, cannot be used to demonstrate sideroblasts (reaction is negative) by this method.[1] Silver staining is not considered to substitute for the Prussian blue reaction in identification of ringed sideroblasts.[1]

There has been little study of marrow iron stores in healthy children. It appears that stainable marrow iron is quite limited in apparently normal children during the first 5 years of life. Thus, iron stains of marrow in early childhood may not be helpful in establishing diagnosis of iron deficiency anemia while presence of classical stainable iron may assist in excluding such diagnosis.[5]

A cost-efficient and noninvasive alternative to bone marrow iron study is the proposed combined determination of zinc protoporphyrin:heme ratio and serum ferritin.[6,7] In a study of the anemia of chronic disease (rheumatoid arthritis) it was concluded that a combination of peripheral blood parameters (MCV, ferritin, and transferrin) could detect iron deficiency without resorting to marrow aspiration.[8]

Footnotes

1. Tham KT, Cousar JB, and Macon WR, "Silver Stain for Ringed Sideroblasts. A Sensitive Method That Differs From Perls' Reaction in Mechanism and Clinical Application," *Am J Clin Pathol*, 1990, 94(1):73-6.
2. Krause JR, Brubaker D, and Kaplan S, "Comparison of Stainable Iron in Aspirated and Needle-Biopsy Specimens of Bone Marrow," *Am J Clin Pathol*, 1979, 72(1):68-70.
3. Cox TC, Bottomley SS, Wiley JS, et al, "X-Linked Pyridoxine-Responsive Sideroblastic Anemia Due to a Thr388-to-Ser Substitution in Erythroid 5-Aminolevulinate Synthase," *N Engl J Med*, 1994, 330(10):675-9.
4. Koduri PR, "Prussian Blue Reaction and Hemophagocytosis: A New Use for an Old Test," *Am J Hematol*, 1995, 49(2):167.
5. Geaghan SM, "Hematologic Values and Appearances In the Healthy Fetus, Neonate, and Child," *Clinics in Lab Medicine: Diagnostic Pediatric Hematology*, Geagham SM, ed, 1999, 19(1):1-37.
6. Labbe RF, "Zinc Protoporphyrin/Heme Ratio as an Indicator of Marrow Iron Stores," *Am J Clin Pathol*, 1991, 95(5):758.
7. Labbe RF and Rettmer RL, "Zinc Protoporphyrin: A Product of Iron-Deficient Erythropoiesis," *Semin Hematol*, 1989, 26(1):40-6.
8. Vreugdenhil G, Baltus CA, Van Eijk HG, et al, "Anaemia of Chronic Disease: Diagnostic Significance of Erythrocyte and Serological Parameters in Iron Deficient Rheumatoid Arthritis Patients," *Br J Rheumatol*, 1990, 29(2):105-10.

References

Krantz SB, "Pathogenesis and Treatment of the Anemia of Chronic Disease," *Am J Med Sci*, 1994, 307(5):353-9.

Lee GE, "Anemia: A Diagnostic Strategy," *Wintrobe's Clinical Hematology*, Volume 1, Chapter 30, Lee GR, Foerster J, Luken J, et al, eds, Baltimore MD: Lippincott Williams & Wilkins, 1999, 927-9.

Perkins S, "Hypochromic Microcytic Anemias," *Practical Diagnosis of Hematologic Disorders*, 3rd ed, Chapter 2, Kjeldsberg C, ed, Chicago, IL: ASCP Press, American Society of Clinical Pathologists, 2000, 29-32.

◆ **Itano Solubility Test** *see* Sickle Cell Tests *on page 486*

◆ **Joint Fluid Analysis** *see* Body Fluid Analysis, Cell Count *on page 408*

◆ **Kawasaki Disease** *see* Thrombopoietin, Serum or Plasma *on page 491*

Kleihauer-Betke

Related Information

Alpha$_1$-Fetoprotein, Amniotic Fluid *on page 96*
Fetal Cell Detection by Flow Cytometry *on page 430*
Fetal Hemoglobin *on page 431*
Prenatal Screen, Immunohematology *on page 855*

Rh$_o$(D) Immune Globulin (Human) *on page 860*
Rosette Test for Fetomaternal Hemorrhage *on page 863*

Synonyms Acid Elution for Fetal Hemoglobin

Applies to Cordocentesis; Permeabilization of Red Blood Cells

Abstract Staining of maternal blood specimen (usually postpartum) for identification of percentage of fetal cells present. Estimation of volume of fetomaternal hemorrhage (FMH) as a guide to necessary dose of Rh(D) immune globulin.

Specimen Whole blood

Container Lavender top (EDTA) tube

Storage Instructions Blood must be less than 6 hours old. Smears must be fixed within 1 hour after preparation.

Causes for Rejection Clotted specimen, gross hemolysis

Special Instructions A cord blood specimen should also be obtained and submitted. It is needed as a source of fetal blood (for use as a positive control).

Reference Interval Full-term newborns: Hb F cells are >90%; normal adults: Hb F cells are <0.01%

Use Determine possible fetomaternal hemorrhage (FMH) in the newborn; aid in diagnosis of certain types of anemia in adults; assess the magnitude of fetal-maternal hemorrhage; calculate dosage of Rh immune globulin (eg, RhoGAM™) to be given. A study by Emery concludes (on the basis of 523 tests performed in 1993) that the Kleihauer-Betke (KB) test should be performed on all screening test (a qualitative fetal cell screening test using chemically modified anti-D antibody and D-positive indicator cells to produce agglutination - rosetting of D-positive fetal cells was utilized) positive Rh-negative mothers of Rh-positive infants and in cases of maternal trauma, unexplained increased maternal alpha-fetoprotein levels, fetal distress with abnormal cardiac tracings, intrauterine fetal death, and in cases of unexplained neonatal anemia.[1] Testing should also be considered in cases of cordocentesis (in which FMH may occur).

Limitations Possibility of the presence of a hemoglobinopathy with increase in Hb F must be considered when this test is used to assess fetal-maternal hemorrhage. Specimens must be obtained prior to transfusion. The KB assay lacks precision, coefficient of variation (CV) has been found to range from 40% to 60% on samples with fetal cells at the 0.2% to 1% level.[2]

Contraindications Known pre-existing elevation of maternal Hb F (eg, mothers with hereditary persistence of fetal hemoglobin)[3,4]

Methodology Acid elution. After fixation with alcohol Hb F remains as a precipitate within the cell while Hb A is soluble in citric acid phosphate buffer. The adult RBCs containing little or no Hb F appear as ghosts under the microscope. Automated (flow cytometric) assays are becoming commercially available. One such assay utilizes anti-Hb F monoclonal antibodies applied to red cells (test sample) that have been glutaraldehyde-fixed and permeabilized by suspension in nonionic detergent (Triton X-100).[5,6] A commercial version (Caltag, Burlingame, CA) has been FDA approved for identification and enumeration of fetal red blood cells. Cytometric tests based on the detection of D antigen and/or CD71 (transferrin receptor) have also been developed but are not ideal for routine detection of fetomaternal hemorrhage. See Fetal Cell Detection by Flow Cytometry *on page 430*.

Additional Information The KB test is helpful in distinguishing some forms of thalassemia from hereditary persistence of fetal hemoglobin (HPFH). The hereditary persistence of fetal hemoglobin reveals a uniform distribution of fetal hemoglobin in each red cell. Δβ-thalassemia, in contrast, demonstrates a heterogeneous distribution of fetal hemoglobin (ie, some cells are stained and others are ghost RBCs).

Some RhoGAM™ failures are due to a failure to suspect and diagnose FMH that may require more than one dose of RhoGAM™. The ultimate purpose is to prevent generation of anti-D antibodies in the postpartum woman and subsequent evolution of hemolytic disease of the newborn (erythroblastosis fetalis). The amount of fetal blood contamination can be calculated. Each vial of Rh immune globulin contains 300 μg of anti-D. This is enough to prevent maternal immunization when the fetal bleed is up to 30 mL of whole blood (15 mL packed cells). One vial of Rh immune globulin is given to the Rh-negative mother for every 30 mL of fetal blood contamination from an Rh-positive fetus.

In cases of maternal hereditary persistence of fetal hemoglobin, a flow cytometric-based method for detection and quantification of fetal Rh(D) positive cells can be used. An indirect immunofluorescent reaction is involved with IgG anti-D as the primary antibody.[3]

A study designed to determine the incidence of FMH following cesarean section utilizing KB testing found some degree of hemorrhage in 18.5% of the study patients. In 2.5%, there was evidence of more than 30 mL of fetal blood lost into the maternal circulation. This finding led to the recommendation that all Rh-negative patients having a C-section be screened (KB test) for fetomaternal hemorrhage.[7]

KB testing should also be considered when cordocentesis may have led to alloimmunization to D antigen.[8] A recent review found a 4.4% incidence of massive FMH (on the basis of KB test results) in a sample of 319 cases of fetal death. There were a total of 69,390 births reviewed in the study period from 1990-1994. In this large number of births, 645 were fetal deaths with weight >500 grams; KB tests were performed on 319 (49.5%). Clinical risk factors did not predict an increased rate of massive FMH. Major fetal anomalies were present in 35.7% of cases of massive FMH. It was recommended (Continued)

Kleihauer-Betke (Continued)

that KB testing be performed in all cases of fetal death irrespective of the presence or absence of risk factors.[9]

Footnotes

1. Emery CL, Morway CF, Chung-Park M, et al, "The Kleihauer-Betke Test. Clinical Utility, Indication, and Correlation in Patients With Placental Abruption and Cocaine Use," *Arch Pathol Lab Med*, 1995, 119(11):1032-7.
2. Duckett JR and Constantine G, "The Kleihauer Technique: An Accurate Method of Quantifying Fetomaternal Haemorrhage?" *Br J Obstet Gynaecol*, 1997, 104(7):845-6.
3. Patton WN, Nicholson GS, Sawers AH, et al, "Assessment of Fetal-Maternal Haemorrhage in Mothers With Hereditary Persistence of Fetal Haemoglobin," *J Clin Pathol*, 1990, 43(9):728-31.
4. Holcomb WL, Gunderson E, and Petrie RH, "Clinical Use of the Kleihauer-Betke Test," *J Perinat Med*, 1990, 18(5):331-7.
5. Davis BH, Olsen S, Bigelow NC, et al, "Detection of Fetal Red Cells in Fetomaternal Hemorrhage Using a Fetal Hemoglobin Monoclonal Antibody by Flow Cytometry," *Transfusion*, 1998, 38(8):749-56.
6. Nelson M, Zarkos K, Popp H, et al, "A Flow-Cytometric Equivalent of the Kleihauer Test," *Vox Sang*, 1998, 75(3):234-41.
7. Feldman N, Skoll A, and Sibai B, "The Incidence of Significant Fetomaternal Hemorrhage in Patients Undergoing Cesarean Section," *Am J Obstet Gynecol*, 1990, 163(3):855-8.
8. Gold E, "Severe Fetal Anemia," Clinical Pathology Rounds, *Lab Med*, 1997, 28(1):21-3.
9. Samadi R, Greenspoon JS, Gviazda I, et al, "Massive Fetomaternal Hemorrhage and Fetal Death: Are They Predictable?" *J Perinatol*, 1999, 19(3):227-9.

References

Kleihauer E, "Determination of Fetal Hemoglobin: Elution Technique," *The Detection of Hemoglobinopathies*, Schmidt RM, al, eds, Cleveland, OH: CRC Press, 1974.

Naulaers G, Barten S, Vanhole C, et al, "Management of Severe Neonatal Anemia Due to Fetomaternal Transfusion," *Am J Perinatol*, 1999, 16(4):193-6.

Salama A, Wittmann MDG, Stelzer A, et al, "Use of the Gel Agglutination Technique for Determination of Fetomaternal Hemorrhage," *Transfusion*, 1998, 38(2):177-80.

Von Stein GA, Munsick RA, Stiver K, et al, "Fetomaternal Hemorrhage in Threatened Abortion," *Obstet Gynecol*, 1992, 79(3):383-6.

♦ **Kleihauer Test** *see* Fetal Cell Detection by Flow Cytometry *on page 430*

♦ **Krabbe Disease** *see* Inherited Diseases of Metabolism and Cell Structure *on page 449*

Lamellar Bodies, Amniotic Fluid

Related Information

Lecithin:Sphingomyelin Ratio, Amniotic Fluid *on page 210*
Phosphatidylglycerol, Amniotic Fluid *on page 251*
Pulmonary Surfactant, Amniotic Fluid *on page 271*

Synonyms Amniotic Fluid Lamellar Bodies; Lamellar Body Count; Lamellar Body Density Count; Lamellar Body Number Density

Abstract Amniotic fluid lamellar body density (lamellar body counts) have been considered to have value as a screen for the assessment of fetal lung maturity.[1,2,3,4,5] The procedure is rapid, inexpensive, and uses cell counting equipment that is usually readily available.

Specimen Fresh amniotic fluid

Container Specimen from amniocentesis must be submitted in a sterile container.

Collection Specimen is obtained at amniocentesis by an obstetrician.

Storage Instructions Keep at room temperature. Specimen will usually be analyzed within 8 hours of sample collection but can be kept refrigerated at 2°C to 8°C for at least 2 weeks or frozen at -20°C for some 4-10 weeks.[4,6] After 30 days, the concentric layers appear loose by electron microscopy with a trend to decrease in number of lamellar bodies.[6]

Causes for Rejection Presence of visible blood, meconium or mucous specimen, specimen not in sterile container

Turnaround Time 1 hour (procedure itself can be performed in 15-20 minutes)

Reference Interval Lamellar body count >30,000/μL (decision threshold) is predictive of pulmonary maturity. Count <10,000/μL is 67% positive predictive value for respiratory distress syndrome.

Use Predict fetal lung maturity and the risk of developing respiratory distress syndrome

Limitations Presence of mucous (as may be present in vaginal pool samples) can produce artifactual increase in lamellar body (LB) counts.[1] Contamination with meconium or lysed blood do not appear to affect LB count.[4] Varying decision thresholds have been recommended as the result of different studies and may relate in part to use of variable centrifugation protocols.[3]

Methodology Lamellar bodies range in size from 1.7-7.3 fL.[6] They are conveniently and accurately counted utilizing the platelet apertures of multi-channel hematology analyzers (flow/impedance method of particle counting). Dependent upon instrument manufacturer, counting aperture size used for platelets is 50-60 μm, and upper limit of volume range used for platelet classification is 20-35 fL. Within-run coefficients of variation have ranged from 1.3% to 3.5% for different count levels.[6]

Additional Information Lamellar bodies are concentrically layered protein, cholesterol, and phospholipid structures, 1-5 μm in diameter, largely some 2 μm across.[1,4] They are produced in the lung by type II pneumocytes and are

the storage form of pulmonary surfactant.[2] As the fetal lung matures, lamellar bodies increase in number with, as expected, increased amniotic fluid phospholipids and lecithin:sphingomyelin ratio. Lamellar bodies have size and volume characteristics similar to platelets which allow the use of readily available multichannel cell counters in their enumeration. A number of studies have shown a high correlation of lamellar body count with traditional phospholipid analytic based methods commonly used in fetal lung maturity testing.[2,3,4,5,7,8] Studies comparing results of different cell counters[1,8] emphasize the need for proper instrument calibration and appropriate cutoff values (the result in part of different aperture sizes used in different counters). There is a recommendation that reference ranges identify the analyzer and method used.[1] When a threshold value of 30,000/μL (or greater) was used to indicate fetal lung maturity, no false-negative results were noted.[8] The significance of numerous false positives could be decreased by use of a separate cutoff value (<10,000/μL) as indicative of risk for respiratory distress syndrome.

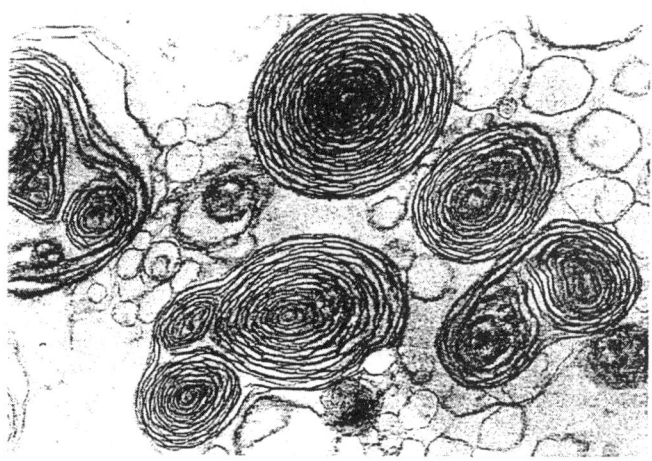

Transmission electron micrograph of lamellar bodies from fresh human amniotic fluid. Uranyl acetate, x 21,000.

From Lafler D, Mendoza A, Cousins L, et al, "Refrigerated and Frozen Amniotic Fluid for Fetal Lung Maturity Testing and Lamellar Body Density Counts," *Lab Med*, 1996, 27(11):770-4.

Footnotes

1. Lafler D, Mendoza A, Poeltler D, et al, "Coulter STK-S vs Abbott Cell-Dyn 3500 for Counting Lamellar Bodies in Amniotic Fluid," *Lab Med*, 1998, 29(5):298-301.
2. Dalence CR, Bowie LJ, Dohnol JC, et al, "Amniotic Fluid Lamellar Body Count: A Rapid and Reliable Fetal Lung Maturity Test," *Obstet Gynecol*, 1995, 86(2):235-9.
3. Ashwood ER, Palmer SE, Taylor JS, et al, "Lamellar Body Counts for Rapid Fetal Lung Maturity Testing," *Obstet Gynecol*, 1993, 81(4):619-24.
4. Dubin SB, "Characterization of Amniotic Fluid Lamellar Bodies by Resistive-Pulse Counting: Relationship to Measures of Fetal Lung Maturity," *Clin Chem*, 1989, 35(4):612-6.
5. Ashwood ER, Oldroyd RG, and Palmer SE, "Measuring the Number of Lamellar Body Particles in Amniotic Fluid," *Obstet Gynecol*, 1990, 75(2):289-92.
6. Lafler D, Mendoza A, Cousins L, et al, "Refrigerated and Frozen Amniotic Fluid for Fetal Lung Maturity Testing and Lamellar Body Density Counts," *Lab Med*, 1996, 27(11):770-4.
7. Pearlman ES, Baiocchi JM, Lease JA, et al, "Utility of a Rapid Lamellar Body Count in the Assessment of Fetal Maturity," *Am J Clin Pathol*, 1991, 95(6):778-80.
8. Bowie LJ, Shammo J, Dohnal JC, et al, "Lamellar Body Number Density and the Prediction of Respiratory Distress," *Am J Clin Pathol*, 1991, 95(6):781-6.

♦ **Lamellar Body Count** *see* Lamellar Bodies, Amniotic Fluid *on page 454*

♦ **Lamellar Body Density Count** *see* Lamellar Bodies, Amniotic Fluid *on page 454*

♦ **Lamellar Body Number Density** *see* Lamellar Bodies, Amniotic Fluid *on page 454*

♦ **LAP** *see* Leukocyte Alkaline Phosphatase *on page 455*

♦ **LAP Score** *see* Leukocyte Alkaline Phosphatase *on page 455*

♦ **LAP Smear** *see* Leukocyte Alkaline Phosphatase *on page 455*

♦ **Large Molecule Diseases** *see* Inherited Diseases of Metabolism and Cell Structure *on page 449*

♦ **Large Platelets** *see* Reticulated Platelet Count *on page 480*

LE Cell Test

Related Information

Anti-DNA *on page 504*
Antinuclear Antibody *on page 507*
Sjögren Antibodies *on page 542*
Smooth Muscle Antibody *on page 543*

Synonyms LE Preparation

Abstract Historically, an important test for systemic lupus erythematosus (SLE), it is currently outmoded.

Patient Preparation Avoid heparin therapy for 2 days prior to collection. Large doses of heparin may increase the incidence of false-negative results.

Specimen Whole blood

Container Green top (heparin) tube; EDTA anticoagulated blood may cause false-negative results

Collection Routine venipuncture. Invert gently to mix. Transport to the laboratory within 30 minutes.

Causes for Rejection Insufficient volume, clotted specimen, patient on heparin

Reference Interval Negative

Use Evaluate autoimmune diseases, specifically SLE (systemic lupus erythematosus). The discovery of the LE cell more than 40 years ago has been important in understanding autoimmune disease. As stated by Tan and associates, however, "It has been superseded by modern ANA tests with greater sensitivity and rapidity, but its fundamental contribution to understanding of ANAs cannot be overlooked."[1] A few authors[2,3] still advocate the use of this test.

Limitations This test is an indirect method for detecting one of the antinuclear antibodies. It is less sensitive than fluorescent antibody techniques for ANA and not specific for lupus erythematosus. Positive tests have been reported in a variety of drug induced lupus syndromes, in rheumatoid arthritis, chronic and active hepatitis, drug hypersensitivity, and other collagen diseases. One negative result should not be considered to rule out the possibility of LE. EDTA anticoagulated blood may cause a false-negative reaction.

Contraindications Patients receiving large doses of heparin or with severe leukopenia/neutropenia

Methodology Blood cells are ruptured by a variety of methods - glass beads have been commonly used. Nuclear material is thereby released to interact with any antibody that may be present. One hour incubation at 37°C allows time for interaction of nuclear material and antibody and for the altered nuclear material to be phagocytosed (a complement dependent process). Buffy coat smears are prepared, stained, and studied for presence of phagocytosed homogenous lavender staining material. Presence of extracellular LE material or formation of rosettes does not add specific diagnostic information.

Performance of this test can be discouraged on the basis of its limited usefulness and exposure of the medical technologist to blood (appropriate precautions should be followed during processing of materials).

Additional Information SLE is a disease of protean clinical manifestations commonly with rash, arthralgia, fever, anemia, leukopenia, thrombocytopenia, and hypocomplementemia, occurring especially in women. The LE slide cell test is relatively insensitive. It is positive in only 60% to 80% of acutely ill cases of LE. A negative LE slide cell test does not exclude the diagnosis of lupus erythematosus. The patient's serum should be studied for antinuclear antibody (ANA). The antibody may be of IgG, A, or M specificity but is most commonly of IgG class. A negative ANA test nearly excludes the diagnosis of LE (>95% sensitivity) if the patient is not being treated with corticosteroid or immunosuppressive drugs. Some drugs (in particular Dilantin®) may relate to lupus erythematosus and cause positive LE slide cell tests. Up to 25% of individuals taking Dilantin® (diphenylhydantoin) develop antinuclear antibodies. See table.

Drugs Capable of Inducing Lupus Syndrome Positive LE Slide Test

Dilantin	Phenelzine sulfate
Ethosuximide	Phenylbutazone
Griseofulvin	Primidone
Hydralazine	Procainamide
Isoniazid	Propylthiouracil
Mesantoin	Reserpine
Methyldopa	Streptomycin
Methylthiouracil	Sulfonamides
Oral contraceptives	Tetracycline
Penicillin	Tridione

Footnotes

1. Tan EM, Robinson CA, and Nakamura RM, "ANAs in Systemic Rheumatic Disease. Diagnostic Significance," *Postgrad Med*, 1985, 78(3):141-2, 145-8.
2. Hidalgo C and Vladutiu AO, "Lupus Erythematosus Cells in Serum and Pleural Fluid of a Patient With Negative Fluorescent Antinuclear Antibody Test," *Am J Clin Pathol*, 1987, 87(5):660-2.
3. Wallace DJ, "Lupus Erythematosus Cell Test," *Am J Clin Pathol*, 1995, 104(1):110-1.

References

Dacie JV and Lewis SM, "Demonstration of LE Cells," *Practical Haematology*, 8th ed, New York, NY: Churchill Livingstone, 1995, 569-71.

Hargraves MM, Richmond H, and Morton R, "Presentation of Two Bone Marrow Elements: The "Tart" Cell and the "LE" Cell," *Proc Staff Meet Mayo Clin*, 1948, 23:25.

Steensma DP, "Fifty Years of Tart Cells," *Mayo Clin Proc*, 1999, 74(9):936-8.

♦ *Legionella dumoffii* see Buffy Coat Smear Study of Peripheral Blood on page 412

♦ **Leigh Syndrome** see Inherited Diseases of Metabolism and Cell Structure on page 449

♦ **LE Preparation** see LE Cell Test on page 454

♦ **Leukemic Reticuloendotheliosis Test** see Tartrate Resistant Leukocyte Acid Phosphatase on page 488

♦ **Leukocyte Acid Phosphatase** see Tartrate Resistant Leukocyte Acid Phosphatase on page 488

♦ **Leukocyte Acid Phosphatase Isoenzymes** see Tartrate Resistant Leukocyte Acid Phosphatase on page 488

Leukocyte Alkaline Phosphatase

Related Information

Bone Marrow on page 410
Breakpoint Cluster Region Rearrangement in CML on page 721
Leukocyte Cytochemistry on page 456
Phlebotomy, Therapeutic on page 849
White Blood Cell Count on page 496

Synonyms LAP; LAP Score; LAP Smear

Abstract A cytochemical reaction (LAP score) useful in differential diagnosis of myeloproliferative diseases, in particular, distinguishing leukemoid reaction from chronic myelogenous leukemia (CML). The LAP score reflects the intensity of alkaline phosphatase (AP) staining (of a neutrophil apparently nongranular but intracytoplasmic component) scored on a scale of 0 to 4+.

Specimen Whole blood

Container Slides with smears of blood

Collection Make six smears on long slides from fingerstick blood. Air dry the slides. Transport to Hematology immediately (ie, within 30 minutes).

Storage Instructions Slides must be fixed with cold 10% formalin methanol or citrated buffered acetone, rinsed, air dried, and frozen within 8 hours (preferably within 30 minutes) after obtaining the blood. After fixation, smears can be stored for up to 8 weeks before staining. The enzyme activity may, in some cases, be stable for up to 1 year when stored at -20°C.

Causes for Rejection Blood collected in EDTA anticoagulant, transit time to the laboratory in excess of 30 minutes, neutrophil count <1000/mm³ in peripheral blood

Reference Interval 15-130 (variable between laboratories)

Use Aid in the differential diagnosis of chronic myelogenous leukemia (CML) versus leukemoid reaction; aid in the evaluation of polycythemia and myelofibrosis

Limitations Pregnancy, increased number of immature forms of neutrophils, and postoperative or "stressful" states are associated with increased scores. The differential must have adequate numbers of mature neutrophilic granulocytes to perform the LAP.

Methodology Enzyme reaction with leukocyte alkaline phosphatase liberating naphthol or a substituted naphthol compound which then couples with fast blue RR or other chromogen to form an insoluble precipitate. Color of the precipitate relates to the type of substituted naphthol substrate and diazonium dye used (color is reagent dependent). Cells are scored as to the degree of phosphatase activity present, 0 to 4+. One hundred cells are counted and the score totaled.

Additional Information Low LAP scores have been associated with CML, myelodysplasia, PNH, thrombocytopenic purpura, and hereditary hypophosphatasia. In chronic phase CML, regardless of the total white count, the score remains low but with therapy or progression of disease, the LAP score may increase. Occasionally, an apparent new myeloproliferative disorder is described. One such is characterized by low LAP score and also by leukocytosis, polycythemia, thrombocytopenia, splenomegaly, and generalized lymphoadenopathy but without Philadelphia chromosome, *bcr* gene rearrangement, or other karyotypic abnormalities.[1] In CML, it has been demonstrated that the mRNA for leukocyte alkaline phosphatase by Northern blotting is undetectable.[2] This suggests either rapid degradation of the message or no transcription of the LAP gene. In chronic neutrophilic leukemia (a rare myeloproliferative disorder with neutrophil granulocytosis and an indolent course) LAP score is normal or increased.

In nonleukemic neutrophilia, the LAP rises as the WBC rises. High LAP scores have been seen in leukemoid reactions, polycythemia vera, myelofibrosis, aplastic anemia, mongolism, hairy cell leukemia, and neutrophilia either physiological or secondary to infection. LAP is also increased in Hodgkin disease. Serial activity can be a useful adjunct in evaluating the activity of Hodgkin disease as well as its response to therapy. Increase in LAP does not occur in cases of sickle cell crisis, possibly due to zinc deficiency (leukocyte alkaline phosphatase is a zinc metalloenzyme) but more likely relating to a mild defect in the hypothalamic-pituitary-adrenal axis with decreased plasma cortisol response in patients in sickle cell crisis.[3]

Footnotes

1. Schofield JR and Robinson WA, "A New Myeloproliferative Syndrome," *Am J Hematol*, 1995, 48(3):186-91.
2. Rambaldi A, Terao M, Bettoni S, et al, "Differences in the Expression of Alkaline Phosphatase mRNA in Chronic Myelogenous Leukemia and Paroxysmal Nocturnal Hemoglobinuria Polymorphonuclear Leukocytes," *Blood*, 1989, 73(5):1113-5.

(Continued)

Leukocyte Alkaline Phosphatase (Continued)

3. Rosenbloom BE, Odell WD, and Tanaka KR, "Pituitary-Adrenal Axis Function in Sickle Cell Anemia and Its Relationship to Leukocyte Alkaline Phosphatase," *Am J Hematol*, 1980, 9(4):373-9.

References

Catovsky D, "Leukocyte Cytochemical and Immunological Techniques," *Practical Haematology*, 8th ed, Chapter 9, Dacie JV and Lewis SM, eds, New York, NY: Churchill Livingstone, 1995, 143-74.

Enright H and McGlave P, "Chronic Myelogenous Leukemia," *Hematology: Basic Principles and Practice*, 3rd ed, Chapter 62, Hoffman R, Benz EJ Jr, Shattil SJ, et al, eds, Philadelphia, PA: Churchill Livingstone, 2000, 1155-71.

Grozdea J, Vergnes H, Cambus JP, et al, "Neutrophil Alkaline Phosphatase Activity in Turner Syndrome," *Acta Haematol*, 1999, 102(4):201-2.

Helbert BJ and Rappaport ES, "Cytochemistry," *Clinical Hematology: Principles, Procedures, Correlations*, 2nd ed, Chapter 29, Stiene-Martin EA, Lotspeich-Steininger CA and Koepke J, eds, Philadelphia, PA: Lippincott-Raven Publishers, 1998, 393-9.

Kaplow LS, "Cytochemistry of Leukocyte Alkaline Phosphatase: Use of Complex Naphthol AS Phosphates in Azo Dye-Coupling Techniques," *Am J Clin Pathol*, 1963, 39:439-49.

Rutenberg AM, Rosales CI, and Bennett JM, "An Improved Histochemical Method for the Demonstration of Leukocyte Alkaline Phosphatase Activity: Clinical Application," *J Lab Clin Med*, 1965, 65(4):698-705.

♦ **Leukocyte Count** *see* White Blood Cell Count *on page 496*

Leukocyte Cytochemistry

Related Information

Synonyms Cytochemistry, Leukocyte

Applies to Acid-Fast, Ziehl-Neelsen, Stain for Intracellular Pigment; Acid Phosphatase Stain With and Without Tartrate; Alpha-Naphthyl Esterase Stain With and Without Fluoride; Amyloid; ASD Chloroacetate Esterase Stain; Beta-Glucuronidase Stain; Leukocyte Immunophenotyping; Megakaryoblasts; Methenamine Silver; Methyl Green-Pyronine; Monocytes; Myeloblasts; Myeloperoxidase (MPO) Stain; Nonspecific Esterase; Oil Red O Stain; PAS Stain; Promyelocytes; Sudan Black B (SBB) Stain

Test Includes Any of the above stains indicated by examination of routinely stained preparations or specific request

Abstract Cytochemical reactions are useful in differential diagnosis of conditions in which leukocytes are involved, in particular, in the study and characterization of acute leukemia. Immunophenotypic and cytochemical studies of the leukemias are generally complementary. Identification of cell antigens using specific individual (or panels of) antibodies with flow cytometry techniques usually provide a more detailed and definitive analysis of cell populations. Cytogenetic analysis may be required to confirm or establish a diagnosis.

Specimen Blood or bone marrow smears, imprints or smears of cell suspensions

Container Green top (heparin) tube

Collection Smears are prepared at the patient's bedside.

Storage Instructions Transport specimen to the laboratory immediately.

Turnaround Time Variable

Reference Interval Interpretation and significance usually requires correlation of cytomorphologic, cytochemical, immunophenotypic, cytogenetic, and clinical features. The French-American-British (FAB) cooperative group classification of acute leukemias requires that SBB or MPO staining be positive in at least 3% of blasts to establish myeloid lineage. If staining is below the 3% level (FAB M0, see below), immunophenotyping must be performed to provide myeloid identification. Generally, intensity of granule staining increases with cell maturation. See Table 1.

Use Cytochemically evaluate neoplasms and abnormal cells in bone marrow, peripheral blood, or other specimens such as imprints; detect amyloidosis; classification of leukemias and plasma cell dyscrasias, in particular the acute myeloid leukemias; evaluate myeloproliferative/lymphoproliferative disorders

Limitations Enzyme cytochemical positive reaction may not have diagnostic specificity in any particular cell or tissue preparation.

Methodology Generally, based on cell cytoplasmic granule enzymatic activity. Test conditions include provision of substrate, which when acted upon by the appropriate enzyme, generates reaction product(s) that react with color reagent(s) allowing visualization (see Leukocyte Alkaline Phosphatase *on page 455*). Sudan black B (SBB) is a lipophilic dye reacting with phospholipids, neutral fats, and steroids. It allows visualization of the phospholipid membranes of myeloid granules. SBB is more sensitive but less specific than MPO in demonstrating granulocytic lineage.

Additional Information See also Tartrate Resistant Leukocyte Acid Phosphatase *on page 488*, for hairy cell leukemia. In the technique of Yam et al for esterase reactions, a single slide preparation is consecutively stained for two different enzyme activities.[1] The nonspecific esterase (α-naphthol acetate substrate - black granulation) is monocyte specific, while the chloroacetate esterase (naphthol ASD chloroacetate - red granulation) is granulocyte specific.[1] These reactions should be helpful in some cases in distinguishing acute myelogenous from acute monocytic leukemia and are of value in distinguishing acute myelomonocytic leukemia from acute myelogenous leukemia and acute monocytic leukemia. In acute myelomonocytic leukemia, both granulocytic and monocytic markers are present simultaneously in the leukemic cells. Nonspecific esterase activity inhibited by fluoride has been described in red cell precursors - including megaloblasts in cases of untreated pernicious anemia, megaloblastoid rubricytes in cases of DiGuglielmo syndrome, and rubricytes in cases of severe untreated iron deficiency. The rubricyte series of cells from normal marrow lack nonspecific esterase activity. The fluoride inhibited nonspecific esterase reaction indicates monocytic origin and is unusual in T- lymphocyte cell malignancy.

Cytochemistry (CC) is especially employed in identification and classification of acute myeloid leukemia (AML). This role of CC is increasingly shared and diluted by the application of immunophenotypic and cytogenetic findings which have led to accelerated activity in reclassification of the hematopoietic malignancies. The accompanying tables are derived from current and proposed classifications of the acute myeloid leukemias, notably those of the World Health Organization (WHO) and the French-American-British Cooperative Group (FAB).[2,3,4,5,6] Seen in this context, time, cost, and performance constraints may limit application of CC.[7,8,9]

Cytochemical stains are generally negative or do not contribute significantly to the diagnosis of acute lymphoblastic leukemia (ALL). In a study designed to assess the value of PAS (periodic acid-Schiff) stain in delineating lymphoblastic and myeloblastic leukemia, it was concluded that a positive PAS reaction combined with negative myeloperoxidase, Sudan black B, and alpha-naphthyl butyrate esterase results continues to have a diagnostic role in differentiating lymphoblastic and myeloblastic leukemia.[10] Another study showed that PAS and iron stain together or PAS and double esterase together was helpful in excluding a diagnosis of myelodysplastic syndrome.[11] Flow cytochemistry has been applied to the differentiation of acute leukemias.[12] Immunocytochemical marker, enzyme and cytokine studies can be applied to the differentiation of macrophages, Langerhans cells, and dendritic cells and their disease processes.[13]

Table 1. Cytochemistry – Normal White Blood Cells

| | MPO/ SBB | Nonspecific Esterase | | Chloroacetate Esterase | PAS | Acid Phos |
		α-N Acetate	α-N Butyrate			
Promyelocyte	+/++	-/±	-	+/++	±	+/++
Myelocyte	++	±		++		
Neutrophil	+++	±		+++	+++	+
Monocyte	-/±	+++*	++/+++*	±	±	++
Lymphocyte	-	-/±	±	-	-/+	-/++
Erythroblast	-	-/±	-	-	-	±
Megakaryocyte	-	+++	±		++	++

*Strongly inhibited by sodium fluoride.

Table 2. Proposed WHO Classification of Acute Myeloid Leukemias (AML)[2,3]

I.	AML with recurrent cytogenetic translocations
	AML with t(8;21) (q22; q22),
	Acute promyelocytic leukemia (AML with t(15;17) (q22; q11-12) and variants
	AML with abnormal bone marrow eosinophils (inv (16) (p13; q22) or t(16;16) (p13; q11)
	AML with 11q23 abnormalities
II.	Acute myeloid leukemia with multilineage dysplasia with or without prior myelodysplastic syndrome
III.	AML, therapy related
	Alkylating agent related
	Epipodophyllotoxin related (some lymphoid)
	Other types
IV.	AML not otherwise categorized (extension of FAB groups)
	M0-M7 (see Table 3)
	Acute basophilic leukemia
	Acute panmyelosis with myelofibrosis
	Acute leukemia and transient myeloproliferative disorder followed by acute megakaryoblastic leukemia in Down syndrome
	Myeloid sarcoma

Table 3. FAB / WHO Morphologic Classification With Cytochemistry of Acute Myeloid Leukemias

Subtype of AML		Morphology*	Cytochemistry†		
			MPO or SBB	CAE	NSE
M0	Myeloblastic minimally differentiated	≥20% myeloblasts without granules	-	-	-
M1	Myeloblastic without maturation	≥20% myeloblasts, some with scant granules <10% with maturation beyond blast stage	+	±	-
M2	Myeloblastic with maturation	≥20% myeloblasts with granules; ≥10% more mature cells; <20% monocytic cells	+	±	-
M3	Acute promyelocytic hypergranular	≥20% myeloblasts and promyelocytes with prominent granules	+++	+++	-
M3v	Acute promyelocytic microgranular (hypogranular) variant	Granules with procoagulant substances → DIC‡			+ in 20% to 25% of cases
M4	Myelomonocytic (MM)	>20% myeloblasts, monoblasts, and promyelocytes	+	+	+ NaF inhibits
M4eo	MM with marrow eosinophilia	>20% monocytes; blood monocyte count >5 x 10³/mm³ if <20% monocytes			
M5a	Monocytic without differentiation	>80% monocytic cells of which >80% are large monoblasts	-	-	+ NaF inhibits
M5b	Monocytic with differentiation	>80% monocyte cells with monoblasts, promonocytes, monocytes			
M6	Erythroleukemia¶	Erythroblasts (megaloblastic) >50% of nucleated marrow cells; >20% of remaining cells - myeloblasts	+	-	±
M7	Megakaryoblastic§	>20% blasts, megakaryoblasts; cytoplasmic budding may be present	-	±	±

*FAB criteria require 30% blasts. WHO proposed classification of 20% to 30% blast as sufficient for lower limit in recognition that some cases with a 20% blast level have similar clinical outcome to those satisfying the higher (30%) FAB criteria.

†MPO = myeloperoxidase; SBB = Sudan black B; CAE = chloroacetate esterase; NSE = nonspecific esterase.

‡Disseminated intravascular coagulation.

¶Cytoplasmic vacuoles, strongly PAS positive may be present.

§On tissue sections, megakaryocytes may be PAS positive. Cytochemistry is nonspecific. Immunologic and/or ultrastructural (electron microscopic) studies may be needed to show platelet peroxidase in the leukemic blasts.

Table 4. Acute Myeloid Leukemias, Immunophenotypic Characteristics, Cytogenetic Abnormalities

FAB Category	Immunophenotype*	Chromosomal Abnormality
M0	CD13, CD33, CD11b, CD15	None unique
M1	CD13, CD33, HLA-DR, CD19	None unique
M2	CD13, CD15, CD33, HLA-DR, CD19	t(8;21) (q22; q22) in 20% to 25% of cases relatively good prognosis
M3	CD13, CD15, CD33	t(15;17), nearly diagnostic retinoic acid-α fusion retinoic acid may induce maturation
M4 M4eo	CD11, CD13, CD14, CD15, CD33, HLA-DR	inv(16); t(16;16) (p13;q22) (seen with m4eo) relatively good prognosis
M5 M5a	CD11b, CD11c, CD13, CD14, CD15, CD33, HLA-DR May show CD34 expression	t(9,11) (p22; q23)
M6	CD71, glycophorin A mixed populations	Clonal abnormalities present in most cases, none specific - 5/5q-, -7/7q- , and +8 are common and are also seen in therapy-induced leukemia
M7	CD33, CD41, CD42, CD61	inv(3), t(3;-) in older infants and children; t(1;22) (p13, q13)

*The CD antigens may be expressed either singly or in combination by the leukemic cells.

Footnotes

1. Yam LT, Li CY, Crosby WH, et al, "Cytochemical Identification of Monocytes and Granulocytes," *Am J Clin Pathol*, 1971, 55(3):283-90.
2. Willman CL, "Acute Leukemias: A Paradigm for the Integration of New Technologies in Diagnosis and Classification," *Mod Pathol*, 1999, 12(2):218-28.
3. Harris NL, Jaffé ES, Diebold J, et al, "The World Health Organization Classification of Hematological Malignancies Report of the Clinical Advisory Committee Meeting, Arlie House, Virginia, November 1997," *Mod Pathol*, 2000, 13(2):193-207.
4. Rosenthal N and Farhi DC, "Special Stains in the Diagnosis of Acute Leukemia," *Clin Lab Med*, 2000, 20(1):29-38.
5. Nguyen AND, Milam JD, Johnson KA, et al, "A Relational Database for Diagnosis of Hematopoietic Neoplasms Using Immunophenotyping by Flow Cytometry," *Am J Clin Pathol*, 2000, 113(1):95-106.
6. McKenna R, "Acute Myeloid Leukemia," *Practical Diagnosis of Hematologic Disorders*, 3rd ed, Chapter 27, Kjeldsberg CR, ed, Chicago, IL: ASCP Press, 2000, 399-430.
7. Kheiri SA, MacKerrell T, Bonagura VR, et al, "Flow Cytometry With or Without Cytochemistry for the Diagnosis of Acute Leukemias?" *Cytometry*, 1998, 34(2):82-6.
8. Nguyen PL, Olszak I, Harris NL, et al, "Myeloperoxidase Detection by Three-Color Flow Cytometry and by Enzyme Cytochemistry in the Classification of Acute Leukemia," *Am J Clin Pathol*, 1998, 110(2):163-9.
9. Cualing H, Kothari R, and Balachander T, "Immunophenotypic Diagnosis of Acute Leukemia by Using Decision Tree Induction," *Lab Invest*, 1999, 79(2):205-12.
10. Snower DP, Smith BR, Munz UJ, et al, "Re-Evaluation of the Periodic Acid-Schiff Stain in Acute Leukemia With Immunophenotypic Analyses," *Arch Pathol Lab Med*, 1991, 115(4):346-50.
11. Seo IS, Li CY, and Yam LT, "Myelodysplastic Syndrome: Diagnostic Implications of Cytochemical and Immunocytochemical Studies," *Mayo Clin Proc*, 1993, 68(1):47-53.
12. Tsakona CP, Kinsey SE, and Goldstone AH, "Use of Flow Cytochemistry Via the H*1 in FAB Identification of Acute Leukaemias," *Acta Haematol*, 1992, 88(2-3):72-7.
13. Cline MJ, "Histiocytes and Histiocytosis," *Blood*, 1994, 84(9):2840-53.

References

Berman E, "Recent Advances in the Treatment of Acute Leukemia: 1999," *Curr Opin Hematol*, Stossel TP, ed, 2000, 7(4):205-11.

Catovsky D, "Leukocyte Cytochemical and Immunological Techniques," *Practical Haematology*, 8th ed, Chapter 9, Dacie JV and Lewis SM, eds, Ney York, NY: Churchill Livingstone, 1995, 143-71.

Dunphy CH, "Comprehensive Review of Adult Acute Myelogenous Leukemia: Cytomorphological, Enzyme Cytochemical, Flow Cytometric Immunophenotypic and Cytogenetic Findings," *J Clin Lab Anal*, 1999, 13(1):19-26.

Glassman AB, "Chromosomal Abnormalities in Acute Leukemias," *Clin Lab Med*, 2000, 20(1):39-48.

Goasguen J and Bennett JM, "The Acute Myeloid Leukemias: Morphology and Cytochemistry," *Hematology: Clinical and Laboratory Practice*, Volume 2, Chapter 77, Bick RL, ed, St Louis, MO: CV Mosby Co, 1993, 1195-216.

Kass L and Elias JM, "Cytochemistry and Immunocytochemistry in Bone Marrow Examination: Contemporary Techniques for the Diagnosis of Acute Leukemia and Myelodysplastic Syndrome," *Hematol Oncol Clin North Am*, 1988, 2(4):537-55.

Kinney MC and Lukeus JN, "Classification and Differentiation of the Acute Leukemias," *Wintrobe's Clinical Hematology*, 10th ed, Chapter 86, Lee GR, Foerster J, Lukens J, et al, eds, Baltimore, MD: Lippincott Williams & Wilkins, 1999, 2209-40.

Krause JR, "Morphology and Classification of Acute Myeloid Leukemias," *Clinics in Laboratory Medicine: Acute Leukemias*, Crisan D, ed, Philadelphia, PA: WB Saunders Co, 2000, 20(1):1-16.

Li CY, Yam LT, and Sun T, *Modern Modalities for the Diagnosis of Hematologic Neoplasms: Color Atlas/Text*, New York, NY: Igaku-Shoin, 1996, 7-19 and 112-40.

Li CY and Yam LT, "Cytochemistry and Immunochemistry in Hematologic Diagnoses," *Hematol Oncol Clin North Am*, 1994, 8(4):665-81.

Manaloor EJ, Neiman RS, Heilman DK, et al, "Immunohistochemistry Can Be Used to Subtype Acute Myeloid Leukemia in Routinely Processed Bone Marrow Biopsy Specimens. Comparison With Flow Cytometry," *Am J Clin Pathol*, 2000, 113(6):814-22.

Nelson DA and Davey FR, "Leukocyte Peroxidase," *Williams Hematology*, 5th ed, Chapter L23, Beutler E, Lichtman MA, Coller BS, et al, eds, New York, NY: McGraw-Hill Inc, 1995, L65-72.

Zipursky A, Brown EJ, Christensen H, et al, "Transient Myeloproliferative Disorder (Transient Leukemia) and Hematologic Manifestations of Down Syndrome," *Clin Lab Med*, 1999, 19(1):157-67.

♦ **Leukocyte Immunophenotyping** see Leukocyte Cytochemistry on page 456

♦ **Lipidoses** see Inherited Diseases of Metabolism and Cell Structure on page 449

♦ **Lumbar Puncture** see Cerebrospinal Fluid Analysis: Overview on page 416

♦ **Lysosomal Storage Diseases** see Inherited Diseases of Metabolism and Cell Structure on page 449

Lysozyme, Blood and Urine

Related Information

Bone Marrow on page 410
Eosinophil Count on page 424
Leukocyte Cytochemistry on page 456
Lymph Node Biopsy on page 67
Urine Collection, 24-Hour on page 47

Synonyms Muramidase, Blood; Muramidase, Urine

Specimen Serum, 24-hour urine

(Continued)

Lysozyme, Blood and Urine *(Continued)*

Container Red top tube; EDTA plasma (lavender top tube) may also be used; 24-hour urine container

Collection Collect urine for 24-hour period on ice, no preservative.

Storage Instructions Separate serum and freeze **immediately** in plastic vial on dry ice. Upon receipt of urine specimen, freeze on dry ice **immediately** in plastic vial.

Reference Interval Serum: 4.0-15.6 µg/mL (0.28-1.10 µmol/L); urine: 0-1.4 µg/mL (0-0.097 µmol/L)[1]

Use Differential diagnosis of leukemia; present in association with some cases of myelogenous and most cases of monocytic leukemia. Serum lysozyme has been proposed as a parameter for monitoring disease progression/regression in cases of proven sarcoidosis.[2]

Revised FAB (French, American, British) criteria indicate that serum or urine lysozyme levels three times normal fulfill one of three criteria for presence of M4/M5 (acute myeloid leukemia with monocytic differentiation) vs M2 (acute myeloblastic leukemia with maturation).[3]

Limitations Test may lack specificity when applied to classification of acute leukemia (occasional false positive in cases of M1, M2, and M6).[3]

Methodology Turbidimetric, immunochemical (nephelometry), enzymatic - colorimetric, radioimmunoassay (RIA), agarose gel diffusion (recommended method),[1] and ELISA[4]

Additional Information Lysozyme, an hydrolytic enzyme - a bacteriolytic glycosidase, when present in large amounts may appear as a far cathodal migrating ("cationic") band on serum or urine protein electrophoresis. Lysozyme has been found in all three human neutrophil granules (azurophil, specific, and gelatinase types).[4] It is elevated in some cases of myelogenous, and most cases of myelomonocytic and monocytic leukemia. The elevation is proportional to the degree of monocytic differentiation and to tumor cell burden and if marked, can result in potassium wasting and hypokalemia.[5] Lysozyme has been found within the granules of normal and leukemic eosinophils by immunoelectron microscopic study. Elevated serum lysozyme may not establish presence of monocytic differentiation in cases of acute myelogenous leukemia with eosinophilia.[6] The level of serum lysozyme has been used as a predictor of CNS involvement in these leukemias.[7] Serum lysozyme has been shown to be elevated in a number of conditions, including tuberculosis and sarcoidosis as well as leukemia.[2] Sensitivity for prediction of sarcoidosis was 79% in a recent study (c.f. that of serum angiotensin-converting enzyme (ACE) at 59% in the same study).[2] The serum lysozyme level increased with the number of organs involved. Serum lysozyme, however, is less specific for sarcoidosis than serum ACE. Utilizing a turbidimetric method for measurement of serum lysozyme activity, there was evidence that such an assay was useful in differentiating infection from rejection in transplant recipients.[8]

Footnotes

1. Schultz AL, "Lysozyme," *Methods in Clinical Chemistry*, Chapter 95, Pesce AJ and Kaplan LA, eds, St Louis, MO: CV Mosby Co, 1987, 742-6.
2. Tomita H, Sato S, Matsuda R, et al, "Serum Lysozyme Levels and Clinical Features of Sarcoidosis," *Lung*, 1999, 177(3):161-7.
3. Sexton C, Buss D, Powell B, et al, "Usefulness and Limitations of Serum and Urine Lysozyme Levels in the Classification of Acute Myeloid Leukemia: An Analysis of 208 Cases," *Leuk Res*, 1996, 20(6):467-72.
4. Lollike K, Kjeldsen L, Sengelov H, et al, "Lysozyme in Human Neutrophils and Plasma. A Parameter of Myelopoietic Activity," *Leukemia*, 1995, 9(1):159-64.
5. Hillman RS and Ault KA, "The Acute Myeloid Leukemias," *Hematology in Clinical Practice: A Guide to Diagnosis and Management*, Chapter 17, 2nd ed, New York, NY: McGraw-Hill, Health Professions Division, 1998, 274.
6. Moscinski LC, Kasnic G Jr, and Saker A Jr, "The Significance of an Elevated Serum Lysozyme Value in Acute Myelogenous Leukemia With Eosinophilia," *Am J Clin Pathol*, 1992, 97(2):195-201.
7. Peterson BA, Brunning RD, Bloomfield CD, et al, "Central Nervous System Involvement in Acute Nonlymphocytic Leukemia. A Prospective Study of Adults in Remission," *Am J Med*, 1987, 83(3):464-70.
8. Jones JW, Su S, Jones MB, et al, "Serum Lysozyme Activity Can Differentiate Infection From Rejection in Organ Transplant Recipients," *J Surg Res*, 1999, 84(2):134-7.

References

Wickenhauser C, Thiele J, Schmitz B, et al, "Polycythemia Vera Megakaryocytes Store and Release Lysozyme to a Higher Extent Than Megakaryocytes in Secondary Polycythemia (Polyglobuly)," *Leuk Res*, 1999, 23(3):299-306.

Wolach B, Gavrieli R, Manor Y, et al, "Leukocyte Function in Chronic Myeloproliferative Disorders," *Blood Cells Mol Dis*, 1998, 24(4):544-51.

♦ **Macrocytes** *see* Peripheral Blood: Differential Leukocyte Count *on page 464*

♦ **Malarial Parasites** *see* Malaria Smear and Tests *on page 458*

Malaria Smear and Tests

Related Information

Synonyms Blood Smear for Malarial Parasites; Malarial Parasites

Applies to Gametocytes; Glutamine, Plasma; Histidine-Rich Protein (HRP-2); Maurer Dots; OptiMAL®; Plasmodium Species; Pseudoreticulocytosis; QBC Tube, Buffy Coat; Schüffner Dots

Test Includes Examination of thick and thin smears

Abstract Malaria is still the most common infectious disease in the world. Its rapid diagnosis in the laboratory is extremely important. With continuing increase in international travel and liberalization of world trade (social and economic homogeneity) the incidence of malaria in the United States and Europe may be expected to increase.

Specimen Fresh blood (no anticoagulant) - fresh fingerstick smears (two or three of each thick and thin film type) preferably made at bedside using clean oil-/grease-free slides. Air dry and fix by brief dip in methyl alcohol. EDTA anticoagulated whole blood should be obtained for saponin lysis.[1]

To make a thick film smear, spread a drop of blood centrally placed on a slide into a square about four times the area of original drop. Spreading is conveniently achieved with the corner of another slide. Ideally, blood should be thinned until small newsprint is just visible.[2]

Container Slides and lavender top (EDTA) tube

Sampling Time Specimen should be drawn immediately before a fever spike is anticipated.

Causes for Rejection Specimen clotted

Special Instructions If the patient has traveled to a malaria endemic area the date and area traveled should be specified on the requisition. Most cases of malaria seen in the U.S. are found in foreign nationals traveling in the United States.

Reference Interval No organisms identified

Use Diagnose malaria, parasitic infestation of blood; evaluate febrile disease of unknown origin

Limitations One negative result does not rule out the possibility of parasitic infestation. If protozoal, filarial, or trypanosomal infection is strongly suspected, test should be performed at least three times with samples obtained at different times in the fever cycle.

Methodology Microscopic examination of thick and thin peripheral blood Romanowsky dye (in particular Giemsa) stained smears. Thick films are more difficult to interpret but greatly increase sensitivity (by concentrating cells and organisms). Thick smears require considerable experience with malaria. They increase the number of cells examined in a given time period by a factor of about 12.[2] The thin/thick film study is a sensitive technique which under ideal circumstances can detect as few as 10 parasites/µL of blood.

Screening for malaria can also be accomplished by fluorescent microscopy using acridine orange or benzothiocarboxypurine.[3,4,5] These methods are sensitive and can provide consistent results without the need for highly experienced observers. DNA hybridization probes for detection of malaria have been described,[6,7] but in one study, sensitivity was not comparable to that obtained with use of thick films.[7] Thin smears, although not as sensitive, are far superior for determining the species of *Plasmodium* on morphological grounds.[8] A rapid and sensitive "magnet test" has been developed.[9]

Malaria Species Infecting Human Red Cells

Plasmodium Species	Type of Malaria	Time, Bite to Symptoms	Length of Cycle (h)
P. vivax	Tertian	10-14 d	45
P. falciparum	Malignant tertian	10-14 d	48
P. ovale	Ovale		48
P. malariae	Quartan	18-42 d	72

Additional Information Malaria is a protozoan parasitic infection caused in humans by four members of the species *Plasmodium*: *P. vivax*, *P. falciparum*, *P. malariae*, and *P. ovale*. The disease is endemic in subtropical/tropical areas of the world, corresponding to the distribution of the mosquito insect vector, members of the genus *Anopheles*, in which the sexual phase of the life cycle transpires. There has been a resurgence of cases in the United States and Europe beginning in the late 1960s and relating importantly to the problems in Vietnam and political/economic unrest on the African continent.

Proper therapy depends upon identification of the specific variety of malaria parasite. Release of trophozoites and RBC debris results in a febrile response. Periodicity of fever correlates with type of malaria (see table). Organisms are most likely to be detected just before onset of fever which is predictable in many cases. Sampling immediately upon onset of fever is the most desirable time to obtain blood. Alternatively in cases negative by these means but with a strong clinical history, multiple sampling at different times in the fever cycle may prove successful. Hemozoin, a component of malarial pigment, is present in mature trophozoites and gametocytes of all human malarial species. It is a polymer of ferriprotoporphyrin and has paramagnetic and birefringent properties. It allows parasitized red cells to separate in a magnetic field forming the basis of the "magnet test" (see above).[9] Malarial parasites are destroyed in AS and SS patients. Resistance to malaria is also seen with glucose-6-phosphate dehydrogenase deficiency, with increase in Hb E and/or F, and with Southeast Asian ovalocytosis.[10] Malarial resistance to *Plasmodium vivax* occurs in Duffy (Fy^a Fy^b) negative individuals.[11]

While stained thin and thick blood smears are not difficult to prepare and have low space and cost requirements, technical expertise in identification of malarial organisms is difficult to assure, especially in those geographic areas of the world where it is most needed. Tests that would not require human detection/identification of malarial organisms by microscopy have been developed and assessed but cost, unfortunately, may limit their broad application. During the past decade, the following have undergone field evaluation:

- QBC tube Buffy coat with acridine orange (could not identify species in 40% of cases)[12]
- Para-Sight™-F test (a laminated nitrocellulose stick using a single drop of blood, with results in about 10 minutes and using antigen capture technique with mouse monoclonal antibody to a portion of histidine-rich protein-2 (HRP-2) of *P. falciparum*.[13,14,15] Rheumatoid factor or post-therapy persistent antigenemia may give false-positive results.
- ICT Malarial Pf™ (for *Plasmodium falciparum*) or Pv™ (for *Plasmodium vivax*) rapid methods for detection and diagnosis using 10 µL whole blood, placed on a sample pad with colloidal gold-labeled antibody to histidine-rich protein (HRP)-2.[16,17] Rheumatoid factor or post-therapy persistent antigenemia may give false-positive results.
- OptiMAL® (based on detection of parasite lactate dehydrogenase), a 15 minute test that is claimed to detect and differentiate *falciparum* from non-*falciparum* malaria.[18]

Changes in Infected RBCs Useful in Identification of Malaria Species

Plasmodium Species	Infected RBC Enlarged	Presence of Schüffner Dots	Presence of Maurer Dots	Multiple Parasites per RBC	Parasite With Double Chromatin Dots	Gametocytes
P. vivax	+	+	—	Rare	Rare	Spherical, compact
P. falciparum	—	—	+	+	+	Crescentic
P. ovale	±	+	—	—	—	Oval, fills ³/₄ cell
P. malariae	—	—	+	—	—	Round, fills ²/₃ cell

The HRP-2 dependent tests may be misleading in post-treatment follow-up studies (to confirm cure) in that many patients have persistent HRP-2 anti-genemia for up to 7-14 days post-therapy even though microscope study and clinical evidence indicates cure. A number of disadvantages of the new generation of alternative tests (as compared to conventional microscopy) are reviewed by Hänscheid.[19]

Reticulocyte methods used by automated routine hematology analyzers that stain intraerythrocytic nucleic acid may give falsely increased reticulocyte counts (pseudoreticulocytosis) in patients with severe malaria infection.[20] Decreased plasma glutamine concentration has been found in a study population of 50 Ghanaian children with acute *falciparum* malaria. Glutamine becomes conditionally essential in catabolic states and likely contributes to clinical sepsis and mortality. After therapy, plasma glutamine concentration increased. It was considered that acute *falciparum* malaria was associated with significant decrease in plasma glutamine levels and associated increase in sepsis and dyserythropoiesis.[21]

Malaria during pregnancy, while potentially the most controllable aspect of global malaria, is not commonly the target of programs to prevent the disease.[22] The need to work with traditional birth attendants, in attempts to provide control in those geographic regions in which the problem exists, has been emphasized.[22]

Footnotes

1. Keffer JH, "Malarial Parasites. Concentration by Saponin Hemolysis," *Tech Bull Regist Med Technol*, 1966, 36:153-5.
2. Dacie JV and Lewis SM, "Preparation and Staining Methods for Blood and Bone-Marrow Films," *Practical Haematology*, 8th ed, Chapter 6, New York, NY: Churchill Livingstone, 1995, 89-96.
3. Rickman LS, Long GW, Oberst R, et al, "Rapid Diagnosis of Malaria by Acridine Orange Staining of Centrifuged Parasites," *Lancet*, 1989, 1(8629):68-71.
4. Long GW, Jones TR, Rickman LS, et al, "Acridine Orange Detection of *Plasmodium falciparum* Malaria: Relationship Between Sensitivity and Optical Configuration," *Am J Trop Med Hyg*, 1991, 44(4):402-5.
5. Makler MT, Ries LK, Ries J, et al, "Detection of *Plasmodium falciparum* Infection With the Fluorescent Dye, Benzothiocarboxypurine," *Am J Trop Med Hyg*, 1991, 44(1):11-6.
6. Barker RH Jr, Suebsaeng L, Rooney W, et al, "Detection of *Plasmodium falciparum* Infection in Human Patients: A Comparison of the DNA Probe Method to Microscopic Diagnosis," *Am J Trop Med Hyg*, 1989, 41(3):266-72.
7. Lanar DE, McLaughlin GL, Wirth DF, et al, "Comparison of Thick Films, In Vitro Culture and DNA Hybridization Probes for Detecting *Plasmodium falciparum* Malaria," *Am J Trop Med Hyg*, 1989, 40(1):3-6.
8. Pammenter MD, "Techniques for the Diagnosis of Malaria," *S Afr Med J*, 1988, 74(2):55-7.
9. Nalbandian RM, Sammons DW, Manley M, et al, "A Molecular-Based Magnet Test for Malaria," *Am J Clin Pathol*, 1995, 103(1):57-64.
10. Gallagher PG and Javalim P, "Red Cell Membrane Disorders," *Hematology: Basic Principles and Practice*, 3rd ed, Chapter 33, Hoffman R, Benz EJ Jr, Shattil SJ, et al, eds, Philadelphia, PA: Churchill Livingstone, 2000, 594.

11. Lee GR, "Acquired Hemolytic Anemias Resulting From Direct Effects of Infections, Chemical or Physical Agents," *Wintrobe's Clinical Hematology*, 10th ed, Chapter 48, Lee GR, Foerster J, Lukens J, et al, eds, Baltimore, MD: Lippincott Williams & Wilkins, 1999, 1289-94.
12. Mak JW, Normaznah Y and Chiang GL, "Comparison of the Quantitative Buffy Coal Techniques With the Conventional Thick Blood Film Technique for Malaria Case Detection in the Field," *Singapore Med J*, 1992, 33(5):452-4.
13. Shiff CJ, Premji Z, and Minjas JN, "The Rapid Manual Para-Sight™-F Test. A New Diagnostic Tool for *Plasmodium falciparum* Infection," *Trans R Soc Trop Med Hyg*, 1993, 87(6):646-8.
14. Tarimo DS, Moshiro C, Mpembeni R, et al, "Field Trial of the Direct Acridine Orange Method and Para-Sight™-F Test for the Rapid Diagnosis of Malaria at District Hospitals in Dar es Salaam, Tanzania," *Trans R Soc Trop Med Hyg*, 1999, 93(5):521-2.
15. Faiz MA, Rashid R, Palit R, et al, "Para-Sight™-F Test Results in Cerebral Malaria Patients Before and After Treatment in Chittagong Medical College Hospital, Bangladesh," *Trans R Soc Trop Med Hyg*, 2000, 94(1):56-7.
16. Araz E, Tanyuksel M, Ardic N, et al, "Performances of a Commercial Immunochromatographic Test for the Diagnosis of Vivax Malaria in Turkey," *Trans R Soc Trop Med Hyg*, 2000, 94(1):55-6.
17. Stow NW, Torrens JK, and Walker J, "An Assessment of the Accuracy of Clinical Diagnosis, Local Microscopy and a Rapid Immunochromatographic Card Test in Comparison With Expert Microscopy in the Diagnosis of Malaria in Rural Kenya," *Trans R Soc Trop Med Hyg*, 1999, 93(5):519-20.
18. Palmer CJ, Validum L, Lindo J, et al, "Field Evaluation of the OptiMAL® Rapid Malaria Diagnostic Test During Antimalarial Therapy in Guyana," *Trans R Soc Trop Med Hyg*, 1999, 93(5):517-8.
19. Hänscheid T, "Diagnosis of Malaria: A Review of Alternatives to Conventional Microscopy," *Clin Lab Haematol*, 1999, 21(4):235-45.
20. Hoffman JJML and Pennings JMA, "Pseudoreticulocytosis as a Result of Malaria Parasites," *Clin Lab Haematol*, 1999, 21(4):257-60.
21. Cowan G, Planche T, Agbenyega T, et al, "Plasma Glutamine Levels and Falciparum Malaria," *Trans R Soc Trop Med Hyg*, 1999, 93(6):616-8.
22. Nahlen BL, "Rolling Back Malaria in Pregnancy," *N Engl J Med*, 2000, 343(9):651-2.

References

British Committee for Standards in Haematology, Malaria Working Party of the General Haematology Task Force, "The Laboratory Diagnosis of Malaria," *Clin Lab Haematol*, 1997, 19(3):165-70.

Carrasquilla G, Banguero M, Sanchez P, et al, "Epidemiologic Tools for Malaria Surveillance in an Urban Setting of Low Endemicity Along the Colombian Pacific Coast," *Am J Trop Med Hyg*, 2000, 62(1):132-71.

Chalandon Y and Kocher A, Images in Clinical Medicine, "Severe Malaria," *N Engl J Med*, 2000, 342(23):1715.

Chen Q, Schlichtherle M, and Wahlgren M, "Molecular Aspects of Severe Malaria," *Clin Microbiol Rev*, 2000, 13(3):439-50.

Fritsche TR and Smith JW, "Medical Parasitology," *Clinical Diagnosis and Management by Laboratory Methods*, 19th ed, Chapter 53, Henry JB, ed, Philadelphia, PA: WB Saunders Co, 1996, 1252-310.

Jakobsen PH, Bygbjerg IC, Theander TG, et al, "Soluble Haemoglobin Is a Marker of Recent *Plasmodium falciparum* Infections," *Immunol Lett*, 1997, 59(1):35-42.

Kurtzhals JAL, Addae MM, Akanmori BD, et al, "Anaemia Caused by Asymptomatic *Plasmodium falciparum* Infection in Semi-immune African Schoolchildren," *Trans R Soc Trop Med Hyg*, 1999, 93(6):623-7.

Makler MT and Gibbins B, "Laboratory Diagnosis of Malaria," *Clin Lab Med*, 1991, 11(4):941-56.

Makono R and Sibanda S, "Review of the Prevalence of Malaria in Zimbabwe With Specific Reference to Parasite Drug Resistance (1984-96)," *Trans R Soc Trop Med Hyg*, 1999, 93(5):449-52.

"Malaria," *CRC Desk Reference for Hematology*, Shinton NK, ed, Boca Raton, FL: CRC Press, 1998, 445-9.

Pasvol G, "Malaria and Resistance Genes - They Work in Wondrous Ways," *Lancet*, 1996, 348(9041):1532-4.

Wahlgren M, "Creating Deaths From Malaria," *Nat Genet*, 1999, 22(2):120-1.

White NJ, "The Treatment of Malaria: Current Concepts, Review Article," *N Engl J Med*, 1996, 335(11):800-6.

◆ **Mediterranean Macrothrombocytopenia** *see* Platelet Count *on page 468*

◆ **Megakaryoblasts** *see* Leukocyte Cytochemistry *on page 456*

◆ **Megakaryocyte Growth and Differentiation Factor** *see* Thrombopoietin, Serum or Plasma *on page 491*

◆ **Megapoietin** *see* Thrombopoietin, Serum or Plasma *on page 491*

◆ **Megathrombocytes** *see* Platelet Histogram Maximum *on page 471*

◆ **Membrane Leukocyte Alkaline Phosphatase** *see* Alkaline Phosphatase, Neutrophil Membrane (mNAP) *on page 402*

◆ **Merosin** *see* Inherited Diseases of Metabolism and Cell Structure *on page 449*

◆ **Mesothelial Cells** *see* Flow Cytometry, Overview *on page 432*

◆ **Metachromatic Leukodystrophy** *see* Inherited Diseases of Metabolism and Cell Structure *on page 449*

◆ **Methenamine Silver** *see* Leukocyte Cytochemistry *on page 456*

◆ **Methyl Green-Pyronine** *see* Leukocyte Cytochemistry *on page 456*

◆ **Methyl Violet Stain for Heinz Bodies** *see* Heinz Body Stain *on page 440*

◆ **MGDF** *see* Thrombopoietin, Serum or Plasma *on page 491*

◆ **Microbuffy Coat Method for Detection of Bacteremia** *see* Bacteremia Detection, Buffy Coat Micromethod *on page 406*

Microfilariae, Peripheral Blood Preparation

Related Information
Bacteremia Detection, Buffy Coat Micromethod *on page 406*
Filariasis Serological Test *on page 608*
Peripheral Blood: Red Blood Cell Morphology *on page 467*

Synonyms Filariasis, Peripheral Blood Preparation; Helminths, Blood; Trypanosomal/Filarial Parasites, Peripheral Blood Preparation; Trypanosomiasis, Peripheral Blood Preparation

Applies to Filarial Infestation; Hemoflagellates

Test Includes Examination of both thick and thin smears, wet preparation

Specimen Fresh blood from fingerstick

Container Slides

Collection Recommended procedure is for specimen to be obtained when patient spikes a fever. Optimal yield results from examination of a daytime specimen (ie, noon), and a night time specimen (ie, midnight). Timing of sampling relates to geographic place of exposure.

Causes for Rejection Specimen clotted

Special Instructions If patient has traveled to an endemic area, the date of travel, the area, and the suspect parasite should be specified.

Reference Interval No parasites identified

Use Diagnose trypanosomiasis or microfilariasis; work up of elephantiasis, parasitic infestation of blood

Limitations One negative result does not rule out the possibility of parasitic infestation. Since some species of blood parasites can be found during the day and others are nocturnal, both day and night specimens enhance identification. Most filariae generate microfilariae which can be found in peripheral blood, but *Onchocerca volvulus* and *Dipetalonema streptocerca* give rise to microfilariae which do not circulate.

Methodology Fresh wet blood film, with a coverslip, in which motile microfilariae cause agitation of adjacent red cells. Stained films are used as well. Buffy coat methods may be applicable.[1] In some cases, diagnosis may be made by aspiration or brush cytology.[2]

Additional Information Anemia, thrombocytopenia and disseminated intravascular coagulation may characterize the clinical course after some forms of therapy.[3] Biopsy of skin and subcutaneous mass is used in diagnosis of *D. streptocerca* and *O. volvulus*. Differential diagnosis of species of circulating microfilariae requires distinction between the presence or absence of a sheath, the pattern of nuclei in the tail and sometimes the history of geographic exposure and time of sampling. The QBC tube (quantitative buffy coat), utilizing tubes precoated with acridine orange) may provide rapid detection of microfilarial organisms but has low sensitivity.[1]

Microfilariae have been identified in specimens from a variety of unusual sites including gastric brushing study of a large antral gastric ulcer, the latter apparently relating to use of nonsteroidal anti-inflammatory drugs.[2]

Footnotes
1. Freedman DO and Berry RS, "Rapid Diagnosis of Bancroftian Filariasis by Acridine Orange Staining of Centrifuged Parasites," *Am J Trop Med Hyg*, 1992, 47(6):787-93.
2. Singh M, Mehrotra R, Shukla J, et al, "Diagnosis of Microfilaria in Gastric Brush Cytology: A Case Report," *Acta Cytol*, 1999, 43(5):853-5.
3. Maddocks S and O'Brien R, Images in Clinical Medicine, "African Trypanosomiasis in Australia," *N Engl J Med*, 2000, 342(17):1254.

References
Dacie JV and Lewis SM, "Blood Parasites in Preparation and Staining Methods for Blood and Bone-Marrow Films," *Practical Haematology*, 8th ed, Chapter 6, New York, NY: Churchill Livingstone, 1995, 93-6.

◆ **Microhematocrit** *see* Hematocrit *on page 441*

◆ **Microviscometer: Polycythemia of the Newborn** *see* Viscosity, Blood *on page 494*

◆ **mNAP** *see* Alkaline Phosphatase, Neutrophil Membrane (mNAP) *on page 402*

◆ **Monge Disease** *see* Red Cell Mass *on page 478*

◆ **Monocytes** *see* Leukocyte Cytochemistry *on page 456*

◆ **Montreal Platelet Syndrome** *see* Platelet Count *on page 468*

◆ **Morphology** *see* Peripheral Blood: Red Blood Cell Morphology *on page 467*

◆ **MPC** *see* Platelet Count *on page 468*

◆ **mpl-Ligand** *see* Thrombopoietin, Serum or Plasma *on page 491*

◆ **MPM** *see* Platelet Count *on page 468*

◆ **MPV** *see* Platelet Count *on page 468*

◆ **MPV** *see* Platelet Histogram Maximum *on page 471*

◆ **MPV** *see* Platelet Sizing *on page 471*

◆ **Mucolipidoses** *see* Inherited Diseases of Metabolism and Cell Structure *on page 449*

◆ **Mucopolysaccharidoses** *see* Inherited Diseases of Metabolism and Cell Structure *on page 449*

◆ **Muramidase, Blood** *see* Lysozyme, Blood and Urine *on page 457*

◆ **Muramidase, Urine** *see* Lysozyme, Blood and Urine *on page 457*

◆ **Murayama Test** *see* Sickle Cell Tests *on page 486*

◆ **Myeloblasts** *see* Leukocyte Cytochemistry *on page 456*

◆ **Myelokathexis** *see* White Blood Cell Count *on page 496*

◆ **Myeloperoxidase (MPO) Stain** *see* Leukocyte Cytochemistry *on page 456*

◆ **NADH Diaphorase** *see* Red Blood Cell Enzyme Deficiency Screen *on page 476*

◆ **NADH Oxidase** *see* Nitroblue Tetrazolium Test *on page 461*

◆ **Nasal Smear for Eosinophils** *see* Eosinophil Smear *on page 428*

◆ **NBT Dye Test** *see* Nitroblue Tetrazolium Test *on page 461*

n-Butanol Stability Test

Related Information
Heinz Body Stain *on page 440*
Hemoglobin, Unstable, Heat Labile Test *on page 447*
Hemoglobin, Unstable - Isopropanol Precipitation Test *on page 448*

Synonyms Unstable Hemoglobins

Applies to Heinz Bodies

Abstract A simple, low-cost test for unstable hemoglobins. The van der Waals bonds of the molecular structure of hemoglobin in n-butanol solvent (a relatively nonpolar environment as compared with water) are weakened and molecular stability is decreased. Under the test conditions, unstable hemoglobins precipitate.

Specimen Whole blood

Container Lavender top (EDTA) tube

Storage Instructions Fresh blood should be used.

Reference Interval Absence of formation of a precipitate at 120 minutes is a negative test for unstable hemoglobin.

Use Screening test for unstable hemoglobins

Limitations False-positive results may occur if the sample contains ≥10% of Hb F. Increased methemoglobin (which may occur with storage) may also cause a false-positive result.

Methodology Patient's washed, packed red blood cells are mixed with phosphate buffer diluted n-butanol at three different temperature ranges (18°C to 20°C, 21°C to 23°C, and 24°C to 26°C). Normal red cells lyse resulting in a clear solution. A positive control (Hb F) and a normal control (Hb A) sample are run with each test. Tubes are observed (at room temperature) at 30-minute intervals for the presence of turbidity (fine flocculation). The normal control should be clear at 120 minutes. The test is continued until the positive control shows a precipitate. Examination of tubes that are clear (negative reaction) the following day will assist in detection of false-negative results.

Additional Information Hemoglobin that is significantly unstable develops marked precipitation at 90 minutes with flocculation at 2 hours. Slightly unstable hemoglobins (Hb E) develop diffuse precipitation, in some cases minimal, at 2 hours. See Hemoglobin, Unstable, Heat Labile Test *on page 447* and Hemoglobin, Unstable - Isopropanol Precipitation Test *on page 448* for additional comments about unstable hemoglobins.

References
Brozovic M and Henthron J, "Investigation of Abnormal Haemoglobins and Thalassemia," *Practical Haematology*, 8th ed, Chapter 14, Dacie JV and Lewis SM, eds, New York, NY: Churchill Livingstone, 1995, 269-70.
Molchanova TP, "A New Screening Test for Unstable Hemoglobins Using n-Butanol and Red Blood Cells," *Hemoglobin*, 1993, 17(1):81-4.

◆ **Neutral β-Galactosidase** *see* Inherited Diseases of Metabolism and Cell Structure *on page 449*

◆ **Neutropenia** *see* White Blood Cell Count *on page 496*

◆ **Nitroblue Tetrazolium Reduction Test** *see* Nitroblue Tetrazolium Test *on page 461*

Nitroblue Tetrazolium Test

Related Information
Flow Cytometry, Overview *on page 432*

Synonyms NBT Dye Test; Nitroblue Tetrazolium Reduction Test; Tetrazolium Reduction Test

Applies to NADH Oxidase; Respiratory Burst; Superoxide Production

Abstract NBT test is used mainly for the diagnosis of chronic granulomatous disease (CGD). In CGD there is failure of the respiratory burst with decreased or absent superoxide production. Reactive oxygen elements (eg, H_2O_2, hypohalous acids, and $\cdot$OH) are produced from superoxide and have potent microbial activity. The condition has a heterogeneous genetic basis, the result of mutations in any of the components of the NADPH oxidase complex (including gp 91-phox, p22-phox, p47-phox, p67-phox, and p40-phox). CGD is characterized by disabled phagocyte NADPH oxidase with inability to efficiently kill phagocytized bacteria.

Specimen Whole blood

Container Green top (heparin) tube

Storage Instructions Specimen cannot be stored (test utilizes live granulocytes).

Causes for Rejection Transit to the laboratory of more than 1 hour

Special Instructions Advance scheduling with the laboratory may be required, as the specimen must be tested while the neutrophils are still viable. Transport to the laboratory **immediately** following collection.

Reference Interval Without *Staphylococcus* activation, 2% to 8% segmented neutrophils reduce dye. In patients with bacterial infection, NBT-positive cells may be increased (>10%).[1]

Use Diagnose chronic granulomatous disease (CGD) of childhood

Limitations The NBT test is unreliable in the differentiation of bacterial from viral and other infections, producing unacceptable false-negative and false-positive results.

Methodology Assessment of reduction of a tetrazolium dye by stimulated and unstimulated neutrophils. Neutrophils reduce the dye to a dark blue-black formazan pigment upon phagocytosis. Flow cytometry and chemiluminescence-based methods may also be applicable.[1,2] Chronic granulomatous disease can be diagnosed using restriction fragment length polymorphism with labeled gene probes.

Additional Information The NBT test is usually a reliable aid in the diagnosis of CGD, in which neutrophils are unable to reduce the NBT dye (which correlates with their inability to kill bacteria). In patients with CGD, the NADPH oxidase system fails to generate superoxide and derived oxygen intermediates, with resultant susceptibility to recurrent bacterial (in particular, *Staphylococcus aureus*) and fungal (in particular, *Aspergillus* sp) infections. Catalase-positive microorganisms are especially aggressive pathogens in CGD patients because catalase degrades hydrogen peroxide (they neutralize their own H_2O_2).

CGD is rare, with an incidence of some 1:500,000 individuals. It manifests shortly after birth as recurrent suppurative infections with skin involvement, infected eczematoid rash, lymphadenitis, multiple abscesses (lung, liver, other viscera, epidural space) and osteomyelitis. Common pathogens are *S. aureus*, *S. serratia*, and *Salmonella* species. Alternate inflammatory response produces granulomas, occasionally bulky, which can lead to gastrointestinal obstruction. Severity of clinical features is variable. Some mild forms of CGD are not evident until adolescence or adulthood.

The heterogeneous nature of CGD derives from multiple different mutations involving different components of the NADPH oxidase enzyme complex. In the inactive state of the oxidase, two membrane-bound components (gp91-phox-phagocyte oxidase and p22-phox) form a unique cytochrome (cytochrome b_{558}), the central redox component of phagocyte oxidase. It is unique in that it has a very low redox potential. With neutrophil phagocytic activation, three cytosolic factors (p47-phox, p67-phox, and p40-phox) translocate from the cytosol and associate with membrane cytochrome b_{558} along with rac1 or rac2 of the p21 ras family of guanosine 5'-triphosphatases.

The graphic shows a model of NADPH oxidase activation.[3]

In this manner the superoxide-generating enzyme complex, respiratory burst oxidase, is formed. Mutations in the gp91-phox gene (x chromosome at p21.1), account for 60% to 65% of cases of CGD. The other 35% to 40% of patients have autosomal recessive mode of inheritance.[4] See table.

One study suggests that peripheral segmented neutrophils from patients with solid cancer (nonlymphomatous tumors) have decreased capacity to reduce NBT dye to formazan when maximally stimulated with endotoxin.[5] NBT reduction in lymphoma patients was comparable to that of controls. It was also found that stimulated NBT reduction apparently declines with age.[5]

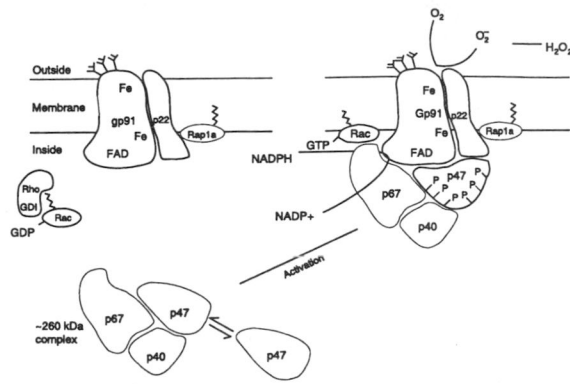

Model of NADPH oxidase activation. Current knowledge of the oxidase suggests that in its dormant state (left side of figure) it is composed of both membrane-bound and cytosolic components. The former include gp91-phox and p22-phox, which together form the cytochrome b heterodimer that also contains the redox centers of the enzyme: FAD and two heme groups (Fe). Rap1a, a low-molecular-weight GTP-binding protein, is also present in the membrane and may functionally associate with the cytochrome. The cytosolic components include p40-phox, p47-phox, and p67-phox, which exist in a complex of 260 kd. A pool of free, monomeric p47-phox is also present in the cytosol prepared from resting neutrophils. In its inactive GDP-bound state, the small GTP-binding protein Rac (Rac2 in human neutrophils) is also cytosolic and is bound to RhoGDP-dissociation inhibitor (GDI). On stimulation (right side of figure), p47-phox, p67-phox, and p40-phox become associated with the plasma membrane primarily through interactions between p47-phox and the subunits of the cytochrome. This translocation process is accompanied by, and perhaps requires (1) the release of Rac from RhoGDI, its conversion to an active (GTP-bound) state, and its association with the plasma membrane, and (2) the multisite phosphorylation of p47-phox. By a mechanism that is not fully understood, binding of the cytosolic components activates the flavocytochrome to catalyze the transfer of electrons from NADPH to oxygen via the FAD and heme redox centers. The compartment labeled "inside" is the cytoplasmic space; "outside" refers either to the extracellular or phagosomal space. (Adapted from Heyworth et al)

Genetic Forms of Chronic Granulomatous Disease

NADPH Oxidase Subunit Involved	Site of Gene Mutation	% of Cases of CGD	Cell Locale
gp91phox	X at p21.1	60% to 65%	Membrane
p47phox	7q 11.23	25%	Cytosol
p67phox	1q 25	5%	Cytosol
p22phox	16q 24	5%	Membrane
p40phox	None known	Unknown	Cytosol

Neutrophil function was found altered (chemotaxis and chemiluminescence decreased) in diabetic patients, especially those with vascular complications and hyperglycemia. While NBT-reducing cells increased after stimulation, there was no difference between patients and controls.[2] In a study of the effect of anesthesia on neutrophil function, halothane, and in particular enflurane, were associated with decreased bactericidal activity in minor and moderately traumatic circumstances, but not with major surgery.[6]

Treatment of CGD patients with recombinant interferon-γ has been shown to result in a near-normal level of superoxide production and return of granulocyte bactericidal capacity to normal control levels. Interferon-γ (rIFN-γ) stimulates progenitor cells and their mature progeny. Colonies of such cells regain the ability to generate superoxide.[7] Therapy with rIFN-γ is considered safe and effective with decrease in the number and severity of infections,[8] but is expensive.[9]

Patients with advanced CGD, who have failed treatment with sulphamethazole trimethoprim, multiple courses of antibiotic/antifungal agents, and interferon-γ therapy may be treated successfully by bone marrow transplant,[9,10] reports of morbidity/mortality not withstanding. Gene transfer studies using viral vectors in murine models,[11,12] and cultured CD34+ hematopoietic progenitor cells[13] have been performed. Peripheral blood stem cells (CD34+) transduced with retrovirus encoding normal p47-phox have been transfused to 5 adults with the p47-phox deficient form of CGD with some success.[14] There is a single report with 24-month follow-up of evident successful allogeneic peripheral blood stem cell transplantation (HLA-matched sister), following nonmyeloablative conditioning and with post-transplant donor (HLA-matched sister) lymphocyte infusions.[15] Engraftment was reported as stable with 100% donor chimerism, normal superoxide production and no graft versus host disease. The NBT test was used in the planning, monitoring, and evaluation of a number of these studies.

Footnotes

1. Paraskevas F, "Phagocytosis," *Wintrobe Clinical Haematology*, Chapter 17, Lee GR, Foerster J, Lukens J, et al, ed, Baltimore, MD: Lippincott Williams & Wilkins, 1999, 426.

2. Delamaire M, Maugendre D, Moreno M, et al, "Impaired Leukocyte Functions in Diabetic Patients," *Diabet Med*, 1997, 14(1):29-34.

3. Heyworth PG, Curnulte JT, and Badereg JA, "Structure and Regulation of the NADPH Oxidase of Phagocytic Leukocytes. Insights From Chronic Granulomatous

(Continued)

Nitroblue Tetrazolium Test *(Continued)*

Disease," *Molecular and Cellular Basis of Inflammation*, Serhan CN and Ward PA, eds, Totowa, NJ: Humana Press, 1999.

4. Patino PJ, Rae J, Noak D, et al, "Molecular Characterization of Autosomal Recessive Chronic Granulomatous Disease Caused by a Defect of the Nicotinamide Adenine Nucleotide Phosphate (Reduced Form) Oxidase Component p67-phox," *Blood*, 1999, 94(7):2505-14.

5. Haim N, Obedeanu N, Meshulam T, et al, "Comparative Study of the Endotoxin-Stimulated Nitroblue Tetrazolium Test in Disease and Health," *J Clin Pathol*, 1978, 31:1249-52.

6. Khan FA, Kamal RS, Mithani CH, et al, "Effect of General Anaesthesia and Surgery on Neutrophil Function," *Anaesthesia*, 1995, 50(9):769-75.

7. Ezekowitz RAB, "Chronic Granulomatous Disease: An Update and a Paradigm for the Use of Interferon-γ as Adjunct Immunotherapy in Infectious Diseases," *Curr Top Microbiol Immunol*, 1992, 181:283-92.

8. Bemiller LS, Roberts DH, Starko KM, et al, "Safety and Effectiveness of Long-Term Interferon Gamma Therapy in Patients With Chronic Granulomatous Disease," *Blood Cells Mol Dis*, 1995, 21(3):239-47.

9. Leung TF, Chik KW, Li CK, et al, "Bone Marrow Transplantation for Chronic Granulomatous Disease: Long-term Follow-up and Review of Literature," *Bone Marrow Transplant*, 1999, 24(5):567-70.

10. Ozsahin BH, vonPlanta M, Müller I, et al, "Successful Treatment of Invasive Aspergillosis in Chronic Granulomatous Disease by Bone Marrow Transplantation, Granulocyte Colony-Stimulating Factor-Mobilized Granulocytes, and Liposomal Amphotericin-B," *Blood*, 1998, 92(8):2719-24.

11. Li LL and Dinauer, "Reconstitution of NADPH Oxidase Activity in Human X-Linked Chronic Granulomatous Disease Myeloid Cells After Stable Gene Transfer Using a Recombinant Adeno-Associated Virus 2 Vector," *Blood Cells Mol Dis*, 1998, 24(4):522-38.

12. Kume A and Dinauer MC, "Gene Therapy for Chronic Granulomatous Disease," *J Lab Clin Med*, 2000, 135(2):122-8.

13. Li F, Linton GF, Sekhsaria S, et al, "CD34+ Peripheral Blood Progenitors as a Target for Genetic Correction of the Two Flavocytochrome b₅₅₈ Defective Forms of Chronic Granulomatous Disease," *Blood*, 1994, 84(1):53-8.

14. Malech HL, Maples PB, Whiting-Theobald N, et al, "Prolonged Production of NADPH Oxidase-Corrected Granulocytes After Gene Therapy of Chronic Granulomatous Disease," *Proc Natl Acad Sci U S A*, 1997, 94(22):12133-8.

15. Nagler A, Ackerstein A, Kapelushnik J, et al, "Donor Lymphocyte Infusion Post-Nonmyeloablative Allogeneic Peripheral Blood Stem Cell Transplantation for Chronic Granulomatous Disease," *Bone Marrow Transplant*, 1999, 24(3):339-42.

References

Curnutte JT and Coates TD, "Disorders of Phagocyte Function and Number," *Hematology: Basic Principles and Practice*, Chapter 41, Hoffman R, Benz EJ Jr, Shattil SJ, et al, eds, Philadelphia, PA: Churchill Livingstone, 2000, 720-62.

Malech HL, Bauer TR Jr, and Hickstein DD, "Prospects for Gene Therapy of Neutrophil Defects," *Semin Hematol*, 1997, 34(4):355-61.

Segal BH, Leto TL, Gallin JI, et al, "Genetic, Biochemical, and Clinical Features of Chronic Granulomatous Disease," *Reviews in Molecular Medicine, Medicine*, 2000, 79(3):170-200.

Winkelstein JA, Marino MC, Johnston RB Jr, et al, "Chronic Granulomatous Disease. Report on a National Registry of 368 Patients," *Medicine*, 2000, 79(3):155-69.

Yu L, Cross AR, Zhen L, et al, "Functional Analysis of NADPH Oxidase in Granulocytic Cells Expressing a Δ488-497 gp91 (phox) Deletion Mutant," *Blood*, 1999, 94(7):2497-504.

♦ **Nitrous Oxide Neuropathy** *see* Sickle Cell Tests *on page 486*

♦ **Nonspecific Esterase** *see* Leukocyte Cytochemistry *on page 456*

♦ **Oil Red O Stain** *see* Leukocyte Cytochemistry *on page 456*

♦ **Opiate Addiction** *see* TGF-β, Serum *on page 490*

♦ **OptiMAL®** *see* Malaria Smear and Tests *on page 458*

Osmotic Fragility

Related Information

Autohemolysis Test *on page 405*
Band 4.2, Red Cell Membrane *on page 406*
Gelation Assay *on page 437*
Glycerol Lysis Test, Acidified, Modified *on page 439*
Osmotic Fragility, Incubated *on page 463*
Peripheral Blood: Red Blood Cell Morphology *on page 467*
Red Blood Cell Indices *on page 477*
Reticulocyte Count *on page 481*

Synonyms Incubated Osmotic Fragility; RBC Fragility; Red Cell Fragility

Applies to Band 3 (Anion Transport Protein); Elliptocytes; Glycophorin C Deficiency; Poikilocytes; Pyropoikilocytosis, Hereditary; Spectrin; Stomatocytes; Xerocytosis

Abstract Osmotic fragility, when increased, is consistent with the presence of spherocytes in the peripheral blood. Spherocytes (spherical-shaped red blood cells) form as a result of loss of red cell membrane surface area relative to intracellular volume. Osmotic fragility is increased when spherocytic red cells are present as occurs with hereditary spherocytosis (HS) a heterogeneous condition clinically and pathologically due to diversity at the molecular level. Abnormal osmotic fragility occurs with, but is not exclusively diagnostic of, hereditary spherocytosis.

Specimen Whole blood

Container Lavender top (EDTA) tube or green top (heparin) tube

Storage Instructions Store refrigerated (4°C) if test performance must be delayed.

Causes for Rejection Hemolysis, clotted specimen, blood more than 6 hours old, oxalate or citrate anticoagulated blood collected

Special Instructions May need to schedule this test in advance.

Reference Interval Hemolysis begins 0.45%, hemolysis complete 0.35%. In some 10% to 20% of individuals with HS, the osmotic fragility curve (unincubated red cells) will be in the normal range. Osmotic fragility test after incubation (see Osmotic Fragility, Incubated *on page 463*) will identify the great majority of these "false-negative" cases.

Use Evaluate hemolytic anemia, especially hereditary spherocytosis; evaluate immune hemolytic states

Limitations Any severe anemia including iron deficiency will yield an abnormal curve. Test measures presence of spherocytes and "spheroidal" cells. Test is **not** specific for hereditary spherocytosis. Trauma-free venipuncture is needed.

Methodology Erythrocytes are placed in graded dilutions of sodium chloride solution; swelling and hemolysis in the lower dilutions provide an index of the resistance of the cells to hypotonic saline. Percent hemolysis is determined using optical density measurements. A modification of osmotic fragility using glycerol and Bis-Tris, is purportedly more sensitive for the diagnosis of hereditary spherocytosis.[1]

Additional Information Hereditary spherocytosis is a common hemolytic anemia with a broad spectrum of severity. Patients have chronic hemolysis but may be clinically asymptomatic or may suffer severe uncompensated hemolysis that responds to splenectomy. HS is the result of inherited defects of the erythrocyte membrane skeleton.[2] A series of proteins interact with each other and form the red cell membrane and interact with lipid of the outer lipid bilayer. Vertical interactions (perpendicular to the membrane) stabilize the lipid bilayer and include spectrin-ankyrin-band 3 interactions and protein 4.1-glycophorin C linkage. Horizontal interactions (parallel to the plane of the membrane) are responsible for structural integrity of the red cell membrane. Horizontal interactions affect the assembly of tetramers from spectrin heterodimers at the spectrin heterodimer site and contact with actin and protein 4.1. HS is considered a disorder of vertical interactions. The lipid bilayer is destabilized, lipid is lost, and the membrane surface area becomes deficient with resultant spherocytosis (see following diagram). Studies have identified structural membrane abnormalities corresponding to four different groups of patients. These are combined spectrin and ankyrin deficiency, the most common defect, followed by band 3 deficiency, isolated spectrin deficiency, and protein 4.2 deficiency.[3,4] See graphic.

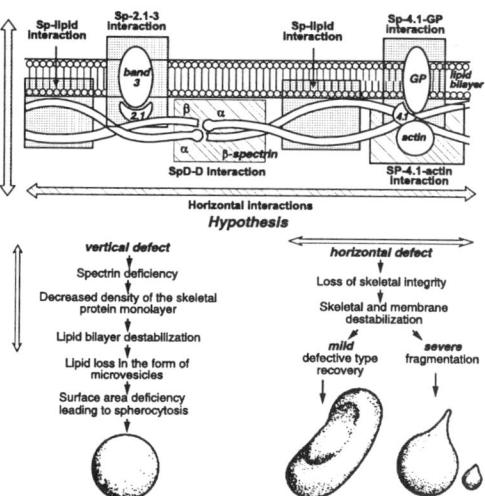

Pathobiology of the red cell lesion in hereditary spherocytosis, elliptocytosis, and pyropoikilocytosis. Left: A defect of vertical interactions as exemplified by the red cell membrane lesions in hereditary spherocytosis. Partial deficiency of spectrin, resulting from either a primary defect of spectrin, and possibly other defects, leads to a reduced density of the skeletal monolayer, leading to destabilization of the membrane lipid bilayer and separation from the underlying skeleton. The bilayer lipids are released from the membrane in the form of microvesicles with loss of cell surface area and spherocytosis. Right: Defect of horizontal interactions as exemplified by the membrane lesion in haemolytic forms of hereditary elliptocytosis pyropoikilocytosis associated with a defect of spectrin self-association.

Adapted from Palek J and Lambert S, "Genetics of the Red Cell Membrane Skeleton," *Seminars in Hematology*, 1990.

HS with uncompensated hemolytic anemia may be associated with reticulocytosis (usually mild to moderate) and mild elevation of serum indirect bilirubin. Patients are susceptible to pigment stones of the gallbladder and to aplastic marrow crises. Spherocytes are more susceptible than are normal red cells to hemolysis in dilute (hypotonic) saline. They show increased osmotic fragility. Spherocytes of any origin (including conditions other than hereditary spherocytosis, eg, autoimmune hemolytic anemia) will cause increased osmotic fragility. Generally, fully expanded cells (eg, spheroidal cells or spherocytes) have increased osmotic fragility while cells with higher surface area to volume ratios (eg, thin cells, hypochromic, target) have decreased osmotic fragility, including some cases of stomatocytosis. See following table for some hematologic findings that may assist in the characterization of some red cell membrane disorders.

Laboratory Differentiation of RBC Membrane Disorders

Test	Result in Patients With:				
	HS	HE	HPP	HST	HX
RBC morphology	Spherocyte	Elliptocyte	Spherocyte, elliptocyte, poikilocyte	Stomatocyte	Target cell
MCV	↑, ↓, or normal	Slightly ↑ or normal	↓	↑	↑ or normal
MCHC	↑	Normal	↑	↓	↑
Osmotic fragility	↑	Normal	↑	↑	↓
Thermal sensitivity	NA	↑, fragments at 47°C-48°C	↑, fragments at 46°C	NA	NA

HS = hereditary spherocytosis; HE = hereditary elliptocytosis; HPP = hereditary pyropoikilocytosis; HST = hereditary stomatocytosis; HX = hereditary xerocytosis; MCV = mean corpuscular volume; MCHC = mean corpuscular hemoglobin concentration; NA = not applicable.

Adapted from Hassoun H, Vassiliadis JN, Murray J, et al, "Hereditary Spherocytosis With Spectrin Deficiency Due to an Unstable Truncated β Spectrin," *Blood*, 1996, 87(6):2538-45.

Osmotic Fragility of Erythrocytes in Various Diseases

Disease	Initial Hemolysis (% saline ±1 SD)	Complete Hemolysis (% saline ±1 SD)	Remarks
Normal	0.44 ±0.02	0.32 ±0.02	
Hereditary spherocytosis	0.68 ±0.14	0.46 ±0.10	Abnormal in all cases; initial hemolysis may occur in 0.85% saline solution
Acquired hemolytic anemia	0.52 ±0.04	0.42 ±0.04	Abnormal in most cases; degree varies with severity
Hemolytic disease caused by ABO incompatibility	0.50 ±0.02	0.40 ±0.02	Abnormal in many cases; degree varies with severity
Hemolytic disease caused by Rh incompatibility	0.60 ±0.06	0.40 ±0.04	Abnormal in many cases; degree varies with severity
Hemolytic anemia caused by drugs	0.50 ±0.04	0.40 ±0.04	Abnormal in most cases during onset; may be normal in later stages
Hemolytic anemia caused by burns	0.50 ±0.04	0.40 ±0.04	Abnormal in about 50% of cases during first few days; usually normal after a few days
Pernicious anemia	0.48 ±0.04	0.36 ±0.02	Occasionally very abnormal; normal in most cases
Congenital nonspherocytic hemolytic anemia	0.44 ±0.02	0.32 ±0.02	Fragility may be increased after blood is incubated
Elliptocytosis, asymptomatic	0.44	0.32	
Elliptocytosis with hemolytic anemia	0.50	0.32	
Thalassemia	0.38 ±0.04	0.20 ±0.06	Complete hemolysis may not be achieved until salt concentration of 0.1% is reached
Sickle cell anemia	0.36 ±0.02	0.20 ±0.04	Abnormal in all cases
Sickle cell trait (S/A)	0.44 ±0.04	0.32 ±0.04	Always normal
Hb C disease	0.34	0.22	Abnormal in almost all cases
Erythremia	0.40 ±0.02	0.28 ±0.02	Not a constant finding
Iron deficiency anemia	0.38 ±0.02	0.28 ±0.02	Typical in severe anemia; not common otherwise
Obstructive jaundice (severe)	0.36 ±0.02	0.28 ±0.04	Decreased fragility usually noted in severely jaundiced patients

Adapted from Miale JB, *Laboratory Medicine: Hematology*, 6th ed, St Louis, MO: Mosby-Year Book Inc, 1982, 584.

The molecular pathology of spherocytosis and other red cell membrane structural protein defects has been partially established and described (see references). Most hereditary hemolytic anemias (including spherocytosis and elliptocytosis) involve mutations of membrane structural proteins, the majority code for abnormal spectrin molecules. In hereditary elliptocytosis, the defect involves horizontal membrane protein interactions which may relate to defective spectrin chains, defective or deficient-based 4.1, glycophorin C deficiency, or presence of abnormal band 3 (anion transport protein).[5] In hereditary pyropoikilocytosis there are two inherited abnormalities, an α-spectrin deficiency (causing defective vertical interactions) and a mutant spectrin that causes atypical horizontal interactions.[5,6] Red cell protein 4.2 deficiency has been described. It has been reported recently in

Japanese individuals who have related anemia and whose red cells show osmotic fragility.[7] (See also Band 4.2, Red Cell Membrane *on page 406*.)

Osmotic fragility is increased in cases of malaria infestation. Both infected and uninfected cells show the increased osmotic fragility. Both osmotic and mechanical fragility of RBCs in patients with multiple sclerosis has been reported as increased.[8] See table.

Decreased osmotic fragility (resistance to lysis) may be seen with iron deficiency (hypochromic cell population), other hemoglobinopathies (especially hemoglobin C disease) likely due to the target cell population, and is characteristic of thalassemia.

Mean osmotic fragility (MOF), found to be significantly increased in hemodialyzed patients prior to dialysis (0.41 ±0.03% vs control 0.39 ±0.02%) corrected after dialysis (MOF 0.38 ±0.03%). MOF was correlated with intact parathyroid hormone level, MOF was higher in patients with a predialysis level >100 pg/dL.[9] The research group concluded that parathyroid hormone likely exerted a major influence on RBC osmotic fragility in chronic renal failure.

See Red Blood Cell Indices *on page 477* for value of histogram of MCHC in detection of hereditary spherocytosis.

Footnotes

1. Vettore L, Zanella A, Molaro GL, et al, "A New Test for the Laboratory Diagnosis of Spherocytosis," *Acta Haematol*, 1984, 72(4):258-63.
2. Palek J, "The Red Cell Skeleton and Haemolytic Anaemias," *Br J Haematol*, 1992, 82(1):260-4.
3. Hassoun H, Vassiliadis JN, Murray J, et al, "Hereditary Spherocytosis With Spectrin Deficiency Due to an Unstable Truncated β Spectrin," *Blood*, 1996, 87(6):2538-45.
4. Gallagher PG and Forget BG, "Hematologically Important Mutations: Spectrin and Ankyrin Variants in Hereditary Spherocytosis," *Blood Cells Mol Dis*, 1998, 24(23):539-43.
5. Gallagher PG and Forget BG, "Hematologically Important Mutations: Band 3 and Protein 4.2 Variants in Hereditary Spherocytosis," *Blood Cells Mol Dis*, 1997, 23(3):417-21.
6. Cochran DL and Burnside LK, "Detecting and Identifying Hereditary Pyropoikilocytosis," *Lab Med*, 1999, 30(1):26-9.
7. Rybicki AC, Qiu JJ, Musto S, et al, "Human Erythrocyte Protein 4.2 Deficiency Associated With Hemolytic Anemia and a Homozygous ^{40}Glutamic Acid → Lysine Substitution in the Cytoplasmic Domain of Band 3 (Band 3^{Montefiore})," *Blood*, 1993, 81(8):2155-65.
8. Schauf CL, Frischer H, and Davis FA, "Mechanical Fragility of Erythrocytes in Multiple Sclerosis," *Neurology*, 1980, 30:323-5.
9. Wu SG, Jeng FR, Wei SY, et al, "Red Blood Cell Osmotic Fragility in Chronically Hemodialyzed Patients," *Nephron*, 1998, 78(1):28-32.

References

Cho MR, Eber SW, Liu SC, et al, "Regulation of Band 3 Rotational Mobility by Ankyrin in Intact Human Red Cells," *Biochemistry*, 1998, 37(51):17828-35.

Delhommeau F, Cynober T, Schischmanoff PO, et al, "Natural History of Hereditary Spherocytosis During the First Year of Life," *Blood*, 2000, 95(2):393-7.

Eber SW, Gonzalez JM, Lux MC, et al, "Ankyrin-1 Mutations Are a Major Cause of Dominant and Recessive Hereditary Spherocytosis," *Nat Genet*, 1996, 13(2):214-8.

Elghetany MT and Davey FR, "Erythrocytic Disorders," *Clinical Diagnosis and Management by Laboratory Methods*, 19th ed, Henry JB, ed, Philadelphia, PA: WB Saunders Co, 1996, 633-5.

Gallagher PG and Jarolim P, "Red Cell Membrane Disorders," *Hematology: Basic Principles and Practice*, 3rd ed, Chapter 33, Hoffman R, Benz EJ Jr, Shattil SJ, et al, eds, Philadelphia, PA: Churchill Livingstone, 2000, 576-610.

Luzzato L and Roper D, "Osmotic Fragility as Measured by Lysis in Hypotonic Saline," *Practical Haematology*, 8th ed, Chapter 13, Dacie JV and Lewis SM, eds, New York, NY: Churchill Livingstone, 1995, 216-20.

Palek J, "Introduction: Red Blood Cell Membrane Proteins, Their Genes and Mutations," *Semin Hematol*, 1993, 30(1):1-3.

Palek J and Jarolim P, "Clinical Expression and Laboratory Detection of Red Blood Cell Membrane Protein Mutations," *Semin Hematol*, 1993, 30(4):249-83.

Pekrun A, Eber SE, Kuhlmey A, et al, "Combined Ankyrin and Spectrin Deficiency in Hereditary Spherocytosis," *Ann Hematol*, 1993, 67(2):89-93.

Yawata Y, "Band 4.2 Abnormalities in Human Red Cells," *Am J Med Sci*, 1994, 307(3):190-203.

Osmotic Fragility, Incubated

Related Information

Autohemolysis Test *on page 405*
Gelation Assay *on page 437*
Glycerol Lysis Test, Acidified, Modified *on page 439*
Osmotic Fragility *on page 402*

Synonyms RBC Fragility; Red Cell Fragility

Abstract The same as the previous test (osmotic fragility) except blood is incubated at 37°C for 24 hours. The test is mainly for diagnosis of hereditary spherocytosis.

Specimen Whole blood

Container Lavender top (EDTA) tube or green top (heparin) tube

Collection Sterile technique must be used.

Causes for Rejection Specimen hemolyzed, specimen clotted, improper anticoagulant (oxalate or citrate), improper venipuncture technique

Use Evaluate hemolytic anemia, particularly hereditary spherocytosis, congenital nonspherocytic hemolytic anemia, thalassemia

Methodology The osmotic fragility test is performed on patient's red blood cells after incubation for 18-24 hours (under sterile conditions) at 37°C. (Continued)

Osmotic Fragility, Incubated *(Continued)*

Additional Information Incubation accentuates increased osmotic fragility. In cases of nonspherocytic hemolytic anemia, fragility may be normal in the unincubated osmotic fragility test but increased after incubation. See graph.

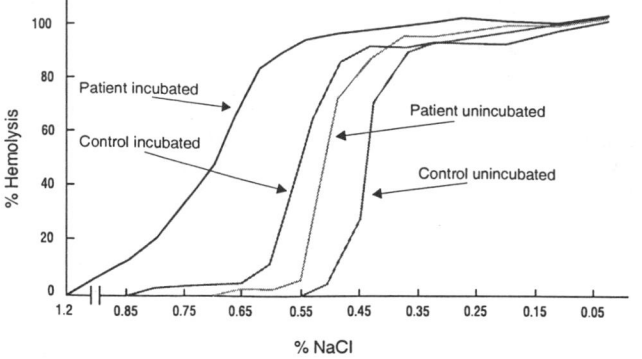

Osmotic fragility of unincubated and incubated RBCs from a normal individual and from a patient with hereditary spherocytosis. Note the increase in fragility produced by incubation of hereditary spherocytosis RBCs.

From Rapaport SI, *Introduction to Hematology*, 2nd ed, Philadelphia, PA: J.B. Lippincott Co., 1987, with permission.

References

Luzzato L and Roper D, "Osmotic Fragility as Measured by Lysis in Hypotonic Saline," *Practical Haematology*, 8th ed, Chapter 13, Dacie JV and Lewis SM, eds, New York, NY: Churchill Livingstone, 1995, 216-20.

- ◆ **Ovalocytes** *see* Band 4.2, Red Cell Membrane *on page 406*

- ◆ **Ovalocytes** *see* Peripheral Blood: Differential Leukocyte Count *on page 464*

- ◆ **Ovalocytes, Smear** *see* Peripheral Blood: Red Blood Cell Morphology *on page 467*

- ◆ **Packed Cell Volume** *see* Hematocrit *on page 441*

- ◆ **Pallidin** *see* Band 4.2, Red Cell Membrane *on page 406*

- ◆ **Pappenheimer Body Stain** *see* Siderocyte Stain *on page 487*

- ◆ **Paracentesis Fluid Analysis** *see* Body Fluid Analysis, Cell Count *on page 408*

- ◆ **Parasites, Red Cells** *see* Peripheral Blood: Differential Leukocyte Count *on page 464*

- ◆ **Paris-Trousseau Syndrome** *see* Platelet Count *on page 468*

- ◆ **Paroxysmal Cold Hemoglobinuria Test** *see* Cold Hemolysin Test *on page 418*

- ◆ **Paroxysmal Nocturnal Hemoglobinuria Test** *see* Ham Test *on page 439*

- ◆ **Parvovirus B19** *see* Cold Hemolysin Test *on page 418*

- ◆ **PAS Stain** *see* Leukocyte Cytochemistry *on page 456*

- ◆ **PCV** *see* Hematocrit *on page 441*

- ◆ **Pelger-Hüet Anomaly** *see* Peripheral Blood: Differential Leukocyte Count *on page 464*

- ◆ **Pericardial Fluid Analysis** *see* Body Fluid Analysis, Cell Count *on page 408*

Peripheral Blood: Differential Leukocyte Count

Related Information

Apoptosis Assays *on page 402*
Bacteremia Detection, Buffy Coat Micromethod *on page 406*
Bone Marrow *on page 410*
Buffy Coat Smear Study of Peripheral Blood *on page 412*
CD4/CD8 Enumeration *on page 511*
Complete Blood Count *on page 419*
Cryoglobulin, Qualitative, Serum and Plasma *on page 524*
Eosinophil Count *on page 424*
Infectious Mononucleosis Screening Test *on page 643*
Leukocyte Cytochemistry *on page 456*
Lymph Node Biopsy *on page 67*
Peripheral Blood: Red Blood Cell Morphology *on page 467*
Platelet Count *on page 468*
Platelet Sizing *on page 471*
White Blood Cell Count *on page 496*

Synonyms Automated Differential; Differential; Differential Smear; Peripheral Differential; White Blood Cell Morphology

Applies to Acanthocytes; Alder-Rielly Anomaly; Auer Rods; Burr Cells; Cabot Rings; *Capnocytophaga canimorsus*; Chédiak-Higashi Anomaly; Dacryocytes; Döhle Bodies; Elliptocytes; Heinz Bodies; Helmet Cells; Howell-Jolly Bodies; Macrocytes; Ovalocytes; Parasites, Red Cells; Pelger-Hüet Anomaly; Platelet Satellitosis; Rouleaux; Schizocytes; Sickle Cells; Spherocytes; Target Cells

Test Includes Relative frequency (%) of and also (in some laboratories) the absolute number of the different types of white blood cells in the peripheral blood, RBC morphology, platelet evaluation

Abstract This procedure, usually a part of the complete blood count, determines the relative and/or absolute number of different types of leukocytes circulating in the peripheral blood. There are significant differences between pediatric and adult reference ranges.

Specimen Whole blood, fresh, anticoagulated (EDTA preferred)

Container Lavender top (EDTA) tube or smears prepared directly from fingerstick or heelstick blood. Heparin or oxalate may produce artifactual distortion of morphology, especially of white blood cells. International Council for Standardization in Hematology recommendation is for use of K_2-EDTA, 1.5-2.2 mg/mL of blood as anticoagulant for blood cell counting and sizing.[1]

Use Determine qualitative and quantitative variations in white cell numbers and morphology, morphology of red cells and platelet evaluation; evaluate anemia, leukemia, infections, inflammatory states, and inherited disorders of red cells, white cells, and platelets; with automated instruments, generation of cell histograms

Limitations Because of sampling, large statistical variation exists, particularly with 100 cell count manual method and with low incidence cells. Day-to-day changes should be interpreted in relation to known method-related variation.

Reference Interval See following tables and tables in White Blood Cell Count *on page 496.*

Leukocyte Values From Birth to Maturity

Age	Leukocyte count (x 10³/mm³)	Neutrophils			Eosinophils	Basophils	Lymphocytes	Monocytes
		Total	Band	Segmented				
At birth	18.1 (9.0-30.0)	11.0 (6.0-26.0) 61%	1.65 9.1%	9.4 52%	0.40 (0.02-0.85) 2.2%	0.10 (0-0.64) 0.6%	5.5 (2.0-11.0) 31%	1.05 (0.40-3.1) 5.8%
12 h	22.8 (13.0-38.0)	15.5 (6.0-28.0) 68%	2.33 10.2%	13.2 58%	0.45 (0.02-0.95) 2.0%	0.10 (0-0.50) 0.4%	5.5 (2.0-11.0) 24%	1.20 (0.40-3.6) 5.3%
24 h	18.9 (9.4-34.0)	11.5 (5.0-21.0) 61%	1.75 9.2%	9.8 52%	0.45 (0.05-1.00) 2.4%	0.10 (0-0.30) 0.5%	5.8 (2.0-11.5) 31%	1.10 (0.20-3.1) 5.8%
1 wk	12.2 (5.0-21.0)	5.5 (1.5-10.0) 45%	0.83 6.8%	4.7 39%	0.50 (0.07-1.10) 4.1%	0.05 (0-0.25) 0.4%	5.0 (2.0-17.0) 41%	1.10 (0.30-2.7) 9.1%
1 mo	10.8 (5.0-19.5)	3.8 (1.0-9.0) 35%	0.49 4.5%	3.3 30%	0.30 (0.07-0.90) 2.8%	0.05 (0-0.20) 0.5%	6.0 (2.5-16.5) 56%	0.70 (0.15-2.0) 6.5%
6 mo	11.9 (6.0-17.5)	3.8 (1.0-8.5) 32%	0.45 3.8%	3.3 28%	0.30 (0.07-0.75) 2.5%	0.05 (0-0.20) 0.4%	7.3 (4.0-13.5) 61%	0.58 (0.10-1.3) 4.8%
1 y	11.4 (6.0-17.5)	3.5 (1.5-8.5) 31%	0.35 3.1%	3.2 28%	0.30 (0.05-0.70) 2.6%	0.05 (0-0.20) 0.4%	7.0 (4.0-10.5) 61%	0.55 (0.05-1.1) 4.8%
6 y	8.5 (5.0-14.5)	4.3 (1.5-8.0) 51%	0.25 3.0%	4.0 48%	0.23 (0-0.65) 2.7%	0.05 (0-0.20) 0.6%	3.5 (1.5-7.0) 42%	0.40 (0-0.8) 4.7%
12 y	8.0 (4.5-13.5)	4.4 (1.8-8.0) 55%	0.25 3.0%	4.2 52%	0.20 (0-0.55) 2.5%	0.04 (0-0.20) 0.5%	3.0 (1.2-6.0) 38%	0.35 (0-0.8) 4.4%
18 y	7.7 (4.5-12.5)	4.4 (1.8-7.7) 57%	0.23 3.0%	4.2 54%	0.20 (0-0.45) 2.6%	0.04 (0-0.20) 0.5%	2.7 (1.0-5.0) 35%	0.40 (0-0.8) 5.2%
21 y	7.4 (4.5-11.0)	4.4 (1.8-7.7) 59%	0.22 3.0%	4.2 56%	0.20 (0-0.45) 2.7%	0.04 (0-0.20) 0.5%	2.5 (1.0-4.8) 34%	0.30 (0-0.8) 4.0%

Adapted from Altman PL and Dittmer DS, eds, *Biology Data Book*, 2nd ed, Volume 3, Bethesda, MD: Federation of American Societies for Experimental Biology, 1974.

Review of Peripheral Blood Smear

Red Cell Variant*†	Clinical Associations
Crenated cell (Echinocyte)	Variant form of normal RBC
Burr cell	DIC, I.V. fibrin deposition
Schizocyte	Microangiopathic hemolytic anemia
Helmet cell	Hypertension
(Schizocyte)	Cardiac valve disease
	Uremia, burns
	Metastatic malignancy
	Severe iron deficiency/bleeding lesion
	Normal newborn
Elliptocyte	Few seen normally
Ovalocyte	Many may mean primary elliptocytosis
	Iron deficiency
	Thalassemia
	Hb S or C
	Other hemolytic anemias
Target cell (Codocyte)	Hemoglobinopathies (S, C, D, thalassemia, esp)
	Iron deficiency
	Liver disease
	LCAT deficiency
Oval macrocyte (Megalocyte)	Megaloblastic anemia
	B_{12}/folate deficiency
	Myeloproliferative disease
	Chemotherapy patients
Spherocyte	Hereditary spherocytosis
	Immune and other hemolytic states
Tear drop cell (Dacryocyte)	Myeloproliferative diseases
	Myelophthisic processes
	Pernicious anemia
	Thalassemia
Sickle cell (Drepanocyte)	Sickle cell disease and variants (ie, sickle/thalassemia, SD disease, SC disease)
Acanthocyte	Abetalipoproteinemia
	Alcoholic cirrhosis with hemolysis
	Pyruvate kinase deficiency
	Postheparin in some individuals[1]
Stomatocyte	Hereditary stomatocytosis
	Alcoholism
	Rh null disease
Schistocyte	Microangiopathic hemolysis
Helmet cell	Cardiac valve disease
Spurr cell	DIC
(Schizocyte) (Keratocyte)	Severe burns
	Uremia
Triangulocytes[2]	Alcoholism
	Rarely, Hb C disease
	Thalassemia
	Nonalcohol liver disease
	TTP
	Antimitotic chemotherapy
Eccentrocytes[3] (Asymmetric distribution of Hb)	G6PD deficiency
Bite cells[4,5]	Heinz body hemolytic anemia
(Degmacyte)	Oxidative hemolysis
	Methemoglobinemia due to phenazopyridine sulfanilamide
	Unstable hemoglobin (eg, Hb Köln)
	Thalassemia
Hemighosts[6]	Severe oxidative injury
	Heinz body hemolytic anemia
	Oxidative hemolysis
Polychromatophil	Increased erythropoiesis
Reticulocyte	Myelophthisic states
Nucleated RBC	Hemolytic states
	Postsplenectomy
Basophilic stippling	Lead poisoning
(Punctate basophilis)	Hemolytic states, other anemias
	Thalassemia
	Pyrimidine-5'-nucleotidase deficiency
Pappenheimer bodies	Some hemolytic anemias
(Siderocytes)	Postsplenectomy
	Some megaloblastic anemias
	Some sideroblastic states
Parasites	Plasmodium (malaria)
	Bartonella
	Microfilaria (not intracellular)
	Whipple's disease bacillus (Tropheryma whippelii)
	Babesia and Babesia-like organisms
	Spirochetes of Borrelia species (relapsing fever)

Review of Peripheral Blood Smear

Red Cell Variant*†	Clinical Associations
Rouleaux of RBCs	Reflects increased protein concentration
	May be associated with multiple myeloma
	Waldenström's macroglobulinemia blue staining background
Howell-Jolly bodies	Hemolytic anemia
(Nuclear fragments)	Hyposplenism/asplenism (splenectomy)
	Megaloblastic anemia
Cabot Ring (Nuclear remnants)	Megaloblastic anemia
Heinz bodies	Some drug sensitive oxidative hemolytic anemias
(Denatured Hb)	Unstable hemoglobinopathies
WBC Abnormalities	**Clinical Associations**
Leukocytosis Increase in % bands (left shift)	Acute reactive state metabolic basis infections (esp bacterial) basis
Toxic granulation	
Toxic vacuolation	
Döhle bodies	Acute infection, esp pneumonia
	Scarlet fever
	Measles,
	Septicemia
	May-Hegglin anomaly
Chediak-Higashi anomaly	Inherited, giant lysosomal granules
Pseudo-Chediak-Higashi anomaly	Few cases of acute myeloid leukemia
Hypersegmented neutrophils	Megaloblastic states as pernicious anemia
Hypogranular neutrophils	Some cases of chronic myelogenous leukemia
Intraleukocyte microorganisms	Bacteria
	Ehrlichia sennetsu (Sennetsu fever)
Intragranulocytic	Ehrlichia species
Intramonocytic and small lymphocytic	Ehrlichia chaffeensis (human ehrlichiosis)
Auer rods (present in blast cells)	Acute myelogenous leukemia
Chediak-Higashi inclusions	Congenital deficiency
	Lysosomal membrane
	Phospholipid
Alder-Reilly anomaly	Mucopolysaccharidosis
Pelger-Huët anomaly (mono and bilobed neutrophils with clumped nuclear chromatin)	Congenital form
	Acquired form - associated with myelogenous leukemia
Howell-Jolly body-like basophilic neutrophil inclusions	AIDS
Monocytes with disorganized cytoplasmic fibrils[7]	AIDS
Neutrophil cytoplasmic inclusion bodies	Human ehrlichiosis
Platelet Abnormalities	**Clinical Associations**
Platelet satellitosis	No definite causal clinical association
Platelet clumping	May cause spurious leukocytosis and thrombocytopenia[8]

[1]Silber R, "Of Acanthocytes, Spurs, Burrs, and Membranes," Blood, 1969, 34:111.

[2]Schumacher HR, Khanna S, and Moyer B, "Letter: Triangulocytes in Alcoholism," JAMA, 1976, 235:2285-6.

[3]Ham TH, Grauel JA, Dunn RF, et al, "Physical Properties of Red Cells as Related to Effects In Vivo. IV. Oxidant Drugs Producing Abnormal Intracellular Concentration of Hemoglobin (Eccentrocytes) With a Rigid Red-Cell Hemolytic Syndrome," J Lab Clin Med, 1973, 82:898-910.

[4]Ward PC, Schwartz BS, and White JG, "Heinz Body Anemia: Bite Cell Variant — A Light and Electron Microscopic Study," Am J Hematol, 1983, 15:135-46.

[5]Greenberg MS, "Heinz Body Hemolytic Anemia: "Bite Cells — A Clue to Diagnosis," Arch Intern Med, 1976, 136:153-5.

[6]Chan TK, Chan WC, and Weed RI, "Erythrocyte Hemighosts: A Hallmark of Severe Oxidative Injury In Vivo," Br J Haematol, 1982, 50:575.

[7]Kass L, "Cytoplasmic Abnormalities in Monocytes From Patients With AIDS," Lab Med, 2001, 32(3):139-42.

[8]Solanki DL and Blackburn BC, "Spurious Leukocytosis and Thrombocytopenia. A Dual Phenomenon Caused by Clumping of Platelets In Vitro," JAMA, 1983, 250:2514-5.

*Established terminology is followed (parentheses) by that of Bessis M et al, introduced on the basis of ultrastructural analyses.

†Some abnormal red cell forms may represent artifact introduced during preparation of the blood smear (especially stomatocytes and elliptocytes, occasionally target-like cells).

Adapted from Bessis M, Blood Smears Reinterpreted, New York, NY: Springer International, 1977.

Adapted from Bessis M, Weed RI, and Leblond PF, Red Cell Shape: Physiology, Pathology, Ultrastructure, New York, NY: Springer Verlag, 1973.

(Continued)

Differential Leukocyte Count

Age	Segs (%)	Bands (%)	Eos (%)	Basos (%)	Lymphs (%)	Monos (%)
Birth	47±15	14.1±4	2.2	0.6	31±5	5.8
12 h	53	15.2	2.0	0.4	24	5.3
24 h	47	14.2	2.4	0.5	31	5.8
1 wk	34	11.8	4.1	0.4	41	9.1
2 wk	29	10.5	3.1	0.4	48	8.8
2 mo	25	8.4	2.7	0.5	57	5.9
6 mo	23	8.8	2.5	0.4	61	4.8
10 mo	22	8.3	2.5	0.4	63	4.6
2 y	25	8.0	2.6	0.5	59	5.0
6 y	43	8.0	2.7	0.6	42	4.7
10 y	46±15	8.0±3	2.4	0.5	38±10	4.3
14 y	48	8.0	2.5	0.5	37	4.7
21 y	51±15	8.0±3	2.7	0.5	34±10	4.0

Adapted from Miale JB, *Laboratory Medicine: Hematology*, 6th ed, St Louis, MO: Mosby-Year Book Inc, 1982.

Methodology One or a combination of methods: manual enumeration of white cells on Wright-stained peripheral blood smear; automated WBC computer image analysis (such instruments are no longer being manufactured); continuous flow system (automated) using cytochemical/light scattering measurements; cell volume (impedance related/conductivity/light scattering) measurements, resultant electronic signals of combined methods are further manipulated with computer-assisted synthesis and derivations.

Additional Information Significantly abnormal findings (automated or manual method) should be the subject of further study and review. Changes in leukocyte fractions are a window to a spectrum of minor to serious physiologic and pathologic changes. Some of these are tabulated in the table and in the tables in the Hematology Introduction *on page 391*.

The past decade has seen significant contributions to the definition of WBC differential reference values. The considerable increase in available data (as compared to that of the 1940-1970 period) cannot be summarized comprehensively in a simple manner. Variations, often not clinically significant, relate to differences in sex, race, physiologic state, and method of analysis. More significant variation is seen with age. A continuous flow cytochemical based automated analytic system (Bayer® Diagnostics, Tarrytown, NY) determines immaturity of the neutrophilic granulocytic series on the basis of a peroxidase reaction. This is not directly comparable to identification of band (stab) population using morphologic criteria. It is possible to detect myeloperoxidase deficiency with this peroxidase reaction-based system. Enumeration of band population is definition dependent. Automated differential determinations may vary between instruments and manual techniques but clinical significance of such differences may be minimal. Black individuals have lower neutrophil values than whites.[2] The greatest variation, both in relative and absolute terms occurs as the result of age. High WBC levels are present in the newborn and lymphocytes are increased in childhood (as compared to adult values). Correlation of the manually performed vs automated differential is somewhat poorer in pediatric as compared to adult populations.[3] Both relative (%) and absolute (actual number of cells/mm³) values need to be considered in relation to the clinical situation.

Current hematology instruments can produce automated differentials by cytochemistry/light scattering or cell volume/conductivity/light scattering techniques. Conductivity measurements utilize a high frequency electromagnetic probe. Leukocytes are separated into granulocytes, lymphocytes, monocytes, eosinophils, and basophil categories and an immaturity index (not exactly bands) of the granulocytes. With modern hematology instruments, manual differential determinations are at least partially redundant. High white counts[4,5] and fever are better indicators of clinical infection than the percentage of bands. This is because of the high variability of manual differential band counts from technologist to technologist. The band count was found superior to the immature to total neutrophil count ratio, the total WBC count, and the neutrophil count in the diagnosis of inflammatory and infective disease when compared to the C-reactive protein level.[6]

Any particular patient (however uncommonly encountered) may present with very few but very significantly abnormal peripheral red or white cells allowing timely diagnosis not possible by other initial methods of evaluation. Some morphologic abnormalities of peripheral blood neutrophils (degree of hypogranulation and of Pelger-Huët-like changes) reflect the degree of marrow dysplasia in myelodysplastic syndromes.[7] Detection of circulating myeloma cells is clinically important as they correlate with disease activity. The cells of multiple myeloma are best detected by the use of sensitive immunofluorescent, flow cytometric, or molecular genetic techniques.[8] Cryoglobulins, while of rare occurrence, may be due to multiple myeloma in some 50% of cases and are also seen as a complication of hepatitis C. Cryoglobulins are circulating immunoglobulins that are reversibly cold precipitable. Clinically, they may be associated with arthralgia, skin lesions, the Raynaud phenomena and liver/kidney changes. Associated laboratory abnormalities include elevated erythrocyte sedimentation rate, positive rheumatoid factor test, and hypocomplementemia. There may be pseudoleukocytosis and pseudothrombocytosis. The routine Wright-stained peripheral blood smear (prepared from blood collected at room temperature) shows neutrophil and monocyte intracytoplasmic vacuole-like inclusions and extracellular globules of lightly pink to slightly basophilic amorphous material in the background.[9,10] These morphologic changes, present on the peripheral blood smear, may be the initial finding in some cases of myeloma and should prompt evaluation for cryoglobulinemia.

The cytoplasmic vacuoles seen in cases of cryoglobulinemia must be distinguished from artifact due to EDTA, and most importantly, from those that occur with overwhelming sepsis. With septicemia, the neutrophil intracytoplasmic vacuoles are clear while those seen with cryoglobulinemia are usually pink to lightly basophilic.[8] Clinical correlation with other findings is essential (eg, presence of "left shift", toxic granulation, Döhle bodies).

A number of other uncommon but potentially critically important conditions may leave footprints on the peripheral blood smear (see table and Buffy Coat Smear Study of Peripheral Blood *on page 412*). A recent example is the report of potentially rapidly fatal septicemia with Waterhouse-Friderichsen syndrome due to *Capnocytophaga canimorsus*. The PBS may show neutrophil toxic granulation with intracytoplasmic and extracellular bacterial rods. This gram-negative microaerophil has been associated with infection and with hemolytic uremic syndrome following animal bites, particularly dogs.[11,12]

Careful study of morphologic abnormalities by experienced laboratory personnel is mandatory. False identification of "look-alike" abnormalities can lead to unnecessary patient morbidity/mortality and/or the expense and inconvenience of additional and inappropriate tests. Pseudo-Chédiak-Higashi syndrome, pseudo-Pelger-Huët anomaly, and Pseudo-Gaucher cells are examples in which the named entities are mimicked by formation of abnormal granules or other changes by a myelodysplastic or myeloproliferative (leukemic) disease process.[13]

EDTA-induced leukoagglutination has been reported but is very uncommon. It has been seen with neutrophils and with both benign and malignant lymphocytes.[14]

Cytoplasmic abnormalities ("disorganized" cytoplasmic fibrils) have been observed in monocytes and found to be associated with clinical AIDS.[15]

See also comments under Additional Information of Peripheral Blood: Red Blood Cell Morphology *on page 467*. See Platelet Count *on page 468* and Platelet Sizing *on page 471* for discussion of platelet morphology and abnormalities.

Footnotes

1. "Recommendations of the International Council for Standardization in Haematology for Ethylenediaminetetraacetic Acid Anticoagulation of Blood for Blood Cell Counting and Sizing," *Am J Clin Pathol*, 1993, 100(4):371-2.
2. Karayalcin G, Rosner F, and Sawitsky A, "Pseudoneutropenia in Blacks: A Normal Phenomenon," *N Y State J Med*, 1972, 72:1815-7.
3. Goyzueta FG, Bailey CJ, and Billett HH, "Automated Differential White Blood Cell Counts in the Young Pediatric Population," *Lab Med*, 1996, 27(1):48-52.
4. Banez EI and Bacaling JH, "An Evaluation of the Technicon® HI Automated Hematology Analyzer in Detecting Peripheral Blood Changes in Acute Inflammation," *Arch Pathol Lab Med*, 1988, 112(9):885-8.
5. Bentley SA, "Alternatives to the Neutrophil Band Count," *Arch Pathol Lab Med*, 1988, 112(9):883-4.
6. Seebach JD, Morant R, Rüegg R, et al, "The Diagnostic Value of the Neutrophil Left Shift in Predicting Inflammatory and Infectious Disease," *Am J Clin Pathol*, 1997, 107(5):582-91.
7. Widell S, Hellström-Lindberg E, Kock Y, et al, "Peripheral Blood Neutrophil Morphology Reflects Bone Marrow Dysplasia in Myelodysplastic Syndromes," *Am J Hematol*, 1995, 49(2):115-20.
8. Witzig TE, "Detection of Malignant Cells in the Peripheral Blood of Patients With Multiple Myeloma: Clinical Implications and Research Applications," *Mayo Clin Proc*, 1994, 69(9):903-7.
9. Maitra A, Ward PC, Kroft SH, et al, "Cytoplasmic Inclusions in Leukocytes: An Unusual Manifestation of Cryoglobulinemia," *Am J Clin Pathol*, 2000, 113(1):107-12.
10. Lesesve JF and Goasguen J, "Cryoglobulin Detection From a Blood Smear Leading to the Diagnosis of Multiple Myeloma," *Eur J Haematol*, 2000, 65(1):77.
11. Mirza I, Wolk J, Toth L, et al, "Waterhouse-Friderichsen Syndrome Secondary to *Capnocytophaga canimorsus* Septicemia and Demonstration of Bacteremia by Peripheral Blood Smear," *Arch Pathol Lab Med*, 2000, 124(6):859-63.
12. Tobe TJ, Franssen CF, Zijlstra JG, et al, "Hemolytic Uremic Syndrome Due to *Capnocytophaga canimorsus* Bacteremia After a Dog Bite," *Am J Kidney Dis*, 1999, 33(6):e5.
13. Bridgen ML and Dalal BI, "Morphologic Abnormalities, Pseudosyndromes, and Spurious Test Results," *Lab Med*, 1999, 30(6):397-403.
14. Deol I, Hernandez AM, and Pierre RV, "Ethylenediamine Tetraacetic Acid-Associated Leukoagglutination," *Am J Clin Pathol*, 1995, 103(3):338-40.
15. Kass L, "Cytoplasmic Abnormalities in Monocytes From Patients With AIDS," *Lab Med*, 2001, 32(3):139-142.

References

Ardron MJ, Westengard JC, and Dutcher TF, "Band Neutrophil Counts Are Unnecessary for the Diagnosis of Infection in Patients With Normal Total Leukocyte Counts," *Am J Clin Pathol*, 1994, 102(5):646-9.

Barenfanger J, Patel PG, Dumler JS, et al, "Identifying Human Ehrlichiosis," *Lab Med*, 1996, 27(6):372-3.

Brouqui P and Raoult D, "Human Ehrlichiosis," *N Engl J Med*, 1994, 330(24):1760-1.

Constantino BT and Cogionis B, "Nucleated RBCs-Significance in the Peripheral Blood Film," *Lab Med*, 2000, 31(4):223-9.

Cornbleet J, "Spurious Results From Automated Hematology Cell Counters," *Lab Med*, 1983, 14(8):509-14.

Elin RJ, Whitis J, and Snyder J, "Infectious Disease Diagnosis From a Peripheral Blood Smear," *Lab Med*, 2000, 31(6):324-8.

Everett ED, Evans KA, Henry RB, et al, "Human Ehrlichiosis in Adults After Tick Exposure. Diagnosis Using Polymerase Chain Reaction," *Ann Intern Med*, 1994, 120(9):730-5.

Gulati GL and Hyun BH, "Blood Smear Examination," *Hematol Oncol Clin North Am*, 1994, 8(4):631-50.

Hope E and Peerschke EI, "Principles of Automated Differential Analysis," *Clinical Hematology and Fundamentals of Hemostasis*, 2nd ed, Chapter 30, Section II, Harmening DM, ed, Philadelphia, PA: FA Davis Co, 1992, 554-67.

Howard MR and Smith RA, "Early Diagnosis of Septicaemia in Preterm Infants From Examination of Peripheral Blood Films," *Clin Lab Haematol*, 1999, 21(5):365-8.

Hoyer JD, "Leukocyte Differential," *Mayo Clin Proc*, 1993, 68(10):1027-8.

Krause JR, "The Automated White Blood Cell Differential: A Current Perspective," *Hematol Oncol Clin North Am*, 1994, 8(4):605-16.

Mollinedo F, Borregaard N, and Boxer LA, "Novel Trends in Neutrophil Structure, Function, and Development," *Immunol Today*, 1999, 20(12):535-7.

Paddock CD, Suchard DP, Grumbach KL, et al, "Brief Report: Fatal Seronegative Ehrlichiosis in a Patient With HIV Infection," *N Engl J Med*, 1993, 329(16):1164-7.

Reed KD, Mitchell PD, Persing DH, et al, "Transmission of Human Granulocytic Ehrlichiosis," *JAMA*, 1995, 273(1):23.

Robertson EP, Lai HW, and Wei DC, "An Evaluation of Leukocyte Analysis on the Coulter STK-S," *Clin Lab Haematol*, 1992, 14(1):53-68.

Saxena S and Wong ET, "Heterogeneity of Common Hematologic Parameters Among Racial, Ethnic and Gender Subgroups," *Arch Pathol Lab Med*, 1990, 114(7):715-9.

Swaim WR, "Laboratory and Clinical Evaluation of White Blood Cell Differential Counts: Comparison of the Coulter VCS, Technicon® H-1, and 800-Cell Manual Method," *Am J Clin Pathol*, 1991, 95(3):381-8.

Winkel P, Statland BE, Saunders AM, et al, "Within-day Physiologic Variation of Leukocyte Types in Healthy Subjects as Assayed by Two Automated Leukocyte Differential Analyzers," *Am J Clin Pathol*, 1981, 75(5):693-700.

Peripheral Blood: Red Blood Cell Morphology

Related Information

Synonyms Blood Smear Morphology; Morphology; Peripheral Smear, Blood; RBC Morphology; RBC Smear; Red Blood Cell Morphology

Applies to Ovalocytes, Smear; Pyropoikilocytosis; Schistocytes, Smear; Sickle Cells, Smear; Spherocytes, Smear; Stippled RBCs, Smear; Thermal Sensitivity Test

Specimen Whole blood

Container Lavender top (EDTA) tube or smears prepared directly from fingerstick or heelstick blood. Heparin or oxalate may produce artifactual distortion especially of white blood cells.

Collection Routine venipuncture. Invert tube gently to mix.

Storage Instructions Refrigerate

Causes for Rejection Clotted or hemolyzed specimen

Reference Interval Normal morphology. It may not be possible to correlate minor changes in RBC morphology (eg, 5% to 10% elliptocytosis) with identifiable disease.

Use Evaluate red cell disorders, white cell disorders, platelet disorders, and correlation of findings with CBC parameters as quality control function

Methodology Study of red blood cell morphology as it presents on Wright stained peripheral blood. Red blood cell indices as determined by automated cell counters (eg, MCV, MCH, MCHC, RDW) also give insight into morphologic red cell abnormalities.

Additional Information Diverse trends at all levels of the medical care system have combined to focus attention on the utility/cost-effectiveness of manual review of the peripheral blood smear (PBS), in particular, as a routine incorporated in the CBC. The CBC has evolved from highly labor intensive to highly capital intensive, while the PBS has remained highly labor intensive. Automated devices continue to expand their repertoire, adding new parameters that digitize and in some cases improve upon information formerly gleaned from study of the PBS (eg, red cell distribution width which quantitates the morphologic observation anisocytosis). There is a trend to perform WBC differential only in cases of abnormal WBC count or only upon specific order. It should be recognized, however, that review of PBS is a part of the quality control cross check system built into each CBC and available to the medical technologist performing the test and to physicians and others who may subsequently question the integrity of the results. Each CBC (when truly complete with review of PBS, WBC differential count, and RBC indices) is a self-contained case individualized quality control unit. Automated counters when confronted with uncertainty (capable of generating spurious results) respond with a set of "flags" some parameters of which can be set or adjusted by laboratory staff professionals.[1] A flagged result indicates the need for manual review of that patient's peripheral blood smear. A large study (467 samples) from various inpatient/outpatient environments found that at a detection limit ≥1% abnormal WBCs, >20% of samples were not correctly flagged (1997 study).[1]

Cost and utilization considerations seem to indicate that review of PBS and differential study of WBCs should be relegated to the occasional special situation (ie, on physician order or to assist with evaluation of an abnormal result from an automated cell counter). This role in itself would necessitate review of some 10% to 30% of CBC studies depending on the type of institution. Computer assisted automated differential analyzers flag and require some 10% to 20% of cases for manual review, also institution variable. While labor intensive, the study of PBS is nearly devoid of capital costs. On the other hand, automated counters are not free of labor costs and are highly capital intensive. These expensive units are not centralized, due in part to the perceived need for "stat" capability. They are, therefore, not efficiently utilized; they are idle for part of the day. In effect a costly instrument is used to screen (CBC without differential) for performance of a low cost but in some respects more definitive test.

Efforts expended on technical and economic aspects of delivering a CBC may cloud the fact that some information may be hidden (eg, presence of target, sickle, or tear drop cells, Howell-Jolly or Pappenheimer bodies, intracellular parasites, and other abnormalities). This data, beneficial to the patient, may be lost without manual study of the PBS. Examples of blood cell morphologic abnormalities (not comprehensive) are given in tabular form in Peripheral Blood: Differential Leukocyte Count *on page 464*. The possibility of confusing ring forms of *Babesia* (an intraerythrocytic protozoan which is also characterized by presence of red cell tetrad forms) with ring forms of the malarial organism *Plasmodium falciparum* is notable.[2,3] While babesiosis is usually transmitted by tick bite, infection can also be caused by transfusion of blood (or blood components) from donors (who themselves are without evident illness).[4] On the other hand, fulminant babesiosis, unresponsive to initial medical therapy (eg, clindamycin and quinine), may show rapid improvement after whole blood exchange transfusion.[5]

The numerous abnormal morphologic red cell forms present potentially on a patient's peripheral blood smear must be identified and correlated with clinical features to determine the need for additional laboratory investigation. An example is the finding of elliptocytes. Occasional elliptocytes (ovalocytes), present on the peripheral smear, may not have meaningful clinical association. Hereditary elliptocytosis (HE) may account for greater numbers of such cells. A study based on morphology of 1000 RBCs per iron deficient patient found that as the percentage of elliptocytes increased, Hb, Hct, RBC count, and MCH levels decreased. As the percentage of tailed poikilocytes increased, Hb, Hct, and RBC count decreased while the RBC distribution width increased.[6] Serum ferritin levels did not correlate with the morphologic abnormalities, severity of anemia, or RBC indices. It was concluded that "...microscopic evaluation of RBC morphology remains an important tool... to evaluate the severity of anemia in patients with iron deficiency."[6] Concerning elliptocytes, their presence on peripheral smear along with spherocytes and schistocytes (micropoikilospherocytes) and with family history of hereditary elliptocytosis may indicate the presence of hereditary pyropoikilocytosis (HPP). A positive thermal sensitivity test (TST) will support diagnosis of this rare condition.[7] The TST is performed by incubating patient's blood for 10 minutes at 46°C. The test is positive if there is marked increase in elongation and fragmentation of the patient's RBCs (see table in Osmotic Fragility *on page 462*). Detection and identification of HPP and differentiation from HE is important for consideration of proper therapy.

Footnotes

1. Thalhammer-Scherrer R, Knöbl P, Korninger L, et al, "Automated Five-Part White Blood Cell Differential Counts. Efficiency of Software-Generated White Blood Cell Suspect Flags of the Hematology Analyzers Sysmex SE-9000, Sysmex NE-8000, and Coulter STK-S," *Arch Pathol Lab Med*, 1997, 121(6):573-7.

2. Quick RE, Herwaldt BL, Thomford JW, et al, "Babesiosis in Washington State: A New Species of *Babesia*?" *Ann Intern Med*, 1993, 119(4):284-90.

3. Persing DH, Herwaldt BL, Glaser C, et al, "Infection With a *Babesia*-Like Organism in Northern California," *N Engl J Med*, 1995, 332(5):298-303.

4. Linden JV, Wong SJ, Chu FK, et al, "Transfusion-Associated Transmission of Babesiosis in New York State," *Transfusion*, 2000, 40(3):285-9.

5. Dorman SE, Cannon ME, Telford III SR, et al, "Fulminant Babesiosis Treated With Clindamycin, Quinine, and Whole-Blood Exchange Transfusion," *Transfusion*, 2000, 40(3):375-80.

6. Rodgers MS, Chang C-C, and Kass L, "Elliptocytes and Tailed Poikilocytes Correlate With Severity of Iron-Deficiency Anemia," *Am J Clin Pathol*, 1999, 111(5):672-5.

7. Cochran DL and Burnside LK, "Detecting and Identifying Hereditary Pyropoikilocytosis," *Clinical Pathology Rounds*, *Lab Med*, 1999, 30(1):26-9.

(Continued)

Peripheral Blood: Red Blood Cell Morphology
(Continued)

References

Gulati GL and Hyun BH, "Blood Smear Examination," *Hematol Oncol Clin North Am*, 1994, 8(4):631-50.

Homer MJ, Aguilar-Delfin I, and Telford SR III, "Babesiasis," *Clin Microbiol Rev*, 2000, 13(3):451-69.

Javidian P, Garshelis L, and Peterson P, "Pathologist Review of the Peripheral Smear: A Mandatory Quality Assurance Activity?" *Clin Lab Med*, 1993, 13(4):853-61.

♦ **Peripheral Blood Stem Cells** *see* CD34+ Hematopoietic Stem Cells by Flow Cytometry *on page 413*

♦ **Peripheral Blood Stem Cell Transplantation** *see* CD34+ Hematopoietic Stem Cells by Flow Cytometry *on page 413*

♦ **Peripheral Differential** *see* Peripheral Blood: Differential Leukocyte Count *on page 464*

♦ **Peripheral Smear, Blood** *see* Peripheral Blood: Red Blood Cell Morphology *on page 467*

♦ **Peritoneal Fluid Analysis** *see* Body Fluid Analysis, Cell Count *on page 408*

♦ **Peritoneal Lavage, Diagnostic** *see* Body Fluid Analysis, Cell Count *on page 408*

♦ **Perls' Reaction** *see* Iron Stain, Bone Marrow *on page 452*

♦ **Perls' Test** *see* Iron Stain, Bone Marrow *on page 452*

♦ **Perl's Test** *see* Siderocyte Stain *on page 487*

♦ **Permeabilization** *see* Flow Cytometry, Overview *on page 432*

♦ **Permeabilization of Red Blood Cells** *see* Kleihauer-Betke *on page 453*

♦ **Peroxisomes** *see* Inherited Diseases of Metabolism and Cell Structure *on page 449*

♦ **Persistent Hyperinsulinemic Hypoglycemia of Infancy** *see* Inherited Diseases of Metabolism and Cell Structure *on page 449*

♦ **PG-M3 Antibody** *see* Promyelocytic Leukemia Assay *on page 474*

♦ **Pickwickian Syndrome** *see* Red Cell Mass *on page 478*

♦ **PI-Linked Antigen** *see* PNH Test (GPI-Anchored Proteins) by Flow Cytometry *on page 472*

♦ **Pink Test** *see* Glycerol Lysis Test, Acidified, Modified *on page 439*

♦ **Plasma/Blood Volume** *see* Blood Volume *on page 407*

♦ **Plasma Free Hemoglobin** *see* Hemoglobin, Plasma *on page 446*

♦ **Plasma Volume Measurement** *see* Blood Volume *on page 407*

♦ **Plasmodium Species** *see* Malaria Smear and Tests *on page 458*

♦ **Platelet Cloud** *see* Reticulated Platelet Count *on page 480*

♦ **Platelet Component Distribution Width** *see* Platelet Count *on page 468*

Platelet Count

Related Information

Activated Partial Thromboplastin Time *on page 328*
Antiphospholipid Antibody (Lupus Anticoagulant and/or Anticardiolipin Antibody) *on page 331*
Blood, Urine *on page 870*
Complete Blood Count *on page 419*
Fanconi Anemia, Chromosome Breakage Study *on page 365*
Peripheral Blood: Differential Leukocyte Count *on page 464*
Platelet Aggregation *on page 348*
Platelet Antibodies *on page 349*
Platelet Antibody, Immunohematologic *on page 852*
Platelets, Apheresis, Donation *on page 853*
Platelet Sizing *on page 471*
Platelet Transfusion *on page 854*
Quinidine, Serum *on page 764*
Reticulated Platelet Count *on page 480*
Thrombopoietin, Serum or Plasma *on page 491*

Synonyms Thrombocyte Count

Applies to Abciximab; Bernard-Soulier Syndrome; CD61; CD62P; Epstein Syndrome; Fechtner Syndrome; Genetic Chronic Thrombocytopenia; Gray Platelet Syndrome; Hereditary Macrothrombocytopenia; May-Hegglin Anomaly; Mean Platelet Component Concentration; Mean Platelet Mass; Mean Platelet Volume; Mediterranean Macrothrombocytopenia; Montreal Platelet Syndrome; MPC; MPM; MPV; Paris-Trousseau Syndrome; Platelet Component Distribution Width; Platelet Mass Distribution Width; PMDW; RBC:Platelet Ratio Method; Sebastian Syndrome; Wiscott-Aldrich Syndrome

Abstract Enumeration of platelets in the circulating peripheral blood. Platelet count is important in the assessment of bleeding, thrombotic, and malignant neoplastic processes, in evaluation of marrow function, and in study of effects of some diseases involving autoimmune mechanisms.

Specimen Whole blood

Container Lavender top (EDTA) tube

Causes for Rejection Clotted specimen, platelet clumping

Reference Interval 150,000-450,000/mm³ (150-450 x 10⁹/L or 150,000-450,000/μL).[1] Platelet count in healthy term infants and in preterm infants weighing <1500 g is comparable to that in adults with use of either venous or capillary blood and by either phase microscopy or automated impedance counting methods.[2] The count gradually rises during the first few months of life (see table).

Platelet Counts in Normal Low Birth Weight Infants (<2500 g) During First Month of Life*

Day	Number of infants	Mean	Range 1000s
0	60	203,000	80-356
3	47	207,000	61-335
5	14	233,000	100-502
7	52	319,000	124-678
10	40	399,000	172-680
14	50	386,000	147-670
21	47	388,000	201-720
28	40	384,000	212-625

*All platelet counts were performed on venous samples. Serial counts were performed on 60 infants within 24 hours of birth and repeated on days 3, 5, 7, 10, 14, 21, and 28.

Adapted from Geaghan SM, "Hematologic Values and Appearances in the Healthy Fetus, Neonate, and Child," *Clin Lab Med*, 1999, 19(1):1-37.

Considerable interlaboratory variation exists, manual vs electronic automated procedures. Count is method dependent; results of manual count have high coefficient of variation as compared to automated methods.[3] Occasional, apparently normal children, in particular those under 24 months of age, may have platelet counts in the 500,000-750,000 range.[4]

Possible Panic Range <50,000/mm³ or >1,000,000/mm³

Use Evaluate, diagnose, and follow up bleeding disorders, purpura/petechiae, drug-induced thrombocytopenia, idiopathic thrombocytopenic purpura, disseminated intravascular coagulation, leukemia, hypercoagulable states, and chemotherapeutic management of malignant disease

Limitations Clumping may cause false low count. Platelet satellitism around neutrophils may cause pseudothrombocytopenia. An IgG autoantibody is apparently involved with specificity against the platelet membrane glycoprotein IIb/IIIa complex and also against the neutrophil Fcγ receptor III (CD16).[5] Formation of circulating platelet-neutrophil complexes (PNCs), however, may have more ominous implications and may also be associated with a decline in platelet count (see Additional Information). Pseudoincrease in automated platelet counts may occur due to hypertriglyceridemia.[6] The increase is in the range of 2-40 x 10⁹/L, a relatively small change if the platelet count is normal but of potential significance with low platelet numbers. The combination of thrombocytopenia and hypertriglyceridemia (as may occur with L-asparaginase treated childhood acute leukemia) may necessitate manual platelet count.[6] RBC (eg, microspherocytes) or WBC fragments including fragmented fragile leukemic cells and neutrophil pseudoplatelets may cause falsely elevated counts.[7] EDTA-induced platelet clumping is a frequent cause of spuriously low platelet counts[8] resulting from various platelet antigen/antibody reactions including antiplatelet with antiphospholipid antibodies[8] and occurring also *in vitro* (eg, IgM autoantibody against 78 kD platelet glycoprotein).[9]

Methodology A variety of automated/semiautomated devices are in use. Counts are performed on platelet-rich plasma or whole blood by optical or impedance matching counting techniques. Carefully controlled phase microscopy manual count is usually considered the reference method but suffers from a wide coefficient of variation (Brecher-Cronkite phase contrast method has CV of 7% to 17%). In a study documenting the reliability of automated platelet counts performed on one commercially available analyzer, the mean of low platelet counts (machine determined) had a CV of 10% while manual counts had a CV of 30%.[10] Automated platelet counts using immunologic markers with detection of fluorescence by flow cytometry have recently become available (see Additional Information).

Additional Information The platelet, of growing practical clinical importance in hemostatic considerations and a variety of medical/surgical processes, is also fundamental to etiologic considerations of arteriosclerotic and malignant disease. Platelets are generally 2-3 microns in diameter but large forms (megathrombocytes) appear when production is increased. The production of platelets is controlled by thrombopoietin (see Thrombopoietin, Serum or Plasma *on page 491*). Platelets survive for 8-10 days and are subject to circadian periodicity, highest platelet counts occurring during midday.[11] Some drugs may increase the platelet count by stimulating thrombopoietin production. Deaths from cardiovascular disease may relate temporally to the circadian rhythm of platelet production.[11]

Careful estimate of platelet number from stained peripheral blood smear can provide useful information. A variety of factors affect the distribution of platelets on a peripheral blood smear, and thus platelet estimates lack precision. Capillary blood platelet counts (compared to venous blood counts) may be significantly underestimated. Platelets are often clumped on smears obtained from capillary blood, contributing to imprecision. A small whole blood clot or very small fibrin clots in the EDTA anticoagulated specimen will usually be associated with clumping of platelets on the slide and with a false low platelet count.

Quantitative platelet disorders have varied etiology. Thrombocytopenia may have an immunologic basis, may be the result of production deficiency due to the effect of drugs or physical agents, abnormal platelet pooling or increased destruction (eg, sequestration by large vascular tumor), or result from a variety of probably nonimmunologic mechanisms (eg, hypersplenism). Decreases may occur after severe bleeding, transfusion, infections, or relating to defective production of or regulation by thrombopoietin. Serum lactate dehydrogenase and platelet count may predict survival in thrombotic thrombocytopenic purpura.[12]

Drugs and chemicals associated with thrombocytopenia, often on an immune mediated basis or as the result of marrow suppression, include quinidine, quinine, heparin, gold salts, sulfas, rifampicin, ASA, digitoxin, apronal, chlorothiazides, chlorpropamide, meprobamate, antihistamines, chloramphenicol, penicillin, DDT, benzol, a variety of other industrial organic chemicals, diphenylhydantoin, PAS, hydrochlorothiazide, phenylbutazone, and a variety of antineoplastic chemotherapeutic agents. ASA acts by acetylating cyclo-oxygenase. A recent review of English language publications concerning drug-induced thrombocytopenia concluded that most reports do not present evidence that the drug has a definite or probable role as a cause of thrombocytopenia.[13] Nearly 65 drugs (many in common use) are tabulated and assigned to level I (definite) or level II (probable) status on the basis of clinical evidence as cause of thrombocytopenia.[13]

Thrombocytosis is less common, but likewise varied in etiology: physiologic (eg, postpartum or after exercise); myeloproliferative syndromes (eg, thrombocythemia, some cases of chronic myelogenous leukemia, myelofibrosis with myeloid metaplasia); rebound following thrombocytopenia, marrow regenerative activity after bleeding episode, hemophilia, iron deficiency; asplenism, infections, inflammatory or malignant disease, in particular, carcinomatosis but also in early (stage IB) cervical carcinoma.[11]

A study of 732 patients with thrombocytosis found 89 (12.3%) with primary and 643 (87.7%) with secondary thrombocytosis.[14] Nearly half (45%) of the primary cases were due to essential thrombocythemia. The other cases of primary thrombocytosis related to myeloproliferative disorders such as chronic myeloid leukemia, polycythemia vera, and osteomyelofibrosis. Secondary thrombocytosis related to tissue damage (42%), infection (24%), malignancy (13%), and chronic inflammation (10%). Cases of primary thrombocytosis were associated with higher platelet counts and both arterial and venous thromboembolic complications. In secondary thrombocytosis, thromboembolic complications involved only the venous system and occurred only when other risk factors were present. These findings stress the importance of determining if thrombocytosis is of primary of secondary

nature.[14] Artifactual serum hyperkalemia and hypercalcemia may occur with essential thrombocythemia, apparently the result of in vitro secretion of calcium from the large number of abnormally activated platelets.[15]

Thrombocytosis in cases of malignancy may relate to the production of cytokines and/or growth factors (eg, interleukin-6, thrombopoietin). Interleukin-6 has been shown to be produced by some malignant cells, notably by a number of different cancer cell lines.[16]

Oral contraceptives may cause slight increase in platelet count. Slight to moderate decrease in platelet count has been noted during pregnancy in most women who have essential thrombocythemia.[17]

Congenital causes of thrombocytopenia include Wiskott-Aldrich syndrome, May-Hegglin anomaly, thrombocytopenia with absent radius, Bernard-Soulier syndrome, and Paris-Trousseau syndrome.[18] Thrombocytopenia, while variable, usually accompanies the inherited giant platelet disorders (IGPDs).[18,19,20,21] See table.

See Platelet Sizing on page 471 for discussion of changes in platelet count and size in pre-eclampsia and the HELLP syndrome (hemolysis, elevated liver tests, and low platelet count).

The management of patients with platelet disorders, in particular the relatively common occurrence of severe thrombocytopenia (often relating to chemotherapy), relies upon accurate true platelet enumeration. Automated methods in current use may not be able to discriminate true platelets from nonplatelet particles (eg, microcytic RBCs, RBC fragments, and other cell debris) as may be generated by a variety of pathologic processes including the tumor lysis syndrome.[7] Two-dimensional optical platelet analysis and immunoplatelet counting have recently become available.[22,23] Two angles of laser light scatter (high-angle 5°C to 15°C plotted on X axis and low-angle 2°C to 3°C events plotted along the Y axis) are used for platelet and red cell analysis on the Advia 120 Hematology System (Bayer®, Tarrytown, NY). Platelets are "sphered and volume (platelet size) and refractive index (platelet density) are simultaneously determined, cell by cell using a flow system with determination of the two angles of light scatter. Optical two-dimensional platelet analysis shows a high degree of correlation with the phase microscopy current reference method[22] (see below concerning "reference method"). In addition to platelet data previously available:

- PLTs: platelet count
- MPV: mean platelet volume
- PCT: platelet-crit
- PDW: platelet distribution width

The Advia 120 also provides the following:
- MPC: mean platelet component concentration
- PCDW: platelet component distribution width
- MPM: mean platelet mass
- PMDW: platelet mass distribution width

Inherited Abnormalities of Platelet Production
Characterized by Large Platelets and Variable Bleeding/Thrombocytopenia

Condition	Inheritance	Clinical Associations	Platelet Abnormality	Molecular Defect
May-Hegglin anomaly	AD	Mild bleeding nephritis, FSP, GHD, MI	Severe thrombocytopenia NA	Possible DMS abnormality
Bernard-Soulier syndrome	AR	Variable bleeding	Ristocetin AGG absent	gpIb-IX-V complex defect
Fechtner syndrome	AD	Variable bleeding, hereditary nephritis, high frequency hearing loss, juvenile glaucoma/cataract, neutrophil inclusions	NA	Possible DMS abnormality
Sebastian syndrome	AD	Variable bleeding, neutrophil inclusions	NA	Unknown
Epstein syndrome	AD	Mild bleeding, nephritis, high frequency hearing loss	AGG with collagen, ADP, decreased thrombin	Unknown
Paris-trousseau syndrome	AD	Mild bleeding	Giant (red on giemsa stain) alpha granules	
Montreal platelet syndrome	AD	Bleeding (bruising and hemorrhage)	Severe thrombocytopenia, spontaneous AGG, decreased AGG to thrombin	Decreased calpain activity
Giant platelet with velocardiofacial syndrome	AR	No bleeding, velopharyngeal insufficiency, conotruneal cardiac defects, learning disability	Decreased platelet lifespan but with normal bleeding time and with normal platelet adhesion and aggregation	Defect of platelet surface glycoprotein; deletion, chromosome 22q11 (gpIb-beta deletion)
Giant platelets with abnormal surface Glycoprotein and mitral valve Insufficiency syndrome	AR	Mild bleeding, mitral valve insufficiency	Moderate thrombocytopenia, slow AGG response to ADP, thrombin, AA	Absence of surface glycoproteins gpIa, gpIc, and gpIIa
Gray platelet syndrome	AD	Mild/moderate bleeding, splenomegaly, Marfan syndrome, pulmonary fibrosis	Decreased AGG with thrombin, collagen, and ristocetin	Alpha-granule defect with abnormal Ca flux and reduced P-selectin and osteonectin
Hereditary macrothrombocytopenia	AD	Mild bleeding, high frequency hearing loss	Mild thrombocytopenia, decreased AGG with epinephrine and AA	Glycophorin A is expressed (a red cell specific protein)
Mediterranean macrothrombocytopenia	Unknown	No bleeding, asymptomatic episodic hemolytic anemia may occur, may have slight spenomegaly	Mild thrombocytosis, may be a benign anomaly, AGG unknown	Unknown
Genetic chronic thrombocytopenia	AD	Neonatal hemorrhage, cephalohematoma (rare), minimal to nil clinical severity	Platelet macrocytosis, normal autologous platelet lifespan (normal platelet survival), no functional platelet abnormalities	Abnormality of platelet release from bone marrow

AD = autosomal dominant; AR = autosomal recessive; AGG = aggregation; NA = normal aggregation; AA = arachidonic acid; DMS = demarcation membrane system; FSP = familial spastic paraplegia; GHD = growth hormone deficiency; MI = myocardial infarction
Adapted from Mhawech P and Saleem A, "Inherited Giant Platelet Disorders," Am J Clin Pathol, 2000, 113:176-90.

(Continued)

Platelet Count (Continued)

The clinical significance of these new parameters must be determined and is complicated by the status of platelet activation. Studies using measurement of platelet CD62P expression by flow cytometry (to establish the absence of sample activation) at time intervals of 20 minutes and 3.5 hours (to simulate "routine" and "urgent" sample test requests) confirm that some platelet parameters change with sample age (in vitro, EDTA anticoagulated).[23] As the MPV increases, MPC decreases, stabilizing at 15-20 minutes. This finding is consistent with previous observations that platelets swell and lose their discoid shape (becoming more spherical) during the first 2 hours of EDTA anticoagulation.[23] Platelet parameters may not be effected similarly by all anticoagulants. Platelet discoid shape tends to persist in sodium citrate resulting in a lower MPC and wider PCDW.[23]

ImmunoPlt (CD61) assay is based on an antiglycoprotein IIIa monoclonal antibody, a flow cytometric assay that has been automated and implemented on the Cell-Dyn 4000 analyzer.[24] The method can provide a rapid result (<5 minutes from closed-tube aspiration to report). For low platelet counts, the CD61-based assay is more accurate and precise than optical scatter or impedance count methods.[25] Immunoplatelet counting methodology, based on the RBC:platelet ratio and using a double-labeling (CD61 and CD41) procedure (with different flow cytometers), has been developed by a multinational interlaboratory task force.[26] The RBC:platelet ratio method for platelet counting is now recommended by the International Council for Standardization in Hematology and the International Society of Laboratory Hematology (Task Force on Platelet Counting) as a reference method for the enumeration of platelets.[27]

Knowledge of the intimate association of platelet number, biomolecular function, fragmentation, and resultant particles and particulate aggregates (eg, platelet/neutrophil aggregates) is expanding to encompass an ever-increasing number of significant problematic clinical situations.[28,29,30,31,32,33] Of particular import is modification of platelet function/reactivity, the use of abciximab (a chimeric monoclonal antibody Fab fragment directed against platelet glycoprotein IIb/IIIa) as an example.[28,34,35,36] Defining the role of platelet-derived microparticles and of platelet-leukocyte-interactions provides new avenues in understanding pathobiology.[37,38,39,40,41,42,43,44]

Footnotes

1. Rowan RM, "Platelet Counting and the Assessment of Platelet Function," *Practical Laboratory Hematology*, Chapter 8, Koepke JA, ed, New York, NY: Churchill Livingstone, 1991, 164.
2. Geaghan SM, "Hematologic Values and Appearances in the Healthy Fetus, Neonate, and Child," *Clin Lab Med*, 1999, 19(1):1-37.
3. Lohmann RC, Crawford LN, and Wood DE, "Proficiency Testing of Platelet Counting in Ontario," *Am J Clin Pathol*, 1992, 98(2):231-6.
4. Novak RW, Tschantz JA, and Krill CE Jr, "Normal Platelet and Mean Platelet Volumes in Pediatric Patients," *Lab Med*, 1987, 18:613-4.
5. Bizzaro N, Goldschmeding R, and von dem Borne AE, "Platelet Satellitism Is FCγ RIII (CD16) Receptor-Mediated," *Am J Clin Pathol*, 1995, 103(6):740-4.
6. Kabutomori O, Iwatani Y, and Kabutomori M, "Effects of Hypertriglyceridemia on Platelet Counts in Automated Hematologic Analysis," *Ann Intern Med*, 1999, 130(5):452.
7. Li S and Salhany KE, "Spurious Elevation of Automated Platelet Counts in Secondary Acute Monocytic Leukemia Associated With Tumor Lysis Syndrome," *Arch Pathol Lab Med*, 1999, 123(11):1111-4.
8. Bizzaro N and Brandalise M, "EDTA-Dependent Pseudothrombocytopenia. Association With Antiplatelets and Antiphospholipid Antibodies," *Am J Clin Pathol*, 1995, 103(1):103-7.
9. De Caterina M, Fratellanza G, Grimaldi E, et al, "Evidence of a Cold Immunoglobulin M Autoantibody Against 78-kD Platelet Glycoprotein in a Case of EDTA-Dependent Pseudothrombocytopenia," *Am J Clin Pathol*, 1993, 99(2):163-7.
10. Lawrence JB, Yomtovian RA, Dillman C, et al, "Reliability of Automated Platelet Counts: Comparison With Manual Method and Utility for Prediction of Clinical Bleeding," *Am J Hematol*, 1995, 48:244-50.
11. de Nicola P and Casale G, "Platelets," *Blood Diseases in the Aged*, Stuttgart, West Germany: Schwer Verlag, 1988, 71-6.
12. Patton JF, Manning KR, Case D, et al, "Serum Lactate Dehydrogenase and Platelet Count Predict Survival in Thrombotic Thrombocytopenic Purpura," *Am J Hematol*, 1994, 47(2):94-9.
13. George JN, Raskob GE, Shah SR, et al, "Drug-Induced Thrombocytopenia: A Systematic Review of Published Case Reports," *Ann Intern Med*, 1998, 129(11):886-90.
14. Greisshammer M, Bangerter M, Sauer T, et al, "Aetiology and Clinical Significance of Thrombocytosis: Analysis of 732 Patients With an Elevated Platelet Count," *J Intern Med*, 1999, 245(3):295-300.
15. Howard MR, Ashwell S, Bond LR, et al, "Artifactual Serum Hyperkalaemia and Hypercalcaemia in Essential Thrombocythaemia," *J Clin Pathol*, 2000, 53(2):105-9.
16. Rodriguez GC, Clarke-Pearson DL, Soper JT, et al, "The Negative Prognostic Implications of Thrombocytosis in Women With Stage IB Cervical Cancer," *Obstet Gynecol*, 1994, 83(3):445-8.
17. Chow EY, Haley LP, and Vickars LM, "Essential Thrombocythemia in Pregnancy: Platelet Count and Pregnancy Outcome," *Am J Hematol*, 1992, 41(4):249-51.
18. Breton-Gorius J, Favier R, Guichard J, et al, "A New Congenital Dysmegakaryocytic Thrombocytopenia (Paris-Trousseau) Associated With Giant Platelet α-Granules and Chromosome 11 Deletion at 11q23," *Blood*, 1995, 85(7):1805-14.
19. Mhawech P and Saleem A, "Inherited Giant Platelet Disorders. Classification and Literature Review," *Am J Clin Pathol*, 2000, 113(2):176-90.
20. Najean Y and Lecompte T, "Genetic Thrombocytopenia With Autosomal Dominant Transmission: A Review of 54 Cases," *Br J Haematol*, 1990, 74(2):203-8.
21. Noris P, Spedini P, Belletti, et al, "Thrombocytopenia, Giant Platelets, and Leukocyte Inclusion Bodies (May-Hegglin Anomaly): Clinical and Laboratory Findings," *Am J Med*, 1998, 104(4):355-60.
22. Kunicka JE, Fischer G, Murphy J, et al, "Improved Platelet Counting Using Two-Dimensional Laser Light Scatter," *Am J Clin Pathol*, 2000, 114(2):283-9.
23. Brummitt DR and Barker HF, "The Determination of a Reference Range for New Platelet Produced by the Bayer® ADVIA™ 120 Full Blood Count Analyzer," *Clin Lab Haematol*, 2000, 22(2):103-7.
24. Harrison P, Horton A, Grant D, et al, "Immunoplatelet Counting: A Proposed New Reference Procedure," *Br J Haematol*, 2000, 108(2):228-35.
25. Gill JE, Davis KA, Cowart WJ, et al, "A Rapid and Accurate Closed-Tube Immunoassay for Platelets on an Automated Hematology Analyzer," *Am J Clin Pathol*, 2000, 114(1):47-56.
26. Harrison P, Ault KA, Chapman S, et al, "An Interlaboratory Study of a Candidate Reference Method for Platelet Counting," *Am J Clin Pathol*, 2001, 115:448-59.
27. International Council for Standardization in Haematology Expert Panel on Cytometry and International Society of Laboratory Hematology Task Force on Platelet Counting, "Platelet Counting by the RBC/Platelet Ratio Method. A Reference Method," *Am J Clin Pathol*, 2001, 115:460-4.
28. Fischman DL and Savage MP, "The Platelet, the Patient, and Periprocedural Infarction During Percutaneous Transluminal Coronary Angioplasty." *JAMA*, 1997, 278(6):518-9.
29. Nomura S, Kagawa H, Ozaki Y, et al, "Relationship Between Platelet Activation and Cytokines in Systemic Inflammatory Response Syndrome Patients With Hematological Malignancies," *Thromb Res*, 1999, 95(5):205-13.
30. Scheuerer B, Ernst M, Dürrbaum-Landmann I, et al, "The CXC-Chemokine Platelet Factor 4 Promotes Monocyte Survival and Induces Monocyte Differentiation into Macrophages," *Blood*, 2000, 95(4):1158-66.
31. Nieuwland R, Berckmans RJ, McGregor S, et al, "Cellular Origin and Procoagulant Properties of Microparticles in Meningococcal Sepsis," *Blood*, 2000, 95(3):930-5.
32. Gawaz M, Dickfeld T, Bogner C, et al, "Platelet Function in Septic Multiple Organ Dysfunction Syndrome," *Intensive Care Med*, 1997, 23(4):379-85.
33. Brus F, van Oeveren W, Okken A, et al, "Number and Activation of Circulating Polymorphonuclear Leukocytes and Platelets Are Associated With Neonatal Respiratory Distress Syndrome Severity," *Pediatrics*, 1997, 99(5):672-80.
34. Poujol C, Durrieu-Jais C, Larrue B, et al, "Accessibility of Abciximab to Megakaryocytes and Endothelial Cells in the Bone Marrow Compartment: Studies on a Patient Receiving Antithrombotic Therapy," *Br J Haematol*. 1999, 107(3):526-31.
35. Massé JM, Perlemuter K, Debili N, et al, "Intracellular Trafficking of the Alpha$_{IIb}$-beta$_3$ Receptor Antagonist, Abciximab, in Normal and Glanzmann's Disease Megakaryocytes," *Br J Haematol*, 1999, 107(4):720-30.
36. Matzdorff AC, Kühnel G, Kemkes-Matthes B, et al, "Effect of Glycoprotein IIb/IIIa Inhibitors on CD62p Expression, Platelet Aggregates, and Microparticles In Vitro," *J Lab Clin Med*, 2000, 135(3):247-55.
37. Warkentin TE, Hayward CP, Boshkov LK, et al, "Sera From Patients With Heparin-Induced Thrombocytopenia Generate Platelet-Derived Microparticles With Procoagulant Activity: An Explanation for the Thrombotic Complications of Heparin-Induced Thrombocytopenia," *Blood*, 1994, 84(11):3691-9.
38. Hughes M, Hayward CP, Warkentin TE, et al, "Morphological Analysis of Microparticle Generation in Heparin-Induced Thrombocytopenia," *Blood*, 2000, 96(1):188-94.
39. Celi A, Lorenzet R, Furie B, et al, "Platelet-Leukocyte-Endothelial Cell Interaction on the Blood Vessel Wall," *Semin Hematol*, 1997, 34(4):327-35.
40. Bengtsson T, Fryden A, Zalavary S, et al, "Platelets Enhance Neutrophil Locomotion: Evidence for a Role of P-Selectin," *Scand J Clin Lab Invest*, 1999, 59(6):439-49.
41. Peters MJ, Dixon G, Kotowicz KT, et al, "Circulating Platelet - Neutrophil Complexes Represent a Subpopulation of Activated Neutrophils Primed for Adhesion, Phagocytosis, and Intracellular Killing," *Br J Haematol*, 1999, 106(2):391-9.
42. Forlow SB, McEver RP, and Nollert MU, "Leukocyte-Leukocyte Interactions Mediated by Platelet Microparticles Under Flow," *Blood*, 2000, 95(4):1317-23.
43. Li N, Goodall AH, and Hjemdahl P, "A Sensitive Flow Cytometric Assay for Circulating Platelet-Leucocyte Aggregates," *Br J Haematol*, 1997, 99(4):808-16.
44. Miyamoto S, Kowalska MA, Marcinkiewicz C, et al, "Interaction of Leukocytes With Platelet Microparticles Derived From Outdated Platelet Concentrates," *Thromb Haemost*, 1998, 80(6):982-8.

References

Ajzenberg N, Dreyfus M, Kaplan C, et al, "Pregnancy-Associated Thrombocytopenia Revisited: Assessment and Follow-up of 50 Cases," *Blood*, 1998, 92(12):4573-80.

Bangerter M, Güthner C, Beneke H, et al, "Pregnancy in Essential Thrombocythaemia: Treatment and Outcome of 17 Pregnancies," *Eur J Haematol*, 2000, 65(3):165-9.

Bizzaro N, "EDTA-Dependent Pseudothrombocytopenia: A Clinical and Epidemiological Study of 112 Cases, With 10-Year Follow-up," *Am J Hematol*, 1995, 50(2):103-9.

Cornbleet PJ and Kessinger S, "Accuracy of Low Platelet Counts on the Coulter S-Plus IV®," *Am J Clin Pathol*, 1985, 83(1):78-80.

García-Suárez J, Burgaleta C, Hernanz N, et al, "HCV-Associated Thrombocytopenia: Clinical Characteristics and Platelet Response After Recombinant Alpha 2b-Interferon Therapy," *Br J Haematol*, 2000, 110(1):98-103.

George JN, El-Harake MA, and Raskob GE, "Chronic Idiopathic Thrombocytopenic Purpura," *N Engl J Med*, 1994, 331(18):1207-11.

Jagadeeswaran P, Sheehan JP, Craig FE, et al, "Identification and Characterization of Zebrafish Thrombocytes," *Br J Haematol*, 1999, 107(4):731-8.

Johnson JR and Samuels P, "Review of Autoimmune Thrombocytopenia: Pathogenesis, Diagnosis, and Management in Pregnancy," *Clin Obstet Gynecol*, 1999, 42(2):317-26.

Kaushansky K, "Thrombopoietin: The Primary Regulator of Platelet Production," *Blood*, 1995, 86(2):419-31.

Kirk RI, Deitch JA, Wu JM, et al, "Resveratrol Decreases Early Signaling Events in Washed Platelets but Has Little Effect on Platelet Aggregation in Whole Blood," *Blood Cells Mol Dis*, 2000, 26(2):144-50.

Kunishima S, Tomiyama Y, Honda S, et al, "Cys97→Tyr Mutation in the Glycoprotein IX Gene Associated With Bernard-Soulier Syndrome," *Br J Haematol*, 1999, 107(3):539-45.

Shcherbina A, Bretscher A, Rosen FS, et al, "The Cytoskeletal Linker Protein Moesin: Decreased Levels in Wiskott-Aldrich Syndrome Platelets and Identification of a Cleavage Pathway in Normal Platelets," *Br J Haematol*, 1999, 106(1):216-23.

Shehata N, Burrows R, and Kelton JG, "Gestational Thrombocytopenia," *Clin Obstet Gynecol*, 1999, 42(2):327-34.

Tefferi A and Hoagland HC, "Issues in the Diagnosis and Management of Essential Thrombocythemia," *Mayo Clin Proc*, 1994, 69(7):651-5.

Uhrynowska M, Niznikowska-Marks M, and Zupanska B, "Neonatal and Maternal Thrombocytopenia: Incidence and Immune Background," *Eur J Haematol*, 2000, 64(1):42-6.

Yoon SY, Li CY, Mesa RA, et al, "Bone Marrow Effects of Anagrelide Therapy in Patients With Myelofibrosis With Myeloid Metaplasia," *Br J Haematol*, 1999, 106(3):682-8.

Zaman A, Hapke R, Flora K, et al, "Factors Predicting the Presence of Esophageal or Gastric Varices in Patients With Advanced Liver Disease," *Am J Gastroenterol*, 1999, 94(11):3292-6.

♦ **Platelet Count, Reticulated** *see* Reticulated Platelet Count *on page 480*

♦ **Platelet Factor 4** *see* TGF-β, Serum *on page 490*

Platelet Histogram Maximum

Related Information
Platelet Count *on page 468*
Platelet Sizing *on page 471*
Platelet Transfusion *on page 854*
Reticulated Platelet Count *on page 480*
Reticulocyte Count *on page 481*

Applies to Megathrombocytes; MPV

Abstract The highest peak of the platelet volume distribution curve applied to the study of thrombocytopenia, is less effected by particulate artifact than the mean platelet volume (MPV). The test is of value in discriminating between decreased platelet production and increased platelet destruction and thus in establishing the presence of idiopathic thrombocytopenic purpura (ITP).

Specimen Whole blood

Container Lavender top (EDTA) tube

Turnaround Time 1-2 hours

Reference Interval Maxima ±SD: ITP: 7.9 ±0.93; hypoproduction: 5.12 ±0.71

Use Differential diagnosis of thrombocytopenia, in particular, differentiation of decreased platelet production from increased platelet destruction

Limitations Appropriate instrumentation for producing a platelet histogram must be available.

Methodology Platelet volume distribution measured by automated platelet counting equipment

Additional Information An increased percentage of large platelets in the peripheral blood reflects increased numbers of marrow megakaryocytes and a state of platelet hyperproduction, as occurs with idiopathic thrombocytopenic purpura (ITP). Few to absent megathrombocytes (platelets larger than 3.0 microns across) are seen with hypoproductive thrombocytopenia (eg, aplastic anemia, chemotherapy). Sensitivity/specificity studies using receiver operating characteristic curves show that the maximum of the platelet histogram is superior to the MPV in the evaluation of thrombocytopenia. Use of the "maximum" avoids the effect of artifacts (debris and/or cell fragments from red cells or leukemic blasts) that artificially change the platelet count and MPV (especially in cases of very low platelet count).

References Reticulated Platelet Count;
Niethammer AG and Forman EN, "Use of the Platelet Histogram Maximum in Evaluating Thrombocytopenia," *Am J Hematol*, 1999, 60(1):19-23.

♦ **Platelet Indices** *see* Platelet Sizing *on page 471*

♦ **Platelet Mass Distribution Width** *see* Platelet Count *on page 468*

♦ **Platelet Satellitosis** *see* Peripheral Blood: Differential Leukocyte Count *on page 464*

Platelet Sizing

Related Information
Complete Blood Count *on page 419*
Peripheral Blood: Differential Leukocyte Count *on page 464*
Peripheral Blood: Red Blood Cell Morphology *on page 467*
Platelet Count *on page 468*
Platelet Transfusion *on page 854*
Reticulated Platelet Count *on page 480*
Thrombopoietin, Serum or Plasma *on page 491*

Synonyms MPV; PDW; Platelet Indices

Applies to May-Hegglin Anomaly

Test Includes MPV (mean platelet volume), platelet count, PDW (platelet distribution width)

Abstract Modern automated cell counters may generate platelet sizing parameters (eg, MPV and PDW) which may be abnormal in some clinical situations. Platelet indices are analogous to red blood cell indices (eg, MCV

and RDW) but have only modest clinical application. MPV and PDW are increased in patients with idiopathic thrombocytopenic purpura (ITP).

Specimen Whole blood

Container Lavender top (EDTA) tube; green top (heparin) tube may cause platelet clumping

Storage Instructions In EDTA anticoagulated whole blood, platelets undergo a change in shape from discoid to spherical (discocyte-to-echinocyte transformation) with increase in apparent volume such that the MPV increases about 20% with time in the first 1-2 hours (*in vitro*), is then stable for 1-3 hours, and then undergoes further increase with time. Thus, MPV should be determined between 1 and 3 hours after the sample is obtained.[1]

Reference Interval See tables for mean platelet volume and platelet "crit" reference values. Overall, MPV reference value for adults is 6.5 to 12 fL. Platelet size normally varies inversely with platelet count.[1]

Platelet Parameters in Males (mean ±SD)*

Age (y)	n	Platelet Count (x 10^3/mm³) (x 10^9/L)	MPV (fL)	PCT (%)
1-5	24	357 ±70	8.6 ±0.7	0.304 ±0.059
6-10	24	351 ±85	8.6 ±0.8	0.300 ±0.058
11-15	16	282 ±63	9.8 ±1.0	0.274 ±0.053
16-20	16	266 ±63	10.2 ±1.1	0.266 ±0.049
21-30	24	238 ±49	9.6 ±0.6	0.277 ±0.045
31-40	12	244 ±56	9.8 ±1.2	0.237 ±0.044
41-50	17	271 ±66	9.4 ±1.0	0.250 ±0.045
51-60	22	258 ±61	9.8 ±1.2	0.248 ±0.045
61-70	29	256 ±53	9.4 ±1.1	0.238 ±0.047
71-86n	23	237 ±49	9.6 ±1.0	0.226 ±0.048

*SI conversion units for platelet count x 10^3/mm³ is platelet count x 10^9/L.

Adapted from Graham SS, Traub B, and Minic IB, "Automated Platelet-Sizing Parameters on a Normal Population," *Am J Clin Pathol*, 1987, 87:365-9.

Platelet Parameters in Females (mean ±SD)*

Age (y)	n	Platelet Count (x 10^3/mm³) (x 10^9/L)	MPV (fL)	PCT (%)
1-5	25	381 ±76	8.9 ±0.8	0.337 ±0.069
6-10	18	336 ±76	9.7 ±1.1	0.326 ±0.080
11-15	31	298 ±72	9.8 ±1.2	0.288 ±0.058
16-20	22	270 ±58	9.7 ±0.7	0.262 ±0.058
21-30	43	270 ±58	9.8 ±1.0	0.261 ±0.046
31-40	30	282 ±56	9.8 ±1.2	0.271 ±0.046
41-50	26	279 ±65	9.8 ±0.9	0.274 ±0.072
51-60	21	285 ±54	9.7 ±0.7	0.276 ±0.045
61-70	30	274 ±61	9.6 ±0.9	0.262 ±0.052
71-83	24	279 ±65	9.5 ±1.0	0.261 ±0.054

*SI conversion units for platelet count x 10^3/mm³ is platelet count x 10^9/L.

Adapted from Graham SS, Traub B, and Minic IB, "Automated Platelet-Sizing Parameters on a Normal Population," *Am J Clin Pathol*, 1987, 87:365-9.

Use Differential diagnosis of hematologic disease; assess platelet function; evaluation of thrombocytopenia; guide the need for platelet transfusion in thrombocytopenic patients

Limitations May be unreliable if platelet count is <10,000/mm³. MPV may be unstable in EDTA. With impedance counting methods, increase in platelet volume may occur with increasing time from venous sampling while MPV may decrease with storage when a light scattering method is used.

Methodology Flow cytometry (FC) with measurement of platelet volume and size parameters by changes in electrical impedance (resistance of an individual cell is proportional to its volume) and microprocessor assisted mathematical analysis. Electrical signals (proportional to particle size) are sorted according to magnitude. Upper and lower thresholds define the central platelet volume distribution (2-20 fL).

Additional Information Large platelets are generally young platelets and have better hemostatic function than average age or old platelets. MPV (in normal subjects) bears an inverse relation to platelet count. MPV rises with increased platelet turnover, due to production of megathrombocytes. MPV and PDW are increased with ITP. MPV tends to be low in reactive thrombocytosis. Use of increased platelet volume may assist in the differential diagnosis of ITP versus acute leukemia. Large platelets are present in the recovery stage of alcohol-induced thrombocytopenia. Platelet size, while often a marker for platelet age, may in some cases reflect altered platelet production (eg, dyspoietic states such as the May-Hegglin anomaly, in which increased platelet volume occurs). Small platelets are seen in the Wiskott-Aldrich syndrome. Autoimmune thrombocytopenia and leukemia may be associated with presence of platelet fragments and decreased platelet volume. Hypersplenetic patients have smaller platelet size. Low MPV may be seen in patients with septic thrombocytopenia and in some cases of myeloproliferative disease after treatment with cytotoxic drugs. In the Bernard-Soulier syndrome, there is thrombocytopenia with large platelets. Large platelets, occasionally with abnormal morphology, occur in the (Continued)

Platelet Sizing (Continued)

myeloproliferative syndromes. Increased MPV may also be seen in hyperthyroidism but only with low platelet count. Generally, the platelet count is normal in hyperthyroidism, MPV is normal, but reticulated platelets are increased, suggestive of increase in thrombopoiesis.[2] Mediterranean macrothrombocytopenia is characterized by low platelet count, large platelets, and a generally normal platelet "crit".[3] Mean platelet volume correlates with bleeding tendency in thrombocytopenic patients.[4] A significantly lower frequency of bleeding occurs with mean platelet volumes >6.4 fL. This measure, then, may be of use in assessing the need for platelet transfusion.

MPV and platelet count are normal and constant between the first trimester and the end of normal pregnancy, but MPV is increased in patients with pre-eclampsia. Platelet count is decreased in cases of pre-eclampsia but was also found to be decreased in 10% of normal pregnancies.[5] Platelet count is decreased in pre-eclamptic women with the HELLP syndrome (hemolysis, elevated liver tests, and low platelet count). Platelets have also been found to decrease in pre-eclamptic women initially with platelet count in the normal range.[6] Increase in MPV has been noted in neonates with coagulase-negative staphylococcal septicemia.[7] Platelet volume has been noted to decrease during cardiopulmonary bypass and to increase in atherosclerotic smokers.[8,9] Increase in MPV due to smoking has been proposed as a risk factor for atherosclerotic disease.[9]

An apparently new hemorrhagic disorder characterized by moderate thrombocytopenia, giant platelets, and markedly prolonged bleeding time has been described.[10] The condition has been considered to represent a new syndrome of thrombocytopenia with giant platelets distinct from Bernard-Soulier, Montreal giant platelets, Swiss cheese platelets, May-Hegglin anomaly, and other described syndromes (see Platelet Count *on page 468*).

A new parameter "PDW$_{residual}$", defined as:

$$PDW_{residual} = PDW_{observed} - PDW_{expected}$$

has been found (combined with the use of platelet count and MPV) to be useful in the differential diagnosis of thrombocytosis, in particular in distinguishing between reactive thrombocytosis and myeloproliferative disease (MPD) (essential thrombocythemia and polycythemia vera). PDW$_{residual}$ was above the 95th percentile in 76% of MPD patients.[11]

Footnotes

1. Morris WW and Davey FR, "Basic Examination of Blood," *Clinical Diagnosis and Management by Laboratory Methods*, 19th ed, Chapter 24, Henry JB, ed, Philadelphia, PA: WB Saunders Co, 1996, 558-9.

2. Stiegler G, Stohlawetz P, Brugger S, et al, "Elevated Numbers of Reticulated Platelets in Hyperthyroidism: Direct Evidence for an Increase of Thrombopoiesis," *Br J Haematol*, 1998, 101(4):656-8.

3. England JM, "Blood Cell Sizing," *Practical Laboratory Hematology*, Chapter 6, Koepke JA, ed, New York, NY: Churchill Livingstone, 1991, 127-8.

4. Eldor A, Avitzour M, Or R, et al, "Prediction of Haemorrhagic Diathesis in Thrombocytopenia by Mean Platelet Volume," *Br Med J (Clin Res Ed)*, 1982, 285(6339):397-400.

5. Ahmed Y, van Iddekinge B, Paul C, et al, "Retrospective Analysis of Platelet Numbers and Volumes in Normal Pregnancy and in Pre-eclampsia," *Br J Obstet Gynaecol*, 1993, 100(3):216-20.

6. Neiger R, Contag SA, and Coustan DR, "Pre-eclampsia Effect on Platelet Count," *Am J Perinatol*, 1992, 9(5-6):378-80.

7. O'Connor TA, Ringer KM, and Gaddis ML, "Mean Platelet Volume During Coagulase-Negative Staphylococcal Sepsis in Neonates," *Am J Clin Pathol*, 1993, 99(1):69-71.

8. Boldt J, Zickmann B, Benson M, et al, "Does Platelet Size Correlate With Function in Patients Undergoing Cardiac Surgery?" *Intensive Care Med*, 1993, 19(1):44-7.

9. Kario K, Matsuo T, and Nakao K, "Cigarette Smoking Increases the Mean Platelet Volume in Elderly Patients With Risk Factors for Atherosclerosis," *Clin Lab Haematol*, 1992, 14(4):281-7.

10. Becker PS, Clavell LA, and Beardsley DS, "Giant Platelets With Abnormal Surface Glycoproteins: A New Familial Disorder Associated WIth Mitral Valve Insufficiency," *J Pediatr Hematol Oncol*, 1998, 20(1):69-73.

11. Osselaer JC, Jamart J, and Scheiff JM, "Platelet Distribution Width for Differential Diagnosis of Thrombocytosis," *Clin Chem*, 1997, 43(6):1072-6.

References

Bithell TC, "Thrombocytopenia Caused by Immunologic Platelet Destruction," *Wintrobe's Clinical Hematology*, 9th ed, Volume 2, Chapter 50, Philadelphia, PA: Lea & Febiger, 1993, 1335.

Graham SS, Traub B, and Mink IB, "Automated Platelet-Sizing Parameters on a Normal Population," *Am J Clin Pathol*, 1987, 87(3):365-9.

Jackson SR and Carter JM, "Platelet Volume: Laboratory Measurement and Clinical Application," *Blood Rev*, 1993, 7(2):104-13.

Mhawech P and Saleem A, "Inherited Giant Platelet Disorders: Classification and Literature Review," *Am J Clin Pathol*, 2000, 113(2):176-90.

Threatte GA, "Usefulness of the Mean Platelet Volume," *Clin Lab Med*, 1993, 13(4):937-50.

♦ **Pleural Fluid Analysis** *see* Body Fluid Analysis, Cell Count *on page 408*

♦ **PMDW** *see* Platelet Count *on page 468*

♦ **Pneumonia, Chronic Eosinophilic** *see* Eosinophil Granule Proteins *on page 426*

♦ **PNH Test** *see* Ham Test *on page 439*

PNH Test (GPI-Anchored Proteins) by Flow Cytometry

Related Information
Flow Cytometry, Overview *on page 432*
Ham Test *on page 439*
Hemosiderin Stain, Urine *on page 876*
Peripheral Blood: Red Blood Cell Morphology *on page 467*
Red Blood Cells, Washed *on page 859*
Sugar Water Test Screen *on page 488*

Synonyms CD55 by Flow Cytometry; CD59 by Flow Cytometry; Flow Cytometric Analysis for Paroxysmal Nocturnal Hemoglobinuria (PNH); Flow Cytometric Test for GPI-Anchored Protein Deficient Cells; PI-Linked Antigen

Applies to CD14; CD16; CD24; CD55 (Decay Accelerating Factor - DAF); CD59 (Membrane Inhibitor of Reactive Lysis - MIRL); CD66b; Glycophorin A; GPI-Anchored Proteins

Test Includes Flow cytometric analysis of peripheral red and/or white blood cells using monoclonal antibodies against glycosyl-phosphatidylinositol anchored proteins, in particular the CD55 (decay accelerating factor - DAF) and/or CD59 (membrane inhibitor of reactive lysis - MIRL, protectin) antigens

Abstract This test determines the presence or absence of the glycosyl-phosphatidylinositol (GPI) anchored protein decay-accelerating factor (DAF, CD55), membrane inhibitor of reactive lysis (MIRL, CD59), and others (individual laboratory dependent). DAF and MIRL are complement regulatory proteins. Their absence accounts for the complement sensitivity of PNH red cells. PNH is characterized by chronic intravascular hemolysis which is the result of abnormal sensitivity of PNH red cells to complement-mediated lysis. Failure of regulation of the alternative pathway of complement activation results in hemolysis (in patients with PNH). The test involves flow cytometric analysis (immunophenotyping) of red cells or white cells (in particular, neutrophils) of peripheral blood utilizing monoclonal antibodies (conjugated with fluorescent dye) to tag the appropriate GPI-anchored proteins. Results of such analyses are considered to define the presence of PNH. Flow cytometry for PNH is an important advance over the Ham (acidified serum) test which in comparison lacks sensitivity as well as specificity and is subject to operational inconsistency.

Specimen 5 mL whole blood

Container Lavender top (EDTA) tube or green top (heparin) tube; consult laboratory as to their specimen container preference.

Storage Instructions Analysis should be performed within 24 hours of specimen collection for optimal results. Test may be performed on samples obtained 48-72 hours prior to analysis. Keep specimen at room temperature. Refrigeration may cause loss of cell surface antigen.

Causes for Rejection Aged and/or cold stored specimens may cause false-positive results.

Turnaround Time 1 day

Special Instructions This relatively recently developed assay[1,2,3,4,5,6] is likely to be performed by a research or reference laboratory. Consult your clinical laboratory for availability and requirements.

Reference Interval Normal individuals (those without PNH) have presence of flow cytometric detected GPI-anchored proteins while patients with PNH have absence of such proteins (and thus are positive for PNH).

Use To establish the presence of cells diagnostic of PNH. Patients with congenital dyserythropoietic anemia (CDA) give a false-positive result (for PNH) with the Ham test[7,8] but test (appropriately) negative for PNH with flow cytometry analysis (CDA patients show presence of GPI-anchored proteins).

Limitations Requires availability of flow cytometer, associated reagents (in particular appropriate monoclonal antibodies and controls), and technical support personnel.

Methodology Flow cytometry (FC) using a variety of fluorescent-tagged monoclonal antibodies to one or more GPI-anchored proteins with accompanying controls. A well-controlled three-color flow cytometric protocol developed and used at the National Heart, Lung, and Blood Institute including delineation of (and commercial sources for) antibody reagents has been published.[9] While GPI protein deficiencies involve the membranes of red cells, granulocytes, monocytes, lymphocytes, and platelets, the neutrophilic granulocyte is the preferred test cell because abnormal granulocytes have normal survival time in the circulation while target (GPI protein deficient) red cells may be variably decreased due to hemolytic activity and/or dilution by transferred normal erythrocytes. One or more of the following membrane antigens may be targeted for analysis in flow cytometry tests for PNH:

- CD59: Membrane inhibitor of reactive lysis (MIRL), also known as "protectin" and MAC inhibiting factor (MAC - the membrane attack complex of complement cascade). CD59 regulates complement activity by inhibiting factors C5b to C8 catalyzed insertion of C9 into lipid bilayers.
- CD55: Decay accelerating factor (DAF) accelerates decay of the classic (C4b2a) and alternative (C3bBb) C3 convertases (release of C2a from C4b and Bb from C3b).
- CD24: A GPI-linked sialoglycoprotein that takes part in signal transduction, B-cell proliferation/differentiation

- CD16: Low affinity receptor for IgG (FcγRIII) with two molecular species one of which (FcγRIIIB) is a GPI-anchored protein. Present on natural killer cell membranes and is required for antibody-dependent cell cytotoxicity.
- CD14: GPI-anchored receptor for the lipopolysaccharide complex (LPS) and the LPS-binding protein. Participates in initiation of the process of endotoxin mediated shock.
- CD66b: Previously CD67; antigens CD66a through CD66e are members of a family of some 17 or more proteins that include carcino-embryonic antigen and nonspecific cross-reacting antigens. CD66b is a GPI-anchored protein present on granulocytes.
- Glycophorin A: A non-GPI-anchored protein marker used for the identification of erythrocytes.
- A variety of mouse IgG and/or IgM monoclonal antibodies for the identification of granulocytes.

Monoclonal antibody CD59 is the preferred single monoclonal antibody to use for GPI-anchored protein deficiency. CD59 is present on granulocytes and is the most deficient GPI protein in cases of PNH in which cells are only partially deficient.

Demonstration of the absence of GPI-anchored protein (one or more) by flow cytometry currently provides the most reliable method for diagnosis of PNH. The method is sensitive and specific and should be used in preference to the Ham test. The Ham and sugar water hemolysis tests detect only PNH erythrocytes which may be variably decreased due to shortened lifespan with resultant false-negative test results.[10]

Additional Information The conundrum of apparently disparate clinical and laboratory features that characterize paroxysmal nocturnal hemoglobinuria (PNH) have been largely (albeit still incompletely) resolved during the past 1-3 decades by significant (and brilliant) advances in delineation of the underlying molecular pathology. The PNH condition has been established as a loss of multiple membrane proteins, all of which share the common feature of being anchored to the cell surface by glycosyl-phosphatidylinositol. See diagram.

Red Cell Membrane and Skeleton

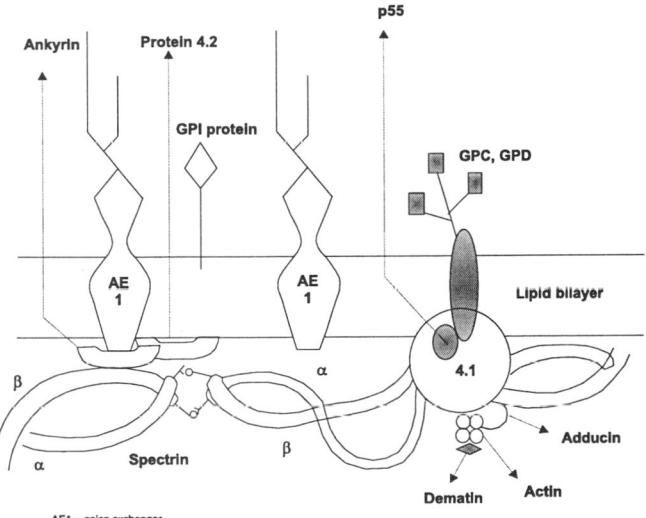

AE1 = anion exchanger
GPI = protein, glycosylphosphatidylinositol anchored protein
GPC = glycophorin C
GPD = glycophorin D

Adapted from McMullin MF, "The Molecular Basis of Disorders of the Red Cell Membrane," *J Clin Pathol*, 1999, 52(4):245-8.

Some 18 proteins are currently identified as deficient in PNH. These include leukocyte alkaline phosphatase, acetylcholinesterase, decay accelerating factor (DAF, CD55), membrane inhibitor of reactive lysis (MIRL, CD59) and FcγRIIIB (CD16b). The absence of CD55 and CD59 account for the susceptibility of erythrocytes to lysis by complement in patients with PNH. PNH is caused by an acquired somatic mutation. The defective gene, identified in 1993, is present on the short arm of the X chromosome (Xp 22.1).[11] The gene, PIG-A (phosphatidylinositol glycan-class A) encodes a protein that is needed for the early synthesis of N-acetylglucosaminylphosphatidlinositol (G1cNAc-PI), an early intermediate in the synthesis of the GPI anchor. The somatic mutation occurs at an early stage in the evolution of a pluripotent hematopoietic stem cell,[11,12] accounting for involvement of multiple cell lines (ie, erythrocytes, neutrophils, monocytes, lymphocytes, and platelet precursors). Variation in the nature of the mutation and the degree of inactivation of PIG-A provide a molecular basis for some of the phenotypic mosaicism seen clinically in patients with PNH.[12] Some 125 PIG-A mutations have been reported.[13,14]

The clinical features of PNH relate (albeit at times somewhat tortuously) to missing GPI-anchored proteins and include intravascular hemolysis, aplastic anemia/pancytopenia, and venous thrombosis.[15] The relationship of PNH to apparently associated bone marrow failure syndromes (in particular myelodysplasia), aplastic anemia, autoimmunity, and apoptosis is

under investigation,[9,10,14,16,17] occasionally with disparate results. Concerning thrombogenesis in PNH, there is evidence that microvesicle formation with externalization of phosphatidylserine (RBC membrane phospholipid redistribution) may accelerate activation of hemostasis and account for a hypercoagulable state, especially after a hemolytic episode.[18] Future therapy may relate to transfer of GPI-anchored proteins to PNH red cells.[19] Genetic instability may underlie the development of PIG-A mutations that lead to clinical PNH.[20]

Footnotes

1. van der Schoot CE, Huizinga TW, van't Veer-Korthof ET, et al, "Deficiency of Glycosyl-Phosphatidylinositol-Linked Membrane Glycoproteins of Leukocytes in Paroxysmal Nocturnal Hemoglobinuria, Description of a New Diagnostic Cytofluorometric Assay," *Blood*, 1990, 76(9):1853-9.
2. Hall SE and Rosse WF, "The Use of Monoclonal Antibodies and Flow Cytometry in the Diagnosis of Paroxysmal Nocturnal Hemoglobinuria," *Blood*, 1996, 87(12):5332-40.
3. Plesner T, Hansen NE, and Carlsen K, "Estimation of PI-Bound Proteins on Blood Cells From PNH Patients by Quantitative Flow Cytometry," *Br J Haematol*, 1990, 75(4):585-90.
4. Hillmen P, Hows JM, and Luzzatto L, "Two Distinct Patterns of Glycosyl-Phosphatidylinositol (GPI) Linked Protein Deficiency in the Red Cells of Patients With Paroxysmal Nocturnal Haemoglobinuria," *Br J Haematol*, 1992, 80(3):399-405.
5. Schubert J, Alvarado M, Uciechowski P, et al, "Diagnosis of Paroxysmal Nocturnal Haemoglobinuria Using Immunophenotyping of Peripheral Blood Cells," *Br J Haematol*, 1991, 79(3):487-92.
6. Shichishima T, Terasawa T, Saitoh Y, et al, "Diagnosis of Paroxysmal Nocturnal Haemoglobinuria by Phenotypic Analysis of Erythrocytes Using Two-Colour Flow Cytometry With Monoclonal Antibodies to DAF and CD59/MACIF," *Br J Haematol*, 1993, 85(2):378-86.
7. Wickramasinghe SN, "Congenital Dyserythropoietic Anaemias: Clinical Features, Haematologic Morphology and New Biochemical Data," *Blood Rev*, 1998, 12(3):178-200.
8. Wickramasinghe SN, "Congenital Dyserythropoietic Anemias," *Curr Opin Hematol*, 2000, 7(2):71-8.
9. Dunn DE, Tanawattanacharoen P, Boccuni P, et al, "Paroxysmal Nocturnal Hemoglobinuria Cells in Patients With Bone Marrow Failure Syndromes," *Ann Intern Med*, 1999, 131(6):401-8.
10. Benz EJ Jr, "Clonal Variation, Autoimmunity, and Neoplasia: An Ecology Lesson From Paroxysmal Nocturnal Hemoglobinuria," *Ann Intern Med*, 1999, 131(6):467-8.
11. Takeda J, Miyata T, Kawagoe K, et al, "Deficiency of the GPI Anchor Caused by a Somatic Mutation in the PIG-A Gene in Paroxysmal Nocturnal Hemoglobinuria," *Cell*, 1993, 73(4):703-11.
12. Endo M, Ware RE, Vreeke TM, et al, "Molecular Basis of the Heterogeneity of Expression of Glycosyl-Phosphatidylinositol Anchored Proteins in Paroxysmal Nocturnal Hemoglobinuria," *Blood*, 1996, 87(6):2546-57.
13. Nafa K, Bessler M, Castro-Malaspina H, et al, "The Spectrum of Somatic Mutations in the PIG-A Gene in Paroxysmal Nocturnal Hemoglobinuria Includes Large Deletions and Small Duplications," *Blood Cells Mol Dis*, 1998, 24(3):370-84.
14. Beutler E and Luzzatto L, "Hemolytic Anemia," *Semin Hematol*, 1999, 36(4 Suppl 7):38-47.
15. Hillmen P, Lewis SM, Bessler M, et al, "Natural History of Paroxysmal Nocturnal Hemoglobinuria," *N Engl J Med*, 1995, 333(19):1253-8.
16. Brodsky RA, Vala MS, Barber JP, et al, "Resistance to Apoptosis Caused by PIG-A Gene Mutations in Paroxysmal Nocturnal Hemoglobinuria," *Proc Natl Acad Sci U S A*, 1997, 94(16):8756-60.
17. Ware RE, Nishimura J, Moody MA, et al, "The PIG-A Mutation and Absence of Glycosyl-Phosphatidylinositol-Linked Proteins Do Not Confer Resistance to Apoptosis in Paroxysmal Nocturnal Hemoglobinuria," *Blood*, 1998, 92(7):2541-50.
18. Ninomiya H, Kawashima Y, Hasegaura Y, et al, "Complement-Induced Procoagulant Alteration of Red Cell Membranes With Microvesicle Formation in Paroxysmal Nocturnal Hemoglobinuria (PNH): Implication for Thrombogenesis in PNH," *Br J Haematol*, 1999, 106(1):224-31.
19. Sloand EM, Maciejewski JP, Dunn D, et al, "Correction of the PNH Defect by GPI-anchored Protein Transfer," *Blood*, 1998, 92(11):4439-45.
20. Purow DB, Howard TA, Marcus SJ, et al, "Genetic Instability and the Etiology of Somatic PIG-A Mutations in Paroxysmal Nocturnal Hemoglobinuria," *Blood Cells Mol Dis*, 1999, 25(5):81-91.

References

Hillmen P and Richards SJ, "Implications of Recent Insight Into the Pathophysiology of Paroxysmal Nocturnal Hemoglobinuria," *Br J Haematol*, 2000, 108(3):470-9.

Hsi ED, "Paroxysmal Nocturnal Hemoglobinuria Testing by Flow Cytometry: Evaluation of the Redquant and Cellquant Kits," *Am J Clin Pathol*, 2000, 114(5):798-806.

McMullin MF, "The Molecular Basis of Disorders of the Red Cell Membrane," *J Clin Pathol*, 1999, 52(4):245-8.

Parker CJ and Lee GR, "Paroxysmal Nocturnal Hemoglobinuria," *Wintrobe's Clinical Hematology*, 10th ed, Chapter 47, Lee GR, Foerster J, Lukens J, et al, eds, Baltimore, MD: Lippincott Williams & Wilkins, 1999, 1264-88.

Rosse WF, "Paroxysmal Nocturnal Hemoglobinuria," *Hematology: Basic Principles and Practice*, 3rd ed, Chapter 20, Hoffman R, Benz EJ Jr, Shattil SJ, et al, eds, Philadelphia, PA: Churchill Livingstone, 2000, 331-42.

Rosse WF, "Paroxysmal Nocturnal Hemoglobinuria as a Molecular Disease," Reviews in Molecular Medicine, *Medicine*, 1997, 76(2):63-93.

Young NS, "The Problem of Clonality in Aplastic Anemia: Dr Dameshek's Riddle, Restated," *Blood*, 1992, 79(6):1385-92.

Promyelocytic Leukemia Assay

Related Information

Bone Marrow *on page 410*
Fluorescence *In Situ* Hybridization *on page 367*
Leukocyte Cytochemistry *on page 456*

Synonyms APL® Cell Test

Applies to PG-M3 Antibody; Retinoic Acid Receptor α Gene (RARα)

Abstract Rapid, low cost immunofluorescence-based assay to detect the presence of acute promyelocytic leukemia (APL®) cells in bone marrow specimens.

Specimen EDTA or heparin anticoagulated bone marrow aspirate specimen

Storage Instructions Cells cryopreserved in liquid nitrogen utilizing controlled freezing of cells suspended in a solution of 90% fetal calf serum and 10% dimethylsulfoxide

Turnaround Time <3 hours when the test is performed on site

Special Instructions Cytopreparations of fresh or thawed cells are prepared. Slides fixed in 1:1 acetone-methanol at -10°C for 1 minute and then air dried. May delay up to 24 hours prior to immunostaining.

Reference Interval Marrow negative for demonstrable APL® cells

Use Demonstration of PG-M3 monoclonal antibody-positive cells (APL® cells) in bone marrow aspirate specimens. Helpful in providing rapid confirmation of a diagnosis of APL® and in differentiation of regenerative myelopoiesis from recurrence of APL®.

Limitations Recently developed procedure, likely to be available on a limited referral basis. Subjective endpoint depends on the assessment of a diffuse, finely speckled pattern of fluorescent PML on cogenic domains.

Contraindications The threshold for detection of APL cells is about 5%, so this assay should not be used to assess post-treatment minimal residual disease.

Methodology Slide/epifluorescence microscopy based immunofluorescence, using the murine monoclonal antibody PG-M3 (identifies the PML-RARα gene rearrangement)

Additional Information APL is characterized by a chromosomal translocation, t(15;17) that creates a chimeric gene, the fusion of the retinoic acid receptor α gene (RARα on chromosome 17) with the PML gene (on chromosome 15). The monoclonal antibody PG-M3, developed against the aminoterminal end of the PML gene product, reacts with some human cell lines and can be used with paraffin-embedded tissue.[1] This test may provide a simple, rapid low-cost alternative to the diagnosis by cytogenetic analysis (karyotyping) or by reverse transcription-polymerase chain reaction.[2]

Footnotes

1. Flenghi L, Fagioloi M, Tomassoni L, et al, "Characterization of a New Monoclonal Antibody (PG-M3) Directed Against the Amino-Terminal Portion of the PML Gene Product: Immunocytochemical Evidence for High Expression of PML Proteins on Activated Macrophages, Endothelial Cells, and Epithelia," *Blood*, 1995, 85(7):1871-80.
2. Miller WH Jr, Kakikuza A, Frankel SR, et al, "Reverse Transcription Polymerase Chain Reaction for the Rearranged Retinoic Acid Receptor Alpha Clarifies Diagnosis and Detects Minimal Residual Disease in Acute Promyelocytic Leukemia," *Proc Natl Acad Sci U S A*, 1992, 89(7):2694-7.

References

Samoszuk MK, Tynan W, Sallash G, et al, "An Immunofluorescent Assay for Acute Promyelocytic Leukemia Cells," *Am J Clin Pathol*, 1998, 109(2):205-10.

♦ **Propidium Iodide** *see* Apoptosis Assays *on page 402*

♦ **Protein 4.2** *see* Band 4.2, Red Cell Membrane *on page 406*

♦ **Protein 4.2**[Lisboa] *see* Band 4.2, Red Cell Membrane *on page 406*

♦ **Prussian Blue Reaction** *see* Iron Stain, Bone Marrow *on page 452*

♦ **Prussian Blue Stain** *see* Iron Stain, Bone Marrow *on page 452*

♦ **Pseudoreticulocytosis** *see* Malaria Smear and Tests *on page 458*

♦ **Pyrimidine-5-Nucleotidase Deficiency** *see* Red Blood Cell Enzyme Deficiency, Quantitative *on page 475*

♦ **Pyropoikilocytosis** *see* Peripheral Blood: Red Blood Cell Morphology *on page 467*

♦ **Pyropoikilocytosis, Hereditary** *see* Autohemolysis Test *on page 405*

♦ **Pyropoikilocytosis, Hereditary** *see* Osmotic Fragility *on page 462*

♦ **Pyruvate Kinase Assay** *see* Pyruvate Kinase Assay, Erythrocytes *on page 474*

Pyruvate Kinase Assay, Erythrocytes

Related Information

Autohemolysis Test *on page 405*
Red Blood Cell Enzyme Deficiency, Quantitative *on page 475*
Red Blood Cell Enzyme Deficiency Screen *on page 476*

Synonyms Pyruvate Kinase Assay

Abstract A deficiency of this glycolytic enzyme is characterized by a decrease in RBC ATP level and resultant nonspherocytic chronic hemolytic anemia. Signs and symptoms usually develop in early childhood and consist of anemia, icterus and splenomegaly. An autosomal recessive condition, parents will be heterozygotes. Hemolytic disease of the newborn may occur.

Specimen Erythrocytes (washed)

Container Yellow top (ACD) tube, green top (heparin) tube, or lavender top (EDTA) tube

Collection Mix tube three times by gentle inversion, place on ice.

Causes for Rejection Specimen not fresh

Special Instructions Notify laboratory before specimen collection. Deliver specimen on ice. Specimen **must** be received in the laboratory within 30 minutes of collection.

Reference Interval Adults: 6-19 μmol NAD(H)$_2$/min/g Hb (37°C)

Use Evaluate chronic hemolytic anemia

Limitations Some patients with pyruvate kinase-deficient variant hemolytic disease may not be identified if the enzyme is assayed only under conditions of substrate saturation.

Methodology Spectrophotometric kinetic assay

Additional Information Pyruvate kinase (PK) deficiency is the most common enzyme defect in anaerobic red cell glycolysis and the most common cause of congenital nonspherocytic hemolytic anemia. Glycolysis is a major energy source for red cells, thus, enzyme deficiency leads to hemolysis. The substrate for anaerobic glycolysis is glucose-6-phosphate (phosphorylated by hexokinase to glucose) which is processed through the Embden-Meyerhof pathway to pyruvate or may undergo oxidative (aerobic) glycolysis in the pentose phosphate pathway. Some 20 enzymes are involved in the anaerobic and oxidative glycolytic pathways. PK is a glycolytic enzyme that converts phosphoenolpyruvate to pyruvate. There are four isoenzymes, M$_1$, M$_2$, L, and R, the latter expressed only in red blood cells. The deficiency is inherited as an autosomal recessive trait, about 400 cases have been reported and about 100 gene mutations have been identified.[1,2,3,4] Missense and splicing mutations occur, as well as insertions and deletions, a missense mutation in codon 510 (CGA; Arg→CAA; Gln) accounts for about 30% of cases in northern Europe and the United States. Clinical characteristics (phenotypic expression) is variable, indicating the influence of environmental interaction and/or additional genetic factors.

PK deficiency causes hemolytic anemia of varying severity. About 33% of patients are symptomatic in the neonatal period with hemolysis and jaundice. Splenomegaly may be present. Exchange transfusion may be required. Subsequently, hemolysis may require transfusion. Hemolysis may be mild and go unnoticed for years. Echinocytes and (if severe hemolysis is present) spherocytes and nucleated red cells may be seen on peripheral smear. Anemia is normochromic/normocytic. Reticulocyte count may be very high (40% to 70%), especially, paradoxically, after splenectomy.

Current assay techniques preclude accurate distinction of all heterozygotes from normals. Specialized PK assays and the determination of red cell 2,3-DPG levels are often helpful in these cases. Most homozygous PK deficient children, younger than 2 years of age, have higher residual PK activities than those found in adult PK deficient homozygotes with comparable levels of reticulocytosis. Reductions of red cell pyruvate kinase activity to <20% of normal indicates hereditary PK deficiency. Application of molecular biologic techniques (polymerase chain reaction and restriction endonuclease analysis) may allow prenatal diagnosis (using amniotic fluid cells and/or cord blood).[5] Slight to moderate decrease of red cell PK activity can be seen in some patients with leukemia and in bone marrow aplasia. Further characterization may be necessary to diagnose hemolytic disease due to PK deficient variants, including doubly heterozygous individuals.

Footnotes

1. McMullin MF, "The Molecular Basis of Disorders of Red Cell Enzymes," *J Clin Pathol*, 1999, 52(4):241-4.
2. Miwa S and Fujii H, "Molecular Basis of Erythroenzymopathies Associated With Hereditary Hemolytic Anemia: Tabulation of Mutant Enzymes," *Am J Hematol*, 1996, 51(2):122-32.
3. Lenzner C, Nürnberg P, Jacobasch G, et al, "Molecular Analysis of 29 Pyruvate Kinase-Deficient Patients From Central Europe With Hereditary Hemolytic Anemia," *Blood*, 1997, 89(5):1793-9.
4. Zanella A, Bianchi P, Baronciani L, et al, "Molecular Characterization of PK-LR Gene in Pyruvate Kinase-Deficient Italian Patients," *Blood*, 1997, 89(10):3847-52.
5. Baronciani L and Beutler E, "Prenatal Diagnosis of Pyruvate Kinase Deficiency," *Blood*, 1994, 84(7):2354-6.

References

Baronciani L and Beutler E, "Molecular Study of Pyruvate Kinase Deficient Patients With Hereditary Nonspherocytic Hemolytic Anemia," *J Clin Invest*, 1995, 95(4):1702-9.

Mentzer WC, "Pyruvate Kinase Deficiency and Disorders of Glycolysis," *Nathan and Oski's Hematology of Infancy and Childhood*, 5th ed, Chapter 17, Nathan DG and Orkin SH, eds, Philadelphia, PA: WB Saunders Co, 1998, 665-703.

Mosca A, Tagarelli A, Paleari R, et al, "Rapid Determination of Erythrocyte Pyruvate Kinase Activity," *Clin Chem*, 1993, 39(3):512-6.

♦ **QBC Tube, Buffy Coat** *see* Malaria Smear and Tests *on page 458*

♦ **QBC Tube (Quantitative Buffy Coat)** *see* Bacteremia Detection, Buffy Coat Micromethod *on page 406*

♦ **Radioactive Vitamin B$_{12}$ Absorption Test With or Without Intrinsic Factor** *see* Schilling Test *on page 483*

♦ **RBC** *see* Red Cell Count *on page 478*

Red Blood Cell Enzyme Deficiency, Quantitative

Related Information

Synonyms Erythrocyte Enzyme Deficiency, Quantitative; RBC Enzymes, Quantitative

Applies to Acatalasemia; Adenosine Deaminase Overproduction; Adenylate Kinase Deficiency; γ-Glutamylcysteine Synthetase; Glutathione Reductase Deficiency, RBC; Heinz Bodies; Pyrimidine-5-Nucleotidase Deficiency

Test Includes Glucose-6-phosphate dehydrogenase (G6PD), pyruvate kinase (PK), and any of over 20 RBC enzymes included in the following reference by E. Beutler.

Abstract Clinical suspicion of red cell enzyme deficiency as a cause of hemolytic anemia but with normal G6PD and PK levels indicates the need to consider use of assays for the more uncommon red cell enzyme deficiencies.

Specimen Erythrocytes; about 1 mL of blood is required for each enzyme assay.

Container Lavender top (EDTA) tube; heparin or acid-citrate-dextrose samples may also be used.

Storage Instructions Normal enzymes are stable for 24 hours at 25°C and for 6-20 days at 4°C.

Causes for Rejection Clotted or hemolyzed specimen

Special Instructions Most of these assays are rarely performed and will need to be sent to a reference laboratory. Ship on wet ice, do not freeze.

Reference Interval G6PD: 8.6-18.6 IU/g hemoglobin; phosphohexoisomerase: 14.7-42.2 IU/g hemoglobin; pyruvate kinase: 2.0-8.8 IU/g hemoglobin

Use Investigation of hemolytic anemia

Limitations False-normal results may occur if testing is performed on a sample obtained just after a hemolytic episode (deficiency may be obscured by the presence of a young, enzyme-rich population of RBCs, reticulocytes, the older enzyme-deficient red cells having been destroyed).

In vitro assay (with optimal pH, substrate concentration, and other conditions) may not reflect *in vivo* enzyme performance. Contamination by leukocytes (that may have enzymes with high specific activity) can cause spurious normal RBC values. Transfused RBCs may mask a deficient state. Mixed reticulocytes and senescent red cells (with reduced enzyme activity) may obscure the level of enzyme deficiency.

Contraindications Sample obtained just after an acute hemolytic episode has occurred

Methodology Standardized methods have been recommended by the International Committee for Standardization in Haematology.[1]

Additional Information See graphic.

The mature red blood cell cannot synthesize protein or lipids and is dependent upon glycolysis to obtain energy from glucose. Glucose is initially phosphorylated by hexokinase with the resultant glucose-6-phosphate (G6P) further processed as substrate for anaerobic glycolysis (Embden-Meyerhof pathway with production of pyruvate and ATP) or alternately G6P is processed in the pentose phosphate pathway (oxidative glycolysis). Of the some 20 enzymes that function in these two major pathways, the two most common enzyme disorders associated with hemolysis are glucose-6-phosphate dehydrogenase (G6PD) deficiency and pyruvate kinase (PK) deficiency.

The following enzymes of the anaerobic glycolytic pathway cause hemolysis when deficient:
• hexokinase (HK)
• glucose phosphate isomerase (GPI)

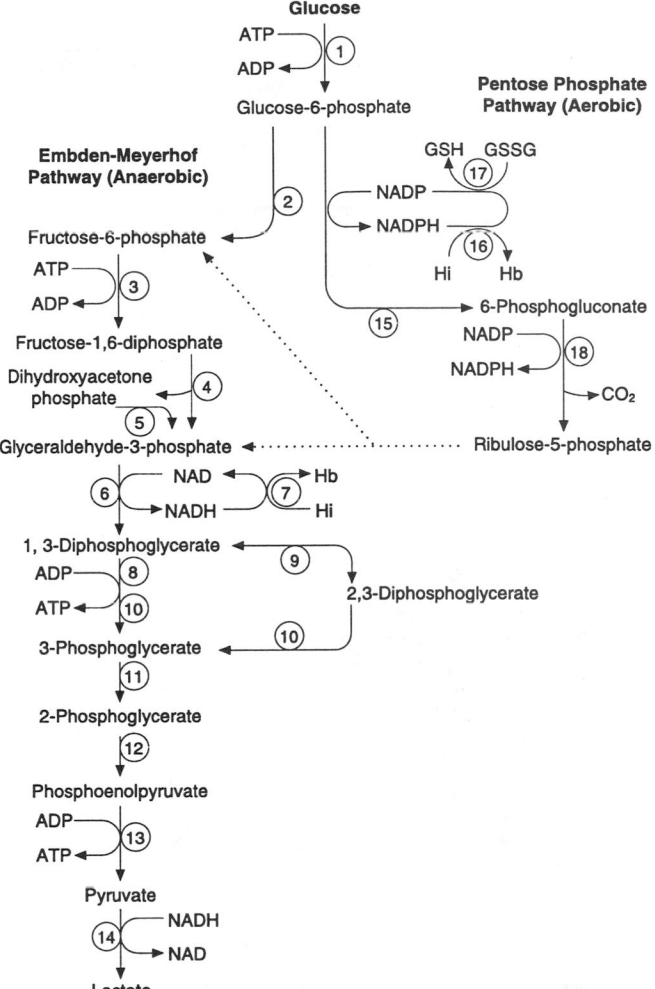

Schematic representation of red cell glycolytic pathways. The enzymes are indicated as follows: (1) hexokinase, (2) glucosephosphate isomerase, (3) phosphofructokinase, (4) aldolase, (5) triose phosphate isomerase, (6) glyceraldehyde-3-phosphate dehydrogenase, (7) NADH-methaemoglobin reductase, (8) phosphoglycerate kinase, (9) diphosphoglyceromutase, (10) diphosphoglycerate phosphatase, (11) phosphoglyceromutase, (12) enolase, (13) pyruvate kinase, (14) lactate dehydrogenase, (15) glucose-6-phosphate dehydrogenase, (16) NADPH-methaemoglobin reductase, (17) glutathione reductase, (18) 6-phosphogluconate dehydrogenase.

Adapted from Luzzatto L, Roper D, Dacie Sir JV, et al, *Practical Haematology*, 8th ed, Chapter 13, New York, NY: Churchill Livingstone, 1995, 226.

• phosphofructokinase (PFK)
• aldolase
• triose phosphate isomerase (TPI)
• phosphoglycerate kinase (PGK)
• enolase
• pyruvate kinase (PK)

Enzymes of the oxidative glycolytic pathway that may cause hemolysis when deficient:
• glucose-6-phosphate dehydrogenase (G6PD)

Abnormalities of red cell nucleotide metabolism:
• pyrimidine-5'-nucleotidase deficiency
• adenylate kinase deficiency
• adenosine deaminase overproduction

Individuals with low levels of RBC G6PD are susceptible to hemolytic episodes after exposure to certain chemicals, drugs, and fava beans. Drugs that may precipitate hemolysis in patients with G6PD deficiency include:
• analgesics/antipyretics: aspirin
• sulfa drugs: sulfapyridine, sulfisoxazole
• antimalarias: primaquine, pentaquine, quinine, nitrofurantoin, Chloromycetin®, quinidine, para-aminosalicylic acid
• others

Deficient or absent RBC enzyme activity may relate to absence of or decreased level of the enzyme, presence of an inactive molecular form or of an isoenzyme with altered activity. In some hematologic diseases (eg, PNH, aplastic anemia and acute leukemia), acquired red cell enzyme deficiency is not infrequently seen. RBC glutathione reductase deficiency bears an association with a variety of chemotherapeutically treated malignant states (Continued)

Red Blood Cell Enzyme Deficiency, Quantitative
(Continued)

(up to 43% in a study of hospitalized patients). Glutathione reductase deficiency also occurs in some cases of malnutrition, liver disease, and sepsis. Disorders of red cell nucleotide metabolism possibly associated with hemolytic anemia:

- pyrimidine-5-nucleotidase deficiency
- adenylate kinase deficiency
- adenosine deaminase overproduction

Glucose-6-phosphate dehydrogenase deficiency, see Glucose-6-Phosphate Dehydrogenase, Quantitative, Blood *on page 437*.

Pyruvate kinase (PK) deficiency, see Pyruvate Kinase Assay, Erythrocytes *on page 474*.

When immune hemolytic anemia, hemoglobinopathy, paroxysmal nocturnal hemoglobinuria, and Wilson disease have been excluded as causes of acute hemolytic anemia, presence of a red cell membrane disorder and/or the following uncommon red cell enzymopathies should be considered in the diagnostic evaluation.

Glucose phosphate isomerase (GPI) deficiency, the 2nd most common glycolytic enzymopathy associated with hemolysis is the 4th most common hereditary enzyme defect of red cells. Some 35 pedigrees, with nearly 50 anemic patients, have been reported. Clinical features are those of PK deficiency. With severe anemia, spiculated microspherocytes may occur after splenectomy. Some cases show stomatocytosis. Reticulocyte levels are high, occasionally reaching the 80% level. Variant forms of the enzyme may be divided into those with increased, normal, or slow electrophoretic mobility. Inheritance is autosomal recessive, as with most of the RBC enzymopathies. Heterozygotes are hematologically normal even though red cell GPI activity is reduced to about 50% of normal.

Pyrimidine 5'-nucleotidase (P5N) deficiency, the 3rd most common cause of red cell enzymopathy associated with hemolysis, is an abnormality of nucleotide metabolism. P5' N catalyzes the degradation of pyrimidine nucleotides with hemolysis apparently resulting from retained aggregates of ribosomes that attach to and cause membrane injury. There is resultant marked basophilic stippling of red cells seen on peripheral blood smear. There is also mild to moderate anemia, reticulocytosis, and hyperbilirubinemia. P5N deficiency has autosomal recessive inheritance, biochemical heterozygotes are hematologically normal.

Phosphoglycerate kinase (PGK) deficiency differs from other glycolytic enzymopathies in that it has x-linked inheritance. Most severely PGK-deficient subjects have neurologic involvement as well as hemolysis, nearly all with clinical involved are male (sex linked disorder). There may be seizures, movement disorders, emotional instability, psychomotor retardation, aphasia and tetraplegia. With milder forms of PGK deficiency there may be only hemolytic anemia or no clinical abnormalities. There have been some 40 or more cases described worldwide.

Adenylate kinase (AK) deficiency is a rare (some 6 pedigrees reported as of 1997) evident cause of chronic hemolytic anemia. The enzyme catalyzes the interconversion of ATP, ADP, and AMP (nucleotide phosphatases) and is important, if not critical, in maintaining nucleotide phosphate pools and availability of ADP for generation of red cell ATP. There are three isoenzymes, AK1, AK2, and AK3. AK1 is present in red cells, skeletal muscle, and brain. The clinical course is characterized by chronic hemolytic anemia (episodically severe), mild jaundice, and splenomegaly with signs and symptoms developing in the first few months of life. There may be severe anemia requiring multiple periodic transfusions. Mental retardation has characterized some cases. There may be concomitant G6PD deficiency.[2] AK1 isozyme (erythrocyte) has been proposed as a marker for hemolysis.[3]

Triosephosphate isomerase (TPI) Deficiency and associated hemolytic anemia have been reported in some 25 individuals, most of whom die before age 5. There is early onset of a severe neurologic affliction with spasticity, motor retardation, and hypotonia. The enzyme catalyzes the interconversion of dihydroxyacetone phosphate (DHP) and glyceraldehyde phosphate with deficiency resulting in accumulation of DHP in red blood cells, skeletal muscle, cerebrospinal fluid, and leukocytes. In addition to neuromuscular involvement and anemia, there may be cardiomyopathy and susceptibility to infection. Molecular genetic analysis for prenatal diagnosis has been described.[4]

Inherited deficiency in an enzyme, γ-glutamylcysteine synthetase (GCS), one of six enzymes in the γ-glutamyl cycle involved in glutathione synthesis, has been reported. Eight patients have been reported as of 2000. They have hemolytic anemia, neonatal jaundice, and low red cell levels of glutathione. Some cases have aminoaciduria and develop neurologic symptoms.[5]

Acatalasemia, a rare condition, with near absence of red cell catalase, has been reported and studied.[6,7] The red cell is the most severely affected cell type in humans. Even when challenged by oxidant drugs, however, red cells are not destroyed, red cell survival is normal, due apparently to compensatory increase in activity of the pentose phosphate shunt.

The numerous other red cell enzyme deficiencies are rare (as are the last two entities above). Adenosine deaminase (ADA) overproduction is unique. Some 14 individuals in 3 families have been reported. The condition is inherited as an autosomal dominant. It is the third of the inherited disorders of erythrocyte nucleotide metabolism. Some patients show stomatocytosis. Hemolysis appears to be due to decreased red cell ATP, the result of redirection of most adenosine metabolism through the overactive ADA reaction. For additional details of RBC enzyme metabolic abnormalities, please see the following references.

Footnotes

1. Beutler E, Blume KG, Kaplan JC, et al, "International Committee for Standardization in Haematology: Recommended Methods for Red-Cell Enzyme Analysis," *Br J Haematol*, 1977, 35(2):331-40.
2. Qualtieri A, Pedace V, Bisconte MG, et al, "Severe Erythrocyte Adenylate Kinase Deficiency Due to Homozygous A→G Substitution at Codon 164 of Human AK1 Gene Associated With Chronic Haemolytic Anaemia," *Br J Haematol*, 1997, 99(4):770-6.
3. Thomas G and Murthy VV, "Erythrocyte Adenylate Kinase Isoenzyme as a Marker for Hemolysis," *J Clin Lab Anal*, 1997, 11(6):351-6.
4. Pekrun A, Neubauer BA, Eber SW, et al, "Triosephosphate Isomerase Deficiency: Biochemical and Molecular Genetic Analysis for Prenatal Diagnosis," *Clin Genet*, 1995, 47(4):175-9.
5. Ristoff E, Augustson C, Geissler J, et al, "A Missense Mutation in the Heavy Subunit of γ-Glutamylcysteine Synthetase Gene Causes Hemolytic Anemia," *Blood*, 2000, 95(7):2193-7.
6. Goth L, Shemirani A, and Kalmar T, "A Novel Catalase Mutation (a GA Insertion) Causes the Hungarian Type of Acatalasemia," *Blood Cells, Molecules, and Diseases*, 2000, 26(2):151-4.
7. Eaton JW and Ma M, "Acatalasemia," *The Metabolic and Molecular Bases of Inherited Disease*, 7th ed, Volume 11, Scriver CR, Beaudet AL, Sly WS, et al, eds, New York, NY: McGraw-Hill, 1995, 2371.

References

Arya R, Layton DM, and Bellingham AJ, "Hereditary Red Cell Enzymopathies," *Blood Rev*, 1995, 9(3):167-75.

Beutler E, "Glucose-6-Phosphate Deficiency and Other Enzyme Abnormalities," *Williams Hematology*, 5th ed, Chapter 54, Beutler E, Lichtman MA, Coller BS, et al, eds, New York, NY: McGraw-Hill Inc, 1995, 564-81.

Beutler E, *Red Cell Metabolism: A Manual of Biochemical Methods*, 3rd ed, New York, NY: Grune and Stratton Inc, 1984.

Brown KA, "Erythrocyte Metabolism and Enzyme Defects," *Lab Med*, 1996, 27(5):329-30.

Glader BE, "Hemolytic Anemia in Children," Diagnostic Pediatric Hematology, Geaghan SM, guest ed, *Clin Lab Med*, 1999, 19(1):87-111.

Layton DM and Bellingham AJ, "Disorders of Erythrocyte Metabolism," *Pediatric Hematology*, 2nd ed, Lilleyman JS, Hann IM, and Blanchette VS, eds, New York, NY: Churchill Livingstone, 1999, 285.

Luzzatto L and Roper D, "Investigation of the Hereditary Haemolytic Anaemias: Membrane and Enzyme Abnormalities," *Practical Hematology*, 8th ed, Dacie Sir JV and Lewis SM, eds, New York, NY: Churchill Livingstone, 1995, 215.

McMullin MF, "The Molecular Basis of Disorders of Red Cell Enzymes," *J Clin Pathol*, 1999, 52(4):241-4.

Mentzer WC, "Pyruvate Kinase Deficiency and Disorders of Glycolysis," *Nathan and Oski's Hematology of Infancy and Childhood*, 5th ed, Chapter 17, Nathan DE and Orkin SH, eds, Philadelphia, PA: WB Saunders Co, 1998, 665-703.

Miwa S and Fujii H, "Molecular Basis of Erythroenzymopathies Associated With Hereditary Hemolytic Anemia: Tabulation of Mutant Enzymes," *Am J Hematol*, 1996, 51(2):122-32.

Red Blood Cell Enzyme Deficiency Screen

Related Information
Anemia Flowchart *on page 392*
Glucose-6-Phosphate Dehydrogenase, Quantitative, Blood *on page 437*
Glucose-6-Phosphate Dehydrogenase Screen, Blood *on page 438*
Heinz Body Stain *on page 440*
Pyruvate Kinase Assay, Erythrocytes *on page 474*
Red Blood Cell Enzyme Deficiency, Quantitative *on page 475*
Reticulocyte Count *on page 481*

Synonyms Erythrocyte Enzyme Deficiency Screen; RBC Enzyme Screen

Applies to Adenylate Kinase Deficiency; γ-Glutamylcysteine Synthetase; Glutathione Reductase; Heinz Bodies; NADH Diaphorase; Triosephosphate Isomerase

Test Includes G6PD qualitative, pyruvate kinase, triosephosphate isomerase, NADH diaphorase (NADH methemoglobin reductase), glutathione reductase. Completeness varies between laboratories.

Specimen Erythrocytes

Container Lavender top (EDTA) tube

Causes for Rejection Clotted or hemolyzed specimen

Reference Interval Enzyme present, reported as normal

Use Detect etiology of hemolytic state, available for and indicated primarily for detection of G6PD deficiency

Limitations Does not detect heterozygotes. False normal results may occur if testing is performed on a sample obtained just after a hemolytic episode.

Additional Information Phenotyping of RBC enzymes has been applied to paternity testing.[1] See Red Blood Cell Enzyme Deficiency, Quantitative *on page 475*

Footnotes

1. Polesky HF, "Applications of Genetic Marker Typing in Disputed Parentage Cases," *Principles of Transfusion Medicine*, Rossi EC, Simon TL, Moss GS, et al, eds, Baltimore, MD: Lippincott Williams & Wilkins, 1996, 849-61.

References

Luzzatto L and Mehta A, "Glucose 6-Phosphate Dehydrogenase Deficiency," *The Metabolic and Molecular Bases of Inherited Disease*, 7th ed, Chapter 111, Scriver CR, Beaudet AL, Sly WS, et al, eds, New York, NY: McGraw-Hill Inc, 1995, 3367-98.

Luzzatto L and Roper D, "Investigation of the Hereditary Haemolytic Anaemias: Membrane and Enzyme Abnormalities," *Practical Haematology*, 8th ed, Chapter 13, New York, NY: Churchill Livingstone, 1995, 215-47.

Tanaka KR and Paglia DE, "Pyruvate Kinase and Other Enzymopathies of the Erythrocyte," *The Metabolic and Molecular Bases of Inherited Disease*, 7th ed, Chapter 114, Scriver CR, Beaudet AL, Sly WS, et al, eds, New York, NY: McGraw-Hill Inc, 1995, 3485-3511.

Red Blood Cell Indices

Related Information

Synonyms Erythrocyte Indices; Indices

Applies to MCH; MCHC; MCV; Mean Corpuscular Hemoglobin; Mean Corpuscular Hemoglobin Concentration; Mean Corpuscular Volume; RBC Indices; RDW; Red Cell Distribution Width

Test Includes MCV, MCH, MCHC, RDW, RBC, Hct, Hb

Abstract The RBC indices are measured or mathematically derived from Hb, Hct, and red blood cell count. The values can be used for quick assessment of anemia and have application in the provision of internal quality control.

Specimen Whole blood

Container Lavender top (EDTA) tube for venipuncture specimen; lavender top Microtainer™ tube for capillary specimen

Collection Routine venipuncture. Invert the tube 5-10 times gently to mix. There must be no clots.

Storage Instructions Specimen cannot be used if stored over 10 hours at room temperature or 18 hours at 4°C refrigerated temperature. Specimen must not be frozen.

Causes for Rejection Hemolyzed or clotted specimen

Reference Interval Because of slight physiologic and machine analytic variation, the following reference values, derived from review of multiple sources, are given as general ranges. For extensive tables of reference ranges delineating variation with age, race, altitude, and analyzer consult texts by Kjeldsberg[1] and Shinton.[2] The upper limit of MCV is important in the evaluation of cobalamin (and possible early or subclinical cobalamin) deficiency. Upper limit for MCV might better be considered >96.[3] See Cobalamin, Serum *on page 150*.

Red Blood Cell Indices

	MCV (fL)	MCH (pg)	MCHC (g/dL)	RDW (%)
Neonates	110-130	31-37	29-37	
1 y	70-86	23-31	30-36	
2-12 y	75-95	24-33	31-37	
12-18 y	78-100	25-35	31-37	
Adult male	80-100	26-34	31-37	11.7-14.2
Adult female	79-98	26-34	30-36	11.7-14.2

Use Evaluate red cell parameters; differential diagnosis of anemia, iron deficiency, hereditary spherocytosis (about 50% of such individuals have MCHC >36%), immune spherocytosis, thalassemia, chronic lead poisoning, folate deficiency, vitamin B₁₂ deficiency, vitamin B₆ deficiency, pernicious anemia, and anemia of pregnancy

Limitations Patients showing both macrocytosis and microcytosis of the red cells may have indices within the reference range because of the averaging method used in determining indices. Patients with autoagglutination will show spurious results. Although MCV is commonly elevated early in pernicious anemia, it may be normal, especially later when micropoikilocytosis develops. In a recent review of the value of MCV in detection of cobalamin (vitamin B₁₂) deficiency (uncertainty over the upper limit of normal for MCV as an acknowledged limiting factor), sensitivity of MCV was less than desirable. At best (patients with established cobalamin deficiency and anemia), sensitivity was 75%, positive predictive value for B₁₂ deficiency ranged (5 different studies) from 0% to 55%.[4]

Methodology The great majority of RBC indices are obtained by the use of microcomputerized, highly automated electronic and pneumatic multichannel analyzers based on aperture-impedance cell sizing and counting (see reference by Koepke).

Additional Information The group of three red cell indices are a productive and economically efficient approach to screening for hematologic abnormality, in particular the compensated and uncompensated anemias. The MCV (mean corpuscular volume) is the size (volume) of the average red cell. The MCH (mean corpuscular hemoglobin) is the weight of hemoglobin in the average red cell. The MCHC (mean corpuscular hemoglobin concentration) is the amount of hemoglobin present in the average red cell as compared to its size. The RBC indices are a valuable guide to the choice of more specific measurements such as serum iron, ferritin, folic acid, and/or vitamin B₁₂ levels. The MCV decreases before MCHC in evolving iron deficiency anemia while the MCHC decreases before the MCV in evolving anemia of chronic disease. In hemolytic anemias, particularly the hemoglobinopathies, the RBC indices are less helpful. Decreased MCV levels may be due to thalassemia minor although they are not specific for this condition; A₂ hemoglobin levels should be studied to follow-up low MCV levels in appropriate clinical settings. Screening for high A₂ hemoglobin levels will discriminate a population of beta-thalassemics with normal MCV levels. Hemoglobin A₂ levels are most useful using the column chromatography method. Technicon® (Bayer® Diagnostics) series H analyzers provide a measure of heterogeneity in hemoglobin concentration of individual red cells (histogram of MCHCs). Decreased cell Hb concentration (increased cell hydration) has been noted to characterize α-thalassemia while both decreased and increased cell Hb concentration (cell hydration and dehydration) characterize β-thalassemia red cells.[5] Cell dehydration as reflected by histogram of MCHCs can also be used to identify most patients with hereditary spherocytosis.[6]

Changes in RBC Indices With Disease

Condition	MCV	MCH	MCHC	RDW
Iron deficiency anemia	↓	↓	↓	↑
Chronic inflammation	↓	N±	N±	N±
Pernicious anemia	↑	N or high N	high N	↑
B₁₂/folate deficiency	↑	N or high N	high N	↑
Hereditary spherocytosis	N or ↓	↑	↑	N±
Hemolytic/aplastic anemia	N±	N±	N±	N±
Anemia secondary to acute blood loss	N±	N±	N±	N±
Polycythemia	N±	N±	N±	N±
Hemochromatosis	↑	↑	↑	N±

A number of conditions (usually characterized by the generation of numerous RBC fragments) may show "relative microcytosis" as reflected by slightly decreased to low normal MCV. This has been described with sickle cell anemia. In children, low MCV for age suggests iron deficiency, lead poisoning, thalassemia syndrome, or very rarely, a pyridoxine-responsive anemia. Examination of the peripheral smear, family history, dietary history, and stool guaiac are helpful in this setting. Megaloblastic hematopoiesis causes <10% of cases of macrocytosis (increase in MCV). Mean values of MCV, MCH, and MCHC (as well as Hb and Hct) are increased in hemochromatosis.[7] MCV may be significantly increased in diabetic ketoacidosis[8] (this is due to plasma hyperosmolarity). The high molar concentration of glucose is the main contributing factor to the increased plasma osmolarity, producing a hypertonic intracellular state of RBCs. When such cells are put into a relatively hypotonic diluent (eg, Coulter cell counting), water enters the cell, it swells and may produce erroneously high MCV. Recognition of increase in MCV may alert the clinician to presence of the hyperosmolar state.[8]

Aluminum toxicity, occurring in uremic patients on chronic hemodialysis, is associated in some cases with decreased MCV, microcytic anemia.[9]

RDW is an electronic measurement of anisocytosis (red cell size variability). RDW is typically elevated in iron deficiency anemia while usually normal in beta thalassemia minor (heterozygous thalassemia). RDW is elevated in beta thalassemia major. In establishing nomograms of hematologic parameters in pregnancy, study of the RDW found that it was significantly increased between 34 weeks of gestation and the onset of labor.[10]

Drugs, in particular DNA inhibiting anti-AIDs therapeutics and other viral antinucleoside therapeutics are the most common cause of macrocytosis (increase in MCV) in the hospitalized urban patient population.[11]

Statistical analysis of RBC indices, notably a set of linear discriminant functions, are said to effectively differentiate between α-thalassemia, β-thalassemia, and iron deficiency anemia with a high degree of accuracy.[12]

Footnotes

1. Kjeldsberg CR, Elenitoba-Johnson K, Foucar K, et al, *Practical Diagnosis of Hematologic Disorders*, 3rd ed, Kjeldsberg CR, ed, Chicago, IL: ASCP Press, 2000.

2. *CRC Desk Reference for Hematology*, 3rd ed, Shinton NK, ed, New York, NY: CRC Press, 1998.

3. Chanarin I and Metz J, "Diagnosis of Cobalamin Deficiency: The Old and the New," *Br J Haematol*, 1997, 97(4):695-700.

4. Oosterhuis WP, Niessen RW, Bossuyt PM, et al, "Diagnostic Value of the Mean Corpuscular Volume in the Detection of Vitamin B₁₂ Deficiency," *Scand J Clin Lab Invest*, 2000, 60(1):9-18.

5. Bunyaratvej A, Fucharoen S, Greenbaum A, et al, "Hydration of Red Cells in Alpha and Beta Thalassemias Differs. A Useful Approach to Distinguish Between These Red Cell Phenotypes," *Am J Clin Pathol*, 1994, 102(2):217-22.

(Continued)

Red Blood Cell Indices (*Continued*)

6. Lux SE and Palek J, "Disorders of the Red Cell Membrane," *Blood: Principles and Practice of Hematology*, Chapter 54, Handin RI, Lux SE, and Stossel TP, eds, Philadelphia, PA: JB Lippincott Co, 1995, 1758.

7. Barton JC, Bertoli LF, and Rothenberg BE, "Peripheral Blood Erythrocyte Parameters in Hemochromatosis: Evidence for Increased Erythrocyte Hemoglobin Content," *J Lab Clin Med*, 2000, 135(1):96-104.

8. van Duijnhoven HL and Treskes M, "Marked Interference of Hyperglycemia in Measurements of Mean (Red) Cell Volume by Technicon® H Analyzers," *Clin Chem*, 1996, 42(1):76-80.

9. Mladenovic J, "Aluminum Inhibits Erythropoiesis *In Vitro*," *J Clin Invest*, 1988, 81(6):1661-5.

10. Shehata HA, Ali MM, Evans-Jones JC, et al, "Red Cell Distribution Width (RDW) Changes in Pregnancy," *Int J Gynaecol Obstet*, 1998, 62(1):43-6.

11. Snower DP and Weil SC, "Changing Etiology of Macrocytosis: Zidovudine as a Frequent Causative Factor," *Am J Clin Pathol*, 1993, 99(1):57-60.

12. Eldibany MM, Totonchi KF, Joseph NJ, et al, "Usefulness of Certain Red Blood Cell Indices in Diagnosing and Differentiating Thalassemia Trait From Iron-Deficiency Anemia," *Am J Clin Pathol*, 1999, 111(5):676-82.

References

Fraser CG, Wilkinson SP, Neville RG, et al, "Biologic Variation of Common Hematologic Laboratory Quantities in the Elderly," *Am J Clin Pathol*, 1989, 92(4):465-70.

Koepke JA, "Quantitative Blood Cell Counting," *Practical Laboratory Hematology*, Chapter 3, Koepke JA, ed, New York, NY: Churchill Livingstone, 1991, 43-60.

Perkins SL, "Examination of the Blood and Bone Marrow," *Wintrobe's Clinical Hematology*, 10th ed, Chapter 2, Lee GR, Foerster J, Lukens J, et al, eds, Baltimore, MD: Lippincott Williams & Wilkins, 1999, 9-35.

Savage DG, Ogundipe A, Allen RH, et al, "Etiology and Diagnostic Evaluation of Macrocytosis," *Am J Med Sci*, 2000, 319(6):343-52.

◆ **Red Blood Cell Morphology** *see* Peripheral Blood: Red Blood Cell Morphology *on page 467*

Red Cell Count

Related Information

Cobalamin, Serum *on page 150*
Complete Blood Count *on page 419*
Erythropoietin, Serum *on page 169*
Ferritin, Serum *on page 173*
Hematocrit *on page 441*
Hemoglobin *on page 442*
Peripheral Blood: Red Blood Cell Morphology *on page 467*
Red Blood Cell Indices *on page 477*
Red Cell Mass *on page 478*
White Blood Cell Count *on page 496*

Synonyms Erythrocyte Count; RBC; Red Blood Cell Count

Specimen Whole blood

Container Lavender top (EDTA) tube for venipuncture specimen; properly filled lavender top Microtainer™ tubes for capillary specimen

Causes for Rejection Hemolyzed or clotted specimen

Reference Interval Male: $4.6-6.0 \times 10^6/mm^3$; female: $3.9-5.5 \times 10^6/mm^3$. See Complete Blood Count *on page 419* for age related normals.

Use Evaluate anemia, polycythemia

Limitations Presence of cold agglutinins may result in falsely low RBC counts. Modern electronic cell counters have a level of precision and accuracy greatly improved over manual counting techniques. With correct threshold setting, properly controlled and functioning instrumentation, reliability, and reproducibility of the RBC count is equivalent to or better than most laboratory tests. Surveys (College of American Pathologists) indicate a coefficient of variation (CV) of 1% to 2%. Some instruments commonly perform with CVs <1%. Between laboratory precision has been reported as 2.8%.

A succinct description of quality assurance methods, including internal quality control (with reference material preparation and data analysis) and external quality assessment for hematologic parameters, is available and recommended.[1]

Methodology Manual hemocytometer chamber count of diluted blood sample or electronic counting and sizing of red cells made to flow through a fine aperture or capillary, microcomputer control and analysis of data developed from changes in impedance or flow past a laser beam

Additional Information Decrease in RBC count may be the result of red cell loss by bleeding or hemolysis (intravascular or extravascular), failure of marrow production (due to a broad variety of causes), or may be secondary to dilutional factors (eg, intravenous fluids). Increase in RBC count may be the result of primary polycythemia (polycythemia vera) or secondary polycythemia (hypoxemia of lung or cardiovascular disease, increased erythropoietin production associated with renal cyst, renal cell carcinoma, cerebellar hemangioblastoma, or high O_2 affinity hemoglobinopathy) including stress polycythemia (hemoconcentration associated with exercise, exertion, fright, etc). The uncommon condition, "inapparent polycythemia vera" is characterized by normal Hb, Hct, and RBC count levels, but increased red cell mass and clinical features of polycythemia vera.[2] RBC count is normally higher in individuals residing at high altitudes.

Footnotes

1. "Quality Assurance," *Practical Hematology*, 8th ed, Chapter 4, Dacie Sir JV and Lewis SM, eds, New York, NY: Churchill Livingstone, 1995, 35-47.

2. Lamy T, Devillers A, Bernard M, et al, "Inapparent Polycythemia Vera: An Unrecognized Diagnosis," *Am J Med*, 1997, 102(1):14-20.

References

Koepke JA, "Quantitative Blood Cell Counting," *Practical Laboratory Hematology*, Chapter 3, New York, NY: Churchill Livingstone, 1991, 43-60.

Morris MW and Davey FR, "Basic Examination of Blood," *Clinical Diagnosis and Management by Laboratory Methods*, 19th ed, Chapter 24, Henry JB, ed, Philadelphia, PA: WB Saunders Co, 1996, 554-6.

◆ **Red Cell Distribution Width** *see* Red Blood Cell Indices *on page 477*

◆ **Red Cell Folate** *see* Folic Acid, RBC *on page 435*

◆ **Red Cell Fragility** *see* Osmotic Fragility *on page 462*

◆ **Red Cell Fragility** *see* Osmotic Fragility, Incubated *on page 463*

Red Cell Mass

Related Information

Blood Volume *on page 407*
Erythropoietin, Serum *on page 169*
Hematocrit *on page 441*
Hemoglobin *on page 442*
Red Cell Count *on page 478*

Synonyms ^{51}Cr-Labeled Red Cell Volume; Red Cell Volume

Applies to Gaisbock Syndrome; Monge Disease; Pickwickian Syndrome

Test Includes Red cell mass, plasma volume, and total blood volume

Abstract In the evaluation of patients with reproducibly high Hb or Hct, it must be determined if there is an absolute increase in the red cell mass. Direct measurement of RBC mass with an isotope dilution method will obtain the necessary definitive data.

Specimen Laboratory will usually manage sampling and reinjecting.

Special Instructions May require scheduling with laboratory in order to procure radioisotope. Patient's weight and height must be made available to the laboratory.

Reference Interval Male: 28.2 ± 4 mL/kg; female: 24.2 ± 2.6 mL/kg.[1] See table for reference values relating to body surface area. At higher elevations (2000-3000 meters above sea level), RBC mass is also higher in otherwise normal individuals (ie, in the $30-32 \pm 6-7$ mL/kg range).

Formulas for Calculating RBC Mass Reference Values From Body Surface Area(s)[2]

Male	Mean normal RCM (mL) = (1486 x S) - 825
	98% limits = ±25%
	Mean normal PV (mL) = 1578 x S
	99% limits = ±25%
Female	Mean normal RCM (mL) = (1.06 x age) + (822 x S)
	99% limits = ±25%
	Mean normal PV (mL) = 1395 x S
	99% limits = ±25%

$S = W^{0.425} \times h^{0.725} \times 0.007184$

S = surface area (m₂)

age = age (years)

h = height (cm)

w = weight (kg)

From International Committee for Standardization in Hematology, "Interpretation of Measured Red Cell Mass and Plasma Volume in Adults," *Br J Haematol*, 1995, 89(4):748-56.

An elevated RCM can be defined as being 25% or more over the normal value predicted for any individual. Blood volume increases gradually over the course of pregnancy.[3]

Determination of elevated RBC volume in mL/kg body weight is confounded by obesity as RBC volume per kg fat is only 1/10 that of total RBC volume of the lean body mass (LBM). Application of biologic impedance measuring devices to directly measure a person's body composition and percentage of fat has allowed normalization of total RBC volume (TRCV) for men and women to mL/kg of LBM. TRCV is 36 mL/kg; when >43 mL/kg LBM, the presence of polycythemia can be considered as established.[4]

Use Determine red cell mass; support the diagnosis of polycythemia vera; monitor therapy with antineoplastic drugs

Limitations Radiation from isotopes used in bone scans, liver scans, brain scans, and other isotope procedures may interfere with red cell mass determination. Application of "normal range" tables based on weight and height must be made cautiously. An individual patient may not be comparable to the normal (eg, severely edematous individuals). Dilutional relationship will be unrepresentative and RBC mass overestimated. Severe edema might also be associated with isotope loss but is especially problematic due to unrepresentative normal range comparisons. Test is expensive and time consuming.

Contraindications Severe active bleeding

Methodology Patient anticoagulated blood sample is obtained, red cells are labeled with ^{51}Cr, washed with buffered saline, resuspended, and then reinjected into the patient. All procedures must use sterile precautions.

Schematic for Normalizing Total RBC Volume From Body Fat Content

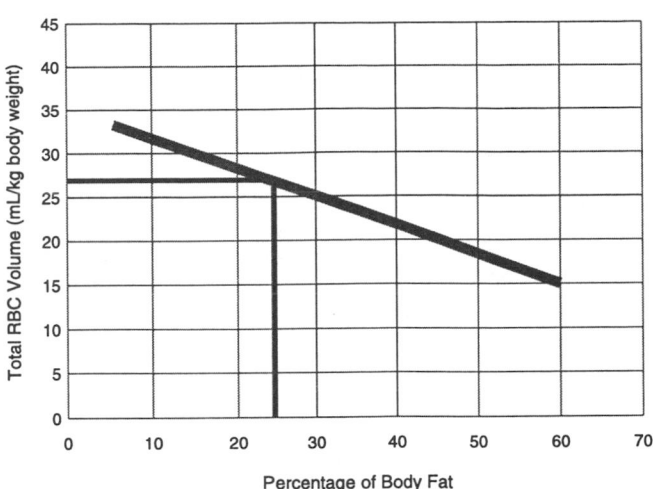

After measuring the percentage of fat, a line is drawn vertically from that number along the x-axis until it intersects the slope. At the intersect with the slope, a horizontal line is drawn to the y-axis, which gives a reading of the normalized TRCV.

Adapted from Berlin NI and Lewis SM, "Measurement of Total RBC Volume Relative to Lean Body Mass for Diagnosis of Polycythemia," *Am J Clin Pathol*, 2000, 114:922-6.

Separate blood samples are obtained prior to injection and at a timed interval (usually 10 or 15 minutes) after injection. RBC mass is calculated on the basis of dilution principle. While other isotope labels are used, ^{51}Cr is the most convenient and widely used. Technetium-99m can be used for red cell mass determination after treatment of patient's red blood cells with stannous ion ($SnCl_2$) before incubation with pertechnetate. This results in the binding of nearly all of the added technetium to patient's red cells. If splenomegaly, heart failure, or a shock state is present, sampling should be delayed for 30 minutes after injection of the isotope labeled red cells to allow for complete mixing and pooling. Repeat sampling at 60 and 90 minutes should also be considered.

Additional Information The assessment of anemia and polycythemia (assessment of whether or not one of these conditions truly exists) depends foremost upon a reliable and direct determination of red cell volume. RBC count, Hb level, and Hct provide only concentration parameters, the measured number or amount relative to the solution in which it exists. In a number of clinical situations (eg, acute blood loss) the RBC count, Hb, and Hct will not reflect the actual decrease or increase in circulating red cell mass. Components (RBC count, etc) do correlate with RBC volume. Due to technical complexity (resulting in high cost and prolonged turnaround time)

CBC is usually used, especially for follow-up or monitoring situations, even though RBC mass study would provide a more meaningful result. Nevertheless, some clinical situations (eg, polycythemia, complicated fluid and electrolyte management problems) will benefit from at least initial red cell volume determination.

Causes of decreased red cell volume include anemia, nutritional (iron, B_{12}, folate deficit, etc), hemolytic (intravascular or extravascular hemolysis); production deficit (marrow failure, drug or chemical related); acute and/or chronic blood loss; acute blood loss (decreased RBC volume may be present with normal or increased Hb/Hct/RBC count); chronic disease (inflammation/infection); radiation, starvation, or severe edema.

Causes of increased red cell volume include: a) polycythemia vera ("primary" polycythemia); b) secondary polycythemia, hypoxia may be due to **lung disease** (eg, emphysema, Pickwickian syndrome), **CV disease** with right to left shunt or due to high altitude, **hemoglobin variants** (eg, high O_2 affinity hemoglobinopathies such as Hb Chesapeake, the first described in 1966, with more than 110 reported by 1996 of which 38 are listed in *Wintrobe's Clinical Hematology* text along with their molecular and biochemical characteristics), methemoglobinemia, carboxyhemoglobinemia (increased CO due to smoking), **erythropoietin producing tumors/cysts**, rarely (eg, renal cyst, renal cell adenocarcinoma, hepatoma, large uterine myomas, cerebellar hemangioblastoma), or **hereditary overproduction of erythropoietin**;[2] and c) stress (relative, spurious, pseudo, benign) polycythemia due to decreased plasma volume, as in cases of severe dehydration, burns, and fluid and electrolyte abnormalities with Addison or Cushing diseases. Relative polycythemia is also seen in a population of "stressed" hypertensive middle aged males. The accompanying table shows relationship between increased and decreased red cell and plasma volumes.

Clinical Effect of Variable Relationship Between Red Cell Volume and Plasma Volume

Red Cell Volume	Plasma Volume	Cause	Effect
Normal	High	Pregnancy Cirrhosis Nephritis Congestive cardiac failure	Pseudoanemia
Normal	Low	Stress Peripheral circulatory failure Dehydration Edema Prolonged bedrest	Pseudopolycythemia
Low	Normal	Anemia	Accurate reflection of degree of anemia
Low	High	Anemia	Anemia less severe than indicated by blood count
Low	Low	Hemorrhage Severe anemia (when hematocrit <0.2)	Anemia more severe than indicated by blood count
High	Normal to low	Polycythemia	Accurate reflection of polycythemia or polycythemia less severe than apparent
High	High	Polycythemia (when hematocrit >0.5)	Polycythemia more severe than apparent
Normal or even high	High	Marked splenomegaly	Pseudoanemia

Adapted from Dacie JV and Lewis SM, *Practical Haematology*, 7th ed, New York, NY: Churchill Livingstone, 1991, 362.

Forms of Erythrocytosis

Relative erythrocytosis or polycythemia (pseudoerythrocytosis)
  Hemoconcentration, stress-induced
  Gaisböck syndrome (spurious or pseudopolycythemia)
Polycythemia (absolute erythrocytosis)
  Primary polycythemia vera
  Inapparent polycythemia vera
  Secondary polycythemia
    Secondary (physiologically appropriate or hypoxic erythrocytosis)
    High-altitude erythrocytosis (Monge disease)
    Pulmonary disease
      Chronic cor pulmonale
      Ayerza syndrome
    Cyanotic congenital heart disease
    Hypoventilation syndromes
      Primary alveolar hypoventilation
      Pickwickian syndrome, Ondine curse
      Positional desaturation
      Sleep apnea
    Abnormal hemoglobins
      Inherited
        High oxygen affinity
        Congenital decrease in 2,3-diphosphoglycerate
      Acquired: drugs and chemicals; carboxyhemoglobinemia
  Secondary to aberrant erythropoietin production or response
  (Physiologically inappropriate polycythemia)
    Tumor
      Renal carcinoma
      Hepatoma
      Cerebellar hemangioblastoma
      Uterine leiomyoma
      Adrenal cortical adenoma/hyperplasia
      Ovarian carcinoma
    Renal disease
      Cysts
      Hydronephrosis
      Bartter syndrome
      Transplantation
    Cobalt
    Androgen abuse
    Erythropoietin abuse
    Familial polycythemia
  Idiopathic polycythemia

A group of patients with clinical features suggestive of polycythemia (splenomegaly with thrombocytosis and/or leukocytosis or portal vein thrombosis and thrombocytosis and/or leukocytosis without splenomegaly) but with normal hemoglobin and hematocrit levels has been described. Red cell
(Continued)

Red Cell Mass (Continued)

mass was increased, but "masked", by accompanying increase in plasma volume resulting in the concept of "inapparent polycythemia."[5]

See also Blood Volume on page 407.

Footnotes

1. Elghetany MT and Davey FR, "Erythrocytic Disorders," Clinical Diagnosis and Management by Laboratory Methods, 19th ed, Chapter 26, Henry JB, ed, Philadelphia, PA: WB Saunders Co, 1996, 661.
2. Pearson TC, Guthrie DL, Simpson J, et al, "Interpretation of Measured Red Cell Mass and Plasma Volume in Adults: Expert Panel on Radionuclides of the International Council for Standardization in Haematology," Br J Haematol, 1995, 89(4):748-56.
3. Thornburg KL, Jacobson SL, and Giraud GD, "Hemodynamic Changes in Pregnancy," Semin Perinatol, 2000, 24(1):11-4.
4. Berlin NI and Lewis SM, "Measurement of Total RBC Volume Relative to Lean Body Mass for Diagnosis of Polycythemia," Am J Clin Pathol, 2000, 114(6):922-6.
5. Lamy T, Devillers A, Bernard M, et al, "Inapparent Polycythemia Vera: An Unrecognized Diagnosis," Am J Med, 1997, 102(1):14-20.

References

Balga I, Solenthaler M, and Furlan M, "Should Whole-Body Red Cell Mass Be Measured or Calculated?" Blood Cells Mol Dis, 2000, 26(1):25-31; discussion 32-6.

Berk PD, "Epilogue: Broader Lessons From the Study of Polycythemia Vera," Semin Hematol, 1997, 34(1):77-80.

Berlin NI, "Seminars in Hematology: Prologue: Polycythemia Vera," Semin Hematol, 1997, 34(1):1-5.

Dacie JV and Lewis SM, Practical Haematology, 8th ed, New York, NY: Churchill Livingstone, 1995, 391-7.

Djulbegovic B, Hadley T, and Joseph G, "A New Algorithm for the Diagnosis of Polycythemia," Am Fam Phys, 1991, 44(1):113-20.

Fairbanks VF, "Commentary: Should Whole-Body Red Cell Mass Be Measured or Calculated?" Blood Cells Mol Dis, 2000, 26(1):32-6.

Leslie WD, Dupont JO, and Peterdy AE, "Effect of Obesity on Red Cell Mass Results," J Nucl Med, 1999, 40(3):422-8.

Means RT, "Polycythemia: Erythrocytosis," Wintrobe's Clinical Hematology, 10th ed, Chapter 59, Lee RG, Foerster J, Lukens J, et al, eds, Baltimore, MD: Lippincott Williams & Wilkins, 1999, 1538-54.

Messinezy M and Pearson TC, "The Classification and Diagnostic Criteria of the Erythrocytoses," Clin Lab Haematol, 1999, 21(5):309-16.

Pollycove M and Tono M, "Blood Volume," Diagnostic Nuclear Medicine, 3rd ed, Volume 2, Chapter 42, Sandler MP, Coleman RE, Wackers FJT, et al, eds, Baltimore, MD: Lippincott Williams & Wilkins, 1996, 827-34.

"Recommended Methods for Measurement of Red Cell and Plasma Volume: International Committee for Standardization in Hematology," J Nucl Med, 1980, 21(8):793-800.

- ♦ **Red Cell Survival** see 51Cr Red Cell Survival on page 422
- ♦ **Red Cell Volume** see Blood Volume on page 407
- ♦ **Red Cell Volume** see Red Cell Mass on page 478
- ♦ **Respiratory Burst** see Nitroblue Tetrazolium Test on page 461
- ♦ **Retic Count** see Reticulocyte Count on page 481

Reticulated Platelet Count

Related Information

Flow Cytometry, Overview on page 432
Platelet Aggregation on page 348
Platelet Count on page 468
Platelet Sizing on page 471

Synonyms Immature Platelets; Large Platelets; Platelet Count, Reticulated; Reticulated Platelet Percentages; Stress Platelets

Applies to Auramine O; CD61 Per CP; Platelet Cloud; Thiazole Orange; TRAP (platelet agonist)

Abstract Results of this test (which is performed on peripheral blood) reflect bone marrow thrombopoietic activity. While requiring use of a flow cytometer, the test has been proposed as a simple and rapid means to distinguish between thrombocytopenia due to excess consumption (destruction) or as a result of inadequate production of platelets. Currently, lack of discriminate ability in patients with platelet counts <50,000/μL and lack of RNA staining specificity may limit clinical application of this test.

Specimen 2 mL EDTA or sodium citrate anticoagulated whole blood; 1 mL anticoagulated blood is sufficient for most flow cytometer based methods (only about 2 μL of blood is required for each pass through the cytometer). Blood shed from a bleeding time wound can actually be analyzed.[1]

Storage Instructions If test is not performed on the sample (kept at room temperature) the same day of collection, use of 1% formaldehyde fixed platelet-rich plasma sample is recommended (stable for up to 7 days in buffer at 4°C).[2]

Turnaround Time 1-2 hours

Reference Interval Method dependent; varies in adults from 1% to 15%

Gestational age (in %, mean ±SD):
- >36 weeks: 4.0 ±2.4
- 30-36 weeks: 4.6 ±1.7
- <30 weeks: 8.8 ±5.1[3]

Use The percentage of reticulated platelets (% RPLT) in peripheral blood, the platelet count, and absolute reticulated platelet count reflect bone marrow megakaryocyte activity (to produce platelets). These parameters have been applied to differentiate thrombocytopenia due to bone marrow failure (decreased platelet production) from increased platelet consumption (destruction). The % of RPLT has been used in the study of platelet engraftment times following peripheral blood progenitor cells compared with bone marrow transplant, in the evaluation of post-transplant thrombocytopenia, (potentially) in the timing of thrombopoietin therapy,[4] and in the evaluation of the effects of drugs and growth factors on thrombopoiesis.

Limitations Requires use of a flow cytometer and cytometer knowledgeable personnel. May require use of formalin-fixed platelets if analysis cannot be performed within 24 hours. With platelet counts <50,000 μL, normal or decreased reticulated platelet level may not reflect decreased thrombopoiesis.[5]

Methodology Platelets from platelet-rich plasma are pelleted, suspended in a buffer, and fixed in 1% formaldehyde. Platelets, resuspended in buffer, are stained with the RNA fluorochrome, thiazole orange (TO), and enumerated by a fluorescence-assisted cell analyzer (flow cytometer). Controls, including simultaneous identification of particles as platelets by use of platelet-specific antibodies and study after treatment with RNase to ensure specificity of the dye for RNA must also be employed.[5,6] A method using the fluorescent dye, auramine O, and a reticulocyte counter has also been described.[7]

The "platelet cloud" includes platelets, red blood cells, and cellular fragments that can have overlapping light scatter profiles. A dual-staining (two color) method has been described that circumvents problems occurring in samples that have a complex "platelet cloud". CD61 Per CP (Becton Dickinson, Oxford, UK) which binds to platelet surface glycoprotein IIIa is used to verify isolation of the platelet cloud (based on the characteristic size) (log forward scatter) and granularity (log side scatter) of platelets. Microparticles and platelets bound to other cells of the blood are not included in this representation of the cloud. Reticulated platelets within the GpIIIa-positive population are identified using a second fluorescence tag (retic count solution) that is seen in a different channel.[8]

Additional Information Reticulated platelets are analogous to reticulated red blood cells (reticulocytes). As such, they are young, ribonucleic acid (RNA) rich and larger than normal adult platelets. The RNA fluorochrome thiazole orange (TO) used to tag these young reticulated platelets renders them highly fluorescent, detected and counted by a flow cytometer, the original method utilizing laser emission at 488 nm (for excitation) and a 530/30 nm band pass filter for fluorescence detection.[9] TO is the same dye used for erythrocyte reticulocyte determination. TO permeates live cell membranes without pretreatment, binds to RNA and DNA, and absorbs/emits at wavelengths similar to fluorescein (509/533).[5] The results of flow cytometric determination of reticulated platelets have been applied to differentiate between thrombocytopenia due to impaired platelet production and that caused by increased platelet destruction (consumption).[2,3,5,6,7,9,10]

Clinical utility of the reticulated platelet level is limited by the observation that at platelet counts <50,000 μL, normal or decreased absolute reticulated platelet levels may not be indicative of decreased thrombopoiesis.[5] As the platelet count falls ≤50,000, platelet survival may be 3 days or less, reticulated platelets account for most of the circulating platelet mass. Reticulated platelets would then be the major targets of destruction, and with marrow thrombopoiesis at maximum levels, a decrease in the absolute level of reticulated platelets would result (at platelet count levels <20,000 μL).[5] Under these circumstances, a decrease in the absolute level of reticulated platelets might not be indicative of decreased thrombopoiesis.

Reticulated platelet count methodology is also complicated by recent studies showing that TO labeling is not entirely mRNA specific.[11,12] TO-positive platelets are lower than normal in dense granule-deficient platelets (Hermansky-Pudlak syndrome and storage pool disease) and are at about the same level as TRAP degranulated platelets (TRAP is a nonenzymatic platelet agonist thrombin receptor activating peptide).[11] Nonspecific labeling by TO is probably due to dense granule nucleotides (such as ADP and ATP) or mitochondrial DNA. The dense granular pool of nucleotides may cause as much as 50% of nonspecific labeling under some conditions.[11] A standardized assay will require control of TO labeling by degranulation or monitoring of labeling by use of RNase.[12] Without such controls, assay results could be clinically misleading. There is also an implication that the higher level of TO fluorescence of young platelets is due to their larger volume and granule content.[13] The reticulated platelet count may not provide significant clinical advantage over the platelet parameter MPV (mean platelet volume), which is provided readily and at low cost by many automated cell counters.[13]

Reticulated platelets are increased in hyperthyroidism, likely reflecting increase in thrombopoiesis[14] (see Platelet Sizing on page 471).

Footnotes

1. Michelson AD, MacGregor H, Barnard MR, et al, "Reversible Inhibition of Human Platelet Activation by Hypothermia In Vivo and In Vitro," Thromb Haemost, 1994, 71(5):633-40.
2. Rinder HM, Munz UJ, Ault KA, et al, "Reticulated Platelets in the Evaluation of Thrombopoietic Disorders," Arch Pathol Lab Med, 1993, 117(6):606-10.
3. Peterec SM, Brennan SA, Rinder HM, et al, "Reticulated Platelet Values in Normal and Thrombocytopenic Neonates," J Pediatr, 1996, 129(2):269-74.
4. Richards EM, Jestice HK, Mahendra P, et al, "Measurement of Reticulated Platelets Following Peripheral Blood Progenitor Cell and Bone Marrow Transplantation: Implications for Marrow Reconstitution and the Use of Thrombopoietin," Bone Marrow Transplant, 1996, 17(6):1029-33.

5. Ault KA, Rinder HM, Mitchell J, et al, "The Significance of Platelets With Increased RNA Content (Reticulated Platelets): A Measure of the Rate of Thrombopoiesis," *Am J Clin Pathol*, 1992, 98(6):637-46.

6. Richards EM and Baglin TP, "Quantitation of Reticulated Platelets: Methodology and Clinical Application," *Br J Haematol*, 1995, 91(2):445-51.

7. Watanabe K, Takeuchi K, Kawai Y, et al, "Automated Measurement of Reticulated Platelets in Estimating Thrombopoiesis," *Eur J Haematol*, 1995, 54(3):163-71.

8. Robinson MS, Mackie IJ, Machin SJ, et al, "Two Colour Analysis of Reticulated Platelets," *Clin Lab Haematol*, 2000, 22(4):211-3.

9. Kienast J and Schmitz G, "Flow Cytometric Analysis of Thiazole Orange Uptake by Platelets: A Diagnostic Aid in the Evaluation of Thrombocytopenic Disorders," *Blood*, 1990, 75(1):116-21.

10. Saxon BR, Blanchette VS, Butchart S, et al, "Reticulated Platelet Counts in the Diagnosis of Acute Immune Thrombocytopenic Purpura," *J Pediatr Hematol Oncol*, 1998, 20(1):44-8.

11. Robinson MS, Mackie IJ, Khair K, et al, "Flow Cytometric Analysis of Reticulated Platelets: Evidence for a Large Proportion of Nonspecific Labeling of Dense Granules by Fluorescent Dyes," *Br J Haematol*, 1998, 100(2):351-7.

12. Harrison P, "Variables Affecting Flow Cytometric Analysis of Reticulated Platelets," *Clin Lab Haematol*, 1997, 19(4):312.

13. Balduini CL, Noris P, Spedini P, et al, "Relationship Between Size and Thiazole Orange Fluorescence of Platelets in Patients Undergoing High-Dose Chemotherapy," *Br J Haematol*, 1999, 106(1):202-7.

14. Stiegler G, Stohlawetz P, Brugger S, et al, "Elevated Numbers of Reticulated Platelets in Hyperthyroidism: Direct Evidence for an Increase of Thrombopoiesis," *Br J Haematol*, 1998, 101(4):656-8.

References

Joutsi-Korhonen L, Sainio S, Riikonen S, et al, "Detection of Reticulated Platelets: Estimating the Degree of Fluorescence of Platelets Stained With Thiazole Orange," *Eur J Haematol*, 2000, 65(1):66-71.

Koh KR, Yamane T, Ohta K, et al, "Pathophysiological Significance of Simultaneous Measurement of Reticulated Platelets, Large Platelets, and Serum Thrombopoietin in Nonneoplastic Thrombocytopenic Disorders," *Eur J Haematol*, 1999, 63(5):295-301.

Koike Y, Yoneyama A, Shirai J, et al, "Evaluation of Thrombopoiesis in Thrombocytopenic Disorders by Simultaneous Measurement of Reticulated Platelets of Whole Blood and Serum Thrombopoietin Concentrations," *Thromb Haemostat*, 1998, 79(6):1106-10.

Michelson AD, "Flow Cytometry: A Clinical Test of Platelet Function," *Blood*, 1996, 87(12):4925-36.

Ryan DH, "Automated Analysis of Blood Cells," *Hematology: Basic Principles and Practice*, 3rd ed, Chapter 156, Hoffman R, Benz EJ Jr, Shattil SJ, et al, eds, Philadelphia, PA: Churchill Livingstone, 2000, 2471.

Tassies D, Reverter JC, and Cases A, "Reticulated Platelets in Uremic Patients: Effect of Hemodialysis and Continuous Ambulatory Peritoneal Dialysis," *Am J Haematol*, 1995, 50(3):161-6.

♦ **Reticulated Platelet Percentages** *see* Reticulated Platelet Count *on page 480*

Reticulocyte Count

Related Information

Synonyms Retic Count

Applies to Highly Fluorescent Reticulocytes; Reticulocyte Maturity Index

Aftercare Reticulocytes are young red blood cells from which the nucleus has been extruded but which still contain some remnants of ribosomal ribonucleic acid. Ribosomes will react with some basic dyes - vital stains (azure B, brilliant cresyl blue, methylene blue) with the formation of a granular and/or filamentous blue precipitate. The number of reticulocytes present in the peripheral blood relates to erythropoietic activity occurring normally largely in the bone marrow. Recently available automated analyzers determine reticulocyte maturity by measuring fluorescence intensity. Highly fluorescent reticulocytes (HFR) percentage allow derivation of the reticulocyte maturity index (RMI), an early predictor of bone marrow regenerative activity, of use in following the results of bone marrow transplantation.[1]

Specimen Whole blood

Container Lavender top (EDTA) tube or green top (heparin) tube for venipuncture specimen; heparinized capillary tube for capillary specimen

Storage Instructions Store EDTA anticoagulated blood at room temperature for up to 48 hours or up to 72 hours at 4°C. Immature reticulocyte fraction (IRF) parameters using the ABX-Pentra 120 Retic are reported as stable for only 8 hours at 4°C and 6 hours at room temperature.[2]

Causes for Rejection Clotted or hemolyzed specimen

Reference Interval Adults: 0.5% to 1.5%; newborns: ≤7%, expressed as a percentage of 1000 RBCs. Normal values at birth (by flow cytometry): 1.6% to 8.3%, mean of 5.3,[3] falling to normal adult level by the end of the second week. The elderly (older than 70 years of age) have a slightly higher percent of reticulocytes than young individuals but still fall within the normal range.[4]

Use Evaluate erythropoietic activity. Increased in acute and chronic hemorrhage, hemolytic anemias. Evaluate erythropoietic response to therapy of various anemias. **The test is underutilized, especially when one considers it is at a pivotal decision-making juncture.** The reticulocyte production index will decide if one is working with a hyperproliferative or nonproliferative anemia, and thus, which tests should be subsequently ordered.

The RMI has application as a criterion for the success of marrow engraftment following bone marrow transplantation. The HFR fraction appears to be the earliest and most sensitive index of engraftment as determined in some 80% of marrow (stem cell, allogenic, and autologous) transplant patients.[5] HFR might also be used as a marker of early response to immunosuppression in the therapy of severe aplastic anemia.[6] Maturity grading indexes vary between methods (counters), each laboratory should determine its own IRF predictive value of hematologic marrow recovery.[1,5]

Limitations In recently transfused patients, reticulocytes may decrease on a dilutional basis due to transfusion. Automated flow cytometry methods using thiazole orange may give spuriously high counts in patients with chronic lymphocytic leukemia, Howell-Jolly bodies, intracellular parasites (including malarial parasites as a cause of pseudoreticulocytosis[7]) large platelets, some drug therapies, erythropoietic protoporphyria, and in patients who have cold agglutinins (see NCCLS Document H44-P). Hb H may cause high or low interference (time dependent) in automated analyzers using new methylene blue. Increase in incubation time from 60-180 minutes results, in some cases of Hb H disease, in falsely elevated reticulocyte counts. This problem is most likely to present with patients of Southeast Asian origin.[8]

Contraindications Patients receiving a large number of blood transfusions

Methodology Manual methods utilize vital stains, new methylene blue is commonly used; brilliant cresyl blue may be used. The decision as to what constitutes a true reticulocyte on examination of a stained slide is experience dependent. College of American Pathologists proficiency surveys show that the manual method lacks precision with coefficient of variation averaging 30% - data from manually performed reticulocyte counts is "highly unreliable."[3] Flow cytometric and other methods using new methylene blue (Coulter STK-S), thioflavin T, thiazole orange, auramine O, acridine orange, ethidium bromide, pyronine Y, or Oxazine 750 (Technicon® H3 - Bayer® Corporation) have been developed that have the advantage of reproducibility.[9] The measured fluorescence is proportional to the amount of RNA in the cell allowing derivation of the reticulocyte maturation index.[10] The assay is a standard part of the repertoire of some multiparameter hematology instruments. Flow cytometry reticulocyte study using thiazole orange allows rapid analysis of 20,000-50,000 red cells per sample with resultant markedly improved reproducibility/precision as compared to manual methods. The Technicon® H3 combines routine CBC with 5-part differential analysis and reticulocyte (r) parameters including r count, and r cellular indices (r mean cell volume, r mean cell hemoglobin concentration, r cell hemoglobin content, and their distribution widths).

Additional Information Demonstration of an increase in the number of circulating reticulocytes provides reliable and inexpensive evidence of increased red cell production. Care should be exercised during interpretation of results that an apparent increase in reticulocytes is not the result of decrease in the number of nonreticulated RBCs (ie, anemia with fewer mature red cells). A variety of corrections have been proposed and are in use. Absolute reticulocyte count = reticulocytes (%) x RBC count. This gives the number of reticulocytes per mm^3 of blood. Reticulocyte index (RI) = reticulocytes (%) x patient Hct/normal Hct or patient RBC/normal RBC or patient Hb/normal Hb. This corrects the reticulocyte count for anemia. Reticulocyte production index (RPI) = RI x (1/maturation time), or RPI = patient's absolute reticulocyte count/normal absolute reticulocyte count x (1/maturation time). Maturation time is usually taken as 2. RPI corrects for the premature release of reticulocytes from the marrow as might occur in cases of brisk hemolysis or significant bleeding. RPI gives a reticulocyte percent value that reliably estimates RBC production.

Current generation automated methods derive a reticulocyte maturity index (RMI) from study of reticulocyte RNA levels. Absolute reticulocyte count with RMI can be applied to classification and evaluation of anemia. Failure of marrow production results in anemia with absence of the expected increase in RPI. Reticulocyte count should be performed prior to transfusion. Image recognition and flow cytometry methods of reticulocyte determination provide greater precision and accuracy compared to the manual method of counting.[11,12]

An evaluation/comparison of three commercially available flow cytometers utilizing thiazole orange for reticulocyte enumeration found comparable performance with acceptable linearity, carryover (zero or near zero) and precision.[13] A multi-institutional study comparing different stains and instruments has also been reported.[14] In a comparison study the Miles (Technicon®) H3 analyzer reticulocyte count results were found acceptable with good precision and linearity.[15] The H3 also determines reticulocyte cellular indices (see Reticulocyte Hemoglobin Content *on page 482*).

Rapid development and availability of multiparameter hematology analyzers with reticulocyte and IRF measurement capability have generated comparison and use studies involving the Cell-Dyn 3500 (Abbott);[1] ABX-Pentra 120 Retic, Sysmex R-2000 and R-3000[5] (TOA Medical Electronics)

(Continued)

Reticulocyte Count (Continued)

reticulocyte counter;[2] GEN-S (Beckman-Coulter); Cell-Dyn 3500 (Abbott); and Cell-Dyn 4000 (Abbott).[16,17,18] A rare case of myelodysplastic syndrome may have anemia with reticulocytosis, thus presenting some features of hemolytic disease.[19]

A method (utilizing the reticulocyte count) for determining if an erythrocytosis is present has been proposed.[20] Patients suspect of polycythemia (with increased hemoglobin level) are studied for quantitative reticulocyte level. A disproportionately high reticulocyte count infers increased red cell production; low plasma volume is unlikely as a cause of the erythrocytosis. If the serum erythropoietin (EPO) level is elevated, then hypoxia or other stimulus is likely. If EPO levels are not increased, a possible defect in the normal mechanism of erythropoietic control may be defined by EPO receptor study (see Erythropoietin Receptor *on page 169*). By these maneuvers, presence of erythrocytosis can be established without the need to measure red cell mass.[20]

Footnotes

1. Grotto HZ, Vigoritto AC, Noronha JF, et al, "Immature Reticulocyte Fraction as a Criterion for Marrow Engraftment. Evaluation of a Semiautomated Reticulocyte Counting Method," *Clin Lab Haematol*, 1999, 21(4):285-7.
2. Lacombe F, Lacoste L, Vial JP, et al, "Automated Reticulocyte Counting and Immature Reticulocyte Fraction Measurement. Comparison of ABX PENTRA 120 Retic, Sysmex R-2000, Flow Cytometry, and Manual Counts," *Am J Clin Pathol*, 1999, 112(5):677-86.
3. Geaghan SM, "Hematologic Values and Appearances in the Healthy Fetus, Neonate, and Child," Diagnostic Pediatric Hematology, *Clin Lab Med*, 1999, 19(1):16-20.
4. Kosower NS, "Altered Properties of Erythrocytes in the Aged," *Am J Hematol*, 1993, 42(3):241-7.
5. d'Onofrio G, Tichelli A, Foures C, et al, "Indicators of Haematopoietic Recovery After Bone Marrow Transplantation: The Role of Reticulocyte Measurements," *Clin Lab Haematol*, 1996, 18(Suppl 1):45-53.
6. Sica S, Sora F, Laurenti L, et al, "Highly Fluorescent Reticulocyte Count Predicts Haematopoietic Recovery After Immunosuppression for Severe Aplastic Anaemia," *Clin Lab Haematol*, 1999, 21(6):387-9.
7. Hoffmann JJ and Pennings JM, "Pseudoreticulocytosis as a Result of Malaria Parasites," *Clin Lab Haematol*, 1999, 21(4):257-60.
8. Lai SK, Yow CMN, and Benzie IFF, "Interference of Hb H Disease in Automated Reticulocyte Counting," *Clin Lab Haematol*, 1999, 21(4):261-4.
9. Metzger DK and Charache S, "Flow Cytometric Reticulocyte Counting With Thioflavin T in a Clinical Hematology Laboratory," *Arch Pathol Lab Med*, 1987, 111(6):540-4.
10. Rowan RM and Cavill I, eds, "The Clinical Usefulness of Measurement of the Reticulocyte Count and Its Maturation Parameters," *Clin Lab Haematol*, 1996, (Suppl 1):1-59.
11. Pappas AA, Owens RB, and Flick JT, "Reticulocyte Counting by Flow Cytometry. A Comparison With Manual Methods," *Ann Clin Lab Sci*, 1992, 22(2):125-32.
12. Serke S and Huhn D, "Improved Specificity of Determination of Immature Erythrocytes (Reticulocytes) by Multiparameter Flow-Cytometry and Thiazole Orange Using Combined Staining With Monoclonal Antibody (Antiglycophorin-A)," *Clin Lab Haematol*, 1993, 15(1):33-44.
13. Van Petegem M, Cartuyvels R, DeSchouwer P, et al, "Comparative Evaluation of Three Flow Cytometers for Reticulocyte Enumeration," *Clin Lab Haematol*, 1993, 15(2):103-11.
14. Davis BH, Bigelow NC, Koepke JA, et al, "Flow Cytometric Reticulocyte Analysis. Multi-institutional Interlaboratory Correlation Study," *Am J Clin Pathol*, 1994, 102(4):468-77.
15. Brugnara C, Hipp MJ, Irving PJ, et al, "Automated Reticulocyte Counting and Measurement of Reticulocyte Cellular Indices. Evaluation of the Miles H*3 Blood Analyzer," *Am J Clin Pathol*, 1994, 102(5):623-32.
16. Yu PH, So CC, Wong KF, et al, "Automated Reticulocyte Counting - An Evaluation of GEN-S, Cell-Dyn 3500 and Cell-Dyn 4000," *Clin Lab Haematol*, 1999, 21(2):145-7.
17. Grimaldi E and Scopacasa F, "Evaluation of the Abbott Cell-Dyn 4000 Hematology Analyzer," *Am J Clin Pathol*, 2000, 113(4):497-505.
18. Kendall R, "Application of Automated Fluorescence Flow Cytometry to Routine Haematological Analysis," *Clin Lab Haematol*, 1997, 19:289-320.
19. Sher GD, Pinkerton PH, Ali MA, et al, "Myelodysplastic Syndrome With Prolonged Reticulocyte Survival Mimicking Hemolytic Disease," *Am J Clin Pathol*, 1994, 101(2):149-53.
20. Cavill I, "Classification and Diagnostic Criteria of the Erythrocytoses," *Clin Lab Haematol*, 2000, 22(2):129-30.

References

Brecher G, "New Methylene Blue as a Reticulocyte Stain," *Am J Pathol*, 1949, 19:895.
Brown BA, *Hematology: Principles and Procedures*, 6th ed, Philadelphia, PA: Lea & Febiger, 1993, 111-6, 279-80, 386-90.
Buttarello M, Bulian P, Farina G, et al, "Flow Cytometric Reticulocyte Counting: Parallel Evaluation of Five Fully Automated Analyzers: An NCCLS-ICSH Approach," *Am J Clin Pathol*, 2001, 115(1):100-11.
Buttarello M, Bulian P, Venudo A, et al, "Laboratory Evaluation of the Miles H*3 Automated Reticulocyte Counter," *Arch Pathol Lab Med*, 1995, 119(12):1141-8.
Davis BH and Bigelow NC, "Automated Reticulocyte Analysis: Clinical Practice and Associated New Parameters," *Hematol Oncol Clin North Am*, 1994, 8(4):617-30.
Davis BH and Bigelow NC, "Flow Cytometric Reticulocyte Analysis and the Reticulocyte Maturity Index," *Ann N Y Acad Sci*, 1993, 677:281-92.
d'Onofrio G, Chirillo R, Zini G, et al, "Simultaneous Measurement of Reticulocyte and Red Blood Cell Indices in Healthy Subjects and Patients With Microcytic and Macrocytic Anemia," *Blood*, 1995, 85(3):818-23.
Houwen B, "Reticulocyte Maturation," *Blood Cells*, 1992, 18(2):167-86.
Koepke J, Broden P, Corash L, et al, "Reticulocyte Counting by Flow Cytometry; Proposed Guidelines," *NCCLS Document H44-P*, 1993, 13.

Shinton NK, ed, "CRC Desk Reference for Hematology," Boca Raton, FL: CRC Press, 1998, 599.

Reticulocyte Hemoglobin Content

Related Information

Flow Cytometry, Overview *on page 432*
Hematocrit *on page 441*
Hemoglobin *on page 442*
Iron and Total Iron Binding Capacity/Transferrin, Serum *on page 203*
Iron Stain, Bone Marrow *on page 452*
Red Blood Cell Indices *on page 477*
Reticulocyte Count *on page 481*
Transferrin Receptor, Soluble, Serum or Plasma *on page 493*

Applies to MCHCr; MCVr

Abstract Reticulocyte hemoglobin content (CHr), one of a number of reticulocyte parameters available from automated flow cytometry based hematology analysis, may have application in the early detection and evaluation of iron deficient erythropoiesis and in monitoring the effectiveness of iron replacement therapy.[1,2,3]

Specimen Whole blood

Container Lavender top (EDTA) or green top (heparin) tube

Storage Instructions Refrigerate specimen immediately after collection.

Causes for Rejection Clotted or hemolyzed specimen

Reference Interval CHr of 26 pg or more. CHr of under 26 pg is associated with other demonstrable features of iron deficiency.[1]

Use Early detection and monitoring of treatment of iron deficiency. Detection of functional iron deficiency in patients treated with recombinant human erythropoietin (rHuEPO).

Limitations The necessary analyzer may not be in immediate close proximity to the patient candidate.

Methodology Flow cytometric technique (eg, Bayer H•3 hematology analyzer) utilizing three parameters:

- low-angle light scatter at 2°C to 3°C (correlates to cell volume)
- high-angle scatter at 5°C to 15°C (correlates to hemoglobin concentration)
- absorbance (correlates to intensity of staining and reflects RNA content)

The EDTA-anticoagulated whole blood specimen is prepared manually by dilution in a reagent that contains a surfactant (spheres the red cells) and a nucleic acid dye (oxazine 750) that stains the reticulocyte on the basis of its RNA content. Fluorescence measurement is not required.

Reticulocytes are divided into three fractions according to the level of maturity. Reticulocyte indices are determined, the mean cell volume (MCVr), mean cell hemoglobin concentration (MCHCr) and the reticulocyte hemoglobin content (CHr). The latter is the most stable. If there is a delay in testing, change in reticulocyte water content may affect the MCVr and MCHCr but not hemoglobin content. The CHr, as well as CH (mean hemoglobin content of red blood cells), is calculated from the product of volume times hemoglobin concentration of single cells.[2,4,5]

Additional Information Reticulocyte hemoglobin content (CHr), if decreased, can provide an early indication of iron deficiency. CHr can identify iron deficient erythropoiesis in some apparently iron sufficient individuals.[6] CHr has been studied in nondialysis patients treated with rHuEPO and found to be a sensitive and specific indicator of functional iron deficiency.[7] With rHuEPO stimulation of erythropoiesis there is high erythroid iron use with shift in the balance between storage and erythroid iron reservoirs. With the intense erythropoietic stimulation the amount of iron immediately available for erythropoiesis may be insufficient, even though whole body iron stores are not depleted. This is a result of the massive transfer of storage iron to erythroid precursors, with such brisk mobilization of iron that storage sites cannot keep up with the demand.[8] Thus, the concept evolves of "functional iron deficiency" occurring despite normal appearing levels of serum ferritin and transferrin saturation. There may be associated poor response to treatment of renal anemia (with rHuEPO) which can be corrected by intravenous administration of iron. CHr at baseline (under 26 pg) predicts iron deficiency defined as a reticulocyte response (rise in corrected reticulocyte index of over 1 within 2 weeks), to a single-dose infusion of iron dextran with more accuracy than other measures of iron response (eg, serum ferritin, transferrin saturation, and percent hypochromic red cells), as determined on study of a small group of rHuEPO-treated hemodialysis patients.[2] Determination that "functional" iron deficiency is present in rHuEPO treated dialysis patients may allow use of a lower erythropoietin dose.

The CHr may prove to have value as a screening test for early iron deficiency (before the onset of anemia), particularly if studies show that adverse effects of iron deficiency (eg, those on the brain such as irreversible mental/motor impairment) begin before anemia develops. As to the prevention of iron deficiency in infants and children, the question arises as to allocation of resources, public health initiatives (better nutritional advice and support vs improvement in laboratory technology).[9]

Footnotes

1. Brugnara C, Zurakowski D, DiCanzio J, et al, "Reticulocyte Hemoglobin Content to Diagnose Iron Deficiency in Children," *JAMA*, 1999, 281(23):2225-30.
2. Fishbane S, Galgano C, Langley RC, et al, "Reticulocyte Hemoglobin Content in the Evaluation of Iron Status of Hemodialysis Patients," *Kidney Int*, 1997, 52(1):217-22.

3. Brugnara C, Laufer MR, Friedman AJ, et al, "Reticulocyte Hemoglobin Content (CHr): Early Indicator of Iron Deficiency and Response to Therapy," *Blood*, 1994, 83(10):3100-1.
4. Buttarello M, Bulian P, Venudo A, et al, "Laboratory Evaluation of the Miles H.3 Automated Reticulocyte Counter. A Comparative Study With Manual Reference Method and Sysmex R-1000," *Arch Pathol Lab Med*, 1995, 119(12):1141-8.
5. d'Onofrio G, Chirillo R, Zini G, et al, "Simultaneous Measurement of Reticulocyte and Red Blood Cell Indices in Healthy Subjects and Patients With Microcytic and Macrocytic Anemia," *Blood*, 1995, 85(3):818-23.
6. Brugnara C, Colella GM, Cremins J, et al, "Production of Iron-Deficient Reticulocytes in Normal Subjects Taking Subcutaneous Recombinant Human Erythropoietin," *Blood*, 1992, 80(10 Suppl 1):280a.
7. Brugnara C, Colella GM, Cremins J, et al, "Effects of Subcutaneous Recombinant Human Erythropoietin in Normal Subjects: Development of Decreased Reticulocyte Hemoglobin Content and Iron-Deficient Erythropoiesis," *J Lab Clin Med*, 1994, 123(5):660-7.
8. Eschbach JW, Egrie JC, Downing MR, et al, "Correction of the Anemia of End-Stage Renal Disease With Recombinant Human Erythropoietin. Results of a Combined Phase I and II Clinical Trial," *N Engl J Med*, 1987, 316(2):73-8.
9. Cohen AR, "Choosing the Best Strategy to Prevent Childhood Iron Deficiency," *JAMA*, 1999, 281(23):2247-8.

References
Brugnara C, "Reticulocyte Cellular Indices: A New Approach in the Diagnosis for Anemias and Monitoring of Erythropoietic Function," *Crit Rev Clin Lab Sci*, 2000, 37(2):93-130.
Goodnough LT, Skikne B, and Brugnara C, "Erythropoietin, Iron, and Erythropoiesis," *Blood*, 2000, 96(3):822-33.
Mittman N, Sreedhara R, Mushnick R, et al, "Reticulocyte Hemoglobin Content Predicts Functional Iron Deficiency in Hemodialysis Patients Receiving rHuEPO," *Am J Kidney Dis*, 1997, 30(6):912-22.

Schilling Test

Related Information

Synonyms Radioactive Vitamin B$_{12}$ Absorption Test With or Without Intrinsic Factor; Vitamin B$_{12}$ Absorption Test

Applies to Intrinsic Factor; R Proteins

Test Includes Measure of B$_{12}$ absorption (based on urinary excretion of a radiolabeled dose), before and after administration of intrinsic factor (two stage procedure). Need for the Schilling test has been called into question on theoretic grounds as well as on practical logistic and operational bases. The most common cause of an abnormal Schilling test is an incomplete urine collection. Economic necessity dictates that most Schilling tests will be performed on an outpatient basis with attendant operational shortcomings (eg, incomplete urine collection, fecal contamination of urine). Acceptance of a urine immunoassay test for intrinsic factor may also impact use of the Schilling test.[1]

Abstract *In vivo* test for pernicious anemia, cobalamin (vitamin B$_{12}$) malabsorption, and integrity of distal small intestine. To understand the complexities of the Schilling test, the complexities of B$_{12}$ absorption require review. After release from food proteins, cobalamin binds to glycoproteins (R-binders) in saliva and gastric juice. In the upper small intestine, pancreatic proteases release B$_{12}$ from the R-proteins. B$_{12}$ then binds to intrinsic factor (IF) secreted by gastric parietal cells. The IF-B$_{12}$ complex resists proteolysis, and in the distal ileum it binds to receptors unique to cells of the ileal mucosal membrane microvilli. A few hours after IF-B$_{12}$ binds to ileal absorptive cells, B$_{12}$ appears in the circulation complexed to transcobalamin II.

Patient Preparation Patient must be fasting from midnight the day of the test. Patient should have received no B vitamins for a period of 3 days before the test.

Aftercare The radiolabeled crystalline cobalamin (^{57}Co) used in the Schilling test generates such a low level of radiation as to be noninjurious to patient, attendants, or the environment.

Container Large gallon (plastic preferred) container that has been counted and shown to be free of contaminating radiation

Sampling Time 24 hours (urine)

Collection 24-hour urine

Storage Instructions Keep specimen on ice or refrigerate.

Causes for Rejection Patient having radioisotope scan prior to test,[2] patient receiving cobalamin (Cbl) prior to the test, patient not fasting, incomplete collection of urine, failure to administer the parenteral B$_{12}$, contamination of urine with stool (which will contain some unabsorbed radiolabeled B$_{12}$). The waiting time between prior radiopharmaceutical administration and the Schilling examination varies considerably, dependent on the isotope previously administered. Only a few days may be involved or over 100 days may be required. Consult recent study and guidelines developed by Zuckier et al.[2]

Reference Interval Normal values vary with the laboratory and procedure used. Generally, >10% excretion in the urine of radioactive B$_{12}$ indicates intact intrinsic factor (IF) function. When only a few percent of B$_{12}$ absorption occurs without IF, with improvement into normal range with exogenous IF, the presence of pernicious anemia is essentially established. Poor absorption (<6% or 7%) with, as well as without, IF suggests intestinal malabsorption.

Use Assess cobalamin absorption in the diagnosis of malabsorption due to the lack of intrinsic factor (eg, Addisonian pernicious anemia), a diagnostic adjunct in other defects of small intestinal absorption; evaluate extent of Crohn disease in terminal ileum. Part I of the Schilling test is ^{57}Co by itself. If abnormal, 5 days later it is repeated with intrinsic factor administered orally at the same time (Part II). If this part of the test is still abnormal, it suggests that the cause is not gastric in origin (PA) but lower in the GI tract.

Limitations If other isotope tests are to be performed, Schilling test should be completed first. The presence of renal dysfunction, pancreatic insufficiency, bacterial overgrowth of intestinal content, antibodies against IF in gastric secretions, myxedema, liver disease, or any other condition resulting in decreased absorption of B$_{12}$ from the GI tract, its concentration in the liver, or its excretion in the urine may result in abnormal values. Incomplete urine collection or fecal contamination may invalidate results.

In elderly individuals with hypochlorhydria, the proteolytic activity of pepsin may be negated by absence of requisite low pH with failure of release of Cbl from food protein and a resultant false-negative stage I Schilling test (normal Stage I results in a Cbl-deficient individual). On the other hand, a modified "food-Cbl" absorption test found that in some healthy elderly individuals there was reduced absorption but normal serum levels.[3] Renal insufficiency, with delay in excretion of labeled Cbl and potential false-positive result may be circumvented by measuring radiolabeled Cbl in plasma samples.

Methodology Patient swallows radiolabeled B$_{12}$ dose and receives a B$_{12}$ intramuscular injection. The patient's urine is collected for 24 hours. The total activity from the B$_{12}$ label is measured and calculated. The percent excretion of vitamin B$_{12}$ is then determined. This is Part I of the Schilling test. If abnormal (<7% to 10% excretion indicating impaired cobalamin absorption), Part II of the test is performed. This is a repeat of Part I, but with oral administration of intrinsic factor.

Additional Information Cobalamin tagged with ^{57}Co without (and on a repeat test, as indicated, with) intrinsic factor is given orally. A large parenteral dose of unlabeled B$_{12}$ is given 1 hour later to load the cyanocobalamin serum binding sites. All orally absorbed (radioactively-tagged) B$_{12}$ will be excreted in the urine. The 24-hour urine is analyzed, radioactive ^{57}Co is counted. This radiopharmaceutical should not be administered to patients who are pregnant or during lactation unless the information to be gained outweighs the potential hazards. The test should not be started within 2-3 days of a therapeutic dose (1000 µg) of B$_{12}$ or previous Schilling test. Bone marrow examinations and B$_{12}$ and folate levels must be obtained before the Schilling test is performed.

Some patients with pernicious anemia may not absorb B$_{12}$ adequately, even when given with IF, reversible after B$_{12}$ therapy, thus complicating the diagnosis of pernicious anemia using the Schilling test. The importance of establishing the diagnosis and commencing life-long B$_{12}$ maintenance therapy (so as to reverse the severe effects of the megaloblastic anemia and nervous system degenerative process - combined systems disease) dictates that a combination of clinical and laboratory findings be considered. The laboratory picture should include appropriate abnormalities of RBC indices (in particular high MCV), presence of anemia, peripheral blood smear findings of oval macrocytes, tear drop shaped RBCs, leukopenia, thrombocytopenia, hypersegmented PMNs, megaloblastic marrow picture, decreased serum B$_{12}$ level, usually increased serum LD, all to be correlated with Schilling test result and the clinical presentation.

The Schilling test may be "overused" in the evaluation of Cbl deficiency and is often normal when more sensitive indicators of early or subclinical functional deficiency (eg, methylmalonic acid (MMA), "metabolic levels" are abnormal (elevated)).[4,5] Homocyst(e)ine levels are increased in both Cbl (Continued)

Schilling Test *(Continued)*

and folate deficiency. See Methylmalonic Acid, Serum, Plasma, Urine, or Amniotic Fluid *on page 224*.

A peroral nonradioactive vitamin B_{12} absorption test has been utilized.[5]

Footnotes

1. Waters HM and Dawson DW, "An Enzyme Immunoassay for Intrinsic Factor in Urine," *Clin Lab Haematol*, 1999, 21(3):169-72.
2. Zuckier LS, Stabin M, Krynyckyi BR, et al, "Effect of Prior Radiopharmaceutical Administration on Schilling Test Performance: Analysis and Recommendations," *J Nucl Med*, 1996, 37(12):1995-9.
3. Scarlett JD, Read H, and O'Dea K, "Protein-Bound Cobalamin Absorption Declines in the Elderly," *Am J Hematol*, 1992, 39(2):79-83.
4. Snow CF, "Laboratory Diagnosis of Vitamin B_{12} and Folate Deficiency," *Arch Intern Med*, 1999, 159(12):1289-98.
5. Magnus E and Müller C, "A New, Peroral Nonradioactive Vitamin B_{12} Absorption Test Compared With the Schilling Test," *Eur J Haematol*, 1995, 54:117-9.

References

Antony AC, "Megaloblastic Anemias," *Hematology: Basic Principles and Practice*, 3rd ed, Chapter 28, Hoffman R, Benz EJ Jr, Shattil SF, et al, eds, Philadelphia, PA: Churchill Livingstone, 2000.

Brigden ML, "Schilling Test Still Useful in Pernicious Anemia?" *Postgrad Med*, 1999, 106(5):37-8.

Carethers M, "Diagnosing Vitamin B_{12} Deficiency, A Common Geriatric Disorder," *Geriatrics*, 1988, 43(3):89-94, 105-7, 111-2.

Pruthi RK and Tefferi A, "Pernicious Anemia Revisited," *Mayo Clin Proc*, 1994, 69(2):144-50.

♦ **Schistocytes, Smear** *see* Peripheral Blood: Red Blood Cell Morphology *on page 467*

♦ **Schizocytes** *see* Peripheral Blood: Differential Leukocyte Count *on page 464*

♦ **Schnitzler Syndrome** *see* Sedimentation Rate, Erythrocyte *on page 484*

♦ **Schüffner Dots** *see* Malaria Smear and Tests *on page 458*

♦ **Schwachman-Diamond Syndrome** *see* White Blood Cell Count *on page 496*

♦ **Sebastian Syndrome** *see* Platelet Count *on page 468*

♦ **Sedimentation Rate** *see* Sedimentation Rate, Erythrocyte *on page 484*

Sedimentation Rate, Erythrocyte

Related Information

C-Reactive Protein, Serum *on page 523*
Fibrinogen *on page 341*
Zeta Sedimentation Ratio *on page 500*

Synonyms ESR; Sedimentation Rate; Westergren Sed Rate

Applies to Schnitzler Syndrome; Sediscan; Seditainer; Starrsed; Test 1; Ves-Matic Analyzer

Abstract The erythrocyte sedimentation rate (ESR) is a generally nonspecific measure of inflammation which is applied to the detection/evaluation of infectious and immune based (in particular rheumatic type) inflammatory disease. It is commonly used to follow management of rheumatology patients. The test is a measure of the acute phase inflammatory response. Test result is derived from the sedimentation of patient's red blood cells through his/her plasma. As such, ESR is accelerated by increase in the plasma level of acute phase proteins of large molecular size, (fibrinogen in particular) and by anemia. Thus, the ESR may reflect both the hyperproteinemia and anemia of inflammatory disease. ESR methodology has undergone modification in order to increase precision and decrease biohazard exposure.

Specimen Whole blood

Container Lavender top (EDTA) tube or citrated plasma in 4:1 dilution (4 volumes of blood to 1 volume of 109 mmol/L of trisodium citrate)

Collection Specimen must be received and test carried out within 4-6 hours of collection.

Storage Instructions Keep specimen at 4°C prior to testing

Causes for Rejection Insufficient blood, clotted, hemolyzed specimen

Turnaround Time 1-2 hours, some recent automated methods can determine an ESR endpoint in as little as 20 minutes

Special Instructions If EDTA anticoagulated blood is used for the standard Westergren method, 1 volume of 109 mmol/L of trisodium citrate is added to 4 volumes of blood just before performing the test.

Reference Interval Male: younger than 50 years of age: 0-15 mm/hour, older than 50 years of age: 0-20 mm/hour; female: younger than 50 years of age: 0-25 mm/hour, older than 50 years of age: 0-30 mm/hour by Westergren method. See reference by Wolfe and Michaud for their extensive study of and application of the ESR in a number of different settings. Their study indicates that in a rheumatology clinic women younger than 60 years of age who have noninflammatory disorders have upper limit of normal for ESR of 38 mm/hour.

Use Evaluate the nonspecific activity of infections, inflammatory states, autoimmune disorders, and plasma cell dyscrasias; in particular to screen for, to assess severity of and follow clinical activity of rheumatic diseases, especially rheumatoid arthritis; important in clinical evaluation of temporal arteritis and polymyalgia rheumatica

Limitations Anemia and paraproteinemia invalidate results; High-thermal-amplitude cold agglutinins cause less rapid sedimentation (lower ESR) as the temperature rises towards 37°C. The ESR is usually reduced in stored blood. Some procedural methods may be associated with hazardous exposure of medical technologists to fresh whole blood.

Methodology Westergren: A 30 cm long glass tube, 2.55 mm in diameter, is filled with mixed sample of blood up to the 200 mm mark of a Westergren tube. Mechanical pipetting device, not mouth pipetting should be used. The test is performed at room temperature (18°C to 25°C). The vertically placed tube, containing patient's blood, is left for 60 minutes in a vibrationless, constant temperature environment away from direct sunlight. After 1 hour the column of clear plasma above the upper limit of sedimenting red cells is measured by reading to the nearest 1 mm. The result is given as number of mm in 1 hour. The Westergren tube must be kept clean and dry before use. Special racks with leveling screws are used to maintain an exact vertical tube placement. Sedimentation is accelerated with rise in temperature.

The ESR is simple in concept and not technically demanding. It is, however, in its classic form, labor intensive, sensitive to environmental conditions and thus subject to poor precision (poor reproducibility). Most significantly, technician/technologist biohazard exposure due to handling of blood is of concern. In the past decade a number of semiautomated/automated procedures have been developed, many in Europe, to replace the classical ESR procedure and its variants. These include the Sediscan (Becton Dickinson), Starrsed (R & R Mechatronics),[1] Ves-Matic and Mini-Ves (Disease Diagnostica Senese), and Test 1 (SIRE Analytical Systems). Most of these are closed systems that puncture the stopper of a blood collection tube to obtain a capillary sample of whole blood upon which red cell sedimentation is measured by infrared microphotometry or photoelectronically utilizing photodiodes/phototransistors. The appropriate anticoagulant must be utilized, specialized blood collection tubes may be necessary. The measurements are converted into comparable Westergren values. Test 1, by using EDTA anticoagulated samples avoids a dilution step (with attendant possible error) and allows use of one sample for multiple hematologic analyses.

Results of comparison studies have been reported as generally favorable[2,3,4] although a few have not been acceptable due to lack of sufficient correlation with Westergren type ESR.[5] Procedure for verification of a modified method has been published.[1,6] Instrumentation for an earlier alternative sedimentation rate method (the ZSR, see Zeta Sedimentation Ratio *on page 500*) was discontinued by its manufacturer but has recently been resurrected in China.[7] Studies in China determined the normal ZSR (326 normal subjects) to be 52.5% ±5.05% while 106 inpatients had ZSR of 68.52% ±5.54%. Comparison with the Westergren method gave agreement of 86.6%. Advantages of the ZSR (as noted previously in Western countries) were rapid result, low sample volume, not affected by anemia, and lack of need for age/sex correction.

Red cell sedimentation rate is expressed in mm/hour, utilizing Westergren type sedimentation tubes. A validation procedure and method for the in laboratory production of a sedimentation rate reference material has been developed for and can be used for quality assurance programs.[8]

Additional Information Elevations in fibrinogen, alpha- and beta-globulins (acute phase reactants), and immunoglobulins increase the sedimentation rate of red cells through plasma. The test is important in the diagnosis and management of temporal arthritis and of polymyalgia rheumatica (PMR), which are nearly always but not uniformly, characterized by a significantly elevated ESR.[9,10,11] One study found normal ESR in 22% of PMR patients,[10] another found an incidence of 7%.[11] Presence of a normal ESR in a PMR-like clinical setting could lead to delay in diagnosis and therapy. Use of the ESR, ZSR, and/or CRP may aid in the differential diagnosis of the anemia of chronic disease vs iron deficiency anemia.[12] ESR is elevated in about 50% of patients with newly diagnosed Hodgkin disease, especially in advanced stage disease.

The ESR, while lacking in specificity, is elevated in a very broad spectrum of conditions characterized by inflammation. The procedure is of low cost and is readily available. ESR results are frequently compared to those of other nonspecific tests relating to inflammatory proteins, such as C-Reactive Protein, Serum *on page 523* and Viscosity, Serum or Plasma *on page 495*. For decades the ESR has played a prominent role in the evaluation and monitoring of rheumatoid inflammatory processes, notably rheumatoid arthritis and its variants including ankylosing spondylitis. A sampling of recent literature indicates that the ESR continues to be actively utilized in this manner being further defined and itself further defining rheumatoid inflammatory conditions and their therapy.[13,14,15,16,17,18,19]

In a study comparing IgM rheumatoid factor (RF) methods, serial measures of RF did correlate with changes in clinical activity but repeat testing to determine clinical status was found to be only a "fair predictor" and to have little utility in clinical practice. ESR and C-reactive Protein (CRP) were found to be more effective in following clinical activity.[13]

In a study comparing the value of ESR vs CRP in measuring disease activity in ankylosing spondylitis (AS) the positive predictive values of both CRP and ESR were low, neither CRP nor ESR was considered superior in assessment of disease activity.[15] On the basis of literature review (1967 through April 1998) it was concluded that neither ESR or CRP is superior in terms of validity and it was considered that acute phase reactants "do not comprehensively represent the disease process" in AS.[16]

An ESR >100 mm/hour, in a patient with back pain, has a likelihood ratio of 55 for presence of a serious underlying cause.[20]

A normal ESR and CRP was "reliable" in predicting absence of infection in a series of patients in need of revision total hip arthroplasty.[17] The ESR increases with age at an annual rate of increase quantified as 0.22 mm/hour.[21]

In addition to inclusion of ESR in evaluation of the common inflammatory conditions, ESR continues to be included in the study of more unusual entities and associations. A small sampling shows reports of elevated ESR in systemic *Bartonella henselae* infection (cat-scratch disease),[22] and in Schnitzler syndrome (severe chronic urticaria, arthralgia, fever and elevated ESR with or without IgM monoclonal gammopathy).[23] See tables.

Table 1. Factors That May Affect Erythrocyte Sedimentation Rate

Factor	Effect on rate
Red blood cell aggregation (plasma proteins raised in infection, inflammation, and malignant conditions)	Increased*
Pregnancy	Increased*
Anemia (decreased hematocrit)	Increased*
Obesity	Possibly increased*
Drug therapy (eg, steroids, anti-inflammatories)	Decreased*
Female sex	Slightly increased*
Old age	Increased*, possibly due to higher prevalence of disease
Red blood cell abnormalities	
Macrocytosis	Increased*
Microcytosis	Decreased
Sickle cell disease	Decreased
Polycythemia	Decreased
Protein abnormalities (hypofibrinogenemia, hypogammaglobulinemia, dysproteinemia with hyperviscosity state)	Decreased

*Upper limit of normal: Age ≤50 years: men: 15 mm/hour, women: 25 mm/hour. Age >50 years: men: 20 mm/hour; women: 30 mm/hour.

Adapted from Sox and Liang, *Postgrad Med*, 1998, 103(5):258.

Table 2. Comparison of Erythrocyte Sedimentation Rate, Plasma Viscosity, and C-Reactive Protein Tests

Test	Advantages	Disadvantages
Erythrocyte sedimentation rate (ESR)	Inexpensive, quick, simple to perform	Affected by anemia and red blood cell size, not sensitive enough for screening
Plasma viscosity	Not affected by anemia or red blood cell size	Cumbersome apparatus, expensive, not widely available
C-reactive protein	Rapid response to inflammation, complementary to ESR	Wide reference range necessitates sequential recording of values, expensive, batch processing may delay individual results

Footnotes

1. Dacie JV Sir and Lewis SM, "Tests for the Acute Phase Response," *Practical Haematology*, 559.
2. Plebani M, De Toni SD, Sanzari MC, et al, "The Test 1 Automated System. A New Method for Measuring the Erythrocyte Sedimentation Rate," *Am J Clin Pathol*, 1998, 110(3):334-40.
3. Giavarina D, Dall'Olio G, and Soffiati G, "Method Comparison of Automated Systems for the Erythrocyte Sedimentation Rate," *Am J Clin Pathol*, 1999, 112(5):721-4.
4. de Jonge N, Sewkaransing I, Slinger J, et al, "Erythrocyte Sedimentation Rate by the Test-1 Analyzer," *Clin Chem*, 2000, 46(6 Pt 1):881-2.
5. Browning AC, Burbidge AA, and Hodgkins PR, "Comparison of the Erythrocyte Sedimentation Rate Measured in the Eye Casualty Department by the Seditainer Method With an Automated System," *Eye*, 1999, 13(Pt 6):754-7.
6. "ICSH Recommendations for Measurement of Erythrocyte Sedimentation Rate," *J Clin Pathol*, 1993, 46(3):198-203.
7. Su J, Peng Z, Li P, et al, "Investigation of the Zeta Reference Values by Chinese-built Zetafuge® and Preliminary Application," *Hua Hsi I Ko Ta Hsueh Hsueh Pao*, 1998, 29(4):431-4.
8. Thomas RD, Westengard JC, Hay KL, et al, "Calibration and Validation for Erythrocyte Sedimentation Tests: Role of the International Committee on Standardization in Hematology Reference Procedure," *Arch Pathol Lab Med*, 1993, 117(7):719-23.
9. Wong RL and Korn JH, "Temporal Arteritis Without an Elevated Erythrocyte Sedimentation Rate," *Am J Med*, 1986, 80(5):959-64.
10. Helfgott SM and Kieval RI, "Polymyalgia Rheumatica in Patients With a Normal Erythrocyte Sedimentation Rate," *Arthritis Rheum*, 1996, 39(2):304-7.
11. Proven A, Gabriel SE, O'Fallon WM, et al, "Polymyalgia Rheumatica With Low Erythrocyte Sedimentation Rate at Diagnosis," *J Rheumatol*, 1999, 26(6):1333-7.
12. Johnson MA, "Iron: Nutrition Monitoring and Nutrition Status Assessment," *J Nutr*, 1990, 120(Suppl 11):1486-91.
13. Wolfe F, "A Comparison of IgM Rheumatoid Factor by Nephelometry and Latex Methods: Clinical and Laboratory Significance," *Arthritis Care Res*, 1998, 11(2):89-93.
14. van Jaarsveld CH, Jacobs JW, van der Veen MJ, et al, "Aggressive Treatment in Early Rheumatoid Arthritis: A Randomised Controlled Trial," *Ann Rheum Dis*, 2000, 59(6):468-77.
15. Spoorenberg A, van der Heijde D, de Klerk E, et al, "Relative Value of Erythrocyte Sedimentation Rate and C-reactive Protein in Assessment of Disease Activity in Ankylosing Spondylitis," *J Rheumatol*, 1999, 26(4):980-4.
16. Ruof J and Stucki G, "Validity Aspects of Erythrocyte Sedimentation Rate and C-reactive Protein in Ankylosing Spondylitis: A Literature Review," *J Rheumatol*, 1999, 26(4):966-70.
17. Spangehl MJ, Masri BA, O'Connell JX, et al, "Prospective Analysis of Preoperative and Intraoperative Investigations for the Diagnosis of Infection at the Sites of Two Hundred and Two Revision Total Hip Arthroplasties," *J Bone Joint Surg*, 1999, 81A(5):672-83.
18. Narvaez J, Nolla-Sole JM, Clavaguera MT, et al, "Long-Term Therapy in Polymyalgia Rheumatica: Effect of Coexistent Temporal Arteritis," *J Rheumatol*, 1999, 26(9):1945-52.
19. Salvarani C, Boiardi L, Mantovani V, et al, "HLA-DRB1 Alleles Associated With Polymyalgia Rheumatica in Northern Italy: Correlation With Disease Severity," *Ann Rheum Dis*, 1999, 58(5):303-8.
20. Lurie JD, Gerber PD, and Sox HC, "A Pain in the Back," *N Engl J Med*, 2000, 343(10):723-6.
21. Brigden ML and Heathcote JC, "Problems in Interpreting Laboratory Tests, What Do Unexpected Results Mean?" *Postgrad Med*, 2000, 107(7):145-62.
22. Ventura A, Massei F, Not T, et al, "Systemic *Bartonella henselae* Infection With Hepatosplenic Involvement," *J Pediatr Gastroenterol Nutr*, 1999, 29(1):52-6.
23. Husak R, Nestoris S, Goerdt S, et al, "Severe Course of Chronic Urticaria, Arthralgia, Fever and Elevation of Erythrocyte Sedimentation Rate: Schnitzler's Syndrome Without Monoclonal Gammopathy?" *Br J Dermatol*, 2000, 142(3):581-2.

References

Agroyannis B, Dalamangas A, Tzanatos H, et al, "Alterations in Echinocyte Transformation and Erythrocyte Sedimentation Rate During Hemodialysis," *Artif Organs*, 1997, 21(4):327-43.

Brigden M, "The Erythrocyte Sedimentation Rate. Still a Helpful Test When Used Judiciously," *Postgrad Med*, 1998, 103(5):257-62, 272-4.

Chen S, Eldor A, Barshtein G, et al, "Enhanced Aggregability of Red Blood Cells of β-Thalassemia Major Patients," *Am J Physiol*, 1996, 270(6 Pt 2):H1951-6.

Danesh J, Collins R, Peto R, et al, "Haematocrit, Viscosity, Erythrocyte Sedimentation Rate: Meta-analyses of Prospective Studies of Coronary Heart Disease," *Eur Heart J*, 2000, 21(7):515-20.

Gambino R, DiRe JJ, Monteleone M, et al, "The Westergren Sedimentation Rate, Using K_3 EDTA," *Am J Clin Pathol*, 1965, 43:173-80.

Game L, Voegel JC, Schaaf P, et al, "Do Physiological Concentrations of IgG Induce a Direct Aggregation of Red Blood Cells: Comparison With Fibrinogen," *Biochim Biophys Acta*, 1996, 1291(2):138-42.

International Committee for Standardization in Haematology, "Guidelines on Selection of Laboratory Tests for Monitoring the Acute Phase Response," *J Clin Pathol*, 1988, 41:1203-12.

Lowe GD, "Should Plasma Viscosity Replace the ESR?" *Br J Haematol*, 1994, 86(1):6-11.

Paulus HE, Ramos B, Wong WK, et al, "Equivalence of the Acute Phase Reactants C-Reactive Protein, Plasma Viscosity, and Westergren Erythrocyte Sedimentation Rate When Used to Calculate American College of Rheumatology 20% Improvement Criteria or the Disease Activity Score in Patients With Early Rheumatoid Arthritis," *J Rheumatol*, 1999, 26(11):2324-31.

Wolfe F and Michaud K, "The Clinical and Research Significance of the Erythrocyte Sedimentation Rate," *J Rheumatol*, 1994, 21(7):1227-37.

Zlonis M, "The Mystique of the Erythrocyte Sedimentation Rate: A Reappraisal of One of the Oldest Laboratory Tests Still in Use," *Clin Lab Med*, 1993, 13(4):787-800.

♦ **Sediscan** *see* Sedimentation Rate, Erythrocyte *on page 484*

♦ **Seditainer** *see* Sedimentation Rate, Erythrocyte *on page 484*

♦ **Selectin** *see* CD34⁺ Hematopoietic Stem Cells by Flow Cytometry *on page 413*

♦ **Septicemia Detection, Buffy Coat Micromethod** *see* Bacteremia Detection, Buffy Coat Micromethod *on page 406*

♦ **Serous Fluid Analysis** *see* Body Fluid Analysis, Cell Count *on page 408*

♦ **Serum Folate** *see* Folic Acid, Serum *on page 435*

♦ **Serum Lysis** *see* Ham Test *on page 439*

♦ **Serum Transferrin Receptor** *see* Transferrin Receptor, Soluble, Serum or Plasma *on page 493*

♦ **Serum Viscosity** *see* Viscosity, Serum or Plasma *on page 495*

♦ **Shindler Disease** *see* Inherited Diseases of Metabolism and Cell Structure *on page 449*

♦ **Sickle Cell Preparation, Metabisulfite Test** *see* Sickle Cell Tests *on page 486*

♦ **Sickle Cells** *see* Peripheral Blood: Differential Leukocyte Count *on page 464*

♦ **Sickle Cell Solubility Test** *see* Sickle Cell Tests *on page 486*

♦ **Sickle Cells, Smear** *see* Peripheral Blood: Red Blood Cell Morphology *on page 467*

Sickle Cell Tests

Related Information

Anemia Flowchart *on page 392*
Fetal Hemoglobin *on page 431*
Hemoglobin *on page 442*
Hemoglobin Electrophoresis *on page 444*
Hemosiderin Stain, Urine *on page 876*
Reticulocyte Count *on page 481*

Synonyms Dithionite Test; Itano Solubility Test; Murayama Test; Sickle Cell Preparation, Metabisulfite Test; Sickle Cell Solubility Test; Sickledex™; Sickle Screen™; Sickle-Sol™; Sickle-Stat™

Applies to Acute Chest Syndrome; Flippase; Floppase; Hemoglobin Munchausen; Hydroxyurea; Nitrous Oxide Neuropathy; Ribonucleotide Reductase Inhibitor; Translocase

Test Includes A variety of similar but usually slightly modified tests have been developed, described, and achieved varying degrees of acceptance. In some institutions a positive is confirmed by performing an alternate confirmatory sickle cell test and/or hemoglobin electrophoresis (the preferred procedure).

Abstract Screening tests for sickle cell anemia and related entities which include hemoglobin S (eg, SC, SD, sickle thalassemia, others). The sickle solubility test, available in slightly different form from a number of commercial sources, is based on the decreased solubility of reduced hemoglobin S in a concentrated phosphate buffer with standardized detection of resultant turbidity. If a sickle screen test is positive, confirmatory studies (eg, Hb electrophoresis) should be performed (see following). There are continuing advances in understanding the mechanisms of pathologic damage in sickle cell disease (SCD) with resultant improvements in management and therapy.

Specimen Whole blood

Container Lavender top (EDTA) tube for venipuncture specimen; lavender top Microtainer™ for capillary specimen

Collection Routine venipuncture. Invert tube gently to mix.

Causes for Rejection Clotted specimen, hemolyzed specimen

Reference Interval Negative

Use Detect sickling hemoglobins; evaluate hemolytic anemia; evaluate undiagnosed hereditary anemia with morphologic (sickle-like) abnormalities on peripheral blood smear

Limitations False-positive solubility test for sickling may be due to polycythemic blood; excess blood in relation to the quantity of reagent; interference by some forms of hyperglobulinemia such as may occur with myeloma, Waldenström macroglobulinemia or cryoglobulinemia (if suspect, test should be repeated using patient's washed red cells); and a variety of abnormal hemoglobins including I, Bart's, $C_{Georgetown}$, Alexandra, C_{Harlem}, Porto Alegre, Memphis/S, $C_{Ziguinchor}$ and S_{Travis}. False-negative solubility test reaction may occur with inadequate quantities of blood from anemic patients (hemoglobin levels <8.0 g/dL); deterioration of reducing agents (detected by negative result on positive control); deterioration of the lytic agent (detected by negativity of positive control); improper illumination and visualization of the line-reader scale and high concentration of Hb F or of phenothiazines that may inhibit the sickle reaction; quantities of hemoglobin S too small to detect, as at birth or with transfusions of nonhemoglobin S units of blood into patients who have sickle blood (or multiunit transfusion including some donor units from sickle cell trait individuals).[1,2] The appearance of hemoglobin S is genetically delayed and is not usually present in sufficient quantity (above ~25%) for a positive screening test result until after 3 months of age. Maximum levels are not reached until about 6 months of age. Solubility tests and sodium metabisulfite test are unlikely to be reliably positive until after 6 months of age. Babies with initial evidence of SS, SC, SD, Sβ⁺, or Sβ⁰ thalassemia should be retested within 6-8 weeks of birth.[3]

Methodology Hb high salt solubility - Sickledex™ and a number of other commercially available products (see Synonyms); alternate: slide test with 2% sodium metabisulfite. The sodium metabisulfite sickling test involves microscopic identification of sickled red blood cells which have formed due to deoxygenation of hemoglobin (in intact red cells) after exposure to the reducing agent, sodium metabisulfite. Use of excessive metabisulfite will cause a false-positive reaction (changes resembling sickling in normal red cells). Poikilocytes may be difficult to differentiate from true sickle cells. Outdated metabisulfite or sickle solubility test reagents may be the cause of false-negative results. Sickle solubility screening procedures have evolved from the Itano solubility test. These tests are based on visual detection of turbidity resulting from decreased solubility of reduced hemoglobin S in a concentrated phosphate buffer solution.

Additional Information Hb S is the result of a single amino acid substitution (valine for the normally present glutamic acid) at the 6th position of the β-globin chain of the hemoglobin molecule. The homozygous state results in sickle cell disease, a condition with significant morbidity and mortality. The heterozygous state causes sickle trait, a condition ordinarily characterized by little or no morbidity. Sickle disease presents a spectrum of clinical severity relating in part to activation of coagulation through loss of normal

membrane phospholipid asymmetry and the appearance of phosphatidylserine (PS) on cell surfaces. Surface PS, a "docking site" for hemostatic proteins, is involved in "flip-flop" activity (leading to increased procoagulant activity) as the red cell membrane skeleton is uncoupled from the lipid bilayer.[4] Aminophospholipid translocase, or "flippase" and "floppase", are involved in the transport of PS and phosphatidylethanolamine from outer to inner and inner to outer red cell membrane surfaces in the maintenance of membrane phospholipid asymmetry. High levels of fetal hemoglobin (F-cell level of some 70%) favor decreased red cell membrane microvesicle formation, PS exposure, and thrombin generation (with normalized levels of prothrombin fragment 1.2)[4] (see Fetal Hemoglobin *on page 431* and Hypercoagulation Panel *on page 345*). Amelioration results from coincidental occurrence of other hemoglobinopathies, notably those with increased levels of Hb F (eg, thalassemia and different types of hereditary persistence of fetal hemoglobin). Variation in clinical expression is also the result of DNA polymorphism in the β-globin gene cluster.[5]

The incidence of sickle cell trait amongst African Americans in the U.S. is 8.5%. Because of possible anterior segment ischemia (a significant complication of retinal detachment surgery) that may occur in otherwise asymptomatic sickle trait individuals, it has been recommended that African-Americans undergo preoperative sickle tests prior to such procedures.[6]

Distinction between Hb S beta-thalassemia and sickle cell anemia is not always possible on clinical, hematologic, or electrophoretic grounds. Thalassemia heterozygotes have hypochromia and microcytosis, but overlap values exist. Differentiation can best be made by family or molecular pathology methods. Regional prevalence in the midwest area of Hb S beta-thalassemia is estimated to be 1:23,000 of the black population. It is recommended that positive sickle cell screen patients be further evaluated with cellulose acetate or agarose gel hemoglobin electrophoresis at pH 8.6, citrate agar gel electrophoresis at pH 6.0, Hb F studies and family studies. Complete characterization may require specialized laboratory studies. Erythrocyte ecdysis (long free filamentous processes stripping away from the surface of red cells) has been described in sickle cell anemia associated with elevated cold agglutinin titer.[7]

Study of peripheral blood smear has utility in detection of sickled red blood cells (RBCs) with classic findings of numerous sickled cells, schistocytes, nucleated red cells, leukocytosis, target cells, and other abnormalities dependent on the degree of hypoxia and stage of the disease (eg, Howell-Jolly bodies if splenic atrophy has occurred). In quiescent periods of sickle disease (Hb SS), however, sickle cells may present irregularly and uncommonly on peripheral smears. Review of routinely stained blood smears has been considered to have no role in the confident identification of abnormal cells in subjects with sickle cell trait (Hb AS). A recent report, however, indicates that on the basis of light microscopy, abnormal cells (defined as elongated RBCs with tapering of opposite ends culminating in a point) can be identified in a majority of patients with sickle cell trait. Ninety-six percent of trait subjects had such abnormal red cells as compared to 4% of controls (96% of the control group had no abnormal RBCs in their peripheral smears).[8]

Survey testing to determine the incidence and significance of hereditary anemias (including the sickle hemoglobinopathies) continues on a worldwide basis.[9,10,11] The application of molecular biologic (DNA) based techniques for population screening is currently cost prohibitive but in future years is likely to be the preferred method for detection of sickle hemoglobinopathies, in particular for detection of the heterozygous states.[12]

A survey of laboratory results, methods and problems in screening for sickle cell disease with emphasis on laboratory responsibilities has been published by the US Department of Health and Human Services.[13]

The rare condition, "hemoglobin Munchausen" has been reviewed.[14]

Significant advances in the therapy of SCD have accompanied increased understanding of the mechanisms responsible for morbidity and mortality.[15,16] Use of hydroxyurea, a ribonucleotide reductase inhibitor (RRI), for induction of Hb F production, has been followed by the search for more effective RRIs and the use of combination therapy.[17] Antiadhesion therapy, with use of monoclonal antibodies to endothelial αVβ3 integrin receptor has been proposed.[18,19] Aggressive therapy of the acute chest syndrome including appropriate use of antibiotic agents and rarely, complete exchange transfusion is described.[15,20] Bone marrow transplant has been used in over 100 cases of SCD with a 75% success (cure) rate,[15,16] but with 10% mortality.[15]

Nitrous oxide may cause a neuropathy similar to that seen with pernicious anemia and has been reported in SCD patients.[21] While serum vitamin B_{12} levels may be reduced and slight macrocytosis may be present, Schilling test may be normal and gastric parietal antibody negative. The neuropathy responds to intramuscular B_{12} and avoidance of nitrous oxide. Presence of SCD may be a contraindication for use of nitrous oxide.[21]

Footnotes

1. Ahmad E and Sykes E, "Low Levels of Hemoglobin S in a White Woman," *Lab Med*, 1999, 30(9):572.
2. Veillon DM, Kaltenbach JE, Hall CG, et al, "Assays for Hemoglobin S," *Lab Med*, 2000, 31(2):68.
3. Brozovic M and Henthorn J, "Investigation of Abnormal Haemoglobins and Thalassaemia," *Practical Haematology*, 8th ed, 1995, Dacie JV Sir and Lewis SM, eds, New York, NY: Churchill Livingstone, 1995, 249.

4. Setty BN, Kulkarni S, Rao AK, et al, "Fetal Hemoglobin in Sickle Cell Disease: Relationship to Erythrocyte Phosphatidylserine Exposure and Coagulation Activation," *Blood*, 2000, 96(3):1119-24.
5. El-Hazmi MA, Bahakim HM, and Warsy AS, "DNA Polymorphism in the Beta-Globin Gene Cluster in Saudi Arabs: Relation to Severity of Sickle Cell Anaemia," *Acta Haematol*, 1992, 88(2-3):61-6.
6. Cartwright MJ, Blair CJ, Combs JL, et al, "Anterior Segment Ischemia: A Complication of Retinal Detachment Repair in a Patient With Sickle Cell Trait," *Ann Ophthalmol*, 1990, 22(9):333-4.
7. Ward PC, Smith CM, and White JG, "Erythrocytic Ecdysis: An Unusual Morphologic Finding in a Case of Sickle Cell Anemia With Intercurrent Cold-Agglutinin Syndrome," *Am J Clin Pathol*, 1979, 72(3):479-85.
8. Wilson CI, Hopkins PL, Cabello-Inchausti B, et al, "The Peripheral Blood Smear in Patients With Sickle Cell Trait: A Morphologic Observation," *Lab Med*, 2000, 31(8):445.
9. Aluoch JR and Aluoch LH, "Survey of Sickle Disease in Kenya," *Trop Geogr Med*, 1993, 45(1):18-21.
10. Ali M and Lafferty J, "The Clinical Significance of Hemoglobinopathies in the Hamilton Region: A Twenty Year Review," *Clin Invest Med*, 1992, 15(5):401-5.
11. Martins MC, Olim G, Melo J, et al, "Hereditary Anaemias in Portugal: Epidemiology, Public Health Significance, and Control," *J Med Genet*, 1993, 30(3):235-9.
12. Steinberg MH, "DNA Diagnosis for the Detection of Sickle Hemoglobinopathies," *Am J Hematol*, 1993, 43(2):110-5.
13. Guideline: Laboratory Screening for Sickle Cell Disease, U.S. Department of Health and Human Services, *Lab Med*, 1993, 24(8):515-22.
14. Ballas SK, "Munchausen Sickle Cell Painful Crisis," *Ann Clin Lab Sci*, 1992, 22(4):226-8.
15. Rosse WF, "New Views of Sickle Cell Disease," *N C Med J*, 1997, 58(1):62-6.
16. Davies SC, "Sickle Cell Disease: Modern Concepts," *Clin Lab Haematol*, 1997, 19(4):309-10.
17. Iyamu WE, Adunyah SE, Fasold H, et al, "Enhancement of Hemoglobin and F-Cell Production by Targeting Growth Inhibition and Differentiation of K562 Cells With Ribonucleotide Reductase Inhibitors (Didox and Trimidox) in Combination With Streptozotocin," *Am J Hematol*, 2000, 63(4):176-83.
18. Harlan JM, "Introduction: Antiadhesion Therapy in Sickle Cell Disease," *Blood*, 2000, 95(2):365-7.
19. Hebbel RP, "Blockade of Adhesion of Sickle Cells to Endothelium by Monoclonal Antibodies," *N Engl J Med*, 2000, 342(25):1910-12.
20. Platt OS, "The Acute Chest Syndrome of Sickle Cell Disease," *N Engl J Med*, 2000, 342(25):1904-7.
21. Ogundipe O, Walker M, Pearson TC, et al, "Sickle Cell Disease and Nitrous Oxide-Induced Neuropathy," *Clin Lab Haematol*, 1999, 21(6):409-12.

References

Ashley-Koch A, Yang Q, and Olney RS, "Sickle Hemoglobin (Hb S) Allele and Sickle Cell Disease: A HuGE Review," *Am J Epidemiol*, 2000, 151(9):839-45.
Bunn HF, "Human Hemoglobins: Sickle Hemoglobin and Other Mutants," *The Molecular Basis of Blood Diseases*, 3rd ed, chapter 7, Stamatoyannopoulos G, Majerus PW, Perlmutter RM, et al, eds, Philadelphia, PA: WB Saunders Co, 2001, 227-73.
Hiti AL, Zent L, Xiang Q, et al, "Beta-Globin Haplotypes From Blood Spots for Follow-up of Newborn Hemoglobinopathy Screening," *Am J Hematol*, 1997, 54(1):76-8.
Homi J, Levee L, Higgs D, et al, "Pulse Oximetry in a Cohort Study of Sickle Cell Disease," *Clin Lab Haematol*, 1997, 19(1):17-22.
Kaul DK, Tsai HM, Liu XD, et al, "Monoclonal Antibodies to Alpha Vbeta3 (7E3 and LM609) Inhibit Sickle Red Blood Cell-Endothelium Interactions Induced by Platelet-Activating Factor," *Blood*, 2000, 95(2):368-74.
Koshy M, "Sickle Cell Disease and Pregnancy," *Blood Rev*, 1995, 9(3):157-64.
Platt OS, Brambilla DJ, Rosse WF, et al, "Mortality in Sickle Cell Disease: Life Expectancy and Risk Factors for Early Death," *N Engl J Med*, 1994, 330(23):1639-44.
Serjeant GR, *Sickle Cell Disease*, 2nd ed, Oxford, England: Oxford U Pr, 1992.
Steinberg MH, "Sickle Cell Anemia and Fetal Hemoglobin," *Am J Med Sci*, 1994, 308(5):259-65.
Vichinsky EP, Neumayr LD, Earles AN, et al, "Causes and Outcomes of the Acute Chest Syndrome in Sickle Cell Disease," *N Engl J Med*, 2000, 342(25):1855-65.

Siderocyte Stain

Related Information
Bone Marrow on page 410
Iron Stain, Bone Marrow on page 452

Synonyms Hemosiderin Stain; Iron Stain; Pappenheimer Body Stain; Perl's Test

Abstract Siderocyte stain (Prussian blue reaction) demonstrates non-haem iron containing granules in non-nucleated red blood cells on smear of peripheral blood. Iron containing granules are called Pappenheimer bodies as seen on Wright stain of peripheral blood smear. Finding of siderocytes has application to the study of sideroblastic anemia-myelodysplastic syndrome and hemolytic anemia.

Specimen Blood: coverslip or slide smears; bone marrow: coverslip smears preferred

Reference Interval Peripheral blood: no siderocytes identified; bone marrow: stainable iron present

Use Detect sideroblastic anemias and hemolytic anemia; semiquantitation of marrow iron stores, evaluation of iron reserve; assist in the diagnosis of iron deficiency and hemosiderosis/hemochromatosis

Limitations Siderocytes may be present in asplenic patients. They occur in large numbers following splenectomy.

Methodology Prussian blue (potassium ferrocyanide) reaction in which a blue colored compound, ferriferocyanide, is formed with the siderotic material (hemosiderin).

Additional Information Siderotic granules represent iron not yet incorporated into hemoglobin and are a water insoluble complex of ferric iron, lipid, protein, and carbohydrate. They occur primarily when there is impaired hemoglobin synthesis (eg, sideroblastic anemia, lead poisoning). Savage et al[1] have shown that 36% of alcoholic patients with bone marrow proven sideroblastic anemia have siderocytes in the peripheral blood. Otherwise, siderocytes are uncommon in the peripheral blood unless a splenectomy has been performed on the patient. Study of marrow iron stains is more important than iron stains of peripheral blood in terms of deciding on questionable causes of anemia. Numerous siderocytes are noted postsplenectomy and in some hemoglobinopathies. They are absent with iron deficiency.

In a normal individual, iron positive granules in circulating (peripheral) red blood cells (siderocytes) are not identified. After splenectomy they may be seen in up to 14% to 15% of red cells. The spleen normally removes such abnormal erythrocytes from peripheral blood. Other abnormalities seen on study of Romanowsky type dye-stained peripheral blood smears from splenectomized patients are target cells, Howell-Jolly bodies, acanthocytes, and Pappenheimer bodies (equivalent to siderotic granules as seen with an iron stain). These features are sufficiently distinctive to allow laboratory diagnosis of clinical splenectomy and may be of special importance in identifying a clinically unsuspected "medical" splenectomy. Siderocytes may be found in the peripheral blood in a variety of hemolytic anemias but not in thalassemia. Splenic activity in removing circulating siderocytes makes correlation of quantitative siderocyte counts with type of hemolysis unreliable.

Footnotes
1. Savage D and Lindenbaum J, "Anemia in Alcoholics," *Medicine (Baltimore)*, 1986, 65(5):322-38.

References
Beutler E, "Blood, Marrow, and Urine Iron Stains," *Williams Hematology*, 5th ed, Chapter L6, Beutler E, Lichtman MA, Coller BS, et al, eds, New York, NY: McGraw-Hill Inc, 1995, L27.
Douglas AS and Dacie JV, "The Incidence and Significance of Iron Containing Granules in Human Erythrocytes and Their Precursors," *J Clin Pathol*, 1953, 6:307.
Grüneberg H, "Siderocytes: A New Kind of Erythrocytes," *Nature*, 1941, 148(3755):469-70.

◆ **Sucrose Hemolysis Test** *see* Sugar Water Test Screen *on page 488*

◆ **Sucrose Lysis Test** *see* Sugar Water Test Screen *on page 488*

◆ **Sudan Black B (SBB) Stain** *see* Leukocyte Cytochemistry *on page 456*

◆ **Sudden Infant Death Syndrome** *see* Fetal Hemoglobin *on page 431*

Sugar Water Test Screen

Related Information
Ham Test *on page 439*
Hemosiderin Stain, Urine *on page 876*
PNH Test (GPI-Anchored Proteins) by Flow Cytometry *on page 472*

Synonyms PNH Test Screen; Sucrose Hemolysis Test; Sucrose Lysis Test

Test Includes Sucrose hemolysis if hemolysis is found in the sugar water screen test

Abstract Screening test for suspected paroxysmal nocturnal hemoglobinuria (PNH). Confirm with PNH Test (GPI-Anchored Proteins) by Flow Cytometry *on page 472*.

Specimen Blood

Container Blue top (sodium citrate) tube

Causes for Rejection Hemolyzed specimens

Reference Interval Absence of hemolysis is the normal condition. If no hemolysis is present, the patient probably does not have PNH provided multiple recent transfusions have not reduced the proportion of abnormal cells. When positive, the test shows lysis of some 10% to 80% of red cells. The screening test is not definitive.

Use Screen for PNH

Limitations False positives may be seen in cases of megaloblastic anemias and autoimmune hemolytic anemias (usually <5% lysis). Some patients with leukemia or myelosclerosis may also have false-positive results (usually mild lysis, <10% of red cells). False-negative results may occur if heparin or EDTA is used as an anticoagulant.

Methodology Washed erythrocytes are exposed to an iso-osmotic solution of sucrose and normal group AB or ABO compatible serum (as a source of complement). Complement will then fix to the cell surface. PNH red cells have unusual susceptibility to complement and will hemolyze under these conditions.

Additional Information If the sugar water test is positive, a subsequent PNH test by flow cytometry is strongly recommended. A negative sugar water test rules out PNH in most instances, provided the proportion of patient cells has not been reduced by previous transfusion. It has been demonstrated that the most complement sensitive cells in PNH are younger RBCs and reticulocytes. Increased sensitivity can be obtained for the assay by separating young RBCs from old by centrifugation.[1]

Patients with aplastic anemia may develop PNH.[2] Patients with PNH may present as pancytopenia and have a dysplastic or aplastic appearing marrow. Patients may develop thrombosis with hypercoagulable state, and may bleed with thrombocytopenia and a disseminated intravascular coagulation-like picture.[3] Renal pathology, clinically including acute renal failure, results at least in part from repeated renal microvascular thrombosis.[4]

The molecular pathology of PNH is partially, if not largely, established and involves a number of PIG-A gene mutations. These affect a glycolipid (glycosyl-phosphatidylinositol anchor for decay accelerating factor (DAF)) or CD59. DAF and CD59 are membrane-regulatory proteins which inhibit complement activation. See Ham Test *on page 439* and PNH Test (GPI-Anchored Proteins) by Flow Cytometry *on page 472*. Deficient or absent CD59 (which regulates assembly of the C9 complement attack complex) results in red cell hemolysis and the hypercoagulable state. Demonstration of decreased red cell (and/or granulocyte) levels of CD59 (see PNH Test (GPI-Anchored Proteins) by flow cytometry) is the preferred test for supporting a diagnosis of PNH.[3,5]

Footnotes
1. Shimoda M and Yawata Y, "An Increased Calcium Accumulation in ATP-dependent Red Cells of the Patients With Paroxysmal Nocturnal Hemoglobinuria," *Am J Hematol*, 1985, 20(4):325-35.
2. Azenishi Y, Ueda E, Machii T, et al, "CD59-Deficient Blood Cells and PIG-A Gene Abnormalities in Japanese Patients With Aplastic Anemia," *Br J Haematol*, 1999, 104(3):523-9.
3. Hillman RS and Ault KA, "The Dysplastic and Sideroblastic Anemias," *Hematology in Clinical Practice: A Guide to Diagnosis and Management*, 2nd ed, Chapter 9, New York, NY: McGraw-Hill, 1998, 151-2.
4. Mooraki A, Boroumand B, Zadeh FM, et al, "Acute Reversible Renal Failure in a Patient With Paroxysmal Nocturnal Hemoglobinuria," *Clin Nephrol*, 1998, 50(4):255-7.
5. Shinton NK, "Paroxysmal Nocturnal Hemoglobinuria," *CRC Desk Reference for Hematology*, Boca Raton, FL: CRC Press, 1998, 528-30.

References
Hartmann RC and Jenkins DE, "The "Sugar Water" Test for Paroxysmal Nocturnal Hemoglobinuria," *N Engl J Med*, 1966, 275(3):155-7.
Rosse WF, "Paroxysmal Nocturnal Hemoglobinuria," *Hematology: Basic Principles and Practice*, 3rd ed, Chapter 20, Hoffman R, Benz EJ Jr, Shattil SJ, et al, eds, Philadelphia, PA: Churchill Livingstone, 2000, 331-42.

◆ **Sulfatidase** *see* Inherited Diseases of Metabolism and Cell Structure *on page 449*

◆ **Sulfonylurea Receptor** *see* Inherited Diseases of Metabolism and Cell Structure *on page 449*

◆ **Superoxide Production** *see* Nitroblue Tetrazolium Test *on page 461*

◆ **Survival of Red Blood Cells** *see* ⁵¹Cr Red Cell Survival *on page 422*

◆ **Survivin** *see* Apoptosis Assays *on page 402*

◆ **Suspension Array Technology** *see* Flow Cytometry, Overview *on page 432*

Syndecan-1, Serum

Related Information
Beta$_2$-Microglobulin, Serum or Urine *on page 509*
Bone Marrow *on page 410*
Immunofixation Electrophoresis, Serum or Urine *on page 530*

Abstract Syndecan is a membrane heparin sulfate proteoglycan. It is involved in cell-matrix adhesion processes, is a low-affinity receptor for heparin-binding growth factors, and in the bone marrow, is a cell surface antigen in early and late stages of B-lymphocyte differentiation. While absent on mature B cells, it is re-expressed on plasma cells. In patients with multiple myeloma, syndecan-1 has been found to be expressed only on myeloma cells.[1] It is also seen on malignant plasma cells circulating in the peripheral blood.[2] The level of syndecan-1, shed from the surface of myeloma cells,[3] has been found to correlate with tumor burden[3] and survival.[4] Serum syndecan-1 level may be of use in prognostic classification of myeloma.[4]

Specimen Serum, 1-2 mL

Container Red top tube

Turnaround Time 4 hours

Reference Interval Median syndecan-1 levels in normal controls was 128 units/mL, 79% of myeloma patients had syndecan-1 levels above the mean level, ±2 SD in the control group (>370 units/mL)

Use Serum syndecan-1 levels correlate with survival in multiple myeloma. Syndecan-1 is considered to represent a new independent prognostic parameter in myeloma.[5]

Methodology Enzyme-linked immunosorbent assay (ELISA), commercially available (Diaclone Research, Besancon, France)[5]

Additional Information Syndecans are a family of transmembrane heparan sulfated proteoglycans. Syndecan-1 is formed of a core protein with side chains of heparan sulfate and chondroitin sulfate. Syndecan-1 is involved in the adhesion of mature plasma cells to stomal cells of bone marrow. Monoclonal antibodies against syndecan-1 are markers for malignant plasma cells and are of use in the purification of myeloma cells.[1] The Nordic Myeloma Study Group has concluded that serum syndecan-1 levels represent a new independent prognostic parameter in multiple myeloma. Their study of 174 myeloma patients found that "low" syndecan-1 levels had a median survival of 44 months, while "high" levels had a median survival of only 20 months.[4] Currently, serum β_2-microglobulin level is the most useful and widely used prognostic indicator in patients with multiple myeloma. Serum syndecan-1 levels show prognostic value in a Cox regression model with β_2-microglobulin.[4] A study from MD Anderson Cancer Center found prognostic value in cytogenetic analysis applied to multiple myeloma.[5] Abnormal karyotypes, however, were found in only 46% of 79 previously untreated myeloma patients. Of patients with abnormal karyotypes, 47% had monosomy or deletion of chromosome 13 with shorter survival (median of 10 months) than subjects with other abnormalities (median survival of 34 months).

Footnotes
1. Wijdenes J, Vooijs WC, Clement C, et al, "A Plasmocyte Selective Monoclonal Antibody (B-B4) Recognizes Syndecan-1," *Br J Haematol*, 1996, 94(2):318-23.
2. Witzig TE, Kimlinger T, Stenson M, et al, "Syndecan-1 Expression on Malignant Cells From the Blood and Marrow of Patients With Plasma Cell Proliferative Disorders and B-Cell Chronic Lymphocytic Leukemia," *Leukemia and Lymphoma*, 1998, 31(1-2):167-75.
3. Dhodapkar MV, Kelly T, Theus A, et al, "Elevated Levels of Shed Syndecan-1 Correlate With Tumour Mass and Decreased Matrix Metalloproteinase-9 Activity in the Serum of Patients With Multiple Myeloma," *Br J Haematol*, 1997, 99(2):368-71.
4. Seidel C, Sundan A, Hjorth M, et al, "Serum Syndecan-1: A New Independent Prognostic Marker in Multiple Myeloma," *Blood*, 2000, 95(2):388-92.
5. Seong C, Delasalle K, Hayes K, et al, "Prognostic Value of Cytogenetics in Multiple Myeloma," *Br J Haematol*, 1998, 101(1):189-94.

References
Davies FE, Jack AS, and Morgan GJ, "The Use of Biological Variables to Predict Outcome in Multiple Myeloma," *Br J Haematol*, 1997, 99(4):719-25.
Jourdan M, Ferlin M, Legouffe E, et al, "The Myeloma Cell Antigen Syndecan-1 Is Lost by Apoptotic Myeloma Cells," *Br J Haematol*, 1998, 100(4):637-46.
Witzig TE, Gertz MA, Lust JA, et al, "Peripheral Blood Monoclonal Plasma Cells as a Predictor of Survival in Patients With Multiple Myeloma," *Blood*, 1996, 88(5):1780-7.

◆ **Target Cells** *see* Peripheral Blood: Differential Leukocyte Count *on page 464*

Tartrate Resistant Leukocyte Acid Phosphatase

Related Information
Leukocyte Cytochemistry *on page 456*
Lymph Node Biopsy *on page 67*

Synonyms Acid Phosphatase, Tartrate Resistant, Leukocytes; Hairy Cell Leukemia Test; Leukemic Reticuloendotheliosis Test; Leukocyte Acid Phosphatase; TRAP Test

Applies to Hairy Cell Leukemia; Leukocyte Acid Phosphatase Isoenzymes; TRAP (Tartrate Resistant Acid Phosphatase)

Test Includes Leukocyte acid phosphatase reaction with and without tartrate inhibition

Abstract Tartrate resistant acid phosphatase (TRAP) positive white cells identified on peripheral blood and/or bone marrow smears along with characteristic findings on study of sections from bone marrow biopsy are largely diagnostic of hairy cell leukemia (HCL).

Specimen Glass microscope slide smears prepared from fresh capillary or heparinized whole blood, fixed immediately (glutaraldehyde-acetone) after preparation

Container Green top (heparin) tube

Storage Instructions Smeared glass slides may be stored at least 1 week prior to assay if fixed immediately after preparation.

Causes for Rejection Smears unfixed, blood not fresh

Reference Interval Most white cells of peripheral blood as well as platelets are acid phosphatase positive, the reaction is inhibited by L(+) tartrate (tartrate sensitive). Tartrate resistant cells are not present in the blood of normal individuals.

Use Diagnose "hairy cell leukemia" ("leukemic reticuloendotheliosis")

Limitations Patients with HCL are often leukopenic with relatively few hairy cells in the peripheral blood.

Methodology Naphthol AS-BI, fast garnet GBC, with and without L(+) tartaric acid

Additional Information There are some six isoenzymes of leukocyte acid phosphatase. Of the six, isoenzyme V is not inhibited by (is resistant to) L(+) tartaric acid. It has been found that the malignant mononuclear cells of leukemic reticuloendotheliosis ("hairy cell leukemia") contain isoenzyme V and are resistant to inhibition by L(+) tartaric acid. There is evidence the reaction is not entirely specific as tartrate resistant acid phosphatase reactions have been reported in cases of prolymphocytic leukemia and malignant lymphoma as well as some cases of infectious mononucleosis.[1] There have also been reports of rare false-negative results (patients with leukemic reticuloendotheliosis having negative tartrate resistant acid phosphatase reactions). Most T-cell lymphoproliferative processes are strongly acid phosphatase positive, tartrate sensitive. In T-cell chronic leukemias the acid phosphatase reaction is variable. A few tartrate resistant acid phosphatase positive cells may be found in normal bone marrow. Osteoclasts are strongly TRAP positive. An assay based on antibody against band V acid phosphatase has been described. The immunoassay has greater specificity[2] than the standard cytochemical procedure. A monoclonal antibody against TRAP (anti-TRAP) has been developed and can be used with paraffin-imbedded tissue.[3] The application of immunophenotypic studies to the diagnosis of HCL has decreased the need for TRAP staining. Hairy cells are B lymphocytes and express the pan-B-cell antigens CD19, CD20, and CD22, they lack CD5 and CD10, but express CD103, considered a sensitive marker for HCL.[4]

Footnotes
1. Brown BA, *Hematology: Principles and Practice*, 6th ed, Philadelphia, PA: Lea & Febiger, 1993, 137-8.
2. Whitaker KB, Cox TM, and Moss DW, "An Immunoassay of Human Band-5 (Tartrate Resistant) Acid Phosphatase That Involves the Use of Antiporcine Uteroferrin Antibodies," *Clin Chem* 1989, 35(1):86-9.
3. Janckila AJ, Cardwell EM, Yam LT, et al, "Hairy Cell Identification by Immunohistochemistry of Tartrate-Resistant Acid Phosphatase," *Blood*, 1995, 85(10):2839-44.
4. "Chronic Lymphocytic Leukemias and Other Lymphoid Leukemias: Hairy Cell Leukemia," *Practical Diagnosis of Hematologic Disorders*, 3rd ed, Chapter 33, Kjeldsberg CR, ed, Chicago, IL: ASCP Press, 2000, 543-4.

References
Catovsky E, "Leukocyte Cytochemical and Immunological Techniques," *Practical Haematology*, 8th ed, Dacie JV Sir and Lewis SM, eds, 1995, 143.
Johnston JB, "Hairy Cell Leukemia," *Wintrobe's Clinical Hematology*, 10th ed, Chapter 94, Lee GR, Foerster J, Lukens J, et al, eds, Baltimore MD: Lippincott Williams & Wilkins, 1999, 2428-46.
Tallman MS, Hakiman D, and Peterson LC, "Hairy Cell Leukemia," *Hematology: Basic Principles and Practice*, 3rd ed, Chapter 73, Hoffman R, Benz EJ Jr, Shattil SJ, et al, eds, New York, NY: Churchill Livingstone, 2000, 1363-72.

♦ **TdT** *see* Terminal Deoxynucleotidyl Transferase *on page 489*

Terminal Deoxynucleotidyl Transferase

Related Information
Bone Marrow *on page 410*
Immunophenotypic Analysis of Tissues by Flow Cytometry *on page 62*
Lymph Node Biopsy *on page 67*

Synonyms TdT; Terminal Deoxyribonucleotidyl Transferase; Terminal Transferase

Abstract An enzyme found in lymphoid thymic cells and a minor (1% to 2%) population thymic related T-cell lymphoid precursors in the bone marrow. Some leukemic cell populations are TdT positive, notably T cell acute lymphoblastic leukemia (TALL), CALL, and some blast cells of chronic myelogenous leukemia in crisis. TdT positivity, however, is not exclusively diagnostic of leukemia.

Specimen Blood or bone marrow (avoid heparin) for leukocyte separation, pelletization, and storage at -20°C. Glass slide smears, air dried, of blood or marrow.

Collection Store dried smears at room temperature for up to 5 days.

Storage Instructions Store leukocyte pellets (long-term) at -20°C.

Reference Interval Peripheral blood: negative for TdT-positive cells; bone marrow: <1.8% TdT-positive cells

Use Classify certain leukemias and lymphomas, normally used to distinguish acute lymphoblastic from nonlymphoblastic leukemia (ALL from AML and from other lymphoproliferative disorders such as adult T cell leukemia); diagnose acute lymphoblastic leukemia, lymphoid blast crisis of chronic myelogenous leukemia, and lymphoblastic lymphomas. A TdT positive result does not exclude acute myeloid leukemia (AML) as the latter is characterized in some 5% to 10% of cases by TdT positive myeloblasts.

Terminal Deoxynucleotidyl Transferase (TdT) in Hematologic Disease

Disease	Percent Positive
Acute lymphoblastic leukemia	>90
Lymphoblastic lymphoma	90
Chronic granulocytic leukemia in blast crisis	30
Acute undifferentiated leukemia	60
Acute nonlymphocytic leukemia	2-5

Adapted from Rubin E, MD and Farber JL, MD, *Pathology*, 2nd ed, Philadelphia, PA: JB Lippincott Co, 1994, 1077.

Limitations TdT-positive blasts are seen commonly in the bone marrow recovery phase postchemotherapy for ALL (a small number of TdT-positive cells cannot be considered as indicative of residual disease or relapse).[1]

Methodology Enzyme-linked immunosorbent assay (ELISA), indirect fluorescent antibody (IFA), peroxidase-antiperoxidase, avidin-biotin, immunoperoxidase, and incorporation of radiolabeled thymidine. A variety of methods for the enzyme assay of Ficoll/Hypaque® separated cell extracts have been described. The radiometric assays are technically difficult and are usually available only in a research setting. Avidin-biotin immunoperoxidase[2] and flow cytometric[3] methods have been developed.

Additional Information TdT acts to catalyze the polymerization of deoxynucleoside triphosphates (by addition to the 3' hydroxyl ends of oligodeoxynucleotides or polydeoxynucleotides without DNA template instructions). Thymus is the primary site of TdT-positive cells and TdT is found in the nucleus of the more primitive T cells. A thymus related population of TdT-positive cells resides in the bone marrow (normally a minor population - 1% to 2%). TdT is increased in more than 90% of the cases of ALL of childhood. This is true for even pre-B cell as well as B-cell ALL.[4] A minor (5% to 10%) population of patients with acute nonlymphoblastic leukemia have TdT-positive blasts. TdT-positive blasts are prominent in some cases of chronic myelogenous leukemia relating to the development of an acute blast phase. TdT-positive cases of blast phase CML correlate with a positive response to chemotherapy (vincristine and prednisone).[5] Combined assessment of nuclear TdT and cell surface antigens may assist in the detection of minimal residual disease after therapy of acute leukemia.[6] A 1991 study of acute myeloid leukemia found that frequency of response to chemotherapy, response duration, and overall survival did not correlate with TdT expression.[7]

TdT assay has been applied to the detection of DNA strand breaks, of importance in the study of apoptosis. See Apoptosis Assays *on page 402*. Substitution of deoxynucleotide by dideoxynucleotide (Digoxigenin DIG™ labeled) allows the fluorescent detection step of the assay to be used in a more quantitative manner (the addition of label to a DNA break is limited to a single nucleotide as chain extension beyond a dideoxynucleotide cannot occur). DNA strand breakage can then be assessed by the mean fluorescence of responding cells as determined by flow cytometry.[8] The assay can be used to evaluate DNA damage occurring in chronic lymphocytic leukemia cells exposed to UV irradiation and the apoptosis-inducing chemotherapeutic agents fludarabine and 2-chloro-2'-deoxyadenosine.[8] Thus, by determining the sensitivity of patient's leukemic lymphocytes to induction of apoptosis, the assay may have value in predicting patient response to therapy.[8]

Footnotes
1. "Acute Lymphoblastic Leukemia," *Practical Diagnosis of Hematologic Disorders*, 3rd ed, Chapter 28, Kjeldsberg C, ed, Chicago, IL: ASCP Press, 2000, 451-2.
2. Miller RT and Groothuis CL, "Improved Avidin-Biotin Immunoperoxidase Method for Terminal Deoxyribonucleotidyl Transferase and Immunophenotypic Characterization of Blood Cells," *Am J Clin Pathol*, 1990, 93(5):670-4.
3. Almasri NM, Iturraspe JA, Benson NA, et al, "Flow Cytometric Analysis of Terminal Deoxynucleotidyl Transferase," *Am J Clin Pathol*, 1991, 95(3):376-80.
4. Michiels JJ, Adriaansen HJ, Hagemeijer A, et al, "TdT Positive B-Cell Acute Lymphoblastic Leukemia (B-ALL) Without Burkitt Characteristics," *Br J Haematol*, 1988, 68(4):423-6.
5. Paciucci PA, Keaveney C, Cuttner J, et al, "Mitoxantrone, Vincristine, and Prednisone in Adults With Relapsed or Primarily Refractory Acute Lymphocytic Leukemia and Terminal Deoxynucleotidyl Transferase Positive Blastic Phase Chronic Myelocytic Leukemia," *Cancer Res*, 1987, 47(19):5234-7.

(Continued)

Terminal Deoxynucleotidyl Transferase (Continued)

6. Drach J, Gattringer C, and Huber H, "Combined Flow Cytometric Assessment of Cell Surface Antigens and Nuclear TdT for the Detection of Minimal Residual Disease in Acute Leukaemia," *Br J Haematol*, 1991, 77(1):37-42.
7. Gucalp R, Paietta E, Weinberg V, et al, "Terminal Transferase Expression in Acute Myeloid Leukaemia: Biology and Prognosis," *Br J Haematol*, 1991, 78(1):48-54.
8. Bromidge TJ, Howe DJ, Johnson SA, et al, "Adaptation of the TdT Assay for Semiquantitative Flow Cytometric Detection of DNA Strand Breaks," *Cytometry*, 1995, 20(3):257-60.

References

Chapman RS, Chresta CM, Herberg AA, et al, "Further Characterization of the *In Situ* Terminal Deoxynucleotidyl Transferase (TdT) Assay for the Flow Cytometric Analysis of Apoptosis in Drug Resistant and Drug Sensitive Leukaemic Cells," *Cytometry*, 1995, 20(3):245-56.

♦ **Terminal Deoxyribonucleotidyl Transferase** *see* Terminal Deoxynucleotidyl Transferase *on page 489*

♦ **Terminal Transferase** *see* Terminal Deoxynucleotidyl Transferase *on page 489*

♦ **Test 1** *see* Sedimentation Rate, Erythrocyte *on page 484*

♦ **Test for Congenital Heinz Body Hemolytic Anemia** *see* Hemoglobin, Unstable, Heat Labile Test *on page 447*

♦ **Tests for Uncommon Inherited Diseases of Metabolism and Cell Structure** *see* Inherited Diseases of Metabolism and Cell Structure *on page 449*

♦ **Tetrazolium Reduction Test** *see* Nitroblue Tetrazolium Test *on page 461*

TGF-β, Serum

Related Information

Apoptosis Assays *on page 402*
Immunoglobulin G Subclasses *on page 536*

Synonyms Transforming Growth Factor β

Applies to Bleomycin-Induced Pulmonary Fibrosis; Chronic Idiopathic Neutropenia; Idiopathic Pulmonary Fibrosis; Opiate Addiction; Platelet Factor 4; SMAD Proteins

Abstract Transforming growth factor β (TGF-β) is an immunoregulatory cytokine, one of a family of polypeptide growth factors. Most cells produce TGF-β and most have TGF-β cell membrane receptors. TGF-β is a multifunctional cytokine with both stimulatory and inhibitory effects on cells, including stimulation of fibroblast proliferation and formation of the extracellular matrix. This cytokine may have an important role in the development of bone marrow fibrosis.

Specimen Serum

Storage Instructions Store at -70°C if assay is to be delayed.

Turnaround Time Days, possibly weeks

Special Instructions Assay is likely to be available only from a research laboratory.

Reference Interval 1.4 ±0.1 ng/mL.[1] Patients with idiopathic myelofibrosis had levels of 53 ±4 ng/mL; those with secondary fibrosis had levels of 37 ±5 ng/mL (results given as mean ±SE).

Use In hematology, evaluation of myelofibrosis (idiopathic and secondary marrow fibrosis); of potential use in evaluation of patients with fibrotic conditions of lung, liver, and/or kidney (eg, idiopathic pulmonary fibrosis and generalized scleroderma)

Methodology Bioassay (growth inhibition of mink lung[1] epithelial cells, CCL 64), appears to measure TGF-β1 isoform; bioassay (suppression of lymphocyte proliferation by thymocytes); radioreceptor assay (inhibition of binding of radiolabeled TGF-β to its receptor); enzyme-linked immunosorbent assay (ELISA), commercially available (Quantikine kit, R & D Systems)[1,2]

Additional Information TGF-βs are pleiotropic factors that have a regulatory role in somatic tissue development and renewal. They are multifunctional signaling molecules. They can have opposite (positive or negative) effects dependent upon the target cell's stage of development or upon its environment. There are three isoforms of TGF-β: TGF-β1, TGF-β2, and TGF-β3, each encoded by a specific gene. Each TGF-β has origin from a precursor molecule and after secretion is stored in the extracellular matrix as a complex of TGF-β, propeptide, and latent TGF-β-binding protein. TGF-β is released from the complex by thrombospondin-1 or by plasmin-mediated cleavage of the complex. TGF-β exerts regulatory influence by binding to cell surface receptors, types I, II, and III. Types I and II receptors include serine-threonine kinases in their intracellular domains that phosphorylate transcription factors known as "SMAD" proteins (1 through 9). After further interaction, type I receptors are phosphorylated, protein kinase activity is stimulated, and the SMAD complex moves into the nucleus where it acts to regulate gene transcription. TGF-β has an important role in cell-cycle regulation and is a potent inhibitor of cell proliferation. TGF-β has a number of effects on tumor cell growth, on fibroblasts, on the induction of fibrotic disease, and on atherosclerosis (acting as an inhibitor of this process). Mutations in the type II receptor gene render smooth muscle/endothelial cells resistant to the antiproliferative and apoptotic effects of TGF-β. The surprisingly broad involvement of TGF-β in these and other human developmental and disease processes are detailed in a recent review.[3]

TGF-β is one of a number of cytokines involved in the regulation of hematopoiesis.[4] TGF-β is elevated in the sera of patients with marrow fibrosis including both idiopathic myelofibrosis and secondary marrow fibrosis.[1,5]

Serum TGF-β1 is increased in patients with chronic idiopathic neutropenia along with increase in serum IgA but decreased IgG3.[6] In a study of thrombopoietin mRNA expression, it was found that platelet factor 4, thrombospondin, and TGF-β were negative modulators of megakaryocytopoiesis.[7]

TGF-β is involved in the regulation of inflammation. Opiate addicts are prone to infections, partly due to opiate-induced macrophage apoptosis which is enhanced by TGF-β (and inhibited by anti-TGF-β antibody).[8] TGF-β inhibits lipopolysaccharide-stimulated expression of inflammatory cytokines.[9]

Some studies of idiopathic pulmonary fibrosis indicate involvement of TGF-β1.[10] In a bleomycin-induced model of lung fibrosis and in a long-term study of patients with idiopathic pulmonary fibrosis interferon, gamma-1b (plus prednisolone) was associated with clinical improvement in the latter, and down regulation of transcription of the gene for TGF-β1 in the former.[10]

Footnotes

1. Rameshwar P, Chang VT, Thacker UF, et al, "Systemic Transforming Growth Factor-Beta in Patients With Bone Marrow Fibrosis - Pathophysiological Implications," *Am J Hematol*, 1998, 59(2):133-42.
2. Sturm A, Schulte C, Schatton R, et al, "Transforming Growth Factor-Beta and Hepatocyte Growth Factor Plasma Levels in Patients With Inflammatory Bowel Disease," *Eur J Gastroenterol Hepatol*, 2000, 12(4):445-50.
3. Blobe GC, Schiemann WP, and Lodish HF, "Role of Transforming Growth Factor β in Human Disease," *N Engl J Med*, 2000, 342(18):1350-8.
4. Fortunel NO, Hatzfeld A, and Hatzfeld JA, "Transforming Growth Factor-β: Pleiotropic Role in the Regulation of Hematopoiesis," *Blood*, 2000, 96(6):2022-36.
5. Rameshwar P, Denny TN, Stein D, et al, "Monocyte Adhesion in Patients With Bone Marrow Fibrosis Is Required for the Production of Fibrogenic Cytokines. Potential Role for IL-1 and TGF-β," *J Immunol*, 1994, 153(6):2819-30.
6. Papadaki HA, Palmblad J, Kapsimali V, et al, "Increased Serum IgA and Decreased IgG3 Strongly Correlate With Increased Serum TGF-β1 Levels in Patients With Nonimmune Chronic Idiopathic Neutropenia of Adults," *Eur J Haematol*, 2000, 65(3):237-44.
7. Sungaran R, Chisholm OT, Markovic B, et al, "The Role of Platelet α-Granular Proteins in the Regulation of Thrombopoietin Messenger RNA Expression in Human Bone Marrow Stromal Cells," *Blood*, 2000, 95(10):3094-101.
8. Singhal PC, Kapasi AA, Franki N, et al, "Morphine-Induced Macrophage Apoptosis: The Role of Transforming Growth Factor-β," *Immunology*, 2000, 100(1):57-62.
9. Imai K, Takeshita A, and Hanazawa S, "Transforming Growth Factor-β Inhibits Lipopolysaccharide-Stimulated Expression of Inflammatory Cytokines in Mouse Macrophages Through Downregulation of Activation Protein 1 and CD14 Receptor Expression," *Infect Immun*, 2000, 68(5):2418-23.
10. Ziesche R, Hofbauer E, Wittmann K, et al, "A Preliminary Study of Long-Term Treatment With Interferon Gamma-1b and Low-Dose Prednisolone in Patients With Idiopathic Pulmonary Fibrosis," *N Engl J Med*, 1999, 341(17):1264-9.

References

Fox HS, "Cytokines and Cell Adhesion Molecules," *Clinical Diagnosis and Management by Laboratory Methods*, 19th ed, Chapter 37, Henry JB, ed, Philadelphia, PA: WB Saunders Co, 1996, 947-8.

Gauldie J, Sime PJ, Xing Z, et al, "Transforming Growth Factor-β Gene Transfer to the Lung Induces Myofibroblast Presence and Pulmonary Fibrosis," *Tissue Repair and Fibrosis. The Role of the Myofibroblast*, Desmouliére A and Tuchweber B, eds, New York, NY: Springer-Verlag, 1999, 93:35-45.

Narani N, Arora PD, Lew A, et al, "Transforming Growth Factor-β Induction of α-Smooth Muscle Actin Is Dependent on the Deformability of the Collagen Matrix," *Curr Top Pathol*, 1999, 93:47-60.

Wahl SM and Dougherty SF, "Measurement of Transforming Growth Factor β," *Current Protocols in Immunology*, Coligan JE, Kruisbeek AM, Margulies DH, et al, eds, 1991, 6.11.1-.6.

Zhou S, Kinzler KW, and Vogelstein B, "Going Mad With *SMADS*," *N Engl J Med*, 1999, 341(15):1144-5.

♦ **Thanatosomes** *see* Apoptosis Assays *on page 402*

♦ **Thermal Sensitivity Test** *see* Peripheral Blood: Red Blood Cell Morphology *on page 467*

♦ **Thiazole Orange** *see* Reticulated Platelet Count *on page 480*

♦ **Thoracentesis Fluid Analysis** *see* Body Fluid Analysis, Cell Count *on page 408*

Thorn Test

Related Information

Corticotropin Stimulation Test (Rapid) *on page 153*
Cortisol, Serum or Plasma *on page 154*
Eosinophil Count *on page 424*

Synonyms Adrenal Function Eosinophil Count

Abstract Eosinophil count is performed before and 4 hours following an injection of ACTH as a biological indicator of adrenocortical function. Relative eosinophilia may reflect functional deficiency of glucocorticoids in cases of partial hypothalamic-pituitary-adrenal failure during severe stress.[1]

Patient Preparation Hold breakfast. Draw blood for initial eosinophil count. Give 250 μg (for standard dose) or 1 μg (for low dose) ACTH intramuscularly. May eat breakfast. Hold lunch. Repeat eosinophil count 4 hours after ACTH is given. May have lunch after second count is taken.

Specimen Whole blood

Container Lavender top (EDTA) tube

Causes for Rejection Patient not fasting

Use This test is of largely historical interest.

Limitations The test is rather antiquated and nonspecific. Addison disease is most appropriately diagnosed using modern ACTH and cortisol levels. Borderline values are further investigated by stimulation tests of the pituitary and adrenals.

Additional Information If adrenal cortical function is normal, the eosinophil count will act as follows: The eosinophil count before the injection will be about twice the value of the eosinophil count after the injection (eg, eosinophil count of 200 before injection vs 100 after injection). If the adrenal cortical function is decreased, eosinophil count before the injection will be approximately the same as the eosinophil count after the injection (eg, eosinophil count before the injection of 200, after the injection, 195). When adrenal cortical function is decreased, it indicates hypoadrenalism (Addison disease). There is evidence that a low-dose Thorn test is better able than the standard dose test to detect relative adrenocortical insufficiency in critically ill patients.[1]

Footnotes

1. Beishuizen A and Vermes I, "Relative Eosinophilia (Thorn Test) as a Bioassay to Judge the Clinical Relevance of Cortisol Values During Severe Stress," *J Clin Endocrinol Metab*, 1999, 84(9):3400.

References

McNeely JC and Brown D, "Laboratory Evaluation of Leukocytes," *Clinical Hematology: Principles, Procedures, Correlations*, Chapter 25, Lotspeich-Steininger CA, Stiene-Martin EA, and Koepke JA, eds, Philadelphia, PA: JB Lippincott Co, 1992, 331.

♦ **Thrombocyte Count** *see* Platelet Count *on page 468*

Thrombopoietin, Serum or Plasma

Related Information

Erythropoietin, Serum *on page 169*
Platelet Count *on page 468*
Platelet Sizing *on page 471*
Reticulated Platelet Count *on page 480*

Synonyms c-mpl-Ligand (ligand for the receptor encoded by the *c-mpl* proto-oncogene); Megakaryocyte Growth and Differentiation Factor; Megapoietin; MGDF; *mpl*-Ligand; TPO

Applies to Hereditary Thrombocythemia; Interleukin 3; Interleukin 6; Interleukin 11; Kawasaki Disease; Steel Factor

Abstract Thrombopoietin, a cytokine glycoprotein, is the primary regulator of marrow megakaryocyte and platelet development. Thrombopoietin levels may indicate whether a patient has thrombocytopenia on the basis of failure of marrow production (decrease in thrombopoietin effect) or increase in peripheral platelet destruction.

Specimen Serum or EDTA plasma; sample requirements may be method dependent. A correlation has been reported between TPO values in serum and plasma (serum TPO = -0.257 + 4.039 x plasma TPO values).[1]

Storage Instructions Stable for up to 6 days in platelet poor and in platelet-rich plasma.[2] For prolonged storage, remove serum from cells and store at -30°C.[1] Free TPO is evidently quite stable. Repeated freeze/thaw (up to nine times) of EDTA plasma did not effect TPO levels. The interval between specimen collection and plasma separation (up to 25 hours) did not effect plasma TPO levels.[3]

Reference Interval

- Male: 0.79 ±0.35 fmol/mL; female: 0.70 ±0.26 fmol/mL[4]
- Cord blood: 3.73 ±1.48 fmol/mL
- 5 days: 4.32 ±0.94 fmol/mL
- 1 month: 3.77 ±1.45 fmol/mL
- 2-11 months: 2.10 ±0.69 fmol/mL
- 1-2 years: 2.23 ±0.89 fmol/mL
- 3-15 years: 1.97 ±0.67 to 1.24 ±0.40 fmol/mL[1]

Mean adult normal value (using plasma) has been noted as 133 pg/mL (range of 57-377).[5]

Use May be helpful in determining the etiology of thrombocytopenia.

Methodology Enzyme-linked immunosorbent assay (ELISA) for recombinant TPO (rhTPO) using a murine monoclonal antibody (Ab) as capture Ab and biotinylated rabbit polyclonal Ab as detector.[2] A number of TPO ELISA assays using serum and/or plasma have been developed. Results/normal ranges may not be directly comparable.[3,4,5,6,7,8] An ELISA Kit is available commercially (R & D Systems, Abington, UK).

This method uses a murine antihuman TPO monoclonal antibody for capture and peroxidase-conjugated anti-TPO-monoclonal antibody for detection.[9]

Additional Information Humoral control of the growth and development of megakaryocytes (and their platelet progeny) has undergone partial definition only gradually over the past 30 some years. Multiple growth factors (protein regulators - cytokines) are involved. The identification and cloning of many human hematopoietic growth factors (and the availability of their recombinant forms) in the 1980s/1990s has allowed new insight into cytokine control of megakaryocytopoiesis. In particular, interleukin-3 (IL-3), granulocyte/monocyte colony stimulating factor (GM-CSF), interleukin-6 (IL-

6), interleukin-11 (IL-11), and others contribute to multifactorial synergistic control of megakaryocytopoiesis (see figure).

The Role of Cytokines in Megakaryocytopoiesis

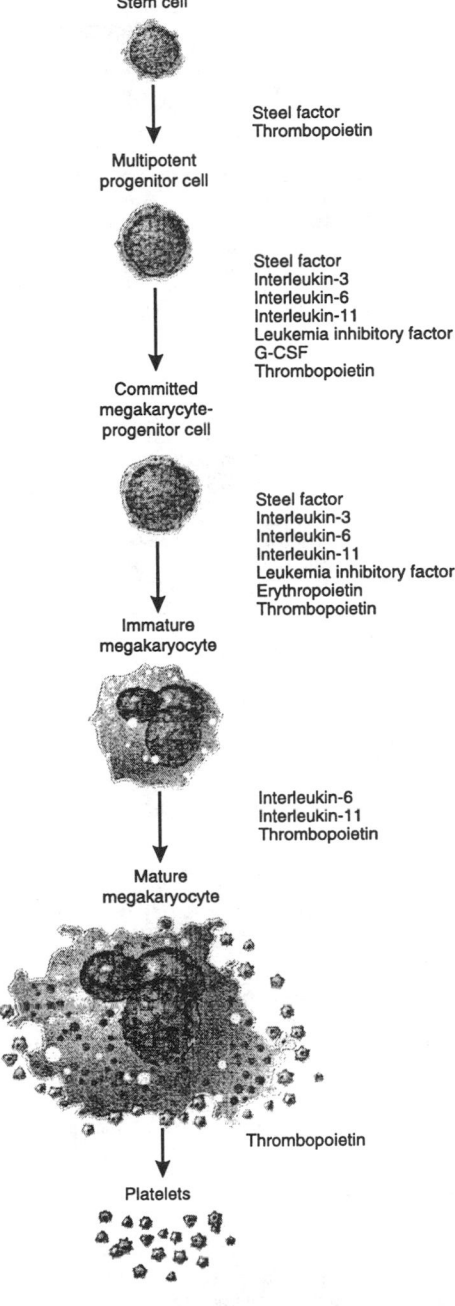

Many stages of megakaryocyte development can be affected by several cytokines *in vitro*, including steel factor (also termed stem-cell factor, mast-cell growth factor, or Kit ligand), interleukin-3, interleukin-6, interleukin-11, granulocyte colony-stimulating factor (G-CSF), erythropoietin, leukemia inhibitory factor, and thrombopoietin. Although these cytokines support several aspects of megakaryocyte development *in vitro*, genetic elimination of only steel factor or thrombopoietin affects megakaryocyte and platelet production *in vivo*.

Adapted from Kaushansky K, "Thrombopoietin," *N Engl J Med*, 1998, 339(11):746-54.

These growth factors, however, are not megakaryocyte/platelet lineage specific and, as in the case of IL-3, individually may not affect *in vivo* platelet production.[10] IL-3 is produced by antigen-activated T lymphocytes consistent with the platelet's role in inflammatory processes (in addition to its essential procoagulant activities). IL-11 has been shown (in mice) to increase megakaryocyte progenitors, nuclear polyploidy, and peripheral platelet counts.[11] Approval has been given for the use of IL-11 in treatment of chemotherapy-induced thrombocytopenia.

Early thrombopoietin (TPO) assays lacked specificity due to the interplay of pleiotropic cytokines (IL-3, IL-11, etc). Doubt about the existence of a lineage-specific megakaryocyte platelet humoral regulator was allayed (Continued)

Thrombopoietin, Serum or Plasma (Continued)

when a transforming oncogene of the virus that induces myeloproliferative leukemia (MPL), in mice, was found also in humans (over time) to have characteristics consistent with the TPO receptor.[6] In particular, antisense oligonucleotides against *c-mpl* RNA were shown to inhibit *in vitro* mega-karyocytopoiesis.[12] Thus, TPO (the ligand) was identified (cloned in 1994) only after its receptor (*c-mpl*) was discovered and cloned.

TPO is now recognized as the lineage specific and most important mega-karyocyte/platelet regulatory protein. TPO is a 90-kDa glycoprotein encoded by a gene located on chromosome 3 (3q 26-27). cDNA for human TPO indicates that it is a polypeptide formed of 353 amino acids. There are two domains. The amino terminal (155 residues with 21% erythropoietin sequence identity) domain binds to the *c-mpl* receptor. The carboxyterminal 177 residues decrease bioavailability after parenteral administration. Two forms of TPO have been produced for clinical study. One form, recombinant human TPO consists of the full-length polypeptide. The other form consists of the receptor-binding region only, chemically modified by the addition of polyethylene glycol (PEG) and referred to as PEG-conjugated recombinant human megakaryocyte growth and development factor, a "pegylated" mole-cule.

Thrombopoietin acts to increase the number and size of megakaryocytes, stimulates polyploidy, stimulates megakaryocyte colony formation, and acts in synergy with other cytokines (including IL-3, IL-11, and erythropoietin) to stimulate megakaryocyte and erythroid progenitor cell growth as well as hematopoietic stem-cell proliferation and survival.[13] With a lag period of some 6-16 days, TPO produces an increase in platelet count and causes increase in platelet activation.

Platelets remove and degrade TPO by receptor binding and internalization. Unbound TPO is quite stable.[3] TPO is degraded in a time-dependent manner and is not recycled to the surface.[2] The resultant plasma survival half-life is some 20-30 hours.[14] Data indicates that the level of TPO is regulated by its binding to platelets and/or megakaryocytes (the platelet/megakaryocyte mass itself is the key regulator of TPO serum/plasma levels).[2] When the platelet mass is normal (remains constant), circulating TPO is at a basal equilibrium level. With decrease in platelet mass (throm-bocytopenia uncompensated by enlarged size of platelets) there is decreased binding of TPO (and subsequent degradation by *c-mpl*-positive cells) with resultant increase in free TPO. Reactive thrombocytosis, conversely, is occasioned by decreased levels of TPO. In chronic idiopathic thrombocytopenic purpura (in which megakaryocytes are increased), TPO levels are normal or decreased.

The existence of receptor (*c-mpl*)-mediated degradation of TPO indicates that in chemotherapy patients platelet transfusions may delay the recovery of megakaryocytes. TPO levels are inversely correlated with the platelet mass. In myelodysplastic syndrome (MDS), TPO levels correlated inversely with the platelet count in refractory anemia (RA) but not in RA with excess of blasts (RAEB) or RA with excess of blasts in transformation (RAEB-T).[15] In a recent study involving 52 MDS patients, while the mean TPO level was increased and levels in patients with RAEB were generally low, TPO levels were heterogeneous and did not correlate with platelet counts.[16]

A study of the mechanism of thrombocytopenia in cirrhosis of the liver (by measuring reticulated platelets and thrombopoietin levels) found that there was decreased TPO production by the liver as well as increase in platelet sequestration in the spleen.[17] Numerous studies attest to the diagnostic value of measuring TPO levels for the evaluation of thrombocytopenia, in which decreased platelet production is associated with increased serum/plasma TPO.[18]

In the term and preterm newborn, changes in the relation of TPO levels to thrombocytopenia are similar to those occurring in adults, TPO levels decreasing with resolution of thrombocytopenia.[19]

Patients with systemic sclerosis (scleroderma) have been reported to have higher TPO levels than normal controls and patients with rheumatoid arthritis, using a commercially available ELISA kit (Quantikine, R & D Systems, Minneapolis, MN). Possibly, TPO-mediated release of growth factors (eg, transforming growth factor-β, interleukin 6, platelet derived-growth factor, and others) induce the fibrosis that is the hallmark of systemic sclerosis.[20]

The relation of TPO levels to myeloproliferative disorders is uncertain and significantly variable. Reactive thrombocytosis and essential thrombocy-themia (a myeloproliferative disorder) are not differentiated by TPO levels. Nevertheless, impaired expression of the thrombopoietin receptor and receptor glycation defects have been described in platelets from patients with polycythemia vera.[21,22] While an inverse correlation between serum TPO level and platelet count in essential thrombocythemia (ET) has been noted,[23] the disease is heterogeneous[24] and an uncertain number of cases apparently do not have a clonal disorder.[25] Hereditary thrombocythemia (HT), not the same disorder as ET, is a rare condition, has a constant association with increased serum/plasma TPO, and in some families, is transmitted as an autosomal dominant trait. Some 12 families with HT have been identified. Sporadic cases of ET with mutation of the thrombopoietin gene are reported.[26,27]

Elevation of serum TPO has been noted to precede thrombocytosis in Kawasaki disease[28] and to occur in thrombocytosis associated with inflam-matory bowel disease.[29] The latter finding may be of pathogenetic signifi-cance to the risk of thromboembolic complications in Crohn disease and ulcerative colitis.[29]

The therapeutic use of thrombopoietin may be limited by concern over inducing thrombocytosis with attendant risk for thrombosis (which may occur in patients with myeloproliferative disorders).[14]

Footnotes

1. Ishiguro A, Nakahata T, Matsubara K, et al, "Age-Related Changes in Thrombo-poietin in Children: Reference Interval for Serum Thrombopoietin Levels," *Br J Haematol*, 1999, 106(4):884-8.
2. Li J, Xia Y, and Kuter D, "Interaction of Thrombopoietin With the Platelet *c-mpl* Receptor in Plasma: Binding, Internalization, Stability and Pharmacokinetics," *Br J Haematol*, 1999, 106(2):345-56.
3. Folman CC, von dem Borne AE, Rensink IH, et al, "Sensitive Measurement of Thrombopoietin by a Monoclonal Antibody Based Sandwich Enzyme-Linked Immu-nosorbent Assay," *Thromb Haemost*, 1997, 78(4):1262-7.
4. Tahara T, Usuki K, Sato H, et al, "A Sensitive Sandwich ELISA for Measuring Thrombopoietin in Human Serum: Serum Thrombopoietin Levels in Healthy Volun-teers and in Patients With Haemopoietic Disorders," *Br J Haematol*, 1996, 93(4):783-8.
5. Moliterno AR, Hankins WD, and Spivak JL, "Impaired Expression of the Thrombo-poietin Receptor by Platelets From Patients With Polycythemia Vera," *N Engl J Med*, 1998, 338(9):572-80.
6. Kojima S, Matsuyama T, Kodera Y, et al, "Measurement of Endogenous Plasma Thrombopoietin in Patients With Acquired Aplastic Anaemia by a Sensitive Enzyme-Linked Immunosorbent Assay," *Br J Haematol*, 1997, 97(3):538-43.
7. Marsh JC, Gibson FM, Prue RL, et al, "Serum Thrombopoietin Levels in Patients With Aplastic Anaemia," *Br J Haematol*, 1996, 95(4):605-10.
8. Emmons RV, Reid DM, Cohen RL, et al, "Human Thrombopoietin Levels Are High When Thrombocytopenia Is Due to Megakaryocyte Deficiency and Low When Due to Increased Platelet Destruction," *Blood*, 1996, 87(10):4068-71.
9. Harrison CN, Gale RE, Pezella F, et al, "Platelet *c-mpl* Expression Is Dysregulated in Patients With Essential Thrombocythaemia but This Is Not of Diagnostic Value," *Br J Haematol*, 1999, 107(1):139-47.
10. Lindemann A, Ganser A, Herrmann F, et al, "Biologic Effects of Recombinant Human Interleukin-3 *In Vivo*," *J Clin Oncol*, 1991, 9(12):2120-7.
11. Neben TY, Loebelenz J, Hayes L, et al, "Recombinant Human Interleukin-11 Stimulates Megakaryocytopoiesis and Increases Peripheral Platelets in Normal and Splenectomized Mice," *Blood*, 1993, 81(4):901-8.
12. Methia N, Louache F, Vainchenker W, et al, "Oligodeoxynucleotides Antisense to the Proto-oncogene *c-mpl* Specifically Inhibit *In Vitro* Megakaryocytopoiesis," *Blood*, 1993, 82(5):1395-401.
13. Kaushansky K, "Thrombopoietin," *N Engl J Med*, 1998, 339(11):746-54.
14. Vadhan-Raj S, Murray LJ, Bueso-Ramos C, et al, "Stimulation of Megakaryocyte and Platelet Production by a Single Dose of Recombinant Human Thrombopoietin in Patients With Cancer," *Ann Intern Med*, 1997, 126(9):673-81.
15. Tamura H, Ogata K, Nakamura K, et al, "Plasma Thrombopoietin (TPO) Levels and Expression of TPO Receptor on Platelets in Patients With Myelodysplastic Syndromes," *Br J Haematol*, 1998, 103(3):778-84.
16. Hellström-Lindberg E, Kanter-Lewensohn L, Nichol J, et al, "Spontaneous and Cytokine-Induced Thrombocytopenia in Myelodysplastic Syndromes: Serum Thrombopoietin Levels and Bone Marrow Morphology," *Br J Haematol*, 1999, 105(4):966-73.
17. Koike Y, Yoneyama A, Shirai J, et al, "Evaluation of Thrombopoiesis in Thrombocy-topenic Disorders by Simultaneous Measurement of Reticulated Platelets of Whole Blood and Serum Thrombopoietin Concentrations," *Thromb Haemost*, 1998, 79(6):1106-10.
18. Porcelijn L, Folman CC, Bossers B, et al, "The Diagnostic Value of Thrombopoietin Level Measurements in Thrombocytopenia," *Thromb Haemost*, 1998, 79(6):1101-5.
19. Albert TS, Meng YG, Simms P, et al, "Thrombopoietin in the Thrombocytopenic Term and Preterm Newborn," *Pediatrics*, 2000, 105(6):1286-91.
20. Ertenli I, Kiraz S, Ertürk H, et al, "Circulating Thrombopoietin in Systemic Scle-rosis," *J Rheumatol*, 1999, 26(1):1939-41.
21. Moliterno AR, Hankins WD, and Spivak JL, "Impaired Expression of the Thrombo-poietin Receptor by Platelets From Patients With Polycythemia Vera," *N Engl J Med*, 1998, 338(9):572-80.
22. Moliterno AR and Spivak JL, "Post-translational Processing of the Thrombopoietin Receptor Is Impaired in Polycythemia Vera," *Blood*, 1999, 94(8):2555-61.
23. Tomita N, Motomura S, Sakai R, et al, "Strong Inverse Correlation Between Serum TPO Level and Platelet Count in Essential Thrombocythemia," *Am J Hematol*, 2000, 63(3):131-5.
24. Nimer SD, "Essential Thrombocythemia: Another "Heterogeneous Disease" Better Understood?" *Blood*, 1999, 93(2):415-6.
25. Harrison CN, Gale RE, Machin SJ, et al, "A Large Proportion of Patients With a Diagnosis of Essential Thrombocythemia Do Not Have a Clonal Disorder and May Be at Lower Risk of Thrombotic Complications," *Blood*, 93(2):417-24.
26. Kondo T, Okabe M, Sanada M, et al, "Familial Essential Thrombocythemia Associ-ated With One-Base Deletion in the 5'-Untranslated Region of the *Thrombopoietin* Gene," *Blood*, 1998, 92(4):1091-6.
27. Ghilardi N, Wiestner A, Kikuchi M, et al, "Hereditary Thrombocythaemia in a Japanese Family Is Caused by a Novel Point Mutation in the Thrombopoietin Gene," *Br J Haematol*, 1999, 107(2):310-6.
28. Ishiguro A, Ishikita T, Shimbo T, et al, "Elevation of Serum Thrombopoietin Precedes Thrombocytosis in Kawasaki Disease," *Thromb Haemost*, 1998, 79(6):1096-100.
29. Heits F, Stahl M, Ludwig D, et al, "Elevated Serum Thrombopoietin and Interleukin-6 Concentrations in Thrombocytosis Associated With Inflammatory Bowel Disease," *J Interferon Cytokine Res*, 1999, 19(7):757-60.

References

Cerutti A, Custodi P, Mduranti, et al, "Circulating Thrombopoietin in Reactive Conditions Behaves Like an Acute Phase Reactant," *Clin Lab Haematol*, 1999, 21(4):271-5.

Drachman JG, "Role of Thrombopoietin in Hematopoietic Stem Cell and Progenitor Regulation," *Curr Opin Hematol*, 2000, 7(3):183-90.

Kaushansky K, "Use of Thrombopoietic Growth Factors in Acute Leukemia," *Leukemia*, 2000, 14(3):505-8.

Kaushansky K, "Thrombopoietin: Understanding and Manipulating Platelet Production," *Annu Rev Med*, 1997, 48:1-11.

Long MW and Hoffman R, "Thrombocytopoiesis," *Hematology: Basic Principles and Practice*, 3rd ed, Chapter 17, Hoffman R, and Benz EJ Jr, Shattil SJ, eds, New York, NY: Churchill Livingstone, 2000, 245-60.

Matsumoto A, Tahara T, Morita H, et al, "Characterization of Native Human Thrombopoietin in the Blood of Normal Individuals and of Patients With Haematologic Disorders," *Thromb Haemost*, 1999, 82(1):24-9.

Schiffer CA, Miller K, Larson RA, et al, "A Double-Blind, Placebo-Controlled Trial of Pegylated Recombinant Human Megakaryocyte Growth and Development Factor as an Adjunct to Induction and Consolidation Therapy for Patients With Acute Myeloid Leukemia," *Blood*, 2000, 95(8):2530-5.

Schulze H, Ballmaier M, Welte K, et al, "Thrombopoietin Induces the Generation of Distinct Stat1, Stat3, Stat5a, and Stat5b Homo- and Heterodimeric Complexes With Different Kinetics in Human Platelets," *Exp Hematol*, 2000, 28(3):294-304.

Stenberg PE and Hill RJ, "Platelets and Megakaryocytes," *Wintrobe's Clinical Hematology*, 10th ed, Volume 1, Chapter 22, Lee GR, Foerster J, Lukens J, et al, eds, Baltimore, MD: Williams & Wilkins, 1999, 637-41.

Tafuri A, Lemoli RM, Petrucci MT, et al, "Thrombopoietin and Interleukin 11 Have Different Modulatory Effects on Cell Cycle and Programmed Cell Death in Primary Acute Myeloid Leukemia Cells," *Exp Hematol*, 1999, 27(8):1255-63.

Vadhan-Raj S, "Clinical Experience With Recombinant Human Thrombopoietin in Chemotherapy-Induced Thrombocytopenia," *Semin Hematol*, 2000, 37(2 Suppl 4):28-34.

Verbeek W, Faulhaber M, Griesinger F, et al, "Measurement of Thrombopoietic Levels: Clinical and Biological Relationships," *Curr Opin Hematol*, 2000, 7(3):143-9.

♦ **TPO** *see* Thrombopoietin, Serum or Plasma *on page 491*

♦ **Transcobalamins** *see* Vitamin B$_{12}$ Unsaturated Binding Capacity *on page 495*

Transferrin Receptor, Soluble, Serum or Plasma

Related Information

Anemia Flowchart *on page 392*
Ferritin, Serum *on page 173*
Hereditary Hemochromatosis DNA Test *on page 709*
Iron and Total Iron Binding Capacity/Transferrin, Serum *on page 203*
Protoporphyrin, Free Erythrocyte *on page 269*
Reticulocyte Hemoglobin Content *on page 482*

Synonyms Circulating Transferrin Receptor; Serum Transferrin Receptor; Soluble Serum Transferrin Receptor; sTfR

Abstract Soluble transferrin receptor (sTfR) has origin from red blood cell precursors (normoblasts) and is found in the circulation. It is a truncated form of the cellular transferrin receptor.[1] As iron deficiency develops, the number of cellular transferrin receptors increases, and this is reflected by an increased plasma concentration of sTfR. The test has application in differentiating iron deficiency anemia (sTfR usually increased) from the anemia of chronic disease (sTfR usually normal). Serum sTfR is also increased in conditions of high turnover erythropoiesis (eg, hemolytic anemia). The role of sTfR in routine clinical practice is not fully defined.

Specimen Serum or plasma

Container Red top tube, lavender top (EDTA) tube, or green top (heparin) tube

Collection Separate from cells within 30 minutes and freeze.

Storage Instructions Specimen is stable for 30 minutes at ambient temperature and indefinitely when frozen. Avoid repeated freeze/thaw cycles.

Causes for Rejection Severe hemolysis, icterus, or lipemia

Reference Interval Check with the testing laboratory as reference intervals and units vary greatly due to intermethod standardization differences (eg, purified tissue receptor vs transferrin receptor complex vs purified soluble serum receptor).

An overall reference interval of 9.6-29.6 nmol/L is reported from a study of 225 healthy, adult subjects without hematological abnormalities.[2] This study found no differences in reference intervals as a function of either age or sex. However, black subjects and inhabitants at high altitude had higher sTfR levels than comparable groups of nonblack subjects and sea level inhabitants.

In another study of 204 nonanemic adults that used a different assay method, an upper reference limit of 2.8 mg/L was reported.[3]

Reference interval data in infants and children are limited. In one study of normal infants 9-15 months of age, mean (±SD) sTfR plasma concentrations of 4.4±1.1 mg/L were reported.[4] In another study of healthy, pubertal boys averaging 11.7-13.6 years of age, mean serum sTfR concentrations ranged from 6.9-8.0 mg/L.[5]

Reference range as provided with a commercially available method "Quantikine sTfR," R&D systems, Minneapolis, MN is 8.8-28.1 nmol/L. Reference range provided with another commercially available method "The Ramco TfR," Ramco Laboratories, Houston, TX is 2.9-8.3 µg/mL.

Use This relatively new test is proposed as a sensitive, early indicator of iron deficiency. A specificity of 100% for iron deficiency was reported from a study of 223 pregnant women.[6] In a study of 51 patients with chronic liver disease, the reported sensitivity for the diagnosis of iron deficiency was 91.6% and the specificity was 84.6%.[7]

In a study of 145 anemic patients, investigators used serum ferritin as a first-line test: ferritin values <25 µg/L were classified as iron deficiency, and ferritin values >300 µg/L were interpreted as excluding the possibility of iron deficiency. sTfR testing was used for patients with ferritin values in between these extremes. An elevated sTfR indicated iron deficiency and a normal sTfR was interpreted as excluding iron deficiency.[8]

Evaluation of iron restricted erythropoiesis. Guide to need for intravenous administration of iron to ensure adequate iron replacement. Of use in prediction of the erythropoietic response to increased erythropoietin dosage (in conjunction with use of serum ferritin and reticulocyte hemoglobin content). Assist in monitoring response to erythropoietin therapy.

The ultimate usefulness of this test may be limited by the large number of conditions, other than iron deficiency, in which elevated values are obtained (see Limitations).

Limitations The differential diagnosis of increased sTfR includes autoimmune hemolytic anemia, recent blood donation, recent blood loss, sickle cell anemia, hereditary spherocytosis, β-thalassemia, α-thalassemia, polycythemia vera, and other hematological malignancies, vitamin B$_{12}$ deficiency, and folic acid deficiency. This broad differential indicates lack of specificity if the test is utilized for general hematologic diagnosis.

Methodology Enzyme-linked immunosorbent assay (ELISA)

Additional Information Transferrin receptor was isolated from the serum in 1990[1] using monoclonal antibodies and immunoaffinity chromatography after report of its initial detection in 1986.[9] The serum receptor, smaller than its cell membrane counterpart, is apparently a soluble fragment of the complete molecule, missing the first 100 amino acid residues, and resulting from proteolytic cleavage by a serine protease.[10] The intact cell transferrin receptor is formed of 1520 amino acid residues and consists of two disulfide-linked monomers with intracellular, transmembrane, and extracellular domains. The soluble fragment consists of the major portion of the extracellular domains of the two monomers, thus, it is a truncated form of the cell tissue receptor.

Investigators have proposed that sTfR values may be used to assess erythropoiesis in patients with sickle cell disease or thalassemia undergoing chronic transfusion therapy.[11,12]

In iron overload states, sTfR values are decreased.[13,14] The clinical utility of this observation is not known.

The measurement of sTfR to assess anemia in rheumatoid arthritis and other inflammatory conditions is superior to traditional tests (eg, ferritin, transferrin, TIBC), because sTfR is unaffected by the acute-phase response. In a recent study, TfR's ability to discriminate between iron deficiency anemia (IDA) and anemia of chronic disease (ACD) using indicators of iron status (serum iron concentration, total iron binding capacity, and % transferrin saturation) and of RBC size (MCV and RDW) was examined. Statistical study, including receiver operating characteristic curve analysis, showed that ability to discriminate decreased in the order: TIBC > TfR > MCV > %TS=RDW > SIC. Area under the curve values for TIBC and TfR were not significantly different.[15] TIBC and TfR measures provided the highest (and similar) ability to discriminate between IDA and ACD, although data is derived from a small sample.

Footnotes

1. Shih YJ, Baynes RD, Hudson BG, et al, "Serum Transferrin Receptor Is a Truncated Form of Tissue Receptor," *J Biol Chem*, 1990, 265(31):19077-81.
2. Allen J, Backstrom KR, Cooper JA, et al, "Measurement of Soluble Transferrin Receptor in Serum of Healthy Adults," *Clin Chem*, 1998, 44(1):35-9.
3. Mast AE, Blinder MA, Gronowski AM, et al, "Clinical Utility of the Soluble Transferrin Receptor and Comparison With Serum Ferritin in Several Populations," *Clin Chem*, 1998, 44(1):45-51.
4. Yeung GS and Zlotkin SH, "Percentile Estimates for Transferrin Receptor in Normal Infants 9-15 Mo of Age," *Am J Clin Nutr*, 1997, 66(2):342-6.
5. Anttila R, Cook JD, and Siimes MA, "Body Iron Stores in Relation to Growth and Pubertal Maturation in Healthy Boys," *Br J Haematol*, 1997, 96:(1)12-8.
6. Akesson A, Bjellerup P, Berglund M, et al, "Serum Transferrin Receptor: A Specific Marker of Iron Deficiency in Pregnancy," *Am J Clin Nutr*, 1998, 68(6):1241-6.
7. Nagral A, Mehta AB, Gomes ATB, et al, "Serum Soluble Transferrin Receptor in the Diagnosis of Iron Deficiency in Chronic Liver Disease," *Clin Lab Haematol*, 1999, 21(2):93-7.
8. Means RT, Allen J, Sears DA, et al, "Serum Soluble Transferrin Receptor and the Prediction of Marrow Aspirate Iron Results in a Heterogeneous Group of Patients," *Clin Lab Haematol*, 1999, 21(3):161-7.
9. Kohgo Y, Nishisato T, Kondo H, et al, "Circulating Transferrin Receptor in Human Serum," *Br J Haematol*, 1986, 64(2):277-81.
10. Baynes RD, Shih YJ, and Cook JD, "Mechanism of Production of the Serum Transferrin Receptor," *Adv Exp Med Biol*, 1994, 356:61-8.
11. Singhal A, Cook JD, Skikne BS, et al, "The Clinical Significance of Serum Transferrin Receptor Levels in Sickle Cell Disease," *Br J Haematol*, 1993, 84(2):301-4.
12. Tancabelic J, Sheth S, Paik M, et al, "Serum Transferrin Receptor as a Marker of Erythropoiesis Suppression in Patients on Chronic Transfusion," *Am J Hematol*, 1999, 60(2):121-5.

(Continued)

Transferrin Receptor, Soluble, Serum or Plasma
(Continued)

13. Khumalo H, Gomo ZA, Moyo VM, et al, "Serum Transferrin Receptors Are Decreased in the Presence of Iron Overload," *Clin Chem*, 1998, 44(1):40-4.

14. Looker AC, Loyevsky M, and Gordeuk VR, "Increased Serum Transferrin Saturation Is Associated With Lower Serum Transferrin Receptor Concentration," *Clin Chem*, 1999, 45(12):2191-9.

15. Wians FH Jr, Urban JE, Keffer JH, et al, "Discriminating Between Iron Deficiency Anemia and Anemia of Chronic Disease Using Traditional Indices of Iron Status vs Transferrin Receptor Concentration," *Am J Clin Pathol*, 2001, 115(1):112-8.

References
Ahluwalia N, Skikne BS, Savin V, et al, "Markers of Masked Iron Deficiency and Effectiveness of EPO Therapy in Chronic Renal Failure," *Am J Kidney Dis*, 1997, 30(4):532-41.

Akesson A, Bjellerup P, and Vahter M, "Evaluation of Kits for Measurement of the Soluble Transferrin Receptor," *Scand J Clin Lab Invest*, 1999, 59:77-82.

Choi JW, Im MW, Pai SH, "Serum Transferrin Receptor Concentrations During Normal Pregnancy," *Clin Chem*, 2000, 46(5):725-7.

Cook JD, "The Measurement of Serum Transferrin Receptor," *Am J Med Sci*, 1999, 318(4):269-76.

Flowers CH and Cook JD, "Dried Plasma Spot Measurements of Ferritin and Transferrin Receptor for Assessing Iron Status," *Clin Chem*, 1999, 45(10):1826-32.

Flowers CH, Skikne BS, Covell AM, et al, "The Clinical Measurement of Serum Transferrin Receptor," *J Lab Clin Med*, 1989, 114(4):368-77.

Goodnough LT, Skikne B, and Brugnara C, "Erythropoietin, Iron, and Erythropoiesis," *Blood*, 2000, 96(3):823-33.

Rees DC, Williams TN, Maitland K, et al, "Alpha Thalassemia Is Associated With Increased Soluble Transferrin Receptor Levels," *Br J Haematol*, 1998, 103(2):365-9.

Skikne BS, "Circulating Transferrin Receptor Assay-Coming of Age," *Clin Chem*, 1998, 44(1):7-9.

Suominen P, Punnonen K, Rajamaki A, et al, "Evaluation of a New Immunoenzymometric Assay for Measuring Soluble Transferrin Receptor to Detect Iron Deficiency in Anemic Patients," *Clin Chem*, 1997, 43(9):1641-6.

♦ **Transforming Growth Factor** β *see* TGF-β, Serum *on page 490*

♦ **Translocase** *see* Sickle Cell Tests *on page 486*

♦ **TRAP (platelet agonist)** *see* Reticulated Platelet Count *on page 480*

♦ **TRAP (Tartrate Resistant Acid Phosphatase)** *see* Tartrate Resistant Leukocyte Acid Phosphatase *on page 488*

♦ **TRAP Test** *see* Tartrate Resistant Leukocyte Acid Phosphatase *on page 488*

♦ **Triosephosphate Isomerase** *see* Red Blood Cell Enzyme Deficiency Screen *on page 476*

♦ **Trypanosomal/Filarial Parasites, Peripheral Blood Preparation** *see* Microfilariae, Peripheral Blood Preparation *on page 460*

♦ **Trypanosomiasis, Peripheral Blood Preparation** *see* Microfilariae, Peripheral Blood Preparation *on page 460*

♦ **TUNEL Assay** *see* Apoptosis Assays *on page 402*

♦ **UBBC** *see* Vitamin B$_{12}$ Unsaturated Binding Capacity *on page 495*

♦ **Umbilical Cord Blood Transplantation** *see* CD34$^+$ Hematopoietic Stem Cells by Flow Cytometry *on page 413*

♦ **Unsaturated Vitamin B$_{12}$ Binding Capacity** *see* Vitamin B$_{12}$ Unsaturated Binding Capacity *on page 495*

♦ **Unstable Hemoglobins** *see* Hemoglobin, Unstable, Heat Labile Test *on page 447*

♦ **Unstable Hemoglobins** *see* Hemoglobin, Unstable - Isopropanol Precipitation Test *on page 448*

♦ **Unstable Hemoglobins** *see* n-Butanol Stability Test *on page 460*

♦ **Ves-Matic Analyzer** *see* Sedimentation Rate, Erythrocyte *on page 484*

Viscosity, Blood

Related Information
Erythropoietin, Serum *on page 169*
Immunoglobulin M *on page 537*
Viscosity, Serum or Plasma *on page 495*

Synonyms Blood Viscosity

Applies to Beckwith-Wiedemann Syndrome; Microviscometer: Polycythemia of the Newborn

Abstract Viscosity refers to the internal friction of a fluid which makes it resistant to flow (as in relation to a solid surface or additional layer of fluid). Whole blood viscosity is the resistance to shearing motion of blood flow and is due, primarily, to circulating red blood cells. Whole blood viscosity is determined by the packed cell volume of erythrocytes (logarithmic relationship, plasma viscosity) aggregation of red blood cells, and deformability of red cells.[1] Hyperviscosity accounts for the symptoms that occur in polycythemia of the newborn.[2]

Specimen Whole blood

Container Green top (heparin) tube

Causes for Rejection Specimen clotted or hemolyzed

Special Instructions While this is an infrequently performed test and may not be routinely available, there is evidence that neonatal hyperviscosity is common,[2] suggesting that the test should be more frequently utilized. Consult the laboratory to determine if the requisite microviscometer can be obtained.

Reference Interval See references for normal range data. Viscosity normally rises with increase in hematocrit and is lower with lower shear rates. Study has shown that umbilical cord and venous hematocrits (not capillary) correlate with microviscometer readings in newborns.[3]

Use Detect hyperviscosity states including especially hyperviscosity in the neonatal period.

Methodology Wells-Brookfield microviscometer;[4] Coulter-Harkness capillary viscometer. Viscosity is measured at low and high shear rates at 37°C.

Additional Information The relatively new fields of haemorheology and clinical haemorheology focus upon the characteristics and resultant clinical effects of the flow behavior of blood. Somer and Meiselman have classified the hematological hyperviscosity syndromes as of polycythemic, sclerocythemic, or plasma type.[5] The polycythemic category includes syndromes the result of erythrocytosis (primary or secondary) or of hyperleukocytic leukemia. Sclerocythemic cases are the result of decreased deformability of red cells (as occur with sickle hemoglobinopathies, other hemolytic anemias, some forms of malaria, and with rigid leukemic cells). In the plasma category are paraproteinemias (eg, multiple myeloma and Waldenström's macroglobulinemia) and reactive polyclonal dysproteinemias.

Neonatal hyperviscosity, usually but not always associated with polycythemia (central hematocrit ≥65%), may be accompanied by a fairly typical clinical picture while many are asymptomatic. Plethora, anorexia, feeding disturbances, hypoglycemia, lethargy, and jitteriness/seizures (CNS symptoms) occur. There may be symptoms and findings suggesting congenital heart disease (CHD) (ie, respiratory distress, cardiac enlargement, and cyanosis). False diagnoses of CHD have been made in such cases. About 50% of such infants have modest hyperbilirubinemia (bilirubin >12 mg/dL). Severe complications include pulmonary hypertension, necrotizing enterocolitis, and renal failure.[2] Blood viscosity of small or large-for-gestational age infants does not differ from average-for-gestational age infants. About 50% of the cases have schistocytes and increased nucleated RBC on peripheral blood smear. There may be thrombocytopenia. The whole blood viscosity test can be used to follow the result of exchange transfusion therapy of neonatal hyperviscosity syndrome. Whole blood viscosity is increased after splenectomy (adults).[6]

The incidence of neonatal polycythemia is increased with:[2]
- high altitude
- small for gestational age infants
- twin-to-twin transfusion
- delayed clamping of the umbilical cord
- infants of diabetic mothers
- 13-, 18-, or 21 trisomy, adrenogenital syndrome, and in Beckwith-Wiedemann syndrome
- exposure to chronic fetal hypoxia

The treatment of symptomatic neonatal hyperviscosity is phlebotomy and replacement with saline/albumin or partial exchange transfusion (to decrease the hematocrit to 50%).[2,7]

Hemorheological cardiovascular risk factors have been shown to improve in as short a period as 2 days following cessation of smoking. Withdrawal of tobacco from heavy smokers was associated with a reduction in high shear rate blood viscosity of 8% with a greater fall in viscosity at low shear rate. Changes in viscosity were the result in part of decreases in packed cell volume, total plasma protein, and fibrinogen concentration.[8]

Footnotes
1. Shinton NK, ed, *CRC Desk Reference for Hematology*, Boca Raton: FL, CRC Press, 1998, 681-2.

2. Stoll BJ and Kliegman RM, "The Fetus and the Neonatal Infant," *Nelson Textbook of Pediatrics*, 16th ed, Chapter 99, Behrman RE, Kliegman RM, and Jenson HB, eds, Philadelphia, PA: WB Saunders Co, 2000, 525-6.

3. Ramamurthy RS and Berlanga M, "Postnatal Alteration in Hematocrit and Viscosity in Normal and Polycythemic Infants," *J Pediatr*, 1987, 110(6):929-34.

4. Wells RE, Denton R, and Merrill EW, "Measurement of Viscosity of Biologic Fluids by Cone Plate Viscometer," *J Lab Clin Med*, 1961, 57(4):646-56.

5. Somer T and Meiselman HJ, "Disorders of Blood Viscosity," *Ann Med*, 1993, 25(1):31-9.

6. Robertson DA, Simpson FG, and Losowsky MS, "Blood Viscosity After Splenectomy," *Br Med J (Clin Res Ed)*, 1981, 283(6291):573-5.

7. Wong W, Fok TF, Lee CH, et al, "Randomised Controlled Trial: Comparison of Colloid or Crystalloid for Partial Exchange Transfusion for Treatment of Neonatal Polycythaemia," *Arch Dis Child*, 1997 77(2):F115-8.

8. Rothwell M, Rampling MW, Cholerton S, et al, "Haemorheological Changes in the Very Short Term After Abstention From Tobacco by Cigarette Smokers," *Br J Haematol*, 1991 79(3):500-3.

References
Crowley JP, Metzger JB, Merrill EW, et al, "Whole Blood Viscosity in Beta Thalassemia Minor," *Ann Clin Lab Sci*, 1992, 22(4):229-35.

Lowe GD, "Blood Rheology, Haemostasis and Vascular Disease," *Haemostasis and Thrombosis*, 3rd ed, Chapter 51, Bloom AL, Forbes CD, Thomas DP, et al, eds, New York, NY: Churchill Livingston, 1994, 1169-88.

Viscosity, Serum or Plasma

Related Information

Immunofixation Electrophoresis, Serum or Urine *on page 530*
Protein Electrophoresis, Serum *on page 267*
Protein Electrophoresis, Urine *on page 268*
Viral Culture, Respiratory Symptoms *on page 694*
Viscosity, Blood *on page 494*

Synonyms Serum Viscosity

Abstract Viscosity of a fluid is its intrinsic resistance to flow due to internal friction between molecular/particles flowing through a tube or vessel.[1,2] Plasma viscosity is the resistance to shearing motion of plasma mainly due to large proteins, fibrinogen, and some immunoglobulins, in particular, those with proximal atrial asymmetry.

Specimen Serum or plasma

Container Red top tube or lavender top (EDTA) tube

Reference Interval See table.

Normal and Abnormal Levels of Viscosity

	Absolute Viscosity		Relative Viscosity
	37°C	25°C	
Distilled water	0.69	0.89	1.00
Plasma viscosity			
Reference range	1.16-1.35	1.50-1.72	1.67-1.94
Population range	1.14-1.50	1.46-1.94	1.65-2.17
Acute reactions	1.35-1.95	1.72-2.51	1.95-2.83
Chronic reactions	1.35-1.55	1.72-2.00	1.95-2.25
?Paraproteinemia	>2.0	>2.5	>2.9
Serum viscosity			
Reference range	1.09-1.23	1.40-1.60	1.57-1.80
Population range	1.08-1.36	1.39-1.60	1.57-1.97
?Paraproteinemia	>1.85	>2.4	>2.7

Reference and population ranges (mean ±2 SD) for plasma and serum viscosity at 37°C and 25°C, and relative to water. The usual zones for plasma viscosity in acute and chronic phase protein reactions are indicated, as are cutoff points above which paraproteins are very likely.

Adapted from *CRC Desk Reference for Hematology*, 3rd ed, Shinton NK, ed, Boca Raton, FL: CRC Press,1998, 682.

Use Evaluate hyperviscosity syndromes associated with monoclonal gammopathy states (myeloma, macroglobulinemia of Waldenström and other dysproteinemias), including occasional cases of rheumatoid arthritis, systemic lupus erythematosus, hyperfibrinogenemia

Limitations Does not measure whole blood viscosity, which increases with high hemoglobin/hematocrit. Subjective endpoint, temperature dependent, large technical error, less than ideal correlation exists between measured viscosity levels and clinical symptoms.

Methodology Viscometer (viscosimeter), Cannon-Feuske, Ostwald viscometers. Water and plasma "flow times" are determined with the use of a viscometer, RBC or WBC pipette, and stopwatch.[3] Test may be performed at room temperature or 37°C. The relative viscosity is expressed as a ratio of plasma "flow time" to water "flow time" Contraves LS30 Viscometer (Contraves AG, Zurich, Switzerland). A viscometer is commercially available which gives an automated measurement of plasma viscosity.[4]

Additional Information Hyperviscosity is most frequent (33% of cases)[5] with IgM monoclonal gammopathy (Waldenström's macroglobulinemia); next with IgA myeloma. When IgG myeloma leads to hyperviscosity IgG levels are usually very significantly elevated. Kappa light chain myeloma may (rarely) be responsible for hyperviscosity syndrome apparently as a result of true polymer formation.[6] A relative viscosity of 6-7 usually results in symptoms of the hyperviscosity syndrome, they have however been described with lower levels of relative viscosity (ie, 4). Results of plasma viscosity obtained with an automated capillary viscometer show good precision and close correlation with the Harkness manual method (standard method selected by the International Committee for Standardization in Hematology).[4]

There is ongoing interest in association of changes in blood/plasma viscosity with inflammatory/rheumatic diseases,[7,8] heart/coronary artery/vascular diseases,[9,10] and contributors (possibly through effects on viscosity) to the genesis of these disease processes.[11] Only a limited sample is included in this listing.

Footnotes

1. Lowe GD, ed, "Blood Rheology and Hyperviscosity Syndromes," *Bailliere Clin Haematol*, 1987, 1(3):597-867.
2. Shinton NK, ed, *CRC Desk Reference for Hematology*, Boca Raton: FL, CRC Press, 1998, 681-2.
3. Wright DJ and Jenkins DE Jr, "Simplified Method for Estimation of Serum and Plasma Viscosity in Multiple Myeloma and Related Disorders," *Blood*, 1970, 36:516-22.
4. Cooke BM and Stuart J, "Automated Measurement of Plasma Viscosity by Capillary Viscometer," *J Clin Pathol*, 1988, 41(11):1213-6.
5. Gandara DR and MacKenzie MR, "Differential Diagnosis of Monoclonal Gammopathy," *Med Clin North Am*, 1988, 72(5):1155-67.

6. Carter PW, Cohen HJ, and Crawford J, "Hyperviscosity Syndrome in Association With Kappa Light Chain Myeloma," *Am J Med*, 1989, 86(5):591-5.
7. Paulus HE, Ramos B, Wong WK, et al, "Equivalence of the Acute Phase Reactants C-reactive Protein, Plasma Viscosity, and Westergren Erythrocyte Sedimentation Rate When Used to Calculate American College of Rheumatology 20% Improvement Criteria or the Disease Activity Score in Patients With Early Rheumatoid Arthritis," *J Rheumatol*, 1999, 26(11):2324-31.
8. Murphy PT, Allen B, and Hutchinson RM, "Plasma Viscosity and Erythrocyte Sedimentation Rate in Suspected Cases of Temporal Arteritis," *Br J Haematol*, 1994, 87(3):671.
9. Danesh J, Collins R, Peto R, et al, "Haematocrit, Viscosity, Erythrocyte Sedimentation Rate: Meta-analyses of Prospective Studies of Coronary Heart Disease," *Eur Heart J*, 2000, 21(7):515-20.
10. Smith FB, Rumley A, Lee AJ, et al, "Haemostatic Factors and Prediction of Ischaemic Heart Disease and Stroke in Claudicants," *Br J Haematol*, 1998, 100(4):758-63.
11. Rothwell M, Rampling MW, Cholerton S, "Haemorheological Changes in the Very Short Term After Abstention From Tobacco by Cigarette Smokers," *Br J Haematol*, 1991, 79(3):500-3.

References

"A 62-Year-Old Man With Epistaxis, Confusion, Renal Failure, and Bilateral Central Retinal-Vein Thrombosis," Case Records of the Massachusetts General Hospital, Case 13-1994, Scully RE, Mark EJ, McNeely WF, et al, eds, *N Engl J Med*, 1994, 330(13):920-7.

Foerster J, "Plasma Cell Dyscrasias: General Considerations," *Wintrobe's Clinical Hematology*, 10th ed, Chapter 98, Section 5, Lee RG, Foerster J, Luken J, et al, eds, Baltimore, MD: Lippincott William & Wilkins, 1999, 2612-30.

Henry JB, *Clinical Diagnosis and Management by Laboratory Methods*, 19th ed, Philadelphia, PA: WB Saunders Co, 1996, 695, 814.

Lowe GD, "Should Plasma Viscosity Replace the ESR?" *Br J Haematol*, 1994, 86(1):6-11.

Lowe GD, "Blood Rheology, Haemostasis and Vascular Disease," *Haemostasis and Thrombosis*, 3rd ed, Chapter 51, Bloom AL, Forbes CD, Thomas DP, et al, eds, New York, NY: Churchill Livingstone, 1994, 1169-88.

Somer T and Meiselman HJ, "Disorders of Blood Viscosity," *Ann Med*, 1993, 25(1):31-9.

Vitamin B$_{12}$ Unsaturated Binding Capacity

Related Information

Cobalamin, Serum *on page 150*
Erythropoietin, Serum *on page 169*
Folic Acid, RBC *on page 435*
Folic Acid, Serum *on page 435*
Homocyst(e)ine, Plasma *on page 193*
Intrinsic Factor Blocking Antibody *on page 537*
Methylmalonic Acid, Serum, Plasma, Urine, or Amniotic Fluid *on page 224*
Parietal Cell Antibody *on page 541*
Schilling Test *on page 483*

Synonyms UBBC; Unsaturated Vitamin B$_{12}$ Binding Capacity; Vitamin B$_{12}$ UBC

Applies to Cobalophilin; Transcobalamins

Specimen Serum is most commonly used by most reference laboratories but use of EDTA plasma avoids increase in binding protein released from granulocytes (see following information).

Container Red top tube

Storage Instructions Refrigerate serum if not delivered to the laboratory immediately. Stable for days. Very stable when stored at -20°C.

Reference Interval 1000-2000 pg/mL binding capacity

Use Differential diagnosis of polycythemia vera from secondary/relative polycythemias; evaluate macrocytic/megaloblastic anemia; diagnose congenital absence of transcobalamin II or cobalophilin (transcobalamin I and III)

Limitations Increased with pregnancy and use of contraceptive hormones. Unrepresentative increase may occur during clotting of blood samples by release of unsaturated binding protein (cobalophilin) from granulocytes.[1] May give low values in samples with low protein content. Usually available only at reference or research laboratories.

Methodology Binding proteins are determined by their B$_{12}$ binding capacity. Uptake of radiolabeled B$_{12}$ is quantitated after saturation of serum transport systems and removal of excess vitamin with albumin or hemoglobin-coated charcoal. DEAE cellulose ion-exchange chromatography and isoelectric focusing are also used (in research environments).

Additional Information Serum transport of vitamin B$_{12}$ is accomplished by normally occurring proteins termed transcobalamins including I (an α-globulin), II (a β-globulin), and III (a group of transport factors - "R-type" binders or binder III - found also in some tissues, saliva, milk, and tears). Transcobalamin cell membrane receptors regulate cellular uptake of the cobalamins. The term "R-type" refers to binding protein with "rapid" mobility on electrophoresis. The term haptocorrin (TCO, I, II, R binder, cobalophyllin) refers to a family of immunologically similar proteins which are variably glycosylated and not all of which have rapid electrophoretic mobility. Transcobalamin I is the major B$_{12}$ transport protein binding 80% to 90% of endogenous cobalamin which is delivered from peripheral tissues to the liver. It bears immunologic identity to granulocyte cobalophilin. Transcobalamin II binds only 10% to 25% of total plasma cobalamin but provides most of the total UBBC of plasma. Thus, transcobalamin II is the carrier protein that provides most of the cobalamin transport within the intravascular (and extracellular) space. Intrinsic factor is the carrier protein within
(Continued)

Vitamin B$_{12}$ Unsaturated Binding Capacity
(Continued)

the gastrointestinal tract. Less than 2% of plasma TC II is saturated at any one point in time. The TC II bound B$_{12}$ is decreased in untreated B$_{12}$ deficiency. As the B$_{12}$ deficient state develops, TC II UBBC increases.[1] See accompanying table for other clinical associations. Isoelectric focusing has shown that the cobalophilins (R-binders) are a microheterogenous group of plasma binding proteins. Cobalophilin is increased in diseases characterized by excess granulocyte production, reactive leukocytosis, chronic myelogenous leukemia, and other myeloproliferative states, in particular polycythemia vera. UBBC levels are increased in >66% of the cases of polycythemia vera. Most cases of secondary/relative polycythemia patients have normal levels of UBBC. High levels occur in some patients with hepatoma. The transcobalamins are normally about 25% saturated with vitamin B$_{12}$. UBBCs of transcobalamins I and II are increased in asymptomatic human immunodeficiency seropositive patients.[2]

Levels and Binding Capacity of Cobalamin-Binding Proteins in Disease

Binder	Disease
Increased TC I (R protein)	Myeloproliferative disorders
	Polycythemia vera
	Myelofibrosis
	Benign neutrophilia
	Chronic myelocytic leukemia
	Hepatoma (occasionally)
	Metastatic cancer
Increased TC II	Myeloproliferative disorders
	Liver disease
	Inflammatory disorders
	Gaucher disease
	Anti-TC II antibodies
Unsaturated cobalamin binders*	
Increased	Transient neutropenia
	Elevated TC I
Decreased	Liver disease
	Elevated serum cobalamin

*UBBC = unsaturated B$_{12}$ binding capacity

Adapted from Babior BM, "Metabolic Aspects of Folic Acid and Cobalamin," *Williams Hematology*, 5th ed, Chapter 35, Beutler E, Lichtman MA, Coller BS, et al, eds, New York, NY: McGraw-Hill Inc, 1995, 390.

TC II deficiency (presents shortly after birth as failure to thrive) is an uncommon condition characterized by vomiting and weakness, pancytopenia, megaloblastic anemia, and serum cobalamin levels that are normal or nearly normal (most serum cobalamin is carried by TC I, an R binder). Some, but not all, patients may develop neurological sequela (mental deficiency and other neurological changes) in particular with inadequate or absent cobalamin therapy.[3] Even more uncommon is R-binder deficiency (absent or deficient TC I) in which serum cobalamin level is decreased but there are no clinical signs of B$_{12}$ deficiency. In such cases TC II cobalamin levels are normal.

Specialized cobalamin analogs have been developed and applied to the imaging of transcobalamin receptors in animal models.[4]

Footnotes
1. Herzlich B and Herbert V, "Depletion of Serum Holotranscobalamin II. An Early Sign of Negative Vitamin B$_{12}$ Balance," *Lab Invest*, 1988, 58(3):332-7.
2. Rule SA, Hooker M, Costello C, et al, "Serum Vitamin B$_{12}$ and Transcobalamin Levels in Early HIV Disease," *Am J Hematol*, 1994, 47(3):167-71.
3. Bibi H, Gelman-Kohan Z, Baumgartner ER, et al, "Transcobalamin II Deficiency With Methylmalonic Aciduria in Three Sisters," *J Inherit Metab Dis*, 1999, 22(7):765-72.
4. Collins DA and Hogenkamp HPC, "Transcobalamin II Receptor Imaging Via Radiolabeled Diethylene-Triaminepentaacetate Cobalamin Analogs," *J Nucl Med*, 1997, 38(5):717-23.

References
Babior BM, "Metabolic Aspects of Folic Acid and Cobalamin," *Williams Hematology*, 5th ed, Chapter 35, Beutler E, Lichtman MA, Coller BS, et al, eds, New York, NY: McGraw-Hill Inc, 1995, 388-90.

Fenton WA and Rosenberg LE, "Inherited Disorders of Cobalamin Transport and Metabolism," *The Metabolic and Molecular Bases of Inherited Disease*, 7th ed, Chapter 102, McGraw-Hill Inc, 1995, 3129-49.

Zittoun J, Farcet JP, Marquet J, et al, "Cobalamin (Vitamin B$_{12}$) and B$_{12}$ Binding Proteins in Hypereosinophilic Syndromes and Secondary Eosinophilia," *Blood*, 1984, 63(4):779-83.

- **Vitamin B$_{12}$ Absorption Test** *see* Schilling Test *on page 483*

- **Vitamin B$_{12}$ UBC** *see* Vitamin B$_{12}$ Unsaturated Binding Capacity *on page 495*

- **VLA-4** *see* CD34$^+$ Hematopoietic Stem Cells by Flow Cytometry *on page 413*

- **VLA-5** *see* CD34$^+$ Hematopoietic Stem Cells by Flow Cytometry *on page 413*

- **Volumetric Glycerol Lysis Test** *see* Glycerol Lysis Test, Acidified, Modified *on page 439*

- **WBC** *see* White Blood Cell Count *on page 496*

- **WBC, Total** *see* White Blood Cell Count *on page 496*

- **Wells Syndrome** *see* Eosinophil Granule Proteins *on page 426*

- **Westergren Sed Rate** *see* Sedimentation Rate, Erythrocyte *on page 484*

White Blood Cell Count

Related Information
Antineutrophil Antibody *on page 835*
Apoptosis Assays *on page 402*
Bone Marrow *on page 410*
CD4/CD8 Enumeration *on page 511*
Chromosome Analysis, Bone Marrow *on page 362*
Complete Blood Count *on page 419*
HIV-1/HIV-2 Antibody Screen and Western Blot *on page 636*
Leukocyte Alkaline Phosphatase *on page 455*
Leukocyte Cytochemistry *on page 456*
Lymph Node Biopsy *on page 67*
Peripheral Blood: Differential Leukocyte Count *on page 464*

Synonyms Leukocyte Count; WBC; WBC, Total; White Count

Applies to Apoptosis *bcl-x*; Congenital Neutropenia; Myelokathexis; Neutropenia; Schwachman-Diamond Syndrome

Abstract This procedure determines the white blood cell concentration in a body fluid, usually peripheral blood. The count is most commonly generated by an automated analyzer using aperture-impedance and/or laser beam technology. Different types of white blood cells (eg, granulocytes, monocytes, lymphocytes, etc) are included in the total count. The results have widespread application to the diagnosis and monitoring of a variety of clinical conditions including infectious, neoplastic, and immunologic disease states.

Specimen Whole blood or other body fluid

Container Lavender top (EDTA) tube

Causes for Rejection Clotted specimen, hemolyzed specimen

Reference Interval Peripheral blood (adult): 4500-11,000/mm^3 (SI: 4.5-11.0 x 10^9/L). There is diurnal variation with lowest level of WBC count in the morning (subject at rest) and with maximum level in the afternoon. With high levels of activity, stress, exercise (associated with release of Adrenalin®), increase in WBC count of 2000-5000/mm^3 is common; rises up to 30,000/mm^3 may occur.[1]

Remarkably, many major textbooks still provide "reference" ranges for hematologic values (including in particular white blood cell or leukocyte count) that were compiled some 50 years ago as "normal" ranges of manual methods. Are such reference values still appropriate in the current age of sophisticated highly automated and microcomputerized multichannel analyzers? In today's texts, there is acknowledged or assumed recognition of EC Albritton's *Standard Values in Blood*, the title of which continues as "Being the First Fascicle of a Handbook of Biological Data."[2] This work was born on January 31, 1949, by a contract from the National Academy of Sciences - National Research Council to the Wright Air Development Center, United States Air Force and was published as a volume of tables in 1952 after being first issued as Air Force Technical Report No. 6039. Table 49 of the 1952 fascicle is entitled "Blood Leukocyte Values, Birth to Maturity: Man" and provides means and ranges... "from smoothed curves plotted from averages (...of means...of ranges) from the literature," the latter not additionally referenced. Values are given "at birth" and also for hours (12 and 24), weeks, and months after birth but with a footnote acknowledging that "values and ranges within the first year are from fragmentary data." Some recent major texts now heed this footnote by leaving "total leukocytes," birth to 1-4 weeks blank with their own footnote indicating "insufficient data for a reliable estimate." Albritton's work includes tables of leukocyte values for different altitudes, pregnancy, laboratory animals, and farm animals.

Some 30 years later (and 20 years ago), a massive, reasonably comprehensive and well referenced set of hematologic data became available but seems little utilized.[3] Series 11, No. 232, data from the National Health Survey, the second National Health and Nutrition Examination Survey - NHANES II (U.S. Department of Health and Human Services Publication No. (PHS) 83-1682) was titled "Hematologic and Nutritional Biochemistry Reference Data for Persons 6 Months to 74 Years of Age: United States," 1976-80. Published in December 1982, it includes data from CBC parameters with white blood cell counts but without white cell subset determinations. Age range is 3-74 years and data is segregated as to "all races," "white," and "black." The sample examined was large, 20,322 individuals, 10,339 females, 9983 males, 17,105 white, 2763 black, and 454 "other." Methods of collection used by mobile examination centers at 64 field locations are detailed, with procedures performed at these sites including Hb by Coulter hemoglobinometer, spun microhematocrit, and red and white cell counts by Coulter Model FN. Red cell indices were computer generated. Thus, an earlier generation of hematology devices of which current analyzers are descendents. Statistical treatment is detailed, data includes mean, standard deviation, and 5th to 95th percentile tables. The considerable data, including references, is distributed over 77 pages. After this prodigious effort, focusing upon the normal ranges for WBC count, all races, 3-74 years of age, the 5th to 95th percentile range is given as 4.5-11.0 x 10⁹/L,[3] essentially the same as derived by Albritton's study 30 years earlier and based on manual methods.[2] NHANES II text summarized findings pertinent to the WBC count as:

- The mean WBC count for females ages 12-24 years (7.1 x 10⁹/L) was significantly lower than that for females ages 3-5 years (7.9 x 10⁹/L). Decrease for males, also significant, was 7.6 x 10⁹/L to 6.9 x 10⁹/L.
- The mean WBC count of males 15-74 years showed no consistent pattern. For females, there was a significant decrease from 7.7 x 10⁹/L at ages 15-17 years to 6.8 x 10⁹/L for age range of 55-74 years.
- Black persons, 3-74 years, had consistently lower mean WBC counts than did whites (0.6-1.3 x 10⁹/L between males and 0.2-1.4 x 10⁹/L between females).
- The difference in age-adjusted mean WBC counts were independent of poverty status.

It would appear that allowing for some minor exceptions, **past reference ranges for the WBC count**, and for that matter, for most parameters of the "complete blood count" **are clinically useful**. Studies from the last decade, utilizing multiparameter automated analyzers, deal with necessarily smaller sample sizes (as compared to the NHANES II study) but result in similar reference ranges.[4,5] Modern investigations generally focus on population subsets such as very-low-birth-weight neonates,[6,7] newborns at term,[8] infants,[9] school-age children,[10,11] and ethnic/sex differences.[12] See accompanying tables for a sample of resultant data.

A 10-year old study of the use of total and differential leukocyte counts in clinically well children found no unsuspected illness as a result of an abnormal total leukocyte count (778 CBC results during a 1-year period) and including 9.8% of 387 clinically well subjects with neutropenia. The high frequency of results outside published normal ranges led the authors of this study to call for a re-evaluation of "normal ranges" for leukocyte counts in pediatric patients.[13] Logistic and efficiency considerations with use of multi-channel analyzers (in spite of low yield in case finding situations) are likely to perpetuate use of total leukocyte and differential counts in such surveys.

WBC normal ranges[2] (SI units: x 10⁹ cells/L):
- birth: 9.0-30.0 cells x 1000/mm³
- 24 hours: 9.4-34.0 cells x 1000/mm³
- 1 month: 5.0-19.5 cells x 1000/mm³
- 1-3 years: 6.0-17.5 cells x 1000/mm³
- 4-7 years: 5.5-15.5 cells x 1000/mm³
- 8-13 years: 4.5-13.5 cells x 1000/mm³
- adults: 4.5-11.0 cells x 1000/mm³

Note: Data largely from Albritton EC, 1952[2]

See the following tables and charts for data from recent reference range studies.

Possible Panic Range On admission <2500/mm³ (SI: 2.5 x 10⁹/L) or >30,000/mm³ (SI: >30.0 x 10⁹/L).

Leukocyte Count, Children 7-14 Years of Age
(at 1869 m Altitude - Turkey)

Age	Median	25th Percentile	97.5th Percentile
7-10 y	8.0	5.1 (4.8-5.4)	14.6 (13.5-15.3)
11-14 y	7.4	4.9 (4.8-5.3)	12.6 (11.6-13.7)
7-14 y			
granulocytes %	54.0	32.8	71.6
lymphocytes %	37.7	21.7	52.7

Adapted from Akdag R, Energin VM, Kalayci AG, et al, "Reference Limits for Routine Haematological Measurements in 7-14-Year Old Children Living at an Intermediate Altitude (1869 m, Erzurum, Turkey)," *Scand J Clin Lab Invest*, 1996, 56(2):103-9.

Total WBC Count, Sex, and Ethnic Subsets:
Geometric Mean and 95% Range
(London, UK)

	Caucasian	Afrocaribbean	African
Male	5.7 (3.6-9.2)	5.2 (2.8-9.5)	4.5 (2.8-7.2)
Female	6.2 (3.5-10.8)	5.7 (3.3-9.85)	5.0 (3.2-7.8)

Adapted from Bain BJ, "Ethnic and Sex Differences in the Total and Differential White Cell Count and Platelet Count," *J Clin Pathol*, 1996, 49(8):664-6.

Total WBC Count, Infants at 2, 5, and 13 Months
(Western Bank, Sheffield, UK)

Age	Mean	Median	95% Range
2 mo	8.9	9.1	5.1-15.4
5 mo	9.9	9.8	5.9-16.6
13 mo	9.7	9.6	5.9-16.1

Adapted from Bellamy GJ, Hinchliffe RF, Crawshaw KC, et al, "Total and Differential Leukocyte Counts in Infants at 2, 5, and 13 Months of Age," *Clin Lab Haematol*, 2000, 22(2):81-7.

Total WBC Count, Schoolchildren, Ages 4-19
(Dublin, Ireland)

Age	Mean	Median	3rd Percentile	97th Percentile
Boys				
4 and 5 y	7.59	7.10	4.80	11.79
7 y	7.00	6.65	4.37	11.06
9 y	6.91	6.80	4.80	10.65
11 y	6.86	6.65	4.00	10.76
13 y	6.30	6.05	3.75	9.83
15 y	6.93	6.50	4.30	12.59
17 and 18 y	6.40	6.10	4.17	10.33
Girls				
4 and 5 y	7.47	7.05	4.9	12.2
7 y	7.37	6.80	5.2	11.2
9 y	7.08	7.00	4.5	9.9
11 y	6.83	6.45	4.8	10.4
13 y	6.89	6.55	4.5	10.8
15 y	6.76	6.50	4.5	10.5
17 and 18 y	6.93	6.85	4.2	10.2

Adapted from Taylor MR, Holland CV, Spencer R, et al, "Haematological Reference Ranges for Schoolchildren," *Clin Lab Haematol*, 1997, 19(1):1-15.

Peripheral (Total) WBC Count and Leukocyte Indexes in
Healthy Newborn Term Infants
(Texas USA, Wilford Hall USAF)

	Healthy Neonates Age: 4 Hours		Effect of Duration of Stage 1 of Labor		# Patients With Abnormal WBCs by Previous Criteria*
	Mean	Range 10% to 90%	<12 h	>12 h	
Total leukocytes	24.06	16.2-31.5	23.6 ±5.8	28.0 ±7.1	43%
ANC	15.62	9.5-21.5	15.3 ±4.5	18.9 ±5.1	63%
I/M	0.21	0.06-0.35			13.5%
I/T	0.16	0.05-0.27			36.3%
Immature neutrophils			2.3 ±1.8	2.6 ±1.5	72.5%

ANC - Absolute neutrophil count.

I/M - Ratio of Immature to mature neutrophils.

I/T - Ratio of immature to total neutrophils.

*See text and Footnotes 23 and 24.

Adapted from Schelonka RL, Yoder BA, desJardins SE, et al, "Peripheral Leukocyte Count and Leukocyte Indexes in Healthy Newborn Term Infants," *J Pediatr*, 1994, 125(4):603-6.

Reference Values, Leukocytes, From Patient Populations
(University Hospital, Groningen, Netherlands)

Age	New		Old		Wintrobe		Miale	
	Male	Female	Male	Female	Male	Female	Male	Female
1-4 y	5.0-12.0		5.0-16.0					
5-49 y	4.0-10.5		5.0-10.0		4.3-10.0		3.8-10.9	
>50 y	4.0-11.0	4.0-10.0	5.0-10.0		4.3-10.0		3.8-10.0	

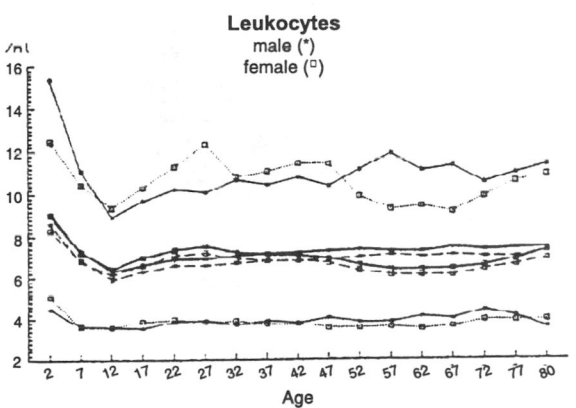

Leukocytes
male (*)
female (□)

Means:
male ——×——
female ——□——

Medians:
male — × —
female — □ —

2½ and 97½ percentiles:
male ·····×·····
female ·····□·····

From Swaanenberg JC, Rutten WP, Holdrinet AC, et al, "The Determination of Reference Values for Hematologic Parameters Using Results Obtained From Patient Populations," *Am J Clin Pathol*, 1987, 88(2):182-91. See text for comments on significance.

(Continued)

White Blood Cell Count (Continued)

Total Leukocytes, 0.025-0.975 Percentiles
(Institute of Clinical Chemistry, Clinical Hospital, Merkura, Zagreb, Croatia)

Age	Range
8-19 y	4.4-11.6
20-70 y	3.4-9.7

Adapted from Flegar-Mestric Z, Nazor A, and Jagarinec N, "Haematological Profile in Healthy Urban Population (8-70 Years of Age)," *Coll Antropol*, 2000, 24(1):185-96.

Postnatal Absolute Neutrophil Count (SD), Appropriate Weight for Gestational Age vs Low Birth Weight for Gestational Age

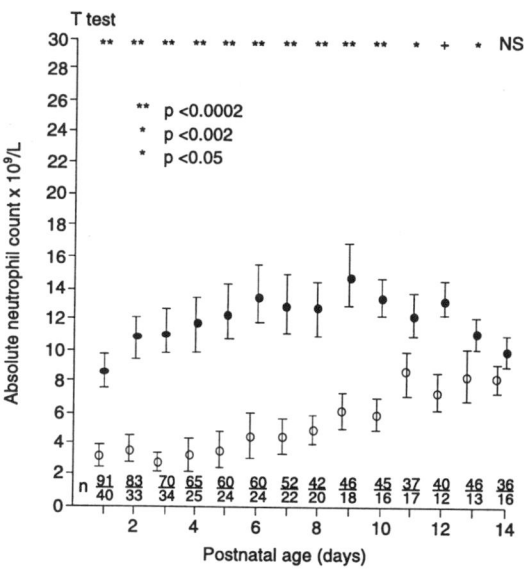

Absolute neutrophil count (SD) during the first 14 days of life in babies of appropriate weight for gestational age (●) and babies who were small for gestational age (○).

Data and chart from McIntosh N et al, 1988, footnote #7.
See text for comments on significance.

Absolute Total Neutrophil Count, Very-Low-Birth-Weight Neonates

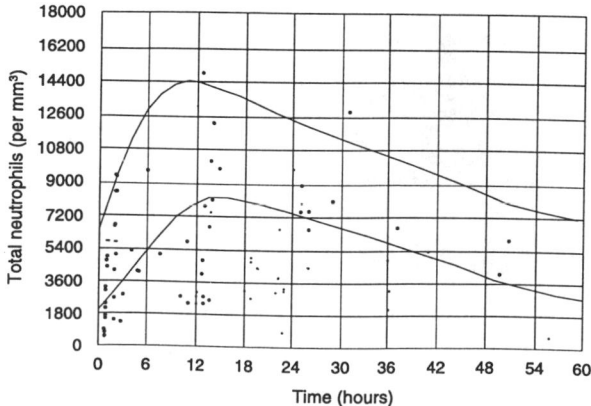

Distribution of ATN counts obtained from "normal" VLBW neonates between birth to 60 hours of age using the reference range of Manroe et al.[23]

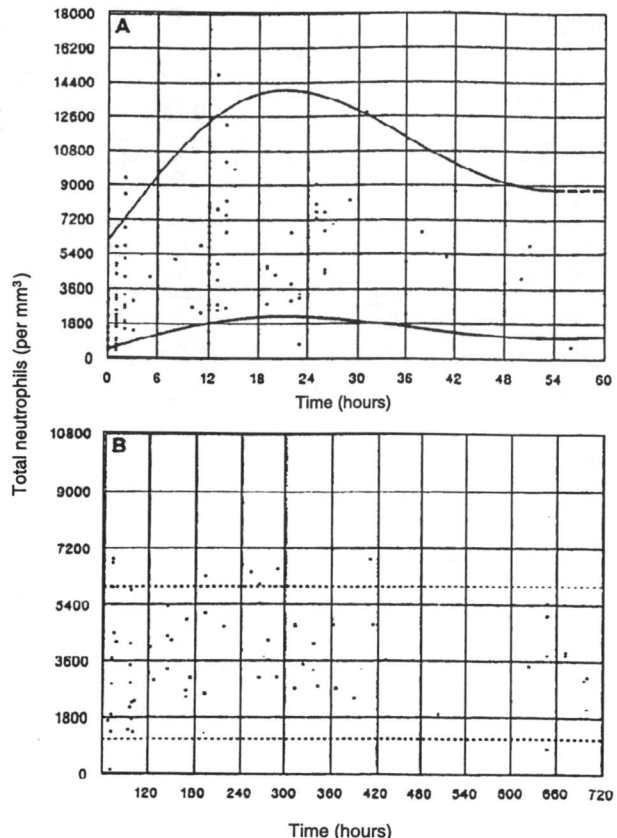

Revised reference ranges for total neutrophil values in VLBW neonates:
   A. from birth to 60 hours of life.
   B. from 61 hours to 28 days of life.

Bold lines (A) and dotted lines (B) represent boundaries of the data.

Data and charts from Mouzinho A et al, 1994, footnote #6.
See text for comments on significance.

Use White cell enumeration; evaluate myelopoiesis, bacterial and viral infections, toxic metabolic processes; diagnose/evaluate leukemic states

Limitations If nucleated RBCs are found in differential count, the white blood count should be corrected. The use of capillary blood samples may give WBC count some 3% to 12% higher values than those obtained with use of venous blood.[9] Electronic machine counters are subject to spurious high WBC counts in a variety of situations including presence of cryoglobulins/cryofibrinogen, clumped platelets (which may cause false elevation of WBC count and thrombocytopenia), fibrin strands, nucleated red blood cells, nonlysed red cells (as in some cases of hemoglobinopathy), EDTA-induced platelet aggregation, and cold agglutinins.[14]

Methodology Manual - hemocytometer counting chambers. Most WBC count determinations are obtained from one channel of a highly automated multichannel electronic and pneumatic analyzer using aperture-impedance and/or aperture conductance and/or laser light scattering technologies. Prior to manual or automated counting, blood is diluted with a solution that lyses red cells. Visual-based manual methods are time-consuming and are less reproducible. Coefficient of variation (CV) is about 10%, compared to machine methods that have CVs in the 1% to 3% range. WBC differential determination is provided by recent generations of analyzers. Excellent performance (precision, linearity, and lack of carryover) has been found on field evaluation of a commonly utilized multichannel device[15] and its recent generation, the Coulter GEN-S.[16] An automated hematology analyzer performs the differential leukocyte count (DLC) using flow-cytochemical technology.[17]

Additional Information The white blood cell count (leukocyte count) in the postmillenium is commonly determined by an automated hematology analyzer. A variety of circulating white cells (neutrophils, lymphocytes, monocytes, eosinophils, basophils) and ordinarily much less commonly encountered elements (eg, plasma cells and CD34+ blastic stem cells) form the normal leukocyte composite. Reference ranges for the total white count are age- and ethnic-dependent. Individual cell components are particularly age-dependent, knowledge of which may have significant clinical relevance. In adults, polymorphonuclear leukocytes (PMNs) are the predominant cell type (normally slightly over 1/2 to 3/4 of circulating white blood cells) while lymphocytes are the most common type of circulating white cell in most infants and children.

PMNs are critical effectors of the acute inflammatory response. They function in host defense by phagocytosing and killing invading microorganisms. Mature PMNs, incapable of cell division, are replenished through myelopoietic activity of the bone marrow, normally in an adult, at the prodigious rate of 10^{11} cells/day.[18]

In **newborn infants** WBC counts from different vascular sources (ie, capillary vs venous vs arterial blood) should not necessarily be considered equivalent. WBC counts from actively crying babies may show leukocytosis with left shift, **possibly erroneously suggesting bacterial infections**. Any stressful situation in newborns, children, or adults which leads to increase in endogenous epinephrine production may cause a rapid (15-30 minutes) increase in WBC count. In the evaluation of infection in newborns and young children, it is recommended that several counts be obtained from a consistent vascular source in resting individuals. A study of within subject and between subject variation has reaffirmed that hematologic parameters have significant individuality. Screening using conventional reference limits may be misleading.[13] Subject specific reference values are likely to have greater clinical utility.[19,20] There is modest progressive leukocytosis (due to neutrophils) throughout **pregnancy** into the third trimester with subsequent decline in white count after about 34 weeks gestation.[21] The count returns to normal about 1 week after delivery.

Elevated WBC count has a broad clinical differential diagnosis. Infections and/or leukemic processes are of special importance. **Acute infections** are usually associated with an increase in neutrophil type WBCs. If the white cells are **lymphocytes**, however, viral illness, leukemic process, and **pertussis** (whooping cough) are candidates for consideration. While pertussis is usually associated with lymphocytosis at the 25,000/mm^3 or so level, some cases (especially in the very young) may be seen, temporarily with 100,000/mm^3 level WBC counts. Paroxysmal cough in a nonimmunized child are important clinical findings.

Included in the broad differential consideration for the cause of neutropenia is collagen-vascular disease, notably lupus erythematosus and other autoimmune neutropenias (see References). Many drugs result in leukopenia including bezafibrate, an antihyperlipidemic fibric acid.[22]

Studies by McIntosth et al[7] and Mouzinho et al[6] draw attention to the differences in absolute total neutrophil counts (ATN) between infants of appropriate weight for gestational age vs infants small for gestational age (extremely low birth-weight or "very low birth-weight neonates" - VLBW neonates). Infants of appropriate weight showed the expected postnatal rise in WBC count but VLBW neonates showed a fall in WBC count for the first 3 days. Some individual VLBW neonates became technically neutropenic. These findings have importance to the possible presence of neutropenia. Some VLBW neonate mothers may have hypertension with associated thrombocytopenia and neutropenia while some VLBW neonates may have chronic intrauterine hypoxia with marrow capacity diverted to red cell production.[7] If neutropenia is not the result of neonatal sepsis, it may predispose to the development of sepsis. The study by Mouzinho et al compares neutrophil values (absolute total neutrophil count - ATN) from VLBW neonates (≤1500 g), in the period 1974-1976 vs the year 1990, a 15-year interval which saw a doubling of VLBW neonate survival from 42% in 1978 to 79% in 1989 creating a different population (greater number <1500 g) neonates. New ATN reference ranges for VLBW neonates had a wider range of distribution than previously reported (Manroe et al)[23] due largely to a decrease in the lower boundary (see chart). Thus, with new ranges in use, fewer VLBW neonates would be considered "neutropenic," again with implications (not yet fully defined) to the recognition and treatment of neonatal sepsis.[6,7,24]

Fat cells (as may accompany connective tissue stores) may cause artifactual elevation of machine white cell counts on specimens from traumatic venous puncture[25] and from bone marrow aspirate material.[26] The H2 analyzer (Bayer-Technicon) showed a curvilinear cluster in the peroxidase channel and two abnormal clusters in the basophil/lobularity channel, lipid induced. Counts from the Coulter GEN-S were much less affected, likely due to the use of a different cell lysis reagent.[26]

Several studies indicate that the baseline WBC count is a predictor of the relative risk of coronary heart disease (CHD) morbidity and mortality independent of cigarette smoking, while the latter increases the white cell count significantly within the normal range.[27] The white count is a direct function of the amount of inhaled smoke. The cause of the associations between leukocyte (essentially neutrophil) count, smoking, and CHD have not been defined.[27]

Mechanisms of neutrophil function, granule development/maturation/function, and mechanisms of neutropenia, in particular as they relate to immune senescence and apoptosis are under active investigation[18,28,29,30,31,32,33,34,35] (see Apoptosis Assays *on page 402*). Apoptosis of bone marrow hematopoietic precursors is increased in myelodysplasia, some 40% of marrow cells undergoing apoptotic cell death.[36] Congenital disorders with severe neutropenia include cyclic neutropenia, myelokathexis, the Schwachman-Diamond syndrome, and severe congenital neutropenia. In these conditions, marrow neutrophil precursors fail to complete differentiation and fail to enter into the peripheral blood (apoptosis implied). In myelokathexis, a rare congenital cause of chronic leukopenia/neutropenia, there is evidence that accelerated apoptosis of marrow myeloid precursors accounts for underproduction of myeloid cells and resultant neutropenia.[36,37] $CD34^+$ cells undergo increased apoptotic cell death as compared to controls due to a decrease in *bcl-x* expression in marrow precursors, with restoration of *bcl-x* level and increase in blood neutrophils after treatment with granulocyte colony-stimulating factor.[37] Neutrophil participation (possibly unique to neutrophils) in a nonapoptotic, non-necrotic form of cell death involving prostaglandin E_2 receptor subtype 3 has been recently proposed.[38] See Apoptosis Assays *on page 402*.

Neutrophils have been considered to play a role in the link between pathways of coagulation and inflammation.[39] The neutrophil membrane has binding sites for proteins of the contact system, provides a platform for assembly of the prothrombinase complex, with affects on neutrophil functions (eg, chemotaxis and degranulation). Neutrophil elastase, in turn, can degrade some coagulation proteins contributing to modulation of thrombotic and fibrinolytic systems.[39]

Footnotes

1. Dacie Sir JV and Lewis SM, eds, "Reference Ranges and Normal Values," *Practical Haematology*, 8th ed, Chapter 2, New York, NY: Churchill Livingstone, 1995, 15-7.
2. American Institute of Biological Sciences, The National Research Council, *Standard Values in Blood*, "Being the First Fascicle of a Handbook of Biological Data," Albritton EC, ed, Philadelphia, PA: WB Saunders Co, 1952.
3. Second National Health and Nutrition Examination Survey (NHANES II), "Hematological and Nutritional Biochemistry Reference Data for Persons 6 Months to 74 Years of Age: United States, 1976-80," *Vital and Health Statistics*, DHHS Publication No. (PHS) 83-1682, data from the National Health Survey, Series 11, No. 232, 1982.
4. Flegar-Mestric Z, Nazor A, and Jagarinec N, "Haematological Profile in Healthy Urban Population (8 to 70 Years of Age)," *Coll Antropol*, 2000, 24(1):185-96.
5. Swaanenburg JC, Rutten WP, Holdrinet AC, et al, "The Determination of Reference Values for Hematologic Parameters Using Results Obtained From Patient Populations," *Am J Clin Pathol*, 1987, 88(2):182-91.
6. Mouzinho A, Rosenfeld CR, Sanchez PJ, et al, "Revised Reference Ranges for Circulating Neutrophils in Very-Low-Birth-Weight Neonates," *Pediatrics*, 1994, 94(1):76-82.
7. McIntosh N, Kempson C, and Tyler RM, "Blood Counts in Extremely Low Birthweight Infants," *Arch Dis Child*, 1988, 63(1):74-6.
8. Schelonka RL, Yoder BA, desJardins SE, et al, "Peripheral Leukocyte Count and Leukocyte Indexes in Healthy Newborn Term Infants," *J Pediatr*, 1994, 125(4):603-6.
9. Bellamy GJ, Hinchliffe RF, Crawshaw KC, et al, "Total and Differential Leukocyte Counts in Infants at 2, 5, and 13 Months of Age," *Clin Lab Haematol*, 2000, 22(2):81-7.
10. Taylor MR, Holland CV, Spencer R, et al, "Haematological Reference Ranges for Schoolchildren," *Clin Lab Haematol*, 1997, 19(1):1-15.
11. Akdag R, Energin VM, Kalayci AG, et al, "Reference Limits for Routine Haematological Measurements in 7-14-Year-Old Children Living at an Intermediate Altitude (1869 m, Erzurum, Turkey)," *Scand J Clin Lab Invest*, 1996, 56(2):103-9.
12. Bain BJ, "Ethnic and Sex Differences in the Total and Differential White Cell Count and Platelet Count," *J Clin Pathol*, 1996, 49(8):664-6.
13. Moyer VA and Grimes RM, "Total and Differential Leukocyte Counts in Clinically Well Children. Information or Misinformation?" *Am J Dis Child*, 1990, 144(11):1200-3.
14. Bowen KL, "Clinical Pathology Rounds: Erroneous Leukocyte Counts and Cold Agglutinins," *Lab Med*, 1997, 28(4):247-50.
15. Warner BA and Reardon DM, "A Field Evaluation of the Coulter STK-S," *Am J Clin Pathol*, 1991, 95(2):207-17.
16. Picard F, Gicquel C, Marnet L, et al, "Preliminary Evaluation of the new Hematology Analyzer Coulter GEN-S in a University Hospital," *Clin Chem Lab Med*, 1999, 37(6):681-6.
17. Bentley SA, Johnson TS, Sohier CH, et al, "Flow-Cytochemical Differential Leukocyte Analysis With Quantitation of Neutrophil Left Shift. An Evaluation of the Cobas-Helios Analyzer," *Am J Clin Pathol*, 1994, 102(2):223-30.
18. Mollinedo F, Borregaard N, and Boxer LA, "Novel Trends in Neutrophil Structure, Function, and Development," *Immunol Today*, 1999, 20(12):535-7.
19. Fraser CG, Wilkinson SP, Neville RG, et al, "Biologic Variation of Common Hematologic Laboratory Quantities in the Elderly," *Am J Clin Pathol*, 1989, 92(4):465-70.
20. Dot D, Miró J, and Feuntes-Arderiu X, "Within-Subject Biological Variation of Hematological Quantities and Analytical Goals," *Arch Pathol Lab Med*, 1992, 116(8):825-6.
21. Balloch AJ and Cauchi MN, "Reference Ranges for Haematology Parameters in Pregnancy Derived From Patient Populations," *Clin Lab Haematol*, 1993, 15(1):7-14.
22. Ariad S and Hechtlinger V, "Bezafibrate-Induced Neutropenia," *Eur J Haematol*, 1993, 50(3):179.
23. Manroe BL, Rosenfeld CR, Weinberg AG, et al, "The Differential Leukocyte Count in the Assessment and Outcome of Early-Onset Neonatal Group B Streptococcal Disease," *J Pediatr*, 1977, 91(4):632-7.
24. Rodwell RL, Leslie AL, and Tudehope DI, "Early Diagnosis of Neonatal Sepsis Using a Hematologic Scoring System," *J Pediatr*, 1988, 112(5):761-7.
25. Whiteway AJ and Bain BJ, "Artifactual Elevation of an Automated White Cell Count Following Femoral Vein Puncture," *Clin Lab Haematol*, 1999, 21(1):65-8.
26. Lesesve JF, Goupil JJ, Latger V, et al, "Artifactual Elevation of the Automated White Cell Count in the Context of a Bone Marrow Aspirate Analysis," *Clin Lab Haematol*, 2000, 22(1):55-8.
27. Faulkner WR, "Smoking, Leukocytes, and Coronary Artery Disease," *Lab Report: A Comprehensive Update on Laboratory Diagnosis*, 1998, 20(204):13-7.
28. Cowland JB and Borregaard N, "The Individual Regulation of Granule Protein mRNA Levels During Neutrophil Maturation Explains the Heterogeneity of Neutrophil Granules," *J Leukoc Biol*, 1999, 66(6):989-95.
29. Smith CW, "Introduction: Functional Polarity of Motile Neutrophils," *Blood*, 2000, 95(8):2459-61.
30. Johnston B and Kubes P, "The Alpha-4-Integrin: An Alternative Pathway for Neutrophil Recruitment?" *Immunol Today*, 1999, 20(12):545-50.
31. Welte K and Boxer LA, "Severe Chronic Neutropenia: Pathophysiology and Therapy," *Semin Hematol*, 1997, 34(4):267-78.
32. Kim SK and Demetri GD, "Chemotherapy and Neutropenia," *Hematol Oncol Clin North Am*, 1996, 10(2):377-95

(Continued)

White Blood Cell Count (Continued)

33. Bain BJ, Phillips D, Thomson K, et al, "Investigation of the Effect of Marathon Running on Leukocyte Counts of Subjects of Different Ethnic Origins: Relevance to the Aetiology of Ethnic Neutropenia," Br J Haematol, 2000, 108(3):483-7.

34. Levy J, Espanol-Boren T, Thomas C, et al, "Clinical Spectrum of X-Linked Hyper-IgM Syndrome," J Pediatr, 1997, 131(1 Pt 1):47-54.

35. Butcher S, Chahel H, and Lord JM, "Aging and the Neutrophil: No Appetite for Killing?" Immunology, 2000, 100(4):411-6.

36. Aprikyan AA, Liles WC, and Dale DC, "Emerging Role of Apoptosis in the Pathogenesis of Severe Neutropenia," Curr Opin Hematol, 2000, 7(3):131-2.

37. Aprikyan AA, Liles WC, Park JR, et al, "Myelokathexis, a Congenital Disorder of Severe Neutropenia Characterized by Accelerated Apoptosis and Defective Expression of bcl-x in Neutrophil Precursors," Blood, 2000, 95(1):320-7.

38. Liu J, Akahoshi T, Jiang S, et al, "Induction of Neutrophil Death Resembling Neither Apoptosis nor Necrosis by ONO-AE-248, a Selective Agonist for PGE$_2$ Receptor Subtype 3," J Leukoc Biol, 2000, 68(2):187-93.

39. Gillis S, Furie BC, and Furie B, "Interactions of Neutrophils and Coagulation Proteins," Semin Hematol, 1997, 34(4):336-42.

References

Carr R, "Neutrophil Production and Function in Newborn Infants," Br J Haematol, 2000, 110(1):18-28.

Cassatella MA and McDonald PP, "Interleukin-15 and its Impact on Neutrophil Function," Curr Opin Hematol, 2000, 7(3):174-7.

Dzik S, Moroff G, and Dumont L, "A Multicenter Study Evaluating Three Methods for Counting Residual WBCs in WBC-Reduced Blood Components: Nageotte Hemocytometry, Flow Cytometry, and Microfluorometry," Transfusion, 2000, 40(5):513-20.

Hartman KR, "Antineutrophil Antibodies of the Immunoglobulin M Class in Autoimmune Neutropenia," Am J Med Sci, 1994, 308(2):102-5.

Hoyer JD, "Leukocyte Differential," Mayo Clin Proc, 1993, 68(10):1027-8.

Shastri KA and Logue GL, "Autoimmune Neutropenia," Blood, 1993, 81(8):1984-95.

Witko-Sarsat V, Rieu P, Descamps-Latscha B, et al, "Neutrophils: Molecules, Functions, and Pathophysiological Aspects," Lab Invest, 2000, 80(5):617-53.

♦ **White Blood Cell Morphology** see Peripheral Blood: Differential Leukocyte Count on page 464

♦ **White Count** see White Blood Cell Count on page 496

♦ **Wiscott-Aldrich Syndrome** see Platelet Count on page 468

♦ **Xerocytosis** see Osmotic Fragility on page 462

♦ **X-Linked Pyridoxine-Responsive Sideroblastic Anemia** see Iron Stain, Bone Marrow on page 452

♦ **Zellweger Syndrome** see Inherited Diseases of Metabolism and Cell Structure on page 449

♦ **Zeta Sedimentation Rate, ESR** see Zeta Sedimentation Ratio on page 500

Zeta Sedimentation Ratio

Related Information

Bacterial Culture, Burn Sites on page 569
C-Reactive Protein, Serum on page 523
Fibrinogen on page 341
Sedimentation Rate, Erythrocyte on page 484
Viscosity, Serum or Plasma on page 495

Synonyms Erythrocyte Sedimentation Rate; Zeta Sedimentation Rate, ESR; ZSR

Test Includes Sedimentation rate expressed in percent

Abstract An automated sedimentation rate method, which however is not entirely analogous to other ESR methods. The ZSR requires a special centrifuge (the Zetafuge® - which is no longer under manufacture) for its performance. This test is not offered by the great majority of clinical laboratories and is performed only occasionally, largely in a research setting.[1]

Aftercare If results are equivocal or inconsistent with clinical impression, the C-reactive protein (CRP), or, the less commonly available plasma viscosity determination are also tests useful in assessment of the acute phase reaction.

Specimen Whole blood

Container Lavender top (EDTA) tube

Collection Specimen must be received within 4 hours of collection.

Causes for Rejection Insufficient blood, clotted specimen, hemolyzed specimen

Reference Interval Younger than 50 years: <55%; 50-80 years: 40% to 60%

Use Nonspecific indicator of infectious disease and inflammatory states, reflects acute phase reactant levels; screen for collagen diseases; screen for and follow activity of rheumatic diseases, especially rheumatoid arthritis

Limitations The ZSR centrifuge is no longer produced. The test is not performed by most clinical laboratories. The majority of laboratories use the manual Westergren sed rate method (see Sedimentation Rate, Erythrocyte on page 484).

Methodology Standardized stress is applied to a column of red cells and the extent of red cell packing is determined.

Additional Information The ZSR is rapidly performed, reproducible, and independent of the hematocrit. Sedimentation rate is increased, generally, in cases of infection/inflammation/tissue necrosis, especially where fibrinogen and inflammatory or macroglobulins are increased. May be increased with pregnancy, malignancy, and dysproteinemias (eg, especially macroglobulinemia and myeloma). Sedimentation rate may be decreased in sickle cell disease and spherocytosis. Poikilocytosis acts to inhibit red cell sedimentation. Use of the ESR, ZSR, and/or CRP may aid in the differentiation of the anemia of chronic disease from iron deficiency.[2] ZSR has been used to monitor disease activity including clinical assessment of rheumatoid arthritis. The erythrocyte sedimentation rate (including the ZSR) is usually markedly elevated in temporal (giant cell) arteritis.

Equipment for performance of the ZSR was discontinued by its American manufacturers but has recently been produced in China.[3] Chinese data indicate that the normal ZSR is 52.5% ±5.1%. ZSR on inpatients was 68.5% ±5.5%. Comparison with the Westergren method gave agreement of 86.6%. As previously noted by laboratories in the West, the ZSR was found advantageous by Chinese users due to provision of a rapid result, use of low sample volume, unaffected by anemia, and lack of need for age/sex correction.[3]

Footnotes

1. Baskurt OK, Temiz A, and Meiselman HJ, "Red Blood Cell Aggregation in Experimental Sepsis," J Lab Clin Med, 1997, 130(2):183-90.

2. Johnson MA, "Iron: Nutrition Monitoring and Nutrition Status Assessment," J Nutr, 1990, 120(Suppl 11):1486-91.

3. Su J, Peng Z, Li P, et al, "Investigation of the Zeta Reference Values by Chinese-Built Zetafuge® and Preliminary Application," Hua Hsi I Ko Ta Hsueh Hsueh Pao, 1998, 29(4):431-4.

References

"Guidelines on Selection of Laboratory Tests for Monitoring the Acute Phase Response. International Committee for Standardization in Haematology (Expert Panel on Blood Rheology)," J Clin Pathol, 1988, 41(11):1203-12.

"Zeta Sedimentation Rate," CRC Desk Reference for Hematology, Shinton NK, ed, Boca Raton, FL: CRC Press, 1998, 695.

♦ **Zinc Protoporphyrin:Heme Ratio** see Iron Stain, Bone Marrow on page 452

♦ **ZSR** see Zeta Sedimentation Ratio on page 500

IMMUNOLOGY

Wayne R. DeMott, MD

David S. Jacobs, MD

Fred V. Plapp, MD, PhD

Dwight K. Oxley, MD

Susan H. Hsu, PhD

Contributor: Eugene S. Olsowka, MD, PhD

The science of immunology includes its cellular and humoral constituents. Its mechanisms have been addressed in recent literature.[1]

This chapter focuses on laboratory tests pertinent to diseases which are known, or believed, to be of immune pathogenesis, including connective tissue diseases, vasculitides, organ-specific autoimmune diseases, autoimmune skin diseases, allergic disorders, transplantation immunology, and immunodeficiency syndromes. In previous editions of *Laboratory Test Handbook*, this chapter was titled, Immunology and Serology, and also included serologic tests used in the diagnosis of infectious diseases – tests which now appear in the chapter, Infectious Diseases.

The traditional approaches used to investigate serologic responses to disease were labor-intensive, as well as insensitive and nonspecific. Automation of serologic tests, broad availability of monoclonal antibody reagents, and dramatic improvements in flow cytometry instrumentation and software have combined to expand the readily available capabilities for immunologic evaluation of many clinical laboratories. Generally, diagnosis of disease by immunoassay involves either the detection of specific antibody or specific antigen. DNA methods have rapidly progressed since the last edition of this book.

The tests for antibodies may detect all classes of immunoglobulins or may be specific for IgG, IgM, or IgA. Detection of autoimmune antibodies may require interpretation of specific patterns. The immunology tests in this chapter include useful assays that may improve diagnosis of specific diseases. We have tried to provide information to orchestrate application of immunologic assays, and to include specifics of each test. Potential problems and applications are briefly addressed.

The authors express appreciation to Dr David F. Keren, who provided numerous additions and enhancements to the Immunology and Serology test listings in the 3rd edition of the *Laboratory Test Handbook*.

Footnotes

1. Schwartz RS, "Advances in Immunology - A New Series of Review Articles," *N Engl J Med*, 2000, 343(1):61-2.

♦ **Aβ42** *see Cerebrospinal Fluid and Plasma β-Amyloid(1-42) on page 513*

♦ **Aβ42 Peptide** *see Cerebrospinal Fluid and Plasma β-Amyloid(1-42) on page 513*

♦ **A Beta(1-42)** *see Cerebrospinal Fluid and Plasma β-Amyloid(1-42) on page 513*

♦ **ACA** *see Centromere/Kinetochore Antibody on page 512*

♦ **Aceruloplasminemia** *see Cerebrospinal Fluid Protein on page 517*

♦ **Acetylcholine Modulating Antibody** *see Acetylcholine Receptor Antibody on page 502*

Acetylcholine Receptor Antibody

Related Information
Antinuclear Antibody *on page 507*
Thyroglobulin Antibody *on page 544*
Thyroperoxidase Autoantibody *on page 545*

Synonyms Acetylcholine Modulating Antibody; Receptor Blocking Antibody; Receptor Modulating Antibody

Applies to Edrophonium Chloride Test; Prostigmin® Test; Rapid Nerve Stimulation Test; Single-Fiber Electromyographic Test

Abstract Myasthenia gravis (MG) is associated with autoantibodies of two types: those that bind to the acetylcholine receptor at sites not involved in acetylcholine binding, and those that block the binding of alpha-bungarotoxin.

About 15% of patients with MG have thymomas: about 3% in those younger than 20 years of age, 35% when older than 45 years of age. Usually symptoms of MG occur before recognition of thymoma, but MG can develop following diagnosis or even resection of thymoma. Thirty-three percent to 50% of patients seen in general hospitals with thymomas have MG. MG is the most common complication associated with thymoma.[1]

Specimen Serum

Container Red top tube or SST™ tube

Storage Instructions Separate serum and freeze in plastic vial

Reference Interval There are substantial interlaboratory differences in reference ranges. AChR binding antibody: <0.03 nmol/L; AChR modulating antibody: 0% to 20%.[2] Some laboratories report semiquantitative results.

Use Confirm the diagnosis of myasthenia gravis; the assay is highly specific for MG (specificity 99.9%); detect subclinical myasthenia gravis in patients with thymoma or graft versus host disease. Changes in the AChR concentration correlate with the clinical severity of MG during therapy with prednisone or with immunosuppressive agents, and following thymectomy. The highest levels of antibody are seen in younger patients.

Limitations AChR are negative in 7% to 34% of subjects with MG, and false negatives are found in 21% to 50% of cases of ocular MG. False negatives are seen in 6% to 25% of cases of generalized MG. Antibody may not be detected during the first 6-12 months after symptoms appear. The test is more likely to be positive in those with moderate to severe MG than in those with mild disease. Biologic false-positive AChR results are found in patients with Eaton-Lambert syndrome, rarely in first-degree relatives of subjects with MG, patients with thymoma without evidence of MG, patients with amyotrophic lateral sclerosis, primary biliary cirrhosis, carcinoma of lung, and in elderly individuals with propensity for autoimmune diseases. Although false positives are described in individuals who have had bone marrow transplantation and following treatment with penicillamine, clinical signs of MG may develop in some patients in those groups.

Contraindications Recent radioactive scan

Methodology The binding-antibody assay provides relatively high sensitivity and specificity. It is a radioimmunoassay (RIA) procedure. Tests done with human acetylcholine-receptor antigen are more sensitive than those performed with rat or ape antigen. Other assays include those for blocking antibody and tests for modulating antibody.

Additional Information The antibodies in patients with MG are believed to block acetylcholine-binding sites, damage the postsynaptic membrane, and accelerate receptor degradation.

Other tests for MG are available.

Footnotes
1. Shimosato Y and Mukai K, "Tumors of the Mediastinum," *Atlas of Tumor Pathology*, Washington DC: Armed Forces Institute of Pathology, American Registry of Pathology, 1997.
2. Mayo Medical Laboratories, *2000 Test Catalog*, Rochester, MN, 38-9.

References
Pachner AR, "Antiacetylcholine Receptor Antibodies Block Bungarotoxin Binding to Native Human Acetylcholine Receptor on the Surface of TE671 Cells," *Neurology*, 1989, 39(8):1057-61.
Siao P and Zuckerberg LR, "A 69-Year Old Man With Myasthenia Gravis and a Mediastinal Mass," Case Records of the Massachusetts General Hospital, Case 15-2000, Scully RE, Mark EJ, McNeely WF, et al, eds, *N Engl J Med*, 2000, 342(20):1508-14.
Spickett G, *Oxford Handbook of Clinical Immunology*, New York, NY: Oxford Press, 1999.

♦ **Acute Phase Reactant** *see C-Reactive Protein, Serum on page 523*

♦ **AD7c-Neuronal Thread Protein** *see Cerebrospinal Fluid and Plasma β-Amyloid(1-42) on page 513*

♦ **Adhesion Molecule CD31** *see HLA Typing, Single Human Leukocyte Antigen on page 529*

♦ **Allergen Profile** *see Allergen Specific IgE Antibody on page 502*

Allergen Specific IgE Antibody

Related Information
Immunoglobulin E *on page 533*

Synonyms Allergen Profile; Allergy Screen; IgE Allergen Specific; Radioallergosorbent Test (RAST®)

Applies to Fish Sensitivity; Immunocapture; Latex Sensitization; Phadenzyme RAST®; Pharmacia CAP; RAST®; Shrimp Sensitivity; UniCAP™

Test Includes *Alternaria tenuis*, Bermuda grass, cat epithelium, common ragweed, *Dermatophagoides farinae*, dog epithelium, egg white, English plantain, house dust, maple, oak, timothy, or specific mini panels of grasses, foods, animal danders, etc, one or multiple allergens from a large library (available commercially) can be chosen for analysis dependent upon clinical guidance.

Abstract Radiolabeled anti-IgE is used to detect binding of patient's IgE to specific allergens present on a paper disk (radioallergosorbent test-RAST). A number of commercial variations are available, some nonradiolabeled (eg, with enzyme-labeled detection system such as used by Phadenzyme RAST®). Absolute specific IgE levels (reported in mass units) are measured by the recently introduced UniCAP™ and Pharmacia CAP systems.[1]

Patient Preparation No radioisotopes administered 24 hours prior to collection of specimen (not applicable to nonisotope-based methods)

Specimen Serum; plasma may be used including heparinized plasma but fibrin, if formed, may cause high interassay variation and increased nonspecific binding.

Container Red top tube

Storage Instructions Separate serum and refrigerate. It is best to let blood clot and retract overnight at 4°C. Store at -20°C.

Turnaround Time Test is commonly performed by a reference laboratory.

Reference Interval Each allergen is scored from 0-4, 0 meaning no IgE detected, 1 meaning a borderline result, and 2-4 increasing IgE antibody against the allergen

Use Detect possible allergic responses to various substances in the environment such as animals, antibiotics, foods, grasses, house dust, mites, insects, insulin, molds, smuts, trees, and weeds. Evaluate hay fever, extrinsic asthma, atopic eczema, respiratory allergy.

Radioallergosorbent (RAST®) test, or its equivalent, is indicated when:
• specific allergic sensitivity is needed to allow immunotherapy ("desensitization shots") to be initiated
• testing for food or chemical sensitivity, in which skin testing is unreliable
• there is a history of severe allergic reaction to skin testing
• testing infants
• evaluating patients who refuse skin tests or who are unable to have them because of dermatopathic conditions
• immunotherapy or other therapeutic measures based on skin testing results have not led to a satisfactory remission of symptoms

Limitations RAST® results should be interpreted in the context of all available clinical and laboratory findings. False-negative results are possible and may reflect the timing of the blood sample relative to the previous adverse reaction. There may be overlap of IgE values between atopic and nonatopic conditions. High levels of total IgE (>3000 IU/mL as may be seen due to parasitic infestation) may result in nonspecific binding and, thus, false-positive RAST® results. Total quantitative IgE level must usually be ordered separately. When the level of total IgE is less than the geometric mean of IgE reference range, RAST® results may not have clinical significance.

Contraindications Recently administered radioisotopes will interfere with the radioisotope based forms of this test, causing spurious results.

RAST® is contraindicated when:
• all skin tests are negative
• the patient has only mild symptoms or can be successfully treated with medication and avoidance
• IgE levels are <10 IU/mL unless there is strong clinical suggestion of allergic disease
• patients have successfully responded to immunotherapy
• evaluating non-IgE mediated disease, such as certain drug and food reactions

Methodology Radioallergosorbent (RAST®) test (a radioimmunoassay). In this procedure specific allergen is adsorbed on a paper disk. Immunospecific IgE, if present in the test (patient's) serum will bind to the disk. Detection is effected by radiolabeled anti-IgE. Different scoring systems comparing test results with the absolute binding of a negative control are in use. A number of commercial variants have been introduced, many with nonradioactive detection systems. Enzyme immunoassay and immunofluorometric-based systems have been developed. While still in use and referred to as recently as 1997 as a "reference research assay,"[2] older methods will likely be replaced by the recently introduced quantitative IgE assays that quantitate specific IgE antibodies in mass units (ie, UniCAP and Pharmacia CAP systems).[1,3] A study of specific IgE laboratory-assay performance (6 laboratories using 5 different test procedures) found overall poor precision and accuracy by 4 of 6 testing facilities. The two laboratories using Pharmacia CAP System-Standard scoring performed nearly as well as the ideal standard.[4] Also, a multiallergen dipstick screening test has been introduced.[5]

Additional Information IgE is elevated 4 to 30 times normal in various diseases, among which atopic disorders and parasitic infections are most prominent. The principal limitation of this test is the wide and overlapping range of IgE values between atopic and nonatopic disease states. A positive value is usually meaningful; a negative value is equivocal. RAST® test is valuable on patients who do not respond to environmental control or conservative medical management and where skin tests are contraindicated.

Over 20 years have passed since RAST® testing has been available. Identification of allergen or allergens in patients with atopic disease may be approached clinically by history, avoidance of the offender, by skin testing and/or by RAST® studies. Numerous reports comparing skin testing and RAST® have accumulated in the literature, generally to assess which method has the better sensitivity/specificity. The results appear to vary with the allergen, that is, the relative performance of the two different methods, skin prick test (SPT) vs allergen specific IgE level, is allergen-dependent. This finding has provided the stimulus for expanded allergen specific comparison studies in the decade of the eighties. A brief summary of a subset of such studies follows.

- With dog and cat as allergens, sensitivity/specificity are similar but negative predictive value of either skin test or RAST® is much greater than positive predictive value.[6]
- Sensitivity of skin test vs RAST® in studies of shrimp allergens is somewhat comparable. There are apparent species-specific shrimp allergens possibly explaining intermittent nature of symptoms in some patients. Test sensitivity may be increased by use of extracts from more than one species of shrimp.[7]
- A comparison of fresh food skin prick tests and RAST® for a variety of vegetables, fruits, and nuts in patients with oral allergy syndrome showed generally variable specificity but better sensitivity with skin testing. RAST® showed better sensitivity only with hazelnut.[8]
- A comparison of RAST® with skin prick testing results in wasp venom allergy found systemic reaction to correlate with a positive paper RAST®. There was relatively good specificity with paper RAST® and skin prick testing, nearly all patients with a systemic reaction had positive paper RAST®.[9]

With the advent of specific IgE quantitative assays (UniCAP and Pharmacia CAP systems), a new round of comparison studies to evaluate the clinical significance of such quantitation is underway.[3] Applications in the area of predicting development of atopic disorders are also important (eg, egg-specific IgE levels in the first year of life vs subsequent aeroallergen sensitization/asthma, mite sensitization in early infancy vs subsequent asthma, and many other applications).[3] A comparison of skin prick test (SPT), Pharmacia CAP RAST®, and intradermal skin tests in cat allergy concluded that the latter "added little to the diagnostic evaluation."[10] Skin prick testing, however, has not been considered "obsolete" for a number (many of them clinical) reasons.[3]

Allergen-specific IgE testing has a large and growing number of applications. A sampling of some more unusual areas includes latex sensitization,[11,12] fish hypersensitivity,[13,14] venom allergy,[15,16,17] cow's milk protein,[18] and toxoplasmosis (IgE immunocapture method).[19]

Footnotes

1. Paganelli R, Ansotegui IJ, Sastre J, et al, "Specific IgE Antibodies in the Diagnosis of Atopic Disease. Clinical Evaluation of a New *In Vitro* Test System, UniCAP, in Six European Allergy Clinics" *Allergy*, 1998, 53(8):763-8.
2. Hamilton RG and Adkinson NF Jr, "Immunological Tests for Diagnosis and Management of Human Allergic Disease: Total and Allergen-Specific IgE and Allergen-Specific IgG," Rose NR, de Macario EC, Folds JD, et al, eds, *Manual of Clinical Laboratory Immunology*, 1997, 881-92.
3. Yunginger JW, Ahlstedt S, Eggleston PA, et al, "Quantitative IgE Antibody Assays in Allergic Diseases," *J Allergy Clin Immunol*, 2000, 105(6 Pt 1):1077-84.
4. Williams PB, Barnes JH, Szeinbach SL, et al, "Analytic Precision and Accuracy of Commercial Immunoassays for Specific IgE. Establishing a Standard," *J Allergy Clin Immunol*, 2000, 105(6 Pt 1):1221-30.
5. Twiggs JT, Gray RL, Pichler K, et al, "Evaluation of Multiallergen Dipstick Screening Test," *Ann Allergy*, 1989, 63(3):225-8.
6. Ferguson AC and Murray AB, "Predictive Value of Skin Prick Tests and Radioallergosorbent Tests for Clinical Allergy to Dogs and Cats," *Can Med Assoc J*, 1986, 134(12):1365-8.
7. Morgan JE, O'Neil CE, Daul CB, et al, "Species-Specific Shrimp Allergens: RAST® and RAST®-Inhibition Studies," *J Allergy Clin Immunol*, 1989, 83(6):1112-7.
8. Ortolani C, Ispano M, Pastorello EA, et al, "Comparison of Results of Skin Prick Tests (With Fresh Foods and Commercial Food Extracts) and RAST® in 100 Patients With Oral Allergy Syndrome," *J Allergy Clin Immunol*, 1989, 83(3):683-900.
9. Heinig JH, Mosbech H, Engel T, et al, "A Comparison of Two RAST® Methods and Skin Prick Testing in the Diagnosis of Wasp Venom Allergy," *Allergy*, 1989, 44(4):260-3.
10. Wood RA, Phipatanakul W, Hamilton RG, et al, "A Comparison of Skin Prick Tests, Intradermal Skin Tests, and RASTs in the Diagnosis of Cat Allergy," *J Allergy Clin Immunol*, 1999, 103(5 Pt 1):773-9.
11. Chen FC, von Dehn D, Büscher U, et al, "Atopy, The Use of Condoms, and a History of Cesarean Delivery: Potential Predisposing Factors for Latex Sensitization in Pregnant Women," *Am J Obstet Gynecol*, 1999, 181(6):1461-4.
12. Grote M, Mahler V, Spitzauer S, et al, "*In Situ* Localization of Latex Allergens in 3 Different Brands of Latex Gloves by Means of Immunogold Field Emission Scanning and Transmission Electron Microscopy," *J Allergy Clin Immunol*, 2000, 105(3):561-9.
13. Bernhisel-Broadbent J, Scanlon SM, and Sampson HA, "Fish Hypersensitivity. I. *In Vitro* and Oral Challenge Results in Fish-Allergic Patients," *J Allergy Clin Immunol*, 1992, 89(3):730-7.
14. Hansen TK, Bindslev-Jensen C, Skov PS, et al, "Codfish Allergy in Adults: IgE Cross-Reactivity Among Fish Species," *Ann Allergy Asthma Immunol*, 1997, 78(2):187-94.
15. Sainte-Laudy J, Sabbah A, Droute M, et al, "Diagnosis of Venom Allergy by Flow Cytometry. Correlation With Clinical History, Skin Tests, Specific IgE, Histamine and Leukotriene C4 Release," *Clin Exp Allergy*, 2000, 30(8):1166-71.
16. Stapel SO, Waanders-Lijster de Raadt J, van Toorenenbergen AW, et al, "Allergy to Bumblebee Venom. II. IgE Cross-Reactivity Between Bumblebee and Honeybee Venom," *Allergy*, 1998, 53(8):769-77.
17. Reimers AR, Weber M, and Müller UR, "Are Anaphylactic Reactions to Snake Bites Immunoglobulin E-Mediated?" *Clin Exp Allergy*, 1999, 30(2):276-82.
18. Sicherer SH and Sampson HA, "Cow's Milk Protein-Specific IgE Concentrations in Two Age Groups of Milk-Allergic Children and in Children Achieving Clinical Tolerance," *Clin Exp Allergy*, 1999, 29(4):507-12.
19. Villena I, Aubert D, Brodard V, et al, "Detection of Specific Immunoglobulin E During Maternal, Fetal, and Congenital Toxoplasmosis," *J Clin Microbiol*, 1999, 37(11):3487-90.

♦ **Allergic Fungal Sinusitis** *see* Immunoglobulin E *on page 533*

♦ **Allergy Screen** *see* Allergen Specific IgE Antibody *on page 502*

♦ **AMA** *see* Antimitochondrial Antibody *on page 505*

♦ **Amphiphysin** *see* Antineuronal Nuclear Antibody, Type 1 (Anti-Hu) *on page 506*

♦ **β-Amyloid$_{42}$** *see* Cerebrospinal Fluid and Plasma β-Amyloid$_{(1-42)}$ *on page 513*

♦ **Amyloid A, Serum** *see* C-Reactive Protein, Serum *on page 523*

♦ **Amyloid Beta Peptide** *see* Cerebrospinal Fluid and Plasma β-Amyloid$_{(1-42)}$ *on page 513*

♦ **Amyloid β-Protein** *see* Cerebrospinal Fluid and Plasma β-Amyloid$_{(1-42)}$ *on page 513*

♦ **Amyloid Precursor Protein (APP), CSF** *see* Cerebrospinal Fluid and Plasma β-Amyloid$_{(1-42)}$ *on page 513*

♦ **ANA** *see* Antinuclear Antibody *on page 507*

♦ **Anaphylatoxins** *see* Complement Components, Overview *on page 520*

♦ **ANCA** *see* Antineutrophil Cytoplasmic Antibody *on page 507*

♦ **ANNA-1** *see* Antineuronal Nuclear Antibody, Type 1 (Anti-Hu) *on page 506*

♦ **ANNA-2** *see* Antineuronal Nuclear Antibody, Type 2 (Anti-Ri) *on page 506*

♦ **Antiactin Antibodies** *see* Smooth Muscle Antibody *on page 543*

♦ **Anti-ASGPR** *see* Smooth Muscle Antibody *on page 543*

♦ **Antibody to Double-Stranded DNA** *see* Anti-DNA *on page 504*

♦ **Antibody to Native DNA** *see* Anti-DNA *on page 504*

Anticardiolipin Antibody

Related Information
Antinuclear Antibody *on page 507*
Antiphospholipid Antibody (Lupus Anticoagulant and/or Anticardiolipin Antibody) *on page 331*
Factor Inhibitors *on page 340*
Hypercoagulation Panel *on page 345*
Prothrombin Time *on page 354*
RPR *on page 677*
Sjögren Antibodies *on page 542*
VDRL, Serum *on page 688*

Applies to Antiphospholipid Antibody; Apolipoprotein H; Catastrophic Antiphospholipid Syndrome; β2-Glycoprotein 1; LA; Lupus Anticoagulant; Retinopathy

Test Includes Detection of IgG, IgM, and IgA antibody to the phospholipid, cardiolipin

Abstract Anticardiolipin antibodies (ACA) belong to the antiphospholipid antibody group of proteins and may have anticoagulant activity (similar to that of lupus anticoagulants). The **antiphospholipid antibody syndrome** is characterized by recurrent clinical events: noninflammatory thrombosis of small or large arteries and/or veins and fetal loss, with demonstrable antiphospholipid antibodies (anticardiolipin antibody or lupus anticoagulant). They are autoantibodies found in subjects with systemic lupus erythematosus and related entities, lupus-like diseases, infectious diseases, and drug reactions. The syndrome is primary if SLE is not present. When patients have SLE and also have antiphospholipid antibodies (with corresponding clinical features) cases are considered as secondary antiphospholipid antibody syndrome.

Specimen Serum

Container Red top tube

(Continued)

Anticardiolipin Antibody *(Continued)*

Storage Instructions Repeated freeze-thaw cycles alters stability of anti-cardiolipin antibodies.[1]

Reference Interval Negative

Use Differential diagnosis of recurrent thromboses, lupus-like syndromes, false-positive VDRL or RPR, recurrent fetal loss, and rarely, severe hemorrhage

Limitations Anticardiolipin levels by enzyme-linked immunosorbent assay (ELISA) are associated with poor reproducibility.

Methodology Enzyme-linked immunosorbent assay (ELISA)[2] for IgG or IgM anticardiolipin antibody

Additional Information Antibody to cardiolipin (the diphosphatidyl glycerol component of many phospholipid membranes) is at least partially cross reactive with the reagin antibody of syphilis and the lupus anticoagulant. The commonality between these diseases is antibody involving phosphate groups (lupus-DNA; VDRL-phospholipid of cardiolipin; and ACA - antibody directed against phospholipids of the coagulation system).

Binding of ACA to phospholipid is mediated by β_2-glycoprotein 1 (also known as apolipoprotein H), a serum protein with anticoagulant properties that may inhibit thrombin generation. Upon binding of β_2-glycoprotein 1 to phospholipid/cardiolipin, resultant change in structural configuration appears to expose new epitopes that stimulate formation of antiphospholipid antibodies.[3] Structural variants (mutants) with functional significance have been described.[4]

Neoepitopes, however, are not universally accepted as the antigenic targets. Pathophysiologic considerations of the recently proposed "catastrophic antiphospholipid syndrome" (CAPS), an accelerated form of primarily microvascular thrombosis as a severe manifestation of the antiphospholipid syndrome and with multiorgan involvement, focus on the role of endothelial cells in promoting a procoagulant state.[5] A sufficient "density" of proteins bound to phospholipid surfaces are required, representing a threshold for antibody binding. Endothelial cells, platelets, and monocytes are "activated" and adhesion molecules are upregulated.

ACA is associated with a host of clinical and laboratory abnormalities. Abnormal tests include thrombocytopenia, reactive VDRL or RPR, SS-A/Ro antibodies, and prolonged activated partial thromboplastin time (APTT) (lupus anticoagulant). Clinically, patients have lupus-like symptoms, often "ANA negative," recurrent venous and arterial thromboses, recurrent fetal loss (usually more than two episodes for a strong association), mitral valve endocarditis, chorea, and epilepsy. The entire constellation represents the antiphospholipid antibody syndrome. The association between thrombosis and recurrent fetal loss and ACA in patients with a prolonged APTT is especially strong in patients in whom ACA is not induced by infection or medication. IgG anticardiolipin is more likely to be influenced by disease activity than is IgM anticardiolipin. Plasmapheresis along with anticoagulant therapy may be used in symptomatic cases. Lupus anticoagulant and anticardiolipin antibodies are found together in about 70% of patients with antiphospholipid antibody syndrome. LA is found in about 20% to 40% and ACA is found in some 45% of subjects with SLE.[3] An increased incidence of antiphospholipid antibodies has been found among patients with monoclonal gammopathy of undetermined significance.[6]

Retinopathy has been shown to be associated with anticardiolipin antibody and with central nervous system lupus.[7] A recent report (based on a small sample size but utilizing 11 different thromboplastins) found no evidence that presence of ACA affects the international normalized ratio.[8] A recently developed ELISA system to detect complement-fixing ability of ACA with reported sensitivity of 78% and specificity of 84% (relative to the occurrence of thrombotic events) is possibly a marker for thrombotic manifestations of the antiphospholipid syndrome.[9] High titers of cerebrospinal fluid IgG-ACA have been shown to occur in symptomatic cerebral lupus patients with evidence of intrathecal synthesis.[10] The presence of ACA in patients with chronic hepatitis C virus (HCV) infection is reportedly significantly higher than in subjects with other inflammatory diseases of the liver (eg, chronic hepatitis B virus infection, primary biliary cirrhosis). The frequency of thrombotic complications was similar in ACA-positive and ACA-negative patients with chronic HCV infection. Sera from all but one ACA-positive HCV patient was negative for phospholipid-dependent anti-β_2-glycoprotein 1 antibodies.[11] Thus, while ACA commonly occurs in patients with chronic HCV infection, it may be without clinical import.

Footnotes

1. Brey RL, Cote SA, McGlasson DL, et al, "Effects of Repeated Freeze-Thaw Cycles on Anticardiolipin Antibody Immunoreactivity," *Am J Clin Pathol*, 1994, 102(5):586-8.

2. Harris EN, Pierangeli S, and Birch D, "Anticardiolipin Wet Workshop Report. Fifth International Symposium on Antiphospholipid Antibodies," *Am J Clin Pathol*, 1994, 101(5):616-24.

3. Kessler CM, "Coagulation Factor Deficiencies," *Cecil Textbook of Medicine*, 21st ed, Volume 1, Goldman L and Bennett JC, eds, Philadelphia, PA: WB Saunders Co, 2000, 1011-2.

4. Gushiken FC, Arnett FC, and Thiagarajan P, "Primary Antiphospholipid Antibody Syndrome With Mutations in the Phospholipid Binding Domain of β_2-Glycoprotein I," *Am J Hematol*, 2000, 65(2):160-5.

5. Triplett DA and Asherson RA, "Pathophysiology of the Catastrophic Antiphospholipid Syndrome (CAPS)," *Am J Hematol*, 2000, 65(2):154-9.

6. Stern JJ, Ng RH, Triplett DA, et al, "Incidence of Antiphospholipid Antibodies in Patients With Monoclonal Gammopathy of Undetermined Significance," *Am J Clin Pathol*, 1994, 101(4):471-4.

7. Ushiyama O, Ushiyama K, Koarada S, et al, "Retinal Disease in Patients With Systemic Lupus Erythematosus," *Ann Rheum Dis*, 2000, 59(9):705-8.

8. Mant MJ, Stang L, and Etches WS, "Warfarin Monitoring in Patients With Anticardiolipin Antibodies, but Without Lupus Anticoagulants," *Thromb Res*, 2000, 99(5):477-82.

9. Munakata Y, Saito T, Matsuda K, et al, "Detection of Complement-Fixing Antiphospholipid Antibodies in Association With Thrombosis," *Thromb Haemost*, 2000, 83(5):728-31.

10. Lai NS and Lan JL, "Evaluation of Cerebrospinal Anticardiolipin Antibodies in Lupus Patients With Neuropsychiatric Manifestations," *Lupus*, 2000, 9(5):353-7.

11. Tanikawa K and Sata M, "High Prevalence of Anticardiolipin Antibodies in Hepatitis C Virus Infection: Lack of Effects on Thrombocytopenia and Thrombotic Complications," *J Gastroenterol*, 2000, 35(4):272-7.

References

Alving BM, Barr CF, and Tang DB, "Correlation Between Lupus Anticoagulants and Anticardiolipin Antibodies in Patients With Prolonged Activated Partial Thromboplastin Times," *Am J Med*, 1990, 88(2):112-6.

Boumpas DT, Fessler BJ, Austin HA 3rd, et al, "Systemic Lupus Erythematosus: Emerging Concepts. Part 2: Dermatologic and Joint Disease, the Antiphospholipid Antibody Syndrome, Pregnancy and Hormonal Therapy, Morbidity and Mortality, and Pathogenesis," *Ann Intern Med*, 1995, 123(1):42-53.

Greisman SG, Thayaparan RS, Godwin TA, et al, "Occlusive Vasculopathy in Systemic Lupus Erythematosus. Association With Anticardiolipin Antibody," *Arch Intern Med*, 1991, 151(2):389-92.

Khamashta MA, Cuadrado MJ, Mujic F, et al, "The Management of Thrombosis in the Antiphospholipid-Antibody Syndrome," *N Engl J Med*, 1995, 332(15):993-7.

Khamashta MA and Hughes GR, "Detection and Importance of Anticardiolipin Antibodies. ACP Broadsheet No 136," *J Clin Pathol*, 1993, 46(2):104-7.

Lockshin MD, "Answers to the Antiphospholipid-Antibody Syndrome?" *N Engl J Med*, 1995, 332(15):1025-7.

Lopez LR, Santos ME, Espinoza LR, et al, "Clinical Significance of Immunoglobulin A Versus Immunoglobulins G and M Anticardiolipin Antibodies in Patients With Systemic Lupus Erythematosus - Correlation With Thrombosis, Thrombocytopenia, and Recurrent Abortion," *Am J Clin Pathol*, 1992, 98(4):449-54.

Male C, Mitchell L, Julian J, et al, "Acquired Activated Protein C Resistance Is Associated With Lupus Anticoagulants and Thrombotic Events in Pediatric Patients With Systemic Lupus Erythematosus," *Blood*, 2001, 97(4):844-9.

Ogawa H, Zhao D, Dlott JS, et al, "Elevated Anti-Annexin V Antibody Levels in Antiphospholipid Syndrome and Their Involvement in Antiphospholipid Antibody Specificities," *Am J Clin Pathol*, 2000, 114(5):619-28.

Anti-DNA

Related Information

Antinuclear Antibody *on page 507*
Complement C3, Serum *on page 519*
Complement, Total, Serum or Body Fluid *on page 522*
Sjögren Antibodies *on page 542*
Smith (Sm) and Ribonucleoprotein (RNP) Antibodies *on page 543*
Topoisomerase I Antibody *on page 546*

Synonyms Antibody to Double-Stranded DNA; Antibody to Native DNA; Anti-Double-Stranded DNA; Anti-ds-DNA; DNA Antibody; n-DNA

Applies to ss-DNA

Replaces Anti-ss-DNA

Test Includes Titers on positive specimens

Abstract IgG autoantibodies to ds-DNA are found characteristically in subjects with systemic lupus erythematosus (SLE) and only rarely with other connective tissue diseases. The other autoantibodies relatively specific for SLE include anti-Sm, which provides less sensitivity. Anti-Ro (SS-A) may be helpful. Antibodies to ds-DNA are found in 60% to 83% of patients with SLE at some time during their disease course;[1] thus, the absence of anti-ds-DNA antibody does not exclude the diagnosis of SLE. Results must be interpreted with other clinical and laboratory observations.

Specimen Serum

Container Red top tube

Storage Instructions Refrigerate immediately. Store at 4°C for up to 72 hours or at -20°C or colder without freezing and thawing indefinitely.

Reference Interval Normal: low levels of antibody or none (units and reference range will depend on laboratory and methodology). Most normal individuals have IgM antibodies to single-stranded DNA (ss-DNA). Such antibodies bear only low affinity for DNA. The specificity of anti-ss-DNA for SLE is substantially less than that of ds-DNA. Anti-ss-DNA is no longer considered useful for clinical diagnosis. IgG antibodies to double-stranded DNA are less common.[1]

One reference laboratory has for IgG ds-DNA antibody:[2]
- negative: <25 IU
- borderline positive: 25-30 IU
- positive: 31-200 IU
- strongly positive: >200 IU

Critical Values Higher values are more specific for active SLE.

Use Confirmatory test for systemic lupus erythematosus (SLE); monitor clinical course and response to treatment: 40% to 60% incidence in SLE in high to moderate titer

Limitations False-positive tests due to antibodies against histones have been reported with use of the *Crithidia luciliae* substrate assay, but are rare using calf thymus DNA.[3] Serum antibodies to single-stranded DNA lack utility for the diagnosis of SLE by virtue of lack of specificity. They are found in SLE, drug-induced SLE, and other entities.

Methodology Most tests are reactive to B DNA, the right-handed form of ds-DNA.[1] Methods include enzyme-linked immunosorbent assay (ELISA), indirect fluorescent antibody (IFA) using *Crithidia luciliae* substrate, radioimmunoassay (RIA), and Farr assay.

Additional Information The ANA may be positive in a number of diseases, some of which have clinical features similar to those of SLE. With ANA reactivity, additional tests can help establish the diagnosis of SLE: tests for autoantibodies to ds-DNA (anti-ds-DNA), to Smith antigen (anti-Sm), and to Ro (SS-A).

Anti-DNA antibody, in practice, refers to antibodies that bind specifically to double stranded DNA. Anti-ds-DNA antibodies may be detected by a radioimmunoassay technique known as Farr assay. The Farr assay is more specific for the diagnosis of SLE than the more commonly used enzyme immunoassays and is the assay which is most likely to predict flares, especially exacerbations of glomerulonephritis,[1] and/or to predict response to therapy. Anti-ds-DNA antibodies have specificity for SLE of nearly 100%. High antibody concentrations are more specific for SLE than are low concentrations just above the upper limit of normal (4 IU/mL). Between 50% and 85% of SLE patients have high titer antibodies. Weakly positive anti-ds-DNA antibodies occur infrequently in other autoimmune disease and in healthy persons.

In addition to diagnosis of SLE, measurement of anti-ds-DNA antibodies is helpful in assessing prognosis and monitoring disease activity in context of the entire clinical picture. Renal disease is more common in patients with high antibody levels. An increase in anti-ds-DNA concentration often precedes flares of disease activity in SLE patients. Because of this association, many physicians measure anti-DNA levels serially. Appropriate testing intervals are every 1-3 months in patients with active disease and every 6-12 months in patients with less active disease. The disease facets most likely to be heralded are flares of glomerulonephritis, vasculitis, or both. Serial tests should be performed in the same laboratory if disease activity is to be reliably monitored over time.

Other tests relevant to SLE and additional to the complements are CBC including platelet count, ESR, urinalysis with urine sediment microscopy, urinary protein excretion, and creatinine. Falling concentrations of C3 and C4 can also predict exacerbation.[1] Rising ESR, falling WBC counts, increasing urinary protein excretion, or observation of microscopic hematuria may also measure disease activity in SLE.[1] Creatinine and creatinine clearance are relatively insensitive to deterioration of glomerular filtration rate in lupus nephritis.[4]

Footnotes

1. Hahn BH, "Antibodies to DNA," *Mechanisms of Disease*, Epstein FH, ed, *N Engl J Med*, 1998, 338(19):1359-68.
2. Mayo Medical Laboratories, *2000 Test Catalogue*, Rochester, MN, 157.
3. Leavelle DE, *Mayo Medical Laboratories Interpretive Handbook*, Rochester, MN: Mayo Medical Laboratories, 1997.
4. Boumpas DT, Austin HA 3d, Fessler BJ, et al, "Systemic Lupus Erythematosus: Emerging Concepts. Part 1: Renal, Neuropsychiatric, Cardiovascular, Pulmonary, and Hematologic Disease," *Ann Intern Med*, 1995, 122(12):940-50.

References

Homburger HA, "Cascade Testing for Autoantibodies in Connective Tissue Diseases," *Mayo Clin Proc*, 1995, 70(2):183-4.

Kavanaugh A, Tomar R, Reveille J, et al, "Guidelines for Clinical Use of the Antinuclear Antibody Test and Tests for Specific Autoantibodies to Nuclear Antigens," *Arch Pathol Lab Med*, 2000, 124(1):71-81.

Keren DF, "Anti-ss-DNA Not Useful, Withdrawn From Survey," *CAP Today*, November 2000, 86.

Moder KG, "Use and Interpretation of Rheumatologic Tests: A Guide for Clinicians," *Mayo Clin Proc*, 1996, 71(4):391-6.

♦ **Anti-Double-Stranded DNA** *see* Anti-DNA *on page 504*

♦ **Anti-ds-DNA** *see* Anti-DNA *on page 504*

♦ **Anti-F Actin** *see* Smooth Muscle Antibody *on page 543*

♦ **Anti-GBM** *see* Glomerular Basement Membrane Antibody *on page 526*

♦ **Antigliadin Antibody** *see* Endomysial Antibodies *on page 525*

♦ **Antiglomerular Basement Membrane Antibody** *see* Glomerular Basement Membrane Antibody *on page 526*

♦ **Antihistidyl Transfer tRNA Synthase** *see* Jo-1 Antibody *on page 538*

♦ **Anti-Hu** *see* Antineuronal Nuclear Antibody, Type 1 (Anti-Hu) *on page 506*

♦ **Anti-Ku** *see* Topoisomerase I Antibody *on page 546*

♦ **Antiliver Cytosol 1 Antibodies** *see* Liver/Kidney Microsomal Type 1 Antibodies *on page 539*

♦ **Antiliver/Kidney Microsomal Antibodies** *see* Liver/Kidney Microsomal Type 1 Antibodies *on page 539*

♦ **Anti-LKM1** *see* Liver/Kidney Microsomal Type 1 Antibodies *on page 539*

Antimitochondrial Antibody

Related Information

Alkaline Phosphatase, Serum *on page 93*
Antineutrophil Antibody *on page 835*
Antineutrophil Cytoplasmic Antibody *on page 507*
Aspartate Aminotransferase, Serum *on page 112*
Bilirubin, Total, Serum *on page 118*
Gamma-Glutamyl Transferase, Serum *on page 179*
Immunoglobulin M *on page 537*
Liver Biopsy *on page 65*
Liver Disease: Laboratory Assessment, Overview *on page 216*
Liver/Kidney Microsomal Type 1 Antibodies *on page 539*
Smooth Muscle Antibody *on page 543*

Synonyms AMA; Mitochondrial Antibody

Abstract Biliary tract diseases which lead to cirrhosis include primary biliary cirrhosis (PBC), primary and secondary sclerosing cholangitis, hepatic diseases associated with chronic inflammatory bowel disease, and duct obstruction. They are characterized by disproportionately increased concentrations of serum alkaline phosphatase.[1] PBC is a chronic progressive autoimmune cholestatic disease in which intrahepatic bile ducts undergo continual destruction with portal inflammation and scarring, leading ultimately to cirrhosis and hepatic failure. Mitochondrial antibodies are found in up to 95% of patients with primary biliary cirrhosis, but may be found in other circumstances as well. They are usually absent in subjects with extrahepatic jaundice. Antimitochondrial antibodies (AMA) have high specificity for PBC when in substantial titer.[2]

Specimen Serum

Container Red top tube

Reference Interval ≤1:20 considered nondiagnostic; patients with PBC usually have titers >1:160; patients with other autoimmune disease often have titers between 1:20 and 1:80.

Use Tests for mitochondrial antibody are needed in differential diagnosis of chronic liver disease and to provide confirmatory evidence for diagnosis of PBC

Limitations AMA is also found in cryptogenic cirrhosis and in 25% to 30% of cases which have been classified as autoimmune hepatitis. AMA is rarely found in patients with extrahepatic biliary obstruction, drug-induced hepatitis, viral hepatitis, alcoholic and other forms of cirrhosis, and hepatic malignancy. There is an incidence of 1% positives in a general hospital population, mostly people with other autoimmune disease. AMA may be found in SLE and other disorders, but usually with lower titers.

AMA titer does not correlate with disease severity.

Methodology Indirect immunofluorescence, enzyme-linked immunosorbent assay (ELISA)

Additional Information PBC is a chronic intrahepatic cholestatic disease found most frequently in women, with an incidence which is highest in the 35- to 60-year age group. The diagnosis of PBC is based upon clinical observations including pruritus and often fatigue, malabsorption of fat soluble vitamins, histopathologic findings on liver biopsy,[1] markedly increased serum alkaline phosphatase activity and cholesterol concentrations, elevated IgM levels, and presence of mitochondrial antibodies.[2] Increases of 5'-nucleotidase and gamma-glutamyl transferase parallel those of alkaline phosphatase. Aminotransferases are increased only two-to fourfold in PBC. In >90% of patients, the key M2 antigen has been identified as the E_2 component of the pyruvate dehydrogenase complex, a mitochondrial enzyme. Enzyme-linked immunosorbent assays developed using pyruvate, branched-chain ketoacid, and alpha-ketoglutarate dehydrogenase promise to add objectivity to analysis of these antibodies.

An overlap syndrome is recognized in which histopathologic features of autoimmune hepatitis accompany antimitochondrial antibodies.[3]

A group of AMA-negative PBC patients all had ANA titers, often high.[4] With pruritus and high serum alkaline phosphatase, autoimmune cholangiopathy resembles primary biliary cirrhosis or primary sclerosing cholangitis but lacks antimitochondrial antibodies.[3] Patients with autoimmune cholangitis do not differ from those with PBC in respects other than negativity for AMA.[2]

Antineutrophil cytoplasmic antibody may prove helpful in the differential diagnosis between PBC and primary sclerosing cholangitis.[5] The following features are useful in this differential diagnosis. See table.

Antimitochondrial Antibody

	PBC	PSC
History of ulcerative colitis, Crohn disease	–	++
Antimitochondrial antibody	+++	±
Antinuclear antibody, double-stranded DNA, smooth muscle antibody	+	±
↑ IgM	+++	–
↑ Alkaline phosphatase	++	++
Endoscopic retrograde cholangiopancreatography findings	+	+++
Long indolent course	+	+++

PBC = primary biliary cirrhosis; PSC = primary sclerosing cholangitis; + = present to a 1+ degree; ++ = present to a 2+ degree; +++ = present to a 3+ degree; – = not present; ± = minimal degree of involvement

Adapted from Ferrell LD, "Liver and Gallbladder Pathology," *The Difficult Diagnosis in Surgical Pathology*, Weidner N, ed, Philadelphia, PA: WB Saunders Co, 1996, 290.

(Continued)

Antimitochondrial Antibody (Continued)

Patients with PBC are likely to have evidence of other autoimmune diseases, including Sjögren syndrome, scleroderma, CREST syndrome, and autoimmune thyroiditis. Subjects with PBC may have reactivity for rheumatoid factor, antismooth muscle antibodies, ANA, or thyroid antibodies. An association with sarcoidosis is recognized, a disease in which positive results of antimitochondrial antibodies is unusual.[6]

The laboratory tests of prognostic relevance in PBC include serum bilirubin, albumin, and prothrombin time. Serum bilirubin is the most important test for prediction of survival in candidates for liver transplantation in PBC.[2] GGT and C-reactive protein are among tests useful to monitor the course of PBC.

Footnotes

1. Ferrel L, "Liver Pathology: Cirrhosis, Hepatitis, and Primary Liver Tumors: Update and Diagnostic Problems," *Mod Pathol*, 2000, 13(6):679-704.
2. Kaplan MM, "Primary Biliary Cirrhosis," *N Engl J Med*, 1996, 335(21):1570-80.
3. Krawitt EL, "Autoimmune Hepatitis," *N Engl J Med*, 1996, 334(14):897-903.
4. Michieletti P, Wanless IR, Katz A, et al, "Antimitochondrial Antibody Negative Primary Biliary Cirrhosis: A Distinct Syndrome of Autoimmune Cholangitis," *Gut*, 1994, 35(2):260-5.
5. Hardarson S, Labrecque DR, Mitros FA, et al, "Antineutrophil Cytoplasmic Antibody in Inflammatory Bowel and Hepatobiliary Diseases. High Prevalence in Ulcerative Colitis, Primary Sclerosing Cholangitis, and Autoimmune Hepatitis," *Am J Clin Pathol*, 1993, 99(3):221-3.
6. Reilly JJ Jr and Mark EJ, "A 49-year-old Woman With Primary Biliary Cirrhosis, Pulmonary Opacities, and a Pleural Effusion," Case Records of the Massachusetts General Hospital, Case 14-1998, Scully RE, Mark EJ, McNeely WF, et al, eds, *N Engl J Med*, 1998, 338(18):1293-301.

References

Berg PA and Klein R, "Antimitochondrial Antibodies in Primary Biliary Cirrhosis and Other Disorders: Definition and Clinical Relevance," *Dig Dis*, 1992, 10(2):85-101.

Brenard R and Geubel AP, "Antimitochondrial and Antinuclear Antibodies in Primary Biliary Cirrhosis: An Update in Relation to Their Biochemical Characterization and Clinical Significance," *Acta Clin Belg*, 1991, 46(5):305-12.

Butler P, Valle F, and Burroughs AK, "Mitochondrial Antigens and Antibodies in Primary Biliary Cirrhosis," *Postgrad Med J*, 1991, 67(791):790-7.

Fussey SP, West SM, Lindsay JG, et al, "Clarification of the Identity of the Major M2 Autoantigen in Primary Biliary Cirrhosis," *Clin Sci*, 1991, 80(5):451-5.

Galperin C and Gershwin ME, "Immunopathogenesis of Gastrointestinal and Hepatobiliary Disease," *JAMA*, 1997, 278(22):1946-55.

Heseltine L, Turner IB, Fussey SP, et al, "Primary Biliary Cirrhosis. Quantitation of Autoantibodies to Purified Mitochondrial Enzymes and Correlation With Disease Progression," *Gastroenterology*, 1990, 99(6):1786-92.

Klein R, Huizenga JR, Gips CH, et al, "Antimitochondrial Antibody Profiles in Patients With Primary Biliary Cirrhosis Before Orthotopic Liver Transplantation and Titres of Antimitochondrial Antibody-Subtypes After Transplantation," *J Hepatol*, 1994, 20(2):181-9.

Klion FM, Fabry TL, Palmer M, et al, "Prediction of Survival of Patients With Primary Biliary Cirrhosis," *Gastroenterology*, 1992, 102(1):310-3.

Neuberger J, Lombard M, and Galbraith R, "Primary Biliary Cirrhosis," *Gut*, 1991, S73-8.

Perros P, Palmer JM, Yeaman SJ, et al, "Antimitochondrial Antibodies in Patients With Graves' Disease May Not Signify Primary Biliary Cirrhosis," *Postgrad Med J*, 1994, 70(819):17-8.

Provenzano G, Diquattro O, Craxi A, et al, "Immunoblotting as a Confirmatory Test for Antimitochondrial Antibodies in Primary Biliary Cirrhosis," *Gut*, 1993, 34(4):544-8.

Yeaman SJ, Fussey SP, Danner DJ, et al, "Primary Biliary Cirrhosis: Identification of Two Major M2 Mitochondrial Autoantigens," *Lancet*, 1988, 1(8594):1067-70.

Yoshida T, Bonkovsky H, Ansari A, et al, "Antibodies Against Mitochondrial Dehydrogenase Complexes in Primary Biliary Cirrhosis," *Gastroenterology*, 1990, 99(1):187-94.

Antineuronal Nuclear Antibody, Type 1 (Anti-Hu)

Related Information

Antineuronal Nuclear Antibody, Type 2 (Anti-Ri) *on page 506*

Synonyms ANNA-1; Anti-Hu

Applies to Amphiphysin; CRMP; PCA-1; PCA-2; PCA-Tr

Abstract Anti-Hu is one of several antibodies detected in the serum of patients with neurologic paraneoplastic syndrome. Anti-Hu antibody causes a subacute syndrome of encephalomyeloradiculopathy, sensory neuropathy, or autonomic neuropathy predominantly affecting the gastrointestinal tract.

Specimen Serum or CSF

Container Red top or SST™ tube

Reference Interval Serum: <1:60; CSF: <1:2

Use The presence of anti-Hu antibody suggests that a middle-aged patient with neurologic symptoms has a paraneoplastic syndrome. The underlying cancer is usually a small cell lung carcinoma. These tumors are not infrequently unsuspected but are found with searching in >80% of subjects. They are often undetected by routine imaging.[1] Clinically, the rapid onset of dementia without focal cerebral signs, but with cerebellar, brain stem, or peripheral nerve dysfunction, suggests paraneoplastic dementia.[2]

Limitations Anti-Hu is not recommended as a screening test for lung cancer. The absence of antibodies does not exclude a paraneoplastic syndrome or cancer.

Methodology Indirect immunofluorescence on sections of cerebellum, Western blot using recombinant protein, and immunohistochemical staining of brain tissue

Additional Information Anti-Hu antibody, an IgG marker, causes a spectrum of paraneoplastic neurologic disorders. Most frequent are pure sensory, predominantly autonomic, and mixed sensorimotor neuropathies. Some patients may present with gastroparesis or intestinal obstruction. When anti-Hu is found in high titer with encephalitis or sensory neuropathy, small cell lung carcinoma is almost always present, but may be difficult to find. Approximately 15% of patients will have another tumor coexisting with small cell lung carcinoma. Most patients have a long history of cigarette smoking. These syndromes occur twice as frequently in women as in men. Occasionally, other primaries are responsible (eg, carcinoma of prostate).

Anti-Hu has been detected in children with intestinal dysmotility, cerebellar ataxia, and brainstem encephalitis with and without peripheral neuroblastoma.

Anti-Hu is not detected in the serum or CSF of healthy individuals. It is found in about 5% to 10% of patients with small cell carcinoma of lung, not complicated by a neurological autoimmune disease.

Other paraneoplastic IgG markers recognized by immunofluorescence include ANNA-2, PCA-1, PCA-2, PCA-Tr, amphiphysin, and CRMP.

Footnotes

1. Posner JB, "Nonmetastatic Effects of Cancer: The Nervous System," *Cecil Textbook of Medicine*, 21st ed, Chapter 195, Goldman L and Bennett JC, eds, Philadelphia, PA: WB Saunders Co, 2000, 1051-4.
2. Lucchinetti CF, Kimmel DW, and Lennon VA, "Paraneoplastic and Oncologic Profiles of Patients Seropositive for Type 1 Antineuronal Nuclear Autoantibodies," *Neurology*, 1998, 50(3):652-7.

References

Benyahia B, Liblau R, Merle-Beral H, et al, "Cell-Mediated Autoimmunity in Paraneoplastic Neurological Syndromes With Anti-Hu Antibodies," *Ann Neurol*, 1999, 45(2):162-7.

Galanis E, Frytak S, Rowland KM, et al, "Neuronal Autoantibody Titers in the Course of Small-Cell Lung Carcinoma and Platinum-Associated Neuropathy," *Cancer Immunol Immunother*, 1999, 48(2-3):85-90.

Lennon VA, "Response in Q&A," *CAP Today*, 2000, 14(9):104.

Patel AM, Davila DG, Peters SG, "Paraneoplastic Syndromes Associated With Lung Cancer," *Mayo Clin Proc*, 1993, 68(3):278-87.

Posner J, "Anti-Yo and Anti-Hu," *Lab Med*, 1999, 30:770.

Sillevis-Smitt P, Manley G, Moll JW, et al, "Pitfalls in the Diagnosis of Autoantibodies Associated With Paraneoplastic Neurologic Disease," *Neurology*, 1996, 46(6):1739-41.

Antineuronal Nuclear Antibody, Type 2 (Anti-Ri)

Related Information

Antineuronal Nuclear Antibody, Type 1 (Anti-Hu) *on page 506*

Synonyms ANNA-2; Anti-Ri

Abstract Anti-Ri is the least common of the paraneoplastic autoantibodies and is usually associated with breast carcinoma.

Specimen Serum or cerebrospinal fluid

Container Red top or SST™ tube for blood

Collection 3 mL serum or 2 mL CSF

Reference Interval Serum: <1:60; CSF: <1:2

Use Detection of anti-Ri antibody in serum or cerebrospinal fluid identifies an otherwise unexplained neurological disorder as autoimmune and paraneoplastic. A positive result prompts a search for an underlying occult malignancy.

Limitations A negative result does not rule out a paraneoplastic syndrome or cancer. Anti-Ri antibodies are seldom detected in patients with breast carcinoma who do not have neurological dysfunction. In patients with ovarian carcinoma, the frequency of antineuronal antibodies is greater than the frequency of paraneoplastic syndromes. The presence of antibody does not necessarily lead to appearance of a paraneoplastic neurological syndrome.[1]

Methodology Western blot, indirect immunofluorescence (IIF)

Additional Information Anti-Ri antibodies are detected most commonly in postmenopausal women who usually present with signs of midbrain, brain stem, cerebellar and/or spinal cord dysfunction. Ocular opsoclonus-myoclonus may be a prominent symptom.

Most patients have a primary carcinoma of the breast. Small cell lung and gynecological cancer are less frequently associated with this syndrome. Treatment of the cancer can lead to decreased antibody titer and improvement of the neurological disorder.

Footnotes

1. Drlicek M, Bianchi G, Bogliun G, et al, "Antibodies of the Anti-Yo and Anti-Ri Type in the Absence of Paraneoplastic Neurological Syndromes: A Long-Term Survey of Ovarian Cancer Patients," *J Neurol*, 1997, 244(2):85-9.

References

Hunter SF, Parisi JE, Mastovich SL, et al, "Chronic Progressive Paraneoplastic Syndrome With Prominent Brainstem and Spinal Cord Involvement Associated With Type-2 Antineuronal Nuclear Antibodies (ANNA-2) and Breast Carcinoma," *J Neuropath Exp Neurol*, 1995, 54:464.

Moll JW, Hooijkaas H, van Goorbergh BC, et al, "Systemic and Antineuronal Autoantibodies in Patients With Paraneoplastic Neurological Disease," *J Neurol*, 1996, 243(1):51-6.

Antineutrophil Cytoplasmic Antibody

Related Information
Antimitochondrial Antibody on page 505
Antinuclear Antibody on page 507
Bronchial Brushings Cytology on page 373
Cryoglobulin, Qualitative, Serum and Plasma on page 524
Glomerular Basement Membrane Antibody on page 526
Kidney Biopsy on page 64
Urinalysis on page 887

Synonyms ANCA

Applies to C-ANCA; Myeloperoxidase Antibody (MPO-ANCA); P-ANCA; Proteinase 3 (PR3)

Abstract
Systemic necrotizing vasculitides are inflammatory diseases of the blood vessels, which are difficult to distinguish from infectious, connective tissue, and degenerative disease. Biopsies may reveal only nonspecific acute or chronic inflammation. Standard laboratory tests such as hemoglobin, WBC, ESR, ANA, and urinalysis have poor predictive value for vasculitis, because none of them is specific for vasculitis. Antineutrophil cytoplasmic antibodies (ANCA) are autoantibodies against several cytoplasmic antigens of neutrophils and monocytes. These antibodies are detected by indirect immunofluorescence microscopy. Two different immunofluorescent staining patterns have been identified, cytoplasmic (C-ANCA) and perinuclear (P-ANCA), which reflect different antigenic specificities. Diagnostically, ANCA tests are helpful adjuncts in the differential diagnosis of systemic vasculitides including Wegener granulomatosis (WG), microscopic polyangiitis, renal-limited vasculitis, Churg-Strauss angiitis, drug-induced ANCA-associated vasculitis, and idiopathic crescentic glomerulonephritis (ICGN). ANCA is best utilized in subjects with WG and microscopic polyangiitis with the combination of indirect immunofluorescence of neutrophils and ELISA for proteinase 3 (PR3)-ANCA and myeloperoxidase (MPO) ANCA.

Specimen Serum

Container Red top tube or SST™ tube

Reference Interval
Absent. Standard units for PR3-ANCA and MPO-ANCA by ELISA are not available.

Use
Diagnostically, ANCA tests are helpful adjuncts in the differential diagnosis of systemic vasculitides, multiple pulmonary nodules, destructive lesions of the upper airways, chronic otitis, and subglottic tracheal stenosis. C-ANCA is most often present in patients with WG, a necrotizing granulomatous inflammatory disease often including giant cells and epitheliod granulomas, involving the upper and/or lower respiratory tract, necrotizing vasculitis of small to medium vessels and necrotizing glomerulonephritis. P-ANCA is present in some patients with WG, but it is less sensitive and specific than the C-ANCA pattern. P-ANCA is most often found in patients with microscopic polyarteritis, crescentic glomerulonephritis, and occasionally inflammatory bowel disease.

Limitations
Although C-ANCA is useful in making the initial diagnosis and in monitoring disease activity, treatment should not be based soley on its presence. False-positive C-ANCA results have been reported in a number of infectious and neoplastic disorders. In a recent study, slightly >50% of the positive C-ANCA results occurred in patients who did not have Wegener granulomatosis as a final diagnosis. A positive or negative ANCA does not obviate the need for a tissue diagnosis in a patient with clinical manifestations suggestive of Wegener granulomatosis.

Heat inactivation of serum leads to false positives.

Criteria for atypical ANCA are described.[1]

Samples should be examined for PR3-ANCA and MPO-ANCA by ELISA, especially those negative by immunofluorescence. However, 5% of samples are positive only by ELISA.

ANCA-negative entities include leukocytoclastic skin vasculitis, Henoch-Schönlein purpura, classical polyarteritis nodosa, Kawasaki disease, Behçet disease, thromboarteritis obliterans, and giant cell (Takayasu) arteritis.[2] About 10% of subjects with WG or microscopic polyangiitis lack positive assays for ANCA.[2]

Methodology
Indirect immunofluorescence using whole buffy coat preparations, enzyme-linked immunosorbent assay (ELISA). Maximum specificity is provided by combined application of both.[3]

Patient's serum is incubated on slides containing ethanol-fixed human neutrophils. If ANCAs are present, they bind to neutrophils and are detected by adding fluorescently-labeled antihuman IgG. Two different immunofluorescent staining patterns have been identified, cytoplasmic (C-ANCA) and perinuclear (P-ANCA), which reflect different antigenic specificities. Antibodies producing a C-ANCA pattern usually bind to proteinase-3, a serine protease in the primary granules of neutrophils. Antibodies producing a P-ANCA pattern recognize one or more positively charged proteins such as myeloperoxidase (MPO), elastase, cathepsin G, lactoferrin, and lysozyme. Immunofluorescence titer is recommended when serum is positive to immunofluorescence and negative in ELISA for PR3 and MPO.[4]

Additional Information
The different staining patterns have diagnostic significance. C-ANCA with PR3 specificity by enzyme-linked immunosorbent assay is detected in 70% to 90% of individuals who have generalized WG.[1,2] ANCA is detectable in only 65% of patients without active renal disease (limited Wegener). The ANCA titer usually decreases with successful therapy, but varies widely from patient to patient. Baseline ANCA titers should be done prior to therapy to serve as a reference point for subsequent serial monitoring.

Evaluation for WG is supported by negative cultures. Bronchial brush and lavage may be useful.[5] Biopsies are pivotal.

P-ANCA is present in some patients with Wegener, but it is much less sensitive and specific than the C-ANCA pattern. In most cases of generalized active WG, C-ANCA with PR3 specificity is found; in up to 25%, P-ANCA with MPO specificity is demonstrated. About 60% of patients with microscopic polyangiitis or pauci-immune segmental necrotizing glomerulonephritis have P-ANCA with MPO specificity and 30% have C-ANCA with PR3 specificity. In a few, antiglomerular basement membrane antibodies are seen. WG and microscopic polyangiitis are more common causes of pulmonary-renal syndrome than antiglomerular basement membrane disease.[1] ANA can cause a false-positive P-ANCA. Therefore, an ANA should be ordered on any specimen with a positive P-ANCA, before the test is interpreted as clinically significant. ELISA for PR3-ANCA and MPO-ANCA are recommended as confirmation of P-ANCA specificity.

Anti-MPO antibodies are present in <1% of patients with systemic rheumatic diseases and are much more specific for vasculitis than the P-ANCA fluorescent pattern.

When asthma and eosinophilia are found with vasculitis, Churg-Strauss syndrome must be suspected.

See tables in Glomerular Basement Membrane Antibody on page 526.

P-ANCA occurs with some cases of autoimmune diseases, including ulcerative colitis more frequently than Crohn disease (about 60% to 70% positivity with ulcerative colitis, 5% to 10% with Crohn disease); autoimmune hepatitis, rheumatoid arthritis, and with SLE. Usually, specificities in such cases are other than MPO.

Footnotes
1. Jayne DR and Rasmussen N, "Treatment of Antineutrophil Cytoplasm Autoantibody-Associated Systemic Vasculitis: Initiatives of the European Community Systemic Vasculitis Clinical Trials Study Group," Mayo Clin Proc, 1997, 72(8):737-47.
2. Jennette JC and Falk RJ, "Small-Vessel Vasculitis," N Engl J Med, 1997, 337(21):1512-23.
3. Lim LC, Taylor JG III, Schmitz JL, et al, "Diagnostic Usefulness of Antineutrophil Cytoplasmic Autoantibody Serology: Comparative Evaluation of Commercial Indirect Fluorescent Antibody Kits and Enzyme Immunoassay Kits," Am J Clin Pathol, 1999, 111(3):363-9.
4. Savige J, Gillis D, Benson E, et al, "International Consensus Statement on Testing and Reporting of Antineutrophil Cytoplasmic Antibodies (ANCA)," Am J Clin Pathol, 1999, 111(4):507-13.
5. Michael CW and Flint A, "The Cytologic Features of Wegener's Granulomatosis," Am J Clin Pathol, 1998, 110(1):110-15.

References
Gibson LE, Daoud MS, Muller SA, et al, "Malignant Pyodermas Revisited," Mayo Clin Proc, 1997, 72(8):734-6.

Kalluri R, Meyers K, Mogyorosi A, et al, "Goodpasture Syndrome Involving Overlap With Wegener's Granulomatosis and Antiglomerular Basement Membrane Disease," J Am Soc Nephrol, 1997, 8(11):1795-800.

Kyndt X, Reumaux D, Bridoux F, et al, "Serial Measurements of Antineutrophil Cytoplasmic Autoantibodies in Patients With Systemic Vasculitis," Am J Med, 1999, 106(5):527-33.

Leff RD, Hellman RN, and Mullany CJ, "Acute Aortic Insufficiency Associated With Wegener Granulomatosis," Mayo Clin Proc, 1999, 74(9):897-9.

Merkel PA, Polisson RP, Chang Y, et al, "Prevalence of Antineutrophil Cytoplasmic Antibodies in a Large Inception Cohort of Patients With Connective Tissue Disease," Ann Intern Med, 1997, 126(11):866-73.

Michael CW and Flint A, "The Cytologic Features of Wegener's Granulomatosis," Am J Clin Pathol, 1998, 110(1):10-5.

Rao JK, Weinberger M, Oddone EZ, et al, "The Role of Antineutrophil Cytoplasmic Antibody (C-ANCA) Testing in the Diagnosis of Wegener Granulomatosis," Ann Intern Med, 1995, 123(12):925-32.

Romain PL and Aretz HT, "A 17½-Year-Old Girl With a Thoracoabdominal Aneurysm," Case Records of the Massachusetts General Hospital, Case 6-1999, Scully RE, Mark EJ, McNeely WF, et al, eds, N Engl J Med, 1999, 340(8):635-41.

Sandborn WJ, Landers CJ, Tremaine WJ, et al, "Association of Antineutrophil Cytoplasmic Antibodies With Resistance to Treatment of Left-Sided Ulcerative Colitis: Results of a Pilot Study," Mayo Clin Proc, 1996, 71(5):431-6.

Schaller JG, Niles JL, and Lerner LH, "A 16-Year-Old Girl With Fever, Rash, and Severe Ocular Disease," Case Records of the Massachusetts General Hospital, Case 20-1999, Scully RE, Mark EJ, McNeely WF, et al, eds, N Engl J Med, 1999, 341(2):110-6.

Schwartz WK and Niles JL, "A 75-Year-Old Woman With Hydrocephalus and Pleocytosis," Case Records of the Massachusetts General Hospital, Case 9-1999, Scully RE, Mark EJ, McNeely WF, et al, eds, N Engl J Med, 1999, 12(340):945-52.

Simms RW and Kirby RE, "A 64-Year-Old Man With Cranial-Nerve Palsies and a Positive Test for Antinuclear Cytoplasmic Antibodies," Case Records of the Massachusetts General Hospital, Case 28-1998, Scully RE, Mark EJ, McNeely WF, et al, eds, N Engl J Med, 1998, 339(11):755-63.

Antinuclear Antibody

Related Information
Anemia Flowchart on page 392
Anticardiolipin Antibody on page 503
Anti-DNA on page 504
(Continued)

Antinuclear Antibody (Continued)

Antiphospholipid Antibody (Lupus Anticoagulant and/or Anticardiolipin Antibody) on page 331
Aspartate Aminotransferase, Serum on page 112
Centromere/Kinetochore Antibody on page 512
Complement C4, Serum on page 520
Complement Components, Overview on page 520
Complement, Total, Serum or Body Fluid on page 522
Factor Inhibitors on page 340
Jo-1 Antibody on page 538
Kidney Biopsy on page 64
Liver Biopsy on page 65
Procainamide, Serum on page 763
Rheumatoid Factor, Serum or Body Fluid on page 541
RPR on page 677
Sjögren Antibodies on page 542
Skin Biopsy on page 71
Smith (Sm) and Ribonucleoprotein (RNP) Antibodies on page 543
Smooth Muscle Antibody on page 543
Topoisomerase I Antibody on page 546
VDRL, Cerebrospinal Fluid on page 688
VDRL, Serum on page 688

Synonyms ANA; FANA

Applies to ENA; Extractable Nuclear Antigens; Nucleolar Antibody

Replaces LE Cell Preparation

Test Includes Titers and pattern of nuclear fluorescence on positive samples

Abstract Antinuclear antibodies (ANA) are a central feature of systemic lupus erythematosus (SLE) and related rheumatic diseases, presently called the connective tissue diseases. ANAs are thought to be directly involved in the pathogenesis of these disorders. The antinuclear antibody (ANA) test provides good sensitivity for SLE, and therefore is often used to screen for autoimmune rheumatic diseases. Nearly all patients with active, untreated SLE have a positive ANA, and a negative ANA effectively rules out SLE.

Specimen Serum

Container Red top tube or SST™ tube

Storage Instructions Store at 4°C for up to 72 hours or -20°C or colder without freezing and thawing for an indefinite time period; -70°C used.[1]

Special Instructions A complete drug history is needed to rule out drug-induced lupus.

Reference Interval Negative; initial serum dilution may vary from laboratory to laboratory. A titer of 1:80 is often reported, but a titer ≥1:160 is considered significant by IFA, and <1:40 is considered negative. Cutoff value ≥3 units on enzyme immunoassay has been recommended.[1] Mayo Medical Laboratories has elected to use ≥1 units for EIA as a positive result, and to use ≥3 units for follow-up tests.[2]

Critical Values A titer ≥1:320 has specificity of almost 97% for SLE or a related disorder.

Use An ANA test should be ordered if the physician feels there is a reasonable clinical suspicion of SLE or another systemic rheumatic disease based on the clinical history, physical findings, and results of other laboratory tests. A large number of diverse conditions in addition to SLE are associated with positive ANA test results, including many chronic inflammatory and infectious diseases and some drugs.

Limitations A substantial number of normal healthy persons have a positive ANA. The prevalence of ANAs among healthy individuals varies with sex and age; older persons, particularly women older than 65 years, more commonly have positive results. Titers are usually low, <5% of healthy people have a titer of ≥1:160. Due to the low prevalence of SLE (50 cases per 100,000 persons) in the general population, the majority of persons randomly discovered to have a positive ANA result do not have SLE. Thus, lack of specificity is recognized. (Anti-ds-DNA and anti-Smith are specific for SLE.)

Repeat testing with ANA is not indicated for prediction of disease activity. Anti-ds-DNA is generally the test of choice to monitor disease progression in SLE, especially for lupus nephritis. C3 and C4 are also useful to monitor patients with SLE.

Drugs inducing proven and possibly causing positive ANA tests and clinical evidence of SLE include acebutolol, p-aminosalicylate, atenolol, captopril, carbamazepine, chlorpromazine, chlorthalidone, ethosuximide, hydralazine, isoniazid, lithium carbonate, mephenytoin, methimazole, α-methyldopa, metoprolol, minocycline, nitrofurantoin, oxprenolol, penicillamine, phenylethylacetylurea, phenytoin, practolol, primidone, procainamide, propylthiouracil, quinidine, sulfonamides, tartrazine, trimethadione, and others.[3]

Methodology Indirect immunofluorescence on HEp-2 cell line or animal tissue, sandwich immunoassay (immunometric assay), enzyme immunoassay[1,2,4,5]

Additional Information The ANA is based on indirect immunofluorescence. Serum is incubated on a slide containing a monolayer of human epithelial cells (HEp-2 cell line). If antibody is present, it binds to cell nuclei. Bound antibody is detected by adding fluorescent antihuman IgG. Positive cells demonstrate bright green fluorescence with a distinct staining pattern. Different laboratories may test patient samples at various initial dilutions

ranging from 1:40-1:160. Positive samples are then diluted and both the fluorescent pattern and titer are reported. The titer is the highest dilution of serum that still shows immunofluorescent nuclear staining.

The four commonly recognized staining patterns are homogenous, speckled, nucleolar, and centromere. Previously, attempts were made to correlate the fluorescent pattern with specific diseases. For example, the **homogenous pattern** was believed to indicate SLE or drug-induced SLE, **nucleolar pattern** scleroderma, **centromere pattern** the CREST syndrome, and **speckled pattern** a wide variety of diseases. During the last several years, however, the clinical importance of the staining pattern has diminished. Considerable overlap exists between the different fluorescent patterns and rheumatic diseases and more specific autoantibody tests have become available.

The clinical usefulness of the ANA is summarized in the following table.

Clinical Utility of ANA	Frequency (%) of Positive ANA
Diseases for which ANA is very useful for diagnosis	
SLE	95-100
Systemic sclerosis (scleroderma)	60-80
Diseases for which ANA is somewhat useful for diagnosis	
Sjögren syndrome	40-70
Idiopathic inflammatory myositis (dermatomyositis or polymyositis)	30-80
Diseases for which ANA is useful for monitoring or prognosis	
Juvenile chronic oligoarticular arthritis with uveitis	20-50
Raynaud phenomenon	20-60
Conditions in which ANA is part of the diagnostic criteria	
Drug-induced SLE	~100
Autoimmune hepatic disease	~100
Mixed connective tissue disease (MCTD)	~100
Diseases for which an ANA is not directly useful in diagnosis, but may be relevant to differential diagnosis	
Rheumatoid arthritis	30-50
Multiple sclerosis	25
Idiopathic thrombocytopenic purpura	10-30
Thyroid disease	30-50
Discoid lupus	5-25
Infectious diseases	Varies widely
Malignancies	Varies widely
Patients with silicone breast implants	15-25
Fibromyalgia	15-25
Relatives of patients with autoimmune diseases	5-25
Normal persons with titer >1:40	20-30
Normal persons with titer >1:160	5

Adapted from Kavanaugh A, Tomar R, Reveille J, et al, "Guidelines of Clinical Use of the Antinuclear Antibody Test and Test for Specific Autoantibodies to Nuclear Antigens," *Arch Pathol Lab Med*, 2000, 124(1):71-81.

ANAs and specific autoantibodies are an integral part of the diagnostic criteria of the American College of Rheumatology for systemic lupus erythematosus (SLE). Nearly all patients (95% to 100%) with active, untreated SLE have a positive ANA.

American College of Rheumatology Classification Criteria for SLE

Malar rash

Discoid rash

Photosensitivity

Oral or nasal ulcers

Arthritis of two or more peripheral joints

Pleuritis or pericarditis

Renal disease with persistent proteinuria (>0.5 g/d or >3+) or cellular casts

Unexplained seizures or psychosis

Hemolytic anemia, leukopenia (WBC <4.0 x 10^9/L), or lymphopenia on two or more occasions

Positive ANA, anti-ds-DNA antibodies, anti-Sm antibodies, or antiphospholipid antibodies

An expansion of this table is available. Raynaud phenomenon, hair loss, FUO, lymphadenopathy and/or splenomegaly, and thromboembolic phenomena are also characteristic of SLE.

Adapted from Bloom BJ and Zukerberg LR, "Case Records of the Massachusetts General Hospital. Weekly Clinicopathological Exercises. Case 14-1999. A 9-Year-Old Girl With Fever and Cervical Lymphadenopathy," Scully RE, Mark EJ, McNeely WF, et al, eds, *N Engl J Med*, 1999, 340(19):1491-7.

Patients who have few signs or symptoms suggestive of SLE have a low pretest probability of having the disease. In these patients, a positive ANA test result does little to increase the probability that the patient has SLE. In fact, positive ANA results in such cases can be misleading and precipitate unnecessary testing, erroneous diagnosis, or even inappropriate therapy. Patients classified as "ANA-negative LE" often demonstrate reactivity to Ro (SS-A).

Patients with **scleroderma (systemic sclerosis)** usually present with a distinct set of clinical signs and symptoms. Sixty to 90% of patients have a positive result. A positive ANA is not required for diagnosis, but can be supportive. A negative result might lead the physician to consider other fibrosing illnesses such as local scleroderma, the CREST syndrome, eosinophilic fasciitis, or scleredema.

Forty to 70% of patients with **Sjögren syndrome** have a positive ANA test result. This finding supports the diagnosis, but is not an absolute requirement. Testing is useful in patients with persistent sicca symptoms or in women who have given birth to a child with congenital heart block.

The ANA is positive in 30% to 70% of patients with **polymyositis** and **dermatomyositis**. A positive result is supportive, but a negative result does not rule out the diagnosis.

A positive ANA result is an integral component of the diagnosis of **drug-induced lupus erythematosus**, **autoimmune hepatitis**, and **mixed connective tissue disease**. Patients must have a positive ANA before these diagnoses can be made. All studies of drug-induced SLE have included a positive ANA result in the definition of the syndrome. Similarly, criteria for the diagnosis of certain types of autoimmune hepatitis and mixed connective tissue disease (MCTD) dictate that the ANA result be positive for diagnosis.

Raynaud phenomenon is diagnosed by physical examination and by specific clinical history. An ANA test does not establish the diagnosis, but may provide prognostic information. Raynaud phenomenon may be associated with several connective tissue diseases including SLE, rheumatoid arthritis, and scleroderma. However, the Raynaud phenomenon is also common among the general population and 80% of these individuals do not develop a systemic rheumatic disease. A positive ANA in a patient with Raynaud phenomenon increases the likelihood of development of a systemic rheumatic disease from 20% to 30%, while a negative result decreases the likelihood to about 7%.

The ANA is not useful in establishing diagnosis of **juvenile chronic arthritis**. However, in children with known disease, a positive ANA result may predict the development of **uveitis**, a serious complication. Approximately 33% of patients with a positive ANA develop uveitis. In such patients, a positive ANA is an indication for screening for uveitis.

An ANA is not necessary for diagnosis of the **antiphospholipid antibody syndrome**. However, approximately half of patients with this syndrome have a positive ANA. Positivity of ANA increases likelihood that the syndrome is secondary to SLE.

Except for subjects with the Raynaud phenomenon, juvenile chronic arthritis, and antiphospholipid antibody syndrome, ANA testing does not provide useful prognostic information. The ANA is not useful in assessment of disease activity. Since the ANA does not provide useful information about prognosis or disease activity, there is no indication for sequentially monitoring the ANA titer. (Serial measurements of anti-ds-DNA are utilized.)

ANA is positive in some individuals with chronic nonviral hepatitis, especially type 1 autoimmune hepatitis, in which antismooth muscle antibodies are also detected. These antibodies may also be found in some instances of primary biliary cirrhosis. In type 2 autoimmune hepatitis, antiliver/kidney microsomal type 1 antibodies are found; ANA and antismooth muscle antibodies are not detected. See table in Smooth Muscle Antibody *on page 543.*

Other tests useful to follow up a reactive ANA, in the appropriate clinical setting, in evaluation of possible autoimmune disease, include Sm, nRNP, Ro (SS-A), La (SS-B), topoisomerase 1 antibody, Scl-70, and Jo-1 antibody.[6]

Footnotes
1. Homburger HA, Cahen YD, Griffiths J, et al, "Detection of Antinuclear Antibodies: Comparative Evaluation of Enzyme Immunoassay and Indirect Immunofluorescence Methods," *Arch Pathol Lab Med*, 1998, 122(11):993-9.
2. Mayo Medical Laboratories, "Update on Serologic Tests for Systemic Rheumatic Diseases: Changes in the Analytical Methods for Antinuclear Antibodies and Anticentromere Antibodies," *Mayo Communique*, 1998, 23(4):1-3.
3. Schur PH, "Systemic Lupus Erythematosus," *Cecil Textbook of Medicine*, 21st ed, Chapter 289, Goldman L and Bennett JC, eds, Philadelphia, PA: WB Sanders Co, 2000, 1509-17.
4. Jaskowski TD, Schroder C, Martins TB, et al, "Screening for Antinuclear Antibodies by Enzyme Immunoassay," *Am J Clin Pathol*, 1996, 105(4):468-73.
5. Reisner BS, DiBlasi J, and Goel N, "Comparison of an Enzyme Immunoassay to an Indirect Fluorescent Immunoassay for the Detection of Antinuclear Antibodies," *Am J Clin Pathol*, 1999, 111(4):503-6.
6. Keren DF, "Anti-ss-DNA Not Useful, Withdrawn From Survey," *CAP Today*, November 2000, 86.

References
Bloom BJ and Zukerberg LR, "A 9-Year-Old Girl With Fever and Cervical Lymphadenopathy," Case Records of the Massachusetts General Hospital, Case 14-1999, Scully RE, Mark EJ, McNeely WF, et al, eds, *N Engl J Med*, 1999, 340(19):1491-7.
Kavanaugh A, Tomar R, Reveille J, et al, "Guidelines of Clinical Use of the Antinuclear Antibody Test and Tests for Specific Autoantibodies to Nuclear Antigens," *Arch Pathol Lab Med*, 2000, 124(1):71-81.

Madaio MP and McCluskey RT, "A 29-Year-Old Woman With Necrotizing Lymphadenitis, the Nephrotic Syndrome, and Acute Renal Failure," Case Records of the Massachusetts General Hospital, Case 33-1998, Scully RE, Mark EJ, McNeely WF, et al, eds, *N Engl J Med*, 1998, 339(18):1308-17.
Moder KG, "Use and Interpretation of Rheumatologic Tests: A Guide for Clinicians," *Mayo Clin Proc*, 1996, 71(4):391-6.
Warrington KJ, Moder KG, and Brutinel WM, "The Shrinking Lungs Syndrome in Systemic Lupus Erythematosus," *Mayo Clin Proc*, 2000, 75(5):467-72.

♦ **Antiparietal Cell Antibody** *see* Parietal Cell Antibody *on page 541*

♦ **Antiphospholipid Antibody** *see* Anticardiolipin Antibody *on page 503*

♦ **Anti-PM-1** *see* Topoisomerase I Antibody *on page 546*

♦ **Anti-PM-Scl** *see* Topoisomerase I Antibody *on page 546*

♦ **Antireticulin Antibody** *see* Endomysial Antibodies *on page 525*

♦ **Anti-Ri** *see* Antineuronal Nuclear Antibody, Type 2 (Anti-Ri) *on page 506*

♦ **Antismooth Muscle Antibody** *see* Smooth Muscle Antibody *on page 543*

♦ **Anti-ss-DNA** *replaced by* Anti-DNA *on page 504*

♦ **Antisynthetases** *see* Jo-1 Antibody *on page 538*

♦ **Antithyroglobulin Antibody** *see* Thyroglobulin Antibody *on page 544*

♦ **Antithyroid Peroxidase Antibody** *see* Thyroperoxidase Autoantibody *on page 545*

♦ **Anti-TPO** *see* Thyroperoxidase Autoantibody *on page 545*

♦ **Anti-U1snRNP** *see* Smith (Sm) and Ribonucleoprotein (RNP) Antibodies *on page 543*

♦ **Apolipoprotein H** *see* Anticardiolipin Antibody *on page 503*

♦ **Apoptosis** *see* CD4/CD8 Enumeration *on page 511*

♦ **Asialoglycoprotein Receptor Antibodies** *see* Smooth Muscle Antibody *on page 543*

♦ ***Aspergillus fumigatus* Precipitating Antibodies** *see* Hypersensitivity Pneumonitis Serology *on page 530*

♦ ***Aspergillus niger* Precipitating Antibodies** *see* Hypersensitivity Pneumonitis Serology *on page 530*

♦ **Autoimmune Lymphoproliferative Syndrome** *see* CD4/CD8 Enumeration *on page 511*

♦ **Bence Jones Protein Test** *replaced by* Immunofixation Electrophoresis, Serum or Urine *on page 530*

♦ **Berger Disease** *see* Immunoglobulin A *on page 532*

♦ **Berylliosis** *see* Lymphocyte Transformation Test *on page 539*

Beta₂-Microglobulin, Serum or Urine

Related Information
Aminoglycosides, Serum *on page 734*
Cadmium, Urine *on page 783*
CD4/CD8 Enumeration *on page 511*
Cerebrospinal Fluid Cytology *on page 376*
HIV-1/HIV-2 Antibody Screen and Western Blot *on page 636*
Zidovudine, Serum or Plasma *on page 771*

Synonyms β₂-Microglobulin

Abstract Beta-2 microglobulin (BMG) is a low molecular weight serum protein derived from cell membranes. It is the light chain component of the class I human leukocyte antigen (HLA) complex. BMG, with a half-life in plasma of ~107 minutes, is filtered by the renal glomerulus, and most of it is reabsorbed by the tubules. Elevated values are found in a large number of diseases, including renal failure (any cause), multiple myeloma, other lymphomas, many neoplasms, chronic inflammation, amyloidosis, and common variable immunodeficiency with granulomatous complications.

Patient Preparation Avoid recent administration of radioisotopes if assay performed by RIA.

Specimen Serum or 24-hour urine

Container Red top tube or SST™ tube, plastic urine container

Storage Instructions Urine BMG is unstable when pH is <5.5.

Reference Interval There are significant interlaboratory differences. One reference laboratory uses the cutoff for serum: <0.27 mg/dL[1].

A standard text uses, for serum, **average** values:[2]
• Neonates: 0.3 mg/dL
• 0-59 years: 0.19 mg/dL
• 60-69 years: 0.21 mg/dL
• >69 years: 0.24 mg/dL

Urine: <120 µg/day

Use Prognosis assessment in multiple myeloma: The serum BMG reflects tumor size, growth rate, and renal function. A value at presentation <0.4 mg/dL has the best prognosis; and a value >2.0 mg/dL has the worst.[3]

Renal tubular function. In the past BMG was measured in urine to assess proximal tubular function, but is rarely used now for that purpose.[4] (Continued)

Beta₂-Microglobulin, Serum or Urine (Continued)

Other. See Additional Information.

Limitations Increased synthesis of BMG in Crohn disease, hepatitis, sarcoidosis, vasculitis, hyperthyroidism, viral infections, and some malignancies decreases the usefulness of serum levels.

Methodology Radioimmunoassay (RIA), enzyme immunoassay (EIA), radial immunodiffusion (RID), nephelometry

Additional Information Serum BMG predicts response in subjects with low grade lymphoma: at 42 months no patient with a level ≥3.0 mg/L was projected to be in remission.[5] Urinary BMG becomes abnormal before serum creatinine in aminoglycoside nephrotoxicity. BMG is increased in AIDS patients with progressive disease, particularly those with opportunistic infection; it decreases in response to therapy. Its use has been combined with CD4 lymphocyte counts to calculate the probability of an HIV-infected person developing AIDS within the next 3 years.

BMG is reported to delineate a subset of subjects with primary amyloidosis whose outcomes are unfavorable, but it is not useful in such patients as an index of response to therapy.[6]

Pretreatment BMG concentrations >2.9 mg/dL are reported to recognize patients with stage I Philadelphia-positive chronic myelogenous leukemia, on interferon-α-based treatment, who are at greater risk of adverse outcome.[7]

Footnotes

1. Mayo Medical Laboratories, *2000 Test Catalogue*, Rochester, MN, 100.
2. Painter PC, Cope JY, and Smith JL, "Reference Information for the Clinical Laboratory," *Tietz Textbook of Clinical Chemistry*, 3rd ed, Philadelphia, PA: WB Saunders Co, 1999, 1826.
3. Riches P, *Clinical Biochemistry*, Marshall WJ and Bangert SK, eds, New York, NY: Churchill Livingstone, 1995, 499-500.
4. Newman DJ and Price CP, "Renal Function and Nitrogen Metabolites," *Tietz Textbook of Clinical Chemistry*, 3rd ed, Philadelphia, PA: WB Saunders Co, 1999, 1260.
5. Litam P, Swan F, Cabanillas F, et al, "Prognostic Value of Serum β-2 Microglobulin in Low-Grade Lymphoma," *Ann Intern Med*, 1991, 114(10):855-60.
6. Gertz MA, Kyle RA, Greipp PR, et al, "Beta 2-Microglobulin Predicts Survival in Primary Amyloidosis," *Am J Med*, 1990, 89(5):609-14.
7. Rodriguez J, Cortes J, Talpaz M, et al, "Serum β-2 Microglobulin Levels Are a Significant Prognostic Factor in Philadelphia Chromosome-Positive Chronic Myelogenous Leukemia," *Clin Cancer Res*, 2000, 6(1):147-52.

References

Klein J and Sato A, "The HLA System. First of Two Parts," *N Engl J Med*, 2000, 343(10):702-9.
Klein J and Sato A, "The HLA System. Second of Two Parts," *N Engl J Med*, 2000, 343(11):782-6.
Lucey PR, McGuire SA, Clerici M, et al, "Comparison of Spinal Fluid β₂-Microglobulin Levels With CD4+ T-Cell Count, *In Vitro* T Helper Cell Function, and Spinal Fluid IgG Parameters in 163 Neurologically Normal Adults Infected With the Human Immunodeficiency Virus Type 1," *J Infect Dis*, 1991, 163(5):971-5.
Roiter I, Da Rin G, De Menis E, et al, "Increased Serum β₂-Microglobulin Concentrations in Hyperthyroid States," *J Clin Pathol*, 1991, 44(1):73-4.

♦ **Buckley syndrome** *see* Immunoglobulin E *on page 533*

♦ **C1** *see* Complement Components, Overview *on page 520*

C1 Esterase Inhibitor, Serum

Related Information

Complement Components, Overview *on page 520*

Synonyms C1 Inactivator; C1 Inhibitor; Esterase Inhibitor; HANE Assay; Hereditary Angioneurotic Edema Test

Applies to C2 Kinin; Esterase, Subunit of C1

Test Includes Total immunoreactive level by immunodiffusion

Abstract C1 inhibitor is decreased in both hereditary and acquired angioedema.

Specimen Plasma

Container Lavender top (EDTA) tube

Storage Instructions Refrigerate

Reference Interval Total: 18-40 mg/dL

Use C1 esterase inhibitor is decreased in acquired and hereditary angioneurotic edema; decrease may be functional or quantitative

Limitations Levels are within normal limits in 15% of patients with the inherited form of the disease.

Methodology A functional (enzymatic) method should be used that tests the ability of a serum to inhibit the esterolytic activity of a preparation of activated C1 (C1 esterase). Some 25% of patient's and family members may have dysfunctional C1 inhibitor molecules with normal serum concentration. Thus, selection of inappropriate test methodology may deny therapy for a potentially fatal condition.[1] Radial immunodiffusion (RID) or nephelometry for measurement of antigenic material (may be used to measure concentration if presence of deficiency has been established). A functional (hemolytic) assay has been described.[2]

Additional Information C1 esterase inhibitor is a serum alpha₂ globulin acute-phase protein and a member of the serpin family of protease inhibitors that is synthesized by hepatocytes, monocytes (of blood), dermal fibroblasts, and vascular endothelium. Its physiologic function is inhibition of the catalytic subunits of the first component of the classic complement pathway (C1r and C1s). Deficiency of C1 esterase inhibitor results in the inappropriate activation of C1 and generation of C2 kinin. The latter molecule increases vascular permeability and is believed to be the mediator of the angioedema observed in patients with C1 esterase inhibitor deficiency. There are resultant recurrent bouts of circumscribed edema involving the subcutaneous tissue, gastrointestinal tract, and respiratory tract. C1 inhibitor plays a central role in regulation of the coagulation and contact (kinin-forming) systems as well as in control of the complement cascade. It inhibits C1r and C1s in the complement system, factor XII and kallikrein in the intrinsic pathway of coagulation, and activates plasminogen to plasmin in the fibrinolytic system (see figure).[3]

Pathogenesis of Hereditary Angioedema

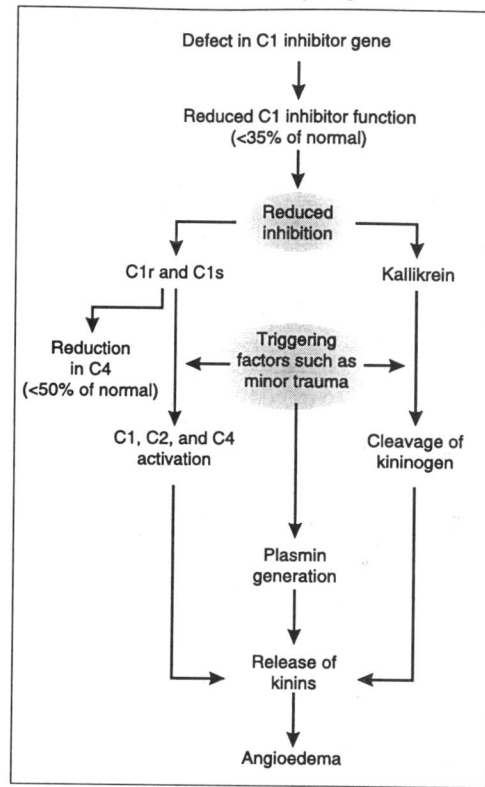

Persons with hereditary angioedema have one normal and one abnormal C1 inhibitor gene, resulting in defective inhibition of C1r, C1s, and kallikrein, the target proteases of C1 inhibitor. Under normal circumstances, this defect is clinically silent. Minor trauma, mental stress, and other unknown triggering factors activate the complement components of the classic pathway (C1, C2, and C4) and cleave high-molecular-weight kininogen in the contact system, as well as generating plasmin, leading to the release of vasoactive peptides that produce the symptoms of angioedema.

Adapted from Cicardi M and Agostoni A, "Hereditary Angioedema," *N Engl J Med*, 1996, 334(25): 1666-7.

Fatality may occur with involvement of airway/lungs. There may be massive swelling involving skin/subcutaneum. GI symptoms include severe abdominal pain, vomiting, and self-limited intestinal obstruction commonly followed by diarrhea.

There are two forms of C1 esterase inhibitor deficiency. The inherited form is usually detected in the first or second decade of life and has an autosomal dominant pattern of inheritance. Pathogenic mutants may be responsible for defective inhibitor molecules.[4] All patients with hereditary angioneurotic edema (HANE) are heterozygous for the deficiency with one normal gene controlling the synthesis of normal C1 inhibitor. This genetic basis, with a variable rate of biosynthesis of C1 inhibitor, may explain the variability in symptoms. The acquired form primarily affects adult or elderly patients with autoimmune or lymphoproliferative disorders, and relates to antibody activity to C1 inhibitor.

In the inherited form of C1 esterase inhibitor deficiency, there is either a quantitative or qualitative defect in the synthesis of the C1 esterase inhibitor protein. The more common form of hereditary angioneurotic edema (85% of cases) is due to an absolute decrease in the synthesis of the C1 esterase inhibitor. The less common form (15% of cases) is due to production of normal quantities of a functionally deficient protein. In both hereditary subtypes, C1 activation proceeds unabated, resulting in normal levels of C1q. Levels of C2 and C4 are decreased because of the uncontrolled activity of C1s. Patients in prolonged remission may have normal C4 levels but with activation of C1 (by incubation of serum at 37°C for 60 minutes) hemolytic (functional) C4 activity will be destroyed (by C1).

Patients with the acquired form of C1 esterase inhibitor deficiency produce immune complexes that consume large amounts of C1q and C1 esterase inhibitor, resulting in quantitative and functional deficiency of the C1 esterase inhibitor and C1q. C2, C3, and C4 levels are reduced in some patients.

Differentiation of Acquired and Hereditary Deficiencies

Type of Deficiency	C1q Levels	C2 and C4 Levels
Inherited	Normal	Decreased
Acquired	Decreased	Decreased

Footnotes

1. Bork K, Siedlecki K, Bosch S, et al, "Asphyxiation by Laryngeal Edema in Patients With Hereditary Angioedema," *Mayo Clin Proc*, 2000, 75(4):349-54.
2. Davis AE III, Aulak KS, Zahedi K, et al, "C1 Inhibitor," *Methods Enzymol*, Volume 223, Part B, San Diego, CA: Academic Press Inc, 1993, 97-120.
3. Cicardi M and Agostoni A, "Hereditary Angioedema," *N Engl J Med*, 1996, 334(25):1666-7.
4. Verpy E, Couture-Tosi E, Eldering E, et al, "Crucial Residues in the Carboxy-Terminal End of C1 Inhibitor Revealed by Pathogenic Mutants Impaired in Secretion or Function," *J Clin Invest*, 1995, 95(1):350-9.

References

Baldwin J, Pence HL, Karibo JM, et al, "C1-Esterase Inhibitor Deficiency: Three Presentations," *Ann Allergy*, 1991, 67(2 Pt 1):107-13.

Burak KW and May GR, "C1 Inhibitor Deficiency and Angioedema of the Small Intestine Masquerading as Crohn's Disease," *Can J Gastroenterol*, 2000, 14(4):349-451.

Caliezi C, Wuillemin WA, Zeerleder S, et al, "C1 Esterase Inhibitor: An Anti-inflammatory Agent and Its Potential Use in the Treatment of Diseases Other Than Hereditary Angioedema," *Pharmacol Rev*, 2000, 52(1):91-112.

Colten HR, "Hereditary Angioneurotic Edema, 1887-1987," *N Engl J Med*, 1987, 317(1):43-4.

Donaldson VH, "Inherited and Acquired C1 Inhibitor Deficiency," Section M, Immunodeficiency Disease, Cunningham-Rundles C, section editor, de Macario EC, volume editor, *Manual of Clinical Laboratory Immunology*, 5th ed, Chapter 102, Washington, DC: ASM Press, American Society of Microbiology, 1997, 841-4.

Greaves M and Lawlor F, "Angioedema: Manifestations and Management," *J Am Acad Dermatol*, 1991, 25(1 Pt 2):155-61.

Markovic SN, Inwards DJ, Frigas EA, et al, "Acquired C1 Esterase Inhibitor Deficiency," *Ann Intern Med*, 2000, 132(2):144-50.

Waytes AT, Rosen FS, and Frank MM, "Treatment of Hereditary Angioedema With a Vapor-Heated C1 Inhibitor Concentrate," *N Engl J Med*, 1996, 334(25):1630-4.

♦ **C1 Inactivator** *see* C1 Esterase Inhibitor, Serum *on page 510*

♦ **C1 Inhibitor** *see* C1 Esterase Inhibitor, Serum *on page 510*

♦ **C1q** *see* Complement Components, Overview *on page 520*

♦ **C1r** *see* Complement Components, Overview *on page 520*

♦ **C1s** *see* Complement Components, Overview *on page 520*

♦ **C2** *see* Complement Components, Overview *on page 520*

♦ **C2 Kinin** *see* C1 Esterase Inhibitor, Serum *on page 510*

♦ **C3** *see* Complement Components, Overview *on page 520*

♦ **C3a** *see* Complement Components, Overview *on page 520*

♦ **C3 Complement** *see* Complement C3, Serum *on page 519*

♦ **C3 Convertase** *see* Complement Components, Overview *on page 520*

♦ **C4** *see* Complement Components, Overview *on page 520*

♦ **C4a** *see* Complement Components, Overview *on page 520*

♦ **C4 Complement** *see* Complement C4, Serum *on page 520*

♦ **C5a** *see* Complement Components, Overview *on page 520*

♦ **C6** *see* Complement Components, Overview *on page 520*

♦ **C7** *see* Complement Components, Overview *on page 520*

♦ **C9** *see* Complement Components, Overview *on page 520*

♦ **Canale-Smith Syndrome** *see* CD4/CD8 Enumeration *on page 511*

♦ **C-ANCA** *see* Antineutrophil Cytoplasmic Antibody *on page 507*

♦ **Catastrophic Antiphospholipid Syndrome** *see* Anticardiolipin Antibody *on page 503*

CD4/CD8 Enumeration

Related Information

Beta$_2$-Microglobulin, Serum or Urine *on page 509*
Complete Blood Count *on page 419*
Flow Cytometry, Overview *on page 432*
HIV-1/HIV-2 Antibody Screen and Western Blot *on page 636*
Human Immunodeficiency Virus Culture *on page 639*
Peripheral Blood: Differential Leukocyte Count *on page 464*
White Blood Cell Count *on page 496*
Zidovudine, Serum or Plasma *on page 771*

Synonyms Immunodeficiency Profile

Applies to Apoptosis; Autoimmune Lymphoproliferative Syndrome; Canale-Smith Syndrome; CD4/CD8 Ratio; CD8; CD28; CD95; Fas-Mediated Cytotoxicity; Flow Cytometry; HAART; Highly Active Antiretroviral Therapy; Idiopathic CD4 Lymphocytopenia; Lymphocyte CD4 Counts; Opportunistic Infection; Perforin-Mediated Cytotoxicity; Space Flight

Test Includes Lymphocyte subpopulation enumeration

Abstract Depletion of CD4$^+$ helper/inducer T lymphocytes is one of the most significant surrogate markers to study progression of human immunodeficiency virus disease.

Specimen Whole blood; peripheral blood leukocytes can be harvested from leukopheresis packs or lymphoid tissue by use of Ficoll-Hypaque density gradient centrifugation. Skin puncture specimens may be used in children or adults with difficult venous access.[1]

Container Green top (heparin) tube

Storage Instructions Blood ideally is delivered to the laboratory immediately; however, whole blood may be held for 24 hours at room temperature prior to assay. Do not refrigerate or freeze sample.

Special Instructions With additional processing, polypropylene centrifuge tubes may be used. Polystyrene or polycarbonate should not be used in order to avoid cell adhesion. If RBC contamination occurs (due to clinical low mean corpuscular hemoglobin content), the red cells can be removed by hypotonic saline or ammonium chloride lysis.

Reference Interval See table.

Lymphocyte	Absolute Count (cells/μL)	Relative %
Mature T cells (CD3)	650-3036	65-92
Helper T cells (CD4)	310-2112	31-64
Suppressor T cells (CD8)	80-1353	8-41
CD4:8 ratio	1.0-1.5	

Use Enumeration of CD4 and CD8 cells is useful in the diagnosis and monitoring of patients with human immunodeficiency virus infections.

Limitations Values can be abnormal if patient is taking steroids or other immunosuppressives, has a severe intercurrent illness, or has had recent surgery requiring general anesthesia; patterns of maturation are disordered and inconsistent in lymphomas.

Methodology Flow cytometry (FC)

Additional Information The introduction of flow cytometry has allowed subclassification of lymphocytes on the basis of function and differentiation. Mature T cells in the peripheral blood usually express either the CD4 or CD8 antigen. CD4$^+$ T cells are functionally defined as T helper cells, while CD8$^+$ cells exhibit either suppressor or cytotoxic activity. Imbalances or deficiencies in the immune system can result from abnormalities in either the CD4 or CD8 population. In cases of Fas deficiency (result of specific Fas mutations) there is nonmalignant but potentially massive proliferation of T lymphocytes that are both CD4$^-$ and CD8$^-$.[2] This condition is generally referred to as the autoimmune lymphoproliferative syndrome (ALPS).[3] It has also been referred to as the Canale-Smith syndrome.[4] Fas (apo-1, CD95) represents a cell surface molecule of the tumor necrosis factor (TNF) group. Interaction of Fas with Fas-L (Fas-ligand) as occurs with prolonged lymphocyte activation leads to lymphocyte cell death by apoptosis.

HIV-1 infection causes significant changes in the number of CD4$^+$ and CD8$^+$ lymphocytes; within 6 months of seroconversion, the CD4 count falls about 30%, while the CD8 count increases by 40%, causing a decrease in the CD4:CD8 ratio. Healthy persons generally have absolute CD4 cell counts of about 1000 cells/μL and a CD4:CD8 ratio >1.0. CD4 counts <400 cells/μL are generally associated with a progression to AIDS. The continuing lymphocyte depletion may relate to one or more mechanisms, including direct killing of CD4 cells by HIV, syncytial formation with removal of both HIV+ and HIV- lymphocytes, immune responses to gp120 adsorbed on uninfected CD4 cells, and induction of programmed cell death (apoptosis) by the interaction of gp120 with CD4 (the HIV receptor).[5] With decrease in the absolute number of CD4 cells, the CD8 population is also affected with change from CD8$^+$ CD28$^+$ to CD8$^+$ CD28$^-$ phenotype, accelerated apoptosis, and increased turnover with chromosome telomere shortening. The generation of Fas-L-expressing CD4$^+$ T cells can lead to apoptosis of both CD4 and CD8 type of lymphocytes.[6] There is direct correlation between the CD4 count and the incidence of development of AIDS within 4 years. Increase in CD4 count from very low levels (CD4 count nadir) to at least 200 cells/mm^3 has been reported to be associated with a decreased rate of disease progression.[7]

The increase in CD8$^+$ cells is not unique to HIV-1 infection, since many viruses and vaccinations cause a transient increase in the CD8 population. It is important to determine absolute numbers of CD4$^+$ and CD8$^+$ cells, not just the CD4:CD8 ratio, in order to distinguish HIV-1 from other viral infections. In postsplenectomy patients, the absolute lymphocyte count may increase such that use of the percent of CD4 lymphocytes may be more reliable.

Rare individuals, occasionally with manifestations of immunodeficiency, have unusually low CD4 levels but no evidence of HIV infection. They have been labeled as cases of "idiopathic CD4 lymphocytopenia" (ICL).[8] These patients often have general lymphocytopenia with decrease in CD8 T cells, B cells, and NK cells, as well as CD4 T cells. Criteria for diagnosis is <300 CD4$^+$ T cells/μL or <20% of peripheral blood lymphocytes on at least two (Continued)

CD4/CD8 Enumeration *(Continued)*

occasions. Existence for hereditary CD4[+] T lymphocytopenia has been proposed in two siblings who suffered mental retardation, bronchiectasis, pansinusitis, warts, and marked decrease in CD4 T cells.[9]

Modest variations in CD4, CD8, and CD4:CD8 ratio occur with age, sex, and race. Absolute lymphocyte count (and each derived subset) peak in infancy and decline with age.[10] The Asian population (in particular males) appears to have lower mean percentages of CD3 and CD4 cells, a lower CD4:CD8 ratio and a lower absolute level of CD4 lymphocytes.[10,11]

Immediately following space flight, altered peripheral leukocyte subsets, serum and urine stress hormone levels, and T-cell cytokine secretion profiles were noted. Nearly all astronauts had increase in the CD4/CD8 T-cell ratio. These changes were considered to result from microgravity exposure and/or the physiologic stresses of landing and readaptation to unit gravity.[12]

Footnotes

1. Cracknell SE, Hinchliffe RF, and Lilleyman JS, "Lymphocyte Subset Counts in Skin Puncture and Venous Blood Compared," *J Clin Pathol*, 1995, 48(12):1137-8.
2. Le Deist F, Emile JF, Rieux-Laucat F, et al, "Clinical, Immunological, and Pathological Consequences of Fas-Deficient Conditions," *Lancet*, 1996, 348(9029):719-23.
3. Straus SE, Sneller M, Lenardo MJ, et al, "An Inherited Disorder of Lymphocyte Apoptosis: The Autoimmune Lymphoproliferative Syndrome," NIH Conference, *Ann Intern Med*, 1999, 130(7):591-601.
4. Drappa J, Vaishnaw AK, Sullivan KE, et al, "Fas Gene Mutations in the Canale-Smith Syndrome, an Inherited Lymphoproliferative Disorder Associated With Autoimmunity," *N Engl J Med*, 1996, 335(22):1643-9.
5. Hoxie JA, "Hematologic Manifestations of HIV Infection," *Hematology: Basic Principles and Practice*, 3rd ed, Chapter 154, Hoffman R, Benz EJ Jr, Shattil SJ, et al, eds, Philadelphia, PA: Churchill Livingstone, 2000, 2430-57.
6. Tateyama M, Oyaizu N, McCloskey TW, et al, "CD4 T Lymphocytes Are Primed to Express Fas Ligand by CD4 Cross-Linking and to Contribute to CD8 T Cell Apoptosis via Fas/FasL Death Signaling Pathway," *Blood*, 2000, 96(1):195-202.
7. Miller V, Mocroft A, Reiss P, et al, "Relations Among CD4 Lymphocyte Count Nadir, Antiretroviral Therapy, and HIV-1 Disease Progression: Results From the EuroSIDA Study," *Ann Intern Med*, 1999, 130(7):570-7.
8. Smith DK, Neal JJ, and Holmberg SD, "Unexplained Opportunistic and CD4+ T-Lymphocytopenia Without HIV Infection," *N Engl J Med*, 1993, 328(6):373-9.
9. Freier S, Kerem E, Dranitzki Z, et al, "Hereditary CD4+ T Lymphocytopenia," *Arch Dis Child*, 1998, 78(4):371-2.
10. Lee BW, Yap HK, Chew FT, et al, "Age- and Sex- Related Changes in Lymphocyte Subpopulations of Healthy Asian Subjects: From Birth to Adulthood," *Cytometry*, 1996, 26(1):8-15.
11. Howard RR, Fasano CS, Frey L, et al, "Reference Intervals of CD3, CD4, CD8, CD4/CD8, and Absolute CD4 Values in Asian and Non-Asian Populations," *Cytometry*, 1996, 26(3):231-2.
12. Crucian BE, Cubbage ML, and Sams CF, "Altered Cytokine Production by Specific Human Peripheral Blood Cell Subsets Immediately Following Space Flight," *J Interferon Cytokine Res*, 2000, 20(6):547-56.

References

Baseler MW, Stevens RA, Lambert LA, et al, "Immunologic Evaluation of Patients With Human Immunodeficiency Virus Infection," Section L Human Immunodeficiency Virus, Lane HC, section editor, *Manual of Clinical Laboratory Immunology*, 5th ed, Rose NR, deMacario EC, Folds JD, et al, eds, Washington, DC: ASM Press, American Society for Microbiology, 1997, 764-72.

Gougeon ML and Montagnier, L, "Programmed Cell Death as a Mechanism of CD4 and CD8 T Cell Deletion in AIDS: Molecular Control and Effect of Highly Active Antiretroviral Therapy," Mechanisms of Cell Death, The Second Annual Conference of the Cell Death Society, *Ann N Y Acad Sci*, New York, NY: New York Academy of Sciences, 1999, 199-209.

Kagan J, Calvelli T, Denny TN, et al, "Guideline for Flow Cytometric Immunophenotyping, a Report From the National Institute of Allergy and Infectious Diseases, Division of AIDS," *Cytometry*, 1993, 14(7):702-15.

Keren DF, Hanson CA, and Hurtubise PE, *Flow Cytometry and Clinical Diagnosis*, Chicago, IL: American Society of Clinical Pathologists, 1994.

Laurence J, "T-Cell Subsets in Health, Infectious Disease, and Idiopathic CD4[+] T Lymphocytopenia," *Ann Intern Med*, 1993, 119(1):55-62.

Nicholson J, Kidd P, Mandy F, et al, "Three-Color Supplement to the NIAID DAIDS Guideline for Flow Cytometric Immunophenotyping," *Cytometry*, 1996, 26(3):227-30.

"Revised Guidelines for the Performance of CD4+ T-Cell Determinations in Persons With Human Immunodeficiency (HIV) Infection," *MMWR Morb Mortal Wkly Rep*, 1994, 43:1-21.

Saah AJ, Spruill C, Hoover DR, et al, "Helper T-Lymphocyte Count. TRAx CD4 Test Kit Versus Conventional Flow Cytometry," *Arch Pathol Lab Med*, 1997, 121(9):960-2.

Shapiro NI, Karras DJ, Leech SH, et al, "Absolute Lymphocyte Count as a Predictor of CD4 Count," *Ann Emerg Med*, 1998, 32(3):323-8.

Stein DS, Lyles RH, Graham NM, et al, "Predicting Clinical Progression or Death in Subjects With Early-Stage Human Immunodeficiency Virus (HIV) Infection: A Comparative Analysis of Quantification of HIV RNA, Soluble Tumor Necrosis Factor Type II Receptors, Neopterin and β2-Microglobulin. Multicenter AIDS Cohort Study," *J Infect Dis*, 1997, 176(5):1161-7.

♦ **CD4/CD8 Ratio** *see* CD4/CD8 Enumeration *on page 511*

♦ **CD8** *see* CD4/CD8 Enumeration *on page 511*

♦ **CD21** *see* Complement, Total, Serum or Body Fluid *on page 522*

♦ **CD28** *see* CD4/CD8 Enumeration *on page 511*

♦ **CD35** *see* Complement, Total, Serum or Body Fluid *on page 522*

CD40-CD40 Ligand

Related Information
Immunoglobulin G Subclasses *on page 536*
Immunoglobulin M *on page 537*

Synonyms CD40:gp50; CD40-L:CD40 Ligand; CD154; gp39; T-BAM; TRAF

Applies to Hyper-IgM Syndrome

Abstract CD40, a cell surface receptor belonging to the tumor necrosis factor-R family, is expressed during all stages of B-cell development. Its ligand (CD40-L, synonym CD154) is expressed largely on activated CD4[+] T cells. CD40-CD40-L is involved in T-cell dependent B-cell responses. Patients with X-linked hyper-IgM syndrome (HIGM) have mutations in their CD40-L gene. CD40-CD40-L interactions have a broad role in immune regulation. CD40-L is involved in host immunity against human immunodeficiency virus (HIV) infection.

Specimen Tissue for frozen section study

Reference Interval Excessive CD40 and/or CD40-L expression indicates immune activation. Absence of expression is consistent with immunodeficiency.

Use Studies of immune regulation and investigation of immunodeficiency, in particular the hyper-IgM syndrome

Limitations CD40-CD40 ligand investigations are currently research level studies and will require advance planning in conjunction with local and/or research laboratories.

Methodology Monoclonal antibody-based direct immunofluorescent methods applied to tissue frozen section, *in vitro* cultured cells, and isolated cells.[1] These methods are of limited availability, generally only in research laboratories. Both CD40 and CD40-L have soluble forms. Enzyme-linked immunosorbent assays for sCD40 and sCD40-L have been developed, but significant clinical applications are not currently available.

Additional Information CD40 plays an important role in T-cell-dependent humoral immune responses. Originally identified and characterized in the mid 1980s (CD40 on B-lymphocytes and CD40 ligand on activated CD4[+] T cells). It is now considered that CD40-CD40-L interactions are of critical import for many immune responses. Applications are evolving in the control of HIV infection and in the therapy of chronic lymphocytic leukemia (CLL).[1,2] CD40 is expressed on monocytes and dendritic cells and is important in the late and final maturation of these antigen-presenting cells. CD40 is also expressed on endothelial cells, fibroblasts, and epithelial cells with their involvement in the inflammatory response.

Studies involving the use of blocking CD40-L antibodies in animal models for autoimmunity (eg, lupus nephritis, diabetes, collagen-induced arthritis, and experimental allergic encephalomyelitis) and in patients (eg, subacute lupus erythematosus) show evidence of beneficial effect.[1] Animal and human studies suggest a role for CD40-CD40-L in transplantation and in chronic inflammation (including atherosclerosis and pulmonary fibrosis).

Development of the acquired immunodeficiency syndrome (AIDS) involves interaction of CD40 ligand and HIV infection. During the later stages of this process, CD40-L expressing CD4[+] T cells become selectively depleted, possibly relating to a gp120-induced signal through CD40 that down regulates CD40-L expression.[2] The resultant acquired CD40-L deficiency contributes to the development of opportunistic infections similar to those seen in congenital CD40-L deficiency.

Footnotes

1. van Kooten C and Banchereau J, "CD40-CD40 Ligand," *J Leukoc Biol*, 2000, 67(1):2-17.
2. Kornbluth RS, "The Emerging Role of CD40 Ligand in HIV Infection," *J Leukoc Biol*, 2000, 68(3):373-82.

References

Ma X and Montaner LJ, "Proinflammatory Response and IL-12 Expression in HIV-1 Infection," *J Leukoc Biol*, 2000, 68(3):383-90.

Wierda WG, Cantwell MJ, Woods SJ, et al, "CD40-Ligand (CD154) Gene Therapy for Chronic Lymphocytic Leukemia," *Blood*, 2000, 96(9):2917-24.

♦ **CD40:gp50** *see* CD40-CD40 Ligand *on page 512*

♦ **CD40-L:CD40 Ligand** *see* CD40-CD40 Ligand *on page 512*

♦ **CD95** *see* CD4/CD8 Enumeration *on page 511*

♦ **CD154** *see* CD40-CD40 Ligand *on page 512*

Centromere/Kinetochore Antibody

Related Information
Antinuclear Antibody *on page 507*
Topoisomerase I Antibody *on page 546*

Synonyms ACA

Abstract Anticentromere antibodies (ACA) are strongly associated with CREST syndrome. They are a subset of antinuclear antibodies.

Patients with scleroderma are categorized primarily into two types of disease: limited and diffuse. Patients with the form of limited disease known as CREST syndrome, a scleroderma variant, tend to have a better prognosis than those with diffuse disease. Subcutaneous **c**alcinosis, **R**aynaud phenomenon, **e**sophageal dysfunction, **s**clerodactyly, and **t**elangiectasia characterize the CREST syndrome (3 of 5 must be evident). Autoantibodies may be useful in differentiating these two types. Limited disease is most commonly associated with the anticentromere pattern of ANA staining.

Specimen Serum

Container Red top tube or SST™ tube

Reference Interval IFA: negative;[1] ELISA: negative

Use Aid in diagnosis of CREST syndrome. Association with diffuse scleroderma is less strong, about 10% to 20%. Anticentromere antibodies are rarely found in systemic lupus erythematosus.

Anticentromere pattern is found in up to a quarter of individuals with idiopathic Raynaud phenomenon.[2] In such patients, the presence of this antibody may predict progression to the CREST syndrome.

Limitations May be absent in some patients with CREST syndrome and many with scleroderma. Positive in 15% of healthy controls; there is greater sensitivity for patients with limited cutaneous disease.[2]

Methodology Indirect immunofluorescent antibody (IFA) detected on HEp-2 tissue culture cell substrate, enzyme immunoassay (EIA)[3]

Additional Information Approximately 60% of patients with limited scleroderma have anticentromere antibodies. They occur more frequently in Caucasians than in African Americans, Hispanics, or Asians. Diffuse scleroderma is associated with antinuclear antibodies (ANA) as well as with Topoisomerase I Antibody *on page 546.* The presence of ACA and topoisomerase I is mutually exclusive.

Limited scleroderma bears association with primary biliary cirrhosis. ACA is found in 10% of subjects with that entity.

Footnotes

1. Moder KG, "Use and Interpretation of Rheumatologic Tests: A Guide for Clinicians," *Mayo Clin Proc*, 1996, 71(4):391-6.
2. Kavanaugh A, Tomar R, Reveille J, et al, "Guidelines for Clinical Use of the Antinuclear Antibody Test and Tests for Specific Autoantibodies to Nuclear Antigens," *Arch Pathol Lab Med*, 2000, 124(1):71-81.
3. Mayo Medical Laboratories, "Update on Serologic Tests for Systemic Rheumatic Diseases: Changes in the Analytical Methods for Antinuclear Antibodies and Anticentromere Antibodies," *Mayo Communique*, 1998, 23(4):1-3.

References

Goldman JA, "Anticentromere Antibody in Patients Without CREST and Scleroderma: Association With Active Digital Vasculitis, Rheumatic and Connective Tissue Disease," *Ann Rheum Dis*, 1989, 48(9):771-5.

Wigley FM, "Scleroderma (Systemic Sclerosis)," *Cecil Textbook of Medicine*, 21st ed, Chapter 290, Goldman L and Bennett JC, eds, Philadelphia, PA: WB Sanders Co, 2000, 1517-22.

♦ **Cerebral Lupus Erythematosus** *see Cerebrospinal Fluid IgG/Albumin Ratio, IgG Index, and IgG Synthesis Rate on page 514*

Cerebrospinal Fluid and Plasma β-Amyloid$_{(1-42)}$

Related Information

AD7c Neural Thread Protein, CSF or Urine *on page 83*
Apolipoprotein E, Plasma *on page 110*
Cerebrospinal Fluid Protein *on page 517*
Cerebrospinal Fluid Protein Electrophoresis *on page 518*
Complement Components, Overview *on page 520*

Synonyms Aβ42; Aβ42 Peptide; A Beta$_{(1-42)}$; β-Amyloid$_{42}$; Amyloid Beta Peptide; Plasma β-Amyloid$_{(1-42)}$

Applies to AD7c-Neuronal Thread Protein; Amyloid β-Protein; Amyloid Precursor Protein (APP), CSF; Creutzfeldt-Jakob Disease; CSF Amyloid Precursor Protein; Gamma Secretase; Presenilin; 14-3-3 Protein Assay; sAβ; Soluble Amyloid Beta; Tau Protein

Abstract Progressive deterioration in cognitive function gradually develops in Alzheimer disease (AD). Extracellular senile plaques and intracellular neurofibrillary tangles accumulate in the brains of affected patients in both familial and sporadic forms. Senile plaques are formed by deposition of β-amyloid peptides, which are toxic to neurons. The predominant form of β-amyloid in AD is β-amyloid$_{42}$ which aggregates more readily than do shorter forms of β-amyloid.[1] CSF levels of β-amyloid$_{(1-42)}$ are decreased in patients with AD.

The explanation for low concentrations of β-amyloid$_{42}$ in CSF in AD, while increased amounts are found in brain, is obscure, but possible explanations are discussed. The lowest concentrations occur in subjects with early-onset AD and in those with Ae4/e4 genotype.[1]

Patient Preparation Patient should be informed, relaxed, and properly positioned for lumbar puncture. Signed consent form is required. Antiseptic agents must be carefully and properly applied to the proposed puncture site. Local anesthetic (to which patient is not allergic) is usually advised.

Aftercare Patient should be maintained supine for a few hours postpuncture in an attempt to avoid postpuncture headache.

Specimen Cerebrospinal fluid, plasma

Collection Lumbar puncture

Storage Instructions Keep specimen refrigerated.

Causes for Rejection Specimen contaminated with blood

Turnaround Time Currently, β-amyloid$_{(1-42)}$, tau protein, and myelin basic protein levels are available only from a few referral, largely research laboratories.

Special Instructions Advance preparation (following the recommendations of research or referral laboratory) should be made prior to obtaining specimen (see Limitations).

Reference Interval CSF cutoff >1130 pg/mL[2]

Critical Values CSF concentrations of β-amyloid are decreased in AD to about 50% of those in controls.[2] Alternatively, the CSF ratio of β-amyloid$_{42}$ to β-amyloid$_{40}$ is increased in AD, early onset autosomal dominant forms.

Use The interest in using amyloid precursor protein derivatives as laboratory markers to help confirm a clinical diagnosis of Alzheimer disease arises from evidence that cerebral accumulation of the β-amyloid$_{(1-42)}$ (Aβ42) peptide occurs in many cases of Alzheimer disease. Low levels are not dependent on disease stage.

Limitations Different sizes of amyloid fragments exist in CSF. Measurement of total β-amyloid fragments does not correlate with the presence of AD and has no clinical utility.

Measurement of plasma Aβ40 levels is not useful in diagnosis of AD,[3] but elevated plasma levels of Aβ$_{(1-42)}$ can be detected several years prior to onset of symptoms in incipient AD.[4] Plasma β-amyloid$_{(1-42)}$ concentrations are increased in patients with Down syndrome, but are similar to levels from other mentally retarded individuals.[5]

Currently, this test is essentially unavailable in the United States from major general reference/research laboratories. The CSF 14-3-3 protein assay (for diagnosis of Creutzfeldt-Jakob disease - see below) is performed as a service by the Laboratory of CNS Studies, NINDS, National Institutes of Health, Bethesda, MD (301-496-4821).

Different groups have used different sets of antibodies.

More autopsy correlative studies are needed.

Methodology Immunoblotting, enzyme-linked immunosorbent assay (ELISA)

Additional Information AD usually begins in the seventh to ninth decades of life, but an early-onset form is well recognized, and histopathologic findings of Alzheimer encephalopathy appear in the brains of patients with Down syndrome. Several studies of Aβ42 in CSF have shown a decrease in the level of β-amyloid peptides in patients with AD compared to age-matched normal or neurologic disease control subjects. The probable biological explanation for a decrease in CSF Aβ42 is that the levels decrease as the peptide becomes increasingly insoluble and deposits in senile plaques.

The amyloid gene encodes a large protein called amyloid precursor protein (APP). Sequential proteolytic cleavages of APP by proteases referred to as beta and gamma secretases result in formation of two sizes of β-amyloid peptides (Aβ), containing 40 or 42 amino acids. Mutations in the amyloid precursor protein and 3 different presenilin genes enhance the cellular production of Aβ42 throughout life by selectively increasing the final cleavage of the APP by beta or gamma secretase. Presenilin is believed to act directly or as a cofactor in the cleavage of amyloid by gamma secretase. Mutations in the APP and presenilin genes are responsible for the relatively infrequent autosomal dominant form of early-onset AD. The E4 allele of apolipoprotein E is a strong susceptibility gene for the development of AD in individuals in their 60s and 70s, apparently affecting age of onset. It appears to somehow enhance Aβ42 aggregation and intracellular deposition. Other risk factors include those with cognitive impairment, family history, and Down syndrome. Elevation of plasma concentration of the 42-residue β-amyloid is found in presymptomatic carriers of mutations which are associated with familial AD.[6]

Combined application with tau protein improves diagnostic classification: high tau levels with low Aβ42 are found in the CSF of most subjects with AD.[7,8,9] Abnormal highly phosphorylated forms of the microtubule-associated tau protein are major constituents of the paired helical filaments that form neurofibrillary tangles in Alzheimer disease. Significant increase of CSF tau protein has been found in AD patients of five different national origins.[10,11,12,13,14] Tau protein in CSF may provide better discrimination of brain dysfunction in those younger than age 70 than in older patients.[15] Traumatic brain injury/environmental insults (with resultant neuronal or axonal injury) may elevate CSF amyloid peptide Aβ42, and correlate with increase in CSF tau protein.[16] There are recent reports of increased CSF tau protein in multiple sclerosis[17] and in normal pressure hydrocephalus.[18] In cases of dementia with Lewy bodies (DLB), the second most common neurodegenerative disease that causes dementia after AD, CSF Aβ42 levels are decreased but CSF tau levels have been reported as normal.[19] These findings in CSF are consistent with studies of DLB brain in which numerous senile plaques but few NFTs are usually found on neuropathologic study.[20]

Decreased CSF β-amyloid$_{(1-42)}$ has been reported in patients with Creutzfeldt-Jakob disease (CJD).[21] Interest has developed in 14-3-3 protein as a possible marker for the *in vivo* diagnosis of CJD.[22,23,24,25] The 14-3-3 proteins are involved in the regulation of protein phosphorylation and the mitogen-activated protein kinase pathway. Apparent false-negative results occur as well as false-positive results as reported in patients with herpes simplex encephalitis, multi-infarct dementia, acute infarction, stroke, subarachnoidal hemorrhage, viral encephalitis, and carcinomatous meningitis.[23,25] A commercial kit for 14-3-3 protein utilizing chemiluminescence is available (Amersham Buchler, Germany); see Limitations concerning a resource performing the 14-3-3 protein assay as a service.

Recently, CSF tau and AD7c-neuronal thread protein (each measured by enzyme-linked immunosorbent assay) have been suggested as biomarkers
(Continued)

Cerebrospinal Fluid and Plasma β-Amyloid(1-42)
(Continued)

for AD (together with reported specificity of 93% and sensitivity of 63%);[26] their utility remains under investigation.

Footnotes

1. Galasko D, "Cerebrospinal Fluid Opens a Window on Alzheimer Disease," *Arch Neurol*, 1999, 56(6):655-6.
2. Andreasen N, Hesse C, Davidsson P, et al, "Cerebrospinal Fluid β-Amyloid(1-42) in Alzheimer Disease: Differences Between Early- and Late-Onset Alzheimer Disease and Stability During the Course of Disease," *Arch Neurol*, 1999, 56(6):673-80.
3. Mehta PD, Pirttila T, Mehta SP, et al, "Plasma and Cerebrospinal Fluid Levels of Amyloid Beta Proteins 1-40 and 1-42 in Alzheimer Disease," *Arch Neurol*, 2000, 57(1):100-5.
4. Mayeux R, Tang MX, Jacobs DM, et al, "Plasma Amyloid Beta-Peptide 1-42 and Incipient Alzheimer's Disease," *Ann Neurol*, 1999, 46(3):412-6.
5. Mehta PD, Dalton AJ, Mehta SP, et al, "Increased Plasma Amyloid Beta Protein 1-42 Levels in Down Syndrome," *Neurosci Lett*, 1998, 241(1):13-6.
6. Skoog I, "Detection of Preclinical Alzheimer's Disease," *N Engl J Med*, 2000, 343(7):502-3.
7. Kanai M, Matsubara E, Isoe K, et al, "Longitudinal Study of Cerebrospinal Fluid Levels of Tau, Aβ1-40, and Aβ1-42(43) in Alzheimer's Disease: A Study in Japan," *Ann Neurol*, 1998, 44(1):17-26.
8. Andreasen N, Minthon L, Vanmechelen E, et al, "Cerebrospinal Fluid Tau and Aβ42 as Predictors of Development of Alzheimer's Disease in Patients With Mild Cognitive Impairment," *Neurosci Lett*, 1999, 273(1):5-8.
9. Hulstaert F, Blennow K, Ivanoiu A, et al, "Improved Discrimination of AD Patients Using β-amyloid(1-42) and Tau Levels in CSF," *Neurology*, 1999, 52(8):1555-62.
10. Arai H, Terajima M, Miura M, et al, "Tau in Cerebrospinal Fluid: A Potential Diagnostic Marker in Alzheimer's Disease," *Ann Neurol*, 1995, 38(4):649-52.
11. Vigo-Pelfrey C, Seubert P, Barbour R, et al, "Elevation of Microtubule-Associated Protein Tau in the Cerebrospinal Fluid of Patients With Alzheimer's Disease," *Neurology*, 1995, 45(4):788-93.
12. Hock C, Golombowski S, Naser W, et al, "Increased Levels of Tau Protein in Cerebrospinal Fluid of Patients With Alzheimer's Disease-Correlation With Degree of Cognitive Impairment," *Ann Neurol*, 1995, 37(3):414-5.
13. Vandermeeren M, Mercken M, Vanmechelen E, et al, "Detection of Tau Proteins in Normal and Alzheimer's Disease Cerebrospinal Fluid With a Sensitive Sandwich Enzyme-Linked Immunosorbent Assay," *J Neurochem*, 1993, 61(5):1828-34.
14. Franciotta D, Di Paolo E, Tinelli C, et al, "Protein Tau in Cerebrospinal Fluid of Patients With Alzheimer Disease," *Clin Chem*, 1998, 44(2):357.
15. Burger nee Buch K, Padberg F, Nolde T, et al, "Cerebrospinal Fluid Tau Protein Shows a Better Discrimination in Young Old (<70 years) Than in Old Old Patients With Alzheimer's Disease Compared With Controls," *Neurosci Lett*, 1999, 277(1):21-4.
16. Emmerling MR, Morganti-Kossmann MC, Kossmann T, et al, "Traumatic Brain Injury Elevates the Alzheimer's Amyloid Peptide A β42 in Human CSF. A Possible Role for Nerve Cell Injury," *Ann N Y Acad Sci*, 2000, 903:118-22.
17. Kapaki E, Paraskevas GP, Michalopoulou M, et al, "Increased Cerebrospinal Fluid Tau Protein in Multiple Sclerosis," *Eur Neurol*, 2000, 43(4):228-232.
18. Kudo T, Mima T, Hashimoto R, et al, "Tau Protein Is a Potential Biological Marker for Normal Pressure Hydrocephalus," *Psychiatry Clin Neurosci*, 2000, 54(2):199-202.
19. Kanemaru K, Kameda N, and Yamanouchi H, "Decreased CSF Amyloid β42 and Normal Tau Levels in Dementia With Lewy Bodies," *Neurology*, 2000, 54(9):1875.
20. Hansen LA, Masliah E, Galasko D, et al, "Plaque-Only Alzheimer Disease Is Usually the Lewy Body Variant, and Vice Versa," *J Neuropathol Exp Neurol*, 1993, 52(6):648-54.
21. Otto M, Esselmann H, Schulz-Schaeffer W, et al, "Decreased β-Amyloid1-42 in Cerebrospinal Fluid of Patients With Creutzfeldt-Jakob Disease," *Neurology*, 2000, 54(5):1099-102.
22. Zerr I, Bodemer M, Gefeller O, et al, "Detection of 14-3-3 Protein in the Cerebrospinal Fluid Supports the Diagnosis of Creutzfeldt-Jakob Disease," *Ann Neurol*, 1998, 43(1):32-40.
23. Hsich G, Kenney K, Gibbs C, et al, "The 14-3-3 Brain Protein in Cerebrospinal Fluid as a Marker for Transmissible Spongiform Encephalopathies," *N Engl J Med*, 1996, 335(13):924-30.
24. Moussavian M, Potolicchio S, and Jones R, "The 14-3-3 Brain Protein and Transmissible Spongiform Encephalopathy," *N Engl J Med*, 1997, 336(12):873-4.
25. Will RG, Zeidler M, Brown P, et al, "Cerebrospinal Fluid Test for New-Variant Creutzfeldt-Jakob Disease," *Lancet*, 1996, 348(9032):955.
26. Kahle PJ, Jakowec M, Teipel SJ, et al, "Combined Assessment of Tau and Neuronal Thread Protein in Alzheimer's Disease CSF," *Neurology*, 2000, 54(7):1498-504.

References

Brown P, "Infections of the Nervous System: F. Transmissible Spongiform Encephalopathies," *Neurology in Clinical Practice*, 3rd ed, Chapter 59, Bradley WG, Daroff RB, Fenichel GM, et al, eds, Boston MA: Butterworth Heinemann, 2000, 1423-30.

Fagan AM, Younkin LH, Morris JC, et al, "Differences in the Aβ40/Aβ42 Ratio Associated With Cerebrospinal Fluid Lipoproteins as a Function of Apolipoprotein E Genotype," *Ann Neurol*, 2000, 48(2):201-10.

Galasko D, Chang L, Motter R, et al, "High Cerebrospinal Fluid Tau and Low Amyloid β42 Levels in the Clinical Diagnosis of Alzheimer Disease and Relation to Apolipoprotein E Genotype," *Arch Neurol*, 1998, 55(7):937-45.

Heutink P, "Untangling Tau-Related Dementia," *Hum Mol Genet*, 2000, 9(6):979-86.

Martin JB, "Molecular Basis of the Neurodegenerative Disorders," *N Engl J Med*, 1999, 340(25):1970-8.

McNamara MJ, Gomez-Isla T, and Hyman BT, "Apolipoprotein E Genotype and Deposits of Abeta40 and Abeta42 in Alzheimer Disease," *Arch Neurol*, 1998, 55(7):1001-4.

Mulder C, Scheltens P, Visser JJ, et al, "Genetic and Biochemical Markers for Alzheimer's Disease: Recent Developments," *Ann Clin Biochem*, 2000, 37(Pt 5):593-607.

Murayama O, Tomita T, Nihonmatsu N, et al, "Enhancement of Amyloid Beta 42 Secretion by 28 Different Presenilin 1 Mutations of Familial Alzheimer's Disease," *Neurosci Lett*, 1999, 265(1):61-3.

Selkoe DJ, "The Origins of Alzheimer's Disease: A Is for Amyloid," *JAMA*, 2000, 283(12):1615-7.

Working Group on Molecular and Biochemical Markers of Alzheimer's Disease, "Molecular and Biochemical Markers of Alzheimer's Disease," *Neurobiol Aging*, 1998, 19(2):109-16.

♦ **Cerebrospinal Fluid IgG** *see* Cerebrospinal Fluid Immunoglobulin G *on page 515*

Cerebrospinal Fluid IgG:Albumin Ratio, IgG Index, and IgG Synthesis Rate

Related Information

Cerebrospinal Fluid Analysis: Overview *on page 416*
Cerebrospinal Fluid Immunoglobulin G *on page 515*
Cerebrospinal Fluid Oligoclonal Bands *on page 516*
Cerebrospinal Fluid Protein *on page 517*
Immunofixation Electrophoresis, Serum or Urine *on page 530*

Synonyms CSF IgG/CSF α_2-Macroglobulin; CSF IgG/CSF Albumin Ratio; CSF IgG:CSF Total Protein Ratio; IgG Ratios and IgG Index, Cerebrospinal Fluid

Applies to Cerebral Lupus Erythematosus; CSF IgG:Albumin Ratio; IgG Synthesis Rate; Oligoclonal Bands, CSF; Subacute Sclerosing Panencephalitis

Test Includes Protein measurements, frequently immunochemical, on CSF and/or serum with determination of ratio or ratios of one protein to another.

Abstract Multiple sclerosis is a relapsing and remitting demyelinating disease of the central nervous system for which there are no specific diagnostic laboratory tests. About 50% of multiple sclerosis patients have elevated CSF protein levels and about 75% have increased gamma globulin. Several tests have been devised to determine if the elevated gamma globulin is the result of intrathecal IgG synthesis. The most useful tests to aid in the diagnosis of multiple sclerosis are detection of oligoclonal bands in the CSF and estimations of the intrathecal synthesis of IgG. The detection of oligoclonal bands is the most helpful of the laboratory tests.[1] Synthesis of IgG in the central nervous system is typically oligoclonal, for reasons that are unknown. Estimates of intrathecal protein synthesis include calculations of IgG index, CSF IgG index, and the IgG synthesis rate. All methods require quantitation of serum and CSF albumin and IgG. The most helpful of the estimates of intrathecal protein synthesis is the IgG index.[2] An abnormal IgG index or IgG synthesis rate (indicative of increased CSF IgG production) is noted in some 90% of cases of clinically definite MS. The IgG synthesis rate is a complex formula which provides no more useful clinical information than the IgG index.[3]

Patient Preparation Patient should be informed, relaxed, and properly positioned for lumbar puncture. Signed consent form is required. Antiseptic agents must be carefully and properly applied to the proposed puncture site. Local anesthetic (to which patient is not allergic) is usually advised.

Aftercare Patient should be maintained supine for a few hours postpuncture in an attempt to avoid postpuncture headache.

Specimen Cerebrospinal fluid and serum; minimum of 0.1-0.5 mL of CSF is required, preferably, 3 mL of CSF and one SST™ tube of blood. Contact referral laboratory for specific specimen requirements.

Container Clean, sterile CSF tube; red top tube or SST™ tube of blood

Collection Tube should be labeled with the number indicating the sequence in which tubes were obtained.

Storage Instructions Store CSF in refrigerator at 4°C.

Causes for Rejection CSF received without concurrently obtained serum, insufficient quantity of CSF, CSF contaminated with blood ("bloody tap")

Special Instructions Before performing lumbar puncture, communicate with laboratory to determine which measurements and ratios are offered or can be obtained on a referral basis. The third tube of routinely obtained three tube set of CSF should be used for these studies. Simultaneous detection of oligoclonal bands by immunofixation or isoelectric focusing is recommended.

Reference Interval Published cutoff data utilizing receiver operator curves for CSF IgG index, CSF IgG:albumin ratio, and CSF IgG synthesis rate (mg/day) listed in the following table are from McMillan et al[2] using rate nephelometry methods with specificity threshold set at 90%. Published information is relevant only to lumbar CSF. Ventricular, cisternal, or cervical CSF may have different reference ranges. Alternative reference ranges from *Tietz Textbook of Clinical Chemistry* include:

- CSF IgG index: <0.7
- CSF IgG:albumin ratio: <0.27
- CSF IgG synthesis rate: -9.9-3.3 mg/day

Values >0.7, 0.27, and 8 mg/day are interpreted as increased.[3] Reference ranges used are dependent upon methodology and ideally are determined by each individual laboratory.

Formula	Specificity	Sensitivity	Cutoff Value	Predictive Value		
				Positive	Negative	
Index	90%	78%	0.7	86	83	96
Ratio	90%	62%	0.22	84	74	87
IgG synthesis rate	90%	47%	15	79	67	78

Cutoff values giving a specificity of 90% with the three formulae using rate nephelometry.

Adapted from McMillan SA, Douglas JP, Droogan AG, et al, "Evaluation of Formulae for CSF IgG Synthesis Using Data Obtained From Two Methods: Importance of Receiver Operator Characteristic Curve Analysis," *J Clin Pathol*, 1996, 49(1):24-8.

Use Oligoclonal bands and estimation of IgG production by the central nervous system are helpful in support of the diagnosis of multiple sclerosis, which is essentially a clinical diagnosis.

Limitations Conditions in which lymphoreticular elements of the CNS produce immunoglobulins may result in oligoclonal IgG synthesis. Such conditions include, but are not limited to, aseptic meningitis, lymphoma, subacute sclerosing panencephalitis (SSPE), sarcoidosis, neurosyphilis, Guillain-Barré syndrome[3], and cerebral lupus erythematosus.[4] These conditions, however, are either uncommon and may be ruled out clinically or by finding a CSF total protein >100 mg/dL, a leukocyte count >50/μL, or a positive test for neurosyphilis. Oligoclonal bands and IgG index are less commonly positive in childhood cases of multiple sclerosis.[5] Contamination of CSF by blood (even by small amounts) may elevate the IgG index and IgG synthesis rate.

Methodology Wide variety of generally immunochemical based methods (eg, rate nephelometry). See also Cerebrospinal Fluid Immunoglobulin G on page 515.

Additional Information Cerebrospinal fluid (CSF) is an ultrafiltrate of plasma lacking the highest molecular weight proteins (ie, IgM and alpha$_2$-macroglobulin). IgG may be synthesized in the CNS and normally comprises <10% of the total CSF protein. Elevated CNS IgG levels can be either a result of local synthesis or diffusion of plasma IgG across an altered blood brain barrier. Patients with demyelinating disorders often have elevated CSF IgG concentrations due to intrathecal synthesis. It is useful to determine the degree of permeability of the blood brain barrier when assessing CSF IgG synthesis, as increased CSF IgG may merely be a function of increased permeability of the blood-brain barrier. Albumin is a protein which is neither synthesized nor metabolized in the CSF compartment. Calculation of the CSF:serum albumin ratio allows one to assess the degree of permeability of the CSF.

The CSF/serum albumin index is calculated as:

$$\text{CSF/serum albumin index} = \text{albumin}_{CSF} / \text{albumin}_S$$

where albumin$_{CSF}$ is expressed in mg/dL and serum albumin (albumin$_S$) is expressed in g/dL. An index value <9 is consistent with an intact barrier.[3] In approximately 70% of multiple sclerosis cases, CSF albumin concentrations are not elevated.

The CSF IgG:albumin ratio is given as:

$$\text{IgG}_{CSF}:\text{albumin}_{CSF}$$

Both IgG$_{CSF}$ and albumin$_{CSF}$ are expressed in mg/dL. This ratio is a method of standardizing the CSF IgG relative to albumin. This formula especially estimates CSF IgG correcting for the permeability of the blood brain barrier.

The CSF IgG index is calculated as:

$$(\text{IgG}_{CSF} / \text{albumin}_{CSF}) / (\text{IgG}_{serum} / \text{albumin}_{serum})$$

where IgG$_{CSF}$ and albumin$_{CSF}$ are expressed in mg/dL and IgG$_S$ and albumin$_S$ are expressed in g/dL. This ratio further refines the estimation of CSF IgG synthesis by estimating IgG as a function of both serum concentration and permeability of the blood brain barrier to albumin and IgG.

Although these ratios are useful clinically, they do not quantify the CNS IgG production rate. Tourtellotte CSF IgG synthesis rate is calculated as follows:

$$5 \left[\left\{ \text{CSF IgG} - \frac{\text{serum IgG}}{369} \right\} - \left\{ (\text{CSF alb} - \frac{\text{serum alb}}{230}) \times \frac{0.43 \, (\text{serum IgG})}{\text{serum alb}} \right\} \right]$$

Where alb = albumin

Protein concentrations are expressed in mg/dL. The numbers 369 and 230 are the average normal serum:CSF ratios for IgG and albumin, respectively, 0.43 is the molecular weight ratio of albumin: IgG and 5 is the daily CSF production expressed in dL. The reference interval is -9.9 to +3.3 mg/day. Negative values are considered normal. Multiple sclerosis patients usually have a synthesis rate >8.0. This calculation is more complex (it rearranges the albumin and IgG values and introduces new constants) and does not provide any more clinical information than the CSF IgG index. Therefore, it is not routinely performed as part of multiple sclerosis panels. In the receiver operator curve study of McMillan et al, the CSF IgG synthesis rate had the lowest sensitivity of any index (47% sensitivity for IgG synthesis rate vs 78% sensitivity for the IgG index and 62% sensitivity for the IgG/albumin ratio).[2] Calculation of the CSF IgG synthesis rate may not be routinely performed as part of a multiple sclerosis panel, depending upon the reference laboratory.

Up to 20% of patients with neurosyphilis, SSPE, chronic fungal meningitis, and Guillain-Barré syndrome may have some of these protein abnormalities.

In a population of 56 HIV-seropositive individuals in which five had AIDS, 30% showed an increase in the CSF:serum albumin/IgG ratio.[6]

Patients with sciatica caused by lumbar disk herniation may leak plasma proteins into the CSF, resulting in increased CSF total protein. Disk patients with paresis may have significant increase in CSF total protein, CSF albumin and IgG, and in the CSF/serum albumin and IgG ratios but not in the IgG index (as compared to patients with lumbar disk herniation but without symptoms).[7]

Footnotes

1. Andersson M, Alvarez-Cermeno J, Bernardi G, et al, "Cerebrospinal Fluid in the Diagnosis of Multiple Sclerosis: A Consensus Report," *J Neurol Neurosurg Psychiatry*, 1994, 57(8):897-902.
2. McMillan SA, Douglas JP, Droogan AG, et al, "Evaluation of Formulae for CSF IgG Synthesis Using Data Obtained From Two Methods: Importance of Receiver Operator Characteristic Curve Analysis," *J Clin Pathol*, 1996, 49(1):24-8.
3. Johnson AM, Rohlfs EM, and Silverman LM, "Proteins," *Tietz Textbook of Clinical Chemistry*, 3rd ed, Chapter 20, Burtis CA and Ashwood ER, eds, Philadelphia, PA: WB Saunders Co, 1999, 515-7.
4. Martinez CE, Rivera GB, and Aguilar LD, "Anticardiolipin Antibodies in Serum and Cerebrospinal Fluid From Patients With Systemic Lupus Erythematosus," *J Investig Allergol Clin Immunol*, 1997, 7(6):596-601.
5. Selcen D, Anlar B, and Renda Y, "Multiple Sclerosis in Childhood: Report of 16 Cases," *Eur Neurol*, 1996, 36(2):79-84.
6. Hall CD, Snyder CR, and Robertson KR, "Cerebrospinal Fluid Analysis in Human Immunodeficiency Virus Infection," *Ann Clin Lab Sci*, 1992, 22(3):139-43.
7. Skouen JS, Larsen JL, and Vollset SE, "Cerebrospinal Fluid Protein Concentrations Related to Clinical Findings in Patients With Sciatica Caused by Disk Herniation," *J Spinal Disord*, 1994, 7(1):12-8.

References

Cavuoti D, Baskin L, and Jialal I, "Detection of Oligoclonal Bands in Cerebrospinal Fluid by Immunofixation Electrophoresis," *Am J Clin Pathol*, 1998, 109(5):585-8.

Krakauer M, Schaldemose, Nielsen H, et al, "Intrathecal Synthesis of Free Immunoglobulin Light Chains in Multiple Sclerosis," *Acta Neurol Scand*, 1998, 98(3):161-5.

Kyle RA and Katzmann JA, "Immunochemical Characterization of Immunoglobulins," Immunoglobulin Methods, Section C, Kyle RA, section ed, *Manual of Clinical Laboratory Immunology*, Nakamura RM, volume ed, 5th ed, Chapter 16, Washington, DC: ASM Press, American Society for Microbiology, 1997, 173-4.

LeVine SM, Lynch SG, Ou CN, et al, "Ferritin, Transferrin and Iron Concentrations in the Cerebrospinal Fluid of Multiple Sclerosis Patients," *Brain Res*, 1999, 821(2):511-5.

McMillan SA, McDonnell GV, Douglas JP, et al, "Evaluation of the Clinical Utility of Cerebrospinal Fluid (CSF) Indices of Inflammatory Markers in Multiple Sclerosis," *Acta Neurol Scand*, 2000, 101(4):239-43.

Olek MS and Dawson DM, "Multiple Sclerosis and Other Inflammatory Demyelinating Diseases of the Central Nervous System," *Neurology in Clinical Practice*, Volume 2, 3rd ed, Chapter 60, Bradley WG, Daroff RB, and Ferichel GM, et al, eds, Boston MA: Butterworth Heinemann, 2000, 1431-65.

Perez L, Alvarez-Cermeño JC, Rodriguez C, et al, "B Cells Capable of Spontaneous IgG Secretion in Cerebrospinal Fluid From Patients With Multiple Sclerosis: Dependency on Local IL-6 Production," *Clin Exp Immunol*, 1995, 101(3):449-52.

Sellebjerg F and Christiansen M, "Qualitative Assessment of Intrathecal IgG Synthesis by Isoelectric Focusing and Immunodetection: Interlaboratory Reproducibility and Interobserver Agreement," *Scand J Clin Lab Invest*, 1996, 56(2):135-43.

Tourtellotte WW, Tavolato B, Parker JA, et al, "Cerebrospinal Fluid Electroimmunodiffusion. An Easy, Rapid, Sensitive, Reliable, and Valid Method for the Simultaneous Determination of Immunoglobulin-G and Albumin," *Arch Neurol*, 1971, 25(4):345-50.

Cerebrospinal Fluid Immunoglobulin G

Related Information

Cerebrospinal Fluid IgG:Albumin Ratio, IgG Index, and IgG Synthesis Rate on page 514
Cerebrospinal Fluid Oligoclonal Bands on page 516
Cerebrospinal Fluid Protein on page 517
Cerebrospinal Fluid Protein Electrophoresis on page 518

Synonyms Cerebrospinal Fluid IgG; CSF Gamma G; CSF IgG; CSF Immunoglobulin; Gamma G, CSF; IgG, CSF; Immunoglobulin G, Cerebrospinal Fluid; Spinal Fluid Globulin; Spinal Fluid Immunoglobulin

Applies to Kappa Light Chains, CSF

Replaces Colloidal Gold Curve

Abstract The pathogenesis of multiple sclerosis (MS) may involve immunoglobulins. Increased concentrations of immunoglobulins may be found in serum, cerebrospinal fluid (CSF), and brain of subjects with multiple sclerosis.[1]

Patient Preparation Patient should be informed, relaxed, and properly positioned for lumbar puncture. Signed consent form is required. Antiseptic agents must be carefully and properly applied to the proposed puncture site. Local anesthetic (to which patient is not allergic) is usually advised. Lumbar puncture is not without potential complications.[2]

Aftercare Patient should be maintained supine for a few hours postpuncture in an attempt to avoid postpuncture headache.

Specimen Cerebrospinal fluid; usually at least 0.1-0.5 mL of CSF is required.

Container Clean, sterile CSF tube

Collection Tube should be labeled with the sequence in which tubes were obtained.

Storage Instructions Store in refrigerator.

Causes for Rejection CSF received without concurrently obtained serum, insufficient quantity of CSF, CSF contaminated with blood ("bloody tap") (Continued)

Cerebrospinal Fluid Immunoglobulin G *(Continued)*

Special Instructions The third tube of a routinely obtained three tube set of CSF should be used for CSF IgG study.

Reference Interval Normal CSF IgG: 3% to 12% of total CSF protein.[3] IgG in CSF is normally <5 mg/dL. There is no evidence of diurnal variation.

Use Evaluate central nervous system involvement by infection, neoplasm, or primary neurologic disease (in particular, multiple sclerosis)

Limitations Normal levels do not exclude disease; clinical correlation is needed. Patients in early phases of multiple sclerosis are those most likely to have normal CSF concentrations of IgG. Free kappa light chains are found less often than are oligoclonal bands, but provide greater specificity for multiple sclerosis than do intact IgG abnormalities.[4]

Methodology Radial immunodiffusion (RID), electroimmunodiffusion, immunofluorometry, immunoprecipitation, immunonephelometry, rate immunonephelometry

Additional Information Cerebrospinal fluid protein is elevated in many conditions which affect the central nervous system primarily or secondarily. In inflammatory or destructive processes in which serum leaks into CSF, both IgG and albumin will be present in the CSF in increased amounts. Since albumin is not, but immunoglobulins are, synthesized in the central nervous system, a relative increase in CSF IgG indicates presence of a process involving the central nervous system primarily, in particular multiple sclerosis.

Clinical evidence of MS includes (but is not limited to) weakness, early fatigue, double vision, numbness and tingling, difficulty with coordination, and dizziness.

While MS patients are maintained on ACTH and/or steroid therapy or during remission, CSF IgG levels decrease but generally remain significantly elevated.

Electrophoresis of CSF may also be enlightening if oligoclonal gamma globulin bands are demonstrated, which also suggests, but is not diagnostic of, multiple sclerosis. See also Cerebrospinal Fluid Oligoclonal Bands *on page 516*.

While CSF laboratory findings alone cannot establish or exclude the diagnosis of MS and CSF total protein or albumin level is normal in most patients, CSF immunoglobulin is usually elevated relative to the other proteins with the implication of intrathecal synthesis. IgG is predominantly increased with excess of IgG lambda and kappa light chains. The IgG level is commonly ratioed to another CSF protein component. The Poser committee diagnostic criteria for MS use CSF laboratory findings to support a diagnosis of MS. A number of IgG ratios and the IgG index have been considered. The IgG index (normal value <0.66) is a "ratio of ratios" and compares CSF with serum parameters as follows:

$$\text{CSF Ig Index} = [\text{IgG}_{CSF}/\text{albumin}_{CSF}] / [\text{IgG}_{serum}/\text{albumin}_{serum}]$$

Tourtellotte's IgG synthesis rate has also been utilized.[5] (Cerebrospinal Fluid IgG:Albumin Ratio, IgG Index, and IgG Synthesis Rate *on page 514*.) Quantitative measures of CNS IgG production are said to be less sensitive than isoelectric focusing of CNS protein (for oligoclonal bands).[6] See Cerebrospinal Fluid Oligoclonal Bands *on page 516*. The use of both oligoclonal bands (sensitivity 90%) and IgG index (sensitivity 80%) test results increases the sensitivity to 95%.[7]

Footnotes

1. Hogancamp WE, Rodriguez M, and Weinshenker BG, "Identification of Multiple Sclerosis-Associated Genes," *Mayo Clin Proc*, 1997, 72(10):965-76.
2. Evans RW, "Complications of Lumbar Puncture," *Neurol Clin*, 1998, 16(1):83-105.
3. Fishman RA, *Cerebrospinal Fluid in Diseases of the Nervous System*, 2nd ed, Philadelphia, PA: WB Saunders Co, 1992, 206-14.
4. Rudick RA, "Multiple Sclerosis and Related Conditions," *Cecil Textbook of Medicine*, 21st ed, Chapter 482, Goldman L and Bennett JC, eds, Philadelphia, PA: WB Saunders Co, 2000, 2141-49.
5. Tourtellotte WW, Stangaitis SM, Walsh MJ, et al, "The Basis of Intra-Blood-Brain-Barrier IgG Synthesis," *Ann Neurol*, 1985, 17(1):21-7.
6. Andersson M, Alvarez-Cermeno J, Bernardi G, et al, "Cerebrospinal Fluid in the Diagnosis of Multiple Sclerosis: A Consensus Report," *J Neurol Neurosurg Psychiatry*, 1994, 57(8):897-902.
7. Kyle RA and Katzmann JA, "Immunochemical Characterization of Immunoglobulins," Section C, Kyle RA, section ed, *Manual of Clinical Laboratory Immunology*, 5th ed, Nakamura RM, volume ed, Washington, DC: ASM Press, American Society for Microbiology, 1997, 172-4.

References

Barna BP, Valenzuela R, and Gupta MK, "Laboratory Analyses of Cerebrospinal Fluid," *Laboratory Handbook of Neuroimmunologic Disease*, Chapter 5, Barna BP, ed, Chicago, IL: American Society of Clinical Pathologists, 1987, 65-104.

Marshall DW, Brey RL, Cahill WT, et al, "Spectrum of Cerebrospinal Fluid Findings in Various Stages of Human Immunodeficiency Virus Infection," *Arch Neurol*, 1988, 45(9):954-8.

Olek MJ and Dawson DM, "Multiple Sclerosis and Other Inflammatory Demyelinating Diseases of the Central Nervous System," *Neurology in Clinical Practice: The Neurological Disorders*, 3rd ed, Volume 2, Chapter 60, Bradley WG, Daroff RB, Fenichel GM, et al, eds, Boston MA: Butterworth-Heinemann, 2000, 1431-65.

Cerebrospinal Fluid Oligoclonal Bands

Related Information

Cerebrospinal Fluid IgG:Albumin Ratio, IgG Index, and IgG Synthesis Rate *on page 514*

Cerebrospinal Fluid Immunoglobulin G *on page 515*
Cerebrospinal Fluid Protein *on page 517*
Cerebrospinal Fluid Protein Electrophoresis *on page 518*

Synonyms Oligoclonal Bands, Cerebrospinal Fluid; Spinal Fluid Oligoclonal Bands

Applies to Myelin Basic Protein; Optic Neuritis; Tau Fraction

Test Includes High-resolution electrophoresis of cerebrospinal fluid (CSF) and serum obtained concurrently

Abstract Oligoclonal bands on CSF electrophoresis are typical of but not pathognomonic for multiple sclerosis.

Patient Preparation Patient should be informed, relaxed, and properly positioned for lumbar puncture. Signed consent form is required. Antiseptic agents must be carefully and properly applied to the proposed puncture site. Local anesthetic (to which patient is not allergic) is usually advised. Fasting serum specimen is preferred (to avoid hyperlipemia).

Aftercare Patient should be maintained supine for a few hours postpuncture in an attempt to avoid postpuncture headache.

Specimen Cerebrospinal fluid (5 mL) and serum obtained concurrently

Container Clean, sterile CSF tube; red top tube or SST™ tube of blood

Storage Instructions Serum and CSF specimens may be kept at room temperature for up to 6 hours or at 4°C to 8°C for up to 24 hours before testing. If there is greater delay, they should be stored at -20°C.

Causes for Rejection CSF contaminated with blood ("bloody tap"), CSF submitted without accompanying serum specimen

Reference Interval Normal CSF has no demonstrable oligoclonal bands.

Use Oligoclonal CSF bands contribute to the diagnosis of inflammatory and autoimmune disease of the CNS. In particular, they are found in 83% to 94% of subjects with clinically definite multiple sclerosis and in 100% of patients with subacute sclerosing panencephalitis (SSPE),[1] and in other degenerative states as well (eg, presenile dementia). SSPE may be the result of long-standing measles infection. With widespread measles vaccination, it has been nearly eradicated.

CSF examination is useful in entities such as neuropsychiatric SLE to exclude infectious meningitis.[2]

Limitations Test has a satisfactorily high level of sensitivity (~90%) for association with multiple sclerosis, but it is not specific. Serum protein electrophoresis must be run concurrently to assure that any CSF bands detected do not have origin in the serum (diffusion of serum bands into the CSF). A few cases of MS may have oligoclonal bands in both serum and CSF; the incidence increases with use of isoelectric focusing.

Although oligoclonal bands have been seen in neuropsychiatric SLE, they lack specificity.[2]

Methodology Thin gel agarose high-resolution electrophoresis, immunofixation electrophoresis, isoelectric focusing; requires concentration of CSF.

Additional Information During CSF protein electrophoresis, IgG in normal spinal fluid migrates as a faint diffuse zone. In demyelinating diseases, IgG migrates as discrete bands called oligoclonal bands. An abnormal result is the finding of two or more oligoclonal bands in the CSF that are not present in a concurrent serum sample. Oligoclonal bands are present in the CSF of 90% of patients with multiple sclerosis. The occurrence of oligoclonal bands in both CSF and serum is seen in CLL, lymphoma, malignancies, autoimmune hepatitis, and viral illnesses.

Oligoclonal bands are not specific for MS but have been described in many other disorders, including subacute sclerosing panencephalitis, syphilis, Jakob-Creutzfeldt disease, encephalitis, Guillain-Barré syndrome, neurosyphilis, stroke, cerebral vasculitis, lupus erythematosus, and neoplasms. Immunoglobulin D oligoclonal bands have been noted in the CSF of some patients with central nervous system tumors.[3] However, in most of these diseases, oligoclonal bands are uncommon, whereas they are present in about 90% or more of patients with MS.

The Optic Neuritis Treatment Trial has found that lumbar puncture (to detect CSF oligoclonal bands) does not add predictive value (5-year risk) of definite MS in patients who have abnormal magnetic resonance imaging (MRI) at the time of onset of monosymptomatic optic neuritis. Testing for oligoclonal bands, however, may assist assessment of risk for MS in patients with normal brain MRI at the onset of optic neuritis.[4]

At least some MS patients have oligoclonal band patterns with EBNA-1 (Epstein Barr virus nuclear antigen-1) specific comigration. Some oligoclonal bands could be absorbed with EBNA-1 antigens. EBNA-1 may be a target epitope for some MS-associated oligoclonal bands.[5]

Oligoclonal banding was present in 26% of asymptomatic, HIV seropositive men.[6]

A symposium through the December 1997 issue of *Mayo Clinic Proceedings* began with a foreward in the July issue.[7]

Myelin basic protein (MBP) assays have also been applied to the diagnosis, evaluation, and post-therapeutic monitoring of multiple sclerosis. The methods suffer from fragmentation and variation of the myelin antigen(s). There have been disparate results of RIA analyses between laboratories and CSF MBP levels are not specific to MS, with a number of entities causing breakdown of myelin, including stroke, hypoxia, trauma, neoplasms, Guillain-Barré syndrome, and other entities. Newer assays have increased sensitivity, specificity would be expected to be low. MBP assay, however, might be used as an indicator of MS disease activity in some circumstances.[8]

Footnotes

1. Fishman RA, *Cerebrospinal Fluid in Diseases of the Nervous System*, 2nd ed, Philadelphia, PA: WB Saunders Co, 1992, 208-10.
2. Boumpas DT, Austin HA 3d, Fessler BJ, et al, "Systemic Lupus Erythematosus: Emerging Concepts. Part 1: Renal, Neuropsychiatric, Cardiovascular, Pulmonary, and Hematologic Disease," *Ann Intern Med*, 1995, 122(12):940-50.
3. Mavra M, Drulovic J, Levic Z, et al, "CNS Tumors: Oligoclonal Immunoglobulin D in Cerebrospinal Fluid and Serum," *Acta Neurol Scand*, 1999, 100(2):117-8.
4. Cole SR, Beck RW, Moke PS, et al, "The Predictive Value of CSF Oligoclonal Banding for MS 5 Years After Optic Neuritis," *Neurology*, 1998, 51(3):885-7.
5. Rand KH, Houck H, Denslow ND, et al, "Are the Oligoclonal Bands (OCBs) in the Cerebrospinal Fluid (CSF) of Patients With Multiple Sclerosis (MS) Directed at Epstein Barr Virus Nuclear Antigen-1 (EBNA-1)?" *Neurology*, 1998, 50:A147-8.
6. Chalmers AC, April BS, and Shephard H, "Cerebrospinal Fluid and Human Immunodeficiency Virus - Findings in Healthy, Asymptomatic, Seropositive Men," *Arch Intern Med*, 1990, 150(7):1538-40.
7. Rodriguez M, "Multiple Sclerosis: Insights Into Molecular Pathogenesis and Therapy," *Mayo Clin Proc*, 1997, 72(7):663-4.
8. Ohta M, Ohta K, Ma J, et al, "Clinical and Analytical Evaluation of an Enzyme Immunoassay for Myelin Basic Protein in Cerebrospinal Fluid," *Clin Chem*, 2000, 46(9):1326.

References

Andersson M, Alvarez-Cermeno J, Bernardi G, et al, "Cerebrospinal Fluid in the Diagnosis of Multiple Sclerosis: A Consensus Report," *J Neurol Neurosurg Psychiatry*, 1994, 57(8):897-902.

Giles PD, Heath JP, and Wroe SJ, "Oligoclonal Bands and the IgG Index in Multiple Sclerosis: Uses and Limitations," *Ann Clin Biochem*, 1989, 26(Pt 4):317-23.

Sorensen PS, "Biological Markers in Body Fluids for Activity and Progression in Multiple Sclerosis," *Mult Scler*, 1999, 5(4):287-90.

Wekerle H, "Immunology of Multiple Sclerosis," *McAlpine's Multiple Sclerosis*, 3rd ed, Chapter 12, Compston A, Ebers G, Lassmann H, et al, eds, New York, NY: Churchill Livingstone, 1998, 379.

Cerebrospinal Fluid Protein

Related Information

Bacterial Antigens, Rapid Detection Methods *on page 562*
Bacterial Culture, Cerebrospinal Fluid *on page 569*
Cerebrospinal Fluid Analysis: Overview *on page 416*
Cerebrospinal Fluid and Plasma β-Amyloid$_{(1-42)}$ *on page 513*
Cerebrospinal Fluid Glucose *on page 140*
Cerebrospinal Fluid IgG:Albumin Ratio, IgG Index, and IgG Synthesis Rate *on page 514*
Cerebrospinal Fluid Immunoglobulin G *on page 515*
Cerebrospinal Fluid Lactic Acid *on page 143*
Cerebrospinal Fluid Oligoclonal Bands *on page 516*
Cerebrospinal Fluid Protein Electrophoresis *on page 518*
Fungal Culture, Cerebrospinal Fluid *on page 611*
Mycobacterial Culture, Cerebrospinal Fluid *on page 656*
VDRL, Cerebrospinal Fluid *on page 688*
Viral Culture, Central Nervous System Symptoms *on page 692*

Synonyms CSF Protein; Protein, Cerebrospinal Fluid; Spinal Fluid Protein

Applies to Aceruloplasminemia; CSF Amino Acids; CSF Leakage; CSF Neopterin; CSF Rhinorrhea; CSF Taurine; Froin Syndrome; O-Sialotransferrin; POEMS Syndrome; Prealbumin, CSF; Tau Fraction

Test Includes Culture, Gram stain, cell count with differential, glucose, and protein are usually ordered together to work up possible meningitis.

Abstract Increased CSF protein may indicate presence of infectious/inflammatory, hemorrhagic, neoplastic or demyelinating disease of the CNS (central nervous system). Great increases may be found in acute bacterial meningitis, including tuberculous meningitis. See Cerebrospinal Fluid Analysis: Overview *on page 416*, in which protein concentrations in various entities are outlined.

Patient Preparation Patient should be informed, relaxed, and properly positioned for lumbar puncture. Signed consent form is required. Antiseptic agents must be carefully and properly applied to the proposed puncture site. Local anesthetic (to which patient is not allergic) is usually advised. If increased intracranial pressure due to a mass lesion (eg, abscess) is suspected, lumbar puncture should be deferred until appropriate neuroimaging study is performed and the issue resolved. Lumbar puncture is not without potential complications.[1]

Aftercare Patient should be maintained supine for a few hours postpuncture in an attempt to avoid postpuncture headache.

Specimen Cerebrospinal fluid, usually at least 0.1-0.5 mL of CSF is required.

Container Clean, sterile CSF tube

Collection Tubes should be labeled with patient's name, hospital number, and date and time of collection.

Storage Instructions Do not store. Must be delivered to clinical laboratory immediately.

Turnaround Time 1-2 hours

Special Instructions Usually three tubes of CSF are collected for count and culture in addition to protein and glucose with collection of 1 mL in each tube labeled #1, #2, #3 in order of collection. **For diagnosis of meningitis, culture and then Gram staining have priority over all other testing,** when only a small quantity of cerebrospinal fluid (CSF) is available. **Cell count with differential deserves the next priority, followed by glucose and total protein.**

Reference Interval Lumbar CSF: 0-1 month: <150 mg/dL (SI: <1.5 g/L); 1-6 months: approximately 30-100 mg/dL (SI: 0.30-1.00 g/L); 6 months and up: approximately 15-45 mg/dL; elderly adults: 15-60 mg/dL (SI: 0.15-0.50 g/L). Ventricular CSF protein is generally lower, 5-15 mg/dL. Cisternal CSF is midway, 15-25 mg/dL. See tables.

Infant Reference Values

CSF Total Protein Levels, First 3 Months of Life		
Analyzer-Vitros 700 (Ortho, formerly Kodak Ektachem)		
Age	mg/dL	SI (g/L)
1-8 d	26-135	0.26-1.35
8-30 d	26-115	0.26-1.15
1-2 mo	18-86	0.18-0.86
2-3 mo	10-74	0.10-0.74

Adapted from Evans RW, "Complications of Lumbar Puncture," *Neurol Clin N America*, 1998, 16(1):83-105.

Protein Analyte

Protein	Molecular Weight	Plasma Concentration (mg/L)	CSF Concentration (mg/L)	Plasma:CSF Ratio
Prealbumin	61,000	238	17.3	14
Albumin	69,000	36,600	155.0	236
Transferrin	81,000	2040	14.4	142
Ceruloplasmin	152,000	366	1.0	366
IgG	150,000	9870	12.3	802
IgA	150,000	1750	1.3	1346
Alpha$_2$ macroglobulin	798,000	2220	2.0	1111
Fibrinogen	340,000	2964	0.6	4940
IgM	800,000	700	0.6	1167
Beta lipoprotein	2,239,000	3728	0.6	6213

Data from Felgenhauser, 1974 as cited by Fishman RA, "Cerebrospinal Fluid in Diseases of the Nervous System," 2nd ed, Philadelphia, PA: WB Saunders Co, 1992 and Swaiman KF and Ashwal S, *Pediatric Neurology: Principles and Practice*, 3rd ed, St Louis, MO: Mosby, 1999.

Hitachi (turbidimetric method) has been found to give values 21% lower, on average, than the Vitros (copper binding Biuret colorimetry based) method.[2]

Use Increased with bacterial meningitis including tuberculous meningitis; brain abscess, meningovascular syphilis, diabetes mellitus, CVA (including cases in which no hemorrhage has occurred), arachnoiditis, dehydration, some major depressive disorders, some patients with sciatica due to lumbar disk herniation, POEMS syndrome (**P**olyneuropathy, **O**rganomegaly, **E**ndocrinopathy, **M** protein, and **S**kin changes), drug effects, and subarachnoid hemorrhage. Protein is normal or **slightly** high in psychiatric disease. Used for differential diagnosis of multiple sclerosis; encephalomyelitis; other degenerative processes causing neurologic disease, some neoplastic diseases, some cases of myxedema and other instances of endocrine disorders, traumatic tap, and in CSF recovered from below the level of an obstruction of the spinal cord.

Decreased CSF protein falls rapidly during the first few months of life, followed by a low plateau in the 20-30 mg/dL general range from age 6 months to 10 years.[2] CSF protein is decreased with dilution from water intoxication, CSF leak (CSF rhinorrhea or otorrhea, leaks following lumbar puncture, other fistulas), with removal of large volumes of CSF, in some patients with benign intracranial hypertension, in some leukemic subjects, and with hyperthyroidism. Low CSF protein is 10-20 mg/dL.

Limitations Fresh blood in the specimen (traumatic tap) will invalidate the protein result; turbid samples may exhibit a positive interference; hemolyzed or xanthochromic specimens may falsely depress results; diabetics may have high CSF protein; ampicillin, gentamicin, and vancomycin increase the apparent CSF protein in at least some cases (method dependent).[3] Problems in the differential diagnosis of multiple sclerosis, meningitis, and other entities are discussed in following paragraphs.

Methodology Quantitative turbidimetric (sulfosalicylic acid, trichloroacetic acid, TCA); colorimetric (Biuret, Folin-Lowry phenol); dye binding (bromcresol green); Kjeldahl technique (reference method); UV spectrophotometry

Additional Information Spinal fluid is an ultrafiltrate of plasma that lacks high molecular weight proteins such as beta lipoprotein, alpha$_2$-macroglobulin, IgM, and polymeric haptoglobins. Thus, most CSF protein is albumin and has origin from plasma. The protein concentration of spinal fluid is <1% of plasma proteins.

Elevation of spinal fluid protein is the most frequently encountered abnormality. The most common causes of altered protein concentration are listed in the table on following page.

Infants have higher protein levels (60-150 mg/dL) due to increased blood brain barrier permeability. Cisternal and ventricular fluids have both lower total protein concentration and leukocyte levels than fluid obtained by lumbar puncture.[4] Ventricular fluid protein level may be <5 mg/dL. Such uneven distribution must be considered when CNS bacterial infection is a possibility.
(Continued)

Cerebrospinal Fluid Protein (Continued)

Increased Protein	Decreased Protein
Inflammation	Water intoxication
Tumor	Leukemia
Demyelinating disorders	CSF leakage
Subarachnoid hemorrhage	Rhinorrhea, otorrhea
Traumatic tap	Hyperthyroidism
Phenothiazine medications	Pneumoencephalography

The significance of elevated CSF protein should be carefully considered, in relation to the clinical findings, in particular if blood is present in the CSF. This could occur at the time of needling the subarachnoid space ("bloody tap") and be clinically misleading, or reflect clinically significant CNS hemorrhage, trauma, vascular anomaly or tumor, and have prime clinical significance.

If the spinal canal is obstructed (eg, by tumor) CSF protein content is increased, apparently the result of absence of reabsorption by arachnoidal villi. High CSF protein levels (several 100 mg/dL) may occur and due to the presence of fibrinogen, the CSF may clot (Froin syndrome).

Patients with elevated CSF protein may require additional analyses (eg, cerebrospinal fluid IgG/albumin index, IgG synthetic rate, and high resolution agarose protein electrophoresis for demonstration of "oligoclonal" bands), in particular if there are clinical findings of multiple sclerosis. (Multiple sclerosis is a clinical diagnosis.) Total protein in CSF is within normal limits in many subjects with MS but may be slightly increased. Protein levels >75 mg/dL bring a diagnosis of MS or other neurologic disease into question.[5]

Protein may be normal or increased in viral meningitis/aseptic meningitis but is usually slightly increased, 50-80 mg/dL. Protein in most cases of viral meningitis is <100 mg/dL.[6] It is usually 100-500 mg/dL in acute bacterial meningitis and is occasionally >1000 mg/dL. Protein was <45 mg/dL in fewer than 2% of a series of 157 patients with acute bacterial meningitis. It is almost always high in tuberculous meningitis.

AIDS patients with primary CNS disease or secondary CNS infections may have elevated CSF protein. Studies of asymptomatic, HIV seropositive individuals, however, have shown that pleocytosis or elevated CSF protein occurs in some 50% of such patients, with 12% to 26% showing oligoclonal banding.[7,8] The percentage of protein abnormalities increases with inclusion of patients with AIDS and AIDS-related complex.[8]

CSF cellular and protein abnormalities occur with 10% to 20% of subjects who have primary syphilis and with 30% to 70% of those with secondary lues.[9]

Lumbar disk herniation with sciatica may be associated with increased CSF total protein (see comments in Cerebrospinal Fluid IgG:Albumin Ratio, IgG Index, and IgG Synthesis Rate on page 514).[10]

Methods have been developed for detection of CSF leakage (as occurs most commonly from the subarachnoid space into nasal or aural cavities). The "marker protein" O-sialotransferrin (also called β_2-transferrin, asialo-transferrin, or the tau fraction) is detected by high resolution agarose electrophoresis and immunofixation or, most recently, by isoelectric focusing on polyacrylamide gel followed by immunofixation of transferrins and silver staining.[11]

There is evidence that mean CSF protein concentration is higher (high normal to slightly increased - mean ±SD of 40.9 ±15.8 mg/dL) in men with major depressive disorder (unipolar or bipolar depression) than in other subjects (in particular, women with similar diagnoses) and in controls.[12,13] The increase is polyclonal on protein electrophoretic study suggesting increased blood-brain capillary permeability.[12] There is also evidence that secretion of prealbumin into CSF may be increased in depression.[14]

Continuing investigation of two dimensional gel protein electrophoresis has led to development of a CSF protein database.[15] Also in the research arena, CSF levels of amino acids and nucleic acid compounds have been of interest, but in some cases with conflicting results due possibly, at least in part, by inappropriate sample handling and processing.[16,17] Research interest has also been focused on CSF as the medium reflecting CNS activity. Methods for numerous uncommon analytes have been developed and molecular biologic techniques are increasingly applied. Mentioned only as examples are aceruloplasminemia (CSF superoxide dismutase activity and lipid peroxidation products measured),[18] CSF apolipoprotein E content of HDL,[19] acute herpes zoster (varicella zoster virus DNA),[20] leptomeningeal metastasis (polymerase chain reaction for tumor-derived K-ras DNA in CSF),[21] and CSF taurine (by HPLC) levels (increased in patients with brain tumors).[22]

Footnotes

1. Evans RW, "Complications of Lumbar Puncture," Neurol Clin, 1998, 16(1):83-105.

2. Biou D, Benoist JF, Nguyen-Thi C, et al, "Cerebrospinal Fluid Protein Concentrations in Children: Age-related Values in Patients Without Disorders of the Central Nervous System," Clin Chem, 2000, 46(3):399-403.

3. Lott JA and Warren P, "Estimation of Reference Intervals for Total Protein in Cerebrospinal Fluid," Clin Chem, 1989, 35(8):1766-70.

4. Gerber J, Tumani H, Kolenda H, et al, "Lumbar and Ventricular CSF Protein, Leukocytes, and Lactate in Suspected Bacterial CNS Infections," Neurology, 1998, 51(6): 1710-4.

5. Rudick RA, "Multiple Sclerosis and Related Conditions," Cecil Textbook of Medicine, 21st ed, Chapter 482, Goldman L and Bennett JC, eds, Philadelphia, PA: WB Saunders Co, 2000, 2141-9.

6. Hammer SM and Connolly KJ, "Viral Aseptic Meningitis in the United States: Clinical Features, Viral Etiologies, and Differential Diagnosis," Curr Clin Top Infect Dis, 1992, 12:1-25.

7. Chalmers AC, Aprill BS, and Shephard H, "Cerebrospinal Fluid and Human Immunodeficiency Virus - Findings in Healthy, Asymptomatic, Seropositive Men," Arch Intern Med, 1990, 150(7):1538-40.

8. Hall CD, Snyder CR, Robertson KR, et al, "Cerebrospinal Fluid Analysis in Human Immunodeficiency Virus Infection," Ann Clin Lab Sci, 1992, 22(3):139-43.

9. Hook EW 3d and Marra CM, "Acquired Syphilis in Adults," N Engl J Med, 1992, 326:1060-9.

10. Skouen JS, Larsen JL, and Vollset SE, "Cerebrospinal Fluid Protein Concentrations Related to Clinical Findings in Patients With Sciatica Caused by Disk Herniation," J Spinal Disord, 1994, 7(1):12-8.

11. Roelandse FW, van der Zwart N, Didden JH, et al, "Detection of CSF Leakage by Isoelectric Focusing on Polyacrylamide Gel, Direct Immunofixation of Transferrins and Silver Staining," Clin Chem, 1998, 44(2):351-2.

12. Samuelson SD, Winokur G, and Pitts AF, "Elevated Cerebrospinal Fluid Protein in Men With Unipolar or Bipolar Depression," Biol Psychiatry, 1994, 35(8):539-44.

13. Pitts AF, Carroll BT, Gehris TL, et al, "Elevated CSF Protein in Male Patients With Depression," Biol Psychiatry, 1990, 28(7):629-37.

14. Jorgensen OS, "Neural Cell Adhesion Molecule and Prealbumin in Cerebrospinal Fluid From Depressed Patients," Acta Psychiatr Scand, 1988, 345:29-37.

15. Yun M, Wu W, Hood L, et al, "Human Cerebrospinal Fluid Protein Database: Edition 1992," Electrophoresis, 1992, 13(12):1002-13.

16. Anesi A, Rondanelli M, and d'Eril GM, "Stability of Neuroactive Amino Acids in Cerebrospinal Fluid Under Various Conditions of Processing and Storage," Clin Chem, 1998, 44(11):2359-60.

17. Millner MM, Franthal W, Thalhammer GH, et al, "Neopterin Concentrations in Cerebrospinal Fluid and Serum as an Aid in Differentiating Central Nervous System and Peripheral Infections in Children," Clin Chem, 1998, 44(1):161-7.

18. Miyajima H, Fujimoto M, Kohno S, et al, "CSF Abnormalities in Patients With Aceruloplasminemia," Neurology, 1998, 51(4):1188-90.

19. Miida T, Yamazaki F, Sakurai M, et al, "The Apolipoprotein E Content of HDL in Cerebrospinal Fluid Is Higher in Children Than in Adults," Clin Chem, 1999, 45(8):1294-6.

20. Haanpää M, Dastidar P, Weinberg A, et al, "CSF and MRI Findings in Patients With Acute Herpes Zoster," Neurology, 1998, 51(5):1405-11.

21. Swinkels DW, deKok JB, Hanselaar A, et al, "Early Detection of Leptomeningeal Metastasis by PCR Examination of Tumor-derived K-ras DNA in Cerebrospinal Fluid," Clin Chem, 2000, 46(1):132-3.

22. d'Eril M, Anesi A, Nauti A, et al, "Increased Taurine Levels in Cerebrospinal Fluid of Patients With Brain Tumors," Clin Chem, 2000, 46(Suppl 6):A166.

References

Kjeldsberg CR and Knight JA, Body Fluids - Laboratory Examination of Amniotic, Cerebrospinal, Seminal, Serous and Synovial Fluids, 3rd ed, Chicago, IL: ASCP Press, American Society of Clinical Pathologists, 1993, 89-102.

Kleine TO and Althaus H, "Detection of Asialo-transferrin and β-trace Protein in Mixtures of Blood Serum and Cerebrospinal Fluid (CSF) as Models for CNS Contamination With Rhinorrhea and Otorrhea," Clin Chem, 2000, 46(Suppl 6):A49-50.

Knight JA, "Advances in the Analysis of Cerebrospinal Fluid," Ann Clin Lab Sci, 1997, 27(2):93-104.

Olek MJ and Dawson DW, "Multiple Sclerosis and Other Demyelinating Disease of the Central Nervous System," Neurology in Clinical Practice: The Neurological Disorders, 3rd ed, Chapter 60, Bradley WG, Daroff RB, Fenichel GM, et al, eds, Boston, MA: Butterworth Heinemann, 2000, (2):1448-9.

Roldán A, Figueras-Aly J, Deulofeu R, et al, "Glycine and Other Neurotransmitter Amino Acids in Cerebrospinal Fluid in Perinatal Asphyxia and Neonatal Hypoxia-Ischemic Encephalopathy," Acta Paediatr, 1999, 88(10):1137-41.

Roos KL, Tunkel AR, and Scheld WM, "Acute Bacterial Meningitis in Children and Adults," Infections of the Central Nervous System, Scheld WM, Whitley RJ, and Durack DT, eds, New York, NY: Raven Press, 1991, 335-409.

Swaiman KF, "Spinal Fluid Examination," Pediatric Neurology: Principles and Practice, 3rd ed, Chapter 10, Swaiman KF and Ashwal S, eds, St Louis, MO: Mosby, 1999, 115-9.

Zunt JR and Marra CM, "Cerebrospinal Fluid Testing for the Diagnosis of Central Nervous System Infection," Neurol Clin, 1999, 17(4):675-89.

Cerebrospinal Fluid Protein Electrophoresis

Related Information

Cerebrospinal Fluid Cytology on page 376
Cerebrospinal Fluid Glucose on page 140
Cerebrospinal Fluid IgG:Albumin Ratio, IgG Index, and IgG Synthesis Rate on page 514
Cerebrospinal Fluid Immunoglobulin G on page 515
Cerebrospinal Fluid Oligoclonal Bands on page 516
Cerebrospinal Fluid Protein on page 517
Immunofixation Electrophoresis, Serum or Urine on page 530
Protein Electrophoresis, Serum on page 267
Protein, Total, Serum on page 269

Synonyms CSF Electrophoresis; Protein Electrophoresis, Spinal Fluid; Spinal Fluid Electrophoresis

Applies to Oligoclonal Bands; Tau Fraction; Transthyretin

Test Includes Total protein

Abstract This is among several studies used in evaluation of patients presenting with signs and/or symptoms of multiple sclerosis (MS), but findings are not exclusively diagnostic of this condition.

Patient Preparation Patient should be informed, relaxed, and properly positioned for lumbar puncture. Signed consent form is required. Antiseptic agents must be carefully and properly applied to the proposed puncture site. Local anesthetic (to which patient is not allergic) is usually advised.

Aftercare Patient should be maintained supine for a few hours postpuncture in an attempt to avoid postpuncture headache.

Specimen Cerebrospinal fluid

Container Clean, sterile CSF tube

Collection Tube should be labeled with the number indicating the sequence in which tubes were obtained.

Storage Instructions Store refrigerated.

Causes for Rejection Insufficient quantity of CSF, CSF contaminated with blood ("bloody tap")

Special Instructions The third tube of routinely obtained three tube set of CSF should be used for protein electrophoretic study.

Reference Interval See table.

Total protein	15-60 mg/dL
Prealbumin	1% to 8%
Albumin	50% to 80%
Alpha$_1$ globulin	2% to 8%
Alpha$_2$ globulin	2% to 12%
Beta globulin	8% to 18%
Gamma globulin	3% to 12%

The second of the two transferrin bands is called the tau band.

Use The primary reason to perform protein electrophoresis is to detect oligoclonal bands, which are most often associated with multiple sclerosis. CSF protein electrophoresis can be used to assist in the detection of CSF leakage (with resultant nasal and aural discharge).[1]

Methodology Cellulose acetate, agarose electrophoresis, "high resolution" agarose gel electrophoresis. The latter is the method of choice in the initial detection and study of oligoclonal bands. A procedure for CSF protein separation by capillary isoelectric focusing has recently been developed.[2]

Additional Information Spinal fluid is an ultrafiltrate of plasma that lacks high molecular weight proteins such as beta lipoprotein, alpha$_2$-macroglobulin, IgM, and polymeric haptoglobulins (see table of protein analytes in *Cerebrospinal Fluid Protein* on page 517). The protein concentration of spinal fluid is <1% of plasma proteins. A normal CSF protein electrophoretic pattern has relatively more prealbumin, less alpha$_2$-globulin, and less gamma globulin than serum from the same individual. Albumin and beta bands appear similar to serum. If the CSF shows presence of a monoclonal band, immunofixation study of patient's serum as well as CSF should be performed (most M-proteins will cross the blood-brain barrier).[3] If a monoclonal band is present in the CSF but none is detected in the serum, presence of central nervous system (CNS) lymphoma or plasmacytoma of the CNS (admittedly rare) should be considered.[3] Cytology study of CSF may be important in establishing a diagnosis.

Footnotes
1. Zaret D, Morrison N, Gulbranson R, et al, "Immunofixation to Quantify β 2-Transferrin in Cerebrospinal Fluid to Detect Leakage of CSF From Skull Injury," *Clin Chem*, 1992, 38(9):1909-12.
2. Manabe T, Miyamoto H, Inoue K, et al, "Separation of Human Cerebrospinal Fluid Proteins by Capillary Isoelectric Focusing in the Absence of Denaturing Agents," *Electrophoresis*, 1999, 20(18):3677-83.
3. Kyle RA, "Sequence of Testing for Monoclonal Gammopathies," *Arch Pathol Lab Med*, 1999, 123(2):114-8.

References
Keren DF, "Clinical Indications for Electrophoresis and Immunofixation," Immunological Methods, Ritchie R, Section ed, *Manual of Clinical Laboratory Immunology*, 5th ed, Nakamura RM, volume ed, Washington, DC: ASM Press, American Society for Microbiology, 1997, 71-2.
Kjeldsberg CR and Knight JA, *Body Fluids - Laboratory Examination of Amniotic, Cerebrospinal, Seminal, Serous and Synovial Fluids*, 3rd ed, Chicago, IL: ASCP Press, American Society of Clinical Pathologists, 1993, 89-102.
Zaret D, Morrison N, Gulbranson R, et al, "Immunofixation to Quantify β 2-Transferrin in Cerebrospinal Fluid to Detect Leakage of CSF From Skull Injury," *Clin Chem*, 1992, 38(9):1909-12.

◆ **CH$_{50}$** *see* Complement, Total, Serum or Body Fluid on page 522

◆ **CH$_{100}$** *see* Complement, Total, Serum or Body Fluid on page 522

◆ **Class I and Class II Genes** *see* HLA Typing, Single Human Leukocyte Antigen on page 529

◆ **Colloidal Gold Curve** *replaced by* Cerebrospinal Fluid Immunoglobulin G on page 515

Complement C3, Serum

Related Information
Anti-DNA on page 504
Complement C4, Serum on page 520
Complement Components, Overview on page 520

Complement, Total, Serum or Body Fluid on page 522

Synonyms C3 Complement

Abstract Complement levels can be a useful index for following autoimmune disease activity. Genetic deficiencies may be associated with pyogenic infections and susceptibility to autoimmune disease.

Specimen Serum

Container Red top tube or SST™ tube

Storage Instructions Allow sample to clot 15-30 minutes at room temperature (cold activation of the complement system with loss of activity may occur at 0°C), then 30-60 minutes at 4°C. Centrifuge at 4°C. Freeze serum at -70°C if assay cannot be run at once.

Reference Interval Fresh serum: 80-170 mg/dL

Use Quantitation of C3 is used to detect individuals with a congenital deficiency or those with immunologic disease in whom complement is consumed at an increased rate. These include chronic hepatitis, certain chronic infections (including hepatitis C virus associated cryoglobulinemic vasculitis), immune complex disease, poststreptococcal and membranoproliferative glomerulonephritis, and others. It is especially useful to assess disease activity in lupus erythematosus (SLE).

Limitations Detects both biologically active and inactive C3. Thus, C3 levels determined by nephelometry may be misleading as the test reagent antisera will react with inactive forms of C3 (eg, nonfunctional split products C3c).[1] Enzyme-linked immunoassays are commercially available and can measure C3 split products iC3b and C3dg which can indicate the extent of complement activation.[1]

Methodology Rate nephelometry

Additional Information C3 is made in the liver and comprises about 70% of the total protein in the complement system. It is central to activation of both the classical and alternate pathways. Increased levels are found in numerous inflammatory states as an acute phase response. CH$_{50}$ (total complement hemolytic activity), C3 and/or C4 may be decreased in cases of systemic lupus erythematosus, especially in cases with lupus nephritis, acute and chronic glomerulonephritis, infective endocarditis, and with disseminated intravascular coagulation (DIC). However, C3 level is a poor indicator of diagnosis or prognosis in many entities. The "nongamma" (C3) Coombs test may detect C3 on red cell membranes in some cases of autoimmune hemolytic anemias, but C3 levels are seldom decreased. In cases of DIC, plasmin attacks C3 directly, and C3 levels have been low. Cases of hereditary C3 deficiency, while rare, have been reported and are characterized clinically by recurrent infections and by immune complex disease, in particular, membranoproliferative glomerulonephritis. Complement components are apparently involved in the efficient clearance of apoptotic cells (by macrophages) in the systemic circulation. Deficiency of early stage complement components may predispose to autoimmunity by abnormal exposure to apoptotic cells.[2] The central role of C3 (classical and alternate pathways) place C3 deficient patients at risk for especially severe infections by the encapsulated organisms, *S. pneumoniae*, *H. influenzae*, and *N. meningitidis* (both gram-positive and gram-negative bacteria). Bacteremia, sinopulmonary infections, meningitis, paronychia, and impetigo may occur. C3 levels have also been found deficient in cases of uremia, chronic liver diseases, anorexia nervosa, and celiac disease.

An undetectable C3 level suggests a congenital C3 deficiency. Decreased levels of both C3 and C4 indicate classical pathway activation. Decreased C3 levels with normal C4 levels indicate alternate pathway activation. Very low or undetectable levels of C4 are often seen in type II cryoglobulinemic vasculitis, which is most commonly associated with hepatitis C infection.[3] C3 levels fluctuate during the course of the disease. Generally, decreased levels of individual complement proteins are due to increased catabolism. Because synthesis of complement proteins increases with inflammatory disease, normal levels do not prove that the complement sequence is not involved in tissue injury. See table.

C3 and C4 Levels in Presence of Decreased Hemolytic Complement Activity

		Normal C4	Decreased C4
Normal C3	Inborn errors (other than C4 or C3)		Inborn C4 deficiency
	Alterations *in vitro* (eg, improper specimen handling)		Immune complex disease
	Coagulation-associated complement consumption		Hypergammaglobulinemic states
			Cryoglobulinemic vasculitis
			Hereditary angioedema
Decreased C3	Inborn C3 deficiency		Active SLE
	Acute glomerulonephritis		Serum sickness
	Membranoproliferative glomerulonephritis		Immune complex disease
	Immune complex disease		Autoimmune/chronic active hepatitis
	Active SLE		Infective endocarditis

A number of genetic defects have been reported as the cause of C3 deficiency, including nonsense mutations with decrease in normal mRNA, deletions, frameshifts (with resultant truncated C3).[1] There is an expanding body of knowledge concerning the role of complement in enhancing the humoral immune response.[4] Attachment of C3 to antigen affects the (Continued)

Complement C3, Serum *(Continued)*

acquired immune response, in particular with respect to the function of B cells including:

- enhancement of antigen uptake and processing by B cells for presentation to antigen-specific T cells
- direct activation of B cells through a CD21/CD19 complex-mediated signaling pathway
- support of B-cell interaction with follicular dendritic cells (involvement of C3d bearing immune complexes in intercellular bridging)
- complement receptor type 2 (CR2, CD21) participation in the determination of B-cell tolerance towards self antigens (with implications to the correlation of early-stage complement deficiency and autoimmune disease)

Lytic activity of the complement system and of complement components is lower in neonates as compared to adults. A recent study of Brazilian children included C3 determination by rate nephelometry.[5] Children (ages 3-14) had generally lower levels than those of North American children and adults. The need to determine reference values for each population being reviewed was emphasized.[5]

Footnotes

1. Giclas PC, "Complement Tests," Section D, "Complement, Immune Complexes, and Cryoglobulin," Giclas PC, section ed, *Manual of Clinical Laboratory Immunology*, 5th ed, Rose NR, de Macario EC, Folds JD, et al, eds, Washington, DC: ASM Press, American Society for Microbiology, 1997, 181-6.
2. Mevorach D, Mascarenhas JO, Gershov D, et al, "Complement-Dependent Clearance of Apoptotic Cells by Human Macrophages," *J Exp Med*, 1998, 188(12):2313-20.
3. Lamprecht P, Gause A, and Gross WL, "Cryoglobulinemic Vasculitis," *Arthritis Rheum*, 1999, 42(12):2507-16.
4. Nielsen CH, Fischer EM, and Leslie RG, "The Role of Complement in the Acquired Immune Response," *Immunology*, 2000, 100(1):4-12.
5. Ferriani VP, Barbosa JE, and de Carvalho IF, "Complement Haemolytic Activity (Classical and Alternative Pathways), C3, C4, and Factor B Titres in Healthy Children," *Acta Paediatr*, 1999, 88(10):1062-6.

References

Densen P, "Complement," *Principles and Practice of Infectious Diseases*, 4th ed, Volume 1, Chapter 6, Mandell GL, Bennett JE, and Dolin R, eds, New York, NY: Churchill Livingstone, 1995, 58-78.

Johnston RB Jr, "Disorders of the Complement System," *Immunologic Disorders in Infants and Children*, 4th ed, Chapter 17, Stiehm ER, ed, Philadelphia, PA: WB Saunders Co, 1996, 490-509.

Winkelstein JA and Ameratunga R, "Genetically Determined Deficiencies of the Complement System: C1, C4, C2, and C3," Section M, "Immunodeficiency Diseases," Cunningham-Rundles C, section ed, *Manual of Clinical Laboratory Immunology*, 5th ed, Chapter 103, Rose NR, de Macario EC, Folds JD, et al, eds, Washington, DC: ASM Press, American Society for Microbiology, 1997, 845-9.

Complement C4, Serum

Related Information

Antinuclear Antibody *on page 507*
Complement C3, Serum *on page 519*
Complement Components, Overview *on page 520*
Complement, Total, Serum or Body Fluid *on page 522*
HLA-B27 *on page 528*

Synonyms C4 Complement

Applies to Complement, Classical Pathway

Specimen Serum

Container Red top tube or SST™ tube

Storage Instructions Allow sample to clot 15-30 minutes at room temperature, then 30-60 minutes at 4°C. Freeze serum at -70°C if assay cannot be run at once.

Reference Interval 18-51 mg/dL

Use Quantitation of C4 is used to detect individuals with congenital deficiency or those with autoimmune diseases such as lupus erythematosus (SLE), rheumatoid arthritis, serum sickness, certain glomerulonephritides, chronic hepatitis, cryoglobulinemia, immune complex disease, and hereditary angioedema. C4 levels are sensitive indicators of SLE and proliferative glomerulonephritis disease activity. C4 may be increased with autoimmune hemolytic anemia.

Limitations Complement proteins are acute phase reactants and have short half-lives. Serum level is a balance of synthesis and catabolism. Serial measurements are more useful than single values.

Methodology Rate nephelometry, functional assays, electrophoretic allotyping and isotyping, gene cloning and sequencing

Additional Information The C4 protein is encoded by two genes (class III region of the major histocompatibility complex). There are two isotypes, C4A and C4B, that differ by four amino acids. C4 is utilized only by the classical pathway, so that it is decreased only when this arm of the complement cascade is activated. In diseases activating the alternate pathway alone, C4 levels will be normal. Total hemolytic activity (CH_{50}), C3, and C4 are frequently decreased in a variety of conditions producing immune complexes. In hereditary angioedema, the lack of C1 esterase inhibitor allows unopposed lysis of C2 and C4 by C1 esterase, so C4 levels will be low. Hereditary C4 deficiency is associated with an increased incidence of

pyogenic bacterial infections, in particular those caused by the encapsulated organism *S. pneumoniae*. See table in Complement C3, Serum *on page 519*.

Neuroinflammation with complement activation is likely importantly involved in the pathogenesis of Alzheimer disease (AD).[1] See also Complement Components, Overview *on page 520*. There is evidence that primary human astrocytes are a source of complement C4 in the human central nervous system.[2]

Serum levels of C3c and C4 are reportedly increased in boys (but not in girls) living in urban areas with high levels of air pollution.[3] Partial deletions of the C4 gene (combined with mild upper respiratory infection) may be a risk factor for sudden infant death.[4] The complement system, including levels of C4, C3, and serum functional hemolytic activity (CH_{50}) is apparently intact in elderly individuals.[5] A number of cutaneous diseases are characterized by association with complete or partial C4 deficiency. Systemic lupus erythematosus and related syndromes occur in patients with complete C4 deficiency.

Footnotes

1. Rogers J, "An IL-1α Susceptibility Polymorphism in Alzheimer's Disease," *Neurology*, 2000, 55(4):464-5.
2. Walker DG, Kim SU, and McGeer PL, "Expression of Complement C4 and C9 Genes by Human Astrocytes," *Brain Res*, 1998, 809(1):31-8.
3. Shima M, Adachi M, Tanaka T, et al, "Serum Complement Levels in Children in Communities With Different Levels of Air Pollution in Japan," *Arch Environ Health*, 1999, 54(4):264-70.
4. Opdal SH, Vege A, Stave AK, et al, "The Complement Component C4 in Sudden Infant Death," *Eur J Pediatr*, 1999, 158(3):210-2.
5. Bellavia D, Frada G, DiFranco P, et al, "C4, BF, C3 Allele Distribution and Complement Activity in Healthy Aged People and Centenarians," *J Gerontol*, 1999, 54(4):B150-3.

References

Bishof NA, Welch TR, and Beischel LS, "C4B Deficiency: A Risk Factor for Bacteremia With Encapsulated Organisms," *J Infect Dis*, 1990, 162(1):248-50.

Lokki ML, Circolo A, Ahokas P, et al, "Deficiency of Human Complement Protein C4 Due to Identical Frameshift Mutations in the C4A and C4B Genes," *J Immunol*, 1999, 162(6):3687-93.

Nousari HC, Kimyai-Asadi A, and Provost TT, "Generalized Lupus Erythematosus Profundus in a Patient With Genetic Partial Deficiency of C4," *J Am Acad Dermatol*, 1999, 41(2 Pt 2):362-4.

Winkelstein JA and Ameratunga R, "Genetically Determined Deficiencies of the Complement System: C1, C4, C2, and C3," Section M, Immunodeficiency Diseases, Cunningham-Rundles C, section ed, *Manual of Clinical Laboratory Immunology*, de Macario EC, volume ed, 5th ed, Chapter 103, Washington, DC: ASM Press, American Society for Microbiology, 1997, 845-9.

◆ **Complement, Classical Pathway** *see* Complement C4, Serum *on page 520*

Complement Components, Overview

Related Information

Antinuclear Antibody *on page 507*
C1 Esterase Inhibitor, Serum *on page 510*
Cerebrospinal Fluid and Plasma β-Amyloid$_{(1-42)}$ *on page 513*
Complement C3, Serum *on page 519*
Complement C4, Serum *on page 520*
Complement, Total, Serum or Body Fluid *on page 522*
HLA-B27 *on page 528*

Applies to Anaphylatoxins; C1; C1q; C1r; C1s; C2; C3; C3a; C3 Convertase; C4; C4a; C5a; C6; C7; C9; Complement Receptors; CR1; CR1 (CD35); CR2; CR2 (CD21); CR3; CR4; Delay Accelerating Factor; Factor B; Factor D; Factor I; HLA Complex; Membrane Attack Complex; Membrane Cofactor Protein; Membrane Inhibitor of Active Lysis; Properdin

Test Includes Quantitation of antigenic (immunologic) and/or functional complement components - C1, C1q, C1r, C1s, C2, C3, C4, C5, C6, C7, C8, C9; factor B; factor D

Abstract The complement system is a major participant in inflammatory reactions. It consists of cascading protein/enzymatic activities with associated receptors and inhibitors. During this process, potent low molecular weight peptide anaphylatoxins (C4a, C3a, and C5a) are generated. Complement components and their deficiency states relate importantly to pyogenic infection, *Neisseria* infection (including, in particular, meningococcal meningitis), and connective tissue disease (eg, systemic lupus erythematosus (SLE)).

Specimen Serum

Container Red top tube

Collection Complement protein components are heat labile. Samples for complement analysis should be allowed to clot 15-30 minutes at room temperature (cold activation may occur at 0°C with loss of activity) and then 30-60 minutes at 4°C. If the assay cannot be run at once, serum should be stored at -70°C. Freezing at -20°C will result in significant loss of complement activity. If sample must be transported or there is delay in processing, a normal control specimen handled in the same manner should also be analyzed.

Reference Interval The following reference values reflect the wide range of complement protein present in most "normal" populations. Null alleles (code for nonsynthesis of complement protein) may be common, as has been shown in the case of C4. Complement proteins are acute phase reactants.

Increased levels may be due to recent clinical or subclinical infections and/or other illnesses. Levels may be elevated during pregnancy or with use of oral contraceptives. It is difficult to establish meaningful reference ranges. Vagaries in test reagent antisera, standardization, and intralaboratory/interlaboratory technical variation make it difficult to interpret an isolated value. Interpretation should be made using reference ranges from a verified "normal" population, samples properly collected and handled by the same laboratory performing the patient's test.

Complement Components

Component	Serum Concentrations (μg/mL)
Classical pathway	
C1q	70-300
C1r	34-100
C1s	30-80
C2	15-30
C4	350-600
Alternative pathway	
Factor B	140-240
Factor D	1-2
Factor I	35
C3	1200-1500
Terminal pathway	
C5	70-85
C6	60-70
C7	55-70
C8	55-80
C9	50-160

Components of the classical complement system may be significantly decreased (on both an immunochemical and a functional basis) in neonates and during the first few weeks of life.[1]

Use Assess patients with hereditary or acquired deficiency of complement components

Methodology Nephelometry, functional analysis in hemolytic system (CH_{50} or total hemolytic assay)

Genetically Determined Complement Deficiencies in Man

Component	Chromosome/ Gene Location*	Approx Number of Patients/ Kindreds	Major Clinical Associations
Activation Pathway			
C1q	1	24/14	Pyogenic infections, SLE, glomerulonephritis
C1r/C1s	12	11/7	
C4	6 (MHC class III)	21/17	Pyogenic infections, SLE, immune complex disease
C2	6 (MHC class III)	109/79	Pyogenic infections, SLE, glomerulonephritis
C3	19	19/14	Severe immune deficiency, SLE, glomerulonephritis
Membrane Attack Complex			
C5	9	27/17	Meningococcal meningitis/sepsis, gonococcal sepsis, SLE
C6	5	77/49	Meningococcal meningitis, SLE (rare)
C7	5	73/50	
C8	9	73/52	
C9	5	18/15	Usually asymptomatic, susceptible to *M. meningitis*
C1 Inhibitor	11	100s/100s	Hereditary angioedema
Factor H	1	13/8	Hemolytic uremic syndrome
Factor I		14/12	Pyogenic infections
Properdin	x-linked recessive	70/23	Meningococcal meningitis, pneumonia

*Inheritance is predominantly autosomal recessive.

SLE = systemic lupus erythematosus

Adapted from:

Sims PJ and Wiedmer T, "Complement Biology," 3rd ed, Chapter 37, *Hematology: Basic Principles and Practice*, Philadelphia, PA: Churchill Livingstone, 2000, 61.

Winkelstein JA, Sullivan KE, and Colten HR, "Genetically Determined Disorders of the Complement System," *The Metabolic and Molecular Basis of Inherited Disease*, 7th ed, Chapter 130, Scriver CR, Beaudet AL, Sly WS, et al, eds, New York, NY: McGraw-Hill, Inc, 1995, 3913.

Additional Information The complement system is an array of over 30 proteins, mostly enzymes, which interact sequentially to produce a number of biologically active products. Most proteins of the complement system are acute phase reactants (of the inflammatory system). Serum levels of C3 (of the "classical" pathway of activation) and of factor B (of the "alternate" pathway of activation) increase by 50% and 200% respectively during an acute phase response. Most complement components are synthesized by the liver[2] but C7 of the membrane attack complex (MAC) is synthesized by bone marrow-derived cells (monocytes/macrophages, platelets, and in particular, granulocytes) as well as fibroblasts, synovial tissue, and endothelial cells.[2,3] Microglial cells of the central nervous system are rich in (synthesize) complement factors and astrocytes produce C7.[4] Only some 10% to 60% of circulating C7 may be produced by hepatic cells.[5] Local synthesis of C7 (in particular by granulocytes and endothelial cells in areas of inflammation) provide for an available pool of C7 and for modulation of membrane attack by the complement system's MAC.[6] A variety of factors regulate complement system activity, including C1 inhibitor, a family of complement receptors (CR1, CR2, CR3, and CR4), C3 convertase stabilizers, and cell surface factors such as membrane cofactor protein (MCP, CD46),[7] delay accelerating factor (DAF, CD55) and importantly, membrane inhibitor of reactive lysis (MIRL, CD59). DAF and MIRL are glycosylphosphatidyl inositol (GPI) anchored proteins, deficient in paroxysmal nocturnal hemoglobinuria (PNH). The gene PIG-A regulates GPI synthesis. PIG-A is defective in PNH (see PNH Test (GPI-Anchored Proteins) by Flow Cytometry *on page 472*).

The C3 gene is present on chromosome 19. Genes for C2, C4A, C4B, and Bf are present on the short arm of chromosome 6 of the major-histocompatibility-complex (MHC), coding for human leukocyte antigen (HLA) gene products, class III region between HLA complex class I and II genes.[8,9] Genes for other complement components and regulators have been identified and are distributed widely on chromosomes 1, 4, 5, 9, 11, 12, and 16 (see table).

Complement is most often "activated" through either the "classical" pathway, beginning with antigen-antibody immune complexes (usually on some biologic surface) or the "alternate" pathway which is largely independent of antigen/antibody reaction and commonly relates to the action of bacterial products. Either mode of activation leads to formation of C3 convertase which then leads to production of the membrane attack complex (MAC). The classical pathway consists of the plasma proteins C1, C4, C2, and C3. C1 is a large complex formed of C1q (one molecule) and C1r and C1s (two molecules of each). C1 assembly requires calcium. C1q has six globular heads that bind immunoglobulin. Only IgG and IgM bind C1q and activate complement. The IgG_3 subset binds C1q efficiently; IgG_4 does not bind C1q. Activated C1 cleaves C4 to C4a and C4b. C4b then binds to the cell membrane beside C1. C2 binds to C4b and is cleaved by C1; C2a remains bound to C4b. C3 is then cleaved. It is activated by C3 convertase (C4b2a) of the classical or C3bBb of the alternative pathways. C3a is removed and the residual C3b undergoes conformational change with exposure of a highly reactive internally situated thiolester bond which is instrumental in further reaction and degradation of C3b on the cell surface, in part by serum proteases. C3b cleavage products attach to the membrane after which C5 is bound and cleaved. The anaphylatoxin C5a is released. C6 is then bound, initiating the terminal path (formation of the membrane attack complex consisting of C5b-poly C9). The MAC cylinder consists of up to 12 C9 molecules. See references by Morgan et al for review of considerable additional established detail concerning the process of complement activation and control. Complement proteins account for about 10% of the serum proteins; C3 is present in the highest concentration (120-150 mg/dL). See figure.

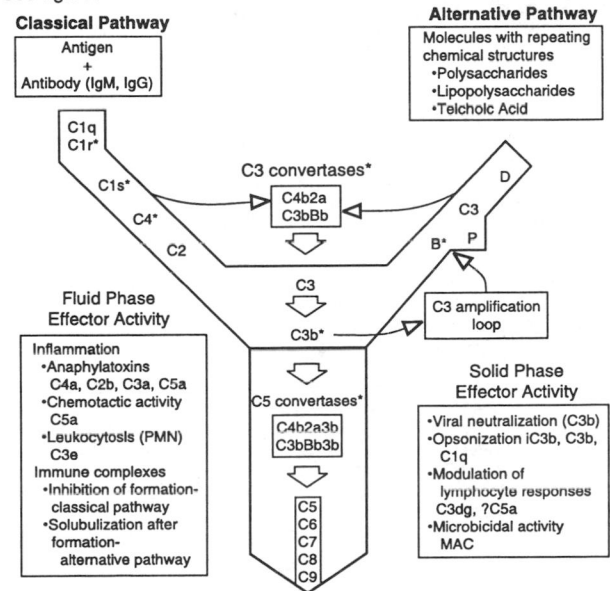

Classical Pathway

Alternative Pathway

Membrane attack complex (MAC) formation and insertion → cell death/lysis

Asterisks (*) indicate sites of downregulation of complement activity.

From Densen P, "Complement," *Principles and Practice of Infectious Diseases*, 4th ed, Chapter 6, Mandell GL, Bennett JE, and Dolin R, eds, New York, NY: Churchill Livingstone, 1995, 58-78.

(Continued)

Complement Components, Overview (Continued)

In the course of activation several byproducts are produced which are active mediators of inflammation. C3a, C3b, C5a, and C5,6,7 are particularly important chemotactic factors and opsonins.

Measurement of total complement activity or components, particularly C3 and C4 which can reflect both complement pathways, may be useful in evaluating the activity of rheumatic disorders in which complement may be involved in pathogenesis. These include SLE, arteritis, and immune arthritis in particular.

Congenital deficiencies of complement components are associated with distinct clinical syndromes (see table).

The most common infections occurring in complement deficient individuals are those due to *Neisseria meningitidis* (some 75% of identified infections). Meningococcal disease may occur with any plasma protein complement deficiency but is most common in C5, C6, C7, C8, C9, or properdin deficiency.

Deficiency of C3 is associated with severe recurrent infections, usually with encapsulated microorganisms. Deficiencies of C1 components, C2 and C4 are associated with rheumatic diseases, including SLE, vasculitis, and dermatomyositis. Some individuals with deficiency may have no evidence of disease.

The most common complement deficiency is C2, which is a homozygous abnormality in 1 in 10,000 to 40,000 individuals, and is heterozygous in 1% to 2% of the general population. Patients with C2 deficiency and SLE often have negative or low titer ANA.

Complement components may drop in patients with active rheumatic diseases, particularly lupus nephritis, sometimes decreasing prior to the clinical attack.

Paleobiology studies indicate that the complement system consists of soluble molecular components that evolved long before the humoral antibody system. The complement system (along with acute-phase proteins and cytokines) represent innate (natural) response to invading microbes, while B-cell secreted immunoglobulins represent acquired/adaptive (antigen-specific antibody based) response leading to elimination of extracellular microorganisms.[10] Innate immunity assists in guiding the adaptive immune response with B-lymphocyte activation determined by coreceptors, including two complement receptors that are expressed on B lymphocytes, CR1 (CD35) and CR2 (CD21).[11]

Innate complement responses have been identified in the brain. Central nervous system inflammation relating to Alzheimer-type degenerative neuropathy involves complement components which are up-regulated in microglia.[12] Activated microglia, failing in attempts to phagocytose senile plaques and extracellular tangles of Alzheimer disease-affected brain, nonspecifically destroy neighboring neurons and their processes (bystander lysis). This process has been seen as one of "autotoxicity", distinct from classic autoimmunity.[13,14]

Footnotes

1. Beurskens F, Schornagel I, Krediet T, et al, "Functional Complement Deficiencies in Newborns," *Clin Exp Immunol*, 1994, 97(Suppl 2):17.
2. Morgan BP and Gasque P, "Extrahepatic Complement Biosynthesis: Where, When and Why?" *Clin Exp Immunol*, 1997, 107(1):1-7.
3. Langeggen H, Pausa M, Johnson E, et al, "The Endothelium Is an Extrahepatic Site of Synthesis of the Seventh Component of the Complement System," *Clin Exp Immunol*, 2000, 121(1):69-76.
4. Morgan BP and Gasque P, "Expression of Complement in the Brain: Role in Health and Disease," *Immunol Today*, 1996,17(10):461-6.
5. Naughton MA, Walport MJ, Würzner R, et al, "Organ-Specific Contribution to Circulating C7 Levels by the Bone Marrow and Liver in Humans," *Eur J Immunol*, 1996, 26(9):2108-12.
6. Wurzner R, "Modulation of Complement Membrane Attack by Local C7 Synthesis," *Clin Exp Immunol*, 2000, 121(1):8-10.
7. Okada N, Liszewski MK, Atkinson JP, et al, "Membrane Cofactor Protein (CD46) Is a Keratinocyte Receptor for the M Protein of the Group A *Streptococcus*," *Proc Natl Acad Sci U S A*, 1995, 92(7):2489-93.
8. Volanakis JE, "Transcriptional Regulation of Complement Genes," *Annu Rev Immunol*, 1995, 13:277-305.
9. Trowsdale J, "Molecular Genetics of HLA Class I and Class II Regions," *HLA and MHC: Genes, Molecules and Function*, Browning MJ, McMichael AJ, eds, Oxford: BIOS Scientific, 1996, 23-38.
10. Delves PJ and Roitt IM, "The Immune System: First of Two Parts," Review Article-Advance in Immunology, *N Engl J Med*, 2000, 343(1):37-49.
11. Fearon D, "The Complement System and Adaptive Immunity," *Semin Immunol*, 1998, 10(5):355-61.
12. Yasojima K, Schwab C, McGeer EG, et al, "Up-Regulated Production and Activation of the Complement System in Alzheimer's Disease Brain," *Am J Pathol*, 1999, 154(3):927-36.
13. McGeer PL and McGeer EG, "Autotoxicity and Alzheimer Disease," Pleasure DE, section ed, *Arch Neurol*, 2000, 57(6):789-90.
14. Honig LS, "Inflammation in Neurodegenerative Disease: Good, Bad, or Irrelevant?" *Arch Neurol*, 2000, 57(6):786-8.

References

Densen P, "Complement," *Principles and Practice of Infectious Diseases*, 4th ed, Volume 1, Chapter 6, Mandell GL, Bennett JE, and Dolin R, eds, New York, NY: Churchill Livingstone, 1995, 58-78.

Eikelenboom P and Veerhuis R, "The Role of Complement and Activated Microglia in the Pathogenesis of Alzheimer's Disease," *Neurobiol Aging*, 1996, 17(5):673-80.

Giclas PC, section ed, Folds JD, volume ed, "Complement, Immune Complexes and Cryoglobulin," *Manual of Clinical Laboratory Immunology*, 5th ed, Part I, Section D, Washington, DC: ASM Press, American Society for Microbiology, 1997, 179-207.

Lambris JD, Reid KB, and Volanakis JE, "The Evolution, Structure, Biology and Pathophysiology of Complement," *Immunol Today*, 1999, 20(5):207-11.

Morgan BP and Harris CL, *Complement Regulatory Proteins*, Academic Press, Inc, 1999.

Nielsen CH, Fischer EM, and Leslie RG, "The Role of Complement in the Acquired Immune Response," *Immunology*, 2000, 100(1):4-12.

O'Banion MK and Finch CE, "Inflammatory Mechanisms and Anti-inflammatory Therapy in Alzheimer's Disease," *Neurobiol Aging*, 1996, 17(5):669-71.

Paraskevas F, "Cell Interactions in the Immune Response," Wintrobe's Clinical Hematology, 10th ed, Chapter 21, Lee GR, Foerster J, Lukens J, et al, eds, Baltimore MD: Lippincott Williams & Wilkins, 1999, 544-614.

Rogers J, Cooper NR, Webster S, et al, "Complement Activation by β-Amyloid in Alzheimer Disease," *Proc Natl Acad Sci U S A*, 1992, 89(21):10016-20.

Rogers J, Webster S, Lue LF, et al, "Inflammation and Alzheimer's Disease Pathogenesis," *Neurobiol Aging*, 1996, 17(5):681-6.

Shen Y, Li R, McGeer EG, et al, "Neuronal Expression of mRNAs for Complement Proteins of the Classical Pathway in Alzheimer Brain," *Brain Res*, 1997, 769(2):391-5.

Sims PJ and Wiedmer T, "Complement Biology," *Hematology: Basic Principles and Practice*, 3rd ed, Chapter 37, Hoffman R, Benz EJ Jr, Shattil SJ, et al, eds, Philadelphia, PA: Churchill Livingstone, 2000, 651-67.

Terai K, Walker DG, McGeer EG, et al, "Neurons Express Proteins of the Classical Complement Pathway in Alzheimer Disease," *Brain Res*, 1997, 769(2):385-90.

Winkelstein JA, Sullivan KE, and Colten HR, "Genetically Determined Disorders of the Complement System," *The Metabolic and Molecular Bases of Inherited Disease*, 7th ed, Volume III, Chapter 130, Scriver CR, Beaudet AL, Sly WS, et al, eds, New York, NY: McGraw-Hill, Inc, 1995, 3911-41.

♦ **Complement Receptors** see Complement Components, Overview on page 520

Complement, Total, Serum or Body Fluid

Related Information
Anti-DNA on page 504
Antinuclear Antibody on page 507
Complement C3, Serum on page 519
Complement C4, Serum on page 520
Complement Components, Overview on page 520

Synonyms CH_{50}; CH_{100}; Total Hemolytic Complement

Applies to CD21; CD35; CR1; CR2; Mannose-Binding Lectin; MASP-1; MASP-2

Test Includes Quantitation of total functional serum complement

Abstract The most frequently occurring alterations of complement are increased levels, since most complement proteins are acute phase reactants. The main clinical application of complement assays is the detection of decreased levels, which may indicate an on-going immunological disorder.

Specimen Serum, synovial fluid, other body fluids

Container Red top tube

Storage Instructions Allow sample to clot 15-30 minutes at room temperature, then 30-60 minutes at 4°C. Store serum at -70°C if assay cannot be run at once. Complement components may degrade if exposed to longer clotting times or higher temperatures.

Reference Interval 25-110 CH_{50} units with some variation between laboratories. Synovial fluid levels are 33% to 50% of serum levels in patients with nonimmune processes.

Use Total hemolytic complement (CH_{50}) is the best functional assay of the complete complement sequence. CH_{50} is often decreased in SLE, glomerulonephritis, and other immune complex diseases. Falling complement levels are associated with increased disease activity. Decrease to undetectable activity may result from an inherited deficiency of one or more complement components.

Limitations A single normal result may be misleading; longitudinal studies are clinically more helpful. Decreased or absent activity may be due to a complement component deficiency but may also result from improper specimen handling (see Storage Instructions).

Methodology Quantitative hemolysis (total complement hemolytic activity (CH_{50})). CH_{50} unit reflects the reciprocal of the dilution of patient's serum required to hemolyze 50% of sheep red blood cells. More recent methods include enzyme-linked immunoabsorbent (ELISA) assays (INCSTAR, Stillwater, MN and Quidel, San Diego, CA) and one involving lysis of liposomes (WAKO Diagnostics, Richmond, VA), used in an automated system. Both the CH_{50} assay (for evaluation of total classical pathway function) and the AH_{50} assay (alternative pathway function) are magnesium dependent.

Additional Information modes of response, **innate (natural)** and **acquired (adaptive)**. Innate responses are fixed and constant while adaptive responses increase and expand with repeat activation. The soluble molecular components of the innate arm include complement, acute-phase proteins, and cytokines (including the series of interferons/interleukins). Acquired responses involve the proliferation of antigen-specific B and T cells and immunoglobulin antigen-specific antibody production.[1] The innate immune system lacks immunologic memory and developed earlier during evolution. The innate system is ancient, appearing in sponges/sea urchins and teleost fishes, well before the evolution of the adaptive arm of immunity with its increasingly efficient antibody production. Innate immunity, however, guides the adaptive arm of the immune response with activation of the B lymphocyte and subsequent specific antibody production determined by coreceptors. These include the two complement receptors that are expressed on B lymphocytes, CR1 (CD35) and CR2 (CD21).[2]

Complement activation occurs by one or more of three mechanisms.
- Classic pathway: activated by antigen/antibody complexes
- Alternative pathway: activated by microbial-cell walls
- Lectin pathway: activated by the interaction of microbial carbohydrates with mannose-binding protein present in the plasma, mannose-binding lectin (MBL)

MBL and its two associated serine proteases (MASP-1 and MASP-2) bring about complement activation by MBL binding to carbohydrate epitopes on the surfaces of pathogenic microorganisms.[3] The sequence of activation in the classical pathway is C1, C4, C2, C3, and C5 to C9. In the alternate pathway, C1, C4, and C2 are bypassed and C3 is activated by an initiating factor (IF), and two substances called Properdin factors D and B. Total hemolytic complement (CH_{50}) is the best functional assay of the complement sequence.

A normal CH_{50} level indicates that all the components, C1 through C9, are present. However, individual complement factors may be depleted 50% to 80% without affecting CH_{50} activity. Depletion of alternative factors is not detected. For this reason, it may be necessary to measure individual complement components.

Body fluid CH_{50} activity should normally be approximately 33% to 50% of the serum value. Decreased CH_{50} titers and complement protein levels may be seen in the joint fluid of patients with rheumatoid arthritis, gout, pseudogout, Reiters syndrome, and gonococcal arthritis. Serum levels in these patients may be normal or increased.

Footnotes
1. Mackay I and Rosen FS, "The Immune System: First of Two Parts," *N Engl J Med*, 2000, 343(1):37-49.
2. Fearon DT, "The Complement System and Adaptive Immunity," *Semin Immunol*, 1998, 10(5):355-66.
3. Wallis R, Drickamer K, "Molecular Determinants of Oligomer Formation and Complement Fixation in Mannose-Binding Proteins," *J Biol Chem*, 1999, 274(6):3580-9.

References
Buyon JP, Tamerius J, Ordorica S, et al, "Activation of the Alternative Complement Pathway Accompanies Disease Flares in Systemic Lupus Erythematosus During Pregnancy," *Arthritis Rheum*, 1992, 35(1):55-61.

Giclas PC, "Complement Tests," *Manual of Clinical Laboratory Immunology*, 5th ed, Section D, Chapter 18, Folds JM, Volume ed, Washington, DC: ASM Press, American Society for Microbiology, 1997, 181-6.

McPherson RA, "Serologic Evaluation of Renal Status," *Clin Lab Med*, 1993, 13(1):69-87.

- ◆ **CR1** see Complement Components, Overview *on page 520*
- ◆ **CR1** see Complement, Total, Serum or Body Fluid *on page 522*
- ◆ **CR1 (CD35)** see Complement Components, Overview *on page 520*
- ◆ **CR2** see Complement Components, Overview *on page 520*
- ◆ **CR2** see Complement, Total, Serum or Body Fluid *on page 522*
- ◆ **CR2 (CD21)** see Complement Components, Overview *on page 520*
- ◆ **CR3** see Complement Components, Overview *on page 520*
- ◆ **CR4** see Complement Components, Overview *on page 520*

C-Reactive Protein, Serum

Related Information
Albumin, Serum *on page 88*
Alpha₁-Antitrypsin, Serum *on page 96*
Bacterial Culture, Sputum *on page 574*
Cholesterol, Total, Serum or Plasma *on page 146*
Haptoglobin, Serum *on page 190*
Hypercoagulation Panel *on page 345*
Lipids, Overview *on page 213*
Sedimentation Rate, Erythrocyte *on page 484*
Transthyretin, Serum *on page 287*
Zeta Sedimentation Ratio *on page 500*

Synonyms CRP

Applies to Acute Phase Reactant; Amyloid A, Serum

Abstract C-reactive protein (CRP) is an acute phase reactant (APR) which begins to increase in serum a few hours after the initiation of an inflammatory process. CRP is a sensitive but nonspecific indicator of acute injury, bacterial infection, or inflammation. Very high CRP values are found in acute myocardial infarction, sepsis, and following surgery. Since 1996 important studies have been published linking serum CRP levels to coronary heart disease risk (see Use). It has not escaped these investigators that such results support the view that inflammation is important in the pathogenesis of atherosclerosis.

Specimen Serum

Container Red top tube

Storage Instructions Do not freeze.

Reference Interval Reference ranges vary, depending on the method used and the reference population. It is important to obtain this information from the laboratory performing the test. In addition, it is important to note that many laboratories offer both a **routine** CRP and a **high-sensitivity** CRP, and that these may have different reference ranges.

In a study of 143 normal blood donors, performed in a university medical center laboratory, and using an in-house enzyme-labeled immunoassay calibrated with WHO reference material, the reference range was **0.08-3.1 mg/L;** there were no significant gender- or age-related differences.[1]

In an assay designated as **high-sensitivity** by a national reference laboratory, the reference range is **0.02-8 mg/L** (with the caveat that 75% of the putatively normal values are <3.2 mg/L).[2]

Listed below are selected data sets from a study of 2291 adult men and 2203 adult women, representing the general population of Augsburg, Germany. A high-sensitivity assay (minimum detectable concentration 0.05 mg/L) was used. For additional results, consult Hutchinson et al.[3]

Central 95% of population distribution, CRP mg/L
Male:
- 25-34 years: 0.08-7.27 CRP mg/L
- 45-54 years: 0.19-13.95 CRP mg/L
- 65-74 years: 0.33-18.47 CRP mg/L

Female:
- 25-34 years: 0.07-17.18 CRP mg/L
- 45-54 years: 0.15-12.12 CRP mg/L
- 65-74 years: 0.30-16.58 CRP mg/L

Other sources use: adults: 0.068-8.2 mg/L;[4] umbilical cord: 0.001-0.035 mg/L.

Within-individual variability is reported to account for 14% of total (biological) variance; thus triplicate sampling is recommended for estimating an individual's personal baseline for risk evaluation.[5]

A threshold <10 mg/L is often proposed as a cutoff for significant inflammatory disease.

Use For several decades the serum CRP has been used, somewhat like the erythrocyte sedimentation rate (ESR), as a useful marker of inflammation, both for early detection and activity monitoring.

Postoperative monitoring: By 4-6 hours after a surgical procedure the serum CRP begins to rise and reaches a peak, in the range of 25-35 mg/L, by 2-3 days after the operation. Postoperative values exceeding this range are associated with significant complications, usually inflammatory processes.[6,7,8] German investigators recommend that patients who have a **preoperative** CRP >5 mg/L not undergo **elective** surgery involving cardiopulmonary bypass because of the increased risk of postoperative sepsis.[9]

Pelvic inflammatory disease (PID): In a study of 51 women receiving antibiotic treatment for PID, the CRP was a more sensitive indicator of clinically assessed severity than was the ESR, the leukocyte count, or body temperature.[10]

Sepsis in critically ill patients: In a study of 23 critically ill patients for a total of 306 patient days, the serum CRP was more accurate than leukocyte count or body temperature in detecting sepsis and providing an index of its severity. A serum CRP >50 mg/L had a sensitivity of 98.5% and a specificity of 75% in the detection of sepsis (defined as a systemic inflammatory response syndrome plus a positive culture from one of these sites: blood, bronchoalveolar lavage, or central venous catheter).[11]

Diagnosis of acute appendicitis: Investigators from Norway have found that there is diagnostic value in adding a serum CRP to three routinely used laboratory tests (WBC, % neutrophils, ESR) for the evaluation of patients with possible acute appendicitis.[12]

Patients with coronary heart disease (CHD): Serum CRP is elevated in patients with acute myocardial infarction (AMI), often to the very high levels seen in severe sepsis and the postoperative state. In a series of 110 patients with an acute coronary syndrome, the mean serum CRP was 5 mg/L among those with a final diagnosis of unstable angina, but was 17.0 mg/L among those with a final diagnosis of AMI.[13]

Risk factor for cardiovascular disease: A possible role for serum CRP as a risk factor (eg, similar to cholesterol, cigarette smoking, hypertension, and diabetes) for coronary heart disease was suggested by a report from the Physician's Health Study. In a subset of 1086 subjects, the risk of a first AMI increased with increasing serum CRP. For men in the highest quartile (serum CRP >2.11 mg/L) the risk was three times the risk in the lowest quartile (serum CRP <0.55 mg/L). The risk was also increased for stroke and peripheral vascular disease.[14,15] A point for emphasis is that these values are well within the reference range for serum CRP. Similar results were reported in a large group of women participating in the Women's Health Study. Women in the highest quartile (mean serum CRP 8.5 mg/L) had a relative risk of 4.4 in comparison with women in the lowest quartile (mean serum CRP 0.6 mg/L).[16] (The CRP method used in the Physician's Health Study was not the same as that used in the Women's Health Study).

Limitations Lipemia or hemolysis may give false-positive results.

Methodology Immunoassays (multiple labels and formats) including enzyme-linked immunosorbent assay (ELISA), immunonephelometry, immunoturbidimetry, radioimmunoassay, immunodiffusion (ID), fluorescence polarization immunoassay (FPIA)

(Continued)

C-Reactive Protein, Serum *(Continued)*
Additional Information

Relationship to obesity. A report from the Third National Health and Nutrition Examination Survey (NHANES III) finds that obese individuals (body-mass index >25 kg/m², including young persons aged 17-39 years, have higher serum CRP levels than nonobese individuals.[17] (This study used a CRP method with a lower detection limit of 2.2. mg/dL, not a high-sensitivity assay.)

Effect of estrogens: In a subset of 493 postmenopausal participants in the Women's Health Study, CRP levels were higher in those taking hormone replacement therapy (estrogen, alone or with progesterone) than in women not taking replacement therapy.[18] A similar finding emerged from the Post-menopausal Estrogen/Progestin Intervention (PEPI) Study. There is suggestive evidence that elevation of high-sensitivity C-reactive protein (within "safe levels" of LDL - 130 mg/dL) is an independent predictor of risk for future cardiovascular events in postmenopausal women.[16] The PEPI subjects had, in addition to the CRP increase, a concomitant decrease in soluble E-selectin; the latter conceivably represents a compensating anti-inflammatory effect.[19]

Footnotes

1. Macy EM, Hayes TE, and Tracy RP, "Variability in the Measurement of C-Reactive Protein in Healthy Subjects: Implications for Reference Intervals and Epidemiological Applications," *Clin Chem*, 1997, 43(1):52-8.
2. Mayo Reference Services Publication, *New Test Announcement*, Rochester, MN: Mayo Medical Laboratories, July 2000.
3. Hutchinson WL, Koenig W, Frohlich M, et al, "Immunoradiometric Assay of Circulating C-Reactive Protein: Age-Related Values in the Adult General Population," *Clin Chem*, 2000, 46(7):934-8.
4. Johnson AM, Rohlfs EM, and Silverman LM, "Proteins," *Tietz Textbook of Clinical Chemistry*, 3rd ed, Burtis CA and Ashwood ER, eds, Philadelphia, PA: WB Saunders Co, 1999, 477-540.
5. Gambino R, "C-Reactive Protein - Undervalued, Underutilized," *Clin Chem*, 1997, 43(11):2017-8.
6. Fischer CL, Gill C, and Forrester MG, "Quantitation of 'Acute-Phase Proteins' Postoperatively. Value in Detection and Monitoring of Complications," *Am J Clin Pathol*, 1976, 66(5):840-6.
7. Ghoneim AT, McGoldrick J, and Ionescu MI, "Serial C-Reactive Protein Measurements in Infective Complications Following Cardiac Operation: Evaluation and Use in Monitoring Response to Therapy," *Ann Thorac Surg*, 1982, 34(2):166-75.
8. Schentag JJ, O'Keefe D, Marmion M, et al, "C-Reactive Protein as an Indicator of Infection Relapse in Patients With Abdominal Sepsis," *Arch Surg*, 1984, 119(3):300-4.
9. Boeken U, Feindt P, Zimmermann N, et al, "Increased Preoperative C-Reactive Protein (CRP)-Values Without Signs of an Infection and Complicated Course After Cardiopulmonary Bypass (CPB)-Operations," *Eur J Cardiothorac Surg*, 1998, 13(5):541-5.
10. Relijic M and Gorisek B, "C-Reactive Protein and the Treatment of Pelvic Inflammatory Disease," *Int J Gynaecol Obstet*, 1998, 60(2):143-50.
11. Povoa P, Almeida E, Moreira P, et al, "C-Reactive Protein as an Indicator of Sepsis," *Intensive Care Med*, 1998, 24(10):1052-6.
12. Hallan S, Asberg A, and Edna TH, "Additional Value of Biochemical Tests in Suspected Acute Appendicitis," *Eur J Surg*, 1997, 163(7):533-8.
13. Mach F, Lovis C, Gaspoz JM, et al, "C-Reactive Protein as a Marker for Acute Coronary Syndromes," *Eur Heart J*, 1997, 18(12):1897-902.
14. Ridker PM, Cushman M, Stampfer MJ, et al, "Inflammation, Aspirin, and the Risk of Cardiovascular Disease in Apparently Healthy Men," *N Engl J Med*, 1997, 336(14):973-9.
15. Ridker PM, Cushman M, Stampfer MJ, et al, "Plasma Concentration of C-Reactive Protein and Risk of Developing Peripheral Vascular Disease," *Circulation*, 1998, 97(5):425-8.
16. Ridker PM, Hennekens CH, Buring JE, et al, "C-Reactive Protein and Other Markers of Inflammation in the Prediction of Cardiovascular Disease in Women," *N Engl J Med*, 2000, 342(12):836-43.
17. Visser M, Bouter LM, McQuillan GM, et al, "Elevated C-Reactive Protein Levels in Overweight and Obese Adults," *JAMA*, 1999, 282(22):2131-5.
18. Ridker PM, Hennekens CH, Rifai N, et al, "Hormone Replacement Therapy and Increased Plasma Concentration of C-Reactive Protein," *Circulation*, 1999, 100(7):713-6.
19. Cushman M, Legault C, Barrett-Connor E, et al, "Effect of Postmenopausal Hormones on Inflammation-Sensitive Proteins: The Postmenopausal Estrogen/Progestin Interventions (PEPI) Study," *Circulation*, 1999, 100(7):717-22.

References

Froehlich M, Imhof A, Berg G, et al, "C-Reactive Protein: Its Correlation With Components of the Insulin Resistance Syndrome," *Circulation*, 1999, 100 (Suppl 1):1-231.
Liuzzo G, Biasucci LM, Gallimore JR, et al, "The Prognostic Value of C-Reactive Protein and Serum Amyloid a Protein in Severe Unstable Angina," *N Engl J Med*, 1994, 331(7):417-24.
Roberts WL, Sedrick R, Moulton L, et al, "Evaluation of Four Automated High-Sensitivity C-Reactive Protein Methods: Implications for Clinical and Epidemiological Applications," *Clin Chem*, 2000, 46(4):461-8.

Cryoglobulin, Qualitative, Serum and Plasma

Related Information

Applies to Cryocrit

Abstract Cryoglobulins are immunoglobulins that reversibly precipitate or form a gel upon exposure to cold temperatures. Cryoglobulins consist of single immunoglobulins or complexes that may fix complement and initiate an inflammatory reaction similar to antigen-antibody complexes. Called "essential" when not related to recognized disease, cryoglobulins are most commonly associated with plasmaproliferative, lymphoproliferative, infectious, and autoimmune disorders.

Cryofibrinogens are fibrin and fibrinogen complexes which precipitate in cold temperatures[1] (see Cryofibrinogen *on page 337*). Other cold-related phenomena involve **cold agglutinins**.

Patient Preparation Patient should be fasting.

Specimen Serum and plasma, the latter to identify cryofibrinogen. If sample volume is small, cryoprecipitates may not be recognized. Even trace quantities can be symptomatic.[1]

Container Red top tube for cryoglobulins and lavender top (EDTA) tube for plasma for cryofibrinogen, each prewarmed to 37°C.

Collection Phlebotomy should be performed using prewarmed 37°C plain red top tube to collect 15 mL blood, for evaluation for cryoglobulins, and EDTA (lavender) tube prewarmed at 37°C to collect 5 mL blood for evaluation for cryofibrinogen.[1] The tubes should be transported to the laboratory immediately in a thermos filled with 37°C water.

Storage Instructions Keep blood at 37°C for 30-60 minutes. Centrifuge at 37°C. Separate serum from cells, recentrifuge serum if possible at 37°C and pour into clean test tube. Do not refrigerate or freeze.

Causes for Rejection Specimen not maintained at 37°C before separation

Reference Interval Negative

Use Cryoglobulins are often associated with macroglobulinemia of Waldenström, myeloma and other lymphoproliferative/plasmaproliferative diseases with monoclonal gammopathies, autoimmune disorders, and chronic infections. Cryoglobulin testing should be ordered if a patient has suggestive clinical symptoms or laboratory findings and/or is known to have one of these diseases.

Limitations Failure to detect cryoglobulin may be due to:
- allowing blood to clot at temperatures below 37°C
- too short of incubation time
- binding to serum lipids

Methodology Precipitation of cryoglobulin at 4°C for 24 hours.[1] If precipitation is not seen, evaluate again in 7 days. After centrifugation, the "cryocrit" of precipitated cryoglobulin can be determined, followed by immunochemical analysis of the precipitate.

Type 1 monoclonal cryoglobulins generally precipitate within 24 hours, but mixed cryoglobulins, especially Type 3, are often present in low concentrations and require prolonged incubation (7 days) at low temperatures for detection. Results are reported as present or absent. If present in sufficient quantity, cryoglobulins can be semiquantitated by performing cryocrit. Immunoglobulin class can be determined by immunofixation.

When precipitation is found in the plasma tube but not in serum, cryofibrinogen is recognized.

Additional Information Cryoglobulins have been classified as type 1, 2, or 3 on the basis of immunoglobulin composition.

Type 1 cryoglobulinemia is often associated with a plasma cell disorder and detectable monoclonal gammopathy. Type 2 is the most common cryoglobulinemia and is often associated with hepatitis C infection. The serum concentration of the monoclonal IgM is sometimes too low to be detected by serum protein electrophoresis. Type 3 consists of mixed polyclonal cryoglobulins, most commonly IgM-IgG complexes. The concentration of the cold precipitating proteins may be too low to detect.

The major antibody is IgM, its antigen IgG. Such activity is usually designated rheumatoid factor.

Type 2 mixed cryoglobulinemia is characterized clinically by a triad of palpable purpura, arthralgias, and weakness. Other features include Raynaud phenomena, renal disease, sensory motor neuropathy, splenomegaly, and anemia. CH_{50} is usually detected along with a significant depression of C4 and slight depression of C3.

The temperature at which precipitation takes place is more clinically relevant than the quantity of precipitation (ie, a cryoglobulin which precipitates only at very low temperatures is less likely to cause clinical difficulties).

Smears made from room temperature blood of subjects with cryoglobulinemia may contain clear, light pink or basophilic substance as cytoplasmic inclusions in leukocytes. Such material is consistent with phagocytosed immunoglobulins. Identification of such bodies may provide an important clue to recognition of cryoglobulinemia.[2]

Other relevant initial laboratory studies include RF, C3, C4, ESR, serum protein electrophoresis, creatinine clearance, and consideration of possible lymphoproliferative or plasmaproliferative neoplastic disease.

Type	Composition	Disease Associations	Signs/Symptoms
1 - Monoclonal IgM or IgG	May be IgA or immunoglobulin light chain; precipitates often in 24 hours	M components with lymphoproliferative, plasmaproliferative diseases including Waldenström macroglobulinemia, myeloma, monoclonal gammopathy of uncertain significance, and B-cell lymphoma	Many patients asymptomatic, others have pain, Raynaud phenomenon, palpable purpura, acrocyanosis, ulceration, on cold exposure
2 - Monoclonal IgM with RF activity and polyclonal IgG	Can cause immune complex disorders; precipitates 1-7 days at 4°C	Hepatitis C, lymphoproliferative diseases, connective tissue diseases including Sjögren syndrome; marked depression C4 with near normal C3	Arthralgias, glomerulonephritis, vasculitis, neuropathy, and palpable purpura
3 - Polyclonal IgM with RF activity and polyclonal IgG	Can cause immune complex disorders; may require 7 days at 4°C to precipitate	Hepatitis C; other chronic infections including HIV, CMV, EBV, bacterial endocarditis, leprosy, spirochetal, fungal, and parasitic diseases; autoimmune disease including SLE, RA, biliary cirrhosis; and inflammatory bowel disease	Less often symptomatic than Type 2

Footnotes

1. "The Challenges of Testing for Cryoglobulins," *Mayo References Services Communique*, March 2000, 1-3.
2. Maitra A, Ward PC, Kroft SH, et al, "Cytoplasmic Inclusions in Leukocytes: An Unusual Manifestation of Cryoglobulinemia," *Am J Clin Pathol*, 2000, 113(1):107-12.

References

Dimitrakopoulos AN, Kordosis T, Hatzakis A, et al, "Mixed Cryoglobulinemia in HIV-1 Infection: The Role of HIV-1," *Ann Intern Med*, 1999, 130(3):226-30.

Gorevic PD, "Cryoglobulinemia," *Internal Medicine*, Chapter 202, Stein JH, ed, St Louis, MO: CV Mosby, 1998 , 1248-50.

Kallemuchikkal U and Gorevic PD, "Evaluation of Cryoglobulins," *Arch Pathol Lab Med*, 1999, 123(2):119-25.

McLaughlin WJ and Schifman RB, Clinical Chemistry No. CC97-1, American Society of Clinical Pathologists, Chicago, IL, 1997.

Seiden MV and Pins MR, "A 69-Year-Old Woman With Lupus Erythematosus and Painful Skin Lesions of the Feet," Case Records of the Massachusetts General Hospital, Case 30-1995, Scully RE, Mark EJ, McNeely WF, et al, *N Engl J Med*, 1995, 333(13):862-8.

♦ **CSF Amino Acids** *see* Cerebrospinal Fluid Protein *on page 517*

♦ **CSF Amyloid Precursor Protein** *see* Cerebrospinal Fluid and Plasma β-Amyloid(1-42) *on page 513*

♦ **CSF Electrophoresis** *see* Cerebrospinal Fluid Protein Electrophoresis *on page 518*

♦ **CSF Gamma G** *see* Cerebrospinal Fluid Immunoglobulin G *on page 515*

♦ **CSF IgG** *see* Cerebrospinal Fluid Immunoglobulin G *on page 515*

♦ **CSF IgG:Albumin Ratio** *see* Cerebrospinal Fluid IgG:Albumin Ratio, IgG Index, and IgG Synthesis Rate *on page 514*

♦ **CSF IgG/CSF α₂-Macroglobulin** *see* Cerebrospinal Fluid IgG:Albumin Ratio, IgG Index, and IgG Synthesis Rate *on page 514*

♦ **CSF IgG/CSF Albumin Ratio** *see* Cerebrospinal Fluid IgG:Albumin Ratio, IgG Index, and IgG Synthesis Rate *on page 514*

♦ **CSF IgG:CSF Total Protein Ratio** *see* Cerebrospinal Fluid IgG:Albumin Ratio, IgG Index, and IgG Synthesis Rate *on page 514*

♦ **CSF Immunoglobulin** *see* Cerebrospinal Fluid Immunoglobulin G *on page 515*

♦ **CSF Leakage** *see* Cerebrospinal Fluid Protein *on page 517*

♦ **CSF Neopterin** *see* Cerebrospinal Fluid Protein *on page 517*

♦ **CSF Protein** *see* Cerebrospinal Fluid Protein *on page 517*

♦ **CSF Rhinorrhea** *see* Cerebrospinal Fluid Protein *on page 517*

♦ **CSF Taurine** *see* Cerebrospinal Fluid Protein *on page 517*

♦ **Delay Accelerating Factor** *see* Complement Components, Overview *on page 520*

♦ **Desmoglein 1** *see* Pemphigus-Like Antibodies *on page 541*

♦ **DNA Antibody** *see* Anti-DNA *on page 504*

♦ **DR3** *see* Smooth Muscle Antibody *on page 543*

♦ **DR4** *see* Smooth Muscle Antibody *on page 543*

♦ **Dysgammaglobulinemia Evaluation** *see* Immunofixation Electrophoresis, Serum or Urine *on page 530*

♦ **Edrophonium Chloride Test** *see* Acetylcholine Receptor Antibody *on page 502*

♦ **EMA** *see* Endomysial Antibodies *on page 525*

♦ **ENA** *see* Antinuclear Antibody *on page 507*

♦ **ENA** *see* Sjögren Antibodies *on page 542*

♦ **ENA** *see* Smith (Sm) and Ribonucleoprotein (RNP) Antibodies *on page 543*

Endomysial Antibodies

Related Information
Gliadin IgG/IgA Antibodies *on page 526*
Skin Biopsy, Immunofluorescence *on page 72*

Synonyms EMA

Applies to Antigliadin Antibody; Antireticulin Antibody; Transglutinase Antibody (Anti-tTG)

Test Includes Detection of IgA antibodies to endomysin using immunofluorescence

Abstract Celiac disease (celiac sprue), or gluten-sensitive enteropathy, is a malabsorptive disease of the jejunum and proximal ileum histopathologically characterized by villous atrophy. High sensitivity as well as specificity of endomysial IgA antibodies for celiac disease offers a worthwhile screening test. Those whose results are positive are candidates for small bowel endoscopic biopsy.

Specimen Serum; a minimum of 0.25 mL is required for pediatric samples

Container Red top tube or SST™ tube

Special Instructions Maintain sterility.

Reference Interval Negative

Use Diagnosis of celiac disease, characterized by diarrhea, flatus, malabsorption, steatorrhea, intestinal cramping, and weight loss. Dermatitis herpetiformis coexists with celiac disease. Testing for endomysial antibodies and for gliadin antibodies is used in evaluation of children in whom a failure to thrive problem is recognized. Testing is also done to monitor adherence to a gluten-free diet.

Limitations A negative result does not completely rule out celiac disease or dermatitis herpetiformis, because patients with mild gluten-sensitive enteropathy may not develop detectable antibody levels. IgA deficiency is found in a significant number of celiac disease patients, who cannot develop IgA endomysial antibodies. Measurement of IgG gliadin antibodies is helpful in making the diagnosis in this situation.

Methodology Indirect immunofluorescence, enzyme-linked immunosorbent assay (EIA)

Additional Information Celiac disease, or gluten enteropathy, is caused by sensitivity to gliadin, a gluten protein, the major constituent of wheat protein and to other cereal proteins in barley, rye, and oats. Celiac disease usually begins at about age 2, soon after the introduction of cereal to the diet. Symptoms may disappear in later childhood or early adolescence despite continued signs of malabsorption. It sometimes appears in the third or fourth decade of life. Gliadin is the alcohol soluble fraction of gluten that actually causes celiac disease. Affected individuals develop villous atrophy of the small intestine and malabsorption that result in diarrhea, growth retardation, delayed puberty, anemia, and osteoporosis. These symptoms resolve following removal of gluten from the diet. The definitive diagnosis of celiac disease requires jejunal biopsies before and after elimination of dietary gluten.

Ingestion of gluten triggers the production of IgG and IgA antibodies to gliadin and IgA antibodies to endomysium. (Endomysium is the sheath of reticular fibrils surrounding each smooth muscle fiber.) The IgA EMA test is both more specific and more sensitive than antigliadin assays. Because of its high specificity for celiac disease, a positive test for endomysial antibodies with an appropriate clinical response to withdrawal of dietary gluten may obviate the need for multiple small bowel biopsies to verify the diagnosis of celiac disease. Endomysial antibody was detected in 87% of celiac patients and 1% of nonceliac patients in a recent study.[1] See Gliadin IgG/IgA Antibodies *on page 526*.

Tissue transglutinase antibodies (anti-tTG) for celiac disease, using enzyme-linked immunosorbent assays (ELISA), may provide useful serologic tests.[2,3] They are not presently widely available.

Dermatitis herpetiformis is a bullous skin disease closely associated with gluten-sensitive enteropathy. Strict adherence to gluten-free diet often induces remission of both the skin and small bowel abnormalities. Endomysial antibodies are also useful in diagnosis of dermatitis herpetiformis.

The titer of IgA-EMA as well as biopsy findings correlate with the severity of gluten-sensitive enteropathy. If patients strictly adhere to a gluten-free diet, the titer of IgA-EMA should begin to decrease within 6-12 months after the onset of dietary therapy.

Cholesterol concentrations which are high to normal may rule out celiac disease. Serum iron <60 μg/dL, ferritin <50 μg/dL, cholesterol <156 mg/dL, and hypochromic anemia (Hb: male <13 g/dL, female <12 g/dL) are anticipated in celiac disease.[4]
(Continued)

Endomysial Antibodies (Continued)

Footnotes

1. Feighery C, Weir DG, Whelan A, et al, "The Diagnosis of Gluten-Sensitive Enteropathy: Is Exclusive Reliance on Histology Appropriate?" *Eur J Gastroenterol Hepatol*, 1998, 10(11):919-25.
2. Sulkanen S, Halttunen T, Laurila K, et al, "Tissue Transglutinase Autoantibody Enzyme-Linked Immunosorbent Assay in Detecting Celiac Disease," *Gastroenterology*, 1998, 115(6):1322-8.
3. Dieterich W, Laag E, Schopper H, et al, "Autoantibodies to Tissue Transglutaminase as Predictors of Celiac Disease," *Gastroenterology*, 1998, 115(6):1317-21.
4. Ciacci C, Cirillo M, Giorgetti G, et al, "Low Plasma Cholesterol: A Correlate of Nondiagnosed Celiac Disease in Adults With Hypochromic Anemia," *Am J Gastroenterol*, 1999, 94(7):1888-91.

References

Beutner EH, Kumar V, and Chorzelski TP, "Screening for Celiac Disease," *N Engl J Med*, 1989, 320(16):1087-9.

Ferreira M, Davies SL, Butler M, et al, "Endomysial Antibody: Is It the Best Screening Test for Coeliac Disease?" *Gut*, 1992, 33(12):1633-7.

Kapuscinska A, Zalewski T, and Chorzelski TP, "Disease Specificity and Dynamics of Changes in IgA Class Antiendomysial Antibodies in Celiac Disease," *J Pediatr Gastroenterol Nutr*, 1987, 6(4):529-34.

Kumar V, Hemedinger E, Chorzelski TP, et al, "Reticulin and Endomysial Antibodies in Bullous Diseases - Comparison of Specificity and Sensitivity," *Arch Dermatol*, 1987, 123(9):1179-82.

Ladinser B, Rossipal E, and Pittschieler K, "Endomysium Antibodies in Coeliac Disease: An Improved Method," *Gut*, 1994, 35(6):776-8.

Lindquist BL, Rogozinski T, Moi H, et al, "Endomysium and Gliadin IgA Antibodies in Children With Coeliac Disease," *Scand J Gastroenterol*, 1994, 29(5):452-6.

Mayo Medical Laboratories, *2000 Test Catalogue*, Rochester, MN.

Patchett SE, Alstead EM, and Kumar PJ, "Case 30-1994: Antiendomysial Antibodies and Celiac Disease," *N Engl J Med*, 1994, 331(26):1776 (letter).

Volta U, Molinaro N, Fusconi M, et al, "IgA Antiendomysial Antibody Test. A Step Forward in Celiac Disease Screening," *Dig Dis Sci*, 1991, 36(6):752-6.

♦ **Eosinophilic Mucin Rhinosinusitis** *see* Immunoglobulin E *on page 533*

♦ **Esterase Inhibitor** *see* C1 Esterase Inhibitor, Serum *on page 510*

♦ **Esterase, Subunit of C1** *see* C1 Esterase Inhibitor, Serum *on page 510*

♦ **Extractable Nuclear Antibodies/Antigens** *see* Sjögren Antibodies *on page 542*

♦ **Extractable Nuclear Antigen (ENA)** *see* Smith (Sm) and Ribonucleoprotein (RNP) Antibodies *on page 543*

♦ **Extractable Nuclear Antigens** *see* Antinuclear Antibody *on page 507*

♦ **Extrinsic Allergic Alveolitis Serology** *see* Hypersensitivity Pneumonitis Serology *on page 530*

♦ **Factor B** *see* Complement Components, Overview *on page 520*

♦ **Factor D** *see* Complement Components, Overview *on page 520*

♦ **Factor I** *see* Complement Components, Overview *on page 520*

♦ **Familial Hibernian Fever** *see* Immunoglobulin D *on page 532*

♦ **Familial Mediterranean Fever** *see* Immunoglobulin D *on page 532*

♦ **FANA** *see* Antinuclear Antibody *on page 507*

♦ **Farmer's Lung Disease Serology** *see* Hypersensitivity Pneumonitis Serology *on page 530*

♦ **Fas-Mediated Cytotoxicity** *see* CD4/CD8 Enumeration *on page 511*

♦ **Fish Sensitivity** *see* Allergen Specific IgE Antibody *on page 502*

♦ **Flow Cytometry** *see* CD4/CD8 Enumeration *on page 511*

♦ **Froin Syndrome** *see* Cerebrospinal Fluid Protein *on page 517*

♦ **GAD65** *see* Glutamic Acid Decarboxylase (GAD65) Antibody *on page 527*

♦ **Gamma G, CSF** *see* Cerebrospinal Fluid Immunoglobulin G *on page 515*

♦ **Gamma Secretase** *see* Cerebrospinal Fluid and Plasma β-Amyloid$_{(1-42)}$ *on page 513*

Gliadin IgG/IgA Antibodies

Related Information

Endomysial Antibodies *on page 525*
Immunoglobulin A *on page 532*
Skin Biopsy *on page 71*
Skin Biopsy, Immunofluorescence *on page 72*

Abstract Celiac disease, or gluten enteropathy, is caused by ingestion of wheat, rye, barley, and oats in patients with hypersensitivity to gliadin, a gluten protein. Ingestion of gluten triggers the production of IgG and IgA antibodies to gliadin and IgA antibodies to endomysium. Measurement of IgG and IgA gliadin and IgA endomysial antibodies (EMA) offers a useful diagnostic approach. The gold standard for diagnosis is the small intestinal biopsy. In **early** stages there is subtotal atrophy with intraepithelial lymphocytes. In **late** stages villous atrophy is total.

Specimen Serum; a minimum of 0.25 mL is required for pediatric samples.

Container Red top tube or SST™ tube

Causes for Rejection Heat-treated specimens, icteric or lipemic specimens, specimens containing microbial contamination[1]

Reference Interval IgA and IgG:[2]

<2 years:
- negative: <50 units/mL
- weak positive: 50-100 units/mL
- positive: >100 units/mL

≥2 years:
- negative: <25 units/mL
- weak positive: 25-50 units/mL
- positive: >50 units/mL

Use Diagnosis of celiac disease, a malabsorptive small intestinal disease characterized by diarrhea, flatus, malabsorption, steatorrhea, intestinal cramping, and weight loss; diagnosis of dermatitis herpetiformis; monitoring adherence to a gluten-free diet

Limitations A negative IgA gliadin antibody result does not completely rule out celiac disease or dermatitis herpetiformis. Measurements of IgG gliadin antibodies are indicated when IgA gliadin antibody is not detected. Antigliadin antibody provides less sensitivity and specificity in comparison to endomysial antibody and histopathologic evaluation.[1]

Methodology Indirect immunofluorescence, enzyme-linked immunosorbent assay (ELISA)

Additional Information IgG antibodies to gliadin are less specific than IgA antibodies. They are needed when the IgA result is negative, because selective IgA deficiency is found in ~10% of patients with celiac disease. Gliadin IgG antibody was detected in 69% of celiac patients and 29% of nonceliac patients. Seven of 13 patients who were endomysial antibody-negative had positive IgG antigliadin antibody.[1] See Endomysial Antibodies *on page 525*.

IgA gliadin antibody levels can be followed to monitor response to a gluten-free diet. If patients strictly adhere to a gluten-free diet, the titer of IgA-gliadin antibodies should begin to decrease towards normal values over the course of several months. Decreasing titers indicate a favorable response. IgG antibodies tend to persist for variable amounts of time on a gluten-free diet.

Background HLA abnormalities are discussed with evidence that gliadin-specific T cells play a critical role in the pathogenesis of celiac disease.[3]

The major complication of celiac disease is the development of enteropathy-associated T-cell lymphoma,[3] which develops in 5% to 10% of cases of gluten-sensitive enteropathy.[4]

Dermatitis herpetiformis is a bullous skin disease closely associated with gluten-sensitive enteropathy. Strict adherence to a gluten-free diet often includes remission of both the skin and small bowel abnormalities. Gliadin antibodies are also useful in diagnosis of dermatitis herpetiformis.

Footnotes

1. Feighery C, Weir DG, Whelan A, et al, "Diagnosis of Gluten-Sensitive Enteropathy: Is Exclusive Reliance on Histology Appropriate?" *Eur J Gastroenterol Hepatol*, 1998, 10(11):919-25.
2. Mayo Medical Laboratories, *2000 Test Catalogue*, Rochester, MN.
3. Galperin C and Gershwin E, "Immunopathogenesis of Gastrointestinal and Hepatobiliary Diseases," *JAMA*, 1997, 278(22):1946-55.
4. Fenoglio-Preiser CM, Noffsinger AE, Stemmerman GN, et al, *Gastrointestinal Pathology: An Atlas and Text*, 2nd ed, Philadelphia, PA: Lippincott-Raven, 1999, 1151.

References

McMillan SA, Haughton DJ, Biggart JD, et al, "Predictive Value for Coeliac Disease of Antibodies to Gliadin, Endomysium, and Jejunum in Patients Attending for Jejunal Biopsy," *BMJ*, 1991, 303(6811):1163-5.

Troncone R and Ferguson A. "Antigliadin ANtibodies," *J Pediatr Gastroenterol Nutr*, 1992, 12:150-8.

"Revised Criteria for Diagnosis of Coeliac Disease. Working Group of European Society of Paediatric Gastroenterology and Nutrition," *Arch Dis Child*, 1990, 65(8):909-11.

Glomerular Basement Membrane Antibody

Related Information

Antineutrophil Cytoplasmic Antibody *on page 507*
Antinuclear Antibody *on page 507*
Blood, Urine *on page 870*
Hemoglobin, Qualitative, Urine *on page 875*
Kidney Biopsy *on page 64*

Synonyms Anti-GBM; Antiglomerular Basement Membrane Antibody; Goodpasture Antibody

Abstract Immunologic aspects of renal disease can be divided into antibody-mediated entities such as Goodpasture syndrome (antiglomerular basement membrane disease) and cell-mediated glomerulonephritis; see tables. Antibodies recognizing the α_3 domain of type IV collagen (the Goodpasture autoantigen) lead to proliferative glomerulonephritis in Goodpasture syndrome,[1] and less commonly, cause pulmonary hemorrhage and idiopathic pulmonary hemosiderosis. Anti-GBM assays are positive in about 95% of patients with Goodpasture syndrome. Immunofluorescent studies of renal biopsy are confirmatory.

Antibody-Mediated Glomerulonephritis

Disease	Special Features
Antiglomerular Basement Membrane Diseases	
Goodpasture syndrome	Pulmonary hemorrhage and renal disease
Anti-GBM GN	No pulmonary disease
Alport disease, status following renal transplantation	Transplant contains "new" antigens
Immune Complex-Mediated Diseases	
IgA nephropathy	Male predominance; no vasculitis; may be related to cirrhosis; dermatitis herpetiformis
Henoch-Schönlein purpura	IgA in GBM and mesangium; systemic vasculitis involving skin, bowel, and kidney
Systemic lupus erythematosus	Photosensitive skin lesions, arthralgias, autoantibodies, other systemic features
Acute postinfectious GN	Recent streptococcal or staphylococcal infection; resolves with supportive care
Type 1 membranoproliferative GN (MPGN)	Mesangiocapillary changes
Type 2 MPGN	GBM dense deposits
Type 3 MPGN	Type 1 MPGN with overlapping features
Membranous GN	Subepithelial deposits; slow progression of renal dysfunction
Fibrillary GN	Membranous GN with 20-mm fibrils

Adapted from Ambrus JL and Sridhar NR, "Immunologic Aspects of Renal Disease," *JAMA*, 1997, 278(22):1938-45.

Cell-Mediated Glomerulonephritis*

Disease	Special Features
Wegener granulomatosis	Granulomatous vasculitis involving upper airways, lungs, and kidneys; often rapidly progressive glomerulonephritis; often positive C-ANCA
Microscopic polyarteritis	Nongranulomatous vasculitis involving skin, lung, and kidney; often rapidly progressive glomerulonephritis; often positive P-ANCA
Churg-Strauss syndrome	Granulomatous vasculitis involving upper airway, peripheral nerves, and bowel; associated asthma and eosinophilia
ANCA-positive glomerulonephritis	No systemic vasculitis; often P-ANCA
Scleroderma	Skin tightening, gastrointestinal dysmotility, Raynaud phenomenon, autoantibodies

*ANCA: antineutrophil cytoplasmic antibodies; C-ANCA: cytoplasmic ANCA; P-ANCA: perinuclear ANCA.

Adapted from Ambrus JL and Sridhar NR, "Immunologic Aspects of Renal Disease," *JAMA*, 1997, 278(22):1938-45.

Specimen Serum

Container Red top tube or SST™ tube

Special Instructions Tissue for immunofluorescence should be transported frozen in liquid nitrogen.

Reference Interval
- Negative: ≤5 EU/mL
- Borderline: 5.1-20.0 EU/mL
- Positive: >20.1 EU/mL

Use Evaluate patients with rapidly progressive microscopic hematuria and proteinuria; glomerulonephritis with or without pulmonary hemorrhage. Elevated levels, often >250 EU/mL, are detected in patients with glomerulonephritis with pulmonary hemorrhage (Goodpasture syndrome), glomerulonephritis without pulmonary involvement, and in idiopathic pulmonary hemosiderosis.

Limitations Weakly positive results (5-30 EU/mL) may occur in some patients without antiglomerular basement membrane antibody-mediated disease. The use of crude basement membrane preparations in a laboratory can lead to lower sensitivity or misdiagnosis.[2]

Methodology Direct (DFA) or indirect fluorescent antibody (IFA), enzyme-linked immunosorbent assay (ELISA)

Additional Information The two principal pathogenic mechanisms of autoimmune renal disease are immune complex mediation and specific autoantibody-mediated damage to fixed renal antigens: the renal glomerular basement membrane, Goodpasture syndrome, and antitubulointerstitial antibodies. Renal failure develops rapidly in Goodpasture syndrome without treatment. Antitubulointerstitial antibodies mediate tubulointerstitial nephritis (eg, following methicillin).

Recurrence in Goodpasture syndrome is rare but does occur.[1]

Other entities which may present with or as Goodpasture syndrome include Wegener granulomatosis, SLE, vasculitis, and Henoch-Schönlein purpura. Low serum complement would support diagnoses of SLE or postinfectious glomerulonephritis. Normal concentrations of complement would support vasculitis or anti-GBM disease; ANCA and anti-GBM antibodies prove helpful. Wegener granulomatosis and anti-GBM antibodies may coexist.[2]

Footnotes
1. Levy JB, Lachmann RH, and Pusey CD, "Recurrent Goodpasture's Disease," *Am J Kidney Dis*, 1996, 27(4):573-8.
2. Kalluri R, Meyers K, Mogyorosi A, et al, "Goodpasture Syndrome Involving Overlap With Wegener's Granulomatosis and Antiglomerular Basement Membrane Disease," *J Am Soc Nephrol*, 1997, 8(11):1795-800.

References
Ambrus JL and Sridhar NR, "Immunologic Aspects of Renal Disease," *JAMA*, 1997, 278(22):1938-45.

Ball JA and Young KR Jr, "Pulmonary Manifestations of Goodpasture's Syndrome. Antiglomerular Basement Membrane Disease and Related Disorders," *Clin Chest Med*, 1998, 19(4):777-91.

Lee SM and Marks EA, "The Emerging Spectrum of IgA-Mediated Renal Diseases: Is There an IgA Variant of Goodpasture's Syndrome?" *Am J Kidney Dis*, 1999, 34(3):565-8.

Savige JA, Dowling J, and Kincaid-Smith P, "Superimposed Glomerular Immune Complexes in Antiglomerular Basement Membrane Disease," *Am J Kidney Dis*, 1989, 14(2):145-53.

Internet Web Sites
rehd.med.upenn.edu:1025/

Glutamic Acid Decarboxylase (GAD65) Antibody

Related Information
Glucose, Fasting, Plasma *on page 183*
Glucose, Postglucose Load, Plasma *on page 185*
Glucose Tolerance Test, Plasma *on page 186*
Islet Cell Antibody *on page 538*
Parietal Cell Antibody *on page 541*
Thyroglobulin Antibody *on page 544*
Thyroperoxidase Autoantibody *on page 545*

Synonyms GAD65

Abstract Antibodies specific for the 65 kDa isoform of glutamic acid decarboxylase (GAD65) appear up to 10 years before the onset of clinical diabetes. Individuals with autoantibodies to GAD65 are at greater risk of developing type 1 diabetes than individuals without these antibodies. (Type 1 is that entity formerly called insulin-dependent diabetes mellitus.) Anti-GAD65 autoantibodies are detectable in the sera of about 75% of patients at the time of diagnosis of type 1 diabetes mellitus and described as a correlate of susceptibility to type 1 diabetes.

GAD65 antibodies characterize the stiff-man syndrome, in which muscle spasms of the back and legs occur with spinal hyperloidosis. It is a marker for a cluster of autoimmune disorders including thyroiditis, Graves disease, pernicious anemia, and vitiligo, as well as for type 1 diabetes susceptibility.

Specimen Serum

Container Red top tube or SST™ tube

Reference Interval <0.02 nmol/L

Use Assess susceptibility to type 1 diabetes mellitus; distinguish subjects with type 2 (noninsulin-dependent) diabetes mellitus who will subsequently evolve with type 1 diabetes; confirm the diagnosis of stiff-man syndrome (Moersch-Woltman syndrome) in 98% of patients[1]

Limitations GAD65 antibodies are detected in 20% of nondiabetic twins who remain disease free extended periods of time and in 8% of healthy individuals.[1]

Methodology Double-antibody radioimmunoassay (RIA), immunoprecipitation assay using a radioactively labeled recombinant human protein antigen, enzyme-linked immunosorbent assay (ELISA), immunofluorescence (IF), Western blot (WB)

Additional Information The enzyme glutamic acid decarboxylase (GAD) is a neurotransmitter-synthesizing enzyme. GAD is present in highest concentration in brain and pancreatic beta cells. Antibodies specific for the 65 kDa isoform of glutamic acid decarboxylase (GAD65) comprise the majority of pancreatic islet cell autoantibodies. Anti-GAD65 antibodies are detected in 75% of patients who have type I (insulin-dependent) diabetes mellitus and 98% of patients who have the rare disorder, stiff-man syndrome.[1] Patients with type 1 diabetes mellitus usually have antibody levels between 0.02 and 20 nmol/L. Levels >20 nmol/L are usually found in patients with stiff-man syndrome and related autoimmune neurologic disorders such as encephalomyelopathy.

The stiff-man syndrome may be a different entity or subgroup from the stiff limb syndrome.[2]

No GAD65 antibody-negative sample was positive for islet cell antibodies in a small series.[1] A positive association exists between GAD65 antibodies and antibodies to gastric parietal cells and thyroperoxidase antibody. It is found in 24% of patients with Lambert-Eaton myasthenic syndrome and in patients with idiopathic acquired cerebellar ataxia.[1]

Most antibody-positive relatives of patients with type I diabetes mellitus do not develop diabetes, but one or more immune markers are usually found among those who do.[3]

Footnotes
1. Walikonis JE and Lennon VA, "Radioimmunoassay for Glutamic Acid Decarboxylase (GAD65) Autoantibodies as a Diagnostic Aid for Stiff-Man Syndrome and a Correlate of Susceptibility to Type 1 Diabetes Mellitus," *Mayo Clin Proc*, 1998, 73(12):1161-6.
2. Barker RA, Revesz T, Thom M, et al, "Review of 23 Patients Affected by the Stiff Man Syndrome: Clinical Subdivision Into Stiff Trunk (Man) Syndrome, Stiff Limb

(Continued)

Glutamic Acid Decarboxylase (GAD65) Antibody
(Continued)

Syndrome, and Progressive Encephalomyelitis With Rigidity," *J Neurol Neurosurg Psychiatry*, 1998, 65(5):633-40.

3. Lernmark A, "Rapid-Onset Type 1 Diabetes With Pancreatic Exocrine Dysfunction," *N Engl J Med*, 2000, 342(5):344-5.

References

Batstra MR, Pina M, Quan J, et al, "Fluctuations in GAD65 Antibodies After Clinical Diagnosis of IDDM in Young Children," *Diabetes Care*, 1997, 20(4):642-4.

Batstra MR, van Driel A, Peterson JS, et al, "Glutamic Acid Decarboxylase Antibodies in Screening for Autoimmune Diabetes: Influence of Comorbidity, Age and Sex on Specificity and Threshold Values," *Clin Chem*, 1999, 45(12):2269-72.

Bazzigaluppi E, Bonfanti R, Bingley PJ, et al, "Capillary Whole Blood Measurement of Islet Autoantibodies," *Diabetes Care*, 1999, 22(2):275-9.

Borg H, Fernlund P, and Sundkvist G, "Protein Tyrosine Phosphatase-Like Protein IA-2-Antibodies Plus Glutamic Acid Decarboxylase 65 Antibodies (GADA) Indicates Autoimmunity as Frequently as Islet Cell Antibodies Assay in Children With Recently Diagnosed Diabetes Mellitus," *Clin Chem*, 1997, 43(12):2358-63.

Christie MR, Roll U, Payton MA, et al, "Validity of Screening for Individuals at Risk for Type I Diabetes by Combined Analysis of Antibodies to Recombinant Proteins," *Diabetes Care*, 1997, 20(6):965-70.

Dozio N, Beretta A, Belloni C, et al, "Low Prevalence of Islet Autoantibodies in Patients With Gestational Diabetes Mellitus," *Diabetes Care*, 1997, 20(1):81-3.

Fuchtenbusch M, Ferber K, Standl E, et al, "Prediction of Type 1 Diabetes Postpartum in Patients With Gestational Diabetes Mellitus by Combined Islet Cell Autoantibody Screening: A Prospective Multicenter Study," *Diabetes*, 1997, 46(9):1459-67.

Hallengren B, Falorni A, Landin-Olsson M, et al, "Islet Cell and Glutamic Acid Decarboxylase Antibodies in Hyperthyroid Patients: At Diagnosis and Following Treatment," *J Intern Med*, 1996, 239(1):63-8.

Hampe CS, Ortqvist E, Rolandsson O, et al, "Species-Specific Autoantibodies in Type 1 Diabetes," *J Clin Endocrinol Metab*, 1999, 84(2):643-8.

Hatziagelaki E, Jaeger C, Petzoldt R, et al, "The Combination of Antibodies to GAD-65 and IA-2ic Can Replace the Islet-Cell Antibody Assay to Identify Subjects at Risk of Type 1 Diabetes Mellitus," *Horm Metab Res*, 1999, 31(10):564-9.

Imagawa A, Hanafusa T, Miyagawa J, et al, "A Novel Subtype of Type 1 Diabetes Mellitus Characterized by a Rapid Onset and an Absence of Diabetes-Related Antibodies," *N Engl J Med*, 2000, 342(5):301-7.

Jaeger C, Brendel MD, Hering BJ, et al, "Progressive Islet Graft Failure Occurs Significantly Earlier in Autoantibody-Positive Than in Autoantibody-Negative IDDM Recipients of Intrahepatic Islet Allografts," *Diabetes*, 1997, 46(11):1907-10.

Littorin B, Sundkvist G, Hagopian W, et al, "Islet Cell and Glutamic Acid Decarboxylase Antibodies Present at Diagnosis of Diabetes Predict the Need for Insulin Treatment. A Cohort Study in Young Adults Whose Disease Was Initially Labeled as Type 2 or Unclassifiable Diabetes," *Diabetes Care*, 1999, 22(3):409-12.

Muir A, "Anti-islet Autoantibodies in Diabetes: Clinical Applications," *J Clin Ligan Assay*, 1998, 21:282-92.

Redondo MJ, Rewers M, Yu L, et al, "Genetic Determination of Islet Cell Autoimmunity in Monozygotic Twin, Dizygotic Twin, and Nontwin Siblings of Patients With Type 1 Diabetes: Prospective Twin Study," *BMJ*, 1999, 318(7185):698-702.

Reijonen H, Elliott JF, van Endert P, et al, "Differential Presentation of Glutamic Acid Decarboxylase 65 (GAD65) T Cell Epitopes Among HLA-DRB1•0401-Positive Individuals," *J Immunol*, 1999, 163(3):1674-81.

Tremble J, Morgenthaler NG, Vlug A, et al, "Human B Cells Secreting Immunoglobulin G to Glutamic Acid Decarboxylase-65 From a Nondiabetic Patient With Multiple Autoantibodies and Graves' Disease: A Comparison With Those Present in Type 1 Diabetes," *J Clin Endocrinol Metab*, 1997, 82(8):2664-70.

Tuomi T, Bjorses P, Falorni A, et al, "Antibodies to Glutamic Acid Decarboxylase and Insulin-Dependent Diabetes in Patients With Autoimmune Polyendocrine Syndrome Type I," *J Clin Endocrinol Metab*, 1996, 81(4):1488-94.

Turner R, Stratton I, Horton V, et al, "UKPDS 25: Autoantibodies to Islet-Cell Cytoplasm and Glutamic Acid Decarboxylase for Prediction of Insulin Requirement in Type 2 Diabetes," UK Prospective Diabetes Study Group, *Lancet*, 1997, 350(9087):1288-93.

Vandewalle CL, Falorni A, Lernmark A, et al, "Associations of GAD65- and IA-2-Autoantibodies With Genetic Risk Markers in New-Onset IDDM Patients and Their Siblings," *Diabetes Care*, 1997, 20(10):1547-52.

Verge CF, Stenger D, Bonifacio E, et al, "Combined Use of Autoantibodies (IA-2 Autoantibody, GAD Autoantibody, Insulin Autoantibody, Cytoplasmic Islet Cell Antibodies) in Type 1 Diabetes: Combinatorial Islet Autoantibody Workshop," *Diabetes*, 1998, 47(12):1857-66.

Yokota I, Shirakawa N, Shima K, et al, "Relationship Between GAD Antibody and Residual Beta-Cell Function in Children After Overt Onset of IDDM," *Diabetes Care*, 1996, 19(1):74-5.

Yu L, Rewers M, Gianani R, et al, "Anti-islet Autoantibodies Usually Develop Sequentially Rather Than Simultaneously," *J Clin Endocrinol Metab*, 1996, 81(12):4264-7.

♦ **β2-Glycoprotein 1** *see* Anticardiolipin Antibody *on page 503*

♦ **Goodpasture Antibody** *see* Glomerular Basement Membrane Antibody *on page 526*

♦ **gp39** *see* CD40-CD40 Ligand *on page 512*

♦ **HAART** *see* CD4/CD8 Enumeration *on page 511*

♦ **HANE Assay** *see* C1 Esterase Inhibitor, Serum *on page 510*

♦ **Hematopoietic Stem Cell Transplant** *see* Tissue Typing *on page 546*

♦ **Hereditary Angioneurotic Edema Test** *see* C1 Esterase Inhibitor, Serum *on page 510*

♦ **HIDS** *see* Immunoglobulin D *on page 532*

♦ **Highly Active Antiretroviral Therapy** *see* CD4/CD8 Enumeration *on page 511*

Histamine, Urine, Plasma, or Whole Blood

Related Information
Immunoglobulin E *on page 533*

Applies to Methylimidazoleacetic Acid

Abstract Histamine is pathogenetically important in anaphylaxis and other allergic states, including urticaria, flushing, asthma-like wheezing, and tachycardia. Histamine release occurs from sensitized basophil and mast cells. In sensitized individuals (ie, persons who have formed immunoglobulin E (IgE) antibodies to an antigen), much of the IgE is bound to specific receptors on basophils and mast cells. When the antigen appears again and combines with cell-bound IgE, histamine is among the vasoactive substances that are released.

Patient Preparation Patient must be on a diet of microbially processed foods, such as cheeses or sauerkraut.

Specimen Urine, plasma, whole blood

Collection Fifty percent acetic acid used as preservative should be added at beginning of 24-hour urine collection to maintain pH 2.0-4.0. Collect plasma or whole blood in EDTA tube.

Storage Instructions Store urine frozen.

Reference Interval The test is not widely available. One reference laboratory uses these reference intervals:[1]
- plasma: 0-6 nmol/L
- whole blood: 200-2000 nmol/L
- urine: 0-321 nmol/g creatinine

Another laboratory assays urine for histamine, with the following reference intervals:[2]
- 24-hour urine: <45 µg/g creatinine
- random urine: <100 µg/g creatinine

Use Assays for histamine are little used outside of research settings. Elevated values are found in systemic mastocytosis, urticaria, anaphylaxis, and following provocative testing.

Limitations Test is not very sensitive. There are false-positive results associated with urinary tract infections. Histamine level alone may not fully reflect the role of histamine in a disease process. Measurement of histamine and its metabolites may be necessary.[3,4]

Methodology Radioimmunoassay (RIA), gas chromatography (GC), fluorometry, radioisotope enzymatic, high performance liquid chromatography (HPLC), chemical ionization mass spectrometry

Additional Information Mast cells produce numerous biologically active materials, including histamine. Histamine may be elevated in myeloproliferative disorders and carcinoid tumors (particularly of gastric origin). Measurement of urinary methylated and other histamine metabolites may be more sensitive and specific. In a study of 25 patients with urticaria pigmentosa, all cases of systemic mastocytosis were identified with investigation of methylimidazoleacetic acid, the major histamine metabolite (>4.1 mg/24 hours) while histamine was elevated in only 50% of cases.[5]

Footnotes
1. ARUP Laboratories, *1999-2000 Users Guide*, 384-5.
2. Mayo Medical Laboratories, *2000 Test Catalog*, Rochester, MN, 292.
3. Green JP, Prell GD, Khandelwal JK, et al, "Aspects of Histamine Metabolism," *Agents Actions*, 1987, 22(1-2):1-15.
4. Khandelwal JK, Hough LB, Mornshow AM, et al, "Measurement of Tele-Methylhistamine and Histamine in Human Cerebrospinal Fluid, Urine, and Plasma," *Agents Actions*, 1982, 12(5-6):583-90.
5. Granerus G and Roupe G, "Increased Urinary Methylimidazoleacetic Acid (MeImAA) as an Indicator of Systemic Mastocytosis," *Agents Actions*, 1982, 12(1-2):29-31.

References

Fleck A and Myers M, "Cellular Aspects of Clinical Biochemistry," *Clinical Biochemistry*, Marshall WJ and Bangert SK, eds, New York, NY: Churchill Livingstone, 1995, 717-38.

Kaplan AP, "Anaphylaxis," *Cecil Textbook of Medicine*, 21st ed, Goldman L and Bennett JC, eds, WB Saunders Co, 2000, 1450-2.

Keyzer JJ, de Monchy JG, van Doormaal JJ, et al, "Improved Diagnosis of Mastocytosis by Measurement of Urinary Histamine Metabolites," *N Engl J Med*, 1983, 309(26):1603-5.

Spickett G, *Oxford Handbook of Clinical Immunology*, Oxford University Press, 1999, 629-39.

♦ **Histocompatibility Testing** *see* Tissue Typing *on page 546*

♦ **HLA-Antigen B27** *see* HLA-B27 *on page 528*

♦ **HLA-B8** *see* Smooth Muscle Antibody *on page 543*

HLA-B27

Related Information
Complement C4, Serum *on page 520*
Complement Components, Overview *on page 520*
HLA Typing, Single Human Leukocyte Antigen *on page 529*
Rheumatoid Factor, Serum or Body Fluid *on page 541*
Tissue Typing *on page 546*
Yersinia enterocolitica Antibody *on page 698*

Synonyms HLA-Antigen B27

Applies to Human Leukocyte Antigen

Test Includes Human leukocyte antigen testing for locus B27

Abstract HLA-B27 is an allele of the human HLA-B locus that is present in a small percentage of the general population. Positive patients have a greater likelihood of developing spondyloarthritis.

Specimen Lymphocytes

Container Yellow top (ACD) tube

Storage Instructions Store at room temperature. Refrigerate for DNA typing.

Special Instructions Sample must be tested as soon as possible unless DNA typing is used.

Reference Interval Negative

Use Evaluate spondyloarthritis, juvenile rheumatoid arthritis, Reiter's syndrome, psoriatic arthritis and anterior uveitis

Methodology Flow cytometry (FC), complement dependent cytotoxicity, DNA-based methods

Additional Information HLA-B27 is present in 3% to 4% of African-Americans, 6% to 8% of Caucasians, and 1% of Asians. HLA-B27 bears a strong association with but is not found in all patients with ankylosing spondylitis (AS; Marie-Strumpell disease); over 90% of such patients are positive. Most, but not all of the current recognized B27 subtypes are associated with AS. The disease-associated B27 alleles share a specific B pocket in the peptide binding groove with a strong specificity for an arginine side chain. This strict selection of peptides is consistent with the role of B27 in the process of binding and presentation of "arthritogenic" peptides. A B27-positive patient with consistent clinical and radiographic findings has ~100 times greater likelihood of having or developing ankylosing spondylitis than has a negative patient. However, the antigen is not causative, and 10% of normal subjects are B27 positive. **This test should not be used as a screening procedure for ankylosing spondylitis.** The antigen is less strongly associated with Reiter syndrome, psoriatic arthritis, juvenile rheumatoid arthritis, and other forms of postinfectious arthritis associated with several other gram-negative organisms. B27 has also been associated with congenital deficiency of C4 and C2, adrenal hyperplasia, and with inflammatory bowel disease.

References

Braun WE and Zachary AA, "The HLA Histocompatibility System in Autoimmune States," *Clin Lab Med*, 1988, 8(2):351-72.

Khan A, "Ankylosing Spondylitis: Clinical Aspects," *The Spondyloarthritides*, Calin A and Taurog JD, eds, Oxford University Press, 1998, 27-40.

Klein J and Sato A, "The HLA System. Second of Two Parts," *N Engl J Med*, 2000, 343(11):782-6.

Lamas JR, Paradela A, Roncal F, et al, "Modulation at Multiple Anchor Positions of the Peptide Specificity of HLA-B27 Subtypes Differentially Associated With Ankylosing Spondylitis," *Arthritis Rheum*, 1999, 42(9):1975-85.

Mear JP, Schreiber KL, Munz C, et al, "Misfolding of HLA-B27 as a Result of its B Pocket Suggests a Novel Mechanism for its Role in Susceptibility to Spondyloarthropathies," *J Immunol*, 1999, 163(12):6665-70.

Wordsworth P, "Genes in the Spondyloarthropathies," *Rheum Dis Clin North Am*, 1998, 24(4):845-63.

♦ **HLA Class II Antigens** *see* Mixed Lymphocyte Culture *on page 540*

♦ **HLA Complex** *see* Complement Components, Overview *on page 520*

♦ **HLA-DP** *see* Mixed Lymphocyte Culture *on page 540*

♦ **HLA-DQ** *see* Mixed Lymphocyte Culture *on page 540*

♦ **HLA-DR** *see* Mixed Lymphocyte Culture *on page 540*

♦ **HLA-DR3** *see* Sjögren Antibodies *on page 542*

♦ **HLA-DRw52** *see* Sjögren Antibodies *on page 542*

♦ **HLA Typing** *see* Tissue Typing *on page 546*

HLA Typing, Single Human Leukocyte Antigen

Related Information

Autopsy *on page 50*
HLA-B27 *on page 528*
Identification DNA Testing *on page 711*
Mixed Lymphocyte Culture *on page 540*
Platelet Transfusion *on page 854*
Rheumatoid Factor, Serum or Body Fluid *on page 541*
Tissue Typing *on page 546*

Synonyms Human Leukocyte Antigen System

Applies to Adhesion Molecule CD31; Class I and Class II Genes; Leukocyte Antigens; Major Histocompatibility Coded Antigens; Major Histocompatibility Complex (MHC); MHC

Test Includes Identification of human leukocyte antigens (HLA) or class I or class II alleles

Abstract The major histocompatibility complex (MHC) exists as a group of closely-linked genes that encode the HLA antigens, which are the major histocompatibility antigens. They determine compatibility between donor and recipient in transplantation, and therefore are expressed as "major." The HLA antigen captures foreign peptides, to present to antigen-binding T-cell receptors.[1] Malfunction of the HLA system exerts effects on a variety of human disorders. Over 200 genes are included in the HLA complex on chromosome 6. Over 40 encode leukocyte antigens.[2] Autoimmune phenomena are prominent features in many of the HLA and disease associations.

Specimen Leukocytes (for serology typing), white cells (for DNA typing)

Container Lavender top (EDTA) tube for DNA testing, yellow top (ACD) tube for serology and DNA testing

Collection Deliver immediately to the laboratory.

Storage Instructions Maintain at room temperature for serology testing. Refrigerate for DNA-based testing.

Special Instructions Test requires viable lymphocytes for serologic testing, either viable or dead cells for DNA testing.

Reference Interval Identification of specific leukocyte antigens, class I and II alleles

Use The HLA system is used as an epidemiologic marker, in paternity exclusion testing, transplantation donor and recipient matching to diminish likelihood of rejection and graft-vs-host disease (GVHD), and for compatible platelet transfusions for refractory patients. Investigation of the HLA system promises applications in immunodiagnosis and in immunotherapy. Many of these antigens have been more or less closely associated statistically with a wide variety of diseases. The most striking association is that of HLA-B27 with ankylosing spondylitis (AS).

Other associations with autoimmune diseases include birdshot retinochoroidopathy, reactive arthropathy including Reiter syndrome, celiac disease, dermatitis herpetiformis, idiopathic membranous glomerulonephritis, Goodpasture syndrome, and pemphigus vulgaris. Lower levels of relative risk include rheumatoid arthritis, Behçet syndrome, systemic lupus erythematosus, insulin-dependent (type 1) diabetes mellitus, idiopathic Addison disease, Graves disease, Hashimoto disease, postpartum thyroiditis, sicca syndrome, myasthenia gravis, and multiple sclerosis.[3]

HFE, a defective class I gene, causes hereditary hemochromatosis.

The HLA system is involved in protection against severe malaria and in other infectious disease problems.[3]

Another significant association is DRB1*-15, DQA1*-0102, and DQB1*-0602 with narcolepsy, a wake disorder.

Limitations The possible mechanisms and clinical significance of many of the disease associations are not well defined. Except AS and narcolepsy, none of these is presently an aid to diagnosis.

Methodology HLA class I typing (A, B, and C loci) conventionally is done by use of a dye exclusion (eosin, trypan blue) method to assess lymphocyte viability after reaction with various HLA-directed antisera and complement (serology); molecular genetic typing methods are increasingly in use.

Loci in class II are designated by three letters. The first, D, indicates the class. The second letter, M, O, P, Q, R, indicates the family, and the third, A or B, the chain: respectively, alpha or beta.[1] HLA class II typing (DR, DQ, and DP) by serological methods similar to those described above; B cells must be used, since many T cells lack class II antigens.

Molecular genetic HLA typing is rapidly replacing serologic methods. The advantages of DNA-based methods are: the sample requirements are less stringent (smaller sample; fingersticks; tissues such as buccal swab, formalin-fixed tissue, or hair follicles can be used); the oligonucleotide typing reagents have specific sequences and can be chemically synthesized in unlimited quantities; these standardized reagents can be used by all HLA laboratories worldwide to obtain consistently-defined HLA types; new alleles not detectable by serology can be identified by DNA methods; and for unrelated hematopoietic stem cell transplant, allelic level matching at DRB1 gene is required. High resolution HLA typing can only be achieved by DNA-based methods.

Molecular HLA typing is based on the amplification of target sequence by using primer pairs designed to flank either the class I or the class II polymorphic regions via polymerase chain reaction (PCR). The DNA-based typing varies, depending on the methods used to detect the amplified products. The commonly used DNA methods are sequence-specific primers (PCR-SSP), sequence-specific oligonucleotide blot hybridization (PCR-SSOP), and sequence-based typing (PCR-SBT).

The PCR-SSP method can provide both antigen level (serological equivalents) or allelic level typing depending on primer pairs used. The PCR/SSOP method also provides antigen level or allelic level typing depending on whether generic or group-specific primer pairs are used in PCR coupled with hybridization of blots with many SSOP probes. Sequence-based typing determines the exact base sequence encoding an HLA allele, and is the gold standard for HLA typing.

Additional Information The HLA system has been generally categorized into class I, class II, and class III gene regions. HLA class I genes including the A, B, and C loci and their respective antigens are expressed on most nucleated cells. The HLA class III genes encode the complement proteins, C2, C4, and factor B of the alternative complement pathway. Classes I and II are involved in immune response. HLA class I and II molecules bind processed self and foreign peptides for presentation to CD8- and CD4-positive T cells, respectively. Most HLA genes are highly polymorphic, which accounts for their recognition in transplantation. Many of the alleles of these genes are in linkage disequilibrium. Many of these antigens have been more or less closely associated statistically with a wide variety of diseases. The most striking association is that of HLA-B27 with ankylosing spondylitis (AS).
(Continued)

HLA Typing, Single Human Leukocyte Antigen
(Continued)

HLA typing is also performed for cadaveric renal transplantation, in conjunction with ABO typing and crossmatching. The degree of HLA mismatch between the recipient and donor is one component of the kidney allocation algorithm. These HLA molecules are the targets of rejection and of GVHD.

The system is useful in exclusion of paternity and in forensic medicine, since the HLA system includes many alleles which can be identified in addition to the many red cell antigenic systems.

Footnotes
1. Kernan NA and DuPont B, "Minor Histocompatibility Antigens and Marrow Transplantation," *N Engl J Med*, 1996, 334(5):323-4.
2. Klein J and Sato A, "The HLA System. First of Two Parts," *N Engl J Med*, 2000, 343(10):702-9.
3. Klein J and Sato A, "The HLA System. Second of Two Parts," *N Engl J Med*, 2000, 343(11):782-6.

References
Bodmer JG, Marsh SG, Albert ED, et al, "Nomenclature for Factors of the HLA System," *Tissue Antigens*, 1997, 49:297-321.
Braun WE and Zachary AA, "The HLA Histocompatibility System in Autoimmune States," *Clin Lab Med*, 1988, 8(2):351-72.
Colvin RB, Bhan AK, and McCluskey RT, *Diagnostic Immunopathology*, New York, NY: Raven Press, 1988, 159.
Hurley CK, Tang J, Ng J, et al, "HLA Typing by Molecular Methods," *Manual of Clinical Laboratory Immunology*, Washington, DC: ASM Press, American Society for Microbiology, 1997, 1098-111.
Petersdorf EW and Hansen JA, "A Comprehensive Approach for Typing Alleles of the HLA-B Locus by Automated Sequencing," *Tissue Antigens*, 1995, 46(2):73-85.
Raulet DH, "Does a Low Level of Expression of HLA Molecules Engender Autoimmunity?" *N Engl J Med*, 1999, 340(4):314-5.
Rodey GE, "HLA Beyond Tears," *Introduction to Human Histocompatibility*, Durango, CO: De Novo, Inc, 2000.
Schreuder GMTh, Hurley CK, Marsh SGE, et al, "The HLA Dictionary 1999: A Summary of HLA-A, -B, -C, -DRB1/3/4/5, -DQB1 Alleles and Their Association With Serologically Defined HLA-A, -B, -C, -DR and -DQ Antigens," *Tissue Antigens*, 1999, 54(4):409-37.

♦ **HSC Transplant** see Tissue Typing *on page 546*

♦ **Human Leukocyte Antigen** see HLA-B27 *on page 528*

♦ **Human Leukocyte Antigens** see Tissue Typing *on page 546*

♦ **Human Leukocyte Antigen System** see HLA Typing, Single Human Leukocyte Antigen *on page 529*

21-Hydroxylase Antibodies, Serum

Related Information
Adrenal Cortex: Laboratory Assessments Overview *on page 84*
Adrenocorticotropic Hormone, Plasma *on page 86*
Corticotropin Stimulation Test (Rapid) *on page 153*
Cortisol, Serum or Plasma *on page 154*
Insulin Tolerance Test *on page 202*
Metyrapone Stimulation Test, Serum *on page 225*
Urinary Cortisol/Creatinine Increment *on page 296*

Abstract Antibodies directed against the microsomal antigen, 21-hydroxylase, serve as a marker of autoimmune destruction of the adrenals.

Specimen Serum

Container Red top tube

Reference Interval <1 unit/mL[1]

Use This test is useful in the evaluation of patients with adrenal insufficiency (AI-Addison disease). A positive result identifies autoimmune destruction as the etiology of the patient's AI.[2]

Footnotes
1. Mayo Reference Services Publication, "21-Hydroxylase antibodies, Serum," *New Test Announcement*, Rochester, MN: Mayo Medical Laboratories, 2000.
2. Tanaka H, Perez MS, Powell M, et al, "Steroid 21-Hydroxylase Autoantibodies: Measurements With a New Immunoprecipitation Assay," *J Clin Endocrinol Metab*, 1997, 82(5):1440-6.

♦ **Hyper-IgM Syndrome** see CD40-CD40 Ligand *on page 512*

♦ **Hyperimmunoglobulin D and Periodic Fever Syndrome** see Immunoglobulin D *on page 532*

♦ **Hyperimmunoglobulin M Syndrome** see Immunoglobulin M *on page 537*

Hypersensitivity Pneumonitis Serology

Related Information
Aspergillus Serology *on page 560*
Bacterial Culture, Sputum *on page 574*
Lymphocyte Transformation Test *on page 539*

Synonyms Extrinsic Allergic Alveolitis Serology; Farmer's Lung Disease Serology

Applies to *Aspergillus fumigatus* Precipitating Antibodies; *Aspergillus niger* Precipitating Antibodies; *Micropolyspora faeni* Precipitating Antibodies;

Thermoactinomyces vulgaris Precipitating Antibodies; *Thermolospora viridis* Precipitating Antibodies

Replaces *Thermoactinomyces* Precipitating Antibodies

Test Includes *Micropolyspora faeni*, *Aspergillus fumigatus*, *Alternaria* species, *Aspergillus niger*, *Thermoactinomyces vulgaris*, *Thermolospora viridis* antigen testing by immunodiffusion of combined antigenic extract.

Abstract The diagnostic term, **hypersensitivity pneumonitis**, applies to patients with interstitial lung disease caused by inhaled organic dusts derived from living sources (*vide supra*) as well as chemical agents (eg, isocyanates and trimellitic anhydride).[1]

Specimen Serum

Container Red top tube

Reference Interval Negative

Use Support the clinical diagnosis of hypersensitivity pneumonitis in those who, following repeated exposure to moist hay or grains, develop cough, chills, dyspnea, and sometimes fever, without bronchospasm.

Limitations A positive test does not establish the diagnosis of hypersensitivity pneumonitis, nor does the absence of precipitins eliminate the diagnosis. Open lung biopsy may be needed to establish the diagnosis.

Methodology Immunodiffusion (ID)

Additional Information Some individuals become sensitized to inhaled antigens and develop acute bronchospastic symptoms 4-6 hours following exposure. Many of these have been diagnosed with disease names indicating the nature of the exposure. They include bird-fancier's disease, farmer's lung, mushroom-picker's disease, silo-filler's disease, maple bark-stripper's disease, paprika-slicer's lung, sauna-taker's lung, as well as bagassosis (particles of sugar cane fiber). Other sources include redwood tree bark, cheese, and dust from air conditioners. The antigenic material is usually an *Aspergillus* species or one of the thermophilic actinomycetes. Individuals with precipitating antibodies may have no symptoms, and patients with severe symptoms may not show antibody while their disease is inactive. Thus, there must be careful correlation of clinical and laboratory results.

Footnotes
1. Samet JM, "Occupational Pulmonary Disorders," *Cecil Textbook of Medicine*, 21st ed, Goldman L and Bennett JC, eds, Philadelphia, PA: WB Saunders Co, 2000, 424.

References
Colby TV, Lombard C, Yousen SA, et al, *Atlas of Pulmonary Surgical Pathology*, Philadelphia, PA: WB Saunders Co, 1991, 260-3.
Sharma OP, "Hypersensitivity Pneumonitis," *Dis Mon*, 1991, 37(7):409-71.

♦ **Idiopathic CD4 Lymphocytopenia** see CD4/CD8 Enumeration *on page 511*

♦ **IF Antibody** see Intrinsic Factor Blocking Antibody *on page 537*

♦ **IFE** see Immunofixation Electrophoresis, Serum or Urine *on page 530*

♦ **IgA Isotypes** see Immunoglobulin A *on page 532*

♦ **IgA, Quantitative** see Immunoglobulin A *on page 532*

♦ **IgD, Quantitative** see Immunoglobulin D *on page 532*

♦ **IgE Allergen Specific** see Allergen Specific IgE Antibody *on page 502*

♦ **IgE Myeloma** see Immunoglobulin E *on page 533*

♦ **IgE, Quantitative** see Immunoglobulin E *on page 533*

♦ **IgG₁** see Immunoglobulin G Subclasses *on page 536*

♦ **IgG₂** see Immunoglobulin G Subclasses *on page 536*

♦ **IgG₃** see Immunoglobulin G Subclasses *on page 536*

♦ **IgG₄** see Immunoglobulin G Subclasses *on page 536*

♦ **IgG, CSF** see Cerebrospinal Fluid Immunoglobulin G *on page 515*

♦ **IgG, Quantitative** see Immunoglobulin G *on page 535*

♦ **IgG Ratios and IgG Index, Cerebrospinal Fluid** see Cerebrospinal Fluid IgG:Albumin Ratio, IgG Index, and IgG Synthesis Rate *on page 514*

♦ **IgG Subclasses** see Immunoglobulin G Subclasses *on page 536*

♦ **IgG Synthesis Rate** see Cerebrospinal Fluid IgG:Albumin Ratio, IgG Index, and IgG Synthesis Rate *on page 514*

♦ **IgM, Quantitative** see Immunoglobulin M *on page 537*

♦ **Immunocapture** see Allergen Specific IgE Antibody *on page 502*

♦ **Immunodeficiency Profile** see CD4/CD8 Enumeration *on page 511*

♦ **Immunoelectrophoresis** replaced by Immunofixation Electrophoresis, Serum or Urine *on page 530*

Immunofixation Electrophoresis, Serum or Urine

Related Information
Bone Marrow *on page 410*
Cerebrospinal Fluid IgG:Albumin Ratio, IgG Index, and IgG Synthesis Rate *on page 514*
Cerebrospinal Fluid Protein Electrophoresis *on page 518*
Immunoglobulin A *on page 532*
Immunoglobulin D *on page 532*

Synonyms IFE

Applies to Dysgammaglobulinemia Evaluation; Isotypes, Light Chains; Kappa Chains; Lambda Chains; Light Chains; MGUS; Monoclonal Gammopathy; M Protein; Paraprotein Evaluation; POEMS Syndrome; Pseudoparaprotein

Replaces Bence Jones Protein Test; Immunoelectrophoresis

Test Includes Identification of monoclonal gammopathies, pathologist interpretation

Abstract A monoclonal protein (M-protein) population is the product of an expanded single clone of B lymphocytes and/or plasma cells that can be detected in serum or urine by protein electrophoresis. Serum protein electrophoresis is the simplest and lowest cost means of excluding the presence of a monoclonal protein but is not particularly sensitive (can detect bands ≤0.5 g/dL). Visual examination of electrophoretic patterns by a pathologist is the most sensitive method of detecting monoclonal proteins, since narrow and/or faint bands may be obscured in densitometric scans. After detection of an M-protein (see Protein Electrophoresis, Serum *on page 267* and Protein Electrophoresis, Urine *on page 268*), it can be further characterized by immunofixation electrophoresis (IFE) as to its immunoglobulin class (G, A, M, D, or E) and/or the light chain type (kappa or lambda). Biclonal, or even triclonal, patterns may occur, reflecting the presence of two or more M-proteins or formation of paraprotein fragments or complexes.

Specimen Serum, urine, or other body fluid, in particular cerebrospinal fluid

Container Red top or SST™ tube, urine container

Collection Urine: No preservative required.

Storage Instructions Separate serum from cells, centrifuge and/or filter urine.

Reference Interval Not applicable; each study should be accompanied by an interpretive report.

Use Evaluate and characterize clinical conditions (eg, plasmacytic, in particular multiple myeloma, lymphocytic, protein infiltrative, or other) that may be associated with monoclonal gammopathy (M-protein) detected initially on protein electrophoretic study of serum, urine, cerebrospinal fluid, or other body fluids. Detect, quantitate, and analyze abnormal specific (but non-M-protein) serum protein populations. Can be used for detection of leakage of CSF into nose or ear, in which a beta-2 transferrin band may be detected by use of an antiserum against human transferrin. There may be problems with sensitivity (a negative result cannot exclude CSF leakage). Congenital atransferrinemia is of rare occurrence, a serum control should be used.

Methodology The immunofixation electrophoresis (IFE) process is, essentially, one of protein electrophoretic separation with detection of the specific protein(s) of interest (the antigen) by appropriate monoclonal or polyclonal antibody (antigen-antibody reaction) followed by a staining procedure for visualization. IFE is most commonly (but not exclusively) applied to the detection and characterization/visualization of monoclonal immunoglobulins which are most frequently associated with a plasma cell proliferation. IFE consists of four steps:

1. Proteins are separated by electrophoresis.
2. Antisera (containing the antibody to the antigen of interest) is rolled over the gel or applied by use of an antibody saturated cellulose acetate strip placed on the gel. Rate of the resultant immunoprecipitation reaction depends on concentration of the reactants, temperature, and ionic characteristics/pH of the buffer.
3. Gel is washed free of soluble nonreacted proteins.
4. The residual immunoprecipitates (usually in the form of bands) are visualized by a protein stain. IFE can also be performed on gel after isoelectric focusing.

Additional Information The differential diagnosis of a monoclonal serum or urine protein includes solitary plasmacytoma, plasma cell myeloma, B-cell lymphoma/leukemia, amyloidosis,[1,2] Waldenström macroglobulinemia, heavy-chain diseases, the POEMS syndrome (**P**eripheral neuropathy, **O**rganomegaly, **E**ndocrine deficiency, **M**onoclonal gammopathy, **S**kin pigmentation and sclerotic bone lesions (sclerosing myeloma)), and a heterogeneous default group called "monoclonal gammopathy of undetermined significance" (MGUS).[3] Serum protein immunofixation is also recommended

Gammopathy	Frequency (%)
IgG	61
IgM	19
IgA	11
Light chain	5
Biclonal	4

for patients with a normal serum protein electrophoresis, but whose clinical symptoms suggest the possibility of amyloidosis, myeloma, or POEMS.

The relative frequency of monoclonal proteins reported in 1994 by Mayo Medical Laboratories is summarized in the table.

Guidelines for evaluation of M-proteins (presented at the College of American Pathologists (CAP) Conference XXXII, May 1998) recommended use of IFE to "define the abnormal protein type" and, in some cases, to detect small M-proteins.[4] A flowchart in Immunoglobulin G *on page 535* may be helpful. Immunoelectrophoresis is "discouraged" and is no longer a listing in the *Laboratory Test Handbook*.

Serum M-proteins have been noted in some kidney transplant recipients. A recent study implicates cytomegalovirus (CMV) and Epstein-Barr virus (EBV) infections in the development of oligomonoclonal immunoglobulins (oligo M-Igs) in transplanted individuals.[5] Oligo M-Igs were noted in 25% of patients postrenal allografting (sample size of 84), 86% had concurrent CMV/EBV infections.

IFE was used to assist in the analysis of a case of simultaneous macroamylasemia and macrolipasemia in a patient with celiac disease. These macroenzymes were formed of polyclonal IgA complexed with amylase and lipase. The changes in IgA levels and enzyme activities led to the conclusion that increase in IgA led to increased macroenzyme formation.[6] An article of the CAP consensus conference[7] indicates that IFE of urine (for monoclonal light chain - Bence Jones protein) should be performed on all patients with a serum M-protein >1.5 g/dL (irrespective of urinary total protein) and/or if a plasma cell proliferative process is suspect. It is advised that kappa and lambda antisera that are "monospecific and potent" for both free and combined (intact immunoglobulin molecule) light chains be used. If urine protein electrophoresis shows a localized globulin spike but IFE is negative for monoclonal light chain, the possibility of gamma heavy-chain disease should be considered and IFE using antisera to IgG (includes γ heavy chains) should be performed.[7] The demonstration of low levels of Bence Jones protein may be different with both sensitivity and specificity problems relating to mechanical concentration and ladder pattern backgrounds (polyclonal free light chains).[8,9,10,11]

There is evidence that urine levels of free light chain can be used to track disease-related B-cell activity in subacute lupus erythematosus.[12] Normally occurring proteins may mimic serum M-proteins in high resolution protein electrophoresis requiring IFE for differentiation. Such "pseudoparaproteins" may have characteristic features (migration positions and appearances) in many cases such that further laboratory or clinical evaluation may not be required.[13]

In the Mayo series, patients with monoclonal proteins had the following (see table) diagnoses at the time of detection.

Disease	% of cases
MGUS	56
Myeloma	22
Amyloid	10
Lymphoma	5
Plasmacytoma	3
CLL	2
Macroglobulinemia	2

The most common M-protein in myeloma is IgG. IgA and IgM are less frequent. The most common M-protein in B-cell lymphoma/leukemia is IgM but cases with IgG or IgA are frequent. The most common M-protein in amyloidosis (unaccompanied by plasma cell myeloma) is either IgG or IgA typically in low concentration (<10 g/L).[14]

Monoclonal gammopathy of unknown significance (MGUS) is common, occurring in 1% of patients >50 years and 3% of patients >70 years. The risk of malignant transformation (eg, development of or transformation into myeloma, lymphoma, or amyloidosis) is 17% at 10 years after detection and 33% at 20 years. Patients with MGUS typically have a serum IgG M-protein <20 g/L or an IgA M-protein <10 g/L.[14] The associated normal polyclonal immunoglobulins are not suppressed, Bence Jones proteinuria is absent, and urine beta-2 microglobulin is <3 mg/dL.

Footnotes

1. Case Records of the Massachusetts General Hospital, Case 3-2000, Scully RE, Mark EJ, McNeely WF, et al, eds, *N Engl J Med*, 2000, 342(4):264-73.
2. Alexanian R, Weber D, and Liu F, "Differential Diagnosis of Monoclonal Gammopathies," *Arch Pathol Lab Med*, 1999, 123(2):108-13.
3. Gertz MA, Lacy MQ, and Dispenzieri A, "Amyloidosis: Recognition, Confirmation, Prognosis, and Therapy," *Mayo Clin Proc*, 1999, 74(5):490-4.
4. Keren DF, Alexanian R, Goeken JA, et al, "Guidelines for Clinical and Laboratory Evaluation of Patients With Monoclonal Gammopathies," *Arch Pathol Lab Med*, 1999, 123(2):106-7.
5. Drouet E, Chapuis-Cellier C, Bosshard S, et al, "Oligomonoclonal Immunoglobulins Frequently Develop During Concurrent Cytomegalovirus (CMV) and Epstein-Barr Virus (EBV) Infections in Patients After Renal Transplantation," *Clin Exp Immunol*, 1999, 118(3):465-72.
6. Zaman Z, Van Orshoven A, Mariën G, et al, "Simultaneous Macroamylasemia and Macrolipasemia," *Clin Chem*, 1994, 40(6):939-42.
7. Kyle RA, "Sequence of Testing for Monoclonal Gammopathies," *Arch Pathol Lab Med*, 1999, 123(2):114-8.

(Continued)

Immunofixation Electrophoresis, Serum or Urine
(Continued)

8. Hess PP, Mastropaolo W, Thompson GD, et al, "Interference of Polyclonal Free Light Chains With Identification of Bence Jones Proteins," *Clin Chem*, 1993, 39(8):1734-8.

9. Harrison HH, "Fine Structure of "Light-Chain Ladders" in Urinary Immunofixation Studies Revealed by ISO-DALT Two-Dimensional Electrophoresis," *Clin Chem*, 1990, 36(8 Pt 1):1526-7.

10. Pascali E, "Bence Jones Proteins Identified by Immunofixation Electrophoresis of Concentrated Urine," *Clin Chem*, 1994, 40(6):945-6.

11. Kaplan IV and Levinson SS, "Misleading Urinary Protein Pattern in a Patient With Hypogammaglobulinemia: Effects of Mechanical Concentration of Urine," *Clin Chem*, 1999, 45(3):417-9.

12. Hopper JE, Golbus J, Meyer C, et al, "Urine Free Light Chains in SLE: Clonal Markers of B-Cell Activity and Potential Link to *In Vivo* Secreted IG," *J Clin Immunol*, 2000, 20(2):123-37.

13. Strobel SL, "The Incidence and Significance of Pseudoparaproteins in a Community Hospital," *Ann Clin Lab Sci*, 2000, 30(3):289-94.

14. Attaelmannan M and Levinson SS, "Understanding and Identifying Monoclonal Gammopathies," *Clin Chem*, 2000, 46(8 Pt 2):1230-8.

References

Bataille R and Harousseau JL, "Multiple Myeloma," *N Engl J Med*, 1997, 336(23):1657-64.

Keren DF, Alexanian R, Goeken JA, et al, "Guidelines for Clinical and Laboratory Evaluation of Patients With Monoclonal Gammopathies," *Arch Pathol Lab Med*, 1999, 123(2):106-7.

Kyle RA, "Plasma Cell Disorders," *Cecil Textbook of Medicine*, 21st ed, Goldman L and Bennett JC, eds, WB Saunders Co, 2000, 977-87.

Kyle RA, "The Monoclonal Gammopathies," *Clin Chem*, 1994, 40(11 Pt 2):2154-61.

Ledue TB and Garfin DE, "Immunofixation and Immunoblotting," Section A, Immunological Methods, Ritchie R, section ed, *Manual of Clinical Laboratory Immunology*, 5th ed, Chapter 8, Nakamura RM, volume ed, Washington, DC: ASM Press, American Society for Microbiology, 1997, 54-64.

Levinson SS, "Urine Protein Electrophoresis and Immunofixation Electrophoresis Supplement One Another in Characterizing Proteinuria," *Ann Clin Lab Sci*, 2000, 30(1):79-84.

Liu D, Read A, and Hjelm NM, "Can Isoelectric Focusing Reduce the Number of Samples Requiring Immunofixation?" *Ann Clin Biochem*, 1999, 36(Pt 6):769-70.

Immunoglobulin A

Related Information

Antibodies to IgA *on page 833*
Immunofixation Electrophoresis, Serum or Urine *on page 530*
Immunoglobulin D *on page 532*
Immunoglobulin G Subclasses *on page 536*
Protein Electrophoresis, Capillary Zone *on page 266*
Protein Electrophoresis, Serum *on page 267*
Protein, Total, Serum *on page 269*
Risks of Transfusion *on page 861*

Synonyms IgA, Quantitative

Applies to Berger Disease; IgA Isotypes

Abstract Immunoglobulin A (IgA) comprises about 13% of serum gamma globulin. It is the major secretory immunoglobulin, with an important role in mucosal immunity. There are two subclasses, IgA_1 and IgA_2. IgA molecules have a half-life of some 6 days. IgA does not fix complement and does not cross the placenta.

Specimen Serum

Container Red top tube

Storage Instructions If there is clinical suspicion of cryoglobulinemia, or of presence of macroglobulins (polymeric IgA M-protein), the sample should be drawn and held at 37°C. See Cryoglobulin, Qualitative, Serum and Plasma *on page 524*. Such samples should not be refrigerated prior to serum separation from clot.

Reference Interval Ranges may vary among laboratories.
Pediatrics: See table.[1]
Adults: 85-385 mg/dL

Age	Male (mg/dL)	Female (mg/dL)
1-30 d	1-20	1-19
31-182 d	7-56	1-59
183-365 d	9-107	15-90
1-3 y	18-171	25-141
4-6 y	60-231	47-206
7-9 y	77-252	41-218
10-12 y	61-269	73-239
13-15 y	42-304	82-296
16-18 y	89-314	90-322

Critical Values In IgA monoclonal gammopathy, concentrations as high as 6.0 g/dL occur.

Use Evaluate humoral immunity; diagnose multiple myeloma; monitor therapy in IgA myeloma; evaluate anaphylaxis associated with transfusion of blood and blood components (see Antibodies to IgA *on page 833*). Association of IgA deficiency with celiac disease is recognized.

Limitations If samples containing cryoglobulins or cold agglutinins are handled at incorrect temperatures, false low values may result. Of individuals subject to anaphylaxis on exposure to IgA, some have deficiency only to certain subclasses of IgA.

Methodology Rate nephelometry, capillary electrophoresis with or without immunosubtraction.[2]

Additional Information IgA, the secretory immunoglobulin, is the primary antibody in saliva, tears, colostrum, and gastrointestinal/respiratory/urinary tract mucosal membrane related fluids. IgA_1 and IgA_2 are the two subclasses of IgA. IgA_1 is 85% of total plasma IgA. IgA usually circulates in the serum as a single 7S unit. In secretions, however, it is a dimer or tetramer linked by a J (for joining) peptide chain.

Increased monoclonal IgA may be produced in lymphoproliferative disorders, especially multiple myeloma and "Mediterranean" lymphoma involving bowel. An IgA monoclonal peak >2 g/dL is a major criterion for IgA myeloma. Of subjects with myeloma, about 25% have monoclonal IgA.[3] Hypercalcemia is a prominent feature of IgA myeloma. The hyperviscosity syndrome is prominent as IgA M-components tend to form polymers. IgA myeloma is the second most common cause of hyperviscosity syndrome.

IgA may be elevated in a wide range of conditions affecting mucosal surfaces, where IgA is largely produced. Some clinically significant IgA deficiencies have concomitant deficiencies of IgG_2 and IgG_4. IgA may be decreased in patients with chronic sinopulmonary disease, in ataxia-telangiectasia, or congenitally. Patients with congenital IgA deficiency are prone to autoimmune diseases, and may develop antibody to IgA and anaphylaxis if transfused; see Antibodies to IgA *on page 833* and Risks of Transfusion *on page 861*. IgA levels may rise with exercise and fall during pregnancy.

IgA deficiency bears association with respiratory and other bacterial infection, especially with IgG_2 deficiency. IgA deficiency relates also to chronic diarrheal disease including giardiasis (hypogammaglobulinemia in general as with common variable immunodeficiency) and autoimmune diseases such as rheumatoid arthritis. In genetically susceptible individuals IgA deficiency may occur following therapy with phenytoin or penicillamine.[4]

Idiopathic IgA nephropathy (Berger disease) is the most common primary glomerulonephritis. About 50% of patients have elevated serum IgA.[5] There are clinical and glomerular histopathologic similarities to the nephritis of Henoch-Schönlein purpura, both may have elevated levels of IgA-fibronectin aggregates. Serum complement is usually normal. Frequently presenting as recurrent painless gross hematuria, often following an acute upper respiratory infection or flu-like episode, the subsequent course is quite variable with some 20% to 50% of cases developing renal failure over the course of many (20-30 years).[6] At the glomerular level, IgA nephropathy is characterized by mesangial deposition of IgA_1 (with possible subsequent deposition of IgG) followed by variable mesangial expansion and proliferation. The precise pathogenesis is unknown and the natural clinical course is quite variable, rendering evaluation of results of therapy and prognosis problematic. IgA nephropathy is likely a spectrum of diseases with a common marker of IgA immune complex mesangial deposition. Unfavorable prognosis is predicted in adult patients by high serum creatinine, severe proteinuria, and arterial hypertension (when encountered as presenting features).[7]

Footnotes

1. Soldin SJ, Bailey J, Beatey J, et al, "Pediatric Reference Ranges for Immunoglobulins G, A, and M on the Behring Nephelometer," *Clin Chem*, 1996, 42(S1):308.

2. Kyle RA, "Sequence of Testing for Monoclonal Gammopathies: Serum and Urine Assays," *Arch Pathol Lab Med*, 1999, 123(2):114-8.

3. Tricot G, "Multiple Myeloma and Other Plasma Cell Disorders," *Hematology: Basic Principles and Practice*, 3rd ed, Chapter 76, Hoffman R, Benz EJ Jr, Shattil SJ, eds, Philadelphia, PA: Churchill Livingstone, 2000, 1398-1416.

4. Cooper MD and Lawton AR III, "Primary Immune Deficiency Diseases," *Harrison's Principles of Internal Medicine*, 14th ed, Chapter 307, Fauci AS, Braunwald E, Isselbacher KJ, et al, eds, New York, NY: McGraw-Hill Inc, 1998, 1783-91.

5. Couser WG, "Glomerular Diseases," *Internal Medicine*, 5th ed, Chapter 116, Stein JH, ed-in-chief, St Louis, MO, 1998, 845.

6. Ambrus JL and Sridhar NR, "Immunologic Aspects of Renal Disease," *JAMA*, 1997, 278(22):1938-45.

7. D'Amico G, "Natural History of Idiopathic IgA Nephropathy: Role of Clinical and Histological Prognostic Factors," *Am J Kidney Dis*, 2000, 36(2):227-37.

References

Fervenza FC, Terreros D, Boutaud A, et al, "Recurrent Goodpasture's Disease Due to a Monoclonal IgA-Kappa Circulating Antibody," *Am J Kidney Dis*, 1999, 34(3):549-55.

Foerster J and Paraskevas F, "Multiple Myeloma," *Wintrobe's Clinical Hematology*, 10th ed, Chapter 99, Lee GR, Foerster J, Lukens J, et al, eds, Baltimore, MD: Lippincott Williams & Wilkins, 1999, 2631-80.

Julian BA, Tomana M, Novak J, et al, "Progress in the Pathogenesis of IgA Nephropathy," *Adv Nephrol Necker Hosp*, 1999, 29:53-72.

Utsunomiya Y, Kawamura T, Abe A, et al, "Significance of Mesangial Expression of α-Smooth Muscle Actin in the Progression of IgA Nephropathy," *Am J Kidney Dis*, 1999, 34(5):902-10.

Immunoglobulin D

Related Information

Cerebrospinal Fluid Oligoclonal Bands *on page 516*
Immunofixation Electrophoresis, Serum or Urine *on page 530*
Immunoglobulin A *on page 532*

Immunoglobulin G *on page 535*

Mevalonic Acid, Urine or Amniotic Fluid *on page 225*

Synonyms IgD, Quantitative

Applies to Familial Hibernian Fever; Familial Mediterranean Fever; HIDS; Hyperimmunoglobulin D and Periodic Fever Syndrome; Mevalonic Acid; PFAPA Syndrome

Abstract Immunoglobulin (Ig) D has a very low serum concentration but is an important lymphocyte membrane receptor, functioning as an antigen receptor and leading to B-lymphocyte activation and antibody production. IgD myeloma is rare but should be a diagnostic consideration when protein studies do not identify one of the more common monoclonal gammopathies. An IgD immune response (with increase in serum IgD or with cerebrospinal fluid IgD oligoclonal bands) may occur in at least some patients with central nervous system (CNS) tumors.

Specimen Serum

Container Red top tube or two microbilirubin tubes

Storage Instructions Store serum at 4°C. May be stored at -20°C for 10-20 years without significant degradation.

Reference Interval 0-14 mg/dL (SI: 0-140 mg/L); IgD is <1% of plasma immunoglobulin (Ig).

Use Investigation of monoclonal gammopathy for diagnosis of IgD myeloma

Limitations Not a screening test

Methodology Radial immunodiffusion (RID), rate nephelometry, radioimmunoassay (RIA), enzyme immunoassay (EIA). Using the latter two sensitive assays, IgD can be detected in the serum of nearly all individuals, whereas with the less sensitive RID procedure, IgD is not detected in some sera.

Additional Information IgD, formed of two heavy chains and two light chains, is a 7S immunoglobulin with a molecular weight of 180 kDa. It has a short half-life of 2.8 days and does not cross the placental barrier. The IgD molecule has been completely sequenced. While IgD has a very low serum concentration, it is a major surface Ig of lymphocytes. There is an unusual hinge region and absence of a disulfide bond, making it susceptible to proteolytic cleavage with subsequent B-cell activation. It functions as an antigen receptor in B-cell activation and may lead to antibody production.

When looking for myeloma, initial investigation usually includes serum protein electrophoresis and quantification of IgG, IgA, IgM, kappa, and lambda. In cases in which an unexplained restriction is seen (not explained by heavy chain studies), an IgD assay should be performed. IgD-producing myelomas are rare, <2% of reported cases.[1] They are usually characterized by a serum M-spike that is small or absent and by heavy light chain proteinuria. With the IgD M-protein and the prominent urine lambda light chain as the only distinctive features, IgD myeloma has been considered a variant of Bence Jones myeloma.[2] The median survival is nearly 2 years, but one-fifth of patients survive for more than 5 years.

A study of unconcentrated cerebrospinal fluid from a variety of central nervous system tumors found oligoclonal IgD bands upon isoelectric focusing (7 of 25 cases). Two patients with CNS malignancy had demonstrable intrathecal synthesis of both IgD and IgG oligoclonal bands. Four patients had a systemic (serum) IgD immune response but no serum oligoclonal bands.[3]

A syndrome, hyperimmunoglobulinemia D and periodic fever (HIDS) was first described just 16 years ago,[4] but has already been characterized at the biomolecular level.[5,6,7] Most patients develop recurrent high fever within the first year of life. The fever lasts from 1-7 days with variable frequency of episodes between patients. There may be associated rash, diarrhea, abdominal pain, arthralgia, vomiting, and headache.[7,8] Mevalonic acid is increased in the urine, during but not between, febrile crises.[6] Investigations by two groups in France and the Netherlands have shown that mutations in MVK, encoding mevalonate kinase, cause HIDS.[5,6] Fibroblasts from HIDS patients have decreased mevalonate kinase activity. The International Hyper IgD Study Group has considered an IgD value >6 mg/dL as elevated.[9] A few cases, considered to represent HIDS, have had normal IgD levels.[10] Serum IgA and IgG subclass 3 are often elevated, IgG subclass 4 may be very low.[8] A syndrome of episodic fever, malaise, aphthous stomatitis, tonsillitis, pharyngitis, and cervical adenopathy (PFAPA syndrome) is also associated with elevated levels of IgD.[11] Two other febrile disorders have been shown to have a genetic basis. Familial Mediterranean fever, an autosomal recessive condition, is caused by mutation in the MEFV gene.[12] Familial Hibernian fever (autosomal dominant familial recurrent fever) is the result of mutations involving the gene for type I tumor necrosis factor receptor.[13] While patients with IgD-related syndromes may be of rare occurrence, many are likely clinically overlooked.

Footnotes

1. Weinlander G, Drach J, Raderer M, et al, "Cytogenetic Analysis and Fluorescence *In Situ* Hybridization in a Case of IgD Multiple Myeloma," *Cancer Genet Cytogenet*, 1998, 105(2):172-6.

2. Blade J and Kyle RA, "Nonsecretory Myeloma, Immunoglobulin D Myeloma, and Plasma Cell Leukemia," *Hematol Oncol Clin North Am*, 1999, 13(6):1259-72.

3. Mavra M, Drulovic J, Levic Z, et al, "CNS Tumours: Oligoclonal Immunoglobulin D in Cerebrospinal Fluid and Serum," *Acta Neurol Scand*, 1999, 100(2):117-8.

4. van der Meer JW, Vossen JM, Radl J, et al, "Hyperimmunoglobulinaemia D and Periodic Fever: A New Syndrome," *Lancet*, 1984, 1(8386):1087-90.

5. Drenth JP, Cuisset L, Grateau G, et al, "Mutations in the Gene Encoding Mevalonate Kinase Cause Hyper-IgD and Periodic Fever Syndrome," *Nat Genet*, 1999, 22(2):178-81.

6. Houten SM, Kuis W, Duran M, et al, "Mutations in MVK, Encoding Mevalonate Kinase, Cause Hyperimmunoglobulinaemia D and Periodic Fever Syndrome," *Nat Genet*, 1999, 22(2):175-7.

7. Valle D, "You Give Me Fever," *Nat Genet*, 1999, 22(2):121-2.

8. Grose C, Schnetzer JR, Ferrante A, et al, "Children With Hyperimmunoglobulinemia D and Periodic Fever Syndrome," *Pediatr Infect Dis J*, 1996, 15(1):72-7.

9. Drenth JP, Boom BW, Toonstra J, et al, "Cutaneous Manifestations and Histologic Findings in the Hyperimmunoglobulinemia D Syndrome," *Arch Dermatol*, 1994, 130(1):59-65.

10. Drenth JP, Haagsma CJ, van der Meer JW, et al, "Hyperimmunoglobulinemia D and Periodic Fever Syndrome. The Clinical Spectrum in a Series of 50 Patients," *Medicine*, 1994, 73(3):133-44.

11. Padeh S, Brezniak N, Zemer D, et al, "Periodic Fever, Aphthous Stomatitis, Pharyngitis, and Adenopathy Syndrome: Clinical Characteristics and Outcome," *J Pediatr*, 1999, 135(1):98-101.

12. The French FMF Consortium, "A Candidate Gene for Familial Mediterranean Fever," *Nat Genet*, 1997, 17(1):25-31.

13. McDermott MF, Aksentijevich I, Galon J, et al, "Germline Mutations in the Extracellular Domains of the 55 kDa TNF Receptor, TNFR1, Define a Family of Dominantly Inherited Autoinflammatory Syndromes," *Cell*, 1999, 97(1):133-44.

References

Bianchi P, MacNamara E, Bergami MR, et al, "Immunochemical Evaluation of Monoclonal Gammopathies: Heavy Chain to Light Chain Ratio Is of Little Practical Value for Detecting IgD Myelomas and Free Light Chains," *Clin Chem*, 1992, 38(2):317-9.

Paraskevas F, "Cell Interactions in the Immune Response," *Wintrobe's Clinical Hematology*, 10th ed, Chapter 21, Lee GR, Foerster J, Lukens J, et al, eds, Baltimore, MD: Lippincott Williams & Wilkins, 1999, 544-614.

Rassenti LZ and Kipps TJ, "Immunoglobulin Genes," Chapter 15, Section C, *Manual of Clinical Laboratory Immunology*, Rose NR, Conway de Macario E, Folds JD, eds, Washington, DC: ASM Press, American Society for Microbiology, 1997, 147-55.

Vladutiu AO, "Immunoglobulin D: Properties, Measurement and Clinical Relevance," *Clin Diagn Lab Immunol*, 2000, 7(2):131-40.

Immunoglobulin E

Related Information

Allergen Specific IgE Antibody *on page 502*

Aspergillus Serology *on page 560*

Eosinophil Count *on page 424*

Histamine, Urine, Plasma, or Whole Blood *on page 528*

Synonyms IgE, Quantitative

Applies to Allergic Fungal Sinusitis; Buckley syndrome; Eosinophilic Mucin Rhinosinusitis; IgE Myeloma; Job Syndrome; Kimura Disease; Organochlorine Compounds

Abstract Allergic individuals often have elevated serum IgE levels. Significant elevations are seen in patients with allergic disease, parasitism, bronchopulmonary aspergillosis, extrinsic asthma, urticaria, atopic eczema, IgE myeloma, and hyperimmunoglobulinemia E *Staphylococcus* abscess syndrome (Buckley syndrome, Job syndrome).

Patient Preparation Avoid exposure to radioisotopes when assay method is RIA.

Specimen Serum

Container Red top tube or SST™ tube

Reference Interval <100 IU/mL (100-700 µg/L with mean of 300 µg/L); age-specific ranges vary by laboratory and method; cord serum, usually <2 IU/mL. Total serum IgE values may be expressed in international units/mL, in weight/volume measures, in terms of molar concentration, or less commonly in SI units. One IU = 2.4 ng of protein, one SI = 1 µg/L. See *Manual of Clinical Laboratory Immunology* reference.

Use Very high IgE levels may be helpful diagnostically. Atopic disease is likely if the total IgE level ≥375 IU/mL. Extreme elevations of 800-25,000 IU/mL are found in asthma associated with severe atopic dermatitis, allergic bronchopulmonary aspergillosis, parasitic infections, IgE myeloma, and Buckley syndrome.

For allergic patients, serial testing may be useful to confirm expected seasonal variations that occur with allergen contact. There is some evidence that elevated serum IgE levels in cord blood are predictive of subsequent development of atopy later in life.[1]

Limitations Total IgE antibody levels can be correlated with clinical allergy only in a general way. Patients with high concentrations of total IgE usually demonstrate sensitivity to many specific allergens. However, many patients with clinical evidence of allergy and detectable allergen-specific IgE have total IgE levels within the reference range. If the total IgE level is very low, atopic disease can usually be excluded. Patients with total IgE level ≤20 IU/mL rarely have detectable specific IgE levels.

Methodology Radioimmunosorbent assay, immunoassay

Additional Information IgE is a monomeric immunoglobulin formed of two epsilon heavy chains and two kappa or lambda light chains (epsilon$_2$kappa$_2$ or epsilon$_2$lambda$_2$). IgE does not fix complement, does not cross the placenta, and has a short serum half-life of 2.4 days. Like other immunoglobulins, it is formed in response to antigenic stimulation. Unlike other immunoglobulins, IgE routinely binds via its Fc region, at least partly through the high-affinity IgE receptor, Fc epsilon RI (FceRI), to the surface membrane of basophils. The FceRI complex provides a receptor for the Fc region of antigen-specific IgE, participates in IgE-mediated antigen presentation, and controls activation of basophils, mast cells, and T cells.[2] Subsequent trapping of antigen with cross-linking by cell-bound IgE molecules triggers basophilic cells to release a variety of bioactive molecules, (Continued)

Immunoglobulin E (Continued)

including histamine, prostaglandin D2, kallikrein, and leukotrienes C, D, and E. These compounds produce the classic allergic reaction. Signs and symptoms of this immediate (type I hypersensitivity) reaction may include, dependent in part on allergen-specific IgE involvement, hives or urticaria, sneezing, rhinorrhea, conjunctival edema with itching and irritation, attacks of shortness of breath/wheezing (asthma), and/or anaphylaxis (difficulty in breathing with potentially catastrophic fall in blood pressure/shock).

Plasma cells that produce IgE are present especially along respiratory and gastrointestinal membranes. They populate regional lymph nodes but are represented only minimally in the spleen and other lymph nodes. In this respect, IgE is similar to IgA and is considered to represent a secretory immunoglobulin. IgE-dependent reactions likely represent protective mechanisms against parasitic invaders. Biologically powerful affector molecules are necessarily involved, requiring tight control to avoid serious pathologic consequences of IgE-dependent inflammation. Recent investigations have partially defined interactions between protein chemical mediators (cytokines) and specific inflammatory cells and their membrane receptors. Definition of this immunoregulatory process has (and will) allow identification of dysregulation on a genetic basis (mutant regulatory molecules and cell membrane receptors). Interleukin-4 (IL-4) and Interleukin-13 (IL-13) are important cytokines that mediate IgE synthesis. IL-4 effects B-lymphocyte switching to IgE antibody production. IL-13 also acts on B cells to produce IgE. CD4+ lymphocytes, the T helper (Th) cells are of at least two phenotypic types, Th1 and Th2. IL-4 stimulates the maturation of T helper cells towards the Th2 phenotype. The Th1 and Th2 type T4 lymphocytes have been identified on the basis of their different patterns of cytokine production. Th1 cells produce IL-2 tumor necrosis factor B, and interferon-gamma (IFN-γ) whereas Th2 cells produce IL-4, IL-5, IL-6, and IL-13. Th1 cells are involved in delayed type hypersensitivity, induction of cytotoxic effector T cells, and through the effect of IFN-γ, strongly suppress IL-4-induced IgE production while Th2 cells support immune reactions in which eosinophils and IgE participate.[3,4] Variants of the interleukin-4 receptor (IL-4R) are under study for their involvement in the hyper-IgE syndrome, severe eczema, and other conditions.[4] In addition to IL-4, IgE synthesis by B cells requires interaction of the B cell surface antigen CD40 with its ligand (CD40-L) which is expressed on activated T cells.[5] There is interest at the pharmacologic level in the mechanisms by which IL-4 and CD40 signaling switch on IgE production. With intervention there is the possibility that the IgE antibody response might be suppressed.[5] See graphics.

The IgE System as a Model of Allergic Inflammation

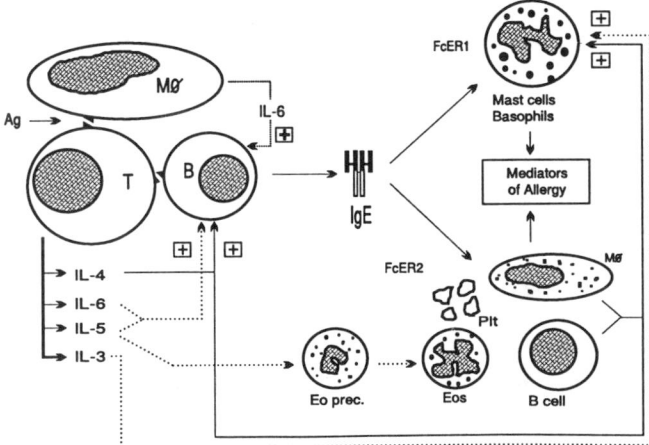

Adapted from Vercelli D and Geha RS, *J Clin Immunol*, 1989, 9:75-83.

Two Types of Helper T Cells

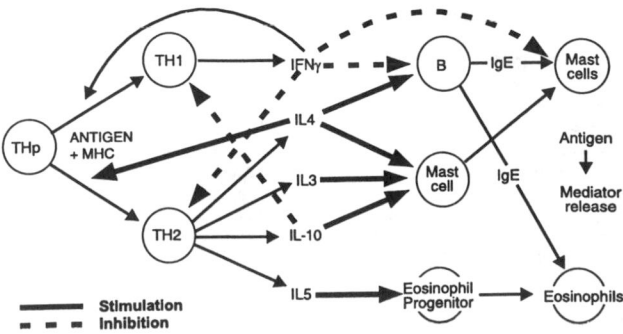

These are distinguished by their cytokine profiles and by their postulated roles in the regulation of IgE synthesis.

Adapted from Mosmann TR and Coffman RL, "T_H1 and T_H2 Cells: Different Patterns of Lymphokine Secretion Lead to Different Functional Properties," *Annu Rev Immunol*, 1989, 7:145.

Further definition of the cellular/molecular mechanisms referred to but briefly above may assist in understanding the involvement of IgE in the following situations:

- Neonatal B cells are capable of being switched to IgE production (if given exogenous IL-4). Minimal production of IgE in the neonatal period is the result of helper T-cell functional immaturity.[6]

- Allergen or parasite specific IgE is detectable in cord plasma of some neonates. Cultured cord blood mononuclear cells from babies of helminth infected African mothers can produce parasite antigen-specific IgE. Such cells from cord blood of North American delivered babies do not have this capability.[7]

- Cord blood from 2050 neonates showed elevated total IgE levels from Slovak regions where cities were polluted with organic chemicals, notably with placental contamination by organochlorine compounds, as compared to placentas delivered in unpolluted rural regions. The evident higher level of allergic sensitization was associated with increased incidence of atopic eczema in the industrial areas.[1]

- The hyper-IgE syndrome (#s 147060 and 2437000 in McKusick's *Mendelian Inheritance in Man (MIM)*, 12th ed, 1998),[8] is a rare multisystem disorder[9] characterized by marked increase in serum levels of IgE (>2000 IU/mL), recurrent staphylococcal skin abscesses, pneumonia often with residual pneumatocoele formation, dental and skeletal abnormalities including facial asymmetry, prominent forehead, broad nasal bridge, mild prognathism, tendency to fracture with minor trauma, hyperextensible joints, and other changes. There is question of cytokine-mediated increased bone resorption.[9] There is usually blood eosinophilia but without correlation to serum IgE levels. Occasionally, an adult with hyper-IgE syndrome has a normal serum IgE result. Referred to in the past as Job syndrome, there is some question as to the existence of variant or incomplete forms of the hyper-IgE syndrome, rendering reports of incidence (generally considered as over 200 case reports) uncertain. There has been recent interest in a mutant form of the IL-4 α-subunit and its possible role in the genesis of this syndrome (IL-4 receptor variant Q576R).[10] A current report, however, indicates that the frequency of Q576R is not increased in the syndrome (as compared to normals) and that the interleukin-4 receptor locus is not linked to the hyper-IgE syndrome.[11] A recent single case report describes a 29 year old woman with multisystem disease including facial features of hyper-IgE syndrome, IgE peak levels of 38,600, eosinophilia but with a Th0 profile.[12] There was restricted cytokine expression and on analysis of T-cell receptor genes evidence of at least one T-cell clonal population was obtained. The authors suggest that "...immunophenotyping and molecular study of peripheral-blood lymphocytes should be performed in patients with this syndrome..."[12]

- Kimura disease, a rare condition characterized in most cases by eosinophilia and elevated IgE levels with enlargement of salivary glands, lymph nodes, and subcutaneous soft tissue. The condition can be confused with lymphoma or infection and requires biopsy study to establish the diagnosis. Atypical follicular hyperplasia with intense eosinophil infiltrate often with foci of necrosis and/or hyaline deposits within follicles and/or polykaryotic giant cells is seen histopathologically.[13] Parasites are not demonstrable. It has been considered that Th2 cytokines are involved in the development of Kimura disease.[14]

- Allelic variants of the IL-4 receptor α-chain (IL-4Rα), notably the R576 IL-4α allele have been reported. R576 IL-4Rα, an evident risk factor for atopy,[15] has been found to act as an allergic asthma susceptibility and disease-modifying gene and has been proposed as a "clinically useful marker of asthma severity."[16]

- Patients with low levels of serum IgE (<2.5 IU/mL), considered to have IgE deficiency (IgE hypogammaglobulinemia) were analyzed and found to have an increased prevalence of multiple immunoglobulin deficits, autoimmune disease, and nonallergic reactive airway disease (as compared to allergy-immunology patients of the same clinic who had normal or elevated IgE levels).[17]

- In the differential diagnosis between allergic fungal sinusitis (AFS) and the proposed "eosinophilic mucin rhinosinusitis" (EMRS), serum total IgE is elevated in both entities but more significantly elevated in AFS patients. IgG₁ deficiency occurred in 50% of evaluated EMRS patients.[18]

- Study of a 12-year old long-term (since birth) survivor of vertically acquired HIV found findings of hyper-IgE syndrome, increased Th2 cytokine production (includes IL-4), maintenance of HIV specific immune response, low viral load and normal CD4 level without antiretroviral therapy. Presence of anti-HIV-specific IgE was interpreted as possibly representing "a protective mechanism against HIV replication..."[19]

- IgE myeloma is rare, some 40 cases having been reported.[20] "Benign" IgE monoclonal gammopathies and biclonal/triclonal gammopathies (with IgE as one component) have been described. A recent survey found that IgE myeloma presents a variety of symptoms that are similar to those of the more common forms of myeloma. Specific or typical symptoms/findings for IgE myeloma were not noted.[20] Bone pain, weight loss, fatigue, dyspnea, and anemia were common. Elevated sedimentation rate is common but a normal ESR does not exclude the diagnosis. Hypercalcemia, hypocalcemia, osteoblastic, osteolytic, or osteosclerotic changes may occur. IgE myeloma generally has a more malignant clinical course than other forms of multiple myeloma.[20]

Footnotes

1. Reichrtova E, Ciznar P, Prachar V, et al, "Cord Serum Immunoglobulin E Related to the Environmental Contamination of Human Placentas With Organochlorine Compounds," *Environ Health Perspect*, 1999, 107(11):895-9.
2. Turner H and Kinet JP, "Signaling Through the High-Affinity IgE Receptor FceRI," *Nature*, 1999, 402 (6760 Suppl):B24-30.
3. Corry DB and Kheradmand F, "Induction and Regulation of the IgE Response," *Nature*, 1999, 402(6760 Suppl):B18-23.
4. Shirakawa I, Deichmann KA, Izuhara I, et al, "Atopy and Asthma: Genetic Variants of IL-4 and IL-13 Signaling," *Immunol Today*, 2000, 21(2):60-4.
5. Bacharier LB and Geha RS, "Molecular Mechanisms of IgE Regulation," *J Allergy Clin Immunol*, 2000, 105(2 Pt 2):S547-58.
6. Holt PG and Jones CA, "Allergy Review Series VI: The Immunology of Fetuses and Infants, The Development of the Immune System During Pregnancy and Early Life," *Allergy*, 2000, 55(8):688-97.
7. King CL, Malhotra I, Mungai P, et al, "B Cell Sensitization to Helminthic Infection Develops *in utero* in Humans," *J Immunol*, 1998, 160(7):3578-84.
8. McKusick VA, *Mendelian Inheritance in Man. Catalogues of Human Genes and Genetic Disorders*, 12th ed, Baltimore, MD: Johns Hopkins University Press, 1998.
9. Grimbacher B, Holland SM, Gallin JI, et al, "Hyper-IgE Syndrome With Recurrent Infections - An Autosomal Dominant Multisystem Disorder," *N Engl J Med*, 1999, 340(9):692-702.
10. Hershey GK, Friedrich MF, Esswein LA, et al, "The Association of Atopy With a Gain-of-Function Mutation in the Alpha Subunit of the Interleukin-4 Receptor," *N Engl J Med*, 1997, 337(24):1720-5.
11. Grimbacher B, Holland SM and Puck JM, "The Interleukin-4 Receptor Variant Q576R in Hyper-IgE Syndrome," letter, *N Engl J Med*, 1998, 338(15):1073-4.
12. Presotto F, Trentin L and Agostini C, "Hyper-IgE Syndrome," *N Engl J Med*, 1999, 341(5):375-7.
13. Karavattathayyil SJ and Krause JR, "Kimura's Disease: A Case Report," *Ear Nose Throat J*, 2000, 79(3):195-6, 199.
14. Katagiri K, Itami S, Hatano Y, et al, "*In Vivo* Expression of IL-4, IL-5, IL-13 and IFN-γ in RNAs in Peripheral Blood Mononuclear Cells and Effect of Cyclosporin A in a Patient With Kimura's Disease," *Br J Dermatol*, 1997, 137(6):972-7.
15. Hershey GK, Friedrich MF, Esswein LA, et al, "The Association of Atopy With a Gain-of-Function Mutation in the Alpha Subunit of the Interleukin-4 Receptor," *N Engl J Med*, 1997, 337(24):1720-5.
16. Rosa-Rosa L, Zimmermann N, Bernstein JA, et al, "The R576 IL-4 Receptor α-Allele Correlates With Asthma Severity," *J Allergy Clin Immunol*, 1999, 104(5):1008-14.
17. Smith JK, Krishnaswamy GH, Dykes R, et al, "Clinical Manifestations of IgE Hypogammaglobulinemia," *Ann Allergy Asthma Immunol*, 1997, 78(3):313-8.
18. Ferguson BJ, "Eosinophilic Mucin Rhinosinusitis: A Distinct Clinicopathological Entity," *Laryngoscope*, 2000, 110(5 Pt 1):799-813.
19. Seroogy CM, Wara DW, Bluth MH, et al, "Cytokine Profile of a Long-Term Pediatric HIV Survivor With Hyper-IgE Syndrome and a Normal CD4 T-Cell Count," *J Allergy Clin Immunol*, 1999, 104(5):1045-51.
20. Kairemo KJ, Lindberg M and Prytz M, "IgE Myeloma: A Case Presentation and a Review of the Literature," *Scand J Clin Lab Invest*, 1999, 59(6):451-6.

References

Buckley RH, "Disorders of the IgE System," *Immunologic Disorders in Infants and Children*, 4th ed, Chapter 13, Stiehm ER, ed, Philadelphia PA: WB Saunders Co, 1996, 409-22.

Hamilton RG and Adkinson NF Jr, "Immunological Tests for Diagnosis and Management of Human Allergic Disease: Total and Allergen-Specific IgE and Allergen-Specific IgG," Section N, Allergic Diseases, Hamilton RG, section ed, *Manual of Clinical Laboratory Immunology*, 5th ed, Chapter 109, deMacario EC, volume ed, Washington, DC: ASM Press, American Society of Microbiology, 1997, 881-92.

Jensen EJ, Dahl R, and Steffensen F, "Bronchial Reactivity to Cigarette Smoke; Relation to Lung Function, Respiratory Symptoms, Serum-Immunoglobulin E and Blood Eosinophil and Leukocyte Counts," *Respir Med*, 2000, 94(2):119-27.

Katz MF and Beer DJ, "T lymphocytes and Cytokine Networks in Asthma: Clinical and Therapeutic Implications," *Adv Intern Medicine*, 1993, 38:189-222.

Marsh DG, Neely JD, Breazeale DR, et al, "Linkage Analysis of IL4 and Other Chromosome 5q31.1 Markers and Total Serum Immunoglobulin E Concentrations," *Science*, 1994, 264(5162):1152-6.

Milgrom H, Fick RB, Su JQ, et al, "Treatment of Allergic Asthma With Monoclonal Anti-IgE Antibody," *N Engl J Med*, 1999, 341(26):1966-73.

Mosmann TR and Coffman RL, "TH1 and TH2 Cells: Different Patterns of Lymphokine Secretion Lead to Different Functional Properties," *Annu Rev Immunol*, 1989, 7:145-73.

Ownby DR, "Allergy Testing: *In Vivo* Versus *In Vitro*," *Pediatr Clin North Am*, 1988, 35(5):995-1009.

Sherrill DL, Stein R, Halonen M, et al, "Total Serum IgE and its Association With Asthma Symptoms and Allergic Sensitization Among Children," *J Allergy Clin Immunol*, 1999, 104(1):28-36.

Van Arsdel PP Jr and Larson EB, "Diagnostic Tests for Patients With Suspected Allergic Disease," *Ann Intern Med*, 1989, 110(4):304-12.

Williams PB, Dolen WK, Koepke JW, "Comparison of Skin Testing and Three *In Vitro* Assays for Specific IgE in the Clinical Evaluation of Immediate Hypersensitivity," *Ann Allergy*, 1992, 68(1):35-45.

Wiltshire S, O'Malley S, Lambert J, et al, "Detection of Multiple Allergen-Specific IgEs on Microarrays by Immunoassay With Rolling Circle Amplification," *Clin Chem*, 2000, 46(12):1990-3.

Immunoglobulin G

Related Information

Immunofixation Electrophoresis, Serum or Urine *on page 530*
Immunoglobulin D *on page 532*
Immunoglobulin G Subclasses *on page 536*
Protein Electrophoresis, Capillary Zone *on page 266*
Protein Electrophoresis, Serum *on page 267*
Protein Electrophoresis, Urine *on page 268*
Protein, Total, Serum *on page 269*

Synonyms IgG, Quantitative

Abstract There are five major types of immunoglobulins classified on the basis of their heavy chain: IgG, IgM, IgA, IgE, and IgD. IgG is present in plasma in the highest concentration. Elevation of all immunoglobulin classes (polyclonal gammopathy) is seen in chronic inflammatory and auto-immune diseases. An increase of a single immunoglobulin (monoclonal gammopathy) may be associated with a benign condition or a malignancy such as plasma cell myeloma or lymphoma. In these latter conditions, other immunoglobulins may be suppressed. Reduced immunoglobulins are seen in various immune deficiency states.

Specimen Serum

Container Red top tube

Storage Instructions Serum specimens may be kept up to 5 days at 2°C to 8°C. For longer period of time prior to analysis freeze samples at temperature of -20°C or less. Do not refreeze thawed specimens.

Samples suspected of having macroglobulins or cryoglobulins should be drawn and held at 37°C. Samples suspected of containing cold agglutinins should not be refrigerated prior to separation of serum from the clot.

Special Instructions Requisition must provide patient's age.

Reference Interval Ranges are individual method and laboratory dependent.
Pediatrics[1]: See table.
Adults: 564-1765 mg/dL

Age	Male (mg/dL)	Female mg/dL
1-30 d	260-986	221-1031
31-182 d	195-643	390-794
183-365 d	184-974	407-774
1-3 y	507-1305	550-1407
4-6 y	571-1550	675-1540
7-9 y	700-1680	589-1717
10-12 y	818-1885	705-1871
13-15 y	709-1861	891-1907

Possible Panic Range Very high levels of immunoglobulin (as occur in some cases of multiple myeloma) may be associated with hyperviscosity and/or hypercalcemia and represent a medical emergency.

Use Quantitate IgG in patient's serum to evaluate humoral immunity; establish diagnosis and monitor therapy in IgG myeloma; evaluate patients, including especially children and those with lymphoma, with propensity to infections. Detection, evaluation, and follow-up of patients with various immunodeficiency states and for hyper-IgM syndrome (in which IgG is usually decreased). In asymptomatic plasma cell myeloma, monoclonal IgG is usually >3 g/dL.[2]

Limitations If samples containing macroglobulins, cryoglobulins, or cold agglutinins are inappropriately handled (prematurely exposed to cold), false low values may result.

Methodology Rate nephelometry, enzyme immunoassay (EIA), capillary electrophoresis with or without immunosubtraction. Capillary zone electrophoresis measures protein by absorbance (proteins are not stained). The electrophoretograms, while similar to those of high resolution gel electrophoresis, are slightly more sensitive. If an M-protein is identified, immunotyping can be performed by immunosubtraction. In this relatively new procedure, the serum is incubated with anti-γ, α, μ, kappa, or lambda conjugated sepharose beads after which the supernatants are studied (again by capillary electrophoresis) to determine which reagent(s) removed the abnormal protein.[3] The immunosubtraction procedure is not technically difficult as it is automated.

Additional Information Immunoglobulin G is the major antibody containing protein fraction of blood. There are four subtypes, of which IgG$_1$ and IgG$_2$ comprise 85% of the total.

The four subclasses of IgG differ in the constant regions of their heavy chains. A patient may have a normal total IgG yet still have a significant decrease in one subclass. IgG$_1$ deficiencies are associated with EBV infections, IgG$_2$ with sinorespiratory infections and infections with encapsulated bacteria, IgG$_3$ with sinusitis and otitis media, and IgG$_4$ with allergies, ataxia telangiectasia, and sinorespiratory infections.

With significant decreases in IgG level, on either a congenital or acquired basis, there is an increased susceptibility to infectious processes ordinarily
(Continued)

Immunoglobulin G *(Continued)*

dealt with by humoral antibody (ie, bacterial infection). Thus, patients with repeated infection should have their immunoglobulins, and specifically IgG, measured. Therapy with exogenous gamma globulins may be efficacious in such patients.

Conversely, IgG levels will be increased in immunocompetent individuals responding to a wide variety of infections or inflammatory insults (indeed, this represents the basis of the serologic diagnosis of infectious diseases). Today, a major cause for a polyclonal increase in IgG is the acquired immunodeficiency syndrome.

Oligoclonal IgG can occur in multiple sclerosis and in some cases of chronic hepatitis, in particular those with features of autoimmune hepatitis in which hypergammaglobulinemia (increased IgG) occurs.[4]

Monoclonal IgG can be demonstrated in ~60% of cases of multiple myeloma. 3 g/dL of monoclonal IgG is a major diagnostic criterion for myeloma. A monoclonal gammopathy may be present when the total IgG value is in the normal range. While many of these patients do not have multiple myeloma, evaluation for such gammopathy and the presence of Bence Jones protein in urine is important. The differential diagnosis of myeloma includes essential monoclonal gammopathy (monoclonal gammopathy of undetermined significance, "MGUS"), which is characterized by lack of symptoms, lack of anemia, lack of bone lesions, monoclonal gammopathy with M component <3.5 g/dL IgG or <2.5 g/dL IgA and marrow plasma cells <10%.

Guidelines for the evaluation of monoclonal gammopathy have been developed by the College of American Pathologists (conference XXXII).[5] The initial study, obtained on all patients with clinical suspicion of a plasma cell dyscrasia, is high resolution electrophoresis of serum/urine. Use of low resolution electrophoretic procedures is discouraged. Immunofixation is recommended to define the abnormal protein, use of the less sensitive immunoelectrophoresis is discouraged. With suspicion of a plasma cell dyscrasia, immunofixation with kappa and lambda light chain antisera is recommended for detection of small M-proteins. Nephelometry is recommended to establish the levels (on initially substantiating the presence of a plasma cell dyscrasia) of immunoglobulins. Use of radial immunodiffusion is discouraged. Additional guidance is provided including evaluation/therapy of the hyperviscosity syndrome and cryoglobulinemia.[5]

A recommended sequence for utilization of serum and urine assays has also been published by the College of American Pathologists as a part of Conference XXXII, see flowchart.[3]

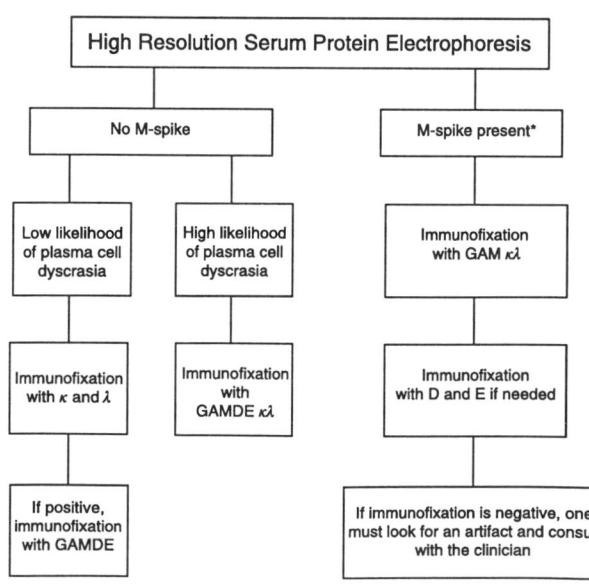

If the M-spike is >1.5 g/dL (15 g/L), a 24-hour urine specimen should be collected for electrophoresis and immunofixation. If the M-spike is >1.5 g/dL (15 g/L), nephelometric measurement of immunoglobulin (Ig) G, IgA, and IgM is indicated.

Adapted from Kyle RA, "Sequence of Testing for Monoclonal Gammopathies: Serum and Urine Assays," *Arch Pathol Lab Med*, 1999,123(2):114-8

Reduction of IgG, usually <300 mg/dL, with normal or increased IgM and IgD levels (the hyper-IgM syndrome), leads to susceptibility to pyogenic and opportunistic (including *P. carinii*, candidal, and mycobacterial) infections. This condition is inherited as X-linked (X-HIM) or autosomal recessive and is due to failure of activated T lymphocytes to express CD40 ligand that binds CD40 on B cells signaling them to proliferate, form lymphoid follicle germinal centers, and develop into memory B cells[6] (see Immunoglobulin M *on page 537*).

Footnotes

1. Soldin SJ, Bailey J, Beatey J, et al, "Pediatric Reference Ranges for Immunoglobulins G, A, and M on the Behring Nephelometer," *Clin Chem*, 1996, 42(S1):308.
2. Weber DM, Dimopoulos MA, Moulopoulos LA, et al, "Prognostic Features of Asymptomatic Multiple Myeloma," *Br J Haematol*, 1997, 97(4):810-4.
3. Kyle RA, "Sequence of Testing for Monoclonal Gammopathies: Serum and Urine Assays," *Arch Pathol Lab Med*, 1999, 123(2):114-8.
4. Krawitt EL, "Autoimmune Hepatitis," *N Engl J Med*, 1996, 334(14):897-903.
5. Keren D, Alexanian R, Goeken JA, et al, "Guidelines for Clinical and Laboratory Evaluation of Patients With Monoclonal Gammopathies," *Arch Pathol Lab Med*, 1999, 123(2):106-7.
6. Levy J, Espanol-Boren T, Thomas C, et al, "Clinical Spectrum of X-Linked Hyper-IgM Syndrome," *J Pediatr*, 1997, 131(1):47-54.

References

Barlogie B, "Plasma Cell Myeloma," *Williams Hematology*, 5th ed, Chapter 114, Beutler E, Lichtman MA, Coller S, et al, eds, New York, NY: McGraw-Hill Inc, 1995, 1109-26.

Jacobson DL, McCutchan JA, Spechko PL, et al, "The Evolution of Lymphadenopathy and Hypergammaglobulinemia Are Evidence for Early and Sustained Polyclonal B Lymphocyte Activation During Human Immunodeficiency Virus Infection," *J Infect Dis*, 1991, 163(2):240-6.

Tricot G, "Multiple Myeloma and Other Plasma Cell Disorders," *Hematology: Basic Principles and Practice*, 3rd ed, Chapter 76, Hoffman R, Benz EJ Jr, Shattil SJ, et al, eds, Philadelphia, PA: Churchill Livingstone, 2000, 1398-1416.

♦ **Immunoglobulin G, Cerebrospinal Fluid** *see* Cerebrospinal Fluid Immunoglobulin G *on page 515*

Immunoglobulin G Subclasses

Related Information
    Immunofixation Electrophoresis, Serum or Urine *on page 530*
    Immunoglobulin A *on page 532*
    Immunoglobulin G *on page 535*
    Protein, Total, Serum *on page 269*

Synonyms IgG Subclasses

Applies to IgG_1; IgG_2; IgG_3; IgG_4

Abstract Approximately 80% of total serum immunoglobulin (Ig) in adults is IgG, which is divided into four subclasses on the basis of structural differences in the hinge region. IgG_3 and IgG_1 are closely related, as are IgG_2 and IgG_4. Impaired synthesis or abnormal loss may cause deficiencies of one or more immunoglobulin subclasses. Selective IgG subclass deficiencies can occur in spite of a normal total IgG level.

Specimen Serum

Container Red top tube or SST™ tube

Storage Instructions Store at 4°C.

Reference Interval IgG_1 is 65%, IgG_2 is 25%, IgG_3 is 6%, and IgG_4 is some 4% of total immunoglobulin G. See tables.

IgG Subclass Levels (mg/dL)

Age	IgG_1	IgG_2	IgG_3	IgG_4
0-1 y	190-620	30-140	9-62	6-63
1-2 y	230-710	30-170	11-98	4-43
2-3 y	280-830	40-240	6-130	3-120
3-6 y	350-810	50-310	9-160	5-180
>6 y	270-1740	30-630	13-320	11-620

Characteristics of IgG Subclasses

Subtype	1	2	3	4
% of total IgG	66	22	8	4
Complement fixation	+	±	++	–
Macrophage FcR binding	++	±	++	+
Crosses placenta	+	±	+	+
Anti-Ig abs (rheumatoid factors)	+	+	–	+
Aggregation with hyperviscosity	–	–	++	–
Retention in sera of patients with generalized hypogammaglobulinemia	–	–	+	–
Average 1/2 life of circulating subtype	21 d	21 d	7-8 d	21 d

Use Study of patients with recurrent bacterial infections. Selective deficiencies may be found among the subclasses in some individuals who suffer repeated infections, especially IgG_1.

Methodology Nephelometry, radial immunodiffusion (RID), enzyme-linked immunosorbent assay (ELISA)

Additional Information IgG antibody responses to certain antigens occur to a greater extent in one type of IgG subclass than another. Therefore, some patients with normal total IgG levels may have problems with pyogenic infections because they do not produce IgG_2 or combinations of IgG_2, IgG_3, and/or IgG_4. IgG_2-deficient patients usually have recurrent respiratory infections. Rarely, severe neutropenia with marrow T-lymphocyte infiltrate (apparently benign) has been noted.[1] Some 120 cases of selective IgG_1-deficient patients have been reported from France. Infections, largely mild to moderate, were predominantly sinorespiratory and caused by the encapsulated bacteria *Pneumococcus* and *Haemophilus*.[2] Some clinically significant IgG subclass deficiencies occur in patients who have IgA deficiency. IgA and IgG$_2$/IgG$_4$ subclass deficiency have been reported with phenytoin therapy.[3] Some 5% of epileptic patients maintained on phenytoin develop an IgA deficiency. Combined IgA and IgG$_2$ deficiency in association with zonisamide therapy has been noted.[4]

Footnotes

1. Lassoued K, Oksenhendler E, Lambin JP, et al, "Severe Neutropenia Associated With IgG$_2$ Subclass Deficiency and Bone Marrow T-Lymphocyte Infiltration," *Am J Hematol*, 1998, 57(3):241-4.
2. Lacombe C, Aucouturier P, Preudhomme JL, "Selective IgG$_1$ Deficiency," *Clin Immunol Immunopathol*, 1997, 84(2):194-201.
3. Ishizaka A, Nakanishi M, Kasahara E, et al, "Phenytoin-Induced IgG$_2$ and IgG$_4$ Deficiencies in a Patient With Epilepsy," *Acta Paediatr*, 1992, 81(8):646-8.
4. Maeoka Y, Hara T, Dejima S, et al, "IgA and IgG$_2$ Deficiency Associated With Zonisamide Therapy: A Case Report," *Epilepsia*, 1997, 38(5):611-3.

References

Check IJ and Papadea C, "Immunoglobulin Quantitation," Immunoglobulin Methods, Kyle RA, section ed, *Manual of Clinical Laboratory Immunology*, Section C, Chapter 14, Nakamura RM, volume ed, Washington, DC: ASM Press, American Society for Microbiology, 1997, 134-46.

Ekdahl K, Braconier JH, and Svanborg C, "Impaired Antibody Response to Pneumococcal Capsular Polysaccharides and Phosphorylcholine in Adult Patients With a History of Bacteremic Pneumococcal Infection," *Clin Infect Dis*, 1997, 25(3):654-60.

Keren DF and Warren JS, *Diagnostic Immunology*, Baltimore, MD: Lippincott Williams & Wilkins, 1992, 109-10.

Kondo N, Inoue R, Kasahara K, et al, "Reduced Expression of the Interferon-Gamma Messenger RNA in IgG$_2$ Deficiency," *Scand J Immunol*, 1997, 45(2):227-30.

Paraskevas F, "Cell Interactions in the Immune Response," *Wintrobe's Clinical Hematology*, 10th ed, Chapter 21, Lee RG, Foerster J, Lukes J, et al, eds, Baltimore MD: Williams and Wilkins, 1999, 544-614.

Shield JP, Strobel S, Levinsky RJ, et al, "Immunodeficiency Presenting as Hypergammaglobulinemia With IgG$_2$ Subclass Deficiency," *Lancet*, 1992, 340(8817):448-50.

Immunoglobulin M

Related Information

Antimitochondrial Antibody *on page 505*
Cold Agglutinin Titer *on page 594*
Cryoglobulin, Qualitative, Serum and Plasma *on page 524*
Immunofixation Electrophoresis, Serum or Urine *on page 530*
Protein Electrophoresis, Capillary Zone *on page 266*
Protein Electrophoresis, Serum *on page 267*
Protein, Total, Serum *on page 269*
Rheumatoid Factor, Serum or Body Fluid *on page 541*
Viscosity, Blood *on page 494*

Synonyms IgM, Quantitative

Applies to Hyperimmunoglobulin M Syndrome

Replaces Macroglobulins, Ultracentrifuge Determination

Abstract With a large molecular mass, about 900 daltons, the distribution of IgM is essentially limited to the vascular compartment.[1] IgM composes 5% to 10% of immunoglobulins. IgM molecules are clinically important as rheumatoid factors, cold agglutinins and as isoagglutinins.

IgM synthesis against intravascular antigens includes that against parasites and red cell surface antigens. It is a complement activator.

Specimen Serum, cerebrospinal fluid

Container Red top tube or SST™ tube, sterile CSF tube

Storage Instructions Samples suspected of having macroglobulins or cryoglobulins should be drawn and held at 37°C. Samples suspected of containing cold agglutinins should not be refrigerated prior to serum separation from clot.

Reference Interval

Pediatrics[2]: See table.
Adults: 53-375 mg/dL

Age	Male (mg/dL)	Female (mg/dL)
1-30 d	12-117	19-104
31-182 d	27-147	9-212
183-365 d	41-197	4-216
1-3 y	63-240	70-298
4-6 y	64-248	81-298
7-9 y	49-231	62-270
10-12 y	58-249	81-340
13-15 y	57-298	69-361
16-18 y	59-291	86-360

Use Evaluate humoral immunity; establish the diagnosis and monitor therapy in macroglobulinemia of Waldenström and other lymphoid and lymphoplasmacytic neoplasms. Differential diagnosis includes plasma cell myeloma (the rare IgM myeloma), essential macroglobulinemia, and other entities. Like IgG and IgA, IgM increase can present as a monoclonal gammopathy.

IgM is increased in primary biliary cirrhosis with high concentrations of serum alkaline phosphatase and with antimitochondrial antibodies.[3]

IgM levels are used to evaluate likelihood of *in utero* infections or acuteness of infection. IgM deficiency is associated especially with gram-negative infections.

Limitations If samples containing macroglobulins, cryoglobulins, or cold agglutinins are handled at incorrect temperatures, false low values may result.

Methodology Rate nephelometry, immunofixation

Additional Information Immunoglobulin M is a pentamer of 7S gamma globulin, and is an efficient complement binder. It is the antibody type produced initially in the immune response and the first immunoglobulin class to be synthesized by a fetus or newborn. IgM antibodies do not cross the placenta. For these reasons the demonstration of IgM-specific antibody is useful in assessing whether a particular infection is acute (in which case IgM antibodies will be present) or chronic (IgG antibodies will predominate) and whether a newborn has a congenital infection (a newborn with IgM antibody is infected; a newborn with IgG antibody has passively acquired maternal antibody, which crossed the placenta).

In the hyper-IgM combined primary immunodeficiency syndrome, there is an absence or low levels of IgG, IgA, and IgE in serum and a marked increase in IgM with neutropenia. Patients with the syndrome develop serious pyogenic infections in which the pathogens are encapsulated bacteria, and intracellular organisms including *Pneumocystis carinii*, *Cryptosporidium parvum*, and *Leishmania*.[4] Macroglobulins produced in Waldenström's disease are IgM, and may produce hyperviscosity syndrome. In contrast, monoclonal IgG or IgA are found in most cases of myeloma. Increased IgM (with other immunoglobulins) may develop in inflammatory/infectious conditions. The majority of rheumatoid factors are IgM. IgM is decreased in congenital or acquired hypogammaglobulinemia, associated with increased, recurrent infection. In patients with bacterial meningitis, CSF IgM is usually elevated along with C-reactive protein.

In macroglobulinemia of Waldenström, weight loss and epistaxis are found, in contrast to essential macroglobulinemia. In the former, hepatosplenomegaly, purpura, and lymphadenopathy occur; IgM is >3 g/dL; and anemia and hyperviscosity are seen.[5]

Footnotes

1. Rich RR, "Human Immune Response," *Internal Medicine*, 5th ed, Chapter 171, Stein JH, ed, St Louis, MO: CV Mosby, 1998, 1108-15.
2. Soldin SJ, Bailey J, Beatey J, et al, "Pediatric Reference Ranges for Immunoglobulins G, A, and M on the Behring Nephelometer," *Clin Chem*, 1996, 42(S1):308.
3. Kaplan MM, "Primary Biliary Cirrhosis," *N Engl J Med*, 1996, 335(21):1570-80.
4. Hadzic N, Pagliuca A, Rela M, et al, "Correction of the Hyper-IgM Syndrome After Liver and Bone Marrow Transplantation," *N Engl J Med*, 2000, 342(5):320-4.
5. Foerster J, "Waldenström Macroglobulinemia," *Wintrobe's Clinical Hematology*, 10th ed, Chapter 100, Lee GR, Foerster J, Lukens J, et al, eds, Baltimore, MD: Lippincott Williams & Wilkins, 1999, 2681-92.

References

Gougeon ML, Morelet L, Doussau M, et al, "Hyper-IgM Immunodeficiency Syndrome: Influence of Lymphokines on *In Vitro* Maturation of Peripheral B Cells," *J Clin Immunol*, 1992, 12(2):92-100.

Jones RG, Aguzzi F, Bienvenu J, et al, "Use of Immunoglobulin Heavy-Chain and Light-Chain Measurements in a Multicenter Trial to Investigate Monoclonal Components: I. Detection," *Clin Chem*, 1991, 37(11):1917-21.

Reddy PS and Corley RB, "The Contribution of ER Quality Control to the Biologic Functions of Secretory IgM," *Immunol Today*, 1999, 20(12):582-8.

Ribeiro MA, Kimura RT, Irulegui I, et al, "Cerebrospinal Fluid Levels of Lysozyme, IgM, and C-Reactive Protein in the Identification of Bacterial Meningitis," *J Trop Med Hyg*, 1992, 95(2):87-94.

Ropper AH and Gorson KC, "Neuropathies Associated With Paraproteinemia," *N Engl J Med*, 1998, 338(22):1601-7.

♦ **Intrinsic Factor Autoantibodies** *see* Parietal Cell Antibody *on page 541*

Intrinsic Factor Blocking Antibody

Related Information

Anemia Flowchart *on page 392*
Cobalamin, Serum *on page 150*
Folic Acid, Serum *on page 435*
Gastric Analysis *on page 180*
Helicobacter pylori Biopsy-Based Tests: The Urease Tests, Culture, Cytology, and PCR *on page 620*
Homocyst(e)ine, Plasma *on page 193*
Methylmalonic Acid, Serum, Plasma, Urine, or Amniotic Fluid *on page 224*
Parietal Cell Antibody *on page 541*
Schilling Test *on page 483*
Vitamin B$_{12}$ Unsaturated Binding Capacity *on page 495*

Synonyms IF Antibody

Abstract A glycoprotein, intrinsic factor (IF), is generated in gastric parietal cells. It tightly binds cyanocobalamin (vitamin B$_{12}$) and facilitates its absorption. About 50% of patients with pernicious anemia (PA) develop antibodies to intrinsic factor. Secretion of IF parallels that of gastric HCl.

Patient Preparation Avoid recent radioactive scan, B$_{12}$ injection within the past week.

Specimen Serum

Container Red top tube or SST™ tube

(Continued)

Intrinsic Factor Blocking Antibody (Continued)

Reference Interval None detected

Use Differentiate pernicious anemia (PA) from other megaloblastic anemias; investigate patients with low vitamin B_{12} levels

Limitations Negative results do not rule out PA.

Methodology Radioimmunoassay (RIA), enzyme-linked immunosorbent assay (ELISA)

Additional Information Pernicious anemia is the most common cause of cobalamin (vitamin B_{12}) deficiency and is associated with antibodies to gastric parietal cells and with anti-intrinsic factor autoantibodies. Two types of antibodies to intrinsic factor have been described. Type 1 antibodies block the binding of cobalamin to intrinsic factor. Type 2 (precipitating antibody) react with the intrinsic factor binding site to ileal receptors. Type 2 antibodies are rarely found in the absence of type 1 antibodies. Fifty percent of patients with pernicious anemia have the type 1 intrinsic factor blocking antibody. About 35% (probably a much greater number) of patients with PA have type II antibodies.[1] Detection of intrinsic factor blocking antibody may be helpful in determination of the cause of a low vitamin B_{12} level. False-positive results are rare; some patients with Graves disease and atrophic gastritis have detectable antibodies.

Although parietal cell antibodies are present in 90% of patients with pernicious anemia, they are less specific than intrinsic factor antibodies.

Footnotes

1. Waters HM, Dawson DW, Howarth JE, et al, "High Incidence of Type II Autoantibodies in Pernicious Anaemia," *J Clin Pathol*, 1993, 46(1):45.

References

Antony AC, "Megaloblastic Anemias," *Hematology: Basic Principles and Practice*, 3rd ed, Chapter 28, Hoffman R, Benz EJ Jr, Shattil SJ, eds, Philadelphia, PA: Churchill Livingstone, 2000, 462-3.

Bunting RW, Bitzer AM, Kenney RM, et al, "Prevalence of Intrinsic Factor Antibodies and Vitamin B_{12} Malabsorption in Older Patients Admitted to a Rehabilitation Hospital," *J Am Geriatr Soc*, 1990, 38(7):743-7.

Galperin C and Gershwin E, "Immunopathogenesis of Gastrointestinal and Hepatobiliary Diseases," *JAMA*, 1997, 278(22):1946-55.

Harty RF and Leibach JR, "Immune Disorders of the Gastrointestinal Tract and Liver," *Med Clin North Am*, 1985, 69(4):675-704.

Jackson BF and Hoffbrand AV, "Investigation of Megaloblastic Anaemia," *Practical Haematology*, 8th ed, Chapter 22, Dacie Sir JV and Lewis SM, New York, NY: Churchill Livingstone, 1995, 430-2.

Islet Cell Antibody

Related Information

Glucose, Postglucose Load, Plasma *on page 185*
Glucose Tolerance Test, Plasma *on page 186*
Glutamic Acid Decarboxylase (GAD65) Antibody *on page 527*
Liver/Kidney Microsomal Type 1 Antibodies *on page 539*

Abstract Islet cell autoantibodies (ICA) were the first markers of islet cell-specific autoimmunity applied to diabetes research. They are detectable in about 80% of patients with new onset type 1 diabetes mellitus. When they occur in high titer in unaffected individuals, they indicate a 40% to 50% risk of developing type 1 diabetes within 5 years.

Specimen Serum

Container Red top tube or SST™ tube of blood

Use Assess risk of developing type 1 diabetes mellitus

Limitations Tremendous variability has existed between laboratories. Not all patients with islet cell antibodies will develop hyperglycemia. The test is often negative at the time of diagnosis in children who develop diabetes before the age of 2 years. The test frequently becomes negative within 2-10 years after the onset of overt disease. This assay is much less sensitive than the assay for glutamic acid decarboxylase antibodies (GAD65).

Methodology Indirect immunofluorescence using fresh frozen human pancreatic tissue

Additional Information ICA can occur in type 2 diabetes.[1] Variability of assays between laboratories has led to confusion in the medical literature about the significance of islet antibodies. This assay should be considered a first generation test for anti-islet cell autoimmunity. However, its usefulness has become debatable following the introduction of the assay for GAD65 antibodies. No GAD65 antibody-negative serum was islet cell antibody positive in a 1998 paper.[2]

Eighty-nine percent of subjects with stiff-man syndrome were detected by ICA, compared to 98% by GAD65.[2]

Many of the citations appended to Glutamic Acid Decarboxylase (GAD65) Antibody *on page 527* address islet cell antibodies as well.

Footnotes

1. Turner R, Stratton I, Horton V, et al, "UKPDS 25: Autoantibodies to Islet-Cell Cytoplasm and Glutamic Acid Decarboxylase for Prediction of Insulin Requirement in Type 2 Diabetes," UK Prospective Diabetes Study Group, *Lancet*, 1997, 350(9087):1288-93.

2. Walikonis JE and Lennon VA, "Radioimmunoassay for Glutamic Acid Decarboxylase (GAD65) Autoantibodies as a Diagnostic Aid for Stiff-Man Syndrome and a Correlate of Susceptibility to Type 1 Diabetes Mellitus," *Mayo Clin Proc*, 1998, 73(12):1161-6.

References

Knip M, Karjalainen J, and Akerblom HK, "Islet Cell Antibodies Are Less Predictive of IDDM Among Unaffected Children in the General Population Than in Sibs of Children With Diabetes," The Childhood Diabetes in Finland Study Group, *Diabetes Care*, 1998, 21(10):1670-3.

Muir A, "Anti-islet Autoantibodies in Diabetes: Clinical Applications," *J Clin Ligan Assay*, 1998, 21:282-92.

♦ **Isotypes, Light Chains** *see* Immunofixation Electrophoresis, Serum or Urine *on page 530*

Jo-1 Antibody

Related Information

Antinuclear Antibody *on page 507*
Muscle Biopsy *on page 69*
Sjögren Antibodies *on page 542*
Topoisomerase I Antibody *on page 546*

Synonyms Antihistidyl Transfer tRNA Synthase

Applies to Antisynthetases

Abstract An autoantibody identifiable in ANA-positive sera, Jo-1 is more common than the other antisynthetases.[1] It is the only myositis-specific antibody presently available for clinical use.[2]

Specimen Serum

Container Red top tube or SST™ tube

Storage Instructions Refrigerate

Reference Interval Negative

Use Marker for idiopathic inflammatory myopathies, including polymyositis and dermatomyositis. Jo-1 antibody is found in ~25% of patients with polymyositis or dermatomyositis, especially those patients in whom disease advances to pulmonary fibrosis.[3]

Methodology Immunoblot assay, polyacrylamide gel electrophoresis

Additional Information Patients with dermatomyositis and polymyositis have inflammatory infiltration and destruction of muscle and other organ systems. Autoantibodies to the antigen, Jo-1, have been associated with pulmonary involvement and arthropathy. The Jo-1 antigen resides on the enzyme, histidyl-tRNA synthetase, which is usually located in the cytoplasm of cells, rather than the nucleus. Antibodies to the Jo-1 antigen are detected in ~25% of adult patients with myositis including polymyositis, dermatomyositis, and overlap syndromes. Jo-1 is detected in polymyositis more frequently than in dermatomyositis.

The enzymes CPK (CK), AST, ALT, and LDH (LD) with isoenzyme LD-5 are useful in evaluation of muscle disease. CK and LD-5 are especially helpful. Electrolytes should be measured in work-up of weakness or myalgia. Some metabolic myopathies can resemble myositis. A broad differential diagnosis exists, which includes dermatomyositis, polymyositis, overlap syndromes, inclusion body myositis, and cancer-associated myositis.[4]

Footnotes

1. Plotz PH, Rider LG, Targoff IN, et al, "Myositis: Immunologic Contributions to Understanding Cause, Pathogenesis, and Therapy," *Ann Intern Med*, 1995, 122(9):715-24.

2. Moder KG, "Use and Interpretation of Rheumatologic Tests: A Guide for Clinicians," *Mayo Clin Proc*, 1996, 71(4):391-6.

3. Lazarus DS and Mark EJ, "A 46-Year-Old Woman With Dermatomyositis, Increasing Pulmonary Insufficiency, and Terminal Right Ventricular Failure," Case Records of the Massachusetts General Hospital, Case 24-1995, Scully RE, Mark, EJ, McNealy WF, et al, eds, *N Engl J Med*, 1995, 333(6):369-77.

4. Smith DR and Weiner HL, "Immunologic Aspects of Neurologic and Neuromuscular Diseases," *JAMA*, 1997, 278(22):1956-61.

References

Homburger HA, "Cascade Testing for Autoantibodies in Connective Tissue Diseases," *Mayo Clin Proc*, 1995, 70(2):183-4.

♦ **Job Syndrome** *see* Immunoglobulin E *on page 533*

♦ **Kappa Chains** *see* Immunofixation Electrophoresis, Serum or Urine *on page 530*

♦ **Kappa Light Chains, CSF** *see* Cerebrospinal Fluid Immunoglobulin G *on page 515*

♦ **Kimura Disease** *see* Immunoglobulin E *on page 533*

♦ **LA** *see* Anticardiolipin Antibody *on page 503*

♦ **La Antibodies** *see* Sjögren Antibodies *on page 542*

♦ **Lambda Chains** *see* Immunofixation Electrophoresis, Serum or Urine *on page 530*

♦ **Latex Sensitization** *see* Allergen Specific IgE Antibody *on page 502*

♦ **LATS** *see* Thyrotropin Receptor Antibody, Serum *on page 545*

♦ **LE Cell Preparation** *replaced by* Antinuclear Antibody *on page 507*

♦ **Leukocyte Antigens** *see* HLA Typing, Single Human Leukocyte Antigen *on page 529*

♦ **Light Chains** *see* Immunofixation Electrophoresis, Serum or Urine *on page 530*

Liver/Kidney Microsomal Type 1 Antibodies

Related Information

Antimitochondrial Antibody *on page 505*
Bilirubin, Total, Serum *on page 118*
Islet Cell Antibody *on page 538*
Liver Biopsy *on page 65*
Liver Disease: Laboratory Assessment, Overview *on page 216*
Parietal Cell Antibody *on page 541*
Smooth Muscle Antibody *on page 543*
Thyroglobulin Antibody *on page 544*
Thyroperoxidase Autoantibody *on page 545*

Synonyms Antiliver/Kidney Microsomal Antibodies; Anti-LKM1

Applies to Antiliver Cytosol 1 Antibodies; P-45011D6; Soluble Liver Antigen (Anti-SLA)

Abstract Chronic liver diseases include **autoimmune hepatitis** characterized by chronic inflammatory changes and autoantibodies. Three diagnostic categories are recognized. **Type 1** is the classical type, corresponding to the entity lupoid hepatitis described in 1950-1951. Type 1 patients have smooth muscle antibodies and/or ANA reactivity. **Type 2** patients lack those antibodies but are characterized by anti-LKM1 antibodies. **Type 3** have antibodies to soluble liver antigen (SLA) and SMA, but lack anti-LKM1. See the table in Smooth Muscle Antibody *on page 543* for clinical and immunologic features.

Specimen Serum

Container Red top tube or SST™ tube

Reference Interval Negative

Use One of the major immunologic tests for autoimmune liver disease, especially in children. Others include smooth muscle antibody, antimitochondrial antibody, and antinuclear antibody.

Methodology Indirect immunofluorescence

Additional Information A fraction of cases of autoimmune hepatitis, autoimmune hepatitis Types 2a and 2b, are positive for these antibodies. These reactive subsets include a number with related immunologic disorders. Type 2a patients are characterized as well by the presence of antiliver cytosol 1 antibodies.[1] Other immunologic disorders in LKM1-positive patients include thyroiditis, diabetes mellitus, hemolytic anemia, arthritis, and ulcerative colitis. Antithyroid, antiparietal cell, and anti-islet antibodies are common.[2] Low IgA levels in serum are often seen.[3]

Only two of 26 cases of recent onset autoimmune hepatitis were reactive with LKM1, while 22 were reactive with smooth muscle antibodies. Each of the two was reported to have titer of 1:320, and one was negative to smooth muscle antibody.[4]

Patients with type 2a are predominantly children, female, lack HCV, and have higher titers of anti-LKM1. Their serum is often reactive for P-45011D6, which is recognized by the antibody LKM1. Patients classified as type 2b are characterized by seroreactivity to HCV, features of chronic viral disease, and infrequent positivity to P-45011D6.

Footnotes

1. Krawitt EL, "Autoimmune Hepatitis," *N Engl J Med*, 1996, 334(14):897-903.
2. Vinayek R and Rakela J, "Acute and Chronic Viral Hepatitis," *Internal Medicine*, 5th ed, Chapter 355, Stein JH, ed, St Louis, MO: Mosby, 1998, 2172-84.
3. Galperin C and Gershwin ME, "Immunopathogenesis of Gastrointestinal and Hepatobiliary Diseases," *JAMA*, 1997, 278(22):1946-55.
4. Burgart LJ, Batts KP, Ludwig J, et al, "Recent-Onset Autoimmune Hepatitis. Biopsy Findings and Clinical Correlations," *Am J Surg Pathol*, 1995, 19(6):699-708.

♦ **Liver/Kidney Microsomes Antibody** *see* Smooth Muscle Antibody *on page 543*

♦ **LKM Antibody** *see* Smooth Muscle Antibody *on page 543*

♦ **Long-Acting Thyroid Stimulator** *see* Thyrotropin Receptor Antibody, Serum *on page 545*

♦ **Lupus Anticoagulant** *see* Anticardiolipin Antibody *on page 503*

♦ **Lymphocyte Blast Transformation** *see* Lymphocyte Transformation Test *on page 539*

♦ **Lymphocyte CD4 Counts** *see* CD4/CD8 Enumeration *on page 511*

♦ **Lymphocyte Crossmatch** *see* Tissue Typing *on page 546*

♦ **Lymphocyte Mitogen Response Test** *see* Lymphocyte Transformation Test *on page 539*

Lymphocyte Transformation Test

Related Information

Aspergillus Serology *on page 560*
Candidiasis Serology *on page 588*
Cell Cycle Analysis by Flow Cytometry *on page 53*
Fanconi Anemia, Chromosome Breakage Study *on page 365*
Hypersensitivity Pneumonitis Serology *on page 530*
Mixed Lymphocyte Culture *on page 540*

Synonyms Lymphocyte Blast Transformation; Lymphocyte Mitogen Response Test; PHA Stimulation

Applies to Berylliosis; Mitogens; Nezelof Syndrome

Abstract Lymphocyte proliferation normally occurs early in an immune response. Lymphocyte transformation assays test the integrity of the early proliferative response using either nonspecific mitogens or specific antigens to induce blastogenesis. Antigen induced lymphocyte proliferation also correlates with previous exposure and acquisition of cellular immunity.

Specimen Whole blood

Container Yellow top (ACD) tube or green top (heparin) tube. Check with the laboratory performing the assay for special instructions.

Causes for Rejection Old specimen, specimen without viable lymphocytes, specimen refrigerated or frozen

Special Instructions Schedule procedure in advance with laboratory. Specimens to evaluate therapy should include three baseline samples.

Reference Interval Mitogen: phytohemagglutinin (PHA), stimulation index >130; mitogen: pokeweed mitogen (PWM), stimulation index >20; mitogen: concanavalin A (con A), stimulation index >40

Use Detect and classify congenital or acquired immunodeficiency disorders, study the integrity of lymphokine production, monitor immunosuppressive or immunoenhancing therapy. Document cellular hypersensitivity reactions to environmental allergens or antigens. Similar methods are used to predict allograft compatibility in the transplantation setting. See Mixed Lymphocyte Culture *on page 540*.

Methodology Most commonly, lymphocyte transformation is measured by the incorporation of tritiated thymidine into lymphocytes. Lymphocytes are isolated from peripheral blood and set up in microtiter plate cultures for a period of 3-7 days with and without mitogen or antigen. Commonly, cell density and mitogen or antigen concentration are varied to establish a dose-response curve. Approximately 6-18 hours prior to harvest, lymphocytes are pulsed with tritiated thymidine. Incorporated thymidine is measured and a stimulation index calculated based on control values.

Flow cytometric assays have also been developed. In these procedures, measurement of S-phase fraction or incorporation of bromodeoxyuridine correlates with blastogenesis. Multiparameter analysis allows assessment of blastogenic response within lymphocyte subpopulations colabeled with selected monoclonal antibodies.

A number of other immunodiagnostic methods (eg, agarose gel double diffusion, immunoenzymetric (IEMA/ELISA) assays, and Western blot analysis) have been developed to demonstrate serum antibodies to respiratory allergens, notably antibody to *Aspergillus* antigens and to organic dust (see Hypersensitivity Pneumonitis Serology *on page 530*).

Additional Information PHA and con A are potent T-cell mitogens while PWM, lipopolysaccharide and staphylococcal protein A are selective B-cell mitogens. Patients with DiGeorge anomaly, Nezelof syndrome, and severe combined immunodeficiency syndrome typically show selectively impaired blastogenic responses to T-cell mitogens, while patients with pure humoral immunodeficiencies generally are characterized by normal responses. Variable blastogenic responses to B-cell selective mitogens are found in humoral immunodeficiency disorders.

Patients with chronic mucocutaneous candidiasis may show relatively normal mitogenic responses with T- and B-cell selective mitogens but have impaired blastogenesis to *Candida* antigen.

Patients with pulmonary berylliosis show beryllium induced lymphocyte blastogenesis. Evidence suggests that blastogenic responses of lymphocytes isolated from bronchoalveolar washings are more closely related to active lung disease than blastogenesis measured in peripheral blood lymphocytes.[1]

Footnotes

1. Newman LS, Bobka C, Schumacher B, et al, "Compartmentalized Immune Response Reflects Clinical Severity of Beryllium Disease," *Am J Respir Crit Care Med*, 1994, 150(1):135-42.

References

Kurup VP and Fink JN, "Immunological Tests for Evaluation of Hypersensitivity Pneumonitis and Allergic Bronchopulmonary Aspergillosis," Allergic Diseases, Hamilton RG, section ed, de Macario EC, volume ed, *Manual of Clinical Laboratory Immunology*, 5th ed, Chapter 112, Section N, Rose NR, de Macario E, Folds JD, et al, eds, Washington, DC: ASM Press, American Society for Microbiology, 1997, 908-15.

Pacheco SE and Shearer WT, "Laboratory Aspects of Immunology," *Pediatr Clin North Am*, 1994, 41(4):623-55.

Sarma PU, Banerjee B, Bir N, et al, "Immunodiagnosis of Allergic Bronchopulmonary Aspergillosis," *Immunol Allergy Clin North Am*, 1998, 18(3):525-47.

Shearer WT, Paul ME, Smith CW, et al, "Laboratory Assessment of Immune Deficiency Disorders," *Immunol Allergy Clin North Am*, 1994, 14(2):265-99.

♦ **Lymphocytotoxic Antibody Screening** *see* Tissue Typing *on page 546*

♦ **Lymphocytotoxicity Assay** *see* Tissue Typing *on page 546*

♦ **Macroglobulins, Ultracentrifuge Determination** *replaced by* Immunoglobulin M *on page 537*

♦ **Major Histocompatibility Coded Antigens** *see* HLA Typing, Single Human Leukocyte Antigen *on page 529*

♦ **Major Histocompatibility Complex** *see* Tissue Typing *on page 546*

♦ **Major Histocompatibility Complex (MHC)** *see* HLA Typing, Single Human Leukocyte Antigen *on page 529*

♦ **Mannose-Binding Lectin** *see* Complement, Total, Serum or Body Fluid *on page 522*

- **MASP-1** *see* Complement, Total, Serum or Body Fluid *on page 522*

- **MASP-2** *see* Complement, Total, Serum or Body Fluid *on page 522*

- **Membrane Attack Complex** *see* Complement Components, Overview *on page 520*

- **Membrane Cofactor Protein** *see* Complement Components, Overview *on page 520*

- **Membrane Inhibitor of Active Lysis** *see* Complement Components, Overview *on page 520*

- **Methylimidazoleacetic Acid** *see* Histamine, Urine, Plasma, or Whole Blood *on page 528*

- **Mevalonic Acid** *see* Immunoglobulin D *on page 532*

- **MGUS** *see* Immunofixation Electrophoresis, Serum or Urine *on page 530*

- **MHC** *see* HLA Typing, Single Human Leukocyte Antigen *on page 529*

- **MHC** *see* Tissue Typing *on page 546*

- **β$_2$-Microglobulin** *see* Beta$_2$-Microglobulin, Serum or Urine *on page 509*

- ***Micropolyspora faeni* Precipitating Antibodies** *see* Hypersensitivity Pneumonitis Serology *on page 530*

- **Microsomal Antibody, Thyroid** *see* Thyroperoxidase Autoantibody *on page 545*

- **Mitochondrial Antibody** *see* Antimitochondrial Antibody *on page 505*

- **Mitogens** *see* Lymphocyte Transformation Test *on page 539*

Mixed Lymphocyte Culture

Related Information
Flow Cytometry, Overview *on page 432*
HLA Typing, Single Human Leukocyte Antigen *on page 529*
Lymphocyte Transformation Test *on page 539*
Tissue Typing *on page 546*

Synonyms Mixed Lymphocyte Culture Reaction; MLR

Applies to HLA Class II Antigens; HLA-DP; HLA-DQ; HLA-DR; Mononuclear Cells

Test Includes Blood lymphocytes (and some monocytes - dendritic cells) from potential donors and the recipient are cultured together and tested for reactivity against each other.

Abstract Mixed lymphocyte culture (MLC) is used primarily to predict histocompatibility in the transplantation setting. Results of the MLC reaction are determined by the D locus of the human leukocyte antigen (HLA) system. If cells share common D loci, they do not activate one another. If the D loci are different, lymphocyte cell activation occurs.

Specimen Leukocytes

Container Green top (heparin) tubes, usually 20-30 mL of **sterile** heparinized blood

Collection Blood must be delivered to the laboratory immediately.

Storage Instructions Do not refrigerate and do not freeze. Specimen must not be exposed to extremes of heat or cold. Specimen should be processed within 24 hours of collection.

Causes for Rejection Lack of sterile collection, specimen not collected in heparin, specimen without viable lymphocytes, specimen refrigerated or frozen

Turnaround Time The classical MLC reaction includes an incubation period of 4-6 days.

Special Instructions Blood specimen must be collected fresh on day of test. Check with the laboratory performing the assay for special instructions.

Reference Interval Response compared with that of simultaneously evaluated normal control; requires interpretation

Use Tissue matching for transplantation, largely bone marrow transplantation; evaluate cellular immunocompetence

Limitations Test will be negative if donor or responder cells have a severe cellular immunodeficiency. Test depends on viability of lymphocytes. With the advent and use of DNA-based HLA typing methods, MCL is used less for donor selection but can be used to follow the transplant recipients posttransplant donor antigen-specific immune status.

Methodology Lymphocytes from two individuals are typically cocultured to measure unidirectional lymphocyte blastogenesis (lymphocyte activation). Lymphocytes from the allograft donor are typically rendered nonresponsive by treating with mitomycin-C or radiation. Responder lymphocytes are derived from the prospective allograft recipient. After several days in culture, proliferating cells are pulsed with tritiated thymidine approximately 6-18 hours prior to harvest. Therefore, measurement of incorporated thymidine is a function of responder (allograft recipient) lymphocyte blastogenesis. The results may be expressed as a relative response (RR) where:

RR = (cpm test - cpm autologous) / (cpm max - cpm autologous) x 100

cpm = counts per minute

See Lymphocyte Transformation Test *on page 539*. In the setting of bone marrow transplantation when graft versus host response is of concern, lymphocytes from the prospective allograft recipient may be rendered unresponsive in order to measure blastogenesis of donor lymphocytes. Multiparameter flow cytometry and other methods have been developed as

variations of MLC. The procedures are less time consuming and avoid use of radioisotopes.[1,2]

Additional Information MLC measures the ability of CD4 positive lymphocytes to recognize HLA class II antigens encoded by the HLA-DR, DQ, and DP loci. Incompatibility of these antigens are among the most potent of blastogenic stimuli. Unidirectional or bidirectional histocompatibility is reflected by little or no blastogenesis. Prominent blastogenic responses predict tissue incompatibility and poor graft survival. Recent advances in molecular genetic typing has also shown high predictive value and assays for the identification of HLA proteins are being replaced by DNA-based typing methods.

The role of a number of cytokines, costimulatory and modulating molecules upon the MLC are under study.[3,4,5,6]

Footnotes
1. Lavergne JA and del Llano AM, "Assessment of Cellular Activation by Flow Cytometric Methods," *Pathobiology*, 1990, 58(2):107-17.
2. Palutke M, KuKuruga D, and Tabaczka P, "A Flow Cytometric Method for Measuring Lymphocyte Proliferation Directly From Tissue Culture Plates Using Ki-67 and Propidium Iodide," *J Immunol Methods*, 1987, 105(1):97-105.
3. Kohka H, Ivagaki H, Yoshino T, et al, "Involvement of Interleukin-18 (IL-18) in Mixed Lymphocyte Reactions (MLR)," *J Interferon Res*, 1999, 19(9):1053-7.
4. Umemoto M, Azuma E, Hirayama M, et al, "Cytokine-Enhanced Mixed Lymphocyte Reaction (MLR) in Cord Blood," *Clin Exp Immunol*, 1998, 112(3):459-63.
5. Scheinecker C, Machold KP, Majdic O, et al, "Initiation of the Autologous Mixed Lymphocyte Reaction Requires the Expression of Costimulatory Molecules B7-1 and B7-2 on Human Peripheral Blood Dendritic Cells," *J Immunol*, 1998, 161(8):3966-73.
6. Tibbetts SA, Chirathaworn C, Nakashima M, et al, "Peptides Derived From ICAM-1 and LFA-1 Modulate T Cell Adhesion and Immune Function in a Mixed Lymphocyte Culture," *Transplantation*, 1999, 68(5):685-92.

References
Auchincloss H Jr, Sykes M, and Sachs DH, "Transplant Immunology," *Fundamental Immunology*, 4th ed, Chapter 36, Paul WE, ed, Philadelphia, PA: Lippincott-Raven, 1999, 1175-235.
"Human Leukocyte Antigen," *CRC Desk Reference for Hematology*, Shinton NK, ed, Boca Raton, FL: CRC Press, 1998, 346-9.
James SP, "Measurement of Proliferative Responses of Cultured Lymphocytes," *Current Protocols in Immunology*, Volume 2, Section II, Coico R, series ed, John Wiley & Sons, Inc, 1994, National Institutes of Health (1991-1999) Supplement 11, 7.10.1-7.10.10.
Margulies DH, "The Major Histocompatibility Complex," *Fundamental Immunology*, 4th ed, Chapter 8, Paul WE, ed, Philadelphia, PA: Lippincott-Raven, 1999, 263-85.
Reinsmoen NL, "Histocompatibility Testing by Immunologic Methods: Cellular Assays," *Transplantation Immunology and Immunogenetics*, Chapter 138, Section R, Leffell MS, section ed, *Manual of Clinical Laboratory Immunology*, deMacario EC, volume ed, Washington, DC: American Society of Microbiology, 1998, 1080-6.
Riley RS, "Basic Principles of Immunodiagnosis," *Clinical Laboratory Medicine*, Chapter 56, Section X, MrClatchey KD, ed, Baltimore, MD: Lippincott Williams & Wilkins, 1994, 1491-4.

- **Mixed Lymphocyte Culture Reaction** *see* Mixed Lymphocyte Culture *on page 540*

- **MLR** *see* Mixed Lymphocyte Culture *on page 540*

- **Molecular Genetic HLA Typing** *see* Tissue Typing *on page 546*

- **Monoclonal Gammopathy** *see* Immunofixation Electrophoresis, Serum or Urine *on page 530*

- **Mononuclear Cells** *see* Mixed Lymphocyte Culture *on page 540*

- **M Protein** *see* Immunofixation Electrophoresis, Serum or Urine *on page 530*

- **Myelin Basic Protein** *see* Cerebrospinal Fluid Oligoclonal Bands *on page 516*

- **Myeloperoxidase Antibody (MPO-ANCA)** *see* Antineutrophil Cytoplasmic Antibody *on page 507*

- **n-DNA** *see* Anti-DNA *on page 504*

- **Nezelof Syndrome** *see* Lymphocyte Transformation Test *on page 539*

- **nRNP** *see* Smith (Sm) and Ribonucleoprotein (RNP) Antibodies *on page 543*

- **Nuclear Ribonucleoprotein** *see* Smith (Sm) and Ribonucleoprotein (RNP) Antibodies *on page 543*

- **Nucleolar Antibody** *see* Antinuclear Antibody *on page 507*

- **Oligoclonal Bands** *see* Cerebrospinal Fluid Protein Electrophoresis *on page 518*

- **Oligoclonal Bands, Cerebrospinal Fluid** *see* Cerebrospinal Fluid Oligoclonal Bands *on page 516*

- **Oligoclonal Bands, CSF** *see* Cerebrospinal Fluid IgG:Albumin Ratio, IgG Index, and IgG Synthesis Rate *on page 514*

- **Opportunistic Infection** *see* CD4/CD8 Enumeration *on page 511*

- **Optic Neuritis** *see* Cerebrospinal Fluid Oligoclonal Bands *on page 516*

- **Organ Donor Tissue Typing** *see* Tissue Typing *on page 546*

- **Organochlorine Compounds** *see* Immunoglobulin E *on page 533*

- **O-Sialotransferrin** *see* Cerebrospinal Fluid Protein *on page 517*

- **P-45011D6** *see* Liver/Kidney Microsomal Type 1 Antibodies *on page 539*

- **P-ANCA** *see* Antineutrophil Cytoplasmic Antibody *on page 507*

- **Paraprotein Evaluation** *see* Immunofixation Electrophoresis, Serum or Urine *on page 530*

Parietal Cell Antibody

Related Information
Anemia Flowchart *on page 392*
Cobalamin, Serum *on page 150*
Folic Acid, RBC *on page 435*
Folic Acid, Serum *on page 435*
Gastric Analysis *on page 180*
Gastrin, Serum *on page 181*
Glutamic Acid Decarboxylase (GAD65) Antibody *on page 527*
Helicobacter pylori Biopsy-Based Tests: The Urease Tests, Culture, Cytology, and PCR *on page 620*
Intrinsic Factor Blocking Antibody *on page 537*
Liver/Kidney Microsomal Type 1 Antibodies *on page 539*
Methylmalonic Acid, Serum, Plasma, Urine, or Amniotic Fluid *on page 224*
Phosphorus, Urine *on page 253*
Schilling Test *on page 483*
Vitamin B_{12} Unsaturated Binding Capacity *on page 495*

Synonyms Antiparietal Cell Antibody

Applies to Intrinsic Factor Autoantibodies

Test Includes Titers are performed if the test is positive.

Abstract The gastric parietal cell secretes intrinsic factor which combines with ingested vitamin B_{12} to facilitate absorption in the ileum. Parietal cells also secrete hydrochloric acid, blood group substances, transforming growth factors (TGFα), and cathepsin. **Autoimmune gastritis** is characterized by disturbance of parietal cell function, resulting in reduced production of gastric acid. Progressive destruction of fundic glands ultimately leads to atrophic gastritis with achlorhydria and vitamin B_{12} (cobalamin) deficiency (pernicious anemia).[1]

Specimen Serum

Container Red top tube or SST™ tube

Storage Instructions Keep specimen cool.

Reference Interval Negative

Use In classical pernicious anemia with complete gastric atrophy, autoantibodies to parietal cells and to intrinsic factor may be identified. Testing for parietal cell antibody is occasionally used in the differential diagnosis of pernicious anemia, atrophic gastritis, and autoimmune gastritis.

Limitations Parietal cell antibodies are not disease specific, because they are also detectable in 30% to 60% of patients with chronic atrophic gastritis, 20% with gastric ulcers, 30% with Sjogren syndrome, 30% of first-degree relatives of patients with pernicious anemia, and 7% of healthy adults.

Patients with common variable immunodeficiency may develop a pernicious anemia-like disorder in which antibodies to intrinsic factor and to parietal cells are not found.

Methodology Indirect immunofluorescence

Additional Information Parietal cells are histologically distinctive. They are pyramidal with eosinophilic to clear cytoplasm.

Antibodies to parietal cells are present in about 90% of adults with pernicious anemia and in up to 60% of subjects with atrophic gastritis; they do not correlate with malabsorption of vitamin B_{12}. They are also present in occasional patients with gastric ulcer or gastric cancer. There is cross positivity of parietal cell and thyroid antibodies in patients with thyroiditis and pernicious anemia. With time, the titer of parietal cell antibodies will decline in some patients with pernicious anemia (possibly related to loss of parietal cells) whereas intrinsic factor antibodies persist.

Anti-intrinsic factor, as well as antiparietal cell autoantibodies, can be detected with substantial frequency in unaffected family members and in subjects who have other autoimmune disorders.[1]

Footnotes
1. Galperin C and Gershwin E, "Immunopathogenesis of Gastrointestinal and Hepatobiliary Diseases," *JAMA*, 1997, 278(22):1946-55.

References
Burman P, Kampe O, Kraaz W, et al, "A Study of Autoimmune Gastritis in the Postpartum Period and at a 5-Year Follow-up," *Gastroenterology*, 1992, 103(3):934-42.
Davidson RJ, Atrah HI, and Sewell HF, "Longitudinal Study of Circulating Gastric Antibodies in Pernicious Anemia," *J Clin Pathol*, 1989, 42(10):1092-5.
Harty RF and Leibach JR, "Immune Disorders of the Gastrointestinal Tract and Liver," *Med Clin North Am*, 1985, 69(4):675-704.

- **PCA-1** *see* Antineuronal Nuclear Antibody, Type 1 (Anti-Hu) *on page 506*

- **PCA-2** *see* Antineuronal Nuclear Antibody, Type 1 (Anti-Hu) *on page 506*

- **PCA-Tr** *see* Antineuronal Nuclear Antibody, Type 1 (Anti-Hu) *on page 506*

Pemphigus-Like Antibodies

Related Information
Skin Biopsy, Immunofluorescence *on page 72*
Viral Culture *on page 689*

Applies to Desmoglein 1

Abstract Patients with pemphigus vulgaris, bullous pemphigoid, paraneoplastic pemphigus, epidermolysis bullosa acquisita have autoantibodies directed against epidermal components.[1,2] *In vitro* testing for these antibodies has been available, but sensitivity and specificity have been poor. Contemporary practice focuses on identification of these autoantibodies by skin biopsy direct immunofluorescence (see Skin Biopsy, Immunofluorescence *on page 72*).

Methodology Enzyme-linked immunosorbent assay (ELISA) for desmoglein 1 antibodies,[3] indirect immunofluorescence on skin sections for desmoglein 1 and 3[4]

Additional Information Autoantibodies against desmoglein 1 are found in serum of patients with endemic pemphigus foliaceus (fogo selvagem) and in some normal individuals in an area of Brazil in which this disease is endemic.[3]

Footnotes
1. Leung DYM, Diaz LA, DeLeo V, et al, "Allergic and Immunologic Skin Disorders," *JAMA*, 1997, 278(22):1914-23.
2. Edelson RL, "Pemphigus-Decoding the Cellular Language of Cutaneous Autoimmunity," *N Engl J Med*, 2000, 343(1):60-1.
3. Warren SJ, Lin MS, Giudice GJ, et al, "The Prevalence of Antibodies Against Desmoglein 1 in Endemic Pemphigus Foliaceus in Brazil," *N Engl J Med*, 2000, 343(1):23-30.
4. Wu H, Wang ZH, Yan A, et al, "Protection Against Pemphigus Foliaceus by Desmoglein 3 in Neonates," *N Engl J Med*, 2000, 343(1):31-5.

- **Perforin-Mediated Cytotoxicity** *see* CD4/CD8 Enumeration *on page 511*

- **PFAPA Syndrome** *see* Immunoglobulin D *on page 532*

- **Phadenzyme RAST®** *see* Allergen Specific IgE Antibody *on page 502*

- **Pharmacia CAP** *see* Allergen Specific IgE Antibody *on page 502*

- **PHA Stimulation** *see* Lymphocyte Transformation Test *on page 539*

- **Plasma β-Amyloid$_{(1-42)}$** *see* Cerebrospinal Fluid and Plasma β-Amyloid$_{(1-42)}$ *on page 513*

- **POEMS Syndrome** *see* Cerebrospinal Fluid Protein *on page 517*

- **POEMS Syndrome** *see* Immunofixation Electrophoresis, Serum or Urine *on page 530*

- **Prealbumin, CSF** *see* Cerebrospinal Fluid Protein *on page 517*

- **Presenilin** *see* Cerebrospinal Fluid and Plasma β-Amyloid$_{(1-42)}$ *on page 513*

- **Progressive Systemic Sclerosis Antibody** *see* Topoisomerase I Antibody *on page 546*

- **Properdin** *see* Complement Components, Overview *on page 520*

- **Prostigmin® Test** *see* Acetylcholine Receptor Antibody *on page 502*

- **Proteinase 3 (PR3)** *see* Antineutrophil Cytoplasmic Antibody *on page 507*

- **14-3-3 Protein Assay** *see* Cerebrospinal Fluid and Plasma β-Amyloid$_{(1-42)}$ *on page 513*

- **Protein, Cerebrospinal Fluid** *see* Cerebrospinal Fluid Protein *on page 517*

- **Protein Electrophoresis, Spinal Fluid** *see* Cerebrospinal Fluid Protein Electrophoresis *on page 518*

- **Pseudoparaprotein** *see* Immunofixation Electrophoresis, Serum or Urine *on page 530*

- **Radioallergosorbent Test (RAST®)** *see* Allergen Specific IgE Antibody *on page 502*

- **Rapid Nerve Stimulation Test** *see* Acetylcholine Receptor Antibody *on page 502*

- **RAST®** *see* Allergen Specific IgE Antibody *on page 502*

- **Receptor Blocking Antibody** *see* Acetylcholine Receptor Antibody *on page 502*

- **Receptor Modulating Antibody** *see* Acetylcholine Receptor Antibody *on page 502*

- **Retinopathy** *see* Anticardiolipin Antibody *on page 503*

- **RF** *see* Rheumatoid Factor, Serum or Body Fluid *on page 541*

Rheumatoid Factor, Serum or Body Fluid

Related Information
Antinuclear Antibody *on page 507*
Body Fluid Chemical Analysis *on page 123*
(Continued)

Rheumatoid Factor, Serum or Body Fluid
(Continued)

Body Fluid Glucose *on page 124*
Body Fluid pH *on page 125*
C-Reactive Protein, Serum *on page 523*
Cryoglobulin, Qualitative, Serum and Plasma *on page 524*
HLA-B27 *on page 528*
HLA Typing, Single Human Leukocyte Antigen *on page 529*
Immunoglobulin M *on page 537*
Sedimentation Rate, Erythrocyte *on page 484*
Synovial Fluid Analysis *on page 323*

Synonyms RF

Applies to Rheumatoid Factor, Synovial Fluid

Replaces Rose-Waaler Test; Singer-Plotz Test

Abstract Rheumatoid arthritis (RA) and juvenile RA are clinical syndromes diagnosed by specific criteria.[1,2] Rheumatoid factor (RF) is an antibody (usually of the IgM class) which reacts with the Fc region of other immunoglobulins (often, but not always, of the IgG class).

Specimen Serum, body fluid

Container Red top or SST™ tube

Reference Interval There are wide interlaboratory differences, some of which are method dependent. One reference laboratory using rate nephelometry has these ranges for adults:[3]
- nonreactive: 0-39 IU/mL
- weakly reactive: 40-79 IU/mL
- reactive: >79 IU/mL

Use

Diagnosis: Approximately 65% to 85% of adult patients with the clinical diagnosis of RA have serologic evidence of RF. Unfortunately, positive serologic results are found in a number of other conditions, including clinically normal persons (see Limitations).

Disease activity monitoring: Serial RF measurements have **not** been useful in monitoring the course of RA. Better tests for this purpose include: C-Reactive Protein, Serum *on page 523* and Sedimentation Rate, Erythrocyte *on page 484*.

Limitations Approximately 3% of the general population has low level RF. The prevalence increases with age, up to 20% in persons older than 65 years old. Only 5% of healthy individuals with a positive RF test will eventually develop rheumatoid arthritis. In higher risk populations, such as first-degree relatives of multicase families, a positive RF test is associated with a much greater risk of developing rheumatoid arthritis. The higher the RF levels, the greater the risk of disease. A long latent period of 4 or more years may occur between detection of RF and development of disease.

A positive RF test is not specific for rheumatoid arthritis. High levels of RF are present in the majority of patients with Sjögren syndrome and essential mixed cryoglobulinemia. RF is present in low titers in other connective tissue diseases, and in a variety of chronic infections and inflammatory disorders. They include subacute bacterial endocarditis, tuberculosis, liver disease, and idiopathic pulmonary fibrosis. Many of these conditions are associated with hypergammaglobulinemia and intense stimulation of the immune system. The specificity of RF for rheumatoid arthritis increases when the RF test is repeatedly positive and present in high titer.

Other laboratory studies which may be useful include erythrocyte sedimentation rate, especially if it remains elevated for a period of weeks. Antinuclear antibody testing and other investigation for the connective tissue diseases may be relevant.

Methodology Latex-human IgG agglutination, sheep RBC-rabbit IgG agglutination, rate nephelometry in which international units are reported

Additional Information RF is typically an immunoglobulin of the IgM or IgG class, but occasionally may be IgA or IgE. RF forms immune complexes with target immunoglobulin within the circulation or joint fluid. These complexes may reach high concentrations and mediate tissue injury.

Approximately 65% to 85% of patients with rheumatoid arthritis have RF in their sera. Seropositive rheumatoid arthritis patients tend to have more severe disease than seronegative patients and high RF titers are often associated with multiple subcutaneous nodules, necrotizing vasculitis, and poorer long-term prognosis. Treatment does not usually alter RF titers; however, they may decrease with gold therapy. Elevated RF titers may not be seen in the serum for the first several months in early rheumatoid arthritis and may be found in the joint fluid before it is seen in the serum.

Up to 35% of patients with rheumatoid arthritis have negative rheumatoid factor tests. Therefore, a negative test does not rule out the diagnosis of rheumatoid arthritis in a patient who otherwise meets clinical criteria. Female patients and patients with elderly onset rheumatoid arthritis are more likely to be seronegative.

RF is present in only 30% of children with juvenile rheumatoid arthritis. Other joint diseases, such as ankylosing spondylitis, Reiters syndrome, Lyme disease, and psoriatic arthritis do not have elevated RF titers.

RF in pleural fluid, with titer ≥320, provides evidence of rheumatoid pleuritis in patients who have established rheumatoid arthritis.

Monographs providing additional information relevant to rheumatoid effusions are included under Related Information; *vide supra*.

Footnotes
1. Desai SP and Isa-Pratt S, *Clinician's Guide to Laboratory Medicine*, Hudson, OH: Lexi-Comp Inc, 2000, 610.
2. Miller ML and Cassidy JT, "Juvenile Rheumatoid Arthritis," *Nelson Textbook of Pediatrics*, 16th ed, Behrman RE, Kliegman RM, and Jenson HB, eds, Philadelphia, PA: WB Saunders Co, 2000, 704-9.
3. *Mayo Medical Laboratories Interpretive Handbook*, Rochester, MN: Mayo Medical Laboratories, 1999, 462.

References
Kalsi J and Isenberg D, "Rheumatoid Factor: Primary or Secondary Event in the Pathogenesis of RA?" *Int Arch Allergy Immunol*, 1993, 102(3):209-15.
Moder KG, "Use and Interpretation of Rheumatologic Tests: A Guide for Clinicians," *Mayo Clin Proc*, 1996, 71(4):391-6.
Ota T and Kobayashi T, "Rheumatoid Factors - Recent Advances in Measurement Techniques, Their Fine Specificities and Mechanisms of Their Production," *Rinsho Byori*, 1993, 41(1):26-35.
Shmerling RH and Delbanco TL, "How Useful Is the Rheumatoid Factor? An Analysis of Sensitivity, Specificity, and Predictive Value," *Arch Intern Med*, 1992, 152(12):2417-20.

♦ **Rheumatoid Factor, Synovial Fluid** *see* Rheumatoid Factor, Serum or Body Fluid *on page 541*

♦ **Ribonucleoprotein Antibodies** *see* Smith (Sm) and Ribonucleoprotein (RNP) Antibodies *on page 543*

♦ **RNA Polymerase III** *see* Topoisomerase I Antibody *on page 546*

♦ **RNP** *see* Smith (Sm) and Ribonucleoprotein (RNP) Antibodies *on page 543*

♦ **RNP Antibodies** *see* Smith (Sm) and Ribonucleoprotein (RNP) Antibodies *on page 543*

♦ **Ro Antibodies** *see* Sjögren Antibodies *on page 542*

♦ **Rose-Waaler Test** *replaced by* Rheumatoid Factor, Serum or Body Fluid *on page 541*

♦ **sAβ** *see* Cerebrospinal Fluid and Plasma β-Amyloid$_{(1-42)}$ *on page 513*

♦ **Scl-70 Antibody** *see* Topoisomerase I Antibody *on page 546*

♦ **Scleroderma Antibody** *see* Topoisomerase I Antibody *on page 546*

♦ **Shrimp Sensitivity** *see* Allergen Specific IgE Antibody *on page 502*

♦ **Singer-Plotz Test** *replaced by* Rheumatoid Factor, Serum or Body Fluid *on page 541*

♦ **Single-Fiber Electromyographic Test** *see* Acetylcholine Receptor Antibody *on page 502*

Sjögren Antibodies

Related Information
Anticardiolipin Antibody *on page 503*
Anti-DNA *on page 504*
Antinuclear Antibody *on page 507*
Bacterial Culture, Conjunctiva *on page 570*
Chlamydia trachomatis Culture *on page 590*
Fungal Culture, Ocular Infections *on page 612*
Jo-1 Antibody *on page 538*
LE Cell Test *on page 454*
Ocular Cytology *on page 385*
Topoisomerase I Antibody *on page 546*
Viral Culture, Eye or Ocular Symptoms *on page 693*

Synonyms La Antibodies; Ro Antibodies; SS-A Antibodies; SS-B Antibodies

Applies to ENA; Extractable Nuclear Antibodies/Antigens; HLA-DR3; HLA-DRw52; Sm; SS-A/Ro; SS-B/La; U₁RNP Antibody

Abstract Sjögren syndrome (SS) is a complex immunologic, autoimmune entity. It includes keratoconjunctivitis sicca, xerostomia, parotid enlargement, and arthritis. A secondary form is found in patients with other diseases regarded as autoimmune. Lymphoproliferative disorders occur. Renal involvement is found in about 40% of those with primary Sjögren syndrome. Antibodies to double-stranded DNA are not found in Sjögren syndrome.

Extractable nuclear antigens (ENA) include nuclear ribonuclear protein (RNP), Smith (Sm), Sjögren syndrome A (SS-A/Ro), and Sjögren syndrome B (SS-B/La).

Specimen Serum

Container Red top or SST™ tube

Storage Instructions Store at 4°C for up to 72 hours **or** -20°C or colder, without freezing and thawing indefinitely.

Reference Interval Negative

Use SS-A (Ro) and SS-B (La) are useful in diagnosis of Sjögren syndrome (especially with vasculitis) and some forms of lupus; may be present in antiphospholipid antibody syndrome

Limitations Some autoantibodies, especially anti-SS-A (Ro), can be found in sera of apparently normal individuals.[1]

Methodology Immunodiffusion (ID). Best detection for anti-SS-B (La) antibodies was by immunoblotting while anti-SS-A (Ro) antibodies were more often detected by enzyme immunoassay (EIA).[1]

Additional Information Antibodies to the ribonucleoprotein SS-A (Ro) are detected in 35% to 60% of SLE patients and antibodies to SS-B/La in about 15% of subjects with SLE. Anti-SS-A autoantibodies have been associated with photosensitivity, sicca symptoms, thrombocytopenia, and subacute cutaneous LE rash. Subacute cutaneous lupus erythematosus is a widespread, nonscarring, often photosensitive, form of cutaneous lupus with mild systemic manifestations and a low frequency of CNS and renal involvement. Anti-SS-A (Ro) antibodies are strongly associated with neonatal lupus. Maternal IgG antibodies cross the placenta, causing disease in the neonate. The two major manifestations of neonatal lupus erythematosus are transient dermatitis and usually irreversible heart block.[2] Photosensitive dermatitis develops after the first few weeks of life and resolves within 6 months, coincident with the clearing of maternal antibodies from the infant's circulation. Heart block is due to binding of SS-A antibodies in conducting system tissue.

Lymphocytic infiltration of exocrine glands, particularly the salivary and lacrimal glands, and other organs characterize Sjögren syndrome. The most common clinical presentation is with sicca symptoms, xerophthalmia, and xerostomia. Peripheral neuropathy, often presenting as paresthesias, occurs in 22%. Autonomic dysfunction is seen.[3]

The autoantibodies strongly associated with Sjögren syndrome are directed against the ribonucleoproteins SS-A (Ro) and SS-B (La). SS-A antibodies are detected in 40% to 60% of patients with Sjögren syndrome when the assays are done by immunodiffusion. The frequency approaches 90% or more when EIA is used. SS-B (La) antibodies occur slightly less frequently and never occur in the absence of SS-A antibodies. The presence of SS-A and SS-B antibodies are used to support the diagnosis of Sjögren syndrome. However, their presence must be interpreted in the proper clinical context because they are also found in patients with SLE and other diseases. These antibodies also provide prognostic information. Patients with these antibodies more often have extraglandular disease including vasculitis, purpura, lymphadenopathy, leukopenia, thrombocytopenia, hypergammaglobulinemia, and the presence of rheumatoid factor.[4]

Other laboratory abnormalities in Sjögren syndrome may include elevation of the ESR, presence of antinuclear antibodies, presence of rheumatoid factor, polyclonal gammopathy, and the presence of cryoglobulins which may include IgM kappa proteins. Hypothyroidism secondary to Hashimoto thyroiditis occurs.[5]

Diagnosis of Sjögren syndrome may be supported by minor salivary gland biopsy (lip biopsy).

Footnotes
1. Bridges AJ, Lorden TE, and Havighurst TC, "Autoantibody Testing for Connective Tissue Diseases. Comparison of Immunodiffusion, Immunoblot, and Enzyme Immunoassay," *Am J Clin Pathol*, 1997, 108(4):406-10.
2. Moder KG, Miller TD, and Tazelaar HD, "Cardiac Involvement in Systemic Lupus Erythematosus," *Mayo Clin Proc*, 1999, 74(3):275-84.
3. Sorajja P, Poirier MK, and Bundrick JB, "Autonomic Failure and Proximal Skeletal Myopathy in a Patient With Primary Sjögren Syndrome," *Mayo Clin Proc*, 1999, 74(7):695-7.
4. Kavanaugh A, Tomar R, Reveille J, et al, "Guidelines for Clinical Use of the Antinuclear Antibody Test and Tests for Specific Autoantibodies to Nuclear Antigens," *Arch Pathol Lab Med*, 2000, 124(1):71-81.
5. Hochberg MC, "Sjögren's Syndrome," *Cecil Textbook of Medicine*, 21st ed, Chapter 291, Goldman LJ and Bennett JC, eds, Philadelphia, PA: WB Saunders Co, 2000, 1522-4.

References
Fox RI, Chan EK, and Kang HI, "Laboratory Evaluation of Patients With Sjögren's Syndrome," *Clin Biochem*, 1992, 25(3):213-22.
Homburger HA, "Cascade Testing for Autoantibodies in Connective Tissue Diseases," *Mayo Clin Proc*, 1995, 70(2):183-4.
Moder K, "Use and Interpretation of Rheumatologic Tests: A Guide for Clinicians," *Mayo Clin Proc*, 1996, 71(4):391-6.
Tengner P, Halse AK, Haga HJ, et al, "Detection of Anti-Ro/SSA and Anti-La/SSB Autoantibody-Producing Cells in Salivary Glands From Patients With Sjögren's Syndrome," *Arthritis Rheum*, 1998, 41(12):2238-48.

◆ **SLA Antibody** see Smooth Muscle Antibody on page 543

◆ **Sm** see Sjögren Antibodies on page 542

◆ **SMA** see Smooth Muscle Antibody on page 543

Smith (Sm) and Ribonucleoprotein (RNP) Antibodies

Related Information
Anti-DNA on page 504
Antinuclear Antibody on page 507

Synonyms Anti-U1snRNP; nRNP; Nuclear Ribonucleoprotein; Ribonucleoprotein Antibodies; RNP; RNP Antibodies; U1 snRNP Antibody

Applies to ENA; Extractable Nuclear Antigen (ENA)

Abstract The Smith (Sm) and nuclear ribonucleoprotein (RNP) antigens are a particulate complex composed of small nuclear RNAs (U-RNAs) and proteins. This complex has also been referred to as **extractable nuclear antigens (ENA)**, since it is soluble in saline. Autoantibodies to Sm and RNP occur respectively in systemic lupus erythematosus and mixed connective

tissue disease. **ENAs** include **SS-A (Ro)** and **SS-B (La)**, nuclear ribonuclear protein (**RNP**), and Smith (**Sm**).

Specimen Serum

Container Red top or SST™ tube

Causes for Rejection Some laboratories will perform ENA testing only on ANA-positive cases to avoid false positives.

Reference Interval Negative

Use Confirm the diagnosis of **systemic lupus erythematosus** (SLE) or **mixed connective tissue disease** (MCTD). In the presence of possible diseases similar to SLE, with ANA positivity, anti-ds-DNA and anti-Sm may be helpful.

Limitations With rare exceptions, these tests should not be ordered if the ANA was negative or weakly positive, because <5% of patients with ANA titers <1:160 will have positive follow-up tests. Sm titers should not be measured as a marker of disease activity or to establish prognosis.

Methodology Immunodiffusion (ID), enzyme-linked immunosorbent assay (ELISA), immunoblotting provided best detection for RNP in a comparison study.[1]

Additional Information The Sm (Smith) and related nuclear ribonucleoproteins (nRNPs) are targets for autoantibodies in SLE. These antigens are present in subcellular organelles called spliceosomes that are composed of peptide containing small RNAs. **Anti-Sm antibodies are only present in 15% to 30% of patients with SLE, but they are highly specific for SLE.** They occur more frequently (60%) in young black females with SLE. They almost never occur in healthy individuals or patients with other diseases. (Anti-Sm antibodies should not be confused with antismooth muscle antibodies detected in autoimmune liver disease.)

Anti-RNP antibodies, which are commonly tested in conjunction with anti-Sm, are found in 30% to 40% of SLE patients but anti-RNP antibodies are not useful to establish the diagnosis of SLE. They lack specificity for SLE. High titers of Sm and RNP antibodies have been reported in patients with less renal and central nervous system disease, though others have refuted these findings. Sm antibodies may disappear with treatment, while RNP antibodies persist.

Many patients present with clinical signs and symptoms that are compatible with more than one systemic rheumatic disease. One such overlap syndrome is **mixed connective tissue disease** (MCTD), an entity in which females predominate. Patients with MCTD have overlapping features of SLE, scleroderma, polymyositis, and rheumatoid arthritis. Arthritis, arthralgia, dyspnea, Raynaud phenomenon, esophageal dysfunction, and myositis are common, but renal involvement is rare. Half or more are RF positive. **Detection of high levels of RNP antibody, in the absence of other antibodies, strongly suggests the diagnosis of MCTD in the appropriate clinical setting.** (Low titers of nRNP are found in SLE, scleroderma, and other diseases.) Isolated pulmonary hypertension and/or severe interstitial lung disease may evolve in patients with MCTD. Two laboratory criteria are necessary to diagnose MCTD: 1) the presence of high titer RNP antibodies and 2) the absence of anti-DNA, anti-Sm, and histone antibodies.

Footnotes
1. Bridges AJ, Lorden TE, and Havighurst TC, "Autoantibody Testing for Connective Tissue Diseases: Comparison of Immunodiffusion, Immunoblot, and Enzyme Immunoassay," *Am J Clin Pathol*, 1997, 108(4):406-10.

References
Kavanaugh A, Tomar R, Reveille J, et al, "Guidelines for Clinical Use of the Antinuclear Antibody Test and Tests for Specific Autoantibodies to Nuclear Antigens," *Arch Pathol Lab Med*, 2000, 124(1):71-81.
Lazarus DS and Mark EJ, "A 46-Year-Old Woman With Dermatomyositis, Increasing Pulmonary Insufficiency and Terminal Right Ventricular Failure," Case Records of the Massachusetts General Hospital, Case 24-1995, Scully RE, Mark EJ, McNeely WF, et al, eds, *N Engl J Med*, 1995, 333(6):369-77.
Moder K, "Use and Interpretation of Rheumatologic Tests: A Guide for Clinicians," *Mayo Clin Proc*, 1996, 71(4):391-6.

Smooth Muscle Antibody

Related Information
Alanine Aminotransferase, Serum on page 87
Alkaline Phosphatase, Serum on page 93
Antimitochondrial Antibody on page 505
Antinuclear Antibody on page 507
Aspartate Aminotransferase, Serum on page 112
Bilirubin, Total, Serum on page 118
Hepatitis C Virus RNA Detection and Quantitation on page 626
LE Cell Test on page 454
Liver Biopsy on page 65
Liver Disease: Laboratory Assessment, Overview on page 216
Liver/Kidney Microsomal Type 1 Antibodies on page 539
Protein Electrophoresis, Serum on page 267

Synonyms Antismooth Muscle Antibody; SMA

Applies to Antiactin Antibodies; Anti-ASGPR; Anti-F Actin; Asialoglycoprotein Receptor Antibodies; DR3; DR4; HLA-B8; Liver/Kidney Microsomes Antibody; LKM Antibody; SLA Antibody; Soluble Liver Antigen Antibody

Abstract Major types of autoimmune liver disease include primary biliary cirrhosis, autoimmune hepatitis, and primary sclerosing cholangitis. The differential diagnosis of these disorders includes chronic viral hepatitis B, D, (Continued)

Smooth Muscle Antibody *(Continued)*

and C, drug-induced chronic hepatitis and Wilson disease. Overlap and outlier syndromes are also recognized. Detection of antimitochondrial and antismooth muscle antibodies (SMA) has become an important facet in the differential diagnosis of chronic liver disease: SMA positivity supports classification as type 1 or 3 autoimmune hepatitis, while antimitochondrial antibodies are found more often and in higher titer in primary biliary cirrhosis.

Specimen Serum

Container Red top or SST™ tube

Storage Instructions Keep specimen cool.

Reference Interval Titers <1:20 are considered negative.

Use Smooth muscle antibody is useful in the differential diagnosis of chronic liver disease. Autoimmune type 1 hepatitis is characterized by autoantibodies (ANA, SMA, and marked polyclonal increases of serum immunoglobulins, high IgG, and often, relationship with other autoimmune entities). Antiliver/kidney microsomal type 1 (anti-LKM-1) and SMA are mutually exclusive. Anti-LKM-1 is found in type 2 autoimmune hepatitis. See table.

Limitations Antismooth muscle antibody is present, usually at titers <1:80, in 35% of patients with primary biliary cirrhosis, and in occasional cases of cryptogenic cirrhosis, infectious mononucleosis, asthma, and neoplasm. Detection of antimitochondrial or antismooth muscle antibodies does not rule out bile duct obstruction.

Methodology Indirect immunofluorescent antibody (IFA)

Additional Information Smooth muscle antibodies are IgG or IgM antibodies that are primarily directed against F-actin. Since F-actin is present in all smooth muscle fibers, these antibodies are not organ specific. Smooth muscle antibodies are found in 50% to 80% of patients with autoimmune hepatitis, with the exception of type 2. It is also associated with positive ANA. Elevated titers are also found in a minority of patients with primary biliary cirrhosis, and patients with cryptogenic cirrhosis. Elevated smooth muscle antibody titers have also been reported in a small number of patients with viral hepatitis, infectious mononucleosis, malignant tumors, alcoholic cirrhosis, and 5% of normal patients.

Antibodies to soluble liver antigens (cytokeratins 8 and 18) can be detected in about 10% of those with type 1 autoimmune hepatitis. Most subjects with autoimmune hepatitis are positive for HLA-B8, DR3, or DR4.

The differential diagnosis of autoimmune liver disease includes hemochromatosis, alpha₁-antitrypsin deficiency, and liver disease secondary to drugs such as alpha methyldopa, nitrofurantoin, and propylthiouracil as well as viral infection and the entities mentioned above.

See Liver/Kidney Microsomal Type 1 Antibodies *on page 539* for a discussion of autoimmune hepatitis subtypes 2a and 2b. See table.

References

Buschenefelde KH, Lohse AW, Meyer zum, "Autoimmune Hepatitis," *N Engl J Med*, 1995, 333(15):1004-5.

Colvin RB, Bhan AK, and McCluskey RT, *Diagnostic Immunopathology*, New York, NY: Raven Press, 1988, 108-10.

Galperin G and Gershwin ME, "Immunopathogenesis of Gastrointestinal and Hepatobiliary Diseases," *JAMA*, 1997, 278(22):1946-55.

Manns MP and Nakamura RM, "Autoimmune Liver Diseases," *Clin Lab Med*, 1988, 8(2):281-301.

Vrethem M, Skogh T, Berlin G, et al, "Autoantibodies Versus Clinical Symptoms in Blood Donors," *J Rheumatol*, 1992, 19(12):1919-21.

♦ **Soluble Amyloid Beta** *see* Cerebrospinal Fluid and Plasma β-Amyloid₍₁₋₄₂₎ *on page 513*

♦ **Soluble Liver Antigen Antibody** *see* Smooth Muscle Antibody *on page 543*

♦ **Soluble Liver Antigen (Anti-SLA)** *see* Liver/Kidney Microsomal Type 1 Antibodies *on page 539*

♦ **Space Flight** *see* CD4/CD8 Enumeration *on page 511*

♦ **Spinal Fluid Electrophoresis** *see* Cerebrospinal Fluid Protein Electrophoresis *on page 518*

♦ **Spinal Fluid Globulin** *see* Cerebrospinal Fluid Immunoglobulin G *on page 515*

♦ **Spinal Fluid Immunoglobulin** *see* Cerebrospinal Fluid Immunoglobulin G *on page 515*

♦ **Spinal Fluid Oligoclonal Bands** *see* Cerebrospinal Fluid Oligoclonal Bands *on page 516*

♦ **Spinal Fluid Protein** *see* Cerebrospinal Fluid Protein *on page 517*

♦ **SS-A Antibodies** *see* Sjögren Antibodies *on page 542*

♦ **SS-A/Ro** *see* Sjögren Antibodies *on page 542*

♦ **SS-B Antibodies** *see* Sjögren Antibodies *on page 542*

♦ **SS-B/La** *see* Sjögren Antibodies *on page 542*

♦ **ss-DNA** *see* Anti-DNA *on page 504*

♦ **Subacute Sclerosing Panencephalitis** *see* Cerebrospinal Fluid IgG:Albumin Ratio, IgG Index, and IgG Synthesis Rate *on page 514*

♦ **Tau Fraction** *see* Cerebrospinal Fluid Oligoclonal Bands *on page 516*

♦ **Tau Fraction** *see* Cerebrospinal Fluid Protein *on page 517*

♦ **Tau Fraction** *see* Cerebrospinal Fluid Protein Electrophoresis *on page 518*

♦ **Tau Protein** *see* Cerebrospinal Fluid and Plasma β-Amyloid₍₁₋₄₂₎ *on page 513*

♦ **T-BAM** *see* CD40-CD40 Ligand *on page 512*

♦ **Tg Ab** *see* Thyroglobulin Antibody *on page 544*

♦ ***Thermoactinomyces* Precipitating Antibodies** *see* Hypersensitivity Pneumonitis Serology *on page 530*

♦ ***Thermoactinomyces vulgaris* Precipitating Antibodies** *replaced by* Hypersensitivity Pneumonitis Serology *on page 530*

♦ ***Thermolospora viridis* Precipitating Antibodies** *see* Hypersensitivity Pneumonitis Serology *on page 530*

Thyroglobulin Antibody

Related Information
Acetylcholine Receptor Antibody *on page 502*
Glutamic Acid Decarboxylase (GAD65) Antibody *on page 527*
Parietal Cell Antibody *on page 541*
Thyroperoxidase Autoantibody *on page 545*
Thyrotropin Receptor Antibody, Serum *on page 545*

Synonyms Antithyroglobulin Antibody; Tg Ab; Thyroid Antithyroglobulin Antibody

Applies to Thyroid Autoantibodies

Test Includes Titers on positive specimens

Autoimmune Hepatitis Subtypes

Characteristics	Type 1	Type 2a	Type 2b	Type 3
Female preponderance	Yes	Uncertain	No	Yes
Age, years	10-20, 45-70	2-14 (adults: 4%)	>40	30-50
Immunologic features				
Serologic profile				
Autoantibody (target antigen)	SMA (actin F and G, tubulin); ANA (centromere, 52-kd, SS-A/Ro, histones, RNPs)	Anti-LKM-1 (cytochrome P-450, IID6 protein); antiliver cytosol 1	Anti-LKM-1; anti-HCV	Anti-SLA (hepatocyte cytokeratins 8 and 18); anti-AMA (PDC-E2)
Remarks	Anti-F-actin antibodies: increase specificity for Type 1 AIH	Anti-LKM-1 presence is mutually exclusive of SMA	Significant number of patients with anti-HV have confirmed HCV RNA in serum	Anti-SLA: increases specificity for Type 3 AIH
Serum IgA levels	Normal	Low	Normal	Normal
Extrahepatic autoimmune syndromes	+	++	−	+++
Progression to cirrhosis	+/++	+++	+++	Uncertain
Remarks	Classic or lupoid hepatitis type	Predominantly children	Predominantly children	Antisoluble liver antigen (anti-SLA)

SMA = antismooth muscle antibodies; **anti-LKM-1** = antiliver-kidney microsomal antibodies; **anti-SLA** = antisoluble liver antigen antibodies; **ANA** = antinuclear antibodies; **AMA** = antimitochondrial antibodies; **HCV** = hepatitis C virus; **RNPs** = ribonucleoproteins; **PDC-E2** = E2 component of pyruvate dehydrogenase; + = present; − = absent. Extrahepatic syndromes include arthritis, thyroid disease, and ulcerative colitis. Type 2 patients suffer more frequent nonhepatic disorders.

Adapted from Galperin C and Gershwin ME, "Immunopathogenesis of Gastrointestinal and Hepatobiliary Diseases," *JAMA*, 1997, 278(22):1946-55.

Abstract Thyroid antibodies include antibodies to thyroglobulin (Tg Ab) and thyroid peroxidase (TPO). Measurement of anti-TPO is a more sensitive test for diagnosis of thyroiditis. The improved sensitivity and specificity of current anti-TPO assays obviates the need to test for Tg Ab. Its measurement is generally no longer recommended.

Specimen Serum

Container Red top or SST™ tube

Reference Interval Hemagglutination: <1:400; IFA: negative; values vary with technology used

Use Because Tg Ab is often found with TPO-Ab in patients with chronic thyroiditis, its measurement adds little. The test may be used to identify sera containing Tg Ab which may interfere with serum globulin testing.[1]

Limitations This test is less sensitive than measuring thyroperoxidase antibody. It should not be ordered as a single test and is presently considered superfluous.[2] A high prevalence of reactivity in adults without evidence of thyroid disease is recognized.

Methodology Passive hemagglutination, indirect fluorescent antibody (IFA), enzyme-linked immunosorbent assay (ELISA), chemiluminescent immunometric techniques

Additional Information Antibodies to thyroglobulin can be detected in 40% to 70% of patients with chronic thyroiditis. Antibodies may also be present in 70% of hypothyroid patients, 40% of patients with Graves disease, and smaller numbers of patients with other autoimmune conditions, particularly pernicious anemia. Normal individuals, especially elderly females, may have antibody.

Footnotes

1. Kaplan LA, ed, The National Academy of Clinical Biochemistry, *Standards of Laboratory Practice: Laboratory Support for the Diagnosis & Monitoring of Thyroid Disease*, 1996.
2. Dayan CM and Daniels GH, "Chronic Autoimmune Thyroiditis," *N Engl J Med*, 1996, 335(2):99-107.

References

Baker JR Jr, Saunders NB, Wartofsky L, et al, "Seronegative Hashimoto Thyroiditis With Thyroid Autoantibody Production Localized to the Thyroid," *Ann Intern Med*, 1988, 108(1):26-30.

Feldt-Rasmussen U, "Analytical and Clinical Performance Goals for Testing Autoantibodies to Thyroperoxidase, Thyroglobulin and Thyrotropin Receptor," *Clin Chem*, 1996, 42(1):160-3.

Harchali AA, Montagne P, Cuilliere ML, et al, "Detection of Antithyroglobulin Autoantibodies With Defined Epitopic Specificity by a Microparticle-Enhanced Nephelometric Immunoassay," *Clin Chem*, 1992, 38(9):1859-64.

Mizukami Y, Michigishi T, Nonomura A, et al, "Pathology of Chronic Thyroiditis: A New Clinically Relevant Classification," *Pathol Annu*, 1994, 29(Pt 1):135-58.

Takaichi Y, Tamai H, Honda K, et al, "The Significance of Antithyroglobulin and Antithyroidal Microsomal Antibodies in Patients With Hyperthyroidism Due to Graves' Disease Treated With Antithyroid Drugs," *J Clin Endocrinol Metab*, 1989, 68(6):1097-100.

Thyroperoxidase Autoantibody

Related Information

Acetylcholine Receptor Antibody *on page 502*
Anemia Flowchart *on page 392*
Free Thyroxine Index *on page 177*
Glutamic Acid Decarboxylase (GAD65) Antibody *on page 527*
Parietal Cell Antibody *on page 541*
T_3 Uptake, Serum or Plasma *on page 279*
Thyroglobulin Antibody *on page 544*
Thyroid Stimulating Hormone, Serum *on page 282*
Thyroxine, Free, Serum *on page 285*
Thyroxine, Serum *on page 286*

Synonyms Antithyroid Peroxidase Antibody; Anti-TPO; Microsomal Antibody, Thyroid; Thyroid Antimicrosomal Antibody; TPO-Ab

Applies to Thyroid Autoantibodies

Abstract Thyroperoxidase (TPO) is the major antigen in antibody-dependent cell-mediated cytotoxicity in thyroid disease.[1] Chronic autoimmune thyroiditis may be subclinical or may present with hypothyroidism and/or goiter. Thyroid antibodies include thyroglobulin and thyroperoxidase (microsomal) antibodies. Measurement of TPO-Ab is a more sensitive test for diagnosis of autoimmune thyroiditis. About 60% of patients with diffuse goiter, hypothyroidism, or both have antithyroglobulin antibodies, while about 95% have TPO-Ab.[2]

The highest incidence of chronic autoimmune thyroiditis correlates with countries in which iodine intake is greatest (eg, U.S.).

Specimen Serum

Container Red top or SST™ tube

Storage Instructions Refrigeration is acceptable for up to 72 hours.

Reference Interval 0-1 units/mL by ELISA

Antimicrosomal titer: normal: <1:100

Anti-TPO concentration:

- normal: <20 IU/mL
- positive (adults): ≥20 IU/mL
- associated with autoimmune thyroiditis, other autoimmune diseases:[1] ≥50 IU/mL

Use TPO-Ab is relevant in the differential diagnosis of hypothyroidism. Its measurement is especially useful in confirmation of the diagnosis of subclinical hypothyroidism in patients with elevated serum TSH concentration and normal free T_4 level. Between 5% and 25% of patients with high titer TPO-Ab convert to overt hypothyroidism each year.

Limitations Caution must be exercised in interpretation of positive results, because 10% of adults may have low titers of thyroid antibodies without symptoms.

Subacute thyroiditis (de Quervain thyroiditis) is not an autoimmune disease.

Results may be invalid in sera from patients with myeloma and IgG levels >4 g/L.

Methodology Enzyme-linked immunosorbent assay (ELISA), thyroperoxidase antibodies by chemiluminometric assay[3]

Additional Information Autoantibodies to thyroid antigens can cause thyroid tissue injury that leads to transient hyperthyroidism and long-term hypothyroidism. TPO-Ab are detectable in about 90% of patients with Hashimoto thyroiditis and are also present in about 75% of cases of Graves disease.[4] Antibody is seldom detectable in nonautoimmune thyroid diseases. The improved sensitivity and specificity of current anti-TPO assays obviates the need to test for antithyroglobulin antibody.

A high incidence of thyroid autoantibodies has been reported in middle age or older subjects who have sarcoidosis, particularly in males.[5]

Development of the fetal brain is adversely affected when mother and fetus are hypothyroid. A major cause of hypothyroidism is autoimmune thyroiditis. Antithyroid peroxidase antibodies were utilized in a 1999 study; 77% of the women in the study with hypothyroidism had high concentrations of anti-TPO.[6]

Footnotes

1. Rodien P, Madec AM, Ruf J, et al, "Antibody-Dependent Cell-Mediated Cytotoxicity in Autoimmune Thyroid Disease: Relationship to Antithyroperoxidase Antibodies," *J Clin Endocrinol Metab*, 1996, 81(7):2595-600.
2. Dayan CM and Daniels GH, "Chronic Autoimmune Thyroiditis," *N Engl J Med*, 1996, 335(2):99-107.
3. Mayo Reference Services Publication, "Thyroperoxidase (TPO) Antibodies, Serum," *New Test Announcement*, Rochester, MN: Mayo Medical Laboratories, November, 1998.
4. Weetman AP, "Grave's Disease," *N Engl J Med*, 2000, 343(17):1236-48.
5. Nakamura H, Genma R, Mikami T, et al, "High Incidence of Positive Autoantibodies Against Thyroid Peroxidase and Thyroglobulin in Patients With Sarcoidosis," *Clin Endocrinol*, 1997, 46(4):467-72.
6. Haddow JE, Palomaki GE, Allan WC, et al, "Maternal Thyroid Deficiency During Pregnancy and Subsequent Neuropsychological Development of the Child," *N Engl J Med*, 1999, 341(8):549-55.

References

Feldt-Rasmussen U, "Analytical and Clinical Performance Goals for Testing Autoantibodies to Thyroperoxidase, Thyroglobulin, and Thyrotropin Receptor," *Clin Chem*, 1996, 42(1):160-3.

Thyrotropin Receptor Antibody, Serum

Related Information

Free Thyroxine Index *on page 177*
T_3 Uptake, Serum or Plasma *on page 279*
Thyroglobulin Antibody *on page 544*
Thyroid Stimulating Hormone, Serum *on page 282*
Thyroperoxidase Autoantibody *on page 545*
Thyroxine, Free, Serum *on page 285*
Thyroxine, Serum *on page 286*

Synonyms LATS; Long-Acting Thyroid Stimulator; Thyroid Stimulating Autoantibody; Thyroid Stimulating Immunoglobulins; TRAb; Ts Antibodies; TSH-Receptor Antibodies; TSIG

Abstract Thyroid stimulating activity additional to thyroid stimulating hormone (TSH) may be found in sera of subjects with Graves disease. This is an autoantibody, with affinity for the thyrotropin receptor located on thyroid secretory cells. It is important in the pathogenesis of Graves disease. This antibody is present in >85% of patients with Graves disease. Historically, it is the entity previously known as the long-acting thyroid stimulator (LATS). Graves disease has three major manifestations: hyperthyroidism, infiltrative ophthalmopathy, and infiltrative dermopathy. Most patients have only one or two of these manifestations, and the most common is hyperthyroidism. The anatomic substrate of Graves hyperthyroidism is diffuse hyperplasia of the thyroid, in contrast to other forms of hyperthyroidism which are characterized by nodules of hyperplastic tissue,
(Continued)

Thyrotropin Receptor Antibody, Serum *(Continued)*

interspersed with regions of uninvolved tissue (Plummer disease) (toxic nodular goiter).

Patient Preparation Recent radioisotope administration must be avoided if test is done by competitive binding radioimmunoassay.

Specimen Serum

Container Red top tube

Reference Interval This test is performed in only a few reference laboratories. Reference values should be obtained directly from the laboratory in order to be useful in patient management; <10% (reported as percent inhibition of TSH binding) is negative in one reference laboratory.[1]

Critical Values In one reference laboratory, values ≥15% provide indication of thyroid antibodies consistent with Graves disease.[1]

Use This assay may provide support in the differential diagnosis between Graves disease and toxic nodular goiter, and may also be used to monitor the role of antithyroid drugs. Despite the importance of the thyrotropin receptor antibody (TRAb) in the pathogenesis of Graves disease, the test is not often used in the clinical management of patients. TRAb is probably most helpful in patients with infiltrative ophthalmopathy or dermopathy without overt hyperthyroidism. In such situations, correct diagnosis requires correlation of physical findings, imaging studies, and laboratory tests.[2]

Limitations Negative values can be secondary to low concentrations of serum proteins or immunoglobulins. Subjects with subclinical Graves disease may have indeterminant values.[1]

Methodology Indirect assay of thyroid cell activation, competitive assay using solubilized porcine TSH receptor

Additional Information The titer of TRAb detected at the time of diagnosis is highly predictive of disease remission. Low titers are indicative of disease remission between 6-18 months following antithyroid drug medication. Conversely, a high antibody titer upon initial diagnosis indicates a low likelihood of disease remission following antithyroid therapy.[3]

Sensitivity in Graves hyperthyroidism is 80% to 99%, depending upon assay methods.[4]

Footnotes

1. Mayo Reference Services Publication, "Thyrotropin Receptor Antibody, Serum," *New Test Announcement*, Rochester, MN: Mayo Medical Laboratories, 1999.
2. Larsen PR, Davies TF, and Hay ID, "The Thyroid Gland," *Williams Textbook of Endocrinology*, 9th ed, Wilson JD, Foster DW, Kronenberg HM, et al, eds, Philadelphia, PA: WB Saunders Co, 1998,389-515.
3. Weiss RL, *ARUP Interpretive Data Guide*, ARUP Laboratories Inc, 1999, 496-7.
4. Weetman AP, "Graves' Disease," *N Engl J Med*, 2000, 343(17):1236-48.

References

Braverman LE, "Evaluation of Thyroid Status in Patients With Thyrotoxicosis," *Clin Chem*, 1996, 42(12):174-8.

Feldt-Rasmussen U, "Analytical and Clinical Performance Goals for Testing Autoantibodies to Thyroperoxidase, Thyroglobulin, and Thyrotropin Receptor," *Clin Chem*, 1996, 42(1):160-3.

Gupta MK, "Thyrotropin-Receptor Antibodies in Thyroid Diseases: Advances in Detection Techniques and Clinical Applications," *Clin Chim Acta*, 2000, 293(1-2):1-29.

Rieu M, Richard A, Rosilio M, et al, "Effects of Thyroid Status on Thyroid Autoimmunity Expression in Euthyroid and Hypothyroid Patients With Hashimoto's Thyroiditis," *Clin Endocrinol (Oxf)*, 1994, 40(4):529-35.

Tissue Typing

Related Information

Synonyms Crossmatch, Lymphocyte; Hematopoietic Stem Cell Transplant; Histocompatibility Testing; HLA Typing; HSC Transplant; Human Leukocyte Antigens; Lymphocyte Crossmatch; Lymphocytotoxic Antibody Screening; Molecular Genetic HLA Typing; Organ Donor Tissue Typing; Tissue Typing, Donor; Transplant Tissue Typing; White Cell Crossmatch

Applies to Lymphocytotoxicity Assay; Major Histocompatibility Complex; MHC

Test Includes Determination of compatibility between recipient and donors for organ or hematopoietic stem cell transplant

Abstract Multiple alloantigenic determinants (epitopes) are found on each HLA molecule, which can be classified as public or private. Donor-specific antibodies may harm the organ transplant.

Specimen Blood from donor, serum from recipient for kidney or hematopoietic stem cell transplant

Container Donor: green top (heparin) tube or preferably yellow top (ACD) tube; recipient: red top tube; DNA testing: lavender top (EDTA) tube. Consult the reference laboratory which will be used.

Storage Instructions Should be tested immediately. Do **not** refrigerate or freeze unless testing by DNA.

Use Tissue typing aids in determination of compatibility of solid organs (transplanted kidneys, hearts, and lungs) and hematopoietic stem cell transplant. HLA-B27 is addressed in a separate listing (HLA-B27 *on page 528*). DR antigens are found in diseases with immune associations. Addison disease is strongly associated with DR3. Juvenile diabetes mellitus (DR3,4 and DQ2,8), myasthenia gravis, and Graves disease also show association

with DR3, as does gluten-sensitive enteropathy. Multiple sclerosis is associated with DR2.

Methodology Lymphocytotoxicity assay, mixed lymphocyte culture (MLC), polymerase chain reaction (PCR), sequence-specific primers (SSP), sequence-specific oligonucleotide probe (SSOP), sequence-based typing (SBT), enzyme-linked immunosorbent assay (ELISA), flow cytometry (FC)

Additional Information HLA antigens are glycoproteins, the product of six closely linked genes on short arm of chromosome 6, usually inherited as an intact unit (haplotype). HLA antigens are the primary determinants of tissue graft acceptance, and thus, the major histocompatibility complex. This same HLA region contains genes of importance to complement and immune responses. The HLA loci are HLA-A, B, C (class I) and DR, DQ, and DP (class II or HLA-D region). A, B, and C antigens are expressed on nearly all nucleated human cells, D region antigens are restricted to B lymphocytes, monocytes, and endothelial cells. HLA antigens are inherited as two sets of six antigens, one set from each parent and are codominantly expressed. These antigens show linkage disequilibrium, that is certain pairs or triplets occur more frequently than expected by chance.

Tissue typing is usually undertaken to assess the "match" between donor and recipient of an organ or hematopoietic stem cell transplantation. Since these antigens are widely expressed in tissue, mismatches result in graft rejection, or graft-vs-host disease. Estimated renal graft survival at 10 years was 52% for HLA-matched transplants, but 37% for HLA-mismatched organs. The estimated half-lives of the transplants were 12.5 and 8.6 years, respectively, in a recently published study. Other factors are relevant as well.[1] DNA-based methods are gradually replacing serologic typing. The HLA lymphocytotoxic antibody screening is also performed by ELISA or flow methods. Many laboratories also perform crossmatch by flow cytometry.

Footnotes

1. Takemoto SK, Terasaki PI, Gjertson DW, et al, "Twelve Years' Experience With National Sharing of HLA-Matched Cadaveric Kidneys for Transplantation," *N Engl J Med*, 2000, 343(15):1078-84.

References

Bray RA, "Flow Cytometry Crossmatching for Solid Organ Transplantation," *Methods Cell Biol*, 1994, 41:103-18.

Duquesnoy RJ, "Histocompatibility Testing in Organ Transplantation," *Lab Med*, 1999, 30(12):796-802.

Helderman JH and Goral S, "The Allocation of Cadaveric Kidneys," *N Engl J Med*, 1999, 341(19):1468-9.

Kao KJ, Scornik JC, and Small SJ, "Enzyme-Linked Immunoassay for Anti-HLA Antibodies - An Alternative to Panel Studies by Lymphocytotoxicity," *Transplantation*, 1993, 55(1):192-6.

Klein J and Sato A, "The HLA System. First of Two Parts," *N Engl J Med*, 2000, 343(10):702-9.

Klein J and Sato A, "The HLA System. Second of Two Parts," *N Engl J Med*, 2000, 343(11):782-6.

Müller-Steinhardt M, Fricke L, Kirchner H, et al, "Monitoring of Anti-HLA Class I and II Antibodies by Flow Cytometry in Patients After Cadaveric Kidney Transplantation," *Clin Transplant*, 2000, 14(1):85-9.

Olerup O and Zetterquist H, "HLA-DR Typing by PCR Amplification With Sequence-Specific Primers in 2 Hours: An Alternative to Serological DR Typing in Clinical Practice Including Donor-Recipient Matching in Cadaveric Transplantation," *Tissue Antigens*, 1992, 39(5):225-35.

Pei R, Wang G, Tarsitani C, et al, "Simultaneous HLA Class I and Class II PRA Screening With Flow Cytometry," *Hum Immunol*, 1998, 59(5):313-22.

Perkins HA, "HLA Typing for Transplantation of Stem Cells From Unrelated Donors," *Lab Med*, 1997, 28(7):451-5.

Schnitzler MA, Hollenbeak CS, Cohen DS, et al, "The Economic Implications of HLA Matching in Cadaveric Renal Transplantation," *N Engl J Med*, 1999, 341(19):1440-6.

♦ **Tissue Typing, Donor** *see Tissue Typing on page 546*

Topoisomerase I Antibody

Related Information

Synonyms Progressive Systemic Sclerosis Antibody; Scl-70 Antibody; Scleroderma Antibody

Applies to Anti-Ku; Anti-PM-1; Anti-PM-Scl; RNA Polymerase III

Abstract Scl-70 is an antigen present on DNA topoisomerase I, which is the nuclear enzyme responsible for twisting and untwisting the DNA helix during gene transcription. Antibodies directed against topoisomerase I usually give a nucleolar ANA pattern.

Progressive systemic sclerosis (diffuse scleroderma) (PSS) is a multisystem disease which includes sclerosis (fibrosis) of skin, gastrointestinal tract, lungs, vessels, heart, and renal parenchyma. Scleroderma may be localized. Topoisomerase I antibody (Scl-70 antibody) is often related to more widespread skin and internal organ disease than is anticentromere antibody. Both antibodies are useful to investigate the differential diagnosis of scleroderma. See Centromere/Kinetochore Antibody *on page 512*. The clinical differential diagnosis of scleroderma includes scleredema, eosino-philic fasciitis, scleromyxedema, as well as CREST syndrome, mixed connective tissue disease, and related entities.[1] Scleroderma overlap syndromes are recognized disorders.[2] Scleroderma is among the disorders called connective tissue diseases.

Specimen Serum

Container Red top tube

Storage Instructions Refrigerate separated serum.

Reference Interval Negative; titers are not usually performed.

Use Aid the differential diagnosis of diffuse scleroderma (progressive systemic sclerosis). The antibody is found in up to a quarter of individuals who have idiopathic Raynaud phenomenon.

Limitations Absence of scleroderma antibody does not exclude diagnosis either of PSS or of CREST syndrome. Sensitivity for the diagnosis of PSS is 34%, specificity >98% to 99%.[3]

Contraindications Once demonstrated, this test need not be repeated.

Methodology Indirect fluorescent antibody (IFA), immunodiffusion (ID), immunoblotting, enzyme immunoassay (EIA)

Additional Information Approximately 25% to 40% of patients with diffuse scleroderma have autoantibodies to Scl-70, mainly IgG. Patients with scle-roderma whose anti-Scl-70 autoantibody result is positive are more likely to have more severe visceral disease, particularly pulmonary fibrosis.[3] Scleroderma patients with anti-Scl-70 antibodies tend to have more widespread skin disease as well. Anti-Scl-70 and anticentromere antibodies seldom coexist in the same individual. Of patients with scleroderma, 60% to 80% have positive ANA.

Other autoantibodies associated with scleroderma include anti-PM-1, anti-Ku, and anti-PM-Scl.

Footnotes

1. Wigley FM, "Scleroderma (Systemic Sclerosis)," *Cecil Textbook of Medicine*, 21st ed, Chapter 290, Goldman L and Bennett JC, eds, Philadelphia, PA: WB Saunders Co, 2000, 1517-22.
2. Landzberg MJ, Roberts DJ, and Mark EJ, "A 38-Year-Old Woman With Increasing Pulmonary Hypertension After Delivery," Case Records of the Massachusetts General Hospital, Case 4-1999, Scully RE, Mark EJ, McNeely WF, et al, eds, *N Engl J Med*, 1999, 340(6):455-64.
3. Kavanaugh A, Tomar R, Reveille J, et al, "Guidelines for Clinical Use of the Antinuclear Antibody Test and Tests for Specific Autoantibodies to Nuclear Antigens," *Arch Pathol Lab Med*, 2000, 124(1):71-81.

References

Homburger HA, "Cascade Testing for Autoantibodies in Connective Tissue Diseases," *Mayo Clin Proc*, 1995, 70(2):183-4.

Moder KG, "Use and Interpretation of Rheumatologic Tests: A Guide for Clinicians," *Mayo Clin Proc*, 1996, 71(4):391-6.

Vazquez-Abad D, Monteon V, Senecal JL, et al, "Analysis of IgG Subclasses of Human Antitopoisomerase I Autoantibodies Suggests Chronic B Cell Stimulation," *Clin Immunol Immunopathol*, 1997, 84(1):65-72.

INFECTIOUS DISEASES

Rebecca T. Horvat, PhD

David S. Jacobs, MD

Dwight Oxley, MD

Daniel R. Hinthorn, MD

Holly Alexander, PhD

Although there have been tremendous gains in the treatment and prevention of infectious diseases during the last few centuries, around the world infectious diseases still remains one of the major causes of morbidity and mortality faced by humans. Diseases due to bacterial, viral and parasitic organisms remain the leading cause of death globally. According to WHO statistics, one of every three deaths around the world in 1997 resulted from an infectious disease.

Tests performed by the diagnostic laboratory are often used to identify an infectious process. A critical step in obtaining a useful laboratory report is the collection and transport of the specimen. The material sent for culture or assay should be collected from the appropriate site with minimal contamination and should be submitted in the appropriate collection container. All specimens should be labeled properly to avoid incorrect results from affecting patient care. Finally, specimens should be promptly transported to the laboratory to prevent overgrowth of organisms or loss of organism viability (especially viral cultures).

A rapid result for diagnosis of infectious disease is essential to both patient management and hospital and public infection control. The Gram stain still remains one of the most rapid results available in infectious disease. However, other rapid tests are gradually being introduced such as antigen and antibody detection methods that have increased sensitivity. A new area of rapid diagnosis in infectious disease is the used of molecular technology. This technology permits rapid detection of fastidious and nonculturable infectious agents. At the current time a complete culture result for bacteriology is usually not available until 48 hours after submission and certain fastidious organisms, mycobacteria and fungal cultures require longer incubations, and results may take as long as 4-6 weeks. Molecular methods have shortened this time to a few days. In addition, molecular techniques can be used to detect antibiotic or antiviral resistance, determine relatedness of microorganisms for epidemiology purposes, and to monitor disease progression after therapy.

As with any progressive work, the contents of this chapter have been based on the scholarship of previous authors. The current authors wish to acknowledge Drs David F. Keren, Larry D. Gray, Christopher J. Papasian, and Bernard L. Kasten for their contributions in previous editions of these chapters.

♦ *Acanthamoeba* *see* Bacterial Culture, Conjunctiva *on page 570*

Acid-Fast Stain

Related Information
Acid-Fast Stain, Modified, *Nocardia* Species *on page 550*
Fine Needle Aspiration Culture *on page 609*
Mycobacteria by DNA Probe *on page 654*
Mycobacterial Culture, Biopsy or Body Fluid *on page 655*
Mycobacterial Culture, Cerebrospinal Fluid *on page 656*
Mycobacterial Culture, Cutaneous and Subcutaneous Tissue *on page 657*
Mycobacterial Culture, Sputum *on page 658*
Mycobacterial Culture, Stool *on page 659*
Mycobacterial Culture, Urine *on page 660*

Synonyms AFB Smear; Atypical *Mycobacterium* Smear; *Mycobacterium* Smear; TB Smear

Applies to Auramine-Rhodamine Stain; Fluorochrome Stain; Kinyoun Stain; Ziehl-Neelsen Stain

Test Includes Acid-fast stain and culture are usually ordered together.

Abstract Acid-fast bacilli are surrounded by a waxy cell wall that is resistant to destaining by acid alcohol. Heat (classic Ziehl-Neelsen), prolonged exposure, or detergent (Tergitol™ Kinyoun method) is required to allow carbolfuchsin stain to penetrate the cell wall. Once stained, acid-fast bacteria resist decolorization with acid alcohol.[1] Auramine O, a fluorochrome stain that binds to mycolic acids, is more sensitive than the Ziehl-Neelsen or Kinyoun methods, especially when low numbers of acid-fast bacilli are present.[2] The acid-fast smear is inexpensive, has high specificity (<100%), but it has low sensitivity. Molecular techniques are less sensitive than acid-fast smear, but if positive allow rapid and specific identification of *Mycobacterium tuberculosis*.

Patient Preparation Same as for mycobacteria culture of given site

Specimen The appropriate specimen for an acid-fast smear is the same as for culture. Specimens may include sputum, bronchopulmonary lavage, tissue including liver biopsy and endometrium, material from fine needle aspiration, bone marrow, CSF, gastric aspiration, urine, and stool. In neonates, smears and cultures of gastric and endotracheal aspirates are useful.[3]

Such specimens should be cultured as well. See mycobacteria culture listings for details.

Causes for Rejection Specimen received on a dry swab

Reference Interval No acid-fast organisms

Use Determine the presence of mycobacteria

Limitations Cultures are more sensitive than smears, therefore, negative acid-fast smears do not exclude a diagnosis of mycobacterial disease. Acid-fast stains are not specific for *M. tuberculosis*; other species in the genus *Mycobacterium* will stain acid-fast, and other organisms will occasionally stain acid-fast (eg, *Nocardia* species, *Rhodococcus equi*).[4] Immunocompromised individuals (eg, those who are HIV positive) may have infection by organisms of the *Mycobacterium avium-intracellulare* complex (MAC). Some laboratories may guess an organism's identity (eg, *M. tuberculosis* vs atypical *Mycobacterium* sp) by its staining characteristics and morphology, but definitive identification can only be accomplished by culture and subsequent phenotypic or genotypic characterization. Occasional strains of rapidly growing mycobacteria may not be acid-fast by fluorochrome stains.[5]

Methodology Acid-fast stain of concentrated or unconcentrated specimen (Ziehl-Neelsen, Kinyoun, or fluorochrome stain).[1] See diagram. Positive smears are quantitated and reported as 1+ (1-9 bacilli/100 fields), 2+ (1-9/10 fields), 3+ (1-9/field), or 4+ (>9/field) acid-fast bacilli seen, based on smears examined at x1000 magnification. Smears screened by the fluorochrome method are multiplied by 10.[1] Use of the cytocentrifuge to concentrate organisms in sputum enhances sensitivity of smears.[6] Specimens should not be evaluated by the criteria used for rejection of sputum specimens for bacterial culture.[7]

Carbolfuchsin
(triaminotriphenylmethane)

Additional Information In recent studies, the sensitivity and specificity of acid-fast staining was approximately 87% and 99.8%, respectively. The sensitivity and specificity of culture was 81.5% and 98.4%, respectively.[8,9,10]

At least 5 mL of **CSF** is recommended for proper acid-fast staining and evaluation.[7]

Molecular target amplification techniques are currently being used with significant success for rapid detection and identification of *Mycobacterium tuberculosis* in clinical specimens.[10,11,12] Certain laboratories may use these techniques as an adjunct to AFB smears. See Mycobacteria by DNA Probe *on page 654*.

Occasionally request for stat AFB stains are performed without prior digestion and concentration, which compromises sensitivity. Discontinuing AFB or respiratory isolation on the basis of a negative stat result is inappropriate. Identification of positive AFB smear 12-18 hours earlier than routine smears may be useful for controlling exposure of healthcare workers.

Footnotes
1. Koneman EW, Allen SD, Janda WM, et al, *Color Atlas and Textbook of Diagnostic Microbiology*, 5th ed, Philadelphia, PA: JB Lippincott Co, 1997, 903-5.
2. Ba F and Rieder HL, "A Comparison of Fluorescence Microscopy With the Ziehl-Neelsen Technique in the Examination of Sputum for Acid-Fast Bacilli," *Int J Tuberc Lung Dis*, 1999, 3(12):1101-5.
3. Cantwell MF, Shehab ZM, Costello AM, et al, "Brief Report: Congenital Tuberculosis," *N Engl J Med*, 1994, 330(15):1051-4.
4. Olson ES, Simpson AJ, Norton AJ, et al, "Not Everything Acid-Fast Is *Mycobacterium tuberculosis* - A Case Report," *J Clin Pathol*, 1998, 51(7):535-6.
5. Joseph SW, Vaichulis EM, and Houk VN, "Lack of Auramine-Rhodamine Fluorescence of Ruyon Group IV Mycobacteria," *Am Rev Respir Dis*, 1967, 95(1):114-5.
6. Saceanu CA, Pfeiffer NC, and McLean T, "Evaluation of Sputum Smears Concentrated by Cytocentrifugation for Detection of Acid-Fast Bacilli," *J Clin Microbiol*, 1993, 31(9):2371-4.
7. Havlik D and Woods GL, "Screening Sputum Specimens for Mycobacterial Culture," *Lab Med*, 1995, 26(6):411-3.
8. Christie JD and Callihan DR, "The Laboratory Diagnosis of Mycobacterial Diseases. Challenges and Common Sense," *Clin Lab Med*, 1995, 15(2):279-306.
9. Merrick ST, Sepkowitz KA, Walsh J, et al, "Comparison of Induced Versus Expectorated Sputum for Diagnosis of Pulmonary Tuberculosis by Acid-Fast Smear," *Am J Infect Control*, 1997, 25(6):463-6.
10. Aslanzadeh J, de la Viuda M, Fille M, et al, "Comparison of Culture and Acid-Fast Bacilli Stain to PCR for Detection of *Mycobacterium tuberculosis* in Clinical Samples," *Mol Cell Probes*, 1998, 12(4):207-11.
11. Miller N, Hernandez SG, and Cleary TJ, "Evaluation of Gen-Probe® Amplified *Mycobacterium tuberculosis* Direct Test and PCR for Direct Detection of *Mycobacterium tuberculosis* in Clinical Specimens," *J Clin Microbiol*, 1994, 32(2):393-7.
12. Woods GL, "Molecular Methods in the Detection and Identification of Mycobacterial Infections," *Arch Pathol Lab Med*, 1999, 123(11):1002-6.

References
Behr MA, Warren SA, Salamon H, et al, "Transmission of *Mycobacterium tuberculosis* From Patients Smear-Negative for Acid-Fast Bacilli," *Lancet*, 1999, 353(9151):444-9.

"Diagnosis and Treatment of Disease Caused by Nontuberculous Mycobacteria," *Am J Respir Crit Care Med*, 1997, 156(2 Pt 2):S1-25.

Dutt AK and Stead WW, "Smear-Negative Pulmonary Tuberculosis," *Semin Respir Infect*, 1994, 9(2):113-9.

Farinha NJ, Razali KA, Holzel H, et al, "Tuberculosis of the Central Nervous System in Children: A 20-Year Survey," *J Infect*, 2000, 41(1):61-8.

Krane JF and Renshaw AA, "Relative Value and Cost-Effectiveness of Cultures and Special Stains in Fine Needle Aspirates of the Lung," *Acta Cytol*, 1998, 42(2):305-11.

Mankin HJ and Wu HC, "A 21-Year-Old African Woman With Thoracolumbar Pain and Fever," Case Records of the Massachusetts General Hospital, Case 9-1996, Scully RE, Mark EJ, McNeely WF, eds, *N Engl J Med*, 1996, 334(12):784-89.

Menzies D, Fanning A, Yuan L, et al, "Tuberculosis Among Health Care Workers," *N Engl J Med*, 1995, 332(2):92-8.

Pfaller MA, "Application of New Technology to the Detection, Identification, and Antimicrobial Susceptibility Testing of Mycobacteria," *Am J Clin Pathol*, 1994, 101(3):329-37.

Smith RL, Yew K, Berkowitz KA, et al, "Factors Affecting the Yield of Acid-Fast Sputum Smears in Patients With HIV and Tuberculosis," *Chest*, 1994, 106(3):684-6.

Sullivan AK, Hannan MM, Azadian BS, et al, "Acid-Alcohol Fast Bacilli in Sputa of HIV-Infected Patients," *Int J STD AIDS*, 10(9):606-8.

Acid-Fast Stain, Modified, *Nocardia* Species

Related Information
Acid-Fast Stain *on page 550*
Actinomyces Culture *on page 551*
Cryptosporidium Direct Staining Procedures *on page 596*
Fine Needle Aspiration Culture *on page 609*
Fungus Smear, Stain *on page 615*
Gram Stain *on page 617*
Nocardia Culture *on page 665*

Synonyms Hank's Stain; *Nocardia* Species Modified Acid-Fast Stain

Test Includes Specific order as modified acid-fast stain is needed. The recovery of *Nocardia* species requires special culture techniques.

Abstract Found in vegetation and soil, *Nocardia* usually infects humans by the pulmonary route. Thus, lung disease is the most common form. Hematogenous dissemination occurs, particularly in immunocompromised individuals.

The organisms are aerobic bacteria, although they produce a fungus-like mycelium.[1] Infections with *Nocardia* species resemble other more common diseases. Because therapy differs, it is important to establish a definitive diagnosis, preferably by culture. The diagnosis of nocardiosis should be considered in unexplained cavitary lung disease, granulomatous lung disease of established cause not responsive to appropriate therapy, brain abscess particularly in the presence of cavitary lung disease, alveolar proteinosis, with mycetoma, and in any patient in whom a disseminated granulomatous disease is considered.

Specimen Appropriate specimen for smear is the same as for culture

Causes for Rejection Specimen received on a dry swab

Reference Interval No acid-fast organisms seen

Use Determine the presence or absence of *Nocardia* species, which can be acid-fast when stained by the modified acid-fast stain. *Actinomyces* and *Streptomyces* species which may be microscopically similar to *Nocardia* on Gram stain, are negative with the modified acid-fast stain. Establish the etiology of maduromycosis and of fever of unknown origin in patients with suspected defects of cellular immunity (eg, AIDS, Hodgkin disease, lymphoma, and so forth).

Limitations *Nocardia* species do not always stain acid-fast by this method. Consequently, the presence of branching, gram-positive bacilli on Gram stain may have greater sensitivity. *Nocardia* species, however, cannot be distinguished from *Actinomyces* species and other closely related organisms by Gram stain. *Nocardia* is variable to positive with Gram staining.

Methodology Kinyoun stain followed by light decolorization with 3% acid alcohol (940 mL of 95% ethanol and 60 mL of concentrated HCl); see the method in the 1998 Isenberg text.[2]

Additional Information *Nocardia* species can cause a spectrum of disease that varies from a self-limited infection to a progressive disease that results in death. Nocardiosis has also been reported with lupus, rheumatoid arthritis, and liver disease. Aggressive diagnostic procedures are often necessary to obtain an appropriate specimen for definitive diagnosis. Elements consistent with *Nocardia* species can be identified presumptively on Gram stain and modified acid-fast stain pending more definitive diagnosis by culture. Examination of sputum with *Nocardia* may show thin, crooked, weakly to strongly gram-positive, modified acid-fast positive, irregularly staining or beaded filaments. Opaque or pigmented sulfur granules may occasionally be present in direct smear of pus. Colonization without apparent infection may occur.

In tissue sections, the filaments are best seen with methenamine silver and Gram staining, less well with PAS and acid-fast preparations.[3]

Footnotes

1. Koneman EW, Allen SD, Janda WM, et al, *Color Atlas and Textbook of Diagnostic Microbiology*, 5th ed, Philadelphia, PA: JB Lippincott Co, 1997, 688-95.

2. Isenberg HD, ed, "Hanks Acid-Fast Stain (Modified) Technique," *Essential Procedures for Clinical Microbiology*, 1998, Washington, DC: American Society for Microbiology, 1998, 277.

3. Drapkin MS and Mark EJ, "A 69-Year-Old Renal Transplant Recipient With Low-Grade Fever and Multiple Pulmonary Nodules," Case Records of the Massachusetts General Hospital, Case 29-2000, Scully RE, Mark EJ, McNeely WF, et al, *N Engl J Med*, 2000, 343(12):870-7.

References

Beaman BL and Beaman L, "*Nocardia* Species: Host Parasite Relationships," *Clin Microbiol Rev*, 1994, 7(2):213-64.

Forbes BA, Sahm DF, and Weissfeld AS, *Bailey and Scott's Diagnostic Microbiology*, 10th ed, St Louis, MO: Mosby, 1998, 890.

McNeil MM and Brown JM, "The Medically Important Aerobic Actinomycetes: Epidemiology and Microbiology," *Clin Microbiol Rev*, 1994, 7(3):357-417.

Olson ES, Simpson AJ, Norton AJ, et al, "Not Everything Acid-Fast Is *Mycobacterium tuberculosis*," *J Clin Pathol*, 1998, 51(7):535-6.

Sridhar MS, Sharma S, Reddy MK, et al, "Clinicomicrobiological Review of *Nocardia* keratitis," *Cornea*, 1998, 17(1):17-22.

♦ **Acid-Fast Stain for Microsporidia** see Microsporidia Diagnostic Procedures on page 652

♦ **Acid-Fast Stain, Modified,** *Cryptosporidium* see *Cryptosporidium* Direct Staining Procedures on page 596

Acid-Fast Stain, Modified, Parasites

Related Information

Acid-Fast Stain on page 550
Cryptosporidium Antigen Detection by EIA on page 596
Cryptosporidium Direct Staining Procedures on page 596
Ova and Parasites, Stool on page 666

Synonyms *Cryptosporidium* Acid-Fast Stain; *Cyclospora* Acid-Fast Stain; *Microsporidium* Acid-Fast Stain

Applies to Cyclosporiasis Detection; *Isospora belli* Detection

Test Includes Modified acid-fast stain on concentrated specimens. Traditional concentration and staining methods used for ova and parasite exams are inadequate for detection of oocysts of *Cyclospora*, *Cryptosporidium*, and *Microsporidium*, and special methods must be used.

Abstract *Cryptosporidium* and *Microsporidium* species are recognized as protozoan pathogens of humans. These pathogens are obligate intracellular parasites. Microsporidia is usually associated with immunocompromised hosts. *Cyclospora* and *Cryptosporidium* are causes of chronic diarrhea and are responsible for water-borne and food-borne outbreaks. The small size and poor staining properties may result in the under-reporting of these infections. For accurate detection, a modified acid-fast stain will usually detect these organisms in stool specimens of infected patients.

Specimen Stool

Causes for Rejection Specimen received on a swab

Reference Interval No acid-fast organisms seen

Use Evaluation of watery diarrhea; determine the presence or absence of the gastrointestinal parasites *Cryptosporidium parvum*, *Cyclospora*

cayetanensis, and *Microsporidium* species (eg, *Enterocytozoon bieneusi*), which are acid-fast when stained by the modified acid-fast stain[1]

Limitations The critical step in this procedure is the destaining reagent, since over-destaining will make the organisms difficult to detect. Formed stool may have artifact material that can be confused with oocysts.

Methodology Kinyoun stain followed by light decolorization with 1% to 3% H_2SO_4. An acid-fast-trichrome stain for *Microsporidium*, *Cryptosporidium parvum*, *Cyclospora cayetanensis*, and *Isospora belli* has been recently described. Further studies will be needed.[2]

Additional Information *Cryptosporidium* and *Cyclospora* can cause diarrheal disease in humans and infection is usually associated with food and water. *Cryptosporidium* infection is associated with traveling, and person-to-person transmission. *Cyclospora cayetanensis* has been associated with prolonged diarrheal disease and can last for 7-8 weeks.[3] It is found in developing countries including Guatemala, Mexico, Peru, and the Caribbean. Microsporidia infection occurs more frequently in immunocompromised hosts, but is being recognized as a cause of diarrheal disease in the immunocompetent individual as well.[3,4] *Cyclospora* oocytes can be found in stool with modified acid-fast stains, phase contrast microscopy, with PCR, and with autofluorescence.[5] Outbreaks have been traced to imported raspberries.[6]

See Ova and Parasites, Stool on page 666.

Footnotes

1. Garcia LS and Bruckner DA, *Diagnostic Medical Parasitology*, 3rd ed, Washington, DC: ASM Press, 1997, 638-45.

2. Reisner BS and Spring J, "Evaluation of a Combined Acid-Fast Trichrome Stain for Detection of Microsporidia and *Cryptosporidium parvum*," *Arch Pathol Lab Med*, 2000, 124(5):777-9.

3. Curry A and Smith HV, "Emerging Pathogens: *Isospora*, *Cyclospora*, and Microsporidia," *Parasitology*, 1998, 117(Suppl):S143-59.

4. Lopez-Velez R, Turrientes MC, Garron C, et al, "Microsporidiosis in Travelers With Diarrhea From the Tropics," *J Travel Med*, 1999, 6(4):223-7.

5. Herwaldt BL and Ackers ML, "An Outbreak in 1996 of Cyclosporiasis Associated With Imported Raspberries," *N Engl J Med*, 1997, 336(22):1548-56.

6. Osterholm MT, "Lessons Learned Again: Cyclosporiasis and Raspberries," *Ann Intern Med*, 1999, 130(3):134-5.

References

Chioralia G, Trammer T, Kampen H, et al, "Relevant Criteria for Detecting Microsporidia in Stool Specimens," *J Clin Microbiol*, 1998, 36(8):2279-83.

Connor BA, Reidy J, and Soave R, "Cyclosporiasis: Clinical and Histopathologic Correlates," *Clin Infect Dis*, 1999, 28(6):1216-22.

Herwalt BL, "*Cyclospora caytanesis*: A Review, Focusing on the Outbreaks of Cyclosporiasis in the 1990s," *Clin Infect Dis*, 2000, 31(4):1040-57.

Kotler DP and Orenstein JM, "Clinical Syndromes Associated With Microsporidiosis," *Adv Parasitol*, 1998, 40:321-49.

♦ **Acquired Immune Deficiency Syndrome Serology** see HIV-1/HIV-2 Antibody Screen and Western Blot on page 636

Actinomyces Culture

Related Information

Acid-Fast Stain, Modified, *Nocardia* Species on page 550
Bacterial Culture, Anaerobes on page 564
Bacterial Culture, Biopsy or Body Fluid on page 565
Fine Needle Aspiration, Deep Masses on page 381
Nocardia Culture on page 665

Synonyms Wound *Actinomyces* Culture

Applies to Intrauterine Device Culture; IUD Culture

Test Includes Anaerobic culture for *Actinomyces* species and direct microscopic examination of Gram stain for sulfur granules and gram-positive branching bacilli

Abstract Actinomycosis is a chronic progressive suppurative disease characterized by the formation of multiple abscesses, draining sinuses, and dense fibrosis. The classic presentations include cervicofacial, thoracic, abdominal, and pelvic infections.

Patient Preparation Cleanse the skin around the opening of a draining sinus or lesion with an alcohol swab, allow to dry, and obtain the specimen from as deep within the sinus or lesion as possible.

Specimen Exudate, material from draining sinus, tissue

Container Anaerobic specimen transport medium or needle and syringe

Collection *Actinomyces* species are fastidious anaerobic organisms. It is, therefore, essential that the specimen be placed into the appropriate anaerobic transport tube and delivered to the laboratory as quickly as possible. All air should be expelled from syringes before transport or transfer. Swabs, if used, should be transported in anaerobic transport medium. With a draining sinus, obtain the specimen by aspirating with needle and syringe as far up the sinus or lesion as possible.

Storage Instructions Specimens should be transported immediately to the laboratory and processed as soon as possible.

Causes for Rejection Specimens exposed to air, specimens which have been refrigerated or have an excessive delay in transit, specimens from sites which have anaerobic bacteria as normal flora (eg, throat, feces, colostomy stoma, rectal swabs, bronchial washes, cervical-vaginal mucosal swabs, sputums, skin and superficial wounds, voided or catheterized urine)

Turnaround Time Cultures with no growth may be reported after 14 days. (Continued)

Actinomyces Culture *(Continued)*

Special Instructions Inform the laboratory that actinomycosis is clinically suspected, to ensure that cultures will be incubated sufficiently long to permit recovery of *Actinomyces* species. The specific site of specimen, current antibiotic therapy, and clinical diagnosis should be provided.

Reference Interval No *Actinomyces* isolated. Most species of *Actinomyces* are normal inhabitants of the mouth, oropharynx, and gastrointestinal tract.

Use Detect infections due to *Actinomyces* species; establish the etiology of suppurative/granulomatous fibrosing disease, chronic draining sinus, and fever of unknown origin (FUO), particularly in immunocompromised patients

Limitations *Actinomyces* species are relatively slow growing and will often fail to grow in the period in which most laboratories incubate routine cultures. Additionally, even when incubated appropriately, recovery of *Actinomyces* species may be hindered by overgrowth with obligate and facultative anaerobic bacteria.

Methodology Anaerobic culture including thioglycolate broth media; no reliable serologic methods are available.

Additional Information In tissue, *Actinomyces* species produce chronic suppuration, commonly with formation of multiple draining sinuses. Microscopic examination of material from such sinuses often reveals tangled masses of filamentous elements and granules called **sulfur granules**. The presence of sulfur granules is highly suggestive of *Actinomyces* infection. The differential diagnosis between actinomycosis and nocardiosis is relevant because treatment of each is different.

If granules are detected on the gauze pad covering a draining sinus, submit the granules to the laboratory for Gram stain and culture; on smear, branching gram-positive rods may be found. They may be similar in appearance to other actinomycetes including species of *Nocardia*, *Streptomyces*, and some *Mycobacterium*.[1] Actinomycetes are not acid-fast by the modified acid-fast stain used for *Nocardia* species. Several species of *Actinomyces* are responsible for human infection. *Actinomyces israelii* is the most significant. *A. naeslundii*, *A. odontolyticus*, *A. viscosus*, and *Arachnia propionica* also have been reported as human pathogens. Pelvic and perirectal infections have been associated with intrauterine devices (IUDs). A classic presentation of actinomycosis is as a painless lump in the jaw.[2] *Actinomyces* may be found in rare instances of recurrent ventral hernia following appendectomy for appendicitis, and in cases of osteomyelitis and prosthetic joint infection.[3] The diagnosis of actinomycosis often requires clinical consideration of this possibility, communication to the laboratory, and persistence on the part of laboratory personnel.

Footnotes

1. Rodloff AC, Hillier AL, and Moncla BJ, "*Peptostreptococcus*, *Propionibacterium*, *Lactobacillus*, *Actinomyces*, and Other Nonspore-Forming Anaerobic Gram-Positive Bacteria," *Manual of Clinical Microbiology*, 7th ed, Washington, DC: ASM Press, American Society for Microbiology, 1999, 672-89.
2. Feder HM Jr, "Actinomycosis Manifesting as an Acute Painless Lump of the Jaw," *Pediatrics*, 1990, 85(5):858-64.
3. Wust J, Steiger U, Vuong H, et al, "Infection of a Hip Prosthesis by *Actinomyces naeslundii*," *J Clin Microbiol*, 2000, 38(2):929-30.

References

Allen SD, Siders JA, and Marler LM, "Current Issues and Problems in Dealing With Anaerobes in the Clinical Laboratory," *Clin Lab Med*, 1995, 15(2):333-64.

Belmont MJ, Behar PM, and Wax MK, "Atypical Presentations of Actinomycosis", *Head Neck*, 1999, 21(3):264-8.

Lippes J, "Pelvic *Actinomyces*: A Review and Preliminary Look at Prevalence," *Am J Obstet Gynecol*, 1999, 180(2 Pt 1):265-9.

McNeil MM and Brown JM, "The Medically Important Aerobic Actinomycetes: Epidemiology and Microbiology," *Clin Microbiol Rev*, 1994, 7(3):357-417.

Smego RA Jr and Foglia G, "Actinomycosis," *Clin Infect Dis*, 1998, 26(6):1255-61.

Zitsch 3rd RP and Bothwell M, "Actinomycosis: A Potential Complication of Head and Neck Surgery," *Am J Otolaryngol*, 1999, 20(4):260-2.

♦ *Actinomyces israelii* see Bacterial Culture, Wounds, Bites *on page 579*

♦ **Adenovirus** see Adenovirus Antibody Titer *on page 552*

Adenovirus Antibody Titer

Related Information

Adenovirus Culture *on page 552*
Bacterial Culture, Conjunctiva *on page 570*
Viral Culture *on page 689*
Viral Culture, Body Fluid *on page 691*
Viral Culture, Respiratory Symptoms *on page 694*
Virus, Direct Detection by Fluorescent Antibody *on page 696*

Synonyms Adenovirus; Serology, Adenovirus Antibodies

Abstract Adenoviruses usually infect respiratory and gastrointestinal epithelia. A definitive diagnosis of adenovirus infection depends on the isolation of the virus from a patient specimen, demonstration of adenovirus antigen or detection of an increased antibody titer (greater than fourfold) during the course of the illness.

Specimen Serum

Container Red top tube

Collection Acute and convalescent sera drawn 2-4 weeks apart

Special Instructions Acute and convalescent sera must be tested simultaneously. Tests should, therefore, not be performed unless both specimens are received.

Reference Interval A fourfold or greater increase in titer in paired sera is indicative of a recent virus infection. Expected value single specimen: <1:8

Use Establish adenovirus as the etiologic agent for respiratory ailments including pneumonia and tonsillitis, fever and chills, gastroenteritis, hemorrhagic cystitis, and keratoconjunctivitis including swimming pool conjunctivitis.

Limitations Adenovirus infections are relatively common and circulating antibody may be long-lasting. Consequently, titers on unpaired sera are essentially uninterpretable.

Methodology Complement fixation (CF), enzyme-linked immunosorbent assay (ELISA), hemagglutination inhibition (HAI), serum neutralization

Additional Information Complement fixation and ELISA measure genus-specific antibodies, while HAI and serum neutralization, which are not widely available, may be used to measure antibody to type-specific determinants. There are 47 different types of adenovirus, and infections may vary from asymptomatic to persistent. Thus, serologic evidence of adenovirus, and even isolation of an adenovirus from a patient, may be coincidental rather than the cause of the patient's present complaints. Genus-reactive tests may be followed by serotype-specific tests, if epidemiologically warranted.

References

Bisno AL, "Acute Pharyngitis," *N Engl J Med*, 2001, 344(3):205-11.

Chien JW and Johnson JL, "Viral Pneumonias. Infection in the Immunocompromised Host," *Postgrad Med*, 2000, 107(2):67-80.

Erdman DD and Hierholzer JC, "Adenoviruses," *Manual of Clinical Laboratory Immunology*, 5th ed, Rose NR, Conway de Macario E, Folds JD, et al, eds, Washington, DC: American Society for Microbiology, 1997, 661-6.

Ginsberg HS, "The Life and Times of Adenoviruses," *Adv Virus Res*, 1999, 54:1-13.

King JC Jr, "Community Respiratory Viruses in Individuals With Human Immunodeficiency Virus Infection," *Am J Med*, 1997, 102(3A):19-24.

Munoz FM, Piedra PA, and Demmler GJ, "Disseminated Adenovirus Disease in Immunocompromised and Immunocompetent Children," *Clin Infect Dis*, 1998, 27(5):1194-200.

Adenovirus Culture

Related Information

Adenovirus Antibody Titer *on page 552*
Bacterial Culture, Conjunctiva *on page 570*
Viral Culture *on page 689*
Viral Culture, Eye or Ocular Symptoms *on page 693*
Viral Culture, Respiratory Symptoms *on page 694*
Viral Culture, Urine *on page 695*
Virus, Direct Detection by Fluorescent Antibody *on page 696*

Synonyms Adenovirus, Rapid Culture; Shell Vial Culture, Adenovirus

Test Includes Culture for adenovirus only; adenovirus is usually detected in a routine/general virus culture. Rapid culture can be done by staining inoculated shell vials with a specific monoclonal antibody.

Abstract The name "adenovirus" is based on viral isolation from adenoids. The virus is best known for its propensity to infect the upper airway, where it may cause an exudative pharyngitis similar to that of Group A *Streptococcus*. It is the most common cause of epidemic conjunctivitis. Forty-seven or more serotypes exist. A definitive diagnosis of adenovirus infection depends on the isolation of the virus from a patient specimen, demonstration of adenovirus antigen or detection of an increased antibody titer (greater than fourfold) during the course of the illness.

Specimen Midstream urine, stool or rectal swabs, nasopharyngeal secretions, eye exudates, throat swab or tissue, cerebrospinal fluid

Container Sterile container. Swabs should be placed into cold viral transport medium.

Storage Instructions Keep specimens cold and moist. Adenoviruses are more stable than are most other viruses; however, specimens should not be stored or refrigerated for long periods of time. Specimens should be delivered immediately to the clinical laboratory.

Turnaround Time Variable (1-14 days) and depends on culture method used and amount of virus in the specimen

Reference Interval No virus isolated

Use Aid in the diagnosis of disease caused by adenovirus (eg, conjunctivitis, cystitis, gastroenteritis, pneumonia, and pharyngoconjunctivitis)

Limitations Rule out or identify adenovirus **only**

Methodology Conventional culture: Inoculation of specimen into cell cultures, incubation of cell cultures, observation for characteristic cytopathic effect (CPE), and identification by fluorescent monoclonal antibody.

Rapid culture: Specimens are centrifuged onto cell cultures grown on coverslips in the bottoms of 1-dram shell vials. Centrifugation greatly accelerates virus attachment and penetration. After incubation for 2 and/or 5 days, fluorescein-labeled monoclonal antibodies are applied to the infected cells to detect viral antigens that are expressed in the membranes of the cells. Characteristic fluorescent foci indicate the presence of virus.

Additional Information Adenoviruses are spread directly by oral transmission or infectious aerosols. Infections with adenoviruses occur throughout the year, especially in people who are grouped together such as those in schools, day care centers, nursing home facilities, and hospitals.[1] Adenoviruses can cause severe respiratory infections in children and immunocompromised adults, which can mimic pertussis and which are sometimes fatal.[2] They cause ocular infections in both children and adults. These include pharyngoconjunctival fever, usually acquired in the summer, sporadic or epidemic keratoconjunctivitis, and acute hemorrhagic conjunctivitis.[2]

Types 40 and 41 are common causes of viral diarrhea in children. Diarrhea and viral shedding can persist for up to 14 days.[3] However, culture of type 40 and 41 is more difficult than culture of other adenoviruses and may not be isolated. Stool specimens can be examined for adenovirus type 40 and 41 using enzyme immunoassay or electron microscopy.[4] It is known to persist in lymphoid tissues. Adenoviruses also have been associated with intussusception.[5]

Serology to detect adenovirus antibodies is available and is often helpful in establishing a diagnosis. DNA amplification is being investigated, but is not widely available.[6]

Footnotes
1. Singh-Naz N, Brown M, and Ganeshananthan M, "Nosocomial Adenovirus Infection: Molecular Epidemiology of an Outbreak," *Pediatr Infect Dis J*, 1993, 12(11):922-5.
2. Carrigan DR, "Adenovirus Infections in Immunocompromised Patients," *Am J Med*, 1997, 102(3A):71-4.
3. Kotloff KL, Losonsky GA, Morris JG Jr, et al, "Enteric Adenovirus Infection and Childhood Diarrhea: An Epidemiologic Study in Three Clinical Settings," *Pediatrics*, 1989, 84(2):219-25.
4. Van H, Wun CC, O'Ryan ML, et al, "Outbreaks of Human Enteric Adenovirus Types 40 and 41 in Houston Day Care Centers," *J Pediatr*, 1992, 120(4 Pt 1):516-21.
5. Munoz FM, Piedra PA, and Demmler GJ, "Disseminated Adenovirus Disease in Immunocompromised and Immunocompetent Children," *Clin Infect Dis*, 1998, 27(5):1194-200.
6. Jackson R, Morris DJ, Cooper RJ, et al, "Multiplex Polymerase Chain Reaction for Adenovirus and Herpes Simplex Virus in Eye Swabs," *J Virol Methods*, 1996, 56(1):41-8.

References
Bisno AL, "Acute Pharyngitis," *N Engl J Med*, 2001, 344(3):205-11.
Ginsberg HS, "The Life and Times of Adenoviruses," *Adv Virus Res*, 1999, 54:1-13.
Hughes JH, "Physical and Chemical Methods for Enhancing Rapid Detection of Viruses and Other Agents," *Clin Microbiol Rev*, 1993, 6(2):150-75.
Khoo SH, Bailey AS, de Jong JC, et al, "Adenovirus Infections in Human Immunodeficiency Virus-Positive Patients: Clinical Features and Molecular Epidemiology," *J Infect Dis*, 1995, 172(3):629-37.
King JC Jr, "Community Respiratory Viruses in Individuals With Human Immunodeficiency Virus Infection," *Am J Med*, 1997, 102(3A):19-24.
Olsen MA, Shuck KM, Sambol AR, et al, "Isolation of Seven Respiratory Viruses in Shell Vials: A Practical and Highly Sensitive Method," *J Clin Microbiol*, 1993, 31(2):422-5.
Wadell G, Allard A, and Hierholzer JC, "Adenoviruses," *Manual of Clinical Microbiology*, 7th ed, Murray PR, Baron EJ, Pfaller MA, et al, eds, Washington, DC: ASM Press, American Society of Microbiology, 1999, 970-82.

Anthrax Detection

Related Information
Bacterial Culture, Blood *on page 566*
Fine Needle Aspiration Culture *on page 609*

Synonyms Bacterial Culture, Anthrax

Test Includes Aerobic culture and Gram stain of specimen

Abstract The reservoir for this gram-positive sporulating *Bacillus* is the soil. It exists in an infected host as a vegetative bacillus, in the environment as a spore. Spores remain viable for years, even decades, and spores are the usual infective form.[1] Bacterial culture for aerobic organisms will provide proper growth conditions for *Bacillus anthracis*; however, it is important to notify the laboratory if this organisms is suspected.

Patient Preparation Varies with source.

Specimen Blood, cerebrospinal fluid, sputum, or cutaneous lesion fluid

Container Sterile container or swab; varies with source

Collection Varies with source

Turnaround Time Varies with specimen. Negative results are typically reported as follows: blood and CSF: 5-7 days; sputum and wounds: 2 days. Preliminary morphologic information for positive cultures (for specimens other than blood and aseptically obtained body fluids) is usually available within 24 hours. Suspicious isolates should be forwarded to a state or local public health laboratory for complete identification.

Use Detect the presence of *Bacillus anthracis* in clinical specimens from humans, grazing animals including cattle, goats, sheep, and other animals

Limitations Patients with inhalation anthrax become ill and die rapidly. Sputum cultures may be obtained but are rarely positive.[2]

Methodology Inoculation of microbiological media, incubation of media at 35°C in ambient or CO_2-enhanced atmospheric conditions. Blood cultures become positive, but unfortunately late in the clinical course.[1,3]

An enzyme-linked immunosorbent assay (ELISA) detects circulating toxin. *Bacillus anthracis* can be found in peripheral blood smears with Wright or Gram stains.[1] Molecular methods may become available.[3]

Additional Information Anthrax is a zoonotic disease that may present as cutaneous, gastrointestinal or pulmonary disease. Although rare, human anthrax does occur throughout the world, including the United States,[4] and is usually acquired by contact with contaminated animals or animal products such as hides, wool, or other fractions. Means of transmission include contact with inoculation of minor lesions, meat ingestion, handling, or inhalation. The last is known as Woolsorter disease. Person-to-person transmission does not occur.

The reader is encouraged to review a splendidly illustrated, recently published review paper.[3]

Anthrax is one of the bacteria that could potentially be used as an agent of biological warfare, and laboratories throughout the U.S. should have procedures in place to make a preliminary identification and to notify the proper authorities if a suspicious isolate is recovered.[1,5] It is recommended that laboratories utilize biosafety level 2 facilities and practices for handling specimens and cultures for *Bacillus anthracis*.[6]

Footnotes
1. Franz DR, Jahrling PB, Friedlander AM, et al, "Clinical Recognition and Management of Patients Exposed to Biological Warfare Agents," *JAMA*, 1997, 278(5):399-411.
2. Shafazand S, Doyle R, Ruoss S, et al, "Inhalational Anthrax: Epidemiology, Diagnosis, and Management," *Chest*, 1999, 116(5):1369-76.
3. Dixon TC, Meselson JG, Guillemin J, et al, "Anthrax," *N Engl J Med*, 1999, 341(11):815-26.
4. "Human Ingestion of *Bacillus anthracis*-Contaminated Meat - Minnesota, August 2000," *MMWR Morb Mortal Wkly Rep*, 2000, 49(36):813-6.
5. "Bioterrorism Readiness Plan: A Template for Healthcare Facilities," APIC Bioterrorism Task Force and CDC Hospital Infections Program Bioterrorism Working Group, 1999, available at: www.apic.org.
6. Richmond JY and McKinney RW, "Biosafety in Microbiological and Biomedical Laboratories," 1999, Washington, DC: U.S. Government Printing Office,

References
"Biological and Chemical Terrorism: Strategic Plan for Preparedness and Response. Recommendations of the CDC Strategic Planning Workgroup," *MMWR Recommend & Rep*, 2000, 49(RR-4):1-14.
"Bioterrorism Alleging Use of Anthrax and Interim Guidelines for Management - United States, 1998," *MMWR Morb Mortal Wkly Rep*, 1999, 48(5):69-74.
Inglesby TV, Henderson DA, Bartlett JG, et al, "Anthrax as a Biological Weapon: Medical and Public Health Management. Working Group on Civilian Biodefense," *JAMA*, 1999, 281(18):1735-45.

♦ **Anti-B19 IgM Antibodies** see *Parvovirus B19 Serology on page 669*

♦ **Antibacterial Activity, Serum** see *Serum Bactericidal Test on page 679*

♦ **Antibiotic-Associated Colitis Toxin Test** see *Clostridium difficile* Toxin Assay and Culture *on page 592*

♦ **Antibody to HAV, IgM** see *Hepatitis A Antibodies, IgM and IgG on page 622*

♦ **Antibody to Hepatitis B Core Antigen** see *Hepatitis B Core Antibody on page 622*

♦ **Antibody to Hepatitis B Surface Antigen** see *Hepatitis B Surface Antibody on page 625*

♦ **Antibody to Hepatitis E** see *Hepatitis E Serology on page 628*

♦ **Antibody to HEV** see *Hepatitis E Serology on page 628*

Antideoxyribonuclease-B Titer, Serum

Related Information
Antistreptolysin O Titer, Serum *on page 559*
Bacterial Culture, Throat, and Antigen Detection Testing for Group A Streptococci *on page 577*
Group A *Streptococcus* Screen, Rapid *on page 617*
Sedimentation Rate, Erythrocyte *on page 484*
Streptozyme *on page 682*

Synonyms Anti-DNase-B Titer; Antistreptococcal DNase-B Titer; Streptodornase

Abstract Detection of an immune response to extracellular products of *S. pyogenes*, such as DNase B, is useful in demonstration of evidence of streptococcal infections in patients without documentation of recent infection, who present with nonsuppurative sequelae such as rheumatic fever or glomerulonephritis.

Specimen Serum

Container Red top tube

Reference Interval Children: preschool: ≤60 units; school: ≤170 units; adults: ≤85 units; a rise in titer of two or more dilution increments between acute and convalescent sera is significant.

Use Document recent streptococcal infection (eg, to evaluate possible rheumatic fever).

Poststreptococcal reactive arthritis is an arthritis which follows β-hemolytic streptococcal infection, in patients lacking criteria for acute rheumatic fever. Increased ASO and anti-DNase titers are useful to confirm recent streptococcal infection for this diagnosis.[1]

Limitations Normal ranges may vary in different populations; test must use a pure source of DNase-B to ensure specificity.

Contraindications Not valid in patients with hemorrhagic pancreatitis

Methodology Colorimetry based on hydrolysis of DNA

Additional Information DNase-B is antigenically the most consistent of four streptococcal DNases. The presence of antibodies to streptococcal DNase is an indicator of recent infection, especially if a rise in titer can be documented. This test has advantages over the ASO test: It is more sensitive to streptococcal pyoderma, it is not as subject to false positives due to liver disease, reagents are not likely to oxidize, and it is not affected by the site of infection. It is positive, like ASO, in about 80% to 85% of patients with streptococcal infections. Application of both tests detects about 95%.[2] Used together, each is helpful. Throat culture is relevant.

Footnotes
1. Aviles RJ, Ramakrishna G, Mohr DN, et al, "Poststreptococcal Reactive Arthritis in Adults: A Case Series," *Mayo Clin Proc*, 2000, 75(2):144-7.
2. Leavelle DE, *Mayo Medical Laboratories Interpretive Handbook*, Rochester, MN: Mayo Medical Laboratories, 1997.

References
Bisno AL, "Acute Pharyngitis," *N Engl J Med*, 2001, 344(3):205-11.
Cunningham MW, "Pathogenesis of Group A Streptococcal Infections," *Clin Microbiol Rev*, 2000, 13(3):470-511.
Efstratiou A, "Group A Streptococci in the 1990s," *J Antimicro Chemother*, 2000, 45(Suppl):3-12.
Olivier C, "Rheumatic Fever - Is It Still a Problem?" *J Antimicro Chemother*, 2000, 45(Suppl):13-21.
Pacifico L, Mancuso M, Properzi E, et al, "Comparison of Nephelometric and Hemolytic Techniques for Determination of Antistreptolysin O Antibodies," *Am J Clin Pathol*, 1995, 103(4):396-9.

♦ **Anti-DNase-B Titer** see Antideoxyribonuclease-B Titer, Serum *on page 554*

♦ **Antigen Detection for *W. bancrofti*** see Filariasis Serological Test *on page 608*

♦ **Anti-HAV, IgM** see Hepatitis A Antibodies, IgM and IgG *on page 622*

♦ **Anti-HB$_c$** see Hepatitis B Core Antibody *on page 622*

♦ **Anti-HB$_e$** see Hepatitis B$_e$ Antibody *on page 624*

♦ **Anti-HB$_s$** see Hepatitis B Surface Antibody *on page 625*

♦ **Anti-HCV, Enzyme Immunoassay (EIA)** see Hepatitis C Virus Serology *on page 627*

♦ **Antimicrobial Combinations - Test for Synergism and Antagonism** see *Antimicrobial Susceptibility Testing, Antimicrobial Combinations on page 556*

♦ **Antimicrobial Drugs** see *Antimicrobial Susceptibility Testing, Aerobic and Facultatively Anaerobic Bacteria on page 554*

♦ **Antimicrobial Removal Device (ARD) Blood Culture** see *Bacterial Culture, Blood on page 566*

Antimicrobial Susceptibility Testing, Aerobic and Facultatively Anaerobic Bacteria

Related Information
Aminoglycosides, Serum *on page 734*
Antimicrobial Susceptibility Testing, Antimicrobial Combinations *on page 556*
Antimicrobial Susceptibility Testing, Fungi *on page 556*
Antimicrobial Susceptibility Testing, Minimum Bactericidal Concentration *on page 557*
Antimicrobial Susceptibility Testing, Mycobacteria *on page 557*
Antimicrobial Susceptibility Testing, Unusual Isolates/Fastidious Organisms *on page 558*
Bacterial Culture, Abscess *on page 562*
Bacterial Culture, Aerobes *on page 563*
Beta-Lactamase Test *on page 581*
Serum Bactericidal Test *on page 679*
Vancomycin, Serum *on page 769*

Synonyms E-Test; Kirby-Bauer Susceptibility Test; MIC; Minimum Inhibitory Concentration Susceptibility Test; Sensitivity Testing, Aerobic and Facultatively Anaerobic Organisms; Susceptibility Testing Aerobic and Facultatively Anaerobic Organisms

Applies to Antimicrobial Drugs; Beta-Lactam Ring; Penicillinase

Test Includes Qualitative or quantitative determination of antimicrobial susceptibility of an isolated organism

Abstract The purpose of antimicrobial susceptibility testing is to determine the antibacterial activity of antimicrobial agents against specific pathogens. These susceptibility assays have been standardized for use in clinical laboratories by the National Committee for Clinical Laboratory Standards (NCCLS).[1,2,3] Standards include use of quality control microorganisms to support reliability and use of standard agar and broth media to diminish variability between laboratories.

Specimen Viable pure culture of a rapidly growing aerobic or facultatively anaerobic organism

Turnaround Time Usually 1 day after recovering an organism from a clinical specimen

Reference Interval Minimal inhibitory concentration (MIC) reported. Results may be qualitatively reported as susceptible (S), intermediate (I), or resistant (R).

Use Determine antimicrobial susceptibility of organisms involved in infectious processes when the susceptibility of the organism cannot be predicted from its identity. The pattern of antibiotic susceptibility is sometimes used to monitor nosocomial infections such as those due to methicillin-resistant *Staphylococcus aureus* and to evaluate or follow the development of resistance to new antimicrobial drugs.[4,5,6]

Limitations Interpretive guidelines developed for antimicrobial susceptibility tests are applicable to most nonfastidious, rapidly growing bacteria (*Staphylococcus* species, *Enterococcus* species, *Pseudomonas aeruginosa*, and members of the *Enterobacteriaceae*), and some common fastidious pathogens (eg, *Streptococcus pneumoniae*, *Haemophilus influenzae*, *Neisseria gonorrhoeae*). Interpretive criteria for less common pathogens (eg, *Neisseria meningitidis*, *Corynebacterium* species, *Nocardia* species, rapidly-growing mycobacteria, *Bacillus* species) have not been standardized.

Methodology Disk diffusion (qualitative) broth dilution, microbroth dilution, agar dilution (quantitative), or gradient diffusion (quantitative) or antimicrobial concentrations are selected to correspond to therapeutically relevant levels. Several automated instruments have been developed to perform routine susceptibility testing of microorganisms.[7]

Additional Information Effective antimicrobial therapy is usually selected with intent to achieve a peak level two to four times the MIC at the site of infection. An antimicrobial level 10 times the MIC is usually sought in urinary tract infections. The "breakpoints" are based on achievable levels of antibiotic in the blood and indicate MICs above which organisms are moderately or very resistant and would not be expected to respond to that antibiotic.

Susceptible: This category implies that an infection due to the strain may be appropriately treated with the dosage of antimicrobial agent recommended for that type of infection and infecting species, unless otherwise contraindicated.

Intermediate: This category provides a "buffer zone," which should prevent small, uncontrolled, technical factors from causing major discrepancies in interpretations (eg, species that should have few or no endpoints in this range, or drugs with *in vitro* results affected by media variation or drugs with narrow pharmacotoxicity margins).

Antimicrobial agents that are excreted via the kidneys can usually be used to treat uncomplicated cystitis due to an organism with intermediate susceptibility. For systemic infections, antimicrobials with intermediate activity should be avoided unless used in combination with a nonantagonistic agent with greater activity against the infecting organism; if such an agent does not exist, use maximal nontoxic dosing of the agent with intermediate activity.

Resistant: Strains falling in this category are not inhibited by the usually achievable systemic concentrations of the agent with normal dosage schedules and/or fall in the range in which specific microbial resistance mechanisms are likely (eg, beta-lactamases), and clinical efficacy has not been reliable in treatment studies. See the following information.

Major Mechanisms of Bacterial Antimicrobial Resistance

Enzymatic inactivation or modification of drug
- β-lactamase hydrolysis of β-lactam ring with subsequent inactivation of β-lactam antibiotics
- Modification of aminoglycosides by acetylating, adenylating, or phosphorylating enzymes
- Modification of chloramphenicol by chloramphenicol acetyltransferase

Decreased drug uptake or accumulation
- Intrinsic or acquired lack of outer membrane permeability
- Faulty or lacking antibiotic uptake and transport system
- Antibiotic efflux system

Altered or lacking antimicrobial target
- Altered penicillin-binding proteins (β-lactam resistance)
- Altered ribosomal target (eg, aminoglycoside, macrolide, and lincomycin resistance)
- Altered enzymatic target (eg, sulfonamide, trimethoprim, rifampin, and quinolone resistance)

Circumvention of drug action consequences
- Hyperproduction of drug targets or competitive substrates (eg, sulfonamide and trimethoprim resistance)

Uncoupling of antibiotic attack and cell death
- Bacterial tolerance and survival in presence of usually bactericidal drugs (eg, β-lactams and vancomycin)

Footnotes

1. National Committee for Clinical Laboratory Standards, "Performance Standards for Antimicrobial Disk Susceptibility Tests," Approved Standard M2-A7, Villanova, PA: National Committee for Clinical Laboratory Standards, 2000.
2. National Committee for Clinical Laboratory Standards, "Methods for Dilution Susceptibility Tests for Bacteria That Grow Aerobically." Approved Standard M7-A5, Villanova, PA: National Committee for Clinical Laboratory Standards, 2000.
3. National Committee for Clinical Laboratory Standards, "Performance Standards for Antimicrobial Testing," Supplemental Tables, NCCLS Document M100-S10 (M7-A5 Aerobic Dilution), Villanova, PA: National Committee for Clinical Laboratory Standards, 2000.
4. Elliott TS and Lambert PA, "Antimicrobial Resistance in the Intensive Care Unit: Mechanisms and Management," *Br Med Bull*, 1999, 55(1):259-76.
5. Cookson BD, "Nosocomial Antimicrobial Resistance Surveillance," *J Hosp Infect*, 1999, 43:S97-103.
6. Gaynes R, "The Impact of Antimicrobial Use on the Emergence of Antimicrobial Resistant Bacteria in Hospitals," *Infect Dis Clin North Am*, 1997, 11(4):757-65.
7. Jorgensen JH, "Selection Criteria for an Antimicrobial Susceptibility Testing System," *J Clin Microbiol*, 1993, 31(11):2841-4.

References

Cockerill FR III, "Conventional and Genetic Laboratory Tests Used to Guide Antimicrobial Therapy," *Mayo Clin Proc*, 1998, 73(10):1007-21.

Hessen MT and Kaye D, "Principles of Selection and Use of Antibacterial Agents. *In Vitro* Activity and Pharmacology," *Infect Dis Clin North Am*, 2000, 14(2):265-79.

Jorgensen JH, "Antimicrobial Susceptibility Testing of Bacteria That Grow Aerobically," *Infect Dis Clin North Am*, 1993, 7(2):393-409.

Rubenstein E, "Antimicrobial Resistance - Pharmacological Solutions," *Infection*, 1999, 27(S):32-4.

Schifman RB, Pindur A, and Bryan JA, "Laboratory Practices for Reporting Bacterial Susceptibility Tests That Affect Antibiotic Therapy," *Arch Pathol Lab Med*, 1997, 121(11):1168-70.

Thompson RL and Wright AJ, "General Principles of Antimicrobial Therapy," *Mayo Clin Proc*, 1998, 73(10):995-1006.

Turnbridge, JD and Jorgensen JH, "Antimicrobial Susceptibility Testing: General Considerations," *Manual of Clinical Microbiology*, 7th ed, Murray PR, Baron EJ, Pfaller MA, et al, eds. Washington, DC: ASM Press, American Society of Microbiology, 1999, 1469-73.

Virk A and Steckelberg JM, "Clinical Aspects of Antimicrobial Resistance," *Mayo Clin Proc*, 2000, 75(2):200-14.

Antimicrobial Susceptibility Testing, Anaerobic Bacteria

Related Information

Antimicrobial Susceptibility Testing, Antimicrobial Combinations *on page 556*

Antimicrobial Susceptibility Testing, Unusual Isolates/Fastidious Organisms *on page 558*

Bacterial Culture, Abscess *on page 562*

Bacterial Culture, Anaerobes *on page 564*

Beta-Lactamase Test *on page 581*

Synonyms Anaerobic Bacterial Susceptibility; E-Test, Anaerobic Bacteria; MIC, Anaerobic Bacteria; Sensitivity Testing, Anaerobic Bacteria; Susceptibility Testing, Anaerobic Bacteria

Abstract Antimicrobial susceptibility testing of anaerobic bacteria is important in selection of therapy for anaerobic infections which lack predictable susceptibility patterns, especially *Bacteroides* species. Most infections are treated empirically due to the time necessary to recover and test anaerobic bacteria.

Specimen A pure culture of the isolated organism to be tested, prepared by the laboratory

Turnaround Time 2-5 days from time organism is isolated and identified

Special Instructions Appropriateness and scope of anaerobic susceptibility testing in a particular clinical setting is supported by laboratory consultation.

Reference Interval See table.

Use Antimicrobial therapy of anaerobic infections is usually empiric because many of these infections are polymicrobic, and because there is an unavoidable delay in provision of results. The major reasons for testing are to determine susceptibility to new antimicrobials, to establish institutional or regional susceptibility patterns which may be used to guide empiric therapy, and to assist in management of infection in individual patients. Circumstances such as anaerobic brain abscess, endocarditis, osteomyelitis, and prosthetic device or vascular graft infections are particularly relevant.[1]

Limitations Anaerobic infections are often polymicrobial (involving aerobic and anaerobic organisms), and are associated with tissue necrosis and abscess formation resulting in impaired delivery of antimicrobial agents to the infection site.[2] Additionally, methods for recovering and identifying anaerobic bacteria are cumbersome and time consuming, resulting in elapsed periods of nearly a week before susceptibility test results are available. These factors, in conjunction with the fact that standardized methods for testing anaerobes are not always reliable and often produce growth patterns that are difficult to interpret, make the usefulness of routine susceptibility testing of anaerobic bacteria questionable.

Contraindications Anaerobic bacterial isolate from patient is not available or fails to give adequate growth for susceptibility testing

Methodology Broth microdilution, macrobroth dilution, and E-Test (gradient diffusion), agar dilution technique, beta-lactamase testing

Additional Information At present, routine susceptibility testing of anaerobic isolates is not recommended.[3] Infections involving anaerobes frequently contain mixed flora, and appropriate drainage rather than antimicrobial therapy seems to be the most crucial factor in the successful treatment of such infections.

Typical Sensitivities of Important Anaerobic Pathogens to Major Classes of Antibiotics

Antibiotic	B. fragilis Group	B. melaninogenicus Group	Fusobacterium	Clostridium	Propionibacterium	Actinomyces	Peptostreptococcus
Penicillin G	– to +	– to +++	++	+ to ++	+++	+++	+++
Antipseudomonal penicillins	++ to +++	+ to +++	+++	+++	+++	+++	+++
Cefoxitin	++	+++	++ to +++	– to ++	+++	+++	+++
Imipenem-cilastatin	+++	+++	++	+++	+++	+++	+++
Combinations of beta-lactam and beta-lactamase inhibitor	+++	+++	+++	+++	+++	+++	+++
Clindamycin	++ to +++	+++	+++	++	+++	+++	+++
Chloramphenicol	+++	+++	+++	+++	+++	+++	+++
Metronidazole	+++	+++	+++	+++	–	–	++ to +++

– denotes that <50% of the strains were susceptible.

+ denotes that 50% to 70% of the strains were susceptible.

++ denote that 70% to 90% of the strains were susceptible.

+++ denote that >90% of the strains were susceptible.

Adapted from Styrt B and Gorbach SL, "Recent Developments in the Understanding of the Pathogenesis and Treatment of Anaerobic Infections," *N Engl J Med*, 1989, Part I, 321:240-6 and Part II, 321:298-302 (review).

(Continued)

Antimicrobial Susceptibility Testing, Anaerobic Bacteria *(Continued)*

Indications for anaerobic susceptibility testing include:
- determination of susceptibility of anaerobes to new antimicrobial agents
- monitoring susceptibility patterns by geographic area
- monitoring susceptibility patterns in local hospitals
- assisting in the management of selected individual patients

Some anaerobes have predictable *in vitro* susceptibility patterns but grow so slowly that by the time isolation and susceptibility testing are completed (6-14 days), results are of little clinical value. Thus, susceptibility testing is generally performed only on anaerobic isolates from blood, pleural fluid, peritoneal fluid, and CSF. In cases of chronic anaerobic infections (septic arthritis, osteomyelitis, etc), susceptibility testing may be done by special request. The physician should contact the laboratory regarding the specific antibiotic(s) to be tested and the testing method available.

Footnotes

1. Finegold SM, "Perspective on Susceptibility Testing of Anaerobic Bacteria," *Clin Infect Dis*, 1997, 25(Suppl 2):S251-3.
2. Aldridge KE, "The Occurrence, Virulence, and Antimicrobial Resistance of Anaerobes in Polymicrobial Infections," *Am J Surg*, 1995, 169(5A Suppl):2S-7S.
3. National Committee for Clinical Laboratory Standards, "Methods for Antimicrobial Susceptibility Testing of Anaerobic Bacteria," Approved Standard, M11-A4, Villanova, PA: National Committee for Clinical Laboratory Standards, 1997.

References

Falagas ME and Siakavellas E, "*Bacteroides, Prevotella,* and *Porphyromonas* species: A Review of Antibiotic Resistance and Therapeutic Options," *Int J Antimicrob Agents*, 2000, 15(1):1-9.

Hecht DW, "Resistance Trends in Anaerobic Bacteria," *Clin Microbiol Newslet*, 2000, 22(6):41-4.

Hecht DW, "Susceptibility Testing of Anaerobic Bacteria," *Manual of Clinical Microbiology*, 7th ed, Murray PR, Baron EJ, Pfaller MA, et al, eds, Washington, DC: ASM Press, American Society of Microbiology, 1999, 1555-62.

Murdoch DA, "Gram-Positive Anaerobic Cocci," *Clin Microbiol Rev*, 1998, 11(1):81-120.

Nguyen MH, Yu VL, Morris AJ, et al, "Antimicrobial Resistance and Clinical Outcome of *Bacteroides*, Bacteremia: Findings of a Multicenter Prospective Observational Trial," *Clin Infect Dis*, 2000, 30(6):870-6.

Rasmussen BA, Bush K, and Tally FP, "Antimicrobial Resistance in Anaerobes," *Clin Infect Dis*, 1997, 24(Suppl 1):S110-20.

Virk A and Steckelberg JM, "Clinical Aspects of Antimicrobial Resistance," *Mayo Clin Proc*, 2000, 75(2):200-14.

Wexler HM, Molitoris E, and Molitoris D, "Susceptibility Testing of Anaerobes: Old Problems, New Options?" *Clin Infect Dis*, 1997, 25(Suppl 2):S275-8.

Antimicrobial Susceptibility Testing, Antimicrobial Combinations

Related Information

Antimicrobial Susceptibility Testing, Aerobic and Facultatively Anaerobic Bacteria *on page 554*

Antimicrobial Susceptibility Testing, Anaerobic Bacteria *on page 555*

Antimicrobial Susceptibility Testing, Unusual Isolates/Fastidious Organisms *on page 558*

Serum Bactericidal Test *on page 679*

Synonyms Antimicrobial Combinations - Test for Synergism and Antagonism; Susceptibility Testing, Antimicrobial Combinations; Synergistic Studies, Antimicrobial

Applies to Fractional Bactericidal Concentration (FBC); Fractional Inhibitory Concentration (FIC); Minimal Bactericidal Concentration (MBC); Minimal Inhibitory Concentration (MIC); Schlichter Test

Test Includes MICs of both antibiotics against patient's organism, determination of synergistic or antagonistic antimicrobial effect of drug combination

Abstract Susceptibility testing of antibiotics in combination, or synergy testing was originally used to predict clinical efficacy of antimicrobial treatment of serious infections. However, the test is complex and difficult to perform and to interpret. Therefore, it is rarely used except in investigation of the spectrum of a new antimicrobial agents.

Specimen A pure culture of the isolated organism to be tested, prepared by the laboratory

Causes for Rejection Organism discarded prior to request for test by physician, organism fails to grow on subculture or is too fastidious to grow under usual conditions of testing

Turnaround Time 2-4 days (depends on antimicrobials assayed and procedure used)

Special Instructions Notify the laboratory to retain organism needed for test.

Reference Interval Additive effect, synergism or antagonism

Use Determine whether the addition of a second antibiotic (B) will increase or decrease the known sensitivity of an organism to antibiotic (A). Some antibiotics have well established synergistic activity such as the use of a cell wall active agent (ie, penicillin and vancomycin) and an aminoglycoside to treat serious infections due to *Enterococcus faecalis*.[1] This test, which is performed by testing for susceptibility to high levels of gentamicin and streptomycin, should be reported routinely for this organism.[2] Other antibacterial agents are tested for their ability to inhibit each other, usually done for experimental purposes during development of new antibiotics.

Limitations This test procedure (other than that done for enterococci) is usually available only from specialized laboratories, predicated upon availability of antibiotic standard for testing. A test cannot be run if an organism fails to grow. The clinical relevance of synergy studies and standardized methods is still being defined.

Methodology Checkerboard titration, time-kill technique, double diffusion testing

Additional Information Laboratory should be notified 24 hours in advance of time when test is to be performed. Patient's organism must be saved at request of physician. Physician must specify antimicrobials to be tested in combination culture, site of isolated organism, and culture date. The MICs of antibiotics to be tested must be known or performed.

Combinations of antimicrobials are often used with intent of achieving a synergistic effect (ie, a demonstrated inhibitory or bactericidal activity that is greater than the sum of the activities of the agents alone). The use of combination therapy is also often undertaken to reduce potential toxicity. A lower dose of each agent may be used (eg, aminoglycosides and a cephalosporin or penicillin). The use of combinations prevents or minimizes the emergence of resistant strains.

Several methods, checkerboard titration, time-kill technique, and diffusion tests, are used in research settings.[3,4] When the checkerboard method is used, the MIC of each antibiotic is determined alone and in combination, and the Fractional Inhibitory Concentration (FIC) is calculated:

$$FIC = \frac{MIC_a \text{ in combination}}{MIC_a \text{ alone}} + \frac{MIC_b \text{ in combination}}{MIC_b \text{ alone}}$$

The combined inhibitory effect may be synergistic (FIC $\leq$0.5), additive (FIC = 1), indifferent (FIC = 2), or antagonistic (FIC $\geq$4) ("a" and "b" are the antimicrobials tested).

In usual clinical practice, testing of enterococci and viridans streptococci isolated from patients with serious infections for high level aminoglycoside resistance is adequate to predict the potential presence or absence of synergism, when these agents are combined with cell wall active agents (eg, cephalosporins, penicillins). Fixed-dose combinations, trimethoprim-sulfamethoxazole and beta-lactam/beta-lactamase inhibitor combinations (eg, amoxicillin-clavulanate or ticarcillin-clavulanate) can be tested because of the standard availability of combination disks and commercially prepared microtiter susceptibility panels which include the combinations.

A clear consensus regarding the usefulness of synergy studies has not yet emerged, primarily because of organism strain differences in response and lack of consensus on choice of laboratory methods. The greatest potential for clinical usefulness exists in patients with sustained profound neutropenia and in patients with endocarditis. The **serum bactericidal test (Schlichter test)** has efficacy to determine potential clinical effects of antimicrobial combinations in an individual patient, particularly in endocarditis and osteomyelitis.

Footnotes

1. Dressel DC, Tornatore-Reuscher MA, Boschman CR, et al, "Synergistic Effect of Gentamicin Plus Ampicillin on Enterococci With Differing Sensitivity to Gentamicin: A Phenotypic Assessment of NCCLS Guidelines," *Diagn Microbiol Infect Dis*, 1999, 35(3):219-25.
2. Swenson JM, Ferraro MJ and Sahm DF, "Multilaboratory Evaluation of Screening Methods for Detection of High-Level Aminoglycoside Resistance in Enterococci," *J Clin Microbiol*, 1995, 33(11):3008-18.
3. Eliopolous GM and Moellering RC Jr, "Antimicrobial Combinations," *Antibiotics in Laboratory Medicine*, 4th ed, Lorian V ed, Baltimore, MD: Lippincott Williams & Wilkins, 1996, 330-96.
4. Mackay ML, Milne K, and Gould IM, "Comparison of Methods for Assessing Synergic Antibiotic Interactions," *Int J Antimicrob Agents*, 2000, 15(2):125-9.

References

Acar JF, "Antibiotic Synergy and Antagonism," *Med Clin North Am*, 2000, 84(6):1391-406.

Bouza E and Munoz P, "Monotherapy Versus Combination Therapy for Bacterial Infections," *Med Clin North Am*, 2000, 84(6):1357-89.

Rand KH, Houck HJ, Brown P, et al, "Reproducibility of the Microdilution Checkerboard Method for Antibiotic Synergy," *Antimicrob Agents Chemother*, 1993, 37(3):613-5.

Virk A and Steckelberg JM, "Clinical Aspects of Antimicrobial Resistance," *Mayo Clin Proc*, 2000, 75(2):200-14.

Antimicrobial Susceptibility Testing, Fungi

Related Information

Amphotericin B, Serum *on page 737*

Antimicrobial Susceptibility Testing, Aerobic and Facultatively Anaerobic Bacteria *on page 554*

Fungal Culture, Biopsy or Body Fluid *on page 610*

Fungal Culture, Blood *on page 610*

Fungal Culture, Skin *on page 612*

Fungal Culture, Sputum *on page 613*

Fungus Smear, Stain *on page 615*

Itraconazole, Serum *on page 753*

Synonyms Fungi Susceptibility Testing; Susceptibility Testing, Fungi

Test Includes Broth dilution or agar dilution testing of antifungal agents. Results may be quantitative or qualitative.

Abstract Fungi have emerged in the last ten years as important nosocomial pathogens. As the incidence of serious fungal infections has increased a number of new antifungal agents have been introduced, thus the need for *in vitro* antifungal susceptibility tests. Susceptibility testing of yeasts is now standardized,[1] but standard methods and clinical relevance of antifungal susceptibility tests for filamentous fungi have not been determined.

Specimen A pure culture of the isolated organism to be tested, prepared by the laboratory

Causes for Rejection Organism disposed of prior to request for testing.

Special Instructions Consult the laboratory to determine availability and choice of methods.

Reference Interval See table.

Interpretive Guidelines (in μg/mL) for *in vitro* Susceptibility Testing of *Candida* Species

Agent	Susceptible	Susceptible-DD*	Intermediate	Resistant
Fluconazole†,‡	≤8	16-32	—	≥64
Itraconazole§	≤0.125	0.25-0.5	—	≥1
Flucytosine	≤4	—	8-16	≥32

*Susceptible-dose dependent; susceptibility depends on achieving maximal possible blood level.

†*Candida krusei* isolates are assumed to be intrinsically resistant to fluconazole.

‡Guidelines based on experience with mucosal infections, but are consistent with limited information for invasive infections.

§Guidelines based on experience with mucosal infections only.

Use Routine antifungal susceptibility testing is clearly unwarranted. In certain clinical circumstances, it may be appropriate to test *Candida* species and *Pseudoallescheria boydii*.[2] Susceptibility of yeasts against amphotericin B is problematic since results fall within a narrow range and therefore, are difficult to categorize. Several yeasts have demonstrated resistance to the azoles (eg, ketoconazole, itraconazole, fluconazole) and susceptibility testing may occasionally be warranted; the dimorphic fungi need not be tested since they are virtually always susceptible.[3]

Limitations Although susceptibility testing of yeasts has recently been standardized, the relationship between test results and patient response to therapy has not been established. In fact, little correlation is found between *in vitro* susceptibility results and clinical results.[3] Susceptibility testing of yeasts against the azoles often produces variable results.[1] Susceptibility testing of filamentous fungi has not been standardized and is quite variable; isolates should be sent to a well respected reference laboratory for testing.

Methodology A standardized broth-dilution method is available for susceptibility testing of yeasts.[1] The availability of a choice of therapeutic agents will continue to cause laboratories to attempt to provide susceptibility data with useful predictive value.

Additional Information Interpretation of *in vitro* susceptibility data for antifungal drugs has been hindered by the absence of standardized test criteria. Thus, it has been extremely difficult to identify a clear relation between *in vitro* minimal inhibitory concentrations and clinical outcome, which is highly dependent on host factors. However, some recent reports suggest that clinically significant resistance exists in some important fungal strains.[3,4] The situation appears more readily resolvable for yeast-like than for filamentous fungi, since the former are more easily quantified by standardized microbiologic techniques.[5,6] The E-Test, a continuous gradient diffusion method, may prove to be useful for susceptibility testing of yeasts. See Antimicrobial Susceptibility Testing, Unusual Isolates/Fastidious Organisms *on page 558*.

Footnotes

1. National Committee for Clinical Laboratory Standards, "Reference Method for Broth Dilution Antifungal Susceptibility Testing for Yeasts," Approved Standard Document M-27-A, Villanova, PA: National Committee for Clinical Laboratory Standards, 1997.
2. Gianinni MA, Pearson T, and Patrick CC, "Fungal Susceptibility Testing," *Pediatr Infect Dis J*, 1999, 18(11):1021-2.
3. Espinel-Ingroff A, White T, and Pfaller MA, "Antifungal Agents and Susceptibility Testing," *Manual of Clinical Microbiology*, 7th ed, Murray PR, Baron EJ, Pfaller MA, et al, eds, Washington, DC: AMS Press, American Society for Microbiology, 1999, 1640-52.
4. Vanden Bossche H, Dromer R, Improvisi L, et al, "Antifungal Drug Resistance in Pathogenic Fungi," *Med Mycol*, 1998, 36(Suppl 1):119-28.
5. Klepser ME, Lewis RE, and Pfaller MA, "Therapy of *Candida* Infections: Susceptibility Testing, Resistance and Therapeutic Options," *Ann Pharmacother*, 1998, 32(12):1353-61.
6. Espinel-Ingroff A, Kish CW Jr, Kerkering TM, et al, "Collaborative Comparison of Broth Macrodilution and Microdilution Antifungal Susceptibility Tests," *J Clin Microbiol*, 1992, 30(12):3138-45.

References

Arikan S, Lozano-Chiu M, Paetznick V, et al, "Microdilution Susceptibility Testing of Amphotericin B, Itraconazole, and Voriconazole Against Clinical Isolates of *Aspergillus* and *Fusarium* species," *J Clin Microbiol*, 1999, 37(12):3946-51.

Espinel-Ingroff A, Barchiesi F, Hazen KC, et al, "Standardization of Antifungal Susceptibility Testing and Clinical Relevance," *Med Mycol*, 1998, 36(Suppl 1):68-78.

Meis J, Petrou M, Bille J, et al, "A Global Evaluation of the Susceptibility of *Candida* Species to Fluconazole by Disk Diffusion. Global Antifungal Surveillance Group," *Diagn Microbiol Infect Dis*, 2000, 36(4):215-23.

Pfaller MA, Rex JH, and Rinaldi MG, "Antifungal Susceptibility Testing. Technical Advances and Potential Clinical Applications," *Clin Infect Dis*, 1997, 24(5):776-84.

Sheehan DJ, Hitchcock CA, and Sibley CM, "Current and Emerging Azole Antifungal Agents," *Clin Microbiol Rev*, 1999, 12(1):40-79.

Antimicrobial Susceptibility Testing, Minimum Bactericidal Concentration

Related Information

Antimicrobial Susceptibility Testing, Aerobic and Facultatively Anaerobic Bacteria *on page 554*

Synonyms MBC; Minimum Bactericidal Concentration; Minimum Lethal Concentration; MLC; Susceptibility Testing, Minimum Bactericidal Concentration

Applies to Tolerance Testing, Antimicrobial

Abstract The minimum bactericidal concentration (MBC) is the concentration of an antibiotic that kills 99%, 99.9%, or 100% of a standardized bacterial inoculum.

Specimen A pure culture of the isolated organism to be tested, prepared by the laboratory

Causes for Rejection Organism discarded prior to request by physician to save the organism for MBC, organism fails to grow on subculture from original plates

Turnaround Time 48 hours after isolation of bacterium to be tested

Special Instructions In order to perform an MBC test, an isolate of the organism of interest must be saved at the request of the physician, often within 48 hours of submission of specimen for initial culture. If the isolate has not been saved, the test cannot be performed. The laboratory should be informed by the physician of the specific source of the culture, culture date, as well as the specific bacterial isolate to be tested and the antimicrobial agent to be tested.

Reference Interval End points are generally reported as μg/mL of antimicrobial agent required to kill 99.9% of colonies.

Use Determine minimum bactericidal concentration, MBC, of an antimicrobial agent. Frequently utilized in endocarditis and osteomyelitis in immunocompromised hosts. Often used in premarket evaluation of new antibiotics but rarely used in clinical practice.

Limitations Results are accurate to plus or minus one dilution. However, technical factors including inoculum, medium, incubation, growth phase, tube type, mixing, and so forth, significantly influence results.

Contraindications Bacterium isolated from patient is not available or fails to grow for susceptibility testing.

Methodology Macrodilution or microdilution technique with subculture. Twofold dilutions of antibiotics are added to broth media that is then inoculated with a standard number of bacteria. After incubation, bacterial growth is monitored. The MIC of the isolate is determined by visually inspecting broth media, while the MBC is determined by plating a portion of each well/tube onto solid media and performing colony counts to determine the percent survival.

Additional Information Tolerance, defined as inhibition of growth without killing, is manifested in the laboratory as an MBC (minimum bactericidal concentration) 32 or more times the MIC (minimum inhibitory concentration). Tolerance is most frequently observed with vancomycin and beta-lactam antibiotics against gram-positive organisms. Although tolerance is frequently observed in the laboratory, it is not often associated with clinical treatment failure. The selection of an endpoint of 99.9% killing is used to avoid the problem of the "persistent phenomenon" where a few highly resistant organisms persist regardless of the concentration of the antimicrobial agent.

References

Cockerill FR III, "Conventional and Genetic Laboratory Tests Used to Guide Antimicrobial Therapy," *Mayo Clin Proc*, 1998, 73(10):1007-21.

Hacek DM, Dressel DC, and Petersen LR, "Highly Reproducible Bactericidal Activity Test Results by Using a Modified National Committee for Clinical Laboratory Standards Broth Macrodilution Technique," *J Clin Microbiol*, 1999, 37(6):1881-4.

James PA, "Comparison of Four Methods for the Determination of MIC and MBC of Penicillin for Viridans Streptococci and the Implications for Penicillin Tolerance," *J Antimicrob Chemother*, 1990, 25(2):209-16.

National Committee for Clinical Laboratory Standards, "Methods for Determining Bactericidal Activity of Antimicrobial Agents," Tentative Guideline M26-T, 1992.

Schentag JJ, "Antimicrobial Action and Pharmacokinetics/Pharmacodynamics: The Use of AUIC to Improve Efficacy and Avoid Resistance," *J Chemother*, 1999, 11(6):426-39.

Antimicrobial Susceptibility Testing, Mycobacteria

Related Information

Antimicrobial Susceptibility Testing, Aerobic and Facultatively Anaerobic Bacteria *on page 554*

Mycobacterial Culture, Biopsy or Body Fluid *on page 655*

Mycobacterial Culture, Cutaneous and Subcutaneous Tissue *on page 657*

Mycobacterial Culture, Sputum *on page 658*

Mycobacterial Culture, Stool *on page 659*

(Continued)

Antimicrobial Susceptibility Testing, Mycobacteria

(Continued)

Mycobacterial Culture, Urine *on page 660*

Synonyms Mycobacteria Susceptibility Testing; Susceptibility Testing, Mycobacteria

Test Includes Panel of antimycobacterial agents tested against clinical isolates at appropriate concentrations

Abstract Susceptibility testing of *Mycobacterium tuberculosis* is important in determining long-term therapy of infections. Broth methods are more rapid and correlate well with the proportion method and have replaced it in many laboratories. Broth-dilution methods are used to test rapidly-growing mycobacteria, but the methods and interpretation have not been standardized.

Specimen A pure culture of the isolated organism to be tested, prepared by the laboratory

Causes for Rejection Specimen not available for testing.

Turnaround Time 4-6 weeks after organism is isolated and identified

Use Determine the susceptibility of the isolated organism to a panel of antimycobacterial agents

Limitations Methodology and interpretive criteria for *M. tuberculosis* is well standardized. Methodology and interpretive criteria for *Mycobacterium* species other than *M. tuberculosis* have not been standardized; consequently, the distinction between susceptible and resistant isolates is often unclear.[1]

Methodology Disk diffusion, agar containing antibiotic, or broth containing antibiotic. Quantitative methods may be required to accurately assess the clinical value of susceptibility data provided when an atypical species, particularly one of the rapidly-growing mycobacteria, is tested. See table.

Antimicrobials Commonly Used for Mycobacterial Susceptibility Testing

Antituberculosis Drugs	
Primary	**Secondary**
Ethambutol	Capreomycin
Isoniazid	Ciprofloxacin
Pyrazinamide	Cycloserine
Rifampin	Ethionamide
Streptomycin	Kanamycin
Other Mycobacterial Isolates*	
Rapidly Growing Mycobacteria*	***Mycobacterium avium-intracellulare* Complex**
Amikacin	Azithromycin OR
Cefoxitin	Clarithromycin
Ciprofloxacin	
Doxycycline	
Imipenem	
Sulfonamides	
Tobramycin	

*Drug regimens will depend on the mycobacterial species identified.

Adapted from Wolinsky E, "Mycobacterial Diseases Other Then Tuberculosis," *Clin Infect Dis*, 1992, 15(1):1-10.

Additional Information Susceptibilities are performed on the first organism isolated from a patient and at 3- to 6-month intervals, if that organism continues to be isolated while the patient is on therapy. Susceptibility tests should be performed in patients with recurrent tuberculosis, as resistant strains are common in recurrent infection. The incidence of tuberculosis increased in the United States between 1985 and 1991. High incidence populations were identified in depressed inner city areas, some rural areas, among new immigrants, in prison inmates, and in HIV-positive patients.[2,3] An increasing number of these isolates were resistant to typical mycobacterial drugs.[3,4] However, since 1992 the number of tuberculosis cases has consistently declined in the U.S., primarily due to the effectiveness of prevention and control measures implemented by the CDC. Such control measures include the rapid and prompt identification of *M. tuberculosis* by the laboratory, preventive therapy in high-risk populations, decreased transmission in correctional facilities, and improved follow-up of tuberculosis patients. In spite of measures taken in the U.S., tuberculosis is very prevalent throughout the world. Failure to take all drugs in a multidrug regimen can lead to a shift toward resistant organisms and treatment failure. Atypical or environmental mycobacteria, particularly strains of the *M. avium* complex, demonstrate variable susceptibility within species. They are frequently resistant to oral therapy.[5,6]

Footnotes

1. Inderfield CB and Salfinger M, "Antimicrobial Agents and Susceptibility Tests: Mycobacteria," *Manual of Clinical Microbiology*, 6th ed, Murray PR, Baron EJ, Pfaller MA, et al, eds, Washington, DC: ASM Press, American Society for Microbiology, 1999, 1601-23.
2. Centers for Disease Control, "Tuberculosis Morbidity - United States, 1991," *MMWR Morb Mortal Wkly Rep*, 1992, 41:240.
3. Beck-Sague C, Dooley Sw, Hutton MD, et al, "Hospital Outbreak of Multidrug-Resistant *Mycobacterium tuberculosis* Infections. Factors in Transmission to Staff and HIV-Infected Patients," *JAMA*, 1992, 268(10):1280-6.
4. Dooley SW, Villarino ME, Lawrence M, et al, "Nosocomial Transmission of Tuberculosis in a Hospital Unit for HIV-Infected Patients," *JAMA*, 1992, 267(19):2632-4.
5. Wolinsky E, "Mycobacterial Diseases Other Than Tuberculosis," *Clin Infect Dis*, 1992, 15(1):1-10.
6. Smith DS, Lindholm-Levy P, Huitt GA, et al, "*Mycobacterium terrae*: Case Reports, Literature Review, and *In Vitro* Antibiotic Susceptibility Testing," *Clin Infect Dis*, 2000, 30(3):444-53.

References

Heifets LB, "Antimycobacterial Drugs," *Semin Respir Infect*, 1994, 9(2):84-103.

Neville K, Bromberg A, Bromberg R, et al, "The Third Epidemic - Multidrug-Resistant Tuberculosis," *Chest*, 1994, 105(1):45-8.

Pfyffer GE, Bonato DA, Ebrahimzadeh A, et al, "Multicenter Laboratory Validation of Susceptibility Testing of *Mycobacterium tuberculosis* Against Classical Second-Line and Newer Antimicrobial Drugs by Using the Radiometric Bactec® 460 Technique and the Proportion Method With Solid Media," *J Clin Microbiol*, 1999, 37(10):3179-86.

Rusch-Gerdes S, Domehl C, Nardi G, et al, "Multicenter Evaluation of the Mycobacteria Growth Indicator Tube for Testing Susceptibility of *Mycobacterium tuberculosis* to First-Line Drugs," *J Clin Microbiol*, 1999, 37(1):45-8.

Siddiqi SH, Heifets LB, Cynamon MH, et al, "Rapid Broth Macrodilution Method for Determination of MICs for *Mycobacterium avium* Isolates," *J Clin Microbiol*, 1993, 31(9):2332-8.

Antimicrobial Susceptibility Testing, Unusual Isolates/Fastidious Organisms

Related Information

Antimicrobial Susceptibility Testing, Aerobic and Facultatively Anaerobic Bacteria *on page 554*

Antimicrobial Susceptibility Testing, Anaerobic Bacteria *on page 555*

Antimicrobial Susceptibility Testing, Antimicrobial Combinations *on page 556*

Synonyms MIC, Fastidious Organisms, Unusual Isolates; Minimum Inhibitory Concentration, Unusual Isolates; Susceptibility Testing, Unusual Isolates/Fastidious Organisms

Applies to E-Test

Test Includes Panel of antibiotics or single antibiotic selected by physician

Abstract Broth-dilution susceptibility testing is used to determine the minimal inhibitory concentration of one or more antibiotics considered for treatment of an infection due to a fastidious organism. It is especially useful when published studies of antimicrobial susceptibility are not available, or when the patient is unable to take the most commonly prescribed antibiotics.

Specimen A pure culture of the isolated organism to be tested, prepared by the laboratory

Causes for Rejection Organism discarded prior to request by physician to save the organism for susceptibility testing. Certain isolates are too fastidious (eg, some anaerobes, some streptococci) to perform susceptibility testing.

Turnaround Time 24-48 hours after isolation of bacterium

Special Instructions An isolate of the organism of interest must be saved at the request of the physician. The request usually must be received by the laboratory within 48 hours of submission of specimen for initial culture, in order to perform an MIC test. Broth dilution minimum inhibitory concentration (MIC) susceptibility can be requested for drugs not in the routine panels. The laboratory should be informed by the physician of the specific source of the culture, culture date, the specific bacterial isolate to be tested, and the antimicrobial agent(s) to be tested.

Reference Interval Minimal inhibitory concentration reported in µg/mL of antimicrobial agent. Results may be qualitatively reported as susceptible (S), intermediate (I), and resistant (R) if interpretive standards are available.

Use Determine minimum inhibitory concentration (MIC) of a given organism to an antimicrobial agent

Limitations The organism may fail to grow in media used for testing. A disk diffusion susceptibility test (Kirby-Bauer susceptibility) is usually reported (susceptible, intermediate, resistant) if interpretive criteria exist. If interpretive criteria do not exist, the MIC or zone size will be reported.

Methodology Broth microdilution or macrodilution technique, disk diffusion. Special methods are required for individual species. These generally include addition of supplement and/or alteration of incubation atmosphere.

Additional Information The terms "fastidious or unusual isolates" refer to organisms that do not grow well on Mueller-Hinton medium or are unusual in that there is insufficient data to document that reliable susceptibility testing can be performed by routine methods. Organisms such as *Haemophilus influenzae* and *Neisseria gonorrhoeae* have developed resistance to beta-lactam antibiotics by plasmid or chromosomal genes mediating the production of beta-lactamase.[1,2] Other organisms, such as *Streptococcus pneumoniae*, have developed chromosomal gene mediated alteration of the penicillin-binding proteins. Because of the emergence of resistance, empiric therapy with penicillin or ampicillin can no longer be relied upon, and susceptibility testing for such "fastidious" organisms may be necessary. Susceptibility testing of group A streptococci to penicillin is not necessary because the organism remains highly susceptible; however, resistance to erythromycin and tetracycline has been reported, and susceptibility testing may be appropriate if these drugs are used to treat serious infections.

The following organisms generally require special susceptibility testing procedures: anaerobes, *Moraxella* (*Branhamella*) *catarrhalis*, *Helicobacter* species, *Corynebacterium* species, *Francisella tularensis*, *Haemophilus influenzae*, *Legionella* species, *Listeria monocytogenes*, *Neisseria meningitidis*, *Neisseria gonorrhoeae*, *Nocardia* species, nonfermentative bacteria, *Streptococcus pneumoniae*, *Streptococcus* species, *Streptococcus* species peridoxal dependent.

Methods for susceptibility testing of the above organisms are reasonably well defined and are designed to vary as little as possible from the well established methods used for rapidly growing "nonfastidious" aerobic organisms.[3] Interpretive standards are available for anaerobes, *H. influenzae*, *N. gonorrhoeae*, some nonfermentative bacteria, *S. pneumoniae*, and *Streptococcus* species. Results for other organisms will usually be reported as an MIC value without further interpretation.[4]

The **gradient diffusion (epsilometer testing) (E test)** is an *in vitro* susceptibility testing method now being used for quantitative determination of susceptibility to antimicrobial agents.[5,6] This test uses a defined continuous antimicrobial gradient on a thin plastic strip. When the E-strip is placed on a confluent lawn of bacteria on agar media, the antimicrobial agent diffuses, producing an organism inhibition ellipse. The intercept of the ellipse with the graded test strip indicates MICs. This testing procedure provides a reliable method to assess antimicrobial sensitivity of fastidious isolates.

Footnotes

1. Doern GV, Brueggemann AB, Pierce G, et al, "Antibiotic Resistance Among Clinical Isolates of *Haemophilus influenzae* in the United States in 1994 and 1995 and Detection of β-Lactamase-Positive Strains Resistant to Amoxicillin-Clavulanate: Results of a National Multicenter Surveillance Study," *Antimicrob Agents Chemother*, 1997, 41(2):292-7.
2. Lind I, "Antimicrobial Resistance in *Neisseria gonorrhoeae*," *Clin Infect Dis*, 1997, 24(Suppl 1):93-7.
3. National Committee for Clinical Laboratory Standards, "Methods for Dilution Susceptibility Tests for Bacteria That Grow Aerobically," Approved Standard M7-A5, Villanova, PA: National Committee for Clinical Laboratory Standards, 2000.
4. National Committee for Clinical Laboratory Standards, "Performance Standards for Antimicrobial Testing," Supplemental Tables, NCCLS Document M100-S10 (M7-A2 Aerobic Dilution), Villanova, PA: National Committee for Clinical Laboratory Standards, 2000.
5. Sanchez ML, Barrett MS, and Jones RN, "The E-Test Applied to Susceptibility Tests for Gonococci, Multiply Resistant Enterococci and *Enterobacterioceae* Producing Potent Beta-Lactamases," *Diagn Microbiol Infect Dis*, 1992, 15(5):459-64.
6. Cockerill FR III, "Conventional and Genetic Laboratory Tests Used to Guide Antimicrobial Therapy," *Mayo Clin Proc*, 1998, 73(10):1007-21.

References

Fox KK, Knapp JS, Holmes KK, et al, "Antimicrobial Resistance of *Neisseria gonorrhoeae* in the United States, 1988-1994; The Emergence of Decreased Susceptibility to Fluoroquinolones," *J Infect Dis*, 1997, 175(6):1396-1403.

Hindler JA and Swenson JM, "Susceptibility Tests of Fastidious Bacteria," *Manual of Clinical Microbiology*, 7th ed, Murray PR, Baron EJ, Pfaller MA, et al, eds, Washington, DC: AMS Press, American Society for Microbiology, 1999, 1544-54.

Jones RN and Pfaller MA, "*In Vitro* Activity of Newer Fluoroquinolones for Respiratory Tract Infections and Emerging Patterns of Antimicrobial Resistance: Data from the SENTRY Antimicrobial Surveillance Program," *Clin Infect Dis*, 2000, 31(Suppl 2):S16-23.

Jorgensen JH and Ferraro MJ, "Antimicrobial Susceptibility Testing: Special Needs for Fastidious Organisms and Difficult-to-Detect Resistance Mechanisms," *Clin Infect Dis*, 2000, 30(5):799-808.

Venglarcik JS 3rd, "*Streptococcus pneumoniae* Antimicrobial Susceptibility Testing," *Pediatr Infect Dis J*, 2000, 19(4):329-31.

♦ **Antistreptococcal DNase-B Titer** *see* Antideoxyribonuclease-B Titer, Serum *on page 554*

Antistreptolysin O Titer, Serum

Related Information

Antideoxyribonuclease-B Titer, Serum *on page 554*
Bacterial Culture, Throat, and Antigen Detection Testing for Group A Streptococci *on page 577*
Group A *Streptococcus* Screen, Rapid *on page 617*
Sedimentation Rate, Erythrocyte *on page 484*
Streptozyme *on page 682*

Synonyms ASO

Abstract Detection of elevated immune responses to extracellular products of *S. pyogenes* (eg, streptolysin O), is useful in demonstration of streptococcal infections in patients without documentation of recent infection, who present with nonsuppurative sequelae such as rheumatic fever or glomerulonephritis. While sequential ASO assays are required, a single increased titer of anti-DNase provides indication of recent streptococcal infection.

Specimen Serum

Container Red top tube

Reference Interval Younger than 2 years of age: usually <50 Todd units; 2-5 years: <100 Todd units; 5-19 years: <166 Todd units; adults: <125 Todd units. A rise in titer of four or more dilution increments between acute and convalescent specimens is considered to be significant regardless of the magnitude of the titer. For a single specimen, ASO titers ≤166 Todd units are considered normal; but higher titers may be "normal" in demographic groups or may be associated with chronic pharyngeal carriage.

Use Used with throat culture, antideoxyribonuclease-B and other investigations to document streptococcal infection including acute pharyngitis, tonsillitis, and scarlet fever. A marked rise in titer or a persistently elevated ASO titer indicates a recent or current infection with beta-hemolytic group A *Streptococcus* (*Streptococcus pyogenes*). Elevated titers are seen in 80% to 85% of patients with acute rheumatic fever and in up to 95% of patients with acute glomerulonephritis, but in patients with glomerulonephritis responses are variable.[1]

Poststreptococcal reactive arthritis is an arthritis which follows β-hemolytic streptococcal infection, in patients lacking criteria for acute rheumatic fever. Increased ASO and antideoxyribonuclease-B titers are useful to confirm recent streptococcal infection for this diagnosis.[2]

Limitations False-positive ASO titers can be caused by increased levels of serum betalipoprotein produced in liver disease and by contamination of the serum with *Bacillus cereus* and *Pseudomonas* species. ASO is not sensitive for the diagnosis of streptococcal pyoderma.[1] Test is subject to false positives due to technical and clinical circumstances.

Methodology Nephelometry (the nephelometric assay may provide optimal sensitivity[3]), hemolysis inhibition, latex agglutination (LA)

Additional Information Streptolysin is a hemolysin produced by group A streptococci. In an infected individual streptolysin O acts as a protein antigen, and the patient mounts an antibody response. A rise in titer begins about 1 week after infection and peaks 2-4 weeks later. In the absence of complications or reinfection, the ASO titer will usually fall to preinfection levels within 6-12 months. Both clinical and laboratory findings should be correlated in reaching a diagnosis.

Other relevant investigations include throat culture, streptozyme, WBC count, and ESR.

Footnotes

1. Todd JK, "Group A *Streptococcus*," *Nelson Textbook of Pediatrics*, 16th ed, Chapter 184, Behrman RE, Kliegman RM, and Jenson HB, eds, WB Saunders Co, 2000, 802-10.
2. Aviles RJ, Ramakrishna G, Mohr DN, et al, "Poststreptococcal Reactive Arthritis in Adults: A Case Series," *Mayo Clin Proc*, 2000, 75(2):144-7.
3. Pacifico L, Mancuso G, Properzi E, et al, "Comparison of Nephelometric and Hemolytic Techniques for Determination of Antistreptolysin O Antibodies," *Am J Clin Pathol*, 1995, 103(4):396-9.

References

Ayoub EM and Harden E, "Immune Response to Streptococcal Antigens: Diagnostic Methods," *Manual of Clinical Laboratory Immunology*, 5th ed, Rose NR, Conway de Macario E, Folds JD, et al, eds, Washington, DC: ASM Press, American Society for Microbiology, 1997, 450-7.

Besada E, Schatz S, and Saremi SS, "Poststreptococcal Uveitis," *Optometry*, 2000, 71(4):233-8.

Cunningham MW, "Pathogenesis of Group A Streptococcal Infections," *Clin Microbiol Rev*, 2000, 13(3):470-511.

Efstratiou A, "Group A Streptococci in the 1990s," *J Antimicro Chemother*, 2000, 45(Suppl):3-12.

Kaplan EL, Rothermel CD, and Johnson DR, "Antistreptolysin O and Antideoxyribonuclease B Titers: Normal Values for Children Ages 2 to 12 in the United States," *Pediatrics*, 1998, 101(1):86-8.

Olivier C, "Rheumatic Fever - Is It Still a Problem?" *J Antimicro Chemother*, 2000, 45(Suppl):13-21.

♦ **Ants** *see* Arthropod Identification *on page 559*

♦ **Arboviral Encephalitis Serology** *see* St Louis Encephalitis Virus Serology *on page 681*

♦ **Arbovirus Antibodies: Arbovirus Titer** *see* Western Equine Encephalitis Virus Serology *on page 697*

♦ **Arboviruses** *see* Encephalitis Viral Serology *on page 604*

♦ **Arbovirus Serology** *see* Encephalitis Viral Serology *on page 604*

♦ **ARD, Blood Culture** *see* Bacterial Culture, Blood *on page 566*

Arthropod Identification

Related Information

Babesiosis Serology *on page 561*
Cerebrospinal Fluid Analysis: Overview *on page 416*
Ehrlichiosis Serology *on page 603*
Lyme Disease DNA Detection *on page 649*
Lyme Disease Serology *on page 650*
Q Fever Serology *on page 673*
Rocky Mountain Spotted Fever Serology *on page 676*
Tularemia Serology *on page 686*

Synonyms Ectoparasite Identification; Insect Identification

Applies to Ants; Beetles; Centipedes; *Cimex* Identification; Crustaceans; *Dermacentor andersoni*; Entomology; Flea Identification; Flies; Hemipterae; Hymenopterae; *Ixodes dammini* Identification; Lepidopterae; Lice Identification; Millipedes; Mite Identification; Nits Identification; *Pediculus humanus* Identification; *Phthirus pubis* Identification; *Sarcoptes scabiei* Skin Scrapings Identification; Scorpions; Skin Scrapings for *Sarcoptes scabiei* Identification; Spiders; Tick-Borne Diseases; Tick Identification

Abstract Arthropoda is a phylum which includes *Arachnida* and *Insecta*, among other classes. Species include parasites and vectors. *Arachnida*
(Continued)

Arthropod Identification *(Continued)*

includes spiders, ticks, mites, and scorpions. *Hymenoptera* include ants, bees, wasps, and hornets.

Tick-borne illnesses include ehrlichiosis, Lyme disease, babesiosis, relapsing fever, tularemia, Rocky Mountain spotted fever, and tick typhus.

Specimen Gross arthropod, skin scrapings

Container Screw-cap tube or screw-cap jar

Collection Arthropods (gross) are to be submitted in alcohol (70%) or formaldehyde in tube or container with secure closure. To establish the diagnosis of scabies, skin scrapings may be collected with a scalpel and a drop of mineral oil. The liquid may be examined directly or alternatively the organism may be teased away from its burrow or papule with a needle or scalpel.

Storage Instructions Maintain specimen at room temperature. Fill the container with preservative as completely as possible to avoid damage to the specimen by air bubbles in the container.

Special Instructions Correct identification of vectors can play a role in clinical diagnosis, especially in instances in which definitive diagnosis may be difficult (eg, Lyme disease).[1,2] Assistance of individuals trained in entomology in specimen identification may be pivotal.[3]

Use Identify arthropods affecting man; establish the presence of ectoparasite infestation. See graphic.

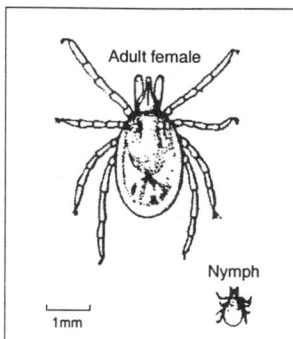

Deer tick (*Ixodes dammini*)

Lyme disease and **babesiosis** may be transmitted to humans by two species of ticks. *Ixodes scapularis* (or *I. dammini*) has been implicated along the Eastern seaboard, and in Southern and North Central states. *I. pacificus* is the most common vector in Western states. In Europe, **Lyme disease** is most often transmitted to humans by *I. ricinus*. *Ehrlichia* sp, known to cause human **ehrlichiosis**, is carried by the tick *Amblyomma americanum*. Other diseases in which ticks are vectors include **Colorado tick fever**, **Rocky Mountain spotted fever**, **tick typhus**, **Q fever**, **tularemia**, and **babesiosis**.

The only vector of louse-borne **relapsing fever** is the body louse. The other variety, endemic relapsing fever, is tick-borne.[4,5]

Tick paralysis, caused by an engorged, attached tick, presents as ascending paralysis. Prompt recovery follows tick removal (see Cerebrospinal Fluid Analysis: Overview *on page 416*). The differential diagnosis includes myasthenia gravis, botulism, or Guillain-Barré syndrome. *Dermacentor andersoni* (the North American wood tick), *D. variabilis* (the common dog tick), and *Ixodes holocyclus* affect humans.[6] *Dermacentor* ticks can harbor *Rickettsia* and transmit Rocky Mountain spotted fever.[7,8]

Scabies is a skin disease in which the itch mite, *Sarcoptes scabiei*, bores into the stratum corneum. Mites act as vectors of **Western equine encephalitis, St Louis encephalitis, murine typhus**, and rickettsialpox. Lice are vectors of **typhus, trench fever**, and **epidemic (louse-borne) relapsing fever**. Mosquitoes are vectors of **malaria, filariasis, viral encephalitis, dengue fever**, and **yellow fever**. Deer flies are vectors of **loiasis** and **tularemia**. Black flies are vectors of **onchocerciasis**. Tsetse flies are vectors of **trypanosomiasis**. Sand flies are vectors of **Leishmaniasis bartonellosis** and **sand fly fever**. Cone-nose (reduvid) (triatomid) bugs are vectors of **Chagas' disease**. Fleas are vectors of **plague, murine typhus, *Rickettsia felis*, *Dypilidium caninum*, *Hymenolepsis diminuta*, and *Bartonella henselae*.[9]

Limitations Of specimens submitted for tick identifications, arthropods included spider beetles, mites, true bugs, lice, and spiders. Ticks are distinguished by four pairs of legs, but antennae of some insects can be confused with legs. Some excellent illustrations are published.[1,3]

Methodology Macroscopic evaluation

Additional Information One outstanding volume we recommend provides useful, extensive tables, maps, transmission cycle diagrams, and color plates of human disease as well as of arthropods, including eggs, nymphs, larvae, and adults.[10]

Footnotes

1. Fix AD, Strickland GT, and Grant J, "Tick Bites and Lyme Disease in an Endemic Setting: Problematic Use of Serologic Testing and Prophylactic Antibiotic Therapy," *JAMA*, 1998, 279(3):206-10.

2. Barbour AG, "Expert Advice and Patient Expectations: Laboratory Testing and Antibiotics for Lyme Disease," *JAMA*, 1998, 279(3):239-40.

3. Falco RC, Fish D, and D'Amico V, "Accuracy of Tick Identification in a Lyme Disease Endemic Area," *JAMA*, 1998, 280(7):602-3.

4. Westenfeld FW, "Clinical Pathology Rounds. Relapsing Fever in a Recent Visitor to Africa," *Lab Med*, 1997, 28(7):436-8.

5. Cooper RI and Neuhauser T, Images in Clinical Medicine, "Borreliosis," *N Engl J Med*, 1998, 338(4):231.

6. Wu ML, Warren DJ, and Jones VA, "Ticked Off: *Ixodes*," *Arch Pathol Lab Med*, 2000, 124(6):925.

7. Felz MW, Smith CD, and Swift TR, "A Six-Year-Old Girl With Tick Paralysis," *N Engl J Med*, 2000, 342(2):90-4.

8. Schaumburg HH and Herskovitz S, "The Weak Child - A Cautionary Tale," *N Engl J Med*, 2000, 342(2):127-9.

9. Schlossberg D, "Arthropods and Leeches," *Cecil Textbook of Medicine*, 21st ed, Goldman L and Bennett JC, eds, Philadelphia PA: WB Sanders Co, 2000, 1995-2000.

10. Peters W, *A Colour Atlas of Arthropods in Clinical Medicine*, London, England: Wolfe Publishing Ltd, 1992.

References

Belongia EA, Reed KD, Mitchell PD, et al, "Clinical and Epidemiological Features of Early Lyme Disease and Human Granulocytic Ehrlichiosis in Wisconsin," *Clin Infect Dis*, 1999, 29(6):1472-7.

Conte JE Jr, "A Novel Approach to Preventing Insect-Borne Diseases," *N Engl J Med*, 1997, 337(11):785-6.

Dalton MT and Haldane DJ, "Unusual Dermal Arthropod Infestations," *Can Med Assoc J*, 1990, 143(2):113-4.

deShazo RD, Williams DF, and Moak ES, "Fire Ant Attacks on Residents in Health Care Facilities: A Report of Two Cases," *Ann Intern Med*, 1999, 131(6):424-9.

Driscoll DM and Tronic B, Images in Clinical Medicine, "*Pediculosis capitis*," *N Engl J Med*, 1996, 335(11):790.

Fritsche TR, "Arthropods of Medical Importance," *Manual of Clinical Microbiology*, 7th ed, Murray PR, Baron EJ, Pfaller MA, et al, eds, Washington, DC: AMS Press, American Society of Microbiology, 1999, 1449-66.

Goddard J, *Physician's Guide to Arthropods of Medical Importance*, Boca Raton, FL: CRC Press, 1993.

Hobbs GD and Harrell RE Jr, "Brown Recluse Spider Bites: A Common Cause of Necrotic Arachnidism," *Am J Emerg Med*, 1989, 7(3):309-12.

Moffitt JE, Yates AB, and Stafford CT, "Allergy to Insect Stings. A Need for Improved Preventive Management," *Postgrad Med*, 1993, 93(8):197-9, 203-4, 207-8.

Persing DH, "The Cold Zone: A Curious Convergence of Tick-Transmitted Diseases," *Clin Infect Dis*, 1997, 25(Suppl 1):S35-42.

Reisman RE, "Venom Hypersensitivity," *J Allergy Clin Immunol*, 1994, 94(4):651-8.

Spach DH, Liles WC, Campbell GL, et al, "Tick-Borne Diseases in the United States," *N Engl J Med*, 1993, 329(13):936-47.

Stack LB, Images in Clinical Medicine, "*Lactodectus mactans*," *N Engl J Med*, 1997, 336(23):1649.

♦ **ART Test** *replaced by* RPR *on page 677*

♦ ***Ascaris lumbricoides*** *see* Ova and Parasites, Stool *on page 666*

♦ **ASO** *see* Antistreptolysin O Titer, Serum *on page 559*

♦ **Aspergillosis antibodies** *see* Aspergillus Serology *on page 560*

Aspergillus Serology

Related Information

Bronchial Washings Cytology *on page 374*
Fungal Culture, Biopsy or Body Fluid *on page 610*
Fungal Culture, Blood *on page 610*
Fungal Culture, Sputum *on page 613*
Hypersensitivity Pneumonitis Serology *on page 530*
Immunoglobulin E *on page 533*
Lymphocyte Transformation Test *on page 539*

Synonyms Aspergillosis antibodies

Applies to Fungus Ball

Test Includes Complement fixing or precipitating antibodies

Abstract *Aspergillus* serology has been used to support a diagnosis of invasive aspergillosis in immunocompromised patients, and as one of the components in testing for hypersensitivity pneumonitis. Aspergillosis in tissue sections is characterized by broad septated hyphae with 45 degree branching angles.

Specimen Serum

Container Red top tube

Special Instructions Acute and convalescent serum specimens are desirable.

Reference Interval Immunodiffusion: no precipitin bands detected; positive: at least one precipitin band detected. **Complement fixation:** titer <1:8 or less than fourfold increase.

Use Confirm the presence of serum precipitating antibodies to *Aspergillus* species

Limitations A negative test does not rule out aspergillosis. Nonspecific precipitin bands could be due to presence of C-reactive protein. Cross reactions may occur in cases of histoplasmosis, coccidioidomycosis and blastomycosis. Bands due to reaction with C-reactive protein can be removed by sodium citrate.

The value of complement fixing antibodies in the diagnosis of pulmonary aspergillosis is not established.

Methodology Immunodiffusion (ID), complement fixation (CF), enzyme-linked immunosorbent assay (ELISA)

Additional Information Aspergillosis immunodiffusion: Sera can be tested against a polyvalent antigen mixture, or a series of species preparations. The greater the number of bands, the greater the likelihood of either a fungus ball or invasive aspergillosis. *Aspergillus* precipitins are seen in 90% of patients with **fungus balls** (aspergillomas), 70% of patients with **allergic bronchopulmonary aspergillosis**, and less often in patients with **invasive aspergillosis**, who usually are immunocompromised, have been on long-term corticosteroids and antibiotics, and often fail to produce detectable antibodies. Invasive pulmonary aspergillosis is a subacute pneumonia, in the periphery of which a thrombosed vessel may be found. Hematogenous dissemination takes place in ~25% of cases.

Fungus balls are saprophytic colonization of pre-existing lung cavities.

Primary criteria for the diagnosis of **allergic bronchopulmonary aspergillosis** include asthma, peripheral blood eosinophilia, immediate skin reactivity and precipitating antibody to *Aspergillus* antigen, elevated serum IgE, pulmonary infiltrates and central bronchiectasis. Secondary criteria include *Aspergillus fumigatus* in sputum, history of expectoration of brown plugs or flecks, and Arthus reaction (late skin reactivity) to *Aspergillus* antigen. Allergic bronchopulmonary aspergillosis is reported in 6% to 20% of patients with asthma and in 5.8% of patients with cystic fibrosis.[1] It is a hypersensitivity reaction which may progress to a fibrotic end stage.[2] Impacted mucin may contain large numbers of eosinophils and Charcot-Leyden crystals.[3] The demonstration of *Aspergillus* antigen in serum for the diagnosis of invasive aspergillosis appears promising but is not widely available.[4]

Saprophytic infections (eg, aspergilloma) are a recognized major category of aspergillosis.

Footnotes

1. Skov M, Koch C, Reimert CM, et al, "Diagnosis of Allergic Bronchopulmonary Aspergillosis (ABPA) in Cystic Fibrosis," *Allergy*, 2000, 55(1):50-8.
2. Hantsch CE and Tanus T, "Allergic Bronchopulmonary Aspergillosis With Adenopathy," *Ann Intern Med*, 1991, 115(7):546-7.
3. Bosken CH, Myers JL, Greenberger PA, et al, "Pathologic Features of Allergic Bronchopulmonary Aspergillosis," *Am J Surg Pathol*, 1988, 12(3):216-22.
4. Buchheidt D, Skladny H, Baust C, et al, "Systemic Infections With *Candida* sp and *Aspergillus* sp in Immunocompromised Patients With Hematological Malignancies: Current Serological and Molecular Diagnostic Methods," *Chemotherapy*, 2000, 46(3):219-28.

References

Caras WE and Pluss JL, "Chronic Necrotizing Pulmonary Aspergillosis: Pathologic Outcome After Itraconazole Therapy," *Mayo Clin Proc*, 1996, 71(1):25-30.

Ho PL and Yuen KY, "Aspergillosis in Bone Marrow Transplant Recipients," *Crit Rev Oncol Hematol*, 2000, 34(1):55-69.

Houser SM and Corey JP, "Allergic Fungal Rhinosinusitis: Pathophysiology, Epidemiology, and Diagnosis," *Otolaryngol Clin North Am*, 2000, 33(2):399-409.

Ledesma D and Pearce WH, Images in Clinical Medicine, "Septic (*Aspergillus*) Embolus," *N Engl J Med*, 2000, 342(14):1015.

Patterson TF, Kirkpatrick WR, White M, et al, "Invasive Aspergillosis. Disease Spectrum, Treatment Practices, and Outcomes. I3 *Aspergillus* Study Group," *Medicine (Baltimore)*, 2000, 79(4):250-60.

Rochester CL and Kradin RL, "A 47-Year-Old Woman With Multilobular Pulmonary Consolidation," Case Records of the Massachusetts General Hospital, Case 39-2000, Scully RE, Mark EJ, McNeely WF, et al, eds, *N Engl J Med*, 2000, 343(25):1876-84.

Sigler L and Kennedy MJ, "*Aspergillus*, *Fusarium*, and Other Opportunistic Moniliaceous Fungi," *Manual of Clinical Microbiology*, 7th ed, Washington, DC: AMS Press, American Society for Microbiology, 1999, 1212-41.

Stevens DA, Kan VL, Judson MA, et al, "Practice Guidelines for Diseases Caused by *Aspergillus*. Infectious Diseases Society of America," *Clin Infect Dis*, 2000, 30(4)696-709.

Thaler SJ and Bailey EM, "A 66-Year-Old Woman With Toxic Epidermal Necrolysis and a Fatal Course," Case Records of the Massachusetts General Hospital, Case 14-1996, Scully RE, Mark EJ, McNeely WF, et al, eds, *N Engl J Med*, 1996, 334(19):1254-61.

Yong S, Attal H, and Chejfec G, "Pseudomembranous Gastritis: A Novel Complication of *Aspergillus* Infection in a Patient With a Bone Marrow Transplant and Graft-Versus-Host Disease," *Arch Pathol Lab Med*, 2000, 124(4):619-24.

♦ **Atypical *Mycobacterium* Smear** see Acid-Fast Stain *on page 550*

♦ **Auramine-Rhodamine Stain** see Acid-Fast Stain *on page 550*

♦ **Australian Antigen** replaced by Hepatitis B Surface Antigen *on page 625*

♦ **Australian Antigen Antibody** replaced by Hepatitis B Surface Antibody *on page 625*

♦ **Autoclave Sterility Check** see Sterility Culture *on page 681*

Babesiosis Serology

Related Information

Anemia Flowchart *on page 392*
Arthropod Identification *on page 559*
Ehrlichiosis Serology *on page 603*
Lyme Disease Serology *on page 650*
Malaria Smear and Tests *on page 458*
Risks of Transfusion *on page 861*

Synonyms Nantucket Fever Serological Test

Applies to *Ixodes dammini*; *Ixodes ricinus*; WA1-Antibody

Abstract *Babesia microti* and *Babesia divergens* are tick-borne intraerythrocytic protozoans, which can cause symptoms resembling those of *Plasmodium falciparum*. Like malaria, it causes hemolytic anemia. Asplenic, immunocompromised, and elderly subjects are especially at risk, but immunocompetent persons can develop the disease. These organisms also cause disease in cattle, including Texas fever. Babesiosis is enzootic in Southern New England, Southern New York, Wisconsin, and Minnesota.

Specimen Serum, blood for smear

Container Red top tube

Storage Instructions Refrigerate at 4°C.

Reference Interval Negative

Critical Values Titers >1:128 are considered consistent with infection. A fourfold increase in titer establishes diagnosis.

Use *Babesia* species serological test is used to diagnose babesiosis and to prevent sequellae. Babesiosis can be transmitted by blood transfusion from asymptomatic donors.[1]

Limitations False reactivity may be seen in patients with malaria. Patients exposed to *Babesia* on the West Coast of the U.S. should be tested for antibodies to the *Babesia* WA1 species rather than the *Babesia microti* antigen due to the lack of cross-reactivity between these organisms.

Methodology Indirect immunofluorescent antibody (IFA), serum. **Note:** Intraerythrocytic ring forms and tetrads can be identified in the peripheral blood film. The ring forms resemble those of *P. falciparum* malaria, but the rare tetrad forms are diagnostic of babesiosis. Organisms can resemble Pappenheimer bodies, which are found in asplenic persons. An acridine orange technique is available. Peripheral blood from a finger puncture can be collected directly on glass slides for thick and thin films. The films are Giemsa stained, and are useful for detection of organisms.

Polymerase chain reaction (PCR) for parasite DNA is under development. To be used on blood specimens,[1] it is more sensitive and as specific as hamster inoculation and direct smear.

Additional Information The geographic distribution of babesiosis is worldwide. Babesiosis is transmitted in nature by hard-bodied ticks. The ticks become infected by feeding on various infected vertebrate animals (cattle, deer, moles, and mice). *Babesia* can also be transmitted to humans by blood transfusions. *Babesia divergens* is the most common species reported in Europe while *B. microti* is the agent most frequently identified in the U.S. Recently, two variants of *Babesia* species have been reported in the U.S. One variant is from the states of Washington and California (WA1 type) and the other is from Missouri (MO-1).

Babesiosis is particularly severe in patients who have undergone splenectomy (and who lack the RBC "pitting" function of the spleen). It may be potentially life-threatening in immunosuppressed persons or those of advanced age. Infections in individuals with normal spleens may often be asymptomatic. The Northern deer tick, *Ixodes scapularis* (*Ixodes dammini*), which transmits one of the *Babesia* species (*B. microti*, a rodent parasite) also transmits Lyme disease. Subjects with either disease should be considered for the other. The preferred host for the tick is the white-tailed deer. Another important vector is *I. ricinus*. Diagnosis of babesiosis is established primarily by examination of peripheral blood smears. A WA1-reactive case was originally misdiagnosed as an instance of *P. falciparum* malaria but intraerythrocytic tetrad forms were recognized.

Footnotes

1. Dobroszycki J, Herwaldt BL, Boctor F, et al, "A Cluster of Transfusion-Associated Babesiosis Cases Traced to a Single Asymptomatic Donor," *JAMA*, 1999, 281(10):927-30.

References

"A 63-Year-Old Man With Fever, Sweats, and Shaking Chills," Case Records of the Massachusetts General Hospital, Case 28-1993, Scully RE, Mark EJ, McNeely WF, et al, eds, *N Engl J Med*, 1993, 329(3):194-9.

Gelfand JA and Callahan MV, "Babesiosis," *Curr Clin Top Infect Dis*, 1998, 18:201-16.

Gorenflot A, Moubri K, Precigout E, et al, "Human Babesiosis," *Ann Trop Med Parasitol*, 1998, 92(4):489-501.

Homer MJ, Aguilar-Delfin I, Telford SR, et al, "Babesiosis," *Clin Microbiol Rev*, 2000, 13(3):451-69.

Krause PJ, Lepore T, Sikand VK, et al, "Atovaquone and Azithromycin for the Treatment of Babesiosis," *N Engl J Med*, 2000, 343(20):1454-8.

Perdrizet GA, Olson NH, Krause PJ, et al, "Babesiosis in a Renal Transplant Recipient Acquired Through Blood Transfusions," *Transplantation*, 2000, 70(1):205-8.

Pershing DH, Herwaldt BL, Glaser C, et al, "Infection With a *Babesia*-Like Organism in Northern California," *N Engl J Med*, 1995, 332(2):298-303.

Pruthi RK, Marshall WF, Wiltsie JC, et al, "Human Babesiosis," *Mayo Clin Proc*, 1995, 70(9):853-62.

Quick RE, Herwaldt BL, Thomford JW, "Babesiosis in Washington State: A New Species of *Babesia*?" *Ann Intern Med*, 1993, 119(4):284-90.

Sweeney CJ, Ghassemi M, Agger WA, et al, "Coinfection With *Babesia microti* and *Borrelia burgdorferi* in a Western Wisconsin Resident," *Mayo Clin Proc*, 1998, 73(4):338-41.

Internet Web Sites

www.astdhpphe.org/infect/babesiosis.html
www.cdc.gov/ncidod/dpd/parasites/babesia/default.htm

♦ **Bacillus cereus Food Poisoning** see Bacterial Culture, Stool *on page 575*

♦ **Bactec®** see Bacterial Culture, Blood *on page 566*

♦ **Bacterial Antigens by Coagglutination** *replaced by* Bacterial Antigens, Rapid Detection Methods *on page 562*

♦ **Bacterial Antigens by Counterimmunoelectrophoresis** *replaced by* Bacterial Antigens, Rapid Detection Methods *on page 562*

♦ **Bacterial Antigens, CSF** *see* Bacterial Antigens, Rapid Detection Methods *on page 562*

Bacterial Antigens, Rapid Detection Methods

Related Information
Bacteremia Detection, Buffy Coat Micromethod *on page 406*
Bacterial Culture, Cerebrospinal Fluid *on page 569*
Cerebrospinal Fluid Analysis: Overview *on page 416*
Cerebrospinal Fluid Glucose *on page 140*
Cerebrospinal Fluid Protein *on page 517*
Cryptococcal Antigen Titer *on page 595*
Gram Stain *on page 617*
Group A *Streptococcus* Screen, Rapid *on page 617*
Group B *Streptococcus* Screen, Rapid *on page 618*
Mycobacterial Culture, Cerebrospinal Fluid *on page 656*
Viral Culture, Central Nervous System Symptoms *on page 692*

Synonyms Latex Agglutination for Bacterial Antigens

Applies to Bacterial Antigens, CSF; Cerebrospinal Fluid Bacterial Antigen Testing

Replaces Bacterial Antigens by Coagglutination; Bacterial Antigens by Counterimmunoelectrophoresis

Test Includes Qualitative determination of the presence of antigens of *H. influenzae*, *S. pneumoniae*, *N. meningitidis*. Test may also identify subgroups of above organisms and may include testing for group B *Streptococcus* and *E. coli* K1 antigen in neonates. Gram staining and culture take precedence over bacterial antigen testing.[1]

Abstract Rapid bacterial antigen tests on CSF can be done by latex agglutination.[1,2] The newer antigen detection systems have a reported sensitivity similar to that of the Gram stain; about 80% of cases have been diagnosed with either technique. However, a study reports that all true-positive latex agglutination CSF specimens showed the causative microorganisms in Gram stain as well. Of 57 latex agglutination positives, 31 were false positives (54%), 22 were true-positive (38%), and four were indeterminant (7%). There was no change in therapy on the basis of any true-positive result. Ten years ago, results of the 31 false positives included prolonged hospitalization, clinical complications, and charges of $175,000 without detected benefit.[3,4] The current cost would be much higher. It is recommended that **these latex agglutination tests are not intended as a substitute for bacterial culture. Confirmatory diagnosis of bacterial meningitis infection is possible only with appropriate culture procedures.** Concentration of antigen depends on variables including the number of bacteria, the duration of infection, and the presence or absence of specific antibodies which may prevent antigen detection.[2]

Patient Preparation Usual aseptic aspiration

Specimen Cerebrospinal fluid

Container Sterile CSF tube

Storage Instructions Do not refrigerate.

Reference Interval Negative

Use Although the test is intended to detect bacterial antigens in CSF for the rapid diagnosis of meningitis, its specific indications remain questionable.

Limitations Antigen detection does not replace Gram stain and culture. The test may be negative in early meningitis. *Staphylococcus aureus* and *Pseudomonas aeruginosa* are not detected by these methods. Most members of the Enterobacteriaceae also fail to react. Group B *Streptococcus* and the *E. coli* K1 antigen are frequently not tested on patients older than 6 months of age. Antigenic cross-reactions are seen. The sensitivity of commercial antigen detection kits remains imperfect. False-negative results occur with low antigen load. Pneumococcal and *Haemophilus* strains not possessing capsular antigens may not be detected by immunological techniques. False positives cause expense and complications.[2,4]

Methodology Latex agglutination (LA) of capsular polysaccharide bacterial antigen

Additional Information The CSF white blood cell count and differential are the best predictors of meningitis.[2] When discussing the differential diagnosis of meningitis, all authors do not include latex agglutination testing in discussion of laboratory results.[5]

Antigen detection methods should never be substituted for culture and Gram stain. Culture and Gram stain must always have priority when limited quantities of CSF are available.[1]

Bacterial antigens may be detected despite previous antibiotic therapy. Positive latex agglutination in patients with negative cultures caused by prior antimicrobial treatment were not found in several studies.[2,4]

Several investigations have shown that PCR may be a very sensitive and specific nonculture method for detection of meningococcal meningitis.[6,7]

The rapid diagnosis of group A and group B *Streptococcus* infection is discussed specifically in Group A *Streptococcus* Screen, Rapid *on page 617* and Group B *Streptococcus* Screen, Rapid *on page 618*.

Footnotes
1. Mein J and Lum G, "CSF Bacterial Antigen Detection Tests Offer no Advantage Over Gram's Stain in the Diagnosis of Bacterial Meningitis," *Pathology*, 1999, 31(1):67-9.
2. Perkins MD, Mirrett S, and Reller LB, "Rapid Bacterial Antigen Detection Is Not Clinically Useful," *J Clin Microbiol*, 1995, 33(6):1486-91.
3. Rodewald LE, Woodin KA, Szilagyi PG, et al, "Relevance of Common Tests of Cerebrospinal Fluid in Screening for Bacterial Meningitis," *J Pediatr*, 1991, 119(3):363-9.
4. Feuerborn SA, Capps WI, and Jones JC, "Use of Latex Agglutination Testing in Diagnosing Pediatric Meningitis," *J Fam Pract*, 1992, 34(2):176-9.
5. Durand ML, Calderwood SB, Weber DJ, et al, "Acute Bacterial Meningitis in Adults - A Review of 493 Episodes," *N Engl J Med*, 1993, 328(1):21-8.
6. Gray SJ, Sobanski MA, Kaczmarski EB, et al, "Ultrasound-Enhanced Latex Immunoagglutination and PCR as Complementary Methods for Nonculture-Based Confirmation of Meningococcal Disease," *J Clin Microbiol*, 1999, 37(6):1797-801.
7. Carrol ED, Thomson AP, Shears P, et al, "Performance Characteristics of the Polymerase Chain Reaction Assay to Confirm Clinical Meningococcal Disease," *Arch Dis Child*, 2000, 83(3):271-3.

References
Hussein AS and Shafran SD, "Acute Bacterial Meningitis in Adults. A 12-Year Review," *Medicine (Baltimore)*, 2000, 79(6):360-8.
Smith AL, "Bacterial Meningitis," *Pediatr Rev*, 1993, 14(1):11-8.
Sobanski MA, Gray SJ, Cafferkey M, et al, "Meningitis Antigen Detection: Interpretation of Agglutination by Ultrasound-Enhanced Latex Immunoassay," *Br J Biomed Sci*, 1999, 56(4):239-46.

Internet Web Sites
www.cdc.gov/ncidod/dbmd/diseaseinfo/meningococcal_g.htm

Bacterial Culture, Abscess

Related Information
Antimicrobial Susceptibility Testing, Aerobic and Facultatively Anaerobic Bacteria *on page 554*
Antimicrobial Susceptibility Testing, Anaerobic Bacteria *on page 555*
Bacterial Culture, Aerobes *on page 563*
Bacterial Culture, Biopsy or Body Fluid *on page 565*
Bacterial Culture, Throat, and Antigen Detection Testing for Group A Streptococci *on page 577*
Bacterial Culture, Wounds, Bites *on page 579*
Body Fluid Chemical Analysis *on page 123*
Fine Needle Aspiration Culture *on page 609*
Fine Needle Aspiration, Deep Masses *on page 381*
Fine Needle Aspiration, Superficial Masses (Palpable) *on page 382*
Mycobacterial Culture, Biopsy or Body Fluid *on page 655*
Mycobacterial Culture, Cutaneous and Subcutaneous Tissue *on page 657*

Applies to Aerobic Culture, Abscess; Anaerobic Culture, Abscess

Test Includes Bacterial culture on a specimen of this type should include a Gram stain as well as aerobic and anaerobic bacterial cultures. At some institutions, culture for anaerobic bacteria must be specifically requested, especially if specimens are submitted on swabs: *vide infra*.

Abstract Common predisposing factors for abscesses include diabetes mellitus, malignant disease, and other entities which are immunocompromising. Most abscesses are caused by mixed bacterial growth that includes both aerobic and anaerobic bacteria. Initial antibiotic coverage should be broad-spectrum to cover these possibilities. Routine culture will not detect slow growing microorganisms such as mycobacteria.

Patient Preparation The site is decontaminated (surgical soap and 70% isopropyl alcohol) to eliminate potentially contaminating aerobic and anaerobic bacteria which colonize many surfaces.

Specimen Fluid, pus, or other material properly obtained from an abscess. Adjacent skin surfaces must not be touched.

Container Specimen may be aspirated into a syringe and capped with an airtight stopper; all air should be expelled from the syringe prior to transport. Alternatively, clinical material may be transferred from the syringe to commercially available vials that contain anaerobic indicators and maintain anaerobic conditions. Specimens may also be transferred to sterile containers that do not maintain anaerobic conditions, but transport to the laboratory should be expedited to maximize survival of anaerobes. Specimens in syringes with needles are not acceptable because of concerns about needlestick injuries. Swabs (even anaerobic swabs) are inferior specimens.

Special transport media (eg, 7H9 broth) should be used if a mycobacterial etiology is suspected.

Collection Contamination with normal flora must be avoided. Some anaerobes will be killed by contact with oxygen for only a few seconds. Ideally, pus obtained by needle aspiration through an intact surface, which has been aseptically prepared, is put directly into an anaerobic transport device or transported directly to the laboratory in the original syringe. Sampling of open lesions is enhanced by deep aspiration using a sterile needle and syringe. Curettings of the base of an open lesion may also provide a good yield. Irrigation should be done with nonbacteriostatic sterile saline. Pulmonary samples are obtained by transtracheal percutaneous needle aspiration by trained physicians or by use of a special sheathed catheter. If swabs must be used, two should be collected; one for culture and one for Gram stain. Specimens collected and transported in syringes should be transported to the laboratory within 30 minutes of collection.

Storage Instructions Syringes should have air expelled and needles removed.

Causes for Rejection Specimens exposed to air, specimens which have been refrigerated, or have an excessive delay in transit have a suboptimal yield.

Clinical Observations Suggestive of Anaerobic Infection

Foul-smelling discharge
Location of infection in proximity to a mucosal surface
Necrotic tissue, gangrene, pseudomembrane formation
Gas in tissues or discharges
Endocarditis with negative routine blood cultures
Infection associated with malignancy or other process producing tissue destruction
Infection related to the use of aminoglycosides (oral, parenteral, or topical)
Septic thrombophlebitis
Bacteremic picture with jaundice
Infection resulting from human or other bites
Black discoloration of blood-containing exudates (may fluoresce red under ultraviolet light in *B. melaninogenicus* infections)
Presence of "sulfur granules" in discharges (actinomycosis)
Classical clinical features of gas gangrene
Clinical setting suggestive for anaerobic infection (septic abortion, infection after gastrointestinal surgery, genitourinary surgery, etc)

Adapted from Bartlett JG," Anaerobic Bacterial Infections of the Lung," *Chest*, 1987, 91:901-9.

Use Define the microbial etiology of the abscess and provide a guide for therapy

Limitations Fastidious anaerobes may not be recovered despite significant efforts to collect and properly submit a specimen. Any specimen submitted for microbial culture can be contaminated with colonizing organisms that are not contributing to disease. Organisms most likely to contaminate specimens of this type include, but are not limited to, *Corynebacterium* species, coagulase-negative staphylococci, alpha-hemolytic streptococci, *Propionibacterium* species, and *Bacillus* species. These organisms are not invariably contaminants, however, and may be pathogenic in certain settings. A Gram stain should always be performed, if sufficient material is obtained, to provide early presumptive information and to help interpret culture results.

Usual laboratory procedure includes screening only for aerobic bacteria and rapidly growing anaerobes (*Bacteroides fragilis*, *Clostridium perfringens*, *Fusobacterium*, and anaerobic gram-positive cocci). Slow-growing *Mycobacterium* species or *Nocardia* species which may cause abscesses will **not** be recovered in routine bacterial cultures even if present, since extended incubation periods or special media are necessary for their isolation. Cultures for these organisms should be specifically requested.

Contraindications Bronchoscopically-obtained specimens are not ideal as the instrument becomes contaminated by organisms which normally inhabit the oropharynx during insertion. Culture of specimens from sites harboring endogenous anaerobic organisms or contaminated by endogenous organisms may be misleading with regard to etiology and selection of appropriate therapy. Special sheathed catheters are available to reduce oropharyngeal flora contamination of bronchial aspirate cultures.

Methodology Aerobic and anaerobic culture, usually with broth and solid media. Special handling to maintain anaerobic conditions is required.

Additional Information Cavitary infected lesions in lung may be caused by mycobacterial, fungal, and parasitic agents. The expression, "**lung abscess**", is usually intended to indicate bacterial infection. **Empyema** indicates a collection of exudate in a body space such as the pleural space. Lung abscess may be secondary to aspiration, a virulent organism such as *Staphylococcus aureus*, or bronchial obstruction.[1] Lung abscess secondary to aspiration is usually solitary, while those complicating septic emboli are often multiple. Obstructive disease with distal abscess is often bronchogenic carcinoma. Ninety percent of lung abscesses involve anaerobes, and 50% include aerobic organisms as well. Aerobes commonly are staphylococci, streptococci, and gram-negatives. Intravenous drug abuse may lead to tricuspid valve endocarditis and septic pulmonary emboli.

Clinically significant specimens for anaerobic culture in patients with pleuropulmonary infections are blood, pleural fluid, transtracheal aspirates, transthoracic pulmonary aspirates, specimens obtained at thoracotomy, and fiberoptic bronchoscopic aspirates using the protected brush or sheathed catheter. Pleural fluid is preferred for patients with empyema.[2] Blood cultures yield positive results in <5% of cases of anaerobic pulmonary infection. Specimens received in anaerobic transport containers are not optimal for fungus cultures.

Serious anaerobic infections are often due to mixed flora, which are pathologic synergists. Anaerobes frequently recovered from closed postoperative wound infections include *Bacteroides fragilis*, ~50%; *Prevotella melaninogenica* (previously *Bacteroides melaninogenicus*), ~25%; *Peptostreptococcus prevotii*, ~15%; and *Fusobacterium* species, ~25%. Aerobes are seldom recovered in pure culture (10% to 15% of cultures). Aerobes and facultative bacteria when present are frequently found in lesser numbers than the anaerobes. Anaerobic infection is most commonly associated with operations involving opening or manipulating the bowel or a hollow viscus

(eg, appendectomy, cholecystectomy, colectomy, gastrectomy, bile duct exploration, etc). The ratio of anaerobes to facultative species is normally about 10:1 in the mouth, vagina, and sebaceous glands and at least 1000:1 in the colon.

See also Bacterial Culture, Anaerobes *on page 564*, Fungal Culture, Biopsy or Body Fluid *on page 610*, and Mycobacterial Culture, Biopsy or Body Fluid *on page 655*.

Footnotes
1. Finegold SM, "Lung Abscess," *Cecil Textbook of Medicine*, 21st ed, Chapter 83, Goldman L and Bennett JC, eds, Philadelphia, PA: WB Saunders Co, 2000, 439-41.
2. Bartlett JG, "Anaerobic Bacterial Infections of the Lung," *Chest*, 1987, 91(6):901-9.

References
Anuradha DE, Saraswathi K, and Gogate A, "Anaerobic Bacteraemia: A Review of 17 Cases," *J Postgrad Med*, 1998, 44(3):63-6.

Brook I and Frazier EH, "Microbiology of Subphrenic Abscesses: A 14-Year Experience," *Am Surg*, 1999, 65(11):1049-53.

Elliott D, Kufera JA, and Myers RA, "The Microbiology of Necrotizing Soft Tissue Infections," *Am J Surg*, 2000, 179(5):361-6.

Holden J, "Collection and Transport of Clinical Specimens for Anaerobic Culture," *Clinical Microbiology Procedures Handbook*, Isenberg HD, ed, Washington, DC: American Society of Microbiology.

Koneman EW, Allen SD, Janda WM, et al, *Color Atlas and Textbook of Diagnostic Microbiology*, 5th ed, New York, NY: Lippincott Raven, 1997.

Nichols RL and Smith JW, "Anaerobes From a Surgical Perspective," *Clin Infect Dis*, 1994, 18(Suppl 4):S280-6.

Stone HH, "Soft Tissue Infections," *Am Surg*, 2000, 66(2):162-5.

Walker CK, Workowski KA, Washington AE, et al, "Anaerobes in Pelvic Inflammatory Disease: Implications for the Centers for Disease Control and Prevention's Guidelines for Treatment of Sexually Transmitted Diseases," *Clin Infect Dis*, 1999, 28(S1):529-36.

Bacterial Culture, Aerobes

Related Information
Anthrax Detection *on page 553*
Antimicrobial Susceptibility Testing, Aerobic and Facultatively Anaerobic Bacteria *on page 554*
Bacterial Culture, Anaerobes *on page 564*
Bacterial Culture, Biopsy or Body Fluid *on page 565*
Bacterial Culture, Blood *on page 566*
Bacterial Culture, Intravascular Device *on page 572*
Bacterial Culture, Middle Ear *on page 573*
Beta-Lactamase Test *on page 581*
Bronchoalveolar Lavage (BAL) *on page 375*
Gram Stain *on page 617*

Synonyms Aerobic Bacterial Culture

Applies to Enterobacteriaceae Culture; *Neisseria* sp; *Pseudomonas* spp; *Staphylococcus aureus*

Test Includes Culture of aerobic or facultative anaerobes contributing to an infectious process and may also include antimicrobial susceptibility testing.

Abstract Culture for aerobic bacteria utilizes methods capable of detecting obligately aerobic (those incapable of reproducing in the absence of oxygen) and facultatively anaerobic (those capable of reproducing in the presence or absence of oxygen) organisms. Obligately anaerobic organisms (those incapable of reproducing in the presence of oxygen) will not be recovered in aerobic cultures.

The overwhelming majority of bacterial pathogens are facultatively anaerobic organisms (eg, all streptococci, enterococci, staphylococci, members of the family Enterobacteriaceae, *Haemophilus influenzae*, *Pasteurella multocida*, *Vibrio* spp). There are relatively few obligately aerobic bacteria that are human pathogens; those that are commonly encountered include *Pseudomonas* spp and most *Neisseria* spp.

A useful overview of aerobic microbiology is that provided by Pezzlo.[1]

Patient Preparation Varies with source.

Specimen Body site, tissue, or fluid associated with infection

Container Sterile container or swab; varies with source

Collection Varies with source.

Turnaround Time Varies with specimen. **Final** reports of negative results are typically available as follows: blood and CSF: 5-7 days; urine: 1 day; sputum and wounds: 2 days; aseptically obtained body fluids: 5 days. **Preliminary** information from positive cultures is usually available within 24 hours; speciation and antimicrobial susceptibility is often available 24 hours later, but certain organisms require more time to identify.

Use Recover and identify obligately aerobic and facultatively anaerobic bacteria suspected of causing infections

Limitations It is often difficult to distinguish contaminating organisms from etiologic agents of infection (see monographs on specific sites, eg, CSF, abscess, blood). Occasionally, organisms may grow slowly, be difficult to isolate in pure culture, or be difficult to identify.

Methodology Inoculation of microbiological media, incubation of media at temperatures varying from 25°C to 42°C (usually 35°C) in ambient or CO_2-enhanced atmospheric conditions

Additional Information *Staphylococcus aureus* causes community- and hospital-acquired infections which are increasing in frequency. The emergence of multidrug-resistant strains has made therapy more difficult. These gram-positive cocci cause diseases which include **toxic shock syndrome**, (Continued)

Bacterial Culture, Aerobes *(Continued)*

staphylococcal scalded skin syndrome, and **food poisoning**. Staphylococcal bacteremia may lead to endocarditis, metastatic infections, or the sepsis syndrome. Patients whose **endocarditis** is related to intravenous drug use are apt to have right-sided disease without antecedent valve disease; endocarditis in such individuals may be a difficult clinical diagnosis. **Metastatic infections** include spread to the skeleton, kidneys, and lungs. *S. aureus* is among the most common pathogens causing **sepsis**. The **toxic shock syndrome** is characterized by high fever, erythematous rash which desquamates, hypotension, and multiorgan disease. A third of all cases presently are nonmenstrual, relating to localized infections.[2]

S. aureus is the most frequent organism in **osteomyelitis**. Other causes include coagulase-negative staphylococci, *Proprionibacterium*, *Enterobacteriaceae*, *Pseudomonas aeruginosa*, streptococci, anaerobic bacteria, *Salmonella*, *Streptococcus pneumoniae*, *Bartonella henselae*, *Pasteurella multocida*, *Eikenella corrodens*, *Aspergillus*, *Mycobacterium avium* complex, *Mycobacterium tuberculosis*, *Candida albicans*, *Brucella*, *Coxiella burnetii*, and various fungi.[2,3]

Pneumonia caused by gram-negative bacilli may be community- or hospital-acquired. The former patient group is composed almost entirely of individuals with chronic diseases (eg, chronic obstructive pulmonary disease, alcoholism, or malignant disease). The second (nosocomial) group is principally found in subjects whose pneumonia is secondary (eg, the postoperative state). Pneumonias caused by gram-negative bacilli are commonly related to aspiration. Blood cultures are useful in diagnosis, especially in those with community-acquired infections. The yield of positive cultures from effusion fluid is about 30%. Bronchoalveolar lavage or bronchial brush techniques are useful.

Footnotes

1. Pezzlo M, "Aerobic Bacteriology," *Essential Procedures for Clinical Microbiology*, Isenberg HD, ed, Washington, DC: ASM Press, American Society for Microbiology, 1998, 37-126.
2. Lowy FD, "*Staphylococcus aureus* Infections," *N Engl J Med*, 1998, 339(8):520-32.
3. Lew DP and Waldvogel FA, "Osteomyelitis," *N Engl J Med*, 1997, 336(14):999-1007.

References

Funke G, "Algorithm for Identification of Aerobic Gram-Positive Rods," *Manual of Clinical Microbiology*, 7th ed, Murray PR, Baron EJ, Pfaller MA, et al, eds, Washington, DC: ASM Press, American Society for Microbiology, 1999, 316-18.

Koneman EW, Allen SD, Janda WM, et al, "The Aerobic Gram-Positive Bacilli," *Color Atlas and Textbook of Diagnostic Microbiology*, 5th ed, New York, NY: Lippincott, 1997, 651-708.

Miller JM and Holmes HT, "Specimen Collection, Transport, and Storage," *Manual of Clinical Microbiology*, 6th ed, Murray PR, Baron EJ, Pfaller MA, et al, eds, Washington, DC: AMS Press, American Society for Microbiology, 1999, 33-63.

Ruoff KL, "Algorithm for Identification of Aerobic Gram-Positive Cocci," *Manual of Clinical Microbiology*, Murray PR, Baron EJ, Pfaller MA, et al, eds, Washington, DC: ASM Press, American Society for Microbiology, 1999, 262-3.

Schreckenberger PC, Janda M, Wong JD, et al, "Algorithms for Identification of Aerobic Gram-Negative Bacteria," *Manual of Clinical Microbiology*, Murray PR, Baron EJ, Pfaller MA, et al, eds, Washington, DC: ASM Press, American Society for Microbiology, 1999, 438-41.

Tuomanen EI, Austrian R, and Masure HR, "Pathogenesis of Pneumococcal Infection," *N Engl J Med*, 1995, 332(19):1280-4.

Bacterial Culture, Anaerobes

Related Information

Actinomyces Culture *on page 551*
Antimicrobial Susceptibility Testing, Anaerobic Bacteria *on page 555*
Bacterial Culture, Abscess *on page 562*
Bacterial Culture, Aerobes *on page 563*
Bacterial Culture, Blood *on page 566*
Botulism Diagnostic Procedures *on page 585*
Clostridium difficile Toxin Assay and Culture *on page 592*
Gram Stain *on page 617*
Tetanus Antibody *on page 682*

Synonyms Anaerobic Bacterial Culture

Test Includes Culture for anaerobic bacteria; Gram stain is usually performed.

Abstract Culture for anaerobic bacteria utilizes methods capable of detecting obligate anaerobes (those incapable of reproducing in the absence of oxygen). Facultatively anaerobic (those capable of reproducing in the presence of oxygen) organisms are also recovered in these cultures, but the primary purpose of anaerobic cultures is to recover obligate anaerobes. Anaerobic bacteria most likely to be identified include *Bacteroides* sp, *Prevotella* sp, *Fusobacterium* sp, *Peptostreptococcus* sp, other streptococci, *Gemella morbillorum*, *Staphylococcus saccharolyticus*, *Veillonella* sp, *Actinomyces* sp, *Eubacterium* sp, *Proprionibacterium* sp, *Bifidobacterium* sp, *Lactobacillus* sp, and *Clostridium* sp.[1]

Specimen Abscess, blood, aseptically obtained body fluid (eg, pleural, peritoneal, synovial), wounds, etc

Container Capped syringe; biopsy; anaerobic transport media, blood culture media

Collection Swabs usually cause unacceptable exposure of anaerobes to oxygen and have a propensity to dry out. Swabs are considered inferior specimens.

Causes for Rejection Specimens from sites in which anaerobic bacteria are normal flora (eg, throat, rectal swabs, urine, bronchial washes, cervicovaginal mucosal swabs, sputums) are unacceptable for anaerobic culture. Specimens that have not been appropriately protected from atmospheric oxygen cannot yield accurate results.

Turnaround Time Varies with specimen. Negative cultures are typically reported as follows: blood cultures: 5-7 days; aseptically obtained body fluids: 5 days; swab specimen: 2-5 days.

Use Recover and identify obligately anaerobic bacteria suspected of causing infections

Infections Which May Be Caused by Anaerobes

Location	Type of Infection
Head and neck	Brain abscess
	Gingivitis
	Chronic sinusitis
	Chronic otitis
	Odontogenic and oropharyngeal space infections
Respiratory tract	Aspiration pneumonia
	Necrotizing pneumonia
	Lung abscess
	Empyema (adults)
Gastrointestinal tract	Peritonitis
	Intra-abdominal abscess
	Liver abscess
Fcmale genital tract	Tubo-ovarian abscess
	Salpingitis (30% to 50% of cases)
	Septic abortion and endometritis
	Bartholin gland abscess
	Bacterial vaginosis
Skin and soft tissue	Crepitant cellulitis
	Necrotizing fascitis
	Myonecrosis (gas gangrene)
	Decubitus ulcer
	Diabetic foot ulcer
	Bite wounds

Adapted from Styrt B and Gorhach SL, "Recent Developments in the Understanding of the Pathogenesis and Treatment of Anaerobic Infections," *N Engl J Med*, 1989, 321:240-6.

Limitations Anaerobic bacterial cultures are intended to recover most common obligately anaerobic bacterial pathogens. Some obligate anaerobes die after very brief exposure to oxygen and are very difficult to recover in culture. Anaerobic bacteria may contaminate clinical specimens that are not collected aseptically; it is often very challenging to distinguish contaminants from etiologic agents of infection.

Contraindications It is usually not relevant to seek anaerobes in acute cholecystitis, acute osteomyelitis, acute otitis media, acute sinusitis, appendicitis, bronchitis, cystitis, meningitis, pharyngitis, primary peritonitis, pyelonephritis, or superficial skin lesions.

Methodology Inoculation of microbiological media suitable for recovering anaerobes and incubation of media at 35°C in an atmosphere lacking oxygen. Biochemical, gas-liquid chromatography (GLC), DNA hybridization, and RNA homology and sequencing define anaerobic genera.

Additional Information Anaerobic bacteria can be involved in all types of bacterial infections, since these bacteria consist of a major part of the indigenous flora of humans. The most common anaerobe encountered in human infections is *Bacteroides fragilis*. A number of other anaerobes also cause human disease (*Prevotella* sp, *Porphyromonas* sp, *Fusobacterium* sp, *Veillonella* sp). Tetanus and botulism are serious diseases due to toxins produced by anaerobes.

C. tetani causes tetanus (see Tetanus Antibody *on page 682*). *C. botulinum* causes botulism (see Botulism Diagnostic Procedures *on page 585*). These organisms elaborate toxins. Clostridial gas gangrene and myonecrosis occur following deep injury, which affects blood supply with carcinoma or with hematologic disorders. Most are caused by *C. perfringens*, the remainder by *C. septicum*, *C. novyi*, *C. histolyticum*, *C. bifermentans*, and *C. fallax*. Bowel disruption and surgery, biliary surgery, retained placenta, prolonged rupture of membranes, and intrauterine fetal demise are among causes of gas gangrene. *C. septicum* is more aerotolerant.[2,3,4]

See Bacterial Culture, Abscess *on page 562*.

Footnotes

1. Koneman EW, Allen SD, Janda WM, et al, *Color Atlas and Textbook of Diagnostic Microbiology*, 5th ed, New York, NY: Lippincott, 1997, 709-84.
2. Stevens DL, "Clostridial Myonecrosis and Other Clostridial Diseases," *Cecil Textbook of Medicine*, 21st ed, Chapter 334, Goldman L and Bennett JC, eds, Philadelphia, PA: WB Saunders Co, 2000, 1668-70.
3. Crawford BE and Rachal TD, "Clinical Pathology Rounds: Spontaneous Myonecrosis Secondary to *Clostridium septicum*," *Lab Med*, 1999, 30(7):444-7.
4. Pelletier JP, Plumbley JA, Rouse EA, et al, "The Role of *Clostridium septicum* in Paraneoplastic Sepsis," *Arch Pathol Lab Med*, 2000, 124(3):353-6.

Clostridial Diseases

Organism	Diagnosis	Clinical Features	Laboratory Features	Toxins
Invasive Infections				
C. perfringens type a	Traumatic gas gangrene	Pain, necrotizing infection, renal impairment, shock	Renal failure; increased CK; gas in tissues	α toxin Theta toxin
C. septicum	Spontaneous gas gangrene	Pain, necrotizing infection, bowel portal	Renal failure; increased CK; gas in tissues	α toxin
C. sordellii	Malignant edema	No pain, no fever, cytotoxin	Leukemoid reaction; hemoconcentration	?
C. tertium	Bacteremia in compromised hosts receiving antibiotics	Bacteremia, shock	Positive blood cultures	?
Gastrointestinal				
C. perfringens type a	Food poisoning	Nausea, vomiting, watery diarrhea	None	Enterotoxin
C. perfringens type c	Necrotizing enterocolitis	Bloody diarrhea, ruptured bowel	None	β toxin
C. septicum	Neutropenic enterocolitis, "typhlitis"	Right lower quadrant pain, abdominal distention	Decreased WBC	Unknown
C. difficile	Pseudomembranous colitis	Water, bloody diarrhea	Stools positive for organism, toxin, blood, and leukocytes	Toxin A Toxin B
Neurologic				
C. tetanii	Tetanus	Spastic paralysis	None	Tetanospasmin
C. botulinum	Botulism	Flaccid paralysis	None	Botulinum toxin (A,B,E,F,G)

Adapted from Stevens DL, "Clostridial Myonecrosis and Other Clostridial Diseases," *Cecil Textbook of Medicine*, 21st ed, Chapter 334, Goldman L and Bennett JC, eds, Philadelphia, PA: WB Saunders Co, 2000, 1668-70.

References
Allen SD, Emory CL, and Siders JA, "Clostridium," *Manual of Clinical Microbiology*, 7th ed, Chapter 46, Murray PR, Baron EJ, Pfaller MA, et al, eds, Washington DC: ASM Press, American Society for Microbiology, 1999, 654-71.

Anuradha DE, Saraswathi K, and Gogate A, "Anaerobic Bacteraemia: A Review of 17 Cases," *J Postgrad Med*, 1998, 44(3):63-6.

Brook I and Frazier EH, "Microbiology of Subphrenic Abscesses: A 14-Year Experience," *Am Surg*, 1999, 65(11):1049-53.

Goldstein EJC, "Diseases Caused by Nonspore-Forming Anaerobic Bacteria," *Cecil Textbook of Medicine*, 21st ed, Chapter 338, Goldman L and Bennett JC, eds, Philadelphia, PA: WB Saunders Co, 2000, 1677-80.

Miller JM and Holmes HT, "Specimen Collection, Transport, and Storage," *Manual of Clinical Microbiology*, 7th ed, Murray PR, Baron EJ, Pfaller MA, et al, eds, Washington, DC: AMS Press, American Society for Microbiology, 1999, 33-63.

Sharp SE, "Commensal and Pathogenic Microorganisms of Humans," *Manual of Clinical Microbiology*, 7th ed, Murray PR, Baron EJ, Pfaller MA, et al, eds, Washington, DC: AMS Press, American Society for Microbiology, 1999, 23-32.

Thurston M, Maida D, and Gannon C, "Oxyrase Cell-Membrane Preparations Simplify Cultivation of Anaerobic Bacteria," *Lab Med*, 2000, 31(9):509-12.

Walker CK, Workowski KA, Washington AE, et al, "Anaerobes in Pelvic Inflammatory Disease: Implications for the Centers for Disease Control and Prevention Guidelines for Treatment of Sexually Transmitted Diseases," *Clin Infect Dis*, 1999, 28(Suppl 1):S29-36.

♦ **Bacterial Culture, Anthrax** *see Anthrax Detection on page 553*

Bacterial Culture, Biopsy or Body Fluid

Related Information
Actinomyces Culture *on page 551*
Bacterial Culture, Abscess *on page 562*
Bacterial Culture, Aerobes *on page 563*
Bacterial Culture, Wounds, Bites *on page 579*
Body Cavity Fluid Cytology *on page 372*
Body Fluid Analysis, Cell Count *on page 408*
Body Fluid Chemical Analysis *on page 123*
Body Fluid pH *on page 125*
Bone Marrow *on page 410*
Brucella Culture *on page 586*
Clostridium difficile Toxin Assay and Culture *on page 592*
Fine Needle Aspiration Culture *on page 609*
Fine Needle Aspiration, Deep Masses *on page 381*
Fine Needle Aspiration, Superficial Masses (Palpable) *on page 382*
Fungal Culture, Biopsy or Body Fluid *on page 610*
Gram Stain *on page 617*
Histopathology *on page 59*
Lymph Node Biopsy *on page 67*
Mycobacterial Culture, Biopsy or Body Fluid *on page 655*
Mycobacterial Culture, Cutaneous and Subcutaneous Tissue *on page 657*
Synovial Fluid Analysis *on page 323*
Viral Culture, Body Fluid *on page 691*
Viral Culture, Tissue *on page 695*

Synonyms Biopsy Aerobic Culture; Body Fluid Aerobic Culture

Applies to Bone Marrow Culture; Synovial Fluid Culture; Tissue Culture

Test Includes Aerobic and anaerobic culture of biopsy or body fluid; may include Gram stain and susceptibility testing on selected pathogens.

Patient Preparation Aseptic preparation of biopsy site or site of body fluid.

Specimen Aseptically aspirated body fluid (excludes cerebrospinal fluid, blood, and urine) or biopsy from normally sterile site. A single specimen will usually suffice for both aerobic and anaerobic cultures.

Container Sterile container with lid, Petri dish, no preservative. Bone marrow aspirates and body fluids may be directly inoculated into blood culture media.

Collection The portion of the biopsy specimen submitted for culture should be separated from the portion submitted for histopathology by the surgeon or pathologist, utilizing sterile technique. Bedside inoculation of blood culture bottles with ascitic fluid improves sensitivity.[1]

Causes for Rejection Specimens in fixative, biopsy specimens from sites which have anaerobic bacteria as normal flora

Turnaround Time Preliminary negative reports can be generated for aerobic bacteria within 1 day and for anaerobic bacteria within 2 days. Final negative results are usually provided after 4-5 days of incubation; if actinomycosis is suspected, however, the specimen may be held for 2 weeks. Positive results may be generated by 18-24 hours (preliminary results for aerobic culture), but final positive results for anaerobic cultures take at least 4 days, and often take considerably longer if speciation and antimicrobial susceptibilities are required (7-14 days).

Special Instructions Blood cultures and cultures from easily obtained sites are indicated before bone marrow cultures.[2]

Use Isolate and identify aerobic and anaerobic bacteria

Limitations Any specimen submitted for bacterial culture can be contaminated with colonizing organisms that are not contributing to disease. *Corynebacterium* spp, *Propionibacterium acnes*, *Bacillus* sp, alpha streptococci, and coagulase-negative staphylococci are usually contaminants and should only be considered pathogens if substantial evidence exists that they are clinically significant (eg, repeated isolation, present in large numbers on Gram stain, more likely pathogens absent). Typical pathogens (such as *E. coli*, *P. aeruginosa*, *Enterococcus* spp, *Bacteroides*, and *Peptostreptococcus* spp) may also contaminate clinical specimens (eg, biopsy specimens of chronically-infected wounds); in order to enhance the value of cultures of this type, it is necessary to carefully debride the site prior to specimen collection and collect viable infected tissue. A Gram stain should always be performed if sufficient material is obtained, to provide early presumptive information and to help interpret culture results.

Specimens collected on swabs, exposed to air, or having excessive travel time to the laboratory may yield less than an optimal yield of obligate anaerobes.

Methodology Aerobic and anaerobic culture

Additional Information Whenever possible, the specimen should be obtained before empiric antimicrobial therapy is started.

Spontaneous bacterial peritonitis is defined as the presence of bacteria in ascitic fluid without an obvious intra-abdominal focus. It is a potentially fatal complication of cirrhosis and ascites. Cases containing increased PMNs in ascitic fluid, culture-negative and culture-positive, are managed similarly and have comparable levels of mortality. Mean PMN count in a 1998 series was 775 (μL). Pathogens included *E. coli*, *Klebsiella pneumoniae*, *Staphylococcus aureus*, *Streptococcus pneumoniae*, and others. Serum albumin >3 g/dL was protective against mortality. Ascitic fluid PMN count >1000/μL was a significant predictor of mortality.[3] The organisms recovered from ascitic fluid of patients with spontaneous **bacterial peritonitis** are usually portions of normal intestinal flora; 92% are monomicrobial.[4] (Continued)

Bacterial Culture, Biopsy or Body Fluid *(Continued)*

Identification of the causative organism is needed for successful therapy of **osteomyelitis**.[5] Swabs of fistulas or ulcers may yield misleading information. Surgical sampling or needle biopsy of infected tissue is needed. See table.

Microorganisms Isolated From Cases of Bacterial Osteomyelitis

Microorganism	Most Common Association
S. aureus (susceptible or resistant to methicillin)	Most frequent microorganism in any type of osteomyelitis
Coagulase-negative staphylococci or propionibacterium	Foreign-body-associated infection
Enterobacteriaceae or *Pseudomonas aeruginosa*	Common in nosocomial infections
Streptococci or anaerobic bacteria	Associated with bites, fist injury caused by contact with another person's mouth, diabetic foot lesions, decubitus ulcers
Salmonella or *Streptococcus pneumoniae*	Sickle cell disease
Bartonella henselae	Human immunodeficiency virus infection
Pasteurella multocida or *Eikenella corrodens*	Bites, human or animal
Aspergillus, Mycobacterium avium complex, or *Candida albicans*	Immunocompromised patients
Mycobacterium tuberculosis	Populations in which tuberculosis is prevalent
Brucella, Coxiella burnetti (chronic Q fever), or other fungi found in specific geographic areas	Areas in which these pathogens are endemic

Adapted from Lew DP and Waldvogel FA. "Osteomyelitis," *N Engl J Med*, 1997, 336(14):999-1007.

The **staphylococcal scalded skin syndrome** is characterized by flaccid bullae, positive Nikolsky sign with the level of cleavage at the granular layer.[6] Unlike *Staphylococcus* or toxic shock syndrome, it is rarely associated with systemic signs. The disease is due to the production of a toxin (exfoliative toxin) by the infecting staphylococci. These bacteria can be isolated from skin lesions.

Footnotes

1. Runyon BA, "Care of Patients With Ascites," *N Engl J Med*, 1994, 330(5):337-42.
2. Volk EE, Miller ML, Kirkley BA, et al, "The Diagnostic Usefulness of Bone Marrow Cultures in Patients With Fever of Unknown Origin," *Am J Clin Pathol*, 1998, 110(2):150-3.
3. Lipka JM, Zibari GB, Dies DF, et al, "Spontaneous Bacterial Peritonitis in Liver Failure," *Am J Surg*, 1998, 64(12):1155-7.
4. Gilbert JA and Kamath PS, "Spontaneous Bacterial Peritonitis: An Update," *Mayo Clin Proc*, 1995, 70(4):365-70.
5. Lew DP and Waldvogel FA, "Osteomyelitis," *N Engl J Med*, 1997, 336(14):999-1007.
6. Schenfeld LA, Images in Clinical Medicine, "Staphylococcal Scalded Skin Syndrome," *N Engl J Med*, 2000, 342(16):1178.

References

Elliott D, Kufera JA, and Myers RA, "The Microbiology of Necrotizing Soft Tissue Infections," *Am J Surg*, 2000, 179(5):361-6.

Koneman EW, Allen SD, Janda WM, et al, *Color Atlas and Textbook of Diagnostic Microbiology*, 5th ed, New York, NY: Lippincott, 1997.

Stone HH, "Soft Tissue Infections," *Am Surg*, 2000, 66(2):162-5.

Bacterial Culture, Blood

Related Information

Synonyms Aerobic Culture, Blood; Anaerobic Culture, Blood; Culture, Blood

Applies to Antimicrobial Removal Device (ARD) Blood Culture; ARD, Blood Culture; Bactec®; Blood Culture, BactAlert®; Blood Culture, Isolator™; Blood Culture, Lysis Centrifugation; Blood Culture With Antimicrobial Removal Device (ARD); *Francisella tularensis* Culture; Isolator™ Blood Culture

Test Includes Isolation of both aerobic and anaerobic microorganisms and antimicrobial susceptibility testing on all significant isolates

Abstract A blood culture is one of the most significant procedures that a laboratory performs. Positive results should be promptly called to the ordering physician. New automated blood culture systems provide continuous monitoring, which allows detection of positive cultures 24 hours/day. A major problem of blood cultures is the possibility of contamination with normal skin flora. Other factors relevant to detection of microbial pathogens in blood include the volume of blood cultured, the number of separate cultures, the extent of dilution, the types of media, the devices selected, the presence of unusual or fastidious organisms, and the presence of antibiotics.

Patient Preparation Blood cultures are often contaminated by skin flora. Such contamination can be markedly reduced by careful attention to skin preparation and antisepsis **prior** to collection of the specimen.

After location of the vein by palpation, the venipuncture site should be cleansed with 70% alcohol (isopropyl or ethyl) and then swabbed in a circular motion concentrically from the center outward using tincture of iodine or a povidone iodine solution. **The iodine should be allowed to dry before the venipuncture is undertaken.** If palpation is required during the venipuncture, the glove covering the palpating finger tip should be disinfected. In iodine-sensitive patients, a double alcohol, green soap, or acetone alcohol preparation may be substituted.

Alcoholic chlorhexidine has recently been recommended for skin preparation.[1]

Aftercare Iodine used in the skin preparation should be carefully removed from the skin after venipuncture.

Specimen Venous blood. The yield of positives is not increased by culturing arterial blood, even in endocarditis.

Blood Culture Collection

Clinical Disease Suspected	Culture Recommendation	Rationale
Sepsis, meningitis osteomyelitis, septic arthritis, bacterial pneumonia	Two to three sets of cultures, each 10-30 mL for adults	Assure sufficient sampling in cases of intermittent or low level bacteremia. Minimize the confusion caused by a positive culture resulting from transient bacteremia or skin contamination.
Fever of unknown origin (eg, occult abscess, empyema, typhoid fever, etc)	Two to three sets of cultures - one from each of two prepared sites, the second or third drawn after a brief time interval (30 minutes). If cultures are negative after 24-48 hours obtain two more sets, preferably prior to an anticipated temperature rise.	The yield after four sets of cultures is minimal. A maximum of three sets per patient per day for 3 consecutive days is recommended.
Endocarditis		
Acute	Obtain two to three blood culture sets within 2 hours, then begin therapy.	95% to 99% of acute endocarditis patients (untreated) will yield a positive in one of the first three cultures.
Subacute	Obtain two to three blood culture sets on day 1, repeat if negative after 24 hours. If still negative or if the patient had prior antibiotic therapy, repeat again.	Adequate sample volume despite low level bacteremia or previous therapy should result in a positive yield.
Immunocompromised host (eg, AIDS)		
Septicemia, fungemia mycobacteremia	Obtain two to three sets of cultures from each of two prepared sites; consider lysis concentration technique to enhance recovery for fungi and mycobacteria.	Low levels of fungemia and mycobacteremia frequently encountered.
Previous antimicrobial therapy		
Septicemia, bacteremia; monitor effect of antimicrobial therapy	Obtain two to three sets of cultures from each of two prepared sites; consider use of antimicrobial removal device (ARD) or increased volume >10 mL/set.	Recovery of organisms is enhanced by dilution, increased sample volume, and removal of inhibiting antimicrobials.

Container Bottles of trypticase soy broth or other standard medium. Recovery may be enhanced by lysis filtration or concentration.[2]

Sampling Time Ideally, three sets of blood cultures should be collected per febrile episode; collection of each set should be separated by at least 1 hour from the previous specimen. Such intervals provide maximum recovery of microorganisms in patients with intermittent bacteremia, and documentation of persistent bacteremia in patients with intravascular infections (eg, endocarditis, intravenous catheter site infections). If multiple sets must be collected simultaneously, draw two sets initially from separate sites, and collect a third set at least 1 hour later. Although three blood culture sets provide optimal yield, the cost-effectiveness of this approach has been challenged and some individuals propose collection of only two sets per febrile episode.

Collection Blood cultures should be drawn prior to initiation of antimicrobial therapy. If more than one culture is ordered, the specimens should be drawn from separately prepared sites. A syringe and needle, transfer set, or pre-evacuated set of tubes containing culture media may be used to collect blood. Collection tubes should be held below the level of the venipuncture to avoid reflux. A sample volume of 10-30 mL in adults or 1-5 mL in children is collected for each set. The likelihood of recovering a pathogen increases as the volume of blood sampled increases;[2] however, **drawing of more than three blood culture sets per bacteremic episode rarely increases yield**. If a syringe and needle or transfer set is used, the top of the blood culture bottle should also be aseptically prepared. See table.

Interpretation of results can be enhanced by collecting blood cultures from more than one site and after a time interval (1 hour). Cultures should be taken as early as possible in the course of a febrile episode.

Storage Instructions Specimens collected in tubes with SPS® (sodium polyanetholesulfonate) should be processed without delay. The specimen should be transferred to appropriate culture media to avoid any possible decrease in yield due to storage or prolonged contact with SPS®. Culture bottles from some automated systems can sit at room temperature for several hours.

Turnaround Time Common laboratory procedure is to issue a final negative culture report after 5-7 days. A preliminary positive culture report based upon Gram stain and primary subculture is usually available at 24-72 hours.

Special Instructions The requisition should indicate current antibiotic therapy, clinical diagnosis, and relevant history. Bird or animal contact may be important [*Chlamydia psittaci*, *Coxiella burnetii* (Q fever), and *Brucella* species].[3]

Reference Interval Negative

Critical Values Positive cultures should be immediately phoned to the nursing station or physician.

Use Isolate, identify, and determine antimicrobial susceptibility of pathogenic organisms causing bacteremia. Blood culture is indicated in community-acquired pneumonia.

The most important single test for diagnosis of infective endocarditis is the blood culture. In the absence of antibiotic therapy, negative blood cultures are found in experienced laboratories in <5% of cases.

The diagnosis of typhoid fever is made by blood culture in 50% to 70% of patients. Bone marrow culture for typhoid is best for patients who have already been given antibiotics; it is reported to be >90% sensitive.[4]

Limitations Prior antibiotic therapy may cause negative blood cultures or delayed growth. Blood cultures from patients suspected of having *Brucella*, tularemia, or *Leptospira* must be requested as special cultures. Consultation with the laboratory for the recovery of these organisms prior to collection of the specimen is recommended. When patients with infective endocarditis have negative bacterial blood cultures, the possibility of a fungal infection should be considered. Yeast often are isolated from routine blood cultures. However, if fungi are specifically suspected, a separate fungal blood culture should be drawn along with each of the routine blood culture specimens. See Fungal Culture, Blood *on page 610* for proper collection of specimen. *Mycobacterium avium-intracellulare* (MAI) is recovered from blood of immunocompromised patients, particularly those with acquired immunodeficiency syndrome (AIDS). Special procedures are required for the recovery of these organisms (ie, lysis filtration concentration or use of a special mycobacteria blood culture medium). Radiometric methods facilitate the recovery of mycobacteria from blood.

Transient bacteremia caused by brushing teeth, bowel movements, or scratching of the skin may cause a positive blood culture, but usually will not cause all of three sets to be positive.

Blood culture contamination produces false-positive results and subjects patients to the side effects of inappropriate therapy. The most common bacterial contaminants in blood cultures include coagulase-negative staphylococci, *Corynebacterium*, *viridans* streptococci, and *Bacillus* species.[5]

Positive blood cultures are among the criteria for the diagnosis of infective endocarditis. A recent paper addresses afebrile blood culture-negative endocarditis. The differential diagnosis includes Whipple disease, *C. burnetii*, *Chlamydia* species, and *Bartonella* species.[6]

Contraindications Use of a 2% iodine preparation is contraindicated in patients sensitive to iodine. Green soap may be substituted for the iodine or alcohol acetone alone may be used. See Patient Preparation; *vide supra*.

Methodology Aerobic and anaerobic culture in broth media with detection of bacterial growth by a variety of methods including visual, radiometric, or infrared monitoring, or blind subculture to solid media. The antimicrobial removal device procedure (ARD) includes use of an adsorbent resin in the aerobic bottle. Resin-containing bottles are also available for several automated detection systems. In the lysis centrifugation procedure, blood is lysed and centrifuged using a Wampole Isolator™ tube or similar method. The sediment is inoculated to media appropriate for growing aerobic and anaerobic bacteria, fungi, and mycobacteria. A method of continuously monitoring media for bacterial growth is available from several commercial sources.

Additional Information Sequential blood cultures in nonendocarditis patients using a 20 mL sample resulted in an 80% positive yield after the first set, a 93% yield after the second set, and a 98% yield after the third set. The volume of blood cultured seems to be more important than the specific culture technique being employed by the laboratory. The isolation of coagulase-negative staphylococci (CNS) poses a critical and difficult clinical dilemma. Although CNS are the most commonly isolated organism from blood cultures, only a few (6.3%) of the isolates represent "true" clinically significant bacteremia.[7] Conversely, CNS are well recognized as a cause of infections involving prosthetic devices, cardiac valves, CSF shunts, dialysis catheters, and indwelling vascular catheters.[7] Ultimately, the physician is responsible for determination of whether an organism is a contaminant or a pathogen. The decision is based on both laboratory and clinical data. Patient data including patient history, physical examination, body temperatures, clinical course, and laboratory data (ie, culture results, white blood cell count, and differential) are relevant. Clinical experience and judgment may play a significant role in resolution of this clinical dilemma.[8] Various sources of contamination include the patient's own skin flora, transient benign bacteremias, and perhaps, disinfection materials.

The use of a lysis centrifugation system has been reported to increase the recovery rate and decrease the time of fungal recovery compared to traditional or biphasic blood culture systems.[9] Recovery of mycobacteria, atypical mycobacteria, and *Legionella* may also be enhanced by lysis filtration.

The use of antimicrobial removal devices (ARD) or resin bottles to attempt to increase the yield of blood cultures drawn from patients on antimicrobial therapy is controversial. Some microorganisms are occasionally not recovered with the use of ARD blood cultures. It is, therefore, advised that at least one culture in a series of three be requested without the use of the ARD bottles. ARD blood cultures are substantially more expensive than routine blood cultures.

The diagnosis of bacterial meningitis is accomplished by blood culture as well as culture and examination of cerebrospinal fluid.[10] Most children with bacterial meningitis are initially bacteremic.[11,12]

Any organism isolated from the blood is usually tested for susceptibility.

Footnotes

1. Mimoz O, Karim A, Mercat A, et al, "Chlorhexidine Compared With Povidone-Iodine as Skin Preparation Before Blood Culture," *Ann Intern Med*, 1999, 131(11):834-7.
2. Mylotte JM and Tayara A, "Blood Cultures: Clinical Aspects and Controversies," *Eur J Clin Microbiol Infect Dis*, 2000, 19(3):157-63.
3. Berbari EF, Cockerill FR, and Steckelberg JM, "Infective Endocarditis Due to Unusual or Fastidious Microorganisms," *Mayo Clin Proc*, 1997, 72(6):532-42.
4. Zenilman JM, "Typhoid Fever," *JAMA*, 1997, 278(10):847-50.
5. Reisner BS, Woods GS, Thomson RB, et al, "Specimen Processing," *Manual of Clinical Microbiology*, 7th ed, Murray PR, Baron EJ, Pfaller MA, et al, eds, Washington, DS: AMS Press, American Society for Microbiology Press, 1999, 65.
6. Raoult D, "Afebrile Blood Culture-Negative Endocarditis," *Ann Intern Med*, 1999, 131(2):144-5.
7. Goldmann DA and Pier GB, "Pathogenesis of Infections Related to Intravascular Catheterization," *Clin Microbiol Rev*, 1993, 6(2):176-92.
8. Kim SD, McDonald LC, Jarvis WR, et al, "Determining the Significance of Coagulase-Negative Staphylococci Isolated From Blood Cultures at a Community Hospital: A Role for Species and Strain Identification," *Infect Control Hosp Epidemiol*, 2000, 21(3):213-7.
9. Reimer LG, Wilson ML, and Weinstein MP, "Update on Detection of Bacteremia and Fungemia," *Clin Microbiol Rev*, 1997, 10(3):444-65.
10. Francke E, "The Many Causes of Meningitis," *Postgrad Med*, 1987, 82(2):175-8, 181-3, 187-8.
11. Klein JO, Feigin RD, and McCracken GH Jr, "Report of the Task Force on Diagnosis and Management of Meningitis," *Pediatrics*, 1986, 78(5 Pt 2):959-82.
12. Feigin RD, McCracken GH Jr, and Klein JO, "Diagnosis and Management of Meningitis," *Pediatr Infect Dis J*, 1992, 11(9):785-814.

References

Bannister ER and Woods GL, "Evaluation of Routine Anaerobic Blood Cultures in the BacT/Alert Blood Culture System," *Am J Clin Pathol*, 1995, 104(3):279-82.

Chien JW, "Making the Most of Blood Cultures. Tips for Optimal Use of This Time-Honored Test," *Postgrad Med*, 1998, 104(1):119-27.

DesJardin JA, Falagas ME, Ruthazer R, et al, "Clinical Utility of Blood Cultures Drawn From Indwelling Central Venous Catheters in Hospitalized Patients With Cancer," *Ann Intern Med*, 1999, 131(9):641-7.

Edmond MB, Wallace SE, McClish DK, et al, "Nosocomial Bloodstream Infections in United States Hospitals: A Three-Year Analysis," *Clin Infect Dis*, 1999, 29(2):239-44.

Farmer PE and Basgoz N, "A 28-Year-Old Man With Gram-Negative Sepsis of Uncertain Cause," Case Records of the Massachusetts General Hospital, Case 8-1999, Scully RE, Mark EJ, McNeely WF, et al, *N Engl J Med*, 1999, (11):869-76.

Glerant JC, Hellmuth D, Schmit JL, et al, "Utility of Blood Cultures in Community-Acquired Pneumonia Requiring Hospitalization: Influence of Antibiotic Treatment Before Admission," *Respir Med*, 1999, 93(3):208-12.

Gomez R and Buescher ES, Images in Clinical Medicine, "Meningococcemia," *N Engl J Med*, 1997, 336(10):707.

(Continued)

567

Bacterial Culture, Blood (Continued)

Hurley JC, "Concordance of Endotoxemia With Gram-Negative Bacteremia. A Meta-analysis Using Receiver Operating Characteristic Curves," *Arch Pathol Lab Med*, 2000, 124(8):1157-64.

Isaacman DJ, Shults J, Gross Tk, et al, "Predictors of Bacteremia in Febrile Children 3-36 Months of Age," *Pediatrics*, 2000, 106(5):977-82.

Luna CM, Videla A, Mattera J, et al, "Blood Cultures Have Limited Value in Predicting Severity of Illness and as a Diagnostic Tool in Ventilator-Associated Pneumonia," *Chest*, 1999, 116(4):1075-84.

Pizzo PA, "Fever in Immunocompromised Patients," *N Engl J Med*, 1999, 341(12):893-90.

Ram S, Mylotte JM, and Pisano M, "Rapid Classification of Positive Blood Cultures: Validation and Modification of a Prediction Model," *J Gen Intern Med*, 1995, 10(12):82-8.

Ryan MR and Murray PR, "Laboratory Detection of Anaerobic Bacteremia," *Clin Lab Med*, 1994, 14(1):107-17.

Sands KE, Bates DW, Lanken PN, et al, "Epidemiology of Sepsis Syndrome in 8 Academic Medical Centers," *JAMA*, 1997, 278(3):234-40.

Schifman RB, Strand CL, Meier FA, et al, "Blood Culture Contamination. A College of American Pathologists Q-Probes Study Involving 640 Institutions and 497,134 Specimens From Adult Patients," *Arch Pathol Lab Med*, 1998, 122(3):216-21.

Segal GS and Chamberlain JM, "Resources Utilization and Contaminated Blood Cultures in Children at Risk for Occult Bacteremia," *Arch Pediatr Adolesc Med*, 2000, 154(5):469-73.

Souvenir D, Anderson DE Jr, Palpant S, et al, "Blood Cultures Positive for Coagulase-Negative Staphylococci: Antisepsis, Pseudobacteremia, and Therapy of Patients," *J Clin Microbiol*, 1998, 36(7):1923-6.

Waterer GW, Jennings SG, and Wunderink RG, "The Impact of Blood Cultures on Antibiotic Therapy in Pneumococcal Pneumonia," *Chest*, 1999, 116(5):1278-81.

Wheeler AP and Bernard GR, "Treating Patients With Severe Sepsis," *N Engl J Med*, 1999, 340(3):207-14.

Bacterial Culture, Bronchoscopy/Bronchial Brush/Bronchoalveolar Lavage Specimen

Related Information
Bacterial Culture, Sputum *on page 574*
Bronchial Brushings Cytology *on page 373*
Bronchial Washings Cytology *on page 374*
Bronchoalveolar Lavage (BAL) *on page 375*
Cytomegalovirus Cytology *on page 380*
Cytomegalovirus Serology *on page 600*
Fungal Culture, Sputum *on page 613*
Mycobacterial Culture, Sputum *on page 658*
Pneumocystis carinii Preparation *on page 386*
Pneumocystis Immunofluorescence *on page 671*
Viral Culture, Respiratory Symptoms *on page 694*

Synonyms Bronchoscopy Specimen Bacterial Culture

Applies to BAL Culture; *Bordetella* spp; Bronchoalveolar Lavage Culture; *Enterobacteriaceae*; *Fusobacterium nucleatum*; *Haemophilus influenzae*; *Klebsiella pneumoniae*; *Legionella* spp; *Moraxella catarrhalis*; *Mycobacterium* spp; *Prevotella melaninogenica*; Quantitative Culture for Respiratory Tract Pathogens; *Staphylococcus aureus*; *Streptococcus pneumoniae*

Test Includes Gram stain; semiquantitative aerobic bacterial culture; anaerobic bacterial cultures also performed on Bartlett catheters

Abstract Defining the bacterial etiology of lower respiratory infections occasionally requires collection of specimens by bronchoscopy/bronchial brushing/bronchoalveolar lavage. The type of specimen collected impacts the information that can be obtained and the way it should be processed in the laboratory. Bronchoscopy specimens are always contaminated with oropharyngeal flora and even use of a protected brush does not eliminate problems of contamination.

Specimen Bronchoscopically obtained specimens for bacterial culture include:
- bronchial washes
- bronchoalveolar lavages (BAL)
- specimens obtained using a protected catheter brush (PCB), also called a Bartlett catheter

Container Bartlett catheters should be submitted in 1 mL of sterile nonbacteriostatic saline in a sterile container. Bronchial washes or bronchoalveolar lavages should be submitted in tightly sealed, sterile containers.

Collection Collected at bronchoscopy by a physician skilled in the procedure. Transport the specimen to the laboratory within 1 hour of collection.

Turnaround Time Complete reports of cultures may require as long as 2-4 days after receipt of culture.

Special Instructions Patient history is important.[1]

Reference Interval Bartlett catheters (in 1 mL saline): $<10^3$ CFU/mL is within the expected level of contamination

Bronchoalveolar lavages: bacteria: $<10^6$ CFU/mL of original specimen; normal total cell count: $4-23 \times 10^6$; differential, 95% alveolar macrophages; 3% lymphocytes; 1% polymorphonuclear cells, 0.2% eosinophils

Bronchial washes: cannot be established; often contaminated heavily with oral flora

Critical Values The presence or absence of intracellular organisms on Gram staining is important: >7% cells containing intracellular organisms appear to correlate with ventilator-assisted pneumonia.[2]

Use Identify the etiology of pulmonary infections. BAL is useful for diagnosis of opportunistic infections in immunosuppressed subjects. Quantitative culture for respiratory tract pathogens: $>10^3$ to 10^4 bacterial colonies/mL BAL fluid supports the diagnosis of acute bacterial pneumonia. Bronchial brush suspension may also require colony counts.[3]

Limitations Contamination with oral pharyngeal secretions causes false-positive aerobic and anaerobic bacterial cultures; quantitative or semiquantitative cultures on bronchoalveolar lavage and Bartlett catheter specimens circumvent this problem. The use of bronchoalveolar lavage for defining the etiology of anaerobic pulmonary infections has not been established. Differentiation of colonization versus infection may be difficult with agents such as *Aspergillus* or *Candida* species which occasionally grow in bacterial cultures.

Methodology Semiquantitative or quantitative aerobic bacterial culture for BALs. Semiquantitative aerobic and anaerobic bacterial cultures on solid media for protected catheter brushes.

Additional Information Bronchoalveolar lavage (BAL) has become an established procedure for defining the etiology of pulmonary infections. It is particularly useful for recovering opportunistic pathogens (eg, *Pneumocystis*, *Histoplasma capsulatum*, *Candida* spp, *Aspergillus* spp, *Mycobacterium* spp) from immunocompromised individuals and in defining the etiology of nosocomial pneumonia in patients undergoing mechanical ventilation.[4,5] It has a role for evaluation of *Legionella*, *Nocardia*, *T. gondii*, viruses including CMV and RSV, adenovirus and herpes simplex virus.[3] The procedure has an acceptable morbidity in immunocompromised and thrombocytopenic patients and is often an initial diagnostic procedure in the immunosuppressed. BAL is performed with a catheter wedged into a segmented bronchus. Bronchial washings or airway washings are collected with a nonwedged, more proximally positioned scope tip. Bronchial washings, therefore, preferentially sample airways. Lavage is preferred for the diagnosis of *Pneumocystis* pneumonia, which is primarily an alveolar process. Limiting lavage to one segment reduces the risk of postprocedural respiratory compromise. Quantitative bacterial cultures of BAL specimens have also proven useful for defining the etiology of acute bacterial pneumonia.[6,7] Blood cultures are indicated in cases of acute pneumonia.[8]

The abundant normal anaerobic flora of the mouth makes **anaerobic cultures** of any specimen contaminated by oral secretions (eg, bronchial washes, sputums) essentially useless for defining the anaerobic bacterial etiology of lower respiratory infection. Only specimens that bypass the mouth should be cultured anaerobically. Transtracheal aspirates meet this need, but in most hospital settings, they are rarely, if ever, collected. They have been replaced by bronchoscopically obtained specimens using a PCB.[9] Specimens obtained by PCB are subject to low level contamination with normal oral flora.

Footnotes

1. Isenberg HD, "Collection, Transport, and Manipulation of Clinical Specimens and Initial Laboratory Concerns," *Essential Procedures for Clinical Microbiology*, Section 1, Washington, DC: ASM Press, American Society for Microbiology, 1998, 3-36.

2. Reisner BS, Woods GL, Thomson RB Jr, et al, "Specimen Processing," *Manual of Clinical Microbiology*, Chapter 5, Murray PR, Baron EJ, Pfaller MA, et al, eds, Washington, DC: ASM Press, American Society for Microbiology, 1999, 64-104.

3. Forbes BA, Sahm DF, and Weissfeld AS, *Bailey and Scott's Diagnostic Microbiology*, 10th ed, St Louis, MO: CV Mosby, 1998.

4. Guerra LF and Baughman RP, "Use of Bronchoalveolar Lavage to Diagnose Bacterial Pneumonia in Mechanically Ventilated Patients," *Crit Care Med*, 1990, 18(2):169-73.

5. Casetta M, Blot F, Antoun S, et al, "Diagnosis of Nosocomial Pneumonia in Cancer Patients Undergoing Mechanical Ventilation: A Prospective Comparison of the Plugged Telescoping Catheter With the Protected Specimen Brush," *Chest*, 1999, 115(6):1641-5.

6. Baselski VS, El-Torky M, Coalson JJ, et al, "The Standardization of Criteria for Processing and Interpreting Laboratory Specimens in Patients With Suspected Ventilator-Associated Pneumonia," *Chest*, 1992, 102(5 Suppl 1):571S-9S.

7. Flanagan PG, Findlay GP, Magee JT, et al, "The Diagnosis of Ventilator-Associated Pneumonia Using Nonbronchoscopic, Nondirected Lung Lavages," *Intensive Care Med*, 2000, 26(1):20-30.

8. Koneman EW, Allen SD, Janda WM, et al, *Color Atlas and Textbook of Diagnostic Microbiology*, 5th ed, Philadelphia, PA: JB Lippincott Co, 1997.

9. Kirkpatrick MB and Bass JB Jr, "Quantitative Bacterial Cultures of Bronchoalveolar Lavage Fluids and Protected Brush Catheter Specimens From Normal Subjects," *Am Rev Respir Dis*, 1989, 139(2):546-8.

References

Barret JP, Ramzy PI, Wolf SE, et al, "Sensitivity and Specificity of Bronchoalveolar Lavage and Protected Bronchial Brush in the Diagnosis of Pneumonia in Pediatric Burn Patients," *Arch Surg*, 1999, 134(11):1243-6;

de Jaeger A, Litalien C, Lacroix J, et al, "Protected Specimen Brush or Bronchoalveolar Lavage to Diagnose Bacterial Nosocomial Pneumonia in Ventilated Adults: A Meta-analysis," *Crit Care Med*, 1999, 27(11):2548-60.

Henderson AJ, "Bronchoalveolar Lavage," *Arch Dis Child*, 1994, 70(3):167-9.

Mertens AH, Nagler JM, Galdermans DI, et al, "Quality Assessment of Protected Specimen Brush Samples by Microscopic Cell Count," *Am J Respir Crit Care Med*, 1998, 157(4 Pt 1):1240-3.

Veber B, Souweine B, Gachot B, et al, "Comparison of Direct Examination of Three Types of Bronchoscopy Specimens Used to Diagnose Nosocomial Pneumonia," *Crit Care Med*, 2000, 28(4):962-8.

Yungbluth M, "The Laboratory Diagnosis of Pneumonia. The Role of the Community Hospital Pathologist," *Clin Lab Med*, 1995, 15(2):209-34.

Bacterial Culture, Burn Sites

Related Information
Bacterial Culture, Wounds, Bites *on page 579*
Gram Stain *on page 617*
Zeta Sedimentation Ratio *on page 500*

Synonyms Burn Culture, Quantitative; Quantitative Burn Culture; Skin Burn Culture, Quantitative

Applies to Biopsy Specimen Culture, Quantitative; Fungus Culture, Burn Sites; Quantitative Culture, Biopsy Specimen

Test Includes Quantitative bacterial counts (colonies/g of tissue) of skin and tissue specimens from burn patients. Identification of bacterial isolates and susceptibility testing when indicated. May also include direct Gram stain smear and histopathology.

Specimen Viable tissue, **not** eschar

Container Sterile container, no fixative

Collection Aseptic technique. Collection of cultures only from surfaces of burns may be misleading.[1] A punch biopsy is recommended by some authorities for quantitative culture.[1,2]

Storage Instructions Transport to the laboratory as soon as possible.

Causes for Rejection Eschar specimen rather than viable tissue, specimen <0.1 g, specimen in fixative

Turnaround Time Quantitative bacterial counts are usually available in 24 hours. Identification of bacterial isolates is usually available in 48 hours.

Special Instructions The laboratory should be informed of the specific site of specimen. The laboratory should be contacted prior to collection of the specimens to ascertain availability and specific procedures required.

Reference Interval No growth to $<10^5$ colonies/g of tissue

Use Determine bacterial identity and quantity of organism present (colonies/g) in tissue or skin specimen from burn patient

Limitations Predictive value for sepsis is limited.

Methodology Culture is performed after weighing the specimen and disruption in a glass homogenizer. Trypticase soy broth is the diluent. Colony counts are reported after 24 and 48 hours of incubation ($35°C$ with CO_2). Fungus cultures are planted on Sabouraud's agar or supplemented Sabouraud's agar and held at $30°C$ for 4 weeks.

Additional Information Major thermal injuries often precipitate a profound multicentric immunologic depression that may predispose patients to sepsis. Impairment of immune function is almost universal in patients with greater than 40% total body surface area burns and in very young or very old patients with far smaller burns.[3] The number of organisms is considered by some to be relevant: $>10^5$ colony-forming units/g of tissue may provide indication of infection, while fewer may indicate only colonization. A semi-quantitative bacteriologic culture procedure for tissue is available.[4] The principal value of quantitative burn-wound biopsies is the demonstration of the predominant burn-wound flora. Agreement of 96% was found between $<10^5$ colonies/g of tissue and the absence of histopathologic invasive infection. The organisms most frequently recovered from burn wounds include *Pseudomonas* spp, *Staphylococcus aureus*, *S. epidermidis*, Enterobacteriaceae, other gram-negative bacilli, *Candida*, and *Aspergillus*.[4]

Footnotes
1. Miller JM and Holmes HT, "Specimen Collection, Transport, and Storage" *Manual of Clinical Microbiology*, Chapter 4, Murray PR, Baron EJ, Pfaller MA, et al, eds, Washington, DC: ASM Press, American Society for Microbiology, 1999, 3-63.
2. Isenberg HD, "Collection, Transport, and Manipulation of Clinical Specimens and Initial Laboratory Concerns," *Essential Procedures for Clinical Microbiology*, Section 1, Washington, DC: ASM Press, American Society for Microbiology, 1998, 3-36.
3. Ninnemann JL, "Trauma, Sepsis, and The Immune Response," *J Burn Care Rehabil*, 1987, 8(6):462-8.
4. Forbes BA, Sahm DF, and Weissfeld AS, "Skin, Soft Tissue, and Wound Infections," *Bailey and Scott's Diagnostic Microbiology*, 10th ed, Chapter 28, St Louis, MO: CV Mosby, 1998, 398-412.

References
Cook N, "Methicillin-Resistant *Staphylococcus aureus* Versus the Burn Patient," *Burns*, 1998, 24(2):91-8.
Greenfield E and McManus AT, "Infectious Complications: Prevention and Strategies for Their Control," *Nurs Clin North Am*, 1997, 32(2):297-309.
Kagan RJ and Warden GD, "Management of the Burn Wound," *Clin Dermatol*, 1994, 12(1):47-56.
Pruitt BA Jr and McManus AT, "Opportunistic Infections in Severely Burned Patients," *Am J Med*, 1984, 76(3A):146-54.
Robson MC, "Quantitative Bacteriology and the Burned Patient," *Quantitative Bacteriology: Its Role in the Armamentarium of the Surgeon*, Heggers JP and Robson MC, eds, Boca Raton, FL: CRC Press Inc, 1991, 97-108.

Bacterial Culture, Cerebrospinal Fluid

Related Information
Bacterial Antigens, Rapid Detection Methods *on page 562*
Bacterial Culture, Blood *on page 566*
Cerebrospinal Fluid Analysis: Overview *on page 416*
Cerebrospinal Fluid Cytology *on page 376*
Cerebrospinal Fluid Glucose *on page 140*
Cerebrospinal Fluid Lactate Dehydrogenase *on page 142*
Cerebrospinal Fluid Lactic Acid *on page 143*
Cerebrospinal Fluid Protein *on page 517*

Enterovirus Polymerase Chain Reaction *on page 606*
Fungal Culture, Cerebrospinal Fluid *on page 611*
Gram Stain *on page 617*
India Ink Preparation *on page 642*
Mycobacterial Culture, Cerebrospinal Fluid *on page 656*
VDRL, Cerebrospinal Fluid *on page 688*
Viral Culture, Central Nervous System Symptoms *on page 692*

Synonyms Cerebrospinal Fluid Culture; CSF Culture; Culture, Cerebrospinal Fluid; Spinal Fluid Culture

Applies to *E. coli; Flavobacterium meningosepticum; Haemophilus influenzae* Group b; *Listeria monocytogenes; Mycobacterium* spp; *Mycobacterium tuberculosis; Neisseria meningitidis; Streptococcus agalactiae; Streptococcus pneumoniae*; Ventricular Fluid Culture

Test Includes Aerobic culture and Gram stain. Many laboratories inoculate specimens onto broth media that can support growth of anaerobic bacteria.

Abstract The major test to be performed on the CNS for meningitis is the bacteriologic culture. Bacteria commonly isolated include *Neisseria meningitidis, Haemophilus influenzae* group B, *Streptococcus pneumoniae, Listeria monocytogenes, Escherichia coli, Streptococcus agalactiae, Flavobacterium meningosepticum*; and *Mycobacterium* sp.[1] The gold standard for the diagnosis of bacterial meningitis is the isolation of a bacterium from the cerebrospinal fluid.[2] Cell count, differential, Gram stain, CSF glucose, and CSF protein also are useful. Blood cultures are often positive with meningitis.

Patient Preparation Aseptic preparation of the aspiration site

Specimen Cerebrospinal fluid

Container Sterile CSF tube

Collection Contamination with normal flora from skin or other body surfaces must be avoided. Risks to the patient of lumbar puncture are described.[3,4] Peripheral blood white cell count and differential are important part of the clinical investigation.

Tubes should be numbered 1, 2, 3 indicating the sequence of collection. Contamination with normal flora from skin or other body surfaces must be avoided. The third tube collected is most suitable for culture, as skin contaminants from the puncture usually are washed out with fluid collected in the first two tubes. Special media are needed if mycobacteria are suspected.

Storage Instructions The specimen should be transported immediately to the laboratory. If the specimen cannot be processed immediately, it should be kept at room temperature or placed in an incubator. Refrigeration inhibits viability of certain anaerobic organisms and may prevent the recovery of common aerobic pathogens, *Neisseria meningitidis* and *Haemophilus influenzae*.

Turnaround Time Gram stain results can be reported within 1 hour. Preliminary culture results are usually available at 24 hours. Identification of pathogens may require 48 hours.

Special Instructions The laboratory should be informed of the specific source of specimen, age of patient, current antibiotic therapy, clinical diagnosis, and time of collection.

Reference Interval No growth

Critical Values Positive Gram stain result

Use Isolate and identify pathogenic organisms causing meningitis, shunt infection, brain abscess, subdural empyema, cerebral or spinal epidural abscess, bacterial endocarditis with embolism. Gram stain with cultures of CSF in suspected bacterial meningitis are fundamental to appropriate diagnosis and treatment.[4]

Limitations Cultures may be negative in partially treated cases of meningitis. Microorganisms such as *Neisseria meningitidis* and *Haemophilus influenzae* are sensitive to temperature shifts. Refrigeration can inhibit their isolation from the specimen. Gram stains should be interpreted with care. Gram-positive organisms may decolorize (ie, stain gram-negative in partially treated cases).

When cultures are negative in the presence of clinical meningitis, identification of positive blood culture(s) with CSF pleocytosis (leukocyte count ≥10 cells/mL of CSF) can support diagnosis.[5]

Contamination of laboratory equipment can lead to mistaken impressions of meningitis, so-called "pseudomeningitis".[6]

Methodology Aerobic culture, agar plates. Use of broth cultures additional to agar plate cultures contributes little to treatment decisions.[7]

Additional Information *Haemophilus influenzae, Neisseria meningitidis*, and *Streptococcus pneumoniae*, commonly isolated organisms, can be serotyped if requested. Infections of cerebrospinal fluid shunts pose a difficult clinical problem. Organisms most commonly cultured from shunts include *S. epidermidis*, other coagulase-negative staphylococci, *S. aureus*, *S. viridans*, streptococci, enterococci, and *H. influenzae*. Culture of CSF or shunt fluid is diagnostic. Removal of the catheter and later replacement are frequently required to eradicate infection.[8]

Bacterial meningitis remains a diagnostic problem. Symptoms suggestive of the diagnosis are those associated with febrile illness (eg, fever, lethargy, and anorexia); meningeal inflammation giving rise to nausea, vomiting, photophobia, and nuchal rigidity, leading to apathy; and encephalopathy with headache, confusion, and seizures. Stupor, coma, and focal neurologic signs indicate a poor prognosis if present before start of therapy.[9] **Mortality of bacterial meningitis** reaches 30%. Prognosis is worse in the very young, very old, in the presence of sickle cell disease, asplenia, and with (Continued)

Bacterial Culture, Cerebrospinal Fluid (Continued)

endocarditis. Complications occur in survivors despite early diagnosis and appropriate use of antimicrobial drugs.[10] Developmental or neurologic sequelae were found in 33% to 40% of survivors.[11,12]

Anaerobic culture on solid media is indicated only if brain abscess, subdural empyema, or epidural abscess is suspected or in the presence of an anaerobic infection at another site. Cerebrospinal fluid is not the specimen of choice in this setting, collection of cerebrospinal fluid may be contraindicated, and anaerobic bacteria are rarely recovered from spinal fluid.[13] Common underlying conditions associated with central nervous system anaerobic infections include otitis media, lung and pleural infections, sinusitis, oral infections (ie, tonsillitis, paratonsillar abscess, dental infections), and congenital heart disease.

Factors of bacterial virulence and impaired host defense are relevant to septicemia. Susceptibility to bacterial meningitis is affected by deficiencies in host defense. Susceptibility relates to age as well.[5]

A majority of untreated patients with bacterial meningitis have a positive Gram stain of CSF, which is used to guide therapy. Indicated in the following table are likely pathogens when the Gram stain is nondiagnostic.[14]

Most Common Pathogens in Patients With Suspected Bacterial Meningitis Who Have a Nondiagnostic Gram Stain of CSF

Group of Patients	Likely Pathogen
Immunocompetent	
<3 mo	S. agalactiae, E. coli, L. monocytogenes
3 mo to <18 y	N. meningitidis, S. pneumoniae, or H. influenzae
18-50 y	S. pneumoniae or N. meningitidis
>50 y	S. pneumoniae, L. monocytogenes, or gram-negative bacilli
With impaired cellular immunity	L. monocytogenes or gram-negative bacilli
With head trauma, neurosurgery, or CSF shunt	Staphylococci, gram-negative bacilli, or S. pneumoniae

Adapted from Quagliarello VJ and Scheld WM, "Treatment of Bacterial Meningitis," N Engl J Med, 1997, 336(10):708-16.

Point-of-care testing may in the future produce substantial improvements in the speed and specificity of the diagnosis of bacterial meningitis.[15]

A variety of infectious diseases additional to meningitis are relevant to bacterial cultures of the CNS. Among these are lesions related to infective endocarditis and other septic emboli; otitis media and abscesses; fungal, viral, parasitic, and other entities. See Cerebrospinal Fluid Analysis: Overview on page 416 and monographs listed above in Related Information.

Footnotes

1. Koneman EW, Allen SD, Janda WM, et al, Color Atlas and Textbook of Diagnostic Microbiology, 5th ed, New York, NY: Lippincott, 1997, 151-2.
2. Smith AL, "Bacterial Meningitis," Pediatr Rev, 1993, 14(1):11-8.
3. Greenlee JE, "Approach to Diagnosis of Meningitis - Cerebrospinal Fluid Evaluation," Infect Dis Clin North Am, 1990, 4(4):583-98.
4. Fishman RA, Cerebrospinal Fluid in Diseases of the Nervous System, 2nd ed, Philadelphia, PA: WB Saunders Co, 1992, 266-7.
5. Aronin SI, Peduzzi P, and Quagliarello VJ, "Community-Acquired Bacterial Meningitis: Risk Stratification for Adverse Clinical Outcome and Effect of Antibiotic Timing," Ann Intern Med, 1998, 129(11):862-9.
6. Southern PM Jr and Colvin DD, "Pseudomeningitis Again - Association With Cytocentrifuge Funnel and Gram Stain Reagent Contamination," Arch Pathol Lab Med, 1996, 120(5):456-8.
7. Sturgis CD, Peterson LR, and Warren JR, "Cerebrospinal Fluid Broth Culture Isolates: Their Significance for Antibiotic Treatment," Am J Clin Pathol, 1997, 108(2):217-21.
8. McLaurin RL and Frame PT, "Treatment of Infections of Cerebrospinal Fluid Shunts," Rev Infect Dis, 1987, 9(3):595-603.
9. Dagbjartsson A and Ludvigsson P, "Bacterial Meningitis: Diagnosis and Initial Antibiotic Therapy," Pediatr Clin North Am, 1987, 34(1):219-30.
10. Feigin RD, McCracken GH Jr, and Klein JO, "Diagnosis and Management of Meningitis," Pediatr Infect Dis J, 1992, 11(9):785-814.
11. McCracken GH Jr, "Current Management of Bacterial Meningitis in Infants and Children," Pediatr Infect Dis J, 1992, 11(2):169-74.
12. Franco SM, Cornelius VE, and Andrews BF, "Long-Term Outcome of Neonatal Meningitis," Am J Dis Child, 1992, 146(5):567-71.
13. Gray LD and Fedorko DP, "Laboratory Diagnosis of Bacterial Meningitis," Clin Microbiol Rev, 1992, 5(2):130-45.
14. Quagliarello VJ and Scheld WM, "Treatment of Bacterial Meningitis," N Engl J Med, 1997, 336(10):708-16.
15. Borriello SP, "Science, Medicine, and the Future. Near Patient Microbiological Tests," BMJ, 1999, 319(7205):298-301.

References

Bell WE, "Bacterial Meningitis in Children - Selected Aspects," Pediatr Clin North Am, 1992, 39(4):651-68.

Hussein AS and Shafran SD, "Acute Bacterial Meningitis in Adults. A 12-Year Review," Medicine (Baltimore), 2000, 79(6):360-8.

Negrini B, Kelleher KJ, and Wald ER, "Cerebrospinal Fluid Findings in Aseptic Versus Bacterial Meningitis," Pediatrics, 2000, 105(2):316-9.

Rajnik M and Ottolini MG, "Serious Infections of the Central Nervous System: Encephalitis, Meningitis, and Brain Abscess," Adolesc Med, 2000, 11(2):401-25.

Rosman NR and Roberts DJ, "Respiratory Distress and Seizure in a Neonate," Case Records of the Massachusetts General Hospital, Case 15-1997, Scully RE, Mark EJ, McNeely WF, et al, eds, N Engl J Med, 1997, 336(20):1439-46.

Scheld WM, Whitley RJ, and Durack DT, Infections of the Central Nervous System, New York, NY: Raven Press, 1991.

Schuchat A, Robinson K, Wenger JD, et al, "Bacterial Meningitis in the United States in 1995. Active Surveillance Team," N Engl J Med, 1997, 337(14):970-6.

Tunkel AR and Scheld WM, "Acute Bacterial Meningitis," Lancet, 1995, 346(8991-2):1675-80.

Bacterial Culture, Conjunctiva

Related Information

Adenovirus Antibody Titer on page 552
Adenovirus Culture on page 552
Bartonella Culture on page 580
Bartonella Serology on page 581
Chlamydia Group Serology on page 589
Chlamydia trachomatis Culture on page 590
Chlamydia trachomatis Direct Antigen Test on page 590
Chlamydia trachomatis Nucleic Acid Detection on page 591
Fungal Culture, Ocular Infections on page 612
Fungus Smear, Stain on page 615
Gram Stain on page 617
Herpes Simplex Virus Antigen Detection on page 630
Herpes Simplex Virus Culture on page 631
Neisseria gonorrhoeae Culture and Smear on page 662
Neisseria gonorrhoeae Nucleic Acid Detection on page 664
Ocular Cytology on page 385
Sjögren Antibodies on page 542
Tularemia Serology on page 686
Varicella-Zoster Virus Culture on page 686
Viral Culture on page 689
Viral Culture, Eye or Ocular Symptoms on page 693

Synonyms Conjunctival Culture

Applies to Acanthamoeba; Chlamydia trachomatis; Corneal Culture; Eye Culture; Haemophilus spp; Moraxella spp; Neisseria gonorrhoeae; Ocular Culture; Pseudomonas aeruginosa; Red Eye; Staphylococcus aureus; Streptococcus pneumoniae; Streptococcus pyogenes

Test Includes Aerobic bacterial culture and smears (Gram and Giemsa) if specifically requested

Abstract Conjunctivitis clinically is characterized by dilation of superficial vessels with hyperemia, edema, and discharge. Purulent exudate suggests bacterial infection. Bacterial conjunctivitis spreads to the other eye within 48 hours. Hyperacute bacterial conjunctivitis is usually related to **gonococcal infection**, is often accompanied by preauricular lymphadenopathy, and may lead to perforation.

The leading cause of **red eye** is viral infection, which may accompany or follow an upper respiratory tract infection, and which is highly contagious. Replicating **adenovirus** is found in 95% of patients with that infection 10 days after appearance of symptoms.

Chlamydial conjunctivitis causes inclusion conjunctivitis, a sexually transmitted disease. Trachoma is caused by Chlamydia.

Allergic conjunctivitis is IgE-mediated.[1]

Patient Preparation Cleanse skin around eye with mild antiseptic. Gently remove make-up and ointment with sterile cotton and saline.

Specimen Eye swab

Container Swab with transport media

Collection The specimen should be transported to the laboratory immediately. Collect the specimen by swabbing; pass moistened swab two times over lower inferior tarsal conjunctival fornix. Avoid eyelid border and lashes. (Culture these separately in a similar fashion if indicated.) Scrapings: Use local anesthetic and platinum spatula. Rub the spatula with scrapings gently over small area on slide. If the specimen is too dry, use a very small amount of nonbacteriostatic sterile water. Scraping should be done by a physician. Swab collection has a better yield for bacteria, while scraping enhances yield of filamentous organisms.[2] The laboratory and the referring physician should consult to avoid misunderstanding regarding the collection, labeling, or handling of specimens (OD=right eye, OS=left eye). Inoculation of prewarmed plates at the time of collection of the specimen (C-streak) is a useful adjunct to optimal culture yield because of the low numbers of organisms usually present.

Storage Instructions Handle carefully; transport to the laboratory immediately.

Special Instructions The laboratory should be informed of the specific source of the specimen, current antibiotic therapy, and suspected clinical diagnosis. The presence or suspicion of orbital cellulitis should be communicated to the laboratory as well.

Reference Interval Normal flora of the eye may include Corynebacterium species (diphtheroids), Staphylococcus epidermidis, saprophytic fungi, Moraxella catarrhalis, Moraxella species, Streptococcus species (nonhemolytic), and gram-negative rods (rare). Abnormal ocular flora include

Haemophilus influenzae, Haemophilus aegyptius, Streptococcus pneumoniae, Staphylococcus aureus, Pseudomonas aeruginosa, Noguchia granulosus, Bacillus subtilis, Neisseria gonorrhoeae, and *Mycobacterium chelonei.*

Use Isolate and identify potentially pathogenic organisms. Pathogens which may cause bacterial conjunctivitis include *H. influenzae, H. aegyptius, Staphylococcus* sp, *Streptococcus pneumoniae,* and *Neisseria gonorrhoeae. Pseudomonas* is the most common bacterial pathogen in those who wear contact lenses. Viral conjunctivitis may be caused by adenovirus, echovirus, and Coxsackievirus.

Causes of keratitis include herpes simplex, adenovirus, *Streptococcus pneumoniae, Staphylococcus aureus, Pseudomonas, Acanthamoeba,* and chemical agents.

Ophthalmia neonatorum, occurring in infants younger than 4 weeks of age, may be caused by chemical irritation (silver nitrate), *Neisseria gonorrhoeae,* or *Pseudomonas.* In the U.S., the most common cause is *Chlamydia trachomatis.* Gram stain and culture are indicated when conjunctivitis develops more than 48 hours after birth. See Related Information above for other diagnostic procedures.

Limitations The procedure will not detect *Chlamydia,* viruses, fungal agents, or mycobacteria which may cause conjunctivitis and/or keratitis. Scrapings are a more useful specimen than a swab for Gram stain.

Methodology Aerobic culture on blood and chocolate agar, incubation at 37°C with CO_2

Additional Information The major modes of transmission of disease to the conjunctiva include the hands, airborne fomites, spread from adjacent adnexal infections, and sexual transmission. Eye infections include eyelid infections, blepharitis, dacryocystitis, orbital cellulitis, conjunctivitis, keratitis, endophthalmitis retinitis, and chorioretinitis. Blepharitis may be caused by a variety of organisms, including *Staphylococcus.* **Pinkeye** is usually caused by adenovirus. It presents as bilateral conjunctivitis with a sudden onset. Herpes simplex and varicella-zoster present as periorbital or corneal infections. Nontuberculous mycobacterial keratitis may occur following trauma or surgery accompanied by the use of local corticosteroids.[3]

Giemsa and Gram stains must specifically be requested. If gonorrhea is suspected, a Thayer-Martin plate should be inoculated. *Acanthamoeba* may be detected with the Calcofluor white stain (see Fungus Smear, Stain *on page 615* for a description of the stain) and grown on nutrient agar overlaid with a lawn of *E. coli;* cultures for *Acanthamoeba* are not available at many institutions.

A minority of patients with cat scratch disease develop Perinaud oculoglandular syndrome, characterized by conjunctivitis and preauricular lymphadenopathy.[4] This syndrome may also occur in oculoglandular tularemia, in which the conjunctiva is the portal of entry.

Differential diagnosis of **red eye** includes subconjunctival hemorrhage, episcleritis, angle-closure glaucoma, acute anterior uveitis, and superficial keratosis. A splendidly illustrated review paper has recently been published.[1]

See also Sjögren Antibodies *on page 542.*

Footnotes

1. Leibowitz HM, "The Red Eye," *N Engl J Med,* 2000, 343(5):345-51.
2. Benson WH and Lanier JD, "Comparison of Techniques for Culturing Corneal Ulcers," *Ophthalmology,* 1992, 99(5):800-4.
3. Bullington RH Jr, Lanier JD, and Font RL, "Nontuberculous Mycobacterial Keratitis. Report of Two Cases and Review of the Literature," *Arch Ophthalmol,* 1992, 110(4):519-24.
4. Ormerod LD and Dailey JP, "Ocular Manifestations of Cat-Scratch Disease," *Curr Opin Ophthalmol,* 1999, 10(3):209-16.

References

Baum J, "Infections of the Eye," *Clin Infect Dis,* 1995, 21:479-88.
Brodovsky SC and Snibson GR, "Corneal and Conjunctival Infections," *Curr Opin Ophthalmol,* 1997, 8(4):2-7.
Fay A and Jakobiec FA, "Diseases of the Visual System," *Cecil Textbook of Medicine,* 21st ed, Chapter 512, Goldman L and Bennett JC, eds, Philadelphia, PA: WB Saunders Co, 2000, 2224-35.
Morrow GL and Abbott RL, "Conjunctivitis," *Am Fam Phys,* 1998, 57(4):735-46.
Olitsky SE and Nelson LB, "Disorders of the Conjunctiva," *Nelson Textbook of Pediatrics,* 16th ed, Chapter 633, Behrman RE, Kliegman RM, and Jenson HB, eds, Philadelphia, PA: WB Saunders Co, 2000, 1911-4.

Bacterial Culture, Genital Specimen

Related Information

Synonyms Genital Culture

Applies to Amnionitis; *Candida* Culture, Genital; Cervical Culture; *Chlamydia trachomatis;* Clue Cells; *E. coli;* Endocervical Culture; Fungisitis; Group B Streptococci; *Listeria monocytogenes; Neisseria gonorrhoeae;* Prostatic Fluid Culture; Vaginal Culture

Abstract The most common pathogens recovered from nonpregnant women are *Chlamydia trachomatis* and *Neisseria gonorrhoeae.* These infections are often asymptomatic and are usually not diagnosed before membrane rupture.[1] The organisms most often found with chorioamnionitis (infections of the fetal membranes) and fetal infection following rupture of the membranes are group B streptococci and *E. coli.* Less frequent pathogens requiring consideration include *Enterococcus* sp, *Gardnerella vaginalis,* and anaerobes (especially *Actinomyces*).[2] Additional organisms to be considered include genital *Mycoplasma, Escherichia coli,* and *Listeria monocytogenes.*[3] Infection of the umbilical cord is **fungisitis.** Infection of the amniotic fluid is **amnionitis.**

An evidence-based health policy report recommends screening certain subsets of sexually active women for genital chlamydial infection.[4]

Collection

Female: Commercially available kits are useful to ensure that the entire spectrum of organisms will be evaluated. Such kits contain a variety of swabs and transport media needed to recover most of the pathogens encountered in cases of sexually transmitted diseases. Rayon-tipped swabs are used to collect cervical, vaginal, and vesicle cultures. Small dacron-tipped swabs are used to collect cultures from the urethra for gonococcal and chlamydial organisms. Separate transport media are necessary for recovery of gonococci, *Chlamydia trachomatis* and herpesvirus, and *Mycoplasma* and *Ureaplasma* sp.[2]

Male: Commercially available kits are useful, as described above. Urethral exudate is cultured for *Neisseria gonorrhoeae* and *Chlamydia trachomatis.* When no exudate can be expressed, insertion of a swab (cotton, rayon, or Dacron) into the distal urethra may be required. Appropriate transport media are essential.

Currently, *Neisseria gonorrhoeae* and *Chlamydia trachomatis* are often diagnosed using the more sensitive, nonculture methods. Specimens for these assays should be collected in the specified kit.

Storage Instructions Recovery of *N. gonorrhoeae* is enhanced by cultures taken at the bedside (onto special medium at room temperature) and delivery to the laboratory within 30 minutes.

Special Instructions The laboratory should be informed of the specific source of specimen, current antibiotic therapy, clinical diagnosis, and time of collection.

Critical Values Recovery of *N. gonorrhoeae* and/or beta-hemolytic group B strep during pregnancy

Use Cultures are often used in the setting of acute sexually transmitted disease. The role of cultures in chorioamnionitis and postpartum endometritis (PPE) is more controversial. In PPE, blood cultures are very useful and are reported to be positive in 10% to 20% of cases.[3] Screening is often recommended for *Chlamydia trachomatis* infection in women.[4]

Limitations Infections with *Chlamydia trachomatis* and *N. gonorrhoeae* are often evaluated using molecular assays. It is important to note that, because of inhibitors, these techniques may be insensitive in pregnant women.[5] *N. gonorrhoeae* is a fastidious organism; if left in the environment, it may not grow in culture at all. *Chlamydia trachomatis* is an intracellular pathogen. Cultures may be negative if the specimen does not contain adequate cells.

Methodology Cultures on modified Thayer-Martin (or equivalent) medium, 5% sheep blood agar, V agar with protease peptone #3 and human blood, anaerobic blood agar (with and without selective agents), Maconkey agar, and other media may be used. Special transport media and culture systems are required for the identification of genital *Mycoplasma* organisms.[2]

Nucleic acid amplification techniques are more sensitive for identification of both *Chlamydia trachomatis* and *Neisseria gonorrhoeae* in urethral exudates, endocervical exudates, and urine specimens.

Monoclonal antibody-based techniques, once very popular, are now used less often.

Additional Information In addition to cultures, nucleic acid amplification, enzyme-linked immunoassays, and direct fluorescent antibody stains may also be used. It should be noted that there is considerable variation in the specificity among these methods. A "one size fits all" approach should be avoided if patient outcomes are to be optimized.

Vaginitis is one of the most commonly encountered complaints of female patients. A significant portion of these appear to be due to specific etiologic agents such as *Candida* species or *Trichomonas vaginalis.* Nonspecific vaginitis, also called bacterial vaginosis, is characterized by an excessive malodorous vaginal discharge associated with a decrease in the number of lactobacilli and an increase in the number of *Gardnerella vaginalis* and other anaerobic bacteria such as *Bacteroides* species, *Prevotella* species, (Continued)

Bacterial Culture, Genital Specimen (*Continued*)

and *Peptostreptococcus* species.[6] Additionally, curved, motile, anaerobic gram-negative bacilli identified as *Mobiluncus* species have been associated with bacterial vaginosis. **Presently, bacterial cultures do not contribute to the diagnosis of bacterial vaginosis.** Minimum diagnostic requirements for bacterial vaginosis include three of the following signs:[7]

• excessive vaginal discharge
• vaginal pH >4.5
• "clue" cells (vaginal epithelial cells covered by small gram-negative rods)
• a fishy amine-like odor in the KOH test (10% KOH added to vaginal discharge)

Candida species are frequently present as normal flora in vagina. A saline wet mount may demonstrate yeast cells or pseudohyphae and may provide rapid diagnostic information. The most common clinical presentation is a characteristic clumpy white cottage cheese appearance with vaginal or vulvar itching. Vaginitis frequently complicates pregnancy and diabetes and is seen with broad spectrum antibiotic therapy, as well as, in conditions which lower host resistance (eg, AIDS).[8]

Listeria monocytogenes causes uterine infection, chorioamnionitis, placental abscesses, neonatal sepsis, abortion, stillbirth, premature birth, and other diseases. A modicum of additional information is included in Bacterial Culture, Stool *on page 575*.

Infections caused by **group B streptococci** (GBS) (***Streptococcus agalactiae***) can include sepsis, meningitis, pneumonia, and mortality among neonates. GBS are the leading bacterial cause of serious U.S. neonatal disease.[9] Acquired by contact with the maternal genital tract during labor and delivery, 80% appear within 7 days of birth. Such neonatal infections may lead to mental retardation, hearing or visual loss. Screening includes both vaginal and anal specimens[9] for culture at 35-37 weeks gestation. In addition to conventional cultures, DNA-based tests have been reported, PCR assays which require only up to ~100 minutes.[10,11]

The high-risk criteria include:
• previous infant with invasive GBS infection
• GBS bacteriuria during the current gestation
• delivery at <37 weeks gestation
• duration of rupture of membranes ≥18 hours
• intrapartum fever ≥100.4°F (≥38°C)[9]

See also Group B *Streptococcus* Screen, Rapid *on page 618* and Fibronectin, Fetal, Cervicovaginal Secretions *on page 174*.

Footnotes

1. Goldenberg RL, Hauth JC, and Andrews WW, "Intrauterine Infection and Preterm Delivery," *N Engl J Med*, 2000, 342(20):1500-7.
2. Koneman EW, Allen SD, Janda WM, et al, *Color Atlas and Textbook of Diagnostic Microbiology*, 5th ed, New York, NY: Lippincott, 1997, 142-7, 871-2.
3. Mead PB, "Infections of the Female Pelvis," *Mandel, Douglas, and Bennett's Principles and Practice of Infectious Diseases*, 5th ed, Mandell GL, Bennett JE, and Dolin R, eds, New York, NY: Churchill Livingstone, 2000, 1235-43.
4. Pimenta J, Catchpole M, Gray M, et al, "Evidence Based Health Policy Report. Screening for Genital Chlamydial Infection," *BMJ*, 2000, 321(7261):629-31.
5. Jensen IP, Thorsen P, and Moller BR, "Sensitivity of Ligase Chain Reaction Assay of Urine From Pregnant Women for *Chlamydia trachomatis*," *Lancet*, 1997, 349(9048):329-30.
6. Catlin BW, "*Gardnerella vaginalis*: Characteristics, Clinical Considerations, and Controversies," *Clin Microbiol Rev*, 1992, 5(3):213-37.
7. Joesoef MR and Schmid GP, "Bacterial Vaginosis: Review of Treatment Options and Potential Clinical Indications for Therapy," *Clin Infect Dis*, 1995, 20(Suppl 1):S72-9.
8. Kinghorn GR, "Vulvovaginal Candidosis," *J Antimicrob Chemother*, 1991, 28(Suppl A):59-66.
9. Centers for Disease Control and Prevention, "Adoption of Perinatal Group B Streptococcal Disease Prevention Recommendations by Prenatal-Care Providers - Connecticut and Minnesota, 1998," *JAMA*, 2000, 283(18):2384-5.
10. Schuchat A, "Neonatal Group B Streptococcal Disease - Screening and Prevention," *N Engl J Med*, 2000, 343(3):209-10.
11. Bergeron MG, Ke D, Ménard C, et al, "Rapid Detection of Group B Streptococci in Pregnant Women at Delivery," *N Engl J Med*, 2000, 343(3):175-9.

References

Carne C, "Sexually Transmitted Infections," *BMJ*, 1998, 317(7151):129-32.
Cline MK, Bailey-Dorton C, and Cayelli M, "Maternal Infections: Diagnosis and Management," *Prim Care*, 2000, 27(1):13-33.
Emmert DH and Kirchner JT, "Sexually Transmitted Diseases in Women. Gonorrhea and Syphilis," *Postgrad Med*, 2000, 107(2):181-4, 189-90, 193-7.
Genc M and Mardh A, "A Cost-Effectiveness Analysis of Screening and Treatment for *Chlamydia trachomatis* Infection in Asymptomatic Women," *Ann Intern Med*, 1996, 124(1 Pt 1):1-7.
McGregor JA and French JI, "Bacterial Vaginosis in Pregnancy," *Obstet Gynecol Surv*, 2000, 55(5 Suppl 1):S1-19.
Schrag SJ, Zywicki S, Farley MM, et al, "Group B Streptococcal Disease in the Era of Intrapartum Antibiotic Prophylaxis," *N Engl J Med*, 2000, 342(1):15-20.

Internet Web Sites

Group B streptococci: www.cdc.gov/ncidod/dbmd/gbs

Bacterial Culture, Intravascular Device

Related Information

Bacteremia Detection, Buffy Coat Micromethod *on page 406*

Bacterial Culture, Aerobes *on page 563*
Bacterial Culture, Blood *on page 566*

Synonyms Intravascular Device Culture

Applies to Broviac Catheters; Catheter Tip Culture; Central Catheters; Exit Site Infections; Hemovac® Tip Culture; Hickman Catheters; Hyperalimentation Line Culture; Intravenous Catheter Culture; Quantitative Tip Culture (QTC); Swan-Ganz Tip Culture; Tunnel Infection

Test Includes Quantitative or semiquantitative culture of an intravascular catheter or blood specimen collected through the catheter; organism identification, and antimicrobial susceptibilities if appropriate

Abstract American hospitals and clinics purchase several million intravascular catheters annually. The patients in whom they are used are at risk for catheter-related sepsis, and about 16,000 central line-associated bloodstream infections occur in ICUs in the U.S. each year. In meta-analysis, average attributable mortality was 3%. Current studies have focused on prevention of such infections.[1,2,3,4] Culture of intravascular devices should be limited to patients who have laboratory confirmed bacteremia or who appear clinically septic, but have no apparent source of infection. In this situation, the intravascular device is investigated as the possible origin of infection. Alternatively, simultaneous line tip and blood cultures are advocated in suspected catheter-related bacteremia.[5] Blood culture may be the best means to ascertain which patients require treatment.[6] Randomly culturing patients who are not bacteremic or who are not clinically septic is unwarranted.

Specimen Tip from intravascular device

Container Sterile container

Collection One or more 2-3 cm segments are often submitted. Alternatively, blood for comparative quantitative cultures may be collected simultaneously from a peripheral vein and from the central venous catheter. See Bacterial Culture, Blood *on page 566*.

Storage Instructions Specimens should be transported to the laboratory within 1 hour of collection for optimal results.

Reference Interval Roll plate semiquantitative cultures yielding <15 colonies, sonicated specimens yielding $<10^4$ colonies of coagulase-negative staphylococci (cutoffs for other organisms are less clear), and comparative quantitative cultures yielding a ratio <10:1 (central venous catheter vs peripheral vein cultures) or <100 CFU/mL (central venous catheter only) suggests that the catheter should not be strongly considered as the cause of sepsis.[7]

Use Infections complicating therapy with indwelling central venous catheters pose a difficult problem.

Limitations Results of intravascular device cultures contribute to the work-up of patients with bloodstream infections who lack an obvious source. These results do not stand alone, however, and all methods described have a significant number of false-positive and false-negative results. Isolated positive line tip cultures without corresponding blood cultures may cause unnecessary investigation.[5]

Methodology Roll plate semiquantitative cultures: Aseptically roll the catheter tip on a blood and/or chocolate agar plate.[5]

Quantitative sonication method: Place catheter segment in 10 mL of tryptic soy broth, sonicate for 1 minute, then vortex for 15 seconds (original specimen). Add 0.1 mL of this specimen to 9.9 mL of saline (diluted specimen) and inoculate separate blood agar plates with 0.1 mL of the original and diluted specimens. Perform colony counts and multiply by 10^2 (original specimen) or 10^4 (diluted specimen) to determine the number of organisms on the catheter.

Comparative quantitative cultures: Follow procedures for collection listed above and process as you would blood cultures using the lysis centrifugation method. Perform colony counts on both specimens.

Sonication technique is considered useful.[8]

Summary of Results of Prospective Studies Using Semiquantitative Techniques to Diagnose Vascular-Access Infections

Organism	No. With Same Organism in Semiquantitative Catheter Culture and Blood Culture
Coagulase-negative staphylococci	27
Staphylococcus aureus	26
Yeast	17
Enterobacter	7
Serratia	5
Enterococcus	5
Klebsiella	4
Streptococcus viridans group	3
Pseudomonas species	2
Proteus	2
Others: *Pseudomonas aeruginosa*, *Yersinia*	1 each

Adapted from Hampton A and Sheretz RJ, "Vascular-Access Infections in Hospitalized Patients," *Surg Clin North Am*, 1988, 68:57-72.

Additional Information Catheter-related sepsis is defined when:

- positive blood cultures collected through the central venous catheter show a tenfold or greater colony count compared with peripheral quantitative blood culture or >100 CFU/mL if only central venous catheter blood culture is available
- no obvious clinical or microbiologic source for the infection is apparent

Exit site infections are defined as purulent drainage or erythema at the catheter exit site. **Tunnel infection** is defined as spreading cellulitis with erythema, tenderness, and swelling of the skin surrounding the subcutaneous tunnel tract of the catheter. Successful therapy of catheter-related infection with antibiotics and local care has required catheter removal to achieve cure, particularly in *Pseudomonas* tunnel infections. *Staphylococcus aureus* and polymicrobial infections also have been more difficult to eradicate. Intraluminal cultures correlate well with catheter tip cultures (87.5% identical) while skin puncture sites were less frequently identical (37.5%).[9] See table on previous page.

When *Staphylococcus aureus* is found in a positive line tip culture, a high likelihood of bacteremia exists.[5]

Footnotes

1. Mermel LA, "Prevention of Intravascular Catheter-Related Infections," *Ann Intern Med*, 2000, 132(5):391-402.
2. Veenstra DL, Saint S, Saha S, et al, "Efficacy of Antiseptic-Impregnated Central Venous Catheters in Preventing Catheter-Related Bloodstream Infection. A Meta-analysis," *JAMA*, 1999, 281(3):261-7.
3. Wenzel RP and Edmond MB, "The Evolving Technology of Venous Access," *N Engl J Med*, 1999, 340(1):48-50.
4. Darouiche RO, Raad II, Heard SO, "A Comparison of Two Antimicrobial-Impregnated Central Venous Catheters," *N Engl J Med*, 1999, 340(1):1-8.
5. Peacock SJ, Eddleston M, Emptage A, et al, "Positive Intravenous Line Tip Cultures as Predictors of Bacteremia," *J Hosp Infect*, 1998, 40(1):35-8.
6. Reisner BS, Woods GL, Thomson RB Jr, et al, "Specimen Processing," *Manual of Clinical Microbiology*, Chapter 5, Murray PR, Baron EJ, Pfaller MA, et al, eds, Washington, DC: ASM Press, American Society for Microbiology, 1999, 64-104.
7. Sherertz RJ, Raad II, Belani A, et al, "Three-Year Experience With Sonicated Vascular Catheter Cultures in a Clinical Microbiology Laboratory," *J Clin Microbiol*, 1990, 28(1):76-82.
8. Jakobsen CJ, Hansen V, Jensen JJ, et al, "Contamination of Subclavian Vein Catheters: An Intraluminal Culture Method," *J Hosp Infect*, 1989, 13(3):253-60.
9. Kelly M, Wunderlich Wciorka LR, McConico S, et al, "Sonicated Vascular Catheter Tip Cultures: Quantitative Association With Catheter-Related Sepsis and the Nonutility of an Adjuvant Cytocentrifuge Gram Stain," *Am J Clin Pathol*, 1996, 105(2):210-5.

References

Crump JA and Collignon PJ, "Intravascular Catheter-Associated Infections," *Eur J Clin Microbiol Infect Dis*, 2000, 19(1):1-8.

Fry DE, Fry RV, and Borzotta AP, "Nosocomial Blood-Borne Infection Secondary to Intravascular Devices," *Am J Surg*, 1994, 167(2):268-72.

Garrison RN and Wilson MA, "Intravenous and Central Catheter Infections," *Surg Clin North Am*, 1994, 74(3):557-70.

Mermel LA, "Prevention of Intravascular Catheter-Related Infections," *Ann Intern Med*, 2000, 132(5):391-402.

Raad I, "Management of Intravascular Catheter-Related Infections," *J Antimicrob Chemother*, 2000, 45(3):267-70.

Bacterial Culture, Middle Ear

Related Information
Bacterial Culture, Aerobes *on page 563*
Bacterial Culture, Conjunctiva *on page 570*
Gram Stain *on page 617*
Respiratory Syncytial Virus Antigen Detection *on page 674*

Synonyms Culture, Ear; Ear Culture

Applies to *Haemophilus influenzae*; Middle Ear Culture; Outer Ear Culture; *Proteus* spp; *Pseudomonas aeruginosa*; *Streptococcus pneumoniae*; Tympanocentesis Culture

Test Includes Gram stain and culture for aerobic bacteria

Abstract The most common bacteria cultured from patients with otitis media include *Streptococcus pneumoniae*, *Streptococcus pyogenes*, and *Haemophilus influenzae*.[1] Symptoms may include fever, which occurs in 30% to 50% of patients.[2]

Patient Preparation Cleanse the site to reduce the background contamination level

Specimen Tympanic membrane aspirate, nasopharyngeal swab; external meatus drainage

Container Sterile tube or Culturette®

Collection Specimen should be transported to the laboratory as soon as possible.

Special Instructions When ear cultures for obligate anaerobic bacteria are needed, consultation with the laboratory may be helpful. The laboratory should be informed if a specific agent such as *Pseudomonas*, *Haemophilus*, or *Candida* is suspected.

Reference Interval Normal flora of the skin of the healthy ear includes *Staphylococcus epidermidis*, *Corynebacterium* species, and *Staphylococcus aureus*

Use Determine the etiologic agent of otitis media

Limitations Superficial swab specimens are insensitive and nonspecific for definition of the etiology of otitis media; their use for this purpose should be discouraged. Initial therapy of this condition should be empiric.

Contraindications The presence of topical ointments or drugs in or on the site to be cultured

Methodology Aerobic and anaerobic bacterial culture of specimens obtained by tympanocentesis; aerobic cultures, only, of swab specimens

Additional Information Acute otitis media is the most common bacterial infection in children. Although acute otitis media is generally recognized as a bacterial infection, viruses play a role in its etiology and outcome.[3]

The most common complication of otitis media is hearing loss. Other complications include mastoiditis, cholesteatoma, perforation, otorrhea, neck abscess, meningitis, extradural abscess, subdural empyema, otogenic brain abscess, and lateral sinus thrombosis.[2]

Correlation of nasopharyngeal cultures with results of tympanocentesis culture is poor; nasopharyngeal cultures lack predictive value in identification of the causative agent of otitis media. Bodor[4,5] and associates have described a good correlation between conjunctival cultures and cultures obtained by tympanocentesis and have described the simultaneous occurrence of conjunctivitis and otitis as a clinical syndrome in children. In decreasing order of frequency, the following organisms have been recovered from tympanocentesis: *S. pneumoniae* (50% to 75%), *H. influenzae* (10% to 30%), *Moraxella (Branhamella) catarrhalis* (5% to 10%), *Streptococcus pyogenes* (5% to 10%), *Staphylococcus aureus* (1% to 5%), *Pseudomonas aeruginosa* (0.1% to 1%). *E. coli*, *Klebsiella pneumoniae*, *Pseudomonas aeruginosa* may be isolated from neonates. Tympanocentesis is not usually required in primary infections. It should be reserved for complicated, recurrent, or chronic otitis media. *Candida* superinfection may complicate therapy for recurring ear infections and may be a cause of persistent otorrhea.[6] Otitis externa is frequently caused by *P. aeruginosa* and less frequently by *Candida* species, *Proteus* species, *S. aureus*, and *Trichophyton* species.

In a recent study, respiratory syncytial virus was the most common virus found in middle ear fluid. Other agents in middle ear fluid included parainfluenza viruses and influenza viruses.[3]

Footnotes

1. Arguedas A, Loaiza C, Perez A, et al, "Microbiology of Acute Otitis Media in Costa Rican Children," *Pediatr Infect Dis J*, 1998, 17(8):680-9.
2. Kenna M, "The Ear," *Nelson Textbook of Pediatrics*, 16th ed, Behrman RE, Kliegman RM, Jenson HB, eds, Philadelphia, PA: WB Saunders Co, 2000, 1938-63.
3. Heikkinen T, Thint M, and Chonmaitree T, "Prevalence of Various Respiratory Viruses in the Middle Ear During Acute Otitis Media," *N Engl J Med*, 1999, 340(4):260-4.
4. Bodor FF, Marchant CD, and Shurin PA, "Bacterial Etiology of Conjunctivitis-Otitis Media Syndrome," *Pediatrics*, 1985, 76(1):26-8.
5. Bodor FF, "Conjunctivitis-Otitis Syndrome," *Pediatrics*, 1982, 69:695-8.
6. Cohen SR and Thompson JW, "Otitic Candidiasis in Children: An Evaluation of the Problem and Effectiveness of Ketoconazole in 10 Patients," *Ann Otol Rhinol Laryngol*, 1990, 99(6 Pt 1):427-31.

References

Gehanno P, Nguyen L, Derriennic M, et al, "Pathogens Isolated During Treatment Failures in Otitis," *Pediatr Infect Dis J*, 1998, 17(10):885-90.

Liederman EM, Post JC, Aul JJ, et al, "Analysis of Adult Otitis Media: Polymerase Chain Reaction Versus Culture for Bacteria and Viruses," *Ann Otol Rhinol Laryngol*, 1998, 107(1):10-6.

Nozicka CA, Hanly JG, Beste DJ, et al, "Otitis Media in Infants Aged 0-8 weeks: Frequency of Associated Serious Bacterial Disease," *Pediatr Emerg Care*, 1999, 15(4):252-4.

Sutton DV, Derkay CS, Darrow DH, et al, "Resistant Bacteria in Middle Ear Fluid at the Time of Tympanotomy Tube Surgery," *Ann Otol Rhinol Laryngol*, 2000, 109(1):24-9.

Bacterial Culture, Nasopharynx

Related Information
Bordetella pertussis Culture *on page 583*
Chlamydia trachomatis Direct Antigen Test *on page 590*
Parainfluenza Virus Culture *on page 668*

Synonyms Nasopharyngeal Culture

Abstract The gold standard for diagnosis of pertussis is isolation of *B. pertussis* in culture.[1]

Specimen Nasopharyngeal swab

Container Sterile wire swab expressed into transport medium or transported directly to the laboratory

Collection Use special nasopharyngeal wire swabs/Calgiswab®. Gently insert swab through nose to posterior nasopharynx; allow to remain for a few seconds and gently remove wire. The specimen should be transported to the laboratory as soon as possible. Swabs must be collected carefully, taking care not to touch the skin.

Turnaround Time Cultures for *B. pertussis* are incubated and examined regularly for 7 days. The tiny colonies grow slowly.

Reference Interval Normal nasopharyngeal flora

Use In clinical practice, suspected infection with *Bordetella pertussis* is the major indication for a nasopharyngeal bacterial culture.[2] Such specimens are also useful for viral diagnosis.
(Continued)

Bacterial Culture, Nasopharynx *(Continued)*

Nasopharyngeal or conjunctival culture provides diagnosis of *C. trachomatis* infection in neonates, some of whom develop neonatal pneumonia and conjunctivitis.

Limitations Results suggesting primary nasopharyngeal infection must be interpreted with caution, because of the variety of potentially pathogenic normal flora and the potential presence of infection in adjacent sites. Cultures for pertussis may be negative in partly immune patients and in subjects who have been treated with amoxicillin or erythromycin.[1]

Contraindications Avoid rayon or cotton swabs, which may contain fatty acids toxic to *Bordetella* spp.[3]

Methodology Aerobic culture following nasopharyngeal aspiration or flexible dacron or alginate swab. DFA testing of isolates enhances recovery. PCR applications are described.

Additional Information Presence or absence of normal flora is usually reported. Normal flora of the nose includes *S. epidermidis* (coagulase-negative *Staphylococcus*), *S. aureus*, *S. pneumoniae*, *H. influenzae*, *S. pyogenes*, *M. catarrhalis*, and *Neisseria* species. Consequently, nasal cultures for such bacteria rarely provide useful clinical information.

A characteristic laboratory feature of pertussis is leukocytosis with absolute lymphocytosis, characterized by small lymphocytes rather than virocytes.

Viruses which may be recovered from the nasopharynx include influenza virus, parainfluenza virus, and respiratory syncytial virus.

Footnotes

1. Long SS, "Pertussis (*Bordetella pertussis* and *B. parapertussis*)," *Nelson Textbook of Pediatrics*, 16th ed, Chapter 195, Kleigman RM and Jenson HB, eds, Philadelphia, PA: WB Saunders Co, 2000, 838-42.
2. Koneman EW, Allen SD, Janda WM, et al, *Color Atlas and Textbook of Diagnostic Microbiology*, 5th ed, New York, NY: Lippincott Raven, 1997, 128-30.
3. Reisner BS, Woods GL, Thomson RB Jr, et al, "Specimen Processing," *Manual of Clinical Microbiology*, Chapter 5, Murray PR, Baron EJ, Pfaller MA, et al, eds, Washington, DC: ASM Press, American Society for Microbiology, 1999, 64-104.

References

Muller FM, Hoppe JE, and Wirsing von Konig CH, "Laboratory Diagnosis of Pertussis: State of the Art in 1997," *J Clin Microbiol*, 1997, 35(10):2435-43.

Bacterial Culture, Sputum

Related Information

Synonyms Sputum Culture

Applies to *Bacteroides* spp; *Bordetella pertussis*; *Chlamydia trachomatis*; *Corynebacterium diphtheriae*; *Enterobacteriaceae*; *Haemophilus influenzae*; *Klebsiella* spp; *Legionella* spp; *Moraxella catarrhalis*; *Mycoplasma pneumoniae*; *Neisseria gonorrhoeae*; *Staphylococcus aureus*; *Streptococcus* β-Hemolytic Group A; *Streptococcus pneumoniae*

Test Includes Gram stain, quantitative scoring for specimen adequacy, and inoculation of culture media (acceptable specimens only); Gram stain and culture of aerobic organisms

Abstract Laboratory evaluation begins with the microscopic examination of a Gram stain of the specimen to guide initial therapy and to determine the suitability of the specimen for culture. Even when meticulous technique is used (see below), sputum is a problematic specimen because of contaminating organisms from the mouth and pharyngeal region. Alternative specimen sources, highly effective in recovering organisms which cause lower respiratory infections, include transtracheal aspirates and specimens obtained via bronchoscopy and bronchoalveolar lavage. Depending on the clinical situation, **blood culture may also be very useful in the diagnosis of bacterial pneumonia.**[1,2] When pleural effusion or empyema exists, it too can be evaluated and cultured if clinically indicated. See Body Fluids topic in the Key Word Index.

Patient Preparation The patient should remove dentures, rinse mouth, and gargle with water. (Mouthwashes, which often contain antibacterial agents, should not be used.) The patient should then cough deeply and expectorate sputum into sterile container.

Container Sterile sputum container, sputum trap, sterile tracheal aspirate or bronchoscopy aspirate tube. Specimens contaminated on the outside of the container pose excessive risk.

Collection Collect expectorated sputum under direct supervision of nurse or physician. Specimen collected, at time of bronchoscopy, by aspiration or by transtracheal aspiration by a physician skilled in the procedure. The specimen should be transported to the laboratory within 1 hour of collection for processing.

Storage Instructions Refrigerate if the specimen cannot be promptly processed.

Causes for Rejection Microscopy provides an index of the magnitude and character of exudate and may permit recognition of abnormalities, such as fungal hyphae or evidence of anaerobic infection. Gram stain is commonly utilized. Two well-validated methods are used to determine the suitability of a sputum specimen for culture. **Bartlett's system**[3] is a grading system (see Table 1) based on the number of neutrophils and squamous epithelial cells, and the presence of mucus. Specimens with a final score ≤0 should be rejected. **Murray and Washington's system**[4] is similar (see Table 2). Specimens with a group of 1 or 2 are invalidated.[1] Van Scoy advocates acceptance for culture even when >10 epithelial cells are found, when >25 PMNs are counted.[5] When patients are neutropenic, only squamous cells are evaluated, and specimens are invalidated if there are >10 squamous cells/lpf.[1,6]

Table 1. Bartlett's Grading System to Assess the Quality of Sputum Samples

Number of Neutrophils/10 x lpf	Grade (indicates intensity of exudate)
<10	0
10-25	+1
>25	+2
Presence of mucus	+1
Number of Epithelial Cells/10 x lpf	**Grade (indicates proportion of saliva)**
10-25	-1
>25	-2
Total*	

lpf = low power field.

*Average the number of epithelial cells and neutrophils in 20-30 10x microscopic fields, then calculate a total. A final score of 0 or less indicates lack of active inflammation or contamination with saliva. Repeat sputum specimens should be requested.

Adapted from Koneman EW, Allen SD, Janda WM, et al, *Color Atlas and Textbook of Diagnostic Microbiology*, 5th ed, New York, NY: Lippincott Raven, 1997.

Table 2. Murray and Washington's Grading System to Assess the Quality of Sputum Samples

	Epithelial Cells/lpf	Leukocytes/lpf
Group 1	25	10
Group 2	25	10-25
Group 3	25	25
Group 4	10-25	25
Group 5	<10	25

lpf = low power field.

Adapted from Koneman EW, Allen SD, Janda WM, et al, *Color Atlas and Textbook of Diagnostic Microbiology*, 5th ed, New York, NY: Lippincott Raven, 1997, 76, 83-4, 128-31.

Consequently, the best expectorated sputum specimens have many PMNs and few to no squamous epithelial cells. Such specimens are likely to include the etiologic agent of the infection in relatively high numbers and comparatively few contaminating organisms from the upper respiratory tract.

Microscopic examination of specimens under oil (1000x total magnification) often provides preliminary morphologic information about the etiologic agent that can be used to guide empiric therapy. Organisms are especially important in Gram stain when phagocytosis is seen. Interpretation of results of bacterial sputum cultures without considering specimen quality (determined by Gram stain) is problematic.

Specimen rejection criteria are not applied when the suspected organisms include *Mycoplasma pneumoniae*, *Legionella* sp, mycobacteria[6] fungi, and viruses.[1]

Turnaround Time Stat Gram stain results usually are available in 15-30 minutes. Identification of pathogens usually requires at least 48 hours for completion.

Special Instructions The most productive sputum is that which represents bronchial secretions. A plug or cast of the infected bronchus may be evident. Such identified portions are inoculated on selective and nonselective media.

Reference Interval Normal upper respiratory flora. Tracheal aspirate and bronchoscopy specimens can be contaminated with normal oral flora. Transtracheal aspiration should have no growth.

Use Sputum cultures are performed to diagnose the etiology of lower respiratory infections, principally pneumonia. Media are selected to support the growth of the most common pathogens causing pneumonia.[7] In adults: *Streptococcus pneumoniae* is the most common cause of community-acquired pneumonia.[8] Other causes include *Haemophilus influenzae*, *Staphylococcus aureus*, many gram-negative rods, *Legionella* spp, and *Moraxella catarrhalis*. In the elderly, *Klebsiella pneumoniae*, and group B streptococci are also included. In critically ill patients, additional possibilities include *Mycoplasma pneumoniae*, *Chlamydia trachomatis*, and *Chlamydia pneumoniae*. In HIV-infected patients, additional possibilities include *Pneumocystis carinii*, cytomegalovirus, *Mycoplasma pneumoniae*, and *Cryptococcus neoformans*. In children, the most common pathogens causing pneumonia are viruses:[9] respiratory syncytial virus and parainfluenza virus type 3.

Limitations Contamination of sputum specimens by organisms normally present in the mouth and pharyngeal area is the principal factor limiting the usefulness of sputum cultures. Therefore, it is imperative that everyone involved in the collection and handling of a sputum specimen exercise meticulous technique; but even when this is done, contamination will occur in some specimens. Such contamination is an example of preanalytical variability (see Maximizing the Information From Laboratory Tests - The Ulysses Syndrome *on page 15*). As pointed out by Koneman et al[1], *Klebsiella pneumoniae* can be part of the nasopharyngeal normal flora and also the cause of acute pneumonia.

Agents such as *Bordetella pertussis*, *Corynebacterium diphtheriae*, *Legionella pneumophila*, *Mycoplasma pneumoniae*, and *Mycobacterium tuberculosis* require special laboratory measures for isolation. Clinical suspicion of involvement by such organisms should be communicated to the laboratory.

The yield from sputum culture in patients with bacteremic *Streptococcus pneumoniae* pneumonia is only about 50%.[2]

Additional Information Alcohol abuse and chronic liver disease are known indicators of poor prognosis in subjects with pneumonia.[10]

C-reactive protein (CRP) has been advocated as an adjunctive means to distinguish bacterial from viral pneumonia. Except for adenovirus and Epstein-Barr virus, viral infections mostly are not associated with CRP increases. In this role, CRP exhibits high sensitivity but specificity of only 60% to 70%.[11]

Footnotes

1. Koneman EW, Allen SD, Janda WM, et al, *Color Atlas and Textbook of Diagnostic Microbiology*, 5th ed, New York, NY: Lippincott, 1997, 76, 83-4, 128-31.
2. Plouffe JF, McNally C, and File TM, "Value of Noninvasive Studies in Community-Acquired Pneumonia," *Infect Dis Clin North Am*, 1998, 12(3):689-99.
3. Bartlett RC, *Medical Microbiology: Quality, Cost, and Clinical Relevance*, New York, NY: John Wiley and Sons, 1974.
4. Murray PR and Washington JA II, "Microscopic and Bacteriologic Analysis of Expectorated Sputum," *Mayo Clin Proc*, 1975, 50(6):339-44.
5. Van Scoy RE, "Bacterial Sputum Cultures. A Clinician's Viewpoint," *Mayo Clin Proc*, 1977, 52(1):39-41.
6. Reisner BS, Woods GL, Thomson RB Jr, et al, "Specimen Processing," *Manual of Clinical Microbiology*, 7th ed, Murray PR, Baron EJ, Pfaller MA, et al, eds, Washington DC: AMS Press, American Society for Microbiology, 1999, 64-104.
7. Donowitz GR and Mandell GL, "Acute Pneumonia," *Mandel, Douglas, and Bennett's Principles and Practice of Infectious Diseases*, 5th ed, Mandell GL, Bennett JE, and Dolin R, eds, New York, NY: Churchill Livingstone, 2000, 717-43.
8. Chenoweth CE, Saint S, Martinez F, et al, "Antimicrobial Resistance in *Streptococcus pneumoniae* Implications for Patients With Community-Acquired Pneumonia," *Mayo Clin Proc*, 2000, 75(11):1161-8.
9. Prober CG, "Pneumonia," *Nelson Textbook of Pediatrics*, 16th ed, Behrman RE, Kliegman RM, and Jenson HB, eds, Philadelphia, PA: WB Saunders Co, 2000, 761-5.
10. Shuster LT and McDougall JC, "Pneumonia Management Guidelines - Why, How, and Where to Start," *Mayo Clin Proc*, 1998, 73(1):96-7.
11. Gonzales R and Sande MA, "Uncomplicated Acute Bronchitis," *Ann Intern Med*, 2000, 133(12):981-91.

References

Almirall J, Bolibar I, Vidal J, et al, "Epidemiology of Community-Acquired Pneumonia in Adults: A Population-Based Study," *Eur Respir J*, 2000, 15(4):757-63.
Bartlett JG and Mundy L, "Community-Acquired Pneumonia," *N Engl J Med*, 1995, 333(24):1618-24.
Hindiyeh M and Carroll KC, "Laboratory Diagnosis of Atypical Pneumonia," *Semin Respir Infect*, 2000, 15(2):101-13.
Juven T, Mertsola J, Waris M, et al, "Etiology of Community-Acquired Pneumonia in 254 Hospitalized Children," *Pediatr Infect Dis J*, 2000, 19(4):293-8.
Ruiz-Gonzalez A, Falguera M, Nogues A, et al, "Is *Streptococcus pneumoniae* the Leading Cause of Pneumonia of Unknown Etiology? A Microbiologic Study of Lung Aspirates in Consecutive Patients With Community Acquired Pneumonia," *Am J Med*, 1999, 106(4):385-90.
Skerrett SJ, "Diagnostic Testing for Community-Acquired Pneumonia," *Clin Chest Med*, 1999, 20(3):531-48.

Bacterial Culture, Stool

Related Information

Synonyms Enteric Pathogens Culture, Routine; Rectal Swab Culture; Stool Culture

Applies to *Aeromonas hydrophila*; *Bacillus cereus* Food Poisoning; *Campylobacter*; *Clostridium difficile*; *Entamoeba histolytica*; Enterohemorrhagic *E. coli*; *Escherichia coli* O157:H7; *Listeria monocytogenes*; Norwalk Virus; *Plesiomonas shigelloides*; Rotavirus; *Salmonella*; Shiga Toxins; *Shigella*; Staphylococcal Food Poisoning; *Vibrio cholerae*; *Vibrio parahaemolyticus*; *Yersinia enterocolitica*

Test Includes May include Gram stain or methylene blue stain for leukocytes

Abstract Gastrointestinal disease may be the presenting and often only symptom for many food-borne pathogens (eg, *Salmonella* and *Campylobacter* species). Devastating disease may be seen (eg, listeriosis, *E. coli* O157:H7, typhoid fever).

In addition to bacterial causes of gastrointestinal disorders, other important entities exist (see Related Information). All infectious agents are not included in this volume and causes of gastrointestinal disease exist which do not directly relate to the clinical laboratory (eg, anatomic abnormalities). Some noninfectious causes of diarrhea can be found in the Key Word Index.

Cultures from outpatients and persons hospitalized for fewer than 3 days should be placed on media which can support the most common enteric pathogens (*Salmonella* spp, *Shigella* spp, and *Campylobacter* spp). Clinical information should be supplied if less common organisms are sought (eg, enterohemorrhagic *Escherichia coli* [most commonly serotype O157], *Yersinia enterocolitica*, *Vibrio* spp, *Aeromonas hydrophila*, *Plesiomonas shigelloides*, and *Listeria monocytogenes*).

Specimen Fresh random stool, rectal swab

Container Stool container, Culturette®

Sampling Time *Escherichia coli* O157:H7, *Salmonella* species, and *Campylobacter jejuni* are most often cultured from stools in summer months.

Collection If stool is collected in a clean bedpan, it must not be contaminated with urine, residual soap, or disinfectants. Swabs of lesions of the rectal wall during proctoscopy or sigmoidoscopy are preferred; *vide infra*.

Rectal swab: Insert the swab past the anal sphincter, move the swab circumferentially around the rectum. Allow 15-30 seconds for organisms to adsorb onto the swab. Withdraw swab, place in Culturette® tube, and crush media compartment.

Storage Instructions Fresh specimens should be promptly delivered to the laboratory and processed within 1-2 hours. If specimen transport or processing will be delayed, the specimen may be preserved in modified Cary-Blair or buffered glycerol-saline media and refrigerated.

Causes for Rejection Most laboratories reject specimens from patients hospitalized more than 3 days. This policy is based on a study by Siegel et al[1] and was confirmed by a study from the College of American Pathologists.[2]

Because of risk to laboratory personnel, specimens sent on a diaper or tissue paper, or specimen contamination of the outside of a transport container may not be acceptable. Specimens containing interfering substances (eg, castor oil, bismuth, Metamucil®, barium), specimens delayed in transit, and those contaminated with urine may not have optimal yield.

Turnaround Time Minimum 48 hours if negative; 72 hours if identification of *Yersinia* is required

Special Instructions The laboratory should be informed of the specific pathogen suspected if not *Salmonella*, *Shigella*, or *Campylobacter*.

Reference Interval Negative for *Campylobacter*, *Salmonella*, and *Shigella*. In endemic areas the isolation of a pathogen may not indicate the only cause of diarrhea.

Use Indications for stool culture include:[3]

- bloody diarrhea
- fever
- tenesmus
- severe or persistent symptoms
- recent travel to a third world country
- known exposure to a bacterial agent
- presence of fecal leukocytes

Limitations An enormous variety of microorganisms have been proven to cause diarrhea, and many others have been associated with diarrhea. Still, (Continued)

Bacterial Culture, Stool (Continued)

even with the most extensive work-ups, a substantial proportion of patients with gastrointestinal disorders fail to yield an etiologic agent. Routine bacterial stool cultures are designed to recover only a few specific organisms; these vary with the laboratory, but usually include *Salmonella*, *Shigella*, *Campylobacter* species, and may include *E. coli* O157:H7. Culture for the last may require special request, unless the stool is bloody.[4] The laboratory should be consulted if other etiologic agents are suspected (eg, *Vibrio* or *Yersinia*), or a more extensive work-up is required. Rectal swab cultures may not be as effective as stool cultures for identifying individuals with small numbers of organisms. *Clostridium difficile* infection is usually diagnosed by toxin assays rather than culture, often supplemented by endoscopy with biopsies.

Contraindications A rectal swab culture is not as effective as a stool culture for detection of the carrier state.

Methodology Aerobic culture on selective media. Isolates (eg, *E. coli* O157:H7 and *Salmonella enterica*) can be subtyped by pulsed-field gel electrophoresis. This approach supports delineation as sporadic cases or as outbreaks.[5,6] See Pulsed-Field Gel Electrophoresis Genotyping *on page 672*. Multilocus enzyme electrophoresis, ribotyping, and pulsed-field gel electrophoresis have been used in analysis of *Listeria* isolates.[7]

Additional Information In patients hospitalized more than 3 days, the most common causes of diarrhea are antibiotic administration, enteral feeding, osmotic diarrhea, and *Clostridium difficile* infection. Therefore, evaluation of such patients should begin with assessing these possibilities (see *Clostridium difficile* Toxin Assay and Culture *on page 592*).

Even when stool cultures are accepted only from patients hospitalized 3 days or less, the diagnostic yield is low.[3] In outpatient settings, screening for fecal leukocytes or blood may improve the yield.[8] On the other hand, implementation of the 3-day rule across all patient groups results in some missed diagnoses of important and treatable bacterial pathogens. With these facts in mind, investigators have recently devised and validated guidelines for exceptions to the 3-day rule.[9]

The following are the proposed guidelines for stool cultures in hospitalized adults (modified 3-day rule):

Obtain stool culture in the presence of:

- community-acquired diarrhea (if onset is 72 hours or less of admission)
- nosocomial diarrhea (if onset is more than 72 hours of admission) **and** at least one of the following: age 65 years or older with pre-existing comorbidity, HIV infection, neutropenia, suspected nosocomial outbreak
- suspected nondiarrheal manifestations of enteric infections

Maximum of two repeat exams in a given patient

In the above information, comorbidity is "...any pre-existing disease that resulted in permanently altered organ function (eg, cirrhosis, end-stage renal failure, chronic obstructive pulmonary disease, active inflammatory bowel disease, leukemia, or hemiparesis due to cerebrovascular accident)."

- Neutropenia is considered a neutrophil count <0.5 x 10^9/L
- Nondiarrheal manifestation of enteric infections includes "...mesenteric lymphadenitis, acalculous cholecystitis, fever of unknown origin, polyarthritis, and erythema nodosum".

In the special case of suspected food poisoning, a variety of diagnostic techniques are available, including latex agglutination and enzyme-linked immunoassays.[10]

Diarrhea is common in patients with the acquired immunodeficiency syndrome (AIDS). It may be caused by classic bacterial pathogens or unusual opportunistic bacteria viral or parasites (eg, *Giardia*, Microsporidia, *Cryptosporidium*, and *Entamoeba histolytica*).[11] Rectal swabs are useful for the diagnosis of *Neisseria gonorrhoeae* and *Chlamydia* infections.

Diarrhea Syndromes Classified by Predominant Features

Syndrome (anatomic site)	Features	Characteristic Etiologies
Gastroenteritis (stomach)	Vomiting	Rotavirus
		Norwalk virus
		Staphylococcal food poisoning
		Bacillus cereus food poisoning
Enteritis (small bowel)	Watery diarrhea Large-volume stools, few in number	Enterotoxigenic *Escherichia coli*
		Vibrio cholerae
		Any enteric microbe
		Inflammatory bowel disease
Dysentery, colitis (colon)	Small-volume stools containing blood and/or mucus and many leukocytes	*Shigella*
		Campylobacter
		Salmonella
		Invasive *E. coli*
		Plesiomonas shigelloides
		Aeromonas hydrophila
		Vibrio parahaemolyticus
		Clostridium difficile
		Entamoeba histolytica
		Inflammatory bowel disease

In acute or subacute diarrhea, three common syndromes are recognized: gastroenteritis, enteritis, and colitis (dysenteric syndrome). With colitis, patients have fecal urgency and tenesmus. Stools are frequently small in volume and contain blood, mucus, and leukocytes. External hemorrhoids are common and painful. Diarrhea of small bowel origin is indicated by the passage of few large volume stools. This is due to accumulation of fluid in the large bowel before passage. **Leukocytes** usually indicate bacterial colonic inflammation or ulcerative colitis rather than a specific pathogen; see Methylene Blue Stain, Stool *on page 313*. Bacterial diarrhea may be present in the absence of fecal leukocytes, and fecal leukocytes may be present in the absence of bacterial or parasitic agents (ie, idiopathic inflammatory bowel disease).[12] See table. Although most bacterial diarrhea is transient (1-30 days), cases of persistent symptoms (10 months) have been reported.[13] Infants younger than 1 year of age with a history of blood in the stool, more than 10 stools in 24 hours, and temperature greater than 39°C have a high probability of having bacterial diarrhea.[14,15] Diarrhea is also a common side effect of long-term antibiotic treatment. Although often associated with *Clostridium difficile*, other bacteria and yeasts have been implicated.[16]

Escherichia coli O157:H7 infection (enterohemorrhagic *E. coli*) is a food-borne pathogen which causes 20,000-40,000 infections in the U.S. annually, including hemorrhagic colitis and most cases of **hemolytic- uremic syndrome**. Most cases have been traced to contaminated cattle products (eg, beef, milk, cheeses) and meat from other animals,[17] but other cases have originated from produce, presumably contaminated by manure. Even unpasteurized juices must be considered potentially hazardous.[18] The hemolytic-uremic syndrome begins with gastroenteritis, most often in children younger than 4 years of age. It is characterized by microangiopathic hemolytic anemia, thrombocytopenia, and acute renal failure. The bacteria produces shiga-like toxins. See Shiga Toxin Test, Direct *on page 680*. The most common symptom of this organism is bloody diarrhea.[4,19,20] The relationship of antibiotic therapy to the hemolytic-uremic syndrome has been recently addressed.[21,22] In addition to bacterial and viral causes of the hemolytic-uremic syndrome, there are hereditary forms, systemic diseases (eg, SLE, glomerulonephritis, pregnancy, transplant rejection), and exposure to drugs and toxins (eg, cyclosporine, tacrolimus, mitomycin, and radiation).[22]

Yersinia enterocolitica may cause inflammation of the distal ileum with mesenteric lymphadenitis and with marked lymphoid hyperplasia. There is necrosis of germinal centers and a clinical presentation which may resemble that of acute appendicitis. Routine stool culture may miss this organism unless the laboratory is aware of clinical suspicion for this possibility. Incubation at cooler temperature and use of selective media are needed.[23] See *Yersinia enterocolitica* Antibody *on page 698*.

Listeria monocytogenes, a food-borne gram-positive bacillus, may cause fever, gastroenteritis, invasive illnesses including uterine infection, chorioamnionitis, placental abscesses, neonatal sepsis, liver abscess, septic arthritis, abortion, stillbirth, premature birth, meningitis, endocarditis, and other lesions in immunocompromised and immunocompetent individuals.[7,24,25] The risk of invasive listeriosis is 500-1000 times greater in those with advanced AIDS.[26] The organism may be found in stool, neonatal meconium, cerebrospinal fluid, blood, amniotic fluid, placenta, respiratory secretions, gastric aspirates, or cutaneous swabs.[27] See also Bacterial Culture, Genital Specimen *on page 571*.

More than 2200 serotypes of **Salmonella** are classified, including *S. typhi*, *S. choleraesuis*, *S. paratyphi*, *S. gallinarum*, *S. pullorum*, and others. They are a cause of gastroenteritis, diarrhea, and other symptoms and signs. Bacteremia, fever, and other clinical presentations are recognized. Early in **typhoid fever** (*S. typhi*), blood cultures are positive and stools negative. In the second phase, blood cultures become negative and stools positive. A stool-positive carrier state exists.

Shigella causes acute infection which predominantly affects the rectosigmoid, called **bacillary dysentery**. Shiga toxin is produced by *S. dysenteriae* 1, and lesser quantities of toxin are produced by other serotypes. Shiga toxin in children causes the hemolytic-uremic syndrome. There is fever and diarrhea, with fecal leukocytes and blood (see Methylene Blue Stain, Stool *on page 313*). The presence of fecal leukocytes occurs in other entities as well (see table). The need for cultures includes the need to distinguish these infected patients from those with ulcerative colitis.[28]

Campylobacter enteritis causes inflammatory diarrhea. *C. jejuni* is the most often recognized community-acquired inflammatory enteritis. Complications may include Guillain-Barré syndrome. Methylene blue stain and/or fecal lactoferrin are useful (see Fecal Lactoferrin *on page 308*). The need for culture includes differential diagnosis from inflammatory bowel disease.[29] Such distinction can usually also be established by competent surgical pathologists examining endoscopic biopsies; both avenues of investigation are desirable.

See Ova and Parasites, Stool *on page 666*.

Footnotes

1. Siegel DL, Edelstein PH, and Nachamkin I, "Inappropriate Testing for Diarrheal Diseases in the Hospital," *JAMA*, 1990, 263(7):979-82.

2. Valenstein P, Pfaller M, and Yungbluth M, "The Use and Abuse of Routine Stool Microbiology: A College of American Pathologists Q-Probes Study of 601 Institutions," Arch Pathol Lab Med, 1996, 120(2):206-11.

3. Fan K, Morris AJ, and Reller LB, "Application of Rejection Criteria for Stool Cultures for Enteric Pathogens," J Clin Microbiol, 1993, 31(8):2233-5.

4. Su C and Brandt LJ, "Escherichia coli O157:H7 Infection in Humans," Ann Intern Med, 1995, 123(9):698-714.

5. Bender JB, Hedberg CW, Besser JM, et al, "Surveillance for Escherichia coli O157:H7 Infections in Minnesota by Molecular Subtyping," N Engl J Med, 1997, 337(6):388-94.

6. Bender JB, Hedberg CW, Boxrud DJ, et al, "Use of Molecular Subtyping in Surveillance for Salmonella enterica Serotype Typhimurium," N Engl J Med, 2001, 344(3):189-95.

7. Dalton CB, Austin CC, Sobell J, et al, "An Outbreak of Gastroenteritis and Fever Due to Listeria monocytogenes in Milk," N Engl J Med, 1997, 336(2):100-5.

8. Siegel D, Cohen PT, Neighbor M, et al, "Predictive Value of Stool Examination in Acute Diarrhea," Arch Pathol Lab Med, 1987, 111(8):715-8.

9. Bauer TM, Lalvani A, Fehrenbach J, et al, "Derivation and Validation of Guidelines for Stool Cultures for Enteropathogenic Bacteria Other Than Clostridium difficile in Hospitalized Patients," JAMA, 2001, 285(3):313-9.

10. Swaminathan B, Beebe J, and Besser J, "Investigation of Food-Borne and Water-Borne Disease Outbreaks," Manual of Clinical Microbiology, 7th ed, Washington, DC: AMS Press, American Society for Microbiology, 1999, 174-91.

11. Angulo FJ and Swerdlow DL, "Bacterial Enteric Infections in Persons Infected With Human Immunodeficiency Virus," Clin Infect Dis, 1995, 21(Suppl 1):S84-93.

12. DuPont HL, "Subacute Diarrhea to Treat or to Wait?" Hosp Pract (Off Ed), 1989, 24(3A)111-8.

13. Clements D, Ellis CJ, and Allan RN, "Persistent Shigellosis - Case Report," Gut, 1988, 29(9):1277-8.

14. Finkelstein JA, Schwartz JS, Torrey S, et al, "Common Clinical Features as Predictors of Bacterial Diarrhea in Infants," Am J Emerg Med, 1989, 7(5):469-73.

15. Cohen MB, "Etiology and Mechanisms of Acute Infectious Diarrhea in Infants in the United States," J Pediatr, 1991, 118(4 Pt 2):S34-9.

16. Bartlett JG, "Antibiotic-Associated Diarrhea," Clin Infect Dis, 1992, 15(4):573-81.

17 Keene WE, Sazie E, Kok J, et al, "An Outbreak of Escherichia coli O157:H7 Infections Traced to Jerky Made From Deer Meat," JAMA, 1997, 277(15):1229-31.

18. Cody SH, Glynn MK, Farrar JA, et al, "An Outbreak of Escherichia coli O157:H7 Infection From Unpasteurized Commercial Apple Juice," Ann Intern Med, 1999, 130(3):202-9.

19. Tarr PI, Fouser LS, Stapleton AE, et al, "Hemolytic-Uremic Syndrome in a Six-Year-Old Girl After a Urinary Tract Infection With Shiga-Toxin-Producing Escherichia coli O103:H2," N Engl J Med, 1996, 335(9):635-8.

20. Rondeau E and Peraldi MN, "Escherichia coli and the Hemolytic Uremic Syndrome," N Engl J Med, 1996, 335(9):660-2.

21. Wong CS, Jelacic S, Habeeb RL, et al, "The Risk of the Hemolytic-Uremic Syndrome After Antibiotic Treatment of Escherichia coli O157:H7 Infections," N Engl J Med, 2000, 342(26):1930-6.

22. Zimmerhackl LB, "E. coli, Antibiotics, and the Hemolytic-Uremic Syndrome," N Engl J Med, 2000, 342(26):1990-1.

23. Ashkenazi S and Cleary TG, "Yersinia enterocolitica," Principles and Practice of Pediatrics, Oski FA, DeAngelis CD, Feigin RD, et al, eds, Philadelphia, PA: JB Lippincott Co, 1994, 1259-61.

24. Southwick FS and Purich DL, "Intracellular Pathogenesis of Listeriosis," N Engl J Med, 1996, 334(12):770-6.

25. Aureli P, Fiorucci GC, Caroli D, et al, "An Outbreak of Febrile Gastroenteritis Associated With Corn Contaminated by Listeria monogytogenes," N Engl J Med, 2000, 342(17):1236-41.

26. Schlech WF III, "Listeria Gastroenteritis - Old Syndrome, New Pathogen," N Engl J Med, 1997, 336(2):130-1.

27. Bille J, Rocourt J, Swaminathan B, et al, "Listeria, Erysipelothrix, and Kurthia," Manual of Clinical Microbiology, Chapter 22, Murray PR, Baron EJ, Pfaller MA, et al, eds, Washington, DC: ASM Press, American Society for Microbiology, 1999, 346-56.

28. Butler T, "Shigellosis," Cecil Textbook of Medicine, 21st ed, Chapter 342, Goldman L and Bennett JC, eds, Philadelphia, PA: WB Saunders Co, 2000, 1685-7.

29. Guerrant RL, "Campylobacter Enteritis," Cecil Textbook of Medicine, 21st ed, Chapter 343, Goldman L and Bennett JC, eds, Philadelphia, PA: WB Saunders Co, 2000, 1687-90.

References

Ackers ML, Puhr ND, Tauxe RV, et al, "Laboratory-Based Surveillance of Salmonella Serotype Typhi Infections in the United States. Antimicrobial Resistance on the Rise," JAMA, 2000, 283(20):2668-73.

Bauer TM, Lalvani A, Fehrenbach J, et al, "Derivation and Validation of Guidelines for Stool Cultures for Enteropathogenic Bacteria Other Than Clostridium difficile in Hospitalized Adults," JAMA, 2001, 285(3):313-9.

Bishop WP and Ulshen MH, "Bacterial Gastroenteritis," Pediatr Clin North Am, 1988, 35(1):69-87.

Blazer MS, "How Safe Is Our Food? Lessons From an Outbreak of Salmonellosis," N Engl J Med, 1996, 334(20):1324-5.

Dunne EF, Fey PD, Kludt P, et al, "Emergence of Domestically Acquired Ceftriaxone-Resistant Salmonella Infections Associated With AmpC β-Lactamase," JAMA, 2000, 284(24):3151-6.

Kolavic SA, Kimura A, Simons SL, et al, "An Outbreak of Shigella dysenteriae Type 2 Among Laboratory Workers Due to Intentional Food Contamination," JAMA, 1997, 278(5):396-8.

Koneman EW, Allen SD, Janda WM, et al, "The Enterobacteriaceae," Color Atlas and Textbook of Diagnostic Microbiology, 5th ed, Philadelphia, PA: Lippincott, 1997, 171-252.

Molbak K, Baggesen DL, Aarestrup FM, et al, "An Outbreak of Multidrug-Resistant, Quinolone-Resistant Salmonella enterica Serotype Typhimurium DT104," N Engl J Med, 1999, 341(19):1420-5.

Murray BE, "Vancomycin-Resistant Enterococcal Infections," N Engl J Med, 2000, 342(10):710-20.

Torok TJ, Tauxe RV, Wise RP, et al, "A Large Community Outbreak of Salmonellosis Caused by Intentional Contamination of Restaurant Salad Bars," JAMA, 1997, 278(5):389-95.

Bacterial Culture, Throat, and Antigen Detection Testing for Group A Streptococci

Related Information

Antideoxyribonuclease-B Titer, Serum on page 554
Antistreptolysin O Titer, Serum on page 559
Bacterial Culture, Abscess on page 562
Bacterial Culture, Blood on page 566
Chlamydia Group Serology on page 589
Corynebacterium diphtheriae Throat Culture on page 594
Gram Stain on page 617
Group A Streptococcus Screen, Rapid on page 617
Infectious Mononucleosis Screening Test on page 643
Neisseria gonorrhoeae Culture and Smear on page 662
Polymerase Chain Reaction on page 713
Streptozyme on page 682

Synonyms Throat Culture

Applies to Beta-Hemolytic Strep Culture, Throat; Group A Beta-Hemolytic Streptococcus Culture, Throat; Rapid Antigen Detection Tests for Group A Streptococci; Strep Throat Screening Culture; Streptococcus pyogenes Culture; Throat Culture for Group A Beta-Hemolytic Streptococcus

Test Includes Evaluation for group A beta-hemolytic streptococci

Abstract The rate of patient visits to physicians for acute pharyngitis is more than twice that of any other infectious disease.[1]

The differential diagnosis of acute pharyngotonsillitis includes a wide range of infectious agents. The most common cause of acute pharyngotonsillitis is viral (adenovirus, Epstein-Barr virus, Coxsackie A, adenovirus, and others) but laboratories rarely receive requests to identify these. The most important bacterial causes are group A streptococci, group C beta-hemolytic streptococci, Neisseria gonorrhoeae, and H. influenzae type b; very rarely Corynebacterium diphtheriae, Chlamydia pneumoniae and Candida albicans cause pharyngitis. Mycoplasma pneumoniae may cause acute pharyngitis. Arcanobacterium haemolyticum is a rarely diagnosed cause of pharyngotonsillitis which may resemble streptococcal pharyngitis.[1]

The point for emphasis here is that when a throat culture is ordered, the laboratory will employ a procedure that is optimized for the growth and identification of group A, beta-hemolytic streptococci only. If any of the other potential pathogens are suspected, the laboratory must be notified so that appropriate procedures will be undertaken.

Patient Preparation Do not swab throat in cases of acute epiglottitis unless provisions to establish an alternate airway are readily available.

Specimen Throat swab

Container Sterile Culturette®; cotton, dacron, or alginate swabs are acceptable.

Collection The specimen should be transported to the laboratory promptly. Both tonsillar pillars and the oropharynx should be swabbed. The tongue should be depressed while the tonsillar pillars and the oropharynx are swabbed. Exudates should be swabbed, and the tongue and uvula should be avoided.

Storage Instructions Refrigerate

Turnaround Time Reports on specimens from which beta-hemolytic streptococci group A have been isolated usually require 24-48 hours for completion. Cultures with no growth are usually reported after 48 hours.

Special Instructions The laboratory should be informed of the specific site of the specimen, the age of patient, current antibiotic therapy, and clinical diagnosis.

Reference Interval See table.

Throat Culture Summary

Organisms Implicated in Infections of the Oropharynx	Organisms Commonly Present in the Normal Oropharynx
Group A, β-hemolytic streptococci	α-hemolytic streptococci
Bordetella pertussis *†	Candida albicans†
Corynebacterium diphtheriae†	Corynebacterium sp (diphtheroids)
Leptotrichia buccalis†	Enterobacteriaceae
Neisseria gonorrhoeae†	Enterococci
Respiratory viruses:†	Haemophilus sp
Adenovirus†	Neisseria meningitidis
Enterovirus†	Nonhemolytic streptococci
Epstein-Barr virus†	Staphylococcus aureus
Parainfluenza virus†	Staphylococcus epidermidis
Reovirus†	Streptococcus pneumoniae
Rhinovirus†	

*Rare because of vaccination.

†Not recovered by routine culture.

Use Isolate and identify beta-hemolytic Group A Streptococcus, which causes pharyngitis, tonsillitis, and scarlet fever

(Continued)

Bacterial Culture, Throat, and Antigen Detection Testing for Group A Streptococci (Continued)

Limitations Delineation between the acutely infected patient and the asymptomatic carrier with intercurrent viral pharyngitis is not made either by culture nor by rapid antigen detection testing.[1]

Methodology Aerobic incubation of sheep's blood agar

Additional Information Group A *Streptococcus* causes 15% to 30% of cases of acute pharyngitis in children and 5% to 10% in adults. It is characterized by the sudden onset of sore throat with pain on swallowing, pharyngeal exudate, tender cervical lymphadenopathy, fever, headache, abdominal pain, nausea, and vomiting. Children younger than age 3 may have coryza and crusting, but usually not exudative pharyngitis. Uncharacteristic features in older subjects include coryza, hoarseness, cough, diarrhea, conjunctivitis, or discrete ulcers.[1,2]

Antigen detection tests are now widely used to diagnose streptococcal pharyngotonsillitis. Such tests have improved sensitivity and high specificity. They can be performed in a physician's office, with the results available immediately. When the results of an antigen detection test are negative, many authorities, including the American Heart Association, the American Academy of Pediatrics,[3,4] and others[1] recommend performing a confirmatory culture, because antigen detection tests are perceived as having less sensitivity (between 80% and 90%[1]) than culture. A large and well-controlled study,[5] which employed an optical immunoassay technique, reported specificities 93% for the immunoassay and 99% for the culture. The sensitivity of optical immunoassays has been reported from <80%, to equivalency with the throat culture. A 2001 paper describes the throat culture as the gold standard for the diagnosis of group A streptococcal pharyngitis with sensitivity ≥90%. Thus, the newer enzyme immunoassay tests, when positive, can be considered equivalent to a positive culture. However, a negative result is only presumptive, to be followed up with a culture.[1] See also Group A *Streptococcus* Screen, Rapid *on page 617*.

Complications of strep throat include peritonsillar abscess, retropharyngeal abscess, cervical lymphadenitis, otitis media, sinusitis, mastoiditis, meningitis, pneumonia, and/or bacteremia. Rheumatic fever can be a nonsuppurative poststreptococcal complication. However the frequency of rheumatic fever has greatly diminished in the U.S.[2]

A resurgence of serious *Streptococcus pyogenes* infection was observed in the late 1980s. Complications including rheumatic fever, sepsis, severe soft tissue invasion, and toxic shock-like syndrome (TSLS) are reported to be most common with the M1 serotype. A unique invasive clone has become a predominant cause of severe streptococcal infections.[6]

Footnotes

1. Bisno AL, "Acute Pharyngitis," *N Engl J Med*, 2001, 344(3):205-11.
2. Ebell MH, Smith MA, Barry HC, et al, "Does This Patient Have Strep Throat?" *JAMA*, 2000, 284(22):2912-8.
3. Dajani A, Taubert K, Ferrieri P, et al, "Treatment of Acute Streptococcal Pharyngitis and Prevention of Rheumatic Fever: A Statement for Health Professionals," Committee on Rheumatic Fever, Endocarditis, and Kawasaki Disease of the Council on Cardiovascular Disease in the Young, the American Heart Association, *Pediatrics*, 1995, 96(4 Pt 1):758-64.
4. Committee on Infectious Diseases, American Academy of Pediatrics, "Group A Streptococcal Infections," *1994 Red Book: Report of the Committee on Infectious Diseases*, 23rd ed, Peter G, ed, Elk Grove Village, IL: American Academy of Pediatrics, 1994, 430-9.
5. Gerber MA, Tanz RR, Kabat W, et al, "Optical Immunoassay Test for Group A Beta-Hemolytic Streptococcal Pharyngitis. An Office-Based, Multicenter Investigation," *JAMA*, 1997, 277(11):899-903.
6. Cleary PP, Kaplan EL, Handley JP, et al, "Clonal Basis for Resurgence of Serious *Streptococcus pyogenes* Disease in the 1980s," *Lancet*, 1992, 339(8792):518-21.

References

Cunningham MW, "Pathogenesis of Group A Streptococcal Infections," *Clin Microbiol Rev*, 2000, 13(3):470-511.

DiMatteo L, "Managing Streptococcal Pharyngitis: A Review of Clinical Decision-Managing Strategies, Diagnostic Evaluation, and Treatment," *J Am Acad Nurse Pract*, 1999, 11(2):57-62.

Pichichero ME, "Group A Beta-Hemolytic Streptococcal Infections," *Pediatr Rev*, 1998, 19(9):291-302.

Pichichero ME, Green JL, Francis AB, et al, "Recurrent Group A Streptococcal Tonsillopharyngitis," *Pediatr Infect Dis J*, 1998, 17(9):809-15.

Sela S and Barzilai A, "Why Do We Fail With Penicillin in the Treatment of Group A Streptococcus Infections?" *Ann Med*, 1999, 31(5):303-7.

Tsevat J and Kotagal UR, "Management of Sore Throats in Children: A Cost-Effectiveness Analysis," *Arch Pediatr Adolesc Med*, 1999, 153(7):681-8.

Bacterial Culture, Urine

Related Information

Chlamydia trachomatis Culture *on page 590*
Fungal Culture, Urine *on page 614*
Gram Stain *on page 617*
Kidney Stone Analysis *on page 877*
Leukocyte Esterase, Urine *on page 878*
Mycobacterial Culture, Urine *on page 660*
Nitrite, Urine *on page 882*
Polymerase Chain Reaction *on page 713*
Urinalysis *on page 887*

Viral Culture on page 689
Viral Culture, Urine on page 695

Applies to Bacterial Culture, Urine, Clean Catch; Bacterial Culture, Urine, Suprapubic Puncture; *E. coli*; *Enterobacteriaceae*; *Enterococcus* spp; *Klebsiella* spp; *Mycobacterium* spp; *Proteus* spp; *Pseudomonas aeruginosa*; *S. epidermidis*; *S. sapronophyticus*; *Staphylococcus aureus*

Test Includes Aerobic culture of clean catch urine; significant bacterial growth is typically defined as ≥10,000 colony forming units/mL

Abstract Urinary tract infections (UTI) caused by bacteria are a common cause of morbidity. Common clinical presentations include the acute dysuric syndrome, acute and chronic cystitis, and acute and chronic pyelonephritis. Diagnostically challenging are patients who are asymptomatic, or who present with acute abdominal pain simulating appendicitis or cholecystitis. *Escherichia coli* causes ~80% to 90%, and *Staphylococcus saprophyticus* ~10% to 20% of bacterial infections in the urinary tract; rare isolates include various species of *Proteus*, *Klebsiella*, *Enterobacter*, and *Enterococcus*.[1] A clean voided urine is the preferred specimen for most situations; urine obtained via suprapubic puncture is sometimes preferred for infants and small children.[2] Catheterization is not recommended unless it is necessary for other indications. Although differences in reference range may be anticipated between urine from indwelling catheters and straight catheterization, the literature fails to make such possible differences clear.[3] Many physicians and nurses have been taught to screen for bacterial UTI using the routine dipstick urinalysis (with or without microscopic examination of the sediment). There is, however, recent very substantial controversy on this issue (see Additional Information).

Complicated infections may include those associated with diabetes mellitus, anatomic abnormalities, instrumentation, nephrolithiasis, and immunosuppression. The list includes effects of medical therapy, patients with HIV, and intravenous drug users.[4]

Diagnosis of urinary tract infections in febrile infants and young children should be based on culture of a properly collected urine specimen.[5]

Patient Preparation Meticulous attention to technique is necessary.

Clean voided urine (midstream urine): Instruct patient to wash hands thoroughly, wash penis or vulva using downward strokes four times with four soapy sponges, then once with sponge wet with warm water. Urethral meatus and perineum must be washed. Each sponge must be discarded after one use. Urinate about 30 mL (1 ounce) of urine directly into toilet or bedpan - stop - position container and take middle portion of urine sample. Screw cap securely on container without touching the inside rim. Apply the completed patient label to the specimen cup. Most patients, with instruction, do better with privacy than with an attendant.

Suprapubic puncture: Aseptic preparation of the aspiration site. Collect the specimen to avoid contamination with normal skin flora. Fluids should be forced prior to collection of the specimen to distend the bladder. Successful suprapubic collection requires a distended bladder; 6-10 hours may be required for the bladder to fill.

Specimen Clean voided urine specimen

Container Sterile plastic urine container or sterile tube

Collection See Patient Preparation.

Clean voided urine: Early morning specimens yield highest bacterial counts from overnight incubation in the bladder. Forced fluids dilute the urine and may cause reduced colony counts. Hair from perineum will contaminate the specimen. The stream from a male may be contaminated by bacteria from beneath the prepuce. Bacteria from vaginal secretions, vulva, or distal urethra may also contaminate the specimen, as may organisms from hands or clothing. Receptacle must be sterile. Provide time and date of urine collection.

Suprapubic puncture: After aseptic preparation of the skin, the specimen is aspirated in a sterile syringe by a physician skilled in the technique.

Storage Instructions Do not store. Deliver to the laboratory without delay. Storage at room temperature is not acceptable; bacteria multiply at room temperature.[3]

Causes for Rejection Specimen collected more than 2 hours before arrival in the laboratory

Reference Interval Positivity depends on the technique of specimen collection, the character of the patient group at risk, specimen handling, and perhaps the presence of comorbid conditions.[3]

Clean voided urine: Clinical decision limits vary with the clinical syndrome. For example, ≥10,000 colony-forming units (cfu)/mL is usually a clinically significant finding in a properly collected specimen. However, for patients with the acute dysuric syndrome, as few as 1000 cfu/mL, and as few as 100 cfu/mL in the presence of pyuria may be significant in young sexually active females.[6,7] In an unselected outpatient male population, it has been suggested that as few as 1000 cfu/mL in voided urine specimens are clinically significant.[3] In a study on risk factors for symptomatic urinary tract infection in young women, urinary tract infection was defined as dysuria, frequency, and/or urgency, and ≥10^2 cfu/mL of a uropathogen, cultured from midstream urine.[6]

Suprapubic puncture: Any growth is clinically significant if proper technique was followed in collecting the specimen.

Use The urine culture is the gold standard for the diagnosis of bacterial UTI. Some physicians screen for UTI by using urinalysis, and proceed with culture only if one or more of the urinalysis results are positive (eg, leukocyte esterase, nitrites, bacteria, or leukocytes on microscopy). See Additional Information.

Limitations Bacteria present in numbers <1000 organisms/mL may not be detected by routine methods. Contamination of urine specimens is reported as 23% from females, 11% from males, but the definition of contamination is problematic[3,8] Failure to recover aerobic organisms from patients with pyuria or positive Gram stains on urinary sediment may indicate the presence of mycobacteria or anaerobes.

Contraindications Foley catheter tips are consistently contaminated with organisms from the urethra.[7]

Methodology Quantitative aerobic culture; usually plated at a 0.001 dilution, allowing detection of organisms in enumeration $\geq 10^3$ CFU/mL.

Additional Information The use of urinalysis alone as a screen for UTI has little support in the recent medical literature. Nunns et al[9] found that culture was unnecessary if **catheterized** urine specimens were negative for nitrite, leukocyte esterase, and protein; however, this was a highly selected group and included 14 patients with proven UTI. An additional study reported that the dipstick urinalysis is "cost-effective" in screening **asymptomatic pregnant** patients for bacteriuria.[10] Several other, and mostly more recent, studies do **not** support urinalysis as a screen for culture. Van Nostrand et al[11] used a stepwise binary logistic regression model with UTI as the dependent variable and various urinalysis components (including microscopic examination) as independent variables. These investigators found that a positive culture result could not be accurately predicted from the results of urinalysis; specifically, 14% of positive cultures would have been missed. Semeniuk et al[12] evaluated 479 ambulatory women with uncomplicated UTI and found that a dipstick screen (no microscopic examination) would have missed 18.9% of patients. Zaman et al[13] found a sensitivity of 57% and specificity of 94% for the leukocyte esterase result; adding the nitrite result increased the sensitivity to 78% and reduced the specificity to 75%. In addition, a semiquantitative microscopic examination had a sensitivity of 83%, and produced a false-positive frequency of 40%. Bartlett et al[14] found that the leukocyte esterase result had a sensitivity of 71.9% in detecting ≥ 3 leukocytes/hpf, and the nitrite result had a sensitivity of 56.7% in detecting the microscopic presence of bacteria. Pels et al[15] reported a wide range of predictive values for urinalysis in different subsets. For pregnant women, Pels et al recommend culture, not urinalysis, to screen for UTI; they found that dipstick screening may be effective in women who are older than 60 years of age or have diabetes.

Certain biologic factors also militate against dipstick results as an accurate screen. Turner et al[16] report that children who are febrile, but free of UTI, often (~43%) have pyuria. Lam[17] found that urines with bacteria, but free of blood and hemoglobin, have false-positive dipstick results for hematuria. Beer et al[18] found positive dipstick results for leukocyte esterase caused by antibiotic administration in patients free of UTI.

A recent authoritative review recommends performing culture **and** urinalysis when evaluating **children** for possible UTI.[19]

In contrast, **renal tuberculosis** causes fever, frequency, urgency, dysuria, and hematuria with pyuria in which usual urine cultures fail to grow organisms.[4]

Footnotes

1. Kunin CM, "Urinary Tract Infections and Pyelonephritis," *Cecil Textbook of Medicine*, 21st ed, Goldman L and Bennett JC, eds, Philadelphia, PA: WB Saunders Co, 2000, 613-7.
2. Gill VJ, Fedorko DP, and Witebsky FG, "The Clinician and the Microbiology Laboratory," *Mandel, Douglas, and Bennett's Principles and Practice of Infectious Diseases*, 5th ed, Mandell GL, Bennett JE, and Dolin R, eds, New York, NY: Churchill Livingstone, 2000, 184-221.
3. Washington JA, "Urine Culture Contamination," *Arch Pathol Lab Med*, 1998, 122(2):120-2.
4. Roberts JA, "Management of Pyelonephritis and Upper Urinary Tract Infections," *Urol Clin North Am*, 1999, 26(4):753-63.
5. American Academy of Pediatrics, "The Diagnosis, Treatment, and Evaluation of the Initial Urinary Tract Infection in Febrile Infants and Young Children (AC9830)," *Pediatrics*, 2000, 103(4):1-17.
6. Hooton TM, Scholes D, Stapleton AE, et al, "A Prospective Study of Asymptomatic Bacteriuria in Sexually Active Young Women," *N Engl J Med*, 1996, 335(7):468-74.
7. Reisner BS, Woods GL, Thomson RB Jr, et al, "Specimen Processing," *Manual of Clinical Microbiology*, Murray PR, Baron EJ, Pfaller MA, et al, eds, Washington, DC: ASM Press, American Society for Microbiology, 1999, 64-104.
8. Valenstein P and Meier F, "Urine Culture Contamination. A College of American Pathologists Q-Probes Study of Contaminated Urine Cultures in 906 Institutions," *Arch Pathol Lab Med*, 1998, 122(2):123-9.
9. Nunns D, Smith ARB, and Hosker G, "Reagent Strip Testing Urine for Significant Bacteriuria in a Urodynamic Clinic," *Br J Urol*, 1995, 76(1):87-9.
10. Nunns D, "Screening and Treatment of Asymptomatic Bacteriuria of Pregnancy to Prevent Pyelonephritis: A Cost-Effectiveness and Cost-Benefit Analysis," *Obstet Gynecol*, 1995, 86(5):119-23.
11. Van Nostrand JD, Junkins AD, and Bartholdi RK, "Poor Predictive Ability of Urinalysis and Microscopic Examination to Detect Urinary Tract Infection," *Am J Clin Pathol*, 2000, 113(5):709-13.
12. Semeniuk H and Church D, "Evaluation of the Leukocyte Esterase and Nitrite Urine Dipstick Screening Tests for Detection of Bacteriuria in Women With Suspected Uncomplicated Urinary Tract Infections," *J Clin Microbiol*, 1999, 37(9):3051-2.
13. Zaman Z, Borremans A, Verhaegen J, et al, "Disappointing Dipstick Screening for Urinary Tract Infection in Hospital Inpatients," *J Clin Pathol*, 1998, 51(6):471-2.
14. Bartlett RC, Zern DA, Ratkiewicz MA, et al, "Reagent Strip Screening for Sediment Abnormalities Identified by Automated Microscopy in Urine From Patients Suspected to Have Urinary Tract Disease," *Arch Pathol Lab Med*, 1994, 118(11):1096-101.
15. Pels RJ, Bor DH, Woolhandler S, et al, "Dipstick Urinalysis Screening of Asymptomatic Adults for Urinary Tract Disorders. II. Bacteriuria," *JAMA*, 1989, 262(9):1220-4.
16. Turner GM and Coulthard MG, "Fever Can Cause Pyuria in Children," *BMJ*, 1995, 311(7010):924.
17. Lam MH, "False Hematuria Due to Bacteria," *Arch Pathol Lab Med*, 1995, 119(8):717-21.
18. Beer JH, Vogt A, Neftel K, et al, "False Positive Results for Leukocytes in Urine Dipstick Test WIth Common Antibiotics," *BMJ*, 1996, 313(7048):25.
19. Johnson CE, "New Advances in Childhood Urinary Tract Infections," *Pediatr Rev*, 1999, 20(10):335-43.

References

Bartkowski DP, "Recognizing UTIs in Infants and Children. Early Treatment Prevents Permanent Damage," *Postgrad Med*, 2001, 109(1):171-2, 177-81.

Ronald A, "Sex and Urinary Tract Infections," *N Engl J Med*, 1996, 335(7):511-2.

Sodeman TM, "A Practical Strategy for Diagnosis of Urinary Tract Infections," *Clin Lab Med*, 1995, 15(2):235-50.

Tambyah PA, Halvorson KT, and Maki DG, "A Prospective Study of Pathogenesis of Catheter-Associated Urinary Tract Infections," *Mayo Clin Proc*, 1999, 74(2):131-6.

Zhanel GG, Nicolle LE, Harding GK, et al, "Prevalence of Asymptomatic Bacteriuria and Associated Host Factors in Women With Diabetes Mellitus," *Clin Infect Dis*, 1995, 21(2):316-22.

Internet Web Sites

www.pediatrics.org/cgi/content/full/103/4/e54

♦ **Bacterial Culture, Urine, Clean Catch** see Bacterial Culture, Urine *on page 578*

♦ **Bacterial Culture, Urine, Suprapubic Puncture** see Bacterial Culture, Urine *on page 578*

Bacterial Culture, Wounds, Bites

Related Information

Bacteremia Detection, Buffy Coat Micromethod *on page 406*
Bacterial Culture, Abscess *on page 562*
Bacterial Culture, Anaerobes *on page 564*
Bacterial Culture, Biopsy or Body Fluid *on page 565*
Bacterial Culture, Burn Sites *on page 569*
Bartonella Serology *on page 581*
Fine Needle Aspiration Culture *on page 609*
Leptospira Culture *on page 648*
Leptospira Serology *on page 649*
Mycobacterial Culture, Biopsy or Body Fluid *on page 655*
Mycobacterial Culture, Cutaneous and Subcutaneous Tissue *on page 657*
Rabies *on page 673*
Tetanus Antibody *on page 682*
Tularemia Serology *on page 686*

Synonyms Bite Culture; Wound Culture

Applies to *Actinomyces israelii*; *Bacteroides* spp; Bites (Cat, Dog, Human); *Clostridium* spp; Decubitus Ulcer Culture; *Enterobacteriaceae*; *Enterococcus*; Foreign Body Culture; Gunshot Wound Culture; *Mycobacterium marinum*; *Nocardia* spp; *Peptostreptococcus*; *Proteus* spp; *Pseudomonas aeruginosa*; Puncture Wound Culture; *Staphylococcus aureus*; *Streptococcus pyogenes*; Surgical Wound Culture

Test Includes Cultures for aerobes and anaerobes; Gram stain is highly desirable (see below). Antimicrobial susceptibility testing may be required.

Abstract Wounds include skin and mucus membrane injuries due to trauma, surgical procedure, decubitus ulcers, bites (human and animal), and foreign bodies. Discovering the cause(s) of a wound infection is problematic when the material submitted for culture includes commensal organisms.

Patient Preparation The skin or mucus membrane should be thoroughly decontaminated with surgical soap and either ethyl or isopropyl alcohol.

Container Syringe and sterile tube

Collection Meticulous technique is required. The ideal specimen is material obtained via needle aspiration into a sterile container, after a thorough surgical prep. Valuable preliminary information about the pathogen(s) present can be obtained if an aliquot can be examined by Gram stain. Swabs produce inferior specimens and their use is discouraged.

Special Instructions Clinical history of wound duration and of travel may be relevant.

Reference Interval No growth

Use Isolate and identify potentially pathogenic organisms from bites and other wounds

Limitations Unless specifically requested by the physician or mandated by the specimen source (ie, genital specimen), fastidious organisms such as *N. gonorrhoeae* may not be isolated. Anaerobic, fungal, and mycobacterial pathogens should be considered, and appropriate cultures requested, if indicated.

Contraindications Culture of contaminated open wounds which have not been cleansed or debrided may prove suboptimal.

Methodology Aerobic and anaerobic cultures

(Continued)

Bacterial Culture, Wounds, Bites (Continued)
Additional Information

Surgical site infections are most commonly due to one of more of the following: *Staphylococcus aureus*, coagulase-negative staphylococci, enterococci, *Escherichia coli, Pseudomonas aeruginosa, Enterobacter* spp, *Proteus mirabilis, Klebsiella pneumoniae*, various streptococci, *Candida albicans, Bacteroides fragilis*, and other gram-positive aerobes.[1,2] Lowry et al[3] have reported postoperative sternal wound infections due to *Legionella pneumophila* and *Legionella dumoffii*, and acquired by exposure to tap water via bathing; such cases can be diagnostic challenges since the patients do not have pneumonia.

Dog and cat bites commonly yield multiple bacterial species, including aerobes and anaerobes.[2] *Pasteurella canis* is the most common isolate from dog bites. *Capnocytophaga canimorsus* is an invasive organism which may threaten immunosuppressed patients bitten by canines.[4] Cat bites most commonly yield *Pasteurella* subspecies, *multocida* and *septica*. Aerobes commonly found include streptococci, staphylococci, *Moraxella*, and *Neisseria*; common anaerobes are *Fusobacterium, Bacteroides, Porphyromonas*, and *Prevotella*. In addition, Talan et al recovered from dog and cat bites several organisms not previously recognized as human pathogens. Three to 18% of dog bites and 28% to 80% of cat bites become infected. Sequellae may include meningitis, endocarditis, septic arthritis, and septic shock.[5]

Human bites commonly cause infections with one or more of the following: *Streptococcus viridans, Staphylococcus* spp, *Eikenella corrodens, Bacteroides* spp, and microaerophilic streptococci.[6] Human bites can transmit HIV, hepatitis B virus, and even lues.[4]

Bat bites should elicit a level of concern.[4] See Rabies *on page 673.*

Marine creatures or exposure to sea water may lead to wounds infected with *Mycobacterium marinum* (see Mycobacterial Culture, Biopsy or Body Fluid *on page 655* and Mycobacterial Culture, Cutaneous and Subcutaneous Tissue *on page 657*).

Footnotes

1. Kernodle DS and Kaiser AB, "Postoperative Infections and Antimicrobial Prophylaxis," *Mandel, Douglas, and Bennett's Principles and Practice of Infectious Diseases*, 4th ed, Mandell GL, Bennett JE, and Dolin R, eds, New York, NY: Churchill Livingstone, 2000, 3177-91.
2. Angood PB, Gingalewski VA, and Andersen DK, "Surgical Complications," *Sabiston Textbook of Surgery: The Biological Basis of Modern Surgical Practice*, 16th ed, Townsend CM, ed, Philadelphia, PA: WB Saunders Co, 2001, 198-225.
3. Lowry PW, Blankenship RJ, Gridley W, et al, "A Cluster of *Legionella* Sternal-Wound Infections Due to Postoperative Topical Exposure to Contaminated Tap Water," *N Engl J Med*, 1991, 324(2):109-13.
4. Fleisher GR, "The Management of Bite Wounds," *N Engl J Med*, 1999, 340(2):138-40.
5. Talan DA, Citron DM, Abrahamian FM, et al, "Bacteriologic Analysis of Infected Dog and Cat Bites." Emergency Medicine Animal Bite Infection Study Group, *N Engl J Med*, 1999, 340(2):85-92.
6. Stewart RM Page CP, "Wounds, Bites, and Stings," *Trauma*, 4th ed, Mattox KL, Feliciano DV, Moore EE, eds, New York, NY: McGraw-Hill Inc, 1999, 1115-35.

References

Barie PS, "Management of Complicated Intra-abdominal Infections," *J Chemother*, 1999, 11(6):464-77.

Elliott D, Kufera JA, and Myers RA, "The Microbiology of Necrotizing Soft Tissue Infections," *Am J Surg*, 2000, 179(5):361-6.

Smith PF, Meadowcroft AM, and May DB, "Treating Mammalian Bite Wounds," *J Clin Pharm Ther*, 2000, 25(2):85-99.

Thomson PD, "Immunology, Microbiology, and the Recalcitrant Wound," *Ostomy Wound Manage*, 2000, 46(1A Suppl):77S-82S.

Bartonella Culture

Related Information

Bartonella Serology *on page 581*
Polymerase Chain Reaction *on page 713*

Synonyms Cat Scratch Bacterial Culture; Culture for Cat Scratch Bacteria; *Rochalimaea* Culture

Abstract *Bartonella* species are small gram-negative rods. Eleven species of *Bartonella* have been recognized but only four have been implicated in human disease. They include *B. quintana* and *B. henselae*. These bacteria are responsible for bacillary angiomatosis, bacillary peliosis hepatis, bacteremia, and cat scratch disease (CSD). Bacillary angiomatosis, characterized by subcutaneous nodules and fever, occurs primarily in subjects with AIDS but has been found as well in immunocompetent patients and in recipients of organ transplants. Cat scratch disease can occur in any patient but most cases occur in children or adolescents. The disease is characterized by swollen lymph nodes 2 weeks after a scratch or bite of a cat. Other symptoms such as low grade fever, tiredness, and headache may accompany the swollen lymph glands.[1] Cat scratch disease is more likely to be associated with *B. henselae* infection.[2]

Specimen Blood, tissue from skin, liver, spleen, or lymph node

Collection Collect blood in either EDTA tubes or Isolator™ blood-lysis tubes.

Causes for Rejection Tissue fixed in formalin

Reference Interval Negative

Limitations Culture may require more than 7 days of incubation. Recovery of isolates from skin specimens may be overgrown with indigenous bacterial skin flora. *B. henselae* is inhibited by the sodium-polyethylene sulfonate used in many blood culture media.

Methodology Culture on 5% to 10% rabbit or horse blood agar plates, chocolate agar, and 5% sheep blood agar. Incubation should be in a humid atmosphere (40% humidity) for 3-4 weeks. *B. henselae* has been isolated in the biphasic Septi-Chek® system after 40 days of incubation. Several isolates have been detected in the Bactec® system with resin-containing broth media and in the BacT/Alert® system. However, Gram stains of the broth are negative but acridine orange stain will detect the bacilli.[3,4]

Additional Information *Bartonella* species are considered emerging pathogens. *Bartonella quintana* infections have been detected among the urban homeless population.[5,6] *Bartonella henselae* is now recognized as the organism associated with cat scratch disease in immunocompetent individuals and bacillary angiomatosis in immunocompromised patients.[7,8] This pleomorphic organism may be recognized with the Warthin-Starry method in tissue sections and can be labeled by immunocytochemistry.[3] Culture of *Bartonella* species is difficult, time consuming, and costly, but several reference laboratories or large local laboratories will offer specific culture for this organism.[9,10] Some routine blood culture systems can also detect *Bartonella* species and an effort can be made when there is clinical suspicion of active infection.[4,11]

Detection of specific DNA sequences has enhanced epidemiologic investigations and polymerase chain reaction amplification in arthropods has provided understanding of such zoonotic infections.[4,11] Molecular detection will likely replace culture as the preferred diagnostic test for *Bartonella* species.

Footnotes

1. Maguina C and Gotuzzo E, "Bartonellosis. New and Old," *Infect Dis Clin North Am*, 2000, 14(1):1-22.
2. Not T, Canciani M, Buratti E, et al, "Serologic Response to *Bartonella henselae* in Patients With Cat Scratch Disease and in Sick and Healthy Children," *Acta Paediatr*, 1999, 88(3):284-9.
3. Spach DH, Kanter AS, Daniels NA, et al, "*Bartonella (Rochalimaea)* Species as a Cause of Apparent Culture-Negative Endocarditis," *Clin Infect Dis*, 1995, 20(4):1044-7.
4. Tierno PM Jr, Inglima K, and Parisi MT, "Detection of *Bartonella (Rochalemaea) henselae* Bacteremia Using BacT/Alert® Blood Culture System," *Am J Clin Pathol*, 1995, 104(5):530-6.
5. Jackson LA and Spach DH, "Emergence of *Bartonella quintana* Infection Among Homeless Persons," *Emerg Infect Dis*, 1996, 2(2):141-4.
6. Brougui P, Lascola B, Roux V, et al, "Chronic *Bartonella quintana* Bacteremia in Homeless Patients," *N Engl J Med*, 1999, 340(3):184-9.
7. Bass JW, Vincent JM, and Person DA, "The Expanding Spectrum of *Bartonella* Infections: II. Cat-Scratch Disease," *Pediatr Infect Dis J*, 1997, 16(2):163-79.
8. Gasquet S, Maurin M, Brouqui P, et al, "Bacillary Angiomatosis in Immunocompromised Patients," *AIDS*, 1998, 12(14):1793-803.
9. La Scola B and Raoult D, "Culture of *Bartonella quintana* and *Bartonella henselae* From Human Samples: A 5-Year Experience (1993 to 1998)," *J Clin Microbiol*, 1999, 37(6):1899-905.
10. Doern GV, "Detection of Selected Fastidious Bacteria," *Clin Infect Dis*, 2000, 30(1):166-73.
11. Koehler JE, Glaser CA, and Tappero JW, "*Rochalimaea henselae* Infection. A New Zoonosis With the Domestic Cat as Reservoir," *JAMA*, 1994, 271(7):531-5.

References

Brouqui P and Raoult D, "Endocarditis Due to Rare and Fastidious Bacteria," *Clin Microbiol Rev*, 2001, 14(1):177-207.

Eggenberger E, "Cat Scratch Disease: Posterior Segment Manifestations," *Ophthalmology*, 2000, 107(5):817-8.

Glaser C, Lewis P, and Wong S, "Pet-, Animal-, and Vector-Borne Infections," *Pediatr Rev*, 2000, 21(7):219-32.

Maurin M, Birtles R, and Raoult D, "Current Knowledge of *Bartonella* Species," *Eur J Clin Microbiol Infect Dis*, 1997, 16(7):487-506.

Ohl ME and Spach DH, "*Bartonella quintana* and Urban Trench Fever," *Clin Infect Dis*, 2000, 31(1):131-5.

Spach DH and Koehler JE, "*Bartonella*-Associated Infections," *Infect Dis Clin North Am*, 1998, 12(1):137-55.

Internet Web Sites

www.astdhpphe.org/infect

www.thebody.com/cdc/oiguide/guidelines12.html

Bartonella Serology

Related Information
Bacterial Culture, Conjunctiva on page 570
Bacterial Culture, Wounds, Bites on page 579
Bartonella Culture on page 580
Lymph Node Biopsy on page 67
Polymerase Chain Reaction on page 713
Skin Biopsy on page 71

Synonyms Bartonella Titer; Rochalimaea Antibodies; Rochalimaea Titer

Applies to Cat Scratch Disease; PCR Assay for Bartonella; PCR Assay for Rochalimaea

Abstract Bartonella, small gram-negative rods, include B. quintana and B. henselae, which are responsible for bacillary angiomatosis, bacillary peliosis hepatis, bacteremia, and cat scratch disease (CSD). **Bacillary angiomatosis**, characterized by subcutaneous nodules and fever, occurs primarily in subjects with AIDS but has been found as well in immunocompetent patients and in recipients of organ transplants.

Cat scratch disease is found in immunocompetent individuals, 80% of whom are younger than 21 years of age.[1] It is associated with B. henselae infection.[2] It presents as an inoculation-site papule in >50% of patients, followed by local lymphadenopathy. Cat scratch or bite is recognized in ~75%. In 4% to 6%, the oculoglandular syndrome of Perinaud develops.

Specimen Serum, separated quickly

Collection Paired serum samples are desirable, one drawn 2-4 weeks after the other. Blood cultures are indicated as well.

Causes for Rejection Plasma, severe lipemia, hemolysis

Reference Interval IgG: <1:64; IgM: <1:16

Critical Values Fourfold increase in titer is meaningful. IgG: ≥1:256; IgM: ≥1:16; provide evidence of recent or present infection

Diseases Associated With Bartonella Species Infection

Cutaneous bacillary angiomatosis
Extracutaneous infection
Bacillary peliosis of the liver (bacillary peliosis hepatitis) and spleen
Fever and bacteremia (Bartonella bacteremic syndrome)
Cat scratch disease (associated only with Bartonella henselae)
Trench fever (associated only with B. quintana)
Endocarditis

Adapted from Maguina C and Gotuzzo E, "Bartonellosis. New and Old," Infect Dis Clin North Am, 2000, 14(1):1-22.

Use Bartonella quintana is a cause of "culture-negative" endocarditis. Culture of the organism is difficult; it is fastidious. Most cases of cat scratch disease are diagnosed on the basis of history, physical findings, histopathologic characteristics, and serology.

Limitations There is cross-reactivity between antibodies to B. quintana and B. henselae.[3] Additionally, some assays will also cross-react with Chlamydia species and Coxiella burnetii.

In a seroprevalence study of individuals at a community clinic serving the homeless and indigent, 20% had B. quintana IgG titers ≥64, by indirect fluorescence antibody assay.[3]

Methodology Indirect fluorescent antibody (IFA), enzyme immunoassay (EIA). A Western blot analysis is described.[4] Polymerase chain reaction amplification is reported, which may be used in formalin-fixed, paraffin-embedded tissue.[3]

Additional Information Although IFA has been very reliable for detecting antibody to Bartonella, recently developed EIAs detect both IgG and IgM with a specificity of 92.5% and sensitivity of 89.6%.[1] Biopsies of skin and lymph node lesions include well described features. The pleomorphic bacilli may be recognized with the Warthin-Starry method in tissue sections[3] and can be labeled by immunocytochemistry.[2] Detection of specific DNA sequences has enhanced epidemiologic investigations and polymerase chain reaction amplification in arthropods has provided understanding of such zoonotic infections.[5,6] Blood cultures can detect Bartonella species and should be obtained when there is a clinical suspicion of active infection.[7]

Footnotes
1. Not T, Canciane M, Buratti E, et al, "Serologic Response to Bartonella henselae in Patients With Cat Scratch Disease and in Sick and Healthy Children," Acta Paediatr, 1999, 88(3):284-9.
2. Min KW, Reed JA, Welch DF, et al, "Morphologically Variable Bacilli of Cat Scratch Disease Are Identified by Immunocytochemical Labeling With Antibodies to Rochalimaea henselae," Am J Clin Pathol, 1994, 101(5):607-10.
3. Patel R, Newell JO, Procop GW, et al, "Use of Polymerase Chain Reaction for Citrate Synthase Gene to Diagnose Bartonella quintana Endocarditis," Am J Clin Pathol, 1999, 112(1):36-40.
4. Litwin CM, Martins TB, and Hill HR, "Immunologic Response to Bartonella henselae as Determined by Enzyme Immunoassay and Western Blot Analysis," Am J Clin Pathol, 1997, 108(2):202-9.
5. Glaser C, Lewis P, Wong S, "Pet-, Animal-, and Vector-Borne Infections," Pediatr Rev, 2000, 21(7):219-32.
6. Koehler JE, Glaser CA, and Tappero JW, "Rochalimaea henselae Infection. A New Zoonosis With the Domestic Cat as Reservoir," JAMA, 1994, 271(7):531-5.

7. Tierno PM Jr, Inglima K, and Parisi MT, "Detection of Bartonella (Rochalimaea) henselae Bacteremia Using BacT/Alert Blood Culture System," Am J Clin Pathol, 1995, 104(5):530-6.

References
Eggenberger E, "Cat Scratch Disease: Posterior Segment Manifestations," Ophthalmology, 2000, 107(5):817-8.
Giladi M and Avidor B, Images in Clinical Medicine, "Cat Scratch Disease," N Engl J Med, 1999, 340(2):108.
Harrison TG and Doshi N, "Serologica Evidence of Bartonella spp Infection in the UK," Epidemiol Infect, 1999, 123(2):233-40.
Karem KL, "Immune Aspects of Bartonella," Crit Rev Microbiol, 2000, 26(3):133-45.
La Scola B and Raoult D, "Culture of Bartonella quintana and Bartonella henselae From Human Samples: A 5-Year Experience (1993 to 1998)," J Clin Microbiol, 1999, 37(6):1899-905.
Lepidi H, Fournier PE, and Raoult D, "Quantitative Analysis of Valvular Lesions During Bartonella Endocarditis," Am J Clin Pathol, 2000, 114(6):880-9.
Maguina C and Gotuzzo E, "Bartonellosis. New and Old," Infect Dis Clin North Am, 2000, 14(1):1-22.
Relman DA, Hoesley C, and Cobbs CG, "Disease Caused by Bartonella Species," Cecil Textbook of Medicine, 21st ed, Chapter 357, Goldman L and Bennett JC, eds, Philadelphia PA: WB Sanders Co, 2000, 1719-23.
Riviello JJ and Rabinov JD, Case Records of the Massachusetts General Hospital, Case 1-1998, Scully RE, Mark EJ, McNeely WF, et al, eds, N Engl J Med, 1998, 338(2):112-9.
Suhler EB, Lauer AK, Rosenbaum JT, "Prevalence of Serologic Evidence of Cat Scratch Disease in Patients With Neuroretinitis," Ophthalmology, 2000, 107(5):871-6.

Internet Web Sites
www.astdhpphe.org/infect/catscratch.html
www.natip.org/cat.html

◆ **Bartonella Titer** see Bartonella Serology on page 581

◆ **bDNA** see Hepatitis C Virus RNA Detection and Quantitation on page 626

◆ **Beetles** see Arthropod Identification on page 559

◆ **Beta-Hemolytic Strep Culture, Throat** see Bacterial Culture, Throat, and Antigen Detection Testing for Group A Streptococci on page 577

Beta-Lactamase Test

Related Information
Antimicrobial Susceptibility Testing, Aerobic and Facultatively Anaerobic Bacteria on page 554
Antimicrobial Susceptibility Testing, Anaerobic Bacteria on page 555
Bacterial Culture, Aerobes on page 563
Neisseria gonorrhoeae Culture and Smear on page 662

Synonyms Cefinase (Nitrocefin) Testing; Cephalosporinase Production Testing; Penicillinase-Producing Organisms Susceptibility Testing; Penicillinase Test

Applies to Beta-Lactam Ring; Cephalosporinases; Haemophilus influenzae Susceptibility Testing; Neisseria gonorrhoeae Susceptibility Testing; Penicillinases

Test Includes Rapid testing of isolated bacterial colonies for the production of beta lactamase

Abstract Certain bacteria produce enzymes that inactivate beta-lactam antibiotics. Some enzymes can hydrolyze penicillin (penicillinases); others hydrolyze cephalosporins (cephalosporinases). Recently, newer beta lactamases have been identified that have an extended spectrum of antimicrobial activity. These enzymes have been named extended-spectrum beta lactamases (ESBL).[1] In all cases, the detection of enzyme production by bacterial isolates is essential in determination of appropriate therapy.

Specimen Isolated colonies of Haemophilus influenzae, Moraxella (Branhamella) catarrhalis, Neisseria gonorrhoeae, enterococci, Staphylococcus aureus, or gram-negative anaerobic rods including Bacteroides fragilis

Use Rapid detection of beta-lactamase production from isolated colonies of Haemophilus influenzae, Neisseria gonorrhoeae, Moraxella catarrhalis, and Enterococcus species. This test can be used to predict resistance to penicillins and some cephalosporins.

All clinically significant isolates of E. coli and Klebsiella species should be tested for the presence of ESBLs.

Limitations Beta-lactamase negative strains may be resistant to penicillins or cephalosporins by other mechanisms. Results of this test do not predict resistance or susceptibility to other antimicrobial agents.

Methodology Paper disk with a chromogenic cephalosporin reagent. The hydrolysis of the beta-lactam ring results in a color change that is quickly detected. The chromogenic assay can detect both penicillinases and cephalosporinases. The acidimetric method uses pH color indicators to detect increased acidity that results when the beta-lactam ring of penicillin is cleaved to yield a penicilloic acid. Penicilloic acid can also reduce iodine that can be detected as the decolorization of a starch-iodine mixture. This method is referred to as the iodometric method.

Extended-spectrum beta lactamases (ESBL): Several methods have been suggested by the National Committee for Clinical Laboratory Standards for the screening and detection of ESBLs.[2] The initial screen uses a broth-based method to detect MIC values >1 μg/mL to selected cephalosporins (cefpodoxime, ceftazidime, cefotaxime, ceftriaxone) or aztreonam. The confirmatory test uses a broth-based method with both
(Continued)

Beta-Lactamase Test (Continued)

cefotaxime and ceftazidime alone and in combination with clavulanic acid. Several commercial tests have been developed to screen and detect *E. coli* and *Klebsiella* species for the presence of ESBLs.[2]

Additional Information The beta-lactamase test can provide clinically useful information when used for organisms in which the primary mechanism of resistance to beta-lactam antibiotics is by means of beta-lactamase enzymes, and in which resistance patterns to other antimicrobial agents is predictable. Consequently, beta-lactamase testing is restricted to a few specific circumstances that meet such criteria. *H. influenzae* and *M. catarrhalis* isolates that produce beta lactamase are resistant to ampicillin, but resistance to other agents is predictable (ie, virtually all isolates are presently susceptible to most second and third generation cephalosporins, beta-lactamase inhibitor combinations, azithromycin, and clarithromycin).[3] *N. gonorrhoeae* isolates that are beta-lactamase positive are resistant to penicillin, but uniformly susceptible to ceftriaxone.[3] Beta-lactamase testing of anaerobic gram-negative bacilli (eg, *Bacteroides*, *Porphyromonas*, and *Prevotella* sp) can be performed using the nitrocefin disk assay.[4,5] However, beta-lactamase testing of anaerobic bacteria has limited clinical utility since a number of anaerobic bacteria can be resistant to beta-lactam antibiotics in the absence of beta lactamases.[6]

Recently, it has been recognized that changes have occurred in the beta lactamases produced by gram-negative bacteria. These new enzymes have a broader spectrum of activity against several beta-lactam antimicrobial agents. These enzymes are not homogeneous (there are many different types) and do not have predictable responses to beta-lactam antibiotics in the laboratory. More important, patients infected with these ESBL producing infections often do not respond to beta-lactam antibiotics, even when routine susceptibility testing indicates a susceptible phenotype. It is important for the laboratory to properly screen and detect these enzymes to prevent placing patients with serious gram-negative infections at risk.[1,2]

Footnotes

1. Thomson KS and Smith Moland E, "Version 2000: The New Beta-Lactamases of Gram-Negative Bacteria at the Dawn of the New Millennium," *Microbes Infect*, 2000, 2(10):1225-35.
2. National Committee for Clinical Laboratory Standards, "Performance Standards for Antimicrobial Susceptibility Testing; 11th Informational Supplement," NCCLS Document M100-S11, Volume 21(1), Wayne, Pennsylvania, 2001.
3. Hindler JA and Swenson JM, "Susceptibility Tests of Fastidious Bacteria," *Manual of Clinical Microbiology*, 7th ed, Murray PR, Baron EJ, Pfaller MA, eds, et al, Washington, DC: AMS Press, American Society for Microbiology, 1999, 1544-54.
4. Uraz G and Turkmen L, "Beta-Lactamase Activity of Anaerobic *Bacteroides* Strains Isolated From Clinical Samples and Their Susceptibility to antimicrobial Agents," *Drug Metabol Drug Interact*, 1999, 15(2-3):181-6.
5. Fosse T, Madinier I, Hitzig C, et al, "Prevalence of Beta-Lactamase-Producing Strains Among 149 Anaerobic Gram-Negative Rods Isolated From Periodontal Pockets," *Oral Microbiol Immunol*, 1999, 14(6):352-7.
6. Hecht DW, "Susceptibility Testing of Anaerobic Bacteria," *Manual of Clinical Microbiology*, 7th ed, Murray PR, Baron EJ, Pfaller MA, eds, et al, Washington, DC: AMS Press, American Society for Microbiology, 1999, 1555-62.

References

Amyes SG and Miles RS, "Extended-Spectrum Beta-Lactamases: The Role of Inhibitors in Therapy," *J Antimicrob Chemother*, 1998, 42(4):415-7.

Dennesen PJ, Bonten MJ, and Weinstein RA, "Multiresistant Bacteria as a Hospital Epidemic Problem," *Ann Med*, 1998, 30(2):176-85.

Doern GV, Brueggemann AB, Pierce G, et al, "Antibiotic Resistance Among Clinical Isolates of *Haemophilus influenzae* in the United States in 1994 and 1995 and Detection of Beta-Lactamase Positive Strains Resistant to Amoxicillin-Clavulanate: Results of a National Multicenter Surveillance Study," *Antimicrob Agents Chemother*, 1997, 41(2):292-7.

Gibb AP and Crichton M, "Cefpodoxime Screening of *Escherichia coli* and *Klebsiella* spp by Vitek for Detection of Organisms Producing Extended-Spectrum Beta-Lactamases," *Diagn Microbiol Infect Dis*, 2000, 38(4):255-7.

Hand WL, "Current Challenges in Antibiotic Resistance," *Adolesc Med*, 2000, 11(2):427-38.

MacKenzie FM and Gould IM, "Extended Spectrum Beta-Lactamases," *J Infect*, 1998, 36(3):255-8.

Walker ES, Neal CL, Laffan E, et al, "Long-Term Trends in Susceptibility of *Moraxella catarrhalis*: A Population Analysis," *J Antimicrob Chemother*, 2000, 45(2):175-82.

Blastomycosis Serology

Related Information

Fungal Culture, Biopsy or Body Fluid *on page 610*
Fungal Culture, Sputum *on page 613*
Fungal Culture, Urine *on page 614*
Fungus Smear, Stain *on page 615*

Synonyms Blastomycosis Antibody Titer

Test Includes Detection of *Blastomyces dermatitidis* specific serology

Abstract Blastomycosis is caused by the dimorphic fungus *Blastomyces dermatitidis*. The disease may present with subacute pneumonia, acute pneumonia, or as disseminated extrapulmonary disease. Extrapulmonary infections can affect the skin, bone, or genitourinary tract (including the prostate), and other sites (eg, CNS). This mold is a natural inhabitant of the soil, and most cases in the United States have occurred around the Great Lakes and Upper Mississippi River. Recently, the CDC recognized two active cases of blastomycoses that were acquired in Colorado. The two patients had both been involved with a prairie dog relocation project and possibly acquired the disease from this activity.[1,2]

Specimen Serum

Container Red top tube

Reference Interval Complement fixation: titers <1:8; immunodiffusion: no precipitin band; enzyme immunoassay: titers <1:32

Use Support the diagnosis of infection due to *Blastomyces dermatitidis*. Acute and convalescent titers are helpful. This diagnosis is established by demonstration of the organisms in smear and/or tissue section by histology or by culture. Skin lesions are found in ~50% of patients, providing access to histopathologic and mycologic diagnosis.[3]

Limitations Failure to demonstrate precipitin antibodies does not rule out blastomycosis. Cross reactions are seen in patients with histoplasmosis and coccidioidomycosis. Skin testing prior to the test may elevate the complement fixation titer. The complement fixation test lacks sensitivity and specificity and gives positive results in <50% of culture proven cases. Complement fixation assays are often cross-reactive.[4] Newer EIA tests for blastomycosis have shown greater sensitivity with no compromise in specificity compared to other tests. EIA for antibody to purified A antigen is 90% sensitive, with some cross reaction with cases of histoplasmosis.[5,6]

Methodology Immunodiffusion (ID), enzyme immunoassay (EIA), radioimmunoassay (RIA). DNA probes are being developed.

Additional Information The EIA assay uses purified antigen A and is 80% to 100% sensitive. False-positive results can occur in patients with histoplasmosis or sporotrichosis.[5,6] Immunodiffusion assays have poor sensitivity but good specificity. Almost 50% of patients infected with *Blastomyces dermatitidis* will have a negative antibody test on initial testing. Several serial samples should be tested to accurately diagnose blastomycosis. A negative serologic result has little value and in no way excludes the existence of blastomycosis. Cross reactions producing lines of partial identity are seen in patients with histoplasmosis and coccidioidomycosis. Repeated testing at 3-week intervals may be needed to secure a diagnosis. After diagnosis is established, falling titers are a good prognostic sign.

The organisms appear as yeast forms with thick, double-contoured cell walls. Budding is broad-based. PAS is among the useful tissue stains.[7]

Extrapulmonary disease occurs in some patients who lack clinical evidence of disease in lungs. Bone and joint involvement is seen in vertebrae and long bones.

Attempts to isolate *B. dermatitidis* from cerebrospinal fluid are usually unsuccessful; brain biopsy is often necessary when the central nervous system is involved. The CSF is characterized usually by lymphocytic pleocytosis and decreased glucose.[3]

Footnotes

1. Centers for Disease Control, "Blastomycosis Acquired Occupationally During Prairie Dog Relocation - Colorado, 1998," *MMWR Morb Mortal Wkly Rep*, 1999, 48(5):98-100.
2. Centers for Disease Control and Prevention, "Blastomycosis Acquired Occupationally During Prairie Dog Relocation - Colorado, 1998," *JAMA*, 1999, 282(1):21-2.
3. Friedman JA, Wijdicks EF, Fulgham JR, et al, "Meningoencephalitis Due to *Blastomyces dermatitidis*: Case Report and Literature Review," *Mayo Clin Proc*, 2000, 75(4):403-8.
4. Dismukes WE, "Blastomycosis," *Cecil Textbook of Medicine*, 21st ed, Chapter 396, Goldman L and Bennett JC, eds, Philadelphia PA: WB Sanders Co, 2000, 1865-6.
5. Lo CY and Notenboom RH, "A New Enzyme Immunoassay Specific for Blastomycosis," *Am Rev Respir Dis*, 1990, 141(1):84:8.
6. Areno JP 4th, Campbell GD Jr, and George RB, "Diagnosis of Blastomycosis," *Semin Respir Infect*, 1997, 12(3):252-62.
7. Wallen EB and Youngberg GA, Images in Clinical Medicine, "Blastomycosis," *N Engl J Med*, 1997, 336(17):1223.

References

Chapman SW, Bradsher RW, Campbell GD, et al, "Practice Guidelines for the Management of Patients With Blastomycosis. Infectious Diseases Society of America," *Clin Infect Dis*, 2000, 30(4):679-83.

Lemos LB, Guo M, and Baliga M, "Blastomycosis: Organ Involvement and Etiologic Diagnosis: A Review of 123 Patients From Mississippi," *Ann Diagn Pathol*, 2000, 4(6):391-406.

McCullough MJ, DiSalvo AF, Clemons KV, et al, "Molecular Epidemiology of *Blastomyces dermatitidis*," *Clin Infect Dis*, 2000, 30(2):328-35.

Pappas PG, "Blastomycosis in the Immunocompromised Patient," *Semin Respir Infect*, 1997, 12(3):243-51.

Saubolle MA, "Fungal Pneumonia," *Semin Respir Infect*, 2000, 15(2):162-77.

Internet Web Sites
www.cdc.gov/ncidod/dbmd/diseaseinfo/blastomycosis_a.htm

♦ **Blood Culture, BactAlert®** *see* Bacterial Culture, Blood *on page 566*

♦ **Blood Culture, *Brucella* Agglutinins** *see Brucella* Culture *on page 586*

♦ **Blood Culture, Isolator™** *see* Bacterial Culture, Blood *on page 566*

♦ **Blood Culture, *Leptospira*** *see Leptospira* Culture *on page 648*

♦ **Blood Culture, Lysis Centrifugation** *see* Bacterial Culture, Blood *on page 566*

♦ **Blood Culture With Antimicrobial Removal Device (ARD)** *see* Bacterial Culture, Blood *on page 566*

♦ **Blood Fungus Culture** *see* Fungal Culture, Blood *on page 610*

♦ **Body Fluid Aerobic Culture** *see* Bacterial Culture, Biopsy or Body Fluid *on page 565*

♦ **Body Fluid Fungus Culture** *see* Fungal Culture, Biopsy or Body Fluid *on page 610*

♦ **Body Fluid Mycobacteria Culture** *see* Mycobacterial Culture, Biopsy or Body Fluid *on page 655*

♦ **Body Fluid Viral Culture** *see* Viral Culture, Body Fluid *on page 691*

♦ **Bone Marrow Culture** *see* Bacterial Culture, Biopsy or Body Fluid *on page 565*

♦ **Bone Marrow Culture for *Brucella*** *see Brucella* Culture *on page 586*

♦ **Bone Marrow Fungus Culture** *see* Fungal Culture, Biopsy or Body Fluid *on page 610*

♦ **Bone Marrow Mycobacteria Culture** *see* Mycobacterial Culture, Biopsy or Body Fluid *on page 655*

♦ ***Bordetella pertussis*** *see* Bacterial Culture, Sputum *on page 574*

♦ ***Bordetella pertussis* Antibodies** *see Bordetella pertussis* Serology *on page 584*

Bordetella pertussis Culture

Related Information
Bacterial Culture, Nasopharynx *on page 573*
Bordetella pertussis Direct Fluorescent Antibody *on page 583*
Bordetella pertussis Serology *on page 584*

Synonyms Nasopharyngeal Culture for *Bordetella pertussis*; Pertussis Culture; Whooping Cough Culture

Replaces Cough Plate Culture for Pertussis; Throat Culture for *Bordetella pertussis*

Test Includes Culture specifically for *Bordetella pertussis* only

Abstract *B. pertussis* is the predominant cause of pertussis (whooping cough) which occurs during a primary infection in unimmunized children. Laboratory diagnosis of pertussis requires both a nasopharyngeal culture and detection of *B. pertussis*-specific IgG or IgM (especially IgM). For optimal culture of *B. pertussis* from nasopharyngeal specimens, the laboratory must be notified since routine agar plates do not support the growth of this organism and special media needs to be prepared or purchased. Even when appropriate culture media are used, positive growth is seen in only 50% of infected patients.

Patient Preparation Patient should not be on antimicrobial therapy prior to the collection of the specimen.

Specimen Nasopharyngeal swab, cough plate optional

Container Flexible calcium alginate swab (Calgiswab®) and Bordet Gengou plate. Transport medium composed of half strength Oxoid charcoal agar CM19 supplemented with 40 µg/mL cephalexin and 10% hemolyzed defibrinated horse blood may be used.[1]

Collection Shape the flexible swab into the contour of the nares. Pass the swab gently through the nose. Leave swab in place near septum and floor of nose for 15-30 seconds. Rotate and remove. The recovery of the organism depends on collection of an adequate specimen. Inoculate the plate or transport medium directly at the bedside.

The following procedure optimizes the laboratory diagnosis of pertussis.

- Collect nasopharyngeal specimens in the early stage of illness. Provision of specimen collection kits facilitates appropriate specimen collection and transportation.
- For swab collected specimens, use a transport medium consisting of half strength Oxoid charcoal agar supplemented with 10% hemolyzed, defibrinated horse blood, and 40 µg/mL cephalexin.
- Inoculate a selective primary plating medium composed of Oxoid charcoal agar, 10% defibrinated horse blood, and 40 µg/mL cephalexin. A nonselective medium without cephalexin may be used in addition to the selective medium.
- Perform direct fluorescent antibody (DFA) tests on appropriately collected nasopharyngeal secretions with *B. pertussis*- and *B. parapertussis*-conjugated antisera to facilitate earlier diagnosis.

- After inoculation of primary plating media, retain swabs in the original transport medium at room temperature. If cultures become overgrown with indigenous bacterial flora or fungi, use swabs to inoculate additional media.
- Identify suspicious isolates with appropriate cultural and biochemical tests. The DFA test performed on growth from isolated colonies is an excellent procedure for confirmatory or definitive identification.

Storage Instructions The specimen should not be refrigerated. It should be transported to the laboratory as soon as possible.

Causes for Rejection Excessive delay in transit to the laboratory results in suboptimal yield.

Turnaround Time Growth of *Bordetella pertussis* requires at least 72 hours for detection.

Special Instructions Consult the laboratory prior to collection of the specimen so that the special isolation medium can be obtained. The laboratory should be made aware of the specific request to screen for *Bordetella pertussis* with information relevant to current antibiotic therapy.

Reference Interval No *B. pertussis* or *B. parapertussis* isolated

Use Isolate and identify *B. pertussis*, and *B. parapertussis*; establish the diagnosis of whooping cough

Limitations Isolation of *Bordetella* species probably has sensitivity of <50% compared to comprehensive serologic testing or detection by PCR.[2,3]

Contraindications Current antibiotic therapy; history of vaccination is a relative contraindication

Methodology Culture on selective medium (selective chocolate agar with 10% defibrinated horse blood and 40 µg/mL cephalexin), presumptive confirmation by direct fluorescent antibody (DFA). Culture after enrichment in transport medium for 48 hours increases yield. Detection by DNA amplification is currently in development and seems to be more sensitive than culture.[2,3]

Additional Information Despite extensive vaccination programs, pertussis is still one of the 10 most common causes of death from infectious disease worldwide. Pertussis causes 350,000 deaths annually, with the majority of deaths occurring in infants. Typical pertussis can be recognized clinically by the distinctive whooping cough that occurs during the paroxysmal stage. However, other infectious agents can cause a pertussis-like disease (*Chlamydia trachomatis*, adenovirus, and respiratory syncytial virus; refer to the Key Word Index). Pertussis is highly contagious and even immunized individuals can become transiently colonized, thus, spreading the organism to unvaccinated individuals.

To prevent infections of pertussis it is important to recognize the disease, avoid further spread, and provide pertussis vaccination to children. Direct fluorescent antibody (DFA) procedures and PCR assays seem to provide more rapid results and are being increasingly used in the diagnosis of *B. pertussis* infection.

Footnotes

1. He Q, Mertsola J, Soini H, et al, "Comparison of Polymerase Chain Reaction With Culture and Enzyme Immunoassay for Diagnosis of Pertussis," *J Clin Microbiol*, 1993, 31(3):642-5.
2. Loeffelholz MJ, Thompson CJ, Long KS, et al, "Comparison of PCR, Culture and Direct Fluorescent-Antibody Testing for Detection of *Bordetella pertussis*," *J Clin Microbiol*, 1999, 37(9):2872-6.
3. Heininger U, Schmidt-Schlapfer G, Cherry JD, et al, "Clinical Validation of a Polymerase Chain Reaction for the Diagnosis of Pertussis by Comparison With Serology, Culture, and Symptoms During a Large Pertussis Vaccine Efficacy Trial," *Pediatrics*, 2000, 105(3):E31.

References

Hallander HO, "Microbiological and Serological Diagnosis of Pertussis," *Clin Infect Dis*, 1999, 28(S2):S99-106.

Hallander HO, Reizenstein E, Renemar B, et al, "Comparison of Nasopharyngeal Aspirates With Swabs for Culture of *Bordetella pertussis*," *J Clin Microbiol*, 1993, 31(1):50-2.

Hindiyeh M and Carroll KC, "Laboratory Diagnosis of Atypical Pneumonia," *Semin Respir Infect*, 2000, 15(2):101-13.

Marchant CD, Loughlin AM, Lett SM, et al, "Pertussis in Massachusetts, 1981-1991: Incidence, Serologic Diagnosis, and Vaccine Effectiveness," *J Infect Dis*, 1994, 169(6):1297-305.

Smith C and Vyas H, "Early Infantile Pertussis: Increasingly Prevalent and Potentially Fatal," *Eur J Pediatr*, 2000, 159(12):898-900.

Stojanov S, Liese J, and Belohradsky BH, "Hospitalization and Complications in Children Under 2 Years of Age With *Bordetella pertussis* Infection," *Infection*, 2000, 28(2):106-10.

Internet Web Sites
www.astdhpphe.org/infect/per.html
www.cdc.gov/nip/publications/pink/pert.pdf

Bordetella pertussis Direct Fluorescent Antibody

Related Information
Bordetella pertussis Culture *on page 583*
Bordetella pertussis Serology *on page 584*

Synonyms *Bordetella pertussis* Smear; Nasopharyngeal Smear for *Bordetella pertussis*; Pertussis DFA

Replaces Cough Plate Culture for Pertussis

Test Includes Detection of *Bordetella pertussis* directly in nasopharyngeal specimens using fluorescent-labeled antibody specific for the organism
(Continued)

Bordetella pertussis Direct Fluorescent Antibody
(Continued)

Abstract Pertussis (whooping cough) is a very contagious disease that occurs worldwide. Pertussis begins as a mild respiratory infection. Within 2 weeks the infection can be recognized by the distinctive whooping cough that occurs during the paroxysmal stage. However, since other infectious agents can also cause a pertussis-like disease (*Chlamydia trachomatis*, adenovirus, and respiratory syncytial virus) it is very important to diagnose pertussis infection quickly in order to prevent further spread of the disease. Direct fluorescent antibody (DFA) procedures as well as PCR assays provide more rapid results than culture and should be used in the diagnosis of *B. pertussis* infection.[1,2,3]

Patient Preparation Patient must not be on antimicrobial therapy.

Specimen Nasopharyngeal swab

Collection Swab is passed through nose gently and into nasopharynx. Stay near septum and floor of nose. Rotate and remove. Specimen must be hand transported to the laboratory immediately following collection.

Storage Instructions Do not refrigerate.

Causes for Rejection Specimen not received in appropriate sterile container or on appropriate isolation medium, specimen more than 2 hours old. Cough plates are unacceptable.

Turnaround Time 24-48 hours

Special Instructions Consult the laboratory prior to collection of the specimen so that the special reagents can be obtained. The laboratory should be made aware of the specific request to screen for *Bordetella pertussis* with information relevant to current antibiotic therapy.

Reference Interval No *B. pertussis* or *B. parapertussis* detected

Use Detect and identify *B. pertussis* and *B. parapertussis*; establish diagnosis of pertussis

Limitations Direct detection assays are always limited by the adequacy of the sample. Bacteria may be difficult to detect if there are few bacteria present in the specimen or too much mucoid material. Direct assay should always be used in conjunction with culture. Negative direct detection assays do not rule out pertussis. Many laboratories do not keep reagents immediately on hand, due to the low incidence in vaccinated populations.

Contraindications Lack of clinical symptoms of pertussis; previous antibiotic therapy; previous history of complete vaccinations that include pertussis vaccine

Methodology Direct fluorescent antibody (DFA) on nasopharyngeal specimen

Additional Information This procedure enables early presumptive identification of *Bordetella pertussis*, the agent of whooping cough. An experienced laboratory will have a 60% sensitivity and 90% specificity when compared with culture.[4,5] Since a low incidence of pertussis infections exists in many countries with comprehensive vaccine programs, laboratory personnel may not be proficient at detection of *B. pertussis* by immunofluorescence, and may not carry the expensive reagents needed for this assay. For many of these reasons the direct fluorescent detection of *B. pertussis* may be replaced soon by more sensitive DNA amplification methods.[1,2,3] However, at the current time, DNA assays are also expensive and are not available in most hospital laboratories. Therefore, currently, culture and identification of *B. pertussis* should be requested as well as pertussis serology for the definitive diagnosis of pertussis.

Footnotes

1. He Q, Mertsola J, Soini H, et al, "Comparison of Polymerase Chain Reaction With Culture and Enzyme Immunoassay for Diagnosis of Pertussis," *J Clin Microbiol*, 1993, 31(3):642-5.
2. Loeffelholz MJ, Thompson CJ, Long KS, et al, "Comparison of PCR, Culture and Direct Fluorescent-Antibody Testing for Detection of *Bordetella pertussis*," *J Clin Microbiol*, 1999, 37(9):2872-6.
3. Heininger U, Schmidt-Schlapfer G, Cherry JD, et al, "Clinical Validation of a Polymerase Chain Reaction for the Diagnosis of Pertussis by Comparison With Serology, Culture, and Symptoms During a Large Pertussis Vaccine Efficacy Trial," *Pediatrics*, 2000, 105(3):E31.
4. Ewanowich CA, Chui LW, Paranchych MG, et al, "Major Outbreak of Pertussis in Northern Alberta, Canada: Analysis of Discrepant Direct Fluorescent-Antibody and Culture Results by Using Polymerase Chain Reaction Methodology," *J Clin Microbiol*, 1993, 31(7):1715-25.
5. Strebel PM, Cochi SL, Farizo KM, et al, "Pertussis in Missouri: Evaluation of Nasopharyngeal Culture, Direct Fluorescent Antibody Testing, and Clinical Case Definitions in the Diagnosis of Pertussis," *Clin Infect Dis*, 1993, 16(2):276-85.

References

Hindiyeh M and Carroll KC, "Laboratory Diagnosis of Atypical Pneumonia," *Semin Respir Infect*, 2000, 15(2):101-3.
Marchant CD, Loughlin AM, Lett SM, et al, "Pertussis in Massachusetts, 1981-1991: Incidence, Serologic Diagnosis, and Vaccine Effectiveness," *J Infect Dis*, 1994, 169(6):1297-305.
Smith C and Vyas H, "Early Infantile Pertussis: Increasingly Prevalent and Potentially Fatal, " *Eur J Pediatr*, 2000, 159(12):898-900.
Stojanov S, Liese J, and Belohradsky BH, "Hospitalization and Complications in Children Under 2 years of Age With *Bordetella pertussis* Infection," *Infection*, 2000, 28(2):106-10.
Tilley PA, Kanchana MV, Knight I, et al, "Detection of *Bordetella pertussis* in a Clinical Laboratory by Culture, Polymerase Chain Reaction, and Direct Fluorescent Antibody Staining; Accuracy and Cost," *Diagn Microbiol Infect Dis*, 2000, 37(1):17-23.

Internet Web Sites

www.cdc.gov/nip/publications/pink/pert.pdf
www.astdhpphe.org/infect/per.html

Bordetella pertussis Serology

Related Information
Bacterial Culture, Sputum *on page 574*
Bordetella pertussis Culture *on page 583*
Bordetella pertussis Direct Fluorescent Antibody *on page 583*

Synonyms *Bordetella pertussis* Antibodies; *Bordetella pertussis* Titer; Pertussis Serology

Test Includes Enzyme-linked immunosorbent assay to detect antibodies to *Bordetella pertussis* and/or pertussis toxin

Abstract Pertussis (whooping cough) is a very contagious acute infectious disease caused by the bacterium, *Bordetella pertussis*. Outbreaks of pertussis occur worldwide. Pertussis is one of the most common childhood diseases and a major cause of childhood mortality. In unimmunized populations, pertussis is responsible for ~350,000 deaths annually. Other infectious agents can also cause a pertussis-like disease (*Chlamydia trachomatis*, adenovirus, and respiratory syncytial virus). Thus, it is important to distinguish pertussis infection from these other infections. This distinction will support prevention of further spread of the disease.

Serologic testing to document either infection with the bacteria or prior immunization is useful in epidemiology and at times can be used for clinical diagnosis. However, the test is not routinely available. Direct fluorescent antibody (DFA) procedures as well as PCR assays provide more rapid results than does serology and should be used in the diagnosis of *B. pertussis* infection.[1,2,3]

Specimen Serum

Container Red top tube

Storage Instructions Refrigerate serum at 4°C.

Reference Interval Less than fourfold rise in titer in paired sera; IgM antibody: negative in unimmunized individual; positive in vaccinated individual.

Use Evaluate acute infection with *Bordetella pertussis*; establish immunity following vaccination for *Bordetella pertussis*

Limitations The clinical role for serologic diagnosis of acute pertussis is severely limited by the time required for seroconversion. There is a lack of association between antibody levels and immunity. Assays are not well standardized.

Methodology Microhemagglutination, complement fixation (CF), toxin neutralization, enzyme-linked immunosorbent assay (ELISA)

Additional Information Serologic testing alone should not be relied upon for clinical confirmation of pertussis. However, patients with acute infection will develop IgG, IgM, and IgA antibodies to febrile agglutinogens. Following vaccination, IgG and IgM antibodies can be demonstrated, except in infants. IgA antibodies do not develop.

Footnotes

1. He Q, Mertsola J, Soini H, et al, "Comparison of Polymerase Chain Reaction With Culture and Enzyme Immunoassay for Diagnosis of Pertussis," *J Clin Microbiol*, 1993, 31(3):642-5.
2. Loeffelholz MJ, Thompson CJ, Long KS, et al, "Comparison of PCR, Culture and Direct Fluorescent-Antibody Testing for Detection of *Bordetella pertussis*," *J Clin Microbiol*, 1999, 37(9):2872-6.
3. Heininger U, Schmidt-Schlapfer G, Cherry JD, et al, "Clinical Validation of a Polymerase Chain Reaction for the Diagnosis of Pertussis by Comparison With Serology, Culture, and Symptoms During a Large Pertussis Vaccine Efficacy Trial," *Pediatrics*, 2000, 105(3):E31.

References

Cherry JD, Beer T, Chartrand SA, et al, "Comparison of Values of Antibody to *Bordetella pertussis* Antigens in Young German and American Men," *Clin Infect Dis*, 1995, 20(5):1271-4.
Hindiyeh M and Carroll KC, "Laboratory Diagnosis of Atypical Pneumonia," *Semin Respir Infect*, 2000, 15(2):101-3.
Marchant CD, Loughlin AM, Lett SM, et al, "Pertussis in Massachusetts, 1981-1991: Incidence, Serologic Diagnosis, and Vaccine Effectiveness," *J Infect Dis*, 1994, 169(6):1297-305.
Smith C and Vyas H, "Early Infantile Pertussis: Increasingly Prevalent and Potentially Fatal," *Eur J Pediatr*, 2000, 159(12):898-900.
Stojanov S, Liese J, and Belohradsky BH, "Hospitalization and Complications in Children Under 2 Years of Age With *Bordetella pertussis* Infection," *Infection*, 2000, 28(2):106-10.
Tilley PA, Kanchana MV, Knight I, et al, "Detection of *Bordetella pertussis* in a Clinical Laboratory by Culture, Polymerase Chain Reaction, and Direct Fluorescent Antibody Staining; Accuracy and Cost," *Diagn Microbiol Infect Dis*, 2000, 37(1):17-23.

Internet Web Sites

www.cdc.gov/nip/publications/pink/pert.pdf
www.astdhpphe.org/infect/per.html

♦ ***Bordetella pertussis* Smear** *see Bordetella pertussis* Direct Fluorescent Antibody *on page 583*

♦ ***Bordetella pertussis* Titer** *see Bordetella pertussis* Serology *on page 584*

♦ ***Bordetella spp*** *see* Bacterial Culture, Bronchoscopy/Bronchial Brush/Bronchoalveolar Lavage Specimen *on page 568*

Borrelia burgdorferi Culture

Related Information

Lyme Disease Serology *on page 650*
Polymerase Chain Reaction *on page 713*

Synonyms Culture for *Borrelia burgdorferi*; Lyme Disease Bacterial Culture

Applies to Lyme Disease

Abstract *Borrelia burgdorferi* is a corkscrew shaped organism that is the causative agent for Lyme disease. *B. burgdorferi* is transmitted to humans by the bite of an infected deer tick (*Ixodes scapularis*). The number of reported cases of Lyme disease has increased in the U.S. since national surveillance began in 1982. There were nearly 17,000 cases reported to the CDC in 1998.[1] Most of the cases were reported from Northeastern and Mid-Atlantic states and two North-Central States.

Specimen Tick taken from patient; skin, blood, cerebrospinal fluid, or joint fluid

Collection Collect blood in either EDTA or serum tubes.

Causes for Rejection Tissue fixed in formalin

Reference Interval Negative

Limitations Culture may often be negative in patients with disease; requires lengthy incubation before bacteria can be detected (4-6 weeks). Recovery of isolates from skin specimens may be overgrown with indigenous bacterial skin flora. Culture of *B. burgdorferi* is less sensitive than PCR or serology, especially in neuroborreliosis.[2]

Methodology Culture in BSKII medium with a neutral pH. Incubation at 30°C to 37°C. Monitor for growth using a darkfield microscope for 4-6 weeks.[3]

Additional Information The diagnosis of Lyme disease is primarily based on clinical findings and elevated serology. Clinical signs and symptoms of Lyme disease include one or more of the following: malaise, fever, headache, myalgias, swollen lymph nodes, and a characteristic skin rash, erythema migrans (EM). Culture provides a definitive diagnosis, but culture is often negative in patients without skin manifestations. A recent study compared PCR, culture, and serology for the diagnosis of Lyme disease. For patients with EM, PCR was positive in 71% of the patients' skin biopsies, and 13% of the urine specimens. Forty-one percent of the patients had positive serology but only 29% of the skin biopsies were positive by culture. In patients with neuroborreliosis, the PCR detected the bacteria only 17% of the time in cerebrospinal fluid and only 7% of the urine specimens. Culture was unable to detect bacteria, but 90% of the patients have specific intrathecal antibody to *B. burgdorferi*.[2] Another study has shown that blood cultures were positive in only 50% of patients with early Lyme disease.[4] Therefore, diagnosis should not depend entirely on culture for *B. burgdorferi*.

Footnotes

1. Orloski KA, Hayes EB, Campbell GL, et al, "Surveillance for Lyme Disease - United States, 1992-1998," *MMWR Morb Mortal Wkly Rep*, 2000, 49(SS3):1-11.

2. Lebech AM, Hansen K, Brandrup F, et al, "Diagnostic Value of PCR for Detection of *Borrelia burgdorferi* DNA in Clinical Specimens From Patients With Erythema Migrans and Lyme Neuroborreliosis," *Mol Diagn*, 2000, 5(2):139-50.

3. Schwan TG, Burgdorfer W, and Rosa PA, "*Borrelia*," *Manual of Clinical Microbiology*, 7th ed, Murray PR, Baron EJ, Pfaller MA, eds, et al, Washington, DC: AMS Press, American Society for Microbiology, 1999, 746-58.

4. Wormser GP, Bittker S, Cooper D, et al, "Comparison of the Yields of Blood Cultures Using Serum or Plasma From Patients With Early Lyme Disease," *J Clin Microbiol*, 2000, 38(4):1648-50.

References

Eppes SC, Nelson DK, Lewis LL, et al, "Characterization of Lyme Meningitis and Comparison With Viral Meningitis in Children," *Pediatrics*, 1999, 103(5Pt1):957-60.

Nadelman RB and Wormser GP, "Lyme Borreliosis," *Lancet*, 1998, 352(9127):557-65.

Oksi J, Marjamaki M, Nikoskelainen J, et al, "*Borrelia burgdorferi* Detected by Culture and PCR in Clinical Relapse of Disseminated Lyme Borreliosis," *Ann Med*, 1999, 31(3):225-32.

Phillips SE, Mattman LH, Hulinska D, et al, "A Proposal for the Reliable Culture of *Borrelia burgdorferi* From Patients With Chronic Lyme Disease, Even From Those Previously Aggressively Treated," *Infection*, 1998, 26(6):364-7.

Strle F, Nadelman RB, Cimperman J, et al, "Comparison of Culture-Confirmed Erythema Migrans Caused by *Borrelia burgdorferi sensu stricto* in New York State and by *Borrelia afzelii* in Slovenia," *Ann Intern Med*, 1999, 130(1):32-6.

Internet Web Sites

www.cdc.gov/ncidod/dvbid/lymeinfo.htm
www.amm.co.uk/pubs/fa_lyme.htm
www.astdhpphe.org/infect/lyme.html

♦ *Borrelia burgdorferi* **DNA Assay** *see* Lyme Disease DNA Detection *on page 649*

♦ *Borrelia burgdorferi* **DNA Probe Test** *see* Lyme Disease DNA Detection *on page 649*

♦ *Borrelia burgdorferi* **PCR** *see* Lyme Disease DNA Detection *on page 649*

♦ *Borrelia burgdorferi* **Sensu Lato Serology** *see* Lyme Disease Serology *on page 650*

Botulism Diagnostic Procedures

Related Information

Bacterial Culture, Stool *on page 575*
Polymerase Chain Reaction *on page 713*
Tetanus Antibody *on page 682*

Synonyms *Clostridium botulinum* Toxin Identification Procedure; Infant Botulism, Toxin Identification; Sudden Death Syndrome

Abstract Botulism is a toxin-mediated disease caused by *Clostridium botulinum*. Botulism is classified into the following four categories:

- food-borne
- wound botulism
- infant botulism
- botulism from intestinal colonization of children older than infants

The anaerobic bacteria produce a potent neurotoxic protein which affects the nervous system without direct bacterial invasion of the CNS. The clinical manifestations of such intoxication include diplopia and dysphagia with descending progression of paralysis, leading to respiratory embarrassment in afebrile patients.

Two clostridial diseases produce exotoxins. While botulism is caused by ingestion of a preformed toxin, the bacteria proliferate at the site of injury in tetanus.

Specimen Vomitus, serum, stool, gastric washings, cerebrospinal fluid or autopsy tissue; food samples

Container Sterile wide-mouth, leakproof, screw-cap jar; red top tube

Storage Instructions Keep refrigerated at 4°C, except for unopened food samples.

Turnaround Time 3-7 days

Special Instructions The laboratory must be notified prior to obtaining specimen in order to prepare for transport of the specimen to the State Health Laboratory or Centers for Disease Control.

Reference Interval No toxin identified, no *Clostridium botulinum* bacteria isolated

Use Diagnose classic food-borne botulism, a neuroparalytic disease; wound botulism (rare), infant botulism, sudden death syndrome, or floppy baby syndrome

Limitations The toxin from *C. botulinum* binds almost irreversibly to individual nerve terminals; thus, serum and cerebrospinal fluid specimens can yield false-negative results.

Aerosolized toxin generally is not identifiable in serum or stool, although it is in cases of food botulism.[1]

Contraindications Due to the difficulty in performance of the diagnostic test and because of the extensive epidemiological studies initiated upon receipt of the specimen, State Department of Health Laboratories require specific clinical symptomatology for botulism testing. The physician may be asked to submit specific forms before a specimen is submitted to the State Department of Health or CDC. Physicians are encouraged to consult their state epidemiologists as soon as botulism is suspected. They should be consulted early to optimize handling of the suspect case. The CDC provides consultation and services to state and local health departments. An emergency number is (404) 639-2888. No reliable source of antitoxin is known beyond the Western Hemisphere.[2]

Methodology Toxin neutralization test in mice, isolation of *Clostridium botulinum* from feces. ELISA may detect toxin on nasal mucosa for 24 hours following inhalation.[1]

Additional Information *C. botulinum* is an obligate anaerobic, spore-forming, gram-positive bacillus that can be recovered from a wide variety of environmental sources. Infant botulism occurs most commonly in the second and third postnatal months and is rarely seen after the sixth month of life. The disease occurs when infants ingest *C. botulinum* spores that germinate and produce botulinum toxin (usually serotypes A or B) within the gastrointestinal tract. The toxin is disseminated hematogenously, enters nerve cells, and irreversibly interferes with release of acetylcholine. Infants seem particularly susceptible to colonization with *C. botulinum* because their gastrointestinal flora is not fully established. By 12 months of age, the human gastrointestinal tract is more resistant to colonization with *C. botulinum*; food-borne disease is usually a result of ingestion of toxin (rather than organisms) in food. The spectrum of disease in infants varies from mild constipation to sudden death. Infant botulism has in fact been implicated as a cause of sudden infant death syndrome (SIDS). The typical course of infant botulism is constipation, followed within 1-3 weeks by lethargy and listlessness, decreased gag reflex, and poor feeding. Ptosis may develop, and the child may have difficulty keeping his head up.[3,4]

Food-borne botulism usually develops 12-36 hours after toxin ingestion. Initial complaints consist of nausea, dry mouth, and diarrhea followed by evidence of cranial nerve dysfunction.[5] The toxin is destroyed by cooking.[2] Food-borne botulism typically occurs in outbreaks that need to be identified and then controlled to prevent further disease.[3]

In wound botulism, spores are introduced into a wound in which they germinate and produce toxin. Clinically, wound botulism lacks the prodromal gastrointestinal disorder of food-borne botulism, but is otherwise similar. Persons who inject illicit drugs, such as black-tar heroin, are at increased risk for wound botulism.
(Continued)

Botulism Diagnostic Procedures *(Continued)*

The differential diagnosis in individual cases includes Guillain-Barré syndrome, myasthenia gravis or tick paralysis (see the Key Word Index). The cause of death is usually respiratory failure.[1]

Intensive surveillance for botulism in the U.S. is maintained by state health departments and the CDC. Prompt recognition of botulism by physicians will help in detection of the disease. A potential exists for the use of botulism as a bioterrorist weapon.[6,7] National governments and terrorist organizations have been reported to maintain stockpiles of botulism toxin. One gram of aerosolized botulism toxin potentially could kill 1.5 million people or more.[2] Botulinum toxin is 100,000 times more toxic than sarin.[1]

Footnotes

1. Franz DR, Jahrling PB, Friedlander AM, et al, "Clinical Recognition and Management of Patients Exposed to Biological Warfare Agents," *JAMA*, 1997, 278(5):399-411.
2. Shapiro RL, Hatheway C, Becher J, "Botulism Surveillance and Emergency Response. A Public Health Strategy for a Global Challenge," *JAMA*, 1997, 278(5):433-5.
3. Urdaneta-Carruyo E, Suranyi A, and Milano M, "Infantile Botulism: Clinical and Laboratory Observations of a Rare Neuroparalytic Disease," *J Paediatr Child Health*, 2000, 36(2):193-5.
4. Rick JR, Ascher DP, and Smith RA, "Infantile Botulism: An Atypical Case of an Uncommon Disease," *Pediatrics*, 1999, 103(5 Pt 1):1038-9.
5. Roberts JA, "Economic Aspects of Food-Borne Outbreaks and Their Control," *Br Med Bull*, 2000, 56(1):133-41.
6. Sabatini M, "Biological Warfare: Would You Recognize an Attack?" *Nurs Spectr (Wash DC)*, 1998, 8(13):8, 24.
7. Leggiadro RJ, "The Threat of Biological Terrorism: A Public Health and Infection Control Reality," *Infect Control Hosp Epidemiol*, 2000, 21(1):53-6.

References

Hatheway CL, "Botulism: The Present Status of the Disease," *Curr Top Microbiol Immunol*, 1995, 195:55-75.

Hayes MT, Soto O, and Ruoff KL, "A 58-Year Old Woman With Multiple Cranial Neuropathies," Case Records of the Massachusetts General Hospital, Case 22-1997, Scully RE, Mark EJ, McNeely WF, et al, eds, *N Engl J Med*, 1997, 337(3):184-90.

McMaster P, Piper S, Schell D, et al, "A Taste of Honey," *J Paediart Child Health*, 2000, 36(6):596-7.

Mechem CC and Walter FG, "Wound Botulism," *Vet Hum Toxicol*, 1994, 36(3):233-7.

Villar RG, Shapiro RL, Busto S, et al, "Outbreak of Type A Botulism and Development of a Botulism Surveillance and Antitoxin Release System in Argentina," *JAMA*, 1999, 281(14):1334-8, 1340.

Wigginton JM and Thill P, "Infant Botulism. A Review of the Literature," *Clin Pediatr (Phila)*, 1993, 32(11):669-74.

Internet Web Sites

vm.cfsan.fda.gov/~mow/chap2.html

www.cdc.gov/ncidod/dbmd/diseaseinfo/botulism_g.htm

♦ **Branched Chain DNA Assay** *see* Human Immunodeficiency Virus, Viral Load Assay *on page 640*

♦ **Breath Testing for *H. pylori*** *see Helicobacter pylori* Serology *on page 621*

♦ **Bronchoalveolar Lavage Culture** *see* Bacterial Culture, Bronchoscopy/ Bronchial Brush/Bronchoalveolar Lavage Specimen *on page 568*

♦ **Bronchoscopy Fungus Culture** *see* Fungal Culture, Sputum *on page 613*

♦ **Bronchoscopy Specimen Bacterial Culture** *see* Bacterial Culture, Bronchoscopy/Bronchial Brush/Bronchoalveolar Lavage Specimen *on page 568*

♦ **Broviac Catheters** *see* Bacterial Culture, Intravascular Device *on page 572*

♦ ***Brucella abortus*** *see* Brucellosis Serology *on page 587*

Brucella Culture

Related Information

Bacterial Culture, Biopsy or Body Fluid *on page 565*
Bacterial Culture, Blood *on page 566*
Brucellosis Serology *on page 587*

Synonyms Blood Culture, *Brucella* Agglutinins; Undulant Fever, Culture

Applies to Bone Marrow Culture for *Brucella*

Abstract Brucellosis is a zoonosis caused by several species of *Brucella*. These bacteria are intracellular pathogens that cause a mild disease or a severe septicemic febrile illness in humans. Transmission of brucellosis is through contaminated milk or milk products or by direct contact with infected animals. *Brucella melitensis* usually infects goats and sheep, *Brucella suis* swine, *Brucella abortus* cattle, and *Brucella canis* infects dogs. Other mammals, insects and ticks may have *Brucella* infections.

Specimen Blood, bone marrow, infected tissues, spleen, liver biopsies; rarely, cerebrospinal fluid, urine, pleural or peritoneal fluid are submitted for *Brucella* culture.

Container Ideally, blood should be collected in biphasic blood culture bottles; if these are not available, blood may be collected in routine blood culture bottles or lysis centrifugation tubes. Specimens other than blood should be collected in a sterile tightly closed container.

Collection Collect prior to antimicrobial therapy, when possible.

Storage Instructions Specimens should be cultured promptly.

Turnaround Time Blood cultures may be held for up to 6 weeks before reporting out negatives.

Special Instructions *Brucella* spp pose a significant infection control hazard to laboratorians and require special procedures for recovery. The organisms are highly infectious by aerosol, and can survive in dust for 6 weeks. In order to ensure that proper precautions and methods are used, **the laboratory must be informed when brucellosis is suspected.**[1,2]

Reference Interval No growth

Use Establish the diagnosis of brucellosis. The organisms infect lung, spleen, liver, central nervous system, bone marrow, testes, the gallbladder, and the skeletal system. They cause vertebral osteomyelitis, large joint infections, and sacroiliitis. Genitourinary infections occur. Endocarditis and CNS infections are rare, but account for most fatalities.[3]

Limitations Diagnosis of brucellosis in the United States is hampered by failure to consider the diagnosis in early acute phases, and laboratorians who have little experience with this fastidious organism. Blood cultures for *Brucella* are useful in acute infection but are rarely positive in subacute or chronic brucellosis; bone marrow should always be cultured when subacute or chronic brucellosis is suspected. It is also reasonable to collect bone marrow in suspected acute brucellosis since it provides positive results faster and with greater frequency than blood cultures.[4]

Methodology Extended incubation in an atmosphere of 5% to 10% CO_2 on media capable of supporting *Brucella* growth. Solid media (usually available in the laboratory) that is capable of supporting growth of *Brucella* spp includes selective buffered charcoal yeast extract agar, Thayer-Martin agar, and chocolate agar containing VCNT.[5] Cultures must be kept for at least 6 weeks, with periodic subculturing.

For culture of blood or other body fluids, a biphasic medium is recommended. If biphasic media is not available, commercial blood culture bottles can be vented and incubated at 35°C to 37°C with subculture to solid media every 4-5 days for 30 days.[6] Lysis centrifugation techniques have also been used with success.

Additional Information Brucellosis is common worldwide. *B. melitensis* occurs particularly in the USSR, Mediterranean, Latin America, Spain, the Arabian Gulf, Indian subcontinent, and parts of Mexico and Central and South America. Brucellosis is rare in the United States with ~100 cases reported annually, primarily in persons who have traveled to endemic areas or have been exposed to animals or laboratory cultures. Clinical suspicion in low prevalence populations is complicated by the fact that human *Brucella* infections have variable incubation periods, insidious or abrupt onset, and no pathognomonic symptoms or signs.[7,8] Clinical suspicion is often based merely on risk factors such as travel to endemic areas or occupational exposure to animals (eg, butchers, abattoir workers, farmers, dairymen, veterinarians) and laboratory workers.

Footnotes

1. Fiori PL, Mastrandrea S, Rappelli P, et al, "*Brucella abortus* Infection Acquired in Microbiology Laboratories," *J Clin Microbiol*, 2000, 38(5):2005-6.
2. Yagupsky P, Peled N, Riesenberg K, et al, "Exposure of Hospital Personnel to *Brucella melitensis* and Occurrence of Laboratory-Acquired Disease in an Endemic Area," *Scand J Infect Dis*, 2000, 32(1):31-5.
3. Franz DR, Jahrling PB, Friedlander AM, et al, "Clinical Recognition and Management of Patients Exposed to Biological Warfare Agents," *JAMA*, 1997, 278(5):399-411.
4. Shapiro DS and Wong JD, "*Brucella*," *Manual of Clinical Microbiology*, 7th ed, Murray PR, Baron EJ, Pfaller MA, et al, eds, Washington, DC: AMS Press, American Society for Microbiology, 1999, 625-31.
5. Doern GV, "Detection of Selected Fastidious Bacteria," *Clin Infect Dis*, 2000, 30(1):166-73.
6. Yagupsky P, Peled N, and Press J, "Use of Bactec® 9240 Blood Culture System for Detection of *Brucella melitensis* in Synovial Fluid," *J Clin Microbiol*, 2001, 39(2):738-9.
7. Georghiou PR and Young EJ, "Prolonged Incubation in Brucellosis," *Lancet*, 1991, 337(8756):1543.
8. Araj GF, "Human Brucellosis: A Classical Infectious Disease With Persistent Diagnostic Challenges," *Clin Lab Sci*, 1999, 12(4):207-12.

References

Alcala L, Munoz P, Rodriguez-Creixems M, et al, "*Brucella* spp Peritonitis," *Am J Med*, 1999, 107(3):300.

Brouqui P and Raoult D, "Endocarditis Due to Rare and Fastidious Bacteria," *Clin Microbiol Rev*, 2001, 14(1):177-207.

Corbel MJ, "Brucellosis: An Overview," *Emerging Infect Dis*, 1997, 3(2):213-21.

Koneman EW, Allen SD, Janda WM, et al, 5th ed, *Color Atlas and Textbook of Diagnostic Microbiology*, Philadelphia, PA: Lippincott, 1997, 433-4.

Moreno S, Ariza J, Espinosa FJ, et al, "Brucellosis in Patients Infected With the Human Immunodeficiency Virus," *Eur J Clin Microbiol Infect Dis*, 1998, 17(5):319-26.

Solera J, Lozano E, Martinez-Alfaro E, et al, "Brucellar Spondylitis: Review of 35 Cases and Literature Survey," *Clin Infect Dis*, 1999, 29(6):1440-9.

Internet Web Sites

www.cdc.gov/ncidod/dbmd/diseaseinfo/brucellosis_g.htm

www.who.int/inf-fs/en/fact173.html

♦ ***Brucella melitensis*** *see* Brucellosis Serology *on page 587*

♦ ***Brucella suis*** *see* Brucellosis Serology *on page 587*

Brucellosis Serology

Related Information
Bacterial Culture, Blood *on page 566*
Brucella Culture *on page 586*

Synonyms Undulant Fever

Applies to *Brucella abortus*; *Brucella melitensis*; *Brucella suis*

Test Includes Positive serum specimens are titered.

Abstract Brucellosis is a febrile zoonotic infection caused by slowly growing, gram-negative intracellular coccobacilli, *Brucella melitensis*, *B. abortus*, *B. suis*, and *B. canis*. In the U.S., ingestion of unpasteurized goat's milk or cheese is associated with most infections. The clinical symptoms of brucellosis are nonspecific and the onset of disease can be acute or insidious. Brucellosis is a systemic disease and may involve any organ.

Specimen Serum, cerebrospinal fluid

Container Red top tube

Sampling Time Acute phase serum should be drawn at presentation.

Special Instructions Paired specimens should be tested together in the same laboratory.

Reference Interval Negative. A fourfold rise in titer on paired (acute and convalescent) sera drawn 14-21 days apart is strongly indicative of the diagnosis. Titers of 1:160 are suggestive of active past or present disease. Ninety percent of patients with titers ≥1:320 have bacteremia.

Use Diagnosis of *Brucella*

Limitations Previous vaccination may have an effect on the titer. Test must be done utilizing a standard antigen prepared from *B. abortus* strain 1119, which will not detect antibodies to *B. canis*. Serologic testing for *B. canis* infection requires use of *B. canis* or *B. ovis* antigen. Testing for *B. canis* is available in some veterinary laboratories. Blocking antibodies may interfere at low titers. There are cross reactions with *Proteus* OX-19, *Yersinia enterocolitica*, *Francisella tularensis*, and *Vibrio cholerae* including cholera vaccination, as well as with skin tests for *Brucella*. Subjects who live where *Brucella* infections are endemic may have titers ≥160. Therefore, documentation by a fourfold rise in titer is advised.

Methodology Tube agglutination (most common), slide agglutination, complement fixation (CF). Enzyme-linked immunosorbent assay (ELISA) is used with serum and with cerebrospinal fluid. Radioimmunoassay (RIA) is available.

Additional Information Cultures of blood, bone marrow, and of specific sites are desirable. Diagnosis of *Brucella* infection by positive cultures is often difficult. Consequently, serologic diagnosis is often the method of choice. *Brucella* agglutinins appear during the second week in acute cases and peak in 3-6 weeks. The *B. abortus* antigen used in the *Brucella* agglutination test is group specific and not species specific. If infection with *B. canis* is possible, a specific test for those antibodies must be done. (*B. canis* rarely causes infection in humans.) Although cross-reactions occur with several other organisms, usually homologous titers will be much higher than the cross reactants. With newer ELISA assays, IgG and IgM antibodies to *Brucella* are used both for initial diagnosis and for follow-up of the patient. After successful treatment of brucellosis, specific IgG may be present for as long as 1 year. A newly developed immunoassay uses the dipstick method to detect serum antibody to *Brucella* species. This assay was found to have a sensitivity of 83% to 95% and a specificity of 94% when compared to culture and agglutination titers.[1] **Diagnosis of brucellosis ideally requires isolation (blood and/or bone marrow cultures)** or cultures from infected sites, but only about 20% of cases are confirmed.

Footnotes
1. Smits HL, Basahi MA, Diaz R, et al, "Development and Evaluation of a Rapid Dipstick Assay for Serodiagnosis of Acute Human Brucellosis," *J Clin Microbiol*, 1999, 37(12):4179-82.

References
Alcala L, Munoz P, Rodriguez-Creixems M, et al, "*Brucella* spp Peritonitis," *Am J Med*, 1999, 107(3):300.
Brouqui P and Raoult D, "Endocarditis Due to Rare and Fastidious Bacteria," *Clin Microbiol Rev*, 2001, 14(1):177-207.
Franz DR, Jahrling PB, Friedlander AM, et al, "Clinical Recognition and Management of Patients Exposed to Biological Warfare Agents," *JAMA*, 1997, 278(5):399-411.
Koneman EW, Allen SD, Janda WM, et al, *Color Atlas and Textbook of Diagnostic Microbiology*, 5th ed, Philadelphia, PA: Lippincott, 1997, 433-4.
Lucero NE, Foglia L, Ayala SM, et al, "Competitive Enzyme Immunoassay for Diagnosis of Human Brucellosis," *J Clin Microbiol*, 1999, 37(10):3245-8.
Mishal J, Ben-Israel N, Levin Y, et al, "Brucellosis Outbreak: Analysis of Risk Factors and Serologic Screening," *Int J Mol Med*, 1999, 4(6):655-8.
Radolf JD, "Southwestern Internal Medicine Conference: Brucellosis: Don't Let It Get Your Goat," *Am J Med Sci*, 1994, 307(1):64-75.
Salata RA, "Brucellosis," *Cecil Textbook of Medicine*, 21st ed, Chapter 356, Goldman L and Bennett JC, eds, Philadelphia PA: WB Sanders Co, 2000, 1717-9.
Shapiro DS and Wong JD, "*Brucella*," *Manual of Clinical Microbiology*, 7th ed, Murray PR, Baron EJ, Pfaller MA, et al, eds, Washington DC: ASM Press, American Society for Microbiology, 1999, 625-31.
"Suspected Brucellosis Case Prompts Investigation of Possible Bioterrorism-Related Activity - New Hampshire and Massachusetts, 1999," *JAMA*, 2000, 284(3):300-1.

Internet Web Sites
www.cdc.gov/ncidod/dbmd/diseaseinfo/brucellosis_g.htm
www.who.int/inf-fs/en/fact173.html

♦ *Brugia malayi* Serology *see* Filariasis Serological Test *on page 608*

♦ *Brugia timori* Serology *see* Filariasis Serological Test *on page 608*

♦ **Bubonic Plague Serology** *see Yersinia pestis* Antibody *on page 698*

♦ **Bunya Virus** *see* California Encephalitis Virus Serology *on page 587*

♦ **Burn Culture, Quantitative** *see* Bacterial Culture, Burn Sites *on page 569*

♦ **Calcofluor White** *see* Fungus Smear, Stain *on page 615*

♦ **California** *see* California Encephalitis Virus Serology *on page 587*

♦ **California Encephalitis (LaCrosse)** *see* Encephalitis Viral Serology *on page 604*

California Encephalitis Virus Serology

Related Information
Bacterial Culture, Cerebrospinal Fluid *on page 569*
Cerebrospinal Fluid Analysis: Overview *on page 416*
Eastern Equine Encephalitis Virus Serology *on page 602*
Encephalitis Viral Serology *on page 604*
St Louis Encephalitis Virus Serology *on page 681*
Viral Culture *on page 689*
Viral Culture, Central Nervous System Symptoms *on page 692*
Western Equine Encephalitis Virus Serology *on page 697*

Applies to Bunya Virus; California; Encephalitis Virus; Jamestown Canyon Virus; LaCrosse Virus; Snowshoe Hare Virus

Abstract These agents are arboviruses causing endemic disease.

Specimen Serum, cerebrospinal fluid

Container Red top tube, sterile container

Collection Acute and convalescent sera drawn 10-14 days apart are required.

Reference Interval Less than fourfold increase in titer in paired sera; IgM in CSF is considered diagnostic of CNS infection.

Use Support diagnosis of California encephalitis serogroup virus infection

Limitations Complement fixing antibodies appear slowly

Methodology Indirect fluorescent antibody (IFA), enzyme-linked immunosorbent assay (ELISA), complement fixation (CF), hemagglutination

Additional Information Infections are often asymptomatic. Symptomatic individuals develop a mild aseptic meningitis or a severe encephalitis. Most of the acute illnesses occur in children younger than 15 years of age. Diagnosis depends primarily on the detection of positive serology. Recent studies are investigating PCR as a potential technique to improve the diagnosis.[1]

Footnotes
1. Huang C, Campbell WP, Grady L, et al, "Diagnosis of Jamestown Canyon Encephalitis by Polymerase Chain Reaction," *Clin Infect Dis*, 1999, 28(6):1294-7.

References
Campbell WP and Huang C, "Sequence Comparisons of Medium RNA Segment Among 15 California Serogroup Viruses," *Virus Res*, 1999, 61(2):137-44.
Johnson AJ, Martin DA, Karabatsos N, et al, "Detection of Antiarboviral Immunoglobulin G by Using A Monoclonal Antibody-Based Capture Enzyme-Linked Immunosorbent Assay," *J Clin Microbiol*, 2000, 38(5):1827-31.
Lundstrom JO, "Mosquito-Borne Viruses in Western Europe: A Review," *J Vector Ecol*, 1999, 24(1):1-39.
McJunkin JE, Khan RR, Tsai TF, "California-La Crosse Encephalitis," *Infect Dis Clin North Am*, 1998, 12(1):83-93.
Rust RS, Thompson WH, Matthews, et al, "La Crosse and Other Forms of California Encephalitis," *J Child Neurol*, 1999, 14(1):1-14.

Internet Web Sites
www.cdc.gov/ncidod/dvbid/arbor/lacfact.htm

♦ *Campylobacter* *see* Bacterial Culture, Stool *on page 575*

♦ *Campylobacter pylori* Serology *see Helicobacter pylori* Serology *on page 621*

♦ *Campylobacter pylori* Urease Test and Culture *see Helicobacter pylori* Biopsy-Based Tests: The Urease Tests, Culture, Cytology, and PCR *on page 620*

Candida Antigen

Related Information
Candidiasis Serology *on page 588*
Fungal Culture, Biopsy or Body Fluid *on page 610*
Fungal Culture, Blood *on page 610*
Fungal Culture, Stool *on page 614*

Synonyms *Candida* antigenemia

Abstract Numerous reports have studied the diagnosis of disseminated candidiasis by detection of *Candida* antigens in serum. Controversies and problems with such diagnostic testing remain; therefore, antigen testing should not be used alone to confirm or rule out disseminated candidiasis.

Specimen Serum

Container Red top tube

Storage Instructions Separate and refrigerate serum at 4°C.

Reference Interval Negative
(Continued)

Candida Antigen (*Continued*)

Use Diagnosis of candidiasis in immunocompromised patients by detection of *Candida* antigens in serum

Limitations *Candida* antigen tests are insensitive, with a high incidence of false-negative as well as false-positive results. Evaluation of these assays has been hampered by difficulty in establishing the diagnosis of disseminated candidiasis by other clinical and laboratory methods.

Methodology Latex agglutination (LA), enzyme-linked immunosorbent assay (ELISA)

Additional Information Detection of disseminated candidiasis is particularly important in immunocompromised patients. Unfortunately, the sensitivity of *Candida* antigen tests is too low to rule out candidiasis. Consequently, a negative result does not preclude the use of empiric antifungal therapy. A positive test is usually reliable but many of these patients also have positive blood cultures. The decision to initiate therapy should not be based only on results of *Candida* serologic assays.[1]

Footnotes

1. Dismukes WE, "Candidiasis," *Cecil Textbook of Medicine*, 21st ed, Chapter 400, Goldman L and Bennett JC, eds, Philadelphia, PA: WB Saunders Co, 2000, 1871-5.

References

Gutierrez J, Maroto C, Peidrola G, et al, "Circulating *Candida* Antigens and Antibodies: Useful Markers of Candidemia," *J Clin Microbiol*, 1993, 31(9):2550-2.

Iwasaki H, Misaki H, Nakamura T, et al, "Surveillance of the Serum *Candida* Antigen Titer for Initiation of Antifungal Therapy After Postremission Chemotherapy in Patients With Acute Leukemia," *Int J Hematol*, 2000, 71(3):266-72.

Monteagudo C, Lopez-Ribot JL, Murgui A, et al, "Immunodetection of CD45 Epitopes on the Surface of *Candida albicans* Cells in Culture and Infected Human Tissues," *Am J Clin Pathol*, 2000, 113(1):59-63.

Morhart M, Rennie R, Ziola B, et al, "Evaluation of Enzyme Immunoassay for *Candida* Cytoplasmic Antigens in Neutropenic Cancer Patients," *J Clin Microbiol*, 1994, 32(3):766-76.

Na BK and Song CY, "Use of Monoclonal Antibody in Diagnosis of Candidiasis Caused by *Candida albicans*: Detection of Circulating Aspartyl Proteinase Antigen," *Clin Diag Lab Immunol*, 1999, 6(6):924-9.

Reiss E and Morrison CJ, "Nonculture Methods for Diagnosis of Disseminated Candidiasis," *Clin Microbiol Rev*, 1993, 6(4):311-23.

Richardson MD and Kokki MH, "New Perspectives in the Diagnosis of Systemic Funal Infections," *Ann Med*, 1999, 31(5):327-35.

Internet Web Sites

www.cdc.gov/ncidod/dbmd/diseaseinfo/candidiasis_g.htm

♦ *Candida* **antigenemia** *see Candida* Antigen *on page 587*

♦ *Candida* **Culture, Genital** *see* Bacterial Culture, Genital Specimen *on page 571*

Candidiasis Serology

Related Information
Candida Antigen *on page 587*
Fungal Culture, Biopsy or Body Fluid *on page 610*
Fungal Culture, Blood *on page 610*
Fungal Culture, Sputum *on page 613*
Fungal Culture, Stool *on page 614*
Fungal Culture, Urine *on page 614*
Fungus Smear, Stain *on page 615*

Test Includes Precipitin test by agar gel diffusion

Specimen Serum

Container Red top tube

Storage Instructions Store serum at 4°C.

Reference Interval Negative. A fourfold increase in titer in paired sera drawn 10-14 days apart is usually indicative of acute infection. Titer >1:8 in the latex agglutination test is presumptive for systemic disease.

Use Evaluate suspected systemic candidiasis

Limitations Cross reactions with the latex agglutination test occur in cases of cryptococcosis and tuberculosis. Negative results do not rule out candidiasis. This test is difficult to interpret because precipitins are found in 20% to 30% of the normal population. Very severe cases of vaginitis or mucocutaneous candidiasis can produce positive results. Clinical correlation must exist for the test to be useful. The decision to initiate therapy should not be based only on results of such assays.[1]

Methodology Latex agglutination (LA), crossed electrophoresis, immunodiffusion (ID), enzyme-linked immunosorbent assay (ELISA)

Additional Information In general, *Candida*-specific antibody tests have limited use in diagnosis. Most healthy patients have some antibody to *Candida* antigen while immunosuppressed individuals usually have a poor response, thus making them at risk for recurrent or disseminated *Candida* infections. Rising titers of agglutinins may be reliable indicators of the presence of candidiasis. Quantitative tests on sera taken at biweekly intervals are of value in monitoring the progress of infection before and after therapy. Although limited data is available, the presence of IgM antibodies appears to provide a good indicator of disseminated candidiasis.

Footnotes

1. Dismukes WE, "Candidiasis," *Cecil Textbook of Medicine*, 21st ed, Chapter 400, Goldman L and Bennett JC, eds, Philadelphia, PA: WB Saunders Co, 2000, 1871-5.

References

Gutierrez J, Maroto C, Peidrola G, et al, "Circulating *Candida* Antigens and Antibodies: Useful Markers of Candidemia," *J Clin Microbiol*, 1993, 31(9):2550-2.

Knoke M, Bernhardt H, Schulz K, et al, "Funguria and *Candida*-Specific Immunoglobulins in Patients With Systemic Candidosis," *Mycoses*, 2000, 43(3-4):145-9.

Rabah R, Kupsky WJ, and Haas JE, "Arteritis and Fatal Subarachnoid Hemorrhage Complicating Occult *Candida* Meningitis: Unusual Presentation in Pediatric Acquired Immunodeficiency Syndrome," *Arch Pathol Lab Med*, 1998, 122(11):1030-3.

Reiss E and Morrison CJ, "Nonculture Methods for Diagnosis of Disseminated Candidiasis," *Clin Microbiol Rev*, 1993, 6(4):311-23.

Internet Web Sites

www.cdc.gov/ncidod/dbmd/diseaseinfo/candidiasis_g.htm

♦ **Cardiolipin Antibodies** *see* RPR *on page 677*

♦ **Cardiolipin Antibodies** *see* VDRL, Cerebrospinal Fluid *on page 688*

♦ **Cardiolipin Antibodies** *see* VDRL, Serum *on page 688*

♦ **Catheter Tip Culture** *see* Bacterial Culture, Intravascular Device *on page 572*

♦ **Cat Scratch Bacterial Culture** *see* Bartonella Culture *on page 580*

♦ **Cat Scratch Disease** *see* Bartonella Serology *on page 581*

♦ **CD4 Count** *see* HIV-1/HIV-2 Antibody Screen and Western Blot *on page 636*

♦ **cDNA** *see* Hepatitis C Virus RNA Detection and Quantitation *on page 626*

♦ **Cefinase (Nitrocefin) Testing** *see* Beta-Lactamase Test *on page 581*

♦ **Centipedes** *see* Arthropod Identification *on page 559*

♦ **Central Catheters** *see* Bacterial Culture, Intravascular Device *on page 572*

♦ **Cephalosporinase Production Testing** *see* Beta-Lactamase Test *on page 581*

♦ **Cephalosporinases** *see* Beta-Lactamase Test *on page 581*

♦ **Cerebrospinal Fluid Bacterial Antigen Testing** *see* Bacterial Antigens, Rapid Detection Methods *on page 562*

♦ **Cerebrospinal Fluid Cryptococcal Latex Agglutination** *see* Cryptococcal Antigen Titer *on page 595*

♦ **Cerebrospinal Fluid Culture** *see* Bacterial Culture, Cerebrospinal Fluid *on page 569*

♦ **Cerebrospinal Fluid Culture, *Leptospira*** *see* Leptospira Culture *on page 648*

♦ **Cerebrospinal Fluid Fungus Culture** *see* Fungal Culture, Cerebrospinal Fluid *on page 611*

♦ **Cerebrospinal Fluid India Ink Preparation** *see* India Ink Preparation *on page 642*

♦ **Cerebrospinal Fluid Mycobacteria Culture** *see* Mycobacterial Culture, Cerebrospinal Fluid *on page 656*

♦ **Cerebrospinal Fluid VDRL** *see* VDRL, Cerebrospinal Fluid *on page 688*

♦ **Cerebrospinal Fluid, Viral Culture** *see* Viral Culture, Body Fluid *on page 691*

♦ **Cerebrospinal Fluid Virus Culture** *see* Viral Culture, Central Nervous System Symptoms *on page 692*

♦ **Cervical *Chlamydia* Culture** *see* Chlamydia trachomatis Culture *on page 590*

♦ **Cervical Culture** *see* Bacterial Culture, Genital Specimen *on page 571*

♦ **Cervical Culture for T-Strain *Mycoplasma*** *see* Genital Culture for Ureaplasma urealyticum *on page 616*

♦ **Cervical Culture for *Ureaplasma urealyticum*** *see* Genital Culture for Ureaplasma urealyticum *on page 616*

♦ **Cervix, Viral Culture** *see* Viral Culture, Urogenital *on page 696*

Chagas' Disease Serological Test

Related Information
Buffy Coat Smear Study of Peripheral Blood *on page 412*
Malaria Smear and Tests *on page 458*
Risks of Transfusion *on page 861*

Applies to *Trypanosoma cruzi*

Abstract American trypanosomiasis (Chagas' disease) is caused by a protozoan, *Trypanosoma cruzi*. The protozoan is transmitted to humans by bloodsucking triatomine insects. Chagas' disease is a life-long infection with the highest incidence found in Brazil, Argentina, Chile, Bolivia, and Venezuela. This disease is found only in the Western hemisphere. Chagas' disease causes the deaths of 50,000 people annually. Chronic disease includes myocarditis, cardiomyopathy, and megadisease of esophagus and colon. It can cause placentitis, and maternal transmission to the fetus leads to congenital Chagas' disease or abortion. Severe recrudescence may occur with immunosuppression (eg, organ transplantation, AIDS). Laboratory workers may also be accidentally infected. The correlation between infectivity and Chagas' antibodies is suboptimal.

Specimen Serum

Container Red top tube

Reference Interval Indirect hemagglutination titer: <1:128; complement fixation titer: <1:8; immunoelectrophoresis titer: <1:64

Use Support the clinical diagnosis of Chagas' disease. In endemic areas, serologic testing is needed in blood banks, since transfusion from donors with chronic infection results in transmission of *T. cruzi* to the recipient in 13% to 23% of cases per contaminated unit.

Limitations False-positive serologic reactions occur in persons with leishmaniasis, malaria, toxoplasmosis, hepatitis, leprosy, syphilis, and collagen diseases. An individual can be serologically negative but still be infectious.

Methodology Indirect hemagglutination (IHA), complement fixation (CF), indirect fluorescent antibody (IFA), direct agglutination, enzyme-linked immunosorbent assay (ELISA), immunoelectrophoresis (IEP). Indirect immunofluorescence is more sensitive than CF. In patients with chronic infection, there may be diminution of CF titers. Radioimmunoprecipitation assay using purified glycoprotein antigens exists.[1]

Additional Information CF shows a high degree of sensitivity in the acute stages of the disease since the CF assay detects IgM. However, IHA is more sensitive but less specific than the CF. Because of the chronicity of Chagas' disease, stable low to moderate titers by IHA or CF are difficult to interpret. Serologic tests return to normal in a large majority of patients 12-24 months after treatment.

Serum from patients with Chagas' heart disease contain antibodies which bind to endocardial, vascular, and interstitial elements of heart tissue. Such an "EVI" factor may be predictive of cardiac Chagas' disease. A serum should test positive by at least two different assays before the results are accepted.[2]

Several cases of transfusion-transmitted Chagas' disease have been reported in the United States. Studies are being conducted to ascertain if screening of the blood supply is necessary in certain areas of the U.S., such as southern California.[3,4]

Wright-Giemsa-stained peripheral blood smears may demonstrate trypomastigotes of *T. cruzi*.[5]

Footnotes

1. Leiby DA, Wendel S, Takaoka DT, et al, "Serologic Testing for *Trypanosoma cruzi*: Comparison of Radioimmunoprecipitation Assay With Commercially Available Indirect Immunofluorescence Assay, Indirect Hemagglutination Assay, and Enzyme-Linked Immunosorbent Assay Kits," *J Clin Microbiol*, 2000, 38(2):639-42.
2. Saez-Alquezar A, Sabino EC, Salles N, et al, "Serological Confirmation of Chagas' Disease by a Recombinant and Peptide Antigen Line Immunoassay: INNO-LIA Chagas," *J Clin Microbiol*, 2000, 38(2):851-4.
3. Brashear RJ, Winkler MA, Schur JD, et al, "Detection of Antibodies to *Trypanosoma cruzi* Among Blood Donors in the Southwestern and Western United States. I. Evaluation of the Sensitivity and Specificity of an Enzyme Immunoassay for Detecting Antibodies to *T. cruzi*," *Transfusion*, 1995, 35(3):213-8.
4. Winkler MA, Brashear RJ, Hall HJ, et al, "Detection of Antibodies to *Trypanosoma cruzi* Among Blood Donors in the Southwestern and Western United States. II. Evaluation of a Supplemental Enzyme Immunoassay and Radioimmunoprecipitation Assay for Confirmation of Seroreactivity," *Transfusion*, 1995, 35(3):219-25.
5. Pan AA and Winkler MA, "The Threat of Chagas' Disease in Transfusion Medicine. The Presence of Antibodies to *Trypanosoma cruzi* in the U.S. Blood Supply," *Lab Med*, 1997, 28(4):269-73.

References

Bahia-Oliveira LM, Gomes JA, Cancado JR, et al, "Immunological and Clinical Evaluation of Chagasic Patients Subjected to Chemotherapy During the Acute Phase of *Trypanosoma cruzi* Infection 14-30 Years Ago," *J Infect Dis*, 2000, 182(2):634-8.

Betonico GN, Miranda EO, Silva DA, et al, "Evaluation of a Synthetic Tripeptide as Antigen for Detection of IgM and IgG Antibodies to *Trypanosoma cruzi* in Serum Samples From Patients With Chagas' Disease or Viral Diseases," *Trans R Soc Trop Med Hyg*, 1999, 93(6):603-6.

♦ **Chickenpox Culture** *see* Varicella-Zoster Virus Culture *on page 686*

♦ **Chickenpox Titer** *see* Varicella-Zoster Virus Serology *on page 687*

Chlamydia Group Serology

Related Information

Bacterial Culture, Conjunctiva *on page 570*
Bacterial Culture, Throat, and Antigen Detection Testing for Group A Streptococci *on page 577*
Chlamydia trachomatis Culture *on page 590*
Chlamydia trachomatis Direct Antigen Test *on page 590*
Chlamydia trachomatis Nucleic Acid Detection *on page 591*
Psittacosis Serology *on page 672*

Test Includes Detection of antibody titer to *Chlamydia* species

Abstract *Chlamydia* are intracellular bacteria which multiply in living host cells. Three *Chlamydia* species are associated with disease in humans: *C. psittaci*, *C. trachomatis*, and *C. pneumoniae*.[1,2] Chronic asymptomatic or persistent infections in humans are common for *C. trachomatis* and *C. pneumoniae*. Because of this, characteristic serology is not useful in the diagnosis of active disease.

Specimen Serum

Container Red top tube

Collection Collect acute phase blood as soon as possible after onset (no later than 1 week). Convalescent blood should be drawn 1-2 weeks after acute (no less than 2 weeks after onset).

Reference Interval Normal individuals without acute disease may have an IgG titer due to past infections. Determination of IgM antibody may indicates acute infection.

Use Evaluation of atypical pneumonia in infants, lymphogranuloma venereum, or psittacosis

Limitations The antigen used in the test is group specific, not species specific. Conjunctivitis, urethritis, and pneumonia of the newborn do not usually induce an antibody response detectable by complement fixation. A very high "background" of immunity in the general population makes interpretation of levels difficult. Due to the low sensitivity, specificity, and predictive value serology is not useful for the diagnosis of active disease.[3]

Methodology Complement fixation (CF), indirect fluorescence antibody (IFA), enzyme immunoassay (EIA)

Additional Information *C. pneumoniae* is a common cause of community-acquired pneumonia, causing 5% to 10% of cases.[4] *Chlamydia pneumoniae* also causes infantile pneumonia, bronchitis, and pharyngitis.[5] Recent reports have associated *C. pneumoniae* with atherosclerotic cardiovascular disease using seroepidemiologic studies.[6,7] However, other reports have not been able to reproduce these results and found that in large studies there was no relationship between infection with *C. pneumoniae* and heart disease.[8,9] Further study is required to definitely confirm that any association exists between infection with *C. pneumoniae* and coronary heart disease.

Chlamydia trachomatis is the most common sexually transmitted bacterial pathogen in the United States. It is gaining increasing recognition as a respiratory pathogen and is also associated with blindness, ophthalmia neonatorum, lymphogranuloma venereum, pelvic inflammatory disease, ectopic pregnancy, urethritis, epididymitis, and infertility.[1] In a patient being evaluated for trachomatis disease, nonserologic methods (culture or PCR) can be used.[10] For genitourinary infections, serologic test for syphilis and culture for *Neisseria gonorrhoeae* are desirable as well.

A relationship of *Chlamydia trachomatis* as a possible risk factor for squamous cell carcinoma of cervix has been postulated.[11] However, a number of important questions remain to be answered.[12]

Footnotes

1. Kirchner JT and Emmert DH, "Sexually Transmitted Diseases in Women. *Chlamydia trachomatis* and Herpes Simplex Infections," *Postgrad Med*, 2000, 107(1):55-8, 61-5.
2. Tompkins LS, Schachter J, Boman J, et al, "Collaborative Multidisciplinary Workshop Report: Detection, Culture, Serology, and Antimicrobial Susceptibility Testing of *Chlamydia pneumoniae*," *J Infect Dis*, 2000, 181:S460-1.
3. Tuuminen T, Palomaki P, and Paavonen J, "The Use of Serologic Tests for the Diagnosis of Chlamydial Infections," *J Microbiol Methods*, 2000, 42(3):265-79.
4. Bartlett JG and Mundy LM, "Community-Acquired Pneumonia," *N Engl J Med*, 1995, 333(24):1618-24.
5. Bisno AL, "Acute Pharyngitis," *N Engl J Med*, 2001, 344(3):205-11.
6. Saikku P, Leinonen M, Tenkanen L, et al, "Chronic *Chlamydia pneumoniae* Infection as a Risk Factor for Coronary Heart Disease in the Helsinki Heart Study," *Ann Intern Med*, 1992, 116(4):273-8.
7. Shimada K, Mokuno H, Watanabe Y, et al, "High Prevalence of Seropositivity for Antibodies to *Chlamydia*-Specific Lipopolysaccharide in Patients With Acute Coronary Syndrome," *J Cardiovasc Risk*, 2000, 7(3):209-13.
8. Wald NJ, Law MR, Morris JK, et al, "*Chlamydia pneumoniae* Infection and Mortality From Ischaemic Heart Disease: Large Prospective Study," *Br Med J*, 2000, 321(7255): 204-7.
9. Danesh J, Whincup P, Walker M, et al, "*Chlamydia pneumoniae* IgG Titres and Coronary Heart Disease: Prospective Study and Meta-analysis," *Br Med J*, 2000, 321(7255):208-13.
10. Dayan L, "*Chlamydia* Detection and Management," *Aust Fam Physician*, 2000, 29(6):522-6.
11. Anttila T, Saikku P, Koskela P, et al, "Serotypes of *Chlamydia trachomatis* and Risk for Development of Cervical Squamous Cell Carcinoma," *JAMA*, 2001, 285(1):47-51.
12. Zenilman JM, "*Chlamydia* and Cervical Cancer: A Real Association?" *JAMA*, 2001, 285(1):81-3.

References

Blanchard TJ and Mabey DC, "Chlamydial Infections," *Br J Clin Pract*, 1994, 48(4):201-5.

Dicker LW, Mosure DJ, Levine WC, et al, "Impact of Switching Laboratory Tests on Reported Results in *Chlamydia trachomatis* Infections," *Am J Epidemiol*, 2000, 151(4):430-5.

Hwange LY, Ross MW, Zack C, et al, "Prevalence of Sexually Transmitted Infections and Associated Risk Factors Among Populations of Drug Abusers," *Clin Infect Dis*, 2000, 31(4):920-6.

Johnson DH and Cunha BA, "Atypical Pneumonias. Clinical and Extrapulmonary Features of *Chlamydia*, *Mycoplasma*, and *Legionella* Infections," *Postgrad Med*, 1993, 93(7):69-72, 75-6, 79-82.

Persson K and Boman J, "Comparison of Five Serologic Tests for Diagnosis of Acute Infections by *Chlamydia pneumoniae*," *Clin Diagn Lab Immunol*, 2000, 7(5):739-44.

Troy CJ, Peeling RW, Ellis AG, et al, "*Chlamydia pneumoniae* as a New Source of Infectious Outbreaks in Nursing Homes," *JAMA*, 1997, 277(15):1214-18.

Tuuminen T, Varjo S, Ingman H, et al, "Prevalence of *Chlamydia pneumoniae* and *Mycoplasma pneumoniae* Immunoglobulin G and A Antibodies in a Healthy Finnish Population as Analyzed by Quantitative Enzyme Immunoassays," *Clin Diagn Lab Immunol*, 2000, 7(5):734-8.

Weinstock H, Dean D, and Bolan G, "*Chlamydia trachomatis* Infections," *Infect Dis Clin North Am*, 1994, 8(4):797-819.

Internet Web Sites

www.cdc.gov/nchstp/dstd/chlamydia_facts.htm

- **Chlamydia Ligase Chain Reaction (LCR)** *see Chlamydia trachomatis Nucleic Acid Detection on page 591*

- **Chlamydia PCR** *see Chlamydia trachomatis Nucleic Acid Detection on page 591*

- **Chlamydia psittaci Antibodies** *see Psittacosis Serology on page 672*

- **Chlamydia psittaci Direct Immunofluorescent Antibody** *see Psittacosis Serology on page 672*

- **Chlamydia psittaci PCR** *see Psittacosis Serology on page 672*

- **Chlamydia psittaci Titer** *see Psittacosis Serology on page 672*

- **Chlamydia trachomatis** *see Bacterial Culture, Conjunctiva on page 570*

- **Chlamydia trachomatis** *see Bacterial Culture, Genital Specimen on page 571*

- **Chlamydia trachomatis** *see Bacterial Culture, Sputum on page 574*

Chlamydia trachomatis Culture

Related Information
Bacterial Culture, Conjunctiva *on page 570*
Bacterial Culture, Genital Specimen *on page 571*
Bacterial Culture, Urine *on page 578*
Cervical/Vaginal Cytology *on page 377*
Chlamydia Group Serology *on page 589*
Chlamydia trachomatis Direct Antigen Test *on page 590*
Chlamydia trachomatis Nucleic Acid Detection *on page 591*
Neisseria gonorrhoeae Culture and Smear *on page 662*
Neisseria gonorrhoeae Nucleic Acid Detection *on page 664*
Viral Culture, Eye or Ocular Symptoms *on page 693*
Viral Culture, Urogenital *on page 696*

Synonyms Lymphogranuloma Venereum Culture; TRIC Agent Culture

Applies to Cervical *Chlamydia* Culture; Eye Swab *Chlamydia* Culture; Urethral *Chlamydia* Culture

Abstract *Chlamydia trachomatis* is an intracellular pathogen and can be cultured in a variety of cell lines. The specificity of *C. trachomatis* culture approaches 100% but the sensitivity is between 70% and 90%. Cell culture is the only test that should be used to establish *C. trachomatis* infection with legal implications (eg, children suspected of being victims of sexual abuse).[1]

Specimen Obtain swab specimens containing columnar epithelial cells of urethra, cervix, rectum, conjunctiva, posterior nasopharynx, or throat.

Container Culturette® (dacron) swabs should be used and placed in *Chlamydia* transport medium.

Collection Urethra: Remove mucous/pus. The swab should be inserted 2-4 cm into the urethra. Use firm pressure to scrape cells from the mucosal surface. If possible repeat with second swab. Patient should not urinate within 1 hour prior to specimen collection.

Cervix: Remove mucous/pus with a Culturette® and use firm and rotating pressure to obtain specimen with another swab. May be combined with a urethral swab into same transport medium. This two-swab method is highly recommended.

Rectum: Sample anal crypts with a Culturette®.

Conjunctiva: Remove mucous and exudate. Use a Culturette® and firm pressure to scrape away epithelial cells from upper and lower lids.

Posterior nasopharynx or throat: Collect epithelial cells by using a Culturette®.

Storage Instructions Deliver inoculated transport medium **immediately** to the laboratory. **Specimens must be refrigerated** if stored for 2 days. Specimen must be frozen at -70°C if stored more than 2 days.

Turnaround Time Cultures with no growth usually are reported after 7 days. Rapid culture methods require 48 hours or more.

Special Instructions Availability and specific specimen collection requirements for *Chlamydia* cultures vary between laboratories.

Reference Interval No *Chlamydia trachomatis* isolated

Use Aid in the diagnosis of infections caused by *Chlamydia trachomatis* (eg, cervicitis, trachoma, conjunctivitis, pelvic inflammatory disease, pneumonia, urethritis, pneumonitis, and sexually transmitted diseases)

Limitations Culture may be negative in presence of *Chlamydia trachomatis* infection. Culture is probably not the gold standard for detection of *C. trachomatis*. The sensitivity of culture is only 70% to 90% because *C. trachomatis* does not always survive transit to the laboratory, and often there is inadequate sampling with (multiple) swabs.[2]

Methodology Inoculation of specimen onto McCoy cell, HeLa-229, or Buffalo green monkey cell culture and subsequent detection of *Chlamydia*-infected cells by monoclonal antibody and immunofluorescence

Additional Information Genital infections due to *C. trachomatis* are the most frequent reportable bacterial sexually transmitted disease in the United States. There are more than 4 million infections reported annually.[3] Many of the cases are asymptomatic or minimally symptomatic. Many will eventually progress to produce serious infections including pelvic inflammatory disease, ectopic pregnancy, and infertility in women.[4,5] Infection with *C. trachomatis* during pregnancy places the newborn infant at risk of pneumonia and conjunctivitis.[4]

This organism infects the endocervical columnar epithelial cells and will not be found in the inflammatory cells. In obtaining the specimen, clean the area of inflammatory cells and then attempt to scrape epithelial cells for culture. Papanicolaou-stained cervical smears are not sufficiently reliable to establish or exclude the presence of *C. trachomatis*. Direct immunofluorescence techniques and enzyme immunoassays are available to detect *C. trachomatis* in clinical specimens. These methods usually provide reliable results in high-prevalence populations and detect both viable and nonviable organisms, but have for the most part been replaced by nucleic acid-based methods. *C. trachomatis* can be detected by using a DNA amplification assays.[6,7,8] These tests appear to be more sensitive than immunoassays and culture.[7] Selection of the most efficient method for recovery of *C. trachomatis* depends upon the incidence in the patient population and the availability of the various methods. Urine culture for *C. trachomatis* is not a sensitive procedure and should not be done. Urine samples can be tested for *C. trachomatis* using PCR or ligase chain reaction (LCR) rather than culture.[6,7]

Culture should be the test-of-choice in cases of child abuse, ascending pelvic infections, rectal and throat infections, and when a test-for-cure is desired.[1]

Footnotes
1. Hammerschlag MR, Ajl S, and Laraque D, "Inappropriate Use of Nonculture Tests for the Detection of *Chlamydia trachomatis* in Suspected Victims of Child Sexual Abuse: A Continuing Problem," *Pediatrics*, 1999, 104(5 Pt 1):1137-9.
2. Jones RB and Batteiger BE, "*Chlamydia trachomatis* (Trachoma, Perinatal Infections, Lymphogranuloma Vernereum, and Other Genital Infections)," *Principles and Practice of Infectious Diseases*, 5th ed, Mandell GL, Bennett JE, and Dolin R, eds, New York, NY: Churchill Livingstone, 2000, 1989-2004.
3. Kirchner JT and Emmert DH, "Sexually Transmitted Diseases in Women. *Chlamydia trachomatis* and Herpes Simplex Infections," *Postgrad Med*, 2000, 107(1):55-65.
4. Andrews WW, Goldenberg RL, Mercer B, et al, "The Preterm Prediction Study: Association of Second-Trimester Genitourinary *Chlamydia* Infection With Subsequent Spontaneous Preterm Birth," *Am J Obstet Gynecol*, 2000, 183(3):662-8.
5. Parker CA and Topinka MA, "The Incidence of Positive Cultures in Women Suspected of Having PID/Salpingitis," *Acad Emerg Med*, 2000, 7(10):1170.
6. Winter AJ, Gilleran G, Eastick K, et al, "Comparison of a Ligase Chain Reaction-Based Assay and Cell Culture for Detection of Pharyngeal Carriage of *Chlamydia trachomatis*," *J Clin Microbiol*, 2000, 38(9):3502-4.
7. Young DC, Craft S, Day MC, et al, "Comparison of Abbott LCx *Chlamydia trachomatis* Assay With Gen-Probe PACE2 and Culture," *Infect Dis Obstet Gynecol*, 2000, 8(2):112-5.
8. Keenan GF, "Polymerase Chain Reaction as a Diagnostic Tool," *Adolesc Med*, 1998, 9(1):35-43.

References
Baveja UK, Hiranandani MK, Talwar P, et al, "Laboratory Techniques for Diagnosis of Chlamydial Infections of the Eye," *J Commun Dis*, 1997, 29(3):247-53.
Brown SL, Peck KR, and Watts DD, "Routine Pharyngeal Cultures May Not Be Useful in Pediatric Victims of Sexual Assault," *J Emerg Nurs*, 2000, 26(4):306-11.
Dayan L, "*Chlamydia* Detection and Management," *Aust Fam Physician*, 2000, 29(6):522-6.
Eckert LO, Suchland RJ, Hawes SE, et al, "Quantitative *Chlamydia trachomatis* Cultures: Correlation of Chlamydial Inclusion-Forming Units With Serovar, Age, Sex, and Race," *J Infect Dis*, 2000, 182(2):540-4.
Guaschino S and DeSeta F, "Update on *Chlamydia trachomatis*," *Ann N Y Acad Sci*, 2000, 900:293-300.
Wilkinson C, Massil H, and Evans J, "An Interface of *Chlamydia* Testing by Community Family Planning Clinics and Referral to Hospital Genitourinary Medicine Clinics," *Br J Fam Plann*, 2000, 26(4):206-9.

Internet Web Sites
www.cdc.gov/nchstp/dstd/chlamydia_facts.htm

Chlamydia trachomatis Direct Antigen Test

Related Information
Bacterial Culture, Conjunctiva *on page 570*
Bacterial Culture, Genital Specimen *on page 571*
Bacterial Culture, Nasopharynx *on page 573*
Cervical/Vaginal Cytology *on page 377*
Chlamydia Group Serology *on page 589*
Chlamydia trachomatis Culture *on page 590*
Chlamydia trachomatis Nucleic Acid Detection *on page 591*
Neisseria gonorrhoeae Culture and Smear *on page 662*
Neisseria gonorrhoeae Nucleic Acid Detection *on page 664*
Ocular Cytology *on page 385*
Viral Culture, Eye or Ocular Symptoms *on page 693*

Synonyms MicroTrak®

Abstract Several tests are available for direct detection of *Chlamydia trachomatis* in a specimen. The tests are based on detection of specific antigen, using either fluorescent monoclonal antibodies or enzyme immunoassays. The sensitivity of these tests reaches >70% and the specificity 97% to 99%. These tests should not be used to establish *C. trachomatis* infection with legal implications (eg, children suspected of being victims of sexual abuse).[1]

Patient Preparation For urogenital specimens, patient should not urinate 1 hour prior to collection.

Specimen Direct smear or urogenital specimen.

Container Single well (8 mm) glass slide, dacron swabs (one large, one small), one cytobrush, methanol fixative (0.5 mL vial). These items are contained in a commonly used direct detection kit (collection pack) known as MicroTrak®.

Collection Endocervical with cytology brush: Nonpregnant women. Use large swab to remove exudate or mucous from exocervix. Insert cytobrush into cervical os past the squamocolumnar junction. Rest 2-3 seconds, rotate brush 360 degrees to gather columnar cells and withdraw brush. Do not touch vaginal walls with brush, and prepare slides immediately by rotating and twisting brush back and forth across center of slide well.

Endocervical with swab: Pregnant women. Use large swab to remove exudate or mucous from exocervix. Insert another large dacron swab until tip is no longer visible, rotate swab 5-10 seconds, and withdraw swab. Do not touch vaginal walls and prepare slides immediately. Firmly roll one side of swab over top half of well. Turn swab over and roll other side over bottom half of slide well.

Urethral: Males. Patient should not urinate 1 hour before sampling. Remove pus or exudate, insert small swab with wire shaft 2-4 cm into penis. Gently rotate swab to dislodge cells, rest swab 2 seconds, withdraw swab, and prepare slide immediately as above.

Rectal: Symptomatic patients only. Use large swab. Insert ~3 cm into anal canal. Move swab from side to side to sample crypts. If fecal contamination occurs, discard swab and obtain another specimen. Prepare slide immediately as above.

Conjunctival: Neonates, symptomatic only. Use large swab to gently remove pus or discharge and discard. If both eyes are sampled, swab less affected eye first. Swab inside of lower, then upper lid, and prepare slide immediately as above.

Nasopharyngeal: Neonates, symptomatic only. Use small swab or nasal aspirator. Collect specimen from posterior nasopharynx using standard collection method. If swab was used, prepare slide immediately. If nasal aspirate was collected, deliver to the laboratory technician or technologist immediately for slide preparation.

All specimens: Allow specimen to air dry. Lay slide flat and flood with methanol fixative. Let entire quantity evaporate. Refold pack without touching fixed specimen.

Storage Instructions Refrigerate slides at 2°C to 8°C or at room temperature (20°C to 30°C) until taken to the laboratory. Slides must be stained within 7 days of collection.

Causes for Rejection Less than 10 columnar or cuboidal epithelial cells on slide

Turnaround Time 24-48 hours

Special Instructions Specify specimen origin. Include all pertinent information, label slide and collection pack.

Reference Interval No *Chlamydia trachomatis* detected

Use Aid in the diagnosis of disease caused by *Chlamydia trachomatis*

Limitations The direct fluorescent antibody procedure is considerably less sensitive than the cell culture procedure and molecular amplification methods.[2,3] The number of cells on the slide can be too low for diagnosis. It is cumbersome and requires a highly skilled microscopist for proper interpretation.

The direct detection of *Chlamydia* in specimens depends largely on the preparation of the cell smear. Smears that are too thick or lumpy can cause false-positive results. Contamination with red blood cells makes the smears difficult to interpret. Smears with too few cells can cause false-negative results. This test detects only *Chlamydia trachomatis* major outer membrane protein (MOMP). The test does not distinguish between living and dead organisms. Therefore, the test does not necessarily serve as a test-of-cure.

Although the endocervix is the preferred site to collect specimens, 10% to 23% of females only have urethral infection.[4]

Methodology The *Chlamydia trachomatis* direct test uses fluorescein-conjugated monoclonal antibodies (reactive with all 15 known serotypes of *C. trachomatis*) to detect elementary bodies in clinical smears or an enzyme immunoassay to detect outer membrane protein.

Additional Information In some populations, up to 45% of women who have gonorrheal infection have chlamydial infection as well.[5] (Other sexually transmitted diseases are included in the Key Word Index).*Chlamydia trachomatis* has been implicated in neonatal/infantile conjunctivitis and afebrile pneumonia. Thirty-three percent to 50% of babies born vaginally to mothers with chlamydial infection of the cervix will be infected; the majority of these neonates will develop inclusion conjunctivitis and/or a respiratory tract infection that can lead to the distinctive (afebrile) pneumonia syndrome. Conjunctivitis in infected neonates usually occurs between the 5th and 12th day after birth. In neonates born to mothers with premature rupture of the membranes, *C. trachomatis* has been detected, in rare cases, as early as the first day following birth.

Footnotes

1. Hammerschlag MR, Ajl S, and Laraque D, "Inappropriate Use of Nonculture Tests for the Detection of *Chlamydia trachomatis* in Suspected Victims of Child Sexual Abuse: A Continuing Problem," *Pediatrics*, 1999, 104 (5 Pt 1):1137-9.
2. Rabenau HF, Kohler E, Peters M, et al, "Low Correlation of Serology With Detection of *Chlamydia trachomatis* by Ligase Chain Reaction and Antigen EIA," *Infection*, 2000, 28(2):97-102.

3. Panuco BCA, Deleon RI, Mendez HJT, et al, "Detection of *Chlamydia trachomatis* in Pregnant Women by the Papanicolaou Technique Enzyme Immunoassay and Polymerase Chain Reaction," *Acta Cytol*, 2000, 44(2):114-23.
4. Chan EL, Brandt K, Stoneham H, et al, "Comparison of the Effectiveness of Polymerase Chain Reaction and Enzyme Immunoassay in Detecting *Chlamydia trachomatis* in Different Female Genitourinary Specimens," *Arch Pathol Lab Med*, 2000, 124(6):840-3.
5. "Gonorrhea and Chlamydial Infections. ACOG Technical Bulletin Number 190- March 1994," *Int J Gynaecol Obstet*, 1994, 45(2):169-74.

References

Baveja UK, Hiranandani MK, Talwar P, et al, "Laboratory Techniques for Diagnosis of Chlamydial Infections of the Eye," *J Commun Dis*, 1997, 29(3):247-53.

Berlau J, Junker U, Groh A, et al, "*In Situ* Hybridization and Direct Fluorescence Antibodies for the Detection of *Chlamydia trachomatis* in Synovial Tissue From Patients With Reactive Arthritis," *J Clin Pathol*, 1998, 51(11):803-6.

Bisno AL, "Acute Pharyngitis," *N Engl J Med*, 2001, 344(3):205-11.

Dayan L, "*Chlamydia* Detection and Management," *Aust Fam Physician*, 2000, 29(6):522-6.

Dicker LW, Mosure DJ, Levine WC, et al, "Impact of Switching Laboratory Tests on Reported Trends in *Chlamydia trachomatis* Infections," *Am J Epidemiol*, 2000, 151(4):430-5.

Guaschino S and DeSeta F, "Update on *Chlamydia trachomatis*," *Ann N Y Acad Sci*, 2000, 900:293-300.

Olsen MA, Sambol AR, and Bohnert VA, "Comparison of the Syva® MicroTrak® Enzyme Immunoassay and Abbott Chlamydiazyme in the Detection of Chlamydial Infections in Women," *Arch Pathol Lab Med*, 1995, 119(2):153-6.

Wilkinson C, Massil H, and Evans J, "An Interface of *Chlamydia* Testing by Community Family Planning Clinics and Referral to Hospital Genitourinary Medicine Clinics," *Br J Fam Plann*, 2000, 26(4):206-9.

Internet Web Sites

www.cdc.gov/nchstp/dstd/chlamydia_facts.htm

♦ *Chlamydia trachomatis* **DNA Detection Test** *see Chlamydia trachomatis* Nucleic Acid Detection *on page 591*

♦ *Chlamydia trachomatis* **Molecular Probe Assay** *see Chlamydia trachomatis* Nucleic Acid Detection *on page 591*

Chlamydia trachomatis Nucleic Acid Detection

Related Information
Bacterial Culture, Conjunctiva *on page 570*
Bacterial Culture, Genital Specimen *on page 571*
Chlamydia Group Serology *on page 589*
Chlamydia trachomatis Culture *on page 590*
Chlamydia trachomatis Direct Antigen Test *on page 590*
Neisseria gonorrhoeae Culture and Smear *on page 662*
Neisseria gonorrhoeae Nucleic Acid Detection *on page 664*
Viral Culture *on page 689*
Viral Culture, Eye or Ocular Symptoms *on page 693*
Viral Culture, Urogenital *on page 696*

Synonyms Amplicor; *Chlamydia* Ligase Chain Reaction (LCR); *Chlamydia* PCR; *Chlamydia trachomatis* DNA Detection Test; *Chlamydia trachomatis* Molecular Probe Assay; DNA Hybridization Test for *Chlamydia trachomatis*; DNA Test for *Chlamydia trachomatis*; PACE2®; ProbeTec ET

Test Includes Detection of *Chlamydia trachomatis* nucleic acid in clinical specimens, either directly or after nucleic acid amplification.

Abstract *Chlamydia trachomatis* is the most common sexually transmitted bacterial infection. In 1998, over 600,000 new cases of genital *Chlamydia* infection was reported to the CDC.[1] It has been estimated that due to under-reporting and asymptomatic infections nearly 4 million new cases may occur annually in the United States. *Chlamydia* infections may be asymptomatic in up to 70% of women and 30% of men. Disease and infection is associated with a high rate of tubal pregnancies, pelvic inflammatory disease, and infertility.[2] *Chlamydia* also causes a severe infection of the eye that, if untreated, may lead to blindness. While in the past, *Chlamydia trachomatis* had been principally diagnosed by culture or immunoassay, the commercial availability of assays employing molecular approaches has significantly altered the standard approach for detection of this agent. In addition to swab specimens of cervix and urethra, the new assays are sufficiently sensitive to detect organism in the urine of infected males.

Specimen Either direct swabs of a potentially infected site or urine may be used depending on the assay. A swab specimen may be collected from the genital/urinary tract of males or females. Some assays have also been approved for detection of *Chlamydia* in urine. Although rectum and the nasal pharynx are also sites that may be infected with *Chlamydia*, swabs of these sites have not been approved for use with molecular assays.

Container Special collection and transport kits are an integral component of the assay and must be used with the appropriate commercial detection assay. A commercial kit typically contains a swab and a transport media or device. Contact the laboratory for appropriate collection kit.

Collection Two swabs are provided in the typical commercial kit for use in females. The cervix or endocervix is first cleaned with one swab and the second swab is used to collect the specimen. The swab is inserted into the endocervical canal and rotated to collect epithelial cells from the infected site. The swab is then placed into transport media and sent to the laboratory. In males, the swab is inserted into the urethral meatus and rotated to collect epithelial cells. The swab is then placed into transport media and sent to the laboratory.
(Continued)

Chlamydia trachomatis Nucleic Acid Detection
(Continued)

Storage Instructions Many of these specimens may be contained at room temperature and sent without freezing to the laboratory. Specimens collected for commercial molecular assays are typically stable for up to 1 week after collection. Contact the laboratory for appropriate instructions.

Causes for Rejection Collection of a specimen from a nonapproved site; some assays cannot detect genomic material if the specimen contains excess blood. Specimens from a suspected sexual abuse case will be rejected.

Turnaround Time Results are usually available within 24 hours.

Reference Interval Negative for *Chlamydia trachomatis*

Use The rapid detection of *C. trachomatis* in clinical specimens. The sensitivity of the test exceeds that for culture and other nonmolecular assays.

Limitations These tests should not be used to establish *C. trachomatis* infection with legal implications (eg, children suspected of being victims of sexual abuse).[3] A major disadvantage to molecular assays is the lack of acceptance by the legal community and court system; currently the results of molecular assays have not been accepted as evidence.

Methodology Several molecular assays have been approved or are under review by the Food and Drug Administration. A test for detection of *Chlamydia trachomatis* was the first PCR test licensed by the FDA in 1993. The PCR detects the presence of *Chlamydia* DNA following extraction, denaturation, and hybridization with a specific DNA probe. The presence of bound probe is detected using an immunochemical technique.[4] The ligase chain reaction procedure incorporates the extraction and denaturation of DNA followed by specific amplification through the ligation of two segments of the target. Detection is similar to that for PCR.[5] The Gen-Probe® assay detects the presence of ribosomal RNA, which is in vast excess to single copy genes of an organism. The probe incorporates a chemiluminescent chemical which upon activation emits light. Recently, the Gen-Probe® assay has incorporated a transcription-based amplification assay that will amplify the ribosomal RNA before detection.[6] Additionally the ProbeTec ET system has been introduced and uses yet a different method of amplification called strand displacement. It simultaneously amplifies and detects *Chlamydia trachomatis* DNA using fluorescence and chemiluminescence.[7] Various instrumentation has been utilized to make the assays automated.

Additional Information The molecular probe assays provide several advantages over traditional culture assays or antibody-based tests. One of the most significant advantages is the ability to detect nonviable organisms since only the presence of nucleic acids is necessary. This latter property also minimizes the need to rapidly transfer the specimen to culture media or cells. The sensitivity of molecular assays exceeds that of culture techniques, depending upon the prevalence of disease and the site of collection. The ability to detect organisms in urine provides an additional advantage over alternative methods and may have a significant impact on public health attempts at limiting the spread of disease.

The presence of plasma cells in the endometrium, endometritis, is associated with *C. trachomatis*. Detection by PCR and by immunohistochemistry is reported.[8]

Whether or not *Chlamydia* plays a role in atherosclerosis remains to be conclusively studied, and the process further elucidated.[9]

Footnotes

1. Centers for Disease Control, "Summary of Notifiable Diseases, United States, 1998," *MMWR Morb Mortal Wkly Rep*, 1999, 47(53):1-93.
2. Guaschino S and DeSeta F, "Update on *Chlamydia trachomatis*," *Ann N Y Acad Sci*, 2000, 900:293-300.
3. Hammerschlag MR, Ajl S, and Laraque D, "Inappropriate use of Nonculture Tests for the Detection of *Chlamydia trachomatis* in Suspected Victims of Child Sexual Abuse: A Continuing Problem," *Pediatrics*, 1999, 104 (5 Pt 1):1137-9.
4. Van Der Pol B, Quinn TC, Gaydos CA, et al, "Multicenter Evaluation of the AMPLICOR and Automated COBAS AMPLICOR CT/NG Tests for Detection of *Chlamydia trachomatis*," *J Clin Microbiol*, 2000, 38(3):1105-12.
5. Winter AH, Gilleran G, Eastick K, et al, "Comparison of a Ligase Chain Reaction-Based Assay and Cell Culture for Detection of Pharyngeal Carriage of *Chlamydia trachomatis*," *J Clin Microbiol*, 2000, 38(9):3502-4.
6. de Barbeyrac B, Geniaux M, Hocke C, et al, "Detection of *Chlamydia trachomatis* in Symptomatic and Asymptomatic Populations With Urogenital Specimens by AMP CT (Gen-Probe™ incorporated) Compared to Others Commercially Available Amplification Assays," *Diagn Microbiol Infect Dis*, 2000, 37(3):181-5.
7. Chan EL, Brandt K, Olienus K, et al, "Performance Characteristics of the Becton Dickinson ProbeTec System for Direct Detection of *Chlamydia trachomatis* and *Neisseria gonorrhoeae* in Male and Female Urine Specimens in Comparison With the Roche Cobas System," *Arch Pathol Lab Med*, 2000, 124(11):1649-52.
8. Paukku M, Puolakkainen M, Paavonen T, et al, "Plasma Cell Endometritis Is Associated With *Chlamydia trachomatis* Infection," *Am J Clin Pathol*, 1999, 112(2):211-5.
9. Shor A and Phillips JI, "*Chlamydia pneumoniae* and Atherosclerosis," *JAMA*, 1999, 282(17):2071-3.

References

Bull SS, Jones CA, Granberry-Owens D, et al, "Acceptability and Feasibility of Urine Screening for *Chlamydia* and Gonorrhea in Community Organizations: Perspectives From Denver and St. Louis," *Am J Public Health*, 2000, 90(2):285-6.

Chan EL, Brandt K, Stoneham H, et al, "Comparison of the Effectiveness of Polymerase Chain Reaction and Enzyme Immunoassay in Detecting *Chlamydia trachomatis* in Different Female Genitourinary Specimens," *Arch Pathol Lab Med*, 2000, 124(6):840-3.

Dayan L, "*Chlamydia* Detection and Management," *Aust Fam Physician*, 2000, 29(6):522-6.

Dicker LW, Mosure DJ, Levine WC, et al, "Impact of Switching Laboratory Tests on Reported Trends in *Chlamydia trachomatis* Infections," *Am J Epidemiol*, 2000, 151(4):430-5.

Keenan GF, "Polymerase Chain Reaction as a Diagnostic Tool," *Adolesc Med*, 1998, 9(1):35-43.

Mahony JB, "Multiplex Polymerase Chain Reaction for the Diagnosis of Sexually Transmitted Diseases," *Clin Lab Med*, 1996, 16(1):61-71.

Pourahmadi F, Taylor M, Kovacs G, et al, "Toward a Rapid, Integrated, and Fully Automated DNA Diagnostic Assay for *Chlamydia trachomatis* and *Neisseria Gonorrhoeae*," *Clin Chem*, 2000, 46(9):1511-3.

Wilkinson C, Massil H, and Evans J, "An Interface of *Chlamydia* Testing by Community Family Planning Clinics and Referral to Hospital Genitourinary Medicine Clinics," *Br J Fam Plann*, 2000, 26(4):206-9.

Internet Web Sites

www.cdc.gov/nchstp/dstd/chlamydia_facts.htm

♦ **Cimex Identification** *see* Arthropod Identification *on page 559*

♦ **Clostridium botulinum Toxin Identification Procedure** *see* Botulism Diagnostic Procedures *on page 585*

♦ **Clostridium difficile** *see* Bacterial Culture, Stool *on page 575*

Clostridium difficile Toxin Assay and Culture

Related Information

Bacterial Culture, Anaerobes *on page 564*
Bacterial Culture, Biopsy or Body Fluid *on page 565*
Bacterial Culture, Stool *on page 575*
Fecal Lactoferrin *on page 308*
Fungal Culture, Stool *on page 614*
Methylene Blue Stain, Stool *on page 313*
Ova and Parasites, Stool *on page 666*
pH, Stool *on page 317*

Synonyms Antibiotic-Associated Colitis Toxin Test; Pseudomembranous Colitis Toxin Assay; Toxin Assay, *Clostridium difficile*

Applies to Toxin A and/or B

Abstract The major cause of antibiotic-associated diarrhea and pseudomembranous colitis is toxigenic *Clostridium difficile*. *C. difficile* associated diarrhea is responsible for the majority of nosocomial diarrhea and contributes to the cost of hospitalization.[1] The *C. difficile* associated with diarrhea usually produce one or two toxins, toxin A and/or toxin B, that can be detected directly in stool specimens.

Specimen Diarrheal stool or proctoscopic specimen; solid stool specimens should not be tested for the presence of toxin. Material for culture may be derived from peritoneum and tissues.[2]

Container Plastic stool container (swabs are inadequate because of small volume)

Sampling Time Repeat testing within 7 days of an initial assay provides helpful information in only ~1% of cases.[3]

Storage Instructions Keep specimen **cold** and transport immediately. Specimens can be frozen if transportation will be delayed.

Turnaround Time 1-2 days

Special Instructions When antibiotic-associated colitis is suspected, a toxin assay rather than a *C. difficile* stool culture should be ordered.

Reference Interval Presence of toxin is suggestive of disease. Isolation of organism (*C. difficile*) may occur in 5% to 21% of normal adults and in 50% of normal newborns.[4] Isolation of the organism without demonstration of toxin production is a nonspecific finding and does not enhance diagnosis of diarrhea.

Use Diagnose antibiotic-related, pseudomembranous colitis caused by toxigenic *C. difficile*; evaluate diarrhea, especially that in patients admitted to the hospital more than 72 hours before onset. Tube-fed patients with diarrhea especially should be tested.[5] *C. difficile* can be pathogenic in extraintestinal tissues.[2]

Limitations The latex agglutination test is simple and rapid, but it does not detect (is not specific for) toxin A, the protein thought to be primarily responsible for pseudomembranous colitis, and thus provides unreliable results. Cytotoxin assays or immunoassays for toxin A are specific but usually have sensitivities <90%. Newer immunoassays will detect both toxin A and toxin B, and the sensitivity of these assays compared to the cytotoxicity assay was 95%.[6] Toxin detection should not be used to screen hospitalized patients without diarrhea. Many hospitalized patients (44% to 63%) can have positive results and remain asymptomatic during their hospital stay.[7]

Methodology Latex agglutination (LA) test to detect toxin, neutralization test in tissue culture (toxin), selective anaerobic culture (organism), enzyme immunoassay (EIA) (toxin A and/or B), fluorogenic immunoassay (toxin)

Additional Information *C. difficile*-associated diarrhea is a common nosocomial infection. Toxigenic strains usually produce two toxins: toxin A, an enterotoxin and toxin B, a cytotoxin that can be detected by cell culture or EIA. Not all *C. difficile* strains are toxigenic, and even toxigenic strains may not produce disease if present in insufficient numbers; consequently, culture for *C. difficile* often produces false-positive results. Strains that do not produce toxins do not cause diarrhea or colitis. The most accurate clinical laboratory test for diagnosis of pseudomembranous colitis appears to be enzyme immunoassays for toxin A/B.[6,8] These assays are more rapid and accessible than cytotoxin assays and are highly specific (99%) and fairly sensitive (87% to 95%).[6,8] Latex agglutination has been widely utilized because it is fast and easy to use. Unfortunately, the assay detects an antigen produced by many microorganisms other than *C. difficile* and probably should not be relied upon to diagnose *C. difficile* disease. Endoscopy with biopsies is rapid, sensitive, and useful in diagnosis and differential diagnosis.

Pseudomembranous colitis attributable to *C. difficile* is usually associated with antimicrobial therapy,[7] anti-AIDS or antineoplastic drugs.[9] The greatest risk of *C. difficile* diarrhea also includes the use of second- and third-generation cephalosporins, clindamycin, ampicillin, and amoxicillin.[10,11] *C. difficile* is an important nosocomial pathogen that may be treated by discontinuing antimicrobial therapy, if possible, or initiating oral metronidazole or vancomycin therapy.[9]

Footnotes

1. Miller JM, Walton JC, and Tordecilla LL, "Recognizing and Managing *Clostridium difficile*-Associated Diarrhea," *Medsurg Nurs*, 1998, 7(6):348-56.
2. Wolf LE, Gorbach SL, and Granowitz EV, "Extraintestinal *Clostridium difficile*: 10 Year' Experience at a Tertiary-Care Hospital," *Mayo Clin Proc*, 1998, 73(10):943-7.
3. Renshaw AA, Stelling JM, and Doolittle MH, "The Lack of Value of Repeated *Clostridium difficile* Cytotoxicity Assays," *Arch Pathol Lab Med*, 1996, 120(1):49-52.
4. Allen SD, Emery CL and Siders JA, "*Clostridium*," *Manual of Clinical Microbiology*, 7th ed, Murray PR, Baron EJ, Pfaller MA, et al, eds, Washington, DC: AMS Press, American Society for Microbiology, 1999, 654-71.
5. Bliss DZ, Johnson S, Savik K, et al, "Acquisition of *Clostridium difficile* and *Clostridium difficile*-Associated Diarrhea in Hospitalized Patients Receiving Tube Feeding," *Ann Intern Med*, 1998, 129(12):1012-9.
6. Aldeen WE, Bingham M, Aiderzada A, et al, "Comparison of the TOX A/B Test to a Cell Culture Cytotoxicity Assay for the Detection of *Clostridium difficile* in Stools," *Diagn Microbiol Infect Dis*, 2000, 36(4):211-3.
7. Kyne L, Warny M, Qamar A, et al, "Asymptomatic Carriage of *Clostridium difficile* and Serum Levels of IgG Antibody Against Toxin A," *N Engl J Med*, 2000, 342(6):390-7.
8. El-Gammal A, Scotto V, Malik S, et al, "Evaluation of the Clinical Usefulness of *C. difficile* Toxin Testing in Hospitalized Patients With Diarrhea," *Diagn Microbiol Infect Dis*, 2000, 36(3):169-73.
9. Alcantara CS and Guerrant RL, "Update on *Clostridium difficile* Infection," *Curr Gastroenterol Rep*, 2000, 2(4):310-4.
10. Gorbach SL, "Antibiotics and *Clostridium difficile*," *N Engl J Med*, 1999, 341(22):1690-1.
11. Johnson S, Samore MH, and Farrow KA, "Epidemics of Diarrhea Caused by a Clindamycin-Resistant Strain of *Clostridium difficile* in Four Hospitals," *N Engl J Med*, 1999, 341(22):1645-51.

References

Barr HS and Surawicz CM, "Pseudomembranous Colitis: An Update," *Can J Gastroenterol*, 2000, 14(1):51-6.
Fedorko DP, Engler HD, O'Shaughnessy EM, et al, "Evaluation of Two Rapid Assays for Detection of *Clostridium difficile* Toxin A in Stool Specimens," *J Clin Microbiol*, 1999, 37(9):3044-7.
Freeman J and Wilcox MH, "Antibiotics and *Clostridium difficile*," *Microbes Infect*, 1999, 1(5):377-84.
Garbutt JM, Littenberg B, Evanoff BA, et al, "Enteric Carriage of Vancomycin-Resistant *Enterococcus faecium* in Patients Tested for *Clostridium difficile*," *Infect Control Hosp Epidemiol*, 1999, 20(10):664-70.
Levy DG, Stergachis A, McFarland LV, et al, "Antibiotics and *Clostridium difficile* Diarrhea in the Ambulatory Care Setting," *Clin Ther*, 2000, 22(1):91-102.
Nicholson G and Jones M, "Laboratory Assessment of Five Enzyme Immunoassay *Clostridium difficile* Toxin Detection Kits," *Br J Biomed Sci*, 1999, 56(3):204-5.
Samore MH, "Epidemiology of Nosocomial *Clostridium difficile* Diarrhea," *J Hosp Infect*, 1999, 43(S):183-90.

Internet Web Sites

www.amm.co.uk/pubs/fa_cdiff.htm

♦ ***Clostridium* spp** *see* Bacterial Culture, Wounds, Bites *on page 579*

♦ **Clue Cells** *see* Bacterial Culture, Genital Specimen *on page 571*

♦ **CMV Antibody** *see* Cytomegalovirus Serology *on page 600*

♦ **CMV Antigen Detection** *see* Cytomegalovirus Antigen Detection *on page 598*

♦ **CMV, Blood Culture** *see* Viral Culture, Blood *on page 691*

♦ **CMV, Buffy Coat Culture** *see* Viral Culture, Blood *on page 691*

♦ **CMV Culture** *see* Cytomegalovirus Culture *on page 598*

♦ **CMV Culture** *see* Viral Culture, Blood *on page 691*

♦ **CMV Culture, Urine** *see* Viral Culture, Urine *on page 695*

♦ **CMV DNA Detection** *see* Cytomegalovirus Nucleic Acid Detection *on page 599*

♦ **CMV-IFA** *see* Cytomegalovirus Serology *on page 600*

♦ **CMV, IgG** *see* Cytomegalovirus Serology *on page 600*

♦ **CMV, IgM** *see* Cytomegalovirus Serology *on page 600*

♦ **CMV pp65 Detection** *see* Cytomegalovirus Antigen Detection *on page 598*

♦ **CMV Quantitation** *see* Cytomegalovirus Nucleic Acid Detection *on page 599*

♦ **CMV Quantitative PCR** *see* Cytomegalovirus Nucleic Acid Detection *on page 599*

♦ **CMV Rapid Culture** *see* Cytomegalovirus Culture *on page 598*

♦ **CMV Shell Vial Culture** *see* Cytomegalovirus Culture *on page 598*

♦ **CMV Titer** *see* Cytomegalovirus Serology *on page 600*

♦ **Coagglutination Test for Group A Streptococci** *replaced by* Group A Streptococcus Screen, Rapid *on page 617*

♦ ***Coccidia*** *see* Cryptosporidium Direct Staining Procedures *on page 596*

♦ ***Coccidioides immitis* Antibody** *see* Coccidioidomycosis Serology *on page 593*

Coccidioidomycosis Serology

Related Information

Fine Needle Aspiration Culture *on page 609*
Fungal Culture, Biopsy or Body Fluid *on page 610*
Fungal Culture, Blood *on page 610*
Fungal Culture, Sputum *on page 613*
Fungus Smear, Stain *on page 615*
Myoglobin, Qualitative, Urine *on page 880*
Sputum Cytology *on page 387*

Synonyms Desert Fever Serology; San Joaquin Fever Serology; Valley Fever Serology

Applies to *Coccidioides immitis* Antibody; Spherulin®

Test Includes Complement fixing or precipitating antibodies

Abstract Coccidioidomycosis is an infection caused by the dimorphic fungus *Coccidioides immitis*. It is endemic in soil of certain regions of Arizona, California, Nevada, New Mexico, Texas, Utah, and Mexico, essentially in a band extending to Argentina. It is endemic in the San Joaquin Valley of California.

Diagnosis depends on identification of *C. immitis* by culture, cytologic,[1] and/or histopathologic examination. Serology can be helpful in the diagnosis of disease when a patient is unable to produce sputum, or in the diagnosis of chronic meningitis due to *C. immitis*. Coccidioidal pneumonia may be a debilitating disease, characterized by protracted fever and fatigue. Progressive infections in the months following initial exposure may signal spread to bone (including thoracic vertebrae, and bones of the skull, hands, feet and tibia); joints (ankles and knees); skin and soft tissues. Meningitis involves the basilar meninges. Upsurges follow dust storms,[2] drought followed by heavy rain,[3] or earthquakes.[4]

Specimen Serum, cerebrospinal fluid

Container Red top tube; clean, sterile CSF tube

Sampling Time Repeated serologic testing during the first 2 months of illness enhances likelihood of diagnosis.[5]

Special Instructions Travel history is relevant.

Reference Interval Negative

Critical Values Increasing titers signal progressive disease.

Possible Panic Range CF antibody titer ≥1:16 may indicate disseminated disease.[6]

Use Diagnose and evaluate the prognosis of coccidioidomycosis. Transmission is by inhalation of arthroconidia (arthrospores). About 100,000 infections occur annually in the U.S., most asymptomatic, others mild, some evolving to dissemination and death. With migration to the Southwestern U.S. and increasing numbers of immunosuppressed individuals, the importance of this infection is increasing. Corticosteroids, chemotherapy, immune modulation for organ transplantation, and the AIDS epidemic all have magnified the relevance of coccidioidomycosis as an opportunistic infection. Reactivation of infection acquired years earlier is seen with suppression of cellular immunity.[5] Since CSF cultures are usually negative, demonstration of antibody in CSF is an important means of diagnosis. Repeat testing may be necessary.[2]

Limitations A negative test does not exclude coccidioidomycosis. When low titers are obtained, a diagnosis of coccidioidomycosis must be based on subsequent serological tests and on clinical and mycological studies. Cross reactions may occur in sera from patients with active histoplasmosis. False-negative results often occur in patients with solitary pulmonary lesions. Subjects with meningeal coccidioidomycosis may not demonstrate elevated serum antibodies.[2] The sensitivity, specificity, and reproducibility of enzyme immunoassay and other new tests have not been standardized.[7]

Methodology Complement fixation (CF), tube precipitin, latex particle agglutination, double immunodiffusion (ID), enzyme-linked immunosorbent assay (ELISA).[5,8]

Spherules are not stained with Gram stain, but are visualized with KOH, calcofluor, and with Papanicolaou stains of respiratory specimens.

Culture with DNA probe is confirmatory.[5]

Additional Information Symptomatic infection of coccidioidomycosis usually presents as a nonspecific illness with fever, cough, headache, and myalgia. Meningitis due to *C. immitis* can lead to permanent neurologic sequelae. Mortality is high in HIV-infected patients with diffuse lung disease. Other high risk groups include those of African-American or Filipino ancestry, diabetics, infants, pregnant women during the third trimester, and patients on immunosuppressive therapy. Seroreactivity may take place (Continued)

Coccidioidomycosis Serology *(Continued)*

before clinically recognized coccidioidomycosis in some HIV-positive individuals.[7]

Serology is a useful approach to the diagnosis of coccidioidal infections. Low titers are usually associated with early, residual, or meningeal coccidioidomycosis with mild and localized disease. Patients with complement fixing (CF) titers ≥1:16 should be evaluated for evidence of pulmonary or extrapulmonary dissemination. Higher CF titers are associated with poorer prognosis when assessing the extent and severity of both acute and chronic coccidioidomycosis. Falling CF titers indicate an improved clinical status. Specific IgM antibodies may be detected early in the course of the disease. Finding CF antibody in CSF makes the diagnosis of coccidioidal meningitis (if fungal osteomyelitis of the base of the skull can be excluded). CSF is characterized by a mononuclear pleocytosis with decreased glucose and increased protein concentration.

The tube precipitin test for IgM antibodies is effective in detection of early disease, 1-3 weeks after infection, but it becomes negative in 1-6 months. CF test for IgG antibodies becomes positive later and remains positive for years. The agar gel test for precipitins is more specific than CF antibody testing, and may be helpful when CF provides low titer reactivity. In immunodiffusion testing, a band of identity with coccidioidin indicates infection but may be negative early. Some individuals continue to produce detectable antibodies up to a year after clinical recovery from active disease. A negative test does not exclude coccidioidomycosis.

Skin testing is not 100% sensitive nor 100% specific, because infected individuals will remain skin-test positive for life,[9] and because anergy may develop.[2]

The Gomori methenamine silver preparation remains useful for tissue section examination.[10]

Footnotes

1. Raab SS, Silverman JF, and Zimmerman KG, "Fine-Needle Aspiration Biopsy of Pulmonary Coccidioidomycosis. Spectrum of Cytologic Findings in 73 Patients," *Am J Clin Pathol*, 1993, 99(5):582-7.
2. Stevens DA, "Coccidioidomycosis," *N Engl J Med*, 1995, 332(16):1077-82.
3. Centers for Disease Control and Prevention, "Coccidioidomycosis - Arizona, 1990-1995," *JAMA*, 1997, 277(2):104-5.
4. Schneider E, Hajjeh RA, Spiegel RA, et al, "A Coccidioidomycosis Outbreak Following the Northridge, Calif, Earthquake," *JAMA*, 1997, 277(11):904-8.
5. Galgiani JN, "Coccidioidomycosis: A Regional Disease of National Importance. Rethinking Approaches for Control," *Ann Intern Med*, 1999, 130(4 Pt 1):293-300.
6. Galgiani J, "*Coccidioides immitis*," *Principles and Practice of Infectious Diseases*, 5th ed, Mandell GL, Bennett JE, and Dolin R, eds, New York, NY: Churchill Livingstone, 2000, 2746-57.
7. Gambino R, "Coccidioidal Seropositivity Precedes Clinically Apparent Coccidioidomycosis," *Lab Rep*, 1995, 17(6):45.
8. Zartarian M, Peterson EM, and de la Maza LM, "Detection of Antibodies to *Coccidioides immitis* by Enzyme Immunoassay," *Am J Clin Pathol*, 1997, 107(2):148-53.
9. Centers for Disease Control and Prevention, "Update: Coccidioidomycosis - California, 1991-1993," *JAMA*, 1994, 272(8):505.
10. Kleinschmidt-DeMasters BK, Mazowiecki M, Bonds LA, et al, "Coccidioidomycosis Meningitis With Massive Dural and Cerebral Venous Thrombosis and Tissue Arthroconidia," *Arch Pathol Lab Med*, 2000, 124(2):310-4.

References

"Coccidioidomycosis in Travelers Returning From Mexico - Pennsylvania, 2000," *JAMA*, 2000, 284(23):2990-1.

Galgiani JN, " Coccidioidomycosis," *Curr Clin Top Infect Dis*, 1997, 3(1):192-9.

Schneider E, Hajjeh RA, Spiegel RA, et al, "A Coccidioidomycosis Outbreak Following the Northridge, California, Earthquake," *JAMA*, 1997, 277(11):904-8.

Vaz A, Pineda-Roman M, Thomas AR, et al, "Coccidioidomycosis: An Update," *Hosp Pract*, 1998, 33(9):105-15.

Internet Web Sites

www.cdc.gov/ncidod/dbmd/diseaseinfo/coccidioidomycosis_a.htm
www.acponline.org

Cold Agglutinin Titer

Related Information

Cold Hemolysin Test *on page 418*
Cryofibrinogen *on page 337*
Cryoglobulin, Qualitative, Serum and Plasma *on page 524*
Immunoglobulin M *on page 537*
Mycoplasma pneumoniae Culture *on page 660*
Mycoplasma pneumoniae DNA Probe Test *on page 661*
Mycoplasma Serology *on page 662*
Red Blood Cells *on page 857*
Risks of Transfusion *on page 861*
Warming, Blood *on page 865*

Applies to i Antigen; I Antigen of Red Cell Membranes; *Mycoplasma pneumoniae* Infection

Abstract *Mycoplasma* infection activates several components of the immune system. In the majority of patients, several classes of antibody are produced. The best recognized are the cold isohemagglutinins that are capable of clumping erythrocytes at 4°C. Cold agglutinins in *M. pneumoniae* infection are IgM antibodies directed against the I antigen on the surface of erythrocytes.

Cold agglutinins are not to be confused with cryoglobulins or cryofibrinogens.

Specimen Serum

Container Red top tube

Storage Instructions After clotting at 37°C, separate serum from cells if specimen is to be stored overnight in refrigerator.

Causes for Rejection Refrigeration of the specimen before separation of serum from cells, specimen not allowed to clot at 37°C

Special Instructions Transport blood immediately to the laboratory.

Reference Interval Negative: less than a fourfold increase in titer or single titer <1:32

Critical Values Single titers ≥64 or a fourfold titer increase in specimens 5 or more days apart are relevant.

Use In primary atypical pneumonia (infection with *Mycoplasma pneumoniae*), IgM antibodies against I antigen of erythrocyte membranes are found in many but not all subjects. Investigate idiopathic cold agglutinin disease.

Limitations False negatives may occur, especially if serum is refrigerated on the clot. False-positive results are associated with rubeola, adenovirus pneumonia, infectious mononucleosis, some connective tissue diseases and tropical diseases. Antibiotic therapy may interfere with antibody formation.

Methodology The highest dilution causing hemagglutination with type O blood cells at 4°C is the cold agglutinin titer.

Additional Information *M. pneumoniae* has I-like antigen specificity. The i and I RBC antigens appear to be ceramide heptasaccharides and decasaccharides. The fetal i RBCs change after birth so that by 18 months red cells carry largely I. The i substance has been found in saliva, milk, amniotic fluid, ovarian cyst fluid, and serum.

Antibody to the I antigen is more specific for *Mycoplasma*, while i antigen is more commonly found in infectious mononucleosis. The most common cause of elevated cold agglutinin in high titers is an infection with *Mycoplasma pneumoniae*. Fifty-five percent of patients with disease have rising titers. In primary atypical *Mycoplasma pneumoniae*, cold agglutinins are demonstrated 1 week after onset; the titer increases in 8-10 days, peaks at 12-25 days, and rapidly falls after day 30.

Cold agglutinins are usually IgM autoantibodies directed against an altered Ii antigen on the human RBCs of *M. pneumoniae* infected patients. These antibodies may be found in patients with cold agglutinin disease or may occur transiently following a number of acute infectious illnesses (Epstein-Barr virus and cytomegalovirus infections). Cold agglutinins of cold agglutinin disease are usually monoclonal IgM kappa. Cold antibodies of IgG, IgA, or IgM type directed against Ii antigens may be found in infectious mononucleosis. Antibodies reacting near physiologic temperatures are more likely to be clinically important. Detection of cold agglutinins may be particularly important in patients in whom cold blood is to be used.

The differential diagnosis of atypical pneumonias, including features of *Chlamydia*, *Mycoplasma*, and *Legionella* infections, has been published.[1,2]

Footnotes

1. Hindiyeh M and Carroll KC, "Laboratory Diagnosis of Atypical Pneumonia," *Semin Respir Infect*, 2000, 15(2):101-13.
2. Gordon RC, "Community-Acquired Pneumonia in Adolescents," *Asolesc Med*, 2000, 11(3):681-95.

References

Baum SG, "*Mycoplasma pneumoniae* and Atypical Pneumonia," *Principles and Practice of Infectious Diseases*, 5th ed, Mandell GL, Bennett JE, and Dolin R, eds, New York, NY: Churchill Livingstone, 2000, 2018-27.

Hadnagy C, "Agewise Distribution of Idiopathic Cold Agglutinin Disease," *Z Gerontol*, 1993, 26(3):199-201.

Silberstein LE, "B-Cell Origin of Cold Agglutinins," *Adv Exp Med Biol*, 1994, 347:193-205.

Tan JS, "Role of Atypical Pneumonia Pathogens in Respiratory Tract Infections," *Can Respir J*, 1999, 6(Suppl A):15A-9A.

Internet Web Sites

my.webmd.com/content/asset/adam_disease_walking_pneumonia

♦ **Conjunctival Culture** *see* Bacterial Culture, Conjunctiva *on page 570*

♦ **Conjunctival Fungus Culture** *see* Fungal Culture, Ocular Infections *on page 612*

♦ **Core Window** *see* Hepatitis B Core Antibody *on page 622*

♦ **Core Window** *see* Hepatitis B$_e$ Antigen *on page 624*

♦ **Corneal Culture** *see* Bacterial Culture, Conjunctiva *on page 570*

♦ ***Corynebacterium diphtheriae*** *see* Bacterial Culture, Sputum *on page 574*

Corynebacterium diphtheriae Throat Culture

Related Information

Bacterial Culture, Throat, and Antigen Detection Testing for Group A Streptococci *on page 577*

Synonyms Diphtheria Culture; Throat Culture for *Corynebacterium diphtheriae*

Applies to Nasopharyngeal Culture for *Corynebacterium diphtheriae*

Abstract *C. diphtheriae* is a gram-positive, nonsporulating bacillus. Infection with toxigenic *C. diphtheriae* is responsible for the disease diphtheria. The organism may be found in the anterior nasal mucosa (nasal diphtheria) or larynx (resembling infectious croup), but classically it is a disease of the oropharynx, pharynx, and tonsils. *C. diphtheriae* is not an invasive pathogen and the organisms remain superficial in the respiratory tract and skin. It may spread to or begin in the larynx and can involve the tracheobronchial tree. Its potent exotoxin is responsible for the virulence of the disease. The major effects of the exotoxin include damage to the heart, kidneys, and nervous system. It can cause circulatory collapse, respiratory failure, myocarditis, and neuritis.

Pharyngeal diphtheria has become a rare disease in the U.S. Found among unimmunized or poorly immunized individuals, it may be suspected on clinical grounds.[1]

Aftercare Observe for laryngospasm following collection of specimen.

Specimen Throat swab, nasopharyngeal swab; culture nose or larynx if clinically appropriate

Container Sterile Mini-Tip Culturette® or flexible calcium alginate swab, Calgiswab®, is recommended for obtaining nasopharyngeal culture.

Collection The tongue should be depressed while both the tonsillar crypts and nasopharynx and throat lesions are swabbed. If a pseudomembrane is present, the swab should be taken from beneath the membrane, or a part of the membrane should be cultured if possible.

Turnaround Time Final reports on specimens from which *C. diphtheriae* has been isolated usually take at least 4 days.

Special Instructions The laboratory should be notified before collection of specimens so that special isolation media can be made available.

Reference Interval No *C. diphtheriae* isolated

Use Isolate *C. diphtheriae* from patients suspected of having diphtheria. The differential diagnosis of pharyngeal diphtheria includes streptococcal pharyngitis, infectious mononucleosis and candidiasis.

Limitations Cultures should be taken from nasopharynx, as well as the throat; culture of both sites increases the chance of recovery of the organism. Stain results are presumptive and are commonly reported out as "gram-positive pleomorphic bacilli suggestive of *C. diphtheriae*". Definitive diagnosis depends on isolation of the organism, because of the similar appearance of other organisms commonly found in the oropharynx. Special microbiological media that are not routinely available in the laboratory are needed for optimal culture of *C. diphtheriae*.

Contraindications Lack of clinical symptoms or signs of diphtheria, valid history of immunization

Methodology Culture on selective medium (Löeffler), cystine tellurite agar, and blood agar; direct smear stained with Löeffler methylene blue stain and/or Gram stain. *C. diphtheriae* may appear as V, Y, or L figures. Metachromatic granules that stain deep blue are also seen.

Additional Information *C. diphtheriae* may occasionally cause skin infections, wound infections, pulmonary infections, and endocarditis and may be recovered from the oropharynx of healthy carriers. *C. diphtheriae* is spread through respiratory secretions by convalescent and healthy carriers. The clinical presentation of respiratory diphtheria includes a grayish-brown pseudomembrane overlying superficial ulcers in the oropharynx. It can involve one or both tonsils, the nares, uvula, soft palate, pharynx, larynx, trachea, and bronchi. It may cause local lymphadenopathy.[1] The organism is noninvasive; however, the exotoxin elaborated in the throat affects primarily the heart, kidneys, and nervous system. Mortality is 10% to 30% in untreated individuals. Only strains of *C. diphtheriae* infected by β-phage are capable of producing toxin that is a peptide, that inhibits protein synthesis in host cells. Nontoxigenic strains are commonly recovered and are capable of producing pharyngitis. Confirmation of exotoxin production requires animal testing and is rarely done for clinical isolates. *C. ulcerans* may also produce a diphtheria-like disease.

Group A beta-hemolytic streptococcal and other secondary infections may occur. Hypoglycemia may be seen secondary to hepatotoxicity.[2]

Footnotes
1. Bisno AL, "Acute Pharyngitis," *N Engl J Med*, 2001, 344(3):205-11.
2. Feigin RD, "Diphtheria," *Principles and Practice of Pediatrics*, 2nd ed, Oski FA, DeAngelis CD, Feigin RD, et al, eds, Philadelphia, PA: JB Lippincott Co, 1994, 1180-3.

References
Bisgard KM, Hardy IR, Popovic T, et al, "Respiratory Diphtheria in the United States, 1980 through 1995," *Am J Public Health*, 1998, 88(5):787-91.

Efstratiou A, Tiley SM, Sangrador A, et al, "Invasive Disease Caused by Multiple Clones of *Corynebacterium diphtheriae*," *Clin Infect Dis*, 1993, 17(1):136.

Farizo KM, Strebel PM, Chen RT, et al, "Fatal Respiratory Disease Due to *Corynebacterium diphtheriae*: Case Report and Review of Guidelines for Management, Investigation, and Control," *Clin Infect Dis*, 1993, 16(1):59-68.

Golaz A, Lance-Parker S, Welty T, et al, "Epidemiology of Diphtheria in South Dakota," *S D J Med*, 2000, 53(7):281-5.

MacGregor RR, "*Corynebacterium diphtheriae*," *Principles and Practice of Infectious Diseases*, 5th ed, Mandell GL, Bennett JE, and Dolin R, eds, New York, NY: Churchill Livingstone, 2000, 2190-8.

Vitek CR, Bogatyreva EY, and Wharton M, "Diphtheria Surveillance and Control in the Former Soviet Untion and the Newly Independent States," *J Infect Dis*, 2000, 181(S1):23-6.

Internet Web Sites
www.amm.co.uk/pubs/fa_diphtheria.htm
www.cdc.gov/nip/publications/pink/dip.pdf

♦ **Cough Plate Culture for Pertussis** *replaced by Bordetella pertussis* Culture on *page 583*

♦ **Cough Plate Culture for Pertussis** *replaced by Bordetella pertussis* Direct Fluorescent Antibody *on page 583*

♦ **Counterimmunoelectrophoresis for Group B Streptococcal Antigen** *replaced by* Group B *Streptococcus* Screen, Rapid *on page 618*

♦ *Coxiella burnetii* **Antibody** *see* Q Fever Serology *on page 673*

♦ *Coxiella burnetii* **Titer** *see* Q Fever Serology *on page 673*

♦ **Coxsackie B Virus Culture** *see* Enterovirus Culture *on page 605*

♦ **Coxsackievirus Culture, Stool** *see* Viral Culture, Stool *on page 695*

Coxsackievirus Serology

Related Information
Enterovirus Culture *on page 605*
Viral Culture *on page 689*
Viral Culture, Blood *on page 691*
Viral Culture, Body Fluid *on page 691*
Viral Culture, Central Nervous System Symptoms *on page 692*
Viral Culture, Respiratory Symptoms *on page 694*

Test Includes Detection of antibody titer to Coxsackie A or B virus

Abstract The majority of infections with Coxsackie A and B, two groups of nonpolio enteroviruses, are asymptomatic or mildly symptomatic. Patients with Coxsackievirus infections can have a variety of symptoms from meningitis, exanthems, pericarditis, myocarditis, hand-foot and mouth syndrome and conjunctivitis.[1] Other nonpolio viruses include echoviruses. Twenty-three Coxsackieviruses group A are recognized and six Coxsackieviruses group B are recognized.

Specimen Serum

Container Red top tube

Sampling Time Acute and convalescent sera drawn at least 14 days apart are required.

Reference Interval Less than a fourfold increase in titer in paired sera

Use Diagnose recent infections with Coxsackie A or Coxsackie B virus

Limitations Documentation of infection by serology is difficult, and diagnosis may depend on culture and other methods. Neutralizing antibodies develop quickly and persist for many years after infection, making demonstration of a rise in titer difficult. Complement fixation test is not sensitive.

Methodology Viral neutralization, complement fixation (CF)

Additional Information Since culture is frequently unrewarding, diagnosis may hinge on serologic studies, however, it is important to collect both acute and convalescent sera in order to reach an accurate diagnosis. The Coxsackie A and B viruses can also be detected directly in the specimens of infected patients (see Viral Culture *on page 689*), especially CSF, tissue, body fluids (pericardial fluid), or eye swabs or scrapings.

Footnotes
1. Modlin JF, "Coxsackieviruses, Echoviruses, and Newer Enteroviruses," *Principles and Practice of Infectious Diseases*, 5th ed, Mandell GL, Bennett JE, and Dolin R, eds, New York, NY: Churchill Livingstone, 2000, 1904-19.

References
Bauer K, "Foot-and-Mouth Disease as Zoonosis," *Arch Virol Suppl*, 1997, 13:95-7.

Melnick JL, "Enteroviruses," *Manual of Clinical Laboratory Immunology*, 4th ed, Volume 2, Chapter 93, Rose NR, Conway de Macario E, Fahey JL, et al, eds, Washington, DC: ASM Press, American Society for Microbiology, 1992, 631-3.

Modlin JF and Rotbart HA, "Group B Coxsackie Disease in Children," *Curr Top Microbiol Immunol*, 1997, 223:53-80.

See DM and Tilles JG, "Viral Myocarditis," *Rev Infect Dis*, 1991, 13(5):951-6.

Internet Web Sites
www.cdc.gov/ncidod/dvrd/hfmd.htm

♦ **CPE** *see* Viral Culture *on page 689*

♦ **Crustaceans** *see* Arthropod Identification *on page 559*

Cryptococcal Antigen Titer

Related Information
Bacterial Antigens, Rapid Detection Methods *on page 562*
Cerebrospinal Fluid Analysis: Overview *on page 416*
Cerebrospinal Fluid Cytology *on page 376*
Fungal Culture, Blood *on page 610*
Fungal Culture, Cerebrospinal Fluid *on page 611*
Fungal Culture, Sputum *on page 613*
Fungus Smear, Stain *on page 615*
India Ink Preparation *on page 642*
Mycobacterial Culture, Cerebrospinal Fluid *on page 656*

Synonyms Cerebrospinal Fluid Cryptococcal Latex Agglutination; Serum Cryptococcal Latex Agglutination

Test Includes Testing patient's serum, CSF, or pleural fluid for the presence of cryptococcal heteropolysaccharide capsular antigen

Abstract Cryptococcosis is caused by *Cryptococcus neoformans*, a yeast-like organism. This ubiquitous fungus is associated with droppings of birds, especially those of pigeons; infection begins with inhalation of the organism. (Continued)

Cryptococcal Antigen Titer *(Continued)*

Cryptococcal antigen testing on spinal fluid is the single most useful diagnostic test for cryptococcal meningitis.[1] (The other diagnostic fundamentals are visualization of the organism and its culture.) Corticosteroids enhance development of this infection. Many of the cases in the U.S. presently are found in AIDS patients, but infection can also occur in immunocompetent individuals.[2] The gold standard is culture of cerebrospinal fluid, blood, or other source.

Specimen Serum or cerebrospinal fluid

Container Red top tube, sterile CSF tube

Reference Interval Negative

Critical Values Initial positive results are phoned immediately to the physician.

Use Diagnose subacute or chronic meningitis, particularly in immunosuppressed patients; rapid diagnosis of cryptococcal meningitis; monitor response of cryptococcal meningitis to therapy. The test for cryptococcal polysaccharide capsular antigen is second only to culture.

Limitations False positives and false negatives occur. Lack of standardization between manufacturers exists; thus, titers from different kits are not comparable. False-positive results may be seen in patients with *Capnocytophaga canimorsus* and disseminated *Trichosporon beigelii* infections. False-positive reactions usually have a titer ≤1:8.

Methodology Latex agglutination (LA) with rheumatoid factor control and in some laboratories pronase pretreatment

Additional Information Serum and CSF are positive in at least 90% of patients with cryptococcal meningitis. Serum and CSF are much less likely to have positive results in cryptococcosis beyond the CNS.[1] Cryptococcal antigen assays are very sensitive and may detect cryptococcal infection in culture-negative patients. Testing for cryptococcal antigen on other body fluids (eg, bronchoalveolar lavage fluid) is not standard and has been shown to be less sensitive when compared with culture.[3] Dismukes notes that in subjects with pleural effusions, fluid may test positive, obviating a more invasive approach.[4] Most commercially available kits employ controls for nonspecific agglutination by rheumatoid factor. Treatment of serum specimens with pronase may improve test results.

Cryptococcosis may be cultured from CSF, blood, and other sources. It causes meningitis; pulmonary, pleural, pericardial, skin, and bone lesions; and affects other organs as well (eg, prostate).

Footnotes

1. Aberg JA, Mundy LM and Powderly WG, "Pulmonary Cryptococcosis in Patients Without HIV Infection," *Chest*, 1999, 115(3):734-40.
2. Shih C, Chen Y, Chang S, et al, "Cryptococcal Meningitis in Non-HIV-Infected Patients," *QJM*, 2000, 93(4):245-51.
3. Kralovic SM and Rhodes JC, "Utility of Routine Testing of Bronchoalveolar Lavage Fluid for Cryptococcal Antigen," *J Clin Microbiol*, 1998, 36(10):3088-9.
4. Dismukes WE, "Cryptococcosis," *Cecil Textbook of Medicine*, 21st ed, Chapter 398, Goldman L and Bennett JC, eds, Philadelphia, PA: WB Saunders Co, 2000, 1867-70.

References

Abadi J, Nachman S, Kressel AB, et al, "Cryptococcosis in Children With AIDS," *Clin Infect Dis*, 1999, 28(2):309-13.

Hajjeh RA, Conn LA, Stephens DS, et al, "Cryptococcosis: Population-Based Multistate Active Surveillance and Risk Factors in Human Immunodeficiency Virus-Infected Persons. Cryptococcal Active Surveillance Group," *J Infect Dis*, 1999, 179(2):449-54.

Jaye DL, Waites KB, Parker B, et al, "Comparison of Two Rapid Latex Agglutination Tests for Detection of Cryptococcal Capsular Polysaccharide," *Am J Clin Pathol*, 1998, 109(5):634-41.

Lai KK and Rosenberg AE, "A 55-Year-Old Man With a Destructive Bone Lesion 17 Months After Liver Transplantation," Case Records of the Massachusetts General Hospital, Case 19-1999, Scully RE, Mark EJ, McNeely WF, et al, eds, *N Engl J Med*, 1999, 340(25):1981-8.

Lu CH, Chang WN, Chang HW, et al, "The Prognostic Factors of Cryptococcal Meningitis in HIV-Negative Patients," *J Hosp Infect*, 1999, 42(4):313-20.

Nosanchuk JD, Shoham S, Fries BC, et al, "Evidence of Zoonotic Transmission of Cryptococcus neoformans From a Pet Cockatoo to an Immunocompromised Patient," *Ann Intern Med*, 2000, 132(3):205-8.

Oursler KA, Moore RD and Chaisson RE, "Risk Factors for Cryptococcal Meningitis in HIV-Infected Patients," *AIDS Res Hum Retroviruses*, 1999, 15(7):625-31.

Saag MS, Graybill RJ, Larsen RA, et al, "Practice Guidelines for the Management of Cryptococcal Disease. Infectious Diseases Society of America," *Clin Infect Dis*, 2000, 30(4):710-8.

Speed B and Dunt D, "Clinical and Host Differences Between Infections With the Two Varieties of *Cryptococcus neoformans*," *Clin Infect Dis*, 1995, 21(1):28-34.

Thomas CJ, Lee JY, Conn LA, et al, "Surveillance of Cryptococcosis in Alabama, 1992-1994," *Ann Epidemiol*, 1998, 8(4):212-6.

Internet Web Sites

www.cdc.gov/ncidod/dbmd/diseaseinfo/cryptococcosis_a.htm

♦ *Cryptosporidium* **Acid-Fast Stain** *see* Acid-Fast Stain, Modified, Parasites *on page 551*

♦ *Cryptosporidium* **Antigen Assay** *see Cryptosporidium* Antigen Detection by EIA *on page 596*

Cryptosporidium Antigen Detection by EIA

Related Information

Acid-Fast Stain, Modified, Parasites *on page 551*
Bacterial Culture, Stool *on page 575*
Cryptosporidium Direct Staining Procedures *on page 596*
Fungus Smear, Stain *on page 615*
Giardia lamblia Antigen Detection *on page 616*
Microsporidia Diagnostic Procedures *on page 652*
Ova and Parasites, Stool *on page 666*

Synonyms *Cryptosporidium* Antigen Assay

Applies to Enzyme Immunoassay, *Cryptosporidium*

Test Includes Direct detection of cryptosporidial antigens in stool specimens

Abstract Human infections caused by the intracellular *Coccidia* parasites, including *Cryptosporidium parvum*, are manifest as diarrhea in both normal and immunocompromised subjects. Symptoms generally begin 2-10 days after exposure and usually last 2 weeks. Disease in immunocompromised individuals is more severe and prolonged. *Cryptosporidium* infection is sometimes the cause of traveler's diarrhea.[1]

Specimen Fresh stool; stool preserved with 10% buffered formalin

Reference Interval Negative for *Cryptosporidium* antigen

Use Establish the diagnosis of cryptosporidiosis; a part of the differential work-up of diarrhea. Cryptosporidiosis is a known cause of severe and chronic diarrhea in immunocompromised patients and has also been associated with food-borne and water-borne outbreaks of disease.

Limitations Test must be specifically requested. Although some assays will simultaneously detect *Giardia lamblia* antigen as well as *Cryptosporidium*, they will not detect other causes of diarrhea. Most commercial assays have high specificity (98% - 100%) and sensitivity (76% - 98%).[2,3]

Methodology Enzyme immunoassay (EIA), direct immunofluorescent antibodies

Additional Information *Cryptosporidium* is a coccidian parasite that can live in the intestines of many animals, including humans. The parasite is able to survive outside the body for long periods of time and is very resistant to chlorine disinfection.

HIV-infected patients with CD4 counts ≤50/mm^3 are especially at risk when exposed to *Cryptosporidium*. Most therapeutic regimens for cryptosporidiosis are not successful unless immunosuppression is reversed. In HIV-positive patients, the prognosis of *C. parvum* correlates with CD4 cell counts; the disease is self-limited when CD4 counts exceed 80/mm^3.

Footnotes

1. Jelinek T, Lotze M, Eichenlaub S, et al, "Prevalence of Infection With *Cryptosporidium parvum* and *Cyclospora cayetanensis* Among International Travellers," *Gut*, 1997, 41(6):801-4.
2. Dagan R, Fraser D, El-On J, et al, "Evaluation of an Enzyme Immunoassay for the Detection of *Cryptosporidium* spp in Stool Specimens From Infants and Young Children in Field Studies," *Am J Trop Med Hyg*, 1995, 52(2):134-8.
3. Chan R, Chen J, York MK, et al, "Evaluation of a Combination Rapid Immunoassay for Detection of *Giardia* and *Cryptosporidium* Antigens," *J Clin Microbiol*, 2000, 38(1):393-4.

References

Clark DP, "New Insights Into Human Cryptosporidiosis," *Clin Microbiol Rev*, 1999, 12(4):554-63.

Clayton F, Heller T, and Kotler DP, "Variation in the Enteric Distribution of Cryptosporidia in Acquired Immunodeficiency Syndrome," *Am J Clin Pathol*, 1994, 102(4):420-5.

Current WL and Garcia LS, "Cryptosporidiosis," *Clin Microbiol Rev*, 1991, 4(3):325-58.

Goldstein ST, Juranek DD, Ravenholt O, et al, "Cryptosporidiosis: An Outbreak Associated With Drinking Water Despite State-of-the-Art Water Treatment," *Ann Intern Med*, 1996, 124(5):459-68.

Ignatius R, Eisenblatter M, Regnath T, et al, "Efficacy of Different Methods for Detection of Low *Cryptosporidium parvum* Oocyst Numbers or Antigen Concentrations in Stool Specimens," *Eur J Clin Microbiol Infect Dis*, 1997, 16(10):732-6.

Mackenzie WR, Hoxie NJ, Proctor ME, et al, "A Massive Outbreak in Milwaukee of Cryptosporidium Infection Transmitted Through the Public Water Supply," *N Engl J Med*, 1994, 331(3):161-7.

Marsh WW, "Infectious Diseases of Gastrointestinal Tract in Adolescents," *Adolesc Med*, 2000, 11(2):263-78.

Nichols GL, "Food-Borne Protozoa," *Br Med Bull*, 2000, 56(1):209-35.

Petersen C, "Cryptosporidiosis in Patients Infected With the Human Immunodeficiency Virus," *Clin Infect Dis*, 1992, 15(6):903-9.

Xiao L, Morgan UM, Fayer R, et al, "*Cryptosporidium* Systematics and Implications for Public Health," *Parasitol Today*, 2000, 16(7):287-92.

Internet Web Sites

www.cdc.gov/ncidod/dpd/parasites/cryptosporidiosis/

Cryptosporidium Direct Staining Procedures

Related Information

Acid-Fast Stain, Modified, *Nocardia* Species *on page 550*
Acid-Fast Stain, Modified, Parasites *on page 551*
Bacterial Culture, Stool *on page 575*
Cryptosporidium Antigen Detection by EIA *on page 596*
Fecal Lactoferrin *on page 308*
Fungus Smear, Stain *on page 615*

Methylene Blue Stain, Stool *on page 313*
Microsporidia Diagnostic Procedures *on page 652*
Ova and Parasites, Stool *on page 666*
Polymerase Chain Reaction *on page 713*

Synonyms *Coccidia*; Stool Examination for *Cryptosporidium*

Applies to Acid-Fast Stain, Modified, *Cryptosporidium*; *Cryptosporidium parvum*; *Cyclospora cayetanensis*; *Isospora belli*; *S. bovihominis*; *S. suihominis*

Test Includes Examination of stool for the presence of *Cryptosporidium* by phase contrast microscopy, modified acid-fast stain, or fluorescent-labeled antibody

Abstract Human infections caused by the intracellular *Coccidia* parasites, including **Cryptosporidium parvum**, are manifest as diarrhea in both normal and immunocompromised subjects. In humans, *Cryptosporidium* can be an enteric pathogen in all age groups, but disease in immunocompromised individuals is more severe and prolonged. AIDS cholangiopathy, characterized by right upper quadrant pain, cholestasis, low-grade fever, and biliary dilatation or papillary stenosis, is caused by *Cryptosporidia, M. avium* complex, CMV, or *Microsporidia*.[1] Methods that utilize modified acid-fast stain or fluorescent antibody are frequently employed in the clinical laboratory, because routine ova and parasite examination will not detect these organisms.

Specimen Fresh stool; stool preserved with 10% formalin or sodium acetate-acetic acid formalin preservative

Reference Interval Negative

Use Establish the diagnosis of cryptosporidiosis by demonstration of the oocysts; can be used as part of the differential work-up of diarrhea, particularly in immunocompromised hosts and suspected AIDS patients. Cryptosporidiasis has been detected in public water supplies and in foodborne outbreaks.[2]

Limitations *Cryptosporidium* is not detected by standard methods used to examine stool specimens for other ova and parasites; special stains are required for its detection, and in many laboratories, *Cryptosporidium* examination must be specifically requested. The organisms are most readily demonstrated in watery diarrheal stools. A single stool specimen may not be sufficient to make the diagnosis, especially if the organisms are present in small numbers.[3] Forms of *Blastocystis hominis* may cause confusion if Giemsa stain is used. Most recommended procedures cannot be performed on polyvinyl alcohol (PVA) preserved specimens.

Methodology Phase contrast microscopy after floatation or sedimentation concentration techniques; modified acid-fast stain on air-dried, methanol-fixed smears (decolorization with 1% H_2SO_4). An acid-fast-trichrome stain is described.[4] A technique utilizing formalin-ethyl acetate and floatation over hypertonic saline is reported to enhance detection of *Cryptosporidium* oocysts.[5] Fluorescent-labeled anti-*Cryptosporidium* antibodies are commercially available and provide excellent sensitivity and specificity.[6]

Additional Information *Cryptosporidium parvum* is a cause of severe and chronic diarrhea in patients with hypogammaglobulinemia and the acquired immune deficiency syndrome.[7] HIV-infected patients with CD4 counts ≤50/mm^3 are especially at risk when exposed to *Cryptosporidium*. Although the organism is widely recognized as a disease of the immunocompromised patient, it can also cause disease in immunocompetent subjects. Animal contact, travel to endemic areas, living in a rural environment, day care attendance by toddlers, and exposure to contaminated public water are recognized as risk factors for the development of cryptosporidiosis.[8,9] A seasonal variation in incidence exists with the highest frequency reported in summer and autumn.

A variety of diagnostic tests are available for detection of *Cryptosporidium* directly in stool specimens. The assays used may be based on the cost of the test and the experience of the technical staff. Modified acid-fast staining provides a relatively lower cost than enzyme immunoassays and immunofluorescent antibody detection.

Footnotes

1. Liberman E and Benedict Yen TS, "Foamy Macrophages in Acquired Immunodeficiency Syndrome Cholangiopathy With *Encephalitozoon intestinalis*," *Arch Pathol Lab Med*, 1997, 121(9):985-88.
2. "Food-Borne Outbreak of Cryptosporidiosis - Spokane, Washington, 1997," Centers for Disease Control and Prevention, *JAMA*, 1998, 280(7):595-6.
3. Ortega YR, "*Cryptosporidium, Cyclospora*, and *Isospora*," *Manual of Clinical Microbiology*, 7th ed, Murray PR, Baron EJ, Pfaller MA, et al, eds, Washington, DC: AMS Press, American Society for Microbiology, 1999, 1406-12.
4. Reisner BS and Spring J, "Evaluation of a Combined Acid-Fast-Trichrome Stain for Detection of Microsporidia and *Cryptosporidium parvum*," *Arch Pathol Lab Med*, 2000 124(5):777-9.
5. Weber R, Bryan RT, and Juranek DD, "Improved Stool Concentration Procedure for Detection of *Cryptosporidium* Oocysts in Fecal Specimens," *J Clin Microbiol*, 1992, 30(11):2869-73.
6. Garcia LS, Shum AC, and Bruckner DA, "Evaluation of a New Monoclonal Antibody Combination Reagent for Direct Fluorescence Detection of *Giardia* Cysts and *Cryptosporidium* Oocysts in Human Fecal Specimens," *J Clin Microbiol*, 1992, 30(12):3255-7.
7. Clark DP, "New Insights Into Human Cryptosporidiosis," *Clin Microbiol Rev*, 1999, 12(4):554-63.
8. Vakil NB, Schwartz SM, Buggy BP, et al, "Biliary Cryptosporidiosis in HIV-Infected People After the Water-Borne Outbreak of Cryptosporidiosis in Milwaukee," *N Engl J Med*, 1996, 334(1):19-23.

9. Mackenzie WR, Hoxie NJ, Proctor ME, et al, "A Massive Outbreak in Milwaukee of *Cryptosporidium* Infection Transmitted Through the Public Water Supply," *N Engl J Med*, 1994, 331(3):161-7.

References

Ignatius R, Eisenblatter M, Regnath T, et al, "Efficacy of Different Methods for Detection of Low *Cryptosporidium parvum* Oocyst Numbers or Antigen Concentrations in Stool Specimens," *Eur J Clin Microbiol Infect Dis*, 1997, 16(10):732-6.
Marsh WW, "Infectious Diseases of Gastrointestinal Tract in Adolescents," *Adolesc Med*, 2000, 11(2):263-78.
Nichols GI, "Food-Borne Protozoa," *Br Med Bull*, 2000, 56(1):209-35.
Petersen C, "Cryptosporidiosis in Patients Infected With the Human Immunodeficiency Virus," *Clin Infect Dis*, 1992, 15(6): 903-9.
Xiao L, Moregan UM, Fayer R, et al, "*Cryptosporidium* Systematics and Implications for Public Health," *Parastiol Today*, 2000, 16(7):287-92.

Internet Web Sites

www.cdc.gov/ncidod/dpd/parasites/cryptosporidiosis/

♦ **Cryptosporidium parvum** *see Cryptosporidium Direct Staining Procedures on page 596*

♦ **Crystal Violet** *see Gram Stain on page 617*

♦ **CSF Culture** *see Bacterial Culture, Cerebrospinal Fluid on page 569*

♦ **CSF Fungus Culture** *see Fungal Culture, Cerebrospinal Fluid on page 611*

♦ **CSF Mycobacteria Culture** *see Mycobacterial Culture, Cerebrospinal Fluid on page 656*

♦ **CSF VDRL** *see VDRL, Cerebrospinal Fluid on page 688*

♦ **CT Guided Needle Aspiration Culture** *see Fine Needle Aspiration Culture on page 609*

♦ **Culture, Blood** *see Bacterial Culture, Blood on page 566*

♦ **Culture, Cerebrospinal Fluid** *see Bacterial Culture, Cerebrospinal Fluid on page 569*

♦ **Culture, Ear** *see Bacterial Culture, Middle Ear on page 573*

♦ **Culture for Borrelia burgdorferi** *see Borrelia burgdorferi Culture on page 585*

♦ **Culture for Cat Scratch Bacteria** *see Bartonella Culture on page 580*

♦ **Cyclospora Acid-Fast Stain** *see Acid-Fast Stain, Modified, Parasites on page 551*

♦ **Cyclospora cayetanensis** *see Cryptosporidium Direct Staining Procedures on page 596*

♦ **Cyclospora Species** *see Ova and Parasites, Stool on page 666*

♦ **Cyclosporiasis Detection** *see Acid-Fast Stain, Modified, Parasites on page 551*

Cysticercosis Serology

Related Information
Ova and Parasites, Stool *on page 666*

Applies to *Taenia solium*

Abstract Cysticercosis may be the most frequent cause of symptomatic epilepsy on the globe.[1] Eggs of *Taenia solium*, the pork tapeworm acquired from contact with contaminated feces, lead to cysticercosis. Cysticercosis, larval forms in tissues, is endemic in Mexico, portions of South America, Africa, and Asia. Neurocysticercosis is the term used for involvement of *T. solium* cysts in the central nervous system.

T. solium is the only tapeworm for which humans are the intermediate host (harboring larval forms) and the definitive host (harboring the adult tapeworm). The human ingests oncospheres (embryos) which are absorbed, then embolize to striated muscle, eyes, and the central nervous system, becoming cysticerci.

Specimen Serum, cerebrospinal fluid

Container Red top tube

Reference Interval Negative

Use Confirm the diagnosis of cysticercosis. Diagnosis is usually established on the basis of clinical presentation and imaging.

Limitations Cross reactions in patients with tapeworm or *Echinococcus* were found before immunoblotting techniques became available. Sensitivity remains limited when there is low parasite burden (ie, false negatives occur). Studies have shown that only 28% of patients with a single parenchymal lesion will have a positive serologic test.[2] The CDC immunoblot is more specific and sensitive than enzyme immunoassay (EIA). The CDC immunoblot is the immunodiagnostic test of choice for confirmation of a clinical or radiologic diagnosis of neurocysticercosis.[2]

Methodology Immunoblotting, enzyme-linked immunosorbent assay (ELISA). The most accurate test is the enzyme-linked immunotransfer blot.[1]

Additional Information Ingestion of eggs of the pork tapeworm (*Taenia solium*) produces cysticercosis, an infection in which larval cysts (cysticerci) are seen in various tissues. Cysticercosis is most commonly found in brain or muscle, in which a space-occupying mass presents with local inflammatory reaction. Serious CNS involvement is often characterized as intracerebral lesions causing mass effects, seizures, or both.[2] The CNS is involved in (Continued)

Cysticercosis Serology (Continued)

90% of patients: CSF pleocytosis is found with increased CSF protein and decreased glucose.

Water or food may become contaminated with eggs, especially in areas in which water purification systems are inadequate. Recently, the number of cases of cysticercosis has increased in the U.S., likely due to increased levels of immigration from Latin America.[2,3] Pigs are intermediate hosts, thus, completion of the parasitic life cycle occurs in regions in which humans live close to pigs and eat pig meat in their diet. Human cysticercosis is acquired by ingestion of *T. solium* eggs from the feces of a *T. solium* carrier, and can occur in patients who do not eat pig meat. Commonly, transmission takes place through consumption of fruits and vegetables that are grown in soil fertilized with contaminated porcine or human waste.[1]

Footnotes

1. Bromfield EB and Vonsattel JP, "A 23-Year-Old Man With Seizures and a Lesion in the Left Temporal Lobe," Case Records of the Massachusetts General Hospital, Case 24-2000, Scully RE, Mark EJ, McNeely WF, et al, *N Engl J Med*, 2000, 343(6):420-7.
2. White AC, "Neurocysticercosis: Updates on Epidemiology, Pathogenesis, Diagnosis, and Management," *Ann Rev Med*, 2000, 51:187-206.
3. Garcia HH and Del Brutto OH, "*Taenia solium* Cysticercosis," *Infect Dis Clin North Am*, 2000, 14(1):97-119.

References

da Silva AD, Quagliato EM and Rossi CL, "A Quantitative Enzyme-Linked Immunosorbent Assay (ELISA) for the Immunodiagnosis of Neurocysticercosis Using a Purified Fraction from *Taenia solium* cysticerci," *Diagn Microbiol Infect Dis*, 2000, 37(2):87-92.

Del Brutto OH, Dolezal M, Castillo PR, et al, "Neurocysticercosis and Oncogenesis," *Arch Med Res*, 2000, 31(2):151-5.

Katti MK, "Assessment of Specificity of a Recombinant 10-kDa Protein Antigen in Differential Diagnosis of Neurocysticercosis," *J Infect Dis*, 2000, 181(5):1870-2.

Ohsaki Y, Matsumoto A, Miyamoto K, et al, "Neurocysticercosis Without Detectable Specific Antibody," *Intern Med*, 1999, 38(1):67-70.

Sotelo J and Del Brutto OH, "Brain Cysticercosis," *Arch Med Res*, 2000, 31(3):3-14.

Wilkins PP, Allan JC, Verastegui M, et al, "Development of a Serologic Assay to Detect *Taenia solium* taeniasis," *Am J Trop Med Hyg*, 1999, 60(2):199-204.

♦ **Cytomegalic Inclusion Virus Titer** see Cytomegalovirus Serology on page 600

Cytomegalovirus Antigen Detection

Related Information

Cytomegalovirus Culture *on page 598*
Cytomegalovirus Cytology *on page 380*
Cytomegalovirus Nucleic Acid Detection *on page 599*
Cytomegalovirus Serology *on page 600*
Virus, Direct Detection by Fluorescent Antibody *on page 696*

Synonyms CMV Antigen Detection; CMV pp65 Detection

Test Includes Detection of CMV antigens in white blood cells

Abstract Active human cytomegalovirus (CMV) infection can be detected by monitoring the presence of the CMV matrix protein (pp65) in peripheral blood leukocytes. The CMV antigenemia assay has been used to quantitate the amount of active CMV in immunocompromised patients who are a high risk for severe CMV infections.[1,2] This assay has been shown to be sensitive and specific for active CMV replication.[2,3]

Specimen Whole blood

Container Green top (heparin) tube, blue top (sodium citrate) tube, acid citrate dextrose or lavender top (EDTA) tube

Collection Transport to laboratory at room temperature within 2 hours of collection. Process specimen within 6 hours of collection.

Storage Instructions Keep at 4°C; do not freeze.

Use Early diagnosis and monitoring of CMV infection in immunocompromised patients

Limitations Labor-intensive; time-consuming due to isolation and counting of white blood cells; microscopist must be well-trained to detect positive cells; a minimum of 50,000 cells should be available on the slide in order to determine a negative result. The assay is not standardized between laboratories. CMV may be present for a time following acute infections. Some patients with CMV antigenemia are asymptomatic. Specimen must be processed quickly (within 6 hours) to detect viral antigen and, thus, the specimen should not be collected during laboratory off-hours.

Methodology Immunocytochemical detection of CMV antigen (lower-matrix phosphoprotein, pp65) in nuclei of peripheral blood mononuclear cells. A recent study used flow cytometry for detection of CMV antigen in leukocytes.[4]

Additional Information The detection of CMV antigen directly in the peripheral blood leukocytes has been proven to be a clinically relevant marker of CMV infection. It currently has widespread use as a clinical tool in the diagnosis and management of CMV infection in immunocompromised patients. It has been compared to viral culture methods and shown to be sensitive (76% to 88%) and specific (99% to 100%). The major disadvantage of the assay are the time-consuming methods, but a recent rapid assay has been introduced that can be completed in approximately 2 hours and requires only 2 mL of blood.[5,6] Another disadvantage of the assay is the

lack of standardization, however, standardization is currently being introduced in an attempt to improve predictability of test results.[7]

Active CMV infection can also be detected by DNA/RNA amplification methods from plasma, serum, and white blood cells, as well as other specimens (eg, CSF, for neurologic syndromes in AIDS patients and others). See Related Information at the beginning of this listing for further tests relevant to CMV.

Footnotes

1. Blank BS, Meenhorst PL, Weverling GJ, et al, "Quantitative pp65-Antigenemia Assay for the Prediction of Human Cytomegalovirus Disease in HIV-Infected Patients," *AIDS*, 1999, 13(18):2533-9.
2. Schirm J, Kooistra A, van Son WJ, et al, "Comparison of the Murex Hybrid Capture CMV DNA (v2.0) Assay and the pp65 CMV Antigenemia Test for the Detection and Quantitation of CMV in Blood Samples from Immunocompromised Patients," *J Clin Virol*, 1999, 14(3):153-65.
3. Weinberg A, Hodges TN, Li S, et al, "Comparison of PCR, Antigenemia Assay, and Rapid Blood Culture for Detection and Prevention of Cytomegalovirus Disease After Lung Transplantation," *J Clin Microbiol*, 2000, 38(2):768-72.
4. Essa S, Pacsa AS, Al-Attiyah R, et al, "The Use of Flow Cytometry for the Detection of CMV-Specific Antigen (pp65) in Leukocytes of Kidney Recipients," *Clin Transplant*, 2000, 14(2):147-51.
5. Visser CE, van Zeijl CJ, de Klerk EP, et al, "First Experiences With an Accelerated CMV Antigenemia Test: CMV Brite Turbo Assay," *J Clin Virol*, 2000, 17(1):65-8.
6. Landry ML and Ferguson D, "2-Hour Cytomegalovirus pp65 Antigenemia Assay for Rapid Quantitation of Cytomegalovirus in Blood Samples," *J Clin Microbiol*, 2000, 38(1):427-8.
7. Verschuuren EA, Harmsen MC, Limburg PC, et al, "Towards Standardization of the Human Cytomegalovirus Antigenemia Assay," *Intervirology*, 1999, 42(5-6):382-9.

References

Caliendo AM, St George K, Kao SY, et al, "Comparison of Quantitative Cytomegalovirus (CMV) PCR in Plasma and CMV Antigenemia Assay: Clinical Utility of the Prototype Amplicor CMV Monitor Test in Transplant Recipients," *J Clin Microbiol*, 2000, 38(6):2122-7.

Chiaramonte S, Pellizzer G, Rassu M, et al, "Role of Antigenemia Assay in the Early Diagnosis and Treatment of CMV Infection in Renal Transplant Patients," *Clin Nephrol*, 2000, 53(4):10-2.

Durlik M, Siennicka J, Litwinska B, et al, "Comparison of Antigenemia (pp65) Assay and Polymerase Chain Reaction in Diagnosis of Cytomegalovirus Infection in Renal Transplant Recipients Treated With ATG," *Transplant Proc*, 2000, 32(6):1350-2.

Goosen VJ, Blok MJ, Christiaans MH, et al, "Early Detection of Cytomegalovirus in Renal Transplant Recipients: Comparison of PCR, NASBA, pp65 Antigenemia, and Viral Culture," *Transplant Proc*, 2000, 32(1):155-8.

Osarogiagbon RU, Defor TE, Weisdorf MA, et al, "CMV Antigenemia Following Bone Marrow Transplantation: Risk Factors and Outcomes," *Biol Blood Marrow Transplant*, 2000, 6(3):280-8.

Rayes N, Oettle H, Schmidt CA, et al, "Preemptive Therapy in CMV-Antigen Positive Patients After Liver Transplantation - A Prospective Trial," *Ann Transplant*, 1999, 4(2):12-7.

Singh N, Paterson DL, Gayowski T, et al, "Cytomegalovirus Antigenemia Directed Preemptive Prophylaxis With Oral Versus I.V. Ganciclovir for the Prevention of Cytomegalovirus Disease in Liver Transplant Recipients: A Randomized, Controlled Trial," *Transplantation*, 2000, 70(5):717-22.

St George K, Boyd MJ, Lipson SM, et al, "A Multisite Trial Comparing Two Cytomegalovirus (CMV) pp65 Antigenemia Test Kits, Biotest CMV Brite and Bartels/Argene CMV Antigenemia," *J Clin Microbiol*, 2000, 38(4):1430-3.

Weill D and Zamora MR, "Comparison of the Efficacy and Cost-Effectiveness of Preemptive Therapy as Directed by CMV Antigenemia and Prophylaxis With Ganciclovir in Lung Transplant Recipients," *J Heart Lung Transplant*, 2000, 19(8):815-6.

Internet Web Sites

www.cdc.gov/ncidod/diseases/cmv.htm

Cytomegalovirus Culture

Related Information

Bronchoalveolar Lavage (BAL) *on page 375*
Cervical/Vaginal Cytology *on page 377*
Cytomegalovirus Antigen Detection *on page 598*
Cytomegalovirus Cytology *on page 380*
Cytomegalovirus Nucleic Acid Detection *on page 599*
Cytomegalovirus Serology *on page 600*
Sputum Cytology *on page 387*
Urinary Tract Cytology *on page 389*
Viral Culture *on page 689*
Viral Culture, Blood *on page 691*
Viral Culture, Urine *on page 695*
Virus, Direct Detection by Fluorescent Antibody *on page 696*

Synonyms CMV Culture; CMV Rapid Culture; CMV Shell Vial Culture; Viral Culture, Cytomegalovirus

Test Includes Shell vial culture will detect CMV only using specific immunofluorescence; CMV is usually detected in a routine virus culture

Abstract Cytomegalovirus (CMV) is an ubiquitous herpes virus which infects 50% to 85% of the adult population, usually asymptomatically. CMV infection is a major problem in immunocompromised patients. CMV is the virus most frequently transmitted to an unborn child. Transmission of CMV to neonates is associated with serious fulminant disease consisting of jaundice, hepatosplenomegaly, and multiorgan involvement. It may be fatal.

Infectious CMV can be shed in body fluids of any previously infected person and, thus, the virus can be isolated from urine, saliva, blood, semen and breast milk. The virus can be shed asymptomatically from individuals infected with CMV, therefore, culture should be performed only in patients at high risk for severe CMV disease.

Specimen Urine, throat, bronchoalveolar lavage, bronchial washings, lung biopsy, whole blood, amniotic fluid

Container Cold viral transport medium for swabs

Collection Urine: A first morning clean catch urine should be submitted in a sterile screw-cap container.

Throat: Rotate swab in both tonsillar crypts and against posterior oropharynx. Place swab in tube of viral transport medium, break off end of swab and tighten cap.

Blood: Collect in a green top Vacutainer® tube containing free heparin.

Storage Instructions Do not freeze. Specimens should be delivered to the laboratory immediately. If freezing is absolutely necessary, most specimens can be frozen by adding an equal amount of 0.4M sucrose-phosphate to the specimen before freezing. White blood cells should be isolated from blood specimens before freezing.

Causes for Rejection Dry specimen, specimen not refrigerated during transport, specimen fixed in formalin

Turnaround Time Variable (1-14 days); negative routine viral cultures are usually not reported for 28 days; CMV rapid culture: 1-3 days

Reference Interval No virus isolated

Use Aid in the diagnosis of disease caused by CMV

Limitations Rapid culture method will only detect specified virus(es); negative culture does not rule out viral infection. CSF cultures are negative in encephalitis and in subjects with AIDS, and are insensitive with CMV myelitis/polyradiculopathy and with ventriculitis in AIDS. CMV culture may be positive in the absence of obvious clinical disease.

Methodology Routine culture detects CMV by cytopathic effect; rapid shell vial specifically detects CMV early viral antigen with immunofluorescence

Additional Information CMV infections are very common in normal individuals and are usually asymptomatic. However, CMV infections are frequently severe and life-threatening in immunocompromised patients, including organ recipients and AIDS patients. CMV is the major viral pathogen following renal transplantation. Blood cultures positive for CMV predict progression. Detection of CMV infection is of utmost importance so that ganciclovir can be started as soon as possible. Culture is not as sensitive as CMV antigen detection or CMV nucleic acid detection, but has high specificity (90% to 73%) when following immunocompromised patients.[1,2]

CMV is the most frequent cause of congenital viral infections in humans and occurs in about 1% of all newborns. CMV can be cultured from amniotic fluid or urine specimens of the newborn.[3] Approximately 90% have no clinical symptoms at birth. Ten percent to 20% of these infants will develop complications before school age. Congenital infection may occur as a result of either primary or recurrent maternal infection. When HIV-infected infants acquire CMV infection in the first 18 months of life, a higher rate of disease progression and central nervous system disease is reported, compared to those infected only with HIV-1.[4]

The rapid shell vial method for detection of CMV was first reported in the early 1980s and has been shown to be more sensitive than and as specific as conventional tube cell culture.[5] Several modifications of the shell vial method have been reported to enhance sensitivity.[6]

Active CMV infection can also be detected by DNA/RNA amplification methods from plasma, serum, and white blood cells, as well as other specimens (eg, CSF, for neurologic syndromes in AIDS patients and others). Specific CMV antigen is also used to detect and monitor active CMV infection. See Related Information at the beginning of this listing for further tests relevant to CMV.

Footnotes
1. Blank BS, Meenhorst PL, Weverling GJ, et al, "Quantitative pp65-Antigenemia Assay for the Prediction of Human Cytomegalovirus Disease in HIV-Infected Patients," *AIDS*, 1999, 13(18):2533-9.
2. Witt DJ, Kemper M, Stead A, et al, "Analytical Performance and Clinical Utility of a Nucleic Acid Sequence-Based Amplification Assay for Detection of Cytomegalovirus Infection," *J Clin Microbiol*, 2000, 38(11):3994-9.
3. Lazzarotto T, Varani S, Guerra B, et al, "Prenatal Indicators of Congenital Cytomegalovirus Infection," *J Pediatr*, 2000, 137(1):90-5.
4. Kovacs A, Schluchter M, Easley K, et al, "Cytomegalovirus Infection and HIV-1 Disease Progression in Infants Born to HIV-1-Infected Women," *N Engl J Med*, 1999, 341(2):77-84.
5. Gleaves CA, Smith TF, Shuster EA, et al, "Comparison of Standard Tube and Shell Vial Cell Culture Techniques for the Detection of Cytomegalovirus in Clinical Specimens," *J Clin Microbiol*, 1985, 21(2):217-21.
6. Li SB and Fong CK, "Detection of Human Cytomegalovirus Early and Late Antigen and DNA Production in Cell Culture and the Effects of Dimethyl Sulfoxide, Dexamethasone, and DNA Inhibitors on Early Antigen Induction," *J Med Virol*, 1990, 30(2):97-102.

References
Demmler GJ, Istas A, Easley KA, et al, "Results of a Quality Assurance Program for Detection of Cytomegalovirus Infection in the Pediatric Pulmonary and Cardiovascular Complications of Vertically Transmitted Human Immunodeficiency Virus Infection Study," *J Clin Microbiol*, 2000, 38(11):3942-5.
Halwachs-Baumann G, Genser B, Danda M, et al, "Screening and Diagnosis of Congenital Cytomegalovirus Infection: A 5-Year Study," *Scand J Infect Dis*, 2000, 32(2):137-42.
Schafer P, Tenschert W, Cremaschi L, et al, "Cytomegalovirus Cultured From Different Major Leukocyte Subpopulations: Association With Clinical Features in CMV Immunoglobulin G-Positive Renal Allograft Recipients," *J Med Virol*, 2000, 61(4):488-96.
Warren WP, Balcarek K, Smith R, et al, "Comparison of Rapid Methods of Detection of Cytomegalovirus in Saliva With Virus Isolation in Tissue Culture," *J Clin Microbiol*, 1992, 30:786-9.

Internet Web Sites
www.cdc.gov/ncidod/diseases/cmv.htm

Cytomegalovirus Nucleic Acid Detection

Related Information
Bronchoalveolar Lavage (BAL) *on page 375*
Cytomegalovirus Antigen Detection *on page 598*
Cytomegalovirus Culture *on page 598*
Cytomegalovirus Cytology *on page 380*
Cytomegalovirus Serology *on page 600*

Synonyms Amplicor® CMV Monitor; CMV DNA Detection; CMV Quantitation; CMV Quantitative PCR; Molecular Assay for CMV Detection; NucliSens CMV pp67

Test Includes Direct detection of cytomegalovirus nucleic acid in white blood cells, plasma, serum, urine, tissue, CSF, and bronchial alveolar lavage fluid. CMV nucleic acid may also be quantitated to determine or evaluate risk of disease or to monitor disease progress.

Abstract Infection with cytomegalovirus (CMV) in the nonimmunosuppressed host is typically asymptomatic or limited to a mononucleosis-like syndrome with fever, pharyngitis, and lymphadenitis. However, CMV disease is a major risk for immunosuppressed individuals. The number of patients who are immunosuppressed as result of therapeutic intervention (bone marrow transplant, solid organ transplant, and/or cancer chemotherapy) has greatly increased in addition to the number of individuals with altered immune functions due to HIV infection. The detection of CMV disease at an early stage is critical for beginning intervention, and several different assays have been developed using culture or antigen detection techniques. Molecular assays for detection of CMV DNA involve the extraction of viral genome from a variety of sources followed by amplification using oligonucleotide primers to specific regions. A number of targets have been described, such as the polymerase gene or immediate early antigen gene. Detection of CMV DNA by amplification procedures has been shown to have a higher sensitivity than either culture techniques or the antigenemia assay.[1,2] Newer techniques have now incorporated quantitation and are useful for predicting significant risk of CMV disease.[3]

Specimen CMV DNA may be extracted from peripheral blood lymphocytes, plasma, serum, bronchoalveolar lavage fluid, urine, cerebrospinal fluid, and various tissues including lung and brain. Most of the commercial assays use plasma (EDTA or citrate dextrose) to monitor the level of CMV nucleic acid.

Container Glass or plastic containers are acceptable; anticoagulants may be used with the exception of heparin

Storage Instructions While freezing is known to reduce the viability of CMV and its isolation by culture techniques, freezing does not impair detection by amplification procedures. Any of the above fluid samples should be rapidly transported to the laboratory. However, if transportation is expected to exceed 2 hours, the sample should be refrigerated, and if transportation exceeds 8 hours, a specimen should be frozen. All tissue samples should be frozen as soon as possible after the biopsy procedure.

Causes for Rejection Collection of blood in heparinized tubes may result in inhibition of amplification.

Turnaround Time 1-3 days

Special Instructions Specimen should **not** be obtained utilizing heparin as an anticoagulant.

Reference Interval An interpretative report usually accompanies results. CMV may be excreted in urine and saliva or be present in blood without clinical symptoms.

Use The detection of CMV DNA is useful to identify patients in whom appropriate therapy could be instituted, including ganciclovir or immune globulin. Quantitative assays may be useful to establish disease risk and to monitor CMV levels after therapy.

Limitations A negative result does not rule out the presence of CMV in all tissues of the body. The cost of the test is high in comparison with culture, CMV antigenemia detection, or serology. Contamination is a risk and results in false-positive results. A variety of amplification techniques is used and results may not be interchangeable.

Methodology DNA is extracted from fluids or tissues followed by amplification using either PCR, transcription-based amplification of mRNA, or signal amplification methods. Quantitation is most frequently based on simple limiting dilution quantification or coamplification of an internal reference template with the same primer binding sequences.

Additional Information Greater than 80% of adults have been exposed to CMV as evidenced by the presence of antibodies. Although in most nonimmunosuppressed individuals infection by CMV is self-limited, one important exception is found in neonates who are infected in utero. Infection of the fetus during the early stages of pregnancy may result in multiorgan failure, CNS abnormalities or paradoxically, continuous CMV excretion in the urine without disease. Amplification methods show good specificity and sensitivity in detecting CMV from urine of infected newborns.[4]
(Continued)

Cytomegalovirus Nucleic Acid Detection
(Continued)

The development of solid organ transplantation and bone marrow or stem cell transplantation has accelerated the need for early CMV detection. When diagnosed early, CMV infection may be effectively treated with ganciclovir and/or immunoglobulin. Amplification assays for detection of CMV have been developed because of the increased sensitivity that such assays provide. The standard assays for CMV detection in the transplant setting include the shell vial assay and the CMV antigenemia assay. In comparison studies, PCR for CMV nucleic acid has shown a higher sensitivity and specificity for disease.[5,6] Quantitative CMV DNA detection assays have been used to demonstrate viral load and correlate with the progression of CMV disease, as well as response to therapy.[7,8] Another approach to improve the correlation of a positive test by PCR with CMV disease has been to use plasma rather than DNA extracted from peripheral blood lymphocytes. Commercial assays for CMV detection by nucleic acid amplification have recently become available.

Footnotes

1. Caliendo AM, St. George K, Kao SY, et al, "Comparison of Quantitative Cytomegalovirus (CMV) PCR in Plasma and CMV Antigenemia Assay: Clinical Utility of the Prototype Amplicor CMV Monitor Test in Transplant Recipients," *J Clin Microbiol*, 2000, 38(6):2122-7.
2. Goossens VJ, Blok MJ, Christiaans MH, et al, "Early Detection of Cytomegalovirus in Renal Transplant Recipients: Comparison of PCR, NASBA, pp65 Antigenemia, and Viral Culture," *Transplant Proc*, 2000, 32(1):155-8.
3. Emery VC, Cope AV, Sabin CA, et al, "Relationship Between IgM Antibody to Human Cytomegalovirus, Virus Load, Donor and Recipient Serostatus, and Administration of Methylprednisolone as Risk Factors for Cytomegalovirus Disease After Liver Transplantation," *J Infect Dis*, 2000, 182(6):1610-5.
4. Schalasta G, Eggers M, Schmid M, et al, "Analysis of Human Cytomegalovirus DNA in Urines of Newborns and Infants by Means of a New Ultrarapid Real-Time PCR-System," *J Clin Virol*, 2000, 19(3):175-85.
5. Witt DJ, Kemper M, Stead A, et al, "Analytical Performance and Clinical Utility of a Nucleic Acid Sequence-Based Amplification Assay for Detection of Cytomegalovirus Infection," *J Clin Microbiol*, 2000, 38(11):3994-9.
6. Goossens VJ, Blok MJ, Christiaans MH, et al, "Early Detection of Cytomegalovirus in Renal Transplant Recipients: Comparison of PCR, NASBA, pp65 Antigenemia, and Viral Culture," *Transplant Proc*, 2000, 32(1):155-8.
7. Lassner D, Geissler F, Bosse S, et al, "Diagnosis and Monitoring of Acute Cytomegalovirus Infection in Peripheral Blood of Transplant Recipients by Nested Reverse Transcriptase Polymerase Chain Reaction (RT-PCR)," *Transpl Int*, 2000, 13(S1):366-71.
8. Machida U, Kami M, Fukui T, et al, "Real-Time Automated PCR for Early Diagnosis and Monitoring of Cytomegalovirus Infection After Bone Marrow Transplantation," *J Clin Microbiol*, 2000, 38(7):2536-42.

References

Boeckh M and Boivin G, "Quantitation of Cytomegalovirus: Methodologic Aspects and Clinical Applications," *Clin Microbiol Rev*, 1998, 11(3):533-54.

Bowen EF, "Cytomegalovirus Reactivation in Patients Infected With HIV: The Use of Polymerase Chain Reaction in Predication and Management," *Drugs*, 1999, 57(5):735-41.

Einsele H and Hebart H, "Cytomegalovirus Infection Following Stem Cell Transplantation," *Haematologica*, 1999, 84(1):46-9.

Hodinka RL, "The Clinical Utility of Viral Quantitation Using Molecular Methods," *Clin Diagn Virol*, 1998, 10(1):25-47.

Rawlinson WD, "Broadsheet. Number 50: Diagnosis of Human Cytomegalovirus Infection and Disease," *Pathology*, 1999, 31(2):109-15.

Rimsza LM, Vela EE, Frutiger YM, et al, "Rapid Automated Combined *In Situ* Hybridization and Immunohistochemistry for Sensitive Detection of Cytomegalovirus in Paraffin-Embedded Tissue Biopsies," *Am J Clin Pathol*, 1996, 106(4):544-8.

Siennicka J, Durlik M, Litwinska B, et al, "Usefulness of Hybridization and PCR Methods in Monitoring of CMV Infection in Renal Transplant Recipients," *Ann Transplant*, 2000, 5(1):21-4.

Stocchi R, Ward KN, Fanin R, et al, "Management of Human Cytomegalovirus Infection and Disease After Allogeneic Bone Marrow Transplantation," *Haematologica*, 1999, 84(1):71-9.

Internet Web Sites

www.cdc.gov/ncidod/diseases/cmv.htm

Cytomegalovirus Serology

Related Information

Bacterial Culture, Bronchoscopy/Bronchial Brush/Bronchoalveolar Lavage Specimen *on page 568*
Bronchoalveolar Lavage (BAL) *on page 375*
Cytomegalovirus Antigen Detection *on page 598*
Cytomegalovirus Culture *on page 598*
Cytomegalovirus Cytology *on page 380*
Cytomegalovirus Nucleic Acid Detection *on page 599*
Newborn Crossmatch and Transfusion *on page 848*
Red Blood Cells, Leukocytes Reduced *on page 858*
Risks of Transfusion *on page 861*
Sputum Cytology *on page 387*
TORCH *on page 683*

Synonyms CMV Antibody; CMV-IFA; CMV Titer; Cytomegalic Inclusion Virus Titer

Applies to CMV, IgG; CMV, IgM

Test Includes Both IgM and IgG antibodies can be tested.

Abstract Human cytomegalovirus (CMV) establishes a latent infection subsequent to the primary acute infection. A primary CMV infection may manifest as an infectious mononucleosis-like disorder, or be asymptomatic. Primary CMV infection can also be associated with interstitial pneumonia, hepatitis, meningoencephalitis, or intrauterine infections. The most common intrauterine infection is congenital CMV infection. In immunocompromised patients, primary as well as reactivated CMV can cause a variety of serious diseases including retinitis, colitis, and pneumonitis.[1]

Specimen Serum

Container Red top tube

Sampling Time Sampling too early after initial infection may miss detection of antibody. Acute and convalescent sera drawn 10-14 days apart are required for IgG CMV testing. A single specimen may be sufficient for IgM testing. For determination of prior exposure to CMV (for transplantation or transfusion), a single specimen for detection of CMV IgG is satisfactory.

Storage Instructions 4°C

Special Instructions Neonatal specimens should be analyzed for specific IgM antibody only.

Reference Interval IgM: <1:8 is considered nondiagnostic. Less than a fourfold increase in CMV-IgG titer in paired sera drawn 10-14 days apart. Negative results from EIA.

Use Determine prior infection with CMV for purposes of organ transplantation, provision of blood and blood fractions to selected recipients, and screening for pregnant women. Investigate patients with mononucleosis-like illness who are Monospot® negative. CMV serology is part of TORCH screen used to test pregnant women.

Limitations Heterophil antibodies and presence of rheumatoid factor may cause false-positive IgM results. Fetal IgM antibody to maternal IgG may also cause false-positive results. False negatives occur. Because of high levels of "background" antibody in adult populations, a single antibody determination is not useful.

Methodology Enzyme immunoassay (EIA), indirect fluorescent antibody (IFA), latex agglutination (LA), hemagglutination (HA)

Additional Information The majority of CMV infections remain undetected, since most infections with CMV are asymptomatic. Individuals infected with CMV will produce antibody to the virus and antibodies can be detected throughout the lifetime of the individual. Several assays have been developed to detect antibody to CMV. EIA is the most commonly used test. Other methods include immunofluorescence assays, hemagglutination, and latex agglutination.

A single titer is rarely significant if past history is unknown. CMV IgM is produced in low levels during reactivated CMV and, thus, does not always indicate primary infection. Likewise, a positive or high titer of CMV IgG should not be interpreted as representing active CMV infection. However, a fourfold or greater rise in CMV titer between acute and convalescent specimens is evidence of infection. A single IgM specific titer >1:8 is also excellent evidence of acute infection. Significant CMV titers are found almost universally in patients with AIDS.

Intrauterine transmission of CMV can occur whether or not prior maternal immunity exists. However, the presence of maternal antibody prior to conception does provide a significant degree of protection against neonatal damage of congenital CMV infection. Sequellae of congenital CMV infections are more severe in primary maternal infections occurring during pregnancy.[2] CMV causes an infectious mononucleosis syndrome clinically indistinguishable from heterophil-positive mononucleosis. CMV is a significant cause of postcardiotomy, post-transplant, and postpump hepatitis syndromes.[1]

Although serology is a useful method to detect CMV infections, the rapid CMV viral culture, CMV antigen or quantitative CMV PCR can more reliably identify symptomatic CMV infections in immunocompromised patients. See Related Information at the beginning of this listing for further tests relevant to CMV.

Footnotes

1. Drago F, Aragone MG, Lugani C, et al, "Cytomegalovirus Infection in Normal and Immunocompromised Humans. A Review." *Dermatology*, 2000, 200(3):189-95.
2. Halwachs-Baumann G, Genser B, Danda M, et al, "Screening and Diagnosis of Congenital Cytomegalovirus Infection: A 5-Year Study," *Scan J Infect Dis*, 2000, 32(2):137-42.

References

Alberola J, Tamarit A, Igual R, et al, "Early Neutralizing and Glycoprotein B (gB)-Specific Antibody Responses to Human Cytomegalovirus (HCMV) in Immunocompetent Individuals With Distinct Clinical Presentations for Primary HCMV Infection," *J Clin Virol*, 2000, 16(2):113-22.

Broers AE, van Der Holt R, van Esser JW, et al, "Increased Transplant-Related Morbidity and Mortality in CMV-Seropositive Patients Despite Highly Effective Prevention of CMV Disease After Allogeneic T-Cell-Depleted Stem Cell Transplantation," *Blood*, 2000, 95(7):2240-5.

Deorari AK, Broor S, Maitreyi RS, et al, "Incidence, Clinical Spectrum, and Outcome of Intrauterine Infections in Neonates," *J Trop Pediatr*, 2000, 46(3):155-9.

Emery VC, Cope AV, Sabin CA, et al, "Relationship Between IgM Antibody to Human Cytomegalovirus, Virus Load, Donor and Recipient Serostatus, and Administration of Methylprednisolone as Risk Factors for Cytomegalovirus Disease After Liver Transplantation," *J Infect Dis*, 2000, 182(6):1610-5.

Holland CA, Ma Y, Moscicki B, et al, "Seroprevalence and Risk Factors of Hepatitis B, Hepatitis C, and Human Cytomegalovirus Among HIV-Infected and High-Risk Uninfected Adolescents: Findings of the REACH Study. Adolescent Medicine HIV/AIDS Research Network." *Sex Transm Dis*, 2000, 27(5):296-303.

Maine GT, Sticker R, Schuler M, et al, "Development and Clinical Evaluation of a Recombinant-Antigen-Based Cytomegalovirus Immunoglobulin M Automated Immunoassay Using the Abbott AxSYM Analyzer," *J Clin Microbiol*, 2000, 38(4):1476-81.

Mustakangas P, Sarna S, Ammala P, et al, "Human Cytomegalovirus Seroprevalence in Three Socioeconomically Different Urban Areas During the First Trimester: A Population-Based Cohort Study," *Int J Epidemiol*, 2000, 29(3):587-91.

Przepiorka D, LeParc GF, Werch J, et al, "Prevention of Transfusion-Associated Cytomegalovirus Infection. Practice Parameter," American Society of Clinical Pathologists, *Am J Clin Pathol*, 1996, 106(2):163-9.

Schafer P, Tenschert W, Cremaschi L, et al, "Cytomegalovirus Cultured From Different Major Leukocyte Subpopulations: Association With Clinical Features in CMV Immunoglobulin G-Positive Renal Allograft Recipients," *J Med Virol*, 2000, 61(4):488-96.

Internet Web Sites
www.cdc.gov/ncidod/diseases/cmv.htm

♦ **Cytomegalovirus Viral Load** *see* Human Immunodeficiency Virus, Viral Load Assay *on page 640*

♦ **Cytopathic Effect** *see* Viral Culture *on page 689*

Darkfield Examination, Leptospirosis

Related Information
Leptospira Culture *on page 648*
Leptospira Serology *on page 649*

Synonyms Darkfield Microscopy, *Leptospira*; Leptospirosis, Darkfield Examination

Applies to Leptospirosis DNA Amplification Method

Test Includes Examination of serum, urine, or CSF for organisms

Abstract Leptospirosis is a bacterial infection that can affect both humans and animals. The general term leptospirosis is preferred to the synonyms, **Weil disease** and **canicola fever**. Culture and serology are recommended for diagnosis; darkfield examination is not. Darkfield microscopic examination of specimens for leptospires can be useful in establishing a rapid diagnosis, but culture and serology are recommended for confirmation of diagnosis.[1]

Specimen Urine, serum, cerebrospinal fluid

Container Sterile plastic urine container, red top tube, or sterile CSF tube

Use Determine the presence of *Leptospira* for the diagnosis of Weil syndrome, hemorrhagic fever with renal syndrome, atypical pneumonia syndrome, aseptic meningitis, and myocarditis including cardiac arrhythmias.

Limitations The concentration of leptospires in blood and CSF is low. Therefore, concentration by centrifugation with sodium oxalate or heparin can be useful. The incidence of false positives is increased because fibrils and cellular extrusions can be mistaken for organisms.

Failure to detect leptospires does not rule out their presence. **Direct examination of blood or urine by darkfield methods frequently results in failure or misdiagnosis.** Culture has much greater value for diagnosis. Saprophytic strains as well as pathogenic ones exist.

Methodology A very small drop of fluid is distributed in a thin layer between a glass coverslip and slide. The typical morphology helicoidal, flexible organisms 6-12 μm long and 0.1 μm in diameter usually with semicircular hooked ends should be observed before a presumptive diagnosis is made.

Additional Information *Leptospira* are present in blood early in course of disease (first week only). After 10-14 days, they may be found in the urine. Urine must be neutral or alkaline. If the urine is acidic, it should be neutralized by diluting with 1% bovine serum albumin. Darkfield microscopy is best used to demonstrate leptospires in specimens in which a high concentration of organisms is present, ie, tissue from animals (guinea pig or hamster), inoculation including blood, peritoneal fluid, or liver suspensions. Urine or kidney suspensions from swine, dogs, and domestic animals may also yield positive darkfield examination.

A DNA amplification method has recently been used to detect leptospires in clinical specimens.[2] This assay seems to be more sensitive and specific than microscopic examination or culture. It is not currently widely available.

Footnotes
1. Lomar AV, Diament D, and Torres JR, "Leptospirosis in Latin America," *Infect Dis Clin North Am*, 2000, 14(1):23-39.
2. Romero EC, Billerbeck AE, Lando VS, et al, "Detection of *Leptospira* DNA in Patients With Aseptic Meningitis by PCR," *J Clin Microbiol*, 1998, 36(5):1453-5.

References
Centers for Disease Control and Prevention, "Outbreak of Acute Febrile Illness Among Participants in EcoChallenge Sabah 2000 - Malaysia," *JAMA*, 2000, 284(13):1646.
Farr RW, "Leptospirosis," *Clin Infect Dis*, 1995, 21(1):1-8.
Guidugli F, Castro AA, and Atallah AN, "Systemic Reviews on Leptospirosis," *Rev Inst Med Trop Sao Paulo*, 2000, 42(1):47-9.
Holk K, Nielsen SV, and Ronne T, "Human Leptospirosis in Denmark 1970-1996: An Epidemiological and Clinical Study," *Scand J Infect Dis*, 2000, 32(5):533-8.

Internet Web Sites
www.amm.co.uk/pubs/fa_leptospir.htm
www.cdc.gov/ncidod/dbmd/diseaseinfo/leptospirosis_g.htm

Darkfield Examination, Syphilis

Related Information
FTA-ABS, Serum *on page 609*

RPR *on page 677*
VDRL, Cerebrospinal Fluid *on page 688*
VDRL, Serum *on page 688*

Synonyms Darkfield Microscopy, Syphilis; Syphilis, Darkfield Examination; *Treponema pallidum* Darkfield Examination

Applies to Syphilis Diagnosis

Abstract The sexually transmitted disease, syphilis, is caused by the spirochete *Treponema pallidum*. *T. pallidum* is a thin organism that cannot be visualized by conventional light microscopy. Darkfield examination is appropriate for the evaluation of chancre (primary lues) and condylomata lata (secondary syphilis).

Patient Preparation The surface of the chancre or condyloma is cleansed by the physician with a swab moistened with saline. This removes exudate and excess bacterial contamination. Serous fluid is then collected from the surface of the chancre, using a small pipette. The fluid is placed on a slide or coverslip. Alternatively, the specimen can be collected by directly touching the slide to the lesion. The objective is to obtain clear exudate from the subsurface of the lesion. It is then examined by darkfield microscopy without further preparation.

Specimen Moist serous fluid from the base of a cleansed, unhealed chancre or condyloma. The youngest lesion available is best. The chance of identification of treponemes decreases with the age of the lesion as it dries and locally heals. *Treponema pallidum* can be found by lymph node aspiration in the secondary stage of lues.

Collection Collect with a pipette and put directly on a glass slide.

Causes for Rejection Healed chancre, previous treatment, ointment, dried-up specimen

Reference Interval Negative

Critical Values Positive darkfield examination, especially from a pregnant patient

Use Determine the presence of characteristic spirochetes to support the diagnosis of primary or secondary syphilis or of congenital syphilis.

Limitations Darkfield examination is of limited value in oral and rectal lesions, because of the normal presence of other, nonpathogenic spirochetes. Dry or bloody specimens render this examination worthless. The specimen should be examined within 15 minutes of collection because the organisms lose motility with decrease in temperature, exposure to oxygen, and desiccation. Experience and professional expertise are required to accurately identify *T. pallidum* by darkfield examination. Artifacts (eg, cotton fibers) can sometimes be mistaken for spirochetes. A negative result does not rule out syphilis.

Contraindications Antibiotic therapy prior to the darkfield examination. The organisms are rapidly cleared following therapy and as the lesion heals.

Methodology Darkfield microscopy. Motile organisms are observed to rotate around their long axis and to bend, snap, and flex along their length at 90 degree angles. A smooth translational back and forth directed movement is also apparent. *Treponema pallidum* has a rapid and purposeful motion as it travels across the microscopic field. The organisms appear as a tight corkscrew characterized by 6-14 coils. The organisms are 1-1.5 times the diameter of an RBC in length (0.10-0.18 μm by 6-20 μm). Nonpathogenic mucosal treponemes are often irregularly coiled, longer than *T. pallidum*, and are characterized by a different kind of motility.[1]

Additional Information *T. pallidum* can be found in skin lesions and lymph nodes in secondary syphilis but are more plentiful in primary chancres. They cannot be grown in culture. The Centers for Disease Control (CDC) and others use fluorescent microscopy with monoclonal or polyclonal anti-*T. pallidum* antibodies for examination of exudates.[1]

A technique for direct detection of *T. pallidum* is specific amplification of DNA.[2] This test is currently only available as a research tool and further studies of its use as a diagnostic test are needed before it is universally available.

Footnotes
1. Hook EW 3d and Marra CM, "Acquired Syphilis in Adults," *N Engl J Med*, 1992, 326(16):1060-9.
2. Risbud A, Chan-Tack K, Gadkari D, et al, "The Etiology of Genital Ulcer Disease by Multiplex Polymerase Chain Reaction and Relationship to HIV Infection Among Patients Attending Sexually Transmitted Disease Clinics in Pune, India," *Sex Transm Dis*, 1999, 26(2):55-62.

References
Behets FM, Brathwaite AR, Hylton-Kong T, et al, "Genital Ulcers: Etiology, Clinical Diagnosis and Associated Human Immunodeficiency Virus Infection in Kingston, Jamaica," *Clin Infect Dis*, 1999, 28(5):1086-90.
Birnbaum NR, Goldschmidt RH, and Buffet WO, "Resolving the Common Clinical Dilemmas of Syphilis," *Am Fam Phys*, 1999, 59(8):2233-46.
Emmert DH and Kirchner JT, "Sexually Transmitted Diseases in Women. Gonorrhea and Syphilis," *Postgrad Med*, 2000, 107(2):181-97.
Hollier LM and Cox SM, "Syphilis," *Semin Perinatol*, 1998, 22(4):323-31.

Internet Web Sites
www.cdc.gov/nchstp/dstd/fact_sheets/syphilis_facts.htm

♦ **Darkfield Microscopy, *Leptospira*** *see* Darkfield Examination, Leptospirosis *on page 601*

♦ **Darkfield Microscopy, Syphilis** *see* Darkfield Examination, Syphilis *on page 601*

♦ **Davidsohn Differential** *replaced by* Infectious Mononucleosis Screening Test *on page 643*

- **Davidsohn Slide Test** *see* Infectious Mononucleosis Screening Test *on page 643*

- **Decubitus Ulcer Culture** *see* Bacterial Culture, Wounds, Bites *on page 579*

- **Delta Agent Serology** *see* Hepatitis D Serology *on page 627*

- **Delta Hepatitis Serology** *see* Hepatitis D Serology *on page 627*

- *Dermacentor andersoni* *see* Arthropod Identification *on page 559*

- **Dermatophyte Fungus Culture** *see* Fungal Culture, Skin *on page 612*

- **Dermatophytoses** *see* KOH Preparation *on page 645*

- **Desert Fever Serology** *see* Coccidioidomycosis Serology *on page 593*

- *Dientamoeba fragilis* *see* Ova and Parasites, Stool *on page 666*

- **Diphtheria Culture** *see Corynebacterium diphtheriae* Throat Culture *on page 594*

- *Diphyllobothrium latum* *see* Ova and Parasites, Stool *on page 666*

- **DNA Detection for *Neisseria gonorrhoeae*** *see* Neisseria gonorrhoeae Nucleic Acid Detection *on page 664*

- **DNA Hybridization Test for *Borrelia burgdorferi*** *see* Lyme Disease DNA Detection *on page 649*

- **DNA Hybridization Test for *Chlamydia trachomatis*** *see* Chlamydia trachomatis Nucleic Acid Detection *on page 591*

- **DNA Hybridization Test for HBV** *see* Hepatitis B DNA Detection *on page 623*

- **DNA Hybridization Test for HPV** *see* Human Papillomavirus DNA Probe Test *on page 641*

- **DNA Hybridization Test for *Mycoplasma pneumoniae*** *see* Mycoplasma pneumoniae DNA Probe Test *on page 661*

- **DNA Probe Test for HBV** *see* Hepatitis B DNA Detection *on page 623*

- **DNA Probe Test for HPV** *see* Human Papillomavirus DNA Probe Test *on page 641*

- **DNA Probe Test for Lyme Disease** *see* Lyme Disease DNA Detection *on page 649*

- **DNA Test for *Chlamydia trachomatis*** *see* Chlamydia trachomatis Nucleic Acid Detection *on page 591*

- **DNA Test for Mycobacteria** *see* Mycobacteria by DNA Probe *on page 654*

- **DNA Test for *Mycoplasma pneumoniae*** *see* Mycoplasma pneumoniae DNA Probe Test *on page 661*

- **Ear Culture** *see* Bacterial Culture, Middle Ear *on page 573*

- **Eastern Equine Encephalitis** *see* Encephalitis Viral Serology *on page 604*

Eastern Equine Encephalitis Virus Serology

Related Information
Bacterial Culture, Cerebrospinal Fluid *on page 569*
California Encephalitis Virus Serology *on page 587*
Cerebrospinal Fluid Analysis: Overview *on page 416*
Encephalitis Viral Serology *on page 604*
St Louis Encephalitis Virus Serology *on page 681*
Viral Culture *on page 689*
Viral Culture, Central Nervous System Symptoms *on page 692*
Western Equine Encephalitis Virus Serology *on page 697*

Synonyms Encephalitis Virus Titer, Eastern Equine

Abstract Eastern equine encephalitis (EEE) virus is an alphavirus that is vector-borne. EEE is limited geographically to the Eastern and Gulf coasts of the United States. Encephalitis due to EEE is a summertime disease spread by mosquitos (*Cusliseta melanura*). EEE is a low incidence disease, with only a few cases occurring each year, but a 50% to 70% fatality rate is recognized.

Specimen Serum or cerebrospinal fluid

Container Red top tube

Sampling Time Acute and convalescent sera drawn 10-14 days apart

Reference Interval Less than a fourfold increase in titer in paired sera

Use Support the diagnosis of Eastern equine encephalitis virus infection

Limitations Absence of IgM antibodies does not rule out the infection. Extensive cross-reactions with related arboviruses (eg, Western equine encephalitis virus and Venezuelan equine encephalitis virus) makes definitive interpretation difficult.

Methodology Complement fixation (CF), hemagglutination inhibition (HAI), virus neutralization testing, enzyme-linked immunosorbent assay (ELISA) for IgM antibodies

Additional Information EEE is an alphavirus carried by a mosquito vector. The mosquitos known to carry EEE breed in fresh water swamps and infect numerous bird species as well as horses. Infected birds typically have a very high titer viremia and act as a reservoir for human infection.

In humans, EEE causes an acute illness which is either fatal or self-limited; chronic illness should suggest a different diagnosis. Syndromes include headache with fever, meningitis, and meningoencephalitis. The other alphavirus agents causing disease in the U.S. are Western equine encephalitis and Venezuelan equine encephalitis. These have been classified as group A arboviruses.

References
Centers for Disease Control, "Eastern Equine Encephalitis Virus - Florida," *JAMA*, 1992, 267(10):1324.

Garen PD, Tsai TF, and Powers JM, "Human Eastern Equine Encephalitis: Immunohistochemistry and Ultrastructure," *Mod Pathol*, 1999, 12(6):646-52.

Johnson AJ, Martin DA, Karabatsos N, et al, "Detection of Antiarboviral Immunoglobulin G by Using a Monoclonal Antibody-Based Capture Enzyme-Linked Immunosorbent Assay," *J Clin Microbiol*, 2000, 38(5):1827-31.

Markoff L, "Alphaviruses," *Principles and Practice of Infectious Diseases*, 5th ed, Mandell GL, Bennett JE, and Dolin R, eds, New York, NY: Churchill Livingstone, 2000, 1703-8.

Tsai TF, "Arboviruses," *Manual of Clinical Microbiology*, 7th ed, Washington, DC: AMS Press, American Society for Microbiology, 1999, 1107-24.

Internet Web Sites
www.cdc.gov/ncidod/dvbid/arbor/arboinfo.htm

- **Eaton Agent Pneumonia** *see* Mycoplasma pneumoniae DNA Probe Test *on page 661*

- **Eaton Agent Titer** *see* Mycoplasma Serology *on page 662*

- **EBNA** *see* Epstein-Barr Virus Serology *on page 607*

- **EB Nuclear Antigen** *see* Epstein-Barr Virus Serology *on page 607*

- **EBV Titer** *see* Epstein-Barr Virus Serology *on page 607*

Echinococcosis Serological Test

Related Information
Bronchoalveolar Lavage (BAL) *on page 375*
Brushings Cytology *on page 376*
Liver Disease: Laboratory Assessment, Overview *on page 216*
Ova and Parasites, Stool *on page 666*
Sputum Cytology *on page 387*

Synonyms *Echinococcus granulosus* Serological Test; *Echinococcus multilocularis* Serological Test; Hydatid Disease Serological Test; Hydatidosis Serological Test

Abstract Echinococcosis is a cestode parasitic disease important in livestock-raising areas in which dogs (the definitive hosts) are used. In humans, larval stages of *E. granulosus*, *E. multilocularis*, or *E. vogeli* cause the infection. *Echinococcus granulosus* causes unilocular cysts. The adult *E. granulosus* resides in the intestine of dogs. Sheep, caribou, deer, moose, pigs, or man are intermediate hosts. The cause of multilocular alveolar disease, a more invasive form, is a larval form of *E. multilocularis*. Polycystic hydatid disease is caused by *E. vogeli*.

Specimen Serum

Container Red top tube

Reference Interval No *Echinococcus*-specific antibody detected

Use Support a diagnosis of echinococcosis or exposure to the cestode. The detection of cysts in liver, lung, bone, or brain, with a positive serology is 88% sensitive and 96% specific for echinococcosis. Sensitivity and specificity of serologic assays is greater for hepatic than for pulmonary infections or for those in other organs.

Limitations Serologic methods for echinococcosis are compromised by nonspecific cross-reactivity with other helminths.[1] Serum from 50% of patients with cysticercosis cross react in this assay. False positives are occasionally seen in patients with cirrhosis and lupus; false negatives with some large cysts, lung cysts, or dead cysts.

Methodology Complement fixation (CF), bentonite flocculation assay (BFA), indirect hemagglutination (IHA), latex agglutination (LA), enzyme-linked immunosorbent assay (ELISA), immunofluorescence assay, immunoblot.

Cytologic methods, including bronchoalveolar lavage, brushings, or sputum can sometimes reveal scolexes or degenerated hooklets in pulmonary cases.[1]

Additional Information Echinococcosis is usually suspected based on imaging studies and confirmed with serological assays. There is generally a rapid decline in antibody after surgical removal of the cyst. If the antibody titer does not decline, there is indication of incomplete cyst removal. Cysts in the liver are more likely to elicit an immune response than those in lungs. The newer ELISA tests are more sensitive than the more traditional hemagglutination and latex assays. A recent Cabot case provides current clinicopathologic and therapeutic information with outstanding illustrations.[1]

Footnotes
1. Kornfeld H and Mark EJ, "A 34-Year-Old Woman With One Cystic Lesion in Each Lung," Case Records of the Massachusetts General Hospital, Case 29-1999, Scully RE, Mark EJ, and McNeely WF et al, eds, *N Engl J Med*, 1999, 341(13):974-82.

References
Baveja UK, Basak S, and Thusoo TK, "Immunodiagnosis of Human Hydatid Disease," *J Commun Dis*, 1997, 29(4):313-9.

Brehm K, Kern P, Hubert K, et al, "Echinococcosis From Every Angle," *Parasitol Today*, 1999, 15(9):35102.

Cohen H, Paolillo E, Bonifacino R, et al, "Human Cystic Echinococcosis in a Uruaguayan Community: A Sonographic, Serologic and Epidemiologic Study," *Am J Trop Med Hyg*, 1998, 59(4):620-7.

Gadea I, Ayala G, Diago MT, et al, "Immunological Diagnosis of Human Cystic Echinococcosis: Utility of Discriminant Analysis Applied to the Enzyme-Linked Immunoelectrotransfer Blot," *Clin Diag Lab Immunol*, 1999, 6(4):504-8.

Grimm F, Maly FE, Lu J, et al, "Analysis of Specific Immunoglobulin G Subclass Antibodies for Serologic Diagnosis of Echinococcosis by a Standard Enzyme-Linked Immunosorbent Assay," *Clin Diag Lab Immunol*, 1998, 5(5):613-6.

Shambesh MA, Craig PS, Macpherson CN, et al, "An Extensive Ultrasound and Serologic Study to Investigate the Prevalence of Human Cystic Echinococcosis in Northern Libya," *Am J Trop Med Hyg*, 1999, 60(3):462-8.

Internet Web Sites
www.cdc.gov/ncidod/dpd/parasites/alveolarhydatid/default.htm

♦ ***Echinococcus granulosus* Serological Test** *see* Echinococcosis Serological Test *on page 602*

♦ ***Echinococcus multilocularis* Serological Test** *see* Echinococcosis Serological Test *on page 602*

♦ **Echovirus Culture** *see* Enterovirus Culture *on page 605*

♦ **Echovirus Culture, Stool** *see* Viral Culture, Stool *on page 695*

♦ ***E. coli*** *see* Bacterial Culture, Cerebrospinal Fluid *on page 569*

♦ ***E. coli*** *see* Bacterial Culture, Genital Specimen *on page 571*

♦ ***E. coli*** *see* Bacterial Culture, Urine *on page 578*

♦ **Ectoparasite Identification** *see* Arthropod Identification *on page 559*

♦ ***Ehrlichia chaffeensis* Antibodies** *see* Ehrlichiosis Serology *on page 603*

Ehrlichiosis Serology

Related Information
Arthropod Identification *on page 559*
Babesiosis Serology *on page 561*
Buffy Coat Smear Study of Peripheral Blood *on page 412*
Lyme Disease Serology *on page 650*
Rocky Mountain Spotted Fever Serology *on page 676*

Synonyms *Ehrlichia chaffeensis* Antibodies; Human Granulocytotropic Ehrlichiosis Serology

Abstract All *Ehrlichia* species are small, intracellular bacteria. The Ehrlichiae are zoonotic agents that are transmitted to both humans and animals via tick bites. They are rickettsia-like bacteria which localize in leukocyte phagosomes. Distinct forms of ehrlichiosis recognized in the United States include **human monocytic ehrlichiosis (HME)** and **human granulocytic ehrlichiosis (HGE)**. Human granulocytic ehrlichiosis was first described in 1994 in Minnesota and Wisconsin.[1] Of the several species of *Ehrlichia*, each infects leukocytoplasm or the cytoplasm of platelets. The disease is an acute febrile illness which resembles Rocky Mountain spotted fever. It can be mild, but about 33% of cases requires hospitalization.

Thrombocytopenia and leukopenia, increased amniotransferase and alkaline phosphatase concentrations or combinations of these abnormalities, found in an acute febrile disease following tickbite, present a differential diagnosis which includes ehrlichiosis, endocarditis, vasculitis, thrombotic thrombocytopenic purpura, and other kinds of septicemia.[2]

Specimen Serum

Container Red top tube

Collection Collect at time of illness, then 2-4 weeks after onset (ie, acute and convalescent samples).

Storage Instructions Refrigerate or freeze serum.

Reference Interval Titer <1:80 with the source of antigen *E. chaffeensis*.

Critical Values Fourfold rise or fall in titer

Use Aid in the diagnosis of ehrlichiosis. Clinical features of ehrlichiosis may include rapid onset of fever with chills (97% of patients), myalgias, headache (81% of patients), and malaise (84% of patients). A rash is seen in only 36% of patients. Abnormal laboratory findings (leukopenia, lymphopenia, neutropenia, thrombocytopenia, increased aspartate transaminase) are found in at least 86% of patients.

Limitations Positive cutoff titer for disease has not been standardized and varies between laboratories performing the test. At times, serologic results are not reproducible[3]

Methodology The most frequently used methodology is indirect fluorescent antibody (IFA) for IgG and IgM antibodies.[4]

Ehrlichia-infected leukocytes can be detected on peripheral blood smears that are stained with Giemsa or Wright stains. Inclusions (morulae) are found in neutrophils in HGE. Wright stain demonstrates *E. chaffeensis* in mononuclear cells and/or atypical lymphocytes.[3] Beautifully reproduced photomicrographs from buffy-coat smears,[5,6] peripheral blood,[7,8,9] and CSF smears[4] are published. Isolation of *E. chaffeensis* can be accomplished with tissue culture methods and can detect bacteria even in patients with negative examination of peripheral blood. PCR provides early diagnosis, before antibodies are demonstrable but is only available through large reference laboratories.[4,10]

Additional Information Nearly 1200 cases have been confirmed in the U.S. with most of the cases of HME occurring in Southeastern and South

Central states. Cases of HGE were found in Northeastern and upper Midwestern states.[11] The organism responsible for HME (*E. chaffeensis*) is most commonly found in the Lone Star tick (*Amblyomma americanum*) while *E. equi*, responsible for HGE, has been found in the deer tick (*Ixodes scapularis*) and the dog tick (*Dermacentor variabilis*). *E. ewingii* was recently described in humans. HGE is found in the Northern U.S., where Lyme disease and babesiosis are endemic. The latter two entities represent an important portion of the clinical differential diagnosis. HME has mimicked thrombotic thrombocytopenic purpura.

Simultaneous ehrlichiosis and Lyme borreliosis have been reported,[6] but reactive Lyme disease serology may occur in subjects with ehrlichiosis.[12]

Footnotes
1. Bakken JS, Dumler JS, Chen SM, et al, "Human Granulocytic Ehrlichiosis in the Upper Midwest United States. A New Species Emerging?" *JAMA*, 1994, 272(2):212-8.
2. Goodman JL, "Ehrlichiosis - Ticks, Dogs, and Doxycycline," *N Engl J Med*, 1999, 341(3):195-6.
3. Dumler JS, "*Ehrlichia*," *Manual of Clinical Microbiology*, 7th ed, Washington, DC: AMS Press, American Society for Microbiology, 1999, 821-30.
4. Buller RS, Arens M, Hmiel SP, et al, "*Ehrlichia ewingii*, a Newly Recognized Agent of Human Ehrlichiosis," *N Engl J Med*, 1999, 341(3):148-55.
5. Glaser C and Johnson E, Images in Clinical Medicine, "Ehrlichiosis," *N Engl J Med*, 1995, 332(21):1417.
6. Nadelman RB, Horowitz HW, Hsieh TC, et al, "Simultaneous Human Granulocytic Ehrlichiosis and Lyme Borreliosis," *N Engl J Med*, 1997, 337(1):27-30.
7. Martin GS, Christman BW, and Standaert SM, "Rapidly Fatal Infection With *Ehrlichia chaffeensis*," *N Engl J Med*, 1999, 341(10):763-4.
8. Dobbenburgh AV, van Dam AP, and Fikrig E, "Human Granulocytic Ehrlichiosis in Western Europe," *N Engl J Med*, 1999, 340(15):1214-5.
9. Walker DH and Dumler JS, "Human Monocytic and Granulocytic Ehrlichioses. Discovery and Diagnosis of Emerging Tick-Borne Infections and the Critical Role of the Pathologist," *Arch Pathol Lab Med*, 1997, 121(8):785-91.
10. Walker DH, "Tick-Transmitted Infectious Diseases in the United States," *Annu Rev Public Health*, 1998, 19:237-69.
11. McQuiston JH, Paddock CD, Holman RC, et al, "The Human Ehrlichioses in the United States," *Emerg Infect Dis*, 1999, 5(5):635-42.
12. Wormser GP, Horowitz HW, Nowakowski J, et al, "Positive Lyme Disease Serology in Patients With Clinical and Laboratory Evidence of Human Granulocytic Ehrlichiosis," *Am J Clin Pathol*, 1997, 107(2):142-7.

References
Bakken JS, "The Discovery of Human Granulocytotropic Ehrlichiosis," *J Lab Clin Med*, 1998, 132(3):175-80.
Belman AL, "Tick-Borne Diseases," *Semin Pediatr Neurol*, 1999, 6(4):249-66.
Fritz CL and Glaser CA, "Ehrlichiosis," *Infect Dis Clin North Am*, 1998, 12(1).123-36.
Jerrad D, "Ehrlichiosis," *J Emerg Med*, 1999, 17(1):27-30.
Kaplan SL, "Newer Pediatric Pathogens," *Adv Pediatr*, 1999, 46:189-206.
Samuels MA and Newell KL, "A 43-Year-Old Woman With Rapidly Changing Pulmonary Infiltrates and Markedly Increased Intracranial Pressure," Case Records of the Massachusetts General Hospital, Case 32-1997, Scully RE, Mark EJ, McNeely WF, et al, eds, *N Engl J Med*, 1997, 337(16):1149-56.
Schutze GE and Jacobs RF, "Human Monocytic Ehrlichiosis in Children," *Pediatrics*, 1997, 100(1):E10.
Schwartz I, Fish D, and Daniels TJ, "Prevalence of the Rickettsial Agent of Human Granulocytic Ehrlichiosis in Ticks From a Hyperendemic Focus of Lyme Disease," *N Engl J Med*, 1997, 337(1):49.
Taege AJ, "Tick Trouble: Overview of Tick-Borne Diseases," *Clev Clin J Med*, 2000, 67(4):241-9.

Internet Web Sites
www.cdc.gov/ncidod/dvrd/ehrlichia/index.htm

Electron Microscopic Examination for Viruses, Stool

Related Information
Bacterial Culture, Stool *on page 575*
Electron Microscopy *on page 54*
Histopathology *on page 59*
Rotavirus, Direct Detection *on page 676*
Skin Biopsy *on page 71*
Viral Culture *on page 689*
Viral Culture, Stool *on page 695*

Synonyms Enteric Viruses by EM; Gastrointestinal Viruses by EM

Applies to Rotavirus Detection by EM; Skin Viral Disease; Viral Disease in Tissue

Abstract Most viruses causing gastroenteritis are readily detected by electron microscopy (EM). Most viruses usually are present in very high concentration ($\geq 10^6$ virus particles/g). Viruses in stool are stable, can be transported, and survive processing for EM.

Specimen Stool from the acute, diarrheal phase of disease; skin lesions; tissues (biopsy/autopsy)

Turnaround Time 1 day to 1 week

Reference Interval Viruses not observed

Use Demonstrate viral particles (eg, rotavirus, Norwalk virus, calcivirus, astrovirus, and coronavirus) in stool specimens from patients with suspected viral gastroenteritis; examination of tissue from biopsy or autopsy in which immunofluorescent and immunoperoxidase staining is negative.

Limitations Generally, EM visualization of viral particles is not as sensitive as is cell culture, except for detection of nonculturable viruses such as
(Continued)

Electron Microscopic Examination for Viruses, Stool *(Continued)*

rotavirus. EM can detect viruses if they are present in concentrations of 10^6 to 10^7 particles/mL. Such sensitivity is appropriate for agents causing diarrhea, but not for detection of other potential pathogens. Very few clinical microbiology/virology laboratories have immediate access to electron microscopes.

Methodology Diluted stool (either with or without being mixed with patient serum) is mixed with an electron-opaque heavy metal solution such as phosphotungstic acid. The stool solution is placed on an electron-lucent grid support and examined by electron microscopy. Virions or virions agglutinated by specific antibodies (if present in serum) appear as a negative image against a black surrounding background.

Additional Information The electron microscopic observation of viruses is the basis for identification. Electron microscopy is a useful procedure when viruses have not been identified by other methods. Many of the viruses detected by electron microscopy are now detected by nucleic acid methods or specific detection of viral antigen.[1,2]

Footnotes

1. James VL, Lambden PR, Caul EO, et al, "Enzyme-Linked Immunosorbent Assay Based on Recombinant Human Group C Rotavirus Inner Capsid Protein (VP6) to Detect Human Group C Rotaviruses in Fecal Samples," *J Clin Microbiol*, 1998, 36(11):3178-81.
2. Nakata S, Honma S, Numata KK, et al, "Members of the Family Caliciviridae (Norwalk Virus and Sapporo Virus) Are the Most Prevalent Cause of Gastroenteritis Outbreaks Among Infants in Japan," *J Infect Dis*, 2000, 181(6):2029-32.

References

"Diagnosis of Infections Caused by Viruses, *Chlamydia*, Rickettsia, and Related Organisms," *Color Atlas and Textbook of Diagnostic Microbiology*, 5th ed, Chapter 21, Koneman EW, Allen SD, Janda WM, et al, eds, Philadelphia, PA: Lippincott, 1997, 1177-293.

Hedberg CW and Osterholm M, "Outbreaks of Food-Borne and Water-Borne Viral Gastroenteritis," *Clin Microbiol Rev*, 1993, 6:199-210.

MacRae J and Srivastava M, "Detection of Viruses by Electron Microscopy: An Efficient Approach," *J Virol Methods*, 1998, 72(1):105-8.

Miller SE, "Diagnosis of Viral Infections by Electron Microscopy," *Diagnostic Procedures for Viral, Rickettsial, and Chlamydial Infections*, 7th ed, Lennette EH, Lennette DA, Lennette ET, eds, Washington, DC: American Public Health Association, 1995, 37-78.

Petric M, "Caliciviruses, Astroviruses, and Other Diarrheic Viruses," *Manual of Clinical Microbiology*, 7th ed, Washington, DC: AMS Press, American Society for Microbiology, 1999, 1005-13.

Putzker M, Sauer H, Kirchner G, et al, "Community Acquired Diarrhea - The Incidence of Astrovirus Infections in Germany," *Clin Lab*, 2000, 46(5-6):269-73.

Internet Web Sites

www.astdhpphe.org/infect/norwalk.html

www.cdc.gov/ncidod/dvrd/nrevss/rotfeat.htm

Encephalitis Viral Serology

Related Information

California Encephalitis Virus Serology *on page 587*
Cerebrospinal Fluid Analysis: Overview *on page 416*
Eastern Equine Encephalitis Virus Serology *on page 602*
St Louis Encephalitis Virus Serology *on page 681*
Viral Culture *on page 689*
Western Equine Encephalitis Virus Serology *on page 697*

Synonyms Arbovirus Serology

Applies to Arboviruses; California Encephalitis (LaCrosse); Eastern Equine Encephalitis; Japanese Encephalitis Virus; Nipah Virus; St Louis Encephalitis Virus; Western Equine Encephalitis; West Nile Virus

Abstract Encephalitogenic arboviruses commonly seen in North America are California encephalitis (that is closely related to LaCrosse), Western equine encephalitis, Eastern equine encephalitis, and St Louis encephalitis viruses. Arboviruses (arthropod-borne viruses) are a taxonomically heterogeneous group of viruses grouped together because they are all transmitted to humans via an arthropod vector. Around the world, a number of different arboviruses can cause encephalitis (ie, Japanese encephalitis, West Nile, Dengue, Sindbis, Semliki forest, Rift Valley Fever, and numerous others).

Specimen Serum

Container Red top tube

Collection Acute and convalescent sera drawn 10-14 days apart

Reference Interval Less than a fourfold titer increase in paired sera. CSF IgM: negative; hemagglutination inhibition: ≤1:80; complement fixation: ≤1:32; immunofluorescence: ≤1:128.

Use Support the diagnosis of infection with encephalitis viruses

Limitations Cross-reacting antibodies from previous infections or from immunization for yellow fever may produce false-positive results, particularly when assays are performed on unpaired sera. Information regarding travel history of the patient will help to more accurately identify the virus responsible for infection.

Additional Information Central nervous system infection by California encephalitis (LaCrosse), Western equine encephalitis, Eastern equine encephalitis, or St Louis encephalitis viruses may manifest as aseptic meningitis, encephalitis, or meningoencephalitis. There is a seasonal distribution for these infections that reflects their mode of transmission to

humans by mosquitos. In the United States, the incidence of arboviral infection is low, as is the prevalence of antibodies to these agents in the general population. Consequently, a positive result in an unpaired specimen is **presumptive** evidence for a recent infection. A fourfold increase in titer or a positive CSF IgM test is confirmatory. Antibody detection is the diagnostic test of choice, as these viruses are essentially nonculturable in routine diagnostic virology laboratories. Any positive serologic results should be reported to the state health departments to monitor for a possible outbreak of viral encephalitis.

In late summer 1999, an outbreak of human encephalitis, due to West Nile (WN) virus, occurred in the northeastern United States. This was the first recognized occurrence of endemic WN infections in North America.[1,2] This outbreak raised concerns regarding the further spread of this virus and the possibility of the introduction of other encephalitis viruses to North America via commercial shipments.

Another outbreak in 1999 highlights the importance of an accurate diagnosis of viral encephalitis. Between June and September of 1999, an outbreak of viral encephalitis was noted in Malaysia among adult pig farmers. These infections were first attributed to Japanese encephalitis (JE) virus infections, but as the investigation continued, it was recognized that a novel viral agent was responsible for the outbreak. The mortality associated with this outbreak was 32%, which is much higher than mortality associated with JE infections[3]. The new virus is now known as Nipah virus and has an extensive host range including pigs, bats, dogs, cats, as well as humans.[4] Investigation into all routes of transmission is still under investigation.

Footnotes

1. Lanciotti RS, Roehrig JT, Deubel V, et al, "Origin of the West Nile Virus Responsible for an Outbreak of Encephalitis in the Northeastern United States," *Science*, 1999, 286(5448):2333-7.
2. Asnis D, Conetta R, Teixeira AA, et al, "The West Nile Virus Outbreak of 1999 in New York: The Flushing Hospital Experience," *Clin Infect Dis*, 2000, 30(3):413-8.
3. Goh KJ, Tan CT, Chew NK, et al, "Clinical Features of Nipah Virus Encephalitis Among Pig Farmers in Malaysia," *N Engl J Med*, 2000, 342(17):1229-35.
4. Chua KB, Bellini WJ, Rota PA, et al, "Nipah Virus: A Recently Emergent Deadly Paramyxovirus," *Science*, 2000, 288(5470):1432-5.

References

Calisher CH, "Medically Important Arboviruses of the United States and Canada," *Clin Microbiol Rev*, 1994, 7(1):89-116.

Tsai TF, "Arboviruses," *Manual of Clinical Microbiology*, 7th ed, Washington, DC: AMS Press, American Society for Microbiology, 1999, 1107-24.

Internet Web Sites

www.cdc.gov/ncidod/dvbid/arbor/arboinfo.htm

- ♦ **Encephalitis Virus** *see* California Encephalitis Virus Serology *on page 587*
- ♦ **Encephalitis Virus Titer, Eastern Equine** *see* Eastern Equine Encephalitis Virus Serology *on page 602*
- ♦ **Encephalitis Virus Titer, St Louis** *see* St Louis Encephalitis Virus Serology *on page 681*
- ♦ **Encephalitis Virus Titer, Western Equine** *see* Western Equine Encephalitis Virus Serology *on page 697*
- ♦ **Endocervical Culture** *see* Bacterial Culture, Genital Specimen *on page 571*
- ♦ **Endocervix, Viral Culture** *see* Viral Culture, Urogenital *on page 696*
- ♦ *Entamoeba histolytica* *see* Bacterial Culture, Stool *on page 575*
- ♦ *Entamoeba histolytica* *see* Ova and Parasites, Stool *on page 666*
- ♦ *Entamoeba histolytica* **Antibody Titer** *see Entamoeba histolytica* Serology *on page 605*

Entamoeba histolytica Antigen Detection

Related Information

Bacterial Culture, Stool *on page 575*
Entamoeba histolytica Serology *on page 605*
Methylene Blue Stain, Stool *on page 313*
Ova and Parasites, Stool *on page 666*

Synonyms Amebiasis Antigen Test

Test Includes Detection of *Entamoeba histolytica* specific antigen in stool

Abstract *Entamoeba histolytica* is a protozoan parasite that is capable of invading the intestinal mucosa, sometimes spreading to the liver. It is the cause of hepatic amebic abscess. It is estimated that approximately 70 thousand deaths per year are due to amebiasis.[1] Infection with *E. histolytica* is more common in conditions of poverty, overcrowding, and inadequate, contaminated water supplies.

Fecal leukocytes may be absent in this type of inflammatory colitis.

Specimen Freshly collected stool

Container Sterile, leakproof, wide-mouth container

Reference Interval Negative

Use This is a method to establish the diagnosis of amebiasis in patients with watery or bloody diarrhea.

Limitations Extraintestinal amebiasis is frequently found without trophozoites or cysts in stool: patients may have a negative stool antigen result.

Methodology Enzyme immunoassay (EIA)

Additional Information The laboratory diagnosis of amebiasis can be made by examination of a permanent stained stool specimen. The detection of ingested red blood cells in the cytoplasm of the trophozoites is diagnostic for pathogenic *E. histolytica*. Antigen detection assays for *E. histolytica* are available. These assays seem to be more sensitive and specific for amebiasis than microscopy.[2,3] However, the **diagnosis is still based on morphologic diagnosis in fecal specimens**[4] (see Ova and Parasites, Stool *on page 666* and *Entamoeba histolytica* Serology *on page 605*).

Endoscopy with biopsies can provide rapid diagnosis in most cases.

Footnotes
1. World Health Organization, "The World Health Report 1998. Life in the 21st Century: A Vision for All," *World Health Organization*, 1998, Geneva, Switzerland.
2. Haque R, Ali IKM, Akther S, et al, "Comparison of PCR, Isoenzyme Analysis, and Antigen Detection for Diagnosis of *Entamoeba histolytica* Infection," *J Clin Microbiol*, 1998, 36(2):449-52.
3. Pillai DR, Keystone JS, Sheppard DC, et al, "*Entamoeba histolytica* and *Entamoeba dispar*: Epidemiology and Comparison of Diagnostic Methods in a Setting of Nonendemicity," *Clin Infect Dis*, 1999, 29(5):1315-8.
4. Ravdin JI, "Amebiasis," *Cecil Textbook of Medicine*, 21st ed, Chapter 428, Goldman L and Bennett JC, eds, Philadelphia, PA: WB Saunders Co, 2000, 1971-3.

References
Colmer-Hamood JA, "Fecal Microscopy Artifacts Mimicking Ova and Parasites," *Lab Med*, 2001, 32(2):80-4.
Espinosa-Cantellano M and Martinez-Palomo A, "Pathogenesis of Intestinal Amebiasis: From Molecules to Disease," *Clin Microbiol Rev*, 2000, 13(2):318-31.
Hashmey R, Genta RM, and White AC Jr, "Parasites and Diarrhea. I: Protozoans and Diarrhea," *J Travel Med*, 1997, 4(1):17-31.
Leber AL, "Intestinal Amebae," *Clin Lab Med*, 1999, 19(3):601-19.

Internet Web Sites
www.cdc.gov/ncidod/dpd/parasites/amebiasis/default.htm

Entamoeba histolytica Serology

Related Information
Bacterial Culture, Blood *on page 566*
Bacterial Culture, Stool *on page 575*
Entamoeba histolytica Antigen Detection *on page 604*
Fecal Lactoferrin *on page 308*
Fine Needle Aspiration Culture *on page 609*
Fine Needle Aspiration, Deep Masses *on page 381*
Methylene Blue Stain, Stool *on page 313*
Ova and Parasites, Stool *on page 666*
Viral Culture, Stool *on page 695*

Synonyms Amebiasis Serological Test; *Entamoeba histolytica* Antibody Titer

Test Includes Detection of antibodies to *Entamoeba histolytica* in serum

Abstract Infection with *Entamoeba histolytica* is found worldwide, but is much more common in tropical and subtropical regions. Humans are the primary reservoir and infection occurs by ingestion of cysts from contaminated food or water. Infection with *E. histolytica* can result in three different presentations. Patients may be asymptomatic, they may have symptomatic invasive intestinal disease, or they may have extraintestinal disease (eg, liver abscess). A positive serologic test is more likely to occur in patients with invasive amebiasis than in asymptomatic individuals.

Patient Preparation Fasting blood sample required

Specimen Serum

Container Red top tube

Sampling Time False negatives occur when symptoms have been of less than 7 days duration.[1]

Reference Interval IHA titer: <1:128; CF titer: <1:8; immunodiffusion test: negative

Critical Values IHA titer ≥1:256

Use Serologic testing for amebiasis is the best single test to distinguish between the two major types of liver abscesses: amebic and pyogenic. Extraintestinal amebiasis is frequently found without trophozoites or cysts in stool.

Limitations Sensitivity is highest in extraintestinal amebiasis, lower in amebic dysentery, and lowest in asymptomatic carriers. Some false positives occur in patients with ulcerative colitis. The utility of the serologic marker is diminished in those parts of the world in which amebiasis is highly endemic with persistence of antibodies; *vide infra*.

Methodology Complement fixation (CF), indirect hemagglutination (IHA), immunodiffusion (ID), indirect immunofluorescent antibody (IFA), enzyme-linked immunosorbent assay (ELISA), rapid latex agglutination, cellulose acetate precipitin (CAP) test

Additional Information Positive serologic tests are seen in 75% of patients with invasive colonic amebiasis, while a positive serology is seen in >90% of patients with amebic liver abscesses.[2] Indirect hemagglutination is positive in 87% to 100% of patients with amebic liver abscesses and >85% of patients with acute amebic dysentery. A recent study has shown that IHA ≥1:512 is a good predictor of *E. histolytica* infection even when the stool antigen is negative.[3] Fewer than 6% of uninfected individuals react in the test. Amebic serology when negative is strong evidence against amebic liver abscess. IHA titers ≥1:128 are considered to be clinically significant, and a fourfold rise in titer is diagnostic of invasive amebic disease. However, IHA titers may remain positive for more than 6 months after successful treatment of amebiasis.[4]

In the presence of liver abscess, fine needle aspiration for culture and cytology may disclose trophozoites at the margin of the lesion.

Footnotes
1. Ravdin JI, "Amebiasis," *Cecil Textbook of Medicine*, 21st ed, Chapter 428, Goldman L and Bennett JC, eds, Philadelphia, PA: WB Saunders Co, 2000 1971-3.
2. Shamsuzzaman SM, Haque R, Hasin SK, et al, "Evaluation of Indirect Fluorescent Antibody Test and Enzyme-Linked Immunosorbent Assay for Diagnosis of Hepatic Amebiasis in Bangladesh," *J Parisitol*, 2000, 86(3):611-5.
3. Pillai DR, Keystone JS, Sheppard DC, et al, "*Entamoeba histolytica* and *Entamoeba dispar*: Epidemiology and Comparison of Diagnostic Methods in a Setting of Nonendemicity," *Clin Infect Dis*, 1999, 29(5):1315-8.
4. Stanley SL Jr, Jackson TF, Foster L, et al, "Longitudinal Study of the Antibody Response to Recombinant *Entamoeba histolytica* Antigens in Patients With Amebic Liver Abscess," *Am J Trop Med Hyg*, 1998, 58(4):414-6.

References
Espinosa-Cantellano M and Martinez-Palomo A, "Pathogenesis of Intestinal Amebiasis: From Molecules to Disease," *Clin Microbiol Rev*, 2000, 13(2):318-31.
Haque R, Ali IM, and Petri WA Jr, "Prevalence and Immune Response to *Entamoeba histolytica* Infection in Preschool Children in Bangladesh," *Am J Trop Med Hyg*, 1999, 60(6):1031-4.
Hashmey R, Genta RM, and White AC Jr, "Parasites and Diarrhea. I: Protozoans and Diarrhea," *J Travel Med*, 1997, 4(1):17-31.
Leber AL, "Intestinal Amebae," *Clin Lab Med*, 1999, 19(3):601-19.

Internet Web Sites
www.cdc.gov/ncidod/dpd/parasites/amebiasis/default.htm

♦ **Enteric Pathogens Culture, Routine** *see* Bacterial Culture, Stool *on page 575*

♦ **Enteric Viruses by EM** *see* Electron Microscopic Examination for Viruses, Stool *on page 603*

♦ ***Enterobacteriaceae*** *see* Bacterial Culture, Bronchoscopy/Bronchial Brush/Bronchoalveolar Lavage Specimen *on page 568*

♦ ***Enterobacteriaceae*** *see* Bacterial Culture, Sputum *on page 574*

♦ ***Enterobacteriaceae*** *see* Bacterial Culture, Urine *on page 578*

♦ ***Enterobacteriaceae*** *see* Bacterial Culture, Wounds, Bites *on page 579*

♦ **Enterobacteriaceae Culture** *see* Bacterial Culture, Aerobes *on page 563*

♦ ***Enterobius vermicularis*** *see* Ova and Parasites, Stool *on page 666*

♦ ***Enterobius vermicularis* Preparation** *see* Pinworm Preparation *on page 670*

♦ ***Enterococcus*** *see* Bacterial Culture, Wounds, Bites *on page 579*

♦ ***Enterococcus* spp** *see* Bacterial Culture, Urine *on page 578*

♦ **Enterohemorrhagic *E. coli*** *see* Bacterial Culture, Stool *on page 575*

♦ **Enterovirus 71** *see* Enterovirus Polymerase Chain Reaction *on page 606*

♦ **Enterovirus 71 Infection** *see* Enterovirus Culture *on page 605*

♦ **Enterovirus, Blood Culture** *see* Viral Culture, Blood *on page 691*

Enterovirus Culture

Related Information
Bacterial Culture, Stool *on page 575*
Cerebrospinal Fluid Analysis: Overview *on page 416*
Coxsackievirus Serology *on page 595*
Enterovirus Polymerase Chain Reaction *on page 606*
Ova and Parasites, Stool *on page 666*
Poliomyelitis I, II, III Serology *on page 671*
Viral Culture *on page 689*
Viral Culture, Blood *on page 691*
Viral Culture, Central Nervous System Symptoms *on page 692*
Viral Culture, Stool *on page 695*
Viral Culture, Urine *on page 695*

Applies to Coxsackie B Virus Culture; Echovirus Culture; Enterovirus 71 Infection; Poliovirus Culture

Test Includes Inoculation of specimen onto several appropriate cell cultures; isolated viruses are identified using specific monoclonal antibodies or neutralization. Some laboratories will use the rapid culture method combined with monoclonal antibodies to reduce the time to detection of enteroviruses.

Abstract Enterovirus infections are among the most common human viral illnesses. Poliovirus, the prototypic enterovirus, was responsible for summer epidemics of paralytic poliomyelitis. Before the introduction of polio vaccines, epidemic polio occurred regularly in the U.S. with approximately 25 cases per 100,000 people annually.[1] Currently, due to widespread vaccination, wild type poliovirus has been eliminated in the Western hemisphere and nearly eliminated in the rest of the world.[1] Other enteroviruses cause a variety of clinical diseases, such as aseptic meningitis in young children, myocarditis, hemorrhagic conjunctivitis, and hand-foot-mouth syndrome (herpangina)(enterovirus 71).[2,3,4,5,6] Many patients are asymptomatic.

Specimen Stool, rectal swab, cerebrospinal fluid, upper and lower respiratory tract specimens, whole blood, throat swab, various organs and tissues (heart, muscle, brain)

Container Sterile container
(Continued)

Enterovirus Culture (Continued)

Sampling Time It is important to obtain specimens very early in the disease; however, virus is shed in the stool for weeks.

Storage Instructions Enteroviruses are rather hardy; however, specimens should be refrigerated or placed into cold virus transport medium and delivered immediately to the clinical laboratory since other viruses that cause similar clinical diseases are not so resilient.

Turnaround Time Negative cultures often are reported after 2 weeks for conventional culture: negative results are reported after 72 hours for rapid culture methods.

Reference Interval No virus isolated

Use Aid in the diagnosis of disease caused by enteroviruses listed in the following table (eg, polio, congenital viral infections, viral pericarditis, and aseptic meningitis)

Limitations Cell culture generally does not support the growth of certain Coxsackie A enteroviruses. Infrequently, aseptic meningitis is caused by Coxsackie A virus types which require animal inoculation for isolation. The isolation of enterovirus in stool specimens may not indicate an active clinical disease.

Methodology Inoculation of specimens into cell culture, incubation of cultures, and observation for characteristic cytopathic effect (CPE). Enteroviruses are stable at pH 3; rhinoviruses are unstable at this pH. Some (usually reference) laboratories can identify specific enteroviruses by using a battery of specific enterovirus-neutralizing antibodies. These antibodies are useful in identifying and typing Coxsackie A, Coxsackie B, echovirus, and poliovirus.

Specimens suspected of containing Coxsackie A virus can be inoculated into suckling mice, which are then observed for flaccid paralysis without encephalitis. Most clinical laboratories do not perform this virus isolation method.

Additional Information Most enteroviral infections are mild and asymptomatic. Clinical diseases in humans range from a slightly increased temperature to severe CNS disease and paralysis (see table).[1] Humans are the only known reservoir for enteroviruses. Thus, infection occurs by direct contact with infected individuals, the oral-fecal route or the respiratory route. Enteroviral infections occur most commonly between July and September. Children are more likely to become infected than are adults.

The detection of enteroviral nucleic acid directly from specimens is a new technique that enables the detection of enteroviruses within a few hours. This assay has been studied in the clinical setting and has been found to have clinical utility. It is currently available in many larger clinical laboratories.[7,8]

Clinical Diseases Caused by Enteroviruses

Cardiovascular	Myocarditis
	Pericarditis
Neurologic	Aseptic meningitis
	Encephalitis
	Poliomyelitis
Respiratory	Common cold
	Stomatitis
	Hand-foot-mouth disease (herpangina)
	Pharyngitis
	Tonsillitis
	Rhinitis
Miscellaneous	Febrile, exanthematous illness
	Acute hemorrhagic conjunctivitis (enterovirus 70, Coxsackie A24)

Adapted from Rotbart HA, "Nucleic Acid Detection Systems for Enteroviruses," *Clin Micro Rev*, 1991, 4:156-8.

Footnotes

1. American Academy of Pediatrics, "Prevention of Poliomyelitis: Recommendations for Use of Only Inactivated Poliovirus Vaccine for Routine Immunization," *Pediatrics*, 1999, 104(6):1404-6.

2. Rotbart HA, "Nucleic Acid Detection Systems for Enteroviruses," *Clin Microbiol Rev*, 1991, 4(2):156-8.

3. Rotbart HA, "Enteroviruses," *Manual of Clinical Microbiology*, 7th ed, Murray PR, Baron EJ, Pfaller MA, et al, eds, Washington, DC: AMS Press, American Society for Microbiology, 1999, 990-8.

4. Ho M, Chen ER, Hsu KH, et al, "An Epidemic of Enterovirus 71 Infection in Taiwan. Taiwan Enterovirus Epidemic Working Group," *N Engl J Med*, 1999, 341(13):929-35.

5. Huang CC, Liu CC, Chang YC, et al, "Neurologic Complications in Children With Enterovirus 71 Infection," *N Engl J Med*, 1999, 341(13):936-42.

6. Dolin R, "Enterovirus 71 - Emerging Infections and Emerging Questions," *N Engl J Med*, 1999, 341(13): 984-5.

7. Hadziyannis E, Cornish N, Starkey C, et al, "Amplicor Enterovirus Polymerase Chain Reaction in Patients With Aseptic Meningitis: A Sensitive Test Limited by Amplification Inhibitors," *Arch Pathol Lab Med*, 1999, 123(10):882-4.

8. Hamilton MS, Jackson MA, and Abel D, "Clinical Utility of Polymerase Chain Reaction Testing for Enteroviral Meningitis," *Pediatr Infect Dis J*, 1999, 18(6):533-7.

References

Grabow WO, Botma KL, de Villiers JC, et al, "Assessment of Cell Culture and Polymerase Chain Reaction Procedures for the Detection of Polioviruses in Wastewater," *Bull World Health Organ*, 1999, 77(12):973-80.

Rotbart HA, McCracken GH Jr, Whitley RJ, et al, "Clinical Significance of Enteroviruses in Serious Summer Febrile Illnesses of Children," *Pediatr Infect Dis J*, 1999, 18(10):869-74.

Sayer MH, "Enterovirus Infections: Diagnosis and Treatment," *Pediatr Infect Dis J*, 1999, 18(12):1033-9.

Internet Web Sites

www.cdc.gov/ncidod/dvrd/entrvirs.htm

♦ **Enterovirus Culture, Stool** *see* Viral Culture, Stool *on page 695*

♦ **Enterovirus Genome Detection** *see* Enterovirus Polymerase Chain Reaction *on page 606*

♦ **Enterovirus Molecular Probe Assay** *see* Enterovirus Polymerase Chain Reaction *on page 606*

Enterovirus Polymerase Chain Reaction

Related Information
Bacterial Culture, Cerebrospinal Fluid *on page 569*
Cerebrospinal Fluid Analysis: Overview *on page 416*
Enterovirus Culture *on page 605*
Polymerase Chain Reaction *on page 713*
Viral Culture *on page 689*

Synonyms Enterovirus Genome Detection; Enterovirus Molecular Probe Assay; Enterovirus RNA Detection; Molecular Probe for Enterovirus

Applies to Enterovirus 71

Test Includes Detection of enterovirus RNA through the generation of a DNA complement followed by amplification

Abstract Enteroviruses cause a wide variety of clinical disease, including upper respiratory tract infection, aseptic meningitis, myocarditis, conjunctivitis, herpangina, and pleurodynia. Enteroviruses account for >80% of U.S. cases of aseptic meningitis. The direct detection of enterovirus RNA in specimens can be accomplished with PCR amplification of the enterovirus genome. The amplification steps are followed by specific hybridization with an oligonucleotide probe which may be identified in a variety of formats, including radiography or an enzymatic reaction. The value of the enterovirus genome assay lies in the ability to identify the likely etiologic agent and allow for conservative management and cessation of other antivirals and antibiotics.[1] Several studies have analyzed PCR assays for enterovirus and have shown excellent sensitivity and specificity as compared to culture.[1,2,3,4] This assay is available in many larger clinical laboratories.

Specimen Blood, cerebrospinal fluid, and selected tissues including lymph nodes and myocardial tissue

Container Blood: lavender top (EDTA) tube; CSF: plastic or glass tube is acceptable

Collection Tissue samples should be snap-frozen immediately and stored at -80°C.

Storage Instructions Specimens should be transported to the laboratory as soon as they become available. If specimens cannot be processed immediately, they should be frozen and maintained at -80°C.

Causes for Rejection Specimens collected using heparin

Turnaround Time 1-3 days

Reference Interval No enterovirus genome detected

Use Identify enterovirus associated with meningitis, myocarditis, and other enterovirus-related diseases

Limitations A negative result does not rule out the presence of enterovirus genome. Inhibitors of the amplification assay may be present which lead to false-negative results. Enteroviral RNA can quickly be digested by RNases present in all specimens. Thus, the specimen should be transported in a timely fashion or handled appropriately to prevent the loss of target RNA. Limited cross-reactivity and amplification of other viruses within the Picornavirus family has been described, including amplification of some rhinovirus serotypes. It is not available in all local regions.

Methodology Enterovirus RNA is extracted from the specimen and a homologous DNA strand is generated using reverse transcriptase. Specific product is amplified using primers that anneal to the conserved 5' nontranslated region of most enteroviruses.

Additional Information The enterovirus genus includes 67 serotypes, including poliovirus 1-3, Coxsackievirus A1-A22, A24, B1-B6, echovirus 1-9, 11-27, 29-33, and enterovirus 68-71, all of which are members of the large Picornaviridae family. To date no specific disease has been accepted to be uniquely associated with any one enterovirus serotype.[5] Many nonpolioenteroviruses are capable of causing the paralytic disease particularly associated with polioviruses. Although enteroviruses are responsible for a wide-spectrum of clinical diseases, neonatal sepsis, aseptic meningitis, poliomyelitis, encephalitis, myocarditis, pulmonary edema, or hemorrhage are the most significant. Enterovirus 71 epidemics have recently been described in which 91% of deaths were in patients age 5 years or younger.[6,7,8] Meningitis, due to enteroviral infections, has a classic pattern of appearance in the late summer and fall in the northern hemisphere.

The PCR assay can be performed quickly and thus positive results for enterovirus RNA have the potential to impact patient management.[1,4,5]

Footnotes

1. Hamilton MS, Jackson MA, and Abel D, "Clinical Utility of Polymerase Chain Reaction Testing for Enteroviral Meningitis," *Pediatr Infect Dis J*, 1999, 18(6):533-7.
2. Hadziyannis E, Cornish N, Starkey C, et al, "Amplicor Enterovirus Polymerase Chain Reaction in Patients With Aseptic Meningitis: A Sensitive Test Limited by Amplification Inhibitors," *Arch Pathol Lab Med*, 1999, 123(10):882-4.
3. Ramers C, Billman G, Hartin M, et al, "Impact of a Diagnostic Cerebrospinal Fluid Enterovirus Polymerase Chain Reaction Test on Patient Management," *JAMA*, 2000, 283(20):2680-5.
4. Spicher VM, Berclaz PY, Cheseaux JJ, et al, "Detection of Enteroviruses in the Cerebrospinal Fluid by Polymerase Chain Reaction: Prospective Study of Impact on the Management of Hospitalized Children," *Clin Pediatr (Phila)*, 2000, 39(4):203-8.
5. Rotbart HA, "Enteroviruses," *Manual of Clinical Microbiology*, 7th ed, Murray PR, Baron EJ, Pfaller MA, et al, eds, Washington, DC: AMS Press, American Society for Microbiology, 1999, 990-8.
6. Ho M, Chen ER, Hsu KH, et al, "An Epidemic of Enterovirus 71 Infection in Taiwan. Taiwan Enterovirus Epidemic Working Group," *N Engl J Med*, 1999, 341(13):929-35.
7. Huang CC, Liu CC, Chang YC, et al, "Neurologic Complications in Children With Enterovirus 71 Infection," *N Engl J Med*, 1999, 341(13):936-42.
8. Dolin R, "Enterovirus 71 - Emerging Infections and Emerging Questions," *N Engl J Med*, 1999, 341(13): 984-5.

References

Grabow WO, Botma KL, de Villiers JC, et al, "Assessment of Cell Culture and Polymerase Chain Reaction Procedures for the Detection of Polioviruses in Wastewater," *Bull World Health Organ*, 1999, 77(12):973-80.

Romero JR, "Reverse-Transcription Polymerase Chain Reaction Detection of the Enteroviruses," *Arch Pathol Lab Med*, 1999, 123(12):1161-9.

Rotbart HA, McCracken GH Jr, Whitley RJ, et al, "Clinical Significance of Enteroviruses in Serious Summer Febrile Illnesses of Children," *Pediatr Infect Dis J*, 1999, 18(10):869-74.

Sayer MH, "Enterovirus Infections: Diagnosis and Treatment," *Pediatr Infect Dis J*, 1999, 18(12):1033-9.

Woods GL, "Picornaviruses," *Diagnostic Pathology of Infectious Disease*, Chapter 13, Malvern, PA: Lea & Febiger, 1993, 105-15.

Internet Web Sites

www.cdc.gov/ncidod/dvrd/entrvirs.htm

♦ **Enterovirus RNA Detection** *see* Enterovirus Polymerase Chain Reaction *on page 606*

♦ **Entomology** *see* Arthropod Identification *on page 559*

♦ **Enveloped Viruses** *see* Viral Culture *on page 689*

♦ **Enzyme Immunoassay, *Cryptosporidium*** *see Cryptosporidium* Antigen Detection by EIA *on page 596*

♦ **Enzyme Immunoassay for Group A *Streptococcus* Antigen** *see* Group A *Streptococcus* Screen, Rapid *on page 617*

♦ **Epstein-Barr Early Antigens** *see* Epstein-Barr Virus Serology *on page 607*

♦ **Epstein-Barr Viral Capsid Antigen** *see* Epstein-Barr Virus Serology *on page 607*

Epstein-Barr Virus Culture

Related Information

Epstein-Barr Virus Serology *on page 607*
Herpesvirus 8 *on page 634*
Heterophil Agglutinins *on page 635*
Infectious Mononucleosis Screening Test *on page 643*
Lymph Node Biopsy *on page 67*
Viral Culture, Blood *on page 691*

Applies to Lymph Node Culture for Epstein-Barr Virus; Lymphocyte Culture for Epstein-Barr Virus

Abstract Although Epstein-Barr virus (EBV) is a human herpesvirus, it is not easily cultured in the laboratory. EBV was originally isolated from Burkitt lymphomas, but subsequently it was found that EBV infects a large majority of adults and is transmitted in saliva. Primary infection with EBV may be asymptomatic or associated with infectious mononucleosis. Viral culture is rarely indicated for diagnostic purposes. See Epstein-Barr Virus Serology *on page 607* for further clinicopathologic information.

Specimen Whole blood, lymph node, spleen, tumor biopsies (eg, portions of nasopharyngeal biopsies), throat garglings, (for isolation of excreted virus)

Container Green top (heparin) tube for blood; sterile container for other specimens

Storage Instructions Blood specimen can be maintained at room temperature but should be immediately transported to the laboratory. Biopsy specimen should be sent to the Virology Laboratory immediately after collection.

Turnaround Time Cultures often are observed for 6 weeks before being reported as negative.

Special Instructions The laboratory always should be notified prior to receipt of specimen.

Reference Interval No growth of EBV in lymphocyte culture

Use Culture for EBV is generally not performed for diagnostic purposes. The demonstration of EBV DNA, RNA, or protein in biopsy tissue is required for the diagnosis of EBV lymphoproliferative disease.[1]

Limitations Cell culture for EBV is not routinely available and not diagnostically practical, because EBV proliferates only in B cells, which often are

difficult to obtain and process. In addition, many asymptomatic individuals can shed virus orally. Cell culture requires at least 4 weeks to detect EBV infection. EB virus culture is unnecessary for most cases of infectious mononucleosis.

Methodology Virus is given opportunity to grow for 4 weeks in a lymphocyte culture. Virus-infected cells will proliferate; if virus is not present, lymphocytes will die. Positive cultures are confirmed for EBV antigens using monoclonal antibodies.

Additional Information Aid in the diagnosis of EBV, which is the cause of a wide spectrum of diseases. These include oral hairy leukoplakia in HIV-infected individuals and some immunosuppressed patients, infectious mononucleosis (IM), undifferentiated nasopharyngeal carcinoma, 40% to 60% of cases of Hodgkin disease, a subset of diffuse large-cell immunoblastic lymphomas in immunocompromised individuals, subsets of peripheral T-cell lymphomas and carcinomas of stomach, rare smooth muscle neoplasms, and Burkitt lymphomas. Almost all CNS lymphomas contain EBV DNA. Found in patients with very low CD4[+] cell counts, EBV DNA by PCR in CSF predicts lymphoma in AIDS patients who have focal brain lesions. Evidence of EBV as well as HHV-8 is often found in AIDS patients with primary effusion lymphoma.[1] An EBV lymphoproliferative syndrome occurs following transplantation and in other settings. The most common syndrome associated with EBV infection is IM.[2] **The diagnosis of IM is based on three pillars: clinical appearance, CBC with differential characterized by lymphocytosis with virocytes, and conventional (Davidsohn) serology.**

Viral serology is the preferred diagnostic method for detection of active or past EBV infections.[3] EBV persists in the lymphoreticular system of EBV-infected individuals. EBV-positive lymphoblast lines can be established from peripheral leukocytes and lymph node cells from those individuals. Epstein-Barr virus can also be detected by immunochemistry and by polymerase chain reaction.[4] See the comparison listings, Epstein-Barr Virus Serology *on page 607*, Heterophil Agglutinins *on page 635*, and Infectious Mononucleosis Screening Test *on page 643*.

Footnotes

1. Cohen JI, "Epstein-Barr Virus Infection," *N Engl J Med*, 2000, 343(7):481-92.
2. Baldanti F, Grossi P, Furione M, et al, "High Levels of Epstein-Barr Virus DNA in Blood of Solid-Organ Transplant Recipients and Their Value in Predicting Post-transplant Lymphoproliferative Disorders," *J Clin Microbiol*, 2000, 38(2):613-9.
3. Lennette ET, "Epstein-Barr Virus," *Manual of Clinical Microbiology*, 7th ed, Murray PR, Baron EJ, Pfaller MA, et al, eds, Washington, DC: AMS Press, American Society for Microbiology, 1999, 912-8.
4. Wu TT, Swerdlow SH, Locker J, et al, "Recurrent Epstein-Barr Virus-Associated Lesions in Organ Transplant Recipients," *Hum Pathol*, 1996, 27(2):157-64.

References

Ambinder RF and Mann RB, "Detection and Characterization of Epstein-Barr Virus in Clinical Specimens," *Am J Pathol*, 1994, 145(2):239-52.

Faulkner GC, Krajewski AS, and Crawford DH, "The Ins and Outs of EBV Infection," *Trends Microbiol*, 2000, 8(4):185-9.

Godshall SE and Kirchner JT, "Infectious Mononucleosis. Complexities of a Common Syndrome," *Postgrad Med*, 2000, 107(7):175-86.

Liebowitz D, "Epstein-Barr Virus - An Old Dog With New Tricks," *N Engl J Med*, 1995, 332(1):55-7.

Epstein-Barr Virus Serology

Related Information

Epstein-Barr Virus Culture *on page 607*
Heterophil Agglutinins *on page 635*
Infectious Mononucleosis Screening Test *on page 643*

Synonyms EBV Titer

Applies to EBNA; EB Nuclear Antigen; Epstein-Barr Early Antigens; Epstein-Barr Viral Capsid Antigen; VCA; VCA Titer; Viral Capsid Antigen

Abstract Since Epstein-Barr virus (EBV) was found in a Ugandan child with Burkitt lymphoma three decades ago, a role of the virus has been shown in several diseases in addition to infectious mononucleosis. These include hairy leukoplakia (a disorder of the tongue), carcinoma of nasopharynx, lymphomas in patients following transplantation, and other neoplastic entities.[1,2] Relationships to some T-cell lymphomas and to Hodgkin disease have been recognized.[3]

Specimen Serum

Container Red top tube

Reference Interval See table.

Epstein-Barr Virus Serology

	Uninfected	Current Infection	Previous Infection
IgG anti-VCA	<1:10 or negative	>1:10 or positive	≥1:10 or positive
IgM anti-VCA*	<1:10 or negative	>1:10 or positive*	≤1:10 or negative
Anti-EBNA	<1:5 or negative	<1:5 or negative	≥1:5 or positive

*An IgM anti-VCA titer >1:10 or positive by EIA is a key reaction indicative of current or recent infection.

(Continued)

Epstein-Barr Virus Serology (Continued)

Use Diagnose Epstein-Barr virus infection; evaluate heterophil-negative mononucleosis, Burkitt lymphoma, lymphoproliferative disease, X-linked lymphoproliferative disease[3]

Limitations Despite much publicity, these tests are neither sensitive nor specific for chronic fatigue syndrome. EBV infects >90% of humans, persisting for their lifetimes,[3] and chronic fatigue is a commonplace complaint. It is unclear if such investigation is useful for the clinical diagnosis of nasopharyngeal carcinoma or post-transplant lymphomas. It is not needed in the diagnosis of hairy leukoplakia, which has a distinct clinical presentation: see recently published photography.[3]

Contraindications The Epstein-Barr viral test need not be done on patients who have heterophil antibodies with the symptoms, physical findings and lymphocyte morphology consistent with infectious mononucleosis.

Methodology Indirect fluorescent antibody (IFA), enzyme-linked immunosorbent assay (ELISA). EBV can be demonstrated in tissue with *in situ* hybridization, immunohistochemistry, and PCR.[2,4]

Additional Information EBV is a ubiquitous human herpesvirus that infects epithelial cells and B lymphocytes. It causes classic infectious mononucleosis and is associated with >90% of the cases of Burkitt lymphoma, nearly 100% of poorly differentiated nasopharyngeal carcinomas, a subset of gastric carcinomas, lymphoproliferative disorders in immunocompromised patients, hairy leukoplakia, non-Hodgkin lymphomas in patients with congenital or acquired immunodeficiency, 40% to 60% of U.S. cases of Hodgkin disease, and smooth muscle tumors in immunosuppressed children.[3,5,6,7]

Although most cases of infectious mononucleosis can be diagnosed on the basis of clinical findings, blood count and morphology, with a positive test for heterophil antibody (infectious mononucleosis screening test). As many as 20% may be heterophil-negative at presentation but the heterophil may become positive when repeated in a few days. In some such cases, a test for EBV antibodies may be useful, as well as investigation for other entities (eg, cytomegalovirus).

The serologic response to EBV includes antibody to early antigen, which is usually short lived, IgM and IgG antibodies to viral capsid antigen (VCA), and antibodies to nuclear antigen (EBNA); of these, VCA is the most useful. A high presenting VCA titer is good evidence for EBV infection. Since titers are generally high by the time a patient is symptomatic, it may not be possible to demonstrate fourfold rise in titer. Since a very high titer may be due to past infection, IgM titers should be measured to establish acute infection. Persistent absence of antibody to viral capsid is good evidence against EBV infection.

Antibody to EBV nuclear antigen (EBNA) usually develops 4-6 weeks after infection. Its presence early during an acute illness should lead one to consider a diagnosis other than EBV infectious mononucleosis.

For the diagnosis of EBV in nasopharyngeal carcinomas, gastric carcinomas, or lymphoproliferative disorders, the presence of the virus can be detected by histochemical staining with monoclonal antibodies or the direct detection of EBV-specific nucleic acid in tissues.[1,2]

See Epstein-Barr Virus Culture *on page 607* and Infectious Mononucleosis Screening Test *on page 643.*

Footnotes

1. Cheung ST, Huang DP, Hui AB, et al, "Nasopharyngeal Carcinoma Cell Line (C66-1) Consistently Harbouring Epstein-Barr Virus," *Int J Cancer*, 1999, 83(1):121-6.
2. Baldanti F, Grossi P, Furione M, et al, "High Levels of Epstein-Barr Virus DNA in Blood of Solid-Organ Transplant Recipients and Their Value in Predicting Post-transplant Lymphoproliferative Disorders," *J Clin Microbiol*, 2000, 38(2):613-9.
3. Cohen JI, "Epstein-Barr Virus Infection," *N Engl J Med*, 2000, 343(7):481-92.
4. Wu TT, Swerdlow SH, Locker J, et al, "Recurrent Epstein-Barr Virus-Associated Lesions in Organ Transplant Recipients," *Hum Pathol*, 1996, 27(2):157-64.
5. McClain KL, Leach CT, Jenson HB, et al, "Association of Epstein-Barr Virus With Leiomyosarcomas in Children With AIDS," *N Engl J Med*, 1995, 332(1):12-8.
6. Lee ES, Locker J, Nalesnik M, et al, "The Association of Epstein-Barr Virus With Smooth-Muscle Tumors Occurring After Organ Transplantation," *N Engl J Med*, 1995, 332(1):19-25.
7. Liebowitz D, "Epstein-Barr Virus - An Old Dog With New Tricks," *N Engl J Med*, 1995, 332(1):55-7.

References

Ambinder RF and Mann RB, "Detection and Characterization of Epstein-Barr Virus in Clinical Specimens," *Am J Pathol*, 1994, 145(2):239-52.

Cohen AH, Sweet SC, Mendeloff E, et al, "High Incidence of Post-transplant Lymphoproliferative Disease in Pediatric Patients With Cystic Fibrosis," *Am J Respir Crit Care Med*, 2000, 161(4 Pt 1):1252-5.

Faulkner GC, Krajewski AS, and Crawford DH, "The Ins and Outs of EBV Infection," *Trends Microbiol*, 2000, 8(4):185-9.

Godshall SE and Kirchner JT, "Infectious Mononucleosis. Complexities of a Common Syndrome," *Postgrad Med*, 2000, 107(7):175-86.

Lo YM, Leung SF, Chan LY, et al, "Plasma Cell-Free Epstein-Barr Virus DNA Quantitation in Patients With Nasopharyngeal Carcinoma. Correlation With Clinical Staging," *Ann N Y Acad Sci*, 2000, 906:99-101.

♦ *Escherichia coli* O157:H7   *see* Bacterial Culture, Stool *on page 575*

♦ **Espundia Serological Test**   *see* Leishmaniasis Serology *on page 647*

♦ **E-Test**   *see* Antimicrobial Susceptibility Testing, Aerobic and Facultatively Anaerobic Bacteria *on page 554*

♦ **E-Test**   *see* Antimicrobial Susceptibility Testing, Unusual Isolates/Fastidious Organisms *on page 558*

♦ **E-Test, Anaerobic Bacteria**   *see* Antimicrobial Susceptibility Testing, Anaerobic Bacteria *on page 555*

♦ **Exit Site Infections**   *see* Bacterial Culture, Intravascular Device *on page 572*

♦ **Eye Culture**   *see* Bacterial Culture, Conjunctiva *on page 570*

♦ **Eye Fungus Culture**   *see* Fungal Culture, Ocular Infections *on page 612*

♦ **Eye Swab *Chlamydia* Culture**   *see Chlamydia trachomatis* Culture *on page 590*

♦ **Eye, Viral Culture**   *see* Viral Culture, Eye or Ocular Symptoms *on page 693*

♦ **FA Smear for *Legionella pneumophila***   *see Legionella* Direct Fluorescent Antibody Smear *on page 646*

Filariasis Serological Test

Related Information

Microfilariae, Peripheral Blood Preparation *on page 460*
Ova and Parasites, Urine *on page 667*

Synonyms Microfilariae Serological Test

Applies to Antigen Detection for *W. bancrofti*; *Brugia malayi* Serology; *Brugia timori* Serology; *Loa loa* Serology; *Mansonella ozzardi* Serology; *Mansonella perstans* Serology; *Mansonella streptocerca* Serology; *Onchocerca volvulus* Serology; *Wuchereria bancrofti* Serology

Abstract Filariasis is a tropical disease that is transmitted by arthropods. Filarial nematodes live in body cavities, subcutaneous tissue, or as adults, in the lymphatics of the host. Infection often leads to lymphatic inflammation and/or chronic lymphatic obstruction. Hydrocoele and elephantiasis develop secondarily in *Wuchereria* infestation. Microfilariae (embryos) are ingested by bloodsucking arthropods, primarily mosquitoes, and develop to an infective phase. It is the microfilaria stage which is accessible for diagnosis. The term filariasis refers to invasion of lymphatics by the nematodes *Wuchereria bancrofti*, *Brugia malayi*, or *Brugia timori*. Although immunodiagnosis may play a little role, the test of choice is a Giemsa-stained blood smear obtained at the appropriate time for detection of the microfilariae. (Nocturnal periodicity is pivotal for diagnosis by blood smear.)

Specimen Serum

Container Red top tube

Reference Interval Varies with laboratory and methodology

Use Questionably useful, intended to support a diagnosis of filariasis, microfilariasis causing elephantiasis.

Limitations **Testing presently lacks sensitivity and specificity.** Cross-reactivity between filarial antigens and antigens of other helminths complicates interpretation of serologic assays. False positives occur in subjects residing in endemic areas.

Methodology Bentonite flocculation assay (BFA), complement fixation (CF), indirect fluorescent antibody (IFA), indirect hemagglutination (IHA), enzyme immunoassay (EIA). A large reference laboratory uses an IgM monoclonal antibody raised against a filarial cattle parasite, *Onchocerca gibsoni*, in a serum antigen detection test for *W. bancrofti*.[1]

Additional Information For screening, an antigen prepared from the dog heartworm, *Dirofilaria immitis*, detects antibody responses to several clinically significant microfilariae, but sensitivity and specificity are poor. Testing with antigen prepared from homologous parasites is more specific but is essentially unavailable. **Morphologic examination of a blood film or hydrocoele fluid remains the foundation of diagnosis.** Patients with other diseases or other types of parasites (helminths) may have antibodies, as may patients with eosinophilic infiltrates in the lungs, perhaps because of unrecognized dirofilariasis. Such cross reactions may be due to antibodies to phosphocholine, a molecule present in many organisms. IgG$_4$ antibodies are not developed to phosphocholine; antibodies of this class are specific for filaria. Eosinophilia and immunoglobulin E may be helpful additional tests.

Footnotes

1. Mayo Reference Services Publication, "Filarial Antigens, Serum," *New Test Announcement*, #82412, Rochester, MN: Mayo Medical Laboratories, 2001.

References

Boatin BA, Toe L, Alley ES, et al, "Diagnosis in Onchocerciasis: Future Challenges," *Ann Trop Med Parasitol*, 1998, 92(Suppl 1):S41-5.

Freedman DO, "Filariasis," *Cecil Textbook of Medicine*, 21st ed, Chapter 434, Goldman L and Bennett JC, eds, Philadelphia, PA: WB Saunders Co, 2000, 1990-5.

Hall LR and Pearlman E, "Pathogenesis of Onchocercal Keratitis (River Blindness)," *Clin Microbiol Rev*, 1999, 12(3):445-53.

Harnett W, Bradley JE, and Garate T, "Molecular and Immunodiagnosis of Human Filarial Nematode Infections," *Parasitology*, 1998, 117(S):S59-71.

Kale OO, "Onchocerciasis: The Burden of Disease," *Ann Trop Med Parasitol*, 1998, 92(Suppl 1):S101-15.

Kron M, Walker E, Hernandez L, et al, "Lymphatic Filariasis in the Philippines," *Parasitol Today*, 2000, 16(8):329-33.

Internet Web Sites

www.astdhpphe.org/infect/lymphfil.html
www.cdc.gov/ncidod/dpd/parasites/lymphaticfilariasis/default.htm

Fine Needle Aspiration Culture

Related Information
  Bacterial Culture, Biopsy or Body Fluid *on page 565*
  Coccidioidomycosis Serology *on page 593*
  Fine Needle Aspiration, Deep Masses *on page 381*
  Fine Needle Aspiration, Superficial Masses (Palpable) *on page 382*
  Fungal Culture, Biopsy or Body Fluid *on page 610*
  Fungal Culture, Sputum *on page 613*
  Mycobacterial Culture, Biopsy or Body Fluid *on page 655*
  Mycobacterial Culture, Cutaneous and Subcutaneous Tissue *on page 657*

Synonyms CT Guided Needle Aspiration Culture; FNA Culture

Applies to Swabs for Culture

Test Includes Culture for bacterial, mycobacterial, or fungal organisms. Gram stain is commonly indicated if sufficient material is available.

Specimen Tissue specimen from the needle biopsy

Container Clean, sterile container

Causes for Rejection Insufficient material for several cultures

Reference Interval No growth

Use Swabs of ulcers or fistulas may provide misleading information when deep infections are evaluated. Culture of abscesses or masses suspected of being infectious, especially tuberculous masses, requires adequate sampling. Fine needle aspiration culture or surgical sampling is needed to obtain critical material for culture (eg, in osteomyelitis).[1] Fine needle aspiration is also used for molecular techniques of infectious disease diagnosis,[2] and often are highly desirable for cytologic evaluation.

Limitations May not obtain sufficient material for culture

Methodology The skin is cleansed to remove any skin residual flora. A needle is guided into the mass through the skin. The specimen is aspirated into the syringe and taken directly to the laboratory for culture and examination.

Additional Information Fine needle aspiration is a simple diagnostic tool used for the evaluation of superficial and deep seated lesions or masses. Cultures from needle aspiration specimens have a high diagnostic yield and avoid invasive procedures. See specimen requirements for each specific type of culture. Note Bacterial Culture, Biopsy or Body Fluid *on page 565*.

Refer to Lymphadenopathy in the Key Word Index.

Footnotes
  1. Lew DP and Waldvogel FA, "Osteomyelitis," *N Engl J Med*, 1997, 336(14):999-1007.
  2. Alkan S, Eltoum IA, Tabbara S, et al, "Usefulness of Molecular Detection of Human Herpesvirus-8 in the Diagnosis of Kaposi Sarcoma by Fine Needle Aspiration," *Am J Clin Pathol*, 1999, 111(1):91-6.

References
  Ellison E, LaPuerta P, and Martin SE, "Supraclavicular Masses: Results of a Series of 309 Cases Biopsied by Fine Needle Aspiration," *Head Neck*, 1999, 21(3):239-46.
  Ellison E, LaPuerta P, and Martin SE, "Fine Needle Aspiration Diagnosis of Mycobacterial Lymphadenitis. Sensitivity and Predictive Value in the United States," *Acta Cytol*, 1999, 43(2):153-7.
  Francis IM, Das DK, Luthra UK, et al, "Value of Radiologically Guided Fine Needle Aspiration Cytology (FNAC) in the Diagnosis of Spinal Tuberculosis: A Study of 29 Cases," *Cytopathology*, 1999, 10(6):390-401.
  Jain M, Sharma S, and Jain TS, "Cryptococcosis of Thoracic Vertebra Simulating Tuberculosis: Diagnosis by Fine-Needle Aspiration Biopsy Cytology - A Case Report," *Diagn Cytopathol*, 1999, 20(6):385-6.
  Zaharopoulos P, "Fine-Needle Aspiration Cytologic Diagnosis of Lymphocutaneous Sporotrichosis: A Case Report," *Diagn Cytopathol*, 1999, 20(2):74-7.

♦ **Flagellates** *see* Ova and Parasites, Stool *on page 666*

♦ *Flavobacterium meningosepticum* *see* Bacterial Culture, Cerebrospinal Fluid *on page 569*

♦ **Flea Identification** *see* Arthropod Identification *on page 559*

♦ **Flies** *see* Arthropod Identification *on page 559*

♦ **Flukes** *see* Schistosomiasis Serology *on page 678*

♦ **Fluorescent Antibody Test, Direct, for Virus** *see* Virus, Direct Detection by Fluorescent Antibody *on page 696*

♦ **Fluorescent Rabies Antibody Test** *see* Rabies *on page 673*

♦ **Fluorescent Treponemal Antibody-Absorption** *see* FTA-ABS, Serum *on page 609*

♦ **Fluorochrome Stain** *see* Acid-Fast Stain *on page 550*

♦ **FNA Culture** *see* Fine Needle Aspiration Culture *on page 609*

♦ **Foreign Body Culture** *see* Bacterial Culture, Wounds, Bites *on page 579*

♦ **Fractional Bactericidal Concentration (FBC)** *see* Antimicrobial Susceptibility Testing, Antimicrobial Combinations *on page 556*

♦ **Fractional Inhibitory Concentration (FIC)** *see* Antimicrobial Susceptibility Testing, Antimicrobial Combinations *on page 556*

♦ *Francisella tularensis* **Antibodies** *see* Tularemia Serology *on page 686*

♦ *Francisella tularensis* **Culture** *see* Bacterial Culture, Blood *on page 566*

♦ *Francisella tularensis* **Culture** *see* Tularemia Serology *on page 686*

♦ **FRA Test** *see* Rabies *on page 673*

FTA-ABS, Serum

Related Information
  Darkfield Examination, Syphilis *on page 601*
  MHA-TP *on page 651*
  RPR *on page 677*
  VDRL, Cerebrospinal Fluid *on page 688*
  VDRL, Serum *on page 688*

Synonyms Fluorescent Treponemal Antibody-Absorption

Applies to Syphilis Serology; *T. pallidum* DNA

Test Includes Serum specimen is absorbed and then tested with immunofluorescence for antibody to *Treponema pallidum*

Abstract The FTA-ABS, like the MHA-TP, is a specific treponemal test. Although more sensitive than the reaginic tests, it is more expensive and more technically sophisticated. (Quantitative nontreponemal or reaginic tests include the VDRL and RPR.)[1] A reactive FTA-ABS in a patient also reactive to a nontreponemal test is highly specific for syphilis[2] (lues). History of primary or secondary syphilis is not obtained from most patients.[3]

Patient Preparation Patient should be fasting if possible.

Specimen Serum

Container Red top tube

Reference Interval Nonreactive. Results are reported as reactive, reactive minimal, equivocal, nonreactive, or atypical fluorescence observed; a titer is not determined.

Possible Panic Range Serodiagnosis of syphilis in pregnancy

Use Confirm the presence of antibodies to *Treponema pallidum* in patients who have tested positive for nontreponemal antibodies by VDRL or RPR screening test and to support a clinical impression of syphilis in patients in whom a nontreponemal test (eg, VDRL, RPR) is nonreactive.

Tertiary syphilis appears in ~30% of untreated patients with syphilis, usually after 10-40 years, but rarely as early as 1 year after infection.[3]

Limitations FTA-ABS test for syphilis is reported positive in the treponemal diseases pinta, yaws and endemic syphilis (bejel), and falsely positive in patients with some diseases associated with increased or abnormal globulins, antinuclear antibodies, lupus erythematosus (beaded pattern), pregnancy, and drug addiction (although drug addicts are likely to have true positives as well). Lyme disease, leprosy, malaria, infectious mononucleosis, relapsing fever, and leptospirosis are also potential causes of false-positive FTA-ABS. Fewer than 1% of healthy individuals will have a false positive.[4] Borderline results are inconclusive and cannot be interpreted; they may indicate a very low level of treponemal antibody or may be due to nonspecific factors. Further follow-up and serological confirmation with the treponemal immobilization test may be helpful. Potential causes of false-positive serologic tests for syphilis are tabulated in VDRL, Serum *on page 688*. Approximately 90% of patients with syphilitic aortitis have a positive treponemal test.[3]

Methodology Indirect fluorescent antibody (IFA) of killed *Treponema* after serum absorption

Additional Information FTA-ABS is a sensitive test in all stages of syphilis, and is the best standard confirmatory test for a serum reactive to a screening test such as RPR or VDRL. Occasionally, patients with ocular syphilis (uveitis) or otosyphilis will have a negative VDRL while their FTA-ABS is positive. FTA-ABS cannot be used to follow disease activity or response to treatment, since it will remain high for years or for life. A modification of the test can detect IgM specific antibodies, which may distinguish true congenital syphilis from placental transfer of maternal antibodies, the **IgM FTA-ABS** test. This modification has ~35% false-negative results with delayed-onset congenital syphilis, and about 10% false positives.[5] Removal of IgG leads to a **19S IgM FTA-ABS test**, a labor-intensive, specific, and sensitive test.[6,7]

When a positive serum FTA-ABS is required before performing CSF VDRL examination, the specificity of the CSF test is markedly improved. The FTA-ABS test is not recommended for testing cerebrospinal fluid; usually the VDRL is done on CSF.

Treponema can be detected by direct immunofluorescence staining with polyclonal conjugates. PCR has been used to detect *T. pallidum* DNA in specimens including cerebrospinal fluid and amniotic fluid. This approach may be highly sensitive and specific but currently has not been standardized.[8]

The most common manifestation of late syphilis is aortitis, which is especially marked proximally. The coronary ostia are involved in 26% of patients, and such involvement may be the only manifestation of luetic aortitis.

Footnotes
  1. Wicher K, Horowitz HW, and Wicher V, "Laboratory Methods of Diagnosis of Syphilis for the Beginning of the Third Millennium," *Microbes Infect*, 1999, 1(12):1035-49.
  2. Emmert DH and Kirchner JT, "Sexually Transmitted Diseases in Women. Gonorrhea and Syphilis," *Postgrad Med*, 2000, 107(2):181-97.
  3. Vlahakes GJ, Hanna GJ, and Mark EJ, "A 46-Year-Old Man With Chest Pain and Coronary Ostial Stenosis," Case Records of the Massachusetts General Hospital, Case 10-1998, Scully RE, Mark EJ, McNeely WF, et al, eds, *N Engl J Med*, 1998, 338(13):897-903.

(Continued)

FTA-ABS, Serum *(Continued)*

4. Larsen SA, Norris SJ, and Pope V, "*Treponema* and Other Host-Associated Spirochetes," *Manual of Clinical Microbiology*, 7th ed, Washington, DC: AMS Press, American Society for Microbiology, 1999, 759-76.

5. Hook EW, "Syphilis," *Cecil Textbook of Medicine*, 21st ed, Chapter 365, Goldman L and Bennett JC, eds, Philadelphia, PA: WB Saunders Co, 2000, 1746-55.

6. "Improvements in Syphilis Testing," *Mayo References Services Communique*, 1999.

7. Mayo Reference Services Publication, "Syphilis G and M, Serum," *New Test Announcement*, #81814, Rochester, MN: Mayo Medical Laboratories, January 1999.

8. Morse SA, Trees DL, Htun Y, et al, "Comparison of Clinical Diagnosis and Standard Laboratory and Molecular Methods for the Diagnosis of Genital Ulcer Disease in Lesotho: Association With Human Immunodeficiency Virus Infection," *J Infect Dis*, 1997, 175(3):583-9.

References

Birnbaum NR, Goldschmidt RH, and Buffett WO, "Resolving the Common Clinical Dilemmas of Syphilis," *Am Fam Phys*, 1999, 59(8):2233-46.

Clyne B and Jerrad DA, "Syphilis Testing," *J Emerg Med*, 2000, 18(3):361-7.

Darville T, "Syphilis," *Pediatr Rev*, 1999, 20(5):160-4.

Genc M and Ledger WJ, "Syphilis in Pregnancy," *Sex Transm Infect*, 2000, 76(2):73-9.

Miller KE and Graves JC, "Update on the Prevention and Treatment of Sexually Transmitted Diseases," *Am Fam Phys*, 2000, 61(2):379-86.

Musher DM and Baughn RE, "Neurosyphilis in HIV-Infected Persons," *N Engl J Med*, 1994, 331(22):1516-7.

Rome ES, "Sexually Transmitted Diseases: Testing and Treating," *Adolesc Med*, 1999, 10(2):231-41.

Young H, "Syphilis. Serology," *Dermatol Clin*, 1998, 16(4):691-8.

Internet Web Sites

www.astdhpphe.org/infect/syphilis.html

www.cdc.gov/nchstp/dstd/fact_sheets/syphilis_facts.htm

Fungal Culture, Biopsy or Body Fluid

Related Information

Amphotericin B, Serum *on page 737*
Antimicrobial Susceptibility Testing, Fungi *on page 556*
Aspergillus Serology *on page 560*
Bacterial Culture, Biopsy or Body Fluid *on page 565*
Blastomycosis Serology *on page 582*
Body Cavity Fluid Cytology *on page 372*
Body Fluid Analysis, Cell Count *on page 408*
Body Fluid Chemical Analysis *on page 123*
Body Fluid pH *on page 125*
Bone Marrow *on page 410*
Candida Antigen *on page 587*
Candidiasis Serology *on page 588*
Coccidioidomycosis Serology *on page 593*
Fine Needle Aspiration Culture *on page 609*
Fine Needle Aspiration, Deep Masses *on page 381*
Fine Needle Aspiration, Superficial Masses (Palpable) *on page 382*
Fungal Culture, Blood *on page 610*
Fungal Culture, Cerebrospinal Fluid *on page 611*
Fungal Culture, Skin *on page 612*
Fungal Culture, Sputum *on page 613*
Fungus Smear, Stain *on page 615*
Histopathology *on page 59*
Histoplasmosis Antibody *on page 635*
Histoplasmosis Antigen *on page 636*
Sporotrichosis Serology *on page 680*
Synovial Fluid Analysis *on page 323*

Synonyms Body Fluid Fungus Culture

Applies to Bone Marrow Fungus Culture; Histoplasmosis; Mucormycosis; Synovial Fluid Fungus Culture; Tissue Fungus Culture

Abstract Infections due to fungi can sometimes be detected in tissue in the absence of culture. However, fungal culture provides a more accurate diagnosis. Ideally, both histopathologic examination and culture should be done together. Fungal cultures of biopsy material are more desirable than cultures from drainage.

Patient Preparation Aseptic preparation of biopsy site or site of body fluid aspiration

Specimen Surgical tissue, bone marrow, biopsy material, sterile body fluid (synovial fluid, peritoneal fluid, pleural fluid, ascites, etc). See tables in Fungal Culture, Sputum *on page 613*.

Collection The portion of the biopsy specimen submitted for culture should be separated in the sterile field in the operating room from the portion submitted for histopathology.

Causes for Rejection Culture specimen in fixative must be rejected for culture; specimen collected on swabs is suboptimal.

Reference Interval No growth

Use Establish the diagnosis of localized or disseminated mycosis; isolate and identify fungi. Tissue sections with special stains provide rapid and often pivotal results, but cultures are mandatory. For instance, staining for *H. capsulatum* provides positive observations in only ~50% to 60% of tissue biopsies.[1] Discrete granulomas were found in 8.5% of gastrointestinal cases, and <20% of liver specimens, in a series of gastrointestinal and hepatic histoplasmosis.[2]

Methodology Culture under aerobic conditions on several media, usually including Sabouraud's and brain heart infusion (BHI), biphasic media with or without lysis concentration technique, frequently incubation at room temperature or at both 30°C and 37°C

Additional Information Optimal isolation of fungi from tissue is accomplished by processing as much tissue as possible. Swabs should not be submitted and every attempt should be made to obtain adequate tissue for culture. Specimen selection tables are provided in Fungal Culture, Sputum *on page 613* and Fungal Culture, Skin *on page 612*. Depending upon the geographic area, *Histoplasma capsulatum*, *Blastomyces dermatitidis*, and *Coccidioides immitis* are the most frequently isolated deep pathogenic fungi. *Candida* species are common opportunistic pathogens in all geographic locations and are the most common opportunistic fungal infections related to the gastrointestinal tract. Immunocompromised patients, transplant patients, and patients with acquired immunodeficiency syndrome (AIDS) are at increased risk for opportunistic mycoses.[3] Isolates such as *Aspergillus* species or zygomycetes may be environmental in origin and must be interpreted in clinical context.

Fungal peritonitis is clinically similar to bacterial peritonitis with pain, fever, and abdominal tenderness. Fungal infections due to *Candida* species (mostly *Candida albicans* and *Candida parapsilosis*), and rare cases of *Aspergillus fumigatus*, *Fusarium*, and *Nocardia asteroides*, have been reported in patients undergoing chronic dialysis. In a series of AIDS patients, culture of bone marrow biopsy detected opportunistic fungal or mycobacterial infections in 25% of the specimens. Only 27% of the culture positive biopsies were associated with bone marrow granulomas. This study concluded that bone marrow examination has limited value in analysis of fungal and mycobacterial infections,[4] but results can be provided rapidly. Neutrophil count <1000/µL is associated with infection by *Candida*, *Aspergillus*, *Mucor*, *Rhizopus*, *Trichosporon*, and *Fusarium* species. T-cell defects and/or impaired cell-mediated immunity are associated with infection by *Candida*, *Cryptococcus neoformans*, *Histoplasma capsulatum*, *Coccidioides immitis*, and *Aspergillus* species. Catheterization (arterial, venous, or urinary) and mechanical disruption of the skin are associated with *Candida* and *Rhodotorula* species infections. Disruption of the natural barrier of the GI tract and respiratory tree by cytotoxic chemotherapy predispose to *Candida* species infections.[5]

Mucormycosis is a complication of diabetes mellitus, especially when it is poorly controlled and in the presence of ketoacidosis.[6] It complicates hematologic malignant disorders, those on immunosuppressive therapy, and patients in azotemia.

Footnotes

1. Klein CJ, Dinapoli RP, Temesgen Z, et al, "Central Nervous System Histoplasmosis Mimicking a Brain Tumor: Difficulties in Diagnosis and Treatment," *Mayo Clin Proc*, 1999, 74(8):803-7.

2. Lamps LW, Molina CP, West AB, et al, "The Pathologic Spectrum of Gastrointestinal and Hepatic Histoplasmosis," *Am J Clin Pathol*, 2000, 113(1):64-72.

3. Buchheidt D, Skladny H, Baust C, et al, "Systemic Infections With *Candida* sp and *Aspergillus* sp in Immunocompromised Patients With Hematological Malignancies: Current Serological and Molecular Diagnostic Methods," *Chemotherapy*, 2000, 46(3):219-28.

4. Marques MB, Waites KB, Jaye DL, et al, "Histologic Examination of Bone Marrow Core Biopsy Specimens Has Limited Value in the Diagnosis of Mycobacterial and Fungal Infections in Patients With the Acquired Immunodeficiency Syndrome," *Ann Diagn Pathol*, 2000, 4(1):1-6.

5. Jagarlamudi R and Kumar L, "Systemic Fungal Infections in Cancer Patients," *Trop Gastroenterol*, 2000, 21(1):3-8.

6. Brown RB and Lau SK, "A 59-Year-Old Diabetic Man With Unilateral Visual Loss and Oculomotor-Nerve Palsy," Case Record of the Massachusetts General Hospital, Case 3-2001, Scully RE, Mark EJ, McNeely WF, et al, eds, *N Engl J Med*, 2001, 344(4):286-93.

References

Ho PL and Yuen KY, "Aspergillosis in Bone Marrow Transplant Recipients," *Crit Rev Oncol Hematol*, 2000, 34(1):55-69.

Hunt SM, Miyamoto RC, Cornelius RS, et al, "Invasive Fungal Sinusitis in the Acquired Immunodeficiency Syndrome," *Otolaryngol Clin North Am*, 2000, 33(2):335-47.

Johnson RA, "The Immune Compromised Host in the Twenty-First Century: Management of Mucocutaneous Infections," *Semin Cutan Med Surg*, 2000, 19(1):19-61.

Malani PN and Kauffman CA, "Prevention and Prophylaxis of Invasive Fungal Sinusitis in the Immunocompromised Patient," *Otolaryngol Clin North Am*, 2000, 33(2):301-12.

Ribes JA, Vanover-Sams CL, and Baker DJ, "Zygomycetes in Human Disesease," *Clin Microbial Rev*, 2000, 13(2):236-301.

Schell WA, "New Aspects of Emerging Fungal Pathogens. A Multifaceted Challenge," *Clin Lab Med*, 1995, 15(2):365-87.

Shafiq M, Schoch PE, Cunha BA, et al, "*Nocardia asteroids* and *Cryptococcus neoformans* Lung Abscess," *Am J Med*, 2000, 109(1):70-1.

Wingard JR, "Fungal Infections After Bone Marrow Transplant," *Biol Blood Marrow Transplant*, 1999, 5(2):55-68.

Fungal Culture, Blood

Related Information

Amphotericin B, Serum *on page 737*
Antimicrobial Susceptibility Testing, Fungi *on page 556*
Aspergillus Serology *on page 560*
Bacterial Culture, Blood *on page 566*
Bacterial Culture, Sputum *on page 574*
Candida Antigen *on page 587*
Candidiasis Serology *on page 588*

Synonyms Blood Fungus Culture

Abstract The most sensitive method for detection of invasive fungal or yeast infections is culture from blood specimens. Many of the yeasts (*Candida* species, *Cryptococcus neoformans*) are commonly isolated from the routine, automated blood culture systems. Laboratories not using an automated blood culture system should use the lysis centrifugation method with culture onto media enriched for fungal and yeast isolation or the biphasic blood culture media. Certain dimorphic fungi (eg, *Histoplasma capsulatum*) are reliably recovered only by the lysis centrifugation method.

Patient Preparation See preparation in Bacterial Culture, Blood *on page 566*.

Specimen Blood

Container Fungal blood culture media (eg, biphasic blood culture media) or lysis centrifugation collecting tubes (Wampole Isolator™)

Collection Remove plastic cap from biphasic bottle, cleanse stoppers with acetone alcohol and 2% iodine. Collect 8 mL blood in a yellow Vacutainer® tube containing 0.35% sodium polyanethol sulfonate as an anticoagulant. Transfer appropriate volume of blood to biphasic medium to achieve an approximate 1:10 dilution of blood in the broth medium. Alternatively, 10 mL of blood is directly collected in an Isolator™ tube.

Special Instructions The laboratory should be informed of current antifungal therapy and clinical diagnosis.

Reference Interval No growth

Use Isolate and identify fungi; establish the diagnosis of fungemia, fungal endocarditis, and disseminated mycosis. Certain yeasts such as *Candida* species can be isolated from conventional bacterial blood cultures; for other agents of systemic mycoses, however, it is essential to perform blood fungal cultures as outlined above.

Limitations Negative fungal blood culture does not exclude disseminated fungal infection (eg, blood cultures are negative in about 50% of individuals with disseminated candidiasis). If disseminated or deep fungal infection is strongly suspected, biopsy of the appropriate tissue and/or bone marrow aspiration for sections and fungus culture should be considered. Blood cultures are not helpful in some fungal diseases (eg, mucormycosis).

Methodology Biphasic (broth and agar) blood culture medium or lysis centrifugation with prompt subculture to solid media are appropriate methodologies. Fungal cultures should be held not less than 4 weeks.

Additional Information Fungemia can be a complication of venous or arterial catheterization, hyperalimentation, the acquired immunodeficiency syndrome (AIDS), and therapy with steroids, antineoplastic drugs, radiation, or broad spectrum antimicrobial agents. Intravenous drug abusers are prone to *Candida* endocarditis.

Fungemia represents a failure of the host defense system. Although many fungal species including *Histoplasma capsulatum*, *Coccidioides immitis*, and *Cryptococcus neoformans* are recoverable from blood cultures, the most common cause of fungemia is *Candida albicans* followed by other *Candida* species including *Torulopsis glabrata*. Most *Candida* species will also grow in routine aerobic bacterial blood cultures. Fungemia may be precipitated by contamination of an indwelling catheter or, in the critically ill and immunocompromised patient, invasion from the gastrointestinal and less frequently the urinary tract.[1]

Rarely, blastospores (budding yeast structures) and pseudohyphae can be seen by examination of Wright stained venous peripheral blood smears. New assays utilizing DNA analysis are being developed to detect *C. albicans* DNA directly in serum and may eventually replace blood culture for the diagnosis of invasive candidiasis.[2]

See also Histoplasmosis Antigen *on page 636*, Histoplasmosis Antibody *on page 635*, Coccidioidomycosis Serology *on page 593*, Candidiasis Serology Test *on page 588*, and *Candida* Antigen *on page 587*.

Histoplasma capsulatum can sometimes be seen in leukocytes in the Wright-stained peripheral blood smears of patients with AIDS. In that circumstance, a calcofluor white stain may be useful.[3,4] They may also be found occasionally, also as intracellular structures, in bone marrow aspirations. Markedly increased serum LDH concentrations provide a clue to the diagnosis of disseminated histoplasmosis in AIDS patients.[5]

Footnotes
1. Edwards JE Jr and Filler SG, "Current Strategies for Treating Invasive Candidiasis: Emphasis on Infections in Non-neutropenic Patients," *Clin Infect Dis*, 1992, 14(Suppl 1):S106-13.
2. Wahyuningsih R, Freisleben HJ, Sonntag HG, et al, "Simple and Rapid Detection of *Candida albicans* DNA in Serum by PCR for Diagnosis of Invasive Candidiasis," *J Clin Microbiol*, 2000, 38(8):3016-21.
3. Edelman M and McKitrick J, Images in Clinical Medicine, "*Histoplasma capsulatum* in a Peripheral Blood Smear," *N Engl J Med*, 2000, 342(1):28.
4. Elin RJ, Whitis J, and Snyder J, "Infectious Disease Diagnosis From a Peripheral Blood Smear," *Lab Med*, 2000, 31(6):324-8.

5. Corcoran GR, Al-Abdely H, Flanders CD, et al, "Markedly Elevated Serum Lactate Dehydrogenase Levels Are a Clue to the Diagnosis of Disseminated Histoplasmosis in Patients With AIDS," *Clin Infect Dis*, 1997, 24(5):942-4.

References
Costa SF, Marinho I, Araujo EA, et al, "Nosocomial Fungaemia: A 2-Year Prospective Study," *J Hosp Infect*, 2000, 45(1):69-72.
Garcia-Prats JA, Cooper TR, Schneider VF, et al, "Rapid Detection of Microorganisms in Blood Cultures of Newborn Infants Utilizing an Automated Blood Culture System," *Pediatrics*, 2000, 105(3 Pt 1):523-7.
Geha DJ and Roberts GD, "Laboratory Detection of Fungemia," *Clin Lab Med*, 1994, 14(1):83-97.
Jagarlamudi R and Kumar L, "Systemic Fungal Infections in Cancer Patients," *Trop Gastroenterol*, 2000, 21(1):3-8.
Wilson ML and Weinstein MP, "General Principles in the Laboratory Detection of Bacteremia and Fungemia," *Clin Lab Med*, 1994, 14(1):69-82.
Yamamura DL, Rotstein C, Nicolle LE, et al, "Candidemia at Selected Canadian Sites: Results From the Fungal Disease Registry, 1992-1994. Fungal Disease Registry of the Canadian Infectious Disease Society," *CMAJ*, 1999, 160(4):493-9.

Fungal Culture, Cerebrospinal Fluid

Related Information

Synonyms Cerebrospinal Fluid Fungus Culture; CSF Fungus Culture; Spinal Fluid Fungus Culture

Abstract Except for *Cryptococcus neoformans*, most fungal infections that have disseminated or localized to the CNS are seen primarily in patients with underlying immunosuppression. Fungi that are yeasts at body temperatures, such as *Histoplasma capsulatum*, *Cryptococcus neoformans*, and *Blastomyces dermatitidis*, have access to the cerebral microcirculation, enabling such organisms to invade the subarachnoid space to produce acute and chronic meningitis. *Candida* species, which exists as both yeasts and pseudofungi at body temperatures, can occasionally be meningeal pathogens.

Cryptococcal meningitis in non-AIDS patients is characterized by hypoglycorrhachia, increased CSF protein and lymphocytic pleocytosis.[1] See Cryptococcal Antigen Titer *on page 595* and India Ink Preparation *on page 642*.

Patient Preparation Aseptic preparation of aspiration site

Specimen Cerebrospinal fluid (see also the table in Fungal Culture, Sputum *on page 613*)

Collection Sterile tubes should be numbered 1, 2, 3 with tube #1 representing the first portion of the sample collected. Contamination from skin or other body surfaces must be avoided. The third tube collected during lumbar puncture is most suitable for culture, as skin contaminants from the puncture usually are washed out with fluid collected in the first two tubes.

Turnaround Time Turnaround time of culture for cryptococcosis is slower than that of rapid latex agglutination tests for antigen.

Reference Interval No growth

Use Diagnosis and etiology of fungal meningitis

Limitations Recovery of fungi from cerebrospinal fluid is directly related to the volume of cerebrospinal fluid available. A minimum of 10 mL is recommended. *Cryptococcus* can be mistaken for small lymphocytes in the counting chamber. Culture of additional specimens increases the chance for recovery.

Methodology Aerobic culture of centrifuged sediment on noninhibitory media usually including Sabouraud's, brain heart infusion agar (BHI) with blood agar at 25°C to 30°C and also frequently at 37°C. Cultures of the centrifuged sediment of large volumes (5-10 mL) of CSF, which may be obtained by repeated lumbar punctures, may lead to positive cultures in 90% to 95% of cryptococcosis patients.[1]

Additional Information The diagnosis of central nervous system fungal infections is frequently complicated by the overlapping array of signs and symptoms which may accompany other clinical entities such as tuberculous meningitis, pyogenic abscess, brain tumor, hypersensitivity or allergic reactions, collagen vascular disease, leptomeningeal malignancy, chemical meningitis, meningeal inflammation secondary to contiguous suppuration, Behçet disease, Mollaret's meningitis, and the uveomeningitic syndromes.[2]

Cryptococcosis may present as indolent to fulminant infection terminating in death within 2 weeks. A rapidly progressive disease seems to correlate (Continued)

Fungal Culture, Cerebrospinal Fluid *(Continued)*

with immunosuppression in the patient.[3] The India ink preparation is positive in 30% to 75% of cases, and the latex agglutination is positive in >95% of cases. Latex agglutination tests performed on serum are often positive in AIDS patients with cryptococcal meningitis. *Cryptococcus neoformans* can be seen with Papanicolaou stain, and its mucinous capsules stain bright red with mucicarmine.[4] The diagnosis of cryptococcal meningitis is sometimes recognized in CSF cytologic studies.

Cryptococcosis is found in other organs as well, including lung, pleura, pericardium, and skin.[5] It may also involve the skeletal system and prostate. See Cryptococcal Antigen Titer *on page 595.*

Results of cultures for **Histoplasma capsulatum** are commonly negative early. Multiple specimens, large volumes (>10 mL) and incubation periods >35 days are indicated. See Histoplasmosis Antibody *on page 635* and Histoplasmosis Antigen *on page 636.*

Footnotes

1. Dismukes WE, "Cryptococcosis," *Cecil Textbook of Medicine*, 21st ed, Chapter 398, Goldman L and Bennett JC, Philadelphia, PA: WB Saunders Co, 2000, 1867-70.
2. Go JL, Kim PE, Ahmadi J, et al, "Fungal Infections of the Central Nervous System," *Neuroimaging Clin N Am*, 2000, 10(2):409-25.
3. Diamond RD, "Cryptococcus neoformans," Principles and Practice of Infectious Diseases, 5th ed, Mandell GL, Bennett JE, and Dolin R, eds, New York, NY: Churchill Livingstone, 2000.
4. Jaster JH and Malecha MJ, Images in Clinical Medicine, "Cryptococcal Meningitis," *N Engl J Med*, 1996, 335(26):1962.
5. Drapkin MS and Mark EJ, "A 69-Year-Old Renal Transplant Recipient With Low Grade Fever and Multiple Pulmonary Nodules," Case Records of the Massachusetts General Hospital, Case 29-2000, Scully RE, Mark EJ, McNeely WF, et al, eds, *N Engl J Med*, 2000, 343(12):870-7.

References

Gripshover BM and Ellner JJ, "Chronic Meningitis," *Principles and Practice of Infectious Diseases*, 4th ed, Mandell GL, Bennett JE, and Dolin R, eds, New York, NY: Churchill Livingstone, 1995.

Jagarlamudi R and Kumar L, "Systemic Fungal Infections in Cancer Patients," *Trop Gastroenterol*, 2000, 21(1):3-8.

Mylonakis E, Paliou M, Sax PE, et al, "Central Nervous System Aspergillosis in Patients With Human Immunodeficiency Virus Infection. Report of 6 Cases and Review," *Medicine (Baltimore)*, 2000, 79(4):269-80.

Tunkel AR, Wispelwey B, and Scheld WM, "Pathogenesis and Pathophysiology of Meningitis," *Infect Dis Clin North Am*, 1990, 4(4):555-81.

Walsh TJ and Chanock SJ, "Diagnosis of Invasive Fungal Infections: Advances in Nonculture Systems," *Curr Clin Top Infect Dis*, 1998, 18:101-53.

Fungal Culture, Ocular Infections

Related Information

Bacterial Culture, Conjunctiva *on page 570*
Fungus Smear, Stain *on page 615*
Ocular Cytology *on page 385*
Viral Culture, Eye or Ocular Symptoms *on page 693*

Synonyms Conjunctival Fungus Culture

Applies to Eye Fungus Culture

Test Includes Culture, and if specimen is adequate, KOH preparation and PAS smear

Abstract Fungal infections of the eye can manifest as either keratitis or endophthalmitis. The filamentous fungi are the most common causes of fungal keratitis.[1] The most common risk factor for fungal keratitis is corneal injury usually caused by vegetative material (eg, branches or straw).[2] Fungal endophthalmitis can occur from exogenous or endogenous routes. Fungal conjunctivitis is not common. *Candida* conjunctivitis can occur in patients receiving corticosteroid eyedrops.

Patient Preparation Avoid contamination with skin flora.

Specimen Scrapings of corneal ulcer, washings of lacrimal duct, wet swabs of conjunctiva. For diagnosis of fungal endophthalmitis vitreous fluid, tissue from a wound, or tissue from the anterior chamber are appropriate.

Collection The physician should collect corneal fragments from the edge and base of the ulcer. Swabs are insufficient.

Reference Interval No growth; normal eye flora can include *Candida* species

Use Establish the presence of keratomycosis or fungal endophthalmitis

Limitations A single negative culture does not rule out the presence of fungal infection. Specimens should be collected from the appropriate site of infection. Conjunctival cultures are inadequate and can be misleading for the diagnosis of fungal keratitis or fungal endophthalmitis.

Deep adjacent fungal infection can cause visual loss.[3]

Methodology Culture on appropriate media usually including Sabouraud's medium, brain heart infusion (BHI), and blood agar incubation at 37°C and 25°C to 30°C

Additional Information The more common causes of keratomycosis include *Fusarium* species, *Candida albicans*, *Aspergillus fumigatus*, *Curvularia* species, *Aspergillus flavus*, other species of *Aspergillus*, *Penicillium*, and *Paecilomyces*. Many of these fungi cause other types of infection as well (eg, the subcutaneous). A keratomycosis-like clinical presentation may also be caused by *Nocardia asteroides* and *Mycobacterium fortuitum*. Keratomycosis is a rare complication of contact lens use.[4] Direct microscopic

observation provides a higher yield than culture for the diagnosis of keratomycosis.[5]

Footnotes

1. Rosa RH Jr, Miller D, and Alfonso EC, "The Changing Spectrum of Fungal Keratitis in South Florida," *Ophthalmology*, 1994, 101(6):1005-13.
2. Wong TY, Ng TP, Fong KS, et al, "Risk Factors and Clinical Outcomes Between Fungal and Bacterial Keratitis: A Comparative Study," *CLOA J*, 1997, 23(4):275-81.
3. Brown RB and Lau SK, "A 59-Year-Old Diabetic Man With Unilateral Visual Loss and Oculomotor-Nerve Palsy," Case Records of the Massachusetts General Hospital, Case 3-2001, Scully RE, Mark EJ, McNeely WF, et al, eds, *N Engl J Med*, 2001, 344(4):286-93.
4. Foroozan R, Eagle RC Jr, and Cohen EJ, "Fungal Keratitis in a Soft Contact Lens Wearer," *CLOA J*, 2000, 26(3):166-8.
5. O'Brien TP, "Keratitis," *Principles and Practice of Infectious Diseases*, 5th ed, Mandell GL, Bennett JE, and Dolin R, eds, New York, NY: Churchill Livingstone, 2000, 1257-67.

References

Fahey DK, Fenton S, Cahill M, et al, "Candida endophthalmitis: A Diagnostic Dilemma," *Eye*, 1999, 13(Pt 4):596-8.

Garg P, Gopinathan U, Choudhary K, et al, "Keratomycosis: Clinical and Microbiologic Experience With Dematiaceous Fungi," *Ophthalmology*, 2000, 107(3):574-80.

O'Day DM and Head WS, "Advances in the Management of Keratomycosis and Acanthamoeba keratitis," *Cornea*, 2000, 19(5):681-7.

Samson CM and Foster CS, "Chronic Postoperative Endophthalmitis," *Int Ophthalmol Clin*, 2000, 40(1):57-67.

Wang MX, Shen DJ, Liu JC, et al, "Recurrent Fungal Keratitis and Endophthalmitis," *Cornea*, 2000, 19(4):558-60.

Fungal Culture, Skin

Related Information

Amphotericin B, Serum *on page 737*
Antimicrobial Susceptibility Testing, Fungi *on page 556*
Fungal Culture, Biopsy or Body Fluid *on page 610*
Fungal Culture, Stool *on page 614*
Fungus Smear, Stain *on page 615*
HIV-1/HIV-2 Antibody Screen and Western Blot *on page 636*
Itraconazole, Serum *on page 753*
KOH Preparation *on page 645*
Mycobacterial Culture, Cutaneous and Subcutaneous Tissue *on page 657*
Skin Biopsy *on page 71*
Sporotrichosis Serology *on page 680*

Synonyms Dermatophyte Fungus Culture; Skin Fungus Culture

Applies to Fungus Culture, Hair and Nails

Test Includes Detection of superficial fungal infections of the skin or hair

Abstract Fungal infections of the skin, nails, and hair are often considered together because these tissues all contain keratin. These dermatophytes are capable of invading the keratinous tissues and are usually unable to penetrate deeper into tissues. These fungi are grouped into categories on the basis of host preference and natural habitat. **Anthropophilic** fungi only infect humans and are transmitted by close human contact. **Geophilic** fungi are associated with soil and **zoophilic** fungi are transmitted to humans by animals or birds. Identification of dermatophytes can assist in controlling infections by identifying the source of infection.

Patient Preparation Select hairs which are broken off and appear diseased, and pluck them with sterile forceps. If diseased hair stubs are not apparent, scrape the edges of a scalp lesion with a sterile scalpel. Cleanse skin lesions first with 70% alcohol to reduce bacteria and saprophytic fungi. Scrape from the outer edges of skin lesions. In infections of the nails, scrape out the friable material beneath the edge of the nails, or scrape or clip off portions of abnormal appearing nail and submit for examination and culture.

Specimen Skin scrapings, exudates, nail clippings, whole nail, debris under nail, hair

Collection Enclose hair specimens, skin scrapings, or nail clippings or scrapings in clean paper envelopes, sterile urine container, or Petri dish. Do not put specimens in cotton-plugged tubes, because the specimen may become trapped among the cotton fibers and lost. Do not put specimen into closed containers, such as rubber-stoppered tubes, because this keeps the specimen moist and allows overgrowth of bacteria and saprophytic fungi. The laboratory should be informed of the fungal species suspected or clinical diagnosis.

Turnaround Time Cultures in which suspicion of systemic fungal infection has been indicated are usually reported upon becoming positive or negative after 4 weeks.

Special Instructions Careful choice of specimens for laboratory study is important. See table. A Wood's lamp is useful in the collection of specimens in tinea capitis infections, since hairs infected by some members of the genus *Microsporum* exhibit fluorescence under a Wood's lamp. However, in tinea capitis due to *Trichophyton* species, infected hairs usually do not fluoresce.

Reference Interval No growth

Use Isolate and identify fungi

Limitations A single negative specimen does not rule out fungal infections. *Malassezia furfur*, which causes pityriasis (formerly tinea) versicolor, frequently fails to grow in routine culture.

Selection of Specimens for the Diagnosis of Superficial Mycosis and Dermatomycosis

Diagnosis	Specimen of Choice
Superficial mycoses	
Piedra	Hair
Tinea nigra	Skin scraping
Tinea versicolor	Skin scraping
Dermatomycoses (cutaneous mycoses)	
Onychomycosis	Nail scraping
Tinea capitis	Hair (black dot)
Tinea corporis	Skin scraping
Tinea pedis	Skin scraping
Tinea cruris	Skin scraping
Candidiasis	
Thrush	Scraping of oral white patches
Diaper dermatitis	Scraping of pustules at margin
Paronychia	Scraping skin around nail
Cutaneous candidiasis	Scraping of pustules at margin
Erosio interdigitalis blastomycetia (coinfection with gram-negative rods)	Scrapings of interdigital space (routine culture also)
Congenital candidiasis	Scraping of scales, pustules and cutaneous debris, cultures of umbilical stump, mouth, urine and stool
Mucocutaneous candidiasis	Scraping of affected area

Methodology Aerobic culture on selective media usually including nonselective Sabouraud's agar incubated at 25°C to 30°C; some laboratories also incubate these cultures at 35°C to 37°C.

Additional Information Tissues that contain keratin (hair, nails, skin, etc) can become infected with dermatophytes, which are a group of related keratinophilic fungi. Infections are generally mild but may be severe as a consequence of the reaction of the patient to products made by the fungus. Yeasts or certain filamentous fungi may cause cutaneous infections that resemble dermatophytoses. *Candida* species also colonize skin. Clinical diagnosis of *Candida* infection involves consideration of predisposing factors such as occlusion, maceration or altered cutaneous barrier function. Signs of *Candida* infection include bright erythema, fragile papulopustules, and satellite lesions. Patients with defects in T-lymphocyte responses, such as AIDS patients or individuals being treated with antineoplastic drugs, are especially susceptible to many fungal infections including superficial mycoses.[1] Most cutaneous fungal infections can be treated with the antifungal azole drugs like ketoconazole, itraconazole, and fluconazole. Severe infections are treated with intravenous amphotericin B. See Sporotrichosis Serology *on page 680.*

Footnotes

1. Johnson RA, "The Immune Compromised Host in the Twenty-First Century: Management of Mucocutaneous Infections," *Semin Cutan Med Surg*, 2000, 19(1):19-61.

References

Elewski BE, "Update on Superficial Fungal Infections. Introduction," *Postgrad Med*, 1999, Spec #5.

Frieden IJ and Howard R, "Tinea Capitis: Epidemiology, Diagnosis, Treatment, and Control," *J Am Acad Dermatol*, 1994, 31(3 Pt 2):S42-6.

Goldstein AO, Smith KM, Ives TJ, et al, "Mycotic Infections. Effective Management of Conditions Involving the Skin, Hair, and Nails," *Geriatrics*, 2000, 55(5):40-52.

Gupta AK and Humke S, "The Prevalence and Management of Onychomycosis in Diabetic Patients," *Eur J Dermatol*, 2000, 10(5):379-84.

Nowak MA and Brodell RT, "Rapid Diagnosis of Superficial Fungal Infections," *Postgrad Med*, 1999, 105(2):179-80.

Rudy SJ, "Superficial Fungal Infections in Children and Adolescents," *Nurse Pract Forum*, 1999, 10(2):56-66.

Fungal Culture, Sputum

Related Information

Amphotericin B, Serum *on page 737*
Antimicrobial Susceptibility Testing, Fungi *on page 556*
Aspergillus Serology *on page 560*
Bacterial Culture, Bronchoscopy/Bronchial Brush/Bronchoalveolar Lavage Specimen *on page 568*
Bacterial Culture, Sputum *on page 574*
Blastomycosis Serology *on page 582*
Bronchoalveolar Lavage (BAL) *on page 375*
Candidiasis Serology *on page 588*
Coccidioidomycosis Serology *on page 593*
Cryptococcal Antigen Titer *on page 595*
Fine Needle Aspiration Culture *on page 609*
Fungal Culture, Biopsy or Body Fluid *on page 610*
Fungal Culture, Stool *on page 614*
Fungal Culture, Urine *on page 614*
Fungus Smear, Stain *on page 615*
Histoplasmosis Antibody *on page 635*
Histoplasmosis Antigen *on page 636*
Itraconazole, Serum *on page 753*
KOH Preparation *on page 645*
Mycobacterial Culture, Sputum *on page 658*
Nocardia Culture *on page 665*
Sporotrichosis Serology *on page 680*
Sputum Cytology *on page 387*
Viral Culture, Respiratory Symptoms *on page 694*

Synonyms Sputum Fungus Culture

Applies to Bronchoscopy Fungus Culture; Fungus Culture, Gastric Aspirate

Abstract Fungal pulmonary infections include *Histoplasma capsulatum*, *Coccidioides immitis*, *Cryptococcus neoformans*, *Blastomyces dermatitidis*, and Mucormycosis. The incidence of fungal infections is largely related to geographic exposure. Cases can occur in normal hosts. Opportunistic fungal pulmonary infections are due to a variety of etiologic agents, which are ubiquitous in the environment. *Candida* and *Aspergillus* species are the most frequently isolated, however, they may be present as the result of contamination from the patient's normal flora or airborne sources. Their presence may represent colonization rather than invasion.

Patient Preparation The patient should be instructed to remove dentures, rinse mouth with water, and cough deeply expectorating sputum into the sputum collection cup.

Specimen First morning sputum, gastric aspirate, induced sputum, aspirated sputum, bronchial aspirate, tracheal aspirate, transtracheal aspirate. See table.

Table 1. Selection of Specimens for the Diagnosis of Systemic and Subcutaneous Mycosis

Diagnosis	Specimen of Choice
Systemic Mycoses	
Aspergillosis	Sputum
	Bronchial aspirate, bronchoalveolar lavage
	Biopsy (lung, sinuses, skin, gastrointestinal)
Blastomycosis	Skin scrapings, biopsy
	Abscess drainage (pus)
	Bone, biopsy
	Urine
	Sputum
	Bronchial aspirate, lung biopsy
Candidiasis	Sputum
	Bronchial aspirate, bronchoalveolar lavage
	Blood
	Cerebrospinal fluid
	Urine
	Stool
Coccidioidomycosis	Sputum
	Bronchial aspirate, bronchoalveolar lavage
	Cerebrospinal fluid
	Urine
	Skin scrapings
	Abscess drainage (pus)
Cryptococcosis	Cerebrospinal fluid
	Sputum
	Abscess drainage (pus)
	Skin scraping, biopsy
	Urine
Mucormycosis	Biopsies, scrapings
	KOH preparations
	Cultures
	Lung, CNS, other sites
Subcutaneous Mycoses	
Chromoblastomycosis	Skin scrapings
	Biopsy (skin)
	Drainage (pus)
Maduromycosis	Drainage (pus)
	Biopsy
(mycetoma)	Abscess drainage
	Biopsy (lesion)
Sporotrichosis	Biopsy (skin, lymph node; with culture)
	Drainage (pus)
	Abscess drainage

Container Sterile sputum cup, sputum trap, sterile tracheal aspirate or bronchoscopy tube

Collection A recommended screening procedure is three first morning specimens submitted on successive days. The specimen can be divided for fungus culture and KOH preparation, mycobacteria culture and smear, and routine bacterial culture and Gram stain if the specimen is of adequate volume. Deeply coughed sputum, transtracheal aspirate, bronchial washing or brushing, or deep tracheal aspirate are preferred specimens.

Turnaround Time Negative cultures are reported after 4 weeks

(Continued)

Fungal Culture, Sputum (Continued)

Reference Interval No growth; normal flora such as yeast from the oropharynx may be present.

Use Oncology patients, transplant patients, and patients with the acquired immunodeficiency syndrome (AIDS) are particularly prone to infection with fungi,[1] including histoplasmosis, for which cultures of respiratory secretions as well as blood fungal cultures and immunologic methods are useful. Diabetics, especially those poorly controlled and in acidosis, may develop mucormycosis.

Limitations The yield may be reduced by bacterial overgrowth during storage or on standing; therefore, fresh sputum is preferred. Negative cultures do not rule out the presence of fungal infection. Simultaneously received specimens may be pooled.

Methodology Culture on selective media usually including supplemented Sabouraud's agar and brain heart infusion (BHI) with antibiotics to reduce bacterial overgrowth

Additional Information Definitive diagnosis of fungal pulmonary disease depends upon the presence of clinical signs of pulmonary infection, a chest x-ray revealing abnormality such as granuloma; laboratory isolation of a potentially significant organism from a suitable specimen; histologic documentation of tissue invasion by the isolated organism. A list of etiologic agents of pulmonary fungal disease has been compiled; see table. In practice a diagnosis sufficient for therapy can frequently be established by observation of hyphae, pseudohyphae, or yeast cells in tissue sections using Gomori methenamine silver or other methods; recovery of the organism from a normally sterile site; repeated isolation of the same suspect organism from the same or different sites; or seroconversion (ie, the development of an immune response to the suspected organism). Even without invasion **Aspergillus** may cause IgE mediated asthma, allergic alveolitis cell mediated hypersensitivity, mucoid impaction, and bronchocentric granulomatosis.[2,3] The differential diagnosis between **chronic necrotizing pulmonary aspergillosis** and **Aspergillus fungus ball** is relevant, because in the former symptoms are present, cavitation is found secondary to lung necrosis, and medical therapy is available.[2] Fungal tracheobronchitis has recently been recognized as a pseudomembranous form involving the circumference of the bronchial wall or as multiple or discrete plaques. The plaques or pseudomembranes are composed of necrotic tissue exudate and fungal hyphae. See *Aspergillus* Serology *on page 560*.

Table 2. Common Pulmonary Fungal Infections

Endemic Fungi	Opportunistic Fungi
Histoplasma capsulatum	Candida albicans
Blastomyces dermatitidis	Candida tropicalis
Coccidioides immitis	Aspergillus niger
Paracoccidioides brasiliensis	Aspergillus fumigatus
	Mucor
	Rhizopus
	Absidia
	Cryptococcus neoformans

Adapted from Haque AK, "Pathology of Common Pulmonary Fungal Infections," *J Thorac Imaging*, 1992, 7:1-11.

Sporotrichosis, widely recognized as a plant saprophyte which infects skin and subcutaneous tissue, causes pulmonary infection as well. It may be acquired from animal handling and exposure, and may be transmitted by domestic cats.[4] See Sporotrichosis Serology *on page 680*.

Footnotes

1. Connolly JE Jr, McAdams HP, Erasmus JJ, et al, "Opportunistic Fungal Pneumonia," *J Thorac Imaging*, 1999, 14(1):51-62.
2. Sharma OP and Chwogule R, "Many Faces of Pulmonary Aspergillosis," *Eur Respir J*, 1998, 12(3):705-15.
3. Caras WE and Pluss JL, "Chronic Necrotizing Pulmonary Aspergillosis: Pathologic Outcome After Itraconazole Therapy," *Mayo Clin Proc*, 1996, 71(1):25-30.
4. Schell WA, "New Aspects of Emerging Fungal Pathogens. A Multifaceted Challenge," *Clin Lab Med*, 1995, 15(2):365-87.

References

Bethlem EP, Capone D, Maranhao B, et al, "Paracoccidioidomycosis," *Cur Opin Pulm Med*, 1999, 5(5):319-25.

Clancy CJ and Nguyen MH, "Acute Community-Acquired Pneumonia Due to *Aspergillus* in Presumably Immunocompetent Hosts: Clues for Recognition of a Rare but Fatal Disease," *Chest*, 1998, 114(2):629-34.

Nunley DR, Ohori P, Grgurich WF, et al, "Pulmonary Aspergillosis in Cystic Fibrosis Lung Transplant Recipients," *Chest*, 1998, 114(5):1321-9.

Patel RG, Patel B, Petrini MF, et al, "Clinical Presentation, Radiographic Findings and Diagnostic Methods of Pulmonary Blastomycosis: A Review of 100 Consecutive Cases," *South Med J*, 1999, 92(3):289-95.

Regnard JF, Icard P, Nicolosi M, et al, "Aspergilloma: A Series of 89 Surgical Cases," *Ann Thorac Surg*, 2000, 69(3):898-903.

Ribes JA, Vanover-Sams CL, and Baker DJ, "Zygomycetes in Human Disease," *Clin Microbial Rev*, 2000, 13(2):236-301.

Roebuck DJ, Fisher DA, and Currie BJ, "Cryptococcosis in HIV Negative Patients: Findings on Chest Radiography," *Thorax*, 1998, 53(7):554-7.

Fungal Culture, Stool

Related Information

Amphotericin B, Serum *on page 737*
Bacterial Culture, Stool *on page 575*
Candidiasis Serology *on page 588*
Clostridium difficile Toxin Assay and Culture *on page 592*
Fecal Lactoferrin *on page 308*
Fungal Culture, Blood *on page 610*
Fungal Culture, Skin *on page 612*
Fungal Culture, Sputum *on page 613*
Fungus Smear, Stain *on page 615*
Methylene Blue Stain, Stool *on page 313*

Synonyms Stool Fungus Culture

Abstract Fungal stool culture is limited to screening for overgrowth of *Candida* species in immunocompromised patients. Overgrowth of yeast can also be detected with conventional bacterial cultures, thus, often a specific request for stool fungal culture is redundant.

Specimen Stool (see also the table in Fungal Culture, Sputum *on page 613*)

Container Plastic stool container or Culturette®

Collection The specimen can be divided for fungus culture, mycobacterial culture, and bacterial culture if the specimen is of adequate volume.

Storage Instructions Caution: Refrigeration will impede recovery of *H. capsulatum*.

Causes for Rejection Specimen containing interfering substances (eg, castor oil, bismuth, Metamucil®, barium) and those contaminated with urine may not have optimal yield.

Reference Interval No growth

Use Establish the presence of fungi, particularly *Candida* species in debilitated hosts, patients receiving antimicrobial chemotherapeutic agents and hyperalimentation

Limitations Use of this test is generally limited to screening for *Candida*. Yeast are normal flora in the stool and they may be isolated in specimens without having any clinical significance. Stool cultures have a low yield and are not recommended for the isolation of systemic fungi, however, *Histoplasma capsulatum* may be recovered from the stool of AIDS patients with disseminated infection. See Fungal Culture, Sputum *on page 613* and Fungal Culture, Skin *on page 612* for fungus culture specimen selection and Fungal Culture, Blood *on page 610* for additional discussion of appropriate specimens.

Methodology Culture on selective media usually including Sabouraud's agar with antibiotics

Additional Information *Candida* can be isolated in up to 65% of stool cultures. Neonates and adults may develop watery diarrhea due to intestinal overgrowth by yeast that readily responds to specific therapy. *Candida* may become disseminated in patients with leukopenia, immunosuppressive therapy, AIDS, corticosteroid therapy, phagocytic defects, hyperalimentation, use of broad spectrum antibiotics, and oral contraceptives. Broad spectrum antibiotics suppress the normal bacterial flora in the gastrointestinal system and allow *Candida* species to overgrow. If the patient is immune suppressed, the use of antibiotics may complicate the patient's clinical situation.

References

Danna PL, Urban C, Bellin E, et al, "Role of *Candida* in Pathogenesis of Antibiotic-Associated Diarrhoea in Elderly Inpatients," *Lancet*, 1991, 337(8740):511-4.

Edwards JE Jr, "*Candida* Species," *Principles and Practice of Infectious Diseases*, 5th ed, Mandell GL, Bennett JE, and Dolin R, eds, New York, NY: Churchill Livingstone, 2000, 2656-74.

Fidel PL, Vazquez JA, and Sobel JD, "*Candida glabrata*: Review of Epidemiology, Pathogenesis and Clinical Disease With Comparison to *C. albicans*," *Clin Microbiol Rev*, 1999, 12(1):80-96.

Ullrich R, Heise W, Bergs C, et al, "Gastrointestinal Symptoms in Patients Infected With Human Immunodeficiency Virus: Relevance of Infective Agents Isolated From Gastrointestinal Tract," *Gut*, 1992, 33(8):1080-4.

Fungal Culture, Urine

Related Information

Bacterial Culture, Urine *on page 578*
Blastomycosis Serology *on page 582*
Candidiasis Serology *on page 588*
Fungal Culture, Blood *on page 610*
Fungal Culture, Sputum *on page 613*
Fungus Smear, Stain *on page 615*
Itraconazole, Serum *on page 753*
Mycobacterial Culture, Urine *on page 660*
Urinary Tract Cytology *on page 389*

Synonyms Urine Fungus Culture

Abstract Use of antibacterial, antineoplastic, and immunosuppressive drugs, corticosteroids, urinary indwelling catheters, urinary tract obstruction, or the presence of diseases such as diabetes mellitus predispose to funguria. *C. albicans* is reported to cause up to 59% of positive urinary fungal cultures. *Candida glabrata* and other *Candida* species account for many of the remainder.[1]

Patient Preparation Usual preparation for clean catch midvoid urine specimen collection. See Bacterial Culture, Urine *on page 578*.

Specimen Urine. See table for fungus culture specimen selection in Fungal Culture, Sputum *on page 613*.

Collection The patient must be instructed to thoroughly cleanse skin and collect midstream specimen.

Causes for Rejection Unrefrigerated specimen more than 2 hours old is subject to overgrowth of normal microorganisms.

Reference Interval $<10^4$ CFU/mL

Use Detect and identify yeasts and fungi in urine specimens. Candiduria associated with hematogenous infections is observed in patients with granulocytopenia, corticosteroid therapy, and with immunosuppression. The source is frequently the gastrointestinal tract or indwelling catheters, particularly with hyperalimentation.[2] Urine is a useful specimen for culture in cryptococcosis, blastomycosis, and candidiasis. In addition to *Candida*, opportunistic pathogens in the genitourinary tract include *Aspergillus* and *Cryptococcus*. Endemic pathogens such as *Histoplasma*, *Blastomyces*, and *Coccidioides* are also encountered.

Limitations A single negative culture does not rule out the presence of fungal infection.

Methodology Specimen is cultured on selective media such as supplemented Sabouraud's agar and/or brain heart infusion (BHI) with antibiotics; conventional bacterial cultures can also detect candiduria.

Additional Information Asymptomatic funguria often ultimately clears spontaneously. However, candiduria with >15,000 colony forming units/mL of urine and with such evidence of dissemination as elevated serum precipitin antibody titers, is associated with increased mortality.[3] Patients with candiduria may or may not have candidemia; positive urine culture for fungi often may be followed by positive blood culture for fungi. Ascending infections occur in patients with diabetes, prolonged antimicrobial therapy, or following instrumentation. Urinary obstruction due to "fungus balls" may occur in diabetes and following renal transplantation.

A blood fungus culture is useful to define invasive disease. However, proof of invasive *Candida* infection requires direct cystoscopic or operative visualization, fungus balls, pyelonephritis, or histopathologic evidence of mucosal invasion. The incidence of genitourinary fungal infections is increasing. They are usually associated with broad spectrum antibiotic therapy, corticosteroid therapy, underlying general debility, and AIDS.

Footnotes

1. Fidel PL, Vazquez JA, and Sobel JD, "*Candida glabrata*: Review of Epidemiology, Pathogenesis and Clinical Disease With Comparison to *C. albicans*," *Clin Microbiol Rev*, 1999, 12(1):80-96.
2. Sobel JD, Kauffman CA, McKinsey D, et al, "Candiduria: A Randomized, Double-Blind Study of Treatment With Fluconazole and Placebo. The National Institute of Allergy and Infectious Disease (NIAID) Mycoses Study Group," *Clin Infect Dis*, 2000, 30(1):19-24.
3. Wong-Beringer A, Jacobs RA, and Guglielmo BJ, "Treatment of Funguria," *JAMA*, 1992, 267(20):2780-5.

References

Benjamin DK Jr, Fisher RG, McKinney RE Jr, et al, "Candidal Mycetoma in the Neonatal Kidney," *Pediatrics*, 1999, 104(5 Pt 1):1126-9.

de Medeiros CR, Dantas da Cunha A Jr, Pasquini R, et al, "Primary Renal Aspergillosis: Extremely Uncommon Presentation in Patients Treated With Bone Marrow Transplantation," *Bone Marrow Transplant*, 1999, 24(1):113-4.

Edwards JE, Jr, "*Candida* Species," *Principles and Practice of Infectious Diseases*, 5th ed, Mandell GL, Bennett JE, and Dolin R, eds, New York, NY: Churchill Livingstone, 2000, 2656-74.

Kauffman CA, Vazquez JA, Sobel JD, et al, "Prospective Multicenter Surveillance Study of Funguria in Hospitalized Patients. The National Institute of Allergy and Infectious Disease (NIAID) Mycoses Study Group," *Clin Infect Dis*, 2000, 30(1):14-8.

Leu HS and Huang CT, "Clearance of Funguria With Short-Course Antifungal Regimens: A Prospective, Randomized, Controlled Study," *Clin Infect Dis*, 1995, 20(5):1152-7.

Rabkin JM, Oroloff SL, Corless CL, et al, "Association of Fungal Infection and Increased Mortality in Liver Transplant Recipients," *Am J Surg*, 2000, 179(5):426-30.

♦ **Fungisitis** *see* Bacterial Culture, Genital Specimen *on page 571*

♦ **Fungi Susceptibility Testing** *see* Antimicrobial Susceptibility Testing, Fungi *on page 556*

♦ **Fungus Ball** *see* Aspergillus Serology *on page 560*

♦ **Fungus Culture, Burn Sites** *see* Bacterial Culture, Burn Sites *on page 569*

♦ **Fungus Culture, Gastric Aspirate** *see* Fungal Culture, Sputum *on page 613*

♦ **Fungus Culture, Hair and Nails** *see* Fungal Culture, Skin *on page 612*

Fungus Smear, Stain

Related Information

Acid-Fast Stain, Modified, *Nocardia* Species *on page 550*
Antimicrobial Susceptibility Testing, Fungi *on page 556*
Bacterial Culture, Conjunctiva *on page 570*
Blastomycosis Serology *on page 582*
Candidiasis Serology *on page 588*
Coccidioidomycosis Serology *on page 593*
Cryptococcal Antigen Titer *on page 595*
Cryptosporidium Direct Staining Procedures *on page 596*
Fungal Culture, Biopsy or Body Fluid *on page 610*
Fungal Culture, Blood *on page 610*
Fungal Culture, Cerebrospinal Fluid *on page 611*
Fungal Culture, Ocular Infections *on page 612*
Fungal Culture, Skin *on page 612*
Fungal Culture, Sputum *on page 613*
Fungal Culture, Stool *on page 614*
Fungal Culture, Urine *on page 614*
Gram Stain *on page 617*
Histoplasmosis Antibody *on page 635*
Histoplasmosis Antigen *on page 636*
India Ink Preparation *on page 642*
KOH Preparation *on page 645*
Skin Biopsy *on page 71*
Sporotrichosis Serology *on page 680*

Applies to Calcofluor White; GMS Stain; Gomori Methenamine Silver Stain; Periodic Acid Schiff (PAS)

Test Includes Detection of fungi by smear only; fungus culture and KOH preparation must usually be ordered separately

Abstract Direct detection of fungal elements in specimens can sometimes provide a definitive diagnosis of mycotic infections. Classic examples are the detection of *Histoplasma capsulatum* in histiocytes from the blood or bone marrow and the detection of wide, ribbon-like hyphae with few separations compatible with zygomycosis.[1,2] A number of different stains have been used to detect fungal elements (KOH, calcofluor, Gram stain, Wright stain, periodic acid-Schiff, methenamine silver, and immunofluorescence).

Patient Preparation Avoid contamination with skin flora.

Specimen The same specimen as required for fungal culture of the specific site. For conjunctiva or cornea, scrapings of corneal ulcer or wet swabs of conjunctiva. Specimen from conjunctiva or cornea should be obtained only by a physician.

Reference Interval No yeast or hyphal elements seen

Use Aid in the diagnosis of fungal disease; used in combination with fungus culture. Calcofluor white stain and KOH preparation may be more sensitive than culture in detection of keratomycosis or invasive fungal infections.

Limitations A negative smear does not rule out the presence of fungal infection. When using calcofluor white stain, background fluorescence may be prominent. Examinations should be done by trained personnel.

Methodology Periodic acid-Schiff stain, Calcofluor white, and Gomori methenamine silver stain are used to identify fungal structures.

Additional Information Calcofluor white dye binds to cellulose and chitin and fluoresces with longwave UV light and shortwave visible light. Fungal elements viewed under UV light demonstrate a brilliant fluorescence that stands out from cells, tissue debris, and background. The preparations can subsequently be overstained with PAS or GMS. Calcofluor white can be used to screen stool specimens for **Microsporidia** spores or can detect *Acanthamoeba* keratitis[3,4] The PAS stain with a light green counterstain demonstrates the yeast forms, spores and the hyphae of fungi as pinkish red on a green background. The filaments of *Actinomyces* and *Nocardia* are not satisfactorily shown but do stain with Gram stain. *Nocardia* is modified acid-fast positive.

Footnotes

1. Deshpande AH and Munshi MM, "Rhinocerebral Mucormycosis Diagnosis by Aspiration Cytology," *Diagn Cytopathol*, 2000, 23(2):97-100.
2. Marques MB, Waites KB, Jaye DL, et al, "Histologic Examination of Bone Marrow Core Biopsy Specimens Has Limited Value in the Diagnosis of Mycobacterial and Fungal Infections in Patients With the Acquired Immunodeficiency Syndrome," *Ann Diagn Pathol*, 2000, 4(1):1-6.
3. Luna VA, Stewart BK, Bergeron DL, et al, "Use of the Fluorochrome Calcofluor White in the Screening of Stool Specimens for Spores of Microsporidia," *Am J Clin Pathol*, 1995, 103(5):656-9.
4. Marines HM, Osato MS, and Font RL, "The Value of Calcofluor White in the Diagnosis of Mycotic and *Acanthamoeba* Infections of the Eye and Ocular Adnexa," *Ophthalmology*, 1987, 94(1):23-6.

References

Connolly JE Jr, McAdams HP, Erasmus JJ, et al, "Opportunistic Fungal Pneumonia," *J Thorac Imaging*, 1999, 14(1):51-62.

Ho PL and Yuen KY, "Aspergillosis in Bone Marrow Transplant Recipients," *Crit Rev Oncol Hematol*, 2000, 34(1):55-69.

Mylonakis E, Paliou M, Sax PE, et al, "Central Nervous System Aspergillosis in Patients With Human Immunodeficiency Virus Infection. Report of 6 Cases and Review," *Medicine (Baltimore)*, 2000, 79(4):269-80.

Nowak MA and Brodell RT, "Rapid Diagnosis of Superficial Fungal Infections," *Postgrad Med*, 1999, 105(2):179-80.

Ribes JA, Vanover-Sams CL, and Baker DJ, "Zygomycetes in Human Disease," *Clin Microbiol Rev*, 2000, 13(2):236-301.

Sharma OP and Chwogule R, "Many Faces of Pulmonary Aspergillosis," *Eur Respir J*, 1998, 12(3):705-15.

St Germain G and Summerbell R, "Identifying Filamentous Fungi," *A Clinical Laboratory Handbook*, Belmont, CA: Star Publishing, 1996.

Walsh TJ and Chanock SJ, "Diagnosis of Invasive Fungal Infections: Advances in Nonculture Systems," *Curr Clin Top Infect Dis*, 1998, 18:101-53.

♦ *Fusobacterium nucleatum* *see* Bacterial Culture, Bronchoscopy/Bronchial Brush/Bronchoalveolar Lavage Specimen *on page 568*

♦ **Gag Gene of HIV** *see* HIV p24 Antigen Detection *on page 637*

♦ **Gastric Biopsy Culture for *Helicobacter pylori*** *see* Helicobacter pylori Biopsy-Based Tests: The Urease Tests, Culture, Cytology, and PCR *on page 620*

♦ **Gastrointestinal Viruses by EM** *see* Electron Microscopic Examination for Viruses, Stool *on page 603*

♦ **GC Culture** *see* Neisseria gonorrhoeae Culture and Smear *on page 662*

♦ **Genital Culture** *see* Bacterial Culture, Genital Specimen *on page 571*

♦ **Genital Culture for *Mycoplasma* T-Strain** *see* Genital Culture for *Ureaplasma urealyticum on page 616*

Genital Culture for *Ureaplasma urealyticum*

Related Information
Bacterial Culture, Genital Specimen *on page 571*
Neisseria gonorrhoeae Culture and Smear *on page 662*

Synonyms Genital Culture for *Mycoplasma* T-Strain; *Mycoplasma* T-Strain Culture, Genital; *Ureaplasma urealyticum* Culture, Genital

Applies to Cervical Culture for T-Strain *Mycoplasma*; Cervical Culture for *Ureaplasma urealyticum*; Urethral Culture for T-Strain *Mycoplasma*

Abstract *Ureaplasma urealyticum* are small bacteria that do not have a cell wall. These bacteria are included in the class Mollicutes. *U. urealyticum* are commonly isolated from the lower genital tract of sexually active adults. Even though these organisms are recovered from asymptomatic patients, *U. urealyticum* does play an etiologic role in genital tract diseases of both men and women.[1,2] It has been associated with spontaneous abortions and neonatal disease.[3]

Specimen Culturette® swab of urethra or cervix

Container Culturette® swab

Collection Contact laboratory to obtain special collection and transport medium. Swab should be agitated in the medium, expressed against the side of the tube, and then removed.

Storage Instructions Keep specimen refrigerated. **Organism is remarkably sensitive to drying**. Swab must be placed promptly into Culturette® and hand delivered to the Microbiology Laboratory. If stored longer than 24 hours, the specimens should be frozen at -70°C.

Turnaround Time 8 days if negative, up to 2 weeks if positive

Special Instructions Specimen should be collected without contact with lubricants, analgesics, or antiseptics.

Reference Interval Less than 10^4 organisms in genital tract

Use Establish the diagnosis of *Ureaplasma urealyticum* infection in suspected cases of nongonococcal urethritis and cervicitis. It is associated with chorioamnionitis and with perinatal morbidity and mortality. It can be isolated from the central nervous system and the lower respiratory tract of infected neonates.

Limitations Culture can be negative in the presence of infection, and the presence of *Ureaplasma urealyticum* or *Mycoplasma hominis* does not always indicate infection, although there is a significant association with symptomatic disease. Culture is offered in a few specialty laboratories.

Methodology Culture on selective media

Additional Information *Ureaplasma* and *Mycoplasma* can be isolated from urethral and genital swabs and from urine of sexually active individuals. Sixty percent or more of all women asymptomatically carry *U. urealyticum* in their genital tract. Usual prevalence of these organisms in patients with urethral symptoms also is high; thus, conclusions regarding the etiologic role of an isolate in a given patient are difficult to make. *U. urealyticum* is usually associated with cases of nongonococcal urethritis.

Footnotes

1. Potts JM, Ward AM, and Rackley RR, "Association of Chronic Urinary Symptoms in Women and *Ureaplasma urealyticum*," *Urology*, 2000, 55(4):486-9.
2. McKee KT Jr, Jenkins PR, Garner R, et al, "Features of Urethritis in a Cohort of Male Soldiers," *Clin Infect Dis*, 2000, 30(4):736-41.
3. Donders GG, Van Bulck B, Caudron J, et al, "Relationship of Bacterial Vaginosis and *Mycoplasma* to the Risk of Spontaneous Abortion," *Am J Obstet Gynecol*, 2000, 183(2):431-7.

References

Cassell GH, Waites KB, Watson HL, et al, "*Ureaplasma urealyticum* Intrauterine Infection: Role in Prematurity and Disease in Newborns," *Clin Microbiol Rev*, 1993, 6(1):69-87.
Eschenbach DA, "*Ureaplasma urealyticum* and Premature Birth," *Clin Infect Dis*, 1993, 17(Suppl 1):S100-6.
Paul VK, Gupta U, Singh M, et al, "Association of Genital *Mycoplasma* Colonization With low Birth Weight," *Int J Gynaecol Obstet*, 1998, 63(2):109-14.
Sethi S, Sharma M, Narang A, et al, "Isolation Pattern and Clinical Outcomes of Genital *Mycoplasma* in Neonates From a Tertiary Care Neonatal Unit," *J Trop Pediatr*, 1999, 45(3):143-5.

♦ **Genital Culture, Virus** *see* Viral Culture, Urogenital *on page 696*

♦ **Genital Lesions** *see* Viral Culture, Dermatological Symptoms *on page 693*

♦ **German Measles Culture** *see* Rubella Virus Culture *on page 678*

♦ **German Measles Serology** *see* Rubella Serology *on page 677*

♦ *Giardia* **EIA** *see* Giardia lamblia Antigen Detection *on page 616*

♦ *Giardia lamblia* *see* Ova and Parasites, Stool *on page 666*

Giardia lamblia Antigen Detection

Related Information
Cryptosporidium Antigen Detection by EIA *on page 596*
Ova and Parasites, Stool *on page 666*

Synonyms *Giardia* EIA; *Giardia lamblia* DFA; *Giardia lamblia* Immunofluorescence

Applies to *Giardia lamblia*-Specific Protein Detection Directly in Stool Specimens

Abstract *Giardia lamblia* is a flagellated enteric protozoan that infects both humans and animals. It is the most common cause of protozoal diarrhea throughout the world. Infection occurs through fecal-oral transmission and ingestion of contaminated food or water. Stool examination for the trophozoites and cysts is the traditional method used for the diagnosis of *G. lamblia* infection. Antigen detection assays are now available and have become the method of choice for diagnosis of diarrhea due to *G. lamblia*.

Specimen Stool

Container Clean dry container with a wide mouth

Collection Collect the specimen directly in the container and submit to the laboratory quickly.

Storage Instructions Maintain specimen at room temperature.

Turnaround Time 24-48 hours

Special Instructions Collect at least three stool specimens 2-3 days apart.

Reference Interval Negative for *G. lamblia* antigen

Use Aid in the diagnosis of giardiasis; evaluation of diarrhea, especially in campers, travelers, children in daycare centers, in male homosexuals, and in immunocompromised individuals

Limitations The assay will only detect *G. lamblia*; other important enteric pathogens will not be detected with this method. Some commercial assays have decreased specificity if the stool is fixed with EcoFix, a formalin and mercury-free fixative.[1]

Methodology Immunofluorescence or enzyme-linked immunoassay (EIA) (as well as conventional trichrome straining)

Additional Information *G. lamblia* antigen assays are comparable in cost to the stool ova and parasite examination. Both immunofluorescence and EIA methods provide sensitivities between 85% to 98% and specificities that exceed 90%.[2,3] All of these assays detect specific *G. lamblia* cyst cell wall proteins which are stable in human stool specimens.[4]

Footnotes

1. Fedorko DP, Williams EC, Nelson NA, et al, "Performance of Three Immunoassays and Two Direct Fluorescence Assays for Detection of *Giardia lamblia* in Stool Specimens Preserved in EcoFix," *J Clin Microbiol*, 2000, 38(7):2781-3.
2. Garcia LS and Shimizu RY, "Evaluation of Nine Immunoassay Kits (Enzyme Immunoassay and Direct Fluorescence) for Detection of *Giardia lamblia* and *Cryptosporidium parvum* in Human Fecal Specimens," *J Clin Microbiol*, 1997, 35(6):1526-9.
3. Aldeen WE, Hale D, Robison AJ, et al, "Evaluation of a Commercially Available ELISA Assay for Detection of *Giardia lamblia* in Fecal Specimens," *Diagn Microbiol Infect Dis*, 1995, 21(2):77-9.
4. Boone JH, Wilkins TD, Nash TE, et al, "Techlab and Alexon *Giardia* Enzyme-Linked Immunosorbent Assay Kits Detect Cyst Wall Protein 1," *J Clin Microbiol*, 1999, 37(3):611-4.

References

Chan R, Chen J, York MK, et al, "Evaluation of a Combination Rapid Immunoassay for Detection of *Giardia* and *Cryptosporidium* Antigens," *J Clin Microbiol*, 2000, 38(1):393-4.
Colmer-Hamood JA, "Fecal Microscopy Artifacts Mimicking Ova and Parasites," *Lab Med*, 2001, 32(2):80-4.
Leber AL and Novak SM, "Intestinal and Urogenital Amebae, Flagellates, and Ciliates," *Manual of Clinical Microbiology*, 7th ed, Washington, DC: AMS Press, American Society for Microbiology, 1999, 1391-405.
Maraha B and Buiting AG, "Evaluation of Four Enzyme Immunoassays for the Detection of *Giardia lamblia* Antigen in Stool Specimens," *Eur J Clin Microbiol Infect Dis*, 2000, 19(6):485-7.

Internet Web Sites

vm.cfsan.fda.gov/~mow/chap22.html
www.astdhpphe.org/infect/giardiasis.html
www.cdc.gov/ncidod/dpd/parasites/giardiasis/default.htm

♦ *Giardia lamblia* **DFA** *see* Giardia lamblia Antigen Detection *on page 616*

♦ *Giardia lamblia* **Immunofluorescence** *see* Giardia lamblia Antigen Detection *on page 616*

♦ *Giardia lamblia*-Specific Protein Detection Directly in Stool Specimens *see* Giardia lamblia Antigen Detection *on page 616*

♦ **GMS Stain** *see* Fungus Smear, Stain *on page 615*

♦ **Gomori Methenamine Silver Stain** *see* Fungus Smear, Stain *on page 615*

♦ **Gonorrhea Culture** *see* Neisseria gonorrhoeae Culture and Smear *on page 662*

♦ **Gonorrhea DNA Detection** *see* Neisseria gonorrhoeae Nucleic Acid Detection *on page 664*

Gram Stain

Related Information

Acid-Fast Stain, Modified, *Nocardia* Species *on page 550*
Anthrax Detection *on page 553*
Bacterial Culture, Aerobes *on page 563*
Bacterial Culture, Anaerobes *on page 564*
Bacterial Culture, Biopsy or Body Fluid *on page 565*
Bacterial Culture, Burn Sites *on page 569*
Bacterial Culture, Cerebrospinal Fluid *on page 569*
Bacterial Culture, Conjunctiva *on page 570*
Bacterial Culture, Middle Ear *on page 573*
Bacterial Culture, Sputum *on page 574*
Bacterial Culture, Throat, and Antigen Detection Testing for Group A Strep-
tococci *on page 577*
Bacterial Culture, Urine *on page 578*
Body Cavity Fluid Cytology *on page 372*
Body Fluid Chemical Analysis *on page 123*
Body Fluid pH *on page 125*
Cerebrospinal Fluid Analysis: Overview *on page 416*
Fungus Smear, Stain *on page 615*
KOH Preparation *on page 645*
Leukocyte Esterase, Urine *on page 878*
Neisseria gonorrhoeae Culture and Smear *on page 662*
Skin Biopsy *on page 71*
Synovial Fluid Analysis *on page 323*
Transfusion Reaction Work-up *on page 864*

Applies to Crystal Violet; Safranin

Abstract The first step in identification of bacterial isolates is study of their Gram stain properties. The Gram stain is a differential stain used to classify bacteria. Gram-positive bacteria retain crystal violet after decolorization and appear deep blue to purple. Gram-negative bacteria do not retain crystal violet after decolorization and are counterstained red by safranin. Gram staining characteristics may be atypical in very young, old, dead, or degenerating cultures.[1]

Patient Preparation Same as for routine culture of specific site

Specimen Duplicate of specimen appropriate for routine culture of the specific site

Collection Collection procedure same as for routine culture of the specific site. Specimen must be collected to avoid contamination with skin, adjacent structures, and nonsterile surfaces.

Critical Values Organisms detected in aseptically obtained specimens

Possible Panic Range Organisms detected in cerebrospinal fluid, especially those within leukocyte cytoplasm; those detected in peripheral blood smears.[2]

Use For many clinical specimens, a direct Gram stain is performed upon specimen receipt. The direct Gram stain reveals information about specimen quality (eg, by comparing numbers of squamous epithelial cells and polymorphonuclear neutrophils in sputum specimens), presence or absence of potential pathogens, and initial presumptive morphologic categorization of potential pathogens (eg, yeasts, gram-positive cocci vs gram-negative bacilli, etc). Gram stain results can provide a guide for initial empiric therapy, and should be correlated with subsequent culture results to help to ascertain the significance of organisms isolated from clinical specimens.

Limitations Although Gram stain results can provide important information shortly after specimen collection, the information provided is presumptive. Organism detection with specimen Gram stain requires that large numbers of potential pathogens be present; consequently, sensitivity with many specimens is <100% and direct Gram stain of blood is unwarranted, because organisms are almost never present in sufficient numbers for detection. Additionally, clinical specimens that are heavily contaminated with normal flora rarely provide diagnostically useful information unless probable pathogens are morphologically distinct from normal flora. Thus, direct Gram stain of throat swabs, stool, and rectal swabs is usually unwarranted. Certain organisms (eg, *Rickettsia* species, *Treponema pallidum*, *Legionella* species, *Mycobacterium* species, *Mycoplasma* species) stain poorly, or not at all with Gram stain.

Methodology Gram stain technique: Fix the material to the slide so that the material does not wash off during the staining procedure. Flood the surface of the slide with crystal violet solution. After 1 minute of exposure to the crystal violet stain, wash the slide thoroughly with distilled water. Flood the slide with Gram iodine solution for 1 minute. After washing, hold the smear between the thumb and forefinger and flood the surface with a few drops of the acetone-alcohol decolorizer until no violet color washes off. Wash with running water and overlay the surface with safranin counterstain for 1 minute. Wash with running water.

Additional Information Culture results, including organism identification and antimicrobial susceptibility, should be correlated to confirm and enhance the initial information provided by Gram stain. The choice of initial empiric antimicrobial therapy should be re-evaluated; and an equally effective, less expensive, narrower spectrum antimicrobial agent should be substituted whenever possible.

Gram stains are usually scanned for the presence or absence of white blood cells (indicative of infection) and squamous epithelial cells (indicative of mucosal contamination). A **sputum specimen** showing >25 squamous epithelial cells/lpf, regardless of the number of white blood cells, indicates that the specimen is grossly contaminated with saliva and bacterial culture should not be performed. Additional sputum specimens should be submitted to the laboratory when evidence of contamination by saliva is revealed. The best correlation of Gram stain and sputum culture occurs with gram-positive cocci in clusters (staphylococci), in chains (streptococci), and small gram-negative bacilli (*Haemophilus*). Lower predictive value is found for gram-negative bacilli.[3] The Gram stain can be a reliable indicator to guide initial antibiotic therapy. Substantial numbers of neutrophils and bacteria consistent with a pulmonary pathogen are appropriate for initial clinical therapeutic decision making, especially when phagocytosis of the organisms is found.[4] Typically a 90% correlation between Gram stain and culture can be achieved.[5] It is imperative that a valid sputum specimen be obtained for Gram stain.

Gram stains revealing an occasional bacterium per high powered field in an uncentrifuged **urine specimen** suggest a colony count of 10,000 bacteria/mL. Bacteria in the majority of fields suggests >100,000 bacteria/mL.

Gram stain is the most valuable diagnostic test in **bacterial meningitis** that is immediately available.[6] Organisms are detectable in 60% to 80% of patients who have not been treated and in 40% to 60% of those who have been given antibiotics.[6] Its sensitivity relates to the number of organisms present. The sensitivity of the Gram stain is greater in gram-positive infections and is only positive in half of the instances of gram-negative meningitis. It is positive even less frequently with listeriosis meningitis or with anaerobic infections.[6] Important causes of bacterial meningitis include *Haemophilus influenzae*, *Streptococcus pneumoniae*, *Neisseria meningitidis*, Group B *Streptococcus*, *Listeria monocytogenes*, and gram-negative bacilli.[7,8] Culture and Gram stain must have priority over antigen detection methods if only a small volume of CSF is available.[9]

Footnotes

1. Koneman EW, Allen SD, Janda WM, et al, *Color Atlas and Textbook of Diagnostic Microbiology*, 4th ed, Philadelphia, PA: JB Lippincott Co, 1992, 21, 24.
2. Gomez R and Buescher ES, Images in Clinical Medicine, "Meningococcemia," *N Engl J Med*, 1997, 336(10):707.
3. Flournoy DJ, "Interpreting the Sputum Gram Stain Report," *Lab Med*, 1998, 29:763-8.
4. Yungbluth M, "The Laboratory Diagnosis of Pneumonia. The Role of the Community Hospital Pathologist," *Clin Lab Med*, 1995, 15(2):209-34.
5. Reimer LG, "Community-Acquired Bacterial Pneumonias," *Semin Respir Infect*, 2000, 15(2):95-100.
6. Greenlee JE, "Approach to Diagnosis of Meningitis - Cerebrospinal Fluid Evaluation," *Infect Dis Clin North Am*, 1990, 4(4):583-98.
7. Schuchat A, Robinson K, Wenger JD, et al, "Bacterial Meningitis in the United States in 1995. Active Surveillance Team," *N Engl J Med*, 1997, 337(14):970-6.
8. Quagliarello VJ and Scheld WM, "Treatment of Bacterial Meningitis," *N Engl J Med*, 1997, 336(10):708-16.
9. Gray LD and Fedorko DP, "Laboratory Diagnosis of Bacterial Meningitis," *Clin Microbiol Rev*, 1992, 5(2):130-45.

References

Chapin-Robertson K, Dahlberg SE, and Edberg SC, "Clinical and Laboratory Analyses of Cytospin-Prepared Gram Stains for Recovery and Diagnosis of Bacteria From Sterile Body Fluids," *J Clin Microbiol*, 1992, 30(2):377-80.
Dunbar SA, Eason RA, Musher DM, et al, "Microscopic Examination and Broth Culture of Cerebrospinal Fluid in Diagnosis of Meningitis," *J Clin Microbiol*, 1998, 36(6):1617-20.
Giacomini G, "Permanent Diagnosis of Bacterial Vaginosis: Gram Stain or Papanicolaou Stain?" *Diagn Cytopathol*, 2000, 23(4):292-3.
McNair RD, MacDonald SR, Dooley SL, et al, "Evaluation of the Centrifuged and Gram-Stained Smear, Urinalysis, and Reagent Strip Testing to Detect Symptomatic Bacteriuria in Obstetric Patients," *Am J Obstet Gynecol*, 2000, 182(5):1076-9.
Tunkel AR and Scheld WM, "Acute Meningitis," *Principles and Practice of Infectious Diseases*, 5th ed, Mandell GL, Bennett JE, and Dolin R, eds, New York, NY: Churchill Livingstone, 2000, 959-97.

♦ **Group A Beta-Hemolytic *Streptococcus* Culture, Throat** *see* Bacterial Culture, Throat, and Antigen Detection Testing for Group A Streptococci *on page 577*

Group A *Streptococcus* Screen, Rapid

Related Information

Antideoxyribonuclease-B Titer, Serum *on page 554*
Antistreptolysin O Titer, Serum *on page 559*
Bacterial Antigens, Rapid Detection Methods *on page 562*
Bacterial Culture, Throat, and Antigen Detection Testing for Group A Strep-
tococci *on page 577*

Synonyms Rapid Detection of *Streptococcus* Group A; *Streptococcus* Group A Latex Screen; Throat Swab for Group A *Streptococcus* Antigen

Applies to Enzyme Immunoassay for Group A *Streptococcus* Antigen

Replaces Coagglutination Test for Group A Streptococci

Abstract *Streptococcus pyogenes*, also known as group A *Streptococcus*, is a common cause of acute bacterial pharyngitis. Rapid antigen detection assays will detect group A *Streptococcus* antigen directly from throat swabs. This assay can be performed in a few minutes, while throat culture requires overnight incubation. The specificity of these newer tests is very high (>95%) and thus, a positive result does not require culture confirmation. In contrast, the sensitivity of these assays is lower than that of throat (Continued)

Group A *Streptococcus* Screen, Rapid *(Continued)*

culture, and negative specimens should have a routine throat culture performed.[1]

Specimen Throat swab; many laboratories request two swabs, one for culture if the rapid screen is negative

Container Rayon or dacron swabs rather than cotton swabs enhance the chance of detection.

Collection Rigorous swabbing of the tonsillar pillars and posterior throat increases the probability of detection of streptococcal antigen.

Special Instructions Some laboratories favor submission of dry swabs for antigen testing. Consult the laboratory for their specific recommendations.

Use Rapidly screen for the presence of group A streptococci using culture independent methods

Limitations Many reviews have indicated a sensitivity of 75% to 80% and a specificity of 95% to 98% for the rapid methods. Sensitivity varies between manufacturers. Some kits are capable of detecting 10^5 colony forming units (CFUs) while others require 10^6-10^7 CFU/mL. Specimens that yield less than 10 colonies on culture usually are negative by rapid method. Adequate specimen collection on younger patients may be difficult, and thus, contribute to the false-negative rate. A positive result can be relied upon as a rational basis to begin therapy. **A negative result is only presumptive, and a culture should be performed to reasonably exclude the diagnosis of group A streptococcal infection.** Careful attention to the details of the method and the use of appropriate controls are required to assume adequate performance. Group A streptococcal antigen disappears rapidly following antibiotic therapy.

Contraindications This test should not be ordered unless results available within 1-2 hours of specimen collection will impact therapeutic decisions.

Methodology The streptococcal group A carbohydrate antigen is extracted from the swab used for collection by use of acid or enzyme reagents. The group A antigen is detected by enzyme immunoassay (EIA) or latex agglutination (LA). A nucleic acid based test has been developed, but is currently not used as a rapid test.[2]

Additional Information Rheumatic fever remains a concern in the United States and serious complications including sepsis, soft tissue invasion, and toxic shock-like syndrome have been reported to be increasing in frequency.[1] Therefore, timely diagnosis and early institution of appropriate therapy remains important. Timely therapy may reduce the acute symptoms and overall duration of streptococcal pharyngitis. The sequelae of post-streptococcal glomerulonephritis and rheumatic fever are diminished by early therapy.

See also Bacterial Culture, Throat, and Antigen Detection Testing for Group A Streptococci *on page 577.*

Footnotes

1. Chen FM, "Culture Confirmation of Negative Rapid Strep Test Results," *J Fam Pract*, 2000, 49(4):371-2.
2. Heiter BJ and Bourbeau PP, "Comparison of the Gen-Probe® Group A *Streptococcus* Test With Culture and a Rapid Streptococcal Antigen Detection Assay for Diagnosis of Streptococcal Pharyngitis," *J Clin Microbiol*, 1993, 31(8):2070-3.

References

Cunningham MW, "Pathogenesis of Group A Streptococcal Infections," *Clin Microbiol Rev*, 2000, 13(3):470-511.

Greiver M, "Practice Tips. Incorporating a Rapid Group A *Streptococcus* Assay With the Sore Throat Score," *Can Fam Physician*, 1999, 45:1181-2.

Needham CA, McPherson KA, and Webb KH, "Streptococcal Pharyngitis: Impact of a High-Sensitivity Antigen Test on Physician Outcome," *J Clin Microbiol*, 1998, 36(12):3468-73.

Pichero ME, Green JL, Francis AB, et al, "Recurrent Group A Streptococcal Tonsillo-pharyngitis," *Pediatr Infect Dis J*, 1998, 17(9):809-15.

Pitetti RD, Drenning SD, and Wald ER, "Evaluation of a New Rapid Antigen Detection Kit for Group A Beta-Hemolytic Streptococci," *Pediatr Emerg Care*, 1998, 14(6):396-8.

Internet Web Sites

www.astdhpphe.org/infect/strepa.html
www.cdc.gov/ncidod/dbmd/diseaseinfo/groupastreptococcal_g.htm

♦ **Group B Streptococci** *see* Bacterial Culture, Genital Specimen *on page 571*

Group B *Streptococcus* Screen, Rapid

Related Information

Bacterial Antigens, Rapid Detection Methods *on page 562*
Bacterial Culture, Cerebrospinal Fluid *on page 569*
Bacterial Culture, Genital Specimen *on page 571*

Synonyms *Streptococcus agalactiae* Latex Screen; *Streptococcus* Group B Latex Screen

Replaces Counterimmunoelectrophoresis for Group B Streptococcal Antigen

Test Includes Culture-independent detection of group B beta *Streptococcus* antigen

Abstract Group B streptococci is found in 5% to 40% of genital and lower gastrointestinal tract specimens of women. In most cases, this constitutes asymptomatic colonization, however, in pregnant women these bacteria can be transmitted to newborns during delivery. Neonates exposed to group

B streptococci may develop disseminated infection that results in a mortality rate of 5% to 10%.

Specimen Cerebrospinal, endocervical, vaginal, or rectal fluid

Container Sterile container, red top tube

Storage Instructions If a specimen for antigen detection cannot be tested immediately, it may be stored at 2°C to 8°C for 1 day or frozen at -20°C for longer storage. Storage is inconsistent with the role of the test for rapid diagnosis.

Turnaround Time About 1 hour stat

Critical Values Positive intrapartum test

Possible Panic Range Positive neonatal test

Use Culture-independent detection of group B *Streptococcus* is used in two settings. First, it is used to diagnose patients (usually in the neonatal period) suspected of group B *Streptococcus* invasive disease. Secondly, it is used as a rapid intrapartum test to identify maternal group B *Streptococcus* carriers who might transmit the organism to their newborn.

Limitations Rapid group B *Streptococcus* detection has a sensitivity range of 70% to 90% in neonatal meningitis. Identification of maternal group B *Streptococcus* carriers using rapid group B *Streptococcus* tests often fails to identify women colonized with low numbers of organisms. A 1996 study showed that rapid immunoassays were not sufficiently accurate for routine use in detecting vaginal colonization with group B *Streptococcus*.[1]

Methodology Latex agglutination (LA), enzyme immunoassay (EIA), PCR assay[2]

Additional Information Group B *Streptococcus* is one of the most common human pathogens in the neonatal period. Neonatal infection follows exposure to maternal genital flora *in utero* through ruptured membranes, or by colonization during passage through the birth canal. Neonatal infection presents as either early or late onset disease (EOD or LOD, respectively). EOD, which occurs within 5 days of birth (mean period to onset of symptoms is 20 hours), manifests as pneumonia and sepsis, occasionally accompanied by meningitis. LOD, which occurs 7 days to 3 months after birth (mean period to onset is 24 days) usually presents as meningitis.

Intrapartum antimicrobial therapy has been shown to be an effective means of reducing the incidence of EOD. It is currently not clear how best to identify individuals who should be treated.[1] An approach to prevention of neonatal group B streptococci has been endorsed by the American College of Obstetricians and Gynecologists and by the American Academy of Pediatrics.[3] Women selected for chemoprophylaxis are determined by the following criteria.

* Positive screening cultures of vaginal and rectal sites at 35-37 weeks gestation
* Women with group B streptococcal bacteriuria during pregnancy
* Women who have previously delivered an infant with group B streptococcal infection
* Women with significant risk factors (eg, onset of labor or membrane rupture earlier than 37 weeks of gestation, rupture of membranes for 18 hours or more before delivery, intrapartum fever)

Use of these guidelines should reduce the number of cases of neonatal group B streptococcal infection, but will not prevent all cases. The development of a group B streptococcal vaccine is being investigated which may aid in eliminating this disease.[4]

See also Bacterial Culture, Genital Specimen *on page 571.*

Footnotes

1. Baker CJ, "Inadequacy of Rapid Immunoassays for Intrapartum Detection of Group B Streptococcal Carriers," *Obstet Gynecol*, 1996, 88(1):51-5.
2. Bergeron MG, Ke D, Ménard C, et al, "Rapid Detection of Group B Streptococci in Pregnant Women at Delivery," *N Engl J Med*, 2000, 343(3):175-9.
3. Centers for Disease Control, "Prevention of Perinatal Group B Streptococcal Disease: A Public Health Perspective," *MMWR Morb Mortal Wkly Rep*, 1996, 45:1-24.
4. Kasper DL, Paoletti LC, Wessels MR, et al, "Immune Response to Type III Group B Streptococcal Polysaccharide-Tetanus Toxoid Conjugate Vaccine," *J Clin Invest*, 1996, 98(5):2308-14.

References

Donders GG, Vereecken A, Salembier G, et al, "Accuracy of Rapid Antigen Detection Test for Group B Streptococci in the Indigenous Vaginal Bacterial Flora," *Arch Gynecol Obstet*, 1999, 263(1-2):34-6.

Patel DM, Leblanc MH, Morrison JC, et al, "Postnatal Penicillin Prophylaxis and the Incidence of Group B Streptococcal Sepsis in Neonates," *South Med J*, 1994, 87(11):1117-20.

Reisner DP, Haas MJ, Zingheim RW, et al, "Performance of a Group B Streptococcal Prophylaxis Protocol Combining High-Risk Treatment and Low-Risk Screening," *Am J Obstet Gynecol*, 2000, 182(6):1335-43.

Simpson AJ, Mawn JA, and Heard SR, "Assessment of Two Methods for Rapid Intrapartum Detection of Vaginal Group B Streptococcal Colonization," *J Clin Pathol*, 1994, 47(8):752-5.

Wust J, Hebisch G, and Peters K, "Evaluation of Two Enzyme Immunoassays for Rapid Detection of Group B Streptococci in Pregnant Women," *Eur J Clin Microbiol Infect Dis*, 1993, 12(2):124-7.

Internet Web Sites

www.astdhpphe.org/infect/strepb.html
www.cdc.gov/ncidod/dbmd/gbs/

♦ **Gunshot Wound Culture** *see* Bacterial Culture, Wounds, Bites *on page 579*

♦ **HAA** *see* Hepatitis B Surface Antigen *on page 625*

♦ *Haemophilus influenzae* *see* Bacterial Culture, Bronchoscopy/Bronchial Brush/Bronchoalveolar Lavage Specimen *on page 568*

♦ *Haemophilus influenzae* *see* Bacterial Culture, Middle Ear *on page 573*

♦ *Haemophilus influenzae* *see* Bacterial Culture, Sputum *on page 574*

♦ *Haemophilus influenzae* **Group b** *see* Bacterial Culture, Cerebrospinal Fluid *on page 569*

♦ *Haemophilus influenzae* **Susceptibility Testing** *see* Beta-Lactamase Test *on page 581*

♦ *Haemophilus* **spp** *see* Bacterial Culture, Conjunctiva *on page 570*

♦ **Hanging Drop Mount for** *Trichomonas* *see* Trichomonas Preparation *on page 685*

♦ **Hank's Stain** *see* Acid-Fast Stain, Modified, *Nocardia* Species *on page 550*

♦ **Hantavirus Pulmonary Syndrome** *see* Hantavirus Serology *on page 619*

Hantavirus Serology

Synonyms Hantavirus Pulmonary Syndrome; Hemorrhagic Fever With Renal Syndrome; Nephropathia Epidemica; Sin Nombre Hantavirus

Test Includes Detection of IgM and IgG antibody specific for the Sin Nombre hantavirus

Abstract An outbreak of severe respiratory illness associated with respiratory failure, shock, and high mortality, hantavirus pulmonary syndrome (HPS), was recognized in 1993 in the southwestern United States. The cause was identified as Sin Nombre hantavirus (SNV). Since this recognition, other cases have been recognized in the Western U.S. and Canada, with related viruses throughout the Western hemisphere. HPS begins with nonspecific symptoms (eg, fever and myalgia), which are followed in 3-6 days by progressive cough and shortness of breath. Common findings during this later stage include tachypnea, tachycardia, fever, and hypotension. Abnormalities on chest radiographs are detected bilaterally, and pleural effusions are common. Hemoconcentration, thrombocytopenia, prolonged activated partial thromboplastin time, an increased proportion of immature granulocytes on the peripheral blood smear, leukocytosis, and elevated levels of serum lactate dehydrogenase and aspartate aminotransferase are found. Serum antibodies are detectable at the time of clinical presentation.[1,2]

In contrast, nephropathia epidemica (NE) is a milder disease in Northern Europe and Russia, and hemorrhagic fever with renal syndrome (HFRS) has been described in Asia. The triad of fever, hemorrhage, and renal failure is characteristic of HFRS. In addition, thrombocytopenia, petechiae, hypotension, proteinuria, and oliguria, and later during convalescence, diuresis occur.

Specimen Serum from acute phase of illness and a follow-up serum specimen 1-3 weeks later.

Container Red top tube for serum antibodies

Storage Instructions Serum can be stored at 4°C up to 1 week; serum should be stored at -70°C after 1 week and during shipping.

Reference Interval No detectable hantavirus IgM or less than a fourfold increase in IgG

Use Confirm the diagnosis of hantavirus pulmonary syndrome, an acute viral rodent-borne zoonosis

Limitations Assays for detection of antibody to hantavirus are generally available only through reference laboratories. Results of serologic tests will not be available quickly enough to establish a diagnosis before treatment.

Methodology Western blot, enzyme-linked immunosorbent assay (ELISA), indirect immunofluorescence (IIF)

Additional Information Hantaviruses are single-stranded RNA viruses of the family Bunyaviridae. Four distinct hantaviruses have been described in North America with over 20 serotypes or genotypes world-wide.[3] Additional hantaviruses may well be found. Rodents serve as the reservoir for hantaviruses, and infected rodents shed the virus in saliva, urine, and feces. Each hantavirus type seems to be specific for a single rodent host. Transmission to humans occurs most often by inhalation of infected rodent excreta, but a rodent bite has also resulted in infection. Among the greatest risks are occupational exposures to rodents in trappers, forestry workers, farmers, or the military. SNV is found in the deer mouse (*Peromyscus maniculatus*) population, which is prevalent in the western United States. Recommendations for prevention include avoidance of contact with rodent urine or saliva. Hantavirus person-to-person transmission has been shown in an outbreak of 18 people in Argentina, some of whom were treating physicians. Hantavirus has been transmitted from viral cultures in laboratory workers.

HPS can be confirmed by detection of hantavirus IgM and IgG serum antibodies, antigen in tissues by demonstration of viral RNA by RT-PCR, or demonstration of viral antigens in pulmonary vascular endothelial cells by immunohistochemical staining.[4] Viral isolation from human specimens is difficult to impossible in HPS but may be accomplished with difficulty in HRFS.

In HFRS, antigen may be detected in neutrophils and PBMC using monoclonal antibodies. Isolation of virus is difficult, unless the specimen is first passaged through laboratory rodents. Two or three passages may be necessary; thus, it is not often useful clinically.

Footnotes

1. Moolenaar RL, Breiman RF, and Peters CJ, "Hantavirus Pulmonary Syndrome," *Semin Respir Infect*, 1997, 12(1):31-9.
2. Goodman DA and Griego LC, "Hantavirus Pulmonary Syndrome: Implications for Critical Care Nurses," *Crit Care Nurse*, 1998, 18(1):18, 23-30.
3. Young JC, Mills JN, Enria DA, et al, "New World Hantaviruses," *Br Med Bull*, 1998, 54(3):659-73.
4. Colby TV, Zaki SR, Feddersen RM, et al, "Hantavirus Pulmonary Syndrome Is Distinguishable From Acute Interstitial Pneumonia," *Arch Pathol Lab Med*, 2000, 124(10)1463-6.

References

Butler JC and Peters CJ, "Hantaviruses and Hantavirus Pulmonary Syndrome," *Clin Infect Dis*, 1994, 19(3):387-95.

Centers for Disease Control and Prevention, "Hantavirus Pulmonary Syndrome - Panama, 1999-2000," *JAMA*, 2000, 283(17):2232-3.

Harper DR and Meyer AS, *Of Mice, Men, and Microbes: Hantavirus*, San Diego, CA: Academic Press, 1999.

McCaughey D and Hart CA, "Hantaviruses," *J Med Microbiol*, 2000, 49(7):587-99.

Mertz GJ, Hjelle BL, and Bryan RT, "Hantavirus Infection," *Disease-a-Month*, 1998, 44(3):89-138.

Nichol ST, Arikawa J, and Kawaoka Y, "Emerging Viral Diseases," *Proc Natl Acad Sci U S A*, 2000, 97(23):12411-2.

Peters CJ, Simpson GL, and Levy H, "Spectrum of Hantavirus Infection: Hemorrhagic Fever With Renal Syndrome and Hantavirus Pulmonary Syndrome," *Annu Rev Med*, 1999, 50:531-45.

Internet Web Sites

www.cdc.gov/ncidod/diseases/hanta/hps/index.htm

www.hantavirus.net/

♦ **HAVAB** *see* Hepatitis A Antibodies, IgM and IgG *on page 622*

♦ **HB_cAb** *see* Hepatitis B Core Antibody *on page 622*

♦ **HB_eAb** *see* Hepatitis B_e Antibody *on page 624*

♦ **HB_eAg** *see* Hepatitis B_e Antigen *on page 624*

♦ **HB_sAb** *see* Hepatitis B Surface Antibody *on page 625*

♦ **HB_sAg** *see* Hepatitis B Surface Antigen *on page 625*

♦ **HB_sAg Ab** *see* Hepatitis B Surface Antibody *on page 625*

♦ **HBV DNA Probe Test** *see* Hepatitis B DNA Detection *on page 623*

♦ **HCV Antibody** *see* Hepatitis C Virus Serology *on page 627*

♦ **HCV Branched DNA** *see* Hepatitis C Virus RNA Detection and Quantitation *on page 626*

♦ **HCV cDNA** *see* Hepatitis C Virus RNA Detection and Quantitation *on page 626*

♦ **HCV RIBA** *see* Hepatitis C Virus RNA Detection and Quantitation *on page 626*

♦ **HDAg** *see* Hepatitis D Serology *on page 627*

Helicobacter pylori Antigen Detection by EIA

Related Information

Helicobacter pylori Biopsy-Based Tests: The Urease Tests, Culture, Cytology, and PCR *on page 620*

Helicobacter pylori Serology *on page 621*

Pepsinogen I and II, Serum or Plasma *on page 246*

Synonyms *Helicobacter* Stool Test

Abstract The *H. pylori* fecal assay by EIA is a noninvasive qualitative test with high sensitivities (81% to 97%) and specificities (98% to 100%).[1] Thus, it compares favorably with other techniques that require invasive procedures of endoscopy or venipuncture. The FDA has approved this test for initial diagnosis and for test of cure.

Specimen Stool

Storage Instructions 2°C to 8°C; freeze if more than a 72-hour delay is anticipated.

Reference Interval Negative

Use Support the diagnosis of *H. pylori* infection in adults. Positives indicate that *H. pylori* antigen is present in stool.

Limitations Confirmation of eradication of *H. pylori* infection is not required. Negative results do not rule out a possibility of *H. pylori* infection. Performance characteristics are not established for patients younger than 18 years of age, for watery, diarrheal stools, or for evaluation of the efficacy of therapy.[2]

Contraindications The use of testing for *H. pylori* in asymptomatic individuals is not generally advised.[2]

Methodology Stool must be mixed to provide representative sampling; enzyme immunoassay (EIA)

Additional Information Aspects of *H. pylori* fecal or stool antigen, compared with other standard diagnostic studies, are shown in the following table.[3]

(Continued)

Helicobacter pylori Antigen Detection by EIA
(Continued)

Diagnostic Tests for *H. pylori*

Test	Advantages	Disadvantages
EIA on stool	Noninvasive	Less experience
Culture	Allows susceptibilities	Insensitive, slow
Serology	Noninvasive, inexpensive	Unreliable for active disease
Urease detection	Results in 2 hours	False positives, endoscopy
Urea breath tests	Rapid, evaluates response	Expensive

Footnotes

1. Weiss RL, ed, *ARUP Interpretive Data Guide*, ARUP Laboratories Inc, 1999, 262.
2. Mayo Reference Services Publication, "*Helicobacter pylori* Stool Antigen," *New Test Announcement*, #81806, Rochester, MN: Mayo Medical Laboratories, 1998.
3. Blaser MJ, "*Helicobacter pylori* and Related Organisms," *Principles and Practice of Infectious Diseases*, 5th ed, Mandell GL, Bennett JE, and Dolin R, eds, New York, NY: Churchill Livingstone, 2000, 2285-93.

References

Graham DY, Rakel RE, Kendrick AM, et al, "Recognizing Peptic Ulcer Disease. Keys to Clinical and Laboratory Diagnosis," *Postgrad Med*, 1999, 105(3):113-28.

Vaira D, Holton J, Menegatti M, et al, "Invasive and Noninvasive Tests for *Helicobacter pylori* Infection," *Aliment Pharmacol Ther*, 2000, 14(Suppl 3):13-22.

Internet Web Sites

www.cdc.gov/ulcer/md.htm
www.helico.com

Helicobacter pylori Biopsy-Based Tests: The Urease Tests, Culture, Cytology, and PCR

Related Information

Cobalamin, Serum *on page 150*
Gastric Analysis *on page 180*
Gastrin, Serum *on page 181*
Helicobacter pylori Antigen Detection by EIA *on page 619*
Helicobacter pylori Serology *on page 621*
Intrinsic Factor Blocking Antibody *on page 537*
Methylmalonic Acid, Serum, Plasma, Urine, or Amniotic Fluid *on page 224*
Parietal Cell Antibody *on page 541*
Pepsinogen I and II, Serum or Plasma *on page 246*
Polymerase Chain Reaction *on page 713*

Synonyms *Campylobacter pylori* Urease Test and Culture; Gastric Biopsy Culture for *Helicobacter pylori*; Urease Test and Culture, *Helicobacter pylori*

Applies to *H. pylori* Breath Tests

Test Includes Screening for the presence of urease activity in gastric biopsies indirectly indicates the presence of *Helicobacter pylori*; culture of the organism from gastric biopsy specimens, and PCR for detection of microorganisms. See *Helicobacter pylori* Serology *on page 621*.

Abstract *H. pylori* is a gram-negative motile microaerophilic spiral-shaped bacillus, frequently associated with gastritis. *H. pylori* infection is associated with gastric atrophy and intestinal metaplasia. It is acquired earlier in life in lower socioeconomic conditions, or in areas with poorer hygiene. It plays a major role in pathogenesis of peptic ulcer disease, but the majority of persons colonized remain asymptomatic. *H. pylori* infection is an independent risk factor for noncardiac gastric adenocarcinoma and gastric mucosa-associated lymphoid-tissue (MALT) lymphomas.[1]

Its urease activity is important in detection and identification. Culture with biopsy is the gold standard for identification of *H. pylori* (formerly, *Campylobacter pylori*).

Specimen Gastric mucosal biopsy

Container Sterile container, **no fixative** for these microbiologic tests

Storage Instructions If specimen cannot be transported immediately to the laboratory, it should be placed in 0.5 mL transport medium (normal saline).

Reference Interval Negative for urease activity, negative culture, biopsy negative for gastritis, and negative for *H. pylori*

Use Establish the presence and possible etiologic role of *Helicobacter pylori* in cases of chronic gastric ulcer, chronic active gastritis, and a relationship with duodenal ulcer

Limitations Culture and urease testing alone, without biopsies for histopathologic examination, may permit occult neoplasms to go undetected.

Methodology Urease test: Gastric biopsies are incubated on slightly buffered medium. A change of phenol red to alkaline (pink color) persisting more than 5 minutes is considered positive and presumptively indicative of the presence of *Helicobacter pylori*, even if the organism cannot be grown in culture. Specimens negative at 30 minutes should be re-examined periodically up to 24 hours. The sensitivity of urease testing leaves something to be desired. Because of such problems, newer tests have been marketed using names such as CLO-test,[2,3] HUT-test, and Pyloritek,[4] providing sensitivity of up to 90% to 99%, specificity of 95% to 99%. The Pyloritek is a rapid test strip designed to provide an answer in 1 hour compared to the 2-24 hours for the other agar-based tests.[5]

Breath isotope methods, measuring bacterial urease by detection of labeled CO_2[3,4,6] and serologic tests for detection of antibody, are also useful if available. The breath test is preferred as a means of documenting presence of active infection and eradication of infection after therapy in the absence of endoscopy.

Culture: Culture media may include enriched chocolate, Thayer-Martin with antibiotics, brain heart infusion (BHI) with 7% horse blood, and Mueller-Hinton with 5% sheep blood. The organism is microaerophilic and grows best in a reduced O_2 atmosphere or in a Campy-Pak™ system at 35°C. Cultures are usually observed for 7 days before being reported as negative. Patchy distribution of *H. pylori* may allow all biopsy-based tests to fail to diagnose the infection.[7] *H. pylori* can be cultured from vomitus and sometimes from cathartic stools.[8]

Biopsies: Biopsies of the middle of the body of the stomach are reported to provide optimal specimens for the diagnosis of *H. pylori*. Biopsies of the greater curvature of the midantrum are suitable to assess colonization. Both the angulus and middle body are suitable sites for biopsy to ascertain extent of atrophic gastritis.[9] Atrophy and intestinal metaplasia are identified most frequently in the antrum.[10] They are regarded as preneoplastic conditions, associated with *H. pylori* infections as well as other entities. The organism may be seen in biopsies stained with Gram stain, hematoxylin-eosin (H&E), Giemsa or Warthin-Starry silver stain. Newer methods include the Genta stain and immunocytochemistry with application of a specific antibody.[11] It is most often recognized in biopsies of the antrum but may also be seen in the fundic mucosa, metaplastic gastric mucosa of esophagus (Barrett esophagus), or duodenum. Biopsy may also establish the diagnosis of carcinoma or lymphoma. *H. pylori* was not found in the gastric mucosa of Meckel's diverticula.[12]

Cytology: Touch cytology preparations (ie, imprints from biopsies) may provide rapid diagnosis and preserve the biopsy specimen for histopathology or culture. The current gold standard for the diagnosis is arbitrarily defined as two specially stained biopsy specimens taken from the antrum. Histopathology may lean toward overdiagnosis when read by less experienced observers.[13]

Smear: A direct smear can be Gram stained.

Sensitivity of methods for detection of *H. pylori*:

- 24-hour urease: 62%
- direct Gram stain: 69%
- culture: 90%
- histopathology: 93%[7]

Polymerase chain reaction (PCR). The most sensitive technique to detect *H. pylori* is considered to be PCR. Either gastric aspirates or biopsy specimens have shown sensitivity and specificity >95%. As a post-treatment diagnostic test, PCR would seem useful, but it has failed to detect treatment failures more often than cultures or other methods. Further, false positives do occur following inadequate cleaning of endoscopes.[14]

Additional Information *Helicobacter pylori* is a major cause of chronic active gastritis. Its association with duodenal ulcer is strong. It is known that more than 90% of subjects who have duodenal ulcer have *H. pylori* infection. Only 50% of patients with Zollinger-Ellison syndrome with duodenal ulcer have *H. pylori*. Of patients with gastric ulcers, 75% to 80% have *H. pylori*.

Most peptic ulcers related to *H. pylori* infection can be treated with antibiotics and medication to suppress gastric acid. Treatment of the infection is not without controversy.[3,6,15,16] It is presently recommended that individuals with ulcer disease be treated, but patients with ulcers are only a subset of carriers of *H. pylori*. Those with MALT lymphomas also need therapy.[17]

Footnotes

1. Zucca E, Bertoni F, Roggero E, et al, "Molecular Analysis of the Progression From *Helicobacter pylori*-Associated Chronic Gastritis to Mucosa-Associated Lymphoid-Tissue Lymphoma of the Stomach," *N Engl J Med*, 1998, 338(12):804-10.
2. McColl K, Murray L, El-Omar E, et al, "Symptomatic Benefit From Eradicating *Helicobacter pylori* Infection in Patients With Nonulcer Dyspepsia," *N Engl J Med*, 1998, 339(26):1869-74.
3. Ohkusa T, Takashimizu I, Fujiki K, et al, "Disappearance of Hyperplastic Polyps in the Stomach After Eradication of *Helicobacter pylori*. A Randomized, Clinical Trial," *Ann Intern Med*, 1998, 129(9):712-5.
4. Fennerty MB, "A Review of Tests for the Diagnosis of *Helicobacter pylori* Infection," *Lab Med*, 1998, 29(9):561-6.
5. Laine L, Lewin D, Naritoku W, et al, "Prospective Comparison of Commercially Available Rapid Urease Tests for the Diagnosis of *Helicobacter pylori* Infection," *Gastrointest Endosc*, 1996, 44:523-6.
6. Talley NJ, Vakil N, Ballard ED II, et al, "Absence of Benefit of Eradicating *Helicobacter pylori* in Patients With Nonulcer Dyspepsia," *N Engl J Med*, 1999, 341(15):1106-11.
7. Glupczynski Y, "Microbiological and Serological Diagnostic Tests for *Helicobacter pylori*: An Overview," *Brit Med Bull*, 1998, 54(1):175-86.
8. Parsonnet J, Shmuely H, and Haggerty T, "Fecal and Oral Shedding of *Helicobacter pylori* From Healthy Infected Adults," *JAMA*, 1999, 282(23):2240-5.
9. Satoh K, Kimura K, Taniguchi Y, et al, "Biopsy Sites Suitable for the Diagnosis of *Helicobacter pylori* Infection and the Assessment of the Extent of Atrophic Gastritis," *Am J Gastroenterol*, 1998, 93(4):569-73.
10. Guarner J, Herrera-Goepfert R, Mohar A, et al, "Gastric Atrophy and Extent of Intestinal Metaplasia in a Cohort of *Helicobacter pylori*-Infected Patients," *Hum Pathol*, 2001, 32(1):31-5.

11. Toulaymat M, Marconi S, Garb J, et al, "Endoscopic Biopsy Pathology of *Helicobacter pylori* Gastritis. Comparison of Bacterial Detection by Immunohistochemistry and Genta Stain," *Arch Pathol Lab Med*, 1999, 123(9):778-81.

12. Fich A, Talley NJ, Shorter RG, et al, "Does *Helicobacter pylori* Colonize the Gastric Mucosa of Meckel's Diverticulum?" *Mayo Clin Proc*, 1990, 65(2):187-91.

13. Metz DC, Furth EE, Faigel DO, et al, "Realities of Diagnosing *Helicobacter pylori* Infection in Clinical Practice: A Case for Noninvasive Indirect Methodologies," *Yale J Biol Med*, 1998, 71(2):81-90.

14. Lage AP, Godfroid E, Fauconnier A, et al, "Diagnosis of *Helicobacter pylori* Infection by PCR: Comparison With Other Invasive Techniques and Detection of cagA Gene in Gastric Biopsy Specimens," *J Clin Microbiol*, 1995, 33:2752-6.

15. Blum AL, Talley NJ, O'Morain C, et al, "Lack of Effect of Treating *Helicobacter pylori* Infection in Patients With Nonulcer Dyspepsia. Omeprazole Plus Clarithromycin and Amoxicillin Effect One Year After Treatment (OCAY) Study Group," *N Engl J Med*, 1998, 339(26):1875-81.

16. Annibale B, Marignani M, Monarca B, et al, "Reversal of Iron Deficiency Anemia After *Helicobacter pylori* Eradication in Patients With Asymptomatic Gastritis," *Ann Intern Med*, 1999, 131(9):668-72.

17. Blaser MJ, "In a World of Black and White, *Helicobacter pylori* Is Gray," *Ann Intern Med*, 1999, 130(8):695-7.

References

Atherton JC and Spiller RC, "The Urea Breath Test for *Helicobacter pylori*," *Gut*, 1994, 35(6):723-5.

Chan WY, Hui PK, Leung KM, et al, "Coccoid Forms of *Helicobacter pylori* in the Human Stomach," *Am J Clin Pathol*, 1994, 102:503-7.

Chen YY, Antonioli DA, Spechler SJ, et al, "Gastroesophageal Reflux Disease Versus *Helicobacter pylori* Infection as the Cause of Gastric Carditis," *Mod Pathol*, 1998, 11(10):950-6.

Corvaglia L, Bontems P, Devaster JM, et al, "Accuracy of Serology and ¹³C-Urea Breath Test for Detection of *Helicobacter pylori* in Children," *Pediatr Infect Dis J*, 1999, 18(11):976-9.

Debongnie JC, Mairesse J, Donnay M, et al, "Touch Cytology. A Quick, Simple, Sensitive Screening Test in the Diagnosis of Infections of the Gastrointestinal Mucosa," *Arch Pathol Lab Med*, 1994, 118(11):1115-8.

Hilzenrat N, Lamoureux E, Weintrub I, et al, "*Helicobacter heilmannii*-Like Spiral Bacteria in Gastric Mucosal Biopsies, Prevalence and Clinical Significance," *Arch Pathol Lab Med*, 1995, 119(12):1149-53.

Lee A, "The *Helicobacter pylori* Genome-New Insights Into Pathogenesis and Therapeutics," *N Engl J Med*, 1998, 338(12):832-3.

Ruiz B, Correa P, Fontham ET, et al, "Antral Atrophy, *Helicobacter pylori* Colonization, and Gastric pH," *Am J Clin Pathol*, 1996, 105(1):96-101.

Van Dam J, Graeme-Cook FM, "A 35-Year-Old Woman With Recurrent Bleeding From a Gastric Ulcer After Treatment for *Helicobacter pylori* Infection," Case Records of the Massachusetts General Hospital, Case 13-1995, Scully RE, Mark EJ, McNeely WF, et al, eds, *N Engl J Med*, 1995, 332(17):1153-9.

Internet Web Sites

www.cdc.gov/ulcer/md.htm
www.helico.com

Helicobacter pylori Serology

Related Information

Gastric Analysis *on page 180*
Helicobacter pylori Antigen Detection by EIA *on page 619*
Helicobacter pylori Biopsy-Based Tests: The Urease Tests, Culture, Cytology, and PCR *on page 620*
Pepsinogen I and II, Serum or Plasma *on page 246*

Synonyms *Campylobacter pylori* Serology

Applies to Breath Testing for *H. pylori*

Test Includes Detection of IgG, IgA, and IgM antibodies specific for *Helicobacter pylori*

Abstract Persons who have peptic ulcer disease commonly are users of nonsteroidal anti-inflammatory agents or have infection with *H. pylori*.[1] Patients with peptic ulcer disease associated with *H. pylori* have elevated levels of serum antibody against this bacterium. *H. pylori* is very strongly associated with duodenal and gastric ulcer and chronic active gastritis. Most instances of chronic gastritis are secondary to *H. pylori* infection. *H. pylori* is an independent risk factor for gastric cancer. Even after treatment, antibodies to *H. pylori* may persist up to a year.

Specimen Serum or plasma

Container Red top tube; some laboratories use lavender top (EDTA) tube or green top (heparin) tube

Collection Acute and convalescent samples may be useful.

Reference Interval Undetectable or lower than cutoff limits in commercial assays

Use Increased antibody levels are associated with *H. pylori* infection, chronic active gastritis, and peptic ulcer. Negative serological results provide evidence against these diagnoses. IgG antibody testing offers a noninvasive alternative to urea breath tests to confirm post-therapeutic eradication of infection,[2] but *vide infra*.

Limitations Serologic findings only provide evidence of past or present infection. A large number of people are infected with the organism but do not have apparent disease.[1] There is strain-to-strain antigenic variability in *H. pylori*, which makes the test potentially insensitive. Sensitivities of commercially available assays range from 59% to 100%, while specificities range from 29% to 100%.[3,4] In comparison, the sensitivity and specificity of histopathologic examination of gastric mucosal biopsy are well above 90%.[5] Serology kits that measured IgA, IgG, and IgM simultaneously or measured

only IgA alone did not perform as well as those that measured IgG antibodies alone. A review of 35 such serology kits showed that serum antibodies accurately detect *H. pylori* infections.[4] Persistence of seropositivity in 72% of treated subjects by a quantitative method and 62% by a qualitative method is reported (ie, seroconversion cannot be regularly anticipated promptly following successful therapy).[6]

A promising development to detect *H. pylori* is the fecal antigen test, which is rapid, easy to use, and noninvasive. Both sensitivity and specificity were about 93%. After therapy, the antigen disappeared from feces in a few days, but the specificity was 79%.[7]

Methodology Enzyme-linked immunosorbent assay (ELISA), IgG antibody titers,[2] antibodies to *H. pylori* cytoxin-associated gene A protein (Cag-A).[8] Presently, the need for evaluation of Cag-A protein is controversial.[9]

Additional Information Large numbers of small, spiral-shaped bacteria, *Helicobacter pylori*, can be cultured from, or seen microscopically (especially with Dieterle or Giemsa stain) in gastric biopsies from most patients with chronic active gastritis and/or peptic ulcers. They can also be found in significant numbers of asymptomatic patients who have histologic gastritis, and from some individuals with no abnormality. Similarly, patients with chronic gastritis usually have elevated titers of IgG antibodies to *H. pylori*. The association of *H. pylori* infection in carcinogenesis of gastric epithelium and primary malignant lymphoma of stomach is recognized. IgG antibody to *H. pylori* is increased in sera of patients with gastric cancer.[10] A gold standard for the presence of *H. pylori* differs depending on the reference, but may include culture of biopsy, urea breath tests, rapid urease tests, PCR, or others. The gastric biopsy specimen is often stained with Giemsa or comparable stain as well as H&E, to demonstrate *H. pylori*. Acridine orange staining and anti-*H. pylori* monoclonal antibody may be used as well.[10]

The Urea Breath Test. Patients ingest a capsule containing radiolabeled carbon urea followed by collection of breath samples at 5-minute intervals for 30 minutes.[11] From the exhaled breath, radioactivity is measured using a scintillation counter. In untreated patients, this technique shows a sensitivity of 100%, specificity of 97%. After therapy, breath testing showed a sensitivity of 100% but specificity of only 86%.[12]

Footnotes

1. Shiotani A, Nurgalieva ZZ, Yamaoka Y, et al, "*Helicobacter pylori*," *Med Clin North Am*, 2000, 84(5):1125-36.

2. Marchildon P, Balaban DH, Sue M, et al, "Usefulness of Serological IgG Antibody Determinations for Confirming Eradication of *Helicobacter pylori* Infection," *Am J Gastroenterol*, 1999, 94(8):2105-8.

3. Taha AS, Reid J, Boothmann P, et al, "Serological Diagnosis of *Helicobacter pylori* - Evaluation of Four Tests in the Presence or Absence of Nonsteroidal Anti-inflammatory Drugs," *Gut*, 1993, 34(4):461-5.

4. Jaheij RJF, Straatman H, Jansen JBMJ, et al, "Evaluation of Commercially Available *Helicobacter pylori* Serology Kits: A Review," *J Clin Microbiol*, 1998; 36:2803-9.

5. Sipponen P, "*Helicobacter pylori*: A Cohort Phenomenon," *Am J Surg Pathol*, 1995, 19(Suppl 1):S30-6.

6. Cutler AF, Prasad VM, and Santogade P, "Four-Year Trends in *Helicobacter pylori* IgG Serology Following Successful Eradication," *Am J Med*, 1998, 105(1):18-20.

7. Vaira D, Holton J, Menegatti, Ricci C et al. "New Immunological Assays for the Diagnosis of *Helicobacter pylori* Infection," *Gut*, 1999, 45(Suppl I):I23-I27.

8. Guarner J, Herrera-Goepfert R, Mohar A, et al, "Gastric Atrophy and Extent of Intestinal Metaplasia in a Cohort of *Helicobacter pylori*-Infected Patients," *Hum Pathol*, 2001, 32(1):31-5.

9. Spechler SJ, Fischbach L, and Feldman M, "Clinical Aspects of Genetic Variability in *Helicobacter pylori*," *JAMA*, 2000, 283(10):1264-6.

10. Endo S, Ohkusa T, Saito Y, et al, "Detection of *Helicobacter pylori* Infection in Early Stage Gastric Cancer: A Comparison Between Intestinal- and Diffuse-Type Gastric Adenocarcinomas," *Cancer*, 1995, 75(9):2203-9.

11. Faigel DO, Childs M, Furth EE, et al, "New Noninvasive Tests for *Helicobacter pylori* Gastritis. Comparison With Tissue-Based Gold Standard," *Dig Dis Sci*, 1996, 41(4):740-8.

12. Metz DC, Furth EE, Faigel DO, et al, "Realities of Diagnosing *Helicobacter pylori* Infection in Clinical Practice: A Case for Non-Invasive Indirect Methodologies," *Yale J of Biol and Med*, 1998, 71:81-90.

References

Crabtree JE, Shallcross TM, Heatley RV, et al, "Evaluation of a Commercial ELISA for Serodiagnosis of *Helicobacter pylori*," *J Clin Pathol*, 1991, 44(4):326-8.

Graham DY, Malaty HM, Evans PG, et al, "Epidemiology of *Helicobacter pylori* in an Asymptomatic Population in the United States. Effect of Age, Race, and Socioeconomic Status," *Gastroenterology*, 1991, 100(6):1495-501.

Hentschel E, Brandstätter G, Dragosics B, et al, "Effect of Ranitidine and Amoxicillin Plus Metronidazole on the Eradication of *Helicobacter pylori* and the Recurrence of Duodenal Ulcer," *N Engl J Med*, 1993, 328(5):308-12.

Hirschl AM, Rathbone BJ, Wyatt JI, et al, "Comparison of ELISA Antigen Preparation Alone or in Combination for Serodiagnosing *Helicobacter pylori* Infections," *J Clin Pathol*, 1990, 43(6):511-3.

Parsonnet J, Hansen S, Rodriguez L, et al, "*Helicobacter pylori* Infection and Gastric Lymphoma," *N Engl J Med*, 1994, 330(18):1267-71.

Roggero E, Zucca E, Pinotti G, et al, "Eradication of *Helicobacter pylori* Infection in Primary Low-Grade Gastric Lymphoma of Mucosa-Associated Lymphoid Tissue," *Ann Intern Med*, 1995, 122(10):767-9.

Sung JJ, Chung SC, Ling TK, et al, "Antibacterial Treatment of Gastric Ulcers Associated With *Helicobacter pylori*," *N Engl J Med*, 1995, 332(3):139-42.

Van Dam J and Graeme-Cook FM, "A 35-Year-Old Woman With Recurrent Bleeding From a Gastric Ulcer After Treatment for *Helicobacter pylori* Infection," Case Records of the Massachusetts General Hospital, Case 13-1995, Scully RE, Mark EJ, McNeely WF, et al, eds, *N Engl J Med*, 1995, 332(17):1153-9.

(Continued)

Helicobacter pylori Serology (Continued)

Internet Web Sites
www.cdc.gov/ulcer/md.htm
www.helico.com

♦ **Helicobacter Stool Test** *see Helicobacter pylori Antigen Detection by EIA on page 619*

♦ **Helminths** *see Ova and Parasites, Stool on page 666*

♦ **Hemadsorbing Virus** *see Influenza Virus Culture on page 644*

♦ **Hemadsorbing Virus** *see Mumps Virus Culture on page 653*

♦ **Hemadsorbing Virus** *see Parainfluenza Virus Culture on page 668*

♦ **Hemipterae** *see Arthropod Identification on page 559*

♦ **Hemorrhagic Fever With Renal Syndrome** *see Hantavirus Serology on page 619*

♦ **Hemovac® Tip Culture** *see Bacterial Culture, Intravascular Device on page 572*

Hepatitis A Antibodies, IgM and IgG

Related Information
Aspartate Aminotransferase, Serum *on page 112*
Bilirubin, Total, Serum *on page 118*
Hepatitis B DNA Detection *on page 623*
Hepatitis: Laboratory Assessment, Overview *on page 629*
Liver Disease: Laboratory Assessment, Overview *on page 216*

Synonyms Antibody to HAV, IgM; Anti-HAV, IgM; HAVAB; Hepatitis A-Specific IgG or IgM Antibody

Test Includes Detection of IgM antibody to hepatitis A virus

Abstract Risk factors for hepatitis A include travel to an endemic area and/or ingestion of contaminated food such as shellfish.

Hepatitis A is an acute self-limited disease in which hallmarks include fever, jaundice, anorexia and diarrhea. Hepatitis A virus (HAV) is a nonenveloped RNA-containing virus. The hepatitis A-specific IgM antibody appears in acute hepatitis A at the clinical onset of symptoms and usually persists 3-6 months, and in 25% of patients for 12 months. It appears at the same time that serum aminotransferase concentrations are increased. Persistence for longer than 1 year suggests a false-positive test, a rare event. Past evidence of HAV infection is found using IgG-specific HAV antibody, or total (IgG + IgM) HAV antibody. Immunization results in HAV IgG antibody. While hepatitis A and E are transmitted by the fecal-oral route, hepatitis B, C, and D are blood-borne, and all viral hepatitis (A-E) are due to very different viral pathogens.

Specimen Serum

Container Red top tube

Storage Instructions Remove serum and freeze.

Reference Interval Negative

Use Differential diagnosis of hepatitis and other causes of jaundice. Presence of IgM antibody to hepatitis A virus is good evidence for acute or subacute hepatitis A. Presence of IgG antibody without IgM demonstrates antibody due to immunization. Usually, testing for IgG HAV is of little value, since antibodies persist for many years.

Methodology Enzyme-linked immunosorbent assay (ELISA), microparticle enzyme immunoassay (MEIA)

Additional Information Hepatitis A is usually transmitted by contaminated food or water. Its incubation period is 2-7 weeks. Fecal excretion of HAV peaks before symptoms develop. If hepatitis A antibody is IgM, the hepatitis A infection is acute. IgM antibody develops within a week of symptom onset, peaks in 3 months, and is usually gone after 6 months. Hepatitis A antibody of IgG type is indicative of old infection, is found in almost half of adults, persists throughout life, and is not usually clinically relevant. Many cases of hepatitis A are subclinical, particularly in children. Presence of IgG antibody to HAV does not exclude acute hepatitis B or hepatitis C.

Hepatitis A rarely causes fulminant disease, but when it does, it is sometimes fatal. Recovery never results in chronic liver disease.[1]

Footnotes
1. Hoofnagle JH, Carithers RL, Shapiro C, et al, "Fulminant Hepatic Failure," *Hepatology*, 1995, 21:240.

References
Appleton H, "Control of Food-Borne Viruses," *Br Med Bull*, 2000, 56(1):172-83.
Kemmer NM and Miskovsky EP, "Hepatitis A," *Infect Dis Clin North Am*, 2000, 14(3):605-15.
Maddrey WC, "Update in Hepatology," *Ann Intern Med*, 2001, 134(3):216-23.
OiConnor JA, "Acute and Chronic Viral Hepatitis," *Adolesc Med*, 2000, 11(2):279-92.
Ryder SD and Beckingham IJ, "ABC of Diseases of Liver, Pancreas, and Biliary System: Acute Hepatitis," *BMJ*, 2001, 322(7279):151-3.
Sacher RA, Peters SM, and Bryan JA, "Testing for Viral Hepatitis. A Practice Parameter," *Am J Clin Pathol*, 2000, 113(1):12-7
Shovein JT, Damazo RJ, and Hyams I, "Hepatitis A: How Benign Is It?" *Am J Nurs*, 2000, 100(3):43-7.

Internet Web Sites
www.cdc.gov/ncidod/diseases/hepatitis/index.htm
www.cdc.gov/ncidod/diseases/hepatitis/slideset/index.htm

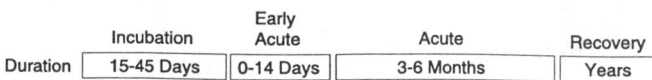

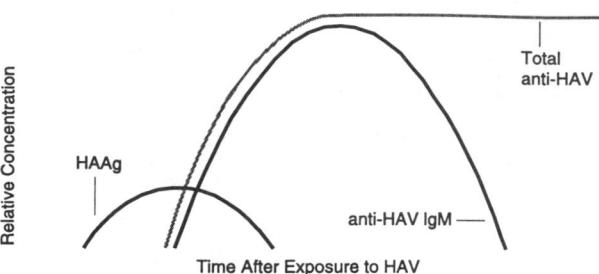

Reprinted from Abbott Diagnostics

♦ **Hepatitis A-Specific IgG or IgM Antibody** *see Hepatitis A Antibodies, IgM and IgG on page 622*

♦ **Hepatitis Associated Antigen** *see Hepatitis B Surface Antigen on page 625*

Hepatitis B Core Antibody

Related Information
Alanine Aminotransferase, Serum *on page 87*
Alkaline Phosphatase, Serum *on page 93*
Aspartate Aminotransferase, Serum *on page 112*
Bilirubin, Direct, Serum *on page 117*
Bilirubin, Total, Serum *on page 118*
Donation, Blood *on page 839*
Hepatitis B DNA Detection *on page 623*
Hepatitis B_e Antibody *on page 624*
Hepatitis B_e Antigen *on page 624*
Hepatitis B Surface Antibody *on page 625*
Hepatitis B Surface Antigen *on page 625*
Hepatitis C Virus Serology *on page 627*
Hepatitis D Serology *on page 627*
Hepatitis: Laboratory Assessment, Overview *on page 629*
Lactate Dehydrogenase, Serum *on page 207*
Liver Biopsy *on page 65*
Liver Disease: Laboratory Assessment, Overview *on page 216*
Polymerase Chain Reaction *on page 713*
Prothrombin Time *on page 354*
Risks of Transfusion *on page 861*

Synonyms Antibody to Hepatitis B Core Antigen; Anti-HB_c; HB_cAb

Applies to Core Window; Hepatitis B Core Antibody, IgM

Test Includes Detection of serologic response to hepatitis B infection; specifically, the antibody response to the core protein

Abstract The onset of hepatitis A is abrupt, while that of hepatitis B is insidious. The onset of hepatitis C is even more insidious and is apt to be subclinical.

For diagnosis of acute hepatitis, hepatitis B core IgM antibody and HB_sAg are helpful. HB_c antibody is found in early acute hepatitis B, in resolved hepatitis B, and in chronic hepatitis B. The IgG antibody directed against hepatitis B virus (HBV) nucleocapsid or core protein, may be the only serologic test that remains positive years after initial infection with hepatitis B.

Specimen Serum

Container Red top tube

Reference Interval Negative

Use Differential diagnosis of hepatitis syndromes. Used, in conjunction with clinical chemistry and other hepatitis B viral serologic markers, to assess the stage of hepatitis B infection. At the onset of symptoms of acute hepatitis B, anti-HB_c IgM becomes detectable and may persist for up to 1 year. With HB_sAg, IgM anti-HB_c is used to confirm the diagnosis of hepatitis B. Occasionally, in chronic hepatitis B, it may persist for life, but has been reported to rarely revert to negative. Anti-HB_c IgG appears shortly after IgM and usually persists for life, but has been reported to rarely revert to negative. Anti-HB_c may be used to screen volunteer blood donors for hepatitis B infection, detecting donors in the window period after HB_sAg has disappeared before anti-HB_s has appeared. Anti-HB_c is used to look for past hepatitis B infections, since immunization for hepatitis B produces antibodies to hepatitis B surface antigen but not antibodies to core antigen. Up to 50% of persons immunized with hepatitis B vaccine may have serum HB_sAg false positive for as long as 2 weeks.[1]

Limitations Weak positives without other positive markers or abnormalities in liver-related enzymes may represent false-positive reactions. The diagnostic significance of this test is increased when it is part of a panel of hepatitis serologic markers (HB$_s$Ag, anti-HB$_s$).

Methodology Enzyme-linked immunosorbent assay (ELISA). IgG and IgM antibodies may be differentiated.

Additional Information Early in hepatitis B before liver enzyme elevation, HBV proliferates without hepatocyte damage. At this stage, HBV DNA, HB$_s$Ag, HB$_e$Ag, and anti-HB$_c$ are detectable. Later, this immune tolerance is replaced by host response and hepatocellular damage of hepatitis. Most individuals clear the infection and have only persisting HB$_s$Ag, anti-HB$_e$, and anti-HB$_c$. The period between the disappearance of HB$_s$Ag and the appearance of HB$_s$Ab is often called the "core window." Anti-HB$_c$ persists for months to years after resolution of acute hepatitis B and persists in cases of chronic infection along with HB$_e$Ag, HBV DNA. Conversely, the absence of IgM core antibody in a patient with a chronic surface antigenemia and symptoms of acute hepatitis suggests acute hepatitis C or supervening delta hepatitis. Either may be quite serious. The majority of patients with reactivation hepatitis will have detectable serum anti-HB$_c$ IgM. See figure.

Hepatitis B Profile

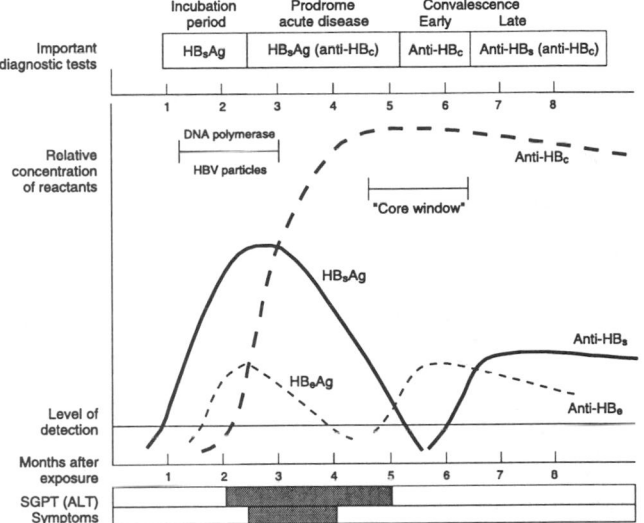

Serologic and clinical patterns observed during acute hepatitis B viral infection. From Hollinger FB and Dreesman GR, *Manual of Clinical Immunology*, 2nd ed, Rose NR and Friedman H, eds, Washington, DC: American Society for Microbiology, 1980, with permission.

The prevalence of hepatitis B in Asia may reach 20%. About 66% of subjects infected with HBV are asymptomatic. Acute hepatitis develops in ~25%. The rest become carriers. Chronic carrier status bears risk for ultimate development of cirrhosis and for hepatoma.[2]

Footnotes

1. Olde C and Garcia M, "Hepatitis B Vaccine as a Cause of False Positive Hepatitis B Surface Antigen," *J Cannt*, 1998, 8(4):20-1.
2. Sacher RA, Peters SM, and Bryan JA, "Testing for Viral Hepatitis. A Practice Parameter," *Am J Clin Pathol*, 2000, 113(1):12-7

References

Befeler AS and Di Bisceglie AM, "Hepatitis B," *Infect Dis Clin North Am*, 2000, 14(3):617-26.

Desforges JF, "Infectious Disease Testing for Blood Transfusions," *NIH Consensus Statement*, 1995, 13(1):1-27.

Grob PJ, "Hepatitis B: Virus, Pathogenesis and Treatment," *Vaccine*, 1998, 16(Suppl):S11-6.

Herrera JL, "Serologic Diagnosis of Viral Hepatitis," *South Med J*, 1994, 87(7):677-84.

Maddrey WC, "Hepatitis B: An Important Public Health Issue," *J Med Virol*, 2000, 61(3):362-6.

Mahoney FJ, "Update on Diagnosis, Management, and Prevention of Hepatitis B Virus Infection," *Clin Microbiol Rev*, 1999, 12(2):351-66.

Sjögren MH, "Serologic Diagnosis of Viral Hepatitis," *Gastroenterol Clin North Am*, 1994, 23(3):457-77.

Zuckerman JN and Zuckerman AJ, "Current Topics in Hepatitis B," *J Infect*, 2000, 41(2):130-6.

Internet Web Sites

www.cdc.gov/ncidod/diseases/hepatitis/index.htm

www.cdc.gov/ncidod/diseases/hepatitis/slideset/index.htm

www2.hepb.org/linksresources.html

♦ **Hepatitis B Core Antibody, IgM** *see* Hepatitis B Core Antibody *on page 622*

Hepatitis B DNA Detection

Related Information

Synonyms DNA Hybridization Test for HBV; DNA Probe Test for HBV; HBV DNA Probe Test; Hepatitis B Viral DNA Assay

Test Includes Use of an HBV specific DNA probe for detection of HBV viral DNA in serum samples or tissue. Sometimes the HBV DNA is amplified by polymerase chain reaction (PCR).

Abstract Chronic viral hepatitis may be due to infection with the human hepadnavirus, hepatitis B (HBV) or hepatitis C. Infection may result in a long-term carrier state of mild to severe chronic liver disease. Two weeks after infection with hepatitis B a large excess of viral protein can be detected in serum (surface antigen of HBV) and is followed by an antibody response to the viral proteins (anti-HB$_s$). The antihepatitis B response will persist in most patients for life. However, about 10% of HBV infections result in a chronic carrier state marked by a lack of anti-HB$_s$, but persistent anti-HB$_c$ and usually HB$_s$Ag. Diagnosis in these cases should be supplemented by additional analysis. Hepatitis B viral DNA can be detected in the serum or liver tissue from these individuals. Recent studies on symptomatic individuals with chronic liver disease of unknown etiology show that >90% are positive when tested for HBV DNA;[1] indicating that current serological testing does not detect all infections due to HBV.

Specimen Serum or plasma, liver tissue

Container Red top tube or lavender top (EDTA) tube, sterile container

Storage Instructions Serum or plasma should be transferred to a plastic tube and kept frozen at -20°C. Tissue should be frozen at -70°C.

Causes for Rejection Samples containing sodium azide cannot be used in this test.

Turnaround Time 4-7 days; turnaround time may vary with individual laboratories.

Reference Interval No HBV viral DNA detected

Use Aids in the diagnosis of HBV versus the other hepatidites; help to establish the stage of disease.[2] HBV DNA is the most sensitive marker for ongoing infection. Its quantification may provide prognostic relevance. It has been used as a measure of response to interferon-alpha-2b therapy.[3]

Methodology A slot-blot DNA hybridization based assay or amplification by polymerase chain reaction (PCR) is used. Quantitation of HBV DNA is also available for monitoring HBV infection.[4,5]

Additional Information The DNA probe assay provides a direct measure of HBV in serum or plasma and correlates with infectivity titers. The information provided from this test should be used in conjunction with serologic tests and HBV antigen detection. HBV DNA and HB$_e$Ag levels decline as the body clears the infection. Viral DNA becomes negative by hybridization techniques, but is often detectable by PCR in the later integrative stage of infection when aminotransferase levels are normal.[6] DNA detection should not replace serologic testing.

Footnotes

1. Overby LR and Houghton M, "Hepatitis Viruses," *Laboratory Diagnosis of Viral Infections*, 2nd ed, Chapter 19, Lennette EH, ed, New York, NY: Marcel Dekker Inc, 1992, 403-41.
2. Brechot C, Degos F, Lugassy C, et al, "Hepatitis B Virus DNA in Patients With Chronic Liver Disease and Negative Tests for Hepatitis B Surface Antigen," *N Engl J Med*, 1985, 312(5):270-6.
3. Sacher RA, Peters SM, and Bryan JA, "Testing for Viral Hepatitis. A Practice Parameter," *Am J Clin Pathol*, 2000, 113(1):12-7
4. Larzul D, Guigue F, Sninsky JJ, et al, "Detection of Hepatitis B Virus Sequences in Serum by Using In Vitro Enzymatic Amplification," *J Virol Methods*, 1988, 20(3):227-37.
5. Kaneko S, Feinstone SM, and Miller RH, "Rapid and Sensitive Method for the Detection of Serum Hepatitis B Virus DNA Using the Polymerase Chain Reaction Technique," *J Clin Microbiol*, 1989, 27(9):1930-3.
6. Lee WM, "Hepatitis B Virus Infection," *N Engl J Med*, 1997, 337:1733-45.

References

Grob PJ, "Hepatitis B: Virus, Pathogenesis and Treatment," *Vaccine*, 1998, 16(Suppl):S11-6.

Herrera JL, "Serologic Diagnosis of Viral Hepatitis," *South Med J*, 1994, 87(7):677-84.

Hytiroglou P, Dash S, Haruna Y, et al, "Detection of Hepatitis B and Hepatitis C Viral Sequences in Fulminant Hepatic Failure of Unknown Etiology," *Am J Clin Pathol*, 1995, 104(5):588-93.

Maddrey WC, "Hepatitis B: An Important Public Health Issue," *J Med Virol*, 2000, 61(3):362-6.

Mahoney FJ, "Update on Diagnosis, Management, and Prevention of Hepatitis B Virus Infection," *Clin Microbiol Rev*, 1999, 12(2):351-66.

(Continued)

Hepatitis B DNA Detection *(Continued)*

Sjögren MH, "Serologic Diagnosis of Viral Hepatitis," *Gastroenterol Clin North Am*, 1994, 23(3):457-77.

Wu PC, Fang JW, Lai CL, et al, "Hepatic Expression of Hepatitis B Virus Genome in Chronic Hepatitis B Virus Infection," *Am J Clin Pathol*, 1996, 105(1):87-95.

Zuckerman JN and Zuckerman AJ, "Current Topics in Hepatitis B," *J Infect*, 2000, 41(2):130-6.

Internet Web Sites

www.cdc.gov/ncidod/diseases/hepatitis/index.htm
www.cdc.gov/ncidod/diseases/hepatitis/slideset/index.htm
www2.hepb.org/linksresources.html

Hepatitis B_e Antibody

Related Information

Synonyms Anti-HB_e; HB_eAb

Test Includes Detection of antibody response to hepatitis e antigen

Abstract Hepatitis B_e antibody (anti-HB_e) appears in early convalescence in hepatitis B. HB_e antigen is a circulating peptide derived from the core hepatitis B gene and demonstrates viral replication. It is used as a marker for increased infectivity when present in serum.[1] **Antibody** to HB_e demonstrates reduced infectivity.

Specimen Serum

Container Red top tube

Reference Interval Negative

Use Differential diagnosis, staging, and prognosis of hepatitis B infection. Anti-HB_e and anti-HB_c together confirm the convalescent stage of hepatitis B after the disappearance of HB surface antigen (HB_sAg).

Limitations Absence of anti-HB_e does not rule out chronic hepatitis B carrier state or infectivity.

Methodology Enzyme immunoassay (EIA)

Additional Information Hepatitis B_e antigen usually is present only when there is circulating serum HBV DNA. The appearance of anti-HB_e indicates a reduced risk of infectivity. Failure of anti-HB_eAg to appear implies disease activity and probable chronicity, and patients with HB_eAb may have chronic hepatitis. Chronic HB_sAg carriers can be positive for either HB_eAg or anti-HB_e, but are less infectious when anti-HB_e is present. Antibody to e antigen can persist for years, but usually disappears earlier than anti-HB_s or anti-HB_c. HB_eAb is not used as the sole serologic marker for hepatitis B infection. See figure in Hepatitis B Core Antibody *on page 622*. Quantitation of HBV DNA, pre-S antigens, and IgM anti-HB_c may prove helpful for monitoring antiviral therapy, particularly in anti-HB_e-positive HB_sAg carriers.[2]

Footnotes

1. Befeler AS and Di Bisceglie AM, "Hepatitis B," *Infect Dis Clin North Am*, 2000, 14(3):617-32.
2. Zoulim F, Mimms L, Floreani M, et al, "New Assays for Quantitative Determination of Viral Markers in Management of Chronic Hepatitis B Virus Infection," *J Clin Microbiol*, 1992, 30(5):1111-9.

References

Grob PJ, "Hepatitis B: Virus, Pathogenesis and Treatment," *Vaccine*, 1998, 16(Suppl):S11-6.
Herrera JL, "Serologic Diagnosis of Viral Hepatitis," *South Med J*, 1994, 87(7):677-84.
Maddrey WC, "Hepatitis B: An Important Public Health Issue," *J Med Virol*, 2000, 61(3):362-6.
Mahoney FJ, "Update on Diagnosis, Management, and Prevention of Hepatitis B Virus Infection," *Clin Microbiol Rev*, 1999, 12(2):351-66.
Sjögren MH, "Serologic Diagnosis of Viral Hepatitis," *Gastroenterol Clin North Am*, 1994, 23(3):457-77.
Zuckerman JN and Zuckerman AJ, "Current Topics in Hepatitis B," *J Infect*, 2000, 41(2):130-6.

Internet Web Sites

www.cdc.gov/ncidod/diseases/hepatitis/index.htm
www.cdc.gov/ncidod/diseases/hepatitis/slideset/index.htm
www2.hepb.org/linksresources.html

Hepatitis B_e Antigen

Related Information

Synonyms HB_eAg

Applies to Core Window; Hepatitis, Chronic Carrier

Test Includes Detection of hepatitis B_e antigen in patient's serum

Abstract Hepatitis B_e antigen (HB_eAg) is a circulating peptide derived from the core hepatitis B gene and demonstrates viral replication. It is used as a marker for increased infectivity when present in serum.[1] HB_eAg appears early in hepatitis B. Infectivity of a patient with hepatitis B virus (HBV) can be evaluated with HB_eAg and HB_sAg. Measurement of serum HBV DNA also provides evidence of infectivity.

Specimen Serum

Container Red top tube

Storage Instructions Serum must be stored frozen or refrigerated, as HB_eAg is thermolabile.

Reference Interval Negative

Use Differential diagnosis, infectivity, and prognosis of hepatitis B infection. Hepatitis B_e antigen is found during the most infectious period of hepatitis B. It is usually found for only 3-6 weeks. With appearance of anti-HB_e and disappearance of HB_eAg, initiation of resolution of hepatitis B can be recognized. Persistence beyond 10 weeks suggests development of the chronic carrier state and chronic hepatitis.

Limitations Absence does not rule out infectivity or chronic hepatitis B carrier state.

Methodology Enzyme immunoassay (EIA)

Additional Information HB_eAg appears in acute hepatitis B about the same time as HB_sAg, when the patient is most infectious. HB_eAg is a proteolytic product of HB_cAg and is found only in HB_sAg positive sera. During the HB_eAg-positive state, usually 3-6 weeks, hepatitis B patients are at increased risk of transmitting the virus to their contacts, including babies born during this period. Exposure to serum or body fluid positive for HB_eAg and HB_sAg is associated with three to five times greater risk of infectivity than when HB_sAg positivity occurs without HB_eAg. Yet nosocomial transmission has been reported from HB_eAg negative persons.[2] Increased transmission from HB_eAg persons is probably related to increased amounts of circulating viral DNA. Persistence of HB_eAg is also associated with chronic liver disease. See figures and also Hepatitis B Core Antibody *on page 622*.

Modes of transmission of HBV include percutaneous (eg, drug use, blood or body fluid exposure in healthcare workers, transfusions); sexual (heterosexual or male homosexual); mother to infant (blood exposure at delivery). Other types of transmission occur as well.[3]

Hepatitis B Serological Profile
Core Window Identification

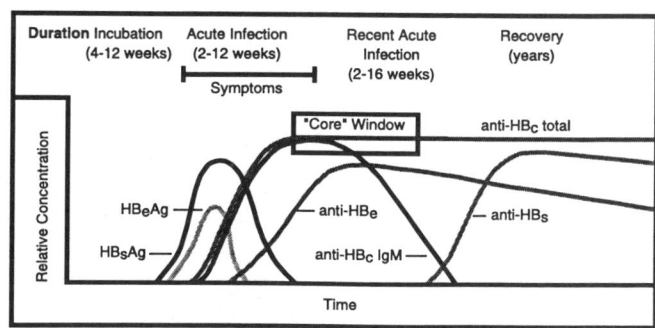

Hepatitis B Chronic Carrier
No Seroconversion

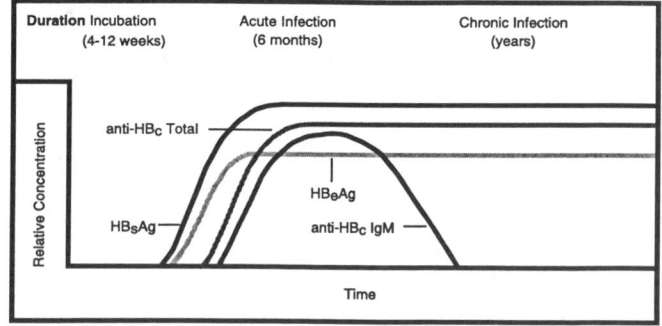

Hepatitis B Chronic Carrier
Late Seroconversion

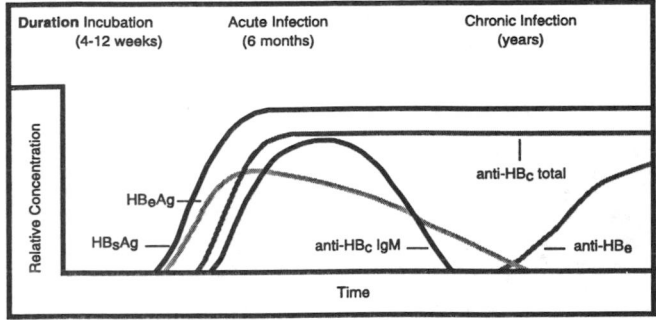

Duration Incubation (4-12 weeks)	Acute Infection (6 months)	Chronic Infection (years)

Relative Concentration

HB$_e$Ag

HB$_s$Ag

anti-HB$_C$ total

anti-HB$_C$ IgM

anti-HB$_e$

Time

Footnotes

1. Befeler AS and Di Bisceglie AM, "Hepatitis B," *Infect Dis Clin North Am*, 2000, 14(3):617-32.
2. Incident Investigation Teams and others, "Transmission of Hepatitis B to Patients From Four Infected Surgeons Without Hepatitis B e Antigen," *N Eng J Med*, 1997, 337:178-84.
3. Lee WM, "Hepatitis B Virus Infection," *Clin Lab Med*, 1997, 337:1733-45.

References

Grob PJ, "Hepatitis B: Virus, Pathogenesis and Treatment," *Vaccine*, 1998, 16(Suppl):S11-6.

Herrera JL, "Serologic Diagnosis of Viral Hepatitis," *South Med J*, 1994, 87(7):677-84.

Maddrey WC, "Hepatitis B: An Important Public Health Issue," *J Med Virol*, 2000, 61(3):362-6.

Mahoney FJ, "Update on Diagnosis, Management, and Prevention of Hepatitis B Virus Infection," *Clin Microbiol Rev*, 1999, 12(2):351-66.

Sjögren MH, "Serologic Diagnosis of Viral Hepatitis," *Gastroenterol Clin North Am*, 1994, 23(3):457-77.

Zuckerman JN and Zuckerman AJ, "Current Topics in Hepatitis B," *J Infect*, 2000, 41(2):130-6.

Internet Web Sites

www.cdc.gov/ncidod/diseases/hepatitis/index.htm
www.cdc.gov/ncidod/diseases/hepatitis/slideset/index.htm
www2.hepb.org/linksresources.html

♦ **Hepatitis B$_s$ Antibody** *see Hepatitis B Surface Antibody on page 625*

Hepatitis B Surface Antibody

Related Information

Aspartate Aminotransferase, Serum *on page 112*
Bilirubin, Total, Serum *on page 118*
Hepatitis B Core Antibody *on page 622*
Hepatitis B DNA Detection *on page 623*
Hepatitis B$_e$ Antibody *on page 624*
Hepatitis B$_e$ Antigen *on page 624*
Hepatitis B Surface Antigen *on page 625*
Hepatitis C Virus RNA Detection and Quantitation *on page 626*
Hepatitis C Virus Serology *on page 627*
Hepatitis D Serology *on page 627*
Hepatitis: Laboratory Assessment, Overview *on page 629*
Liver Biopsy *on page 65*
Liver Disease: Laboratory Assessment, Overview *on page 216*
Polymerase Chain Reaction *on page 713*

Synonyms Antibody to Hepatitis B Surface Antigen; Anti-HB$_s$; HB$_s$Ab; HB$_s$Ag Ab; Hepatitis B$_s$ Antibody

Applies to Hepatitis Vaccine

Replaces Australian Antigen Antibody

Test Includes Detection of serologic response to hepatitis B infection or hepatitis B immunization; specifically, antibody response to surface protein

Abstract Hepatitis B surface antibody (anti-HB$_s$) develops following resolved hepatitis B. It is responsible for immunity.

Highly effective vaccines are used throughout the world and may eventually lead to eradication of hepatitis B. Detection of antibody to HB$_s$ antigen in a vaccinated patient is associated with protective immunity.

Specimen Serum

Container Red top tube

Reference Interval Varies with clinical circumstance

Use Presence of hepatitis B surface antibody indicates past infection with resolution of previous hepatitis B infection, in which case anti-HB$_c$ is also present, or, if no other hepatitis B markers are present, vaccination against hepatitis B. Anti-HB$_s$ may be monitored serially in individuals who are at increased risk for further exposure to hepatitis B (ie, dentists, hygienists, hemodialysis personnel, phlebotomists, etc). Hepatitis B surface antibody is used to evaluate the need to repeat hepatitis B vaccination or to give hepatitis B immune globulin after needlestick injury.

Limitations Presence of anti-HB$_s$ is not an absolute indicator of resolved hepatitis, nor of protection from future infection. Since there are different serologic subtypes of hepatitis B virus, it is possible (and has been reported) for a patient to have antibody to one surface antigen type and to be acutely infected with virus of a different subtype. Thus, a patient may have coexisting HB$_s$Ag and HB$_s$Ab. Transfused individuals or hemophiliacs receiving plasma components may give false-positive tests for antibody to hepatitis B surface antigen, and passively acquired reactivity from transfusion or globulin therapy does not indicate immunity. Most individuals vaccinated with HBV vaccine develop anti-HB$_s$, although some do not.

Methodology Enzyme immunoassay (EIA)

Additional Information Anti-HB$_s$ usually can be detected several weeks to several years after HB$_s$Ag is no longer found, and it usually persists for life after acute infection has resolved. It may disappear in some patients with only antibody to hepatitis B core remaining. See figure in Hepatitis B Core Antibody *on page 622*. Patients with this antibody are not infectious. Presence of anti-HB$_s$ without the presence of HB$_s$Ag is evidence for immunity from reinfection, with virus of the same subtype (*vide supra*). Anti-HB$_s$ can be induced by vaccination with hepatitis vaccine. This vaccine is safe and effective in protecting most recipients from acute hepatitis B. Vaccine recipients tested for HB$_s$Ag during the 2 weeks after immunization may test positive transiently from the vaccine itself.

References

Barash C, Conn MI, DiMarino AJ, et al, "Serologic Hepatitis B Immunity in Vaccinated Health Care Workers," *Arch Intern Med*, 1999, 159(13):1481-3.

Grob PJ, "Hepatitis B: Virus, Pathogenesis and Treatment," *Vaccine*, 1998, 16(Suppl):S11-6.

Herrera JL, "Serologic Diagnosis of Viral Hepatitis," *South Med J*, 1994, 87(7):677-84.

Incident Investigation Teams, et al, "Transmission of Hepatitis B to Patients From Four Infected Surgeons Without Hepatitis B$_e$ Antigen," *N Engl J Med*, 1997, 337:178-84.

Maddrey WC, "Hepatitis B: An Important Public Health Issue," *J Med Virol*, 2000, 61(3):362-6.

Mahoney FJ, "Update on Diagnosis, Management, and Prevention of Hepatitis B Virus Infection," *Clin Microbiol Rev*, 1999, 12(2):351-66.

Sjögren MH, "Serologic Diagnosis of Viral Hepatitis," *Gastroenterol Clin North Am*, 1994, 23(3):457-77.

Zuckerman JN and Zuckerman AJ, "Current Topics in Hepatitis B," *J Infect*, 2000, 41(2):130-6.

Internet Web Sites

www.cdc.gov/ncidod/diseases/hepatitis/index.htm
www.cdc.gov/ncidod/diseases/hepatitis/slideset/index.htm
www2.hepb.org/linksresources.html

Hepatitis B Surface Antigen

Related Information

Alanine Aminotransferase, Serum *on page 87*
Aspartate Aminotransferase, Serum *on page 112*
Bilirubin, Total, Serum *on page 118*
Blood and Fluid Precautions, Specimen Collection *on page 40*
Hepatitis B Core Antibody *on page 622*
Hepatitis B DNA Detection *on page 623*
Hepatitis B$_e$ Antibody *on page 624*
Hepatitis B$_e$ Antigen *on page 624*
Hepatitis B Surface Antibody *on page 625*
Hepatitis C Virus RNA Detection and Quantitation *on page 626*
Hepatitis C Virus Serology *on page 627*
Hepatitis D Serology *on page 627*
Hepatitis: Laboratory Assessment, Overview *on page 629*
Heterophilic Antibodies *on page 191*
Liver Biopsy *on page 65*
Liver Disease: Laboratory Assessment, Overview *on page 216*
Risks of Transfusion *on page 861*

Synonyms HAA; HB$_s$Ag; Hepatitis Associated Antigen

Applies to Hepatitis B, Window Stage; Hepatitis, Chronic Carrier

Replaces Australian Antigen; Serum Hepatitis Marker

Test Includes Detection of hepatitis B surface antigen in patient's serum

Abstract For evaluation of acute hepatitis, serologic testing is recommended for HB$_s$Ag, anti-HB$_s$, anti-HB$_c$ (IgM), and HAV (IgM). HB$_s$Ag, anti-HB$_c$, HB$_e$Ag and HBV DNA each appear even before liver enzyme elevation. Other causes of acute hepatitis include Epstein Barr infection and cytomegalovirus. Persistence of HB$_s$Ag longer than 6 months indicates a chronic carrier state or chronic hepatitis. Hepatitis A, B, C, or D may cause fulminant hepatitis, especially if two viruses coinfect. Hepatitis C also causes chronic hepatitis. In the presence of positivity to HB$_s$Ag anti-HDV is advised in patients with travel history to the Mediterranean, intravenous drug abuse or multiple transfusions.[1] Other useful tests include the transaminases; see Liver Disease: Laboratory Assessment, Overview *on page 216*.

Specimen Serum

Container Red top tube

Reference Interval Negative

Use Screen blood donors (HB$_s$Ag-positive individuals are rejected); differential diagnosis of hepatitis; evaluate risk in needlestick injuries in healthcare facilities, and guide use of hepatitis B immune globulin. Hepatitis B surface antigen is the earliest indicator of acute hepatitis B infection and is found, as
(Continued)

Hepatitis B Surface Antigen (Continued)

well, in chronic carriers. The presence of HB$_s$Ag without positivity for IgM anti-HB$_c$ is suggestive of active chronic hepatitis B or carrier status.[1]

Limitations Patients who are negative for HB$_s$Ag may still have acute type B viral hepatitis. There is sometimes a "window" stage when HB$_s$Ag has become negative and the patient has not yet developed the antibody (anti-HB$_s$Ag). On such occasions the anti-HB$_s$Ag (IgM) is usually positive; and the patient should be treated as potentially infectious until anti-HB$_s$Ag is detected, at which time immunity is probable. In cases with strong clinical suspicion of viral hepatitis, serologic testing should not be limited to detecting HB$_s$Ag but should include a battery of tests to evaluate different stages of acute and convalescent hepatitis. These should include a test for hepatitis A antibody (IgM), and HB$_s$Ag, anti-HB$_s$, anti-HB$_c$ (IgM), and hepatitis C virus (anti-HCV).

Methodology Enzyme immunoassay (EIA)

Additional Information Hepatitis B virus (HBV) is a DNA virus with a protein coat, surface antigen (HB$_s$Ag), and a core consisting of nucleoprotein (HB$_c$Ag is the core antigen). There are eight different serotypes. Early in infection, HB$_s$Ag, HBV DNA, and DNA polymerase can all be detected in serum.

Transmission is parenteral, sexual or perinatal. The incubation period of hepatitis B is 2-6 months. HB$_s$Ag can be detected 1-7 weeks **before** liver enzyme elevation or the appearance of clinical symptoms. Three weeks after the onset of acute hepatitis about 50% of the patients will still be positive for HB$_s$Ag, while at 17 weeks only 10% are positive. The best available markers for infectivity are HB$_s$Ag and HB$_e$Ag. The presence of anti-HB$_s$ and anti-HB$_e$ is associated with noninfectivity. The chronic carrier state is indicated by the persistence of HB$_s$Ag and/or HB$_e$Ag over long periods (6 months to years) without seroconversion to the corresponding antibodies. Such a condition has the potential to lead to serious liver damage, but may be an isolated asymptomatic serologic phenomenon, especially for persons who acquired disease as neonates. There is also increased risk of hepatoma. Persistence of HB$_s$Ag, without anti-HB$_s$, with combinations of positivity of anti-HB$_{core}$, HB$_e$Ag, or anti-HB$_e$ indicate infectivity and need for investigation for chronic persistent or chronic aggressive hepatitis. See figure in Hepatitis B Core Antibody on page 622.

Chronic carrier states are found in up to 10% of cases. Some remain healthy, but evolution to chronic persistent hepatitis, chronic active hepatitis, cirrhosis, and hepatoma represent major problems of this disease. Prevention of hepatitis B for those at risk is available via vaccination,[2] as well as treatment for some chronic carriers.[3]

Footnotes

1. Sacher RA, Peters SM, and Bryan JA, "Testing for Viral Hepatitis. A Practice Parameter," *Am J Clin Pathol*, 2000, 113(1):12-7
2. Mahoney FJ, Burkholder BT, and Matson CC, "Prevention of Hepatitis B Virus Infection," *Am Fam Phys*, 1993, 47(4):865-72.
3. Kaplan MM, "Twelve Questions Physicians Often Ask," *Consultant*, 1993, 33(3):145-52.

References

Grob PJ, "Hepatitis B: Virus, Pathogenesis and Treatment," *Vaccine*, 1998, 16(Suppl):S11-6.

Herrera JL, "Serologic Diagnosis of Viral Hepatitis," *South Med J*, 1994, 87(7):677-84.

Lee WM, "Hepatitis B Virus Infection," *N Engl J Med*, 1997, 337(24):1733-45.

Maddrey WC, "Hepatitis B: An Important Public Health Issue," *J Med Virol*, 2000, 61(3):362-6.

Mahoney FJ, "Update on Diagnosis, Management, and Prevention of Hepatitis B Virus Infection," *Clin Microbiol Rev*, 1999, 12(2):351-66.

Sjögren MH, "Serologic Diagnosis of Viral Hepatitis," *Gastroenterol Clin North Am*, 1994, 23(3):457-77.

Zuckerman JN and Zuckerman AJ, "Current Topics in Hepatitis B," *J Infect*, 2000, 41(2):130-6.

Internet Web Sites

www.cdc.gov/ncidod/diseases/hepatitis/index.htm
www.cdc.gov/ncidod/diseases/hepatitis/slideset/index.htm
www2.hepb.org/linksresources.html

♦ **Hepatitis B Viral DNA Assay** *see* Hepatitis B DNA Detection on page 623

♦ **Hepatitis B Viral Load** *see* Human Immunodeficiency Virus, Viral Load Assay on page 640

♦ **Hepatitis B, Window Stage** *see* Hepatitis B Surface Antigen on page 625

♦ **Hepatitis C Amplification** *see* Hepatitis C Virus RNA Detection and Quantitation on page 626

♦ **Hepatitis, Chronic Carrier** *see* Hepatitis B$_e$ Antigen on page 624

♦ **Hepatitis, Chronic Carrier** *see* Hepatitis B Surface Antigen on page 625

♦ **Hepatitis C PCR** *see* Hepatitis C Virus RNA Detection and Quantitation on page 626

♦ **Hepatitis C Viral Load** *see* Human Immunodeficiency Virus, Viral Load Assay on page 640

Hepatitis C Virus RNA Detection and Quantitation

Related Information

Alanine Aminotransferase, Serum on page 87
Alkaline Phosphatase, Serum on page 93
Aspartate Aminotransferase, Serum on page 112
Bilirubin, Direct, Serum on page 117
Bilirubin, Total, Serum on page 118
Donation, Blood on page 839
Hepatitis B DNA Detection on page 623
Hepatitis B$_e$ Antibody on page 624
Hepatitis B$_e$ Antigen on page 624
Hepatitis B Surface Antibody on page 625
Hepatitis B Surface Antigen on page 625
Hepatitis C Virus Serology on page 627
Hepatitis D Serology on page 627
Hepatitis: Laboratory Assessment, Overview on page 629
Lactate Dehydrogenase, Serum on page 207
Liver Biopsy on page 65
Liver Disease: Laboratory Assessment, Overview on page 216
Polymerase Chain Reaction on page 713
Prothrombin Time on page 354
Risks of Transfusion on page 861
Smooth Muscle Antibody on page 543

Synonyms HCV Branched DNA; HCV cDNA; HCV RIBA; Hepatitis C Amplification; Hepatitis C PCR; Hepatitis RT-PCR

Applies to bDNA; cDNA

Test Includes Amplification of viral DNA (or amplification of HCV-specific probe) to detect and/or quantitate HCV RNA in plasma.

Abstract The onset of hepatitis C is often insidious.

At present, 6 HCV genotypes and 50 subtypes have been described for this RNA virus. Genotypes 1, 2, and 3 are found worldwide. Genotype 4 is principally in Egypt and Zaire, genotype 5 in South Africa, and genotype 6 in Asia. Variations in the six major types are designated with letters a, b, c, etc.[1,2]

Second generation nucleotide assays (RT-PCR, bDNA) show similar sensitivities. Each of these detect HCV RNA of the serotypes commonly found in the U.S. In chronic HCV infections, types 2 and 3, when associated with low levels of viremia by RT-PCR or bDNA, predict a more sustained response to therapy after treatment with interferon and ribavirin. Genotype 1b may be found in cases with aggressive disease by histopathology, and may result in more aggressive liver disease following liver transplantation. The gold standard for demonstrating HCV genotypes is the cDNA, based on subtype-specific point mutations in PCR-amplified cDNA.

Specimen Serum or liver tissue

Container Red top tube; tissue in a sterile container or sealed plastic bag

Storage Instructions Serum should be collected within 2 hours of specimen collection. Store or ship serum a -20°C. Tissue should be stored or shipped a t -70°C.

Causes for Rejection Serum samples not separated within 2 hours of collection; tissue specimens that have thawed during storage or shipping

Turnaround Time 4-7 days; may vary between different laboratories

Reference Interval No HCV viral RNA detected

Use Aid in the diagnosis of HCV infection, predict responsiveness to therapy, and monitor therapy; useful in the differential diagnosis of severe autoimmune hepatitis and hepatitis C.[3]

Limitations HCV RNA degrades quickly and may cause a false-negative result if specimens are not handled properly.

Methodology Viral RNA is extracted from serum or tissue and after transcription the genetic material is amplified using PCR. Quantitation of the HCV RNA is also available either by direct binding with detection by branched chain DNA (bDNA) probes or by quantitation of the RT-PCR product.

Additional Information Hepatitis C now infects 4 million people in the U.S. and 100 million world-wide. Before 1990-92, acquisition was by blood transfusions, but now 60% of HCV infections are acquired through sharing intravenous or intranasal drug paraphernalia. The initial diagnosis is by checking antibody to HCV. After that is found, HCV genotyping and quantitative viral load testing are done to aid in the decision to treat. Untreated, about 85% of people remain persistently positive. Hepatitis C leads to ascites, esophageal varices, hepatic encephalopathy, cirrhosis, liver failure, and hepatocellular cancer.[4] Genotypes 1b and 4 cause more aggressive liver disease and respond less to therapy, compared to other types.

Footnotes

1. Cheney DP, Chopra S, and Graham C, "Hepatitis C," *Infect Dis Clin North Am*, 2000, 14(3):633-42.
2. Zein NN, "Clinical Significance of Hepatitis C Virus Genotypes," *Clin Microbiol Rev*, 2000, 13(2):223-35.
3. Krawitt EL, "Autoimmune Hepatitis," *N Engl J Med*, 1996, 334(14):897-903.
4. Thomas DL, Astemborski J, Rai RM, et al, "The Natural History of Hepatitis C Virus Infection: Host, Viral, and Environmental Factors," *JAMA*, 2000, 284(4):450-6.

References

Boyer N and Marcellin P, "Pathogenesis, Diagnosis and Management of Hepatitis C," *J Hepatol*, 2000, 32(Suppl 1):98-112.

Gross JB, "Clinician's Guide to Hepatitis C," *Mayo Clin Proc*, 1998, 73:355-61.

Jacob S, Baudy D, Jones E, et al, "Comparison of Quantitative HCV RNA Assays in Chronic Hepatitis C," *Am J Clin Pathol*, 1997:362-7.

Liang TJ, Rehermann B, Seeff LB, et al, "Pathogenesis, Natural History, Treatment, and Prevention of Hepatitis C," *Ann Intern Med*, 2000, 132:296-305.

Reesink HW, ed, *Hepatitis C Virus*, 2nd ed, Farmington, CT: Karger, 1998.

Yokosuka O, Kojima H, Imazeki F, et al, "Spontaneous Negativation of Serum Hepatitis C Virus RNA Is a Rare Event in Type C Chronic Liver Diseases: Analysis of HCV RNA in 320 Patients Who Were Followed for More Than 3 Years," *J Hepatol*, 1999, 31(3):394-9.

Internet Web Sites
www.cdc.gov/ncidod/diseases
www.hepatitis-central.com/index.html

Hepatitis C Virus Serology

Related Information

Synonyms HCV Antibody

Applies to Anti-HCV, Enzyme Immunoassay (EIA); Recombinant Immunoblot Assay; RIBA; Second Generation EIA; Third Generation EIA

Test Includes Detection of antibody specific for hepatitis C virus in serum

Abstract A small, enveloped single-stranded RNA virus, hepatitis C causes disease which often is asymptomatic. Although it can be self-limited, long-term chronic sequellae are well known. Chronic disease is seen in 50% to 85% of patients. Cirrhosis evolves in ~20% to 30% of patients whose chronic infection persists for longer than 20 years. In the U.S., HCV is responsible for 20% of cases of acute hepatitis, 60% of cases of chronic hepatitis, and 30% of cases of cirrhosis.[1] Antibody tests, especially third generation EIAs, become positive 6-8 weeks after exposure to HCV with 97% sensitivity in drug abusers. The presence of antibody indicates infection, not necessarily immunity. Confirmation of a positive EIA may be with the RIBA (recombinant immunoblot assay) or by HCV reverse transcriptase polymerase chain reaction (RT-PCR) or HCV bDNA testing (*vide infra*). Nearly 50% of blood donors who test EIA positive do not have detectable HCV RNA nor a positive RIBA, and are considered false positive.

Specimen Serum

Container Red top tube

Sampling Time HCV RNA appears within days of exposure, before ALT concentrations become increased.

Reference Interval Negative

Use Differential diagnosis of acute and chronic hepatitis; screen blood units for transfusion safety; evaluate patients with essential mixed cryoglobulinemia, membranoproliferative glomerulonephritis, and porphyria cutanea tarda.[2] Individuals who received blood transfusions before 1992 should be tested.

In an individual with abnormal ALT and positive risk factors, anti-HCV is highly suggestive of current infection.

Limitations False-positive HCV Immunoassays are found in 0.2% of pregnant women while true positives are 0.8%.[3] Associations with false-positive tests include recent immunization against influenza virus, hypergammaglobulinemia, rheumatoid factor, and connective tissue disorders. By virtue of problems of low specificity, ELISA-positive specimens require confirmation with recombinant immunoblot assay, RIBA.

Lack of anti-HCV does not exclude a possibility of HCV hepatitis. Antibodies may not be detectable early.[4]

Methodology Enzyme immunoassay (EIA) is confirmed with RIBA for anti-HCV. A positive or indeterminate result in a setting of low prevalence is checked with HCV RT-PCR. RT-PCR is the most sensitive test, but is available only in larger laboratories. A positive EIA in a setting of high prevalence (IVDA, intranasal cocaine use, transfusions before 1992, liver disease, body piercings, multiple sexual partners, STDs, or long-term sex partner who is HCV positive) should be evaluated directly with HCV RNA.

Additional Information When specific testing for HCV became available about 1989, the numbers of new cases annually dropped from 175,000 to about 30,000. Yet, additional cases keep occurring, chiefly from sharing paraphernalia in intravenous or intranasal drug use. In developed countries, most HCV infections are found in injection drug users, persons in younger age groups.[5,6] HCV is rarely transmitted by sexual contact, much less often than HBV. However, transmission rates for multiple partners, unprotected intercourse, and coinfection with other sexually transmitted diseases may increase risk of sexual transmission as high as 20%.[1] The risk of transmission from mother to infant is <5%. The risk of acquisition from a random needlestick in hospital workers is about 0.1%. When the needle has been used in an HCV-positive individual, the risk increases to 5% or 10%. Other risk factors include used razor blades, body piercing and tattooing.[1] There is no postexposure prophylaxis presently available.

ALT concentrations characteristically fluctuate widely in patients with chronic hepatitis C, and are usually normal in about a third. Correlation between the severity of hepatitis and serum ALT concentrations has been inconsistent.

Disappearance of virus is sustained only in 10% to 15% of patients.[7]

Death in patients with hepatitis C includes those with end-stage liver disease. Others die with complications of HIV infection, drug overdose, sepsis, pneumonia, endocarditis, homicide, suicide, and accidental trauma.[5]

Footnotes
1. "The Ongoing Battle With Hepatitis C," *Mayo Reference Services Communique*, April 2000.
2. Gumber SC and Chopra S, "Hepatitis C: A Multifaceted Disease. Review of Extrahepatic Manifestations," *Ann Intern Med*, 1995, 123(8):615-20.
3. Ward C, Tudor-Williams G, Cotzias T, et al, "Prevalence of Hepatitis C Among Pregnant Women Attending an Inner London Obstetric Department: Uptake and Acceptability of Named Antenatal Testing," *Gut*, 2000, 47(2):277-80.
4. Sacher RA, Peters SM, and Bryan JA, "Testing for Viral Hepatitis. A Practice Parameter," *Am J Clin Pathol*, 2000, 113(1):12-7
5. Thomas DL, Astemborski J, Rai RM, et al, "The Natural History of Hepatitis C Virus Infection: Host, Viral, and Environmental Factors," *JAMA*, 2000, 284(4):450-6.
6. Alter MJ, Mast EE, Moyer LA, et al, "Hepatitis C," *Infect Dis Clin North Am*, 1998, 12(1):13-26.
7. Gross JB, "Clinician's Guide to Hepatitis C," *Mayo Clin Proc*, 1998, 73(4):355-60.

References
Boyer N and Marcellin P, "Pathogenesis, Diagnosis and Management of Hepatitis C," *J Hepatol*, 2000, 32 (Suppl 1):98-112.
Brody RI, Eng S, Melamed J, et al, "Immunohistochemical Detection of Hepatitis C Antigen by Monoclonal Antibody TORDJI-22 Compared With PCR Viral Detection," *Am J Clin Pathol*, 1998, 110(1):32-7.
"Centers for Disease Control, Recommendations for Prevention and Control of Hepatitis C Virus (HCV) Infection and HCV-Related Chronic Disease," *MMWR Morb Mortal Wkly Rep*, 1998, 47(RR-19): 1-39.
Cheney DP, Chopra S, and Graham C, "Hepatitis C," *Infect Dis Clin North Am*, 2000, 14(3):633-42.
Christensen PB, Groenbaek K, and Krarup HB, "Transfusion-Acquired Hepatitis C: The Danish Lookback Experience. The Danish HCV [hepatitis C virus] Lookback Group," *Transfusion*, 1999, 39(2):188-93.
Costes V, Durand L, Pageaux GP, et al, "Hepatitis C Virus Genotypes and Quantification of Serum Hepatitis C RNA in Liver Transplant Recipients. Relationship With Histologic Outcome of Recurrent Hepatitis C," *Am J Clin Pathol*, 1999, 111(2):252-8.
Erali M, Ashwood ER, and Hillyard DR, "Performance Characteristics of the COBAS Amplicor Hepatitis C Virus Monitor Test, Version 2.0," *Am J Clin Pathol*, 2000, 114(2):180-7.
Gross JB, "Clinician's Guide to Hepatitis C," *Mayo Clin Proc*, 1998, 73:355-61.
Jacob S, Baudy D, Jones E, et al, "Comparison of Quantitative HCV RNA Assays in Chronic Hepatitis C," *Am J Clin Pathol*, 1997:362-7.
Khella SL, Frost S, Hermann GA, et al, "Hepatitis C Infection, Cryoglobulinemia, and Vasculitic Neuropathy. Treatment With Interferon Alfa: Case Report and Literature Review," *Neurology*, 1995, 45(3 Pt 1):407-11.
Liang TJ, Rehermann B, Seeff LB, et al, "Pathogenesis, Natural History, Treatment, and Prevention of Hepatitis C," *Ann Intern Med*, 2000, 132:296-305.
Moyer LA, Mast EE, and Alter MJ, "Hepatitis C: Part I. Routine Serologic Testing and Diagnosis," *Am Fam Phys*, 1999, 59(1):79-88, 91-2.
Park YN, Boros P, Zhang DY, et al, "Serum Hepatitis C Virus RNA Levels and Histologic Findings in Liver Allografts With Early Recurrent Hepatitis C," *Arch Pathol Lab Med*, 2000, 124(11):1623-7.
Tobler LH, Tegtmeier G, Stramer SL, et al, "Lookback on Donors Who Are Repeatedly Reactive on First-Generation Hepatitis C Virus Assays:Justification and Rational Implementation," *Transfusion*, 2000, 40(1):15-24.
Zein NN, "Clinical Significance of Hepatitis C Virus Genotypes," *Clin Microbiol Rev*, 2000, 13(2):223-35.

Internet Web Sites
www.cdc.gov/hepatitis

Hepatitis D Serology

Related Information

Synonyms Delta Agent Serology; Delta Hepatitis Serology

Applies to HDAg

Abstract Hepatitis delta agent (HDV) was first described in 1977. HDV always occurs in a person infected with hepatitis B (HBV). Patients coinfected with HDV and HBV have fulminant hepatitis more often than patients infected only with HBV, and have increased risk for chronic hepatitis, cirrhosis, and hepatocellular carcinoma.[1]

(Continued)

Hepatitis D Serology *(Continued)*

Specimen Serum

Container Red top tube

Reference Interval Negative

Use Differential diagnosis of chronic, recurrent, and acute viral hepatitis. Testing for serological markers of HDV should be considered when a patient shows clinical signs of acute or fulminant hepatitis, or when deterioration takes place in chronic hepatitis B infection.

Limitations False-positive EIA results have been reported in patients with lipemia or high titer rheumatoid factor. Delta antigen is only found transiently, in the late incubation period. Most of the immunoassays lack desirable levels of sensitivity.[1]

Methodology Enzyme-linked immunosorbent assay (ELISA), HDV molecular hybridization technology is being evaluated. Northern blot analysis is done in a limited number of laboratories. Total (IgG and IgM) and IgM antidelta antibody assays are available. IgM predominates in acute infection, disappearing before HB$_s$Ag is cleared. IgM and IgG antidelta are found in high titer in chronic delta hepatitis.[1]

Additional Information Hepatitis D virus ("delta" agent) is an incomplete RNA virus, or viroid, that can only infect livers already infected by hepatitis B virus. HDV may occur, therefore, as a coinfection with acute HBV hepatitis, which usually resolves, or as a superinfection in chronic HBV infection, following which HDV also causes chronic hepatitis. It cannot occur in an HB$_s$Ag-negative individual. It uses HBV surface antigen as its viral envelope. IgG and IgM antibodies to HDV develop 5-7 weeks after infection. IgM antibody is most useful in distinguishing those patients with active liver disease. IgM anti-HDV is transient and is rapidly replaced by IgG anti-HDV, which persists and is associated with hepatitis. Generally, laboratories use total anti-HDV ELISAs containing both IgM and IgG for diagnostic purposes. HDAg can be detected in serum or liver biopsies but is technically demanding and offers little to diagnosis. Studies of liver transplants in patients with end-stage liver disease due to hepatitis B/D have shown, through serial biopsies post-transplant, that HDV viral reinfection occurs within 1 week but without damage. Not until HBV proliferation occurs several weeks to months later does one find histopathologic and clinical changes.[2]

Transmission of this defective virus is mostly by injection drug use, and less commonly through sexual transmission. Among HBV-infected users of injection drugs, seroprevalence of HDV is 20% to 53%.[3]

Hepatitis D Superinfection

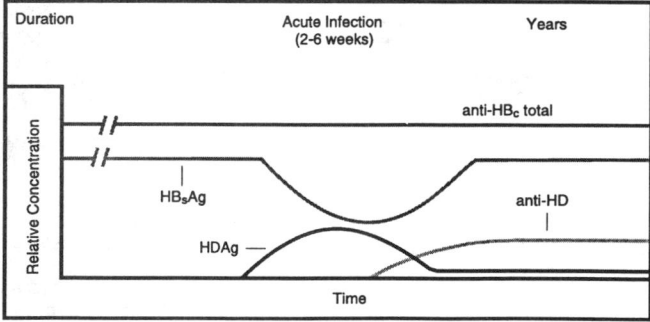

Reprinted from Abbott Diagnostics

Hepatitis D Coinfection

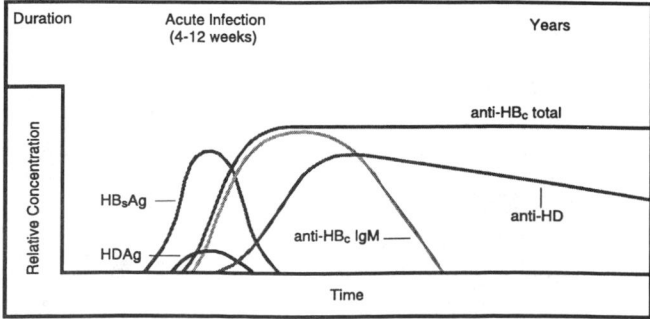

Reprinted from Abbott Diagnostics

Footnotes

1. Sacher RA, Peters SM, and Bryan JA, "Testing for Viral Hepatitis. A Practice Parameter," *Am J Clin Pathol*, 2000, 113(1):12-7.
2. Davies SE, Lau JY, O'Grady JG, et al, "Evidence That Hepatitis D Virus Needs Hepatitis B Virus to Cause Hepatocellular Damage," *Am J Clin Pathol*, 1992, 98(6):554-8.

3. Shapiro CN, "Transmission of Hepatitis Viruses," *Ann Intern Med*, 1994, 120(1):82-4 (editorial).

References

Alter MJ and Hedler SE, "Delta Hepatitis Infection in North America," *Hepatitis Delta Virus, Molecular Biology, Pathogenesis, and Clinical Aspects*, Hadziyannis SJ, Tyler JM, and Bonino F, eds, New York, NY: Wiley-Liss, 1993.

Maddrey WC, "Update in Hepatology," *Ann Intern Med*, 2001, 134(3):216-23.

Modahl LE and Lai MM, "Hepatitis Delta Virus: The Molecular Basis of Laboratory Diagnosis," *Crit Rev Clin Lab Sci*, 2000, 37(1):45-92.

Najm W, "Viral Hepatitis: How to Manage Type C and D Infections," *Geriatrics*, 1997, 52(5):28-30, 33-4, 37.

Ryder SD and Beckingham IJ, "ABC of Diseases of Liver, Pancreas, and Biliary System: Acute Hepatitis," *BMJ*, 2001, 322(7279):151-3.

Tepper MI and Gully PR, "Viral Hepatitis: Know Your D, E, F, and Gs," *CMAJ*, 1997, 156(12):1735-8.

Internet Web Sites

www.cdc.gov

Hepatitis E Serology

Related Information

Aspartate Aminotransferase, Serum *on page 112*
Bilirubin, Total, Serum *on page 118*
Hepatitis A Antibodies, IgM and IgG *on page 622*
Hepatitis B Core Antibody *on page 622*
Hepatitis B DNA Detection *on page 623*
Hepatitis B$_e$ Antibody *on page 624*
Hepatitis B$_e$ Antigen *on page 624*
Hepatitis B Surface Antibody *on page 625*
Hepatitis B Surface Antigen *on page 625*
Hepatitis C Virus RNA Detection and Quantitation *on page 626*
Hepatitis C Virus Serology *on page 627*
Hepatitis D Serology *on page 627*
Liver Disease: Laboratory Assessment, Overview *on page 216*

Synonyms Antibody to Hepatitis E; Antibody to HEV; HEV Antibody

Test Includes Detection of IgM and IgG antibody specific for hepatitis E

Abstract Hepatitis E causes an acute, self-limited hepatitis similar to hepatitis A. This virus is also transmitted fecal-orally, predominantly in the Indian subcontinent, Mexico, the Middle East, and Southeast and Central Asia. The usual vehicle is contaminated water. Food and personal contact have also been implicated. Although most hepatitis E occurs in sporadic cases, it has been known to cause epidemics in tropical and subtropical regions.

During early hepatitis E infection, IgM antibody can be detected beginning 1-4 weeks after exposure. IgG antibodies follow soon afterwards.

Specimen Blood, serum

Container Red top tube

Reference Interval Negative

Use Hepatitis E serology provides help in evaluation of the etiology of hepatitis in travelers who do not have hepatitis A, B, C, or other common causes of elevation of transaminases. The pathogenesis of hepatitis E is similar to that of hepatitis A. Its symptoms are commonly more severe.[1]

Methodology ELISA and Western blot technology may be used, with ELISA methods being a little better. A positive IgM titer remains present for as long as 3 months in 50% of patients. A rising titer, or a very high titer of IgG is also diagnostic. Apparently, some individuals do not develop antibody to hepatitis E. Reasons for this are unclear.

Hepatitis E reverse transcriptase PCR (RT-PCR) technology is available, but is of limited value because no chronic illness occurs. A positive test by HEV RT-PCR is not the same as infectivity, because the PCR is more sensitive at measuring HEV than is clinical infectivity.

Additional Information Seroprevalence in endemic regions varies between 3% and 27%, while in nonendemic regions seroprevalence has ranged between 1% and 28%. Acquisition of antibody seems to occur predominantly during the teenage years.

An exception to self-limited disease is appearance of fulminant disease during the third trimester of pregnancy. A high incidence of spontaneous abortion occurs in infected mothers.

Footnotes

1. Sacher RA, Peters SM, and Bryan JA, "Testing for Viral Hepatitis. A Practice Parameter," *Am J Clin Pathol*, 2000, 113(1):13-7.

References

Goncales HS, Pinho JR, Moreira RC, et al, "Hepatitis E Virus Immunoglobulin G Antibodies in Different Populations in Campinas, Brazil," *Clin Diag Lab Immunol*, 2000, 7(5):813-6.

Krawczynski K, Aggarwal R, and Kamili S, "Hepatitis E," *Infect Dis Clin North Am*, 2000, 14(3):669-80.

Kwo PY, Schlauder GG, and Carpenter HA, "Acute Hepatitis E by a New Isolate Acquired in the United States," *Mayo Clin Proc*, 1997, 72:1133-6.

Purcell RH and Emerson SU, "Hepatitis E Virus," *Principles and Practice of Infectious Diseases*, 5th ed, Mandell GL, Bennett JE, and Dolin R, eds, New York, NY: Churchill Livingstone, 2000.

Internet Web Sites

www.hepnet.com

www.cdc.gov

Hepatitis: Laboratory Assessment, Overview

Related Information

Synonyms Viral Hepatitis

Abstract Broadly defined, hepatitis is inflammation of liver parenchyma. A large number of infectious agents, metabolic diseases, drugs, toxic exposures, and immune derangements are included in the differential diagnosis. Some of these are addressed in the monographs, Liver Disease: Laboratory Assessment, Overview *on page 216* and in Liver Biopsy *on page 65*. The Key Word Index entry, Liver, with the entities and assays it includes, may be useful. Algorithms in the listings Bilirubin, Total, Serum *on page 118* and Aspartate Aminotransferase, Serum *on page 112* may be helpful. The listings Aspartate Aminotransferase, Serum *on page 112* and Alanine Aminotransferase, Serum *on page 87* include information relevant to the differential diagnosis of hepatitis. Aminotransferases (transaminases) may reach 100 times the upper poles of their reference ranges. With jaundice, total and direct bilirubin increase in proportion one to the other in hepatitis. The prothrombin time is close to normal in uncomplicated cases. Prothrombin time more than 4 seconds above the upper limit of reference range may indicate hepatic failure. Alkaline phosphatase is not usually greatly increased with hepatitis. Serum LDH more than slightly or moderately increased may signal an alternative diagnosis (eg, infectious mononucleosis or neoplastic disease). An abrupt onset of hepatitis suggests hepatitis A rather than hepatitis B or C. The onset of hepatitis C is classically insidious.

Algorithm 1. Serologic Testing in Suspected Acute Viral Hepatitis

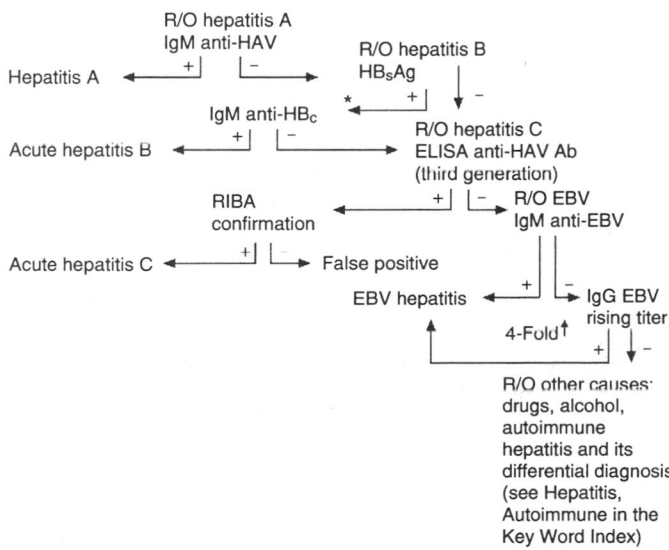

*Refer also to Algorithm 2. EBV = Epstein-Barr virus; ELISA = enzyme-linked immunosorbent assay; HAV = hepatitis A virus; anti-HB$_c$ = antibody to hepatitis B core; HB$_s$Ag = hepatitis B surface antigen; R/O = rule out; RIBA = recombinant immunoblot assay.

Adapted from Sacher RA, Peters SM, and Bryan JA, "Testing for Viral Hepatitis," *Am J Clin Pathol*, 2000, 113(1):13-7.

Chronic hepatitis by definition means increased serum transaminases (aminotransferases) for longer than 6 months, but fluctuation is seen. Fluctuation between abnormal and normal especially characterizes the course of hepatitis C. The differential diagnosis of possible chronic hepatitis includes hepatitis B, C, and D; alcoholism; autoimmune hepatitis; drug-induced chronic hepatitis; hemochromatosis; alpha$_1$ antitrypsin deficiency; and Wilson disease.[1] See the Key Word Index. A valuable review of the histopathologic characteristics of chronic hepatitis has recently been published.[2] Chemical injury and drugs are also included in the differential diagnosis.[3]

If HB$_s$Ag is positive in evaluation of chronic hepatitis B, testing for HB$_e$Ag is advocated to ascertain the presence of active viral replication. If appropriate viral hepatitis markers are not found, other evaluation is indicated, including work-up for autoimmune hepatitis. See the listing for Hepatitis (Autoimmune) in the Key Word Index, in which a list of assays is included.

Viral Hepatitis Summary

Hepatitis Type	Clinical Features	AST, ALT	Serologic Findings	
			Acute Disease	Immunity
A (RNA)	Acute self-limiting; fecal-oral transmission; no carrier state	Markedly elevated, 3+ to 4+	IgM anti-HAV	IgG anti-HAV
B (DNA)	Acute or chronic; often asymptomatic; 5% infected blood and body fluids	1+ to 3+ (acute); variable, chronic	IgM anti-HB$_c$; HB$_s$Ag; HB$_e$ Ag; HBV DNA	IgG anti-HB$_s$; anti-HB$_e$
C (RNA)	Usually chronic	Mild to moderate elevation, even in acute cases	Total anti-HCV; HCV RNA	Unknown
D (RNA)	Requires HBV coinfection; acute or chronic; rare in U.S.	Often markedly elevated	IgM anti-HDV; total anti-HDV; may require multiple assays	Unknown
E (RNA)	Epidemic similar to HAV; acute self-limiting; waterborne and enteric; transmission in India and Southeast Asia	Variable	Testing not widely available	Unknown
G (RNA)	Close homology to HCV; high prevalence (2% of U.S. donors); usually mild disease, if at all; disease spectrum uncertain	Variable	HGV-RNA and EIA (reference laboratory only)	Unknown
Non A-E, exclude EBV, CMV	Possibly acute or chronic	Variable	None	Unknown

CMV: cytomegalovirus; EBV: Epstein-Barr virus; EIA: enzyme immunoassay; HAV: hepatitis A virus; anti-HB$_c$: antibody to hepatitis B core; anti-HB$_e$: antibody to hepatitis B$_e$ antigen; HB$_e$Ag: hepatitis B$_e$ antigen; anti-HB$_s$: antibody to hepatitis B surface antigen; HB$_s$Ag: hepatitis B surface antigen; HBV: hepatitis B virus; HCV: hepatitis C virus; HDV: hepatitis D virus; HGV: hepatitis G virus

Adapted from Sacher RA, Peters SM, and Bryan JA, "Testing for Viral Hepatitis. A Practice Parameter," *Am J Clin Pathol*, 2000, 113(1):12-7.

Algorithm 2. Serologic Testing in Suspected Chronic Viral Hepatitis

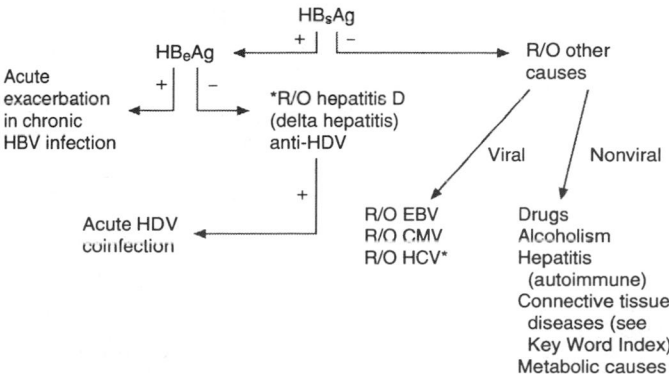

Rule out acute HAV, HBV, and HCV infection; see Algorithm 1.
*See text. CMV = cytomegalovirus; EBV = Epstein-Barr virus; HAV = hepatitis A virus; HB$_s$Ag = hepatitis B surface antigen; HBV = hepatitis B virus; HB$_e$Ag = hepatitis B$_e$ antigen; HCV = hepatitis C virus; HDV = hepatitis D virus; R/O = rule out.

Adapted from Sacher RA, Peters SM, and Bryan JA, "Testing for Viral Hepatitis," *Am J Clin Pathol*, 2000, 113(1):13-7.

(Continued)

Herpes Simplex Antibody (Continued)

Footnotes

1. Sacher RA, Peters SM, Bryan JA, "Testing for Viral Hepatitis. A Practice Parameter," *Am J Clin Pathol*, 2000, 113(1):12-7.
2. Ishak KG, "Pathologic Features of Chronic Hepatitis. A Review and Update," *Am J Clin Pathol*, 2000, 113(1):40-55.
3. Zimmerman HJ, "Hepatotoxicity: The Adverse Effects of Drugs and Other Chemicals on the Liver," 2nd ed, Baltimore, MD: Lippincott, Williams & Wilkins, 1999.

References

Centers for Disease Control and Prevention, "Revision of Acute Hepatitis Panel," *MMWR Morb Mortal Wkly Rep*, 2000, 49:424.

OiConnor JA, "Acute and Chronic Viral Hepatitis," *Adolesc Med*, 2000, 11(2):279-92.

Ryder SD and Beckingham IJ, "ABC of Diseases of Liver, Pancreas, and Biliary System: Acute Hepatitis," *BMJ*, 2001, 322(7279):151-3.

Internet Web Sites

www.ama-assn.org/ama/pub/category/3113.html

♦ **Hepatitis RT-PCR** *see* Hepatitis C Virus RNA Detection and Quantitation *on page 626*

♦ **Hepatitis Vaccine** *see* Hepatitis B Surface Antibody *on page 625*

♦ **Herpes 1 and 2** *see* Herpes Simplex Antibody *on page 630*

Herpes Simplex Antibody

Related Information

Herpes Simplex Virus Antigen Detection *on page 630*
Herpes Simplex Virus Culture *on page 631*
Herpes Simplex Virus DNA Detection *on page 632*
Herpesvirus Cytology *on page 383*
Polymerase Chain Reaction *on page 713*
TORCH *on page 683*
Viral Culture *on page 689*

Synonyms Herpes 1 and 2; Herpesvirus hominis 1 and 2; HSV Antibodies

Test Includes IgG and IgM antibodies

Specimen Serum, cerebrospinal fluid

Container Red top tube, sterile CSF tube

Sampling Time Most useful after the fourth day of illness in herpes simplex virus encephalitis[1] (HSV antibodies are not useful in diagnosing herpes simplex virus encephalitis).

Reference Interval Interpretation depends on whether episode is initial or reinfection. Generally, IgG: <1:5; IgM: <1:10.

Critical Values Increased IgM antibodies or a fourfold rise in titer may indicate recent infection.

Use Determine a patient's previous infection with herpes simplex virus 1 or 2. Neonatal herpes is most often caused by type 2 HSV. Clinical use is for assessing pregnant women for possible neonatal problems with TORCH antibodies, and in identification of seropositive organ transplant recipients. Identification of seronegative pregnant women, near term, who have seropositive partners, has been addressed. Infants who are born to seronegative mothers who acquire primary genital HSV type 2 infection are at more risk than are infants born to seropositive mothers with recurrent genital herpesvirus infection. Primary cases late in gestation are regarded as especially dangerous.[2]

Limitations Extensive background antibody in the population, and cross reaction of HSV-1 and HSV-2 responses have made this test useful mostly in epidemiology. False negatives occur. HSV PCR on cerebrospinal fluid is preferred for diagnosis of herpes simplex encephalitis.[3]

Methodology Indirect fluorescent antibody (IFA), hemagglutination, complement fixation (CF), enzyme immunoassay (EIA), Western blot assay, Western blot or solid-phase enzyme-linked immunosorbent assay (ELISA) for detecting type-specific epitopes (gG or gC). Recent studies suggest peptide 55 may be superior to gG or gC in giving fewer false positives.

Recently, Martins et al have reported comparisons of four enzyme immunoassays for determination of type-specific antibodies to HSV. Specificity without cross reactivity was found in one of the assays.[2]

Additional Information A primary HSV-1 or HSV-2 infection will produce a classical rising antibody titer. Use of antiviral drugs may blunt the antibody response. However, because exposure to herpesvirus is almost universal, the presence of antibodies to HSV is usually not helpful. Collecting paired sera to delineate rising titers generally adds nothing to clinical management, and thus, **herpes serology cannot usually be recommended in routine clinical cases**. Herpes serology has not so far been useful in determining whether Caesarean delivery should be undertaken in pregnant patients with possible herpetic lesions. Nor is herpes serology helpful in the diagnosis of a very sick infant with possible congenital herpes. Virus culture and PCR are preferred, but therapy should not be withheld even for the results of these tests. Because of the fulminant course, even IgM antibody is not present in time to contribute to care. See Herpes Simplex Virus DNA Detection *on page 632*.

Use of type-specific antibody to herpes simplex virus directed towards the gG or gC epitopes can reliably differentiate between HSV-1 and HSV-2. This test remains technically difficult, so use should be targeted. A positive HSV culture with a negative antibody study indicates a primary infection. Pregnant women who sustain a first episode of genital herpes as shown by antibodies are at high risk for vertical transmission. Absence of antibodies and persistently culture-negative genital ulcers excludes HSV as the cause.[4]

Footnotes

1. Uren EC, Johnson PD, Montanaro J, et al, "Herpes Simplex Virus Encephalitis in Pediatrics: Diagnosis by Detection of Antibodies and DNA in Cerebrospinal Fluid," *Pediatr Infect Dis J*, 1993, 12(12):1001-6.
2. Martins TB, Woolstenhulme RD, Jaskowski TD, et al, "Comparison of Four Enzyme Immunoassays With a Western Blot Assay for the Determination of Type-Specific Antibodies to Herpes Simplex Virus," *Am J Clin Pathol*, 2001, 115(2):272-7.
3. Lakman FD, Whitley RJ, and the NIAIS, CA5G, "Diagnosis of Herpes Simplex Encephalitis: Application of Polymerase Chain Reaction to Cerebrospinal Fluid From Brain-Biopsied Patients and Correlation With Disease," *J Infect Dis*, 1995, 171:857-63.
4. Cowan FM, "Testing for Type-Specific Antibody to Herpes Simplex Virus - Implications for Clinical Practice," *J Antimicrob Chemother*, 2000, 45(Topic T3):9-13.

References

Arvin AM and Prober CG, "Herpes Simplex Virus," *Manual of Clinical Microbiology*, 7th ed, Murray PR, Baron EJ, Pfaller MA, et al, eds, Washington, DC: ASM Press, American Society for Microbiology, 1999, 878-87.

Ashley R and Wald A, "Genital Herpes: Review of the Epidemic and Potential Use of Type-Specific Serology," *Clin Microbiol Rev*, 1999, 12(1):1-8.

Benedetti JK, Zeh J, and Corey L, "Clinical Reactivation of Genital Herpes Simplex Virus Infection Decreases in Frequency Over Time," *Ann Intern Med*, 1999, 131(1):14-20.

Brown ZA, Selke S, Zeh J, et al, "The Acquisition of Herpes Simplex Virus During Pregnancy," *N Engl J Med*, 1997, 337(8):509-15.

Corey L and Handsfield HH, "Genital Herpes and Public Health. Addressing a Global Problem," *JAMA*, 2000, 283(6):791-4.

Frenkel LM, Garratty EM, Shen JP, et al, "Clinical Reactivation of Herpes Simplex Virus Type 2 Infection in Seropositive Pregnant Women With No History of Genital Herpes," *Ann Intern Med*, 1993, 118(6):414-8.

Ito Y, Ando Y, Kimura H, et al, "Polymerase Chain Reaction-Proved Herpes Simplex Encephalitis in Children," *Ped Infect Dis J*, 1998, 17:29-32.

Langenberg AG, Corey L, Ashley RL, et al, "A Prospective Study of New Infections With Herpes Simplex Virus Type 1 and Type 2. Chiron HSV Vaccine Study Group," *N Engl J Med*, 1999, 341(19):1432-8.

Oladepo DK, Klapper PE, and Marsden HS, "Peptide Based Enzyme-Linked Immunoassays for Detection of Anti-HSV-2 IgG in Human Sera," *J Virol Methods*, 2000, 87(1-2):63-70.

Wald A, Zeh J, Selke S, et al, "Virologic Characteristics of Subclinical and Symptomatic Genital Herpes Infections," *N Engl J Med*, 1995, 333(12):770-5.

Internet Web Sites

www.cdc.gov/nchstp/dstd/genital_herpes_facts.htm

Herpes Simplex Virus Antigen Detection

Related Information

Bacterial Culture, Conjunctiva *on page 570*
Bacterial Culture, Genital Specimen *on page 571*
Herpes Simplex Antibody *on page 630*
Herpes Simplex Virus Culture *on page 631*
Herpes Simplex Virus DNA Detection *on page 632*
Herpesvirus Cytology *on page 383*
Ocular Cytology *on page 385*
Oral Cavity Cytology *on page 386*
Polymerase Chain Reaction *on page 713*
Skin Biopsy *on page 71*
Urinary Tract Cytology *on page 389*
Viral Culture *on page 689*
Viral Culture, Dermatological Symptoms *on page 693*
Viral Culture, Urogenital *on page 696*
Virus, Direct Detection by Fluorescent Antibody *on page 696*

Synonyms Herpes Simplex Virus by DFA; Herpes Simplex Virus, Direct Immunofluorescence; HSV Antigen Detection, Direct

Applies to Herpes Simplex Virus Antigen Detection by PCR

Test Includes Direct (nonculture) detection of HSV-infected cells in smears of specimens

Specimen Basal cells of a freshly unroofed lesion rolled onto a clean microscope slide; tissue biopsy of brain; cornea; cerebrospinal fluid

Sampling Time Preferably within 3 days of lesion eruption. Specimens taken after 5 days are less likely to contain viral particles.

Collection Cells from the bottom of an ulcer or vesicle should be scraped with a swab, scalpel, or curette. Swabs should be **rolled** (**not** smeared) across a small area of the slide several times, and cells scraped with a scalpel should be gently dabbed onto the slide. The best specimen is a collection of the cells at the base of an intact vesicle. Cells from a diseased cornea can also be used. **The smear should be air dried at room temperature**. The success of direct detection procedures depends on the careful preparation of cell smears. If an EIA method is used, collect specimens as described for HSV viral culture.

Storage Instructions Do not store the specimen. Send it to the laboratory immediately.

Turnaround Time Hours

Special Instructions Operative biopsy specimens and spinal fluid specimens for fluorescent antibody (FA) testing should be **processed immediately**. The laboratory should be **notified in advance** when either of these specimen types will be sent for FA.

Reference Interval No herpes simplex virus-infected cells detected

Critical Values Detection of HSV antigen in CSF is a critical value.

Use Rapid detection of herpes simplex virus

Limitations The efficiency of detection of HSV material depends in great part on the collection of a sufficiently large number of intact infected cells from the lesion. Specimen smears that are too thick can retain or trap the fluorescent reagent and make the test difficult to interpret. If at all possible, it is important to obtain cells from the base of an intact vesicle. Fluorescent antibody staining of cells from an early lesion is 80% sensitive in acute vesicles, but only 60% to 75% sensitive in resolving lesions. The presence of infected cells decreases as the lesion heals, and crusted lesions may have little or no herpes antigenic material remaining. Antigen detection methods have excellent specificity ~98%, thus a high positive predictive value, but are less sensitive than culture.

Methodology Direct fluorescent antibody (DFA) or enzyme immunoassay (EIA)

Additional Information In general, this test is only ~70% as sensitive as cell culture. In critical situations, clinicians should consider using both methods. Air-dried preparations on slides can also be stained with Giemsa, Pap, Wright, or Diff-Quik™ stains (Tzanck), however, these stains are not always specific for HSV. See Herpesvirus Cytology *on page 383.* Fixed preparations (usually 95% ethanol) can also be stained with the Papanicolaou or immunoperoxidase methods. Smears fixed with hairspray and subsequently stained with the Papanicolaou stain usually are excellent preparations. The detection of HSV DNA by PCR in CSF and lesion fluid is becoming available. It is more sensitive than detection of specific antibody for early diagnosis of herpes simplex encephalitis (97% to 99% sensitivity) and provides 95% to 100% specificity.[1]

Polymerase chain reaction was more sensitive than immunocytochemical techniques for detection of herpes simplex virus in formalin-fixed, paraffin-embedded tissue sections from cases of diffuse interstitial pneumonia.[2]

Footnotes
1. ARUP Laboratories, "Herpes Simplex Virus," April 1999.
2. Oda Y, Katsuda S, Okada Y, et al, "Detection of Human Cytomegalovirus, Epstein-Barr Virus, and Herpes Simplex Virus in Diffuse Interstitial Pneumonia by Polymerase Chain Reaction and Immunohistochemistry," *Am J Clin Pathol*, 1994, 102(4):495-502.

References
Arvin AM and Prober CG, "Herpes Simplex Virus," *Manual of Clinical Microbiology*, 7th ed, Murray PR, Baron EJ, Pfaller MA, et al, eds, Washington, DC: AMS Press, American Society of Microbiology, 1999, 878-87.
Corey L and Handsfield HH, "Genital Herpes and Public Health. Addressing a Global Problem," *JAMA*, 2000, 283(6):791-4.

Internet Web Sites
www.cdc.gov/nchstp/dstd/genital_herpes_facts.htm

♦ **Herpes Simplex Virus Antigen Detection by PCR** *see* Herpes Simplex Virus Antigen Detection *on page 630*

♦ **Herpes Simplex Virus by DFA** *see* Herpes Simplex Virus Antigen Detection *on page 630*

Herpes Simplex Virus Culture

Related Information
Bacterial Culture, Conjunctiva *on page 570*
Bacterial Culture, Genital Specimen *on page 571*
Herpes Simplex Antibody *on page 630*
Herpes Simplex Virus Antigen Detection *on page 630*
Herpes Simplex Virus DNA Detection *on page 632*
Herpesvirus Cytology *on page 383*
Neisseria gonorrhoeae Culture and Smear *on page 662*
Ocular Cytology *on page 385*
Oral Cavity Cytology *on page 386*
Polymerase Chain Reaction *on page 713*
Viral Culture *on page 689*
Viral Culture, Central Nervous System Symptoms *on page 692*
Viral Culture, Dermatological Symptoms *on page 693*
Viral Culture, Eye or Ocular Symptoms *on page 693*
Viral Culture, Urogenital *on page 696*
Virus, Direct Detection by Fluorescent Antibody *on page 696*

Synonyms HSV-1 and HSV-2 Culture; HSV Culture

Applies to Viral Culture, Eye; Viral Culture, Genital; Viral Culture, Skin

Test Includes Culture for HSV only; HSV also is detected in a routine viral culture; rapid method includes specific staining with a fluorescent monoclonal antibody

Abstract Herpes simplex viruses cause a wide variety of lesions. Labial or genital herpes are usually less severe. More severe forms of infection include herpetic dendritic eye ulcers, neonatal herpes, or encephalitis, entities which lead to serious sequelae and are often fatal. Herpes infections may be severe in subjects who are immunocompromised. Culture is the method of choice for many clinical presentations, such as vesicles. Classic primary HSV-1 infection includes herpetic gingivostomatitis, which may be accompanied by fever and local lymphadenopathy. HSV-1 also causes conjunctivitis, keratitis, and sporadic encephalitis.

About 85% of instances of primary genital HSV infections are caused by HSV-2, and 99% of recurrent disease is HSV-2. Neonatal herpes, a serious complication of HSV infection, is usually caused by exposure during vaginal delivery. When the mother has a primary infection at delivery, the attack rate is greater than half. Untreated neonates with disseminated infection suffer mortality rates >70%.[1] Most HSV-2 seropositive individuals intermittently shed virus from mucosal surfaces, and represent reservoirs for spread to uninfected sex partners.[2]

Specimen Vesicle fluid, swab of base of lesion, tissue biopsy, nasopharyngeal swab, tonsillar swab, oropharyngeal swab, conjunctival swab, cervical swab, urine, cerebrospinal fluid

Container Cold viral transport medium for swabs

Collection All specimens should be kept cold and moist. Specimens should be collected in the acute stage of the disease, preferably within 3 days and no longer than 7 days after the onset of illness. Spinal fluid specimens should be submitted in the usual sterile tube; no special transport medium is necessary. All other specimens should be collected on a sterile swab as described and the swab should be placed into cold viral transport medium immediately after collection.

Endocervical: Swab cervix with a rolling/scraping motion to assure obtaining epithelial cells.

Vesicular lesion: Wash vesicles with sterile saline. Carefully open several vesicles and soak up vesicular fluid with swab. If vesicles are absent, vigorously swab base of lesion (specimen should be collected during first 3 days of eruption. Specimens collected later in the course of disease rarely yield virus).

Conjunctival: Using a moistened swab, firmly rub conjunctiva using sufficient force to obtain epithelial cells.

Throat, respiratory, oral: Rotate swab in both tonsillar crypts and against posterior oropharynx.

Storage Instructions Specimens should be delivered to the laboratory and handed to a technologist within 30 minutes of collection. Outpatient specimens: If transport is to be delayed more than 30 minutes after collection, specimen **must** be refrigerated (held at 4°C to 8°C) until it can be transported to the laboratory. If inoculation onto cell cultures is not possible within 48 hours, specimens should be frozen at -70°C. Do not freeze at -20°C.

Turnaround Time Routine culture: 1-5 days; rapid culture: 16 hours to 2 days

Special Instructions Special viral transport medium must be obtained from the laboratory prior to collection of specimen.

Reference Interval No virus isolated

Critical Values Detection of HSV in CSF is a critical value.

Use Aid in the diagnosis of disease caused by HSV. These include gingivostomatitis, herpes labialis, genital herpes, skin lesions, keratoconjunctivitis, neonatal herpes, aseptic meningitis, and encephalitis. Genital transmission of HSV infection to sexual partners and neonates involves subclinical shedding of HSV by women with genital herpes. Such shedding is detectable by viral culture.[3] Culture can provide evidence of acyclovir resistance,[4] and detect potential for transmission of HSV to neonates.[5]

Limitations Standard methods suffer 30% false negatives for identification of those neonates who subsequently develop neonatal herpes.[5] Sensitivity of PCR assay for HSV detection is greater than that of culture methods.[6]

Methodology Inoculation of specimen into cell cultures, incubation of cultures, observation for characteristic cytopathic effect (CPE), and identification of HSV by fluorescein-labeled monoclonal antibodies specific for type 1 or 2. In the shell vial isolation technique, the specimen is centrifuged on a tissue culture cell layer, incubated for 12-18 hours, and stained with direct immunofluorescent staining for HSV-1 and HSV-2; characteristic fluorescent foci indicate the presence of virus.

Additional Information HSV-1 can be cultured from CSF in herpes meningitis but only rarely can be cultured from the CSF in encephalitis. The HSV PCR is usually positive in encephalitis. HSV-2 may be isolated from CSF in neonatal meningitis.

Of other diagnostic approaches for herpes simplex virus encephalitis, PCR is more sensitive for early diagnosis than detection of CSF antibody.[7] Virus can also be isolated from urine in patients with primary genital HSV infections concurrent with cystitis. HSV shedding, as determined by HSV culture, occurs on 3% of days, even in immunocompetent persons. For compromised hosts with HIV, shedding occurs even more often. Transmission may occur at such times when infected persons are unaware of their status.[8]

Serology for detection of herpes simplex virus is available (*vide supra*), but the results usually are of value only in the diagnosis of primary HSV infections. Unless special tests are used, there is much cross reaction between the antibodies to HSV-1 and HSV-2.

Immunocompromised patients can develop disseminated HSV infections. These infections are characterized by a persistent, severe mucocutaneous infection involving the mouth, face, genital, or perianal areas. Sometimes such infections spread to organs such as the liver, lungs, adrenal glands, and bone marrow. Genital herpes infection has been suggested to be a possible risk factor for HIV-1 transmission.[9]
(Continued)

Herpes Simplex Virus Culture *(Continued)*

Culture is useful for diagnosis of unusual lesions, such as herpetic glossitis in immunocompromised patients. The buccal mucosa, floor of the mouth, and soft palate may be infected as well.[10] Otherwise, herpes simplex lesions in the mouth are not common in immunocompetent persons, except for primary herpetic gingivostomatitis.

Footnotes

1. Arvin AM and Prober CG, "Herpes Simplex Virus," *Manual of Clinical Microbiology*, 7th ed, Murray PR, Baron EJ, Pfaller MA, et al, eds, Washington, DC: AMS Press, American Society of Microbiology, 1999, 878-87.
2. Corey L and Handsfield HH, "Genital Herpes and Public Health. Addressing a Global Problem," *JAMA*, 2000, 283(6):791-4.
3. Wald A, Zeh J, Selke S, et al, "Virologic Characteristics of Subclinical and Symptomatic Genital Herpes Infections," *N Engl J Med*, 1995, 333(12):770-5.
4. Kost RG, Hill EL, Tigges M, et al, "Brief Report: Recurrent Acyclovir-Resistant Genital Herpes in an Immunocompetent Patient," *N Engl J Med*, 1993, 329(24):1777-82.
5. Cone RW, Hobson AC, Brown Z, et al, "Frequent Detection of Genital Herpes Simplex Virus DNA by Polymerase Chain Reaction Among Pregnant Women," *JAMA*, 1994, 272(10):792-6.
6. Wald A, Zeh J, Selke S, et al, "Reactivation of Genital Herpes Simplex Virus Type 2 Infection in Asymptomatic Seropositive Persons," *N Engl J Med*, 2000, 342(12):844-50.
7. "Herpes Simplex Virus Encephalitis in Pediatrics: Diagnosis by Detection of Antibodies and DNA in Cerebrospinal Fluid," *JAMA*, 1993, 12(12):1001-6.
8. Koelle DM and Wald A, "Herpes Simplex Virus: The Importance of Asymptomatic Shedding," *J Antimicrob Chemother*, 2000, 45(T3):1-8.
9. Hook EW 3d, Cannon RO, Nahmias AJ, et al, "Herpes Simplex Virus Infection as a Risk Factor for Human Immunodeficiency Virus Infection in Heterosexuals," *J Infect Dis*, 1992, 165(2):251-5.
10. Grossman ME, Stevens AW, and Cohen PR, "Brief Report: Herpetic Geometric Glossitis," *N Engl J Med*, 1993, 329(25):1859-60.

References

Banks TA and Rouse BT, "Current Approaches and Future Directions in the Treatment of Herpesvirus Infections," *Infect Med*, 1994, 11(2):148-57.

Benedetti JK, Zeh J, and Corey L, "Clinical Reactivation of Genital Herpes Simplex Virus Infection Decreases in Frequency Over Time," *Ann Intern Med*, 1999, 131(1):14-20.

Corey L and Handsfield HH, "Genital Herpes and Public Health. Addressing a Global Problem," *JAMA*, 2000, 283(6):791-4.

Langenberg AG, Corey L, Ashley RL, et al, "A Prospective Study of New Infections With Herpes Simplex Virus Type 1 and Type 2. Chiron HSV Vaccine Study Group," *N Engl J Med*, 1999, 341(19):1432-8.

Internet Web Sites

www.cdc.gov/nchstp/dstd/genital_herpes_facts.htm

♦ **Herpes Simplex Virus, Direct Immunofluorescence** *see* Herpes Simplex Virus Antigen Detection *on page 630*

Herpes Simplex Virus DNA Detection

Related Information

Herpes Simplex Antibody *on page 630*
Herpes Simplex Virus Antigen Detection *on page 630*
Herpes Simplex Virus Culture *on page 631*
Herpesvirus Cytology *on page 383*
Polymerase Chain Reaction *on page 713*
Viral Culture *on page 689*

Synonyms HSV DNA Detection; Molecular Assay for HSV Detection

Test Includes Direct detection of herpes simplex virus (HSV) nucleic acid in cells, blood, or CSF. HSV may also be detected in cytologic specimens or tissue samples obtained by biopsy.

Abstract Herpes simplex virus (HSV) types 1 and 2 are distinct from other members of the Herpesviridae family, VZV, CMV, EBV, HHV-6, and HHV-8. HSV infects epithelial cells and is responsible for causing vesicular lesions, followed by small ulcers and crusts. It may involve the mouth, intestinal tract, urogenital tract, or central nervous system. HSV establishes a latent infection of nerve dorsal root ganglion cells from which it reactivates, travels retrograde through axons, and reinfects epithelial cells. Transmission is through direct contact and the virus may be spread to the newborn via the birth canal.[1,2] HSV is a common sexually transmitted disease. Infection may cause a wide variety of clinical diseases including encephalitis, for which timely diagnosis and treatment is critical. Differentiation from other causes of CNS disease is important for appropriate therapy with intravenous acyclovir. Detection of HSV may be accomplished by a variety of molecular techniques including amplification, such as by PCR, or through *in situ* hybridization. HSV may be detected by culture in only 40% to 70% of genital lesions and in only 25% to 40% of neonates with encephalitis. Detection of HSV by PCR has been shown to have greater sensitivity than routine culture methods.[1] As with culture techniques, it is possible to distinguish HSV-1 from HSV-2. Molecular assays such as *in situ* hybridization have been used to establish the presence of latent infection, when the virus is not replicating.

Culture is the method of choice for many acute clinical presentations.

Specimen Bronchial alveolar lavage fluid, cerebrospinal fluid, vesicle fluid, blood or serum, and various tissues including lung and brain, depending on the site involved

Container Sterile containers are acceptable; lavender top (EDTA) tube for blood

Storage Instructions While freezing may reduce the viability of HSV and its isolation by culture techniques, freezing does not impair detection by amplification procedures. Any of the above fluid samples should be rapidly transported to the laboratory. However, if transportation is expected to exceed 2 hours, the sample should be refrigerated and if transportation exceeds 8 hours, a specimen should be frozen. All tissue samples should be frozen as soon as possible after the biopsy procedure.

Causes for Rejection Blood collected in heparinized tubes results in inhibition of amplification

Turnaround Time 1-3 days

Reference Interval Most laboratories provide an interpretative report.

Critical Values Detection of HSV DNA in CSF

Use Useful for rapidly identifying active infection with HSV. Untreated, herpes encephalitis and neonatal herpes are fatal, or cause severe morbidity in a majority of patients. Neurologic sequelae are common. PCR is considered the most reliable means of precision of a laboratory diagnosis of CNS HSV,[3] but *vide infra*. Most HSV encephalitis is caused by HSV type 1. HSV meningitis is more frequent than is HSV encephalitis, and usually is caused by type 2. Recurrent HSV meningitis may be responsible for most instances of recurrent lymphocytic meningitis.[3]

Limitations A negative result does not rule out the presence of HSV in all tissues of the body or even in the sample submitted for analysis, since factors such as degradation of the nucleic acid or interference with amplification by substances that may be present.[4] HSV detection by PCR has shown a relatively low specificity when compared with viral culture. False-positive results are possible.

Methodology Techniques in common use are PCR and *in situ* hybridization. The molecular amplification assay utilizes specific primers which may be to a variety of viral gene sequences including polymerase, capsid antigen, or nonstructural genes such as VP-16. For the PCR assay, DNA is extracted from fluids or tissues using a standard lysis buffer followed by phenol-chloroform extraction and amplification. Alternatively, protocols exist for the direct amplification of HSV DNA following the lysis of cells by boiling or detergent without phenol extraction. For *in situ* hybridization, sections of tissue are cut and placed on glass slides, followed by incubation with a labeled probe. The target of *in situ* hybridization may be either DNA or RNA, the latter allowing for the study of the state of activity of the virus.

Additional Information More than 80% of adults have been exposed to HSV, as evidenced by the presence of serum antibodies. Although in most nonimmunosuppressed individuals infection by HSV is self-limited, one important exception is found in individuals who develop encephalitis (HSE). Thirty-three percent of adults who develop herpes encephalitis have primary infection. Of those who have herpes antibodies at the onset of encephalitis, >90% have not had recurrent labial herpes.[1] Neonates who are infected by passage through the birth canal may have skin, eye, and mucous membrane involvement leading to dissemination and encephalitis. Amplification assays for detection of HSV have been developed because of the increased sensitivity that these assays provide. The standard noninvasive approach (without brain biopsy) to diagnosis of HSE shows that serum antibodies, usually positive, are not helpful except as an adjunct to show individuals who have primary herpes infection with negative serum antibodies. Intrathecal synthesis of HSV antibodies, as compared to serum antibody titers, is of limited usefulness. HSV cultures are usually negative in HSE, but may be positive in HSV meningitis or meningoencephalitis of the immunosuppressed hosts. HSV PCR, which has shown a higher sensitivity than culture, is the noninvasive diagnostic technique of choice. Brain biopsy with culture, and histopathology are useful in diagnosis of HSE, and help to exclude clinical syndromes that mimic HSE. Studies have confirmed the ability of PCR to detect HSV DNA when culture results are negative.[2]

Immunocompromised patients may suffer severe reactivation of HSV.

Footnotes

1. Skoldenberg B, "Herpes Simplex Encephalitis," *Scand J Infect Dis*, 1996, 100:8-13.
2. Cone RW, Hobson AC, Palmer J, et al, "Extended Duration of Herpes Simplex Virus DNA in Genital Lesions Detected by the Polymerase Chain Reaction," *J Infect Dis*, 1991, 164(4):757-60.
3. Storch GA, "Identifying HSV Infections of the CNS," *Lab Med*, 2000, 31(6):316-7.
4. Arvin AM and Prober CG, "Herpes Simplex Virus," *Manual of Clinical Microbiology*, 7th ed, Murray PR, Baron EJ, Pfaller MA, et al, eds, Washington, DC: ASM Press, American Society for Microbiology, 1999, 878-87.

References

Benedetti JK, Zeh J, and Corey L, "Clinical Reactivation of Genital Herpes Simplex Virus Infection Decreases in Frequency Over Time," *Ann Intern Med*, 1999, 131(1):14-20.

Corey L and Handsfield HH, "Genital Herpes and Public Health: Addressing a Global Problem," *JAMA*, 2000, 283(6):791-4.

Fleming DT, McQuillan GM, Johnson RE, et al, "Herpes Simplex Virus Type 2 in the United States," *N Engl J Med*, 1997, 337(16):1105-11.

Langenberg AG, Corey L, Ashley RL, et al, "A Prospective Study of New Infections With Herpes Simplex Virus Type 1 and Type 2, Chiron HSV Vaccine Study Group," *N Engl J Med*, 1999, 341(19):1432-8.

Internet Web Sites

www.cdc.gov/nchstp/dstd/genital_herpes_facts.htm

Herpesvirus 6 Culture

Related Information

Herpesvirus 6 DNA Detection *on page 633*
Herpesvirus 6, IgG and IgM Antibodies, Quantitative *on page 633*
Viral Culture, Blood *on page 691*

Synonyms HHV-6 Culture; Human Herpesvirus 6 Culture

Test Includes Culture and identification of HHV-6 isolates

Abstract Recognized only in 1986, HHV-6 infection in the first 2 years of life results in acute febrile illness, including roseola infantum. Infection in adults occurs primarily in immunocompromised individuals, transplant patients, or those with HIV infection. A T-cell lymphotropic virus, it includes HHV-6A and HHV-6B.

Specimen Blood

Container Green top (heparin) tube or lavender top (EDTA) tube

Storage Instructions Transport to laboratory at room temperature. Do not freeze.

Turnaround Time Positive cultures can be detected after 7-10 days; negative cultures are reported after 21 days of culture

Use Confirm the diagnosis of active HHV-6 infection

Limitations Culture for HHV-6 is not routinely done, except in the setting of an illness suspected to be due to HHV-6. Most people encounter HHV-6 during the first 2 years of life and have persisting antibody. However, a fourfold increase in antibody suggests recent disease. Culture for HHV-6 is tedious and requires at least 3 weeks of culture. A rapid shell vial method for culture of HHV-6 allows detection of the virus in 1-3 days, with a sensitivity of 86% and specificity of 100%.

Methodology Peripheral blood mononuclear cells are cultivated with stimulated cord blood lymphocytes or stimulated peripheral blood lymphocytes. In positive cultures, characteristic cytopathic effect can be observed after 7-10 days of culture.

Additional Information HHV-6 occurs in two forms: HHV-6A and HHV-6B. These two variants differ in the cells they infect: 6A infects either blood lymphocytes or transformed T cells, while 6B infects only peripheral blood lymphocytes. PCR can differentiate A from B. Generally, there is much antigenic cross reaction, but specific monoclonal antibodies can be made. HHV-6A is more virulent in cell culture. Most importantly, HHV-6A has not been linked definitively to disease while HHV-6B has. Usually, any disease caused by HHV-6B is referred to as due merely to HHV-6.

HHV-6 causes a common childhood disease called roseola infantum (exanthem subitum). Roseola infantum is mild, with fever for several days followed by appearance of a rash. On occasion, complications such as seizures and/or encephalitis can occur.

Other illness include febrile seizures in infants, encephalitis and other neurologic disorders, heterophil-negative infectious mononucleosis syndrome, and hepatitis that may even be fulminant at times.

References

Cone RW, Hackman RC, Huang ML, et al, "Human Herpesvirus 6 in Lung Tissue From Patients With Pneumonitis After Bone Marrow Transplantation," *N Engl J Med*, 1993, 329(3):156-61.

Dockrell DH, Smith TF, and Paya CV, "Human Herpesvirus 6," *Mayo Clin Proc*, 1999, 74:163-70.

Penchansky L and Jordan JA, "Transient Erythroblastopenia of Childhood Associated With Human Herpesvirus Type 6, Variant B," *Am J Clin Pathol*, 1997, 108(2):127-32.

Pruksananonda P, Hall CB, Insel RA, et al, "Primary Human Herpesvirus 6 Infection In Young Children," *N Engl J Med*, 1992, 326(22):1445-50.

Internet Web Sites

www.emedicine.com

Herpesvirus 6 DNA Detection

Related Information

Herpesvirus 6 Culture *on page 633*
Herpesvirus 6, IgG and IgM Antibodies, Quantitative *on page 633*
Polymerase Chain Reaction *on page 713*

Synonyms HHV-6 DNA Detection; HHV-6 PCR; Human Herpesvirus 6 DNA Detection

Test Includes Direct detection of human herpesvirus type 6 nucleic acid in peripheral blood mononuclear cells or CSF. HHV-6 may also be detected in tissue samples obtained by biopsy or in bronchial lavage fluids.

Abstract Human herpesvirus 6 (HHV-6) is antigenically and genetically distinct from other members of the Herpesviridae family, including HSV-1 and HSV-2, VZV, CMV, and EBV, but it is related genetically to CMV. Although HHV-6A and HHV-6B have been identified, only the 6B form of HHV-6 has been confirmed as a cause of disease. It may cause roseola infantum (exanthem subitum), an illness with high fever for 3-5 days. Subsequently, a rash abruptly appears. It also causes a primary febrile infection without rash. Other associations include febrile convulsions in infants, encephalitis, a heterophil-negative mononucleosis syndrome indistinguishable from that caused by HHV-7, or hepatitis. It is also associated with several other conditions in immunosuppressed individuals, including interstitial pneumonitis, encephalitis, and hepatitis.[1] The most common means for directly detecting HHV-6 is through polymerase chain reaction, although shell viral cultures may be used.

Specimen Bronchoalveolar lavage fluid, cerebrospinal fluid, lymphocytes and monocytes, and various tissues including liver and lung

Container Sterile containers are acceptable; lavender top (EDTA) tube for blood sample

Storage Instructions Freezing does not impair detection by amplification procedures. Samples should be rapidly transported to the laboratory. If transportation is expected to exceed 2 hours, the sample should be refrigerated, and if transportation exceeds 8 hours, a specimen should be frozen. All tissue samples should be frozen as soon as possible following biopsy.

Causes for Rejection Collection of blood in heparinized tubes results in inhibition of amplification

Turnaround Time 1-3 days

Special Instructions Specimens should **not** be obtained utilizing heparin as an anticoagulant.

Reference Interval Most laboratories provide an interpretative report. It should be recognized that detection of HHV-6 in a tissue may reflect latently infected cells rather than active infection.

Critical Values Detection of HHV-6 DNA in CSF is a critical value.

Use Rapid identification of a causative agent for clinical symptoms and signs, including fever, encephalitis, an infectious mononucleosis-like syndrome or hepatitis, which may indicate need for appropriate therapy.

Limitations A negative result does not rule out the presence of HHV-6 in all tissues of the body, or even in the sample submitted for analysis. Limitations include factors such as degradation of nucleic acid or interference with amplification by substances which may be present.

Similarly, a positive result supports, but does not completely prove, that disease is caused by HHV-6 because it is so common and persistent. By 1 year of age, 66% of blood specimens from children are positive by PCR. The virus persists in T cells, but it could be found in only 4 of 220 healthy blood donors.[2]

Methodology Molecular amplification of HHV-6 DNA using polymerase chain reaction (PCR)

Additional Information Primary infection by HHV-6 is self-limited in most nonimmunosuppressed individuals. However, encephalitis has been reported as a complication. In bone marrow transplant patients, pneumonitis may occur with HHV-6, and may be associated with cytomegalovirus infection.[2,3] Amplification assays for detection of HHV-6 have been developed because of the difficulty in isolating the virus and the high sensitivity that PCR provides. CSF has been found to be positive for HHV-6 by PCR from patients with exanthem subitum and evidence of encephalitis.[4] The full clinical spectrum of disease may not yet be known. In addition to encephalitis and pneumonitis, infection is also associated with lymphadenopathy and an infectious mononucleosis syndrome.[5] HHV-6 shares other features with EBV and CMV, including latency and reactivation. Transmission is thought to occur through close contact, especially with mothers or other children, since the virus can be detected in the saliva of asymptomatic individuals. The knowledge that HHV-6 may be found in asymptomatic individuals emphasizes the importance of correlation of detection of HHV-6 DNA with clinical symptoms. Detection of the virus does not necessarily provide evidence of causation of disease.

Footnotes

1. Dockrell DH, Smith TF, and Paya CV, "Human Herpesvirus 6," *Mayo Clin Proc*, 1999, 74:163-70.
2. Carrigan DR, Drobyski WR, Russlor SK, et al, "Interstitial Pneumonitis Associated With Human Herpesvirus-6 Infection After Marrow Transplantation," *Lancet*, 1991, 338(8760):147-9.
3. Cone RW, Hackman RC, Huang ML, et al, "Human Herpesvirus 6 in Lung Tissue From Patients With Pneumonitis After Bone Marrow Transplantation," *N Engl J Med*, 1993, 329(3):156-61.
4. Kondo K, Nagafuji H, Hata A, et al, "Association of Human Herpesvirus 6 Infection of the Central Nervous System With Recurrence of Febrile Convulsions," *J Infect Dis*, 1993, 167(5):1197-200.
5. Stoeckle MY, "The Spectrum of Human Herpesvirus 6 Infection: From Roseola Infantum to Adult Disease," *Annu Rev Med*, 2000, 51:423-30.

References

Campadelli-Fiume G, Mirandola P, Menotti L, "Human Herpesvirus 6: An Emerging Pathogen," *Emerg Infect Dis*, 1999, 5(3):353-66.

Clark DA, "Human Herpesvirus 6," *Rev Med Virol*, 2000, 10(3):155-73.

Knox KK, Brewer JH, Henry JM, et al, "Human Herpesvirus 6 and Multiple Sclerosis: Systemic Active Infections in Patients With Early Disease," *Clin Infect Dis*, 2000, 31(4):894-903.

Leach CT, "Human Herpesvirus-6 and -7 Infections in Children: Agents of Roseola and Other Syndromes," *Curr Opin Pediatr*, 2000, 12(3):269-74.

Internet Web Sites

www.emedicine.com

Herpesvirus 6, IgG and IgM Antibodies, Quantitative

Related Information

Herpesvirus 6 Culture *on page 633*
Herpesvirus 6 DNA Detection *on page 633*
Infectious Mononucleosis Screening Test *on page 643*

Synonyms HHV-6, IgM, IgG; Human Herpesvirus 6, IgG and IgM Antibodies, Quantitative

Test Includes Detection and quantitation of antibodies to human herpesvirus 6 (HHV-6)

(Continued)

Herpesvirus 6, IgG and IgM Antibodies, Quantitative (Continued)

Abstract Human herpesvirus 6 (HHV-6) is a herpes DNA virus with affinity for T lymphocytes. It usually infects infants between age 6 months and 2 years. The primary infection is roseola infantum, but HHV-6 is also the most common cause of febrile convulsions. Adult infections are usually recognized in immunocompromised hosts. Such infections may include several syndromes with fever, rash, pneumonitis, encephalitis, and other findings.

Specimen Serum

Container Red top tube or serum separator tube

Collection Acute and convalescent specimens are recommended. Specimens should be free from bacterial contamination and hemolysis.

Storage Instructions Refrigerate serum.

Causes for Rejection Gross lipemia

Use IgM HHV-6 may aid in the diagnosis of acute or recent infection with HHV-6.

Methodology Indirect fluorescent antibody (IFA)

Additional Information Although HHV-6A and HHV-6B have been identified, only the 6B form of HHV-6 has been confirmed to cause disease. Primary infection occurs as roseola infantum (exanthem subitum) a febrile illness with high fever which lasts for 3-5 days. Subsequently, a rash abruptly appears. It is also a cause of a primary infection with fever without rash. HHV-6B also causes febrile convulsions in infants, encephalitis, a heterophil-negative mononucleosis syndrome indistinguishable from that caused by HHV-7, or hepatitis, sometimes fulminant. HHV-6 is shed in saliva and urine. Whether or not it is also shed in breast milk in not presently clear.

HHV-6 antibodies are very common. Most healthy children have antibody by age 2 or 3 years. Since the virus persists in lymphocytes indefinitely, nearly all adults have antibody, although seropositivity may decrease with age. Because of this frequency, confirmation of HHV-6 etiology in several diseases in which it is considered is difficult.

References

Buchwald D, Cheney PR, Peterson DL, et al, "A Chronic Illness Characterized by Fatigue, Neurologic and Immunologic Disorders, and Active Human Herpesvirus Type 6 Infection," *Ann Intern Med*, 1992, 116(2):103-13.

Campadelli-Fiume G, Mirandola P, Menotti L, "Human Herpesvirus 6: An Emerging Pathogen," *Emerg Infect Dis*, 1999, 5(3):353-66.

Clark DA, "Human Herpesvirus 6," *Rev Med Virol*, 2000, 10(3):155-73.

Dockrell DH, Smith TF, and Paya CV, "Human Herpesvirus 6," *Mayo Clin Proc*, 1999, 74:163-170

Hall CB, Long CE, Schnabel KC, et al, "Human Herpesvirus-6 Infection in Children. A Prospective Study of Complications and Reactivation," *N Engl J Med*, 1994, 331(7):432-8.

Leach CT, "Human Herpesvirus-6 and -7 Infections in Children: Agents of Roseola and Other Syndromes," *Curr Opin Pediatr*, 2000, 12(3):269-74.

Straus SE, "Human Herpesvirus Types 6 and 7," *Principles and Practice of Infectious Diseases*, 5th ed, Mandell GL, Bennett JE, and Dolin R, eds, New York, NY: Churchill Livingstone, 2000, 1613-8.

Stoeckle MY, "The Spectrum of Human Herpesvirus 6 Infection: From Roseola Infantum to Adult Disease," *Annu Rev Med*, 2000, 51:423-30.

Internet Web Sites

www.emedicine.com

Herpesvirus 7

Synonyms HHV-7; Human Herpesvirus 7

Abstract Human herpesvirus 7 (HHV-7) is a recently described herpesvirus found in peripheral blood mononuclear cells (PBMC). It is closely related to HHV-6. HHV-7 antibodies are specific for the virus.

Methodology HHV-7 PCR has recently been described.[1] Antibodies can be detected using immunofluorescence.

Additional Information HHV-7 infections commonly occur in childhood, 1 or 2 years later than HHV-6 infections. By age 5 years, nearly everyone has had exposure to this virus. It has been reported to cause exanthem subitum in children who already had antibody for HHV-6, suggesting this syndrome may be produced by each virus. HHV-7 seems to downregulate expression of CD4 on T lymphocytes, potentially causing host problems in controlling infections. Rare cases of encephalitis and hepatitis have been reported in association with HHV-7.

Footnotes

1. Hoang MP, Barton Rogers B, Dawson B, "Quantitation of 8 Human Herpesviruses in Peripheral Blood of Human Immunodeficiency Virus-Infected Patients and Healthy Blood Donors by Polymerase Chain Reaction," *Am J Clin Pathol*, 1999, 111(5):655-9.

References

Campadelli-Fiume G, Mirandola P, Menotti L, "Human Herpesvirus 6: An Emerging Pathogen," *Emerg Infect Dis*, 1999, 5(3):353-66.

Leach CT, "Human Herpesvirus-6 and -7 Infections in Children: Agents of Roseola and Other Syndromes," *Curr Opin Pediatr*, 2000, 12(3):269-74.

Straus SE, "Human Herpesvirus Types 6 & 7," *Principles and Practice of Infectious Diseases*, 5th ed, Mandell GL, Bennett JE, and Dolin R, eds, New York, NY: Churchill Livingstone, 2000, 1616-7.

Tsukazaki T, Yoshida M, Namba H, et al, "Development of a Dot Blot Neutralizing Assay for HHV-6 and HHV-7 Using Specific Monoclonal Antibodies," *J Virol Methods*, 1998, 73(2):141-9.

Internet Web Sites

www.emedicine.com

Herpesvirus 8

Related Information

Body Cavity Fluid Cytology *on page 372*
Body Fluid Lactate Dehydrogenase *on page 125*
Epstein-Barr Virus Culture *on page 607*
Epstein-Barr Virus Serology *on page 607*
Fine Needle Aspiration, Deep Masses *on page 381*
Fine Needle Aspiration, Superficial Masses (Palpable) *on page 382*
Polymerase Chain Reaction *on page 713*
Skin Biopsy *on page 71*

Synonyms HHV-8; Human Herpesvirus Type 8; Kaposi Sarcoma-Associated Herpesvirus; KSHV

Abstract **Kaposi sarcoma** was originally described over a century ago, but the HHV-8 virus has only recently been identified.

Surveys show HHV-8-specific antibody in up to 10% of healthy U.S. blood donors, 2% to 4% of hemophiliacs, 20% to 30% of HIV-positive gay men without Kaposi sarcoma (KS), 70% to 90% of patients with KS, and almost 100% of immunocompetent patients with the disease.[1]

Infection rates of HHV-8 are parallel with the incidence of KS: low in the U.S. and much of Europe and Asia; intermediate in Mediterranean countries, with the highest rates in Uganda, Zambia, and South Africa. KS is the most frequent neoplasm in patients with AIDS. KS is much more frequent among males than females who are HIV positive. Nonhomosexual HIV-infected individuals (eg, hemophiliacs, heterosexual injection drug users) also have a lower prevalence. The genome of HHV-8 has been found in KS tumor cells from AIDS patients and as well in specimens from KS patients who are HIV negative.

Container Red top tube or SST™ tube for HHV-8 IgG antibody

Use Diagnose HHV-8 with or without KS.

KS, an angioproliferative disease, was originally described as an uncommon entity by a Hungarian physician in 1872, many decades before AIDS was recognized. In addition to its classic form, KS is prevalent among individuals with AIDS and in patients treated with immunosuppressives associated with organ transplantation. HHV-8 is transmitted through renal allografts. It is a risk factor for transplantation-associated KS.[2] HHV-8 antibodies can be used to assess organ transplant patients. Subjects positive for HHV-8 antibodies, who are recipients of an organ transplanted from a donor positive for HHV-8, are at increased risk for post-transplantation development of KS.[3]

The risk of KS is 73,000 times greater in homosexual patients with AIDS.

HHV-8 is found as well in **body cavity-based B-cell lymphoma (primary effusion lymphoma)**, and some plasma cell forms of multicentric Castleman disease. In primary-effusion lymphoma, malignant peritoneal, pericardial, or pleural effusions occur without lymph node involvement or identification of a distinctive, conventional neoplastic mass. It is aggressive.[4]

Limitations Some authorities have criticized lack of sensitivity among the serologic tests.[5] When only low concentrations of IgG are present, in the acute phase, false negatives may be seen.[3]

Although KSHV DNA is found in only about 50% of infected patients with standard PCR assays, PCR and Southern blot hybridization assay can detect viral DNA in essentially all lesions of KS.[1]

Methodology Second generation serological assays, indirect immunofluorescence assay,[3,6] KSHV PCR,[7] quantitative PCR[8]

Additional Information HHV-8 is a Kaposi sarcoma tumor virus prevalent in southern Europe and in Africa. It is virologically similar to EBV, is persistent in the body after infection, reproduces in peripheral blood mononuclear cells, and may be found in saliva. This virus may be even more prevalent than suspected previously. The use of HHV-8 lytic-cycle antigens has shown nearly all KS patients are positive, as are 90% of HIV-infected gay men, 20% of HIV-positive intravenous drug addicts (IVDA), up to 25% of healthy adults, and 8% of children.

KSHV is a sexually transmitted disease, but other means of transmission predominate elsewhere (eg, in Africa, infection can occur in childhood). Maternal-infant transmission is seen in countries in which HHV-8 infection is endemic.

The risk of transmission through transfusion is unknown at this time, but is unequivocally lower than that of HIV.[1]

Footnotes

1. Antman K and Chang Y, "Kaposi's Sarcoma," *N Engl J Med*, 2000, 342(14):1027-38.
2. Regamey N, Tamm M, Wernli M, et al, "Transmission of Human Herpesvirus 8 Infection From Renal-Transplant Donors to Recipients," *N Engl J Med*, 1998, 339(19):1358-63.
3. Mayo Reference Services Publication, "Human Herpesvirus-8 Antibodies, IgG, Serum," *New Test Announcement*, #81971, Rochester, MN: Mayo Medical Laboratories, September 2000.
4. Jones D, Ballestas ME, Kaye KM, et al, "Primary-Effusion Lymphoma and Kaposi's Sarcoma in a Cardiac-Transplant Recipient," *N Engl J Med*, 1998, 339(7):444-9.
5. Jaffe HW and Pellett PE, "Human Herpesvirus 8 and Kaposi's Sarcoma - Some Answers, More Questions," *N Engl J Med*, 1999, 340(24):1912-3.

6. Sitas F, Carrara H, Beral V, et al, "Antibodies Against Human Herpesvirus 8 in Black South African Patients With Cancer," *N Engl J Med*, 1999, 340(24):1863-71.

7. Alkan S, Eltoum IA, Tabbara S, et al, "Usefulness of Molecular Detection of Human Herpesvirus-8 in the Diagnosis of Kaposi Sarcoma by Fine-Needle Aspiration," *Am J Clin Pathol*, 1999, 111(1):91-6.

8. Hoang MP, Rogers BB, Dawson DB, et al, "Quantitation of 8 Human Herpesviruses in Peripheral Blood of Human Immunodeficiency Virus-Infected Patients and Healthy Blood Donors by Polymerase Chain Reaction," *Am J Clin Pathol*, 1999, 111(5):655-9.

References

Gómez-Román JJ, Ocejo-Vinyals JG, Sánchez-Velasco P, et al, "Presence of Human Herpesvirus 8 DNA Sequences in Renal Transplantation-Associated Pleural Kaposi Sarcoma," *Arch Pathol Lab Med*, 1999, 123(12):1269-73.

Ho M, "Human Herpesvirus 8 - Let the Transplantation Physician Beware," *N Engl J Med*, 1998, 339(19):1391-2.

Kedes DH, Ganem D, Ameli N, et al, "The Prevalence of Serum Antibody to Human Herpesvirus 8 (Kaposi Sarcoma-Associated Herpesvirus) Among HIV-Seropositive and High-Risk HIV-Seronegative Women," *JAMA*, 1997, 277(6):478-81.

Martin JN, Ganem DE, Osmond DH, et al, "Sexual Transmission and the Natural History of Human Herpesvirus 8 Infection," *N Engl J Med*, 1998, 338(14):948-54.

Moore PS, "The Emergence of Kaposi's Sarcoma-Associated Herpesvirus (Human Herpesvirus 8)," *N Engl J Med*, 2000, 343(19):1411-3.

Pauk J, Huang ML, Brodie SJ, et al, "Mucosal Shedding of Human Herpesvirus 8 in Men," *N Engl J Med*, 2000, 343(19):1369-77.

Schulz TF, "Kaposi's Sarcoma-Associated Herpesvirus (Human Herpesvirus 8): Epidemiology and Pathogenesis," *JAC*, 2000, 45(Topic T3):15-27.

Straus SE, "Human Herpesvirus Type 8 (Kaposi's Sarcoma-Associated Herpesvirus)," *Principles and Practice of Infectious Diseases*, 5th ed, Mandell GL, Bennett JE, and Dolin R, eds, New York, NY: Churchill Livingstone, 2000, 1618-21.

Internet Web Sites

www.emedicine.com

♦ **Herpesvirus hominis 1 and 2** *see* Herpes Simplex Antibody *on page 630*

♦ **Herpes Zoster Serology** *see* Varicella-Zoster Virus Serology *on page 687*

Heterophil Agglutinins

Related Information

Epstein-Barr Virus Culture *on page 607*
Epstein-Barr Virus Serology *on page 607*
Infectious Mononucleosis Screening Test *on page 643*

Applies to Paul-Bunnell-Davidsohn Test

Test Includes Differentiation and quantitation of antibodies associated with infectious mononucleosis from the Forssman as well as other heterophil antibodies.

Specimen Serum

Container Red top tube

Reference Interval Negative agglutination

Use Detect heterophil antibodies related to infectious mononucleosis. **This test has largely been replaced by rapid screening tests. See Infectious Mononucleosis Screening Test** *on page 643* **and Epstein-Barr Virus Serology** *on page 607.*

Limitations Rare patients may have positive heterophil agglutinins after a negative rapid screening test. Ten percent of cases of true EBV mononucleosis may have negative heterophil agglutinins. These may be diagnosed with EBV specific tests.

Methodology Differential serum absorption and agglutination of sheep red blood cells

Additional Information Heterophil agglutinins clump sheep erythrocytes. They develop in infectious mononucleosis, other conditions including serum sickness, and in some normal individuals. To diagnose infectious mononucleosis, an absorption of serum is done, with guinea pig kidney (which binds serum sickness and Forssman antibodies but not infectious mononucleosis antibodies) and bovine red cells (which bind infectious mononucleosis and serum sickness antibodies but not Forssman antibodies). Absorption of patient's serum with guinea pig kidney leaves agglutination, but absorption with beef red cells allows no agglutination. This differential absorption procedure is the Paul-Bunnell-Davidsohn test. In present usage horse erythrocytes are used in place of sheep cells in many laboratories. In the presumptive test, a positive test in the presence of consistent clinical and/or hematologic findings confirms the diagnosis of infectious mononucleosis. Such antibodies may persist for up to 2 years. Approximately 10% to 20% of mononucleosis syndromes are heterophil-negative. In some of these, antibody to specific Epstein-Barr viral antigen can be demonstrated. See Epstein-Barr Virus Serology *on page 607.* Children may have heterophil-negative infectious mononucleosis. Others cases resembling infectious mononucleosis may be due to CMV, HHV-6, or toxoplasmosis. Although this classic test has excellent specificity, its performance is time consuming. False-positive tests occur and may lead to diagnostic confusion.

References

Bruu AL, Hjetland R, Holter E, et al. "Evaluation of 12 Commercial Tests for Detection of Epstein-Barr Virus-Specific and Heterophil Antibodies," *Clin Diag Lab Immunol*, 2000, 7(3):451-6.

Godshall SE and Krichner JT, "Infectious Mononucleosis," *Postgrad Med*, 2000, 107(7):175-186.

Horwitz CA, Henle W, Henle G, et al, "Persistent Falsely Positive Rapid Tests for Infectious Mononucleosis. Report of Five Cases With 4-6 Year Follow-up Data," *Am J Clin Pathol*, 1979, 72(5):807-11.

Schooley RT, "Epstein-Barr Virus (Infectious Mononucleosis)," *Principles and Practice of Infectious Diseases*, 5th ed, Mandell GL, Bennett JE, and Dolin R, eds, New York, NY: Churchill Livingstone, 2000, 1599-612.

Internet Web Sites

www.emedicine.com

♦ **Heterophil Antibody** *see* Infectious Mononucleosis Screening Test *on page 643*

♦ **HEV Antibody** *see* Hepatitis E Serology *on page 628*

♦ **HHV-6 Culture** *see* Herpesvirus 6 Culture *on page 633*

♦ **HHV-6 DNA Detection** *see* Herpesvirus 6 DNA Detection *on page 633*

♦ **HHV-6, IgM, IgG** *see* Herpesvirus 6, IgG and IgM Antibodies, Quantitative *on page 633*

♦ **HHV-6 PCR** *see* Herpesvirus 6 DNA Detection *on page 633*

♦ **HHV-7** *see* Herpesvirus 7 *on page 634*

♦ **HHV-8** *see* Herpesvirus 8 *on page 634*

♦ **Hickman Catheters** *see* Bacterial Culture, Intravascular Device *on page 572*

♦ *Histoplasma* **Antibodies** *see* Histoplasmosis Antibody *on page 635*

♦ *Histoplasma capsulatum* **Antigen** *see* Histoplasmosis Antigen *on page 636*

♦ **Histoplasmosis** *see* Fungal Culture, Biopsy or Body Fluid *on page 610*

Histoplasmosis Antibody

Related Information

Bacteremia Detection, Buffy Coat Micromethod *on page 406*
Bronchoalveolar Lavage (BAL) *on page 375*
Fungal Culture, Biopsy or Body Fluid *on page 610*
Fungal Culture, Blood *on page 610*
Fungal Culture, Cerebrospinal Fluid *on page 611*
Fungal Culture, Sputum *on page 613*
Fungus Smear, Stain *on page 615*
Histoplasmosis Antigen *on page 636*

Synonyms *Histoplasma* Antibodies

Test Includes Reaction with yeast and mycelial antigens

Abstract Antibodies to *H. capsulatum* may be found in 20% to 80% of individuals who live in endemic areas of the Ohio, Missouri, and Mississippi River valleys. Use of serology to diagnose histoplasmosis is **not reliable**. Results are positive in >90% of cases of acute pulmonary disease, 70% to 90% in cavitary lung disease, but only 30% to 50% in acute disseminated disease. Serologic testing should be interpreted in conjunction with other tests.

Specimen Serum, cerebrospinal fluid

Container Red top tube, sterile CSF tube, plastic urine container

Collection Acute and convalescent sera are recommended, especially when acute titers are only presumptive. Specimens taken 3-4 weeks apart are desirable.

Reference Interval Less than a fourfold change in titer between acute and convalescent samples

Use Diagnose chronic/self-limited histoplasmosis. Fungal stains and cultures of sputum, bone marrow examination and culture, *Histoplasma* antigen, or *Histoplasma* PCR are also needed for such patients.

Limitations Other diagnostic approaches are preferable. A negative result does not rule out histoplasmosis, nor do all who have encountered the fungus develop CF antibodies. False negatives occur in normals and in immunosuppressed individuals.[1] Histoplasmin skin testing may interfere with results, giving a positive test for mycelial phase antibodies. Testing with both myecelial and yeast phase antigens must be performed. Antibodies cross react with other fungi. Anticomplementary sera cannot be tested for complement fixing antibodies. The latex agglutination test gives some false positives, and must be confirmed with another procedure.

Contraindications Previous skin testing, made from supernatant of myecelial growth

Methodology Immunodiffusion (ID), complement fixation (CF), latex agglutination (LA), enzyme immunoassay (EIA)

Additional Information A serum titer ≥1:16 for *Histoplasma* mycelial antigen, or serum titer ≥1:32 for yeast antigen provide evidence of active disease. Increasing titers in complement fixation provide evidence of active infection.[2] Titers between 1:8 to 1:32 are less diagnostic, and require clinical and other laboratory correlation. Immunodiffusion tests to detect H and M bands are useful. H bands are beta-glucosidases, found infrequently in disease (<10%) but, if present, indicate active infection. M bands are similar to catalase and are commonly (>80%) found in normals after exposure to *Histoplasma*. The latex agglutination test detects IgM antibodies and is positive early in disease, but not in late, chronic, or recurrent infection. Complement fixation is more sensitive than immunodiffusion.

In addition to histoplasmosis in immunologically intact individuals, this fungal infection is a serious opportunistic infection in patients with AIDS (Continued)

Histoplasmosis Antibody (Continued)

(occasionally as its first manifestation). Organisms can sometimes be found in leukocytes in Wright-stained peripheral blood films in patients with AIDS.[3] (A calcofluor white stain may prove useful).[4]

Giemsa or methenamine silver preparations of bone marrow, mucosal ulcers, biopsies of liver, lung, skin, lymph nodes, or bronchoalveolar lavage may provide rapid diagnosis; and cultures are required as well, especially of blood, bone marrow, sputum, urine and portions of biopsies. Isolates can be identified by DNA probe.[5]

Clinical central nervous system involvement occurs in 10% to 20% of cases of disseminated histoplasmosis; with autopsy, the prevalence reaches 75%. Meningitis and cerebral mass lesions occur. Serologic tests reach 92% sensitivity (serum) and 80% (CSF). Serologic positivity may be prolonged, making application of serologic methods for detection of relapse difficult.[6]

Footnotes

1. Williams B, Fojtasek M, Connolly-Stringfield P, et al, "Diagnosis of Histoplasmosis by Antigen Detection During an Outbreak in Indianapolis, Ind," *Arch Pathol Lab Med*, 1994, 118(12):1205-8.
2. Wu LA and Thomas CF, "35-Year-Old Man With Fever, Hemoptysis, and Lymphadenopathy," *Mayo Clin Proc*, 2000, 75(6):651-4.
3. Edelman M and McKitrick J, Images in Clinical Medicine, "*Histoplasma capsulatum* in a Peripheral Blood Smear," *N Engl J Med*, 2000, 342(1):28.
4. Elin RJ, Whitis J, and Snyder J, "Infectious Disease Diagnosis From a Peripheral Blood Smear," *Lab Med*, 2000, 31(6):324-8.
5. "A 38-Year-Old Man With AIDS and the Recent Onset of Diarrhea, Hematochezia, Fever, and Pulmonary Infiltrates," Case Records of the Massachusetts General Hospital, Case 4-1994, Scully RE, Mark EJ, McNeely WF, et al, eds, *N Engl J Med*, 1994, 330(4):273-80.
6. Klein CJ, Dinapoli RP, Temesgen Z, et al, "Central Nervous System Histoplasmosis Mimicking a Brain Tumor: Difficulties in Diagnosis and Treatment," *Mayo Clin Proc*, 1999, 74(8):803-7.

References

Deepe GS, "*Histoplasma capsulatum*," *Principles and Practice of Infectious Diseases*, 5th ed, Mandell GL, Bennett JE, and Dolan R, eds, New York, NY: Churchill Livingstone, 2000, 2718-33.

Wheat J, "Histoplasmosis. Experience During Outbreaks in Indianapolis and Review of the Literature," *Medicine*, 1997, 76(5):339-54.

Internet Web Sites

www.cdc.gov

www.emedicine.com

Histoplasmosis Antigen

Related Information

Fungal Culture, Biopsy or Body Fluid *on page 610*
Fungal Culture, Blood *on page 610*
Fungal Culture, Cerebrospinal Fluid *on page 611*
Fungal Culture, Sputum *on page 613*
Fungus Smear, Stain *on page 615*
Histoplasmosis Antibody *on page 635*

Applies to *Histoplasma capsulatum* Antigen

Abstract Less helpful in chronic pulmonary or self-limited forms of histoplasmosis, in which cultures and serologic tests are needed. Antigen tests are useful in subjects with severe disease including disseminated histoplasmosis.

Specimen Serum, urine, cerebrospinal fluid[1,2]

Container Red top tube, urine container, sterile CSF tube

Reference Interval <1.0 EIA

Use Detection of *Histoplasma* antigen occurs in 90% of cases in the urine of non-AIDS patients with disseminated infection, and 75% of persons with acute pulmonary histoplasmosis. Antigenemia is found in <50% of patients. In those with AIDS, antigenuria is detected in 95% and antigenemia in 85%.[2] The immunoassay for *Histoplasma* glycoprotein antigen, the precise nature of which remains unknown, has proven diagnostically useful in a variety of clinical settings (particularly in AIDS patients), and is also useful for monitoring response to therapy. Biopsies, examination of peripheral blood smears for organisms, blood cultures, and serology are also indicated for investigation of disseminated histoplasmosis.[3]

Limitations The test is now widely performed. It occasionally produces false-negative results with less severe forms of histoplasmosis, and may give false-negative results in patients with proven disseminated disease.[3]

Cross reactions have occurred in patients who have other fungal infections due to similar antigens, including blastomycosis, paracoccidioidomycosis, and penicillosis, but not with *Aspergillus*, *Candida*, or *Cryptococcus*. Rheumatoid factor may cause a false-positive antigen test.

Methodology Microtiter plates with anti-*H. capsulatum* antibody;[3] enzyme immunoassay (EIA) for *Histoplasma* polysaccharide antigen

Additional Information Ninety percent of patients with progressive disseminated histoplasmosis have positive antigen, 40% who have cavitary lung disease, but only 20% who have acute pulmonary histoplasmosis.[4] In the clinical setting of suspected histoplasmosis, fungal cultures and antibodies are desirable.

Footnotes

1. Klein CJ, Dinapoli RP, Temesgen Z, et al, "Central Nervous System Histoplasmosis Mimicking a Brain Tumor: Difficulties in Diagnosis and Treatment," *Mayo Clin Proc*, 1999, 74(8):803-7.

2. Wu LA and Thomas CF, "35-Year-Old Man With Fever, Hemoptysis, and Lymphadenopathy," *Mayo Clin Proc*, 2000, 75(6):651-4.
3. Wheat J, "Histoplasmosis. Experience During Outbreaks in Indianapolis and Review of the Literature," *Medicine*, 1997, 76(5):339-54.
4. Deepe GS, "*Histoplasma capsulatum*," *Principles and Practice of Infectious Diseases*, 5th ed, Mandell GL, Bennett JE, and Dolin R, eds, New York, NY: Churchill Livingstone, 2000, 2718-33.

References

"A 38-Year-Old Man With AIDS and the Recent Onset of Diarrhea, Hematochezia, Fever, and Pulmonary Infiltrates," Case Records of the Massachusetts General Hospital, Case 4-1994, Scully RE, Mark EJ, McNeely WF, et al, eds, *N Engl J Med*, 1994, 330(4):273-80.

Limaye AP, Connolly PA, Sagar M, et al, "Transmission of *Histoplasma capsulatum* by Organ Transplantation," *N Engl J Med*, 2000, 343(16):1163-6.

Wheat LJ, Connolly-Stringfield P, Blair R, et al, "Histoplasmosis Relapse in Patients With AIDS: Detection Using *Histoplasma capsulatum* Variety *capsulatum* Antigen Levels," *Ann Intern Med*, 1991, 115(12):936-41.

Internet Web Sites

www.apha.org/public_health/aids.htm

www.emedicine.com

www.hivatis.org

HIV-1/HIV-2 Antibody Screen and Western Blot

Related Information

Antiphospholipid Antibody (Lupus Anticoagulant and/or Anticardiolipin Antibody) *on page 331*
Beta$_2$-Microglobulin, Serum or Urine *on page 509*
CD4/CD8 Enumeration *on page 511*
Donation, Blood *on page 839*
Fungal Culture, Skin *on page 612*
HIV p24 Antigen Detection *on page 637*
HTLV-I/II Antibody *on page 638*
Human Immunodeficiency Virus Culture *on page 639*
Human Immunodeficiency Virus DNA Amplification *on page 639*
Neisseria gonorrhoeae Culture and Smear *on page 662*
Ova and Parasites, Stool *on page 666*
Risks of Transfusion *on page 861*
Toxoplasmosis Serology *on page 684*
White Blood Cell Count *on page 496*
Zidovudine, Serum or Plasma *on page 771*

Synonyms Acquired Immune Deficiency Syndrome Serology; AIDS Screen; HIV Antibody; Human Immunodeficiency Virus 1/2 Serology; Western Blot Test for HIV Antibody

Applies to CD4 Count; Recombinant Antigen Immunoblot Assay; Western Blot

Test Includes Detection of antibody to HIV by ELISA and confirmation of positives by Western blot

Abstract Present screening tests for HIV antibodies are ELISA procedures which use recombinant antigen products. Different antibodies are detected. Both the sensitivity and specificity of these tests are extremely high, but positive results on a screen should be repeated using a new specimen. If positive a second time they should be confirmed with a Western blot procedure. Because of the grave implications of a positive result, it is recommended that a second sample be assayed to eliminate false positives due to switched samples or sample contamination. Before patients develop antibody (window phase) in early disease, detection of HIV nucleic acid by PCR or branched DNA assays can be used for diagnosis.

A second virus that causes AIDS, HIV-2, was recognized in 1986. HIV-2 is very closely related to HIV-1 with 40% nucleic acid homology. HIV-2 is endemic in West Africa, however, it has spread to other countries. Occasional cases have been confirmed in the United States.[1] It produces the same clinical disease as HIV-1, although the incubation period before clinical AIDS develops in HIV-2 may be longer than in HIV-1.

Patient Preparation In some states test may not be done or results revealed without express written or informed consent of the patient or guardian.

Specimen Serum or plasma; some test systems use saliva or urine

Container Red top tube or lavender top (EDTA) tube

Special Instructions Blood and body fluid precautions must be observed.

Reference Interval Negative

Use Document exposure to HIV-1 and HIV-2; screen blood and blood fractions for transfusion; screen organ transplant donors; test patients after documented needlestick exposure of healthcare personnel.

Screening for AIDS infection in low risk populations will be hampered by false-positive results. Although the combined false-positive rate of sequential ELISA and Western blot testing may be very low (0.005% estimated in one article) testing large numbers of individuals in a population with a very low prevalence of disease will generate large numbers of false-positive results. The predictive value of a positive test will be low, and many individuals will be unnecessarily alarmed. Thus, mass screening is not recommended.[2]

Patients in high risk groups (men who have sex with men, gay or bisexual men, I.V. drug abusers and their sexual contacts, male and female prostitutes, hemophiliacs exposed to large amounts of nonheat processed factor VIII) should be tested by standard protocol.[2]

Long-term nonprogressors (LTNP) These are persons who have had HIV-1 for sufficient duration to have developed low CD4 cells or an opportunistic infection but did not. Such persons have been evaluated for the mechanism of delayed viral growth. Chemokine receptors (eg. CCR5, CXCR4, and several others) are essential coreceptors for HIV to infect CD4 receptor-bearing cells. Most individuals that are LTNPs have a variant cytokine receptor. These persons have HIV-1 antibody with positive WB, but HIV loads are typically very low or undetectable, even without antiretroviral therapy.[2]

Limitations Positive screening tests must be confirmed by more specific follow-up procedures. If the Western blot or immunofluorescent antibody for HIV-1 is negative or indeterminate with a positive HIV-1/HIV-2 serology, further testing is required for HIV-2. This may include HIV-2 EIA and HIV-2 Western blot. Antibody is not protective against disease, but indicates infection with the virus. There are cross reactions in some test systems due to histocompatibility antigen mismatches (in particular, antibodies to HLA-DR4). Cross reactions have been observed to other viral antigens as well. A recent influenza vaccination can result in reactivity against p24 antigen and give a false-positive enzyme-linked immunosorbent assay.

Because screening tests are not completely sensitive or specific, a positive anti-HIV-1/HIV-2 result must be interpreted cautiously, taking into account the prevalence of AIDS in the population being tested. As prevalence decreases, false positives increase, and the predictive value of a positive result decreases.

Serology cannot be used to determine if an infant born to an HIV-positive mother is infected, because of the maternal transfer of antibodies. These infants should be tested using molecular assays or culture.

Contraindications Some states require informed consent.

Methodology Enzyme-linked immunosorbent assay (ELISA), Western blot, indirect fluorescent antibody (IFA). Other test systems include HIV-1/HIV-2 combination ELISA kit, SUDS (single use diagnostic system) HIV diagnostic kit.

Additional Information Human immunodeficiency virus (HIV-1) is the etiologic agent of AIDS. Acute infection is characterized by a flu-like illness, or no symptoms. Generally, following infection with the virus, there is local replication of the virus in regional lymph nodes and the viral nucleic acid can be detected in the plasma. By ~17 days after infection, viral replication can be detected by p24 antigen test or by PCR for genomic DNA. By ~23 days, the antibody to the HIV virus can be detected in the serum or plasma.

HIV preferentially binds to and infects CD4 (T4,helper) lymphocytes. HIV also binds to monocytes and macrophages, and infection of bronchial macrophages may explain the frequency of *Pneumocystis* infections in AIDS patients. HIV probably enters the CNS by means of infected monocytes crossing the blood-brain barrier.

Other tests used in HIV-positive patients include quantitation of CD4 (T4 helper) and CD8 (suppressor) lymphocytes. AIDS is present when the absolute CD4 count <200/mm^3 is found. Alternatively, AIDS may be diagnosed when one of many opportunistic infections or tumors is diagnosed.

The third generation ELISA assay, using HIV-1 env and gag proteins and HIV-2 env proteins, is now the standard for screening and detects IgM, IgA, and IgG anti-HIV. This reduces the window period in early HIV. Confirmation with Western blot (WB) is still required.

Rapid testing with results in 30 minutes, can be done using the single use diagnostic system (SUDS). Results may be used in STD clinics or emergency departments, but require follow-up with standard HIV testing for positives. HIV-2 antibodies are **not** detected.

Oral mucosa transudate test (OMT)[3] uses a cotton pad placed between cheek and gum for 5 minutes under direct supervision. The pad is tested by a special micro-ELISA system. WB is needed to confirm positives.

Urine based HIV tests to detect HIV-1 antibodies may be useful when serum specimens are nearly impossible to obtain. But a positive must be confirmed by standard serum tests, ELISA and WB.

HIV home bleed test systems allow individuals to prick their own fingers, place three drops of blood on a card, and mail it to the manufacturer where an ELISA is performed anonymously. Positive results are followed by telephone counseling. Other systems have an indicator to show positives on the card 5 minutes after blood is placed on the card. False positives and negatives remain problems with these systems.

In the **Western blot procedure**, electrophoretically separated HIV proteins are overlaid with patient's serum. Antibodies present will bind to antigen, and the bound antibody is then visualized using a labeled antibody to human immunoglobulin. The standard of the Association of State and Territorial Public Health Laboratories was adopted by the Centers for Disease Control in 1989 and is now the most widely accepted definition of a positive Western blot. Criteria require the Western blot to contain at least two of the following three bands: p24, gp41, and gp 160/120. The presence of other band patterns is termed indeterminate and should be followed up with subsequent testing. The Western blot is a complex procedure, requiring great technical expertise and informed interpretation. False-positive rates may be in the range of 1% to 2%. False-negative rates are not well established. A disadvantage of WB is the high percentage of "indeterminate" patterns - neither positive nor negative. As many as 40% of repeat reactive specimens will have an indeterminate pattern. IFA, in contrast, reveals a

<5% indeterminate pattern. Thus, for confirmatory testing IFA is more specific. On the other hand, it is more difficult and expensive than WB.[4,5,6]

See Human Immunodeficiency Virus, Viral Load Assay *on page 640.*

Footnotes

1. Schim van der Loeff MF and Aaby P, "Towards a Better Understanding of the Epidemiology of HIV-2," *AIDS*, 1999, 13(Suppl A):S69-84.
2. Hidalgo JA, MacArthur RD, and Crane LR, "An Overview of HIV Infection and AIDS: Etiology, Pathogenesis, Diagnosis, Epidemiology, and Occupational Exposure," *Semin Thorac Cardiovasc Surg*, 2000, 12(2):130-9.
3. Merson MH, Feldman EA, Bayer R, et al, "Rapid Self Testing for HIV Infection," *Lancet*, 1996, 349(9048):352-3.
4. Centers for Disease Control, "Interpretation and Use of the Western Blot Assay for Serodiagnosis of Human Immunodeficiency Virus Type 1 Infections," *MMWR Morb Mortal Wkly Rep*, 1989, 38(Suppl 7):1-7.
5. Consortium for Retrovirus Serology Standardization, "Serologic Diagnosis of Human Immunodeficiency Virus Infection by Western Blot Testing," *JAMA*, 1988, 260(5):674-9.
6. O'Gorman MR, Weber D, Landis SE, et al, "Interpretive Criteria of the Western Blot for Serodiagnosis of Human Immunodeficiency Virus Type 1 Infection," *Arch Pathol Lab Med*, 1991, 115(10):26-30.

References

Belshe RB, Clements ML, Keefer MC, et al, "Interpreting HIV Serodiagnostic Test Results in the 1990s: Social Risks of HIV Vaccine Studies in Uninfected Volunteers," *Ann Intern Med*, 1994, 121(8):584-9.

Burke DS, Brundage JF, Redfield RR, et al, "Measurement of the False Positive Rate in a Screening Program for Human Immunodeficiency Virus Infections," *N Engl J Med*, 1988, 319(15):961-4.

Carpenter CC, Cooper DA, Fischl MA, et al, "Antiretroviral Therapy in Adults. Updated Recommendations of the International AIDS Society - USA Panel," *JAMA*, 2000, 283(3):381-90.

Craven DE, Steger KA, La Chapelle R, et al, "Factitious HIV Infection: The Importance of Documenting Infection," *Ann Intern Med*, 1994, 121(10):763-6.

Cumming PD, Wallace EL, Schorr JB, et al, "Exposure of Patients to Human Immunodeficiency Virus Through the Transfusion of Blood Components That Test Antibody-Negative," *N Engl J Med*, 1989, 321(14):941-6.

De Cock KM, Porter A, Kouadio J, et al, "Cross-Reactivity on Western Blots in HIV-1 and HIV-2 Infections," *AIDS*, 1991, 5(7):859-63.

"HIV Subtypes: Implications for Epidemiology, Pathogenicity, Vaccines and Diagnostics," *AIDS*, 1997, 11(15):17-36.

"Human Immunodeficiency Virus (HIV) Infection. American College of Physicians and Infectious Diseases Society of America," *Ann Intern Med*, 1994, 120(4):310-9.

Imagawa DT, Lee MH, Wolinsky SM, et al, "Human Immunodeficiency Virus Type 1 Infection in Homosexual Men Who Remain Seronegative for Prolonged Periods," *N Engl J Med*, 1989, 320(22):1458-62.

Leitman SF, Klein HG, Melpolder JJ, et al, "Clinical Implications of Positive Tests for Antibodies to Human Immunodeficiency Virus Type 1 in Asymptomatic Blood Donors," *N Engl J Med*, 1989, 321(14):917-24.

Misrahi M, Teglas JP, Nicole N, et al, "CCR5 Chemokine Receptor Variant in HIV-1 Mother-to-Child Transmission and Disease Progression in Children," *JAMA*, 1998, 279(4):317-8.

Nuwayhid NF, "Laboratory Tests for Detection of Human Immunodeficiency Virus Type I Infection," *Clin Diag Lab Immunol*, 1995, 2(6):637-45.

O'Brien TR and Goedert JJ, "Chemokine Receptors and Genetic Variability," *JAMA*, 1998, 279(4):317-8.

Pomerantz RJ, "HIV/AIDS," *Clin Lab Med*, 1994, 14(2).

Quinn TC, "Screening for HIV Infection - Benefits and Costs," *N Engl J Med*, 1992, 327(7):486-8.

Internet Web Sites

www.apha.org/public_health/aids.htm
www.emedicine.com
www.hivatis.org

♦ **HIV-1 Viral Load Assay** *see* Human Immunodeficiency Virus, Viral Load Assay *on page 640*

♦ **HIV Antibody** *see* HIV-1/HIV-2 Antibody Screen and Western Blot *on page 636*

♦ **HIV Burden** *see* Human Immunodeficiency Virus, Viral Load Assay *on page 640*

♦ **HIV Core Antigen** *see* HIV p24 Antigen Detection *on page 637*

♦ **HIV Culture** *see* Human Immunodeficiency Virus Culture *on page 639*

♦ **HIV DNA Amplification Assay** *see* Human Immunodeficiency Virus DNA Amplification *on page 639*

♦ **HIV DNA PCR Test** *see* Human Immunodeficiency Virus DNA Amplification *on page 639*

♦ **HIV Genotyping** *see* Human Immunodeficiency Virus, Resistance (Susceptibility) Testing *on page 640*

♦ **HIV Load** *see* Human Immunodeficiency Virus, Viral Load Assay *on page 640*

HIV p24 Antigen Detection

Related Information

HIV-1/HIV-2 Antibody Screen and Western Blot *on page 636*
Human Immunodeficiency Virus Culture *on page 639*
Human Immunodeficiency Virus DNA Amplification *on page 639*
Risks of Transfusion *on page 861*
Viral Culture *on page 689*
(Continued)

HIV p24 Antigen Detection (Continued)

Synonyms HIV Core Antigen; HIV p24 gag; p24 Antigen Detection

Applies to Gag Gene of HIV

Test Includes Detection of HIV p24 antigen in serum, plasma, or cerebrospinal fluid

Abstract Detection of p24 antigen of the human immunodeficiency virus (HIV) in serum of blood donors will shorten the time needed to detect HIV infection to ~2 weeks after initial infection. The plasma or serum level of HIV p24 antigen is also useful as a marker of AIDS progression.

Specimen Serum, plasma, or cerebrospinal fluid

Container Red top tube, sterile CSF tube

Special Instructions In some states written or informed patient consent is a prerequisite for the test.

Reference Interval Negative

Use Diagnose recent acute infection with HIV; may also be of prognostic significance in AIDS, if antigen becomes positive during infection, after having been negative. (This assay is also used to detect active HIV replication in viral culture supernatants.)

Limitations Test is not as sensitive as culture or nucleic acid amplification assays for detecting HIV infection.

Methodology Enzyme immunoassay (EIA)

Additional Information The p24 antigen is a 24 kD protein product of the **gag** gene of HIV. As a viral rather than host product, it appears concomitant with initial infection, and then generally becomes undetectable during periods of viral latency. It reappears with renewed viral replication; the reappearance of p24 antigen in serum generally heralds progression of clinical disease in AIDS. Measuring antigen may also be useful to assess therapy. Recent studies indicate that an acid dissociation procedure that disrupts the p24 antigen-antibody complexes can increase the sensitivity of the procedure up to fivefold. This may improve its diagnostic utility,[1] especially for neonatal testing. The detection of p24 antigen in serum precedes seroconversion by a few days.[2,3] In July, 1995, the FDA's Blood Product Advisory Committee (BPAC) had advised against the test for several reasons. First, the cost of the additional test would be about $80 million nationally and would prevent as few as 10 HIV transmissions. Second, until 1996 there was not an FDA-licensed test that could be automated or performed in the time the other seven infectious disease tests were completed. Despite the above arguments, in early 1996, the FDA required all blood for transfusion be screened for the HIV p24 antigen.

A new EIA has been developed recently that will simultaneously detect HIV p24 antigen and HIV antibody in a direct assay format. This assay has been evaluated for large scale blood screening.[4]

Footnotes

1. Bollinger RC Jr, Kline RL, Francis HL, et al, "Acid Dissociation Increases the Sensitivity of p24 Antigen Detection for the Evaluation of Antiviral Therapy and Disease Progression in Asymptomatic HIV-Infected Persons," *J Infect Dis*, 1992, 165(5):913-6.
2. Busch MP, Lee LL, Satten GA, et al, "Time Course of Detection of Viral and Serologic Markers Preceding Human Immunodeficiency Virus Type 1 Seroconversion: Implications for Screening of Blood and Tissue Donors," *Transfusion*, 1995, 35:91-7.
3. Martinez-Martinez P, Martin del Barrio E, DeBenito J, et al, "New Lineal Immunoenzymatic Assay for Simultaneous Detection of p24 Antigen and HIV Antibodies," *Eur J Clin Microbiol Infect Dis*, 1999, 18(8):591-4.
4. van Binsbergen J, Siebelink A, Jacobs A, et al, "Improved Performance of Seroconversion With a 4th Generation HIV Antigen/Antibody Assay," *J Virol Methods*, 1999, 82(1):77-84.

References

Le Pont F, Costagliola D, Rouzioux C, et al, "How Much Would the Safety of Blood Transfusion Be Improved by Including p24 Antigen in the Battery of Tests?" *Transfusion*, 1995, 35(7):542-7.

Nadal D, Boni J, Kind C, et al, "Prospective Evaluation of Amplification-Boosted ELISA for Heat-Denatured p24 Antigen for Diagnosis and Monitoring of Pediatric Human Immunodeficiency Virus Type 1 Infection," *J Infect Dis*, 1999, 180(4):1089-95.

Ortigao-de-Sampaio MB, Abreu TF, Linhares-de-Carvalho MI, et al, "Surrogate Markers of Disease Progression in HIV-Infected Children in Rio de Janeiro, Brazil," *J Trop Pediatr*, 1999, 45(5):299-302.

Internet Web Sites

www.who.int/health-topics/hiv.htm

♦ **HIV p24 gag** *see* HIV p24 Antigen Detection *on page 637*

♦ **HIV Phenotyping** *see* Human Immunodeficiency Virus, Resistance (Susceptibility) Testing *on page 640*

♦ **HIV, Quantitation** *see* Human Immunodeficiency Virus, Viral Load Assay *on page 640*

♦ **HIV Resistance** *see* Human Immunodeficiency Virus, Resistance (Susceptibility) Testing *on page 640*

♦ **HIV RT-PCR** *see* Human Immunodeficiency Virus DNA Amplification *on page 639*

♦ **HIV RT-PCR** *see* Human Immunodeficiency Virus, Viral Load Assay *on page 640*

♦ **HIV Susceptibility** *see* Human Immunodeficiency Virus, Resistance (Susceptibility) Testing *on page 640*

♦ **Hookworm** *see* Ova and Parasites, Stool *on page 666*

♦ **HPV DNA Probe Test** *see* Human Papillomavirus DNA Probe Test *on page 641*

♦ **HPV Hybrid Capture Assay** *see* Human Papillomavirus DNA Probe Test *on page 641*

♦ **HPV Screen** *see* Human Papillomavirus DNA Probe Test *on page 641*

♦ **HPV Type** *see* Human Papillomavirus DNA Probe Test *on page 641*

♦ ***H. pylori* Breath Tests** *see* Helicobacter pylori Biopsy-Based Tests: The Urease Tests, Culture, Cytology, and PCR *on page 620*

♦ **HSV-1 and HSV-2 Culture** *see* Herpes Simplex Virus Culture *on page 631*

♦ **HSV Antibodies** *see* Herpes Simplex Antibody *on page 630*

♦ **HSV Antigen Detection, Direct** *see* Herpes Simplex Virus Antigen Detection *on page 630*

♦ **HSV Culture** *see* Herpes Simplex Virus Culture *on page 631*

♦ **HSV DNA Detection** *see* Herpes Simplex Virus DNA Detection *on page 632*

HTLV-I/II Antibody

Related Information

Donation, Blood *on page 839*
HIV-1/HIV-2 Antibody Screen and Western Blot *on page 636*
Human Immunodeficiency Virus DNA Amplification *on page 639*
Risks of Transfusion *on page 861*

Synonyms Human T-Cell Leukemia Virus Type I and Type II; Human T-Lymphotropic Virus Type I Antibody

Test Includes Screening test with confirmation of positives

Abstract Human T-lymphotropic virus type I (HTLV-I) and type II (HTLV-II) are human retroviruses which are associated with adult T-cell leukemias and lymphomas as well as HTLV-associated myelopathy.

Specimen Serum

Container Red top tube

Reference Interval Negative

Use Screen blood and blood fractions for transfusion; evaluation of injection drug users; differential diagnosis of spastic paraparesis. HTLV-I is associated with adult T-cell lymphoblastic leukemia (ALL) and B-cell chronic lymphocytic leukemia. HTLV-II has been associated with a chronic HTLV-associated neurologic disorder.

Limitations The combined assay for anti HTLV-I/II is used mainly to screen blood donors. The assay cross reacts with only 80% of patients with antibody to HTLV-II.[1] The 20% of blood donors who are not detected by the assay for HTLV-II are not believed to be at sufficiently high risk to transmit the disease to warrant a separate assay.

Methodology Screen: enzyme immunoassay (EIA); confirmation: Western blot (WB) or radioimmunoprecipitation (RIPA). Western blot is associated with a large number of indeterminate results, neither positive nor negative.[2]

Additional Information HTLV-I is a pathogenic retrovirus found in Japan, the Caribbean, Eastern South America, West and Central Africa, and Papua New Guinea/Melanesia. Viral infection can be asymptomatic for prolonged periods (20 years) but is strongly associated with myelopathies and adult T-cell leukemia. Fewer than 5% of those infected with HTLV-I develop myelopathies or leukemia even after 20 years. Adult T-cell leukemia is an aggressive malignancy often associated with skin infiltrates and hypercalcemia. The viruses are tropic for T4 lymphocytes and are passed by sexual contact, blood fractions, injection drug abuse, from mother to fetus, and by breast milk. Pretransfusion testing for antibody to HTLV-I is now mandated by blood banks in order to avoid transfusion transmitted HTLV-I infection from asymptomatic infected donors. Retrospective studies from the American Red Cross have concluded that about 700 individuals per year received HTLV-I/II blood prior to 1988 when donor testing began. This risk is extremely low (0.024% per unit). Currently, two large studies of more than 600,000 U.S. blood donors showed seropositivity rate of 0.05%.[3] Early seroconverters have antibodies to the C-terminal region of gp46 (envelope protein) and to gag p19 and p24. The clinical course of HTLV-I infection, and the meaning of a positive serology are not yet well understood. Indeed, a recent study of hemophiliacs who were transfused regularly with plasma or its derivatives found no evidence of HTLV-I/II antibody in 179 patients.

HTLV-II appears to have a lower association with neoplasia than HTLV-I. The rare neoplasms associated with HTLV-II involve CD8 T lymphocytes. T-cell CD8 tumors may be related to HTLV-II, HTLV-I, or EBV. Co-infection of HIV with HTLV-II has been associated with cutaneous T-cell lymphoma. In contrast, most reports of co-infection with HTLV-I and HIV suggest a more favorable prognosis than for infection with HIV alone.[4]

Footnotes

1. CDCP and USPHS Working Group, "Guidelines for Counseling Persons Infected With Human T-lymphotropic Virus Type I (HTLV-I) and Type II (HTLV-II)," *Ann Intern Med*, 1993, 118(6):448-54.
2. Zaaijer HL, Cuypers HT, Dudok de Wit C, et al, "Results of 1-Year Screening of Donors in the Netherlands for Human T-lymphotropic Virus (HTLV) Type I: Significance of Western Blot Patterns for Confirmation of HTLV Infection," *Transfusion*, 1994, 34(10):877-80.

3. Ifthikharuddin JJ and Rosenblatt JD, "Human T-cell Lymphotropic Viruses Types I & II," *Principles and Practice of Infectious Diseases*, 5th ed, Mandell GL, Bennett JE, and Dolin R, eds, New York, NY: Churchill Livingstone, 2000, 1862-73.

4. Poiesz B, Dube D, Dube S, et al, "HTLV-II Associated Cutaneous T-Cell Lymphoma in a Patient With HIV-1 Infection," *N Engl J Med*, 2000, 342:930-6.

References

Blattner WA, "Human Retroviruses: Their Role in Cancer," *Proc Assoc Am Physicians*, 1999, 111(6):563-72.

Chen YM, Gomez-Lucia E, Okayama A, et al, "Antibody Profile of Early HTLV-I Infection," *Lancet*, 1990, 336(8725):1214-6.

Dow BC, "Noise in Microbiological Screening Assays," *Transfus Med*, 2000, 10(2):97-106.

Edlich RF, Arnette JA, and Williams FM, "Global Epidemic of Human T-Cell Lymphotropic Virus Type-I (HTLV-I)," *J Emerg Med*, 2000, 18(1):109-19.

Glynn SA, Murphy EL, Wright DJ, et al, "Laboratory Abnormalities in Former Blood Donors Seropositive for Human T-lymphotropic Virus Types 1 and 2: A Prospective Analysis," *Arch Pathol Lab Med*, 2000, 124(4):550-5.

Sullivan MT, Williams AE, Fang CT, et al, "Transmission of Human T-Lymphotropic Virus Types I and II by Blood Transfusion," *Arch Intern Med*, 1991, 151(10):2043-8.

Internet Web Sites

www.apha.org/public_health/aids.htm
www.emedicine.com
www.hivatis.org

Human Immunodeficiency Virus Culture

Related Information

CD4/CD8 Enumeration *on page 511*
HIV-1/HIV-2 Antibody Screen and Western Blot *on page 636*
HIV p24 Antigen Detection *on page 637*
Human Immunodeficiency Virus DNA Amplification *on page 639*
Zidovudine, Serum or Plasma *on page 771*

Synonyms AIDS Virus Culture; HIV Culture; HTLV-III Culture

Specimen Whole blood (20-40 mL), cerebrospinal fluid (10 mL), other body fluids, biopsies.[1] See special precautions in Specimen Collection Introduction *on page 35*.

Container Green top (heparin) tube for blood, sterile container for CSF and other fluids

Collection Routine venipuncture. Invert the tubes several times after drawing the blood to be sure the blood is thoroughly mixed with the heparin.

Storage Instructions Do not freeze or refrigerate blood specimen. Some laboratories require that the specimen be received in the laboratory the same day the specimen is obtained.

Causes for Rejection Specimen leaking from container, blood frozen or refrigerated

Turnaround Time Positive cultures are usually reported after two consecutive positive reverse transcriptase assays. Blood cultures are usually incubated 4 weeks and some laboratories incubate CSF cultures 8 weeks before reporting as negative.

Reference Interval No virus isolated

Use Test for active HIV infection, especially in infants

Limitations This test has largely been replaced by the HIV PCR. The use of cultures for HIV is now a tool for investigation. A negative culture cannot be assumed to rule out the presence of the virus. Fresh human lymphocytes are needed for growth of HIV. These cells are costly and more difficult to maintain than are cell lines. Many laboratories do not have the capability of HIV culture. Culture of HIV poses a risk to laboratory personnel.

Methodology Growth of virus in lymphocyte culture and subsequent (indirect) testing for presence of virus in culture supernatant fluids by enzyme immunoassay (EIA) or reverse transcriptase assay

Additional Information Serology for detection of HIV antibodies is widely available and is the diagnostic tool favored along with confirmation of specificity by Western blot.[2] HIV PCR has become the standard technique to demonstrate viral presence. HIV can be cultured from plasma or peripheral blood mononuclear cells (PBMCs). PBMCs are cocultured with lymphocytes from an HIV-negative donor using cell stimulation with phytohemagglutinin and interleukin-2. Weekly samples of supernatant are analyzed for p24 antigen to reveal viral growth. Growth usually occurs within 3 weeks. This is a highly specific, difficult test. It has been used to detect HIV infection in neonates, but was positive in only 50% of infected newborns during the first month of life. PCR may be more sensitive than culture and has become the favored test.

Footnotes

1. Clarke JR, Williamson JD, Mitchell DM, "Comparative Study of the Isolation of Human Immunodeficiency Virus From the Lung and Peripheral Blood of AIDS Patients," *J Med Virol*, 1993, 39(3):196-9.

2. Abb J, "Diagnostic and Prognostic Significance of Testing for HIV Antigen," *Clin Immunol Newslet*, 1988, 9:85-7.

References

Corrigan GE, Al-Khalili L, Malmsten A, et al, "Differences in Reverse Transcriptase Activity Versus p24 Antigen Detection in Cell Culture, When Comparing a Homogeneous Group of HIV Type 1 Subtype B Viruses With a Heterogeneous Group of Divergent Strains," *AIDS Res Hum Retroviruses*, 1998, 14:347-52.

Crowe SM and Sonza S, "HIV-1 Can Be Recovered From a Variety of Cells Including Peripheral Blood Monocytes of Patients Receiving Highly Active Antiretroviral Therapy: A Further Obstacle to Eradication," *J Leukoc Biol*, 2000, 68(3):345-50.

Fiscus SA, Welles SI, Spector SA, et al, "Length of Incubation Time for Human Immunodeficiency Virus Cultures," *J Clin Microbiol*, 1995, 33:246-7.

Nielsen K and Bryson YJ, "Diagnosis of HIV Infection in Children," *Pediatr Clin North Am*, 2000, 47(1):39-63.

Panther LA, Tucker L, Xu C, et al, "Genital Tract Human Immunodeficiency Virus Type 1 Shedding and Inflammation and HIV-1 Env Diversity in Perinatal HIV-1 Transmission," *J Infect Dis*, 2000, 181:555-63.

Internet Web Sites

www.apha.org/public_health/aids.htm
www.emedicine.com
www.hivatis.org

Human Immunodeficiency Virus DNA Amplification

Related Information

HIV-1/HIV-2 Antibody Screen and Western Blot *on page 636*
HIV p24 Antigen Detection *on page 637*
HTLV-I/II Antibody *on page 638*
Human Immunodeficiency Virus Culture *on page 639*
Polymerase Chain Reaction *on page 713*
Viral Culture, Tissue *on page 695*

Synonyms HIV DNA Amplification Assay; HIV DNA PCR Test; Human Immunodeficiency Virus (HIV) Proviral DNA by Polymerase Chain Reaction Amplification; PCR for HIV DNA

Applies to HIV RT-PCR

Test Includes HIV proviral DNA is detected by amplifying specific DNA sequences from peripheral blood lymphocytes and subsequent hybridization with a specific HIV DNA probe.

Abstract Human immunodeficiency virus (HIV) contains an RNA genome that will incorporate into host DNA as proviral DNA. The target cells of this virus are the CD4 (T4) T-lymphocytes (helper T cells) and monocytes/macrophage populations, and lymph node dendritic cells; however, during infection, few such peripheral blood cells contain HIV.[1] To detect the incorporated viral genome, the DNA must be amplified. This procedure specifically increases the amount of DNA from within the HIV genome, and the amplified DNA product is detected by specific binding to an HIV probe. The DNA detection assay is used for the diagnosis of HIV in infants. It is also used as a method to recover the HIV genome when the HIV viral load is undetectable in plasma.

Specimen Peripheral blood lymphocytes from 10-20 mL whole blood

Container Two yellow top (ACD) or lavender top (EDTA) tubes should be collected. Consult the laboratory performing the test.

Storage Instructions Tubes of blood can be sent directly to the laboratory at ambient temperature and should arrive within 48 hours of collection.

Causes for Rejection Specimens with inadequate volume or more than 48 hours old may be rejected.

Turnaround Time 2 weeks is usually required. Turnaround time may vary with individual laboratories.

Reference Interval No HIV viral DNA detected in peripheral blood lymphocytes.

Use HIV detection in patients with unusual or indeterminant HIV serology. It may also be useful in patients with immunodeficiency syndromes characterized by a negative HIV serology and Western blot tests. It can be used in infants who have positive maternal antibody.

Methodology DNA amplification is used, polymerase chain reaction (PCR).[2] DNA is extracted from peripheral blood lymphocytes. The amplified HIV DNA is confirmed by hybridization with an HIV-specific DNA probe. Hybridization with the HIV DNA probe can be detected using autoradiography or enzymatic detection procedures.

Additional Information The initial step in diagnosis of HIV infection is dependent on the detection of specific antibodies. The antibody screening test commonly used is the enzyme-linked immunosorbent assay (ELISA) with a confirmatory Western or immunoblot. These serologic assays will identify individuals with prior exposure to HIV or passively obtained antibody such as babies born to HIV-positive mothers. In addition, serologic tests may not identify patients with recent active infection. Due to this problem, other tests have also been used to document the presence of HIV, such as viral antigen assays, viral culture, and the detection of viral DNA.[1,2] Viral culture of HIV is a prolonged procedure taking 3-4 weeks; it suffers from a lack of sensitivity in that HIV cannot be consistently isolated from seropositive patients.[3] Studies using *in situ* hybridization have shown that (Continued)

Human Immunodeficiency Virus DNA Amplification
(Continued)

few peripheral blood mononuclear cells may actually harbor HIV proviral DNA (1 in 10,000).[1] This makes it difficult to directly assay for HIV proviral DNA. Thus, DNA amplification assays have been developed to detect HIV DNA. The assay most commonly used is the polymerase chain reaction (PCR), which can amplify a single copy of DNA by 10^5 to 10^6 fold.[4] The PCR test for HIV DNA is useful in resolution of unsatisfactory HIV antibody test results and in determination of the status of children born to mothers with positive HIV serology[2] without the need for viral culture. It has been superseded largely by the plasma HIV RT-PCR.

Footnotes
1. Harper ME, Marselle LM, Gallo RC, et al, "Detection of Lymphocytes Expressing Human T-lymphotropic Virus Type III in Lymph Nodes and Peripheral Blood From Infected Individuals by *In Situ* Hybridization," *Proc Natl Acad Sci U S A*, 1986, 83(3):772-6.
2. Lindegren ML, Byers RH, Thomas P, et al, "Trends in Perinatal Transmission of HIV/AIDS in the United States," *JAMA*, 1999, 282(6):531-8.
3. Crowe SM and Sonza S, "HIV-1 Can Be Recovered From a Variety of Cells Including Peripheral Blood Monocytes of Patients Receiving Highly Active Antiretroviral Therapy: A Further Obstacle to Eradication," *J Leukoc Biol*, 2000, 68(3):345-50.
4. Saiki RK, Gelfand DH, Stoffel S, et al, "Primer-Directed Enzymatic Amplification of DNA With a Thermostable DNA Polymerase," *Science*, 1988, 239(4839):487-91.

References
Engels EA, Rosenberg PS, O'Brien TR, et al, "Plasma HIV Viral Load in Patients With Hemophilia and Late-Stage HIV Diseases: A Measure of Current Immune Suppression," *Ann Intern Med*, 1999, 131(4):256-64.

International Perinatal HIV Group, "The Mode of Delivery and the Risk of Vertical Transmission of Human Immunodeficiency Virus Type 1," *N Engl J Med*, 1999, 340(13):977-87.

Kane B, "Beyond HIV Viral Load Testing," *Ann Intern Med*, 1999, 131:637-8.

Internet Web Sites
www.apha.org/public_health/aids.htm
www.emedicine.com
www.hivatis.org

♦ **Human Immunodeficiency Virus (HIV) Proviral DNA by Polymerase Chain Reaction Amplification** *see* Human Immunodeficiency Virus DNA Amplification *on page 639*

Human Immunodeficiency Virus, Resistance (Susceptibility) Testing

Synonyms HIV Genotyping; HIV Phenotyping; HIV Resistance; HIV Susceptibility

Applies to Susceptibility of HIV-1 Virus to Antiviral Therapy

Test Includes Genotypic or phenotypic susceptibility studies

Abstract Resistance of HIV to antiretroviral medications that the patient is taking is a common cause of treatment failure and results in increased viral load. Use of genotypic or phenotypic susceptibility tests may be used to help select change of therapy in failing regimens.

Specimen Plasma

Container Lavender top (EDTA) tube or SPS® tube

Turnaround Time Consult reference laboratory.

Use Detect mutations in HIV that correlate with therapy failure

Limitations The test system evaluates the predominant viruses present in the specimen. HIV exists as complex mixtures of virus with multiple strains being present, often with varying susceptibilities. Resistance demonstrated by testing is useful evidence to avoid that therapeutic agent. Lack of resistance on the test may not confer susceptibility. Assays for resistance may provide information only on the predominant circulating variants, and may miss minor variants.[1] Such minor variants may predominate when antiviral therapy effectively controls the previously predominant virus. The cost of testing can be high.

Methodology Genotyping requires the amplification of the reverse transcriptase gene and/or the protease gene followed by detection of mutations. Mutations can be detected by direct sequencing (costly) or by blotting techniques such as Line Probe Assay (LIPA).[2]

Phenotyping requires growth of the HIV isolate and testing the viral replication with various drugs in tissue culture.

Additional Information There are many reasons HIV therapy fails, including missing doses of complex drug schedules, lack of adsorption of certain drugs due to interference from foods or other medications, and low serum or tissue levels of medications due to metabolism interactions, usually at the P-450 level. When the HIV viral load increases to significant levels, HIV susceptibility testing has become an important adjunct in selected individuals.

When change of therapy is contemplated, along with the history of each of the antiretroviral drugs the patient has taken, knowledge of resistance to these and sometimes to other drugs the patient has not taken is provided in either the genotype or phenotype susceptibilities. This allows rational selection of a probable effective regimen. Interpretation of genotype susceptibility testing is complicated by the need to know which codon changes are likely to convey resistance to each medication. Interpretation of phenotype susceptibility is more readily understandable by giving the susceptibility or resistance pattern of the predominantly tested virus.

Knowledge of resistance to commonly used therapies of the major classes of highly active antiretroviral therapy (HAART) helps select optimal choices for initial therapy, or determine which modifications are needed because of increasing viral load during therapy.

Footnotes
1. Hirsch MS, Conway B, D'Aquila RT, et al, "Antiretroviral Drug Resistance Testing in Adults With HIV Infection," *JAMA*, 1998, 279(24):1984-91.
2. Wilson JW, Bean P, Robins T, et al, "Comparative Evaluation of Three Human Immunodeficiency Virus Genotyping Systems: The HIV-Genotyp® Method, the HIV PRT GeneChip Assay, and the HIV-1 RT Line Probe Assay," *J Clin Microbiol*, 2000, 38(8):3022-8.

References
Alcorn TM and Faruki H, "HIV Resistance Testing: Methods, Utility, and Limitations," *Mol Diagn*, 2000, 5(3):159-68.

O'Brien WA, "Resistance Against Reverse Transcriptase Inhibitors," *Clin Infect Dis*, 2000, 30(S2):S185-92.

Omrani AS and Pillay D, "Multidrug Resistant HIV-1," *J Infect*, 2000, 41(1):5-11.

Romano G, Kasten M, and Giordano A, "Current Understanding of AIDS Pathogenesis," *Anticancer Res*, 1999, 19(4B):3157-66.

Internet Web Sites
www.apha.org/public_health/aids.htm
www.emedicine.com
www.hivatis.org

♦ **Human Immunodeficiency Virus Type I, Subtype/Clade B** *see* Human Immunodeficiency Virus, Viral Load Assay *on page 640*

Human Immunodeficiency Virus, Viral Load Assay

Synonyms HIV-1 Viral Load Assay; HIV Burden; HIV Load; Quantitative HIV PCR

Applies to Branched Chain DNA Assay; Cytomegalovirus Viral Load; Hepatitis B Viral Load; Hepatitis C Viral Load; HIV, Quantitation; HIV RT-PCR; Human Immunodeficiency Virus Type I, Subtype/Clade B; Human Papillomavirus Viral Load

Test Includes Amplification of HIV nucleic acid from plasma and quantitation based on internal standard

Abstract Serial HIV viral load monitoring is the current standard of care for persons with HIV disease, both for initiation of therapy, and for revision of therapy due to less-than-acceptable response. The HIV viral load detects cell-free plasma viral RNA by using amplification techniques such as PCR or bDNA. These quantitative techniques are very sensitive, allowing detection of virus as low as 50 Eq/mL. During therapy, viral loads are usually quite stable, and often become undetectable (lower limits of assays are usually <50 or <400 Eq/mL). Small transient increases in viral loads may occur when the therapy is adequate, but a progressive increase in loads over an interval of 1-3 months, or a single high viral load (>10,000) is taken to mean that a revision in therapy may be appropriate.

Aftercare Patients require in-depth discussion and counseling to learn to cope with changes in numbers, both of HIV loads and CD4 lymphocyte counts.

Specimen Blood, plasma

Container Lavender top (EDTA) tube or SPS® tube

Causes for Rejection HIV-1 plasma viral load testing performed as initial screening for diagnosis of HIV may show false-positive results. Reject such specimens unless the pretest chance for HIV is high, and the viral load is also high (>100,000 Eq/mL).[1] Plasma should be separated from clot within 3-4 hours and frozen to prevent a false decrease in viral load.

Use Monitor progression of HIV disease and detect therapy failure

Limitations False positives do occur in persons without HIV infection if the HIV viral load is used as a screening test.

Contraindications Informed consent is required in many areas.

Methodology Usually reverse-transcriptase polymerase chain reaction (RT-PCR) technology (Roche Amplicor Monitor, Basel, Switzerland) or branched chain DNA assay (Chiron Quantiplex, Emeryville, California) is used.

Additional Information To determine the rapidity of HIV disease progression, quantitation of serum virus is performed. The viral load with the CD4 lymphocyte counts are used together to determine whether therapy should be initiated in early illness, and whether therapy should be changed later. These recommendations are subject to change as information accumulates on the balance between risk of developing AIDS versus risk of problems with medications. Plasma HIV-1 RNA load correlates with rapidity of progression to AIDS after seroconversion.[2] Very low viral loads are associated with long-term disease-free states even without antiretroviral therapy.[3] The goal of highly active antiretroviral therapy (HAART) of HIV is to reduce the viral load to an undetectable level (<50 copies/mL). This is believed to prevent acquisition of resistance mutations.[4] See table.

The use of screening ELISA followed by Western blot has a very low false-positive rate (approximately 0.0006%). Antibodies are not detectable for about 3-4 weeks after exposure to the virus. In persons who will seroconvert, the HIV quantitative load may be detected by day 4-11 after exposure, and primary seroconversion HIV syndromes may occur toward the end of that time. This has led to the use of the quantitative HIV test to detect early

HIV infection. However, commercial assays now available are not approved for use in antibody-negative patients. When used in this manner, both the number of viral copies and the time after presumed exposure should be considered. Viral loads, when the person is not HIV infected, have been reported to be low (<2000) (ie, false-positive viral loads). An infected person would be expected to have a viral load in excess of 10,000 and usually much greater, if the viral load were used to screen for HIV.

HIV viral loads have also been correlated with transmission of virus to others in heterosexual contacts, as well as maternal transmission during childbirth. In Africa, among heterosexual couples, there was no HIV transmission when the viral loads were <1500 copies HIV-1 RNA/mL.[5]

Indications for the Initiation of Antiretroviral Therapy in the Chronically HIV-1 Infected Patient

Clinical Category	CD4[4] T-Cell Count	Plasma HIV RNA	Recommendation
Symptomatic (AIDS, severe symptoms)	Any value	Any value	Treat
Asymptomatic, AIDS	CD4+ T cells <200/mm³	Any value	Treat
Asymptomatic	CD4+ >200/mm³ but <350/mm³	Any value	Offer treatment
Asymptomatic	CD4+ T cells >350/mm³	>30,000 (bDNA) or >55,000 (RT-PCR)	Consider therapy
Asymptomatic	CD4+ T cells >350/mm³	<30,000 (bDNA) or <55,000 (RT-PCR)	Defer therapy. Many experts would defer therapy and observe, recognizing that the 3-year risk of developing AIDS in untreated patients is <15%.

Clinical benefit has been demonstrated in controlled trials only for patients with CD4+ T cells <200/mm³. However, most experts would offer therapy at a CD4+ T-cell threshold <350/mm³. All decisions to initiate therapy should be based on prognosis for disease-free survival in the absence of treatment, the potential benefits and risks of therapy, and the willingness of the patient to accept therapy.

Adapted from "DHHS Guidelines for the Use of Antiretroviral Agents in HIV-Infected Adults and Adolescents," *The HIV/AIDS Treatment Information Service (ATIS)*, 2001.

Footnotes

1. Rich JD, Merriman NA, Mylonakis E, et al, "Misdiagnosis of HIV Infection by HIV-1 Plasma Viral Load Testing: A Case Series," *Ann Intern Med*, 1999, 130(1):37-9.
2. Mellors JW, Kingsley LA, Rinaldo CR, et al, "Quantitation of HIV-1 RNA in Plasma Predicts Outcome After Seroconversion," *Ann Intern Med*, 1995, 122(8):573-9.
3. Learmont JC, Geczy AF, Mills J, et al, "Immunologic and Virologic Status After 14 to 18 Years of Infection With an Attenuated Strain of HIV-1," A Report From the Sydney Blood Bank Cohort, *N Engl J Med*, 1999, 340(22):1715-22.
4. Hirsch MS, Conway B, D'Aquila RT, et al, "Antiretroviral Drug Resistance Testing in Adults With HIV Infection: Implications for Clinical Management," International AIDS Society - USA Panel, *JAMA*, 1998, 279(24):1984-91.
5. Quinn TC, Wawer MJ, Sewankambo N, et al, "Viral Load and Heterosexual Transmission of Human Immunodeficiency Virus Type 1," Rakai Project Study Group, *N Engl J Med*, 2000, 342(13):921-9.

References

Bagasra O, Steiner RM, and Ballas SK, "Viral Burden and Disease Progression in HIV-1-Infected Patients With Sickle Cell Anemia," *Am J Hematol*, 1998, 59(3):199-207.

Helbert M and Breuer J, "Monitoring Patients With HIV Disease," *J Clin Pathol*, 2000, 53(4):266-72.

Henry K, "The Case for More Cautious, Patient-Focused Antiretroviral Therapy," *Ann Intern Med*, 2000, 132(4):306-11.

Laufer M and Scott GB, "Medical Management of HIV Disease in Children," *Pediatr Clin North Am*, 2000, 47(1):127-53.

Nolte FS, "Impact of Viral Load Testing on Patient Care," *Arch Pathol Lab Med*, 1999, 123(11):1011-4.

Internet Web Sites

www.apha.org/public_health/aids.htm
www.emedicine.com
www.hivatis.org

Human Papillomavirus DNA Probe Test

Related Information

bcl-2 Gene Rearrangement *on page 720*
Cervical/Vaginal Cytology *on page 377*
Histopathology *on page 59*
p53, Functional Assay/Sequencing *on page 728*
Polymerase Chain Reaction *on page 713*
Viral Culture, Tissue *on page 695*
Viral Culture, Urogenital *on page 696*

Synonyms DNA Hybridization Test for HPV; DNA Probe Test for HPV; HPV DNA Probe Test; HPV Hybrid Capture Assay; HPV Screen; HPV Type; ViraPap®; ViraType®

Test Includes Screening specimens for the presence of HPV DNA and optional determination of the specific type(s) of HPV present in positive specimens

Abstract The diagnosis of human papillomavirus (HPV) infections is usually clinical, made during the physical examination. But because of the variety of

diseases HPV causes, and because some forms of HPV do not exhibit examination abnormalities, cytology, histopathology, and HPV nucleic antigen tests may be needed. HPV of the uterine cervix is venereally transmitted. It causes koilocytosis, condyloma acuminatum, squamous intraepithelial lesion (SIL), cervical intraepithelial neoplasia (CIN), and cervical carcinoma.[1] See Cervical/Vaginal Cytology *on page 377*. HPV infections of the cervix frequently cause low-grade SIL and are commonplace in young, sexually active women. Such infections often resolve spontaneously, but some progress. Risk factors which support progression are thought to include cell-mediated immunity and reproduction factors, as well as HPV type and intensity.[2]

HPV infections of the uterine cervix are associated with >90% of invasive squamous cell carcinomas and with variants. Such variants include large cell keratinizing, large cell nonkeratinizing, and small cell carcinomas. HPV-positive lymphoepithelioma-like carcinoma of the uterine cervix has recently been reported.[3] Although a substantial incidence of HPV infection in sexually active young women is recognized, a role for conservative management has been discussed.[4]

HPV has been detected in certain tumors of the upper airway. Many other such viral infections probably have little oncogenic potential.

Patient Preparation At least 2 days must elapse between the time acetic acid or iodine preparations are used and the time swab specimens are taken. Biopsies can be taken immediately after the use of acetic acid or iodine.

Specimen Cervical swab, cervical biopsy, vulvar biopsy

Container Specific tubed transport medium provided by the laboratory. Do **not** substitute.

Sampling Time At the time of clinical suspicion of HPV infection

Collection Use **specific** swab provided by the laboratory to collect endocervical and ectocervical cells similar to the manner in which Pap smear cells are taken. Obtain biopsy in usual manner. Biopsies **must** be ≤3 mm. Cervical cells also can be taken by **scraping** the cervix with an appropriate spatula. Place swabs, scrapings, and biopsies into specific transport medium. **Important**: Collection of a sufficiently large number of epithelial cells is mandatory. However, scraping/removal of cells to the point of bleeding should not be done, because visible blood in specimen might reduce the chance of detection of HPV.

Storage Instructions Freeze biopsies in transport medium immediately. Swab or scrape specimens can be stored at room temperature for several days, but for simplicity, can be frozen immediately.

Causes for Rejection Some laboratories reject visibly bloody specimens.

Turnaround Time Usually 4 days to 2 weeks, but depends on laboratory protocol and lability of reagents

Reference Interval HPV has been found in genital lesions of both normal and symptomatic persons.[5,6] HPV has been detected in patients whose exfoliative cytology smears are morphologically normal.[7]

Use Theoretically useful in making decisions regarding treatment, follow-up visits and tests, management, and prognosis of patients with possible HPV infections, including proliferative, atypical lesions of the uterine cervix and the anorectal mucosa. Such lesions include carcinomas and their precursors. A role for HPV DNA testing for patients with equivocal results of cervical/vaginal cytologic evaluation exists.[1,8]

Limitations

- Detects only a few of the 75 genotypes of HPV, of which 20 have been isolated from the female genital tract.
- Can be negative with accompanying cytological changes.
- Can be positive without accompanying cytological changes; by Southern blot hybridization, HPV DNA is found in ~15% of morphologically normal cervices.
- Viral integration is not always found in invasive carcinoma of uterine cervix.
- Can give false-negative results if specimens are visibly bloody or if an insufficient sample of HPV-infected cells is obtained.
- Latent viral infection does not cause morphologic abnormalities.
- A fraction of patients with high-risk HPV infection have only low-grade lesions when biopsied.
- A wide variety of HPV types is found in CIN 1.
- Can give borderline results.
- The number of viral copies in invasive carcinoma of cervix may be <100 copies/cell.[9]
- Expensive

Although HPV plays an important role in the development of genital cancers, especially in women, but also in men, the cost-effectiveness of HPV DNA detection and typing has not yet been defined. In addition, only a small percent of persons infected with oncogenic types actually develop neoplasia.[7,10] Part of the explanation for this may be that in benign HPV lesions, the viral DNA is extrachromosomal. When HPV DNA is present in cancer, it is usually integrated.

Methodology Disruption and digestion of specimen, attachment of specimen DNA to filters, and probing denatured (HPV) DNA with commercially available nucleic acid probes which are specific for HPV types 6, 11, 16, 18, 31, 33, and 35. Amplification by polymerase chain reaction (PCR) is also used to detect HPV types in cervical and anorectal specimens. *In situ* hybridization (ISH), as well as PCR, is used,[11] but the threshold at which HPV DNA is detected by ISH is less than that by PCR.[3]
(Continued)

Human Papillomavirus DNA Probe Test *(Continued)*

Additional Information More than 75 HPV types have been recognized, with much overlap in epithelial tumors of the skin or mucus membranes produced by various types. The diseases include plantar warts, common warts on the hands, flat warts, genital condyloma acuminata, recurrent respiratory papilloma, oral epithelial hyperplasia of Heck, and conjunctival papillomas. Neoplastic lesions include conjunctival carcinomas.

Certain types are associated with cervical neoplasia, including types 16, 18, 31, or 45. The presence of HPV types 6/11, 16/18, and 31/33/35 has been associated with "low" (condyloma), "high," and "moderate" risk of development of cervical cancer, respectively.[7,12,13] HPV 16 is found in 20% of CIN 1, 40% of CIN 2, and 66% of CIN 3, and is found in about 50% of the invasive squamous cell carcinomas of the cervix. HPV 18 is found in about 20% of invasive cervical squamous cell carcinomas. Less frequently, a dozen other types may be associated with malignancy, especially carcinoma of the cervix. The utility of HPV typing continues to be studied. Not all HPV-infected subjects develop cervical carcinoma, even when infected with oncogene types 16, 18, 31, 33, or 35.[7] The standard of care does not include typing of HPV as part of patient management, but does include the clinical identification and treatment of sites of involvement of female genital skin and mucus membranes. The HPV viral load of HPV 16 in cervical carcinoma *in situ* appears to correlate with development of cervical carcinoma (*in situ*).[10]

Footnotes

1. Cuzick J, "Human Papillomavirus Testing for Primary Cervical Cancer Screening," *JAMA*, 2000, 283(1):108-9.
2. Schiffman MH and Brinton LA, "The Epidemiology of Cervical Carcinogenesis," *Cancer*, 1995, 76(Suppl 10):1888-901.
3. Noel JC, Lespagnard L, Fayt I, et al, "Evidence of Human Papilloma Virus Infection but Lack of Epstein-Barr Virus in Lymphoepithelioma-Like Carcinoma of Uterine Cervix: Report of Two Cases and Review of the Literature," *Hum Pathol*, 2001, 32(1):135-8.
4. Ho GY, Bierman R, Beardsley L, et al, "Natural History of Cervicovaginal Papillomavirus Infection in Young Women," *N Engl J Med*, 1998, 338(7):423-8.
5. Meanwell CA, Cox MF, Blackledge G, et al, "HPV 16 DNA in Normal and Malignant Cervical Epithelium: Implications for the Aetiology and Behavior of Cervical Neoplasia," *Lancet*, 1987, 1(8535):703-7.
6. de Villiers EM, Wagner D, Schneider A, et al, "Human Papillomavirus Infections in Women With and Without Abnormal Cervical Cytology," *Lancet*, 1987, 2(8561):703-6.
7. Chua KL and Hjerpe A, "Persistence of Human Papillomavirus (HPV) Infections Preceding Cervical Carcinoma," *Cancer*, 1996, 77(1):121-7.
8. Manos MM, Kinney WK, Hurley LB, et al, "Identifying Women With Cervical Neoplasia. Using Human Papillomavirus DNA Testing for Equivocal Papanicolaou Results," *JAMA*, 1999, 281(17):1605-10.
9. Van den Brule A, Snijders P, Meijer C, et al, "PCR Based Detection of Genital HPV Genotypes: An Update and Future Perspective," *Papillomavirus Reviews: Current Research on Papillomavirus*, Lacey C, ed, Leeds, UK: Leeds University Press, 1996, 181-9.
10. Josefsson AM, Magnusson PK, Ylitalo N, et al, "Viral Load of Human Papillomavirus 16 and Determinant for Development of Cervical Carcinoma *In Situ*: A Nested Case-Control Study," *Lancet*, 2000, 355(9222):2189-93.
11. Shroyer KR, Brookes CG, Markham NE, et al, "Detection of Human Papillomavirus in Anorectal Squamous Cell Carcinoma. Correlation With Basaloid Pattern of Differentiation," *Am J Clin Pathol*, 1995, 104(3):299-305.
12. zurHausen H and Schneider A, "The Role of Papillomaviruses in Human Anogenital Cancer," *The Papovaviridae*, Volume 2, Salzmann NP and Howley PM, eds, New York, NY: Plenum, 1987, 245-63.
13. Shah KV and Buscema J, "Genital Warts, Papillomaviruses, and Genital Malignancies," *Annu Rev Med*, 1988, 39:371-9.

References

Bonnez W and Reichman RC, "Papillomaviruses," *Principles and Practice of Infectious Diseases*, 5th ed, Mandell GL, Bennett JE, and Dolin R, eds, New York, NY: Churchill Livingstone, 2000, 1630-44.

Crum CP and Roche JK, "Molecular Pathology of the Lower Female Genital Tract - The Papillomavirus Model," *Am J Surg Pathol*, 1990, 14(Suppl 1):26-33.

Herrington CS, Evans MF, Gray W, et al, "Morphological Correlation of Human Papillomavirus Infection of Matched Cervical Smears and Biopsies From Patients With Persistent Mild Cervical Cytological Abnormalities," *Hum Pathol*, 1995, 26(9):951-5.

Milde-Langosch K, Schreiber C, Becker G, et al, "Human Papillomavirus Detection in Cervical Adenocarcinoma by Polymerase Chain Reaction," *Hum Pathol*, 1993, 24(6):590-4.

Shroyer KR, Brookes CG, Markham NE, et al, "Detection of Human Papillomavirus in Anorectal Squamous Cell Carcinoma. Correlation With Basaloid Pattern of Differentiation," *Am J Clin Pathol*, 1995, 104(3):299-305.

Internet Web Sites

hpv-web.lanl.gov

www.niaid.nih.gov/factsheets/stdhpv.htm

♦ **Human Papillomavirus Viral Load** *see* Human Immunodeficiency Virus, Viral Load Assay *on page 640*

♦ **Human T-Cell Leukemia Virus Type I and Type II** *see* HTLV-I/II Antibody *on page 638*

♦ **Human T-Lymphotropic Virus Type I Antibody** *see* HTLV-I/II Antibody *on page 638*

♦ **Hydatid Disease Serological Test** *see* Echinococcosis Serological Test *on page 602*

♦ **Hydatidosis Serological Test** *see* Echinococcosis Serological Test *on page 602*

♦ *Hymenolepis nana* *see* Ova and Parasites, Stool *on page 666*

♦ **Hymenopterae** *see* Arthropod Identification *on page 559*

♦ **Hyperalimentation Line Culture** *see* Bacterial Culture, Intravascular Device *on page 572*

♦ **i Antigen** *see* Cold Agglutinin Titer *on page 594*

♦ **I Antigen of Red Cell Membranes** *see* Cold Agglutinin Titer *on page 594*

♦ **IgG Antibodies to Rubella** *see* Rubella Serology *on page 677*

♦ **IgM and IgG Specific for Yellow Fever Virus** *see* Yellow Fever *on page 697*

♦ **IgM Antibodies to Rubella** *see* Rubella Serology *on page 677*

♦ **IM Serology** *see* Infectious Mononucleosis Screening Test *on page 643*

India Ink Preparation

Related Information

Bacterial Culture, Cerebrospinal Fluid *on page 569*
Cerebrospinal Fluid Analysis: Overview *on page 416*
Cerebrospinal Fluid Cytology *on page 376*
Cryptococcal Antigen Titer *on page 595*
Fungal Culture, Blood *on page 610*
Fungal Culture, Cerebrospinal Fluid *on page 611*
Fungus Smear, Stain *on page 615*

Synonyms Cerebrospinal Fluid India Ink Preparation

Applies to Mucicarmine Staining for *Cryptococcus*

Test Includes Staining of CSF sediment with India ink to detect the polysaccharide capsule surrounding the yeast

Abstract *Cryptococcus neoformans* is the most common central nervous system fungal disease in both immunocompetent hosts and patients with the acquired immunodeficiency syndrome (AIDS). Skin, lungs, spleen, kidneys, liver, and/or bone may also be infected. Pigeon droppings act as a year-round vector for dispersion of encapsulated yeast cells.

Patient Preparation Same as for culture of specific site

Specimen Cerebrospinal fluid

Storage Instructions Do **not** refrigerate.

Reference Interval No *Cryptococcus* identified

Critical Values Presence of encapsulated yeast

Use Establish a diagnosis of cryptococcal meningitis; organisms may be identified in cytologic preparations with Papanicolaou stain as well as with India ink.

Limitations This technique is only 30% to 75% sensitive in cases of cryptococcal meningitis. Cultures and rapid latex agglutination (LA) methods are more sensitive than direct preparations; therefore, the India ink preparation may be negative when the culture or LA test is positive. Many laboratories have abandoned the use of the India ink preparation in favor of LA. In facilities in which the LA test is not available, microscopic examination of centrifuged CSF stained with Giemsa, periodic acid - Schiff and/or Gram stain are more sensitive than India ink stain for the rapid detection of cryptococcal meningitis.[1] The mucinous capsules of *Cryptococcus* appear bright red on mucicarmine staining.[2] (Mucicarmine is available in almost all histopathology laboratories.)

Leukocytes in the specimen may be mistaken for yeast cells leading to a false-positive result,[3] and overall there is a substantial incidence of false positives.

Methodology Wet mount with India ink (nigrosin) for contrast. Centrifugation may concentrate organisms and improve sensitivity (10-20 minutes at 1500 g). Some sources of India ink are better than others for this purpose. Finer particles are desirable. Addition of 2% chromium mercury to the India ink preparation allows for the identification of characteristic structures of the organism.[4]

Footnotes

1. Sato Y, Osabe S, Kuno H, et al, "Rapid Diagnosis of Cryptococcal Meningitis by Microscopic Examination of Centrifuged Cerebrospinal Fluid Sediment," *J Neurol Sci*, 1999, 164(1):72-5.
2. Jaster JH and Malecha MJ, Images in Clinical Medicine, "Cryptococcal Meningitis," *N Engl J Med*, 1996, 335(26):1962.
3. Thiruchelvan N, Wuu KY, Arseculeratne SN, et al, "A Pseudo-Cryptococcal Artifact Derived From Leukocytes in Wet India Ink Mounts of Centrifuged Cerebrospinal Fluid," *J Clin Pathol*, 1998, 51(3):246-8.
4. Zerpa R, Huicho L, and Guillen A, "Modified India Ink Preparation for *Cryptococcus neoformans* in Cerebrospinal Fluid Specimens," *J Clin Microbiol*, 1996, 34(9):2290-1.

References

Perfect JR, Wong B, Chang YC, et al, "*Cryptococcus neoformans*: Virulence and Host Defenses," *Med Mycol*, 1998, 36(S1):79-86.

Roebuck DJ, Fisher DA, and Currie BJ, "Cryptococcosis in HIV-Negative Patients: Findings on Chest Radiography," *Thorax*, 1998, 53(7):554-7.

Internet Web Sites

www.cdc.gov/ncidod/dbmd/diseaseinfo/cryptococcosis_a.htm

♦ **Infant Botulism, Toxin Identification** *see* Botulism Diagnostic Procedures *on page 585*

Infectious Mononucleosis Screening Test

Related Information
Complete Blood Count *on page 419*
Cytomegalovirus Serology *on page 600*
Epstein-Barr Virus Culture *on page 607*
Epstein-Barr Virus Serology *on page 607*
Herpesvirus 6 DNA Detection *on page 633*
Heterophil Agglutinins *on page 635*
Heterophilic Antibodies *on page 191*
Lactate Dehydrogenase Isoenzymes, Serum *on page 206*
Lactate Dehydrogenase, Serum *on page 207*
Lymph Node Biopsy *on page 67*
Peripheral Blood: Differential Leukocyte Count *on page 464*

Synonyms Davidsohn Slide Test; Heterophil Antibody; IM Serology; Monospot™ Test; Monosticon® Dri-Dot® Test

Replaces Davidsohn Differential; Paul-Bunnell Davidsohn Test

Test Includes Screening for the presence of heterophil antibodies

Abstract The first patients described with infectious mononucleosis in 1926, had fever, sore throat, and lymphadenopathy. Abnormal lymphocytes were recognized, and the patients recovered spontaneously.[1]

Heterophil antibodies agglutinate sheep erythrocytes. They were first described in association with infectious mononucleosis (IM) by Paul and Bunnell in 1932.[2] These antibodies are usually detected at the onset of illness. A delayed appearance of heterophil antibodies may be associated with a prolonged illness.

Most cases involve patients 15-24 years of age.

Specimen Serum

Container Red top tube

Reference Interval Negative

Use Infectious mononucleosis (IM) is a self-limiting disease caused by the Epstein-Barr virus (EBV), characterized clinically by fever, cervical lymphadenitis, tonsillopharyngitis, and not infrequently, hepatosplenomegaly. Petechiae may be found on the palate. About 5% of patients are jaundiced.

Limitations Correlation with clinical findings is imperative since false-positive and negative results have been reported. About 10% of the adult population with IM will not develop heterophil antibodies. Failure to develop heterophil antibodies occurs even more frequently in younger children. In such instances, the presence of EBV antibodies is relevant. Less than 2% false positives have been reported with Hodgkin disease, lymphoma, acute lymphocytic leukemia, infectious hepatitis, pancreatic carcinoma, cytomegalovirus, Burkitt lymphoma, rheumatoid arthritis, malaria, and rubella. Rare unexplained positive horse cell screening tests have been reported with negative differential absorptions. Overall, the heterophil test has 95% specificity.

Methodology Heterophil antibodies are IgM. They can agglutinate sheep or horse red blood cells. In IM, heterophil antibodies can be absorbed by beef erythrocytes but not by guinea pig kidney. The classical present tests were introduced by Dr Israel Davidsohn. The rapid slide test is widely used.[3] It has essentially replaced the older Paul-Bunnell-Davidsohn technique, which is more sensitive but time consuming.

Additional Information The IM heterophil antibody appears in the serum of patients by the sixth to tenth day of illness. Highest titers are usually found in the second to third week. Antibody levels may remain detectable as briefly as 1 week, or persist for as long as a year; usual persistence is 4-8 weeks. The level of antibody activity is not correlated with the severity of disease or the degree of lymphocytosis. A positive test with the appropriate clinical and hematologic setting is sufficient to make the diagnosis of IM. If there is a clinical mononucleosis syndrome, but the screening test is negative, consider tests for EBV specific antibodies, CMV, HHV-6, and toxoplasmosis antibodies. Consider especially repeating this test after a short delay. Laboratory criteria for IM include peripheral blood lymphocytosis, >50% of WBCs with at least 10% of lymphocytes appearing reactive ("reactive lymphs") ie, virocytes. Serologic, hematologic, and clinical criteria all ideally should be met for diagnosis. The peripheral blood smear should be carefully examined.

Other tests often elevated in IM include aminotransferase with disproportionately greater elevations of LDH and alkaline phosphatase. The isomorphic pattern is found with LDH isoenzyme separation. Hemoglobin is usually normal in IM, while platelets are rarely worse than slightly diminished, findings in contrast to those of leukemia. Complications occur in some individuals.

Cold agglutinins, cryoglobulins, ANA, or rheumatoid factor may be increased in IM. A very useful review paper with diagrams of Epstein-Barr virus infections and clinical photographs has recently been published.[4]

The differential diagnosis includes streptococcal pharyngitis, CMV infection and rubella, and the acute retroviral syndrome. The last is a manifestation of HIV.[5] Herpesvirus 6 can cause a heterophil-negative mononucleosis syndrome.

Several commercial kits are available and exhibit varied sensitivities and specificities.[6,7]

Footnotes
1. Auwaerter PG, "Infectious Mononucleosis in Middle age," *JAMA*, 1999, 281(5):454-9.
2. Paul JR and Bunnell W, "The Presence of Heterophil Antibodies in Infectious Mononucleosis," *Am J Med Sci*, 1932, 183:90-104.
3. Lee CL, Davidsohn I, and Slaby R, "Horse Agglutinins in Infectious Mononucleosis," *Am J Clin Pathol*, 1968, 49:3-11.
4. Cohen JI, "Epstein-Barr Virus Infection," *N Engl J Med*, 2000, 343(7):481-92.
5. Bisno AL, "Pharyngitis," *N Engl J Med*, 2001, 344(3):205-11.
6. Rogers R, Windust A, and Gregory J, "Evaluation of a Novel Dry Latex Preparation for Demonstration of Infectious Mononucleosis Heterophil Antibody in Comparison With Three Established Tests," *J Clin Microbiol*, 1999, 37(1):95-8.
7. Elgh F and Linderholm M, "Evaluation of Six Commercially Available Kits Using Purified Heterophil Antigen for the Rapid Diagnosis of Infectious Mononucleosis Compared With Epstein-Barr Virus-Specific Serology," *Clin Diagn Virol*, 1996, 7(1):17-21.

References
Brigden ML, Au S, Thompson S, et al, "Infectious Mononucleosis in an Outpatient Population; Diagnostic Utility of 2 Automated Hematology Analyzers and the Sensitivity and Specificity of Hoagland's Criteria in Heterophil-Positive Patients" *Arch Pathol Lab Med*, 1999, 123(10):875-81.
Field PR and Dwyer DE, "Difficulties With the Serologic Diagnosis of Infectious Mononucleosis: A Review of the RCPA Quality Assurance Programs," *Pathology*, 1996, 28(3):270-6.
Hickey SM and Strasburger VC, "What Every Pediatrician Should Know About Infectious Mononucleosis in Adolescents," *Pediatr Clin North Am*, 1997, 44(6):1541-56.
Lennette ET, "Epstein-Barr Virus," *Manual of Clinical Microbiology*, 7th ed, Chapter 68, Murray PR, Baron EJ, Pfaller MA, et al, eds, Washington, DC: AMS Press, American Society for Microbiology, 1999, 912-18.

♦ **Influenza A and B Antibodies** *see* Influenza A and B Serology *on page 643*

♦ **Influenza A and B Antigen Testing** *see* Influenza Virus Culture *on page 644*

Influenza A and B Serology

Related Information
Influenza Virus Culture *on page 644*
Viral Culture, Respiratory Symptoms *on page 694*
Virus, Direct Detection by Fluorescence Antibody *on page 696*

Synonyms Influenza A and B Antibodies; Influenza A and B Titer

Test Includes IgG and IgM antibody titers to influenza A and/or B

Abstract Influenza type A and B viruses belong to the family Orthomyxoviridae. Infection with influenza is usually an acute, self-limiting, febrile illness that occurs in outbreaks seasonally (winter months in temperate climates). At times pandemics of influenza have occurred due to the emergence of a new virus to which the worldwide population lacks immunity.

Specimen Serum

Container Red top tube

Collection Acute and convalescent sera drawn 10-14 days apart are required.

Reference Interval Less than a fourfold increase in titer in paired sera; IgG <1:10, IgM <1:10

Use Although serologic diagnosis has been seldom practical or necessary during an influenza epidemic, serologic typing is valuable for epidemiology. Presence of specific IgM antibody indicates acute infection.

Methodology Complement fixation (CF), hemagglutination inhibition (HAI), single radial immunodiffusion (RID), enzyme-linked immunosorbent assay (ELISA)

See Virus, Direct Detection by Fluorescent Antibody *on page 696*.

Additional Information Virus-specific antibody can be detected in serum in the second week after a primary infection with influenza. These titers usually peak by 4 weeks. The antibody response is more rapid after reinfection.

The majority of neutralizing antibodies are directed against the hemagglutinin antigen and usually persist for months to years. Complement-fixing antibodies usually react with the influenza ribonucleoprotein and are type specific. These antibodies decline rapidly in weeks to months, since they are predominantly IgM.

Serology is useful in measuring the immunogenicity of annual vaccines.

Virus can be detected by culture; see Influenza Virus Culture *on page 644*.

References
Belshe RB, "Influenza Prevention and Treatment: Current Practices and New Horizons," *Ann Intern Med*, 1999, 131(8):621-4.
Betts RF, "Influenza Virus," *Principles and Practice of Infectious Diseases*, 4th ed, Mandell GL, Bennett JE, Dolin R, eds, New York, NY: Churchill Livingstone Inc, 1995.
Nelson JK, Shields MD, Stewart MC, et al, "Investigation of Seroprevalence of Respiratory Virus Infections in an Infant Population With a Multiantigen Fluorescence Immunoassay Using Heelprick Blood Samples Collected on Filter Paper," *Pediatr Res*, 1999, 45(6):799-802.
Pertmer TM and Robinson HL, "Studies on Antibody Responses Following Neonatal Immunization With Influenza Hemagglutinin DNA or Protein," *Virology*, 1999, 257(2):406-14.
(Continued)

Influenza A and B Serology *(Continued)*

Internet Web Sites
www.amm.co.uk/pubs/fa_influenza.htm
www.astdhpphe.org/infect/flu.html
www.cdc.gov/ncidod/diseases/flu/fluvirus.htm
www.who.int/health-topics/influenza.htm

♦ **Influenza A and B Titer** *see* Influenza A and B Serology *on page 643*

Influenza Virus Culture

Related Information
Bacterial Culture, Bronchoscopy/Bronchial Brush/Bronchoalveolar Lavage Specimen *on page 568*
Bronchial Washings Cytology *on page 374*
Bronchoalveolar Lavage (BAL) *on page 375*
Influenza A and B Serology *on page 643*
Parainfluenza Virus Culture *on page 668*
Viral Culture *on page 689*
Viral Culture, Respiratory Symptoms *on page 694*
Virus, Direct Detection by Fluorescent Antibody *on page 696*

Applies to Hemadsorbing Virus; Influenza A and B Antigen Testing

Test Includes Rapid culture for influenza A and B using specific monoclonal antibodies and immunofluorescence. Currently, some laboratories provide a rapid culture that will detect seven of the most common respiratory viruses (parainfluenza type 1, 2, and 3; influenza Type A and type B; adenovirus; and respiratory syncytial virus) in a single culture. Conventional viral culture is useful in that it may detect other viruses not detected by the rapid culture, and provides for influenza surveillance that is useful in typing for vaccine development.

Abstract Influenza causes a highly contagious acute respiratory disease.[1] Epidemics occur almost every year, typically from December to March in the Northern Hemisphere and from May to August in the Southern Hemisphere. Annual vaccination with trivalent vaccine has been shown to reduce the severity of illness.[2] Several antiviral agents are available for the treatment and prevention of influenza viral infections.[3,4]

Antigen testing of nasopharyngeal secretions is available.

Rapid (15-20 minutes) immunoassays, suitable for use in physician offices and clinics, detect influenza A and B viral antigens in nasal, nasopharyngeal, and sputum specimens.[4]

Specimen Throat or nasopharyngeal swab, bronchial washings, bronchoalveolar lavage; sputum specimens are not appropriate for isolation of influenza virus.

Use ≥1 mL of nasopharyngeal aspirate for influenza A and B antigen.[5]

Container Viral transport medium; cold virus transport medium for swabs

Sampling Time Specimens should be collected within 3 days of the onset of illness.

Storage Instructions Specimens should be placed into viral transport medium and kept cold at all times. Specimens should be delivered immediately to the laboratory. Do not freeze specimens.

Causes for Rejection Dry specimen; specimen submitted on bacterial Culturettes®; sputum, drainages of bile, pus, or exudate specimens

Turnaround Time 1-2 days for rapid (shell vial) culture; 2 weeks for conventional tube culture

Reference Interval No virus isolated

Use Isolate and identify influenza virus as an etiologic agent in croup, bronchitis, primary viral pneumonia, and combined influenza and bacterial pneumonia. Isolation permits surveillance of epidemic viral strains and aids in selection of influenza strains used in the production of the annual vaccine.

Influenza may cause complications in patients with other disorders, including bronchopulmonary disease, heart disease, and those with compromised immune status.

Limitations Negative culture does not rule out a viral etiology.

Methodology

Routine culture: Inoculation of specimens into cell cultures, incubation of cultures, observation for characteristic cytopathic effect (CPE), and identification/speciation by methods such as hemadsorption and fluorescent monoclonal antibodies specific for influenza virus A or B.

Rapid culture: Inoculation of cells in a shell vial, centrifugation, culture, and staining with an immunofluorescent monoclonal antibody.

Immunoassay procedures are available for nasal aspiration testing.

Additional Information The influenza pandemic of 1918 killed 21-40 million people, including 675,000 in the U.S. A book review providing a medical perspective is recommended.[6,7]

Influenza is transmitted from person to person by inhalation of aerosols, especially in crowded conditions. In the U.S., the Centers for Disease Control (CDC), in collaboration with the World Health Organization (WHO), conducts ongoing surveillance to monitor influenza activity. This surveillance assists the WHO in detecting antigenic changes in the influenza strains.[3] Information is available from the CDC regarding influenza surveillance and vaccination composition through the toll-free CDC phone number (888) 232-3228, fax (888) 232-3299 (request document number 361100), or

through the CDC web site, http://www.cdc.gov/ncidod/diseases/flu/weekly.htm.

The shell vial technique for rapid (within 24 hours) detection of viruses has been adopted to detect influenza A and B viruses.[4,8] Serology for detection of influenza antibodies is available. See Influenza A and B Serology *on page 643*.

In a year 2000 report, 99.8% were type A and 0.2% were type B.[9]

Footnotes
1. Yungbluth M, "The Laboratory Diagnosis of Pneumonia. The Role of the Community Hospital Pathologist," *Clin Lab Med*, 1995, 15(2):209-34.
2. CDC, "Prevention and Control of Influenza: Recommendations of the Advisory Committee on Immunization Practices (ACIP)," *MMWR Morb Mortal Wkly Rep*, 1999, 48(RR-4):1-22.
3. Zambon M, "Cell Culture for Surveillance on Influenza," *Dev Biol Stand*, 1999, 98:65-71.
4. Magnard C, Valette M, Aymard M, et al, "Comparison of Two Nested PCR, Cell Culture, and Antigen Detection for the Diagnosis of Upper Respiratory Tract Infections Due to Influenza Viruses," *J Med Virol*, 1999, 59(2):215-20.
5. Mayo Reference Services Publication, "Influenza A and B Antigen, Nasopharyngeal Aspirate," *New Test Announcement* #81856, Rochester, MN: Mayo Medical Laboratories, December 1998.
6. Hostetter MK, "Influenza 1918: The Worst Epidemic in American History," *N Engl J Med*, 1999, 341(9):703 (book review - see Footnote 7).
7. Iezzoni L, *Influenza 1918: The Worst Epidemic in American History*, New York, NY: TV Books, 1999.
8. Shih SR, Tsao KC, Ning HC, et al, "Diagnosis of Respiratory Tract Viruses in 24 Hours by Immunofluorescent Staining of Shell Vial Cultures Containing Madin-Darby Canine Kidney (MDCK) Cells," *J Virol Methods*, 1999, 81(1-2):77-81.
9. Centers for Disease Control and Prevention, "Update: Influenza Activity - United States, 1999-2000 Season," *JAMA*, 2000, 283(13):1681-2.

References
Bachman CA, Doyle WJ, and Skoner DP, "Influenza A Virus-Induced Acute Otitis Media," *J Infect Dis*, 1995, 172(5):1348-51.
Guarner J, Shieh WJ, Dawson J, et al, "Immunohistochemical and *In Situ* Hybridization Studies of Influenza A Virus Infection in Human Lungs," *Am J Clin Pathol*, 2000, 114(2):227-33.
Izurieta HS, Thompson WW, Kramarz P, et al, "Influenza and the Rates of Hospitalization for Respiratory Disease Among Infants and Young Children," *N Engl J Med*, 2000, 342(4):232-9.
Kohn MA, Farley TA, Sundin D, et al, "Three Summertime Outbreaks of Influenza Type A," *J Infect Dis*, 1995, 172(1):246-9.
Neuzil KM, Mellen BG, Wright PF, et al, "The Effect of Influenza on Hospitalizations, Outpatient Visits, and Courses of Antibiotics in Children," *N Engl J Med*, 2000, 342(4):225-31.
Ruiz M, Ewig S, Marcos MA, et al, "Etiology of Community-Acquired Pneumonia: Impact of Age, Comorbidity, and Severity," *Am J Respir Crit Care Med*, 1999, 160(2):397-405.
Sintchenko V and Dwyer DE, "The Diagnosis and Management of Influenza. An Update," *Aust Fam Physician*, 1999, 28(4):313-7.
Ziegler T and Cox NJ, "Influenza Viruses," *Manual of Clinical Microbiology*, 7th ed, Murray PR, Baron EJ, Pfaller MA, et al, eds, Washington, DC: AMS Press, American Society for Microbiology, 1999, 928-35.

Internet Web Sites
www.amm.co.uk/pubs/fa_influenza.htm
www.astdhpphe.org/infect/flu.html
www.cdc.gov/ncidod/diseases/flu/fluvirus.htm
www.who.int/health-topics/influenza.htm

♦ **Influenza Virus, Direct Detection** *see* Virus, Direct Detection by Fluorescent Antibody *on page 696*

♦ **Insect Identification** *see* Arthropod Identification *on page 559*

♦ **Intestinal Helminths** *see* Schistosomiasis Serology *on page 678*

♦ **Intrauterine Device Culture** *see* Actinomyces Culture *on page 551*

♦ **Intravascular Device Culture** *see* Bacterial Culture, Intravascular Device *on page 572*

♦ **Intravenous Catheter Culture** *see* Bacterial Culture, Intravascular Device *on page 572*

♦ **Isolator™ Blood Culture** *see* Bacterial Culture, Blood *on page 566*

♦ *Isospora* *see* Ova and Parasites, Stool *on page 666*

♦ *Isospora belli* *see* Cryptosporidium Direct Staining Procedures *on page 596*

♦ *Isospora belli* **Detection** *see* Acid-Fast Stain, Modified, Parasites *on page 551*

♦ **IUD Culture** *see* Actinomyces Culture *on page 551*

♦ *Ixodes dammini* *see* Babesiosis Serology *on page 561*

♦ *Ixodes dammini* **Identification** *see* Arthropod Identification *on page 559*

♦ *Ixodes ricinus* *see* Babesiosis Serology *on page 561*

♦ **Jamestown Canyon Virus** *see* California Encephalitis Virus Serology *on page 587*

♦ **Japanese Encephalitis Virus** *see* Encephalitis Viral Serology *on page 604*

- ♦ **Kahn Test** *replaced by* RPR *on page 677*

- ♦ **Kahn Test** *replaced by* VDRL, Serum *on page 688*

- ♦ **Kala-azar Serological Test** *see* Leishmaniasis Serology *on page 647*

- ♦ **Kaposi Sarcoma-Associated Herpesvirus** *see* Herpesvirus 8 *on page 634*

- ♦ **Kinyoun Stain** *see* Acid-Fast Stain *on page 550*

- ♦ **Kirby-Bauer Susceptibility Test** *see* Antimicrobial Susceptibility Testing, Aerobic and Facultatively Anaerobic Bacteria *on page 554*

- ♦ **Klebsiella pneumoniae** *see* Bacterial Culture, Bronchoscopy/Bronchial Brush/Bronchoalveolar Lavage Specimen *on page 568*

- ♦ **Klebsiella spp** *see* Bacterial Culture, Sputum *on page 574*

- ♦ **Klebsiella spp** *see* Bacterial Culture, Urine *on page 578*

- ♦ **Kline Test** *replaced by* RPR *on page 677*

- ♦ **Kline Test** *replaced by* VDRL, Serum *on page 688*

KOH Preparation

Related Information
Fungal Culture, Skin *on page 612*
Fungal Culture, Sputum *on page 613*
Fungus Smear, Stain *on page 615*
Gram Stain *on page 617*
Skin Biopsy *on page 71*

Synonyms Potassium Hydroxide Preparation

Applies to Dermatophytoses; Tinea Barbae; Tinea Capitis; Tinea Corporis; Tinea Cruris; Tinea Manuum; Tinea Pedis; Tinea Unguium

Test Includes Potassium hydroxide (KOH) hydrolysis of proteinaceous debris, cells, and so forth before microscopic examination under 10x and 40x objectives

Specimen The appropriate specimen for KOH preparation is the same as for culture. See specific site fungus culture listing for details. See the specimen selection tables provided in Fungal Culture, Skin *on page 612* and Fungal Culture, Sputum *on page 613*.

Special Instructions The laboratory should be informed of the specific source of the specimen and the clinical diagnosis. Aseptic technique should be used to collect the specimen. Use sterile scissors, forceps, and nail clippers and disinfect the specimen site with 70% alcohol before collection.

Reference Interval No fungus elements identified

Use Determine the presence of fungi in skin, nails, or hair. Exudates from abscesses, sinus tracts, aspirates, etc, can be examined by KOH preparation and also smeared for Gram stain.

Limitations Cultures are usually more sensitive than KOH preparations. The test may require overnight incubation for complete disintegration of hair, nail, or skin debris.

Methodology 10% KOH with gentle heat, alternately 10% to 20% KOH and 40% dimethyl sulfoxide (DMSO)

Additional Information Fungal infections of the keratinized tissues such as skin, nails, and hair are called dermatophytoses. Different fungus species may cause similar diseases. Dermatophyte infections are named for the anatomic location of the fungal infection (infections of the nails are called tinea unguium; infections of the feet are called tinea pedis; infections of the palms and fingers are called tinea manuum; infections of the groin are called tinea cruris; infections of the face, trunk, and limbs are called tinea corporis; infections of the scalp, hair, eyebrows, and eyelashes are called tinea capitis; and infections of the beard or moustache are called tinea barbae).

Recent reports have emphasized the changing pattern of tinea capitis, particularly the fact that infection due to *Trichophyton tonsurans* has become increasingly common. When present it causes a less discrete, more diffuse pattern of alopecia. It is negative by Wood's light examination. The "black dot", a remnant of a broken infected hair shaft, is a good source for diagnostic material which should be sought with a magnifying glass and collected with forceps. Scale and pulled hairs are also useful specimens.[1,2] Diagnostic specimens should be collected before antifungal therapy is instituted. Topical steroids should not be prescribed until fungal infection is excluded.

Footnotes
1. Kemna ME and Elewski BE, "A U.S. Epidemiologic Survey of Superficial Fungal Diseases," *J Am Acad Dermatol*, 1996, 35(4):539-42.
2. Schwinn A, Ebert J, and Brocker EB, "Frequency of *Trichophyton rubrum* in Tinea Capitis," *Mycoses*, 1995, 38(1-2):1-7.

References
Chapman SW and Daniel CR 3rd, "Cutaneous Manifestations of Fungal Infections," 1994, 8(4):879-910.
Kane J and Summerbell RC, "*Trichophyton, Microsporum, Epidermophyton*, and Agents of Superficial Mycoses," 7th ed, Murray PR, Baron EJ, Pfaller MA, et al, eds, Washington, DC: American Society for Microbiology, 1999, 1275-94.
St Germain G and Summerbell R, "Identifying Filamentous Fungi," *A Clinical Laboratory Handbook*, Belmont, CA: Star Publishing, 1996.

- ♦ **KSHV** *see* Herpesvirus 8 *on page 634*

- ♦ **LaCrosse Virus** *see* California Encephalitis Virus Serology *on page 587*

- ♦ **Latex Agglutination for Bacterial Antigens** *see* Bacterial Antigens, Rapid Detection Methods *on page 562*

- ♦ **L. bosemanii** *see* Legionella Direct Fluorescent Antibody Smear *on page 646*

- ♦ **L. bosemanii** *see* Legionella Serology *on page 646*

- ♦ **L. dumoffii** *see* Legionella Direct Fluorescent Antibody Smear *on page 646*

- ♦ **L. dumoffii** *see* Legionella Serology *on page 646*

- ♦ **Legionella Antigen, Urine** *see* Legionella Urine Antigen *on page 647*

Legionella Culture

Related Information
Bacterial Culture, Biopsy or Body Fluid *on page 565*
Bacterial Culture, Sputum *on page 574*
Bronchoalveolar Lavage (BAL) *on page 375*
Fine Needle Aspiration Culture *on page 609*
Legionella Direct Fluorescent Antibody Smear *on page 646*
Legionella Serology *on page 646*
Legionella Urine Antigen *on page 647*
Psittacosis Serology *on page 672*
Q Fever Serology *on page 673*

Synonyms Legionnaires' Disease Agent

Applies to *Legionella* DNA Probe; *Legionella pneumophila* Latex Agglutination

Test Includes Culture and frequently direct fluorescent antibody (DFA) smear for *Legionella* spp

Abstract Legionnaires' disease is a systemic disease with pneumonia as the prominent clinical finding. During the 1976 American Legion convention in Philadelphia, an epidemic of pneumonia caused 34 deaths. Currently, it is estimated that each year 8000-18,000 people in the U.S. are infected with *Legionella* sp and approximately 5% to 30% of these patients die from the disease (see CDC website below). Sputum characterized by acute inflammatory features, without a classical pattern of bacteria, may represent *Legionella*. Extrapulmonary disease occurs more frequently in immunosuppressed patients. *Legionella* may cause extrapulmonary infections, including abscesses.

Legionella is most likely to be found in warm water (eg, water heaters, complex plumbing systems).[1]

Specimen Lung tissue, other body tissue, pleural fluid, other body fluid, transtracheal aspiration, bronchoalveolar lavage, bronchial brushing, sputum, content of abscess

Turnaround Time Positive results require 2-5 days. Primary plates are often held for 7-14 days before a final negative report is issued.

Special Instructions Clinical suspicion of *Legionella* infection should be reported to the laboratory.

Reference Interval No *Legionella* recovered

Use Isolate and identify *Legionella pneumophila*; evaluation of pneumonia, including primary atypical pneumonia. Legionnaires' disease is among entities considered as building-related illnesses.[2]

Limitations Sputum (expectorated), bronchial aspirates, and other specimens having normal flora are subject to bacterial overgrowth and are not as desirable as transtracheal aspirates, pleural fluid, and biopsy material for culture. Sensitivity of cultures is generally ~80% and specificity approaches 100%.[3,4]

Methodology Culture on selective and nonselective media (buffered charcoal yeast extract). *Legionella* requires L-cysteine and ferric salt supplementation of growth media. Growth cannot be anticipated on conventional media.

Additional Information Laboratory diagnosis of *Legionella* infection can be attempted with three distinct methodological approaches.[3,4,5] First, a rapid diagnosis can be attained by culture-independent methods that detect bacterial products in clinical specimens (eg, direct fluorescent antibody tests on respiratory specimens, DNA amplification, radioimmunoassay, or enzyme immunoassays on urine specimens). The sensitivity of these methods is usually between 70% and 90%, and specificity exceeds 95%. Second, indirect fluorescence antibody methods can be used to detect the patient's antibody response to *Legionella* spp. Serologic methods have sensitivities of 70% to 80% and specificities exceeding 95%, but their clinical utility is limited by the retrospective nature of most serologic methods. Finally, *Legionella* cultures can be performed; *Legionella* cultures have sensitivities and specificities of approximately 80% and 100%, respectively. Culture for *Legionella* may require 2 weeks of incubation before a result is available, thus it is not helpful in making clinical decisions. Other nonculture tests are more useful for the rapid diagnosis of Legionnaires' disease.

Legionella infections have been associated with reservoirs, water distribution systems, cooling systems, and hot water systems. Recently, passengers of a cruise ship contracted Legionnaires' disease from the on board water supply.[6]

Over 34 species in the Legionellaceae family of bacteria have been discovered since *Legionella pneumophila* was first recognized. Thirteen species have been implicated as causes of human pneumonia. See table.

The differential diagnosis includes psittacosis and Q fever.
(Continued)

Legionella Culture *(Continued)*

Clinical Clues to the Diagnosis of Legionnaires' Disease

- Gram stain of respiratory secretions reveals numerous neutrophils, but few organisms
- Presence of hyponatremia (serum sodium ≤130 mmol/L)
- Failure to respond to β-lactam and aminoglycoside antibiotics
- Occurrence in hospital where potable water system is known to be contaminated with *Legionella*
- History of smoking and alcohol use
- Pleuritic chest pain
- Fever malaise, myalgia, headache

Adapted from Harrison TG and Taylor AG, "Timing of Seroconversion in Legionnaires' Disease," *Lancet*, 1988, 2(8614):795.

Footnotes

1. Edelstein PH, "Legionellosis," *Cecil Textbook of Medicine*, 21st ed, Chapter 323, Goldman L and Bennett JC, eds, Philadelphia, PA: WB Saunders Co, 2000, 1616-19.
2. Menzies D and Bourbeau J,"Building-Related Illnesses," *N Engl J Med*, 1997, 337(21):1524-31.
3. Plouffe JF, McNally C, and File TM Jr, "Value of Noninvasive Studies in Community-Acquired Pneumonia," *Infect Dis Clin North Am*, 1998, 12(3):689-99.
4. Roig J, Domingo C, and Morera J, "Legionnaires' Disease," *Chest*, 1994, 105(6):1817-25.
5. Koide M and Saito A, "Diagnosis of *Legionella pneumophila* Infection by Polymerase Chain Reaction," *Clin Infect Dis*, 1995, 21(1):199-201.
6. Castellani Pastoris M, Lo Monaco R, et al, "Legionnaires' Disease on a Cruise Ship Linked to the Water Supply System: Clinical and Public Health Implications," *Clin Infect Dis*, 1999, 28(1):33-8.

References

Bernstein JM, "Treatment of Community-Acquired Pneumonia-IDSA Guidelines. Infectious Diseases Society of America," *Chest*, 1999, 115(3S):9S-13S.

Breiman RF and Butler JC, "Legionnaires' Disease: Clinical, Epidemiological, and Public Health Perspectives," *Semin Respir Infect*, 1998, 13(2):84-9.

Centers for Disease Control, "Legionnaires' Disease Associated With Potting Soil - California, Oregon, and Washington, May-June 2000," *MMWR Morb Mortal Wkly Report*, 2000, 49:7778.

Cunha BA, "Clinical Features of Legionnaires' Disease," *Semin Respir Infect*, 1998, 13(2):116-27.

Shelton BG, Kerbel W, Witherell L, et al, "Review of Legionnaires' Disease," *AIHAJ*, 2000, 61(5):738-42.

Waterer GW, Baselski VS, and Wunderink RG, "*Legionella* and Community-Acquired Pneumonia: A Review of Current Diagnostic Tests From a Clinician's Viewpoint," *Am J Med*, 2001, 110(1):41-8.

Weir SC, Fischer SH, Stock F, et al, "Detection of *Legionella* by PCR in Respiratory Specimens Using a Commercially Available Kit," *Am J Clin Pathol*, 1998, 110(9):295-300.

Winn WC, "*Legionella*," *Manual of Clinical Microbiology*, Chapter 37, 7th ed, Murray PR, Baron EJ, Pfaller MA, et al, eds, Washington, DC: AMS Press, American Society for Microbiology, 1999, 572-85.

Internet Web Sites

www.amm.co.uk/pubs/fa_legionnaires.htm
www.astdhpphe.org/infect/legion.html
www.cdc.gov/ncidod/dbmd/diseaseinfo/legionellosis_g.htm

♦ *Legionella* Detection by PCR *see Legionella* Direct Fluorescent Antibody Smear *on page 646*

Legionella Direct Fluorescent Antibody Smear

Related Information

Bacterial Culture, Sputum *on page 574*
Bronchoalveolar Lavage (BAL) *on page 375*
Legionella Culture *on page 645*
Legionella Serology *on page 646*
Legionella Urine Antigen *on page 647*

Synonyms FA Smear for *Legionella pneumophila*; *Legionella pneumophila* Direct FA Smear; Legionnaires' Disease Direct Fluorescent Antibody Smear

Applies to *L. bosemanii*; *L. dumoffii*; *Legionella* Detection by PCR; *L. gormanii*; *L. jordanis*; *L. longbeachae*; *L. micdadei*

Abstract Direct fluorescent antibody (DFA) used to detect organisms directly in specimens for rapid diagnosis of *Legionella* pneumonia.

Specimen Lung tissue, pleural fluid, other body fluid, transtracheal aspirate, sputum, bronchial washing, bronchoalveolar lavage, abscess content

Container Sterile container

Reference Interval No *Legionella* species detected

Use Determine the presence of *Legionella* organisms in direct smear of specimen by fluorescent antibody, providing rapid diagnosis of primary atypical pneumonia. Monoclonal antibody is available.

Limitations DFA is not as sensitive as culture and false-positive results occur due to cross-reactions with other bacterial infections and with environmental *Legionella* species. False-positive reactions can occur with other bacterial species, especially gram-negative bacteria.[1,2] Sensitivity ranges for various respiratory specimens are as follows:

- sputum: 18% to 33%
- tracheal aspirates: 33% to 40%
- bronchoalveolar lavage: 66%

Since culture has a higher sensitivity, DFA should never replace culture for the diagnosis of *Legionella* infections. It is not helpful for all species of *Legionella*.

Methodology Direct fluorescent antibody (DFA); detection of *Legionella* by PCR in respiratory specimens is available.[3]

Additional Information Community-acquired and nosocomial infections caused by multiple serogroups of *Legionella* are increasingly recognized. Culture is now possible on buffered charcoal yeast extract agar. However, the demonstration of organisms in sputum, tissue, or brushings is a rapid means to make a diagnosis. It also has the advantage of applicability to specimens contaminated with other bacteria. Development of monoclonal antibodies has increased sensitivity and specificity. A combination of both culture and antigen detection is recommended. A direct FA should not be ordered alone; it should always be accompanied by a request for *Legionella* culture. Direct fluorescence antibody staining can be done on tissue specimens as well.

Footnotes

1. Andersen LP and Bangsborg J, "Cross Reactions Between *Legionella* and *Campylobacter* Species," *Lancet*, 1992, 340(8813):245.
2. Boswell TC, "Serological Cross Reaction Between *Legionella* and *Campylobacter* in the Rapid Microaggglutination Test," *J Clin Pathol*, 1996, 49(7):584-6.
3. Weir SC, Fischer SH, Stock F, et al, "Detection of *Legionella* by PCR in Respiratory Specimens Using a Commercially Available Kit," *Am J Clin Pathol*, 1998, 110(3):295-300.

References

Chow JW and Yu VL, "*Legionella*: A Major Opportunistic Pathogen in Transplant Recipients," *Semin Respir Infect*, 1998, 13(2):132-9.

Plouffe JF, McNally C, and File TM Jr, "Value of Noninvasive Studies in Community-Acquired Pneumonia," *Infect Dis Clin North Am*, 1998, 12(3):689-99.

Roig J, Domingo C, and Morera J, "Legionnaires' Disease," *Chest*, 1994, 105(6):1817-25.

Shelton BG, Kerbel W, Witherell L, et al, "Review of Legionnaires' Disease," *AIHAJ*, 2000, 61(5):738-42.

Waterer GW, Baselski VS, and Wunderink RG, "*Legionella* and Community-Acquired Pneumonia: A Review of Current Diagnostic Tests From a Clinician's Viewpoint," *Am J Med*, 2001, 110(1):41-8.

Internet Web Sites

www.amm.co.uk/pubs/fa_legionnaires.htm
www.astdhpphe.org/infect/legion.html
www.cdc.gov/ncidod/dbmd/diseaseinfo/legionellosis_g.htm

♦ *Legionella* DNA Probe *see Legionella* Culture *on page 645*

♦ *Legionella pneumophila* Antibodies *see Legionella* Serology *on page 646*

♦ *Legionella pneumophila* Direct FA Smear *see Legionella* Direct Fluorescent Antibody Smear *on page 646*

♦ *Legionella pneumophila* Latex Agglutination *see Legionella* Culture *on page 645*

♦ *Legionella pneumophila*, Serogroup 1 Antigen, Urine *see Legionella* Urine Antigen *on page 647*

♦ *Legionella pneumophila* Titer *see Legionella* Serology *on page 646*

Legionella Serology

Related Information

Bacterial Culture, Sputum *on page 574*
Legionella Culture *on page 645*
Legionella Direct Fluorescent Antibody Smear *on page 646*
Legionella Urine Antigen *on page 647*

Synonyms *Legionella pneumophila* Antibodies; *Legionella pneumophila* Titer; Legionnaires' Disease Antibodies; Legionnaires', Indirect Fluorescent Antibody Titer

Applies to *L. bosemanii*; *L. dumoffii*; *L. gormanii*; *L. jordanis*; *L. longbeachae*; *L. micdadei*; Pneumonia, Atypical Agents

Test Includes Detection of antibody (IgG or IgM) to *Legionella pneumophila*

Abstract Detection of antibodies to the *Legionella* species is useful for epidemiologic purposes to determine prevalence, but is only rarely employed for the diagnosis of suspected cases of *Legionella* pneumonia. The differential diagnosis of the atypical pneumonias includes *Chlamydia pneumoniae*, Legionnaires' disease, *Mycoplasma* pneumonia, and rickettsial pneumonia.[1] *Legionella*, *Mycoplasma pneumoniae*, and *Chlamydia pneumoniae* collectively cause 10% to 20% of cases of pneumonia. Antibody detection for Legionnaires' disease from a random sample is unlikely to be useful.

Specimen Serum, acute and convalescent

Container Red top tube

Collection It is recommended to draw a convalescent sample 10-14 days after acute sample is drawn.

Reference Interval Less than a fourfold change in titer between acute and convalescent samples; <1:256 in a single sample

Use Determine the prevalence of disease; possibly for the retrospective diagnosis of *Legionella* infection; study of primary atypical pneumonia

Limitations It is important to test for both IgG and IgM; when this is done, overall sensitivity is ~80%. Specificity is fairly high (approaching 95%), but predictive values may be low in low prevalence populations. Serologic diagnosis is often retrospective and should be considered presumptive. Antibody may persist for years. False positives are found due to serologic cross-reactions with numerous bacteria such as *Pseudomonas* species, *Burkholderia* species, and other gram-negative bacteria.[1,2] Seroconversion may be delayed.

Methodology Indirect fluorescent antibody (IFA) assay using serogroup 1: Philadelphia, Knoxville, serogroup 2: Togus, serogroup 3: Los Angeles, serogroup 4: Bloomington. When available a polyvalent antigen, which includes serogroup 1-6, is utilized. Latex agglutination (LA).

Additional Information A fourfold rise in titer to >1:128 is evidence of recent infection. A single titer ≥1:256 is evidence of infection at an undetermined time in the past. However, due to the relatively high prevalence of antibodies to *Legionella pneumophila*, acute and convalescent titers are preferred to a single sample. Most seroconversions can be documented within 3 weeks of onset.

Footnotes
1. Musso D and Raoult D, "Serological Cross-Reactions Between *Coxiella burnetii* and *Legionella micdadei*," *Clin Diagn Lab Immunol*, 1997, 4(2):208-12.
2. Boswell TC, "Serological Cross Reaction Between *Legionella* and *Campylobacter* in the Rapid Microagglutination Test," *J Clin Pathol*, 1996, 49(7):584-6.

References
Bartlett JG and Mundy LM, "Community-Acquired Pneumonia," *N Engl J Med*, 1995, 333(24):1618-24.
Chow JW and Yu VL, "*Legionella*: A Major Opportunistic Pathogen in Transplant Recipients," *Semin Respir Infect*, 1998, 13(2):132-9.
Shelton BG, Kerbel W, Witherell L, et al, "Review of Legionnaires' Disease," *AIHAJ*, 2000, 61(5):738-42.
Tateda K, Murakami H, Ishii Y, et al, "Evaluation of Clinical Usefulness of the Microplate Agglutination Test for Serological Diagnosis of *Legionella pneumoniae*," *J Med Microbiol*, 1998, 47(4):325-8.
Waterer GW, Baselski VS, and Wunderink RG, "*Legionella* and Community-Acquired Pneumonia: A Review of Current Diagnostic Tests From a Clinician's Viewpoint," *Am J Med*, 2001, 110(1):41-8.

Internet Web Sites
www.amm.co.uk/pubs/fa_legionnaires.htm
www.astdhpphe.org/infect/legion.html
www.cdc.gov/ncidod/dbmd/diseaseinfo/legionellosis_g.htm

♦ ***Legionella* spp** see Bacterial Culture, Bronchoscopy/Bronchial Brush/Bronchoalveolar Lavage Specimen *on page 568*

♦ ***Legionella* spp** see Bacterial Culture, Sputum *on page 574*

Legionella Urine Antigen

Related Information
Legionella Culture *on page 645*
Legionella Direct Fluorescent Antibody Smear *on page 646*
Legionella Serology *on page 646*

Synonyms *Legionella* Antigen, Urine; Legionnaires' Disease Urine Antigen

Applies to *Legionella pneumophila*, Serogroup 1 Antigen, Urine

Test Includes Detection of excreted *Legionella pneumophila* serogroup 1 antigen in urine

Abstract *Legionella* antigen can be detected in urine to diagnose *Legionella* infections more rapidly than other techniques.

Specimen Urine

Container Sterile urine container

Reference Interval Negative

Use Antigen detection in urine provides an additional rapid approach to diagnosis of infections due to *Legionella pneumophila* serogroup 1; work-up of primary atypical pneumonia. Other *Legionella* species are not detected with this assay.

Limitations Commercially available enzyme immunoassays have a specificity >99% and sensitivity of 70% to 90%. Concentration of the urine increases the sensitivity.[1] Latex agglutination tests have a specificity of 85% to 99% and sensitivity of 55% to 90%. Antigen excretion in urine may persist for months after recovery from infection. This test should be obtained in conjunction with other, more proven, laboratory tests such as *Legionella* culture and/or antibody assays. It is not useful for detection of all species of *Legionella*.[2]

Methodology Enzyme immunoassay (EIA) or latex agglutination (LA)

Additional Information The rapid detection of *Legionella* antigen in urine is currently recommended to assist in establishing a diagnosis of *Legionella* infection.[3] The commercially available tests have an acceptable sensitivity and specificity. However, as with many diagnostic tests, a negative test does not definitively rule out *Legionella*. *Legionella* antigen may be detected in urine for months after the acute infection; thus a positive result with these assays does not always indicate a current infection.

Footnotes
1. Dominguez JA, Gali N, Pedroso P, et al, "Comparison of the Binax *Legionella* Urinary Antigen Enzyme Immunoassay (EIA) With the Biotest *Legionella* Urine Antigen EIA for detection of *Legionella* Antigen in Both Concentrated and Nonconcentrated Urine Samples," *J Clin Microbiol*, 1998, 36(9):2718-22.

2. Edelstein PH, "Legionellosis," *Cecil Textbook of Medicine*, 21st ed, Chapter 323, Goldman L and Bennett JC, eds, Philadelphia, PA: WB Saunders Co, 2000, 1616-19.
3. Bernstein JM, "Treatment of Community-Acquired Pneumonia-IDSA Guidelines. Infectious Diseases Society of America," *Chest*, 1999, 115(3S):9S-13S.

References
Lepine LA, Jernigan DB, Butler JC, et al, "A Recurrent Outbreak of Nosocomial Legionnaires' Disease Detected by Urinary Antigen Testing: Evidence for Long-Term Colonization of a Hospital Plumbing System," *Infect Control Hosp Epidemiol*, 1998, 19(12):905-10.
Plouffe JF, File TM, Breiman RF, et al, "Re-evaluation of the Definition of Legionnaires' Disease: Use of the Urinary Antigen Assay. Community Based Pneumonia Incidence Study Group," *Clin Infect Dis*, 1995, 20(5):1286-91.
Plouffe JF, McNally C, and File TM Jr, "Value of Noninvasive Studies in Community-Acquired Pneumonia," *Infect Dis Clin North Am*, 1998, 12(3):689-99.
Shelton BG, Kerbel W, Witherell L, et al, "Review of Legionnaires' Disease," *AIHAJ*, 2000, 61(5):738-42.
Waterer GW, Baselski VS, and Wunderink RG, "*Legionella* and Community-Acquired Pneumonia: A Review of Current Diagnostic Tests From a Clinician's Viewpoint," *Am J Med*, 2001, 110(1):41-8.

Internet Web Sites
www.amm.co.uk/pubs/fa_legionnaires.htm
www.astdhpphe.org/infect/legion.html
www.cdc.gov/ncidod/dbmd/diseaseinfo/legionellosis_g.htm

♦ **Legionnaires' Disease Agent** see *Legionella* Culture *on page 645*

♦ **Legionnaires' Disease Antibodies** see *Legionella* Serology *on page 646*

♦ **Legionnaires' Disease Direct Fluorescent Antibody Smear** see *Legionella* Direct Fluorescent Antibody Smear *on page 646*

♦ **Legionnaires' Disease Urine Antigen** see *Legionella* Urine Antigen *on page 647*

♦ **Legionnaires', Indirect Fluorescent Antibody Titer** see *Legionella* Serology *on page 646*

♦ ***Leishmania braziliensis* Serological Test** see Leishmaniasis Serology *on page 647*

♦ ***Leishmania donovani* Serological Test** see Leishmaniasis Serology *on page 647*

Leishmaniasis Serology

Related Information
Bone Marrow *on page 410*
Chagas' Disease Serological Test *on page 588*
Lymph Node Biopsy *on page 67*
Protein Electrophoresis, Serum *on page 267*
Skin Biopsy *on page 71*

Synonyms Espundia Serological Test; Kala-azar Serological Test; *Leishmania braziliensis* Serological Test; *Leishmania donovani* Serological Test; *Leishmania tropica* Serological Test; Oriental Sore Serological Test

Abstract Infections with *Leishmania* species are commonly zoonotic and in certain parts of the world leishmaniasis is endemic. Visceral leishmaniasis (kala-azar) is typically caused by *Leishmania donovani* which parasitizes macrophage infections found in spleen, bone marrow, liver, and lymph nodes. Other infections include cutaneous leishmaniasis (*L. tropica*, *L. major*, *L. aethiopica*) and new world cutaneous leishmaniasis (*L. mexicana*, *L. braziliensis*, *L. venezuelensis*, *L. peruviana*), and mucocutaneous leishmaniasis (espundia) caused by *L. braziliensis*.

Specimen Serum

Container Red top tube

Reference Interval Negative

Use Serology is helpful in epidemiology studies but is less than adequate to support the clinical diagnosis of visceral, cutaneous, or mucocutaneous leishmaniasis.

Limitations Cross reactivity with Chagas' disease; false positives in malaria. Sensitivity of serologic tests for cutaneous leishmaniasis is poor. Serologic diagnosis often is insufficient in subjects infected with HIV virus.[1]

Methodology Indirect hemagglutination (IHA), indirect fluorescent antibody (IFA), complement fixation (CF), enzyme-linked immunosorbent assay (ELISA), immunodot assay. Of these, the enzyme-linked immunosorbent assay (ELISA) presently is considered the most sensitive.[1] Direct agglutination detecting IgM is a sensitive test for acute disease. Recently developed competitive ELISA assays have been shown to be more sensitive than microscopy, especially early in the disease.[2]

Additional Information Recent estimates show that as many as 350 million people are at risk of acquiring leishmaniasis and 112 million are currently infected.[3] *Leishmania* species are intracellular parasites that are transmitted to humans by bites from phlebotomine sand flies. Occasionally, nonvector transmissions have been reported through blood transfusions, sexual intercourse, organ transplantation, and congenital transmission.

Serodiagnosis of visceral leishmaniasis is more reliable than serodiagnosis of cutaneous disease, although there has been improvement by use of recombinant proteins in the ELISA.[4]

Massive polyclonal IgG gammopathy on serum protein electrophoresis is characteristic of kala-azar. Leukopenia, thrombocytopenia, and anemia are
(Continued)

Leishmaniasis Serology (Continued)

found. **Bone marrow aspiration** provides diagnostic organisms in kala-azar.[5] **Skin biopsies** for stains, culture, and histopathology are useful in cutaneous and mucocutaneous leishmaniasis. *L. tropica*, which usually causes cutaneous disease, produced visceral infection in soldiers returning from Desert Storm.[6]

Diagnosis of visceral leishmaniasis remains dependent on detection of *L. donovani* in specimens in some settings.

Footnotes

1. Albrecht H, Sobottka I, Emminger C, et al, "Visceral Leishmaniasis Emerging as an Important Opportunistic Infection in HIV-Infected Persons Living in Areas Nonendemic for *Leishmania donovani*," *Arch Pathol Lab Med*, 1996, 120:189-98.
2. Chatterjee M, Jaffe CL, Sundar S, et al, "Diagnostic and Prognostic Potential of a Competitive Enzyme-Linked Immunosorbent Assay for Leishmaniasis in India," *Clin Diagn Lab Immunol*, 1999, 6(4):550-4.
3. World Health Organization, "Control of the Leishmaniases," *WHO Tec Rep Ser*, 1990, 793:155.
4. Jensen AT, Gasin S, Moller T, et al, "Serodiagnosis of *Leishmania donovani* Infections: Assessment of Enzyme-Linked Immunosorbent Assays Using Recombinant *L. donovani* Gene B Protein (GBP) and a Peptide Sequence of *L. donovani* GBP," *Trans R Soc Trop Med Hyg*, 1999, 93(2):157-60.
5. Garcia Bueno MJ and Herraez J, Images in Clinical Medicine, "Visceral Leishmaniasis," *N Engl J Med*, 1996, 335(14):1034.
6. Magill AJ, Grögl M, Gasser RA Jr, et al, "Visceral Infection Caused by *Leishmania tropica* in Veterans of Operation Desert Storm," *N Engl J Med*, 1993, 328(19):1383-7.

References

Belli A, Garcia D, Palacios X, et al, "Widespread Atypical Cutaneous Leishmaniasis Caused by *Leishmania (L.) chagasi* in Nicaragua," *Am J Trop Med Hyg*, 1999, 61(3):380-5.

Berenguer J, Gomez-Campdera F, Padilla B, et al, "Visceral Leishmaniasis (Kala-Azar) in Transplant Recipients: Case Report and Review," *Transplantation*, 1998, 65(10):1401-4.

Grimaldi G Jr and Tesh RB, "Leishmaniases of the New World: Current Concepts and Implications for Future Research," *Clin Microbiol Rev*, 1993, 6(3):230-50.

Kagan IG and Maddison SE, "Serodiagnosis of Parasitic Diseases," *Manual of Clinical Laboratory Immunology*, 4th ed, Volume 2, Chapter 79, Rose NR, Conway de Macario E, Fahey JL, et al, eds, Washington, DC: ASM Press, American Society for Microbiology, 1992, 529-43.

Kenner JR, Aronson NE, Bratthauer GL, et al, "Immunohistochemistry to Identify *Leishmania* Parasites in Fixed Tissues," *J Cutan Pathol*, 1999, 26(3):130-6

Meinecke CK, Schottelius J, Oskam L, et al, "Congenital Transmission of Visceral Leishmaniasis (Kala Azar) From an Asymptomatic Mother to Her Child," *Pediatrics*, 1999, 104(5):e65.

Internet Web Sites

www.cdc.gov/ncidod/dpd/parasites/leishmania/default.htm

♦ ***Leishmania tropica* Serological Test** *see* Leishmaniasis Serology *on page 647*

♦ ***Lepidopterae*** *see* Arthropod Identification *on page 559*

♦ ***Leptospira* Antibodies** *see Leptospira* Serology *on page 649*

Leptospira Culture

Related Information

Bacterial Culture, Blood *on page 566*
Bacterial Culture, Wounds, Bites *on page 579*
Darkfield Examination, Leptospirosis *on page 601*
Leptospira Serology *on page 649*

Applies to Blood Culture, *Leptospira*; Cerebrospinal Fluid Culture, *Leptospira*

Abstract Leptospires are spiral-shaped bacteria that can be found as free-living organisms in freshwater, soil, or mud, or they live in association with animal hosts. The bacteria can infect a variety of wild and domestic animals which excrete the organisms in urine. Leptospirosis results from the direct or indirect exposure to the urine of infected animals. The bacteria enter the body through breaks in the skin or through the mucous membranes and conjunctivae. Clinical manifestations can vary from a mild self-limiting illness to a fulminating fatal illness including hepatorenal failure (Weil syndrome).

Patient Preparation Thoroughly instruct the patient in the proper collection technique for a midvoid urine specimen; avoid contamination with skin flora since the normal urine contaminants will overgrow leptospires in the specimen. See also Bacterial Culture, Urine *on page 578* and Bacterial Culture, Blood *on page 566* for detailed instructions.

Specimen Urine, indicate midvoid, catheter or suprapubic puncture specimen; **blood** and **cerebrospinal fluid** may also be cultured

Container Sterile, urine container; for blood, lavender top (EDTA) Vacutainer® or green top (heparin) Vacutainer®. Avoid collecting blood in citrate solutions, which may inhibit the growth of leptospires.

Collection Specimen should be transported to the laboratory within 1 hour of collection. For midvoid urine culture, patient should be instructed to clean skin thoroughly, do not collect first portion of stream, **collect midportion of stream**, and do not collect final portion of stream. Catheter or suprapubic puncture specimen may also be used. If possible, specimens should be collected prior to antibiotic treatment and while the patient is febrile.

Storage Instructions Specimens should not be refrigerated. They should be left at room temperature. Urine with an acid pH should be alkalinized if it cannot be set up immediately.

Turnaround Time 4-8 weeks

Special Instructions The laboratory should be informed of the specific request for *Leptospira* culture, collection time, current antibiotic therapy, and date of onset of illness. Urine must be alkaline; *Leptospira* do not survive for more than a few hours in acid urine. Repeated cultures may be required.

Reference Interval No *Leptospira* isolated

Use Diagnose leptospirosis (Weil disease)

Limitations Other organisms are not isolated or identified. The organism is slow growing; results of cultures may be prolonged.

Contraindications Leptospiremia occurs during the septicemic acute phase of infection. This phase last 4-7 days after which organisms are not recoverable from blood.

Methodology Specimen is inoculated onto specially prepared media containing rabbit serum or albumin and fatty acids. Incubation is for 4-6 weeks in the dark at 28°C to 29°C. Cultures are examined with darkfield or phase microscopy for motile leptospires at weekly intervals; growth occurs 1-3 cm below the surface.

Additional Information Leptospirosis in humans is usually associated with exposure to water or soil contaminated by infected animal urine. Outbreaks have been associated with canoeing, rafting, and swimming in contaminated lakes and rivers.[1,2,3] In 1995, a large epidemic of leptospirosis, affecting nearly 2000 people, occurred in Nicaragua following heavy rainfall and flooding.[4] This particular epidemic was associated with pulmonary hemorrhage, a severe form of leptospirosis. In addition to recreational and accidental exposure, occupational exposure of veterinarians, dairymen, swineherds, abattoir workers, miners, fish and poultry processors, and those who work in rat-infested environments are at increased risk.

The septicemic phase of the disease lasts from 4-7 days. During this first week of disease the most reliable means of detecting leptospires is by direct culture of blood or spinal fluid on appropriate media. The initial phase is followed by a quiescent period of 1-3 days. The last phase of the disease is the immune phase in which as many as 40% of the patients will have meningitis and the majority will have *Leptospira* in the urine. Urine can remain positive for several months. Concentration of *Leptospira* in human urine is low and shedding may be intermittent. Therefore, repeated isolation attempts should be made. Serology (acute and early convalescent) is recommended. Direct darkfield examination is no longer recommended. Urine culture and serology are recommended during and after the immune phase.

Pleocytosis with <500 cells/mm³, normal glucose, and slightly increased protein are found in the CSF.

Serum aspartate aminotransferase, alanine aminotransferase, and alkaline phosphatase are increased 2-3 times and associated with predominantly conjugated hyperbilirubinemia. Myositis with increased CK is found in about 50% of patients.[5]

Immunocytochemical demonstration of *Leptospira* is beautifully illustrated in a 1997 paper.[6]

Footnotes

1. Jackson LA, Kaufmann AF, Adams WG, et al, "Outbreak of Leptospirosis Associated With Swimming," *Pediatr Infect Dis J*, 1993, 12:48-54.
2. CDC, "Outbreak of Leptospirosis Among White-Water Rafters - Costa Rica, 1996," *MMWR Morb Mortal Wkly Rep*, 1997, 46(25):577-79.
3. CDC, "Outbreak of Acute Febrile Illness Among Athletes Participating in Triathlons - Wisconsin and Illinois - 1998," *MMWR Morb Mort Wkly Rep*, 1998, 47:585-8.
4. Zaki SR, Shieh WJ, and the Epidemic Working Group, "Leptospirosis Associated With Outbreak of Acute Febrile Illness and Pulmonary Haemorrhage, Nicaragua, 1995. The Epidemic Working Group at Ministry of Health in Nicaragua," *Lancet*, 1996, 347(9000):535-6.
5. Petrie WA Jr, "Leptospirosis," *Cecil Textbook of Medicine*, 21st ed, Chapter 369, Goldman L and Bennett JC, eds, Philadelphia, PA: WB Saunders Co, 2000, 1761-3.
6. Schwartz DA, "Emerging and Reemerging Infections. Progress and Challenges in the Subspecialty of Infectious Disease Pathology," *Arch Pathol Lab Med*, 1997, 121(8):776-84.

References

Centers for Disease Control and Prevention, "Outbreak of Acute Febrile Illness Among Participants in EcoChallenge Sahah 2000 - Malaysia," *JAMA*, 2000, 284(13):1646.

Farr RW, "Leptospirosis," *Clin Infect Dis*, 1995, 21(1):1-8.

Guidugli F, Castro AA, and Atallah AN, "Systemic Reviews on Leptospirosis," *Rev Inst Med Trop Sao Paulo*, 2000, 42(1):47-9.

Holk K, Nielsen SV, and Ronne T, "Human Leptospirosis in Denmark 1970-1996: An Epidemiological and Clinical Study," *Scand J Infect Dis*, 2000, 32(5):533-8.

Weyant RS, Bragg SL, and Kaufmann AF, "*Leptospira* and Leptonema," *Manual of Clinical Microbiology*, 7th ed, Murray PR, Baron EJ, Pfaller MA, et al, eds, Washington, DC: AMS Press, American Society for Microbiology, 1999, 739-45.

Internet Web Sites

www.amm.co.uk/pubs/fa_leptospir.htm

www.cdc.gov/ncidod/dbmd/diseaseinfo/leptospirosis_g.htm

♦ ***Leptospira* Serodiagnosis** *see Leptospira* Serology *on page 649*

Leptospira Serology

Related Information
Bacterial Culture, Wounds, Bites on page 579
Darkfield Examination, Leptospirosis on page 601
Leptospira Culture on page 648

Synonyms Leptospira Antibodies; Leptospira Serodiagnosis

Test Includes Testing of patient's serum for antibodies against Leptospira species

Abstract Leptospirosis is a disease that occurs in all parts of the world. The disease can present as a mild flu-like form or as a severe fatal disease characterized by renal failure, liver dysfunction, and hemorrhages (Weil syndrome). Culture of blood, cerebrospinal fluid, and urine for organisms is strongly recommended but serologic diagnosis is often needed for confirmation when cultures are negative.

Specimen Serum

Container Red top tube

Sampling Time Acute and convalescent sera drawn 10-14 days apart are suggested. Agglutinins peak at 3-4 weeks of illness.

Reference Interval Negative. A fourfold increase in titer in paired sera is diagnostic of infection.

Critical Values IgM titer ≥1:100 provides evidence of recent or active disease

Use Diagnose leptospirosis (Weil disease) by demonstrating rising antibody titers. Antibody appears at the end of the first week of illness and peaks at 3-4 weeks, after which it slowly disappears.

Limitations The antigens used in the test are from the serovars most commonly causing disease, but there are many other serovars that might not be detected. A battery of antigens should be used.

Methodology Microscopic agglutination test (MAT), macroagglutination, complement fixation (CF), hemagglutination, enzyme-linked immunosorbent assay (ELISA), LEPTO dipstick

Additional Information Leptospirosis is an acute febrile zoonotic illness caused primarily by Leptospira interrogans, a large spirochete with more than 180 serologic variants. Patients with extensive animal contact or contact with contaminated water are particularly at risk. Although leptospires can be cultured from blood or urine during the first week of illness, this interval is often missed.

Recently, a quick and easy dipstick assay was developed for detection of Leptospira-specific IgM in human sera. The dipstick was coated with antigen from Leptospira biflexa. When compared with ELISA for detection of Leptospira IgM antibodies, the specificity was 92% to 94% and sensitivity was 60% for patients in the acute phase and 87% for patients in the convalescent phase of disease.[1,2]

An association between patients with leptospirosis and anticardiolipin antibodies exists which may induce vascular endothelial injury in severe cases.[3]

Leptospirosis in pregnant women is associated with abortion.

Footnotes
1. Gussenhoven GC, van der Hoorn MA, Goris MG, et al, "LEPTO Dipstick, a Dipstick Assay for Detection of Leptospira-Specific Immunoglobulin M Antibodies in Human Sera," J Clin Microbiol, 1997, 35(1):92-7.
2. Smits HL, Ananyina YV, Chereshsky A, et al, "International Multicenter Evaluation of the Clinical Utility of a Dipstick Assay for Detection of Leptospira-Specific Immunoglobulin M Antibodies in Human Serum Specimens," J Clin Microbiol, 1999, 37(9):2904-9.
3. Rugman FP, Pinn G, Palmer MF, et al, "Anticardiolipin Antibodies in Leptospirosis," J Clin Pathol, 1991, 44(6):517-9.

References
Centers for Disease Control and Prevention, "Outbreak of Acute Febrile Illness Among Participants in EcoChallenge Sahah 2000 - Malaysia," JAMA, 2000, 284(13):1646.
Farr RW, "Leptospirosis," Clin Infect Dis, 1995, 21(1):1-8.
Guidugli F, Castro AA, and Atallah AN, "Systemic Reviews on Leptospirosis," Rev Inst Med Trop Sao Paulo, 2000, 42(1):47-9.
Holk K, Nielsen SV, and Ronne T, "Human Leptospirosis in Denmark 1970-1996: An Epidemiological and Clinical Study," Scand J Infect Dis, 1996, 32(5):533-8.
Larsen SA, Pope V, and Quan TJ, "Immunologic Methods for the Diagnosis of Spirochetal Diseases," Manual of Clinical Laboratory Immunology, 4th ed, Volume 2, Chapter 73, Rose NR, Conway de Macario E, Fahey JL, et al, eds, Washington, DC: ASM Press, American Society for Microbiology, 1992, 467-81.
Levett PN and Whittington CU, "Evaluation of the Indirect Hemagglutination Assay for Diagnosis of Acute Leptospirosis," J Clin Microbiol, 1998, 36(1):11-4.

Internet Web Sites
www.amm.co.uk/pubs/fa_leptospir.htm
www.cdc.gov/ncidod/dbmd/diseaseinfo/leptospirosis_g.htm

♦ **Leptospirosis, Darkfield Examination** see Darkfield Examination, Leptospirosis on page 601

♦ **Leptospirosis DNA Amplification Method** see Darkfield Examination, Leptospirosis on page 601

♦ **L. gormanii** see Legionella Direct Fluorescent Antibody Smear on page 646

♦ **L. gormanii** see Legionella Serology on page 646

♦ **Lice Identification** see Arthropod Identification on page 559

♦ **Listeria monocytogenes** see Bacterial Culture, Cerebrospinal Fluid on page 569

♦ **Listeria monocytogenes** see Bacterial Culture, Genital Specimen on page 571

♦ **Listeria monocytogenes** see Bacterial Culture, Stool on page 575

♦ **L. jordanis** see Legionella Direct Fluorescent Antibody Smear on page 646

♦ **L. jordanis** see Legionella Serology on page 646

♦ **L. longbeachae** see Legionella Direct Fluorescent Antibody Smear on page 646

♦ **L. longbeachae** see Legionella Serology on page 646

♦ **L. micdadei** see Legionella Direct Fluorescent Antibody Smear on page 646

♦ **L. micdadei** see Legionella Serology on page 646

♦ **Loa loa Serology** see Filariasis Serological Test on page 608

♦ **Lumbar Puncture Hazards** see Viral Culture, Central Nervous System Symptoms on page 692

♦ **Lyme Borreliosis Serology** see Lyme Disease Serology on page 650

♦ **Lyme Disease** see Borrelia burgdorferi Culture on page 585

♦ **Lyme Disease Antibody Detection** see Lyme Disease Serology on page 650

♦ **Lyme Disease Bacterial Culture** see Borrelia burgdorferi Culture on page 585

Lyme Disease DNA Detection

Related Information
Borrelia burgdorferi Culture on page 585
Lyme Disease Serology on page 650

Synonyms Borrelia burgdorferi DNA Assay; Borrelia burgdorferi DNA Probe Test; Borrelia burgdorferi PCR; DNA Hybridization Test for Borrelia burgdorferi; DNA Probe Test for Lyme Disease; Lyme Disease PCR

Test Includes DNA from the spirochete Borrelia burgdorferi is amplified from a patient specimen or tick and specific DNA hybridization is used to detect the amplified product.

Abstract Lyme disease is a tick-borne zoonosis caused by infection with the spirochete Borrelia burgdorferi. It was first recognized in the U.S. in Wisconsin in 1969. Since that time, Lyme disease has been recognized as the most common vector-borne disease in North America and Eurasia.[1,2] Epidemics tend to occur in the spring and fall when a tick vector, Ixodes ricinus, is proliferating. Ticks transmit the spirochete to humans through bites. The diagnosis of Lyme disease is difficult due to the insensitivity and unreliability of serologic diagnostic tests. The detection of Borrelia burgdorferi genetic material by amplifying DNA directly in serum, spinal fluid, synovial fluid, skin biopsy, and urine can often confirm the diagnosis of Lyme disease when serologic tests are equivocal.[3]

Specimen Serum or plasma, cerebrospinal fluid, skin biopsy, synovial fluid, urine

Container Red top tube or lavender top (EDTA) tube for blood samples. Spinal fluid and synovial fluid should be collected in a sterile container. Plastic container is used for urine. Skin biopsy should be frozen quickly and should not be fixed with formalin.

Sampling Time Specimens should be collected before antibiotic therapy is initiated.

Storage Instructions All specimens should be sent to the laboratory immediately or kept at 4°C until shipped to the laboratory. Once in the laboratory, serum or plasma should be transferred to a sealed plastic tube.

Causes for Rejection Samples containing sodium azide cannot be used in this test

Turnaround Time 1 week

Reference Interval No Borrelia burgdorferi DNA detection

Use Detect the presence of the spirochete Borrelia burgdorferi genomic material in patients with signs and symptoms of Lyme disease

Methodology Patient specimens are treated to isolate DNA and rid the sample of substances that inhibit amplification of DNA. The DNA is then amplified using specific primers for Borrelia burgdorferi sequences. The amplified DNA is then confirmed to be B. burgdorferi by hybridization with a DNA probe, which can be accomplished by a variety of methods. At the current time, DNA amplification methods have not been standardized for routine diagnosis of Lyme disease. Thus, specificity and sensitivity may vary between assays.

Additional Information Transmission of Borrelia burgdorferi, a pathogenic spirochete, to humans occurs primarily by way of infected Ixodid ticks, including I. dammini, I. pacificus, Ixodes ricinus complex, and others. The signs and symptoms of Lyme disease vary, but the most common clinical manifestation following the bite of an infected tick is a distinctive skin lesion, erythema chronicum migrans. This initial stage of Lyme disease is benign and is usually successfully treated with oral antibiotics. Symptoms sometimes persist or reappear after antibiotic treatment. The later stage disease may include chronic progressive encephalomyelitis, chronic severe arthritis, (Continued)

Lyme Disease DNA Detection (Continued)

as well as various cardiac manifestations.[4] Direct microscopic detection of *Borrelia burgdorferi* is difficult; therefore the most widely used indicator of infection is the detection of *Borrelia burgdorferi*-specific antibody. Lyme disease serologic testing suffers from lack of specificity and reproducibility. Infected patients appear to have spirochetes in their tissues, serum, or spinal fluids. Amplification of *Borrelia burgdorferi* DNA detects the organism in a specific and sensitive assay from patient specimens. A test for direct detection of *Borrelia burgdorferi* DNA would enable detection of dissemination of the spirochete early in the course of infection.[5,6] Thus, appropriate antibiotic therapy can be initiated. It also allows for monitoring of patients during and after chemotherapy.[6] This is a valuable diagnostic tool since recognition of Lyme disease is often complicated by the variety of clinical signs and presentations.

Footnotes

1. Dennis DT, "Epidemiology, Ecology, and Prevention of Lyme Disease," *Lyme Disease*, Rahn DW, Evans J, eds, Philadelphia, PA: American College of Physicians, 1998, 7-34.
2. O'Connell S, Granstrom M, Gray JS, et al, "Epidemiology of European Lyme Borreliosis," *Zentralbl Bakteriol*, 1998, 287:229-40.
3. Brettschneider S, Bruckbauer H, Klugbauer N, et al, "Diagnostic Value of PCR for Detection of *Borrelia burgdorferi* in Skin Biopsy and Urine Samples From Patients With Skin Borreliosis," *J Clin Microbiol*, 1998, 36(9):2658-65.
4. Tugwell P, Dennis DT, Weinstein A, et al, "Laboratory Evaluation in the Diagnosis of Lyme Disease," *Ann Intern Med*, 1997, 127(12):1109-23.
5. Nocton JJ, Bloom BJ, Rutledge BJ, et al, "Detection of *Borrelia burgdorferi* DNA by Polymerase Chain Reaction in Cerebrospinal Fluid in Lyme Neuroborreliosis," *J Infect Dis*, 1996, 174(3):623-7.
6. Oksi J, Marjamaki M, Nikoskelainen J, et al, "*Borrelia burgdorferi* Detected by Culture and PCR in Clinical Relapse of Disseminated Lyme Borreliosis," *Ann Med*, 1999, 31(3):225-32.

References

Misonne MC and Hoet PP, "Species-Specific Plasmid Sequences for PCR Identification of the Three Species of *Borrelia burgdorferi* Sensu Lato Involved in Lyme Disease," *J Clin Microbiol*, 1998, 36(1):269-72.

Mouritsen CL, Wittwer CT, Litwin CM, et al, "Polymerase Chain Reaction Detection of Lyme Disease. Correlation With Clinical Manifestations and Serologic Responses," *Am J Clin Pathol*, 1996, 105(5):647-54.

Nadelman RB and Wormser GP, "Lyme Borreliosis," *Lancet*, 1998, 352(9127):557-65.

Nocton JJ, Dressler F, Rutledge BJ, et al, "Polymerase Chain Reaction *Borrelia burgdorferi* Synovial Fluid," *N Engl J Med*, 1994, 330(4):229-34.

Wang G, van Dam AP, Schwartz I, et al, "Molecular Typing of *Borrelia burgdorferi* Sensu Lato: Taxonomic, Epidemiological, and Clinical Implications," 1999, 12(4):633-53.

Internet Web Sites

www.amm.co.uk/pubs/fa_lyme.htm
www.astdhpphe.org/infect/lyme.html
www.cdc.gov/ncidod/dvbid/lymeinfo.htm

♦ **Lyme Disease PCR** see Lyme Disease DNA Detection on page 649

Lyme Disease Serology

Related Information

Arthropod Identification on page 559
Babesiosis Serology on page 561
Borrelia burgdorferi Culture on page 585
Ehrlichiosis Serology on page 603
Lyme Disease DNA Detection on page 649
Synovial Fluid Analysis on page 323

Synonyms *Borrelia burgdorferi* Sensu Lato Serology; Lyme Borreliosis Serology; Lyme Disease Antibody Detection; Serodiagnosis of Lyme Disease

Test Includes Detection of serological response to *Borrelia burgdorferi*

Abstract Lyme disease is a zoonosis due to *Borrelia burgdorferi*, transmitted to humans by tick bites. *B. burgdorferi* infection is often characterized by a characteristic skin lesion (erythema migrans) which occurs in 60% to 80% of patients. Weeks to months later some patients develop arthralgia, meningoencephalitis, or myocarditis.[1] The clinical presentation and exposure in an endemic area support clinical and laboratory integration and are critical to accurate diagnosis.[1] Early, clinical identification of erythema migrans is helpful. Therapy may be appropriate in seronegative individuals with clinical evidence of Lyme disease.

Physicians should interpret tests for *B. burgdorferi* in an appropriate clinical context.[2] The positive predictive value of Lyme disease serology is greater when testing takes place more than 12 months following onset.[3]

Specimen Serum or cerebrospinal fluid

Container Red top tube, sterile CSF tube

Sampling Time Brown et al, of the FDA, note that early in Lyme disease, test sensitivities are low and serologic testing is not considered useful.[3]

Reference Interval Values vary among laboratories

Use Serologic evaluation has a very limited role in evaluation of possible Lyme disease; investigate arthritis, rash, encephalopathy, polyneuropathy, carditis. The use of these serologic tests is to support the clinical diagnosis of Lyme disease.[3] **Negative serologic results should never be used as a reason to withhold antibiotic treatment when Lyme disease is suspected.**

Limitations False positives occur in patients infected with tick-borne relapsing fever, human granulocytic ehrlichiosis,[4] syphilis, leptospirosis, or periodontal disease,[5] and seronegative results early in the disease are frequent. Positives remain so for years after successful treatment.[6] Serologic evidence should not be the sole criterion for a diagnosis of Lyme disease; rather, it deserves consideration with clinical evaluation and risk of exposure. Positive serologic results in apparently healthy subjects are likely to be false positives.

Antibodies against Lyme disease antigens can interfere with the ANA test.

Commercial test kit performance has recently been addressed. Interlaboratory results, given these results, have been reported to provide poor agreement. Test performance varies among tests.[2] Incorrect diagnosis of Lyme disease in a subject with babesiosis may delay optimal therapy for that patient.[3]

Contraindications Lyme disease serology does not become positive until weeks or more following a tick bite; *vide supra*.[3] Patients who have only the nonspecific symptoms of myalgia, fatigue, and arthralgia need not be tested for Lyme disease.[2]

Methodology Indirect immunofluorescent antibody (IFA), enzyme-linked immunosorbent assay (ELISA), Western blot assay. A two-test approach for detection of active Lyme disease and of previous infection is recommended by the Centers for Disease Control. The specimen should first be tested using a sensitive enzyme immunoassay (EIA) or immunofluorescent antibody (IFA) followed by Western blot of positive or equivocal specimens.[7]

Additional Information Lyme disease is a multisystem disorder, with rash and arthritis as conspicuous symptoms. It is caused by *Borrelia burgdorferi*, a spirochete transmitted by the bite of ticks of the *Ixodes ricinus* complex. In the Eastern U.S. *I. scapularis* is the vector; it is also the vector for human granulocytic ehrlichiosis and for babesiosis.[8] In the Western U.S., *I. pacificus* has been found to transmit Lyme disease. Assay is available for IgG and IgM antibody in both serum and CSF. In early disease, a negative assay does not exclude the diagnosis because of the low sensitivity of the serologic assays. Further, response may be mitigated by antibiotics. Most patients with chronic disease usually have strong serologic responses to *B. burgdorferi* antigens. Recently developed immunoassays using recombinant outer surface protein C (22 kDa), flagellin protein (14 kDa), as well as a high molecular weight protein, p83, seem to have increased sensitivity when compared to use of an EIA with sonicated antigen from *B. burgdorferi*. All positive EIA or IFA results should be confirmed using a Western blot assay and detection of antibodies specific for *B. burgdorferi* proteins.[9]

Cultivation of *B. burgdorferi* from skin lesions suggestive of erythema migrans is described,[10] but culture is difficult because of need for a special bacteriologic medium and a long observation period required. Culture for *B. burgdorferi* is not done in a routine clinical laboratory.

Neurologic manifestations are found in about 15% of subjects. CSF pleocytosis is found in many but not all patients who have cranial nerve or meningeal involvement.[11] Increased lymphocytes may be found in cerebrospinal fluid. *Borrelia*-specific DNA using PCR assay is useful for diagnosis of neuroborreliosis.[12] See Lyme Disease DNA Detection on page 649.

Recently, two Lyme disease vaccines have been developed, LYMErix™ (SmithKline Beecham Pharmaceuticals) and ImuLyme™ (Pasteur Merieux Connaught). Only LYMErix™ has been licensed by the U.S. Food and Drug Administration. Both vaccines use the *B. burgdorferi* outer-surface protein A (rOspA) as the immunogen.[13,14] The Advisory Committee on Immunization Practices for the CDC has indicated that the Lyme disease vaccine does not protect all individuals against infection with the *B. burgdorferi* bacteria and that vaccinated persons should continue to practice personal protective measures when participating in outdoor activities that put them at risk for tick bites.[15] Specific guidelines are available.[15]

Identification of ticks is not always simple. Physicians are advised to seek assistance from sources trained in entomology.[16]

Footnotes

1. Nadelman RB and Wormser GP, "Lyme Borreliosis," *Lancet*, 1998, 352(9127):557-65.
2. Wormser GP, Aguero-Rosenfeld ME, and Nadelman RB, "Lyme Disease Serology: Problems and Opportunities," *JAMA*, 1999, 282(1):79-80.
3. Brown SL, Hansen SL, and Langone JJ, "Role of Serology in the Diagnosis of Lyme Disease," *JAMA*, 1999, 282(1):62-6
4. Wormser GP, Horowitz HW, Nowakowski J, et al, "Positive Lyme Disease Serology in Patients With Clinical and Laboratory Evidence of Human Granulocytic Ehrlichiosis," *Am J Clin Pathol*, 1997, 107(2):142-7.
5. Magnarelli LA, Miller JN, Anderson JF, et al, "Cross-Reactivity of Nonspecific Treponemal Antibody in Serologic Tests for Lyme Disease," *J Clin Microbiol*, 28(6):1276-9.
6. Steere AC, Taylor E, McHugh GL, et al, "The Overdiagnosis of Lyme Disease," *JAMA*, 1993, 269(14):1812-6.
7. Centers for Disease Control, "Notice to Readers Recommendations for Test Performance and Interpretation From the Second National Conference on Serologic Diagnosis of Lyme Disease," *MMWR Morb Mortal Wkly Rep*, 1995, 44(31):590-1.
8. Dennis DT, Nekomoto TS, Victor JC, et al, "Reported Distribution of *Ixodes scapularis* and *Ixodes pacificus* (Acari: Ixodidae) in the United States," *J Med Entomol*, 1998, 35(5):629-38.
9. Kaiser R and Rauer S, "Advantage of Recombinant Borrelial Proteins for Serodiagnosis of Neuroborreliosis," *J Med Microbiol*, 1999, 48(1):5-10.
10. Mitchell PD, Reed KD, Vandermause MF, et al, "Isolation of *Borrelia burgdorferi* From Skin Biopsy Specimens of Patients With Erythema Migrans," *Am J Clin Pathol*, 1993, 99(1):104-7.

11. Kaslow RA, "Current Perspective on Lyme Borreliosis," *JAMA*, 1992, 267(10):1381-3.

12. Kaiser R and Rauer S, "Serodiagnosis of Neuroborreliosis: Comparison of Reliability of Three Confirmatory Assays," *Infection*, 1999, 27 (3):177-82.

13. Steere AC, Sikand VK, Meurice F, et al, "Vaccination Against Lyme Disease With Recombinant *Borrelia burgdorferi* Outer-Surface Lipoprotein A With Adjuvant. Lyme Disease Vaccine Study Group," *N Engl J Med*, 1998, 339(4):209-15.

14. Sigal LH, Zahradnik JM, Levin P, et al, "A Vaccine Consisting of Recombinant *Borrelia burgdorferi* Outer-Surface Protein A to Prevent Lyme Disease. Recombinant Outer-Surface Protein A Lyme Disease Vaccine Study Consortium," *N Engl J Med*, 1998, 339(4):216-22.

15. Centers for Disease Control, "Recommendations for the Use of Lyme Disease Vaccine, Recommendations of the Advisory Committee on Immunization Practices (ACIP)," *MMWR Morb Mortal Wkly Rep*, 1999, 48:RR-7.

16. Falco RC, Fish D, and D'Amico V, "Accuracy of Tick Identification in a Lyme Disease Endemic Area," *JAMA*, 1998, 280(7):602-3.

References

Barbour AG, "Expert Advice and Patient Expectations: Laboratory Testing and Antibiotics for Lyme Disease," *JAMA*, 1998, 279(3):239-40.

Engstrom SM, Shoop E, and Johnson RC, "Immunoblot Interpretation Criteria for Serodiagnosis of Early Lyme Disease," *J Clin Microbiol*, 1995, 33(2):419-27.

Fix AD, Strickland GT, and Grant J, "Tick Bites and Lyme Disease in an Endemic Setting: Problematic Use of Serologic Testing and Prophylactic Antibiotic Therapy," *JAMA*, 1998, 279(3):206-10.

Gardner P, "Long-Term Outcomes and Management of Patients With Lyme Disease," *JAMA*, 2000, 283(5):658-9.

Rahn DW, "Lyme Disease - Where's the Bug?" *N Engl J Med*, 1994, 330(4):282-3.

Sweeney CJ, Ghassemi M, Agger WA, et al, "Coinfection With Babesia Microti and *Borrelia Burgdorferi* in a Western Wisconsin Resident," *Mayo Clin Proc*, 1998, 73(4):338-41.

Trevejo RT, Krause PJ, Sikand VK, et al, "Evaluation of Two-Test Serodiagnostic Method for Early Lyme Disease in Clinical Practice," *J Infect Dis*, 1999, 179(4):931-8.

Internet Web Sites

www.amm.co.uk/pubs/fa_lyme.htm
www.astdhpphe.org/infect/lyme.html
www.cdc.gov/ncidod/dvbid/lymeinfo.htm

♦ **Lymph Node Culture for Epstein-Barr Virus** *see* Epstein-Barr Virus Culture *on page 607*

♦ **Lymphocyte Culture for Epstein-Barr Virus** *see* Epstein-Barr Virus Culture *on page 607*

♦ **Lymphogranuloma Venereum Culture** *see* Chlamydia trachomatis Culture *on page 590*

♦ **Lysogenic Bacteriophages** *see* Shiga Toxin Test, Direct *on page 680*

♦ ***Mansonella ozzardi* Serology** *see* Filariasis Serological Test *on page 608*

♦ ***Mansonella perstans* Serology** *see* Filariasis Serological Test *on page 608*

♦ ***Mansonella streptocerca* Serology** *see* Filariasis Serological Test *on page 608*

♦ **Maximum Bactericidal Dilution** *see* Serum Bactericidal Test *on page 679*

♦ **Mazzini** *replaced by* RPR *on page 677*

♦ **Mazzini** *replaced by* VDRL, Serum *on page 688*

♦ **MBC** *see* Antimicrobial Susceptibility Testing, Minimum Bactericidal Concentration *on page 557*

♦ **MBD** *see* Serum Bactericidal Test *on page 679*

♦ **Measles Culture, 3-Day** *see* Rubella Virus Culture *on page 678*

Measles Serology

Related Information

Viral Culture *on page 689*
Viral Culture, Respiratory Symptoms *on page 694*

Synonyms Rubeola Antibodies

Applies to Rubeola Serology, CSF

Test Includes Antibodies specific for rubeola, either IgG and IgM, in patient's serum or cerebrospinal fluid

Abstract Measles is an acute viral disease which causes generalized infection involving the respiratory tract and lymphoreticular tissues. It includes a papular eruption, lymphadenopathy, cough, and fever. Due to the widespread use of childhood immunization, measles has been nearly eliminated in most developed countries, including the U.S.[1,2]

Specimen Serum or cerebrospinal fluid

Container Red top tube, sterile CSF tube

Reference Interval Less than fourfold rise in IgG titer, absent IgM titer; IgG: <1:5; IgM: <1:10; hemagglutination inhibition >1:10, neutralization >1:20 indicates immunity

Use Serologic study can be useful in establishing that an individual has immunity subsequent to vaccination. In many individuals **detectable** immunity does not persist. In acute illness, hemagglutinating and neutralizing

antibody peak 2 weeks after the rash appears. It is necessary to demonstrate rising titers over 2 weeks, or identify IgM antibody to establish diagnosis. Very high serum titers in the absence of acute illness, or high CSF titer, are seen in subacute sclerosing panencephalitis. Protective antibody levels of antibodies to measles, mumps, and rubella have been assessed by oral fluid sampling.[3]

Limitations The presence of measles-specific IgG in a single serum specimen indicates past or present infection or past vaccination.

Methodology The most commonly used assay is the enzyme-linked immunosorbent assay (ELISA). Less frequently used methods are hemagglutination inhibition (HAI) and viral neutralization (NT).

Additional Information Measles (rubeola) is caused by a paramyxovirus, and is rapidly spread from person-to-person via aerosol. Occasional small epidemics have occurred in vaccinated populations and revaccination appears to be of value. Due to massive immunization of children, measles is no longer an indigenous disease in the U.S. Most (71%) of the 100 cases reported to the CDC in 1998 were associated with internationally imported cases.[2] Information on childhood immunizations including the combination measles, mumps, and rubella vaccine can be found in the CDC publication "Combination Vaccines for Childhood Immunizations, Recommendations of the Advisory Committee on Immunization Practices (ACIP), the American Academy of Pediatrics (AAP), and the American Academy of Family Physicians (AAFP)".[4]

Footnotes

1. Peltola H, Heinonen OP, Valle M, et al, "The Elimination of Indigenous Measles, Mumps, and Rubella From Finland by a 12-Year, Two-Dose Vaccination Program," *N Engl J Med*, 1994, 331(21):1397-1402.

2. Centers for Disease Control, "Epidemiology of Measles - United States, 1998," *MMWR Morb Mortal Wkly Rep*, 1999, 48(34):749-53.

3. Thieme T, Piacentini S, Davidson S, et al, "Determination of Measles, Mumps, and Rubella Immunization Status Using Oral Fluid Samples," *JAMA*, 1994, 272(3):219-21.

4. CDC, "Combination Vaccines for Childhood Immunizations, Recommendations of the Advisory Committee on Immunization Practices (ACIP), the American Academy of Pediatrics (AAP), and the American Academy of Family Physicians (AAFP)," *MMWR Morb Mortal Wkly Rep*, 1999, 48(RR-5):1-15.

References

Bellini WJ, Rota JS, and Rota PA, "Virology of Measles Virus," *J Infect Dis*, 1994, 170(Suppl 1):S15-S23.

Helfand RF, Kebede S, Gary HE Jr, et al, "Timing of Development of Measles-Specific Immunoglobulin M and G After Primary Measles Vaccination," *Clin Diagn Lab Immunol*, 1999, 6(2):178-80.

Osterhaus AD, de Vries P, and van Binnedijk RS, "Measles Vaccines: Novel Generations and New Strategies," *J Infect Dis*, 1994, 170(Suppl 1):S42-S55.

Whittle H, Aaby P, Samb B, et al, "Poor Serologic Responses Five to Seven Years After Immunization With High and Standard Titer Measles Vaccines," *Pediatr Infect Dis*, 1999, 18(1):53-7.

Internet Web Sites

www.astdhpphe.org/infect/measles.html
www.cdc.gov/nip/publications/pink/meas.pdf
www.who.int/vaccines-diseases/research/virus1.htm

♦ **Measles Serology, 3-day** *see* Rubella Serology *on page 677*

♦ **Measles Virus, Direct Detection** *see* Virus, Direct Detection by Fluorescent Antibody *on page 696*

MHA-TP

Related Information

Darkfield Examination, Syphilis *on page 601*
FTA-ABS, Serum *on page 609*
RPR *on page 677*
VDRL, Cerebrospinal Fluid *on page 688*
VDRL, Serum *on page 688*

Synonyms Microhemagglutination-*Treponema pallidum*

Applies to Syphilis Enzyme Immunoassay; Syphilis Serology

Test Includes Detection of serologic response specific for *Treponema pallidum*

Abstract In the diagnosis and management of patients with syphilis, the MHA-TP is used as a treponemal-specific (confirmatory) test for syphilis. The FTA-ABS and the MHA-TP are the standard treponemal tests. A reactive treponemal test in a subject also reactive in a nontreponemal test is highly specific.[1]

Patient Preparation Patient should be fasting if possible.

Specimen Serum

Container Red top tube

Storage Instructions Remove serum from clot and freeze to ship.

Causes for Rejection Plasma collected

Reference Interval Nonreactive

Critical Values Results reported as nonreactive, inconclusive, or reactive

Possible Panic Range Positive serodiagnosis of syphilis in pregnancy

Use Confirmatory serologic test for syphilis

Limitations The test cannot be used to test CSF specimens. The test has decreased sensitivity in early (primary) stages of syphilis, but in the secondary and latent stages of syphilis, the sensitivity is equal to that of the FTA-ABS tests. THe MHA-TP assay gives fewer false-positive results than the other treponemal test methods. False positives may occur in patients with
(Continued)

MHA-TP *(Continued)*

systemic lupus, infectious mononucleosis, drug addiction, collagen disease, or lepromatous leprosy. Potential causes of false-positive serologic tests for syphilis are tabulated in VDRL, Serum *on page 688*.

Methodology Hemagglutination - sensitized sheep cells are coated with *T. pallidum* antigen

Additional Information This is a *Treponema*-specific test and should not be used as a screening test except in late stages of syphilis. It is as sensitive and specific as FTA-ABS in all stages of syphilis except primary, in which it is less sensitive. It provides fewer false positives than the FTA-ABS.[1] It is positive with treponemal infections other than syphilis (bejel, pinta, yaws). Historically, it was thought that the treponemal tests, FTA-ABS and MHA-TP, would remain positive even after effective treatment; however, with newer antibiotic treatments in immunocompetent patients with first-episode syphilis, 13% of the patients had nonreactive MHA-TP after 36 months.[2] In general, it is not clear whether treponemal-specific serologic assays will determine if a patient has been adequately treated for syphilis.

EIA, IgG and IgM, is a recently available method. IgM EIA is reported to be useful for diagnosis of congenital syphilis. IgG EIA is reported to be a reliable test which can replace the MHA-TP or FTA-ABS.[2,3]

PCR may be useful for congenital syphilis but currently is only available in a few reference and research laboratories.[4,5]

Footnotes

1. Larsen SA, Steiner BM, and Rudolph AH, "Laboratory Diagnosis and Interpretation of Tests for Syphilis," *Clin Microbiol Rev*, 1995, 8(1):1-21.
2. Singh AE and Romanowski B, "Syphilis: Review and Emphasis on Clinical, Epidemiologic, and Some Biologic Features," *Clin Microbiol Rev*, 1999, 12(2):187-209.
3. Reisner BS, Mann LM, Tholcken CA, et al, "Use of the *Treponema pallidum*-Specific Captia Syphilis IgG Assay in Conjunction With the Rapid Plasma Reagin to Test for Syphilis," *J Clin Microbiol*, 1997, 35(5):1141-3.
4. Centurion-Lara A, Castro C, Shaffer JM, et al, "Detection of *Treponema pallidum* by a Sensitive Reverse Transcriptase PCR," *J Clin Microbiol*, 1997, 35(6):1348-52.
5. Pietravalle M, Pimpinelli F, Maini A, et al, "Diagnostic Relevance of Polymerase Chain Reaction Technology for *T. pallidum* in Subjects With Syphilis in Different Phases of Infection," *New Microbiol*, 1999, 22(2):99-104.

References

Augenbraun MH, Rolfs R, Johnson R, et al, "Treponemal Specific Tests for the Serodiagnosis of Syphilis. Syphilis and HIV Study Group," *Sex Transm Dis*, 1998, 25(10):549-52.

Romanowski B, Sutherland R, Fick GH, et al, "Serologic Response to Treatment of Infectious Syphilis," *Ann Intern Med*, 1991, 114(12):1005-9.

Young H, "Syphilis Serology," *Dermatol Clinic*, 1998, 16(4):691-8.

Internet Web Sites

www.amm.co.uk/pubs/fa_leptospir.htm

www.cdc.gov/ncidod/dbmd/diseaseinfo/leptospirosis_g.htm

♦ **MIC** *see* Antimicrobial Susceptibility Testing, Aerobic and Facultatively Anaerobic Bacteria *on page 554*

♦ **MIC, Anaerobic Bacteria** *see* Antimicrobial Susceptibility Testing, Anaerobic Bacteria *on page 555*

♦ **MIC, Fastidious Organisms, Unusual Isolates** *see* Antimicrobial Susceptibility Testing, Unusual Isolates/Fastidious Organisms *on page 558*

♦ **Microfilariae Serological Test** *see* Filariasis Serological Test *on page 608*

♦ **Microhemagglutination-***Treponema pallidum* *see* MHA-TP *on page 651*

♦ **Microsporidia** *see* Ova and Parasites, Stool *on page 666*

Microsporidia Diagnostic Procedures

Related Information

Bacterial Culture, Stool *on page 575*
Cryptosporidium Direct Staining Procedures *on page 596*
Electron Microscopy *on page 54*
Ova and Parasites, Stool *on page 666*
Ova and Parasites, Urine *on page 667*

Synonyms Acid-Fast Stain for Microsporidia; Microsporidia Immunofluorescent Assay; Stool Examination for Microsporidia

Test Includes Examination of stool, body fluids, or biopsy for Microsporidia using special stains, immunofluorescence, or electron microscopy

Abstract Microsporidiosis refers to diseases produced by Microsporidia, a group of primitive, obligate intracellular protozoan parasites belonging to the phylum Microspora. Five different genera (*Enterocytozoon, Encephalitozoon, Nosema, Septata, Pleistophora*) have been implicated in human infections. They are best known as causes of diarrhea in patients with AIDS and also cause acute bilateral keratoconjunctivitis, sinonasal disease, bronchiolitis, pneumonia, infection of biliary and pancreatic ducts, acalculus cholecystitis, and other disease states.[1]

Specimen Feces, urine, sputum, corneal or conjunctival scrapings, biopsy tissue, cerebrospinal fluid

Collection Biopsies should be fixed in formalin as soon as possible.

Special Instructions If microsporidiosis is suspected, consult with the laboratory. These organisms may not be detected with usual stains.

Use A part of the differential diagnostic work-up of diarrhea and other Microsporidia-associated diseases in immunocompromised patients, particularly AIDS patients

Limitations Detection of Microsporidia is entirely dependent on the adequacy of the specimen, staining and preparation of the specimen, and experience of the person who examines the specimen. They are small organisms and easily missed in biopsies and cytology specimens as well as in stool specimens by light microscopy. Conventional H&E and Papanicolaou stains do not lend themselves to recognition of these organisms.

Methodology Organisms can be detected in stained cytologic smears, tissue biopsies, and stool.

Microsporidia do not stain well with either H&E or the Papanicolaou stains. There are several good stains for Microsporidia; however, not all of them stain the five major species of Microsporidia. Microsporidia in paraffin-embedded tissues are seen with a tissue Gram stain (Brown and Hopps stain, Brown and Brenn stain, Steiner stains, chromotrope methods). Microsporidia in plastic-embedded tissues stain well with toluidine blue and with methylene blue-azure II-basic fuchsin.

Microsporidia in cytologic centrifugation, smears and scraping preparations usually stain well with Gram stain for specimens with little or no bacterial contamination. In these preparations, most Microsporidia and bacteria are dark purple; some Microsporidia are gram-negative or gram-variable. Weber's modified trichrome (chromotrope-based) stain works well with specimens with bacterial contamination; Microsporidia are magenta-pink and the background (including bacteria) is blue-green. When large numbers of bacteria are present, the Weber chromotrope stain is also useful.[1]

Some laboratories use Giemsa stain for stool smears and body fluids. Calcofluor white is useful for screening stools for Microsporidia spores.[2] Gram stain is useful for demonstration of spores in sputum.[3] Most strains cause Microsporidia to appear as extremely fat bacteria which have a uniform oval shape, do not show budding, contain polar densities, and have a central clear band or area. Positive controls are needed for each of the methods.[3] Immunofluorescence staining techniques, which include labeled antibody to Microsporidia, appear to work well in detecting Microsporidia in clinical specimens and in differentiating infections due to certain Microsporidia. Some Microsporidia have been cultured *in vitro*, but routine culture for Microsporidia is not yet practical. PCR has been successfully utilized and is available in some reference and research laboratories.[1]

Additional Information Microsporidiosis can be considered an emerging infectious disease that was first recognized in HIV-infected patients. These parasites have been recognized as one of the major causes of AIDS enteropathy, especially in homosexual patients.[4] The diarrhea in these patients is of gradual onset and can persist for months. The stools are usually watery without blood or mucus, and undigested food may be seen in feces. The diarrhea may lead to dehydration, hypokalemia, and hypomagnesemia.[5] Some HIV patients may have coinfections with other enteric pathogens such as cryptosporidia, atypical mycobacteria, or cytomegalovirus.[6]

A few infections have been noted in immunocompetent hosts, however, infections in immunocompetent individuals are rare and are usually mild or subclinical.[4,7]

Footnotes

1. Schwartz DA, Sobottka I, Leitch GJ, et al, "Pathology of Microsporidiosis: Emerging Parasitic Infections in Patients With Acquired Immunodeficiency Syndrome," *Arch Pathol Lab Med*, 1996, 120(2):173-88.
2. Luna VA, Stewart BK, Bergeron DL, et al, "Use of the Fluorochrome Calcofluor White in the Screening of Stool Specimens for Spores of Microsporidia," *Am J Clin Pathol*, 1995, 103(5):656-9.
3. Long EG and Christie JD, "The Diagnosis of Old and New Gastrointestinal Parasites," *Clin Lab Med*, 1995, 15(2):307-31.
4. Sandfort J, Hannemann A, Gelderblom H, et al, "*Enterocytozoon bieneusi* Infection in an Immunocompetent Patient Who Had Acute Diarrhea and Who Was Not Infected With the Human Immunodeficiency Virus," *Clin Infect Dis*, 1994, 19(3):514-6.
5. Asmuth DM, De Girolami PC, Federman M, et al, "Clinical Features of Microsporidiosis in Patients With AIDS," *Clin Infect Dis*, 1994, 18(5):819-25.
6. Garcia LS, Shimizu RY, and Bruckner DA, "Detection of Microsporidial Spores in Fecal Specimens From Patients Diagnosed With Cryptosporidiosis," *J Clin Microbiol*, 1994, 32(7):1739-41.
7. Raynaud L, Delbac R, Broussolle V, et al, "Identification of *Encephalitozoon intestinalis* in Travelers With Chronic Diarrhea by Specific PCR Amplification," *J Clin Microbiol*, 1998, 36(1):37-40.

References

Chioralia G, Trammer T, Kampen H, et al, "Relevant Criteria for Detecting Microsporidia in Stool Specimens," *J Clin Microbiol*, 1998, 36(8):2279-83.

Conteas CN, Sowerby T, Berlin GW, et al, "Fluorescence Techniques for Diagnosing Intestinal Microsporidiosis in Stool, Enteric Fluid, and Biopsy Specimens From Acquired Immunodeficiency Syndrome Patients With Chronic Diarrhea," *Arch Pathol Lab Med*, 1996, 120(9):847-53.

Croppo GP, Visvesvara GS, Leitch GJ, et al, "Identification of the Microsporidian *Encephalitozoon hellem* Using Immunoglobulin G Monoclonal Antibodies," *Arch Pathol Lab Med*, 1998, 122(2):182-6.

Franzen C and Muller A, "Molecular Techniques for Detection, Species Differentiation and Phylogenetic Analysis of Microsporidia," *Clin Microbiol Rev*, 1999, 12(2):243-85.

Goodgame R, Stager C, Marcantel B, et al, "Intensity of Infection in AIDS-Related Intestinal Microsporidiosis," *J Infect Dis*, 1999, 180(3):929-32.

Joste NE, Rich JD, Busam KJ, et al, "Autopsy Verification of *Encephalitozoon intestinalis* (Microsporidiosis) Eradication Following Albendazole Therapy," *Arch Pathol Lab Med*, 1996, 120(2):199-203.

Lamps LW, Bronner MP, Vnencak-Jones CL, et al, "Optimal Screening and Diagnosis of Microsporidia in Tissue Sections: A Comparison of Polarization, Special Stains, and Molecular Techniques," *Am J Clin Pathol*, 1998, 109(4):404-10.

Moura H, Schwartz DA, Bornay-Llinares F, et al, "A New and Improved Quick-Hot Gram-Chromotrope Technique That Differentially Stains Microsporidian Spores in Clinical Samples, Including Paraffin-Embedded Tissue Sections," *Arch Pathol Lab Med*, 1997, 121(8):888-93.

Schwartz DA, "Emerging and Reemerging Infections. Progress and Challenges in the Subspecialty of Infectious Disease Pathology," *Arch Pathol Lab Med*, 1997, 121(8):776-84.

Soule JB, Halverson AL, Becker RB, et al, "A Patient With Acquired Immunodeficiency Syndrome and Untreated *Encephalitozoon (Septata) intestinalis* Microsporidiosis Leading to Small Bowel Perforation. Response to Albendazole," *Arch Pathol Lab Med*, 1997, 121(8):880-7.

Weber R and Bryan RT, "Microsporidial Infections in Immunodeficient and Immunocompetent Patients," *Clin Infect Dis*, 1994, 19(3):517-21.

Weber R, Deplazes P, Flepp M, et al, "Cerebral Microsporidiosis Due to *Encephalitozoon cuniculi* in a Patient With Human Immunodeficiency Virus Infection," *N Engl J Med*, 1997, 336(7):474-8.

Weiss LM and Vossbrinck CR, "Microsporidiosis: Molecular and Diagnostic Aspects," *Adv Parasitol*, 1998, 40:351-95.

Yachnis AT, Berg J, Martinez-Salazar A, et al, "Disseminated Microsporidiosis Especially Infecting the Brain, Heart, and Kidneys. Report of a Newly Recognized Pansporoblastic Species in Two Symptomatic AIDS Patients," *Am J Clin Pathol*, 1996, 106(4):535-43.

Internet Web Sites
www.cdc.gov/ncidod/dpd/parasites/microsporidia/default.htm

Mumps Serology

Related Information

Synonyms Mumps Antibodies

Test Includes Detection of serologic response to mumps infection or vaccination

Abstract Mumps is caused by a paramyxovirus and man is the only known reservoir. Mumps is a self-limited illness characterized by parotitis, high fever, and fatigue. In the U.S. and many other developed countries, mumps has decreased dramatically due to the mumps vaccine. It is recommended that children 12-15 months of age receive the trivalent vaccine that contains live, attenuated measles, mumps, and rubella. A second dose of vaccine should be administered at 4-6 or 11-12 years of age.[1,2]

Specimen Serum

Container Red top tube

Sampling Time Acute and convalescent sera drawn 10-14 days apart are required to diagnose natural mumps infection.

Reference Interval A fourfold or greater increase in titer is indicative of recent mumps infection in complement fixation test; normal IgG is <1:5 and IgM is <1:10; a positive IgM indirect fluorescent test and IgG ≥1:5 are indicative of recent infection; demonstrable IgG usually provides indication of immunity and/or prior exposure

Use Support for the diagnosis of mumps virus infection; document previous exposure to mumps virus or mumps vaccination; detection of mumps-specific IgM is useful for the diagnosis of acute disease

Limitations Several test systems that detect IgG are not specific for mumps and may cross-react with other paramyxovirus antibodies. Cross-reactions between mumps and parainfluenza viruses have not been observed for IgM antibody.[3]

Methodology Complement fixation (CF), enzyme-linked immunosorbent assay (ELISA), indirect fluorescent antibody (IFA), hemagglutination inhibition (HAI), hemolysis-in-gel, virus neutralization

Additional Information Complications of mumps include aseptic meningitis, encephalitis, orchitis, oophoritis, and pancreatitis. Serologic study may be undertaken to confirm a diagnosis in acute disease or to demonstrate established immunity. For diagnosis in an acute illness, measuring IgM antibody is simple, accurate, and rapid. The laboratory diagnosis of mumps can be achieved by viral isolation, detection of viral antigen directly in specimen, detection of viral genome, or by serologic methods. Since the introduction of the trivalent mumps, measles, and rubella vaccine in 1967, the number of mumps infections has decreased in the U.S. to only 308 in 1999. Several problems still exist in the delivery of vaccinations. There are still some populations that do not accept immunization to prevent disease. The number of vaccines and the complexity of vaccination schedules make delivering vaccinations difficult, and often the immunization provider is likely to change during the course of a child's vaccination series. In order to improve vaccination coverage, the CDC has recently published a report on vaccine-preventable diseases.[4]

Footnotes
1. Peltola H, Heinonen OP, Valle M, et al, "The Elimination of Indigenous Measles, Mumps, and Rubella From Finland by a 12-Year, Two-Dose Vaccination Program," *N Engl J Med*, 1994, 331(21):1397-1402.

2. CDC, "Combination Vaccines for Childhood Immunizations, Recommendations of the Advisory Committee on Immunization Practices (ACIP), the American Academy of Pediatrics (AAP), and the American Academy of Family Physicians (AAFP)," *MMWR Morb Mortal Wkly Rep*, 1999, 48:RR-5.

3. Swierkosz EM, "Mumps Virus," *Manual of Clinical Microbiology*, 7th ed, Chapter 74, Murray PR, Baron EJ, Pfaller MA, et al, eds, Washington, DC: AMS Press, American Society for Microbiology, 1999, 959-63.

4. CDC, "Vaccine-Preventable Diseases: Improving Vaccination Coverage in Children, Adolescents, and Adults," *MMWR Morb Mortal Wkly Rep*, 1999, 48:RR-8.

References
Black FL, "Measles and Mumps," *Manual of Clinical Laboratory Immunology*, 4th ed, Chapter 89, Rose NR, Conway de Macario E, Fahey JL, et al, eds, Washington, DC: ASM Press, American Society for Microbiology, 1992, 596-9.

Costello MJ, Smernoff NT, and Yungbluth M, "Laboratory Diagnosis of Viral Respiratory Tract Infections," *Lab Med*, 1993, 24(3):150.

Narita M, Matsuzono Y, Takekoshi Y, et al, "Analysis of Mumps Vaccine Failure by Means of Avidity Testing for Mumps Virus-Specific Immunoglobulin G," *Clin Diagn Lab Immunol*, 1998, 5(6):799-803.

Pipkin PA, Afzal MA, Heath AB, et al, "Assay of Humoral Immunity to Mumps Virus," *J Virol Methods*, 1999, 79(2):219-25.

Internet Web Sites
web.health.gov/communityguide
www.astdhpphe.org/infect/mumps.html
www.cdc.gov/nip/publications/pink/mumps.pdf

Mumps Virus Culture

Related Information

Applies to Hemadsorbing Virus

(Continued)

Mumps Virus Culture (Continued)

Test Includes Mumps virus is isolated from routine viral cultures usually after 3-7 days of incubation

Abstract Due to immunization, the number of mumps infections has decreased in the U.S. as well as around the world.[1,2] Humans are the only known natural host of the mumps virus and a carrier state in humans has not been reported. Thus it is possible that this viral disease can be eliminated from humans by mass vaccination.

Specimen Saliva, urine, cerebrospinal fluid, viral swab of Stensen's duct

Container Sterile container for urine and CSF; tube with cold viral transport medium for swabs

Sampling Time At or within 5 days of the onset of illness

Collection It is desirable to collect specimens as early in the disease as possible.

Saliva, 9 days before onset to 8 days after onset. In young patients, saliva is collected by a suitable suction device or by swabbing, especially the area around the orifices of the Stensen's duct. The swabs must immediately be placed into cold viral transport medium.

Cerebrospinal fluid (CSF) from patients with meningoencephalitis should be collected within 6 days after onset. CSF is obtained in the usual manner and should be put into a sterile test tube.

Virus is also excreted in urine for as long as 14 days after the onset of illness. For urine specimens, preferably collect the first voided morning urine in a sterile container.

All specimens must immediately be placed on ice and sent to the laboratory.

Storage Instructions Do **not** freeze at -20°C. Storage at -20°C rapidly inactivates the mumps virus. If inoculation is delayed by more than 48 hours, specimens should be frozen at -70°C.

Turnaround Time Variable (3-14 days) and depends on methods used and amount of virus in the specimen. Negative results are reported at 14 days.

Reference Interval No virus isolated

Use Aid in the diagnosis of disease caused by mumps virus, especially meningitis

Limitations Negative viral culture does not rule out the involvement of mumps virus in disease process.

Methodology Inoculation of specimen into cell cultures, incubation of cultures, observation for characteristic cytopathic effect (CPE), and identification by methods such as hemadsorption and fluorescent monoclonal antibodies

Additional Information Although virus isolation is the most certain means for establishing the laboratory diagnosis, serologic methods are also useful and technically easier. Demonstration of IgM antibodies in acute serum is diagnostic of primary infection. In most instances, the diagnosis of mumps is made on the basis of exposure, history of immunization (or lack of immunization), and the presence of parotid swelling. The white blood cell and differential counts are usually normal with maybe a slight leukopenia.

The incidence of mumps infections has dramatically declined since the introduction of the mumps vaccine in 1967. All children from 12-15 months of age should receive the trivalent vaccine that contains live, attenuated measles, mumps, and rubella. A second dose of vaccine should be administered at 4-6 or 11-12 years of age.[1,2] Most states require evidence of immunization to mumps before children can attend school.

Footnotes

1. Peltola H, Heinonen OP, Valle M, et al, "The Elimination of Indigenous Measles, Mumps, and Rubella From Finland by a 12-Year, Two-Dose Vaccination Program," *N Engl J Med*, 1994, 331(21):1397-1402.

2. CDC, "Combination Vaccines for Childhood Immunizations, Recommendations of the Advisory Committee on Immunization Practices (ACIP), the American Academy of Pediatrics (AAP), and the American Academy of Family Physicians (AAFP)," *MMWR Morb Mortal Wkly Rep*, 1999, 48:RR-5.

References

Germann D, Gorgievski M, Strohle A, et al, "Detection of Mumps Virus in Clinical Specimens by Rapid Centrifugation Culture and Conventional Tube Cell Culture," *J Virol Methods*, 1998, 73(1):59-64.

Hierholzer JC, Bingham PG, Castells E, et al, "Time-Resolved Fluoroimmunoassays With Monoclonal Antibodies for Rapid Identification of Parainfluenza Type 4 and Mumps Viruses," *Arch Virol*, 1993, 130(3-4):335-52.

Swierkosz EM, "Mumps Virus," *Manual of Clinical Microbiology*, 7th ed, Chapter 74, Murray PR, Baron EJ, Pfaller MA, et al, eds, Washington, DC: AMS Press, American Society for Microbiology, 1999, 959-63.

Internet Web Sites

www.astdhpphe.org/infect/mumps.html

www.cdc.gov/nip/publications/pink/mumps.pdf

♦ **Mumps Virus Culture, Urine** see Viral Culture, Urine on page 695

♦ **Mumps Virus, Direct Detection** see Virus, Direct Detection by Fluorescent Antibody on page 696

Mycobacteria by DNA Probe

Related Information

Acid-Fast Stain on page 550

Adenosine Deaminase, CSF, Pleural Fluid, Pericardial Fluid, Peritoneal Fluid on page 83
Mycobacterial Culture, Biopsy or Body Fluid on page 655
Mycobacterial Culture, Cerebrospinal Fluid on page 656
Mycobacterial Culture, Cutaneous and Subcutaneous Tissue on page 657
Mycobacterial Culture, Sputum on page 658
Mycobacterial Culture, Stool on page 659
Mycobacterial Culture, Urine on page 660

Synonyms DNA Test for Mycobacteria; Mycobacteria DNA Detection Test; PCR for *M. tuberculosis*

Applies to Amplification of Genetic Material Specific for Mycobacteria

Test Includes Direct detection of mycobacterial DNA in patient specimens or after primary culture

Abstract It has been estimated that world-wide the number of people infected with *Mycobacterium tuberculosis* (TB) each year is ~8 million.[1] In the U.S., the number of tuberculosis cases dramatically increased between 1985 and 1992. This increased frequency of TB infection was due in part to transmission to and between patients with acquired immune deficiency syndrome, patients with malignant disorders and immunosuppression, I.V. drug users, prison inmates, refugees and immigrants, nursing home residents, and the homeless population.[2] Since 1992, the number of cases has consistently declined, primarily due to the prevention and control measures instituted by the CDC. One of these measures was the use of new and improved laboratory methods to both culture and detect TB. In the past, the lack of a rapid method to detect *M. tuberculosis* was a major obstacle in establishing effective infection control. Following exposure, baseline and 12-week follow-up tuberculin skin tests (PPD) are included in standard assessment protocols. However, tuberculin testing is unreliable in immunocompromised individuals (eg, those with HIV infection). Culture and identification of this organism can take up to 8 weeks and direct staining procedures are insensitive. Thus, the ability to detect specific mycobacterial DNA directly from the patient specimen with provision of early diagnosis has great advantages in diagnosis, treatment, and prevention of spread to others. Nucleic acid tests are also available to determine the species of *Mycobacterium* after isolation by culture. Many of the culture confirmation nucleic acid tests for *Mycobacterium* are available in larger clinical laboratories.

Specimen Sputum, pleural fluid, cerebrospinal fluid, bronchial aspirates, urine, and tissue biopsy or isolate from growth of acid-fast bacteria

Container Sputum, pleural fluid, and cerebrospinal fluid should be collected and transported in a tightly sealed plastic container such as a sputum cup or a sterile bronchoscopy tube. This container should be transferred into a secondary sealed container for transport.

Collection Samples should be collected as for mycobacteria culture. Sputum should be collected as early in the morning as possible, preferably before the morning meal. First morning urine should be collected.

Storage Instructions The specimens should be kept refrigerated if not immediately processed. Do not freeze.

Causes for Rejection External contamination of containers poses a risk to laboratory personnel and may be rejected. Samples that are left at room temperature for more than 12 hours may be rejected due to overgrowth of other bacteria.

Turnaround Time Approximately 24-72 hours

Reference Interval No *M. tuberculosis* nucleic acid detected

Use Rapid detection and identification of *M. tuberculosis* in clinical specimens. Use of PCR in search of mycobacterial DNA is superior to the Ziehl-Neelsen and auramine-rhodamine stains for acid-fast bacilli and is helpful to distinguish TB from sarcoidosis in paraffin-embedded tissue.

Limitations A potential for false-positive results exists with molecular assays due to cross contamination of specimens. False negatives may occur as well due to inhibitors in the specimen. **Nonviable mycobacterial DNA can lead to positive PCR. Thus, this assay cannot be used to monitor the efficacy of therapy.** The currently available nucleic acid assays do not differentiate among members of the *M. tuberculosis* complex (*M. tuberculosis*, *M. bovis*, *M. bovis* BCG, *M. africanum*, *M. microti*, and *M. canetti*).

Methodology Culture confirmation: DNA probe is used to detect species specific rRNA from cultured acid-fast bacteria. After hybridization the enzyme on the unbound probe is removed and the bound probe with protected enzyme is detected by chemiluminescence.

Specific amplification of *Mycobacterium tuberculosis* nucleic acid by polymerase chain reaction (PCR) or transcription-based amplification is currently FDA approved for direct detection in respiratory specimens from untreated patients.[3,4] Several other nucleic acid amplification assays are currently being evaluated for their clinical utility for direct detection of mycobacteria.[5,6,7] Of great interest is the development of a DNA probe array assay that will accurately detect and identify various species of mycobacteria in clinical specimens and will also detect specific antimicrobial resistance genes within a single platform.[8] At the current time, these DNA assays are not available in conventional diagnostic laboratories.

Additional Information Mycobacteria are aerobic rod-shaped bacteria noted for their very slow growth. The laboratory diagnosis of mycobacterial disease is currently based on a positive acid-fast stain and on laboratory culture of the mycobacterial organism. The most common isolates in the

United States are *Mycobacterium tuberculosis* and species within the *Mycobacterium avium* complex. Because of the long culture periods required, therapeutic decisions are often made before a laboratory diagnosis is available. To improve upon the detection of mycobacteria, DNA detection assays have been developed that have increased sensitivity and specificity when compared with culture assays and have a decreased turnaround time.[3,4] Specimens may be smear negative, culture negative, but PCR positive, especially cerebrospinal fluid.

Footnotes

1. Ginsberg AM, "The Tuberculosis Epidemic. Scientific Challenges and Opportunities," *Public Health Rep*, 1998, 113(2):128-36.
2. Rieder HL, Cauthen GM, Kelly GD, et al, "Tuberculosis in the United States," *JAMA*, 1989, 262(3):385-9.
3. Choi YJ, Hu Y, and Mahmood A, "Clinical Significance of a Polymerase Chain Reaction Assay for the Detection of *Mycobacterium tuberculosis*," *Am J Clin Pathol*, 1996, 105(2):200-4.
4. Pfyffer GE, Kissling P, Jahn EM, et al, "Diagnostic Performance of Amplified *Mycobacterium tuberculosis* Direct Test With Cerebrospinal Fluid, Other Nonrespiratory, and Respiratory Specimens," *J Clin Microbiol*, 1996, 34(4):834-41.
5. Shah JS, Liu J, Buxton D, et al, "Q-Beta Replicase-Amplified Assay for Detection of *Mycobacterium tuberculosis* Directly From Clinical Specimens," *J Clin Microbiol*, 1995, 33(6):1435-41.
6. Tortoli E, Lavinia F, and Simonette MT, "Evaluation of a Commercial Ligase Chain Reaction Kit (Abbott LCX) for Direct Detection of *Mycobacterium tuberculosis* in Pulmonary and Extrapulmonary Specimens," *J Clin Microbiol*, 1997, 35(9):2424-6.
7. Ichiyama S, Ito Y, Sugiura F, et al, "Diagnostic Value of the Strand Displacement Amplification Method Compared to Those of Roche Amplicor PCR and Culture for Detecting Mycobacteria in Sputum Samples," *J Clin Microbiol*, 1997, 35(12):3082-5.
8. Troesch A, Nguyen H, Miyada CG, et al, "*Mycobacterium* Species Identification and Rifampin Resistance Testing With High-Density DNA Probe Arrays," *J Clin Microbiol*, 1999, 37(1):49-55.

References

Alland D, Kalkut GE, Moss AR, et al, "Transmission of Tuberculosis in New York City. An Analysis by DNA Fingerprinting and Conventional Epidemiologic Methods," *N Engl J Med*, 1994, 330(24):1710-6.

Attorri S, Dunbar S, and Clarridge JE, "Assessment of Morphology for Rapid Presumptive Identification of *Mycobacterium tuberculosis* and *Mycobacterium kansasii*," *J Clin Microbiol*, 2000, 38(4):1426-9.

Bradley SP, Reed SL, and Catanzaro A, "Clinical Efficacy of the Amplified *Mycobacterium tuberculosis* Direct Test for the Diagnosis of Pulmonary Tuberculosis," *Am J Respir Crit Care Med*, 1996, 153:1606-10.

Centers for Disease Control, "Diagnosis of Tuberculosis by Nucleic Acid Amplification Methods Applied to Clinical Specimens," *MMWR Morb Mortal Wkly Rep*, 1993, 42:686.

Della-Latta P and Whittier S, "Comprehensive Evaluation of Performance, Laboratory Application, and Clinical Usefulness of Two Direct Amplification Technologies for the Detection of *Mycobacterium tuberculosis* Complex," *Am J Clin Pathol*, 1998, 110(3):301-10.

French AL, Welbel SF, Dietrich SE, et al, "Use of DNA Fingerprinting to Assess Tuberculosis Infection Control," *Ann Intern Med*, 1998, 129(11):856-61.

Haas DW, "Current and Future Applications of Polymerase Chain Reaction for *Mycobacterium tuberculosis*," *Mayo Clin Proc*, 1996, 71(3):311-3.

Hardman WJ, Benian GM, Howard T, et al, "Rapid Detection of Mycobacteria in Inflammatory Necrotizing Granulomas From Formalin-Fixed, Paraffin-Embedded Tissue by PCR in Clinically High-Risk Patients With Acid-Fast Stain and Culture-Negative Tissue Biopsies," *Am J Clin Pathol*, 1996, 106(3):384-9.

Kapur V, Li LL, Hamrick MR, et al, "Rapid *Mycobacterium* Species Assignment and Unambiguous Identification of Mutations Associated With Antimicrobial Resistance in *Mycobacterium tuberculosis* by Automated DNA Sequencing," *Arch Pathol Lab Med*, 1995, 119(2):131-8.

Kiechle FL, "DNA Technology, The Clinical Laboratory and the Future," *Arch Pathol Lab Med*, 2001, 125(1):78-6.

Noordhoek GT, Kolk AH, Bjune G, et al, "Sensitivity and Specificity of PCR for Detection of *Mycobacterium tuberculosis*: A Blind Comparison Study Among Seven Laboratories," *J Clin Microbiol*, 1994, 32(2):277-84.

Popper HH, Winter E, and Höfler G, "DNA of *Mycobacterium tuberculosis* in Formalin-Fixed, Paraffin-Embedded Tissue in Tuberculosis and Sarcoidosis Detected by Polymerase Chain Reaction," *Am J Clin Pathol*, 1994, 101(6):738-41.

Raviglione MC, Snider DE, and Kochi A, "Global Epidemiology of Tuberculosis. Morbidity and Mortality of a Worldwide Epidemic," *JAMA*, 1995, 273:220-6.

Salian NV, Rish JA, Eisenach KD, et al, "Polymerase Chain Reaction to Detect *Mycobacterium tuberculosis* in Histologic Specimens," *Am J Respir Crit Care Med*, 1998, 158(4):1150-5.

Smith MB, Bergmann JS, Onoroto M, et al, "Evaluation of the Enhanced Amplified *Mycobacterium tuberculosis* Direct Test for Direct Detection of *Mycobacterium tuberculosis* Complex in Respiratory Specimens," *Arch Pathol Lab Med*, 1999, 123(11):1101-3.

"Update: Nucleic Acid Amplification Tests for Tuberculosis," *JAMA*, 2000, 284(7):826.

Internet Web Sites

www.astdhpphe.org/infect/tb.html
www.cdc.gov/nchstp/tb/faqs/qa.htm
www.who.int/health-topics/tb.htm

♦ **Mycobacteria Culture, Bronchial Aspirate** *see* Mycobacterial Culture, Sputum *on page 658*

♦ **Mycobacteria Culture, Gastric Aspirate** *see* Mycobacterial Culture, Sputum *on page 658*

♦ **Mycobacteria DNA Detection Test** *see* Mycobacteria by DNA Probe *on page 654*

♦ **Mycobacteria, DNA Probe** *see* Mycobacterial Culture, Sputum *on page 658*

Mycobacterial Culture, Biopsy or Body Fluid

Related Information

Acid-Fast Stain *on page 550*
Adenosine Deaminase, CSF, Pleural Fluid, Pericardial Fluid, Peritoneal Fluid *on page 83*
Antimicrobial Susceptibility Testing, Mycobacteria *on page 557*
Bacterial Culture, Abscess *on page 562*
Bacterial Culture, Biopsy or Body Fluid *on page 565*
Body Cavity Fluid Cytology *on page 372*
Body Fluid Analysis, Cell Count *on page 408*
Body Fluid Chemical Analysis *on page 123*
Body Fluid pH *on page 125*
Bone Marrow *on page 410*
Bronchial Washings Cytology *on page 374*
Fine Needle Aspiration Culture *on page 609*
Fine Needle Aspiration, Deep Masses *on page 381*
Fine Needle Aspiration, Superficial Masses (Palpable) *on page 382*
Histopathology *on page 59*
Mycobacteria by DNA Probe *on page 654*
Mycobacterial Culture, Cutaneous and Subcutaneous Tissue *on page 657*
Mycobacterial Culture, Sputum *on page 658*
Synovial Fluid Analysis *on page 323*
Viral Culture, Body Fluid *on page 691*

Synonyms AFB Culture, Biopsy; AFB Culture, Body Fluid; Body Fluid Mycobacteria Culture; TB Culture, Biopsy; TB Culture, Body Fluid

Applies to Bone Marrow Mycobacteria Culture; Tissue Mycobacteria Culture

Test Includes Preparation of the tissue specimen by grinding and/or mincing and inoculation of appropriate media. The culture media and temperature used will support the growth of most known pathogenic mycobacterial species except for *Mycobacterium leprae*.

Abstract In addition to *Mycobacterium tuberculosis*, a number of nontuberculous mycobacteria can cause granulomatous inflammatory diseases. In a recent study, mycobacteria were cultured from biopsies that contained necrotizing granulomas, nonnecrotizing granulomas, or acute inflammation. Tissue with fibrotic or hyalinized granulomas, nonspecific chronic inflammation, nonspecific reactive or reparative changes, or malignancy failed to yield a positive culture.[1]

Specimen Surgical tissue, bone marrow, biopsy material, endometrial curettings, aspirated fluid; **swab specimens are not acceptable specimens.**

Container Sterile container

Collection Utilizing sterile technique, the portion of the surgical specimen submitted for culture should be separated from the portion submitted for histopathology. Up to a liter of ascitic fluid is needed to achieve 80% sensitivity for mycobacterial culture.[2]

Causes for Rejection Specimen collected on a swab

Turnaround Time Negative cultures are reported after 8 weeks.

Reference Interval No growth

Use Isolate and identify mycobacteria; establish the etiology of granulomatous disease, fever of unknown origin (FUO) particularly in immunocompromised patients

Limitations Transbronchial biopsy cultures may be of assistance in diagnosing tuberculosis in sputum smear negative cases; however, sputum and bronchial washing cultures have a higher yield.[3]

Mycobacterium marinum may cause a localized cutaneous lesion that may be nodular, verrucous, ulcerative, or sporotrichoid, and which may rarely involve deeper structures. If it is suspected, the laboratory must be notified so that the culture may be incubated at an appropriate temperature (30°C);[4] *vide infra*. *M. haemophilum*, which has been recovered in a variety of biopsy specimens from immunosuppressed patients, also requires special media and conditions to grow; inform the laboratory if this organism is suspected.

Methodology Culture on specialized selective media, usually including Löwenstein-Jensen (LJ) and Middlebrook 7H11, incubated at 35°C with 5% to 10% CO_2. Cutaneous and subcutaneous tissues are incubated at room temperature to enhance recovery of *M. marinum* and *M. ulcerans*. If *M. haemophilum* is suspected, blood containing medium is inoculated and incubated at room temperature in 10% CO_2.[5] Mycobacteria are definitively identified and may be tested for antimicrobial susceptibility. Radiometric (Bactec®) and DNA probe methods are utilized by some laboratories to provide rapid detection and identification of mycobacteria.

With the emergence of multidrug-resistant *Mycobacterium tuberculosis* strains, isolates are submitted for antimicrobial susceptibility testing. A specific request is required by some laboratories (see Antimicrobial Susceptibility Testing, Mycobacteria *on page 557*). Susceptibility testing of mycobacteria is frequently referred to specialized laboratories.

Additional Information Occult infections with **atypical mycobacteria**, particularly *Mycobacterium avium* and *Mycobacterium intracellulare*, occur in patients with acquired immune deficiency syndrome (AIDS).[6] In some institutions, the incidence of isolation of non-*Mycobacterium tuberculosis* species, specifically *M. avium-intracellulare* (*M. avium* complex), may exceed the rate of isolation of *M. tuberculosis*. Mycobacteria have been recovered from several types of tissue in which the characteristic granulomatous reaction has been absent.[1] Optimal isolation of mycobacteria from
(Continued)

Mycobacterial Culture, Biopsy or Body Fluid
(Continued)

tissue is accomplished by processing as much tissue as possible for culture.

Mycobacterium marinum infection occurs in patients who have been exposed to the organism following cutaneous abrasion or penetrating injury while cleaning aquariums, clearing barnacles, using heated swimming pools, and with other aquatic exposures. *M. marinum* infections have followed alligator or crocodile bites.[4] A striking photograph was published not long ago.[7] See Mycobacterial Culture, Cutaneous and Subcutaneous Tissue *on page 657*.

Mycobacterium ulcerans is associated with an ulcerating infection. These infections have been found almost exclusively in the tropics, especially in Africa and Australia. The disease is usually painless with a lump developing under the skin at the site of a previous trauma. Within a few weeks an ulcer develops at the site of the lump.[8]

Rapidly growing mycobacteria have been implicated in cases of sternal wound infection, early prosthetic valve endocarditis, infections complicating mammary augmentation surgery, and other cutaneous/subcutaneous infections.[9,10] *M. fortuitum* is most commonly implicated in these infections. Rapidly growing mycobacteria grow on routine bacterial culture media within incubation periods used in routine bacterial cultures. Such organisms can be misidentified as "diphtheroids" and disregarded as contaminants.

Tuberculous spondylitis represents 50% to 60% of all cases of skeletal tuberculosis. It is seen in children in developing countries and adults older than 50 years of age in the United States and Europe. Frequently, several vertebrae are involved and adjacent psoas muscle or paravertebral abscesses are not uncommon ("cold abscesses"). The diagnosis of vertebral tuberculosis should be considered in all cases of unexplained spondylitis.[11]

Pleural effusions yield positive cultures in cases of pulmonary tuberculosis in about 25% of cases. The diagnostic yield increased to ~90% when biopsy specimens are cultured as well. Sensitivity is enhanced more when thoracoscopic biopsies are obtained.[12] The diagnosis of peritoneal tuberculosis is difficult and is usually made at laparotomy or after a considerable delay. Tuberculosis should be considered in any patient with **ascitic fluid** and chronic abdominal pain.[2,13]

A discussion in a 1998 Case Records of the Massachusetts General Hospital presentation observed a reported high sensitivity and excellent specificity of adenosine deaminase for detection of *M. tuberculosis* in pleural or peritoneal fluid, and observed the prediction of some authorities that the current gold standard for diagnosis of tuberculous peritonitis (a peritoneal biopsy) may eventually be replaced by this analyte.[2] Pericardial tuberculosis accounts for <5% of extrapulmonary tuberculosis and frequently requires biopsy for diagnosis. See table.

Predisposing Clinical Conditions and Site of Involvement of Non-*M. tuberculosis* Mycobacterial Infections

Site	Predisposing Clinical Conditions	Species
Disseminated	Immunodeficiency/malignancy	M. avium-intracellulare M. kansasii
Gastrointestinal tract/ disseminated	Acquired immunodeficiency syndrome	M. avium-intracellulare
Lung	Chronic pulmonary disease	M. avium-intracellulare M. kansasii
Lymph nodes	Pediatric age group	M. avium-intracellulare M. scrofulaceum
Peritonitis	Chronic ambulatory peritoneal dialysis	M. fortuitum M. chelonae
Skeleton	Immunodeficiency/malignancy	M. avium-intracellulare M. kansasii
Skin and soft tissue	Percutaneous trauma/abrasion	M. fortuitum M. chelonae
	Immunodeficiency/malignancy	M. haemophilum

The differential diagnosis of tuberculosis sometimes includes sarcoidosis, both from a clinical and histopathologic perspective.[14]

Footnotes

1. Tang YW, Procop GW, Zheng X, et al, "Histologic Parameters Predictive of Mycobacterial Infection," *Am J Clin Pathol*, 1998, 109(3):331-4.
2. Sheets EE and Smith RN, "A 31-Year-Old Woman With a Pleural Effusion, Ascites, and Persistent Fever Spikes," Case Records of the Massachusetts General Hospital, Case 3-1998, Scully RE, Mark EJ, McNeely WF, et al, *N Engl J Med*, 1998, 338(4):248-54.
3. Saceanu CA, Pfeiffer NC, and McLean T, "Evaluation of Sputum Smears Concentrated by Cytocentrifugation for Detection of Acid-Fast Bacilli," *J Clin Microbiol*, 1993, 31(9):2371-4.
4. Hernandez-Martin A, Fonseca E, Gonzalez A, et al, "Sporotrichoid Cutaneous Infection Caused by *Mycobacterium marinum*," *Pediatr Infect Dis J*, 1999, 18(7):656-8.
5. Straus WL, Ostroff SM, Jernigan DB, et al, "Clinical and Epidemiologic Characteristics of *Mycobacterium haemophilum*, an Emerging Pathogen in Immunocompromised Patients," *Ann Intern Med*, 1994, 120(2):118-25.
6. Ellner JJ, Goldberger MJ, and Parenti DM, "*Mycobacterium avium* Infection and AIDS: A Therapeutic Dilemma in Rapid Evaluation," *J Infect Dis*, 1991, 163(6):1326-35.
7. Ramakrishnan L, Images in Clinical Medicine, "*Mycobacterium marinum* Infection of the Hand," *N Engl J Med*, 1997, 337(9):612.
8. Goutzamanis JJ and Gilbert GL, "*Mycobacterium ulcerans* Infection in Australian Children: Report of Eight Cases. A Review," *Clin Infect Dis*, 1995, 21(5):1186-92.
9. Wallace RJ, Musser JM, Hull SI, et al, "Diversity and Sources of Rapidly Growing Mycobacteria Associated With Infections Following Cardiac Surgery," *J Infect Dis*, 1989, 159(4):708-16.
10. Wallace RJ, Steele LC, Labidi A, et al, "Heterogeneity Among Isolates of Rapidly Growing Mycobacteria Responsible for Infections Following Augmentation Mammoplasty Despite Case Clustering in Texas and Other Southern Coastal States," *J Infect Dis*, 1989, 160(2):281-8.
11. Mankin HJ and Wu HC, "A 21-Year-Old African Woman With Thoracolumbar Pain and Fever," Case Records of the Massachusetts General Hospital, Case 9-1996, Scully RE, Mark EJ, McNeely WF, eds, *N Engl J Med*, 1996, 334(12):784-89.
12. Drapkin MS and Mark EJ, "A 38-Year-Old Man With Fever, Cough, and a Pleural Effusion," Case Records of the Massachusetts General Hospital, Case 25-1996, Scully RE, Mark EJ, McNeely WF, eds, *N Engl J Med*, 1996, 335(7):499-505.
13. Ellison E, Lapuerta P, and Martin SE, "Cytologic Features of Mycobacterial Pleuritis: Logistic Regression and Statistical Analysis of a Blinded, Case-Controlled Study," *Diagn Cytopathol*, 1998, 19(3):173-6.
14. Newman LS, Rose CS, and Maier LA, "Sarcoidosis," *N Engl J Med*, 1997, 336(17):1224-34.

References

Das DK, "Fine-Needle Aspiration Cytology in the Diagnosis of Tuberculous Lesions," *Lab Med*, 2000, 31(11):425-32.

"Diagnosis and Treatment of Disease Caused by Nontuberculous Mycobacteria. The Official Statement of the American Thoracic Society was Approved by the Board of Directors, March 1997. Medical Section of the American Lung Association," *Am J Respir Crit Care Med*, 1997, 156(2 Pt 2):S1-25.

Husson RN and Mark EJ, "A 10-Month-Old Girl With Fever, Upper-Lobe Pneumonia and a Pleural Effusion," Case Records of the Massachusetts General Hospital, Case 23-1999, Scully RE, Mark EJ, McNeely WF, et al, eds, *N Engl J Med*, 1999, 341(5):353-60.

Hussong J, Peterson LR, Warren JR, et al, "Detecting Disseminated *Mycobacterium avium* Complex Infections in HIV-Positive Patients: The Usefulness of Bone Marrow Trephine Biopsy Specimens, Aspirate Cultures, and Blood Cultures," *Am J Clin Pathol*, 1998, 110(6):806-9.

Levendoglu-Tugal O, Munoz J, Brudnicki A, et al, "Infections Due to Nontuberculous Mycobacteria in Children With Leukemia," *Clin Infect Dis*, 1998, 27(5):1227-30.

Mayer KH and Rosenberg AE, "A 49-Year-Old Man With the Acquired Immunodeficiency Syndrome and a Tibial Lesion," Case Records of the Massachusetts General Hospital, Case 23-2000, Scully RE, Mark EJ, McNeely WF, et al, eds, *N Engl J Med*, 2000, 343(4):281-7.

O'Brien DP, Currie BJ, and Krause VL, "Nontuberculous Mycobacterial Disease in Northern Australia: A Case Series and Review of the Literature," *Clin Infect Dis*, 2000, 31(4):958-68.

Olivier KN, "Nontuberculous Mycobacterial Pulmonary Disease," *Curr Opin Pulm Med*, 1998, 4(3):148-53.

Suskind DL, Handler SD, Tom LW, et al, "Nontuberculous Mycobacterial Cervical Adenitis," *Clin Pediatr (Phila)*, 1997, 36(7):403-9.

Weitzul S, Eichhorn PJ, and Pandya AG, "Nontuberculous Mycobacterial Infections of the Skin," *Dermatol Clin*, 2000, 18(2):359-77.

Internet Web Sites

www.astdhpphe.org/infect/tb.html
www.cdc.gov/nchstp/tb/faqs/qa.htm
www.who.int/health-topics/tb.htm

Mycobacterial Culture, Cerebrospinal Fluid

Related Information

Acid-Fast Stain *on page 550*
Adenosine Deaminase, CSF, Pleural Fluid, Pericardial Fluid, Peritoneal Fluid *on page 83*
Bacterial Antigens, Rapid Detection Methods *on page 562*
Bacterial Culture, Cerebrospinal Fluid *on page 569*
Bacterial Culture, Wounds, Bites *on page 579*
Cerebrospinal Fluid Analysis: Overview *on page 416*
Cerebrospinal Fluid Cytology *on page 376*
Cerebrospinal Fluid Glucose *on page 140*
Cerebrospinal Fluid Protein *on page 517*
Cryptococcal Antigen Titer *on page 595*
Fungal Culture, Cerebrospinal Fluid *on page 611*
Mycobacteria by DNA Probe *on page 654*
Viral Culture, Central Nervous System Symptoms *on page 692*

Synonyms Cerebrospinal Fluid Mycobacteria Culture; CSF Mycobacteria Culture; Spinal Fluid Mycobacteria Culture

Test Includes Culture for mycobacteria; may include acid-fast stain if requested.

Abstract Conventional cultures and direct acid-fast stain for mycobacteria rarely detect the bacteria in cerebrospinal fluid and, thus, are of limited value in the diagnosis of tuberculosis meningitis. Because of the low number of organisms in meningitis due to *M. tuberculosis*, the direct acid-fast stain is usually negative. Currently, the best laboratory assay for detection of *M. tuberculosis* in cerebrospinal fluid is one of the nucleic acid amplification assays such as PCR or transcription mediated amplification.[1,2] See Mycobacteria by DNA Probe *on page 654* and Adenosine Deaminase, CSF, Pleural Fluid, Pericardial Fluid, Peritoneal Fluid *on page 83.*

Patient Preparation Usual sterile preparation

Specimen Cerebrospinal fluid; 10 mL is optimum, 5 mL the minimum volume

Reference Interval No growth

Use Investigate cases of meningitis with subacute/subchronic or chronic onset, cases in which a history of contact with tuberculosis, or cases in which abnormal CSF findings (decreased glucose, increased protein, increased WBC) suggest mycobacterial meningitis.

Limitations Recovery of mycobacteria is directly related to the volume of specimen available for culture; 5-10 mL is recommended for optimal yield. Recovery of organisms can require 4-6 weeks. Usually CSF glucose ≤60 mg/dL (3.3 mmol/L) and CSF WBC is increased; if not, culture is unlikely to be useful.[3]

Methodology Culture in broth media, such as 7H9, is recommended for primary mycobacterial isolation, which generally yields a more rapid detection of positive cultures. Additionally, solid media that supports the growth of most mycobacteria (Löwenstein-Jensen (LJ) or Middlebrook 7H11) may also be used.

Additional Information Early in the course, neutrophils may predominate in the CSF, and they may predominate in patients with generalized tuberculosis in the acquired immune deficiency syndrome.[4] Lymphocytes, mononuclear cells, and granulocytes are found later. Rarely does the cell count exceed 1000 cells/mm³. The CSF is clear and colorless early; later, a pellicle forms on standing. Low CSF glucose, <40 mg/dL, can be observed. Increased protein is often >300 mg/dL. Other factors raising the index of suspicion include subacute or chronic onset, positive tuberculin skin test, previous active tuberculosis, significant recent exposure to tuberculosis, and suspicion of tuberculosis on imaging procedures. Acid-fast organisms can be identified only rarely on centrifuged sediments.

Untreated tuberculous meningitis is fatal, usually within 3 weeks of presentation. African-Americans, Hispanics, and the elderly are most frequently affected. Alcohol abuse, drug abuse, steroid therapy, head trauma, pregnancy, and AIDS all may increase risk. Despite therapy, mortality is high, ~30%. Evaluation of contacts is recommended. Atypical mycobacteria species can also cause meningitis, primarily in immunosuppressed and elderly patients.[5]

Footnotes

1. Seth P, Ahuja GK, Bhanu NV, et al, "Evaluation of Polymerase Chain Reaction for Rapid Diagnosis of Clinically Suspected Tuberculous Meningitis," *Tuber Lung Dis*, 1996, 77(4):353-7.
2. Lang AM, Feris-Iglesias J, Pena C, et al, "Clinical Evaluation of the Gen-Probe® Amplified Direct Test for Detection of *Mycobacterium tuberculosis* Complex Organisms in Cerebrospinal Fluid," *J Clin Microbiol*, 1998, 36(8):2191-4.
3. Christie JD and Callihan DR, "The Laboratory Diagnosis of Mycobacterial Diseases. Challenges and Common Sense," *Clin Lab Med*, 1995, 15(2):279-306.
4. Smith MB, Boyars MC, Veasey S, et al, "Generalized Tuberculosis in the Acquired Immune Deficiency Syndrome. A Clinicopathologic Analysis Based on Autopsy Findings," *Arch Pathol Lab Med*, 2000, 124(9):1267-74.
5. Wayne LG and Sramek HA, "Agents of Newly Recognized or Infrequently Encountered Mycobacterial Diseases," *Clin Microbiol Rev*, 1992, 5(1):1-25.

References

Bell WE, "Bacterial Meningitis in Children - Selected Aspects," *Pediatr Clin North Am*, 1992, 39(4):651-68.
Berenguer J, Moreno S, Laguna F, et al, "Tuberculous Meningitis in Patients Infected With the Human Immunodeficiency Virus," *N Engl J Med*, 1992, 326(10):668-72.
Kelly JJ, Horowitz EA, Destache CJ, et al, "Diagnosis and Treatment of Complicated Tubercular Meningitis," *Pharmacotherapy*, 1999, 19(10):1167-72.
Sheets EE and Smith RN, "A 31-Year-Old Woman With a Pleural Effusion, Ascites, and Persistent Fever Spikes," *Case Records of the Massachusetts General Hospital*, Case 3-1998, Scully RE, Mark EJ, McNeely WF, et al, *N Engl J Med*, 1998, 338(4):248-54.
Wolinsky E, "Mycobacterial Diseases Other Than Tuberculosis," *Clin Infect Dis*, 1992, 15(1):1-10.

Internet Web Sites

www.astdhpphe.org/infect/tb.html
www.cdc.gov/nchstp/tb/faqs/qa.htm
www.who.int/health-topics/tb.htm

Mycobacterial Culture, Cutaneous and Subcutaneous Tissue

Related Information

Synonyms Skin Mycobacteria Culture; TB Culture, Skin

Applies to *Mycobacterium avium-intracellulare*; *Mycobacterium fortuitum* Complex; *Mycobacterium marinum*; *Mycobacterium ulcerans*

Test Includes Culture and identification of acid-fast bacteria. This will include a direct acid-fast smear of specimen.

Abstract Cutaneous or subcutaneous manifestations of mycobacterial infection may result from either direct inoculation or hematogenous dissemination of infecting organisms. A variety of *Mycobacterium* spp may cause infections of this type; they are most likely to occur in patients at risk due to immunosuppression (eg, *M. tuberculosis*, *M. haemophilum*, *M. kansasii*), poverty and geographic exposure (eg, *M. leprae*, *M. ulcerans*), prior surgical treatment (eg, *M. fortuitum*), or hobbies or occupational exposure (eg, *M. marinum*).

Container Sterile tube containing 0.5 mL sterile saline

Turnaround Time Positive cultures may be detected as early as 2-3 days for a rapid growing mycobacteria and as long as 8 weeks in specimens with a very low number of organisms. Negative cultures are usually reported after 6-8 weeks.

Reference Interval No growth

Use Isolate and identify mycobacteria

Limitations For optimal yield, scrapings, curettings, or biopsy tissue rather than swabs of lesions should be submitted to the laboratory. Mycobacteria adhere tightly to material on a swab and thus are difficult to remove from the swab. The yield on cultures is proportional to the volume of specimen submitted. *M. leprae* does not grow in culture.

Methodology Acid-fast stain of smear prepared from clinical specimen, culture of specimen on appropriate media (eg, Lowenstein-Jensen, Middlebrook 7H11 solid media, liquid media such as 7H12 or 7H9). Incubation at both 35°C and 25°C to 30°C. Hemin-containing media such as chocolate agar incubated at 25°C to 30°C is required to recover *M. haemophilum*.[1] Identification is based on growth rate, colony morphology (rough vs smooth), development of pigment, color of pigment, and whether or not the pigment is induced by light. Other biochemical and nucleic acid tests can be used to confirm the identification.

Additional Information *Mycobacterium marinum* causes granulomatous cutaneous lesions. Lesions are similar to those seen with sporotrichosis and follow lymphatics; see Mycobacterial Culture, Biopsy or Body Fluid *on page 655*. Diagnosis of *Mycobacterium marinum* infection is frequently delayed. A careful clinical history addressing occupational or recreational activities usually yields important clues to the diagnosis (eg, swimming pool or seawall abrasions, barnacle scrapes, fish fin punctures, exposure to tropical salt water fish tanks).[2]

Members of the *Mycobacterium fortuitum* complex (*M. fortuitum* and *M. chelonae*) can cause surgical wound infections and cutaneous abscesses and osteomyelitis in trauma victims and debilitated hosts. The organisms are not fastidious and may grow well on routine blood or chocolate agar. The key clinical feature is that symptoms of infection, localized cellulitis, or abscess formation appear 4-6 weeks after traumatic injury or surgery.[3] It is important to identify these organisms to the species level because the different species have differences in drug susceptibility patterns.[1]

Mycobacterium ulcerans causes a chronic granulomatous skin lesion called Buruli ulcer. *M. ulcerans* may also be saprophytic, colonizing cutaneous ulcers associated with circulatory insufficiency and diabetes. *M. ulcerans* is uncommon in North America. It is most frequently isolated in Australia and Africa.

Isolates of *Mycobacterium avium-intracellulare* (MAI) have been reported from skin lesions of patients with the acquired immunodeficiency syndrome (AIDS).[4] *Mycobacterium kansasii* can also cause cutaneous infections in immunosuppressed patients.[5]

Cutaneous tuberculosis has been found in patients with neoplastic or immunosuppressive diseases. The most common clinical presentations are lupus vulgaris, scrofuloderma, tuberculids, tuberculous verrucosa cutis, and tuberculous gumma. Patients may present with more than one clinical form of cutaneous disease.[6,7] *M. haemophilum* produces disseminated cutaneous disease and infections of the bones, joints, and lymphatics in immunocompromised individuals.[8]

The atypical or environmental mycobacteria are frequently resistant to oral antituberculosis therapy. There is wide variation in susceptibility within species. Susceptibility testing should be considered.

Footnotes

1. Metchcock B, Nolte FS, and Wallace RJ Jr, "*Mycobacterium*," *Manual of Clinical Microbiology*, 7th ed, Murray PR, Baron EJ, Pfaller MA, et al, eds, Washington, DC: AMS Press, American Society for Microbiology, 1999, 399-437.
2. Hernandez-Martin A, Fonseca E, Gonzalez A, et al, "Sporotrichoid Cutaneous Infection Caused by *Mycobacterium marinum*," *Pediatr Infect Dis J*, 1999, 18(7):656-8.
3. Escalonilla P, Esteban J, Soriano ML, et al, "Cutaneous Manifestations of Infection by Nontuberculous Mycobacteria," *Clin Exp Dermatol*, 1998, 23(5):214-21.
4. Bedlow AJ, Vittay GI, Stephenson J, et al, "Deep Cutaneous Infection With *Mycobacterium avium-intracellulare* Complex in an Immunosuppressed Patient With Dermatomyositis," *Br J Dermatol*, 1998, 139(5):920-2.
5. Czelusta A and Moore AY, "Cutaneous *Mycobacterium kansasii* Infection in a Patient With Systemic Lumus Erythematosus: Case Report and Review," *J Am Acad Dermatol*, 1999, 40(2 Pt 2):359-63.
6. Kumar B and Muralidhar S, "Cutaneous Tuberculosis: A Twenty-Year Prospective Study," *Int J Tuberc Lung Dis*, 1999, 3(6):494-500.
(Continued)

Mycobacterial Culture, Cutaneous and Subcutaneous Tissue *(Continued)*

7. Ramesh V, Misra RS, Beena KR, et al, "A Study of Cutaneous Tuberculosis in Children," *Pediatr Dermatol*, 1999, 16(4):264-9.

8. Straus WL, Ostroff SM, Jernigan DB, et al, "Clinical and Epidemiologic Characteristics of *Mycobacterium haemophilum*, an Emerging Pathogen in Immunocompromised Patients," *Ann Intern Med*, 1994, 120(2):118-25.

References

O'Brien DP, Currie BJ, and Krause VL, "Nontuberculous Mycobacterial Disease in Northern Australia: A Case Series and Review of the Literature," *Clin Infect Dis*, 2000, 31(4):958-68.

Wayne LG and Sramek HA, "Agents of Newly Recognized or Infrequently Encountered Mycobacterial Diseases," *Clin Microbiol Rev*, 1992, 5(1):1-25.

Weitzul S, Eichhorn PJ, and Pandya AG, "Nontuberculous Mycobacterial Infections of the Skin," *Dermatol Clin*, 2000, 18(2):359-77.

Wolinsky E, "Mycobacterial Diseases Other Than Tuberculosis," *Clin Infect Dis*, 1992, 15(1):1-10.

Internet Web Sites

www.astdhpphe.org/infect/tb.html
www.cdc.gov/nchstp/tb/faqs/qa.htm
www.who.int/health-topics/tb.htm

Mycobacterial Culture, Sputum

Related Information

Acid-Fast Stain *on page 550*
Antimicrobial Susceptibility Testing, Mycobacteria *on page 557*
Bacterial Culture, Bronchoscopy/Bronchial Brush/Bronchoalveolar Lavage Specimen *on page 568*
Bacterial Culture, Sputum *on page 574*
Bronchoalveolar Lavage (BAL) *on page 375*
Fungal Culture, Sputum *on page 613*
Mycobacteria by DNA Probe *on page 654*
Mycobacterial Culture, Biopsy or Body Fluid *on page 655*
Mycobacterial Culture, Cutaneous and Subcutaneous Tissue *on page 657*
Mycobacterial Culture, Stool *on page 659*
Mycobacterial Culture, Urine *on page 660*
Nocardia Culture *on page 665*
Sputum Cytology *on page 387*

Synonyms AFB Culture, Sputum; Sputum Mycobacteria Culture; TB Culture, Sputum

Applies to Mycobacteria Culture, Bronchial Aspirate; Mycobacteria Culture, Gastric Aspirate; Mycobacteria, DNA Probe

Test Includes Mycobacteria (AFB) stain, culture, and identification

Abstract Tuberculosis is a pulmonary disease caused by *Mycobacterium tuberculosis*. It is spread from person to person by airborne droplets that are generated when a patient with pulmonary tuberculosis coughs. Pulmonary tuberculosis is a slowly progressing disease characterized by intense inflammation, necrosis, and caseation. Patients can be latently infected with *M. tuberculosis* for many years, have a positive skin test but remain asymptomatic. These patients are not infectious and have only a 10% risk for development of active tuberculosis.

The World Health Organization (WHO) estimates there are over 8 million new cases of tuberculosis in the world each year.[1] Causes of the enormous global burden of tuberculosis include poor control in Southeast Asia, Sub-Saharan Africa, and Eastern Europe, and include the high incidence of *M. tuberculosis* and HIV coinfection in parts of Africa.[2] In the U.S., cases of tuberculosis are found more commonly in populations that are medically underserved, homeless persons, elderly, prison inmates, alcoholics, people who inject illegal drugs, and foreign-born people from areas of high tuberculosis prevalence.[3] In 1998, the tuberculosis cases among immigrants accounted for 42% of the total tuberculosis cases in the U.S. reported to the CDC. In addition, recent outbreaks of multidrug-resistant tuberculosis has increased the demand for the rapid diagnosis and culture of tuberculosis. Diagnosis of *M. tuberculosis* by DNA probe and polymerase chain reaction permits rapid detection.[3] Molecular typing methods have been used to determine the person-to-person transmission of tuberculosis and play an important role in epidemiology of this disease.[4,5,6,7,8,9,10,11,12] Transmission of tuberculosis has recently been described in a jail,[13,14] by bronchoscopes,[15,16,17] transfer from a cadaver to an embalmer,[18] through medical waste,[19] and from a child.[20]

Patient Preparation The patient should be instructed to remove dentures, rinse mouth with water, and then cough deeply expectorating sputum into the sputum collection cup.

Specimen First morning sputum or induced sputum, fasting gastric aspirate, bronchial aspirate, tracheal aspirate, transtracheal aspirate. In neonates, gastric and endotracheal aspirates may be used but are not optimal.[21]

Container Sputum cup, sputum trap, sterile tracheal aspirate or bronchoscopy tube

Sampling Time In children, gastric aspiration should be done early in the morning as the child awakens before the stomach empties, collect samples on three separate mornings.

Collection A newly recommended screening procedure includes two first morning specimens submitted on successive days.[21] The patient should be instructed to brush his/her teeth and/or rinse mouth well with water before attempting to collect the specimen to reduce the possibility of contamination of the specimen with food particles, oropharyngeal secretions, and so forth. After the specimen has been collected, it should be examined to make sure it contains a sufficient quantity (at least 5 mL) of thick mucus (**not saliva**). If a two-part collection system has been used, only the screw-cap tube should be submitted to the laboratory. (The outer container is considered contaminated and its transport through the hospital or by courier constitutes a health hazard!) The specimen should be properly labeled and accompanied by properly completed requisition. The specimen can be divided in the laboratory for fungal, mycobacterial, and routine cultures.

Storage Instructions The specimen should be refrigerated if it cannot be promptly processed. If a gastric aspirate cannot be processed immediately, its pH should be neutralized for storage.

Turnaround Time Negative cultures are reported after 6-8 weeks; *vide infra*.

Special Instructions Early morning specimen is preferred. Since at least 5 mL of sputum (**not saliva**) is required, the specimen may be collected over a 1- to 2-hour period in order to obtain a sufficient quantity. It should not be collected over the entire day, to avoid overgrowth of other bacteria in the specimen.

Reference Interval No growth

Use Diagnose pulmonary tuberculosis or other *Mycobacterium* species from expectorated sputum, induced sputum, nasotracheal aspiration, or, if necessary, gastric aspiration, bronchoscopy, or bronchoalveolar lavage. Tuberculosis must be considered in patients who have chronic cough and fever, regardless of results of tuberculin testing, especially in the presence of HIV infection.[6]

Limitations Bronchial washings are frequently diluted with topical anesthetics and irrigating fluids, but bronchoscopy still provides a high yield of positive specimens. Postbronchoscopy expectorated specimens may provide a better yield of organisms than those obtained during the procedure. Gastric aspirates yield organisms in <50% of cases of *M. tuberculosis* infection in children. Acid-fast stain of gastric aspirate has a sensitivity of 19% and a specificity of 100%. Acid-fast smear of gastric aspirates provides a useful clinical diagnosis only if positive and indicates a high tuberculosis burden within the respiratory tract.[22] The relative yield of mycobacteria from clinical specimens is prebronchoscopy sputum > bronchial washings > postbronchoscopy sputum > bronchial biopsy.

Severe limitations are recognized with traditional diagnostic approaches for mycobacteria. Poor sensitivity of smears (45%) and prolonged times required for culture have complicated emerging problems of tuberculosis in immunocompromised individuals and of multidrug-resistant organisms.[21] A positive culture results currently require 7-20 days, even with the newer culture systems.[23] It is recommended that a direct molecular assay be used on acid-fast smear positive specimens to detect *M. tuberculosis* complex. The sensitivity of this assay is ~95% and the specificity is 100%.[24,25]

Methodology Concentration and decontamination by exposure to acid or alkaline agents, mycolytic agents, and centrifugation. Broth media, such as Middlebrook 7H9 or 7H11, is required for the initial isolation of mycobacteria. Several commercial systems are available for the rapid culture of mycobacteria in broth media and usually use a broth similar to 7H9 supplemented with various growth factors and antimicrobial agents. It is useful to also include a solid medium such as Löwenstein-Jensen (LJ) or Middlebrook 7H11 agar plate in addition to the broth medium for isolation of mycobacteria.

Identification of culture isolates may be accomplished by traditional biochemical methods or by gas liquid chromatography. The method more commonly used is the DNA probe technology using chemiluminescent-labeled DNA probes. The probes can provide a rapid confirmation of the species of mycobacteria isolated.

Additional Information The incidence of tuberculosis increased in the United States between 1985 and 1991. High incidence populations were identified in depressed inner city areas, some rural areas, amongst new immigrants, in prison inmates, and in HIV-positive patients. However, since 1992 the number of tuberculosis cases has consistently declined in the U.S., primarily due to the effectiveness of prevention and control measures implemented by the CDC. These control measures include the rapid and prompt identification of *M. tuberculosis* by the laboratory, preventive therapy in high-risk populations, decreased transmission in correctional facilities, and improved follow-up of tuberculosis patients. In spite of measures taken in the U.S., tuberculosis is very prevalent throughout the world. One out of every three people are infected with *M. tuberculosis* and ~3 million deaths are attributed to tuberculosis annually.[1]

The emergence of *M. tuberculosis* and *M. avium-intracellulare* infections in patients with the acquired immunodeficiency syndrome has contributed to the increasing need for rapid, accurate diagnosis of mycobacterial infections. When tuberculosis occurs as a first or case-defining opportunistic infection, 75% to 100% of HIV-positive patients have pulmonary disease. After the diagnosis of AIDS has been made, 25% to 70% of HIV-associated tuberculosis patients have an extrapulmonary site of infection.[26]

In an ambulatory inner city population, two specimens processed for acid-fast stain and culture identified all cases of active tuberculosis within the time required for culture. The most infective cases were identified immediately by the acid-fast stain. Tuberculin tests and chest x-rays were also performed but did not significantly increase the number of cases identified in this population.[27]

M. kansasii is uncommon as an environmental contaminant. Implication of *M. avium-intracellulare* as a pathogen usually requires at least one of the following criteria:

- clinical evidence of a disease process that can be explained by atypical mycobacterial infection
- repeated isolation of the same mycobacterial species from sputum over a period of weeks to months
- exclusion of other possible etiologies
- biopsy demonstrating acid-fast bacilli or diagnostic histopathologic changes[28]

Nosocomial transmission of multidrug-resistant *Mycobacterium tuberculosis* has been noted to occur from patient to patient and from patient to health-care worker. Acid-fast bacilli isolation precautions and adherence to appropriate infection control procedures are recommended.[29,30]

While *M. tuberculosis* is contagious and is usually transmitted from person to person, most of the other disease-causing mycobacteria are not characterized by person-to-person spread. There bacteria are found in the environment and are considered opportunistic pathogens. They include *M. avium*, *M. intracellulare*, *M. asiaticum*, *M. flavescens*, *M. fortuitum* complex, *M. gordonae*, *M. haemophilum*, *M. kansasii*, *M. malmoense*, *M. marinum*, *M. scrofulaceum*, *M. simiae*, *M. smegmatis*, and *M. xenopi*.

See Mycobacteria by DNA Probe *on page 654*.

Footnotes

1. Ginsberg AM, "The Tuberculosis Epidemic. Scientific Challenges and Opportunities," *Public Health Rep*, 1998, 113(2):128-36.
2. Dye C, Scheele S, Dolin P, et al, "Global Burden of Tuberculosis. Estimated Incidence, Prevalence, and Mortality by Country," *JAMA*, 1999, 282(7):677-86.
3. Barnes PF and Barrows SA, "Tuberculosis in the 1990s," *Ann Intern Med*, 1993, 119(5):400-10.
4. Small PM, Hopewell PC, Singh SP, et al, "The Epidemiology of Tuberculosis in San Francisco. A Population-Based Study Using Conventional and Molecular Methods," *N Engl J Med*, 1994, 330(24):1703-9.
5. Alland D, Kalkut GE, Moss AR, et al, "Transmission of Tuberculosis in New York City. An Analysis by DNA Fingerprinting and Conventional Epidemiologic Methods," *N Engl J Med*, 1994, 330(24):1710-6.
6. Hamburg MA and Frieden TR, "Tuberculosis Transmission in the 1990s," *N Engl J Med*, 1994, 330(24):1750-1.
7. Jasmer RM, Hahn JA, Small PM, et al, "A Molecular Epidemiologic Analysis of Tuberculosis Trends in San Francisco, 1991-1997," *Ann Intern Med*, 1999, 130(12):971-8.
8. Bishai WR, Graham NM, Harrington S, et al, "Molecular and Geographic Patterns of Tuberculosis Transmission After 15 Years of Directly Observed Therapy," *JAMA*, 1998, 280(19):1679-84.
9. Barnes PF, "Reducing Ongoing Transmission of Tuberculosis," *JAMA*, 1998, 280(19):1702-3.
10. Bifani PJ, Mathema B, Liu Z, et al, "Identification of a W Variant Outbreak of *Mycobacterium tuberculosis* via Population-Based Molecular Epidemiology," *JAMA*, 1999, 282(24):2321-7.
11. Valway SE, Sanchez MP, Shinnick TF, et al, "An Outbreak Involving Extensive Transmission of a Virulent Strain of *Mycobacterium tuberculosis*," *N Engl J Med*, 1998, 338(10):633-9.
12. Chin DP, Crane CM, Diul MY, et al, "Spread of *Mycobacterium tuberculosis* in a Community Implementing Recommended Elements of Tuberculosis Control," *JAMA*, 2000, 283(22):2968-74.
13. Jones TF, Craig AS, Valway SE, et al, "Transmission of Tuberculosis in a Jail," *Ann Intern Med*, 1999, 131(8):557-63.
14. Reichman LB, "On Target: A Tuberculosis Control Strategy Whose Time Has Come," *Ann Intern Med*, 1999, 131(8):617-8.
15. Agerton T, Valway S, Gore B, et al, "Transmission of a Highly Drug-Resistant Strain (Strain W1) of *Mycobacterium tuberculosis*. Community Outbreak and Nosocomial Transmission via a Contaminated Bronchoscope," *JAMA*, 1997, 278(13):1073-7.
16. Michele TM, Cronin WA, Graham NM, et al, "Transmission of *Mycobacterium tuberculosis* by a Fiberoptic Bronchoscope. Identification by DNA Fingerprinting," *JAMA*, 1997, 278(13):1093-5.
17. Wenzel RP and Edmond MB, "Tuberculosis Infection After Bronchoscopy," *JAMA*, 1997, 278(13):1111.
18. Sterling TR, Pope DS, Bishai WR, et al, "Transmission of *Mycobacterium tuberculosis* From a Cadaver to an Embalmer," *N Engl J Med*, 2000, 342(4):246-8.
19. Johnson KR, Braden CR, Cairns KL, et al, "Transmission of *Mycobacterium tuberculosis* From Medical Waste," *JAMA*, 2000, 284(13):1683-8.
20. Curtis AB, Ridzon R, Vogel R, et al, "Extensive Transmission of *Mycobacterium tuberculosis* From a Child," *N Engl J Med*, 1999, 341(20):1491-5.
21. Stone BL, Burman WJ, Hildred MV, et al, "The Diagnostic Yield of Acid-Fast Bacillus Smear-Positive Specimens," *J Clin Microbiol*, 1997, 35(4):1030-1.
22. Bahammam A, Choudhri S, and Long R, "The Validity of Acid-Fast Smears of Gastric Aspirates as an Indicator of Pulmonary Tuberculosis," *Int J Tuberc Lung Dis*, 1999, 3(1):62-7.
23. Somoskovi A and Magyar P, "Comparison of the Mycobacteria Growth Indicator Tube With MB Redox, Lowenstein-Jensen, and Middlebrook 7H11 Media for Recovery of Mycobacteria in Clinical Specimens," *J Clin Microbiol*, 1999, 37(5):1366-9.
24. "Rapid Diagnostic Tests for Tuberculosis - What Is the Appropriate Use? American Thoracic Society Workshop," *Am J Respir Crit Care Med*, 1997, 155(5):1804-14.
25. Barnes PF, "Rapid Diagnostic Tests for Tuberculosis, Progress but no Gold Standard," *Am J Respir Crit Care Med*, 1997, 155(5):1497-8.
26. Centers for Disease Control, "USPHS/IDSA Guidelines for the Prevention of Opportunistic Infections in Persons Infected With Human Immunodeficiency Virus," *MMWR Morb Mortal Wkly Rep*, 1997, 46(RR12):1-46.
27. Tenover FC, Crawford JT, Huebner RE, et al, "The Resurgence of Tuberculosis: Is Your Laboratory Ready?" *J Clin Microbiol*, 1993, 31(4):767-70.
28. Wayne LG and Sramek HA, "Agents of Newly Recognized or Infrequently Encountered Mycobacterial Diseases," *Clin Microbiol Rev*, 1992, 5(1):1-25.

References

Al-Moamary MS, Black W, Bessuille E, et al, "The Significance of the Persistent Presence of Acid-Fast Bacilli in Sputum Smears in Pulmonary Tuberculosis," *Chest*, 1999, 116(3):726-31.

American Thoracic Society, "Diagnosis and Treatment of Disease Caused by Nontuberculous Mycobacteria," *Am J Respir Crit Care Med*, 1997, 156(2 Pt 2):S1-25.

Bergmann JS, Fish G, and Woods GL, "Evaluation of the BBL MGIT (Mycobacterial Growth Indicator Tube) AST SIRE System for Antimycobacterial Susceptibility Testing of *Mycobacterium tuberculosis* to 4 Primary Antituberculous Drugs," *Arch Pathol Lab Med*, 2000, 124(1):82-6.

Bloch KC, Zwerling L, Pletcher MJ, et al, "Incidence and Clinical Implications of Isolation of *Mycobacterium kansasii*: Results of a 5-Year, Population-Based Study," *Ann Intern Med*, 1998, 129(9):698-704.

Della-Latta P and Whittier S, "Comprehensive Evaluation of Performance, Laboratory Application, and Clinical Usefulness of Two Direct Amplification Technologies for the Detection of *Mycobacterium tuberculosis* Complex," *Am J Clin Pathol*, 1998, 110(3):301-10.

Divinagracia RM, Harkin TJ, Bonk S, et al, "Screening by Specialists to Reduce Unnecessary Test Ordering in Patients Evaluated for Tuberculosis," *Chest*, 1998, 114(3):681-4.

El-Solh AA, Nopper J, Abdul-Khoudoud MR, et al, "Clinical and Radiographic Manifestations of Uncommon Pulmonary Nontuberculous Mycobacterial Disease in AIDS Patients," *Chest*, 1998, 114(1):138-45.

Griffith DE, "Mycobacteria as Pathogens of Respiratory Infection," *Infect Dis Clin North Am*, 1998, 12(3):593-611.

Jacobson K, Garcia R, Libshitz H, et al, "Clinical and Radiological Features of Pulmonary Disease Caused by Rapidly Growing Mycobacteria in Cancer Patients," *Eur J Clin Microbiol Infect Dis*, 1998, 17(9):615-21.

Olivier KN, "Nontuberculous Mycobacterial Pulmonary Disease," *Curr Opin Pulm Med*, 1998, 4(3):148-53.

Raviglione MC, Snider DE Jr, and Kochi A, "Global Epidemiology of Tuberculosis. Prevalence and Mortality of a Worldwide Epidemic," *JAMA*, 1995, 273(3):220-6.

Sharp SE, Lemes M, Sierra SG, et al, "Löwenstein-Jensen Media. No Longer Necessary for Mycobacterial Isolation," *Am J Clin Pathol*, 2000, 113(6):770-3.

Smith MB, Bergmann JS, Onoroto M, et al, "Evaluation of the Enhanced Amplified *Mycobacterium tuberculosis* Direct Test for Direct Detection of *Mycobacterium tuberculosis* Complex in Respiratory Specimens," *Arch Pathol Lab Med*, 1999, 123(11):1101-3.

Torrens JK, Dawkins P, Conway SP, et al, "Nontuberculous Mycobacteria in Cystic Fibrosis," *Thorax*, 1998, 53(3):182-5.

Woods GL, "Tuberculosis. Role of the Clinical Laboratory in Providing Rapid Diagnosis and Assessment of Disease Activity," *Am J Clin Pathol*, 1994, 101(6):679-80.

Internet Web Sites

www.astdhpphe.org/infect/tb.html
www.cdc.gov/nchstp/tb/faqs/qa.htm
www.cdc.gov/ncidod/dbmd/diseaseinfo/mycobacteriumavium_t.htm
www.who.int/health-topics/tb.htm

Mycobacterial Culture, Stool

Related Information

Acid-Fast Stain *on page 550*
Antimicrobial Susceptibility Testing, Mycobacteria *on page 557*
Bacterial Culture, Stool *on page 575*
Fecal Lactoferrin *on page 308*
Methylene Blue Stain, Stool *on page 313*
Mycobacteria by DNA Probe *on page 654*
Mycobacterial Culture, Sputum *on page 658*
Mycobacterial Culture, Urine *on page 660*

Synonyms AFB Culture, Stool; Stool Mycobacterial Culture; TB Culture, Stool

Test Includes The detection of mycobacterial organisms from stool specimens after processing and decontaminating the specimen

Abstract The isolation of *Mycobacterium avium* complex from stool specimens in AIDS patients indicates gastrointestinal infections and may be predictive of the development of disseminated infection.[1,2] Although *M. tuberculosis* can be isolated from a stool specimen, it is not the specimen of choice for diagnosis of tuberculosis.

Specimen 1-2 g formed stool, 5 mL liquid stool[3]

Storage Instructions If the specimen cannot be processed immediately by the laboratory, it should be refrigerated.

Turnaround Time Negative cultures are usually reported after 8 weeks.

Reference Interval No growth

Use Isolate and identify mycobacteria, especially *M. avium* complex in subjects with AIDS.

Limitations Isolation of *M. tuberculosis* from feces does not necessarily imply intestinal tuberculosis. Mycobacteria in feces are most likely from sputum swallowed by patients with pulmonary disease. The recovery of *M. gordonae*, "the tap water bacillus," from stool occurs occasionally and is not considered a pathogen. The recovery of mycobacteria from stool is technically limited by the rapid overgrowth of normal intestinal bacterial flora. **Stool is rarely the specimen of choice** for the primary diagnosis of (Continued)

Mycobacterial Culture, Stool *(Continued)*

mycobacterial infection and should only be cultured from immunocompromised patients.

Methodology Culture on selective media usually including Löwenstein-Jensen (LJ) and Middlebrook 7H11 media with antibiotics after decontamination of the specimen by a procedure similar to that used for sputum cultures. Many laboratories screen by smear before culturing, however, the sensitivity of direct smears of stool specimens is only 32% to 34% when compared to culture results.[4] In some laboratories, if the smear is negative, culture is not performed.

Additional Information The increasing recognition of mycobacterial infections in patients with the acquired immunodeficiency syndrome (AIDS) has resulted in increased awareness of the potential to recover clinically significant mycobacteria from stool. Patients with AIDS are often found to be colonized with *M. avium-intracellulare*.[1] If a stool culture is positive for *Mycobacterium* spp, dissemination often follows.[2] Isolation of mycobacteria from stool indicates disseminated disease, and cultures from blood, bone marrow, and lymph nodes are usually also positive for the same mycobacterial isolate.[5]

Footnotes

1. Havlik JA Jr, Metchock B, Thompson SE, et al, "A Prospective Evaluation of *Mycobacterium avium* Complex Colonization of the Respiratory and Gastrointestinal Tracts of Persons With Human Immunodeficiency Virus Infection," *J Infect Dis*, 1993, 168(4):1045-8.
2. Horsburgh CR Jr, Metchock B, McGowan JE Jr, et al, "Clinical Implications G of Recovery of *Mycobacterium avium* Complex From the Stool or Respiratory Tract of HIV-Infected Individuals," *AIDS*, 1992, 6(5):512-4.
3. Reisner BS, Woods GL, Thomson RB Jr, et al, "Specimen Processing," *Manual of Clinical Microbiology*, 7th ed, Chapter 5, Murray PR, Baron EJ, Pfaller M, et al, eds, Washington, DC: ASM Press, American Society for Microbiology, 1999, 64-104.
4. Morris A, Reller LB, Salfinger M, et al, "Mycobacteria in Stool Specimens: The Nonvalue of Smears for Predicting Culture Results," *J Clin Microbiol*, 1993, 31:1385-7.
5. Wolinsky E, "Mycobacterial Diseases Other Than Tuberculosis," *Clin Infect Dis*, 1992, 15(1):1-10.

References

Gradon JD, Timpone JG, and Schnittman SM, "Emergence of Unusual Opportunistic Pathogens in AIDS: A Review," *Clin Infect Dis*, 1992, 15(1):134-57.

Mwachari C, Batchelor BI, Paul J, et al, "Chronic Diarrhoea Among HIV-Infected Adult Patients in Nairobi, Kenya," *J Infect*, 1998, 37(1):48-53.

Pankhurst CL, Luo N, Kelly P, et al, "Intestinal Mycobacteria in African AIDS Patients," *Lancet*, 1995, 345(8949):585.

Yajko DM, Nassos PS, Sanders CA, et al, "Comparison of Four Decontamination Methods for Recovery of *Mycobacterium avium* Complex From Stools," *J Clin Microbiol*, 1993, 31(2):302-6.

Internet Web Sites

www.astdhpphe.org/infect/tb.html

www.cdc.gov/nchstp/tb/faqs/qa.htm

www.cdc.gov/ncidod/dbmd/diseaseinfo/mycobacteriumavium_t.htm

www.who.int/health-topics/tb.htm

Mycobacterial Culture, Urine

Related Information

Acid-Fast Stain *on page 550*
Antimicrobial Susceptibility Testing, Mycobacteria *on page 557*
Bacterial Culture, Urine *on page 578*
Fungal Culture, Urine *on page 614*
Mycobacteria by DNA Probe *on page 654*
Mycobacterial Culture, Biopsy or Body Fluid *on page 655*
Mycobacterial Culture, Sputum *on page 658*
Mycobacterial Culture, Stool *on page 659*
Viral Culture, Urine *on page 695*

Synonyms AFB Culture, Urine; TB Culture, Urine; Urine Mycobacteria Culture

Abstract Active extragenitourinary tuberculosis is found in fewer than 10% of subjects who have genitourinary tuberculosis.

Patient Preparation Usual preparation for clean catch midvoid urine specimen collection. See Bacterial Culture, Urine *on page 578* for detailed information.

Specimen At least 40 mL of first morning voided urine

Collection Three first morning voided urine specimens should be submitted. The specimen may be divided for fungus culture, mycobacteria culture and AFB stain, and routine bacterial culture and Gram stain if the specimen is of adequate volume for all tests requested.

Turnaround Time Negatives are reported after 6-8 weeks.

Reference Interval No growth

Use Isolate and identify mycobacteria from the urinary tract. Most patients with genitourinary tuberculosis have symptoms of urinary tract disease, but some are asymptomatic.

Limitations Positive acid-fast stained smears are not diagnostic, because of the presence of *Mycobacterium smegmatis* in genital secretions of normal patients.

Contraindications A 24-hour pooled urine and catheter bag specimens are unacceptable because of increased chance of bacterial contamination.

Methodology Culture in broth media, such as 7H9, and on solid media that supports the growth of mycobacteria (Löwenstein-Jensen in Middlebrook 7H11).

Additional Information If mycobacteria are cultured, isolates can be definitively identified, and susceptibility testing performed on request. Although it has been thought that tuberculosis of the urinary tract should be suspected when hematuria and pyuria occur without recovery by routine culture of usual urinary tract pathogens (sterile pyuria), concomitant infections with ordinary pathogens are not rare. Mycobacteria cultures of the urine are ~90% sensitive. The kidney is the most frequent site of such genitourinary infection; prostate, salpinx, and endometrial involvement also occurs. Continuing tuberculous bacilluria may cause cystitis with frequency. Genitourinary infections with atypical mycobacteria, particularly *M. kansasii* and *M. avium-intracellulare*, occur.[1] Mycobacterial genitourinary tract infections represented about 20% of extrapulmonary tuberculosis cases.[2] This proportion will probably increase as more infections with *M. tuberculosis* and *M. avium-intracellulare* are identified in patients with the acquired immunodeficiency syndrome (AIDS). Urine cultures were reported positive in 77% of HIV-positive patients with extrapulmonary tuberculosis, but detection of *M. tuberculosis* DNA by amplification seems to be more sensitive than culture.[3,4]

Footnotes

1. Wayne LG and Sramek HA, "Agents of Newly Recognized or Infrequently Encountered Mycobacterial Diseases," *Clin Microbiol Rev*, 1992, 5(1):1-25.
2. Alvarez S and McCabe WR, "Extrapulmonary Tuberculosis Revisited: A Review of Experience at Boston City and Other Hospitals," *Medicine*, 1984, 63(1):25-55.
3. Sechi LA, Pinna MP, Sanna A, et al, "Detection of *Mycobacterium tuberculosis* by PCR Analysis of Urine and Other Clinical Samples from AIDS and non-HIV-Infected Patients," *Mol Cell Probes*, 1997, 11(4):281-5.
4. Pfyffer GE, Kissling P, Jahn EMI, et al, "Diagnostic Performance of Amplified *Mycobacterium tuberculosis* Direct Test With Cerebrospinal Fluid, Other Nonrespiratory, and Respiratory Specimens," *J Clin Microbiol*, 1996, 34(4):834-41.

References

Metchock BG, Nolte FS, and Wallace RJ Jr, "*Mycobacterium*," *Manual of Clinical Microbiology*, 7th ed, Chapter 25, Murray PR, Baron EJ, Pfaller M, et al, eds, Washington, DC: ASM Press, American Society for Microbiology, 1999, 399-437.

Internet Web Sites

www.astdhpphe.org/infect/tb.html

www.cdc.gov/nchstp/tb/faqs/qa.htm

www.who.int/health-topics/tb.htm

♦ **Mycobacteria Susceptibility Testing** *see* Antimicrobial Susceptibility Testing, Mycobacteria *on page 557*

♦ **Mycobacterium avium-intracellulare** *see* Mycobacterial Culture, Cutaneous and Subcutaneous Tissue *on page 657*

♦ **Mycobacterium fortuitum Complex** *see* Mycobacterial Culture, Cutaneous and Subcutaneous Tissue *on page 657*

♦ **Mycobacterium marinum** *see* Bacterial Culture, Wounds, Bites *on page 579*

♦ **Mycobacterium marinum** *see* Mycobacterial Culture, Cutaneous and Subcutaneous Tissue *on page 657*

♦ **Mycobacterium Smear** *see* Acid-Fast Stain *on page 550*

♦ **Mycobacterium spp** *see* Bacterial Culture, Bronchoscopy/Bronchial Brush/ Bronchoalveolar Lavage Specimen *on page 568*

♦ **Mycobacterium spp** *see* Bacterial Culture, Cerebrospinal Fluid *on page 569*

♦ **Mycobacterium spp** *see* Bacterial Culture, Urine *on page 578*

♦ **Mycobacterium tuberculosis** *see* Bacterial Culture, Cerebrospinal Fluid *on page 569*

♦ **Mycobacterium ulcerans** *see* Mycobacterial Culture, Cutaneous and Subcutaneous Tissue *on page 657*

♦ **Mycoplasma Antibodies** *see* Mycoplasma Serology *on page 662*

♦ **Mycoplasma Culture** *see* Mycoplasma pneumoniae Culture *on page 660*

♦ **Mycoplasma pneumoniae** *see* Bacterial Culture, Sputum *on page 574*

Mycoplasma pneumoniae Culture

Related Information

Bacterial Culture, Sputum *on page 574*
Cold Agglutinin Titer *on page 594*
Mycoplasma pneumoniae DNA Probe Test *on page 661*
Mycoplasma Serology *on page 662*

Synonyms Mycoplasma Culture

Test Includes Culture for *Mycoplasma* organisms only

Abstract *Mycoplasma* organisms are smaller than conventional bacteria and are included in the class Mollicutes. These bacteria are the smallest free-living organisms known. Unlike other prokaryotes, the *Mycoplasma* bacteria do not have a cell wall; rather they have a trilayered cell membrane. Due to the lack of a cell wall, these organisms are not susceptible to killing by beta-lactam antibiotics and do not take up stains used in the Gram-staining technique.

Mycoplasma pneumoniae commonly causes respiratory infections. Most involve the upper respiratory tract, but pneumonia and other manifestations can occur as well. Diagnostic testing for *M. pneumoniae* is not easy because these organisms are not detected by routine bacterial culture. Other methods (eg, serologic or DNA detection) should be specifically requested.

Specimen Throat or nasopharyngeal swabs, sputum, bronchoalveolar lavage

Collection If throat or nasopharyngeal swabs are used, the site must be sampled vigorously to obtain as many cells as possible. Throat or nasopharyngeal swabs should be placed **immediately** in special transport medium (often obtained from the laboratory) and sent immediately to the laboratory. All specimen should be kept at 4°C during transport.

Storage Instructions If storage longer than 24 hours is needed, the specimen should be frozen at -70°C.

Turnaround Time 2-3 weeks

Reference Interval No *Mycoplasma pneumoniae* identified

Use Aid in the diagnosis of pneumonia or other respiratory diseases caused by *Mycoplasma pneumoniae*

Limitations The culture procedure is not often used because it is slow and somewhat insensitive; 2-3 weeks or more are often required for isolation and definitive identification of positive cultures.

Methodology Isolates are cultured in special broth and on special agar media and are identified by biochemical tests and ability to hemolyze erythrocytes. However, the most commonly used and currently recommended method of diagnosis is serology, to measure acute and convalescent antibody levels to *M. pneumoniae* or amplification of specific *Mycoplasma pneumoniae* nucleic acid sequences.

Mycoplasma pneumoniae
Clinical Manifestations of Infection

Respiratory	Pneumonia
	Pharyngitis
	Otitis media
	Bullous myringitis
	Sinusitis
	Laryngotracheobronchitis
	Bronchiolitis
	Nonspecific upper respiratory symptoms
Neurologic	Meningoencephalitis
	Encephalitis
	Transverse myelitis
	Cranial neuropathy
	Poliomyelitis-like syndrome
	Psychosis
	Cerebral infarction
	Guillain-Barré syndrome
Cardiac	Pericarditis
	Myocarditis
	Complete heart block
	Congestive heart failure
	Myocardial infarction
Gastrointestinal	Pancreatitis
	Hepatic dysfunction
Hematologic	Autoimmune hemolytic anemia
	Bone marrow suppression
	Thrombocytopenia
	Disseminated intravascular coagulation
Musculoskeletal	Myalgias
	Arthralgias
	Arthritis
Genitourinary	Glomerulonephritis
	Tubulointerstitial nephritis
	Tubo-ovarian abscess
Immunologic	Depressed cellular immunity and neutrophil chemotaxis

Adapted rom Broughton RA, "Infections Due to *Mycoplasma pneumoniae* in Childhood," *Pediatr Infect Dis J*, 1986, 71-85.

Additional Information *Mycoplasma pneumoniae* causes ~20% of all community-acquired pneumonia in the general population.[1,2] *Mycoplasma pneumoniae* infection is acquired via the respiratory route from small-particle aerosols or large droplets of secretions. The organism can penetrate the mucociliary barrier of respiratory epithelium and produce cellular injury and ciliostasis which may account for the prolonged cough observed clinically. Most infections are observed in older children and young adults, but recent studies have noted occasional epidemics in older persons and children younger than 5 years of age.[1,2]

Cold agglutinins and *Mycoplasma pneumoniae* serology have been the mainstays of diagnosis because of the limitations and long turnaround time

for cultures. Immunofluorescence techniques and immunoassays to detect antibodies specific for *M. pneumoniae* are available and are the recommended diagnostic methods. A DNA amplification method has recently become available.[3,4] A number of reference laboratories offer this test as a rapid alternative to culture. See *Mycoplasma pneumoniae* DNA Probe Test on page 661.

Footnotes
1. Foy HM, "Infections Caused by *Mycoplasma pneumoniae* and Possible Carrier State in Different Populations of Patients," *Clin Infect Dis*, 1993, 17(S1):37-46.
2. Taylor-Robinson D, "Infections Due to Species of *Mycoplasma* and *Ureaplasma*: An Update," *Clin Infect Dis*, 1996, 23(4):671-84.
3. Tong CY, Donnelly C, Harvey G, et al, "Multiplex Polymerase Chain Reaction for the Simultaneous Detection of *Mycoplasma pneumoniae*, *Chlamydia pneumoniae*, and *Chlamydia psittaci* in Respiratory Samples," *J Clin Pathol*, 1999, 52(4):257-63.
4. Dorigo-Zetsma JW, Zaat SA, Wertheim-van Dillen PM, et al, "Comparison of PCR, Culture, and Serological Tests for Diagnosis of *Mycoplasma pneumoniae* Respiratory Tract Infection in Children," *J Clin Microbiol*, 1999, 37(1):14-7.

References
Cimolai N, Wenstey D, Seear M, et al, "*Mycoplasma pneumoniae* as a Cofactor in Severe Respiratory Infections," *Clin Infect Dis*, 1995, 21:1182-5.
Cimolai N, "*Mycoplasma pneumoniae* Respiratory Infection," *Pediatr Rev*, 1998, 19(10):327-31.
Ewing S and Torres A, "Severe Community-Acquired Pneumonia," *Clin Chest Med*, 1999, 20(3):575-87.
Foy HM, "*Mycoplasma pneumoniae* Pneumonia: Current Perspectives," *Clin Infect Dis*, 1999, 28(2):237.
Ruuskanen O and Mertsola J, "Childhood Community-Acquired Pneumonia," *Semin Respir Infect*, 1999,14(2):163-72.

Internet Web Sites
my.webmd.com/content/asset/adam_disease_walking_pneumonia

◆ **Mycoplasma pneumoniae DNA Detection Test** see *Mycoplasma pneumoniae* DNA Probe Test on page 661

Mycoplasma pneumoniae DNA Probe Test

Related Information
Cold Agglutinin Titer *on page 594*
Mycoplasma pneumoniae Culture *on page 660*
Mycoplasma Serology *on page 662*

Synonyms DNA Hybridization Test for *Mycoplasma pneumoniae*; DNA Test for *Mycoplasma pneumoniae*; *Mycoplasma pneumoniae* DNA Detection Test

Applies to Eaton Agent Pneumonia

Test Includes Direct detection of *Mycoplasma pneumoniae* nucleic acids in clinical specimens

Abstract Synonyms for infections due to this agent include Eaton agent pneumonia, and this bacteria causes a portion of primary atypical pneumonia cases. Respiratory infections due to *Mycoplasma pneumoniae* are difficult to assess because current laboratory techniques lack sensitivity or require long periods of time (3 weeks) for results. Serological procedures are the most widely used diagnostic tests.[1] Cold agglutinins are also used to diagnose *M. pneumoniae*; however, only ~50% of infected patients become positive.[2] Culture of this microorganism is rarely done due to the difficulty of recovery and the long incubation time required for growth. A rapid and sensitive test for the diagnosis of *M. pneumoniae* infection is important, since effective antibiotic therapy is available. The nucleic acid based test is a sensitive method for rapid diagnosis of respiratory infections of *M. pneumoniae*.

Specimen Sputum, throat swab, bronchial wash, lung biopsy

Container Special DNA transport medium may be provided by the laboratory. For some specimens (eg, sputum, bronchial wash or biopsy), a sterile container is acceptable. Sterile viral swabs placed in specific *Mycoplasma* media (eg, SP4, 10 B, or 2SP) can be used to collect throat specimens.

Collection Sputum specimens should be collected early in the day so they can be sent directly to the laboratory.

Storage Instructions The specimens should be maintained at room temperature or refrigerated. Do not freeze.

Turnaround Time 1-2 days

Reference Interval Negative for *Mycoplasma pneumoniae*

Use Rapid detection of *Mycoplasma pneumoniae* in clinical specimens from respiratory sites.

Limitations This assay cannot determine whether or not the microorganism is viable. The organism may persist for varying lengths of time following acute infection. As with other molecular tests, costs and the potential for intralaboratory contamination must be controlled.

Methodology This test detects *Mycoplasma pneumoniae* nucleic acid directly from respiratory specimens. It requires lysis of the cells in the specimen and release of the *Mycoplasma pneumoniae*-specific RNA or DNA. The lysed specimens are then hybridized with a specific DNA probe. Detection of the bound probe is assessed by use of a labeled DNA probe.

Additional Information A wide range of clinical manifestations of *Mycoplasma pneumoniae* respiratory infections is recognized, from mild infection to severe pneumonia. This microorganism causes approximately 20% of community-acquired lower respiratory infection. Mortality is rare and infection is usually self-limited.[3,4] Laboratory diagnosis of *Mycoplasma pneumoniae* is usually based on measurement of specific antibodies in paired sera (Continued)

INFECTIOUS DISEASES: *MYCOPLASMA* SEROLOGY

Mycoplasma pneumoniae DNA Probe Test
(Continued)

and/or isolation of the organism by culture. Culture isolation of the fastidious *Mycoplasma pneumoniae* is tedious, labor intensive, and usually requires several weeks.[4] Serological assays remain the most commonly used tests for both diagnosis and epidemiology.[1] The DNA detection assay for *Mycoplasma pneumoniae* has been found to have a specificity and sensitivity which match culture and antibody assays.[5,6] The advantage of this test is the rapid turnaround time, which facilitates treatment with appropriate antibiotics.

Footnotes

1. Duffy MF, Whithear KG, Noormohammadi AH, et al, "Indirect Enzyme-Linked Immunosorbent Assay for Detection of Immunoglobulin G Reactive With a Recombinant Protein Expressed From the Gene Encoding the 116-Kilodalton Protein of *Mycoplasma pneumoniae*," *J Clin Microbiol*, 1999, 37(4):1024-9.
2. Cassell GH, Gambill G, and Duffy L, "ELISA in Respiratory Infections of Humans," *Molecular and Diagnostic Procedures in Mycoplasmology*, Tully JG, Razin S, eds, New York, NY: Academic Press, Inc, 1996, 123-36.
3. Foy HM, "Infections Caused by *Mycoplasma pneumoniae* and Possible Carrier State in Different Populations of Patients," *Clin Infect Dis*, 1993, 17(S1):37-46.
4. Taylor-Robinson D, "Infections Due to Species of *Mycoplasma* and *Ureaplasma*: An Update," *Clin Infect Dis*, 1996, 23(4):671-84.
5. Tong CY, Donnelly C, Harvey G, et al, "Multiplex Polymerase Chain Reaction for the Simultaneous Detection of *Mycoplasma pneumoniae*, *Chlamydia pneumoniae*, and *Chlamydia psittaci* in Respiratory Samples," *J Clin Pathol*, 1999, 52(4):257-63.
6. Dorigo-Zetsma JW, Zaat SA, Wertheim-van Dillen PM, et al, "Comparison of PCR, Culture, and Serological Tests for Diagnosis of *Mycoplasma pneumoniae* Respiratory Tract Infection in Children," *J Clin Microbiol*, 1999, 37(1):14-7.

References

Foy HM, "*Mycoplasma pneumoniae* Pneumonia: Current Perspectives," *Clin Infect Dis*, 1999, 28(2):237.
Yungbluth M, "The Laboratory Diagnosis of Pneumonia. The Role of the Community Hospital Pathologist," *Clin Lab Med*, 1995, 15(2):209-34.

Internet Web Sites

my.webmd.com/content/asset/adam_disease_walking_pneumonia

♦ *Mycoplasma pneumoniae* Infection *see* Cold Agglutinin Titer *on page 594*

♦ *Mycoplasma pneumoniae* Titer *see* Mycoplasma Serology *on page 662*

Mycoplasma Serology

Related Information

Bacterial Culture, Sputum *on page 574*
Cold Agglutinin Titer *on page 594*
Mycoplasma pneumoniae Culture *on page 660*
Mycoplasma pneumoniae DNA Probe Test *on page 661*

Synonyms Eaton Agent Titer; *M. pneumoniae* Titer; *Mycoplasma* Antibodies; *Mycoplasma pneumoniae* Titer; Pleuropneumonia-like Organism (PPLO) Titer; Walking Pneumonia Titer

Test Includes Detection of serologic response to *Mycoplasma pneumoniae* infection

Abstract *Mycoplasma* lacks the rigid cell walls of other bacteria, thus, they do not react with Gram stain. They are fastidious and smaller than some viruses. *Mycoplasma pneumoniae* accounts for up to 20% of hospitalized adults with community-acquired pneumonia, and a larger percentage of those treated as outpatients.[1] Pneumonias caused by atypical organisms most commonly include chlamydial and mycoplasmal pneumonia, and Legionnaires' disease.

Specimen Serum

Container Red top tube

Sampling Time Acute and convalescent sera drawn 10-14 days apart are desirable.

Reference Interval Negative. IgG <1:10, IgM <1:10. A fourfold increase in titer in paired sera, drawn 2-4 weeks apart, is a definitive diagnosis. Increase in IgG titer in paired sera may be helpful, but high IgG titer usually indicates prior exposure. IgM titer is needed for evaluation in community-acquired pneumonia.

Use Support the diagnosis of *Mycoplasma pneumoniae* infection and investigate atypical pneumonia. Although the most common agent which causes croup is the parainfluenza virus, other viruses and *M. pneumoniae* can be etiologic. The frequency of cases of pharyngitis caused by *Mycoplasma* is uncertain.[2]

Limitations False positives occur when antibody from prior infection is detected, which is especially a problem in patients older than 40 years of age.[3] The complement fixation procedures are based on lipid extracts of the organism, which cross react with antigens in other bacteria, human tissues, and some plants.[3] False positives can occur in patients with cross-reactive autoantibodies. False negatives are found when testing is done too early and may be found in immunocompromised individuals. Rational implementation requires interprocedure comparisons, as well as understanding of the population served.[4]

The numerous commercial enzyme immunoassays (EIA) are not equivalent, due to variations in the antigen preparation, EIAs are more sensitive

than complement fixation. Newer EIAs use recombinant antigens that have less cross reactions, which increases the specificity of the assay.[4,5]

Elevated cold agglutinins have been used to indicate acute *M. pneumoniae* disease, but this test lacks sensitivity. Titers ≥1:64 are considered significant. All patients with *Mycoplasma* infections do not have cold agglutinins. Cold agglutinins are IgM antibodies against the I antigen of red cells.

Methodology Complement fixation (CF), indirect fluorescent antibody (IFA), enzyme immunoassay (EIA), specific IgM antibody by agglutination, IgM anti-P1 immunoblotting, microtiter procedure utilizing anti-*M. pneumoniae* IgM[5]

Additional Information *Mycoplasma pneumoniae* is a cause of "primary atypical pneumonia." The *Mycoplasma* organisms are more difficult to culture than ordinary bacteria and thus serologic confirmation of the diagnosis is often desirable. A fourfold or greater rise in titer occurs in about 80% of cases. Serologic tests for antibody to *M. pneumoniae* are more specific and more sensitive than the cold agglutinin titer. Demonstration of specific IgG and IgM antibody by immunofluorescence is rapid, sensitive, and specific. IgM antibody indicates acute infection.

ESR and C-reactive protein are often abnormal.

See also *Mycoplasma pneumoniae* DNA Probe Test *on page 661* and *Mycoplasma pneumoniae* Culture *on page 660*.

Footnotes

1. Foy HM, "Infections Caused by *Mycoplasma pneumoniae* and Possible Carrier State in Different Populations of Patients," *Clin Infect Dis*, 1993, 17(S1):S37-S46.
2. Bisno AL, "Acute Pharyngitis," *N Engl J Med*, 2001, 344(3):205-11.
3. Cassell GH, Gambill G, and Duffy L, "ELISA in Respiratory Infections of Humans," *Molecular and Diagnostic Procedures in Mycoplasmology*, Tully JG, Razin S, eds, New York, NY: Academic Press, Inc, 1996, 123-36.
4. Cimolai N and Cheong AC, "An Assessment of a New Diagnostic Indirect Enzyme Immunoassay for the Detection of Anti-*Mycoplasma pneumoniae* IgM," *Am J Clin Pathol*, 1996, 105:205-9.
5. Duffy MF, Whithear KG, Noormohammadi AH, et al, "Indirect Enzyme-linked Immunosorbent Assay for Detection of Immunoglobulin G Reactive With a Recombinant Protein Expressed From the Gene Encoding the 116-Kilodalton Protein of *Mycoplasma pneumoniae*," *J Clin Microbiol*, 1999, 37(4):1024-9.

References

Cimolai N, "*Mycoplasma pneumoniae* Respiratory Infection," *Pediatr Rev*, 1998, 19(10):327-31.
Clyde WA Jr, "*Mycoplasma* Infections," *Harrison's Principles of Internal Medicine*, 13th ed, Isselbacher KJ, Braunwald E, Wilson JD, et al, eds, New York, NY: McGraw-Hill Inc, 1994, 757-9.
File TM, Tan JS, and Plouffe JF, "The Role of Atypical Pathogens: *Mycoplasma pneumoniae*, *Chlamydia pneumoniae*, and *Legionella pneumophila* in Respiratory Infection," *Infect Dis Clin N Amer*, 1998, 12(3):569-592.
Foy HM, "*Mycoplasma pneumoniae* Pneumonia: Current Perspectives," *Clin Infect Dis*, 1999, 28(2):237.
Johnson DH and Cunha BA, "Atypical Pneumonias. Clinical and Extrapulmonary Features of *Chlamydia*, *Mycoplasma*, and *Legionella* Infections," *Postgrad Med*, 1993, 93(7):69-72, 75-6, 79-82.

Internet Web Sites

my.webmd.com/content/asset/adam_disease_walking_pneumonia

♦ *Mycoplasma* T-Strain Culture, Genital *see* Genital Culture for *Ureaplasma urealyticum on page 616*

♦ **Nantucket Fever Serological Test** *see* Babesiosis Serology *on page 561*

♦ **Nasopharyngeal Culture** *see* Bacterial Culture, Nasopharynx *on page 573*

♦ **Nasopharyngeal Culture for *Bordetella pertussis*** *see* Bordetella pertussis Culture *on page 583*

♦ **Nasopharyngeal Culture for *Corynebacterium diphtheriae*** *see* Corynebacterium diphtheriae Throat Culture *on page 594*

♦ **Nasopharyngeal Smear for *Bordetella pertussis*** *see* Bordetella pertussis Direct Fluorescent Antibody *on page 583*

♦ **Negri Bodies** *see* Rabies *on page 673*

♦ *Neisseria gonorrhoeae* *see* Bacterial Culture, Conjunctiva *on page 570*

♦ *Neisseria gonorrhoeae* *see* Bacterial Culture, Genital Specimen *on page 571*

♦ *Neisseria gonorrhoeae* *see* Bacterial Culture, Sputum *on page 574*

Neisseria gonorrhoeae Culture and Smear

Related Information

Bacterial Culture, Conjunctiva *on page 570*
Bacterial Culture, Genital Specimen *on page 571*
Beta-Lactamase Test *on page 581*
Cervical/Vaginal Cytology *on page 377*
Chlamydia trachomatis Culture *on page 590*
Chlamydia trachomatis Direct Antigen Test *on page 590*
Chlamydia trachomatis Nucleic Acid Detection *on page 591*
Genital Culture for *Ureaplasma urealyticum on page 616*
Gram Stain *on page 617*
Herpes Simplex Virus Culture *on page 631*
HIV-1/HIV-2 Antibody Screen and Western Blot *on page 636*

Neisseria gonorrhoeae Nucleic Acid Detection *on page 664*
RPR *on page 677*
Synovial Fluid Analysis *on page 323*
VDRL, Serum *on page 688*

Synonyms GC Culture; Gonorrhea Culture

Test Includes Selective culture for *Neisseria gonorrhoeae*; Gram stain of specimen from normally sterile site and male urethral swabs

Abstract Gonorrhea is a sexually-transmitted disease. *N. gonorrhoeae* can be vertically transmitted during birth. Most gonococcal infections are uncomplicated genital tract infections that can be effectively treated with antimicrobial agents. Of concern is the large number of asymptomatic infections in both men and women. If untreated, gonococcal infection may develop into epididymitis, prostatitis, or urethral stricture. In women, untreated gonorrhea may cause pelvic inflammatory disease manifested as endometritis, salpingitis, pelvic peritonitis, or tubo-ovarian abscesses. A small percentage of patients (1% to 3%) will develop disseminated gonococcal infection.[1,2]

Patient Preparation Preparation same as for clean catch urine. See Bacterial Culture, Urine *on page 578* for detailed information. *Neisseria gonorrhoeae* is very sensitive to lubricants and disinfectants. If possible, avoid collecting urethral specimens until at least 1 hour after urination.

Specimen Body fluid, discharge, pus, swab of genital lesions, urethral discharge (best when available for men); endocervix (best when available for female); throat swab, rectal swab; sediment of first 10 mL of centrifuged urine collected at least 2 hours after last micturition, or first few drops of urine voided into a sterile cup for "first voided urine specimen" for asymptomatic males, or first void overnight urine, centrifuged.

Container Swab with transport medium, a dacron or rayon swab should be used, cotton swabs may be used only if the cotton is treated to neutralize toxicity, sterile container for tissue or pus. The best method for growth of *N. gonorrhoeae* is to directly plate the specimen on Transgrow, Jembec™, or Thayer-Martin medium immediately after collection.

Collection

Urethral discharge: Collect male urethral discharge by endourethral swab after stripping toward the orifice to express exudate.

Rectal swab: Collect anorectal specimens from the crypts just inside the anal ring. Direct visualization with anoscopy is useful. Insert the swab past the anal sphincter. Move the swab circumferentially around the anal crypts. Allow 15-30 seconds for organisms to adsorb onto the swab.

Prostatic fluid yields fewer positives than culture of urethral discharge.

Urethral or vaginal cultures are indicated from females when endocervical culture is not possible.

Urethra in women: Massage the urethra against the pubic symphysis to express discharge or use endourethral swab.

Vagina: Obtain the specimen from the vaginal vault. Allow 15-30 seconds for organisms to adsorb onto the swab.

Selection of Culture Sites for the Isolation of *Neisseria gonorrhoeae*

Culture Site	Diagnostic Sensitivity (%)
Female (nonhysterectomized) Primary site Endocervical canal	86-96
Secondary sites Vagina	55-90
Urethra	60-86
Anal canal	70-85
Oropharynx	50-70
Female (hysterectomized) Primary site Urethra	88.9
Secondary sites Vagina	55.7
Anal canal	40.7
Male (heterosexuals) Primary site Urethra	94-98 (symptomatic) 84 (asymptomatic)
Male (homosexuals) Primary sites Urethra	60-98
Anal canal	40-85
Oropharynx	50-70

Adapted from Ehret JM and Knapp JS, "Gonorrhea," *Clin Lab Med*, 1989, 9:445-80.

Endocervical/cervical: Gently compress cervix between speculum blades to express any endocervical exudate. Swab in a circular pattern.

Bartholin gland: Express exudate from duct. Abscesses should be aspirated with needle and syringe.

Oropharyngeal and tonsillar specimens are obtained via swab, preferably under direct vision.

Specimens should be transported to the laboratory within 1 hour of collection or plated on appropriate media in the examination room.

Storage Instructions Specimen should not be refrigerated or exposed to a cold environment. Growth of the organism is less likely following refrigeration. If the specimen is directly inoculated on Thayer-Martin medium, it should be transported to the laboratory as soon as possible and placed directly in CO_2 incubator or candle jar.

Turnaround Time Gram stain results are usually available in less than 1 hour. Cultures from which *N. gonorrhoeae* is isolated usually require 48 hours for completion.

Reference Interval Gram stain: no intracellular gram-negative diplococci seen; no *Neisseria gonorrhoeae* isolated

Critical Values Positive culture for *Neisseria gonorrhoeae* during pregnancy, or in young children or neonates

Use Isolate and identify *Neisseria gonorrhoeae*; establish the diagnosis of gonorrhea

Limitations Cultures are usually screened only for *Neisseria gonorrhoeae*. Other organisms are usually not identified. Overgrowth by *Proteus* and yeast may make it impossible to rule out presence of *N. gonorrhoeae*. The vancomycin in Thayer-Martin media may inhibit some strains of *N. gonorrhoeae* and the trimethoprim in New York City media may inhibit the growth of other strains of *N. gonorrhoeae*.

Methodology Culture on selective medium, Thayer-Martin, or New York City (NYC). DNA probes, monoclonal antibodies, enzyme immunoassays (EIA), and chromogenic substrate assays are used as alternatives or adjuncts to culture in some laboratories.

Additional Information Gram stain smear has a high sensitivity in a symptomatic male with urethral discharge (95% to 99%). Endocervical Gram stain is of little value in the female as the sensitivity is lower (50%), and endemic normal flora have a similar morphologic appearance, causing false positives. The Gram stain smear will detect 75% of gonococcal conjunctivitis and 10% to 20% of gonococcal skin lesions. It is of no value in pharyngitis. Anal and throat cultures are recommended for individuals engaging in anal or oral sex. Cervical cultures have a sensitivity of 80% to 90%. Although demonstration of gram-negative diplococci in leukocytes in a urethral smear from a symptomatic male is presumptive evidence of gonorrhea and is sufficiently diagnostic to initiate therapy, culture confirmation should be considered if available.

Sensitivity and Specificity of Gram Stains for Diagnosis of Gonorrhea

Specimen Source	Sensitivity (%)	Specificity (%)
Female Endocervical canal	45-65	90-97
Vagina	Not studied	–
Urethra	16	–
Anal canal	Not recommended	–
Pharynx	Not recommended	–
Male Urethra (symptomatic)	95-99	97-98
Urethra (asymptomatic)	50-70	86
Anal canal (with mucopurulent discharge)	40-80	87-100
Pharynx	Not recommended	–

Adapted from Ehret JM and Knapp JS, "Gonorrhea," *Clin Lab Med*, 1989, 9:445-80.

Serologic tests for syphilis (VDRL, RPR), HIV, Cervical/Vaginal Cytology, and a diagnostic test for *Chlamydia* should be performed in patients suspected of having gonorrhea. As many as 45% of women with gonorrheal infection have chlamydial infection as well.[1,2] Thayer-Martin medium and transport systems are available in most laboratories. Aseptically obtained body fluids from patients with suspected gonococcal arthritis should be inoculated to chocolate agar; isolates may fail to grow on selective media.

The major viral sexually transmitted diseases also include HIV, genital herpes, human papillomavirus, *Chlamydia*, syphilis, and hepatitis B.

Laboratories may presumptively identify *Neisseria gonorrhoeae* from clinical specimens if the following criteria are met.

- The specimen is from a genital source.
- The patient is presumed to be sexually active.

(Continued)

Neisseria gonorrhoeae Culture and Smear
(Continued)

- The organism grows on selective medium, is oxidase positive, and is morphologically consistent with *Neisseria gonorrhoeae* (ie, gram-negative diplococci with adjacent sides flattened).

If any of these criteria are not met, the organism must be definitively identified using stricter definitions. **Thus, organisms from the throat or rectum, or isolates from nonsexually active (eg, infants or young children) individuals should never be presumptively identified using the criteria listed above.**[3] In these cases, identification of *N. gonorrhoeae* must be made with two test systems that use different methods for identification (acid production and biochemical tests or use of monoclonal antibodies specific for *N. gonorrhoeae* or use of specific nucleic acid probes). Many of the rapid biochemical methods for identifying *Neisseria gonorrhoeae* are based on three or four biochemical reactions and use a very limited database. These kits are only acceptable for genital specimens from sexually active patients.

Nongonococcal urethritis may be caused by *Ureaplasma urealyticum*, *Corynebacterium genitalium* type 1, *Trichomonas vaginalis*, *Chlamydia trachomatis*, herpes simplex virus, and rarely, *Candida albicans*.

Footnotes

1. Centers for Disease Control and Prevention, "1998 Guidelines for the Treatment of Sexually Transmitted Diseases," *Morbid Mortal Weekly Rep*, 1998, 47(RR1):59-63.
2. "Gonorrhea and Chlamydial Infections. ACOG Technical Bulletin Number 190-March 1994," *Int J Gynaecol Obstet*, 1994, 45(2):169-74.
3. Whittington WL, Rice RJ, Biddle JW, et al, "Incorrect Identification of *Neisseria gonorrhoeae* From Infants and Children," *Pediatr Infect Dis J*, 1988, 7(1):3-10.

References

Angulo JM and Espinoza LR, "Gonococcal Arthritis," *Compr Ther*, 1999, 25(3):155-62.

Baron EJ, Cassell GH, Duffy LB, et al, "Cumitech 17A: Laboratory Diagnosis of Female Genital Tract Infections," Baron EJ, ed, Washington, DC: American Society for Microbiology, 1993.

Centers for Disease Control and Prevention, "Gonorrhea - United States, 1998," *JAMA*, 2000, 284(2):173-4.

Evangelista AT and Beilstein HR, "Cumitech 4A: Laboratory Diagnosis of Gonorrhea," Abramson C, ed, Washington, DC: American Society for Microbiology, 1993.

Gunn RA, Rolfs RT, Greenspan JR, et al, "The Changing Paradigm of Sexually Transmitted Disease Control in the Era of Managed Health Care," *JAMA*, 1998, 279(9):680-4.

Ingram DL, Everett VD, Flick LAR, et al, "Vaginal Gonococcal Cultures in Sexual Abuse Evaluations: Evaluation of Selective Criteria for Preteenaged Girls," *Pediatrics*, 1997, 99(6):E8.

Olsen CC, Schwebke JR, Benjamin WH Jr, et al, "Comparison of Direct Inoculation and Copan Transport Systems for Isolation of *Neisseria gonorrhoeae* From Endocervical Specimens," *J Clin Microbiol*, 1999, 37(11):3583-5.

Internet Web Sites

www.cdc.gov/ncidod/dastlr/gcdir/gono.html
www.medinfo.ufl.edu/year2/mmid/bms5300/bugs/neigonor.html

♦ *Neisseria gonorrhoeae* **DNA Detection Test** *see Neisseria gonorrhoeae* Nucleic Acid Detection *on page 664*

♦ *Neisseria gonorrhoeae* **Molecular Probe Assay** *see Neisseria gonorrhoeae* Nucleic Acid Detection *on page 664*

Neisseria gonorrhoeae Nucleic Acid Detection

Related Information

Bacterial Culture, Conjunctiva *on page 570*
Bacterial Culture, Genital Specimen *on page 571*
Chlamydia trachomatis Culture *on page 590*
Chlamydia trachomatis Direct Antigen Test *on page 590*
Chlamydia trachomatis Nucleic Acid Detection *on page 591*
Neisseria gonorrhoeae Culture and Smear *on page 662*

Synonyms DNA Detection for *Neisseria gonorrhoeae*; Gonorrhea DNA Detection; *Neisseria gonorrhoeae* DNA Detection Test; *Neisseria gonorrhoeae* Molecular Probe Assay

Test Includes Detection of *Neisseria gonorrhoeae* nucleic acid in clinical specimens

Abstract *Neisseria gonorrhoeae* is one of the most common sexually transmitted infections. Gonorrhea infections are commonly asymptomatic. Disease and infection in women is associated with a high rate of tubal pregnancies, pelvic inflammatory disease and infertility. While in the past, *Neisseria gonorrhoeae* was principally diagnosed by culture, the commercial availability of assays employing molecular approaches has significantly altered the standard approach for detection of this agent. Molecular assays, either direct detection or after amplification, have greatly decreased the time for identification of *N. gonorrhoeae* and has increased the sensitivity of detection. *N. gonorrhoeae* is fastidious, and optimal growth conditions must be maintained for its recovery. Although the cost of molecular assays is typically greater than that of culture, the molecular probe is recommended for situations in which specimens must be transported to an off-site laboratory for testing.[1,2] In recognition of common dual infections by *Chlamydia* and gonorrhea, commercial assays have been developed which permit detection of these organisms with a single swab or specimen. Numerous assays have been developed using nucleic acid amplification methods for detection of the *N. gonorrhoeae* bacterial genome.[2,3,4] One commercial

assay, the Gen-Probe® PACE 2 assay, detects ribosomal RNA of the organism (rRNA) without amplification.[2] In addition to use on swab specimens of cervix and urethra, the new assays are sufficiently sensitive to detect organisms in the urine of infected individuals, especially male patients.

Patient Preparation For urethral specimens, the patient should not have urinated for 1 hour prior to collection.

Specimen Either direct swabs of a potentially infected site or urine may be used depending on the assay. A swab specimen may be collected from the genital/urinary tract of males or females. Commercial assays have also been approved for detection of gonorrhea from urine. Although the rectum and the nasopharynx are also sites that may be infected by gonorrhea, swabs of these sites have not been approved for use with molecular assays.

Container Special collection and transport kits are an integral component of the assay and must be used with the appropriate commercial detection assay. A commercial kit typically contains a swab and transport media or device.

Collection Two swabs are provided in the typical commercial kit for use in females. The cervix or endocervix is first cleaned with one swab and the second swab is used to collect the specimen. The swab is inserted into the endocervical canal and rotated to collect epithelial cells from the infected site. The swab is then placed into transport media and sent to the laboratory. In males, the swab is inserted into the urethral meatus and rotated to collect epithelial cells. The swab is then placed into transport media and sent to the laboratory.

Use of urine in some of the amplification assays requires first voided urine. The patient should not have urinated for 2 hours prior to collection of urine for testing.

Storage Instructions Some specimens may be stored at room temperature or refrigerated and sent without freezing to the laboratory. Specimens collected for commercial molecular assays are typically stable for up to 1 week after collection. Urine specimens should be refrigerated immediately after collection.

Causes for Rejection Collection of a specimen from a nonapproved site, excessively bloody specimens (for some assays)

Turnaround Time Results are typically available within 24-48 hours of receipt of the specimen.

Reference Interval Negative for *Neisseria gonorrhoeae*

Use This test provides for the rapid detection of *N. gonorrhoeae* in a wide variety of clinical specimens. The sensitivity of the test exceeds that for culture and other nonmolecular assays.

Limitations Gonococcal nucleic acid can be detected for up to 3 weeks after successful treatment; thus, these assays cannot be used to determine cure. Results by molecular assays have not been accepted as evidence by the courts and legal system. For these purposes, a culture is required. Antimicrobial resistance in *N. gonorrhoeae* cannot be detected by the commercial probe assays.

Some of the amplification assays produce false-positive results due to the detection of nonpathogenic strains of *Neisseria* which are known to be normal human flora.

Methodology Several molecular assays have been approved or are under review by the Food and Drug Administration. Most of the assays utilize a nucleic amplification step, either by PCR, ligase chain reaction, or transcription-based amplification of RNA. After amplification, the specific products are detected using various immunochemical methods or chemiluminescence.[3,4] One commercial assay utilizes a signal amplification of RNA:DNA hybrids captured on a solid matrix.[5] The Gen-Probe® assay directly detects the presence of ribosomal RNA which is in vast excess to single copy genes of an organism without amplification. The probe incorporates a chemiluminescent chemical which upon activation emits light.[6] Various instrumentation is utilized by each of the methodologies, and various aspects of the assay have been automated.

Additional Information Gonorrhea is one of the most important sexually transmitted diseases in the United States. Infection is characterized by acute urethritis in males and as cervicitis in females.[7] The molecular probe assays provide several advantages over traditional culture assays or antibody-based tests. One of the most significant advantages is the ability to detect nonviable organisms, since only the presence of nucleic acids is necessary. This latter property also minimizes the need to rapidly transfer the specimen to culture media.[1] The sensitivity of molecular assays may either equal or significantly exceed that of culture techniques, depending upon the prevalence of disease and the site of collection.[1] Detection of organisms in urine provides an additional advantage over alternative methods, and may have a significant impact on public health attempts at limiting the spread of disease.

Footnotes

1. Koumans EH, Johnson RE, Knapp JS, et al, "Laboratory Testing for *Neisseria gonorrhoeae* by Recently Introduced Nonculture Tests: A Performance Review With Clinical and Public Health Considerations," *Clin Infect Dis*, 1998, 27(5):1171-80.
2. Limberger RJ, Biega R, Evancoe A, et al, "Evaluation of Culture and Gen-Probe® PACE 2 Assay for Detection of *Neisseria gonorrhoeae* and *Chlamydia trachomatis* in Endocervical Specimens Transported to a State Health Laboratory," *J Clin Microbiol*, 1992, 30(5):1162-6.
3. Farrell DJ, "Evaluation of AMPLICOR *Neisseria gonorrhoeae* PCR Using cppB Nested PCR and 16S rRNA PCR," *J Clin Microbiol*, 1999, 37(2):386-90.

4. Xu K, Glanton V, Johnson SR, et al, "Detection of *Neisseria gonorrhoeae* Infection by Ligase Chain Reaction Testing of Urine Among Adolescent Women With and Without *Chlamydia trachomatis* Infection," *Sex Transm Dis*, 1998, 25(10):533-8.

5. Schachter J, Hook EW 3rd, McCormack WM, et al, "Ability of the Digene Hybrid Capture II Test to Identify *Chlamydia trachomatis* and *Neisseria gonorrhoeae* in Cervical Specimens," *J Clin Microbiol*, 1999, 37(11):3668-71.

6. Panke ES, Yang LI, Leist PA, et al, "Comparison of Gen-Probe® DNA Probe Test and Culture for the Detection of *Neisseria gonorrhoeae* in Endocervical Specimen," *J Clin Microbiol*, 1991, 29(5):883-8.

7. Molodysky E, "Urethritis and Cervicitis," *Aust Fam Physician*, 1999, 28(4):333-8.

References

Brown TJ, Yen-Moore A, and Tyring SK, "An Overview of Sexually Transmitted Diseases. Part I," *J Am Acad Dermatol*, 1999, 41(4):511-32.

Burstein GR, Waterfield G, Joffe A, et al, "Screening for Gonorrhea and *Chlamydia* by DNA Amplification in Adolescents Attending Middle School Health Centers. Opportunity for Early Intervention," *Sex Transm Dis*, 1998, 25(8):395-402.

Carroll KC, Aldeen WE, Morrison M, et al, "Evaluation of the Abbott LCx Ligase Chain Reaction Assay for Detection of *Chlamydia trachomatis* and *Neisseria gonorrhoeae* in Urine and Genital Swab Specimens From a Sexually Transmitted Disease Clinic Population," *J Clin Microbiol*, 1998, 36(6):1630-3.

Iwen PC, Walker RA, Warren KL, et al, "Effect of Off-Site Transportation on Detection of *Neisseria gonorrhoeae* in Endocervical Specimens," *Arch Pathol Lab Med*, 1996, 120(11):1019-22.

Lin JS, Donegan SP, Heeren TC, et al, "Transmission of *Chlamydia trachomatis* and *Neisseria gonorrhoeae* Among Men With Urethritis and Their Female Sex Partners," *J Infect Dis*, 1998, 178(6):1707-12.

Modarress KJ, Cullen AP, Jaffurs WJ Sr, et al, "Detection of *Chlamydia trachomatis* and *Neisseria gonorrhoeae* in Swab Specimens by the Hybrid Capture II and PACE 2 Nucleic Acid Probe Tests," *Sex Transm Dis*, 1999, 26(5):303-8.

Uhrin M, "Molecular Diagnostics. The Polymerase Chain Reaction and Its Use in the Diagnosis of *Chlamydia trachomatis* and *Neisseria gonorrhoeae*," *Gac Med Mex*, 1997, 133(S1):133-7.

Internet Web Sites

www.cdc.gov/ncidod/dastlr/gcdir/gono.html
www.medinfo.ufl.edu/year2/mmid/bms5300/bugs/neigonor.html

♦ **Neisseria gonorrhoeae Susceptibility Testing** see Beta-Lactamase Test on page 581

♦ **Neisseria meningitidis** see Bacterial Culture, Cerebrospinal Fluid on page 569

♦ **Neisseria sp** see Bacterial Culture, Aerobes on page 563

♦ **Nephropathia Epidemica** see Hantavirus Serology on page 619

♦ **Nipah Virus** see Encephalitis Viral Serology on page 604

♦ **Nits Identification** see Arthropod Identification on page 559

Nocardia Culture

Related Information

Acid-Fast Stain, Modified, *Nocardia* Species on page 550
Actinomyces Culture on page 551
Cerebrospinal Fluid Analysis: Overview on page 416
Fine Needle Aspiration Culture on page 609
Fungal Culture, Sputum on page 613
Mycobacterial Culture, Sputum on page 658

Applies to Sputum *Nocardia* Culture

Test Includes Culture for *Nocardia* spp and direct microscopic examination of clinical specimens by Gram stain and/or modified acid-fast stains

Abstract *Nocardia* infections in humans are rare and usually occur in patients who are severely immunocompromised or in patients with a traumatic injury.[1] Human nocardial infections may be divided into six categories based on body site involved, and clinical and pathological characteristics:

- pulmonary nocardiosis
- systemic nocardiosis
- central nervous system nocardiosis
- extrapulmonary, localized nocardiosis
- cutaneous, subcutaneous, and lymphocutaneous nocardioses
- mycetoma

The usual portal of entry is the lung and skin manifestations may be complications of disseminated disease and should not always be attributed to local inoculation.

Specimen Pus, tissue, cerebrospinal fluid or other body fluid, aspirate, sputum

Special Instructions Consultation with laboratory prior to collection of the specimen is recommended when nocardiosis is suspected clinically. **Culture should be specifically ordered as "Culture for *Nocardia*."**

Reference Interval No *Nocardia* species isolated

Critical Values *Nocardia* species recovered from a central nervous system specimen

Use Establish the diagnosis of nocardiosis or mycetoma; identify its etiologic agent

Limitations *Nocardia* species will not be recovered by routine bacterial culture techniques because of its relatively slow growth. Growth of *Nocardia* may be obscured by overgrowth of other organisms in mixed culture (ie, sputum). The diagnosis may not be made unless the laboratory is advised of the clinical suspicion of nocardiosis. *Nocardia* species are not strongly gram-positive, but their branching pattern when visible is helpful. A modified

acid-fast stain (see Acid-Fast Stain, Modified, *Nocardia* Species on page 550) is needed, since *Nocardia* are weakly acid-fast and may not be found with conventional acid-fast staining. Staining may be positive when cultures fail. *Nocardia* species are variably acid-fast and may be frequently confused with *Actinomyces* species or saprophytic fungi in Gram stains of clinical specimens. Routine blood cultures do not detect *Nocardia* species.

Methodology Aerobic culture on various bacterial culture media including blood and chocolate agars. *Legionella* culture media (selective and nonselective buffered charcoal yeast agar) will support the recovery of *Nocardia*.[2] *Nocardia* species can also be cultured on noninhibitory fungal or mycobacterial media. Cultures are usually held for 10-30 days, when the laboratory is aware of clinical suspicion of nocardiosis.

Additional Information *Nocardia* species are aerobic, gram-positive bacteria which are filamentous and relatively slow growing. *N. asteroides*, *N. brasiliensis*, *N. farcinica*, *N. nova*, *N. otitidiscaviarum* (formerly *N. caviae*), and *N. transvalensis* are human pathogens.[3] Many laboratories do not distinguish organisms in the *N. asteroides* complex (ie, *N. asteroides*, *N. nova*, *N. farcinica*) from one another, and identify all these organisms as *N. asteroides*. Human infection is seen most frequently in patients whose immune systems are suppressed by HIV infection, lymphoreticular malignancy, or chemotherapy.[4] However, pulmonary nocardiosis may occur in immunocompetent patients.[5,6] The clinical picture may be similar to that observed with systemic mycobacterial or fungal infections. Infections may be acute, subacute, or chronic; and they may be disseminated or localized to cutaneous sites or the respiratory tract.[4] Metastatic infection in brain, bone, joints, soft tissue, heart, kidneys, skin, or subcutaneous infection in the presence of pulmonary involvement is suggestive of nocardiosis. Organisms in the *N. asteroides* complex are the species most commonly recovered from clinical specimens; they are usually associated with respiratory infections. *N. brasiliensis* is the species usually associated with mycetoma.[7]

In >50% of patients with nocardiosis, the pleural space, the pericardial cavity, or both are involved.[8]

Prognosis is dependent on early diagnosis, treatment with appropriate antimicrobials, and the course of the underlying disease.

Footnotes

1. McNeil MM and Brown JM, "The Medically Important Aerobic Actinomycetes: Epidemiology and Microbiology," *Clin Microbiol Rev*, 1994, 7(3):357-417.

2. Kerr E, Snell H, Black BL, et al, "Isolation of *Nocardia asteroides* From Respiratory Specimens by Using Selective Buffered Charcoal-Yeast Extract Agar," *J Clin Microbiol*, 1992, 30(5):1320-2.

3. Brown JM, McNeil MM, and Desmond EP, "*Nocardia, Rhodococcus, Gordona, Actinomadura, Streptomyces,* and Other Actinomycetes of Medical Importance," *Manual of Clinical Microbiology*, 7th ed, Murray PR, Baron EJ, Pfaller MA, et al, eds, Washington, DC: AMS Press, American Society for Microbiology, 1999, 370-98.

4. Beaman BL and Beaman L, "*Nocardia* Species: Host-Parasite Relationships," *Clin Microbiol Rev*, 1994, 7(2):213-64.

5. Menendez R, Cordero PJ, Santos M, et al, "Pulmonary Infection With *Nocardia* Species: A Report of 10 Cases and Review," *Eur Respir J*, 1997, 10(7):1542-6.

6. Gaude GS, Hemashettar BM, Bagga AS, et al, "Clinical Profile of Pulmonary Nocardiosis," *Indian J Chest Dis Allied Sci*, 1999, 41(3):153-7.

7. Lerner PI, "Nocardiosis," *Clin Infect Dis*, 1996, 22(6):891-903.

8. Drapkin MS and Mark EJ, "A 69-Year-Old Renal Transplant Recipient With Low-Grade Fever and Multiple Pulmonary Nodules," Case Records of the Massachusetts General Hospital, Case 29-2000, Scully RE, Mark EJ, McNeely WF, et al, eds, *N Engl J Med*, 2000, 343(12):870-7.

References

Cremades MJ, Menendez R, Santos M, et al, "Repeated Pulmonary Infection by *Nocardia asteroides* Complex in a Patient With Bronchiectasis," *Respiration*, 1998, 65(3):211-3.

Exmelin L, Malbruny B, Vergnaud M, et al, "Molecular Study of Nosocomial Nocardiosis Outbreak Involving Heart Transplant Recipients," *J Clin Microbiol*, 1996, 34(4):1014-6.

Forbes BA, Sahm DF, and Weissfeld AS, "*Nocardia, Streptomyces, Rhodococcus, Oerskovia,* and Similar Organisms," *Bailey and Scott's Diagnostic Microbiology*, 10th ed, Chapter 57, St Louis, MO: Mosby, 1998, 672-7.

Oerlemans WG, Jansen EN, Prevo RL, et al, "Primary Cerebellar Nocardiosis and Alveolar Proteinosis," *Acta Neurol Scand*, 1998, 97(2):138-41.

Sharma S and Sridhar MS, "Diagnosis and Management of *Nocardia* Keratitis," *J Clin Microbiol*, 1999, 37(7).2389.

Wilson JP, Turner HR, Kirchner KA, et al, "Nocardial Infections in Renal Transplant Recipients," *Medicine (Baltimore)*, 1989, 68(1):38-57.

Internet Web Sites

www.cdc.gov/ncidod/dbmd/diseaseinfo/nocardiosis_t.htm

♦ **Nocardia Species Modified Acid-Fast Stain** see Acid-Fast Stain, Modified, *Nocardia* Species on page 550

♦ **Nocardia spp** see Bacterial Culture, Wounds, Bites on page 579

♦ **Norwalk Virus** see Bacterial Culture, Stool on page 575

♦ **NucliSens CMV pp67** see Cytomegalovirus Nucleic Acid Detection on page 599

♦ **Ocular Culture** see Bacterial Culture, Conjunctiva on page 570

♦ **Onchocerca volvulus Serology** see Filariasis Serological Test on page 608

♦ **Oriental Sore Serological Test** see Leishmaniasis Serology on page 647

♦ **Outer Ear Culture** see Bacterial Culture, Middle Ear on page 573

Ova and Parasites, Stool

Related Information

Synonyms Parasites, Stool; Parasitology Examination, Stool; Stool Exam for Ova and Parasites

Applies to Amebiasis; *Ascaris lumbricoides*; *Balantidium coli*; *Blastocystis hominis*; *Cyclospora* Species; *Dientamoeba fragilis*; *Diphyllobothrium latum*; *Entamoeba histolytica*; *Enterobius vermicularis*; Flagellates; *Giardia lamblia*; Helminths; Hookworm; *Hymenolepis nana*; *Isospora*; Microsporidia; *Schistosoma* Species; *Strongyloides stercoralis*; *Taenia* Species; *Trichuris trichiura*

Test Includes Gross appearance, direct wet mounts, saline and iodine, concentration procedure, hematoxylin smear or trichrome smear. Many laboratories do not do all possible tests on all specimens (eg, most laboratories do not routinely examine for *Cryptosporidium* or *Cyclospora* without direct orders by a physician).[1] Evaluation for intestinal parasites would include cysts and trophozoites of protozoa and larvae, ova and adults (including proglottids).[2]

Abstract World travel has resulted in global exposure of naïve patients to intestinal parasites. In industrialized countries, intestinal protozoal infections were once rare, but these infections are now seen with increased frequency. The two most common protozoal infections seen worldwide are *Giardia lamblia* and *Entamoeba histolytica*. The symptoms produced by pathogenic intestinal protozoa are similar (eg, diarrhea, cramping, abdominal pain). These symptoms are neither specific nor diagnostic. Additionally, clinical symptoms can vary depending on the type of protozoal infection and the immune status of the patient. The definitive diagnosis of intestinal protozoal infections has depended on the microscopic examination of stool specimens. The procedures normally consist of a direct wet mount, a concentrated wet mount which is used to separate parasites from fecal debris, and a permanent stained smear.[3] See *Giardia lamblia* Antigen Detection *on page 616*, *Entamoeba histolytica* Antigen Detection *on page 604*, and *Entamoeba histolytica* Serology *on page 605*.

Patient Preparation Specimens obtained with a warm saline enema or Fleet® Phospho®-Soda are acceptable. Specimens obtained with mineral oil, bismuth, or magnesium compounds are unsatisfactory. Wait 1 week or more after barium procedures or laxative administration before collecting stools for ova and parasite examination.

Aftercare Warning: Any stool collected by or from the patient may harbor pathogens which are **immediately infective.** Use extreme caution when *Entamoeba histolytica*, *Hymenolepis nana*, *Cryptosporidium*, and *Taenia* species are suspected or reported. Gloves should be used when collecting stool specimens and hands should be washed after collecting specimens.

Specimen Fresh or preserved random stool or duodenal aspirate. Examination of duodenal content may permit diagnosis of *Giardia*, *Cryptosporidium*, and larvae *Strongyloides*. If pinworm is suspected, a Scotch® Tape preparation should be submitted to the laboratory instead of stool (see Pinworm Preparation *on page 670*).

Container Use a clean, dry plastic stool container with a wide mouth. The collection procedure of choice is to provide patients with collection devices that contain polyvinyl alcohol (PVA) and formalin into which they can place fresh stool. Zinc sulfate can replace mercuric chloride in PVA. Sodium acetate-acetic acid-formalin (SAF) fixative also avoids use of mercury.[3] Preservation of the feces specimen assures that ova and trophozoites will be well preserved for examination.

Collection Unpreserved specimen should be delivered within 30 minutes to 1 hour of collection to the laboratory. Stools which can be processed by the laboratory in less than 1 hour need not be preserved. Direct wet preparation exams for motile trophozoite observation can only be performed on fresh stools.

Mushy, loose, or watery stools which cannot reach the laboratory within 1 hour should be preserved in formalin or merthiolate-iodine-formalin (MIF) and/or polyvinyl alcohol (PVA). PVA will preserve the trophozoite stage of

protozoa. The MIF kit will preserve protozoan cysts, helminth eggs, and larvae. It is intended to be sent home with the patient and mailed back to the laboratory.

OVA AND PARASITES, AMEBAE

Amebae found in human stool specimens.

OVA AND PARASITES, COCCIDIA

Ciliate, coccidia, and *B. hominis* found in human stool specimens.

OVA AND PARASITES, FLAGELLATES

Flagellates found in human stool specimens.

Parasite	Cyclical Peak
Ascaris lumbricoides	Constant
Dientamoeba fragilis	Irregular
Diphyllobothrium latum	Irregular
Entamoeba histolytica	7-10 days
Giardia lamblia	3-7 days
Hookworm	Constant
Trichuris trichiura	Constant
Schistosoma species	Irregular

Adapted from Miller JM and Holmes HT, "Specimen Collection, Transport and Storage," *Manual of Clinical Microbiology*, 7th ed, Murray PR, Baron EJ, Pfaller MA, et al, eds, Washington, DC: American Society for Microbiology, 1999, 33-63.

Formalin will preserve protozoan cysts and larvae and the eggs of helminths. Formed stools may be preserved in formalin or refrigerated in a secure container until they can be transported to the laboratory.

Examination of a single specimen per day has been recommended with examination of additional specimens if indicated. Cartwright notes that successful diagnoses are made in 92% of patients when two specimens are examined. A third specimen provides a relatively low additional yield, in a population bearing a high prevalence of ova and parasites.[4] The shedding of parasites in the stool varies and may be intermittent and in cases of high suspicion (travel in endemic countries) several specimens should be collected over 7-10 days (see table).

Storage Instructions Liquid specimens should be brought directly to the laboratory. Wet mounts should be performed immediately, and the specimen placed in PVA and/or MIF preservatives to maintain ova and trophozoite states.

Causes for Rejection Patients who develop diarrhea after 3 days of hospitalization rarely have bacterial or parasitic diseases identified by routine examination.[5] The most frequent etiologic agent implicated in this setting is *Clostridium difficile*.[5]

The third stool specimen, if collected over 3-7 days apart will detect 98.8% of protozoal pathogens.[6]

Because of risk to laboratory personnel, specimens sent on diaper or tissue paper, specimen contaminating outside of transport container may not be acceptable. Specimen containing interfering substances (eg, castor oil, bismuth, Metamucil®, barium, specimens delayed in transit, and those contaminated with urine) will not have optimal yield. Stool specimens that are extremely hard (nonpuncturable) will not yield a useful parasitic examination.

Special Instructions Geographic and travel history is helpful to the Parasitology Laboratory in order to examine the specimen for likely parasites.

Reference Interval No parasites seen

Use Establish the diagnosis of intestinal parasitic infestation or infection. Watery or bloody stools with variable numbers of fecal leukocytes may harbor amebas.

Major causes of diarrhea include *Cryptosporidium* and *Giardia*, spread in daycare centers and through municipal water supplies.[2]

Limitations A negative result does not rule out the possibility of parasitic infestation. Stool examination for *Giardia* may be negative in early stages of infection, in patients who shed organisms cyclically, and in chronic infections.[7] The sensitivity of microscopic methods for detection of *Giardia* range from 46% to 95%. *Giardia* are found predominantly in the upper small intestine. Tests for *Giardia* antigen may have a much higher yield.[7] The enzyme-linked immunosorbent assay for detection of *Giardia* antigen in stool has a sensitivity of 89% to 100% (see *Giardia lamblia* Antigen Detection *on page 616*).[8,9] Differential diagnosis of pathogens from artifacts, accidental parasites and spurious infection may be challenging. A very useful paper has recently been published.[10]

Contraindications Parasite exams on stool from **patients hospitalized more than 3 days are not productive and should not be ordered unless special circumstances exist.** Administration of barium, bismuth, Metamucil®, castor oil, mineral oil, tetracycline therapy, administration of antiamebic drugs within 1 week prior to test. Purgation contraindicated for pregnancy, ulcerative colitis, cardiovascular disease, child younger than 5 years of age, appendicitis or possible appendicitis.

Stool must be collected directly into a dry container or into fixative. Urine and water destroy amebas.

Methodology Wet mounts and trichrome stains after concentration are routine. Immunologic techniques, including direct immunofluorescent assay or enzyme immunoassay, are helpful for *Cryptosporidium* species. Immunologic techniques are used for *Giardia lamblia*.

An acid-fast-trichrome stain for *Microsporidium*, *Cryptosporidium parvum*, *Cyclospora cayetanensis*, and *Isospora belli* is described. Further studies will be needed.[11]

It is difficult to sufficiently emphasize the importance of a calibrated ocular micrometer. It supports classification of observed structures as artifacts or pathogens.[10]

Additional Information The proper collection, preservation, and transport of specimens are of primary importance in acquiring an accurate and reliable identification of intestinal parasites. Certain parasites cannot be seen in stools containing barium, and urine or water in the specimen can destroy the amebas structures. Optimal diagnostic yield is obtained by the examination of fresh, warm stool by an experienced technologist. Amebic cysts, *Giardia* cysts, and helminth eggs can be recovered from formed stools. Mushy or liquid stools (either normally passed or obtained by purgation) often yield trophozoites. Of the pathogenic protozoa, *E. histolytica* and *G. lamblia* are the two most common infections identified worldwide. An accurate diagnosis of infestation is critical for the management of these diseases as well as the prevention of new protozoal infections. The observation of erythrophagocytic trophozoites in bloody, mucoid stools provides optimal evidence of the presence of invasive **amebiasis**. Such forms are best examined from fresh, warm stool. A smear stained by trichrome or iron hematoxylin is confirmatory. *E. histolytica* is recognized in endoscopic biopsies in only 50% of the cases. Amebas are not always present in the stools of patients who have amebic abscess of liver.[2] In such patients, serologic tests are more reliable (see *Entamoeba histolytica* Serology *on page 605*).

Treatment of intestinal protozoal infections with antiprotozoal drugs is very effective and drug resistance has not been identified. Recurrent infection is usually due to reinfection rather than resistance to treatment.[12]

Parasites identified in the stool of **immunocompromised subjects** (eg, AIDS patients) include *Cryptosporidium*, *Microsporidia*, *Entamoeba histolytica*, *Giardia lamblia*, *Isospora belli*, and *Strongyloides stercoralis*.[13,14]

Microsporidia are obligate intracellular spore-forming protozoa. *Enterocytozoon bieneusi*, a *Microsporidia* species, is a common cause of chronic diarrhea in HIV-positive persons.[14]

Cyclospora cayetanensis, a coccidian parasite, causes gastroenteritis. Its oocysts can be found in stool with modified acid-fast stains, wet mounts under phase contrast microscopy, and with autofluorescence.[15,16]

Therapy has recently been reviewed.[17]

Footnotes

1. "Food-Borne Outbreak of Cryptosporidiosis - Spokane, Washington, 1997," Centers for Disease Control and Prevention, *JAMA*, 1998, 280(7):595-6.
2. Rosenblatt JE, "Laboratory Diagnosis of Parasitic Infections," *Mayo Clin Proc*, 1994, 69(8):779-80.
3. National Committee for Clinical Laboratory Standards, "Procedures for the Recovery and Identification of Parasites From the Intestinal Tract," 1997, Approved Guideline M28-A, National Committee for Clinical Laboratory Standards, Villanova, Pa.
4. Cartwright CP, "Utility of Multiple-Stool-Specimen Ova and Parasite Examinations in a High-Prevalence Setting," *J Clin Microbiol*, 1999, 37(8):2408-11.
5. Valenstein P, Pfaller M, and Yungbluth M, "The Use and Abuse of Routine Stool Microbiology: A College of American Pathologists Q-Probes Study of 601 Institutions," *Arch Pathol Lab Med*, 1996, 120(2):206-11.
6. Hiatt RA, Markell EK, and Ng E, "How Many Stool Examinations Are Necessary to Detect Pathogenic Intestinal Protozoa?" *Am J Trop Med Hyg*, 1995, 53(1):36-9.
7. Chappell CL and Matson CC, "*Giardia* Antigen Detection in Patients With Chronic Gastrointestinal Disturbances," *J Fam Pract*, 1992, 35(1):49-53.
8. Donowitz AM, Kokke FT, and Saidi R, "Evaluation of Patients With Chronic Diarrhea," *N Engl J Med*, 1995, 332(11):725-9.
9. Aldeen WE, Carroll K, Robinson A, et al, "Comparison of Nine Commercially Available Enzyme-Linked Immunosorbent Assays for Detection of *Giardia lamblia* in Fecal Specimens," *J Clin Microbiol*, 1998, 36(5):1338-40.
10. Colmer-Hamood JA, "Fecal Microscopy Artifacts Mimicking Ova and Parasites," *Lab Med*, 2001, 32(2):80-4.
11. Reisner BS and Spring J, "Evaluation of a Combined Acid-Fast-Trichrome Stain for Detection of Microsporidia and *Cryptosporidium parvum*," *Arch Pathol Lab Med*, 2000, 124(5):777-9.
12. Leber AL and Novak SM, "Intestinal and Urogenital Amebae, Flagellates, and Ciliates," *Manual of Clinical Microbiology*, 7th ed, Murray PR, Baron EJ, Pfaller MA, et al, eds, Washington, DC: AMS Press, American Society for Microbiology, 1999, 1391-1405.
13. Garcia LS and Shimizu R, "Diagnostic Parasitology: Parasitic Infections and the Compromised Host," *Lab Med*, 1993, 24:205-15.
14. Asmuth DM, De Girolami PC, Federman M, et al, "Clinical Features of Microsporidiosis in Patients With AIDS," *Clin Infect Dis*, 1994, 18(5):819-25.
15. Herwaldt BL and Ackers ML, "An Outbreak in 1996 of Cyclosporiasis Associated With Imported Raspberries," *N Engl J Med*, 1997, 336(22):1548-56.
16. Osterholm MT, "Lessons Learned Again: Cyclosporiasis and Raspberries," *Ann Intern Med*, 1999, 130(3):234-5.
17. Rosenblatt JE, "Antiparasitic Agents," *Mayo Clin Proc*, 1999, 74(11):1161-75.

References

Blaum JM and Omura EF, Images in Clinical Medicine, "Cutaneous Larva Migrans," *N Engl J Med*, 1998, 338(24):1733.

Brennick J and Mattia A, Images in Clinical Medicine, "*Strongyloides stercoralis* Infestation," *N Engl J Med*, 1996, 334(18):1173.

Brigden ML, "A Practical Work-up for Eosinophilia. You Can Investigate the Most Likely Causes Right in Your Office," *Postgrad Med*, 1999, 105(3):193-4, 199-202, 207-10.

Franzen C, Müller A, Salzberger B, et al, "Uvitex 2B Stain for the Diagnosis of *Isospora belli* Infections in Patients With the Acquired Immunodeficiency Syndrome," *Arch Pathol Lab Med*, 1996, 120:1023-25.

Kabani A, Cadrain G, Trevenen C, et al, "Practice Guidelines for Ordering Stool Ova and Parasite Testing in a Pediatric Population," *Am J Clin Pathol*, 1995, 104(3):272-8.

Long EG and Christie JD, "The Diagnosis of Old and New Gastrointestinal Parasites," *Clin Lab Med*, 1995, 15(2):307-31.

Orihel TC and Ash LR, *Parasites in Human Tissues*, Chicago, IL: ASCP Press, 1995.

Reed SL, "Amebiasis: An Update," *Clin Infect Dis*, 1992, 14(2):385-93.

Reitano M, Masci JR, and Bottone EJ, "Amebiasis: Clinical and Laboratory Perspective," *Crit Rev Clin Lab Sci*, 1991, 28(5-6):357-85.

Sun T, "Current Topics in Protozoal Diseases," *Am J Clin Pathol*, 1994, 102(1):16-29.

Sun T, Ilardi CF, Asnis D, "Light and Electron Microscopic Identification of *Cyclospora* Species in the Small Intestine: Evidence of the Presence of Asexual Life Cycle in Human Host," *Am J Clin Pathol*, 1996, 105(2):216-20.

Walker JC, "Parasitology. Diagnostic Techniques in the Laboratory," *Med J Aust*, 1993, 158(12):824-9.

Wolfe MS, "Giardiasis," *Clin Microbiol Rev*, 1992, 5(1):93-100.

Wu M L-c, Kuksuk LK and Olinger EJ, "Enterobius Vermicularis," Images in Pathology, *Arch Pathol Lab Med*, 2000, 124(4):647-8.

Internet Web Sites

www.cdc.gov/ncidod/diseases/list_parasites.htm

Ova and Parasites, Urine

Related Information

(Continued)

Ova and Parasites, Urine *(Continued)*

Schistosomiasis Serology *on page 678*
Urinary Tract Cytology *on page 389*

Synonyms Parasites, Urine; Urine for Parasites; Urine for *Schistosoma haematobium*

Applies to Schistosomiasis

Test Includes Wet preparation and concentration procedure

Abstract Urine specimens can be examined for the identification of certain parasitic infections such as *Schistosoma haematobium*, filarial infections, and *Trichomonas vaginalis*.

Specimen Early voided midday urine

Container Sterile, plastic urine container

Collection For *Trichomonas vaginalis*, collect freshly passed urine and immediately transport to the laboratory within 1 hour without refrigeration so that the sediment can be examined for motile trophozoites. For *Schistosoma haematobium*, the terminal portion of the urine specimen may contain numerous eggs trapped in mucus and pus. Peak egg excretion occurs between noon and 3 PM; samples collected during this time, or during a 24-hour urine collection (without preservatives) may be obtained for examination.

Storage Instructions Do **not** refrigerate.

Special Instructions The laboratory should be informed of the parasite clinically suspected. Geographic travel history may be useful.

Reference Interval No parasites identified

Use Detect parasitic infestation, particularly *Trichomonas*, filarial, or *Schistosoma haematobium*. Eggs of *Enterobius vermicularis* are sometimes present in urine as the result of fecal contamination, but are best investigated as described in Pinworm Preparation *on page 670.*

Limitations A single negative result does not rule out the possibility of parasitic infestation.

Additional Information Immunodiagnostic tests including enzyme-linked immunosorbent assay and immunoblot tests have been used to diagnose schistosomiasis in some centers.[1,2] However, egg counts from urine specimens continue to be used routinely in most endemic countries due to cost constraints. The infection intensity, as measured by egg output, is thought to reflect the severity of infection. The patient should have a geographic history consistent with schistosomiasis to warrant undertaking screening the urine.

Footnotes

1. Tsang VC and Wilkins PP, "Immunodiagnosis of Schistosomiasis. Screen With FAST-ELISA and Confirm With Immunoblot," *Clin Lab Med*, 1991, 11(4):1029-39.
2. Kahama AI, Nibbeling HA, van Zeyl RJ, et al, "Detection and Quantification of Soluble Egg Antigen in Urine of *Schistosoma haematobium*-Infected Children From Kenya," *Am J Trop Med Hyg*, 1998, 59(5):769-74.

References

Leber AL and Novak SM, "Intestinal and Urogenital Amebae, Flagellates, and Ciliates," *Manual of Clinical Microbiology*, 7th ed, Murray PR, Baron EJ, Pfaller MA, et al, eds, Washington, DC: AMS Press, American Society for Microbiology, 1999, 1391-1405.

Mkoji GM, Muchemi GK, Kipesha FS, et al, "*Shistosoma mansoni* Ova in Urine of Children From an Endemic Area of Kenya: A Short Report," *East Afr Med J*, 1998, 75(9):558-9.

Vester U, Kardorff R, Traore M, et al, "Urinary Tract Morbidity Due to *Schistosoma haematobium* Infection in Mali," *Kidney Int*, 1997, 52(2):478-81.

Internet Web Sites

www.cdc.gov/ncidod/diseases/list_parasites.htm

♦ **p24 Antigen Detection** *see* HIV p24 Antigen Detection *on page 637*

♦ **PACE2®** *see Chlamydia trachomatis* Nucleic Acid Detection *on page 591*

♦ **Parainfluenza 1, 2, and 3 Virus Culture** *see* Parainfluenza Virus Culture *on page 668*

Parainfluenza Viral Serology

Related Information

Parainfluenza Virus Culture *on page 668*
Viral Culture *on page 689*
Viral Culture, Eye or Ocular Symptoms *on page 693*
Viral Culture, Respiratory Symptoms *on page 694*
Virus, Direct Detection by Fluorescent Antibody *on page 696*

Test Includes Antibody titers to parainfluenza virus types 1, 2, 3, and 4

Abstract Human parainfluenza viruses have been isolated throughout the world.[1,2] They are known to cause a wide variety of both lower and upper respiratory infections.[3] This group of viruses also routinely causes otitis media, pharyngitis, conjunctivitis, and the common cold. All four types of human parainfluenza viruses can reinfect individuals throughout their lives. Thus, immunity does not confer lifetime protection.

Specimen Serum

Container Red top tube

Sampling Time Acute and convalescent sera drawn 10-14 days apart are recommended.

Reference Interval A single low titer or a less than fourfold change in titer in paired sera is considered normal.

Use Support the diagnosis of parainfluenza virus infection. Serologic studies are of value in epidemiology.

Limitations Need for convalescent specimen delays diagnosis. Heterotypic rises in parainfluenza titers may occur in infections with other viruses such as mumps. Infant antibody response may be undetectable. Parainfluenza viral serology is not recommended for clinical diagnostic purposes.

Methodology Complement fixation (CF), hemagglutination inhibition (HAI), enzyme-linked immunosorbent assay (ELISA)

Additional Information Since the demonstration of a fourfold rise in antibody titer requires testing a convalescent specimen, serologic diagnosis is seldom useful in clinical management of an acute illness. This is especially so since the rise may occur even in an infection caused by some other virus such as mumps. **Rapid diagnosis during acute illness may be accomplished by demonstrating viral antigen in smears or tissue by immunofluorescence.** Parainfluenza culture is available; see Parainfluenza Virus Culture *on page 668.* Since parainfluenza virus may respond to ribavirin, prompt accurate diagnosis could become important, particularly in the immunocompromised host.

Footnotes

1. Ng W, Rajaduai VS, Pradeepkumar VK, et al, "Parainfluenza Type 3 Viral Outbreak in a Neonatal Nursery," *Ann Acad Med Singapore*, 1999, 28(4):471-5.
2. Nelson JK, Shields MD, Stewart MC, et al, "Investigation of Seroprevalence of Respiratory Virus Infections in an Infant Population With a Multiantigen Fluorescence Immunoassay Using Heel-Prick Blood Samples Collected on Filter Paper," *Pediatr Res*, 1999, 45(6):799-802.
3. Marx A, Gary HE Jr, Marston BJ, et al, "Parainfluenza Virus Infection Among Hospitalized for Lower Respiratory Tract Infection," *Clin Infect Dis*, 1999, 29(1):134-40.

References

Fedova D, Novotny J, and Kubinova I, "Serological Diagnosis of Parainfluenza Virus Infections: Verification of the Sensitivity and Specificity of the Haemagglutination-Inhibition (HI), Complement Fixation (CF), Immunofluorescence (IFA) Tests, and Enzyme Immunoassay (ELISA)," *Acta Virol*, 1992, 36(3):304-12.

Waner JL, "Parainfluenza Viruses," *Manual of Clinical Microbiology*, 7th ed, Murray PR, Baron EJ, Pfaller MA, et al, eds, Washington, DC: AMS Press, American Society for Microbiology, 1999, 936-41.

Parainfluenza Virus Culture

Related Information

Bacterial Culture, Nasopharynx *on page 573*
Influenza Virus Culture *on page 644*
Parainfluenza Viral Serology *on page 668*
Viral Culture *on page 689*
Viral Culture, Respiratory Symptoms *on page 694*
Virus, Direct Detection by Fluorescent Antibody *on page 696*

Synonyms Parainfluenza 1, 2, and 3 Virus Culture

Applies to Hemadsorbing Virus

Test Includes Culture and identification of parainfluenza viruses. Often includes the concurrent culture for other respiratory viruses (influenza, adenovirus, and respiratory syncytial viruses)

Abstract Parainfluenza viruses types 1, 2, and 3 are the most common cause of croup (laryngotracheitis) in infants and children. An acute self-limited upper airway disease of children, croup presents with barking cough, inspiratory stridor, and hoarseness.[1] Parainfluenza viruses are second only to respiratory syncytial virus as a cause of serious infantile respiratory diseases. Several vaccines are in the process of development to prevent the severe respiratory tract infections in infants and children caused by parainfluenza viruses.[2,3]

Specimen Throat or nasopharyngeal swab, nasopharyngeal washes and secretions

Container Viral transport medium; cold viral transport medium for swabs

Collection Place swabs into cold viral transport medium and keep cold. With infants and small children a soft catheter or suction device (syringes and suction bulbs) can be used to collect nasal secretions from far back in the nose (best specimens). Another excellent method is to introduce 3-7 mL of sterile saline into the child's posterior nasal cavity and immediately aspirate the fluid. **Note:** Do not use **cold** sterile saline when aspirating samples. Warm to room temperature.

Storage Instructions Keep specimens ice cold after collection, but **do not freeze specimens at -20°C.** Specimens that cannot be inoculated into cell culture within 48 hours should be frozen at -70°C.

Turnaround Time Conventional culture: 5-14 days; rapid culture: 2-4 days

Reference Interval No virus isolated

Critical Values Positive results in a child younger than 5 years of age

Use Disease caused by parainfluenza virus includes croup (laryngotracheitis), other respiratory illness including laryngitis and pneumonia; bronchopneumonia and bronchiolitis occur in infants. The differential diagnosis includes epiglottitis, bacterial tracheitis, and retropharyngeal abscess. Reinfections with parainfluenza viruses are common and generally result in a less acute disease resembling the common cold.

Limitations Negative viral culture does not rule out viral etiology; rapid methods will only detect specified virus(es)

Methodology Routine culture: Inoculation of specimens into cell cultures, incubation of cultures, observation for hemadsorption or characteristic cytopathic effect (CPE), and identification/speciation by fluorescent monoclonal antibodies specific for types 1, 2, or 3 or by virus neutralization. Rapid culture: Inoculation of cells in shell vial and detection of specific virus with an immunofluorescent monoclonal antibody.

Rapid recognition of viral antigen in nasopharyngeal secretions by immuno-fluorescent and ELISA methods is available with varying levels of sensitivity.

Additional Information Parainfluenza viruses are rarely isolated from healthy individuals, thus their detection is usually diagnostic. Conventional and rapid cultures will generally detect other respiratory viruses in addition to the parainfluenza viruses. Currently, the standard for many laboratories is to do a rapid shell vial assay for detection of several respiratory viruses. This test will detect influenza A and B virus, respiratory syncytial virus, and parainfluenza virus 1, 2, and 3.[4] Some laboratories may also start a conventional culture as a back-up to the rapid culture. Serology for detection of parainfluenza antibodies is available, but the results are often difficult to interpret and results are not available in a timely fashion.

Several studies have shown the successful detection of parainfluenza viruses in clinical specimens by using nucleic acid amplification techniques; however, these assays are currently only available from research laboratories.[5,6]

Footnotes
1. Rosencrans JA, "Viral Croup: Current Diagnosis and Treatment," *Mayo Clin Proc*, 1998, 73(11): 1102-7.
2. Skiadopoulos MH, Tao T, Surman SR, et al, "Generation of a Parainfluenza Virus Type 1 Vaccine Candidate by Replacing the HN and F Glycoproteins of the Live-Attenuated PIV3 cp45 Vaccine Virus With Their PIV1 Counterparts," *Vaccine*, 1999, 18(5-6):503-10.
3. Ewasyshyn M, Cates G, Jackson G, et al, "Prospects for a Parainfluenza Virus Vaccine," *Pediatr Pulmonol Suppl*, 1997, 16:280-1.
4. Shih SR, Tsao KC, Ning HC, et al, "Diagnosis of Respiratory Tract Viruses in 24 h by Immunofluorescent Staining of Shell Vial Cultures Containing Madin-Darby Canine Kidney (MDCK) Cells," *J Virol Methods*, 1999, 81(1-2):77-81.
5. Corne JM, Green S, Sanderson G, et al, "A Multiplex RT-PCR for the Detection of Parainfluenza Viruses 1-3 in Clinical Samples," *J Virol Methods*, 1999, 82(1):9-18.
6. Echevarria JE, Erdman DD, Swierkosz EM, et al, "Simultaneous Detection and Identification of Human Parainfluenza Viruses 1, 2, and 3 From Clinical Samples by Multiplex PCR," *J Clin Microbiol*, 1998, 36(5):1388-91.

References
Beekmann SE, Engler HD, Collins AS, et al, "Rapid Identification of Respiratory Viruses: Impact on Isolation Practices and Transmission Among Immunocompromised Pediatric Patients," *Infect Control Hosp Epidemiol*, 1996, 17(9):581-6.

Chan PW, Goh AY, Chua KB, et al, "Viral Aetiology of Lower Respiratory Tract Infection in Young Malaysian Children," *J Paediatr Child Health*, 1999, 35(3):287-90.

Murphy BR and Collins PL, "Current Status of Respiratory Syncytial Virus (RSV) and Parainfluenza Virus Type 3 (PIV3) Vaccine Development: Memorandum From a Joint WHO/NIAID Meeting," *Bull World Health Organ*, 1997, 75(4):307-13.

Reed G, Jewett PH, Thompson J, et al, "Epidemiology and Clinical Impact of Parainfluenza Virus Infections in Otherwise Healthy Infants and Young Children <5 Years Old," *J Infect Dis*, 1997, 175(4):807-13.

Waner JL, "Parainfluenza Viruses," *Manual of Clinical Microbiology*, 7th ed, Murray PR, Baron EJ, Pfaller MA, et al, eds, Washington, DC: AMS Press, American Society for Microbiology, 1999, 936-41.

♦ **Parainfluenza Virus, Direct Detection** *see* Virus, Direct Detection by Fluorescent Antibody *on page 696*

♦ **Parasites, Stool** *see* Ova and Parasites, Stool *on page 666*

♦ **Parasites, Urine** *see* Ova and Parasites, Urine *on page 667*

♦ **Parasitology Examination, Stool** *see* Ova and Parasites, Stool *on page 666*

Parvovirus B19 DNA

Related Information
Parvovirus B19 Serology *on page 669*

Test Includes Detection of parvovirus B19 by nucleic acid amplification most commonly using polymerase chain reaction (PCR) and detection of PCR products

Abstract Infections with parvovirus B19 can be asymptomatic or cause mild nonspecific symptoms. The most common manifestation caused by parvovirus B19 is erythema infectiosum, an illness of children, also known as fifth disease. The more serious clinical manifestations of parvovirus B19 include arthralgias, severe anemia, fetal hydrops, severe pancytopenia, and thrombocytopenic purpura.[1,2] These serious manifestations are generally seen in patients with underlying conditions such as sickle cell anemia, organ or bone marrow transplantation, or those who are immunocompromised. Replication of parvovirus B19 is in erythroid progenitor cells in marrow.

Specimen Serum, amniotic fluid, tissue, bone marrow aspirate

Container Red top tube for serum and amniotic fluid, EDTA tube for bone marrow, fresh frozen tissue

Use Parvovirus B19 infection is associated with stillbirth, arthritis, aplastic crisis and fifth disease. This test may be positive in patients who do not produce antibodies against parvovirus B19 (eg, the immunocompromised).

Methodology Amplification of virus specific nucleic acid and detection of specific products of amplification.[3] A quantitative assay to detect parvovirus B19 DNA is currently being developed.[4]

Additional Information Parvovirus B19 is a DNA virus that can cause a wide spectrum of disease including self-limited erythema infectiosum, bone marrow failure, and fetal death. In most people, the low titer viremia which begins about 1 week after exposure and persists for 7-10 days is associated with mild symptoms and a red cell aplasia which may be subclinical.

The clinical presentation may include facial rash in ≥50% of patients. Because the virus destroys red blood cell precursors, there is a reduction in erythrocyte production. This transient aplastic crisis may be particularly severe in patients with hemoglobinopathies associated with decreased erythrocyte lifespan (sickle cell disease, spherocytosis, and β-thalassemia).

Parvovirus B19 DNA can be detected in serum of infected patients 6 days after infection. Viremia usually peaks 2-3 days later and may last for 1 week. After that time, the viral titer declines and low levels of parvovirus B19 DNA can be detected for several months only with nucleic acid amplification techniques.[5] The presence of parvovirus DNA provides definite evidence of recent infection.

Footnotes
1. Marchand S, Tchernia G, Hiesse C, et al, "Human Parvovirus B19 Infection in Organ Transplant Recipients," *Clin Transplant*, 1999, 13(1 Pt 1):17-24.
2. Kido S, Ito Y, Nishimura N, et al, "Human Parvovirus B19-Associated Thrombocytopenic Purpura," *Acta Paediatr Jpn*, 1998, 40(5):486-8.
3. Zerbini M, Gallinella G, Manaresi E, et al, "Standardization of a PCR-ELISA in Serum Samples: Diagnosis of Active Parvovirus B19 Infection," *J Med Virol*, 1999, 59(2):239-44.
4. Boggino H and Payne DA, "Quantitative Direct Probe Method for the Detection of Parvovirus B19," *J Clin Lab Anal*, 2000, 14(1):38-41.
5. Musiani M, Zerbini M, Gentilomi G, et al, "Parvovirus B19 Clearance From Peripheral Blood After Acute Infection," *J Infect Dis*, 1995, 172(5):1360-3.

References
Abkowitz JL, Brown KW, Wood RW, et al, "Clinical Relevance of Parvovirus B19 as a Cause of Anemia in Patients With Human Immunodeficiency Virus Infection," *J Infect Dis*, 1997, 176(1):269-73.

Brown KE and Young NS, "Parvovirus B19 Infection and Hematopoiesis," *Blood Rev*, 1995, 9(3):176-82.

Dieck D, Schild RL, Hansmann M, et al, "Prenatal Diagnosis of Congenital Parvovirus B19 Infection: Value of Serological and PCR Techniques in Maternal and Fetal Serum," *Prenat Diagn*, 1999, 19(12):1119-23.

Lundqvist A, Tolfvenstam T, Bostic J, et al, "Clinical and Laboratory Findings in Immunocompetent Patients With Persistent Parvovirus B19 DNA in Bone Marrow," *Scand J Infect Dis*, 1999, 31(1):11-6.

Vadlamudi G, Rezuke WN, Ross JW, et al, "The Use of Monoclonal Antibody R92F6 and Polymerase Chain Reaction to Confirm the Presence of Parvovirus B19 in Bone Marrow Specimens of Patients With Acquired Immunodeficiency Syndrome," *Arch Pathol Lab Med*, 1999, 123(9):768-73.

Internet Web Sites
www.amm.co.uk/pubs/fa_parvovirus.htm
www.cdc.gov/ncidod/diseases/parvovirus/b19&preg.htm
www.cdc.gov/ncidod/diseases/parvovirus/b19.htm

Parvovirus B19 Serology

Related Information
Bone Marrow *on page 410*
Parvovirus B19 DNA *on page 669*

Synonyms Anti-B19 IgG Antibodies; Anti-B19 IgM Antibodies

Test Includes Assays for parvovirus B19 may include detection of IgM and IgG antibodies

Abstract Detection of antibodies specific for parvovirus B19 are used to diagnose recent infections and to determine immune status. In normal hosts, specific IgM antibodies can be detected during the second week of infection and can be detected for 4-6 months after an active infection. Specific IgG antibodies appear shortly after IgM and can persist for years. In immunocompromised patients, the immune response to parvovirus B19 may be normal, altered, or even absent.

Specimen Serum, amniotic fluid for IgM antibody. In the presence of hydrops, amniocentesis and fetal blood sampling are advocated.[1]

Container Red top tube

Sampling Time B19-specific IgM antibodies appear 10-14 days after onset and persist for only 4-6 months. Collect acute and convalescent sera for IgG antibodies.

Storage Instructions Separate serum and freeze.

Reference Interval <0.80 is usually negative for IgG and IgM.

Use Such serologic testing is employed in investigation of maculopapular rash with fever, arthralgias, red cell aplastic crisis in subjects with hemolytic anemias; work-up of fetal hydrops and spontaneous abortion

Limitations The absence of antiparvovirus B19 antibodies cannot exclude infection.[2] Immunocompromised patients may show poor antibody response. Unpaired sera tested for IgG are of little use for diagnosis of infection, as 2% to 15% of children younger than 5 years of age, 15% to 60% 5-19 years of age, and up to 60% of adults have circulating IgG antibodies specific for parvovirus B19. IgM antibodies rise rapidly after infection and remain elevated for 4-6 months. Detection of IgM antibodies provides strong evidence for recent infection. Fetal blood sampling prior to 22 weeks of gestation often produces false-negative IgM results. Some cross-reactions with patient sera containing rubella virus-specific IgM.

Methodology Radioimmunoassay (RIA), indirect enzyme immunoassay (EIA) for IgG, or immunoblot assay (Western blot) for detection of IgM antibodies to parvovirus B19

Additional Information Parvovirus B19 is a DNA virus and can cause a wide spectrum of disease, ranging form outbreaks of self-limiting erythema infectiosum (fifth disease) to bone marrow failure and to fetal death.[3] Intrauterine transfusion has been suggested when there is evidence of B19
(Continued)

Parvovirus B19 Serology (Continued)

parvovirus-associated anemia and hydrops. Although application of specific IgM to parvovirus B19 is useful in detecting recent infections during pregnancy, a study noted false-positive B19 IgM results and found that a sensitive and specific PCR has more diagnostic value.[4] The low-titer parvovirus B19 viremia, which begins ~1 week after exposure and lasts 7-10 days, is usually associated with mild symptoms and subclinical red cell aplasia. Because the virus destroys erythroid precursors, which leads to a reduction in normal red blood cell production, infection with parvovirus B19 can cause aplastic crisis in patients already at maximum red cell production and in those with increased red cell destruction (sickle cell disease, β-thalassemia, and spherocytosis). In immunocompromised patients, parvovirus B19 infection can cause life-threatening anemia or thrombocytopenic purpura.[5] It is a known cause of chronic reticulocytopenic anemia in HIV-infected individuals.[6] IgG antibody production usually occurs 18-24 days after exposure and is probably immune-complex mediated. The presence of IgM antibodies to parvovirus B19 provide definite evidence of recent infection.

Parvovirus infection can also be confirmed with immunocytochemistry, electron microscopy, and the presence of large intranuclear inclusions in bone marrow specimens. Such inclusions are vividly illustrated in recent publications.[2,6] See also Parvovirus B19 DNA on page 669.

Footnotes

1. Ghidini A and Lynch L, "Prenatal Diagnosis and Significance of Fetal Infections," West J Med, 1993, 159(3):366-73.
2. Vadlamudi G, Rezuke WN, Ross JW, et al, "The Use of Monoclonal Antibody R92F6 and Polymerase Chain Reaction to Confirm the Presence of Parvovirus B19 in Bone Marrow Specimens of Patients With Acquired Immunodeficiency Syndrome," Arch Pathol Lab Med, 1999, 123(9):768-73.
3. Valeur-Jensen AK, Pedersen CB, Westergaard T, et al, "Risk Factors for Parvovirus B19 Infection in Pregnancy," JAMA, 1999, 281(12):1099-105.
4. Dieck D, Schild RL, Hansmann M, et al, "Prenatal Diagnosis of Congenital Parvovirus B19 Infection: Value of Serological and PCR Techniques in Maternal and Fetal Serum," Prenat Diagn, 1999, 19(12):1119-23.
5. Kido S, Ito Y, Nishimura N, et al, "Human Parvovirus B19-Associated Thrombocytopenic Purpura," Acta Paediatr Jpn, 1998, 40(5):486-8.
6. Borkowski J, Amrikachi M, and Hudnall SD, "Fulminant Parvovirus Infection Following Erythropoietin Treatment in a Patient With Acquired Immunodeficiency Syndrome," Arch Pathol Lab Med, 2000, 124(3):441-5.

References

Hemauer A, Gigler A, Searle K, et al, "Seroprevalence of Parvovirus B19 NS1-Specific IgG in B19-Infected and Uninfected Individuals and in Infected Pregnant Women," J Med Virol, 2000, 60(1):48-55.

Jones LP, Erdman DD, and Anderson LJ, "Prevalence of Antibodies to Human Parvovirus B19 Nonstructural Protein in Persons With Various Clinical Outcomes Following B19 Infection," J Infect Dis, 1999, 180(2):500-4.

Kerr JR, McQuaid S, and Coyle PV, "Expression of P Antigen in Parvovirus B19-Infected Bone Marrow," N Engl J Med, 1995, 332(2):128.

Lin KH, You SL, Chen CJ, et al, "Seroepidemiology of Human Parvovirus B19 in Taiwan," J Med Virol, 1999, 57(2):169-73.

Schmid ML, McWhinney PH, Will EJ, et al, "Parvovirus B19 and Glomerulonephritis in a Healthy Adult," Ann Intern Med, 2000, 132(8):682.

Seishima M, Kanoh H, and Izumi T, "The Spectrum of Cutaneous Eruptions in 22 Patients With Isolated Serological Evidence of Infection by Parvovirus B19," Arch Dermatol, 1999, 135(12):1556-7.

Internet Web Sites

www.amm.co.uk/pubs/fa_parvovirus.htm
www.cdc.gov/ncidod/diseases/parvovirus/b19&preg.htm
www.cdc.gov/ncidod/diseases/parvovirus/b19.htm

♦ **Paul-Bunnell-Davidsohn Test** see Heterophil Agglutinins on page 635

♦ **Paul-Bunnell Davidsohn Test** replaced by Infectious Mononucleosis Screening Test on page 643

♦ **P. carinii** see Pneumocystis Immunofluorescence on page 671

♦ **PCR Assay for Bartonella** see Bartonella Serology on page 581

♦ **PCR Assay for Rochalimaea** see Bartonella Serology on page 581

♦ **PCR Detection** see Pneumocystis Immunofluorescence on page 671

♦ **PCR for HIV DNA** see Human Immunodeficiency Virus DNA Amplification on page 639

♦ **PCR for M. tuberculosis** see Mycobacteria by DNA Probe on page 654

♦ **Pediculus humanus Identification** see Arthropod Identification on page 559

♦ **Penicillinase** see Antimicrobial Susceptibility Testing, Aerobic and Facultatively Anaerobic Bacteria on page 554

♦ **Penicillinase-Producing Organisms Susceptibility Testing** see Beta-Lactamase Test on page 581

♦ **Penicillinases** see Beta-Lactamase Test on page 581

♦ **Penicillinase Test** see Beta-Lactamase Test on page 581

♦ **Peptostreptococcus** see Bacterial Culture, Wounds, Bites on page 579

♦ **Periodic Acid Schiff (PAS)** see Fungus Smear, Stain on page 615

♦ **Pertussis Culture** see Bordetella pertussis Culture on page 583

♦ **Pertussis DFA** see Bordetella pertussis Direct Fluorescent Antibody on page 583

♦ **Pertussis Serology** see Bordetella pertussis Serology on page 584

♦ **Phthirus pubis Identification** see Arthropod Identification on page 559

Pinworm Preparation

Related Information

Ova and Parasites, Stool on page 666
Ova and Parasites, Urine on page 667

Synonyms Enterobius vermicularis Preparation; Scotch® Tape Test

Test Includes Detection of pinworm eggs from the perianal region

Abstract The human pinworm, Enterobius vermicularis, has a worldwide distribution. The parasite primarily infects young children.[1] The eggs of the parasite rapidly develop to the infective stage and they can persist for long periods in the environment, which can lead to dissemination of the infection between children. The adult female worm migrates out of the anal orifice at night and lays its eggs in the perianal area. The eggs adhere to the skin of the perianal area and can be detected by the use of a cellulose tape pressed to the perianal area. This scotch tape is then examined under the microscope for the presence of the E. vermicularis eggs.

Specimen Scotch® Tape slide preparation of perianal region

Container Scotch® Tape slide must be submitted in a covered container. Commercial kit products are also available for collection of pinworm specimens. **Caution:** Pinworm eggs are very infectious.

Collection The specimen is best obtained early in the morning before a bowel movement or bath. This collection procedure is essential if valid results are expected. Clear Scotch® Tape should be used; the nontransparent type is unsatisfactory. An 8 cm (3 in) piece of cellophane tape is placed over the end of a glass slide sticky side out. The anal folds are spread apart and the mucocutaneous junction is firmly pressed in all four quadrants. The tape is then pressed over the slide and the specimen is transported to the laboratory in a carefully sealed container. Refer to diagram. It is important to provide clear instructions, because these specimens are often collected at home.

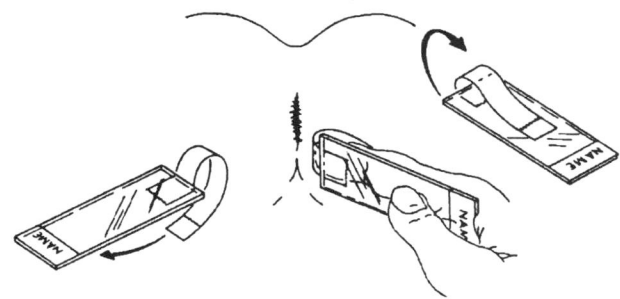

Cellophane tape slide preparation. Attach 3" piece of cellophane tape to undersurface of clear end of microscope slide, which has previously been identified (ground-glass end). Press sticky surface of tape against perianal skin. Then roll back tape onto slide, sticky surface down. Wash hands and nails well. From Bauer JD, Clinical Laboratory Methods, 9th ed, St Louis, MO: Mosby-Year Book Inc, 1982, 989.

Causes for Rejection Use of nontransparent Scotch® Tape, Scotch® Tape on both sides of the slide, specimen which is not inside a covered container, use of frosted slide, tape sent sticky side up. Specimens which are not properly contained pose excessive risk to laboratory personnel since the eggs of E. vermicularis are extremely contagious.

Reference Interval No pinworm eggs (Enterobius vermicularis) identified. Positives reported as few, moderate, or many eggs identified.

Use Detect cases of pinworm infestation (enterobiasis), Enterobius vermicularis parasitic infestation

Limitations Examination for pinworm only. One negative result does not rule out possibility of parasitic infestation. Examinations on multiple days may be required to diagnose infection. Stool specimens are not usually satisfactory for pinworm studies.

Contraindications Specimen collection at improper time

Methodology Microscopy

Additional Information The most satisfactory means of diagnosing pinworm infection is by the recovery of eggs or female worms from the perianal region. Only 5% to 10% of infected persons have demonstrable eggs in their stools. If fecal material is submitted for examination, only the surface should be sampled. Enterobiasis often is present in multiple family members. Therefore, it is recommended that all members of the family be tested. The responsible parent should be instructed how to collect samples, using one kit per individual. Female worms or parts of them may be demonstrated on the tape by microscopic examination. The number of positive specimens on different days correlates with the severity of disease. Eggs, if present, may be immature, embryonated (with viable or dead larvae), or (if the specimen is several days or more old) empty egg shells will be present. Enterobius vermicularis has been reported as a rare cause of appendicitis, salpingitis, epididymitis, vulvovaginitis, and hepatic granuloma. Diagnosis at colonoscopy has been reported.

Footnotes

1. Juckett G, "Common Intestinal Helminthes," *Am Fam Phys*, 1995, 52(7):2039-48, 2051-2.

References

al-Rufaie HK, Rix GH, Perez Clemente MP, et al, "Pinworms and Postmenopausal Bleeding," *J Clin Pathol*, 1998, 51(5):401-2.

Cook GC, "*Enterobius vermicularis* Infection," *Gut*, 1994, 35(9):1159-62.

Herrstrom P, Fristrom A, Karlsson A, et al, "*Enterobius vermicularis* and Finger Sucking in Young Swedish Children," *Scand J Prim Health Care*, 1997, 15(3):146-8.

Nabulsi M, Shararah N, and Khalil A, "Perinatal *Enterobius vermicularis* Infection," *Int J Gynaecol Obstet*, 1998, 60(3):285-6.

Russell LJ, "The Pinworm, *Enterobius vermicularis*," *Prim Care*, 1991, 18(1):13-24.

Tanowitz HB, Weiss LM, and Wittner M, "Diagnosis and Treatment of Common Intestinal Helminths. II: Common Intestinal Nematodes," *Gastroenterologist*, 1994, 2(1):39-49.

Internet Web Sites

www.cdc.gov/ncidod/dpd/parasites/pinworm/default.htm

◆ **Plague Serology** *see Yersinia pestis* Antibody *on page 698*

◆ **Plesiomonas shigelloides** *see* Bacterial Culture, Stool *on page 575*

◆ **Pleuropneumonia-like Organism (PPLO) Titer** *see Mycoplasma* Serology *on page 662*

◆ **Pneumocystis carinii Direct Detection** *see Pneumocystis* Immunofluorescence *on page 671*

Pneumocystis Immunofluorescence

Related Information

Bacterial Culture, Bronchoscopy/Bronchial Brush/Bronchoalveolar Lavage Specimen *on page 568*
Bacterial Culture, Sputum *on page 574*
Blood Gases and pH, Arterial *on page 119*
Bronchoalveolar Lavage (BAL) *on page 375*
Pneumocystis carinii Preparation *on page 386*
Polymerase Chain Reaction *on page 713*
Sputum Cytology *on page 387*

Synonyms *Pneumocystis carinii* Direct Detection

Applies to *P. carinii*; PCR Detection

Test Includes Direct and indirect immunofluorescence for detection of *Pneumocystis carinii* in clinical specimens

Abstract The most common lung complication in untreated AIDS patients is pneumonia caused by *Pneumocystis carinii*, but *P. carinii* causes diseases in other patients as well. Most are immunocompromised, but some do not present identifiable risk factors. Entities associated with *P. carinii* pneumonia in patients without HIV infection include systemic corticosteroid therapy, malignant hematologic diseases, transplantation, inflammatory disorders, and solid tumors.[1] The extrapulmonary organs most often affected are lymph nodes, liver, spleen, and bone marrow. Hypoxemia is a pivotal marker.[2]

Specimen Tissue, sputum, bronchoalveolar lavage

Container Sterile container

Special Instructions Tissue specimens should be received fresh or snap-frozen.

Reference Interval No organisms observed

Use Diagnose *Pneumocystis carinii* pneumonia

Limitations A negative result does not exclude the diagnosis.

Methodology Indirect (IFA) and direct fluorescent antibody (DFA). See *Pneumocystis carinii* Preparation *on page 386*.

Additional Information Pneumonia due to *Pneumocystis carinii* (PCP) usually only occurs in immunosuppressed patients, primarily patients with advanced HIV infection. The prevalence of PCP has declined due to improved treatment of patients infected with HIV; however, detection of PCP in a patient may warrant HIV testing, since it is often the first sign of immunosuppression.

Diagnosis depends primarily on seeing either cysts in tissue or cytology preparations. The *Pneumocystis* cell wall contains chitin and glucan polymers, and thus stains that are used to detect fungi (eg, methenamine silver, toluidine blue, calcofluor) can be used to detect *P. carinii*. An advantage of silver stains includes detection of various fungal infections. Direct immunofluorescence is more sensitive than silver stains and can be completed more rapidly. PCR detection of *P. carinii* is more sensitive than conventional cytologic stains or immunofluorescence.[3,4]

Up to 20% of cases are fatal, even with treatment. Serum LD is more increased in subjects with *Pneumocystis carinii* than in those with other pulmonary disorders in HIV, and >90% of patients have <200 CD4 cells at diagnosis.[2]

Footnotes

1. Yale SH and Limper AH, "*Pneumocystis carinii* Pneumonia in Patients Without Acquired Immunodeficiency Syndrome: Associated Illness and Prior Corticosteroid Therapy," *Mayo Clin Proc*, 1996, 71(1):5-13.

2. Feinberg JE and Satler FR, "*Pneumocystis carinii* Pneumonia," *Cecil Textbook of Medicine*, 21st ed, Chapter 402, Goldman L and Benett JC, eds, Philadelphia, PA: WB Saunders Co, 2000, 1877-83.

3. Leibovitz E, Pollack H, Moore T, et al, "Comparison of PCR and Standard Cytological Staining for Detection of *Pneumocystis carinii* From Respiratory Specimens

From Patients With or at High Risk for Infection by Human Immunodeficiency Virus," *J Clin Microbiol*, 1995, 33(11):3004-7.

4. Huang SN, Fischer SH, O'Shaughnessy E, et al, "Development of a PCR Assay for Diagnosis of *Pneumocystis carinii* Pneumonia Based on Amplification of the Multicopy Major Surface Glycoprotein Gene Family," *Diagn Microbiol Infect Dis*, 1999, 35(1):27-32.

References

Amin MB, Mezger E, and Zarbo RJ, "Detection of *Pneumocystis carinii*: Comparative Study of Monoclonal Antibody and Silver Impregnation," *Am J Clin Pathol*, 1992, 98(1):13-8

Bédos JP, Hignette C, Lucet JC, et al, "Serum Carcinoembryonic Antigen: A Prognostic Marker in HIV-Related *Pneumocystis carinii* Pneumonia," *Scand J Infect Dis*, 1992, 24(3):309-15.

Blumenfeld W, Miller CN, Chew KL, et al, "Correlation of *Pneumocystis carinii* Cyst Density With Mortality in Patients With Acquired Immunodeficiency Syndrome and *Pneumocystis* Pneumonia," *Hum Pathol*, 1992, 23(6):612-8.

Boswell SL and van Gorder M, "A 38-Year-Old Man With the Acquired Immunodeficiency Syndrome and Cavitary Pulmonary Lesions," Case Records of the Massachusetts General Hospital, Case 27-1997, Scully RE, Mark EJ, McNeely WF, et al, eds, *N Engl J Med*, 1997, 337(9):619-27.

Crans CA Jr and Boiselle PM, "Imaging Features of *Pneumocystis carinii* Pneumonia," *Crit Rev Diagn Imaging*, 1999, 40(4):251-84.

Homer KS, Wiley EL, Smith AL, et al, "Monoclonal Antibody to *Pneumocystis carinii*: Comparison With Silver Stain in Bronchial Lavage Specimens," *Am J Clin Pathol*, 1992, 97(5):619-24.

Kiska DL, Bartholoma NY, and Forbes BA, "Acceptability of Low-Volume, Induced Sputum Specimens for Diagnosis of *Pneumocystis carinii* Pneumonia," *Am J Clin Pathol*, 1998, 109(3):335-7.

Metersky ML, Aslenzadeh J, and Stelmach P, "A Comparison of Induced and Expectorated Sputum for the Diagnosis of *Pneumocystis carinii* Pneumonia," *Chest*, 1998, 113(6):1555-9.

Salzman SH, "Bronchoscopic Techniques for the Diagnosis of Pulmonary Complications of HIV Infection," *Semin Respir Infect*, 1999, 14(4):318-26.

Sepkowitz KA, Brown AE, Telzak EE, et al, "*Pneumocystis carinii* Pneumonia Among Patients Without AIDS at a Cancer Hospital," *JAMA*, 1992, 267(6):832-7.

Torres J, Goldman M, Wheat LJ, et al, "Diagnosis of *Pneumocystis carinii* Pneumonia in Human Immunodeficiency Virus-Infected Patients With Polymerase Chain Reaction: A Blinded Comparison to Standard Methods," *Clin Infect Dis*, 2000, 30(1):141-5.

Wilkin A and Feinberg J, "*Pneumocystis carinii* Pneumonia: A Clinical Review," *Am Fam Phys*, 1999, 60(6):1699-708, 1713-4.

Internet Web Sites

www.cdc.gov/ncidod/dpd/parasites/pneumocystis/default.htm

◆ **Pneumonia, Atypical Agents** *see Legionella* Serology *on page 646*

Poliomyelitis I, II, III Serology

Related Information

Cerebrospinal Fluid Analysis: Overview *on page 416*
Enterovirus Culture *on page 605*
Viral Culture *on page 689*
Viral Culture, Stool *on page 695*

Synonyms Poliovirus Titer

Test Includes Detection of antibodies to poliovirus in patient's serum

Abstract The eradication of poliomyelitis by vaccination is the aim of the World Health Organization (WHO) Poliomyelitis Eradication Initiative (PEI).[1] Due to ongoing efforts to provide vaccination throughout the world, a dramatic reduction of cases of poliomyelitis has been noted in regions of the world which were once endemic for polio.[2] Currently, wild type poliovirus is rarely found in the Western hemisphere and nearly eliminated in the rest of the world. Unfortunately, a recent case (October 1999) of poliomyelitis in the Qinghai province of China was identified by culture as wild type poliovirus type 1.[3] Before this case, the last indigenous wild type poliovirus was isolated in China in 1994. Thus, although poliovirus infection is now rare, it has not been completely eradicated. Thus, the differential diagnosis of individuals with acute aseptic meningitis, with or without paralysis, should consider poliomyelitis if the patient has not been immunized.

Specimen Serum

Container Red top tube

Sampling Time Acute and convalescent sera drawn 10-14 days apart are required to test for neutralizing antibody for each of the three polioviral types.

Reference Interval Presence of neutralizing antibody indicates adequate immunization; normal <1:8

Possible Panic Range A fourfold increase in neutralizing antibody titer in paired sera is diagnostic of poliomyelitis. Specific IgM neutralizing antibody is diagnostic as well. Any suspected case of poliomyelitis should be reported to the local health department as well as to the CDC.

Use Support for the diagnosis of acute poliovirus infection, documentation of previous exposure to poliovirus (complement fixing antibodies); documentation of immunization (neutralizing antibodies)

Limitations Complement-fixing antibodies can be broadly cross-reactive with other enteroviruses.

Methodology Viral neutralization, complement fixation (CF)

Additional Information Poliovirus, an enterovirus, may also be cultured, producing a characteristic cytopathic effect in tissue culture. Culture is more

(Continued)

Poliomyelitis I, II, III Serology (Continued)

suitable than serology for diagnosis of acute infection. Amplification of poliovirus genome has also been investigated and can be used to diagnose poliovirus versus nonpoliovirus enteroviruses.[4]

Footnotes

1. Kim-Farley RJ, "Global Immunization. The Expanded Programme on Immunization Team," 1992, *Ann Rev Public Health*, 13:223-37.
2. "Progress Toward Poliomyelitis Eradication - Africa," 1996, *MMWR Morb Mortal Wkly Rep*, 46(15):321-5.
3. "Importation of Wild Poliovirus Into Qinghai Province - China," *MMWR Morb Mortal Wkly Rep*, 2000, 49(6):113-4.
4. Kilpatrick DR, Nottay B, Yang CF, et al, "Serotype-Specific Identification of Poliovirus by PCR Using Primers Containing Mixed-Base or Deoxyinosine Residues at Positions of Codon Degeneracy," *J Clin Microbiol*, 1998, 36(2):352-7.

References

American Academy of Pediatrics, "Prevention of Poliomyelitis: Recommendations for Use of Only Inactivated Poliovirus Vaccine for Routine Immunization," *Pediatrics*, 1999, 104(6):1404-6.

Centers for Disease Control and Prevention, "Developing and Expanding Contributions of the Global Laboratory Network for Poliomyelitis Eradication, 1997-1999," *JAMA*, 2000, 283(13):1683-4.

John TJ, "The Final Stages of the Global Eradication of Polio," *N Engl J Med*, 2000, 343(11):806-7.

Melnick JL, "Enteroviruses," *Manual of Clinical Laboratory Immunology*, 4th ed, Volume 2, Chapter 93, Rose NR, de Macario EC, Fahey JL, et al, eds, Washington, DC: ASM Press, American Society for Microbiology, 1992, 631-3.

Soto NE and Lutwick LI, "Poliovirus Immunizations. What Goes Around, Comes Around," *Infect Dis Clin North Am*, 1999, 13(1):265-78.

Internet Web Sites

www.astdhpphe.org/infect/polio.html
www.cdc.gov/nip/publications/vis/vis-polio.pdf
www.who.int/health-topics/poliomyelitis.htm

♦ **Poliovirus Culture** *see* Enterovirus Culture *on page 605*

♦ **Poliovirus Culture, Stool** *see* Viral Culture, Stool *on page 695*

♦ **Poliovirus Titer** *see* Poliomyelitis I, II, III Serology *on page 671*

♦ **Potassium Hydroxide Preparation** *see* KOH Preparation *on page 645*

♦ *Prevotella melaninogenica* *see* Bacterial Culture, Bronchoscopy/Bronchial Brush/Bronchoalveolar Lavage Specimen *on page 568*

♦ **ProbeTec ET** *see Chlamydia trachomatis* Nucleic Acid Detection *on page 591*

♦ **Prostate, Viral Culture** *see* Viral Culture, Urogenital *on page 696*

♦ **Prostatic Fluid Culture** *see* Bacterial Culture, Genital Specimen *on page 571*

♦ *Proteus* OX-19 *replaced by* Rocky Mountain Spotted Fever Serology *on page 676*

♦ *Proteus* spp *see* Bacterial Culture, Middle Ear *on page 573*

♦ *Proteus* spp *see* Bacterial Culture, Urine *on page 578*

♦ *Proteus* spp *see* Bacterial Culture, Wounds, Bites *on page 579*

♦ **Pseudomembranous Colitis Toxin Assay** *see Clostridium difficile* Toxin Assay and Culture *on page 592*

♦ *Pseudomonas aeruginosa* *see* Bacterial Culture, Conjunctiva *on page 570*

♦ *Pseudomonas aeruginosa* *see* Bacterial Culture, Middle Ear *on page 573*

♦ *Pseudomonas aeruginosa* *see* Bacterial Culture, Urine *on page 578*

♦ *Pseudomonas aeruginosa* *see* Bacterial Culture, Wounds, Bites *on page 579*

♦ *Pseudomonas* spp *see* Bacterial Culture, Aerobes *on page 563*

Psittacosis Serology

Related Information
Chlamydia Group Serology *on page 589*

Synonyms *Chlamydia psittaci* Antibodies; *Chlamydia psittaci* Titer

Applies to *Chlamydia psittaci* Direct Immunofluorescent Antibody; *Chlamydia psittaci* PCR

Test Includes Detection of antibody specific for *Chlamydia psittaci*

Abstract Human psittacosis is usually contracted from exposure to birds, including domestic fowl. Infection in birds usually involves the intestinal tract and the organism is shed in the feces, which can contaminate the environment.[1] *C. psittaci* is a prevalent zoonotic infection which can cause diseases in many domestic mammals.

Specimen Serum

Container Red top tube

Collection Acute and convalescent samples are needed.

Reference Interval Less than a fourfold increase in titer in paired sera

Use Diagnose psittacosis; serology is the best available laboratory diagnostic test for psittacosis.

Limitations The microimmunofluorescence test is technically difficult to perform properly but can be useful for identifying the infecting species or serovar. Complement fixation tests identify antibody to an antigen common to all members of the genus but do not provide information on the species or serovar involved. Consequently, a fourfold rise in CF antibody titer provides evidence that a chlamydial infection occurred, but it cannot distinguish psittacosis from other chlamydial infections. Interpretation of complement fixation test results performed on unpaired sera is complicated by high "background" levels of antibody in the general population. The presence of IgG titer may indicate prior exposure. Assays are only performed in large reference laboratories or research facilities.

Methodology Complement fixation (CF), enzyme immunoassay (EIA), microimmunofluorescence which has been improved with application of monoclonal antibodies. Direct immunofluorescent antibody can be applied to respiratory secretions.[2] PCR can be useful.[2,3]

Additional Information Most patients with psittacosis develop high titers of complement fixing antibody and in the appropriate clinical setting a single very high titer may be strongly supportive of the diagnosis. Specific IgM antibody can sometimes be demonstrated.

Direct detection of *Chlamydia psittaci* can be accomplished by direct immunofluorescent antibody staining of respiratory secretions with monoclonal antibodies or by PCR.[2,3]

C. psittaci is generally very stable and can persist in the environment for months without losing viability. Culture for *C. psittaci* is available from some reference laboratories, however, care should be taken when collecting the specimen. The organism, difficult to isolate, is contagious and dangerous.

Footnotes

1. Schlossberg D, Delgado J, Moore MM, et al, "An Epidemic of Avian and Human Psittacosis," *Arch Intern Med*, 1993, 153(22):2594-6.
2. Oldach DW, Gaydos CA, Mundy LM, et al, "Rapid Diagnosis of *Chlamydia psittaci* Pneumonia," *Clin Infect Dis*, 1993, 17(3):338-43.
3. Tong CY and Sillis M, "Detection of *Chlamydia pneumoniae* and *Chlamydia psittaci* in Sputum Samples by PCR," *J Clin Pathol*, 1993, 46(4):313-7.

References

Blanchard TJ and Mabey DC, "Chlamydial Infections," *Br J Clin Pract*, 1994, 48(4):201-5.

Hedberg K, White KE, Hedberg CW, et al, "Persistence of *Chlamydia* Complement-Fixation Antibody After an Outbreak of Psittacosis," *J Infect Dis*, 1993, 167(2):502-3.

Peeling RW and Brunham RC, "Chlamydiae as Pathogens: New Species and New Issues," *Emerg Infect Dis*, 1996, 2(4):307-19.

Russell EG, "Evaluation of Two Serologic Tests for the Diagnosis of Chlamydial Respiratory Disease," *Pathology*, 1999, 31(4):403-5.

Internet Web Sites

www.cdc.gov/ncidod/dbmd/diseaseinfo/psittacosis_t.htm

Pulsed-Field Gel Electrophoresis Genotyping

Synonyms Bacterial Genome Restriction Fragment Polymorphism; Bacterial Genotyping; Pulse-Field Genotyping

Test Includes Analysis of individual bacterial isolates by careful isolation of high molecular weight DNA, digestion with a restriction enzyme, and electrophoresis in a special pulsed-field gel electrophoresis (PFGE) apparatus that separates high molecular weight DNA fragments

Abstract Genetic analysis of bacteria is usually performed to determine if bacterial isolates associated with an outbreak are genetically related. The technique has been used to distinguish contamination of food products to detect a common source of infection,[1] dissemination of antibiotic resistant bacterial strains between different hospitals,[2] to study bacterial isolates associated with a specific clinical syndrome,[3] and, most commonly, to detect nosocomial spread of common bacterial infections within a hospital or healthcare system.[4]

Specimen Bacterial isolates from an outbreak

Storage Instructions Most bacterial isolates can be stored frozen at -20°C for several months or at -70°C for years before testing

Turnaround Time Usually 1-2 weeks

Reference Interval Results are expressed as percent of relatedness between at least two different bacterial isolates.

Use Identification of an outbreak of closely related bacterial infections, usually for epidemiologic purposes

Limitations There is currently no gold standard for clonal typing methods. Clonal typing of bacterial genetic material by PFGE takes from 4-7 days to complete analysis. This technique requires specialized electrophoresis equipment.[5] Certain common strains of bacteria, such as methicillin-resistant *Staphylococcus aureus* and *E. coli* O157:H7, represent small genetic subsets of strains within the species and isolates unrelated epidemiologically may show very similar genetic patterns.[6]

Methodology Bacterial DNA is obtained by embedding organisms into agarose plugs and then gently lysing the bacterial cell wall and digesting the bacterial proteins with enzymes. The bacterial DNA obtained in this way provides unsheared DNA that can be enzymatically cut at very specific sites with restriction enzymes known to cut DNA at infrequent sites. The DNA is digested within the agarose plugs to protect the DNA from excessive handling which may break the large DNA genome. The fragments resulting from restriction enzyme digestion will range from 10-800 kilobases. These fragments can be separated in a specialized agarose gel electrophoresis in which the orientation of the electrical field is changed periodically, or pulsed, rather than kept constant.[5] After staining the agarose gel for DNA (usually with ethidium bromide) a DNA "banding" pattern can be distinguished. Bacterial strains may contain from 5-20 distinct, well resolved "bands". Each band represents a specific product of DNA digestion and the pattern of all bands is used to compare two or more isolates for genetic relatedness or clonality. Criteria have been established for interpreting strain patterns and can be used to evaluate a possible outbreak.[7]

Additional Information Generally, bacterial species show a substantial amount of genetic diversity, and clinical isolates are usually quite divergent genetically. By using PFGE, an investigator can determine the likely relatedness between bacterial isolates of the same species. PFGE has been used with a wide variety of microorganisms and seems to be highly discriminatory and reproducible. Currently, PFGE is the typing method of choice for most of the commonly encountered bacterial pathogens such as staphylococci, enterococci, and common gram-negative rods such as bacteria from the family *Enterobacteriaceae* and *Pseudomonas aeruginosa*.

Footnotes

1. Maguire HC, Seng C, Chambers S, et al, "*Shigella* Outbreak in a School Associated With Eating Canteen Food and Person to Person Spread," *Commun Dis Public Health*, 1998, 1(4):279-80.
2. Horvat RT, Potter LM, and Bartholomew WR, "Clonal Dissemination of Vancomycin-Resistant Enterococci and Comparison of Susceptibility Testing Methods," *Diagn Microbiol Infect Dis*, 1998, 30(4):235-41.
3. Saiman L, Jakob K, Holmes KW, et al, "Molecular Epidemiology of Staphylococcal Scalded Skin Syndrome in Premature Infants," *Pediatr Infect Dis*, 1998, 17(4):329-34.
4. Guyot A, Barrett SP, Threlfall EJ, et al, "Molecular Epidemiology of Multi-Resistant *Escherichia coli*," *J Hosp Infect*, 1999, 43(1):39-48.
5. Birren B and Lai E, *Pulsed Field Gel Electrophoresis: A Practical Guide*, San Diego, CA: Academic Press, Inc, 1993.
6. Kreiswirth B, Kornblum J, Arbeit RD, et al, "Evidence for a Clonal Origin of Methicillin Resistance in *Staphylococcus aureus*," *Science*, 1993, 259(5092):227-30.
7. Tenover FC, Arbeit RD, Goering RV, et al, "Interpreting Chromosomal DNA Restriction Patterns Produced by Pulsed-Field Gel Electrophoresis: Criteria for Bacterial Strain Typing," *J Clin Microbiol*, 1995, 33(9):2233-9.

References

Arakawa E, Murase T, Matsushita S, et al, "Pulsed-Field Gel Electrophoresis-Based Molecular Comparison of *Vibrio* Cholerae O1 Isolates From Domestic and Imported Cases of Cholera in Japan," *J Clin Microbiol*, 2000, 38(1):424-6.
Boyce JM, "Vancomycin-Resistant *Enterococcus*. Detection, Epidemiology, and Control Measures," *Infect Dis Clin North Am*, 1997, 11(2):367-84.
Morrison D, Woodford N, Barrett SP, et al, "DNA Banding Pattern Polymorphism in Vancomycin-Resistant *Enterococcus faecium* and Criteria for Defining Strains," *J Clin Microbiol*, 1999, 37(4):1084-91.
Vanderlinde PB, Fegan N, Mills L, et al, "Use of Pulse Field Gel Electrophoresis for the Epidemiological Characterization of Coagulase Positive *Staphylococcus* Isolated from Meat Workers and Beef Carcasses," *Int J Food Microbiol*, 1999, 48(2):81-5.

♦ **Pulse-Field Genotyping** *see* Pulsed-Field Gel Electrophoresis Genotyping *on page 672*

♦ **Puncture Wound Culture** *see* Bacterial Culture, Wounds, Bites *on page 579*

Q Fever Serology

Related Information
Arthropod Identification *on page 559*
Bone Marrow *on page 410*
Liver Biopsy *on page 65*

Synonyms *Coxiella burnetii* Antibody; *Coxiella burnetii* Titer

Abstract *Coxiella burnetii*, originally called *Rickettsia burneti*, is a pleomorphic coccobacillus with a gram-negative cell wall, which, however, does not stain with the Gram stain. It is an obligate intracellular pathogen. The primary reservoirs for Q fever are cattle, sheep, and goats. Exposure to ruminants and to raw milk is relevant for this zoonosis. Originally described in Australia, its distribution is worldwide. It is also called Balkan grippe. The organism withstands heat and drying, survives on inanimate surfaces, and can persist in the environment long after an infected animal has vacated an area.[1] It is highly infectious.

The clinical characteristics include fever with interstitial pneumonitis, but no exanthem. Its complications include granulomatous hepatitis, osteomyelitis, endocarditis, and lymphocytic meningitis. It infects vascular aneurysms and prostheses. A broad clinical spectrum exists, from subclinical to fatal. The organism is extremely infectious. Transmission is by inhalation of the organism[2], by intradermal inoculation, and by transfusion of contaminated blood. Person to person transmission has been documented but it is rare. Sixty percent of infected patients are asymptomatic and the majority of symptomatic patients experience only a mild disease without need for hospitalization.[3]

It is a potential biological warfare agent.[1]

Specimen Serum

Container Red top tube

Sampling Time Acute and convalescent samples are recommended, the latter 2-4 weeks from onset. CF antibodies to phase-1 antigen are found in 7-10 days.

Reference Interval Titer: <1:10; comparison of acute and convalescent titers is of greatest diagnostic value

Critical Values Titer ≥1:10; fourfold or greater increase in titer provides evidence of recent infection

Use Support the diagnosis of Q fever, a disease in which respiratory abnormalities are common. Consider Q fever in the presence of fever with negative blood cultures. Increased AST and/or ALT are seen, and two to threefold increases are found in 50% to 75% of patients.

Limitations Reagents prepared from fresh isolates (phase I organisms) react differently from those from multiply-passaged organism, a laboratory artifact (phase II). Enzyme-linked immunosorbent assay (ELISA) is more sensitive than indirect immunofluorescent antibody (IFA) or complement fixation (CF) assay. Serology tests for the diagnosis of Q fever have not been standardized.

Methodology Complement fixation (CF), indirect immunofluorescent antibody (IFA), enzyme-linked immunosorbent assays (ELISA). Monoclonal antibodies can detect *C. burnetii* in paraffin tissue blocks[4,5]

Additional Information Serology is preferable to culture for detection of infection with *C. burnetii*. Nucleic acid amplification has also been used to detect *C. burnetii* in blood specimens of infected patients.[5] Sera from patients with Q fever do not react in the Weil-Felix test with *Proteus* antigen. Convalescent sera react best with phase II organism (see above), but sera from chronic persistent infection react best with phase I organisms. Chronic Q fever is uncommon and tends to affect patients with valvular heart disease. Cross reactions with *Legionella* have been described.

Footnotes

1. Franz DR, Jahrling PB, Friedlander AM, et al, "Clinical Recognition and Management of Patients Exposed to Biological Warfare Agents," *JAMA*, 1997, 278(5):399-411.
2. Tissot-Dupont H, Torres S, Nezri M, et al, "A Hyperendemic Focus of Q Fever Related to Sheep and Wind," *Am J Epidemiol*, 1999, 150(1):67-74.
3. Marrie TJ and Raoult D, "Q Fever - A Review and Issues for the Next Century," *Int J Antimicrob Agents*, 1997, 8:145-61.
4. Raoult D, Laurent JC, and Mutillod M, "Monoclonal Antibodies to *Coxiella burnetii* for Antigenic Detection in Cell Cultures and In Paraffin-Embedded Tissues," *Am J Clin Pathol*, 1994, 101(3):318-20.
5. Musso D and Raoult D, "*Coxiella burnetii* Blood Cultures From Acute and Chronic Q-Fever Patients," *J Clin Microbiol*, 1995, 33(12):3129-32.

References

Anguita M, Ciudad M, Gallardo A, et al, "Infectious Endocarditis Due to Q Fever. A Report of 4 New Cases," *Rev Esp Cardiol*, 1993, 46(8):506-8.
Htwe KK, Yoshida T, Hayashi S, et al, "Prevalence of Antibodies to *Coxiella burnetii* in Japan," *J Clin Microbiol*, 1993, 31(3):722-3.
Levy PY, Carrieri P, and Raoult D, "*Coxiella burnetii* Pericarditis: Report of 15 Cases and Review," *Clin Infect Dis*, 1999, 29(2):393-7.
Maurin M and Raoult D, "Q Fever," *Clin Microbiol Rev*, 1999, 12(4):518-53.
Ropper AH and Caliendo AM, "An 18-Year Old Man With Severe Headache, Pleocytosis, and Ataxia," Case Records of the Massachusetts General Hospital, Case 38-1996, Scully RE, Mark EJ, McNeely WF, et al, eds, *N Engl J Med*, 1996, 335(24):1829-34.
Soriano F, Camacho MT, Ponte C, et al, "Serological Differentiation Between Acute (Late Control) and Endocarditis Q Fever," *J Clin Pathol*, 1993, 46(5):411-4.
Yale SH, de Groen PC, Tooson JD, et al, "Unusual Aspects of Acute Q Fever-Associated Hepatitis," *Mayo Clin Proc*, 1994, 69(8):769-73.

Internet Web Sites
www.cdc.gov/ncidod/dvrd/qfever/index.htm

♦ **Quantitative Burn Culture** *see* Bacterial Culture, Burn Sites *on page 569*

♦ **Quantitative Culture, Biopsy Specimen** *see* Bacterial Culture, Burn Sites *on page 569*

♦ **Quantitative Culture for Respiratory Tract Pathogens** *see* Bacterial Culture, Bronchoscopy/Bronchial Brush/Bronchoalveolar Lavage Specimen *on page 568*

♦ **Quantitative HIV PCR** *see* Human Immunodeficiency Virus, Viral Load Assay *on page 640*

♦ **Quantitative Tip Culture (QTC)** *see* Bacterial Culture, Intravascular Device *on page 572*

♦ **Rabbit Fever Antibodies** *see* Tularemia Serology *on page 686*

♦ **Rabid Animals** *see* Rabies *on page 673*

Rabies

Related Information
Bacterial Culture, Wounds, Bites *on page 579*
Virus, Direct Detection by Fluorescent Antibody *on page 696*

Synonyms Rabid Animals

Applies to Fluorescent Rabies Antibody Test; FRA Test; Negri Bodies

Test Includes Microscopy for Negri bodies, human skin biopsy using direct immunofluorescent antibody

Abstract Rabies has been recognized as a fatal infection in humans and animals for more than 25 centuries. It is usually transmitted through the bite of a rabid animal or exposure to rabid bats. Individuals with a high risk of contact with rabid animals (eg, veterinarians, animal control officers) should consider vaccination against rabies. Human exposure to bats, followed by skunks, foxes, and dogs, has been responsible for all but a single case of rabies acquired in the United States. Animal bites carry risk of infection 50-
(Continued)

Rabies (Continued)

100 times that of a scratch.[1] From 1980 to 1996 there have been only 32 cases of human rabies diagnosed in the U.S.[2]

Specimen Head of large animal or entire small animal suspected of rabies. Use gloves and mask when handling an animal carcass suspected of rabies.

Human diagnosis is possible through laboratory investigation of cerebrospinal fluid, serum, saliva, biopsy of brain, corneal impressions or nuchal skin.

Container Double-sealed container

Collection A 6-8 mm full thickness wedge or punch biopsy specimen from the neck containing as many hair follicles as possible should be sampled, snap frozen, and shipped frozen at -70°C to a reference laboratory. Consult with reference laboratory for shipping instructions. False-negative results occur, especially after the development of neutralizing antibodies.[3]

Storage Instructions Ideally, animal brain should be examined in the fresh state. Transport using wet ice or place in absorbent material, then in two plastic bags, or, place half the brain in 50% glycerol, half in 10% formalin, depending on instructions from state laboratory. The local state laboratory must be consulted. Rabies virus may also be demonstrated by immunofluorescence in skin biopsies of patients suspected of having rabies (*vide infra*).

Causes for Rejection Unlabeled or improperly packaged specimen, formalin fixation of tissue, samples not shipped at -20°C

Use Diagnose rabies; investigate patients with pain and paresthesias at bite sites; evaluate animal bites and exposure to possibly rabid animals for candidacy for rabies immune globulin and/or rabies vaccine.[4,5]

Limitations Negri bodies (viral inclusions in neurons) are found in about 90% of rabid animals. All tests are not positive in all cases.

Contraindications Formalin fixation precludes fluorescent antibody application

Methodology The preferred diagnostic test for rabies is the direct immunofluorescent antibody (DFA) for detection of rabies virus antigen in brain or skin tissue;[6] Negri bodies can be seen in H&E; nucleotide sequence analysis, PCR testing of saliva and skin. Inoculation of mice with suspension of brain tissue is not available in conventional clinical laboratories.

Additional Information Human exposure to bats, followed by skunks, foxes, and dogs has been responsible for most of the cases of rabies in the U.S.[5] Thus, animals at high risk for rabies include bats, skunks, raccoons, dogs, cats, foxes, and to a lesser extent, jackals, wolves, bobcats, bears, coyotes, mongooses, weasels, groundhogs, and any escaped wild animal including American bison.[7] Twenty-one of 24 cases of human rabies diagnosed in the U.S. since 1981 are associated with variants of rabies virus related to bats. A clear history of bite was only documented in six.[8] Bites of rabbits, squirrels, hamsters, guinea pigs, gerbils, chipmunks, rats, mice, and other rodents have seldom if ever resulted in human rabies in the United States and are regarded as low risk.

Domestic animals suspected of rabies should be kept alive in quarantine if possible. Animal bites, when unprovoked, are more likely to transmit rabies.[5] Survival of an animal for 10 days makes rabies unlikely. Signs of rabies among wild carnivorous animals cannot be reliably interpreted; any such animal that bites or scratches a person should be killed at once and the head submitted for rabies testing.

Although a dog bite along the U.S.-Mexican border is considered a rabies exposure until proven otherwise, such bites in other portions of the U.S. may not require immediate prophylaxis while the animal is confined and observed for 10 days. Dogs in the U.S. are at extremely low risk for rabies. Most Americans infected with rabies were exposed in foreign countries. Several reports have noted cases of rabies despite pre-exposure prophylaxis with human diploid cell vaccine or postexposure therapy.[9,10] Around the world, almost all rabies follows a rabid animal bite exposure. However, rabies virus can enter through nonbite exposure, such as an open wound, or by inhalation of aerosolized bat urine (eg, cave explorers) or by corneal transplantation. The table lists location of exposure to rabid canine bites and extent of exposure as it relates to mortality rates.

Representative Mortality Rates in Nonvaccinated Individuals Following Exposure to Rabid Canines

Location of Exposure	Extent of Exposure	Mortality (%)
Face	Bites (multiple and severe)	60
Other part of head	Bites (multiple and severe)	50
Face	Bite (single)	30
Fingers/hand	Bite (severe)	15
Face	Bites (multiple and superficial)	10
Hand	Bites (multiple and superficial)	5
Trunk/legs	Scratch	3
Hands/exposed skin	Bleeding and superficial wound	2
Skin covered by clothes	Superficial wound	0.5
Recent wound	Saliva	0.1
Wounds >24 h old	Saliva	0.0

Adapted from Whitley RJ and Middlebrooks M, "Rabies," *Infections of the Central Nervous System*, Chapter 7, Scheld WM, Whitley RJ, and Durack DT, eds, New York, NY: Raven Press, 1991, 134.

Antemortem rabies virus has been isolated from human saliva, brain tissues, CSF, urine sediment, and tracheal secretions. Rabies virus may also be demonstrated by immunofluorescent rabies antibody staining of skin biopsy tissue. The most reliable and reproducible of the immunofluorescent studies that can aid in patient diagnosis is biopsy of the neck skin.

Footnotes
1. Bosgoz N and Frosch M, "A 32-Year-Old Woman With Pharyngeal Spasms and Paresthesias After a Dog Bite," Case Records of the Massachusetts General Hospital, Case 21-1998, Scully RE, Mark EJ, McNeely WF, et al, eds, *N Engl J Med*, 1998, 339(2):105-12.
2. Moran GJ, Talan DA, Mower W, et al, "Appropriateness of Rabies Postexposure Prophylaxis Treatment for Animal Exposures," *JAMA*, 2000, 284(8):1001-7.
3. Bernard KW and Fishbein DB, "Rabies Virus," *Principles and Practice of Infectious Diseases*, Chapter 140, Mandell GL, Douglas RG Jr, and Bennett JE, eds, New York, NY: Churchill Livingstone, 1990, 1291-1301.
4. Hanlon CA, Olson JG, and Clark CJ, "Article I: Prevention and Education Regarding Rabies in Human Beings. National Working Group on Rabies Prevention and Control," *J Am Vet Med Assoc*, 1999, 215(9):1276-80.
5 "Human Rabies Prevention," *MMWR Morb Mortal Wkly Rep*, 1999, 48(RR-1):1-21.
6. Trimarchi CV and Debbie J, "The Fluorescent Antibody in Rabies," *The Natural History of Rabies*, 2nd ed, Baer GM, ed, Boca Raton, FL: CRC Press, 1991, 219-33.
7. Stoltenow CL, Solemsass K, Niezgoda M, et al, "Rabies in an American Bison From North Dakota," *J Wildl Dis*, 2000, 36(1):169-71.
8. "Human Rabies - Texas and New Jersey, 1997," *MMWR Morb Mortal Wkly Rep*, 1998, 47:41-5.
9. Hemachudha T, Mitrabhakdi E, Wilde H, et al, "Additional Reports of Failure to Respond to Treatment After Rabies Exposure in Thailand," *Clin Infect Dis*, 1999, 28(1):143-4.
10. Gacouin A, Bourhy H, Renaud JC, et al, "Human Rabies Despite Postexposure Vaccination," *Eur J Clin Microbiol Infect Dis*, 1999, 18(3):233-5.

References
Centers for Disease Control and Prevention, "Human Rabies - California, Georgia, Minnesota, New York, and Wisconsin, 2000," *JAMA*, 2001, 285(2):158-60.
Centers for Disease Control and Prevention, "Human Rabies - Quebec, Canada, 2000," *JAMA*, 2001, 285(2):160-1.
Centers for Disease Control and Prevention, "Public Health Response to a Potentially Rabid Bear Cub - Iowa, 1999," *JAMA*, 2000, 283(2):192-3.
Crawford-Miksza LK, Wadford DA, and Schnurr DP, "Molecular Epidemiology of Enzootic Rabies in California," *J Clin Virol*, 1999, 14(3):207-19.
David D, Rupprecht CE, Smith J, et al, "Human Rabies in Israel," *Emerg Infect Dis*, 1999, 5(2):306-8.
De Mattos CC, De Mattos CA, Loza-Rubio E, et al, "Molecular Characterization of Rabies Virus Isolates From Mexico: Implications for Transmission Dynamics and Human Risk," *Am J Trop Med Hyg*, 1999, 61(4):587-97.
Fleisher GR, "The Management of Bite Wounds," *N Engl J Med*, 1999, 340(2):138-40.
Haupt W, "Rabies - Risk of Exposure and Current Trends in Prevention of Human Cases," *Vaccine*, 1999, 17(13-14):1742-9.
Mrak RE and Young L, "Rabies Encephalitis in Humans: Pathology, Pathogenesis and Pathophysiology," *J Neuropathol Exp Neurol*, 1994, 53(1):1-10.
Smith JS, "Rabies," *Clin Microbiol Newslet*, 1999, 21(3):17-23.
"Upate: Raccoon Rabies Epizootic - United States and Canada, 1999," *MMWR Morb Mortal Wkly Rep*, 2000, 49(2):31-5.
Whitley RJ and Kimberlin DW, "Viral Encephalitis," *Pediatr Rev*, 1999, 20(6):192-8.

Internet Web Sites
www.amm.co.uk/pubs/fa_rabies.htm
www.astdhpphe.org/infect/rabies.html
www.cdc.gov/ncidod/dvrd/rabies

◆ **Rabies Virus, Direct Detection** see Virus, Direct Detection by Fluorescent Antibody *on page 696*

◆ **Rapid Antigen Detection Tests for Group A Streptococci** see Bacterial Culture, Throat, and Antigen Detection Testing for Group A Streptococci *on page 577*

◆ **Rapid Detection of *Streptococcus* Group A** see Group A *Streptococcus* Screen, Rapid *on page 617*

◆ **Rapid Plasma Reagin Test** see RPR *on page 677*

◆ **Recombinant Antigen Immunoblot Assay** see HIV-1/HIV-2 Antibody Screen and Western Blot *on page 636*

◆ **Recombinant Immunoblot Assay** see Hepatitis C Virus Serology *on page 627*

◆ **Rectal Swab Culture** see Bacterial Culture, Stool *on page 575*

◆ **Red Eye** see Bacterial Culture, Conjunctiva *on page 570*

Respiratory Syncytial Virus Antigen Detection

Related Information
Bacterial Culture, Middle Ear *on page 573*
Respiratory Syncytial Virus Culture *on page 675*
Respiratory Syncytial Virus Serology *on page 675*
Viral Culture, Respiratory Symptoms *on page 694*
Virus, Direct Detection by Fluorescent Antibody *on page 696*

Synonyms RSV Antigen; RSV Direct Immunofluorescence

Test Includes Detection of RSV antigen in specimens using enzyme immunoassay (EIA) or immunofluorescence (IFA)

Abstract Respiratory syncytial virus (RSV), an RNA virus, was first isolated in 1956. It is a common cause of acute lower respiratory disease in infants and young children. Clinical symptoms due to RSV include bronchiolitis and pneumonia. Forty percent of infected children younger than 2 years of age develop lower respiratory tract disease. Hypoxemia is common. In infants and young children, RSV is the most frequent cause of hospitalization for lower respiratory tract infection.[1]

Specimen Nasopharyngeal secretions (nasal washings or aspirates) are preferred; nasopharyngeal swab is acceptable.

Collection Swabs must be placed in cold viral transport medium. Soft catheters and suction devices can be used to collect nasal secretions. Nasal washings are done by carefully introducing sterile saline (3-7 mL) into the nasal cavity and aspirating the fluid. **Do not use cold sterile saline when aspirating samples. Warm to room temperature.**

Storage Instructions Can be transported at room temperature without loss of viral antigens.

Turnaround Time 1 day; some laboratories may have a few hours turn-around time

Critical Values Positive results

Use Rapid diagnosis of bronchiolitis, lower respiratory disease caused by RSV, and other disease including otitis media

Limitations Specimens with <100 cells on the slide will yield an insensitive result when detecting RSV by immunofluorescence; immunofluorescence requires experienced personnel to read results.

Methodology Enzyme-linked immunosorbent assay (ELISA), direct fluorescent antibody (DFA) recognize about 85% of cases.

Additional Information RSV direct EIAs have become the most frequently used method of detecting RSV infections. RSV is very labile and cell culture infectivity is lost rapidly when the virus is kept at 37°C. The detection of RSV antigen allows for detection of virus in specimens in which virus is not culturable. EIA and IFA are considered more sensitive than culture. Specimen handling requirements are not as stringent as those required for culture. The EIAs used to detect RSV antigen are simple, objective, and quick.

Footnotes

1. Izurieta HS, Thompson WW, Kramarz P, et al, "Influenza and the Rates of Hospitalization for Respiratory Disease Among Infants and Young Children," *N Engl J Med*, 2000, 342(4):232-9.

References

Baker KA and Ryan ME, "RSV Infection in Infants and Young Children. What's New in Diagnosis, Treatment, and Prevention?" *Postgrad Med*, 1999, 106(7):97-9, 103-4, 107-8 passim.

Choy G, "A review of Respiratory Syncytial Virus Infection in Infants and Children," *Home Care Provid*, 1998, 3(6):306-11.

Falsey AR, Cunningham CK, Barker WH, et al, "Respiratory Syncytial Virus and Influenza A Infections in the Hospitalized Elderly," *J Infect Dis*, 1995, 172(2):389-94.

Hall CB, "Respiratory Syncytial Virus: A Continuing Culprit and Conundrum," *J Pediatr*, 1999, 135(2 Pt 2):2-7.

Jones BL, Clark S, Curran ET, et al, "Control of an Outbreak of Respiratory Syncytial Virus Infection in Immunocompromised Adults," *J Hosp Infect*, 2000, 44(1):53-7.

Simoes EA, "Respiratory Syncytial Virus Infection," *Lancet*, 1999, 354(9181):847-52.

Walker TA, Khurana S, and Tilden SJ, "Viral Respiratory Infections," *Pediatr Clin North Am*, 1994, 41(6):1365-81.

Internet Web Sites

www.astdhpphe.org/infect/rsv.html
www.cdc.gov/ncidod/dvrd/nrevss/rsvfeat.htm

Respiratory Syncytial Virus Culture

Related Information

Respiratory Syncytial Virus Antigen Detection *on page 674*
Respiratory Syncytial Virus Serology *on page 675*
Viral Culture, Respiratory Symptoms *on page 694*
Virus, Direct Detection by Fluorescent Antibody *on page 696*

Synonyms RSV Culture

Test Includes Conventional culture or rapid culture using specific monoclonal antibodies for respiratory syncytial virus (RSV). May also include concurrent culture for other respiratory viruses (influenza, adenovirus, and parainfluenza viruses).

Abstract Respiratory syncytial virus (RSV) is the most common viral agent causing infant lower respiratory illnesses. By the first year of life, 50% of infants have experienced an RSV infection. Common symptoms are fever, wheezing, lower respiratory tract congestion, cough, and rhinorrhea. In healthy adult individuals, the mortality rates due to RSV are relatively low.

Specimen Throat or nasopharyngeal swab, nasopharyngeal washes and secretions. Sputum is not an appropriate specimen for detection of RSV in viral culture.

Container Cold viral transport medium for swabs

Collection Place swabs into cold viral transport medium and keep cold. Infants and small children: soft catheters and suction devices (syringes and suction bulbs) can be used to collect nasal secretions from far back in the nose (best specimens). Another excellent method is to introduce 3-7 mL of sterile saline into the child's posterior nasal cavity and immediately aspirate the fluid. Do not use **cold** sterile saline when aspirating samples. Warm to room temperature.

Storage Instructions Respiratory syncytial virus is extremely labile and will lose as much as 90% of cell culture infectivity when left at room temperature

---

for 24 hours.[1] **Do not freeze specimens at -20°C.** Send specimens to the laboratory **as soon as possible**. Although less than optimal conditions, specimens can be stored up to 48 hours at 4°C. If necessary specimen can be quickly frozen at -70°C, but freezing will cause loss of infectivity.

Turnaround Time Conventional culture: 1-14 days; rapid culture: 1-2 days

Reference Interval No virus isolated

Critical Values Positive results

Use Culture supports diagnosis of respiratory disease caused by respiratory syncytial virus.

Limitations Culture is not available in many clinical laboratories. Rapid methods will only detect specified virus(es), negative culture does not rule out RSV infection. RSV is a very thermolabile virus and may not survive transport to the laboratory or extreme conditions. Thus, false-negative cultures occur.

Methodology Inoculation of specimen into cell cultures, incubation of cultures, observation for characteristic cytopathic effect in 2-7 days, and identification by fluorescent monoclonal antibodies specific for respiratory syncytial virus. The use of a rapid shell vial culture technique is reported to yield positive culture results overnight.[2,3]

Additional Information In healthy individuals, the mortality rate due to RSV infection is low; however, in patients with respiratory or cardiac compromise, immune dysfunction, and the elderly, the mortality rate is high (~37%).[4,5]

Many laboratories offer enzyme immunoassay (EIA) tests for the direct detection of RSV in patient nasopharyngeal swab specimens. In general, these tests are very rapid, sensitive, and specific. Serology can detect antibodies to respiratory syncytial virus, but antigen detection from nasopharyngeal washings is better for patient care.[4]

The detection of RSV nucleic acid in clinical specimens is available through some laboratories but has not been widely evaluated. Some studies have shown a 94% sensitivity and a specificity >99% when compared to RSV culture.[6]

Footnotes

1. Tristram DA and Welliver RC, "Respiratory Syncytial Virus," *Manual of Clinical Microbiology*, 7th ed, Murray PR, Baron EJ, Pfaller MA, et al, eds, Washington, DC: AMS Press, American Society for Microbiology, 1999, 942-50.

2. Mathey S, Nicholson D, Ruhs S, et al, "Rapid Detection of Respiratory Viruses by Shell Vial Culture and Direct Staining by Using Pooled and Individual Monoclonal Antibodies," *J Clin Microbiol*, 1992, 30(3):540-4.

3. Shih SR, Tsao KC, Ning HC, et al, "Diagnosis of Respiratory Tract Viruses in 24 h by Immunofluorescence Staining of Shell Vial Cultures Containing Madin-Darby Canine Kidney (MDCK) Cells," *J Virol Methods*, 1999, 81(1-2):77-81.

4. Falsey AR, Cunningham CK, Barker WH, et al, "Respiratory Syncytial Virus and Influenza A Infections in the Hospitalized Elderly," *J Infect Dis*, 1995, 172(2):389-94.

5. Whimbey E, Couch RB, and Englund JA, "Respiratory Syncytial Virus Pneumonia in Hospitalized Adult Patients With Leukemia," *Clin Infect Dis*, 1995, 21(2):376-9.

6. Tang YW, Heimgartner PJ, Tollefson SJ, et al, "A Colorimetric Microtiter Plate PCR System Detects Respiratory Syncytial Virus in Nasal Aspirates and Discriminates Subtypes A and B," *Diagn Microbiol Infect Dis*, 1999, 34(4):333-7.

References

Baker KA and Ryan ME, "RSV Infection in Infants and Young Children. What's New in Diagnosis, Treatment, and Prevention?" *Postgrad Med*, 1999, 106(7):97-9, 103-4, 107-8 passim.

Choy G, "A Review of Respiratory Syncytial Virus Infection in Infants and Children," *Home Care Provid*, 1998, 3(6):306-11.

Hall CB, "Respiratory Syncytial Virus: A Continuing Culprit and Conundrum," *J Pediatr*, 1999, 135(2 Pt 2):2-7.

Hemming VG, Prince GA, Groothuis JR, et al, "Hyperimmune Globulins in Prevention and Treatment of Respiratory Syncytial Virus Infections," *Clin Microbiol Rev*, 1995, 8(1):22-33.

Jones BL, Clark S, Curran ET, et al, "Control of an Outbreak of Respiratory Syncytial Virus Infection in Immunocompromised Adults," *J Hosp Infect*, 2000, 44(1):53-7.

Ottolini MG and Hemming VG, "Respiratory Syncytial Viral Infection: An Old Problem Presents New Challenges," *Infect Med*, 1994, 11(5):342, 347-54, 360.

Simoes EA, "Respiratory Syncytial Virus Infection," *Lancet*, 1999, 354(9181):847-52.

Yungbluth M, "The Laboratory Diagnosis of Pneumonia. The Role of the Community Hospital Pathologist," *Clin Lab Med*, 1995, 15(2):209-34.

Internet Web Sites

www.astdhpphe.org/infect/rsv.html
www.cdc.gov/ncidod/dvrd/nrevss/rsvfeat.htm

Respiratory Syncytial Virus Serology

Related Information

Respiratory Syncytial Virus Antigen Detection *on page 674*
Respiratory Syncytial Virus Culture *on page 675*
Viral Culture, Respiratory Symptoms *on page 694*
Virus, Direct Detection by Fluorescent Antibody *on page 696*

Synonyms RSV Antibodies

Test Includes Detection of antibodies specific for RSV

Abstract In a primary infection, RSV-specific IgM appears after 5-8 days and persists for several weeks. Detectable increases in RSV-specific IgG antibody titers occur 2-4 weeks after symptomatic infections. Thus, during an acute infection, serology is less sensitive than direct antigen detection or cell culture methods.[1]

Specimen Serum

Container Red top tube

(Continued)

Respiratory Syncytial Virus Serology (Continued)

Special Instructions Acute and convalescent specimens are recommended.

Reference Interval IgG: less than fourfold rise in titer; IgM: negative

Use Detect specific RSV antibody in patients suspected of having RSV

Limitations Young infants have maternal IgG antibody and may have a false positive. A fourfold rise in IgG titers cannot be detected in half of the children younger than 6 months of age. Enzyme immunoassays may use different antigen sources. No serologic assay has been standardized for detection of RSV infection.

Methodology Complement fixation (CF), enzyme immunoassay (EIA), virus-neutralization assay, immunofluorescence assay

Additional Information RSV is a common cause of acute respiratory disease, including serious disease among older persons. Complications, especially in infants and children with underlying cardiopulmonary disease, and the immunocompromised, include bronchiolitis and pneumonia. Nosocomial outbreaks can occur.

Presence of neutralizing antibody is the only antibody associated with protection against RSV infection. However, EIA is more rapidly performed and some EIAs can be as sensitive as neutralization assays. Diagnosis of RSV by RSV-specific IgG depends on demonstration of a rise in antibody titer over a 2- to 3-week period. As such, the test is seldom useful in planning clinical care in an acute illness or in control of nosocomial infections. For rapid diagnosis of RSV, the demonstration of viral antigen in nasopharyngeal washings is more useful. See Respiratory Syncytial Virus Antigen Detection *on page 674* and Respiratory Syncytial Virus Culture *on page 675*.

Footnotes

1. Tristram DA and Welliver RC, "Respiratory Syncytial Virus," *Manual of Clinical Microbiology*, 7th ed, Murray PR, Baron EJ, Pfaller MA, et al, eds, Washington, DC: AMS Press, American Society for Microbiology, 1999, 942-50.

References

Falsey AR, Cunningham CK, Barker WH, et al, "Respiratory Syncytial Virus and Influenza A Infections in the Hospitalized Elderly," *J Infect Dis*, 1995, 172(2):389-94.

Hall CB, "Respiratory Syncytial Virus: A Continuing Culprit and Conundrum," *J Pediatr*, 1999, 135(2 Pt 2):2-7.

Jones BL, Clark S, Curran ET, et al, "Control of an Outbreak of Respiratory Syncytial Virus Infection in Immunocompromized Adults," *J Hosp Infect*, 2000, 44(1):53-7.

Simoes EA, "Respiratory Syncytial Virus Infection," *Lancet*, 1999, 354(9181):847-52

Internet Web Sites

www.astdhpphe.org/infect/rsv.html

www.cdc.gov/ncidod/dvrd/nrevss/rsvfeat.htm

♦ **RIBA** see Hepatitis C Virus Serology *on page 627*

♦ ***Rickettsia rickettsii* Serology** see Rocky Mountain Spotted Fever Serology *on page 676*

♦ ***Rochalimaea* Antibodies** see Bartonella Serology *on page 581*

♦ ***Rochalimaea* Culture** see Bartonella Culture *on page 580*

♦ ***Rochalimaea* Titer** see Bartonella Serology *on page 581*

Rocky Mountain Spotted Fever Serology

Related Information

Anemia Flowchart *on page 392*

Arthropod Identification *on page 559*

Ehrlichiosis Serology *on page 603*

Synonyms *Rickettsia rickettsii* Serology

Replaces Proteus OX-19

Abstract Transmitted by ticks, this acute, febrile disease is characterized by headache, fever, weakness, and (in ~90% of cases) a centipetal macular eruption beginning on wrists and ankles. Rocky Mountain spotted fever (RMSF) is a life-threatening illness, even in previously healthy patients and if left untreated, the case fatality rate is 20% to 25%.[1] The disease is caused by *Rickettsia rickettsii*, obligate intracellular, gram-negative, pleomorphic bacteria that cannot be detected by routine microbiological culture. In the United States, RMSF is seen most frequently in a narrow geographic band from North Carolina to Oklahoma. Serologic diagnosis is generally the only test performed for detection of RMSF.

Specimen Serum

Container Red top tube

Sampling Time Paired sera 7-10 days apart is recommended.[1] A titer >1:128 can often be detected during the second week of illness.

Special Instructions Acute and convalescent specimens are recommended.

Reference Interval Less than a fourfold increase in titer in paired sera; IgG <1:32, IgM <1:8 indicates that RMSF is unlikely

Critical Values Fourfold increase to specific rickettsial antigen is diagnostic

Possible Panic Range IgG: ≥1:128

Use Diagnose Rocky Mountain spotted fever

Limitations Diagnostic IgG titers may persist for years and IgM titers as high as 1:64 have occasionally been demonstrated a year after infection. IgG titer may be negative early in disease. Consequently, convincing serologic diagnosis can only be demonstrated with increasing titers or an IgM titer ≥1:128; the threshold for therapeutic intervention is often considerably less than that which is required for a convincing serologic diagnosis. False-positive reactions occur during pregnancy, particularly in the last two trimesters. False positives are also occasionally seen with other *Rickettsia* in the spotted fever group. Patients treated with antibiotics early in the illness may not develop serologic responses. The disease may progress rapidly.

Methodology Indirect immunofluorescent antibody (IFA) and enzyme-linked immunosorbent assay (ELISA) are highly sensitive. Latex agglutination (LA) is helpful in early convalescence. Solid phase dot immunoassays, such as serum dipsticks, have become available. Immunohistologic methods are also in use. A direct fluorescent test is available to demonstrate the *Rickettsia* in tissue or in circulating endothelial cells. As many as 71% of patients with RMSF also develop antibodies against cardiolipin and endothelial cells.

Complement fixation (CF) and microagglutination methods are no longer in general use due to their lack of sensitivity.

More recently, PCR techniques have been used to detect *R. rickettsii* DNA in patients' specimens. PCR studies can be used for rapid diagnosis but are available only in research laboratories or large reference laboratories.

Additional Information RMSF occurs primarily from April through October, when ticks are active. It is a disease of variable clinical manifestation and some cases present with few or no "spots". All laboratory tests used to aid in the diagnosis are important, since there is good specific therapy available, and if left untreated the disease has serious outcomes. Serologic diagnosis may be made promptly enough to direct therapy. Tests for IgM specific antibody are helpful in early disease, since they appear 3-8 days after infection.

The differential diagnosis includes ehrlichiosis. Clinically, the rash may be confused with those of meningococcemia, typhus, and measles.

Footnotes

1. Drage LA, "Life-Threatening Rashes: Dermatologic Signs of Four Infectious Diseases," *Mayo Clin Proc*, 1999, 74(1):68-72.

References

Abramson JS and Givner LB, "Rocky Mountain Spotted Fever," *Pediatr Infect Dis J*, 1999, 18(6):539-40.

Akinbami L, "Rocky Mountain Spotted Fever," *Pediatr Rev*, 1998, 19(5):171-2.

Belman AL, "Tick-Borne Diseases," *Semin Pediatr Neurol*, 1999, 6(4):249-66.

Samuels MA and Newell KL, "43-Year-Old Woman With Rapidly Changing Pulmonary Infiltrates and Markedly Increased Intracranial Pressure," Case Records of the Massachusetts General Hospital, Case 32-1997, Scully RE, Mark EJ, McNeely WF, et al, eds, *N Engl J Med*, 1997, 337(16):1149-56.

Sexton DJ and Kirkland KB, "Rickettsial Infections and the Central Nervous System," *Clin Infect Dis*, 1998, 26(1):247-8.

Shapiro ED, "Tick-Borne Diseases," *Adv Pediatr Infect Dis*, 1997, 13:187-218.

Thorner AR, Walker DH, and Petri WA Jr, "Rocky Mountain Spotted Fever," *Clin Infect Dis*, 1998, 27(6):1353-9.

Walker DH, "Tick-Transmitted Infectious Diseases in the United States," *Annu Rev Public Health*, 1998, 19:237-69.

Internet Web Sites

www.astdhpple.org/infect/rms.html

www.cdc.gov/ncidod/dvrd/rmsf/index.htm

♦ **Rotavirus** see Bacterial Culture, Stool *on page 575*

♦ **Rotavirus Antigen Detection** see Rotavirus, Direct Detection *on page 676*

♦ **Rotavirus Detection by EM** see Electron Microscopic Examination for Viruses, Stool *on page 603*

Rotavirus, Direct Detection

Related Information

Bacterial Culture, Stool *on page 575*

Electron Microscopic Examination for Viruses, Stool *on page 603*

Ova and Parasites, Stool *on page 666*

Polymerase Chain Reaction *on page 713*

Viral Culture, Stool *on page 695*

Synonyms Rotavirus Antigen Detection

Applies to Viral Antigen Detection, Direct, Stool

Test Includes Direct (nonculture) detection of rotavirus in stool specimens

Abstract Human rotavirus is a major cause of pediatric diarrhea. Infection is acquired by the fecal-oral route. Infections due to group A rotaviruses occur all over the world. Group B rotaviruses have been detected primarily in China. Group C rotaviruses also occur worldwide but have been detected only sporadically.[1] Generally the incubation period is 1-2 days and the onset is abrupt. Symptoms include vomiting, diarrhea, fever, and abdominal pain. Loss of fluids is the most severe result of rotavirus infection and can lead to severe dehydration. Transmission is mainly fecal-oral.[2]

Specimen Stool from the acute, diarrheal phase of disease; rectal swab

Sampling Time 3-5 days after onset

Collection Several specimens during the course of illness should be submitted in an attempt to eliminate false-negative results.

Reference Interval No virus detected

Use Evaluation of patients in whom viral gastroenteritis is suspected; differential diagnosis of acute onset winter gastroenteritis, diarrhea, emesis. Among infants and small children worldwide, rotavirus infections are the most common cause of severe gastroenteritis.[3]

Limitations Commercially available EIA kit for detection of rotavirus in stool leads to false positives when used in healthy neonates, but results in symptomatic subjects are reliable.

Methodology Latex agglutination (LA), enzyme immunoassay (EIA), enzyme-linked immunosorbent assay (ELISA), radioimmunoassay (RIA), dot blot technology. RIA and dot blot are definitive procedures but less widely used. Enzyme immunoassay (EIA) is the preferred diagnostic method with a sensitivity of 63% to 100% and specificities of 100% for group A rotaviruses.[4] In general, these assays detect the highly conserved internal capsid protein of the group A rotavirus.

Additional Information Rotavirus is a common cause of pediatric gastroenteritis. Young children between 6 months-3 years of age exhibit the most severe effects of the disease. The illness is most likely to occur in winter, is highly contagious, involves 5-8 days of diarrhea, and is rarely fatal.[4] Patients should also be evaluated for possible bacterial gastroenteritis. If available, electron microscopy or polymerase chain reaction are useful techniques for detection of rotavirus in stool specimens. Other viral agents causing gastroenteritis are enteric adenoviruses, caliciviruses, astroviruses, coronaviruses, and Norwalk and Norwalk-like viruses.

Footnotes

1. Gouvea V, Allen JR, Glass RI, et al, "Detection of Group B and C Rotaviruses by Polymerase Chain Reaction," *J Clin Microbiol*, 1991, 29:519-23.
2. Christensen ML, "Rotaviruses," *Manual of Clinical Microbiology*, 7th ed, Murray PR, Baron EJ, Pfaller MA, et al, eds, Washington, DC: AMS Press, American Society for Microbiology, 1999, 999-1004.
3. Centers for Disease Control and Prevention, "Laboratory-Based Surveillance for Rotavirus - United States, July 1996-June 1997," *JAMA*, 1998, 279(3):192.
4. Steele JC Jr, "Rotavirus," *Clin Lab Med*, 1999, 19(3):691-703.

References

Belhorn T, "Rotavirus Diarrhea," *Curr Probl Pediatr*, 1999, 29(7):198-207.
Centers for Disease Control and Prevention, "Laboratory-Based Surveillance for Rotavirus - United States, July 1996-June 1997," *JAMA*, 1998, 279(3):192.
Desselberger U, "Rotavirus Infections: Guidelines for Treatment and Prevention," *Drugs*, 1999, 58(3):447-52.
Parashar UD, Chung MA, Holman RC, et al, "Use of State Hospital Discharge Data to Assess the Morbidity From Rotavirus Diarrhea and to Monitor the Impact of a Rotavirus Immunization Program: A Pilot Study in Connecticut," *Pediatrics*, 1999, 104(3 Pt 1):489-94.

Internet Web Sites

vm.cfsan.fda.gov/~mow/chap33.html
www.astdhpphe.org/infect/rot.html
www.cdc.gov/ncidod/dvrd/nrevss/rotfeat.htm

RPR

Related Information
Anticardiolipin Antibody *on page 503*
Bacterial Culture, Genital Specimen *on page 571*
Darkfield Examination, Syphilis *on page 601*
FTA-ABS, Serum *on page 609*
MHA-TP *on page 651*
Neisseria gonorrhoeae Culture and Smear *on page 662*
VDRL, Cerebrospinal Fluid *on page 688*
VDRL, Serum *on page 688*

Synonyms Rapid Plasma Reagin Test

Applies to Cardiolipin Antibodies; Syphilis Serology

Replaces ART Test; Kahn Test; Kline Test; Mazzini; Wassermann

Test Includes Detection of nontreponemal antibodies that accompany syphilis infections. Reactive specimens are titered and then tested with a treponemal-specific test such as FTA-ABS.

Abstract Antibodies that develop in response to *T. pallidum* infection are classified as nontreponemal antibodies and treponemal-specific antibodies. The nontreponemal antibodies react with lipoidal material such as cardiolipin. Such antibodies can be produced in other conditions (eg, autoimmune diseases and pregnancy).

Specimen Serum

Container Red top tube

Reference Interval Negative

Use Screening test for syphilis

Limitations This is a nontreponemal test and is associated with false-positive reactions due to intercurrent infections, pregnancy, drug addiction, autoimmune disease, increased age, Gaucher disease, malignancy, and a number of viral, protozoal, and *Mycoplasma* infections.[1] Potential causes of false-positive serologic tests for syphilis are tabulated in VDRL, Serum *on page 688*. This test cannot be performed on cerebrospinal fluid.

The VDRL and RPR are insensitive early (in the primary phase) and late (latent and tertiary phases).

Methodology Flocculation test to detect reagin antibody

Additional Information RPR is a screening test for syphilis and detects antibodies to cardiolipin, cholesterol, and lecithin, also called reagin. Such antibodies usually develop after 4-6 weeks of initial infection, peak during the secondary phase of disease, and then decrease with time. They also decrease and usually disappear with treatment. The RPR is more sensitive than the VDRL and the ART for determining efficacy of treatment. Ninety-three percent of patients with primary syphilis have positive tests. RPR titers are usually higher in HIV-infected patients than in those who do not have HIV infection and at times fail to elicit specific treponemal antibodies as

detected by fluorescent assays such as FTA.[2] HIV bears a close epidemiologic relationship to syphilis.[3]

Because of the many causes of false-positive tests, any reactive serum should be tested by a treponemal-specific test, preferably MHA-TP or FTA-ABS for confirmation. The RPR should not be done on cerebrospinal fluid. False-negative tests may occur at birth in some infants with recently acquired congenital syphilis. Therefore, especially in areas where the disease is prevalent, a serologic test for syphilis should be included in evaluation of febrile infants even if they had a negative screen at birth. False negatives may also be due to the prozone effect. Therefore, dilution should be performed on serum of pregnant women at risk for sexually transmitted diseases and in areas with high syphilis prevalence when screening tests are negative.[4]

Because most infants with congenital syphilis lack signs of infection, tests for both nontreponemal and treponemal antibodies are needed for diagnosis. "Reagin" refers to antibody which cross reacts with extracts of cardiac muscle and treponemal cell wall components. Such nontreponemal tests are subject to false positives. Serial serologic testing during pregnancy with maternal and neonatal serologic studies at delivery is desirable for detection of neonates at risk. In instances of negative tests even following dilutions, serology should be repeated within several weeks when suspicion of congenital syphilis exists.

Footnotes

1. Singh AE and Romanowski B, "Syphilis: Review With Emphasis on Clinical, Epidemiologic, and Some Biologic Features," *Clin Microbiol Rev*, 1999, 12(2):187-209.
2. Erbelding EJ, Vlahov D, Nelson KE, et al, "Syphilis Serology in Human Immunodeficiency Virus Infection: Evidence for False-Negative Fluorescent Treponemal Testing," *J Infect Dis*, 1997, 176(5):1397-400.
3. Dibbern DA and Ray SC, "Recrudescence of Treated Neurosyphilis in a Patient With Human Immunodeficiency Virus," *Mayo Clin Proc*, 1999, 74(1):53-6.
4. Sheffield JS and Wendel GD Jr, "Syphilis in Pregnancy," *Clin Obstet Gynecol*, 1999, 42(1):97-106.

References

Augenbraun MH and Rolfs R, "Treatment of Syphilis, 1998: Nonpregnant Adults," *Clin Infect Dis*, 1999, 28(S1):S21-8.
Birnbaum NR, Goldschmidt RH, and Buffett WO, "Resolving the Common Clinical Dilemmas of Syphilis," *Am Fam Phys*, 1999, 59(8):2233-40.
Darville T, "Syphilis," *Pediatr Rev*, 1999, 20(5):160-4.
Desforges JF, "Infectious Disease Testing for Blood Transfusions," *NIH Consensus Statement*, 1995, 13(1):1-27.
Miller KE and Graves JC, "Update on the Prevention and Treatment of Sexually Transmitted Diseases," *Am Fam Phys*, 2000, 61(2):379-86.
Peate I, "Syphilis: Signs, Symptoms, Treatment and Nursing Management," *Br J Nurs*, 1998, 7(14):817-23.
Thomas DL and Quinn TC, "Serologic Testing for Sexually Transmitted Diseases," *Infect Dis Clin North Am*, 1993, 7(4):793-824.
van Voorst Vader PC, "Syphilis Management and Treatment," *Dermatol Clin*, 1998, 16(4):699-711.
Young H, "Syphilis. Serology," *Dermatol Clin*, 1998, 16(4):691-8.

Internet Web Sites

www.cdc.gov/nchstp/dstd/fact_sheets/syphilis_facts.htm

♦ **RSV Antibodies** *see* Respiratory Syncytial Virus Serology *on page 675*

♦ **RSV Antigen** *see* Respiratory Syncytial Virus Antigen Detection *on page 674*

♦ **RSV Culture** *see* Respiratory Syncytial Virus Culture *on page 675*

♦ **RSV Direct Immunofluorescence** *see* Respiratory Syncytial Virus Antigen Detection *on page 674*

Rubella Serology

Related Information
Rubella Virus Culture *on page 678*
TORCH *on page 683*

Synonyms German Measles Serology; Measles Serology, 3-day; Three-Day Measles Serology

Applies to IgG Antibodies to Rubella; IgM Antibodies to Rubella

Test Includes Detection of serologic response to rubella infection or vaccination

Abstract Rubella infection is found only in humans. Also known as German measles, it is an RNA virus. Infection is usually characterized by a macular exanthem, lymphadenopathy, pharyngitis, and conjunctivitis. The incubation period is 14-21 days but subclinical or asymptomatic infections are common. Severe transplacental infections can occur in the first trimester.

Specimen Serum, fetal blood

Container Red top tube

Collection Acute and convalescent samples for IgG.

Reference Interval Absence of antibody indicates susceptibility to rubella. IgG, IgM: negative. **Postvaccination:** positive.

Critical Values Presence of IgM antibody indicates acute infection or vaccination. Fourfold increase in IgG titer may indicate acute infection.

Possible Panic Range Evidence of susceptibility in a pregnant woman recently exposed to rubella

Use Prenatal diagnosis of congenital rubella infection (IgM); evaluate immune status
(Continued)

Rubella Serology (Continued)

Limitations Most laboratories perform rubella serology as a qualitative test to determine susceptibility to infection and do not determine titers. This presents a problem when trying to diagnose infection by increasing IgG titers; special arrangements need to be made with the laboratory if titers are required for diagnosis. Rubella-specific antibodies are transferred from the mother to the child in utero and thus the detection of rubella-specific antibody in a child younger than 6 months of age may give a false-positive result.[1] Rubella-specific IgM may persist for some months after vaccination.[2]

Methodology Indirect fluorescent antibody (IFA), hemagglutination, radioimmunoassay (RIA), complement fixation (CF), latex agglutination (LA), enzyme immunoassay (EIA)

Additional Information When acquired *in utero*, rubella virus can lead to fetal demise, cataracts, malformation, deafness, and mental retardation. For this reason the federal government and many states support programs to immunize women against rubella before they have children. There has been a resurgence of congenital rubella in the early 1990s and more widespread screening for rubella serology is recommended.

The role of serologic testing for antibodies to rubella is different in different clinical settings. The simplest and most straight forward application is an assessment of immunity. If a woman has antibodies against rubella, there should be no concern about infection during subsequent pregnancy. If she is not immune, and is not pregnant, she should receive the rubella vaccine.

This test may also be used in the management of a pregnant woman who has been exposed to rubella. In this situation, it must be determined if the patient is susceptible, has an acute infection, and evaluate the risk to the fetus. Management of such a case requires individualized expert consultation.

An infant born with an illness which may be congenital rubella should also be evaluated for rubella titers. Problems here include evaluation of whether antibody represents passively acquired immunity by transplacental passage or is indicative of true neonatal infection. In this setting, determination of the immunoglobulin class is particularly important, since IgM antibodies do not pass the placental barrier. The presence of rubella-specific IgM antibody strongly supports congenital infection.

Footnotes

1. Linder N, Sirota L, Aboudy Y, et al, "Placental Transfer of Maternal Rubella Antibodies to Full-Term and Preterm Infants," *Infection*, 1999, 27(3):203-7.
2. Thomas HIJ, Morgan-Capner P, Roberts A, et al, "Persistent Rubella-Specific IgM Reactivity in the Absence of Recent Primary Rubella and Rubella Reinfection," *J Med Virol*, 1992, 36:188-92.

References

Bar-Oz B, Ford-Jones L, and Koren G, "Congenital Rubella Syndrome. How Can We Do Better?" *Can Fam Physician*, 1999, 45:1865-9.

Bullens D, Smets K, and Vanhaesebrouck P, "Congenital Rubella Syndrome After Maternal Reinfection," *Clin Pediatr (Phila)*, 2000, 39(2):113-6.

Craig SC, Broughton G 2nd, Bean J, et al, "Rubella Outbreak, Fort Bragg, North Carolina, 1995: A Clash of Preventive Strategies," *Milit Med*, 1999, 164(9):616-8.

"Consensus Conference on Measles," *Can Commun Dis Rep*, 1993, 19(10):72-9.

Ghidini A and Lynch L, "Prenatal Diagnosis and Significance of Fetal Infections," *West J Med*, 1993, 159(3):366-73.

Skendzel LP, "Rubella Immunity. Defining the Level of Protective Antibody," *Am J Clin Pathol*, 1996, 106(2):170-4.

Internet Web Sites

www.astdhpphe.org/infect/rubella.html

Rubella Virus Culture

Related Information

Rubella Serology *on page 677*

Viral Culture *on page 689*

Synonyms German Measles Culture; Measles Culture, 3-Day; Three-Day Measles Culture

Test Includes Isolation and identification of rubella virus in cell culture; detection of an outbreak of rubella infections

Abstract Rubella infection was one of the viral diseases targeted by the CDC for eradication by the end of the year 2000, because it is specifically a human disease with no animal reservoir.[1] In the United States, the incidence of rubella infections has been very low since 1994. This has been primarily due to the wide use of mumps-measles-rubella (MMR) immunization in children. However, several recent outbreaks of rubella have occurred in populations which were not vaccinated, such as people who have immigrated to the United States from countries in which vaccination for rubella is not common.[2,3] Culture for rubella is used to identify an outbreak in conjunction with specific rubella serology.

Specimen Two throat swabs, 10 mL urine, cerebrospinal fluid, tissues, amniotic fluid

Container Sterile container or viral transport medium

Sampling Time Virus is more likely to be isolated if specimen is collected within 5 days after onset of illness.

Storage Instructions Specimens should not be stored. Specimens should be delivered immediately to the laboratory. If unavoidable delays occur the specimen can be stored at 4°C for up to 3 days, but there is a loss of infectivity when culture is delayed.

Turnaround Time Positive cultures are usually detected in 3-7 days.

Reference Interval No virus isolated

Critical Values Any positive culture, especially from amniotic fluid. **All positive cultures should be immediately reported to the state health department.**

Use Aid in the diagnosis of disease caused by rubella virus

Limitations Because of the length of time for positive detection, the isolation of rubella virus is usually of little help in the diagnosis of rubella. Exceptions may be in cases of severe rubella complications, epidemiological purposes, and fatality. Serological diagnosis is much more useful.

Methodology Cell culture, isolation, and confirmation/identification by antibody-specific neutralization

Additional Information Pregnant women, who become infected with rubella, have a very high risk of the virus crossing the placenta and infecting the fetus. Congenital rubella infections have disastrous effects, causing fetal death, premature delivery, and severe congenital defects including deafness and congenital heart disease. Neonates with congenital rubella excrete rubella virus in nasopharyngeal secretions and urine for many months after birth. These children pose a risk to susceptible pregnant women.[4] Serology is available for diagnostic purposes. Usually immune status can be determined by examining a single serum sample.

Footnotes

1. Fenner F, "Candidate Viral Diseases for Elimination or Eradication," *Bull World Health Organ*, 1998, 76(Suppl 2):68-70.
2. Centers for Disease Control, "Rubella Outbreak - Westchester County, New York, 1997-1998," *MMWR Morb Mortal Wkly Rep*, 1999, 48(26):560-3.
3. Centers for Disease Control, "Rubella Among Hispanic Adults - Kansas, 1998, and Nebraska, 1999," *MMWR Morb Mortal Wkly Rep*, 2000, 49(11):225-8.
4. Herrman KL, "Rubella Virus," *Laboratory Diagnosis of Viral Infections*, Lennette EH, ed, New York, NY: Marcel Dekker Inc, 1992, 731-47.

References

Chernesky MA and Mahony JB, "Rubella Virus," *Manual of Clinical Microbiology*, 7th ed, Murray PR, Baron EJ, Pfaller MA, et al, eds, Washington, DC: AMS Press, American Society for Microbiology, 1999, 964-9.

Internet Web Sites

www.astdhpphe.org/infect/rubella.html

Schistosomiasis Serology

Related Information

Ova and Parasites, Stool *on page 666*

Ova and Parasites, Urine *on page 667*

Urinalysis *on page 887*

Urinary Tract Cytology *on page 389*

Synonyms Bilharziasis

Applies to Flukes; Intestinal Helminths

Abstract In excess of 250 million people have schistosomiasis (bilharziasis) and it is associated with death in 200,000 cases per year.[1] The three major species of these blood flukes are *Schistosoma haematobium*, *S. mansoni*, and *S. japonicum*. **Identification of ova in rectal or bladder biopsy is definitive.**

Specimen Serum

Container Red top tube

Reference Interval Negative

Use Support a clinical diagnosis of schistosomiasis in selected cases

Limitations Serological testing does not differentiate between recently acquired infection and chronic multiple exposures and so is simply reported as positive or negative. Test does not differentiate between intestinal and vesical schistosomiasis. Serologic diagnosis is now sensitive and specific, but its present role in clinical decision making appears limited to instances in which ova cannot be found in fecal or urine specimens, or rectal or vesical biopsy. Cross-reactions with other helminths such as *Ancylostoma* species and *Ascaris lumbricoides* can occur.

Methodology Indirect fluorescent antibody (IFA) using sections of adult worms, enzyme-linked immunosorbent assay (ELISA) with egg antigen, indirect hemagglutination (IHA). An immunoblot test has recently been used to differentiate recent from chronic schistosomiasis from *Schistosoma mansoni*.[2]

Additional Information Schistosomiasis worldwide is one of the greatest public health challenges, and one of the most common parasitic diseases (the most common cause of hematuria, for example). The details of protective immunity to *Schistosoma* species infection are not fully understood or defined, thus, the **demonstration of eggs in bladder or bowel biopsy** is a more sensitive and definitive test. *Schistosoma mansoni* ova in tissue sections are acid-fast.[3] Their broad lateral spines are characteristic. **The examination of stool and urine for eggs is a mainstay of diagnosis.**

Eosinophil counts add little to screening and are inferior to stool examination and serology.[4]

A photomicrograph of an ovum of *Schistosoma haematobium* in urine sediment, with its characteristic terminal spine, was recently published.[5]

Footnotes
1. Lucey DR and Maquire JH, "Schistosomiasis," *Infect Dis Clin North Am*, 1993, 7:635-53.
2. Valli LC, Kanamura HY, DaSilva RM, et al, "*Schistosomiasis mansoni*: Immunoblot Analysis to Diagnose and Differentiate Recent and Chronic Infection," *Am J Trop Med Hyg*, 1999, 61(2):302-7.
3. Recht LD and Louis DN, "A 30-Year-Old Man With a Generalized Tonic-Clonic Seizure and a Left Temporal-Lobe Mass," Case Records of the Massachusetts General Hospital, Case 39-1969, Scully RE, Mark EJ, McNeely WF, et al, eds, *N Engl J Med*, 1996, 335(25):1906-14.
4. Libman MD, Mac Lean JD, and Gyorkos TW, "Screening for Schistosomiasis, Filariasis, and Strongyloidiasis Among Expatriates Returning From the Tropics," *Clin Infect Dis*, 1993, 17(3):353-9.
5. Kaplan BS and Meyers K, Images in Clinical Medicine, "*Schistosoma haematobium*," *N Engl J Med*, 2000, 3443(15):1085.

References
Blute RD Jr and Oliva E, "A 32-Year-Old Man With a Lesion of the Urinary Bladder," Case Records of the Massachusetts General Hospital, Case 31-2000, Scully RE, Mark EJ, McNeely WF, et al, eds, *N Engl J Med*, 2000, 343(15):1105-11.
Hamilton JV, Klinkert M, and Doenhoff MJ, "Diagnosis of Schistosomiasis: Antibody Detection, With Notes on Parasitological and Antigen Detection Methods," *Parasitology*, 1998, 117(S1):41-57.
Hernandez MG, Hafalla JC, Acosta LP, et al, "Paramyosin Is a Major Target of the Human IgA Response Against *Schistosoma japonicum*," *Parasite Immunol*, 1999, 21(12):641-7.
Li YS, Ross AG, Sleigh AC, et al, "Antibody Isotype Responses, Infection, and Reinfection for *Schistosoma japonicum* in a Marshland Area of China," *Acta Trop*, 1999, 73(2):79-92.
Salah F, Demerdash Z, Shaker Z, et al, "A Monoclonal Antibody Against *Schistosoma haematobium* Soluble Egg Antigen: Efficacy for Diagnosis and Monitoring of Cure of *S. haematobium* Infection," *Parasitol Res*, 2000, 86(1):74-80.
Woolhouse ME and Hagan P, "Seeking the Ghost of Worms Past," *Nat Med*, 1999, 5(11):1225-7.

Internet Web Sites
www.cdc.gov/ncidod/dpd/parasites/schistosomiasis/default.htm
www.who.int/health-topics/schisto.htm

Serum Bactericidal Test

Related Information
Antimicrobial Susceptibility Testing, Aerobic and Facultatively Anaerobic Bacteria *on page 554*
Antimicrobial Susceptibility Testing, Antimicrobial Combinations *on page 556*

Synonyms Antibacterial Activity, Serum; Bacterial Inhibitory Level, Serum; Maximum Bactericidal Dilution; MBD; Schlichter Test; Serum Antibacterial Titer; Serum Bactericidal Level; Serum Inhibitory Titer; Susceptibility Testing, Serum Bactericidal Dilution Method

Applies to SBD; Serum Bactericidal Dilution; Serum Inhibitory Dilution; SID

Test Includes Assay of serum or body fluid for antimicrobial activity

Abstract This method is used to assess bactericidal activity of serum from patients treated for critical infections, such as endocarditis or osteomyelitis, or for the assessment of new antimicrobial agents. A recent study examined the reproducibility of this assay and found that 94% were reproducible ± one dilution.[1]

Patient Preparation Sterile aspiration of body fluid

Specimen Peak and trough serum from patient and bacterial isolate causing infection (prepared by laboratory)

Container Red top tube; sterile tube for body fluid

Sampling Time Both peak and trough levels should be obtained. The peak level is the level 60 minutes after completing an intravenous or intramuscular dose and 90 minutes after an oral dose.[2] With vancomycin, the peak occurs 2 hours after an intravenous dose. Trough levels are obtained immediately before the next dose. If more than one antibiotic is administered, an attempt should be made to draw the peak and trough specimens around a dose when antibiotics are administered simultaneously. If this is not feasible, draw the specimens around the dose of the more frequently administered agent.

Collection Specimen should be transported to the laboratory within 1 hour of collection. Label specimens with time and date collected, time of last antimicrobial infusion (start and completion of infusion), and whether the specimen is a peak or trough.

Storage Instructions Separate serum from cells and freeze at -70°C if test will not be performed within 2 hours.

Causes for Rejection Bacterial isolate discarded before request for bactericidal testing, serum specimen allowed to sit at room temperature for more than 2 hours

Turnaround Time 2-3 days

Special Instructions If a serum bactericidal test is desired, the physician should request that the laboratory save the patient's isolate within 48 hours of submission of the specimen for initial culture. **If the isolate has not been saved, the test cannot be performed.** The laboratory should be informed of current antibiotic therapy including date and time of last dosage, route of administration on all antimicrobial agents patient is receiving, and clinical diagnosis.

Reference Interval Peak and trough titers ≥1:32 and ≥1:8, respectively, are considered adequate. Peak and trough titers ≤1:2 are considered inadequate. Titers between these ranges are considered intermediate.[2]

Use Determine the maximum bactericidal dilution (MBD) and/or serum bactericidal dilution (SBD) of serum or body fluid after administration of antibiotic(s). This is the last serum/body fluid dilution which is bactericidal for the patient's infecting organism. This titer is useful in monitoring total therapeutic effect. Frequently, it is used to evaluate the adequacy of therapy in endocarditis, osteomyelitis, and suppurative arthritis.[3,4]

The serum bactericidal test has been applied experimentally to detect antimicrobial activity in cerebrospinal fluid, joint fluid, and amniotic fluid. It is also useful in determining whether serum antimicrobial activity remains adequate after a shift from parenteral to oral therapy. Serum bactericidal titers are useful in evaluation of synergy between antibiotics after administration of the drugs.

Limitations Technical and biological variables affecting test performance make interpretation of test results difficult. Some antimicrobial agents lose activity quickly at room temperature and if not stored appropriately, the assay results are not accurate.

Methodology Serial dilution of patient's serum with Mueller-Hinton broth, 1:1 final ratio recommended, supplemented if necessary. Each dilution is incubated with a standard inoculum of the patient's isolate and assessed for inhibitory and bactericidal activity.[2]

Additional Information Results reflect the combined effect of all antimicrobial agents present in the patient's serum (or body fluid) on the infecting organism(s). Results are accurate to ±1 dilution. Maximum inhibitory dilution (MID) or serum inhibitory dilution (SID) may also be reported. An apparently adequate ratio may represent a highly susceptible organism responding to a relatively low blood level or a moderately resistant organism responding to an unexpectedly high blood level. A serum inhibitory titer might suggest an adequate therapeutic level but would give no clue to potential toxicity, when an extremely narrow margin exists between a therapeutically adequate dose and a possibly toxic one (eg, aminoglycosides).

Footnotes
1. Hacek DM, Dressel DC, and Peterson LR, "Highly Reproducible Bactericidal Activity Test Results by Using a Modified National Committee for Clinical Laboratory Standards for Broth Macrodilution Technique," *J Clin Microbiol*, 1999, 37(6):1881-4.
2. National Committee for Clinical Laboratory Standards, *Methodology for the Serum Bactericidal Test, Approved Guideline M21-A*, in press, Villanova, PA: National Committee for Clinical Laboratory Standards, 2000.
3. Peltola H, Unkila-Kallio L, and Kallio MJ, "Simplified Treatment of Acute Staphylococcal Osteomyelitis of Childhood. The Finnish Study Group," *Pediatrics*, 1997, 99(6):846-50.
4. Somekh E, Heifets L, Dan M, et al, "Penetration and Bactericidal Activity of Cefixime in Synovial Fluid," *Antimicrob Agents Chemother*, 1996, 40(5):1198-200.

References
Dan M, Zabeeda D, and Poch F, "Comparative Serum Bactericidal Activity Against *Pseudomonas aeruginosa* of Six Antipseudomonal Agents," *Chemotherapy*, 1995, 41(5):323-9.
Schaadt RD, Batts DH, Daley-Yates PT, et al, "Serum Inhibitory Titers and Serum Bactericidal Titers for Human Subjects Receiving Multiple Doses of the Antimicrobial
(Continued)

Serum Bactericidal Test (Continued)

Oxazolidinone Eperezolid and Linezolid," *Diagn Microbiol Infect Dis*, 1997, 28(4):201-4.

Schentag JJ, "Antimicrobial Action and Pharmacokinetics/Pharmacodynamics: The Use of AUIC to Improve Efficacy and Avoid Resistance," *J Chemother*, 1999, 11(6):426-39.

Schentag JJ, Birmingham MC, Paladino JA, et al, "In Nosocomial Pneumonia, Optimizing Antibiotics Other Than Aminoglycosides Is a More Important Determinant of Successful Clinical Outcome and a Better Means of Avoiding Resistance," *Semin Respir Infect*, 1997, 12(4):278-93.

◆ **Serum Cryptococcal Latex Agglutination** *see* Cryptococcal Antigen Titer *on page 595*

◆ **Serum Hepatitis Marker** *replaced by* Hepatitis B Surface Antigen *on page 625*

◆ **Serum Inhibitory Dilution** *see* Serum Bactericidal Test *on page 679*

◆ **Serum Inhibitory Titer** *see* Serum Bactericidal Test *on page 679*

◆ **Shell Vial Culture, Adenovirus** *see* Adenovirus Culture *on page 552*

◆ **Shiga Toxins** *see* Bacterial Culture, Stool *on page 575*

Shiga Toxin Test, Direct

Related Information
Bacterial Culture, Stool *on page 575*
Clostridium difficile Toxin Assay and Culture *on page 592*

Synonyms Verotoxin Detection

Applies to Lysogenic Bacteriophages

Test Includes Detection of *E. coli* O157:H7 by assay for the Shiga-like toxin directly in stool or after isolation of a bacterial isolate

Abstract In the late 1970s, the *E. coli* serotype O157:H7 was recognized as a human pathogen and was associated with severe bloody diarrhea and the hemolytic-uremic syndrome. This serotype of *E. coli* bacteria produces a Shiga-like toxin that is similar to the Shiga toxin expressed by *Shigella dysenteriae*.[1] The production of the toxin, or the genes encoding the toxin, can be detected by a variety of methods, and some are commercially available.

Specimen Stool, food, or bacterial isolate

Container Sterile container

Reference Interval No toxin detected

Critical Values Positive detection of Shiga-like toxin

Use The toxin assay can be used to detect toxin-producing strains after they have been isolated,[2] directly from patient specimens such as stool,[3] directly from food (especially meat),[4] or from fecal specimens of food animals such as cattle.[5]

Limitations These assays are still new and have not been fully evaluated in the routine clinical laboratory. Results from such assays should be confirmed by the isolation of a Shiga-toxin producing *E. coli*. Some of the commercial assays may have false-positive results with *Pseudomonas aeruginosa*.[6]

Methodology There are a variety of methods available, from enzyme immunoassays (EIA)[1,6] and latex agglutination,[2] to genetic detection methods.[3,4,5]

Additional Information Certain strains of *E. coli* have the ability to produce toxins (verotoxins or Shiga-like toxins) that closely resemble the Shiga toxin of *Shigella dysenteriae*. Two distinct toxins, Shiga toxin 1 (stx1) and Shiga toxin 2 (stx2), have been identified. Any individual isolate may produce either the stx1 or the stx2, or both.[1] The genes of both toxins are encoded on lysogenic bacteriophages which may play a role in the spread of the Shiga toxin to other *E. coli*, as well as other members of the *Enterobacteriaceae* family.[7] The detection of this toxin or the genes required for toxin production can be used to predict the presence of this bacteria.

Since *E. coli* isolates that produce the Shiga-like toxin are associated with severe hemorrhagic colitis and/or the life-threatening hemolytic uremic syndrome (HUS), any laboratory detection of this toxin should be considered clinically important and should be immediately reported to the attending physician and the state health department.

Footnotes

1. Nataro JP and Kaper JB, "Diarrheagenic *Escherichia coli*," *Clin Microbiol Rev*, 1998, 11(1):142-201.

2. Karmali MA, Petric M, and Bielaszewska M, "Evaluation of a Microplate Latex Agglutination Method (Verotoxin Assay) for Detecting and Characterizing Verotoxins (Shiga Toxins) From *Escherichia coli*," *J Clin Microbiol*, 1999, 37(2):396-9.

3. Louie M, Read S, Simor AE, et al, "Application of Multiplex PCR for Detection of Non-O157 Verocytotoxin-Producing *Escherichia coli* in Bloody Stools: Identification of Serogroups O26 and O111," *J Clin Microbiol*, 1998, 36(11):3375-7.

4. Gilgen M, Hubner P, Hofelein C, et al, "PCR-Based Detection of Verotoxin-Producing *Escherichia coli* (VTEC) in Ground Beef," *Res Microbiol*, 1998, 149(2):145-54.

5. Chen S, Xu R, Yee A, et al, "An Automated Fluorescent PCR Method for Detection of Shiga Toxin-Producing *Escherichia coli* in Foods," *Appl Environ Microbiol*, 1998, 64(11):4210-6.

6. Kehl KS, Havens P, Behnke CE, et al, "Evaluation of the Premier EHEC Assay for Detection of Shiga Toxin-Producing *Escherichia coli*," *J Clin Microbiol*, 1997, 35(8):2051-4.

7. Beutin L, Zimmermann S, and Gleier K, "Human Infections With Shiga Toxin-Producing *Escherichia coli* Other Than Serogroup O157 in Germany," *Emerg Infect Dis*, 1998, 4(4):635-9.

References

Acheson DWK and Jaeger JL, "Shiga Toxin-Producing *Escherichia coli*," *Clin Microbiol*, 1999, 21(23):183-8.

Banatvala N, DeBeukelaer MM, Griffin PM, et al, "Shiga-Like Toxin-Producing *Escherichia coli* O111 and Associated Hemolytic-Uremic Syndrome: A Family Outbreak," *Pediatr Infect Dis J*, 1996, 15(11):1008-11.

Bolton FJ and Aird H, "Verocytotoxin-Producing *Escherichia coli* O157: Public Health and Microbiological Significance," *Br J Biomed Sci*, 1998, 55(2):127-35.

Kawamura N, Yamazaki T, and Tamai H, "Risk Factors for the Development of *Escherichia coli* O157:H7 Associated With Hemolytic Uremic Syndrome," *Pediatr Intern*, 1999, 41(2):218-22.

Paton JC and Paton AW, "Pathogenesis and Diagnosis of Shiga Toxin-Producing *Escherichia coli* Infections," *Clin Microbiol Rev*, 1998, 11(3):450-79.

Internet Web Sites

vm.cfsan.fda.gov/~mow/chap15.html
www.amm.co.uk/pubs/fa_vte.htm

◆ ***Shigella*** *see* Bacterial Culture, Stool *on page 575*

◆ **Shingles Culture** *see* Varicella-Zoster Virus Culture *on page 686*

◆ **SID** *see* Serum Bactericidal Test *on page 679*

◆ **Sin Nombre Hantavirus** *see* Hantavirus Serology *on page 619*

◆ **Skin Burn Culture, Quantitative** *see* Bacterial Culture, Burn Sites *on page 569*

◆ **Skin Fungus Culture** *see* Fungal Culture, Skin *on page 612*

◆ **Skin Mycobacteria Culture** *see* Mycobacterial Culture, Cutaneous and Subcutaneous Tissue *on page 657*

◆ **Skin Scrapings for *Sarcoptes scabiei* Identification** *see* Arthropod Identification *on page 559*

◆ **Skin Viral Disease** *see* Electron Microscopic Examination for Viruses, Stool *on page 603*

◆ **Snowshoe Hare Virus** *see* California Encephalitis Virus Serology *on page 587*

◆ **Spherulin®** *see* Coccidioidomycosis Serology *on page 593*

◆ **Spiders** *see* Arthropod Identification *on page 559*

◆ **Spinal Fluid Culture** *see* Bacterial Culture, Cerebrospinal Fluid *on page 569*

◆ **Spinal Fluid Fungus Culture** *see* Fungal Culture, Cerebrospinal Fluid *on page 611*

◆ **Spinal Fluid Mycobacteria Culture** *see* Mycobacterial Culture, Cerebrospinal Fluid *on page 656*

Sporotrichosis Serology

Related Information
Fungal Culture, Biopsy or Body Fluid *on page 610*
Fungal Culture, Sputum *on page 613*
Fungus Smear, Stain *on page 615*
Skin Biopsy *on page 71*

Abstract Sporotrichosis is a fungal disease classically beginning in the distal extremity, often at a site of inoculation as a painless papule. It spreads proximally, involving lymphatics (lymphangitic sporotrichosis). The organisms in tissue and in 37°C culture exist as small oval to round yeast with single or multiple buds. They are often difficult or impossible to see in tissue sections. Extracutaneous disease includes monarticular arthritis. Pulmonary sporotrichosis is much less frequently found than osteoarticular infection. **Optimally, diagnosis is made by culture of biopsy material, rather than by culture of drainage or by serology.**[1]

Specimen Serum or cerebrospinal fluid

Container Red top tube; sterile CSF tube

Reference Interval Latex agglutinating titer: <1:4; ELISA: <1:16 in serum, <1:8 in CSF. Depending upon laboratory and method, antibody titers up to 1:40 may be found in normal subjects.

Critical Values Titer ≥1:4 may provide evidence for sporotrichosis. Titers greater than 1:128, rising titers, and persistent elevation are common with pulmonary or systemic disease. Positive reaction in CSF is diagnostic, and is particularly useful in chronic meningitis caused by this organism, which is difficult to culture from spinal fluid.

Use Support the diagnosis of sporotrichosis, especially extracutaneous disease

Limitations A negative test result does not rule out infection. Serial titers are not prognostically useful. There are occasional low titer false positives from nonfungal disease. This test is not widely available and is not standardized.

Methodology Tube agglutination, latex agglutination (LA), enzyme-linked immunosorbent assay (ELISA), immunoblot analysis

Additional Information Sporotrichosis is usually acquired by traumatic implantation of the dimorphic fungus *Sporothrix schenckii*, a plant saprophyte. Rose gardening, sphagnum moss, and hay bales have been implicated in some cases.[2,3] The disease is found in gardeners and florists, among others. The first signs of infection appear after an average incubation period of 3 weeks; the initial lesion may appear as a small ulcer or a small, hard movable, nontender and nonattached subcutaneous nodule. Disease progresses along lymphatic channels that drain the area of the initial lesion. Less frequent forms of sporotrichosis include pulmonary, osteoarticular, central nervous system, and disseminated disease. Immunosuppression, including the acquired immunodeficiency syndrome (AIDS), increases the probability of hematogenous dissemination, particularly to skin and bone.

False-negative cultures are not unknown.

The clinical differential diagnosis of **nodular lymphangitis** includes sporotrichosis, as well as *Nocardia brasiliensis*, *Mycobacterium kansasii*, *Mycobacterium marinum*, *Leishmania braziliensis*, and *Francisella tularensis*.[4]

Footnotes

1. Schell WA, Salkin IF, Pasarell L, et al, "*Bipolaris*, *Exophiala*, *Scedosporium*, *Sporothrix* and Other Dematiaceous Fungi," *Manual of Clinical Microbiology*, 7th ed, Murray PR, Baron EJ, Pfaller MA, et al, eds, Washington, DC: AMS Press, American Society for Microbiology, 1999, 1295-1317.
2. Hajjeh R, McDonnell S, Reef S, et al, "Outbreak of Sporotrichosis Among Tree Nursery Workers," *J Infect Dis*, 1997, 176(2):499-504.
3. Dooley DP, Bostic PS, and Beckius ML, "Spook House Sporotrichosis. A Point-Source Outbreak of Sporotrichosis Associated With Hay Bale Props in a Halloween Haunted-House," *Arch Intern Med*, 1997, 157(16):1885-7.
4. Smego RA Jr, Castiglia M, and Asperilla MO, "Lymphocutaneous Syndrome. A Review of Non-Sporothrix Causes," *Medicine (Baltimore)*, 1999, 78(1):38-63.

References

Bennett JE, "*Sporothrix schenckii*," *Principles and Practice of Infectious Diseases*, 3rd ed, Mandell GL, Douglas RG Jr, and Bennett JE, eds, New York, NY: Churchill Livingstone, 1990, 1972-5.

Davis BA, "Sporotrichosis," *Dermatol Clin*, 1996, 14(1):69-76.

Purvis RS, Diven DG, Drechsel RD, et al, "Sporotrichosis Presenting as Arthritis and Subcutaneous Nodules," *J Am Acad Dermatol*, 1993, 28(5 Pt 2):879-84.

Werner AH and Werner BE, "Sporotrichosis in Man and Animal," *Int J Dermatol*, 1994, 33(10):692-700.

Wescott BL, Nasser A, and Jarolim DR, "*Sporothrix* Meningitis," *Nurse Pract*, 1999, 24(2):90-8

Internet Web Sites

www.cdc.gov/ncidod/dbmd/diseaseinfo/sporotrichosis_g.htm

♦ **Sputum Culture** *see* Bacterial Culture, Sputum *on page 574*

♦ **Sputum Fungus Culture** *see* Fungal Culture, Sputum *on page 613*

♦ **Sputum Mycobacteria Culture** *see* Mycobacterial Culture, Sputum *on page 658*

♦ **Sputum *Nocardia* Culture** *see Nocardia* Culture *on page 665*

♦ **S. sapronophyticus** *see* Bacterial Culture, Urine *on page 578*

♦ **S. suihominis** *see Cryptosporidium* Direct Staining Procedures *on page 596*

♦ **Staphylococcal Food Poisoning** *see* Bacterial Culture, Stool *on page 575*

♦ **Staphylococcus aureus** *see* Bacterial Culture, Aerobes *on page 563*

♦ **Staphylococcus aureus** *see* Bacterial Culture, Bronchoscopy/Bronchial Brush/Bronchoalveolar Lavage Specimen *on page 568*

♦ **Staphylococcus aureus** *see* Bacterial Culture, Conjunctiva *on page 570*

♦ **Staphylococcus aureus** *see* Bacterial Culture, Sputum *on page 574*

♦ **Staphylococcus aureus** *see* Bacterial Culture, Urine *on page 578*

♦ **Staphylococcus aureus** *see* Bacterial Culture, Wounds, Bites *on page 579*

Sterility Culture

Synonyms Autoclave Sterility Check

Abstract

Methods of Sterilization and Disinfection include:
- Moist heat is used in autoclaves, utilizing steam under pressure.
- Dry heat ovens can sterilize items such as glassware.
- Chemical agents such as ethylene oxide can be used to sterilize heat-sensitive structures, and other substances can be used as well.
- Boiling at 100°C for 15 minutes.
- Pasteurization destroys food pathogens.
- Ionizing radiation[1]

The sterilization process should be monitored by biological methods.

Specimen Three strips (one control and two test strips); Attest® biologic indicator tube

Container Sterility test envelope

Collection The two test strips should be placed separately in the center of the two largest packs, in the largest loads or in areas of the load that is least likely to come up to sterilizing temperature. Do not place the strips on open shelves, on the peripheral, or the exterior surface of a pack.

Special Instructions One strip (control strip) must not be autoclaved or steam sterilized. The two other strips (test strips) must be placed in the center of the load to be sterilized.

Reference Interval No growth in test strips; growth in control strip

Use Confirm that adequate sterilization conditions have been attained; sterilizer function check

Limitations Manufacturers instructions should be followed carefully. It may be necessary to add water (500 mL) to sealed plastic biohazard bags. See bag manufacturer's instructions.

Methodology Indicator strips impregnated with spores of *Bacillus stearothermophilus* are used with steam autoclaves, and *Bacillus subtilis* variety *niger* are used for ethylene oxide sterilizers.

Additional Information Biological indicators must be used at least once weekly with the steam autoclaves and in every load with the ethylene oxide sterilizer.

The following citations are only introductory.

Footnotes

1. Forbes BA, Sahm DF, and Weissfeld AS, "Laboratory Safety," *Bailey and Scott's Diagnostic Microbiology*, 10th ed, Chapter 2, St Louis, MO: Mosby, 1998, 20-38.

References

Allison DG, "A Review: Taking the Sterile Out of Sterility," *J Appl Microbiol*, 1999, 87(6):789-93.

Isenberg HD, ed, "Autoclave (Steam Sterilizer)," *Essential Procedures for Clinical Microbiology*, Washington, DC: ASM American Society for Microbiology, 1998, 712-4.

Isenberg HD, ed, "Culture of Biological Indicators of Sterilization Processes," *Essential Procedures for Clinical Microbiology*, Washington, DC: ASM American Society for Microbiology, 1998, 684-92.

Peacock R, "Ethylene Oxide Sterilization: The Way Ahead," *Med Device Technol*, 1999, 10(6):24-6.

Reichert M and Schultz JK, "Is it Sterile? How Do You Know?" *OR Manager*, 1999, 15(10):32-2.

Rutala WA, "Disinfection, Sterilization, and Waste Disposal," *Prevention and Control of Nosocomial Infections*, 2nd ed, Wenzel RP, ed, Baltimore, MD: Lippincott Williams & Wilkins, 1993, 460-95.

♦ **St Louis Encephalitis Virus** *see* Encephalitis Viral Serology *on page 604*

St Louis Encephalitis Virus Serology

Related Information

Arthropod Identification *on page 559*
Bacterial Culture, Cerebrospinal Fluid *on page 569*
California Encephalitis Virus Serology *on page 587*
Cerebrospinal Fluid Analysis: Overview *on page 416*
Eastern Equine Encephalitis Virus Serology *on page 602*
Encephalitis Viral Serology *on page 604*
Viral Culture *on page 689*
Viral Culture, Central Nervous System Symptoms *on page 692*
Western Equine Encephalitis Virus Serology *on page 697*

Synonyms Encephalitis Virus Titer, St Louis

Applies to Arboviral Encephalitis Serology

Abstract St Louis encephalitis virus causes fever with headache, aseptic meningitis, and encephalitis. Viral transmission includes birds and mosquitoes. Severity of illness increases with age. Patients older than 60 years of age bear the highest frequency of encephalitis.

Specimen Serum or cerebrospinal fluid

Container Red top tube, sterile CSF tube

Sampling Time Acute and convalescent sera drawn 10-14 days apart are recommended.

Reference Interval A less than fourfold increase in titer in paired sera; HI titer: <1:10; CF titer: <1:8; plaque reduction: <70%; no IgM antibody in CSF

Use To support the diagnosis of St Louis encephalitis virus infection in individuals with CSF pleocytosis. The patient's age, season of the year, place of residence, and exposure are important in the differential diagnosis.

Limitations Cross reactivity between alphavirus group and flavivirus group; false reactions from yellow fever vaccination. (The yellow fever virus is found in the family Flaviviridae, as is the St Louis encephalitis virus.)

Methodology Complement fixation (CF), hemagglutination inhibition (HAI), indirect immunofluorescent antibody, enzyme-linked immunosorbent assay (ELISA) for IgM or IgG in CSF or serum antibodies

Additional Information Arboviruses, such as St Louis encephalitis, are the most frequent cause of epidemic encephalitides in the United States.[1] In the elderly, the disease may be confused with a cerebrovascular accident. In most cases, demonstration of IgM antibody in CSF rapidly establishes a diagnosis of arboviral encephalitis.

Footnotes

1. Day JF and Curtis GA, "Blood Feeding and Oviposition by Culex Nigripalpus (Diptera: Culicidae) Before, During, and After a Widespread St. Louis Encephalitis Virus Epidemic in Florida," *J Med Entomol*, 1999, 36(2):176-81.

References

Monath TP, "Flavivirus (Yellow Fever, Dengue, and St Louis Encephalitis)," *Principles and Practice of Infectious Diseases*, 3rd ed, Mandell GL, Douglas RG Jr, and Bennett JE, eds, New York, NY: Churchill Livingstone, 1990, 1248-51.

Tsai TF and Kuno G, "Arboviruses," *Manual of Clinical Laboratory Immunology*, 5th ed, Rose NR, Conway de Macario E, Folds JD, et al, eds, Washington, DC: ASM Press, American Society for Microbiology, 1997, 729-36.

Internet Web Sites

www.astdhpphe.org/infect/sle.html

(Continued)

St Louis Encephalitis Virus Serology *(Continued)*

www.cdc.gov/ncidod/dvbid/arbor/sle_qa.htm

- ◆ **Stool Culture** *see* Bacterial Culture, Stool *on page 575*
- ◆ **Stool Exam for Ova and Parasites** *see* Ova and Parasites, Stool *on page 666*
- ◆ **Stool Examination for *Cryptosporidium*** *see* Cryptosporidium Direct Staining Procedures *on page 596*
- ◆ **Stool Examination for Microsporidia** *see* Microsporidia Diagnostic Procedures *on page 652*
- ◆ **Stool Fungus Culture** *see* Fungal Culture, Stool *on page 614*
- ◆ **Stool Mycobacterial Culture** *see* Mycobacterial Culture, Stool *on page 659*
- ◆ **Strep Throat Screening Culture** *see* Bacterial Culture, Throat, and Antigen Detection Testing for Group A Streptococci *on page 577*
- ◆ ***Streptococcus agalactiae*** *see* Bacterial Culture, Cerebrospinal Fluid *on page 569*
- ◆ ***Streptococcus agalactiae* Latex Screen** *see* Group B *Streptococcus* Screen, Rapid *on page 618*
- ◆ ***Streptococcus* β-Hemolytic Group A** *see* Bacterial Culture, Sputum *on page 574*
- ◆ ***Streptococcus* Group A Latex Screen** *see* Group A *Streptococcus* Screen, Rapid *on page 617*
- ◆ ***Streptococcus* Group B Latex Screen** *see* Group B *Streptococcus* Screen, Rapid *on page 618*
- ◆ ***Streptococcus pneumoniae*** *see* Bacterial Culture, Bronchoscopy/Bronchial Brush/Bronchoalveolar Lavage Specimen *on page 568*
- ◆ ***Streptococcus pneumoniae*** *see* Bacterial Culture, Cerebrospinal Fluid *on page 569*
- ◆ ***Streptococcus pneumoniae*** *see* Bacterial Culture, Conjunctiva *on page 570*
- ◆ ***Streptococcus pneumoniae*** *see* Bacterial Culture, Middle Ear *on page 573*
- ◆ ***Streptococcus pneumoniae*** *see* Bacterial Culture, Sputum *on page 574*
- ◆ ***Streptococcus pyogenes*** *see* Bacterial Culture, Conjunctiva *on page 570*
- ◆ ***Streptococcus pyogenes*** *see* Bacterial Culture, Wounds, Bites *on page 579*
- ◆ ***Streptococcus pyogenes* Culture** *see* Bacterial Culture, Throat, and Antigen Detection Testing for Group A Streptococci *on page 577*
- ◆ **Streptodornase** *see* Antideoxyribonuclease-B Titer, Serum *on page 554*

Streptozyme

Related Information
Antideoxyribonuclease-B Titer, Serum *on page 554*
Antistreptolysin O Titer, Serum *on page 559*
Bacterial Culture, Throat, and Antigen Detection Testing for Group A Streptococci *on page 577*

Abstract Streptozyme is one of the serologic tests which detect immune response to extracellular products of *S. pyogenes*.[1]

Specimen Serum

Container Red top tube

Reference Interval <100 streptozyme units

Use Screening for antibodies to streptococcal antigens NADase, DNase, streptokinase, streptolysin O, and hyaluronidase. With throat culture (the most useful laboratory test for pharyngitis/tonsillitis),[2] this test is useful for evaluation of patients suspected of having poststreptococcal sequelae. They include rheumatic fever following *Streptococcus pyogenes* infection.

Limitations A single determination is less useful than a series. May not be as sensitive in children as in adults. A disadvantage of the test is that borderline antibody elevations, which could be clinically significant particularly in children, may not be detected.

Methodology Hemagglutination

Additional Information Streptozyme is a screening test for antibodies to several streptococcal antigens. It has the advantages of detecting several antibodies in a single assay (although which one has been detected cannot be ascertained), of being technically quick and easy, and of being unaffected by several factors producing false positives in the ASO test. A serially rising titer is more significant than a single determination.

Footnotes
1. Ruoff K, Whiley RA, and Beighton D, "*Streptococcus*," *Manual of Clinical Microbiology*, 7th ed, Chapter 17, Murray PR, Baron EJ, Pfaller MA, et al, eds, Washington, DC: ASM Press, American Society for Microbiology, 1999, 283-96.
2. Todd JK, "Group A *Streptococcus*," *Nelson Textbook of Pediatrics*, 16th ed, Chapter 184, Behrman RE, Kliegman RM, and Jenson HB, eds, Philadelphia, PA: WB Saunders Co, 2000, 802-10.

References
Ayoub EM and Harden E, "Immune Response to Streptococcal Antigens: Diagnostic Methods," *Manual of Clinical Laboratory Immunology*, 5th ed, Rose NR, Conway de Macario E, Folds JD, et al, eds, Washington, DC: ASM Press, American Society for Microbiology, 1997, 450-7.
Bisno AL, "Group A Streptococcal Infections and Acute Rheumatic Fever," *N Engl J Med*, 1991, 325(11):783-93.

Internet Web Sites
www.astdhpphe.org/infect/strepa.html
www.cdc.gov/ncidod/dbmd/diseaseinfo/groupastreptococcal_g.htm

- ◆ ***Strongyloides stercoralis*** *see* Ova and Parasites, Stool *on page 666*
- ◆ **Sudden Death Syndrome** *see* Botulism Diagnostic Procedures *on page 585*
- ◆ **Surgical Wound Culture** *see* Bacterial Culture, Wounds, Bites *on page 579*
- ◆ **Susceptibility of HIV-1 Virus to Antiviral Therapy** *see* Human Immunodeficiency Virus, Resistance (Susceptibility) Testing *on page 640*
- ◆ **Susceptibility Testing Aerobic and Facultatively Anaerobic Organisms** *see* Antimicrobial Susceptibility Testing, Aerobic and Facultatively Anaerobic Bacteria *on page 554*
- ◆ **Susceptibility Testing, Anaerobic Bacteria** *see* Antimicrobial Susceptibility Testing, Anaerobic Bacteria *on page 555*
- ◆ **Susceptibility Testing, Antimicrobial Combinations** *see* Antimicrobial Susceptibility Testing, Antimicrobial Combinations *on page 556*
- ◆ **Susceptibility Testing, Fungi** *see* Antimicrobial Susceptibility Testing, Fungi *on page 556*
- ◆ **Susceptibility Testing, Minimum Bactericidal Concentration** *see* Antimicrobial Susceptibility Testing, Minimum Bactericidal Concentration *on page 557*
- ◆ **Susceptibility Testing, Mycobacteria** *see* Antimicrobial Susceptibility Testing, Mycobacteria *on page 557*
- ◆ **Susceptibility Testing, Serum Bactericidal Dilution Method** *see* Serum Bactericidal Test *on page 679*
- ◆ **Susceptibility Testing, Unusual Isolates/Fastidious Organisms** *see* Antimicrobial Susceptibility Testing, Unusual Isolates/Fastidious Organisms *on page 558*
- ◆ **Swabs for Culture** *see* Fine Needle Aspiration Culture *on page 609*
- ◆ **Swan-Ganz Tip Culture** *see* Bacterial Culture, Intravascular Device *on page 572*
- ◆ **Synergistic Studies, Antimicrobial** *see* Antimicrobial Susceptibility Testing, Antimicrobial Combinations *on page 556*
- ◆ **Synovial Fluid Culture** *see* Bacterial Culture, Biopsy or Body Fluid *on page 565*
- ◆ **Synovial Fluid Fungus Culture** *see* Fungal Culture, Biopsy or Body Fluid *on page 610*
- ◆ **Synovial Fluid, Viral Culture** *see* Viral Culture, Body Fluid *on page 691*
- ◆ **Syphilis, Darkfield Examination** *see* Darkfield Examination, Syphilis *on page 601*
- ◆ **Syphilis Diagnosis** *see* Darkfield Examination, Syphilis *on page 601*
- ◆ **Syphilis Enzyme Immunoassay** *see* MHA-TP *on page 651*
- ◆ **Syphilis Serology** *see* FTA-ABS, Serum *on page 609*
- ◆ **Syphilis Serology** *see* MHA-TP *on page 651*
- ◆ **Syphilis Serology** *see* RPR *on page 677*
- ◆ **Syphilis Serology** *see* VDRL, Cerebrospinal Fluid *on page 688*
- ◆ **Syphilis Serology** *see* VDRL, Serum *on page 688*
- ◆ ***Taenia solium*** *see* Cysticercosis Serology *on page 597*
- ◆ ***Taenia* Species** *see* Ova and Parasites, Stool *on page 666*
- ◆ **TB Culture, Biopsy** *see* Mycobacterial Culture, Biopsy or Body Fluid *on page 655*
- ◆ **TB Culture, Body Fluid** *see* Mycobacterial Culture, Biopsy or Body Fluid *on page 655*
- ◆ **TB Culture, Skin** *see* Mycobacterial Culture, Cutaneous and Subcutaneous Tissue *on page 657*
- ◆ **TB Culture, Sputum** *see* Mycobacterial Culture, Sputum *on page 658*
- ◆ **TB Culture, Stool** *see* Mycobacterial Culture, Stool *on page 659*
- ◆ **TB Culture, Urine** *see* Mycobacterial Culture, Urine *on page 660*
- ◆ **TB Smear** *see* Acid-Fast Stain *on page 550*

Tetanus Antibody

Related Information
Bacterial Culture, Anaerobes *on page 564*

Bacterial Culture, Wounds, Bites *on page 579*
Botulism Diagnostic Procedures *on page 585*

Synonyms Tetanus Immunostatus

Test Includes Detection of tetanus toxoid-specific antibody in serum

Abstract Two of the genus *Clostridium* elaborate toxins. In tetanus, *Clostridium tetani* proliferates at the site of a deep or penetrating injury. *C. tetani* is a gram-positive, spore-forming obligate anaerobe found in soil and in the gastrointestinal tracts of animals. In developed countries, tetanus is rare with only 33 cases reported in the United States in 1999.[1] However, over one million cases still occur annually worldwide with a 20% to 50% mortality.[2] Immunity to tetanus is seen in response to tetanus toxoid immunization but this immunity wanes with age.[3] Booster immunizations are recommended to maintain adequate immunity to the toxin. Adverse reactions such as local pain and tenderness at the site of injection have been reported to be associated with tetanus toxoid immunizations.

Specimen Serum

Container Red top tube

Reference Interval Hemagglutinating antibody present; hemagglutination concentrations >0.01 units/mL and EIA results >0.15 IU/mL are considered protective.[4]

Use Assess immunocompetence and patients at risk for tetanus and epidemiology studies. Acute spastic paralysis is caused by tetanospasmin, a neurotoxin, better known as tetanus toxin.

Contraindications Not valid in an unimmunized individual or in patients who have recently received tetanus antitoxin serum.

Methodology Hemagglutination, enzyme immunoassay (EIA)

Additional Information In developed countries, most individuals have been immunized against tetanus and assessing whether they have antibody to tetanus antigen is a way to document intact humoral immunity. Serologic studies have no place in management of clinical tetanus. Since the tests are too slow, too insensitive, and do not correlate with the course of disease or response to treatment. Indeed, clinical tetanus has been reported in patients with high antitetanus titers. Only 12% of individuals older than age 49 years were considered immune in a survey done in Spain.[5]

See Bacterial Culture, Anaerobes *on page 564*.

Footnotes
1. Centers for Disease Control, "Notifiable Diseases/Deaths in Selected Cities Weekly Information," *MMWR Morb Mortal Wkly Rep*, 2000, 48(51):1183-90.
2. Sanford JP, "Tetanus - Forgotten but Not Gone," *N Engl J Med*, 1995, 332(12):812-3.
3. Murphy SM, Hegarty DM, Feighery CS, et al, "Tetanus Immunity in Elderly People," *Age Ageing*, 1995, 24(2):99-102.
4. Gergen PJ, McQuillan GM, Kiely M, et al, "A Population-Based Serologic Survey of Immunity to Tetanus in the United States," *N Engl J Med*, 1995, 332(12):761-6.
5. Cilla G, Saenz-Dominguez JR, Montes M, et al, "Immunity Against Tetanus in Adults Over the Age of 49 Years," *Med Clin*, 1994, 103(15):571-3.

References
Arnon SS, "Tetanus," *Nelson Textbook of Pediatrics*, 16th ed, Chapter 29, Behrman RE, Kliegman RM, and Jenson HB, eds, Philadelphia, PA: WB Saunders Co, 2000, 878-81.
Jones IG, Tyrrell H, Hill A, et al, "Randomized Controlled Trial of Combined Diphtheria, Tetanus, Whole Cell Pertussis Vaccine Administered in the Same Syringe and Separately With *Haemophilus influenzae* Type B Vaccine at Two and Four Months of Age," *Vaccine*, 1998, 16(1):109-13.
Kruger S, Seyfarth M, Sack K, et al, "Defective Immune Response to Tetanus Toxoid in Hemodialysis Patients and its Association With Diphtheria Vaccination," *Vaccine*, 1999, 17(9-10):1145-50.
Okada K, Ueda K, Morokuma K, et al, "Comparison of Antibody Titers in Eleven- to Twelve-Year Old Japanese School Children Six Years After Administration of Acellular and Whole Cell Pertussis Vaccines Combined With Diphtheria-Tetanus Toxoid," *Pediatr Infect Dis J*, 1998, 17(12):1167-9.
O'Malley CD, Smith N, Braun R, et al, "Tetanus Associated With Body Piercing," *Clin Infect Dis*, 1998, 27(5):1343-4.
Saikh KU, Sesno J, Brandler P, et al, "Are DNA-Based Vaccines Useful for Protection Against Secreted Bacterial Toxins? Tetanus Toxin Test Case," *Vaccine*, 1998, 16(9-10):1029-38.
Soyletir G, Yagci A, Topkaya A, et al, "Detection of Antitetanus Antibodies in Turkish Population," *Trop Doct*, 1999, 29(3):161-3.

Internet Web Sites
www.astdhpphe.org/infect/tetanus.html
www.cdc.gov/nip/publications/pink/tetanus.pdf

♦ **Tetanus Immunostatus** *see* Tetanus Antibody *on page 682*

♦ **Third Generation EIA** *see* Hepatitis C Virus Serology *on page 627*

♦ **Three-Day Measles Culture** *see* Rubella Virus Culture *on page 678*

♦ **Three-Day Measles Serology** *see* Rubella Serology *on page 677*

♦ **Throat Culture** *see* Bacterial Culture, Throat, and Antigen Detection Testing for Group A Streptococci *on page 577*

♦ **Throat Culture for *Bordetella pertussis*** *replaced by* Bordetella pertussis Culture *on page 583*

♦ **Throat Culture for *Corynebacterium diphtheriae*** *see* Corynebacterium diphtheriae Throat Culture *on page 594*

♦ **Throat Culture for Group A Beta-Hemolytic *Streptococcus*** *see* Bacterial Culture, Throat, and Antigen Detection Testing for Group A Streptococci *on page 577*

♦ **Throat Swab for Group A *Streptococcus* Antigen** *see* Group A Streptococcus Screen, Rapid *on page 617*

♦ **Tick-Borne Diseases** *see* Arthropod Identification *on page 559*

♦ **Tick Identification** *see* Arthropod Identification *on page 559*

♦ **Tinea Barbae** *see* KOH Preparation *on page 645*

♦ **Tinea Capitis** *see* KOH Preparation *on page 645*

♦ **Tinea Corporis** *see* KOH Preparation *on page 645*

♦ **Tinea Cruris** *see* KOH Preparation *on page 645*

♦ **Tinea Manuum** *see* KOH Preparation *on page 645*

♦ **Tinea Pedis** *see* KOH Preparation *on page 645*

♦ **Tinea Unguium** *see* KOH Preparation *on page 645*

♦ **Tissue Culture** *see* Bacterial Culture, Biopsy or Body Fluid *on page 565*

♦ **Tissue Fungus Culture** *see* Fungal Culture, Biopsy or Body Fluid *on page 610*

♦ **Tissue Mycobacteria Culture** *see* Mycobacterial Culture, Biopsy or Body Fluid *on page 655*

♦ **Tolerance Testing, Antimicrobial** *see* Antimicrobial Susceptibility Testing, Minimum Bactericidal Concentration *on page 557*

TORCH

Related Information
Cytomegalovirus Serology *on page 600*
Herpes Simplex Antibody *on page 630*
Rubella Serology *on page 677*
Toxoplasmosis Serology *on page 684*

Synonyms TORCH Screen; TORCH Titer

Test Includes Detection of antibody specific for toxoplasmosis, rubella, cytomegalovirus, and herpes simplex virus

Abstract Although the acronym TORCH serves to enhance awareness of congenital infections, the disease entities must be considered separately rather than collectively.[1] The entities are **TO**xoplasmosis, **R**ubella, **C**ytomegalovirus, **H**erpes.

Specimen Serum

Container Red top tube

Collection Paired specimens drawn 2-4 weeks apart or a single sample for monitoring immunity in pregnant females

Reference Interval IgG: less than a fourfold increase in titer; IgM: negative

Use Screen for serologic response to toxoplasmosis, rubella, cytomegalovirus, and herpesvirus infection, important in pregnant mothers and newborn infants for evaluation of possible congenital infection

Limitations The presence of IgG antibodies in maternal blood indicates prior exposure to that specific agent through natural infection or immunization (rubella). Since the prevalence of antibodies to HSV and CMV is very high in the general population, a single positive IgG antibody to these agents is of little diagnostic value regardless of titer. Fetal or neonatal IgG antibodies merely indicate transplacental transfer of maternal antibodies. Negative serologic results do not exclude infection.

Methodology Indirect fluorescent antibody (IFA), enzyme-linked immunosorbent assay (ELISA), IgG and IgM specificity

Additional Information *Toxoplasma*, rubella, cytomegalovirus, and herpes simplex are all causes of potentially catastrophic congenital infections, which can be quickly fatal or lead to chronic sequelae including hepatitis, encephalitis, and failure to thrive. In the fulminant case serologic diagnosis is of little use since the disease outstrips the immune response and even IgM antibody cannot be demonstrated in time to be clinically useful. However, in the disease that becomes manifest weeks to months after birth, demonstration of IgM antibody or rising titers of IgG antibody can confirm a diagnosis of specific infection. The presence of IgM-specific antibody in cord, fetal, or neonatal blood indicates congenital infection. **It should be emphasized that TORCH testing is of very limited usefulness. Results must be interpreted in conjunction with complete clinical information, and such testing in no way substitutes for careful clinical examination and judgment.** TORCH testing should not be applied indiscriminately to pregnant women or infants with nondescript illnesses. See individual listings for more detailed information and websites.

Footnotes
1. Stamos JK and Rowley AH, "Timely Diagnosis of Congenital Infections," *Pediatr Clin North Am*, 1994, 41(5):1017-33.

References
Crino JP, "Ultrasound and Fetal Diagnosis of Perinatal Infection," *Clin Obstet Gynecol*, 1999, 42(1):71-80.
Cullen A, Brown S, Cafferkey M, et al, "Current Use of the TORCH Screen in the Diagnosis of Congenital Infection," *J Infect*, 1998, 36(2):185-8.
Greenough A, "The TORCH Screen and Intrauterine Infections," *Arch Dis Child*, 1994, 70(3 Spec No):163-5
Helfgott A, "TORCH Testing in HIV-infected Women," *Clin Obstet Gynecol*, 1999, 42(1):149-62.
Newton ER, "Diagnosis of Perinatal TORCH Infections," *Clin Obstet Gynecol*, 1999, 42(1):59-70.

- **TORCH Screen** *see* TORCH *on page 683*

- **TORCH Titer** *see* TORCH *on page 683*

- **Toxin A and/or B** *see* Clostridium difficile Toxin Assay and Culture *on page 592*

- **Toxin Assay, *Clostridium difficile*** *see* Clostridium difficile Toxin Assay and Culture *on page 592*

- ***Toxoplasma* Antibodies** *see* Toxoplasmosis Serology *on page 684*

Toxoplasmosis Serology

Related Information
Buffy Coat Smear Study of Peripheral Blood *on page 412*
HIV-1/HIV-2 Antibody Screen and Western Blot *on page 636*
TORCH *on page 683*

Synonyms *Toxoplasma* Antibodies; Toxoplasmosis Titer

Replaces Sabin-Feldman Dye Test

Test Includes IgG and IgM antibody specific for *Toxoplasma gondii*

Abstract *Toxoplasma gondii* is an intracellular protozoan parasite that infects both humans and animals. The organism has a worldwide distribution and human infections are very common; serologic studies indicate that approximately a third to a half of the United States population has been infected with *T. gondii*. Most human infections follow an asymptomatic chronic course, however, severe disseminated infections occur, particularly in immunocompromised hosts.[1,2] Human infection is most commonly acquired by ingestion of oocysts in undercooked meat, but contamination of food or drink with oocysts from cat feces is also an important mode of human infection. It can be transmitted through the placenta.

Toxoplasmosis infection is especially important in two clinical situations: infections transmitted to the fetus, and as the most common opportunistic infection of the central nervous system in patients with acquired immunodeficiency syndrome (AIDS).[1,3] It is also important in organ transplantation.[4]

Detection of the organism by stains and cultures in specimens from cerebrospinal fluid and amniotic fluid is not reliable.

Specimen Serum, cerebrospinal fluid, amniotic fluid. Amniocentesis with ultrasonography and fetal blood sampling can lead to correct diagnosis in ~92% of patients.[5]

Container Red top tube

Collection Acute and convalescent serum specimens are recommended at 3-week interval.

Reference Interval IgG: less than a fourfold increase in titer; IgM: negative

Use Support the diagnosis of toxoplasmosis; document past exposure and/or immunity to *Toxoplasma gondii*. The absence of IgG is useful: it provides evidence of lack of infection.

Limitations There is a high prevalence of IgG antibody to *Toxoplasma* in most populations. Although a single high titer is frequently used to suggest active infection, it is unreliable because titers may persist at high levels for years in healthy people. Diagnosis of neonatal infection may be difficult because infection outstrips demonstrable antibody response. Toxoplasmosis occurs in advanced AIDS. The absence in such patients of anti-*Toxoplasma* antibodies on immunofluorescence assay does not exclude the diagnosis.[1] Distinction between chronic active, inactive, and past infection may be obscure. Many different tests are available and false-positive and false-negative results are seen with these tests to varying degrees. Serologic responses in the presence of immunodeficiency lack reliability.[4] Polymerase chain reaction (PCR), when positive, provides indication of the presence of *T. gondii* DNA, but negative PCR does not rule out the presence of active disease.[6]

Methodology Indirect fluorescent antibody (IFA), enzyme-linked immunosorbent assay (ELISA). The Sabin Feldman dye test remains in use as a reference method and for interlaboratory standardization.[7] PCR used for prenatal diagnosis of congenital *T. gondii* infection is reported as safe, rapid, and accurate with a sensitivity of 81% and a specificity reported as 96%.[8]

The diagnosis has been made by observation of tachyzoites in Wright-stained peripheral blood smears, and with immunocytochemistry applied to skin biopsy for panniculitis.[4]

Additional Information *Toxoplasma gondii* is a protozoan parasite endemic in cats and oocysts are excreted by them. The oocysts shed in cat feces can be in large numbers (100,000 per gram of feces) and can survive in the environment for several months. Humans are easily exposed to oocysts, either in caring for pets or in casual environmental contact. The majority of individuals develop antibody without any clinical disease, and a self-limited lymphadenitis is the most common clinical presentation in symptomatic infection.

Congenital toxoplasmosis and infection in immunocompromised hosts (especially AIDS or transplant patients) are more serious, and can produce a fatal cerebritis or disseminated illness. The median CD4 cell count in subjects with AIDS and toxoplasmosis, at presentation, was 50/mm³.[1]

Congenital toxoplasmosis can now be diagnosed *in utero* by detection of IgM antibody in fetal blood. Diagnosis is supported by high or rising IgG antibody titer, or the demonstration of IgM antibody. The recent availability of IgA anti-*Toxoplasma* may be useful in detection of congenital toxoplasmosis. However, IgM is still the established technique. Neonatal screening

by IgM capture immunoassay, with confirmation by specific IgG and IgM antibodies in neonatal and maternal serum is described.[3]

IgG antibodies usually appear within 1-2 weeks of infection, peak within 1-2 months, fall at variable rates, and persist for life. Diagnosis of congenital infection is made by demonstrating specific IgM or IgA in serum obtained by periumbilical blood sampling or at birth; contamination with maternal blood can be excluded by assaying for β-hCG and coagulation factors, as well as by the Kleihauer test. IgG in neonatal of fetal blood merely indicates transplacental transfer of maternal antibody. Amniotic fluid can be tested.[6]

Intrathecal production suggesting CNS infection can be determined as follows: C = (antibody titer in CSF x IgG concentration in serum) / (antibody titer in serum x IgG concentration in CSF). Intrathecal production is probable when C is ≥8. *Toxoplasma gondii* tachyzoites have been seen in ventricular cerebrospinal fluid; two cases of 6090 CSF specimens were reported.[9]

Footnotes
1. Lanska DJ, "Epidemiology of Human Immunodeficiency Virus Infection and Associated Neurologic Illness," *Semin Neurol*, 1999, 19(2):105-11.
2. Dietrich U, Maschke M, Dorfler A, et al, "MRI of Intracranial Toxoplasmosis After Bone Marrow Transplantation," *Neuroradiology*, 2000, 42(1):14-8.
3. Naessens A, Jenum PA, Pollak A, et al, "Diagnosis of Congenital Toxoplasmosis in the Neonatal Period: A Multicenter Evaluation," *J Pediatr*, 1999, 135(6):714-9.
4. Arnold SJ, Kinney MC, McCormick MS, et al, "Disseminated Toxoplasmosis. Unusual Presentations in the Immunocompromised Host," *Arch Pathol Lab Med*, 1997, 121(8):869-73.
5. Stamos JK and Rowley AH, "Timely Diagnosis of Congenital Infections," *Pediatr Clin North Am*, 1994, 41(5):1017-33
6. Mayo Reference Services Publication, "*Toxoplasma gondii* by Polymerase Chain Reaction (PCR), Amniotic Fluid or Spinal Fluid," *New Test Announcement*, #81795, Rochester, MN: Mayo Medical Laboratories, January 1999.
7. Reiter-Owona I, Petersen E, Joynson D, et al, "The Past and Present Role of the Sabin-Feldman Dye Test in the Serodiagnosis of Toxoplasmosis," *Bull World Health Organ*, 1999, 77(11):929-35.
8. Foulon W, Pinon JM, Stray-Pedersen B, et al, "Prenatal Diagnosis of Congenital Toxoplasmosis: A Multicenter Evaluation of Different Diagnostic Parameters," *Am J Obstet Gynecol*, 1999, 181(4):843-7.
9. Brogi E, and Cibas ES, "Cytologic Detection of *Toxoplasma gondii* Tachyzoites in Cerebrospinal Fluid," *Am J Clin Pathol*, 2000, 114(6):951-955.

References
Aubert D, Maine GT, Villena I, et al, "Recombinant Antigens to Detect *Toxoplasma gondii*-Specific Immunoglobulin G and Immunoglobulin M in Human Sera by Enzyme Immunoassay," *J Clin Microbiol*, 2000, 38(3):1144-50.
Cohen BA, "Neurologic Manifestations of Toxoplasmosis in AIDS," *Semin Neurol*, 1999, 19(2):201-11.
Djurkovic-Djakovic O, Romand S, Nobre R, et al, "Serologic Rebounds After One-Year-Long Treatment for Congenital Toxoplasmosis," *Pediatr Infect Dis J*, 2000, 19(1):81-3.
Li S, Maine G, Suzuki Y, et al, "Serodiagnosis of Recently Acquired *Toxoplasma gondii* Infection With a Recombinant Antigen," *J Clin Microbiol*, 2000, 38(1):179-84.
Meisheri YV, Mehta S, Patel U, et al, "A Prospective Study for Seroprevalence of Toxoplasmosis in General Population and in HIV/AIDS Patients in Bombay, India," *J Postgrad Med*, 1997, 43(4):93-7.
Robert-Gangneux F, Commerce V, Tourte-Schaefer C, et al, "Performance of a Western Blot Assay to Compare Mother and Newborn Anti-*Toxoplasma* Antibodies for the Early Neonatal Diagnosis of Congenital Toxoplasmosis," *Eur J Clin Microbiol Infect Dis*, 1999, 18(9):648-54.
Zufferey J, Hohlfeld P, Bille J, et al, "Value of the Comparative Enzyme-Linked Immunofiltration Assay for Early Neonatal Diagnosis of Congenital *Toxoplasma* Infection," *Pediatr Infect Dis J*, 1999, 18(11):971-5.

Internet Web Sites
www.amm.co.uk/pubs/fa_toxoplasma.htm
www.astdhpphe.org/infect/toxo.html
www.cdc.gov/ncidod/dpd/parasites/toxoplasmosis/default.htm

- **Toxoplasmosis Titer** *see* Toxoplasmosis Serology *on page 684*

- ***T. pallidum* DNA** *see* FTA-ABS, Serum *on page 609*

- ***Treponema pallidum* Darkfield Examination** *see* Darkfield Examination, Syphilis *on page 601*

- **TRIC Agent Culture** *see* Chlamydia trachomatis Culture *on page 590*

- **Trichinellosis Serology** *see* Trichinosis Serology *on page 684*

Trichinosis Serology

Related Information
Ova and Parasites, Stool *on page 666*

Synonyms Trichinellosis Serology

Abstract The parasite, *Trichinella spiralis*, is the agent of human trichinosis and is a parasite of carnivores. There is little host specificity and cysts have been detected in such diverse products as pork meat, bear meat, boar meat, and badger meat.[1,2,3] Ingestion of undercooked meat products containing the encysted larvae is responsible for human infections.

Specimen Serum

Container Red top tube

Sampling Time Measurable antibody titers are not usually reached until 2-3 weeks after infestation. Paired specimens collected 1-2 months apart are recommended.

Reference Interval Negative; <1:16 by ELISA; less than a fourfold increase in paired titer; dependent upon laboratory and method

Use Screen for antibodies to *Trichinella spiralis* to establish the diagnosis of trichinosis. Ingestion of undercooked pork, bear, or wild animal meat containing larvae may lead to myalgias, fever, myocardial infestation, neurological symptoms, and peripheral blood eosinophilia. ESR may be increased with infestation.

Limitations Low titers may represent antibody from previous rather than current infection. Antibody remains detectable for 2-3 years. The test may have a high false-negative rate of 15% to 22% during the first period of the infection. Sensitivity and specificity of testing depends on the type of antigen used (excretory/secretory or crude somatic antigens).

Methodology Bentonite flocculation test (BFT), indirect fluorescent antibody (IFA), complement fixation (CF), latex agglutination (LA), enzyme-linked immunosorbent assay (ELISA)

Additional Information The bentonite flocculation test is sensitive and specific but is not often used in the diagnostic laboratory. Antibody becomes detectable 3 weeks after infection, reaches peak concentrations at ~3 months, and then declines slowly so that most individuals will test negative 2-3 years after the initial infection.[4] Immunofluorescence is more sensitive for detection of light infection in pigs.

In humans, finding cysts in a muscle biopsy can also make a diagnosis or trichinosis. As an incidental finding, trichinosis was not infrequently found in pharyngeal striated muscle adhering to tonsillectomy specimens.

Footnotes

1. Rodriguez-Osorio M, Abad JM, de Haro T, et al, "Human Trichinellosis in Southern Spain: Serologic and Epidemiologic Study," *Am J Trop Med Hyg*, 1999, 61(5):834-7.
2. Suzdaltsev AA, Verkhovtsev VN, Spiridonov AM, et al, "Trichinosis Outbreak After Ingestion of Barbecued Badger," *Int J Infect Dis*, 1999, 3(4):216.
3. Gamble HR, Brady RC, Bulaga LL, et al, "Prevalence and Risk Association for *Trichinella* Infection in Domestic Pigs in the Northeastern United States," *Vet Parasitol*, 1999, 82(1):59-69.
4. Mahannop P, Setasuban P, Morakote N, et al, "Immunodiagnosis of Human Trichinellosis and Identification of Specific Antigen for *Trichinella spiralis*," *Int J Parasitol*, 1995, 25(1):87-94.

References

Ben GJM, Malmassari SL, Nunez GG, et al, "Evaluation of an Enzymatic Immunohistochemical Technique in Human Trichinellosis," *J Helminthol*, 1997, 71(4):299-303.

Gamble HR, "Parasites Associated With Pork and Pork Products," *Rev Sci Tech*, 1997, 16(2):496-506.

Ko RC, "A Brief Update on the Diagnosis of Trichinellosis," *Southeast Asian J Trop Med Public Health*, 1997, 28(S1):91-8.

Moorhead A, Grunenwald PE, Dietz VJ, et al, "Trichinellosis in the United States, 1991-1996: Declining but Not Gone," *Am J Trop Med Hyg*, 1999, 60(1):66-9.

Wakelin D, "Immune Responses to Intestinal Parasites: Protection, Pathology and Prophylaxis," *Parasitologia*, 1997, 39(4):269-74.

Internet Web Sites

www.cdc.gov/ncidod/dpd/parasites/trichinosis/default.htm

♦ *Trichomonas* Culture *see Trichomonas* Preparation *on page 685*

Trichomonas Preparation

Related Information

Bacterial Culture, Genital Specimen *on page 571*
Cervical/Vaginal Cytology *on page 377*
Ova and Parasites, Urine *on page 667*

Synonyms Hanging Drop Mount for *Trichomonas*; *Trichomonas vaginalis* Culture; *Trichomonas vaginalis* Wet Preparation

Applies to *Trichomonas* Culture; Urethral *Trichomonas* Smear; Urine *Trichomonas* Wet Mount

Test Includes Wet mount and microscopic examination. Pap smear and/or culture may also be performed.

Abstract The pathogenic flagellate, *Trichomonas vaginalis*, is primarily a sexually transmitted protozoan disease that infects the urogenital tracts of both men and women. The incidence of *Trichomonas* varies depending on the population studied, but estimates range from 0.25% to 5.1%.[1,2]

Specimen Vaginal, cervical, or urethral swabs, prostatic fluid, urine sediment

Container Sterile tube containing 1 mL of sterile nonbacteriostatic saline or specific media for *Trichomonas*

Collection The specimen should be collected using a speculum without lubricant. The mucosa of the posterior vagina may be swabbed, or the secretions may be collected with a pipette. The swab should be expressed into saline for transport. The specimen should be examined as soon as possible.

Storage Instructions Do not refrigerate. Transport immediately to the laboratory so that viable motile organisms may be examined.

Turnaround Time Same day; 48 hours if culture is performed

Special Instructions Provide the specific source of the specimen to the laboratory.

Reference Interval Negative: no trichomonads identified; positive: demonstration of actively motile flagellates and/or positive culture

Use Establish the presence of *Trichomonas vaginalis*

Limitations The specimen is examined for *Trichomonas vaginalis* only. A separate swab (Culturette®) must be collected for culture or DNA detection

of *Neisseria gonorrhoeae*, if required. Culture or DNA analysis for *Chlamydia trachomatis* requires an additional specimen (urine or cervical swab) or a specific *Chlamydia* culture swab. One negative result does not rule out the possibility of *Trichomonas vaginalis* infection. The wet mount is negative in 30% to 50%[3] of women with trichomoniasis. The most important factor affecting sensitivity is the time between collection of the specimen and examination in the laboratory. Culture is not available in many laboratories.

Contraindications Douching within 3 days prior to specimen collection

Methodology Wet mount microscopic examination within 1 hour of collection; Pap smear; culture in Diamond's, Trichosol, or Hollanders liquid medium; use of a commercial culture system such as InPouch TV[4]; direct immunofluorescent technique with monoclonal antibody

Additional Information The absence of the classical yellow, frothy discharge does not exclude trichomoniasis. Up to 50% of women are asymptomatic carriers and the majority of men are asymptomatic. In males, a milky white fluid discharge and urethral irritation present for more than 4 weeks is frequently associated with urethritis caused by *T. vaginalis*. *Trichomonas vaginalis* infection was more common than *Neisseria gonorrhoeae* or *Chlamydia trachomatis* in men 30 years and older.[2] Neonates usually acquire *T. vaginalis* during vaginal births and 2% to 17% of female babies acquire trichomoniasis by direct vulvovaginal contamination.

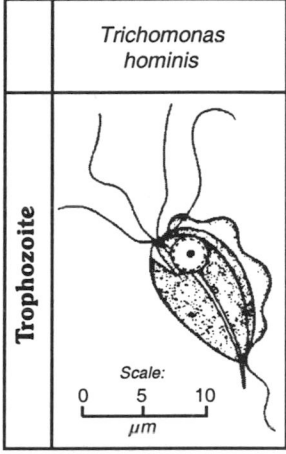

From Brooks MM and Melvin DM, *Morphology of Diagnostic Stages of Intestinal Parasites of Humans*, 2nd ed, Atlanta, GA: U.S. Department of Health and Human Services, Publication No. 84-8116, Centers for Disease Control, 1984, with permission.

Culture may yield positive results when wet preparations are negative. The high rate of false negatives, ~40%, and false positives observed with stained preparations (Pap smears) requires that confirmation by wet mount or culture be considered when the reported results are inconsistent with the clinical findings.[3] Immunofluorescence tests, nucleic acid assays, and latex agglutination tests have been developed but are generally not commercially available.[5]

Footnotes

1. Bowden FJ, Paterson BA, Mein J, et al, "Estimating the Prevalence of *Trichomonas vaginalis, Chlamydia trachomatis, Neisseria gonorrhoeae* and Human Papillomavirus Infection in Indigenous Women in Northern Australia," *Sex Transm Infect*, 1999, 75(6):431-4.
2. Joyner JL, Douglas JM Jr, Ragsdale S, et al, "Comparative Prevalence of Infection With *Trichomonas vaginalis* Among Men Attending a Sexually Transmitted Diseases Clinic," *Sex Transm Dis*, 2000, 27(4):236-40.
3. Ohlemeyer CL, Hornberger LL, Lynch DA, et al, "Diagnosis of *Trichomonas vaginalis* in Adolescent Females: InPouch TV Cultures Versus Wet-Mount Microscopy," *J Adolesc Health*, 1998, 22(3):205-8.
4. Levi MH, Torres J, Pina C, et al, "Comparison of the InPouch TV Culture System and Diamond's Modified Medium for Detection of *Trichomonas vaginalis*," *J Clin Microbiol*, 1997, 35(12):3308-10.
5. Madico G, Quinn TC, Rompalo A, et al, "Diagnosis of *Trichomonas vaginalis* Infection by PCR Using Vaginal Swab Samples," *J Clin Microbiol*, 1998, 36(11):3205-10.

References

Beverly AL, Venglarik M, Cotton B, et al, "Viability of *Trichomonas vaginalis* in Transport Medium," *J Clin Microbiol*, 1999, 37(11):3749-50.

Blake DR, Duggan A, and Joffe A, "Use of Spun Urine to Enhance Detection of *Trichomonas vaginalis* in Adolescent Women," *Arch Pediatr Adolesc Med*, 1999, 153(12):1222-5.

Donders GG, Bosmans E, Dekeersmaecher A, et al, "Pathogenesis of Abnormal Vaginal Bacterial Flora," *Am J Obstet Gynecol*, 2000, 182(4):872-8.

Kostara I, Carageorgiou H, Varonos D, et al, "Growth and Survival of *Trichomonas vaginalis*," *J Med Microbiol*, 1998, 47(6):555-60.

Internet Web Sites

www.cdc.gov/ncidod/dpd/parasites/trichomonas/default.htm

♦ **Trichomonas vaginalis Culture** *see Trichomonas* Preparation *on page 685*

♦ **Trichomonas vaginalis Wet Preparation** *see Trichomonas* Preparation *on page 685*

♦ **Trichuris trichiura** *see* Ova and Parasites, Stool *on page 666*

♦ **Trypanosoma cruzi** *see* Chagas' Disease Serological Test *on page 588*

Tularemia Serology

Related Information
Arthropod Identification *on page 559*
Bacterial Culture, Blood *on page 566*
Bacterial Culture, Wounds, Bites *on page 579*

Synonyms *Francisella tularensis* Antibodies; Rabbit Fever Antibodies

Applies to *Francisella tularensis* Culture

Abstract *Francisella tularensis*, a small gram-negative pleomorphic rod, found in wild rabbits and in a number of other animals, may be transmitted to man by direct contact, by inhalation, and by ticks and deer flies. Often the diagnosis of tularemia is made in the absence of a positive culture for *F. tularensis* by detection of increased titers of specific antibodies.

Specimen Serum (culture from blood, sputum, skin, mucosa)

Container Red top tube

Sampling Time Paired sera collected 2-3 weeks apart are recommended.

Special Instructions Since *F. tularensis* is a risk to laboratory personnel, the clinical possibility of this entity should be addressed.

Reference Interval Agglutination titer: <1:40; ELISA: <1:500; less than a fourfold increase in paired titer

Critical Values A single serologic result with a titer ≥1:160 in a subject having clinical tularemia or a fourfold rise in titer is diagnostic.

Use Investigation of illness characterized by an ulcerative lesion at a site of inoculation, with regional lymphadenopathy, fever, and pneumonia. Conjunctivitis occurs in a minority of cases; it is seen with preauricular lymphadenopathy, Perinaud oculoglandular syndrome.

Limitations There is serologic cross reactivity with *Brucella* species, *Proteus* OX-19, and *Yersinia* species. IgM and IgG titers may remain elevated (1:20-1:80) for over a decade after infection, limiting the value of unpaired specimens; single titers may be misleading. Cell-mediated immunity is also important in host response to *F. tularensis*.

Methodology Agglutination, hemagglutination, enzyme-linked immunosorbent assay (ELISA), culture

Additional Information Antibodies to *F. tularensis* develop 2-3 weeks after infection and peak in 4-5 weeks. Although antibodies may cross react with *Brucella* those titers will generally be much lower. Rising titers over a 2-week interval are the best indicator of recent infection. In the United States there are approximately 100-200 cases reported annually with 1-4 deaths. The Centers for Disease Control and Prevention defines tularemia as an illness characterized by several distinct forms.[1]

• **Ulceroglandular:** cutaneous ulcers with regional lymphadenopathy
• **Glandular:** regional lymphadenopathy with no ulcer
• **Oculoglandular:** conjunctivitis with preauricular lymphadenopathy
• **Oropharyngeal:** stomatitis, pharyngitis, or tonsillitis and cervical lymphadenopathy
• **Intestinal:** intestinal pain, vomiting, and diarrhea
• **Pneumonic:** primary pleuropulmonary disease
• **Typhoidal:** febrile illness without early localizing signs and symptoms

Although laboratory diagnosis of tularemia is often established by serologic methods, *F. tularensis* may be recovered in culture from a variety of clinical specimens. Isolation is hazardous and sometimes difficult. Blood cultures are often negative. Liver and spleen can be affected and endocarditis can occur. **Agglutinins represent the key laboratory evaluation in many cases.** *F. tularensis* is an extremely hazardous infectious agent responsible for several laboratory acquired infections. **If tularemia is clinically suspected, contact the laboratory so that appropriate precautions can be taken.** *F. tularensis* is listed as a potential biologic agent that can be used as a weapon. An effective response to such biological weapons requires an increased index of suspicion for the syndromes of tularemia.[2,3]

Nodular lymphangitis occurs with sporotrichosis, *Nocardia brasiliensis*, *Mycobacterium marinum*, *Leishmania braziliensis*, and *Francisella tularensis*. A painful ulcer at the initial site is suggestive of tularemia in such cases.[4]

Footnotes
1. Centers for Disease Control and Prevention, "Case Definitions for Infectious Conditions Under Public Health Surveillance," *Morbid Mortal Weekly Rep*, 1997, 46(RR-10):53-4.
2. Leggiadro RJ, "The Threat of Biological Terrorism: A Public Health and Infection Control Reality," *Infect Control Hosp Epidemiol*, 2000, 21(1):53-6.
3. Franz DR, Jahrling PB, Friedlander AM, et al, "Clinical Recognition and Management of Patients Exposed to Biological Warfare Agents," *JAMA*, 1997 278(5):399-411.
4. Kostman JR and Di Nubile MJ, "Nodular Lymphangitis: A Distinctive but Often Unrecognized Syndrome," *Ann Intern Med*, 1993, 118(11):883-8.

References
Billings AN, Rawlings JA, and Walker DH, "Tick-Borne Diseases in Texas: A 10-Year Retrospective Examination of Cases," *Tex Med*, 1998, 94(12):66-76.

McGovern TW, Christopher GW, and Eitzen EM, "Cutaneous Manifestations of Biological Warfare and Related Threat Agents," *Arch Dermatol*, 1999, 135(3):311-22.

Shapiro ED, "Tick-Borne Diseases," *Adv Pediatr Infect Dis*, 1997, 13:187-218.

Shapiro DS and Mark EJ, "A 60-Year-Old Farm Worker With Bilateral Pneumonia," Case Records of the Massachusetts General Hospital, Case 14-2000, Scully RE, Mark EJ, McNeely WF, et al, eds, *N Engl J Med*, 2000, 342(19):1430-8.

Spach DH, Liles WC, Campbell GL, et al, "Tick-Borne Diseases in the United States," *N Engl J Med*, 1993, 329(13):936-47.

Steinemann TL, Sheikholeslami MR, Brown HH, et al, "Oculoglandular Tularemia," *Arch Ophthalmol*, 1999, 117(1):132-3.

Tarnvik A, Sandstrom G, and Sjostedt A, "Infrequent Manifestations of Tularemia in Sweden," *Scand J Infect Dis*, 1997, 29(5):443-6.

Internet Web Sites
www.cdc.gov/ncidod/dvbid/tularemi.htm

♦ **Tunnel Infection** *see* Bacterial Culture, Intravascular Device *on page 572*

♦ **Tympanocentesis Culture** *see* Bacterial Culture, Middle Ear *on page 573*

♦ **Undulant Fever** *see* Brucellosis Serology *on page 587*

♦ **Undulant Fever, Culture** *see* Brucella Culture *on page 586*

♦ **Ureaplasma urealyticum Culture, Genital** *see* Genital Culture for *Ureaplasma urealyticum on page 616*

♦ **Urease Test and Culture, Helicobacter pylori** *see* Helicobacter pylori Biopsy-Based Tests: The Urease Tests, Culture, Cytology, and PCR *on page 620*

♦ **Urethral Chlamydia Culture** *see Chlamydia trachomatis* Culture *on page 590*

♦ **Urethral Culture for T-Strain Mycoplasma** *see* Genital Culture for *Ureaplasma urealyticum on page 616*

♦ **Urethral Trichomonas Smear** *see Trichomonas* Preparation *on page 685*

♦ **Urethra, Viral Culture** *see* Viral Culture, Urogenital *on page 696*

♦ **Urine for Parasites** *see* Ova and Parasites, Urine *on page 667*

♦ **Urine for Schistosoma haematobium** *see* Ova and Parasites, Urine *on page 667*

♦ **Urine Fungus Culture** *see* Fungal Culture, Urine *on page 614*

♦ **Urine Mycobacteria Culture** *see* Mycobacterial Culture, Urine *on page 660*

♦ **Urine Trichomonas Wet Mount** *see Trichomonas* Preparation *on page 685*

♦ **Vaginal Culture** *see* Bacterial Culture, Genital Specimen *on page 571*

♦ **Valley Fever Serology** *see* Coccidioidomycosis Serology *on page 593*

♦ **Varicella Immunization** *see* Varicella-Zoster Virus Serology *on page 687*

Varicella-Zoster Virus Culture

Related Information
Bacterial Culture, Conjunctiva *on page 570*
Herpesvirus Cytology *on page 383*
Varicella-Zoster Virus Serology *on page 687*
Viral Culture *on page 689*
Viral Culture, Central Nervous System Symptoms *on page 692*
Viral Culture, Dermatological Symptoms *on page 693*
Virus, Direct Detection by Fluorescent Antibody *on page 696*

Synonyms Chickenpox Culture; Shingles Culture; VZV Culture

Applies to Alpha-Herpesviruses; Varicella-Zoster Virus DNA; Viral Culture, Rash; Viral Culture, Skin

Test Includes Rapid culture by detection of virus using immunofluorescence staining with specific monoclonal antibody. Varicella-zoster virus (VZV) can be detected in a routine viral culture.

Abstract Varicella or chickenpox in children and herpes zoster or shingles (reactivated latent infection) in adults are caused by varicella-zoster virus. Severe sharp persistent pain (postherpetic neuralgia) following zoster can be debilitating. Deaths have been noted to occur from primary infection with varicella even though this disease is preventable with the availability of an effective vaccine.[1] The diagnosis is usually made clinically, without laboratory tests.

Specimen Swab specimens from the base of fresh, unroofed lesions, vesicle fluid, vesicle scrapings; blood or bronchial washings (immunocompromised patients). Although VZV cannot be cultured from cerebrospinal fluid (CSF), PCR has detected varicella-zoster viral DNA there, and CSF antibody has been detected. In addition, acute and convalescent sera should be collected at appropriate times to document a clinically significant rise in antibody titer. (See Varicella-Zoster Virus Serology *on page 687*).

Container Cold viral transport medium for swab specimens; green top (heparin) tube for blood; sterile CSF tube; syringe or sterile capillary pipet can be used to collect vesicular fluid

Sampling Time Specimens should be collected during the acute phase of the disease (within 3 days of lesion eruption).

Collection Unroofed lesions should be cleaned before specimens are taken. Vesicular fluid from several vesicles can be pooled in a single syringe and sent to the laboratory undiluted. Alternatively, the bases of several freshly unroofed lesions can be vigorously sampled with a sterile swab which should then be placed into cold viral transport medium and sent to the laboratory as soon as possible.

Storage Instructions Keep specimens cold and moist. **Do not freeze specimens at -20°C.** VZV is extremely labile. If immediate inoculation onto cell cultures is not possible, specimens should be frozen quickly at -70°C. Freezing at -70°C will reduce infectivity 10% to 30%.

Turnaround Time Conventional culture: 1-14 days; rapid culture: 2-5 days

Reference Interval No virus isolated

Critical Values Positive culture from CSF or blood

Use Aid in the diagnosis of disease caused by varicella-zoster virus (ie, chickenpox and shingles). Varicella-zoster virus is a single virus which causes two diseases: **chickenpox** (varicella) in primary infection and, after reactivation from latency, **shingles** (zoster) in adults. Laboratory testing may rarely be needed in the differential diagnosis of skin lesions and for resolution of other questions.

Limitations Rapid method will only detect specified virus(es), negative culture does not rule out other viral infections. VZV is extremely labile and many times cannot be isolated from specimens that have been transported and/or stored in adverse conditions. Cell culture of VZV is less sensitive than direct antigen detection of VZV by immunofluorescence. PCR for VZV DNA is even more sensitive, but it is expensive.[2] VZV DNA can be found in blood mononuclear cells up to 6 weeks after the rash of herpes zoster.[3]

Methodology Routine culture: Inoculation of specimens into cell cultures, incubation of cultures, observation for characteristic cytopathic effect (CPE), and identification by fluorescent monoclonal antibody

Rapid culture: Specimens are centrifuged onto cell cultures grown on coverslips in the bottoms of 1-dram shell vials. Centrifugation greatly accelerates virus attachment and penetration. After incubation, fluorescein-labeled monoclonal antibodies are applied to the infected cells to detect viral antigens. Characteristic fluorescent foci indicate the presence of virus.

Additional Information Varicella-zoster virus is a common virus found around the world. Diseases caused by VZV are usually self-limited. However, the primary VZV infection can be life-threatening in pregnant persons, immunocompromised persons, children who receive cancer therapy following organ transplantation, and in fetuses exposed during pregnancy. Complications include dissemination, pneumonitis, myocarditis, cardiomyopathy, hepatitis, Guillain-Barré syndrome, myelitis, ventriculitis, granulomatous arteritis, vasculopathy, and meningoencephalitis.[3] Ophthalmic complications have recently been reviewed.[4] Congenital chickenpox can result in neonatal systemic disease and/or congenital malformations. Congenital varicella syndrome occurs in 2% of infected neonates. People suffering from AIDS can have prolonged reactivated VZV infections.[5] In bone marrow transplant recipients, 23% to 40% of patients develop active VZV reactivation and many times these infections are without skin involvement.[6] Zoster occurs mostly in elderly and immunocompromised individuals.[3]

Serology for detection of VZV antibodies is available. See Varicella-Zoster Virus Serology *on page 687*. Rapid turnaround time of serological tests can be especially important in detecting the presence of antibody (prior exposure) in pregnant women who have been exposed to individuals with chickenpox. In such cases, VZV-specific immunoglobulin should be given within 3 days (maximum) of exposure.

Footnotes

1. Centers for Disease Control and Prevention, "Varicella - Related Deaths - Florida, 1998," *Morbid Mortal Weekly Rep*, 1999, 48(18):379-81.
2. Sauerbrei A, Eichhorn U, Schalke M, et al, "Laboratory Diagnosis of Herpes Zoster," *J Clin Virol*, 1999, 14(1):31-6.
3. Gilden DH, Kleinschmidt-DeMasters BK, LaGuardia JJ, et al, "Neurologic Complications of the Reactivation of Varicella-Zoster Virus," *N Engl J Med*, 2000, 342(9):635-45.
4. Leisegang TJ, "Varicella Zoster Viral Disease," *Mayo Clin Proc*, 1999, 74(10):983-8.
5. Glesby MJ, Moore RD, and Chaisson RE, "Clinical Spectrum of Herpes Zoster in Adults Infected With Human Immunodeficiency Virus," *Clin Infect Dis*, 1995, 21(2):370-5.
6. Rogers SY, Irving W, Harris A, et al, "Visceral Varicella-Zoster Infection After Bone Marrow Transplantation Without Skin Involvement and the use of PCR for Diagnosis," *Bone Marrow Transplant*, 1995, 15(5):805-7.

References

Choo PW, Donahue JG, Manson JE, et al, "The Epidemiology of Varicella and its Complications," *J Infect Dis*, 1995, 172(3):706-12.
Cohen JI, Brunell PA, Straus SE, et al, "Recent Advances in Varicella-Zoster Virus Infection," *Ann Intern Med*, 1999, 130(11):922-32.
Houston SH, Sinnott JT 4th, Murphy SJ, et al, "Chickenpox in Pregnancy," *Infect Med*, 1994, 11(8):564-8.
Isaacs D, "Neonatal Chickenpox," *J Paediatr Child Health*, 2000, 36(1):76-7.
Lipton SA and Ma MJ, "A 37-Year-Old Man With AIDS, Neurologic Deterioration, and Multiple Hemorrhagic Cerebral Lesions," Case Records of the Massachusetts General Hospital, Case 36-1996, Scully RE, Mark EJ, McNeely WF, et al, eds, *N Engl J Med*, 1996, 335(21):1587-95.
McCarter YS and Ratkiewicz IN, "Comparison of Virus Culture and Direct Immunofluorescent Staining of Cytocentrifuged Virus Transport Medium for Detection of Varicella-Zoster Virus in Skin Lesions," *Am J Clin Pathol*, 1998, 109(5):631-3.

Internet Web Sites

www.cdc.gov/ncidod/srp/varicella.htm

www.who.int/vaccines-diseases/diseases/pp_varicella.htm

♦ **Varicella-Zoster Virus, Direct Detection** *see* Virus, Direct Detection by Fluorescent Antibody *on page 696*

♦ **Varicella-Zoster Virus DNA** *see* Varicella-Zoster Virus Culture *on page 686*

Varicella-Zoster Virus Serology

Related Information

Herpesvirus Cytology *on page 383*
Polymerase Chain Reaction *on page 713*
Varicella-Zoster Virus Culture *on page 686*
Viral Culture *on page 689*
Virus, Direct Detection by Fluorescent Antibody *on page 696*

Synonyms Chickenpox Titer; VZV Serology; Zoster Titer

Applies to Alpha-Herpesviruses; Herpes Zoster Serology; Varicella Immunization

Test Includes IgG, IgM antibodies

Abstract Varicella-zoster is one of eight herpesviruses that infects humans. It produces two clinical syndromes. **Chickenpox**, the manifestation of primary exposure, is usually benign in immunocompetent children, but may have severe complications in adults and the immunosuppressed. However, a recent report from CDC documented fatal cases of primary varicella in children.[1] Following primary infection, PCR and *in situ* hybridization have identified VZV, primarily within the neurons of the cranial nerve and dorsal root ganglia. **Shingles** or **herpes zoster** occurs when the latent VZV infection is reactivated, leading to rash and sharp, lancinating radicular pain. Facial lesions can be accompanied by keratitis, a potential cause of blindness.

Diagnosis of chickenpox and shingles is usually based upon history and physical examination. In those rare cases in which VZV infection cannot be clinically distinguished from similar infections (eg, disseminated herpes simplex infection vs disseminated zoster), the diagnostic test of choice is viral culture.[2] Serologic tests are used primarily to confirm recent or past infections that are unlikely to produce positive culture results.

Specimen Serum, amniotic fluid, cerebrospinal fluid (CSF)

Container Red top tube

Sampling Time Acute and convalescent sera drawn 10-14 days apart are recommended. A single specimen is satisfactory to establish immune status. Antibodies to VZV are not usually detected until 1-3 days after the exanthem appears.[3]

Special Instructions Both PCR and antibody analysis are recommended for CSF evaluation.[4]

Reference Interval Diagnosis of infection: A single low titer or less than a fourfold increase in IgG titer in paired sera; undetectable antibody by fluorescent antibody to membrane antigen test. **Immune status:** IgG alone is sufficient. Reactive result indicates immunity (either from infection or vaccination) but does not assure protection from shingles.

Critical Values Negative serology in an adult or pregnant female exposed to varicella-zoster virus

Use Occasionally, to establish diagnosis of varicella-zoster infection; more often used to determine adult susceptibility or immunity to infection

Limitations Complement fixation test is insensitive and has heterologous reactions with herpesvirus. Primary or secondary infections with other herpesviruses may produce significant VZV titer increases in individuals who have previously had chickenpox.[5] A positive low titer may not correlate with protection. Zoster can develop despite substantial antibody titers.[3] Antibodies to VZV persist in serum in most adults.[4]

VZV antigens can be detected on smears from the base of the vesicle by immunologic staining with monoclonal antibodies.

Methodology Fluorescent antibody to membrane antigen (FAMA), hemagglutination, anticomplement immunofluorescence, enzyme-linked immunosorbent assay (ELISA). Molecular techniques (eg, PCR) will become methods of choice for VZV when methods become widely available.[2,4] Detection of viral DNA in amniotic fluid by PCR may prove to be useful.[6]

Additional Information More than 85% of adults who do not recall having chickenpox are seropositive for this virus.[2] Although most cases of varicella or zoster are clinically unambiguous, serology may rarely be useful in the differential diagnosis of other blistering illnesses or when infection shows an unusual complication, such as hepatitis. IgG antibodies can be detected 9 days after the onset of rash in primary varicella and 10 days after reactivation or zoster. IgM antibodies can be detected after 6-7 days and peak at ~14 days. It may also be important to establish whether an individual is susceptible when clinical history is unclear, or when varicella immune globulin may be needed, as in the immunocompromised host or cancer patient on toxic chemotherapy. Zoster is more common with aging and may occur in spite of significant antibody titers, demonstrating that cell-mediated immunity is critical. Varicella pneumonia in adults is the most frequent severe complication.[7] Viral myocarditis occurs and may progress to dilated cardiomyopathy, experimentally and clinically.[8] Pregnant and postpartum women are at increased risk of VZV pneumonia.[6] Some seronegative women may have primary infection while pregnant. The risk of fetal damage in the presence of maternal varicella infection in the first 20 weeks of pregnancy is ~2%, and life-threatening illness may develop in the mother. (Continued)

Varicella-Zoster Virus Serology *(Continued)*

Neonatal infection is possible if the mother contracts the infection in the last 3 weeks of gestation. Serious cases of VZV are treated with acyclovir.

A vaccine consisting of live-attenuated varicella is now available and is recommended by the CDC for children between the ages of 1-6 years of age, persons who work in an environment where transmission of VZV is likely such as day care center, teachers, residents and staff in institutional settings, college students, prison inmates, and military personnel. Additionally, the vaccine is recommended for nonpregnant women of childbearing years and international travelers who are unsure of past exposure. Patients who are immunocompromised (eg, childhood leukemics) and other susceptible individuals should also be immunized.[9] Positive serology should be indicative of protection.

See Varicella-Zoster Virus Culture *on page 686.*

Footnotes

1. Centers for Disease Control and Prevention, "Varicella - Related Deaths - Florida, 1998," *Morbid Mortal Weekly Rep*, 1999, 48(18):379-81.
2. Cohen PR, "Tests for Detecting Herpes Simplex Virus and Varicella-Zoster Virus Infections," *Dermatol Clin*, 1994, 12(1):51-68.
3. Leisegang TJ, "Varicella Zoster Viral Disease," *Mayo Clin Proc*, 1999, 74(10):983-8.
4. Gilden DH, Kleinschmidt-DeMasters BK, LaGuardia JJ, et al, "Neurologic Complications of the Reactivation of Varicella-Zoster Virus," *N Engl J Med*, 2000, 342(9):635-45.
5. Oladepo DK, Klapper PE, Percival D, et al, "Serological Diagnosis of Varicella-Zoster Virus in Sera With Antibody-Capture Enzyme-Linked Immunosorbent Assay of IgM," *J Virol Methods*, 2000, 84(2):169-73.
6. Isaacs D, "Neonatal Chickenpox," *J Paediatr Child Health*, 2000, 36(1):76-7.
7. Feldman S, "Varicella-Zoster Virus Pneumonitis," *Chest*, 1994, 106(Suppl 1):22S-7S.
8. Tsintsof A, Delprado WJ, and Keogh AM, "Varcella Zoster Myocarditis Progressing to Cardiomyopathy and Cardiac Transplantation," *Br Heart J*, 1993, 70(1):93-5.
9. Centers for Disease Control and Prevention, "Prevention of Varicella Updated Recommendations of the Advisory Committee on Immunization Practices (ACIP)," *Morbid Mortal Weekly Rep*, 1999, 48(RR-06):1-5.

References

Brunell PA and Wood D, "Varicella Serological Status of Healthcare Workers as a Guide to Whom to Test or Immunize," *Infect Control Hosp Epidemiol*, 1999, 20(5):355-7.

Chartrand SA, "Varicella Vaccine," *Pediatr Clin North Am*, 2000, 47(2):373-94.

Cohen JI, Brunell PA, Straus SE, et al, "Recent Advances in Varicella-Zoster Virus Infection," *Ann Intern Med*, 1999, 130(11):922-32.

Gil A, Gonzalez A, Dal-Re R, et al, "Prevalence of Antibodies Against Varicella Zoster, Herpes Simplex (Types 1 and 2), Hepatitis B and Hepatitis A Viruses Among Spanish Adolescents," *J Infect*, 1998, 36(1):53-6.

Katial RK, Ratto-Kim S, Sitz KV, et al, "Varicella Immunity: Persistent Serologic Nonresponse to Immunization," *Ann Allergy Asthma Immunol*, 1999, 82(5):431-4.

Niederhauser VP, "Varicella: The Vaccine and the Public Health Debate," *Nurse Pract*, 1999, 24(3):74-84.

Qureshi F and Jacques SM, "Maternal Varicella During Pregnancy: Correlation of Maternal History and Fetal Outcome With Placental Histopathology," *Hum Pathol*, 1996, 27(2):191-5.

Sauerbrei A, Eichhorn U, Schalke M, et al, "Laboratory Diagnosis of Herpes Zoster," *J Clin Virol*, 1999, 14(1):31-6.

Smith TF, Wold AD, Espy MJ, et al, "New Developments in the Diagnosis of Viral Diseases," *Infect Dis Clin North Am*, 1993, 7(2):183-201.

Straus SE, "Overview: The Biology of Varicella-Zoster Virus Infection," *Ann Neurol*, 1994, 35(Suppl):4-8.

Internet Web Sites

www.cdc.gov/ncidod/srp/varicella.htm
www.who.int/vaccines-diseases/diseases/pp_varicella.htm

♦ **VCA** *see* Epstein-Barr Virus Serology *on page 607*

♦ **VCA Titer** *see* Epstein-Barr Virus Serology *on page 607*

VDRL, Cerebrospinal Fluid

Related Information

Bacterial Culture, Cerebrospinal Fluid *on page 569*
Cerebrospinal Fluid Analysis: Overview *on page 416*
Cerebrospinal Fluid Protein *on page 517*
Darkfield Examination, Syphilis *on page 601*
FTA-ABS, Serum *on page 609*
MHA-TP *on page 651*
RPR *on page 677*
VDRL, Serum *on page 688*

Synonyms Cerebrospinal Fluid VDRL; CSF VDRL

Applies to Cardiolipin Antibodies; Syphilis Serology

Test Includes Titer of reactive specimens

Abstract Throughout the world, syphilis is a common sexually transmitted disease despite effective therapy. About 66% of the syphilis cases reported in the U.S. are diagnosed at the latent stage. Additionally, many cases are not diagnosed until the patient is suffering from neurosyphilis. A reactive CSF VDRL test result is acceptable to establish the diagnosis of neurosyphilis, although the sensitivity is only 50% to 60%.[1] A nonreactive test is inconclusive.

Specimen Cerebrospinal fluid

Container Clean, sterile CSF container

Special Instructions Do not heat inactivate the CSF.

Reference Interval Nonreactive

Use Test for neurosyphilis; VDRL, CSF is the only laboratory test for neurosyphilis approved by the Centers for Disease Control. It is very specific. The sensitivity of the CSF VDRL for the diagnosis of neurosyphilis is ~90%.[2]

Limitations A negative VDRL on CSF does not rule out the diagnosis of neurosyphilis;[3] further investigation when clinically appropriate may include a serum FTA-ABS.

Methodology Flocculation test detects reagin, antibody to nontreponemal antigen

Additional Information Central nervous system syphilis may be asymptomatic. Neurosyphilis includes **meningeal syphilis**, which is usually found within a year of infection. Its characteristics include headache, stiff neck, nausea and vomiting, sometimes with cranial nerve involvement. **Syphilitic meningitis** can be localized (**gumma**). **Meningovascular syphilis** is found 4-7 years after infection. **General paresis** or **tabes dorsalis** occur late, frequently decades after infection. Uveitis, retinitis, luetic optic neuritis may occur with or without syphilitic meningitis. Optic atrophy is usually found with tabes dorsalis.[4] The diagnosis of neurosyphilis is excluded if the serum FTA-ABS result is nonreactive.[1]

A positive VDRL in a spinal fluid uncontaminated by serum is essentially diagnostic of neurosyphilis. However, a negative test may occur in 30% of patients with tabes dorsalis, and was positive in only 69% to 92% of patients who had active neurosyphilis.[2,3] The CSF VDRL may take years to become nonreactive after adequate therapy.

Criteria for neurosyphilis include CSF cell count >5 mononuclear cells/mm³ and CSF total protein >40 mg/dL.[5]

Patients with HIV may develop neurosyphilis following therapy that is usually considered adequate. In AIDS patients, serial CSF VDRL determinations may be needed when neurosyphilis is suspected. By requiring either a positive serum RPR or FTA-ABS, seropositivity of CSF VDRL could increase to 90%.[6]

Footnotes

1. Smith GP and Kjeldsberg CR, "Cerebrospinal, Synovial, and Serous Body Fluids," *Clinical Diagnosis and Management by Laboratory Methods*, 20th ed, Henry JB, ed, Philadelphia, PA: WB Saunders Co, 2001, 403-24.
2. Luger AF, Schmidt BL, and Kaulich M, "Significance of Laboratory Findings for the Diagnosis of Neurosyphilis," *Int J STD AIDS*, 2000, 11(4):224-34.
3. Woods GL, "Update on Laboratory Diagnosis of Sexually Transmitted Diseases," *Clin Lab Med*, 1995, 15(3):665-84.
4. Hook EW 3d and Marra CM, "Acquired Syphilis in Adults," *N Engl J Med*, 1992, 326:1060-9.
5. Larsen SA, Steiner BM, and Rudolph AH, "Laboratory Diagnosis and Interpretation of Tests for Syphilis," *Clin Microbiol Rev*, 1995, 8(1):1-21.
6. Flood JM, Weinstock HS, Guroy ME, et al, "Neurosyphilis During the AIDS Epidemic, San Francisco, 1985-1992," *J Infect Dis*, 1998, 177(4):931-40.

References

Albright RE Jr, Christenson RH, Emlet JL, et al, "Issues in Cerebrospinal Fluid Management. CSF Venereal Disease Research Laboratory Testing," *Am J Clin Pathol*, 1991, 95(3):397-401.

Birnbaum NR, Goldschmidt RH, and Buffet WO, "Resolving the Common Clinical Dilemmas of Syphilis," *Am Fam Phys*, 1999, 59(8):2233-46.

Desforges JF, "Infectious Disease Testing for Blood Transfusions," *NIH Consensus Statement*, 1995, 13(1):1-27.

Horowitz HW, Valsamis MP, Wicher V, et al, "Brief Report: Cerebral Syphilitic Gumma Confirmed by the Polymerase Chain Reaction in a Man With Human Immunodeficiency Virus Infection," *N Engl J Med*, 1994, 331(22):1488-91.

Janier M, Chastang C, Spindler E, et al, "A Prospective Study of the Influence of HIV Status on the Seroconversion of Serological Tests for Syphilis," *Dermatology*, 1999, 198(4):362-9.

Quinn P and Weisberg L, "Cerebral Syphilitic Gumma," *N Engl J Med*, 1997, 336(14):1027.

Internet Web Sites

www.cdc.gov/nchstp/dstd/fact_sheets/syphilis_facts.htm

VDRL, Serum

Related Information

Anticardiolipin Antibody *on page 503*
Antiphospholipid Antibody (Lupus Anticoagulant and/or Anticardiolipin Antibody) *on page 331*
Bacterial Culture, Genital Specimen *on page 571*
Darkfield Examination, Syphilis *on page 601*
FTA-ABS, Serum *on page 609*
MHA-TP *on page 651*
Neisseria gonorrhoeae Culture and Smear *on page 662*
Risks of Transfusion *on page 861*
RPR *on page 677*
VDRL, Cerebrospinal Fluid *on page 688*

Synonyms Venereal Disease Research Laboratory Test, Serum

Applies to Cardiolipin Antibodies; Syphilis Serology

Replaces Kahn Test; Kline Test; Mazzini; Wassermann

Test Includes Determination of serologic response to *Treponema* infection

Abstract The diagnosis of syphilis can present a difficult dilemma. Nontreponemal serologic tests can be used for screening but can be negative if performed in the primary stage. The VDRL serum test may also be falsely negative in late syphilis. Prozone reactions are seen. False-positive results are also recognized: they are defined as a reproducible reactive test in an individual without clinical or historical evidence of lues, whose FTA-ABS or MHA-TP is negative.[1]

Specimen Serum

Container Red top tube

Collection The CDC recommends that when screening for congenital syphilis the mother's serum should be tested rather than cord blood.

Causes for Rejection Plasma cannot be used

Reference Interval Nonreactive

Possible Panic Range Positive results in pregnancy should be confirmed by a treponemal test.

Use VDRL is a reaginic (nontreponemal) test for syphilis. It is a screening test for syphilis that may also be used to assess adequacy of treatment. The differential diagnosis of a genital ulcer includes herpes, although classically herpetic lesions are vesicular and multiple.[1] VDRL is recommended in all expectant mothers at the beginning of pregnancy and near term to avoid congenital syphilis.

Limitations False-positive results may be found in advancing age, during pregnancy, malaria, infectious mononucleosis, infectious hepatitis, leprosy, brucellosis, SLE, atypical pneumonia, typhus, and other entities.[2] See table. Reactive tests due to related treponemal infections also occur: *T. pallidum* subspecies *pertenue*, which causes yaws; *T. carateum* which causes pinta and *T. pallidum* subspecies *endemicum*, the cause of nonvenereal or endemic syphilis. False-negative results occur early in primary syphilis when the chancre is still present, and also occur in late syphilis.[3] The serum VDRL may be negative in as many as 40% of subjects who have tabes dorsalis, while the specific tests (eg, FTA-ABS) remain reactive.[2]

False-positive results may occur in newborns. In young females, a chronic false-positive VDRL may signal future development of autoimmune disorders, including SLE or thyroiditis.[1]

False-negative tests due to prozone phenomenon are identified by testing with diluted serum. This should be performed in individuals who test negative despite high clinical suspicion. False negative RPR and VDRL tests are seen early, in the primary stage, and in late syphilis (latent, tertiary), and in the elderly.[4]

Treponemal tests (eg, FTA-ABS) become reactive before nontreponemal (reaginic) tests such as VDRL.[2] A positive result in cord blood may be due to passive transfer from mother's blood. (Maternal IgG antibodies cross the placenta. The diagnosis of congenital syphilis utilizes IgM antibodies).

Potential Causes of False-Positive Serologic Tests for Syphilis

	Infectious Causes	Noninfectious Causes
Reaginic or nontreponemal tests (RPR, VDRL)		
Bacterial	Pneumococcal pneumonia	Pregnancy
	Scarlet fever	Chronic liver disease
	Leprosy	Advanced cancer
	Lymphogranuloma venereum	Intravenous drug use
	Relapsing fever	Multiple myeloma, other types of malignancy, other entities causing immunoglobulin abnormalities
	Bacterial endocarditis	Advancing age
	Malaria	Connective tissue diseases, (eg, SLE)
	Rickettsial disease	Multiple blood transfusions
	Psittacosis	Narcotic addiction
	Leptospirosis	Technical error
	Chancroid	
	Tuberculosis	
	Mycoplasmal pneumonia	
	Trypanosomiasis	
Viral	Vaccinia (vaccination)	
	Chickenpox	
	HIV	
	Measles	
	Infectious mononucleosis	
	Mumps	
	Viral hepatitis	
Treponemal tests (FTA-ABS, MHA-TP)	Lyme disease	Systemic lupus erythematosus
	Leprosy	Rheumatoid arthritis
	Malaria	Biliary cirrhosis
	Infectious mononucleosis	
	Rat bite fever	
	Relapsing fever	
	Leptospirosis	

Adapted from Hook EW 3d and Marra CM, "Acquired Syphilis in Adults," *N Engl J Med*, 1992, 326:1060-9.

Methodology Flocculation procedure detecting the presence of reagin, antibody to nontreponemal cardiolipin antigen

Additional Information Despite false-positive results, the VDRL remains an extremely useful screening test for syphilis. The VDRL becomes positive 2 weeks after the chancre appears, and by 6 weeks, 90% of cases are positive. By 9-12 weeks, in the secondary stage, 100% of patients should be reactive. (The secondary stage includes rash, mucocutaneous lesions, and lymphadenopathy). The latent stage follows. With therapy the VDRL reverts to negative. Even without treatment the VDRL may become negative years after infection. Thus, the VDRL may be negative in tertiary syphilis. Only about 40% of patients with syphilitic aortitis have a positive nontreponemal test.[4] The VDRL test can be done on CSF and is useful in the diagnosis of neurosyphilis (see VDRL, Cerebrospinal Fluid *on page 688*). Positive VDRL results should be confirmed with a *Treponema*-specific test. The VDRL is recommended as a screen for uveitis or unexplained ocular inflammation.

The diagnosis of syphilis in persons infected with HIV may be difficult: lack of serologic response in a patient with confirmed syphilis is seen and rapid progression in spite of treatment occurs.[5] The presence of syphilis bears positive association with risk of HIV acquisition.

Footnotes
1. Hook EW 3d, "Syphilis," *Cecil Textbook of Medicine*, 21st ed, Chapter 365, Goldman L and Bennett JC, eds, Philadelphia, PA: WB Saunders Co, 2000, 1746-55.
2. Hook EW 3d and Marra CM, "Acquired Syphilis in Adults," *N Engl J Med*, 1992, 326:1060-9.
3. Birnbaum NR, Goldschmidt RH, and Buffett WO, "Resolving the Common Clinical Dilemmas of Syphilis," *Am Fam Physician*, 1999, 59(8):2233-56.
4. Vlahakes GJ, Hanna GJ, and Mark EJ, "A 46-Year-Old Man With Chest Pain and Coronary Ostial Stenosis," Case Records of the Massachusetts General Hospital, Case 10-1998, Scully RE, Mark EJ, McNeely WF, et al, eds, *N Engl J Med*, 1998, 338(13): 897-903.
5. Janier M, Chastang C, Spindler E, et al, "A Prospective Study of the Influence of HIV Status on the Seroconversion of Serological Tests for Syphilis," *Dermatology*, 1999, 198(4):362-9.

References
Bordon J, Martinez-Vazquez C, de la Fuente-Aguado J, et al, "Response to Standard Syphilis Treatment in Patients Infected With Human Immunodeficiency Virus," *Eur J Clin Microbiol Infect Dis*, 1999, 18(10):729-32.
Flood JM, Weinstock HS, Guroy ME, et al, "Neurosyphilis During the AIDS Epidemic, San Francisco, 1985-1992," *J Infect Dis*, 1998, 177(4):931-40.
Gwanzura L, Latif A, Bassett M, et al, "Syphilis Serology and HIV Infection in Harare, Zimbabwe," *Sex Transm Infect*, 1999, 75(6):426-30.
Kaur H and Marshalla R, "Seroepidemiology of HIV, HBV, HCV and Treponemal Infections," *J Commun Dis*, 1998, 30(1):29-31.
Kilmarx PH, Black CM, Limmpakarnjanarat K, et al, "Rapid Assessment of Sexually Transmitted Diseases in a Sentinel Population in Thailand: Prevalence of Chlamydial Infection, Gonorrhoea, and Syphilis Among Pregnant Women - 1996," *Sex Transm Infect*, 1998, 74(3):189-93.
Larsen SA, Steiner BM, and Rudolph AH, "Laboratory Diagnosis and Interpretation of Tests for Syphilis," *Clin Microbiol Rev*, 1995, 8(1):1-21.
Luger AF, Schmidt BL, and Kaulich M, "Significance of Laboratory Findings for the Diagnosis of Neurosyphilis," *Int J STD AIDS*, 2000, 11(4):224-34.
Musher DM and Baughn RE, "Neurosyphilis in HIV-Infected Persons," *N Engl J Med*, 1994, 331(22):1516-7.

Internet Web Sites
www.cdc.gov/nchstp/dstd/fact_sheets/syphilis_facts.htm

◆ **Venereal Disease Research Laboratory Test, Serum** *see* VDRL, Serum *on page 688*

◆ **Ventricular Fluid Culture** *see* Bacterial Culture, Cerebrospinal Fluid *on page 569*

◆ **Verotoxin Detection** *see* Shiga Toxin Test, Direct *on page 680*

◆ **Vesicle Viral Culture** *see* Viral Culture, Dermatological Symptoms *on page 693*

◆ ***Vibrio cholerae*** *see* Bacterial Culture, Stool *on page 575*

◆ ***Vibrio parahaemolyticus*** *see* Bacterial Culture, Stool *on page 575*

◆ **Viral Antigen Detection, Direct, Stool** *see* Rotavirus, Direct Detection *on page 676*

◆ **Viral Capsid Antigen** *see* Epstein-Barr Virus Serology *on page 607*

Viral Culture

Related Information
(Continued)

Viral Culture (Continued)

Applies to CPE; Cytopathic Effect; Enveloped Viruses

Test Includes Inoculation of specimen onto appropriate cell cultures; isolated viruses are identified using specific monoclonal antibodies, neutralization, or hemadsorption

Abstract The primary technique for many viral infections is the isolation of virus in tissue culture cells. For other viral infections serologic diagnosis, direct antigen detection in body fluids or tissues, or nucleic acid detection is the method of choice for diagnosis. As with any diagnostic test there are advantages and disadvantages to each method. For viral culture, specimens must be collected within the first few days of an illness and specimens should be brought to the laboratory in viral holding medium as quickly as possible. This helps to ensure adequate sensitivity of viral culture.

Specimen Whole blood, cerebrospinal fluid, dermal, ocular, genital, mucosal, respiratory, oral, stool, rectal, urine, tissue, biopsy. See table.

Viruses Typically Isolated From Clinical Specimens

Specimen	Virus*
Blood	CMV, enteroviruses†,#, HSV#, VZV#
CSF and CNS tissues	Enteroviruses, mumps virus, HSV, CMV
Dermal lesions	HSV, VZV, adenovirus, enteroviruses
Eye	HSV, VZV, adenovirus, enteroviruses, CMV, *Chlamydia*
Genital	HSV, CMV, *Chlamydia*
Mucosal	HSV, VZV
Oral	HSV, VZV
Rectal	HSV, VZV, enterovirus
Respiratory tract	
upper	Adenovirus, rhinovirus, influenza, parainfluenza, enteroviruses, RSV, reovirus, HSV
lower	Adenovirus, influenza, parainfluenza, RSV, CMV•
Sputum not acceptable	
Stool	Enteroviruses, adenoviruses
Tissues	CMV, HSV, enteroviruses
Urine	CMV, adenovirus, enteroviruses, mumps

*Abbreviations:

  HSV — herpes simplex virus

  CMV — cytomegalovirus

  VZV — varicella-zoster virus

  RSV — respiratory syncytial virus

†Enteroviruses: Coxsackievirus, poliovirus, echovirus, and enterovirus.

#Rarely isolated.

•Usually in immunocompromised hosts.

Container Viral transport medium for swabs; sterile screw-cap tube or container for fluids, feces, nasal washings, urine, or biopsy (without preservative); green top (heparin) tube for blood, bone marrow, and buffy coat. **Keep all specimens at 4°C and moist. Do not freeze specimen at -20°C especially in a frost-free freezer.**

Collection Specimen should be collected during the acute phase of the disease, as follows.

Blood: 5 mL whole blood in heparinized tube

Cerebrospinal fluid: Collect 1 mL CSF aseptically in a sterile dry screw-cap vial. Spinal fluid and throat washings must be kept cold and must not be frozen. **Keep cold and bring to the laboratory immediately.**

Skin lesions: Open the vesicle and absorb exudate into a dry swab, and/or vigorously scrape base of freshly exposed lesion with a swab to obtain cells which contain viruses. If enough vesicle fluid is available, aspirate the fluid with a fine-gauge needle and tuberculin syringe, and place fluid into cold viral transport medium. Use Virocult® or Culturette® swabs for specimen collection. **Keep cold and bring to the laboratory immediately.** Calcium alginate swabs are toxic to *Chlamydia* and many enveloped viruses. **Do not use calcium alginate swabs for viral or chlamydial isolation.**

Eye swab or scraping: Use a Virocult® or Culturette® swab to collect conjunctival material or take conjunctival scrapings with a fine sterile spatula and transfer the scraping to a viral transport medium. **Keep cold and bring to the laboratory immediately.** Calcium alginate swabs are toxic to *Chlamydia* and many enveloped viruses. **Do not use calcium alginate swabs for viral or chlamydial isolation.**

Genital swab: See skin. **Keep cold and bring to the laboratory immediately.**

Throat swab: Carefully rub the posterior wall of the nasopharynx with a dry, sterile swab. Avoid touching the tongue or buccal mucosa. Use Virocult® or Culturette® swabs for specimen collection. **Keep cold and bring to the laboratory immediately.**

Feces: Collect 4-8 g of feces (about the size of a thumbnail), and place in a clean, leakproof container. Stool specimens should not be placed into viral transport medium or frozen. **Do not** dilute the specimen (into virus transport medium) or use preservatives. **Keep cold and bring to the laboratory immediately.**

Rectal swab: Insert a sterile swab 2-4 inches into the rectum and rub the mucosa. Use Virocult® or Culturette® swabs for specimen collection. **Keep cold and bring to the laboratory immediately.** Swab may be placed into cold virus transport medium.

Urine: Collect clean-catch, midstream urine in a leakproof, sterile container. Urine specimens for CMV culture **must not** be frozen; they should be packed with an ice pack or snow gel, but not with dry ice. **Keep cold and bring to the laboratory immediately.**

Tissue: Use a fresh set of sterile instruments to collect each tissue. Place each specimen in its own dry, sterile nontoxic leakproof container. Identify each tissue with patient's name, type of tissue, and date collected. **Keep cold and bring tissue to the laboratory immediately.**

Storage Instructions Specimen must be kept cold and moist, and must be delivered to the laboratory as soon as possible. If a longer period is required, specimen should be stored or transported according to the laboratory that will receive the specimen. **Do not freeze specimens at -20°C;** if absolutely necessary store specimens at 4°C to 6°C up to 96 hours after collection. For longer storage, freeze the specimen quickly at -70°C. Specimens to be cultured for influenza virus and cytomegalovirus should be sent on wet ice or with an ice pack.

Causes for Rejection Dry specimen, specimen not refrigerated during transport, specimen fixed in formalin, unlabeled specimen

Turnaround Time The presence of viruses is usually suggested by the characteristic cytopathic effect (CPE) they cause when they infect cell cultures. CPE (and, therefore, positive results) can be observed as soon as 1 day and as late as 28 days postinoculation of the cell culture.[1] Virus grown in rapid cultures from shell-vials can be detected as early as 24 hours after inoculation.[2,3]

Special Instructions Culture, serological tests, antigen detection, and nucleic acid detection for certain specific viruses are available. Contact the laboratory to determine availability of tests. When possible, the serological tests should be requested at same time as culture. Acute and convalescent blood samples (5 mL) are required for serologic studies. Requisition **must** state specific virus(s) suspected, source of specimen, age of patient, current antibiotic therapy, relevant vaccinations, and pertinent clinical history.

Reference Interval No virus isolated

Use Aid in the diagnosis of viral diseases (eg, AIDS, aseptic meningitis, conjunctivitis, congenital viral infections, keratitis, chickenpox, shingles, viral pneumonia, and some diseases characterized by skin vesicles and rashes)

Limitations Many common viruses are not culturable (see table). For many such viral diseases, serologic testing is required. Recovery of virus from sites where it may be found in the absence of disease may not be the causative agent of disease. Negative viral culture does not rule out a viral etiology. Some positive cultures are sent to State Health Laboratory for specific virus identification.

Viruses That Are Nonculturable or Require Animal Inoculation or Special Culture Technique

Arenaviruses	Hepatitis D
Astrovirus	Hepatitis E
Calicivirus	Lassa
California encephalitis	Marburg
Coronaviruses	*Molluscum contagiosum*
Coxsackievirus type A	Norwalk agent
Dengue	Papillomaviruses
Eastern equine encephalitis	Parvoviruses
Ebola	Polyomavirus
Filoviruses	Rabies
Hantavirus (Muerto Canyon)	Rotaviruses
Hepatitis A	St Louis encephalitis
Hepatitis B	Western equine encephalitis
Hepatitis C	Yellow fever

Methodology Inoculation of specimen into cell cultures, incubation of cultures, observation for characteristic cytopathic effect (CPE), and identification by methods such as hemadsorption and fluorescent monoclonal antibodies. If specific viruses such as HSV, CMV, VZV, influenza, RSV, parainfluenza, or adenovirus are suspected, the laboratory might be able to use rapid (1-2 days) culture (shell vial) methods to detect these viruses.[2,3]

Additional Information

Viral cultures: Viruses are obligate intracellular organisms that require cell culture techniques for growth. The detection and identification of viruses associated with infection is important for patient management, such as choice of antiviral therapy, and for epidemiology. Some viral infections can be detected by identification of viral antigens without culture. Other diagnostic methods are the detection of specific viral nucleic acid and the detection of a specific antibody response in the patient. The laboratory diagnosis of viral diseases is changing rapidly; consultation with the laboratory for currently used methods is recommended.

In general, specimens for viral culture should be collected in the acute stage of the illness, kept moist, and refrigerated immediately. Always check with the laboratory to coordinate shipping/transfer times and expected arrival times. Viruses that are enveloped (herpesviruses, myxoviruses, and paramycoviruses such as RSV) are not stable outside the body. However, these viruses can survive transit for at least 24-48 hours if they are kept at 4°C. Many viruses do not survive freezing at -20°C. For example, herpes simplex virus titer can decease by 100-fold with a single freeze-thaw cycle. Every measure should be taken to ensure the proper collection and transport of specimens for viral cultures.

Footnotes

1. Yolken RH, "Laboratory Diagnosis of Viral Infections," *Practical Diagnosis of Viral Infections*, Galasso GJ, Whitley RJ, Merigan TC, eds, New York, NY: Raven Press, 1993, 17-67.
2. Shih SR, Tsao KC, Ning HC, et al, "Diagnosis of Respiratory Tract Viruses in 24 Hours by Immunofluorescent Staining of Shell Vial Cultures Containing Madin-Darby Canine Kidney (MDCK) Cells," *J Virol Methods*, 1999, 81(1-2):77-81.
3. Navarro-Mari JM, Sanbonmatsu-Gamez S, Perez-Ruiz M, et al, "Rapid Detection of Respiratory Viruses by Shell Vial Assay Using Simultaneous Culture of Hep-2, LLC-MK2, and MDCK Cells in a Single Vial," *J Clin Microbiol*, 1999, 37(7):2346-7.

References

Casteels A, Naessens A, Gordts F, et al, "Neonatal Screening for Congenital Cytomegalovirus Infections," *J Perinat Med*, 1999, 27(2):116-21.

Chien JW and Johnson JL, "Viral Pneumonias: Epidemic Respiratory Viruses," *Postgrad Med*, 2000, 107(3):41-52.

Pugh RN, Omar RI, and Hossain MM, "Varicella Infection and Pneumonia Among Adults," *Int J Infect Dis*, 1998, 2(4):205-10.

Raj P, "Classification of Medically Important Viruses I: DNA Viruses," *Clin Microbiol Newslet*, 1994, 16(16):121-4.

Raj P, "Classification of Medically Important Viruses II: RNA Viruses," *Clin Microbiol Newslet*, 1994, 16(17):129-34.

Riley LE, "Herpes Simplex Virus," *Semin Perinatol*, 1998, 22(4):284-92.

Sintchenko V and Dwyer DE, "The Diagnosis and Management of Influenza: An Update," *Aust Fam Physician*, 1999, 28(4):313-7.

Zambon M, "Cell Culture for Surveillance on Influenza," *Dev Biol Stand*, 1999, 98:65-74.

♦ **Viral Culture, Biopsy** see Viral Culture, Tissue on page 695

Viral Culture, Blood

Related Information
Bacterial Culture, Blood on page 566
Coxsackievirus Serology on page 595
Cytomegalovirus Culture on page 598
Enterovirus Culture on page 605
Epstein-Barr Virus Culture on page 607
Herpesvirus 6 Culture on page 633
Viral Culture on page 689

Synonyms CMV, Blood Culture; CMV, Buffy Coat Culture; CMV Culture; Enterovirus, Blood Culture

Test Includes Usually includes both rapid shell vial isolation technique (to detect CMV early antigen) and/or conventional cell culture for all major viruses

Abstract It is rare to detect virus from blood specimens, but when a virus such as varicella-zoster or herpes simplex is isolated from a blood specimen it usually indicates a serious condition. The most commonly isolated virus from blood is cytomegalovirus (CMV) in immunocompromised patients. Detection of CMV in leukocytes is more indicative of active CMV infection than is the detection of CMV shedding in the urine or respiratory specimens. Other herpesviruses have occasionally been isolated from blood of patients.

Patient Preparation Cleanse skin with 70% isopropyl alcohol. Apply povidone-iodine in concentric circles. **Note:** Iodine should remain in contact with skin for at least 1 minute prior to venipuncture to ensure complete antisepsis. Remove iodine with 70% isopropyl alcohol in concentric circles after venipuncture. Obtain 3-6 mL of blood.

Specimen Whole blood

Container Green top (heparin) tube. Some laboratories request that blood be collected in citrate anticoagulant or EDTA. Alternatively, a blood specimen can be obtained in a heparinized syringe. The heparin should be sterile and free of preservative.

Sampling Time Collect blood during early acute phase of infection.

Storage Instructions Do not store specimen. Send to the laboratory immediately.

Turnaround Time Shell vial rapid isolation: 1-2 days; conventional culture: 2 days to 4 weeks

Use Aid in the diagnosis of systemic viral infections, especially CMV (eg, transplantation-associated viral diseases and congenital viral diseases)

Limitations Blood (serum in particular) is generally not a good specimen from which to recover viruses. Detection of CMV depends on adequate numbers of white blood cells. After bone marrow transplantation there are episodes of leukopenia and the sensitivity of culture is greatly decreased during such episodes. CMV loses infectivity after freezing at -20°C, and best results are noted when the specimen is inoculated quickly after collection.

Methodology Inoculation of peripheral blood cells or serum into cell cultures (either shell vials or tube cultures), identification of virus by cytopathic effect (CPE) and monoclonal antibodies

Additional Information Infections with CMV can be detected in white blood cells, especially from immunocompromised patients.[1] Recent studies have shown that the detection of CMV nucleic acid in white blood cells or serum from bone marrow transplant patients is superior to detection of virus in culture.[2,3] Such tests are currently available in most larger reference laboratories and some laboratories can perform quantitation of viral DNA. A table in Viral Culture on page 689 provides further information.

Footnotes

1. Patel R, Klein DW, Espy MJ, et al, "Optimization of Detection of Cytomegalovirus Viremia in Transplantation Recipients by Shell Vial Assay," *J Clin Microbiol*, 1995, 33(11):2984-6.
2. Matsunaga T, Sakamaki S, Ishigaki S, et al, "Use of PCR Serum in Diagnosing and Monitoring Cytomegalovirus Reactivation in Bone Marrow Transplant Patients," *Int J Hematol*, 1999, 69(2):105-11.
3. Zipeto D, Morris S, Hong C, et al, "Human Cytomegalovirus (CMV) DNA in Plasma Reflects Quantity of CMV DNA Present in Leukocytes," *J Clin Microbiol*, 1995, 33(10):2607-11.

References

Blok MJ, Goossens VJ, Vanherle V, et al, "Diagnostic Value of Monitoring Human Cytomegalovirus Late pp67 mRNA Expression in Renal-Allograft Recipients by Nucleic Acid Sequence-Based Amplification," *J Clin Microbiol*, 1998, 36(5):1341-6.

Flechner SM, Avery RK, Fisher R, et al, "Monitoring of CMV Infection After Renal Transplantation: Serology, Culture, and Viral DNA Detection by Hybrid Capture," *Transplant Proc*, 1999, 31(1-2):1255-7.

Hodinka RL, "Human Cytomegalovirus," *Manual of Clinical Microbiology*, 7th ed, Murray PR, Baron EJ, Pfaller MA, et al, eds, Washington, DC: AMS Press, American Society for Microbiology, 1999, 888-99.

Internet Web Sites
www.cdc.gov/ncidod/diseases/cmv.htm

Viral Culture, Body Fluid

Related Information
Adenovirus Antibody Titer on page 552
Bacterial Culture, Biopsy or Body Fluid on page 565
Body Cavity Fluid Cytology on page 372
Body Fluid Analysis, Cell Count on page 408
Body Fluid Chemical Analysis on page 123
Body Fluid Glucose on page 124
Body Fluid Lactate Dehydrogenase on page 125
Body Fluid pH on page 125
Coxsackievirus Serology on page 595
Fungal Culture, Biopsy or Body Fluid on page 610
Mycobacterial Culture, Biopsy or Body Fluid on page 655
Viral Culture on page 689

Synonyms Body Fluid Viral Culture

Applies to Amniotic Fluid, Viral Culture; Cerebrospinal Fluid, Viral Culture; Synovial Fluid, Viral Culture

Test Includes Isolation of all major viruses using conventional cell culture

Abstract Viruses are seldom isolated from synovial or pericardial fluid. Often when a virus causes pericarditis or arthritis, it is no longer present when symptoms are diagnosed. Viruses are most commonly isolated from fluids such as cerebrospinal fluid, amniotic fluid, and pleural fluid. Body fluids generally contain a sufficient amount of proteins to protect the viruses from lysis and thus virus transport media are not required.

Specimen Body fluids (eg, cerebrospinal fluid, pleural fluid, pericardial fluid, amniotic fluid)

Collection Specimens obtained aseptically. **Do not place fluids into virus transport medium.** Keep specimens cold (2°C to 8°C) because viruses isolated from body fluids are often labile. Transport to the laboratory as soon as possible.

Turnaround Time Variable (1-28 days)

Reference Interval No virus isolated

Use Aid in the differential diagnosis of systemic viral diseases

Limitations Some enteroviruses (Coxsackie A) cannot be isolated from routine viral culture. Recent studies have shown that detection of viral nucleic acid has better sensitivity than viral culture, especially on cerebrospinal fluid.[1,2] Often, only a few virus-infected cells are present in fluids. Therefore, larger amounts of fluid are required for a productive viral isolation and specimens should be placed onto cell cultures as soon as possible. If bacteria are suspected, a separate specimen must be submitted. (Continued)

Viral Culture, Body Fluid *(Continued)*

Methodology Inoculation of specimen into cell cultures, incubation of cultures, observation for characteristic cytopathic effect (CPE), and identification/speciation by methods such as hemadsorption and fluorescent monoclonal antibodies. If specific viruses such as HSV, CMV, VZV, or adenovirus are suspected, the laboratory might be able to use rapid (1-2 days) culture (shell vial) methods.

Additional Information See the table in Viral Culture *on page 689.*

Footnotes

1. Lakeman FD and Whitley RJ, "Diagnosis of Herpes Simplex Encephalitis: Application of Polymerase Chain Reaction to Cerebrospinal Fluid From Brain-Biopsied Patients and Correlation With Disease. National Institute of Allergy and Infectious Disease Collaborative Antiviral Study Group," *J Infect Dis*, 1995, 171(4):857-63.
2. Romero JR, "Reverse-Transcription Polymerase Chain Reaction Detection of the Enteroviruses," *Arch Pathol Lab Med*, 1999, 123(12):1161-9.

References

Chien JW and Johnson JL, "Viral Pneumonias: Infection in the Immunocompromised Host," *Postgrad Med*, 2000, 107(2):67-80.

Nairn C and Clements GB, "A Study of Enterovirus Isolations in Glasgow From 1977 to 1997," *J Med Virol*, 1999, 58(3):304-12.

Riley LE, "Herpes Simplex Virus," *Semin Perinatol*, 1998, 22(4):284-92.

Smith TF, "Rapid Diagnosis of Viral Infections," *Adv Exp Med Biol*, 1990, 263:115-21.

Internet Web Sites

www.cdc.gov/ncidod/dvrd/hfmd.htm

♦ **Viral Culture, Brain** *see* Viral Culture, Central Nervous System Symptoms *on page 692*

♦ **Viral Culture, Brain** *see* Viral Culture, Tissue *on page 695*

♦ **Viral Culture, Bronchial** *see* Viral Culture, Tissue *on page 695*

♦ **Viral Culture, Bronchial Wash** *see* Viral Culture, Respiratory Symptoms *on page 694*

Viral Culture, Central Nervous System Symptoms

Related Information

Bacterial Antigens, Rapid Detection Methods *on page 562*
Bacterial Culture, Cerebrospinal Fluid *on page 569*
California Encephalitis Virus Serology *on page 587*
Cerebrospinal Fluid Analysis: Overview *on page 416*
Cerebrospinal Fluid Cytology *on page 376*
Cerebrospinal Fluid Glucose *on page 140*
Cerebrospinal Fluid Immunoglobulin G *on page 515*
Cerebrospinal Fluid Oligoclonal Bands *on page 516*
Cerebrospinal Fluid Protein *on page 517*
Cerebrospinal Fluid Protein Electrophoresis *on page 518*
Coxsackievirus Serology *on page 595*
Eastern Equine Encephalitis Virus Serology *on page 602*
Enterovirus Culture *on page 605*
Fungal Culture, Cerebrospinal Fluid *on page 611*
Herpes Simplex Virus Culture *on page 631*
Mumps Serology *on page 653*
Mumps Virus Culture *on page 653*
Mycobacterial Culture, Cerebrospinal Fluid *on page 656*
Polymerase Chain Reaction *on page 713*
St Louis Encephalitis Virus Serology *on page 681*
Varicella-Zoster Virus Culture *on page 686*
Viral Culture *on page 689*
Western Equine Encephalitis Virus Serology *on page 697*

Synonyms Cerebrospinal Fluid Virus Culture

Applies to Lumbar Puncture Hazards; Viral Culture, Brain; Viral Culture, CSF

Test Includes Isolation of all culturable viruses using conventional cell culture

Abstract Viral meningitis is the most important cause of aseptic meningitis, a condition which has several clinical presentations and which has both infectious and noninfectious etiologies. Enteroviruses most often cause meningitis in the late summer and are the most common cause of aseptic meningitis in the United States. Patients are usually children and young adults. Enteroviruses include polioviruses, Coxsackieviruses, and echoviruses. Several recent reviews discuss criteria for distinguishing viral meningitis from bacterial meningitis.[1,2,3] The presence of polymorphonuclear cells in the cerebrospinal fluid (CSF) does not rule out viral meningitis. By definition, the cerebrospinal fluid in aseptic meningitis has pleocytosis and is culture-negative for bacteria.[2]

Specimen Cerebrospinal fluid (do not put into virus transport medium), brain biopsy, lesions, throat or throat washings, stool, urine

Container Sterile CSF tube; sterile screw-cap container for biopsy, tissue, urine, or throat washing; sterile viral transport medium for swab specimens

Sampling Time As soon as possible after the onset of symptoms. Many viruses are more likely to be cultured when samples are obtained early.

Collection Specimen should be collected during the acute phase of the disease, as follows.

Cerebrospinal fluid: Collect 1 mL CSF aseptically in a sterile dry screw-cap vial. **Keep cold and bring to the laboratory immediately.**

The following specimens may be useful for diagnosis of CNS viral infection:

Eye swab or scraping

Skin lesions: Vigorously scrape base of freshly exposed lesion with a swab to obtain cells that contain viruses. Alternatively, open the vesicle and absorb exudate into a dry swab. If enough vesicle fluid is available, aspirate the fluid with a fine gauge needle and tuberculin syringe, and place the fluid into cold viral transport medium. Use Virocult® or Culturette® swabs for specimen collection. **Keep cold and bring to the laboratory immediately.** The clinical appearance of herpes zoster or the vesicles of herpes simplex may suggest the diagnosis. See Herpesvirus Cytology *on page 383* Viral Culture, Dermatological Symptoms *on page 693*, and Skin Biopsy *on page 71*.

Throat swab: May be useful for identification of Coxsackie B, mumps, adenovirus, and herpes simplex. Epstein-Barr virus may be recovered from throat washings but is difficult to culture. Infectious mononucleosis screening test should be done with examination of the peripheral blood smear.

Feces: An enterovirus may be recovered.

Urine: Mumps virus and cytomegalovirus may be recovered.

Storage Instructions Keep all viral specimens cold and moist. Transport to the laboratory immediately. Enteroviruses are relatively stable from -70°C to 4°C but are labile if allowed to dry or to be at room temperature for several hours. Specimens suspected of having varicella-zoster virus should never be frozen at -20°C or left at room temperature. Freezing at -20°C for 24 hours results in 99% reduction in viral isolation.

Turnaround Time Variable (1-28 days)

Reference Interval No virus isolated

Critical Values Growth of virus in CSF

Use Determine etiological agent of viral CNS diseases (eg, aseptic meningitis, meningoencephalitis, polio, and encephalitis)

Limitations The CSF findings in tuberculous meningitis may simulate those of viral meningitis, especially herpes simplex and mumps. Negative viral culture does not rule out viral etiology. Other methods such as nucleic acid amplification have now been shown to be more sensitive than culture.[3,4,5]

The arboviruses (arthropod-borne) and the reoviruses are not considered culturable; infection can be detected indirectly by identifying specific antibodies (see Encephalitis Viral Serology *on page 604*, Eastern Equine Encephalitis Virus Serology *on page 602*, California Encephalitis Virus Serology *on page 587*, St Louis Encephalitis Virus Serology *on page 681*, and Western Equine Encephalitis Virus Serology *on page 697*).

Methodology Inoculation of specimen into cell cultures, incubation of cultures, observation for characteristic cytopathic effect, and identification/speciation by methods such as hemadsorption and fluorescent monoclonal antibodies. Several specific viruses can be isolated using a rapid (1-2 days) culture (shell vial) method. Polymerase chain reaction is a pivotal method of detection of CNS infections such as those caused by herpesvirus.

Bacterial culture, Gram stain, cell count, glucose, and protein are needed to rule out bacterial meningitis, and blood culture is very strongly recommended.

Additional Information The seasonal peak of viral meningitis in late summer is clinically significant in differential diagnosis.[3] The significance of seasonal curves for viral meningitis (more frequent in summer) versus bacterial meningitis is greater than most physicians recognize.[3] Meningitis caused by human immunodeficiency virus, Epstein-Barr virus, cytomegalovirus, or herpes simplex lacks seasonal variation. Mumps meningitis is usually self-limited and benign. As with lymphocytic choriomeningitis and herpes simplex meningoencephalitis, hypoglycorrhachia may be found.

In the differential diagnosis between viral and bacterial meningitis, markedly elevated CSF leukocyte count ($>1180/mm^3$) and protein concentration (>220 mg/dL) favor bacterial meningitis. Spanos reported that in one group of studied patients no patient with acute viral meningitis had glucose <30.6 mg/dL, but 43% of the patients with acute bacterial meningitis had glucose levels this low.[6] Although aseptic meningitis is usually characterized by mononuclear leukocytes, polymorphonuclear leukocytes may predominate early in the disease.[1,2] Hammer and Connolly summarized **the typical CSF laboratory test profile in viral aseptic meningitis as one with leukocyte count $<500/mm^3$ with lymphocyte predominance, protein <100 mg/dL, and normal glucose.**[7]

The outcome of chronic idiopathic meningitis is usually benign, but the following studies should be considered: cultures for viruses, mycobacteria, fungi, and bacteria; cerebrospinal fluid syphilis serology; nucleic acid amplification for enteroviruses and herpes simplex; arbovirus serology and cerebrospinal fluid cytology.[2]

Complications of lumbar puncture (LP) are between 0.19% and 0.43%, reaching up to 35.5% when minor complications are included. Instances of meningitis and local infection are described following LP in subjects with bacteremia, who may be at risk for meningeal seeding during the puncture.[8] Repeat lumbar puncture may fail to identify patients who require further therapy.[8]

Nonviral causes of aseptic meningitis include meningeal carcinomatosis, collagen diseases, sarcoidosis, drugs (including antineoplastic agents and immunosuppressants, and materials used in radiology units), Mollaret's meningitis and many other entities.[1]

See the table in Viral Culture on page 689 for the appropriate specimen that should be collected based on the suspected viral infection.

Footnotes

1. Negrini B, Kelleher KJ, and Wald ER, "Cerebrospinal Fluid Findings in Aseptic Versus Bacterial Meningitis," Pediatrics, 2000, 105(2):316-9.
2. Dedicoat M and Muir D, "Viral Meningitis - or Encephalitis?" Practitioner, 1998, 242(1587):489-92.
3. Sawyer MH, "Enterovirus Infections: Diagnosis and Treatment," Pediatr Infect Dis J, 1999, 18(12):1033-9.
4. Hamilton MS, Jackson MA, and Abel D, "Clinical Utility of Polymerase Chain Reaction Testing for Enteroviral Meningitis," Pediatr Infect Dis J, 1999, 18(6):533-7.
5. Poggio GP, Rodriguez C, Cisterna D, et al, "Nested PCR for Rapid Detection of Mumps Virus in Cerebrospinal Fluid From Patients With Neurological Diseases," J Clin Microbiol, 2000, 38(1):274-8.
6. Spanos A, Harrell FE Jr, and Durack DT, "Differential Diagnosis of Acute Meningitis - An Analysis of the Predictive Value of Initial Observations," JAMA, 1989, 262(19):2700-7.
7. Hammer SM and Connolly KJ, "Viral Aseptic Meningitis in the United States: Clinical Features, Viral Etiologies, and Differential Diagnosis," Curr Clin Top Infect Dis, 1992, 12:1-25.
8. Fishman RA, Cerebrospinal Fluid in Diseases of the Nervous System 2nd ed, Philadelphia, PA: WB Saunders Co, 1992, 266, 277-343.

References

Bumbalough MR and Welch-Coleman L, "Aseptic Herpetic Meningitis: An Uncommon Genital Herpes Sequelae," Nurse Pract, 1999, 24(7):84-8.
Coyle PK, "Overview of Acute and Chronic Meningitis," Neurol Clin, 1999, 17(4):691-710.
Greenlee JE, "Approach to Diagnosis of Meningitis - Cerebrospinal Fluid Evaluation," Infect Dis Clin North Am, 1990, 4(4):583-98.
Huang CC, Liu CC, Chang YC, et al, "Neurologic Complications in Children With Enterovirus 71 Infection," N Engl J Med, 1999, 341(13):936-42.
Norris CM, Danis PG, and Gardner TD, "Aseptic Meningitis in the Newborn and Young Infant," Am Fam Phys, 1999, 59(10):2761-70.
Read SJ and Kurtz JB, "Laboratory Diagnosis of Common Viral Infections of the Central Nervous System by Using a Single Multiplex PCR Screening Assay," J Clin Microbiol, 1999, 37(5):1352-5.
Vieth UC, Kunzelmann M, Diedrich S, et al, "An ECHO Virus 30 Outbreak With a High Meningitis Attack Rate Among Children and Household Members at Four Day-Care Centers," Eur J Epidemiol, 1999 15(7):655-8.
Waisman Y, Lotem Y, Hemmo M, et al, "Management of Children With Aseptic Meningitis in the Emergency Department," Pediatr Emerg Care, 1999, 15(5):314-7.

Internet Web Sites

www.astdhpphe.org/infect/sle.html
www.astdhpphe.org/infect/wee.html
www.cdc.gov/ncidod/dvbid/arbor/arboinfo.htm
www.cdc.gov/ncidod/dvbid/arbor/lacfact.htm
www.cdc.gov/ncidod/dvbid/arbor/sle_qa.htm
www.cdc.gov/ncidod/dvrd/entrvirs.htm

◆ **Viral Culture, CSF** see Viral Culture, Central Nervous System Symptoms on page 692

◆ **Viral Culture, Cytomegalovirus** see Cytomegalovirus Culture on page 598

Viral Culture, Dermatological Symptoms

Related Information

Herpes Simplex Virus Antigen Detection on page 630
Herpes Simplex Virus Culture on page 631
Varicella-Zoster Virus Culture on page 686
Viral Culture on page 689
Viral Culture, Tissue on page 695
Viral Culture, Urogenital on page 696

Synonyms Vesicle Viral Culture; Viral Culture, Lesion; Viral Culture, Pustule; Viral Culture, Rash; Viral Culture, Skin/Dermatological Specimen; Viral Culture, Skin Scrapings; Viral Culture, Ulcer

Applies to Genital Lesions

Test Includes Usually includes both rapid shell vial isolation technique and conventional cell culture for all culturable viruses; isolated viruses are identified using specific monoclonal antibodies.

Abstract Viral agents most commonly associated with skin lesions are herpes simplex virus (HSV), type 1 and 2, and varicella zoster virus (VZV). These viruses are prevalent worldwide. Both viruses establish latency after a primary infection and can react to cause lesions when a host becomes immunosuppressed. Among bone marrow transplant patients, up to 40% will develop reactivated VZV infections.[1] HSV commonly causes recurrent mucocutaneous lesions, but may also be associated with infections of the eye, encephalitis, pneumonia, and perinatal disease.

Patient Preparation Do not prep skin with alcohol, iodine, or Betadine® prior to collection.

Specimen Scraping, swab, fluid of lesion

Container Viral transport medium for swabs

Sampling Time Preferably within 3 days of dermatological symptoms

Collection Specimen should be collected during the acute phase of the disease, as follows. **Skin lesions:** Open the vesicle and absorb exudate into a dry swab, and/or vigorously scrape base of freshly exposed lesion

---

with a swab to obtain cells which contain viruses. If enough vesicle fluid is available, aspirate the fluid with a fine-gauge needle and tuberculin syringe, and place the fluid into cold viral transport medium. Use Virocult® or Culturette® swabs for specimen collection. **Keep cold and bring to the laboratory immediately,** especially if varicella-zoster virus is suspected. Calcium alginate swabs are toxic to *Chlamydia* and many enveloped viruses. **Do not use calcium alginate swabs for viral or chlamydial isolation.**

Reference Interval No virus isolated

Critical Values Isolation of varicella-zoster virus (VZV) from any adult patient or hospitalized patient or genital herpes simplex virus (HSV) from pregnant woman

Use In rare clinical situations, viral culture is used to determine the etiological agent of dermatological infections. Orf viruses cause a skin disorder of sheep and goats which may occasionally be transmitted to humans. Parapoxvirus particles of orf can be seen by electron microscopy.[2]

Limitations False-negative results are common. Crusted lesions do not contain viral particles. For all practical purposes, measles virus is not culturable from patients' skin rash.

Methodology Inoculation of specimen into cell cultures, incubation of cultures, observation for characteristic cytopathic effect (CPE), and identification/speciation by fluorescent monoclonal antibodies. If specific viruses such as HSV, VZV, or adenovirus are suspected, most laboratories will use rapid (1-2 days) culture (shell vial) methods to detect these viruses.

Additional Information Virus shedding diminishes rapidly after the onset of illness; therefore, it is important to collect specimens early.

If a systemic disease is associated with a rash, throat swab, rectal swab, stool, or serum can be taken for the isolation of other viruses (eg, enteroviruses, mumps virus, measles virus, and rubella virus). A table in Viral Culture on page 689 provides additional information.

Footnotes

1. Wilson A, Sharp M, Koropchak CM, et al, "Subclinical Varicella-Zoster Virus Viremia, Herpes Zoster, and T Lymphocyte Immunity to Varicella-Zoster Viral Antigens After Bone Marrow Transplantation," J Infect Dis, 1992, 165(1):119-26.
2. Roingeard P and Machet L, Images in Clinical Medicine, "Orf Skin Ulcer," N Engl J Med, 1997, 337(16):1131.

References

Arvin AM, "Varicella-Zoster Virus," Clin Microbiol Rev, 1996, 9(3):361-81.
Nahass GT, Goldstein BA, Zhu W, et al, "Comparison of Tzanck Smear, Viral Culture, and DNA Diagnostic Methods in Detection of Herpes Simplex and Varicella-Zoster Infection (PCR)," JAMA, 1992, 268(18):2541-4.
Pugh RN, Omar RI, and Hossain MM, "Varicella Infection and Pneumonia Among Adults," Int J Infect Dis, 1998, 2(4):205-10.
Riley LE, "Herpes Simplex Virus," Semin Perinatol, 1998, 22(4):284-92.
Sauerbrei A, Eichhorn U, Schalke M, et al, "Laboratory Diagnosis of Herpes Zoster," J Clin Virol, 1999, 14(1):31-6.
Whallett EJ and Pahor AL, "Herpes and the Head and Neck: The Difficulties in Diagnosis," J Laryngol Otol, 1999, 113(6):573-7.

Internet Web Sites

www.amm.co.uk/pubs/fa_herpes.htm
www.cdc.gov/ncidod/srp/varicella.htm
www.nfid.org/factsheets/herpes.html
www.who.int/vaccines-diseases/diseases/pp_varicella.htm

◆ **Viral Culture, Eye** see Herpes Simplex Virus Culture on page 631

Viral Culture, Eye or Ocular Symptoms

Related Information

Adenovirus Culture on page 552
Bacterial Culture, Conjunctiva on page 570
Chlamydia trachomatis Culture on page 590
Chlamydia trachomatis Direct Antigen Test on page 590
Chlamydia trachomatis Nucleic Acid Detection on page 591
Enterovirus Culture on page 605
Herpes Simplex Virus Culture on page 631
Viral Culture on page 689

Synonyms Eye, Viral Culture

Test Includes Usually includes both rapid shell vial isolation technique and conventional cell culture for all culturable viruses; isolated viruses are identified using specific monoclonal antibodies.

Abstract The leading cause of a red eye is viral conjunctivitis, which usually affects one eye before the other.[1] Conjunctivitis is the most common eye infection and can be found in patients of all ages. Several viruses can infect the eye. Among the most common viral infections of the eye are adenovirus, influenza viruses, herpes simplex viruses (HSV), varicella-zoster virus (VZV), and cytomegalovirus (CMV) infections. Infection of the cornea, keratitis, is a much more serious infection and if left untreated can result in loss of eyesight.

Patient Preparation Local anesthesia might be necessary. Corneal and sclera specimens should be taken only by an ophthalmologist or other properly trained physician.

Specimen Conjunctival scrapings or swabs, eye exudate, vitreous washings, corneal biopsy

Container Cold and sterile viral transport medium for swabs; sterile container for washings or biopsy
(Continued)

Viral Culture, Eye or Ocular Symptoms *(Continued)*

Collection Pus should be removed with a sterile swab. Obtain conjunctival scrapings with a sterile spatula. Collect eye exudate by rubbing palpebral conjunctiva with sterile moist swab and place the swab into cold viral transport medium. Conjunctivitis due to *Chlamydia trachomatis* should be collected with a swab and media specific for chlamydial infections; see *Chlamydia* listings.

Storage Instructions Specimen should be kept cold and transported to the laboratory immediately.

Special Instructions Viral conjunctivitis is highly contagious.[1]

Reference Interval No virus isolated

Use Determine etiological agent of viral ocular infections (eg, conjunctivitis and keratitis)

Methodology Inoculation of specimen into cell cultures, incubation of cultures, observation for characteristic cytopathic effect, and identification/speciation by fluorescent monoclonal antibodies. If specific viruses such as HSV, CMV, VZV, influenza, or adenovirus are suspected, the laboratory might be able to use rapid (1-2 days) culture (shell vial) methods to detect these viruses; see appropriate listings.

Additional Information Viral serology can be helpful to establish a diagnosis. See the table in Viral Culture *on page 689*.

Footnotes
1. Leibowitz HM, "The Red Eye," *N Engl J Med*, 2000, 343(5):345-51.

References
Arvin AM, "Varicella-Zoster Virus," *Clin Microbiol Rev*, 1996, 9(3):361-81.

Davis JL, "Differential Diagnosis of CMV Retinitis," *Ocul Immunol Inflamm*, 1999, 7(3-4):159-66.

Kowalski RP, Karenchak LM, Romanowski EG, et al, "Evaluation of the Shell Vial Technique for Detection of Ocular Adenovirus. Community Ophthalmologist of Pittsburgh, Pennsylvania," *Ophthalmology*, 1999, 106(7):1324-7.

Pavan-Langston D, "Major Ocular Viral Infections," *Practical Diagnosis of Viral Infections*, Galasso GJ, Whitley RJ, Merigan TC, eds, New York, NY: Raven Press, 1993, 69-108.

Riley LE, "Herpes Simplex Virus," *Semin Perinatol*, 1998, 22(4):284-92.

Sauerbrei A, Eichhorn U, Schalke M, et al, "Laboratory Diagnosis of Herpes Zoster," *J Clin Virol*, 1999, 14(1):31-6.

Whallett EJ and Pahor AL, "Herpes and the Head and Neck: The Difficulties in Diagnosis," *J Laryngol Otol*, 1999, 113(6):573-7.

Internet Web Sites
www.amm.co.uk/pubs/fa_herpes.htm
www.cdc.gov/nchstp/dstd/chlamydia_facts.htm
www.cdc.gov/ncidod/diseases/cmv.htm
www.cdc.gov/ncidod/srp/varicella.htm
www.nfid.org/factsheets/herpes.html
www.who.int/vaccines-diseases/diseases/pp_varicella.htm

♦ **Viral Culture, Genital** *see* Herpes Simplex Virus Culture *on page 631*

♦ **Viral Culture, Genital** *see* Viral Culture, Urogenital *on page 696*

♦ **Viral Culture, Heart** *see* Viral Culture, Tissue *on page 695*

♦ **Viral Culture, Kidney** *see* Viral Culture, Tissue *on page 695*

♦ **Viral Culture, Lesion** *see* Viral Culture, Dermatological Symptoms *on page 693*

♦ **Viral Culture, Lung** *see* Viral Culture, Tissue *on page 695*

♦ **Viral Culture, Muscle** *see* Viral Culture, Tissue *on page 695*

♦ **Viral Culture, Nasopharyngeal** *see* Viral Culture, Respiratory Symptoms *on page 694*

♦ **Viral Culture, Pulmonary Biopsy** *see* Viral Culture, Respiratory Symptoms *on page 694*

♦ **Viral Culture, Pustule** *see* Viral Culture, Dermatological Symptoms *on page 693*

♦ **Viral Culture, Rash** *see* Varicella-Zoster Virus Culture *on page 686*

♦ **Viral Culture, Rash** *see* Viral Culture, Dermatological Symptoms *on page 693*

Viral Culture, Respiratory Symptoms

Related Information
Adenovirus Antibody Titer *on page 552*
Adenovirus Culture *on page 552*
Bacterial Culture, Bronchoscopy/Bronchial Brush/Bronchoalveolar Lavage Specimen *on page 568*
Bacterial Culture, Nasopharynx *on page 573*
Bacterial Culture, Sputum *on page 574*
Bronchial Washings Cytology *on page 374*
Bronchoalveolar Lavage (BAL) *on page 375*
Coxsackievirus Serology *on page 595*
Fungal Culture, Sputum *on page 613*
Influenza Virus Culture *on page 644*
Mycobacterial Culture, Sputum *on page 658*
Parainfluenza Viral Serology *on page 668*
Parainfluenza Virus Culture *on page 668*
Respiratory Syncytial Virus Antigen Detection *on page 674*
Respiratory Syncytial Virus Culture *on page 675*
Respiratory Syncytial Virus Serology *on page 675*
Sputum Cytology *on page 387*
Viral Culture *on page 689*
Virus, Direct Detection by Fluorescent Antibody *on page 696*

Synonyms Viral Culture, Bronchial Wash; Viral Culture, Nasopharyngeal; Viral Culture, Pulmonary Biopsy; Viral Culture, Throat Swab

Test Includes Usually includes both rapid shell vial isolation technique and conventional cell culture for all culturable viruses; isolated viruses are identified using specific monoclonal antibodies.

Abstract Viral agents cause 20% to 62% of community-acquired pneumonias. The most common viral agents are influenza viruses, parainfluenza virus, rhinoviruses, and respiratory syncytial virus (RSV).[1,2] Pneumonia due to adenovirus is less common.

Patient Preparation Local anesthesia might be necessary

Specimen Throat swab; throat washing; nasopharyngeal washing, aspirates, or secretions; bronchial washings or lavage; lung biopsy

Container Cold and sterile viral transport medium for swabs; sterile container for washings and aspirates.

Sampling Time As soon as possible after onset of illness

Collection Methods are the same as those used for collecting most respiratory specimens (see Specimen) except that sputum is not an acceptable specimen for viral isolation. If respiratory syncytial virus or parainfluenza virus is suspected, see collection techniques for these viruses.

Storage Instructions Keep specimen cold and moist. Transport to the laboratory immediately. Can be stored at 4°C up to 48 hours. If longer storage is required freeze quickly at -70°C. **Do not freeze at -20°C.**

Turnaround Time Variable (1-14 days)

Reference Interval No virus isolated

Use Determine etiological agent of respiratory infections. Viruses to be considered include influenza virus, parainfluenza virus, rhinovirus, RSV, adenovirus, cytomegalovirus (CMV), and reovirus. Immunocompromised patients can also have respiratory infection due to HSV or VZV.

Limitations Presence of nonculturable, disease-causing virus (eg, encephalitis, hepatitis, and gastroenteritis viruses); invasive procedures. Many asymptomatic persons carry and shed viruses that might not be related to illness.

Methodology Inoculation of specimen into cell cultures, incubation of cultures, observation for characteristic cytopathic effect (CPE), and identification/speciation by methods such as hemadsorption and the use of fluorescent monoclonal antibodies. Many laboratories use rapid (1-2 days) culture (shell vial) methods to detect respiratory viruses. Identification is based on reaction with a specific fluorescent-monoclonal antibody.[3,4]

Rapid immunoassays for use in medical offices and clinics detect influenza A and B antigens in respiratory secretions.[5]

Additional Information See the table in Viral Culture *on page 689*. It is well to contact the Virology Laboratory, to inform the staff if influenza or parainfluenza is suspected. Using mixtures of monoclonal antibodies and shell vial cultures, the rapid detection of several respiratory viruses can be made within 24 hours.[3,4]

Footnotes
1. Juven T, Mertsola J, Waris M, et al, "Etiology of Community-Acquired Pneumonia in 254 Hospitalized Children," *Pediatr Infect Dis J*, 2000, 19(4):293-8.
2. McCracken GH Jr, "Etiology and Treatment of Pneumonia," *Pediatr Infect Dis J*, 2000, 19(4):373-7.
3. Shih SR, Tsao KC, Ning HC, et al, "Diagnosis of Respiratory Tract Viruses in 24 Hours by Immunofluorescent Staining of Shell Vial Cultures Containing Madin-Darby Canine Kidney (MDCK) Cells," *J Virol Methods*, 1999, 81(1-2):77-81.
4. Navarro-Mari JM, Sanbonmatsu-Gamez S, Perez-Ruiz M, et al, "Rapid Detection of Respiratory Viruses by Shell Vial Assay Using Simultaneous Culture of Hep-2, LLC-MK2, and MDCK Cells in a Single Vial," *J Clin Microbiol*, 1999, 37(7):2346-7.
5. Magnard C, Valette M, Aymard M, et al, "Comparison of Two Nested PCR, Cell Culture, and Antigen Detection for the Diagnosis of Upper Respiratory Tract Infections Due to Influenza Viruses," *J Med Virol*, 1999, 59(2):215-20.

References
Chien JW and Johnson JL, "Viral Pneumonias. Epidemic Respiratory Viruses," *Postgrad Med*, 2000, 107(3):41-52.

Chien JW and Johnson JL, "Viral Pneumonias. Infection in the Immunocompromised Host," *Postgrad Med*, 2000, 107(2):67-80.

Gant V and Parton S, "Community-Acquired Pneumonia," *Curr Opin Pulm Med*, 2000, 6(3):226-33.

Hendley JO, "Clinical Virology of Rhinoviruses," *Adv Virus Res*, 1999, 54:453-66.

Pugh RN, Omar RI, and Hoosain MM, "Varicella Infection and Pneumonia Among Adults," *Int J Infect Dis*, 1998, 2(4):205-10.

Ruuskanen O and Mertsola J, "Childhood Community-Acquired Pneumonia," *Semin Respir Infect*, 1999, 14(2):163-72.

Sintchenko V and Dwyer DE, "The Diagnosis and Management of Influenza. An Update," *Aust Fam Physician*, 1999, 28(4):313-7.

Internet Web Sites
www.amm.co.uk/pubs/fa_influenza.htm
www.astdhpphe.org/infect/flu.html
www.astdhpphe.org/infect/rsv.html
www.cdc.gov/ncidod/diseases/flu/fluvirus.htm
www.cdc.gov/ncidod/dvrd/nrevss/rsvfeat.htm
www.who.int/health-topics/influenza.htm

♦ **Viral Culture, Skin** *see* Herpes Simplex Virus Culture *on page 631*

♦ **Viral Culture, Skin** see Varicella-Zoster Virus Culture on page 686

♦ **Viral Culture, Skin/Dermatological Specimen** see Viral Culture, Dermatological Symptoms on page 693

♦ **Viral Culture, Skin Scrapings** see Viral Culture, Dermatological Symptoms on page 693

Viral Culture, Stool

Related Information
Bacterial Culture, Stool on page 575
Electron Microscopic Examination for Viruses, Stool on page 603
Entamoeba histolytica Serology on page 605
Enterovirus Culture on page 605
Fecal Lactoferrin on page 308
Poliomyelitis I, II, III Serology on page 671
Rotavirus, Direct Detection on page 676
Viral Culture on page 689
Yersinia enterocolitica Antibody on page 698
Yersinia pestis Antibody on page 698

Applies to Adenovirus Culture, Stool; Coxsackievirus Culture, Stool; Echovirus Culture, Stool; Enterovirus Culture, Stool; Poliovirus Culture, Stool

Test Includes After extensive preparation of the specimen it is cultured for the isolation of all culturable viruses using conventional cell culture.

Abstract The viruses usually isolated from the stool are enteroviruses, and surveillance cultures for enterovirus are sometimes performed to determine outbreaks. However, enteroviruses can be isolated in the absence of disease and thus the recovery of the virus has limited diagnostic specificity. Many viruses that cause gastrointestinal diseases cannot be cultured (eg, rotavirus, Norwalk agent, adenovirus type 40-41). Cytomegalovirus can cause gastrointestinal disease in immunocompromised patients.

Specimen Stool or rectal swab. Freshly passed stool is preferable to a rectal swab.

Collection Collect stools into plastic screw-cap container; do not use cardboard or waxed containers.

Insert swab gently into rectum and hold there for 10-15 seconds, moisten with contents of Culturette® bulb, and send to the laboratory in cold viral transport medium.

Storage Instructions Keep specimens cold.

Turnaround Time Variable (usually 1-14 days)

Reference Interval No virus isolated

Use Identify carriage or excretion of a virus in stool; isolate and identify an enterovirus which could be the cause of aseptic (nonbacterial) meningitis. The viruses most likely to be isolated from stool specimen are those which are extremely hardy and which do not have a lipid membrane envelope (eg, enterovirus, polio, Coxsackie, and echoviruses).

Limitations Cannot detect the presence of nonculturable, disease-causing virus (eg, Norwalk group, calicivirus, and rotaviruses). Some bacterial toxins in fecal specimens, such as *Clostridium difficile* toxin A, can mimic viral cytopathic effect (CPE) in many cell lines, leading to false positives.

Methodology Inoculation of specimen into cell cultures, incubation of cultures, observation for characteristic cytopathic effect, and identification/speciation by methods such as hemadsorption and fluorescent monoclonal antibodies

Additional Information Isolation of virus from stool specimens may be of diagnostic help. It is important to be aware of viral shedding to avoid transmission to other people. Children recently vaccinated against polio can shed poliovirus in the stool for months after vaccination. Children convalescing from upper respiratory illness or aseptic meningitis can shed virus in the stool for weeks. See the table in Viral Culture on page 689 for viruses most likely to be isolated from stool specimens. Many viruses responsible for diarrhea, such as rotavirus, can be detected only with immunoassays or electron microscopy.

References
Bhan MK, Raj P, Bhandari N, et al, "Role of Enteric Adenoviruses and Rotaviruses in Mild and Severe Acute Enteritis," *Pediatr Infect Dis J*, 1988, 7(5):320-3.
Blacklow NR and Greenberg HB, "Viral Gastroenteritis," *N Engl J Med*, 1991, 325(4):252-64.
Coyle PK, "Overview of Acute and Chronic Meningitis," *Neurol Clin*, 1999, 17(4):691-710.
Hammer SM and Connolly KJ, "Viral Aseptic Meningitis in the United States: Clinical Features, Viral Etiologies, and Differential Diagnosis," *Curr Clin Top Infect Dis*, 1992, 12:1-25.
Nairn C and Clements GB, "A Study of Enterovirus Isolations in Glasgow From 1977 to 1997," *J Med Virol*, 1999, 58(3):304-12.
Spanos A, Harrell FE Jr, and Durack DT, "Differential Diagnosis of Acute Meningitis - An Analysis of the Predictive Value of Initial Observations," *JAMA*, 1989, 262(19):2700-7.

Internet Web Sites
vm.cfsan.fda.gov/~mow/chap33.html
www.astdhpphe.org/infect/rot.html
www.cdc.gov/ncidod/dvrd/entrvirs.htm
www.cdc.gov/ncidod/dvrd/nrevss/rotfeat.htm

♦ **Viral Culture, Throat Swab** see Viral Culture, Respiratory Symptoms on page 694

Viral Culture, Tissue

Related Information
Bacterial Culture, Biopsy or Body Fluid on page 565
Bone Marrow on page 410
Human Immunodeficiency Virus DNA Amplification on page 639
Human Papillomavirus DNA Probe Test on page 641
Mycobacterial Culture, Biopsy or Body Fluid on page 655
Mycobacterial Culture, Cutaneous and Subcutaneous Tissue on page 657
Skin Biopsy on page 71
Viral Culture on page 689
Viral Culture, Dermatological Symptoms on page 693

Applies to Viral Culture, Biopsy; Viral Culture, Brain; Viral Culture, Bronchial; Viral Culture, Heart; Viral Culture, Kidney; Viral Culture, Lung; Viral Culture, Muscle; Viral Culture, Trachea

Test Includes Usually includes both rapid shell vial isolation technique and conventional cell culture for all culturable viruses; isolated viruses are identified using specific monoclonal antibodies

Abstract After a virus has infected a patient, it can spread from the site of inoculation to other organs or produce systemic disease. Some of the more commonly involved organs are liver, lymph nodes, skin, kidney, heart, muscle, central nervous system, or bone marrow.

Specimen Biopsy, swab, brush, or scrape specimen from any suspect organ, site, lesion, or tissue

Container Sterile, screw-cap container

Sampling Time As soon as possible after onset of illness

Collection Specimen should be collected during the acute phase of the disease, as follows.

Tissue: Use a fresh set of sterile instruments to collect each tissue. Place each specimen in a dry, sterile nontoxic leakproof container. Identify each tissue with patient's name, type of tissue, and date collected. **Keep cold and bring tissue to the laboratory immediately.**

Tracheal or bronchial tissue or brushings: If possible, brushes should be placed into cold viral transport medium.

Storage Instructions Specimens should be kept cold and moist. If specimen is to be stored longer than 48 hours it should be frozen at -70°C. **Do not freeze at -20°C.** Tissues can be put into viral transport medium.

Turnaround Time Variable (usually 1-14 days)

Reference Interval No virus isolated

Use Aid in the diagnosis of disseminated viral diseases (eg, encephalitis and meningitis)

Limitations Presence of nonculturable, disease-causing virus (eg, encephalitis, hepatitis, and gastroenteritis viruses); collection of specimen requires invasive procedures

Methodology Inoculation of specimen into cell cultures, incubation of cultures, observation for characteristic cytopathic effect (CPE), and identification/speciation by methods such as hemadsorption and fluorescent monoclonal antibodies. If specific viruses such as herpes simplex virus (HSV), cytomegalovirus (CMV), varicella-zoster virus (VZV), or adenovirus are suspected, the laboratory might be able to use rapid (1-2 days) culture (shell vial) methods to detect these viruses.

Additional Information See the table in Viral Culture on page 689 for the viruses most likely to be isolated from clinical specimens and for the list of viruses not routinely cultured. Viral DNA can now be detected using nucleic acid amplification procedures or in situ hybridization. These techniques are very sensitive and specific. In some viral diseases, such tests can be diagnostically useful (eg, hepatitis, human immunodeficiency virus). However, other viruses can reside in the host in a latent form without causing disease (cytomegalovirus, herpes simplex virus, varicella-zoster virus). Such latent viruses can produce false-positive results if amplification of DNA for these viruses is used in a diagnostic test on tissue.

References
Arvin AM, "Varicella-Zoster Virus," *Clin Microbiol Rev*, 1996, 9(3):361-81.
Casteels A, Naessens A, Gordts F, et al, "Neonatal Screening for Congenital Cytomegalovirus Infections," *J Perinat Med*, 1999, 27(2):116-21.
Pugh RN, Omar RI, and Hossain MM, "Varicella Infection and Pneumonia Among Adults," *Int J Infect Dis*, 1998, 2(4):205-10.
Riley LE, "Herpes Simplex Virus," *Semin Perinatol*, 1998, 22(4):284-92.
Wilson A, Sharp M, Koropchak CM, et al, "Subclinical Varicella-Zoster Virus Viremia, Herpes Zoster, and T Lymphocyte Immunity to Varicella-Zoster Viral Antigens After Bone Marrow Transplantation," *J Infect Dis*, 1992, 165(1):119-26.

♦ **Viral Culture, Trachea** see Viral Culture, Tissue on page 695

♦ **Viral Culture, Ulcer** see Viral Culture, Dermatological Symptoms on page 693

Viral Culture, Urine

Related Information
Adenovirus Culture on page 552
Bacterial Culture, Urine on page 578
Cytomegalovirus Culture on page 598
Enterovirus Culture on page 605
Mumps Virus Culture on page 653
(Continued)

Viral Culture, Urine (Continued)

Mycobacterial Culture, Urine *on page 660*
Urinary Tract Cytology *on page 389*
Viral Culture *on page 689*
Viral Culture, Blood *on page 691*

Applies to CMV Culture, Urine; Mumps Virus Culture, Urine

Test Includes Usually includes both rapid shell vial isolation technique and conventional cell culture for all culturable viruses; isolated viruses are identified using specific monoclonal antibodies.

Specimen Urine

Sampling Time Shedding of CMV can be intermittent. Therefore, several specimens should be collected, if possible.

Collection Clean catch, midstream urine in sterile, screw-cap container

Storage Instructions Refrigerate if delay of more than 1 hour in transit to the laboratory. Specimen may be stored up to 72 hours at 4°C before inoculation onto cell culture. **Do not freeze specimens at -20°C**. Some viruses are inactivated by freezing at -20°C. Specimens that need to be stored longer than 72 hours can be frozen at -70°C or below in the presence of 30% sorbitol.[1]

Turnaround Time Variable (1-28 days)

Reference Interval No virus isolated

Use The viruses most frequently isolated from urine are CMV, mumps, and adenoviruses.

Limitations Urine can be toxic for cell cultures and can result in inconclusive results

Methodology Inoculation of specimen into cell cultures, incubation of cultures, observation for characteristic cytopathic effect, and identification/speciation by hemadsorption and/or fluorescent monoclonal antibodies. If specific viruses such as cytomegalovirus (CMV) or adenovirus are suspected, the laboratory might be able to use rapid (1-2 days) culture (shell vial) methods to detect these viruses.

Additional Information The isolation of CMV from a blood specimen is a better indication of active infection than isolation of CMV in urine. Although mumps infections are rare in the U.S. due to vaccination of children, after an active infection the mumps virus can be isolated from urine up to 2 weeks after onset of disease[1]. See the table in Viral Culture *on page 689*.

Footnotes

1. Swierkosz EM, "Mumps Virus," *Manual of Clinical Microbiology*, 7th ed, Murray PR, Baron EJ, Pfaller MA, et al, eds, Washington, DC: AMS Press, American Society for Microbiology, 1999, 959-63.

References

Flechner SM, Avery RK, Fisher R, et al, "Monitoring of CMV Infection After Renal Transplantation: Serology, Culture, and Viral DNA Detection by Hybrid Capture," *Transplant Proc*, 1999, 31(1-2):1255-7.

Hodinka RL, "Human Cytomegalovirus," *Manual of Clinical Microbiology*, 7th ed, Murray PR, Baron EJ, Pfaller MA, et al, eds, Washington, DC: AMS Press, American Society for Microbiology, 1999, 888-99.

Internet Web Sites

www.cdc.gov/ncidod/diseases/cmv.htm
www.cdc.gov/ncidod/dvrd/entrvirs.htm

Viral Culture, Urogenital

Related Information

Bacterial Culture, Genital Specimen *on page 571*
Chlamydia trachomatis Culture *on page 590*
Chlamydia trachomatis Nucleic Acid Detection *on page 591*
Cytomegalovirus Culture *on page 598*
Herpes Simplex Virus Antigen Detection *on page 630*
Herpes Simplex Virus Culture *on page 631*
Human Papillomavirus DNA Probe Test *on page 641*
Mycobacterial Culture, Biopsy or Body Fluid *on page 655*
Mycobacterial Culture, Urine *on page 660*
Urinary Tract Cytology *on page 389*
Viral Culture *on page 689*
Viral Culture, Dermatological Symptoms *on page 693*

Synonyms Genital Culture, Virus; Viral Culture, Genital

Applies to Cervix, Viral Culture; Endocervix, Viral Culture; Prostate, Viral Culture; Urethra, Viral Culture

Test Includes Usually includes both rapid shell vial isolation technique and conventional cell culture for all culturable viruses; isolated viruses are identified using specific monoclonal antibodies.

Abstract One of the most common viruses isolated from urogenital specimens is herpes simplex viruses (HSV). The classic presentation of primary herpes simplex infection is the appearance of several painful genital vesicles. Generally, primary infections are also associated with fever and inguinal lymphadenopathy. Many individuals do not have symptoms with recurrent infections but may shed infectious viruses from the genital site. This asymptomatic shedding poses a serious risk to the developing fetus and newborn.[1,2]

Specimen Cervical, urethral, and genital lesions, surgical and biopsy tissue

Container Sterile and cold viral transport medium

Sampling Time As soon as possible after the eruption of vesicles or lesions, preferably within 3 days of lesion eruption. Only occasionally can HSV be isolated as late as 7-10 days after onset.

Collection Use a Culturette® swab, spatula, or scalpel blade to scrape away cells from the base of freshly unroofed lesions, and place the swab or collected cells immediately into cold viral transport medium. Vesicular fluid is an excellent specimen, and can be collected by using a tuberculin syringe and a 26-gauge needle. Rinse contents of syringe into cold viral transport medium.

Storage Instructions Keep all specimens cold and moist. Specimens which cannot be inoculated onto cell cultures within 48 hours should be frozen at -70°C.

Turnaround Time Variable (1-14 days)

Reference Interval No virus isolated

Critical Values Positive viral culture for HSV during pregnancy.[1,2]

Use Aid in the diagnosis of viral entities including sexually transmitted diseases. The detection of virus such as HSV or cytomegalovirus (CMV) in pregnant women is important to prevent the complications of neonatal infections.[1] Infants are at risk of infection during delivery even if the mother is asymptomatic. Human papillomavirus (HPV) causes genital warts and some strains of HPV are associated with carcinoma of cervix. HPV can only be detected using nucleic acid methods or *in situ* hybridization.

Limitations Some methods detect only HSV in genital specimens; some disease-causing virus (eg, papillomavirus) are nonculturable (see the table in Viral Culture *on page 689*).

Methodology Inoculation of specimen into cell cultures, incubation of cultures, observation for characteristic cytopathic effect, and identification/speciation by fluorescent monoclonal antibodies. If specific viruses such as HSV, CMV, or adenovirus are suspected, the laboratory might be able to use rapid (1-2 days) culture (shell vial) methods to detect these viruses.

Additional Information In the United States, sexually transmitted herpes simplex infections have increased since the 1970s. Many of the infected women are of childbearing age and may possibly transmit the virus to a fetus or newborn. Treatment options for HSV are available and recommended for pregnant women infected with HSV.[3]

Urogenital, dermal, oral, and mucosal specimens often yield the same viruses. See the table in Viral Culture *on page 689*.

Footnotes

1. Brown Z, Selke S, Zeh J, et al, "Acquisition of Herpes Simplex Virus During Pregnancy," *N Engl J Med*, 1997, 337(8):509-15.
2. Brown ZA, "Genital Herpes Complicating Pregnancy," *Dermatol Clin*, 1998, 16(4):805-10.
3. Scott LL, "Prevention of Perinatal Herpes: Prophylactic Antiviral Therapy?" *Clin Obstet Gynecol*, 1999, 42(1):134-48.

References

American College of Obstetricians and Gynecologists, "ACOG Practice Bulletin: Management of Herpes in Pregnancy. Number 8 October 1999. Clinical Management Guidelines for Obstetrician-Gynecologists," *Int J Gynaecol Obstet*, 2000, 68(2):165-73.

Corey L, "Herpes Simplex Virus," *Principles and Practice of Infectious Diseases*, 5th ed, Mandell GL, Bennett JE, and Dolin R, eds, New York, NY: Churchill Livingstone, 2000, 1564-80.

McNamee K, "Patient Education. What You Should Know About Genital Herpes," *Aust Fam Physician*, 1999, 28(11):1168.

Preboth M, "ACOG Practice Bulletin on Management of Herpes in Pregnancy. American College of Obstetricians and Gynecologists," *Am Fam Phys*, 2000, 61(2):556-61.

Riley LE, "Herpes Simplex Virus," *Semin Perinatol*, 1998, 22(4):284-92.

Wald A, Zeh J, Selke S, et al, "Reactivation of Genital Herpes Simplex Virus Type 2 Infection in Asymptomatic Seropositive Persons," *N Eng J Med*, 2000, 342(12):844-50.

Internet Web Sites

www.amm.co.uk/pubs/fa_herpes.htm
www.nfid.org/factsheets/herpes.html

♦ **Viral Disease in Tissue** *see* Electron Microscopic Examination for Viruses, Stool *on page 603*

♦ **Viral Hepatitis** *see* Hepatitis: Laboratory Assessment, Overview *on page 629*

♦ **ViraPap®** *see* Human Papillomavirus DNA Probe Test *on page 641*

♦ **ViraType®** *see* Human Papillomavirus DNA Probe Test *on page 641*

Virus, Direct Detection by Fluorescent Antibody

Related Information

Adenovirus Antibody Titer *on page 552*
Adenovirus Culture *on page 552*
Cytomegalovirus Antigen Detection *on page 598*
Cytomegalovirus Culture *on page 598*
Herpes Simplex Virus Antigen Detection *on page 630*
Herpes Simplex Virus Culture *on page 631*
Influenza A and B Serology *on page 643*
Influenza Virus Culture *on page 644*
Mumps Serology *on page 653*
Mumps Virus Culture *on page 653*
Parainfluenza Viral Serology *on page 668*
Parainfluenza Virus Culture *on page 668*
Rabies *on page 673*
Respiratory Syncytial Virus Antigen Detection *on page 674*

Respiratory Syncytial Virus Culture *on page 675*
Respiratory Syncytial Virus Serology *on page 675*
Varicella-Zoster Virus Culture *on page 686*
Varicella-Zoster Virus Serology *on page 687*
Viral Culture *on page 689*
Viral Culture, Respiratory Symptoms *on page 694*

Synonyms Fluorescent Antibody Test, Direct, for Virus; Virus Fluorescent Antibody Test

Applies to Influenza Virus, Direct Detection; Measles Virus, Direct Detection; Mumps Virus, Direct Detection; Parainfluenza Virus, Direct Detection; Rabies Virus, Direct Detection; Varicella-Zoster Virus, Direct Detection

Test Includes Direct (nonculture) detection of virus-infected cells using immunofluorescence

Abstract Direct detection methods can provide a rapid diagnosis of viral infections (eg, herpes simplex (HSV), influenza A and B, varicella-zoster virus (VZV), respiratory viruses).

Specimen Impression smears of tissues, lesion scrapings and swabs, frozen sections, cell suspensions, upper respiratory tract swabs; Use ≥1 mL of nasopharyngeal aspirate for influenza A and B antigen.[1]

Storage Instructions Refrigerate nasopharyngeal aspirations.

Turnaround Time Less than 1 day

Special Instructions Make at least four impression smears or place four frozen sections on four separate slides. Cell suspensions should be centrifuged, resuspended to slight turbidity, and applied to prewelled slides.

Reference Interval No virus detected

Possible Panic Range Positive detection of rabies

Use Useful in the rapid diagnosis of HSV, VZV, respiratory syncytial virus (RSV), parainfluenza, influenza, adenovirus, cytomegalovirus (CMV), measles, mumps, and rabies infections

Limitations It is possible for the test to be negative in the presence of viral infection. Expertly trained and experienced personnel, excellent quality reagents, and adequate numbers of cells are required for accurate detection of virus. **Contact laboratory prior to requesting test to determine if laboratory offers a direct test for the viruses suspected.** Generally, this test is not as sensitive as cell culture.

Methodology Monoclonal antibody reagents and immunofluorescence microscopy are used to detect viruses/viral antigens in specimen cells.

Additional Information Direct detection of viruses in respiratory secretions can be diagnostically helpful because cell culture results often take several days to weeks.[2]

Polymerase chain reaction (PCR) is available and has acceptable sensitivity for CMV and other entities.

Footnotes
1. Mayo Reference Services Publication, "Influenza A and B Antigen, Nasopharyngeal Aspirate," *New Test Announcement*, #81856, Rochester, MN: Mayo Medical Laboratories, December 1998.
2. Landry ML and Ferguson D, "SimulFluor Respiratory Screen for Rapid Detection of Multiple Respiratory Viruses in Clinical Specimens by Immunofluorescence Staining," *J Clin Microbiol*, 2000, 38(2):708-11.

References
Baker KA and Ryan ME, "RSV Infection in Infants and Young Children. What's New in Diagnosis, Treatment and Prevention?" *Postgrad Med*, 1999, 106(7):97-108.
Coyle PV, Desai A, Wyatt D, et al, "A Comparison of Viral Isolation, Indirect Immunofluorescence and Nested Multiplex Polymerase Chain Reaction for the Diagnosis of Primary and Recurrent Herpes Simplex Type 1 and Type 2 Infections," *J Virol Methods*, 1999, 83(1-2):75-82.
Scicchitano LM, Shetterly B, and Bourbeau PP, "Evaluation of Light Diagnostics SimulFluor HSV/VZV Immunofluorescence Assay," *Diagn Microbiol Infect Dis*, 1999, 35(3):205-8.

♦ **Virus Fluorescent Antibody Test** *see* Virus, Direct Detection by Fluorescent Antibody *on page 696*

♦ **VZV Culture** *see* Varicella-Zoster Virus Culture *on page 686*

♦ **VZV Serology** *see* Varicella-Zoster Virus Serology *on page 687*

♦ **WA1-Antibody** *see* Babesiosis Serology *on page 561*

♦ **Walking Pneumonia Titer** *see* Mycoplasma Serology *on page 662*

♦ **Wassermann** *replaced by* RPR *on page 677*

♦ **Wassermann** *replaced by* VDRL, Serum *on page 688*

♦ **Western Blot** *see* HIV-1/HIV-2 Antibody Screen and Western Blot *on page 636*

♦ **Western Blot Test for HIV Antibody** *see* HIV-1/HIV-2 Antibody Screen and Western Blot *on page 636*

♦ **Western Equine Encephalitis** *see* Encephalitis Viral Serology *on page 604*

Western Equine Encephalitis Virus Serology

Related Information
Arthropod Identification *on page 559*
Bacterial Culture, Cerebrospinal Fluid *on page 569*
California Encephalitis Virus Serology *on page 587*
Cerebrospinal Fluid Analysis: Overview *on page 416*
Eastern Equine Encephalitis Virus Serology *on page 602*

Encephalitis Viral Serology *on page 604*
St Louis Encephalitis Virus Serology *on page 681*
Viral Culture *on page 689*
Viral Culture, Central Nervous System Symptoms *on page 692*

Synonyms Arbovirus Antibodies: Arbovirus Titer; Encephalitis Virus Titer, Western Equine

Abstract In North America, Western equine encephalitis (WEE) is a disease of summer and it usually causes disease in states west of the Mississippi. Infants are susceptible and are at risk for sequelae. WEE often causes infantile convulsions. The case fatality rate is 3% to 5%. Transmission is via the mosquito vector *Culex tarsalis*. The pathogenesis of WEE resembles that of Eastern equine encephalitis (EEE). Clinical features are also similar to those of St Louis encephalitis.

Specimen Serum or cerebrospinal fluid

Container Red top tube, sterile CSF tube

Collection Acute and convalescent specimens are recommended.

Reference Interval Less than a fourfold increase in titer in paired sera; HAI titer: <1:10; CF titer: <1:8; **no IgM antibody in serum or cerebrospinal fluid (CSF)**

Use Establish the diagnosis of Western equine encephalitis virus infection; differential diagnosis includes St Louis encephalitis (SLE). Generally an encephalitis antibody panel is tested that includes WEE, EEE, SLE, and California encephalitis virus.

Limitations Cross reactions can occur to Eastern equine encephalitis (EEE) virus.

Methodology Diagnosis is best established by detection of specific IgM antibody, particularly in CSF. Complement fixation, hemagglutination inhibition (HAI), neutralization, indirect fluorescent antibody (IFA), enzyme-linked immunosorbent assay are available. Alphaviruses share antigenic relationships.

Additional Information The initial signs and symptoms of WEE infection resemble those of enterovirus infections. Symptoms of WEE infection include fever, aseptic meningitis, and meningoencephalitis. The CSF leukocyte count is 10-300 /mm^3. Virus has been recovered from CSF, blood, and brain and recent developments show that when the patient is viremic, specific nucleic acid can be detected by polymerase chain reaction (PCR) from serum, tissue, or CSF.[1]

This alphavirus disease is usually most severe in infants and children.

Footnotes
1. Linssen B, Kinney RM, Aguilar P, et al, "Development of Reverse Transcription-PCR Assays Specific for Detection of Equine Encephalitis Viruses," *J Clin Microbiol*, 2000, 38(4):1527-35.

References
Kramer LD and Fallah HM, "Genetic Variation Among Isolates of Western Equine Encephalomyelitis Virus From California," *Am J Trop Med Hyg*, 1999, 60(4):708-13.
Markoff L, "Alphavirus," *Principles and Practice of Infectious Diseases*, 5th ed, Mandell GL, Bennett JE, and Dolin R, eds, New York, NY: Churchill Livingstone, 2000, 1703-8.
Nasci RS and Moore CG, "Vector-Borne Disease Surveillance and Natural Disasters," *Emerg Infect Dis*, 1998, 4(2):333-4.

Internet Web Sites
www.astdhpphe.org/infect/wee.html
www.cdc.gov/ncidod/dvbid/arbor/arboinfo.htm

♦ **West Nile Virus** *see* Encephalitis Viral Serology *on page 604*

♦ **Whooping Cough Culture** *see Bordetella pertussis* Culture *on page 583*

♦ **Wound Actinomyces Culture** *see* Actinomyces Culture *on page 551*

♦ **Wound Culture** *see* Bacterial Culture, Wounds, Bites *on page 579*

♦ ***Wuchereria bancrofti* Serology** *see* Filariasis Serological Test *on page 608*

Yellow Fever

Related Information
Arthropod Identification *on page 559*
Bilirubin, Total, Serum *on page 118*
Hepatitis D Serology *on page 627*
Hepatitis: Laboratory Assessment, Overview *on page 629*
Prothrombin Time *on page 354*

Synonyms Yellow Fever Antibody Titer

Applies to IgM and IgG Specific for Yellow Fever Virus

Abstract Yellow fever is classified among the viral hemorrhagic fevers, a group which also includes hantavirus pulmonary syndrome and others.

The first clinical description of the disease caused by yellow fever (YF) was in 1648. The virus was probably spread to the Western hemisphere by trading vessels from West Africa that were infested with YF infected *Aedes aegypti*. Currently, YF is transmitted in parts of sub-Saharan Africa and South America. The disease has never been documented in Asia. *A. aegypti* mosquitoes are infected after feeding on viremic humans spread the infection in subsequent feeding attempts. This method of transmission is responsible for epidemic (urban) YF. The illness due to YF ranges in severity from a mild self-limited disease to hemorrhagic fever which is fatal in 50% of cases.

A. aegypti also spreads dengue fever.
(Continued)

Yellow Fever *(Continued)*

The differential diagnosis includes hepatitis, including hepatitis D.

Specimen Serum

Container Red top tube

Sampling Time Acute and convalescent phases; *vide infra.*

Storage Instructions Refrigerate at 4°C.

Reference Interval Negative

Critical Values Fourfold or greater change in titer; *vide infra.*

Use Diagnose yellow fever; document vaccination

Limitations Patients from areas of the world where there are numerous flavivirus infections (eg, Africa) can have cross-reactive antibodies that give low positive values.

Methodology Enzyme immunoassay (EIA), indirect immunofluorescent antibody (IFA), complement fixation (CF), reverse transcriptase PCR

Additional Information Yellow fever has been a disease of public health importance since the 15th century. At various times in human history it has caused epidemics of disease in the Americas, Africa, and Europe. Yellow fever is an arboviral infection with epidemiologic transmission cycles between monkeys, mosquitoes, and humans. The disease, characterized by fever, headache, and myalgias, follows an incubation period of 3-6 days. The symptoms begin abruptly, accompanied by facial flushing and a relative bradycardia (Faget's sign). Laboratory abnormalities include leukopenia, thrombocytopenia, prolongation of prothrombin time and PTT, proteinuria, increased serum total and conjugated bilirubin, AST, ALT, and creatinine. Resolution of this period of infection is the end of the illness in most patients. However, in others, the fever will fade for a few hours to several days to be followed by symptoms that include high fever, headache, back pain, nausea, vomiting, abdominal pain, and somnolence. This phase of the illness is dominated by icteric hepatitis and a hemorrhagic diathesis.[1]

The liver is characterized by classical midzone necrosis with Councilman bodies and vacuolar fatty changes. Liver biopsy is usually considered contraindicated by virtue of possible uncontrolled bleeding.

Effective vaccines are available for the prevention of yellow fever. Travelers (including children) to endemic areas are encouraged to receive these vaccinations before visiting countries with high prevalence of YF.[2,3]

Patients tested for serology will usually have positive results from 7-10 days after the onset of illness. IgM ELISA is detected in high titer only for a short interval following infection; thus, a single convalescent serum specimen is reliable for this method. In secondary infections, the IgM and IgG ELISA is usually detected as early as 4-5 days after the onset of illness.

Footnotes

1. Tsai TF, "Flaviviruses (Yellow Fever, Dengue, Dengue Hemorrhagic Fever, Japanese Encephalitis, St Louis Encephalitis, Tick-Borne Encephalitis)," *Principles and Practice of Infectious Diseases*, 5th ed, Mandell GL, Bennett JE, and Dolin R, eds, New York, NY: Churchill Livingstone, 2000.
2. Sood SK, "Immunization for Children Traveling Abroad," *Pediatr Clin North Am*, 2000, 47(2):435-48.
3. Dick L, "Travel Medicine: Helping Patients Prepare for Trips Abroad," *Am Fam Phys*, 1998, 58(2):383-402.

References

Centers for Disease Control and Prevention, "Fatal Yellow Fever in a Traveler Returning From Venezuela, 1999," *JAMA*, 2000, 283(17):2230-2.

Coker AO, Isokpehi RD, Thomas BN, et al, "Zoonotic Infections in Nigeria: Overview From a Medical Perspective," *Acta Trop*, 2000, 76(1):59-63.

Jong EC, "Travel Immunizations," *Med Clin North Am*, 1999, 83(4):903-22.

Robertson SE, Hull BP, Tomori O, et al, "Yellow Fever: A Decade of Reemergence," *JAMA*, 1996, 276(14):1157-62.

Shope RE, "Introduction to Hemorrhagic Fever Viruses," *Cecil Textbook of Medicine*, 21st ed, Chapter 391, Goldman L and Bennett JC, eds, Philadelphia, PA: WB Saunders Co, 2000, 1840-8.

Tomori O, "Impact of Yellow Fever on the Developing World," *Adv Virus Res*, 1999, 53:5-34.

Internet Web Sites

www.astdhpphe.org/infect/yellow.html

www.cdc.gov/ncidod/dvbid/yellowf.htm

♦ **Yellow Fever Antibody Titer** *see* Yellow Fever *on page 697*

♦ *Yersinia enterocolitica* *see* Bacterial Culture, Stool *on page 575*

Yersinia enterocolitica Antibody

Related Information

Bacterial Culture, Blood *on page 566*

Bacterial Culture, Stool *on page 575*

HLA-B27 *on page 528*

Risks of Transfusion *on page 861*

Viral Culture, Stool *on page 695*

Test Includes Detection of antibody (IgG, IgM, and IgA) specific for *Yersinia enterocolitica*

Abstract Reservoirs of *Y. enterocolitica* are a variety of animals including pigs, goats, sheep, dogs, and cats. Transmission may include milk, pork, and water. Usually the organisms are ingested, but the infection can also be acquired by transfusion (red cells, platelets). Diarrhea due to *Y. enterocolitica* is infrequent in the United States but is more common in Europe. Often

the differential diagnosis includes appendicitis. *Y. enterocolitica* and *Y. pseudotuberculosis* may cause similar clinical presentations.[1]

Specimen Serum

Container Red top tube

Collection Acute and convalescent specimens are recommended.

Reference Interval Titer <1:160

Critical Values Antibodies may not be detectable for the first week of symptoms, but then rise rapidly to high titers (1:1280 is diagnostic).

Use Useful in diagnosis of *Yersinia enterocolitica* infection, which is characterized by mesenteric lymphadenitis and/or terminal ileitis with abdominal pain, gastroenteritis, and diarrhea. Bloody diarrhea may occur. It manifests often as enterocolitis in children younger than 5 years of age. Arthritis and other extraintestinal complications may occur; yersiniosis is considered within the differential diagnosis of rheumatic and collagen diseases.[1] Such arthritis usually is seen in individuals who are HLA-B27 positive.[2] It is a cause of liver abscesses; 60% of such patients were associated with hemochromatosis.[2] Most infections are self-limited.

Limitations Present serodiagnostic techniques are described as having only limited value due to high seroprevalence in certain healthy populations.[3]

Methodology Enzyme immunoassay (EIA); agglutination with serotypes 03, 08, and 09. Serologic diagnosis enjoys wider application in Europe than in the U.S.[2]

Additional Information Detection of *Yersinia*-specific antibody should be used in conjunction with culture to confirm a diagnosis of yersiniosis. After recovery of infection, low titers (1:40 or 1:80) may persist for years. **When stool is sent to the laboratory for culture, request for culture of this organism is usually needed so that an enrichment technique can be utilized.**

The most common manifestation of *Y. enterocolitica* infection is enterocolitis accompanied by fever, diarrhea and abdominal pain that may last 1-3 weeks. A reactive polyarthritis has been recognized in 10% to 30% of adults and may begin a few days to a month after diarrhea.[4]

Footnotes

1. Smego RA, Frean J, and Koornhof HJ, "Yersiniosis I: Microbiological and Clinicoepidemiological Aspects of Plague and Nonplague *Yersinia* Infections," *Eur J Clin Microbiol Infect Dis*, 1999, 18(1):1-15.
2. Morris JG Jr, "*Yersinia* Infections," *Cecil Textbook of Medicine*, 21st ed, Chapter 348, Goldman L and Bennett JC, eds, Philadelphia, PA: WB Saunders Co, 2000, 1700-1.
3. Maki-Ikola O, Heesemann J, Toivanen A, et al, "High Frequency of *Yersinia* Antibodies in Healthy Populations in Finland and Germany," *Rheumatol Int*, 1997, 16(2):227-9.
4. van der Heijden IM, Res PC, Wilbrink B, et al, "*Yersinia enterocolitica*: A Cause of Chronic Polyarthritis," *Clin Infect Dis*, 1997, 25(4):831-7.

References

Katz JA, "At the Focal Point. *Yersinia enterocolitica*," *Gastrointest Endosc*, 1998, 48(1):61.

Koornhof HJ, Smego RA Jr, and Nicol M, "Yersiniosis. II: The Pathogenesis of *Yersinia* Infections," *Eur J Clin Microbiol Infect Dis*, 1999, 18(2):87-112.

Tiddia F, Cherchi GB, Pacifico L, et al, "*Yersinia enterocolitica* Causing Suppurative Arthritis of the Shoulder," *J Clin Pathol*, 1994, 47(8):760-1.

Tuohy AM, O'Gorman M, Byington C, et al, "*Yersinia enterocolitica* Mimicking Crohn's Disease in a Toddler," *Pediatrics*, 1999, 104(3):e36.

Verhaegen J, Charlier J, Lemmens P, et al, "Surveillance of Human *Yersinia enterocolitica* Infections in Belgium: 1967-1996," *Clin Infect Dis*, 1998, 27(1):59-64.

Internet Web Sites

vm.cfsan.fda.gov/~mow/chap5.html

www.cdc.gov/ncidod/dbmd/diseaseinfo/yersinia_g.htm

Yersinia pestis Antibody

Related Information

Bacterial Culture, Blood *on page 566*

Bacterial Culture, Sputum *on page 574*

Fine Needle Aspiration Culture *on page 609*

Viral Culture, Stool *on page 695*

Synonyms Bubonic Plague Serology; Plague Serology

Applies to *Yersinia pestis* Culture

Test Includes Detection of antibody specific for *Yersinia pestis*

Abstract *Yersinia pestis* (*Pasteurella pestis* until 1970) is the etiologic agent of plague. Epidemic bubonic plague has been described historically and was responsible for the deaths of 25% of Europe's population in the Middle Ages. Currently, epidemics occur throughout the world with at least 2000 cases reported annually.[1] The cycle can be stable (enzootic) or epidemic (epizootic) in rodent populations. A recent concern is the possibility that *Y. pestis* may be used as a biological weapon.[2] The forms of plague include lymphadenitis (bubonic plague), septicemic, pneumonic, cutaneous, and meningeal. Recognition of these clinical presentations of plague is important in order to provide appropriate therapy, prevent deaths, and control an outbreak.

Specimen Serum

Container Red top tube

Storage Instructions Acidified serum may be stored in a refrigerator

Special Instructions In cases of suspected plague, the Centers for Disease Control and Prevention, Vector-borne Infectious Diseases, Fort Collins, CO (970) 221-6400 should be contacted at once. Sera must be inactivated and absorbed with sheep erythrocytes prior to testing.

Reference Interval Titer <1:16

Critical Values A fourfold or greater increase in titer or a single titer >1:16 indicates exposure to *Y. pestis* and should be immediately reported to the physician and the CDC.

Use Confirm the diagnosis of plague

Methodology Passive hemagglutination on acute and convalescent serum

Additional Information A hemagglutination titer ≥1:16 is presumptive evidence of an immunologic response to *Yersinia pestis*, the plague bacillus. Seeing the stained organism in clinical material (aspiration of a bubo, sputum) can also make diagnosis, using Gram stain or fluorescent antibody. Blood, bubo (lymph node) aspiration, and other materials can be cultured on special request.

Plague occurs west of the 100th meridian (North Dakota to Texas) in the U.S.

Footnotes

1. Titball RW and Leary SE, "Plague," *Br Med Bull*, 1998, 54(3):625-33.
2. Inglesby TV, Dennis DT, Henderson DA, et al, "Plague as a Biological Weapon: Medical and Public Health Management. Working Group on Civilian Biodefense." *JAMA*, 2000, 283(17):2281-90.

References

Duschet P, "The Threat of Biological Warfare," *Arch Dermatol*, 1999, 135(11):1417-8.

Gage KL, Dennis DT, Orloski KA, et al, "Cases of Cat-Associated Human Plague in the Western US, 1977-1998," *Clin Infect Dis*, 2000, 30(6).

Koornhof HJ, Smego RA Jr, and Nicol M, "Yersiniosis. II: The Pathogenesis of *Yersinia* Infections," *Eur J Clin Microbiol Infect Dis*, 1999, 18(2):87-112.

Morris JG Jr, "*Yersinia* Infections," *Cecil Textbook of Medicine*, 21st ed, Chapter 348, Goldman L and Bennett JC, eds, Philadelphia, PA: WB Saunders Co, 2000, 1700-1.

Ratsitorahina M, Chanteau S, Rahalison L, et al, "Epidemiological and Diagnostic Aspects of the Outbreak of Pneumonic Plague in Madagascar," *Lancet*, 2000, 355(9198):111-3.

Smego RA, Frean J, and Koornhof HJ, "Yersiniosis I: Microbiological and Clinicoepidemiological Aspects of Plague and Nonplague *Yersinia* Infections," *Eur J Clin Microbiol Infect Dis*, 1999, 18(1):1-15.

Internet Web Sites

www.astdhpphe.org/infect/plague.html

www.cdc.gov/ncidod/dvbid/plagindex.htm

♦ ***Yersinia pestis* Culture** *see Yersinia pestis* Antibody *on page 698*

♦ **Ziehl-Neelsen Stain** *see* Acid-Fast Stain *on page 550*

♦ **Zoster Titer** *see* Varicella-Zoster Virus Serology *on page 687*

MOLECULAR GENETIC TESTING

Karen Stephens, PhD

Jonathan F. Tait, MD

David S. Jacobs, MD

Uttam Garg, PhD

The first DNA-based genetic tests became available in the mid 1980s. Since then, the field has expanded rapidly, and today there are clinical tests available for hundreds of diseases[1]. The number of tests will continue to increase as information from the Human Genome Project is translated into new diagnostic procedures. DNA-based genetic testing is also moving out of specialized genetics clinics and is becoming more common in general clinical practice.

The new DNA-based genetic tests represent a genuine advance, but they also pose new challenges for patients, for the physicians providing them to patients, and for the laboratories offering these test services. On the one hand, news reports of genetic breakthroughs can create unrealistic expectations for the availability or utility of new genetic tests. On the other hand, both public and professional groups have raised various concerns about the quality, appropriateness, and potential misuse of genetic testing. Although most evidence to date indicates that molecular-genetic testing is accurate and has a low frequency of adverse events,[2] and does not lead to discrimination in health insurance coverage decisions,[3] some caution is appropriate, particularly for certain tests that are either controversial or have major impact on life events. This introduction provides some general guidance on factors to consider for effective and responsible use of genetic tests.

APPROACH TO TESTING

Molecular-genetic tests are highly heterogeneous; some can be ordered and used as part of a panel of general laboratory tests (eg, testing for genetic thrombophilia in a patient presenting with venous thrombosis), while others require careful pretest preparation and post-test follow-up for patient and family (eg, tests for Huntington disease or hereditary risk for breast and ovarian cancer).

A general approach is as follows.

Pretest Evaluation and Counseling

- Evaluate the indication for testing - diagnostic versus presymptomatic versus carrier testing. The nature of testing and counseling procedures can often differ when the same laboratory test is used for different clinical indications.

- Assess need for specialized genetic counseling. Directories of specialized genetics clinics are available online.[1]

- Assess clinical and psychosocial appropriateness of testing.

- Address confidentiality concerns. Patients may be concerned about disclosure of information to relatives, or its impact on insurability or employability.

- For some presymptomatic tests, it may be appropriate to first confirm the presence of a detectable mutation in an affected relative.

- Obtain informed consent. Explain the nature of the test procedure, the expected outcomes, the risks, benefits, and alternatives. Specific items to cover vary greatly from test to test, but can include:

  - clinical utility of results

  - alternatives to testing (ie, risk calculation for carrier status, diagnosis on clinical grounds instead of diagnostic testing)

  - sensitivity, specificity, cost, and turnaround time

  - possible psychological risks and impact on family members

  - irrevocable nature of results

  - possible risks to insurance and employment

Post-test Counseling and Follow-up

This will also vary greatly from test to test, but factors to consider include:

- How and when to give results. Tests with a major impact on life events should usually be given in person, and presence of a support person may be helpful.

- Psychological and emotional impact of test results.

- Clinical follow-up and referral required for the disease or predisposition in question.

- Counseling of at-risk family members. Particularly for a family newly diagnosed with a genetic disease, counseling or referral of relatives is important. Some genetic diseases such as hemochromatosis are highly treatable, and other relatives may be spared by timely diagnosis. Reproductive decisions may also be affected. At the same time, one does not want to encourage testing for its own sake; each family member needs to decide what is best for himself or herself.

- Confidentiality concerns. Patients may consider some test results especially sensitive, and may wish to apply a higher standard of confidentiality than is normally the case for healthcare information.

SPECIAL SITUATIONS AND ETHICAL ISSUES

For tests that have major impact on medical care or life planning, some clinical circumstances call for special care before testing is performed:

- Adoptees. There may be pressure from the adoptive parents or the adoption agency to determine if the child carries a disease present or suspected in the birth parents. In evaluating these requests, one should ask whether testing serves the best interests of the child. For example, presymptomatic testing for an untreatable adult-onset disease may provide no clinical benefit to the adoptee. Guidelines for genetic testing during adoption have been provided recently.[4]

- Testing of children for adult-onset diseases. Testing for adult-onset diseases that are currently not treatable or preventable may provide no benefit to a child, and may be harmful if it leads to discriminatory treatment in school, family, or community. If a test result primarily affects adult decisions such as choice of career, insurance coverage, marriage, or reproductive options, testing may be best postponed until a child can make his or her own decision as an adult.[5]

- Persons with impaired ability to give consent. Caution should be exercised in performing predictive testing on people such as the mentally handicapped, critically ill patients, or prisoners.

- Persons at 25% risk for an autosomal dominant disease. The person requesting testing should be aware that a positive result will reveal the status of the parent at 50% risk, and be encouraged to reach a prior understanding with the parent about how testing will be done and who will have access to the information.

ALTERNATIVES TO TESTING

Because of the technical limitations, complexity or expense of some molecular-genetic tests, it is appropriate to consider alternatives to testing. Depending on the circumstances, one or more of the following alternatives might be most appropriate for a given individual or family. Discussion and choice of alternatives is often well handled by specialized genetics clinics.

- Information and reassurance. This may be helpful for some people who perceive their risk of a genetic disease to be unrealistically high, or who have unrealistic expectations about the utility of a given genetic test result. This situation commonly occurs with many of the current tests that detect genetic predisposition to a variety of cancers; these tests are generally applicable only to a small subset of people with very strong family histories of cancer, and clinically proven surveillance or preventive strategies based on test results are not necessarily available.

- Diagnosis on clinical grounds or by other test methods. In some instances, other laboratory methods provide a better means for initial diagnosis. For example, screening for thalassemia carriers is still best done with a combination of hemoglobin electrophoresis and quantitation, red-cell indices, and special staining for intraerythrocytic inclusions. DNA-based tests are reserved for confirmation or for prenatal diagnosis. Similarly, conventional clinical chemistry testing provides the best initial screening test for hereditary hemochromatosis.

- Risk estimates. For families with known genetic diseases, it is often possible to estimate an individual's risk of carrying the mutant gene based on simple pedigree analysis. For people without a known family history, their risk of carrying a mutant gene can often be estimated from the population frequency of that gene in their particular ethnic group.

  For some forms of cancer, empirical risk estimates can be provided based on analysis of a patient's known risk factors. An example would be analysis of the risk of breast cancer.[6]

- DNA banking. This simple, low-cost alternative is often useful in the setting of terminally ill patients with undiagnosed diseases. DNA can be safely stored for years, thus preserving the option of future genetic diagnosis for an individual or family. For example, patients terminally ill with cancer of suspected genetic origin can store their DNA to allow future diagnosis for their at-risk relatives

ELECTRONIC REFERENCES ON GENETIC DISEASES AND GENETIC TESTING

The GeneTests web site provides a directory of laboratories providing clinical or research-based testing for genetic diseases, and directories of clinics providing specialized services for genetic diseases.[1] GeneClinics provides a series of brief reviews on many genetic diseases.[7] Online Mendelian Inheritance in Man (OMIM) provides an encyclopedic reference source on genetic diseases of all kinds.[8] The American Society of Human Genetics provides a series of policy statements on ethical, legal and social issues related to genetic testing.[9]

Footnotes

1. Anonymous, *GeneTests: Directory of Genetic Testing Laboratories* [database online] Children's Health System, 1999, available at: http://www.genetests.org/
2. Hofgartner WT and Tait JF, "Frequency of Problems During Clinical Molecular-Genetic Testing," *Am J Clin Pathol*, 1999; 112:14-21.
3. Hall MA and Rich SS, "Laws Restricting Health Insurers' Use of Genetic Information: Impact on Genetic Discrimination," *Am J Hum Genet*, 2000, 66:293-307.
4. Anonymous, "Genetic Testing in Adoption," The American Society of Human Genetics Social Issues Committee and The American College of Medical Genetics Social, Ethical, and Legal Issues Committee, *Am J Hum Genet*, 2000, 66:761-7.
5. "Points to Consider: Ethical, Legal, and Psychosocial Implications of Genetic Testing in Children and Adolescents," American Society of Human Genetics Board of Directors, American College of Medical Genetics Board of Directors, *Am J Hum Genet*, 1995, 57:1233-41.
6. Armstrong K, Eisen A, and Weber B, "Assessing the Risk of Breast Cancer," *N Engl J Med* 2000, 342:564-71.
7. Anonymous, *GeneClinics: Medical Genetics Knowledge Base* [database online] 1995, available at: http://www.geneclinics.org/ (updated weekly).
8. Anonymous, *Online Mendelian Inheritance in Man, OMIM (TM)*, McKusick-Nathans Institute for Genetic Medicine, Johns Hopkins University (Baltimore, MD) and National Center for Biotechnology Information, National Library of Medicine (Bethesda, MD), 2000, available at: http://www.ncbi.nlm.nih.gov/omim/
9. American Society of Human Genetics, *Society Policy Statements and Reports*, available at: http://www.faseb.org/genetics/ashg/policy/pol-00.htm

♦ **ADPKD** *see* Autosomal Dominant Polycystic Kidney Disease DNA Detection *on page 704*

♦ **Adult Polycystic Kidney Disease Inheritance Determination** *see* Autosomal Dominant Polycystic Kidney Disease DNA Detection *on page 704*

♦ **Ataxia** *see* Spinocerebellar Ataxia Type 1 DNA Test *on page 714*

♦ **Ataxin-1** *see* Spinocerebellar Ataxia Type 1 DNA Test *on page 714*

♦ **Ataxin-2** *see* Spinocerebellar Ataxia Type 2 DNA Test *on page 715*

♦ **Ataxin-3** *see* Spinocerebellar Ataxia Type 3 DNA Test *on page 716*

♦ **Ataxin-7** *see* Spinocerebellar Ataxia Type 7 DNA Test *on page 717*

♦ **Autosomal Dominant Cerebellar Ataxia Type III [ADCA III]** *see* Spinocerebellar Ataxia Type 7 DNA Test *on page 717*

♦ **Autosomal Dominant Cerebellar Ataxia Type III [ADCA III] (subset of)** *see* Spinocerebellar Ataxia Type 6 DNA Test *on page 716*

♦ **Autosomal Dominant Cerebellar Ataxia Type I [ADCA I] (subset of)** *see* Spinocerebellar Ataxia Type 1 DNA Test *on page 714*

♦ **Autosomal Dominant Cerebellar Ataxia Type I [ADCA I] (subset of)** *see* Spinocerebellar Ataxia Type 2 DNA Test *on page 715*

♦ **Autosomal Dominant Cerebellar Ataxia Type I [ADCA I] (subset of)** *see* Spinocerebellar Ataxia Type 3 DNA Test *on page 716*

Autosomal Dominant Polycystic Kidney Disease DNA Detection

Related Information
Chorionic Villus Sampling, Chromosome and Genetic Abnormality Analysis *on page 361*
Kidney Biopsy *on page 64*
Polymerase Chain Reaction *on page 713*

Synonyms ADPKD; Adult Polycystic Kidney Disease Inheritance Determination; Genetic Detection of Presymptomatic Adult Polycystic Kidney Disease; Molecular Diagnosis of Polycystic Kidney Disease; Polycystic Kidney Disease, Autosomal Dominant; Polycystic Kidney Disease, Prenatal Diagnosis

Test Includes This test can detect DNA linkage association with the major genetic mutation (autosomal dominant polycystic kidney disease locus 1, ADPKD1) on chromosome 16. This gene is tightly linked with adult polycystic kidney disease, presently designated autosomal dominant PKD.

Abstract Autosomal dominant polycystic kidney disease (ADPKD) is a heterogenous disorder characterized by the development of myriads of renal cysts. The disease results from mutations in either of two genes, PKD1 or PKD2. The genes code for polycystin-1 and polycystin-2 respectively. Symptoms usually develop between the ages of 30-40 years, but they can begin earlier. Most of the cases have mutations in PKD1 gene, which is been located on chromosome 16.[1] PKD2 gene is located on chromosome 4, and mutations in this gene results in a less severe form of ADPKD. Individuals in families affected with this entity can now have genetic studies performed to determine their risk for developing the disease. Patients at high risk can then be followed closely. Such testing must be done only with genetic counseling.

Specimen Blood, amniotic fluid, chorionic villus, or tissue

Container Blood should be collected in yellow top (ACD) Vacutainer® tube; amniotic fluid and chorionic villus should be collected in a sterile manner and transferred to a sterile tube for transport or to a T25 culture flask; amniotic cells can be sent after culturing or can be sent directly to the laboratory.

Sampling Time Amniotic fluid should be collected between the 17th and 18th week of pregnancy. Chorionic villus specimens should be collected between the 8th and 12th week of gestation.

Storage Instructions All specimens should be sent to the laboratory **immediately** after collection, preferably by overnight delivery. All specimens should be kept at room temperature or refrigerated, never frozen.

Causes for Rejection Any amniotic fluid specimen that is bloody may be contaminated with maternal blood and is unsuitable for this test, any specimen that has been frozen before processing cannot be tested

Turnaround Time Results are usually available in 1-2 weeks.

Special Instructions A complete family pedigree and clinical information are generally needed. Prior testing of family members is usually necessary for prenatal testing.

Reference Interval The laboratory generally provides an interpretive report that includes a risk analysis.

Use This test is indicated for a family with history of autosomal dominant polycystic disease. For this purpose it is necessary to have a family pedigree that includes all medical histories. This test is also indicated for prenatal diagnosis in couples known to be carriers of the much less common recessive form of polycystic kidney disease, which has been called infantile PKD, which is strongly associated with hepatic fibrosis and pulmonary maldevelopment. This test requires genetic testing of several family members (often as many as seven or eight) to determine the characteristics of the mutation.

Limitations DNA linkage analysis for polycystic kidney disease can detect the inheritance pattern associated with one of the major genes responsible

for the disease. However, a negative result does not rule out the possibility that an individual may carry another mutation causing polycystic kidney disease, or even be affected with polycystic kidney disease. However, the test can greatly lower that probability. Such testing is available only in a few reference laboratories.

PKD1 gene analysis is complicated by the existence of highly homologous loci on chromosome 16. Approximately 70% of the gene length is replicated 3-4 times with sequence homology >95%.

Methodology DNA is isolated from the specimen. Several regions on chromosome 16 close to and flanking the ADPKD1 gene are examined using Southern blotting techniques. Restriction enzyme sites on the DNA close to the disease gene are examined. Genetic linkage analysis uses specific DNA probes to follow the inheritance of a gene associated with disease. This requires testing several members of a family, including both affected and unaffected individuals, preferably from several generations. The DNA probes used to follow the gene must be located very close to the disease gene and must show differences in the size of DNA that results from restriction enzyme digestion (polymorphic) between individuals from the same family (see figure). This allows for distinction between all the possible different chromosomes 16 that an individual could inherit; it can be determined from this information which chromosome is associated with disease. If these polymorphic sites are located very close to the disease gene then they are called "informative". The accuracy of genetic linkage analysis is greater if DNA probes on both sides of the disease gene are informative. The genetic linkage analysis for polycystic kidney disease uses flanking markers very closely associated with ADPKD1, the gene associated with the disease. Thus, in families in which this mutation is found, linkage analysis can very accurately predict inheritance of the disease gene (ADPKD1).

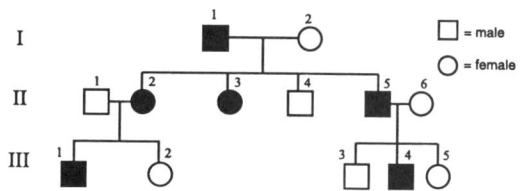

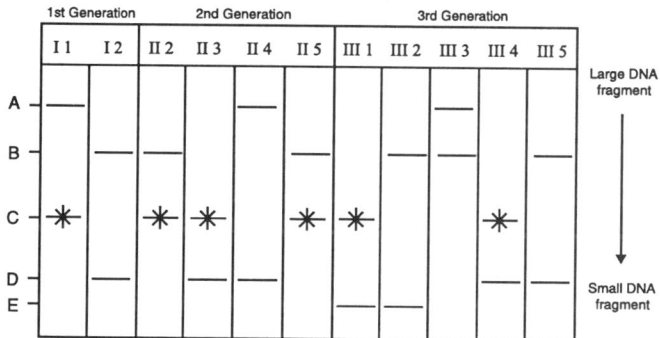

DNA is digested with restriction enzymes to make smaller pieces of DNA. This DNA is then electrophoresed in an agarose gel to separate DNA of different sizes (large to small). After transfer to a membrane, the DNA is hybridized with a radioactive or fluorescent DNA probe and hybridized DNA bands are visible with autoradiography or autoluminography. Inheritance patterns are noted that associate with disease (✳). Open symbols are normal individuals and shaded symbols are affected individuals.

In recent years, polymerase chain reaction (PCR) has also been used in genetic analysis of PKD genes. A very long transcript (14.5 Kb), including an unusual 2.5 Kb polypyrimidine tract in the middle of the gene, makes PCR very challenging. Long-range PCR protocols have overcome several problems associated with the long gene.[1]

Additional Information Polycystic kidney diseases (PKD) are common genetic disorders responsible for ~10% of all cases requiring long-term dialysis or renal transplantation. PKD may be recessive or dominant. The incidence of ADPKD is 1 in 500-1000 individuals.[2] At least three different loci, PKD1 and PKD2 and non-PKD1/PKD2 have been identified for ADPKD.[3]

Due to dominant inheritance of ADPKD, each child born of an affected parent has a 50% chance of inheritance of the disease gene. Polycystic kidney disease is characterized by progressive increase and enlargement of numerous fluid-filled renal cysts. The growth of such cysts causes progressive impairment, which usually leads to irreversible renal failure in middle age. In 40% to 70% of patients, cysts are also present in the liver. They are encountered sporadically in the pancreas, spleen, subarachnoid space, and pineal gland, and other abnormalities are described as well. The mechanism of cyst formation and the biochemical defect of the disease are currently not known. Although no specific treatment is available for ADPKD, supportive management and renal transplant are highly effective.

Mutations in PKD1 gene are the most common cause of ADPKD. PKD1 gene should not be confused with PKD1-like loci, which are 97% identical to PKD1. The 14.5 Kb PKD1 transcript encodes a 4304 amino acid protein.[4]

Molecular analysis of PKD1 gene allows preasymptomatic diagnosis in individuals younger than 30 years of age and helps in establishing prognosis and follow-up.

Footnotes

1. Watnick T and Germino GG, "Molecular Basis of Autosomal Dominant Polycystic Kidney Disease," *Semin Nephrol*, 1999, 19(4):327-43.
2. Grantham JJ, "Polycystic Kidney Disease: I. Etiology and Pathogenesis," *Hosp Pract*, 1992, 27(3):51-9.
3. Murcia NS, Woychik RP, and Avner ED, "The Molecular Biology of Polycystic Kidney Disease," *Pediatr Nephrol*, 1998, 12(9):721-6.
4. "Polycystic Kidney Disease: The Complete Structure of the PKD1 Gene and its Protein. The International Polycystic Kidney Disease Consortium," *Cell*, 1995, 81(2):289-98.

References

Bear JC, Parfrey PS, Morgan JM, et al, "Autosomal Dominant Polycystic Kidney Disease: New Information for Genetic Counseling," *Am J Med Genet*, 1992, 43(3):548-53.

Gabow PA, "Autosomal Dominant Polycystic Kidney Disease," *N Engl J Med*, 1993, 329(5):332-42.

Hanaoka K, Qian F, Boletta A, et al, "Coassembly of Polycystin-1 and -2 Produces Unique Cation-Permeable Currents," *Nature*, 2000, 408(6815):990-4.

Koptides M and Deltas CC, "Autosomal Dominant Polycystic Kidney Disease: Molecular Genetics and Molecular Pathogenesis," *Hum Genet*, 2000, 107(2):115-26.

Murcia NS, Sweeney WE Jr, and Avner ED, "New Insights Into the Molecular Pathophysiology of Polycystic Kidney Disease," *Kidney Int*, 1999, 55(4):1187-97.

Peral B, Gamble V, Strong C, et al, "Identification of Mutations in the Duplicated Region of the Polycystic Kidney Disease 1 Gene (PKD1) by a Novel Approach," *Am J Hum Genet*, 1997, 60(6):1399-410.

Thomas R, McConnell R, Whittaker J, et al, "Identification of Mutations in the Repeated Part of the Autosomal Dominant Polycystic Kidney Disease Type 1 Gene, PKD1, by Long-Range PCR," *Am J Hum Genet*, 1999, 65(1):39-49.

Ye M and Grantham JJ, "The Secretion of Fluid by Renal Cysts From Patients With Autosomal Dominant Polycystic Kidney Disease," *N Engl J Med*, 1993, 329(5):310-3.

Cystic Fibrosis DNA Detection

Related Information

Amniotic Fluid, Chromosome and Genetic Abnormality Analysis *on page 360*

Chloride, Sweat *on page 144*

Chorionic Villus Sampling, Chromosome and Genetic Abnormality Analysis *on page 361*

Polymerase Chain Reaction *on page 713*

Synonyms *CFTR* Gene Mutation Analysis; Cystic Fibrosis, Carrier Testing; Cystic Fibrosis, Prenatal Diagnosis; Genetic Testing, Cystic Fibrosis; Molecular Diagnosis, Cystic Fibrosis; Mutation Testing, Cystic Fibrosis

Applies to CFTR; Chorionic Villus Biopsies; Cystic Fibrosis Transmembrane Conductance Regulator; Delta F508

Test Includes Detection of the 10-30 most common mutations causing cystic fibrosis

Abstract Cystic fibrosis (CF) is an autosomal recessive disease caused by mutations in a gene called *CFTR* (cystic fibrosis transmembrane conductance regulator). About 4% of the Caucasian population are carriers. There are nearly 1000 known mutations in the *CFTR* gene, but the 10 most common mutations account for about 80% to 85% of all mutations in Caucasians. DNA-based testing can be used to diagnose cystic fibrosis, to detect carriers of the disease, and to perform prenatal diagnosis. It is also useful in the evaluation of fetuses with ultrasound findings suspicious for cystic fibrosis, and in the evaluation of men with infertility due to congenital absence of the vas deferens. It is occasionally used in the evaluation of patients with idiopathic chronic pancreatitis. Failure to detect gene mutations of CF does not rule out the diagnosis. CF is characterized by a broad spectrum of disease severity.[1]

Specimen 3-10 mL whole blood, 10-20 mL amniotic fluid, 1 T25 flask of cultured amniocytes or chorionic villi, 5-10 mg wet chorionic villi

Container Lavender top (EDTA) or yellow top (ACD) tube; avoid use of tubes containing heparin anticoagulants, which can interfere with polymerase chain reaction analysis. Amniotic fluid and chorionic villus biopsies should be collected in a sterile manner and transferred to a sterile tube for transport. Syringes and tubes should not contain additives that interfere with cell culture methods.

Sampling Time Blood samples can be taken at any time. Amniotic fluid should be collected between the 14th and 16th week of gestation. Chorionic villus specimens should be collected between the 8th and 12th week of gestation.

Storage Instructions Store blood samples refrigerated or at room temperature. Do not freeze. Blood samples should normally be received in the testing laboratory within 4 days of collection to ensure adequate yield of DNA. Transport amniotic fluid or chorionic villus biopsy samples to the laboratory immediately.

Turnaround Time 7-14 days

Special Instructions To provide optimal interpretation and risk calculation, the testing laboratory needs to know the patient's diagnosis, ethnic background, and family history/pedigree. Such information can support customization of mutation panels to augment sensitivity of DNA testing. When testing is being performed for carrier detection, pretest counseling should explain the meaning and limitations of testing, including the imperfect sensitivity for detection of carriers. Post-test counseling should explain the significance of the result and describe the post-test risk that an individual couple may have with a child with CF.

Reference Interval A normal result is the absence of detectable mutations (see Limitations). An abnormal result is the detection of either one or two mutations. The laboratory usually provides an interpretive report, which includes a risk estimate where appropriate (eg, for carrier testing).

Use Indications for testing include:

Diagnosis of suspected CF: Detection of two mutant alleles confirms the diagnosis of CF. In the Caucasian population, about 70% to 80% of patients with CF have two detectable mutations, about 20% to 30% have one detectable mutation, and about 1% to 2% have no detectable mutations.

Carrier detection in patient with family history of CF and in his/her reproductive partner: Detection of one mutant allele indicates carrier status, and is useful for reproductive planning. In the northern European Caucasian population, about 85% to 90% of carriers have one detectable mutation.

Carrier detection in parents of fetus with echogenic bowel: CF is one explanation for the presence of echogenic bowel detected by ultrasound during the 2nd trimester. To help rule out this explanation, both parents can be tested for *CFTR* mutations. If a fetal sample is already being obtained for other purposes (eg, chromosome analysis), the fetal sample can be tested directly.

Prenatal diagnosis in a fetus at risk for CF: When both parents carry known mutations in the *CFTR* gene, their fetus can be tested to determine if it has inherited one or both mutant alleles.

Evaluation of infertile men with congenital bilateral absence of the vas deferens: This clinical syndrome is often caused by "mild" mutations in the *CFTR* gene that do not manifest as classical CF with pulmonary and pancreatic symptoms. Detection of *CFTR* mutant alleles can be useful to these patients in deciding on reproductive options, and for genetic counseling of their relatives regarding their risk of being carriers of CF.

Evaluation of individuals with progressive pulmonary infection, with other evidence of possible CF.

Evaluation of patients with pancreatic exocrine deficiency; evaluation of patients with idiopathic chronic pancreatitis: Some 15% to 35% of patients with idiopathic chronic pancreatitis have at least one detectable *CFTR* mutation.

DNA testing may be useful when results of pilocarpine iontophoresis sweat test are negative or equivocal, especially in subjects with clinical features of CF.[1]

Limitations Current technology will detect 10-80 of the most common CF mutations, which account for 80% to 90% of the mutant alleles in the Caucasian population. Thus, a negative result does not rule out the possibility that an individual is a CF carrier but can lower that probability by a factor of 5-10. Similarly, detection of zero mutations does not completely rule out CF, but makes the diagnosis unlikely. The pitfalls in genetic analysis for CF have been reviewed by Chmiel et al.[2]

Sweat chloride analysis can provide additional information in the diagnosis of CF (see Chloride, Sweat *on page 144*), and is particularly useful when the DNA test for CF is negative.

Methodology DNA is isolated from the specimen and several regions in the *CFTR* gene are amplified using polymerase chain reaction (PCR). Mutations are detected by gel electrophoresis of amplified DNA, by restriction-enzyme digestion, or by hybridization with oligonucleotide probes specific for the mutations.

Additional Information The *CFTR* is a large gene, about 250 kilobases long, and is located on chromosome 7q31. It encodes a transmembrane protein of 1480 amino acids called the CF transmembrane conductance regulator (CFTR). This protein is a regulated chloride channel present in the epithelia of the lung, the exocrine pancreas, and sweat glands. Mutations in the *CFTR* gene can prevent proper expression of the protein, or can impair its function as a chloride channel.

The most common mutation causing CF is called ΔF508 (deltaF508), which deletes a phenylalanine (F) residue at amino acid 508. This mutation accounts for about 70% to 75% of *CFTR* mutant alleles in Caucasians, while the 10 next most common mutations account for about 10% of the *CFTR* mutant alleles. Nearly 1000 other mutations are known, most very
(Continued)

Cystic Fibrosis DNA Detection (Continued)

rare or limited to a single family. Currently available clinical test procedures focus on the 10-80 most common mutations, and thus do not detect rare or novel mutations that may be present.

In a recent study of patients with rhinosinusitis, the proportion of patients with a CF mutation was higher than in a control group. Nine of 10 CF carriers had the polymorphism M470V. M470V homozygotes were over-represented.[3]

Footnotes

1. Hilman BC and Constantinesco M, "Role of DNA Testing in Cystic Fibrosis," *Lab Med*, 1999, 30(1):48-55.
2. Chmiel JF, Drumm ML, Konstan MW, et al, "Pitfall in the Use of Genotype Analysis as the Sole Diagnostic Criterion for Cystic Fibrosis," *Pediatrics*, 1999, 103(4 Pt 1):823-6.
3. Wang XJ, Moylan B, Leopold DA, et al, "Mutation in the Gene Responsible for Cystic Fibrosis and Predisposition to Chronic Rhinosinusitis in the General Population," *JAMA*, 2000, 284(14):1814-9.

References

Chillon M, Casals T, Mercier B, et al, "Mutations in the Cystic Fibrosis Gene in Patients With Congenital Absence of the Vas Deferens," *N Engl J Med*, 1995, 332(22):1475-80.

Cohn JA, Friedman KJ, Noone PG, et al, "Relation Between Mutations of the Cystic Fibrosis Gene and Idiopathic Pancreatitis," *N Engl J Med*, 1998, 339(10):653-8.

Cystic Fibrosis Foundation, *Clinical Practice Guidelines for Cystic Fibrosis*, Bethesda, MD, 1997.

Durie PR, "Pancreatitis and Mutations of the Cystic Fibrosis Gene," *N Engl J Med*, 1998, 339(10):687-8.

Estivill X, Bancells C, and Ramos C, "Geographic Distribution and Regional Origin of 272 Cystic Fibrosis Mutations in European Populations. The Biomed CF Mutation Analysis Consortium," *Hum Mutat*, 1997, 10(2):135-54.

Mickle JE and Cutting GR, "Clinical Implications of Cystic Fibrosis Transmembrane Conductance Regulator Mutations," *Clin Chest Med*, 1998, 19(3):443-58.

Riordan JR, Rommens JM, Kerem B, et al, "Identification of the Cystic Fibrosis Gene: Cloning and Characterization of Complementary DNA," *Science*, 1989, 245(4922):1066-73.

Schwartz MJ. "DNA Diagnosis of Cystic Fibrosis," *Ann Clin Biochem*, 1998, 35:584-610.

Sharer N, Schwarz M, Malone G, et al, "Mutations of the Cystic Fibrosis Gene in Patients With Chronic Pancreatitis," *N Engl J Med*, 1998, 339(10):645-52.

Slotnick RN and Abuhamad AZ, "Prognostic Implications of Fetal Echogenic Bowel," *Lancet*, 1996, 347(8994):85-7.

Stern RC, "The Diagnosis of Cystic Fibrosis," *N Engl J Med*, 1997, 336(7):487-91.

Zielenski J, Rozmahel R, Bozon D, et al, "Genomic DNA Sequence of the Cystic Fibrosis Transmembrane Conductance Regulator (CFTR) Gene," *Genomics*, 1991, 10:214-28.

Zielenski J and Tsui LC, "Cystic Fibrosis: Genotypic and Phenotypic Variations," *Annu Rev Genet*, 1995, 29:777-807.

Internet Web Sites

www.genet.sickkids.on.ca/cftr/

odp.od.nih.gov/consensus/cons/106/106_statement.htm

◆ **Cystic Fibrosis, Prenatal Diagnosis** *see* Cystic Fibrosis DNA Detection *on page 705*

◆ **Cystic Fibrosis Transmembrane Conductance Regulator** *see* Cystic Fibrosis DNA Detection *on page 705*

◆ **Delta F508** *see* Cystic Fibrosis DNA Detection *on page 705*

◆ **DM1 Gene Mutation Analysis** *see* Myotonic Dystrophy DNA Test *on page 712*

◆ **DNA Amplification** *see* Polymerase Chain Reaction *on page 713*

◆ **DNA Analysis for Parentage Evaluation** *see* Identification DNA Testing *on page 711*

DNA Banking

Related Information

Polymerase Chain Reaction *on page 713*

Synonyms DNA Storage

Test Includes Isolation and storage of DNA specimens for future diagnostic testing

Abstract Understanding of the molecular basis of disease is proceeding at a rapid rate, and will continue to progress at an even faster rate in the future with the success of the Human Genome Project. Advances expected from this project include an increase in diagnostic tests for inherited diseases and further characterization of genetic abnormalities associated with neoplasms. Such information may also elucidate the influence of the environment on genetic material. Thus, the storage of DNA from individuals or tumors will be invaluable both to scientists and to individuals interested in their family history of disease. Presently, DNA applications are increasingly being used in the forensic field as well. Several states in the U.S. have policies in place for collection and storage of DNA from convicted offenders.

Specimen Whole blood, tissue, cultured cells, buccal swabs, hair follicles, blood spots

Container Blood should be collected in yellow top (ACD) or lavender top (EDTA) tubes; tissue should be frozen at -70°C; amniotic cells, fibroblasts, or lymphocytes should be grown in appropriate media in T25 tissue culture flasks. As DNA diagnostic techniques have become very sensitive, buccal swabs, hair follicles and blood spots on filter paper have become acceptable samples for DNA banking.

Collection 5-10 mL of blood should be collected. 0.1-1 g specimen should be obtained, which should then be put into a sealable plastic freezer bag and frozen at -70°C. It should be kept frozen until shipped to the laboratory. Cell cultures should be grown to confluency and tightly sealed before shipping. Buccal cells are collected on cotton swabs and smeared onto glass slides and dried. Blood can be spotted onto filter paper and dried before shipping to the laboratory.

Storage Instructions Store tissue at -70°C or on dry ice. Samples can be stored at -70°C for an unlimited amount of time. Peripheral blood should be stored and shipped at 4°C. Do **not** freeze blood.

Causes for Rejection Thawing of the tissue specimen during transport to the laboratory or before shipping

Use The storage of DNA isolated from individuals provides purified genetic material that can be used either for identification or for future diagnostic testing.

Limitations Inappropriate shipping or processing

Methodology DNA is released and isolated from white blood cells, tissue, or cultured cells by lysing the cells and extracting the cell lysate with phenol and chloroform. Purified, intact DNA is precipitated with salt in the presence of alcohol. Other methods of DNA purification are also available. The DNA is then stored indefinitely at -70°C, usually at two separate facilities. Buccal cells, hair follicles, and blood spots are stored without DNA extraction and can be directly used for polymerase chain reaction (PCR).

Additional Information There has been remarkable progress recently in the field of diagnostic molecular biology. The new tests currently being developed will analyze DNA for the diagnosis of genetic diseases and may facilitate the genetic testing of future generations. This enables individuals to have access to their genetic heritage, which could be crucial to future family testing. Some of the other tests being developed will be used to diagnose certain cancers and metabolic diseases; thus, it can sometimes be prudent to bank DNA from certain unusual neoplasms. Tissue from such tumors can be used to isolate DNA that can be stored for years at -70°C, permitting investigation of the genetics of such neoplasms in the future. Stored DNA is always the property of the person from whom it was isolated. When family testing for either a genetic disease or tumor characterization is desired, signed permission is usually required before the sample is released. If the person owning the DNA is deceased, then its disposition is under the control of a legal guardian or heir. All information received from DNA tests performed on any DNA sample is completely confidential and is released only to the individual requesting the test (through an appropriate medical professional). Anonymous genetic testing at academic institutions is a common practice.

References

Butler D, "Tensions Grow Over Access to DNA Bank," *Nature*, 1998, 391(6669):727.

Farkas DH, Kaul KL, Wiedbrauk DL, et al, "Specimen Collection and Storage for Diagnostic Molecular Pathology Investigation," *Arch Pathol Lab Med*, 1996, 120(6):591-6.

Harty LC, Garcia-Closas M, Rothman N, et al, "Collection of Buccal Cell DNA Using Treated Cards," *Cancer Epidemiol Biomarkers Prev*, 2000, 9(5):501-6.

Knoppers BM, Hirtle M, Lormeau S, et al, "Control of DNA Samples and Information," *Genomics*, 1998, 50(3):385-401.

McEwen JE, "Forensic DNA Data Banking by State Crime Laboratories," *Am J Hum Genet*, 1995, 56(6):1487-92.

McEwen JE and Reilly PR, "A Survey of DNA Diagnostic Laboratories Regarding DNA Banking," *Am J Hum Genet*, 1995, 56(6):1477-86.

McQueen MJ, "Ethical and Legal Issues in the Procurement, Storage and Use of DNA," *Clin Chem Lab Med*, 1998, 36(8):545-9.

Polesky HF, "Impact of Molecular (DNA) Testing on Determination of Parentage," *Arch Pathol Lab Med*, 1999, 123(11):1060-2.

Steinberg KK, Sanderlin KC, Ou CY, et al, "DNA Banking in Epidemiologic Studies," *Epidemiol Rev*, 1997, 19(1):156-62.

◆ **DNA Fingerprinting** *see* Identification DNA Testing *on page 711*

◆ **DNA Storage** *see* DNA Banking *on page 706*

◆ **DNA Testing** *see* Identification DNA Testing *on page 711*

◆ **Duchenne/Becker Muscular Dystrophy Carrier Detection** *see* Duchenne/Becker Muscular Dystrophy DNA Detection *on page 706*

Duchenne/Becker Muscular Dystrophy DNA Detection

Related Information

Aldolase, Plasma or Serum *on page 89*

Alpha$_1$-Fetoprotein, Amniotic Fluid *on page 96*

Amniotic Fluid, Chromosome and Genetic Abnormality Analysis *on page 360*

Chorionic Villus Sampling, Chromosome and Genetic Abnormality Analysis *on page 361*

Creatine Kinase, Serum *on page 158*

Muscle Biopsy *on page 69*

Myotonic Dystrophy DNA Test *on page 712*

Polymerase Chain Reaction *on page 713*

Synonyms Duchenne/Becker Muscular Dystrophy Carrier Detection; Duchenne/Becker Muscular Dystrophy, Prenatal Diagnosis; Genetic Detection of Duchenne/Becker Muscular Dystrophy; Molecular Diagnosis of Duchenne/Becker Muscular Dystrophy; Mutation Test for Duchenne/Becker Muscular Dystrophy

Applies to Dystrophin

Abstract Duchenne and Becker progressive muscular dystrophies are X-linked recessive disorders caused by mutations in the dystrophin gene.[1] Most of the cases are familial but sporadic cases are seen. The dystrophin gene has been located on Xp21.3-p21.2. In a majority of the cases, diagnosis can be made by molecular testing without muscle biopsy. The remaining cases are diagnosed by clinical findings, family history, serum creatine kinase concentration, and muscle biopsy. Duchenne muscular dystrophy (DMD) progresses more rapidly than Becker muscular dystrophy (BMD). Approximately 70% of males with DMD and 85% of males with BMD have deletions or duplications of one or more exons of the dystrophin gene.

Patient Preparation Consultation with a medical geneticist is desirable.

Specimen Whole blood, amniotic fluid, chorionic villus

Container Blood should be collected in yellow top (ACD) Vacutainer® tubes, blood collected in lavender top (EDTA) Vacutainer® tubes is also acceptable; amniotic fluid and chorionic villus should be collected in a sterile manner and transferred to a sterile tube for transport or to a T25 culture flask.

Sampling Time Amniotic fluid should be collected between the 14th and 17th week of pregnancy. Chorionic villus specimens should be dissected free of maternal tissue and blood clot. Transport medium is needed.

Storage Instructions All specimens should be sent to the laboratory immediately after collection, preferably by overnight delivery. All specimens should be kept at room temperature or refrigerated, never frozen.

Causes for Rejection Amniotic fluid specimens that are bloody may be unsuitable.

Turnaround Time Approximately 1 week

Special Instructions A complete family pedigree and clinical information are needed. Prior testing of family members is usually necessary for prenatal testing.

Reference Interval An interpretive report which includes a risk analysis is usually provided.

Use This test is indicated for patients and families with history of Duchenne or Becker muscular dystrophy. This test is also indicated for prenatal diagnosis in females known to be carriers. It is helpful for diagnosis of neonates suspected of Duchenne or Becker muscular dystrophy.

Limitations DNA analysis for Duchenne or Becker muscular dystrophy can only detect ~80% of the abnormalities responsible for the disease. Thus, a negative result does not rule out the possibility that an individual is a muscular dystrophy carrier or affected, but can lower that probability. Gonadal mosaicism occurs in about 10% of cases.

Methodology DNA is isolated from the specimen and several regions within the dystrophin gene are detected, using Southern blotting techniques. The DNA in each exon can be examined. Because of the large size of the gene, several different Southern blots are required. Multiplex polymerase chain reaction (PCR) is used to detect many of the most common deletions. Several of the DNA regions can be amplified in the same PCR and a change (either loss or varied mobility) in the DNA fragments indicates an abnormality. Such changes can be detected visually after gel electrophoresis and staining DNA with ethidium bromide. Examinations of 18 exons in this way detects up to 98% of the deletions identifiable by cDNA hybridization.[2] In affected families in which there is no detectable deletion, linkage analysis can be done using Southern blotting to detect linkage to several known mutations. Capillary electrophoresis for carrier status identification has been described.[3]

Additional Information Duchenne muscular dystrophy, the most common of the childhood dystrophies, is the most severe type of progressive primary muscular degeneration. A crippling muscle disorder, it is associated with an abnormality in band 1 of region 2 of the short arm on the X chromosome, a locus designated Xp21.3-p21.2. In most cases, it is clinically evident by 5 years and wheelchair dependency occurs before 13 years of age. The mean age of diagnosis is 4 years 10 months.[4,5] CK is very high during its early phase. Cardiac involvement leads to ECG abnormalities; heart failure and arrhythmias may occur. Cardiomyopathy may be severe.[1] Some degree of nonprogressive cognitive impairment is common in children with DMD.[6]

Becker muscular dystrophy is a milder form with a similar clinical course, as of Duchenne muscular dystrophy, but followed at a much slower rate.

Wheelchair dependency, if present, occurs after 16 years of age. Preservation of neck flexor muscle strength in BMD differentiates from DMD. Despite milder skeletal involvement, heart failure is a common cause of morbidity and mortality.[7] Signs and symptoms in carriers of DMD and BMD are shown in the previous table. A complete cardiac evaluation is recommended at least once in all carriers.[8] CK bears a less marked increase in BMD as compared to DMD.

The gene responsible for these disorders has been cloned and the protein product has been identified as the dystrophin protein, a muscle cytoskeletal protein. This protein was found to be 427 kilodalton (kDa). The gene spans 2-4 mb of DNA and is comprised of 79 exons. It has at least four promoters. It is the largest known human gene.

When deletion is not identified, linkage analysis is usually successful in provision of risk assessment. In cases with a positive family history but with no detectable mutation, a more intensive search using restriction fragment length polymorphism (RFLP)-linkage analysis can be done to determine the existence of known point mutations or alterations not detected by the other assay. This requires the participation of several family members, both affected and unaffected, to correlate the inheritance pattern of the RFLPs with inheritance of disease.[9]

Muscle biopsy with dystrophin analysis may be needed in selected patients.[10]

Footnotes

1. Oldfors A, Eriksson BO, Kyllerman M, et al, "Dilated Cardiomyopathy and the Dystrophin Gene: An Illustrated Review," *Br Heart J*, 1994, 72(4):344-8.
2. Beggs AH, Koenig M, Boyce FM, et al, "Detection of 98% of DMD/BMD Gene Deletions by Polymerase Chain Reaction," *Hum Genet*, 1990, 86(1):45-8.
3. Fortina P, Cheng J, Shoffner MA, et al, "Diagnosis of Duchenne/Becker Muscular Dystrophy and Quantitative Identification of Carrier Status by Use of Entangled Solution Capillary Electrophoresis," *Clin Chem*, 1997, 43(5):745-51.
4. Bushby KM, "The Limb-Girdle Muscular Dystrophies - Multiple Genes, Multiple Mechanisms," *Hum Mol Genet*, 1999, 8(10):1875-82.
5. Zaludek I, Bonelli RM, Koltringer P, et al, "Early Diagnosis in Duchenne Muscular Dystrophy," *Lancet*, 1999, 353(9168):1975.
6. Moizard MP, Billard C, Toutain A, et al, "Are Dp71 and Dp140 Brain Dystrophin Isoforms Related to Cognitive Impairment in Duchenne Muscular Dystrophy?" *Am J Med Genet*, 1998, 80(1):32-41.
7. Cox GF and Kunkel LM, "Dystrophies and Heart Disease," *Curr Opin Cardiol*, 1997, 12(3):329-43.
8. Hoogerwaard EM, Bakker E, Ippel PF, et al, "Signs and Symptoms of Duchenne Muscular Dystrophy and Becker Muscular Dystrophy Among Carriers in The Netherlands: A Cohort Study," *Lancet*, 1999, 353(9170):2116-9.
9. Fassati A, Tedeschi S, Bordoni A, et al, "Rapid Direct Diagnosis of Deletions Carriers of Duchenne and Becker Muscular Dystrophies," *Lancet*, 1994, 344(8918):302-3.
10. Richards S and Iannaccone ST, "Dystrophin and DNA Diagnosis in a Large Pediatric Muscle Clinic," *J Child Neurol*, 1994, 9(2):162-6.

References

Clemens PR, Fenwick RG, Chamberlain JS, et al, "Carrier Detection and Prenatal Diagnosis in Duchenne and Becker Muscular Dystrophy Families, Using Dinucleotide Repeat Polymorphisms," *Am J Hum Genet*, 1991, 49(5):951-60.

Cox GF and Kunkel LM, "Dystrophies and Heart Disease," *Curr Opin Cardiol*, 1997, 12(3):329-43.

Felisari G, Martinelli BF, Bardoni A, et al, "Loss of Dp140 Dystrophin Isoform and Intellectual Impairment in Duchenne Dystrophy," *Neurology*, 2000, 55(4):559-64.

Ferlini A, Sewry C, Melis MA, et al, "X-Linked Dilated Cardiomyopathy and the Dystophin Gene," *Neuromuscul Disord*, 1999, 9(5):339-46.

Hoogerwaard EM, van der Wouw PA, Wilde AA, et al, "Cardiac Involvement in Carriers of Duchenne and Becker Muscular Dystrophy," *Neuromuscul Disord*, 1999, 9(5):347-51.

Mansfield ES, Robertson JM, Lebo RV, et al, "Duchenne/Becker Muscular Dystrophy Carrier Detection Using Quantitative PCR and Fluorescence-Based Strategies," *Am J Med Genet*, 1993, 48(4):200-8.

Palmucci L, Mongini T, Chiado-Piat L, et al, "Dystrophinopathy Expressing as Either Cardiomyopathy or Becker Dystrophy in the Same Family," *Neurology*, 2000, 54(2):529-30.

Rininsland F and Reiss J, "Microlesions and Polymorphisms in the Duchenne/Becker Muscular Dystrophy Gene," *Hum Genet*, 1994, 94(2):111-6.

Shomrat R, Gluck E, Legum C, et al, "Relatively Low Proportion of Dystrophin Gene Deletions in Israeli Duchenne and Becker Muscular Dystrophy Patients," *Am J Med Genet*, 1994, 49(4):369-73.

Sjoberg G, Edstrom L, Lendahl U, et al, "Myofibers From Duchenne/Becker Muscular Dystrophy and Myositis Express the Intermediate Filament Nestin," *J Neuropathol Exp Neurol*, 1994, 53(4):416-23.

Yazaki M, Yoshida K, Nakamura A, et al, "Clinical Characteristics of Aged Becker Muscular Dystrophy Patients With Onset After 30 Years," *Eur Neurol*, 1999, 42(3):145-9.

Internet Web Sites

www.mdausa.org
www.muscular-dystrophy.org

◆ **Duchenne/Becker Muscular Dystrophy, Prenatal Diagnosis** see Duchenne/Becker Muscular Dystrophy DNA Detection on page 706

◆ **Dystrophia Myotonica** see Myotonic Dystrophy DNA Test on page 712

◆ **Dystrophin** see Duchenne/Becker Muscular Dystrophy DNA Detection on page 706

◆ **Episodic Ataxia Type 1** see Spinocerebellar Ataxia Type 6 DNA Test on page 716

Signs and Symptoms in Carriers of Duchenne and Becker Muscular Dystrophy

	DMD Carriers	BMD Carriers
No symptoms/signs	76%	81%
Muscle weakness*	19%	14%
Myalgia/cramps	5%	5%
Left ventricle dilation	19%	16%
Dilated cardiomyopathy	8%	0

*Mild to moderate weakness.

- **Familial Hemiplegic Migraine** *see* Spinocerebellar Ataxia Type 6 DNA Test on page 716

- **FMR1 Mutation Analysis** *see* Fragile X Syndrome DNA Test *on* page 708

- **FMRI Protein** *see* Fragile X Syndrome DNA Test *on* page 708

- **FMRP** *see* Fragile X Syndrome DNA Test *on* page 708

- **Fragile X, Carrier Detection** *see* Fragile X Syndrome DNA Test *on* page 708

- **Fragile X Mental Retardation Syndrome** *see* Fragile X Syndrome DNA Test *on* page 708

- **Fragile X Mutation Analysis** *see* Fragile X Syndrome DNA Test *on* page 708

- **Fragile X, Prenatal Diagnosis** *see* Fragile X Syndrome DNA Test *on* page 708

Fragile X Syndrome DNA Test

Related Information

Amniotic Fluid, Chromosome and Genetic Abnormality Analysis *on* page 360

Chorionic Villus Sampling, Chromosome and Genetic Abnormality Analysis *on* page 361

Chromosome Analysis, Blood *on* page 361

Polymerase Chain Reaction *on* page 713

Synonyms FMR1 Mutation Analysis; Fragile X, Carrier Detection; Fragile X Mental Retardation Syndrome; Fragile X Mutation Analysis; Fragile X, Prenatal Diagnosis; FRAXA Syndrome; Genetic Detection of Fragile X Syndrome; Martin-Bell Syndrome; Molecular Diagnosis of Fragile X Syndrome; Mutation Test for Trinucleotide Repeat Disorder, Fragile X

Applies to FMRI Protein; FMRP; FRAXE Syndrome

Test Includes Determination of the number of CGG trinucleotide repeats in the noncoding region of the FMR1 (fragile X mental retardation 1) gene and the methylation status of the FMR1 promoter region

Abstract Fragile X syndrome is the most common cause of inherited mental retardation. Recent population studies using DNA testing have provided a more accurate prevalence of 1:5000 males and about half that in females. A clinical diagnosis is often difficult. Males with fragile X syndrome have characteristics that can vary with age, including motor and speech delays, cognitive impairment, atypical craniofacial features, and certain behaviors. Affected females exhibit a similar but generally less severe phenotype.

Fragile X syndrome is inherited in an X-linked dominant fashion with reduced penetrance. The syndrome is caused by an absence or decreased amount of the protein encoded by the FMR1 (fragile X mental retardation 1) gene (chromosome locus Xq27). A diagnosis of fragile X syndrome, or of carrier status, requires a DNA test that detects two specific abnormalities of the FMR1 gene: an abnormally large number of CGG trinucleotide repeats and aberrant methylation of the promoter region. Normal FMR1 alleles have ≤45 CGG repeats with unmethylated promoter regions and produce a normal amount of fragile X protein. Normal alleles do not change when transmitted from parent to child. Abnormal full mutation FMR1 alleles have >200 CGG repeats and aberrant methylation of the promoter region, which silences the gene resulting in no protein production. All mothers of affected sons are carriers of either a full mutation or a premutation FMR1 allele. Premutation FMR1 alleles have between 45 and ~200 CGG repeats, are not methylated, and produce a sufficient amount of protein to result in a normal phenotype. Premutation FMR1 alleles do not change when transmitted by an unaffected carrier father. In contrast, premutation alleles can change to a full mutation when transmitted by an unaffected carrier mother. Therefore, premutation carrier mothers, but not fathers, are at risk of having an affected child. All sons, but only 30% to 50% of daughters, with a full mutation are affected. Unaffected daughters that are heterozygous for a full mutation presumably have skewed X inactivation ratios that permit production of sufficient FMR1 protein. Regardless of phenotype, all women carriers of full mutations are at 100% risk of having an affected son and about 50% risk of having an affected daughter.

Patient Preparation Because the genetics of fragile X syndrome are complicated, a pretest consultation with a medical geneticist is advisable, particularly for carrier and prenatal risk assessment.

Specimen Whole blood, amniotic fluid; chorionic villus samples are not optimal for this test (see Limitations)

Container Collect anticoagulated blood in either a lavender top (EDTA) tube or yellow top (ACD) Vacutainer®. Avoid use of heparin anticoagulants, which can interfere with polymerase chain reactions and endonuclease restriction enzyme activity. Amniotic fluid and chorionic villus samples should be collected in a sterile manner and transferred to a sterile tube for transport. **Note:** If a routine cytogenetic analysis is being performed simultaneously to screen for chromosomal abnormalities, an additional blood sample in sodium heparin (green top) is required (see Chromosome Analysis, Blood *on* page 361).

Sampling Time Blood samples can be taken at any time. Amniotic fluid samples should be collected at or after 16 weeks gestation. Chorionic villus samples should be collected between 8 and 12 weeks gestation.

Storage Instructions Blood samples can be stored and shipped at room temperature or refrigerated (4°C); do not freeze. Blood samples should be received in the testing laboratory within 4 days of the draw to ensure an adequate DNA yield. Amniotic fluid and chorionic villus samples should be maintained at room temperature and sent to the testing laboratory immediately after collection, preferably by overnight delivery, to ensure successful cell culture.

Causes for Rejection Frozen samples, whole blood in heparin anticoagulant (green top) or other inappropriate collection tube, amniotic fluid sample bloody, chorionic villus sample lacking viable chorionic villi

Turnaround Time 7-14 days

Reference Interval An interpretive report is usually provided that includes a risk analysis when appropriate. There are important exceptions to the reference ranges below (see Limitations). Normal FMR1 alleles have ≤45 CGG repeats. Premutation FMR1 alleles have 46-200 CGG repeats. Premutations, which do not cause fragile X syndrome but can expand to a full mutation upon transmission through the maternal germline, are generally observed in asymptomatic carrier males and females. Full mutation FMR1 alleles have both >200 CGG repeats and abnormal methylation. Full mutations are generally observed in symptomatic males and females, and also in some asymptomatic females.

Use Testing is indicated for males or females with developmental delay, autism, or mental retardation, especially if they show other features or behaviors commonly associated with fragile X syndrome and/or have a positive family history of fragile X or undiagnosed mental retardation. In addition to fragile X DNA testing, these patients should undergo a full genetic evaluation that also includes testing for chromosomal abnormalities (see Chromosome Analysis, Blood *on* page 361). Carrier testing is indicated for individuals seeking reproductive counseling with a family history of fragile X syndrome or undiagnosed mental retardation. Testing should be considered for the fetus of a mother who is a known carrier of an FMR1 premutation or full mutation. In addition, it may be appropriate to perform the DNA test for individuals that were tested previously by the less sensitive method of cytogenetic detection of a folate-sensitive fragile site at chromosome X band q27.3, particularly if the patients' phenotype is discordant with the cytogenetic testing result.

Limitations Rare cases (<1%) of fragile X syndrome that are caused by a deletion of, or point mutation in, the FMR1 gene will not be detected by this test. The number of CGG repeats in full mutation FMR1 alleles does not predict disease severity or cognitive ability. The probability that a premutation allele will expand upon transmission and result in fragile X syndrome depends upon the number of CGG repeats, gender of parent, and gender of the child. The available probability estimates should be used with caution due to the small sample size. Premutation and full mutation alleles cannot be defined solely by the number of CGG repeats, methylation status must be determined. This is because there are individuals with alleles that do not follow the usual patterns, such as alleles with $(CGG)_{45-200}$ that are methylated or alleles with $(CGG)_{>200}$ that are not methylated. In addition, some individuals are mosaic for cells with alleles that differ in CGG length and/or methylation. Some mentally retarded males with a $(CGG)_{>200}$ allele and methylation mosaicism are "high-functioning" compared to typical fragile X patients, presumably because the unmethylated alleles can produce a small amount of fragile X protein. FMR1 premutation alleles with $(CGG)_{46-55}$ are rare and are sometimes referred to as "gray zone" alleles. Such alleles do not cause fragile X syndrome, but can have a propensity for slight expansion of a few CGG repeats upon transmission; risk of expansion to a full mutation in one transmission is considered to be very low. Chorionic villus samples are not optimal for testing because methylation of the FMR1 gene may not yet be established in the tissue.

Methodology Genomic DNA is amplified by polymerase chain reaction, using primers that flank the CGG repeat region, and sized after electrophoresis (see Polymerase Chain Reaction *on* page 713). This method detects normal and premutation sized FMR1 alleles and determines the number of CGG repeats present. Both large (>150) CGG alleles and methylation status are detected by digesting the genomic DNA with EcoRI and EagI restriction endonucleases, the latter of which is sensitive to methylation status. DNA fragments are electrophoresed and transferred to a Southern membrane that is hybridized to a small fragment of the FMR1 gene. The pattern of DNA fragments reveals the methylation status of all alleles and determines the number of CGG repeats in large sized alleles. Recently, new polymerase chain reaction methods have been reported that permit detection of the methylation status of an allele; in the future this method may replace Southern blot analysis.

Additional Information The normal functions of the FMR1 protein, FMRP, are under investigation. *In vitro*, FMRP binds selective mRNA molecules and associates with ribosomes as a component of a messenger ribonucleoprotein particle. These data suggest that loss of FMRP function would be disruptive to RNA metabolism, however, the *in vivo* target mRNAs are yet to be identified. In addition to the FMR1 gene, there is another gene on the X chromosome, called FMR2, which upon expansion and methylation, can cause a rare form of mental retardation called FRAXE syndrome. DNA testing for FRAXE syndrome is available and may be an appropriate follow-up for selected FMR1-negative subjects. A listing of laboratories that perform FMR1 and/or FRAXE DNA testing can be found at GeneTests® (see Websites).

Recently, a few laboratories have begun testing for protein product of FMR1, FMRP. In some patients, assessment of FMRP has been proposed as a potential prognostic indicator of disease severity.[1]

Footnotes

1. Tassone F, Hagerman RJ, Ikle DN, et al, "FMRP Expression as a Potential Prognostic Indicator in Fragile X-Syndrome," *Am J Med Genet*, 1999, 84(3):250-61.

References

Curry CJ, Stevenson RE, Aughton D, et al, "Evaluation of Mental Retardation: Recommendations of a Consensus Conference: American College of Medical Genetics," *Am J Med Genet*, 1997, 72(4):468-77.

Jin P and Warren ST, "Understanding the Molecular Basis of Fragile X Syndrome," *Hum Mol Genet*, 2000, 9(6):901-8.

Kooy RF, Willemsen R, and Oostra BA, "Fragile X Syndrome at the Turn of the Century," *Mol Med Today*, 2000, 6(5):193-8.

Nolin SL, Lewis FA 3rd, Ye LL, et al, "Familial Transmission of the FMR1 CGG Repeat," *Am J Hum Genet*, 1996, 59(6):1252-61.

Tarleton J and Saul RA (updated 5/26/2000), "Fragile X Syndrome," *GeneClinics: Medical Genetics Knowledge Base* (database online), University of Washington, Seattle.

Wohrle D, Salat U, Glaser D, et al, "Unusual Mutations in High Functioning Fragile X Males: Apparent Instability of Expanded Unmethylated CGG Repeats," *J Med Genet*, 1998, 35(2):103-11.

Internet Web Sites

www.genetests.org

www.geneclinics.org/profiles/fragilex

Hereditary Hemochromatosis DNA Test

Related Information

Synonyms Hemochromatosis, C282Y/Cys282Tyr Mutation; Hemochromatosis, DNA Testing; Hemochromatosis, H63D/His63Asp Mutation; Hemochromatosis, S65C/Ser63 Cys Mutation; *HFE* Genotyping

Applies to *HFE* gene

Test Includes Detection of the two most common mutations in the *HFE* gene, C282Y (nucleotide 845G→A) and H63D (nucleotide 187C→G)

Abstract Hereditary hemochromatosis (HH) is an autosomal recessive disease that is very common among people of European ethnicity. Among Caucasians, about 1 in 400 has the disease and about 1 in 10 is a carrier. DNA-based testing can diagnose hemochromatosis in people with persistently elevated serum transferrin-iron saturation values. Testing is also useful in the differential diagnosis of liver diseases with increased iron loading and for evaluating at-risk relatives in families with hemochromatosis. In northern European patients with a diagnosis of hereditary hemochromatosis, about 80% to 90% have two copies of a mutation in the HLA-linked *HFE* gene referred to as C282Y. A second mutation, H63D, occurs in a smaller percentage of these patients (40% to 70% of non-C282Y cases of HH) and is associated with a much lower penetrance (likelihood of developing clinical disease). Since the C282Y mutation is very uncommon in Asian and African populations, this test is less useful in people from those ethnic backgrounds.

The classical signs of hemochromatosis include the triad of cirrhosis, diabetes mellitus and skin bronzing. It is now recognized that these late manifestations are preventable with early recognition and treatment.[1]

Specimen 3-10 mL whole blood

Container Lavender top (EDTA) tube or yellow top (ACD) tube; avoid tubes containing heparin anticoagulants, which interfere with polymerase chain reaction analysis

Sampling Time Blood samples can be collected at any time.

Storage Instructions Store samples refrigerated or at room temperature. Do not freeze. Blood samples should normally be received in the testing laboratory within 4 days of collection to ensure adequate yield of DNA.

Turnaround Time 7-14 days

Special Instructions Providing the following information helps the laboratory provide an interpretive report: clinical diagnosis; ethnic background (Caucasian, Asian, African, etc); relevant laboratory values: serum iron, TIBC, and ferritin; presence or absence of a family history of hemochromatosis; presence or absence of a history of therapeutic phlebotomy.

Reference Interval

- Normal: absence of any detectable mutations
- Carrier status: detection of a single mutation
- Hereditary hemochromatosis or a genetic predisposition to develop the disease: detection of two mutations

Use Indications for testing include:

Evaluation of suspected hemochromatosis: When asymptomatic patients have persistently elevated values for transferrin-iron saturation on two separate fasting blood samples, they should be evaluated further for possible hereditary hemochromatosis. Patients with clinical signs or symptoms suggesting hemochromatosis should also be evaluated. Molecular-genetic testing is being used increasingly for diagnostic purposes; detection of two mutant alleles will confirm the diagnosis in the setting of elevated biochemical iron measurements. Liver biopsy is still appropriate as a diagnostic test for patients who lack two *HFE* mutations, and is also useful for prognosis in patients who have already developed liver disease.

Testing at-risk relatives in families known to carry mutant alleles in the *HFE* gene: It is generally appropriate to evaluate first-degree and other relatives of an index case to determine if they are also at risk for the disease.[2] Usually, siblings have a 1 in 4 risk of having the disease, while Caucasian parents and offspring usually have a 1 in 20 chance of being affected. Early detection and treatment of the disease by therapeutic phlebotomy can prevent development of significant organ damage.

Differential diagnosis of liver diseases with increased iron loading: Genetic testing can be useful in ruling out hereditary hemochromatosis as a causative factor in patients with cirrhosis who have other risk factors such as alcohol abuse or chronic viral hepatitis.

Limitations Expression of C282Y/C282Y homozygosity is not invariable; individuals have been reported who are homozygous for this mutation who fail to meet clinical criteria for the diagnosis of hereditary hemochromatosis. Hepatic fibrosis is not usually found before age 40 without a cofactor, eg, excessive ethanol consumption or hepatitis C infection. Age and phenotypic expression are relevant.[3,4]

The penetrance of the H63D allele is much less than that of the C282Y allele. No more than 2% of people with a C282Y/H63D or H63D/H63D genotype develop clinically significant iron overload. Thus, most asymptomatic patients with these genotypes may only require periodic monitoring of serum ferritin every few years, and few will require therapeutic phlebotomy.

All homozygotes for the major hemochromatosis mutation are not detected by screening for transferrin saturation and ferritin concentrations.[1]

This test is not useful for the diagnosis of neonatal or juvenile hemochromatosis, which are due to mutations in different genes.

Methodology DNA from portions of the *HFE* gene is amplified by polymerase chain reaction (PCR). Mutations are detected by restriction-enzyme digestion or by hybridization with oligonucleotide probes specific for the mutations. Analysis by automated capillary electrophoresis is described.[5]

Additional Information The *HFE* gene is located in the HLA cluster on chromosome 6p21. It encodes a cell-surface protein of 321 amino acids that has structural similarity to HLA class I molecules. The normal protein forms a heterodimer with β-2-microglobulin; this heterodimer interacts with the transferrin receptor and may modulate its affinity for transferrin. The C282Y (Continued)

Hereditary Hemochromatosis DNA Test (Continued)

mutation disrupts an important disulfide bond in the *HFE* protein, and thereby prevents expression of the protein on the cell surface.

Other conditions relating to hemochromatosis include increased ALT and AST without other identifiable cause, hemochromatotic arthropathy,[2] cardiomyopathy, hyperpigmentation (bronzing), hypothyroidism, testicular atrophy and abnormalities of the anterior pituitary and pancreas.

Non-HFE-related iron overload conditions include juvenile hemochromatosis (see above), African iron overload, iron overload in African-Americans, aceruloplasminemia, and Hallervorden-Spatz disease (a degenerative neurologic disorder).[6]

Footnotes

1. Beutler E, Felitti V, Gelbart T, et al, "The Effect of *HFE* Genotypes on Measurements of Iron Overload in Patients Attending a Health Appraisal Clinic," *Ann Intern Med*, 2000, 133(5):329-37.
2. Bulaj ZJ, Ajioka RS, Phillips J, et al, "Disease-Related Conditions in Relatives of Patients With Hemochromatosis," *N Engl J Med*, 2000, 343(21):1529-35.
3. Tavill AS, "Clinical Implications of the Hemochromatosis Gene," *N Engl J Med*, 1999, 341(10):755-6.
4. Olynyk JK, Cullen DJ, and Aquilia S, "A Population-Based Study of the Clinical Expression of the Hemochromatosis Gene," *N Engl J Med*, 1999, 341(10):718-24.
5. Lubin IM, Yamada NA, Stansel RM, et al, "*HFE* Genotyping Using Multiplex Allele-Specific Polymerase Chain Reaction and Capillary Electrophoresis," *Arch Pathol Lab Med*, 1999, 123(12):1177-81.
6. Andrews NC, "Iron Metabolism: Iron Deficiency and Iron Overload," *Annual Review of Genomics and Human Genetics*, Volume 1, Palo Alto, CA: Annual Reviews, 2000, 75.

References

Adams PC and Valberg LS, "Screening Blood Donors for Hereditary Hemochromatosis: Decision Analysis Model Comparing Genotyping to Phenotyping," *Am J Gastroenterol*, 1999, 94(6):1593-1600.

Bacon BR, Olynyk JK, Brunt EM, et al, "*HFE* Genotype in Patients With Hemochromatosis and Other Liver Diseases," *Ann Intern Med*, 1999, 130(12):953-62.

Beutler E, Gelbart T, West C, et al, "Mutation Analysis in Hereditary Hemochromatosis," *Blood Cells Mol Dis*, 1996, 22(2):187-94.

Brandhagen DJ, Fairbanks VF, Batts KP, et al, "Update on Hereditary Hemochromatosis and the *HFE* Gene," *Mayo Clin Proc*, 1999, 74(9):917-21.

Bulaj ZJ, Griffen LM, Jorde LB, et al, "Clinical and Biochemical Abnormalities in People Heterozygous for Hemochromatosis," *N Engl J Med*, 1996, 335(24):1799-805.

Cullen LM, Anderson GJ, Ramm GA, et al, "Genetics of Hemochromatosis," *Annu Rev Med*, 1999, 50:87-98.

El-Serag HB, Inadomi JM, and Kowdley KV, "Screening for Hereditary Hemochromatosis in Siblings and Children of Affected Patients," *Ann Intern Med*, 2000, 132(4):261-9.

Feder JN, Gnirke A, Thomas W, et al, "A Novel MHC Class I-Like Gene Is Mutated in Patients With Hereditary Haemochromatosis," *Nat Genet*, 1996, 13(4):399-408.

Franks AL and Burke W, "Will the Real Hemochromatosis Please Stand Up?" *Ann Intern Med*, 1999, 130(12):1018-9.

Klein J and Sato A, "The HLA System," Mackay I and Rosen FS, eds, *N Engl J Med*, 2000, 343(11):782-6.

Mura C Raguenes O, and Férec C, "*HFE* Mutations Analysis in 711 Hemochromatosis Probands: Evidence for S65C Implication in Mild Form of Hemochromatosis," *Blood*, 1999, 93(8):2502-5.

Pietrangelo A, Montosi G, Totaro A, et al, "Hereditary Hemochromatosis in Adults Without Pathogenic Mutations in the Hemochromatosis Gene," *N Engl J Med*, 1999, 341(10):725-32.

Pirisi M, Scott CA, Avellini C, et al, "Iron Deposition and Progression of Disease in Chronic Hepatitis C," *Am J Clin Pathol*, 2000, 113(4):546-54.

Press RD, Flora K, Gross C, et al, "Hepatic Iron Overload: Direct *HFE* (HLA-H) Mutation Analysis Versus Quantitative Iron Assays for the Diagnosis of Hereditary Hemochromatosis," *Am J Clin Pathol*, 1998, 109(5):577-84.

Ramrakhiani S and Bacon BR, "Hemochromatosis: Advances in Molecular Genetics and Clinical Diagnosis," *J Clin Gastroenterol*, 1998, 27(1):41-6.

Snover DC, "Hepatitis C, Iron, and Hemochromatosis Gene Mutations," *Am J Clin Pathol*, 2000, 113(4):475-8.

Witte DL, Crosby WH, Edwards CQ, et al, "Practice Guideline Development Task Force of the College of American Pathologists. Hereditary Hemochromatosis," *Clin Chim Acta*, 1996, 245(2):139-200.

Internet Web Sites

www.geneclinics.org/profiles/hemochromatosis/

♦ **HFE gene** see Hereditary Hemochromatosis DNA Test on page 709

♦ **HFE Genotyping** see Hereditary Hemochromatosis DNA Test on page 709

♦ **Huntingtin** see Huntington Disease DNA Test on page 710

♦ **Huntington Disease 2 DNA Test** see Huntington Disease DNA Test on page 710

Huntington Disease DNA Test

Related Information

Polymerase Chain Reaction on page 713

Synonyms Genetic Detection of HD; HD DNA Test; HD Gene Mutation Analysis; Huntingtin; Huntington Disease 2 DNA Test; Molecular Diagnosis of Huntington Disease; Mutation Test for Trinucleotide Repeat Disorder

Test Includes Determination of the number of CAG trinucleotide repeats in the HD (alias IT-15) gene at chromosome 4 band p16.

Abstract Huntington disease is a progressive disorder of the central nervous system characterized primarily by motor, cognitive, and psychiatric disturbances. HD is commonly an adult disease with the average onset from 35-44 years of age. Severe disease, however, has been reported in juveniles who present with marked rigidity, intellectual decline, and prominent motor and cerebellar symptoms.[1,2] Affected, or genetically predisposed, individuals typically have one normal HD allele and one mutant allele. In all cases, the mutant allele has an abnormally large number of a naturally-occurring CAG trinucleotide repeat motif in the HD gene. The DNA test detects 100% of cases by measuring the number of CAG repeats in each HD allele. The number of CAG repeats is polymorphic in the normal population but is always ≤26; normal alleles are stable and show no changes in CAG repeat number upon transmission to offspring. The presence of ≥40 CAG repeats indicates that an individual has, or is genetically predisposed to develop, Huntington disease. Mutant alleles with ≥40 CAG repeats are often unstable upon transmission, with offspring having an increased or decreased number of repeats; increases are more common with paternal transmission. Nearly all cases of juvenile HD are associated with paternal transmission. In patient population studies, a greater number of CAG repeats is generally correlated with an earlier age at onset and more severe disease. This explains why, in some families, the disease appears to be more severe in affected individuals of the most recent generation. However, because the age at onset, progression, and severity is variable, the number of CAG repeats cannot reliably predict the clinical course of the disease in an individual case. HD is an autosomal dominant disorder; each child of an affected, or asymptomatic individual carrying a mutant HD allele, has a 50% chance of inheriting the mutant gene.

Patient Preparation Testing of asymptomatic at-risk adults is predictive testing and the patient should have formal genetic counseling to explain the meaning, benefits, and risks of testing.

Aftercare For asymptomatic at-risk adults, post-test genetic counseling is appropriate to explain the test result and its significance.

Specimen Whole blood (3-10 mL)

Container Collect anticoagulated blood in either a lavender top (EDTA) tube or yellow top (ACD) Vacutainer® tube. Avoid use of heparin anticoagulants, which can interfere with polymerase chain reactions and endonuclease restriction enzyme activity.

Storage Instructions Blood samples can be stored and shipped at room temperature or refrigerated (4°C); do not freeze. Blood samples should be received in the testing laboratory within 4 days of draw to ensure an adequate DNA yield.

Causes for Rejection Frozen samples, whole blood in heparin anticoagulant (green top) or other inappropriate collection tube

Turnaround Time 7-14 days

Special Instructions To provide an optimal test interpretation, the testing laboratory needs to know the clinical diagnosis, family history, and whether DNA testing has confirmed the clinical diagnosis of an affected family member.

Reference Interval Normal HD alleles have <26 CAG repeats. Affected individuals have ≥40 CAG repeats. An asymptomatic adult with an HD allele with ≥40 CAG repeats is predicted to develop Huntington disease. Alleles with between 27-35 CAG repeats do not cause disease in the carrier individual, but these alleles can be unstable with the CAG repeats increasing in number to the abnormal pathogenic range upon transmission to offspring.[3] Alleles with between 36 and 39 CAG repeats show reduced penetrance and may or may not cause Huntington disease. Juvenile HD cases typically have about 80-250 CAG repeats.[1,2]

Use Testing is useful to rule out or confirm a clinical diagnosis in individuals with progressive motor disability, cognitive decline, or personality changes, particularly if there is a positive family history of such manifestations. Testing of asymptomatic adults at-risk for Huntington disease should be preceded by formal genetic counseling to explain the meaning, benefits, and risks of testing. Testing can be used to identify which progenitor in a family carries the HD mutation; this is important information for genetic counseling and the identification of other at-risk family members. Consensus holds that testing of asymptomatic at-risk children under the legal age, for an adult onset disorder for which no treatment exists, is not appropriate.[4] The reasons should be discussed and explained in detail during formal genetic counseling to parents requesting testing of asymptomatic at-risk children. Children who present with symptoms usually benefit from having a specific diagnosis established. Prenatal testing is available, but should be preceded by formal genetic counseling to discuss difficult ethical issues related to testing for a (typically) adult-onset disease.

Limitations The number of CAG repeats cannot reliably predict disease onset, severity, or cognitive ability in an individual patient. In cases with juvenile onset with typically larger numbers of CAG repeats, it is more difficult for the testing laboratory to detect the large mutant allele. In these cases, concerns about allele size detection should be discussed with the testing laboratory, especially when only a single sized allele is observed in an affected child (ie, an apparent HD homozygote).

Methodology Polymerase chain reaction (PCR). A segment of the HD gene is amplified from the patient's DNA, using primers that flank the CAG repeat region of the gene. After electrophoresis, the number of repeats is calculated from the product size. This reaction can detect both normal and mutant HD alleles.

Additional Information Huntington disease has a prevalence of about 5 per 100,000 in populations of Western European descent; frequencies vary by geography and ethnic background. The normal function of huntingtin, the protein product of the HD gene, is not known. The CAG trinucleotide repeat motif is located in the coding region of the gene and encodes a tract of polyglutamine residues. Abnormally long polyglutamine tracts confer an unknown new function to huntingtin; how this "gain-of-function" causes the disease is not clear. HD testing is widely available; a list of clinical laboratories that perform this test can be found at GeneTests® (http://www.genetests.org).

Footnotes

1. Telenius H, Kremer HP, Theilmann J, et al, "Molecular Analysis of Juvenile Huntington Disease: The Major Influence on (CAG)n Repeat Length Is the Sex of the Affected Parent," *Hum Mol Genet*, 1993, 2(10):1535-40.
2. Nance MA, Mathias-Hagen V, Breningstall G, et al, "Analysis of a Very Large Trinucleotide Repeat in a Patient With Juvenile Huntington's Disease," *Neurology*, 1999, 52(2):392-4.
3. "The American College of Medical Genetics/American Society of Human Genetics Huntington Disease Genetic Testing Working Group. ACMG/ASHG Statement. Laboratory Guidelines for Huntington Disease Genetic Testing," *Am J Hum Genet*, 1998, 62:1243-7.
4. "American Society of Human Genetics Board of Directors, American College of Medical Genetics Board of Directors. Points to Consider: Ethical, Legal, and Psychological Implications of Genetic Testing in Children and Adolescents," *Am J Hum Genet*, 1995, 57:1233-41.

References

Andrew SE, Goldberg YP, Kremer B, et al, "The Relationship Between Trinucleotide (CAG) Repeat Length and Clinical Features of Huntington's Disease," *Nat Genet*, 1993, 4(4):398-403.

Brandt J, Bylsma FW, Gross R, et al, "Trinucleotide Repeat Length and Clinical Progression in Huntington's Disease," *Neurology*, 1996, 46(2):527-31.

Huq AHMM and Hayden MR, "Huntington Disease," GeneClinics: Medical Genetics Knowledge Base, updated September 30, 1998, available at: http://www.geneclinics.org/profiles/huntington/details.html.

Kremer B, Goldberg P, Andrew SE, et al, "A Worldwide Study of the Huntington's Disease Mutation. The Sensitivity and Specificity of Measuring CAG Repeats," *N Engl J Med*, 1994, 330(20):1401-6.

Nance MA, "Huntington Disease: Clinical, Genetic, and Social Aspects," *J Geriatr Psychiatry Neurol*, 1998, 11(2):61-70

Snell RG, MacMillan JC, Cheadle JP, et al, "Relationship Between Trinucleotide Repeat Expansion and Phenotypic Variation in Huntington's Disease," *Nat Genet*, 1993, 4(4):393-7.

Internet Web Sites

www.genetests.org

Identification DNA Testing

Related Information

Chain-of-Custody Protocol *on page 785*
HLA Typing, Single Human Leukocyte Antigen *on page 529*
Polymerase Chain Reaction *on page 713*
Tissue Typing *on page 546*

Synonyms DNA Analysis for Parentage Evaluation; DNA Fingerprinting; DNA Testing; Genetic Identification by DNA Fingerprinting; Paternity Testing by DNA Testing; RFLP Analysis for Parentage Evaluation

Test Includes Identification of individuals by using DNA polymorphic regions

Abstract The progress in the field of DNA technology and Human Genome Project has resulted in tremendous knowledge about the genetic material that makes each individual unique. The human genome is made up of about 120 million base pairs organized into 46 different chromosomes. The DNA from both maternal and paternal sources may be normal, but will have slight variations in character. These variations can be detected and used to map heredity much like the variations in blood group antigens and the human leukocyte antigen (HLA) system. By using between 20-30 different polymorphic sites on different chromosomes, identity or parentage can be established with up to 99.99% exclusion probability. Other DNA identification applications include identification of suspects in forensic cases, and origin and migration history of modern humans.

Patient Preparation Patient should receive no transfusions 90 days prior to testing.

Specimen Peripheral whole blood, tissue, amniotic fluid, semen, or cultured cells; dried blood, hair and skin scrapings are frequently used in forensic cases.

Collection Blood should be collected in a yellow top (ACD) tube or lavender top (EDTA) tube; tissue should be frozen at -70°C; amniotic cells, fibroblasts, or lymphocytes should be grown in appropriate media in T25 tissue culture flasks. Collection in heparin tubes should be avoided as heparin interferes in polymerase chain reaction. Dried blood, hair and skin scrapings are collected in a plastic sealable bag.

Storage Instructions Store tissue at -70°C or on dry ice. Peripheral blood should be stored and shipped at 4°C. Do **not** freeze blood. Dried blood, hair and skin scraping can be stored at room temperature.

Causes for Rejection If the tissue specimen thaws out during transport to the laboratory or before shipping, DNA may not be obtained from the specimen. Blood samples that have been frozen and thawed will yield low quality DNA. Specimens inadequately identified will be rejected.

Turnaround Time 2-4 weeks. Samples of DNA can be stored for an unlimited amount of time.

Reference Interval The laboratory bears an obligation to communicate results in confidence. The test provides a 99.99% exclusion probability.

Use The analysis of highly polymorphic regions of human DNA can clarify the relationships between individuals and verify the identity of unknown individuals (such as suspects in criminal investigations or unidentified victims of murder).

Limitations Failure to obtain DNA from the blood, tissue, or cultured cells due to inappropriate shipping or processing

Methodology DNA is released and isolated from the white blood cells, tissue, or cultured cells by lysing the cells and extracting the cell lysate with phenol and chloroform. Purified, intact DNA is precipitated with salt in the presence of alcohol. The DNA is then digested with various restriction enzymes and electrophoresed through an agarose gel. DNA is then transferred to a solid support such as a nylon membrane and hybridized with a radioactive or fluorescent DNA probe. After washing the unhybridized DNA probe off the membrane, the target DNA is exposed to x-ray or fluorescence sensitive film to detect the polymorphic regions of DNA. Certain regions of the human genome show a high degree of polymorphism in that >85% of the population show heterogeneity. These regions are highly informative in determining DNA identification. When human DNA in these regions is digested with different restriction enzymes, the size and pattern of the DNA fragments will vary with each individual. This pattern is an inherited trait and if the appropriate family members are tested, the inheritance pattern can be established. This is important in determining the paternity of a child or if a set of twins is heterozygous or monozygous. This can also help establish the identity of an unknown criminal or victim.

Frequently, enough material as a source of DNA is not available at the crime scene. When the quantity of DNA (eg, from dried blood, hair and skin scraping) is very small, the polymerase chain reaction is used to amplify DNA before identification by digestion by restriction enzymes. See Polymerase Chain Reaction *on page 713*.

Additional Information The genetic material of humans is highly polymorphic, and an individual's genotype represents a unique pattern which determines that person's identity and heredity. The only exception to this rule is identical twins, since they are derived from a single fertilized egg and hence have the same DNA profile. As a general rule, DNA is constant in all tissues of the body (even prenatal samples such as amniotic cells and chorionic villi specimens). DNA isolated from any specimen from an individual will be identical, which can prove to be very valuable in forensic evidence.

DNA typing provides a valuable tool for establishing family relationships and associations between forensic specimens (dried blood, semen, hair, skin scrapings, etc) and criminal suspects. Southern blots using a panel of DNA probes specific for several polymorphic DNA regions can produce a composite profile, which is unique to an individual and can be traced through families to establish relationships. DNA identification can be used for many applications such as paternity identification, identification of military casualties, clarifying parentage of infants possibly switched at birth or abducted, immigration disputes dealing with relationships, determination of sexual abuse and rape, as well as other criminal investigations.

Healthcare professionals are often involved in collecting specimens. Great care should be taken in the collection and storage of these specimens to prevent contamination and to preserve the evidence which may be crucial to any legal case.

References

Baird ML, "Use of DNA Identification for Forensic and Paternity Analysis," *J Clin Lab Anal*, 1996, 10(6), 350-8.

Debenham PG, "Probing Identity: The Changing Face of DNA Fingerprinting," *Trends Biotechnol*, 1992, 10(3):96-102.

Mao L, "Microsatellite Analysis. Applications and Pitfalls," *Ann N Y Acad Sci*, 2000, 906:55-62.

Reeder DJ, "Impact of DNA Typing on Standards and Practice in the Forensic Community," *Arch Pathol Lab Med*, 1999, 123(11):1063-5.

Schneider PM, "Basic Issues in Forensic DNA Typing," *Forensic Sci Int*, 1997, 88(1):17-22.

Taroni F and Aitken CG, "DNA Evidence, Probabilistic Evaluation and Collaborative Tests," *Forensic Sci Int*, 2000, 108(2):121-43.

Weedn VW, "Forensic DNA Tests," *Clin Lab Med*, 1996, 16(1):187-96.

Myotonic Dystrophy DNA Test

Related Information

Amniotic Fluid, Chromosome and Genetic Abnormality Analysis *on page 360*
Chorionic Villus Sampling, Chromosome and Genetic Abnormality Analysis *on page 361*
Creatine Kinase, Serum *on page 158*
Duchenne/Becker Muscular Dystrophy DNA Detection *on page 706*
Glucose, Fasting, Plasma *on page 183*
Muscle Biopsy *on page 69*
Polymerase Chain Reaction *on page 713*

Synonyms DM1 Gene Mutation Analysis; Dystrophia Myotonica; Genetic Detection of Myotonic Dystrophy; Molecular Diagnosis of Myotonic Dystrophy; Mutation Test for Trinucleotide Repeat Disorder, Myotonic Dystrophy; Myotonia Atrophica; Myotonic Dystrophy, Prenatal Diagnosis; Myotonic Muscular Dystrophy; Steinert Disease

Applies to Congenital Myotonic Dystrophy

Test Includes Determination of the number of CTG trinucleotide repeats in the DM1 (dystrophia myotonica 1) gene at chromosome 19 band 13.3

Abstract Myotonic dystrophy is the most common form of muscular dystrophy in adults , with the prevalence of 1 in 10-20,000. It is an autosomal dominant myotonic myopathy that can also affect the eyes, heart, gastrointestinal, endocrine, and central nervous systems. Weakness in extremities usually begins distally, progressing slowly, ultimately affecting proximal limb-girdle muscles. Normal sensory examination is characteristic. Affected, or genetically predisposed, individuals have one normal DM1 allele and one mutated allele. In virtually all cases, the mutation is an abnormal number of repeats of a naturally-occurring CTG trinucleotide motif in the DM1 gene. The DNA test provides a definitive diagnosis by measuring the number of CTG repeats in each DM1 allele. The number of CTG repeats is polymorphic in the normal population and varies from 5-37; normal alleles in this size range do not change upon transmission to offspring. The presence of 50 or more CTG repeats indicates that an individual has, or is genetically predisposed to develop, myotonic dystrophy. Alleles with ≥50 repeats can be unstable upon transmission; the number of repeats can increase or decrease, with increases being much more common. In patient population studies, a greater number of CTG repeats was roughly correlated with an earlier age at onset and more severe disease. This explains why, in some families, the disease appears to be more severe in individuals of the most recent generation. Neonates with severe congenital myotonic dystrophy, characterized by hypotonia, muscle weakness, respiratory insufficiency, and developmental/mental delay, typically have DM1 alleles with about 1000 or more CTG repeats. Congenital

myotonic dystrophy is inherited almost exclusively from an affected, or presymptomatic carrier, mother. The probability that a woman's abnormal DM1 allele will expand sufficiently to cause the congenital form of the disease in her child cannot be predicted, but the probability does appear to increase if the mother's DM1 allele has >300 CTG repeats and/or she has a previous child with congenital disease.

Patient Preparation For asymptomatic and prenatal testing, pretest counseling with a medical geneticist or genetic counselor is recommended to explain the meaning, benefits, and risks of testing.

Aftercare For asymptomatic and prenatal testing, post-test genetic counseling is recommended to explain the test result and its significance.

Specimen Whole blood (3-10 mL), amniotic fluid (10-20 mL), chorionic villus (3-5 mg wet weight), or one T25 flask of cultured amniocytes or chorionic villus

Container Collect anticoagulated blood in either a lavender top (EDTA) tube or yellow top (ACD) Vacutainer®. Avoid use of heparin anticoagulants, which can interfere with polymerase chain reactions and endonuclease restriction enzyme activity. Amniotic fluid and chorionic villus samples should be collected in a sterile manner and transferred to a sterile tube for transport.

Storage Instructions Blood samples can be stored and shipped at room temperature or refrigerated (4°C); do not freeze. Blood samples should be received in the testing laboratory within 4 days of the draw to ensure an adequate DNA yield. Amniotic fluid and chorionic villus samples should be maintained at room temperature and sent to the testing laboratory immediately after collection, preferably by overnight delivery, to ensure successful cell culture.

Causes for Rejection Frozen samples, whole blood in heparin anticoagulant (green top) or other inappropriate collection tube, amniotic fluid sample bloody, chorionic villus sample lacking viable chorionic villi

Turnaround Time 7-14 days

Special Instructions To provide an optimal test interpretation, the testing laboratory needs to know the clinical diagnosis, the family history or pedigree, and whether DNA testing has confirmed the clinical diagnosis of an affected family member.

Reference Interval Normal DM1 alleles have ≤37 CTG repeats. Abnormal mutant DM1 alleles have from 50 to >2000 CTG repeats. Rarely, DM1 alleles with 38-49 CTG repeats are detected; these are considered intermediate or premutation alleles. Individuals with premutation alleles are not known to develop myotonic dystrophy. Upon transmission, however, a premutation allele can expand to >50 CTG repeats and cause myotonic dystrophy in offspring.

Use Testing is useful to confirm or clarify a clinical diagnosis, to perform asymptomatic testing for adults at risk for myotonic dystrophy, and to perform prenatal testing for fetuses at risk for myotonic dystrophy. Asymptomatic children under the legal age should not be tested. Testing can be used to identify which progenitor in a family carries the DM1 mutation; this is important information for genetic counseling and the identification of other at-risk family members. In addition, DNA testing is part of the differential diagnosis of neonates with unexplained hypotonia, poor feeding, and/or respiratory difficulties, and of children with developmental delay and myopathic facies. This test is used occasionally to evaluate unexplained perioperative pulmonary complications, which occur at increased frequency in affected individuals,[1] and idiopathic polyhydramnios, which can be associated with an affected fetus.[2]

Limitations The number of CTG repeats cannot reliably predict disease onset, severity, or cognitive ability in an individual patient. This is because there are significant overlaps in the number of CTG repeats in congenital, childhood, adult and late onset cases. Prenatal testing cannot reliably predict whether a fetus will have the severe congenital form of the disease based on the number of CTG repeats in the DM1 gene of the fetus. This test will not detect rare cases of myotonic dystrophy-like disease (probably <1% of clinical cases) that are caused by mutations at the DM2 locus on chromosome 3.[3]

Methodology Polymerase chain reaction (PCR). A segment of the DM1 gene is amplified from genomic DNA, using primers that flank the CTG region of the gene. After electrophoresis, the number of repeats is calculated from the product size. This reaction can detect both normal and mutated DM1 alleles with <200 CTG repeats. Alleles with a greater number of CTG repeats are generally detected by Southern blot and hybridization to a fragment of the DM1 gene. The fragment size is indicative of the number of CTG repeats.

Additional Information Every affected individual has inherited an abnormally expanded DM1 gene from one of their parents; new mutations are not known to occur in this gene. Myotonic dystrophy occurs worldwide, with a prevalence of about 1 in 10-20,000. The DM1 protein is a serine-threonine protein kinase whose normal functions are not known. The CTG trinucleotide repeat motif is located in the 3' untranslated part of the DM1 gene; how CTG expansion affects DM1 gene expression and causes the disease is not clear. There is evidence that long CTG repeat tracts in DM1 affect the expression of several nearby genes; whether these genes contribute to the myotonic dystrophy phenotype remains to be determined. A listing of laboratories that perform myotonic dystrophy (DM1) DNA testing can be found at GeneTests® (see Websites).

Other characteristics of the disease include cataracts, testicular atrophy, intellectual impairment, difficulties with ventilation and hypoxia. Dysphagia, cardiac conduction defects, and endocrine problems occur. Serum CK is normal to moderately high.

Footnotes

1. Mathieu J, Allard P, Gobeil G, et al, "Anesthetic and Surgical Complications in 219 Cases of Myotonic Dystrophy," *Neurology*, 1997, 49(6):1646-50.
2. Esplin MS, Hallam S, Farrington PF, et al, "Myotonic Dystrophy Is a Significant Cause of Idiopathic Polyhydramnios," *Am J Obstet Gynecol*, 1998, 179(4):974-7.
3. Ranum LP, Rasmussen PF, Benzow KA, et al, "Genetic Mapping of a Second Myotonic Dystrophy Locus," *Nat Genet*, 1998, 19(2):196-8.

References

Adams C (updated 8/4/99), "Myotonic Dystrophy," *GeneClinics: Medical Genetics Knowledge Base* (database online), University of Washington, Seattle.

Cobo AM, Poza JJ, and Martorell L, "Contribution of Molecular Analyses to the Estimation of the Risk of Congenital Myotonic Dystrophy," *J Med Genet*, 1995, 32(2):105-9.

Groenen P and Wieringa B, "Expanding Complexity in Myotonic Dystrophy," *Bioessays*, 1998, 20(11):901-12.

The International Myotonic Dystrophy Consortium (IDMC), "New Nomenclature and DNA Testing Guidelines for Myotonic Dystrophy Type 1 (DM1)," *Neurology*, 2000, 54(6):1218-21.

Internet Web Sites

www.genetests.org

www.geneclinics.org/profiles/myotonic-d

Polymerase Chain Reaction

Related Information

Synonyms DNA Amplification; PCR

Test Includes Amplification of target DNA sequences as much as a millionfold

Abstract The polymerase chain reaction (PCR) is a technique with unlimited potential use in the medical laboratory. The major diagnostic applications of PCR include disease detection by mutational analysis and detection and identification of bacteria and viruses. It was developed at the Cetus Corporation in Emeryville, California, and was first described for use in the prenatal diagnosis of sickle cell anemia. The PCR technique permits over a millionfold amplification of target DNA in several hours. The amplification of target DNA is achieved by repetition of three steps: denaturation of target DNA, annealing (binding) of primers to specific sequences, and elongation of primers.

Specimen The specimen for the PCR assay will depend on the type of analysis. For example, prenatal diagnosis will require amniotic fluid or chorionic villus biopsy (see Amniotic Fluid, Chromosome and Genetic Abnormality Analysis *on page 360*), whole blood will be required for human immunodeficiency virus (HIV) detection, other specimens such as cerebrospinal fluid, sputum, serum, biopsies, or discharge from wounds for other infectious agents, or solid tissue by biopsy for cancer diagnosis. With the improved PCR assays, DNA purification is generally not required.

Collection Varies with type of specimen

Use The use of the technique to amplify short fragments of DNA is limited only by one's imagination. The uses in the laboratory include prenatal diagnosis of sickle cell anemia, hemoglobin Bart's hydrops fetalis, thalassemias, 21-hydroxylase deficiency, Down syndrome, Marfan syndrome, fragile X syndrome, hemophilia, cystic fibrosis, and muscular dystrophy, as well as oncogene activation in the case of lymphoma and chronic myelogenous leukemia. Numerous infectious agents such as *Mycobacterium* species, the agent of Lyme disease, bacteria, and viruses have been detected using this amplification technique.

Limitations Because PCR is very sensitive, the potential for contamination is great. The tests must be carefully monitored with appropriate controls (especially negative controls). The most common cause of contamination is from the products previously amplified in the laboratory. **Never open the tubes containing amplified product in the same room being used for PCR reactions.** The PCR technique requires knowledge of at least partial base sequence (where primers bind) of the DNA of interest to be amplified.

Methodology From the sequence data of target DNA, oligonucleotide primers approximately 18-25 nucleotides in length can be constructed using oligonucleotide synthesizers. These primers generally flank a 100-2000 base sequence of the DNA sequence of interest. The primers are constructed so that the primers bind (anneal) to opposite strands of the target double helix. A special DNA polymerase, purified from *Thermus aquaticus* (*Taq*), is used because it can withstand the many denaturing, reannealing, and elongation cycles without the need for replenishment. The reaction requires the target DNA, the primers, *Taq* polymerase, and the four deoxynucleotide triphosphates. The mixture is heated several minutes to 95°C to separate the target DNA double strands. The primers are then allowed to bind to the target DNA at 50°C to 60°C and the polymerase reaction allowed to proceed for several minutes at 72°C. This cycle of denaturation, annealing, and elongation is repeated over and over, as many as 25-35 times, amplifying the sequence between the primers hundreds of thousands to millions of times (see figure on following page). The amplified DNA can then be detected by agarose electrophoresis followed by ethidium bromide staining. The amplified bands can be seen with a UV light and photographed for analysis. The amplified DNA can also be detected by other techniques, such as hybridization or direct measurement of fluorescence, if fluorescent primers and deoxynucleotides are used.

DNA can be extracted from paraffin-embedded tissue for PCR analysis. Such tissue is best fixed in 10% formalin. Genotype can be ascertained by selective ultraviolet radiation fractionation.

Blood spotted on to filter paper, saliva, and tissue extract can be directly used as a source of DNA.

Additional Information The technique is continuously being expanded and refined for more uses. The current PCR techniques can amplify DNA sequences over 10 kilobases. Reverse transcription PCR has been useful in detection of a number of viral diseases. The procedure is automated with programmable heating blocks to cycle the reaction automatically. The technique has unprecedented sensitivity, being able to use nanogram quantities of target DNA, and could theoretically be used to amplify the DNA from a single cell. Other amplification reactions (eg, ligase chain reaction) are also being developed for use in the diagnostic laboratory. In the past, PCR was being used only for qualitative analysis, but in recent years, PCR is increasingly being used for quantitative analyses, such as for measuring viral load in a sample.

(Continued)

Polymerase Chain Reaction (Continued)

Polymerase Chain Reaction Cycles

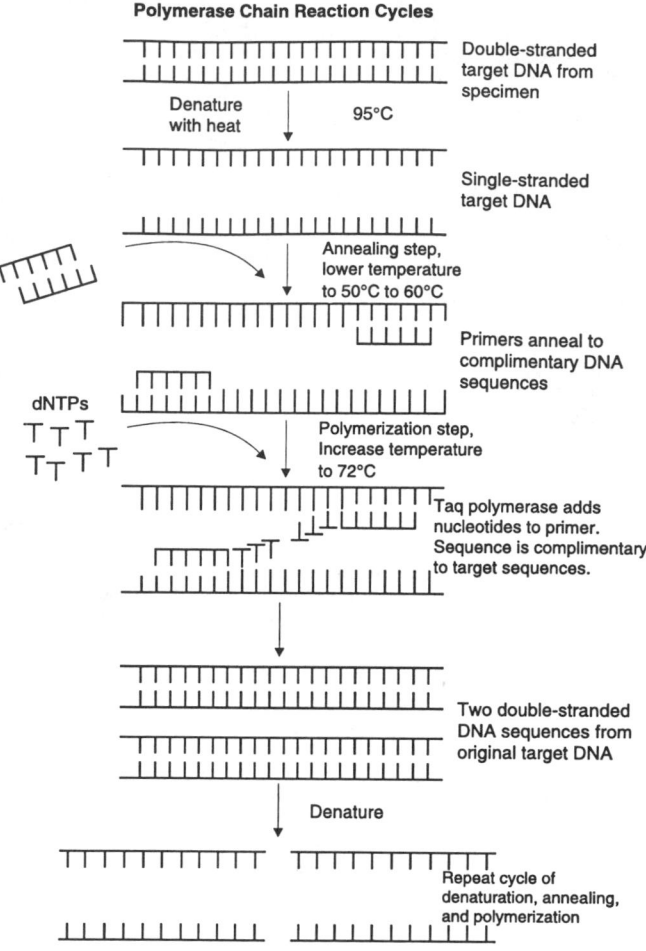

Double-stranded target DNA from specimen

Denature with heat — 95°C

Single-stranded target DNA

Annealing step, lower temperature to 50°C to 60°C

Primers anneal to complimentary DNA sequences

dNTPs

Polymerization step, Increase temperature to 72°C

Taq polymerase adds nucleotides to primer. Sequence is complimentary to target sequences.

Two double-stranded DNA sequences from original target DNA

Denature

Repeat cycle of denaturation, annealing, and polymerization

References

Baumforth KR, Nelson PN, Digby JE, et al, "Demystified...the Polymerase Chain Reaction," *Mol Pathol*, 1999, 52(1):1-10.

Crotty PL, Staggs RA, Porter PT, et al, "Quantitative Analysis in Molecular Diagnostics," *Hum Pathol*, 1994, 25(6):572-9.

Kogan SC, Doherty M, and Gitschier J, "An Improved Method for Prenatal Diagnosis of Genetic Diseases by Analysis of Amplified DNA Sequences. Application to Hemophilia A," *N Engl J Med*, 1987, 317(16):985-90.

Kiechle FL, "DNA Technology in the Clinical Laboratory," *Arch Pathol Lab Med*, 1999, 123(12):1151-3.

Lo YM, Hjelm NM, Fidler C, et al, "Prenatal Diagnosis of Fetal RhD Status by Molecular Analysis of Maternal Plasma," *N Engl J Med*, 1998, 339(24):1734-8.

Loda M, "Polymerase Chain Reaction-Based Methods for the Detection of Mutations in Oncogenes and Tumor Suppressor Genes," *Hum Pathol*, 1994, 25(6):564-71.

Mies C, "Molecular Biological Analysis of Paraffin-Embedded Tissues," *Hum Pathol*, 1994, 25(6):555-60.

Naber SP, "Molecular Pathology - Diagnosis of Infectious Disease," *N Engl J Med*, 1994, 331(18):1212-5.

Post JC and Ehrlich GD, "The Impact of the Polymerase Chain Reaction in Clinical Medicine," *JAMA*, 2000, 283(12):1544-6.

Rogers BB, "Nucleic Acid Amplification and Infectious Disease," *Hum Pathol*, 1994, 25(6):590-3.

Saiki RK, Chang, CA, Levenson CH, et al, "Diagnosis of Sickle Cell Anemia and β-Thalassemia With Enzymatically Amplified DNA and Nonradioactive Allele-Specific Oligonucleotide Probes," *N Engl J Med*, 1988, 319(9):537-41.

Saiki RK, Gelfand DH, Stoffel S, et al, "Primer-Directed Enzymatic Amplification of DNA With Thermostable DNA Polymerase," *Science*, 1988, 239(4839):487-9.

Shibata D, "Extraction of DNA From Paraffin-Embedded Tissue for Analysis by Polymerase Chain Reaction: New Tricks From an Old Friend," *Hum Pathol*, 1994, 25(6):561-3.

White TJ, "The Future of PCR Technology: Diversification of Technologies and Applications," *Trends Biotechnol*, 1996, 14(12):478-83.

Worman HJ, "Molecular Biological Methods in Diagnosis and Treatment of Liver Diseases," *Clin Chem*, 1997, 43(8 Pt 2):1476-86.

♦ **RFLP Analysis for Parentage Evaluation** *see* Identification DNA Testing *on page 711*

♦ **SCA1** *see* Spinocerebellar Ataxia Type 1 DNA Test *on page 714*

♦ **SCA1 DNA Test** *see* Spinocerebellar Ataxia Type 1 DNA Test *on page 714*

♦ **SCA1 Gene Mutation Analysis** *see* Spinocerebellar Ataxia Type 1 DNA Test *on page 714*

♦ **SCA2** *see* Spinocerebellar Ataxia Type 2 DNA Test *on page 715*

♦ **SCA2 DNA Test** *see* Spinocerebellar Ataxia Type 2 DNA Test *on page 715*

♦ **SCA2 Gene Mutation Analysis** *see* Spinocerebellar Ataxia Type 2 DNA Test *on page 715*

♦ **SCA3** *see* Spinocerebellar Ataxia Type 3 DNA Test *on page 716*

♦ **SCA3 Gene Mutation Analysis** *see* Spinocerebellar Ataxia Type 3 DNA Test *on page 716*

♦ **SCA6** *see* Spinocerebellar Ataxia Type 6 DNA Test *on page 716*

♦ **SCA6 Gene Mutation Analysis** *see* Spinocerebellar Ataxia Type 6 DNA Test *on page 716*

♦ **SCA7** *see* Spinocerebellar Ataxia Type 7 DNA Test *on page 717*

♦ **SCA7 Gene Mutation Analysis** *see* Spinocerebellar Ataxia Type 7 DNA Test *on page 717*

♦ **Spinocerebellar Ataxia, Cuban Type** *see* Spinocerebellar Ataxia Type 2 DNA Test *on page 715*

Spinocerebellar Ataxia Type 1 DNA Test

Related Information
Polymerase Chain Reaction *on page 713*

Synonyms Ataxia; Ataxin-1; Autosomal Dominant Cerebellar Ataxia Type I [ADCA I] (subset of); Genetic Detection of SCA1; Molecular Diagnosis of Spinocerebellar Ataxia Type 1; Mutation Test for Trinucleotide Repeat Disorder; SCA1; SCA1 DNA Test; SCA1 Gene Mutation Analysis

Test Includes Determination of the number of CAG trinucleotide repeats in the SCA1 gene at chromosome 6 band p23.

Abstract Spinocerebellar ataxia type 1 (SCA1) is an inherited progressive ataxia, often associated with extrapyramidal signs and peripheral neuropathy. This is commonly an adult disease with the average onset in the 4th decade, but onset in childhood has been reported. Affected, or genetically predisposed, individuals have one normal SCA1 allele and one mutant allele. In all cases, the mutant allele has an abnormally large number of a naturally-occurring CAG trinucleotide repeat motif in the SCA1 gene. The DNA test detects 100% of cases by measuring the number of CAG repeats in each SCA1 allele. Because the clinical manifestations are nonspecific, SCA1 cannot be reliably distinguished from other hereditary ataxias.[1] The diagnosis depends on the DNA test. The number of CAG repeats is polymorphic in the normal population and varies from 6-36; normal alleles in this size range do not change upon transmission to offspring. The presence of ≥45 CAG repeats indicates that an individual has, or is genetically predisposed to develop, spinocerebellar ataxia type 1. Mutant alleles with ≥45 CAG repeats are often unstable upon transmission and the child has an increased or decreased number of repeats, with increases being more common. In patient population studies, a greater number of CAG repeats was generally correlated with an earlier age at onset and more severe disease. This explains why, in some families, the disease appears to be more severe in affected individuals of the most recent generation.[2] However, because SCA1 age at onset, progression, and severity is variable, the number of CAG repeats cannot reliably predict the clinical course of the disease in an individual case. SCA1 is an autosomal dominant disorder; each child of an affected, or asymptomatic carrier, has a 50% chance of inheriting the mutant gene.

Patient Preparation Testing of asymptomatic, at-risk adults is predictive testing and the patient should have formal genetic counseling to explain the meaning, benefits, and risks of testing.

Aftercare For asymptomatic at-risk adults, post-test genetic counseling is appropriate to explain the test result and its significance.

Specimen Whole blood (3-10 mL)

Container Collect anticoagulated blood in either a lavender top (EDTA) tube or yellow top (ACD) Vacutainer® tube. Avoid use of heparin anticoagulants, which can interfere with polymerase chain reactions and endonuclease restriction enzyme activity.

Storage Instructions Blood samples can be stored and shipped at room temperature or refrigerated (4°C); do not freeze. Blood samples should be received in the testing laboratory within 4 days of draw to ensure an adequate DNA yield.

Causes for Rejection Frozen samples, whole blood in heparin anticoagulant (green top) or other inappropriate collection tube

Turnaround Time 7-14 days

Special Instructions To provide an optimal test interpretation, the testing laboratory needs to know the clinical diagnosis, family history, and whether DNA testing has confirmed the clinical diagnosis of an affected family member.

Reference Interval Normal SCA1 alleles have ≤36 CAG repeats. Abnormal mutant SCA1 alleles have ≥44 CAG repeats. Cases with an SCA1 allele of 37-44 CAG repeats should be considered for additional analyses. It is generally thought that normal SCA1 alleles are stabilized by the presence of CAT trinucleotide repeats that interrupt the CAG tract.[3] Tests exist that detect the presence or absence of the CAT repeat interrupts, which may modify the risk of individuals carrying these uncommon "intermediate" sized SCA1 alleles.

Use Testing is useful to rule out or confirm a clinical diagnosis and to perform asymptomatic testing for adults at risk for spinocerebellar ataxia type 1. Consensus holds that testing of asymptomatic at-risk children under the legal age, for an adult-onset disorder for which no treatment exists, is not appropriate.

Limitations The number of CAG repeats cannot reliably predict disease onset, severity, or cognitive ability in an individual patient. SCA1 mutations appear to account for very few, if any, cases of idiopathic sporadic cerebellar ataxia.[4]

Methodology Polymerase chain reaction (PCR). A segment of the SCA1 gene is amplified from the patient's DNA using primers that flank the CAG repeat region of the gene. After electrophoresis, the number of repeats is calculated from the product size. This reaction can detect both normal and mutant SCA1 alleles.

Additional Information Spinocerebellar ataxia type 1 has an incidence of about 1-2 in 100,000 individuals, but varies significantly by geography and with ethnic background. In the U.S., SCA1 mutations are found in about 5% to 6% of patients in the autosomal dominant cerebellar ataxia (ADCA) population. The protein product of the SCA1 gene, ataxin-1, is expressed in many tissues of the body, but its normal function is not known. The CAG trinucleotide repeat motif is located in the coding region of the gene and encodes a tract of polyglutamine residues. Abnormally long polyglutamine tracts confer an unknown new function to ataxin-1; how this "gain-of-function" causes the disease remains to be elucidated. SCA1 testing is widely available; a list of clinical laboratories that perform this test can be found at GeneTests® (http://www.genetests.org). Prenatal testing is available, but should be preceded by formal genetic counseling to discuss difficult ethical issues regarding testing for a typically adult onset disease.

Footnotes

1. Bird TD, "Hereditary Ataxia Overview," GeneClinics: Medical Genetics Knowledge Base, September 25, 2000, available at: http://www.geneclinics.org/profiles/ataxias/details.html.
2. Ranum LP, Chung MY, Banfi S, et al, "Molecular and Clinical Correlations in Spinocerebellar Ataxia Type 1: Evidence for Familial Effects on the Age at Onset," Am J Hum Genet, 1994, 55(2):244-52.
3. Chung MY, Ranum LP, Duvick LA, et al, "Evidence for a Mechanism Predisposing to Intergenerational CAG Repeat Instability in Spinocerebellar Ataxia Type 1," Nat Genet, 1993, 5(3):254-8.
4. Schols L, Szymanski S, Peters S, et al, "Genetic Background of Apparently Idiopathic Sporadic Cerebellar Ataxia," Hum Genet, 2000, 107(2):132-7.

References

Brandt V and Zoghbi HY, "Spinocerebellar Ataxia Type 1," GeneClinics: Medical Genetics Knowledge Base, updated June 12, 1998, available at: http://www.geneclinics.org/profiles/sca1/details.html.
Moseley ML, Benzow KA, Schut LJ, et al, "Incidence of Dominant Spinocerebellar and Friedreich Triplet Repeats Among 361 Ataxia Families," Neurology, 1998, 51(6):1666-71.
Orr HT, "The Ins and Outs of a Polyglutamine Neurodegenerative Disease: Spinocerebellar Ataxia Type 1 (SCA1)," Neurobiol Dis, 2000, 7(3):129-34.
Zoghbi HY, "Spinocerebellar Ataxia Type 1," Clin Neurosci, 1995, 3(1):5-11.

Internet Web Sites

www.genetests.org
www.geneclinics.org/profiles/ataxias/details.html
www.geneclinics.org/profiles/sca1/details.html
www.ataxia.org

Spinocerebellar Ataxia Type 2 DNA Test

Related Information

Polymerase Chain Reaction *on page 713*

Synonyms Ataxin-2; Autosomal Dominant Cerebellar Ataxia Type I [ADCA I] (subset of); Genetic Detection of SCA2; Molecular Diagnosis of Spinocerebellar Ataxia Type 2; Mutation Test for Trinucleotide Repeat Disorder; Olivopontocerebellar Atrophy, Holguin; SCA2; SCA2 DNA Test; SCA2 Gene Mutation Analysis; Spinocerebellar Ataxia, Cuban Type

Test Includes Determination of the number of CAG trinucleotide repeats in the SCA2 gene at chromosome 12 band q24.

Abstract Spinocerebellar ataxia type 2 is an inherited, slowly progressive gait ataxia, often associated with slow saccadic eye movement, peripheral neuropathy, decreased deep tendon reflexes, dystonia or chorea, and/or dementia. SCA2 is commonly an adult disease with the average onset in the 3rd to 4th decade, but severe disease has been reported in at-risk neonates.[1] Affected, or genetically predisposed, individuals have one normal SCA2 allele and one mutant allele. In all cases, the mutant allele has an abnormally large number of a naturally-occurring CAG trinucleotide repeat motif in the SCA2 gene. The DNA test detects 100% of cases by measuring the number of CAG repeats in each SCA2 allele. Because the clinical manifestations are nonspecific, SCA2 cannot be reliably distinguished from other hereditary ataxias.[2] The diagnosis depends on the DNA test. The number of CAG repeats is polymorphic in the normal population and varies from 14-31; normal alleles in this size range do not change upon transmission to offspring. The presence of ≥35 CAG repeats indicates that an individual has, or is genetically predisposed to develop, SCA2. Mutant alleles with ≥35 CAG repeats are often unstable upon transmission, and the child has an increased or decreased number of repeats, with increases being more common. In patient population studies, a greater number of

CAG repeats was generally correlated with an earlier age at onset and more severe disease. This explains why, in some families, the disease appears to be more severe in affected individuals of the most recent generation. However, because SCA2 age at onset, progression, and severity is variable, the number of CAG repeats cannot reliably predict the clinical course of the disease in an individual case. SCA2 is an autosomal dominant disorder; each child of an affected, or asymptomatic individual carrying the mutant SCA2 allele, has a 50% chance of inheriting the mutant gene.

Patient Preparation Testing of asymptomatic at-risk adults is predictive testing and the patient should have formal genetic counseling to explain the meaning, benefits, and risks of testing.

Aftercare For asymptomatic at-risk adults, post-test genetic counseling is appropriate to explain the test result and its significance.

Specimen Whole blood

Container Collect anticoagulated blood in either a lavender top (EDTA) tube or yellow top (ACD) Vacutainer® tube. Avoid use of heparin anticoagulants, which can interfere with polymerase chain reactions and endonuclease restriction enzyme activity.

Storage Instructions Blood samples can be stored and shipped at room temperature or refrigerated (4°C); do not freeze. Blood samples should be received in the testing laboratory within 4 days of draw to ensure an adequate DNA yield.

Causes for Rejection Frozen samples, whole blood in heparin anticoagulant (green top) or other inappropriate collection tube

Turnaround Time 7-14 days

Special Instructions To provide an optimal test interpretation, the testing laboratory needs to know the clinical diagnosis, family history, and whether DNA testing has confirmed the clinical diagnosis of an affected family member.

Reference Interval Normal SCA2 alleles have 14-31 CAG repeats. Abnormal mutant SCA2 alleles in adults have 35 to about 64 CAG repeats. Affected neonates, with a family history of SCA2, have 200-400 CAG repeats.[1] SCA2 alleles with between 32-35 CAG repeats are considered "intermediate" because they may or may not be associated with clinical symptoms.

Use Testing is useful to rule out or confirm a clinical diagnosis and to perform asymptomatic testing for adults at risk for spinocerebellar ataxia type 2. Consensus holds that testing of asymptomatic at-risk children under the legal age, for an adult onset disorder for which no treatment exists, is not appropriate. Children presenting with symptoms usually benefit from having a specific diagnosis established.

Limitations The number of CAG repeats cannot reliably predict disease onset, severity, or cognitive ability in an individual patient. In cases with neonatal or childhood onset with typically larger numbers of CAG repeats, it is more difficult for the testing laboratory to detect the large mutant allele. In these cases, concerns about allele size detection should be discussed with the testing laboratory, especially when only a single sized allele is observed in an affected child (ie, an apparent SCA2 homozygote). SCA2 mutations appear to account for very few cases of idiopathic sporadic cerebellar ataxia.

Methodology A segment of the SCA2 gene is amplified from the patient's DNA, using primers that flank the CAG repeat region of the gene. After electrophoresis, the number of repeats is calculated from the product size. This reaction can detect both normal and mutant SCA2 alleles. For neonatal and childhood onset cases, where the number of CAG repeats may be very great, analysis by Southern blot may be necessary to detect the large mutant SCA2 allele.

Additional Information In the United States, SCA2 mutations are found in 15% of patients in the autosomal dominant cerebellar ataxia (ADCA) population;[3,4] frequency varies by geography and ethnic background. The normal function of the protein product of the SCA2 gene, ataxin-2, is not known. The CAG trinucleotide repeat motif is located in the coding region of the gene and encodes a tract of polyglutamine residues. Abnormally long polyglutamine tracts confer an unknown new function to ataxin-2; how this "gain-of-function" causes the disease is not clear. SCA2 testing is widely available; a list of clinical laboratories that perform this test can be found at GeneTest® (http://www.genetests.org). Prenatal testing is available, but should be preceded by formal genetic counseling to discuss difficult ethical issues related to testing for a (typically) adult-onset disease.

Footnotes

1. Babovic-Vuksanovic D, Snow K, Patterson MC, et al, "Spinocerebellar Ataxia Type 2 (SCA2) in an Infant With Extreme CAG Repeat Expansion," Am J Med Genet, 1990, 79(5).383-7.
2. Bird TD, "Hereditary Ataxia Overview," GeneClinics: Medical Genetics Knowledge Base, September 25, 2000, available at: http://www.geneclinics.org/profiles/ataxias/details.html.
3. Moseley ML, Benzow KA, Schut LJ, et al, "Incidence of Dominant Spinocerebellar and Friedreich Triplet Repeats Among 361 Ataxia Families," Neurology, 1998, 51(6):1666-71.
4. Riess O, Laccone FA, Gispert S, et al, "SCA2 Trinucleotide Expansion in German SCA Patients," Neurogenetics, 1997, 1(1):59-64.

References

Burk K, Globas C, Bosch S, et al, "Cognitive Deficits in Spinocerebellar Ataxia 2," SPINBrain, 1999, 122(Pt 4):769-7.
Cancel G, Durr A, Didierjean O, et al, "Molecular and Clinical Correlations in Spinocerebellar Ataxia 2: A Study of 32 Families," Hum Mol Genet, 1997, 6(5):709-15.

(Continued)

Spinocerebellar Ataxia Type 2 DNA Test (Continued)

Geschwind DH, Perlman S, Figueroa CP, et al, "The Prevalence and Wide Clinical Spectrum of the Spinocerebellar Ataxia Type 2 Trinucleotide Repeat in Patients With Autosomal Dominant Cerebellar Ataxia," *Am J Hum Genet*, 1997, 60(4):842-50.

Pulst SM, "SpinOcerebellar Ataxia Type 2," GeneClinics: Medical Genetics Knowledge Base, July 11, 1998, available at: http://www.geneclinics.org/profiles/sca2/details.html.

Internet Web Sites

www.genetests.org

www.geneclinics.org/profiles/ataxias/details.html

www.geneclinics.org/profiles/sca2/details.html

Spinocerebellar Ataxia Type 3 DNA Test

Related Information

Polymerase Chain Reaction *on page 713*

Synonyms Ataxin-3; Autosomal Dominant Cerebellar Ataxia Type I [ADCA I] (subset of); Azorean Ataxia; Genetic Detection of SCA3; Machado-Joseph Disease; MJD; MJD DNA Test; MJD Gene Mutation Analysis; Molecular Diagnosis of Spinocerebellar Ataxia Type 3; Mutation Test for Trinucleotide Repeat Disorder; Olivopontocerebellar Ataxia 3; SCA3; SCA3 Gene Mutation Analysis

Test Includes Determination of the number of CAG trinucleotide repeats in the MJD gene at chromosome 14 band q21

Abstract Spinocerebellar ataxia type 3 (SCA3) is an inherited progressive gait ataxia, often associated with pyramidal and extrapyramidal signs, lid retraction, nystagmus, decreased saccade velocity, amyotrophy, fasciculations, and sensory loss. SCA3 is commonly an adult disease with the average onset in the 4th decade, but childhood onset has been reported. Affected, or genetically predisposed, individuals have one normal MJD allele and one mutant allele. In all cases, the mutant allele has an abnormally large number of a naturally-occurring CAG trinucleotide repeat motif in the MJD gene. The DNA test detects 100% of cases by measuring the number of CAG repeats in each MJD allele. Because the clinical manifestations are nonspecific, SCA3 cannot be reliably distinguished from other hereditary ataxias.[1] The diagnosis depends on the DNA test. The number of CAG repeats is polymorphic in the normal population and varies from 12-47; normal alleles in this size range do not change upon transmission to offspring. The presence of 55 to about 86 CAG repeats indicates that an individual has, or is genetically predisposed to develop, spinocerebellar ataxia type 3. Mutant alleles with ≥55 CAG repeats are often unstable upon transmission and the child has an increased or decreased number of repeats, with increases being more common. In patient population studies, a greater number of CAG repeats was generally correlated with an earlier age at onset and more severe disease. This explains why, in some families, the disease appears to be more severe in affected individuals of the most recent generation. However, because SCA3 age at onset, progression, and severity is variable, the number of CAG repeats cannot reliably predict the clinical course of the disease in an individual case. SCA3 is an autosomal dominant disorder; each child of an affected, or asymptomatic individual carrying the mutant SCA3 allele, has a 50% chance of inheriting the mutant gene.

Patient Preparation Testing of asymptomatic at-risk adults is predictive testing and the patient should have formal genetic counseling to explain the meaning, benefits, and risks of testing.

Aftercare For asymptomatic at-risk adults, post-test genetic counseling is appropriate to explain the test result and its significance.

Specimen Whole blood

Container Collect anticoagulated blood in either a lavender top (EDTA) tube or yellow top (ACD) Vacutainer® tube. Avoid use of heparin anticoagulants, which can interfere with polymerase chain reactions and endonuclease restriction enzyme activity.

Storage Instructions Blood samples can be stored and shipped at room temperature or refrigerated (4°C); do not freeze. Blood samples should be received in the testing laboratory within 4 days of draw to ensure an adequate DNA yield.

Causes for Rejection Frozen samples, whole blood in heparin anticoagulant (green top) or other inappropriate collection tube

Turnaround Time 7-14 days

Special Instructions To provide an optimal test interpretation, the testing laboratory needs to know the clinical diagnosis, family history, and whether DNA testing has confirmed the clinical diagnosis of an affected family member.

Reference Interval Normal MJD alleles have 12-47 CAG repeats. Abnormal mutant MJD alleles have 55-86 CAG repeats.

Use Testing is useful to rule out or confirm a clinical diagnosis and to perform asymptomatic testing for adults at risk for SCA3. Consensus holds that testing of asymptomatic at-risk children under the legal age, for an adult onset disorder for which no treatment exists, is not appropriate. Children presenting with symptoms usually benefit from having a specific diagnosis established.

Limitations The number of CAG repeats cannot reliably predict disease onset, progression, or severity in an individual patient. MJD mutations appear to account for very few, if any, cases of idiopathic sporadic cerebellar ataxia.[2]

Methodology Polymerase chain reaction (PCR). A segment of the MJD gene is amplified from the patient's DNA, using primers that flank the CAG repeat region of the gene. After electrophoresis, the number of repeats is calculated from the product size. This reaction can detect both normal and mutant MJD alleles.

Additional Information In the United States, MJD mutations are found in 21% of patients in the autosomal dominant cerebellar ataxia (ADCA) population; frequency varies by geography and ethnic background. The normal function of the protein product of the MJD gene, ataxin-3, is not known. The CAG trinucleotide repeat motif is located in the coding region of the gene; each CAG repeat encodes a glutamine residue. In affected individuals, abnormally long polyglutamine tracts confer an unknown new function to ataxin-3; how this "gain-of-function" causes the disease is not clear. Testing for SCA3 disease is widely available; a list of clinical laboratories that perform this test can be found at GeneTests® (http://www.genetests.org). Prenatal testing is available, but should be preceded by formal genetic counseling to discuss difficult ethical issues regarding testing for a typically adult onset disease. Management of patients remains supportive, since there is no specific treatment available.

Footnotes

1. Bird TD, "Hereditary Ataxia Overview," GeneClinics: Medical Genetics Knowledge Base, September 25, 2000, available at: http://www.geneclinics.org/profiles/ataxias/details.html.

2. Moseley ML, Benzow KA, Schut LJ, et al, "Incidence of Dominant Spinocerebellar and Friedreich Triplet Repeats Among 361 Ataxia Families," *Neurology*, 1998, 51(6):1666-71.

References

Subramony SH, McDaniel O, Smith S, "Spinocerebellar Ataxia Type 3," GeneClinics: Medical Genetics Knowledge Base, updated October 1, 1998, available at: http://www.geneclinics.org/profiles/sca3/details.html.

Sudarsky L and Coutinho P, "Machado-Joseph Disease," *Clin Neurosci*, 1995, 3(1):17-22.

Takiyama Y, Igarashi S, Rogaeva EA, et al, "Evidence for Intergenerational Instability in the CAG Repeat in the MJD1 Gene and for Conserved Haplotypes at Flanking Markers Amongst Japanese and Caucasian Subjects With Machado-Joseph Disease," *Hum Mol Genet*, 1995, 4(7):1137-46.

Internet Web Sites

www.genetests.org

www.geneclinics.org/profiles/ataxias/details.html

www.geneclinics.org/profiles/sca3/details.html

Spinocerebellar Ataxia Type 6 DNA Test

Related Information

Polymerase Chain Reaction *on page 713*

Synonyms Autosomal Dominant Cerebellar Ataxia Type III [ADCA III] (subset of); CACNA1A Gene Mutation Screening; Genetic Detection of SCA6; Molecular Diagnosis of Spinocerebellar Ataxia Type 6; Mutation Test for Trinucleotide Repeat Disorder; SCA6; SCA6 Gene Mutation Analysis

Applies to Episodic Ataxia Type 1; Familial Hemiplegic Migraine

Test Includes Determination of the number of CAG trinucleotide repeats in the CACNA1A (calcium channel alpha 1A subunit; previously called CACNL1A4; alias SCA6) gene at chromosome 19 band p13.

Abstract Spinocerebellar ataxia type 6 (SCA6) is a slowly progressive cerebellar ataxia with the mean onset in the 5th to 6th decade. Occasionally, patients with SCA6 present with episodic ataxia. Affected, or genetically predisposed, individuals have one normal CACNL1A4 allele and one mutant allele. In >99% of cases, the mutant allele has an abnormally large number of a naturally-occurring CAG trinucleotide repeat motif in the CACNL1A4 gene. The DNA test measures the number of CAG repeats in each CACNL1A4 allele. Because the clinical manifestations are nonspecific, SCA6 cannot be reliably distinguished from other hereditary ataxias.[1] The diagnosis depends on the DNA test. The number of CAG repeats is polymorphic in the normal population and varies from 4-19. The presence of ≥21 CAG repeats indicates that an individual has, or is genetically predisposed to develop, spinocerebellar ataxia type 6. SCA6 is an autosomal dominant disorder; each child of an affected, or asymptomatic individual carrying the mutant SCA6 allele, has a 50% chance of inheriting the mutant gene. In contrast to other hereditary spinocerebellar ataxias,[1] mutant SCA6 alleles are relatively stable and rarely show changes in CAG repeat number upon transmission to offspring.

Patient Preparation Testing of asymptomatic at-risk adults is predictive testing and the patient should have formal genetic counseling to explain the meaning, benefits, and risks of testing.

Aftercare For asymptomatic at-risk adults, post-test genetic counseling is appropriate to explain the test result and its significance.

Specimen Whole blood

Container Collect anticoagulated blood in either a lavender top (EDTA) tube or yellow top (ACD) Vacutainer® tube. Avoid use of heparin anticoagulants, which can interfere with polymerase chain reactions and endonuclease restriction enzyme activity.

Storage Instructions Blood samples can be stored and shipped at room temperature or refrigerated (4°C); do not freeze. Blood samples should be received in the testing laboratory within 4 days of draw to ensure an adequate DNA yield.

Causes for Rejection Frozen samples, whole blood in heparin anticoagulant (green top) or other inappropriate collection tube

Turnaround Time 7-14 days

Special Instructions To provide an optimal test interpretation, the testing laboratory needs to know the clinical diagnosis, family history, and whether DNA testing has confirmed the clinical diagnosis of an affected family member.

Reference Interval Normal CACNA1A alleles have 3-19 CAG repeats. Abnormal mutant CACNA1A alleles have ≥21 CAG repeats; the largest abnormal allele reported to date had 30 repeats. CACNA1A alleles with 20 CAG repeats are very rare and may be associated with late onset or episodic disease.[2]

Use Testing is useful to rule out or confirm a clinical diagnosis and to perform asymptomatic testing for adults at risk for SCA6. SCA6 testing is also useful in assessment of apparently idiopathic sporadic cerebellar ataxia, particularly cases with late onset.[3]

Limitations The number of CAG repeats cannot reliably predict disease onset, progression, or severity in an individual patient. This test will not detect the <1% of SCA6 cases that are caused by a mutation in a single nucleotide outside of the CAG repeat region. This test cannot detect the mutations in the CACNA1A that cause episodic ataxia type 2 or familial hemiplegic migraine (see Additional Information).

Methodology Polymerase chain reaction (PCR). A segment of the CACNA1A gene is amplified from the patient's DNA, using primers that flank the CAG repeat region of the gene. After electrophoresis, the number of repeats is calculated from the product size. This reaction can detect both normal and mutant CACNA1A alleles.

Additional Information In the United States, CACNA1A mutations are found in 15% of patients in the autosomal dominant cerebellar ataxia (ADCA) population;[4] frequency varies by geography and ethnic background. The CACNA1A gene encodes the alpha 1A subunit of a voltage-dependent calcium channel. The CAG trinucleotide repeat motif is located in the coding region of the gene; each CAG repeat encodes a glutamine residue. In affected individuals, abnormally long polyglutamine tracts confer an unknown new function to the alpha 1A subunit of the calcium channel; how this "gain-of-function" causes the disease is not clear but alteration in calcium channel function has been reported. Testing for SCA6 disease is widely available; a list of clinical laboratories that perform this test can be found at GeneTest® (http://www.genetests.org). Prenatal testing is available, but should be preceded by formal genetic counseling to discuss difficult ethical issues related to testing for a (typically) adult-onset disease.

Mutations outside the CAG repeat region of the CACNA1A gene cause two related disorders, episodic ataxia type 1 (EA2) and familial hemiplegic migraine (FHM).[5] In EA2 there is a high prevalence of mutations that predict a prematurely truncated calcium channel protein.[6] In FHM, there is a high prevalence of single base pair mutations that alter a single amino acid residue.[7] Management of patients remains supportive, since there is no specific treatment available.

Footnotes

1. Bird TD, "Hereditary Ataxia Overview," GeneClinics: Medical Genetics Knowledge Base, September 25, 2000, available at: http://www.geneclinics.org/profiles/ataxias/details.html.

2. Jodice C, Mantuano E, Veneziano L, et al, "Episodic Ataxia Type 2 (EA2) and Spinocerebellar Ataxia Type 6 (SCA6) Due to CAG Repeat Expansion in the CACNA1A Gene on Chromosome 19p," *Hum Mol Genet*, 1997, 6(11):1973-8.

3. Schols L, Szymanski S, Peters S, et al, "Genetic Background of Apparently Idiopathic Sporadic Cerebellar Ataxia," *Hum Genet*, 2000, 107(2):132-7.

4. Moseley ML, Benzow KA, Schut LJ, et al, "Incidence of Dominant Spinocerebellar and Friedreich Triplet Repeats Among 361 Ataxia Families," *Neurology*, 1998, 51(6):1666-71.

5. Tournier-Lasserve E, "CACNA1A Mutations. Hemiplegic Migraine, Episodic Ataxia Type 2, and the Others," *Neurology*, 1999, 53(1):3-4.

6. Denier C, Ducros A, Vahedi K, et al, "High Prevalence of CACNA1A Truncations and Broader Clinical Spectrum in Episodic Ataxia Type 2," *Neurology*, 1999, 52(9):1816-21.

7. Ducros A, Denier C, Joutel A, et al, "Recurrence of the T666M Calcium Channel CACNA1A Gene Mutation in Familial Hemiplegic Migraine With Progressive Cerebellar Ataxia," *Am J Hum Genet*, 1999, 64(1):89-98.

References

Geschwind DH, Perlman S, Figueroa KP, et al, "Spinocerebellar Ataxia Type 6: Frequency of the Mutation and Genotype-Phenotype Correlations," *Neurology*, 1997, 49(5):1247-51.

Gomez CM, "Spinocerebellar Ataxia Type 6," GeneClinics: Medical Genetics Knowledge Base, available at http://www.geneclinics.org/profiles/sca6/details.html.

Gomez CM, Thompson RM, Gammack JT, et al, "Spinocerebellar Ataxia Type 6: Gaze-Evoked and Vertical Nystagmus, Purkinje Cell Degeneration, and Variable Age of Onset," *Ann Neurol*, 1997, 42(6):933-50.

Jen J, "Calcium Channelopathies in the Central Nervous System," *Curr Opin Neurobiol*, 1999, 9(3):274-80.

Stevanin MS, Durr A, David G, et al, "Clinical and Molecular Features of Spinocerebellar Ataxia Type 6," *Neurology*, 1997, 49(5):1243-46.

Zuchenko O, Bailey J, Bonnern P, et al, "Autosomal Dominant Cerebellar Ataxia (SCA6) Associated With Small Polyglutamine Expansions in the Alpha 1A-Voltage-Dependent Calcium Channel," *Nature Genet*, 1997, 15:62-9.

Internet Web Sites

www.genetests.org

www.geneclinics.org/profiles/ataxias/details.html

www.geneclinics.org/profiles/sca6/details.html

Spinocerebellar Ataxia Type 7 DNA Test

Related Information

Polymerase Chain Reaction *on page 713*

Synonyms Ataxin-7; Autosomal Dominant Cerebellar Ataxia Type III [ADCA III]; Genetic Detection of SCA7; Hereditary Ataxia With Retinal Degeneration; Molecular Diagnosis of Spinocerebellar Ataxia Type 7; Mutation Test for Trinucleotide Repeat Disorder; Olivopontocerebellar Atrophy III [OPCA III]; OPCA With Retinal Degeneration; SCA7; SCA7 Gene Mutation Analysis

Test Includes Determination of the number of CAG trinucleotide repeats in the SCA7 gene at chromosome 3 band p21-p12.

Abstract Spinocerebellar ataxia type 7 (SCA7) is an inherited progressive cerebellar ataxia, often associated with retinal dystrophy with progressive central visual loss. SCA7 is commonly an adult disease with the average onset in the 3rd to 4th decade, but aggressive disease in neonates and children has been reported. Affected, or genetically predisposed, individuals have one normal SCA7 allele and one mutant allele. In all cases, the mutant allele has an abnormally large number of a naturally-occurring CAG trinucleotide repeat motif in the SCA7 gene. The DNA test detects 100% of cases by measuring the number of CAG repeats in each SCA7 allele. The number of CAG repeats is polymorphic in the normal population and varies from 4-19; normal alleles in this size range do not change upon transmission to offspring. The presence of 37 to >300 CAG repeats indicates that an individual has, or is genetically predisposed to develop, spinocerebellar ataxia type 7. Mutant alleles with ≥37 CAG repeats are often unstable upon transmission and the child has an increased or decreased number of repeats, with increases being more common. In patient population studies, a greater number of CAG repeats was generally correlated with an earlier age at onset and more severe disease. This explains why, in some families, the disease appears to be more severe in affected individuals of the most recent generation; in extreme cases, the child may be diagnosed before the parent or grandparent is showing signs of the disorder. However, because SCA7 age at onset, progression, and severity is variable, however, the number of CAG repeats cannot reliably predict the clinical course of the disease in an individual case. SCA7 is an autosomal dominant disorder; each child of an affected, or asymptomatic individual carrying the mutant SCA7 allele, has a 50% chance of inheriting the mutant gene.

Patient Preparation Testing of asymptomatic at-risk adults is predictive testing and the patient should have formal genetic counseling to explain the meaning, benefits, and risks of testing.

Aftercare For asymptomatic at-risk adults, post-test genetic counseling is appropriate to explain the test result and its significance.

Specimen Whole blood

Container Collect anticoagulated blood in either a lavender top (EDTA) tube or yellow top (ACD) Vacutainer® tube. Avoid use of heparin anticoagulants, which can interfere with polymerase chain reactions and endonuclease restriction enzyme activity.

Storage Instructions Blood samples can be stored and shipped at room temperature or refrigerated (4°C); do not freeze. Blood samples should be received in the testing laboratory within 4 days of draw to ensure an adequate DNA yield.

Causes for Rejection Frozen samples, whole blood in heparin anticoagulant (green top) or other inappropriate collection tube

Turnaround Time 7-14 days

Special Instructions To provide an optimal test interpretation, the testing laboratory needs to know the clinical diagnosis, family history, and whether DNA testing has confirmed the clinical diagnosis of an affected family member.

Reference Interval Normal SCA7 alleles have 4-19 CAG repeats. Abnormal mutant SCA7 alleles have 37 to >300 CAG repeats. SCA7 alleles with 28-36 CAG repeats are extremely rare and difficult to interpret.

Use Testing is useful to confirm a clinical diagnosis in an adult with cerebellar ataxia, retinopathy, and a family history of autosomal dominant ataxia. The DNA test can clarify a diagnosis in an adult presenting with visual loss as the initial sign, or alternatively, in adults presenting initially with only cerebellar ataxia. In children presenting with combined retinal disease and ataxia, the DNA test is useful to distinguish SCA7 from lipid storage diseases, ceroid lipofuscinoses, and mitochondrial encephalopathies. Testing of asymptomatic at-risk children under the legal age, for an adult-onset disorder for which no treatment exists, is not appropriate. Children presenting with symptoms usually benefit from having a specific diagnosis established.

Limitations The number of CAG repeats cannot reliably predict disease onset, severity, or cognitive ability in an individual patient. In cases with neonatal or childhood onset with typically larger numbers of CAG repeats, it is more difficult for the testing laboratory to detect the large mutant allele. In these cases, concerns about allele size detection should be discussed with the testing laboratory, especially when only a single sized allele is observed in an affected child (ie, an apparent SCA7 homozygote). SCA7 mutations appear to account for very few, if any, cases of idiopathic sporadic cerebellar ataxia.[1]

Methodology Polymerase chain reaction (PCR). A segment of the SCA7 gene is amplified from the patient's DNA, using primers that flank the CAG repeat region of the gene. After electrophoresis, the number of repeats is calculated from the product size. This reaction can detect both normal and (Continued)

Spinocerebellar Ataxia Type 7 DNA Test *(Continued)*

mutant SCA7 alleles. For neonatal and childhood onset cases, the number of CAG repeats can be very great; analysis by Southern blot may be necessary to detect the large mutant SCA7 allele.

Additional Information In the United States, SCA7 mutations are found in 4% of patients in the autosomal dominant cerebellar ataxia (ADCA) population; frequency varies by geography and ethnic background.[2] The normal function of the protein product of the SCA7 gene, ataxin-7, is not known. The CAG trinucleotide repeat motif is located in the coding region of the gene; each CAG repeat encodes a glutamine residue. In affected individuals, abnormally long polyglutamine tracts confer an unknown new function to ataxin-7; how this "gain-of-function" causes the disease is not clear. Testing for SCA7 disease is widely available; a list of clinical laboratories that perform this test can be found at GeneTest® (http://www.genetests.org). Prenatal testing is available, but should be preceded by formal genetic counseling to discuss difficult ethical issues related to testing for a (typically) adult-onset disease. Management of patients remains supportive, since there is no specific treatment available.

Footnotes

1. Schols L, Szymanski S, Peters S, et al, "Genetic Background of Apparently Idiopathic Sporadic Cerebellar Ataxia," *Hum Genet*, 2000, 107(2):132-7.

2. Moseley ML, Benzow KA, Schut LJ, et al, "Incidence of Dominant Spinocerebellar and Friedreich Triplet Repeats Among 361 Ataxia Families," *Neurology*, 1998, 51(6):1666-71.

References

Benton CS, de Silva R, Rutledge SL, et al, "Molecular and Clinical Studies in SCA-7 Define a Broad Clinical Spectrum and the Infantile Phenotype," *Neurology*, 1998, 51(4):1081-6.

Bird TD, "Hereditary Ataxia Overview," GeneClinics: Medical Genetics Knowledge Base, September 25, 2000, available at: http://www.geneclinics.org/profiles/ataxias/details.html.

Giunti P, Stevanin G, Worth PF, et al, "Molecular and Clinical Study of 18 Families With ADCA II: Evidence for Genetic Heterogeneity and de novo Mutation," *Am J Hum Genet*, 1999, 64(6):1594-1603.

Gouw LG, Castaneda MA, McKenna CK, et al, "Analysis of the Dynamic Mutation in the SCA7 Gene Shows Marked Parental Effects on CAG Repeat Transmission," *Hum Mol Genet*, 1998, 7(3):525-32.

Gouw LG and Ptacek LJ, "Spinocerebellar Ataxia Type 7," GeneClinics: Medical Genetics Knowledge Base, available at: http://www.geneclinics.org/profiles/sca7/details.html.

O'Sullivan-Smith C, Bennett RL, and Bird TD, "Spinocerebellar Ataxia: Making an Informed Choice About Genetic Testing," available at: http://depts.washington.edu/neurogen/AtaxiaBrochure99.pdf.

Internet Web Sites

www.genetests.org

www.geneclinics.org/profiles/ataxias/details.html

depts.washington.edu/neurogen/AtaxiaBrochure99.pdf

♦ **Steinert Disease** *see* Myotonic Dystrophy DNA Test *on page 712*

MOLECULAR ONCOLOGY

Diane L. Persons, MD

Wayne R. DeMott, MD

David S. Jacobs, MD

Contributors:

Beiyun Chen, MD, PhD

Uttam Garg, PhD

Research that is defining the molecular blueprints of malignancy has uncovered a bewildering array of gene-based mechanisms. Involvement of proto-oncogenes, oncogenes, tumor suppressor genes, molecular signaling mechanisms, and control of apoptosis includes, importantly, gene expression/transcription of effector proteins, and their interaction and collaboration as multimeric complexes. Malignant transformation usually requires activation of multiple proto-oncogenes and involvement of tumor suppressor genes (the multiple hit hypothesis). The activation of proto-oncogenes and oncogenes may be the result of point mutation, deletion, recombination, insertional mutation, chromosomal translocation, gene amplification, and/or abnormal expression of oncogene-encoded cell growth factors.[1] The pathway to malignant transformation includes interwoven viral DNA and damaged DNA resultant from environmental carcinogens. DNA-related molecular testing procedures have evolved in tandem with implications to the diagnosis of malignant neoplasia, but in particular with clinical applications in therapy, monitoring of therapy, and prognosis.

The genetic control and containment of cell maturation and proliferation is subverted and deranged with the onset of tumorigenesis. Tissue growth and molding during organogenesis is dependent upon orderly maturation of cells and also upon their timely elimination (demise). As noted above, a number of gene-based processes are involved in malignant transformation. Proto-oncogenes are derived from normal components of the genome, but may be activated to oncogenes. The viral oncogenes *abl*, *erb-B*, *ets*, *mos*, *myc*, *myb*, *H-ras*, *K-ras* and *Sis* include four with proto-oncogenes that may have a role in human malignancy (*myc*, *ras*, *abl* and *erb-B*). Proto-oncogenes encode proteins involved in normal growth and differentiation that can be activated (eg, by mutation or other genetic mechanism) to oncogenes which can then be activated to transform cells.

By negative regulation of transcription factors, by inhibition of apoptotic cell death, or by other mechanisms, tumor suppressor genes (eg, retinoblastoma (*RB*), and *p53* genes) lead to the development of malignancy. The proto-oncogene *bcl-2* is considered to act as a suppressor of programmed cell death (direct action in the prevention of apoptosis). *RB* and *p53* genes both encode nuclear phosphoproteins, the degree of phosphorylation fluctuating with the cell cycle. The phosphoprotein pRB exerts growth inhibition only in its hypophosphorylated form. In some tumors, presence of mutated *p53* is indicative of short survival and of resistance to chemotherapy.[2] Thus, the clinical interest in demonstrating expression/overexpression of *p53*.

The test listings in this chapter deal largely with molecular oncology and are certainly not comprehensive. A common thread is the often uncertain application and utility that these costly analyses may have in clinical environments. In screening situations, cost savings may be claimed, not only in terms of human concern and suffering but also in the identification of individuals who may benefit from preventive measures. The expense of some procedures may detract from compliance with recommended screening strategies, even when significant benefit is evident. Illustrative is the current status of screening for hereditary nonpolyposis colorectal cancer (HNPCC). A study from Finland concludes (on the basis of a 15-year trial in families with HNPCC) that screening by colonoscopy at 3-year intervals more than halves the risk of colorectal cancer, prevents death, and decreases overall mortality by about 65%.[3] Over half (57%) of members of HNPCC families, however, were found to have declined genetic testing.[4] Hopefully, new technology may improve (lower) the cost:benefit ratio.

Footnotes

1. Fitzgerald PJ, *From Demons and Evil Spirits to Cancer Genes: The Development of Concepts Concerning the Causes of Cancer and Carcinogenesis*, Washington, DC: The American Registry of Pathology, 2000, 207-40.

2. Soussi T, "The p53 Tumor Suppressor Gene: From Molecular Biology to Clinical Investigation," *Ann N Y Acad Sci*, 2000, 910:121-37.

3. Jarvinen HJ, Aarnio M, Mustonen H, et al, "Controlled 15-year Trial on Screening for Colorectal Cancer in Families With Hereditary Nonpolyposis Colorectal Cancer," *Gastroenterology*, 2000, 118(5):829-34.

4. Lerman C, Hughes C, Trock BJ, et al, "Genetic Testing in Families With Hereditary Nonpolyposis Colon Cancer," *JAMA*, 1999, 281(17):1618-22.

- ◆ **Amsterdam Criteria** *see* Colon Cancer, Hereditary Nonpolyposis Type *on page 724*
- ◆ **Angelman Syndrome** *see* Gene Rearrangement for Leukemia and Lymphoma *on page 725*
- ◆ **B-Cell Lymphomas** *see bcl-2* Gene Rearrangement *on page 720*
- ◆ ***bcl-2* Gene Analysis** *see bcl-2* Gene Rearrangement *on page 720*

bcl-2 Gene Rearrangement

Related Information
Apoptosis Assays *on page 402*
Gene Rearrangement for Leukemia and Lymphoma *on page 725*
Human Papillomavirus DNA Probe Test *on page 641*
Lymph Node Biopsy *on page 67*
p53, Functional Assay/Sequencing *on page 728*
Polymerase Chain Reaction *on page 713*

Synonyms *bcl-2* Gene Analysis; Southern Blot of *bcl-2* Gene Rearrangement

Applies to B-Cell Lymphomas; Oncogenes

Test Includes Identification of unique DNA bands associated with the *bcl-2* oncogene rearrangement in B-cell lymphomas

Abstract The *bcl-2* oncogene codes for a protein that is located in mitochondria of the cell. The *bcl-2* protein regulates cell death, and when it is overexpressed the cell is resistant to the "natural" death cycle, called apoptosis. Rearrangement of the *bcl-2* gene with the B-cell receptor genes is found in a number of different B-cell lymphomas. This translocation can be identified cytogenetically as t(14;18) in follicular lymphoma (FL), its original relationship, or large diffuse lymphomas.[1]

Specimen 0.1 g or more of frozen tissue, specifically from the involved area of the lymph node or tumor. Polymerase chain reaction protocols are available for use with tissue that has been formalin fixed/paraffin embedded.

Container Tissue must be shipped on dry ice or in 95% ethanol.

Collection Tissue must be carefully cut from the surgically removed tumor and contain at least 10% of tumor cells from the involved area.

Storage Instructions Tissue can be stored in a -70°C freezer until shipped.

Causes for Rejection Tissue samples that have thawed during transit cannot be used for DNA analysis.

Turnaround Time Results are usually available within 10 days to 2 weeks.

Reference Interval No rearrangement of *bcl-2* is normal.

Use Detect *bcl-2* rearrangement in B-cell lymphomas, in both frozen and paraffin sections. It is used most commonly to distinguish follicular lymphoma from follicular hyperplasia in lymphoid tissue. Reactive follicles are negative for *bcl-2*. The rearrangement is found in FL, large diffuse B-cell lymphomas, and undifferentiated lymphomas. Usually a reciprocal translocation with the J_H region on chromosome 14 is involved, thus forming t(14;18). Abnormal expression of *bcl-2* has also been identified in solid malignant neoplasms. In association with HPV, it may play a role in early stages of tumorigenesis of the uterine cervix.[2]

Limitations Rearrangement will not be found if the tissue is not from the involved tumor. Tissue samples that are too small will not yield enough DNA to do an accurate Southern blot analysis. The method is not useful to distinguish follicular lymphomas from other lymphoma cell types.

Methodology DNA is extracted from the clinical sample and digested with restriction enzymes. The digested fragments of DNA are electrophoresed in an agarose gel and then transferred to a nylon membrane (Southern blotting). The DNA on the membrane is hybridized with a labeled DNA probe specific for the *bcl-2* gene. Hybridization of the *bcl-2* probe is detected using autoradiography or enzymatic color development. Clinical samples are always compared to a normal control sample that does not have a *bcl-2* rearrangement. Hybridization to a DNA fragment different from the control sample typically indicates a rearranged *bcl-2* gene. PCR with conventional gel electrophoresis is now commonly used.

In immunohistochemical application, *bcl-2* is best recovered after fixation in B5 or Bouin fixed tissues, unless microwaved.

Additional Information The protein (p26 Bcl-2) coded for by the oncogene, *bcl-2*, acts by suppressing the cell death program or apoptosis.[3] Its role involves control of cell growth. The gene *bcl-x_L*, a homolog of *bcl-2*, encodes for p29 Bcl-x_L, also an antiapoptotic protein. p26 Bcl-2 and p29 Bcl-x_L localize on the outer mitochondrial membrane, smooth endoplasmic reticulum, and perinuclear membrane.[4] Their antiapoptotic effect results from inhibition of the mitochondrial permeability transition with increase in the generation of reactive oxygen species and by blocking the release of cytochrome c into the cytoplasm.[5,6] BAX, BAK, and BAD are proapoptotic members of the *bcl-2* family and can form heterodimers with Bcl-2 or Bcl-x_L. When the Bcl-2:BAX ratio is low (due to increase in BAX) cell death is caused by anticancer drug therapy.[7] Low levels of BAX may result in a poor response to chemotherapy[8] (see diagram).

Apoptosis occurs in all cells but is especially important in immune and hematopoietic cells, which have a high cell turnover rate. When the *bcl-2* gene is overexpressed, it will act to prevent apoptosis and may thus render cells resistant to cell death by irradiation and certain chemotherapeutic agents.[9,10] A translocation between immunoglobulin genes (heavy chain or light chain genes) and *bcl-2* results in the overexpression of *bcl-2* protein and thus the expansion of B cells due to suppression of cell death. This

translocation is found in some 85% of patients with follicular lymphoma. It is found in some cases of chronic lymphocytic leukemia, acute lymphoblastic leukemia, and small noncleaved cell lymphoma as well as cases of Hodgkin lymphoma[11] and myeloid neoplasms. The t(14;18) is rarely detected in monocytoid B-cell lymphoma and MALT lymphomas. Some 25% to 35% of cases of FL undergo transformation to a more aggressive diffuse subtype of lymphoma (actuarial risk of histologic transformation, 60% to 70% at 10 years).[12] This change is usually accompanied by the mutation/deletion of the p53 gene (and less commonly by alterations of the *c-myc* gene) in addition to the pre-existent *bcl-2* abnormality. Transformation has also been associated with inactivation of p16 by deletion, mutation or hypermethylation.[13] Overexpression of *bcl-2* is not pathognomic for lymphomas. It is found in 10% of reactive lymph nodes, and in some normal cells (eg, lymphoid and myeloid precursors, medullary thymocytes, most T cells, nongerminal center B cells, and plasma cells). It is not expressed in reactive germinal centers.

Increased *bcl-2* protein is reported in some carcinomas of prostate.[14] Immunostaining for *bcl-2* was not associated with outcome upon study of 90 meningiomas for *bcl-2* expression. *bcl-2* positivity, however, was more common in malignant meningiomas as compared to low-grade tumors.[15]

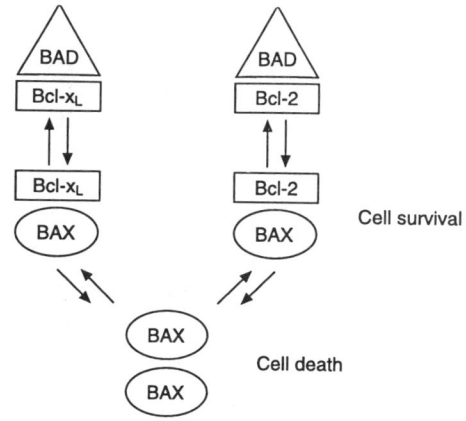

≥50% of BAX heterodimerized with
bcl-2 or *bcl-x_L* = survival

BAD is a regulator of apoptosis. BAD displaces BAX from *bcl-2*/BAX or *bcl-x_L*/BAX heterodimers, allowing more BAX/BAX homodimer formation, which promotes death.

Adapted from Yang E and Korsmeyer SJ, "Molecular Thanatopsis: A Discourse on the BCL-2 Family and Cell Death," *Blood*, 1996, 88(2):386-401.

Footnotes

1. Weiss LM, Warnke RA, Sklar J, et al, "Molecular Analysis of the t(14;18) Chromosomal Translocation in Malignant Lymphomas," *N Engl J Med*, 1987, 317(19):1185-9.
2. Saegusa M, Takano Y, Hashimura M, et al, "The Possible Role of *bcl-2* Expression in the Progression of Tumors of the Uterine Cervix," *Cancer*, 1995, 76(11):2297-303.
3. Cohen JJ, "Programmed Cell Death in the Immune System," *Adv Immunol*, 1991, 50:55-85.
4. Yang E and Korsmeyer SJ, "Molecular Thanatopsis: A Discourse on the *bcl-2* Family and Cell Death," *Blood*, 1996, 88(2):386-401.
5. Yang J, Liu X, Bhalla K, et al, "Prevention of Apoptosis by *bcl-2*: Release of Cytochrome c From Mitochondria Blocked," *Science*, 1997, 275(5303):1129.
6. Kluck RM, Bossy-Wetzel E, Green DR, et al, "The Release of Cytochrome c From Mitochondria: A Primary Site for *bcl-2* Regulation of Apoptosis," *Science*, 1997, 275(5303):1132.
7. Kim CN, Wang X, Huang Y, et al, "Overexpression of Bcl-x_L Inhibits Ara-C-Induced Mitochondrial Loss of Cytochrome c and Other Perturbations That Activate the Molecular Cascade of Apoptosis," *Cancer Res*, 1997, 57(15):3115-20.
8. Krajewski S, Blomqvist C, Franssila K, et al, "Reduced Expression of Proapoptotic Gene *BAX* Is Associated With Poor Response Rates to Combination Chemotherapy and Shorter Survival in Women With Metastatic Breast Adenocarcinoma," *Cancer Res*, 1995, 55(19):4471-8.
9. Strasser A, Harris AW, and Cory S, "*bcl-2* Transgene Inhibits T-Cell Death and Perturbs Thymic Self-Censorship," *Cell*, 1992, 67(5):889-99.
10. Sentman CL, Shutter JR, Hockenbery D, et al, "*bcl-2* Inhibits Multiple Forms of Apoptosis but Not Negative Selection in Thymocytes," *Cell*, 1992, 67(5):879-88.
11. Lones MA, Pinkus GS, Shintaku IP, et al, "*bcl-2* Oncogene Protein Is Preferentially Expressed in Reed-Sternberg Cells in Hodgkin Disease of the Nodular Sclerosis Subtype," *Am J Clin Pathol*, 1994, 102(4):464-7.
12. Kroft SH, Domiati-Saad R, Finn WG, et al, "Precursor B-Lymphoblastic Transformation of Grade I Follicle Center Lymphoma," *Am J Clin Pathol*, 2000, 113(3):411-8.
13. Pinyol M, Cobo F, Bea S, et al, "p16(INK4a) Gene Inactivation by Deletions, Mutations, and Hypermethylation Is Associated With Transformed and Aggressive Variants of non-Hodgkin's Lymphomas," *Blood*, 1998, 91(8):2977-84.
14. Kallakury BV, Figge J, Leibovich B, et al, "Increased *bcl-2* Protein Levels in Prostatic Adenocarcinoma Are Not Associated With Rearrangements in the 2.8 kb Major Breakpoint Region or With *p53* Protein Accumulation," *Mod Pathol*, 1996, 9(1):41-7.

15. Abramovich CM and Prayson RA, "Apoptotic Activity and *bcl-2* Immunoreactivity in Meningiomas. Association With Grade and Outcome," *Am J Clin Pathol*, 2000, 114(1):84-92.

References

Bagg A and Kallakury BV, "Molecular Pathology of Leukemia and Lymphoma," *Am J Clin Pathol*, 1999, 112(1 Suppl 1):S76-92.

Bhalla KN, Gerson SL, Grant S, et al, "Pharmacology and Molecular Mechanism of Action or Resistance of Antineoplastic Agents: Current Status and Future Potential," *Hematology: Basic Principles and Practice*, 3rd ed, Chapter 50, Hoffman R, Benz EJ Jr, Shattil SJ, et al, eds, New York, NY: Churchill Livingstone, 2000, 885-9

Corbally N, Grogan L, Keane MM, et al, "*bcl-2* Rearrangement in Hodgkin Disease and Reactive Lymph Nodes," *Am J Clin Pathol*, 1994, 101(6):756-60.

Cornfield DB, Mitchell DM, Almasri NM, et al, "Follicular Lymphoma Can Be Distinguished From Benign Follicular Hyperplasia by Flow Cytometry Using Simultaneous Staining of Cytoplasmic *bcl-2* and Cell Surface CD20," *Am J Clin Pathol*, 2000, 114(2):258-63.

Crisan D, "*bcl-2* Gene Rearrangements in Lymphoid Malignancies," *Clin Lab Med*, 1996, 16(1):23-47.

Gaidano G and Dalla-Favera, "Pathobiology of non-Hodgkin Lymphomas," *Hematology: Basic Principles and Practice*, 3rd ed, Chapter 66, Hoffman R, Benz EJ, Shattil SJ, et al, eds, Philadelphia, PA: Churchill Livingstone, 2000, 1213-29.

Inghirami G and Frizzera G, "Role of the *bcl-2* Oncogene in Hodgkin Disease," editorial, *Am J Clin Pathol*, 1994, 101(6):681-3.

Mies C, "Molecular Biological Analysis of Paraffin-Embedded Tissues," *Hum Pathol*, 1994, 25(6):555-60.

Pezzella F and Gatter K, "What Is the Value of *bcl-2* Protein Detection for Histopathologists?" *Histopathology*, 1995, 26(1):89-93.

Salomoni P, Condorelli F, Sweeney SM, et al, "Versatility of BCR/ABL-Expressing Leukemic Cells in Circumventing Proapoptotic BAD Effects," *Blood*, 2000, 96(2):676-84.

Warnke RA, Weiss LM, Chan JK, et al, "Tumors of the Lymph Nodes and Spleen," *Atlas of Tumor Pathology*, 3rd Series, Fascicle 14, Washington, DC: Armed Forces Institute of Pathology, 1995.

Breakpoint Cluster Region Rearrangement in CML

Related Information

Bone Marrow on page 410
Chromosome Analysis, Blood on page 361
Chromosome Analysis, Bone Marrow on page 362
Leukocyte Alkaline Phosphatase on page 455
Leukocyte Cytochemistry on page 456
Polymerase Chain Reaction on page 713

Synonyms bcr; bcr/abl Translocation; bcr/c-abl Translocation; Breakpoint Cluster Rearrangement; Chronic Myelogenous Leukemia; Gene Rearrangement, bcr

Applies to Bone Marrow Transplantation; Chronic Neutrophilic Leukemia; Oncogenes; Philadelphia Chromosome; Tyrphostins

Test Includes DNA detection of chromosomal translocation associated with chronic myelogenous leukemia (CML)

Abstract Chronic myelogenous leukemia (CML) is a myeloproliferative disorder characterized by the transformation of pluripotent hematopoietic stem cells. Ninety percent to 95% of the CML cases have a translocation between chromosome 9 and chromosome 22. This chromosomal translocation results in an abnormal gene rearrangement that can be detected using nucleic acid technology. The translocation involves a rearrangement of the breakpoint cluster region (bcr) gene located on chromosome 22 with the c-abl oncogene on chromosome 9.

Specimen Blood or bone marrow

Container Blood should be collected in a lavender top (EDTA) Vacutainer® tube; bone marrow should be collected in a syringe with heparin or transferred to a green top (heparin) tube or lavender top (EDTA) tube.

Turnaround Time 1-2 weeks

Reference Interval No rearrangement observed

Use This test is used for the confirmation of CML along with bone marrow examination, cytogenetics, and leukocyte alkaline phosphatase score.

The bcr/c-abl rearrangement assay is clinically useful for:
- confirmation of Philadelphia chromosome-positive CML
- diagnosis of Philadelphia-negative CML
- diagnosis and monitoring of CML blast crisis during and after chemotherapy and bone marrow transplantation
- detection of remission and early detection of relapse (for the characterization and monitoring of chronic myelogenous leukemia)

Methodology Leukocyte DNA is extracted, cut with restriction enzymes, electrophoresed in agarose, and then transferred to membranes using the Southern blot method. The membrane is hybridized with a gene probe that will bind only to the target bcr gene on the membrane. The banding pattern is developed by autoradiography or color detection methods. Detection of this translocation is also accomplished by reverse transcription polymerase chain reaction (RT-PCR). The RNA from patients' cells is extracted and transcribed into copy DNA (cDNA). The cDNA is then amplified by PCR with specific primers to detect the bcr-abl translocation.[1]

Additional Information Chronic myelogenous leukemia is a malignant clonal disorder of hematopoietic stem cells, characterized by increase in myeloid cells (and in many cases erythroid cells and platelets) in the peripheral blood, and by marked predominantly myeloid hyperplasia in the bone marrow. It affects males and females in a ratio of 1.5:1 with a peak incidence between 40 and 60 years of age and a median age at presentation of 53 years. All ages (including children) may be affected.

CML is characterized by a reciprocal translocation between chromosomes 9 and 22, producing the Philadelphia chromosome. The c-abl gene (a cellular oncogene - the Abelson proto-oncogene) is the human homologue of a gene for a murine oncogenic virus, the Abelson murine leukemia virus, that maps to chromosome 9q34. The hybrid bcr/c-abl gene is transcribed into an abnormal messenger RNA, which is translated into an abnormal tyrosine kinase of 210,000 molecular weight instead of the normal 145,000 molecular weight protein. More than 90% of patients with CML have the Philadelphia chromosome by cytogenetic analysis as well as rearrangement of bcr c-abl. Most patients with clinically documented CML that lack the Philadelphia chromosome still have the bcr/c-abl rearrangement. A small number of patients do not have the Philadelphia chromosome as the bcr/c-abl rearrangement. During reassessment many of these patients have a myelodysplastic syndrome, usually chronic myelomonocytic leukemia. A very small number of patients with clinical CML remain both Philadelphia chromosome negative and bcr/c-abl negative.

Cytogenetically the Philadelphia chromosome has been found in 20% to 25% of adults and 5% of children with acute lymphoblastic leukemia (ALL) and 2% of patients with acute myelogenous leukemia (AML).[2] The Philadelphia chromosome from ALL cases appears similar to CML Philadelphia chromosomes in cytogenetic analysis. However, the two chromosomes result from distinct molecular rearrangements that can be analyzed and detected with DNA analysis. Some ALL Philadelphia chromosomes have been found to be identical to the CML Philadelphia chromosome even at the molecular level. These ALL cases are generally regarded as the blast crisis of CML. Some laboratories perform a DNA amplification assay, polymerase chain reaction (PCR), for detection of this translocation. This may assist in the detection of minimal residual disease.[3]

In addition to the bcr-abl hybrid gene-encoded p210 tyrosine kinase, additional fusion proteins (p230 bcr-abl and p190 bcr-abl) have been described. The role of these proteins and certain of their domains in determining leukemic phenotype is under active investigation as is their interaction with signaling molecules to effect growth factor independence and inhibition of apoptosis.[4,5] The fusion protein p230 bcr-abl has been linked to the phenotype of chronic neutrophilic leukemia.[6]

Current therapy (for cure) is dependent upon bone marrow transplantation from sibling or volunteer donors.[7] Autologous transplantation, even with the use of chemotherapy,[8] antisense oligonucleotides,[9,10] or ribozymes,[11] to purge the (autologous) marrow of Ph+ cells has produced only short-lived cytogenetic responses in some patients.[4] The use of tyrphostins (to effect specific inhibition of abl tyrosine kinase [CGP57148P], now called Stl-571, a 2-phenylaminopyrimidine derivative) has been through phase I/II trials, has produced responses in interferon refractory CML patients, and appears to be a major advance in therapy.[12,13,14]

Footnotes

1. Tilzer LL and Concepcion EG, "Detection of the Gene Rearrangement in Chronic Myelogenous Leukemia With Biotinylated Gene Probes," *Am J Clin Pathol*, 1989, 91(4):464-7.
2. Kurzrock R, Gutterman J, and Talpaz M, "The Molecular Genetics of Philadelphia Chromosome-Positive Leukemias," *N Engl J Med*, 1988, 319(15):990-8.
3. Lee MS, Chang KS, Freireich EJ, et al, "Detection of Minimal Residual bcr/abl Transcripts by a Modified Polymerase Chain Reaction," *Blood*, 1988, 72(3):893-7.
4. Chopra R, Pu QQ, and Elefanty AG, "Biology of bcr-abl," *Blood Rev*, 1999, 13(4):211-29.
5. Horita M, Andreu EJ, Benito A, et al, "Blockade of the bcr-abl Kinase Activity Induces Apoptosis of Chronic Myelogenous Leukemia Cells by Suppressing Signal Transducer and Activator of Transcription 5-Dependent Expression of bcl-x_L," *J Exp Med*, 2000, 191(6):977-84.
6. Pane F, Frigeri F, Sindona M, et al, "Neutrophilic-Chronic Myeloid Leukemia: A Distinct Disease With a Specific Molecular Marker (bcr-abl With C3/A2 Junction)," *Blood*, 1996, 88(7):2410-4.
7. Hansen JA, Gooley TA, Martin PJ, et al, "Bone Marrow Transplants From Unrelated Donors for Patients With Chronic Myeloid Leukemia," *N Engl J Med*, 1998, 338(14):962-8.
8. Carlo-Stella C, Mangoni L, Piovani D, et al, "Selection of Philadelphia-Negative Progenitors From Chronic Myelogenous Leukemia," *Bone Marrow Transplant*, 1994, 14(Suppl 3):S45-8.
9. Pigneux A, Mahon FX, Jazwiec B, et al, "Effect of Antisense Oligonucleotides on CD34+ Cells From Chronic Myeloid Leukemia," *Leuk Lymphoma*, 2000, 36(5-6):569-78.

(Continued)

Breakpoint Cluster Region Rearrangement in CML
(Continued)

10. de Fabritiis P, Petti MC, Montefusco E, et al, "*bcr-abl* Antisense Oligodeoxynucleotide *In Vitro* Purging and Autologous Bone Marrow Transplantation for Patients With Chronic Myelogenous Leukemia in Advanced Phase," *Blood*, 1998, 91(9):3156-62.

11. Snyder DS, Wu Y, McMahon R, et al, "Ribozyme Mediated Inhibition of a Philadelphia Chromosome-Positive Acure Lymphoblastic Leukemia Cell Line Expressing the p190 *bcr-abl* Oncogene," *Biol Blood Marrow Transplant*, 1997, 3(4):179-86.

12. Druker BJ, Sawyers CJ, Talpaz M, et al, "Phase I Trial of a Specific *abl* Tyrosine Kinase Inhibitor CGP57148 in Interferon Refractory Chronic Myelogenous Leukemia," Abstract 24, Proceedings of ASCO, Atlanta, May 1999,

13. Deininger MW, Vieira S, Mendiola R, et al, "*bcr-abl* Tyrosine Kinase Activity Regulates the Expression of Multiple Genes Implicated in the Pathogenesis of Chronic Myeloid Leukemia," *Cancer Res*, 2000, 60(7):2049-55.

14. Stewart AK and Schuh AC, "White Cells 2: Impact of Understanding the Molecular Basis of Haematological Malignant Disorders on Clinical Practice," *Lancet*, 2000, 355(9213):1447-53.

References

Crisan D and Carr ER, "*bcr/abl* Gene Rearrangement in Chronic Myelogenous Leukemia and Acute Leukemias," *Lab Med*, 1992, 23:730-6.

Cross NC, Melo JV, Feng L, et al, "An Optimized Multiplex Polymerase Chain Reaction (PCR) for Detection of BCR-ABL Fusion mRNAs in Haematological Disorders," *Leukemia*, 1994, 8(1):186-9.

Faderl S, Talpaz M, Estrov Z, et al, "The Biology of Chronic Myeloid Leukemia," *N Engl J Med*, 1999, 341(3):164-72.

Groffen J, de Jong R, Haataja L, et al, "Phosphorylation Substrates and Altered Signalling in Leukemias Caused by *bcr-abl*," *Leukemia*, 1999, 13(Suppl 1):S81-S82.

Hehlmann R, Hochhaus A, Berger U, et al, "Current Trends in the Management of Chronic Myelogenous Leukemia," *Ann Hematol*, 2000, 79(7):345-54.

Herens C, Tassin F, Lemaire V, et al, "Deletion of the 5'-*abl* Region: A Recurrent Anomaly Detected by Fluorescence *In Situ* Hybridization in About 10% of Philadelphia-Positive Chronic Myeloid Leukaemia Patients," *Br J Haematol*, 2000, 110(1):214-6.

Horton Y, Ford A, Mackie MJ, et al, "Rapid Detection of *bcr-abl* and *pml-rara* Using Fluorescence *In Situ* Hybridization in Cytospin Preparations," *Clin Lab Haematol*, 2000, 22(2):97-101.

Laurent E, Talpaz M, Wetzler M, et al, "Cytoplasmic and Nuclear Localization of the 130 and 160 kDa *bcr* Proteins," *Leukemia*, 2000, 14(11):1892-7.

Roumiantsev S, de Aos IE, Varticovski L, et al, "The Src Homology 2 Domain of *bcr-abl* Is Required for Efficient Induction of Chronic Myeloid Leukemia-Like Disease in Mice but Not for Lymphoid Leukemogenesis or Activation of Phosphatidylinositol 3-Kinase," *Blood*, 2001, 97(1):4-13.

Salomoni P, Condorelli F, Sweeney SM, et al, "Versatility of BCR/ABL-Expressing Leukemic Cells in Circumventing Proapoptotic BAD Effects," *Blood*, 2000, 96(2):676-84.

Sawyers CL, "Chronic Myeloid Leukemia," *N Engl J Med*, 1999, 340(17):1330-40.

Sawyers CL and Witte ON, "Mechanisms of Leukemogenesis," *The Molecular Basis of Blood Diseases*, 3rd ed, Chapter 26, Stamatoyannopoulos G, Majerus PW, Perlmutter RM, et al, eds, Philadelphia, PA: WB Saunders Co, 2001, 832-60.

Stiewe T, Parssanedjad K, Esche H, et al, "E1A Overcomes the Apoptosis Block in *bcr-abl*⁺ Leukemia Cells and Renders Cells Susceptible to Induction of Apoptosis by Chemotherapeutic Agents," *Cancer Res*, 2000, 60(14):3957-64.

Talpaz M, Qiu X, Cheng K, et al, "Autoantibodies to *abl* and *bcr* Proteins," *Leukemia*, 2000, 14(9):1661-6.

Breast Cancer, Hereditary, BRCA1, BRCA2

Related Information
Breast Biopsy *on page 51*
CA 15-3, Serum *on page 127*
p53, Functional Assay/Sequencing *on page 728*
Polymerase Chain Reaction *on page 713*

Synonyms BRCA1; BRCA2; Familial Breast/Ovarian Cancer

Test Includes This molecular test involves end-to-end sequencing and/or protein truncation assay to detect carriers of mutations in the gene.

Abstract Mutations in BRCA1 and BRCA2 are characterized by predisposition to breast and ovarian cancers, but such mutations are rare in sporadic carcinoma of breast. About 5% of patients with carcinoma of breast have a pattern of autosomal dominant inheritance. Most of these patients have mutations of either BRCA1 or BRCA2 genes, which can exist and be passed to offspring by males as well as females. BRCA1 and BRCA2 are the two major susceptibility genes for breast carcinoma. Germline mutations of BRCA2 may cause fewer cases of breast carcinoma in young women

Table 1. Family History Risk Factors for Carrying a BRCA1 or BRCA2 Mutation

Known BRCA1 or BRCA2 mutation
Breast and/or ovarian cancer
Two or more family members <50 years with breast cancer
Male breast cancer
One or more family members <50 years with breast cancer plus Ashkenazi ancestry
Ovarian cancer plus Ashkenasi ancestry

Adapted from Armstrong K, Eisen A, and Weber B, "Assessing the Risk of Breast Cancer," *N Engl J Med*, 2000, 342(8):564-71.

than do those of BRCA1.[1] Complex interactions include patient age, family history, and other factors relevant to consideration for testing or interpretation of results.[2] Of cases of early-onset familial carcinoma of breast, a substantial proportion are related to BRCA1 or BRCA2 mutations.[3] See table.

Patient Preparation Pretest education and counseling should always be provided prior to orders for molecular genetic testing.

Specimen Whole blood

Container Blue top (sodium citrate) tube or yellow top (ACD) tube. Struewing et al used fingerstick procedures and collection cards.[4]

Storage Instructions All specimens should be sent to the laboratory **immediately** after collection, preferably by overnight delivery. All specimens should be kept at room temperature or refrigerated, never frozen.

Causes for Rejection Lysed or frozen blood sample

Turnaround Time Results are available in phases: top three mutations: 2-3 weeks; exon 11: 8 additional weeks; rest of the gene: 6-10 weeks

Use This test is indicated for families with a history of autosomal dominant early-onset breast/ovarian cancer (ie, identification of those with high risk). Genetic testing is appropriate when carcinoma of breast develops in younger women, especially in those with positive family history of breast and/or ovarian cancer, in first degree relatives, and/or women whose blood relatives bear BRCA1 or BRCA2 mutations.[5] Genetic testing can identify those who carry a mutation bearing serious risk from those who do not.

Limitations Statistical prophesies can lead to irreversible decisions (eg, prophylactic mastectomy or oophorectomy). Better data from controlled clinical trials will accumulate in future years. A role for modifying factors influencing whether or not a given BRCA mutation leads to carcinoma may include genetic, hormonal, dietary, or environmental influences. Other genes may cause carcinoma through different mechanisms. "Without facts about these other variables, the fortune tellers are reading a pretty cloudy crystal ball,"[6] an observation made in 1997. The advances made by 2001 are remarkable.[3]

Statistical models used in projections relevant to BRCA1 and BRCA2 have assumed that all carcinomas are the same and comparable to those in subjects without BRCA1 and BRCA2 mutations.

Patients with BRCA1- or BRCA2-associated carcinoma of breast recognize a degree of increased risk for contralateral breast neoplasm; many may consider prophylactic contralateral mastectomy and tamoxifen. Women with these mutations may consider prophylactic oophorectomy. The effect of such interventions on projected life-expectancy has been studied, but risks and uncertanties are recognized.[7]

Contraindications Routine widespread screening for such mutations is wasteful, and not warranted in the general U.S. population.[2,6]

Methodology Referral to a center providing specialized genetic counseling for BRCA testing is recommended. Call 1-800-422-6337.[8]

DNA and/or RNA are isolated from the specimen. A protein truncation assay will detect mutations that cause shortened protein products.[9] Regions within the BRCA1 gene are amplified by PCR and sequenced in entirety.

Additional Information Breast cancer is one of the most common diseases in women. The lifetime risk for a woman in the United States to develop breast cancer is 1 in 9 (11%). The risk for BRCA1/BRCA2 mutation increases with the strength of the family history and with earlier ages of onset (premenopausal). Although the occurrence of breast cancer **in families** may be due to chance alone or shared environment, the inheritance of a gene mutation increasing susceptibility to breast cancer is the most common reason. In October 1994, BRCA1, the first gene conferring an increased risk for the development of breast and ovarian cancer, was cloned.[10] It is estimated that 1 in 200 to 1 in 400 women carry BRCA1 mutations. Mutations in BRCA1 are thought to be responsible for about 50% of all inherited breast cancer and about 85% to 90% of breast/ovarian family histories.[11] The lifetime risk for breast cancer in a woman who has inherited a mutation in BRCA1 is about 85% by age 85 as opposed to 11% for women in the general population, and the risk for ovarian cancer is up to 45% by age 70 compared to 1% in the general population.[12] (See Table 2.) Once breast cancer has been diagnosed, the risk for carcinoma in the contralateral breast in the presence of hereditary breast cancer is about 60%. Breast and ovarian cancer survival rates are significantly better when diagnosis occurs in an early, localized stage.

When a BRCA1 or BRCA2 mutation is identified in a family, asymptomatic, at-risk women should be offered testing. Women found to carry the mutation should be encouraged to undergo earlier and more intensive surveillance for breast cancer, which is expected to lead to earlier detection and improved outcome. Some women may consider the option of prophylactic surgery (mastectomy and/or oophorectomy). BRCA1/BRCA2 testing can help rule out family members who, because they do not carry the mutation, do not require increased surveillance.

Different groups of genes are expressed by tumors with BRCA1 and those with BRCA2 mutations.[13]

Men who carry a BRCA1 mutation appear not to be at great risk for breast cancer but male carriers of BRCA1 or BRCA2 are at increased risk for prostate cancer.[4] The risk of prostate carcinoma is ~16% by age 70.[4] Men with BRCA2 are at risk for male carcinoma of breast.

See Breast Biopsy *on page 51.*

Table 2. The BRCA1 and BRCA2 Genes

Characteristic	BRCA1	BRCA2
Underlies what percentage of breast cancer in the population	2% to 3%	2% to 3%
Frequency in population Jewish individuals	1/345 1%	Unknown 1.2%
Chromosome location	17	13
Breast cancer risk if woman carries gene and has:		
Strong family history	50% by age 50 70% to 90% by age 70	Same as BRCA1
Limited pedigree or no family history	Uncertain; probably about 50%	Same as BRCA1
Ovarian cancer risk if woman carries gene and has:		
Strong family history	30% by age 50 20% to 45% by age 70	About 15%
Limited pedigree or no family history	Unknown	Unknown
Risk of male breast cancer	Low	6% to 7%

Some published papers provide somewhat different estimates of risk. BRCA genes may behave differently in different women.

Adapted from Muss HB, "Breast Cancer and Differential Diagnosis of Benign Nodules," *Cecil Textbook of Medicine,* 21st ed, Chapter 258, Goldman L and Bennett JC, Philadelphia, PA: WB Saunders Co, 2000, 1373-80.

Footnotes

1. Krainer M, Silva-Arrieta S, FitzGerald MG, et al, "Differential Contributions of *BRCA1* and *BRCA2* to Early-Onset Breast Cancer," *N Engl J Med,* 1997, 336(20):1416-21.
2. Newman B, Mu H, Butler LM, et al, "Frequency of Breast Cancer Attributable to *BRCA1* in a Population-Based Series of American Women," *JAMA,* 1998, 279(12):915-21.
3. Golub TR, "Genome-Wide Views of Cancer," *N Engl J Med,* 2001, 344(8):601-2.
4. Struewing JP, Hartge P, Wacholder S, et al, "The Risk of Cancer Associated With Specific Mutations of *BRCA1* and *BRCA2* Among Ashkenazi Jews," *N Engl J Med,* 1997, 336(20):1401-8.
5. Muss HB, "Breast Cancer and Differential Diagnosis of Benign Nodules," *Cecil Textbook of Medicine,* 21st ed, Chapter 258, Goldman L and Bennett JC, eds, Philadelphia, PA: WB Saunders Co, 2000, 1373-80.
6. Healy B, "BRCA Genes - Bookmaking, Fortunetelling, and Medical Care," *N Engl J Med,* 1997, 336(20):1448-9.
7. Schrag D, Kuntz KM, Garber JE, et al, "Life Expectancy Gains From Cancer Prevention Strategies for Women With Breast Cancer and *BRCA1* or *BRCA2* Mutations," *JAMA,* 2000, 283(5):617-24.
8. Armstrong K, Eisen A, and Weber B, "Assessing the Risk of Breast Cancer," *N Engl J Med,* 2000, 342(8):564-71.
9. Hogervorst FB, Cornelis RS, Bout M, et al, "Rapid Detection of BRCA1 Mutations by the Protein Truncation Test," *Nat Genet,* 1995, 10(2):208-12.
10. Miki Y, Swensen J, Shattuck-Eidens D, et al, "A Strong Candidate for the Breast and Ovarian Cancer Susceptibility Gene BRCA1," *Science,* 1994, 266(5182):66-71.
11. Narod SA, Ford D Devilee P, et al, "An Evaluation of Genetic Heterogeneity in 145 Breast-Ovarian Cancer Families. Breast Cancer Linkage Consortium," *Am J Hum Genet,* 1995, 56(1):254-64.
12. Easton DF, Ford D, and Bishop DT, "Breast and Ovarian Cancer Incidence in BRCA1-Mutation Carriers. Breast Cancer Linkage Consortium," *Am J Hum Genet,* 1995, 56(1):265-71.
13. Hedenfalk I, Duggan D, Chen Y, et al, "Gene-Expression Profiles in Hereditary Breast Cancer," *N Engl J Med,* 2001, 344(8):539-48.

References

Boyd J, Sonoda Y, Federici MG, et al, "Clinicopathologic Features of *BRCA*-Linked and Sporadic Ovarian Cancer," *JAMA,* 2000, 283(17):2060-5.

Castilla LH, Couch FJ, Erdos MR, et al, "Mutations in the BRCA1 Gene in Families With Early-Onset Breast and Ovarian Cancer," *Nat Genet,* 1994, 8(4):387-91.

Couch FJ, DeShano ML, Blackwood MA, et al, "*BRCA1* Mutations in Women Attending Clinics That Evaluate the Risk of Breast Cancer," *N Engl J Med,* 1997, 336(20):1409-15.

Frank TS, "Laboratory Determination of Hereditary Susceptibility to Breast and Ovarian Cancer," *Arch Pathol Lab Med,* 1999, 123(11):1023-6.

Friedman LS, Ostermeyer EA, Szabo CI, et al, "Confirmation of BRCA1 by Analysis of Germline Mutations Linked to Breast and Ovarian Cancer in Ten Families," *Nat Genet,* 1994, 8(4):399-404.

Greene MH, "Genetics of Breast Cancer," *Mayo Clin Proc,* 1997, 72:54-65.

Lerman C, Daly M, Masny A, et al, "Attitudes About Genetic Testing for Breast-Ovarian Cancer Susceptibility," *J Clin Oncol,* 1994, 12(4):843-50.

National Advisory Council for Human Genome Research, "Statement on Use of DNA Testing for Presymptomatic Identification of Cancer Risk," *JAMA,* 1994, 271(10):785.

Shattuck-Eidens D, McClure M, Simard J, et al, "A Collaborative Survey of 80 Mutations in the BRCA1 Breast and Ovarian Cancer Susceptibility Gene. Implications for Presymptomatic Testing and Screening," *JAMA,* 1995, 273(7):535-41.

Simard J, Tonin P, Durocher F, et al, "Common Origins of BRCA1 Mutations in Canadian Breast and Ovarian Cancer Families," *Nat Genet,* 1994, 8(4):392-8.

Wooster R, Neuhausen SL, Mangion J, et al, "Localization of a Breast Cancer Susceptibility Gene, BRCA2, to Chromosome 13q12-13," *Science,* 1994, 265(5181):2088-90.

Internet Web Sites

www.geneclinics.org/profiles/brca1

cancernet.nci.nih.gov/genesrch.shtml

A description of laboratory methods used is available through the National Auxiliary Publications Service (NAPS) and the Breast Cancer Information Core site (http://www.nhgri.nih.gov/Intramural_research/Lab transfer/Bic/).[3]

See NAPS document no. 05401 for 5 pages of supplementary material. Order from NAPS, c/o Microfiche Publications, P.O. box 3513, Grand Central Station, New York, NY 10163-3513. Remit in advance (in US funds only) $11.65 for photocopies or $5 for microfiche. Outside the U.S., add postage of $4.50 for up to 20 pages, $5.50 for over 20 pages, or $1.50 for microfiche. There is a $15 invoicing charge on all orders filled before payment.

♦ **Catch 22 Syndrome** *see* Gene Rearrangement for Leukemia and Lymphoma *on page 725*

♦ **Chemotherapy-Associated Hair Loss** *see p53,* Functional Assay/Sequencing *on page 728*

Chromosomal Translocations, Molecular Detection

Related Information

bcl-2 Gene Rearrangement *on page 720*
Bone Marrow *on page 410*
Breakpoint Cluster Region Rearrangement in CML *on page 721*
Chromosome Analysis, Blood *on page 361*
Chromosome Analysis, Bone Marrow *on page 362*
Gene Rearrangement for Leukemia and Lymphoma *on page 725*
Polymerase Chain Reaction *on page 713*

Synonyms Translocations, Chromosomal

Applies to GeneChip; Light Cycler; Microarray Technology; Prism 7700 Sequence Detector; Reverse Transcriptase - PCR; RT-PCR

Test Includes Identification of specific chromosomal translocations by polymerase chain reaction (PCR) or reverse transcriptase-polymerase chain reaction (RT-PCR) or Southern blot assay using cDNA probe

Abstract Many malignant solid tumors and leukemia/lymphomas often exhibit recurrent chromosomal translocations. These translocations may be unique for a particular type of tumor and thus provide definitive or confirmatory evidence for a specific diagnosis with implications for therapy and prognosis. Detection of specific chromosomal translocations can also play a role in post-treatment monitoring.

Specimen Peripheral whole blood, leukocytes, or bone marrow aspirate for leukemia/lymphoma; fresh and snap frozen tissue containing viable tumor cells for solid tumors/lymphoma; formalin-fixed paraffin-embedded tissue block may be used by some laboratories. The tissue must have been fixed promptly after excision and in some cases may not be subjected to prolonged formalin fixation.

Container Lavender top (EDTA) tube for liquid sample

Storage Instructions Transport to the laboratory immediately on ice or frozen; or store at -20°C (preferably -70°C) until transport.

Causes for Rejection Transport at room temperature, frozen tissue thawed during transit

Turnaround Time 3-5 days from receipt of specimen[1]

Reference Interval Chromosomal translocation should be absent in normal tissue. Report may include an illustration and/or interpretive report.

Use Molecular detection of specific chromosomal translocation in hematopoietic malignancies and in solid tumors when the involved genes are known to provide diagnostic and prognostic information; monitor patients after therapy

Limitations The sequences at the breakpoint regions on both chromosomes involved in the translocation must be known for molecular detection. Sampling of necrotic area in a tumor is a technical limitation.

Methodology For analysis by PCR, genomic DNA is extracted from the sample. PCR is performed using specific primers flanking the breakpoint involved in chromosomal translocation.

For analysis by RT-PCR, total RNA is extracted from the sample. Complementary DNA (cDNA) is produced using reverse transcriptase. Then the cDNA is subjected to PCR with specific primers flanking the breakpoint region.

Negative and positive controls are included with each set of analyses.

Automated, quantitative PCR instruments have been introduced (Applied Biosystems Inc Prism 7700 Sequence Detector, ABI, Foster City, CA, and Roche LightCycler, Roche, Indianapolis, IN). They utilize fluorescent oligonucleotide probe technology. Quantitation of nucleic acid targets is based on changes in fluorescence emission during the generation of specific PCR products.[1] Nucleotide microarray (GeneChip) technology is being applied to the detection of gene fusion.[1] These quantitative PCR methods may expedite the detection and quantitation of residual leukemia at the molecular level.[2] Molecular analysis extends cytogenetic assessment of the leukemias by providing improved sensitivity and specificity. Some 30% to 40% of pediatric B-cell ALL patients have nonrandom translocation fusion genes. Some cases (eg, *TEL-AML1* fusion) may be undetected by conventional chromosomal analysis (karyotyping).[1]

Additional Information The following table lists common chromosomal translocations in leukemia/lymphoma and solid tumors that may be detected by molecular methods (eg, PCR and RT-PCR).

The following is a list of genetic abnormalities that may occur in the pediatric acute leukemias.

Chromosomal translocations are of common occurrence in acute leukemias. The translocation usually results in the abnormal juxtaposition of one
(Continued)

Chromosomal Translocations, Molecular Detection
(Continued)

gene to another with creation of a unique "fusion gene". Such a chimeric gene, after transcription, results in a hybrid mRNA that produces a chimeric protein. Fusion proteins may disrupt growth or cell death in lymphoid or myeloid developing precursors with resultant leukemia. Another mechanism of leukemogenesis is post-translocation activation of a proto-oncogene with resultant overexpression of the oncogenic protein.[1] Translocations and other gene abnormalities often correlate with clinical features and in particular with severity and prognosis. As an example, in a case of acute lymphocytic leukemia, it would be of clinical significance to identify a 12;21 translocation (which results in fusion of the *TEL* and *AML1* genes), as such cases have a relatively favorable outcome with conventional chemotherapy but are subject to late relapse. For an excellent discussion of the chromosome/gene abnormalities relating to acute lymphoblastic and myeloid pediatric leukemias with clinical associations, the recent review by Bartolo and Viswanatha is recommended.[1] Translocations involving the *MLL* gene (chromosome 11q23) occur in 5% to 10% of human leukemias, fusion involving over 30 different partner genes. The clinical presentation and outcome of such cases is highly variable.[3]

Diagnosis	Chromosomal Translocation
Chronic myelogenous leukemia (CML)	t(9;22)(q34;q11)
Acute lymphoblastic leukemia (ALL)	t(9;22)(q34;q11) t(12;21)(p13;q22) t(1;19)(q23;p13)
Acute myeloid leukemia (AML)	t(8;21)(q22;q22) t(15;17)(q22;q12) inv(16)(p13;q22)
Lymphoma	t(14;18)(q32;q21) t(11;14)(q13;q32) t(2;5)(p23;q35)
Ewing sarcoma/peripheral neuroectodermal tumor	t(11;22)(q24;q12) t(21;22)(q22;q12)
Desmoplastic small round cell tumor	t(11;22)(p13;q12)
Myxoid/round cell liposarcoma	t(12;16)(q13;p11) t(12;22)(q13;q12)
Extraskeletal myxoid chondrosarcoma	t(9;22)(q22;q12) t(9;17)(q22;q11)
Malignant melanoma of soft parts/clear cell sarcoma	t(12;22)(q13;q12)
Synovial sarcoma	t(X;18)(p11;q11)
Alveolar rhabdomyosarcoma	t(2;13)(q35;q14) t(1;13)(p36;q14)
Dermatofibrosarcoma protuberans	t(17;22)(q22;q13)
Congenital fibrosarcoma	t(12;15)(p13;q25)

Cytogenetic Loci	Disease	Gene(s) Involved
t(9;22)(q34;q11)	B-precursor ALL	*BCR-ABL*
t(1;19)(q23;p13.3)	Pre-B-cell ALL	*E2A-PBX1*
t(12;21)(p13;q22)	P-precursor ALL	*TEL-AML1*
t(4;11)(q21;q23)	B-precursor/mixed lineage ALL	*MLL-AF4*
t(11;19)(q23;p13.3)	B-precursor/mixed lineage ALL	*MLL-ENL*
t(15;17)(q22;q12)	AML-M3 (promyelocytic)	*PML-RARα*
t(8;21)(q22;q22)	AML-M2	*AML1-ETO*
inv(16)(p13;q22); t(16;16)(p13;q22)	AML-M4Eo	*CBFβ-MYH11*
t(9;11)(p21;q23)	AML-M4 or -M5, some ALL	MLL-AF9
t(6;9)(p23;q24)	AML-M2 or M4	DEK-CAN

Footnotes
1. Bartolo C and Viswanatha DS, "Molecular Diagnosis in Pediatric Acute Leukemias," *Clin Lab Med*, 2000, 20(1):139-82.
2. Eckert C, Landt O, Taube T, et al, "Potential of LightCycler Technology for Quantification of Minimal Residual Disease in Childhood Acute Lymphoblastic Leukemia," *Leukemia*, 2000, 14(2):316-23.
3. Gore L, Ess J, Bitter MA, et al, "Protean Clinical Manifestations in Children With Leukemias Containing *MLL-AF10* Fusion," *Leukemia*, 2000, 14(2):2070-5.

References
Cassinat B, Zassadowski F, Balitrand N, et al, "Quantitation of Minimal Residual Disease in Acute Promyelocytic Leukemia Patients With t(15;17) Translocation Using Real-Time RT-PCR," *Leukemia*, 2000, 14(2):324-8.

Hayashi Y, "The Molecular Genetics of Recurring Chromosome Abnormalities in Acute Myeloid Leukemia," *Semin Hematol*, 2000, 37(4):368-80.

Hokland P and Pallisgaard N, "Integration of Molecular Methods for Detection of Balanced Translocations in the Diagnosis and Follow-up of Patients With Leukemia," *Semin Hematol*, 2000, 37(4):358-67.

Kurzrock R and Talpaz M, *Molecular Biology in Cancer Medicine*, 2nd ed, London, UK: Martin Dunitz Ltd, 1999.

Ladanyi M and Bridge JA, "Contribution of Molecular Genetic Data to the Classification of Sarcomas," *Hum Pathol*, 2000, 31(5):532-8.

Wattjes MP, Krauter J, Nagel S, et al, "Comparison of Nested Competitive RT-PCR and Real-Time RT-PCR for the Detection and Quantification of AML1/MTG8 Fusion

Transcripts in t(8;21) Postive Acute Myelogenous Leukemia," *Leukemia*, 2000, 14(2):329-35.

♦ **Chronic Myelogenous Leukemia** *see* Breakpoint Cluster Region Rearrangement in CML *on page 721*

♦ **Chronic Neutrophilic Leukemia** *see* Breakpoint Cluster Region Rearrangement in CML *on page 721*

Colon Cancer, Hereditary Nonpolyposis Type

Related Information
Carcinoembryonic Antigen, Serum *on page 135*
Chromosome Analysis, Lymph Node and Solid Tumor *on page 364*
Occult Blood, Stool *on page 315*

Synonyms Hereditary Nonpolyposis Colon Cancer; HNPCC Gene Testing; Lynch Syndrome; Nonpolyposis Type Colon Cancer

Applies to Amsterdam Criteria; Muir-Torre Syndrome

Test Includes This molecular test involves end-to-end sequencing of four genes in a sequential fashion: *hMLH1*, *hMSH2*, *hPMS1*, and *hPMS2*.

Abstract Polyposis and nonpolyposis syndromes include HNPCC as well as other entities. HNPCC is an autosomal-dominant syndrome with early onset of colonic carcinoma (usually proximally situated) and with increased risk for malignancy at other (extracolonic GI and GU) sites.

Mutations in at least four mismatch repair genes (MSH2[1], MLH1[2], PMS1, PMS2) are known to cause hereditary nonpolyposis colon cancer (HNPCC). Sequencing is the most accurate method for detection of mutations. Ninety percent of HNPCC mutations are found in MSH2 and MLH1.

Specimen Whole blood

Container Blue top (sodium citrate) tube or yellow top (ACD) tube

Storage Instructions All specimens should be sent to the laboratory **immediately** after collection, preferably by overnight delivery. All specimens should be kept at room temperature or refrigerated, never frozen.

Causes for Rejection Lysed or frozen blood sample

Turnaround Time Results are available in phases: MSH2: 6 weeks; MLH1: 6 additional weeks; PMS1 and PMS2 together: 4 additional weeks

Use The laboratory generally provides an interpretive report based upon direct sequencing analysis and/or the protein truncation assay. This test is indicated for families with a history of nonpolyposis colon cancer in an autosomal dominant pattern.

Limitations Because the genes for HNPCC have only recently been identified, HNPCC testing is much newer and is generally available only in investigational settings. Such settings provide the structure needed to assure that patients are adequately informed of the risks and benefits of testing and orchestrate the provision of genetic counseling. Such testing is costly. The cost of detecting gene mutations associated with HNPCC in a family depends on the number of genes which need to be sequenced. On the basis of telephone interview, it appears that over half (57%) of subjects (members of HNPCC families) declined genetic testing, with an important barrier to test acceptance being the presence of depression symptoms.[3]

Methodology Mutation analysis of mismatch repair genes. DNA is isolated from the specimen. Regions within the MSH2, MLH1, PMS1, and PMS2 genes are amplified by PCR and sequenced in entirety.

Additional Information Colorectal carcinoma (CRC) ranks second as a cause of cancer deaths in the United States. Some 130,200 persons in the U.S. are diagnosed with colorectal carcinoma annually, and approximately 56,300 will die from the disease.[4] A positive family history of CRC increases risk. The empiric risk increases with the strength of the family history and with earlier ages of onset. As a result, increased surveillance in first degree relatives of an individual with CRC is currently recommended for early detection of CRC. Five-year survival rates are substantially higher for localized CRC. Survival in asymptomatic patients is greater. About 15% to 20% of CRC may be due to an autosomal dominant mutation. Two of the types of inherited CRC are hereditary nonpolyposis colon cancer (HNPCC) and familial adenomatous polyposis coli (FAP). HNPCC is characterized by CRC in the absence of large numbers of polyps, early age of onset (mean 40-45 years of age), mucinous and poorly differentiated tumors, and an excess of tumors in the proximal colon. (Carcinoma develops early in polyps associated with HNPCC.) The lifetime risk for CRC in individuals who inherit a mutation associated with HNPCC is >90%. In addition, individuals with type II HNPCC are at increased risk for extracolonic cancers including tumors of endometrium, stomach, pancreaticobiliary system, ovary, small intestine, skin, bone marrow, larynx, and upper urological tract.[5] Because there are no distinguishing characteristics of HNPCC, historically the diagnosis has been made on the basis of the family history. The "Amsterdam Criteria" were developed to provide a uniform clinical method of diagnosis.[6] These criteria include histologically-verified CRC in three or more relatives, one of whom is a first-degree relative of the other two; CRC in at least two generations; and at least one CRC diagnosed before the age of 50. The limitations of the Amsterdam Criteria as a means of diagnosis became apparent upon the identification of the genes responsible for HNPCC. Mutations have been found in families that do not meet the Amsterdam Criteria, in particular, with the *hMSH6* gene.[7] Germline mutations in *hMSH6* are rare (possibly nonexistent) in HNPCC families that meet the Amsterdam Criteria. However, germline mutations in the *hMSH6* gene were reported in 8.1% of probands with colorectal cancer and a family history of cancer that fell short of the Amsterdam Criteria.[8] In addition, studies have shown that the presence of other cancers in the family including endometrial, ovarian, and ureteral tumors provides a strong indicator of HNPCC.

In 1993, the first HNPCC gene (MSH2)[1] was cloned, with the second gene (MLH1) cloned shortly thereafter in 1994.[2] Mutations of MSH2 and MLH1 account for 90% of HNPCC. Two additional HNPCC genes (PMS1 and PMS2) were cloned in 1994.[9] These genes encode DNA mismatch repair proteins that appear to function within a multimeric complex (to repair base pair mismatches and heteroduplex loops that develop during new DNA synthesis).[10] The significance of hMSH6 germline mutations is undergoing analysis. This highly polymorphic gene and its mutations (including missense, frameshifts, and splice-site types) appears to be associated with later-onset colon cancer with weaker familial phenotypes and not with families having clinical features of classic HNPCC.[8,10] With loss of the DNA mismatch repair system, genomic instability occurs with hypermutability (microsatellite instability). The latter is linked to about 90% of the cancers in HNPCC but also occurs in some 15% of sporadic tumors.[7] The identification of mutations in any of these genes permits accurate diagnosis of HNPCC. Once a mutation has been identified in a family at risk, presymptomatic relatives should be offered testing. If a relative is found to carry the mutation, annual colonoscopy is recommended. Colonoscopy is recommended over sigmoidoscopy especially in these individuals because of the predilection for right-sided tumors in HNPCC. Due to the high incidence of multiple synchronous and metachronous cancers, subtotal colectomy is recommended in affected individuals. In an individual who has already had partial resection, aggressive surveillance of the remaining colon is warranted.

A variant of HNPCC is the Muir-Torre syndrome in which sebaceous gland lesions exhibit microsatellite instability as do the colonic and endometrial tumors from these HNPCC patients.[11]

Footnotes

1. Fishel R, Lescoe MK, Rao MR, et al, "The Human Mutator Gene Homolog MSH2 and Its Association With Hereditary Nonpolyposis Colon Cancer," Cell, 1993, 75(5):1027-38.
2. Papadopoulos N, Nicolaides NC, and Wei YF, "Mutation of a mutL Homolog in Hereditary Colon Cancer," Science, 1994, 263(5153):1625-9.
3. Lerman C, Hughes C, Trock BJ, et al, "Genetic Testing in Families With Hereditary Nonpolyposis Colon Cancer," JAMA, 1999, 281(17):1618-22.
4. American Cancer Society, Cancer Facts and Figures - 2000, Atlanta, GA: American Cancer Society, 2000.
5. Marra G and Boland CR, "Hereditary Nonpolyposis Colorectal Cancer. The Syndrome, the Genes, and Historical Perspectives," J Natl Cancer Inst, 1995, 87(15):1114-25.
6. Baba S, "Hereditary Nonpolyposis Colorectal Cancer," Dis Colon Rectum, 1997, 40(10 Suppl):S86-S95.
7. Boland CR, "Molecular Genetics of Hereditary Nonpolyposis Colorectal Cancer," Ann N Y Acad Sci, 2000, 910:50-9.
8. Kolodner RD, Tytell JD, Schmeits JL, et al, "Germ-Line msh6 Mutations in Colorectal Cancer Families," Cancer Res, 1999, 59(20):5068-74.
9. Nicolaides NC, Papadopoulos N, Liu B, et al, "Mutations of Two PMS Homologues in Hereditary Nonpolyposis Colon Cancer," Nature, 1994, 371(6492):75-80.
10. Boland CR, "Roles of the DNA Mismatch Repair Genes in Colorectal Tumorigenesis," Int J Cancer, 1996, 69(1):47-9.
11. Swale VJ, Quinn AG, Wheeler JM, et al, "Microsatellite Instability in Benign Skin Lesions in Hereditary Nonpolyposis Colorectal Cancer Syndromes," J Invest Dermatol, 1999, 113(6):901-5.

References

Bronner CE, Baker SM, Morrison PT, et al, "Mutation in the DNA Mismatch Repair Gene Homologue hMLH1 Is Associated With Hereditary Nonpolyposis Colon Cancer," Nature, 1994, 368(6468):258-61.

Burke W, Petersen G, Lynch P, et al, "Recommendations for Follow-up Care of Individuals With an Inherited Predisposition to Cancer. Hereditary Nonpolyposis Colon Cancer," JAMA, 1997, 277(11):915-9.

Dicato M, Berchem G, Duhem C, et al, "The Biology of Colorectal Cancer," Semin Oncol, 2000, 27(5):2-9.

Hanski C, Scherübl, and Mann B, Colorectal Cancer. New Aspects of Molecular Biology and Immunology and Their Clinical Applications, Volume 910, New York, NY: The New York Academy of Sciences, 2000.

Hawk E, Lubet R, Limburg P, et al, "Chemoprevention in Hereditary Colorectal Cancer Syndromes," Cancer, 1999, 86(11 Suppl):2551-63.

Järvinen HJ, Aarnio M, Mustonen H, et al, "Controlled 15-Year Trial on Screening for Colorectal Cancer in Families With Hereditary Nonpolyposis Colorectal Cancer," Gastroenterology, 2000, 118(5):829-34.

Kinney AY, DeVellis BM, Skrzynia C, et al, "Genetic Testing for Colorectal Carcinoma," Focus Group Responses of Individuals With Colorectal Carcinoma and First-Degree Relatives, Cancer, 2001, 91(1):57-65.

Kinzler KW and Vogelstein B, "Lessons From Hereditary Colorectal Cancer," Cell, 1996, 87(2):159-70.

Lynch HT, Smyrk T, and Lynch JF, "Overview of Natural History, Pathology, Molecular Genetics and Management of HNPCC (Lynch Syndrome)," Int J Cancer, 1996, 69(1):38-43.

Iffit K, "Genetic Prognostic Markers for Colorectal Cancer," N Engl J Med, 2000, 342(2):124-5.

O'Leary TJ, "Molecular Diagnosis of Hereditary Nonpolyposis Colorectal Cancer," JAMA, 1999, 282(3):281.

Petersen GM, Brensinger JD, Johnson KA, et al, "Genetic Testing and Counseling for Hereditary Forms of Colorectal Cancer," Cancer, 1999, 86(11 Suppl):2540-50.

Shibata D and Aaltonen LA, "Genetic Predisposition and Somatic Diversification in Tumor Development and Progression," Advances in Cancer Research, Volume 80, Vande Woude GF and Klein G, eds, San Diego, CA: Academic Press, 2001, 83-114.

Syngal S, Fox EA, Li C, et al, "Interpretation of Genetic Test Results for Hereditary Nonpolyposis Colorectal Cancer. Implications for Clinical Predisposition Testing," JAMA, 1999, 282(3):247-53.

Wijnen J, Vasen H, Khan PM, et al, "Clinical Findings With Implications for Genetic Testing in Families With Clustering of Colorectal Cancer," N Engl J Med, 1998, 339(8):511-8.

Wijnen J, Vasen H, Khan PM, et al, "Seven New Mutations in hMSH2, and HNPCC Gene, Identified by Denaturing Gradient-Gel Electrophoresis," Am J Hum Genet, 1995, 56(5):1060-6.

♦ **Constant Region of T-Cell Receptor** see Gene Rearrangement for Leukemia and Lymphoma on page 725

♦ **E2F-1** see p53, Functional Assay/Sequencing on page 728

♦ **Ectrodactyly, Ectodermal Dysplasia and Facial Clefts (EEC) Syndrome** see p53, Functional Assay/Sequencing on page 728

♦ **Familial Breast/Ovarian Cancer** see Breast Cancer, Hereditary, BRCA1, BRCA2 on page 722

♦ **Familial Medullary Thyroid Carcinoma/Multiple Endocrine Neoplasia** see Multiple Endocrine Neoplasia/Familial Medullary Thyroid Carcinoma on page 727

♦ **Gene Array Technology** see Gene Rearrangement for Leukemia and Lymphoma on page 725

♦ **GeneChip** see Chromosomal Translocations, Molecular Detection on page 723

♦ **GeneChip p53 Assay** see p53, Functional Assay/Sequencing on page 728

♦ **Gene Rearrangement, bcr** see Breakpoint Cluster Region Rearrangement in CML on page 721

Gene Rearrangement for Leukemia and Lymphoma

Related Information
bcl-2 Gene Rearrangement on page 720
Body Cavity Fluid Cytology on page 372
Bone Marrow on page 410
Chromosomal Translocations, Molecular Detection on page 723
Chromosome Analysis, Lymph Node and Solid Tumor on page 364
Flow Cytometry, Overview on page 432
Fluorescence In Situ Hybridization on page 367
Histopathology on page 59
Immunoperoxidase Procedures on page 60
Immunophenotypic Analysis of Tissues by Flow Cytometry on page 62
Leukocyte Cytochemistry on page 456
Lymph Node Biopsy on page 67
Polymerase Chain Reaction on page 713
Skin Biopsy on page 71

Synonyms Leukemia Gene Rearrangement; Lymphocyte T-Cell Receptor Gene Rearrangement; Lymphoma Gene Rearrangement

Applies to Angelman Syndrome; Catch 22 Syndrome; Constant Region of T-Cell Receptor; Gene Array Technology; Joining Region of B-Cell Receptor; Kappa Light Chains; Lambda Light Chains; Newborn Aneuploidy Detection; Prader-Willi Syndrome; Velocardiofacial Syndrome; Williams Syndrome

Test Includes Detection of unique DNA rearrangements associated with T- and B-cell leukemias and lymphomas

Abstract Molecular biology techniques allow for detection of receptor gene rearrangement in germline DNA of maturing T or B cells. As lymphoid cells mature they go through rearrangements of variable, joining, and constant DNA coding regions of immunoglobulin or T-cell receptors. Such recombinations allow for almost unlimited diversity of immune responses, allowing response to literally millions of antigens. Lymphoma and lymphocytic leukemia are neoplastic disorders, diagnosis of which sometimes requires demonstration of clonal expansion of lymphoid cells. In the typical case, demonstration of clonality may be satisfied immunophenotypically by demonstration of surface T- and B-cell markers. When immunophenotypic methods fail to demonstrate clonality, the detection of T-cell and B-cell receptor gene rearrangements may be an invaluable test in cases in which morphologic diagnosis is difficult.

Specimen Peripheral whole blood for leukemia or lymphoma cells. **Unfixed, fresh or frozen lymph node biopsy** of suspected lymphoma is obtained during surgery for histopathologic diagnosis, immunophenotyping, and gene rearrangement assay. Other tissue (eg, skin biopsies, gastrointestinal tissue, and bone marrow) may also be studied for presence of variant gene rearrangement. Use of paraffin-embedded tissue is possible in some laboratories. Consultation with the laboratory (or laboratories) performing or providing referral of the specimen is critical **PRIOR** to sampling of blood, marrow, and/or tissue.

Container Lavender top (EDTA) tube for fresh whole blood sample

Storage Instructions Isolated white cells, lymph nodes, or tissue can be frozen at -70°C until DNA is extracted.

Causes for Rejection Insufficient DNA isolated. Muscle tissue yields little DNA for analysis.

Turnaround Time PCR: 2-4 days; Southern blot: 10 days to 3 weeks
(Continued)

Gene Rearrangement for Leukemia and Lymphoma
(Continued)

Reference Interval No unique rearrangement of genes for T- and B-cell receptors is found in normal white blood cells. An interpretive report is usually included with results.

Use Gene rearrangement analysis may be used to supplement and complement the results of more conventional studies that rely on histopathologic, cytogenetic, and/or immunophenotypic techniques in difficult diagnoses of leukemia/lymphoma. Gene rearrangement studies have revealed that (of cases previously considered non-B, non-T cell) most lymphoid leukemias are pre-B cell in origin rather than non-B, non-T cell. Such leukemic cells have rearrangements of genes coding for B-cell receptors, but are too immature to express cytoplasmic or surface immunoglobulins. Lymphoid leukemia and lymphoma may be of T-cell phenotype, as indicated by the use of probes designed to detect rearrangements of genes coding for T-cell receptors. Rarely, lymphoid neoplasms may have rearrangements of both T- and B-cell genes.[1]

Table 1: Comparison of Conventional Karyotypic (Cytogenetic) Analysis With Molecular (PCR-Based) Analysis

	Karyotypic Analysis	Molecular Analysis
Requirement for fresh, viable, dividing cells	Yes	No
Average turnaround time	2-3 wk	2-4 d
Ability to detect submicroscopic abnormalities	No	Yes
Ability to detect numeric abnormalities	Yes	No
Approximate sensitivity for minimal disease detection (%)	5-10	0.001-1

Adapted from Bagg A and Kallakury B, "Molecular Pathology of Leukemia and Lymphoma," *Am J Clin Pathol*, 1999, 112(Suppl 1):S76-S92.

Table 2: Examples of Non-neoplastic Disorders Associated With Clonal Antigen Receptor Gene Rearrangements

Autoimmune diseases
Sjögren syndrome
Rheumatoid arthritis
Immunodeficiency states
Congenital
Post-transplantation immunosuppression
Human immunodeficiency virus
Miscellaneous immunologic dysregulation
Castleman disease
Angioimmunoblastic lymphadenopathy
Dermatologic disorders
Lymphomatoid papulosis
Acute lichenoid pityriasis

Adapted from Bagg A and Kallakury B, "Molecular Pathology of Leukemia and Lymphoma," *Am J Clin Pathol*, 1999, 112(Suppl 1):S76-S92.

Limitations Some tissues yield little DNA or DNA that is degraded. Lymph nodes with <1% tumor cells cannot provide evidence of gene rearrangements when the Southern blotting method is used. Conventional cytogenetic and molecular (PCR-based) analyses are complimentary in many respects, but karyotypic analysis is unable to detect submicroscopic abnormalities (see Table 1).[2] Result of PCR analysis, positive for antigen receptor gene rearrangement, may not always be associated with malignancy. Disorders with immunologic dysregulation may occur with antigen receptor rearrangements (see Table 2).[2]

Methodology Genomic DNA is extracted and then digested with restriction endonucleases. Digested DNA is electrophoresed in agarose gel and then transferred to nylon membrane (Southern blotting). DNA is exposed to labeled gene probes. Specificity of most probes **is nearly perfect**. Detection of rearrangements thus may help to demonstrate clonality (neoplastic nature) of an atypical lymphoid lesion. Membrane containing hybridized DNA-probe complexes are examined for bands after autoradiography or color detection to ascertain if germline or unique gene rearrangements are present.

While detection of rearrangements by Southern blot hybridization is more definitive, initial testing using polymerase chain reaction (PCR) based procedures for immunoglobulin or T-cell receptor gene rearrangement is recommended. PCR studies, technically more efficient, may be used to establish the presence of a clonal B- or T-cell proliferative process and yield results in 3-4 days, versus 2-3 weeks for Southern blot analysis. In many laboratories, PCR serves as the first test followed by Southern blotting if results are negative or uninterpretable. Guidelines for interpretation and use of molecular pathology-based procedures in the diagnosis of lymphomas and leukemias have been published.[2]

A new approach in the use of PCR for detection of T-cell receptor beta chain rearrangement has been described. Family-specific JP primers are utilized with the resulting PCR products analyzed by high resolution GeneScan technique.[3]

Additional Information These procedures are useful to determine whether T- or B-cell gene rearrangements exist in lymphoid neoplasms. Most commonly used probes are for the joining region of B-cell receptors (J_H) and the constant region of the T-cell receptor (C_BT). B-cell maturation may be further categorized by determining if kappa and/or lambda light chain genes have undergone rearrangement, using probes directed against their constant or joining DNA regions. Gene rearrangements may be detected in minute quantities of tissue, sometimes as little as 200 mg. The assays are sensitive such that gene rearrangements may be detected in larger specimens even if the percentage of cancer cells is 1%. Gene rearrangement studies are invaluable adjunctive tests that may provide evidence of clonality in an atypical lymphoid infiltrate when other methods fail. Application of PCR to detection of minimal residual disease is of increasing import. There is need for standardization.[2] General consensus holds that in both pediatric and adult acute lymphocytic leukemia (ALL), a level >0.1% leukemic cells at the end of induction chemotherapy is strongly predictive of subsequent marrow relapse. Continuing rearrangement of antigen receptor (AR) loci in ALL may confound interpretation. A number of variables must be considered.[2] PCR for AR gene rearrangements may, in some conditions (eg, B-cell precursor acute lymphoblastic leukemia) avoid misleading results of flow cytometric monitoring (by immunophenotypic analysis) of post-therapy bone marrow specimens.[4] The application of gene array technology to the study of lymphoid neoplasms found that the gene clusterin is present specifically in anaplastic large-cell lymphoma.[5]

Footnotes

1. Farkas DH, "The Southern Blot: Application to the B- and T-Cell Gene Rearrangement Test," *Lab Med*, 1992, 23(11):723-9.
2. Bagg A and Kallakury BL, "Molecular Pathology of Leukemia and Lymphoma," *Am J Clin Pathol*, 1999, 112(Suppl 1):S76-S92.
3. Assaf C, Hummel M, Dippel E, et al, "High Detection Rate of T-Cell Receptor Beta Chain Rearrangements in T-Cell Lymphoproliferations by Family Specific Polymerase Chain Reaction in Combination With the GeneScan Technique and DNA Sequencing," *Blood*, 2000, 96(2):640-6.
4. Kallakury BV, Hartman DP, Cossman J, et al, "Post-therapy Surveillance of B-Cell Precursor Acute Lymphoblastic Leukemia. Value of Polymerase Chain Reaction and Limitations of Flow Cytometry," *Am J Clin Pathol*, 1999, 111(6):759-66.
5. Wellmann A, Thieblemont C, Pittaluga S, et al, "Detection of Differentially Expressed Genes in Lymphomas Using cDNA Arrays: Identification of Clusterin as a New Diagnostic Marker for Anaplastic Large-Cell Lymphomas," *Blood*, 2000, 96(2):398-404.

References

Alkan S, Cosar E, Ergin M, et al, "Detection of T-Cell Receptor-γ Gene Rearrangement in Lymphoproliferative Disorders by Temperature Gradient Gel Electrophoresis," *Arch Pathol Lab Med*, 2001, 125(2):202-7.

Avet-Loiseau H, Daviet A, Brigaudeau C, et al, "Cytogenetic, Interphase, and Multicolor Fluorescence *In Situ* Hybridization Analyses in Primary Plasma Cell Leukemia: A Study of 40 Patients at Diagnosis, on Behalf of the Intergroupe Francophone du Myélome and the Groupe Francais de Cytogénétique Hématologique," *Blood*, 2001, 97(3):822-5.

Bartolo C and Viswanatha DS, "Molecular Diagnosis in Pediatric Acute Leukemias," *Clin Lab Med*, 2000, 20(1):139-82.

Beishuizen A, Verhoeven MA, Mol EJ, et al, "Detection of Immunoglobulin Heavy-Chain Gene Rearrangements by Southern Blot Analysis: Recommendations for Optimal Results," *Leukemia*, 1993, 7(12):2045-53.

Biondi A, Cimino G, Pieters R, et al, "Biological and Therapeutic Aspects of Infant Leukemia," *Blood*, 2000, 96(1):24-33.

Coad JE, Olson DJ, Lander TA, et al, "Molecular Assessment of Clonality in Lymphoproliferative Disorders: I. Immunoglobulin Gene Rearrangements," *Mol Diagn*, 1996, 1(4):335-55.

Coad JE, Olson DJ, Lander TA, et al, "Molecular Assessment of Clonality in Lymphoproliferative Disorders: II. T-Cell Receptor Gene Rearrangements," *Mol Diagn*, 1998, 2(1):69-81.

Eckert C, Landt O, Taube T, et al, "Potential of LightCycler Technology for Quantification of Minimal Residual Disease in Childhood Acute Lymphoblastic Leukemia," *Leukemia*, 2000, 14(2):316-23.

Griesser H, "Gene Rearrangements and Chromosomal Translocations in T-Cell Lymphoma: Diagnostic Applications and Their Limits," *Virchows Arch*, 1995, 426(4):323-38.

Heaney ML and Golde DW, "Myelodysplasia," *N Engl J Med*, 1999, 340(21):1649-60.

Kirsch IR and Kuehl WM, "Lymphopoiesis: Gene Rearrangements in Lymphoid Cells," *The Molecular Basis of Blood Diseases*, 3rd ed, Part III, Stamatoyannopoulos G, Majerus PW, Perlmutter RM, et al, eds, Philadelphia PA: WB Saunders Company, 2001, 389-430.

Krause JR, "Clinical Use of B- and T-Cell Gene Rearrangement Analysis in Hematopoietic Disorders," *Clin Lab Med*, 1996, 16(1):1-21.

Krauter J, Peter W, Pascheberg U, et al, "Detection of Karyotypic Aberrations in Acute Myeloblastic Leukaemia: A Prospective Comparison Between PCR/FISH and Standard Cytogenetics in 140 Patients With *de novo* AML," *Br J Haematol*, 1998, 103(1):72-8.

Löwenberg B, Downing JR, and Burnett A, "Acute Myeloid Leukemia," *N Engl J Med*, 1999, 341(14):1051-61.

Nakao M, Janssen JW, Seriu T, et al, "Rapid and Reliable Detection of N-ras Mutations in Acute Lymphoblastic Leukemia by Melting Curve Analysis Using LightCycler Technology," *Leukemia*, 2000, 14(2):312-5.

Schröck E, du Manoir S, Veldman T, et al, "Multicolor Spectral Karyotyping of Human Chromosomes," *Science*, 1996, 273(5274):494-7.

Wilkens L, Tchinda J, Burkhardt D, et al, "Analysis of Hematologic Diseases Using Conventional Karyotyping, Fluorescence *In Situ* Hybridization (FISH), and Comparative Genomic Hybridization (CGH)," *Hum Pathol*, 1998, 29(8):833-9.

Multiple Endocrine Neoplasia/Familial Medullary Thyroid Carcinoma

Related Information
Calcitonin, Serum or Plasma *on page 129*
Calcium, Serum *on page 131*
Catecholamines, Fractionation, Urine *on page 139*
Metanephrines, Urine or Plasma *on page 223*
Pancreatic Polypeptide, Human, Serum or Plasma *on page 242*
Parathyroid Hormone, Serum *on page 243*
Polymerase Chain Reaction *on page 713*

Synonyms Familial Medullary Thyroid Carcinoma/Multiple Endocrine Neoplasia; MEN 2A; MEN 2B; MEN2/FMTC; RET Gene Testing

Applies to Multiple Endocrine Neoplasia (MEN), Types 2A, 2B; RET Proto-oncogene

Test Includes This molecular test can detect point mutations in the RET gene.

Abstract Medullary thyroid carcinoma (MTC) is an entity distinct from papillary or follicular carcinoma of thyroid. It may be sporadic as well as familial. See Calcitonin, Serum or Plasma *on page 129*. MTC is the major cause of death in individuals with MEN 2A and with familial medullary thyroid carcinoma (FMTC).

Mutations in the RET proto-oncogene associated with FMTC and multiple endocrine neoplasia (type 2A and 2B) (MEN 2A and 2B) were first described in 1993.[1] Mutations are detected by polymerase chain reaction (PCR) followed by restriction digestion or enzyme sequencing the DNA of the RET gene. Testing for RET mutations in all individuals with MTC has been recommended since September of 1994[2] and has become the clinically accepted approach to the diagnosis of MEN 2 and FMTC. RET analysis followed by linkage analysis in the absence of RET mutations identify subjects with MEN 2A and FMTC.[3]

Specimen Whole blood

Container Blue top (sodium citrate) tube or yellow top (ACD) tube or EDTA tube. Avoid collection in heparin tube; heparin inhibits PCR.

Storage Instructions All specimens should be sent to the laboratory **immediately** after collection, preferably by overnight delivery. All specimens should be kept at room temperature or refrigerated, never frozen.

Causes for Rejection Lysed or frozen blood sample

Turnaround Time Results are usually available in 3 weeks.

Use The laboratory generally provides an interpretive report based upon direct sequencing analysis. This test is indicated for families with a history of MEN 2A or MEN 2B or FMTC (autosomal dominant). Hyperparathyroidism also occurs in MEN type 2A (see Parathyroid Hormone, Serum *on page 243*).

Limitations If a high-risk affected individual tests negative for RET mutations, an inherited form of cancer may still exist and appropriate genetic counseling should be provided. This evaluation is costly.

Methodology DNA is isolated from peripheral blood leukocytes. Regions within the RET gene (exons 10, 11, 13, 14, and 16) are amplified by PCR and sequenced in entirety.

Additional Information Medullary thyroid carcinoma (MTC) is a malignancy of the calcitonin-secreting cells (C cells) of the thyroid and accounts for about 10% of thyroid cancer. One in 5000 individuals is affected with MTC each year; about 50% of patients have metastases at the time of diagnosis. The historical 10-year survival is about 50%. About 20% of MTC occurs as part of one of three familial syndromes: multiple endocrine neoplasia type 2A (MEN 2A) characterized by MTC, pheochromocytoma (~50%), and hyperparathyroidism (~10%); multiple endocrine neoplasia type 2B (MEN 2B) consisting of MTC, pheochromocytoma (~50%), ganglioneuromatosis, and marfanoid habitus; and familial medullary thyroid carcinoma syndrome (FMTC) characterized by MTC alone. All are autosomal dominantly inherited. They are caused by germline mutations in the RET proto-oncogene, which is located in the pericentromeric region of chromosome 10, band q11.2.[3] Virtually everyone who inherits a mutation in RET will develop MTC. Prior to the identification of the RET gene in 1993, it was the standard of practice to perform annual biochemical screening on all individuals in definite or suspected FMTC, MEN 2A, and MEN 2B families. Because it is not possible to distinguish sporadic from familial tumors histopathologically and because the family history is often unreliable, biochemical screening has been performed on first-degree relatives of many individuals affected with apparently sporadic MTC. Such screening has been performed annually from 5 years of age to about 40 years to detect C-cell hyperplasia (the precursor of medullary thyroid carcinoma) as early as possible, followed by total thyroidectomy. Pentagastrin stimulation testing yields false positives, false negatives, and equivocal results requiring test repetition.[4] See Calcitonin, Serum or Plasma *on page 129*. The majority of cases of MTC are **not familial**, and in those families in which it is inherited, 50% of first-degree relatives would be expected not to have inherited the gene. DNA testing for mutations in the RET gene in all individuals with MTC accurately diagnoses a heritable form of MTC in >90% of cases and identifies family members who have inherited the mutation.[5] Family members who have not inherited the mutation require no further screening. It is recommended that those family members who do inherit the mutation undergo thyroidectomy. Additionally, with the knowledge that such individuals are at risk for other MEN 2-associated tumors, biochemical screening for premorbid detection of pheochromocytoma and hyperparathyroidism can be initiated.

The risk of C-cell disease, pheochromocytoma, and hyperparathyroidism was higher in subjects with codon 634 mutations than in patients with other mutations in a series of 348 patients and family members at risk. Codon 634 is often involved in MEN 2A.[3]

Footnotes
1. Donis-Keller H, Dou S, Chi D, et al, "Mutations in the RET Proto-Oncogene Are Associated With MEN 2A and FMTC," *Hum Mol Genet*, 1993, 2(7):851-6.
2. Utiger RD, "Medullary Thyroid Carcinoma, Genes, and the Prevention of Cancer," *N Engl J Med*, 1994, 331(13):870-1.
3. Heshmati HM, Gharib H, Khosla S, et al, "Genetic Testing in Medullary Thyroid Carcinoma Syndromes: Mutation Types and Clinical Significance," *Mayo Clin Proc*, 1997, 72(5):430-6.
4. Lips CJ, Landsvater RM, Höppener JW, et al, "Clinical Screening as Compared With DNA Analysis in Families With Multiple Endocrine Neoplasia Type 2A," *N Engl J Med*, 1994, 331(13):828-35.
5. Chi DD, Toshima K, Donis-Keller H, et al, "Predictive Testing for Multiple Endocrine Neoplasia Type 2A (MEN 2A) Based on the Detection of Mutations in the RET Proto-Oncogene," *Surgery*, 1994, 116(2):124-33.

References
Eng C, "The RET Proto-oncogene in Multiple Endocrine Neoplasia Type 2 and Hirschsprung's Disease," *N Engl J Med*, 1996, 335(13):943-51.

Eng C, Clayton D, Schuffenecker I, et al, "The Relationship Between Specific RET Proto-oncogene Mutations and Disease Phenotype in Multiple Endocrine Neoplasia Type 2," International RET Mutation Consortium Analysis, *JAMA*, 1996, 276(19):1575-9.

Pacak K, Linehan M, Eisenhofer G, et al, "Recent Advances in Genetics, Diagnosis, Localization, and Treatment of Pheochromocytoma," *Ann Intern Med*, 2001, 134(4):315-29.

Xue F, Yu H, Maurer LH, et al, "Germline RET Mutations in MEN 2A and FMTC and Their Detection by Simple DNA Diagnostic Tests," *Hum Mol Genet*, 1994, 3(4):635-8.

Zedenius J, Wallin G, and Hamberger B, "Somatic and MEN 2A De Novo Mutations Identified in the RET Proto-Oncogene by Screening of Sporadic MTCs," *Hum Mol Genet*, 1994, 3(8):1259-62.

- ♦ **Nonpolyposis Type Colon Cancer** *see* Colon Cancer, Hereditary Nonpolyposis Type *on page 724*

- ♦ **Nuclear Phosphoprotein p53** *see* p53, Functional Assay/Sequencing *on page 728*

- ♦ **Oncogenes** *see* bcl-2 Gene Rearrangement *on page 720*

- ♦ **Oncogenes** *see* Breakpoint Cluster Region Rearrangement in CML *on page 721*

- ♦ **p110RB1** *see* Retinoblastoma Gene DNA Detection *on page 729*

p53, Functional Assay/Sequencing

Related Information
Apoptosis Assays *on page 402*
Breast Biopsy *on page 51*
Breast Cancer, Hereditary, BRCA1, BRCA2 *on page 722*
Histopathology *on page 59*
Human Papillomavirus DNA Probe Test *on page 641*
Immunoperoxidase Procedures *on page 60*
Polymerase Chain Reaction *on page 713*
Retinoblastoma Gene DNA Detection *on page 729*

Synonyms Growth Suppressor/Oncoprotein p53; Nuclear Phosphoprotein *p53*; *p53* Tumor Suppressor Gene

Applies to Chemotherapy-Associated Hair Loss; E2F-1; Ectrodactyly, Ectodermal Dysplasia and Facial Clefts (EEC) Syndrome; GeneChip p53 Assay; Li-Fraumeni Syndrome; mdm 2; *p63*; *p73*; Rb-mdm2-p53 Trimeric Complex

Test Includes Functional gene assay of *p53* and sequencing of the gene for ascertainment of mutations.

Abstract The *p53* gene is located on the short arm of chromosome 17 (17p13.1) and codes for a nuclear protein that plays a role in the regulation of cell growth and division. *p53* is a tumor suppressor gene and a sequence-specific transactivator (a transcriptional regulator). Mutations of *p53* have been implicated in many inherited and sporadic forms of cancer, including premalignant conditions,[1,2] and are particularly common in bladder, breast, colorectal, lung cancer, brain tumors, and adrenocorticocarcinoma in children. Li-Fraumeni syndrome, a rare autosomal dominant disorder, is characterized by a germline mutation of *p53* and high incidence of malignancies of the breast, soft tissue, and brain. Functional and sequencing assays are available to assess *p53* mutations providing information which can be used to monitor and manage disease.

Specimen 30 mL whole blood; 100 mg solid tumor, frozen or paraffin-embedded; body fluids including bladder washings may be appropriate as specimens;[3] other specimens including feces

Container Yellow top (ACD) tube for blood

Storage Instructions Transport whole blood at ambient temperature to the laboratory immediately. Fresh solid tumor should be frozen and transported on dry ice.

Turnaround Time 3-4 weeks

Reference Interval The *p53* functional assay will detect mutations located within codons 67 and 347 (the DNA-binding domain) of the *p53* gene, where >95% of *p53* mutations have been found. Sequence analysis will provide a complete analysis of the *p53* sequence. Interpretative reports are usually provided by laboratories.

Use Detection of *p53* mutations in families at high risk of developing cancer (Li-Fraumeni syndrome) and as a prognostic parameter in patients with cancer (particularly gastrointestinal, including esophagus, stomach, gallbladder, colon, and rectum;[4,5,6,7,8] lung,[9,10] urinary bladder,[3,11] ovary,[12,13] breast,[14,15] and prostate[16]). *p53* has been detected in a variety of gynecologic tumors.[17,18,19,20] Some studies have shown that *p53* mutations are associated with short survival and resistance to chemo- or radiation-induced DNA damage (colorectal carcinoma).

Association with tumor progression is reported with immunocytochemistry in mucinous borderline tumors of ovary. *p53* accumulation was found in some but not most mucinous, serous, and endometrioid carcinomas.

Limitations The functional assay cannot detect mutations outside of codons 67 and 347 including mutations in the regulatory domains. Association of *p53* mutations with *in situ* bladder tumors which bear a propensity for progression and with high grade or advanced bladder neoplasms is recognized, but *p53* mutations may occur late in the natural history of some tumors. About 40% of carcinomas of bladder lack *p53* mutations.[10,21]

Methodology RNA is extracted and converted back to its DNA blueprint (using reverse transcriptase) in the functional assay. The DNA is inserted into yeast cells where the yeast will grow if the DNA is coding for normal protein. If there is a mutation within codons 67 and 347 (which includes the DNA binding domain) of *p53* gene, yeast will not grow. Polymerase chain reaction-single-strand conformational polymorphism (PCR-SSCP) has been utilized for detection of *p53* mutations in exons 5 through 9.[3] Sequencing of the complete *p53* gene may also be performed.

Monoclonal antibodies PAb1801, PAb421, and DO-7 (DAKO, Carpinteria, California) may be used for immunohistochemistry. They react with the *p53* gene product. The *p53* phosphoprotein is barely detectable in the nucleus of normal cells. With damage to DNA, *p53* can arrest the cell cycle, allowing repair of DNA or progression to apoptosis. Inactive mutant *p53* protein is more stable than wild type *p53* and accumulates in the nucleus of neoplastic cells. Positive immunostaining indicates presence of an abnormal *p53* gene and gene product. Frozen sections or paraffin-embedded tissues may be used.

Additional Information Most human tumors have defects in the *p53* or retinoblastoma (RB) pathways. In human malignancy, *p53* is the most commonly mutated gene. *p53* is a tumor suppressor gene, at least in part due to its role in the induction of apoptosis in response to DNA damage. The *p53* gene is a key regulator in many cellular processes, including cell cycle control, DNA repair, genome stability, apoptosis (programmed cell death), differentiation, cell senescence, and angiogenesis.[22] Conformation-specific monoclonal antibodies have shown that single point mutations in *p53* can change the conformation of the entire resultant protein molecule. p53 is a sequence-specific transactivator, containing an acidic domain near its N-terminus similar to those in other transcription factors, and an activation sequence that functions in both yeast and mammalian cells and is situated within codons 1 and 42.

A host of interactions between p53 and other cell-cycle regulating and apoptotic-inducing molecules are under investigation. Rb is also an important cell cycle regulator and is implicated in the genesis of malignancy. Rb exerts control over the progression of the cell cycle from G1 to S phase by binding to and inactivating the E2F transcription factors. Within the cell, Rb is regulated via phosphorylation (mediated by cell cycle-dependent kinases and cyclins with inhibition by the cell cycle inhibitor, p21$^{cipl/wafl}$). The latter gene (*p21$^{cipl/wafl}$*) is a *p53* target gene and thus, *p53* is implicated in the upstream control and regulation of Rb. The *mdm2* gene is also a *p53* target. The oncoprotein mdm2, once induced by *p53* can then interact with and inhibit p53 as well as target it for degradation, thus establishing a negative feedback loop involving *p53* activity.[23] These and other observations have led to the concept of a Rb-mdm2-p53 trimeric complex that governs the apoptotic function of *p53* (see diagram).

Pathways to p53-Induced Apoptosis

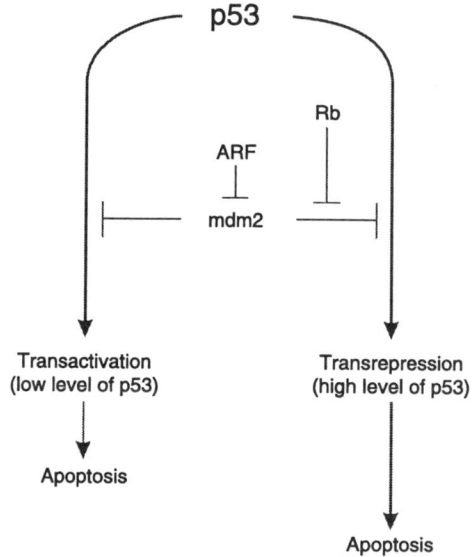

Adapted from Yap DB, Hsieh JK, Chan FS, et al, "mdm2: A Bridge Over the Two Tumor Suppressors, p53 and Rb," *Oncogene*, 1999, 18(53):7681-9.

The identification and study of two homologues of *p53*, *p63*, and *p73*, indicate that they are members of a family of transcription factors. Members of this family have amino acid sequence identity up to 63% in the DNA-binding domain. They (*p53* and *p73*) are both induced by DNA damage and *p73* can activate *p53*-regulated genes as well as suppress growth or induce apoptosis.[24] Both *p63* and *p73* are involved in the regulation of normal development. Mice that are *p63* deficient have developmental abnormalities. In humans, heterozygous germline mutations in *p63* cause the EEC syndrome (ectodactyly, ectodermal dysplasia, and facial clefts). The genes *p63* and *p73* are rarely mutated in human cancer. For this and a variety of reasons, they should probably not be considered as tumor suppressors.[25] The transcription factor E2F-1 can induce apoptosis, using both *p53*-dependent and independent pathways to kill cells. There is evidence that activation of *p73* provides a means for E2F-1 to induce cell death in the absence of *p53*.[26] Disruption of the gene for E2F-1 causes increase in T cells and splenomegaly through a mechanism in which *p73* serves to integrate T-cell receptor-activation-induced cell death (a function not shared by *p53*).[27]

Chemotherapy, stimulating hair follicle epithelial apoptosis, results in hair loss. The process is *p53* dependent. Mice that are *p53*-deficient do not show hair loss or apoptosis of hair follicle epithelium after receiving cyclophosphamide. These findings raise the possibility of pharmacologic initiatives (local *p53* inhibition) in attempts to protect against chemotherapy-associated hair loss.[28] Ultraviolet-induced DNA damage which may act to inhibit *p53* transcriptional activity might also receive consideration.[29]

The GeneChip *p53* assay has been applied to the analysis of *p53* mutation in a cancer of the colon. An accumulation of *p53* mutations was noted, a sample from the primary site having a mutation at codon 273 in exon 8 (of chromosome 17) while a sample of the tumor from a hepatic metastasis had two point mutations, one at codon 217 in exon 6 as well as the exon 8 abnormality.[30]

Footnotes

1. Wong NA, Mayer NJ, MacKell S, et al, "Immunohistochemical Assessment of Ki67 and *p53* Expression Assists the Diagnosis and Grading of Ulcerative Colitis-Related Dysplasia," *Histopathology*, 2000, 37(2):108-14.
2. Woodward TA, Klingler PD, Genko PV, et al, "Barrett's Esophagus, Apoptosis and Cell Cycle Regulation: Correlation of *p53* With Bax, Bcl-2 and p21 Protein Expression," *Anticancer Res*, 2000, 20(4):2427-32.
3. Vet JAM, Hessels D, Marras SAE, et al, "Comparative Analysis of *p53* Mutations in Bladder Washings and Histologic Specimens," *Am J Clin Pathol*, 1998, 110(5):647-52.
4. Ikeguchi M, Oka S, Gomyo Y, et al, "Combined Analysis of *p53* and Retinoblastoma Protein Expressions in Esophageal Cancer," *Ann Thorac Surg*, 2000, 70(3):913-7.
5. Danesi DT, Spano M, Fabiano A, et al, "Flow Cytometric DNA Ploidy, *p53*, PCNA, and c-erbB-2 Protein Expressions as Predictors of Survival in Surgically Resected Gastric Cancer Patients," *Cytometry*, 2000, 42(1):27-34.
6. Kanthan R, Radhi JM, and Kanthan SC, "Gallbladder Carcinomas: An Immunoprognostic Evaluation of *p53*, Bcl-2, CEA and Alpha-Fetoprotein," *Can J Gastroenterol*, 2000, 14(3):181-4.
7. McKay JA, Douglas JJ, Ross VG, "Expression of Cell Cycle Control Proteins in Primary Colorectal Tumors Does Not Always Predict Expression in Lymph Node Metastases," *Clin Cancer Res*, 2000, 6(3):1113-8.
8. Schwander O, Schiedeck TH, Bruch HP, et al, "Apoptosis in Rectal Cancer: Prognostic Significance in Comparison With Clinical Histopathologic, and Immunohistochemical Variables," *Dis Colon Rectum*, 2000, 43(9):1227-36.
9. Schneider PM, Praeuer HW, Stoeltzing O, et al, "Multiple Molecular Marker Testing (*p53*, C-Ki-ras, c-erbB-2) Improves Estimation of Prognosis in Potentially Curative Resected Nonsmall Cell Lung Cancer," *Br J Cancer*, 2000, 3(4):473-9.
10. Tammemagi MC, McLaughlin JR, Mullen JB, et al, "A Study of Smoking, *p53* Tumor Suppressor Gene Alterations and Nonsmall Cell Lung Cancer," *Ann Epidemiol*, 2000, 10(3):176-85.
11. Fleshner N, Kapusta L, Ezer D, et al, "*p53* Nuclear Accumulation Is Not Associated With Decreased Disease-Free Survival in Patients With Node Positive Transitional Cell Carcinoma of the Bladder," *J Urol*, 2000, 164(4):1177-82.
12. Ben-Hur H, Gurevich P, Ben-Arie A, et al, "Apoptosis and Apoptosis-Related Proteins (Fas, Fas ligand, bcl-2, *p53*) in Macrophages of Human Ovarian Epithelial Tumors," *Eur J Gynaecol Oncol*, 2000, 21(2):141-5.
13. Harlozinska A, Bar J, and Montenarh M, "Analysis of the Immunoreactivity of Three Anti-*p53* Antibodies and Estimation of the Relations Between *p53* Status and MDM2 Protein Expression in Ovarian Carcinomas," *Anticancer Res*, 2000, 20(2A):1049-56.
14. Zellars RC, Hilsenbeck SG, Clark GM, et al, "Prognostic Value of *p53* for Local Failure in Mastectomy-Treated Breast Cancer Patients," *J Clin Oncol*, 2000, 18(9):1906-13.
15. Silver SA and Tavassoli FA, "Pleomorphic Carcinoma of the Breast: Clinicopathological Analysis of 26 Cases of an Unusual High-Grade Phenotype of Ductal Carcinoma," *Histopathology*, 2000, 36(6):505-14.
16. Borre M, Stausbol-Gron B, and Overgaard J, "*p53* Accumulation Associated With bcl-2, the Proliferation Marker MIB-1 and Survival in Patients With Prostate Cancer Subjected to Watchful Waiting," *J Urol*, 2000, 164(3 Pt 1):716-21.
17. Chen HY, Hsu CT, Lin WC, et al, "Prognostic Value of *p53* Expression in Stage IB1 Cervical Carcinoma," *Gynecol Obstet Invest*, 2000, 49(4):266-71.
18. Hellstrom AC, Blegen H, Malec M, et al, "Recurrent Fallopian Tube Carcinoma: TP53 Mutation and Clinical Course," *Int J Gynecol Pathol*, 2000, 19(2):145-51.
19. Rosen AC, Ausch C, Klein M, et al, "*p53* Expression in Fallopian Tube Carcinomas," *Cancer Lett*, 2000, 156(1):1-7.
20. Inoue M, Fujita M, Enomoto T, et al, "Immunohistochemical Analysis of *p53* in Gynecologic Tumors," *Am J Clin Pathol*, 1994, 102(5):665-70.
21. Hruban RH, van der Riet P, Erozan YS, et al, "Brief Report: Molecular Biology and the Early Detection of Carcinoma of the Bladder - the Case of Hubert H. Humphrey," *N Engl J Med*, 1994, 330(18):1276-8.
22. May P and May E, "Twenty Years of *p53* Research: Structural and Functional Aspects of the *p53* Protein," *Oncogene*, 1999, 18(53):7621-36.
23. Yap DB, Hsieh JK, Chan FS, et al, "mdm2: A Bridge Over the Two Tumour Suppressors, *p53* and Rb," *Oncogene*, 1999, 18(53):7681-9.
24. Levrero M, De Laurenzi V, Costanzo A, et al, "The *p53/p63/p73* Family of Transcription Factors: Overlapping and Distinct Functions," *J Cell Sci*, 2000, 113(Pt 10):1661-70.
25. Kaelin WG Jr, "The *p53* Gene Family," *Oncogene*, 1999, 18(53):7701-5.
26. Irwin M, Marin MC, Phillips AC, et al, "Role for the *p53* Homologue p73 in E2F-1-Induced Apoptosis," *Nature*, 2000, 407(6804):645-8.
27. Lissy NA, Davis PK, Irwin M, et al, "A Common E2F-1 and p73 Pathway Mediates Cell Death Induced by TCR Activation," *Nature*, 2000, 407(6804):642-5.
28. Botchkarev VA, Komarova EA, Siebenhaar F, et al, "*p53* Is Essential for Chemotherapy-Induced Hair Loss," *Cancer Res*, 2000, 60(18):5002-6.
29. Zhu Q, Wani MA, El-Mahdy M, et al, "Modulation of Transcriptional Activity of *p53* by Ultraviolet Radiation: Linkage Between *p53* Pathway and DNA Repair Through Damage Recognition," *Mol Carcinog*, 2000, 28(4):215-24.
30. Takahasi Y, Nagata T, Asai S, et al, "Detection of Aberrations of 17p and *p53* Gene in Gastrointestinal Cancers by Dual (Two-Color) Fluorescence In Situ Hybridization and GeneChip *p53* Assay," *Cancer Genet Cytogenet*, 2000, 121(1):38-43.

References

Atencio IA, Ramachandra M, Shabram P, et al, "Calpain Inhibitor 1 Activates *p53*-Dependent Apoptosis in Tumor Cell Lines," *Cell Growth Differ*, 2000, 11(5):247-53.
Brito-Babapulle V, Hamoudi R, Matutes E, et al, "*p53* Allele Deletion and Protein Accumulation Occurs in the Absence of *p53* Gene Mutation in T-Prolymphocytic Leukaemia and Sézary Syndrome," *Br J Haematol*, 2000, 110(1):180-7.
Eguchi S, Kohara N, Komuta K, et al, "Mutations of the *p53* Gene in the Stool of Patients With Resectable Colorectal Cancer," *Cancer*, 1996, 77(8 Suppl):1707-10.
Fitzgerald PJ, "The Oncogene," Chapter 20, and "Suppressor Genes," Chapter 21, *From Demons and Evil Spirits to Cancer Genes*, Washington, DC: American Registry of Pathology, Armed Forces Institute of Pathology, 2000, 207-24, 225-40.
Harris CC and Hollstein M, "Clinical Implications of the *p53* Tumor-Suppressor Gene," *N Engl J Med*, 1993, 329(18):1318-27.
Ishioka C, Frebourg T, Yan YX, et al, "Screening Patients for Heterozygous *p53* Mutations Using a Functional Assay in Yeast," *Nat Genet*, 1993, 5(2):124-9.
Jackson-Grusby L, Beard C, Possemato R, et al, "Loss of Genomic Methylation Causes *p53*-Dependent Apoptosis and Epigenetic Deregulation," *Nat Genet*, 2001, 27(1):31-9.
König EA, Kusser WC, Day C, et al, "*p53* Mutations in Hairy Cell Leukemia," *Leukemia*, 2000, 14(4):706-11.
Kinzler KW and Vogelstein B, "Cancer Therapy Meets *p53*," *N Engl J Med*, 1994, 331(1):49-50.
Matlashewski G, "*p53*: Twenty Years on, Meeting Review," *Oncogene*, 1999, 18(53):7618-20.
Murakami K, Mitomi H, Yamashita K, et al, "*p53*, but Not c-Ki-*ras*, Mutations and Down-Regulation of p21^{WAF1/CIP1} and Cyclin D1 Are Associated With Malignant Transformation in Gastric Hyperplastic Polyps," *Am J Clin Pathol*, 2001, 115(2):224-34.
Shimizu T, Tanaka S, Haruma K, et al, "Growth Characteristics of Rectal Carcinoid Tumors," *Oncology*, 2000, 59(3):229-37.
Soussi T, "The *p53* Tumor Suppressor Gene: From Molecular Biology to Clinical Investigation," *Ann N Y Acad Sci*, 2000, 910:121-37

♦ **p53 Tumor Suppressor Gene** *see* p53, Functional Assay/Sequencing *on page 728*

♦ **p63** *see* p53, Functional Assay/Sequencing *on page 728*

♦ **p73** *see* p53, Functional Assay/Sequencing *on page 728*

♦ **Philadelphia Chromosome** *see* Breakpoint Cluster Region Rearrangement in CML *on page 721*

♦ **Prader-Willi Syndrome** *see* Gene Rearrangement for Leukemia and Lymphoma *on page 725*

♦ **Prism 7700 Sequence Detector** *see* Chromosomal Translocations, Molecular Detection *on page 723*

♦ **Rb1 Gene** *see* Retinoblastoma Gene DNA Detection *on page 729*

♦ **Rb-mdm2-p53 Trimeric Complex** *see* p53, Functional Assay/Sequencing *on page 728*

♦ **RB Tumor Suppressor Gene** *see* Retinoblastoma Gene DNA Detection *on page 729*

♦ **RET Gene Testing** *see* Multiple Endocrine Neoplasia/Familial Medullary Thyroid Carcinoma *on page 727*

Retinoblastoma Gene DNA Detection

Related Information
Apoptosis Assays *on page 402*
Histopathology *on page 59*
p53, Functional Assay/Sequencing *on page 728*
Polymerase Chain Reaction *on page 713*

Synonyms p110^{RB1}; *Rb*1 Gene; RB Tumor Suppressor Gene

Test Includes Restriction fragment length polymorphism (RFLP) analysis and/or polymerase chain reaction (PCR) amplification followed by sequencing of the gene to ascertain mutations.

Abstract The retinoblastoma (*Rb*1) gene is the prototype tumor suppressor gene. Located on chromosome 13q14, the gene encodes a nuclear protein that participates in the control of cell proliferation and progression through the cell cycle. Deletion or inactivation of both *Rb* alleles plays an essential role in the development of retinoblastoma, a tumor of retinoblasts affecting newborns and young children. Somatic inactivation of *Rb* is also found in other tumors not associated with retinoblastoma, including astrocytomas, several sarcomas, small cell and squamous cell carcinoma of lung, and carcinomas of breast, bladder, prostate, and parathyroid.[1]

Specimen 30 mL whole blood; 100 mg solid tumor, frozen; amniotic cells grown in appropriate media

Container Blood: Yellow top (ACD) tube; amniotic cells: T25 tissue culture flask

Storage Instructions Transport whole blood at ambient temperature to the laboratory immediately. Store solid tumor at -70°C.

Turnaround Time 3-4 weeks

Reference Interval The laboratory usually provides an interpretive report.

Use DNA tests make it possible to predict the occurrence of tumors in offspring and siblings of patients with retinoblastoma. DNA testing is useful in several settings. Identification of unaffected relatives of patients with retinoblastoma who are carriers of the germline defect aids in accurate risk assessment. DNA testing can be performed in newborns of affected or carrier parents to determine if the newborn carries the mutation. If a mutation is present, more frequent examination for detection of the tumor is warranted. Although successful treatment is available for early diagnosed retinoblastomas, patients remain at risk for nonocular tumors. Because of these risks, prenatal diagnosis can be offered to families with germline mutations.

(Continued)

Retinoblastoma Gene DNA Detection *(Continued)*

Limitations Failure to obtain DNA from the blood, tissue, or cultured cells due to inappropriate shipping or processing.

Methodology Southern blot analysis with restriction fragment length polymorphism (RFLP) is used to detect loss of an *Rb* allele. Amplification by polymerase chain reaction followed by RFLP, single-strand conformation polymorphism analysis, and/or sequencing to detect loss of an *Rb* allele and/or function mutation.[1,2]

Expression of the retinoblastoma gene product (pRB) can also be studied by immunochemistry.

Additional Information Retinoblastoma occurs in either a hereditary (40% of cases) or a nonhereditary (sporadic) form (60% of cases). Hereditary predisposition to retinoblastoma is caused by a germline mutation at the *Rb*1 locus. The germline mutation is transmitted in an autosomal dominant fashion with 90% penetrance. Retinoblastoma develops following a somatic mutation or deletion affecting the remaining *Rb* allele. Bilateral disease occurs in the majority of hereditary cases and patients have an increased risk for developing nonocular tumors (mainly osteosarcoma) in later life. In nonhereditary retinoblastoma, the tumor is usually unilateral and arises following successive somatic mutations affecting the two *Rb* alleles.

The role of the *RB* tumor suppressor gene in tumor initiation and progression is currently being studied in numerous tumors unrelated to retinoblastoma (see above). Such studies may produce prognostic information useful in tumors additional to retinoblastoma.

The *Rb* gene product, pRB, plays an important role in regulating the cell cycle ($G_1 \rightarrow S$ checkpoint), in control of cell cycle progression. Cyclin-dependent protein kinases (Cdks) and cyclins are involved. Regulation is complex and involves activating phosphorylations and dephosphorylations. pRB and its family members are targets of the Cdks. The *Rb* family (including p130 and p107) controls gene expression as mediated by the E2F family of transcription factors. pRB is a nuclear phosphoprotein that may be in an active (underphosphorylated) or inactive (hyperphosphorylated) state. The active form of pRB slows the movement of cells from the G_1 to the S phase of the cell cycle. With growth factor stimulation, pRB is inactivated by phosphorylation and the cell cycle advances across the $G_1 \rightarrow$ S checkpoint. The cells divide and M phase occurs along with removal of phosphate groups from pRB by cellular phosphatases (returning pRB to its dephosphorylated form - see diagram). Recently, p107 and p130, close relatives of the regulatory protein pRB have been identified. These proteins function as relays between cellular signals that control proliferation and nuclear transcription. They are involved in multiple stages of the cell differentiation process, including protection from apoptosis (E2F-1 has the ability to induce apoptosis). The possible function of p107 and p130 in tumor suppression is under investigation.[3]

The combined loss of *p53* protein and pRB expression have been reported to indicate relatively favorable prognosis in squamous cell carcinoma of the esophagus.[4] Low E2F-1 expression and p16[INK4A] inactivation may serve to indicate prognosis in patients who have diffuse large B-cell lymphoma.[5]

Footnotes

1. Cryns VL, Thor A, Xu HJ, et al, "Loss of the Retinoblastoma Tumor-Suppressor Gene in Parathyroid Carcinoma," *N Engl J Med*, 1994, 330(11):757-61.
2. Shimizu T, Toguchida J, Kato MV, et al, "Detection of Mutations of the RB1 Gene in Retinoblastoma Patients by Using Exon-by-Exon PCR-SSCP Analysis," *Am J Hum Genet*, 1994, 54(5):793-800.
3. Jiang H, Karnezis AN, Tao M, et al, "pRB and p107 Have Distinct Effects When Expressed in pRB-Deficient Tumor Cells at Physiologically Relevant Levels," *Oncogene*, 2000, 19(34):3878-87.
4. Ikeguchi M, Oka S, Gomyo Y, et al, "Combined Analysis of p53 and Retinoblastoma Protein Expressions in Esophageal Cancer," *Ann Thorac Surg*, 2000, 70(3):913-7.
5. Møller MB, Kania PW, Ino Y, et al, "Frequent Disruption of the RB1 Pathway in Diffuse Large B-Cell Lymphoma: Prognostic Significance of E2F-1 and p16[INK4A]," *Leukemia*, 2000, 14(5):898-904.

References

Claudio PP, Caputi M, and Giordano A, "The *Rb2*/p130 Gene: The Latest Weapon in the War Against Lung Cancer?" *Clin Cancer Res*, 2000, 6(3):754-64.

Fitzgerald PJ, "The Oncogene," Chapter 20, and "Suppressor Genes," Chapter 21, *From Demons and Evil Spirits to Cancer Genes*, Washington, DC: American Registry of Pathology, Armed Forces Institute of Pathology, 2000, 207-24, 225-40.

Lipinski MM and Jacks T, "The Retinoblastoma Gene Family in Differentiation and Development," *Oncogene*, 1999, 18(55):7873-82.

Lowy DR and Wolff L, "Molecular Oncology: Molecular Aspects of Oncogenesis," *The Molecular Basis of Blood Diseases*, 3rd ed, Part VI, Chapter 25, Stamatoyannopoulos G, Majerus PW, Perlmutter RM, et al, eds, Philadelphia, PA: WB Saunders Company, 2001, 792-3, 821.

Mulligan G and Jacks T, "The Retinoblastoma Gene Family: Cousins With Overlapping Interests," *Trends Genet*, 1998, 14(6):223-9.

Cotran RS, Kumar V, and Collins T, *Robbins Pathologic Basis of Disease*, 6th ed, Chapter 6 "Genetic Disorders" and Chapter 8 "Neoplasia," Philadelphia, PA: WB Saunders Company, 1999, 139-87, 260-327.

Sherr CJ, "Cancer Cell Cycles," *Science*, 1996, 274(5293):1672-7.

Zhang SY, Liu SC, Al-Saleem LF, et al, "E2F-1: A Proliferative Marker of Breast Neoplasia," *Cancer Epidemiol Biomarkers Prev*, 2000, 9(4):395-401.

♦ **RET Proto-oncogene** *see* Multiple Endocrine Neoplasia/Familial Medullary Thyroid Carcinoma *on page 727*

♦ **Reverse Transcriptase - PCR** *see* Chromosomal Translocations, Molecular Detection *on page 723*

♦ **RT-PCR** *see* Chromosomal Translocations, Molecular Detection *on page 723*

♦ **Southern Blot of *bcl-2* Gene Rearrangement** *see bcl-2* Gene Rearrangement *on page 720*

♦ **Translocations, Chromosomal** *see* Chromosomal Translocations, Molecular Detection *on page 723*

♦ **Tyrphostins** *see* Breakpoint Cluster Region Rearrangement in CML *on page 721*

♦ **Velocardiofacial Syndrome** *see* Gene Rearrangement for Leukemia and Lymphoma *on page 725*

♦ **Williams Syndrome** *see* Gene Rearrangement for Leukemia and Lymphoma *on page 725*

RB and Restriction Point Control of Cell Cycle Progression

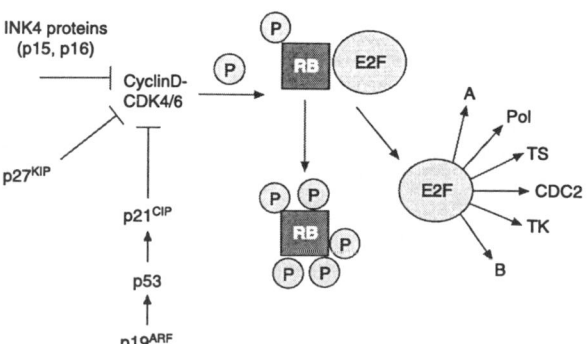

Hypophosphorylated RB binds to the transcription factor E2F, resulting in transcriptional repression of E2F-regulated genes. When RB is hyperphosphorylated by cyclin D-CDK4/6, E2F is released and triggers expression of genes such as DNA polymerase-α (pol), thymidine kinase (TK), thymidylate synthase (TS), CDC2, cyclin A, and cyclin B. The kinase activity of cyclin D-CDK4/6 is negatively regulated by INK4 proteins such as p15 and p16 as well as p21 and p27.

Adapted from Lowy DR and Wolff L, "Molecular Oncology: Molecular Aspects of Oncogenesis," *The Molecular Basis of Blood Disease*, 3rd ed, Part VI, Stamatoyannopoulos G, Majerus PW, Perlmutter RM, et al, Philadelphia PA: WB Sanders Company, 2001, 792.

THERAPEUTIC DRUG MONITORING

Uttam Garg, PhD

David S. Jacobs, MD

Harold J. Grady, PhD

John Foxworth, PharmD

Charles W. Gorodetzky, MD, PhD

Contributors:
Eugene S. Olsowka, MD, PhD
Daniel H. Jacobs, MD

Optimal dosing of many drugs can be achieved by measurement of blood drug levels (therapeutic drug monitoring - TDM). This strategy requires that three prerequisites be satisfied.

1. Therapeutic and dose-related toxic effects are initiated through interaction of the drug with specific receptors on the cells of the target issue.

2. Therapeutic/toxic effects are proportional to drug concentration at the receptor site, which is represented by the free or unbound concentration at that site.

3. Concentration of free drug at the receptor site is directly proportional to the free drug concentration in the serum and, in most cases, to the total drug concentration.

Exceptions to the relationship concerning total drug concentration occur when the drug is highly protein bound. Changes in the fraction bound are produced by various physiological or pathological processes.

Although many drugs are safely and effectively administered without TDM, it is useful to monitor blood levels when one or more of the following conditions apply:

- The drug has a narrow therapeutic range
- The drug exhibits large intra- or interindividual variation
- The drug does not produce the desired therapeutic effect or produces toxicity when empiric dosing is used
- Concurrent disease alters drug utilization
- Noncompliance is suspected
- Drug interactions may have taken place
- Medicolegal verification is desired
- Bioavailability of the drug is suspect
- The therapeutic or toxic effect cannot be easily determined by clinical observation

The availability of a rapid and accurate assay method is necessary for TDM. For the most part, current laboratory methods meet these requirements. Current methods usually employ **enzyme immunoassay techniques (EIA)** although a few of the older radioimmunoassays are still used. Sensitivity of immunoassays has been tremendously increased by use of **fluorescent** and **chemiluminescent labels**. A few current methods require extraction and **high performance liquid chromatography (HPLC) or gas chromatography (GC)**. Methods must be validated with respect to accuracy, precision, specificity, limit of detection, linear dynamic range, and robustness. The concept of robustness refers to the method's stability in the presence of changes in components of the system, such as reagent lot. Also important is the practice of measuring and reporting values for any active metabolites.

It is common practice to use TDM to monitor many of the drugs in the following classes:

- antibiotics
- antiasthmatics
- anticonvulsants
- antipsychotics
- antidepressants
- antiarrhythmics
- immunosuppressants
- analgesics

The serum drug concentration achieved is a consequence of a wide variety of processes. The study of the interrelationships of such processes and their consequences is **pharmacokinetics**. An appreciation of some pharmacokinetic principles helps in the Interpretation of serum drug levels. The aim of TDM is to achieve a steady-state drug concentration within the therapeutic range. This is achieved by controlling a dosage regimen which consists of two parts, the **dose rate** (amount of drug given per dose) and the **dose interval** (how often this amount is given). When starting (or changing) a dosage regimen, it is necessary to wait a period of time to allow for establishment of a stable concentration (steady-state = C). To do so without the use of a loading dose usually requires about five to six half-lives ($t_{1/2}$). The elimination half-life is the time required for the serum level to change from one value to half that value. Increasing the dose rate will increase the steady-state concentration while increasing the dose interval will increase the **peak/trough ratio**. The peak value is the highest value obtained after a given dose, and the trough is the lowest value which usually occurs just before the next dose. Blood samples for TDM are normally drawn at either peak or trough or both. For proper interpretation of TDM values, the sampling time and the time of the last dose must be known and recorded on the order and the report. Without this information, appropriate reference ranges cannot be chosen. **Trough** samples (used for most drugs) are usually drawn just before the next dose. **Peak** samples are drawn at various times depending upon the route of administration or the formulation of the oral dose. For most drugs, for intravenous administration, peak samples are drawn 30-60 minutes after completion of the infusion. For intramuscular administration, the peak time is 2-4 hours after dosing. For oral dosing, 2-3 hours following administration can usually be used for peak sampling except for sustained-release products. Exceptions to the use of only trough samples are many drugs, including aminoglycoside antibiotics and theophylline, which are sampled at both peak and trough.

Any of the following factors may influence the serum level achieved after a given dosage regimen.

- patient age
- genetic variability
- disease processes
- compliance
- absorption

- distribution
- metabolism
- excretion
- drug tolerance
- toxicity

In the drug listings in this chapter, therapeutic ranges are given when TDM is applicable. Separate ranges apply to peak and trough values and are so labeled. The following pharmacokinetic parameters are listed when applicable:

- $T_{1/2}$ (elimination half-life)
- Vd (volume of distribution)
- PB (protein binding)

In the text of the individual monographs, special items concerning toxicity, sampling time, drug-drug interactions, and other helpful clinical and laboratory data are presented. Tables summarizing some of the above information for several classes of drugs can be found in this introduction *on page 733*. Three other important kinetic parameters can be calculated from the above: the **elimination rate constant** (K), the **clearance** (Cl), and the **dose** (D) required to produce a chosen **steady-state concentration** (C_{SS}).

- $K = 0.693/T_{1/2}$
- $Cl = K \times Vd$
- $Css = D/(Cl \times \text{dosage interval})$

A number of drugs are highly protein bound (80% to 90%) by serum albumin and an alpha globulin. It is the "free", or unbound, concentration of the drug that is in equilibrium with intracellular free drug. It determines the pharmacological effect, the rate of liver metabolism, and the amount of parent drug presented to the kidney for excretion. Decreases in binding can occur because of competition for protein binding sites by bilirubin and metabolites accumulating because of renal insufficiency. Increase in free drug will result, but increased liver metabolism and/or renal excretion will reasonably soon bring concentrations back down to near the previous level. The total drug concentration will, however, decrease and may be deceptively low. Increasing the drug level by changing dosage regimen under such circumstances could cause toxicity. Analysis of free or unbound drug level would be the ideal solution, and is available in some laboratories for a number of drugs. Somewhat labor-intensive and expensive, it is not a common practice. In situations not involving changes in protein binding, total drug concentration is useful and almost always proportional to the free value. Certain classes of drugs may require specialized knowledge concerning drug interactions and level of efficacy of the individual members of that group, as illustrated by the following discussion of antiepileptics. Antiepileptic drugs (AED) are titrated clinically to prevent seizures and other adverse effects. Some patients require drug levels outside the classical therapeutic range. Thus, some dosing may be empiric, rather than based on the AED level. Empiric dosage may be based on therapeutic response rather than patient weight. With drugs of this class, changes in serum levels may not always be related to efficacy or toxicity. For example, phenytoin and carbamazepine may mutually lower the level of the other drug without decrease in efficacy. A table of indications and adverse effects is included in the monograph Antiepileptic Drugs, New, Overview *on page 738*.

It is also true that undesirable side effects can occur with drug levels in the therapeutic range. Both desktop and large automated laboratory systems are available for TDM analysis; essentially all provide acceptable accuracy and precision.

Also see the Chemistry Introduction for the table, International Unit (SI Unit) Conversion *on page 75*.

References

Bates DW, "Improving the Use of Therapeutic Drug Monitoring,"*Ther Drug Monit*, 1998, 20(5):550-5.

Bowers L, Shaw L, et al, "Therapeutic Drug Monitoring Conference," *Clin Chem*, 1998, 44:369-436.

Burtis C and Ashwood E, *Tietz Textbook of Clinical Chemistry*, 3rd ed, Philadelphia, PA: WB Saunders, 1999.

Devlin J, ed, *High Throughput Drug Screening*, New York, NY: Marcel Dekker, 1997.

Hardman J and Limbird L, eds, *Goodman and Gilman's: The Pharmacological Basis of Therapeutics*, 9th ed, New York, NY: McGraw-Hill, 1996.

Kaplan A, Linder M, et al, "NACB Symposium on Standards of Laboratory Practice in Therapeutic Drug Monitoring, " *Clin Chem*, 1998, 44:1072-140.

Kaplan L and Pesce A, *Clinical Chemistry: Theory, Analysis, and Correlation*, 3rd ed, St Louis, MO: Mosby, 1996.

Soldin SJ and Steele BW, "Mini Review: Therapeutic Drug Monitoring in Pediatrics," *Clin Biochem*, 2000, 33:333-5.

Table A. Class of Drug — Anticonvulsants

Drug	Therapeutic Range	Toxic Level	Half-Life	Time to Sample	Protein Binding (%)	Active Metabolites	Route of Excretion	Influence on Hepatic Drug Metabolizing Enzymes
Carbamazepine	8-12 µg/mL	>12 µg/mL	15-40 h	3-8 d	60-80	10,11-N-epoxide	Hepatic	Inducer
Clonazepam	10-50 ng/mL	>100 µg/mL	20-60 h	5-10 d	80-90	7-Amino		None
Ethosuximide	40-100 µg/mL	>150 µg/mL	25-70 h	10-13 d	0-5		Hepatic	
Felbamate	20-100 µg/mL		20-23 h		20-25			Inducer and inhibitor
Gabapentin	1-2 µg/mL		5-7 h		<3			None
Lamotrigine	2-4 µg/mL		24-30 h		50-60			None
Mephenytoin	25-40 µg/mL	>50 µg/mL	8 h	2 d	20-50	5-Ethyl, 5-phenyl-hydantoin		
Phenobarbital	20-40µg/mL	>40 µg/mL	50-140 h	20 d	40-50		Hepatic	Inducer
Phenytoin	10-20 µg/mL	>25 µg/mL	20-40 h		85-95			Inducer
Primidone	5-12 µg/mL	>12 µg/mL	4-12 h	5 d	0-20	Phenobarbital		Inducer
Valproic acid	50-100 µg/mL	>200 µg/mL	8-15 h	4 d	85-95		Renal	Inhibitor

See also the table comparing anticonvulsants in the listing, Antiepileptic Drugs, New, Overview *on page 738*.

Table B. Class of Drug — Antibiotics

Drug	Therapeutic Range*	Toxic Level	Half-Life	Time to Sample (after starting)	Protein Binding %	Route of Excretion
Amikacin	P: 15-30 µg/mL†; T: 5-10 µg/mL	T: >8 µg/mL	2-3 h	15 h	4	Renal
Chloramphenicol	P: 10-25 µg/mL; T: <5 µg/mL	P: >25 µg/mL	1.5-5 h‡	10-15 h‡	50-60	Renal§
Gentamicin	P: 4-10 µg/mL†; T: <2 µg/mL	T: >2 µg/mL	2-3 h	15 h	10	Renal
Tobramycin	P: 4-10 µg/mL†; T: <2 µg/mL	T: >2 µg/mL	2-3 h	15 h	10	Renal
Vancomycin¶	P: 20-40 µg/mL; T: 5-10 µg/mL	P: >80 µg/mL	4 h	24 h	55	Renal

P = peak, T = trough.
*Dependent upon site of infection and individual MIC of drug. See individual drugs.
†Higher peak levels will be attained with once daily dosing.
‡Varies substantially with age.
§Hepatic inactivation very important.
¶Routine monitoring of serum vancomycin levels is necessary.

Table C. Class of Drug — Cardiac Drugs

Drug	Therapeutic Range	Toxic Level	Half-Life	Time to Sample	Protein Binding %	Active Metabolites	Route of Excretion	Major Drug Interactions
Digitoxin	18-35 ng/mL	>35 ng/mL	150-250 h		90-95	Digoxin	Hepatic	
Digoxin	0.8-2.0 ng/mL	>2.5 ng/mL	20-60 h	5 d	20-25		Renal	Quinidine
Disopyramide	2.8-3.2 µg/mL	>7.0 µg/mL	4-10 h	30 h	30-70	N-desisopropyl disopyramide	Renal	
Lidocaine	1.5-5.0 µg/mL	>6.0µg/mL	1.5-2 h	5-10 h	60-80	MEGX	Hepatic	Phenobarbital
Procainamide	4-10 µg/mL	>12 µg/mL	2-6 h	20 h	10-20	N-acetylprocainamide	Renal	
Propranolol	50-100 ng/mL	>1000 ng/mL	4-6 h	30 h	90-95	4-Hydroxy-propranolol	Hepatic	
Quinidine	2-5 µg/mL	>8 µg/mL	6-8 h	24 h	70-90	3-Hydroxy-quinidine	Hepatic	Digitalis

- **Acalix®** *see* Diltiazem, Serum or Plasma *on page 747*

- **Accenon** *see* Ethotoin, Serum *on page 749*

- **Adapin®** *see* Antidepressants, Cyclic, Serum *on page 737*

- **Adapin®** *see* Doxepin, Serum *on page 748*

- **Adumbran®** *see* Oxazepam, Serum *on page 759*

- **Albecet®** *see* Amphotericin B, Serum *on page 737*

- **Aliseum®** *see* Diazepam, Serum *on page 745*

- **Allegron®** *see* Nortriptyline, Serum *on page 758*

- **Allocar®** *see* Digoxin, Serum *on page 746*

- **Almartyn®** *see* Flecainide, Serum or Plasma *on page 749*

- **Alupram®** *see* Diazepam, Serum *on page 745*

- **Alurate®** *see* Barbiturates, Quantitative, Serum or Plasma *on page 739*

- **Amazin®** *see* Chlorpromazine, Serum *on page 743*

- **AmBisome®** *see* Amphotericin B, Serum *on page 737*

- **Amethopterin** *see* Methotrexate, Serum or Plasma *on page 756*

- **Amfebutamone** *see* Bupropion, Serum or Plasma *on page 740*

- **Amikacin, Serum** *see* Aminoglycosides, Serum *on page 734*

Aminoglycosides, Serum

Related Information

Beta₂-Microglobulin, Serum or Urine *on page 509*
Magnesium, Serum *on page 221*
Vancomycin, Serum *on page 769*

Applies to Amikacin, Serum; Gentamicin, Serum; Tobramycin, Serum

Abstract Aminoglycoside antibiotics are used primarily in combination with other drugs (often beta-lactams or vancomycin) in order to treat infections caused by aerobic gram-negative bacilli. They are used to treat susceptible nontuberculous mycobacterial and nocardial infections.[1] When used in combination with penicillins and some of their derivatives, aminoglycosides may have synergistic bactericidal activity against gram-positive cocci such as *Staphylococcus aureus* and *Enterococcus faecalis*, as well as some gram-negative aerobic rods, such as *Pseudomonas aeruginosa*. High-level resistance of *Enterococcus* species to aminoglycosides is not rare. Since aminoglycoside transport through cell walls depends on oxygen (among other things), they are not active against anaerobic organisms. Once through the cell wall, the drug binds irreversibly to the 30s and 50s ribosomes and interferes with protein synthesis.

Applications include therapy of severe abdominal infections, urinary tract infections, bacteremia, and endocarditis. They are also used for prophylaxis, particularly against endocarditis.[2]

Gentamicin and tobramycin have been effectively used with broad spectrum β-lactams to treat *P. aeruginosa* infections in children with cancer and cystic fibrosis.[3]

Specimen Serum

Container Red top tube

Sampling Time Peak: it is acceptable to administer the drug intravenously over 30-60 minutes and either obtain a peak level right away, or alternatively, 30 minutes after the infusion is complete. Generally, peak sample is drawn after 30 minutes to allow drug distribution. Realize that in some patients the half-life may be <2 hours (eg, burn patients, young healthy patients, pregnant women) and that this group may clear a substantial amount of aminoglycoside over a very short time period. **Trough** levels should be drawn immediately prior to the next dose. When the drug is administered intramuscularly, specimens may be drawn 60-90 minutes later (**peak**) and just prior to the next dose (**trough**). Specimens should be drawn at steady-state, which is achieved after the same dose has been administered at the same interval for 5 half-lives of the drug. Missed doses, early or late doses, or a change in a patient's status (such as acute renal failure) may result in misleading serum sample results. Since the half-life can vary greatly from "normal" in any individual patient (see below) because of increasing patient age, or loss of renal function, etc, one should estimate both the patient's creatinine clearance (Cockcroft-Gault equation is useful) and elimination half-life initially, and then develop a plan for the loading dose, maintenance dose, and serum concentration monitoring (when indicated) based on the **individual** being treated.

A newer method of aminoglycoside dosing is gaining favor and is extensively used in many centers.[4] It involves the technique of single daily dosing of aminoglycosides, in which 5.0-7.5 mg/kg of tobramycin or gentamicin (or 15 mg/kg of amikacin) are given by I.V. infusion over 1 hour every 24 hours to patients with good renal function. This results in very high peak concentrations (near 16-24 μg/mL for tobramycin or gentamicin, and near 15-64 μg/mL for amikacin). The trough concentrations are near zero (<1 μg/mL) in appropriately selected patients, because >5 half-lives will have passed between the peak and the trough (a little less than 24 hours) and virtually all the drug will have been eliminated from the blood. The method results in at least equivalent efficacy to other dosing methods, without additional toxicity

(perhaps less nephrotoxicity). The rationale is that the higher the peak concentration is over the MIC of the pathogen, the greater the rate of killing. The aminoglycoside binds irreversibly to the ribosome, and remains there (so called "postantibiotic effect"), which allows sustained killing even when the **blood** concentration falls to low or undetectable levels. The high peak concentration also creates a larger blood-tissue gradient, favoring movement of aminoglycoside into tissue down a concentration gradient. It is important to recognize that once-daily doses in patients with poor renal function have been used for many years, and that in those patients, the purpose is to gain a therapeutic peak (eg, 4-10 μg/mL for gentamicin), and a low trough before the next dose is given. These patients have a much flatter decay line, and clear the drug much more slowly than an ideal candidate for single daily large-dose aminoglycoside treatment, where the half-life is likely to be about 2 hours. In the latter instance, every dose of the drug becomes a loading dose because the previous day's dose is essentially gone before the next dose is administered.

Collection Obtain cultures before the first dose when possible. Aminoglycosides are inactivated *in vitro* when in the same tube (or I.V. bag) by extended-spectrum penicillins such as carbenicillin and piperacillin. Amikacin is the least affected.

Storage Instructions Separate within 1 hour of collection and refrigerate or freeze until assayed. Must be frozen if a β-lactam antibiotic is also present, because of potential inactivation of aminoglycosides.

Reference Interval

- Amikacin: peak: 15-30 μg/mL, trough: 5-10 μg/mL
- Gentamicin: peak: 4-10 μg/mL, trough: 1-2 μg/mL
- Tobramycin: peak: 4-10 μg/mL, trough: 1-2 μg/mL

Possible Panic Range

- Amikacin: toxic: peak: >35 μg/mL (SI: >74 μmol/L), trough: >8 μg/mL (SI: >17 μmol/L)
- Gentamicin or tobramycin: peak: >12 μg/mL (>25 μmol/L), trough: >2 μg/mL (SI: >4 μmol/L),

Use Peak levels are necessary to assure adequate therapeutic level for the organism being treated. Monitoring trough levels may reduce the risk of nephrotoxicity in selected patients. Monitoring of single daily dose aminoglycosides is controversial, and may not be necessary because the peaks are expected to be very high, and troughs are near zero when this technique is employed in proper candidates for this therapy (eg, those with very good renal function).

Indications and dosing were recently reviewed.[1,3]

Limitations High peak levels may not have strong correlation with toxicity, especially when produced by single daily dosing. Therapeutic peak levels need to be weighed against the minimal inhibitory concentration of the drug against the organism treated. In general, a concentration at the site of infection at least 4 times greater than the MIC of the organism is recommended.

Methodology Enzyme immunoassay (EIA), fluorescence polarization immunoassay (FPIA), or similar nonisotopic immunoassays are methods of choice.

Additional Information

- Half-life: 0.5 to >24 hours (longer with decreased renal function)
- Volume of distribution: 0.4-1.3 L/kg (adults)
- Protein binding: minimal

Aminoglycosides are cleared by the kidney (no metabolism) and may accumulate in renal proximal tubular cells. Nephrotoxicity may relate to the length of time that trough levels exceed 2 μg/mL (SI: >4 μmol/L) for gentamicin and tobramycin, and 10 μg/mL (SI: >17 μmol/L) for amikacin. Creatinine levels should be monitored every 2-3 days as an indicator of impending renal toxicity, or as a sign of a decline in renal function independent of the aminoglycosides, but signaling a need for reduction in dosage of the aminoglycoside. These drugs can potentially be nephrotoxic, against which the best defense is careful dosing and monitoring. Other factors (eg, very ill patients at risk for organ dysfunction, hypotension, nephrotoxic drugs including pressor agents, contrast dye, amphotericin B, etc) may play a role as well. Aminoglycosides are cleared by hemodialysis as well.

Aminoglycosides may also cause irreversible ototoxicity that is manifested clinically as hearing loss (first expressed as high-tone loss) and tinnitus. Vestibular function may be adversely affected as well. Aminoglycoside ototoxicity is relatively uncommon. Clinical trials in which levels were carefully monitored and dosing adjusted failed to show correlation between auditory toxicity and plasma aminoglycoside levels. In situations in which dosing is not monitored and adjusted, however, sustained high levels may be associated with ototoxicity. The association is not clear and once-daily dosing regimens that produce high peak concentrations do not seem to enhance toxicity. In some patients, a mutation in 125 ribosomal RNA gene has been attributed to aminoglycoside ototoxicity.[5]

Footnotes

1. Edson RS and Terrell CL, "The Aminoglycosides," *Mayo Clin Proc*, 1999, 74(5):519-28.
2. Gonzalez LS 3rd and Spencer JP, "Aminoglycosides: A Practical Review," *Am Fam Phys*, 1998, 58(8):1811-20.
3. Henry NK, Hoecker JL, and Rhodes KH, "Antimicrobial Therapy for INfants and Children: Guidelines for the Inpatient and Outpatient Practice of Pediatric Infectious Diseases," *Mayo Clin Proc*, 2000, 75(1):86-97.

4. Barclay ML, Kirkpatrick CM, and Begg EJ, "Once Daily Aminoglycoside Therapy. Is It Less Toxic Than Multiple Daily Doses and How Should It Be Monitored?" *Clin Pharmacokinet*, 1999, 36(2):89-98.

5. Fischel-Ghodsian N, "Genetic Factors in Aminoglycoside Toxicity," *Ann N Y Acad Sci*, 1999, 884:99-109.

References

Begg EJ, Barclay ML, and Kirkpatrick CJ, "The Therapeutic Monitoring of Antimicrobial Agents," *Br J Clin Pharmacol*, 1999, 47(1):23-30.

Forge A and Schacht J, "Aminoglycoside Antibiotics," *Audiol Neurootol*, 2000, 5(1):3-22.

Isoherranen N and Soback S, "Chromatographic Methods for Analysis of Aminoglycoside Antibiotics," *J AOAC Int*, 1999, 82(5):1017-45.

Lortholary O, Tod M, Cohen Y, et al, "Aminoglycosides," *Med Clin North Am*, 1995, 79(4):761-87.

Sanchez-Alcaraz A, Vargas A, Quintana MB, et al, "Therapeutic Drug Monitoring of Tobramycin: Once-Daily Versus Twice-Daily Dosage Schedules," *J Clin Pharm Ther*, 1998, 23(5):367-73.

Schutze GE, Lowry JA, and Kearns GL, "Monitoring of Aminoglycoside Serum Concentrations," *Pediatr Infect Dis J*, 2000, 19(5):489-90.

◆ **Aminophylline** *see* Theophylline, Serum *on page 766*

Amiodarone, Serum

Related Information
Digoxin, Serum *on page 746*
Lidocaine, Serum or Plasma *on page 754*
Liver Biopsy *on page 65*
Procainamide, Serum *on page 763*
Quinidine, Serum *on page 764*
Theophylline, Serum *on page 766*

Synonyms Cordarone®

Test Includes Desethylamiodarone

Abstract Amiodarone is an antiarrhythmic characterized by substantial toxicity and prolonged half-life. Some of its adverse effects are potentially fatal. Its level should be monitored. It is used for atrial fibrillation and life-threatening recurrent ventricular arrhythmias which have not responded to alternative therapy in patients at risk for sudden death. Aggravation of arrhythmia has usually taken place in subjects with hypokalemia or those receiving another antiarrhythmic agent. Close monitoring of chest films, pulmonary function, liver, thyroid, and cardiac status (including EKG) is recommended.

Specimen Serum

Container Red top tube

Sampling Time Steady-state plasma concentrations are reached in 50-300 days. Time to peak serum concentrations is 4-7 hours after an oral dose.[1] Use trough levels for monitoring.

Reference Interval 1.0-2.5 μg/mL (SI: 1.6-3.9 μmol/L) (parent); desethyl metabolite is active and is present in equal concentration to parent drug.

Possible Panic Range Adverse effects at >2.5 μg/mL (SI: >4.0 μmol/L) (parent) and >5.0 μg/mL (SI: >7.0 μmol/L) (both)

Use Compliance and toxicity assessment; used for rhythm abnormalities

Limitations Life-threatening side effects and management difficulties occur, but unlike other antiarrhythmic agents amiodarone has not been shown to increase mortality. Wide interpatient variability in dose concentration relationships limits usefulness of serum concentrations.[1]

Contraindications Amiodarone decreases the hepatic enzyme activity needed to metabolize many drugs. This results in a decrease in clearance and therefore an increase in concentration, which may result in toxicity. Serum concentrations and pharmacologic effects of the following drugs may be increased by amiodarone: cyclosporine, digitalis, flecainide, lidocaine, phenytoin, procainamide, quinidine, theophylline, and warfarin type oral anticoagulants.

Methodology High performance liquid chromatography (HPLC)

Additional Information
- Half-life: 250-1200 hours or more
- Volume of distribution: 20-100 L/kg
- Protein binding: 95% to 97%

Amiodarone is a class III antiarrhythmic agent approved for the treatment of life-threatening ventricular tachyarrhythmias.[2] It is also used in prevention of recurrences of atrial fibrillation and is more effective than sotalol and propafenone.[3] Because of potential toxicity, the serum level of this drug should be monitored.[4] Its major elimination is by hepatic metabolism. Negligible renal excretion occurs. Use of the drug is restricted because of its many side effects, including pulmonary fibrosis (hypersensitivity pneumonitis or interstitial/alveolar pneumonitis), adult respiratory distress syndrome (ARDS), and pulmonary phospholipidosis (which occurs in subjects on amiodarone and which are not proof of drug-induced pulmonary injury). Other side effects include neuromuscular weakness, peripheral neuropathy, exacerbation of arrhythmia, tremor, thyroid dysfunction and interaction with other drugs. It contains 37% iodine by weight. Up to 5% to 10% of patients on the drug develop hypothyroidism or hyperthyroidism. It may cause increased thyroxine levels and decreased T_3. TSH levels may be useful for diagnosis of thyroid complications. Amiodarone thyrotoxicosis occurs more frequently in areas of low iodine intake.[5] Potassium or magnesium deficiency should be corrected. AST and ALT should be monitored on a regular basis,

because side effects of amiodarone include liver complications, and it is cleared by hepatic metabolism. Increased aminotransferase and alkaline phosphatase levels are found in 25% of subjects. Increased serum concentrations of AST and ALT may be three times normal. If serum AST or ALT concentrations go beyond normal or double in a patient with an elevated baseline, then reduction of dosage or withdrawal should be considered. When liver biopsy has been performed, the histopathological appearance of the liver has been that of nonalcoholic steatohepatitis with phospholipidosis (phospholipidosis is found on electron microscopy). Steatosis occurs less often. Malloy bodies of alcoholic hyaline type occur infrequently. Cirrhosis develops in 33% of patients who have such lesions.[6]

The drug is embryotoxic. Skin complications are recognized.[7] Cardiac rate, rhythm, and ECG also should be monitored regularly.

Because pulmonary toxicity is the most serious noncardiac complication, chest radiographs are recommended.[1]

Amiodarone can potentiate effects of warfarin, elevating prothrombin time. It can elevate serum digoxin level, levels of other antiarrhythmic drugs including quinidine, procainamide, mexiletine, and propafenone. There are effects with anesthetics, β-blockers, or calcium channel blockers.[1] Serum level of amiodarone is decreased by concomitant administration of cholestyramine or phenytoin and increased by cimetidine.

Footnotes
1. Podrid PJ, "Amiodarone: Reevaluation of an Old Drug," *Ann Intern Med*, 1995, 122(9):689-700.

2. Kudenchuk PJ, Cobb LA, Copass MK, et al, "Amiodarone for Resuscitation After Out-of-Hospital Cardiac Arrest Due to Ventricular Fibrillation," *N Engl J Med*, 1999, 341(12):871-8.

3. Roy D, Talajic M, Dorian P, et al, "Amiodarone to Prevent Recurrence of Atrial Fibrillation. Canadian Trial of Atrial Fibrillation Investigators," *N Engl J Med*, 2000, 342(13):913-20.

4. Keyler DE, Van De Voort JT, Howard JE, et al, "Monitoring Blood Levels of Selected Drugs. Remember to Factor in the Many Confounding Variables," *Postgrad Med*, 1998, 103(3):209-12, 215-9, 223-4.

5. Loh KC, "Amiodarone-Induced Thyroid Disorders: A Clinical Review," *Postgrad Med J*, 2000, 76(893):133-40.

6. Zimmerman HJ, "Psychotropic and Anticonvulsant Agents," *Hepatotoxicity - The Adverse Effects of Drugs and Other Chemicals on the Liver*, 2nd ed, Chapter 18, Philadelphia, PA: Lippincott Williams & Wilkins, 1999, 483-516.

7. Primka EJ 3rd, Liranzo MO, Bergfeld WF, et al, "Amiodarone-Induced Linear IgA Disease," *J Am Acad Dermatol*, 1994, 31(5 Pt 1):809-11.

References
Breithardt G, "Amiodarone in Patients With Heart Failure," editorial, *N Engl J Med*, 1995, 333(2):121-2.

Daoud EG, Strickberger SA, Man KC, et al, "Preoperative Amiodarone as Prophylaxis Against Atrial Fibrillation After Heart Surgery," *N Engl J Med*, 1997, 337(25):1785-91.

Disch DL, Greenberg ML, Holzberger PT, et al, "Managing Chronic Atrial Fibrillation: A Markov Decision Analysis Comparing Warfarin, Quinidine, and Low-Dose Amiodarone," *Ann Intern Med*, 1994, 120(6):449-57.

Evans SJ, Myers M, Zaher C, et al, "High Dose Oral Amiodarone Loading: Electrophysiologic Effects and Clinical Tolerance," *J Am Coll Cardiol*, 1992, 19(1):169-73.

Gonzales ER, Kannewurf BS, and Ornato JP, "Intravenous Amiodarone for Ventricular Arrhythmias: Overview and Clinical Use," *Resuscitation*, 1998, 39(1-2):33-42. 33-42.

Murphy MT and Wilkoff BL, "What Internists Should Know About Amiodarone," *Cleve Clin J Med*, 1998, 65(3):159-66.

Physicians' Desk Reference (PDR), 48th ed, Mont Vale, NJ: Medical Economics Data, 1994, 2528-31.

Roden DM, "Pharmacokinetics of Amiodarone: Implications for Drug Therapy," *Am J Cardiol*, 1993, 72(16):45F-50F.

Stevenson WG and Stevenson LW, "Atrial Fibrillation in Heart Failure," *N Engl J Med*, 1999, 341(12):910-1.

◆ **Amitriptyline and Nortriptyline** *see* Antidepressants, Cyclic, Serum *on page 737*

Amitriptyline, Serum

Related Information
Antidepressants, Cyclic, Serum *on page 737*
Nortriptyline, Serum *on page 758*

Synonyms Elavil®; Endep®; Etrafon®; Limbitrol®; Triavil®

Applies to Pamelor®

Test Includes Nortriptyline levels

Abstract Amitriptyline is a tricyclic antidepressant indicated for the relief of symptoms of endogenous depression. Nortriptyline is a major active metabolite.

Specimen Serum or plasma

Container Red top tube, green top (heparin) tube

Sampling Time Trough levels at steady-state (100-200 hours)

Causes for Rejection Specimen collected in gel tube

Reference Interval Amitriptyline: 80-200 ng/mL (SI: 289-722 nmol/L); nortriptyline: 50-150 ng/mL (SI: 190-570 nmol/L); combined: 120-250 ng/mL

Critical Values >300 ng/mL (SI: >1080 nmol/L); amitriptyline + nortriptyline: >500 ng/mL

Possible Panic Range ≥1000 ng/mL
(Continued)

Amitriptyline, Serum (Continued)

Use Therapeutic monitoring and toxicity assessment. Amitriptyline is a tricyclic antidepressant that blocks the re-uptake of serotonin and norepinephrine at nerve endings. It possesses high anticholinergic activity, sedation and cardiovascular toxicity. It has quinidine-like effects on cardiac conduction.

Limitations Use of therapeutic drug monitoring is controversial for this drug. Some data indicate no definite correlation of concentration and clinical outcome and/or severity of side effects. Severity of overdose is better correlated with an EKG finding of QRS widening. Nortriptyline to amitriptyline ratio may be useful.

Methodology Immunoassay, high performance liquid chromatography (HPLC), gas chromatography (GC)

Additional Information
- Half-life: 20-40 hours
- Volume of distribution: 10-36 L/kg
- Protein binding: 85% to 95%

It is cleared by the liver alone and is extensively metabolized to many polar compounds. The most important metabolite is the N-desmethyl metabolite, nortriptyline, which is itself an important antidepressant. Please see Nortriptyline, Serum *on page 758* for more information. A second active metabolite is 10-hydroxynortriptyline.

Amitriptyline is completely absorbed but undergoes some first-pass elimination. The bioavailability of amitriptyline is 40% to 60% with a peak concentration 2-6 hours after an oral dose.

Anticholinergic side effects are common with this drug. They are not severe and may diminish with continued therapy or can be treated with other pharmacologic and nonpharmacologic therapies. Anticholinergic side effects are more troublesome in the elderly. Sedation may also decrease with continued use. Amitriptyline can lower the seizure threshold and cause orthostasis and arrhythmias. Its cardiovascular effects are more common in patients with underlying cardiovascular disorders.

Drug interactions are common with the tricyclic antidepressants. Their elimination is sensitive to decreases in enzyme activity caused by cimetidine, corticosteroids, disulfiram, fluoxetine, and antipsychotics, resulting in unexpectedly increased concentrations of amitriptyline. Enzyme (P-450) inducers (eg, phenytoin, chloral hydrate, smoking, and the barbiturates) will result in unexpectedly decreased amitriptyline concentrations. Additive anticholinergic side effects occur when tricyclics are combined with antihistamines, anti-Parkinson drugs, and antipsychotics. The cardiovascular effects of the tricyclics are additive with any of the class IA antiarrhythmics (quinidine, procainamide, disopyramide). Direct-acting sympathomimetics (epinephrine, norepinephrine, phenylephrine) are potentiated by tricyclics. Monoamine oxidase (MAO) inhibitors and thyroid hormones potentiate the toxicity of tricyclics. Hyperthermia, delirium, convulsions, coma, and fatalities have occurred with the combination of MAO inhibitors and tricyclics. These drugs have been used in combination in refractory cases of depression. The tricyclics can also affect other drugs. The antihypertensive effects of the central α-agonists (clonidine, methyldopa, guanethidine) are reversed when combined with tricyclics. Anticoagulation effects of warfarin may be potentiated by the tricyclics.

Tricyclic antidepressants should be avoided in pregnant and lactating women because the safety of these drugs has not been established in these subjects. Geriatric patients are especially susceptible to orthostasis, urinary retention, constipation, and sedation. Tricyclic antidepressants are commonly seen in overdose situations. Cardiovascular, anticholinergic, and central nervous system toxicities can be lethal.

Certain studies have shown that certain antidepressants and stimulants are equally effective for adults with attention deficit hyperactivity disorder (ADHD). Antidepressants may offer a safe first-line treatment for adults with ADHD.

References
Bryson HM and Wilde MI, "Amitriptyline. A Review of its Pharmacological Properties and Therapeutic Use in Chronic Pain States," *Drugs Aging*, 1996, 8(6):459-76.

Geller B, Reising D, Leonard HL, et al, "Critical Review of Tricyclic Antidepressant Use in Children and Adolescents," *J Am Acad Child Adolesc Psychiatry*, 1999, 38(5):513-6.

Higgins ES, "A Comparative Analysis of Antidepressants and Stimulants for the Treatment of Adults With Attention-Deficit Hyperactivity Disorder," *J Fam Pract*, 1999, 48(1):15-20.

Hulten BA, Heath A, Knudsen K, et al, "Amitriptyline and Amitriptyline Metabolites in Blood and Cerebrospinal Fluid Following Human Overdose," *J Toxicol Clin Toxicol*, 1992, 30(2):181-201.

Katz MM, Koslow SH, Maas JW, et al, "Identifying the Specific Clinical Actions of Amitriptyline: Interrelationships of Behavior, Affect, and Plasma Levels in Depression," *Psychol Med*, 1991, 21(3):599-611.

Linder MW and Keck PE Jr, "Standards of Laboratory Practice: Antidepressant Drug Monitoring. National Academy of Clinical Biochemistry," *Clin Chem*, 1998, 44(5):1073-84.

♦ **Amobarbital** *see* Barbiturates, Quantitative, Serum or Plasma *on page 739*

♦ **Amoxapine and 8-Hydroxyamoxapine** *see* Antidepressants, Cyclic, Serum *on page 737*

Amoxapine, Serum or Plasma

Related Information
Antidepressants, Cyclic, Serum *on page 737*
Disopyramide, Serum or Plasma *on page 747*
Fluoxetine, Serum *on page 750*
Phenytoin, Serum or Plasma *on page 761*
Procainamide, Serum *on page 763*
Prolactin, Serum *on page 262*
Quinidine, Serum *on page 764*

Synonyms Asendin®; Demolox®; Moxadil®; Omnipres®

Applies to Loxapine

Test Includes 8-OH-amoxapine

Abstract Amoxapine is a second generation antidepressant. It acts by blocking reuptake of norepinephrine in a more selective manner than the tricyclic antidepressants.

Specimen Serum or plasma

Container Red top tube or green top (heparin) tube

Sampling Time Trough level at steady-state. Time to steady-state is 35-50 hours.

Reference Interval Amoxapine 20-100 ng/mL (SI: 64-319 nmol/L); 8-OH-amoxapine 150-300 ng/mL (SI: 478-956 nmol/L); both 200-400 ng/mL (SI: 637-1275 nmol/L)

Critical Values >600 ng/mL (SI: >1913 nmol/L)

Possible Panic Range ≥1000 ng/mL

Use Toxicity assessment. Amoxapine is a heterocyclic antidepressant that blocks the reuptake of serotonin and norepinephrine at nerve endings.

Methodology High performance liquid chromatography (HPLC), gas chromatography (GC). Amoxapine and its metabolite can be qualitatively detected by thin layer chromatography (TLC).

Additional Information
- Half-life: 8-15 hours
- Volume of distribution: 1.0-1.2 L/kg
- Protein binding: 80% to 90%; highly bound to tissues also

The drug is a demethylated derivative of loxapine, a neuroleptic used to treat schizophrenia. It possesses anticholinergic activity, sedative effects, and cardiovascular toxicity. It has quinidine-like effects on cardiac conduction. It is cleared by the liver alone and is hydroxylated to form two active metabolites: 7-hydroxy- and 8-hydroxy-amoxapine. The 7-OH metabolite has dopamine-blocking activity giving it a neuroleptic effect similar to haloperidol.

Amoxapine is completely and quickly absorbed. The peak concentration occurs 1-4 hours after an oral dose, with a bioavailability of 46% to 82%.

Anticholinergic side effects are common with this drug. They are not severe and may diminish with continued therapy or can be treated with other pharmacologic and nonpharmacologic therapies. Anticholinergic side effects are more troublesome in the elderly. Sedation may also decrease with continued use. Amoxapine can lower the seizure threshold and cause orthostasis and arrhythmias. Its cardiovascular effects are more common in patients with underlying cardiovascular disorders.

Drug interactions are common with the tricyclic antidepressants. Concomitant treatment with cimetidine, fluoxetine, and antipsychotics produce unexpectedly high concentrations of amoxapine. Enzyme inducers (eg, phenytoin, chloral hydrate, smoking, and the barbiturates) will decrease amoxapine concentrations. Additive anticholinergic side effects occur when cyclics are combined with antihistamines, anti-Parkinson drugs, and antipsychotics. The cardiovascular effects are additive with any of the class IA antiarrhythmics (quinidine, procainamide, disopyramide). Direct-acting sympathomimetics (epinephrine, norepinephrine, phenylephrine) are potentiated by cyclics. Monoamine oxidase inhibitors (MAOIs) and thyroid hormones potentiate the toxicity of cyclics. Hyperthermia, delirium, convulsions, coma, and fatalities have occurred with the combination of MAOIs and cyclics. These drugs have been used in combination in refractory cases of depression. The cyclics can also effect other drugs. The antihypertensive effects of the central α-agonists (clonidine, methyldopa, guanethidine) are reversed when combined with cyclics. Anticoagulation effects of warfarin may be potentiated by the cyclics.

Cyclic antidepressants should be avoided in pregnant and lactating women because the safety of these drugs for these patients has not been established. The 7-hydroxy metabolite has been detected in the breast milk of nursing mothers. Geriatric patients are especially susceptible to orthostasis, urinary retention, constipation, and sedation. The cyclic antidepressants are commonly seen in overdose situations. Cardiovascular, anticholinergic, and central nervous system toxicities can be lethal.

Adverse Reactions of Amoxapine
- Anticholinergic: extrapyramidal effects, tardive dyskinesia, blurred vision
- Cardiovascular: hypotension, sinus tachycardia; relatively low cardiac toxicity as compared to other tricyclic antidepressants
- Central nervous system: drowsiness, dizziness/vertigo, nervousness, insomnia, seizures, Parkinson-like symptoms, chorea (extrapyramidal), tardive dyskinesia, fever
- Dermatologic: rash, toxic epidermal necrolysis
- Endocrine & metabolic: amenorrhea, galactorrhea

- Gastrointestinal: constipation, dry mouth
- Hematologic: leukopenia/neutropenia (agranulocytosis, granulocytopenia)
- Ocular: oculogyric crisis (extrapyramidal)
- Miscellaneous: neuroleptic malignant syndrome, pancreatitis

Signs and symptoms of acute overdose include grand mal convulsions, photosensitivity, insomnia, hyperprolactinemia, cognitive dysfunction, nystagmus, acidosis, coma, supraventricular arrhythmias, hematuria, incomplete right bundle-branch block, renal failure (acute) (neurotoxic effects may be permanent), myoglobinuria, hematuria.

References

Anton RF Jr and Burch EA Jr, "Amoxapine Versus Amitriptyline Combined With Perphenazine in the Treatment of Psychotic Depression," *Am J Psychiatry*, 1990, 147(9):1203-8.

Fenton J, "Amoxapine," *The Laboratory and the Poisoned Patient*, Washington, DC: AACC Press, American Association of Clinical Chemistry, 1998, 50-3.

Hue B, Palomba B, Giacardy-Paty M, et al, "Concurrent High-Performance Liquid Chromatographic Measurement of Loxapine and Amoxapine and of Their Hydroxylated Metabolites in Plasma," *Ther Drug Monit*, 1998, 20(3):335-9.

Merigian KS, Browning RG, and Leeper KV, "Successful Treatment of Amoxapine-Induced Refractory Status Epilepticus With Propofol," *Acad Emerg Med*, 1995, 2(2):128-33.

♦ **Amphocil®** *see* Amphotericin B, Serum *on page 737*

♦ **Amphotec®** *see* Amphotericin B, Serum *on page 737*

♦ **Amphotericin B Cholesteryl Complex** *see* Amphotericin B, Serum *on page 737*

♦ **Amphotericin B Colloidal Dispersion** *see* Amphotericin B, Serum *on page 737*

♦ **Amphotericin B Desoxycholate** *see* Amphotericin B, Serum *on page 737*

♦ **Amphotericin B Lipid Complex** *see* Amphotericin B, Serum *on page 737*

Amphotericin B, Serum

Related Information

Flucytosine, Serum *on page 750*
Itraconazole, Serum *on page 753*
Potassium, Urine *on page 259*

Synonyms Albecet®; AmBisome®; Amphocil®; Amphotec®; Amphotericin B Cholesteryl Complex; Amphotericin B Colloidal Dispersion; Amphotericin B Desoxycholate; Amphotericin B Lipid Complex; Fungizone®; Liposomal Amphotericin B

Abstract Amphotericin B desoxycholate is an antifungal agent that is available for intravenous or intrathecal administration. Although amphotericin was initially prepared solely as a colloidal mixture, it is also currently available in various lipid forms designed to reduce toxicity.[1] These newer agents may offer reduced nephrotoxicity, but are not known to be more effective and are more expensive. Amphotericin B is used for aspergillosis, blastomycosis, candidiasis, coccidioidomycosis, cryptococcosis, histoplasmosis, mucormycosis, paracoccidioidomycosis (*Blastomyces brasiliensis*), and many other fungal infections. Liposomal amphotericin B is available for the treatment of visceral leishmaniasis.[2] Newer, less toxic agents (eg, azoles) are available for use in some instances. However, for many serious fungal infections, amphotericin B is the drug of choice despite its toxic potential.

There is also a form of amphotericin B oral suspension available for oral usage in treatment of oral candidiasis. Amphotericin B colloidal dispersion is now available and is somewhat less nephrotoxic. Liposomal amphotericin B has also been shown to be less toxic and somewhat more effective.

Specimen Serum

Container Red top tube

Reference Interval Therapeutic: peak serum concentrations of 0.5-2 µg/mL are seen after a dose of 0.4-0.6 mg/kg.

Use Little utility in monitoring serum levels for potential toxicity and correlation with *in vitro* susceptibility data (see Limitations)

Limitations Poor penetration of the drug into CSF is recognized. Amphotericin B causes electrolyte imbalance, including hypokalemia and hypomagnesemia.[3]

Routine monitoring of amphotericin B concentrations is not indicated; studies have not correlated serum concentrations with efficacy or toxicity. In usual clinical use, it is probably more prudent to follow serum creatinine, potassium, bicarbonate, magnesium concentrations, and CBC than to perform amphotericin B assays. Assays for amphotericin B are performed in only a few reference laboratories.

Methodology High performance liquid chromatography (HPLC),[4] bioassay

Additional Information

- Half-life: 15 days
- 95% protein bound, mainly to lipoproteins
- Volume of distribution: 4 L/kg

Amphotericin B irreversibly binds to sterols in fungal cell membranes, increasing the permeability of the cell membrane. It is not significantly absorbed after oral administration; the oral preparation for oral candidiasis works through direct contact. A 1 mg test dose is recommended by the manufacturer, but is probably not necessary and is usually not performed. Amphotericin is not excreted unchanged by the kidneys but its metabolism is not understood. Dose reductions are not necessary until creatinine clearance falls to <10 mL/minute, and even then may not be necessary.

The drug may be found in blood up to 4 weeks and urine up to 4-8 weeks after administration. Amphotericin B is not removed by hemodialysis.

Amphotericin B therapy frequently induces fever, chills, and nausea. Liposomal amphotericin B preparation seems to have fewer side effects as compared to conventional preparation.[5] Approximately 80% of patients develop increased serum creatinine concentrations. When creatinine levels exceed 3.0 µg/mL, it is often advised to withhold amphotericin B until creatinine levels fall. Patients may suffer mild renal tubular acidosis, accompanied by hypokalemia and hypomagnesemia. Sodium loading, if the patient's clinical status will allow it (500 mL normal saline pre- and postinfusion), may reduce nephrotoxicity, and avoidance of other nephrotoxins (contrast media, cisplatin, etc) is advised as well. Anemia may develop over time, and is caused by decreased erythropoietin release. Susceptibility testing is not widely available, not well-standardized, and is not known to accurately predict clinical response.

Footnotes

1. Robinson RF and Nahata MC, "A Comparative Review of Conventional and Lipid Formulation of Amphotericin B," *J Clin Pharm Ther*, 1999, 24(4):249-57.
2. Meyerhoff A, "U.S. Food and Drug Administration Approval of AmBisome® (liposomal Amphotericin B) for Treatment of Visceral Leishmaniasis," *Clin Infect Dis*, 1999, 28(1):42-8.
3. Warny LD and Brophy DF, "Amiloride for the Prevention of Amphotericin B-Induced Hypokalemia and Hypomagnesemia," *Ann Pharmacother*, 2000, 34(1):94-7.
4. Eldem T and Arican-Cellat N, "High Performance Liquid Chromatographic Determination of Amphotericin B in a Liposomal Pharmaceutical Product and Validation of the Assay," *J Chromatogr Sci*, 2000, 38(8):338-44.
5. Walsh TJ, Finberg RW, Arndt C, et al, "Liposomal Amphotericin B for Empirical Therapy in Patients With Persistent Fever and Neutropenia," National Institute for Allergy and Infectious Diseases Mycoses Study Group, *N Engl J Med*, 1999, 340(10):764-71.

References

Herbrecht R, Letscher V, Andres E, et al, "Safety and Efficacy of Amphotericin B Colloidal Dispersion. An Overview," *Chemotherapy*, 1999, 45(Suppl 1):67-76.

Rapp RP, Gubbins PO, and Evans ME, "Amphotericin B Lipid Complex," *Ann Pharmacother*, 1997, 31(10):1174-86.

Rosenblatt JE, "Antiparasitic Agents," *Mayo Clin Proc*, 1999, 74(11):1161-75.

Starke JR, Mason EO Jr, Kramer WG, et al, "Pharmacokinetics of Amphotericin B in Infants and Children," *J Infect Dis*, 1987, 155(4):766-74.

Terrell CL and Hughes CE, "Antifungal Agents Used for Deep-Seated Mycotic Infections," *Mayo Clin Proc*, 1992, 67(1):69-91.

Wong-Beringer A, Jacobs RA, and Guglielmo BJ, "Lipid Formulations of Amphotericin B: Clinical Efficacy and Toxicities," *Clin Infect Dis*, 1998, 27(3):603-18.

♦ **Amytal®** *see* Barbiturates, Quantitative, Serum or Plasma *on page 739*

♦ **Ancobon®** *see* Flucytosine, Serum *on page 750*

♦ **Anestacon®** *see* Lidocaine, Serum or Plasma *on page 754*

♦ **Angilol®** *see* Propranolol, Serum *on page 763*

♦ **Anticoagulants, Oral** *see* Warfarin *on page 770*

Antidepressants, Cyclic, Serum

Related Information

Amitriptyline, Serum *on page 735*
Amoxapine, Serum or Plasma *on page 736*
Diazepam, Serum *on page 745*
Doxepin, Serum *on page 748*
Fluoxetine, Serum *on page 750*
Imipramine, Serum or Plasma *on page 752*
Maprotiline, Serum *on page 755*
Nortriptyline, Serum *on page 758*
Phenobarbital, Serum or Plasma *on page 760*
Phenothiazines, Serum or Urine *on page 760*
Phenytoin, Serum or Plasma *on page 761*
Sertraline, Serum *on page 765*
Trazodone, Serum or Plasma *on page 768*

Synonyms CAD; Cyclic Antidepressants

Applies to Adapin®; Amitriptyline and Nortriptyline; Amoxapine and 8-Hydroxyamoxapine; Aventyl®; Desipramine; Doxepin and Nordoxepine; Etrafon®; Fluoxetine and Norfluoxetine; Imipramine and Desipramine; Maprotiline; Norpramin®; Nortriptyline; Pamelor®; Pertofrane®; Presamine®; Protriptyline; Sinequan®; TAD; TCA; Tetracyclic Antidepressants; Tofranil®; Trazodone; Tricyclic Antidepressants; Vivactil®

Abstract Drugs in this class are widely used as antidepressants. They are frequently involved in suicidal ingestion and responsible for a large percentage of drug-related deaths. The central nervous system and cardiovascular system are primarily affected in toxicity of the cyclic antidepressants. Drowsiness, seizures, coma, and cardiac dysrhythmias occur. Hypoventilation and anticholinergic findings are seen.[1]

Specimen Serum or plasma

Container Red top tube, green top (heparin) tube; avoid serum separator tubes as drugs tend to bind to gel.

(Continued)

Antidepressants, Cyclic, Serum (Continued)

Sampling Time Steady-state specimen after 1 week of dose schedule; draw specimen 12 hours after the last dose.

Storage Instructions Remove serum within 2 hours of drawing. Samples are stable for 24 hours at room temperature, 4 weeks at 4°C, and more than 1 year at -20°C.

Causes for Rejection Specimen collected in gel tube

Special Instructions Order individual drug level or tricyclic overdose screen

Reference Interval See table.

Cyclic Antidepressants Therapeutic and Toxic Levels

Drug/Active Metabolite	Range (ng/mL)	Toxic Level (ng/mL)	Half-life (h) (Drug/Metabolite)
Amitriptyline + nortriptyline	120-250	>500	20-40/20-90
Amoxapine + 8-hydroxyamoxapine	200-400	>600	8-15/25-40
Desipramine	75-300	>500	20-90
Doxepin + nordoxepine	150-250	>500	10-25/35-55
Fluoxetine + norfluoxetine	300-1200	>2000	24-72/170-360
Imipramine + desipramine	100-300	>500	5-25/20-90
Maprotiline	200-400	>1000	25-30
Nortriptyline	50-150	>500	20-60
Protriptyline	70-250	>500	60-90
Trazodone	800-1600	>5000	6-15

Use Concentrations play a role in therapeutic monitoring. Blood levels may be useful for diagnosis of toxicity but not in projection of severity of exposure.

Limitations Immunoassays for cyclic antidepressants (toxic overdose) do not distinguish between parent compounds and active metabolites. Immunoassays are available for amitriptyline, nortriptyline, desipramine, and imipramine. A number of drugs, including alimenazine, diphenhydramine, doxepin, carbamazepine, chlorpromazine, and cyclobenzaprine interfere in immunoassays. Drug-drug interactions occur; hydrocortisone, neuroleptics, methylphenidate, cimetidine, and oral contraceptives produce higher levels by inhibiting metabolism of tricyclics by the liver. Barbiturates, chloral hydrate, and glutethimide lower plasma tricyclic levels by stimulating liver microsomal activity. Interactions with fluoxetine are recognized. Cigarette smoking also lowers steady-state plasma levels, apparently by a similar hepatic enzyme induction mechanism. Plasma levels do not always correlate with clinical effectiveness.

Contraindications Patient taking more than one cyclic antidepressant, patient taking phenothiazines or monoamine oxidase inhibitors

Methodology Immunoassay, gas chromatography (GC), gas chromatography/mass spectrometry (GC/MS), high performance liquid chromatography (HPLC). Fluorescence polarization immunoassay (FPIA), originally designed for toxicology screen, has been adapted to TDM. Point-of-care test from Biosite Diagnostics, San Diego, CA is also available.

Additional Information Cyclic antidepressants (CAs) are metabolized to secondary active compounds. These agents are useful in treating clinical depression, and enuresis (imipramine). However, they have a narrow therapeutic window, and great individual variations in blood levels associated with dosage. African-Americans usually have 50% higher blood level than whites for same dose schedule. Symptoms of overdose may mimic those of condition for which agent was prescribed. The most important of the more serious or toxic effects of CAs is cardiotoxicity. Arrhythmias and conduction defects with precipitation of congestive heart failure and possibly myocardial infarction are common at combined levels >1000 ng/mL. Widening of the QRS interval to >100 msec is highly suggestive of a TAD overdose, QRS wide. Total tricyclic concentrations reflect the severity of overdose; however, the better clinical correlation is with an EKG finding of QRS widening.

CAs represent a frequent and serious problem in both unintentional and intentional overdosage. Reports of poor correlations between plasma levels and toxic clinical manifestations indicate that QRS duration >100 msec may provide the most reliable indicator of toxicity. It has been reported that the ratio of parent to metabolite (P:M) is useful in monitoring. Ratios >2 are associated with acute overdose. In contrast, P:M ratios <2 are more consistent with high steady-state plasma levels following therapeutic dosages (although EKG or other clinical evidence of toxicity may be present). Variations in blood levels between doses are comparatively small. Peak levels occur 4-8 hours after oral ingestion. A level dose of medication should be prescribed for at least 2 weeks to obtain steady plasma levels. Monitoring of CA plasma levels is useful in a number of situations. Older patients may develop higher steady-state plasma levels than younger individuals. In geriatric patients, conventional doses may lead to toxic levels. Toxic plasma levels of cyclic drugs may be dangerous in cardiac disease patients. Recommended lower and higher plasma levels for the different CAs are evolving and are discussed in the literature. A recent study of levels in children and adolescents has emphasized the lack of correlation between oral dose and plasma concentration and has found that the incidence of side effects and therapeutic effect in treatment of enuresis relates to concentration of circulating drug.

Footnotes

1. Rodgers GC Jr and Maryunas NJ, "Poisonings: Drugs, Chemicals, and Plants," *Nelson Textbook of Pediatrics*, 16th ed, Chapter 722, Behrman RE, Kliegman RM, and Jenson HB, eds, Philadelphia, PA: WB Saunders Co, 2000, 2160-71.

References

Bergstrom RF, Peyton AL, and Lemberger L, "Quantification and Mechanism of the Fluoxetine and Tricyclic Antidepressant Interaction," *Clin Pharmacol Ther*, 1992, 51(3):239-48.

Boyce P and Judd F, "The Place for the Tricyclic Antidepressants in the Treatment of Depression," *Aust N Z J Psychiatry*, 1999, 33(3):323-7.

Brasfield KH, "Practical Psychopharmacologic Considerations in Depression," *Nurs Clin North Am*, 1991, 26(3):651-63.

Caravati EM and Bossart PJ, "Demographic and Electrocardiographic Factors Associated With Severe Tricyclic Antidepressant Toxicity," *J Toxicol Clin Toxicol*, 1991, 29(1):31-43.

Frommer DA, Kulig KW, Marx JA, et al, "Tricyclic Antidepressant Overdose: A Review," *JAMA*, 1987, 257(4):521-6.

Geller B, Reising D, Leonard HL, et al, "Critical Review of Tricyclic Antidepressant Use in Children and Adolescents," *J Am Acad Child Adolesc Psychiatry*, 1999, 38(5):513-6.

Hulten BA, Adams R, Askenasi R, et al, "Predicting Severity of Tricyclic Antidepressant Overdose," *J Toxicol Clin Toxicol*, 1992, 30(12):161-70.

Krishel S and Jackimczyk K, "Cyclic Antidepressants, Lithium, and Neuroleptic Agents. Pharmacology and Toxicology," *Emerg Med Clin North Am*, 1991, 9(1):53-86.

Lavoie FW, Gansert GG, and Weiss RE, "Value of Initial ECG Findings and Plasma Drug Levels in Cyclic Antidepressant Overdose," *Ann Emerg Med*, 1990, 19(6):696-700.

Linder MW and Keck PE Jr, "Standards of Laboratory Practice: Antidepressant Drug Monitoring. National Academy of Clinical Biochemistry," *Clin Chem*, 1998, 44(5):1073-84.

Newton EH, Shih RD, and Hoffman RS, "Cyclic Antidepressant Overdose: A Review of Current Management Strategies," *Am J Emerg Med*, 1994, 12(3):376-9.

Williams JW Jr, Mulrow CD, Chiquette E, et al, "A Systematic Review of Newer Pharmacotherapies for Depression in Adults: Evidence Report Summary," *Ann Intern Med*, 2000, 132(9):743-56.

Antiepileptic Drugs, New, Overview

Related Information

Phenobarbital, Serum or Plasma on page 760

Applies to Felbamate; Felbatol®; Gabapentin; Gabitril®; Keppra®; Lamictal®; Lamotrigine; Levetiracetam; Neurontin®; Oxcarbazepine; Sabril®; Sabrilex®; Tiagabine; Topamax®; Topiramate; Trileptal®; Vigabatrin; Zonegran™; Zonisamide Excegran®

Abstract A number of new antiepileptic drugs have reached the market in the past 10 years. Very little hard information exists regarding the therapeutic plasma ranges of these drugs. Some of these drugs may become candidates for therapeutic monitoring.[1] Such monitoring may be useful in assessing compliance or in evaluating circumstances in which therapeutic or toxic effects are difficult to interpret. Many investigators feel that these drugs are not candidates for routine monitoring at this time due to lack of solid information on therapeutic ranges and dose-related side effects. Because community hospitals do not perform these levels routinely, at this time, assays in the emergency setting have a limited role. In the case of felbamate, for which hepatotoxicity and aplastic anemia are reported,[2,3] identification of metabolites that are thought to play a role in toxicity might predict patients susceptible to fatality. Assays for aldehyde carbamate and aldehyde-derived mercaptouric acids have been proposed for patients choosing to remain on felbamate therapy.[4]

Specimen Usually plasma or serum

Container Green top (heparin) tube or red top tube

Storage Instructions Usually stored and shipped frozen.

Turnaround Time 2-4 days for reference laboratories

Reference Interval Some are provided by the reference laboratories performing the test; use range given by the laboratory that analyzed the sample.

Use When assay is appropriate, to follow therapy and assess toxicity and compliance

Limitations Sufficient data from large studies is not yet available for these drugs.

Methodology Usually gas chromatography (GC) or high performance liquid chromatography (HPLC)

Additional Information The following table lists some currently used antiepileptic drugs, indications, and adverse effects.[5] Several recent articles discuss the use and problems concerning monitoring of these new drugs. Some are listed in the following references.

Footnotes

1. Tomson T and Johannessen SI, "Therapeutic Monitoring of the New Antiepileptic Drugs," *Eur J Clin Pharmacol*, 2000, 55(10):697-705.

2. Pennell PB, Ogaily MS, and Macdonald RL, "Aplastic Anemia in a Patient Receiving Felbamate for Complex Partial Seizures," *Neurology*, 1995, 45(3 Pt 1):456-60.

3. O'Neil MG, Perdun CS, Wilson MB, et al, "Felbamate-Associated Fatal Acute Hepatic Necrosis," *Neurology*, 1996, 46(5):1457-9.

4. Thompson CD, Barthen MT, Hopper DW, et al, "Quantification in Patient Urine Samples of Felbamate and Three Metabolites: Acid Carbamate and Two Mercapturic Acids," *Epilepsia*, 1999, 40(6):769-76.
5. Sirven JI, "Acute and Chronic Seizures in Patients Older Than 60 Years," *Mayo Clin Proc*, 2001, 76:175-83.

References

Cramer JA, Fisher R, Ben-Menachem E, et al, "New Antiepileptic Drugs: Comparison of Key Clinical Trials," *Epilepsia*, 1999, 40(5):590-600.

Dichter MA and Brodie MJ, "New Antiepileptic Drugs," *N Engl J Med*, 1996, 334(24):1583-90.

Gatti G, Bonomi I, Jannuzzi G, et al, "The New Antiepileptic Drugs: Pharmacological and Clinical Aspects," *Curr Pharm Des*, 2000, 6(8):839-60.

Lima JM, "The New Drugs and the Strategies to Manage Epilepsy," *Curr Pharm Des*, 2000, 6(8):873-8.

Perucca E, "Is There a Role for Therapeutic Drug Monitoring of New Anticonvulsants?" *Clin Pharmacokinet*, 2000, 38(3):191-204.

Perucca E, "The Clinical Pharmacokinetics of the New Antiepileptic Drugs," *Epilepsia*, 1999, 40(Suppl 9):S7-13.

Ross EL, "The Evolving Role of Antiepileptic Drugs in Treating Neuropathic Pain," *Neurology*, 2000, 55(5 Suppl 1):S41-6.

Antiepileptic Drugs in Current Use

Drug	Indication	Adverse Effect
Carbamazepine	SPS, CPS, 2 GTC	Diplopia, dizziness, idiosyncratic aplastic anemia, rash, hyponatremia, osteoporosis
Diazepam	Acute seizures	Hypotension, respiratory depression, sedation, tolerance
Clonazepam	Myoclonic, atonic, 1 GTC	Hypotension, respiratory depression, sedation, tolerance
Ethosuximide	Absence seizures	Sedation, GI distress
Felbamate	SPS, CPS, 1 and 2 GTC, atonic, absence	Dizziness, headache, idiosyncratic hepatic failure or aplastic anemia, insomnia, weight loss
Gabapentin	SPS, CPS, 2 GTC	Fatigue, transient GI distress
Lamotrigine	SPS, CPS, 1 and 2 GTC	Dizziness, headache, rash
Levetiracetam	SPS, CPS, 1 and 2 GTC	Somnolence, coordination difficulties
Oxacarbazepine	SPS, CPS, 1 and 2 GTC	Dizziness, diplopia, ataxia, hyponatremia
Phenobarbital	SPS, CPS, 1 and 2 GTC	Cognitive effects, respiratory depression, sedation
Phenytoin	SPS, CPS, 1 and 2 GTC	Ataxia, gingival hyperplasia, hirsutism, lymphadenopathy, nystagmus, osteoporosis
Primidone	SPS, CPS, 1 and 2 GTC	Sedation, depression, dizziness
Tiagabine	SPS, CPS, 1 and 2 GTC	GI distress, cognitive effects
Topiramate	SPS, CPS, 1 and 2 GTC	Impaired memory, weight loss, word-finding difficulty
Vigabatrin	SPS, CPS, 2 GTC, infantile spasms	Visual field defects, psychiatric symptoms, somnolence, fatigue
Zonisamide	SPS, CPS, 1 and 2 GTC	Somnolence, dizziness, agitation, difficulty concentrating, weight loss

CPS = complex partial seizure; GI = gastrointestinal; 1 GTC = primary generalized tonic-clonic seizure; 2 GTC = secondary generalized seizure; SPS - simple partial seizure

Adapted from Sirven JI, "Acute and Chronic Seizures in Patients Older Than 60 Years," *Mayo Clin Proc*, 2001, 76:175-83.

♦ **Antisacer®** see Phenytoin, Serum or Plasma *on page 761*

♦ **A-Poxide®** see Chlordiazepoxide, Serum *on page 742*

♦ **Aprobarbital** see Barbiturates, Quantitative, Serum or Plasma *on page 739*

♦ **Apsolol®** see Propranolol, Serum *on page 763*

♦ **Asendin®** see Amoxapine, Serum or Plasma *on page 736*

♦ **Atensine®** see Diazepam, Serum *on page 745*

♦ **Athrombin-K®** see Warfarin *on page 770*

♦ **Auranofin** see Gold, Serum *on page 751*

♦ **Aurothioglucose** see Gold, Serum *on page 751*

♦ **Aventyl®** see Antidepressants, Cyclic, Serum *on page 737*

♦ **Aventyl® Hydrochloride** see Nortriptyline, Serum *on page 758*

♦ **Azidothymidine** see Zidovudine, Serum or Plasma *on page 771*

♦ **AZT** see Zidovudine, Serum or Plasma *on page 771*

♦ **Azupamil®** see Verapamil, Serum or Plasma *on page 769*

♦ **Barbita®** see Phenobarbital, Serum or Plasma *on page 760*

♦ **Barbiturate Screen, Urine** see Barbiturates, Quantitative, Serum or Plasma *on page 739*

Barbiturates, Quantitative, Serum or Plasma

Related Information
Barbiturates, Qualitative, Urine *on page 781*
Diazepam, Serum *on page 745*
Ethanol, Blood, Urine, and Other Sources *on page 789*
Methylphenobarbital, Serum *on page 757*
Phenobarbital, Serum or Plasma *on page 760*

Applies to Alurate®; Amobarbital; Amytal®; Aprobarbital; Barbiturate Screen, Urine; Blue Angels; Butabarbital; Butalbital; Butisol Sodium®; Fiorinal®; Gemonil®; Lotusate®; Luminal®; Mebaral®; Mephobarbital; Metharbital; Nembutal®; Pentobarbital; Phenobarbital; Red Devils; Secobarbital; Seconal™; Talbutal; Yellow Jackets

Abstract Measurement of barbiturates as a class is usually used for drug-of-abuse testing or as evidence for toxicity. Urine sample is generally used for barbiturate abuse testing. Certain barbiturates (eg, secobarbital, amobarbital, phenobarbital, pentobarbital) are measured in the blood for therapeutic drug monitoring purposes. See individual listings for details.

Specimen Plasma or serum

Container Lavender top (EDTA) tube; green top (heparin) tube; red top tube (avoid serum separator tube)

Sampling Time Trough

Reference Interval Therapeutic: short-acting (secobarbital): 1-5 µg/mL (SI: 4.2-21.0 µmol/L); intermediate-acting (amobarbital): 5-15 µg/mL (SI: 22-66 µmol/L); long-acting (phenobarbital): 15-40 µg/mL (SI: 65-172 µmol/L) for seizure control

Critical Values Toxic: short-acting: >10 µg/mL (SI: >43 µmol/L); intermediate-acting: >20 µg/mL (SI: >86 µmol/L); long-acting: >40 µg/mL (SI: >172 µmol/L)

Use Evaluate barbiturate toxicity, drug abuse, therapeutic levels; if barbiturates are suspected in a drug overdose, determination of long-, medium-, or short-acting may influence treatment

Limitations Only barbiturates as a class will be identified by immunoassays.

Methodology Gas chromatography (GC), high performance liquid chromatography (HPLC), immunoassay

Additional Information To monitor therapeutic phenobarbital level see Phenobarbital, Serum or Plasma *on page 760*. Barbiturates are sedative hypnotics and frequent drugs of abuse, alone and in combination with alcohol and/or amphetamines. If overdosage occurs, coma and death may result. Generally, the implication of any concentration is more serious for short-acting barbiturates than for long-lasting ones. The toxic or lethal blood level varies with many factors and cannot be provided with certainty. Lethal blood levels determined at autopsy may be as low as 60 µg/mL (SI: 258 µmol/L) for long-acting (barbital and phenobarbital) and 10 µg/mL (SI: 43 µmol/L) for intermediate- and short-acting barbiturates (amobarbital, butabarbital, butalbital, pentobarbital, secobarbital). In the presence of alcohol or other depressant drugs (eg, benzodiazepines), lethal concentrations may be lower. Addicts, however, may tolerate levels with no ill effect, which would be acutely toxic to a nonaddicted individual. The long-acting drugs are metabolized slowly and depend primarily on the kidney for elimination. The short- and intermediate-acting drugs are metabolized primarily by the liver and are much less dependent on the kidney for excretion. Only barbital is dependent mainly on renal excretion for termination of its pharmacological action. Individual barbiturates can be identified and separated from each other by HPLC or GC.

Barbiturates can be assayed in **urine** and **gastric contents**. For most immunoassays, the presence of barbiturates in urine is presumptively positive at a level ≥300 ng/mL. Levels above this cutoff can occur from medical use of these drugs as well as from abuse. The presence of these drugs should be confirmed. The most commonly abused barbiturates are secobarbital (red devils), pentobarbital (yellow jackets), and amobarbital (blue angels). Short and intermediate acting barbiturates can be detected in urine 24-72 hours following ingestion, longer-acting drugs up to 7 days.

References
Alvarez N, "Barbiturates in the Treatment of Epilepsy in People With Intellectual Disability," *J Intellect Disabil Res*, 1998, 42(Suppl 1):16-23.

Cannon RD, Wong SH, Cock SB, et al, "Comparison of the Serum Barbiturate Fluorescence Polarization Immunoassay by the COBAS INTEGRA to a CG/MS Method," *Ther Drug Monit*, 1999, 21(5):553-8.

Moyer TP, "Therapeutic Drug Monitoring," *Tietz Textbook of Clinical Chemistry*, 3rd ed, Burtis CA and Ashwood ER, eds, Philadelphia, PA: WB Saunders Co, 1999, 862-905.

Stirling LC, Kurowska A, and Tookman A, "The Use of Phenobarbitone in the Management of Agitation and Seizures at the End of Life," *J Pain Symptom Manage*, 1999, 17(5):363-8.

♦ **Bay Clor®** see Chlorpromazine, Serum *on page 743*

♦ **Baylocaine®** see Lidocaine, Serum or Plasma *on page 754*

♦ **Beaden®** see Propranolol, Serum *on page 763*

♦ **Bedranol®** see Propranolol, Serum *on page 763*

♦ **Benozil®** see Flurazepam, Serum *on page 751*

♦ **Berkolol®** *see* Propranolol, Serum *on page 763*

♦ **Berkomine®** *see* Imipramine, Serum or Plasma *on page 752*

♦ **Bespar®** *see* Buspirone, Serum *on page 740*

♦ **Biocoryl®** *see* Procainamide, Serum *on page 763*

♦ **Biquin®** *see* Quinidine, Serum *on page 764*

♦ **Blue Angels** *see* Barbiturates, Quantitative, Serum or Plasma *on page 739*

♦ **Botanical Dietary Supplements** *see* Digoxin, Serum *on page 746*

♦ **Britiazim®** *see* Diltiazem, Serum or Plasma *on page 747*

Bupropion, Serum or Plasma

Related Information
Antidepressants, Cyclic, Serum *on page 737*

Synonyms Amfebutamone; Wellbutrin®; Zyban™

Abstract An antidepressant that decreases the reuptake of serotonin, norepinephrine, and dopamine. It is not a monoamine oxidase inhibitor and is not related to tricyclic or tetracyclic antidepressants. It is also used as an aid to smoking cessation.

Specimen Serum or plasma

Container Plain red top tube or lavender top (EDTA) tube

Sampling Time Trough

Storage Instructions Freeze sample.

Turnaround Time 2-4 days

Reference Interval Therapeutic: 50-100 ng/mL

Critical Values Levels >170 ng/mL are associated with seizures.

Possible Panic Range >300 ng/mL

Use Monitor therapy; evaluate possible toxicity

Methodology Gas chromatography (GC), high performance liquid chromatography (HPLC)

Additional Information
- Half-life: 14 hours
- Volume of distribution: 30-60 L/kg
- Protein binding: 70% to 90%

Bupropion is metabolized to hydroxybupropion, an active metabolite with a half-life of 20 hours. The other two metabolites, threohydrobupropion and erythrohydrobupropion are also active. Use of the drug is contraindicated in patients with seizure disorders.

References
Britton J and Jarvis MJ, "Bupropion: A New Treatment for Smokers. Nicotine Replacement Treatment Should Also Be Available on the NHS," *BMJ*, 2000, 321(7253):65-6.

Holm KJ and Spencer CM, "Bupropion: A Review of its Use in the Management of Smoking Cessation," *Drugs*, 2000, 59(4):1007-24.

Horst WD and Preskorn SH, "Mechanisms of Action and Clinical Characteristics of Three Atypical Antidepressants: Venlafaxine, Nefazodone, Bupropion," *J Affect Disord*, 1998, 51(3):237-54.

Settle EC, "Bupropion Sustained Release: Side Effect Profile," *J Clin Psychiatry*, 1998, 59(Suppl 4):32-6.

Sweet RA, Pollock BG, Kirshner M, et al, "Pharmacokinetics of Single- and Multiple-Dose Bupropion in Elderly Patients With Depression," *J Clin Pharmacol*, 1995, 35(9):876-84.

♦ **BuSpar®** *see* Buspirone, Serum *on page 740*

Buspirone, Serum

Related Information
Antidepressants, Cyclic, Serum *on page 737*
Lithium, Serum *on page 754*

Synonyms Bespar®; BuSpar®

Abstract This is an anxiolytic drug that antagonizes serotonin receptors, without affecting benzodiazepine-GABA receptors. It is also used in the treatment of panic disorder, manic depressive disorder, and obsessive compulsive disorder.[1]

Specimen Serum

Container Red top plain tube; do not use gel separation tubes.

Sampling Time Peak specimen 40-90 minutes postdose; trough specimen just before a dose, following 5 half-lives.

Reference Interval Peak: 100-800 ng/mL; trough: 40-350 ng/mL

Use Monitor therapy

Methodology Gas chromatography (GC), high performance liquid chromatography (HPLC), radioimmunoassay (RIA)

Additional Information
- Half-life: 2-3 hours
- Volume of distribution: 3-8 L/kg
- Protein binding: 95%

Buspirone undergoes extensive first-pass metabolism, with absolute bioavailability of only 4%. One of the major metabolites of buspirone, 1-pyrimidinyl piperazine (1-PP), is pharmacologically active.[2] Coadministration of buspirone with verapamil, diltiazem, erythromycin, or itraconazole increases plasma concentration of buspirone. Rifampin decreases plasma concentration of buspirone by almost tenfold.[2]

Adverse effects of buspirone include bradycardia, dizziness, headache, ataxia, and nausea. There is no specific treatment for buspirone toxicity.[3]

Footnotes
1. Apter JT and Allen LA, "Buspirone: Future Directions," *J Clin Psychopharmacol*, 1999, 19(1):86-93.
2. Mahmood I and Sahajwalla C, "Clinical Pharmacokinetics and Pharmacodynamics of Buspirone, an Anxiolytic Drug," *Clin Pharmacokinet*, 1999, 36(4):277-87.
3. Leikin JB and Paloucek FP, *Poisoning and Toxicology Compendium*, Hudson, OH: Lexi-Comp Inc, 1998, 160.

♦ **Butabarbital** *see* Barbiturates, Quantitative, Serum or Plasma *on page 739*

♦ **Butalbital** *see* Barbiturates, Quantitative, Serum or Plasma *on page 739*

♦ **Butisol Sodium®** *see* Barbiturates, Quantitative, Serum or Plasma *on page 739*

♦ **CAD** *see* Antidepressants, Cyclic, Serum *on page 737*

Caffeine, Serum

Related Information
Theophylline, Serum *on page 766*

Synonyms Coffee Break®; Dexitac®; Durvitan®; Magnum®; Max Alert Magnum®; Mole®; No-Doz®; Pep Back®; Percoffedrinol N®; Percutafeine®; Pick-me-up®; Pro-Plus®; Stay Awake®; Vivarin®

Abstract Caffeine is a methylxanthine structurally related to theophylline. It is used clinically with other measures to treat idiopathic apnea of prematurity. It is used as a stimulant to prevent drowsiness and fatigue, and as an analgesic adjuvant. The principal sources are coffee, tea, and soft drinks. It is a metabolite of theophylline in infants.

Specimen Serum

Container Red top tube

Collection Indicate exact time of blood drawn and relationship to last theophylline or caffeine dose on request.

Reference Interval None present. The therapeutic range in the treatment of neonatal apnea is 8-14 µg/mL (SI: 41-72 µmol/L).

Possible Panic Range Toxic: >50 µg/mL (SI: >155 µmol/L); **fatal:** >100 µg/mL (SI: >512 µmol/L)

Use Monitor total xanthine concentration in newborns receiving theophylline. Clinical endpoints (eg, cessation of apnea) should be used for therapeutic decision making.

Methodology High performance liquid chromatography (HPLC), immunoassay, gas chromatography (GC), capillary electrophoresis

Additional Information
- Half-life (adults): 3-5 hours; up to 100 hours in neonates
- Volume of distribution: 0.7 L/kg; 0.8 L/kg in neonates
- Protein binding: 35%

Caffeine is one of the most widely used mind-altering substances. It is found in numerous beverages (cocoa, coffee, cola, tea) and prescription and nonprescription medications. Xanthines, caffeine, and theophylline are used to treat neonatal apnea. Idiopathic apnea of prematurity begins on the second to seventh day of life.[1] Due to the very long half-life of caffeine in neonates, this drug is gaining in popularity for treatment of neonatal apnea. Unlike its metabolism in adults, theophylline in neonates is extensively metabolized to caffeine. Caffeine is well absorbed in adults after oral administration with peak concentrations occurring in 15-45 minutes after administration. Caffeine overdoses are rare.

In the presence of liver disease, the half-life is increased and may lead to toxicity. In addition, zero-order kinetics prevail following an overdose due to saturation of metabolic enzymes. Overdose may cause seizures (rare), irritability, headache, and cardiac arrhythmias.

Physical dependence may develop upon repeated use. Withdrawal symptoms include headache and fatigue.

Footnotes
1. Stoll BJ and Kliegman RM, "Respiratory Tract Disorders," *Nelson Textbook of Pediatrics*, 16th ed, Behrman RE, Kliegman RM, and Jenson HB, eds, Philadelphia, PA: WB Saunders Co, 2000, 496-510.

References
Baselt RC, *Disposition of Toxic Drugs and Chemicals in Man*, 5th ed, Foster City, CA: Chemical Toxicology Institute, 2000, 120-3.

Dobrocky P, Bennett PN, and Notarianni LJ, "Rapid Method for the Routine Determination of Caffeine and Its Metabolites by HPLC," *J Chromatogr*, 1994, 652(1):104-8.

Fenton J, "Caffeine," *The Laboratory and the Poisoned Patient*, Washington, DC: AACC Press, American Association of Clinical Chemistry, 1998, 101-3.

Lewin NA, "Caffeine," *Toxicological Emergencies*, Goldfrank LR, et al, eds, Norwalk, CT: Appleton-Century-Crofts, 1994, 55-62.

Massey LK, "Caffeine and the Elderly," *Drugs Aging*, 1998, 13(1):43-50.

Moyer TP, "Therapeutic Drug Monitoring," *Tietz Textbook of Clinical Chemistry*, 3rd ed, Burtis CA and Ashwood ER, eds, Philadelphia, PA: WB Saunders Co, 1999, 862-905.

Nurminen ML, Niittynen L, Korpela R, et al, "Coffee, Caffeine and Blood Pressure: A Critical Review," *Eur J Clin Nutr*, 1999, 53(11):831-9.

Pesce AJ, Rashkin M, and Kotagal U, "Standards of Laboratory Practice: Theophylline and Caffeine Monitoring. National Academy of Clinical Biochemistry," *Clin Chem*, 1998, 44(5):1124-8.

♦ **Calan®** *see* Verapamil, Serum or Plasma *on page 769*

◆ **Carbamazepine** *see* Phenytoin, Serum or Plasma *on page 761*

Carbamazepine-10,11-Epoxide, Serum

Related Information
Carbamazepine, Serum *on page 741*

Synonyms Carbamazepine Metabolite

Test Includes Carbamazepine and carbamazepine-10,11-epoxide

Abstract Carbamazepine-10,11-epoxide is the active metabolite of carbamazepine. Occasional cases of carbamazepine toxicity occur with normal levels of carbamazepine due to accumulation of 10,11-epoxide.[1,2]

Specimen Serum

Container Red top tube

Reference Interval 0.8-3.2 mg/L. High level: In patients on chronic carbamazepine therapy, the addition of valpromide or progabide produces clinical toxicity with high levels of metabolite and normal levels of parent compound.[3]

Limitations Valproic acid, an anticonvulsant chemically related to valpromide, may increase the epoxide:carbamazepine ratio by eliminating excretion of the epoxide. Since most cases of fatal valproate hepatotoxicity occur in young children on multiple anticonvulsants, the combination of valproate and carbamazepine is not recommended in the susceptible population. Phenytoin may also increase the ratio of epoxide:parent compound.[4,5]

Methodology High performance liquid chromatography (HPLC), fluorescence polarization immunoassay (FPIA)

Additional Information Carbamazepine-induced thrombocytopenia is probably due to carbamazepine-10,11-epoxide.[5,6]

Footnotes
1. Pisani F, Fazio A, Oteri G, et al, "Sodium Valproate and Valpromide: Differential Interaction With Carbamazepine in Epileptic Patients," *Epilepsia*, 1986, 27(5):548-52.
2. Moyer TP, "Therapeutic Drug Monitoring," *Tietz Textbook of Clinical Chemistry*, 3rd ed, Burtis VA and Ashwood ER, eds, Philadelphia, PA: WB Saunders Co, 1999, 862-905.
3. Meijer JW, Binnie CD, Debets RM, et al, "Possible Hazard of Valpromide-Carbamazepine Combination Therapy in Epilepsy," *Lancet*, 1984, 1(8380):802.
4. Theodore WH, Narang PK, Holmes MD, et al, "Carbamazepine and its Epoxide: Relation of Plasma Levels to Toxicity and Seizure Control," *Ann Neurol*, 1989, 25:194-6.
5. Albright PS and Bruni J, "Effects of Carbamazepine and its Epoxide Metabolite on Amygdala-Kindled Seizures in Rats," *Neurology*, 1984, 34(10):1383-6.
6. Kimura M, Yoshimo K, Maeoka Y, et al, "Carbamazepine-Induced Thrombocytopenia and Carbamazepine-10,11-Epoxide: A Case Report," *Psychiatry Clin Neurosci*, 1995, 49(1):69-70.

References
Divanoglou D, Orologas A, Iliadis S, et al, "Pharmacokinetic Behaviour of Carbamazepine and its Main Metabolite-10,11 Epoxide of Carbamazepine in Monotherapy or in Combination With Other Antiepileptic Drugs," *Eur J Neurol*, 1998, 5(4):397-400.
Potter JM and Donnelly A, "Carbamazepine-10,11-Epoxide in Therapeutic Drug Monitoring," *Ther Drug Monit*, 1998, 20(6):652-7.
So EL, Ruggles KH, Cascino GD, et al, "Seizure Exacerbation and Status Epilepticus Related to Carbamazepine-10,11-epoxide," *Ann Neurol*, 1994, 35(6):743-6.

◆ **Carbamazepine Metabolite** *see* Carbamazepine-10,11-Epoxide, Serum *on page 741*

Carbamazepine, Serum

Related Information
Carbamazepine-10,11-Epoxide, Serum *on page 741*
Homocyst(e)ine, Plasma *on page 193*
Phenytoin, Serum or Plasma *on page 761*
Theophylline, Serum *on page 766*
Valproic Acid, Serum or Plasma *on page 768*
Verapamil, Serum or Plasma *on page 769*
Warfarin *on page 770*

Synonyms Carbamazepinum; Carbategretal®; Carbatrol®; Carbazep®; CBZ; Epitrol®; Tegretol®; Tegretol® XR

Applies to P-450 System

Abstract Carbamazepine is a first-line antiepileptic drug for generalized and partial seizures. It is also used for control of neurogenic pain from trigeminal neuralgia and diabetic neuropathy. It has been successfully used in the treatment of bipolar disease and other psychiatric and neurologic illnesses. It has a distinctive pharmacokinetic property of inducing the hepatic enzymes responsible for increase in its own clearance, called "autoinduction."

Patient Preparation Levels should be drawn before next oral dose with patient at steady-state.

Specimen Serum

Container Red top tube

Sampling Time A consistent sampling time, ideally a trough level, should be used to monitor patients on chronic therapy. Time to reach steady-state is 3-8 days.

Reference Interval 8-12 µg/mL (SI: 34-51 µmol/L); with other anticonvulsants: 4-8 µg/mL

THERAPEUTIC DRUG MONITORING: CARBAMAZEPINE, SERUM

Critical Values Disturbances of vision (nystagmus, diplopia), gait (ataxia), along with drowsiness, dizziness, and headache are commonly seen at concentrations >12 µg/mL.

Possible Panic Range >12 µg/mL. Central nervous system toxicity may occur progressively with levels near or above the high end of the reference range.

Use Monitor for compliance, efficacy, or possible toxicity. Carbamazepine has concentration-related toxicities and concentration-unrelated toxicities. Monitor for efficacy with change of formulation.

Limitations See Carbamazepine-10,11-Epoxide, Serum *on page 741*.

Contraindications Half-life of warfarin is shortened; coadministration of monoamine oxidase inhibitors are not recommended. Carbamazepine should be used cautiously in subjects with bone marrow depression. It should not be used in most circumstances if the absolute neutrophil count (ANC) is <1500. It may cross-react in those with hypersensitivity to tricyclic antidepressants.

Methodology Enzyme immunoassay (EIA), fluorescence polarization immunoassay (FPIA), gas-liquid chromatography (GLC), high performance liquid chromatography (HPLC)

Additional Information
- Half-life: 15-40 hours
- Volume of distribution: 0.8-1.8 L/kg
- Protein binding: 60% to 80%

Carbamazepine is only commercially available in oral formulations. It is absorbed slowly and is about 80% bioavailable. Plasma concentrations peak at about 6 hours after an oral dose. Carbamazepine is totally cleared hepatically and has one active metabolite, the 10,11-epoxide. Carbamazepine induces the hepatic enzymes that are responsible for its clearance. Clearance increases with time. The enzymes are fully "induced" within 4-6 weeks after starting the drug. Since clearance is increasing, half-life correspondingly decreases. The average half-life of carbamazepine before autoinduction is about 25-40 hours and 15-25 hours after autoinduction. Along with inducing the enzymes used to metabolize its own metabolism, it also increases the enzyme activity and therefore clearance of many other drugs, including many anticonvulsants. Side effects, principally nausea, prevent oral "loading" of carbamazepine.

Low level: The most common cause of a low level is noncompliance. The addition of anticonvulsants which induce the P-450 system, such as phenytoin, primidone, and phenobarbital, may decrease carbamazepine levels without causing seizures. (The P-450 system is a pivotal liver enzymatic system which processes and degrades drugs.) The withdrawal of phenytoin from the regimen of a patient on carbamazepine may increase the level and still cause seizures. Because of autoinduction of metabolism, patients in the first 2 months of therapy may have diminishing levels and be at ongoing risk for seizures. Occasionally, patients may have toxicity when levels are within the reference range. **High level:** Drugs which inhibit the P-450 system, including isoniazid, fluoxetine, propoxyphene, verapamil, and stiripentol can cause a precipitous rise in carbamazepine levels and clinical toxicity, usually within 48 hours. Danazol may cause a delayed toxicity. The addition of cimetidine, erythromycin, lithium, triacetyloleandomycin, and valproic acid can also cause toxicity. High or low levels may also be caused by switching from a brand formulation to a generic or vice-versa; generics may have variable amounts of active drug compared to brands, and this variability can engender toxic or subtherapeutic levels.

Leukopenia is the most common hematologic side effect, with incidences as high as 10% being reported, and may be dose-related. The most serious, blood dyscrasias, aplastic anemia (1 in 50,000 patients), agranulocytosis, and hepatitis, are rare and not concentration-related. In most patients, leukopenia is transient in nature and may be dose-related. Hypersensitivity reactions include Stevens-Johnson syndrome and osteomalacia. Cardiac conduction effects can occur, including sinus bradycardia and tachycardia. Hyponatremia[1] is more common in older patients. Patients in the first month of pregnancy are at increased risk of neural tube defects. Carbamazepine causes hyperhomocysteinemia.[2]

The most common side effect is morbilliform rash, developing in about 10% of patients.[1]

Women of childbearing age prescribed this medication should take supplemental folic acid.[3] See Phenobarbital, Serum or Plasma *on page 760* for more information.

Carbamazepine may interfere with the actions of theophylline, oral contraceptives, oral anticoagulants, or doxycycline. Carbamazepine may induce the metabolism of phenytoin, benzodiazepines, ethosuximide, valproic acid, corticosteroids, and thyroid hormones; synergistic anticonvulsant effect with propranolol.

Carbamazepine increases BUN, AST, ALT, ammonia, bilirubin, and alkaline phosphatase and decreases calcium, sodium, T_3, and T_4 in test samples.

Rarely, therapeutic doses may cause progressive dystonia.[4]

Two new preparations, Tegretol® XR and Carbatrol®, are extended-release formulations of carbamazepine that are formulated for twice-a-day dosing. Therapeutic monitoring of carbamazepine levels is appropriate.

Footnotes
1. Brodie MJ and Dichter MA, "Antiepileptic Drugs," *N Engl J Med*, 1996, 334(3):168-75.
(Continued)

Carbamazepine, Serum *(Continued)*

2. Verrotti A, Pascarella R, Trotta D, et al, "Hyperhomocysteinemia in Children Treated With Sodium Valproate and Carbamazepine," *Epilepsy Res*, 2000, 41(3):253-7.
3. Hernández-Diaz S, Werler MM, Walker AM, et al, "Folic Acid Antagonists During Pregnancy and the Risk of Birth Defects," *N Engl J Med*, 2000, 343(22):1608-14.
4. Haslem RHA, "Movement Disorders," *Nelson Textbook of Pediatrics*, 16th ed, Chapter 606, Behrman RE, Kliegman RM, and Jenson HB, eds, Philadelphia, PA: WB Saunders Co, 2000, 1839-43.

References

Arroyo S and Sander JW, "Carbamazepine in Comparative Trials: Pharmacokinetic Characteristics Too Often Forgotten," *Neurology*, 1999, 53(6):1170-4.

Feldkamp J, Becker A, Witte OW, et al, "Long-Term Anticonvulsant Therapy Leads to Low Bone Mineral Density - Evidence for Direct Drug Effects of Phenytoin and Carbamazepine on Human Osteoblast-Like Cells," *Exp Clin Endocrinol Diabetes*, 2000, 108(1):37-43.

Gal P and Reed MD, "Medications," *Nelson Textbook of Pediatrics*, 16th ed, Chapter 728, Behrman RE, Kliegman RM, and Jenson HB, eds, Philadelphia, PA: WB Saunders Co, 2000, 2235-304.

Grimsley SR, Jann MW, Carter JG, et al, "Increased Carbamazepine Concentrations After Fluoxetine Coadministration," *Clin Pharmacol Ther*, 1991, 50(1):10-5.

Leikin JB and Paloucek FP, *Poisoning and Toxicology Compendium*, Hudson, OH: Lexi-Comp Inc, 1998.

Levy RH, Dreifuss FE, Mattson RH, et al, *Antiepileptic Drugs*, 3rd ed, New York, NY: Raven Press, 1989.

Lifshitz M, Gavrilov V, and Sofer S, "Signs and Symptoms of Carbamazepine Overdose in Young Children," *Pediatr Emerg Care*, 2000, 16(1):26-7.

Liu H and Delgado MR, "A Comprehensive Study of the Relation Between Serum Concentrations, Concentration Ratios, and Level/Dose Ratios of Carbamazepine and Its Metabolite With Age, Weight, Dose, and Clearances in Epileptic Children," *Epilepsia*, 1994, 35(6):1221-9.

Persinger MA, "Subjective Improvement Following Treatment With Carbamazepine (Tegretol®) for a Subpopulation of Patients With Traumatic Brain Injuries," *Percept Mot Skills*, 2000, 90(1):37-40.

Tibballs J, "Acute Toxic Reaction to Carbamazepine: Clinical Effects and Serum Concentrations," *J Pediatr*, 1992, 121(2):295-9.

♦ **Carbamazepinum** *see* Carbamazepine, Serum *on page 741*

♦ **Carbategretal®** *see* Carbamazepine, Serum *on page 741*

♦ **Carbatrol®** *see* Carbamazepine, Serum *on page 741*

♦ **Carbazep®** *see* Carbamazepine, Serum *on page 741*

♦ **Cardioquin®** *see* Quinidine, Serum *on page 764*

♦ **Cardioreg®** *see* Digoxin, Serum *on page 746*

♦ **Cardizem®** *see* Diltiazem, Serum or Plasma *on page 747*

♦ **Catapres®** *see* Clonidine, Serum or Plasma *on page 744*

♦ **CBZ** *see* Carbamazepine, Serum *on page 741*

♦ **Cerebrospinal Fluid Methotrexate** *see* Methotrexate, Serum or Plasma *on page 756*

♦ **Chan Su** *see* Digoxin, Serum *on page 746*

Chloramphenicol

Synonyms Chloromycetin®; Mychel-S®

Abstract The use of chloramphenicol has greatly diminished in recent years because of the introduction of a wide array of less toxic alternative agents. It is still appropriate to use this agent to treat certain rickettsial infections in selected patients, or in carefully selected penicillin-allergic patients with bacterial meningitis. The most feared side effect of this drug, aplastic anemia, is idiopathic, and is therefore not serum concentration related.

Specimen Serum

Container Red top tube

Sampling Time Collect trough level immediately before next dose; peak level 1-2 hours after oral dose, 30 minutes after I.V. dose (time to peak can be variable).

Storage Instructions Freeze processed specimen

Reference Interval Therapeutic: 10-25 µg/mL (SI: 31-77 µmol/L); trough: <5 µg/mL (SI: <15 µmol/L)

Critical Values Toxic: >25 µg/mL (SI: >77 µmol/L)

Use Monitor drug therapy; monitoring for potential toxicity. See Table B in the Therapeutic Drug Monitoring Introduction *on page 733*.

Limitations There are no data that correlate serum concentrations with efficacy. Trough concentrations have not been associated with efficacy or toxicity. Reversible dose-related (nonidiosyncratic) bone marrow depression may occur with serum/plasma concentrations >25 µg/mL (SI: >77 µmol/L). Idiosyncratic (nondose-related and serum-concentration independent) bone marrow aplasia is a rare event (1 in 20,000 or more treatment courses) that usually occurs weeks to months after completion of therapy, but may occur during the course of therapy. Hematologic studies (leukocyte count with differential, reticulocyte count, platelet count, hemoglobin) should be performed before and during therapy.

Methodology High performance liquid chromatography (HPLC), gas-liquid chromatography (GLC), immunoassay

Additional Information
- Half-life (adults): 1.5-4.1 hours
- Volume of distribution: 0.9 L/kg
- Protein binding: 50% to 60%

Chloramphenicol is an effective antibacterial agent which unfortunately has both idiosyncratic and dose-related toxicities. Half-life is increased in infants and patients with hepatic and renal disease. Chloramphenicol inhibits bacteria by binding to the 50 s subunit of the 70 s bacterial ribosome, which blocks attachment of aminotransfer RNA to the ribosome.

Hematologic toxicities of chloramphenicol have limited its use. They can be manifested as concentration-related, reversible bone marrow suppression, or rare, irreversible idiosyncratic aplastic anemia. Concentration-related bone marrow suppression has been associated with peak concentrations >25 µg/mL. Reversible bone marrow suppression begins with reticulocytopenia and a decrease in hemoglobin. With continued use, thrombocytopenia and neutropenia may occur. The more feared aplastic anemia is not concentration related. There may be a genetic predisposition to this adverse effect. There may be an increased incidence of leukemia in survivors of this toxicity. Gray baby syndrome is the other dreaded adverse effect seen with chloramphenicol use. This toxicity generally occurs in infants, but may occur in susceptible adults (those with hepatic dysfunction). In infants, there is a limited ability to conjugate chloramphenicol with glucuronide, which inactivates the parent compound. This syndrome includes vomiting, ashen gray color, abdominal distention, metabolic acidosis, and about a 40% mortality rate.

Chloramphenicol is a hepatic enzyme inhibitor. It decreases the clearance of many drugs, including warfarin, tolbutamide, chlorpropamide, and phenytoin. Chloramphenicol clearance is increased by some enzyme inducers including phenobarbital, phenytoin, and rifampin. Laboratory guidelines for monitoring antimicrobial drugs have been reviewed.[1]

Footnotes
1. Hammett-Stabler CA and Johns T, "Laboratory Guidelines for Monitoring of Antimicrobial Drugs," National Academy of Clinical Biochemistry, *Clin Chem*, 1998, 44(5):1129-40.

References

Kasten MJ, "Clindamycin, Metronidazole, and Chloramphenicol," *Mayo Clin Proc*, 1999, 74(8):825-33.

Niessen WM, "Analysis of Antibiotics by Liquid Chromatograph-Mass Spectrometry," *J Chromatogr A*, 1998, 812(1-2):53-75.

Smilack JD, Wilson WR, and Cockerill FR 3d, "Tetracyclines, Chloramphenicol, Erythromycin, Clindamycin, and Metronidazole," *Mayo Clin Proc*, 1991, 66(12);1270-80.

Yunis AA, "Chloramphenicol: Relation of Structure to Activity and Toxicity," *Annu Rev Pharmacol Toxicol*, 1988, 28:83-100.

Chlordiazepoxide, Serum

Related Information
Benzodiazepines, Qualitative, Urine *on page 782*
Diazepam, Serum *on page 745*

Synonyms A-Poxide®; Equibral®; Librax®; Libritabs®; Librium®; Methaminodiazepoxide Hydrochloride; Mitran®; Resposan-10®; SK-Lygen®; Smail®; Solium®; Tropium®

Abstract The benzodiazepines and the tricyclic antidepressants are used in patients with panic disorder. Chlordiazepoxide is a widely prescribed benzodiazepine drug used as a sedative-hypnotic (tranquilizer) prescribed for anxiety and panic. The drug is also used for withdrawal symptoms of acute alcoholism and for preoperative apprehension.

Specimen Serum

Container Red top tube

Sampling Time Trough levels at steady state (40-60 hours); collect for peak level 4 hours after oral dosing.

Storage Instructions Process immediately; avoid exposure to light; freeze if not analyzed immediately.

Reference Interval Therapeutic: 0.7-1.0 µg/mL (SI: 2.3-3.3 µmol/L)

Critical Values Toxic: >5 µg/mL (SI: >17 µmol/L)

Use Monitor therapeutic drug level for compliance; determine toxic level

Methodology High performance liquid chromatography (HPLC), thin-layer chromatography (TLC), gas chromatography (GC), fluorometry

Additional Information
- Half-life: 8-12 hours, longer with renal disease, up to 30-63 hours with cirrhosis
- Volume of distribution: 0.2-0.4 L/kg
- Protein binding: 90% to 95%

This antianxiety agent is commonly used in suicide attempts. Chlordiazepoxide is slowly absorbed and may take several hours to reach a peak plasma level. The drug is metabolized by the liver and is excreted by the kidneys. The drug is highly (90%) protein bound. Overdosage with the benzodiazepines is frequent, but serious sequelae are rare. However, there is an additive effect when used with other CNS depressants (eg, ethanol and barbiturates). If a patient is comatose after a drug ingestion, chlordiazepoxide **alone** is not a sufficient explanation. Metabolism results in the production of four active metabolites. Toxicity is manifested by ataxia, sedation, coma, cardiac arrhythmias, hypotension, and seizures.

References

Baselt RC, *Disposition of Toxic Drugs and Chemicals in Man*, 5th ed, Foster City, CA: Chemical Toxicology Institute, 2000, 153-6.

Closser MH and Brower KJ, "Treatment of Alprazolam Withdrawal With Chlordiazepoxide Substitution and Taper," *J Subst Abuse Treat*, 1994, 11(4):319-23.

Fraser AD, "Use and Abuse of the Benzodiazepines," *Ther Drug Monit*, 1998, 20(5):481-9.

Garretty DJ, Wolff K, and Hay A, "Microextraction of Chlordiazepoxide and its Primary Metabolites, Desmethylchlordiazepoxide and Demoxepam, From Plasma and Their Measurement by Liquid Chromatography," *Ann Clin Biochem*, 1998, 35:(Pt 4)528-33.

Giri AK and Banerjee S, "Genetic Toxicology of Four Commonly Used Benzodiazepines: A Review," *Mutat Res*, 1996, 340(2-3):93-108.

Minder EI, "Toxicity in a Case of Acute and Massive Overdose of Chlordiazepoxide and its Correlation to Blood Concentration," *J Toxicol Clin Toxicol*, 1989, 27(1-2):117-27.

♦ **Chloromycetin®** *see* Chloramphenicol *on page 742*

♦ **Chlorpromazine** *see* Phenothiazines, Serum or Urine *on page 760*

Chlorpromazine, Serum

Related Information
Antiphospholipid Antibody (Lupus Anticoagulant and/or Anticardiolipin Antibody) *on page 331*
Bilirubin, Total, Serum *on page 118*
Phenothiazines, Serum or Urine *on page 760*

Synonyms Amazin®; Bay Clor®; Dozine®; Hibanil®; Largactil®; Ormazine®; Prozil®; Repazine®; Thorazine®

Applies to Phenothiazines

Abstract This is an aliphatic phenothiazine used as an antipsychotic and sedative agent. The drug is also used for intractable hiccups and to control nausea and vomiting.

Specimen Serum

Container Red top Vacutainer®

Sampling Time Trough (serum) at steady state (150 hours)

Collection Serum

Storage Instructions Refrigerate

Reference Interval Therapeutic: 50-300 ng/mL (SI: 157-942 nmol/L)

Critical Values Toxic: >750 ng/mL (SI: >2355 nmol/L)

Use Screen for chlorpromazine in urine; evaluate possibility of chlorpromazine poisoning or drug toxicity (serum)

Limitations Urine test is not specific for chlorpromazine; it may detect other phenothiazines if present.

Contraindications The drug should not be used in the presence of nervous system depressants such as alcohol, barbiturates, and narcotics.

Methodology Gas-liquid chromatography (GLC), high performance liquid chromatography (HPLC)

Additional Information
- Half-life: 30 hours
- Volume of distribution: 20 L/kg
- Protein binding: 95% to 98%

Due to the complex metabolism of this drug, the pharmacokinetics are variable and follow a multiphasic pattern. Attempts to correlate drug levels with clinical responses have not been successful. Chlorpromazine in overdose causes drowsiness, fainting, hypotension or hypertension, tachycardia, tremor, dizziness, hypoglycemia, coma, and other signs and symptoms. A wide spectrum of adverse reactions is recognized. They include hypotension, tachycardia, cardiac arrhythmias, sedation, seizures, photosensitivity, and other phenomena. Deaths from accidental poisonings are rare.

Chlorpromazine may have endocrinopathic, hematologic, hepatic and CNS consequences. **Endocrinopathic** consequences may include amenorrhea with blocked ovulation with increased urinary estrogens, decreased urinary gonadotropins and progestins. Galactorrhea, gynecomastia, and inappropriate antidiuretic hormone activity occur. Other endocrinopathic consequences may be associated with decreased serum growth hormone, increased metabolism by hepatic microsomes (decreased thyroxine, T_4), increased metabolism and decreased organ uptake of norepinephrine (increased VMA), altered steroid metabolism, or an inhibition of hypothalamic corticotropin-releasing hormone and decreased ACTH secretion. **Hematologic** consequences may be associated with hemolytic anemia as well as occasional neutropenia, agranulocytosis, and granulocytopenia. Some patients taking this drug develop antiphospholipid antibodies. However, no predisposition to thromboembolism was noted. Increase in antinuclear antibodies has been noted. **Hepatic** sensitivity occurs in 1% of patients and is the prototype of hepatocanalicular cholestasis. Several hundred cases had been reported by 1962. It may resemble extrahepatic obstructive jaundice and can lead to laparotomy. It is characterized by an approximately threefold increase in alkaline phosphatase, slight to moderate increases in AST and ALT, and frequently, eosinophilia as well as increased bilirubin. A pseudoprimary biliary cirrhosis clinical picture is uncommon but well described.[1]

Central nervous system reactions include extrapyramidal changes, confusion, and tardive dyskinesia.

False-positive pregnancy tests may occur in patients on chlorpromazine. Chlorpromazine causes false positives for phenylketonuria, amylase, uroporphyrins, urobilinogen. It may cause positive direct Coombs reaction and may interfere with determinations of BUN and vitamin B_{12}.

Chlorpromazine has an additive effect with other CNS-depressing agents. Chlorpromazine may increase valproic acid serum concentrations; when given with piperazine, seizures may occur. Antacids, cimetidine may interfere with chlorpromazine absorption. Nortriptyline or propranolol may increase chlorpromazine levels. Salicylamide and acetanilide may displace chlorpromazine from its protein binding. H_2-antagonists decrease absorption of chlorpromazine.

Footnotes
1. Zimmerman HJ, "Psychotropic and Anticonvulsant Agents," *Hepatotoxicity: The Adverse Effects of Drugs and Other Chemicals on the Liver*, 2nd ed, Chapter 18, Philadelphia, PA: Lippincott Williams & Wilkens, 1999, 483-516.

References
Baselt RC, *Disposition of Toxic Drugs and Chemicals in Man*, 5th ed, Foster City, CA: Chemical Toxicology Institute, 2000, 173-7.

Boehme C and Strobel HW, "High Performance Liquid Chromatographic Methods for the Analysis of Haloperidol and Chlorpromazine Metabolism *In Vitro* by Purified Cytochrome P-450 Isoforms," *J Chromatogr B Biomed Sci Appl*, 1998, 718(2):259-66.

Friedman NL, "Hiccups: A Treatment Review," *Pharmacotherapy*, 1996, 16(6):986-95.

Gocke E, "Review of the Genotoxic Properties of Chlorpromazine and Related Phenothiazines," *Mutat Res*, 1996, 366(1):9-21.

Howanitz E, Pardo M, Smelson DA, et al, "The Efficacy and Safety of Clozapine Versus Chlorpromazine in Geriatric Schizophrenia," *J Clin Psychiatry*, 1999, 60(1):41-4.

Lillicrap DP, Pinto M, Benford K, et al, "Heterogeneity of Laboratory Test Results for Antiphospholipid Antibodies in Patients Treated With Chlorpromazine and Other Phenothiazines," *Am J Clin Pathol*, 1990, 93(6):771-5.

Zucker S, Zarrabi HM, Schubach WH, et al, "Chlorpromazine-Induced Immunopathy: Progressive Increase in Serum IgM," *Medicine (Baltimore)*, 1990, 69(2):92-100.

♦ **Chrysotherapy** *see* Gold, Serum *on page 751*

♦ **Cibalith-S®** *see* Lithium, Serum *on page 754*

♦ **Ciclosporin** *see* Cyclosporine, Blood *on page 744*

♦ **Cin-Quin®** *see* Quinidine, Serum *on page 764*

♦ **Citrovorum Factor** *see* Methotrexate, Serum or Plasma *on page 756*

Clonazepam, Serum

Related Information
Benzodiazepines, Qualitative, Urine *on page 782*
Diazepam, Serum *on page 745*

Synonyms Iktorivil®; Klonopin™; Rivatril®

Abstract The drug is in the class of benzodiazepines, which are used as tranquilizers. This drug is effective in prevention of absence seizures, myoclonic jerks, and tonic-clonic seizures. Its use is mostly for refractory myoclonic seizures.[1] It is useful in reducing tardive dyskinesia.[2,3]

Specimen Serum

Container Red top tube

Sampling Time Serum peak levels occur ~2 hours after oral administration. The apparent half-life after a single oral dose is 20-40 hours. Use trough for monitoring. Steady-state concentration is reached in 5-10 days.

Storage Instructions Separate serum and freeze. Protect from sunlight.

Reference Interval Therapeutic: 10-50 ng/mL (SI: 32-158 nmol/L)

Critical Values >80 ng/mL

Possible Panic Range >100 ng/mL (SI: >255 nmol/L)

Use Monitor drug level and toxicity

Methodology Gas-liquid chromatography (GLC) with electron capture detection, high performance liquid chromatography (HPLC)

Additional Information
- Half-life: 20-60 hours; active metabolites have longer half-lives than the parent drug; half-lives are increased in the elderly
- Volume of distribution: 2-6 L/kg
- Protein binding: 80% to 90%.

Therapeutic effect is not well correlated with serum levels. Effect of CNS depressants may be augmented by concomitant use of clonazepam. It exhibits synergistic effect with barbiturates and alcohol. See Table A in the Therapeutic Drug Monitoring Introduction *on page 733*.

Footnotes
1. Brodie MJ and Dichter MA, "Drug Therapy: Antiepileptic Drugs," *N Engl J Med*, 1996, 334(3):168-75.
2. Thaker GK, Nguyen JA, Strauss ME, et al, "Clonazepam Treatment of Tardive Dyskinesia: A Practical GABAmimetic Strategy," *Am J Psychiatry*, 1990, 147(4):445-51.
3. Gerding LB and Labbate LA, "Use of Clonazepam in an Elderly Bipolar Patient With Tardive Dyskinesia: A Case Report," *Ann Clin Psychiatry*, 1999, 11(2):87-9.

References
Baselt RC and Cravey RH, *Disposition of Toxic Drugs and Chemicals in Man*, 5th ed, Foster City, CA: Chemical Toxicology Institute, 2000, 194-6.

Morishita S and Aoki S, "Clonazepam in the Treatment of Prolonged Depression," *J Affect Disord*, 1999, 53(3):275-8.

Sallustio BC, Kassapidis C, and Morris RG, "High Performance Liquid Chromatography Determination of Clonazepam in Plasma Using Solid-Phase Extraction," *Ther Drug Monit*, 1994, 16(2):174-8.

♦ **Clonidine Hydrochloride** *see* Clonidine, Serum or Plasma *on page 744*

Clonidine, Serum or Plasma

Related Information
Diltiazem, Serum or Plasma *on page 747*
Propranolol, Serum *on page 763*

Synonyms Catapres®; Clonidine Hydrochloride

Abstract Clonidine is an antihypertensive. It is also used as a stimulant in a test for growth hormone release and a suppressant in a test for catecholamine release. Occasionally it is used for the treatment of attention-deficit/hyperactivity disorder,[1] smoking cessation,[2] and opiate withdrawal.

Specimen Plasma, serum

Container Lavender top (EDTA) tube for plasma; do not use gel separator tube for serum

Sampling Time Trough

Storage Instructions Refrigerate. Ship at room temperature.

Turnaround Time 2-4 days

Reference Interval 1-3 ng/mL

Critical Values >4 ng/mL

Use Monitor therapy or evaluate toxicity

Contraindications Unsafe in patients with porphyria

Methodology Gas chromatography (GC), gas chromatography/mass spectrometry (GS/MS)

Additional Information
- Half-life: 5-20 hours
- Volume of distribution: 1.5-2.5 hours
- Protein binding: 20% to 40%

Clonidine is metabolized by the liver to inactive metabolites which are eliminated through urine and feces.[3] Adverse reactions include bradycardia, orthostatic hypotension, drowsiness, dizziness, constipation, xerostomia, and nausea. In overdose situations, naloxone is used as an antidote.[3] Clonidine may cause increase in serum cortisol and decrease in epinephrine and norepinephrine.

Footnotes
1. Silver LB, "Alternative (Nonstimulant) Medications in the Treatment of Attention-Deficit/Hyperactivity Disorder in Children," *Pediatr Clin North Am*, 1999, 46(5):965-75.
2. Gourlay SG, Stead LF, and Benowitz NL, "Clonidine for Smoking Cessation," *Cochrane Database Syst Rev*, 2000, 2:CD58.
3. Leikin JB and Palouček FP, *Poisoning and Toxicology Compendium*, Hudson, OH: Lexi-Comp Inc, 1998, 197-8.

References
Cline JC and Connelly J, "Intravenous Clonidine for Hypertensive Emergencies," *Am J Health Syst Pharm*, 1999, 56(6):572-4.
Epstein M, "Diagnosis and Management of Hypertensive Emergencies," *Clin Cornerstone*, 1999, 2(1):41-54.
Lenz T, Ross A, Schumm-Daeger P, et al, "Clonidine Suppression Test Revisited," *Blood Press*, 1998, 7(3):153-9.

♦ **Co-Dax®** *see* Doxepin, Serum *on page 748*

♦ **Coffee Break®** *see* Caffeine, Serum *on page 740*

♦ **Combivir®** *see* Zidovudine, Serum or Plasma *on page 771*

♦ **Comizial®** *see* Phenobarbital, Serum or Plasma *on page 760*

♦ **Compazine®** *see* Phenothiazines, Serum or Urine *on page 760*

♦ **Cordarone®** *see* Amiodarone, Serum *on page 735*

♦ **Cordilox®** *see* Verapamil, Serum or Plasma *on page 769*

♦ **Corramedan®** *see* Digitoxin, Serum *on page 745*

♦ **Coumadin®** *see* Warfarin *on page 770*

♦ **CSA** *see* Cyclosporine, Blood *on page 744*

♦ **CyA** *see* Cyclosporine, Blood *on page 744*

♦ **Cyclic Antidepressants** *see* Antidepressants, Cyclic, Serum *on page 737*

♦ **Cyclosporine A** *see* Cyclosporine, Blood *on page 744*

Cyclosporine, Blood

Related Information
Itraconazole, Serum *on page 753*
Phenytoin, Serum or Plasma *on page 761*
Tacrolimus, Whole Blood *on page 765*
Verapamil, Serum or Plasma *on page 769*

Synonyms Ciclosporin; CSA; CyA; Neoral®; Sandimmune®

Applies to Cyclosporine A

Abstract Cyclosporine is a cyclic polypeptide widely used as an immunosuppressant, especially following organ transplants. It has revolutionized transplantation surgery, providing 10% to 15% improvement in allograft survival. It has serious problems relevant to toxicity.

Cyclosporine use is associated with alterations in helper and effector T lymphocytes and with natural killer cells.

Specimen Whole blood

Container Lavender top (EDTA) tube

Sampling Time Trough levels should be obtained 12-18 hours after oral dose (chronic usage), 12 hours after intravenous dose, or immediately prior to next dose.

Collection Draw from a different line than that through which the dose was given.

Reference Interval 100-300 ng/mL for renal transplant; 200-350 ng/mL for cardiac, hepatic, and pancreatic transplant (12 hours after oral dose). Since cyclosporine binds to erythrocytes and lipoproteins, measuring whole blood concentrations is preferred. Therapeutic ranges are poorly defined. They relate to the organ transplanted, time following transplantation, and organ function. They are method and specimen dependent.

Critical Values >400 ng/mL

Use Monitor blood level in management of immunosuppression for organ transplant recipients. The agent is used extensively to control rejection of organ transplants, especially of liver, heart, bone marrow, and kidney. It is used with corticosteroids to prevent graft-versus-host disease, and with other drugs (eg, tacrolimus).

Monitoring of blood levels is imperative because the pharmacokinetics of cyclosporine are complex and vary over time in the same patient; thus, blood levels cannot be well predicted from dosing schedules. Furthermore, this drug has a narrow therapeutic window and significant toxicity at levels above that range.

Absorption of cyclosporine in the form of Sandimmune® is highly variable. The newer, microemulsion form of cyclosporine (Neoral®) has more reproducible absorption.

Limitations Results are method dependent - some measure multiple metabolites as well as parent drug. Single assays are not as informative as a series over time.

Methodology Radioimmunoassay (RIA), high performance liquid chromatography (HPLC), fluorescence polarization immunoassay (FPIA), enzyme immunoassay (EIA)[1]

Additional Information
- Half-life: 8-24 hours
- Volume of distribution: 4-6 L/kg
- Protein binding: 90%
- Time to reach steady state: 2-6 days

Cyclosporine is an immunosuppressive agent derived from *Tolypocladium inflatum gams*, a fungus originally isolated from a Norwegian soil sample. The exact mechanism of action of the drug is not known, but it appears to interfere with T-helper cell function and secretion of lymphokines. It is not myelosuppressive.

Renal toxicity with eventual renal failure is the most severe complication. Cyclosporine diminishes glomerular filtration rate. Other assays to assess renal function: BUN and creatinine clearance should be considered along with cyclosporine levels, since toxicity may begin even with "acceptable" blood levels. Other important toxic effects include hypertension (in >90% of heart transplant recipients in the first year), convulsions, tremors, pulmonary edema, and an increased risk of lymphoma.

There are many drugs which affect cyclosporine pharmacokinetics, the most common being those which inhibit or induce P-450 enzyme system. Drugs which enhance the potential toxicity of cyclosporine, and which are also likely to be administered to a transplant recipient, include acyclovir, aminoglycoside antibiotics, amphotericin B, cephalosporins, furosemide, ketoconazole, and trimethoprim-sulfa. **Agents which raise cyclosporine levels** by decreasing biotransformation include amphotericin B, cimetidine, erythromycin, and methylprednisolone. Other drugs which lead to increased concentrations of cyclosporine include androgens, diltiazem, ketoconazole, methotrexate, nicardipine, oral contraceptives, and verapamil. Drugs which increase hepatic metabolism and thus **lower cyclosporine levels** include carbamazepine, ethotoin, intravenous trimetheprim-sulfa, mephenytoin, phenobarbital, phenytoin, primidone, and rifampin.

Because results will vary depending on whether the assay is done on whole blood or serum/plasma, and on the method and cyclosporine antibody employed (monospecific or polyspecific), it is best for a given patient's specimens to be analyzed at a single laboratory to eliminate as many assay-dependent variables as possible. If switching of laboratories is unavoidable, it is advisable to have a few specimens run in parallel in the second laboratory prior to changing. HPLC is a preferred method as it measures parent drug and is independent of metabolite interferences. However, it is cumbersome and is not readily available.

The clinical use of cyclosporine is difficult and requires experience and judgment. A drug blood level is only one of many pieces in the puzzle of transplant medicine. Electrolytes including magnesium and measures of renal and hepatic function are also needed.

Footnotes
1. Hamwi A, Veitl M, Männer G, et al, "Evaluation of Four Automated Methods for Determination of Whole Blood Cyclosporine Concentrations," *Am J Clin Pathol*, 1999, 112(3):358-65.

References
Abella I, "Pharmacoeconomics of Neoral®, a New Formulation of Cyclosporine, in Renal Transplantation," *Transplant Proc*, 1996, 28(6):3131-4.
Frei U, "Overview of the Clinical Experience With Neoral® in Transplantation," *Transplant Proc*, 1999, 31(3):1669-74.

Hamwi A, Salomon A, Steinbrugger R, et al, "Cyclosporine Metabolism in Patients After Kidney, Bone Marrow, Heart-Lung, and Liver Transplantation in the Early and Late Post-transplant Periods," *Am J Clin Pathol*, 2000, 114(4):536-43.

Ho S, Clipstone N, Timmermann L, et al, "The Mechanism of Action of Cyclosporin A and FK506," *Clin Immunol Immunopathol*, 1996, 80(3 Pt 2):S40-5.

Holt DW and Johnston A, "Cyclosporin A: Analytical Methodology and Factors Affecting Therapeutic Drug Monitoring," *Ther Drug Monit*, 1995, 17(6):625-30.

Holt DW, Johnston A, Kahan BD, et al, "New Approaches to Cyclosporine Monitoring Raise Further Concerns About Analytical Techniques," *Clin Chem*, 2000, 46(6 Pt 1):872-4.

Kahan BD, Welsh M, and Rutzky LP, "Challenges in Cyclosporine Therapy: The Role of Therapeutic Monitoring by Area Under the Curve Monitoring," *Ther Drug Monit*, 1995, 17(6):621-4.

Keown PA and Primmett DR, "Cyclosporine: The Principal Immunosuppressant for Renal Transplantation," *Transplant Proc*, 1998, 30(5):1712-5.

Kovarik JM and Koelle EU, "Cyclosporin Pharmacokinetics in the Elderly," *Drugs Aging*, 1999, 15(3):197-205.

Levy GA, "Neoral® Therapy in Liver Transplantation," *Transplant Proc*, 1996, 28(4):2225-8.

Lindholm A, "Cyclosporine A: Clinical Experience and Therapeutic Drug Monitoring," *Ther Drug Monit*, 1995, 17(6):631-7.

Moyer TP, "Therapeutic Drug Monitoring," *Tietz Textbook of Clinical Chemistry*, 3rd ed, Burtis CA and Ashwood ER, eds, Philadelphia, PA: WB Saunders Co, 1999, 862-905.

Noble S and Markham A, "Cyclosporin. A Review of the Pharmacokinetic Properties, Clinical Efficacy and Tolerability of a Microemulsion-Based Formulation (Neoral®)," *Drugs*, 1995, 50(5):924-41.

Oellerich M, Armstrong VW, Schultz E, et al, "Therapeutic Drug Monitoring of Cyclosporine and Tacrolimus. Update on Lake Louise Consensus Conference on Cyclosporin and Tacrolimus," *Clin Biochem*, 1998, 31(5):309-16.

Shihab FS, "Cyclosporine Nephropathy: Pathophysiology and Clinical Impact," *Semin Nephrol*, 1996, 16(6):536-47.

♦ **Cystodigin®** *see* Digitoxin, Serum *on page 745*

♦ **Dalcaine®** *see* Lidocaine, Serum or Plasma *on page 754*

♦ **Dalmane®** *see* Flurazepam, Serum *on page 751*

♦ **Demolox®** *see* Amoxapine, Serum or Plasma *on page 736*

♦ **Depacon®** *see* Valproic Acid, Serum or Plasma *on page 768*

♦ **Depakene®** *see* Valproic Acid, Serum or Plasma *on page 768*

♦ **Depakote®** *see* Valproic Acid, Serum or Plasma *on page 768*

♦ **Depakote® XR** *see* Valproic Acid, Serum or Plasma *on page 768*

♦ **Depamide®** *see* Valproic Acid, Serum or Plasma *on page 768*

♦ **Deprax®** *see* Trazodone, Serum or Plasma *on page 768*

♦ **Deralin®** *see* Propranolol, Serum *on page 763*

♦ **Desipramine** *see* Antidepressants, Cyclic, Serum *on page 737*

♦ **Desipramine** *see* Imipramine, Serum or Plasma *on page 752*

♦ **Desoxyphenobarbital** *see* Primidone, Serum or Plasma *on page 762*

♦ **Desyrel®** *see* Trazodone, Serum or Plasma *on page 768*

♦ **Dexitac®** *see* Caffeine, Serum *on page 740*

♦ **Diastat®** *see* Diazepam, Serum *on page 745*

♦ **Diazemuls®** *see* Diazepam, Serum *on page 745*

Diazepam, Serum

Related Information
Antidepressants, Cyclic, Serum *on page 737*
Barbiturates, Quantitative, Serum or Plasma *on page 739*
Benzodiazepines, Qualitative, Urine *on page 782*
Ethanol, Blood, Urine, and Other Sources *on page 789*

Synonyms Aliseum®; Alupram®; Atensine®; Diastat®; Diazemuls®; Di-Tran®; Lamra®; Solis®; Stesolid®; Tensium®; T-Quil®; Valium®; Valrelease®; Vatran®; Vazepam®; Vivol®; Zetran®

Abstract This is a benzodiazepine used as a sedative-hypnotic (tranquilizer) to treat anxiety, panic attacks, and muscle spasms. It is also frequently used to control seizures in emergency situations. It is a commonly abused benzodiazepine and is detectable in urine by benzodiazepine screening.

Specimen Serum

Container Red top tube

Sampling Time For peak level, 1 hour after oral dose or 15 minutes after I.V.

Storage Instructions Do not freeze

Reference Interval Therapeutic: diazepam: 0.2-1.0 μg/mL (SI: 0.7-3.5 μmol/L), N-desmethyldiazepam (nordiazepam): 0.1-0.5 μg/mL (SI: 0.35-1.8 μmol/L)

Critical Values Toxic: sum of diazepam plus N-desmethyldiazepam >3.0 μg/mL

Possible Panic Range Total of diazepam and nordiazepam >5 μg/mL (SI: >18 μmol/L) is toxic.

Use Therapeutic monitoring and toxicity assessment; diazepam is a muscle relaxant and antianxiety drug. Its uses include management of panic disorders, provision of preoperative sedation, alcohol withdrawal, and status epilepticus.[1] Because its active half-life in the CNS is much shorter than its serum half-life, longer-acting benzodiazepines (eg, lorazepam) may be preferred for treating status epilepticus.

Contraindications Cross-sensitivity with other benzodiazepines is described. It should not be used in comatose individuals, or those with pre-existing depression or narrow angle glaucoma. It should not be used in pregnant women.[1]

Methodology Enzyme immunoassay (EIA), fluorescent immunoassay, high performance liquid chromatography (HPLC), gas-liquid chromatography (GLC)

Additional Information
• Half-life: 20-50 hours; bioactive half-life in CNS: 55 minutes
• Volume of distribution: 1.0-1.5 L/kg
• Protein binding: 96% to 99%

Peak blood levels are achieved within an hour after oral dose. The major metabolite (N-desmethyldiazepam) has a half-life in adults of 50-99 hours. It is also the major metabolite of Tranxene® and prazepam. Diazepam may exhibit synergism with barbiturates, tricyclic antidepressants, and monoamine oxidase inhibitors. Toxicity may be additive with other central nervous system depressants, and ethanol enhances the absorption of diazepam itself. Many cases of overdose are seen but few fatalities result from use of this drug alone. A frequent finding is a combination of this drug and ethanol.

Diastat® is a rectal formulation of diazepam, 20 mg suppository, that is used by patients for emergency control of seizures.

Diazepam may cause false-negative urinary glucose determinations when using Clinistix® or Diastix®; it may inhibit thyroxine binding and may increase plasma testosterone.

The mechanism of action appears to be enhancing gamma aminobutyric acid effect. The side effects in toxic situations include outbursts of anger, behavior problems, depression, hallucinations, and memory impairment. Occasionally, status epilepticus can be precipitated.[2]

Footnotes
1. Leikin JB and Paloucek FP, *Poisoning and Toxicology Compendium*, Hudson, OH: Lexi-Comp Inc, 1998.
2. Al Tahan A, "Paradoxic Response to Diazepam in Complex Partial Status Epilepticus," *Arch Med Res*, 2000, 31(1):101-4.

References
Greenblatt DJ, Ehrenberg BL, Gunderman J, et al, "Pharmacokinetic and Electroencephalographic Study of Intravenous Diazepam, Midazolam, and Placebo," *Clin Pharmacol Ther*, 1989, 45(4):356-65.

Iwase H, Gondo K, Koike T, et al, "Novel Precolumn Deproteinization Method Using a Hydroxyapatite Cartridge for the Determination of Theophylline and Diazepam in Human Plasma by High Performance Liquid Chromatography With Ultraviolet Detection," *J Chromatogr B Biomed Appl*, 1994, 655(1):73-81.

Mitchell WG, Conry JA, Crumrine PK, et al, "An Open-Label Study of Repeated Use of Diazepam Recal Gel (Diastat®) for Episodes of Acute Breakthrough Seizures and Clusters: Safety, Efficacy, and Tolerance. North American Diastat® Group," *Epilepsia*, 1999, 40(11):1610-7.

♦ **Dicorynan®** *see* Disopyramide, Serum or Plasma *on page 747*

♦ **Digacin** *see* Digoxin, Serum *on page 746*

♦ **Digitalis** *see* Digitoxin, Serum *on page 745*

♦ **Digitalis Glycosides** *see* Digoxin, Serum *on page 746*

♦ **Digitalis-Like Immunoreactive Substances** *see* Digoxin, Serum *on page 746*

♦ **Digitoxine®** *see* Digitoxin, Serum *on page 745*

Digitoxin, Serum

Related Information
Digoxin, Serum *on page 746*

Synonyms Corramedan®; Cystodigin®; Digitalis; Digitoxine®; Digitrin®; Lanotoxin®; Nativelle®; Purodigin®; Tardigal®

Abstract One of a group of plant glycosides used in the treatment of congestive heart failure, digitoxin is infrequently used (compared to digoxin). It must not be confused with **digoxin** when serum levels are ordered. This drug is not commercially available in the United States,[1] however, it is in use in other parts of the world.

Specimen Serum

Container Red top tube

Sampling Time 6-12 hours after dose

Storage Instructions Separate serum and store in refrigerator.

Reference Interval Therapeutic: 18-35 ng/mL (SI: 24-46 nmol/L)

Critical Values Levels >35 ng/mL (SI: >46 nmol/L) are associated with clinical toxicity in 80% of patients.

Use Therapeutic monitoring and toxicity assessment. See Table C in the Therapeutic Drug Monitoring Introduction *on page 733*.

Limitations Do not order digitoxin level on a patient receiving digoxin. Serious errors will result. Digitoxin is very rarely used.
(Continued)

Digitoxin, Serum (Continued)

Contraindications Patient on **digoxin** or recent radioactive tracer (if RIA is used)

Methodology Radioimmunoassay (RIA), gas-liquid chromatography (GLC), high performance liquid chromatography (HPLC)

Additional Information
- Half-life: 150-250 hours
- Volume of distribution: 0.7 L/kg
- Protein binding: 90% to 95%

Optimal sampling time after dosage is 6 hours. Optimal resampling time after change in dosage is 48-96 hours. Be sure the patient is not on **digoxin** instead of **digitoxin**. There is cross reactivity between the two drugs and the levels reported will not be valid, and in fact could be misleading and catastrophic. Digitalis leaf has both digoxin and digitoxin as active components. Digitoxin is the best test for evaluation of toxicity in a patient taking **digitalis leaf**, but neither test is truly satisfactory. There is considerable overlap in the upper therapeutic ranges with levels which may be toxic. **Digitoxin levels must be correlated with clinical and other chemical data.** Numerous factors modify the effect of cardiac glycosides, including serum potassium, calcium, magnesium, and cardiac blood flow. Hypokalemia, hypomagnesemia, and hypercalcemia all potentiate toxicity from cardiac glycosides. In hospitalized elderly patients, digitoxin was less toxic as compared to digoxin, in a recent study.[2] Decreased GI absorption of digitoxin is seen with antacids, cholestyramine, colestipol; increased hepatic metabolism occurs with phenytoin, phenobarbital, phenylbutazone, isoniazid, ethambutol, rifampin, spironolactone, and aminoglycosides. Decreased protein binding occurs with phenylbutazone, sulfadimethoxine, phenobarbital, clofibrate, and tolbutamide. Digitoxin increases levels of verapamil. Digibind® (antidigoxin Fab fragments) will increase serum digitoxin level tenfold; digitoxin can interfere with urinary 17-hydroxycorticosteroid assay. Digoxin-like immunoreactive substance (DLIS), an endogenous natriuretic substance, may cause false elevation.

Footnotes
1. McEvoy G, ed, *American Hospital Formulary Service Drug Information*, American Society of Health System Pharmacists, Bethesda, MD: Cardiac Drugs, 1999, 1354.
2. Roever C, Ferrante J, Gonzalez EC, et al, "Comparing the Toxicity of Digoxin and Digitoxin in a Geriatric Population: Should an Old Drug Be Rediscovered?" *South Med J*, 2000, 93(2):199-202.

References
Bayer MJ, "Recognition and Management of Digitalis Intoxication: Implications for Emergency Medicine," *Am J Emerg Med*, 1991, 9(2 Suppl 1):29-34.

Dasgupta A and Hart AP, "Rapid Detection of Oleander Poisoning Using Fluorescence Polarization Immunoassay for Digitoxin. Effect of Treatment With Digoxin-Specific Fab Antibody Fragment (Ovine)," *Am J Clin Pathol*, 1997, 108(4):411-6.

Dasgupta A, Wells A, and Datta P, "Effect of Digoxin Fab Antibody on the Measurement of Total and Free Digitoxin by Fluorescence Polarization and a New Chemiluminescent Immunoassay," *Ther Drug Monit*, 1999, 21(2):251-5.

Kulick DL and Rahimtoola SH, "Current Role of Digitalis Therapy in Patients With Congestive Heart Failure," *JAMA*, 1991, 265(22):2995-7.

Taboulet P, Baud FJ, Bismuth C, et al, "Acute Digitalis Intoxication - Is Pacing Still Appropriate?" *Clin Toxicol*, 1993, 31:261-73.

♦ **Digitrin®** *see Digitoxin, Serum on page 745*

Digoxin, Serum

Related Information
Amiodarone, Serum *on page 735*
Digitoxin, Serum *on page 745*
Flecainide, Serum or Plasma *on page 749*
Magnesium, Serum *on page 221*
Potassium, Serum or Plasma *on page 258*
Quinidine, Serum *on page 764*
Verapamil, Serum or Plasma *on page 769*

Synonyms Allocar®; Cardioreg®; Digacin; Lanocor®; Lanoxicaps®; Lanoxin®; Lenoxin®; Purgoxin®

Applies to Botanical Dietary Supplements; Chan Su; Digitalis Glycosides; Digitalis-Like Immunoreactive Substances; Kyushin; Liu-Shan-Wan

Abstract Digoxin is a widely-used cardiac glycoside used in management of atrial fibrillation with rapid ventricular response, and in treatment of heart failure. A 200-year old controversy exists relevant to clinical use of digitalis. Digoxin is generally thought to ameliorate symptoms of heart failure and to improve exercise tolerance. It is an old, effective, inexpensive inotropic drug without an increased risk of death when intelligently used. Opponents of the drug recognize that it may be difficult to distinguish death **with** heart failure from death **of** failure.[1]

Specimen Serum

Container Red top tube

Sampling Time Blood specimen must be drawn **at least** 6 hours after the administration of the last dose.[2] The steady-state is usually reached in 5 days. After this time, a steady-state estimate is best obtained by a specimen drawn just before next dose.

Storage Instructions Separate serum and refrigerate.

Causes for Rejection Patient on a cardiac glycoside other than digoxin, recently administered radioisotopes if RIA is used for assay, hemolysis, sample collected in serum integrator gel tube

Reference Interval Therapeutic: adults: 0.8-2.0 ng/mL (SI: 1.0-2.6 nmol/L). Some have used 0.5 ng/mL as the lower end of the reference range.[3] The reference range may be higher in neonates. Adverse effects can take place within the therapeutic range.[1]

Critical Values Toxic: >2.5 ng/mL (SI: >3.2 nmol/L). The lethal dose is about double the level causing minor toxic manifestations.[4] In patients with hypokalemia or hypomagnesemia, toxicity may occur at a level <2 ng/mL. The most common manifestations of suspected toxicity are ventricular fibrillation, tachycardia, supraventricular arrhythmia, and second- or third-degree atrioventricular block.[3]

Possible Panic Range >3.0 ng/mL (SI: >3.8 nmol/L). See Table C in the Therapeutic Drug Monitoring Introduction *on page 733*.

Use The clinical use of digoxin is driven by relief of persistent symptoms. Its use by the knowledgeable physician is often in concert with other drugs (eg, angiotensin-converting-enzyme inhibitors and beta-adrenergic blockers).

Digoxin levels are useful for diagnosis and prevention of digoxin toxicity; for prevention of underdosage; and for patients with implanted pacemakers, especially patients on digoxin who are elderly, and/or who have renal failure, and/or who have been given quinidine.[4] See Quinidine, Serum *on page 764*.

Indications recently published include clinical suspicion of subtherapeutic response, prior toxicity, evaluation of high-risk patients, following initiation of digoxin therapy, dosage readjustment when patients reach steady state, inpatient admission level and regular monitoring of outpatients each 10 months.[5] Although digoxin does not diminish overall mortality, it reduces hospitalization rates overall and is considered useful for worsening heart failure.[3] However, it increases risk of hospitalization for other cardiovascular causes.[1]

Limitations Digitoxin should not be confused with **digoxin**. Since there is cross reactivity between the two drugs, **results will not be valid if digoxin is measured when the patient is taking digitoxin**. All other digitalis derivatives will also cross react with this test and give invalid results. Toxic levels of digitoxin when assayed as digoxin give low results.

Serum concentrations have not been proven to correlate with drug efficacy. The wide reference range may obscure benefit:risk ratios.

Falsely normal or low levels may occur in patients recently given radioactive isotopes, when the method used is radioimmunoassay (RIA). RIA was the predominant method 10 years ago, but it has been largely replaced by enzyme immunoassay (EIA) and fluorescence polarization immunoassay (FPIA) methods. Endogenous digitalis-like immunoreactive substances (DLIS) are found in digoxin-free patients with a variety of clinical states associated with salt and fluid retention, such as renal failure, hepatic failure, low renin hypertension, and pregnancy. They are also present at birth in neonates and infants. These compounds (DLIS) cross react with digoxin-specific immunoassays and give falsely elevated plasma digoxin concentrations. Current assay methods (as below) do not entirely avoid this interference. Some assay methods give a falsely lowered digoxin concentration in the presence of DLIS.[6]

Methodology Enzyme immunoassay (EIA), fluorescence polarization immunoassay (FPIA), microparticle enzyme immunoassay (MEIA), chemiluminescent assay (CLIA)[7], radioimmunoassay (RIA)

Additional Information
- Half-life: 20-60 hours
- Volume of distribution: 7 L/kg
- Protein binding: 20% to 25%

Digoxin is indicated for long-term management of congestive heart failure and control of supraventricular tachyarrhythmias. It exerts a positive inotropic effect on the heart by inhibition of the Na-K-ATPase system. Approximately 75% of an oral dose is bioavailable. There is great variation in bioavailability between different manufacturers (60% to 100%). The average volume of distribution is 7 L/kg and is decreased in patients on quinidine, with renal failure, and hypothyroidism. Plasma concentrations do not accurately reflect pharmacologic effects of the drug until it is completely distributed. If obtained before complete distribution, concentration will be misleading. Digoxin is cleared primarily by the kidneys. The average half-life is 48 hours for a patient whose renal function is normal.

Be sure the patient is not on **digitoxin** instead of **digoxin**. Digitoxin is also an active component of digitalis leaf. Ninety percent of nontoxic patients have levels ≤2.0 ng/mL (SI: ≤2.6 nmol/L), 87% of toxic patients have levels >2.0 ng/mL. Levels >3.0 ng/mL in adults are strongly suggestive of overdosage. However, **digitalis levels must always be interpreted in light of clinical data**. Older, smaller patients require less digoxin. Proportionally lower loading doses are advocated in the elderly.[4] The most common cause of digitalis intoxication is potassium depletion. The primary cause of digoxin toxicity in the aged is decreased renal function. Maintenance doses should be adjusted to the glomerular filtration rate (GFR).[6] Renal failure, hypercalcemia, alkalosis, myxedema, hypomagnesemia, recent MI and other heart disease, hypokalemia, and hypoxia may increase sensitivity to the toxic effects of digoxin. Renal function and serum electrolytes should be frequently checked in patients receiving digoxin. Potassium-depleting diuretics are a major contributing factor to digitalis toxicity.

Quinidine may cause elevation of digoxin level by decreasing its excretion.[8] It is recommended that serum digoxin concentration be measured before initiation of quinidine therapy and again in 4-6 days. **Verapamil** and amiodarone cause increased digoxin levels, also by decrease in clearance. (Clearance parallels GFR.) Other drugs which decrease its clearance include cyclosporine, spironolactone, and propafenone.

When confronted with unexpectedly low digoxin levels, consider noncompliance, thyroid disease, malabsorption, and reduced intestinal blood flow from mesenteric arteriosclerosis. **Drugs** which diminish its bioavailability include metoclopramide, cholestyramine, colestipol, kaolin-pectin, neomycin, and sulfasalazine. Other agents that decrease digoxin levels include antacids, bran and para-aminosalicylic acid (PAS). Consider, as well, congestive failure and anticholinergic drug effects when low digoxin levels are encountered. Other drug interactions include antacids, cathartics, neomycin, phenytoin, and metoclopramide which may decrease absorption of digoxin. Indomethacin, diltiazem, erythromycin, tetracycline, itraconazole, nicardipine, triamterene, and spironolactone may increase digoxin serum concentration; penicillamine may decrease pharmacologic effects of digoxin. Propantheline and atropine may increase digoxin absorption.

Fab fragments of digoxin-specific antibodies are available for the treatment of serious digoxin toxicities.[9] Digibind® (antidigoxin Fab fragments-digoxin immune Fab) will increase total serum digoxin level about 50-fold.

Patients with **digitalis resistance** may require larger doses and may have higher than usual serum levels (eg, patients with hyperthyroidism).

Extracts of Chan Su, an over-the-counter Chinese medicine used as a cardiotonic agent, demonstrate significant digoxin-like immunoreactivity by FPIA and MEIA, but not by CLIA. Positive interference with serum digoxin with FPIA and negative interference by MEIA was described. Interference could be eliminated with monitoring of free digoxin concentrations. Chan Su is a component of Liu-Shan-Wan and Kyushin. Chinese herbal tea may contain Chan Su. Chan Su at high doses causes cardiac arrhythmia, seizure, and coma.[7]

Botanical dietary "supplements," so-called, contaminated by digitalis lanata have led to high-degree atrioventricular block (complete heart block).[10]

Footnotes

1. Packer M, "End of the Oldest Controversy in Medicine. Are We Ready to Conclude the Debate on Digitalis?" *N Engl J Med*, 1997, 336(8):575-6.
2. Williamson KM, Thrasher KA, Fulton KB, et al, "Digoxin Toxicity: An Evaluation in Current Clinical Practice," *Arch Intern Med*, 1998, 158(22):2444-9.
3. Garg R, Gorlin R, Smith T, et al, The Digitalis Investigation Group, "The Effect of Digoxin on Mortality and Morbidity in Patients With Heart Failure," *N Engl J Med*, 1997, 336(8):525-33.
4. Montamat SC, Cusack BJ, and Vestal RE, "Management of Drug Therapy in the Elderly," *N Engl J Med*, 1989, 321(5):303-9.
5. Canas F, Tanasijevic MJ, Maluf N, et al, "Evaluating the Appropriateness of Digoxin Level Monitoring," *Arch Intern Med*, 1999, 159(4):363-8.
6. Dasgupta A and Trejo O, "Suppression of Total Digoxin Concentrations by Digoxin-Like Immunoreactive Substances in the MEIA Digoxin Assay," *Am J Clin Pathol*, 1999, 111(3):406-10.
7. Dasgupta A, Biddle DA, Wells A, et al, "Positive and Negative Interference of the Chinese Medicine Chan Su in Serum Digoxin Measurement. Elimination of Interference by Using a Monoclonal Chemiluminescent Digoxin Assay or Monitoring Free Digoxin Concentration," *Am J Clin Pathol*, 2000, 114(2):174-9.
8. Mordel A, Halkin H, Zulty L, et al, "Quinidine Enhances Digitalis Toxicity at Therapeutic Serum Digoxin Levels," *Clin Pharmacol Ther*, 1993, 53(4):457-62.
9. Williams RH and Erickson T, "Evaluating Digoxin and Theophylline Intoxication in the Emergency Setting," *Lab Med*, 29(3):158-62.
10. Slifman NR, Obermeyer WR, Aloi BK, et al, "Contamination of Botanical Dietary Supplements by *Digitalis lanata*," *N Engl J Med*, 1998, 339(12):806-11.

References

Cauffield JS, Gums JG, and Grauer K, "The Serum Digoxin Concentration: Ten Questions to Ask," *Am Fam Phys*, 1997, 56(2):495-503, 509-10.

Cohen AF, Kroon R, Schoemaker R, et al, "Influence of Gastric Acidity on the Bioavailability of Digoxin," *Ann Intern Med*, 1991, 115(7):540-5.

Cohn JN, "Heart Failure: Future Treatment Approaches," *Am J Hypertens*, 2000, 13(5 Pt 2):74S-78S.

Cohn JN, "The Management of Chronic Heart Failure," *N Engl J Med*, 1996, 335(7):490-8.

Dasgupta A and Scott J, "Unexpected Suppression of Total Digoxin Concentrations by Cross-Reactants in the Microparticle Enzyme Immunoassay. Elimination of Interference by Monitoring Free Digoxin Concentration," *Am J Clin Pathol*, 1998, 110(1):78-82.

Datta P and Larsen F, "Specificity of Digoxin Immunoassays Toward Digoxin Metabolites," *Clin Chem*, 1994, 40(7 Pt 1):172-3.

Haji SA and Movahed A, "Update on Digoxin Therapy in Congestive Heart Failure," *Am Fam Phys*, 2000, 62(2):409-16.

Johnson MR, "Congestive Heart Failure: Diuretics, Digitalis, and Vasodilator Therapy," *Current Therapy in Critical Care Medicine*, 3rd ed, Parrillo JF, ed, St Louis, MO: Mosby Yearbook, Inc, 1997, 109-15.

Martin-Suarez A, Lanao JM, Calvo MV, et al, "Digoxin Pharmacokinetics in Patients With High Serum Digoxin Concentrations," *J Clin Pharm Ther*, 1993, 18(1):63-8.

Reddy S, Benatar D, Gheorghiade M, "Update on Digoxin and Other Positive Inotropic Agents for Chronic Heart Failure," *Curr Opin Cardiol*, 1997, 12(3):233-41.

Smith TW, "Digoxin in Heart Failure," *N Engl J Med*, 1993, 329(1):51-3.

Trejo O and Dasgupta A, "Unexpected Suppression of Digoxin Concentration by DLIS in the MEIA Assay: Elimination of Interference by Monitoring Free-Digoxin Concentration," *Am J Clin Pathol*, 1998, 110:(1)113-4.

Tsang P and Gerson B, "Digoxin Monitoring in the Geriatric Patient," *Drug Monitoring and Toxicology*, 1991, 12.

Tuncok Y, Hazan E, Oto O, "Relationship Between High Serum Digoxin Levels and Toxicity," *Int J Clin Pharmacol Ther*, 1997, 35(9):366-8.

Withering W, "An Account of the Foxglove," London, England: Paternoster-Row, 1785.

♦ **Dilantin®** *see* Phenytoin, Serum or Plasma *on page 761*

♦ **Dilocaine®** *see* Lidocaine, Serum or Plasma *on page 754*

Diltiazem, Serum or Plasma

Related Information
Clonidine, Serum or Plasma *on page 744*
Propranolol, Serum *on page 763*

Synonyms Acalix®; Britiazim®; Cardizem®; Latiazem Hydrochloride

Abstract Diltiazem is a calcium channel blocker used in the treatment of angina pectoris, hypertension, and supraventricular arrhythmias. The drug is extensively metabolized and primarily excreted in the urine.

Specimen Serum or plasma (EDTA)

Sampling Time Trough

Storage Instructions Store in refrigerator. Ship at room temperature.

Turnaround Time 2-3 days

Reference Interval 50-200 ng/mL

Use Monitor therapy

Methodology Gas-liquid chromatography (GLC), high performance liquid chromatography (HPLC)

Additional Information
- Half-life: 4-6 hours
- Volume of distribution: 4-8 L/kg
- Protein binding: 70% to 90%

Serious toxic effects include arrhythmias, shortness of breath, and fatigue due to heart failure. The common, less severe side effects are headache, drowsiness, swelling of feet and ankles, constipation, and nausea.

Diltiazem causes increase in serum concentration of the following drugs when administered concomitantly: buspirone, carbamazepine, digoxin, cyclosporine, propranolol, and theophylline.

References
Pool PE, "Anomalies in the Dosing of Diltiazem," *Clin Cardiol*, 2000, 23(1):18-23.

Sage PR, Kiosoglous AJ, Wuttke RD, et al, "Early Treatment With Verapamil or Diltiazem in Patients With Acute Myocardial Infarction: Safety and Possible Beneficial Effects," *Cardiovasc Drugs Ther*, 1999, 13(4):309-13.

Smith DH, Neutel JM, Weber MA, et al, "Comparisons of the Effects of Different Long-Acting Delivery Systems on the Pharmacokinetics and Pharmacodynamics of Diltiazem," *Am J Hypertens*, 1999, 12(10 Pt 1):1030-7.

Weir MR, "Diltiazem: Ten Years of Clinical Experience in the Treatment of Hypertension," *J Clin Pharmacol*, 1995, 35(3):220-32.

♦ **Dimipressin®, Iprogen®** *see* Imipramine, Serum or Plasma *on page 752*

♦ **Dintoina®** *see* Phenytoin, Serum or Plasma *on page 761*

♦ **Diphenylan Sodium®** *see* Phenytoin, Serum or Plasma *on page 761*

♦ **Diphenylhydantoin** *see* Phenytoin, Serum or Plasma *on page 761*

♦ **Dipropylacetic Acid** *see* Valproic Acid, Serum or Plasma *on page 768*

Disopyramide, Serum or Plasma

Related Information
Nortriptyline, Serum *on page 758*
Phenytoin, Serum or Plasma *on page 761*
Verapamil, Serum or Plasma *on page 769*

Synonyms Dicorynan®; Napamide®; Norpace®; Rhythmodan®; Ritmilen®

Abstract Disopyramide is a class IA antiarrhythmic agent. It is used in prevention of atrial flutter and fibrillation, and to prevent ventricular tachycardia and fibrillation.

Specimen Serum or plasma

Container Red top tube, green top (heparin) tube, or lavender top (EDTA) tube

Sampling Time Collect specimen 2-3 hours after an oral dose of disopyramide for peak. Draw trough just before next dose. Trough level is the best guide for dosing. Time to peak serum concentration is 30 minutes to 3 hours.

Special Instructions Other cardiac medications should be made known to the laboratory.

Reference Interval Therapeutic: trough: atrial arrhythmias: 2.8-3.2 µg/mL (SI: 8.3-9.4 µmol/L), ventricular arrhythmias: 3.3-5.0 µg/mL (SI: 9.7-15.0 µmol/L)

Critical Values Toxic: >7.0 µg/mL (SI: >20.6 µmol/L)

Possible Panic Range Fatalities are seen with concentrations >20.0 µg/mL. Bradycardia and asystole occur.

Use Therapeutic monitoring

Limitations Arrhythmias may occur at low levels. Disopyramide exhibits nonlinear binding in the therapeutic range. This combined with the fact that disopyramide is administered as a racemic mixture, makes total concentration difficult to correlate with pharmacodynamic effects.

Methodology Enzyme or fluorescent immunoassay, high performance liquid chromatography (HPLC)

Additional Information
- Half-life: 4-10 hours
- Volume of distribution: 0.7-0.9 L/kg
- Protein binding: 20% to 60% (inversely proportional to concentration)

(Continued)

Disopyramide, Serum or Plasma (Continued)

Disopyramide shares electrophysiologic properties with quinidine and procainamide. More than 80% of oral dose is absorbed and only a small fraction of the drug undergoes first-pass metabolism. Fifty percent of the drug is excreted unchanged in the urine. Some of the remainder is metabolized by the liver to inactive products. Dosage must be modified (dosage intervals prolonged) in patients with renal failure, and dosage interval relates to creatinine clearance. Serious toxic effects are depression of myocardial contractility and disturbances in myocardial conduction. Other effects include dry mouth, constipation, urinary hesitancy, and blurred vision. Metabolite N-desisopropyl disopyramide is also pharmacologically active, with activity approximately 25% that of disopyramide. Concomitant treatment with phenytoin may lead to decreased serum levels of disopyramide. There may be cumulative effects with other class I antiarrhythmic drugs (lidocaine, procainamide).

Disopyramide may cause decrease in glucose levels in test samples.

References
Duff HJ, Mitchell LB, Nath CF, et al, "Concentration-Response Relationships of Disopyramide in Patients With Ventricular Tachycardia," Clin Pharmacol Ther, 1989, 45(5):542-7.

Hasegawa J, Mori A, Yamamoto R, et al, "Disopyramide Decreases the Fasting Serum Glucose Level in Man," Cardiovasc Drugs Ther, 1999, 13(4):325-7.

Moyer TP, "Therapeutic Drug Monitoring," Tietz Textbook of Clinical Chemistry, 3rd ed, Chapter 26, Burtis CA and Ashwood ER, eds, Philadelphia, PA: WB Saunders Co, 1999, 862-905.

Witek A, Zawisza P, and Przyborowski L, "Determination of Disopyramide in Plasma by High Performance Liquid Chromatography," J Pharm Biomed Anal, 1994, 12(3):425-7.

- **Ditan®** see Phenytoin, Serum or Plasma on page 761
- **Di-Tran®** see Diazepam, Serum on page 745
- **Divalproex Sodium** see Valproic Acid, Serum or Plasma on page 768
- **Doxepin and Nordoxepine** see Antidepressants, Cyclic, Serum on page 737

Doxepin, Serum

Related Information
Antidepressants, Cyclic, Serum on page 737

Synonyms Adapin®; Co-Dax®; Novoxapin®; Sinequan®; Triadapin®

Test Includes Doxepin and desmethyldoxepine (nordoxepine)

Abstract This is a tricyclic antidepressant, dibenzoxepin analogue of amitriptyline. It is used for various forms of depression, often with psychotherapy. It is used for anxiety disorders, and a topical preparation is used for pruritus.

Specimen Serum or plasma

Container Red top tube or green top (heparin) tube

Sampling Time Trough levels at steady-state (50-125 hours). Time to peak serum concentration is 2-4 hours.

Causes for Rejection Specimen collected in gel tube

Reference Interval Sum of doxepin and desmethyldoxepin: 150-250 ng/mL (SI: 540-900 nmol/L)

Critical Values Toxic: >500 ng/mL (SI: >1800 nmol/L). Fatal cases are associated with values >10,000 ng/mL.

Use Therapeutic monitoring (compliance) and toxicity assessment

Methodology Immunoassay, high performance liquid chromatography (HPLC), gas chromatography (GC)

Additional Information
- Half-life: 10-25 hours
- Volume of distribution: 10-30 L/kg
- Protein binding: 75% to 85%

Doxepin, a tricyclic antidepressant, is a tertiary amine structural analog of amitriptyline with similar but less potent neurotransmitter effects and considerably less cardiotoxicity. Doxepin is metabolized to the active metabolite desmethyldoxepin (nordoxepine). Doxepin serum levels peak at 2-6 hours after an oral dose. The parent drug has a low bioavailability and steady-state is reached in 2-8 days. Geriatric patients respond well to doxepin.

Doxepin has side effects similar to other tricyclic antidepressants. The most common side effects are dry mouth, urinary retention, blurred vision, and constipation. These effects are due to anticholinergic properties of the drug. Respiratory depression, hypotension, coma, cardiac arrhythmias, and tachycardia occur in severe intoxication.

Topical form of doxepin is used for the relief of pruritus associated with eczema.

Doxepin increases glucose and catecholamine levels.

References
Caravati EM and Bossart PJ, "Demographic and Electrocardiographic Factors Associated with Severe Tricyclic Antidepressant Toxicity," J Toxicol Clin Toxicol, 1991, 29(1):31-43.

Deuschle M, Hartter S, Hiemke C, et al, "Doxepin and its Metabolites in Plasma and Cerebrospinal Fluid in Depressed Patients," Psychopharmacology, 1997, 131(1):19-22.

Geller B, Reising D, Leonard HL, et al, "Critical Review of Tricyclic Antidepressant Use in Children and Adolescents," J Am Acad Child Adolesc Psychiatry, 1999, 38(5):513-6.

Millikan LE, "Treating Pruritus. What's New in Safe Relief of Symptoms?" Postgrad Med, 1996, 99(1):173-6, 179-84.

Milstein S, Buetikofer J, Dunnigan A, et al, "Usefulness of Disopyramide for Prevention of Upright Tilt-Induced Hypotension-Bradycardia," Am J Cardiol, 1990, 65(20):1339-44.

Newton EH, Shih RD, and Hoffman RS, "Cyclic Antidepressant Overdose: A Review of Current Management Strategies," Am J Emerg Med, 1994, 12(3):376-9.

Sandor P, Baker B, Irvine J, et al, "Effectiveness of Fluoxetine and Doxepin in Treatment of Melancholia in Depressed Patients," Depress Anxiety, 1998, 7(2):69-72.

- **Dozic®** see Haloperidol, Serum or Plasma on page 752
- **Dozine®** see Chlorpromazine, Serum on page 743
- **Duo-Trach®** see Lidocaine, Serum or Plasma on page 754
- **Durvitan®** see Caffeine, Serum on page 740
- **Elavil®** see Amitriptyline, Serum on page 735
- **Elixophyllin®** see Theophylline, Serum on page 766
- **Endep®** see Amitriptyline, Serum on page 735
- **Enphenemalum** see Methylphenobarbital, Serum on page 757
- **Epanutin®** see Phenytoin, Serum or Plasma on page 761
- **Epilim®** see Valproic Acid, Serum or Plasma on page 768
- **Epinat®** see Phenytoin, Serum or Plasma on page 761
- **Epitrol®** see Carbamazepine, Serum on page 741
- **Equagesic®** see Meprobamate, Serum on page 756
- **Equanil®** see Meprobamate, Serum on page 756
- **Equibral®** see Chlordiazepoxide, Serum on page 742
- **Ergenyl®** see Valproic Acid, Serum or Plasma on page 768
- **Eskalith®** see Lithium, Serum on page 754

Ethchlorvynol, Serum or Plasma

Synonyms Placidyl®

Abstract This is a sedative hypnotic which is dangerous if not carefully monitored. In overdose, it may produce deep coma, severe respiratory depression, hypotension, and bradycardia.[1]

Specimen Serum or plasma

Container Red top tube or green top (heparin) tube

Sampling Time The peak blood level is attained in 1.5 hours; use trough samples for therapeutic drug monitoring.

Reference Interval 2-8 µg/mL (SI: 14-55 µmol/L)

Possible Panic Range Toxic: levels >20 µg/mL (SI: >138 µmol/L) are associated with severe sedation, coma, respiratory depression, hypotension, bradycardia, and hypothermia

Use Monitor therapeutic drug level

Methodology High performance liquid chromatography (HPLC), gas chromatography (GC), spectrophotometry. A color test with TLC and a spot test are available.[1]

Additional Information
- Half-life: 10-20 hours
- Volume of distribution: 4 L/kg
- Protein binding: 60%

Ethchlorvynol is a nonbarbiturate sedative-hypnotic drug. The peak blood level is attained in 1.5 hours. The half-life increases to 100 hours when high levels of drug are present. Most of the drug is metabolized in the liver. Exaggerated hypnotic effects occur if taken with ethanol. Can be detected in urine but only small amounts of the parent drug are present. Should be used cautiously in combination with oral anticoagulants. Effect is potentiated by alcohol.

Footnotes
1. Porter WH, "Clinical Toxicology," Tietz Textbook of Clinical Chemistry, 3rd ed, Chapter 27, Burtis CA and Ashwood ER, eds, Philadelphia, PA: WB Saunders Co, 1999, 906-81.

References
Baselt RC, Disposition of Toxic Drugs and Chemicals in Man, 5th ed, Foster City, CA: Chemical Toxicology Institute, 2000.

Gomolin I, "Ethchlorvynol," Clin Toxicol Rev, 1980, 2:1-2.

"Hypnotic Drugs," Med Lett Drugs Ther, 2000, 42(1084):71-2.

Winek CL, Wahba WW, and Winek CL Jr, "Body Distribution of Ethchlorvynol," J Forensic Sci, 1989, 34(3):687-90.

Yell RP, "Ethchlorvynol Overdose," Am J Emerg Med, 1990, 8(3):246-50.

Ethosuximide, Serum or Plasma

Related Information
Phenobarbital, Serum or Plasma on page 760
Phenytoin, Serum or Plasma on page 761

Synonyms Suxinutin®; Zarontin®; Zartalin®

Abstract Ethosuximide is the drug of choice for uncomplicated absence seizures. Ethosuximide is less toxic than other succinimides, notably methsuximide and phensuximide. If patients have absence seizures plus other seizure types, valproic acid is usually used.

Specimen Serum or plasma

Container Red top tube or green top (heparin) tube

Sampling Time Peak or trough levels may be used to monitor therapy, because blood levels are fairly constant. The trough specimen is more likely to provide useful information relevant to efficacy.[1]

Reference Interval 40-100 µg/mL (SI: 284-710 µmol/L)

Possible Panic Range >150 µg/mL (SI: >1062 µmol/L); toxicity may manifest with lethargy or psychotic behavior; significant drug interactions are uncommon. At steady-state, each 1 mg/kg will result in a serum rise of 2 µg/mL. See Table A in the Therapeutic Drug Monitoring Introduction *on page 733*.

Use Monitor for compliance, efficacy, or possible toxicity

Limitations Ethosuximide has relatively few serious adverse effects with chronic administration. Dose-related adverse effects, including photophobia and lethargy, sometimes may be avoided by slowly titrating the drug to effective levels. Other side effects include nausea, vomiting, anorexia, headache, and dizziness. Blood dyscrasias may occur and respond to decreasing the dose or stopping the drug. If patients have other seizure types in addition to absence seizures, ethosuximide may exacerbate the other seizure types.

Methodology Enzyme immunoassay (EIA), fluorescence polarization immunoassay (FPIA), gas-liquid chromatography (GLC), high performance liquid chromatography (HPLC)

Additional Information
- Half-life: 25-70 hours
- Volume of distribution: 0.7 L/kg
- Protein binding: 0% to 5%

Side effects usually involve the central nervous system (eg, lethargy, dizziness, ataxia) and the gastrointestinal tract (eg, nausea, vomiting, abdominal pain). Such effects do not regularly correlate with high drug concentrations.[2]

See table in Antiepileptic Drugs, New, Overview *on page 738*.

Footnotes
1. Moyer TP, "Therapeutic Drug Monitoring," *Tietz Textbook of Clinical Chemistry*, 3rd ed, Burtis CA and Ashwood ER, eds, Philadelphia, PA: WB Saunders Co, 1999, 862-905.
2. Brodie MJ and Dichter MA, "Antiepileptic Drugs," *N Engl J Med*, 1996, 334(3):168-75.

References
Baselt RC and Cravey RH, "Ethosuximide," *Disposition of Toxic Drugs and Chemicals in Man*, 5th ed, Foster City, CA: Chemical Toxicology Institute, 2000, 331-3.
Capovilla G, Beccaria F, Veggioti P, et al, "Ethosuximide Is Effective in the Treatment of Epileptic Negative Myoclonus in Childhood Partial Epilepsy," *J Child Neurol*, 1999, 14(6):395-400.
Chen SH, Wu HL, Shen MC, et al, "Trace Analysis of Ethosuximide in Human Plasma With a Chemically Removable Derivatizing Reagent and High-Performance Liquid Chromatography," *J Chromatogr B Biomed Sci Appl*, 1999, 729(1-2):111-7.
Wallace SJ, "Myoclonus and Epilepsy in Childhood: A Review of Treatment With Valproate, Ethosuximide, Lamotrigine, and Zonisamide," *Epilepsy Res*, 1998, 29(2):147-54.

Ethotoin, Serum

Related Information
Mephenytoin, Serum *on page 756*
Phenytoin, Serum or Plasma *on page 761*

Synonyms Accenon; Ethylphenylhydantoin; Peganone®

Test Includes Ethotoin. Antiepileptic activity is due to parent compound.

Abstract Ethotoin is occasionally used as an adjunctive anticonvulsant. Patients suffer dose-related gingival hyperplasia and hirsutism less often than with phenytoin.

Specimen Serum

Container Red top tube

Reference Interval 14-34 µg/mL

Use Ethotoin is used for generalized tonic-clonic or complex-partial seizures.[1]

Contraindications Abnormalities of liver, hematologic disorders

Additional Information Like phenytoin, ethotoin has zero-order kinetics and small dosage changes may produce large changes in clinical response. Teratogenicity may occur, particularly since ethotoin is usually combined with other anticonvulsants. The half-life of ethotoin is approximately 5-10 hours (dose dependent), necessitating four times daily dosing. Most common side effect is a bitter taste.

Test interactions include an increase in alkaline phosphatase and a decrease in calcium.

Footnotes
1. Leikin JB and Palourek FP, *Poisoning and Toxicology Compendium*, Hudson, OH: Lexi-Comp Inc, 1998.

References
Baselt RC, *Disposition of Toxic Drugs and Chemicals in Man*, 5th ed, Foster City, CA: Chemical Toxicology Institute, 2000, 333-4.

Kupferberg HJ, "Other Hydantoins: Mephenytoin and Ethotoin," *Antiepileptic Drugs*, 3rd ed, Levy RH, Dreifuss FE, Mattson RH, et al, eds, New York, NY: Raven Press, 1989, 257-65.

- ◆ **Ethylenediamine** *see* Theophylline, Serum *on page 766*
- ◆ **Ethylphenylhydantoin** *see* Ethotoin, Serum *on page 749*
- ◆ **Etrafon®** *see* Amitriptyline, Serum *on page 735*
- ◆ **Etrafon®** *see* Antidepressants, Cyclic, Serum *on page 737*
- ◆ **Etrafon®** *see* Phenothiazines, Serum or Urine *on page 760*
- ◆ **5-FC** *see* Flucytosine, Serum *on page 750*
- ◆ **Felbamate** *see* Antiepileptic Drugs, New, Overview *on page 738*
- ◆ **Felbatol®** *see* Antiepileptic Drugs, New, Overview *on page 738*
- ◆ **Fenilcal®** *see* Phenobarbital, Serum or Plasma *on page 760*
- ◆ **Fenitoina** *see* Phenytoin, Serum or Plasma *on page 761*
- ◆ **Fenytoin®** *see* Phenytoin, Serum or Plasma *on page 761*
- ◆ **Fiorinal®** *see* Barbiturates, Quantitative, Serum or Plasma *on page 739*
- ◆ **FK-506** *see* Tacrolimus, Whole Blood *on page 765*

Flecainide, Serum or Plasma

Related Information
Amiodarone, Serum *on page 735*
Digoxin, Serum *on page 746*
Propranolol, Serum *on page 763*

Synonyms Almartyn®; Tambocor®

Abstract Flecainide is a class IC antiarrhythmic drug. FDA recommends that the drug be reserved for life-threatening ventricular arrhythmias unresponsive to conventional therapy.

Specimen Serum or plasma

Container Red top tube (preferred) or green top (heparin) tube; do not use serum separator tube.

Sampling Time Draw sample just prior to dose (trough).

Storage Instructions Separate serum or plasma within 2 hours of the time the specimen was drawn from the patient.

Special Instructions Collect sample immediately prior to next dose for trough levels.

Reference Interval Therapeutic: trough: 0.2-1.0 µg/mL (SI: 0.5-2.4 µmol/L)

Critical Values Levels >1.0 µg/mL (SI: >2.4 µmol/L) have been related to higher incidence of adverse experiences. Monitor with ECG (QRS width, QTc prolongation, presence of first-degree or greater heart block) as well as with serum concentrations.

Use Therapeutic monitoring and toxicity assessment (toxic effects - hypotension, asystole - proportional to dose and concentration). Monitoring is required in subjects with severe renal failure or severe hepatic disease, and is recommended strongly in patients also on amiodarone. It may be helpful in persons with congestive heart failure and also in patients with moderate renal disease.

Methodology High performance liquid chromatography (HPLC), fluorescence polarization immunoassay (FPIA)

Additional Information
- Half-life (normal adult): 7-19 hours
- Volume of distribution: 5-13 L/kg
- Protein binding: 40% to 50% to plasma protein, primarily alpha-1-acid glycoprotein

Flecainide is a class IC antiarrhythmic drug approved for the suppression of ventricular arrhythmias. IC agents have three primary electrophysiological effects. Potent inhibition of the fast sodium channels depresses the upstroke of the action potential, which is manifested as a decrease in the maximal rate of phase 0 depolarization (conduction). Secondly, the IC agents significantly slow His-Purkinje conduction and cause QRS widening. Finally, these agents shorten the action potential of Purkinje fibers without affecting the surrounding myocardial tissue.

The drug is well absorbed orally. Plasma half-life averages 20 hours in adults although in children it has been reported to be 8 hours. Steady-state concentrations are achieved in 3-5 days. Since 10% to 50% of the drug is eliminated in the urine as unchanged drug, impaired renal function will significantly prolong the plasma half-life. Half-life is also increased with congestive heart failure. Clearance of flecainide can be accelerated by phenobarbital and rifampin. One hepatically produced metabolite of flecainide, m-O-dealkylated flecainide, has some electrophysiologic activity, but it is much less than that of the parent compound. Coadministration with digoxin increases serum digoxin concentrations by about 15% to 25%; coadministration with propranolol increases both drugs' serum concentrations (flecainide's by about 20%, propranolol's by about 30%), and the possibility of adverse negative inotropic effects should be considered. Elevations of serum alkaline phosphatase and also transaminases have been reported.

Flecainide was one of the agents used in the CAST study (cardiac arrhythmia suppression trial), which evaluated several antiarrhythmic agents in suppression of asymptomatic premature ventricular contractions
(Continued)

Flecainide, Serum or Plasma *(Continued)*

(PVCs) in postmyocardial infarction patients. This agent was associated with a higher mortality than that found in patients taking placebo.

References

Capucci A, Villani GQ, Piepoli MF, et al, "The Role of Oral 1C Antiarrhythmic Drugs in Terminating Atrial Fibrillation," *Curr Opin Cardiol*, 1999, 14(1):4-8.

Evers J, Eichelbaum M, and Kroemer HK, "Unpredictability of Flecainide Plasma Concentrations in Patients With Renal Failure: Relationship to Side Effects and Sudden Death," *Ther Drug Monit*, 1994, 16(4):349-51.

Roden DM and Woosley RL, "Drug Therapy. Flecainide," *N Engl J Med*, 1986, 315(1):36-41.

Valdes R Jr, Jortani SA, and Gheorghiade M, "Standards of Laboratory Practice: Cardiac Drug Monitoring," *Clin Chem*, 1998, 44(5):1096-109.

Flucytosine, Serum

Related Information

Amphotericin B, Serum *on page 737*
Itraconazole, Serum *on page 753*

Synonyms Ancobon®; 5-FC; 5-Fluorocytosine

Abstract Flucytosine is a synthetic antifungal agent often used in conjunction with amphotericin B, for treatment of fungal (primarily cryptococcal) meningitis, candidiasis, and chromoblastomycosis. Neutropenia and thrombocytopenia may be seen in patients treated with flucytosine. The drug should be used with caution in patients with renal insufficiency.

Specimen Serum

Container Red top tube

Sampling Time Peak concentrations: 30-60 minutes after last dose; trough: just prior to dose. Peak samples may be most informative in patients with renal failure if obtained 2 hours after a dose (absorption is delayed in these patients).

Reference Interval Therapeutic: 25-100 µg/mL (SI: 194-775 µmol/L) (50-100 mcg/mL in general, 25-60 µg/mL in immunocompromised patients)

Possible Panic Range ≥100-125 µg/mL (SI: 775-970 µmol/L)

Use Monitor weekly for bone marrow toxicity, if patient has normal renal function, more often if renal function is abnormal (diminution of renal function can lead to toxic levels)

Limitations Serum levels do not correlate well with clinical toxicity.

Methodology High performance liquid chromatography (HPLC), gas chromatography/mass spectrometry (GC/MS)

Additional Information

- Half-life: 3-8 hours (much longer in patients with renal dysfunction)
- Protein binding: 2% to 4%
- Volume of distribution: 0.68 L/kg (perhaps 50% less in patients with renal failure)

Flucytosine by itself is not antifungal. It penetrates fungal cells, where it is deaminated to the cytotoxic agent fluorouracil by the fungal enzyme cytosine deaminase (mammalian cells do not convert flucytosine to fluorouracil). Acting as an antimetabolite, fluorouracil competes with uracil, interfering with pyrimidine metabolism and eventually disrupting both RNA and protein synthesis. Resistance develops quickly when flucytosine is used alone.

Clinical use of flucytosine is associated with significant frequency of life-threatening bone marrow suppression which occurs most often when blood levels are >100 µg/mL (SI: >775 µmol/L) for 2 or more weeks. Bone marrow suppression is usually reversible and is most likely to occur in patients with underlying hematologic disorders or in patients undergoing myelosuppressive therapy.

Elevated drug levels may predispose patients to abdominal pain, probably by adversely affecting rapidly reproducing cells in the gastrointestinal tract. The severe side effects include hepatotoxicity and bone marrow depression. As the drug and metabolites are excreted through the kidneys, decreased renal function will increase toxicity.

References

Luna B, Drew RH, and Perfect JR, "Agents for Treatment of Invasive Fungal Infections," *Otolaryngol Clin North Am*, 2000, 33(2):277-99.

Patel R, "Antifungal Agents. Part I. Amphotericin B Preparations and Flucytosine," *Mayo Clin Proc*, 1998, 73(12):1205-25.

Terrell CL and Hughes CE, "Antifungal Agents Used for Deep-Seated Mycotic Infections," *Mayo Clin Proc*, 1992, 67(1):69-91.

Vermes A, Guchelaar HJ, and Dankert J, "Flucytosine: A Review of its Pharmacology, Clinical Indications, Pharmacokinetics, Toxicity, and Drug Interactions," *J Antimicrob Chemother*, 2000, 46(2):171-9.

Vermes A, van Der Sijs H, and Guchelaar HJ, "Flucytosine: Correlation Between Toxicity and Pharmacokinetics Parameters," *Chemotherapy*, 2000, 46(2):86-94.

♦ **5-Fluorocytosine** *see* Flucytosine, Serum *on page 750*

♦ **Fluoxetine and Norfluoxetine** *see* Antidepressants, Cyclic, Serum *on page 737*

Fluoxetine, Serum

Related Information

Amoxapine, Serum or Plasma *on page 736*
Antidepressants, Cyclic, Serum *on page 737*
Imipramine, Serum or Plasma *on page 752*

Prolactin, Serum *on page 262*

Synonyms Fontex; Prozac®

Test Includes Fluoxetine and norfluoxetine

Abstract This is a **nontricyclic** antidepressant with a long half-life and an active metabolite. It is the most frequently prescribed antidepressant in the U.S. The drug is also used for premenstrual dysphoria. Interactions with tricyclic antidepressants and monoamine oxidase inhibitors are well recognized.

Specimen Serum or plasma

Container Red top tube or green top (heparin) tube; do not use serum separator tube

Sampling Time Trough at steady state (10-15 days)

Reference Interval Fluoxetine: 100-800 ng/mL (SI: 289-2314 nmol/L); norfluoxetine: 100-600 ng/mL (SI: 289-1735 nmol/L); combined: 300-1200 ng/mL

Critical Values >2000 ng/mL (SI: >5784 nmol/L) (fluoxetine and norfluoxetine). Although overdose of this drug alone is not often critical, overdose with a tricyclic antidepressant, lithium, carbamazepine, monoamine oxidase inhibitors, or other coadministered drugs may be significant.

Use Therapeutic monitoring and toxicity assessment

Methodology High performance liquid chromatography (HPLC), gas chromatography (GC)

Additional Information

- Half-life: 2-3 days (norfluoxetine: 7-9 days)
- Volume of distribution: 12-42 L/kg
- Protein binding: 90% to 98%

Fluoxetine is an antidepressant that is a potent, selective inhibitor of serotonin reuptake with minimal effect on norepinephrine and dopamine. It is metabolized via demethylation to the active norfluoxetine. Because of extensive tissue binding, the parent drug and the active metabolite norfluoxetine have very long half-lives. Fluoxetine may be helpful for subjects with moderate depression treated as outpatients. The overall toxicity of the drug is considerably less than that of the tricyclics.

Symptoms of overdose include ataxia, sedation, and coma. Respiratory depression may occur, especially with coingestion of alcohol or other drugs.

A report links fluoxetine use with reversible galactorrhea and prolactin increase.[1]

Footnotes

1. Peterson MC, "Reversible Galactorrhea and Prolactin Elevation Related to Fluoxetine Use," *Mayo Clin Proc*, 2001, 76(2):215-6.

References

Borys DJ, Setzer SC, Ling LJ, et al, "The Effects of Fluoxetine in the Overdose Patient," *J Toxicol Clin Toxicol*, 1990, 28(3):331-40.

Cook IA, Leuchter AF, Witte E, et al, "Neurophysiologic Predictors of Treatment Response to Fluoxetine in Major Depression," *Psychiatry Res*, 1999, 85(3):263-73

Cookson J and Duffett R, "Fluoxetine: Therapeutic and Undesirable Effects," *Hosp Med*, 1998, 59(8):622-6.

Fenton J, "Fluoxetine," *The Laboratory and the Poisoned Patient*, Washington, DC: AACC Press, American Association of Clinical Chemistry, 1998, 175-77.

Gidal BE, Anderson GD, Seaton TL, et al, "Evaluation of the Effect of Fluoxetine on the Formation of Carbamazepine Epoxide," *Ther Drug Monit*, 1993, 15(5):405-9.

Gram L, "Fluoxetine," *N Engl J Med*, 1994, 331(20):1354-61.

Norman TR, Gupta RK, Burrows GD, et al, "Relationship Between Antidepressant Response and Plasma Concentrations of Fluoxetine and Norfluoxetine," *Int Clin Psychopharmacol*, 1993, 8(1):25-9.

Richelson E, "Pharmacokinetic Drug Interactions of New Antidepressants: A Review of the Effects on the Metabolism of Other Drugs," *Mayo Clin Proc*, 1997, 72(9):835-47.

Romano S, Judge R, Dillon J, et al, "The Role of Fluoxetine in the Treatment of Premenstrual Dysphoric Disorder," *Clin Ther*, 1999, 21(4):615-33; discussion 613.

Stokes PE and Holtz A, "Fluoxetine Tenth Anniversary Update: The Progress Continues," *Clin Ther*, 1997, 19(5):1135-250.

Fluphenazine, Serum

Related Information

Haloperidol, Serum or Plasma *on page 752*
Phenothiazines, Serum or Urine *on page 760*

Synonyms Moditen®; Permitil®; Prolixin®

Abstract Fluphenazine is a high potency phenothiazine antipsychotic agent.

Specimen Serum

Container Red top tube

Reference Interval 0.3-3.0 ng/mL (SI: 0.6-6.0 ng/mL)

Critical Values >50 ng/mL (SI: >98 nmol/L)

Use Therapeutic monitoring and toxicity assessment

Methodology High performance liquid chromatography (HPLC),[1] gas chromatography (GC), radioimmunoassay (RIA)

Additional Information

- Half-life (see below)
- Protein binding: 91% to 99%

Fluphenazine is a phenothiazine derivative used in the treatment of psychotic disorders. Its dose in milligrams (equivalent to 100 mg of chlorpromazine) is 1-1.5 mg. It is available as the HCl salt (tablets, concentrated solution, elixir, and injectable), and long-acting enanthate and decanoate salts for injection. The elimination half-life varies with the salt form (HCl about 15 hours, enanthate about 3.5-4 days, decanoate about 7-10 days). It has a very high potential to cause extrapyramidal side effects, but a low potential to cause sedation, anticholinergic, or cardiovascular side effects. Fluphenazine blocks postsynaptic dopamine receptors in the mesolimbic system and increases dopamine turnover by blockade of the D_2 somatodendritic autoreceptor. Plasma concentrations during oral therapy should be measured 12 hours after the evening dose and before any morning dose. Plasma concentrations during decanoate therapy should be measured immediately before the next injection. Fluphenazine plasma concentrations are generally observed to be between 0.3-3.0 ng/mL in responders. Fluphenazine is highly plasma protein-bound (91% to 99%), predominantly to alpha$_1$-acid glycoprotein. The drug crosses the placenta and may be excreted into breast milk, although insufficient data are available. Metabolism in the liver is extensive, with metabolites contributing ~50% of antipsychotic activity. There is some conjugation with glucuronide which, along with unconjugated metabolites, are excreted in the urine. Some excretion may occur via the biliary tract and feces.

Footnotes

1. Luo JP, Hubbard JW, and Midha KK, "Sensitive Method for the Simultaneous Measurement of Fluphenazine Decanoate and Fluphenazine in Plasma by High-Performance Liquid Chromatography With Coulometric Detection," *J Chromatogr B Biomed Sci Appl*, 1997, 688(2):303-8.

References

Adams CE and Eisenbruch M, "Depot Fluphenazine for Schizophrenia," *Cochrane Database Syst Rev*, 2000, (2):CD000307.

Chouinard G, Annable L, and Campbell W, "A Randomized Clinical Trial of Haloperidol Decanoate and Fluphenazine Decanoate in the Outpatient Treatment of Schizophrenia," *J Clin Psychopharmacol*, 1989, 9(4):247-53.

Cooper JK, Hawes EM, Hubbard JW, et al, "An Ultrasensitive Method for the Measurement of Fluphenazine in Plasma by High Performance Liquid Chromatography With Coulometric Detection," *Ther Drug Monit*, 1989, 11(3):354-60.

Levinson DF, Simpson GM, Singh H, et al, "Fluphenazine Dose, Clinical Response, and Extrapyramidal Symptoms During Acute Treatment," *Arch Gen Psychiatry*, 1990, 47(8):761-8.

Marder SR, Midha KK, Van Putten T, et al, "Plasma Levels of Fluphenazine in Patients Receiving Fluphenazine Decanoate. Relationship to Clinical Response," *Br J Psychiatry*, 1991, 158:658-65.

Midha KK, Hubbard JW, Marder SR, et al, "Impact of Clinical Pharmacokinetics on Neuroleptic Therapy in Patients With Schizophrenia," *J Psychiatry Neurosci*, 1994, 19(4):254-64.

Midha KK, Marder SR, Jaworski TJ, et al, "Clinical Perspectives of Some Neuroleptics Through Development and Application of Their Assays," *Ther Drug Monit*, 1993, 15(3):179-89.

Flurazepam, Serum

Related Information

Benzodiazepines, Qualitative, Urine *on page 782*

Synonyms Benozil®; Dalmane®; Staurodorm®

Abstract This drug is a sedative-hypnotic of the benzodiazepine class with a wide therapeutic window. The drug is generally used for short-term treatment of insomnia. It is administered orally in doses of 15-30 mg and is very rarely monitored with blood levels.

Specimen Serum

Container Red top tube

Reference Interval Therapeutic: 0-4 ng/mL (SI: 0-9 nmol/L); metabolite N-desalkylflurazepam: 20-110 ng/mL (SI: 43-240 nmol/L)

Possible Panic Range Toxic: 200 ng/mL (SI: 500 nmol/L)

Use Monitor therapeutic drug level (rarely), toxicity assessment

Methodology Thin-layer chromatography (TLC), high performance liquid chromatography (HPLC), immunoassay

Additional Information

- Half-life: parent drug: 3-6 hours; metabolite (N-desalkylflurazepam): 50-100 hours
- Volume of distribution: 15-30 L/kg
- Protein binding: 96% to 98%

Mechanism of action is probably due to increased action of gamma-amino butyric acid. Most common side effect is daytime drowsiness, ataxia, dizziness, and slurred speech. The major urinary metabolite is N-1-hydroxyethyl flurazepam, which is also active. Cimetidine may decrease and enzyme P-450 inducers may increase the metabolism of flurazepam. Most immunoassays for benzodiazepine class detect overdoses. Acute overdose results in apnea, respiratory depression, ataxia, and nystagmus.

References

Fenton J, "Benzodiazepines," *The Laboratory and the Poisoned Patient*, Washington, DC: AACC Press, American Association of Clinical Chemistry, 1998, 85-9.

Fraser AD, "Use and Abuse of the Benzodiazepines," *Ther Drug Monit*, 1998, 20(5):481-9.

Giri AK and Banerjee S, "Genetic Toxicology of Four Commonly Used Benzodiazepines: A Review," *Mutat Res*, 1996, 340(2-3):93-108.

Greenblatt DJ, Harmatz JS, Engelhardt N, et al, "Pharmacokinetic Determinants of Dynamic Differences Among Three Benzodiazepine Hypnotics. Flurazepam, Temazepam, and Triazolam," *Arch Gen Psychiatry*, 1989, 46(4):326-32.

Salzman C, "Addiction to Benzodiazepines," *Psychiatr Q*, 1998, 69(4), 251-61.

Schweizer E and Rickels K, "Benzodiazepine Dependence and Withdrawal: A Review of the Syndrome and its Clinical Management," *Acta Psychiatr Scand Suppl*, 1998, 393:95-101.

Gold, Serum

Synonyms Auranofin; Aurothioglucose; Chrysotherapy; Gold Sodium Thiomalate; Myochrysine®; Ridaura®; Sodium Aurothiomalate; Solganal®

Abstract Gold is sometimes used as a treatment for rheumatoid arthritis, but its value is being questioned because of serious side effects and availability of more efficacious therapies.

Specimen Serum

Container Red top tube

Reference Interval Normal: 0-0.1 µg/mL (SI: 0-0.5 µmol/L); therapeutic: 1.0-3.0 µg/mL (SI: 5.1-15.2 µmol/L)

Use Complex gold compounds have been advocated in the treatment of severe, progressive rheumatoid arthritis as second-line medications since the 1920s.[1] It is also used selectively for juvenile rheumatoid arthritis, lupus erythematosus, and other inflammatory conditions.[2] Gold compounds have been used to treat psoriatic arthritis, but clinical response to gold therapy may be inferior to methotrexate.[3]

Limitations Blood levels do not correlate with therapeutic or toxic effects.[4] A relationship is not recognized between urinary gold and response to therapy. Hair and nail gold concentrations have not been helpful.

Methodology Atomic absorption spectrometry (AA)

Additional Information Gold is most often used in forms to which it is attached to a sulphur moiety. Water soluble gold salts are rapidly absorbed after intramuscular injection with therapeutic levels occurring within 6 hours after injection.[4] Symptoms of general toxicity include fever, nausea, vomiting, diarrhea, proteinuria, hematuria, and blood dyscrasias.[1] Aplastic anemia is one of the most feared side effects.[5] One review of the literature on gold therapy from 110 reports found that gold was being used to treat rheumatoid arthritis (81%), bronchial asthma (6%), pemphigus (5%), and other processes (9%). Serious side effects included gold-induced pulmonary disease, skin rash, peripheral eosinophilia, liver dysfunction, and proteinuria. Only the presence of pemphigus or liver dysfunction correlated with a bad outcome.[6] There are important metabolic differences between the three oxidation states of gold (0, I, and III).[4]

The following values are for gold sodium thiomalate, which is one of the most used gold compounds.

- Half-life: 5-10 days
- Volume of distribution: 0.1 L/kg
- Protein binding: 95%

Footnotes

1. Goetz CG, Kompoliti K, and Washburn K, "Neurotoxic Agents," *Clinical Neurology*, Volume 2, Joynt RJ and Griggs RC, eds, Philadelphia, PA: Lippincott and Williams Co, 1998, 22-3.
2. Jones G and Brooks PM, "Injectible Gold Compounds: An Overview," *Br J Rheumatol*, 1996, 35(11):1154-8.
3. Lacaille D, Stein HB, Raboud J, et al, "Longterm Therapy of Psoriatic Arthritis: Intramuscular Gold or Methotrexate?" *J Rheumatol*, 2000, 27(8):1922-7.
4. Merchant B, "Gold, the Noble Metal and the Paradoxes of its Toxicology," *Biologics*, 1998, 26(1):49-59.
5. *Goldfrank's Toxilogical Emergencies*, 6th ed, Chapters 14 and 24, Goldfrank LR, Flomenbaum NE, Lwein NA, et al, eds, Stamford CT: Appleton and Lange Co, 1998, 232-3, 416.
6. Tomioka R and King TE, "Gold-Induced Pulmonary Disease: Clinical Features, Outcome, and Differentiation From Rheumatoid Lung," *Am J Respir Crit Care Med*, 1997, 155(3):1011-20.

References

Biasi D, Caramaschi P, Carletto A, et al, "Combination Therapy With Hydroxychloroquine, Gold Sodium Thiomalate and Methotrexate in Early Rheumatoid Arthritis. An Open 3-Year Study," *Clin Rheumatol*, 2000, 19(6):505-7.

Hostynek JJ, "Gold: An Allergen of Growing Significance," *Food Chem Toxicol*, 1997, 35(8):839-44.

Menninger H, Herborn G, Sander O, et al "A 36 Month Comparative Trial of Methotrexate and Gold Sodium Thiomalate in the Treatment of Early Active and Erosive Rheumatoid Arthritis," *Br J Rheumatol*, 1998, 37(10):1060-8.

Messori L, Abbate F, Marcon G, et al, "Gold(III) Complexes as Potential Antitumor Agents: Solution Chemistry and Cytotoxic Properties of Some Selected Gold(III) Compounds," *J Med Chem*, 2000, 43(19):3541-8.

Russell MA, Langley M, Truett AP, et al, "Lichenoid Dermatitis After Consumption of Gold-Containing Liquor," *J Am Acad Dermatol*, 1997, 36(5 Pt 2):841-4.

♦ **GX** *see* Lidocaine, Serum or Plasma *on page 754*

♦ **Haldol®** *see* Haloperidol, Serum or Plasma *on page 752*

♦ **Haldol® Decanoate** *see* Haloperidol, Serum or Plasma *on page 752*

♦ **Haloneural®** *see* Haloperidol, Serum or Plasma *on page 752*

Haloperidol, Serum or Plasma

Related Information
Amphetamine, Qualitative, Urine *on page 779*
Chlorpromazine, Serum *on page 743*
Lithium, Serum *on page 754*

Synonyms Dozic®; Fortunan®; Haldol®; Haldol® Decanoate; Haloneural®; Serenace®

Abstract This drug is an antipsychotic agent. It is used in the treatment of Tourette syndrome, severe behavioral problems in children, and for emergency sedation of severely agitated or delirious patients. It is extensively metabolized and should be monitored. Adverse effects include sedation, extrapyramidal effects, and hypotension. Rare cases of hepatic dysfunction and leukopenia have been reported.

Specimen Serum or plasma

Container Red top tube or green top (heparin) tube

Sampling Time Time to peak serum concentration: Oral: 3-6 hours; I.M.: 10-20 minutes; I.M. (long-acting): 3-9 days

Reference Interval 5-20 ng/mL (SI: 10-40 nmol/L) (psychotic disorders - less for Tourette syndrome and mania)

Critical Values >42 ng/mL (SI: >84 nmol/L) (variable)

Use Therapeutic monitoring and toxicity assessment. Haloperidol is an antipsychotic tranquilizer used to control acute and chronic psychotic disorders, for the control of Tourette syndrome, and for the treatment of severe behavior problems in hyperactive children. Haloperidol should be monitored to assess and optimize dosing regimens and maintenance therapy, since the relationship between dosage and serum levels at steady-state can be highly variable. The drug should also be monitored to assess adverse reactions and changes associated with coadministered drugs.

Methodology Radioimmunoassay (RIA), high performance liquid chromatography (HPLC), gas chromatography (GC)

Additional Information
- Half-life: 15-40 hours
- Volume of distribution: 18-30 L/kg
- Protein binding: 90%

Haloperidol is metabolized by dealkalization, oxidation, and conjugation; the hydroxy derivative is active but concentrations are very low. Haloperidol may increase serum tricyclic concentrations; increase the toxicity of lithium; inhibit hypertensive action; and antagonize the stimulant effect of amphetamines. Haloperidol has toxicity similar to that of phenothiazines. Among the most dangerous effects of haloperidol overdose are cardiovascular alterations including myocardial depression and EKG changes such as depression of T and ST waves.

Haloperidol acute overdose may cause hyperglycemia, hypoglycemia, arrhythmias, exacerbation or precipitation of myasthenia gravis, and other signs, symptoms, and abnormalities.

References
Blin O, "A Comparative Review of New Antipsychotics," *Can J Psychiatry*, 1999, 44(3):235-44.

Goff DC, Midha KK, Brotman AW, et al, "Elevation of Plasma Concentrations of Haloperidol After the Addition of Fluoxetine," *Am J Psychiatry*, 1991, 148(6):790-2.

Kudo S and Ishizaki T, "Pharmacokinetics of Haloperidol: An Update," *Clin Pharmacokinet*, 1999, 37(6):435-56.

Lawson GM, "Monitoring of Serum Haloperidol," *Mayo Clin Proc*, 1994, 69(2):189-90.

Leroux JM, Jacquet M, Pommery J, et al, "Correlation of Clinical Response and Plasma Levels of Haloperidol and Reduced Haloperidol in Schizophrenia," *Prog Neuropsychopharmacol Biol Psychiatry*, 1994, 18(2):347-53.

Rifkin A, Doddi S, Karajgi B, et al, "Dosage of Haloperidol for Schizophrenia," *Arch Gen Psychiatry*, 1991, 48(2):166-70.

Ulrich S, Wurthmann C, Brosz M, et al, "The Relationship Between Serum Concentration and Therapeutic Effect of Haloperidol in Patients With Acute Schizophrenia," *Clin Pharmacokinet*, 1998, 34(3):227-63.

Yoshikawa H, Watanabe T, Abe T, et al, "Haloperidol-Induced Rhabdomyolysis Without Neuroleptic Malignant Syndrome in a Handicapped Child," *Brain Dev*, 2000, 22(4):256-8.

♦ **Hexamidinum** *see* Primidone, Serum or Plasma *on page 762*

♦ **Hibanil®** *see* Chlorpromazine, Serum *on page 743*

♦ **Ikacor®** *see* Verapamil, Serum or Plasma *on page 769*

♦ **Iktorivil®** *see* Clonazepam, Serum *on page 743*

♦ **Imipramine and Desipramine** *see* Antidepressants, Cyclic, Serum *on page 737*

Imipramine, Serum or Plasma

Related Information
Antidepressants, Cyclic, Serum *on page 737*
Doxepin, Serum *on page 748*
Fluoxetine, Serum *on page 750*
Warfarin *on page 770*

Synonyms Berkomine®; Dimipressin®; Iprogen®; Janimine®; Pertofrane®; Presamine®; SK-Pramine®; Tofranil®; Tofranil-PM®

Applies to Desipramine; Norpramin®

Test Includes Desipramine levels

Abstract Imipramine is a tricyclic antidepressant used in the treatment of endogenous depression. It is metabolized to desipramine, an active metabolite. Both parent drug and the metabolite should be monitored.

Specimen Serum or plasma

Container Red top tube or green top (heparin) tube

Sampling Time Trough levels at steady-state (30-90 hours)

Reference Interval Imipramine and desipramine: 100-300 ng/mL (SI: 350-1070 nmol/L). Metabolism may be impaired in geriatric patients.

Critical Values >500 ng/mL (SI: 1780 nmol/L)

Possible Panic Range 1000 ng/mL (SI: 3570 nmol/L)

Use Therapeutic monitoring and toxicity assessment of imipramine, a cyclic antidepressant that blocks the reuptake of serotonin and norepinephrine at nerve endings. It possesses high anticholinergic activity, sedation and cardiovascular toxicity. It has quinidine-like effects on cardiac conduction.

Contraindications Cyclic antidepressants should be avoided in pregnant and lactating women because these drugs have not been established to be safe. Geriatric patients are especially susceptible to orthostasis, urinary retention, constipation, and sedation. The cyclic antidepressants are commonly seen in overdose situations. Cardiovascular, anticholinergic, and central nervous system toxicities can be lethal. Concomitant use of MAO inhibitors is contraindicated.

Methodology Immunoassay, high performance liquid chromatography (HPLC), gas chromatography (GC)

Additional Information
- Half-life: 6-18 hours
- Volume of distribution: 9-23 L/kg
- Protein binding: 60% to 95%

Imipramine is cleared by the liver alone and is extensively metabolized to many polar compounds. The most important metabolite is desipramine, which is itself an important antidepressant.

Imipramine is completely absorbed but undergoes some first-pass elimination. Bioavailability is 22% to 77% with a peak concentration 2-6 hours after an oral dose. Imipramine reaches steady-state in about 2-4 days.

Anticholinergic side effects such as blurred vision, dry mouth, constipation, and urinary retention are common with this drug. They are not severe and may diminish with continued therapy or can be treated with other pharmacologic and nonpharmacologic therapies. Anticholinergic side effects are more troublesome in the elderly. Sedation may also decrease with continued use. Imipramine can also lower the seizure threshold and cause orthostasis and arrhythmias. The cardiovascular effects are more common in patients with underlying cardiovascular disorders. Recently, hyperpigmentation has been associated with long-term use of imipramine.

Drug interactions are common with the tricyclic antidepressants. Concomitant treatment with cimetidine, fluoxetine, and antipsychotics produce unexpectedly elevated concentrations of imipramine. Enzyme inducers (eg, phenytoin, chloral hydrate, smoking, and the barbiturates) decrease imipramine concentrations. Additive anticholinergic side effects occur when cyclics are combined with antihistamines, anti-Parkinson drugs, and antipsychotics. The cardiovascular effects of the tricyclics are additive with any of the class IA antiarrhythmics (quinidine, procainamide, disopyramide). Direct-acting sympathomimetics (epinephrine, norepinephrine, phenylephrine) are potentiated by tricyclics. Monoamine oxidase inhibitors (MAOIs) and thyroid hormones potentiate the toxicities of tricyclics. Hyperthermia, delirium, convulsions, coma, and fatalities have occurred with the combination of MAOIs and tricyclics. These drugs have been used in combination in refractory cases of depression. The tricyclics can also affect other drugs. The antihypertensive effects of the central α-agonists (clonidine, methyldopa, guanethidine) are reversed when combined with tricyclics. Anticoagulation effects of warfarin may be potentiated by the tricyclics.

References
Fawcett J and Barkin RL, "Efficacy Issues With Antidepressants," *J Clin Psychiatry*, 1997, 58(Suppl 6):32-9.

Geller B, Reising D, Leonard HL, et al, "Critical Review of Tricyclic Antidepressant Use in Children and Adolescents," *J Am Acad Child Adolesc Psychiatry*, 1999, 38(5):513-6.

Kline JA, De Stefano AA, Schroeder JD, et al, "Magnesium Potentiates Imipramine Toxicity in the Isolated Rat Heart," *Ann Emerg Med*, 1994, 24(2):224-32.

Linder MW and Keck PE Jr, "Standards of Laboratory Practice: Antidepressant Drug Monitoring. National Academy of Clinical Biochemistry," *Clin Chem*, 1998, 44(5):1073-84.

Mavissakalian MR and Ryan MT, "Rational Treatment of Panic Disorder With Antidepressants," *Ann Clin Psychiatry*, 1998, 10(4):185-95.

Ming ME, Bhawan J, Stefanato CM, et al, "Imipramine-Induced Hyperpigmentation: Four Cases and a Review of the Literature," *J Am Acad Dermatol*, 1999, 40(2 Pt 1):159-66.

Perry PJ, Zeilmann C, and Arndt S, "Tricyclic Antidepressant Concentrations in Plasma: An Estimate of Their Sensitivity and Specificity as a Predictor of Response," *J Clin Psychopharmacol*, 1994, 14(4):230-40.

Spina E, Avenoso A, Campo GM, et al, "Decreased Plasma Concentrations of Imipramine and Desipramine Following Cholestyramine Intake in Depressed Patients," *Ther Drug Monit*, 1994, 16(4):432-4.

Swanson JR, Jones GR, Krasselt W, et al, "Death of Two Subjects Due to Imipramine and Desipramine Metabolite Accumulation During Chronic Therapy: A Review of the Literature and Possible Mechanisms," *J Forensic Sci*, 1997, 42(2):335-9.

♦ **Inderal®** *see* Propranolol, Serum *on page 763*

♦ **INH** *see* Isoniazid, Serum or Plasma *on page 753*

♦ **Interleukin Production** *see* Tacrolimus, Whole Blood *on page 765*

♦ **Iproveratril Hydrochloride** *see* Verapamil, Serum or Plasma *on page 769*

Isoniazid, Serum or Plasma

Related Information
Alanine Aminotransferase, Serum *on page 87*
Aspartate Aminotransferase, Serum *on page 112*
Bilirubin, Total, Serum *on page 118*
Liver Disease: Laboratory Assessment, Overview *on page 216*

Synonyms INH; Isonicotinic Acid Hydrazide; Laniazid®; Nydrazid®

Abstract Introduced in 1952, isoniazid is one of the drugs of choice in the therapy and prophylaxis of tuberculosis.[1,2] Use of this drug has increased in recent years in the United States due to resurgence of tuberculosis.[3,4]

Specimen Serum or plasma

Container Serum: red top tube; plasma: green top (heparin) tube

Sampling Time Trough

Storage Instructions Refrigerate. Ship in plastic container in dry ice.

Turnaround Time 2-5 days

Reference Interval Therapeutic: 2-5 µg/mL; toxic: >20 µg/mL

Use Evaluate therapy or possible toxicity

Methodology Gas-liquid chromatography (GLC), high performance liquid chromatography (HPLC)

Additional Information
- Half-life: 1-1.5 hours (fast acetylators); 2-4 hours (slow acetylators)
- Volume of distribution: 0.6 L/kg
- Protein binding: zero

Mild overdose causes nausea and vomiting. Peripheral neuropathy is seen in moderate overdose. Severe overdose causes refractory seizures, metabolic acidosis (from lactic acid and beta-hydroxybutyric acid), and deep coma.[5] Severe and sometimes fatal hepatitis associated with isoniazid therapy may occur and may develop even after many months of treatment.

Isoniazid increases serum phenytoin and carbamazepine when coadministered. Isoniazid increases serum transaminases and bilirubin.

Footnotes
1. Aguado JM, Pulido F, Moreno S, et al, "Isoniazid Prophylaxis for High Risk Patients With Anergy and HIV Infection," *N Engl J Med*, 1997, 337(23):1696-7.
2. Tulsky JP, Pilote L, Hahn JA, et al, "Adherence to Isoniazid Prophylaxis in the Homeless: A Randomized Controlled Trial," *Arch Intern Med*, 2000, 160(5):697-702.
3. Amsterdam D, "The Laboratory Diagnosis of Tuberculosis in a Period of Resurgence: Challenge for the Laboratory," *Clin Lab Sci*, 1996, 9(4):207-12.
4. Wallace D, "The Resurgence of Tuberculosis," *Lancet*, 1996, 347(9008):1115-6.
5. Fenton J, "Isoniazid," *The Laboratory and the Poisoned Patient*, Washington, DC: AACC Press, 1998, 204-6.

References
Riska PF, Jacobs WR Jr, Alland D, et al, "Molecular Determinants of Drug Resistance in Tuberculosis," *Int J Tuberc Lung Dis*, 2000, 4(2 Suppl 1):S4-10.

Self TH, Chrisman CR, Baciewicz AM, et al, "Isoniazid Drug and Food Interactions," *Am J Med Sci*, 1999, 317(5):304-311.

Smith PJ, van Dyk J, Fredericks A, et al, "Determination of Rifampicin, Isoniazid, and Pyrazinamide by High Performance Liquid Chromatography After Their Simultaneous Extraction From Plasma," *Int J Tuberc Lung Dis*, 1999, 3(11 Suppl 3):S325-8; discussion S351-2.

♦ **Isonicotinic Acid Hydrazide** *see* Isoniazid, Serum or Plasma *on page 753*

♦ **Isoptin®** *see* Verapamil, Serum or Plasma *on page 769*

Itraconazole, Serum

Related Information
Amphotericin B, Serum *on page 737*
Cyclosporine, Blood *on page 744*
Flucytosine, Serum *on page 750*
Tacrolimus, Whole Blood *on page 765*

Synonyms Sporanox®

Abstract Itraconazole is an orally administered triazole antifungal agent with a broad spectrum of activity, including most pathologic fungi. Efficacy in candidiasis, blastomycosis, *Blastomyces brasiliensis* (paracoccidioidomycosis), chromoblastomycosis, coccidioidomycosis, cryptococcosis, histoplasmosis, sporotrichosis, maduramycotic mycetomas, and many cases of *Aspergillus* infections is described.[1,2] It has also been effective as adjunctive therapy in patients with corticosteroid-dependent allergic bronchopulmonary aspergillosis.[3] Its role in clinical medicine is still evolving. It appears likely that this agent will become widely accepted due to its low toxicity

compared with other antifungal agents and its broad spectrum of activity. The role for monitoring serum levels has not been established.

Specimen Serum

Container Red top tube

Sampling Time 4-5 hours after an oral dose. Steady-state concentrations are achieved after approximately 5-10 days. This wide range exists because the elimination of itraconazole is dose-dependent (longer elimination half-life with higher serum concentrations).

Reference Interval Therapeutic: varies with methodology; see Additional Information. Tissue levels are 3- to 20-fold higher than plasma concentrations. Only negligible concentrations were reported in CSF and urine.[4]

Use Serum therapeutic levels may be useful if poor absorption is suspected, or in cases of therapeutic failure or relapse.

Limitations *In vitro* susceptibility testing of fungi against itraconazole is method dependent and may not accurately predict clinical success. Consequently, monitoring levels and adjusting dosage to attain therapeutic concentrations as determined by minimum inhibitory concentrations may not be helpful. Itraconazole tablets are best absorbed when taken with food and acidic drinks like cola; the itraconazole solution is best absorbed if taken in fasted state. Itraconazole bioavailability is decreased when the drug is given with H_2 antagonists and didanosine (ddl) (alkaline preparation); phenytoin and rifampin may decrease itraconazole concentrations by inducing its metabolism. Conversely, itraconazole is an inhibitor of the cytochrome P-450 system. Concentrations and clinical activities of sulfonylurea agents (especially tolbutamide) may increase when administered with itraconazole. Coadministration of terfenadine, cisapride, and astemizole may cause dangerous interactions, which may result in prolonged QTc intervals and life-threatening dysrhythmias. Lovastatin concentrations may increase dramatically, resulting in rhabdomyolysis; midazolam and triazolam concentrations may increase substantially when these benzodiazepines are coadministered with itraconazole. **Note:** These are some of the most important drug-drug interactions, there are others. Also note that in the U.S., terfenadine is not available, and cisapride has limited availability, but some patients taking itraconazole may still have access to these agents. Assays for itraconazole are performed only in a few reference laboratories.

Methodology Bioassay, high performance liquid chromatography (HPLC)

Additional Information Itraconazole is a triazole compound (3 nitrogen atoms), which inhibits ergosterol synthesis with ergosterol being the main sterol in the fungal cell wall. This drug interacts with C-14 alpha demethylase (which is dependent on fungal cytochrome P-450) and thereby limits lanosterol conversion to ergosterol.[5] Itraconazole has affinity for mammalian P-450 enzymes also, thus resulting in important drug-drug interactions (eg, rifampin, oral contraceptives, H_2 receptor blockers, warfarin, cyclosporine).[4] Ergosterol depletion alters membrane fluidity and causes increased permeability of the cell wall. Half-life is dose-dependent (longer half-life with higher serum concentrations) and ranges from 24-42 hours. More than 99% binds to plasma proteins. Itraconazole is metabolized mainly in the liver to ~30 metabolites. One of these, hydroxy-itraconazole, has antifungal activity. Serum levels as determined by bioassay are ~10 times the levels determined by HPLC, presumably because bioassay also detects an active metabolite.

Footnotes
1. Zuckerman JM and Tunkel AR, "Itraconazole: A New Triazole Antifungal Agent," *Infect Control Hosp Epidemiol*, 1994, 15(6):397-410.
2. Warnock DW, "Itraconazole Pulse: An Overview of Current Use," *Hosp Med*, 1998, 59(4):309-11.
3. Stevens DA, Schwartz HJ, Lee JY, et al, "A Randomized Trial of Itraconazole in Allergic Bronchopulmonary Aspergillosis," *N Engl J Med*, 2000, 342(11):756-62.
4. Negroni R and Arechavala AI, "Itraconazole: Pharmacokinetics and Indications," *Arch Med Res*, 1993, 24(4):387-93.
5. Leyden J, "Pharmacokinetics and Pharmacology of Terbinafine and Itraconazole," *J Am Acad Dermatol*, 1998, 38(5 Pt 3):S42-7.

References
Andriole VT, "Current and Future Therapy of Invasive Fungal Infections," *Curr Clin Top Infect Dis*, 1998, 18:19-36.

Bennett JE, "Diagnosis and Therapy of Fungal Infections," *Harrison's Principles of Internal Medicine*, 13th ed, Isselbacher KJ, Braunwald E, Wilson JD, et al, eds, New York, NY: McGraw-Hill Inc, 1994, 854-6.

Como JA and Dismukes WE, "Oral Azole Drugs as Systemic Antifungal Therapy," *N Engl J Med*, 1994, 330(4):263-72.

Poirier JM and Cheymol G, "Optimisation of Itraconazole Therapy Using Target Drug Concentrations," *Clin Pharmacokinet*, 1998, 35(6):461-73.

Terrell CL and Hughes CE, "Antifungal Agents Used for Deep-Seated Mycotic Infections," *Mayo Clin Proc*, 1992, 67(1):69-91.

♦ **Janimine®** *see* Imipramine, Serum or Plasma *on page 752*

♦ **Keppra®** *see* Antiepileptic Drugs, New, Overview *on page 738*

♦ **Kiditard®** *see* Quinidine, Serum *on page 764*

♦ **Kinidin®** *see* Quinidine, Serum *on page 764*

♦ **Klonopin™** *see* Clonazepam, Serum *on page 743*

♦ **Kyushin** *see* Digoxin, Serum *on page 746*

♦ **Lamictal®** *see* Antiepileptic Drugs, New, Overview *on page 738*

♦ **Lamotrigine** *see* Antiepileptic Drugs, New, Overview *on page 738*

♦ **Lamra®** *see* Diazepam, Serum *on page 745*

- **Laniazid®** see Isoniazid, Serum or Plasma *on page 753*
- **Lanocor®** see Digoxin, Serum *on page 746*
- **Lanotoxin®** see Digitoxin, Serum *on page 745*
- **Lanoxicaps®** see Digoxin, Serum *on page 746*
- **Lanoxin®** see Digoxin, Serum *on page 746*
- **Largactil®** see Chlorpromazine, Serum *on page 743*
- **Latiazem Hydrochloride** see Diltiazem, Serum or Plasma *on page 747*
- **Lenoxin®** see Digoxin, Serum *on page 746*
- **Leptilan®** see Valproic Acid, Serum or Plasma *on page 768*
- **Levetiracetam** see Antiepileptic Drugs, New, Overview *on page 738*
- **Librax®** see Chlordiazepoxide, Serum *on page 742*
- **Libritabs®** see Chlordiazepoxide, Serum *on page 742*
- **Librium®** see Chlordiazepoxide, Serum *on page 742*
- **Lidocaine Metabolite** see Monoethylglycinexylidide, Serum *on page 758*

Lidocaine, Serum or Plasma

Related Information
Amiodarone, Serum *on page 735*
Monoethylglycinexylidide, Serum *on page 758*
Tocainide, Serum or Plasma *on page 767*

Synonyms Anestacon®; Baylocaine®; Dalcaine®; Dilocaine®; Duo-Trach®; LidoPen®; Lignocaine; Nervocaine®; Norocaine®; Octocaine®; Xylocaine®

Applies to GX

Abstract Lidocaine is a class IB antiarrhythmic and a local anesthetic. It is extensively metabolized to two active metabolites, monoethylglycinexylidide (MEGX) and glycinexylidide (GX).

Specimen Serum or plasma

Container Red top tube, green top (heparin) tube, or lavender top (EDTA) tube

Sampling Time Draw specimens 12 hours after initiating therapy for arrhythmia prophylaxis, then every 24 hours thereafter. Obtain specimens every 12 hours when cardiac or hepatic insufficiency exists.

Collection Avoid collection tubes with stoppers containing the plasticizer, TBEP.

Reference Interval Therapeutic: 1.5-5.0 µg/mL (SI: 6.4-21.4 µmol/L), up to 6.0 µg/mL (SI: 25.6 µmol/L) if necessary.

Critical Values At levels >6.0 µg/mL (SI: >25.6 µmol/L), there may be seizure activity. See Table C in the Therapeutic Drug Monitoring Introduction *on page 733*.

Possible Panic Range Toxic: >8.0 µg/mL (SI: >34.2 µmol/L); levels >15.0 µg/mL (SI: 64.5 µmol/L) are associated with **fatalities**.

Use Monitor therapeutic drug level. Lidocaine is used especially in acute arrhythmias, including premature ventricular contractions and prevention of ventricular arrhythmias.[1]

Limitations Cross reactions with other drugs occur. Certain blood collection tubes have been shown to lead to falsely low results; see Collection. Serum levels are more useful as a gauge for toxicity than for efficacy.

Methodology Enzyme immunoassay (EIA), gas-liquid chromatography (GLC), high performance liquid chromatography (HPLC), fluorescent polarization immunoassay (FPIA)

Additional Information
- Half-life: 1.5-2 hours
- Volume of distribution: 1.0-1.5 L/kg
- Protein binding: 60% to 80%

Lidocaine is used in therapy of ventricular but not supraventricular arrhythmias. It is unique as its activity is directed solely at the His-Purkinje network without affecting S-A and A-V nodal conduction. Oral absorption is rapid, but it is a high extraction or "first-pass" drug; therefore lidocaine is not bioavailable when given orally. It is 60% to 80% serum protein bound and lidocaine becomes more highly bound after myocardial infarction. The volume of distribution is also variable. Lidocaine undergoes two compartment distribution. The initial volume is 0.5 L/kg; but as the drug distributes to the tissues, the eventual volume at steady-state is 1.3 L/kg. Volumes are increased in patients with cirrhosis and decreased in patients with congestive heart failure (CHF). Because of the two compartment distribution lidocaine exhibits, its loading dose is unique. The initial dose is based upon the initial volume of distribution. That first dose will distribute quickly into the tissues, therefore, subsequent mini loading doses are needed until the maintenance infusion produces the desired concentration. Due to high extraction coefficient and first-pass metabolism (90% is metabolized by the liver), lidocaine is not given orally, but is administered intramuscularly or intravenously. Since it is a high extraction drug, it is liver blood flow dependent for clearance; therefore, patients who have CHF, arrhythmias, acute myocardial infarction, or cirrhosis will have a decreased clearance. Impaired renal function should have little impact upon clearance. With clearance and volume being variable, half-life is variable as well.

Adverse effects can be concentration related in many cases. Central nervous system effects such as confusion, dizziness, or blurred vision can be seen at the high end of the therapeutic range. Seizures, cardiovascular depression, tremors, and coma are seen usually at levels >8 µg/mL. Such effects may be due to an accumulation of metabolites, particularly MEGX. Elderly patients with CHF or acute myocardial infarct are at highest risk for these toxicities.

Measurement of MEGX has been proposed as a marker of hepatic function.

Interactions occur with drugs that change liver blood flow or plasma protein binding. Beta-blockers and cimetidine decrease liver blood flow, causing increased lidocaine levels. Anticonvulsants, quinidine, and oral contraceptives can change the plasma protein binding of lidocaine, causing toxicity. Other cardiovascular drugs can potentiate the cardiovascular effects of lidocaine when given concomitantly.

Footnotes
1. Moyer TP, "Therapeutic Drug Monitoring," *Tietz Textbook of Clinical Chemistry*, 3rd ed, Burtis CA and Ashwood ER, eds, Philadelphia, PA: WB Saunders Co, 1999, 862-905.

References
Alexander JH, Granger CB, Sadowski Z, et al, "Prophylactic Lidocaine Use in Acute Myocardial Infarction: Incidence and Outcomes From Two International Trials. The Gusto-I and Gusto-IIb Investigators," *Am Heart J*, 1999, 137(5):799-805.
Klein J, Fernandez D, Gazarian M, et al, "Simultaneous Determination of Lidocaine, Prilocaine, and Prilocaine Metabolite O-Toluidine in Plasma by High Performance Liquid Chromatography," *J Chromatogr B Biomed Appl*, 1994, 655(1):83-8.
Palmisano JM, Meliones JN, Crowley DC, et al, "Lidocaine Toxicity After Subcutaneous Infiltration in Children Undergoing Cardiac Catheterization," *Am J Cardiol*, 1991, 67(7):647-8.

- **LidoPen®** see Lidocaine, Serum or Plasma *on page 754*
- **Lignocaine** see Lidocaine, Serum or Plasma *on page 754*
- **Limbitrol®** see Amitriptyline, Serum *on page 735*
- **Liposomal Amphotericin B** see Amphotericin B, Serum *on page 737*
- **Lithane®** see Lithium, Serum *on page 754*

Lithium, Serum

Related Information
Antidepressants, Cyclic, Serum *on page 737*
Haloperidol, Serum or Plasma *on page 752*
Sodium, Serum or Plasma *on page 275*
Theophylline, Serum *on page 766*
Thyroid Stimulating Hormone, Serum *on page 282*
Thyroxine, Serum *on page 286*
Verapamil, Serum or Plasma *on page 769*

Synonyms Cibalith-S®; Eskalith®; Lithane®; Lithobid®; Lithonate®; Lithotabs®; PFI-Lith®; Phasal®

Abstract Lithium is used in the treatment of the manic phase of affective disorders, mania and particularly for manic-depressive illness. It should be monitored because it has a narrow therapeutic window. Its mood stabilizing effects are poorly understood but are believed to be centrally mediated.

Aftercare Follow urine osmolality, EKGs, thyroid profile, BUN, creatinine, and sodium. Avoid sodium depletion.

Specimen Serum; concentrations can be measured in plasma, urine, and other body fluids.

Container Red top tube

Sampling Time Draw sample 12 hours after the last dose. Steady-state occurs at 90-120 hours.

Storage Instructions Refrigerate.

Causes for Rejection Specimen collected in tube containing lithium heparin, hemolysis

Reference Interval Therapeutic: 0.6-1.2 mEq/L (SI: 0.6-1.2 mmol/L), for acute mania; 0.8-1.0 mEq/L (SI: 0.8-1.0 mmol/L) for protection against future episodes in most patients with bipolar disorder. A higher rate of relapse is described in subjects who are maintained at levels <0.4 mEq/L (SI: 0.4 mmol/L).[1]

Possible Panic Range Warning levels: 1.2-1.5 mEq/L; toxic: >1.5 mEq/L (SI: >1.5 mmol/L). Toxicity can become serious when levels rise to levels ≥2.5 mEq/L (SI: ≥2.5 mmol/L). Intoxication is characterized by muscle rigidity, hyperactive deep tendon reflexes, and epileptic seizures.[2] Levels >4.0 mEq/L (SI: >4.0 mmol/L) are associated with coma, death. A narrow therapeutic index exists for lithium. See table.

Lithium (Acute Ingestion)

Serum Level	Symptoms
1.5-2.5 mEq/L	Polyuria, blurred vision, weakness, lethargy, dizziness, increased reflexes, fasiculations
2.5-3.0 mEq/L	Myoclonic twitching, incontinence, stupor, restlessness, coma
>3.0 mEq/L	Seizures, hypotension, cardiac arrhythmias

Use Monitor therapeutic drug level, support compliance, avoid intoxicating levels; evaluate coma

Limitations Lithium toxicity, including severe neurotoxic effects, can occur with normal serum lithium levels. Instances of acute intoxication may be accompanied by high serum lithium levels without clinical evidence of neurotoxic effects. Lithium penetrates neurons slowly.[3] Thiazides can cause significant rise in serum lithium.

Methodology Flame photometry, atomic absorption spectrophotometry (AA), ion-selective electrode (ISE). Instruments have recently been evaluated.[4]

Additional Information

- Half-life: 18-24 hours
- Volume of distribution: 0.7-1.0 L/kg
- Protein binding: 0%
- Bioavailability: 100%
- Elimination: unchanged, >98% renal
- Peak concentration: 2-5 hours

Lithium as lithium carbonate or citrate is used as a psychoactive agent in the treatment of manic depressive disorders. These oral products are completely absorbed and are completely bioavailable. Peak concentrations occur 1-2 hours after a dose of regular lithium and 4-5 hours after a dose of the sustained-release form. Lithium distribution has two compartments. Concentrations measured during the initial phase do not correlate with efficacy or toxicity. Lithium is cleared by the kidney. It is filtered at the glomerulus and actively reabsorbed at the proximal tubule much like sodium and other electrolytes and vitamins. This is important for potential drug and food interactions. The clearance of lithium is increased in pregnancy and when sodium supplements are given. The clearance is decreased in renal impairment, dehydration, and when patients are hyponatremic. Patients should try to maintain a consistent intake of sodium while on this drug.

Acute lithium toxicity is neuro- and nephrotoxic. Concentration-related side effects include weakness, muscle weakness, tremor, and confusion. Gastrointestinal effects such as nausea and vomiting can be lessened if the patient is given an extended release product.

There are many drugs that can alter the clearance of lithium. Drugs that decrease clearance of lithium include thiazide diuretics, ACE inhibitors, and some nonsteroidal anti-inflammatory agents. Drugs that can increase the clearance of lithium and decrease the concentration are acetazolamide, theophylline, caffeine, and osmotic diuretics. Lithium therapy requires daily monitoring of serum lithium levels until the proper dose schedule is determined.

A fully developed case of intoxication is characterized by coma to semicoma, rigidity, hyperactive reflexes and seizures at times. There is a high incidence of pulmonary complications. It is advisable to perform periodic plasma sodium determinations. Low plasma sodium levels are associated with lithium retention; high levels with lithium elimination. Varying degrees of nephrogenic diabetes insipidus have been reported to occur in 33% of lithium treated patients. Lithium significantly inhibits antidiuretic-hormone-induced water transport in kidney. Lithium interferes with solute and water absorption from the gastrointestinal system producing nausea, vomiting, diarrhea, and abdominal pain. These symptoms may occur at any time, at any serum level. They most commonly occur during early treatment stages and usually clear spontaneously or by adjustment of dosage. Chronic lithium administration has a goitrogenic effect on 4% of lithium-treated patients. Lithium administration results in slightly decreased serum T_4 levels and transiently elevated levels of TSH in nearly 33% of these patients. Thyroxine treatment before or during lithium treatment has been proposed.[5,6] Lithium affects the cardiac conduction system by incomplete substitution for other cations, especially sodium and potassium. These electrolyte changes account for the usually unimportant and reversible T-wave depressions observed in 10% to 20% of patients on lithium therapy. Other interactions include possible effects upon calcium, glucose, magnesium, potassium, bicarbonate, BUN, and bromide levels, leukopenia, and thrombocytopenia.

Footnotes

1. Gelenberg AJ, Kane JM, Keller MB, et al, "Comparison of Standard and Low Serum Levels of Lithium for Maintenance Treatment of Bipolar Disorder," *N Engl J Med*, 1989, 321(22):1489-93.
2. Moyer TP, "Therapeutic Drug Monitoring," *Tietz Textbook of Clinical Chemistry*, 3rd ed, Burtis CA and Ashwood ER, eds, Philadelphia, PA: WB Saunders Co, 1999, 862-905.
3. Stern R, "Lithium in the Treatment of Mood Disorders," *N Engl J Med*, 1995, 332(2):127-8.
4. Sampson M, Ruddel M, and Elin RJ, "Lithium Determinations Evaluated in Eight Analyzers," *Clin Chem*, 1994, 40(6):869-72.
5. Spoov J and Lahdelma L, "Should Thyroid Augmentation Precede Lithium Augmentation - A Pilot Study," *J Affect Disord*, 1998, 49(3):235-9.
6. Bauer M, Hellweg R, Graf KJ, et al, "Treatment of Refractory Depression With High-Dose Thyroxine," *Neuropsychopharmacology*, 1998, 18(6):444-55.

References

Chamberlain S, Hahn PM, Casson P, et al, "Effect of Menstrual Cycle Phase and Oral Contraceptive Use on Serum Lithium Levels After a Loading Dose of Lithium in Normal Women," *Am J Psychiatry*, 1990, 147(7):907-9.

De Maio D, Buffa G, Riva M, et al, "Lithium Ratio, Phospholipids and the Incidence of Side Effects," *Prog Neuropsychopharmacol Biol Psychiatry*, 1994, 18(2):285-93.

Gangadhar B, Subnash MN, Umapathy C, et al, "Lithium Toxicity at Therapeutic Serum Levels," *Br J Psychiatry*, 1993, 163:695.

Groleau G, "Lithium Toxicity," *Emerg Med Clin North Am*, 1994, 12(2):511-31.

Harvey NS and Merriman S, "Review of Clinically Important Drug Interactions With Lithium," *Drug Saf*, 1994, 10(6):455-63.

Krishel S and Jackimczyk K, "Cyclic Antidepressants, Lithium, and Neuroleptic Agents. Pharmacology and Toxicology," *Emerg Med Clin North Am*, 1991, 9(1):53-86.

Manji HK, Hsiao JK, Risby ED, et al, "The Mechanisms of Action of Lithium. I. Effects on Serotoninergic and Noradrenergic Systems in Normal Subjects," *Arch Gen Psychiatry*, 1991, 48(6):505-12.

Price LH and Heninger GR, "Lithium in the Treatment of Mood Disorders," *N Engl J Med*, 1994, 331(9):591-8.

Sadosty AT, Groleau GA, and Atcherson MM, "The Use of Lithium Levels in the Emergency Department," *J Emerg Med*, 1999, 17(5):887-91.

Schweyen DH, Sporka MC, and Burnakis TG, "Evaluation of Serum Lithium Concentration Determinations," *Am J Hosp Pharm*, 1991, 48(7):1536-7.

Timmer RT and Sands JM, "Lithium Intoxication," *J Am Soc Nephrol*, 1999, 10(3):666-74.

- ◆ **Lithobid®** *see* Lithium, Serum *on page 754*
- ◆ **Lithonate®** *see* Lithium, Serum *on page 754*
- ◆ **Lithotabs®** *see* Lithium, Serum *on page 754*
- ◆ **Liu-Shan-Wan** *see* Digoxin, Serum *on page 746*
- ◆ **Lotusate®** *see* Barbiturates, Quantitative, Serum or Plasma *on page 739*
- ◆ **Loxapine** *see* Amoxapine, Serum or Plasma *on page 736*
- ◆ **Ludiomil®** *see* Maprotiline, Serum *on page 755*
- ◆ **Luminal®** *see* Barbiturates, Quantitative, Serum or Plasma *on page 739*
- ◆ **Luminal®** *see* Phenobarbital, Serum or Plasma *on page 760*
- ◆ **Lyphocin®** *see* Vancomycin, Serum *on page 769*
- ◆ **Magnum®** *see* Caffeine, Serum *on page 740*
- ◆ **Majsolin®** *see* Primidone, Serum or Plasma *on page 762*
- ◆ **Maprotiline** *see* Antidepressants, Cyclic, Serum *on page 737*

Maprotiline, Serum

Related Information

Antidepressants, Cyclic, Serum *on page 737*

Synonyms Ludiomil®

Abstract Maprotiline is a tetracyclic antidepressant with a long half-life. Like the tricyclics, maprotiline is an inhibitor of the reuptake of norepinephrine. It is metabolized to an active metabolite, desmethyl maprotiline. In addition to desmethylmaprotiline, another metabolite, maprotiline-N-oxide, is also reported to be pharmacologically active.

Specimen Serum

Container Red top tube

Sampling Time Peak serum values are reached in 12 hours and steady-state is achieved in 5-10 days.

Storage Instructions Separate serum from clot and refrigerate.

Reference Interval 200-400 ng/mL (SI: 721-1442 nmol/L)

Critical Values >1000 ng/mL (SI: >3605 nmol/L)

Use Evaluate toxicity and therapeutic drug monitoring

Methodology High performance liquid chromatography (HPLC), gas chromatography (GC)

Additional Information

- Half-life: Maprotiline: 27-58 hours; active metabolite desmethyl maprotiline: 60-90 hours
- Volume of distribution: 15-35 L/kg
- Protein binding: 80% to 90%

Maprotiline is a tetracyclic antidepressant prescribed for depression, chronic schizophrenia, idiopathic pain, and potentially for drug abuse withdrawal. Maprotiline is often used in patients who do not respond to tricyclics. The drug is taken orally at an average adult dose of 75-300 mg/day (50-75 mg/day in elderly patients). Maprotiline is a very potent inhibitor of the reuptake of norepinephrine to the presynaptic nerve terminal. The drug possesses moderate anticholinergic activity and cardiovascular toxicity. It also may lower seizure control. It has a higher incidence of seizures than the tricyclic antidepressants, trazodone, fluoxetine, and fluvoxamine. The adverse effects include vertigo, blurred vision, seizures, drowsiness, and urinary retention. It should not be given in combination with MAO inhibitors.

References

Fukuchi H, Kitaura T, Miyake K, et al, "Association Between Dosage and Serum Concentration of Antidepressants," *Clin Pharm*, 1990, 9(1):45-9.

Isotani H and Kameoka K, "Hypoglycemia Associated With Maprotiline in a Patient With Type 1 Diabetes," *Diabetes Care*, 1999, 22(5):862-3.

Namera A, Watanabe T, Yashiki M, et al, "Simple Analysis of Tetracyclic Antidepressants in Blood Using Headspace-Solid-Phase Microextraction and GC/MS," *J Anal Toxicol*, 1998, 22(5):396-400.

Pisani F, Spina E, and Oteri G, "Antidepressant Drugs and Seizure Susceptibility: From *In Vitro* Data to Clinical Practice," *Epilepsia*, 1999, 40(Suppl 10):S48-56.

Rotzinger S, Bourin M, Akimoto Y, et al, "Metabolism of Some "Second"- and "Fourth"-Generation Antidepressants: Iprindole, Viloxazine, Bupropion, Mianserin, Maprotiline, Trazodone, Nefazodone, and Venlafaxine," *Cell Mol Neurobiol*, 1999, 19(4):427-42.

Schnyder U and Koller-Leiser A, "A Double-Blind, Multicentre Study of Paroxetine and Maprotiline in Major Depression," *Can J Psychiatry*, 1996, 41(4):239-44.

♦ **Max Alert Magnum®** *see* Caffeine, Serum *on page 740*

♦ **Mebaral®** *see* Barbiturates, Quantitative, Serum or Plasma *on page 739*

♦ **Mebaral®** *see* Methylphenobarbital, Serum *on page 757*

♦ **MEGX** *see* Monoethylglycinexylidide, Serum *on page 758*

♦ **Mellaril®** *see* Phenothiazines, Serum or Urine *on page 760*

Mephenytoin, Serum

Related Information
Ethotoin, Serum *on page 749*
Phenytoin, Serum or Plasma *on page 761*

Synonyms Mesantoin®; Methoin; Methylphenylethylhydantoin; Phenantoin; Sedantoinal®

Applies to 5-Phenyl-5-Ethylhydantoin (Nirvanol®)

Abstract Mephenytoin has a pharmacologic effect similar to that of phenytoin. Mephenytoin has serious toxicity but less dose-related effects compared to phenytoin. This drug is generally used only for patients refractory to or unable to tolerate other anticonvulsants.

Patient Preparation Baseline blood counts and differential counts should be obtained prior to initiation of therapy and monitored periodically.[1]

Specimen Serum

Container Red top tube

Sampling Time Consistent sampling time. Steady-state is reached in ~40 hours.

Reference Interval 25-40 μg/mL for the sum of the parent drug and 5-phenyl-5-ethylhydantoin metabolite, which is usually present at a higher level than the parent compound

Possible Panic Range Toxic level about 50 μg/mL (SI: 230 μmol/L). See Table A in the Therapeutic Drug Monitoring Introduction *on page 733*.

Use Monitor for compliance, efficacy, and possible toxicity. Mephenytoin may be suited for patients who respond to phenytoin but who cannot tolerate dose-related side effects. It is used for treatment of tonic-clonic and partial seizures.

Limitations Unlike phenytoin, cognitive side effects, cerebellar symptoms, gingival hypertrophy, and hirsutism do not occur as commonly with increasing dosage. The main active metabolite, 5-ethyl-5-phenylhydantoin, is a biologically active anticonvulsant with a half-life of 100 hours.

Contraindications Indications for discontinuation of drug include WBC <1600.

Methodology Gas chromatography (GC)

Additional Information
• Half-life: parent compound: ~8 hours, metabolite: >100 hours
• Protein binding: 20% to 50%

Mephenytoin, like phenytoin, has zero-order kinetics so that small changes in dosage may produce large changes in clinical response. Acute overdosage results in sedation and eventually coma. Most adverse effects are not dose-related, but are due to the accumulation of arene-oxide intermediates. They include rash, hepatotoxicity, blood dyscrasias, systemic lupus erythematosus, periarteritis nodosa, and fever. The drug is considered more highly toxic than other hydantoins.

Test interactions include increased serum alkaline phosphatase and decreased calcium.

Footnotes
1. Product Information: Mesantoin®, Mephenytoin, East Hanover, NJ: Sandoz Pharmaceuticals Corporation, 1995.

References
Ko JW, Desta Z, and Flockhart DA, "Human N-Demethylation of (S)-Mephenytoin by Cytochrome P-450s 2C9 and 2B6," *Drug Metab Dispos*, 1998, 26(8):775-8.
Leikin JB and Paloucek FP, *Poisoning and Toxicology Compendium*, Hudson, OH: Lexi-Comp Inc, 1998.

♦ **Mephobarbital** *see* Barbiturates, Quantitative, Serum or Plasma *on page 739*

♦ **Mephobarbital** *see* Methylphenobarbital, Serum *on page 757*

♦ **Mephobarbitone** *see* Methylphenobarbital, Serum *on page 757*

♦ **Meprobam®** *see* Meprobamate, Serum *on page 756*

Meprobamate, Serum

Synonyms Equagesic®; Equanil®; Meprobam®; Meprospan®; Miltown®; Neuramate®; Tenavoid®

Abstract Meprobamate is a sedative-anxiolytic, producing effects similar to those of the benzodiazepines and barbiturates. It is a schedule IV controlled substance.

Specimen Serum

Container Red top tube

Reference Interval Sedative dose: 6-12 μg/mL (SI: 28-55 μmol/L)

Critical Values Toxic: >60 μg/mL (SI: >275 μmol/L)

Possible Panic Range Coma is associated with levels >70 μg/mL (SI: >321 μmol/L); **fatalities** can occur at >142 μg/mL (SI: >650 μmol/L); lethal: 200 μg/mL (SI: 916 μmol/L)

Use Therapeutic monitoring and toxicity assessment. Meprobamate is a propanediol carbamate sedative and tranquilizer, having pharmacological effects similar to barbiturates. Respiratory depression, coma, and cardiovascular collapse characterize overdosage.

Methodology Gas-liquid chromatography (GLC), gas chromatography/mass spectrometry (GC/MS), high performance liquid chromatography (HPLC). Thin-layer chromatography (TLC) is used for qualitative analysis in overdose situations.

Additional Information
• Half-life: 6-15 hours
• Volume of distribution: 0.5-1.0 L/kg
• Protein binding: 20%

Meprobamate is well absorbed from the gastrointestinal tract and reaches its peak concentration in 2-3 hours. It may also be detected in urine or gastric juice. Carisoprodol is a noncontrolled muscle relaxant that is metabolized to meprobamate and may be considered a drug of abuse.

Adverse effects in overdose include hypotension, drowsiness, dizziness, hangover, and seizures. A benzodiazepine antagonist, flumazenil, has been used as an antidote in overdose cases.

References
Gaillard Y, Billault F, and Pepin G, "Meprobamate Overdosage: A Continuing Problem. Sensitive GC/MS Quantitation After Solid Phase Extraction in 19 Fatal Cases," *Forensic Sci Int*, 1997, 86(3):173-80.
Kintz P and Mangin P, "Determination of Meprobamate in Human Plasma, Urine, and Hair by Gas Chromatography and Electron Impact Mass Spectrometry," *J Anal Toxicol*, 1993, 17(7):408-10.
Lambert WE, De Leenheer AP, Van Bocxlaer JF, et al, "Meprobamate Intoxication: Rare and Difficult to Find," *J Toxicol Clin Toxicol*, 1992, 30(4):683-4.
Logan BK, Case GA, and Gordon AM, "Carisoprodol, Meprobamate, and Driving Impairment," *J Forensic Sci*, 2000, 45(3):619-23.
Reeves RR, Carter OS, Pinkofsky HB, et al, "Carisoprodol (Soma): Abuse Potential and Physician Unawareness," *J Addict Dis*, 1999, 18(2):51-6.
Trenque T, Lamiable D, Millart H, et al, "Gas Chromatographic Determination of Meprobamate in Human Plasma," *J Chromatogr*, 1993, 615(2):343-6.

♦ **Meprospan®** *see* Meprobamate, Serum *on page 756*

♦ **Mesantoin®** *see* Mephenytoin, Serum *on page 756*

♦ **Mesoridazine** *see* Phenothiazines, Serum or Urine *on page 760*

♦ **Metabolites of Primidone** *see* Primidone, Serum or Plasma *on page 762*

♦ **Methaminodiazepoxide Hydrochloride** *see* Chlordiazepoxide, Serum *on page 742*

♦ **Metharbital** *see* Barbiturates, Quantitative, Serum or Plasma *on page 739*

♦ **Methoin** *see* Mephenytoin, Serum *on page 756*

Methotrexate, Serum or Plasma

Related Information
C-Reactive Protein, Serum *on page 523*

Synonyms Amethopterin; Folex®; Mexate®; MTX; Rheumatrex®

Applies to Cerebrospinal Fluid Methotrexate; Citrovorum Factor

Abstract Methotrexate (MTX) is used as a single agent or as a component of chemotherapeutic drug combinations. It is an anticancer drug acting through competitively inhibiting folic acid reductase, an enzyme necessary for cellular replication. A role for MTX is recognized as a part of therapy of acute lymphoblastic leukemia; small cell carcinoma of lung; and carcinomas of urinary bladder, breast, and head and neck. In high dosage with leucovorin rescue, it is among drugs used for osteogenic sarcoma. Low-dose methotrexate is also used in a number of other diseases, such as rheumatoid arthritis, psoriatic arthritis, polymyositis, and Reiter syndrome. It has a limited role in management of inflammatory bowel disease. Methotrexate should be monitored in patients receiving high-dose therapy (>100 mg/m²). Since methotrexate is extremely toxic, leucovorin, a folate analogue, is generally used to rescue host cells. This rescue makes possible administration of much higher doses of methotrexate than would otherwise be possible.

MTX can cause granulomatous pneumonitis and dose-dependent hepatic fibrosis.

Specimen Serum or plasma

Container Red top tube, green top (heparin) tube, or lavender top (EDTA) tube

Sampling Time Varies according to dosing protocol. Time to peak serum concentration: oral: within 1-2 hours; parenteral: within 30-60 minutes.

Storage Instructions Separate serum or plasma and freeze.

Reference Interval Therapeutic range is dependent upon therapeutic approach. **"High dose"** regimens produce drug levels between 0.1-1 μmol/L, 24-72 hours after drug infusion.

Critical Values Plasma concentrations >1.0 μmol/L, 48 hours postinfusion are associated with increased toxicity. Leucovorin rescue is not complete until plasma concentrations fall below this level.

Possible Panic Range Toxic: low-dose therapy: >0.02 μmol/L; high-dose therapy: >1 μmol/L, 48 hours postdose

Use Monitor therapeutic drug level of methotrexate; evaluate potential toxicity

Limitations Adverse effects limit the application of methotrexate in some individuals. It has recently been compared with etanercept for management of early rheumatoid arthritis.[1]

Methodology Enzyme immunoassay (EIA), fluorescence polarization immunoassay (FPIA), radioimmunoassay (RIA), high performance liquid chromatography (HPLC)

Additional Information
- Half-life: distribution: 0.5-1 hour; elimination: 5-9 hours
- Volume of distribution: 0.4-1.0 L/kg
- Protein binding: 50% to 70%

Methotrexate, a structural analogue of folic acid, is an antimetabolite that combines with dihydrofolate reductase. It therefore interferes with the synthesis of tetrahydrofolic acid, necessary for DNA synthesis. It is excreted unchanged in the urine in 12 hours when kidney function is adequate and the patient is hydrated. Urinary alkalinization is recommended. Toxicity includes mucosa of the gastrointestinal tract and bone marrow depression with megaloblastosis. Concomitant salicylate administration increases incidence of toxicity, due to diminished renal tubular excretion. The initial half-life is 2-4 hours, but the total body clearance (terminal) half-life is 8-15 hours.

Drugs can interfere with the clearance or absorption of MTX. Antibiotics may decrease its absorption. Salicylates, sulfonamides, probenecid, and nonsteroidal anti-inflammatory drugs may block the renal clearance of methotrexate, increasing its serum concentration.

Signs of fatal MTX toxicity include extensive erosions in the oral cavity and other mucous membranes, gastrointestinal hemorrhage, interstitial pneumonia, and progressive renal insufficiency. Accompanying laboratory findings may include agranulocytosis, thrombocytopenia, anemia, and hyperbilirubinemia. MTX use is contraindicated in patients with severe renal or hepatic impairment, pre-existing myelosuppression, and pleural/peritoneal effusions.

Increased AST and ALT concentrations are found in some patients with rheumatoid arthritis who are taking methotrexate.[1]

Infliximab combined with methotrexate has provided clinical benefit in subjects with persistently active rheumatoid arthritis.[2]

Footnotes
1. Bathon JM, Martin RW, Fleischmann RM, et al, "A Comparison of Etanercept and Methotrexate in Patients With Early Rheumatoid Arthritis," *N Engl J Med*, 2000, 343(22):1586-93.
2. Lipsky PE, van der Heijde DM, St Clair EW, et al, "Infliximab and Methotrexate in the Treatment of Rheumatoid Arthritis," *N Engl J Med*, 2000, 343(22):1594-602.

References
Bertino JR and Salmon SE, "Principles of Cancer Therapy," *Cecil Textbook of Medicine*, 21st ed, Goldman L and Bennett JC, eds, Philadelphia, PA: WB Saunders Co, 2000, 1060-74.
Brooks PJ, Spruill WJ, Parish RC, et al, "Pharmacokinetics of Methotrexate Administered by Intramuscular and Subcutaneous Injections in Patients With Rheumatoid Arthritis," *Arthritis Rheum*, 1990, 33(1):91-4.
Fossa SD, Heilo A, and Bormer O, "Unexpectedly High Serum Methotrexate Levels in Cystectomized Bladder Cancer Patients With an Ileal Conduit Treated With Intermediate Doses of the Drug," *J Urol*, 1990, 143(3):498-501.
Kremer JM, "Methotrexate and Emerging Therapies," *Rheum Dis Clin North Am*, 1998, 24(3):651-8.
McIvor A, "Charcoal Hemoperfusion and Methotrexate Toxicity," *Nephron*, 1991, 58(3):378.
Minocha A, Dean HA, and Pittsley RA, "Liver Cirrhosis in Rheumatoid Arthritis Patients Treated With Long-Term Methotrexate," *Vet Hum Toxicol*, 1993, 35(1):45-8.
Olsen EA, "The Pharmacology of Methotrexate," *J Am Acad Dermatol*, 1991, 25(2 Pt 1):306-18.
Shiroky JB, Neville C, Esdaile JM, et al, "Low-Dose Methotrexate With Leucovorin (Folinic Acid) in the Management of Rheumatoid Arthritis. Results of a Multicenter Randomized, Double-Blind, Placebo-Controlled Trial," *Arthritis Rheum*, 1993, 36(6):795-803.
Treon SP and Chabner BA, "Concepts in Use of High-Dose Methotrexate Therapy," *Clin Chem*, 1996, 42(8 pt 2):1322-9.
Wallace CA, Bleyer WA, Sherry DD, et al, "Toxicity and Serum Levels of Methotrexate in Children With Juvenile Rheumatoid Arthritis," *Arthritis Rheum*, 1989, 32(6):677-81.
Wernick R and Smith DL, "Central Nervous System Toxicity Associated With Weekly Low-Dose Methotrexate Treatment," *Arthritis Rheum*, 1989, 32(6):770-5.

Methylphenobarbital, Serum

Related Information
Barbiturates, Quantitative, Serum or Plasma *on page 739*
Phenobarbital, Serum or Plasma *on page 760*

Synonyms Enphenemalum; Gemonil®; Mebaral®; Mephobarbital; Mephobarbitone

Abstract Mephobarbital is metabolized to phenobarbital, which accounts for most pharmacologic effects. However, mephobarbital has slightly different pharmacokinetics than phenobarbital.

Specimen Serum

Container Red top tube

Sampling Time Consistent sampling time. Steady-state is reached between 8-10 days.

Reference Interval In humans, most of the drug is converted to phenobarbital, and many methods of determination have difficulty distinguishing

between the drug and the metabolite. Determination of the total phenobarbital then gives an approximation of antiepileptic drug (AED) level of the parent compound. Very little data exists on reference values for methylphenobarbital. Phenobarbital level should be in the range of 15-40 µg/mL.

Critical Values See Phenobarbital, Serum or Plasma *on page 760*. Levels >80 µg/mL correlate with decreased mental status.

Use Mephobarbital is used for prophylactic management of tonic-clonic (grand mal) seizures and for absence (petit mal) seizures.

Methodology Gas-liquid chromatography (GLC), gas chromatography/mass spectrometry (GC/MS)

Additional Information
- Half-life: 45-55 hours
- Volume of distribution: 2-3 L/kg
- Protein binding: 40% to 60%

Like other barbiturates, methylphenobarbital is extensively metabolized in the liver, by demethylation, to phenobarbital. About 75% of a single dose is converted to phenobarbital in 24 hours.

Methylphenobarbital has a more linear response between dosage and blood phenobarbital level than does phenobarbital. The limitations and adverse effects of the two drugs are likely to be very similar. Test interactions include an increase in alkaline phosphatase and ammonia, and a decrease in bilirubin and calcium.

References
Ceccato A, Boulanger B, Chiap P, et al, "Simultaneous Determination of Methylphenobarbital Enantiomers and Phenobarbital in Human Plasma by On-Line Coupling of an Achiral Precolumn to a Chiral Liquid Chromatographic Column," *J Chromatogr A*, 1998, 819(1-2):143-53.
Leikin JB and Paloucek FP, *Poisoning and Toxicology Compendium*, Hudson, OH: Lexi-Comp Inc, 1998.
Willis J, Nelson A, Black FW, et al, "Barbiturate Anticonvulsants: A Neuropsychological and Quantitative Electroencephalographic Study," *J Child Neurol*, 1997, 12(3):169-71.

♦ **Methylphenylethylhydantoin** *see* Mephenytoin, Serum *on page 756*

♦ **Mexate®** *see* Methotrexate, Serum or Plasma *on page 756*

Mexiletine, Serum

Related Information
Phenobarbital, Serum or Plasma *on page 760*
Phenytoin, Serum or Plasma *on page 761*
pH, Urine *on page 882*
Theophylline, Serum *on page 766*

Synonyms Mexltll®

Abstract Mexiletine is a class 1B antiarrhythmic agent used to treat ventricular arrhythmia. It is structurally similar to lidocaine, but is orally active. It has also been used in treatment-resistant bipolar disorder[1] and as an analgesic used in diabetic neuropathy.

Specimen Serum

Container Red top tube

Sampling Time Draw 2-4 hours after last dose for peak level. Draw immediately prior to next dose for trough levels.

Reference Interval Therapeutic: 0.75-2.0 µg/mL (SI: 4-11 µmol/L)

Possible Panic Range >2.0 µg/mL (SI: >9 µmol/L). Levels >20 µg/mL (SI: >90 µmol/L) are associated with seizures.

Use Therapeutic monitoring and toxicity assessment. Mexiletine is a class I antiarrhythmic approved for treatment of serious ventricular arrhythmias. It has no active metabolites. Toxic effects include dizziness, vomiting, confusion, tremor, bradycardia, and hypotension. At very high concentrations, it causes seizures.

Methodology Fluorometry, high performance liquid chromatography (HPLC), gas chromatography (GC)

Additional Information
- Half-life: 7-15 hours
- Volume of distribution: 5-7 L/kg
- Protein binding: 60% to 70%

Half-life is urine pH dependent. Acidic urine accelerates elimination. Hepatic impairment prolongs the elimination half-life of mexiletine.

Mexiletine can increase serum theophylline levels. Phenobarbital, phenytoin, rifampin, and other hepatic enzyme inducers may lower mexiletine plasma levels; cimetidine may increase mexiletine levels. Antacids, narcotics, or anticholinergics may decrease rate of absorption; metoclopramide may increase rate of absorption. Drugs or diets which affect urine pH can increase or decrease excretion of mexiletine. Use with beta-blockers or calcium channel blockers may depress cardiac function. Phenytoin or rifampin can enhance mexiletine metabolism.

Footnotes
1. Schaffer A, Levitt AJ, and Joffe RT, "Mexiletine in Treatment-Resistant Bipolar Disorder," *J Affect Disord*, 2000, 57(1-3):249-53.

References
Frank SE, Snyder JT, "Survival Following Severe Overdose With Mexiletine, Nifedipine, and Nitroglycerin," *Am J Emerg Med*, 1991, 9(1):43-6.
Gottlieb SS and Weinberg M, "Comparative Hemodynamic Effects of Mexiletine and Quinidine in Patients With Severe Left Ventricular Dysfunction," *Am Heart J*, 1991, 122(5):1368-74.

(Continued)

Mexiletine, Serum *(Continued)*

Jarvis B and Coukell AJ, "Mexiletine. A Review of Its Therapeutic Use in Painful Diabetic Neuropathy," *Drugs*, 1998, 56(4):691-707.

Ji SG, Kong QH, Li XL, et al, "Gas Chromatographic Determination of Mexiletine in Human Plasma With Flame Ionization Detection After Reaction With Carbon Disulfide," *Biomed Chromatogr*, 1993, 7(4):196-9.

Labbe L and Turgeon J, "Clinical Pharmacokinetics of Mexiletine," *Clin Pharmacokinet*, 1999, 37(5):361-84.

Leiken JB and Paloucek FP, *Poisoning and Toxicology Compendium*, Hudson, OH: Lexi-Comp Inc, 1998, 391-2.

Manolis AS, Deering TF, Cameron J, et al, "Mexiletine: Pharmacology and Therapeutic Use," *Clin Cardiol*, 1990, 13(5):349-59.

♦ **Mexitil®** *see* Mexiletine, Serum *on page 757*

♦ **Miltown®** *see* Meprobamate, Serum *on page 756*

♦ **Mitran®** *see* Chlordiazepoxide, Serum *on page 742*

♦ **Moditen®** *see* Fluphenazine, Serum *on page 750*

♦ **Mole®** *see* Caffeine, Serum *on page 740*

♦ **Molipaxin®** *see* Trazodone, Serum or Plasma *on page 768*

Monoethylglycinexylidide, Serum

Related Information
Lidocaine, Serum or Plasma *on page 754*
Liver Disease: Laboratory Assessment, Overview *on page 216*

Synonyms MEGX

Applies to Lidocaine Metabolite

Test Includes This is the major active metabolite of lidocaine. It is monitored along with lidocaine as an antiarrhythmic agent.

Abstract Monitored with lidocaine as an antiarrhythmic agent. This drug may also be used to assess donor and recipient organ liver function.

Specimen Serum

Container Red top tube

Sampling Time 15 minutes after subtherapeutic, intravenous dose of 1 mg/kg lidocaine when used for lidocaine clearance test. When monitored for therapy, 30 minutes after loading dose; if no loading dose, 5-7 hours after initiation of therapy.

Reference Interval >50 μg/L (SI: >170 nmol/L) when used as liver function test. Lower values are found in women under 45 years of age not on contraceptives.[1]

Critical Values MEGX concentrations <25 μg/L indicate significant liver insufficiency and values <10 μg/L warrant liver transplant.[2]

Use MEGX is the major metabolite of lidocaine and may be used to assess donor and recipient liver function in transplantation of this organ in adults and children. It may be useful in evaluation of liver disease.[3,4] It may have a role as a test in evaluation of shock.[5] Conversion of lidocaine to MEGX after a 1.0 mg/kg dose should result in a level >50 μg/L.

Methodology High performance liquid chromatography (HPLC), gas chromatography (GC)

Additional Information Plasma half-life is 2 hours.

Footnotes
1. Oellerich M, Schutz E, Polzien F, et al, "Influence of Gender on the Monoethylglycinexylidide Test in Normal Subjects and Liver Donors," *Ther Drug Monit*, 1994, 16(3):225-31.
2. Ercolani G, Grazi GL, Calliva R, et al, "The Lidocaine (MEGX) Test as an Index of Hepatic Function: Its Clinical Usefulness in Liver Surgery," *Surgery*, 2000, 127(4):464-71.
3. Forte G, Rocco P, Costanzo A, et al, "Monoethylglycinexylidide Production as a Measure in Predicting Hepatic Histology," *Ital J Gastroenterol*, 1994, 26(4):159-62.
4. Huang YS, Lee SD, Deng JF, et al, "Measuring Lidocaine Metabolite - Monoethylglycinexylidide as a Quantitative Index of Hepatic Function in Adults With Chronic Hepatitis and Cirrhosis," *J Hepatol*, 1993, 19(1):140-7.
5. Chandel B, Shapiro MJ, Kurtz M, et al, "MEGX (Monoethylglycinexylidide): A Novel *In Vivo* Test to Measure Early Hepatic Dysfunction After Hypovolemic Shock," *Shock*, 1995, 3(1):51-3.

References
Abdel-Rehim M, Bielenstein M, Askemark Y, et al, "High-Performance Liquid Chromatography - Tandem Electrospray Mass Spectrometry for the Determination of Lidocaine and Its Metabolites in Human Plasma and Urine," *J Chromatogr B Biomed Sci Appl*, 2000, 741(2):175-88.

Fukuda T, Kakiuchi Y, Miyabe M, et al, "Plasma Lidocaine, Monoethylglycinexylidine, and Glycinexylidide Concentrations After Epidural Administration in Geriatric Patients," *Reg Anesth Pain Med*, 2000, 25(3):268-73.

Wang JS, Backman JT, Taavitsainen P, et al, "Involvement of CYP1A2 and CYP3A4 in Lidocaine N-Deethylation and 3-Hydroxylation in Humans," *Drug Metab Dispos*, 2000, 28(8):959-65.

♦ **Moxadil®** *see* Amoxapine, Serum or Plasma *on page 736*

♦ **MTX** *see* Methotrexate, Serum or Plasma *on page 756*

♦ **Mychel-S®** *see* Chloramphenicol *on page 742*

♦ **Mylepsin®** *see* Primidone, Serum or Plasma *on page 762*

♦ **Myochrysine®** *see* Gold, Serum *on page 751*

♦ **Mysoline®** *see* Primidone, Serum or Plasma *on page 762*

♦ **N-Acetyl Procainamide** *see* Procainamide, Serum *on page 763*

♦ **NAPA** *see* Procainamide, Serum *on page 763*

♦ **Napamide®** *see* Disopyramide, Serum or Plasma *on page 747*

♦ **Nativelle®** *see* Digitoxin, Serum *on page 745*

♦ **Nembutal®** *see* Barbiturates, Quantitative, Serum or Plasma *on page 739*

♦ **Neoral®** *see* Cyclosporine, Blood *on page 744*

♦ **Nervocaine®** *see* Lidocaine, Serum or Plasma *on page 754*

♦ **Neuramate®** *see* Meprobamate, Serum *on page 756*

♦ **Neurontin®** *see* Antiepileptic Drugs, New, Overview *on page 738*

♦ **No-Doz®** *see* Caffeine, Serum *on page 740*

♦ **Norocaine®** *see* Lidocaine, Serum or Plasma *on page 754*

♦ **Norpace®** *see* Disopyramide, Serum or Plasma *on page 747*

♦ **Norpramin®** *see* Antidepressants, Cyclic, Serum *on page 737*

♦ **Norpramin®** *see* Imipramine, Serum or Plasma *on page 752*

♦ **Nortrilen®** *see* Nortriptyline, Serum *on page 758*

♦ **Nortriptyline** *see* Antidepressants, Cyclic, Serum *on page 737*

Nortriptyline, Serum

Related Information
Amitriptyline, Serum *on page 735*
Antidepressants, Cyclic, Serum *on page 737*
Disopyramide, Serum or Plasma *on page 747*
Phenytoin, Serum or Plasma *on page 761*
Procainamide, Serum *on page 763*
Quinidine, Serum *on page 764*
Warfarin *on page 770*

Synonyms Allegron®; Aventyl® Hydrochloride; Nortrilen®; Norval®; Pamelor®

Abstract Nortriptyline is a tricyclic antidepressant. It has analgesic properties, and is included in the group of adjuvant analgesic drugs. It is used as a prophylactic agent for migraine.

Specimen Serum

Container Red top tube

Sampling Time Trough levels at steady state (100-300 hours)

Storage Instructions Separate serum and refrigerate.

Causes for Rejection Sample collected in gel tube

Reference Interval Therapeutic: 50-150 ng/mL (SI: 190-570 nmol/L)

Critical Values Toxic: >500 ng/mL (SI: >1900 nmol/L)

Possible Panic Range ≥1000 ng/mL

Use Monitor therapeutic drug level; evaluate toxicity, overdoses. Nortriptyline is a derivative and metabolite of amitriptyline and is used to treat endogenous depression.

Contraindications Cyclic antidepressants should be avoided in pregnant and lactating women because these drugs have not been established to be safe. It is contraindicated with narrow-angle glaucoma. Geriatric patients are especially susceptible to orthostasis, urinary retention, constipation, and sedation.

Methodology High performance liquid chromatography (HPLC), liquid chromatography,[1] fluorescence polarization immunoassay (FPIA),[2] enzyme immunoassay (EIA)

Additional Information
- Half-life: 20-60 hours (pharmacokinetic parameters may have wide ranges for the tricyclic antidepressants)
- Volume of distribution: 15-23 L/kg
- Protein binding: 90% to 95%

Nortriptyline, primarily detoxified in the liver, may be associated with cholestasis and cholestatic jaundice. Hematologic consequences include agranulocytosis, purpura, and thrombocytopenia. Other side effects include a host of GI, endocrinologic, allergic, anticholinergic, cardiovascular, and neurologic disorders. Fulminant hepatic failure may be idiosyncratic.[3]

Nortriptyline is completely absorbed but undergoes some first-pass elimination. The bioavailability of nortriptyline is 45% to 70% with a peak concentration 2-6 hours after an oral dose. It is 90% bound to plasma proteins and is also highly bound to tissues.

As with other tricyclic antidepressants, anticholinergic side effects are common with this drug. They are not severe and may diminish with continued therapy or can be treated with other pharmacologic and nonpharmacologic therapies. Anticholinergic side effects are more troublesome in the elderly. However, nortriptyline and desipramine appear to be the best tolerated tricyclics in the elderly.[4] Sedation may also decrease with continued use. Nortriptyline can also lower the seizure threshold and cause orthostasis, postural hypotension, and arrhythmias. Cardiovascular effects are more common in patients with underlying cardiovascular disorders.

Drug interactions are common with the tricyclic antidepressants. Concomitant treatment with cimetidine, fluoxetine, and antipsychotics produce unexpectedly increased concentrations of nortriptyline. Enzyme inducers (eg, phenytoin, chloral hydrate, smoking, and the barbiturates) will decrease nortriptyline concentrations. Additive anticholinergic side effects occur when tricyclics are combined with antihistamines, anti-Parkinson drugs, and anti-psychotics. The cardiovascular effects of the tricyclics are additive with any of the class IA antiarrhythmics (quinidine, procainamide, disopyramide). Direct-acting sympathomimetics (epinephrine, norepinephrine, phenyleph-rine) are potentiated by tricyclics. Monoamine oxidase inhibitors (MAOI) and thyroid hormones potentiate the toxicities of tricyclics. Hyperthermia, delirium, convulsions, coma, and fatalities have occurred with the combina-tion of MAOIs and tricyclics. These drugs have been used in combination in refractory cases of depression. The tricyclics can also affect other drugs. The antihypertensive effects of the central α-agonists (clonidine, methyl-dopa, guanethidine) are reversed when combined with tricyclics. Warfarin anticoagulation effects may be potentiated by the tricyclics.

Test interactions include possible increase in glucose and elevation of plasma norepinephrine levels and plasma epinephrine levels threefold to fivefold. EMIT assays for nortriptyline may give false-positive in the pres-ence of high concentrations of diphenhydramine, thioridazine, chlorproma-zine, alimenazine, carbamazepine, cyclobenzaprine, or perphenazine.

The tricyclic antidepressants are commonly seen in overdose situations. Cardiovascular, anticholinergic and central nervous system toxicities can be lethal. Treatment includes supportive measures and removal of ingested drug by emesis or gastric lavage. This drug is not removed by dialysis due to its large volume of distribution.

Footnotes

1. el-Yazigi A and Raines DA, "Concurrent Liquid Chromatographic Measurement of Fluoxetine, Amitriptyline, Imipramine, and Their Active Metabolites Norfluoxetine, Nortriptyline, and Desipramine in Plasma," *Ther Drug Monit*, 1993, 15(4):305-9.
2. Adamczyk M, Fishpaugh JR, Harrington CA, et al, "Immunoassay Reagents for Psychoactive Drugs. Part 4. Quantitative Determination of Amitriptyline and Nortrip-tyline by Fluorescence Polarization Immunoassay," *Ther Drug Monit*, 1994, 16(3):298-311.
3. Berkelhammer C, Kher N, Berry C, et al, "Nortriptyline-Induced Fulminant Hepatic Failure," *J Clin Gastroenterol*, 1995, 20(1):54-6.
4. Gareri P, Stilo G, Bevacqua I, et al, "Antidepressant Drugs in the Elderly," *Gen Pharmacol*, 1998, 30(4):465-75.

References

Baselt RC, *Disposition of Toxic Drugs and Chemicals in Man*, 5th ed, Foster City, CA: Chemical Toxicology Institute, 2000, 630-33.
Feldman MD, "Therapeutic Blood Monitoring of Tricyclic Antidepressants," *South Med J*, 1994, 87(1):101.
Jerling M and Alvan G, "Nonlinear Kinetics of Nortriptyline in Relation to Nortriptyline Clearance as Observed During Therapeutic Drug Monitoring," *Eur J Clin Pharmacol*, 1994, 46(1):67-70.
Jerling M, Bertilsson L, and Sjoqvist F, "The Use of Therapeutic Drug Monitoring Data to Document Kinetic Drug Interactions: An Example With Amitriptyline and Nortripty-line," *Ther Drug Monit*, 1994, 16(1):1-12.
Kehoe WA, Harralson AF, Jacisin JJ, et al, "Sources of Prediction Error When Using a Bayesian Method to Evaluate Nortriptyline Serum Concentrations," *J Clin Pharmacol*, 1994, 34(8):842-7.
Linder MW and Keck PE Jr, "Standards of Laboratory Practice: Antidepressant Drug Monitoring. National Academy of Clinical Biochemistry," *Clin Chem*, 1998, 44(5):1073-84.
Lipper B and Gaynor BD, "Value of Serum Tricyclic Antidepressant Levels With Massive Nortriptyline Overdose and Persistent Hypotension," *Am J Emerg Med*, 1995, 13(1):107.
Lipper B, Bell A, and Gaynor B, "Recurrent Hypotension Immediately After Seizures in Nortriptyline Overdose," *Am J Emerg Med*, 1994, 12(4):452-3.
Nair NP, Amin M, Holm P, et al, "Moclobemide and Nortriptyline in Elderly Depressed Patients. A Randomized, Multicentre Trial Against Placebo," *J Affect Disord*, 1995, 33(1):1-9.
Reynolds CF 3rd, Frank E, Perel JM, et al, "Nortriptyline and Interpersonal Psycho-therapy as Maintenance Therapies for Recurrent Major Depression: A Randomized Controlled Trial in Patients Older Than 59 Years," *JAMA*, 1999, 281(1):39-45.

Oxazepam, Serum

Related Information

Synonyms Adumbran®; Serax®; Serenid® Forte

Abstract Oxazepam is a benzodiazepine used as an antianxiety agent with alcohol withdrawal and as an anticonvulsant for management of simple partial seizures. It is an active metabolite of several other benzodiazepines that are used therapeutically. Benzodiazepines, including oxazepam, are commonly abused among drug addicts.[1]

Specimen Serum

Container Red top tube

Sampling Time Collect specimen immediately prior to next dose unless specified otherwise.

Storage Instructions Separate serum and refrigerate.

Reference Interval 0.2-1.4 µg/mL (SI: 0.7-4.9 µmol/L)

Use Monitor therapeutic drug level; evaluate toxicity

Contraindications Hypersensitivity to benzodiazepines; CNS depression; narrow angle glaucoma

Methodology Gas-liquid chromatography (GLC), high performance liquid chromatography (HPLC)[2] with fluorescence detection[3]

Additional Information
- Half-life: ~4-12 hours
- Volume of distribution: 0.5-2.0 L/kg
- Protein binding: 95% to 98%

Oxazepam, a benzodiazepine derivative, is related to chlordiazepoxide and shares many of its qualities. It does, however, have a shorter duration of action and causes fewer adverse effects. It is rapidly eliminated by urinary excretion as a glucuronide conjugate. Oxazepam is used to manage tension and anxiety and to aid in the control of acute withdrawal symptoms in chronic alcoholism. Peak plasma levels are achieved in 2-4 hours. Adverse effects are mild and infrequent. They include drowsiness, vertigo, ataxia, headache, tremor, slurred speech, nausea, hypotension, and leuko-penia. Simultaneous alcohol ingestion potentiates some of the effects of benzodiazepines.

Footnotes

1. Garretty DJ, Wolff K, Hay AW, et al, "Benzodiazepine Misuse by Drug Addicts," *Ann Clin Biochem*, 1997, 34(Pt 1):68-73.
2. Goldnik A, Gajewska M, and Jaworska M, "Determination of Oxazepam and Diaz-epam in Body Fluids by HPLC," *Acta Pol Pharm*, 1993, 50(6):421-2.
3. Berrueta LA, Gallo B, and Vicente F, "Analysis of Oxazepam in Urine Using Solid-Phase Extraction and High Performance Liquid Chromatography With Fluorescence Detection by Postcolumn Derivatization," *J Chromatogr*, 1993, 616(2):344-8.

References

Baselt RC, *Disposition of Toxic Drugs and Chemicals in Man*, 5th ed, Foster City, CA: Chemical Toxicology Institute, 2000, 641-2.
Moshkowitz M, Pines A, Finkelstein A, et al, "Skin Blisters as a Manifestation of Oxazepam Toxicity," *J Toxicol Clin Toxicol*, 1990, 28(3):383-6.
Schmider J, Standhart H, Deuschle M, et al, "A Double-Blind Comparison of Lora-zepam and Oxazepam in Psychomotor Retardation and Mutism," *Biol Psychiatry*, 1999, 46(3):437-41.
Weinberg AD, Pals JK, Marinelli FC, et al, "Oxazepam Overdose Associated With Ethanol Ingestion: Treatment With a Benzodiazepine Antagonist," *Am J Crit Care*, 1994, 3(6):464-6.

Phenobarbital, Serum or Plasma

Related Information

Antidepressants, Cyclic, Serum *on page 737*
Antiepileptic Drugs, New, Overview *on page 738*
Barbiturates, Quantitative, Serum or Plasma *on page 739*
Benzodiazepines, Qualitative, Urine *on page 782*
Cyclosporine, Blood *on page 744*
Ethosuximide, Serum or Plasma *on page 748*
Folic Acid, RBC *on page 435*
Folic Acid, Serum *on page 435*
Methylphenobarbital, Serum *on page 757*
Mexiletine, Serum *on page 757*
Phenothiazines, Serum or Urine *on page 760*
Phenytoin, Serum or Plasma *on page 761*
Primidone, Serum or Plasma *on page 762*
Quinidine, Serum *on page 764*
Theophylline, Serum *on page 766*
Valproic Acid, Serum or Plasma *on page 768*
Verapamil, Serum or Plasma *on page 769*
Warfarin *on page 770*

Synonyms Barbita®; Comizial®; Fenilcal®; Gardenal®; Luminal®; Phenemal; Phenemalum; Phenobarb; Phenobarbitone; Phenylethylmalonylurea; Solfoton®; Stental Extentabs®

Abstract Phenobarbital is indicated for generalized tonic-clonic and partial seizures.

Specimen Serum or plasma

Container Red top tube, green top (heparin) tube, or lavender top (EDTA) tube

Sampling Time Consistent sampling time is desirable but less important than for other anticonvulsants, due to its long half-life. The time to reach steady-state is 17-24 days in adults and 8-15 days in children.

Reference Interval Infants and children: 15-30 µg/mL (SI: 65-129 µmol/L); **adults:** 20-40 µg/mL (SI: 86-172 µmol/L). See Table A in the Therapeutic Drug Monitoring Introduction *on page 733*. **Low level:** Most common cause is noncompliance. Other causes include drug interactions, including antipsychotic medication, chloramphenicol, acetazolamide, and phenytoin. Infants and children may be fast metabolizers. **High level:** addition of valproic acid to regimen inhibits phenobarbital metabolism (parahydroxylation) and should be accompanied by a cut in phenobarbital dosage. In newborns, unlike older infants, very long half-lives are found which may be associated with high levels.

Critical Values Toxic: >40 µg/mL (SI: >172 µmol/L) but if given intravenously, life-threatening side effects can occur with much lower levels, and patients should be monitored. Toxic effects are mostly neurologic. Adults present with lethargy and coma; children may present with irritability or hyperactivity. Levels >80 µg/mL (SI: >344 µmol/L) are associated with coma. **Fatal:** 50-130 µg/mL (SI: 215-559 µmol/L).

Use Monitor patients for compliance, efficacy, and possible toxicity. Mephobarbital and primidone are metabolized to phenobarbital and, therefore, patients taking these drugs will have detectable levels of phenobarbital on therapeutic monitoring. See table of anticonvulsants in Antiepileptic Drugs, New, Overview *on page 738*.

Methodology Enzyme immunoassay (EIA), fluorescence polarization immunoassay (FPIA), gas-liquid chromatography (GLC), high performance liquid chromatography (HPLC), capillary electrochemical enzyme immunoassay[1]

Additional Information

- Half-life: children: 40-70 hours; adults: 50-140 hours
- Volume of distribution: 0.5-1.0 L/kg
- Protein binding: 40% to 50%

Phenobarbital can affect the metabolism of phenytoin, ethosuximide, and increase the clearance and elimination of carbamazepine, valproic acid, clonazepam, vitamin D and K, cimetidine, dicumarol, chloramphenicol, theophylline, oral anticoagulants (warfarin), cyclosporine, and oral contraceptives; where appropriate, the use of these drugs in patients on phenobarbital should be monitored clinically and through the laboratory.

Phenobarbital may decrease the serum concentration or effect of phenylbutazone, griseofulvin, doxycycline, beta-blockers, theophylline, corticosteroids, tricyclic antidepressants, quinidine, haloperidol, and phenothiazines, valproic acid, methylphenidate, chloramphenicol, propoxyphene. Furosemide may inhibit the metabolism of phenobarbital with resultant increase in phenobarbital serum concentration. Valproic acid and salicylates may also increase phenobarbital concentration. Phenobarbital and benzodiazepines or other CNS depressants may cause an increase of CNS and respiratory depression (especially with I.V. loading doses of phenobarbital). Pyridoxine may reduce serum phenobarbital levels.

Drugs that antagonize folic acid include antiepileptic drugs (AEDs): carbamazepine, phenytoin, phenobarbital, primidone, and non-AEDs: trimethoprim and triamterene. These drugs may increase the baseline rate of neural tube defects in mothers when used in the first month of pregnancy, before the neural tube closes. Use of these drugs during the second or third month following the last menstrual period can increase the relative risk of cardiovascular defects, oral clefts, and urinary tract defects. The use of folic acid supplements from the time of conception can reduce the incidence of such birth defects. Consequently, all women of childbearing age prescribed the above medicines should also take supplemental folic acid.[2]

Phenobarbital may increase alkaline phosphatase, ammonia, and gamma-glutamyl transferase and may decrease bilirubin and calcium in test samples. The most common side effects are nystagmus, ataxia, rash, and hypoprothrombinemia. Overdose causes nervous system and cardiovascular depression.

Footnotes

1. Zhang J, Heineman WR, and Halsall HB, "Capillary Electrochemical Enzyme Immunoassay (CEEI) for Phenobarbital in Serum," *J Pharm Biomed Anal*, 1999, 19(1-2):145-52.
2. Hernández-Diaz S, Werler MM, Walker AM, et al, "Folic Acid Antagonists During Pregnancy and the Risk of Birth Defects," *N Engl J Med*, 2000, 343(22):1608-14.

References

Ammann H and Vinet B, "Accuracy, Precision, and Interferences of Three Modified EMIT Procedures for Determining Serum Phenobarbital, Urine Morphine, and Urine Cocaine Metabolite With A Cobas-Fara," *Clin Chem*, 1991, 37(12):2139-41.
Brodie MJ and Dichter MA, "Antiepileptic Drugs," *N Engl J Med*, 1996, 334(3):168-75.
Lerman-Sagie T and Lerman P, "Phenobarbital Still Has a Role in Epilepsy Treatment," *J Child Neurol*, 1999, 14(12):820-1.
Painter MJ, Minnigh MB, Gaus L, et al, "Neonatal Phenobarbital and Phenytoin Binding Profiles," *J Clin Pharmacol*, 1994, 34(4):312-7.
Painter MJ, Scher MS, Stein AD, et al, "Phenobarbital Compared With Phenytoin for the Treatment of Neonatal Seizures," *N Engl J Med*, 1999, 341(7):485-9.
Winter M, "Phenobarbital," *Basic Clinical Pharmacokinetics*, 3rd ed, Koda-Kimble MA and Young L, eds, Vancouver, WA: Applied Therapeutics, Inc, 1994.

♦ **Phenobarbitone** *see* Phenobarbital, Serum or Plasma *on page 760*

♦ **Phenothiazines** *see* Chlorpromazine, Serum *on page 743*

Phenothiazines, Serum or Urine

Related Information

Antidepressants, Cyclic, Serum *on page 737*
Chlorpromazine, Serum *on page 743*
Fluphenazine, Serum *on page 750*
Phenobarbital, Serum or Plasma *on page 760*

Applies to Chlorpromazine; Compazine®; Etrafon®; Mellaril®; Mesoridazine; Ormazine®; Prochlorperazine; Prolixin®; Serentil®; Stelazine®; Thioridazine; Thorazine®; Trifluoperazine

Abstract The drugs in this class are used as antipsychotic agents and tranquilizers. These are tricyclic compounds with some properties in common with tricyclic antidepressants. In addition, they are used to control nausea or vomiting. Some phenothiazines are potent analgesics (eg, methotrimeprazine). Recently, some phenothiazines have been proposed for use against multidrug-resistant tuberculosis.[1]

Specimen Serum or urine

Container Red top tube, urine container

Sampling Time Obtain serum at least 3 hours after last dose.

Special Instructions In overdose situations, phenothiazines can also be measured in urine and gastric contents. Qualitative detection of drug or metabolites is usually sufficient.

Reference Interval Therapeutic: chlorpromazine: 50-300 ng/mL (SI: 157-942 nmol/L), thioridazine: 1.0-1.5 µg/mL (SI: 2.7-4.1 µmol/L), fluphenazine: 2-4 ng/mL; therapeutic response and blood levels have not been established for trifluoperazine.

Possible Panic Range Toxic: chlorpromazine: >750 ng/mL (SI: >2350 nmol/L), thioridazine: >10 ng/mL (SI: >27 nmol/L), trifluoperazine: >50 ng/mL (SI: >104 nmol/L), fluphenazine: >20 ng/mL

Use Evaluate possibility of phenothiazine toxicity

Limitations Suboptimal assay accuracy and number of drug metabolites make clinical application infrequent. **These drugs are not usually monitored, because poor correlation exists between serum level and pharmacologic effect.**

Methodology Thin-layer chromatography (TLC), gas-liquid chromatography (GLC), radioimmunoassay (RIA), high performance liquid chromatography (HPLC), spectrophotometry. The ferric, perchloric, nitric (FPN) spot test is frequently used for phenothiazine screening.[2]

Additional Information

- Half-life: 20-50 hours
- Volume of distribution: 15-25 L/kg
- Protein binding: 70% to 90%

Phenothiazines are tranquilizers frequently used in the treatment of psychoses. They may act by antagonizing postsynaptic dopamine receptors. There are three different classes of phenothiazines: aliphatic (chlorpromazine), piperidine (thioridazine), and piperazine (fluphenazine). All are effective in therapy in appropriate doses, but differ in frequency, type, and severity of side effects. Phenothiazine toxicity principally involves the central nervous and cardiovascular systems. Side effects include drowsiness, ataxia, respiratory depression, hypotension, tachycardia, cardiac arrest, bone marrow depression. There is also a "dysphoric" response by some patients. Phenothiazines have anticholinergic symptoms similar to those of the tricyclic antidepressants. Toxicity is increased by coingestion of opioids, tricyclic antidepressants, barbiturates, benzodiazepines, and alcohol. Sudden infant death syndrome has been associated with phenothiazine toxicity.[3,4]

The piperazine prochlorperazine (Compazine®) is widely used as an antiemetic.

Chlorpromazine and thioridazine cause false positives for phenylketonuria, uroporphyrins, and urobilinogen. Phenothiazines cause increase in serum glucose (physiologic).

Footnotes

1. Gerin M, Patrice S, Begin D, et al, "A Study of Ethylene GI Conventional Therapy for the Initial Management of Suspected Multidrug Resistant Tuberculosis. A Call for Studies," *Int J Antimicrob Agents*, 2000, 14(3):173-6.
2. Porter WH, "Clinical Toxicology," *Tietz Textbook of Clinical Chemistry*, 3rd ed, Chapter 27, Burtis CA and Ashwood ER, eds, Philadelphia, PA: WB Saunders Co, 1999, 906-81.
3. Pollard AJ and Rylance G, "Inappropriate Prescribing of Promethazine in Infants," *Arch Dis Child*, 1994, 70(4):357.
4. Dyer KS and Woolf AD, "Use of Phenothiazines as Sedatives in Children: What Are the Risks?" *Drug Saf*, 1999, 21(2):81-90.

References

Adamczyk M, Fishpaugh JR, Harrington CA, et al, "Immunoassay Reagents for Psychoactive Drugs. Part 3. Removal of Phenothiazine Interferences in the Quantification of Tricyclic Antidepressants," *Ther Drug Monit*, 1993, 15:(5)436-9.

Eshel G, Usher M, Barr J, et al, "Phenothiazine Treatment and Respiratory Distress Syndrome in a Child," *J Toxicol Clin Toxicol*, 1994, 32(2):191-7.

Gex-Fabry M, Balant-Gorgia AE, Balant LP, et al, "Therapeutic Drug Monitoring Databases for Postmarketing Surveillance of Drug-Drug Interactions: Evaluation of a Paired Approach for Psychotropic Medication," *Ther Drug Monit*, 1997, 19(1):1-10.

Jones GR, "Successful Cancer Therapy With Promethazine: The Rationale," *Med Hypotheses*, 1996, 46(1):25-9.

Krishel S and Jackimczyk K, "Cyclic Antidepressants, Lithium, and Neuroleptic Agents. Pharmacology and Toxicology," *Emerg Med Clin North Am*, 1991, 9(1):53-86.

Levinson DF, Simpson GM, Singh H, et al, "Fluphenazine Dose, Clinical Response, and Extrapyramidal Symptoms During Acute Treatment," *Arch Gen Psychiatry*, 1990, 47(8):761-8.

Marder SR, Midha KK, Van Putten T, et al, "Plasma Levels of Fluphenazine in Patients Receiving Fluphenazine Decanoate. Relationship to Clinical Response," *Br J Psychiatry*, 1991, 158:658-65.

Midha KK, Hubbard JW, Marder SR, et al, "Impact of Clinical Pharmacokinetics on Neuroleptic Therapy in Patients With Schizophrenia," *J Psychiatry Neurosci*, 1994, 19(4):254-64.

Midha KK, Marder SR, Jaworski TJ, et al, "Clinical Perspectives of Some Neuroleptics Through Development and Application of Their Assays," *Ther Drug Monit*, 1993, 15(3):179-89.

Motohashi N, Kurihara T, Satoh K, et al, "Antitumor Activity of Benzo(a)phenothiazines," *Anticancer Res*, 1999, 19(3A):1837-42.

Ryan PM, "Epidemiology, Etiology, Diagnosis, and Treatment of Schizophrenia," *Am J Hosp Pharm*, 1991, 48(6):1271-80.

♦ **5-Phenyl-5-Ethylhydantoin (Nirvanol®)** *see* Mephenytoin, Serum *on page 756*

♦ **Phenylethylmalonamide** *see* Primidone, Serum or Plasma *on page 762*

♦ **Phenylethylmalonylurea** *see* Phenobarbital, Serum or Plasma *on page 760*

Phenytoin, Free, Serum or Plasma

Related Information

Phenytoin, Serum or Plasma *on page 761*

Synonyms Free Dilantin®; Free Phenytoin

Abstract Measurement of free phenytoin may be clinically important in situations associated with altered binding of phenytoin or decrease in albumin.

Specimen Serum or plasma

Container Red top tube or lavender top (EDTA) tube

Reference Interval 1-2 µg/mL (SI: 4-8 µmol/L)

Critical Values >5 µg/mL

Possible Panic Range Toxicity may be progressive >2 µg/mL.

Limitations Free drug levels are not useful when total phenytoin level is <3 µg/mL. Even in severe hepatorenal syndrome, free fraction is seldom >50%.

Additional Information

- Half-life (adults): 20-40 hours
- Volume of distribution: 0.6-0.7 L/kg
- Protein binding: 85% to 95% (significant interindividual variation exists)

Phenytoin is 90% bound to serum proteins, but only the free fraction circulates through plasma membranes and is biologically active. Because of rapid equilibration between free and bound portions of drugs, free levels are potentially important only in antiepileptic drugs (AEDs) that are highly bound (ie, phenytoin but not carbamazepine). Measurement of the free fraction is not cost-effective on a routine outpatient basis, but may be clinically relevant in exceptional circumstances associated with alterations in the binding of phenytoin. There is significant interindividual variation in free phenytoin. In one study, the free phenytoin fraction ranged from 7% to 35%.[1] Binding kinetics may be altered in uremia, hepatic disease, late pregnancy or postpartum, cases of head injury associated with a hypermetabolic state, and certain instances of polypharmacy, described below.[2,3] Free phenytoin concentration is increased in patients with HIV.[4] Determination of free levels may also be helpful in overdosages, since only the free portion can be cleared by dialysis.

Most phenytoin is excreted into bile as inactive metabolites which are then reabsorbed by the intestines and excreted into the urine. In renal disease, total phenytoin levels may generate falsely low values, leading to inaccurate dosing. Dialysis may increase the amount of free phenytoin available.[5] In hepatic disease, phenytoin competes with endogenous bilirubin for binding sites, and thus the need for a free level may be greatest if the total bilirubin level is high and albumin low. Available liver function tests are not predictive of free phenytoin levels in patients with liver disease.[3]

Drugs which compete for binding sites on albumin and which may displace phenytoin include valproic acid, acetazolamide, high doses of salicylic acid, phenylbutazone, ceftriaxone, nafcillin, and sulfamethoxazole.[6] In a clinical setting in which one of these drugs is used with phenytoin and toxicity is suspected despite normal phenytoin levels, a free level may be useful.

The free phenytoin level can be approximated by the total phenytoin level in cerebrospinal fluid or saliva or other body fluids that are albumin-poor.[7]

Footnotes

1. Burt M, Anderson DC, Kloss J, et al, "Evidence-Based Implementation of Phenytoin Therapeutic Drug Monitoring," *Clin Chem*, 2000, 46(8 Pt 1):1132-5.
2. Griebel ML, Kearns GL, Fiser DH, et al, "Phenytoin Protein Binding in Pediatric Patients With Acute Traumatic Injury," *Crit Care Med*, 1990, 18(4):385-91.
3. Dasgupta A, Dennen DA, Dean R, et al, "Prediction of Free Phenytoin Levels Based on Total Phenytoin/Albumin Ratios," *Am J Clin Pathol*, 1991, 95(2):253-6.
4. Dasgupta A and McLemore JL, "Elevated Free Phenytoin and Free Valproic Acid Concentrations in Serum of Patients Infected With Human Immunodeficiency Virus," *Ther Drug Monit*, 1998, 20(1):63-7.
5. Dasgupta A and Abu-Alfa A, "Increased Free Phenytoin Concentrations in Predialysis Serum Compared to Postdialysis Serum in Patients With Uremia Treated With Hemodialysis: Role of Uremic Compounds," *Am J Clin Pathol*, 1992, 98(1):19-25.
6. Dasgupta A, Dennen DA, Dean R, et al, "Displacement of Phenytoin From Serum Protein Carriers by Antibiotics: Studies With Ceftriaxone, Nafcillin, and Sulfamethoxazole," *Clin Chem*, 1991, 37(1):98-100.
7. Liu H and Delgado MR, "Therapeutic Drug Concentration Monitoring Using Saliva Samples. Focus on Anticonvulsants," *Clin Pharmacokinet*, 1999, 36(6):453-70.

References

Jarzabek JI and Kampa IS, "Adaptation of Total Phenytoin Reagent Pack for Measuring Free Phenytoin Levels With the Abbott AxSYM Immunoassay Analyzer," *Ther Drug Monit*, 1999, 21(1):134-6.

Lenn N and Robertson M, "Clinical Utility of Unbound Antiepileptic Drug Blood Levels in the Management of Epilepsy," *Neurology*, 1992, 42(5):988-90.

May TW, Rambeck B, Jurges U, et al, "Comparison of Total and Free Phenytoin Serum Concentrations Measured by High-Performance Liquid Chromatography and Standard TDx Assay: Implications for the Prediction of Free Phenytoin Serum Concentrations," *Ther Drug Monit*, 1998, 20(6):619-23.

Tomson T, Lindbom U, and Ekqvist B, "Epilepsy and Pregnancy: A Prospective Study of Seizure Control in Relation to Free and Total Plasma Concentrations of Carbamazepine and Phenytoin," *Epilepsia*, 1994, 35(1):122-30.

Zarghi A, Gholami K, and Hessami M, "Determination of Phenytoin in Human Plasma by Gas Chromatography," *Boll Chim Farm*, 1999, 138(10):508-10.

Phenytoin, Serum or Plasma

Related Information

Amiodarone, Serum *on page 735*
Amoxapine, Serum or Plasma *on page 736*
Antidepressants, Cyclic, Serum *on page 737*
Carbamazepine, Serum *on page 741*
Cyclosporine, Blood *on page 744*
Disopyramide, Serum or Plasma *on page 747*
Ethosuximide, Serum or Plasma *on page 748*
Imipramine, Serum or Plasma *on page 752*
Mephenytoin, Serum *on page 756*
Mexiletine, Serum *on page 757*
Nortriptyline, Serum *on page 758*
Phenobarbital, Serum or Plasma *on page 760*
Phenytoin, Free, Serum or Plasma *on page 761*
Primidone, Serum or Plasma *on page 762*
Quinidine, Serum *on page 764*
Theophylline, Serum *on page 766*
Valproic Acid, Serum or Plasma *on page 768*

Synonyms Antisacer®; Dilantin®; Dintoina®; Diphenylan Sodium®; Diphenylhydantoin; Ditan®; Epanutin®; Epinat®; Fenitoina; Fenytoin®; Fosphenytoin

Applies to Carbamazepine; Phenobarbital; Primidone

Abstract Phenytoin is effective for generalized tonic-clonic and partial seizures and status epilepticus. Valproic acid, carbamazepine, and phenytoin are effective for tonic-clonic seizures. The drugs of choice for partial seizures are carbamazepine and phenytoin.[1] Serum levels should be monitored for assessing compliance, toxicity, and efficacy. Recently, a new phosphate ester prodrug of phenytoin, called **fosphenytoin** (Cerebyx®) was introduced as a therapeutic form of phenytoin. It has increased aqueous solubility for intramuscular injection and less cardiovascular toxicity than phenytoin if given intravenously.[2,3] Fosphenytoin may be preferred for the treatment of status epilepticus.

Specimen Serum or plasma

Container Red top tube or lavender top (EDTA) tube

Sampling Time In monitoring patients maintained on chronic therapy, a trough level or consistent sampling time should be used.
(Continued)

Phenytoin, Serum or Plasma *(Continued)*

Special Instructions Designate the drug in use in a particular patient: fosphenytoin concentrations cannot be accurately assayed by immunoassays for phenytoin.[4]

Reference Interval Although 10-20 µg/mL (SI: 40-79 µmol/L) is commonly utilized, toxicity is measured clinically and some patients require levels outside the suggested therapeutic range. Free phenytoin: 1-2 µg/mL (SI: 4-8 µmol/L).

Patients treated for status epilepticus should have levels at or slightly above the upper limit of range as defined above. **Low level:** The most common cause of a low level is noncompliance. Absorption problems are most important in young infants (younger than 3 months) or occasionally in patients given phenobarbital, charcoal, or antacids at the same time as the phenytoin. Pediatric and some adult patients (fast metabolizers), who have breakthrough seizures at the end of the day, require more than once-daily dosing. Patients on corticosteroids may require more than once-a-day dosing. Patients with feeding tubes may have difficulty attaining and maintaining therapeutic levels. Some formulations other than Kapseals® may require more than once-daily dosing, and changing formulations can cause changes in levels. Pregnancy or intercurrent illness such as mononucleosis can cause subtherapeutic levels with seizures.

The addition of carbamazepine to a patient taking phenytoin can lower or raise phenytoin levels but usually does not cause seizures. Disulfiram administration can increase phenytoin metabolism, lower levels, and may cause seizures. Patients can have lower than expected values if intravenous formulations are given with fluids containing glucose, which precipitates in solution with phenytoin. **High levels:** In patients chronically controlled on phenytoin who become clinically toxic without a change in dose, toxicity can be brought on by a change in formulation, drug interaction, or intercurrent infection. Drugs which can precipitate phenytoin toxicity include chloramphenicol, tricyclic antidepressants, fluconazole, levodopa, and others (see Additional Information). Small dose changes or changes in formulation (including change from one brand to another or to a generic) can cause large changes in antiepileptic drug (AED) levels and toxicity, because phenytoin manifests zero-order kinetics.

Possible Panic Range Toxic: 25-50 µg/mL (SI: 100-200 µmol/L); lethal: >100 µg/mL (SI: >400 µmol/L). Toxicity may manifest progressively outside reference range (or occasionally within it) with ataxia, dizziness, nystagmus, diplopia, and paradoxical seizures. Patients can have life-threatening complications with intravenous administration with normal levels including arrhythmias and hypotension; such patients should be placed on a cardiac monitor during intravenous administration of drug, which is administered at a rate of 25-50 mg/minute or less. Use of intravenous fosphenytoin does not require cardiac monitoring and may be given more rapidly.

Use Monitor for compliance, efficacy, and possible toxicity. Phenytoin and phenobarbital are equally, but incompletely effective, as neonatal anticonvulsants. Seizures are controlled in <50% with either drug used alone.[5]

Limitations See Phenytoin, Free, Serum or Plasma *on page 761*. A systemic allergic reaction characterized by fever, rash, lymphadenopathy, and eosinophilia may include granulomatous features. Necrosis of hepatocytes and cholestasis may occur, a drug-induced hypersensitivity hepatitis. A syndrome including infectious mononucleosis-like features is recognized.[6,7]

Methodology Routine: Enzyme multiplied immunoassay technique (EMIT), enzyme-linked immunosorbent assay (ELISA), and fluorescence polarization immunoassay (FPIA). A nonlinear relationship between fosphenytoin level and observed cross-reactivity prevents estimation of fosphenytoin concentrations by immunoassays intended for phenytoin. Fosphenytoin can be rapidly converted to phenytoin *in vitro* by alkaline phosphatase.[4]

Additional Information

- Half-life: adults: 20-40 hours, children: ~10 hours
- Volume of distribution: 0.6-0.7 L/kg
- Protein binding: 85% to 95%

Ninety percent of phenytoin is bound to serum proteins. Only the unbound fraction is biologically active. Primary site of action is thought to be the motor cortex, where the promotion of a sodium "efflux" from neurons probably stabilizes the threshold of the neuron against hyperexcitability. Most of a dose of phenytoin is excreted into the bile as inactive metabolites which are then reabsorbed from the intestines and excreted into the urine. Despite normal levels, phenytoin may interfere with the actions of other drugs, including cyclosporine, oral anticoagulants, oral contraceptives, and theophylline; appropriate laboratory monitoring of some of these agents is advised.

The incidence of serious fetal malformations is slightly increased in children of epileptic mothers. The risk increases with the number of antiepileptic drugs, >20% with four drugs.[1] The risks in women of childbearing age should be balanced against the risks of increased seizures.

Phenytoin, phenobarbital, primidone, and carbamazepine, enzyme-inducing antiepileptic drugs, can cause transient deficiency of vitamin K-dependent clotting factors in the neonate. Expectant mothers on these drugs should be given vitamin K in the last several weeks of gestation, and to babies given vitamin K immediately after birth, to avoid neonatal central nervous system hemorrhage.[1]

Women of childbearing age prescribed this medication should take supplemental folic acid.[8] See Phenobarbital, Serum or Plasma *on page 760* for more information.

Phenytoin may decrease the serum concentration or effectiveness of other drugs including valproic acid, carbamazepine, ethosuximide, primidone, corticosteroids, chloramphenicol, rifampin, doxycycline, quinidine, mexiletine, disopyramide, dopamine, or nondepolarizing skeletal muscle relaxants. Protein binding of phenytoin can be affected by valproic acid or salicylates. Serum phenytoin concentrations may be increased by cimetidine, disulfiram, trazodone, ethanol, halothane, phenylbutazone, azapropazone, ibuprofen, amiodarone, imipramine, miconazole, metronidazole, nifedipine, chloramphenicol, INH, trimethoprim, or sulfonamides and decreased by rifampin, cisplatin, vinblastine, bleomycin, folic acid, continuous NG feeds, oxacillin, or nitrofurantoin.

Footnotes

1. Brodie MJ and Dichter MA, "Drug Therapy: Antiepileptic Drugs," *N Engl J Med*, 1996, 334(3):168-75.
2. Armstrong EP, Sauer KA, and Downey MJ, "Phenytoin and Fosphenytoin: A Model of Cost and Clinical Outcomes," *Pharmacotherapy*, 1999, 19(7):844-53.
3. Roberts WL, De BK, Coleman JP, et al, "Falsely Increased Immunoassay Measurements of Total and Unbound Phenytoin in Critically Ill Uremic Patients Receiving Fosphenytoin," *Clin Chem*, 1999, 45(6 Pt 1):829-37.
4. Dasgupta A, Warner BF, and Datta P, "Use of Alkaline Phosphatase to Correct the Underestimation of Fosphenytoin Concentration in Serum Measured by Phenytoin Immunoassays," *Am J Clin Pathol*, 1999, 111(4):557-62.
5. Painter MJ, Scher MS, Stein AD, et al, "Phenobarbital Compared With Phenytoin for the Treatment of Neonatal Seizures," *N Engl J Med*, 1999, 341(7):485-9.
6. Lee WM, "Drug-Induced Hepatotoxicity," *N Engl J Med*, 1995, 333(17):1118-27.
7. Collins RD, Casey TT, Glick AD, et al, "Lymph Nodes," *Diagnostic Surgical Pathology*, 2nd ed, Chapter 17, Sternberg SS, ed, New York, NY: Raven Press, 1994, 673-734.
8. Hernández-Diaz S, Werler MM, Walker AM, et al, "Folic Acid Antagonists During Pregnancy and the Risk of Birth Defects," *N Engl J Med*, 2000, 343(22):1608-14.

References

Bachmann KA and Belloto RJ Jr, "Differential Kinetics of Phenytoin in Elderly Patients," *Drugs Aging*, 1999, 15(3):235-50.
Dasgupta A, Handy BC, and Datta P, "Mathematical Models to Calculate Fosphenytoin Concentrations in the Presence of Phenytoin Using Phenytoin Immunoassays and Alkaline Phosphatase," *Am J Clin Pathol*, 2000, 113(1):87-92.
Lindow J and Wijdicks EF, "Phenytoin Toxicity Associated With Hypoalbuminemia in Critically Ill Patients," *Chest*, 1994, 105(2):602-4.
Phelps SJ, Baldree LA, and Boucher BA, "Neuropsychiatric Toxicity of Phenytoin: Importance of Monitoring Phenytoin Levels," *Clin Pediatr (Phila)*, 1993, 32(2):107-10.
Walton NY, Uthman BM, El Yafi K, et al, "Phenytoin Penetration Into Brain After Administration of Phenytoin or Fosphenytoin," *Epilepsia*, 1999, 40(2):153-6.

♦ **Phyllocontin®** *see* Theophylline, Serum *on page 766*

♦ **Pick-me-up®** *see* Caffeine, Serum *on page 740*

♦ **Placidyl®** *see* Ethchlorvynol, Serum or Plasma *on page 748*

♦ **Presamine®** *see* Antidepressants, Cyclic, Serum *on page 737*

♦ **Presamine®** *see* Imipramine, Serum or Plasma *on page 752*

♦ **Primaclone** *see* Primidone, Serum or Plasma *on page 762*

♦ **Primidone** *see* Phenytoin, Serum or Plasma *on page 761*

Primidone, Serum or Plasma

Related Information

Antiepileptic Drugs, New, Overview *on page 738*
Carbamazepine, Serum *on page 741*
Folic Acid, RBC *on page 435*
Folic Acid, Serum *on page 435*
Phenobarbital, Serum or Plasma *on page 760*
Phenytoin, Serum or Plasma *on page 761*
Urinalysis *on page 887*
Valproic Acid, Serum or Plasma *on page 768*

Synonyms Desoxyphenobarbital; Hexamidinum; Majsolin®; Mylepsin®; Mysoline®; Primaclone; Prysolin®

Applies to Metabolites of Primidone; PEMA; Phenobarbital:Primidone Ratio; Phenylethylmalonamide

Test Includes Phenobarbital, PEMA

Abstract Primidone is indicated for generalized tonic-clonic and partial seizures. Concurrent monitoring of its major active metabolite, phenobarbital, is necessary. A second metabolite, phenylethylmalonamide, also exerts activity.

Specimen Serum or plasma

Container Red top tube, green top (heparin) tube, or lavender top (EDTA) tube

Sampling Time Trough sampling is preferable. Consistent sampling time is desirable. Levels of phenobarbital and PEMA can be measured simultaneously.

Reference Interval Children younger than 5 years of age: 7-10 µg/mL (SI: 32-46 µmol/L); adults: 5-12 µg/mL (SI: 23-55 µmol/L). Phenobarbital concentration should also be used to guide dosing. Phenobarbital, serum: 15-40 µg/mL.

Critical Values At levels >12 µg/mL (SI: >55 µmol/L) primidone produces CNS depression, vertigo, visual disturbances, areflexia, somnolence, and lethargy. Clinical toxicity correlates with primidone rather than metabolite concentrations. In overdosage, a biphasic peak may be seen with highest toxicity a few hours after ingestion and again 48 hours afterwards. Crystalluria is a feature of overdosage.

Possible Panic Range >15 µg/mL (SI: >69 µmol/L). See Table A in the Therapeutic Drug Monitoring Introduction *on page 733.*

Use Monitor efficacy, compliance, and possible toxicity

A table comparing antiepileptic drugs is included in Antiepileptic Drugs, New, Overview *on page 738.*

Methodology Enzyme immunoassay (EIA), fluorescent immunoassay, gas-liquid chromatography (GLC), high performance liquid chromatography (HPLC)

Additional Information
- Half-life: adults: 4-12 hours; children: 4-6 hours
- Volume of distribution: 0.5-1.0 L/kg
- Protein binding: 20%

Since phenobarbital requires a longer interval (48 hours) to achieve therapeutic blood levels, checking its levels can be used to determine chronic compliance. The phenobarbital:primidone ratio normally is 2.5, can be higher (4.3 mean) in patients on other anticonvulsants (phenytoin, carbamazepine) and lower than normal among patients discontinued from those medicines or who are chronically noncompliant. Primidone decreases the effects of oral anticoagulants. Primidone may increase alkaline phosphatase and decrease calcium.

Both primidone and phenobarbital undergo renal biotransformation and excretion. Patients with renal impairment have higher levels and need lower dosage.

All women of childbearing age prescribed this medication should also take supplemental folic acid.[1] See Phenobarbital, Serum or Plasma *on page 760* for more information.

Primidone has been used for the treatment of refractory bipolar disorders. In one study, 50% of the patients responded to the drug.[2]

Footnotes
1. Hernández-Díaz S, Werler MM, Walker AM, et al, "Folic Acid Antagonists During Pregnancy and the Risk of Birth Defects," *N Engl J Med*, 2000, 343(22):1608-14.
2. Shafer LC, Schaffer CB, and Caretto J, "The Use of Primidone in the Treatment of Refractory Bipolar Disorder," *Ann Clin Psychiatry*, 1999, 11(2):61-6.

References
Brodie MJ and Dichter MA, "Antiepileptic Drugs," *N Engl J Med*, 1996, 334(3):168-75.
El-Masri HA and Portier CJ, "Physiologically Based Pharmacokinetics Model of Primidone and its Metabolites Phenobarbital and Phenylethylmalonamide in Humans, Rats, and Mice," *Drug Metab Dispos*, 1998, 26(6):585-94 (published erratum *Drug Metab Dispos*, 1998, 26(12):1222).
Meyer MC, Straughn AB, Mhatre RM, Et al, "Lack of *In Vivo/In Vitro* Correlations for 50 mg and 250 mg Primidone Tablets," *Pharm Res*, 1998, 15(7):1085-9.

Procainamide, Serum

Related Information
Amiodarone, Serum *on page 735*
Antinuclear Antibody *on page 507*
Nortriptyline, Serum *on page 758*
Quinidine, Serum *on page 764*

Synonyms Biocoryl®; Novocainamidum; Novocamid®; Procaine Amide Hydrochloride; Procanbid®; Procan® SR; Pronestyl®; Pronestyl-SR®; Retard®; Rhythmin®

Applies to N-Acetyl Procainamide; NAPA

Test Includes Procainamide and its metabolite, N-acetyl procainamide (NAPA)

Abstract This drug is class 1A antiarrhythmic with an active metabolite, N-acetyl procainamide (NAPA). Both should be measured for therapeutic drug monitoring.

Specimen Serum

Container Red top tube

Sampling Time Oral treatment: peak: 75 minutes after dose; trough: immediately before next dose. I.V. treatment: immediately after loading dose; 2, 6, 12, and 24 hours after starting I.V. maintenance.

Special Instructions One sample is an inadequate basis for evaluating dosing. Three steady-state levels should be obtained during one dosing interval. For therapeutic drug monitoring, consistently use the same time interval between sampling and dose administration when comparing results from serial samples.

Reference Interval Therapeutic: procainamide: 4.0-10.0 µg/mL (SI: 17-42 µmol/L), NAPA: 10-30 µg/mL, sum of procainamide and N-acetyl procainamide: <30 µg/mL (SI: <127 µmol/L). Optimal ranges must be ascertained for individual patients with ECG monitoring.

Possible Panic Range Toxic: procainamide: >12 µg/mL (SI: >59.5 µmol/L); sum of procainamide and N-acetyl procainamide: >30 µg/mL (SI: >127 µmol/L). See Table C in the Therapeutic Drug Monitoring Introduction *on page 733.*

Use Monitor therapeutic drug level. Procainamide may be used in instances instead of quinidine. The reverse is also true.

Limitations Severely hemolyzed, lipemic, or icteric specimens interfere with methods other than HPLC and GC.[1] **Evaluation of toxicity must be made with consideration of patient's clinical status.**

Long-term administration leads to the development of a positive antinuclear antibody test in 50% of patients. A lupus erythematosus-like syndrome may evolve in 20% to 30% of patients. If a positive antinuclear antibody titer develops, the benefits versus risks of continued procainamide therapy should be assessed.

Methodology Enzyme immunoassay (EIA), fluorescence polarization immunoassay (FPIA), enzyme-multiplied immunoassay (EMIT), high performance liquid chromatography (HPLC), gas chromatography (GC)

Additional Information
- Half-life: procainamide: 2-6 hours, NAPA: 8 hours
- Volume of distribution: 2-4 L/kg
- Protein binding: 10% to 20%
- Bioavailability: close to 100% in 85% of patients

The cardiac actions of this drug are similar to those of quinidine. It is used in a variety of arrhythmias. Procainamide usually is rapidly absorbed from the gastrointestinal tract. Peak blood levels are reached within 1 hour. Optimal plasma sampling time after oral dosage is 1-2 hours. Optimal sampling time after I.V. administration of dose is 30 minutes. The drug is converted by the liver to its active metabolite, NAPA. Rate of metabolism is genetically determined (slow and fast acetylator types) contributing to significant inter-individual variability. Fast metabolizers have a NAPA concentration equal to or greater than procainamide 3 hours after dosing. Impairment of renal function has pronounced effect on drug disposition, especially for NAPA. Patients with severe renal dysfunction generally have prolonged and highly variable half-life characteristics. Elimination half-life may be prolonged in geriatric subjects and patients with congestive heart failure.[2] Blood dyscrasias occurs at a rate of ~0.5%. Several cases of psychosis have been reported.[3]

Footnotes
1. Sherwin JE, "Procainamide and N-Acetylprocainamide," *Clinical Chemistry Theory, Analysis, and Correlation*, 3rd ed, Kaplan LA and Pesce AJ, eds, St Louis, MO: CV Mosby Co, 1996, 610-11.
2. Montamat SC, Cusack BJ, and Vestal RE, "Management of Drug Therapy in the Elderly," *N Engl J Med*, 1989, 321(5):303-9.
3. Bizjak ED, Nolan PE Jr, Brody EA, et al, "Procainamide-Induced Psychosis: A Case Report and Review of the Literature," *Ann Pharmacother*, 1999, 33(9):948-51.

References
Gold MR, O'Gara PT, Buckley MJ, et al, "Efficacy and Safety of Procainamide in Preventing Arrhythmias After Coronary Artery Bypass Surgery," *Am J Cardiol*, 1996, 78(9):975-9.
Grimm W, Cho JG, and Marchlinski FE, "Effects of Incremental Doses of Procainamide in Patients With Sustained Uniform Ventricular Tachycardia," *J Cardiovasc Electrophysiol*, 1994, 5(4):313-22.
Interian A Jr, Zaman L, Velez-Robinson E, et al, "Paired Comparisons of Efficacy of Intravenous and Oral Procainamide in Patients With Inducible Sustained Ventricular Tachyarrhythmias," *J Am Coll Cardiol*, 1991, 17(7):1581-6.
Jacobs LO, Andrews TC, Pederson DN, et al, "Effect of Intravenous Procainamide on Direct-Current Cardioversion of Atrial Fibrillation," *Am J Cardiol*, 1998, 82(2):241-2.
McLaughlin K, Gholoum B, Guiraudon C, et al, "Rapid Development of Drug-induced Lupus Nephritis in the Absence of Extrarenal Disease in a Patient Receiving Procainamide," *Am J Kidney Dis*, 1998, 32(4):698-702.
Valdes R Jr, Jortani SA, Gheorghiade M, et al, "Standards of Laboratory Practice: Cardiac Drug Monitoring. National Academy of Clinical Biochemistry," *Clin Chem*, 1998, 44(5):1096-109.
Yamaji A, Kataoka K, Oishi M, et al, "Simultaneous Determination of Procainamide and N-Acetylprocainamide in Serum by Gas Chromatography With Nitrogen-Selective Detection," *J Chromatogr*, 1987, 415(1):143-7.

- **Procaine Amide Hydrochloride** *see* Procainamide, Serum *on page 763*
- **Procanbid®** *see* Procainamide, Serum *on page 763*
- **Procan® SR** *see* Procainamide, Serum *on page 763*
- **Prochlorperazine** *see* Phenothiazines, Serum or Urine *on page 760*
- **Prograf®** *see* Tacrolimus, Whole Blood *on page 765*
- **Prolixin®** *see* Fluphenazine, Serum *on page 750*
- **Prolixin®** *see* Phenothiazines, Serum or Urine *on page 760*
- **Pronestyl®** *see* Procainamide, Serum *on page 763*
- **Pronestyl-SR®** *see* Procainamide, Serum *on page 763*
- **Pro-Plus®** *see* Caffeine, Serum *on page 740*

Propranolol, Serum

Related Information
Flecainide, Serum or Plasma *on page 749*

Synonyms Angilol®; Apsolol®; Beaden®; Bedranol®; Berkolol®; Deralin®; Inderal®

Abstract Propranolol is a relatively short-acting beta-blocker. It is used in the management of angina pectoris, arrhythmias, and hypertension. It is also used in the treatment of pheochromocytoma, essential tremor, migraine headache, and thyrotoxic periodic paralysis. African-Americans are more sensitive to propranolol that Caucasians.[1]
(Continued)

Propranolol, Serum *(Continued)*

Specimen Serum

Container Red top tube

Sampling Time Trough: immediately prior to next dose

Reference Interval Therapeutic: 50-100 ng/mL (SI: 190-390 nmol/L) at end of dose interval

Possible Panic Range >1000 ng/mL (SI: >3860 nmol/L); **fatal:** >2000 ng/mL (SI: >7702 nmol/L). See Table C in the Therapeutic Drug Monitoring Introduction *on page 733.*

Use Monitor therapeutic drug level in patients with cardiac arrhythmias, angina pectoris, and hypertension; evaluate for potential toxicity

Limitations See Flecainide, Serum or Plasma *on page 749.*

Contraindications Uncompensated congestive heart failure, cardiogenic shock, bradycardia, and asthma[1,2]

Methodology Fluorescence polarization immunoassay (FPIA), enzyme immunoassay (EIA), gas-liquid chromatography (GLC), high performance liquid chromatography (HPLC)

Additional Information
- Half-life: 4-6 hours
- Volume of distribution: 3-4 L/kg
- Protein binding: 90% to 95%

Propranolol is well absorbed after oral administration. For therapeutic drug monitoring, consistently use the same time interval between sampling and dose administration when comparing results from serial samples. A number of metabolites have been identified with at least one, 4-hydroxyl propranolol, having pharmacologic activity. Adverse effects of this drug include precipitation of heart failure, bronchospasm, bradycardia, and hypoglycemia. Hyperthyroidism exerts an age-dependent inducing effect on the metabolism of propranolol.

Propranolol is more effective than standard antiarrhythmic agents in the treatment of chloral hydrate-induced cardiac toxicity.[3]

Phenobarbital and rifampin may increase propranolol clearance and may decrease its activity. Cimetidine may reduce propranolol clearance and may increase its effects.

Propranolol may increase thyroxine, cholesterol, and glucose in test samples.

Footnotes
1. Leikin JB and Paloucek FP, *Poisoning and Toxicology Compendium*, Hudson, OH: Lexi-Comp Inc, 1998, 475-6.
2. Fallowfield JM and Marlow HF, "Propranolol Is Contraindicated in Asthma," *BMJ*, 1986, 313(7070);1486.
3. Zahedi A, Grant MH, and Wong DT, "Successful Treatment of Chloral Hydrate Cardiac Toxicity With Propranolol," *Am J Emerg Med*, 1999, 17(5):490-1.

References

Aranow WS, Ahn C, and Kronzon I, "Effect of Propranolol Versus No Propranolol on Total Mortality Plus Nonfatal Myocardial Infarction in Older Patients With Prior Myocardial Infarction, Congestive Heart Failure, and Left Ventricular Ejection Fraction ≥40% Treated With Diuretics Plus Angiotensin-Converting Enzyme Inhibitors," *Am J Cardiol*, 1997, 80(2):207-9.

Reith DM, Dawson AH, Epid D, et al, "Relative Toxicity of Beta Blockers in Overdose," *J Toxicol Clin Toxicol*, 1996, 34(3):273-8.

Walle T, Walle UK, Cowart TD, et al, "Pathway-Selective Sex Differences in the Metabolic Clearance of Propranolol in Human Subjects," *Clin Pharmacol Ther*, 1989, 46(3):257-63.

Quinidine, Serum

Related Information

Synonyms Biquin®; Cardioquin®; Cin-Quin®; Kiditard®; Kinidin®; Quinaglute® Dura-Tabs®; Quinalan®; Quinidex® Extentabs®; Quini® Durules®; Quinora®; Systodin®

Abstract Quinidine is a class 1 antiarrhythmic agent that is frequently used for management of life-threatening ventricular and supraventricular arrhythmias. A great many drug interactions and narrow therapeutic window make quinidine a candidate for laboratory monitoring.

Specimen Serum

Container Red top tube. The stoppers on some tubes contain plasticizers which affect measured drug levels.

Sampling Time Trough: collect just before next dose. Steady state is reached between 30 and 40 hours.

Causes for Rejection Sample collected in gel barrier tube

Special Instructions Serum concentration **must be correlated** with patient's clinical status.

Reference Interval Therapeutic: 2-5 µg/mL (SI: 6.2-15.4 µmol/L). Patient dependent therapeutic response occurs at levels of 3-6 µg/mL (SI: 9.2-18.5 µmol/L). Optimal therapeutic level is method dependent.[1]

Possible Panic Range Toxic: >8 µg/mL (SI: >24.7 µmol/L). Some patients may have toxic effects a levels near of just above the upper limit of therapeutic range. Levels >14 µg/L associated with cardiac toxicity. See Table C in the Therapeutic Drug Monitoring Introduction *on page 733.*

Use Therapeutic monitoring for quinidine is to provide documentation for adequate dosage[1] as well as toxicity assessment.

Limitations An assay method should be used which also detects active metabolites, in particular dihydroquinidine. Cross reactions occur with EMIT and fluorescence polarization methods.

Methodology Enzyme-multiplied immunoassay technique (EMIT), fluorescence polarization immunoassay (FPIA), high performance liquid chromatography (HPLC),[1,2] gas chromatography (GC)

Additional Information
- Half-life: 6-8 hours
- Volume of distribution: 2-3 L/kg
- Protein binding: 70% to 90%

Absorption of quinidine is complete and rapid. Peak concentrations are reached in 1.5-2 hours after oral intake. With slow preparations (quinidine gluconate) peak levels are reached 4-5 hours after intake.[3] Optimal resampling time after change in dosage is 1-2 days. **Doses >250 mg/day of quinidine result in increased serum digoxin concentrations about 2.5 times the digoxin concentration before quinidine is added.** The new steady-state digoxin concentration occurs in 7-14 days, with signs of toxicity beginning to appear in 3-7 days after initiation of quinidine therapy. Therefore, **serum digoxin concentrations should be measured before initiation of quinidine therapy and again in 4-6 days.** Measure trough because of variability of peak interval. Concomitant administration of **phenytoin** increases hepatic metabolism, and therefore decreases half-life and serum quinidine concentrations. Verapamil, amiodarone, alkalinizing agents, and cimetidine may increase quinidine serum concentrations; phenobarbital, and rifampin may decrease quinidine serum concentrations. Beta-blockers and quinidine may cause increased bradycardia; quinidine may enhance coumarin anticoagulants. Quinidine is among the most common causes of thrombocytopenia (~1 patient/1000 at risk). Typically, platelet counts with quinidine-induced thrombocytopenia are <10,000/mm³, with petechiae, purpura and sometimes intracranial hemorrhage.[4] Cimetidine impairs elimination of quinidine; quinidine and verapamil may result in severe hypotension; nifedipine may reduce serum quinidine levels and quinidine is reported to inhibit nifedipine metabolism.[5] A useful table of drug interactions has recently been published.[6] Clearance may be diminished in the elderly. **Renal failure** prolongs apparent half-life, perhaps through accumulation of fluorescent metabolites. Quinidine clearance depends on both liver and renal function. Severe heart failure prolongs half-life, as does decreased liver or renal function.

Psoriasiform eruption and pneumonitis[7] have been reported.

Footnotes
1. Meineke I, Rohde S, and Gundert-Remy U, "An Inexpensive and Sensitive Method for the Determination of Quinidine in Plasma by High Performance Liquid Chromatography With Ultraviolet Detection," *Ther Drug Monit*, 1995, 17(1):75-8.
2. Brandsteterova E, Romanova D, Kralikova D, et al, "Automatic Solid-Phase Extraction and High Performance Liquid Chromatographic Determination of Quinidine in Plasma," *J Chromatogr A*, 1994, 665(1):101-4.
3. Moyer TP, "Therapeutic Drug Monitoring," *Tietz Textbook of Clinical Chemistry*, 3rd ed, Burtis CA and Ashwood ER, eds, Philadelphia, PA: WB Saunders Co, 1999, 884-5.
4. Cines DB and Laposata M, "A 70-Year-Old Woman With Atrial Fibrillation and the Rapid Onset of Hemorrhagic Manifestations," Case Records of the Massachusetts General Hospital, Case 15-1995, Scully RE, Mark EJ, McNeely WF, et al, eds, *N Engl J Med*, 1995, 332(20):1363-70.
5. Bowles SK, Reeves RA, Cardozo L, et al, "Evaluation of the Pharmacokinetic and Pharmacodynamic Interaction Between Quinidine and Nifedipine," *J Clin Pharmacol*, 1993, 33(8):727-31.
6. Grace AA and Camm AJ, "Quinidine," *N Engl J Med*, 1998, 338(1):35-45.
7. Poukkula A and Paakko P, "Quinidine-Induced Reversible Pneumonitis," *Chest*, 1994, 106(1):304-6.

References

Allen LaPointe NM and Li P, "Continuous Intravenous Quinidine Infusion for the Treatment of Atrial Fibrillation or Flutter: A Case Series," *Am Heart J*, 2000, 139(1 Pt 1):114-21.

Bonavita GJ, Pires LA, Wagshal AB, et al, "Usefulness of Oral Quinidine-Mexiletine Combination Therapy for Sustained Ventricular Tachyarrhythmias as Assessed by Programmed Electrical Stimulation When Quinidine Monotherapy Has Failed," *Am Heart J*, 1994, 127(4 Pt 1):847-51.

Capucci A, Aschieri D, Villani GO, "Clinical Pharmacology of Antiarrhythmic Drugs," *Drugs Aging*, 1998, 13(1):51-70.

Capucci A, Boriani G, Rubino I, et al, "A Controlled Study on Oral Propafenone Versus Digoxin Plus Quinidine in Converting Recent Onset Atrial Fibrillation to Sinus Rhythm," *Int J Cardiol*, 1994, 43(3):305-13.

Eisenman DP and McKegney FP, "Delirium at Therapeutic Serum Concentrations of Digoxin and Quinidine," *Psychosomatics*, 1994, 35(1):91-3.

Gillis AM, Mitchell LB, Wyse DG, et al, "Quinidine Pharmacodynamics in Patients With Arrhythmia: Effects of Left Ventricular Function," *J Am Coll Cardiol*, 1995, 25(5):989-94

Oberg KC, O'Toole MF, Gallastegui JL, et al, ""Late" Proarrhythmia Due to Quinidine," *Am J Cardiol*, 1994, 74(2):192-4.

- ◆ **Quini® Durules®** see Quinidine, Serum *on page 764*

- ◆ **Quinora®** see Quinidine, Serum *on page 764*

- ◆ **Red Devils** see Barbiturates, Quantitative, Serum or Plasma *on page 739*

- ◆ **Red Man Syndrome** see Vancomycin, Serum *on page 769*

- ◆ **Repazine®** see Chlorpromazine, Serum *on page 743*

- ◆ **Resposan-10®** see Chlordiazepoxide, Serum *on page 742*

- ◆ **Retard®** see Procainamide, Serum *on page 763*

- ◆ **Retrovir®** see Zidovudine, Serum or Plasma *on page 771*

- ◆ **Rheumatrex®** see Methotrexate, Serum or Plasma *on page 756*

- ◆ **Rhythmin®** see Procainamide, Serum *on page 763*

- ◆ **Rhythmodan®** see Disopyramide, Serum or Plasma *on page 747*

- ◆ **Ridaura®** see Gold, Serum *on page 751*

- ◆ **Ritmilen®** see Disopyramide, Serum or Plasma *on page 747*

- ◆ **Rivatril®** see Clonazepam, Serum *on page 743*

- ◆ **Sabril®** see Antiepileptic Drugs, New, Overview *on page 738*

- ◆ **Sabrilex®** see Antiepileptic Drugs, New, Overview *on page 738*

- ◆ **Sandimmune®** see Cyclosporine, Blood *on page 744*

- ◆ **Secobarbital** see Barbiturates, Quantitative, Serum or Plasma *on page 739*

- ◆ **Seconal™** see Barbiturates, Quantitative, Serum or Plasma *on page 739*

- ◆ **Securon®** see Verapamil, Serum or Plasma *on page 769*

- ◆ **Sedantoinal®** see Mephenytoin, Serum *on page 756*

- ◆ **Serax®** see Oxazepam, Serum *on page 759*

- ◆ **Serenace®** see Haloperidol, Serum or Plasma *on page 752*

- ◆ **Serenid® Forte** see Oxazepam, Serum *on page 759*

- ◆ **Serentil®** see Phenothiazines, Serum or Urine *on page 760*

- ◆ **Sertraline Hydrochloride** see Sertraline, Serum *on page 765*

Sertraline, Serum

Related Information
Antidepressants, Cyclic, Serum *on page 737*
Trazodone, Serum or Plasma *on page 768*

Synonyms Sertraline Hydrochloride; Zoloft®

Abstract Sertraline, an antidepressant, is a serotonin reuptake inhibitor. It is also being evaluated for use in obesity and obsessive-compulsive disorder.[1]

Specimen Serum

Container Red top tube

Reference Interval 30-200 ng/mL

Critical Values >500 ng/mL

Use Treatment of major depression

Contraindications Do not use in combination with monoamine oxidase inhibitors.

Methodology High performance liquid chromatography (HPLC), gas chromatography (GC)

Additional Information
- Half-life: 24 hours
- Volume of distribution: 20 L/kg
- Protein binding: high: 98% to 99%
- Bioavailability: oral: 36%
- Time to peak plasma concentration: 8-12 hours

Sertraline acts by inhibiting serotonin reuptake. The drug has less sedating and anticholinergic effects as compared to tricyclic antidepressants. Sertraline is a relatively safe drug due to its lack of interaction with norepinephrine, dopamine, monoamine oxidase, and cholinergic receptors, as well as its almost complete lack of cardiovascular activity. The signs and symptoms which develop in sertraline overdose are minor and of short duration. These symptoms include tremor, lethargy, nausea, and vomiting. One study of 42 overdose patients reported that 10 had no symptoms, and the others (who consumed up to 160 times the therapeutic dose) had tremors, lethargy, nausea, agitation, confusion, and vomiting.[2]

Sertraline has significant first-pass metabolism. The major metabolite, desmethylsertraline, is weakly active with a half-life of 66 hours.

The common drug-drug interactions include amitriptyline, astemizole, carbamazepine, cimetidine, clorgyline, clozapine, dexfenfluramine, erythromycin, fenfluramine, flecainide, fluphenazine, fosphenytoin, hypericum, iproniazid, isocarboxazid, lamotrigine, metoclopramide, moclobemide, nialamide, pargyline, phenelzine, phenytoin, procarbazine, propafenone, propranolol, rizatriptan, selegiline, sibutramine, sumatriptan, terfenadine, toloxatone, tramadol, tranylcypromine, warfarin, zolmitriptan, and zolpidem.

Footnotes
1. Kronig MH, Apter J, Asnis G, et al, "Placebo-Controlled, Multicenter Study of Sertraline Treatment for Obsessive-Compulsive Disorder," *J Clin Psychopharmacol*, 1999, 19(2):172-6.
2. Lau GT and Horowitz BZ, "Sertraline Overdose," *Acad Emerg Med*, 1996, 3(2):132-6.

References
Edwards JG and Anderson I, "Systematic Review and Guide to Selection of Selective Serotonin Reuptake Inhibitors," *Drugs*, 1999, 57(4):507-33.

Gupta RN and Dziurdzy SA, "Therapeutic Monitoring of Sertraline," *Clin Chem*, 1994, 40(3):498-9.

Klein-Schwartz W and Anderson B, "Analysis of Sertraline-Only Overdose," *Am J Emerg Med*, 1996, 14(5):456-8.

Pigott TA and Seay SM, "A Review of the Efficacy of Selective Serotonin Reuptake Inhibitors in Obsessive-Compulsive Disorder," *J Clin Psychiatry*, 1999, 60(2):101-6.

Richelson E, "Pharmacokinetic Drug Interactions of New Antidepressants: A Review of the Effects on the Metabolism of Other Drugs," *Mayo Clin Proc*, 1997, 72(9):835-47.

Shelton RC, "The Role of Sertraline in the Management of Depression," *Clin Ther*, 1994, 16(5):768-82.

- ◆ **Sinequan®** see Antidepressants, Cyclic, Serum *on page 737*

- ◆ **Sinequan®** see Doxepin, Serum *on page 748*

- ◆ **SK-Lygen®** see Chlordiazepoxide, Serum *on page 742*

- ◆ **SK-Pramine®** see Imipramine, Serum or Plasma *on page 752*

- ◆ **Slo-Phyllin®** see Theophylline, Serum *on page 766*

- ◆ **Smail®** see Chlordiazepoxide, Serum *on page 742*

- ◆ **Sodium Aurothiomalate** see Gold, Serum *on page 751*

- ◆ **Solfoton®** see Phenobarbital, Serum or Plasma *on page 760*

- ◆ **Solganal®** see Gold, Serum *on page 751*

- ◆ **Solis®** see Diazepam, Serum *on page 745*

- ◆ **Solium®** see Chlordiazepoxide, Serum *on page 742*

- ◆ **Sporanox®** see Itraconazole, Serum *on page 753*

- ◆ **Staurodorm®** see Flurazepam, Serum *on page 751*

- ◆ **Stay Awake®** see Caffeine, Serum *on page 740*

- ◆ **Stelazine®** see Phenothiazines, Serum or Urine *on page 760*

- ◆ **Stental Extentabs®** see Phenobarbital, Serum or Plasma *on page 760*

- ◆ **Stesolid®** see Diazepam, Serum *on page 745*

- ◆ **Sustaire®** see Theophylline, Serum *on page 766*

- ◆ **Suxinutin®** see Ethosuximide, Serum or Plasma *on page 748*

- ◆ **Systodin®** see Quinidine, Serum *on page 764*

Tacrolimus, Whole Blood

Related Information
Cyclosporine, Blood *on page 744*
Itraconazole, Serum *on page 753*

Synonyms FK-506; Prograf®

Applies to Interleukin Production

Abstract Tacrolimus is a potent immunosuppressant used in renal, liver, heart, lung, bone marrow, and small bowel transplants.

Specimen Whole blood

Container Lavender top (EDTA) tube

Sampling Time Trough levels should be obtained 12-18 hours after oral dose or immediately prior to next dose.

Collection Do not draw the sample from the line used to administer the drug.

Reference Interval Trough (in whole blood): 3-20 ng/mL. Trough blood concentrations of 4-10 ng/mL for liver transplantation, 6.0-12 ng/mL for renal transplantation, 10.0-18.0 ng/mL for pancreas transplantation, and 10.0-20.0 ng/mL for bone marrow transplantation are recommended.[1] Since tacrolimus binds to erythrocytes and lipoproteins, measurement of whole blood concentrations is preferred. Plasma levels are 2% to 20% of whole blood level.

Use Monitor the adequacy of drug dosage levels in management of immunosuppression for organ transplant recipients. The agent is used extensively to suppress rejection of autologous organ grafts.

(Continued)

Tacrolimus, Whole Blood *(Continued)*

Methodology Enzyme-linked immunosorbent assay (ELISA), microparticle enhanced immunoassay (MEIA), high performance liquid chromatography (HPLC), liquid chromatography with detection by tandem mass spectrometry (LC/MS/MS)[1]

Additional Information
- Half-life: 10-14 hours
- Volume of distribution: 1.5 L/kg
- Protein binding: 99%
- Time to reach steady state: 2-3 days

Tacrolimus is a 822-kDa macrolid antibiotic extracted from the soil fungus, *Streptomyces tsukubaensis*, and was discovered at Mt Tsukuba in northern Japan in 1984. On a molar basis, it is 10- to 100-fold more potent than cyclosporine. The exact mechanism of action of the immunosuppressant properties of the drug is not well known, but it appears to interfere with T-helper cell function and secretion of lymphokines to decrease interleukin production.

The absorption of tacrolimus is highly variable with bioavailability varying from 5% to 67%. The plasma protein binding of tacrolimus is ~99% and is independent of concentration over a range of 5-50 ng/mL. Tacrolimus is bound to albumin and alpha-1-acid glycoprotein, and has a high level of association with erythrocytes. The distribution of tacrolimus between whole blood and plasma depends on several factors, such as hematocrit, temperature at the time of plasma separation, drug concentration, interaction with other drugs, and plasma protein concentration.

As with cyclosporine, renal toxicity with eventual renal failure is the most severe complication. Other assays to assess renal function (ie, BUN, creatinine clearance) should be ordered along with tacrolimus level, since toxicity may begin even with "acceptable" blood levels. In particular, to avoid excess nephrotoxicity, tacrolimus should not be used simultaneously with cyclosporine. Tacrolimus or cyclosporine should be discontinued at least 24 hours prior to initiating the other. Other common toxicities include neurotoxicity and hypertension.

Tacrolimus is extensively metabolized by the mixed-function oxidase system, primarily the cytochrome P-450 system (CYP3A). There are many drugs which affect tacrolimus pharmacokinetics, the most common being those which inhibit or induce the P-450 enzyme system. Drugs which increase tacrolimus concentrations include bromocriptine, cimetidine, cisapride, clarithromycin, clotrimazole, cyclosporine, danazol, diltiazem, erythromycin, fluconazole, itraconazole, ketoconazole, methylprednisolone protease inhibitors, metoclopramide, nicardipine, nifedipine, troleandomycin, and verapamil. Drugs which increase hepatic metabolism and thus lower tacrolimus levels include carbamazepine, ethotoin, mephenytoin, phenobarbital, phenytoin, primidone, rifampin, and intravenous trimethoprim-sulfa.

Footnotes
1. *Mayo Medical Laboratories*, Rochester, MN, 2000.

References
Busuttil RW and Holt CD, "Tacrolimus Is Superior to Cyclosporine in Liver Transplantation," *Transplant Proc*, 1998, 30(5):2174-8.

de Mattos AM, Olyaei AJ, and Bennett WM, "Nephrotoxicity of Immunosuppressive Drugs: Long-Term Consequences and Challenges for the Future," *Am J Kidney Dis*, 2000, 35(2):333-46.

Gummert JF, Ikonen T, and Morris RE, "Newer Immunosuppressive Drugs: A Review," *J Am Soc Nephrol*, 1999, 10(6):1366-80.

Linder MW and Elin RJ, "Implications of Methodologic Bias for Therapeutic Drug Monitoring," *Arch Pathol Lab Med*, 1999, 123(10):931-2.

Oellerich M, Armstrong VW, Schutz E, et al, "Therapeutic Drug Monitoring of Cyclosporine and Tacrolimus. Update on Lake Louise Consensus Conference on Cyclosporine and Tacrolimus," *Clin Biochem*, 1998, 31(5):309-16.

Shapiro R, "Tacrolimus in Pediatric Renal Transplantation: A Review," *Pediatr Transplant*, 1998, 2(4):270-6.

Spencer CM, Goa KL, and Gillis JC, "Tacrolimus. An Update of its Pharmacology and Clinical Efficacy in the Management of Organ Transplantation," *Drugs*, 1997, 54(6):925-75.

Trull AK, "Therapeutic Monitoring of Tacrolimus," *Ann Clin Biochem*, 1998, 35(Pt 2):167-80.

Undre NA, Stevenson P, and Schafer A, "Pharmacokinetics of Tacrolimus: Clinically Relevant Aspects," *Transplant*, 1999, 31(7A):21S-24S.

Young DS, *Effects of Drugs on Clinical Laboratory Tests*, 5th ed, Volume 1: Listing by Test, Washington, DC: AACC Press, American Association of Clinical Chemistry, 2000, Section 3, 734-6.

♦ **TAD** *see* Antidepressants, Cyclic, Serum *on page 737*

♦ **Talbutal** *see* Barbiturates, Quantitative, Serum or Plasma *on page 739*

♦ **Tambocor®** *see* Flecainide, Serum or Plasma *on page 749*

♦ **Tardigal®** *see* Digitoxin, Serum *on page 745*

♦ **TCA** *see* Antidepressants, Cyclic, Serum *on page 737*

♦ **Tegretol®** *see* Carbamazepine, Serum *on page 741*

♦ **Tegretol® XR** *see* Carbamazepine, Serum *on page 741*

♦ **Tenavoid®** *see* Meprobamate, Serum *on page 756*

♦ **Tensium®** *see* Diazepam, Serum *on page 745*

♦ **Tetracyclic Antidepressants** *see* Antidepressants, Cyclic, Serum *on page 737*

♦ **Theo-Dur®** *see* Theophylline, Serum *on page 766*

♦ **Theolair™** *see* Theophylline, Serum *on page 766*

Theophylline, Serum

Related Information
Amiodarone, Serum *on page 735*
Caffeine, Serum *on page 740*
Carbamazepine, Serum *on page 741*
Lithium, Serum *on page 754*
Mexiletine, Serum *on page 757*
Phenobarbital, Serum or Plasma *on page 760*
Phenytoin, Serum or Plasma *on page 761*
Verapamil, Serum or Plasma *on page 769*

Synonyms Aminophylline; Elixophyllin®; Ethylenediamine; Phyllocontin®; Slo-Phyllin®; Sustaire®; Theo-Dur®; Theolair™; Theospan®; Truphylline®

Abstract Used for over 80 years, theophylline is an a bronchodilator useful in asthma and chronic obstructive pulmonary disease (COPD). Its characteristics include immunomodulatory and anti-inflammatory properties.[1] For asthma, it is used in conjunction with inhaled beta-2 agonists. The drug is tolerated well when serum concentrations are kept within therapeutic range. It is used in neonates for idiopathic apnea/bradycardia. Atrioventricular nodal block induced by adenosine, produced by ischemic myocardium, is reported to respond to theophylline. Theophylline, a methylxanthine derivative, antagonizes cardiac actions of adenosine. It is useful for bradyarrhythmias.

Specimen Serum

Container Red top tube

Sampling Time Measure **trough** and **peak**. Draw blood at 2 hours after most recent dose for rapid dissolution preparations; 4-6 hours after sustained release preparations. See table. If toxicity is suspected, draw a level any time during a continuous I.V. infusion, or 2 hours after an oral dose.

Guidelines for Drawing Theophylline Serum Levels

Dosage Form	Time to Draw Level
P.O. liquid, fast-release tab	Peak: 1 h post 4th dose
	Trough: just before 4th dose
P.O. slow-release product	Peak: 4 h post 3rd dose
	Trough: just before 3rd dose

Time to peak serum concentration:
- oral: 1 hour
- uncoated tablets: 2 hours
- chewable tablets: 1-1.5 hours
- enteric-coated tablets: 5 hours
- extended-release capsules and tablets: 4-7 hours, in overdoses up to 27 hours
- retention enema: 1-2 hours

Theophylline levels should be initially drawn after 2 days of therapy; repeat levels are indicated 2 days after each increase in dosage or weekly if on a stabilized dosage.

Storage Instructions Refrigerate (do not freeze) a minimum of 0.5 mL serum.

Reference Interval
Therapeutic:
- asthma: 10-20 μg/mL (SI: 56-111 μmol/L); about 65% of available maximal bronchodilatory effect occurs with levels of 10 μg/mL. The role for low-dose theophylline in subjects with chronic asthma (levels 5-10 μg/mL) requires further study. Levels of 10-15 μg/mL are appropriate for management of COPD, and 8-12 μg/mL may prove to be adequate.[1]
- neonatal apnea: 6-13 μg/mL (SI: 33-72 μmol/L)

Possible Panic Range >20 μg/mL (SI: >111 μmol/L); toxicity can take place at 15 μg/mL. High probability of seizures when levels are >40 μg/mL. Chronic overmedication may induce greater risk, even when serum concentrations are in levels considered the range of mild toxicity. In this group, patient age is a sensitive predictor of toxicity. The drug should be used cautiously in elderly subjects and patients on other medications.[2,3]

Use Monitor therapeutic drug level; detect noncompliance and subtherapeutic levels; attempt to predict theophylline toxicity if possible. Theophylline remains a useful drug in a number of ways. It is a glucocorticoid-sparing agent.[1]

Limitations Elderly, acutely ill subjects, and patients with severe respiratory problems, pulmonary edema, or liver dysfunction are at greater risk of toxicity because of reduced drug clearance. Interactions with other drugs (including antibiotics) with other shortcomings has led to decline in use of theophylline,[1,4] and its use has declined with the advent of potent steroid inhalants for the treatment of asthma.

Contraindications Uncontrolled arrhythmias, hypersensitivity to ethylenediamine are contraindications to use of this drug.

Methodology Enzyme immunoassay (EIA), high performance liquid chromatography (HPLC), gas chromatography (GC)

Additional Information For adult nonsmoker:

- Half-life: 6-10 hours in normal adults
- Volume of distribution: 0.4-0.6 L/kg
- Protein binding: 50% to 60%

In order to improve aqueous solubility, formulation as a complex or salt is common. Aminophylline, the ethylenediamine salt, is widely used. Aminophylline is 85% anhydrous theophylline by weight.

The drug is extensively metabolized with peak serum levels reached 4 hours after oral dose. Troleandomycin and erythromycin may slow theophylline elimination.

Changes in diet may affect the elimination of theophylline. Theophylline may decrease the effects of phenytoin, lithium, and neuromuscular blocking agents. Theophylline increases the excretion of lithium and may have synergistic toxicity with sympathomimetics. Cimetidine, allopurinol, erythromycin, propranolol, influenza virus vaccine, ciprofloxacin, oral contraceptives, amiodarone, clindamycin, and lincomycin may **increase** theophylline concentrations.

A higher incidence of toxicity is recognized in patients with hepatic cirrhosis and hepatitis. Prolonged half-life occurs in premature infants. **Dosage should be reduced in these situations.**

By contrast, half-life is shortened in smokers and is variable with phenobarbital administration; higher doses are tolerated also in acidemia. Smokers on the average are reported to need 1.5-2 times as much of the drugs as nonsmokers to achieve the same effects. Marijuana smoking, rifampin, carbamazepine, phenobarbital, phenytoin, and aminoglutethimide may **decrease** theophylline concentrations. Optimal resampling time after change in dosage is 48 hours for adults, 1-2 days for children. The half-life varies between individuals. See table.

Theophylline Half-Life

Half-life (h)	Patient Population
6-10	Normal healthy adults
2-9	Children
15-58	Premature infants
18-24	Severe congestive heart failure
29	Cirrhosis

Several studies have questioned the correlation between the blood concentration and toxic effect of theophylline.[5] Theophylline may cause tachycardia and serious arrhythmias even at therapeutic serum concentrations.[6] Lack of symptoms in young patients receiving chronic therapy, but having levels >20 µg/mL, has been reported.[7] As some theophylline is converted to caffeine, and caffeine has activity similar to theophylline, monitoring of caffeine concentrations may be indicated if toxicity is suspected and theophylline concentrations are within normal range.

Serum levels should be interpreted in light of the patient's clinical status and use of other medications.

Toxic effects and signs and symptoms of acute overdose include nausea, vomiting, abdominal pain, tremors, esophageal ulceration, palpitation, anorexia, diuresis, skin rash, insomnia, irritability, atrial fibrillation, tachycardia, paroxysmal supraventricular tachycardia, convulsions, hypotension, visual hallucinations, hypokalemia, hypercalcemia, lactic acidosis, feces discoloration (black), and death.

Footnotes

1. Vassallo R and Lipsky JJ, "Theophylline: Recent Advances in the Understanding of its Mode of Action and Uses in Clinical Practice," *Mayo Clin Proc*, 1998, 73(4):346-54.
2. Shannon M, "Predictors of Major Toxicity After Theophylline Overdose," *Ann Intern Med*, 1993, 119(12):1161-7.
3. Shannon M, "Life-Threatening Events After Theophylline Overdose: A 10-Year Prospective Analysis," *Arch Intern Med*, 1999, 159(9):989-94.
4. Young DS, *Effects of Drugs on Clinical Laboratory Tests*, 5th ed, Volume 1: Listing by Test, Washington, DC: AACC Press, American Association of Clinical Chemistry, 2000, Section 3, 743-50.
5. Aitken ML and Martin TR, "Life-Threatening Theophylline Toxicity Is Not Predictable by Serum Levels," *Chest*, 1987, 91(1):10-4.
6. Bittar G and Friedman HS, "The Arrhythmogenicity of Theophylline. A Multivariate Analysis of Clinical Determinants," *Chest*, 1991, 99(6):1415-20.
7. Melamed J and Beaucher WN, "Minor Symptoms Are Not Predictive of Elevated Theophylline Levels in Adults on Chronic Therapy," *Ann Allergy Asthma Immunol*, 1995, 75(6 Pt 1):516-20.

References

Anderson W, Youl B, and Mackay IR, "Acute Theophylline Intoxication," *Ann Emerg Med*, 1991, 20(10):1143-5.

Bectolet BD, McMurtrie EB, Hill JA, et al, "Theophylline for the Treatment of Atrioventricular Block After Myocardial Infarction," *Ann Intern Med*, 1995, 123(7):509-11.

Butts JD, Secrest B, and Berger R, "Nonlinear Theophylline Pharmacokinetics. A Preventable Cause of Iatrogenic Theophylline Toxic Reactions," *Arch Intern Med*, 1991, 151(10):2073-7.

Emerman CL, Devlin C, and Connors AF, "Risk of Toxicity in Patients With Elevated Theophylline Levels," *Ann Emerg Med*, 1990, 19(6):643-8.

Epstein PE, "Hemlock or Healer? The Mercurial Reputation of Theophylline," *Ann Intern Med*, 1993, 119(12):1216-7.

Greenberger PA, Cranberg JA, Ganz MA, et al, "A Prospective Evaluation of Elevated Serum Theophylline Concentrations to Determine if High Concentrations Are Predictable," *Am J Med*, 1991, 91(1):67-73.

Huang D, O'Brien RG, Harman E, et al, "Does Aminophylline Benefit Adults Admitted to the Hospital for an Acute Exacerbation of Asthma?" *Ann Intern Med*, 1993, 119(12):1155-60.

Kips JC, Peleman RA, and Pauwels RA, "The Role of Theophylline in Asthma Management," *Curr Opin Pulm Med*, 1999, 5(2):88-92.

Page CP, "Recent Advances in Our Understanding of the Use of Theophylline in the Treatment of Asthma," *J Clin Pharmacol*, 1999, 39(3):237-40.

Pesce AJ, Rashkin M, and Kotagal U, "Standards of Laboratory Practice: Theophylline and Caffeine Monitoring," National Academy of Clinical Biochemistry, *Clin Chem*, 1998, 44(5):1124-8.

Pesek CA, Cooley R, Narkiewicz K, et al, "Theophylline Therapy for Near-Fatal Cheyne-Stokes Respiration. A Case Report," *Ann Intern Med*, 1999, 130(5):427-30.

Self TH, Chafin CC, and Soberman JE, "Effect of Disease States on Theophylline Serum Concentrations: Are We Still Viligant?" *Am J Med Sci*, 2000, 319(3):177-82.

Schiff G, Regde H, LaCloche L, et al, "Inpatient Theophylline Toxicity: Preventable Factors," *Ann Intern Med*, 1991, 114(9):748-53.

Suissa S, Ernst P, Benayoun S, et al, "Low-Dose Inhaled Corticosteroids and the Prevention of Death From Asthma," *N Engl J Med*, 2000, 343(5):332-6.

Weinberger M and Hendeles L, "Theophylline in Asthma," *N Engl J Med*, 1996, 334(21):1380-8.

♦ **Theospan®** see Theophylline, Serum *on page 766*

♦ **Thioridazine** see Phenothiazines, Serum or Urine *on page 760*

♦ **Thorazine®** see Chlorpromazine, Serum *on page 743*

♦ **Thorazine®** see Phenothiazines, Serum or Urine *on page 760*

♦ **Thrombran®** see Trazodone, Serum or Plasma *on page 768*

♦ **Tiagabine** see Antiepileptic Drugs, New, Overview *on page 738*

♦ **Tobramycin, Serum** see Aminoglycosides, Serum *on page 734*

Tocainide, Serum or Plasma

Related Information
Lidocaine, Serum or Plasma *on page 754*

Synonyms Tonocard®; Xylotocan®

Abstract Tocainide is a class 1B antiarrhythmic agent closely related to lidocaine, but dissimilar from quinidine, procainamide, and disopyramide. In contrast to lidocaine, tocainide undergoes negligible first pass metabolism.

Specimen Serum or plasma

Container Red top tube or green top (heparin) tube; avoid serum separator tube

Sampling Time Peak: 1-1.5 hours after administration; trough: just before next dose

Reference Interval Therapeutic: 6-15 µg/mL (SI: 32-78 µmol/L)

Possible Panic Range >15 µg/mL (SI: >78 µmol/L)

Use Therapeutic monitoring and toxicity assessment

Methodology High performance liquid chromatography (HPLC), gas chromatography (GC)

Additional Information

- Half-life: 10-15 hours
- Volume of distribution: 2-4 L/kg
- Protein binding: 10% to 20%
- Bioavailability: ~100%

Adverse effects of tocainide are mainly neurological (faintness, tremor) and following overdose coma, seizures, edema and respiratory arrest can occur. Many patients receiving recommended dosage develop agranulocytosis, bone marrow depression, leukopenia, and aplastic anemia. Metabolites are inactive.

Decreased effect/levels with cimetidine and rifampin; similar effects occur with phenobarbital or phenytoin. Tocainide is eliminated through the kidneys. Patients with renal insufficiency have prolonged half-life of tocainide.

References

Denaro CP and Benowitz NL, "Poisoning Due to Class 1B Antiarrhythmic Drugs. Lignocaine, Mexiletine, and Tocainide," *Med Toxicol Adverse Drug Exp*, 1989, 4(6):412-28.

Gelfand MS, Yunus F, White FL, "Bone Marrow Granulomas, Fever, Pancytopenia, and Lupus-Like Syndrome Due to Tocainide," *South Med J*, 87(8):839-41.

Gottlieb SS, Kukin ML, Medina N, et al, "Comparative Hemodynamic Effects of Procainamide, Tocainide, and Encainide in Severe Chronic Heart Failure," *Circulation*, 1990, 81(3):860-4.

Loi CM, Wei X, Parker BM, et al, "The Effect of Tocainide on Theophylline Metabolism," *Br J Clin Pharmacol*, 1993, 35(4):437-40.

Manolis AS, Smith E, Payne D, et al, "Randomized Double-Blind Study of Intravenous Tocainide Versus Lidocaine for Suppression of Ventricular Arrhythmias After Cardiac Surgery," *Clin Cardiol*, 1990, 13(3):177-81.

Moyer TP, "Therapeutic Drug Monitoring," *Tietz Textbook of Clinical Chemistry*, 3rd ed, Burtis CA and Ashwood ER, eds, Philadelphia, PA: WB Saunders Co, 1999, 885.

Roden DM and Woosley RL, "Drug Therapy. Tocainide," *N Engl J Med*, 1986, 315(1):41-4.

(Continued)

Tocainide, Serum or Plasma *(Continued)*

Wei X, Dai R, Zhai S, et al, "Inhibition of Human Liver Cytochrome P-450 1A2 by the Class IB Antiarrhythmics Mexiletine, Lidocaine, and Tocainide," *J Pharmacol Exp Ther*, 1999, 289(2):853-8.

- ♦ **Tofranil®** *see* Antidepressants, Cyclic, Serum *on page 737*
- ♦ **Tofranil®** *see* Imipramine, Serum or Plasma *on page 752*
- ♦ **Tofranil-PM®** *see* Imipramine, Serum or Plasma *on page 752*
- ♦ **Tonocard®** *see* Tocainide, Serum or Plasma *on page 767*
- ♦ **Topamax®** *see* Antiepileptic Drugs, New, Overview *on page 738*
- ♦ **Topiramate** *see* Antiepileptic Drugs, New, Overview *on page 738*
- ♦ **T-Quil®** *see* Diazepam, Serum *on page 745*
- ♦ **Trazodone** *see* Antidepressants, Cyclic, Serum *on page 737*

Trazodone, Serum or Plasma

Related Information
Antidepressants, Cyclic, Serum *on page 737*

Synonyms Deprax®; Desyrel®; Molipaxin®; Thrombran®; Trittico®

Abstract This drug is an antidepressant chemically unrelated to the tricyclic or tetracyclic antidepressants. The mechanism of action involves inhibition of reuptake of serotonin and norepinephrine.

Specimen Serum or plasma

Container Red top tube or green top (heparin) tube

Sampling Time Trough: at steady state (20-40 hours)

Reference Interval Therapeutic: 800-1600 ng/mL

Critical Values >5000 ng/mL

Use Therapeutic monitoring and toxicity assessment

Methodology High performance liquid chromatography (HPLC), gas chromatography (GC)

Additional Information
- Half-life: 4-8 hours
- Volume of distribution: 0.9-1.5 L/kg
- Protein binding: 85% to 95%

Trazodone is a structurally unique antidepressant that is pharmacologically different from other antidepressants. The toxicities observed in tricyclic overdose (neuro- and cardiotoxicity and respiratory depression) are not commonly seen with trazodone although it does have unique side effects including akathisia, allergic reactions, chest pain, delayed urine flow, early and delayed menses, hypersalivation, hypomania, and priapism, among others. Acute toxicity causes seizures and hyponatremia.[1,2] Trazodone use is contraindicated in hypersensitivity to trazodone, carcinoid syndrome, and initial recovery phase of myocardial infarction.

Trazodone may antagonize the antihypertensive effects of clonidine and methyldopa; it may increase concentrations of phenytoin or digoxin.

Peak plasma concentrations with average daily dosing is reached in 2-4 hours.

Footnotes
1. Balestrieri G, Cerudelli B, Ciaccio S, et al, "Hyponatremia and Seizure Due to Overdose of Trazodone," *BMJ*, 1992, 304(6828):686.
2. Vanpee D, Laloyaux P, and Gillet JB, "Seizure and Hyponatremia After Overdose of Trazodone," *Am J Emerg Med*, 1999, 17(4):430-1.

References
DeVane CL, "Differential Pharmacology of Newer Antidepressants," *J Clin Psychiatry*, 1998, 59(Suppl 20):85-93.

Haria M, Fitton A, and McTavish D, "Trazodone. A Review of its Pharmacology, Therapeutic Use in Depression and Therapeutic Potential in Other Disorders," *Drugs Aging*, 1994, 4(4):331-55.

Hull M, Jones R, and Bendall M, "Fatal Hepatic Necrosis Associated With Trazodone and Neuroleptic Drugs," *BMJ*, 1994, 309(6951):378.

Maes M, Vandoolaeghe E, and Desnyder R, "Efficacy of Treatment With Trazodone in Combination With Pindolol or Fluoxetine in Major Depression," *J Affect Disord*, 1996, 41(3):201-10.

Mills KC, "Trazodone Toxicity: Current Concepts," *Top Emerg Med*, 1993, 15:37-46.

Ohkubo T, Osanai T, Sugawara K, et al, "High Performance Liquid Chromatographic Determination of Trazodone and 1-M-Chlorophenylpiperazine With Ultraviolet and Electrochemical Detector," *J Pharm Pharmacol*, 1995, 47(4):340-4.

Rotzinger S, Bourin M, Akimoto Y, et al, "Metabolism of Some "Second"- and "Fourth"-Generation Antidepressants: Iprindole, Viloxazine, Bupropion, Mianserin, Maprotiline, Trazodone, Nefazodone, and Venlafaxine," *Cell Mol Neurobiol*, 1999, 19(4):427-42.

- ♦ **Triadapin®** *see* Doxepin, Serum *on page 748*
- ♦ **Triavil®** *see* Amitriptyline, Serum *on page 735*
- ♦ **Tricyclic Antidepressants** *see* Antidepressants, Cyclic, Serum *on page 737*
- ♦ **Trifluoperazine** *see* Phenothiazines, Serum or Urine *on page 760*
- ♦ **Trileptal®** *see* Antiepileptic Drugs, New, Overview *on page 738*
- ♦ **Trittico®** *see* Trazodone, Serum or Plasma *on page 768*

- ♦ **Tropium®** *see* Chlordiazepoxide, Serum *on page 742*
- ♦ **Truphylline®** *see* Theophylline, Serum *on page 766*
- ♦ **Valium®** *see* Diazepam, Serum *on page 745*
- ♦ **Valkote®** *see* Valproic Acid, Serum or Plasma *on page 768*
- ♦ **Valproate Semisodium** *see* Valproic Acid, Serum or Plasma *on page 768*
- ♦ **Valproate Sodium** *see* Valproic Acid, Serum or Plasma *on page 768*

Valproic Acid, Serum or Plasma

Related Information
Ammonia, Plasma *on page 102*
Carbamazepine, Serum *on page 741*
Phenobarbital, Serum or Plasma *on page 760*
Phenytoin, Serum or Plasma *on page 761*
Primidone, Serum or Plasma *on page 762*

Synonyms Depacon®; Depakene®; Depakote®; Depakote® XR; Depamide®; Dipropylacetic Acid; Divalproex Sodium; Epilim®; Ergenyl®; Leptilan®; 2-Propylpentanoic Acid; 2-Propylvaleric Acid; Valkote®; Valproate Semisodium; Valproate Sodium

Applies to Phenobarbital

Abstract Valproic acid is useful for many seizure types, including primary generalized tonic-clonic, partial, complex partial, myoclonic, atonic, and mixed seizures. It is described as the drug of choice for tonic-clonic seizures and spike wave discharges, and for subjects with other types of generalized epilepsy, especially myotonic jerks and absence seizures.[1] It is the drug of choice for mixed absence and generalized seizures and for the epileptic syndromes of juvenile myoclonic epilepsy and generalized tonic-clonic seizures on awakening. It also is used for some psychiatric conditions including bipolar affective disorder and for prophylaxis of migraine headaches.

Specimen Serum or plasma

Container Red top tube or green top (heparin) tube

Sampling Time Trough values drawn just before next dose or consistent sampling time in chronic monitoring. Steady-state levels are reached in 2-3 days.

Reference Interval 50-100 µg/mL (SI: 350-690 µmol/L).[1] Some patients require higher levels for seizure control. **Low levels:** The most important cause is noncompliance. Phenytoin, phenobarbital, primidone, and carbamazepine decrease the half-life of valproic acid by inducing the P-450 system.

Critical Values Toxic concentration >200 µg/mL (SI: >1390 µmol/L). Seizure control may improve at levels >100 µg/mL (SI: >690 µmol/L), but toxicity may occur at levels of 100-150 µg/mL (SI: 690-1040 µmol/L). Patients with hypoalbuminemia may become toxic within the normal range due to the nonlinear protein saturation pharmacokinetic characteristics of valproic acid. In these patients, measurement of free valproic acid is desirable.[2] See Table A in the Therapeutic Drug Monitoring Introduction *on page 733*.

Use Monitor for compliance, efficacy, and possible toxicity

Limitations Since valproic acid is highly bound, drugs that compete for protein binding sites can increase the amount of free valproic acid (biologically active fraction). These include dicumarol, high dose salicylates, and phenylbutazone. If toxicity is suspected and total valproic acid level is normal, a free valproic acid level should be obtained.

Contraindications Pregnant women on valproic acid are at risk for a higher incidence of neural tube defects and transient vitamin K-dependent clotting factors in the neonate.[1]

Methodology Enzyme immunoassay (EIA), fluorescent immunoassay, gas-liquid chromatography (GLC), high performance liquid chromatography (HPLC)

Additional Information
- Half-life (adult): 8-15 hours
- Volume of distribution: 0.1-0.5 L/kg
- Protein binding: 85% to 95%

Valproic acid (VPA) is a broad spectrum antiepileptic that may work by increasing or enhancing the inhibitory neurotransmitter γ-aminobutyric acid (GABA) in the brain. VPA is commercially available in oral formulations, in the acid form, and also as a sodium salt. Both forms are absorbed rapidly and almost completely. Depacon is an intravenous formulation of valproic acid. The bioavailability is 85% to 100%. Food slows absorption. VPA is 90% to 96% bound to albumin, depending upon the concentration of VPA. The free fraction increases as the concentration increases due to nonlinear or capacity-limited binding. This is due to changes in protein binding and the nonlinear binding seen with high concentrations of this drug. The higher the concentration the higher the free fraction and thus the larger the volume of distribution. VPA is almost entirely cleared hepatically and is a low extraction drug, so its clearance is dependent upon enzyme activity and plasma protein binding. The clearance of VPA is also age dependent, children clearing the drug more rapidly than adults. The clearance of valproic acid is also very susceptible to alterations in enzyme activity for its clearance. Valproic acid inhibits the hepatic P-450 enzymes that are responsible for the clearance of other drugs. Hepatic failure has occurred during the first 6 months of therapy. Hepatotoxicity may be preceded by nonspecific symptoms such as malaise, weakness, lethargy, anorexia, and vomiting. Hepatotoxicity may be fatal, but is idiosyncratic and not preventable by routinely monitoring liver enzymes. Hepatotoxicity occurs in very young children, most often those on multiple anticonvulsants. Children younger than age 6 are at increased risk of fatal hepatotoxicity.[3] Valproate-induced cytopenias may be dose-related and warrant monitoring of complete blood counts during therapy.[4] Encephalopathy with hyperammonemia without liver function test abnormalities may occur. About 20% of patients on valproic acid have hyperammonemia without liver damage.[1] Pancreatitis may occur in individuals of any age. Hematologic toxicities may include a variety of types of abnormality and may be dose-dependent and respond to dosage reduction.[5]

Footnotes

1. Brodie MJ and Dichter MA, "Antiepileptic Drugs," *N Engl J Med*, 1996, 334(3):168-75.
2. Haroldson JA, Kramer LE, Wolff DL, et al, "Elevated Free Fractions of Valproic Acid in a Heart Transplant Patient With Hypoalbuminemia," *Ann Pharmacother*, 2000, 34(2):183-7.
3. Konig SA, Siemes H, and Blaker F, "Severe Hepatotoxicity During Valproate Therapy: An Update and Report of Eight New Fatalities," *Epilepsia*, 1994, 35(5):1005-15.
4. Watts RG, Emanuel PD, Zuckerman KS, et al, "Valproic Acid-Induced Cytopenias: Evidence for a Dose-Related Suppression of Hematopoiesis," *J Pediatr*, 1990, 117(3):495-9.
5. Acharya S and Bussel JB, "Hematologic Toxicity of Sodium Valproate," *J Pediatr Hematol Oncol*, 2000, 22(1):62-5.

References

Addy D, "Serum Valproate Concentrations and Control of Seizures," *J Pediatr*, 1992, 121(5 Pt 1):835-6.
Davis LL, Ryan W, Adinoff B, et al, "Comprehensive Review of the Psychiatric Uses of Valproate," *J Clin Psychopharmacol*, 2000, 20(1 Suppl 1):1S-17S.
Engel J, *Seizures and Epilepsy*, Contemporary Neurology Series, Philadelphia, PA: FA Davis Co, 1989.
Franssen EJ, van Essen GG, Protman AT, et al, "Valproic Acid Toxicokinetics: Serial Hemodialysis and Hemoperfusion," *Ther Drug Monit*, 1999, 21(3):289-92.
Kulick SK and Kramer DA, "Hyperammonemia Secondary to Valproic Acid as a Cause of Lethargy in a Postictal Patient," *Ann Emerg Med*, 1993, 22(3):610-2.
Loscher W, "Valproate: A Reappraisal of its Pharmacodynamic Properties and Mechanisms of Action," *Prog Neurobiol*, 1999, 58(1):31-59.
Warner A, Privitera M, and Bates D, "Standards of Laboratory Practice: Antiepileptic Drug Monitoring. National Academy of Clinical Biochemistry," *Clin Chem*, 1998, 44(5):1085-95.
Winter ME, "Valproic Acid," *Basic Clinical Pharmacokinetics*, 3rd ed, Koda-Kimble MA and Young LY, eds, Vancouver, WA: Applied Therapeutics Inc, 1994.

♦ **Valrelease®** *see* Diazepam, Serum *on page 745*
♦ **Vancocin®** *see* Vancomycin, Serum *on page 769*
♦ **Vancoled®** *see* Vancomycin, Serum *on page 769*

Vancomycin, Serum

Related Information
Aminoglycosides, Serum *on page 734*

Synonyms Lyphocin®; Vancocin®; Vancoled®

Applies to Red Man Syndrome

Abstract Vancomycin is a glycopeptide antimicrobial agent with potent activity against most gram-positive bacteria, including some gram-positive rods. It is often bactericidal (not against enterococcal species) and interferes with cell wall synthesis. Its blockade of pepidoglycan synthesis facilitates uptake of aminoglycosides, explaining the synergism of gentamicin with vancomycin.[1] Due to emergence of vancomycin-resistant bacteria, its use is often reserved for gravely ill patients.[2,3]

Specimen Serum, body fluid

Container Red top tube, sterile fluid container

Sampling Time Both peak and trough are measured. **Peak:** 15 minutes to 1 hour after completion of infusion; **trough:** immediately prior to next dose.

Storage Instructions Separate serum using aseptic technique and place in freezer.

Causes for Rejection Specimen more than 4 hours old

Reference Interval Therapeutic: peak: 20-40 µg/mL (SI: 14-27 µmol/L) (depends in part on minimum inhibitory concentration of organism being treated); trough: 5-10 µg/mL (SI: 3.4-6.8 µmol/L)

Critical Values Trough concentrations ≥10 µg/mL may be associated with nephrotoxicity, but a relationship of nephrotoxicity to vancomycin use is controversial.

Possible Panic Range Toxic: >80 µg/mL (SI: >54 µmol/L). See Table B in the Therapeutic Drug Monitoring Introduction *on page 733*.

Use Several recent publications have recommended that **routine** monitoring of serum vancomycin levels is unnecessary. Specific situations in which determination of vancomycin levels **might** be helpful include:

- patients receiving vancomycin/aminoglycoside combinations
- anephric patients undergoing hemodialysis who receive infrequent doses of vancomycin (**Note:** Vancomycin is cleared much more efficiently by contemporary hemodialysis techniques than it was in the past.)

- patients receiving unusually high doses of vancomycin (eg, for treatment of meningitis due to penicillin-resistant pneumococci)
- patients with rapidly changing renal function

Limitations Monitoring serum vancomycin concentration has not been correlated with improved efficacy or decreased toxicity. Vancomycin pharmacokinetics are sufficiently predictable that adequate serum drug concentrations can be obtained with dosing methods that take into account the patient's age, weight, and renal function.

Methodology High performance liquid chromatography (HPLC), gas-liquid chromatography (GLC), enzyme immunoassay (EIA), fluorescence polarization (FPIA). Immunoassays are routinely used.

Additional Information
- Half-life: 4-8 hours (much longer in patients with renal insufficiency); 90% of an intravenous dose is eliminated by glomerular filtration over 24 hours. Concentrations in bile can reach half those in plasma. Cerebrospinal fluid levels reach 1% to 30% of those in plasma, respectively, in the absence or presence of inflammation in the meninges.[1]
- Volume of distribution: 0.62-0.80 L/kg, increased by female sex, obesity, and increasing age[1]
- Protein binding: 55% (range: 44% to 82%)

Vancomycin is bactericidal and appears to exert its effect by binding to precursor units of bacterial cell walls (second stage of cell wall synthesis), thereby inhibiting wall synthesis. Such binding occurs at an earlier step than that of penicillin. The net result is an alteration of bacterial cell wall permeability. In addition, RNA synthesis is inhibited. In the past (1950s) its use was associated with nephrotoxicity, but as the drug became more and more purified during the manufacturing process, that side effect has become very rare. Concomitant use of aminoglycosides may slightly increase the risk. Likewise, ototoxicity also seems to be rare, and may be associated only with very high serum concentrations (80-100 µg/mL). In order to avoid histamine release (which can cause pruritus; erythema of head, neck, and torso; back and/or chest muscle spasm; angioneurotic edema; flushed skin ("red man syndrome"); or hypotension), the intravenous infusion should be administered over at least 1 hour. Vancomycin must not be administered intramuscularly, due to severe pain at the injection site.

Oral doses are poorly bioavailable. Vancomycin is currently used in its intravenous form to treat a variety of gram-positive bacterial infections, particularly those due to methicillin-resistant staphylococcal species but also *Corynebacterium jeikeium* (JK) and enterococcal species. It is sometimes used in patients who are infected with susceptible bacterial species, including staphylococcal and streptococcal infections, when the patient also has penicillin and cephalosporin allergy. Additionally, vancomycin is often used in its oral form to treat pseudomembranous colitis due to *Clostridium difficile*. The emergence of vancomycin-resistant enterococcal species (especially *Enterococcus faecium*) in many hospitals has created substantial oversight motivation to minimize this practice (as well as inappropriate intravenous usage of vancomycin, a fairly widespread practice). *C. difficile* colitis should be treated initially with oral metronidazole. When vancomycin is administered orally, serum vancomycin levels are undetectable due to poor absorption from the gastrointestinal tract. Falsely elevated vancomycin serum concentrations may occur in patients with renal dysfunction.

Footnotes
1. Palmer-Toy DE, "Therapeutic Monitoring of Vancomycin," *Arch Pathol Lab Med*, 2000, 124(2):322-3.
2. Perl TM, "The Threat of Vancomycin Resistance," *Am J Med*, 1999, 106(5A):26S-37S.
3. Murray BE, "Drug Therapy: Vancomycin-Resistant Enterococcal Infection," *N Engl J Med*, 2000, 342(10):710-21.

References
Cantu TG, Yamanaka-Yuen NA, and Lietman PS, "Serum Vancomycin Concentrations: Reappraisal of Their Clinical Value," *Clin Infect Dis*, 1994, 18(4):533-43.
Li JTC, Markus PJ, Osmon DR, et al, "Reduction of Vancomycin Use in Orthopedic Patients With a History of Antibiotic Allergy," *Mayo Clin Proc*, 2000, 75(9):902-6.
Moellering RC Jr, "Monitoring Serum Vancomycin Levels: Climbing the Mountain Because It Is There?" *Clin Infect Dis*, 1994, 18(4):544-6.
Smith PF and Morse GD, "Accuracy of Measured Vancomycin Serum Concentrations in Patients With End-Stage Renal Disease," *Ann Pharmacother*, 1999, 33(12):1329-35.
Tam VH, Moore GE, Triller DM, et al, "Vancomycin Peak Serum Concentration Monitoring," *J Intraven Nurs*, 1999, 22(6):336-42.
Wilhelm MP and Estes L, "Symposium on Antimicrobial Agents - Part XII. Vancomycin," *Mayo Clin Proc*, 1999, 74(9):928-35.

♦ **Vatran®** *see* Diazepam, Serum *on page 745*
♦ **Vazepam®** *see* Diazepam, Serum *on page 745*
♦ **Veramex®** *see* Verapamil, Serum or Plasma *on page 769*

Verapamil, Serum or Plasma

Related Information
Digoxin, Serum *on page 746*
Disopyramide, Serum or Plasma *on page 747*
Quinidine, Serum *on page 764*

Synonyms Azupamil®; Calan®; Cordilox®; Ikacor®; Iproveratril Hydrochloride; Isoptin®; Securon®; Veramex®; Verelan®

Applies to Norverapamil
(Continued)

Verapamil, Serum or Plasma *(Continued)*

Test Includes Verapamil and norverapamil (metabolite levels)

Abstract Verapamil is an antihypertensive, antianginal calcium channel antagonist with an active metabolite, norverapamil. It has a role in management of cardiomyopathy. It is used as an antiarrhythmic drug, including therapy of tachyarrhythmias. It has also been used as prophylaxis of bipolar disorders in pregnant women, reduction of severity of tardive dyskinesia, and Tourette syndrome.

Specimen Serum or plasma

Container Red top tube (preferred) or green top (heparin) tube. Do not use serum separator tubes.

Sampling Time Peak: 1-2 hours after last dose

Storage Instructions Centrifuge, separate, and freeze serum (plasma) in a plastic container.

Reference Interval Therapeutic: 50-250 ng/mL (SI: 100-510 nmol/L) for parent; under normal conditions norverapamil concentration is the same as parent drug.

Critical Values >250 ng/mL (SI: >510 nmol/L); toxicity proportional to verapamil concentration

Possible Panic Range Toxic: >845 ng/mL; **fatal:** >2000 ng/mL. A ratio of verapamil/norverapamil >2.3 may be a predictor for fatal outcome.

Use Therapeutic monitoring and toxicity assessment

Limitations Clinical assessment of signs and symptoms is often preferable to use of drug concentrations. Verapamil is commercially available as a racemic mixture. The (S-) enantiomer is the isomer with the greatest pharmacological activity. These enantiomers exhibit stereoselective absorption, binding, and clearance. This makes for a very complex pharmacokinetic picture. It also makes it very difficult to associate measured verapamil concentrations with effect when it cannot differentiate the active (S) enantiomer from the relatively inactive (R) enantiomer.

Methodology Fluorometry, high performance liquid chromatography (HPLC), gas chromatography (GC)

Additional Information
- Half-life: 3-5 hours
- Volume of distribution: 4-6 L/kg
- Protein binding: 85% to 95%

Verapamil is an antiarrhythmic, antihypertensive drug whose main metabolite is norverapamil, which has about 20% of the activity of the parent drug. Verapamil is a calcium channel blocker. Coadministration of verapamil and beta-blockers should be approached with caution. Verapamil increases serum digoxin concentrations 50% to 70%. Toxicity may result when verapamil is used with carbamazepine or lithium.

Increased cardiovascular adverse effects occur with beta-adrenergic blocking agents (especially when administered intravenously), digoxin, quinidine, and disopyramide. Verapamil may increase serum concentrations of digoxin, quinidine, carbamazepine, theophylline, and cyclosporine necessitating a decrease in dosage. Phenobarbital and rifampin may decrease verapamil serum concentrations by increasing its clearance.

Route of metabolism: hepatic.

References

Brogden RN and Benfield P, "Verapamil: A Review of its Pharmacological Properties and Therapeutic Use in Coronary Artery Disease," *Drugs*, 1996, 51(5):792-819.

Carter BL, Noyes MA, and Demmler RW, "Differences in Serum Concentrations of and Responses to Generic Verapamil in the Elderly," *Pharmacotherapy*, 1993, 13(4):359-68.

Hansen JF and Mellemgaard K, "Angina Pectoris, Myocardial Infarction, and Verapamil," *J Am Coll Cardiol*, 1999, 34(3):957-8.

Hla KK, Latham AN, and Henry JA, "Influence of Time of Administration on Verapamil Pharmacokinetics," *Clin Pharmacol Ther*, 1992, 51(4):366-70.

Hosie J, Hosie G, and Meredith PA, "The Effects of Age on the Pharmacodynamics and Pharmacokinetics of Two Formulations of Verapamil," *J Cardiovasc Pharmacol*, 1989, 13(Suppl 4):S60-2.

Jespersen C, "Verapamil in Acute Myocardial Infarction. The Rationales of the VAMI and DAVIT III Trials," *Cardiovasc Drugs Ther*, 1999, 13(4):301-7.

Pritza DR, Bierman MH, and Hammeke MD, "Acute Toxic Effects of Sustained-Release Verapamil in Chronic Renal Failure," *Arch Intern Med*, 1991, 151(10):2081-4.

Ramoska EA, Spiller HA, and Myers A, "Calcium Channel Blocker Toxicity," *Ann Emerg Med*, 1990, 19(6):649-53.

Tom PA, Morrow CT, and Kelen GD, "Delayed Hypotension After Overdose of Sustained Release Verapamil," *J Emerg Med*, 1994, 12(5):621-5.

- ♦ **Verelan®** *see* Verapamil, Serum or Plasma *on page 769*

- ♦ **Vigabatrin** *see* Antiepileptic Drugs, New, Overview *on page 738*

- ♦ **Vitamin K** *see* Warfarin *on page 770*

- ♦ **Vivactil®** *see* Antidepressants, Cyclic, Serum *on page 737*

- ♦ **Vivarin®** *see* Caffeine, Serum *on page 740*

- ♦ **Vivol®** *see* Diazepam, Serum *on page 745*

Warfarin

Related Information

Amiodarone, Serum *on page 735*
Carbamazepine, Serum *on page 741*
Imipramine, Serum or Plasma *on page 752*
Nortriptyline, Serum *on page 758*
Phenobarbital, Serum or Plasma *on page 760*
Protein C *on page 351*
Protein S *on page 352*
Prothrombin Time *on page 354*
Quinidine, Serum *on page 764*

Synonyms Athrombin-K®; Coumadin®; Panwarfin®

Applies to Anticoagulants, Oral; Vitamin K

Abstract Warfarin is an oral anticoagulant. Serum warfarin concentrations are seldom useful in managing therapy. International normalized ratios (INR), a process which normalizes PT results for variations in reagent activity, and less frequently now, prothrombin times (PTs) are far more helpful than serum warfarin concentrations in assessing clinical efficacy/ toxicity, and in predicting improved patient outcomes (eg, reduction of strokes in older patients with atrial fibrillation when the patient's INR is maintained within a specific recommended range).

Specimen Serum or plasma

Container Red top tube, lavender top (EDTA) tube

Reference Interval Therapeutic: 2-5 μg/mL (SI: 6.5-16 μmol/L)

Possible Panic Range Toxic: >10 μg/mL (SI: >32.4 μmol/L)

Use Selective therapeutic monitoring and toxicity assessment. Plasma concentrations are infrequently used in clinical practice. An example of an application might be in addressing a patient who claims to be compliant in taking warfarin, but whose PT remains normal. A much more appropriate toxicity assessment is to consider the INR, and the presence or absence of active bleeding in a particular patient.

Limitations This test **does not** measure bishydroxycoumarin and should not be used to monitor this drug.

Methodology High pressure liquid chromatography (HPLC) with fluorescence detection, gas-liquid chromatography (GLC), UV spectrophotometry

Additional Information
- Half-life: 36-42 hours
- Volume of distribution: 0.14 L/kg
- Protein binding: 97%+

The coumarins, a class of compounds which include warfarin (Coumadin®), act as anticoagulants because they inhibit vitamin K epoxide reductase, which results in depletion of reduced vitamin K (vitamin KH_2). This depletion limits gamma-carboxylation of glutamate residues on the N-terminal regions of vitamin K-dependent proteins. This gamma-carboxylation normally permits factors II, VII, IX, and X to undergo a factor-activating conformational change in the presence of calcium, which allows the factors to complex with cofactors on phospholipid surfaces. Warfarin also limits carboxylation of the regulatory anticoagulant proteins C and S, and thereby impairs their function.

Commercial warfarin consists of a racemic mixture of two optically active enantiomers (R) and (S), each of which is metabolized by different isoenzymes of the hepatic cytochrome P-450 enzyme system. The S enantiomer is metabolized (hydroxylated) mainly by the cytochrome P-450 (CYP2C9) to the metabolite 7-hydroxywarfarin. THe (S) enantiomer is about five times as active as the (R) form. There are many potentially important and even dangerous drug-drug and drug-food interactions for warfarin; one reference is listed below (Wells). In general, certain other drugs may displace warfarin from its albumin binding sites, thereby increasing the free-drug concentration as well as activity, increase (eg, rifampin) or decrease (eg, trimethoprim-sulfamethoxazole) hepatic metabolism of warfarin, or alter warfarin absorption from the GI tract (eg, cholestyramine). Some drugs (eg, cimetidine), preferentially impair metabolism of the (R) enantiomer, resulting in a very modest effect on the INR. Nonsteroidal anti-inflammatory drugs (aspirin and many others) decrease platelet aggregation and may also create gastric erosions which, in turn, may bleed vigorously. Warfarin-food interactions include those when large amounts of vitamin K are ingested (eg, certain vegetables), decreasing the anticoagulant effect of warfarin.

Hereditary resistance has been reported.

Warfarin is used for chronic oral anticoagulation in a variety of clinical settings. Monitoring warfarin therapy by adjusting the INR to lie within the recommended range for the disorder treated (eg, 2.0-3.0 for treatment of deep venous thrombosis) is currently recommended.

Warfarin is highly bioavailable and is very highly bound (≥97%) to albumin.

The volume of distribution of warfarin is relatively small, 0.14 L/kg (roughly equivalent to the albumin space). It crosses the placenta and is a known teratogen, but is not found in breast milk. Warfarin is hydroxylated by the liver, which produces inactive metabolites. Other important side effects associated with warfarin include bleeding, skin necrosis (thrombosis of venules and capillaries in subcutaneous fat), and purple toe syndrome (cholesterol emboli). Patients receiving warfarin should not be given I.M. drug injections due to the risk of bleeding at the injection site.

Dosing warfarin is more complex than with many drugs, because the steady-state effect is delayed beyond the accumulation of the (S) enantiomer over five half-lives. This is because the half-lives of the vitamin K-dependent coagulation factors II, VII, IX, and X play a vital role in the effect of the drug, and must decline over five of their own individual half-lives to a new (relatively depleted) steady-state. This occurs most rapidly for factor VII, which has the shortest half-life of all these factors (about 6 hours). This in contrast to the half-life of factor II, about 60 hours. This explains why large loading doses of warfarin are not used, and do not work to hasten the anticoagulant effect. A current review of outpatient management of individuals on warfarin is available.[1]

Additional relevant information is included in the Coagulation chapter, especially in Prothrombin Time *on page 354*.

Footnotes

1. Beckey NP, "Outpatient Management of Patients on Warfarin," *Lippincotts Prim Care Pract*, 1999, 3(3):280-9.

References

Cai WM, Hatton J, Pettigrew LC, et al, "A Simplified High Performance Liquid Chromatographic Method for Direct Determination of Warfarin Enantiomers and Their Protein Binding in Stroke Patients," *Ther Drug Monit*, 1994, 16(5), 509-12.

Cropp JS and Bussey HI, "A Review of Enzyme Induction of Warfarin Metabolism With Recommendations for Patient Management," *Pharmacotherapy*, 1997, 17(5):917-28.

Hirsh J, Dalen JE, Anderson DR, et al, "Oral Anticoagulants: Mechanism of Action, Clinical Effectiveness, and Optimal Therapeutic Range," *Chest*, 1998, 114(5 Suppl):445S-69S.

Hylek EM, Heiman H, Skates SJ, et al, "Acetaminophen and Other Risk Factors for Excessive Warfarin Anticoagulation," *JAMA*, 1998, 279(9):657-62.

Porter RS and Sawyer WT, "Warfarin," *Applied Pharmacokinetics: Principles of Therapeutic Drug Monitoring*, 3rd ed, Evans WE, Schentag JJ, and Jusko WJ, eds, Vancouver, WA: Applied Therapeutics Inc, 1992.

Riley RS, Rowe D, and Fisher LM, "Clinical Utilization of the International Normalized Ratio (INR)," *J Clin Lab Anal*, 2000, 14(3):101-14.

Wells PS, Holbrook AM, Crowther NR, et al, "Interaction of Warfarin With Drugs and Food," *Ann Intern Med*, 1994, 121(9):676-83.

◆ **Wellbutrin®** *see* Bupropion, Serum or Plasma *on page 740*

◆ **Xylocaine®** *see* Lidocaine, Serum or Plasma *on page 754*

◆ **Xylotocan®** *see* Tocainide, Serum or Plasma *on page 767*

◆ **Yellow Jackets** *see* Barbiturates, Quantitative, Serum or Plasma *on page 739*

◆ **Zarontin®** *see* Ethosuximide, Serum or Plasma *on page 748*

◆ **Zartalin®** *see* Ethosuximide, Serum or Plasma *on page 748*

◆ **Zetran®** *see* Diazepam, Serum *on page 745*

Zidovudine, Serum or Plasma

Related Information

Beta₂-Microglobulin, Serum or Urine *on page 509*
CD4/CD8 Enumeration *on page 511*
HIV-1/HIV-2 Antibody Screen and Western Blot *on page 636*
Human Immunodeficiency Virus Culture *on page 639*

Synonyms Azidothymidine; AZT; Combivir®; Retrovir®

Abstract Azidothymidine (AZT) or zidovudine was the first FDA-approved drug for the treatment of human immunodeficiency virus (HIV) infection, the cause of AIDS. The drug is also used for the prevention of mother-to-child HIV-1 transmission.[1] The drug is a competitive inhibitor of HIV reverse transcriptase; after metabolism, the zidovudine triphosphate derivative is incorporated into viral DNA in place of thymidine triphosphate. When this occurs, DNA synthesis is prematurely terminated, because the 3'-azido group of zidovudine prevents further 5'- to 3'-phosphodiester linkages. The drug may also decrease production of its competitor, thymidine triphosphate.

Patient Preparation Coadministration of hydrochlorothiazide and sulfapyridine cause misleading AZT results.

Specimen Serum or plasma

Container Red top tube preferred, green top (heparin) tube acceptable

Sampling Time Trough level, just before next dose

Collection Volume needed is method dependent (0.1-1 mL).

Storage Instructions Refrigerate; label as infectious material.

Causes for Rejection Incorrect specimen sampling time; use of SST™ tube

Reference Interval Peak serum level at serum-state after 200 mg dose: ~1.5 µg/mL. Nadir serum concentration (just before the next dose) is <0.02 µg/mL.

Critical Values Not clear; acute overdoses of up to 50 grams in children and adults have been reported without fatalities.

Possible Panic Range Peak concentrations >1.8 µg/mL may provide evidence of increased risk of toxicity.

Use Not established for routine clinical use. Monitoring may be useful to establish compliance or, in subjects with renal impairment, to adjust dosage. Evaluation of serum concentration may be useful to guide dosage and support patient motivation (complex dosage regimens require patient education and motivation.) Otherwise, monitoring can probably be limited to pharmacokinetic studies as well as investigations of the efficacy of antiretroviral therapy.

Methodology High performance liquid chromatography (HPLC), radioimmunoassay (RIA), fluorescence polarization immunoassay (FPIA)

Additional Information

- Half-life: 1 hour
- Volume of distribution: 1.4 L/kg
- Protein binding: 25%

Zidovudine is usually administered orally at a total daily dose of 600 mg (300 mg twice daily or 200 mg three times a day). Peak serum concentrations are attained within 0.4-1.5 hours after ingestion. An intravenous form is also available. The main metabolite is a glucuronide derivative with no antiviral activity, that is produced in the liver and excreted through the kidneys. The major toxicity associated with zidovudine use is hematologic suppression which may manifest as anemia, leukopenia, and/or granulocytopenia. Macrocytic anemia is very common. Monitoring appropriate hematologic parameters is the most reasonable approach toward evaluation of toxicity; serum levels currently contribute little to evaluating toxic effects of zidovudine. Other fairly common side effects include nausea, headache, malaise, asthenia, and insomnia. Hepatic steatosis and lactic acidosis are among risks of toxicity. Hepatic and renal failure increase serum levels. While zidovudine lessened disease progression in the first year, the effect was not sustained and there was no improvement in long-term survival for subjects on this drug.

Zidovudine is used to prevent mother-to-child HIV-1 transmission. Previously, it had been thought that perinatal exposure to zidovudine caused cardiac abnormalities. However, recent data shows that zidovudine is not associated with abnormalities in left ventricular structure or function in infants exposed to the drug in the perinatal period.[2]

Footnotes

1. Peckham C and Newell ML, "Preventing Vertical Transmission of HIV Infection," *N Engl J Med*, 2000, 343(14):1036-7.

2. Lipshultz SE, Easley KA, Orav EJ, et al, "Absence of Cardiac Toxicity of Zidovudine in Infants. Pediatric Pulmonary and Cardiac Complications of Vertically Transmitted HIV Infection Study Group," *N Engl J Med*, 2000, 343(11):759-66.

References

Crouch RA and Arras JD, "AZT Trials and Tribulations," *Hastings Cent Rep*, 1998, 28(6):26-34.

Lallemant M, Jourdain G, Le Coeur S, et al, "A Trial of Shortened Zidovudine Regimens to Prevent Mother-to-Child Transmission of Human Immunodeficiency Virus Type 1," *N Engl J Med*, 2000, 343(14):982-90.

Leikin JB and Paloucek FP, *Poisoning and Toxicology Compendium*, Hudson, OH: Lexi-Comp Inc, 1988, 571-2.

Sperling R, "Zidovudine," *Infect Dis Obstet Gynecol*, 1998, 6(5):197-203.

Mayo Reference Services Publication, "Zidovudine, Serum," *New Test Announcement*, Rochester, MN: Mayo Medical Laboratories, December 1999.

◆ **Zoloft®** *see* Sertraline, Serum *on page 765*

◆ **Zonegran™** *see* Antiepileptic Drugs, New, Overview *on page 738*

◆ **Zonisamide Excegran®** *see* Antiepileptic Drugs, New, Overview *on page 738*

◆ **Zyban™** *see* Bupropion, Serum or Plasma *on page 740*

TOXICOLOGY/DRUGS OF ABUSE

Uttam Garg, PhD

David S. Jacobs, MD

Eugene S. Olsowka, MD, PhD

Harold J. Grady, PhD

Leland B. Baskin, MD

Jasbir Singh, PhD

Contributor: Wayne R. DeMott, MD

TOXICOLOGY

Modern toxicology is employed to resolve environmental, clinical, and forensic problems. Most medical laboratory toxicology concerns the identification of substances involved in acute or chronic poisoning of man. The laboratory is frequently asked to perform a comprehensive drug screen, often when little or no clue from the history and/or physical examination is available concerning the toxin. The term "comprehensive" is a relative one, since no hospital laboratory can truly screen for all possible toxic substances. Two available systems, a thin-layer chromatographic method called Toxi-Lab®, and an automated high performance liquid chromatographic instrument called Remedi®, can screen for several hundred drugs. Most often, they are supplemented with immunoassays for drugs of abuse, acetaminophen, and tricyclic antidepressants. Most of the time, qualitative identification of the toxic substance in a timely manner (1-2 hours) is the most useful, although in a few cases (eg, acetaminophen, salicylates, methanol, and ethylene glycol), a quantitative response is valuable. Quantitative measurement, usually carried out on serum/plasma, is most often used for the following drugs:

- acetaminophen
- salicylate
- carboxyhemoglobin (whole blood)
- digoxin (usually from TDM)
- ethanol, methanol, isopropanol, ethylene glycol

- heavy metals
- iron
- theophylline (usually from TDM)
- phenytoin (usually from TDM)

Of the other anticonvulsants, carbamazepine, primidone, phenobarbital, and valproic acid are most commonly monitored, although others may also be measured.

The laboratory can be most helpful when it has all the information available concerning possible substances involved. The dialogue between the laboratory and the treating physician should be reciprocal and ongoing as the situation develops. Forms designed by the laboratory for requests for toxicological analyses should ask for as much of this detail as possible. Toxicology and Therapeutic Drug Monitoring (TDM) overlap when drug levels significantly above the therapeutic range are involved. It should be noted that at such levels the usual values for elimination rates (half-lives) may not apply, because when enzyme systems become saturated typical first-order kinetics are no longer valid.

DRUGS OF ABUSE

The drugs or drug classes most commonly listed as drugs of abuse include:

- amphetamine/methamphetamine
- barbiturates
- benzodiazepines
- cannabinoids (marijuana or THC)
- cocaine

- opiates (heroin, morphine, codeine)
- phencyclidine (PCP)
- methadone
- methaqualone
- propoxyphene

These drugs are measured under one of two circumstances. One is the overdose situation in which the analysis is treated as any toxicological sample. The second involves testing for the presence of a drug in clinically well persons. Most of the following discussion applies to the latter situation. Analysis for such drugs in clinically-well subjects frequently involves two sequential tests, the first a screening procedure, and the second a confirmatory test performed only on positive screens. The screening test must have good sensitivity but may lack some specificity, while the confirmatory test must be both sensitive and specific and involve a different chemical principle. When used strictly for clinical purposes, the screening test result may be used without confirmation if an occasional false-positive will do no serious harm. However, when medicolegal or forensic application is a possibility, confirmation is essential. It is also extremely important for forensic applications that the sample be accompanied by a chain-of-custody document which will assure the integrity of the sample through the process of collection, delivery, receipt, and analysis (see the Toxicology/Drugs of Abuse Introduction *on page 777* for a chain-of-custody form). Most often, samples without such a document lack forensic value, regardless of the quality of the analysis. The sample for analysis of drugs of abuse is urine, because of the ease of collection and because concentrations of drugs and metabolites are usually higher than in serum/plasma or saliva. Laboratory reports for detection of drugs of abuse in well persons are generally not quantitative and are usually expressed as "positive" or "negative." For each drug, a predetermined threshold or cutoff value has been agreed upon by scientific and regulatory groups. Results equal to the cutoff or above are considered positive and all other values negative. Thus, a report of "negative" does not necessarily mean absence of the drug, but rather a result less than the cutoff. Cutoff values for a given drug are often different for the screening evaluation than for the confirmatory test. For a few drugs (eg, marijuana and opiates), several different cutoff values are in current use. When such specimens are sent to reference laboratories, one must verify that the cutoff they use will satisfy needs. A sample having either a negative screening test or positive screening test followed by a negative confirmatory test is reported as negative. When screening in the overdose situation, quantitative estimates are sometimes given when values are well above the cutoff. In a number of cases, metabolites, rather than the parent drug, are the substances actually measured in screening and confirmatory testing.

A federal agency is responsible for regulation of laboratories involved in analysis of drugs of abuse for federal employees and for companies operating under federal control. It is the Substance Abuse and Mental Health Services Administration (SAMHSA). This agency has set up strict guidelines for sample handling, measurement, and reporting of drugs of abuse in urine. This aspect of federal control of drugs-of-abuse testing was formerly under the National Institute for Drug Abuse (NIDA), which continues to perform other functions in this area. SAMHSA certifies laboratories following a rigorous proficiency testing and inspection procedure. Only SAMHSA-certified laboratories may perform drugs-of-abuse testing for federal agencies or for firms contracting with federal agencies. Only five drugs are on the SAMHSA panel: amphetamine/methamphetamine, cannabinoids, cocaine, opiates, and phencyclidine. Other drugs may be measured by SAMHSA-certified laboratories but are not part of the certification. The College of American Pathologists (CAP), under CAP-Forensic Urine Drug Testing program, also accredits laboratories for toxicology and drugs-of-abuse testing, using similar proficiency testing and inspection procedures. SAMHSA and CAP guidelines for all aspects of drugs-of-abuse testing are goals to which all good drug laboratories aspire. A majority of the laboratories screening for drugs of abuse employ enzyme immunoassay (EIA) methodology, which has adequate sensitivity and, in most cases, reasonable specificity. The amphetamine/methamphetamine class produces the most problems with false-positives, caused by interference from over-the-counter antiallergy and anticold medications. They, of course, will give negative confirmatory tests. Thin-layer chromatography (TLC) is occasionally used to screen (and rarely to confirm), but it provides only borderline sensitivity for some drugs. Confirmatory testing is frequently done by gas chromatography/mass spectrometry (GC/MS), which is clearly the method of choice and is considered the "gold standard." For drugs-of-abuse entries in this chapter, the cutoff values for screening and confirmation are listed.

Urine collection procedures for drugs-of-abuse testing should incorporate certain checks and precautions to preserve sample integrity. The collection room should not have warm water available, and the stool water should be colored with a dye. If the specimen is to be used for forensic purposes, witnessed voiding is preferred. The temperature within 4 minutes of collection should be between 90°F and 99°F. Later measurement of pH should be between 5 and 9, creatinine ≥5 mg/dL, and the specific gravity (refractometer) ≥1.003. Any unusual colors, odors, or physical appearance should be noted.

Also see the Chemistry Introduction for the table, International Unit (SI Unit) Conversion on page 75.

References

Baselt RC, *Disposition of Toxic Drugs and Chemicals in Man*, 5th ed, Foster City, CA: Chemical Toxicology Institute, 2000.

Burtis CA and Ashwood ER, *Tietz Textbook of Clinical Chemistry*, 3rd ed, Philadelphia, PA: WB Saunders Co, 1999.

Ellenhorn K, Schonwald S, et al, *Ellenhorn's Medical Toxicology*, 2nd ed, Baltimore, MD: Williams and Wilkins, 1997.

Kaplan LA and Pesce AJ, *Clinical Chemistry: Theory Analysis and Correlation*, 3rd ed, St. Louis, MO: Mosby, 1996.

Klaasen CD, *Casarette and Doull's Toxicology*, 5th ed, New York, NY: McGraw Hill, 1996.

Leikin J and Paloucek F, *Poisoning and Toxicology Compendium*, Hudson, OH: Lexi-Comp Inc, 1998.

Sipes G, McQueen C, and Gandolfi A, *Comprehensive Toxicology*, 7 volumes, New York, NY: Elsevier Science Inc, 1997.

Web Sites

www.aapcc.org

www.health.org

www.samsha.gov

www.soft-tox.org

The following table lists the Poison Control Centers (source: http://www.aapcc.org). Centers listed in **bold** are certified by the American Association of Poison Control Centers.

State	Poison Control Center	Phone
Alabama	**Alabama Poison Center**	800-462-0800 - Emergency (AL only) 205-345-0600
	Regional Poison Control Center	800-292-6678 - Emergency (AL only) 205-933-4050
Alaska	Anchorage Poison Control Center	800-478-3193 - Emergency 907-261-3193
Arizona	**Arizona Poison & Drug Info Center**	800-362-0101 - Emergency (AZ only) 520-626-6016
	Samaritan Regional Poison Center	800-362-0101 (AZ only) 602-253-3334
Arkansas	Arkansas Poison & Drug Information Center	800-376-4766 - Emergency 800-641-3805 - TDD/TTY
California	**California Poison Control System - Fresno/Madera Division**	800-876-4766 - Emergency (CA only) 800-972-3323 - TDD/TTY
	California Poison Control System - Sacramento Division	800-876-4766 - Emergency (CA only) 800-972-3323 - TDD/TTY
	California Poison Control System - San Francisco Division	800-876-4766 - Emergency (CA only) 800-876-4766 - TDD/TTY
	California Poison Control System - San Diego Division	800-876-4766 - Emergency (CA only) 800-972-3323 - TDD/TTY
Colorado	**Rocky Mountain Poison & Drug Center**	800-332-3073 - Emergency (CO only/outside metro area) 303-739-1123 (Denver metro)
Connecticut	**Connecticut Poison Control Center**	800-343-2722 - Emergency (CT only) 860-679-3456 860-679-4346 - TDD/TTY
Delaware	**The Poison Control Center**	800-722-7112 - Emergency 215-386-2100 215-590-2100
District of Columbia	**National Capital Poison Center**	202-625-3333 - Emergency 202-362-8563 - TTY
Florida	**Florida Poison Information Center - Jacksonville**	800-282-3171 - Emergency (FL only) 904-244-4480 800-282-3171 - TDD/TTY (FL only)
	Florida Poison Information Center - Miami	800-282-3171 - Emergency (FL only) 305-585-5253
	Florida Poison Information Center - Tampa	800-282-3171 - Emergency (FL only) 813-253-4444
Georgia	**Georgia Poison Center**	800-282-5846 - Emergency 404-616-9000 404-616-9287 - TDD
Hawaii	Hawaii Poison Center	808-941-4411 - Emergency
Idaho	**Rocky Mountain Poison & Drug Center**	800-860-0620 - Emergency (ID only)
Illinois	**Illinois Poison Center**	800-942-5969 - Emergency (IL only) 312-906-6185 - TDD/TTY
Indiana	**Indiana Poison Center**	800-382-9097 - Emergency (IN only) 317-929-2323 317-929-2336 - TTY
Iowa	Iowa Statewide Poison Control Center	800-352-2222 - Emergency 712-277-2222
Kansas	Mid-America Poison Control Center	800-332-6633 - Emergency (KS only) 913-588-6633 913-588 6639 - TDD
Kentucky	**Kentucky Regional Poison Center**	800-722-5725 - Emergency 502-589-8222
Louisiana	**Louisiana Drug and Poison Information Center**	800-256-9822 - Emergency (LA only)
Maine	Maine Poison Control Center	800-442-6305 - Emergency (ME only) 207-871-2950 877-299-4447 - TDD/TTY (ME only) 207-871-2879
Maryland	**Maryland Poison Center**	800-492-2414 - Emergency (MD only) 410-706-7701 410-706-1858 - TDD
	National Capital Poison Center	202-625-3333 - Emergency 202-362-8563 - TTY
Massachusetts	Regional Center for Poison Control and Prevention Serving Massachusetts & Rhode Island	800-682-9211 - Emergency (MA & RI only) 617-232-2120 888-244-5313 - TDD/TTY
Michigan	**Children's Hospital of Michigan**	800-764-7661 - Emergency (MI only) 313-745-5711 800-356-3232 - TDD
	DeVos Children's Hospital - Regional Poison Center	800-764-7661 - Emergency (MI only) 800-356-3232 -TTY
Minnesota	**Hennepin Regional Poison Center**	800-222-1222 - Emergency (MN only) 800-POISON1 (SD only) 612-904-4691 - TTY
Mississippi	Mississippi Regional Poison Control Center	601-354-7660 - Emergency
Missouri	**Cardinal Glennon Children's Hospital**	800-366-8888 - Emergency 314-772-5200
Montana	**Rocky Mountain Poison & Drug Center**	800-525-5042 - Emergency (MT only)
Nebraska	**The Poison Center**	800-955-9119 - Emergency (NE & WY only) 402-955-5555
Nevada	Oregon Poison Center	503-494-8968 - Emergency
	Rocky Mountain Poison & Drug Center	800-446-6179 - Emergency (NV only)
New Hampshire	New Hampshire Poison Information Center	800-562-8236 - Emergency (NH only) 603-650-8000
New Jersey	**New Jersey Poison Information and Education System**	800-POISON-1 - Emergency (NJ only) 973-926-8008 - TDD/TTY

State	Poison Control Center	Phone
New Mexico	New Mexico Poison & Drug Information Center	800-432-6866 - Emergency (NM only) 505-272-2222
New York	Central New York Poison Center	800-252-5655 - Emergency (NY only) 315-476-4766
	Finger Lakes Regional Poison & Drug Info Center	800-333-0542 - Emergency (NY only) 716-275-3232 716-273-3854 - TTY
	Hudson Valley Regional Poison Center	800-336-6997 - Emergency (NY only) 914-366-3030
	Long Island Regional Poison & Drug Information Center	516-542-2323 - Emergency 516-663-2650 516-924-8811 - TDD (Suffolk) 516-747-3323 - - TDD (Nassau)
	New York City Poison Control Center	800-210-3985 - Emergency 212-340-4494 212-POI-SONS 212-VEN-ENOS 212-689-9014 - TDD
	Western New York Regional Poison Control Center	800-888-7655 - Emergency 716-878-7654
North Carolina	Carolinas Poison Center	800-848-6946 - Emergency 704-355-4000
North Dakota	North Dakota Poison Information Center	800-732-2200 - Emergency (ND, MN, SD only) 701-234-5575
Ohio	Central Ohio Poison Center	800-682-7625 - Emergency (OH only) 800-762-0727 (Dayton, OH only) 614-228-2272 - TTY
	Cincinnati Drug & Poison Information Center	800-872-5111 - Emergency (OH only) 513-558-5111
	Greater Cleveland Poison Control Center	888-231-4455 - Emergency (OH only) 216-231-4455
Oklahoma	Oklahoma Poison Control Center	800-764-7661 - Emergency (OK only) 405-271-5454 405-271-1122 - TDD/TTY
Oregon	Oregon Poison Center	800-452-7165 - Emergency (OR only) 503-494-8968
Pennsylvania	Central Pennsylvania Poison Center	800-521-6110 - Emergency 717-531-6111 717-531-8335 - TTY
	Pittsburgh Poison Center	412-681-6669 - Emergency
	The Poison Control Center	800-722-7112 - Emergency 215-386-2100 215-590-2100
Rhode Island	Regional Center for Poison Control and Prevention - Serving Massachusetts & Rhode Island	800-682-9211 - Emergency (MA & RI only) 617-232-2120 888-244-5313 - TDD/TTY
South Carolina	Palmetto Poison Center	800-922-1117 - Emergency (SC only) 803-777-1117
South Dakota	Hennepin Regional Poisoin Center	800-POISON1 - Emergency (SD only) 612-904-4691 - TTY
Tennessee	Middle Tennessee Poison Center	800-288-9999 - Emergency (TN only) 615-936-2034 (Greater Nashville) 615-936-2047 - TDD
	Southern Poison Center	800-288-9999 - Emergency (TN only) 901-528-6048
Texas	Central Texas Poison Center	800-POISON-1 - Emergency (TX only) 254-724-7401
	North Texas Poison Center	800-764-7661 - Emergency (TX only)
	South Texas Poison Center	800-764-7661 - Emergency (TX only) 800-764-7661 - TDD/TTY (TX only)
	Southeast Texas Poison Center	800-764-7661 - Emergency (TX only) 409-765-1420
	Texas Panhandle Poison Center	800-764-7661 - Emergency (TX only)
	West Texas Regional Poison Center	800-764-7661 - Emergency (TX only)
Utah	Utah Poison Control Center	800-456-7707 - Emergency (UT only) 801-581-2151
Vermont	Vermont Poison Center	877-658-3456 - Emergency 802-658-3456
Virginia	Blue Ridge Poison Center	800-451-1428 - Emergency (VA only) 804-924-5543
	National Capital Poison Center	202-625-3333 - Emergency 202-362-8563 - TTY
	Virginia Poison Center	800-552-6337 - Emergency 804-828-9123
Washington	Washington Poison Center	800-732-6985 - Emergency (WA only) 206-526-2121 206-517-2394 - TDD 800-572-0638 - TDD (WA only)
West Virginia	West Virginia Poison Center	800-642-3625 - Emergency (WV only)
Wisconsin	Children's Hospital of Wisconsin Poison Center	800-815-8855 - Emergency (WI only) 414-266-2222
	University of Wisconsin Hospital & Clinics	800-815-8855 - Emergency (WI only) 608-262-3702
Wyoming	The Poison Center	800-955-9119 - Emergency (NE & WY only) 402-955-5555

CHAIN-OF-CUSTODY FORM

External chain-of-custody forms vary significantly from laboratory to laboratory, depending on the legal requirements. A typical form covers the following aspects. The following form is a combination requisition and external chain-of-custody form. The strip at the bottom peels off and is used to seal the specimen. The number on the strip appears on all copies of the form and serves to positively associate the form with the sample.

ACCOUNT NAME AND ADDRESS

LABORATORY NAME

TOXICOLOGY

LIG NO.

ACC NO.

COLLECTOR / EMPLOYMENT REPRESENTATIVE IDENTIFICATION

ADDRESS

MEDICAL REVIEW OFFICER'S NAME & ADDRESS

MEDICATIONS WITHIN LAST 30 DAYS

REASON FOR TESTING

1 ☐ PRE-EMPLOYMENT
2 ☐ FOLLOW-UP
3 ☐ REASONABLE CAUSE
4 ☐ RETURN ON DUTY
5 ☐ POST-ACCIDENT
6 ☐ RANDOM
7 ☐ OTHER (SPECIFY)_____

PROFILES

DRUGS OF ABUSE SCREEN
DRUGS OF ABUSE SCREEN (with confirmation)
BLOOD ALCOHOL
URINE ALCOHOL
OTHER (specify):

TEMPERATURE (to be read within 4 minutes of collection)

TEMPERATURE WITHIN RANGE (90° to 100°F / 32° to 38°C)   ☐ Yes   ☐ No

---

TO BE COMPLETED BY COLLECTOR

NAME _____   COLLECTION FACILITY _____

I CERTIFY THAT THE SPECIMEN IDENTIFIED ON THIS FORM IS THE SPECIMEN PRESENTED TO ME BY THE DONOR SIGNING THIS FORM, AND THAT THE SPECIMEN BEARS AN IDENTIFICATION NUMBER IDENTICAL TO THE NUMBER BELOW, AND THAT IT HAS BEEN COLLECTED, LABELED, AND SEALED WITH THE SECURITY LABEL.

SIGNATURE   DATE / TIME   PHONE

TO BE COMPLETED BY DONOR

I _____ HEREBY CONSENT TO HAVE A SPECIMEN OF MY URINE AND/OR BLOOD TAKEN, AND I UNDERSTAND THAT IT WILL BE USED FOR DRUG
PRINT NAME

ANALYSIS BY THE LABORATORY. THE RESULTS OF THE TESTS ON MY SPECIMEN WILL THEN BE MADE AVAILABLE TO THE ABOVE NAMED COMPANY/EMPLOYER FOR EMPLOYMENT EVALUATION ONLY.

IN ADDITION, I HEREBY ACKNOWLEDGE THAT THE SPECIMEN LABELED WITH THE IDENTIFICATION NUMBER BELOW IS MY OWN, AND THE SPECIMEN WAS LABELED AND SEALED IN MY PRESENCE.

IN ADDITION, I ACKNOWLEDGE THAT THE FOLLOWING PRESCRIPTION AND/OR NONPRESCRIPTION MEDICATIONS ARE THE ONLY MEDICATIONS I HAVE TAKEN WITHIN THE LAST 7 DAYS:

I HEREBY RELEASE ALL TESTING FACILITIES, THE ABOVE NAMED EMPLOYER/COMPANY, THEIR EMPLOYEES, AGENTS, AND REPRESENTATIVES FROM ANY AND ALL LIABILITY ARISING FROM THE RELEASE OF THE INFORMATION DISCOVERED FROM MY TEST.

SIGNATURE OF DONOR   DATE / TIME

CHAIN OF CUSTODY: TO BE INITIATED BY THE COLLECTOR AND COMPLETED AS NECESSARY THEREAFTER

DATE MO. DAY YR.	SPECIMEN RELEASED BY	SPECIMEN RECEIVED BY	PURPOSE OF CHANGE
/ /	DONOR - NO SIGNATURE	Signature / Name	PROVIDE SPECIMEN FOR TESTING
/ /	Signature / Name	Signature / Name	
/ /	Signature / Name	Signature / Name	
/ /	Signature / Name	Signature / Name	
/ /	Signature / Name	Signature / Name	
/ /	Signature / Name	Signature / Name	
/ /	Signature / Name	Signature / Name	

LAB USE ONLY

SEAL INTACT   YES   NO   VOLUME   SPECIMEN IS   ☐ ACCEPTED   ☐ NOT SUITABLE FOR ANALYSIS

COMMENTS

Peel and place over CAP   Specimen ID Number: 123456

- ♦ **Abuse Screen** *see* Drugs of Abuse Testing, Urine *on page 788*

- ♦ **Acephen®** *see* Acetaminophen, Serum *on page 778*

- ♦ **Aceta®** *see* Acetaminophen, Serum *on page 778*

- ♦ **Acetaldehyde Adducts** *see* Ethanol, Blood, Urine, and Other Sources *on page 789*

Acetaminophen, Serum

Related Information

Alanine Aminotransferase, Serum *on page 87*
Aspartate Aminotransferase, Serum *on page 112*
Liver Biopsy *on page 65*
Liver Disease: Laboratory Assessment, Overview *on page 216*
Warfarin *on page 770*

Synonyms Acephen®; Aceta®; Anacin-3®; Apacet®; Banesin®; Dapa®; Datril®; Dorcol®; Feverall™; Genapap®; Halenol®; Liquiprin®; Meda-Cap®; Myapap® Drops; Neopap®; Panadol®; Paracetamol; Redutemp®; Ridenol®; Snaplets-FR® Granules; Tempra®; Tylenol®; Ty-Pap; Uni-Ace®

Applies to Acetanilide; Phenacetin

Abstract Acetaminophen is an analgesic-antipyretic available singly or in combination with a number of other medications such as codeine, acetylsalicylic acid, and caffeine. It is the most frequently ingested medication in the U.S., and is frequently seen in the deliberate overdose situation. In addition to suicidal overdose, acetaminophen-related hepatic necrosis is recognized in a "therapeutic misadventure" scenario. The alcohol-acetaminophen syndrome, in which an alcoholic uses acetaminophen in doses exceeding those recommended (4 g/24 hours), is characterized by a direct toxic reaction. It may be the most common form of acute liver failure.[1] Fasting also is a cofactor for toxicity. The prognosis depends on the amount ingested and the time of presentation.

More than 200 formulations containing acetaminophen are available in the U.S.

Specimen Serum

Container Red top tube

Sampling Time If ingestion time is known, the sample should be drawn 4 hours after ingestion.

Reference Interval Acetaminophen, serum: 10-30 μg/mL (SI: 66-169 μmol/L). (Multiply by 6.62 to convert to μmol/L.)

Critical Values Toxic: >150 μg/mL (SI: >990 μmol/L) (4 hours postingestion); >50 μg/mL (SI: >330 μmol/L) (12 hours postingestion). See nomogram.

Use Evaluation of possible toxicity, therapeutic monitoring, or compliance assessment. Acetaminophen causes dose-related centrilobular (zone 3) hepatic necrosis. It can lead to hepatic necrosis in patients with enhanced susceptibility, even in therapeutic doses.[2] In normal individuals, its toxic effect is predictable when quantities exceeding recommended doses are taken.[1]

Methodology UV spectrophotometry, immunoassay, gas-liquid chromatography (GLC), or high performance liquid chromatography (HPLC). Immunoassay is the most commonly used method.

Additional Information

- Half-life: adults: 1-3 hours; neonates: 2-5 hours
- Volume of distribution: 0.95 L/kg
- Protein binding: 20% to 50%

Acetaminophen is an analgesic and antipyretic with limited anti-inflammatory properties. It is used for headache, fever, and relief of pain in patients who cannot tolerate aspirin or those with bleeding disorders, peptic ulcer disease, or for those at high risk of bleeding or morbidity from bleeding. Acetaminophen is the analgesic/antipyretic of choice in children 13 years of age or younger due to the association of aspirin with possible development of Reye syndrome.

Acetaminophen is rapidly absorbed from the GI tract. Peak plasma concentrations are reached in 30-60 minutes after a therapeutic dose. However, following overdose, the peak plasma concentration may not be reached for 4 hours or more. Acetaminophen is metabolized to several inactive sulfate and glucuronide conjugated forms. There is an intermediate metabolite, N-acetyl-p-benzoquinoneimine, that may be responsible for the hepatic toxicity seen with high doses and prolonged use of acetaminophen. Acetanilide and phenacetin owe much of their analgesic effect to their metabolite, acetaminophen.

Acetaminophen is called a "silent" killer because symptoms may not appear 24-48 hours after ingestion and unfortunately, well after the time that an antidote can be effective. The main site of toxicity is the liver, in which damage can occur with untreated ingestion of 140 mg/kg (7.5 g in an adult). In an acute overdose situation, the following Rumack nomogram will help to determine necessity of acetylcysteine treatment and likelihood of hepatotoxicity. The first sample for drug level should not be drawn until at least 4 hours after ingestion. This allows for complete absorption, but a longer interval may be required in a patient with alcoholic liver disease or other underlying hepatic disease. Acetaminophen toxicity can be underestimated in such patients.[3] Using the Rumack nomogram, if the concentration of acetaminophen at 4 hours postingestion, is above the broken line, an entire course of the antidote, acetylcysteine, is necessary. If the concentration at

that time falls below the broken line, treatment with acetylcysteine may not be needed. Acetylcysteine is recommended for late use by most authors.[4] If a patient presents within 6 hours of ingestion, gastrointestinal decontamination procedures can be started while awaiting the results of the acetaminophen concentration. If the patient presents more than 6 hours after ingestion, a loading dose of acetylcysteine should be given empirically if the patient has ingested >140 mg/kg of acetaminophen. Chronic ingestion is more difficult to evaluate. If a patient has been consuming >140 mg/kg/24 hours for more than 1-2 days, treatment with acetylcysteine should be started. Early treatment is especially recommended in pregnant subjects.[5] The nomogram is not intended for extended release preparations.

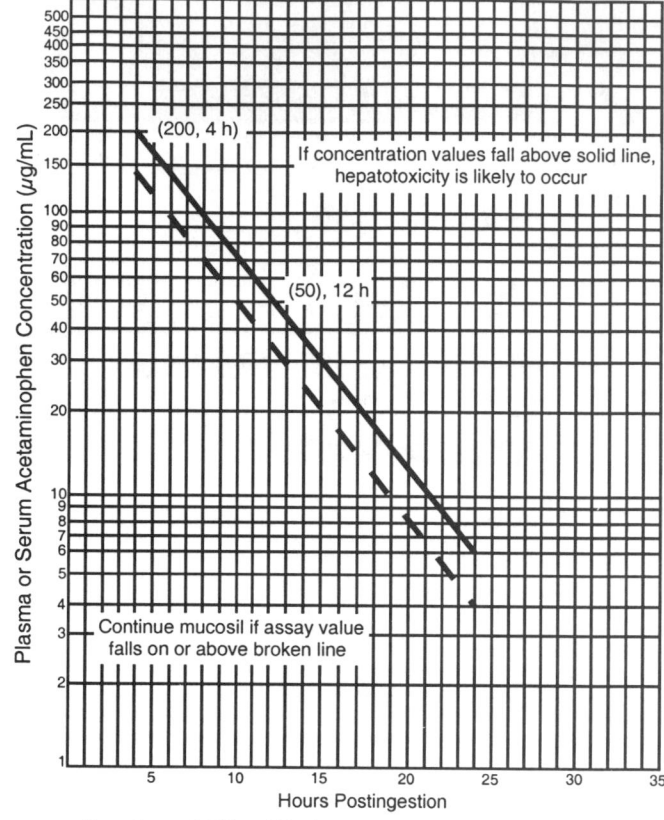

From Rumack BH and Matthews H, "Acetaminophen Poisoning and Toxicity," *Pediatrics*, 1975, 55:871-6, with permission.

Hepatic toxicity may appear 3-5 days after ingestion of a toxic dose. Toxic levels require monitoring with AST, ALT, bilirubin, glucose, creatinine, prothrombin time, partial thromboplastin time, complete blood count, and electrolytes, as well as acetaminophen concentrations for at least 4 days. Extreme increases in AST and ALT distinguish alcohol-acetaminophen syndrome or intentional overdose from alcoholic or viral hepatitis.[1] Serum aminotransferase concentrations >3500 IU/L are characteristic of acetaminophen toxicity. The highest AST level in one series was 34,720 IU/L.[4] Serum levels drawn before 4 hours may not represent peak levels. The hepatotoxicity of acetaminophen is related to the formation of one or more highly reactive metabolites in the liver. When hepatic glutathione is depleted, secondary to starvation and/or chronic ethanol ingestion, toxic metabolites fail to be conjugated and cause hepatic injury. Chronic alcoholics, binge drinkers, and patients taking medications that induce the P-450 system are at greater risk of developing acetaminophen toxicity. Impaired hepatic metabolism may be found in the elderly. Orally administered N-acetylcysteine (Mucomyst®) given through a nasogastric tube immediately and for 48 hours has been shown to provide dramatic protection against acetaminophen hepatotoxicity by replenishment of glutathione. Treatment with N-acetylcystine after 15 hours of overdose, particularly in high-risk patients, is questionable.[6]

Acetaminophen potentiates the anticoagulant activity of warfarin,[7] and is a cause of overcoagulation.[8]

Footnotes

1. Lee WM, "Drug-Induced Hepatotoxicity," *N Engl J Med*, 1995, 333(17):1118-27.

2. Zimmerman HJ, *Hepatotoxicity: The Adverse Effects of Drugs and Other Chemicals on the Liver*, 2nd ed, Philadelphia, PA: Lippincott Williams & Wilkins, 1999.

3. Cheung L, Potts RG, and Meyer KC, "Acetaminophen Treatment Nomogram," *N Engl J Med*, 1994, 330(26):1907-8.

4. Schiødt FV, Rochling FA, Casey DL, et al, "Acetaminophen Toxicity in an Urban County Hospital," *N Engl J Med*, 1997, 337(16):1112-7.

5. Riggs BS, Bronstein AC, Kulig K, et al, "Acute Acetaminophen Overdose During Pregnancy," *Obstet Gynecol*, 1989, 74(2):247-53.

6. Jones AL, "Mechanism of Action and Value of N-acetylcystine in the Treatment of Early and Late Acetaminophen Poisoning: A Critical Review," *J Toxicol Clin Toxicol*, 1998, 36(4):277-85.

7. Bell WR, "Acetaminophen and Warfarin: Undesirable Synergy," *JAMA*, 1998, 279(9):702-3.

8. Hylek EM, Heiman H, Skates SJ, et al, "Acetaminophen and Other Risk Factors for Excessive Warfarin Anticoagulation," *JAMA*, 1998, 279(9):657-62.

References
Ashbourne JF, Olson KR, and Khayam-Bashi H, "Value of Rapid Screening for Acetaminophen in All Patients With Intentional Drug Overdose," *Ann Emerg Med*, 1989, 18(10):1035-8.

Baselt RC, "Acetaminophen," *Disposition of Toxic Drugs and Chemicals in Man*, 5th ed, Foster City, CA: Chemical Toxicology Institute, 2000, 4-8.

Janes J and Routledge PA, "Recent Developments in the Management of Paracetamol (Acetaminophen) Poisoning," *Drug Saf*, 1992, 7(3):170-7.

Kumar S and Rex DK, "Failure of Physicians to Recognize Acetaminophen Hepatotoxicity in Chronic Alcoholics," *Arch Intern Med*, 1991, 151(6):1189-91.

Lewis RK and Paloucek FP, "Assessment and Treatment of Acetaminophen Overdose," *Clin Pharm*, 1991, 10(10):765-74.

Lieber CS, "Medical Disorders of Alcoholism," *N Engl J Med*, 1995, 333(16):1058-65.

Montamat SC, Cusack BJ, and Vestal RE, "Management of Drug Therapy in the Elderly," *N Engl J Med*, 1989, 321(5):303-9.

Rumack BH and Matthew H, "Acetaminophen Poisoning and Toxicity," *Pediatrics*, 1975, 55(6):871-6.

Salgia AD and Kosnik SD, "When Acetaminophen Use Becomes Toxic. Treating Acute Accidental and Intentional Overdose," *Postgrad Med*, 1999, 105(4):81-90.

Smilkstein MJ, Knapp GL, Kulig KW, et al, "Efficacy of Oral N-acetylcysteine in the Treatment of Acetaminophen Overdose. Analysis of the National Multicenter Study (1976 to 1985)," *N Engl J Med*, 1988, 319(24):1557-62.

Tighe TV and Walter FG, "Delayed Toxic Acetaminophen Level After Initial Four Hour Nontoxic Level," *J Toxicol Clin Toxicol*, 1994, 32(4):431-4.

♦ **Acetanilide** see Acetaminophen, Serum *on page 778*

♦ **Acetone** see Volatile Screen, Blood or Urine *on page 809*

♦ **Acetylcholinesterase** see Organophosphate Pesticides, Urine, Blood, or Serum *on page 804*

♦ **6-0-Acetyl Morphine** see Morphine, Urine *on page 802*

♦ **Acetylsalicylic Acid, Blood** see Salicylate, Serum or Plasma *on page 806*

♦ **Actacode** see Codeine, Urine *on page 786*

♦ **Adam** see 3,4 Methylenedioxymethamphetamine, Urine *on page 801*

♦ **Advil®** see Ibuprofen, Serum *on page 793*

♦ **Alcohol** see Ethanol, Blood, Urine, and Other Sources *on page 789*

♦ **Amobarb** see Barbiturates, Qualitative, Urine *on page 781*

Amphetamine, Qualitative, Urine

Related Information
Chain-of-Custody Protocol *on page 785*
Drugs of Abuse Testing, Urine *on page 788*
Haloperidol, Serum or Plasma *on page 752*
Methamphetamine, Qualitative, Urine *on page 799*

Synonyms Bennies; Crystal; Dexedrine®; Dexies; Ferndex®; Speed; Uppers

Test Includes Amphetamine, methamphetamine

Abstract Amphetamine is a sympathomimetic amine. This group of agents exerts alpha- and beta-adrenergic effects and are chemically related to catecholamines. Amphetamine is used as a central nervous system stimulant for the management of hyperkinetic syndromes and narcolepsy. It is also used in the treatment of obesity. Due to euphoric effects, it has a high potential for abuse and the use of amphetamine for weight reduction has been curtailed. It is a DEA schedule II drug.

Specimen Random urine

Collection If forensic, observe precautions (see the Introduction *on page 773*).

Storage Instructions Refrigerate

Causes for Rejection If forensic, failure to meet temperature requirements and/or tests for unusual urine dilution (specific gravity or creatinine) or alteration

Turnaround Time Usually 1-2 hours for screen if done in-house. Confirmation, 1-3 days.

Special Instructions If forensic, use Chain-of-Custody form. See the Chain-of-Custody form in the Introduction *on page 773*.

Reference Interval Negative (less than cutoff)

Critical Values Substance Abuse and Mental Health Services Administration (SAMHSA) cutoff: screen: 1000 ng/mL; confirmation: 500 ng/mL. For methamphetamine, a positive report requires methamphetamine ≥500 ng/mL and amphetamine (a metabolite) ≥200 ng/mL in the same sample.

Use Drug abuse evaluation; toxicity assessment; patient compliance; therapeutic drug monitoring

Limitations Some over-the-counter cold and antiallergy medications may cross react in certain immunoassay screens; confirmation by a different, more sensitive and specific method (eg, GC/MS) is necessary. False-positive and false-negative results diminish the value of urine screening, leading to need for confirmation.

Methodology Screen: fluorescence polarization immunoassay (FPIA),[1] radioimmunoassay (RIA), enzyme immunoassay (EIA), gas chromatography (GC), thin-layer chromatography (TLC), high performance liquid chromatography (HPLC).

Confirmation: gas chromatography/mass spectrometry (GC/MS). To distinguish illicit from legitimate use, there is frequently a need to distinguish d and l enantiomers. This is achieved by using stereospecific column or special derivatizing agents.[2]

Additional Information
- Half-life: 10-20 hours (usual urine pH); 5-10 hours (acidic urine)
- Volume of distribution: 3-4 L/kg
- Protein binding: 10% to 40%
- Urine detection time for amphetamine and methamphetamine: 2-4 days

For the amphetamine class, the material detected is the parent drug. Amphetamines are stimulants that tend to increase alertness and physical activity. Methamphetamine is more frequently abused because its more pronounced central effects are preferred. See Methamphetamine, Qualitative, Urine *on page 799*. Some drivers use amphetamines to counteract the drowsiness or "down" feeling caused by sleeping pills or alcohol. In pure form, they are yellowish crystals that are manufactured into tablets or capsules. Abusers also sniff the crystals, make a solution and inject it. Can be detected in urine as early as 3 hours after use and persists for as long as 24-48 hours.

Amphetamine and methamphetamine facilitate the release of catecholamines, including dopamine and norepinephrine. These drugs increase heart and breathing rate and blood pressure, dilate pupils, and decrease appetite. The user can experience a dry mouth, sweating, headache, blurred vision, dizziness, sleeplessness, and anxiety. Extremely high doses can cause people to flush or become pale; they can cause a rapid or irregular heartbeat, tremors, loss of coordination, and even physical collapse. Individuals who use a large dose over a long period of time may develop an amphetamine psychosis: seeing, hearing, and feeling things that do not exist, having irrational thoughts or beliefs and feeling that people are out to get them. People in this extremely suspicious state frequently exhibit bizarre and sometimes violent behavior. There is no specific antidote for amphetamine overdose and the treatment is generally supportive. Tolerance to the drug is developed after repeated use. Life-threatening overdoses are rare.

In interpretation of methamphetamine and amphetamine concentrations, positive test knowledge of legitimate and illicit sources is important. Amphetamines are sometimes prescribed as weight-reducing medicines. Many substances (amphetaminil, benzphetamine, clobenzorex, deprenyl, dimethylamphetamine, ethylamphetamine, famprofazone, fencamine, fenethylline, tenproporex, furfenorex, mefenorex, mesocarb, and prenylamine) which are available as prescription drugs, are metabolized in the body to methamphetamine or amphetamine.[3]

Footnotes

1. Turner GJ, Colbert DL, and Chowdry BZ, "A Broad Spectrum Immunoassay Using Fluorescence Polarization for the Detection of Amphetamines in Urine," *Ann Clin Biochem*, 1991, 28(Pt 6):588-94.

2. Tetlow VA and Merrill J, "Rapid Determination of Amphetamine Stereoisomer Ratios in Urine by Gas Chromatography-Mass Spectrometry," *Ann Clin Biochem*, 1996, 33(Pt 1):50-4.

3. Musshoff F, "Illegal or Legitimate Use? Precursor Compounds to Amphetamine and Methamphetamine," *Drug Metab Rev*, 2000, 32(1):15-44.

References
Ellenhorn MJ, Schonwald S, Ordog G, et al, "Amphetamines and Designer Drugs," *Ellenhorn's Medical Toxicology: Diagnosis and Treatment of Human Poisoning*, Baltimore, MD: Lippincott Williams & Wilkins, 1997, 340-55.

Gillogley KM, Evans AT, Hansen RL, et al, "The Perinatal Impact of Cocaine, Amphetamine, and Opiate Use Detected by Universal Intrapartum Screening," *Am J Obstet Gynecol*, 1990, 163(5 Pt 1):1535-42.

Grinstead GF, "Ranitidine and High Concentrations of Phenylpropanolamine Cross React in the EMIT Monoclonal Amphetamine/Methamphetamine Assay," *Clin Chem*, 1989, 35(9):1998-9.

Hughes R, Hughes A, Levine B, et al, "Stability of Phencyclidine and Amphetamines in Urine Specimens," *Clin Chem*, 1991, 37(12):2141-2.

Jones AL, Jarvie DR, McDermid G, et al, "Hepatocellular Damage Following Amphetamine Intoxication," *J Toxicol Clin Toxicol*, 1994, 32(4):435-44.

Levine B, "Amphetamines/Sympathomimetic Amines," *Principles of Forensic Toxicology*, Washington, DC: AACC Press, American Association of Clinical Chemistry, 1999, 265-85.

Martz W and Schutz HW, "Synthetic Sweetener Cyclamate as a Potential Source of False-Positive Amphetamine Results in the TDx System," *Clin Chem*, 1991, 37(11):2016-7.

Williams RH, Erickson T, and Broussard LA, "Evaluating Sympathomimetic Intoxication in an Emergency Setting," *Lab Med*, 2000, 31(9):497-507.

♦ **Amphetamines** see Drugs of Abuse Testing, Urine *on page 788*

♦ **Anacin®** see Salicylate, Serum or Plasma *on page 806*

♦ **Anacin-3®** see Acetaminophen, Serum *on page 778*

♦ **Angel Dust** see Phencyclidine, Qualitative, Urine *on page 804*

♦ **Antifreeze** see Ethylene Glycol, Serum or Plasma *on page 790*

♦ **Apacet®** see Acetaminophen, Serum *on page 778*

♦ **Arsenate** see Arsenic, Urine *on page 781*

♦ **Arsenic, Gastric Content** *see* Arsenic, Urine *on page 781*

♦ **Arsenic, Hair** *see* Arsenic, Hair, Nails *on page 780*

Arsenic, Hair, Nails

Related Information
Arsenic, Serum or Plasma *on page 780*
Arsenic, Urine *on page 781*
Heavy Metal Screen, Blood *on page 792*
Heavy Metal Screen, Urine *on page 792*

Synonyms Arsenic, Hair; Arsenic, Nails; As^{3+} (As III); As^{5+} (As V); As, Quantitative

Applies to Hair Analysis; Mee's Lines

Abstract Well known as a means of doing away with one's undesirable acquaintances, this toxic heavy metal is incorporated into keratin, including that of hair and nails. Its presence there in abnormal concentrations is evidence of chronic poisoning. Characteristics of arsenic include high affinity for cysteine, explaining its affinity for keratin, leading to its concentration in hair and nails and its relationship to tumors of the skin (among other sites). In addition to hyperkeratosis, hypopigmentation and hyperpigmentation, transverse striae of fingernails (Mee's lines) may be seen.[1] (Mee's lines can be found as well following intoxication with cadmium, lead, thallium and mercury.)

Chronic exposure to arsenic commonly involves insecticides, industrial sources[2,3] or contamination of food, water,[4,5,6] soil,[7] or medications. Evidence of chronic arsenic poisoning may be manifested 2-8 weeks after ingestion.

Specimen Clean hair or nails, ≥0.5 g

Container Clean envelope or heavy metal-free screw top plastic container

Collection Extreme care is necessary to avoid surface contamination. Hair from the nape of the neck indicates more recent ingestion, while axillary or pubic hair provides evidence of earlier exposure (6-12 months before).[8] Toenails are preferable to fingernails; they are less prone to surface contamination.

Special Instructions Hair should be clean, free of oil and tonic; clip close. Nails should be thoroughly washed, dried, and clipped close to cuticle.

Reference Interval Up to 1 μg/g (SI: 0.13 nmol/g)

Critical Values Values >100 μg/g (SI: >13.4 nmol/g) of hair are considered toxic

Use Diagnose chronic arsenic exposure and intoxication; accumulation of arsenic takes place in bones, hair, and nails since arsenic is laid down in keratin soon after ingestion.

Limitations Urine arsenic concentration is a better indication of recent exposure.

Hair mineral analysis from a number of commercial laboratories was recently found to be unreliable. No CLIA specialty area for hair analysis is available. No approved proficiency testing program for hair mineral analysis exists. For substances other than mercury and arsenic, little or no experimental evidence supports application of hair as a true biologically active marker. Hair analysis for nutritional balance is regarded as generally unreliable.[9,10] A current *JAMA* editorial recommends that patients be advised of the economic consequences of purchases of vitamins or other nutritional supplements from either the laboratory or the practitioner ordering hair analysis tests (for substances other than arsenic or mercury) and the uncertainty of any possible medical consequences based on hair analysis laboratory values.[10]

Methodology Inductively-coupled plasma-mass spectrometry (ICP-MS), electrothermal atomic absorption spectrometry (AA), neutron activation analysis. Standard methods for hair analysis for a number of substances do not exist. Appropriate reference ranges for clinical significance of nutritional importance are not available.[10]

Additional Information Arsenic binds to protein sulfhydryl groups. Variations in arsenic hair levels may be due to geographic location and exposure to industrial waste and drinking water. Complications of chronic arsenic exposure include carcinomas of skin; associations with carcinoma of lung[11] and transitional cell carcinoma of bladder[11,12,13,14] and kidney[15] are also recognized.[16]

The arsenic-related carcinomas of skin include basal cell carcinoma[17] and squamous cell carcinoma including those of Bowen type.[18,19,20] A relationship to Merkel cell carcinoma is also perceived.[21,22] (Merkel cell carcinoma is an uncommon, aggressive neuroendocrine neoplasm of skin). Arsenic-related keratoderma is also recognized.[23]

In 1995, the Toxicology Crime Laboratory of the United States FBI reported toxic levels of arsenic from the hairs of Napoleon Bonaparte, confirming a 1960 report from the University of Glasgow. Napoleon suffered chronic arsenic poisoning on St Helena.[24]

Footnotes
1. Quecedo E, Sanmartin O, Febrer MI, et al, "Mees' Lines: A Clue for the Diagnosis of Arsenic Poisoning," *Arch Dermatol*, 1996, 132(3):349-50.
2. Lubin JH, Pottern LM, Stone BJ, et al, "Respiratory Cancer in a Cohort of Copper Smelter Workers: Results From More Than 50 Years of Follow-up," *Am J Epidemiol*, 2000, 151(6):554-65.
3. Mohamed KB, "Occupational Contact Dermatitis From Arsenic in a Tin-Smelting Factory," *Contact Dermatitis*, 1998, 38(4):224-5.

4. Cantor KP, "Arsenic in Drinking: How Much Is Too Much?," *Epidemiology*, 1996, 7(2):113-5.
5. Karagas MR, Tosteson TD, Blum J, et al, "Measurement of Low Levels of Arsenic Exposure: A Comparison of Water and Toenail Concentrations," *Am J Epidemiol*, 2000, 152(1):84-90.
6. Tondel M, Rahman M, Magnuson A, et al, "The Relationship of Arsenic Levels in Drinking Water and the Prevalence Rate of Skin Lesions in Bangladesh," *Environ Health Perspect*, 1999, 107(9):727-9.
7. Hwang YH, Bornschein RL, Grote J, et al, "Urinary Arsenic Excretion as a Biomarker of Arsenic Exposure in Children," *Arch Environ Health*, 1997, 52(2):139-47.
8. Moyer TP, "Toxic Metals," *Tietz Textbook of Clinical Chemistry*, 3rd ed, Burtis CA and Ashwood ER, eds, Philadelphia, PA: WB Saunders, Co, 1999, 982-98.
9. Seidel S, Kreutzer R, Smith D, et al, "Assessment of Commercial Laboratories Performing Hair Mineral Analysis," *JAMA*, 2001, 285(1):67-72.
10. Steindel SJ and Howanitz PJ, "The Uncertainty of Hair Analysis for Trace Metals," *JAMA*, 2001, 285(1):83-5.
11. Smith AH, Goycoolea M, Haque R, et al, "Marked Increase in Bladder and Lung Cancer Mortality in a Region of Northern Chile Due to Arsenic in Drinking Water," *Am J Epidemiol*, 1998, 147(7):660-9.
12. Chow NH, Guo YL, Lin JS, et al, "Clinicopathological Features of Bladder Cancer Associated With Chronic Exposure to Arsenic," *Br J Cancer*, 1997, 75(11):1708-10.
13. Steinmaus C, Moore L, Hopenhayn-Rich C, et al, "Arsenic in Drinking Water and Bladder Cancer," *Cancer Invest*, 2000, 18(2):174-82.
14. Hopenhayn-Rich C, Biggs ML, Fuchs A, et al, "Bladder Cancer Mortality Associated With Arsenic in Drinking Water in Argentina," *Epidemiology*, 1996, 7(2):117-24.
15. Guo HR, Chiang HS, Hu H, et al, "Arsenic in Drinking Water and Incidence of Urinary Cancers," *Epidemiology*, 1997, 8(5):545-50.
16. Smith AH, Lingas EO, and Rahman M, "Contamination of Drinking-Water by Arsenic in Bangladesh: A Public Health Emergency," *Bull World Health Organ*, 2000, 78(9):1093-103.
17. Boonchai W, Walsh M, Cummings M, et al, "Expression of p53 in Arsenic-Related and Sporadic Basal Cell Carcinoma," *Arch Dermatol*, 2000, 136(2):195-8.
18. Matsui M, Nishigori C, Toyokuni S, et al, "The Role of Oxidative DNA Damage in Human Arsenic Carcinogenesis: Detection of 8-Hydroxy-2'-Deoxyguanosine in Arsenic-Related Bowen's Disease," *J Invest Dermatol*, 1999, 113(1):26-31.
19. Hsu CH, Yang SA, Wang JY, et al, "Mutational Spectrum of p53 Gene in Arsenic-Related Skin Cancers From the Blackfoot Disease Endemic Area of Taiwan," *Br J Cancer*, 1999, 80(7):1080-6.
20. Wong SS, Tan KC, and Goh CL, "Cutaneous Manifestations of Chronic Arsenicism: Review of Seventeen Cases," *J Am Acad Dermatol*, 1998, 38(2 Pt 1):179-85.
21. Lien HC, Tsai TF, Lee YY, et al, "Merkel Cell Carcinoma and Chronic Arsenicism," *J Am Acad Dermatol*, 1999, 41(4):641-3.
22. Tsuruta D, Hamada T, Mochida K, et al, "Merkel Cell Carcinoma, Bowen's Disease and Chronic Occupational Arsenic Poisoning," *Br J Dermatol*, 1998, 139(2):291-4.
23. Navarro B, Sayas MJ, Atienza A, et al, "An Unhappily Married Man With Thick Soles," *Lancet*, 1996, 347(9015):1596.
24. Weider B and Fournier JH, "Activation Analyses of Authenticated Hairs of Napoleon Bonaparte Confirm Arsenic Poisoning," *Am J Forensic Med Pathol*, 1999, 20(4):378-82.

References
Bartolome B, Cordoba S, Nieto S, et al, "Acute Arsenic Poisoning: Clinical and Histopathological Features," *Br J Dermatol*, 1999, 141(6):1106-9.
Germolec DR, Spalding J, Yu HS, et al, "Arsenic Enhancement of Skin Neoplasia by Chronic Stimulation of Growth Factors," *Am J Pathol*, 1998, 153(6):1775-85.
Hei TK, Liu SX, and Waldren C, "Mutagenicity of Arsenic in Mammalian Cells: Role of Reactive Oxygen Species," *Proc Natl Acad Sci U S A*, 1998, 95(14):8103-7.
Hertz-Picciotto I, Arrighi HM, and Hu SW, "Does Arsenic Exposure Increase the Risk for Circulatory Disease?" *Am J Epidemiol*, 2000, 151(2):174-81.
Mayo Medical Laboratories, 2000 Test Catalogue, Rochester, MN, 87.
Santra A, Maiti A, Das S, et al, "Hepatic Damage Caused by Chronic Arsenic Toxicity in Experimental Animals," *J Toxicol Clin Toxicol*, 2000, 38(4):395-405.
Westveer AE, Trestrail JH, and Pinizzotto AJ, "Homicidal Poisoning in the United States: An Analysis of the Uniform Crime Reports From 1980 Through 1989," *Am J Forensic Med Pathol*, 1996, 17(4):282-8.
Woollons A and Russell-Jones R, "Chronic Endemic Hydroarsenicism," *Br J Dermatol*, 1998, 139(6):1092-6.

♦ **Arsenic, Nails** *see* Arsenic, Hair, Nails *on page 780*

Arsenic, Serum or Plasma

Related Information
Arsenic, Hair, Nails *on page 780*
Arsenic, Urine *on page 781*
Heavy Metal Screen, Blood *on page 792*
Heavy Metal Screen, Urine *on page 792*

Synonyms As

Applies to Hair Analysis; Heavy Metal Screen, Arsenic

Abstract Arsenic is a toxic heavy metal. It exists in various forms. Arsine gas, As^{3+}, and As^{5+} are toxic forms; organic forms are less toxic. Arsenic is found in soil and rocks. Major sources of human exposure are arsenic in food resulting from broad use of arsenical insecticides and from drinking water,[1] especially well water.[2] Acute arsenic toxicity follows accidental ingestion, industrial accidents, suicide or homicide. For children, 2 mg/kg body weight can cause lethal arsenic poisoning. Adamsite and Lewisite, war gases of World War I, are arsenic compounds.

Container Trace metal-free containers, royal blue top (EDTA) Monoject® trace element tube

Sampling Time Half-life of inorganic arsenic in blood is 4-6 hours and that of its methylated metabolites, 20-30 hours.[3]

Collection See Blood Collection Methods for Trace Elements in the Trace Elements Introduction *on page 811.*

Causes for Rejection Containers not metal-free

Reference Interval <70 µg/L (SI: 0.93 µmol/L)

Critical Values Poisoning: 100-500 µg/L (SI: 1.33-6.65 µmol/L)

Use Blood arsenic is for the diagnosis of acute poisoning only; use urine for chronic poisoning. Acute arsenic poisoning may be signaled by the abrupt onset of vomiting and diarrhea.

Limitations Short half-life in blood, 4-6 hours. **Serum or plasma is the least useful specimen, except in acute poisoning.** With acute intoxication, the total concentration of As was 7- to 350-fold less than that of the organs in an autopsy of death from arsenic trioxide.[4] Sample collection after food can cause As elevation.

Methodology Inductively-coupled plasma-mass spectrometry (ICP-MS), electrothermal atomic absorption spectrometry (AA)

Additional Information
- Half-life: 4-6 hours
- Volume of distribution: 0.2 L/kg

Whole blood and serum have been used for arsenic determination. Blood levels of arsenic have a short half-life and the half-lives of the methylated metabolites are only 20-30 hours after exposure. Urine arsenic concentration is a better measure of chronic arsenic poisoning. In addition to insecticides, pesticides, rodenticides, weed killers, paint, and wood preservatives contain inorganic arsenic. See Arsenic, Hair, Nails *on page 780.*

Arsenic can be absorbed through the gastrointestinal tract, by inhalation, and by penetration of the skin.

Arsine gas (AsH_3), combining with the globin chain in red cells, causes hemolysis with hemoglobinuria and hematuria. Acute renal failure may cause death.

Although valence three arsenic (As^{3+}) is more toxic than valence five (As^{5+}), arsenic trioxide has provided remission of acute promyelocytic leukemia.[5,6]

Arsenic intoxication causes hypotension, tachycardia, conduction blocks, dysrhythmias, changes of mental status, rhabdomyolysis, pulmonary edema, encephalopathy, seizures, neuropathy, hepatic and renal dysfunction, hemolytic anemia, and bone marrow toxicity. Chronic toxicity manifests cutaneous changes, including alopecia, hyperkeratosis, and hyperpigmentation.[7] See Arsenic, Hair, Nails *on page 780.*

Footnotes
1. Tsai SM, Wang TN, and Ko YC, "Mortality for Certain Diseases in Areas With High Levels of Arsenic in Drinking Water," *Arch Environ Health,* 1999, 54(3):186-93.
2. Graeme KA and Pollack CV, "Heavy Metal Toxicity, Part I: Arsenic and Mercury," *J Emerg Med,* 1998, 16(1):45-56.
3. Moyer TP, "Toxic Metals," *Tietz Textbook of Clinical Chemistry,* 3rd ed, Burtis CA and Ashwood ER, eds, Philadelphia, PA: WB Saunders Co, 1999, 982-98.
4. Benramdane L, Accominotti M, Fanton L, et al, "Arsenic Speciation in Human Organs Following Fatal Arsenic Trioxide Poisoning - A Case Report," *Clin Chem,* 1999, 45(2):301-6.
5. Soignet SL, Maslak P, Wang ZG, et al, "Complete Remission After Treatment of Acute Promyelocytic Leukemia With Arsenic Trioxide," *N Engl J Med,* 1998, 339(19):1341-8.
6. Huang SY, Chang CS, Tang JL, et al, "Acute and Chronic Arsenic Poisoning Associated With Treatment of Acute Promyelocytic Leukaemia," *Br J Haematol,* 1998, 103(4):1092-5.
7. Piamphongsant T, "Chronic Environmental Arsenic Poisoning," *Int J Dermatol,* 1999, 38(6):401-10.

References
Campbell BG, "Broadsheet Number 48: Mercury, Cadmium and Arsenic: Toxicology and Laboratory Investigation," *Pathology,* 1999, 31(1):17-22.
Klaasen C, ed, *Casarett and Doull's Toxicology,* 5th ed, New York, NY: Macmillan Publishing, 1996, 696-9.
Mathieu D, Mathieu-Nolf M, Germain-Alonso M, et al, "Massive Arsenic Poisoning - Effect of Hemodialysis and Dimercaprol on Arsenic Kinetics," *Intensive Care Med,* 1992, 18(1):47-50.
Zhang X, Cornelis R, de Kimpe J, et al, "Study of Arsenic-Protein Binding in Serum of Patients on Continuous Ambulatory Peritoneal Dialysis," *Clin Chem,* 1998, 44(1):141-7.

Arsenic, Urine

Related Information
Arsenic, Hair, Nails *on page 780*
Arsenic, Serum or Plasma *on page 780*
Heavy Metal Screen, Blood *on page 792*
Heavy Metal Screen, Urine *on page 792*
Urine Collection, 24-Hour *on page 47*

Synonyms As^{3+} (As III); As^{5+} (As V); As, Quantitative, Urine

Applies to Arsenate; Arsenic, Gastric Content; Arsenite; Dimethylarsine; DMA; MMA; Monomethylarsine

Test Includes Organic forms of arsenic can also be evaluated.

Abstract This toxic heavy metal appears in urine and stools. Its excretion rate in urine is used to determine toxicity. Arsenic exists in various inorganic and organic forms, of which arsine gas, As^{3+}, and As^{5+} are most toxic. As^{3+} and As^{5+} are partially detoxified to monomethylarsine (MMA) and dimethylarsine (DMA) and excreted in urine.

Patient Preparation Patient should avoid seafood for 48 hours before collection is begun. Organic arsenic may be found especially in shellfish, cod, and haddock.[1] Seafood may contain arsenic as high as 10 mg/lb.

Specimen 24-hour urine

Container Acid-washed plastic container, no preservative, no metal cap or insert

Sampling Time Following ingestion, urine As^{3+} and As^{5+} peak at ~10 hours and return to normal in 20-30 hours. The metabolites, MMA and DMA, are important >24 hours following ingestion, peaking at 40-60 hours, disappearing after 6-20 days.[1]

Collection Collect a 24-hour urine specimen, on ice, with care to avoid specimen contact with metal.

Storage Instructions 4°C and -20°C are suitable storage temperatures for urine specimens for up to 2 months.[2]

Reference Interval Ranges for urine arsenic levels can be variable among different laboratories. A general guideline is given: normal: <120 µg/24 hours (SI: >1.59 µmol/L); chronic exposure: 100-200 µg/L (SI: 1.3-2.6 µmol/L).

Critical Values Toxic: >850 µg/L (SI: >11.3 µmol/L).

Use Evaluate recent exposure to arsenic, arsenic toxicity

Limitations Spot levels, if normal, may not rule out arsenic poisoning.[3] Seafood, particularly shellfish, can increase urinary As to as much as 2000 µg/L.[4]

Methodology Inductively-coupled plasma-mass spectrometry (ICP-MS),[5] chromatography/atomic emission spectroscopy, atomic absorption spectrometry (AA). Methods are intended to distinguish between organic, nontoxic forms and inorganic, toxic forms.

Additional Information 25 mL acidified gastric washing is acceptable for arsenic analysis; gastric content normally contains no arsenic. Random urine samples are acceptable.

Sources of As intoxication are briefly outlined in Arsenic, Hair, Nails *on page 780.* Other reported sources include bird's nest soup.[6]

Arsenic is radiopaque. Abdominal x-rays may prove helpful, but usually are not.[3]

Footnotes
1. Moyer TP, "Toxic Metals," *Tietz Textbook of Clinical Chemistry,* 3rd ed, Burtis CA and Ashwood ER, eds, Philadelphia, PA: WB Saunders Co, 1999, 982-98.
2. Feldmann J, Lai VW, Cullen WR, et al, "Sample Preparation and Storage Can Change Arsenic Speciation in Human Urine," *Clin Chem,* 1999, 45(11):1988-97.
3. Brayer AF, Callahan CM, and Wax PM, "Acute Arsenic Poisoning From Ingestion of "Snakes"," *Pediatr Emerg Care,* 1997, 13(6):394-6.
4. Graeme KA and Pollack CV, "Heavy Metal Toxicity, Part I: Arsenic and Mercury," *J Emerg Med,* 1998, 16(1):45-56.
5. Mayo Medical Laboratories, *2000 Test Catalogue,* Rochester, MN, 87.
6. Luong KV and Nguyen LT, "Organic Arsenic Intoxication From Bird's Nest Soup," *Am J Med Sci,* 1999, 317(4):269-71.

References
Amdur MO, Doull J, and Klaasen CD, ed, *Casarett and Doull's Toxicology: The Basic Science of Poisons,* 5th ed, New York, NY: McGraw-Hill, 1996, 696-9..
Dang TM, Tran QT, and Vu KV, "Determination of Arsenic in Urine by Atomic Absorption Spectrophotometry for Biological Monitoring of Occupational Exposure to Arsenic," *Toxicol Lett,* 1999, 108(2-3):179-83.
Ihrig MM, Shalat SL, and Baynes C, "A Hospital-Based Case-Control Study of Stillbirths and Environmental Exposure to Arsenic Using an Atmospheric Dispersion Model Linked to a Geographical Information System," *Epidemiology,* 1998, 9(3):290-4.
Peters GR, McCurdy RF, and Hindmarsh JT, "Environmental Aspects of Arsenic Toxicity," *Crit Rev Clin Lab Sci,* 1996, 33(6):457-93.

♦ **Arsenite** *see* Arsenic, Urine *on page 781*

♦ **As** *see* Arsenic, Serum or Plasma *on page 780*

♦ **As³⁺ (As III)** *see* Arsenic, Hair, Nails *on page 780*

♦ **As³⁺ (As III)** *see* Arsenic, Urine *on page 781*

♦ **As⁵⁺ (As V)** *see* Arsenic, Hair, Nails *on page 780*

♦ **As⁵⁺ (As V)** *see* Arsenic, Urine *on page 781*

♦ **ASA, Blood** *see* Salicylate, Serum or Plasma *on page 806*

♦ **Ascriptin®** *see* Salicylate, Serum or Plasma *on page 806*

♦ **Aspergum®** *see* Salicylate, Serum or Plasma *on page 806*

♦ **Aspirin, Blood** *see* Salicylate, Serum or Plasma *on page 806*

♦ **As, Quantitative** *see* Arsenic, Hair, Nails *on page 780*

♦ **As, Quantitative, Urine** *see* Arsenic, Urine *on page 781*

♦ **Astramorph™ PF** *see* Morphine, Urine *on page 802*

♦ **Banesin®** *see* Acetaminophen, Serum *on page 778*

♦ **Barbiturates** *see* Drugs of Abuse Testing, Urine *on page 788*

Barbiturates, Qualitative, Urine

Related Information
Chain-of-Custody Protocol *on page 785*
(Continued)

Barbiturates, Qualitative, Urine *(Continued)*

Synonyms Amobarb; Butalbital; Mephobarb; Pentobarb; Phenobarb; Secobarb

Test Includes Identification and confirmation of barbiturates in urine

Abstract Barbiturates are sedative hypnotics which are also drugs of abuse. Overdose causes CNS depression. The effects of barbiturates are augmented by other CNS depressants such as ethanol and benzodiazepines.

Specimen Random urine

Collection If forensic, observe precautions (see the Introduction *on page 773*).

Storage Instructions Refrigerate specimen.

Causes for Rejection If forensic, failure to meet temperature requirements or test for unusual urine dilution or adulteration

Special Instructions Chain-of-custody documentation required for samples submitted for pre-employment, random employee testing, and forensic purposes. See the Introduction *on page 773* for the Chain-of-Custody form.

Reference Interval Less than cutoff

Critical Values Cutoff: screen: 300 ng/mL, confirmation: 50 or 100 ng/mL

Use Urine drugs-of-abuse testing, pre-employment screens, random drug testing.

Limitations Short- and intermediate-acting barbiturates can be detected in urine 24-72 hours following ingestion, longer-acting drugs up to 7 days.

Methodology Enzyme immunoassay (EIA), fluorescence polarization immunoassay (FPIA), gas chromatography/mass spectrometry (GC/MS)

Additional Information Barbiturates are nonselective CNS depressants that may be used as sedative-hypnotics or anticonvulsants. They are capable of producing all levels of CNS mood effects from sedation to hypnosis to deep coma and anesthesia. Sensory cortex functions, cerebellar functions, and motor activity are decreased. Secobarbital and pentobarbital are short-term hypnotics and lose effectiveness after about 2 weeks of continued usage. Withdrawal symptoms from any barbiturate may be severe and may include convulsions and delirium. The presence of barbiturates in urine is presumptively positive at a level >300 ng/mL using secobarbital as a standard and can indicate prescribed or abused intake of this class of drugs. The presence of these drugs should be confirmed by a specific method.

References

Burtis CA and Ashwood ER, *Tietz Textbook of Clinical Chemistry*, Philadelphia, PA: WB Saunders Co, 1999, 945-50.

Hall BJ and Brodbelt JS, "Determination of Barbiturates by Solid-Phase Microextraction (SPME) and Ion Trap Gas Chromatography-Mass Spectrometry," *J Chromatogr A*, 1997, 777(2):275-82.

Martin-Biosca Y, Sagrado S, Villanueva-Camanas RM, et al, "Determination of Barbiturates in Urine by Micellar Liquid Chromatography and Direct Injection of Sample," *J Pharm Biomed Anal*, 1999, 21(2):331-8.

Maurer HH, "Identification and Differentiation of Barbiturates and Their Metabolites in Urine," *J Chromatogr*, 1990, 530:307-26.

♦ **Bennies** *see* Amphetamine, Qualitative, Urine *on page 779*

♦ **Benzedrine®** *see* Methamphetamine, Qualitative, Urine *on page 799*

♦ **Benzodiazepines** *see* Drugs of Abuse Testing, Urine *on page 788*

♦ **Benzodiazepine, Serum and Urine** *see* Benzodiazepines, Qualitative, Urine *on page 782*

Benzodiazepines, Qualitative, Urine

Related Information

Chain-of-Custody Protocol *on page 785*
Chlordiazepoxide, Serum *on page 742*
Clonazepam, Serum *on page 743*
Diazepam, Serum *on page 745*
Drugs of Abuse Testing, Urine *on page 788*
Flunitrazepam, Urine *on page 791*
Flurazepam, Serum *on page 751*
Oxazepam, Serum *on page 759*
Phenobarbital, Serum or Plasma *on page 760*

Synonyms Tranquilizers (Valium®, Librium®, Dalmane®, Tranxene®, Klonopin™, Ativan®, Serax®, Centrax®, Restoril®, Xanax®, Halcion®, Versed®, Doral®, etc)

Applies to Benzodiazepine, Serum and Urine

Test Includes Alprazolam, chlordiazepoxide, clorazepate, diazepam, lorazepam, oxazepam, flurazepam, temazepam, triazolam, clonazepam, midazolam

Abstract These drugs are sedative-hypnotics, anticonvulsants, and anxiolytics. They are used by more Americans than any other single prescription drug due to their efficacy, safety, low addiction potential, and minimal side effects. Suicidal overdoses are not uncommon.

Specimen Random urine

Storage Instructions Refrigerate or freeze if not analyzing immediately

Reference Interval None present unless prescribed. When used as drug-of-abuse screen, negative (less than cutoff).

Critical Values Screening cutoff: 300 ng/mL (generally as oxazepam); Confirmation cutoff: typically 200 ng/mL, may vary between laboratories

Use Drug abuse evaluation, toxicity assessment

Methodology Immunoassay, thin-layer chromatography (TLC), high performance liquid chromatography (HPLC), gas chromatography (GC), gas chromatography/mass spectrometry (GC/MS)

Additional Information

- Half-life: 3-150 hours, depending on a particular benzodiazepine
- Volume of distribution (for most): 2-5 L/kg
- Protein binding (for most): 90% to 95%

Benzodiazepines are a class of chemically-related central nervous depressants used as sedative-hypnotics to treat sleep disorders, anxiety, alcohol withdrawal, and seizure disorders. This drug class in low doses can cause sedation, drowsiness, blurred vision, fatigue, mental depression, and loss of coordination. In higher doses or used chronically, they can cause confusion, slurred speech, hypotension, and diminished reflexes. Chronic use may produce a physical dependence and a withdrawal syndrome which can last for weeks. Elderly patients are particularly prone to sedation and central nervous system effects, and therefore are given lower doses of the drug.[1] Urine should be screened for benzodiazepines in suspected overdose cases, or as part of an abused drug program. These drugs have a relatively low potential for abuse.[2] They are, however, frequently found with other drugs in emergency room drug screens. Immunoassay screens detect a broad range of drugs and their metabolites in this class using either oxazepam or nordiazepam as calibrators and controls. Using the latter, the test is more specific and more sensitive for detection of flurazepam. Positive screen results (>300 ng/mL of urine metabolites) should be confirmed by an alternate technique. When a screening cutoff of 300 ng/mL is used, certain potent benzodiazepines such as triazolam and flunitrazepam may not be detected.

Despite their widespread use, abuse of benzodiazepines is relatively infrequent and is more likely to occur in individuals who abuse other drugs or alcohol. Benzodiazepine's CNS depressive effect is synergistic with barbiturate or alcohol use.[3] Treatment for benzodiazepine overdose is supportive. Because benzodiazepines are extensively bound to protein, hemoperfusion is not very effective. Flumazenil, a benzodiazepine antagonist, is frequently used and improves the clinical situation.[4,5]

A radioreceptor assay for benzodiazepine concentrations in serum is described.[6]

Footnotes

1. Greenblatt DJ, Harmatz JS, Shapiro L, et al, "Sensitivity to Triazolam in the Elderly," *N Engl J Med*, 1991, 324(24):1691-8
2. Cole JO and Chiarello RJ, "The Benzodiazepines as Drugs of Abuse," *J Psychiatr Res*, 1990, 24(Suppl 2):135-44.
3. Harris RA, Mihic SJ, and Valenzuela CF, "Alcohol and Benzodiazepines: Recent Mechanistic Studies," *Drug Alcohol Depend*, 1998, 51(1-2):155-64.
4. Cone AM and Stott SA, "Flumazenil," *Br J Hosp Med*, 1994, 51(7):346-8.
5. Mullins ME, "First-Degree Atrioventricular Block in Alprazolam Overdose Reversed by Flumazenil," *J Pharm Pharmacol*, 1999, 51(3):367-70.
6. Nishikawa T, Suzuki S, Ohtani H, et al, "Benzodiazepine Concentrations in Sera Determined by Radioreceptor Assay for Therapeutic-Dose Recipients," *Am J Clin Pathol*, 1994, 102(5):605-10.

References

Baker MI and Oleen MA, "The Use of Benzodiazepines Hypnotics in the Elderly," *Pharmacotherapy*, 1988, 8(4):241-7.

Beck O, Lafolie P, Hjemdahl P, et al, "Detection of Benzodiazepine Intake in Therapeutic Doses by Immunoanalysis of Urine: Two Techniques Evaluated and Modified for Improved Performance," *Clin Chem*, 1992, 38(2):271-5.

Fitzgerald RL, Rexin DA, and Herold DA, "Detecting Benzodiazepines: Immunoassays Compared With Negative Chemical Ionization Gas Chromatography/Mass Spectrometry," *Clin Chem*, 1994, 40(3):373-80.

Fraser AD, "Use and Abuse of Benzodiazepines," *Ther Drug Monit*, 1998, 20(5):481-9.

Jones CE, Wians FH Jr, Martinez LA, et al, "Benzodiazepines Identified by Capillary Gas Chromatography-Mass Spectrometry With Specific Ion Screening Used to Detect Benzophenone Derivatives," *Clin Chem*, 1989, 35(7):1394-8.

Montamat SC, Cusack BJ, and Vestal RE, "Management of Drug Therapy in the Elderly," *N Engl J Med*, 1989, 321(5):303-9.

Report of a Committee of the Institute for Behavior and Health, Inc., "Abuse of Benzodiazepines: The Problem and the Solutions," *Am J Drug Alcohol Abuse*, 1988, 14(Suppl 1):1-69.

Smith DE and Landry MJ, "Benzodiazepine Dependency Discontinuation: Focus on the Chemical Dependency Detoxification Setting and Benzodiazepine-Polydrug Abuse," *J Psychiatr Res*, 1990, 24(Suppl 2):145-56.

Woods JH and Winger G, "Current Benzodiazepine Issues," *Psychopharmacology (Berl)*, 1995, 118(2):107-15.

Yaster M, Kost-Byerly S, Berde C, et al, "The Management of Opioid and Benzodiazepine Dependence in Infants, Children, and Adolescents," *Pediatrics*, 1996, 98(1):135-40.

♦ **Benzoylecgonine** *see* Cocaine (Cocaine Metabolite), Qualitative, Urine or Hair *on page 785*

♦ **Bhang** *see* Cannabinoids (Marijuana Metabolites), Qualitative, Urine *on page 783*

♦ **Bufferin®** *see* Salicylate, Serum or Plasma *on page 806*

♦ **Bullets** *see* Chain-of-Custody Protocol *on page 785*

♦ **Butalbital** *see* Barbiturates, Qualitative, Urine *on page 781*

Cadmium, Urine

Related Information
Beta$_2$-Microglobulin, Serum or Urine *on page 509*
Heavy Metal Screen, Blood *on page 792*
Heavy Metal Screen, Urine *on page 792*
Mercury, Blood *on page 797*
Urine Collection, 24-Hour *on page 47*

Synonyms Cd, Blood; Cd, Urine

Abstract A silvery white transitional metal, cadmium belongs to the same family as zinc and mercury. Almost the entire output of cadmium in the United States is obtained as a byproduct of the refining of zinc ores. Cadmium is used in industry in alloys, electroplating, ceramics, soldering, and batteries. The compound cadmium sulfide is an important yellow pigment known as cadmium yellow. Cadmium and cadmium compounds are highly toxic with cumulative effects similar to those of mercury. Exposure is predominantly occupational, predominantly from mining and smelting. Some exposure may be had from smoking, as tobacco products may contain cadmium.[1]

Specimen 24-hour urine is recommended for chronic exposure

Container Plastic (preferably polycarbonate) urine container

Collection A 24-hour urine specimen must be collected in a metal-free container and be properly labeled, capped, and sealed. Addition of HCl (10 mL concentrated acid) in the collection container is preferred.

Storage Instructions Refrigerate urine.

Causes for Rejection Specimen allowed to contact metal or dusts containing metals

Reference Interval
- Urine: nonsmoker: <1 µg/L (SI: <8.9 nmol/L) or <1 µg/g creatinine
- Whole blood: nonsmoker: 0.3-1.2 µg/L (SI: 2.7-10.7 nmol/L), smoker: 0.6-3.9 µg/L (SI: 5.3-34.7 nmol/L)

Urinary values in the range of 100-3000 µg/L indicate toxic exposure.[2] Current WHO-based exposure limit is 5 µg/g creatinine in urine.[3]

Possible Panic Range Levels >10 µg/L (SI: >88.97 µmol/L) in whole blood and values >15 µg/g creatinine indicate severe exposure.[2]

Use Evaluate cadmium toxicity in industrial exposure to cadmium fumes or cadmium ingestion

Limitations Blood or urine levels of cadmium may reflect current exposure and may be used as bioindicators of recent exposure.[4] Once exposure ceases, these levels may not provide a good indicator of remaining body burden.[6]

Methodology Inductively-coupled plasma spectrometry (ICPS), atomic absorption spectrometry (AAS)

Additional Information The major route of absorption of many heavy metals, including cadmium, is by inhalation.[5] Inhalation of cadmium fumes produces an acute chemical pneumonitis which can produce pulmonary edema and respiratory failure. Long-term exposure may lead to emphysema (with decreased alpha$_1$-antitrypsin). In studies in Eastern and Western Germany, active cigarette smoking was found to be the dominant factor affecting blood and urine cadmium levels.[6] Environmental and occupational exposure played only a minor role in the exposure model for German adults.[6] Results from the NHANES III studies in the United States reveal that urinary cadmium increased with age (*vide infra*) and with smoking. Approximately 2.3% of the U.S. population have urinary cadmium concentrations >2 µg/g creatinine and 0.2% >5 µg/g creatinine - the World Health Organization recommended exposure limit.[5]

Acute cadmium toxicity may cause hepatic failure. Primary hepatic injury appears to be caused by the binding of the Cd^{+2} to sulfhydryl groups on critical molecules in hepatic mitochondria. Thiol group inactivation leads to oxidative stress, mitochondrial permeability changes, and mitochondrial dysfunction.[7] Endothelial damage may also further cause ischemic hepatic changes. Kupffer cell activation via immune stimulation may also lead to further liver damage.[7,8]

Chronic cadmium toxicity leads to progressive renal dysfunction with proteinuria of slow onset. Because of slow excretion and constant exposure, cadmium values increase with age. Body cadmium elimination half-life may be greater than 20 years. When renal tubular toxicity is suspected, urinary β$_2$-microglobulin and retinol-binding proteins are useful.

Cadmium is a suspected human prostatic carcinogen[9] and it accumulates in the pancreas.[10] Major risk factors for pancreatic cancer (smoking, increasing age, occupational exposure to metal working and pesticides) are all associated with increased risk of exposure to cadmium. Meta-analysis of cohorts with high exposure to cadmium reveals an increased risk for pancreatic cancer.[10] Cadmium is highly neurotoxic in animals. Cross-sectional epidemiologic study of cadmium workers found an excess of neurological complaints before microproteinuria occurs. Such complaints include decreased performance on visual motor tasks, decreased symbol digit substitution performance, decreased simple reaction times and increased complaints of disturbances in equilibrium, peripheral neuropathy, and concentrating abilities.[11]

Footnotes
1. Moyer TP, "Toxic Metals," *Tietz Textbook of Clinical Chemistry*, Chapter 28, Burtis CA and Ashwood ER, eds, Philadelphia, PA: WB Saunders Co, 1999, 988.

2. Painter PC, Cope JY, and Smith JL, "Reference Information for the Clinical Laboratory," *Tietz Textbook of Clinical Chemistry*, Chapter 50, Burtis CA and Ashwood ER, eds, Philadelphia, PA: WB Saunders Co, 1999, 1803.
3. Paschal DC, Burt V, Caudill SP, et al, "Exposure of the U.S. Population Aged 6 Years and Older to Cadmium: 1988-1994," *Arch Environ Contam Toxicol*, 2000, 38(3):377-83.
4. Shimbo S, Zhang ZW, Moon CS, et al, "Correlation Between Urine and Blood Concentrations, and Dietary Intake of Cadmium and Lead Among Women in the General Population of Japan," *Int Arch Occup Environ Health*, 2000, 73(3):163-70.
5. Howard P and Billings CG, "Dynamics and Clinical Effects of Nonferrous Metals in the Human Body," *Monaldi Arch Chest Dis*, 2000, 55(1):70-3.
6. Hoffmann K, Becker K, Friedrich C, et al, "The German Environmental Survey 1990/1992 (GerES II): Cadmium in Blood, Urine, and Hair of Adults and Children," *J Expo Anal Environ Epidemiol*, 2000, 10(2):126-35.
7. Rikans LE and Yamano T, "Mechanisms of Cadmium-Mediated Acute Hepatotoxicity," *J Biochem Mol Toxicol*, 2000, 14(2):110-7.
8. Marth E, Barth S, and Jelovcan S, "Influence of Cadmium on the Immune System. Description of Stimulating Reactions," *Cent Eur J Public Health*, 2000, 8(1):40-4.
9. Achanzar WE, Achanzar KB, Lewis JG, et al, "Cadmium Induces c-myc, p53, and c-jun Expression in Normal Human Prostate Epithelial Cells as a Prelude to Apoptosis," *Toxicol Appl Pharmacol*, 2000, 164(3):291-300.
10. Schwartz GG and Reis IM, "Is Cadmium a Cause of Human Pancreatic Cancer?" *Cancer Epidemiol Biomarkers Prev*, 2000, 9(2):139-45.
11. Viaene MK, Masschelein R, Leenders J, et al, "Neurobehavioural Effects of Occupational Exposure to Cadmium: A Cross Sectional Epidemiological Study," *Occup Environ Med*, 2000, 57(1):19-27.

References
Akesson A, Stal P, and Vahter M, "Phlebotomy Increases Cadmium Uptake in Hemochromatosis," *Environ Health Perspect*, 2000, 108(4):289-91.
Barbee JY and Prince TS, "Acute Respiratory Distress Syndrome in a Welder Exposed to Metal Fumes," *South Med J*, 1999, 92(5):510-2.
Baselt RC, *Disposition of Toxic Drugs and Chemicals in Man*, 5th ed, Foster City, CA: Chemical Toxicology Institute, 2000, 117-9.
Berglund M, Akesson A, Bjellerup P, et al, "Metal-Bone Interactions," *Toxicol Lett*, 2000, 112-3:219-25.
Fels LM, "Risk Assessment of Nephrotoxicity of Cadmium," *Ren Fail*, 1999, 21(3-4):275-81.
Jarup L, Berglund M, Elinder CG, et al, "Health Effects of Cadmium Exposure - A Review of the Literature and a Risk Estimate," *Scand J Work Environ Health*, 1998, 24(Suppl 1):1-51.
Klaassen CD, Liu J, and Choudhuri S, "Metallothionein: An Intracellular Protein to Protect Against Cadmium Toxicity," *Annu Rev Pharmacol Toxicol*, 1999, 39:267-94.
Prozialeck WC, "Evidence That E-cadherin May Be a Target for Cadmium Toxicity in Epithelial Cells," *Toxicol Appl Pharmacol*, 2000, 164(3):231-49.
Staessen JA, Kuznetsova T, Roels HA, et al, "Exposure to Cadmium and Conventional and Ambulatory Blood Pressures in a Prospective Population Study," Public Health and Environmental Exposure to Cadmium Study Group, *Am J Hypertens*, 2000, 13(2):146-56.
Stoica A, Katzenellenbogen BS, and Martin MB, "Activation of Estrogen Receptor-Alpha by the Heavy Metal Cadmium," *Mol Endocrinol*, 2000, 14(4):545-53.

♦ **Cannabinoid:Creatinine Ratio** *see* Cannabinoids (Marijuana Metabolites), Qualitative, Urine *on page 783*

♦ **Cannabinoids** *see* Drugs of Abuse Testing, Urine *on page 788*

Cannabinoids (Marijuana Metabolites), Qualitative, Urine

Related Information
Chain-of-Custody Protocol *on page 785*
Drugs of Abuse Testing, Urine *on page 788*
Ethanol, Blood, Urine, and Other Sources *on page 789*

Synonyms Bhang; Cannabis; Carboxy THC; Ganja; Hashish; Hemp; Marijuana; 11-Nor-9-Carboxy-Delta-9-Tetrahydrocannabinol; Pot; THC (Delta-9-*trans*-Tetrahydrocannabinol)

Applies to Cannabinoid:Creatinine Ratio; *Cannabis sativa*; Tetrahydrocannabinol (THC); THC-Carboxylic Acid

Abstract Marijuana is the most common illicit drug used by children and adolescents in the United States. Despite growing concerns by the medical profession about the physical and psychological effects of its active ingredient, delta-9-tetrahydrocannabinol, survey data continues to show that increasing numbers of young people are using the drug as they become less concerned about its danger. The main active ingredient of marijuana (cannabinoids) is tetrahydrocannabinol (THC). Its behavioral effects include feelings of euphoria, relaxation, altered time perception, lack of concentration, impaired memory, and paranoia. It is metabolized to THC-carboxylic acid, which is detected in the urine. The name comes from the source of marijuana, the plant *Cannabis sativa*.

Specimen Random urine

Collection For employee screening or forensic purpose, use precautions during collection (see the Introduction *on page 773*).

Causes for Rejection Evidence of urine dilution or alteration

Special Instructions If forensic, use chain-of-custody protocol and form. See Chain-of-Custody Protocol *on page 785* and the Chain-of-Custody form in the Introduction *on page 773*.

Reference Interval Negative (less than cutoff)

Critical Values Substance Abuse and Mental Health Services Administration (SAMHSA) screening cutoff: 50 ng/mL (20 ng/mL in some laboratories); confirmation cutoff: 15 ng/mL
(Continued)

Cannabinoids (Marijuana Metabolites), Qualitative, Urine *(Continued)*

Use Drug abuse evaluation, toxicity assessment

Limitations Cannabinoids are rapidly metabolized from blood. Urine is the best specimen for screening although blood (serum or plasma) and saliva have been used. Cannabinoids can adhere to plastic.

Methodology Enzyme immunoassay (EIA), fluorescence polarization immunoassay (FPIA), thin-layer chromatography (TLC), gas chromatography/mass spectrometry (GC/MS)

Additional Information
- Half-life: 20-40 hours
- Volume of distribution: 4-19 L/kg

A positive screen for cannabinoids indicates the presence of cannabinoid metabolites. 11-nor-9-carboxy-delta-9-THC (carboxy THC) is the major metabolite in urine but its presence is not proportional to time of exposure, amount, or impairment. Unless the screen is confirmed by GC/MS, a positive result is presumptive and an unconfirmed screen should not be used to test employees. Urine may contain carboxy THC for 7-10 days after light or moderate use and as long as a month to 6 weeks after heavy use. Rapid storage of THC metabolites in body fat occurs after use. These substances are then released from storage sites slowly over time.

A marijuana cigarette is made form the dried particles of the plant, *Cannabis sativa*. The immediate effects of smoking marijuana include a faster heartbeat and pulse rate, bloodshot eyes, and a dry mouth and throat. The drug can impair or reduce short-term memory, alter sense of time, and reduce the ability to do things which require concentration, swift reactions and coordination, such as driving and operating machinery.

Driving experiments show that marijuana affects a wide range of skills needed for safe driving. Thinking and reflexes are slowed, making it difficult for drivers to respond to sudden unexpected events. Furthermore, a driver's ability to "track" through curves, brake quickly, and maintain speed and proper distance between vehicles is affected. Research shows that such skills are impaired for at least 4-6 hours after smoking a single marijuana cigarette. If a driver drinks alcohol along with using marijuana, the risks of a vehicular collision greatly increase. When monitoring urine cannabinoids over time to determine continued user abstinence, using the cannabinoid:creatinine ratio eliminates substantial variation from changes in urine dilution.[1]

When conventional antiemetic agents fail, the use of tetrahydrocannabinol (THC) to relieve nausea and vomiting associated with cancer chemotherapy has been described.[2] Use of marijuana for medicinal use is currently highly debatable.[3,4,5]

Footnotes
1. Lafoli P, Beck O, Hjemdahl P, et al, "Using Relation Between Urinary Cannabinoid and Creatinine Excretions to Improve Monitoring of Abuser Adherence to Abstinence," *Clin Chem*, 1994, 40(1):170-1.
2. Gonzalez-Rosales F and Walsh D, "Intractable Nausea and Vomiting Due to Gastrointestinal Mucosal Metastases Relieved by Tetrahydrocannabinol (Dronabinol)," *J Pain Symptom Manage*, 1997, 14(5):311-4.
3. DuPont RL, "Examining the Debate on the Use of Medical Marijuana," *Proc Assoc Am Physicians*, 1999, 111(2):166-72.
4. Marmor JB, "Medical Marijuana," *West J Med*, 1998, 168(6):540-3.
5. Watson SJ, Benson JA Jr, and Joy JE, "Marijuana and Medicine: Assessing the Science Base: A Summary of the 1999 Institute of Medicine Report," *Arch Gen Psychiatry*, 2000, 57(6):547-52.

References

Chiang CN and Barnett G, "Marijuana Pharmacokinetics and Pharmacodynamics," *Cocaine, Marijuana, Designer Drugs: Chemistry, Pharmacology and Behavior,* Redda KK, Walker CA, and Barnell G, eds, Boca Raton, FL: CRC Press, 1989, 113-26.

ElSohly MA and ElSohly HN, "Marijuana: Analysis and Detection of Use Through Urinalysis," *Cocaine, Marijuana, Designer Drugs: Chemistry, Pharmacology and Behavior,* Redda KK, Walker CA, and Barnett G, eds, Boca Raton, FL: CRC Press, 1989, 145-62.

Heyman RB, Anglin TM, Copperman SM, et al, "American Academy of Pediatrics. Committee on Substance Abuse. Marijuana: A Continuing Concern for Pediatricians," *J Pediatr*, 1999, 104(4 Pt 1):982-5.

Huestis MA, Mitchell JM, and Cone EJ, "Lowering the Federally-Mandated Cannabinoid Immunoassay Cutoff Increases True-Positive Results," *Clin Chem*, 1994, 40(5):729-33.

Rouse BA, "Epidemiology of Illicit and Abused Drugs in the General Population, Emergency Department Drug-Related Episodes, and Arrestees," *Clin Chem*, 1996, 42(8 Pt 2):1330-6.

Schucket MA, "Cannabinols," *Drug and Alcohol Abuse*, New York, NY: Plenum, 1989, 143-57.

Wells DJ and Barnhill MT Jr, "Comparative Results With Five Cannabinoid Immunoassay Systems at the Screening Threshold of 100 Micrograms/L," *Clin Chem*, 1989, 35(11):2241-3.

Zuckerman B, Frank DA, Hingson R, et al, "Effects of Maternal Marijuana and Cocaine Use on Fetal Growth," *N Engl J Med*, 1989, 320(12):762-8.

- **Cannabis** see Cannabinoids (Marijuana Metabolites), Qualitative, Urine on page 783
- *Cannabis sativa* see Cannabinoids (Marijuana Metabolites), Qualitative, Urine on page 783

- **Carbamate Toxicity** see Organophosphate Pesticides, Urine, Blood, or Serum on page 804
- **Carbon Monoxide** see Carboxyhemoglobin, Blood on page 784
- **Carboxyhemoglobin** see Methemoglobin, Whole Blood on page 800

Carboxyhemoglobin, Blood

Related Information
Blood Gases and pH, Arterial on page 119
Cotinine, Serum, Plasma, or Urine on page 787
Cyanide, Blood on page 787
Methemoglobin, Whole Blood on page 800
Myoglobin, Qualitative, Urine on page 880
Nicotine, Serum or Plasma on page 802
Point-of-Care Testing on page 43

Synonyms Carbon Monoxide; CO; COHb

Applies to Methylene Chloride; Oximeters, Pulse

Test Includes COHb is sometimes included in Blood Gases, but may be ordered as a separate test.

Abstract A byproduct of incomplete combustion of hydrocarbons, carbon monoxide (CO) is a colorless, tasteless, and odorless gas. It binds tightly to hemoglobin (Hb) to form COHb, reducing oxygen-carrying capacity of blood. The affinity of Hb for CO is 200-250 times that of oxygen. Carbon monoxide poisoning is seen from smoke inhalation, suicide attempt and accidental exposure. It is the most common cause of poisoning death in the U.S.

This test measures hemoglobin-bound carbon monoxide. The percent bound measures the extent of carbon monoxide toxicity.

Patient Preparation In suspected carbon monoxide poisoning, the specimen should be collected immediately.

Specimen Whole blood, venous or arterial

Container Green top (heparin) tube or lavender top (EDTA) tube, depending upon laboratory methods

Sampling Time Draw before the patient is started on oxygen, if possible.

Collection Keep tube capped

Storage Instructions Refrigerate immediately after collection. Do not remove cap. Carboxyhemoglobin is stable 4 months in a filled, well-capped tube.

Reference Interval
- **Nonsmoker:** <3%
- **Smoker:** 1-2 packs/day: 4% to 5%, >2 packs/day: 8% to 10%

Carboxyhemoglobin in the **newborn** may run to 10% to 12%. Carbon monoxide is a metabolic product of hemoglobin catabolism. The increased turnover of hemoglobin in the newborn together with decreased efficiency of the infant's respiratory system may and does lead to higher levels of carboxyhemoglobin.

The effects of COHb are magnified in the placental circulation. The fetus, with a normal arterial oxygen saturation of only 75% to 80%, is sensitive to even small changes in oxygen tension.[1]

Critical Values Exposure to CO concentrations 80-140 ppm for 1-2 hours can lead to COHb results of 3% to 6%; in some patients, even these levels can precipitate angina and cardiac arrhythmias.[1] Toxic concentration is 20%; lethal is >50%.

Possible Panic Range Disturbance of judgment, headache, and dizziness occur at 10% to 30%; coma at 50% to 60%; **fatality** occurs at 30% to 60% or more, and rapid death at level of 80%.

Use Determine the extent of carbon monoxide poisoning, toxicity in individuals exposed to exhausts or indoor combustion including heating, cooking, or fumes of gasoline-powered motors and tools, or incomplete combustion of wood or natural gas. It may be secondary to a defective furnace, water heater, cracked heat exchanger, chimney blockage, improperly functioning space heater or fireplace.[2] Check on effect of smoking on the patient; work up headache, weakness, dizziness, nausea, irritability, mental impairment, vomiting, vertigo, dyspnea, syncope, neurologic deficits, pulmonary edema, unstable angina, ischemia of myocardium, metabolic acidosis, collapse, coma, convulsions. Work up persons exposed to fires and smoke inhalation. Classically described cherry red lips, cyanosis, and retinal hemorrhages are not often found.[3]

Limitations CO binds to cytochrome oxidase, interfering with cellular respiration. Thus, although COHb assays provide information on exposure to CO, they do not always consistently correlate with symptoms or prognosis.[4]

Due to spectral interference, some spectrophotometric methods give falsely high values of COHb when fetal hemoglobin is present in the sample.[5]

Arterial blood gases may be of limited value in treatment decisions for carbon monoxide poisoning.[6]

Carbon monoxide levels are of limited value in screening for smoking, since CO is cleared rapidly and is not specific to smoking. Individuals who inhale cigar smoke have markedly increased concentrations of COHb.[7] Better tests for tobacco use include cotinine or nicotine.

Methodology Spectrophotometry.[6] Gas chromatography is used to measure CO. When blood is treated with potassium ferricyanide, COHb is converted to methemoglobin, releasing CO in gas phase.

Additional Information Carboxyhemoglobin is useful in judging the extent of carbon monoxide toxicity and in considering the effect of smoking on the patient. A direct correlation has been claimed between CO level and symptoms of atherosclerotic diseases, intermittent claudication, angina, and myocardial infarction. Exposure may occur not only from smoking but also from exposure to automobile exhaust gases and gases from various engines. Coal gas contains carbon monoxide. A solvent found in paint removers, methylene chloride, is absorbed through skin and lungs and is metabolized to CO. This test may be included when blood gases are ordered, when there is sufficient sample, and when assay is available. Carboxyhemoglobin leads to hypoxia and lactic acidosis. Myoglobinuria may develop. Natural gas does not contain CO but CO is produced after combustion.

A danger of missed diagnosis of CO intoxication is continued exposure of the patient and others to a toxic environment.[8] The cherry red color of CO poisoning is not consistently seen. CO intoxication may contribute to the risk of myocardial infarction.

A strong correlation is present between carboxyhemoglobin levels and psychometric testing abnormalities. Psychometric testing measures actual neurologic disability and may therefore better define carboxyhemoglobin poisoning severity than blood CO level. A delayed neuropsychiatric syndrome is recognized.[4]

The half-life of carboxyhemoglobin at room air is ~6 hours. The half-life with 100% O_2 administration, at atmospheric pressure, is 80 minutes. With O_2 at three atmospheres, the half-life is 24 minutes.

Diagnosis may be facilitated with blood obtained at the scene by emergency medical technicians and/or analysis of exhaled breath by fire department personnel.

Pulse oximetry has not been able to distinguish carboxyhemoglobin from oxyhemoglobin at the wavelengths used by most oximeters.[4,9]

Footnotes

1. Hsia CC, "Respiratory Function of Hemoglobin," *N Engl J Med*, 1998, 338(4):239-47.
2. Perera RD, "The Dangers of Carbon Monoxide," *N Engl J Med*, 1995, 332(13):894.
3. Ernst A and Zibrak JD, "Carbon Monoxide Poisoning," *N Engl J Med*, 1998, 339(22):1603-8.
4. Centers for Disease Control and Prevention, "Carbon Monoxide Poisoning - Weld County, Colorado, 1993," *JAMA*, 1994, 272(19):1489-90.
5. Porter WH, "Clinical Toxicology," *Tietz Textbook of Clinical Chemistry*, 3rd ed, Burtis CA and Ashwood ER, eds, Philadelphia, PA: WB Saunders Co, 1999, 918.
6. Matsuoka T, "Determination of Methemoglobin and Carboxyhemoglobin in Blood by Rapid Colorimetry," *Biol Pharm Bull*, 1997, 20(11):1208-11.
7. Iribarren C, Tekawa IS, Sidney S, et al, "Effect of Cigar Smoking on the Risk of Cardiovascular Disease, Chronic Obstructive Pulmonary Disease, and Cancer in Men," *N Engl J Med*, 1999, 340(23):1773-80.
8. Crawford R, Campbell DG, and Ross J, "Carbon Monoxide Poisoning in the Home: Recognition and Treatment," *BMJ*, 1990, 301(6758):1161.
9. "Carbon Monoxide Poisoning Associated With Use of LPG-Powered (Propane) Forklifts in Industrial Settings - Iowa, 1998" *MMWR Morb Mortal Wkly Rep*, 1999, 48(49):1121-4.

References

Heckerling PS, Leikin JB, Maturen A, et al, "Screening Hospital Admissions From the Emergency Department for Occult Carbon Monoxide Poisoning," *Am J Emerg Med*, 1990, 8(4):301-4.

Jaffé FA, "Pathogenicity of Carbon Monoxide," *Am J Forensic Med Pathol*, 1997, 18(4):406-10.

Kales S, "Carbon Monoxide Intoxication," *Am Fam Phys*, 1993, 48(6):1100-4.

Mahoney JJ, Vreman HJ, Stevenson DK, et al, "Measurement of Carboxyhemoglobin and Total Hemoglobin by Five Specialized Spectrophotometers (CO-oximeter) in Comparison With Reference Methods," *Clin Chem*, 1993, 39(8):1693-1700.

Shenoi R, Stewart G, Rosenberg N, et al, "Screening for Carbon Monoxide in Children," *Pediatr Emerg Care*, 1998, 14(6):399-402.

Thom SR and Keim LW, "Carbon Monoxide Poisoning: A Review Epidemiology, Pathophysiology, Clinical Findings, and Treatment Options Including Hyperbaric Oxygen Therapy," *J Toxicol Clin Toxicol*, 1989, 27(3):141-56.

Tibbles PM and Edelsberg JS, "Hyperbaric-Oxygen Therapy," *N Engl J Med*, 1996, 334(25):1642-8.

Varon J, Marik PE, Fromm RE Jr, et al, "Carbon Monoxide Poisoning: A Review for Clinicians," *J Emerg Med*, 1999, 17(1):87-93.

Weaver LK, "Carbon Monoxide Poisoning," *Crit Care Clin*, 1999, 15(2):297-317.

Zijlstra WG, Buursma A, and Meeuwsen-van-der-Roest WP, "Absorption Spectra of Human Fetal and Adult Oxyhemoglobin, Deoxyhemoglobin, Carboxyhemoglobin, and Methemoglobin," *Clin Chem*, 1991, 37(9):1633-8.

♦ **Carboxy THC** *see* Cannabinoids (Marijuana Metabolites), Qualitative, Urine *on page 783*

♦ **Cd, Blood** *see* Cadmium, Urine *on page 783*

♦ **Cd, Urine** *see* Cadmium, Urine *on page 783*

♦ **Centralgine®** *see* Meperidine, Serum or Urine *on page 796*

Chain-of-Custody Protocol

Related Information

Barbiturates, Qualitative, Urine *on page 781*
Drugs of Abuse Testing, Urine *on page 788*
Flunitrazepam, Urine *on page 791*

Meperidine, Serum or Urine *on page 796*
Methamphetamine, Qualitative, Urine *on page 799*
Morphine, Urine *on page 802*

Synonyms Chain-of-Evidence Form; Specimen Chain-of-Custody Protocol

Applies to Bullets; Medical Legal Specimens

Abstract A procedure to ensure sample integrity from collection through transport, receipt, sampling, and analysis. It is associated with a chain-of-custody form. See Chain-of-Custody form in the Introduction *on page 773*. Similar forms are used (chain-of-evidence) for other forensic materials such as guns, bullets, chemicals, etc.

Specimen Usually urine for drugs-of-abuse-related monitoring; blood for alcohol testing

Container Plastic urine cup with locking lid covered by seal which is signed or initialed (if for drugs of abuse)

Collection See the Introduction *on page 773*.

Causes for Rejection Sample container not sealed or labeled

Special Instructions Form requires signature of sample donor as well as that of the person receiving the sample at the collection site.

Reference Interval Normal: all seals intact and chain-of-custody form completed.

Use Chain-of-custody is a legal term that describes a method to maintain sample integrity in the collection, handling, and storage of urine or other samples.

Additional Information The chain-of-custody protocol is a clerical and custodial service offered by the laboratory to document specimen transfer and provide for extended specimen storage. A written record of specimen transfer from patient, to analyst, to storage and disposal is maintained on all specimens covered by chain-of-custody. All drug screens, blood alcohols, most bullets, or any other tests or objects that have medicolegal significance should be accompanied by chain-of-custody and a written release form.

References

"Mandatory Guidelines for Federal Workplace Drug Testing Programs," *Fed Regist*, 1994, 59:29916-31.

Smith ML, Bronner WE, Shimomura ET, et al, "Quality Assurance in Drug Testing Laboratories," *Clin Lab Med*, 1990, 10(3):503-16.

Wu AH, Bristol B, Sexton K, et al, "Adulteration of Urine by Urine Luck," *Clin Chem*, 1999, 45(7):1051-7.

Internet Web Sites

www.health.org/workplace

♦ **Chain-of-Evidence Form** *see* Chain-of-Custody Protocol *on page 785*

♦ **Cholinesterase, True** *see* Organophosphate Pesticides, Urine, Blood, or Serum *on page 804*

♦ **Cinnabar** *see* Mercury, Blood *on page 797*

♦ **CN⁻** *see* Cyanide, Blood *on page 787*

♦ **CO** *see* Carboxyhemoglobin, Blood *on page 784*

♦ **Cocaine** *see* Drugs of Abuse Testing, Urine *on page 788*

Cocaine (Cocaine Metabolite), Qualitative, Urine or Hair

Related Information

Chain-of-Custody Protocol *on page 785*
Drugs of Abuse Testing, Urine *on page 788*
Ethanol, Blood, Urine, and Other Sources *on page 789*
Myoglobin, Qualitative, Urine *on page 880*

Synonyms Coke; Crack; Dama Blanca; Erythroxylon Coca; Free Base; Gold Dust; Liquid Lady; Methylbenzoylecgonine; Nose Candy; Rock; Snow; Toot; White Lady

Applies to Benzoylecgonine

Abstract A Schedule II controlled substance, cocaine can be smoked or administered intranasally, orally, or intravenously. It is derived from the leaves of *Erythroxylon coca*. Prominent metabolites of cocaine are benzoylecgonine and ecgonine methyl ester. The former is a substance generally measured in urine to detect the use of cocaine.

Specimen Urine; hair can also be analyzed, reflecting long-term exposure.

Collection If forensic, observe precautions concerning surreptitious dilution or alteration.

Storage Instructions Refrigerate

Causes for Rejection If forensic, failure to meet temperature requirements immediately after collection and/or tests for unusual dilution (specific gravity, urine creatinine) or alteration.

Special Instructions If forensic, use chain-of-custody protocol and form. See Chain-of-Custody Protocol *on page 785* and the Chain-of-Custody form in the Introduction *on page 773*.

Reference Interval Negative (less than cutoff)

Critical Values Urine: Substance Abuse and Mental Health Services Administration (SAMHSA) screening cutoff: 300 ng/mL; confirmation cutoff: 150 ng/mL for benzoylecgonine. Toxic cutoff: >1000 ng/mL (SI: >3300 nmol/L); hair: >1.2 ng/mL.[1]

Use Evaluate cocaine use and toxicity; work up as part of a drug screen *(Continued)*

Cocaine (Cocaine Metabolite), Qualitative, Urine or Hair (Continued)

Methodology Screen: enzyme immunoassay (EIA), fluorescence polarization immunoassay (FPIA), thin-layer chromatography (TLC); confirmation: gas chromatography/mass spectrometry (GC/MS). Hair can be analyzed by RIA.

Additional Information
- Half-life: cocaine: 1 hour, benzoylecgonine: 4-9 hours; ecgonine methylester: 3-4 hours; ethylcocaine: about 2 hours
- Volume of distribution: 3-5 L/kg

Cocaine is a highly abused drug which is most frequently detected in the urine as the metabolite, benzoylecgonine, and usually as part of a multiclass drug panel. In pre-employment drug screening or in forensic samples, the presence of cocaine (benzoylecgonine) should be confirmed by GC/MS.

Cocaine is a central nervous system stimulant. It usually appears as a fine crystal-like powder which is the hydrochloride or sulfate salt and as such is "snorted" (inhaled through the nose). When mixed with sodium bicarbonate and converted to free base, it appears as hard pieces called "crack" which can be smoked. This is currently a very prevalent form of the drug.

The effects of the drug begin within minutes and peak within 15-20 minutes. Increase in norepinephrine causes classic adrenergic effects, including mydriasis (marked dilatation of the pupils), hypertension, tachycardia, and tachypnea. The dangers of cocaine use vary, depending on how the drug is taken, the dose, and the individual. Some regular users report feelings of restlessness, irritability, anxiety, and sleeplessness. In some people even low doses of cocaine may create psychological problems. People who use high doses of cocaine over a long period of time may become paranoid or experience what is called a cocaine psychosis. This may include hallucinations of touch, sight, taste, and smell. Benzoylecgonine is detectable in urine within 2-3 hours and for a period of 1-3 days (much longer, up to 3 weeks in heavy users).

Individuals with pseudocholinesterase deficiency may be at special risk when cocaine is used.

Alcohol inhibits cocaine degradation, enhancing its hepatotoxicity.[2] Cocaine and alcohol are commonly used in combination, resulting in production of cocaethylene or ethylcocaine and increased euphoria, cardiotoxicity, and behavioral effects.

Up to a third of all instances of stroke in young adults relate to drug use including amphetamines, phenylpropanolamine, phencyclidine, methylphenidate, and opiates, as well as cocaine, but cocaine has become the most common drug implicated in such events.

Reckless drivers not intoxicated with alcohol may be intoxicated with cocaine and/or marijuana. Appropriate toxicologic testing has been recommended.[3]

Complications of cocaine use may include cocaine-excited delirium, somnolence, coma, shock, disseminated intravascular coagulation, myonecrosis, arrhythmia, myocardial ischemia, infarction, and sudden death. Noncardiogenic pulmonary edema occurs. Cocaine use may cause rhabdomyolysis, hyperthermia, acute renal failure, and adverse effects on fetal growth and development. Cocaine is hepatotoxic.[4] It causes microvesicular steatosis and necrosis.[5] Its abuse has been associated with arterial dissection.[6]

Since hair grows at about 13 mm/month, results of hair analysis reflect longer-term exposure than can urine testing, indicating exposure over periods of weeks or months.[1,7]

Footnotes
1. Ness RB, Grisso JA, Hirschinger N, et al, "Cocaine and Tobacco Use and the Risk of Spontaneous Abortion," *N Engl J Med*, 1999, 340(5):333-9.
2. "A 32-Year-Old Man With the Sudden Onset of a Right-Sided Headache and Left Hemiplegia and Hemianesthesia," Case Records of the Massachusetts General Hospital, Case 27-1993, Scully RE, Mark EJ, McNeely WF, et al, eds, *N Engl J Med*, 1993, 329(2):117-24.
3. Brookoff D, Cook CS, Williams C, et al, "Testing Reckless Drivers for Cocaine and Marijuana," *N Engl J Med*, 1994, 331(8):518-22.
4. Lee WM, "Drug-Induced Hepatotoxicity," *N Engl J Med*, 1995, 333(17):1118-27.
5. Zimmerman HJ, *Hepatotoxicity: The Adverse Effects of Drugs and Other Chemicals on the Liver*, 2nd ed, Philadelphia, PA: Lippincott Williams & Wilkins, 1999.
6. Eskander KE, Brass NS, and Gelfand ET, "Cocaine Abuse and Coronary Artery Dissection," *Ann Thorac Surg*, 2001, 71(1):340-1.
7. Mills JL, "Cocaine, Smoking, and Spontaneous Abortion," *N Engl J Med*, 1999, 340(5):380-1.

References
Angell M and Kassirer JP, "Alcohol and Other Drugs - Toward a More Rational and Consistent Policy," *N Engl J Med*, 1994, 331(8):537-9.

Baskin LB, Morgan DL, and Parupia JY, "A Rapid Immunoassay for Drugs of Abuse and Tricyclic Antidepressants," *Lab Med*, 1996, 27(3):193-7.

Brogan WC 3d, Lange RA, Glamann DB, et al, "Recurrent Coronary Vasoconstriction Caused by Intranasal Cocaine; Possible Role for Metabolites," *Ann Intern Med*, 1992, 116(7):556-61.

Casanova OQ, Lombardero N, Behnke M, et al, "Detection of Cocaine Exposure in the Neonate. Analysis of Urine, Meconium, and Amniotic Fluid From Mothers and Infants Exposed to Cocaine," *Arch Pathol Lab Med*, 1994, 118(10):988-93.

Chan KM, Matthews WS, Saxena S, et al, "Frequency of Cocaine and Phencyclidine Detection at a Large Urban Public Teaching Hospital," *J Anal Toxicol*, 1993, 17(5):299-303.

Hatsukami DK and Fischman MW, "Crack Cocaine and Cocaine Hydrochloride. Are the Differences Myth or Reality?" *JAMA*, 1996, 276(19):1580-8.

Hippenstiel MJ and Gerson B, "Optimization of Storage Conditions for Cocaine and Benzoylecgonine in Urine: A Review," *J Anal Toxicol*, 1994, 18(2):104-9.

Kain ZN, Kain TS, and Scarpelli EM, "Cocaine Exposure in Utero: Perinatal Development and Neonatal Manifestations - Review," *Clin Toxicol*, 1992, 30:607-36.

Karch SB, "The History of Cocaine Toxicity," *Hum Pathol*, 1989, 20(11):1037-9.

Leshner AI, "Molecular Mechanisms of Cocaine Addiction," *N Engl J Med*, 1996, 335(2):128-9.

Preston KL, Silverman K, Schuster CR, et al, "Use of Quantitative Urinalysis in Monitoring Cocaine Use," *NIDA Res Monogr*, 1997, 175:253-65.

Roberts JR and Greenberg MI, "Cocaine Washout Syndrome," *Ann Intern Med*, 2000, 132(8):679-80.

Romberg RW and Past MR, "Reanalysis of Forensic Urine Specimens Containing Benzoylecgonine and THC-COOH," *J Forensic Sci*, 1994, 39(2):479-85.

Uszenski RT, Gillis RA, and Schaer GL, "Additive Myocardial Depressant Effects of Cocaine and Ethanol," *Am Heart J*, 1992, 124(5):1276-83.

Warner EA, "Cocaine Abuse," *Ann Intern Med*, 1993, 119(3):226-33.

Williams RH, Erickson T, and Broussard LA, "Evaluating Sympathomimetic Intoxication in an Emergency Setting," *Lab Med*, 2000, 31(9):497-507.

Zuckerman B, Frank DA, Hingson R, et al, "Effects of Maternal Marijuana and Cocaine Use on Fetal Growth," *N Engl J Med*, 1989, 320(12):762-8.

♦ **Codate** *see* Codeine, Urine *on page 786*

♦ **Codeine** *see* Morphine, Urine *on page 802*

♦ **Codeine Phosphate** *see* Codeine, Urine *on page 786*

♦ **Codeine Sulfate** *see* Codeine, Urine *on page 786*

Codeine, Urine

Related Information
Drugs of Abuse Testing, Urine *on page 788*
Morphine, Urine *on page 802*
Opiates, Qualitative, Urine *on page 803*

Synonyms Actacode; Codate; Codeine Phosphate; Codeine Sulfate; Codlin; Methylmorphine; Paveral; Tricodein

Applies to Morphine; Norcodeine

Test Includes Part of opiate screen

Abstract Codeine occurs naturally in opium but is produced commercially by 3-O-methylation of morphine. It is used as a narcotic analgesic and in lower doses as an antitussive in patients older than 2 years of age. It is present in numerous proprietary preparations combined with non-narcotic analgesics (eg, aspirin and acetaminophen) and antihistamines. It is a drug of abuse.

Specimen Urine

Sampling Time Random

Storage Instructions Refrigerate specimen

Special Instructions If forensic, use precautions in collection and chain-of-custody form. See Chain-of-Custody Protocol *on page 785* and the Chain-of-Custody form in the Introduction *on page 773*.

Reference Interval Negative (below cutoff)

Critical Values Substance Abuse and Mental Health Services Administration (SAMHSA) cutoffs: screen (total opiates): 2000 ng/mL; confirmation: 2000 ng/mL

Use Codeine toxicity may include central nervous system and respiratory depression, constipation and gastrointestinal cramping. Adverse effects of codeine include miosis, increased intracranial pressure, antidiuretic hormone release, and physical and psychological dependence. Assay is used as well to detect drug-of-abuse.

Limitations Codeine may contaminate heroin, and may be detected in urine following use of heroin. The urinary codeine:morphine ratio may be calculated, but may be misleading.[1]

Methodology Enzyme immunoassay (EIA), thin-layer chromatography (TLC) for screen, gas chromatography/mass spectrophotometry (GC/MS) for confirmation

Additional Information
- Half-life: 2.5-4.0 hours
- Volume of distribution: 3-4 L/kg
- Protein binding: 10% to 30%

Codeine, made by the methylation of morphine, is similar to morphine in uses, actions, contraindications, and adverse reactions. About $^1/_6$ to $^1/_{10}$ as potent as morphine, it is used to manage mild to moderate pain. A small amount of codeine (~10%) is converted to morphine, which accounts for analgesic properties of codeine. Thus, both codeine and morphine may be detected in the urine. This is important in drug screening programs, as the detection of morphine in the urine may be due to legitimate use of codeine. Another common source of codeine and morphine is consumption of poppy seeds.[2] To avoid false positives, SAMHSA has recently increased screen and confirmation cutoff to 2000 ng/mL.[3] This has resulted in >300% reduction in the confirmed-positive rate for codeine and morphine.[4] In low doses, it is an antitussive. After an oral dose, the onset of action is 15-30 minutes, and peak levels are reached in 1-1.5 hours. Codeine is excreted mainly in the urine as norcodeine and free and conjugated morphine.

Footnotes
1. Porter WH, "Clinical Toxicology," *Tietz Textbook of Clinical Chemistry*, 3rd ed, Chapter 27, Burtis CA and Ashwood ER, eds, Philadelphia, PA: WB Saunders Co, 1999, 906-81.

2. Meadway C, George S, and Braithwaite R, "Opiate Concentrations Following the Ingestion of Poppy Seed Products - Evidence for the Poppy Seed Defense," *Forensic Sci Int*, 1998, 96(1):29-38.

3. Substance Abuse and Mental Health Administration. "Mandatory Guidelines for Workplace Programs: Revision to Mandatory Guidelines," *Fed Regist*, 1998, 63:483.

4. Fraser AD and Worth D, "Experience With a Urine Opiate Screening and Confirmation Cutoff of 2000 ng/mL," *J Anal Toxicol*, 1999, 23(6):549-51.

References

Cone EJ, Dickerson S, Paul BD, et al, "Forensic Drug Testing for Opiates: Urine Testing for Heroin, Morphine, and Codeine With Commercial Opiate Immunoassays," *J Anal Toxicol*, 1993, 17(3):156-64.

Lin Z, Lafolie P, and Beck O, "Evaluation of Analytical Procedures for Urinary Codeine and Morphine Measurements," *J Anal Toxicol*, 1994, 18(3):129-33.

◆ **Codlin** *see* Codeine, Urine *on page 786*

◆ **COHb** *see* Carboxyhemoglobin, Blood *on page 784*

◆ **Coke** *see* Cocaine (Cocaine Metabolite), Qualitative, Urine or Hair *on page 785*

◆ **Contac®** *see* Methamphetamine, Qualitative, Urine *on page 799*

Cotinine, Serum, Plasma, or Urine

Related Information

Carboxyhemoglobin, Blood *on page 784*
Nicotine, Serum or Plasma *on page 802*
Toxicology Screen, Serum *on page 808*
Toxicology Screen, Urine *on page 808*

Applies to Nicotine

Abstract Nicotine, one of the most toxic of all poisons, is a neural stimulant found in most tobacco products including transdermal patches and Nicorette® gum. Cotinine is the proximal metabolite of nicotine.

Specimen Urine, serum, or plasma

Container Sterile urine container for urine; red top tube for serum; lavender top (EDTA) tube for plasma

Storage Instructions Cotinine is stable in serum at 36°C for up to 6 weeks or several years at -60°C.

Reference Interval Values >100 ng/mL in serum have been reported as indicative of active smoking.[1] The following ranges of serum cotinine concentration were used to stratify smoking status in one study during pregnancy:

• nonsmoker: <15 ng/mL
• light smoker: 15-100 ng/mL
• heavy smoker: >100 ng/mL[2]

Reported urine ranges vary from investigator to investigator with most concurring that passive exposure to cigarette smoke results in urine values <100 ng/mL.[3] Urine values set at 300 ng/mL would rule out passive smoke inhalation. Generally, a ratio of 1:100 exists between cotinine concentrations in passive smokers and active smokers.[4]

Use Useful in situations in which smoking status assessment is of interest: evaluation of the impact of smoking cessation programs, monitoring of pregnancy and of other groups at risk, assessment of occupational exposure to industrial pollutants, validation of phase I clinical trails, selection and control of life insurance candidates, and monitoring of environmental tobacco exposure (passive smoking)

Limitations Interferences due to drugs with a pyridine ring (eg, nicotinic acid, isoniazid, and nicotinamide). Presence of nicotine in some foods (eg, eggplant, potatoes, and tomatoes[2]) that might give rise to increased cotinine levels in vegetarians. Only gas chromatography, high performance liquid chromatography, and some immunoassay methods are sensitive enough for the determination of passive smoke inhalation or environmental tobacco smoke exposure. Urinary cotinine and serum cotinine measurements only provide information on smoking and passive exposure for the 3 days prior to specimen collection and assay.

Methodology Gas chromatography (GC), high performance liquid chromatography (HPLC), colorimetric assay, immunoassay

Additional Information Cotinine, the major metabolite of nicotine in the tobacco user, is further oxidized to trans-3-hydroxycotinine. Conversion of nicotine to cotinine is thought to be the rate-limiting step in nicotine metabolism. Nicotine and cotinine appear to be metabolized by the same enzyme.[5]

Short-term administration of cotinine in doses that result in mean serum concentrations an order of magnitude greater than that of smokers (>2500 ng/mL) are well tolerated by normal subjects during nicotine abstinence[6] and are without effects on body weight, food intake, or significant cardiovascular effects. Cotinine, when given alone during cigarette withdrawal, has no effects on withdrawal symptoms, but blocks the beneficial effect of the nicotine patch.[7]

The longer half-life of cotinine, 16-20 hours versus 1 hour for nicotine, makes it a more reliable marker for active smoking and environmental tobacco exposure than nicotine. It has been recommended as a useful screening tool for predicting poor pregnancy outcomes.[8]

A positive urine reaction forbears association with abortion risk.[9,10]

Footnotes

1. Suadicani P, Hein HO, and Gyntelberg F, "Mortality and Morbidity of Potentially Misclassified Smokers," *Int J Epidemiol*, 1997, 26(2):321-7.

2. Ford RP, Schuter PJ, and Tappin DM, "Changes in Cotinine Levels During Pregnancy," *Aust N Z J Obstet Gynaecol*, 1998, 38(1):50-5.

3. Haufroid V and Lison D, "Urinary Cotinine as a Tobacco-Smoke Exposure Index: A Minireview," *Int Arch Occup Environ Health*, 1998, 71(3):162-8.

4. Scherer G and Richter E, "Biomonitoring Exposure to Environmental Tobacco Smoke (ETS): A Critical Reappraisal," *Hum Exp Toxicol*, 1997, 16(8):449-59.

5. Benowitz NL and Jacobs P 3rd, "Metabolism of Nicotine to Cotinine Studied by a Dual Stable Isotope Method," *Clin Pharmacol Ther*, 1994, 56(5):483-93.

6. Hatsukami DK, Grillo M, Pentel PR, et al, "Safety of Cotinine in Humans: Physiologic, Subjective, and Cognitive Effect," *Pharmacol Bioch Behav*, 1997, 57(4):643-50.

7. Hatsukami DK, Pentel PR, Jensen J, et al, "Cotinine: Effects With and Without Nicotine," *Psychopharmacology*, 1998, 135(2):141-50.

8. Mathews F, Smith R, Yukdin P, et al, "Are Cotinine Assays of Value in Predicting Adverse Pregnancy Outcome?" *Ann Clin Biochem*, 1999, 36(Pt 4):468-76.

9. Mills JL, "Cocaine, Smoking and Spontaneous Abortion," *N Engl J Med*, 1999, 340(5):380-1.

10. Ness RB, Grisso JA, Hirschinger N, et al, "Cocaine and Tobacco Use and the Risk of Spontaneous Abortion," *N Engl J Med*, 1999, 340(5):333-9.

References

Baranowski J, Pochopien G, and Baranowska I, "Determination of Nicotine, Cotinine and Caffeine in Merconium Using High Performance Liquid Chromatography," *J Chromatogr B Biomed Sci Appl*, 1998, 707(1-2):317-21.

Baselt RC, *Disposition of Toxic Drugs and Chemicals in Man*, 5th ed, Foster City, CA: Chemical Toxicology Institute, 2000, 608-12.

Bernert JT Jr, Turner WE, Pirkle JL, et al, "Development and Validation of Sensitive Method for Determination of Serum Cotinine in Smokers and Nonsmokers by Liquid Chromatography/Atmospheric Pressure Ionization Tandem Mass Spectrometry," *Clin Chem*, 1997, 43(12):2281-91.

Caraballo RS, Giovino GA, Pechacek TF, et al, "Racial and Ethnic Differences in Serum Cotinine Levels of Cigarette Smokers," *JAMA*, 1998, 280(2):135-9.

Cope GF, "Simple Colorimetric Procedures to Determine Smoking Status," *Clin Chem*, 1999, 45(4):585.

Hariharan M and VanNoord T, "Liquid-Chromatographic Determination of Nicotine and Cotine in Urine From Passive Smokers: Comparison With Gas Chromatography With a Nitrogen-Specific Detector," *Clin Chem*, 1991, 37(7):1276-80.

Hutchinson J, Yousef T, and Taylor R, "Rapid Method for the Simultaneous Measurement of Nicotine and Cotinine in Urine and Serum by Gas Chromatography-Mass Spectrometry," *J Chromatogr B Biomed Sci Appl*, 1998, 708(1-2):87-93.

Kidwell DA, Holland JC, and Athanaselis S, "Testing for Drugs of Abuse in Saliva and Sweat," *J Chromatogr B Biomed Sci Appl*, 1998, 713(1):111-35.

Oddoze C, Dubus JC, Badier M, et al, "Urinary Cotinine and Exposure to Parental Smoking in a Population of Children With Asthma," *Clin Chem*, 1999, 45(4):505-9.

Oddoze C, Pauli AM, and Pastor J, "Rapid and Sensitive High Performance Liquid Chromatographic Determination of Nicotine and Cotinine in Nonsmoker Human and Rat Urines," *J Chromatogr B Biomed Sci Appl*, 1998, 708(1-2):95-101.

Slotkin TA, "Fetal Nicotine or Cocaine Exposure: Which One Is Worse?" *J Pharmacol Exp Ther*, 1998, 285(3):931-45.

Smith RF, Mather HM, and Ellard GA, "Assessment of Simple Colorimetric Procedures to Determine Smoking Status of Diabetic Subjects," *Clin Chem*, 1998, 44(2):275-80.

◆ **Crack** *see* Cocaine (Cocaine Metabolite), Qualitative, Urine or Hair *on page 785*

◆ **Crank** *see* Methamphetamine, Qualitative, Urine *on page 799*

◆ **Crystal** *see* Amphetamine, Qualitative, Urine *on page 779*

◆ **Crystal** *see* Methamphetamine, Qualitative, Urine *on page 799*

◆ **Crystal Joint** *see* Phencyclidine, Qualitative, Urine *on page 804*

◆ **Cyanide** *see* Thiocyanate, Serum, Plasma, or Urine *on page 807*

Cyanide, Blood

Related Information

Blood Gases and pH, Arterial *on page 119*
Blood Gases and pH, Capillary *on page 121*
Blood Gases and pH, Venous *on page 122*
Carboxyhemoglobin, Blood *on page 784*
Hemoglobin *on page 442*
Lactic Acid, Whole Blood or Plasma *on page 208*
Thiocyanate, Serum, Plasma, or Urine *on page 807*

Synonyms CN⁻; Hydrocyanic Acid; Potassium or Sodium Cyanide

Abstract This highly toxic substance is one of the oldest poisons known. It binds to cytochrome oxidase and prevents cellular respiration, causing tissue hypoxia, severe lactic acidosis, and death. Pharmacokinetic estimates vary widely, probably depending on the circumstances of poisoning.

Specimen Whole blood, since cyanide is concentrated in erythrocytes. Venous blood may appear bright red.

Container Lavender top (EDTA) tube preferred; red top (for serum) may be used in some settings.

Sampling Time Stat

Storage Instructions Fill tube to capacity and keep tightly closed; analyze as soon as possible.

Reference Interval

Whole blood cyanide:[1,2]

• nonsmoker: 0.016 mg/L (SI: 0.61 μmol/L)
• smoker: 0.041 mg/L (SI: 1.57 μmol/L)
• toxic: >1.0 mg/L (SI: >38.4 μmol/L)
• coma: >2.5 mg/L (SI: >96.1 μmol/L)

(Continued)

Cyanide, Blood (Continued)

- death: >3.0 mg/L (SL: >115.4 µmol/L)

Serum cyanide:[1]

- nonsmoker: 0.004 mg/L (SI: 0.15 µmol/L)
- smoker: 0.006 mg/L (SI: 0.23 µmol/L)
- toxic: >0.1 mg/L (SI: >3.84 µmol/L)

Use Establish the diagnosis of cyanide poisoning. Symptoms of toxicity include headache, agitation, vomiting, and confusion. A scent of bitter almonds is suggestive, but not all individuals can detect it.

Methodology Photometric, ion-specific potentiometry

Additional Information Cyanide is found in insecticides, rodenticides, vermicides, metal polishes, and electroplating baths. Other sources include ore refining, laetrile, synthetic rubber manufacturing, and the seeds of cherries, plums, peaches, apricots, pears, apples, crab apples, chokeberries, and lima beans. Some cyanide poisoning occurs among victims of fires, since plastic construction materials produce cyanide from combustion. In such situations, carbon monoxide poisoning may coexist with cyanide poisoning. Fires which involve urea foam insulation may produce hydrocyanic acid, which may be inhaled.

Footnotes

1. Painter PC, Cope JY, and Smith JL, "Reference Information for the Clinical Laboratory," *Tietz Textbook of Clinical Chemistry*, 3rd ed, Burtis CA and Ashwood ER, eds, Philadelphia, PA: WB Saunders Co, 1999, 1809.
2. Schwartz GR, *Principles and Practice of Emergency Medicine*, Baltimore, MD: Lippincott Williams & Wilkins, 1999, 1665-6.

References

Barillo DJ, Goode R, and Esch V, "Cyanide Poisoning in Victims of Fire: Analysis of 364 Cases and Review of the Literature," *J Burn Care Rehabil*, 1994, 15(1):46-57.

Baselt RC, "Disposition of Toxic Drugs and Chemicals in Man," 5th ed, Foster City, CA: Chemical Toxicology Institute, 2000, 221-5.

Beasley DM and Glass WI, "Cyanide Poisoning: Pathophysiology and Treatment Recommendations," *Occup Med*, 1998, 48(7):427-31.

Fenton J, "The Laboratory and the Poisoned Patient," Washington, DC: AACC Press, American Association of Clinical Chemistry, 1998, 141-4.

Hall AH and Rumack BH, "Hydroxocobalamin/Sodium Thiosulfate as a Cyanide Antidote," *J Emerg Med*, 1987, 5(2):115-21.

Kruszyna R, Kruszyna HG, and Smith RP, "A Spectrophotometric Method for Estimating Methemoglobin Concentration in the Presence of Cyanide," *Am J Emerg Med*, 1993, 11(6):642-3.

Laforge M, Buneaux F, Houeto P, et al, "A Rapid Spectrophotometric Blood Cyanide Determination Applicable to Emergency Toxicology," *J Anal Toxicol*, 1994, 18(3):173-5.

Lundquist P and Sorbo B, "Rapid Determination of Toxic Cyanide Concentrations in Blood," *Clin Chem*, 1989, 35(4):617-9.

Moore SJ, Ho IK, and Hume AS, "Severe Hypoxia Produced by Concomitant Intoxication With Sublethal Doses of Carbon Monoxide and Cyanide," *Toxicol Appl Pharmacol*, 1991, 109(3):412-20.

- ◆ **Cyclohexamine** see Phencyclidine, Qualitative, Urine on page 804
- ◆ **Cytochrome b₅ Reductase (NADH-metHb Reductase)** see Methemoglobin, Whole Blood on page 800
- ◆ **Dama Blanca** see Cocaine (Cocaine Metabolite), Qualitative, Urine or Hair on page 785
- ◆ **Dapa®** see Acetaminophen, Serum on page 778
- ◆ **Darvocet-N®** see Propoxyphene, Serum or Urine on page 805
- ◆ **Darvon®** see Propoxyphene, Serum or Urine on page 805
- ◆ **Datril®** see Acetaminophen, Serum on page 778
- ◆ **DAU** see Drugs of Abuse Testing, Urine on page 788
- ◆ **DAU-10** see Drugs of Abuse Testing, Urine on page 788
- ◆ **Delta Aminolevulinic Acid Dehydratase** see Lead, Blood on page 793
- ◆ **Demerol®** see Meperidine, Serum or Urine on page 796
- ◆ **Desoxyephedrine Hydrochloride** see Methamphetamine, Qualitative, Urine on page 799
- ◆ **Desoxyn®** see Methamphetamine, Qualitative, Urine on page 799
- ◆ **Dexedrlne®** see Amphetamine, Qualitative, Urine on page 779
- ◆ **Dexedrine®** see Methamphetamine, Qualitative, Urine on page 799
- ◆ **Dexies** see Amphetamine, Qualitative, Urine on page 779
- ◆ **Dima-Fen®** see Fenfluramine, Serum on page 791
- ◆ **Dimetapp®** see Methamphetamine, Qualitative, Urine on page 799
- ◆ **Dimethylarsine** see Arsenic, Urine on page 781
- ◆ **DMA** see Arsenic, Urine on page 781
- ◆ **d-Methamphetamine** see Methamphetamine, Qualitative, Urine on page 799
- ◆ **Doe** see Methamphetamine, Qualitative, Urine on page 799
- ◆ **Dolantin®** see Meperidine, Serum or Urine on page 796
- ◆ **Dolantina®** see Meperidine, Serum or Urine on page 796
- ◆ **Dolantine®** see Meperidine, Serum or Urine on page 796

- ◆ **Dolophine®** see Methadone, Urine on page 798
- ◆ **Dolosal®** see Meperidine, Serum or Urine on page 796
- ◆ **Dorcol®** see Acetaminophen, Serum on page 778
- ◆ **Drug Screen, Comprehensive Drug Panel or Analysis** see Toxicology Screen, Serum on page 808
- ◆ **Drug Screen, Comprehensive Panel or Analysis, Urine** see Toxicology Screen, Urine on page 808

Drugs of Abuse Testing, Urine

Related Information

Amphetamine, Qualitative, Urine on page 779
Barbiturates, Qualitative, Urine on page 781
Benzodiazepines, Qualitative, Urine on page 782
Cannabinoids (Marijuana Metabolites), Qualitative, Urine on page 783
Chain-of-Custody Protocol on page 785
Cocaine (Cocaine Metabolite), Qualitative, Urine or Hair on page 785
Electrolyte Panel, Serum on page 168
Ethanol, Blood, Urine, and Other Sources on page 789
Flunitrazepam, Urine on page 791
Glucose, Random, Plasma on page 186
Methadone, Urine on page 798
Methamphetamine, Qualitative, Urine on page 799
Methaqualone, Urine on page 800
Morphine, Urine on page 802
Opiates, Qualitative, Urine on page 803
Osmolality, Serum on page 236
Phencyclidine, Qualitative, Urine on page 804
Propoxyphene, Serum or Urine on page 805
Toxicology Screen, Urine on page 808

Synonyms Abuse Screen; DAU; DAU-10; NIDA Screen; Pre-employment Drug Screen

Applies to Amphetamines; Barbiturates; Benzodiazepines; Cannabinoids; Cocaine; Ethanol, Urine; Methadone; Methaqualone; Opiates; Phencyclidine; Propoxyphene

Test Includes Screens for commonly abused drugs and classes of abused drugs - amphetamines, barbiturates, benzodiazepines, cannabinoids, cocaine, methadone, methaqualone, opiates, phencyclidine, propoxyphene. In some laboratories, urine ethanol is included.

Abstract The usual drug-of-abuse screening panel consists of the 10 drugs listed above. Substance Abuse and Mental Health Services Administration (SAMHSA) screen includes only the following 5 drugs: marijuana metabolite, cocaine metabolite, opiates, phencyclidine, and amphetamines.

Specimen Urine

Collection If forensic, observe precautions and follow chain-of-custody protocol.

Storage Instructions Refrigerate

Causes for Rejection If forensic, failure to meet temperature requirements and tests for unusual urine dilution or alteration

Turnaround Time Screen: 1-2 hours if done in-house; confirmation: 1-2 days

Special Instructions Specify the drug or drugs suspected in an emergency situation. If forensic, use chain-of-custody protocol and form. See Chain-of-Custody Protocol on page 785 and the Chain-of-Custody form in the Introduction on page 773.

Reference Interval Negative (less than cutoff)

Critical Values See individual drug entries for cutoff values.

Use Screen for drug overdose and toxicity; screen for the presence of drugs of abuse

Limitations This test provides only **qualitative** detection of drugs. Quantitation of drug levels is not included and is not recommended because urine levels are time and clearance dependent, and are not directly related to toxic symptoms seen clinically. In a nonclinical setting (eg, pre-employment drug screening, etc), the sample should be collected under chain-of-custody, and all positive screens must be confirmed by a different, more sensitive method, preferably GC/MS. The transportation industry [Department of Transportation (DOT)] and Federal employers test certain employees by screening for five classes of drugs only (amphetamines, cannabinoids, cocaine, opiates, phencyclidine) and confirms all positive results with GC/MS. Substance Abuse and Mental Health Services Administration (SAMHSA) requires adherence to mandatory guidelines for workplace drugs of abuse testing.[1] Any agent identified in a screening test **must be confirmed** by a test specific for that drug (GC/MS).

Methodology Screen: immunoassay, gas chromatography (GC), thin-layer chromatography (TLC), high performance liquid chromatography (HPLC); confirmation: gas chromatography/mass spectrometry (GC/MS)

Additional Information For specific drug classes see the listing by specific drug name.

Adulteration of a specimen remains a major challenge. Common tactics to beat the test include substitution of urine, dilution of specimen, or addition of some chemical to the specimen to interfere with the immunoassay or destroy the drug. Direct observation of urine collection is the best safeguard against adulteration, but generally not performed due to hesitation relevant to intrusion of individual privacy and dignity. Most laboratories perform other tests (eg, temperature check, pH, specific gravity, creatinine) to rule out specimen adulteration.

Footnotes

1. Substance Abuse and Mental Health Administration. "Mandatory Guidelines for Workplace Programs: Revision to Mandatory Guidelines," *Fed Regist*, 1994, 59:29916-31.

References

Compton PA, Ling W, Wesson Dr, et al, "Urine Toxicology as an Outcome Measure in Drug Abuse Clinical Trials: Must Every Sample Be Analyzed?" *J Addict Dis*, 1996, 15(2):85-92.

Cone EJ, "New Developments in Biological Measures of Drug Prevalence," *NIDA Res Monogr*, 1997, 167:108-29.

Eskridge KD and Guthrie SK, "Clinical Issues Associated With Urine Testing of Substances of Abuse," *Pharmacotherapy*, 1997, 17(3):497-510.

Fraser AD, "Urine Drug Testing for Social Service Agencies in Nova Scotia, Canada," *J Forensic Sci*, 1998, 43(1):194-6.

Gerson B and Subramaniam S, "Drug Testing as Part of the War on Drugs," *Clin Lab Med*, 1998, 18(4):781-803.

O'Neal CL, Crough DJ, and Fatah AA, "Validation of Twelve Chemical Spot Tests for the Detection of Drugs of Abuse," *Forensic Sci Int*, 2000, 109(3):189-201.

Ostrea EM Jr, "Testing for Exposure to Illicit Drugs and Other Agents in the Neonate: A Review of Laboratory Methods and the Role of Meconium Analysis," *Curr Probl Pediatr*, 1999, 29(2):37-56.

Taylor EH, Oertli EH, Wolfgang JW, et al, "Accuracy of Five On-Site Immunoassay Drugs-of-Abuse Testing Devices," *J Anal Toxicol*, 1999, 23(2):119-24.

"Testing of Drugs of Abuse in Children and Adolescents," American Academy of Pediatrics Committee on Substance Abuse, *Pediatrics*, 1996, 98(2 Pt 1):305-7.

- ◆ **Duramorph®** *see* Morphine, Urine *on page 802*

- ◆ **E** *see* 3,4 Methylenedioxymethamphetamine, Urine *on page 801*

- ◆ **Easprin®** *see* Salicylate, Serum or Plasma *on page 806*

- ◆ **Ecotrin®** *see* Salicylate, Serum or Plasma *on page 806*

- ◆ **Ecstasy** *see* Methamphetamine, Qualitative, Urine *on page 799*

- ◆ **Ecstasy** *see* 3,4 Methylenedioxymethamphetamine, Urine *on page 801*

- ◆ **Elephant Tranquilizers** *see* Phencyclidine, Qualitative, Urine *on page 804*

- ◆ **E-Lor®** *see* Propoxyphene, Serum or Urine *on page 805*

- ◆ **Empirin®** *see* Salicylate, Serum or Plasma *on page 806*

- ◆ **Epimorph Dolcontin®** *see* Morphine, Urine *on page 802*

- ◆ **Eptadone®** *see* Methadone, Urine *on page 798*

- ◆ **Erythroxylon Coca** *see* Cocaine (Cocaine Metabolite), Qualitative, Urine or Hair *on page 785*

- ◆ **1,2-Ethanediol** *see* Ethylene Glycol, Serum or Plasma *on page 790*

- ◆ **Ethanol** *see* Volatile Screen, Blood or Urine *on page 809*

- ◆ **Ethanol, Blood** *see* Ethanol, Blood, Urine, and Other Sources *on page 789*

Ethanol, Blood, Urine, and Other Sources

Related Information

Acetaminophen, Serum *on page 778*
Alanine Aminotransferase, Serum *on page 87*
Alkaline Phosphatase, Serum *on page 93*
Anion Gap, Serum, Plasma, or Urine *on page 106*
Aspartate Aminotransferase, Serum *on page 112*
Cannabinoids (Marijuana Metabolites), Qualitative, Urine *on page 783*
Carbohydrate-Deficient Transferrin, Serum *on page 134*
Cocaine (Cocaine Metabolite), Qualitative, Urine or Hair *on page 785*
Drugs of Abuse Testing, Urine *on page 788*
Ethylene Glycol, Serum or Plasma *on page 790*
Gamma-Glutamyl Transferase, Serum *on page 179*
Gamma Hydroxybutyrate, Serum or Urine *on page 791*
Ketone Bodies, Blood *on page 205*
Lactic Acid, Whole Blood or Plasma *on page 208*
Liver Disease: Laboratory Assessment, Overview *on page 216*
Osmolality, Serum *on page 236*
Volatile Screen, Blood or Urine *on page 809*

Synonyms Alcohol; Ethanol, Blood; Ethyl Alcohol, Blood; EtOH

Applies to Acetaldehyde Adducts; FAEEs; Fatty Acid Ethyl Esters; 5-Hydroxytryptophol/5-HIAA; Phosphatidylethanol

Abstract Ethyl alcohol (EtOH) is a central nervous system depressant. This is the most commonly encountered toxic substance in forensic toxicology and is perhaps the most widely used psychoactive drug.[1] Whole blood ethanol values are often required in law enforcement.

38.4% of all U.S. traffic fatalities are alcohol related.[2] About 50% of patients who are admitted to level I trauma centers secondary to motor vehicle accidents are legally intoxicated.[3] In moderate EtOH consumption, EtOH levels are generally not detectable 5-6 hours following the last ingestion.[4]

Patient Preparation Do not use alcohol wipe to clean venipuncture site. Hexachlorophene-based, iodine-based, or mercury-based antiseptics not containing alcohol may be used.

Specimen Whole blood, serum or plasma, urine. Saliva is used in some settings. Vitreous humor is utilized in forensic necropsy cases. Expired air by breath analysis provides advantages and disadvantages.[4]

Container Red top tube, gray top (sodium fluoride) tube recommended for medicolegal specimens and prolonged storage; plastic urine container

Sampling Time The American College of Surgeons Committee on Trauma has determined that blood alcohol concentrations in patients admitted to level I trauma centers is "essential diagnostic testing".[2]

Collection Do not prepare venipuncture site with an alcohol swab. When police agencies bring an individual in for blood ethanol levels, medical and laboratory people should at all times be aware of their state statutes.[1]

Storage Instructions Refrigerate in a tightly stoppered tube.

Special Instructions Concentrations of ethanol are 12% to 18% higher in serum and plasma than in whole blood. For forensic purposes, only whole blood values are used.

Reference Interval

Blood: negative. While mg/dL are usually used for medical purposes, percentages (g/dL) are usually used for legal needs [eg, driving while intoxicated (DWI)] statutes. In most laboratories, values <5-10 mg/dL (SI: <1-2 mmol/L) are considered negative. Endogenous alcohol production in the gastrointestinal tract might reach 0.005%, while cutoffs between 0.01% and 0.02% are commonplace. Signs of impairment can be observed at levels of 30-80 mg/dL (SI: 0.03% to 0.08%).[5]

Urine: <5-10 mg/dL is considered negative. It is generally accepted that urine alcohol measurements cannot be used to determine impairment in the U.S. However, a challenge to this claim has been made.[6] Urine ethanol levels are legally acceptable in some parts of Europe.

Critical Values Fatal blood concentration is usually considered to be >400 mg/dL (SI: >86.8 mmol/L). Lethal blood levels vary greatly and may be substantially lower when ingested with hypnotics or tranquilizers. Whole blood levels of 300 mg/dL (SI: 65.1 mmol/L) are associated with coma and can be associated with fatalities. In the U.S., levels ≥80-100 mg/dL (0.08% to 0.1%) are considered evidence of impairment for driving. The concentration which defines intoxication is lower in some other countries.[4] Each state statute provides a specific concentration.

Individuals should not be released without accompaniment with EtOH concentrations reaching ≥0.02% (20 mg/dL) (4.34 mmol/L), by virtue of possible impairment and physical injury.[5] Ethanol is metabolized at 10-25 mg/dL/hour.[4]

Possible Panic Range ≥300 mg/dL (SI: ≥65.1 mmol/L)

Use Quantitation of ethanol level is important both for medical and for legal purposes. It is used to diagnose alcohol intoxication and to screen for alcoholism. Persons in rehabilitation programs may be subject to serious penalties.

EtOH concentrations are used to monitor intravenous ethanol treatment for methanol and ethylene glycol intoxication. Ethanol must be tested as a possible cause of coma of unknown etiology, since alcohol intoxication may mimic diabetic coma, cerebral trauma, and drug overdose.

Limitations Certain other alcohols (in high concentration) can interfere with enzymatic methods. The rate of dehydrogenation of isopropanol (2-propanol) is 6%, of methanol and ethylene glycol about 3% to 4%, and that of n-propanol (1-propanol) is 36% of that of ethanol. However, manufacturers of kits for ethanol determination indicate interference is less than these values (about 1%). Diabetics with increased acetone concentrations may be in jeopardy of false-positive concentrations, depending upon cutoff levels.[5] Gas chromatography is the most specific methodology because it can separate, identify, and quantitate each type of alcohol present. Freezing point osmometry and enzymatic analysis can together determine the presence of volatile intoxicants and can determine causes of metabolic intoxication.

A laboratory disclaimer, "for medical purposes only", does not limit interpretation by qualified or underqualified experts.[5]

Methodology Electrochemical oxidation, enzymatic analysis (alcohol dehydrogenase), freezing point osmometry, gas chromatography (GC), infrared spectrometry. GC is the method of choice. A useful tabular presentation of markers and methods has recently been published.[4]

Additional Information Ethanol is absorbed rapidly from the GI tract. Peak blood levels usually occur within 40-70 minutes on an empty stomach. Food in the stomach can decrease the absorption of alcohol. Ethanol is metabolized by the liver to acetaldehyde. Once peak blood ethanol levels are reached, disappearance is linear by zero-kinetics; a 70 kg man metabolizes 7-10 g of ethanol/hour (15 ±5 mg/dL/hour). The plasma:whole blood ratio varies from 1.10-1.35 with an average of about 1.20. The urine:blood ratio is considered to be about 1.3 but is quite variable. Symptoms of intoxication in the presence of low alcohol levels could indicate a serious acute medical problem requiring immediate attention. The half-lives and effectiveness of certain drugs (eg, barbiturates and benzodiazepines) are increased in the presence of ethanol. Urine ethanol can be measured by enzymatic analysis and gas chromatography and is tested for in abused drug screening programs. Ethanol ingestions are discussed in Osmolality, Serum *on page 236*; Anion Gap, Serum, Plasma, or Urine *on page 106*; and Ketone Bodies, Blood *on page 205*. Breath alcohol analyzers are used by law enforcement personnel; their results are accepted as legal evidence of intoxication. They must not be used less than 15 minutes after the last (Continued)

Ethanol, Blood, Urine, and Other Sources
(Continued)

ethanol ingestion.[7] The blood:breath ratio has a mean value of about 2200. The U.S. Department of Transportation has mandated breath alcohol testing for commercial transportation employees. If the concentration is between 20-40 mg/dL, an employee is not allowed to resume safety-sensitive duties for 8 hours (24 hours for motor vehicle drivers). If the concentration is >40 mg/dL, the employee is suspended and referred for professional evaluation.

Because saliva is easy and collection is noninvasive, increased interest in saliva ethanol testing has developed. The average saliva:blood ratio is 1:1. There are presently several test devices available for saliva EtOH measurements (STC Diagnostics and Roche Diagnostic Systems).

FAEEs, long-term markers of EtOH intake, permit recognition of ingestion of intoxicating quantities of EtOH the prior day. Methods are complex.[4]

5-Hydroxytryptophol/5-HIAA ratio in urine may represent a marker of recent ingestion of EtOH. Methods are complex.[4]

Acetaldehyde adducts measurements are discussed.[4]

Phosphatidylethanol may become a marker for longer term EtOH use. Method is tedious.[4]

Electrolyte and acid-base problems found with ethanol abuse include hypophosphatemia, hypomagnesemia, hypocalcemia, hypokalemia, hypoglycemia, metabolic acidosis, diminished urinary excretion of uric acid, secondary hyperuricemia, and compensatory respiratory alkalosis.[8] See Liver Disease: Laboratory Assessment, Overview *on page 216*. The ethanol-acetaminophen syndrome is addressed in Acetaminophen, Serum *on page 778*.

Acetaminophen, EtOH, and fasting cause synergistic effects. Only 2.5-4 g/day of acetaminophen, at therapeutic dosage, can cause liver injury in alcoholics.[9]

Cardiomyopathy may follow 10 years of heavy drinking.

The site of collection for postmortem blood collection yields a potential for variability; sampling of vitreous humor for alcohol may provide the most reliable results, that from the left ventricle the least dependable.[10]

Recently, alcohol use has been reported as a risk factor for bicycling injury. Elevated blood ethanol concentrations were found in 33% of fatally injured bicyclists aged 15 years or older.[11]

Footnotes
1. Li G, "Child Injuries and Fatalities From Alcohol-Related Motor Vehicle Crashes: Call for a Zero-Tolerance Policy," *JAMA*, 2000, 283(17):2291-2.
2. Krahn LE, "Recognizing an Opportunity: Screening for Alcohol Disorders After Motor Vehicle Crashes," *Mayo Clin Proc*, 2000, 75(3):229-30.
3. Maxson PM, Berge KH, Hall-Flavin DK, et al, "Detectable Blood Alcohol After a Motor Vehicle Crash and Screening for Alcohol Abuse/Dependence," *Mayo Clin Proc*, 2000, 75(3):231-4.
4. Laposata M, "Assessment of Ethanol Intake. Current Tests and New Assays on the Horizon," *Am J Clin Pathol*, 1999, 112(4):443-50.
5. Manno JE, "Reporting Blood Ethanol Levels," *Lab Med*, 2000, 31(8):429-30.
6. Jones AW, "Lack of Association Between Urinary Creatinine and Ethanol Concentrations and Urine/Blood Ratio of Ethanol in Two Successive Voids From Drinking Drivers," *J Anal Toxicol*, 1998, 22(3):184-90.
7. Simpson G, "Accuracy and Precision of Breath Alcohol Measurements for a Random Subject in the Postabsorptive State," *Clin Chem*, 1987, 33(2 Pt 1):261-8.
8. De Marchi S, Cecchin E, Basile A, et al, "Renal Tubular Dysfunction in Chronic Alcohol Abuse - Effects of Abstinence," *N Engl J Med*, 1993, 329(26):1927-34.
9. Lieber CS, "Medical Disorders of Alcoholism," *N Engl J Med*, 1995, 333(16):1058-65.
10. Sylvester PA, Wong NA, Warren BF, et al, "Unacceptably High Site Variability in Postmortem Blood Alcohol Analysis," *J Clin Pathol*, 1998, 51(3):250-2.
11. Li G, Baker SP, Smialek JE, et al, "Use of Alcohol as a Risk Factor for Bicycling Injury," *JAMA*, 2001, 285(7):893-6.

References
Blume SB, "Women and Alcohol," *JAMA*, 1986, 256(11):1467-70.

Dubowski KM, Gadsden RH, and Poklis A, "The Stability of Ethanol in Human Whole Blood Controls: An Interlaboratory Evaluation," *J Anal Toxicol*, 1997, 21(6):486-91.

Keim ME, Bartfield JM, Raccio-Roback N, et al, "Blood Ethanol Estimation: A Comparison of Three Methods," *Acad Emerg Med*, 1996, 3(1):85-7.

Koob GF, "Drug Abuse and Alcoholism," *Adv Pharmacol*, 1998, 42:969-77.

O'Connor PG and Schottenfeld RS, "Patients With Alcohol Problems," *N Engl J Med*, 1998, 338(9):529-602.

Osterloh JD, Kelly TJ, Khayam-Bashi H, et al, "Discrepancies in Osmolal Gaps and Calculated Alcohol Concentrations," *Arch Pathol Lab Med*, 1996, 120(7):637-41.

Quinlan KP, Brewer RD, Sleet DA, et al, "Characteristics of Child Passenger Deaths and Injuries Involving Drinking Drivers," *JAMA*, 2000, 283(17):2249-52.

Rainey PM, "Relation Between Serum and Whole Blood Ethanol Concentrations," *Clin Chem*, 1993, 39(11 Pt 1):2288-92.

Rivara FP, Mueller BA, Somes G, et al, "Alcohol and Illicit Drug Abuse and the Risk of Violent Death in the Home," *JAMA*, 1997, 278(7):569-75.

Swift RM, "Drug Therapy for Alcohol Dependence," *N Engl J Med*, 1999, 340(19):1482-90.

Tietz Textbook of Clinical Chemistry, 3rd ed, Burtis CA and Ashwood ER, eds, Philadelphia, PA: WB Saunders Co, 1999, 922-7.

♦ **Ethanol, Urine** *see* Drugs of Abuse Testing, Urine *on page 788*

♦ **Ethyl Alcohol, Blood** *see* Ethanol, Blood, Urine, and Other Sources *on page 789*

♦ **Ethyl and Methyl Thiocyanate (Thanite® and Lethane®)** *see* Thiocyanate, Serum, Plasma, or Urine *on page 807*

Ethylene Glycol, Serum or Plasma

Related Information
Anion Gap, Serum, Plasma, or Urine *on page 106*
Osmolality, Calculated, Serum or Plasma *on page 234*
Osmolality, Serum *on page 236*
Oxalate, Urine *on page 238*
Urinalysis *on page 887*
Volatile Screen, Blood or Urine *on page 809*

Synonyms 1,2-Ethanediol

Applies to Antifreeze; Glycolate, Plasma

Abstract A highly toxic commercial chemical used as a radiator antifreeze and for commercial chemical synthesis. Ethylene glycol by itself is only mildly toxic. Metabolic acidosis and renal failure are due to toxicity of ethylene glycol metabolites.

Specimen Serum or plasma

Container Red top tube or green top (heparin) tube

Reference Interval Negative

Critical Values Toxic: ≥50 mg/dL

Possible Panic Range Values between 300-400 mg/L have been observed in **fatal** cases. Levels at 50 mg/dL with metabolic acidosis or with renal failure indicate a need for hemodialysis, and therapeutic ethanol is recommended at concentrations >20 mg/dL. Survival has taken place with levels of 650 mg/dL (SI: 100 mmol/L).

Use Detect and quantitate ingestion of ethylene glycol. Urinary ethylene glycol measurements may be helpful in screening for chronic industrial exposure such as inhalation and cutaneous absorption.[1]

Limitations Elevated serum lactate and lactate dehydrogenase may interfere in enzymatic assay for ethylene glycol.[2] Because of the short half-life of this compound, low serum concentrations may be misleading if sampling is delayed. Assays are not readily available.

Methodology Gas-liquid chromatography (GLC), photometry, fluorometry, enzymatic assay (automated)[3]

Additional Information
- Half-life: 3-6 hours; 16-18 hours with ethanol therapy
- Volume of distribution: 0.8 L/kg

Ethylene glycol is a colorless, odorless, sweet tasting compound. It has been utilized in suicide attempts, as a substitute for ethanol. Children and domestic animals are attracted to ethylene glycol because its sweetness and odor invite ingestion. 1.5 mL/kg is lethal but rapid treatment may prevent serious organ damage. Toxicity is manifested by CNS depression (1-12 hours after ingestion), cardiopulmonary symptoms (12-24 hours after ingestion), and renal damage (24-72 hours after ingestion), but toxicity may be delayed by the concurrent ingestion of ethanol.[4] Delayed sequellae may occur as late as 10 days after ingestion.[5] Toxicity is due to the accumulation of metabolites, principally glycolate with oxalate appearing as a minor metabolite. In addition to elevated serum ethylene glycol, hypocalcemia, severe high anion gap metabolic acidosis (low chloride, low bicarbonate, low pH), and osmolal gap elevation are observed. Lactic acid production takes place. See Anion Gap, Serum, Plasma, or Urine *on page 106*; Osmolality, Calculated, Serum or Plasma *on page 234*; and Osmolality, Serum *on page 236*.

Poisoning may occur without osmolal gap changes for the following reasons:
- an accurate serum osmolality may not be available
- values for calculated serum osmolarities vary depending on the formula used
- ethylene glycol has a high molecular weight such that even toxic amounts may only contribute minimally to the overall serum osmolality
- little ethylene glycol may be present because it has been metabolized

Osmolal and anion gap increases can be present in patients with very low serum glycol levels. Rarely, the findings of calcium oxalate monohydrate crystals in the urine may be a clue to the diagnosis of ethylene glycol poisoning without other symptoms.[6] Microscopic hematuria is found in some patients.[7]

When antifreeze contains sodium fluorescein (intended to support identification of radiator leakage), urine, or gastric content can be screened with a Wood's lamp.

Plasma concentration of glycolate as well as urinary oxalate excretion, the most important metabolites of ethylene glycol, can be measured.[7]

Clinical and biochemical similarities of ethylene glycol poisoning and methanol poisoning are recognized.[8]

Footnotes
1. Gerin M, Patrice S, Begin D, et al, "A Study of Ethylene Glycol Exposure and Kidney Function of Aircraft Deicing Workers," *Int Arch Occup Envirin Health*, 1997, 69(4):255-65.
2. Eder AF, Dowdy YG, Gardiner JA, et al, "Serum Lactate and Lactate Dehydrogenase in High Concentrations Interfere in Enzymatic Assay of Ethylene Glycol," *Clin Chem*, 1996, 42(9):1489-91.

3. Standefer J and Blackwell N, "Enzymatic Method for Measuring Ethylene Glycol With a Centrifugal Analyzer," *Clin Chem*, 1991, 37(10 Pt 1):1734-6.

4. Ammar KA and Heckerling PS, "Ethylene Glycol Poisoning With a Normal Anion Gap Caused by Concurrent Ethanol Ingestion: Importance of the Osmolal Gap," *Am J Kidney Dis*, 1996, 27(1):130-3.

5. Lewis LD, Smith BW, and Mamourian AC, "Delayed Sequelae After Acute Overdoses or Poisonings: Cranial Neuropathy Related to Ethylene Glycol Ingestion," *Clin Pharmacol Ther*, 1997, 61(6):692-9.

6. Glaser DS, "Utility of the Serum Osmol Gap in the Diagnosis of Methylene or Ethylene Glycol Ingestion," *Ann Emerg Med*, 1996, 27(3):343-6.

7. Brent J, McMartin K, Phillips S, et al, "Fomepizole for the Treatment of Ethylene Glycol Poisoning," *N Engl J Med*, 1999, 340(11):832-8.

8. Jacobsen D, "New Treatment for Ethylene Glycol Poisoning," *N Engl J Med*, 1999, 340(11):879-81.

References

Androgué HJ and Madias NE, "Management of Life-Threatening Acid-Base Disorders," First of Two Parts, *N Engl J Med*, 1998, 338(1):26-34.

Boyer EW, Mejia M, Woolf A, et al, "Severe Ethylene Glycol Ingestion Treated Without Hemodialysis," *Pediatrics*, 2001, 107(1):172-3.

Burkhart KK and Kulig KW, "The Other Alcohols. Methanol, Ethylene Glycol, and Isopropanol," *Emerg Med Clin North Am*, 1990, 8(4):913-28.

de Chazal I, Houghton B, and Frock J, "The Sweet Killer. Can You Recognize the Symptoms of Ethylene Glycol Poisoning?" *Postgrad Med*, 1999, 106(4):221-4, 227, 230.

Dasgupta A, Blackwell W, Gregio J, et al, "Gas Chromatographic-Mass Spectrometric Identification and Quantitation of Ethylene Glycol in Serum After Derivatization With Perflourooctanoyl Chloride: A Novel Derivative," *J Chromatogr B Biomed Sci Appl*, 1995, 666(1):63-70.

Jarvie DR and Simpson D, "Simple Screening Tests for the Emergency Identification of Methanol and Ethylene Glycol in Poisoned Patients," *Clin Chem*, 1990, 36(11):1957-61.

Livesey JF, Perkins SL, Tokessy NE, et al, "Simultaneous Determination of Alcohols and Ethylene Glycol in Serum by Packed- or Capillary-Column Gas Chromatography," *Clin Chem*, 1995, 41(2):300-5.

Walder AD and Tyler CK, "Ethylene Glycol Antifreeze Poisoning," *Anaesthesia*, 1994, 49(11):964-7.

Wisse B, Thakur S, and Baran D, "Recovery From Prolonged Metabolic Acidosis due to Accidental Ethylene Glycol Poisoning," *Am J Kidney Dis*, 1999, 33(2):E4.

Yao HH and Porter WH, "Simultaneous Determination of Ethylene Glycol and its Major Toxic Metabolite, Glycolic Acid, in Serum by Gas Chromatography," *Clin Chem*, 1996, 42(2):292-7.

◆ **EtOH** *see* Ethanol, Blood, Urine, and Other Sources *on page 789*

◆ **Excedrin®** *see* Ibuprofen, Serum *on page 793*

◆ **FAEEs** *see* Ethanol, Blood, Urine, and Other Sources *on page 789*

◆ **Fatty Acid Ethyl Esters** *see* Ethanol, Blood, Urine, and Other Sources *on page 789*

Fenfluramine, Serum

Synonyms Dima-Fen®; Pesos®; Ponderx®; Pondimin®; Ponflural®

Abstract Fenfluramine is an anorectic agent which has been withdrawn from the U.S. market; however, it is available in other countries.

Specimen Serum

Container Red top tube

Reference Interval Therapeutic: 0.05-0.15 µg/mL

Critical Values >6.5 µg/mL

Methodology Thin-layer chromatography (TLC), gas chromatography (GC); in overdose situations, immunoassay for amphetamine may give a positive result with fenfluramine.

Additional Information
- Half-life: 11-20 hours
- Volume of distribution: 15 L/kg
- Protein binding: 34%

Fenfluramine is a sympathomimetic amine, structurally related to amphetamine. However, unlike amphetamine, it does not have a stimulatory effect on the CNS. On September 12, 1997, the FDA announced new summary information concerning abnormal echocardiogram findings in asymptomatic patients seen in five centers. These patients had been treated with fenfluramine or dexfenfluramine for up to 24 months, most often in combination with phenteramine. Abnormal echocardiogram findings were noted in 92 of 291 subjects, including 40 reports of mitral regurgitation (moderate or greater). Connolly, et al, reported 24 cases of valvular heart disease in women treated with fenfluramine-phenteramine combination.[1] Graham and Green reported additional cases in the same issue of *The New England Journal of Medicine*.[2] Those requiring further information can call 1-800-892-2718.

Acute overdose causes tachycardia, asystole, ventricular fibrillation, respiratory failure, mydriasis, nystagmus, seizures, and coma. Treatment is mostly supportive.

Footnotes

1. Connolly HM, Crary JL, McGoon MD, et al, "Valvular Heart Disease Associated With Fenfluramine-Phenteramine," *N Engl J Med*, 1997, 337(9):581-8.

2. Graham DJ and Green L, "Further Cases of Valvular Heart Disease Associated With Fenfluramine-Phenteramine," *N Engl J Med*, 1997, 337(9):635.

References

Derby LE, Myers MW, and Jick H, "Use of Dexfenfluramine, Fenfluramine, and Phenteramine and the Risk of Stroke," *Br J Clin Pharmacol*, 1999, 47(5):565-9.

Mast ST, Jollis JG, Ryan T, et al, "The Progression of Fenfluramine-Associated Valvular Heart Disease Assessed by Echocardiography," *Ann Intern Med*, 2001, 134:261-6.

Schembre DB and Boynton KK, "Appetite-Suppressant Drugs and Primary Pulmonary Hypertension," *N Engl J Med*, 1997, 336(7):510-1.

Spiller HA, Klein-Schwartz W, Weber J, et al, "Retrospective Multicenter Evaluation of Fenfluramine and Dexfenfluramine Ingestion," *J Toxicol Clin Toxicol*, 1997, 35(5):492-3.

Vivero LE, Anderson PO, and Clark RF, "A Close Look at Fenfluramine and Dexfenfluramine," *J Emerg Med*, 1998, 16(2):197-205.

◆ **Ferndex®** *see* Amphetamine, Qualitative, Urine *on page 779*

◆ **Feverall™** *see* Acetaminophen, Serum *on page 778*

Flunitrazepam, Urine

Related Information

Benzodiazepines, Qualitative, Urine *on page 782*
Chain-of-Custody Protocol *on page 785*
Drugs of Abuse Testing, Urine *on page 788*
Gamma Hydroxybutyrate, Serum or Urine *on page 791*

Synonyms Rohypnol®

Abstract Flunitrazepam is a benzodiazepine with sedative and hypnotic activities. The drug is prohibited in the United States and is now used for illicit purposes only, but it is available in other parts of the world. The drug has been identified as an agent used for date rape.

Specimen Random urine

Storage Instructions Refrigerate or freeze if not analyzing immediately.

Special Instructions If forensic, use chain-of-custody protocol and form. See Chain-of-Custody Protocol *on page 785* and the Chain-of-Custody form in the Introduction *on page 773*.

Reference Interval None present; confirmation cutoff: 200 ng/mL

Methodology Enzyme immunoassay (EIA), radioimmunoassay (RIA), gas chromatography/mass spectrometry (GC/MS), high performance liquid chromatography (HPLC)

Additional Information
- Half-life: 9-25 hours
- Protein binding: 80% to 90%
- Volume of distribution: 3.5-5.5 L/kg

The drug is known to impair short-term memory. In an overdose, the drug may cause myocardial depression, hypotension, lethargy, ataxia, nausea, diarrhea, tremor, and apnea. It is frequently coadministered by heroin abusers. In one study, 14 of 40 descendants who died from heroin overdose were found to be positive for flunitrazepam. Poor correlation exists between blood levels and impairment.

The drug is not detected by commonly used benzodiazepine screening assays. Specific immunoassays and GC/MS are needed to detect very small quantities of the drug.

References

Anglin D, Spears KL, and Hutson HR, "Flunitrazepam and Its Involvement in Date or Acquaintance Rape," *Acad Emerg Med*, 1997, 4(4):323-6.

Deinl I, Mahr G, and von Meyer L, "Determination of Flunitrazepam and Its Metabolites in Serum and Urine by HPLC After Mixed Mode Solid-Phase Extraction," *J Anal Toxicol*, 1998, 22(3):197-202.

Drummer OH, Syrjanen ML, and Cordner SM, "Deaths Involving the Benzodiazepine Flunitrazepam," *Am J Forensic Med Pathol*, 1993, 14(3):238-43.

ElSohly MA, Feng S, Salamone SJ, et al, "A Sensitive GC/MS Procedure for the Analysis of Flunitrazepam and Its Metabolites in Urine," *J Anal Toxicol*, 1997, 21(5):335-40.

ElSohly MA and Salamone SJ, "Prevalence of Drugs Used in Cases of Alleged Sexual Assault," *J Anal Toxicol*, 1999, 23(3):141-6.

Gulledge C, Phillips J, and Hammett-Stabler C, "New Kids on the Block An Update on Selected Club Drugs," *Therapeutic Drug Monitoring and Clinical Toxicology Division Newsletter*, 2000, 15(4):1-6.

Hollinger MA, "Rohypnol®: The Date Rape Drug," *Forensic Exam*, 1997, 6:15-7.

Mullins ME, "Laboratory Confirmation of Flunitrazepam in Alleged Cases of Date Rape," *Acad Emerg Med*, 1999, 6:966-8.

Schwartz RH, Milteer R, and LeBeau MA, "Drug Facilitated Sexual Assault (Date Rape)," *South Med J*, 2000, 93(6):558-61.

Simmons MM and Cupp MJ, "Use and Abuse of Flunitrazepam," *Ann Pharmacother*, 1998, 32(1):117-9.

Waltzman ML, "Flunitrazepam: A Review of "Roofies"," *Pediatr Emerg Care*, 1999, 15(1):59-60.

◆ **Free Base** *see* Cocaine (Cocaine Metabolite), Qualitative, Urine or Hair *on page 785*

◆ **Gamma Aminobutyric Acid** *see* Gamma Hydroxybutyrate, Serum or Urine *on page 791*

Gamma Hydroxybutyrate, Serum or Urine

Related Information

Chain-of-Custody Protocol *on page 785*
Drugs of Abuse Testing, Urine *on page 788*
Ethanol, Blood, Urine, and Other Sources *on page 789*
Flunitrazepam, Urine *on page 791*
(Continued)

Gamma Hydroxybutyrate, Serum or Urine

(Continued)

Synonyms Georgia Home Boy; GHB; Grievous Bodily Harm; Liquid Ecstasy; Liquid X; Scoop; Somatomax®

Applies to Gamma Aminobutyric Acid

Abstract Gamma hydroxybutyrate (GHB) is an endogenous metabolite of gamma aminobutyric acid (GABA) that was originally synthesized as an anesthetic. In 1990, it was briefly approved by the Food and Drug Administration (FDA) for use as a hypnotic and to promote weight loss and muscular development. GHB has been withdrawn from the U.S. market and is now used only for illicit purposes. However, its precursors, gamma butyrolactone and 1,4 butanediol are available in health food stores. It is one of the commonly used date-rape drugs.

Specimen Serum or urine

Container Red top tube for serum

Collection If forensic, observe precautions.

Storage Instructions Refrigerate

Special Instructions If forensic, use chain-of-custody protocol and form. See Chain-of-Custody Protocol *on page 785* and the Chain-of-Custody form in the Introduction *on page 773*.

Reference Interval Negative (less than cutoff)

Critical Values Blood levels:
- deep sleep/coma: >260 µg/mL
- moderate sleep: 156-260 µg/mL
- light sleep: 52-156 µg/mL

Use Evaluate GHB toxicity; drug of abuse testing. In some countries, it is used for treatment of narcolepsy, alcohol dependence, and opiate dependence.

Limitations The assay of GHB is not available in all laboratories. Relationship between blood levels and symptoms is not well established.

Methodology Gas chromatography (GC), gas chromatography/mass spectrometry (GC/MS)

Additional Information
- Half-life: 0.3-1 hour
- Volume of distribution: 0.5 L/kg
- Protein binding: 0%

In recent years, there has been an increase in the number of reports of the use of GHB, often in conjunction with alcohol, to commit sexual assault. When added to the victim's drink, the victim becomes semiconscious or unconscious. In a recent study of alleged sexual assault cases, GHB was found in the urine of 48 of 1179 (4.1%) alleged sexual assault victims. Out of these 48 victims, 16 were also positive for alcohol.

GHB toxicity causes CNS depression, amnesia, hypotonia, GI symptoms, loss of consciousness, depressed respiration, tremor, and seizures. It acts synergistically with ethanol to intensify CNS and respiratory depression. There is no specific treatment for GHB toxicity; supportive treatment is given.

Its effects are potentiated by benzodiazepines and neuroleptics, leading to further sedation.[1]

GHB has been used by body-builders and weight lifters as it stimulates growth hormone release by facilitating slow-wave sleep.

Footnotes
1. Gulledge C, Phillips J, and Hammett-Stabler C, "New Kids on the Block: An Update on Selected Club Drugs," *Therapeutic Drug Monitoring and Clinical Toxicology Division Newsletter*, 2000, 15(4):1-6.

References
Bismuth C, Dally S, and Borron SW, "Chemical Submission: GHB, Benzodiazepines, and Other Knock Out Drops," *J Toxicol Clin Toxicol*, 1997, 35(6):595-8.
Chin RL, Sporer KA, Cullison B, et al, "Clinical Course of Gamma-Hydroxybutyrate Overdose," *Ann Emerg Med*, 1998, 31(6):716-22.
Cioffi L, "Gamma Hydroxybutyrate," *Clin Toxicol Rev*, 1997, 19(5):1-2.
Couper FJ and Logan BK, "Determination of Gamma-Hydroxybutyrate (GHB) in Biological Specimens by Gas Chromatography-Mass Spectrometry," *J Anal Toxicol*, 2000, 24(1):1-7.
Dyer JE and Andrews KM, "Gamma Hydroxybutyrate Withdrawal," *J Toxicol Clin Toxicol*, 1997, 35(5):553-4.
Elian AA, "A Novel Method for GHB Detection in Urine and its Application in Drug-Facilitated Sexual Assaults," *Forensic Sci Int*, 2000, 109(3):183-7.
ElSohly MA and Salamone SJ, "Prevalence of Drugs Used in Cases of Alleged Sexual Assault," *J Anal Toxicol*, 1999, 23(3):141-6.
Ingels M, Rangan C, Bellezzo J, et al, "Coma and Respiratory Depression Following the Ingestion of GHB and its Precursors: Three Cases," *J Emerg Med*, 2000, 19(1):47-50.
Li J, Stokes SA, and Woeckener A, "A Tale of Novel Intoxication: A Review of the Effects of Gamma Hydroxybutyric Acid With Recommendations for Management," *Ann Emerg Med*, 1998, 31(6):729-36.
Schwartz RH, Milteer R, and LeBeau MA, "Drug Facilitated Sexual Assault (Date Rape)," *South Med J*, 2000, 93(6):558-61.
Stephens BG and Baselt RC, "Driving Under the Influence of GHB?" *J Anal Toxicol*, 1994, 18(6):357-8.
Williams H, Taylor R, and Roberts M, "Gamma-Hydroxybutyrate (GHB): A New Drug of Misuse," *Ir Med J*, 1998, 91(2):56-7.

Heavy Metal Screen, Blood

Related Information
Arsenic, Hair, Nails *on page 780*
Arsenic, Serum or Plasma *on page 780*
Arsenic, Urine *on page 781*
Cadmium, Urine *on page 783*
Heavy Metal Screen, Urine *on page 792*
Mercury, Blood *on page 797*
Mercury, Urine *on page 798*
Molybdenum, Blood *on page 821*
Thallium, Urine or Blood *on page 807*

Synonyms Metals, Blood; Poisonous Metals, Blood; Toxic Metals, Blood

Test Includes Antimony, arsenic, bismuth, boron, cadmium, cobalt, copper, lead, mercury, selenium, tellurium, thallium, zinc

Abstract Used principally to detect arsenic, cadmium, mercury, and lead poisoning. See individual entries for detailed information.

Specimen Whole blood (EDTA) plus serum

Container Special metal-free tube and red top tube

Storage Instructions Refrigerate: do not spin down.

Special Instructions Check with laboratory performing the assay to determine what elements will be detected and for special instructions.

Reference Interval See individual test listings.

Use Screen for heavy metal poisoning

Methodology Atomic absorption spectrometry (AA), inductively-coupled plasma (ICP)

Additional Information See individual test listings.

References
Baldwin DR and Marshall WJ, "Heavy Metal Poisoning and its Laboratory Investigation," *Ann Clin Biochem*, 1999, 36(Pt 3):267-300.
Barceloux DG, "Nickel," *J Toxicol Clin Toxicol*, 1999, 37(2):239-58.
Graeme KA and Pollack CV Jr, "Heavy Metal Toxicity, Part I: Arsenic and Mercury," *J Emerg Med*, 1998, 16(1):45-56.
Graeme KA and Pollack CV Jr, "Heavy Metal Toxicity, Part II: Lead and Metal Fume Fever," *J Emerg Med*, 1998, 16(2):171-7.
Madden EF and Fowler BA, "Mechanisms of Nephrotoxicity From Metal Combinations: A Review," *Drug Chem Toxicol*, 2000, 23(1):1-12.

Heavy Metal Screen, Urine

Related Information
Arsenic, Hair, Nails *on page 780*
Arsenic, Serum or Plasma *on page 780*
Arsenic, Urine *on page 781*
Cadmium, Urine *on page 783*
Heavy Metal Screen, Blood *on page 792*
Mercury, Blood *on page 797*
Mercury, Urine *on page 798*
Molybdenum, Blood *on page 821*
Thallium, Urine or Blood *on page 807*

Synonyms Metal Screen; Metals, Toxic; Poisonous Metals, Urine; Toxic Metals, Urine

Applies to Hair Analysis

Test Includes Arsenic, mercury, lead (could also include nickel and cadmium)

Abstract Used most often to detect arsenic, mercury, lead, and cadmium poisoning. See individual entries for detailed information.

Specimen 24-hour urine

Container Plastic, acid-washed urine container (preferably polyethylene), no preservative, 20-25 mL 6 N HCl (low metal content)

Storage Instructions Refrigerate

Reference Interval Arsenic: <50 µg/L; lead: <80 µg/L; mercury: <20 µg/L; nickel: <25 µg/L; cadmium: <10 µg/L

Use Screen for heavy metal poisoning and toxic exposure; urine lead analysis is useful for organic lead exposure and to monitor chelation. Blood is preferred for inorganic lead exposure monitoring.

Limitations Hair analysis should be used for arsenic and mercury poisoning or exposure, especially if one is interested in determining chronic exposure. Hair should be clean, free of oil, and clipped (0.5 g for As; 2 g for Hg) as close as possible. (Shortcomings of hair analysis for other substances are addressed in Arsenic, Hair, Nails *on page 780*).

Recent ingestion of seafood can cause misleading increases of urine arsenic.

Methodology Atomic absorption spectrometry (AA), inductively-coupled plasma (ICP)

Additional Information Please see Heavy Metal Screen, Blood *on page 792* for further information. See also the Trace Elements listings.

References

Baldwin DR and Marshall WJ, "Heavy Metal Poisoning and its Laboratory Investigation," *Ann Clin Biochem*, 1999, 36(Pt 3):267-300.

Fukui Y and Miki M, "Urinary Lead as a Possible Surrogate of Blood Lead Among Workers Occupationally Exposed to Lead," *Int Arch Occup Environ Health*, 1999, 72(8):516-20.

Graeme KA and Pollack CV Jr, "Heavy Metal Toxicity, Part I: Arsenic and Mercury," *J Emerg Med*, 1998, 16(1):45-56.

Graeme KA and Pollack CV Jr, "Heavy Metal Toxicity, Part II: Lead and Metal Fume Fever," *J Emerg Med*, 1998, 16(2):171-7.

Philip AT and Gerson B, "Lead Poisoning - Part II. Effects and Assay," *Clin Lab Med*, 1994, 14(3):651-70.

◆ **Hemp** *see* Cannabinoids (Marijuana Metabolites), Qualitative, Urine *on page 783*

◆ **Heroin** *see* Morphine, Urine *on page 802*

◆ **Heroin** *see* Opiates, Qualitative, Urine *on page 803*

◆ **Heroin Detoxification** *see* Methadone, Urine *on page 798*

◆ **Heroin Metabolite, Urine** *see* Morphine, Urine *on page 802*

◆ **Hg, Blood** *see* Mercury, Blood *on page 797*

◆ **Hg, Urine** *see* Mercury, Urine *on page 798*

◆ **Hog** *see* Phencyclidine, Qualitative, Urine *on page 804*

◆ **Hydrocyanic Acid** *see* Cyanide, Blood *on page 787*

◆ **5-Hydroxytryptophol/5-HIAA** *see* Ethanol, Blood, Urine, and Other Sources *on page 789*

◆ **Ibuprin®** *see* Ibuprofen, Serum *on page 793*

Ibuprofen, Serum

Related Information

Anion Gap, Serum, Plasma, or Urine *on page 106*
Complete Blood Count *on page 419*
Electrolyte Panel, Serum *on page 168*
Glucose, Fasting, Plasma *on page 183*
Lactic Acid, Whole Blood or Plasma *on page 208*
Urinalysis *on page 887*

Synonyms Advil®; Excedrin®; Genpril®; Haltran®; Ibuprin®; Ibuprohm®; Medipren®; Menadol®; Midol®; Motrin®; Nuprin®; Pamprin®; Rufen®; Trendar®; Unipro®

Abstract Ibuprofen is a leading non-narcotic, nonsteroidal analgesic and anti-inflammatory agent. As compared to acetylsalicylic acid, it has less intense effects of gastrointestinal irritation and bleeding. In neonates, it is also used in the treatment of patent ductus arteriosus.[1]

Specimen Serum

Turnaround Time 1-3 hours if assay is available in-house

Critical Values See nomogram.

Use Evaluate possible toxicity

Limitations Assays for ibuprofen are not readily available.

Methodology Thin layer chromatography (TLC), high performance liquid chromatography (HPLC),[2] gas chromatography (GC)

Additional Information
- Half-life: 0.9-2.5 hours
- Volume of distribution: 0.14 L/kg
- Protein binding: 99%

Ibuprofen is used in the management of mild to moderate pain and inflammation in conditions such as dysmenorrhea; headache including tension-type headache and migraine; postoperative pain; dental pain; musculoskeletal and joint disorders such as ankylosing spondylitis, osteoarthritis, and rheumatoid arthritis including juvenile chronic arthritis; periarticular disorders such as bursitis and tenosynovitis; pain in sickle cell disease; and soft-tissue disorders such as sprains and strains. It is also used to reduce fever. Ibuprofen has also been used as an alternative to indomethacin in the treatment of patent ductus arteriosus. It acts by inhibiting prostacyclin synthesis, by blocking the activity of cyclo-oxygenase. Ibuprofen is less toxic as compared to salicylates and acetaminophen. Side effects of ibuprofen are predominantly gastritis; they include nausea, epigastric pain, diarrhea, vomiting, dizziness, blurred vision, and edema. Single doses have caused severe anaphylactic reactions in persons allergic to ibuprofen. Some patients develop coma, metabolic acidosis, and renal failure after ibuprofen overdose. Overdose treatment includes gut decontamination and supportive therapy. The following nomogram predicts ibuprofen toxicity (Hall, et al 1992).

Ibuprofen Toxicity Nomogram

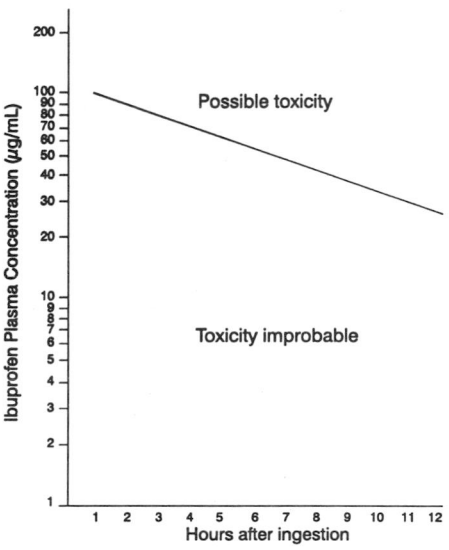

Adapted from Hall AH, Smolinske SC, Stover B, et al, "Ibuprofen Overdose in Adults," *J Toxicol Clin Toxicol*, 1992, 30:34.

Other tests recommended in ibuprofen toxicity include electrolytes, CBC, renal function tests, blood gases, urinalysis to rule out hematuria or proteinuria, and stool guaiac test for GI bleed. Severe toxicity has resulted in hyponatremia and hypophosphatemia. It can cause fulminant hepatitis.

Footnotes

1. Casalaz D, "Ibuprofen Versus Indomethacin for Closure of Patent Ductus Arteriosus," *N Engl J Med*, 2001, 344(6):457-8.
2. Canaparo R, Muntoni E, Zara GP, et al, "Determination of Ibuprofen in Human Plasma by High-Performance Liquid Chromatography: Validation and Application in Pharmacokinetic Study," *Biomed Chromatogr*, 2000, 14(4):219-26.

References

Atta MG and Whelton A, "Acute Renal Papillary Necrosis Induced by Ibuprofen," *Am J Ther*, 1997, 4(1):55-60.

Bernard GR, Wheeler AP, Russell JA, et al, "The Effects of Ibuprofen on the Physiology and Survival of Patients With Sepsis. The Ibuprofen in Sepsis Study Group," *N Engl J Med*, 1997, 336(13):912-8.

Davies NM, "Clinical Pharmacokinetics of Ibuprofen. The First 30 Years," *Clin Pharmacokinet*, 1998, 34(2):101-54.

Fenton J, "Ibuprofen," *The Laboratory and the Poisoned Patient*, Washington, DC: AACC Press, American Association of Clinical Chemistry, 1998, 188-92.

Hall AH, Smolinske SC, Stover B, et al, "Ibuprofen Overdose in Adults," *J Toxicol Clin Toxicol*, 1992, 30(1):23-37.

Hall AH, Smolinske SC, Conrad FL, et al, "Ibuprofen Overdose: 126 Cases," *Ann Emerg Med*, 1986, 15(11):1308-13.

Harchelroad F and Riviello R, "Disorders of Magnesium and Phosphorus in Acute Ibuprofen Ingestion," *Acad Emerg Med*, 1997, 4(5):451.

◆ **Ibuprohm®, Medipren®** *see* Ibuprofen, Serum *on page 793*

◆ **Ice** *see* Methamphetamine, Qualitative, Urine *on page 799*

◆ **Insecticides** *see* Organophosphate Pesticides, Urine, Blood, or Serum *on page 804*

◆ **Isonipecaine Hydrochloride** *see* Meperidine, Serum or Urine *on page 796*

◆ **Isopropanol** *see* Volatile Screen, Blood or Urine *on page 809*

◆ **Kay Jay** *see* Phencyclidine, Qualitative, Urine *on page 804*

◆ **Killer Weed** *see* Phencyclidine, Qualitative, Urine *on page 804*

Lead, Blood

Related Information

Anemia Flowchart *on page 392*
(Continued)

Lead, Blood *(Continued)*

Synonyms Pb, Blood

Applies to Delta Aminolevulinic Acid Dehydratase; Lead, Hair

Abstract A heavy metal, lead can cause chronic or acute toxicity by ingestion, inhalation, or even skin contact. It created disease in the days of the Roman Empire and continues to do so. The hematopoietic system, nervous system, and renal tubular epithelial cells are most affected. The central nervous system is especially sensitive to organic compounds containing lead. In recent decades, lead exposure has significantly decreased in the general population. However, risk of lead exposure continues to be associated with low socioeconomic status, poor nutrition, and low dietary calcium, iron, and zinc.[1] Children may absorb up to 50% of dietary intake, and have greater likelihood of lead exposure.[2]

Specimen Whole blood; venous blood is recommended. Hair can be used as a marker of lead exposure.[3] Nails are also used.

Container Special lead-free tube with heparin; trace metal Vacutainer® tubes containing lithium heparin can be used. EDTA is satisfactory.

Collection See Blood Collection Methods for Trace Elements in the Trace Elements Introduction *on page 811*. Cleansing the site for capillary puncture is needed to avoid contamination if capillary collection is required. Venipuncture is preferred.

Storage Instructions Do not separate red cells.

Causes for Rejection Improper draw

Special Instructions Avoid contact with leaded glass during collection

Reference Interval Children: <10 µg/dL (whole blood) (SI: <0.5 µmol/L). The blood lead level of preindustrial humans is estimated at about 0.016 µg/dL.[4] **Adults:** WHO has defined whole blood levels >30 µg/dL (1.5 µmol/L) as indicative of significant exposure. Lead levels >60 µg/dL (3 µmol/L) require chelation therapy. Due to possible contamination during collection, elevated levels should be confirmed with a second specimen before action is instituted. American Academy of Pediatrics has the recommendations in the following table for venous blood lead management.[5]

Recommended Follow-up Services, According to Diagnostic Blood Lead Level (BLL)

BLL (µg/dL)	Action
<10	No action required
10-14	Obtain a confirmatory venous BLL within 1 month. If still within this range, provide education to decrease blood lead exposure, and repeat BLL test within 3 months.
15-19	Obtain a confirmatory venous BLL within 1 month. If still within this range, take a careful environmental history, provide education to decrease blood lead exposure and to decrease lead absorption, and repeat BLL test within 2 months.
20-44	Obtain a confirmatory venous BLL within 1 week. If still within this range, conduct a complete medical history (including an environmental evaluation and nutritional assessment) and physical examination, provide education to decrease blood lead exposure and to decrease lead absorption, and either refer the patient to the local health department or provide case management that should include a detailed environmental investigation with lead hazard reduction and appropriate referrals for support services. If BLL is >25 µg/dL, consider chelation (not currently recommended for BLLs <45 µg/dL) after consultation with clinicians experienced in lead toxicity treatment.
45-69	Obtain a confirmatory venous BLL within 2 days. If still within this range, conduct a complete medical history (including an environmental evaluation and nutritional assessment) and physical examination, provide education to decrease blood lead exposure and to decrease lead absorption, and either refer the patient to the local health department or provide case management that should include a detailed environmental investigation with lead hazard reduction and appropriate referrals for support services. Begin chelation therapy in consultation with clinicians experienced in lead toxicity treatment.
≥70	Hospitalize the patient and begin medical treatment immediately in consultation with clinicians experienced in lead toxicity therapy. Obtain a confirmatory BLL immediately. The rest of the management should be as noted for management of children with BLLs between 45 and 69 µg/dL

In 1997, CDC recommended a basic three-question questionnaire for parents as a starting point to evaluate risk for lead exposure.

1. Does your child live in or regularly visit a house that was built before 1950? This question can apply to a facility such as home day-care or the home of a babysitter or relative.

2. Does your child live in or regularly visit a house built before 1978 with recent or ongoing renovations or remodeling (within the last 6 months)?
3. Does your child have a sibling or playmate who has or did have lead poisoning?

Screen all children whose parent/guardian responds "yes" or "don't know" to any question.

OSHA uses a lead level of 40 µg/dL for occupational exposure. Lead level >40 µg/dL requires the employer to notify the worker in writing within 5 days. The employee should be removed from work and enter a chelation program if lead level is >60 µg/dL, or with certain other circumstances.[1] In an occupational setting, OSHA requires both whole-blood lead and erythrocyte zinc protoporphyrin testing. Average levels in 1995 were 2.8 µg/dL.

Hair lead content is normally <5 µg/g.

Possible Panic Range >70 µg/dL (SI: >3.34 µmol/L) in acute lead poisoning; toxicity at lower levels in chronic poisoning

Use Blood lead concentrations are used to detect recent lead exposure, but do not necessarily measure lead body burden from past chronic exposure. Levels are used to evaluate lead exposure, toxicity, and poisoning (plumbism). Screening is indicated on the basis of responses to risk questions (*vide supra*) and in differential diagnosis of severe anemia, seizures, abdominal pain, and unexplained illness.

Limitations In chronic lead exposure, blood levels do not correlate with the severity of toxicity. The EDTA lead mobilization test or x-ray fluorescence may be needed for diagnosis of lead nephropathy.[6,7,8]

Great care is required to avoid contamination in the collection of specimens for lead analysis.

Free erythrocyte protoporphyrin and zinc protoporphyrin may be helpful with blood lead level to assess the stage of plumbism (acute vs chronic toxicity). Free erythrocyte protoporphyrin is insensitive to blood lead levels <35 µg/dL.

Methodology Electrothermal atomic absorption spectrometry (AA), anodic stripping voltammetry, inductively-coupled plasma atomic emission spectroscopy, inductively coupled plasma-mass spectrometry (ICP-MS), x-ray fluorescence spectroscopy. Filter paper methods for screening are becoming available.[9]

Additional Information Lead can also be measured in tissue and urine. Another test used to evaluate lead intoxication is the erythrocyte zinc protoporphyrin (ZPP) concentration. ZPP is not thought to be an adequate indicator for lead toxicity at lead blood levels <25 µg/dL, and therefore is not currently recommended by CDC for lead screening in children 6 years of age and younger. Normal values for ZPP are 17-77 µg/dL. See Delta (5)-Aminolevulinic Acid, Urine *on page 165* and Porphyrins, Quantitative, Urine *on page 255*. Inhibition of erythrocyte **delta aminolevulinic acid dehydratase** is also a measure of lead toxicity, but is not inhibited until blood lead levels are >15-20 µg/dL. However, a blood lead assay is the definitive test for recent acute exposure. Blood lead concentrations are evidence of **recent** exposure but do not indicate the body burden from past exposure. See Lead, Urine *on page 795* for lead mobilization test.

Lead expresses its toxicity by several mechanisms and the toxicity follows a progressive pattern, as shown in the following figure.

Of sources of lead poisoning in children, paint is still the most important. A single paint chip can contain as much as 10,000 µg of lead. Although the lead content of paints for household application has been limited to <0.5% since 1972, older paint is still in place on wood and even in adjacent soil and dust (pica). Artists' paints and products for other applications still contain lead.[2]

Use of candles with lead-containing wicks may cause lead poisoning. Thirty percent of candles in a survey contained metallic wicks; of these, 10% contained lead (overall 3% lead-wick prevalence).[10]

Other sources of lead include air, soil, dust, drinking water, food (especially in lead-soldered cans), solder, storage batteries, ammunition, other metal objects, gasoline additives, other chemicals, and imported Asian products including third world cosmetics. Weak acids (eg, fruit juice, vinegar) can leach lead from some ceramic containers and from leaded crystal.[2] Other sources, including Mexican remedies for "empacho", home abortifacients, herbal medicines, folk remedies, and moonshine are published as well. Occupational exposure is important in adults.[4] Retained bullets in the body are a source of plumbism. The surface areas of the missile(s), location, presence of synovial fluid, and length of time in the body are relevant.[3] A branch of the CDC, the National Institute for Occupational Safety and Health (NIOSH), provides recommendations for prevention of occupational lead poisoning. Occupational exposure includes battery workers, welders, lead and other smelter workers, pottery makers, printers, those who paint and repair old houses, those who work on firing ranges, and employees in types of manufacturing.

Lead absorption is influenced by iron deficiency. Greater than 90% of absorbed lead is deposited in the skeleton and in teeth. Plumbism has been identified with lead poisoning in pets.[11] Bone lead concentration can be estimated with K x-ray fluorescence[12] or L x-ray fluorescence.[13]

Effects of lead are mediated by its ability to complex sulfhydryl groups and other ligands in enzyme systems. Lead toxicity occurs secondary to environmental, occupational, or recreational activities. Acute exposures are commonly associated with symptoms of anorexia, malaise, nausea, vomiting, and abdominal pain (lead colic). Fecal discoloration (black or red) may occur. Constipation, anemia, tremor, headache, coma, hearing loss, tinnitus, alopecia, and bradycardia may be seen. Severe exposures can result in encephalopathy and death; chronic exposures manifest with hypertension, arthralgias, teratogenesis, and impotence. Microcytic hypochromic anemia and basophilic stippling are characteristic, but basophilic stippling occurs in lead toxicity as well as in lead poisoning. It only appears in about 2% of erythrocytes and is not found in all cases of lead poisoning. It does not correlate with severity of plumbism. Fanconi syndrome (aminoaciduria, glycosuria, hyperphosphaturia with hypophosphatemia, and proteinuria) may be found with renal dysfunction/failure. Nuclear inclusions in renal tubular cells are found.

Central nervous system effects include ataxia, neuropsychiatric symptoms, encephalopathy, headache, learning disabilities, lethargy, mood and/or mental status changes, and seizures. Lead causes peripheral neuropathy in which wrist drop and foot drop are characteristic. Recently, lead has been associated with a number of affected surfaces for both deciduous and permanent teeth in all age groups, even after adjusting for sociodemographic characteristics, diet, and dental care.[14] Gastrointestinal effects include abdominal colic, constipation, nausea, and vomiting. Saturnine gout, mentioned in Uric Acid, Serum *on page 293*, is hyperuricemia from interstitial nephritis of chronic lead exposure.

Lead crosses the placenta; cord blood concentrations are 85% to 90% those of the mother.

Effects of Inorganic Lead on Children and Adults-- Lowest Observable Adverse Effect Levels

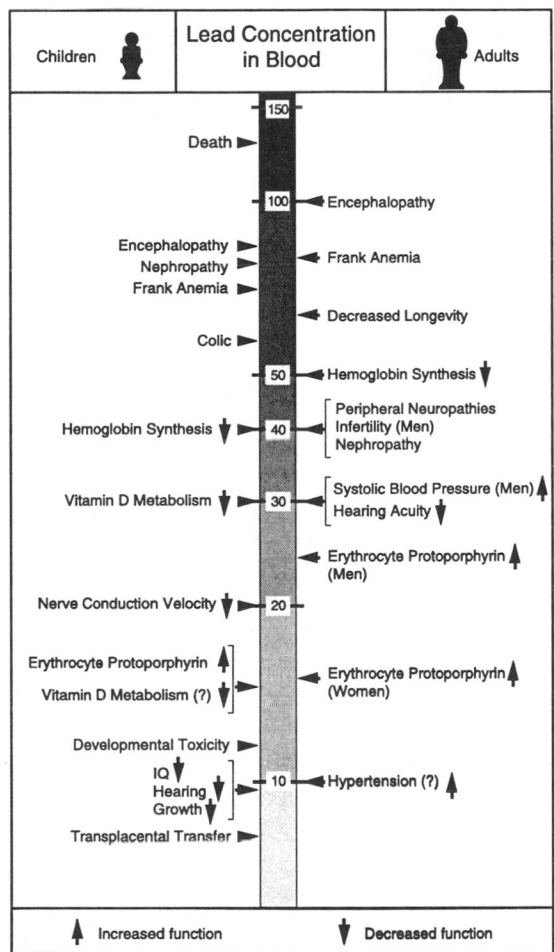

Note that blood levels are usually >40 µg/dL when anemia is recognized (ie, an apparently normal CBC does not rule out plumbism).

Adapted from U.S. Department of Health and Human Services, Royce SE and Needleman HL, eds, "Case Studies in Environmental Medicine: Lead Toxicity," Agency for Toxic Substances and Disease

Footnotes

1. Goyer RA, "Result of Lead Research: Prenatal Exposure and Neurological Consequences," *Environ Health Perspect*, 1996, 104(10):1050-4.
2. Moyer TP, "Toxic Metals," *Tietz Textbook of Clinical Chemistry*, 3rd ed, Burtis CA and Ashwood ER, eds, Philadelphia, PA: WB Saunders Co, 1999, 982-8.
3. Deppisch WM, Centeno JA, Gemmel DJ, et al, "Andrew Jackson's Exposure to Mercury and Lead: Poisoned President?" *JAMA*, 1999, 282(6):569-71.
4. Philip AT and Gerson B, "Lead Poisoning. Part I. Incidence, Etiology, and Toxicokinetics," *Clin Lab Med*, 1994, 14(2):423-44.
5. Etzel RA, Balk SJ, and Beaver CF, eds, "Screening for Elevated Blood Lead Levels. American Academy of Pediatrics Committee on Environmental Health," *Pediatrics*, 1998, 101(6):1072-8.

6. Batuman V, "Lead Nephropathy, Gout, and Hypertension," *Am J Med Sci*, 1993, 305(4):241-7.
7. Lin J-L, Ho HH, and Yu CC, "Chelation Therapy for Patients With Elevated Body Lead Burden and Progressive Renal Insufficiency," *Ann Intern Med*, 1999, 130(1):7-13.
8. Kim R, Rotnitzky A, Sparrow D, et al, "A Longitudinal Study of Low-Level Lead Exposure and Impairment of Renal Function," *JAMA*, 1996, 275(15):1177-81.
9. Stanton NV, Maney JM, and Jones R, "Evaluation of Filter Paper Blood Lead Methods: Results of a Pilot Proficiency Testing Program," *Clin Chem*, 1999, 45(12):2229-35.
10. Sobel HL, Lurie P, and Wolfe SM, "Lead Exposure From Candles," *JAMA*, 2000, 284(2):180.
11. Dowsett R and Shannon M, "Childhood Plumbism Identified After Lead Poisoning in Household Pets," *N Engl J Med*, 1994, 331(24):1661-2.
12. Kosnett MJ, Becker CE, Osterloh JD, et al, "Factors Influencing Bone Lead Concentration in a Suburban Community Assessed by Noninvasive K X-ray Fluorescence," *JAMA*, 1994, 271(3):197-203.
13. Landrigan PJ and Todd AC, "Direct Measurement of Lead in Bone: A Promising Biomarker," *JAMA*, 1994, 271(3):239-40.
14. Moss ME, Lanphear BP, and Auinger P, "Association of Dental Caries and Blood Lead Levels," *JAMA*, 1999, 281(24):2294-8.

References

Beritic T, "Misconceptions About Blood Lead Concentrations," *Br J Ind Med*, 1993, 50(12):1123-4.

Bernard BP and Becker CE, "Environmental Lead Exposure and the Kidney," *J Toxicol Clin Toxicol*, 1988, 26(1-2):1-34.

"Blood Lead Levels in Young Children - United States and Selected States, 1996-1999," *MMWR Morb Mortal Wkly Rep*, 2000, 49(50):1133-7.

Braithwaite RA and Brown SS, "Clinical and Subclinical Lead Poisoning: A Laboratory Perspective," *Hum Toxicol*, 1988, 7(5):503-13.

Brody DJ, Pirkle JL, Kramer RA, et al, "Blood Lead Levels in the U.S. Population. Phase I of the Third National Health and Nutritional Examination Survey," *JAMA*, 1994, 272(4):277-83.

Hu H, Aro A, Payton M, et al, "The Relationship of Bone and Blood Lead to Hypertension," *JAMA*, 1996, 275(15):1171-6.

Labbe RF, Vreman HJ, and Stevenson DK, "Zinc Protoporphyrin: A Metabolite With a Mission," *Clin Chem*, 1999, 45(12):2060-72.

Markowitz ME and Rosen JF, "Need for the Lead Mobilization Test in Children With Lead Poisoning," *J Pediatr*, 1991, 119(2):305-10.

Matte TD, "Reducing Blood Lead Levels: Benefits and Strategies," *JAMA*, 1999, 281(24):2340-2.

Mushak P, Davis JM, Crocetti AF, et al, "Prenatal and Postnatal Effects of Low-Level Lead Exposure: Integrated Summary of a Report to the U.S. Congress on Childhood Lead Poisoning," *Environ Res*, 1989, 50(1):11-36.

Piomelli S, "Childhood Lead Poisoning in the '90s," *Pediatrics*, 1994, 93(3):508-10.

Rempel D, "The Lead-Exposed Worker," *JAMA*, 1989, 262(4):532-4.

Royce SE and Needleman HL, eds, "Case Studies in Environmental Medicine: Lead Toxicity," Agency for Toxic Substances and Disease Registry, 1990.

Staessen JA, Lauwerys RR, Buchet JP, et al, "Impairment of Renal Function With Increasing Blood Lead Concentrations in the General Population," *N Engl J Med*, 1992, 327(3):151-6.

Tong S, Baghurst PA, Sawyer MG, et al, "Declining Blood Lead Levels and Changes in Cognitive Function During Childhood," *JAMA*, 1998, 280(22):1915-9.

Williams RH and Erickson T, "Evaluating Lead and Iron Intoxication in an Emergency Setting," *Lab Med*, 1998, 29(4):224-31.

◆ **Lead Excretion Ratio** *see* Lead, Urine *on page 795*

◆ **Lead, Hair** *see* Lead, Blood *on page 793*

◆ **Lead Mobilization Test** *see* Lead, Urine *on page 795*

Lead, Urine

Related Information

Anemia Flowchart *on page 392*
Delta (5)-Aminolevulinic Acid, Urine *on page 165*
Ferritin, Serum *on page 173*
Iron and Total Iron Binding Capacity/Transferrin, Serum *on page 203*
Lead, Blood *on page 793*
Porphyrins, Quantitative, Urine *on page 255*
Protoporphyrin, Free Erythrocyte *on page 269*

Synonyms Pb, Urine

Applies to Lead Excretion Ratio; Lead Mobilization Test

Abstract This test is used to assess lead body burden (lead mobilization test), not to diagnose lead poisoning. The kidneys represent the most important mechanism of lead excretion, but only slight loss through the kidneys takes place without chelation therapy (eg, with BAL, EDTA, or dimercaprol analogues).

Patient Preparation Patient should be instructed to use a specially cleaned plastic urinal or bedpan

Specimen 24-hour urine is preferred; in an emergency, random specimens may be acceptable

Container Plastic (preferably polyethylene) acid-washed (nitric acid) urine container copiously rinsed with appropriate (nontap deionized) water

Collection Avoid a catheter if possible.

Storage Instructions Record total volume. Acidify to pH 2 with concentrated HCl or add 20 mL 6N HCl to the 24-hour volume.

Causes for Rejection Specimen allowed to contact glass or metal, specimen not collected in acid-washed containers

Special Instructions Indicate if a chelating agent has been administered (Continued)

Lead, Urine (Continued)

Reference Interval ≤80 µg/24 hours (SI: ≤0.39 µmol/day)

Critical Values >125 µg/24 hours (SI: >0.60 µmol/day) is considered excessive and associated with toxicity; values of 80-125 µg/24 hours (SI: 0.39-0.60 µmol/day) are inconclusive

Use Evaluate lead exposure and toxicity before and following chelation therapy

Limitations The value of urinary lead levels without prior administration of a chelating agent is questionable. Blood lead concentrations provide the best correlation with toxicity.

Methodology Electrothermal atomic absorption (AA), inductively-coupled plasma atomic emission spectroscopy, inductively-coupled plasma-mass spectrometry (ICP-MS)

Additional Information Lead is poorly excreted and is found in lower concentrations in urine than in blood. Urine is not the appropriate specimen for screening potential toxicity. Urine lead mobilization tests (postchelation therapy) are good indicators of lead body burden. Children with blood lead levels between 25-40 µg/dL should be evaluated by a lead mobilization test to determine need for chelation therapy. Those with levels >40 µg/dL should receive chelation therapy.[1] The **lead mobilization test (LMT)** is performed by administering 500 mg/m² of CaNa₂-ethylenediaminetetraacetic acid (EDTA) and then collecting urine for 8 hours; a positive result is defined as a ratio of urinary lead/dose EDTA >0.6 (µg lead/mg EDTA given) or a total urinary excretion >200 µg of lead. Details are published.[2]

The **lead excretion ratio (LER)** is calculated by dividing the amount of lead excreted (in µg/24 hours) by the amount of Ca EDTA given (in mg). A ratio >0.60 is considered positive for the LER. Blood for lead and free erythrocyte protoporphyrin should be obtained before chelation. Unstimulated urinary excretion at rates >0.19 µg lead/mg creatinine may also be used to indicate need for chelation therapy.[3]

Serum ferritin or serum iron and total iron binding capacity/transferrin are needed because iron deficiency enhances absorption and toxicity of lead.[2]

Footnotes
1. Markowitz ME and Rosen JF, "Need for the Lead Mobilization Test in Children With Lead Poisoning," *J Pediatr*, 1991, 119(2):305-10.
2. Philip AT and Gerson B, "Lead Poisoning. Part II. Effects and Assay," *Clin Lab Med*, 1994, 14(3):651-70.
3. Berger OG, Gregg DJ, and Succop PA, "Using Unstimulated Lead Excretion to Assess the Need for Chelation in the Treatment of Lead Poisoning," *J Pediatr*, 1990, 116(1):46-51.

References
Cory-Slechta DA, "Lead Exposure During Advanced Age: Alterations in Kinetics and Biochemical Effects," *Toxicol Appl Pharmacol*, 1990, 104(1):67-78.

D'Haese PC, Lamberts LV, Liang L, et al, "Elimination of Matrix and Spectral Interferences in the Measurement of Lead and Cadmium in Urine and Blood by Electrothermal Atomic Absorption Spectrometry With Deuterium Background Correction," *Clin Chem*, 1991, 37(9):1583-8.

Gulson BL, Jameson CW, Mahaffey KR, et al, "Pregnancy Increases Mobilization of Lead From Maternal Skeleton," *J Lab Clin Med*, 1997, 130(1):51-62.

Paloucek FP, "Lead Poisoning," *Am Pharm*, 1993, NS33(11):81-8, quiz 88-90.

♦ **Liquid Ecstasy** *see* Gamma Hydroxybutyrate, Serum or Urine *on page 791*

♦ **Liquid Lady** *see* Cocaine (Cocaine Metabolite), Qualitative, Urine or Hair *on page 785*

♦ **Liquid X** *see* Gamma Hydroxybutyrate, Serum or Urine *on page 791*

♦ **Liquiprin®** *see* Acetaminophen, Serum *on page 778*

♦ **l-Methamphetamine** *see* Methamphetamine, Qualitative, Urine *on page 799*

♦ **LSD** *see* Lysergic Acid Diethylamide, Urine *on page 796*

♦ **LSD-2** *see* Lysergic Acid Diethylamide, Urine *on page 796*

♦ **Lude®** *see* Methaqualone, Urine *on page 800*

♦ **Ludes** *see* Methaqualone, Urine *on page 800*

Lysergic Acid Diethylamide, Urine

Related Information
Drugs of Abuse Testing, Urine *on page 788*
Phencyclidine, Qualitative, Urine *on page 804*

Synonyms LSD; LSD-2

Abstract LSD is one of the most potent hallucinogenic agents and is currently a DEA schedule I drug. It is a drug of abuse. It has no appropriate clinical role.

Specimen Urine; levels can be done on blood specimens as well.

Storage Instructions Refrigerate

Special Instructions If forensic, observe precautions and use chain-of-custody protocol.

Reference Interval None present in normal urine; confirmation cutoff: 0.5 ng/mL

Possible Panic Range 4-8 ng/mL

Methodology Immunoassay, gas chromatography (GC), high performance liquid chromatography (HPLC), gas chromatography/mass spectrophotometry (GC/MS) for confirmation

Additional Information
- Half-life: 3-4 hours
- Volume of distribution: 0.28 L/kg
- Protein binding: 90%
- Onset of action: oral: 20-90 minutes, I.V.: 10 minutes
- Duration of action: 6-8 hours

LSD is an indole derivative, an indolamine. (Other drugs in this class include mescaline). Only the D-isomer is active. LSD is usually administered by drug abusers as the tartrate salt in oral doses of 50-250 µg. The drug may be given as a sugar cube, on filter and blotting paper, or as a tablet or capsule. LSD prevents the inhibitory effect of serotonin, resulting in increased neuronal firing and distortion of perception and orientation.

Fatalities due to LSD are very rare, as the doses required for hallucination are much lower than the amounts that cause fatalities. Signs and symptoms of LSD overdose include hallucinations, delusions, rhabdomyolysis, fear, tremors, delirium, and psychosis. There is no specific antidote for LSD; overdose treatment is supportive. LSD "trips" are ordinarily self-limiting, but can lead to respiratory arrest. Measurement of creatine kinase in patients who are extremely agitated or with seizures is useful.

The detection of LSD in the laboratory is challenging due to very low concentrations of LSD in body fluids. Several manufacturers now make ultrasensitive immunoassay kits, which can detect LSD as low as 0.1 ng/mL. LSD is metabolized to 2-oxo-3-hydroxy-LSD. The metabolite is present in higher concentration in urine and is detected for longer periods of time.

References
Abraham HD and Aldridge AM, "Adverse Consequences of Lysergic Acid Diethylamide," *Addiction*, 1993, 88(10):1327-34.

Batzer W, Ditzler T, and Brown C, "LSD Use and Flashbacks in Alcoholic Patients," *J Addict Dis*, 1999, 18(2):57-63.

Behan WM, Bakheit AM, Behan PO, et al, "The Muscle Findings in the Neuroleptic Malignant Syndrome Associated With Lysergic Acid Diethylamide," *J Neurol Neurosurg Psychiatry*, 1991, 54(8):741-3.

Fenton J, "Lysergic Acid Diethylamide," *The Laboratory and the Poisoned Patient*, Washington, DC: AACC Press, American Association of Clinical Chemistry, 1998, 225-8.

Li Z, McNally AJ, Wang H, et al, "Stability Study of LSD Under Various Storage Conditions," *J Anal Toxicol*, 1998, 22(6):520-5.

Markel H, Lee A, Holmes RD, et al, "LSD Flashback Syndrome Exacerbated by Selective Serotonin Reuptake Inhibitor Antidepressants in Adolescents," *J Pediatr*, 1994, 125(5 Pt 1):817-9.

Poch GK, Klette KL, and Anderson C, "The Quantitation of 2-oxo-3-Hydroxy Lysergic Acid Diethylamide (O-H-LSD) in Human Urine Specimens, a Metabolite of LSD: Comparative Analysis Using Liquid Chromatography-Selected ion Monitoring Mass Spectrometry and Liquid Chromatography-Ion Trap Mass Spectrometry," *J Anal Toxicol*, 2000, 24(3):170-9.

Reuschel SA, Eades D, and Foltz RL, "Recent Advances in Chromatographic and Mass Spectrometric Methods of LSD and Its Metabolites in Physiological Specimens," *J Chromatogr B Biomed Sci Appl*, 1999, 733(1-2):145-59.

Ritter D, Cortese CM, Edwards LC, et al, "Interference With Testing for Lysergic Acid Diethylamide," *Clin Chem*, 1997, 43(4):635-7.

♦ **Marijuana** *see* Cannabinoids (Marijuana Metabolites), Qualitative, Urine *on page 783*

♦ **MDMA** *see* Methamphetamine, Qualitative, Urine *on page 799*

♦ **MDMA** *see* 3,4 Methylenedioxymethamphetamine, Urine *on page 801*

♦ **Measurin®** *see* Salicylate, Serum or Plasma *on page 806*

♦ **Meda-Cap®** *see* Acetaminophen, Serum *on page 778*

♦ **Medical Legal Specimens** *see* Chain-of-Custody Protocol *on page 785*

♦ **Mee's Lines** *see* Arsenic, Hair, Nails *on page 780*

♦ **Mee's Lines** *see* Thallium, Urine or Blood *on page 807*

♦ **Menadol®** *see* Ibuprofen, Serum *on page 793*

Meperidine, Serum or Urine

Related Information
Chain-of-Custody Protocol *on page 785*
Codeine, Urine *on page 786*
Drugs of Abuse Testing, Urine *on page 788*
Morphine, Urine *on page 802*
Propoxyphene, Serum or Urine *on page 805*

Synonyms Centralgine®; Demerol®; Dolantin®; Dolantina®; Dolantine®; Dolosal®; Isonipecaine Hydrochloride; Pethidine Hydrochloride

Applies to Normeperidine

Test Includes This test is included in the comprehensive Urine Drug Screen.

Abstract Meperidine is a synthetic narcotic analgesic with about one-tenth the potency of morphine. It produces less smooth muscle spasm, constipation, and depression of the cough reflex than morphine. It causes delirium and is a drug of abuse.

Specimen Serum or urine

Container Red top tube, plastic urine container

Sampling Time Trough for serum

Storage Instructions Refrigerate

Special Instructions If forensic, use chain-of-custody protocol and form. See Chain-of-Custody Protocol *on page 785* and the Chain-of-Custody form in the Introduction *on page 773.*

Reference Interval Serum: 70-500 ng/mL (SI: 0.28-2.0 µmol/L); urine: negative when not on therapy. Patients with therapeutic blood levels can have a urine meperidine level up to 10 µg/mL.

Critical Values Serum toxic levels: >1000 ng/mL (SI: >4.0 nmol/L)

Possible Panic Range Serum levels: >5000 ng/mL (SI: >20 nmol/L)

Use Evaluate toxicity; detect an abused drug. Meperidine is a shorter-acting synthetic morphine-like compound used in the management of moderate to severe pain and as an adjunct to anesthesia and preoperative sedation.

Limitations Therapeutic levels are not detected by enzyme-multiplied immunoassay technique (EMIT), thin-layer chromatography, and enzyme immunoassay. Use HPLC or gas chromatography (GC) methods to detect therapeutic concentrations.

Contraindications This drug is contraindicated in individuals with renal dysfunction or those on monoamine oxidase inhibitors.

Methodology Gas chromatography (GC) or high performance liquid chromatography (HPLC). High concentrations in overdose can be detected by thin-layer chromatography (TLC).

Additional Information
- Half-life: 2-4 hours
- Volume of distribution: 3-4 L/kg
- Protein binding: 40% to 60%

Analgesic effects after oral ingestion or I.M. injection peak in 1 hour. It is biotransformed to normeperidine, which is a toxic metabolite. Adverse effects include tachycardia, CNS and respiratory depression, nausea and vomiting, hypotension, bradycardia, miosis, increased intracranial pressure, and physical and psychological dependence. When evaluating therapeutic levels, order Meperidine, Serum. It causes increase in carbon dioxide partial pressure and decrease in blood pH. An increase in serum glucose is also noted.

References

Clark RF, Wei EM, and Anderson PO, "Meperidine: Therapeutic Use and Toxicity," *J Emerg Med*, 1995, 13(6):797-802.

Johnson MD, Hurley RJ, Gilbertson LI, et al, "Continuous Microcatheter Spinal Anesthesia With Subarachnoid Meperidine for Labor and Delivery," *Anesth Analg*, 1990, 70(6):658-61.

Volles DF and McGory R, "Pharmacokinetic Considerations," *Crit Care Clin*, 1999, 15(1):55-75.

♦ **Mephobarb** *see* Barbiturates, Qualitative, Urine *on page 781*

Mercury, Blood

Related Information

Cadmium, Urine *on page 783*
Heavy Metal Screen, Blood *on page 792*
Heavy Metal Screen, Urine *on page 792*
Mercury, Urine *on page 798*

Synonyms Cinnabar; Hg, Blood; Organic Mercury; Quicksilver

Applies to Hair Analysis; Methylmercury; Vermilion

Abstract Mercury, also known as quicksilver, is a highly toxic transitional metal belonging to the same family as zinc and cadmium. It is liquid in its elemental form at room temperature and is most commonly found in sulfide form, known as cinnabar. Mercuric sulfide is a common antiseptic and pigment known as vermilion. The surface of the earth and atmosphere are constantly exposed to elemental mercury, a product of the natural "out gassing" of rock. Elemental mercury is toxic if inhaled or injected, but may safely pass through the digestive tract if small amounts are swallowed. Blood analysis for mercury is used principally for evaluation of toxicity from organic mercury, found in wood preservatives, paints, fungicides, cosmetics, foods, seeds, and in contaminated fish. The mercury catastrophe in Minamata Bay, Japan, involved ingestion of methylmercury-contaminated fish. This highly toxic form of mercury derived from methylation of mercuric salt wastes dumped into the regional waters by various industries around Minamata Bay.

Specimen Whole blood

Container Special metal-free EDTA tube

Collection See Blood Collection Methods for Trace Elements in the Trace Elements Introduction *on page 811.*

Causes for Rejection Failure to collect blood in a special metal-free container or exposure to metal containing dusts

Special Instructions Whole blood is analyzed.

Reference Interval Whole blood: 0.6-59 µg/mL (SI: 3-294 nmol/L).[1] Normally whole blood mercury is <10 µg/L, but this number varies widely in a large population of healthy unexposed individuals.[2]

Critical Values >50 µg/L (SI: 250 nmol/L) if exposure is to alkyl mercury compounds and >200 µg/L (SI: 1000 nmol/L) if exposure is to Hg^{+2} compounds.[2]

Possible Panic Range >100.0 µg/L (SI: 500 nmol/L)

Use Evaluate for mercury toxicity, neurological findings related to organic mercurials, inhalation of mercury vapors. Such vapors are efficiently

absorbed through lungs and are very hazardous, leading to pulmonary distress as well as damage to the central nervous system, kidneys, and gastrointestinal tract (*vide infra*).

Limitations Methyl mercury must be measured in whole blood or erythrocytes. Inorganic mercury is best evaluated by urine mercury levels. Once exposure ceases, these levels may not provide a good indicator of remaining body burden.[3] There are marked variations by different investigators[4] in mercury levels considered toxic.

Methodology Electrothermal atomic absorption (AA), gold electrode deposition, gas chromatography (GC)

Additional Information Organic methyl mercury is an important environmental mercurial contaminant. It was discovered that elemental mercury could be oxidized into inorganic mercury (Hg^{+2}) and then into organic mercury (methylmercury) from industrial wastes. Organic mercury then accumulates in large amounts in predator fish, and thus, into the human food chain. Ingestion of mercury-laden fish in Minamata Bay led to severe neurologic deficits.[5]

The major physical forms of mercury to which humans are exposed are (elemental) mercury vapor and methylmercury compounds. Mercury vapor emitted in the atmosphere from varied sources is oxidized into inorganic mercurial salts (Hg^{+2}). Inorganic mercury is subject to microbial conversion into methylmercury compounds (CH_3Hg X) which accumulate in the food chain in freshwater fish and seafood.[6] Acute mercury poisoning, usually due to aspiration of elemental mercury vapors, is seen most commonly in industrial smelting or gold ore processing, requiring the use of gold-mercury amalgams with distillation.[7,8] Severe acute poisoning leads to pulmonary distress with acute pneumonitis, hemoptysis, and cyanosis. Mechanical ventilation is often required. Permanent sequelae may include irreversible lung impairment[4] and pulmonary fibrosis.[9] Inhalation of elemental mercury from mercury-silver dental amalgams is an insignificant exposure risk, as it is estimated that 490 dental amalgam surfaces are required for enough elemental and ionic mercury to be given off to meet maximum exposure thresholds.[10]

Inorganic mercury (Hg^{+2}) causes toxological effects similar to its other family member, cadmium. Both metals are potent chelators of proteins and enzymes. They bind avidly to sulfhydryl groups, leading to oxidative stress, which disrupts the metabolism and biological activities of many proteins, including depletion of intracellular glutathione.[11] Inorganic mercury is corrosive to the GI tract. Exposure may lead to renal failure and infarcts of brain and kidneys.[12] No specific lesions may be seen in the brain of those poisoned by inorganic mercurial compounds. Organic mercurials, however, are potent neurotoxins affecting primarily central nervous tissue with loss of neurons; reactive glial proliferation; microcavitation; vascular congestion; petechial hemorrhage; and edema in the calcarine, precentral, postcentral, transverse temporal cortex and cerebellar cortex.[12]

Half-life of inorganic mercury is 24 days and of methylmercury (organic mercury) is 54 days. Hair analysis may be used for poisoning or chronic exposure. It should be clean and clipped as close to the scalp as possible. Hair analysis is further discussed in Arsenic, Hair, Nails *on page 780.*

Other studies for possible mercury poisoning include BUN, creatinine, and urinalysis.

Footnotes

1. Painter PC, Cope JY, and Smith JL, "Reference Information for the Clinical Laboratory," *Tietz Textbook of Clinical Chemistry*, Chapter 50, Burtis CA and Ashwood ER, eds, Philadelphia, PA: WB Saunders Co, 1999, 1825.

2. Moyer TP, "Toxic Metals," *Tietz Textbook of Clinical Chemistry*, Chapter 28, Burtis CA and Ashwood ER, eds, Philadelphia, PA: WB Saunders Co, 1999, 992-3.

3. Howard P and Billings CG, "Dynamics and Clinical Effects of Nonferrous Metals in the Human Body," *Monaldi Arch Chest Dis*, 2000, 55(1):70-3.

4. Graeme KA and Pollack CV, "Heavy Metal Toxicity, Part I: Arsenic and Mercury," 1998, 16(1):45-56.

5. Uchino M, Okajima T, Eto K, et al, "Neurologic Features of Chronic Minamata Disease (Organic Mercury Poisoning) Certified at Autopsy," *Intern Med*, 1995, 34(8):744-7.

6. Clarkson TW, "The Toxicology of Mercury," *Crit Rev Clin Lab Sci*, 1997, 34(4):369-403.

7. Solis MT, Yuen E, Cortez PS, et al, "Family Poisoned by Mercury Vapor Inhalation," *Am J Emerg Med*, 2000, 18(5):599-602.

8. Donoghue AM, "Mercury Toxicity Due to Smelting of Placer Gold Recovered by Mercury Amalgam," *Occup Med (Lond)*, 1998, 48(6):413-5.

9. Lim HE, Shim JJ, Lee SY, et al, "Mercury Inhalation Poisoning and Acute Lung Injury," *Korean J Intern Med*, 1998, 13(2):127-30.

10. Jones DW, "Exposure of Absorption and the Crucial Question of Limits for Mercury," *J Can Dent Assoc*, 1999, 65(1):42-6.

11. Quig D, "Cysteine Metabolism and Metal Toxicity," *Altern Med Rev*, 1998, 3(4):262-70.

12. Eto K, Takizawa Y, Akagi H, et al, "Differential Diagnosis Between Organic and Inorganic Mercury Poisoning in Human Cases - the Pathological Point of View," *Toxicol Path*, 1999, 27(6):664-71.

References

Cavalleri A and Gobba F, "Reversible Color Vision Loss in Occupational Exposure to Metallic Mercury," *Environ Res*, 1998, 77(2):173-7.

Davis LE, "Unregulated Potions Still Cause Mercury Poisoning," *West J Med*, 2000, 173(1):19.

Knobeloch LM, Ziarnik M, Anderson HA, et al, "Imported Seabass as a Source of Mercury Exposure: A Wisconsin Case Study," *Environ Health Perspect*, 1995, 103(6):604-6.

(Continued)

Mercury, Blood (Continued)

Magos L, "Three Cases of Methylmercury Intoxication Which Eluded Correct Diagnosis," *Arch Toxicol*, 1998, 72(11):701-5.

Mason HJ and Calder IM, "The Correction of Mercury Concentrations in Untimed, Random Samples," *Occup Environ Med*, 1994, 51(4):287.

Maynou C, Mathieu-Nolf M, Mesdagh H, et al, "Accidental Subcutaneous Injection of Elemental Mercury. A Case Report," *Acta Orthop Belg*, 2000, 66(3):292-6.

McRill C, Boyer LV, Flood TJ, et al, "Mercury Toxicity Due to Use of a Cosmetic Cream," *J Occup Environ Med*, 2000, 42(1):4-7.

Myers GJ, Davidson PW, Cox C, et al, "Twenty-Seven Years Studying the Human Neurotoxicity of Methylmercury Exposure," *Environ Res*, 83(3):275-85.

Siegler RW, Nierenberg DW, Hickey WF, et al, "Fatal Poisoning From Liquid Dimethylmercury: A Neuropathologic Study," *Hum Pathol*, 1999, 30(6):720-3.

Zabinski Z, Dabrowski Z, Moszczynski P, et al, "The Activity of Erythrocyte and Basic Indices of Peripheral Blood Erythrocytes From Workers Chronically Exposed to Mercury Vapous," *Toxicol Ind Health*, 2000, 16(2):58-64.

Mercury, Urine

Related Information

Heavy Metal Screen, Blood *on page 792*
Heavy Metal Screen, Urine *on page 792*
Mercury, Blood *on page 797*
Urine Collection, 24-Hour *on page 47*

Synonyms Hg, Urine

Abstract See Mercury, Blood *on page 797*.

Specimen 24-hour urine

Container Plastic (preferably polyethylene) acid-washed container, no preservative

Storage Instructions Store in special metal-free container. If HCl is used as a preservative, it must be of high quality analytical grade; technical grades of HCl may be contaminated by mercury.[1]

Causes for Rejection Failure to collect blood in a special metal-free container or exposure to metal-containing dusts

Reference Interval 24-hour urine: <20 μg/L (SI: <100 nmol/L).[2]

Critical Values Significant exposure is indicated when daily urine mercury reaches 50 μg/day.[3]

Possible Panic Range >150 μg/L (SI: >748.5 nmol/L); symptoms are found with levels >600 μg/L (>3000 nmol/L); lethal urine levels: >800 μg/L (SI: >3992 nmol/L).[2]

Use Urine mercury is best used for evaluation of inorganic mercury exposure. Mercuric salts are present in some cathartics such as calomel, topically applied medicines, plastics, and some foods. Neurologic sequellae of mercury poisoning include intention tremor and neurological symptoms known as "mad hatter disease." This expression applied to workers making felt hats who were exposed to mercury vapor and inorganic mercury salts. Urinary excretion of Hg is used to monitor therapy.

Limitations Organic mercury is found mostly in red cells and is lipid soluble. Urine mercury may not be useful for evaluating pure organic mercury poisoning. Once exposure ceases, urine levels may not represent a good indicator of remaining body burden.[4] There are marked variations in the mercury levels considered toxic by different investigators.[5]

Methodology Electrothermal atomic absorption (AA), gold electrode deposition, gas chromatography (GC)

Additional Information Organic methylmercury is an important environmental contaminant. It was discovered that elemental mercury could be oxidized into inorganic mercury (Hg^{+2}) and then into organic mercury (methylmercury) from industrial wastes dumped into Minimata Bay (Japan). Organic mercury then accumulates in large amounts in predator fish, and thus, the human food chain. Ingestion of mercury-laden fish in Minimata Bay led to severe neurologic deficits.[6]

The major physical forms of mercury to which humans are exposed are (elemental) mercury vapor and methylmercury compounds. Mercury vapor emitted in the atmosphere from varied sources is oxidized into inorganic mercurial salts (Hg^{+2}). Inorganic mercury is subject to microbial conversion into methylmercury compounds ($CH_3Hg\ X$) which accumulate in the food chain in freshwater fish and seafood.[7] Acute mercury poisoning, usually due to aspiration of elemental mercury vapors, is seen most commonly in industrial smelting or gold ore processing, requiring the use of gold-mercury amalgams with distillation.[8,9] Severe acute poisoning leads to pulmonary distress with acute pneumonitis, hemoptysis, and cyanosis. Mechanical ventilation is often required. Permanent sequelae may include irreversible lung impairment[5] and pulmonary fibrosis.[10]

Inorganic mercury (Hg^{+2}) causes toxicological effects similar to its other family member, cadmium. Both metals are potent chelators of proteins and enzymes. They bind avidly to sulfhydryl groups, leading to oxidative stress, which disrupts the metabolism and biological activities of many proteins, including depletion of intracellular glutathione.[11] Inorganic mercury is corrosive to the GI tract. Exposure may lead to renal failure and infarcts of brain and kidneys.[12] No specific lesions may be seen in the brain of those poisoned by inorganic mercurial compounds. Organic mercurials, however, are potent neurotoxins affecting primarily central nervous tissue with loss of neurons; reactive glial proliferation; microcavitation; vascular congestion; petechial hemorrhage; and edema in the calcarine, precentral, postcentral, transverse temporal cortex and cerebellar cortex.[12] Industrial and agricultural exposure usually includes inhalation of vapor, which is efficiently absorbed, oxidized to mercuric form and excreted in urine and feces. Ingestion is the major route for mercuric salts, with urine excretion.

Hg crosses the placenta and can cause profound damage to the fetus, including mental retardation.[4]

Footnotes

1. Wax PM, Goldfarb A, and Cernichiari E, "Mercury Contamination of Heavy Metal Collection Containers," *Vet Hum Toxicol*, 2000, 42(1):22-5.
2. Painter PC, Cope JY, and Smith JL, "Reference Information for the Clinical Laboratory," *Tietz Textbook of Clinical Chemistry*, Chapter 50, Burtis CA and Ashwood ER, eds, Philadelphia, PA: WB Saunders Co, 1999, 1803.
3. Moyer TP, "Toxic Metals," *Tietz Textbook of Clinical Chemistry*, Chapter 28, Burtis CA and Ashwood ER, eds, Philadelphia, PA: WB Saunders Co, 1999, 992-3.
4. Howard P and Billings CG, "Dynamics and Clinical Effects of Nonferrous Metals in the Human Body," *Monaldi Arch Chest Dis*, 2000, 55(1):70-3.
5. Graeme KA and Pollack CV, "Heavy Metal Toxicity, Part I: Arsenic and Mercury," 1998, 16(1):45-56.
6. Uchino M, Okajima T, Eto K, et al, "Neurologic Features of Chronic Minamata Disease (Organic Mercury Poisoning) Certified at Autopsy," *Intern Med*, 1995, 34(8):744-7.
7. Clarkson TW, "The Toxicology of Mercury," *Crit Rev Clin Lab Sci*, 1997, 34(4):369-403.
8. Solis MT, Yuen E, Cortez PS, et al, "Family Poisoned by Mercury Vapor Inhalation," *Am J Emerg Med*, 2000, 18(5):599-602.
9. Donoghue AM, "Mercury Toxicity Due to Smelting of Placer Gold Recovered by Mercury Amalgam," *Occup Med (Lond)*, 1998, 48(6):413-5.
10. Lim HE, Shim JJ, Lee SY, et al, "Mercury Inhalation Poisoning and Acute Lung Injury," *Korean J Intern Med*, 1998, 13(2):127-30.
11. Quig D, "Cysteine Metabolism and Metal Toxicity," *Altern Med Rev*, 1998, 3(4):262-70.
12. Eto K, Takizawa Y, Akagi H, et al, "Differential Diagnosis Between Organic and Inorganic Mercury Poisoning in Human Cases - the Pathological Point of View," *Toxicol Path*, 1999, 27(6):664-71.

References

Aikoh H and Shibahara T, "Determination of Mercury Levels in Human Urine and Blood by Ultraviolet-Visible Spectrophotometry," *Analyst*, 1993, 118(10):1329-32.

Barregard L, Quelquejeu G, Sallsten G, et al, "Dose-Dependent Elimination Kinetics for Mercury in Urine: Observations in Subjects With Brief but High-Level Exposure," *Int Arch Occup Environ Health*, 1996, 68(5):345-8.

Cavalleri A and Gobba F, "Reversible Color Vision Loss in Occupational Exposure to Metallic Mercury," *Environ Res*, 1998, 77(2):173-7.

Cianciola ME, Echeverria D, Martin MD, et al, "Epidemiological Assessment of Measures Used to Indicate Low-Level Exposure to Mercury Vapor (Hg)," *J Toxicol Environ Health*, 1997, 52(1):19-33.

Davis LE, "Unregulated Potions Still Cause Mercury Poisoning," *West J Med*, 2000, 173(1):19.

Knobeloch LM, Ziarnik M, Anderson HA, et al, "Imported Seabass as a Source of Mercury Exposure: A Wisconsin Case Study," *Environ Health Perspect*, 1995, 103(6):604-6.

Magos L, "Three Cases of Methylmercury Intoxication Which Eluded Correct Diagnosis," *Arch Toxicol*, 1998, 72(11):701-5.

Mason HJ and Calder IM, "The Correction of Mercury Concentrations in Untimed, Random Samples," *Occup Environ Med*, 1994, 51(4):287.

Maynou C, Mathieu-Nolf M, Mesdagh H, et al, "Accidental Subcutaneous Injection of Elemental Mercury. A Case Report," *Acta Orthop Belg*, 2000, 66(3):292-6.

McRill C, Boyer LV, Flood TJ, et al, "Mercury Toxicity Due to Use of a Cosmetic Cream," *J Occup Environ Med*, 2000, 42(1):4-7.

Myers GJ, Davidson PW, Cox C, et al, "Twenty-Seven Years Studying the Human Neurotoxicity of Methylmercury Exposure," *Environ Res*, 83(3):275-85.

Siegler RW, Nierenberg DW, Hickey WF, et al, "Fatal Poisoning From Liquid Dimethylmercury: A Neuropathologic Study," *Hum Pathol*, 1999, 30(6):720-3.

Zabinski Z, Dabrowski Z, Moszczynski P, et al, "The Activity of Erythrocyte and Basic Indices of Peripheral Blood Erythrocytes From Workers Chronically Exposed to Mercury Vapous," *Toxicol Ind Health*, 2000, 16(2):58-64.

♦ **Metals, Blood** *see* Heavy Metal Screen, Blood *on page 792*

♦ **Metal Screen** *see* Heavy Metal Screen, Urine *on page 792*

♦ **Metals, Toxic** *see* Heavy Metal Screen, Urine *on page 792*

♦ **Metasedin®** *see* Methadone, Urine *on page 798*

♦ **Meth** *see* Methamphetamine, Qualitative, Urine *on page 799*

♦ **Methadone** *see* Drugs of Abuse Testing, Urine *on page 788*

Methadone, Urine

Related Information

Antidiuretic Hormone, Plasma *on page 107*
Chain-of-Custody Protocol *on page 785*
Drugs of Abuse Testing, Urine *on page 788*
Opiates, Qualitative, Urine *on page 803*
Propoxyphene, Serum or Urine *on page 805*

Synonyms Dolophine®; Eptadone®; Metasedin®; Physeptone®; Symoron®

Applies to Heroin Detoxification; Naloxone

Abstract This drug is a synthetic opiate agonist used during World War II as a morphine substitute. Structurally related to propoxyphene, it is used for detoxification of opiate addicts. It is a drug of abuse.

Specimen Urine

Storage Instructions Refrigerate

Special Instructions If forensic, use chain-of-custody protocol and form. See Chain-of-Custody Protocol *on page 785* and the Chain-of-Custody form in the Introduction *on page 773*.

Reference Interval Negative (less than cutoff); when used therapeutically for pain, plasma levels are in the range of 0.10-0.40 µg/mL (SI: 0.32-1.29 µmol/L).

Critical Values Cutoff for urine screening: 300 ng/mL; confirmation: typically 200 ng/mL, variable between laboratories

Use Evaluate toxicity and detection as drug of abuse. Methadone is a drug of abuse and is included in most drug-of-abuse screening panels.

Methodology Thin-layer chromatography (TLC), fluorescent immunoassay, and enzyme immunoassay (EIA) for screening, gas chromatography/mass spectrometry (GC/MS) for confirmation

Additional Information
- Half-life: 15-25 hours
- Volume of distribution: 4-6 L/kg
- Protein binding: 85% to 95%

Methadone is a synthetic diphenylheptane derivative. It produces less sedation and euphoria than does morphine and its effects are cumulative. Methadone is highly addictive, but the withdrawal symptoms are less intense. Onset of action is 30-60 minutes after an oral dose and 10-20 minutes following parenteral administration. Adverse effects include marked sedation after repeated administration, CNS and respiratory depression, nausea and vomiting, bradycardia, hypotension, increased intracranial pressure, miosis, antidiuretic hormone release, and physical and psychological dependence. Treatment for overdose is supportive and administration of the opioid antagonist naloxone.

This drug is used in the management of narcotic (particularly heroin) detoxification maintenance programs. Methadone maintenance programs have effectively reduced heroin dependency and are available in most countries. Once tolerance is developed, it may be used continually with less harmful side effects. Reduction in criminality and AIDS has been associated with methadone maintenance programs.

It can be detected for 2-4 days in urine.

References
Calsyn DA, Saxon AJ, and Barndt DC, "Urine Screening Practices in Methadone Maintenance Clinics. A Survey of How the Results Are Used," *J Nerv Ment Dis*, 1991, 179(4):222-7.
Dawe S, Harnett PH, Staiger P, et al, "Parent Training Skills and Methadone Maintenance: Clinical Opportunities and Challenges," *Drug Alcohol Depend*, 2000, 60(1):1-11.
Garrido MJ and Troconiz IF, "Methadone: A Review of its Pharmacokinetic/Pharmacodynamic Properties," *J Pharmacol Toxicol Methods*, 1999, 42(2):61-6.
Karch SB and Stephens BG, "Toxicology and Pathology of Deaths Related to Methadone: Retrospective Review," *West J Med*, 2000, 172(1):11-4.
Molyneux E, Ahern R, and Baldwin B, "Accidental Ingestion of Methadone," *BMJ*, 1991, 303(6807):922-3.
Murray JB, "Effectiveness of Methadone Maintenance for Heroin Addiction," *Psychol Rep*, 1998, 83(1):295-302.
Schmidt N, Brune K, Sittl R, et al, "Rapid Determination of Methadone in Plasma, Cerebrospinal Fluid, and Urine by Gas Chromatography and Its Application to Routine Drug Monitoring," *Pharm Res*, 1993, 10(3):441-4.
Specka M, Finkbeiner T, Lodemann E, et al, "Cognitive-Motor Performance of Methadone-Maintained Patients," *Eur Addict Res*, 2000, 6(1):8-19.
Strain EC, Bigelow GE, Liebson IA, et al, "Moderate- vs High-Dose Methadone in the Treatment of Opioid Dependence: A Randomized Trial," *JAMA*, 1999, 281(11):1000-5.
Wolff K, Hay AW, and Raistrick D, "Plasma Methadone Measurements and Their Role in Methadone Detoxification Programs," *Clin Chem*, 1992, 38(3):420-5.
Wolff K, Sanderson M, Hay AW, et al, "Methadone Concentrations in Plasma and Their Relationship to Drug Dosage," *Clin Chem*, 1991, 37(2):205-9.
Wu CH and Henry JA, "Deaths of Heroin Addicts Starting on Methadone Maintenance," *Lancet*, 1990, 335(8686):424.

♦ **Methampex®** *see Methamphetamine, Qualitative, Urine on page 799*

Methamphetamine, Qualitative, Urine

Related Information
Amphetamine, Qualitative, Urine *on page 779*
Chain-of-Custody Protocol *on page 785*
Drugs of Abuse Testing, Urine *on page 788*

Synonyms Crank; Crystal; Desoxyephedrine Hydrochloride; Desoxyn®; Doe; Ecstasy; Go; Ice; Meth; Methampex®; Methedrine®; Speed; Zip

Applies to Benzedrine®; Contac®; Dexedrine®; Dimetapp®; d-Methamphetamine; l-Methamphetamine; MDMA; Methylenedioxymethamphetamine; Phentermine; Phenylpropanolamine; Pseudoephedrine; Sine-Off®; Sudafed®; Vicks Inhaler®

Test Includes Amphetamine, methamphetamine

Abstract The d-isomer of this drug is used therapeutically as an anorectic agent and as therapy for hyperactive children. It is a drug of abuse as well. Methamphetamine and amphetamine, classified as Schedule II controlled substances, stimulate the central and sympathetic nervous systems. Methamphetamine is highly addictive and is widely abused.

Specimen Random urine

Collection If forensic, observe precautions.

Storage Instructions Refrigerate

Causes for Rejection If forensic, failure to meet temperature check and reasonable urine creatinine concentration

Special Instructions If forensic, use chain-of-custody protocol and form. See Chain-of-Custody Protocol *on page 785* and the Chain-of-Custody form in the Introduction *on page 773*.

Reference Interval Negative (less than cutoff); therapeutic, serum: 20-30 ng/mL

Critical Values Substance Abuse and Mental Health Services Administration (SAMHSA) cutoff: screen: 1000 ng/mL; confirmation: 500 ng/mL. For methamphetamine, a positive report requires methamphetamine ≥500 ng/mL and amphetamine (a metabolite) ≥200 ng/mL in the same sample.

Use Evaluate for drug abuse; assess toxicity, including hyperpyrexia, rhabdomyolysis, pulmonary edema, intracranial hemorrhage.[1]

Limitations Screening test may give false positives with common cold and antiallergy medications.

Methodology Screening: enzyme immunoassay (EIA), fluorescence polarization immunoassay (FPIA), thin-layer chromatography (TLC); confirmation: gas chromatography/mass spectrometry (GC/MS), gas-liquid chromatography (GLC), high performance liquid chromatography (HPLC)

Additional Information
- Half-life: 10-30 hours, dependent on urinary pH (urine alkalinization increases the half-life of sympathomimetic amines, acidification decreases it)
- Volume of distribution: 3-4 L/kg
- Protein binding: 10% to 40%

In this class, the most abused drug is d-methamphetamine. The optical isomer, l-methamphetamine, has less pronounced central effects and is used as a nasal decongestant in Vicks Inhaler® (legal, over-the-counter). Amphetamine isomers are present in Dexedrine® and Benzedrine®. These drugs are self-administered orally, intravenously, or by smoking; smokable forms include "ice" and "crystal". It can be detected in urine within 3 hours of use. The parent drugs are the substances detected by the screening tests. Over-the-counter medication for colds and allergies (Contac®, Dimetapp®, Sine-Off®, Sudafed®) contain phenylpropanolamine or pseudoephedrine which, at high concentrations, may give a positive EIA screening test when the polyclonal antibody is used. This antibody also detects methylenedioxymethamphetamine (MDMA), a controlled substance classed as an hallucinogen and "designer" drug.[2] The above medications are generally not detected with the monoclonal EIA test. Confirmation by GC/MS rules out these false positives. In order to rule out the false-positive given by l-methamphetamine (legal nasal decongestant), a chiral column or procedure, which separates the "l" and "d" isomers, must be used in the GC/MS confirmation.[3] See Amphetamine, Qualitative, Urine *on page 779* for a discussion of physiological effects.

Methamphetamine, a sympathomimetic amine, is chemically related to ephedrine and amphetamine. Amphetamine is among the active metabolites of methamphetamine. Methamphetamine and amphetamine are used in the management of obesity, to treat certain depressive reactions, and as adjunctive therapy for narcolepsy, epilepsy, attention deficit disorders, and postencephalitic parkinsonism. Methamphetamine is readily absorbed by the GI tract and the effects last from 6-12 hours. Adverse effects include tremor, insomnia, nervousness, anxiety, euphoria or dysphoria, hyper- or hypotension, arrhythmias, circulatory collapse, and nausea and vomiting. Methamphetamine has greater CNS efficacy than D-amphetamine, most likely because of its greater ability to penetrate CNS.

In interpretation of methamphetamine and amphetamine, positive test knowledge of legitimate and illicit sources is important. Amphetamines are sometimes prescribed as weight-reducing agents. Many substances (amphetaminil, benzphetamine, clobenzorex, deprenyl, dimethylamphetamine, ethylamphetamine, famprofazone, fencamine, fenethylline, fenproporex, furfenorex, mefenorex, mesocarb, and prenylamine) which are available as prescription drugs, are metabolized in the body to methamphetamine or amphetamine.[4]

Footnotes
1. Gulledge C, Phillips J, and Hammett-Stabler C, "New Kids on the Block: An Update on Selected Club Drugs," *Therapeutic Drug Monitoring and Clinical Toxicology Division*, 2000, 15(4):1-6.
2. Bost RD, "3,4-Methylenedioxymethamphetamine (MDMA) and Other Amphetamine Derivatives," *J Forensic Sci*, 1988, 33(2):576-87.
3. Jirovsky D, Lemr K, Sevcik J, et al, "Methamphetamine - Properties and Analytical Methods of Enantiomer Determination," *Forensic Sci Int*, 1998, 96(1):61-70.
4. Musshoff F, "Illegal or Legitimate Use? Precursor Compounds to Amphetamine and Methamphetamine," *Drug Metab Rev*, 2000, 32(1):15-44.

References
DePace A, Verebey K, and ElSohly M, "Capillary Gas-Liquid Chromatography Separation of Phenethylamines in Amphetamine-Positive Urine Samples," *J Forensic Sci*, 1990, 35(6):1431-5.
Derlet RW and Heischober B, "Methamphetamine. Stimulant of the 1990s?" *West J Med*, 1990, 153(6):625-8.
Ellenhorn MJ, Schonwald S, Ordog G, et al, "Amphetamines and Designer Drugs," *Ellenhorn's Medical Toxicology: Diagnosis and Treatment of Human Poisoning*, Baltimore, MD: Lippincott Williams & Wilkins, 1997, 340-55.
Gan BK, Baugh D, Liu RH, et al, "Simultaneous Analysis of Amphetamine, Methamphetamine, and 3,4-Methylenedioxymethamphetamine (MDMA) in Urine Samples by Solid-Phase Extraction, Derivatization, and Gas Chromatography/Mass Spectrometry," *J Forensic Sci*, 1991, 36(5):1331-41.

(Continued)

Methamphetamine, Qualitative, Urine (Continued)

Levine B, "Amphetamines/Sympathomimetic Amines," *Principles of Forensic Toxicology*, Washington, DC: AACC Press, American Association of Clinical Chemistry, 1999, 265-85.

Williams RH, Erickson T, and Broussard LA, "Evaluating Sympathomimetic Intoxication in an Emergency Setting," *Lab Med*, 2000, 31(9):497-507.

♦ **Methanol** see Volatile Screen, Blood or Urine on page 809

♦ **Methaqualone** see Drugs of Abuse Testing, Urine on page 788

Methaqualone, Urine

Related Information

Chain-of-Custody Protocol on page 785
Drugs of Abuse Testing, Urine on page 788

Synonyms Lude®; Ludes; Quaalude®; Sopor™

Abstract This drug is a sedative-hypnotic and is currently a DEA schedule I drug. It is a drug of abuse which was taken off the U.S. market in 1984.

Specimen Serum, urine

Container Red top tube, plastic urine container

Special Instructions If forensic, use chain-of-custody protocol and form. See Chain-of-Custody Protocol on page 785 and the Chain-of-Custody form in the Introduction on page 773.

Reference Interval Urine: negative (less than cutoff)

Critical Values Cutoff for urine: screen: 300 ng/mL; confirmation: typically 200 ng/mL, variable between laboratories

Possible Panic Range Serum values >8 μg/mL (SI: >32 nmol/L) associated with unconsciousness; toxic: >10 μg/mL (SI: >40 nmol/L)

Use Evaluate for toxicity, evaluate for drug abuse

Methodology Immunoassay, capillary chromatography, gas-liquid chromatography (GLC), UV spectrophotometry, fluorometry, gas chromatography/mass spectrophotometry (GC/MS)

Additional Information

- Half-life: 10-40 hours
- Volume of distribution: 5-7 L/kg
- Protein binding: 70% to 90%

Methaqualone is a nonbarbiturate sedative-hypnotic. It is rapidly absorbed from the GI tract. Hyperexcitability, coma, and cardiovascular and respiratory depression characterize overdose. Once a common drug of abuse, in recent years the use of methaqualone has decreased.[1] The street preparations may be adulterated with other pharmacoactive substances. It is extensively metabolized and screening methods must detect metabolites. Enzyme-multiplied immunoassay technique (EMIT) and Abuscreen ONLINE (Roche Diagnostics) detect four of the most common metabolites.

Methaqualone can be extracted under weak alkaline, neutral, or weak acidic conditions and can be identified and quantified by GC without derivatization.

Footnotes

1. ElSohly MA and Salamone SJ, "Prevalence of Drugs Used in Cases of Alleged Sexual Assault," *J Anal Toxicol*, 1999, 23(3):141-6.

References

Baselt RC, *Disposition of Toxic Drugs and Chemicals in Man*, 5th ed, Foster City, CA: Chemical Toxicology Institute, 2000, 536-8.

Beebe DK and Walley E, "Substance Abuse: The Designer Drugs," *Am Fam Phys*, 1991, 43(5):1689-98.

Brenner C, Hui R, Passarelli J, et al, "Comparison of Methaqualone Excretion Patterns Using Abuscreen ONLINE and EMIT II Immunoassays and GC/MS," *Forensic Sci Int*, 1996, 79(1):31-41.

Buckner JC and Mandell W, "Risk Factors for Depressive Symptomatology in a Drug Using Population," *Am J Public Health*, 1990, 80(5):580-5.

Plaut O, Girod, and Staub C, "Analysis of Methaqualone in Biological Matrices by Micellar Electrokinetic Capillary Chromatography, Comparison With Gas Chromatography-Mass Spectrometry," *Forensic Sci Int*, 1998, 92(2-3):219-27.

♦ **MetHb** see Methemoglobin, Whole Blood on page 800

♦ **Methedrine®** see Methamphetamine, Qualitative, Urine on page 799

Methemoglobin, Whole Blood

Related Information

Carboxyhemoglobin, Blood on page 784
Hemoglobin on page 442
Phlebotomy, Therapeutic on page 849

Synonyms MetHb

Applies to Carboxyhemoglobin; Cytochrome b5 Reductase (NADH-metHb Reductase); Hb M; Phenylhydroxylamine; Reduced Hemoglobin; Sulfhemoglobin

Abstract Methemoglobin (metHb) is a form of hemoglobin in which the iron has been oxidized from the normal ferrous (Fe^{++}) to the ferric (Fe^{+++}) state. MetHb cannot bind oxygen to act as an oxygen carrier. The cyanosis of methemoglobinemia is characteristically central rather than peripheral. Central cyanosis with little dyspnea and with tachycardia is an indication for evaluation of metHb.

Specimen Whole blood

Container Green top (heparin) tube

Collection A drop of blood containing metHb, placed on filter paper, appears chocolate brown, when compared to an adjacent drop of normal blood.

Storage Instructions Keep tube on ice. pH dependent. Should be run within 8 hours, or false negatives may occur. Run as promptly as possible after draw. Studies have shown up to 10% drop in 4 hours, up to 16% drop in 8 hours, in samples kept on ice. Such studies have not been extensive. May be drawn into sodium fluoride-containing tubes and immediately frozen at 0°C to -4°C prior to analysis.

Reference Interval Up to 1% of total hemoglobin. Smokers have a slightly higher percent metHb than do nonsmokers.

Possible Panic Range Headache and other symptoms occur at levels >30%. Methemoglobinemia levels >70% may be lethal.

Use MetHb may cause cyanosis, especially in the presence of normal arterial gases, cyanosis unresponsive to oxygen administration and may cause a distinctive chocolate brown color of blood. Testing for metHb is used to evaluate polycythemia and hemoglobinopathies; to work up dyspnea and headache; to work up "poppers" and "sniffers"; to evaluate drug or chemical toxicity, since most instances of methemoglobinemia are so acquired. Examination for metHb is used to monitor patients on high dose nitrate therapy. Its measurement in CSF may detect small cerebral and subdural hematomas.[1]

Limitations Sulfhemoglobin, methylene blue, and Evans blue dye may interfere with some co-oximeters. MetHb exhibits pH sensitivity.

Methodology Co-oximetry, spectrophotometry. Hb M variants are best detected by electrophoresis, because spectrophotometry is unreliable due to their abnormal ferrihemoglobin spectra.

Additional Information MetHb is an inactive, oxidized form of hemoglobin (Hb) which does not contribute to the oxygen-carrying capacity of blood. Therefore, arterial %O_2 saturation will be inappropriately low for a given inhaled air oxygen concentration and p_aO_2, if the calculation for %O_2 saturation is based on total Hb. Concentrations of metHb of over 10% to 25% of Hb will cause cyanosis. The most common cause of cyanosis is the presence of excessive reduced Hb which becomes clinically apparent (as a bluish discoloration of skin and mucous membranes) when the capillary level is >5 g/dL. It is the absolute level (rather than the relative level in %) that results in cyanosis (and accounts for its prominence in polycythemia). MetHb may produce cyanosis at levels as low as 2.0 g/dL, while sulfhemoglobin may be responsible for cyanosis at levels of 0.5 g/dL. Carboxyhemoglobin produces a cherry red color, noted especially in mucous membranes, classically "cherry red lips". Cyanosis appears with metHb levels of 10% to 25%, but symptoms are minimal until metHb rises to 35% to 40%, at which patients may experience fatigue, dizziness, dyspnea, headache, and tachycardia. At the 60% level, lethargy and stupor may occur; levels >70% in adults may be fatal.

Methemoglobinemia may be hereditary or acquired. Polycythemia is occasionally present as a compensatory mechanism. Most instances of methemoglobinemia are acquired, from drugs and chemicals. Nitro and amino groups are especially involved, eg, aniline and derivatives, nitrites, nitroglycerin, nitrate salts in burn patients, flutamide, metoclopramide, phenazopyridine, dapsone (perhaps the most common cause of drug-induced methemoglobinemia), phenacetin, acetophenetidin, prilocaine, some sulfonamides, sulfones, chlorates, primaquine, quinones, large doses of ferrous sulfate, and many other drugs and some intestinal bacteria.[1] The aniline ring is found in many medications including virtually all local anesthetic agents. Methemoglobinemia has been recognized from topically applied anesthetic spray.[2] Well water containing nitrate is the most common cause of methemoglobinemia in the newborn. Methemoglobinemia has been reported after exposure to automobile exhaust fumes.[3] Phenylhydroxylamine, a metabolite of a substance found in artificial fingernail solution, is among the most potent producers of metHg.[4]

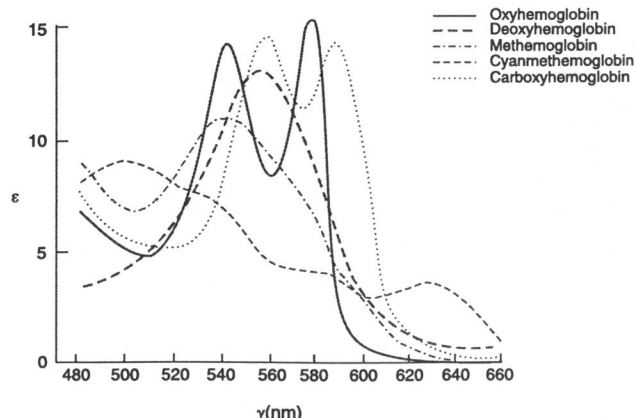

Absorption spectra of oxyhemoglobin (HBO2), deoxyhemoglobin (Hb), methemoglobin (hemiglobin [Hi]), and cyanmethemoglobin (hemiglobincyanide [HiCN]).

From Bunn HF, Forget BG, and Ranney HM, *Human Hemoglobins*, Philadelphia, PA: WB Saunders Co, 1977, 2.

Hereditary methemoglobinemia is uncommon. The most common phenotype is due to a deficiency of red cell NADH-methemoglobin reductase (diaphorase, also termed cytochrome b_5 reductase), which is inherited as an autosomal recessive trait. Homozygotes have metHb levels of 15% to 20%. Heterozygotes are apt to develop toxic methemoglobinemia when exposed to substances which can oxidize hemoglobin iron. Each group carries decreased methemoglobin reductase.[2] Methemoglobinemia may also be the result of certain hemoglobins with an abnormal tendency to stabilize Fe^{+++} in the oxidized state, including members of the Hb M (for methemoglobin) family including Hb M Saskatoon, M Boston, M-Iwate, M Hyde Park, M Akita, and M Milwaukee. Furthermore, these hemoglobins are resistant to reduction by the methemoglobin reductase system. With an autosomal dominant mode of inheritance, they may be associated with clinical cyanosis. Several other hemoglobins that have an abnormal susceptibility to Fe oxidation (eg, Hb Kansas, Hb Seattle, and Hb Warsaw) with variable clinical effects, including cyanosis in some cases but not including clinical methemoglobinemia (these are not M hemoglobins), have been reported.[5,6]

A study of postmortem metHb levels showed a range of 0.8% to 57% in individuals who, clinically, should have had normal antemortem concentrations. There was no correlation with antemortem circumstances, autopsy findings, or interval of time from death to autopsy.[7]

Footnotes

1. Trbojevic-Cepe M, Vogrinc Z, and Brinar V, "Diagnostic Significance of Methemoglobin Determination in Colorless Cerebrospinal Fluid," *Clin Chem*, 1992, 38(8 Pt 1):1404-8.
2. Dinneen SF, Mohr DN, and Fairbanks VF, "Methemoglobinemia From Topically Applied Anesthetic Spray," *Mayo Clin Proc*, 1994, 69(9):886-8.
3. Laney RF and Hoffman RS, "Methemoglobinemia Secondary to Automobile Exhaust Fumes," *Am J Emerg Med*, 1992, 10(5):426-8.
4. Kao L, Leikin JB, Crockett M, et al, "Methemoglobinemia From Artificial Fingernail Solution," *JAMA*, 1997, 278(7):549-50.
5. Honig GR, Telfer MC, Rosenblum BB, et al, "Hb Warsaw (β42 Phe → Val): An Unstable Hemoglobin With Decreased Oxygen Affinity. I. Hematologic and Clinical Expression," *Am J Hematol*, 1989, 32(1):36-41.
6. Weatherall DJ, Clegg JB, Higgs DR, et al, "The Hemoglobinopathies," *The Metabolic and Molecular Bases of Inherited Disease*, 7th ed, Chapter 113, Scriver CR, Beaudet AL, Sly WS, et al, eds, New York, NY: McGraw-Hill, Inc, 1995, 3440-3.
7. Reay DT, Insalaco SJ, and Eisele JW, "Postmortem Methemoglobin Concentrations and Their Significance," *J Forensic Sci*, 1984, 29(4):1160-3.

References

Benz EJ Jr, "Hemoglobin Variants Associated With Hemolytic Anemia, Altered Oxygen Affinity, and Methemoglobinemias," *Hematology: Basic Principles and Practice*, 3rd ed, Chapter 31, Hoffman R, Benz EJ Jr, Shattil SJ, et al, eds, Philadelphia, PA: Churchill Livingstone, 2000, 554-61.

"Centers for Disease Control and Prevention. Prilocaine-Induced Methemoglobinemia - Wisconsin, 1993," *JAMA*, 1994, 272(18):1403-4.

Comly HH, "Landmark Article Sept 8, 1945: Cyanosis in Infants Caused by Nitrates in Well-Water," *JAMA*, 1987, 257(20):2788-92.

Dean BS, Lopez G, and Krenzelok EP, "Environmentally-Induced Methemoglobinemia in an Infant," *J Toxicol Clin Toxicol*, 1992, 30(1):127-33.

Johnson CJ, Bonrud PA, Dosch TL, et al, "Fatal Outcome of Methemoglobinemia in an Infant," *JAMA*, 1987, 257(20):2796-7.

Johnson WS, Hall AH, and Rumack BH, "Cyanide Poisoning Successfully Treated Without Therapeutic Methemoglobin Levels," *Am J Emerg Med*, 1989, 7(4):437-40.

Khan NA and Kruse JA, "Methemoglobinemia Induced by Topical Anesthesia. A Case Report and Review," *Am J Med Sci*, 1999, 318:415-8.

Lukens JN, "Landmark Perspective: The Legacy of Well-Water Methemoglobinemia," *JAMA*, 1987, 257(20):2793-5.

Lukens JN and Lee GR, "Unstable Hemoglobin Disease," *Wintrobe's Clinical Hematology*, 10th ed, Chapter 52, Lee GR, Foerster J, Lukens J, et al, eds, Baltimore, MD: Lippincott Williams & Wilkins, 1999, 1398-404.

Mansouri A and Lurie AA, "Concise Review: Methemoglobinemia," *Am J Hematol*, 1993, 42(1):7-12.

Wentworth P, Madan R, Wilson B, et al, "Toxic Methemoglobinemia in a 2-Year-Old Child," *Lab Med*, 1999, 30(5):311-15.

Williamson D, "The Unstable Haemoglobins," *Blood Rev*, 1993, 7(3):146-63.

Wright RO, Lewander WJ, and Woolf AD, "Methemoglobinemia: Etiology, Pharmacology and Clinical Management," *Ann Emerg Med*, 1999, 34(5):645-56.

3,4 Methylenedioxymethamphetamine, Urine

Related Information

Amphetamine, Qualitative, Urine *on page 779*
Chain-of-Custody Protocol *on page 785*
Drugs of Abuse Testing, Urine *on page 788*

Methamphetamine, Qualitative, Urine *on page 799*

Synonyms Adam; E; Ecstasy; MDMA; X; XTC

Applies to Methylenedioxyamphetamine; Methylenedioxyethamphetamine

Abstract 3,4 methylenedioxymethamphetamine (MDMA) is a derivative of methamphetamine. It produces a relaxed, euphoric state with heightened feelings within 20-40 minutes of oral intake. However, memory and working skills are impaired. Recently, due to its widespread use as a recreational drug in rave parties and dance clubs,[1,2] the U.S. Drug Enforcement Administration placed the drug in Schedule I. In 1999, U.S. Customs seized 5.4 million hits of MDMA, 720% increase from 1998.[3]

Specimen Random urine

Collection If forensic, observe precautions. See the Introduction *on page 773*

Storage Instructions Refrigerate

Causes for Rejection If forensic, failure to meet temperature requirements and/or tests for unusual urine dilution (specific gravity or creatinine) or adulteration

Turnaround Time Usually 1-2 hours for screen if done in-house; confirmation in 1-3 days

Reference Interval Negative (less than cutoff)

Possible Panic Range Blood levels >1000 ng/mL

Use Evaluate drug abuse; assess toxicity

Limitations When screened by immunoassays for amphetamines, MDMA or MDA concentrations must be 5-20 times higher than cutoff values for amphetamine assay to cause positive results.

Methodology

Screen: immunoassays directed towards methamphetamine or amphetamine analysis, gas chromatography (GC), thin-layer chromatography (TLC), high performance liquid chromatography (HPLC)

Confirmation: gas chromatography/mass spectrometry (GC/MS)

Additional Information

- Half-life: 6-10 hours, longer in alkaline urine
- % excreted unchanged in urine: 65%

MDMA is metabolized to an active metabolite 3,4 methylenedioxyamphetamine (MDA). Both MDMA and MDA have marked sympathomimetic activities similar to amphetamines.[4] They cause CNS stimulation, peripheral vasoconstriction, tachycardia, and pupillary dilation. Overdoses result in convulsions, hyperthermia, and behavioral changes.[5] Severe complications include rhabdomyolysis, intravascular coagulation, arrhythmias, seizures, acute renal failure, and hepatonecrosis.[6,7] Acute cholestatic hepatitis has been associated with MDMA.[8] Blood levels do not correlate well with toxicity. Follow serum electrolytes, renal and hepatic function tests, CPK, complete blood count, platelet counts, and coagulation studies in patients with severe toxicity. There is no specific antidote for MDMA or MDA; overdose management is supportive.

The repeated use of the drug causes physical and psychological independence.[9]

Footnotes

1. Pedersen W and Skrondal A, "Ecstasy and New Patterns of Drug Use: A Normal Population Study," *Addiction*, 1999, 94(11):1695-706.
2. Schwartz RH and Miller NS, "MDMA (Ecstasy) and the Race: A Review," *Pediatrics*, 1999, 100(4):705-8.
3. Group CEW, "Epidemiologic Trends in Drug Abuse: Highlights and Executive Summary," *NIDA Res Monogr*, Volume 1, Bethesda, MD. 2000.
4. Baselt RC, *Disposition of Toxic Drugs and Chemicals in Man*, 5th ed, Foster City, CA: Chemical Toxicology Institute, 2000, 562-3.
5. Levine B, "Amphetamines/Sympathomimetic Amines," *Principles of Forensic Toxicology*, 1999, 265-85.
6. Ramcharan S, Meenhorst PL, Otten JM, et al, "Survival After Massive Ecstasy Overdose," *J Toxicol Clin Toxicol*, 1998, 37(6):727-3.
7. Mueller PD and Korey WS, "Death by Ecstasy: The Serotonin Syndrome?" *Ann Emerg Med*, 1998, 32(3 Pt 1):377-80.
8. Jonas MM and Graeme-Cook FM, "A 17-Year-Old Girl With Marked Jaundice and Weight Loss," Case Records of the Massachusetts General Hospital, Case 6-2001, Scully RE, Mark EJ, McNeely WF, et al, eds, *N Engl J Med*, 2001, 344(8):591-9.
9. Jansen KL, "Ecstasy (MDMA) Dependence," *Drug Alcohol Depend*, 1999, 53(2):121-4.

References

Andreu V, Mas A, Bruguera M, et al, "Ecstasy: A Common Cause of Severe Acute Hepatotoxicity," *J Hepatol*, 1998, 29(3):394-7.

Gulledge C, Phillips J, and Hammett-Stabler C, "New Kids on the Block An Update on Selected Club Drugs," *Therapeutic Drug Monitoring and Clinical Toxicology Division Newsletter*, 2000, 15(4):1-6.

McGuire P, "Long-Term Psychiatric and Cognitive Effects of MDMA Use," *Toxicol Lett*, 2000, 112-3:153-6.

Morland J, "Toxicity of Drug a Abuse - Amphetamine Designer Drugs (Ecstasy): Mental Effects and Consequences of Single Dose Use," *Toxicol Lett*, 2000, 112-3:147-52.

Rochester JA and Kirchner JT, "Ecstasy (3,4-Methylenedioxymethamphetamine): History, Neurochemistry, and Toxicology," *J Am Board Fam Pract*, 1999, 12(2):137-42.

Weir E, "Raves: A Review of the Culture, the Drugs, and the Prevention of Harm," *CMAJ*, 2000, 162(13):1843-8.

♦ **Methyl Salicylate** *see* Salicylate, Serum or Plasma *on page 806*

♦ **Midol®** *see* Ibuprofen, Serum *on page 793*

♦ **Mist** *see* Phencyclidine, Qualitative, Urine *on page 804*

♦ **MMA** *see* Arsenic, Urine *on page 781*

♦ **Monomethylarsine** *see* Arsenic, Urine *on page 781*

♦ **Morphine** *see* Codeine, Urine *on page 786*

Morphine, Urine

Related Information
Chain-of-Custody Protocol *on page 785*
Codeine, Urine *on page 786*
Drugs of Abuse Testing, Urine *on page 788*
Opiates, Qualitative, Urine *on page 803*

Synonyms Astramorph™ PF; Duramorph®; Epimorph Dolcontin®; Heroin Metabolite, Urine; MS Contin®; MSIR®; MST®; OMS®; Oramorph SR®; RMS®; Roxanol™; Roxanol SR™; Sevredol®; Statex®

Applies to 6-0-Acetyl Morphine; Codeine; Heroin; Naloxone; Opium

Test Includes Codeine, heroin metabolite (6-O-acetyl morphine), hydromorphone (Dilaudid®), oxycodone

Abstract This drug is widely used therapeutically as an analgesic. Morphine itself is not an extensively used drug of abuse but two derivatives, heroin and codeine, are.

Storage Instructions Refrigerate sample

Special Instructions If forensic, use chain-of-custody protocol and form. See Chain-of-Custody Protocol *on page 785* and the Chain-of-Custody form in the Introduction *on page 773*.

Reference Interval Negative (less than cutoff)

Critical Values Substance Abuse and Mental Health Services Administration (SAMHSA) cutoff: screen (total opiates): 2000 ng/mL; confirmatory: morphine: 2000 ng/mL. For clinical purposes, many laboratories use a cutoff of 300 ng/mL.

Use Concentrations are measured to evaluate toxicity or detect drug of abuse. Heroin is metabolized to morphine, but morphine detection may only suggest heroin use. To **prove** heroin use, 6-O-acetyl morphine must be identified in the urine.

Methodology Enzyme immunoassay (EIA), fluorescent immunoassay, gas-liquid chromatography/mass spectroscopy (GLC/MS)

Additional Information
- Half-life: 2-4 hours (adults), 5-13 hours (neonates)
- Volume of distribution: 2-4 L/kg
- Protein binding: 30% to 40%

Morphine, the major phenanthrene alkaloid of opium, is used for relief of moderate to severe acute and chronic pain after non-narcotic analgesics have failed. It is also used as preanesthetic medication, to relieve the pain of myocardial infarction and to relieve the dyspnea of acute left ventricular failure and pulmonary edema. Peak analgesia is achieved 50-90 minutes after subcutaneous administration and 20 minutes after I.V. injection. Ninety percent of morphine is found in the urine after 24 hours, either free or in the glucuronide conjugated form. Adverse effects include CNS depression, nausea and vomiting, hypotension, bradycardia, histamine release, increased intracranial pressure, miosis, respiratory depression, antidiuretic hormone release, and physical and psychological dependence. Naloxone is a specific antidote. Morphine is generally detectable for 1-2 days after use.[1]

Ingestion of poppy seeds (bagels, pastries including Danish) can cause positive opiate screens at 300 ng/mL[2] or more.[1] In an attempt to address this problem, SAMHSA has recently increased the cutoff of morphine and codeine to 2000 ng/mL.[3]

Morphine may cause an increase in serum levels of ALT, AST, and amylase.

Footnotes
1. Porter WH, "Clinical Toxicology," *Tietz Textbook of Clinical Chemistry*, 3rd ed, Chapter 27, Burtis CA and Ashwood ER, eds, Philadelphia, PA: WB Saunders Co, 1999, 906-81.
2. Selavka CM, "Poppy Seed Ingestion as a Contributing Factor to Opiate-Positive Urinalysis Results: The Pacific Perspective," *J Forensic Sci*, 1991, 36(3):685-96
3. Substance Abuse and Mental Health Administration, "Mandatory Guidelines for Workplace Programs: Revision to Mandatory Guidelines," *Fed Regist*, 1998, 63:483.

References
Baselt RC, *Disposition of Toxic Drugs and Chemicals in Man*, 5th ed, Foster City, CA: Chemical Toxicology Institute, 2000, 589-92.
Cone EJ, Dickerson S, Paul BD, et al, "Forensic Drug Testing for Opiates: Urine Testing for Heroin, Morphine, and Codeine With Commercial Opiate Immunoassays," *J Anal Toxicol*, 1993, 17(3):156-64.
Gill AM, Cousins A, Nunn AJ, et al, "Opiate-Induced Respiratory Depression in Pediatric Patients," *Ann Pharmacother*, 1996, 30(2):125-9.
Lin Z, Lafolie P, and Beck O, "Evaluation of Analytical Procedures for Urinary Codeine and Morphine Measurements," *J Anal Toxicol*, 1994, 18(3):129-33.
McQuay HJ, Carroll D, Faura CC, et al, "Oral Morphine in Cancer Pain: Influences on Morphine and Metabolite Concentration," *Clin Pharmacol Ther*, 1990, 48(3):236-44.
Osborne R, Joel S, Trew D, et al, "Morphine and Metabolite Behavior After Different Routes of Morphine Administration: Demonstration of the Importance of the Active Metabolite Morphine-6-Glucuronide," *Clin Pharmacol Ther*, 1990, 47(1):12-9.
Portenoy RK, Khan E, Layman M, et al, "Chronic Morphine Therapy for Cancer Pain: Plasma and Cerebrospinal Fluid Morphine and Morphine-6-Glucuronide Concentrations," *Neurology*, 1991, 41(9):1457-61.
Portenoy RK, Thaler HT, Inturrisi CE, et al, "The Metabolite Morphine-6-Glucuronide Contributes to the Analgesia Produced by Morphine Infusion in Patients With Pain and Normal Renal Function," *Clin Pharmacol Ther*, 1992, 51(4):422-31.
Rop PP, Fornaris M, Salmon T, et al, "Concentrations of Heroin, 06-Monoacetylmorphine, and Morphine in a Lethal Case Following an Oral Heroin Overdose," *J Anal Toxicol*, 1997, 21(3):232-5.
"Toxicity and Pharmacokinetics of Morphine and Morphine-6-Glucuronide," *Br J Anaesth*, 1991, 67(3):362-3.
Zakowski MI, Ramanathan S, Sharnick S, et al, "Uptake and Distribution of Bupivacaine and Morphine After Intrathecal Administration in Parturients: Effects of Epinephrine," *Anesth Analg*, 1992, 74(5):664-9.

♦ **Motrin®** *see* Ibuprofen, Serum *on page 793*

♦ **MS Contin®** *see* Morphine, Urine *on page 802*

♦ **MSIR®** *see* Morphine, Urine *on page 802*

♦ **MST®** *see* Morphine, Urine *on page 802*

♦ **Myapap® Drops** *see* Acetaminophen, Serum *on page 778*

♦ **Naloxone** *see* Methadone, Urine *on page 798*

♦ **Naloxone** *see* Morphine, Urine *on page 802*

♦ **Narcotics** *see* Opiates, Qualitative, Urine *on page 803*

♦ **Neopap®** *see* Acetaminophen, Serum *on page 778*

♦ **Nicotine** *see* Cotinine, Serum, Plasma, or Urine *on page 787*

Nicotine, Serum or Plasma

Related Information
Carboxyhemoglobin, Blood *on page 784*
Cotinine, Serum, Plasma, or Urine *on page 787*
Toxicology Screen, Serum *on page 808*
Toxicology Screen, Urine *on page 808*

Abstract Nicotine, one of the most toxic of all poisons, is a neural stimulant found in most tobacco products including transdermal patches and Nicorette® gum.

Specimen Serum or plasma

Container Red top tube

Storage Instructions Store at -20°C for 1 week.

Reference Interval Serum concentrations >50 ng/mL may be associated with toxicity. Mean plasma concentration after smoking one cigarette: 5-30 ng/mL.[1]

Possible Panic Range Plasma concentrations >13,000 ng/mL have been associated with **fatality**.[1]

Use Work-up of acute poisoning in children ingesting cigarettes or cigarette butts

Limitations Most clinical laboratories do not offer this test; thus, it may not be offered on a stat basis, limiting its clinical usefulness to documentation of nicotine poisoning.

Methodology Gas chromatography (GC), high performance liquid chromatography (HPLC), immunoassay, colorimetric assay

Additional Information
- Half-life: 24-84 minutes
- Volume of distribution: 1.0 L/kg

Nicotine, an alkaloid obtained from the leaves of the tobacco plant *Nicotiana tabacum*, is ubiquitous at low levels in the environment due to smoking. Nicotine stimulates the sympathetic nervous system by activation of nicotinic acetylcholine receptors localized on peripheral postganglionic sympathetic nerve endings and the adrenal medulla. Acute toxicity may include, but is not limited to: nausea, cyanosis, insomnia, hyponatremia, blurred vision, hyperventilation, nystagmus, dementia, abdominal pain, apnea, and respiratory depression.[2,3,4,5] Poisoning in children can result from ingestion of two whole cigarettes or six cigarette butts.

Chronic exposure to nicotine in the form of cigarette smoke also has other deleterious effects including exacerbation of atherogenesis. Nicotine, through the intracardiac release of norepinephrine, induces a beta-adrenoceptor-mediated increase in heart rate and contractility, and an alpha-adrenoceptor-mediated increase in coronary vasomotor tone. The ensuing simultaneous increase in oxygen demand and coronary resistance is postulated to exert a detrimental effect on oxygen balance of the heart, especially in patients with coronary arterial disease.[6] Nicotine stimulates the release of catecholamines, while other smoke byproducts injure arterial walls and promote atherogenesis. Smoking also potentiates thrombosis by decreasing the concentration of plasma fibrinogen and altering the activity of platelets.[7] These proatherogenic effects are seen in lesser degrees in passive smokers.[7]

Footnotes
1. Gourlay SG and Benowitz NL, "Arteriovenous Differences in Plasma Concentration of Nicotine and Catecholamines and Related Cardiovascular Effects After Smoking, Nicotine Nasal Spray, and Intravenous Nicotine," *Clin Pharmacol Ther*, 1997, 62(4):453-63.
2. Ballard T, Ehlers J, Freund E, et al, "Green Tobacco Sickness: Occupational Nicotine Poisoning in Tobacco Workers," *Arch Environ Health*, 1995, 50(5):384-9.

3. Sisselman SG, Mofenson HC, and Caraccio TR, "Childhood Poisonings From Ingestion of Cigarettes," *Lancet*, 1996, 347(8995):200-1.
4. "Ingestion of Cigarettes and Cigarette Butts by Children - Rhode Island, January 1994 - July 1996," *MMWR Morb Mortal Wkly Rep*, 1997, 46(6):125-8.
5. Ross MP, Revolinski D, and Taurman L, "Green Tobacco Sickness Among Adults in Kentucky," *Vet Hum Toxicol*, 1994, 36:360.
6. Haas M and Kubler W, "Nicotine and Sympathetic Neurotransmission," *Cardiovasc Drugs Ther*, 1997, 10(6):657-65.
7. Powell JT, "Vascular Damage From Smoking: Disease Mechanisms at the Arterial Wall," *Vasc Med*, 1998, 3(1):21-8.

References

Baranowski J, Pochopien G, and Baranowska I, "Determination of Nicotine, Cotinine and Caffeine in Merconium Using High Performance Liquid Chromatography," *J Chromatogr B Biomed Sci Appl*, 1998, 707(1-2):317-21.
Baselt RC, "Disposition of Toxic Drugs and Chemicals in Man," 5th ed, Foster City, CA: Chemical Toxicology Institute, 2000, 608-12.
Hariharan M and VanNoord T, "Liquid-Chromatographic Determination of Nicotine and Cotine in Urine From Passive Smokers: Comparison With Gas Chromatography With a Nitrogen-Specific Detector," *Clin Chem*, 1991, 37(7):1276-80.
Hutchinson J, Yousef T, and Taylor R, "Rapid Method for the Simultaneous Measurement of Nicotine and Cotinine in Urine and Serum by Gas Chromatography-Mass Spectrometry," *J Chromatogr B Biomed Sci Appl*, 1998, 708(1-2):87-93.
Nystrom L, Pettersson M, and Rangermark C, "Simple and Sensitive Method for Determination of Nicotine in Plasma by Gas Chromatography," *J Chromatogr B Biomed Sci Appl*, 1997, 701(1):124-8.
Oddoze C, Pauli AM, and Pastor J, "Rapid and Sensitive High Performance Liquid Chromatographic Determination of Nicotine and Cotinine in Nonsmoker Human and Rat Urines," *J Chromatogr B Biomed Sci Appl*, 1998, 708(1-2):95-101.
Pérez-Stable EJ, Herrera B, Jacob P, et al, "Nicotine Metabolism and Intake in Black and White Smokers," *JAMA*, 1998, 280(2):152-6.
Scherer G and Richter E, "Biomonitoring Exposure to Environmental Tobacco Smoke (ETS): A Critical Reappraisal," *Hum Exp Toxicol*, 1997, 16(8):449-59.
Smith RF, Mather HM, and Ellard GA, "Assessment of Simple Colorimetric Procedures to Determine Smoking Status of Diabetic Subjects," *Clin Chem*, 1998, 44(2):275-80.

♦ **NIDA Screen** see Drugs of Abuse Testing, Urine *on page 788*

♦ **Nipride®** see Thiocyanate, Serum, Plasma, or Urine *on page 807*

♦ **Nitroprusside** see Thiocyanate, Serum, Plasma, or Urine *on page 807*

♦ **11-Nor-9-Carboxy-Delta-9-Tetrahydrocannabinol** see Cannabinoids (Marijuana Metabolites), Qualitative, Urine *on page 783*

♦ **Norcodeine** see Codeine, Urine *on page 786*

♦ **Normeperidine** see Meperidine, Serum or Urine *on page 796*

♦ **Norpropoxyphene** see Propoxyphene, Serum or Urine *on page 805*

♦ **Nose Candy** see Cocaine (Cocaine Metabolite), Qualitative, Urine or Hair *on page 785*

♦ **Novrad®** see Propoxyphene, Serum or Urine *on page 805*

♦ **Nuprin®** see Ibuprofen, Serum *on page 793*

♦ **6-O-Acetyl Morphine** see Opiates, Qualitative, Urine *on page 803*

♦ **Oil of Wintergreen** see Salicylate, Serum or Plasma *on page 806*

♦ **OMS®** see Morphine, Urine *on page 802*

♦ **Opiates** see Drugs of Abuse Testing, Urine *on page 788*

Opiates, Qualitative, Urine

Related Information
Bacterial Culture, Blood *on page 566*
Chain-of-Custody Protocol *on page 785*
Codeine, Urine *on page 786*
Drugs of Abuse Testing, Urine *on page 788*
Morphine, Urine *on page 802*

Applies to Heroin; Narcotics; 6-O-Acetyl Morphine; Poppy Seeds

Test Includes Morphine, codeine, hydrocodone (Hycodan®), hydromorphone (Dilaudid®), oxycodone, oxymorphone

Abstract Opioids are among the most common and effective analgesics for the treatment of mild to severe pain. They have a high potential for addiction, leading to physical and psychological dependence. Opioids include derivatives of the poppy plant, semisynthetic substances, and synthetic compounds. The qualitative detection of urine opiates is used almost exclusively to demonstrate presence of drugs of abuse in this class. Morphine and codeine are commonly used therapeutically for pain.

Specimen Random urine

Collection If forensic, observe precautions (see the Introduction *on page 773*).

Storage Instructions Refrigerate

Special Instructions If forensic, use chain-of-custody protocol and form. See Chain-of-Custody Protocol *on page 785* and the Chain-of-Custody form in the Introduction *on page 773*.

Reference Interval Negative (less than cutoff)

Critical Values Substance Abuse and Mental Health Services Administration (SAMHSA) cutoff: screen: 2000 ng/mL; confirmation: 2000 ng/mL for codeine and morphine. For clinical purposes, many laboratories use a cutoff of 300 ng/mL.

Use Opiates are narcotic drugs used medically to relieve pain; they also have a high potential for abuse. Some opiates come from a resin taken from the seed pod of the Asian poppy. This group of drugs includes opium, morphine, and codeine. Other opiates are synthesized or manufactured (eg, heroin). Opium appears as dark brown chunks or as a powder, and may be smoked or eaten. Heroin can be a white or brownish powder which may be dissolved in water and injected.

A qualitative urine screen for opiates is performed in suspected overdose cases or as part of a drugs-of-abuse program.

Withdrawal from opioids may be manifested by tachycardia, hypertension, fever, insomnia, muscle cramping, miosis, lacrimation, perspiration, nausea, and vomiting.[1]

Limitations In most immunoassays a number of narcotic drugs can cross react to give a positive screen. Every effort should be made to confirm, by an analytically different and more sensitive method, all presumptive positive opiate screens. See above.

Methodology Screening: immunoassay, thin-layer chromatography (TLC), high performance liquid chromatography (HPLC), gas chromatography (GC); confirmation: gas chromatography/mass spectrometry (GC/MS)

Additional Information For morphine:
• Half-life: 2-4 hours (adults), 5-13 hours (neonates)
• Volume of distribution: 2-4 L/kg
• Protein binding: 30% to 40%

The test is most sensitive for morphine and codeine, but other drugs will cross react in an immunoassay and give positive results (eg, hydrocodone, hydromorphone). All presumptive positive assays should be confirmed, preferably by GC/MS. Morphine is a prescribed drug for pain relief, a metabolite of heroin, a metabolite of codeine, and a constituent of poppy seeds. Its presence in urine, even after confirmation, must be interpreted very carefully. Ingestion of poppy seeds (bagels, pastries including Danish) can cause positive opiate screens at a 300 ng/mL cutoff.[2] Due to this, SAMHSA has recently increased the cutoff of morphine and codeine to 2000 ng/mL.[3] The intake of heroin by the user can only be proved by the detection of 6-O-acetyl morphine by the urine confirmatory test.

Opiates tend to relax the user. When the opiates are injected, the user feels an immediate "rush." Other initial and unpleasant effects include restlessness, nausea, and vomiting. The user may go "on the nod," going back and forth from feeling alert to drowsy. With very large doses, the user cannot be awakened, pupils become smaller, and the skin becomes cold, moist, and bluish in color. Furthermore, breathing slows down and death may occur. Clearance may be slower in geriatric patients.

Complications of intravenous drug use include HIV, hepatitis B and C, and bacterial endocarditis. *Staphylococcus aureus* is the most commonly isolated pathogen in endocarditis, which in this group most commonly infects the tricuspid valve. Other complications include bacterial pneumonia, pulmonary talc granulomatosis, septic pulmonary embolism, abscesses, and nephropathy.[1]

Footnotes
1. Samet JH, "Drug Abuse and Dependence," *Cecil Textbook of Medicine*, 21st ed, Chapter 17, Goldman L and Bennett JC, eds, Philadelphia, PA: WB Saunders Co, 2000, 54-9.
2. Selavka CM, "Poppy Seed Ingestion as a Contributing Factor to Opiate Positive Urinalysis Results: The Pacific Perspective," *J Forensic Sci*, 1991, 36(3):685-96.
3. "Substance Abuse and Mental Health Administration. Mandatory Guidelines for Workplace Programs: Revision to Mandatory Guidelines," *Fed Regist*, 1998, 63:483.

References
Barsan W, "Narcotic Agents," *Ann Emerg Med*, 1986, 15:1019-20.
Cone EJ, Dickerson S, Paul BD, et al, "Forensic Drug Testing for Opiates. Urine Testing for Heroin, Morphine, and Codeine With Commercial Opiate Immunoassays," *J Anal Toxicol*, 1993, 17(3):156-64.
Ellenhorn MJ, Schonwald S, Ordog G, et al, "The Opiates," *Medical Toxicology*, Baltimore, MD: Lippincott Williams & Wilkins, 1997, 405-47.
Gillogley KM, Evans AT, Hansen RL, et al, "The Perinatal Impact of Cocaine, Amphetamine, and Opiate Use Detected by Universal Intrapartum Screening," *Am J Obstet Gynecol*, 1990, 163(5 Pt 1):1535-42.
Meatherall R, "GC/MS Confirmation of Codeine, Morphine, 6-Acetylmorphine, Hydrocodone, Hydromorphone, Oxycodone, and Oxymorphone in Urine," *J Anal Toxicol*, 1999, 23(3):177-86.
Paul BD, Shimomura ET, and Smith ML, "A Practical Approach to Determine Cutoff Concentrations for Opiate Testing With Simultaneous Detection of Codeine, Morphine, and 6-Acetylmorphine in Urine," *Clin Chem*, 1999, 45(4):510-9.
Pettitt BC Jr, Dyszel SM, and Hood LV, "Opiates in Poppy Seed: Effect on Urinalysis Results After Consumption of Poppy Seed Cake-Filling," *Clin Chem*, 1987, 33(7):1251-2.
Storrow AB, Wians FH Jr, Mikkelsen SL, et al, "Does Naloxone Cause a Positive Urine Opiate Screen?" *Ann Emerg Med*, 1994, 24(6):1151-3.

♦ **Opium** see Morphine, Urine *on page 802*

♦ **Oramorph SR®** see Morphine, Urine *on page 802*

♦ **Organic Mercury** see Mercury, Blood *on page 797*

Organophosphate Pesticides, Urine, Blood, or Serum

Related Information
Amylase, Serum *on page 102*

Applies to Acetylcholinesterase; Carbamate Toxicity; Cholinesterase, True; Insecticides; Pesticides; Pralidoxime; Pseudocholinesterase

Test Includes Azinphos-methyl, carbophenthion, chlorpyrifos, coumaphos, diazinon, dichlorvos, dimethoate, ethion, fenchlorphos, fenthion, fonofos, malathion, metasystox, methyl parathion, mevinphos, *p*-nitrophenol, para-oxon, parathion, phorate, terbufos

Abstract The organophosphates and the carbamates are the insecticide groups which represent the greatest hazards. Organochlorines are presently rarely used.[1] Organophosphorus insecticide poisoning is a major global health problem with ~3 million poisonings or more and 220,000 deaths annually. These agents cause poisoning by irreversibly inhibiting acetylcholinesterase. Organophosphate poisoning causes CNS intoxication and polyneuropathy.

There are two cholinesterase enzymes in blood: **acetylcholinesterase** (also called true cholinesterase) in red cells; and **"pseudocholinesterase"** (acylcholine acylhydrolase) in serum. Organophosphates inhibit both enzymes, but the toxic effect on the serum enzyme, pseudocholinesterase, is more rapid and intense, so that it is somewhat more useful in the initial diagnosis of organophosphate toxicity. Red cell acetylcholinesterase is often preferred for evaluating chronic organophosphate exposure; red cell acetylcholinesterase levels normalize more slowly than do serum pseudocholinesterase values.

Specimen Urine and blood or serum

Container Lavender top (EDTA) tube or red top tube

Storage Instructions Freeze sample if analysis cannot be performed immediately.

Use Determine occupational, accidental, and intentional poisoning. Insecticides are among the most toxic pesticides and cause most pesticide intoxication.

Organophosphates produce a triphasic effect. In the first phase, there is an accumulation of acetylcholine at muscarinic and nicotinic receptors. Muscarinic receptor stimulation causes increase in secretions, including salivation and lacrimation, bronchoconstriction, and bradycardia. This phase is life-threatening and requires immediate medical attention. The second phase occurs after 2-4 days and is characterized by muscle weakness and cranial nerve palsies. Delayed polyneuropathy usually occurs after 2-4 weeks and causes motor weakness of peripheral muscles with a variable sensory component.

Limitations Organophosphate assays are not readily available. Correlation between severity of toxicity and the amount of pesticide metabolite in urine is poor.

Methodology High performance thin layer chromatography (HPTLC). Urinary metabolites, the di-alkyl-phosphates, can be measured in urine by gas chromatography. It may be necessary to measure multiple metabolites.

Additional Information Organophosphates inhibit acetylcholinesterase in plasma and RBCs. Therefore, determination of both serum pseudocholinesterase and red blood cell cholinesterase activities is preferred. Acute toxicity is better measured by using the serum enzyme and chronic by measuring true cholinesterase in red cells. Depression >50% of baseline activity is generally associated with severe symptoms. Correlation between cholinesterase levels and clinical effects in milder poisonings may be poor. Monitor 12-lead EKG and serum pancreatic amylase levels in patients with significant poisoning. Patients who have increased serum amylase levels and those who develop a prolonged QT interval or PVCs are more likely to develop respiratory insufficiency and have a worse prognosis.

Treatment of organophosphate poisoning includes atropine treatment and suctioning of oral secretions as required until atropinization is achieved. (Atropine is a physiologic antidote, used to treat muscarinic effects.) Pralidoxime (Protopam®, 2-PAM), a specific antidote, should be administered to seriously ill organophosphate-poisoned patients. If induction of paralysis with muscle-relaxing agents is required for intubation, succinylcholine should be avoided because of potential prolonged duration of paralysis secondary to pseudocholinesterase inhibition by the organophosphate.

The chemical terrorist agents Sarin, Soman, Tabun, and VX are organophosphate nerve gases.

Footnotes
1. Keifer MC, "The Clinical Laboratory in the Diagnosis of Overexposure to Agrochemicals," *Lab Med*, 1998, 29(11):689-95.

References
Futagami K, Narazaki C, and Kataoka Y, "Application of High Performance Thin-Layer Chromatography for the Detection of Organophosphorus Insecticides in Human Serum After Acute Poisoning," *J Chromatogr B Biomed Sci Appl*, 1997, 704(1-2):369-73.

Matsumiya N, Tanaka M, Iwai M, et al, "Elevated Amylase Is Related to the Development of Respiratory Failure in Organophosphate Poisoning," *Hum Exp Toxicol*, 1996, 15(3):250-3.

Moretto A and Lotti M, "Poisoning by Organophosphorus Insecticides and Sensory Neuropathy," *J Neurol Neurosurg Psychiatry*, 1998, 64(4):463-8.

Senanayake N and Karalliedde L, "Neurotoxic Effects of Organophosphorus Insecticides. An Intermediate Syndrome," *N Engl J Med*, 1987, 316(13):761-3.

Sofer S, Tal A, and Shahak E, "Carbamate and Organophosphate Poisoning in Early Childhood," *Pediatr Emerg Care*, 1989, 5(4):222-5.

Yamashita M, Yamashita M, Tanaka J, et al, "Human Mortality in Organophosphate Poisonings," *Vet Hum Toxicol*, 1997, 39(2):84-5.

Yilmazlar A and Ozyurt G, "Brain Involvement in Organophosphate Poisoning," *Environ Res*, 1997, 74(2):104-9.

♦ **Oximeters, Pulse** *see* Carboxyhemoglobin, Blood *on page 784*

♦ **Pamprin®** *see* Ibuprofen, Serum *on page 793*

♦ **Panadol®** *see* Acetaminophen, Serum *on page 778*

♦ **Paracetamol** *see* Acetaminophen, Serum *on page 778*

♦ **Paveral** *see* Codeine, Urine *on page 786*

♦ **Pb, Blood** *see* Lead, Blood *on page 793*

♦ **Pb, Urine** *see* Lead, Urine *on page 795*

♦ **PCP** *see* Phencyclidine, Qualitative, Urine *on page 804*

♦ **Peace Pills** *see* Phencyclidine, Qualitative, Urine *on page 804*

♦ **Peace Weed** *see* Phencyclidine, Qualitative, Urine *on page 804*

♦ **Pentobarb** *see* Barbiturates, Qualitative, Urine *on page 781*

♦ **Pesos®** *see* Fenfluramine, Serum *on page 791*

♦ **Pesticides** *see* Organophosphate Pesticides, Urine, Blood, or Serum *on page 804*

♦ **Pethidine Hydrochloride** *see* Meperidine, Serum or Urine *on page 796*

♦ **Phenacetin** *see* Acetaminophen, Serum *on page 778*

♦ **Phencyclidine** *see* Drugs of Abuse Testing, Urine *on page 788*

Phencyclidine, Qualitative, Urine

Related Information
Chain-of-Custody Protocol *on page 785*
Drugs of Abuse Testing, Urine *on page 788*
Lysergic Acid Diethylamide, Urine *on page 796*

Synonyms Angel Dust; Crystal Joint; Elephant Tranquilizers; Goon; Hog; Kay Jay; Killer Weed; Mist; PCP; Peace Pills; Peace Weed; Rocket Fuel; Sheets; Sherm; Snorts; Soma®; Supergrass; Wickistick

Applies to Cyclohexamine; Phenylcyclohexylpyrrolidine; Phenylcyclopentylpiperidine; Thienylcyclohexylpiperidine

Abstract This is a widely used drug of abuse which was formerly sold as a veterinary tranquilizer. All legal manufacture and sale has been stopped. It is classified by DEA as a Schedule II controlled substance. It has no appropriate clinical role. Acute intoxication with phencyclidine may be life threatening. A hallucinogen, it causes psychosis and other symptoms and signs. It has been implicated in violent behavior.

Specimen Random urine

Collection If forensic, observe precautions (see Introduction *on page 773*).

Storage Instructions Refrigerate; stable for 1 year.[1]

Special Instructions If forensic, use chain-of-custody protocol and form. See Chain-of-Custody Protocol *on page 785* and the Chain-of-Custody form in the Introduction *on page 773*.

Reference Interval Negative (less than cutoff)

Critical Values Cutoff: screen: 25 ng/mL; confirmation: 25 ng/mL

Possible Panic Range Excitation: 20-30 ng/mL; coma: 30-100 ng/mL; seizures, **fatalities:** >500 ng/mL

Use Evaluate presence of phencyclidine, drug abuse, PCP toxicity; determine phencyclidine involvement in unexplained psychoses

Limitations Adulteration with bleach can cause false-negative urine immunoassays for phencyclidine. Doxylamine can cause a false-positive urine gas chromatographic result.

Methodology Immunoassay, thin-layer chromatography (TLC), gas chromatography (GC), gas chromatography/mass spectrometry (GC/MS). Immunoassays are very specific and detect PCP at 25 ng/mL (SI: 100 nmol/L) or higher.

Additional Information
- Half-life: 10-50 hours, depending on urine pH (it is water soluble and lipophilic)
- Volume of distribution: 5-7 L/kg
- Protein binding: 65% to 80%

Phencyclidine is most often called "angel dust." It was first developed as an anesthetic in the 1950s. It was taken off the market for human use because it sometimes caused hallucinations. PCP is available in a number of forms. It can be a pure white crystal-like powder, a tablet, liquid, spray, or capsule, and it can be swallowed, smoked (alone or with marijuana), sniffed, or injected. Although PCP is illegal, it is easily manufactured. A number of PCP analogues including cyclohexamine, phenylcyclohexylpyrrolidine, phenylcyclopentylpiperidine, and thienylcyclohexylpiperidine are manufactured as street drugs.

PCP combinations usually involve other drugs, most frequently cocaine, ethanol, and opiates.

PCP, classified as a dissociative anesthetic, exhibits stimulant, depressant, hallucinogenic, and analgesic properties. Effects depend on how much of the drug is taken, the way it is used, and the individual. Small amounts act as a stimulant, speeding up body functions. For many users, PCP changes how they see their own bodies and things around them. Speech, muscle coordination, and vision are affected; sense of touch and pain are dulled; and body movements are slowed. Time seems to "space out." Effects include increased heart rate and blood pressure, flushing, sweating, dizziness, and numbness. When large doses are taken, effects include drowsiness, convulsions, and coma. Taking large amounts of PCP can also cause death from repeated convulsions, heart and lung failure, or ruptured central nervous system blood vessels. PCP can be detected for 7 days after administration; 2-4 weeks in chronic users.

Footnotes

1. Grieshaber A, Costantino A, and Lappas N, "Stability of Phencyclidine in Stored Blood Samples," *J Anal Toxicol*, 1998, 22(6):515-9.

References

Baselt RC, *Disposition of Toxic Drugs and Chemicals in Man*, 5th ed, Foster City, CA: Chemical Toxicology Institute, 2000, 676-9.

Brust JC, "Other Agents. Phencyclidine, Marijuana, Hallucinogens, Inhalants, and Anticholinergics," *Neurol Clin*, 1993, 11(3):555-61.

Chan KM, Matthews WS, Saxena S, et al, "Frequency of Cocaine and Phencyclidine Detection at a Large Urban Public Teaching Hospital," *J Anal Toxicol*, 1993, 17(5):299-303.

Ellenhorn MJ, Schonwald S, Ordog G, et al, "Phencyclidine," *Medical Toxicology*, Baltimore, MD: Lippincott Williams & Wilkins, 1997, 401-4.

Gooch JC, Gallacher G, Wright JG, et al, "Detection of Phencyclidine in Urine Using a Polarization Fluoroimmunoassay," *Analyst*, 1994, 119(8):1797-800.

Milhorn HT Jr, "Diagnosis and Management of Phencyclidine Intoxication," *Am Fam Phys*, 1991, 43(4):1293-302.

Rogowski R and Krenzelok E, "Averting The Medical, Social, and Legal Implications of a False Positive Phencyclidine Determination," *J Toxicol Clin Toxicol*, 1997, 35:551.

Schneider S, Kuffer P, and Wennig R, "Determination of Lysergide (LSD) and Phencyclidine in Biosamples," *J Chromatogr B Biomed Sci Appl*, 1998, 713(1):189-200.

Wessinger WD and Owens SM, "Phencyclidine Dependence: The Relationship of Dose and Serum Concentrations to Operant Behavioral Effects," *J Pharmacol Exp Ther*, 1991, 258(1):207-15.

◆ **Phenobarb** *see* Barbiturates, Qualitative, Urine *on page 781*

◆ **Phentermine** *see* Methamphetamine, Qualitative, Urine *on page 799*

◆ **Phenylcyclohexylpyrrolidine** *see* Phencyclidine, Qualitative, Urine *on page 804*

◆ **Phenylcyclopentylpiperidine** *see* Phencyclidine, Qualitative, Urine *on page 804*

◆ **Phenylhydroxylamine** *see* Methemoglobin, Whole Blood *on page 800*

◆ **Phenylpropanolamine** *see* Methamphetamine, Qualitative, Urine *on page 799*

◆ **Phosphatidylethanol** *see* Ethanol, Blood, Urine, and Other Sources *on page 789*

◆ **Physeptone®** *see* Methadone, Urine *on page 798*

◆ **Poisonous Metals, Blood** *see* Heavy Metal Screen, Blood *on page 792*

◆ **Poisonous Metals, Urine** *see* Heavy Metal Screen, Urine *on page 792*

◆ **Ponderx®** *see* Fenfluramine, Serum *on page 791*

◆ **Pondimin®** *see* Fenfluramine, Serum *on page 791*

◆ **Ponflural®** *see* Fenfluramine, Serum *on page 791*

◆ **Poppy Seeds** *see* Opiates, Qualitative, Urine *on page 803*

◆ **Pot** *see* Cannabinoids (Marijuana Metabolites), Qualitative, Urine *on page 783*

◆ **Potassium or Sodium Cyanide** *see* Cyanide, Blood *on page 787*

◆ **Potassium Thiocyanate (KSCN)** *see* Thiocyanate, Serum, Plasma, or Urine *on page 807*

◆ **Pralidoxime** *see* Organophosphate Pesticides, Urine, Blood, or Serum *on page 804*

◆ **Pre-employment Drug Screen** *see* Drugs of Abuse Testing, Urine *on page 788*

◆ **Propacet®** *see* Propoxyphene, Serum or Urine *on page 805*

◆ **Propoxyphene** *see* Drugs of Abuse Testing, Urine *on page 788*

Propoxyphene, Serum or Urine

Related Information

Chain-of-Custody Protocol *on page 785*
Drugs of Abuse Testing, Urine *on page 788*
Methadone, Urine *on page 798*

Synonyms Darvocet-N®; Darvon®; E-Lor®; Genagesic®; Novrad®; Propacet®; Wygesic®

Applies to Norpropoxyphene

Test Includes Quantitation of propoxyphene and metabolite norpropoxyphene

Abstract Propoxyphene is a narcotic analgesic that is somewhat less potent than codeine. It is structurally and pharmacologically close to methadone. It is used clinically with nonopioid analgesics. It is biotransformed to norpropoxyphene, a potentially toxic metabolite. Overdoses may lead to seizures. This is also a drug of abuse and is generally included in the drug of abuse panel.

Specimen Serum (TDM), urine (drugs of abuse)

Container Red top tube, urine container

Sampling Time Urine: random; serum: trough

Special Instructions If forensic, use chain-of-custody protocol and form. See Chain-of-Custody Protocol *on page 785* and the Chain-of-Custody form in the Introduction *on page 773*.

Reference Interval Therapeutic: serum: 0.1-0.4 µg/mL (SI: 0.3-1.2 µmol/L) (therapeutic ranges published vary between laboratories and may not correlate with clinical effect); urine (for drugs of abuse): negative (less than cutoff)

Critical Values Cutoff for urine: screen: 300 ng/mL; confirmation: 200 ng/mL

Possible Panic Range Toxic: serum: >0.5 µg/mL (SI: >1.5 µmol/L); minimal fatal: 1.0 µg/mL (SI: 2.9 µmol/L)

Use Therapeutic monitoring, toxicity assessment, and drug-of-abuse testing

Limitations Diphenhydramine, a commonly used over-the-counter medication, can interface with immunoassays.[1]

Methodology Immunoassay, gas chromatography (GC), high performance liquid chromatography (HPLC), gas chromatography/mass spectrometry (GC/MS)

Additional Information

- Half-life: 8-24 hours
- Volume of distribution: 10-25 L/kg
- Protein binding: 70% to 80%

Propoxyphene is an analgesic structurally similar to methadone. It has been used clinically since 1957 and is often formulated with acetaminophen. The d and l isomers have different uses, the former as an analgesic and the latter as an antitussive. Its metabolite, norpropoxyphene is also pharmacologically active. Toxic effects include nausea, vomiting, and progressive central nervous system depression. Toxicity is additive with ethanol and other CNS depressants such as barbiturates and benzodiazepines. Toxicity can be neutralized by narcotic antagonists such as naloxone. Peak serum level occurs 2 hours postoral dose. Propoxyphene can also be measured in urine as part of a drug of abuse screen.

Recent data show that propoxyphene is one of the most common inappropriately prescribed drugs for the elderly.[2]

Footnotes

1. Schneider S and Wennig R, "Interference of Diphenhydramine With the EMIT II Immunoassay for Propoxyphene," *J Anal Toxicol*, 1999, 23(7):637-8.
2. Aparasu RR and Sitzman SJ, "Inappropriate Prescribing for Elderly Outpatients," *Am J Health Syst Pharm*, 1999, 56(5):433-9.

References

Baselt RC, "Disposition of Toxic Drugs and Chemicals in Man," 5th ed, Foster City, CA: Chemical Toxicology Institute, 2000, 740-4.

Henricson K, Carlsten A, Ranstam J, et al, "Utilization of Codeine and Propoxyphene: Geographic and Demographic Variations in Prescribing, Prescriber and Recipient Categories," *Eur J Clin Pharmacol*, 1999, 55(8):605-11.

King JW and King LJ, "Propoxyphene and Norpropoxyphene Quantitation in the Same Solid-Phase Extraction Using Toxi Lab Spec VC MP3 System," *J Anal Toxicol*, 1994, 18(4):217-9.

Kurlan R, Majumdar L, Deeley C, et al, "A Controlled Trial of Propoxyphene and Naltrexone in Patients With Tourette's Syndrome," *Ann Neurol*, 1991, 30(1):19-23.

Perin ML, "Problems With Propoxyphene," *Am J Nurs*, 2000, 100(6):22.

Schnitzer TJ, "Non-NSAID Pharmacologic Treatment Options for the Management of Chronic Pain," *Am J Med*, 1998, 105(1B):45S-52S.

◆ **Pseudocholinesterase** *see* Organophosphate Pesticides, Urine, Blood, or Serum *on page 804*

◆ **Pseudoephedrine** *see* Methamphetamine, Qualitative, Urine *on page 799*

◆ **Quaalude®** *see* Methaqualone, Urine *on page 800*

◆ **Quicksilver** *see* Mercury, Blood *on page 797*

◆ **Reduced Hemoglobin** *see* Methemoglobin, Whole Blood *on page 800*

◆ **Redutemp®** *see* Acetaminophen, Serum *on page 778*

◆ **Ridenol®** *see* Acetaminophen, Serum *on page 778*

◆ **RMS®** *see* Morphine, Urine *on page 802*

◆ **Rock** *see* Cocaine (Cocaine Metabolite), Qualitative, Urine or Hair *on page 785*

◆ **Rocket Fuel** *see* Phencyclidine, Qualitative, Urine *on page 804*

◆ **Rohypnol®** *see* Flunitrazepam, Urine *on page 791*

◆ **Roxanol™** *see* Morphine, Urine *on page 802*

◆ **Roxanol SR™** *see* Morphine, Urine *on page 802*

◆ **Rufen®** *see* Ibuprofen, Serum *on page 793*

Salicylate, Serum or Plasma

Related Information

Anion Gap, Serum, Plasma, or Urine *on page 106*
Glucose, Random, Plasma *on page 186*
Lactic Acid, Whole Blood or Plasma *on page 208*
pH, Blood *on page 247*
pH, Urine *on page 882*
Potassium, Serum or Plasma *on page 258*

Synonyms Acetylsalicylic Acid, Blood; Anacin®; ASA, Blood; Ascriptin®; Aspergum®; Aspirin, Blood; Bufferin®; Easprin®; Ecotrin®; Empirin®; Measurin®; Salicylic Acid, Blood; Synalgos®; ZORprin®

Applies to Methyl Salicylate; Oil of Wintergreen

Abstract This is the active product produced from aspirin (acetylsalicylic acid) in the body. It is an analgesic, antipyretic and anti-inflammatory drug. Salicylate is one of the top 10 drugs associated with fatalities in 1998.[1] Chronic salicylism in pediatric patients causes greater morbidity than acute poisoning, caused by dosing errors and/or dehydration.[2]

Acute poisoning may include hypokalemia, respiratory alkalosis, dehydration, metabolic acidosis, and hepatotoxicity. Pulmonary and cerebral edema may develop.[3]

Specimen Serum or plasma

Container Red top tube or lavender top (EDTA) tube

Sampling Time Time to peak serum concentration is about 1-2 hours. Optimal sampling time after dosage is 4-6 hours.

Reference Interval Therapeutic: ~10 mg/dL (SI: ~0.72 mmol/L) for analgesic; 15-20 mg/dL (SI: 1.09-1.45 mmol/L) for anti-inflammatory properties

Possible Panic Range Mild toxicity: ~30 mg/dL (SI: 2.17 mmol/L) (tinnitus, dizziness); severe toxicity: >80 mg/dL (SI: >3.62 mmol/L) (CNS effects)

Use Monitor therapeutic drug level, evaluate aspirin toxicity. Most organ systems are affected by salicylate toxicity.

Methodology Photometry, fluorometry, immunoassay, high performance liquid chromatography (HPLC), gas-liquid chromatography (GLC)

Additional Information

- Half-life: 2-3 hours
- Volume of distribution: 0.1-0.3 L/kg
- Protein binding: 90% to 95%

In patients on chronic therapy, small dose changes may produce disproportionate changes in serum level. Serum half-life is 2-3 hours on low-dose therapy, about 10 hours on high-dose treatment but reaches 15-30 hours as higher doses increase elimination half-life. Optimal resampling time after change in dosage is 6 hours. Use of antacids, which increase renal excretion, can lower serum levels. Steady-state concentrations for an individual patient are not adequately predicted from nomograms or standard dose schedules. In salicylate poisoning the following symptoms may occur: initial respiratory alkalosis, mixed respiratory alkalosis and increased anion gap metabolic acidosis, sometimes with ketosis and possible elevated plasma glucose (see table).

Serum Salicylate: Clinical Correlations

Serum Salicylate Concentration (mg/dL)	Desired Effects	Adverse Effects/ Intoxication
~10	Antiplatelet Antipyresis Analgesia	GI intolerance and bleeding, hypersensitivity, hemostatic defects
15-30	Anti-inflammatory	Mild salicylism
25-40	Treatment of rheumatic fever	Nausea/vomiting, hyperventilation, salicylism, flushing, sweating, thirst, headache, diarrhea, and tachycardia
>40		Respiratory alkalosis, hemorrhage, excitement, confusion, asterixis, pulmonary edema, convulsions, tetany, metabolic acidosis, fever, coma, cardiovascular collapse, renal and respiratory failure

Patients in chronic salicylate toxicity may not exceed levels in the therapeutic range; their levels may be 10-20 mg/dL.[3]

In children, the alkalosis phase is very short. Glucose should be measured when salicylate levels are >25 mg/dL (SI: >1.81 mmol/L) are detected. Salicylate can be done on urine or gastric juice. The Done nomogram is used to estimate severity of toxicity based on blood level 6 hours or more after a single-dose ingestion, but cannot be used for chronic intoxication.[2] See nomogram.

The level measured 6 hours or more following ingestion is plotted. Specimens drawn earlier may not reflect the peak. The nomogram is not useful when accumulation over several ingestions exists. Urine becomes acidic with salicylate intoxication. Urine pH and volume hourly, with urine protein quantitation, plasma pH, potassium and other electrolytes, prothrombin time, AST, ALT, serum bilirubin, and arterial blood gases are advocated for care of serious pediatric salicylate poisoning. The metabolic acidosis includes lactic acid. Ketone bodies may be detected. Both hyperglycemia

and hypoglycemia may occur. Low CNS glucose can evolve in the presence of normal blood glucose. Salicylates are believed to play a role in the hepatonecrosis of Reye syndrome in children. They are no longer recommended for use in children and alternative antipyretic use has increased, especially in young children.

Signs and symptoms of **acute overdose** may include nausea, vomiting, dehydration, hyperpnea, oliguria, and tinnitus. **Severe poisoning** can include coma, convulsions, severe hyperpnea, and metabolic acidosis.

Symptoms of **chronic salicylism** include fever, vomiting, and tachypnea. It is likely following doses in excess of 100 mg/kg/day for 2 days of more.[2]

Serum Salicylate Level and Severity of Intoxication Single Dose Acute Ingestion Nomogram

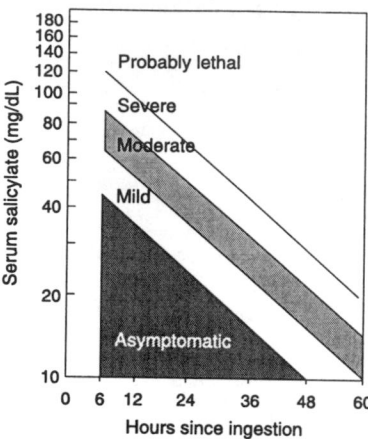

Nomogram relating serum salicylate concentration and expected severity of intoxication at varying intervals following the ingestion of a single dose of salicylate.
From Done AK, "Aspirin Overdosage: Incidence, Diagnosis, and Management," *Pediatrics*, 1978, 62:890-7 with permission.

Phases of Salicylate Poisoning

- Phase I (up to 12 hours after ingestion): Tachypnea and hyperventilation predominate (respiratory alkalosis) with increased renal loses of sodium, potassium, and bicarbonate, resulting in an alkaline urinary and serum pH.
- Phase II (12-24 hours after ingestion): Urine becomes more acid as intracellular potassium decreases; while children <4 years of age may develop a pure metabolic acidosis, older patients will have significant respiratory compensation and thus serum pH can be alkalotic; coagulation abnormalities may occur.
- Phase III (over 24 hours after ingestion): Severe potassium and bicarbonate depletion occurs with renal hydrogen ion excretion; acidosis. Infants may reach this phase within 6 hours.

Platelet adhesiveness becomes decreased. There is an increased bleeding potential with concomitant warfarin therapy. Salicylate may increase lithium and methotrexate concentrations by decreasing renal clearance and may increase nephrotoxicity of cyclosporine. It may decrease diuretic and hypotensive effects of thiazides, loop diuretics, ACE inhibitors, and beta-blockers.

Salicylate causes false-negative results for glucose oxidase urinary glucose tests (Clinistix®), false positives using the cupric sulfate method (Clinitest®). It may interfere with VMA, 5-HIAA, xylose tolerance test, and some thyroid testing.

Footnotes

1. Litovitz TL, Klein-Schwartz W, Caravati EM, et al, "1998 Annual Report of the American Association of Poison Control Centers Toxic Exposure Surveillance System," *Am J Emerg Med*, 1999, 17(5):435-87.
2. Mariscalco MM, "Salicylism," *Oski's Pediatrics: Principles and Practice*, 3rd ed, McMillan JA, De Angelis CD, Feigin RD, et al, eds, Philadelphia, PA: JB Lippincott Co, 1999, 623-5.
3. Rodgers GC Jr and Matyunas NJ, "Poisonings: Drugs, Chemicals, and Plants," *Nelson Textbook of Pediatrics*, Chapter 722, Behrman RE, Kliegman HM, and Jensen HB, eds, Philadelphia, PA: WB Saunders Co, 2000, 2160-71.

References

Androgué HJ and Madias NE, "Management of Life-Threatening Acid-Base Disorders," First of Two Parts, *N Engl J Med*, 1998, 338(1):26-34.

Bailey RB and Jones SR, "Chronic Salicylate Intoxication. A Common Cause of Morbidity in the Elderly," *J Am Geriatr Soc*, 1989, 37(6):556-61.

Chapman BJ and Proudfoot AT, "Adult Salicylate Poisoning: Deaths and Outcome in Patients With High Plasma Salicylate Concentrations," *Q J Med*, 1989, 72(268):699-707.

Done AK, "Aspirin Overdosage: Incidence, Diagnosis, and Management," *Pediatrics*, 1978, 62(5 Pt 2 Suppl):890-7.

Dugandric RM, Tierney MG, and Dickinson GE, "Evaluation of the Done Nomogram in the Management of Acute Salicylate Intoxication," *Ann Emerg Med*, 1989, 18(11):1186-90.

Fenton J, *The Laboratory and the Poisoned Patient: A Guidebook for Interpreting Laboratory Data*, Washington, DC: AACC Press, 1998, 304-9.

Higgins RM, Connolly JO, and Hendry BM, "Alkalinization and Hemodialysis in Severe Salicylate Poisoning: Comparison of Elimination Techniques in the Same Patient," *Clin Nephrol*, 1998, 50(3):178-83.

Hood VL and Tannen RL, "Protection of Acid-Base Balance by pH Regulation of Acid Production," *N Engl J Med*, 1998, 339(12):819-26.

Kuhn MM, "Drug Overdose: Salicylates," *Crit Care Nurse*, 1992, 12(1):16, 25-7.

Lemesh RA, "Accidental Chronic Salicylate Intoxication in an Elderly Patient: Major Morbidity Despite Early Recognition," *Vet Hum Toxicol*, 1993, 35(1):34-6.

Mayer AL, Sitar DS, and Tenenbein M, "Multiple-Dose Charcoal and Whole-Bowel Irrigation Do Not Increase Clearance of Absorbed Salicylate," *Arch Intern Med*, 1992, 152(2):393-6.

Merigian KS and Blaho K, "Diagnosis and Management of the Drug Overdose Patient," *Am J Ther*, 1997, 4(2-3):99-113.

Montgomery H, Porter JC, and Bradley RD, "Salicylate Intoxication Causing a Severe Systemic Inflammatory Response and Rhabdomyolysis," *Am J Emerg Med*, 1994, 12(5):531-2.

Pierce RP, Gazewood J, and Blake RL Jr, "Salicylate Poisoning From Enteric-Coated Aspirin. Delayed Absorption May Complicate Management," *Postgrad Med*, 1991, 89(5):61-2, 64.

Sallis RE, "Management of Salicylate Toxicity," *Am Fam Phys*, 1989, 39(3):265-70.

Vane JR and Botting RM, "Mechanism of Action of Aspirin-Like Drugs," *Semin Arthritis Rheum*, 1997, 26(6 Suppl 1):2-10.

♦ **Salicylic Acid, Blood** *see* Salicylate, Serum or Plasma *on page 806*

♦ **Scoop** *see* Gamma Hydroxybutyrate, Serum or Urine *on page 791*

♦ **Secobarb** *see* Barbiturates, Qualitative, Urine *on page 781*

♦ **Sevredol®** *see* Morphine, Urine *on page 802*

♦ **Sheets** *see* Phencyclidine, Qualitative, Urine *on page 804*

♦ **Sherm** *see* Phencyclidine, Qualitative, Urine *on page 804*

♦ **Sine-Off®** *see* Methamphetamine, Qualitative, Urine *on page 799*

♦ **Snaplets-FR® Granules** *see* Acetaminophen, Serum *on page 778*

♦ **Snorts** *see* Phencyclidine, Qualitative, Urine *on page 804*

♦ **Snow** *see* Cocaine (Cocaine Metabolite), Qualitative, Urine or Hair *on page 785*

♦ **Soma®** *see* Phencyclidine, Qualitative, Urine *on page 804*

♦ **Somatomax®** *see* Gamma Hydroxybutyrate, Serum or Urine *on page 791*

♦ **Sopor™** *see* Methaqualone, Urine *on page 800*

♦ **Specimen Chain-of-Custody Protocol** *see* Chain-of-Custody Protocol *on page 785*

♦ **Speed** *see* Amphetamine, Qualitative, Urine *on page 779*

♦ **Speed** *see* Methamphetamine, Qualitative, Urine *on page 799*

♦ **Statex®** *see* Morphine, Urine *on page 802*

♦ **Sudafed®** *see* Methamphetamine, Qualitative, Urine *on page 799*

♦ **Sulfhemoglobin** *see* Methemoglobin, Whole Blood *on page 800*

♦ **Supergrass** *see* Phencyclidine, Qualitative, Urine *on page 804*

♦ **Symoron®** *see* Methadone, Urine *on page 798*

♦ **Synalgos®** *see* Salicylate, Serum or Plasma *on page 806*

♦ **Tempra®** *see* Acetaminophen, Serum *on page 778*

♦ **Tetrahydrocannabinol (THC)** *see* Cannabinoids (Marijuana Metabolites), Qualitative, Urine *on page 783*

Thallium, Urine or Blood

Related Information
Heavy Metal Screen, Blood *on page 792*
Heavy Metal Screen, Urine *on page 792*
Urine Collection, 24-Hour *on page 47*

Applies to Mee's Lines

Abstract A highly toxic metal, thallium belongs to the aluminum family of metals. A byproduct of lead smelting, thallium salts are used in photomultiplier tubes, infrared detectors and transmitters, lens and glass making, and in rockets and flares. Thallium salts burn with a bright green color. Thallium sulfate, odorless and tasteless, until recently has been a component of insecticides and rodenticides. Thallium has been excluded as a rodenticide in the U.S. since 1972. It may be found in grain. Trace amounts of radioactive thallium (^{201}Tl) are used as a contrast agent (tracer) in radiology for localizing tumors and visualizing heart functions.

Patient Preparation The patient should be instructed to use a plastic bedpan or urinal if necessary, not metal.

Specimen 24-hour urine, serum

Container Special metal-free EDTA tube or metal-free plastic urine container. See Trace Metal Introduction *on page 811*.

Causes for Rejection Specimen allowed to contact metal or dusts with metal, use of nonmetal-free containers

Reference Interval Urine: <2 μg/L (SI: <9.8 nmol/L); serum: <0.5 μg/L (SI: <24.5 nmol/L)[1]

Critical Values Serum value in most normal individuals is <10 μg/L or 10 ng/mL (SI: 49 nmol/L); daily urine excretion in most normal individuals is <10 μg/day (SI: 48.9 nmol/day).[2] Spot urinary thallium concentration in normal unexposed individuals is <1.5 μg/L.[3]

Possible Panic Range Blood values from 100-8000 μg/L (SI: 0.5-39.1 mmol/L) are indicative of severe exposure.[1] Toxicity may be associated with blood levels of 100 μg/L (SI: 0.5 nmol/L) or urine values >200 μg/L (SI: 978 nmol/L).

Use Diagnose thallium exposure and toxicity, including alopecia with neuropathy which may resemble that of Guillain-Barré syndrome, and abdominal colic.

Limitations There are marked variations in heavy metal levels considered toxic by different investigators.

Methodology Graphite furnace atomic absorption spectrometry (GFAAS), inductively-coupled plasma-mass spectrometry (ICP-MS)

Additional Information Thallium is almost 100% absorbed from the GI tract and, like potassium, distributes throughout the body. Thallium salts have been used in the past as a depilatory and are absorbed through the skin. Thallium poisoning symptoms initially begin with generalized nausea, vomiting, abdominal pain, diarrhea, and gastrointestinal bleeding. Other nonspecific clinical findings include polyneuritis, encephalitis, delirium, ophthalmologic symptoms, convulsions, shock, and coma. Alopecia and painful ascending peripheral neuropathy are the most characteristic components of a thallium "toxidrome."[4] Because of the delayed development of alopecia (several weeks after poisoning), the diagnosis of thallotoxicosis is often initially overlooked until the alopecia appears. Mee's lines (transverse white lines on the nails) appear on the hands and feet 1 month after exposure, but are not specific for thallium poisoning.[4] Other dermatological findings include crusted eczematous lesions, hypohydrosis, anhydrosis, palmar erythema, painful glossitis, stomatitis, and hair discoloration.[5]

Severe thallium poisoning may be caused by 1 g or 8 mg/kg body weight. The lethal dose is reported to be 12 mg/kg body weight.[3] When death occurs from acute exposure, it is usually the result of coma, respiratory paralysis, or cardiac arrest. Elimination half-life for individuals with thallium poisoning is 1.7 days.[4]

Thallium salts have varied pathogenic mechanisms. At the cellular level, thallous ions (Tl$^+$) have an ionic radius somewhat similar to K$^+$, and the two ions act interchangeably in many biological membrane systems.[6] Thallous ions, thus, accumulate where there is a high K$^+$ concentration. In low concentrations, thallous ions may replace K$^+$ ions in potassium-dependent enzyme systems and stimulate these systems. Higher thallous ionic concentrations have a paradoxical inhibiting effect.[4] Thallium ions, like mercury and cadmium, have a marked affinity for sulfhydryl groups and may poison key mitochondrial sulfhydryl-containing enzymes. Thiol group inactivation may lead to oxidative stress, mitochondrial permeability changes, and mitochondrial dysfunction. Thallium also adversely affects protein synthesis in animals by damaging the 60S subunit of ribosomes.[4]

Footnotes
1. "Reference Information for the Clinical Laboratory," *Tietz Textbook of Clinical Chemistry*, Chapter 50, Burtis CA and Ashwood ER, eds, Philadelphia, PA: WB Saunders Co, 1999, 1835.
2. Moyer TP, "Toxic Metals," *Tietz Textbook of Clinical Chemistry*, Chapter 28, Burtis CA and Ashwood ER, eds, Philadelphia, PA: WB Saunders Co, 1999, 995-6.
3. Proctor NH and Hughes JP, *Chemical Hazards of the Workplace*, 4th ed, Hathaway GJ, Proctor NH, and Hughes JP, eds, New York, NY: Van Nostrand Rteinhold Co, 1996, 595-6.
4. Mercurio M and Hoffman RS, "Thallium." *Goldfrank's Toxicologic Emergencies*, 6th ed, Goldfrank LR, Flomenbaum NE, Lewin NA, et al, eds, Stamford, CT: Appleton and Lange, 1998, 1349-57.
5. Tromme I, Van Neste D, Dobbelaere F, et al, "Skin Signs in the Diagnosis of Thallium Poisoning," *J Dermatol*, 1998, 138(2):321-5.
6. Low PA, Smith BE, Clarke Stevens J, et al, "Diseases of Peripheral Nerves," *Clinical Neurology*, Volume 4, Joynt RJ and Griggs RC, eds, Philadelphia, PA: Lippincott and Williams Co, 1998, 136-7.

References
Meggs W, Morasco R, Shih R, et al, "Effects of Prussian Blue and N-acetylcysteine on Thallium Toxicity," *Vet Hum Toxicol*, 1994, 36:364.
Sabbioni E, Minoia C, Ronchi A, et al, "Trace Element Reference Values in Tissues From Inhabitants of the European Union. VIII. Thallium in the Italian Population," *Sci Total Environ*, 1994, 158(1-3):227-36.

♦ **THC-Carboxylic Acid** *see* Cannabinoids (Marijuana Metabolites), Qualitative, Urine *on page 783*

♦ **THC (Delta-9-*trans*-Tetrahydrocannabinol)** *see* Cannabinoids (Marijuana Metabolites), Qualitative, Urine *on page 783*

♦ **Thienylcyclohexylpiperidine** *see* Phencyclidine, Qualitative, Urine *on page 804*

Thiocyanate, Serum, Plasma, or Urine

Related Information
Carboxyhemoglobin, Blood *on page 784*
Cyanide, Blood *on page 787*

Synonyms Ethyl and Methyl Thiocyanate (Thanite® and Lethane®); Potassium Thiocyanate (KSCN)

(Continued)

Thiocyanate, Serum, Plasma, or Urine (Continued)

Applies to Cyanide; Nipride®; Nitroprusside

Abstract Thiocyanate is a relatively inert metabolite of the antihypertensive drug, nitroprusside. It is also a product of cyanide metabolism, a byproduct of cigarette smoking, and is found in the serum and urine of individuals consuming cassava beans. The most common cause of cyanide poisoning is smoke inhalation. Other sources include a rodenticide and an acrylic nail remover.[1]

Specimen Serum or plasma, urine

Container Red top tube, lavender top (EDTA) tube, plastic urine container

Reference Interval Serum, nonsmoker: 1-4 µg/mL (SI: 0.02-0.07 mmol/L), smoker: up to 10 µg/mL (SI: up to 0.17 mmol/L); urine: nonsmoker: 1-4 mg/24 hours (SI: 0.02-0.07 mmol/day), smoker: 7-17 mg/24 hours (SI: 0.12-0.30 mmol/day)

Possible Panic Range Serum: >35 µg/mL (SI: >0.60 mmol/L); 200 µg/mL (SI: 3.44 mmol/L) is lethal

Use Follow exposure to cyanide; evaluation of clearance of thiocyanate; monitor nitroprusside toxicity and smoking or nonsmoking compliance. Urine thiocyanate may be used to follow chronic poisoning in those consuming cassava beans.

Limitations Because of rapid metabolism of the drug, results are usually meaningless in the clinical setting of acute CN⁻ exposure by the time they are reported.

Methodology Photometry, chromatography, ion chromatography with fluorescence and ultraviolet detection. Amperometric determination after ion chromatography.

Additional Information Thiocyanate is a major metabolite of cyanide; it is produced in the liver by the enzyme rhodanase. Thiocyanate is present in healthy subjects. It is a component of cigarette smoke. It can arise from the drug nitroprusside, which is sometimes used to control acute hypertension. Thiocyanate toxicity may occur with long-term nitroprusside use (7-10 days with normal renal function and 3-6 days with renal impairment).[2,3] When thiosulfate is given to treat cyanide toxicity, thiocyanate toxicity may occur. Toxic manifestations may include psychotic behavior, agitation, and convulsions. Subclinical poisoning in children of families consuming cassava beans includes ankle clonus.

Home fires in which urea foam insulation burns produce hydrocyanic acid and formaldehyde.

Footnotes

1. Haddad LM, "Acute Poisoning," *Cecil Textbook of Medicine*, 21st ed, Chapter 98, Goldman L and Bennett JC, eds, Philadelphia, PA: WB Saunders Co, 2000, 515-22.
2. Baselt RC, *Disposition of Toxic Drugs and Chemicals in Man*, 5th ed, Foster City, CA: Chemical Toxicology Institute, 2000, 608-12.
3. Apple FS, Lowe MC, Googins MK, et al, "Serum Thiocyanate Concentrations in Patients With Normal or Impaired Renal Function Receiving Nitroprusside," *Clin Chem*, 1996, 42(11):1878-9.

References

Balistreri WF, A-Kader HH, Setchell KD, et al, "New Methods for Assessing Liver Function in Infants and Children," *Ann Clin Lab Sci*, 1992, 22(3):162-74.

Casella IG, Guascito MR, and De Bendetto GE, "Electrooxidation of Thiocyanate on the Copper-Modified Gold Electrode and its Amperometric Determination by Ion Chromatography," *Analyst*, 1998, 123(6):1359-63.

Chinaka S, Takayama N, Michigami Y, et al, "Simultaneous Determination of Cyanide and Thiocyanate in Blood by Ion Chromatography With Fluorescence and Ultraviolet Detection," *J Chromatography B Biomed Sci Appl*, 1998, 713(2):353-9.

Cliff J, Nicala D, Saute F, et al, "Ankle Clonus and Thiocyanate, Linamarin, and Inorganic Sulphate Excretion in School Children in Communities With Konzo, Mozambique," *J Trop Pediatr*, 1999, 45(3):139-42.

Galanti LM, "Specificity of Salivary Thiocyanate as Marker of Cigarette Smoking Is Not Affected by Alimentary Sources," *Clin Chem*, 1997, 43(1):184-5.

Hall AH and Rumack BH, "Clinical Toxicology of Cyanide," *Ann Emerg Med*, 1986, 15(9):1067-74.

Haque MR and Brandbury JH, "Simple Method for Determination of Thiocyanate in Urine," *Clin Chem*, 1999, 45(9):1459-64.

van Dalen CJ, Whitehouse MW, Winterbourn CC, et al, "Thiocyanate and Chloride as Competing Substrates for Myeloperoxidase," *Biochem J*, 1997, 327(Pt 2):487-92.

Vesey CJ, McAllister H, and Langford RM, "A Safer Method for the Measurement of Plasma Thiocyanate," *J Anal Toxicol*, 1999, 23(2):134-6.

♦ **Toot** *see* Cocaine (Cocaine Metabolite), Qualitative, Urine or Hair *on page 785*

♦ **Toxic Metals, Blood** *see* Heavy Metal Screen, Blood *on page 792*

♦ **Toxic Metals, Urine** *see* Heavy Metal Screen, Urine *on page 792*

Toxicology Screen, Serum

Related Information

Cotinine, Serum, Plasma, or Urine *on page 787*
Nicotine, Serum or Plasma *on page 802*
Toxicology Screen, Urine *on page 808*

Synonyms Drug Screen, Comprehensive Drug Panel or Analysis

Test Includes Acetaminophen (Tylenol®); acetone; alcohol (ethyl, methyl, isopropyl); amitriptyline (Elavil®); amobarbital (Amytal®); butabarbital (Butisol®); butalbital (Fiorinal®); caffeine; carbamazepine (Tegretol®); carisoprodol (Soma®); desipramine (Norpramin®); diltiazem (Cardizem®); diphenhydramine (Benadryl®); doxepin (Sinequan®); ephedrine; fluoxetine (Prozac®); glutethimide (Doriden®); ibuprofen; imipramine (Tofranil®); mephobarbital (Mebaral®); meprobamate (Equanil®) methaqualone (Quaalude®); nicotine; nortriptyline (Aventyl®); pentobarbital (Luminal®); phenobarbital; phenytoin (Dilantin®); salicylate (Aspirin®); secobarbital (Seconal™); theophylline (Theo-Dur®); thiopental (Pentithal®); tricyclic antidepressants; varies with the laboratory

Abstract This toxicology screen is carried out by performing individual quantitative tests for each drug or by thin layer chromatography or semiquantitative automated high performance liquid chromatography (Remedi®). Many times urine qualitative screening is faster and more useful in toxicologic emergencies, but both may be needed. Immunoassays are also frequently employed due to their fast turnaround time.

Specimen Serum or plasma

Container Red top tube or lavender top (EDTA) tube

Special Instructions Do **not** collect blood in heparinized tubes.

Reference Interval See individual drug listing for therapeutic and toxic ranges.

Use Monitor toxic/overdose situations; most desirable to analyze in conjunction with urine toxicology testing; used to quantitate drug identified qualitatively in urine

Limitations This is not a drugs-of-abuse screen. Evidence for presence of a drug/drug metabolite (screening, qualitative) in the case of most groups of therapeutic agents and drugs of abuse will be found in urine rather than serum. See Toxicology Screen, Urine *on page 808*. All agents identified in a screening test should be confirmed with a specific test.

Methodology Spot tests, immunoassay, thin-layer chromatography (TLC), gas chromatography (GC), high performance liquid chromatography (HPLC), colorimetry, spectrophotometry

Additional Information If only documentation of exposure to toxic drugs or drugs of abuse is desired, a urine drug screen is the most economical approach. See Toxicology Screen, Urine *on page 808*. When Toxicology Screen, Serum is ordered, the individual drugs are quantitated in serum. When Toxicology Screen, Urine is ordered, qualitative identification is carried out.

References

Clark R and Harchelroad F, "Toxicology Screening of the Trauma Patient. A Changing Profile," *Ann Emerg Med*, 1991, 20(2):151-3.

Elliott SP and Hale KA, "Applications of an HPLC-DAD Drug-Screening System Based on Retention Indices and UV Spectra," *J Anal Toxicol*, 1998, 22(4):279-89.

Giorgi DF and Jagoda A, "Poisoning and Overdose," *Mt Sinai J Med*, 1997, 64(4-5):283-91.

Litovitz TL, Klein-Schwartz W, Caravati EM, et al, "1998 Annual Report of the American Association of Poison Control Centers Toxic Exposure Surveillance System," *Am J Emerg Med*, 1999, 17(5):435-87.

Mahoney JD, Gross PL, Stern TA, et al, "Quantitative Serum Toxic Screening in the Management of Suspected Drug Overdose," *Am J Emerg Med*, 1990, 8(1):16-22.

Merigian KS and Blaho K, "Diagnosis and Management of the Drug Overdose Patient," *Am J Ther*, 1997, 4(2-3):99-113.

Puopolo PR, Volpicelli SA, Johnson DM, et al, "Emergency Toxicology Testing (Detection, Confirmation, and Quantification) of Basic Drugs in Serum by Liquid Chromatography With Photodiode Array Detection," *Clin Chem*, 1991, 37(12):2124-30.

Schwartz JG, Zollars R, Okorodudu AO, et al, "Accuracy of Common Drug Screen Tests," *Am J Emerg Med*, 1991, 9(2):166-70.

Wiley JF 2d, "Difficult Diagnoses in Toxicology: Poisons Not Detected By the Comprehensive Drug Screen," *Pediatr Clin North Am*, 1991, 38(3):725-37.

Toxicology Screen, Urine

Related Information

Cotinine, Serum, Plasma, or Urine *on page 787*
Drugs of Abuse Testing, Urine *on page 788*
Nicotine, Serum or Plasma *on page 802*
Toxicology Screen, Serum *on page 808*

Synonyms Drug Screen, Comprehensive Panel or Analysis, Urine

Test Includes A variety of qualitative screens are in use. Sensitivity and specificity vary and are method dependent. Screens should detect drugs (qualitatively) in the following classes: amphetamines, analgesics, anticonvulsants, antidepressants, antihistamines, cardiacs, narcotics, sedative/hypnotics, tranquilizers, volatiles, and drugs of abuse.

Acetaminophen (Tylenol®); acetone; alcohol (ethyl, methyl, isopropyl); amitriptyline (Elavil®); amobarbital (Amytal®); amphetamines; benzodiazepines; benztropine (Cogentin®); butabarbital (Butisol®); butalbital (Fiorinal®), caffeine, carbamazepine (Tegretol®); carisoprodol (Soma®); cocaine (as metabolite); codeine; cyclobenzaprine (Flexeril®); desipramine (Norpramin®); dextromethorphan (DN®); diltiazem (Cardizem®); diphenhydramine (Benadryl®); doxepin (Sinequan®); ephedrine; fluoxetine (Prozac®); glutethimide (Doriden®); heroin (as monoacetylmorphine); ibuprofen; imipramine (Tofranil®); lidocaine (Xylocaine®); loxapine (Loxitane®); maprotiline (Ludiomil®); meperidine (Demerol®); mephobarbital (Mebaral®); meprobamate (Equanil®); methadone; methamphetamine; methaqualone (Quaalude®); morphine; naproxen (Naprosyn®); nicotine; nortriptyline (Aventyl®); oxycodone (Percodan®); pentazocine (Talwin®); pentobarbital (Nembutal®); phencyclidine (PCP®); phenobarbital (Luminal®); phenylpropanolamine, phenytoin (Dilantin®); propoxyphene (Darvon®); propranolol; protriptyline (Vivactyl®); pseudoephedrine; salicylate (Aspirin®); secobarbital (Seconal™); sertraline (Zoloft®); THC metabolite (marijuana); theophylline

(Theo-Dur®); thiopental (Pentothal®); trazodone (Desyrel®); trimipramine (Surmontil®) are generally included in the urine drug screen

Abstract This is a qualitative screen which with thin-layer chromatography, gas chromatography, or automated high performance liquid chromatography can detect any of several hundred drugs (Remedi®). Immunoassays are generally also used in conjunction with other methods.

Specimen Random urine

Storage Instructions Keep refrigerated.

Special Instructions Specify the drug or drugs suspected.

Reference Interval None detected or negative (less than cutoff for drugs of abuse)

Use Screen for drug abuse, drug toxicity alone or in conjunction with serum/plasma testing. For typical drugs-of-abuse screening, see Drugs of Abuse Testing, Urine *on page 788.*

Limitations Test provides **only** qualitative detection of drugs, unless laboratory automatically confirms and quantitates drugs detected as a part of the "screening" procedure. Quantitation of urine drug levels is usually not included and is not recommended because urine levels are time and clearance dependent and are not directly related to toxic symptoms seen clinically. Some drugs and/or metabolites are not detected or optimally detected in urine, again relating to method. Serum may be preferable because of clinical and at times technical/kinetic factors (eg, barbiturates, phenytoin). Sensitivity is of the order of 0.5-1.0 µg/mL for TLC of urine. Newer methods such as GC and HPLC are more sensitive. Some substances should be quantitated in blood or serum (eg, iron overdose, methanol, acetaminophen, salicylate, carbon monoxide, ethanol, digoxin, lithium, theophylline, and methemoglobin).

Methodology A variety of methods or combination of methods are in fairly common use and include thin-layer chromatography (TLC), colorimetry/spectrophotometry, enzyme immunoassay technique (EIA), enzyme-multiplied immunoassay technique (EMIT), gas chromatography (GC), fluorescence polarization immunoassay (FPIA), gas chromatography/mass spectrometry (GC/MS), high performance liquid chromatography (HPLC).

Additional Information For specific drug blood levels see the listing by specific generic drug name for drug desired. Some toxins (eg, metals, volatiles, gaseous compounds) may require specific methodology (eg, atomic absorption spectrophotometry, gas chromatography). Also see Toxicology Screen, Serum *on page 808.*

References

Catrou PG and Khazanie P, "Limited Toxicology Screening: End of a Controversy," *Am J Clin Pathol*, 1996, 105(5):527-8.

Dawson AH and Whyte IM, "Therapeutic Drug Monitoring in Drug Overdose," *Br J Clin Pharmacol*, 1999, 48(3):278-83.

Elliott SP and Hale KA, "Applications of an HPLC-DAD Drug-Screening System Based on Retention Indices and UV Spectra," *J Anal Toxicol*, 1998, 22(4):279-89.

Giorgi DF and Jagoda A, "Poisoning and Overdose," *Mt Sinai J Med*, 1997, 64(4-5):283-91.

Litovitz TL, Klein-Schwartz W, Caravati EM, et al, "1998 Annual Report of the American Association of Poison Control Centers Toxic Exposure Surveillance System," *Am J Emerg Med*, 1999, 17(5):435-87.

Mahoney JD, Gross PL, Stern TA, et al, "Quantitative Serum Toxic Screening in the Management of Suspected Drug Overdose," *Am J Emerg Med*, 1990, 8(1).16-22.

Merigian KS and Blaho K, "Diagnosis and Management of the Drug Overdose Patient," *Am J Ther*, 1997, 4(2-3):99-113.

Vernon DD and Gleich MC, "Poisoning and Drug Overdose," *Crit Care Clin*, 1997, 13(3):647-67.

♦ **Toxicology, Volatiles** *see* Volatile Screen, Blood or Urine *on page 809*

♦ **Tranquilizers (Valium®, Librium®, Dalmane®, Tranxene®, Klonopin™, Ativan®, Serax®, Centrax®, Restoril®, Xanax®, Halcion®, Versed®, Doral®, etc)** *see* Benzodiazepines, Qualitative, Urine *on page 782*

♦ **Trendar®** *see* Ibuprofen, Serum *on page 793*

♦ **Tricodein** *see* Codeine, Urine *on page 786*

♦ **Tylenol®** *see* Acetaminophen, Serum *on page 778*

♦ **Ty-Pap** *see* Acetaminophen, Serum *on page 778*

♦ **Uni-Ace®** *see* Acetaminophen, Serum *on page 778*

♦ **Unipro®** *see* Ibuprofen, Serum *on page 793*

♦ **Uppers** *see* Amphetamine, Qualitative, Urine *on page 779*

♦ **Vermilion** *see* Mercury, Blood *on page 797*

♦ **Vicks Inhaler®** *see* Methamphetamine, Qualitative, Urine *on page 799*

Volatile Screen, Blood or Urine

Related Information

Anion Gap, Serum, Plasma, or Urine *on page 106*
Ethanol, Blood, Urine, and Other Sources *on page 789*
Ethylene Glycol, Serum or Plasma *on page 790*
Ketone Bodies, Blood *on page 205*
Ketones, Urine *on page 877*
Osmolality, Calculated, Serum or Plasma *on page 234*
Osmolality, Serum *on page 236*

Synonyms Toxicology, Volatiles

Applies to Acetone; Ethanol; Isopropanol; Methanol

Test Includes Determination of volatiles by GLC including acetone, ethanol, isopropanol, and methanol. Some laboratories also include ethylene glycol.

Abstract This screening profile measures ethanol and other possible volatiles.

Specimen Serum or plasma, urine, gastric fluid

Container Red top tube, gray top (sodium fluoride) tube; tightly stoppered container for urine and gastric fluid

Collection All containers should be tightly stoppered and transported on ice. The gray (oxalate/fluoride) tube top is recommended for medicolegal collections and if storage is prolonged. Sodium fluoride (50 mg) can be added as a preservative to urine and gastric samples. Other anticoagulants (eg, heparin EDTA) are acceptable.

Causes for Rejection Specimen leakage

Reference Interval None detected

Possible Panic Range Blood: acetone, methanol, isopropanol >50 mg/dL (SI: acetone: >8.6 mmol/L, methanol: >15.6 mmol/L, isopropanol: >8.32 mmol/L); ethanol: >200 mg/dL (SI: >43.4 mmol/L); urine: acetone, methanol, isopropanol >50 mg/dL (SI: acetone: >8.6 mmol/L, methanol: >15.6 mmol/L, isopropanol: 8.32 mmol/L); ethanol: >160 mg/dL (SI: >34.7 mmol/L). Urine levels do not correlate well with blood levels.

Use Evaluate methanol and isopropanol toxicity, and alcohol drug abuse

Methodology Gas-liquid chromatography (GLC)

Additional Information See Ethanol, Blood, Urine, and Other Sources *on page 789* for more information on ethanol. Both methanol and isopropanol are more intoxicating than ethanol. Like ethanol, methanol exhibits zero order elimination kinetics. Methanol is converted to formaldehyde and formic acid, which causes retinal damage leading to metabolic acidosis and blindness. Treatment may include infusion of ethanol to inhibit methanol metabolism or treatment with alcohol dehydrogenase inhibitors. Isopropanol is converted to acetone.

In most of the laboratories, ethylene glycol is not part of volatile screen. This fact should be made clear to hospital staff and ordering physicians.

References

Burkhart KK and Kulig KW, "The Other Alcohols. Methanol, Ethylene Glycol, and Isopropanol," *Emerg Med Clin North Am*, 1990, 8(4):913-28.

Church AS and Witting MD, "Laboratory Testing in Ethanol, Methanol, Ethylene Glycol, and Isopropanol Toxicities," *J Emerg Med*, 1997, 15(5):687-92.

Hammett-Stabler CA, "Fomepizole, a New Treatment for Methanol and Ethylene Glycol Poisoning," *Ther Drug Monit Toxicol*, 1999, 20:31-2.

Jarvie DR and Simpson D, "Simple Screening Tests for the Emergency Identification of Methanol and Ethylene Glycol in Poisoned Patients," *Clin Chem*, 1990, 36(11):1957-61.

Lacouture PG, Heldreth DD, Shannon M, et al, "The Generation of Acetonemia/Acetonuria Following Ingestion of a Subtoxic Dose of Isopropyl Alcohol," *Am J Emerg Med*, 1989, 7(1):38-40.

Litovitz T, "The Alcohols: Ethanol, Methanol, Isopropanol, Ethylene Glycol," *Pediatr Clin North Am*, 1986, 33(2):311-23.

♦ **White Lady** *see* Cocaine (Cocaine Metabolite), Qualitative, Urine or Hair *on page 785*

♦ **Wickistick** *see* Phencyclidine, Qualitative, Urine *on page 804*

♦ **Wygesic®** *see* Propoxyphene, Serum or Urine *on page 805*

♦ **X** *see* 3,4 Methylenedioxymethamphetamine, Urine *on page 801*

♦ **XTC** *see* 3,4 Methylenedioxymethamphetamine, Urine *on page 801*

♦ **Zip** *see* Methamphetamine, Qualitative, Urine *on page 799*

♦ **ZORprin®** *see* Salicylate, Serum or Plasma *on page 806*

TRACE ELEMENTS

Eugene S. Olsowka, MD, PhD

Knowledge of trace elements in human toxicity, nutrition, and trace element-related disease states has lagged behind similar knowledge in veterinary medicine, but there have recently been substantial advances.

All trace elements are toxic if given in excessive amounts, and some metals such as thallium, lead, mercury, cadmium, and arsenic, classically known as "heavy metals", are covered in the chapter Toxicology/Drugs of Abuse. Other elements having major aspects of clinical interest, included in this chapter, are drawn together by the common thread of either being essential to human health or by the need to monitor them on a regular basis in certain clinical situations (eg, aluminum: patients in chronic renal failure with potential aluminum exposure).

Many essential trace elements have specific binding proteins, and all bind nonspecifically to various serum proteins. Knowledge of such binding characteristics is often essential to properly interpret trace element analyses.

BLOOD COLLECTION METHODS FOR TRACE ELEMENTS

Since at least 1971, reports have appeared detailing trace metal contamination or alteration of blood and serum samples by blood collection needles, syringes, and vacuum tubes. Problems have included the leaching of chromium or manganese from metal needles; the contamination of the sample by the glass or the rubber parts of syringes or by the rubber stopper; or the adsorption with time of selenium or lead onto ordinary glass blood tubes, leading to falsely low levels for these elements.

Because of such problems, the gold-standard methods that evolved are:

- draw the sample through a plastic catheter preplaced in the vein
- use a syringe (acid-leached, all plastic) that allowed centrifugation in the syringe, or transfer of the blood to a plastic centrifuge tube, and
- transfer or store serum or blood sample in a special acid-leached plastic vial

Although these methods provide reliable results, they are cumbersome for clinical practice. Alternative methods have been sought.

For several years, Becton Dickinson has marketed a "trace metal" royal blue top tube which has been found satisfactory for most analyses **but not for chromium, manganese, aluminum, and selenium**. Recently, Sherwood Medical Company has marketed a trace metal evacuated blood collection tube that, for clinical purposes, has been found satisfactory for aluminum, arsenic, cadmium, copper, chromium, iron, lead, magnesium, manganese, mercury, selenium, and zinc. Although slight alterations in lead, aluminum, and manganese were noted over a 24-hour period of time of contact, these tubes appear satisfactory for usual clinical practice in which brief contact time is anticipated. They are recommended for these analyses.

Specifically, if using a vacuum device for drawing blood, use trace metal-free certified blood collection tubes. Powder-free gloves should be worn during blood collection. If several tubes of blood are to be drawn together, draw all trace metal tubes first so as not to contaminate the needle by puncture of the ordinary Vacutainer® stoppers. (Vacutainer® rubber stoppers are heavily contaminated by several trace metals.)

Not reliable are ordinary "red top" clot tubes or the use of needles with metal hubs or syringes with rubber plungers. Directions for obtaining blood samples are briefly summarized for each specific test.

Acknowledgment is given for helpful advice from Phillip H. Stoltenberg, MD, for review of the entries for serum copper and urine copper; and to H. Ray Adams, PhD[1] and Edward D. Harris, PhD,[2] for review of the entire chapter in a prior edition. We are grateful to Dr Glen Willie, the author of earlier editions, for his superlative efforts.

TRACE ELEMENTS INTRODUCTION

Footnotes

1. H. Ray Adams, PhD, Chief of General Chemistry and Toxicology, Department of Pathology, Texas A&M University Health Science Center College of Medicine, Scott & White Clinic, and Memorial Hospital, Temple, Texas.
2. Edward D. Harris, PhD, Professor of Biochemistry and Biophysics, Texas A&M University, Bryan-College Station, Texas.

References

Jackson MJ, "Diagnosis and Detection of Deficiencies of Micronutrients: Minerals," *Br Med Bull*, 1999, 55(3):634-42.
Moyer TP, Mussmann GV, and Nixon DE, "Blood-Collection Device for Trace and Ultra-Trace Metal Specimens Evaluated," *Clin Chem*, 1991, 37:709-14.
Subramanian KS, "Storage and Preservation of Blood and Urine for Trace Element Analysis," *Biol Trace Element Res*, 1995, 49:187-210.

♦ **Al, Bone** *see Aluminum, Bone and Bone Biopsy on page 813*

♦ **Al, Serum** *see Aluminum, Serum on page 814*

Aluminum, Bone and Bone Biopsy

Related Information
Aluminum, Serum *on page 814*
Calcium, Serum *on page 131*
Deferoxamine Infusion Test *on page 819*
Histopathology *on page 59*
Osteocalcin, Serum or Plasma *on page 237*
Parathyroid Hormone, Serum *on page 243*
Vitamin D, Serum *on page 300*

Synonyms Al, Bone

Applies to Bone Biopsy; Bone Histomorphometry; Histomorphometry

Test Includes Aluminum measured on anterior iliac crest bone biopsy specimen

Abstract Aluminum, one of the most common elements in the earth's crust, is a potentially toxic metal, interfering with bone mineralization in individuals with dialysis-dependent renal failure. The human body is protected from aluminum accumulation in normal individuals because the gut is rather impervious to aluminum, and almost all of the aluminum that is absorbed is excreted. Long-term hemodialysis with aluminum contaminants in the dialysate and long-term parenteral nutritional support with trace aluminum contamination in parenteral solutions (especially in those individuals with chronic renal insufficiency) are the two major causes of aluminum-related osteodystrophy and are causes of progressive dementia.

Patient Preparation Tetracycline and Declomycin® fluoresce differently under ultraviolet light and can be separately distinguished under the microscope so as to indicate the amount of bone formed between the two tetracycline labels. Tetracycline and Declomycin® should be taken between meals, and all antacids, calcium supplements, and phosphate binders should be avoided on the days when these labels are taken. Days 1, 2 (2 days): tetracycline 500 mg twice daily, midmorning and midafternoon; days 3-12: no tetracycline; days 13, 14, 15, 16 (4 days): Declomycin® 300 mg twice daily, midmorning and midafternoon; days 17, 18 (2 days): no tetracycline; day 19, 20, or 21: do bone biopsy. The dates and times of labels and of biopsy should be recorded and submitted with the specimen to facilitate interpretation.

Specimen The patient's skeleton is prelabeled with tetracycline (see Patient Preparation). The timing of the labels and the day of the biopsy are critical to standardize the time between tetracycline labels (which fluoresce) and the day of biopsy. The biopsy specimen is a **0.8 cm diameter core of bone** taken under local or general anesthesia full thickness from the anterior iliac crest in a standardized fashion, with a hollow bone biopsy instrument so as to obtain both layers of cancellous bone as well as internal trabecular bone.

Container Acid-washed plastic vial containing 95% ethanol. (**Do not fix the specimen in formalin.) Avoid decalcification of the bone biopsy specimen.**

Special Instructions Bone aluminum is usually measured in concert with bone histomorphometry and is performed by prearrangement with a reference laboratory specializing in bone histomorphometry. These instructions assume bone histomorphometry will also be performed in parallel with bone aluminum determination.

Reference Interval Bone aluminum: <15 µg/g dry weight[1] (see figure). Bone aluminum relates to total body burden of aluminum, whereas **serum aluminum** may be only recently elevated in heavy exposure and may not correlate with aluminum-related bone disease (ARBD). Conversely, individuals with industrial exposure to aluminum might have normal serum aluminum concentrations.[2]

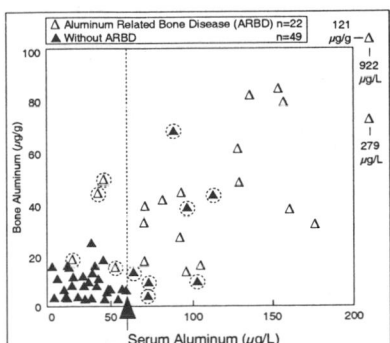
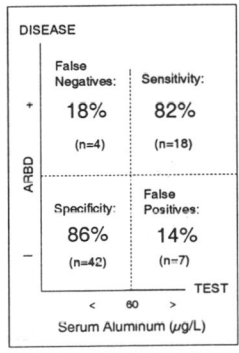

Relationship between serum aluminum, bone aluminum, and aluminum-related bone disease (ARBD). The sensitivity and specificity of a serum aluminum value of 60 µg/L (↑) in the detection of ARBD is illustrated. ▲ without ARBD; △ with ARBD as diagnosed by histochemistry, histology, and bulk analysis; Ⓐ false-positive; Ⓐ false negatives.

Histomorphometry normal values:[3]
- trabecular bone: 3% nonmineralized, 97% mineralized
- osteoid covers 25% bone surface, lined with osteoblasts
- osteoclasts 4% of trabecular surface

Variations from normal histomorphometry are interpreted by the pathologist as compatible with pure osteitis fibrosa, pure osteomalacia, aplastic bone disease, or mixed bone disease. Bone resorption and turnover may be determined. The measured distance between the two tetracycline labels allows calculation of bone formation rate, which is reduced in aluminum-related bone disease. Many feel that an aluminum stain, however, is most specific for aluminum-related bone disease if aluminum is detected on the mineralization front, blocking calcium deposition and resulting in osteomalacia.[4] The rate of bone formation is inversely related to the amount of aluminum present.

Use Diagnose or confirm ARBD in patients with renal failure (with or without dialysis) or in those receiving parenteral nutrition. Aluminum bone disease among parenteral nutrition patients has become much less of a clinical problem, as nutritional products for intravenous use have been improved. Parenteral nutrition solutions prepared with purified amino acids rather than from casein hydrolysate have diminished the incidence of ARBD. Intravenous albumin products may still be a significant source of aluminum.[5] Patients with ARBD may have coexisting other types of bone disease from hyperparathyroidism or osteomalacia related to lack of vitamin D.

Limitations Histomorphometry does not always correlate with total bone aluminum content. Secondary hyperparathyroidism provides relative protection from clinical aluminum bone disease, despite the presence of substantial aluminum stored in bone. Stainable aluminum at the osteoid mineralization front is taken by some authors as the most sensitive indicator of aluminum bone disease, but it is present in many aluminum exposed patients who are without symptoms. Bone aluminum correlates best with aluminum bone disease, but not as well with aluminum-related microcytic anemia, encephalopathy, or other forms of aluminum toxicity.

Contraindications Bone biopsy should be done with caution in the presence of a coagulopathy; history of allergy to tetracyclines precludes tetracycline labeling.

Methodology Atomic absorption (AA), graphite furnace flameless atomic absorption with Zeeman background correction, electrothermal atomic absorption spectroscopy, liquid protein chromatography with inductively-coupled plasma-mass spectroscopy (ICP-MS)

Additional Information Aluminum interferes with normal bone formation by several mechanisms, including direct reduction of osteoblast function and population; reduction of parathyroid hormone release down-regulating bone turnover and in the presence of citrate, direct inhibition of calcium phosphate crystal growth. Bone serves as a store of aluminum, and aluminum from bone can be released back to the blood and other tissues during stress, illness, hyperthyroidism, or failed renal transplant, precipitating aluminum encephalopathy. Aluminum storage occurs in all other tissues of the body, being found in the highest concentrations in bile, blood, urine, lung, and to lesser degrees in other tissues.[6] Renal osteodystrophy includes high turnover bone lesions; its classical histopathologic form is osteitis fibrosa, caused by secondary hyperparathyroidism and deficiency of 12,25-dihydroxycholecalciferol. The severity of clinical manifestations of bone disease correlates with histological features of the bone lesions and the time spent on dialysis.[7] The most common cause of osteomalacia is aluminum intoxication and other heavy metals related to management of renal disease.[8]

Stability of serum aluminum concentrations in one study of dialysis patients has remained constant.[9] This study reports a reduction of bone aluminum content and that ARBD has disappeared despite no change of trends in oral exposure to aluminum. This result suggests that the optimal control of aluminum content in dialysis fluids may be a major factor for controlling aluminum intoxication seen in chronic renal failure patients on dialysis. Mean serum aluminum concentrations correlate highly with mean dialysis fluid aluminum concentrations when dialysis aluminum content is >4 µg/L (SI: 148 nmol/L).[10]

Footnotes

1. D'Haese PC, Clement JP, Elseviers MM, et al, "Value of Serum Aluminum Monitoring in Dialysis Patients: A Multicentre Study," *Nephrol Dial Transplant*, 1990, 5(11):45-53.
2. De Kom JF, Dissels HM, Van Der Voet GB, et al, "Serum Aluminum Levels of Workers in the Bauxite Mines," *J Toxicol Clin Toxicol*, 1997, 35(6):645-51.
3. Visser WJ and Van de Vyver FL, "Aluminum-Induced Osteomalacia in Severe Chronic Renal Failure (SCRF)," *Clin Nephrol*, 1985, 24(1 Suppl):S30-6.
4. McCarthy JT, Kurtz SB, and McCall JT, "Elevated Bone Aluminum Content in Dialysis Patients Without Osteomalacia," *Mayo Clin Proc*, 1985, 60(5):315-20.
5. May JC, Rains TC, Yu LJ, et al, "Aluminum Content of Source Plasma and Sodium Citrate Anticoagulant," *Vox Sang*, 1992, 62(2):65-9.
6. Di Paolo N, Masti A, Comparini IB, et al, "Uremia, Dialysis and Aluminum," *Int J Artif Organs*, 1997, 20(10):547-52.
7. Duarte ME, Peixoto AL, Pacheco AS, et al, "The Spectrum of Bone Disease in 200 Chronic Hemodialysis Patients: A Correlation Between Clinical, Biochemical and Histological Findings," *Rev Paul Med*, 1998, 116(5):1790-7.
8. Hruska KA and Teitelbaum SL, "Renal Osteodystrophy," *N Engl J Med*, 1995, 333(3):166-74.
9. Mazzaferro S, Perruzza I, Costantini S, et al, "Relative Roles of Intestinal Absorption and Dialysis-Fluid-Related Exposure in the Accumulation of Aluminum in Haemodialysis Patients," *Nephrol Dial Transplant*, 1997, 12(12):2679-82.
10. Fernández Martín JL, Canteros A, and Serrano M, "Prevention of Aluminum Exposure Through Dialysis Fluids. Analysis of Changes in the Last 8 Years," *Nephrol Dial Transplant*, 1998, 13(Suppl 3):78-81.

(Continued)

Aluminum, Bone and Bone Biopsy *(Continued)*

References

Guillard O, Pineau A, Fauconneau B, et al, "Biological Levels of Aluminum After Use of Aluminum-Containing Bone Cement in Post-Otoneurosurgery," *J Trace Elem Med Biol*, 1997, 11(1):53-6.

Hdez-Jaras J, Galán A, and Sánchez P, "Accidental Aluminum Intoxication in Patients Undergoing Acetate-Free Biofiltration," *Nephron*, 1998, 78(3):274-7.

Lin JL, Yang YJ, Yang SS, et al, "Aluminum Utensils Contribute to Aluminum Accumulation in Patients With Renal Disease," *Am J Kidney Dis*, 1997, 30(5):653-8.

Mjöberg B, Hellquist E, Mallmin H, et al, "Aluminum, Alzheimer's Disease and Bone Fragility," *Acta Orthop Scand*, 1997, 68(6):511-4.

Ubara Y, "Bone Histomorphometrical Analysis in Patients on Long-Term Dialysis Treatment for More Than Ten Years," *Osaka City Med J*, 1998, 44(2):133-53.

Aluminum, Serum

Related Information

Aluminum, Bone and Bone Biopsy *on page 813*
Calcium, Serum *on page 131*
Deferoxamine Infusion Test *on page 819*
Heavy Metal Screen, Blood *on page 792*
Heavy Metal Screen, Urine *on page 792*
Red Blood Cell Indices *on page 477*

Synonyms Al, Serum

Abstract Aluminum, a lightweight, silvery metal, is never found alone but it commonly occurs as aluminum silicate or as a silicate of aluminum mixed with other metals. Bauxite, an impure hydrated aluminum oxide, is the commercial source of aluminum and its compounds. The potential toxicity of aluminum includes microcytic hypochromic anemia and its role in progressive dementia and osteodystrophy.

Specimen Serum, dialysis fluid, urine, cerebrospinal fluid

Container Special metal-free collection tubes should be used; acid-washed plastic vials for other samples. See the Trace Elements Introduction *on page 811*.

Collection Draw any trace metal tube prior to any other type of blood sample to prevent contamination of needle by regular rubber stoppers. Use powder-free gloves.

Causes for Rejection Contamination by aluminum, aluminum contact, dust, or use of ordinary collection tubes or stoppers. Urine must not be contaminated by stool, as a large amount of unabsorbed aluminum remains in feces.

Special Instructions The patient should take no aluminum-containing antacids or medicines (eg, Amphojel®, Basaljel®, Gelusil®, Maalox®, Mylanta®, Sucralfate, etc) for 24 hours prior to obtaining specimens.

Reference Interval Serum (normal patient): 0-6 ng/mL (SI: 0-0.22 µmol/L) (may vary with laboratory); serum (dialysis patients): up to 40 ng/mL (SI: <1.48 µmol/L) without apparent acute effects; urine: 0-32 ng/day (SI: 0-1.2 µmol/day); dialysate: <0.01 mg/L (AAMI standards)[1]

Critical Values >100 ng/mL (SI: >3.7 µmol/L) possible CNS toxicity, >200 ng/mL (SI: >7.4 µmol/L) probable multisystem toxicity

Use Monitor patients for prior and ongoing exposure to aluminum. Patients at risk include:

- infants on parenteral fluids, particularly parenteral nutrition
- burn patients through administration of intravenous albumin, particularly with coexisting renal failure
- adult and pediatric patients with chronic renal failure, who accumulate aluminum readily from medications and dialysate
- adult parenteral nutrition patients (less so, recently)
- persons with industrial exposure

Monitor dialysate and water to prepare dialysate to prevent aluminum toxicity in dialysis patients. Research use: investigation of amyotrophic lateral sclerosis (in Guam) and Alzheimer disease.

Limitations Serum levels rise and fall after each dose of aluminum-containing phosphate binder or sucralfate. If renal function is normal, renal clearance of aluminum is prompt, with urine levels rising quickly after a course of aluminum-containing antacid is begun and elevated levels persisting for over a week. Urine levels rise after a dose of deferoxamine given for any reason. The degree of rise in serum aluminum after deferoxamine is regarded as reflecting total body aluminum burden (see Deferoxamine Infusion Test *on page 819*) but serum concentrations can fall with deferoxamine as well. Serum aluminum levels <40 ng/mL (SI: <1.48 µmol/L) or even <20 ng/mL (SI: <0.74 µmol/L) do not exclude serious toxicity in dialysis patients and aluminum accumulation in bone leading to osteodystrophy.[2] As aluminum exposure of dialysis patients by medications has fallen in recent years, there is a tendency to move the lower limit of normal down toward 10 ng/mL (SI: 0.38 µmol/L) or 12 ng/mL, even for dialysis patients. Aluminum antacids, aluminum hydroxide, lithium, and sulfacrate can cause an increase.[3]

Methodology Atomic absorption (AA), inductively-coupled plasma atomic emission spectrometry, electrothermal atomic absorption spectroscopy (ETAAS), graphite furnace atomic absorption spectroscopy with Zeeman correction (GFAAS); *vide infra*

Additional Information Aluminum toxicity has been recognized in many settings. Risk factors include heavy or prolonged exposure, poor renal function, chronic citrate intake which enhances aluminum absorption, or a previously accumulated bone burden which may be released in stress or illness. A recent study of bauxite miners exposed to aluminum revealed no significant differences in serum aluminum concentration when compared to unexposed workers[4] suggesting that the kidneys may play a large role in regulation of body burdens of aluminum in normal individuals. Signs and symptoms of possible chronic intoxication include:

- encephalopathy (stuttering, gait disturbance, myoclonic jerks, seizures, coma, abnormal EEG)
- osteomalacia or aplastic bone disease (associated with painful spontaneous fractures, hypercalcemia, tumorous calcinosis)
- proximal myopathy
- increased risk of infection
- increased left ventricular mass and decreased myocardial function
- microcytic anemia
- with very high levels, sudden death

The gastrointestinal tract is relatively impervious to aluminum, absorption normally being only about 2%. Aluminum is absorbed by a mechanism related to that for calcium. Gastric acidity, organic acids, and oral citrate favor absorption, and H_2-blockers reduce absorption. As is true for several trace elements, transferrin is the primary protein binder and carrier for aluminum in the plasma, where 80% is protein bound and 20% is free or complexed to small molecules such as citrate. A recent study utilizing inductively-coupled plasma-mass spectroscopy (ICP-MS) identified transferrin as the only significant aluminum binding protein in unspiked uremic sera.[5] Peripheral cells appear to take up aluminum from transferrin rather than from citrate. Serum aluminum correlates with encephalopathy; red cell aluminum correlates with microcytic anemia;[6] and bone aluminum correlates with aluminum bone disease. Basal PTH, when elevated, appears to protect bone and thereby favor CNS toxicity. Factors favoring one form of toxicity over another are not well understood. There is evidence that aluminum may play a role in Alzheimer disease and that aluminum may contribute to osteodystrophy in some nonuremic individuals.[7] Prolonged intravenous feeding of preterm infants with solutions containing aluminum is associated with impaired neurologic development.[8]

In a study of dialysis related bone disease from Brazil,[9] the spectrum of renal osteodystrophy consisted mainly of high turnover bone lesions (74.5%) including osteitis fibrosa in 57.5% of the patients. Patients with mild bone disease were noted to be dependent on dialysis for shorter periods of time and were mostly asymptomatic. Patients with aluminum-related bone disease (16.5%) had the greatest aluminum exposure, either orally or parenterally, and together with patients with high turnover mixed disease, were the most symptomatic. The severity of the clinical manifestations of bone disease correlated with the histopathologic features of bone lesion and to the time spent on dialysis.

Footnotes

1. Recommended Maximum Promulgated by the Association for Advancement of Medical Instrumentation, 1990, 33330 Washington Blvd, Suite 4000, Arlington, VA.
2. van Landeghem GF, D'Haese PC, Lamberts LV, et al, "Low Serum Aluminum Values in Dialysis Patients With Increased Bone Aluminum Levels," *Clin Nephrol*, 1998, 50(2):69-76.
3. Young DS, *Effects of Drugs on Clinical Laboratory Tests*, 5th ed, Volume 1: Listing by Test, Washington, DC: AACC Press, American Association of Clinical Chemistry, 2000, Section 3, 858.
4. De Kom JF, Dissels HM, Van Der Voet GB, et al, "Serum Aluminum Levels of Workers in the Bauxite Mines," *J Toxicol Clin Toxicol*, 1997, 35(6):645-51.
5. Soldado Cabezuelo AB, Montes Bayón M, Blancon González E, et al, "Speciation of Basal Aluminum in Human Serum by Fast Protein Liquid Chromatography With Inductively-Coupled Plasma Mass Spectrometric Detection," *Analyst*, 1998, 123(5):865-9.
6. Abreo K, Brown ST, Sella M, et al, "Application of An Erythrocyte Aluminum Assay in the Diagnosis of Aluminum-Associated Microcytic Anemia in Patients Undergoing Dialysis and Response to Deferoxamine Therapy," *J Lab Clin Med*, 1989, 113(1):50-7.
7. Mjöberg B, Hellquist E, Mallmin H, et al, "Aluminum, Alzheimer's Disease and Bone Fragility," *Acta Orthop Scand*, 1997, 68(6):511-4.
8. Bishop NJ, Morley R, Day JP, et al, "Aluminum Neurotoxicity in Preterm Infants Receiving Intravenous Feeding Solutions," *N Engl J Med*, 1997, 336(22):1557-61.
9. Duarte ME, Peixoto AL, Pacheco AS, et al, "The Spectrum of Bone Disease in 200 Chronic Hemodialysis Patients: A Correlation Between Clinical, Biochemical, and Histological Findings," *Rev Paul Med*, 1998, 116(5):1790-7.

References

Alfrey AC, LeGendre GR, and Kaehny WD, "The Dialysis Encephalopathy Syndrome. Possible Aluminum Intoxication," *N Engl J Med*, 1976, 294(4):184-8.

Blanusa M, Prester L, Crnogorac M, et al, "Aluminum in Water for Preparation of Dialysate and in Serum of Dialysed Patients," *Arh Hig Rada Toksikol*, 1997, 48(2):197-204.

Chappuis P, Poupon J, and Rousselet F, "A Sequential and Simple Determination of Zinc, Copper, and Aluminum in Blood Samples by Inductively-Coupled Plasma Atomic Emission Spectrometry," *Clin Chim Acta*, 1992, 206(3):155-65.

Di Paolo N, Masti A, Comparini IB, et al, "Uremia, Dialysis and Aluminum," *Int J Artif Organs*, 1997, 20(10):547-52.

Hdez-Jaras J, Galá A, and Sánchez P, "Accidental Aluminum Intoxication in Patients Undergoing Acetate-Free Biofiltration," *Nephron*, 1998, 78(3):274-7.

Mazzaferro S, Perruzza I, Costantini S, et al, "Relative Roles of Intestinal Absorption and Dialysis-Fluid-Related Exposure in the Accumulation of Aluminum in Haemodialysis Patients," *Nephrol Dial Transplant*, 1997, 12(12):2679-82.

Phelps KR, Naylor K, Brien TP, et al, "Encephalopathy After Bladder Irrigation With Alum: Case Report and Literature Review," *Am J Med Sci*, 1999, 318(3):181-5.

Russo LS, Beale G, Sandroni S, et al, "Aluminum Intoxication in Undialysed Adults With Chronic Renal Failure," *J Neurol Neurosurg Psychiatry*, 1992, 55(8):697-700.

- ◆ **Beta-Monooxygenase, Dopamine** *see* Copper, Serum *on page 816*

- ◆ **Bone Biopsy** *see* Aluminum, Bone and Bone Biopsy *on page 813*

- ◆ **Bone Histomorphometry** *see* Aluminum, Bone and Bone Biopsy *on page 813*

Chromium, Serum

Related Information
Glucose Tolerance Test, Plasma *on page 186*
Heavy Metal Screen, Blood *on page 792*
Heavy Metal Screen, Urine *on page 792*
Protein, Quantitative, Urine *on page 883*
Protein, Semiquantitative, Urine *on page 885*
Urinalysis *on page 887*

Synonyms Cr, Serum

Applies to Glucose Tolerance Factor

Abstract Chromium is a lustrous, hard, steel-gray metal, resistant to tarnish and corrosion. It is used as a catalyst to harden steel alloys, to produce stainless steel, and in galvanizing, tanning, dying, and chemical manufacturing. Chromium deficiency may lead to insulin resistance and hyperlipidemia while chromium poisoning may result in vertigo, gastric irritation, conjunctivitis, vomiting, convulsions, shock, coma, and proximal tubule dysfunction. There are two forms of chromium found in biological systems: hexavalent chromium (Cr(VI)) and trivalent chromium (Cr(III)). Hexavalent chromium is more toxic.[1]

Patient Preparation Patient should be fasting for basal level.

Specimen Serum

Container Special metal-free collection tube. See the Trace Elements Introduction *on page 811*.

Sampling Time A morning fasting sample should be obtained. A glucose load, due to the insulin response it induces, drives chromium levels lower. In the nocturnal total parenteral nutrition patient, the sample should be drawn "fasting" in the afternoon, before the glucose-containing TPN solution is started for the evening.

Collection Use powder-free gloves. Follow specific instructions of laboratory to which sample will be submitted. Contact with steel, dust, ordinary glassware, or plastic is to be avoided as these may contain enough chromium to contaminate the specimen. Draw blood through indwelling plastic intracath needle. Some siliconized stainless steel needles have also been found to be acceptable as is the B-D #5175 20-gauge stainless steel needle, or the Terumo or Abbott butterfly needles. Draw trace-metal sample prior to any other blood samples. Remove serum with an all-plastic pipette (no internal metal parts) and store serum in plastic vial. Leeching plastic containers in 10% nitric acid for 48 hours removes trace-metal contamination if special purpose vials are not available. The containers are then rinsed three times with twice distilled water and air dried in a dust-free environment prior to use.

Storage Instructions Some reference laboratories request specimens to be frozen and sent on dry ice.

Causes for Rejection Improper collection or storage with contact by steel, dust, or ordinary Vacutainer® tubes

Reference Interval 0.05-0.15 ng/mL (SI: 1-3 nmol/L).[2] Some laboratories report much higher "normal ranges" because the methods and/or collection techniques in use are inadequate to prevent substantial contamination. If a laboratory reports "<1 ng/mL" or some similar figure without a lower level for normal, the value can be relied upon to discover toxic states, perhaps, but not deficiency states. Serum levels of 10 ng/mL correspond to short-term atmospheric exposure limit of 0.1 mg/m³ of chromium trioxide.[3] Serum levels even higher would be expected in acute systemic toxicity. Almost a twofold diurnal variation is noted in serum chromium levels, with the level highest in the morning and falling after each meal as insulin levels rise. Serum chromium levels are about 60% of normal in diabetic patients, which overlaps the normal range.

Use Evaluate suspected chromium toxicity or exposure; follow patients receiving chromium in parenteral nutrition solutions; evaluate acquired glucose intolerance in refeeding programs; evaluate insulin resistance in the nonseptic patient during parenteral nutrition

Limitations Extreme attention to detail is needed to achieve reliable results; for many laboratories today, a high serum level more often may reflect sample contamination rather than excess chromium exposure. Any reported levels in biological materials prior to about 1979 are suspect, as the available methods did not provide sufficient sensitivity to separate normal values from the "blank." Reported levels were off by by one order of magnitude. All pipettes must have plastic tips and no exposed internal metal parts. It is essential that work to be done in the laboratory must be under a laminar flow class 100 work station, free from exposed stainless steel to avoid airborne contamination. Even with these precautions, different laboratories may report different normal ranges. The reader is encouraged to seek out a paper by Chan et al detailing the technical aspects of chromium assay.[4]

Methodology Stable isotope dilution, isotope ratio mass spectroscopy; graphite furnace atomic absorption spectroscopy. The publication by Chan et al details inductively-coupled plasma-mass spectroscopy (ICP-MS) which is more sensitive than other methods and does not require specimen predigestion.[4]

Additional Information Determination of the amount of chromium in the serum or urine of normal persons is extremely difficult, due to the very low concentrations present which are in the 0.1 ng/mL range, equivalent to one part in 10 billion.

Chromium is felt to be an essential element in humans, with trivalent chromium (chromium III) purported to be an integral part of "glucose tolerance factor," a partially characterized complex that is thought to contain nicotinic acid and a small oligopeptide complexed to chromium III. This organic moiety is considered necessary for insulin action on the cell surface. Deficiency of chromium can cause an acquired insulin resistance or diabetes mellitus with associated hyperlipidemia in otherwise well-nourished patients. The classic cases, however, were reported prior to the availability of accurate assay techniques and reported levels were tenfold or more higher than our current reference range. Chromium deficiency with associated glucose intolerance and fasting hypoglycemia has been most often observed during refeeding of malnourished famine victims. In infants, one or more oral doses of 250 µg of chromium have been curative. Chromium deficiency associated glucose intolerance has been observed in long-term parenteral nutritional support when inadequate chromium was supplemented.[5] Neuropathy, encephalopathy, and abnormalities of amino acid profile (serum low in branched-chain amino acids and high in aromatic amino acids) have been noted in chromium deficiency.[6]

Pure metallic chromium is nontoxic. Trivalent chromium (chromium III) is poorly absorbed and much less toxic than hexavalent chromium (chromium VI). Monitoring for industry-related toxicity has relied on air samples largely for total and hexavalent chromium, the major type of concern. Workers are potentially exposed in tanneries, mines, metal plating, welding, photography, paint, dye, and explosives industries. Skin exposure may lead to dermatitis, and respiratory exposure to bronchitis, asthma, and lung cancer. Hair contains 1000-fold more chromium than serum or urine and hair chromium content correlates with industrial exposure.[7] Intermediate levels of long-term exposure may cause tubular proteinuria in industrial workers.[8]

Chromium supplementation has been shown to improve glucose tolerance and improve insulin efficiency in glucose intolerant (but not in normal or overtly diabetic) patients on diets equivalent to the lower quartile of ordinary chromium intake in the United States.[9] The implication is that many individuals in the U.S. population have a marginal chromium intake, and that the bulk of observed cases of glucose intolerance are due to chromium deficiency. In the United States, addition of 150 µg of Cr(III) in the daily diet improved glucose tolerance in type II diabetics.[1] Others have carefully looked for an effect of "organic chromium" as is found in yeast, but have found no effects on glucose tolerance, insulin levels, or glycosylated hemoglobin in stable elderly patients with glucose intolerance.[10] This of course has not deterred a brisk sale of chromium tablets through the health food stores. We may anticipate even more self-medication and supplementation in the future, and greater medical interest in this trace metal. For adults, 50-200 ng/day is safe and adequate intake.[1] A need for chromium in most individuals is unproven.

Iron competitively inhibits the binding of chromium III to transferrin. Iron overloaded patients with hemochromatosis poorly retain a radioactive tracer dose of chromium III. It has been suggested that chromium deficiency at a cellular level may play a role in the development of diabetes in hemochromatosis.[11]

Footnotes

1. Milne DB, "Trace Elements," *Tietz Textbook of Clinical Chemistry*, 3rd ed, Burtis CA and Ashwood ER, eds, Philadelphia, PA: WB Saunders Co, 1999, 1029-55.
2. Chappuis P, Poupon J, Deschamps JF, et al, "Physiological Chromium Determination in Serum by Zeeman Graphite Furnace Atomic Absorption Spectrometry. A Serious Challenge," *Biol Trace Elem Res*, 1992, 32:85-91.
3. Baruthio F, "Toxic Effects of Chromium and Its Compounds," *Biol Trace Elem Res*, 1992, 32:145-53.
4. Chan S, Gerson B, Reitz RE, et al, "Technical and Clinical Aspects of Spectrometric Analysis of Trace Elements in Clinical Samples," *Clin Lab Med*, 1998, 18(4):615-29.
5. Jeejeebhoy KN, Chu RC, Marliss EB, et al, "Chromium Deficiency, Glucose Intolerance, and Neuropathy Reversed by Chromium Supplementation, in a Patient Receiving Long-Term Total Parenteral Nutrition," *Am J Clin Nutr*, 1977, 30(4):531-8.
6. Freund H, Atamian S, and Fischer JE, "Chromium Deficiency During Total Parenteral Nutrition," *JAMA*, 1979, 241(5):496-8.
7. Randall JA and Gibson RS, "Hair Chromium as an Index of Chromium Exposure of Tannery Workers," *Br J Ind Med*, 1989, 46(3):171-5.
8. Wedeen RP and Qian L, "Chromium-Induced Kidney Disease," *Environ Health Perspect*, 1991, 92:71-4.
9. Anderson RA, Polansky MM, Bryden NA, et al, "Supplemental-Chromium Effects on Glucose, Insulin, Glucagon, and Urinary Chromium Losses in Subjects Consuming Controlled Low-Chromium Diets," *Am J Clin Nutr*, 1991, 54(5):909-16.
10. Uusitupa MI, Mykkanen L, Siitonen O, et al, "Chromium Supplementation in Impaired Glucose Tolerance of Elderly: Effects on Blood Glucose, Plasma Insulin, C-Peptide and Lipid Levels," *Br J Nutr*, 1992, 68(1):209-16.
11. Sargent T, Lim TH, and Jenson RL, "Reduced Chromium Retention in Patients With Hemochromatosis, A Possible Basis of Hemochromatotic Diabetes," *Metabolism*, 1979, 28(1):70-9.

References

Morris BW, MacNeil S, Stanley K, et al, "The Inter-relationship Between Insulin and Chromium in Hyperinsulinaemic Euglycaemic Clamps in Healthy Volunteers," *J Endocrinol*, 1993, 139(2):339-45.

Veillon C, "Chromium," *Methods Enzymol*, 1988, 158:334-43.

Vincent JB, "The Biochemistry of Chromium," *J Nutr*, 2000, 130(4):715-8.

Chromium, Urine

Related Information
Glucose Tolerance Test, Plasma *on page 186*
Heavy Metal Screen, Blood *on page 792*
Heavy Metal Screen, Urine *on page 792*
Urine Collection, 24-Hour *on page 47*

Synonyms Cr, Urine

Abstract Urine chromium levels are extremely low, and until recently, not reliable. Urine chromium assay is used to look for chromium toxicity in cases of potential exposure. Chromium is found in a number of oxidation states but only the trivalent state and the hexavalent state occur in biological systems. Hexavalent chromium (Cr(VI)) is more toxic than trivalent chromium (Cr(III)).[1] As testing becomes more reliable, new applications of the test will arise to determine chromium III nutritional adequacy or deficiency states. See Chromium, Serum *on page 815*, for signs and symptoms of toxicity and deficiency states and for additional references.

Specimen 24-hour urine

Container Plastic metal-free container. To prepare, leech 48 hours in 10% nitric acid and wash with distilled water that has had no contact with metal. Dry in quiet air in a metal-free environment free of dust, dirt, or potential contaminants.

Collection Care must be taken to avoid contact with metal. Use plastic urinal, prepared as above. Stool contamination must be avoided.

Causes for Rejection Improper collection, contact with metal, dust or dirt; use of ordinary urine container without acid washing, stool contamination

Reference Interval <1 μg/24 hours[1]. Reference ranges vary with the laboratory; ranges have declined with improved methods of avoiding contamination and assay. Two- to threefold increases of urine chromium may reflect supplementation or excess losses. Levels elevated to tenfold and higher have been seen in exposed asymptomatic tannery workers. Spot levels of chromium in urine of 30 ng/g creatinine correspond to the short-term atmospheric exposure limit of 0.1 mg/m^3 of chromium trioxide in industrial exposure situations.[2]

Use Evaluate industrial exposure, suspected toxicity; or in conjunction with serum levels, to attempt to detect suspected chromium deficiency, especially in a recent onset of glucose intolerance

Limitations Levels are so low in normal individuals (on the order of one part in 10 billion in urine) that many laboratories are not able to detect the lower limit of normal, and thus report "less than" some set level as being normal. Thus, for many laboratories, the test can only be used to detect toxicity. Contamination of the specimen may result in a tenfold or more increase in urine concentration being reported, making potential urine contamination the major limiting factor in the test.

Methodology Atomic absorption (AA), neutron activation, inductively-coupled plasma-mass spectroscopy (ICP-MS). ICP-MS holds promise as the most sensitive assay technique currently available and does not require predigestion. Interested readers are encouraged to seek out review of the topic.[3]

Additional Information The main excretory pathway for chromium III is renal. Estimated safe and adequate, oral intake recommended by the U.S. National Academy of Sciences range from 50-200 μg/day,[4] but in the U.S. 90% of people have a mean intake of 25-33 μg/day. Such intake recommendations likely derive from the 1980s when average estimated intake was determined to be 50-100 μg/day. With increasingly accurate assays, new recommended ranges may have to be set lower. Absorption of chromium III is on the order of 0.5%, by radioisotope studies. One hospital pharmacy supplies 12 μg of chromium from MTE5® trace mineral parenteral nutrition supplement per day. We are unaware of a large survey.

As improved methods have progressively reduced the lower level of detection, urine chromium levels have been found to be correlated with glucose metabolism. Studies[5] have demonstrated the metabolic relationships between serum insulin, serum glucose, and serum chromium III in fasting and postprandial states and the relationship of the postprandial state to urine chromium concentration. Diabetic patients lose threefold more chromium in the urine than nondiabetics, and despite increased intestinal absorption, diabetic patients on ordinary diets are unable to maintain the normal serum range. Chromium loss is not specifically related to micro- or macroalbuminuria and precedes the onset of diabetic nephropathy. Urine chromium rises threefold 40 minutes after a carbohydrate meal, especially with carbohydrates that stimulate higher insulin levels. Serum chromium concentrations after a meal decline more than expected for pure urinary loss alone. Thus, it appears that glucose stimulates insulin to take chromium to a cellular location, which favors increased renal excretion.

Footnotes
1. Milne DB, "Trace Elements," *Tietz Textbook of Clinical Chemistry*, 3rd ed, Burtis CA and Ashwood ER, eds, Philadelphia, PA: WB Saunders Co, 1999, 1239-55.
2. Baruthio F, "Toxic Effects of Chromium and Its Compounds," *Biol Trace Elem Res*, 1992, 32:145-53.
3. Chan S, Gerson B, Reitz RE, et al, "Technical and Clinical Aspects of Spectrometric Analysis of Trace Elements in Clinical Samples," *Clin Lab Med*, 1998, 18(4):615-29.
4. National Research Council, *Recommended Dietary Allowances*, 10th ed, National Academy of Sciences.
5. Morris BW, Blumsohn A, Mac Neil S, et al, "The Trace Element Chromium - A Role in Glucose Homeostasis," *Am J Clin Nutr*, 1992, 55(5):989-91.

Copper, Serum

Related Information
Ceruloplasmin, Serum *on page 143*
Copper, Urine *on page 818*
Heavy Metal Screen, Blood *on page 792*
Heavy Metal Screen, Urine *on page 792*
Iron and Total Iron Binding Capacity/Transferrin, Serum *on page 203*
Liver Biopsy *on page 65*
Liver Disease: Laboratory Assessment, Overview *on page 216*
Zinc, Serum *on page 824*

Synonyms Cu, Serum

Applies to Beta-Monooxygenase, Dopamine; Metallothionein; Transcuprein; Zinc Administration

Abstract Copper is a red-brown transition metal belonging to the same atomic family as silver and gold. An essential trace element, copper is a cofactor of several key enzyme systems and is required for hemoglobin synthesis. It circulates bound to ceruloplasmin and is excreted into the bile (see Ceruloplasmin, Serum *on page 143*).

Specimen Serum, cerebrospinal fluid, tissue

Container Royal blue top, trace metal-free, tube which contains no anticoagulant. See the Trace Elements Introduction *on page 811*.

Collection Use powder-free gloves. Draw tube prior to any other blood samples. After centrifugation, pour serum into a metal-free vial for transport to reference laboratory. CSF can be transferred directly to a royal blue top tube.

For liver tissue, follow directions of reference laboratory. Handling instructions have been published.[1] Red blood cell copper has a similar value to serum; thus, hemolysis does not interfere with serum copper determination.

Causes for Rejection Contamination by copper, contact with dust, or the use of ordinary collection needles, tubes, or stoppers

Reference Interval Serum: Approximately 0.7-1.5 μg/mL (SI: 11-24 μmol/L). Mean levels are slightly higher in women and children. There is diurnal variation with peak levels in the morning. Cerebrospinal fluid: 6-35 ng/mL (SI: 94-551 nmol/L).[2] Levels in CSF are elevated up to threefold in the neurotoxicity of Wilson disease. Liver tissue: 9-45 ng/g dry weight.

Use Serum copper is used, along with serum ceruloplasmin and urine copper to screen for Wilson disease and to monitor adequate supplementation of parenteral or enteral nutrition, especially when copper deficiency may be suspected because of ongoing gastrointestinal losses (see table).

It is also used in the differential diagnoses of primary biliary cirrhosis and primary sclerosing cholangitis.

It is used to verify suspected copper deficiency in premature infants when they are acutely ill and may not be able to assimilate copper in their prescribed diets. It is used in diagnosis of Indian childhood cirrhosis (ICC) and to follow such children following penicillamine chelation therapy. It is used to verify acute copper intoxication. Serum copper is low in Menkes syndrome and occipital horn syndrome (OHS). Serum and urine copper are used to follow copper status in acrodermatitis enteropathica, in which high-dose oral zinc therapy puts the patient at risk for symptomatic copper deficiency. Serum ceruloplasmin and serum copper tend to parallel each other in normal individuals and therefore do not provide independent information. Copper deficiency is an important etiology of iron resistant anemia in patients receiving total parenteral nutrition.[3]

Limitations Since ceruloplasmin is an acute-phase reactant protein which binds a large portion of serum copper, both serum copper and ceruloplasmin increase with inflammatory conditions and estrogen exposure. Serum copper is therefore elevated in pregnancy, in patients on contraceptive drugs, in rheumatoid arthritis, and in a number of other inflammatory pathologic entities. Serum copper may be increased with carbamazepine, phenobarbital, phenytoin, and valproic acid.[4] It may be low in the presence of low serum proteins as in nephrosis, malabsorption, and malnutrition without necessarily reflecting true liver copper stores and may be reduced under the influence of ACTH or glucocorticoid therapy.[4] Although serum copper levels are usually ordered to work up possible cases of Wilson disease, Menkes syndrome, and Indian childhood cirrhosis, serum copper alone is of only limited value.

Methodology Atomic absorption (AA), inductively-coupled plasma atomic emission spectrometry

Additional Information Our understanding of copper as an essential trace element in human nutrition and a factor in several diseases has advanced substantially over the past few years. An excellent review of the nutritional aspects of copper is available.[5]

Copper is a component of many metalloenzymes including:
- ascorbate oxidase
- cytochrome C oxidase
- superoxide dismutase
- tyrosinase
- dopamine β-hydroxylase
- lysyl oxidase
- factor V
- an unknown enzyme that cross-links keratin in hair

Disorders of Copper Metabolism

	Deficiency, Nutritional	Menkes Syndrome	Acute Copper Toxicity	ICC and Chronic Copper Toxicity	Wilson Disease	Smoking, Inflammatory Conditions, Pregnancy, Estrogens
Serum copper	↓	↓	↑, ↑↑	↑	N or ↓	↑, ↑↑
Serum ceruloplasmin	↓	↓	N (early)	↑	Usually ↓; may be N in individuals <20 y	↑, ↑↑
Urine copper	↓	↑		↑	↑, ↑↑	N
CSF copper					N or ↑	N
Liver copper	↓	↓	N (early)	↑, ↑↑	↑↑	N

N = normal, ↑ = increase, ↑↑ = large increase, ↓ = decrease, ICC = Indian childhood cirrhosis.

- ceruloplasmin, a ferroxidase in serum which also seems to serve as a major transport protein for copper (see Ceruloplasmin, Serum *on page 143*).

Inorganic copper is a very reactive and potent intracellular toxin with complicated metabolism. Copper is absorbed in the stomach and duodenum by a process regulated by metallothionein (MT). MT synthesis, induced by copper, binds copper within intestinal mucosal cells effectively trapping it within mucosal cells. Such cells are sloughed into the intestinal lumen and lost into the stool unabsorbed. Thus, copper absorption is partially self-limiting.

Both copper and zinc induce tissue levels of MT. Zinc is less avidly bound by MT than copper, but zinc is the better inducer of MT. Small increases of zinc in the diet markedly inhibit copper absorption by stimulating synthesis of MT. Zinc also has direct action on copper uptake by blocking transport into intestinal mucosal cells independent of changes in intracellular MT. Vitamins containing large doses of zinc cause copper deficiency. Cadmium and iron may also inhibit copper absorption through similar mechanisms. Molybdenum decreases absorption by forming insoluble copper-molybdenum-sulfur compounds. This interaction has been used in the detoxification of certain patients with Wilson disease by giving oral molybdenum-sulfur compounds.

After absorption, copper appears in the blood, loosely bound to albumin and also as copper-histidine. The liver and other organs take up copper via membrane-bound ligands. In the liver, copper is used to synthesize ceruloplasmin, which appears within serum a few hours later. Copper uptake by peripheral tissues is dependent upon the fraction of copper in the blood that is incorporated into ceruloplasmin rather than that fraction bound to histidine or albumin. About 65% of copper in peripheral blood exists in the form of ceruloplasmin.

Copper is largely eliminated from the body by secretion into bile. Biliary excretion increases when copper stores are plentiful. Copper secreted into the bile as ceruloplasmin resists absorption limiting further uptake. Renal tubular reabsorption of filtered copper is efficient; thus, normally only a small fraction of copper is lost in urine. Overflow losses in the urine are proportional to copper stores, except when abnormal urine losses occur as in burns, intravenous administration of amino acids, Menkes syndrome, and with chelating drugs.

This complicated metabolic pathway explains many features of known human diseases involving copper. Oral zinc administration inhibits copper absorption and may cause copper deficiency states. Oral zinc may be used to treat copper overloading, including Wilson disease,[6] or may inadvertently cause copper deficiency[7] by stimulating excess MT synthesis. Even after oral zinc therapy is discontinued, high total body zinc stores may continue to block oral copper absorption via induction of MT.

The genes for Wilson disease and Menkes disease have been cloned. In Wilson disease there is a defective P-type copper transporting ATPase, which leads to tissue maldistribution of copper.[8] There is secondary failure of ceruloplasmin synthesis (poor incorporation of copper into ceruloplasmin) leading to increases of loosely bound albumin-copper in blood, which allows copper deposition into peripheral tissues and brain tissue. Reduced ceruloplasmin synthesis additionally decreases biliary excretion of copper[9] leading to toxic hepatic copper accumulation. In later stages, the liver can release so much loosely bound copper into the blood that acute encephalopathy, acute red blood cell hemolysis, and acute renal failure may result.

In both Wilson disease and Indian childhood cirrhosis (ICC), there are inherited and environmental factors that lead to toxic accumulation of hepatic copper. ICC had been considered an illness of toxic exposure of the child to milk boiled in brass vessels, when vessels were not tinned sufficiently and frequently enough to prevent exposure to brass. Indeed, the incidence of ICC drops markedly as a community discards brass utensils. There is now however, good evidence that, like Wilson disease, ICC is primarily a genetic disease. In ICC, the basal production and metal-induced synthesis of MT is defective although glucocorticoid-induced MT synthesis is normal. Although copper accumulates in the liver, pathology of the liver in ICC is distinct from that of Wilson disease. ICC has been reported in both Europe and the United States, where excess copper intake could not be proven.[10]

Copper deficiency from any cause markedly reduces ceruloplasmin synthesis rates and blood ceruloplasmin levels, leading to a microcytic or normocytic anemia secondary to blocks in iron metabolism. Copper deficiency anemia fails to respond to iron, but brisk reticulocytosis follows copper administration. Copper deficiency can cause a scurvy-like bone disease (probably due to decreased lysyl oxidase), depigmentation (probably due to decreased tyrosinase), growth failure, and neutropenia.

Menkes disease is a severe X-linked copper deficiency syndrome usually presenting by the age of 3 months. The gene product is also a P-type copper transporting ATPase. When defective, it results in copper accumulation in intestinal mucosa and kidney with failure to deliver adequate copper to liver and peripheral tissues, resulting in functional copper deficiency. There is also increased urine copper loss due to failure of renal tubular reabsorption. Copper deficiency affects bone formation, pigmentation, CNS development, growth, and arterial connective tissues. Oral or intravenous inorganic copper is ineffective in treatment, and the condition is usually fatal. Several reports[11] of intravenous copper-histidine (plus intermittent penicillamine) to prevent copper overload are encouraging, but difficult to interpret. Some cases of Menkes syndrome are more severe than others and each family studied has a different point mutation in the MNK gene. A recently described diagnostic test reflects deficiency of the copper enzyme dopamine β-monooxygenase, but additional strategies still are needed.[12]

Occipital horn syndrome (OHS) (Ehlers-Danlos syndrome type IX) has been confirmed as an inherited disorder of copper metabolism. It may be allelic to Menkes disease. It is usually recognized by its characteristic physical features, but can be confirmed by serum copper, serum ceruloplasmin, and fibroblast lysyl oxidase activity, all of which are low. Intestinal absorption of copper is poor.

There are at least two situations in which ceruloplasmin may not parallel total serum copper. In acute copper toxicity, in which there may not have been time for increased ceruloplasmin synthesis, free or loosely bound copper is elevated, total serum copper may be elevated, and ceruloplasmin may still be normal. In Wilson disease, with chronic low levels of ceruloplasmin, more copper in serum may be loosely bound and (total) serum copper may be normal rather than low. In this situation, it is especially important to measure both total serum copper and ceruloplasmin. High **urine copper** is also a feature of Wilson disease secondary to decreased excretion into bile. Because no combination of noninvasive tests has proven 100% sensitive and specific for Wilson disease, molecular genetics will likely be more frequently used in diagnosis within families.

The demand for sensitive noninvasive tests for Wilson disease, especially for children in families in which the disease is known to occur, has stimulated search for newer indices of copper metabolism. Urine copper after penicillamine load has been proposed.[13]

Elevations in liver tissue copper found in Wilson disease may occur also in other types of liver disease, especially primary biliary cirrhosis.[11] Liver tissue copper levels remain the gold standard for diagnosis of Wilson disease and Indian childhood cirrhosis (ICC), although it is not 100% specific. Increased liver tissue copper levels are diagnostic in cases of Wilson disease or ICC previously diagnosed in a sibling because both diseases are inherited disorders, and other differential considerations such as primary biliary cirrhosis are rare. Wilson disease can be distinguished from chronic copper intoxication in normal individuals by serum ceruloplasmin and the finding that values for free copper in serum and urine of normal individuals tend to normalize in an environment without copper in tap water.[14] Liver copper content is used to confirm Menkes syndrome and may be useful in evaluating liver disease of uncertain etiology. Liver copper rises with time in biliary cirrhosis, but does not confirm the diagnosis. The liver biopsy diagnosis of Wilson disease has been reviewed.[1] See Liver Biopsy *on page 65*.

The combination of increased hepatic copper and low ceruloplasmin occurs only in Wilson disease and normal infants, who are born at term with increased copper stores and develop normal ceruloplasmin levels by 3-6 months of age. Since copper stores rise during the last trimester of pregnancy, premature infants may not have elevated liver copper stores.

Footnotes

1. Ludwig J, Moyer TP, and Rakela J, "The Liver Biopsy Diagnosis of Wilson's Disease: Methods in Pathology," *Am J Clin Pathol*, 1994, 102(4):443-6.
(Continued)

Copper, Serum (Continued)

2. Weisner B, Hartard C, and Dieu C, "CSF Copper Concentration: A New Parameter for Diagnosis and Monitoring Therapy of Wilson's Disease With Cerebral Manifestation," *J Neurol Sci*, 1987, 79(1-2):229-37.

3. Spiegel JE and Willenbucher RF, "Rapid Development of Severe Copper Deficiency in a Patient With Crohn's Disease Receiving Parenteral Nutrition," *JPEN J Parenter Enteral Nutr*, 1999, 23(3):169-72.

4. Young DS, *Effects of Drugs on Clinical Laboratory Tests*, 5th ed, Volume 1: Listing by Test, Washington, DC: AACC Press, American Association of Clinical Chemistry, 2000, Section 3, 222.

5. Barceloux DG, "Copper," *J Toxicol Clin Toxicol*, 1999, 37(2):217-30.

6. Brewer GJ, Dick RD, and Yuzbasiyan-Gurkan V, et al, "Treatment of Wilson's Disease With Zinc. XIII: Therapy With Zinc in Presymptomatic Patients From the Time of Diagnosis," *J Lab Clin Med*, 1994, 123(6):849-58.

7. Hoffman HN, Phyliky RL, and Fleming CR, "Zinc-Induced Copper Deficiency," *Gastroenterology*, 1988, 94(2):508-12.

8. Ferenci P, "Wilson's Disease," *Ital J Gastroenterol Hepatol*, 1999, 31(5):416-25.

9. Lee HH, Hill GM, Sikha VK, et al, "Pancreaticobiliary Secretion of Zinc and Copper in Normal Persons and Patients With Wilson's Disease," *J Lab Clin Med*, 1990, 116(3):283-8.

10. Weiss M, Muller-Höcker J, Wiebecke B, et al, "First Description of 'Indian Childhood Cirrhosis' in A Non-Indian Infant in Europe," *Acta Paediatr Scand*, 1989, 78(1):152-6.

11. Nadal D and Baerlocher K, "Menkes' Disease: Long-Term Treatment With Copper and D-Penicillamine," *Eur J Pediatr*, 1988, 147(6):621-5.

12. Kaler SG, "Diagnosis and Therapy of Menkes' Syndrome, A Genetic Form of Copper Deficiency," *Am J Clin Nutr*, 1998, 67(5 Suppl):1029S-34S.

13. Martins da Costa C, Baldwin D, Portmann B, et al, "Value of Urinary Copper Excretion After Penicillamine Challenge in the Diagnosis of Wilson's Disease," *Hepatology*, 1992, 15(4):609-15.

14. Salvatore F, Sacchetti L, and Castaldo G, "Multivariate Discriminant Analysis of Biochemical Parameters for the Differentiation of Clinically Confounding Liver Diseases," *Clin Chim Acta*, 1997, 257(1):41-58.

References

Cox DW, "Genes of the Copper Pathway," *Am J Hum Genet*, 1995, 56(4):828-34.

Dalekos GN, Ringstad J, Savaidis, et al, "Zinc, Copper, and Immunological Markers in the Circulation of Well-Nourished Patients With Ulcerative Colitis," *Eur J Gastroenterol Hepatol*, 1998, 10(4):331-7.

Eife R, Weiss M, Barros V, et al, "Chronic Poisoning by Copper in Tap Water: I. Copper Intoxications With Predominantly Gastrointestinal Symptoms," *Eur J Med Res*, 1999, 4(6):219-23.

Hsiung CS, Andrade JD, Costa R, et al, "Minimizing Interferences in the Quantitative Multielement Analysis of Trace Elements in Biological Fluids by Inductively-Coupled Plasma Mass Spectrometry," *Clin Chem*, 1997, 43(12):2303-11.

Kaler SG, Gallo LK, Proud VK, et al, "Occipital Horn Syndrome and a Mild Menkes' Phenotype Associated With Splice Site Mutations at the MNK Locus," *Nat Genet*, 1994, 8(2):195-202.

Kiss JE, Berman D, and Van Thiel D, "Effective Removal of Copper by Plasma Exchange in Fulminant Wilson's Disease," *Transfusion*, 1998, 38(4):327-31.

Olivares M, Pizarro F, Speisky H, et al, "Copper in Infant Nutrition: Safety of World Health Organization Provisional Guideline Value for Copper Content of Drinking Water," *J Pediatr Gastroenterol Nutr*, 1998, 26(3):251-7.

Pfeil SA and Lynn DJ, "Wilson's Disease: Copper Unfettered," *J Clin Gastroenterol*, 1999, 29(1):22-31.

Rukgauer M, Klein J, Kruse Jarres JD, "Reference Values for the Trace Elements Copper, Manganese, Selenium, and Zinc in the Serum/Plasma of Children, Adolescents, and Adults," *J Trace Elem Med Biol*, 1997, 11(2):92-8.

Terrés Martos C, Navarro Alarcó[n M, Martín-Lagos F, et al, "Determination of Copper Levels in Serum of Healthy Subjects by Atomic Absorption Spectrometry," *Sci Total Environ*, 1997, 198(1):97-103.

Vulpe CD and Packman S, "Cellular Copper Transport," *Ann Rev Nutr*, 1995, 15:293-322.

Wakai S, Ishikawa Y, Nagaoka M, et al, "Central Nervous System Involvement and Generalized Muscular Atrophy in Occipital Horn Syndrome: Ehlers-Danlos Type IX. A First Japanese Case," *J Neurol Sci*, 1993, 116(1):1-5.

Waslen TA, Houston CS, and Tchang S, "Menkes' Kinky-Hair Disease: Radiologic Findings in a Patient Treated With Copper Histidinate," *Can Assoc Radiol J*, 1995, 46(2):114-7.

Winzerling JJ and Law JH, "Comparative Nutrition of Iron and Copper," *Annu Rev Nutr*, 1997, 17:501-26.

Yuzbasiyan-Gurkan V, Johnson V, and Brewer GJ, "Diagnosis and Characterization of Presymptomatic Patients With Wilson's Disease and the Use of Molecular Genetics to Aid in the Diagnosis," *J Lab Clin Med*, 1991, 118(5):458-65.

Copper, Urine

Related Information

Ceruloplasmin, Serum *on page 143*
Copper, Serum *on page 816*
Heavy Metal Screen, Blood *on page 792*
Heavy Metal Screen, Urine *on page 792*
Liver Biopsy *on page 65*
Liver Disease: Laboratory Assessment, Overview *on page 216*
Urine Collection, 24-Hour *on page 47*

Synonyms Cu, Urine

Abstract Copper is an essential trace element in human nutrition and a component of many metalloenzymes. Although the biliary system is the major pathway of copper excretion, some copper is excreted in urine. Urine copper may be used as an aid to detect copper deficiency, Wilson disease,

Menkes disease, Indian childhood cirrhosis (ICC), and chronic or acute copper toxicity.

Patient Preparation If a bedpan or urinal is necessary for collection, it must be made of plastic. Stool contamination must be avoided.

Specimen 24-hour urine

Container Acid-washed (metal-free) urine collection containers must be used; no preservatives.

Collection Collect in acid-washed plastic container, preferably polyethylene. Acidify to pH 2 with hydrochloric or nitric acid. Avoid contamination by dust or dirt.

Causes for Rejection Specimen allowed to contact metal or feces

Reference Interval 15-60 μg/24 hours (SI: 0.22-0.9 μmol/day). See figure.

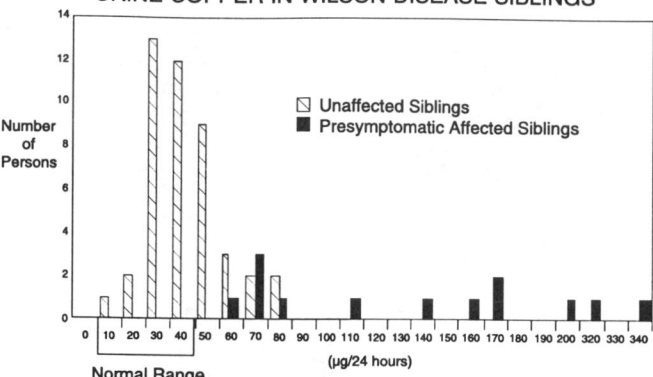

URINE COPPER IN WILSON DISEASE SIBLINGS

From Yuzbasiyan-Gurkan V, Johnson V, and Brewer GS, "Diagnosis and Characterization of Presymptomatic Patients With Wilson's Disease and the Use of Molecular Genetics to Aid in the Diagnosis," *J Lab Clin Med*, 1991, 118(5):458-65, with permission.

Use Increased urinary copper is found in Wilson disease, Menkes syndrome, Indian childhood cirrhosis (ICC), and in chronic and acute copper toxicity states. The test is also used to follow the effectiveness of chelation therapy for Wilson disease, check copper balance in patients with Wilson disease on oral zinc therapy, or check patients receiving parenteral copper as part of parenteral nutrition. It is also used for the differential diagnosis of primary biliary cirrhosis and primary sclerosing cholangitis.

Limitations Increased urinary copper may occur in ICC or with chronic active hepatitis; Wilson disease and chronic hepatitis may also resemble one another. Thus, in addition to urinary copper excretion, other tests such as ceruloplasmin, serum copper, and sometimes liver biopsy are needed. Copper excretion by the kidneys is abnormally increased with high-dose intravenous histidine or mixed amino acids, as in total parenteral nutrition. Captopril and other medications may chelate copper and increase urinary excretion which is usually only a tiny fraction of total daily balance. Urinary copper may be increased with cisplatin, dimercaprol, and with penicillamine or trientine in patients with Wilson disease.[1] For comparison of urine copper in Wilson disease sibships, see figure. Over time, biliary cirrhosis leads to copper accumulation, and since biliary excretion of copper is blocked, urinary excretion rises, potentially leading to diagnostic confusion with Wilson disease. Serum ceruloplasmin and liver biopsy aid in differential diagnosis between Wilson disease and biliary cirrhosis.

Methodology Atomic absorption (AA), inductively-coupled plasma atomic emission spectrometry

Additional Information Chronic copper poisoning has been described as a hypercupric state characterized by increased free copper in the serum and urine of individuals. Elevated total serum copper, though not specific, can suggest this diagnosis. Chronic copper poisoning can be distinguished from Wilson disease by normal levels of ceruloplasmin and the fact that free serum and urinary copper tend to normalize in an environment free of copper in tap water (such as a hospital).[2] Cases of chronic copper poisoning masquerading as gastrointestinal illness (nausea, vomiting, and diarrhea) have been described in Germany.[3] Changes in dietary copper were reported to have no effects on serum copper, ceruloplasmin, osteocalcin (marker of bone formation) nor urinary creatinine in young volunteer men. However, markers for bone resorption (urinary Pyr/Cr and Dpyr/Cr) increased when dietary copper was decreased for several weeks and vice versa.[4] Further information is provided in Copper, Serum *on page 816* and Ceruloplasmin, Serum *on page 143*.

Footnotes

1. Young DS, *Effects of Drugs on Clinical Laboratory Tests*, 5th ed, Volume 1: Listing by Test, Washington, DC: AACC Press, American Association of Clinical Chemistry, 2000, Section 3, 222.

2. Eife R, Weiss M, Müller Höcker M, et al, "Chronic Poisoning by Copper in Tap Water: II. Copper Intoxications With Predominantly Systemic Symptoms," *Eur J Med Res*, 1999, 4(6)224-8.

3. Eife R, Weiss M, Barros V, et al, "Chronic Poisoning by Copper in Tap Water: I. Copper Intoxications With Predominantly Gastrointestinal Symptoms," *Eur J Med Res*, 1999, 4(6):219-23.

4. Baker A, Harvey L, Majask Newman G, et al, "Effect of Dietary Copper Intakes on Biochemical Markers of Bone Metabolism in Healthy Adult Males," *Eur J Clin Nutr*, 1999, 53(5):408-12.

References

Gozzo ML, Colacicco L, Callà C, et al, "Determination of Copper, Zinc, and Selenium in Human Plasma and Urine Samples by Potentiometric Stripping Analysis and Constant Current Stripping Analysis," *Clin Chim Acta*, 1999, 285(1-2):53-68.

Hsiung CS, Andrade JD, Costa R, et al, "Minimizing Interferences in the Quantitative Multielement Analysis of Trace Elements in Biological Fluids by Inductively-Coupled Plasma Mass Spectrometry," *Clin Chem*, 1997, 43(12):2303-11.

Petrukhin K and Gilliam TC, "Genetic Disorders of Copper Metabolism," *Curr Opin Pediatr*, 1994, 6(6):698-701.

Pfeil SA and Lynn DJ, "Wilson's Disease: Copper Unfettered," *J Clin Gastroenterol*, 1999, 29(1):22-31.

Yuzbasiyan-Gurkan V, Johnson V, and Brewer GJ, "Diagnosis and Characterization of Presymptomatic Patients With Wilson's Disease and the Use of Molecular Genetics to Aid in the Diagnosis," *J Lab Clin Med*, 1991, 118(5):458-65.

Zucker SD and Flieder A, "A 23-Year-Old Man With Fulminant Hepatorenal Failure of Uncertain Cause," Case Records of the Massachusetts General Hospital, Case 1-1997, Scully RE, Mark EJ, McNeely WF, et al, eds, *N Engl J Med*, 1997, 336(2):118-25.

♦ **Cr, Serum** *see* Chromium, Serum *on page 815*

♦ **Cr, Urine** *see* Chromium, Urine *on page 816*

♦ **Cu, Serum** *see* Copper, Serum *on page 816*

♦ **Cu, Urine** *see* Copper, Urine *on page 818*

Deferoxamine Infusion Test

Related Information
Aluminum, Bone and Bone Biopsy *on page 813*
Aluminum, Serum *on page 814*
Iron and Total Iron Binding Capacity/Transferrin, Serum *on page 203*

Test Includes Determination of serum aluminum prior to and 48 hours postinfusion of deferoxamine

Abstract This test is advocated in suspected aluminum toxicity, especially among dialysis patients with known aluminum exposure, who lack diagnostically elevated serum aluminum concentrations. It is best used to exclude aluminum bone disease, which a negative test will do. A positive test requires confirmation by bone histomorphometry (see Aluminum, Bone and Bone Biopsy *on page 813*). The test is felt to better reveal the total body burden of aluminum than does serum aluminum, which is more sensitive to recent exposure. Urine aluminum cannot be effectively used in patients with renal failure.

Specimen Serum

Container Special metal-free Sherwood Monoject™ trace element blood collection tube #8881-307006. See the Trace Elements Introduction *on page 811*.

Collection Use B-D #5175 20-gauge stainless steel needle, or Terumo or Abbot butterfly needle. Draw any trace metal tubes prior to collecting other blood samples. Serum is separated and stored or submitted to reference laboratory for analysis of aluminum (see Aluminum, Serum *on page 814*).

Causes for Rejection Failure to collect the specimen using the special collection kit or failure to store specimen in special acid-washed plastic vials; known contamination of specimen with dust or dirt

Special Instructions Most patients for whom this test is indicated are on dialysis, and the test is done in conjunction with their dialysis procedure (hemodialysis or peritoneal dialysis). The patient is instructed to stop any aluminum-containing antacids 3 days prior to the test. The first blood sample is obtained, then 0.5 g deferoxamine is administered in 100 mL 0.9% sodium chloride intravenously during the last 2 hours of dialysis through the venous blood line. Forty-eight hours later, prior to the next hemodialysis, a second blood sample is drawn. The timing is the same for peritoneal dialysis patients, for whom peritoneal dialysis is halted during the 48-hour period.

Reference Interval The test is considered positive if the second sample more than triples the first, or exceeds it by 150 ng/mL (SI: 5.6 μmol/L)[1,2]

Critical Values Serum levels >200 ng/mL (SI: >7.4 μmol/L) can be associated with development of aluminum neurotoxicity.

Use Screen patients with known aluminum exposure and abnormal (but not diagnostically elevated) serum aluminum levels for high body burden of aluminum, which is known to be correlated with aluminum bone disease. Patients with serum aluminum levels ≤75 ng/mL (SI: <2.8 μmol/L) are less likely to benefit from the test[3], and patients with persistent serum aluminum levels >150 ng/mL (SI: >5.6 μmol/L) should probably go directly to bone biopsy for confirmation of bone aluminum burden.

Limitations Use of this test is controversial. Originally proposed as a 2 g deferoxamine infusion test,[4] complications have been reported, including permanent visual disturbances after a single 2 g dose.[5,6] Due to multiple reported complications (ocular, auditory, anaphylaxis, hematopoietic, infectious) of high dose deferoxamine therapy for iron overload in thalassemia and for aluminum overload and toxicity in chronic renal failure, therapeutic doses have generally been reduced. The 0.5 g dose infusion test[2] has so far not been reported to cause complications. Some authors endorse the use of an infusion test,[7] others do not. By restricting its use to patients who probably have a moderate but not extreme body burden of aluminum, the test will help select patients needing further study by bone biopsy, a more invasive procedure.[8] The test appears to be more sensitive and specific with greater positive predictive value when serum parathormone levels are

decreased.[7] Sensitivity is suboptimal; false-negative results are seen in many patients. Serum aluminum values in children appear to be a better estimation of total aluminum body burden than does the deferoxamine challenge test.[9]

Iron status influences response to the deferoxamine test. Patients with high iron levels will have less increase in serum aluminum after challenge with deferoxamine, causing false negative results.[10]

Contraindications When there is a heavy bone burden of aluminum, often reflected by high basal levels, the serum aluminum may acutely rise to toxic levels after deferoxamine dose is given as "challenge" test or as treatment, and encephalopathy may worsen. In cases of actual or anticipated intolerance to deferoxamine, hemoperfusion over specially treated charcoal (an aluminum removal device) would be an alternative treatment modality.

Methodology Atomic absorption (AA), or inductively-coupled plasma atomic emission spectrometry

Additional Information Deferoxamine is the chelator of choice for acute and chronic iron overload from multiple transfusions as may occur in severe chronic anemias (eg, thalassemias). It chelates iron by forming a stable complex that prevents the iron from entering into further chemical reactions.[11] Deferoxamine has also been used successfully to promote aluminum excretion or removal and to provide symptomatic and objective improvement in the treatment of aluminum-associated neurotoxicity and/or bone abnormalities (osteomalacia and osteodystrophy) in patients with chronic renal failure undergoing hemodialysis.[12] The ability of deferoxamine to bind aluminum forms the basis of the Deferoxamine Infusion Test.

The finding of inverse correlations between basal (and deferoxamine stimulated) serum aluminum and serum iron and serum transferrin concentrations suggests that iron deficiency may increase aluminum accumulation in renal dialysis patients.[13] Aplastic bone lesions are the most common form of renal osteodystrophy. Aluminum accumulation has been implicated in only 33% of renal osteodystrophies leading to a suggestion that suppressed parathyroid function may play a role in renal osteodystrophy.[14] Deferoxamine may be used in long-term treatment of both iron and aluminum overload in chronic renal dialysis patients. The amount and time of administration of deferoxamine and time to dialysis can be used to selectively favor chelation of iron or aluminum.[15,16]

Footnotes
1. Yaqoob M, Ahmad R, Roberts N, et al, "Low-Dose Desferrioxamine Test for the Diagnosis of Aluminum-Related Bone Disease in Patients on Regular Haemodialysis," *Nephrol Dial Transplant*, 1991, 6(1):484-6.
2. De Broe ME, D'Haese PC, Elseviers MM, et al, "Aluminum and End-Stage Renal Failure," *Nephrology*, 1988, 2:1086-116.
3. de Vernejoul MC, Marchais S, London G, et al, "Deferoxamine Test and Bone Disease in Dialysis Patients With Mild Aluminum Accumulation," *Am J Kidney Dis*, 1989, 14(2):124-30.
4. Milliner DS, Nebeker HG, Ott SM, et al, "Use of the Deferoxamine Infusion Test in the Diagnosis of Aluminum-Related Osteodystrophy," *Ann Intern Med*, 1984, 101(6):775-9.
5. Bene C, Manzler A, Bene D, et al, "Irreversible Ocular Toxicity From Single "Challenge" Dose of Deferoxamine," *Clin Nephrol*, 1989, 31(1):45-8.
6. Ravelli M, Scaroni P, Mombelloni S, et al, "Acute Visual Disorders in Patients on Regular Dialysis Given Desferrioxamine as a Test," *Nephrol Dial Transplant*, 1990, 5(11):945-9.
7. McCarthy JT, Milliner DS, and Johnson WJ, "Clinical Experience With Desferrioxamine in Dialysis Patients With Aluminum Toxicity," *Q J Med*, 1990, 74(275):257-76.
8. DeVita MV, Rasenas LL, Bansal M, et al, "Assessment of Renal Osteodystrophy in Hemodialysis Patients," *Medicine*, 1992, 71(5):284-90.
9. Roodhooft AM, van de Vyver FL, D'Haese PC, et al, "Aluminum Accumulation in Children on Chronic Dialysis: Predictive Value of Serum Aluminum Levels and Desferrioxamine Infusion Test," *Clin Nephrol*, 1987, 28(3):125-9.
10. Cannata JB, Fernandez-Martin JL, Diaz-Lopez B, et al, "Influence of Iron Status in the Response to the Deferoxamine Test," *J Am Soc Nephrol*, 1996, 7(1):135-9.
11. "Desferal® Vials," *MicroMedix Healthcare Series*, Volume 106, 2000.
12. "Desferroxamine Mesylate," *AHFS Drug Information 2000*, McEvoy GK, ed, 2000, 2722-5.
13. Huang JY, Huang CC, Lim PS, et al, "Effect of Body Iron Stores on Serum Aluminum Level in Hemodialysis Patients," *Nephron*, 1992, 61(2):158-62.
14. Hercz G, Pei Y, Greenwood C, et al, "Aplastic Osteodystrophy Without Aluminum: The Role of "Suppressed" Parathyroid Function," *Kidney Int*, 1993, 44(4):860-6.
15. Canavese C, Salomone M, Pacitti A, et al, "Concomitant Iron and Aluminum Mass Transfer Following Deferoxamine Infusion During Hemofiltration," *Am J Kidney Dis*, 1991, 17(2):179-84.
16. Andriani M, Nordio M, and Saporiti E, "Estimation of Statistical Moments for Desferrioxamine and its Iron and Aluminum Chelates: Contribution to Optimisation of Therapy in Uremic Patients," *Nephron*, 1996, 72(2):218-24.

References
Cohen A, Martin M, Mizanin J, et al, "Vision and Hearing During Deferoxamine Therapy," *J Pediatr*, 1990, 117(2 Pt 1):326-30.

"Deferoxamine Mesylate," 64:00 Heavy Metal Antagonists, *AHFS Drug Information®*, 2000, 2722-5.

"Deferoxamine Mesylate," *Physician's Desk Reference*, 54th ed, Montvale, NJ: Medical Economics Inc, 2000, 2012-3.

Fournier A, Yverneau PH, Hue P, et al, "Adynamic Bone Disease in Patients With Uremia," *Curr Opin Nephrol Hypertens*, 1994, 3(4):396-410.

Kraemer HJ and Breithaupt H, "Quantification of Desferrioxamine, Ferrioxamine and Aluminoxamine by Post-Column Derivatization High-Performance Liquid Chromatography. Nonlinear Calibration Resulting From Second-Order Reaction," *J Chromatogr B Biomed Sci Appl*, 1998, 710(1-2):191-204.

(Continued)

Deferoxamine Infusion Test (Continued)

Menendez Fraga P, Fernandez Martin JL, Blanco Gonzalez E, et al, "Low Percentage of Aluminoxamine and Ferrioxamine in Uremic Serum After Desferrioxamine Administration," *Clin Chem*, 1998, 44(6):1262-8.

Styles LA and Vichinsky EP, "Ototoxicity in Hemoglobinopathy Patients Chelated With Desferrioxamine," *J Pediatr Hematol Oncol*, 1996, 18(1):42-5.

Wills MR and Savory J, "Aluminum and Chronic Renal Failure: Sources, Absorption, Transport, and Toxicity," *Crit Rev Clin Lab Sci*, 1989, 27(1):59-107.

♦ **Glucose Tolerance Factor** *see* Chromium, Serum *on page 815*

♦ **Histomorphometry** *see* Aluminum, Bone and Bone Biopsy *on page 813*

♦ **Hypoxanthine, Urine** *see* Molybdenum, Blood *on page 821*

Manganese, Serum or Blood

Related Information
Heavy Metal Screen, Blood *on page 792*
Heavy Metal Screen, Urine *on page 792*
Manganese, Urine *on page 820*

Synonyms Mn, Serum

Abstract Manganese, essential to life in many species, is part of many human enzyme systems. Most manganese is concentrated in mitochondria. It is considered essential for human nutrition, even though no well-documented example of a manganese deficiency state has been found in humans.[1] Deficiency states can be produced in experimental animals. Manganese is routinely included in enteral formulae and as a "multiple trace metals" additive for parenteral formulas. As true for all of the trace elements, manganese is present in very small quantities in biological samples. Serum concentrations may be increased by more than tenfold if contamination occurs during collection and storage.

Specimen Serum, whole blood

Container Special metal-free blood collection tube. See the Trace Elements Introduction *on page 811*.

Collection Use powder-free gloves. Draw this and any other trace metal blood sample first before using needle to perforate rubber stopper of ordinary blood tube. For isolation of serum, allow time for clotting and centrifuge. Carefully pour serum into special plastic metal-free vial or transfer with acid-washed all-plastic pipet, being careful not to disturb the clot, or buffy coat. Store sample frozen if it is to be transported to reference laboratory.

Causes for Rejection Failure to collect specimen with special collection kit or store serum in special metal-free plastic vials

Reference Interval Serum: 0.43-0.76 ng/mL (SI: 7.8-13.8 nmol/L)[2]; whole blood: 10-11 ng/mL (SI: 190-200 nmol/L).[3] Levels are about threefold higher in very low birth weight babies at birth and fall slightly over the first 3 months of life. Other reference ranges have been recommended for ages 1 month to 18 years and 22-75 years.[4]

Critical Values Exposed manganese workers who developed signs of manganese toxicity had whole blood manganese levels of 20-400 ng/mL when measured during ongoing exposure.[5] A protective limit of 100 μg/m³ average annual exposure has been recommended in long-term ferroalloy workers.[6] In this cohort of exposed workers, the mean blood manganese concentration was 9.18 μg/L compared to 5.74 μg/L in nonexposed individuals.

Use Follow manganese therapy in parenteral nutrition, especially in liver disease, or when there are excessive gastrointestinal losses; evaluate suspected manganese industrial toxicity or exposure. Toxicity occurs in miners following prolonged exposure to manganese dioxide aerosols. Toxic inhalation may cause so-called "manganic madness", involving Parkinson-like characteristics with extrapyramidal movement disorders;[1] *vide infra*.

Limitations Like several other trace metals that are concentrated in the cellular elements of blood, whole blood manganese or red blood cell manganese may better reflect total body manganese stores than do serum levels in healthy individuals. Monocyte manganese has been reported to be a better marker of manganese nutritional status.[3] In evaluating toxicity, serum concentrations may return to normal while elevated cerebral manganese concentrations and neurologic damage persist.[7] Serum manganese concentrations may be increased in children with cholestatic liver disease who are on parenteral nutritional support[8] and in chronic liver failure[9] but reduced in heroin addicts in proportion to the duration of heroin intake.[10] Manganese levels are 60% lower than normal in hemodialysis patients. Plasma uptake of manganese is reduced by concomitant ingestion of calcium but increased by concomitant ingestion of zinc.[11]

Methodology Neutron activation is the most sensitive procedure but does not lend itself to clinical testing. Atomic absorption (AA) spectrophotometry with Zeeman background correction is currently the preferred method.

Additional Information In the serum, essentially all manganese is transported bound to transferrin. Transferrin receptors on the cell internalize the manganese as efficiently as iron transferrin complexes. Once in the cell, manganese is 80% bound to ferritin.[12]

Manganese is implicated as a cofactor in many important cellular enzyme systems, especially mitochondrial superoxide dismutase. *In vitro*, magnesium or even cobalt, iron, calcium, or zinc may substitute for manganese in some of these enzyme systems. From animal studies, manganese deficiency is involved in osteoporosis and skeletal deformities. In humans, low blood concentrations are associated with epilepsy[13] (regardless of type of

anticonvulsant) and reported with the skeletal deformities of Perthes disease.[14] Some have argued that the late hip dislocations in infants may be related to the low manganese content in cow's milk.

Manganese toxicity causes nausea, vomiting, headache, and psychiatric disturbances with central nervous system damage manifested by disorientation, memory loss, anxiety, compulsive laughing or crying, dementia, and psychosis. In the more chronic form, manganese toxicity resembles Parkinson disease with akinesia, rigidity, tremors, and mask-like faces. Normalization of serum levels may or may not reverse neurological damage. T1 weighted magnetic resonance imaging have revealed enhanced signals in the globus pallidus in a pediatric patient who had markedly increased serum manganese.[15] Autopsy of a patient with similar increased T1 weighted signals in the basal ganglia confirmed an increase in manganese concentrations in these areas.[7]

Several medications are thought to chelate manganese, including valproate, and hydralazine. Dialysis lowers manganese levels and patients on hemodialysis usually have lower basal serum levels. Ninety-nine percent of manganese excretion occurs with bile in the feces. When intake is limited, excretion into the urine and feces may fall more than tenfold. Manganese levels rise two to four times normal (without signs of toxicity) in jaundiced children given standard amounts of manganese in parenteral nutrition.

Footnotes

1. Mason JB, "Consequences of Altered Micronutrient Status," *Cecil Textbook of Medicine*, 21st ed, Goldman L and Bonnett JC, eds, Philadelphia, PA: WB Saunders Co, 2000, 1170-8.
2. Neve J and Leclercq N, "Factors Affecting Determinations of Manganese in Serum by Atomic Absorption Spectrometry," *Clin Chem*, 1991, 37(5):723-8.
3. Matsuda A, Kimura M, Takeda T, et al, "Changes in Manganese Content of Mononuclear Blood Cells in Patients Receiving Total Parenteral Nutrition," *Clin Chem*, 1994, 40(5):829-32.
4. Rukgauer M, Klein J, and Kruse-Jarres JD, "Reference Values for the Trace Elements Copper, Manganese, Selenium, and Zinc in the Serum/Plasma of Children, Adolescents, and Adults," *J Trace Elem Med Biol*, 1997, 11(2):92-8.
5. Wang JD, Huang CC, Hwang YH, et al, "Manganese Induced Parkinsonism: An Outbreak Due to an Unrepaired Ventilation Control System in a Ferromanganese Smelter," *Br J Ind Med*, 1989, 46(12):856-9.
6. Lucchini R, Apostoli P, Perrone C, et al, "Long-Term Exposure to 'Low Levels' of Manganese Oxides and Neurofunctional Changes in Ferroalloy Workers," *Neurotoxicity*, 1999, 20(2-3):287-97.
7. Alves G, Thiebot J, Tracqui A, et al, "Neurologic Disorders Due to Brain Manganese Deposition in a Jaundiced Patient Receiving Long-Term Parenteral Nutrition," *JPEN J Parenter Enteral Nutr*, 1997, 21(1):41-5.
8. Reynolds AP, Kiely E, and Meadows N, "Manganese in Long-Term Paediatric Nutrition," *Arch Dis Child*, 1994, 71(6):527-8.
9. Hauser RA, Zesiewicz TA, Martinez C, et al, "Blood Manganese Correlates With Brain Magnetic Resonance Imaging Changes in Patients With Liver Disease," *Can J Neurol Sci*, 1996, 23(2):95-8.
10. Elnimr T, Hashem A, and Assar R, "Heroin Dependence Effects on Some Major and Trace Elements," *Biol Trace Elem Res*, 1996, 54(2):153-62.
11. Freeland-Graves JH and Lin PH, "Plasma Uptake of Manganese as Affected by Oral Loads of Manganese, Calcium, Milk, Phosphorous, Copper, and Zinc," *J Amer Coll Nutr*, 1991, 10(1):38-43.
12. Suarez N and Eriksson H, "Receptor-Mediated Endocytosis of a Manganese Complex of Transferrin Into Neuroblastoma (SHSY5Y) Cells in Culture," *J Neurochem*, 1993, 61(1):127-31.
13. Carl GF, Keen CL, Gallagher BB, et al, "Association of Low Blood Manganese Concentrations With Epilepsy," *Neurology*, 1986, 36(12):1584-7.
14. Hall AJ, Margetts BM, Barker DJ, et al, "Low Blood Manganese Levels in Liverpool Children With Perthes' Disease," *Paediatr Perinat Epidemiol*, 1989, 3(2):131-6.
15. Ono J, Harada K, Kodaka R, et al, "Manganese Deposition in the Brain During Long-Term Total Parenteral Nutrition," *JPEN J Parenter Enteral Nutr*, 1995, 19(4):310-2.

References

Ferraz HB, Bertolucci PHF, Pereira JS, et al, "Chronic Exposure to the Fungicide Maneb May Produce Symptoms and Signs of CNS Manganese Intoxication," *Neurology*, 1988, 38(4):550-3.

Kondakis XG, Makris N, Leotsinidis M, et al, "Possible Health Effects of High Manganese Concentration in Drinking Water," *Arch Environ Health*, 1989, 44(3):175-8.

Milne DB, "Trace Elements," *Tietz Textbook of Clinical Chemistry*, 3rd ed, Burtis CA and Ashwood ER, eds, Philadelphia, PA: WB Saunders Co, 1999, 1044-5.

Manganese, Urine

Related Information
Heavy Metal Screen, Blood *on page 792*
Heavy Metal Screen, Urine *on page 792*
Manganese, Serum or Blood *on page 820*
Urine Collection, 24-Hour *on page 47*

Synonyms Mn, Urine

Abstract Urine manganese is used in conjunction with serum manganese to evaluate possible toxicity or deficiency of manganese.[1] An essential mineral which, in high concentration, can cause neurological damage similar to that of Parkinson disease. See Manganese, Serum or Blood *on page 820* for signs and symptoms of deficiency and toxicity, and for additional references.

Specimen 24-hour or random ("spot") urine. Consider simultaneous determination of urine creatinine, especially on "spot" samples.

Container Acid-washed plastic urine container, avoid contamination by stool, dust, and metal.

Causes for Rejection Contamination by metal, stool, or dust

Reference Interval <2.0 µg/L (SI: <36 nmol/L) (97.5% confidence).[2] Varies with laboratory. Level may fall to 0.2 µg/L (tenfold) in experimental deficiency.[1] Some of the best data on industrial exposure have been normalized to the creatinine content of urine or to µg/hour excretion due to the impracticality of 24-hour urine samples in the industrial setting.[3] Ten free-living, nonexposed young men in Wisconsin had urinary excretion varying from approximately 0.17-0.66 µg/g creatinine.[2] Levels higher than this but <9.0 µg/g creatinine may reflect increased exposure, not necessarily at a toxic level.[4] Another group of factory workers exposed to manganese, some of whom were symptomatic with parkinsonian signs, had urine levels of manganese varying from 11.2-216.0 µg/L.[5] Bile and feces are the main routes of excretion, accounting for 99% of excretion when intake is low, and excretion rather than absorption appears to be regulated. Urine losses appear to be overflow losses, representing a higher fraction of total loss when intake is high.

Use Confirm manganese exposure, toxicity, or poisoning by documentation of excessive urine excretion. Also used to individualize manganese dosing in long-term parenteral nutrition, especially in liver disease, when biliary excretion is low, or with excessive gastrointestinal losses, such as in short bowel syndrome. Used to follow the success of chelation therapy with para-aminosalicylate sodium in manganism.

Limitations Levels in urine are so low that considerable error may be introduced by contamination. Manganese toxicity may leave residual neurologic damage after serum and urine levels have returned to normal. Manganese has a cumulative mechanism of toxicity.[6]

Methodology Atomic absorption (AA) with Zeeman background correction

Additional Information As much as twofold diurnal variation is present in urine manganese, especially in workers occupationally exposed to manganese. Low urinary manganese excretion may play a role in liver manganese overload in alcoholics.[7] Hair manganese content has been utilized as a biological index for exposure in manganese refinery employees.[8] Elevated serum prolactin concentrations have been reported in occupationally exposed individuals.[9]

Footnotes

1. "Manganese Deficiency in Humans: Fact or Fiction?" *Nutr Rev*, 1988, 46(10):348-52.
2. Greger JL, Davis CD, Suttie JW, et al, "Intake, Serum Concentrations, and Urinary Excretion of Manganese by Adult Males," *Am J Clin Nutr*, 1990, 51(3):457-61.
3. Roels HA, Ghyselen P, Buchet JP, et al, "Assessment of the Permissible Exposure Level to Manganese in Workers Exposed to Manganese Dioxide Dust," *Br J Ind Med*, 1992, 49(1):25-34.
4. Siqueira ME, Hirata MH, and Adballa DS, "Studies on Some Biochemical Parameters in Human Manganese Exposure," *Med Lav*, 1991, 82(6):504-9.
5. Hua MS and Huang CC, "Chronic Occupational Exposure to Manganese and Neurobehavioral Function," *J Clin Exp Neuropsychol*, 1991, 13(4):495-507.
6. Lucchini R, Apostoli P, Perrone C, et al, "Long-Term Exposure to "Low Levels" of Manganese Oxides and Neurofunctional Changes in Ferroalloy Workers," *Neurotoxicity*, 1999, 20(2,3):287-97.
7. Rodriguez-Moreno F, Gonzalez-Reimers E, and Santolaria-Fernandez F, "Zinc, Copper, Manganese and Iron in Alcoholic Liver Disease," *Alcohol* 1997, 14(1):39-44.
8. Foo SC, Khoo NY, Heng A, et al, "Metals in Hair as Biological Indices for Exposure," *Int Arch Occup Environ Health*, 1993, 65(1 Suppl):S83-6.
9. Mutti A, Bergamaschi E, Alinovi R, et al, "Serum Prolactin in Subjects Occupationally Exposed to Manganese," *Ann Clin Lab Sci*, 1996, 26(1):10-17.

References

Milne DB, "Trace Elements," *Tietz Textbook of Clinical Chemistry*, 3rd ed, Burtis CA and Ashwood ER, eds, Philadelphia, PA: WB Saunders Co, 1999, 1044-5.
Walter RM, Uriu-Hare JY, Olin KL, et al, "Copper, Zinc, Manganese, and Magnesium Status and Complications of Diabetes Mellitus," *Diabetes Care*, 1991, 14(11):1050-6.

♦ **Metallothionein** *see* Copper, Serum *on page 816*

♦ **Metallothionein** *see* Zinc, Serum *on page 824*

♦ **Methionine, Serum** *see* Molybdenum, Blood *on page 821*

♦ **Mn, Serum** *see* Manganese, Serum or Blood *on page 820*

♦ **Mn, Urine** *see* Manganese, Urine *on page 820*

♦ **Mo, Blood** *see* Molybdenum, Blood *on page 821*

Molybdenum, Blood

Related Information

Heavy Metal Screen, Blood *on page 792*
Heavy Metal Screen, Urine *on page 792*
Uric Acid, Serum *on page 293*

Synonyms Mo, Blood

Applies to Hypoxanthine, Urine; Methionine, Serum; Molybdopterin; S-Sulfocysteine, Urine; Sulfite, Test; Xanthine, Urine

Abstract Molybdenum is vital to human health through its inclusion in at least three human enzymes: xanthine oxidase, aldehyde oxidase, and sulfite oxidase. The active site of each of these binds molybdenum in the form of a cofactor "molybdopterin," a pterin ring similar to folic acid which tightly complexes molybdenum.[1] It is nontoxic, but heavy exposures have been associated with increased serum uric acid.

Specimen Whole blood, serum, plasma

Container In lieu of authoritative recommendations regarding potential molybdenum contamination from blood-drawing vacuum containers and stoppers, the same methods for containers and blood collection for other trace metals should be employed. If other samples are to be collected at the same blood draw, draw the trace metal tube first so as not to contaminate the needle by puncture through ordinary rubber stoppers. Use powder-free gloves. See the Trace Metals Introduction *on page 811*.

Reference Interval Whole blood molybdenum: <60 ng/mL (SI: 625 nmol/L); lower limit not established. Blood level parallels molybdenum intake. Apparently normal individuals vary over a 100-fold from 0.5-60 ng/mL (SI: 5-625 nmol/L), depending on molybdenum intake. 170 ng/mL (SI: 1771 nmol/L) appears to border on the toxic level based on the report below. Seventy-five percent of people in the United States have levels ≤5 ng/mL (SI: 52 nmol/L), but some geographical areas show 70% of the population >5 ng/mL. In children 2-12 years of age, the plasma molybdenum concentrations have been reported to vary from <1 to 3 ng/mL (SI: 10-31 nmol/L) with plasma concentration of 1.75 ng/mL ±0.8 ng/mL (mean ±SD) (SI: 18 nmol/L ±8.3 nmol/L). There are no age nor sex differences.[2]

Limitations Data are new and sketchy for this trace metal, and clinical syndromes poorly defined. Serum or plasma molybdenum norms are still being developed. Levels in apparently healthy people vary enormously based on intake, and blood levels are only significant when extremely high or extremely low levels (yet undefined) are encountered. Two reported methods have listed lowest levels of detection from 1-3 ng/mL[3,4] in serum and plasma.

Methodology Neutron activation; graphite furnace atomic absorption (AA) spectrophotometry after extraction into 8-hydroxyquinoline[4]

Additional Information Molybdenum interferes with copper metabolism, especially in the presence of dietary sulfides by the formation of insoluble copper thiomolybdenates in the gut lumen; absorbed thiomolybdenates may also interfere with copper metabolism. High levels of tungsten in the diet compete with molybdenum in experimental animals so that total body molybdenum deficiency can be created by loading with tungsten. So far this has not been reported to occur in humans, but there is no reason not to anticipate molybdenum deficiency should chronic tungsten exposure occur. The clinical syndromes so far reported for humans involving molybdenum include:

Molybdenum cofactor deficiency: This is a recessively inherited error of metabolism involving failure to synthesize molybdopterin. It is diagnosed by noting combined xanthine oxidase deficiency (low serum uric acid <1 mg/dL, increased urine hypoxanthine and xanthine) and sulfite oxidase deficiency (marked by increased urinary sulfite, decreased to absent urine inorganic sulfate, increased urinary S-sulfocysteine). These patients have severe neurologic abnormalities from infancy on the basis of the sulfite oxidase deficiency including seizures, anterior lens dislocations, opisthotonos, decreased brain weight, decreased brain myelin, and usually death prior to 1 year of age.[5] Molybdenum is virtually absent from the liver of such patients, suggesting that molybdopterin is an important storage form of molybdenum in soft tissues. Molybdenum may not be retained at all in soft tissue without molybdenum cofactor. Serum molybdenum in this disease is reported to be normal. Screening test to detect this among neonates with intractable seizures is the urine sulfite test.

Parenteral nutrition-associated molybdenum deficiency: One case of molybdenum deficiency has been reported in this setting in a 24-year-old man with Crohn disease.[6] Biochemical abnormalities were only corrected by the addition of molybdenum to the total parenteral nutrition (TPN). The biochemical abnormalities were essentially similar to those listed above for molybdenum cofactor deficiency: increased urinary sulfite, thiosulfate, xanthine, and hypoxanthine; decreased urinary sulfate and uric acid. In addition, unlike reported cases of molybdenum cofactors deficiency, this patient showed increased serum levels of methionine. The patient suffered night blindness, tachycardia, tachypnea, central scotomata, and irritability leading to coma over 24-48 hours while on TPN. Symptoms disappeared when amino acid administration was stopped, but reoccurred with either amino acid infusion or bisulfite infusion until molybdenum was added to the TPN.

Molybdenum toxicity: This has only rarely been reported. Two situations are known to expose human populations chronically to excess molybdenum: industrial exposure and through the food chain in areas of the world with high local soil molybdenum. Two villages in Armenia have a high frequency of patients with hepatosplenomegaly, "kidney disease," and an inflammatory arthritis of the knees and small joints of the hands and feet, associated with joint erythema, edema, and deformity. Serum levels of uric acid are modestly elevated and whole blood molybdenum is markedly elevated: 310 ±20 ng/mL (SI: 3231 ±208 nmol/L) versus 60 ±10 ng/mL (SI: 625 ±104 nmol/L) control. Dietary intake for these patients is estimated to be 10-15 mg/day versus 0.15-0.5 mg/day recommended. Asymptomatic subjects in the same villages also with high molybdenum intakes have lower but still markedly elevated blood molybdenum concentrations of 170 ±10 ng/mL (SI: 1772 ±104 nmol/L).[1] Serum molybdenum concentrations are increased in patients with chronic renal failure. Dialysis reduces serum molybdenum concentrations but serum molybdenum still remains high when compared to patients with good renal function. High serum molybdenum may contribute to dialysis related arthritis.[7] Serum molybdenum concentrations are elevated in liver disease including but not limited to
(Continued)

Molybdenum, Blood (Continued)

chronic active hepatitis, cirrhosis, alcoholic liver disease, liver metastases, and gallstones.

Footnotes

1. Rajagopalan KV, "Molybdenum: An Essential Trace Element in Human Nutrition," *Annu Rev Nutr*, 1988, 8:401-27.
2. Gropper SS and Yannicelli S, "Plasma Molybdenum Concentrations in Children With and Without Phenylketonuria," *Biol Trace Elem Res*, 1993, 38(3):227-31.
3. Lavi N and Alfassi ZB, "Determination of Trace Amounts of Cadmium, Cobalt, Chromium, Iron, Molybdenum, Nickel, Selenium, Titanium, Vanadium, and Zinc in Blood and Milk by Neutron Activation Analysis," *Analyst*, 1990, 115(6):817-22.
4. Morrice PC, Humphries WR, and Bremner I, "Determination of Molybdenum in Plasma Using Graphite Furnace Atomic Absorption Spectrometry," *Analyst*, 1989, 114(12):1667-9.
5. Johnson JL, Waud WR, Rajagopalan KV, et al, "Inborn Errors of Molybdenum Metabolism: Combined Deficiencies of Sulfite Oxidase and Xanthine Dehydrogenase in a Patient Lacking the Molybdenum Cofactor," *Proc Natl Acad Sci U S A*, 1980, 77(6):3715-9.
6. Abumrad NN, Schneider AJ, Steel D, et al, "Amino Acid Intolerance During Prolonged Total Parenteral Nutrition Reversed by Molybdate Therapy," *Am J Clin Nutr*, 1981, 34:2551-9.
7. Hosokawa S and Yoshida O, "Clinical Studies on Molybdenum in Patients Requiring Long-Term Hemodialysis," *ASAIO J*, 1994, 40(3):M445-9.

References

Bougle D, Foucault D, Voirin J, et al, "Molybdenum in the Premature Infant," *Biol Neonate*, 1991, 59(4):201-3.

Gou W, Li JY, King H, et al, "Diet and Blood Nutrient Correlations With Ischemic Heart, Hypertensive Heart, and Stroke Mortality in China," *Asia Pac J Public Health*, 1992-1993, 6(4):200-9.

Lugowski SJ, Smith DC, McHugh AD, et al, "Determination of Chromium, Cobalt and Molybdenum in Synovial Fluid by GFAAS," *J Trace Elem Electrolytes Health Dis*, 1991, 5(1):23-9.

Sardesai VM, "Molybdenum: An Essential Trace Element," *Nutr Clin Pract*, 1993, 8(6):277-81.

♦ **Molybdopterin** see Molybdenum, Blood *on page 821*

♦ **Penicillamine** see Zinc, Serum *on page 824*

Selenium, Serum

Related Information

Heavy Metal Screen, Blood *on page 792*
Heavy Metal Screen, Urine *on page 792*
Selenium, Urine *on page 823*

Synonyms Se, Serum

Applies to Selenocysteine; Selenoprotein P

Abstract Selenium is an important essential trace element in human nutrition. It is a constituent of glutathione peroxidase and iodothyronine deiodinases. It is thought to play a protective role in human carcinogenesis and cardiovascular disease.

Specimen Serum, plasma, whole blood. Hair may be analyzed: hair concentrations of selenium correlate with those of blood.[1]

Container Trace metal-free blood collection tube. See the Trace Elements Introduction *on page 811*.

Collection Draw blood into special trace metal vacuum tube. Centrifuge and pour serum into special plastic metal-free vial for transport. Use powder-free gloves.

Causes for Rejection Failure to obtain specimen using special trace element blood collection kit or store specimen in special metal-free plastic vials

Reference Interval Serum: 95-165 ng/mL (SI: 1203-2090 nmol/L). Approximately 40% higher for whole blood. Serum reflects recent intake; red cells reflect more remote intake. Whole blood therefore reflects an average of recent and remote intake of selenium. (Selenium-dependent glutathione peroxidase activity reflects selenium available for enzyme synthesis - see below.)

Critical Values Levels >500 ng/mL (SI: >6332 nmol/L) are associated with toxicity

Use Monitor selenium nutritional status, **especially in long-term parenteral nutrition**. Studies have indicated no factor or factors that can accurately predict serum levels to preclude need for measurement. May be used diagnostically in cardiomyopathy of unknown cause, especially where nutritional factors are suspected. Monitor selenium status in children with propionic acidemia who are at risk of deficiency on their special diets. Monitor for acute toxicity states, characterized clinically by nausea, diarrhea, mental alterations, peripheral neuropathy, and loss of hair and nails.[1]

Limitations Some controversy exists regarding the "best" marker for selenium status. Since selenium as selenomethionine is incorporated nonspecifically into protein, serum and whole blood selenium concentration increases with increasing selenium intake to different degrees, depending on inorganic or organic sources of selenium. Glutathione peroxidase activity is more sensitive to deficiency but the test is not well standardized and therefore not reproducible from laboratory to laboratory. Hair selenium may be contaminated by selenium-containing shampoo. Serum selenium level correlates best with intake and therefore with both deficiency and toxicity states, but a wide range of serum levels is compatible with apparent good health. Selenoprotein P, a selenium-rich plasma protein originally described in rats has been found to be the major selenoprotein in human plasma.[2] It appears to be at least as sensitive as other indices in common use. Determination of selenium in body fluids may suffer from problems like severe background noise, matrix effects, preatomization losses, and spectral interference.

Drugs which may cause decreased serum selenium concentrations include carbamazepine, phenytoin, and valproic acid. Ascorbic acid and indapamide may cause an increase in serum selenium concentrations.[3]

Methodology Graphite furnace atomic absorption spectrophotometry (GFAAS), high performance liquid chromatography (HPLC) with inductively-coupled plasma-mass spectrophotometry (HPLC-ICP-MS), electrothermal atomic absorption spectrophotometry (ETAAS) with electrodeless discharge lamp and automatic Zeeman-effect background correction. A simple, rapid and accurate atomic absorption spectrophotometric method suitable for routine chemical analysis using matched matrix and Pd-Ni modifier has been described.[4]

Additional Information Selenium is part of the enzyme that converts T_4 to the active thyroid hormone T_3. It is also part of selenium-dependant gluta-thione peroxidase, an important antioxidant in blood and tissue. Multiple cases of selenium deficiency have been reported, mostly among patients given parenteral nutrition without selenium supplementation. Deficiency also occurs endemically in places where soil selenium is low, and low levels are thus present throughout the food chain. Endemic cretinism[5,6] Balkan nephropathy,[7] Keschan disease[8] (endemic dilated cardiomyopathy), and Kashin-Back disease[9] (endemic deforming osteoarthritis) are probably all caused by endemic selenium deficiency causing the host to poorly tolerate an additional environmental stress (cretinism: iodine deficiency; the others: unknown local toxins). Low selenium blood levels have been shown to be a risk factor for peripartum cardiomyopathy in sub-Sahara Africa.[10] Simple deficiency is marked by whitening of the nailbeds, erythrocyte macrocytosis, cardiomyopathy, painful weak muscles, skin and hair depigmentation, and elevations of transaminase and creatinine kinase.[9,11,12] Cardiomyopathy may be mild and asymptomatic or fulminant and fatal.

Selenium consumed in foods and supplements exists in a number of different forms including selenomethionine, selenocysteine, selenate, and selenite. The bioavailability of selenium depends upon the form consumed. Selenomethionine is retained in tissue proteins to a greater extent than selenocysteine and the inorganic forms selenate and selenite.[13] Factors which influence the bioavailability of selenium include dietary composition, selenium status, and physiological status. Stable selenium isotope injection studies in rats[14] have delineated part of the metabolism of selenite. Selenite is taken up by erythrocytes and reduced to selenide which then reappears in plasma in a form bound selectively to albumin. Thirty minutes after injection the labeled selenium disappears from the plasma and starts to appear slowly as selenoprotein P and glutathione peroxidase, which attain maximal concentrations 6 hours after injection. Movement between various compartments probably depends upon the exact selenium status at the time of injection. The distribution of selenium has been determined in 21 healthy volunteers; 53% of selenium is associated with selenoprotein P, 39% is associated with glutathione peroxidase, and the remainder is associated with albumin.[15] Selenoprotein P has been proposed as a sensitive index of selenium status.[2]

Selenium toxicity can occur endemically, again due to high soil levels, or through accidental or industrial exposure. Symptoms include garlic breath, odor, thick brittle fingernails, dry brittle hair, red swollen skin of the hands and feet, and nervous system abnormalities of numbness, convulsions, or paralysis. Selenium in serum is mostly represented by selenoprotein P. However, when mild deficiency is induced by reducing oral intake of selenium in volunteers by 50%, glutathione peroxidase levels fall and serum selenium levels fall, yet the level of selenoprotein P remains normal.

Selenium is excreted from bile in feces, in sweat and skin losses, and the remaining 50% to 70% in urine. Significant breath losses occur only in toxic states. Dosages in renal failure need not be modified. Symptoms of the deficiency syndrome may rapidly appear after surgery or other stress following a long asymptomatic but chronic deficiency state.

Selenium is depressed in HIV infection,[16] critical illness,[17] kwashiorkor, inflammatory bowel disease,[18] renal failure, hemodialysis status, low protein diet, phenylketonuria, maple syrup urine disease (possibly all in part related to poor protein intake), low birth weight,[19] and premature infants with inadequate selenium intake. Levels are increased mostly with the use of glucocorticoids.[20]

Therapeutic trials for selenium indicate preventive effects for colorectal, lung, and prostate carcinomas.[21,22]

Footnotes

1. Mason JB, "Consequences of Altered Micronutrient Status," *Cecil Textbook of Medicine*, 21st ed, Chapter 231, Goldman L and Bennett JC, eds, Philadelphia, PA: WB Saunders Co, 2000, 1176.
2. Hill KE, Xia Y, Akesson B, et al, "Selenoprotein P Concentration in Plasma Is an Index of Selenium Status in Selenium Deficient and Selenium-Supplemented Chinese Subjects," *J Nutr*, 1996, 126(1):138-45.
3. Young DS, *Effects of Drugs on Clinical Laboratory Tests*, 5th ed, Volume 1: Listing by Test, Washington: DC, AACC Press, 2000, Section 3, 710.
4. Lin TH, Tseng WC, and Cheng SY, "Direct Determination of Selenium in Human Plasma and Seminal Plasma by Graphite Furnace Atomic Absorption Spectrophotometry and Clinical Application," *Biol Trace Elem Res*, 1998, 64(1-3):133-49.

5. Arthur JR, "The Role of Selenium in Thyroid Hormone Metabolism," *Can J Physiol Pharmacol*, 1991, 69(11):1648-52.

6. Contempré B, Vanderpas J, and Dumont JE, "Cretinism, Thyroid Hormones, and Selenium," *Mol Cell Endocrinol*, 1991, 81(1-3):C193-5.

7. Maksimović ZJ, "Selenium Deficiency and Balkan Endemic Nephropathy," *Kidney Int Suppl*, 1991, 34:S12-4.

8. Lockitch G, Taylor GP, Wong LTK, et al, "Cardiomyopathy Associated With Nonendemic Selenium Deficiency in a Caucasian Adolescent," *Am J Clin Nutr*, 1990, 52(3):572-7.

9. Levander OA, "A Global View of Human Selenium Nutrition," *Annu Rev Nutr*, 1987, 7:227-50.

10. Cenac A, Simonoff M, Moretto P, et al, "A Low Plasma Selenium Is a Risk Factor for Peripartum Cardiomyopathy. A Comparative Study in Sahelian Africa," *Int J Cardiol*, 1992, 36(1):57-9.

11. Kien CL and Ganther HE, "Manifestations of Chronic Selenium Deficiency in a Child Receiving Total Parenteral Nutrition," *Am J Clin Nutr*, 1983, 37(2):319-28.

12. Brown MR, Cohen HJ, Lyons JM, et al, "Proximal Muscle Weakness and Selenium Deficiency Associated With Long-Term Parenteral Nutrition," *Am J Clin Nutr*, 1986, 43(4):549-54.

13. Thomson CD, "Selenium Speciation in Human Body Fluids," *Analyst*, 1998, 123(5):827-31.

14. Suzuki KT and Itoh M, "Metabolism of Selenite Labeled With Enriched Stable Isotope in the Bloodstream," *J Chromatogr B Biomed Sci Appl*, 1997, 692(1):15-22.

15. Harrison I, Littlejohn D and Fell GS, "Distribution of Selenium in Human Blood Plasma and Serum," *Analyst*, 1996, 121(2):189-94.

16. Cirelli A, Ciardi M, De Simone C, et al, "Serum Selenium Concentration and Disease Progress in Patients With HIV Infection," *Clin Biochem*, 1991, 24(2):211-4.

17. Hawker FH, Stewart PM, and Snitch PJ, "Effects of Acute Illness on Selenium Homeostasis," *Crit Care Med*, 1990, 18(4):442-6.

18. Fernández-Bañares F, Mingorance MD, Esteve M, et al, "Serum Zinc, Copper, and Selenium Levels in Inflammatory Bowel Disease: Effect of Total Enteral Nutrition on Trace Element Status," *Am J Gastroenterol*, 1990, 85(12):1584-9.

19. Lockitch G, Jacobson B, Quigley G, et al, "Selenium Deficiency in Low Birth Weight Neonates: An Unrecognized Problem," *J Pediatr*, 1989, 114(5):865-70.

20. Marano G, Fischioni P, Graziano C, et al, "Increased Serum Selenium Levels in Patients Under Corticosteroid Treatment," *Pharmacol Toxicol*, 1990, 67(2):120-2.

21. Clark LC, Combs GF Jr, Turnbull BW, et al, "Effects of Selenium Supplementation for Cancer Prevention in Patients With Carcinoma of the Skin: A Randomized Controlled Trial," *JAMA*, 1996, 276(24):1957-63.

22. Colditz GA, "Selenium and Cancer Prevention: Promising Results Indicate Further Trials Required," *JAMA*, 1996, 276(4):1984-85.

References

Corvilain B, Contempré B, Longombe AO, et al, "Selenium and the Thyroid: How the Relationship Was Established," *Am J Clin Nutr*, 1993, 57(2 Suppl):244S-8S.

Mihailovic MB, Avramovic DM, Jovanovic IB, et al, "Blood and Plasma Selenium Levels and GSH-Px Activities in Patients With Arterial Hypertension and Chronic Heart Disease," *J Envir Path Tox Oncol*, 1998, 17(3-4):285-9.

Pentel P, Fletcher D, and Jentzen J, "Fatal Acute Selenium Toxicity," *J Forensic Sci*, 1985, 30(2):556-62.

Robberecht H and Deelstra H, "Factors Influencing Blood Selenium Concentration Values: A Literature Review," *J Trace Elem Electrolytes Health Dis*, 1994, 8(3-4):129-43.

Ruiz C, Alegria A, Barbera R, et al, "Selenium, Zinc, and Copper in Plasma of Patients With Type 1 Diabetes Mellitus in Different Metabolic Control States," *J Trace Elem Med Biol*, 1998, 12(2):91-5.

Rukgauer M, Klein J, and Kruse-Jarres JD, "Reference Values for the Trace Elements Copper, Manganese, Selenium, and Zinc in the Serum/Plasma of Children, Adolescents and Adults," *J Trace Elem Med Biol*, 1997, 11(2):92-8.

Yu MW, Horng IS, Hsu KH, et al, "Plasma Selenium Levels and Risk of Hepatocellular Carcinoma Among Men With Chronic Hepatitis Virus Infection," *Am J Epidemiol*, 1999, 150(4):367-74.

Selenium, Urine

Related Information

Heavy Metal Screen, Blood *on page 792*
Heavy Metal Screen, Urine *on page 792*
Selenium, Serum *on page 822*
Urine Collection, 24-Hour *on page 47*

Synonyms Se, Urine

Abstract Urine selenium is used in conjunction with serum selenium to assess selenium nutrition or potential toxic exposure. Like other 24-hour urine collections of an essential element, this reflects recent intake, assuming the patient is in selenium balance.

Specimen 24-hour urine

Container Acid-washed plastic urine container

Collection Avoid contamination by hair, since some patients use selenium-containing shampoos.

Causes for Rejection Failure to store urine in acid-washed plastic containers

Reference Interval Levels <15 µg/L or >150 µg/L (SI: <190 µmol/L or >1900 µmol/L) probably represent unusually low or high intake without necessarily representing illness. Values vary widely and in apparently healthy U.S. citizens they have been reported to vary from 7 µg/L (SI: 89 µmol/L) (24-hour sample) to 231 µg/L (SI: 2925 µmol/L). Intake is partly determined by local soil content of selenium and use of local vegetables as food. Healthy persons in New Guinea have been reported with levels as low as 0.9 µg/L (SI: 11.4 µmol/L) but similar patients have rapidly developed symptomatic selenium deficiency when placed on total parenteral nutrition lacking selenium. Urine levels of 7 µg/L have been reported from China in areas where selenium deficiency is symptomatic. Levels >880 µg/L (SI: >11,144 µmol/L) have been seen in chronic selenosis and >600 µg/L (SI: 7599 µmol/L) during the first 24 hours after acute selenium intoxication. Levels >500 µg/L (SI: 6332 µmol/L) probably represent toxicity. See the comprehensive review by Robberecht and Deelstra.[1] Some authors or laboratories report as µg/day.

Use Monitor nutritional therapy, especially parenteral nutrition; monitor potential toxic exposure

Limitations Selenomethionine is retained in tissue proteins to a greater degree than selenocysteine and the inorganic forms, but the selenium in selenomethionine is not necessarily immediately available for incorporation into functional selenoproteins.[2] A number of other factors besides chemical form may also influence the bioavailability and distribution of selenium, including dietary composition, selenium status, and physiological status. Spot urine selenium is of little value, as urine selenium goes up after each meal depending on selenium intake. Fasting urine samples may give a reasonable estimate of urinary output of selenium on a population basis. Twenty-four hour urines are necessary for diagnosis of deficiency.[3] Urinary excretion may be lower in children, elderly people and pregnant women.[4]

Methodology Atomic absorption (AA), gas chromatography/mass spectrometry (GC/MS)

Additional Information In the case of selenium, skin and stool losses are significant and amount to 30% to 50% of total losses; nevertheless, urine losses often represent overflow losses and can help indicate whether recent intake has been adequate or possibly toxic. When selenium intake is low to normal, <140 µg/day, 24-hour urine may not reflect the 24-hour intake of the previous day. This is especially true when the body stores are low and selenium is retained to fill body stores.[4] At higher levels of intake, the 24-hour urine is well correlated with intake and can be used as evidence of excess intake, adequate intake, or prior toxic exposure. When selenium supplementation normalizes serum selenium and whole blood selenium, and then selenium supplementation is stopped, urine selenium falls back toward baseline much faster than blood or serum levels.[5] Urine selenium has recently been found to be correlated with 24-hour urine urea in critically ill patients. This probably reflects catabolism of protein and release of body stores of selenium, though details of the selenium intake of the patients (proportional to protein intake in tube-fed patients) were not provided.[6] Impaired hepatic production of selenoproteins and other selenium containing compounds is the most likely explanation for reduced serum selenium concentrations in patients with chronic liver disease.[5]

Red cell glutathione peroxidase may be monitored as an index of selenium status. Levels will be depressed in deficiency but will not be elevated in toxicity.

Footnotes

1. Robberecht HJ and Deelstra HA, "Selenium in Human Urine: Concentration Levels and Medical Implications," *Clin Chim Acta*, 1984, 136(2-3):107-20.

2. Thomson CD, "Selenium Speciation in Human Body Fluids," *Analyst*, 1998, 123(5):827-31.

3. Thomson CD, Smith TE, Butler KA, et al, "An Evaluation of Urinary Measures of Iodine and Selenium Status," *J Trace Elem Med Biol*, 1996, 10(4):214-22.

4. Sanz Alaejos M and Diaz Romero C, "Urinary Selenium Concentrations," *Clin Chem*, 1993, 39(10):2040-52.

5. Välimäki M, Alfthan G, Vuoristo M, et al, "Effects of Selenium Supplementation on Blood and Urine Selenium Levels and Liver Function in Patients With Primary Biliary Cirrhosis," *Clin Chim Acta*, 1991, 196(1):7-15.

6. Hawker FH, Stewart PM, and Snitch PJ, "Effects of Acute Illness on Selenium Homeostasis," *Crit Care Med*, 1990, 18(4):442-6.

References

Ducros V and Favier A, "Gas Chromatographic-Mass Spectrometric Method for the Determination of Selenium in Biological Samples," *J Chromatogr*, 1992, 583(1).35-44.

Gokmen IG and Abdelqader E, "Determination of Selenium in Biological Matrices Using a Kinetic Catalytic Method," *Analyst*, 1994, 119(4):703-8.

Horng CJ, Tsai JL, and Lin SR, "Determination of Urinary Arsenic, Mercury, and Selenium in Steel Production Workers," *Biol Trace Elem Res*, 1999, 70(1):29-40.

Navarro-Alarcon M, Lopez-Garcia De La Serrana H, Perez-Valero V, et al, "Serum and Urine Selenium Concentration in Patients With Cardiovascular Diseases and Relationship to Other Nutritional Indexes," *Ann Nutr Metab*, 1999, 43(1):30-6.

Suzuki KT, Itoh M, and Ohmichi M, "Detection of Selenium-Containing Biological Constituents by High-Performance Liquid Chromatography-Plasma Source Mass Spectrometry," *J Chromatogr B Biomed Sci Appl*, 1995, 666(1):13-9.

Thomson CD, "Clinical Consequences and Assessment of Low Selenium Status," *N Z Med J*, 1991, 104(919):376-7.

♦ **Selenocysteine** *see* Selenium, Serum *on page 822*

♦ **Selenoprotein P** *see* Selenium, Serum *on page 822*

♦ **Se, Serum** *see* Selenium, Serum *on page 822*

♦ **Se, Urine** *see* Selenium, Urine *on page 823*

♦ **S-Sulfocysteine, Urine** *see* Molybdenum, Blood *on page 821*

♦ **Sulfite, Test** *see* Molybdenum, Blood *on page 821*

♦ **Thymulin Assay** *see* Zinc, Serum *on page 824*

♦ **Transcuprein** *see* Copper, Serum *on page 816*

♦ **Xanthine, Urine** *see* Molybdenum, Blood *on page 821*

♦ **Zinc Administration** *see* Copper, Serum *on page 816*

Zinc, Serum

Related Information
Albumin, Serum *on page 88*
Copper, Serum *on page 816*
Heavy Metal Screen, Blood *on page 792*
Heavy Metal Screen, Urine *on page 792*
Zinc, Urine *on page 825*

Synonyms
Zn, Serum

Applies to
Metallothionein; Penicillamine; Thymulin Assay

Abstract Zinc (Zn) is an essential trace element in human nutrition. Zinc is found in over 100 enzymes. It has effects on growth, development, weight loss, immune function, and central nervous system function. Serum zinc concentrations are not a reliable indicator of zinc status, especially in the elderly.[1] Zinc and copper are competitive for intestinal absorption.

Specimen Serum or plasma

Container Use powder-free gloves. Collect blood in metal-free tubes. Avoid contact with rubber. Separate serum and store in metal-free plastic vial. See the Trace Elements Introduction *on page 811*.

Collection Avoid hemolysis or stasis: red cell zinc concentrations are about 10 times those of serum.

Causes for Rejection Failure to collect specimen with special collection kit or store serum in special metal-free plastic vials

Reference Interval 66-110 µg/dL (SI: 10.0-16.8 µmol/L). Serum zinc, when low in an apparently healthy (nonstressed, nonseptic) patient who has normal serum albumin, is evidence for low zinc stores, especially if urine zinc is also low, or there is known excessive unregulated zinc loss (diarrhea, nephrotic syndrome, etc).

Use Evaluate suspected nutritional inadequacy, especially in enteral or parental nutrition, critically ill or burn patients; cases of diabetes or delayed wound healing; growth retardation; follow therapy in confirmed or potential deficiency states, for example when higher intravenous zinc doses are used to balance ongoing ostomy, biliary, or diarrheal losses as in total parenteral nutrition (TPN); follow oral zinc therapy in Wilson disease; confirm acrodermatitis enteropathica and follow therapy; evaluate possible zinc toxicity or metal fume fever in possible exposure situations (poisoning, industrial exposure).

Limitations One should not interpret a normal serum zinc as evidence for adequate zinc stores, as serum zinc is insensitive and may be normal even after symptoms of zinc deficiency have surfaced. Levels may be low in fever, sepsis, inflammation, exogenous corticosteroids, oral contraceptives, pregnancy, stress, or myocardial infarct reflecting mobilization from serum to the liver by interleukin. Serum concentrations are usually low in uremia with normal tissue levels. Levels may be high in familial hyperzincemia without toxicity or high zinc stores. Albumin is a binding protein for zinc and levels are usually low in cases of hypoalbuminemia of all causes.

Drugs which may decrease serum zinc concentrations include carbamazepine, phenytoin, prednisone, and valproic acid. Those which may cause increased serum zinc concentrations include zurzuofin, chlorthalidone, oral contraceptives, and penicillamine.[2]

Methodology Atomic absorption spectrometry (AA). A simple and sensitive colorimetric method utilizing a cationic porphyrin has been described.[3]

Additional Information Many potential markers have been examined in the search for the ideal index of zinc status. The simplest of these is serum zinc concentration, which is reduced in moderate to severe zinc deficiency. It is not sensitive to mild deficiency states and is depressed in situations often parallel with reductions of serum albumin, its major binding protein. Other more sensitive tests each have their own problems in clinical use.[4,5,6] Serum zinc remains useful in the nonelderly if knowledge of zinc metabolism is applied in interpretation.

Both primary and conditioned nutritional deficiency is fairly common worldwide, as well as in the United States, and has been described in a large variety of clinical situations: premature infants born with low hepatic stores; in breast-fed premature and full-term infants[7] whose mother's milk is lower than normal in zinc; in growing children, especially boys, whose height velocity has increased while under zinc therapy; in prepubertal boys who display delayed sexual maturity, especially in association with diets low in animal protein and high in phytates from grains (which reduce gastrointestinal zinc absorption); in malabsorption and diarrheal states; in diabetes, nephrotic syndrome, cirrhosis (in each of these hyperzincuria occurs), in AIDS and ARC;[8] in burn patients,[9] and those receiving high doses of oral histidine or intravenous amino acids[10] (as in TPN, especially cysteine or histidine) associated with hyperzincuria; and in geophagia (in which zinc absorption is reduced). Pharmacological doses of folate increase stool losses of zinc, and may increase infectious complications of pregnancy. The most severe cases of zinc deficiency have occurred in acrodermatitis enteropathica (see below), and in the early days of total parenteral nutrition, when zinc was not specifically included in the formulation.

Pregnant women are at higher risk of developing acquired zinc deficiency due to high uptake of zinc by the fetus. Also, excessive iron and folic acid, generally prescribed in pregnancy, interfere in zinc absorption.

Babies with the disease of zinc malabsorption known as acrodermatitis enteropathica usually first develop their characteristic facial and diaper rash

when weaned. Untreated, symptoms progress and include growth retardation, diarrhea, impaired T-cell immunity, poor wound healing, infections, delayed testicular development in adolescence, and early death. Parenteral or enteral zinc corrects the condition. The classic disease is associated with low serum and urine zinc, but some cases have a normal serum zinc.[11] These cases nevertheless respond to zinc supplementation.

Zinc absorption appears to be partially regulated through binding receptors on small intestinal mucosal cells, shared with copper and with cross competition by copper. Metallothioneine (MT) also regulates zinc absorption. It is induced by zinc and binds excess intracellular zinc. Binding to MT prevents further uptake of zinc into the body and the zinc is sloughed along with the small bowel mucosal cells. When oral intake of zinc falls, stool excretion, sweat excretion, and eventually urinary excretion are reduced.[7] Normally, urine losses are a small proportion of total losses. Typically healthy nonstressed adults come into neutral zinc balance with 10-20 mg oral zinc and positive zinc balance with 3 mg intravenous zinc per day.

Serum metallothioneine can help to distinguish reductions in serum zinc due to redistribution (sepsis, stress) from that due to nutritional inadequacy.[6] Both serum zinc and metallothioneine concentrations are reduced in nutritional inadequacy (reduced pool size) while low serum zinc concentration with high serum metallothioneine concentration reflects a redistribution of zinc stores. WBC zinc and assay of thymulin (a zinc dependent thymic hormone)[12] have been proposed to serve as a marker for zinc status. IL-1 production or lymphocyte ecto 5'-nucleotidase activity may also be used to assess zinc status. None of these have yet proven sensitive in all situations.

Zinc deficiency in adolescents and adults is marked by slow growth or weight loss, altered taste, delayed puberty, dwarfism, impaired dark adaptation, central scotomata, alopecia, emotional instability, tremors, cerebellar ataxia, and a bullous-pustular rash over sacral areas. Candidiasis reflects impaired T-cell function. Thymulin apo-hormone is present but inactive due to lack of zinc. Lymphopenia may occur in severe deficiency and death may follow an overwhelming infection. Marginal cases of zinc deficiency may only reveal subtle abnormalities such as normocytic anemia.[13] A case report of a 11-year-old boy with a serum zinc concentration >200 µmol/L but with symptoms consistent with zinc deficiency (hepatosplenomegaly, rashes, stunted growth, anemia, and impaired immune function) since birth may represent a previously unrecognized inborn error of zinc metabolism.[14]

Oral zinc supplementation interferes with copper absorption and chronic oral zinc supplementation may precipitate copper deficiency. Copper status should be monitored for patients on long-term zinc therapy.

Footnotes
1. Artacho R, Ruiz-Lopez MD, Gamez C, et al, "Serum Concentration and Dietary Intake of Zn in Healthy Institutionalized Elderly Subjects," *Sci Total Environ*, 1997, 205(2-3):159-65.
2. Young DS, *Effects of Drugs on Clinical Laboratory Tests*, 5th ed, Volume 1: Listing by Test, Washington, DC: AACC Press, American Association of Clinical Chemistry, 2000, Section 3, 858.
3. Makino T, "A Simple and Sensitive Colorimetric Assay of Zinc in Serum Using Cationic Porphyrin," *Clin Chim Acta*, 1999, 282(1-2):65-76.
4. Peretz A, Nève J, Jeghers O, et al, "Interest of Zinc Determination in Leukocyte Fractions for the Assessment of Marginal Zinc Status," *Clin Chim Acta*, 1991, 203(1):35-46.
5. Sandstead HH, "Assessment of Zinc Nutriture," *J Lab Clin Med*, 1991, 118:299-300.
6. King JC, "Assessment of Zinc Status," *J Nutr*, 1990, 120(Suppl 11):1474-9.
7. Khoshoo V, Kjarsgaard J, Krafchick B, et al, "Zinc Deficiency in A Full-Term Breast-Fed Infant: Unusual Presentation," *Pediatrics*, 1992, 89(6 Pt 1):1094-5.
8. Odeh M, "The Role of Zinc in Acquired Immunodeficiency Syndrome," *J Intern Med*, 1992, 231(5):463-9.
9. Boosalis MG, Solem LD, Cerra FB, et al, "Increased Urinary Zinc Excretion After Thermal Injury," *J Lab Clin Med*, 1991, 118(6):538-45.
10. Zlotkin SH, "Nutrient Interactions With Total Parenteral Nutrition: Effect of Histidine and Cysteine Intake on Urinary Zinc Excretion," *J Pediatr*, 1989, 114(5):859-64.
11. Mack D, Koletzko B, Cunnane S, et al, "Acrodermatitis Enteropathica With Normal Serum Zinc Levels: Diagnostic Value of Small Bowel Biopsy and Essential Fatty Acid Determination," *Gut*, 1989, 30(10):1426-9.
12. Prasad AS, Meftah S, Abdallah J, et al, "Serum Thymulin in Human Zinc Deficiency," *J Clin Invest*, 1988, 82(4):1202-10.
13. Nishiyama S, Irisa K, Matsubasa T, et al, "Zinc Status Relates to Hematological Deficits in Middle-Aged Women," *J Am Coll Nutr*, 1998, 17(3):291-5.
14. Sampson B, Kovar IZ, Rauscher A, et al, "A Case of Hyperzincemia With Functional Zinc Depletion: A New Disorder?" *Pediatr Res*, 1997, 42(2):219-25.

References
Alfrey AC, "Essential Trace Elements," *The Kidney: Physiology and Pathophysiology*, 2nd ed, Seldin DW and Giebisch G, eds, New York, NY: Raven Press, 1992, 2993-3003.

Hashim Z, Woodhouse L, and King JC, "Interindividual Variation in Circulating Zinc Concentrations Among Healthy Adult Men and Women," *Int J Food Sci Nutr*, 1996, 47(5):383-90.

Prasad AS, "Zinc: An Overview," *Nutrition*, 1995, 11(1 Suppl):93-9.

Rukgauer M, Klein J, and Kruse-Jarres JD, "Reference Values for the Trace Elements Copper, Manganese, Selenium, and Zinc in the Serum/Plasma of Children, Adolescents, and Adults," *J Trace Elem Med Biol*, 1997, 11(2):92-8.

Ruz M, Cavan KR, Bettger WJ, et al, "Development of a Dietary Model for the Study of Mild Zinc Deficiency in Humans and Evaluation of Some Biochemical and Functional Indices of Zinc Status," *Am J Clin Nutr*, 1991, 53(5):1295-303.

Sandstead HH, "Understanding Zinc: Recent Observations and Interpretations." *J Lab Clin Med*, 1994, 124(3):322-7.

Zapata CL, Simoes TM, and Donangelo CM, "Erythrocyte Metallothionein in Relation to Other Biochemical Zinc Indices in Pregnant and Nonpregnant Women," *Biol Trace Elem Res*, 1997, 57(2):115-24.

Zima T, Mestek O, Nemecek K, et al, "Trace Elements in Hemodialysis and Continuous Ambulatory Peritoneal Dialysis Patients," *Blood Purification*, 1998, 16(5):253-60.

Zinc, Urine

Related Information

Heavy Metal Screen, Blood *on page 792*
Heavy Metal Screen, Urine *on page 792*
Urine Collection, 24-Hour *on page 47*
Zinc, Serum *on page 824*

Synonyms Zn, Urine

Abstract Although zinc is mainly eliminated from the body by fecal excretion, minor quantities are excreted in urine. High urine, but low serum zinc, may be associated with hepatic cirrhosis, neoplastic disease, or increased catabolism. Low urine and serum zinc concentrations may be caused by zinc deficiency.

Specimen 24-hour urine

Container Acid-washed plastic urine container

Collection Use 10 mL concentrated hydrochloric acid as a preservative for 24-hour collection.

Storage Instructions Keep on ice or refrigerated. Laboratory will measure and record volume and remove aliquot for analysis.

Causes for Rejection Failure to collect specimen in metal-free (acid-washed) container, specimen allowed to contact rubber

Special Instructions Avoid contact with rubber during collection such as through rubber catheter. If a urinary catheter is absolutely essential, as in burn patients, consider the use of a silicone catheter, which has been shown to release less zinc than other types. Most catheters contribute zinc to the collection, some to a substantial degree. For critical or research cases, it is advisable to document acceptability of the catheter prior to use.[1]

Reference Interval Normal subjects: 0.14-0.80 mg/24 hours (SI: 2.1-12.2 µmol/24 hours). Compliant patients on oral zinc therapy for Wilson disease: >2.00 mg/24 hours (SI: 30.6 µmol/24 hours).[2]

Use Evaluate zinc toxicity; evaluate low serum zinc levels; evaluate compliance in oral zinc therapy of Wilson disease. Low urine zinc levels in the presence of depressed serum zinc tend to confirm zinc deficiency. Urinary zinc excretion is sensitive only to extreme changes in dietary zinc intake[3] and may be useful as an additional marker of changes in bone metabolism and in monitoring estrogen replacement therapy in osteoporosis.[4,5] Urinary zinc excretion has been proposed as an alternate approach to detection of renal tubular dysfunction.[6]

Limitations Zinc deficiency is usually accompanied by decreased urine zinc excretion. Zinc deficiency, however, may be in part due to excess urine losses, especially in cirrhosis, viral hepatitis, hemolytic anemias, sickle cell disease, alcoholism, diabetes, chronic renal diseases, or parenteral nutrition.

Drugs which may cause an increase in urinary zinc concentration include bendroflumethiazide, bumetanide, chlorthalidone, cisplatin, furosemide, hydrochlorothiazide, naproxen, penicillamine, and triamterene.[7]

Methodology Atomic absorption spectrometry (AA), potentiometric stripping analysis and constant current stripping analysis, inductively-coupled plasma-mass spectrometry (ICP-MS)

Additional Information Urinary zinc excretion is increased in patients with exocrine pancreatic insufficiency,[8] in people exposed to mercury vapor,[9] and those with various types of immune system activation including stress and trauma, allograft recipients,[10] cancer,[6] and alcoholic liver disease.[11] Significant losses of zinc are seen in patients with familial hypercholesterolemia undergoing regular therapeutic apheresis.[12]

Footnotes

1. de Haan KEC and Woroniecka UD, "Bladder Catheters and Zinc Contamination of Urine," *Clin Chem*, 1989, 35(5):888.

2. Brewer GJ, Dick RD, and Yuzbasiyan-Gurkan V, et al, "Treatment of Wilson's Disease With Zinc. XIII. Therapy With Zinc in Presymptomatic Patients From the Time of Diagnosis," *J Lab Clin Med*, 1994, 123(6):849-58.

3. Verus AP and Samman S, "Urinary Zinc as a Marker of Zinc Intake: Results of a Supplementation Trial in Free-Living-Men," *Eur J Clin Nutr*, 1994, 48(3):219-21.

4. Herzberg M, Lusky A, Blondre J, et al, "The Effect of Estrogen Replacement Therapy on Zinc in Serum and Urine," *Obstet Gynecol*, 1996, 87(6):1035-40.

5. Relea P, Revilla M, Ripolli E, et al, "Zinc, Biochemical Markers of Nutrition and Type I Osteoporosis," *Age Ageing*, 1995, 24(4):303-7.

6. Melichar B, Jandil P, Malir F, et al, "Association Between Renal Tubular Cell Dysfunction and Increased Urinary Zinc Excretion in Cancer Patients," *Scand J Clin Lab Invest*, 1995, 55(2):149-52.

7. Young DS, *Effects of Drugs on Clinical Laboratory Tests*, 5th ed, Volume 1: Listing by Test, Washington, DC: AACC Press, American Association of Clinical Chemistry, 2000, Section 3, 858.

8. Dutta SK, Procaccino F, and Aamodt R, "Zinc Metabolism in Patients With Exocrine Pancreatic Insufficiency," *J Am Coll Nutr*, 1998, 17(6):556-63.

9. Sallsten G and Barregard L, "Urinary Excretion of Mercury, Copper, and Zinc in Subjects Exposed to Mercury Vapour," *Biometals*, 1997, 10(4):357-61.

10. Melichar B, Aichberger C, Artner-Dworzak E, et al, "Immune Activation and Enhanced Urinary Zinc Concentrations in Allograft Recipients," *Presse Med*, 1994, 23(15):702-6.

11. Rodriguez-Moreno F, Gonzalez-Reimers E, Santolaria-Fernandez F, et al, "Zinc, Copper, Manganese, and Iron in Chronic Alcoholic Liver Disease," *Alcohol*, 1997, 14(1):39-44.

12. Jackson GE, Blewet R, Rodgers AL, et al, "Trace Metal Excretion in Patients With Homozygous Hypercholesterolemia," *J Trace Elem Med Biol*, 1999, 13(1-2):62-7.

References

Golik A, Zaidenstein R, Dishi V, et al, "Effects of Captopril and Enalapril on Zinc Metabolism in Hypertensive Patients," *J Am Coll Nutr*, 1998, 17(1):75-8.

Gozzo ML, Colacicco L, Calla C, et al, "Determination of Copper, Zinc, and Selenium in Human Plasma and Urine Samples by Potentiometric Stripping Analysis and Constant Current Stripping Analysis," *Clin Chim Acta*, 1999, 285(1-2):53-68.

Henderson LM, Brewer GJ, Dressman JB, et al, "Use of Zinc Tolerance Test and 24-Hour Urinary Zinc Content to Assess Oral Zinc Absorption," *J Am Coll Nutr*, 1996, 15(1):79-83.

Hsiung CS, Andrade JD, Costa R, et al, "Minimizing Interferences in the Quantitative Multielement Analysis of Trace Elements in Biological Fluids by Inductively-Coupled Plasma Mass Spectrometry," *Clin Chem*, 1997, 43(12):2203-11.

Milne DB, "Trace Elements," *Tietz Textbook of Clinical Chemistry*, 3rd ed, Burtis CA and Ashwood ER, eds, Philadelphia, PA: WB Saunders Co, 1999, 1037-41.

Rodriguez E and Diaz C, "Iron, Copper, and Zinc Levels in Urine: Relationship to Various Individual Factors," *J Trace Elem Med Biol*, 1995, 9(4):200-9.

♦ **Zn, Serum** *see* Zinc, Serum *on page 824*

♦ **Zn, Urine** *see* Zinc, Urine *on page 825*

TRANSFUSION MEDICINE
(BLOOD BANK)

Geralyn Meny, MD

David S. Jacobs, MD

Malcolm Beck, FIMLS

The close of the 20st century has witnessed a rush to eliminate transfusion-transmissible disease – a process which was spurred by the introduction of the human immunodeficiency virus (HIV) into the blood supply and which continues today. The following screening tests have been implemented as a means to reduce the risk of transfusion-transmitted disease.

Test	Year Introduced
Syphilis	~1939
Hepatitis B surface antigen	1971
Anti-CMV	1981
Anti-HIV	1985
Antihepatitis B core	1986
ALT	1986
Anti-HTLV I	1989
Anti-HCV	1990
Anti-HIV 1/2	1992
Anti-HTLV I/II	1995
HIV p24 antigen	1996
HIV genomic nucleic acid test (IND)*	1999
HCV genomic nucleic acid test (IND)*	1999

*Investigational use, however, utilized by most blood collection organizations.

In addition to the numerous infectious disease tests, extensive donor questioning also reduces risks of transfusion-transmitted disease. These efforts have increased the safety of the blood supply for patients. It is also important to remember the blood donor. Apheresis and whole blood donation must continue to be safe procedures. For example, donors should be monitored for 15-20 minutes postdonation for signs or symptoms of untoward effects before release. Physicians and surgeons, re-examining their usage of blood, have gradually come to realize that blood transfusion and the maintenance of arbitrary hemoglobin levels are not as important as they were once thought to be. Physicians and surgeons should obtain informed consent for transfusion. It is desirable that patients understand why transfusions of blood and components may be necessary, the risks involved (in appropriate perspective), and ways of reducing the risks. A few states (California, New Jersey, and Pennsylvania) require by law informed consent from patients planning to undergo a medical procedure which may involve a transfusion.

Obviously, such information should be available to the patient well ahead of the anticipated event, so that there will be time to arrange alternatives to address the patient's concerns. Many blood services now have informative brochures about blood transfusion, its risks, and the alternatives. These materials can be placed in clinics and physicians' offices to provide a basis for informed consent for blood transfusion.

Important: The availability of such brochures does not absolve the physician from responsibility to obtain and document informed consent.

PREPARATION FOR TRANSFUSION

1. **Sample Collection.** Ask the patient his or her name and check this against the information on the identification band. At the patient's bedside, label the sample tube with two unique forms of patient identification, such as the patient's full name and hospital number; also include date and identity of the collector. Other information may be locally required. The same identification must be placed on a requisition form. If the Blood Bank uses a special transfusion identification system, collect the sample and label it appropriately.

   If an identification plate is used, information on the patient's identification plate must agree fully with that on the wristband or the sample should not be drawn. Adjust procedures for emergencies or disasters with great care to avoid the increased likelihood of mix-ups that is inherent in such situations.

   - The patient's identification band should remain attached to an accessible part of the patient's body and should not be removed except by established procedure. If the band has been removed for an unauthorized reason, the identification procedure must be repeated and another sample obtained.
   - Any identification discrepancies or problems must be corrected promptly.

   Clerical error is the most common cause of blood incompatibility and transfusion reactions which follow. Full and correct labeling **at the bedside** is essential for all samples of blood drawn for the Blood Bank. The Blood Bank must not be permitted to accept unlabeled tubes or those with unattached or loose identification, no matter who presents them. Specimen identification requirements are outlined in a listing bearing that name in the specimen collection chapter.

2. **Issuing Blood.** Unless there is some good reason to do otherwise, the oldest unit crossmatched for a patient is dispensed first. But if a patient has autologous and/or directed as well as allogeneic (homologous) units, issue them in this order: first autologous, then directed, and last allogeneic.

The selected unit is removed from the refrigerator. It is carefully inspected for clots, hemolysis, or discoloration. Any unit of abnormal appearance is quarantined.

Identifying information on a transfusion request form and blood bag tag should be matched according to established procedures prior to issuing blood. Information may include the following:

- patient's name, hospital number, other identifying data
- patient's ABO and Rh type
- donor blood ABO and Rh type
- donor number, expiration date, component being issued
- crossmatch result (if applicable)
- result of antibody screen

Any discrepancies must be resolved before blood is released. Date and time of issue must be documented.

With some exceptions (emergencies, major surgery), only one unit of blood at a time should be issued for a patient receiving elective transfusions. Otherwise, the second unit may remain at room temperature for an extended period.

Personnel should never be allowed to pick up two units for two or more different patients at the same time.

ADMINISTRATION OF BLOOD AND BLOOD COMPONENTS

1. Except in urgent situations, avoid starting transfusions at night for three reasons. First, hospital staffing is thinner at night, making it harder to keep a close watch on patients being transfused. Second, patients need sleep. Third, any untoward reaction will awaken the patient and create turmoil on the ward.

2. If possible, before picking up the blood from the Blood Bank, an intravenous infusion of isotonic saline using a Y-type blood-recipient set having a standard clot filter should be started. A needle of 19-gauge or bigger should be used. Smaller needles and special sets may be necessary for infants and children. The saline should be run at a slow drip. With an already existing I.V., the needle gauge and the I.V. site should be checked. The I.V. tubing should be changed, if necessary. If solutions other than isotonic saline have been running, a saline flush is indicated.

Do not use any other solution or medications which may cause decreased survival of stored blood. Ringer's, for example, may cause formation of small clots that block the needle. Hypotonic solutions, particularly those containing dextrose, may cause lysis. For similar reasons of pharmacologic incompatibility, no medications should be added to stored blood or to tubing containing blood, unless it is flushed with saline before and after the medication.

Check other I.V. medications that may have to be given and try to reschedule them before or after the blood transfusion. If necessary, other I.V.s can be given into another extremity.

3. The intended recipient must be correctly identified.

- All information on the transfusion form must be compared with that on the patient's identification band or bands, and on the donor blood unit. Make sure that everything conforms.

4. The blood unit must be inspected for hemolysis, discoloration, or other abnormal appearance. In case of anything out of the ordinary, the Blood Bank must be consulted before the transfusion is begun.

5. Vital signs, including temperature, must be recorded.

6. Do not attempt to vent plastic blood containers.

7. Once the blood unit is obtained from the Blood Bank, it should be mixed thoroughly by repeatedly inverting the bag, and started at once. The blood must be returned to the Blood Bank without delay if anything interferes with starting the transfusion.

8. **Do not store blood**, even temporarily, in conventional refrigerators on nursing stations, in operating rooms, emergency departments, or anywhere other than in blood storage units that are specially designated and continuously monitored. To do so violates all accreditation standards and federal regulations.

9. Hang the blood.
- Mix gently.
- Carefully insert the plastic cannula of the infusion set to avoid puncturing the wall of the bag.
- In the case of CPDA-1 red blood cells, lower the unit and allow 50-100 mL of saline to run into the bag. This allows easier and faster infusion. Additive unit red blood cells do not require this step.

10. Special blood filters may be indicated for some patients. See Filters for Blood *on page 842.*

11. The time the blood is started should be recorded.

12. Remain with and observe the patient for at least the first 5 minutes. Take vital signs again at 15 minutes and at the end of the transfusion. The patient should be checked frequently.

13. Infusion generally should not exceed 2 hours for one unit of RBCs. If there is danger of pulmonary edema or congestive heart failure, or if there is a possible immunologic problem or a history of reactions, the time may be extended to 4 hours. If circumstances require even slower transfusion, it may be better to ask the Blood Bank to divide the unit in half and provide it as two transfusions.

14. After the transfusion, dispose of the empty blood bags as per established procedure. If necessary, the residual small amounts of blood can be very useful in the event of reaction.

RELEASE OF BLOOD SET UP FOR TRANSFUSION, THEN NOT USED

1. Blood issued for transfusion and then not used can be used for another patient as long as:

    - the unit has not been entered or punctured
    - the unit (red cells or whole blood) have not been allowed to warm above 10°C or cool below 1°C
    - records indicate that the blood has been reissued and that it has been inspected prior to reissue
    - At least one sealed segment of integral donor tubing has remained attached to the container

2. When blood has been set up for a patient but not used, most hospitals must limit the time it can be held for that patient. Otherwise, there is a likelihood the blood would be held indefinitely and would outdate, because someone forgot to notify the Blood Bank that the patient no longer needed a transfusion. The time limit may vary according to the needs of the institution, but is usually 24-48 hours, or 24 hours after an indicated surgical procedure.

    The foregoing policy should be automatic, but not absolute. Clinicians must have the option of requesting that units be held longer for specific clinical indications, provided those indications do not lead to increased adverse effects of transfusion. The availability of a validated computer crossmatch system allows better utilization of available inventory for patients who have no clinically significant antibodies detected by antibody screening and history review. For such patients, a postcrossmatch time limitation will become a moot point.

    Another exception may be when antigen-negative units have been obtained (often with great difficulty) for a patient with a particular blood group antibody. The likelihood of a continuing need will dictate that such units be reserved for the patient.

3. Patients receiving a series of transfusions are at particular risk of forming blood group antibodies that could cause future transfusion reactions. Because such antibodies can form quickly and unpredictably, standards require that a crossmatch sample be valid only for 3 days, after which a new one must be obtained. This is particularly important in patients who have either been pregnant or had transfusions within the past 3 months. The rule may be waived for those who have not had either such event, but the Blood Bank seldom is provided with such information.

    Both the foregoing rules (ie, the 1-day hold of blood and the 3-day hold of crossmatch samples) are best written into standard policies so as to form part of the operating routine. Requests for exceptions should be the responsibility of the clinical physician and should be referred to the Blood Bank physician for evaluation.

TRANSFUSIONS IN TRAUMA AND OTHER EMERGENCIES

Transfusions may be needed at once in an emergency, in which delay may result in loss of life. In such a case, somewhat different procedures are essential and some steps, such as the crossmatch, may have to be dispensed within the interest of time. All abbreviated procedures increase the risk to the patient, but to varying degrees.

In this discussion, understand that "blood" usually means red blood cells (previously also known as "packed cells"). Whole blood may be the preferred transfusion medium in acute blood loss or in hypovolemic shock, but it is seldom presently available. Experience has shown that emergencies and massive surgical procedures can be effectively treated with red blood cells and appropriate plasma expanders.

The following procedures are suggested for different periods of time available.

1. **No sample, blood needed now.** Give type O Rh-negative red cells (packed cells) without delay and a blood sample requested. If O Rh-negative blood is in short supply, the physician should be informed and O Rh-positive red cells (packed cells) issued. Better a live, immunized patient than a dead one without antibodies. As soon as the patient's own blood type is known, type-specific units can be issued.

2. **Blood sample provided, blood needed in 5-10 minutes.** Give blood of the patient's own type without cross-match. If any blood is needed before the typing is finished, use two units of O Rh-negative red cells (packed cells) immediately, with type-specific to follow.

In both the foregoing situations, it is important for all persons involved to understand that **blood issued in this manner may turn out to be incompatible with the recipient.** The patient's physician must be notified as soon as possible if any test (eg, antibody screen or crossmatch) subsequently becomes positive or reactive.

3. **Blood sample provided, blood needed in 15-30 minutes.** It may be possible to complete the antibody screen (and crossmatches) within this time, depending on the technique used and number of units issued. If the antibody screen is completed and no clinically significant antibodies detected, chances are results on the crossmatches will be the same.

4. **Afterwards.** Complete all serologic testing, including the antibody screen and all crossmatches so that the patient's record will be complete. Documentation must be received on whose authority this departure from normal transfusion protocol was performed. Many hospitals require an Emergency Release form to document the original request.

5. **Additional guidelines.** Blood Bank and Emergency Department should develop policies and procedures together, so that surprises do not emerge during emergencies. Such topics include the importance of sample pickup, identification, and the principles of blood selection. The emergency department should be notified of times of blood shortage.

A well-designed emergency identification system is vital, since the patient's identity may be unknown and since some of the usual precautions cannot be used. The system must also be applicable to the multiple trauma situation (imagine dealing with 4 or 5 people from an accident, all with the same surname) and to the mass casualty disaster.

If red top tubes are used, remember that blood samples do not clot immediately, and there may be difficulty with fibrin shreds in incompletely clotted samples.

The community's supply of O Rh-negative blood should not be exhausted on a single massive trauma case. It is reasonable to switch to Rh-positive early, particularly in the case of a male or female of nonchildbearing age, in whom the effects of immunization are more manageable. This, too, can be part of an understanding between the Blood Bank and the Emergency Department. The Blood Bank physician should always make sure that such decisions are appropriately documented with the names of the deciding parties.

See listing, Uncrossmatched Blood, Emergency *on page 865*.

GUIDELINES FOR OUTPATIENT TRANSFUSION

With some minor exceptions, mostly concerning the timing of the blood sample and crossmatch, outpatient transfusions are handled as are those for inpatients. The precautions are the same, and if the hospital clinic staff is not accustomed to dealing with transfusions, it must be trained to do so.

1. **Informed consent.** The patient should give informed consent. In 1995, the Joint Commission on Accreditation of Healthcare Organizations added the requirement for blood transfusion informed consent to its standards for hospital accreditation. Follow state or local guidelines as to the frequency of required informed consent.

2. **Pretransfusion testing.** Positive identification procedures must be followed for outpatients. There must be no doubt about the identity of the patient and the sample. Alternative methods for identification have been developed, including photographic identification such as a driver's license. If the patient has been pregnant or transfused with allogeneic red cells in the preceding 3 months, a sample shall be obtained within 3 days of the scheduled transfusion.

3. **Quantity to be transfused.** Since most of these patients have chronic conditions, and many are elderly, it may not be possible or desirable to infuse their units rapidly. For these reasons, it is seldom practical to give more than two units in 1 day.

4. **Observation.** The patient should be observed continuously for the first 15 minutes, frequently thereafter. After the transfusion is completed, the patient should remain under observation for at least 30 minutes. If the transfusion is performed in a clinic, it is better that a relative or friend be available to accompany the patient home.

Staff should report any untoward reaction at once to the clinic physician or the patient's physician (see Transfusion Reaction Work-up *on page 864* and Risks of Transfusion *on page 861*). In such a case, the transfusion should be stopped and a saline drip allowed to continue. The Blood Bank should be notified promptly.

5. **Instructions.** It is potentially useful to have a set of printed instructions or an informative brochure to provide to patients.

6. **Follow-up.** The patient's physician should inform the Blood Bank of any delayed untoward reactions to the transfusion, or of any evidence of transfusion-associated infectious disease. It may be helpful to see that the physician gets a copy of the *Circular of Information for the Use of Human Blood and Blood Components*, prepared jointly by the American Association of Blood Banks, America's Blood Centers, and American Red Cross, which should be obtainable from the community blood center or hospital transfusion service.

QUALITY ASSURANCE

Transfusion services and blood centers strive for quality improvement as a means to improve patient outcome. Physicians practicing in hospitals and using blood services are likely to find their transfusion practices monitored by an institutional Transfusion Review Committee. This is a requirement of the Joint Commission on Accreditation of Health Care Organizations (JCAHO). The commission requires detailed records of transfusion practices, including indications, single-unit transfusions, transfusion, transfusion reactions, and clinical effectiveness. Other accrediting agencies, such as the American Association of Blood Banks (AABB) and the College of American Pathologists (CAP), sponsor inspection and accreditation programs. The Health Care Financing Administration (HCFA), through its CLIA '88 regulation, requires laboratories to follow a quality assurance program, which both CAP and AABB provide. The Food and Drug Administration (FDA), as noted in 21 CFR 211, requires an independent quality assurance unit with responsibility for the overall quality of the finished "product", so called. Development and use of quality and operational systems, guided by a quality program, is changing the approach from error detection to prevention, to improve the safety and adequacy of the blood supply.

Current concern over adverse effects, cost, and potential litigious climate of transfusion medicine all justify an important role for quality assurance procedures. The physician must not only strive to become educated about transfusion medicine and follow established transfusion criteria, but is urged to document in every patient's clinical records the rationale for using blood or its components in the clinically existing circumstances.

The authors and editors express appreciation to two outstanding authors of this chapter in earlier editions, Dr Douglas W. Huestis and Dr David C. Jenkins.

Summary Chart of Blood Components

Component	Major Indications	Action	Not Indicated for –	Special Precautions	Hazards	Rate of Infusion
Whole blood	Symptomatic anemia with large volume deficit	Restoration of oxygen-carrying capacity, restoration of blood volume	Condition responsive to specific component	Must be ABO-identical Labile coagulation factors deteriorate within 24 hours after collection	Infectious diseases; graft-vs-host disease; septic/toxic, allergic, febrile reactions; circulatory overload	For massive loss, fast as patient can tolerate
Red blood cells; red blood cells, adenine-saline added	Symptomatic anemia	Restoration of oxygen carrying capacity	Pharmacologically treatable anemia Coagulation deficiency	Must be ABO-compatible	Infectious diseases; graft-vs-host disease; septic/toxic, allergic, febrile reactions	As patient can tolerate but less than 4 hours
Red blood cells, leukocytes removed	Symptomatic anemia, febrile reactions from leukocyte antibodies	Restoration of oxygen-carrying capacity	Pharmacologically treatable anemia Coagulation deficiency	Must be ABO-compatible	Infectious diseases; graft-vs-host disease; septic/toxic, allergic reaction (unless plasma also removed, eg, by washing)	As patient can tolerate but less than 4 hours
Fresh frozen plasma	Deficit of labile and stable plasma coagulation factors and TTP	Source of labile and nonlabile plasma factors	Condition responsive to volume replacement	Should be ABO-compatible	Infectious diseases; allergic reactions; circulatory overload	Less than 4 hours
Liquid plasma, plasma, and thawed plasma	Deficit of stable coagulation factors	Source of nonlabile factors	Deficit of labile coagulation factors or volume replacement	Should be ABO-compatible	Infectious diseases, allergic reactions	Less than 4 hours
Cryoprecipitated AHF	Hemophilia A,* von Willebrand disease,* hypofibrinogenemia, factor XIII deficiency	Provides factor VIII, fibrinogen, vWF, factor XIII	Conditions not deficient in contained factors	Frequent repeat doses may be necessary	Infectious diseases, allergic reactions	Less than 4 hours
Platelets; platelets, pheresis	Bleeding from thrombocytopenia or platelet function abnormality	Improves hemostasis	Plasma coagulation deficits and some conditions with rapid platelet destruction (eg, ITP)	Should not use microaggregate filters	Infectious diseases; graft-vs-host disease; septic/toxic, allergic, febrile reactions	Less than 4 hours
Granulocytes, pheresis	Neutropenia with infection	Provides granulocytes	Infection responsive to antibiotics	Must be ABO-compatible, do not use microaggregate filters	Infectious diseases; graft-vs-host disease; allergic, febrile reactions	One apheresis unit over 2- to 4-hour period – closely observe for reactions

*Use when virus-inactivated concentrates are not available.

Modified from *Circular of Information for the Use of Human Blood and Blood Components*, American Association of Blood Banks, America's Blood Centers, and American Red Cross, 2000.

References

American Association of Blood Banks, *Standards for Hematopoietic Progenitor Cell Services*, 2nd ed, Bethesda, MD: American Association of Blood Banks Press, 2000, 1-81.

AuBuchon JP, "Optimizing the Cost-Effectiveness of Quality Assurance in Transfusion Medicine," *Arch Pathol Lab Med*, 1999, 123(7):603-6.

Belanger AC, "Joint Commission on Accreditation of Healthcare Organizations' Expectations for Transfusion Medicine in Healthcare Organizations," *Arch Pathol Lab Med*, 1999, 123(6):472-4.

Blumberg N, "The Costs and Consequences of Management Fads and Politically Driven Regulatory Oversight: The Case of Blood Transfusion," *Arch Pathol Lab Med*, 1999, 123(7):580-4.

Carmel R and Shulman IA, "Blood Transfusion in Medically Treatable Chronic Anemia. Pernicious Anemia as a Model for Transfusion Overuse," *Arch Pathol Lab Med*, 1989, 113(9):995-7.

Code of Federal Regulations, Title 21 CFR Parts 200-299, 600-799, Washington, DC: U.S. Government Printing Office, 1998.

Joint Commission of Accreditation of Healthcare Organizations, *Comprehensive Accreditation Manual for Hospitals*, Oakbrook Terrace, IL, 1999.

Goldman RL, "The Reliability of Peer Assessments of Quality of Care," *JAMA*, 1992, 267(7):958-60.

Goodnough LT and Audet AM, "Utilization Review for Red Cell Transfusion. Are We Just Going Through the Motions?" *Arch Pathol Lab Med*, 1996, 120(9):802-3.

Gustafson M, "Blood Safety: The Food and Drug Administration's Role," *Arch Pathol Lab Med*, 1999, 123(6):475-7.

Hamlin WB, "Requirements for Accreditation by the College of American Pathologists Laboratory Accreditation Program," *Arch Pathol Lab Med*, 1999, 123(6):465-7.

Hanson M, "The Ps and Qs of Quality Systems," *Arch Pathol Lab Med*, 1999, 123(7):576-9.

Lam HT, Schweitzer SO, Petz L, et al, "Are Retrospective Peer-Review Transfusion Monitoring Systems Effective in Reducing Red Blood Cell Utilization?" *Arch Pathol Lab Med*. 1996, 120(9):810-16.

Marconi M, Almini D, Pizzi N, et al, "Quality Assurance of Clinical Transfusion Practice by Implementation of the Privilege of Blood Prescriptions and Computerized Prospective Audit of Blood Requests," *Transfus Med*, 1996, 6(1):11-9.

McCurdy K and Gregory K, *Blood Bank Regulations: A to Z*, 2nd ed, Bethesda, MD: American Association of Blood Banks, 1999.

Menitove J, ed, *Standards for Blood Banks and Transfusion Services*, 20th ed, Bethesda, MD: American Association of Blood Banks, 2000.

Otter J and Cooper ES, "What Do the Accreditation Organizations Expect? American Association of Blood Banks," *Arch Pathol Lab Med*, 1999, 123(6):468-71.

Sazama K, "College of American Pathologists Conference XXXIII on Transfusion Medicine Performance Improvement," *Arch Pathol Lab Med*, 1999, 123(8):680-1.

Sherman LA, "Outcomes in Transfusion," *Arch Pathol Lab Med*, 1999, 123(7):599-602.

Shulman IR, Saxena S, Ramer L, et al, "Assessing Blood Administering Practices," *Arch Pathol Lab Med*, 1999, 123(7):595-8.

Smith DM and Otter J, "Performance Improvement in a Hospital Transfusion Service. The American Association of Blood Banks' Quality Systems Approach," *Arch Pathol Lab Med*, 1999, 123(7):585-91.

Toy P, "Guiding the Decision to Transfuse: Interventions That Do and Do Not Work," *Arch Pathol Lab Med*, 1999, 123(7):592-4.

Vengelen-Tyler V, *Technical Manual*, 13th ed, Bethesda, MD: American Association of Blood Banks Press, 1999, 1-36.

Wanamaker V, "Health Care Financing Administration/Clinical Laboratory Improvement Amendments of 1988," *Arch Pathol Lab Med*, 1999, 123(6):4 78-81.

Web Sites

Hematopoietic Progenitor Cells
American Association of Blood Banks: www.aabb.org
Bone Marrow Donors Worldwide: www.bmdw.org
Cord Blood Donor Foundation: www.cordblooddonor.org
International Society for Hematotherapy and Graft Engineering: www.ishage.org
The Blood and Marrow Transplant Newsletter Web Site: www.bmtnews.org
The National Marrow Donor Program (NMDP): www.marrow.org
TransWeb: www.transweb.org

Recalls/Withdrawals/Safety Issues
Center for Biologics Evaluation and Research: www.fda.gov/cber
The Pennsylvania Society of Health-System Pharmacists: www.pshp.org

Transfusion Medicine (General)
American Association of Blood Banks: www.aabb.org
American Red Cross: www.redcross.org
America's Blood Centers: www.americasblood.org
International Council for Commonality in Blood Banking Automation, Inc: www.iccbba.com
National Institutes of Health: www.nih.org

- ◆ **ABO Group and Rh Type** *see* Pretransfusion Testing *on page 856*

- ◆ **Acid Elution Test** *see* Rosette Test for Fetomaternal Hemorrhage *on page 863*

- ◆ **Acute Normovolemic Hemodilution** *see* Autologous Transfusion, Intraoperative Blood Salvage *on page 836*

- ◆ **Adverse Effects** *see* Risks of Transfusion *on page 861*

- ◆ **Adverse Effects** *see* Transfusion Reaction Work-up *on page 864*

- ◆ **Adverse Reactions** *see* Risks of Transfusion *on page 861*

- ◆ **Adverse Reactions** *see* Transfusion Reaction Work-up *on page 864*

- ◆ **AHF, Lyophilized** *see* Factor VIII Concentrate *on page 841*

Albumin and Plasma Protein Fraction for Infusion

Related Information
Albumin, Serum *on page 88*
Fibrinogen *on page 341*
Prothrombin Time *on page 354*

Applies to Normal Serum Albumin (Human); Plasma Protein Fraction (Human) (PPF)

Abstract A commercially prepared derivative of donor plasma, human albumin is 96% pure. The manufacturing process and heat inactivation for 10 hours at 60°C destroys viruses. Albumin is available as either 5% or 25% (weight/volume). For volume expansion alone, hydroxyethyl starch or electrolyte solutions are much cheaper and often suitable. **Plasma protein fraction (PPF)** is 83% albumin.

Patient Preparation Dosage and administration: Give a 500 mL dose (10-20 mL/kg in children) rapidly for shock. Hypotension may be seen at rapid rates of administration with PPF (see Limitations). In the absence of shock, administer at a rate of 1-2 mL/minute.

Aftercare Follow blood pressure after rapid administration.

Use A volume expander used mostly for replacement of colloid in emergencies such as burns, pancreatitis, shock due to trauma, hemorrhage, or surgery; adult respiratory distress syndrome; with removal of ascitic fluid and for hypotension related to hemodialysis. Used as standard replacement in therapeutic plasma exchange. The 25% albumin is used in patients who are not dehydrated, but it may be used with large volumes of normal saline or lactated Ringer's solution.

Limitations Does not contain clotting factors; brief retention; not effective for nutritional objectives. **Side effects and hazards**: Fast administration can cause fluid overload, especially with the hyperosmotic 25 g/dL albumin. Letters published recently deserve consideration. Although albumin is concentrated about fivefold in 25% albumin, the electrolytes are not. When diluted with water or dextrose in water, fluid electrolytes become proportionally low. Large volumes of such fluid infused rapidly may lead to hyponatremia and cerebral swelling.

Hemolysis may occur when sterile water is used to dilute 25% albumin.[1]

Additional saline must be given to patients who are dehydrated. PPF may contain Hageman factor fragments that can cause hypotension on rapid infusion (>10 mL/minute). PPF may also lead to anaphylaxis in IgA-deficient patients. It is expensive. There are periodic shortages.

Contraindications Cardiac failure with congestion; not suitable for nutritional support

Additional Information Albumin is not "salt-poor". Sodium content is 100-160 mmol/L; PPF has 130-160 mmol/L. No filter is needed during infusion. No antibodies are present. In plasma exchange, replacement can usually be part albumin and part isotonic saline.[2]

Footnotes
1. Kravath RE, "More on Dangerous Dilution of 25% Albumin," *N Engl J Med*, 1998, 339(9):634.
2. Trissel LA and Manasse HR, "More on Dangerous Dilution of 25% Albumin," *N Engl J Med*, 1998, 339(9):634-5.

References
Alexander MR, Alexander B, Mustion AL, et al, "Therapeutic Use of Albumin: 2," *JAMA*, 1982, 247:831-3.
Erstad BL, Gales BJ, and Rappaport WD, "The Use of Albumin in Clinical Practice," *Arch Intern Med*, 1991, 151:901-11.
Swisher SN and Petz LD, "Plasma and Plasma Derivatives," *Clinical Practice of Transfusion Medicine*, 3rd ed, Petz LK, Swisher SN, Kleinman S, et al, eds, New York, NY: Churchill Livingstone, 1996, 947-65.
Triulzi DJ, *Blood Transfusion Therapy. A Physician's Handbook*, 6th ed, Bethesda, MD: American Association of Blood Banks Press, 1999, 45-7.

- ◆ **Allogeneic Blood Transfusion** *replaced by* Autologous Transfusion, Intraoperative Blood Salvage *on page 836*

- ◆ **Allogeneic Blood Transfusion** *see* Donation, Blood *on page 839*

- ◆ **Alloimmunization, Leukocyte** *see* Filters for Blood *on page 842*

- ◆ **ANH** *see* Autologous Transfusion, Intraoperative Blood Salvage *on page 836*

Antibodies to IgA

Related Information
Frozen Red Blood Cells *on page 842*
Immunoglobulin A *on page 532*
Plasma, Fresh Frozen *on page 851*
Plasma, Frozen, Donor Retested *on page 851*
Platelet Transfusion *on page 854*
Red Blood Cells *on page 857*
Red Blood Cells, Washed *on page 859*
Risks of Transfusion *on page 861*
Transfusion Reaction Work-up *on page 864*

Synonyms Anti-immunoglobulin A; IgA Antibodies

Abstract While 1 in 600 individuals are IgA deficient, IgA anaphylactic transfusion reactions occur infrequently, in approximately 1 in 20,000 to 47,000 transfusions.[1] Antibodies to IgA may be found in sera of individuals who have anaphylactic reactions. Most, but not all, of these individuals are IgA deficient and some authors have questioned the need for screening for IgA levels in diagnosis of anaphylactic reactions.[2]

IgA-deficient individuals who have developed anti-A can only accept plasma fractions prepared from donors completely lacking IgA.[3]

Patient Preparation If possible, delay transfusion in patients who have had an anaphylactic reaction until a pretransfusion sample can be tested for the presence of antibodies to IgA. If antibodies are present, transfuse with IgA-deficient or autologous blood components. Frozen, thawed-deglycerolized red blood cells, washed red blood cells,[4] or washed platelets[5] may be used. Consult manufacturer's package insert prior to infusion of any plasma derivative (eg, immunoglobulin, factor concentrate) and use only those noted to be IgA deficient.

Aftercare Signs and symptoms may occur up to as long as 1 hour after transfusion and are related to cutaneous (hives, pruritus, sweating, flushing of face, angioedema), respiratory (dyspnea, laryngeal edema, wheezing, stridor), gastrointestinal (cramps, nausea, vomiting, diarrhea), and cardiovascular (hypotension, light-headedness, shock, sternal pain, syncope, collapse, arrhythmia) systems.[1,3] For anaphylactic reactions, the transfusion must be stopped and I.V. line kept open with normal saline. For less severe reactions (without marked hypotension), subcutaneous epinephrine (0.3-0.5 mL of a 1:1000 solution, repeated every 20-30 minutes, up to 3 doses) may be administered. Intravenous aminophylline (6 mg/kg loading dose) may be administered for bronchospasm. Normal saline may be administered for volume expansion and oxygen for patients in respiratory distress. For severe hypotension, intravenous epinephrine (0.5 mL of a 1:10,000 solution, repeated every 5-10 minutes as needed) may be administered. Endotracheal intubation may be necessary.[2] Save blood component, notify Blood Bank, and perform transfusion reaction work-up (see Transfusion Reaction Work-up *on page 864*).

Specimen Serum

Container Red top tube or SST™ tube

Sampling Time Ideally, utilize specimen obtained prior to transfusion of blood component or derivative implicated in the anaphylactic reaction.

Turnaround Time Results of testing for antibody to IgA may not be available prior to the decision to transfuse again, as this test is sent to specialized reference laboratories.

Reference Interval Anti-IgA: negative

Use Evaluate anaphylactic adverse effect of transfusion

Limitations Pre-existing antibodies to other serum proteins may exist which also cause anaphylaxis.[6] Thus, a negative test for antibodies to IgA does not mean that the patient may not suffer another anaphylactic reaction. In such rare cases, transfusion of routine (unwashed) blood components under close medical supervision has been advocated. If no reaction occurs, routine transfusions can be continued. If another reaction occurs, continue with washed blood components.[2] In some individuals, more than a single washing is required. In some cases, frozen deglycerolized red cells can be given slowly, but washed cells, cell-free plasma, or plasma protein fraction cause reaction. Such individuals tolerate blood from donors known to lack IgA.[3]

Detection of antibodies to IgA in a nontransfused individual by passive hemagglutination assays does not reliably predict risk of an anaphylactic transfusion reaction.

Methodology A test utilized to detect the presence of antibodies to IgA is passive hemagglutination inhibition. Positive tests are followed by neutralization to confirm specificity. Other methods of antibody identification include ELISA or radioimmunoassay.

Screening assays for IgA levels include rate nephelometry, Ouchterlony double diffusion, or electrophoresis. Samples identified as having undetectable IgA levels by the above methods should be confirmed by a more sensitive method, such as passive hemagglutination inhibition or radioimmunoassay.

Additional Information Exposure to blood fractions containing IgA in IgA-deficient individuals may induce IgG or IgE antibodies, which can cause anaphylactic reactions.[3,7] Immunoglobulin preparations may contain some IgA and lead to serious reactions. Mollison describes an individual without history of prior pregnancies or transfusion, who developed cyanosis and severe hypotension following infusion of as little as 10 mL of blood. This individual had a potent IgG complement-fixing anti-IgA.[3]

(Continued)

Antibodies to IgA *(Continued)*

IgA **red cell** autoantibodies are also recognized. They may be idiopathic or associated with neoplasms.[8]

Footnotes

1. Sandler SG, Mallory D, Malamut D, et al, "IgA Anaphylactic Transfusion Reactions," *Transfus Med Rev*, 1995, 9(1):1-8.
2. Vamvakas EC and Pineda AA, "Allergic and Anaphylactic Reactions," *Transfusion Reactions*, Popovsky MA, ed, Bethesda, MD: American Association of Blood Banks Press, 1996, 81-124.
3. Mollison PL, Engelfriet CP, Contreras M, et al, "Some Unfavorable Effects of Transfusion," *Blood Transfusion in Clinical Medicine*, 10th ed, Chapter 15, Oxford, UK: Blackwell Scientific Publications, 1997, 487-508.
4. Baroti Toth C, Kramer J, Pinter J, et al, "IgA Content of Washed Red Blood Cell Concentrates," *Vox Sang*, 1998, 74(1):13-4.
5. Sloand EM, Fox SM, Banks SM, et al, "Preparation of IgA-Deficient Platelets," *Transfusion*, 1990, 30:332-6.
6. Lambin P, Le Pennec PY, Hauptmann G, et al, "Adverse Transfusion Reactions Associated With a Precipitating Anti-C4 Antibody of Anti-Rodgers Specificity," *Vox Sang*, 1984, 47:242-49.
7. Insel RA and Quaidoo EA, "Disorders of Lymphocyte Function," *Hematology: Basic Principles and Practice*, 3rd ed, Hoffman R, Benz EJ Jr, Shattil SJ, et al, eds, New York, NY: Churchill Livingstone, 2000, 762-82.
8. Sokol RJ, Booker DJ, Stamps R, et al, "IgA Red Cell Autoantibodies and Autoimmune Hemolysis," *Transfusion*, 1997, 37(2):175-81.

Antibody Detection/Identification, Red Cell

Related Information

Antibody Titer *on page 834*
Antiglobulin Test, Indirect *on page 835*
Hemolytic Disease of the Newborn, Antibody Identification *on page 846*
Pretransfusion Testing *on page 856*
Transfusion Reaction Work-up *on page 864*

Synonyms Irregular Antibody Detection/Identification; Unexpected Antibody Detection/Identification

Applies to Autoimmune Hemolytic Anemia Work-up; Investigation of Hemolytic Disease of the Newborn

Test Includes Absorption/elution procedures to distinguish between auto- and alloantibodies; antibody titration studies; red cell antigen typing

Abstract The incidence of immunization to red cell antigens has been determined to be in the order of 1% to 1.5% in the population at large. It is much higher in certain subgroups (eg, sickle cell patients). It is mandatory, therefore, that pretransfusion testing includes an antibody screen. The finding of a positive antibody screen requires further testing with an extended panel of phenotyped red cells to establish the identity of the antibody.

Specimen Blood

Container One red top tube and one lavender top (EDTA) tube is usually sufficient (complex cases may require additional specimen).

Causes for Rejection Gross hemolysis, sample collected in wrong tube (eg, serum separator tube), improper labeling

Turnaround Time Highly variable, depends on complexity of case

Special Instructions Provide Blood Bank with diagnosis, medications, and history of prior pregnancy and transfusions.

Use The object of antibody detection is to detect and subsequently identify clinically important red cell antibodies. Thus, antibody screening is a routine pretransfusion test. Antibody detection and identification also play an important role in the investigation protocols for hemolytic disease of the newborn (HDN), hemolytic anemia, and transfusion reactions.

Limitations Antibody directed to low incidence or "private" antigens, which may not be represented on the testing cell panel, will not be detected. On some occasions, antibody levels are too low for detection.

Contraindications A blood sample taken shortly after massive transfusion or exchange transfusion will not be representative of the patient's blood. In these cases, a limited pretransfusion testing protocol may be implemented.

Methodology Patients' sera are screened for unexpected red cell antibodies by testing against an abbreviated red cell panel selected to contain all the clinically important antigens. The tests are carried out by a variety of techniques with the expectation that all clinically significant antibodies will be detected. Antibody identification is performed in the same way but with extended panels of fully phenotyped red cells.

In cases of HDN and hemolytic anemia, testing may need to be performed with antibody eluted from autologous or test red cells. The presence of autoantibody may mask the serologic expression of underlying alloantibody. In these cases, absorption procedures may be necessary to remove the autoantibody. Autoabsorption and elution studies may require the provision of further blood samples from the patient.

A solid phase method has been described, but failed to detect some antibodies.[1]

Additional Information Specificity and serological characteristics of red cell antibodies are the usual determinants of clinical significance. Determination of antibody specificity permits the appropriate selection of donor blood for compatibility tests.

It is customary to screen for unexpected antibodies associated with HDN early in pregnancy. All positive screen results require antibody identification to permit assessment of clinical significance. Titration of antibody levels throughout the course of the pregnancy may indicate the likelihood of HDN.

Similarly, antibody characterization may assist in the diagnosis of autoimmune hemolytic anemia.

See Anemia, Hemolytic in the Key Word Index.

Footnotes

1. Nagamine K, Kiyokawa T, Aochi H, et al, "A Simple Solid-Phase Method for the Identification of Red Cell-Bound Antibodies Without Elution," *Am J Clin Pathol*, 1996, 106(3):365-9.

References

Issitt PD and Anstee DJ, *Applied Blood Group Serology*, 4th ed, Durham, NC: Montgomery Scientific Publications, 1998, 877-905, 1045-95.
Vengelen-Tyler V, *Technical Manual*, 13th ed, Bethesda, MD: American Association of Blood Banks Press, 1999, 495-512.

Antibody Titer

Related Information

Antibody Detection/Identification, Red Cell *on page 834*
Prenatal Screen, Immunohematology *on page 855*

Synonyms Unexpected Antibody Titer

Applies to Hemolytic Disease of the Newborn, Antibody Titer

Test Includes Known positive antibody screen and identification

Specimen Serum

Container Red top tube

Storage Instructions Keep serum frozen to permit subsequent parallel titrations.

Causes for Rejection Gross hemolysis, sample collected in a serum separator tube, improper labeling

Possible Panic Range Increase of titration value over previous level (at least two dilutions)

Use Antibody titration is an attempt to quantitate antibody by testing serial twofold dilutions against a selected red cell. Results are expressed as the reciprocal of the highest dilution showing serologic activity. Comparative titrations can demonstrate a change in antibody levels over time. This information may be valuable in prenatal studies of Rh-negative mothers with anti-D or other antibody associated with hemolytic disease of the newborn (HDN). Decisions to perform amniocentesis may be based to some extent on maternal antibody titration results.

Limitations Manual titration methods are inherently subjective. It is important that successive studies of the same patient be performed in the same laboratory by a standardized technique with the red cells from the same donor, if possible; if not, then with cells of the same phenotype. The use of semiautomated pipettes is highly advised.

Contraindications Antibody screening test is negative or antibody identification indicates that the detected antibody is not associated with HDN; or paternal red cell studies show that father lacks the offending antigen.

Methodology Serial (usually doubling) dilutions of the serum are tested against red cells of the appropriate phenotype by a technique that demonstrates activity of the antibody. The end-point is recorded as the reciprocal of the highest dilution expressing activity.

Additional Information Although an indirect antiglobulin titration end-point of 16-32 or higher has been considered significant for anti-D, it does not follow that this result is significant in the case of other alloantibody specificities. Failure to demonstrate a rising titer of maternal alloantibody through the course of pregnancy does not necessarily preclude HDN.

References

Vengelen-Tyler V, *Technical Manual*, 13th ed, Bethesda, MD: American Association of Blood Banks Press, 1999, 415-6.

♦ **Antiglobulin-Augmented Lymphotoxicity Assay** *see* Platelet Transfusion *on page 854*

Antiglobulin Test, Direct

Related Information

Anemia Flowchart *on page 392*
Cord Blood Screen *on page 838*
Hemosiderin Stain, Urine *on page 876*
Pretransfusion Testing *on page 856*
Rh₀(D) Immune Globulin (Human) *on page 860*
Transfusion Reaction Work-up *on page 864*

Synonyms Antihuman Globulin; Coombs Test, Direct; DAT; Direct Antiglobulin Test; Direct Coombs Test

Applies to Antiglobulin Test, Direct, Complement; Sensitization

Test Includes Direct antiglobulin testing with monospecific antihuman globulin reagents, red cell elution, and antibody identification

Abstract The direct antiglobulin test (DAT) utilizes reagent antihuman globulin to detect nonagglutinating antibodies bound *in vivo* to the surface of red cells. The test may be performed with polyspecific reagent that will detect red cell bound IgG and complement components (C3) or with monospecific anti-IgG/anticomplement reagents. The DAT is of special value in the diagnosis of hemolytic disease of the newborn (HDN) and autoimmune hemolytic anemia. The simultaneous presence of antibodies to erythrocytes, causing AHA, and antibodies to platelets, causing idiopathic thrombocytopenic purpura (ITP) is known as Evans syndrome. Evans syndrome can be drug-induced or idiopathic, like AHA and ITP.

Specimen Blood (cord blood for the investigation of HDN)

Container One red top tube (cord blood) for HDN investigation; one lavender top (EDTA) tube and one red top tube in other cases. The DAT should be performed on an EDTA (lavender) top tube to avoid artifactual complement activation (see Limitations). Therefore, do not request a red top tube for non-HDN investigations.

Causes for Rejection Gross hemolysis, sample not in EDTA tube (other than HDN testing), improper labeling

Special Instructions Provide diagnosis, transfusion history, obstetric history, and medication list to the Blood Bank.

Reference Interval Negative

Use Polyspecific antiglobulin reagent detects red cell bound immunoglobulin (especially IgG) as well as complement components. The DAT is commonly utilized in the investigation of antibody-induced hemolysis (eg, HDN, auto-immune hemolytic anemia, and transfusion reaction).

Limitations The finding of red cell bound IgG or complement components is not invariably associated with in vivo hemolysis. It is well known that a small percentage of normal blood donors present with positive direct antiglobulin tests. The most frequent cause of a positive DAT in nonhemolysing patients is associated with drug-induced antibodies. Whole blood samples should not be refrigerated before testing. At low temperature, cold autoantibodies present in many sera can activate complement. Artifactual complement activation can be avoided by the exclusive use of EDTA specimens for direct antiglobulin testing.

Methodology Red cells washed free of extraneous immunoproteins are exposed to antihuman globulin and anticomplement components (C3) as polyspecific or monospecific reagents. Agglutination indicates sensitization.

Additional Information The direct antiglobulin (Coombs) test will detect red cells sensitized with IgG in cases of HDN and warm antibody hemolytic anemia. The appropriate reagent will detect red cells sensitized with complement C3 components in cases of cold antibody hemolytic anemia. The test is usefully applied in other cases of suspected in vivo hemolysis, such as transfusion reactions and drug-induced hemolytic anemia.

Interpretation of a positive DAT includes clinical history, diagnosis, and drug exposure. Mechanisms of positive DAT include warm autoantibodies, hypergammaglobulinemia, and passively acquired antibodies. Warm auto-immune hemolytic anemias are usually mediated by IgG, less frequently by IgG with C3 and uncommonly with C3 alone.[1]

Footnotes
1. Chambers LA and Cook SS, "Clinical Pathology Rounds: An Unexpected Positive Direct Antiglobulin Test," Lab Med, 1996, 27(2):89-91.

References
Churchill WH and Nguyen PL, "A 32-Year-Old Man With IgG Antibody and Coombs'-Positive Hemolytic Anemia Resistant to Corticosteroid Therapy," Case Records of the Massachusetts General Hospital, Case 13-1997, Scully RE, Mark EJ, McNeely WF, et al, eds, N Engl J Med, 1997, 336(17):1235-41.

Garratty G, "Drug-Induced Immune Hemolytic Anemia," Immunobiology of Transfusion Medicine, New York, NY: Marcel Dekker, 1994, 523-51.

Issitt PD and Anstee DJ, Applied Blood Group Serology, 4th ed, Durham, NC: Montgomery Scientific Publications, 1998, 115-63, 1019.

Vengelen-Tyler V, Technical Manual, 13th ed, Bethesda, MD: American Association of Blood Banks Press, 1999, 419-49.

♦ **Antiglobulin Test, Direct, Complement** see Antiglobulin Test, Direct on page 834

Antiglobulin Test, Indirect

Related Information
Anemia Flowchart on page 392
Antibody Detection/Identification, Red Cell on page 834
Hemolytic Disease of the Newborn, Antibody Identification on page 846
Prenatal Screen, Immunohematology on page 855
Pretransfusion Testing on page 856

Synonyms Indirect Coombs Test

Abstract The indirect antiglobulin test (IAT) was developed to demonstrate the presence of nonagglutinating IgG alloantibodies in patient's serum or plasma.

Specimen Blood

Container Red top tube or lavender top (EDTA) tube

Causes for Rejection Gross hemolysis, sample collected in serum separator tube, improper labeling

Reference Interval Negative

Use The indirect antiglobulin test (IAT) is a reliable screening procedure for clinically relevant antibodies in patient sera. Effective in detection of alloantibodies (99.6% detection), the IAT is used in antibody screening and identification tests in prenatal evaluations. It is used in investigation of hemolytic conditions, and especially in routine pretransfusion compatibility testing.

Limitations Antibodies directed to low incidence "private" antigens may not be represented on the screening or identification panels and will not be detected. At the time of testing, antibody levels may be below detectable limits.

Methodology This is a two-stage test system. In the first stage, IgG antibody in patient's serum sensitizes test red cell sample (panel cell or donor unit). Red cell bound antibody is detected in the second stage by the use of anti-IgG antiglobulin reagent.

Gel test applications for IAT were recently reviewed. An issue of false-positive gel reactions was resolved with use of EDTA plasma. Rare instances of unsatisfactory detection by gel technology have been reported. The gel test was endorsed for community hospital use in a recent paper in a reputable journal.[1]

Additional Information The difference between the direct and indirect antiglobulin (Coombs) test is that the direct test is used to demonstrate in vivo red cell sensitization with antibody whereas the indirect test is used to demonstrate the presence of antibody in a patient's serum or plasma through in vitro sensitization.

Since its introduction in 1945, the indirect antiglobulin test became the most widely used test for detection and identification of irregular IgG antibodies. It is a simple test with high sensitivity capable of detecting as few as 100-200 molecules of IgG per cell. However, its one serious drawback has proved to be the difficulty of automating this two-staged test. It is not surprising that newer, semiautomated test systems (eg, solid-phase assays and gel tests[1]) are being increasingly used.

Footnotes
1. Cate JC IV and Reilly N, "Evaluation and Implementation of the Gel Test for Indirect Antiglobulin Testing in a Community Hospital Laboratory," Arch Pathol Lab Med, 1999, 123(8):693-7.

References
Issitt PD and Anstee DJ, Applied Blood Group Serology, 4th ed, Durham, NC: Montgomery Scientific Publications, 1998, 115-12.

Vengelen-Tyler V, Technical Manual, 13th ed, Bethesda, MD: American Association of Blood Banks Press, 1999, 392-3.

♦ **Antihemophilic Factor (Human)** see Factor VIII Concentrate on page 841

♦ **Antihuman Globulin** see Antiglobulin Test, Direct on page 834

♦ **Anti-immunoglobulin A** see Antibodies to IgA on page 833

Antineutrophil Antibody

Related Information
Antimitochondrial Antibody on page 505
Transfusion Reaction Work-up on page 864
White Blood Cell Count on page 496

Synonyms Granulocyte Antibody; Neutrophil Antibody

Applies to Granulocyte Agglutination Test; Granulocyte Immunofluorescence Test; Monoclonal Antibody Specific Immobilization of Granulocyte Antigens; Neutropenia

Test Includes For **autoimmune neutropenia:** neutrophil antibody identification and direct neutrophil testing. For **neonatal alloimmune neutropenia:** maternal antibody identification, crossmatching between maternal serum and paternal neutrophils and maternal and paternal neutrophil typing.

Abstract Neutrophil autoantibodies, both alloantibodies and autoantibodies, have been associated with a variety of clinical syndromes. **Autoimmune neutropenia** in adults may be idiopathic or may occur secondary to other diseases such as systemic lupus erythematosus. Autoimmune neutropenia in children, most frequently occurring between ages 6 months to 2 years, is relatively benign.[1] Maternal antibodies directed against fetal neutrophil allo-antigens cause **neonatal alloimmune neutropenia**. Medications should be considered as a cause of immune-mediated neutropenia.[2] Febrile, nonhemolytic transfusion reactions may be caused by neutrophil antibodies, although they are more frequently caused by HLA antibodies or passive transfer of cytokines. Either neutrophil or HLA antibodies may also induce transfusion-related acute lung injury (TRALI) (see Risks of Transfusion on page 861).

Aftercare Neonatal autoimmune neutropenia is relatively benign and may be managed with antibiotics only.[1] Other conditions (eg, drug-induced or neonatal alloimmune neutropenia) may be more life-threatening (secondary to increased risk of infection) and treatment may include intravenous immunoglobulin, granulocyte colony-stimulating factor and plasma exchange, in addition to antibiotics.

Specimen For autoimmune neutropenia: serum and neutrophils from patient. For neonatal alloimmune neutropenia: maternal serum and neutrophils, paternal neutrophils.

Container Red top tube (serum), lavender top (EDTA) (whole blood - provides neutrophils)

Sampling Time Always check with the laboratory performing testing as frequently cases must be scheduled.

Storage Instructions Serum may be separated and stored frozen, but neutrophils may not survive for long periods of time. Check with testing laboratory prior to collection.

Reference Interval Negative

Limitations Premature infants and patients with certain clinical conditions (eg, chronic myelogenous leukemia) may have depression of granulocyte antigens.

Methodology Granulocyte agglutination test (GAT), granulocyte immunofluorescence test (GIFT), monoclonal antibody specific immobilization of granulocyte antigens (MAIGA). A combination of tests is usually beneficial.[3]

Footnotes
1. Bux J, Gehrens G, Jaeger G, et al, "Diagnosis and Clinical Course of Autoimmune Neutropenia in Infancy: Analysis of 240 Cases," Blood, 1998, 91(1):181-6.
(Continued)

Antineutrophil Antibody (Continued)

2. Meyer O, Gaedicke G, and Salama A, "Demonstration of Drug-Dependent Antibodies in Two Patients With Neutropenia and Successful Treatment With Granulocyte Colony-Stimulating Factor," *Transfusion*, 1999, 39(5):527-30.

3. Bux J and Chapman J, "Report on the Second International Granulocyte Serology Workshop," *Transfusion*, 1997, 37(9):977-83.

References

Vengelen-Tyler V, *Technical Manual*, 13th ed, Bethesda, MD: American Association of Blood Banks Press, 1999, 339-56.

Stroncek DF, "Granulocyte Immunology: Is There a Need to Know?" *Transfusion*, 1997, 37(9):886-8.

♦ **Antiplatelet Antibody** *see* Platelet Antibody, Immunohematologic *on page 852*

Apheresis, Therapeutic

Related Information

Low Density Lipoprotein Cholesterol *on page 218*
Plasma Exchange *on page 850*
Platelets, Apheresis, Donation *on page 853*
Sickle Cell Tests *on page 486*

Synonyms Cytapheresis, Therapeutic; Cytoreduction; Plasmapheresis; Therapeutic Cytapheresis

Applies to Erythrocytapheresis; Granulocytapheresis; Leukapheresis, Therapeutic; Photopheresis; Red Cell Exchange; Stem Cell Collection

Test Includes ABO, Rh, antibody screen, and/or crossmatch if appropriate in the following instances: Red cells must be selected and crossmatched for a red cell exchange. Fresh frozen plasma must be selected and thawed if chosen as a replacement solution.

Abstract Selective removal of a pathologic component of a patient's blood to assist in the treatment of a disease. Separation techniques are varied and include manual (whole blood bags) and automated instruments (centrifugation, membrane filtration, and adsorption). With the numerous automated instruments available, manual techniques are seldom used.

Patient Preparation Excellent venous access is a daily requirement. Indwelling dual- or triple-lumen central venous catheters suitable for apheresis procedures are frequently necessary. Hypotension secondary to hypovolemia will become a concern if the extracorporeal volume exceeds 15% of the patient's blood volume. Patients taking angiotensin-converting-enzyme (ACE) inhibitors may be prone to marked hypotension prior to routine or immunosorption treatment. Such therapy should be removed from their medication if possible.[1] Understanding which drugs being given to the patient will be altered by the procedure is relevant, so that dosage can be adjusted accordingly (withhold administration for 1 hour before and after procedure if possible). Obtain and document informed consent.

Aftercare Monitor patient for signs and symptoms of reduced ionized calcium (tingling, perioral paresthesias, cardiac arrhythmias) and hypotension secondary to hypovolemia. Hypocalcemia may be managed by decreasing the inlet flow rate or administering intravenous calcium.[2]

Collection Carried out by Blood Bank personnel in apheresis area or patient's room

Causes for Rejection Decision to perform this procedure is shared between Clinical and Blood Bank physicians. Guidelines for evidence of therapeutic efficacy have been developed by the American Association of Blood Banks and the American Society for Apheresis.[3]

Special Instructions Usually done on a scheduled basis, the procedure can be emergent. Consult with a Blood Bank physician. Emergent procedures may include those for patients with thrombotic thrombocytopenic purpura with end-organ dysfunction; presence of monoclonal gammopathy (paraproteinemia) with significant hyperviscosity; and acute leukemia with an extremely high circulating blast count (>100 x 10^9/L) and evidence of leukostasis.[4]

Use During therapeutic plasmapheresis, plasma containing the pathologic substance is removed and replaced with crystalloids, albumin, or fresh frozen plasma. A combination of replacement fluids is often used. Usually 1-1.5 plasma volumes are exchanged. Selective removal of pathologic substances in plasma via adsorption columns (eg, dextran sulfate removal of LDL cholesterol and staphylococcal protein A removal of IgG antibodies) eliminates the need for replacement fluid. Remove abnormal red cells and replace with normal red cells in sickle cell disease with crisis or in hypertransfusion regimens. Reduce platelets in thrombocythemic patients or leukocytes in hyperleukocytic leukemia. Treat cutaneous T-cell lymphoma via photopheresis (separate lymphocytes, add psoralens, and treat the cells with ultraviolet irradiation prior to returning white cells to patient).[5]

Limitations The extent of each procedure will be determined by the Blood Bank physician in consultation with the clinical physician and is especially important if the patient is pediatric, elderly, clinically unstable, has poor vascular access, or has a condition for which apheresis is of unknown benefit.

Footnotes

1. Owen HG and Brecher ME, "Atypical Reactions Associated With the Use of Angiotensin-Converting Enzyme Inhibitors and Apheresis," *Transfusion*, 1994, 34:891-4.

2. Owen HG and Brecher ME, "Management of the Therapeutic Apheresis Patient," *Apheresis: Principles and Practice*, McLeon BC, Price TH, Drew MJ, eds, Bethesda, MD: American Association of Blood Banks Press, 1997, 223-49.

3. Vengelen-Tyler V, *Technical Manual*, 13th ed, Bethesda, MD: American Association of Blood Banks Press, 1999, 134-47.

4. Leitman S and Strauss R, "Questions and Answers - What Are the Indications for Emergency Hemapheresis?" *J Clin Apheresis*, 1991, 6:64.

5. Lim HW and Edelson RL, "Photopheresis for Treatment of Cutaneous T-Cell Lymphoma," *Hematol Oncol Clin North Am*, 1995, 9(5):1117-26.

References

"Clinical Applications of Therapeutical Apheresis," *J Clin Apheresis*, 2000, 15:1-159 (special issue).

McLeod BC, Price TH, and Drew MJ, "Apheresis Principles and Practice," Bethesda, MD: American Association of Blood Banks Press, 1997.

♦ **Autoimmune Hemolytic Anemia Work-up** *see* Antibody Detection/Identification, Red Cell *on page 834*

Autologous Transfusion, Intraoperative Blood Salvage

Related Information

Autologous Transfusion, Preoperative Deposit *on page 837*

Synonyms Acute Normovolemic Hemodilution; ANH; Blood Salvage, Intraoperative Autologous Transfusion

Applies to Intraoperative Cell Salvage; Normovolemic Hemodilution; Postoperative Cell Salvage

Replaces Allogeneic Blood Transfusion

Special Instructions Collection and recovery services require the coordinated efforts of a multidiscipline team composed of surgeons, anesthesiologists, transfusion medicine specialists, and personnel trained in the use of the equipment. In some regions, trained personnel and equipment are provided by the community blood center.

Methodology Although **preoperative** autologous blood collection is the best-known way of avoiding a transfusion of homologous blood, a patient's own blood may be saved and returned **during** the operation or immediately **afterwards**.

Three procedures are available.

1. **Intraoperative hemodilution (acute normovolemic hemodilution):** Blood is withdrawn into standard blood bags containing anticoagulant after the induction of anesthesia but before the surgical incision is made. Crystalloids or colloids can support the blood volume. Autologous units collected during acute normovolemic hemodilution (ANH) are returned at the conclusion of the surgical procedure (within 8 hours if stored at room temperature and 24 hours if stored in a monitored refrigerator). Recombinant erythropoietin has been used to increase its effectiveness.[1]

 - Patients should be selected for ANH if the following criteria are met:[2] the likelihood of transfusion exceeds 10%; the preoperative hemoglobin is at least 12 g/dL; lack of severe hypertension; lack of infection/bacteremia; and lack of clinically significant coronary, pulmonary, renal, or liver disease.

 - This procedure may diminish the need for allogeneic transfusions. The blood procured requires no testing, diminishing costs. Since the units removed remain in the operating room, mixup of units is diminished. Risk of bacterial contamination is almost eliminated.[3]

2. **Intraoperative cell salvage:** This procedure describes the technique of collecting and reinfusing blood lost by a patient during surgery, for procedures such as liver transplantation, repair of scoliosis, cardiac and vascular surgery. Many instruments collect shed blood, washing it in normal saline and concentrating the red blood cells. Most of the plasma and platelets are removed. Devices that neither wash nor concentrate blood prior to infusion increase the risk of adverse effects. A specially trained operator is required. Other systems usually involve collection of shed blood into a container from which it is returned to the patient through a filter. Without a wash step, such systems risk transfusion of thromboplastic debris admixed with the collected blood. Other risks include aspiration of tumor cells, the presence of infectious agents, or other constraints. The procedure is contraindicated in the presence of bacterial contamination; the equivalent of at least two units of blood must be recovered to reach cost-effective levels.[3] Its use in the presence of bacterial contamination and malignant disease is a contraindication in the British Committee for Standards in Hematology (BCSH) Guidelines for Cell Salvage.[1]

3. **Postoperative cell salvage:** Blood from mediastinal drainage and from other sterile operative sites is collected and reinfused, with or without washing. Reinfusion must be initiated within 6 hours of collection or the blood must be discarded.[4] Recovered blood is dilute and somewhat hemolyzed. The quantities salvaged are often too small to be cost-effective. The safety and benefit of postoperative cell salvage have been questioned.[3]

Additional Information Hospitals must establish documented policies, procedures, labeling requirements, and quality plans to assure proper patient identification, collection and infusion, sterility, and storage conditions. Such policies should be approved by appropriate departments of surgery, operating room committees where they exist, as well as by directors of transfusion services.

Footnotes

1. Duguid JK, "Autologous Blood Transfusion," *Clin Lab Haematol*, 1999, 21(6):371-6.

2. Vengelen-Tyler V, *Technical Manual*, 13th ed, Bethesda, MD: American Association of Blood Banks Press, 1999, 119-28.

3. Goodnough LT, Brecher ME, Kanter MH, et al, "Transfusion Medicine. Second of Two Parts - Blood Conservation," *N Engl J Med*, 1999, 340(7):525-33.

4. Menitove JE, *Standards for Blood Banks and Transfusion Services*, 19th ed, Bethesda, MD: American Association of Blood Banks Press, 1999, 78-9.

References

"Transfusion Alert: Use of Autologous Blood," National Heart, Lung, and Blood Institute Expert Panel on the Use of Autologous Blood, *Transfusion*, 1995, 35(8):703-11.

Autologous Transfusion, Preoperative Deposit

Related Information

Autologous Transfusion, Intraoperative Blood Salvage *on page 836*
Donation, Blood *on page 839*
Donation, Blood, Directed *on page 840*
Erythropoietin, Serum *on page 169*

Synonyms Autotransfusion; PAD; Predeposit Autologous Donation; Transfusion, Autologous

Applies to Cryopreservation; Erythropoietin; Normovolemic Hemodilution

Test Includes ABO group and Rh type of the unit are performed by the collecting facility. If the unit will be transfused outside of the collecting facility, tests for hepatitis B surface antigen, HIV-1 antigen, anti-HIV-1, anti-HIV-2, anti-HCV, antihepatitis B core, anti-HTLV-I, anti-HTLV-II, and a serologic test for syphilis must be performed on the first unit of blood collected within a 30-day period. Each unit must be labeled "autologous donor" and a special label "for autologous use only" is required. In addition, a "biohazard" label is required if any of the above tests are confirmed positive, or found repeat reactive only and confirmatory testing is not completed.[1,2] Up to 50% of the blood collected in PAD programs is discarded.[3]

Abstract This procedure includes removal of blood or components from a donor/patient for subsequent autologous transfusion. Autologous transfusion alleviates concern about the safety and availability of blood for transfusion. Blood collected from a patient is reserved for that patient for elective surgery. There is no risk of transmission of hepatitis, HIV, or other donor-related infectious diseases, nor of reaction to serum proteins or red cell antigens. But risks do exist, both during donation (donor reactions, anemia of donation) and subsequent reinfusion (identification mixup, bacterial contamination, volume overload). Not all patients are suitable candidates.

Categories of autologous programs:
- preoperative phlebotomy (the principal type discussed in this listing)
- immediate preoperative phlebotomy with hemodilution, also known as acute normovolemic hemodilution
- intraoperative cell salvage
- postoperative salvage

Note that combinations of the above techniques may be used to limit the patient's exposure to allogeneic transfusion.

Patient Preparation Patients should generally be in good health prior to donation. Although it has generally been recommended that supplemental iron usually should be prescribed by the patient's primary physician and administered **prior to** collection of the first unit, this procedure has recently been questioned for noniron-deficient patients who are undergoing modest autologous blood donation without erythropoietin therapy.[4] Nevertheless, supplemental iron therapy continues to be recommended to all patients making preoperative autologous donations at a large tertiary care center.[5]

Aftercare Continued replacement of iron is important. Increase fluid intake on the days of donation. Immediately after donation of blood, the patient/donor should remain lying down for a few minutes. When moved to a chair **with assistance**, the donor/patient should remain seated for 15-30 minutes and offered a drink (eg, orange juice and often cookies). The bandage can be removed 2-4 hours after application.

Container Each unit must be labeled "autologous donor" and a special label "for autologous use only" is required. In addition, a "biohazard" label is required if any of the above tests are confirmed positive, or found repeat reactive only and confirmatory testing is not completed.

Collection Documented requests for autologous collection must be received from the patient's primary physician. Sufficient numbers of units should ideally be collected prior to surgery to avoid exposure to allogeneic blood. Two-unit collections via red cell apheresis may be an option. Collections should also be scheduled far enough in advance of surgery to avoid anemia, through compensatory erythropoiesis.

The final collection should occur no sooner than 72 hours prior to scheduled surgery.

Adverse donor reactions are 12 times as high as those associated with voluntary donations.[3]

Storage Instructions Keep blood unit(s) in a monitored Blood Bank refrigerator for up to 42 days. For longer storage, blood may be frozen within 5 days of collection if such facilities are available.

Causes for Rejection Criteria vary. Some criteria which disqualify donors for homologous donation do not apply to autologous donation.

The following are rejection criteria for participation in a preoperative autologous donation program:[6]
- active infection/bacteremia
- significant aortic stenosis
- unstable angina

- uncontrollable seizure disorder
- myocardial infarction or cerebral vascular accident within 6 months of donation
- significant cardiac or pulmonary disease without clearance for donation by treating physician
- high-grade left main coronary artery disease
- cyanotic heart disease

Other possible criteria for rejection of a proposed autologous donor include:
- pregnancy - autologous blood is seldom indicated in an uncomplicated pregnancy. Policies should be developed, nonetheless, for situations in which blood may be needed for the infant or in women with multiple or high-incidence antibodies.
- uncontrolled hypertension

In all cases, the patient's primary physician and the Blood Bank physician share responsibility for acceptance of a patient and collection of the autologous blood.

Special Instructions Usually done by appointment with Blood Bank. Physician should write out a prescription giving the date of the intended surgery, providing the goal of how many units are to be drawn, and indicating that the patient has been given a prescription for oral iron. An order for Type and Screen is desirable to cover unanticipated blood needs that might exceed the amount of autologous blood.

Use Alleviates concerns regarding risk of transfusion-transmitted disease and alloimmunization in elective surgery. Autologous transfusion may be the only suitable source of compatible blood for patients with extremely rare blood types, patients with antibodies to high incidence antigens, or patients with antibodies to multiple antigens.

Limitations Blood collected for autologous transfusion cannot regularly be used for anyone else, because rigid criteria for donor selection are not always required.[1] There is usually a charge for each unit of blood collected, even though it may not be transfused. Combined with advances in the safety of allogeneic transfusion, the cost-effectiveness of the procedure has recently been questioned.[7] Preoperative donations diminish presurgical hemoglobin, which may result in the need for additional transfusion.

PAD is not needed for all surgical procedures.[8]

Autologous predeposit programs do not alleviate all risks of transfusion. As incredible as it seems, autologous blood has been issued to the wrong intended recipient. Bacterial contamination of units has not been eliminated.[9] Air embolism has been reported.[10] Up to 90% of PAD units go unused when intended for such procedures as hysterectomy, vaginal delivery, or prostatic TUR.[3]

Contraindications While the safety of cardiac patients as predeposit autologous donors is supported,[11] others have noted a higher severe reaction rate during autologous donation.[12] A U.S. Supreme Court decision (Bragdon vs Abbott) may make it illegal to deny autologous blood services to individuals protected under the Americans with Disabilities Act (ADA), including those who test positive for HIV.[13]

Methodology Similar to conventional blood donation

Additional Information Some general considerations of a preoperative autologous blood program follow.
- Guidelines are needed to establish or improve a program.[14]
- The patient should take iron for at least 1 week prior to the first donation, particularly if multiple units are needed.
- Units of blood are normally collected at weekly intervals, although if only 2 units are needed they can be collected via apheresis at a single collection in eligible donors.
- Autologous donation stimulates erythropoietin production.
- Use of recombinant human erythropoietin may further assist recovery during autologous donation. Its use may be integrated into a set of guidelines.[5] Patients who benefited from use of human recombinant erythropoietin with iron include those with iron deficiency and those with rheumatoid arthritis, but its application with PAD remains unproven. It is costly.[15]
- Criteria to monitor appropriate use of autologous blood should be established. The most important indicator of appropriate use is how well it reduces demand for allogeneic blood.[7]
- Surgery for which PAD is intended must be appropriately scheduled to permit needed intervals between donations.

Footnotes

1. Menitove JE, *Standards for Blood Banks and Transfusion Services*, 20th ed, Bethesda, MD: American Association of Blood Banks Press, 2000, 31:58-60.

2. Vengelen-Tyler V, *Technical Manual*, 13th ed, Bethesda, MD: American Association of Blood Banks Press, 1999, 112-9.

3. Goodnough LT, Brecher ME, Kanter MH, et al, "Transfusion Medicine, Second of Two Parts: Blood Conservation," *N Engl J Med*, 1999, 340(7):525-33.

4. Weisbach V, Skoda P, Rippel R, et al, "Oral or Intravenous Iron as an Adjuvant to Autologous Blood Donation in Elective Surgery: A Randomized, Controlled Study," *Transfusion*, 1999, 39(5):465-72.

5. Nuttall GA, Santrach PJ, Oliver WC Jr, et al, "Possible Guidelines for Autologous Red Blood Cell Donations Before Total Hip Arthroplasty Based on the Surgical Blood Order Equation," *Mayo Clin Proc*, 2000, 75(1):10-7.

6. Thomas MJG, Gillon J, and Desmond MJ, "Preoperative Autologous Blood Donation," *Transfusion*, 1996, 36(7):633-9.

7. Etchason J, Petz L, Keeler E, et al, "The Cost Effectiveness of Preoperative Autologous Blood Donations," *N Engl J Med*, 1995, 332(11):719-24.

8. Kanter MH, van Maanen D, Anders KH, et al, "Preoperative Autologous Blood Donations Before Elective Hysterectomy," *JAMA*, 1996, 276(10):798-801.

(Continued)

Autologous Transfusion, Preoperative Deposit
(Continued)

9. Klein HG, "Transfusion Safety: Avoid Unnecessary Bloodshed," *Mayo Clin Proc*, 2000, 75(1):5-7.
10. Linden JV, "Errors in Transfusion Medicine," *Arch Pathol Lab Med*, 1999, 123(7):563-65.
11. Adegboyega PA, "Comparative Safety of Blood Collection in High-Risk Autologous Donors Versus Non-High-Risk Autologous and Directed Donors in a Hospital Setting," *Am J Clin Pathol*, 1995, 103(3):374-5.
12. Popovsky MA, Whitaker B, and Arnold NL, "Severe Outcomes of Allogeneic and Autologous Blood Donations: Frequency and Characterization," *Transfusion*, 1995, 35(9):734-7.
13. "The ADA, HIV, and Autologous Blood Donation," Association Bulletin 98-5, Bethesda, MD: American Association of Blood Banks Press, 1998.
14. Autologous Transfusion Committee, "Guidelines for Blood Recovery and Reinfusion in Surgery and Trauma," Bethesda, MD: American Association of Blood Banks Press, 1997.
15. Duguid JK, "Autologous Blood Transfusion," *Clin Lab Haematol*, 1999, 21(6):371-6.

References
Cohen JA and Brecher ME, "Preoperative Autologous Blood Donation: Benefit or Detriment? A Mathematical Analysis," *Transfusion*, 1995, 35(8):640-4.
Domen RE, "Autologous Blood Donation by Patients Who Have Undergone Solid Organ Transplantation," *Am J Clin Pathol*, 1998, 110(1):102-5.
Lee SJ, Liljas B, Churchill WJ, et al, "Perceptions and Preferences of Autologous Blood Donors," *Transfusion*, 1998, 38(8):757-63.
"Transfusion Alert: Use of Autologous Blood. National Heart, Lung, and Blood Institute Expert Panel on the Use of Autologous Blood," *Transfusion*, 1995, 35(8):703-11.
Vamvakas EC and Moore SB, "Total Potential Frequency of Autologous Blood Transfusion in Olmsted County, Minnesota," *Mayo Clin Proc*, 1995, 70(1):37-44.

♦ **Autotransfusion** see Autologous Transfusion, Preoperative Deposit on page 837

♦ **Blood Components, Irradiated** see Irradiated Blood Components on page 846

♦ **Blood Donation** see Donation, Blood on page 839

♦ **Blood Donation, Designated** see Donation, Blood, Directed on page 840

♦ **Blood Grouping and Rh Typing** see Pretransfusion Testing on page 856

♦ **Blood Salvage, Intraoperative Autologous Transfusion** see Autologous Transfusion, Intraoperative Blood Salvage on page 836

♦ **Bone Marrow Transplant, Allogeneic** see Hematopoietic Progenitor Cells, Marrow on page 844

♦ **Bone Marrow Transplant, Autologous** see Hematopoietic Progenitor Cells, Marrow on page 844

♦ **CD34** see Hematopoietic Progenitor Cells, Peripheral Blood on page 845

♦ **CD34 Analysis** see Hematopoietic Progenitor Cells, Marrow on page 844

♦ **Clot Filters** see Filters for Blood on page 842

♦ **Coombs Test, Direct** see Antiglobulin Test, Direct on page 834

Cord Blood Screen

Related Information
Antibody Detection/Identification, Red Cell on page 834
Antiglobulin Test, Direct on page 834
Bilirubin, Amniotic Fluid, Delta A450 on page 116
Bilirubin, Neonatal, Serum on page 117
Hemolytic Disease of the Newborn, Antibody Identification on page 846
Kleihauer-Betke on page 453
Newborn Crossmatch and Transfusion on page 848
Prenatal Screen, Immunohematology on page 855
Rh Genotype on page 860
Rh₀(D) Immune Globulin (Human) on page 860
Rosette Test for Fetomaternal Hemorrhage on page 863

Synonyms Type and Screen, Coombs, Cord Blood

Test Includes ABO group, Rh type, direct antiglobulin test (DAT); evaluation of hemolytic disease of the newborn (HDN) in cases of positive DAT

Abstract Collection of a specimen of blood from the umbilical cord is standard practice at delivery. The test panel comprising the cord blood screen is designed to indicate the presence of HDN, to guide decisions regarding treatment options, and to assess the need for administration of postpartum Rh immune globulin. The Rh type of the mother is relevant.[1]

Specimen Cord blood

Container One lavender top (EDTA) tube and one red top tube

Collection Mix contents of EDTA tube well and do not overfill.

Causes for Rejection Gross hemolysis, sample collected in serum separator tube, improper labeling

Use The cord blood sample will be tested for ABO and Rh type and DAT. If the DAT is positive, both cord blood and maternal samples should be investigated for serological evidence of HDN. Antepartum RhIG can cause a weak-positive DAT; further testing is indicated. If mother and baby are

---

ABO incompatible, an eluate will demonstrate anti-A, anti-B, or both from neonatal red cells.

No testing may be required except to establish the candidacy of the mother to receive RhIG or unless a question of HDN arises. Thus, storing samples is usually necessary,[2] especially if the mother is known to be Rh(D) negative. Infants of mothers who are Rh negative should be typed for Rh₀(D), with a test for weak D, using the antiglobulin phase.[1]

Limitations Wharton's jelly may interfere with the determination of ABO blood group as well as with the DAT. (Repeat testing from capillary blood may be done.) ABO red cell grouping of neonates cannot be confirmed by serum (reverse) grouping. It may prove difficult to establish the Rh type of cord red cells heavily sensitized with IgG maternal antibodies. The presence of large numbers of maternal red cells in a cord blood sample can confuse the interpretation of blood grouping results. Similarly, serological results can be complicated in newborns that received intrauterine blood transfusion. The administration of antenatal Rh immune globulin may complicate interpretation of cord blood DAT results. Studies on paternal blood may be indicated when no antibody can be detected in the maternal serum or eluate from infant's DAT-positive red cells. The antibody in such a case may be directed to a paternal "private" antigen of low incidence (many low-incidence blood group antigens were discovered in cases of HDN).

Additional Information The fetomaternal relationship presents special immunohematological problems for the Blood Bank Laboratory. The results of initial cord blood screening tests will indicate the need for additional studies to determine the likelihood of HDN or the need for Rh immunoprophylaxis. A positive DAT is an important indicator of HDN. A positive result will evolve into antibody identification studies of maternal serum or infant red cell eluate. Antibody specificity is an important guide to disease severity. Most severe HDN is caused by anti-D alone or in combination with anti-C or anti-E. The next grade of severity is caused by antibodies to other Rh antigens (notably anti-c) or by antibodies to antigens in other blood group systems (eg, anti-K). IgG antibodies to antigens of the ABO system cause the lowest grade of HDN severity. ABO HDN can occur in any pregnancy, even the first. The DAT is often negative and the infant is rarely symptomatic at birth.

Administration of postpartum Rh immune globulin depends on maternal Rh₀(D) status, presence or absence of maternal alloimmunization, and the results of infant Rh(D) type. See Rh₀(D) Immune Globulin (Human) on page 860. Rh negative nonimmunized women who are candidates for RhIG, who deliver an Rh-positive baby, should be screened for fetomaternal hemorrhage to ascertain whether a single dose of RhIG is adequate.

See Kleihauer-Betke on page 453 and Rosette Test for Fetomaternal Hemorrhage on page 863. Flow cytometry and enzyme-linked antiglobulin tests are available.[1]

Footnotes
1. Hartwell EA, "Use of Rh Immune Globulin. ASCP Practice Parameter," *Am J Clin Pathol*, 1998, 110(3):281-92.
2. Snyder EL and Shoos-Lipton K, "Prevention of Hemolytic Disease of the Newborn Due to Anti-D," *American Association of Blood Banks Bulletin #98-2*, February 16, 1998.

References
Vengelen-Tyler V, *Technical Manual*, 13th ed, Bethesda, MD: American Association of Blood Banks Press, 1999, 502-4.

Cryoprecipitate

Related Information
Activated Partial Thromboplastin Time on page 328
Factor Inhibitors on page 340
Factor VIII Concentrate on page 841
Fibrinogen on page 341
Kidney Stone Analysis on page 877
Plasma, Fresh Frozen on page 851
Prothrombin Time on page 354
von Willebrand Factor on page 357

Synonyms Cryoprecipitated Antihemophilic Factor

Applies to Cryopreservation; Fibrin Glue; Fibrinogen Therapy; Hemophilia A Therapy; von Willebrand Disease Therapy

Abstract Cryoprecipitate is a labile component containing factor VIII:C, von Willebrand factor (factor VIII:vWF), fibrinogen, factor XIII, and fibronectin. Cryoprecipitate is the only concentrated available source of fibrinogen for patients with clinical deficiencies of that factor (eg, disseminated intravascular coagulation (DIC)).

A crossmatch is not necessary. Many units are sometimes needed. One concentrate per 5 kg body weight may serve as a rough guide to initial dosage.

Patient Preparation Prothrombin time, PTT, and fibrinogen assay to document indication (eg, hemophilia). ABO group (ABO compatible cryoprecipitate is preferred). Rh type need not be considered. Cryoprecipitate should be used only if viral-inactivated factor VIII concentrates are not available for patients with hemophilia A or von Willebrand disease.

Dosage and administration: Rapid administration of about 10 mL of diluted cryoprecipitate per minute is used as a loading dose for hemophilia, followed by a smaller dose at 12-hour intervals,[1] depending on clinical circumstances. In pooling, single containers can be rinsed with 0.9% saline, so that the volume of six units of cryoprecipitate is 100-150 mL. In the presence of circulating anticoagulants, larger doses or other special measures may be indicated.[1] Factor VIII activity should be >80 IU/bag.[2]

A 70 kg patient should have an increase of about 2.5% AHF for each bag of cryoprecipitate given.[3] For minor bleeding, dosage raising the patient's level to 30% to 50% may be used. For major surgical procedures, a preoperative dose should be sufficient to raise the level to 80% to 100%, followed by postoperative maintenance calculated to keep the level constantly >50% for 10-14 days.

In treatment of **von Willebrand disease**, smaller amounts given less often will usually suffice.[1] When using cryoprecipitate, the factor VIII levels achieved from a calculated dose will vary. Use of a factor VIII concentrate which contains vWF is preferred to cryoprecipitate for most von Willebrand patients (those requiring treatment with plasma fractions).[4]

Cryoprecipitate must be given through a filter.

To treat **hypofibrinogenemia**, one bag can be expected to raise plasma fibrinogen level about 7-10 mg/dL. A bag of cryoprecipitate provides at least 150 mg of fibrinogen.[1]

Cryoprecipitate may also be used as a source of topical **"fibrin glue,"** which can stop local bleeding especially in cardiothoracic surgery.[5] It can be derived from autologous techniques.[6] Topical thrombin and calcium chloride convert the fibrinogen in the cryoprecipitate to fibrin. The volume of the individual units of cryoprecipitate used for the fibrin glue should not exceed 15 mL.

Aftercare Factor VIII assay and activated partial thromboplastin time can serve as controls in therapy of hemophilia A and von Willebrand disease, and fibrinogen levels and thrombin time when hypofibrinogenemia is being treated.[1] Ristocetin cofactor, factor VIII antigen, and vWF multimer are useful in monitoring cases of von Willebrand disease.

Specimen Blood

Container One red top tube or one lavender top (EDTA) tube

Storage Instructions (For blood component) Cryoprecipitate requires frozen storage, without thawing, for up to 1 year at -18°C or below. Before infusion, thaw for up to 15 minutes in a water bath at 37°C in a plastic overwrap, so that the precipitate is dissolved. Pool multiple units before administration. Once thawed, store at room temperature. Cryoprecipitate ideally should be transfused within 2 hours or less, but not more than 6 hours after thawing and not more than 4 hours after pooling. Once thawed it cannot be refrozen.

Causes for Rejection (Of patient sample): Gross hemolysis, sample placed in a serum separator tube, specimen tube not properly labeled

Use Treatment of deficiency of coagulation factor VIII (hemophilia A), von Willebrand disease, and hypofibrinogenemic states only if viral-inactivated concentrates are not available. Replacement of fibrinogen should be considered when levels decrease to <100 mg/dL and patient is bleeding. The physician making such decisions should be aware of the coefficient of variation for fibrinogen levels in the laboratory being used. Prolongation of the thrombin time may support indications for infusion of fibrinogen as cryoprecipitate. Fibrin surgical adhesive ("fibrin glue") derived from cryoprecipitate can stop local bleeding during surgery. Cryoprecipitate is useful as a temporary treatment of bleeding tendency in uremia.[7] It also provides factor XIII.

Limitations Cryoprecipitate is a poor source of factors II, V, IX, X, and XI.[3]

Contraindications Do not use, unless laboratory or clinical studies indicate a specific coagulation defect for which cryoprecipitate is appropriate.

Additional Information Hazards: The risk of hepatitis and other viral infections is less than that of nonviral-inactivated concentrate because each bag comes from a single donor. Febrile and allergic reactions may occur.[1] Large volumes of ABO incompatible cryoprecipitate may result in a positive direct antiglobulin test with mild hemolysis.[1] Presence of acquired inhibitors to factor VIII makes treatment with cryoprecipitate difficult or impossible. Factor VIII concentrates will be needed for such patients.

Footnotes

1. *Circular of Information for the Use of Human Blood and Blood Components*, American Association of Blood Banks, America's Blood Centers, American Red Cross, 1998, 20-2.
2. Ness PM and Perkins HA, "Cryoprecipitate as a Reliable Source of Fibrinogen Replacement," *JAMA*, 1979, 241:1690-1.
3. Huestis DW, Bove JR, and Case J, *Practical Blood Transfusion*, 4th ed, Boston, MA: Little, Brown and Co, 1988, 320-1.
4. Fresh Frozen Plasma, Cryoprecipitate and Platelets Administration Practice Guidelines Development Task Force of the American Pathologists, "Practice Parameter for the Use of Fresh Frozen Plasma, Cryoprecipitate, and Platelets," *JAMA*, 1994, 271:777-81.
5. Alving BM, Weinstein MJ, Finlayson JS, et al, "Fibrin Sealant: Summary of a Conference on Characteristics and Clinical Uses," *Transfusion*, 1995, 35(9):783-90.
6. Reiner AP, "Fibrin Glue Increasingly Popular for Topical Surgical Hemostasis," *Lab Med*, 1999, 30(3):189-92.
7. Bolan CD and Alving BM, "Pharmacologic Agents in the Management of Bleeding Disorders," *Transfusion*, 1990, 30:541-51.

References

Blood Transfusion Therapy: A Physician's Handbook, 6th ed, Bethesda, MD: American Association of Blood Banks Press, 1999.
Martinez J, "Quantitative and Qualitative Disorders of Fibrinogen," *Hematology: Basic Principles and Practice*, 3rd ed, Chapter 112, Hoffman R, Benz EJ Jr, Shattil SJ, et al, eds, New York, NY: Churchill Livingstone, 2000, 1924-36.

Donation, Blood

Related Information

Synonyms Blood Donation; Phlebotomy, Blood Donor

Applies to Allogeneic Blood Transfusion

Test Includes Each donation intended for allogeneic use must be typed for ABO and Rh. Donors with a history of transfusion or pregnancy must be tested for unexpected antibodies. Each donation must be tested for syphilis; hepatitis B surface antigen; human immunodeficiency virus (HIV) antigen; antibodies to HIV-1, HIV-2, hepatitis B core antigen (HB$_c$), hepatitis C virus (HCV), and human T-cell lymphotrophic virus (HTLV-I/II).[1] A variety of tests, such as a Western blot or a recombinant immunoblot assay, may be performed in an attempt to confirm any initially positive infectious disease screening test. Although frequently performed, tests for alanine aminotransferase (ALT),[2] antibodies to cytomegalovirus (CMV), and nucleic acid testing for detection of HIV and HCV viral particles are not required.

Abstract Accurate information volunteered by the blood donor during the health assessment, together with infectious disease testing, are necessary for the exclusion of donors whose blood may transmit infectious diseases to recipients.

Patient Preparation Donors should be at least 18 years of age. Depending on state law, donors between 17 and 18 may donate with or without parental consent. The upper age limit usually is decided by the Blood Bank physician. Donor should weigh at least 110 pounds, should have a light meal before donation, no alcoholic beverages for 12 hours, **be in generally good health**, and afebrile. Donor reactions may be precipitated by emotional factors. Personnel should be cheerful and the donor room pleasant.[3] The donor should be asked about drugs being taken (eg, antihypertensives).

Aftercare Donors should be asked about their occupations, since fainting can be especially hazardous for some (eg, bus drivers, air crew).[4] Activities are restricted for certain hazardous occupations for 24 hours. Donor reactions occur, but are rarely severe.[5] Vasovagal reactions occur in 2% to 5% of blood donors, a figure unchanged in the past half century. Severe reactions occur in about 1 per 1000 donations.[6] The vasovagal attack can be provoked in some individuals by the sight of blood, and withdrawal of sufficient blood can lead to such effects. Fainting is more common on the first donation, in persons of small size, among females, and relates to the volume of blood withdrawn.[4,7]

(Continued)

Donation, Blood *(Continued)*

Immediately after donation of blood, the donor should remain lying down for several minutes. He/she should never be left alone. When moved to a chair with assistance, the donor should remain seated for at least 15 minutes and should be offered refreshments (eg, orange juice, and often cookies). The donor should be observed for at least 15 minutes and should be encouraged not to leave earlier than 20 minutes following completion of the donation.[3,4]

The delayed syncopal reaction may take place up to an hour following donation.[7] On occasion, they seem idiosyncratic, independent of any identifiable neglect.[8]

Specimen Blood

Container Blood bag of appropriate configuration

Collection Drawn by Blood Bank personnel

Causes for Rejection History of hepatitis or yellow jaundice, history of HB_sAg or HIV positive, drug addiction involving injection, male-to-male sexual activity, sex for money or drugs, coronary heart disease, residence in the United Kingdom for a total of 6 months or longer between 1980-1996: permanently deferred. Temporary deferments include hypotension, hypertension, anemia (hemoglobin <12.5 g/dL), positive syphilis serology (STS), travel to malaria endemic areas, exposure to hepatitis, pregnancy, childbirth within the last week, recent surgery, recent transfusion, tattoo within 12 months, inmate of penal or mental institution, and certain other medical conditions. FDA advisors suggested that individuals who have received transplanted tissue from animals (xenotransplant recipients) be forbidden to donate blood or plasma fractions.[9] Use of vitamins, thyroid preparations, or oral contraceptives does **not** disqualify donors. However, many other drugs, medications, and even immunizations can either temporarily or permanently defer a donor. Contact a Blood Bank physician for further information. Blood Banks must present would-be donors with educational materials explaining the risk of HIV/AIDS in blood transfusion and encouraging confidential self-deferment (confidential unit exclusion) by those at risk of HIV/AIDS or whenever a donor's blood is unsuitable for transfusion.

Special Instructions The patient's arm should be examined for scarred veins and/or many small puncture marks, possible signs of drug addiction.[8]

Use Obtain blood and its components for allogeneic transfusion to patients.

Limitations Once every 56 days. Donations not to exceed six in any 12-month period. Truthful information must be provided by the prospective donor.

Contraindications Donation is not advised for those who must immediately return to a hazardous activity (eg, heavy machinery operation), because delayed reaction may occur. The exercise of common sense and good judgment are advised. Adverse consequences of donation are much less among experienced donors than in those who are donating for the first time.[7]

Methodology Donors are selected based upon a medical history and a limited physical examination. Both are performed on the date of donation. The medical history questions may be completed by the donors themselves or obtained by a qualified interviewer. Questions pertaining to HIV-associated risk behaviors should be presented to the donors by a qualified interviewer.

Additional Information The word "allogeneic" denotes identical species but with antigenic difference. Allogeneic transfusions are more often called "homologous". The expression is used in contrast to autologous transfusion, in which antigenic differences do not exist.

Footnotes

1. Desforges JF, "Infectious Disease Testing for Blood Transfusion," *NIH Consensus Statement*, 1995, 13(1):1-27.
2. Busch MP, Korelitz JJ, Kleinman SH, et al, "Declining Value of Alanine Aminotransferase in Screening of Blood Donors to Prevent Post-transfusion Hepatitis B and C Virus Infection," *Transfusion*, 1995, 35(11):903-10.
3. Churchill WH and Kurtz SR, *Transfusion Medicine*, Chapter 2, Boston, MA: Blackwell Scientific Publications, 1989, 26.
4. Mollison PL, Engelfriet CP, Contreras M, et al, "The Withdrawal of Blood," *Blood Transfusion in Clinical Medicine*, 10th ed, Chapter 1, Oxford, UK: Blackwell Scientific Publication, 1997, 1-36.
5. Newman DH, "Donor Reactions and Injuries From Whole Blood Donations," *Transfus Med Rev*, 1997, 11:64-75.
6. Klein HG, "Transfusion Safety," *Mayo Clin Proc*, 2000, 75:769-70.
7. Huestis DW, Bove JR, and Case J, *Practical Blood Transfusion*, 4th ed, Boston, MA: Little, Brown and Co, 1988.
8. Heustis DW, personal communication, 1999.
9. Wilson K and Wilson F, "FDA Advisors Recommend That Xenotransplant Recipients Not Donate Blood," *Lab Med*, 2000, 31(3):127.

References

Kasprisin CA and Laird-Fryer B, *Blood Donor Collection Practices*, Bethesda, MD: American Association of Blood Banks, 1993.

Klein HG, "Will Blood Transfusion Ever Be Safe Enough?" *JAMA*, 2000, 284(2):238-40.

Kleinman S and Williams AE, "Donor Selection Procedures: Is it Possible to Improve Them?" *Transfus Med Rev*, 1998, 12(4):288-302.

Menitove JE, *Standards for Blood Banks and Transfusion Services*, 20th ed, Bethesda, MD: American Association of Blood Banks Press, 2000, 9-70.

Mollison PL, Engelfriet CP, Contreras M, et al, *Blood Transfusion in Clinical Medicine*, 10th ed, Oxford, UK: Blackwell Scientific Publication, 1997, 300-4.

Ownby HE, Kong F, Watanabe K, et al, "Analysis of Donor Return Behavior. Retrovirus Epidemiology Donor Study," *Transfusion*, 1999, 39(10):1128-35.

Scott EP, "The Safety of Blood Donation - Is It What It Should Be?" *Transfusion*, 1995, 35(9):717-8.

Donation, Blood, Directed

Related Information

Autologous Transfusion, Preoperative Deposit *on page 837*
Donation, Blood *on page 839*
Irradiated Blood Components *on page 846*

Synonyms Blood Donation, Designated; Directed Blood Donation

Test Includes Donor phlebotomy, ABO grouping, Rh typing, antibody screen, HB_sAg, anti-HB$_c$, anti-HTLV-I, anti-HTLV-II, HIV-1 Ag, anti-HIV-1, anti-HIV-2, anti-HCV, and a serologic test for syphilis. Nucleic acid testing for hepatitis C and HIV may also be performed.

Abstract The designation of friends or relatives to provide blood donations, which was initiated secondary to the public's concerns about the safety of the blood supply due to HIV. Currently, there are certain circumstances where it may be important to utilize designated donor(s) for a designated recipient (eg, patients with rare blood types or difficulty finding compatible blood components due to alloimmunization).

Patient Preparation Donors must meet all the requirements of a regular blood donor.

Aftercare Activities are restricted as for a routine blood donation. Reactions occur occasionally, as with any other donations.

Collection As for regular blood donors, although in some instances, the frequency of donation may be increased if the donor is certified by a physician to be in good health.[1]

Causes for Rejection As for regular blood donation (see Donation, Blood *on page 839*).

Special Instructions The attending physician should specify to the Blood Bank which blood component(s) he/she wishes prepared from each donation. These instructions, along with the name of the patient, the date of the surgery, and the name of the hospital must be relayed **prior** to arrival of the donor for phlebotomy.

Use Obtain blood or components for later use by a designated patient. Some intended recipients have a highly emotional fixation and are not moved by logic. Although the procedure is an administrative nuisance, it does make the patient feel better about transfusions.

Limitations Friends or family members recruited to be directed donors may not meet the eligibility requirements to give blood. If eligibility requirements are met and a unit is obtained, the unit may still not be made available because infectious disease testing requirements were not passed.

Other limitations include the following.

- Directed donors cannot supply blood in an emergency.
- Blood from directed donations generally cannot be available in less than 72 hours.
- Directed donations are neither safer nor riskier than regular volunteer blood donations.[2,3]
- More units are likely needed than the directed donor(s) can provide (because of differences in ABO/Rh types and donor loss due to other incompatibilities/ineligibilities).
- Graft-vs-host disease occurs occasionally in immunocompetent recipients of directed donations from blood relatives. Thus, all cellular components should be gamma irradiated with 15-25 Gy.[4]
- Husband-to-wife transfusions incur increased likelihood of hemolytic disease of the newborn.
- Directed donors risk losing the anonymous position of the conventional (homologous) donor and may become subject to legal complications.
- Administrative costs increase when directed donors are requested, because added efforts are required.

Additional Information Some states have enacted laws which state that a directed donation service must be offered on a nonemergency basis.

Footnotes

1. *Code of Federal Regulations*, 21CFR620.3(f), Washington, DC: U.S. Government Printing Office, 1999.
2. Pink J, Thomson A, and Wylie B, "Infectious Disease Markers in Autologous and Directed Donations," *Transfus Med*, 1994, 4:135-8.
3. "Transfusion Alert: Use of Autologous Blood. National Heart, Lung, and Blood Institute Expert Panel on the Use of Autologous Blood," *Transfusion*, 1995, 35:703-11.
4. Menitove JE, *Standards for Blood Banks and Transfusion Services*, 20th ed, Bethesda, MD: American Association of Blood Banks Press, 2000, 48.

References

Mollison PL, Engelfriet CP, and Contreras M, *Blood Transfusion in Clinical Medicine*, 10th ed, Oxford, UK: Blackwell Scientific Publication, 1997, 12.

Wagner FF and Flegel WA, "Transfusion-Associated Graft-Versus-Host Disease: Risk Due to Homozygous HLA Haplotypes," *Transfusion*, 1995, 35(4):284-91.

♦ **Donor Blood Transfusion** *see* Red Blood Cells *on page 857*

♦ **Donor Blood Transfusion** *see* Red Blood Cells, Leukocytes Reduced *on page 858*

♦ **Donor Plasmapheresis** *see* Plasmapheresis, Donor *on page 852*

♦ **Emergency Blood** *see* Uncrossmatched Blood, Emergency *on page 865*

♦ **Emergency Issue of Uncrossmatched Blood** *see* Uncrossmatched Blood, Emergency *on page 865*

- ♦ **Emergency Transfusion** *see* Uncrossmatched Blood, Emergency *on page 865*
- ♦ **Erythrocytapheresis** *see* Apheresis, Therapeutic *on page 836*
- ♦ **Erythropoietin** *see* Autologous Transfusion, Preoperative Deposit *on page 837*
- ♦ **Exchange Transfusion** *see* Hemolytic Disease of the Newborn, Antibody Identification *on page 846*
- ♦ **Exchange Transfusion** *see* Newborn Crossmatch and Transfusion *on page 848*
- ♦ **Exsanguinating Emergency** *see* Uncrossmatched Blood, Emergency *on page 865*

Factor VIII Concentrate

Related Information
Activated Partial Thromboplastin Time *on page 328*
Coagulation Factor Assays *on page 335*
Cryoprecipitate *on page 838*
Factor Inhibitors *on page 340*
Factor IX Concentrate *on page 841*
Parvovirus B19 DNA *on page 669*
Parvovirus B19 Serology *on page 669*
Plasma, Fresh Frozen *on page 851*
Plasma, Frozen, Solvent Detergent-Treated *on page 851*
von Willebrand Factor *on page 357*

Synonyms AHF, Lyophilized; Antihemophilic Factor (Human)

Abstract Factor VIII concentrates are typically prepared as derivatives from pools of plasma, which undergo further processing to inactivate contaminating viruses. Virus-inactivating procedures include the use of heat, chemical solvents and detergents, and affinity column purification. Concentrates may be produced using recombinant DNA technology.[1,2] These factor VIII concentrates, which have been prepared to decrease or remove the risk of viral transmission, should be utilized in place of cryoprecipitate in patients who require factor VIII replacement (eg, patients with hemophilia A).

Patient Preparation Perform factor VIII assays to calculate dosage or, in emergencies, use the activated partial thromboplastin time (aPTT) as a therapeutic guide.

Reference Interval The half-life for factor VIII concentrates is ~12 hours in the absence of inhibitors or active bleeding.

Use Treatment of acute bleeding and prevention of bleeding in patients with deficiency of clotting factor VIII (hemophilia A) and with low-titer factor VIII inhibitors. Some factor VIII concentrates (eg, Alphanate®, Humate-P®) can be used to treat patients with von Willebrand disease because they contain von Willebrand factor.[3]

Limitations The presence of inhibitors to factor VIII makes treatment more difficult. The most common target of monospecific-acquired anticoagulant antibodies is factor VIII. Conditions associated with such antibodies include systemic lupus erythematosus, rheumatoid arthritis, psoriasis, pemphigus vulgaris, gestation, lymphoproliferative diseases, plasma cell disorders, and use of penicillin, sulfas, chloramphenicol, and phenytoin. Idiopathic causes are recognized as well.[4] Porcine factor VIII is available for patients with factor VIII inhibitors.[5] In bleeding patients with inhibitors, very large doses of human factor VIII or factor IX complex (prothrombin complex) have been administered with varying degrees of success.[6] Refer to physicians experienced in the treatment of such cases.

Contraindications Normal coagulation studies or bleeding unrelated to factor VIII deficiency. Not all factor VIII concentrates are suitable for treatment of von Willebrand disease.

Additional Information The antihemophilic factor concentrates marketed in the U.S. have recently been tabulated, with information relevant to purification methods and virus inactivation/removal methods.[7] The activated partial thromboplastin time is useful for both hemophilia and von Willebrand disease and may be more readily available than are factor assays. All these tests can guide therapy, as can the clinical response of the patient.

Calculation of dosage: Each bottle is labeled with the quantity of factor VIII coagulant activity it contains in terms of International Units (IU). 1 mL of normal plasma contains 1 IU of factor VIII coagulant activity. The initial dose (30% to 100%) varies depending upon the clinical circumstance, in general, with deeper hemorrhage and hemarthrosis requiring higher levels of activity. The following formula[8] may be used:

plasma volume (PV, mL) = 40 mL/kg x body weight (kg)
desired units of factor VIII = PV x [desired level (%) - initial level (%)] divided by 100

Alternately, 1 factor VIII unit/kg body weight may raise the factor VIII level by 2%.

Administration: Factor VIII concentrates are prepared lyophilized and must be aseptically reconstituted using the manufacturer's diluent. Filter prior to administration. Administer as quickly as possible after reconstitution.

Hazards: Currently available factor VIII concentrates (excluding cryoprecipitate) utilize manufacturing procedures to reduce the risk of viral transmission and have not been associated with HIV transmission.[8] All viruses, however, particularly the nonlipid enveloped viruses (eg, hepatitis A and

parvovirus B19), may not be inactivated by these treatments. Due to the presence of anti-A or anti-B, development of a positive direct antiglobulin test with resulting hemolysis is possible.

Footnotes
1. Hay CR, Lee CA, and Savidge G, "A Postmarketing Safety and Efficacy Assessment of a Monoclonal Antibody Purified High-Purity Factor VIII Concentrate," *Haemophilia*, 1996, 2:32-6.
2. Schwartz RS, Abildgaard CF, Aledort LM, et al, "Human Recombinant DNA-Derived Antihemophilic Factor (Factor VIII) in the Treatment of Hemophilia A. Recombinant Factor VIII Study Group," *N Engl J Med*, 1990, 323:1800-5.
3. Berntorp E and Nilsson IM, "Use of High-Purity Factor VIII Concentrate (Humate-P®) in von Willebrand Disease," *Vox Sang*, 1989, 56:212-7.
4. Grosset ABM and Rodgers GM, "Acquired Coagulation Disorders," *Wintrobe's Clinical Hematology*, 10th ed, Volume 2, Chapter 69, Lee GR, Forester J, Lukens J, et al, eds, Baltimore, MD: Lippincott Williams & Wilkins, 1999, 1233-80.
5. Rubinger M, Houston DS, Schwetz N, et al, "Continuous Infusion of Porcine Factor VIII in the Management of Patients With Factor VIII Inhibitors," *Am J Hematol*, 1997, 56(2):112-8.
6. Hoyer LW, "Acquired Anticoagulants," *Williams' Hematology*, 5th ed, Beutler E, Lichtman MA, Coller BS, et al, eds, New York, NY: McGraw-Hill, 1995, 423-34.
7. Drohan WN and Clark DB, "Preparation of Plasma-Derived and Recombinant Human Plasma Proteins," *Hematology: Basic Principles and Practice*, 3rd ed, Chapter 139, Hoffman R, Benz EJ Jr, Shattil SJ, et al, eds, New York, NY: Churchill Livingstone, 2000, 2273-82.
8. *Blood Transfusion Therapy: A Physician's Handbook*, 6th ed, Bethesda, MD: American Association of Blood Banks Press, 1999, 37-40.

References
DiMichele D and Neufeld EJ, "Hemophilia. A New Approach to an Old Disease," *Hematol Oncol Clin North Am*, 1998, 12(6):1315-44.

Factor IX Concentrate

Related Information
Activated Partial Thromboplastin Time *on page 328*
Coagulation Factor Assays *on page 335*
Factor Inhibitors *on page 340*
Plasma, Fresh Frozen *on page 851*
Plasma, Frozen, Solvent Detergent-Treated *on page 851*

Synonyms Prothrombin Complex Concentrates

Abstract Factor IX is also called hemophilia B factor, Christmas factor, and plasma thromboplastin component.

Factor IX concentrates for the treatment of hemophilia B are available using recombinant technology or monoclonal antibody purification, thus, reducing the risk of viral transmission.[1,2] Factor IX complex contains factors II, VII, IX, and X.

Second generation factor IX concentrates are essentially free of the other vitamin K-dependent coagulation factors, and are designated coagulation factor IX (human).[3]

Patient Preparation Perform factor IX assay to calculate dosage before administration.

Reference Interval The half-life for factor IX concentrates is ~24 hours in the absence of inhibitors or active bleeding.

Use Treatment of acute bleeding and prevention of bleeding in patients with deficiency of clotting factor IX (hemophilia B).

Limitations Patients with factor inhibitors may be treated with factor IX complex concentrate. These should be used with caution in patients with liver disease. Disseminated intravascular coagulation and thrombosis are among the risks. Factor IX concentrates appear to be less thrombogenic than factor IX complex. Rapid infusion of factor IX complex may induce side effects, including fever, chills, headaches, nausea, and flushing.

Contraindications Do not use in liver disease. Do not use in vitamin K deficiency, for which vitamin K preparations are appropriate, or in patients with overdose of coumarin. See Plasma, Fresh Frozen *on page 851*.

Calculation of dosage: Each bottle of factor IX is labeled in terms of activity units, with one unit equivalent to that found in 1 mL of normal human plasma. The dose required depends upon the type and severity of bleeding. A formula used for calculating factor VIII dose can also be used to calculate factor IX dose (see Factor VIII Concentrate *on page 841*). However, double the number of units to be given since half of the infused factor IX disappears immediately after the infusion for unknown reasons.

Administration: Factor IX concentrates are prepared lyophilized and must be aseptically reconstituted using the manufacturer's diluent. Filter prior to administration. Administer as quickly as possible after reconstitution.

Additional Information Factor IX concentrates and related fractions marketed in the U.S. have recently been tabulated.[3]

Footnotes
1. White G, Shapiro A, Ragni M, et al, "Clinical Evaluation of Recombinant Factor IX," *Semin Hematol*, 1998, 35(2 Suppl 2):33-8.
2. Kasper CK, Lusher JM, and the Transfusion Practices Committee, "Recent Evolution of Clotting Factor Concentrates for Hemophilia A and B," *Transfusion*, 1993, 33:422-34.
3. Drohan WN and Clark DB, "Preparation of Plasma-Derived and Recombinant Human Plasma Proteins," *Hematology: Basic Principles and Practice*, 3rd ed, Chapter 139, Hoffman R, Benz EJ Jr, Shattil SJ, et al, eds, New York, NY: Churchill Livingstone, 2000, 2273-82.

(Continued)

Factor IX Concentrate (Continued)

References

Blood Transfusion Therapy: A Physician's Handbook, 6th ed, Bethesda, MD: American Association of Blood Banks Press, 1999, 41-3.

Greenberg CS and Orthner CL, "Blood Coagulation and Fibrinolysis," Wintrobe's Clinical Hematology, 10th ed, Volume 1, Chapter 24, Lee GR, Forester J, Lukens J, et al, eds, Baltimore, MD: Lippincott Williams & Wilkins, 1999, 684-764.

♦ **Factor V Replacement** see Plasma, Fresh Frozen on page 851

♦ **Factor V Replacement** see Plasma, Frozen, Donor Retested on page 851

♦ **Factor V Replacement** see Plasma, Frozen, Solvent Detergent-Treated on page 851

♦ **Factor VII Replacement** see Plasma, Fresh Frozen on page 851

♦ **Factor VII Replacement** see Plasma, Frozen, Donor Retested on page 851

♦ **Factor VII Replacement** see Plasma, Frozen, Solvent Detergent-Treated on page 851

♦ **Factor IX Replacement** see Plasma, Fresh Frozen on page 851

♦ **Factor IX Replacement** see Plasma, Frozen, Donor Retested on page 851

♦ **Factor IX Replacement** see Plasma, Frozen, Solvent Detergent-Treated on page 851

♦ **Factor X Replacement** see Plasma, Fresh Frozen on page 851

♦ **Factor X Replacement** see Plasma, Frozen, Donor Retested on page 851

♦ **Factor X Replacement** see Plasma, Frozen, Solvent Detergent-Treated on page 851

♦ **Factor XI Replacement** see Plasma, Fresh Frozen on page 851

♦ **Factor XI Replacement** see Plasma, Frozen, Donor Retested on page 851

♦ **Factor XI Replacement** see Plasma, Frozen, Solvent Detergent-Treated on page 851

♦ **Febrile Transfusion Reaction** see Filters for Blood on page 842

♦ **Fetalscreen™** see Rosette Test for Fetomaternal Hemorrhage on page 863

♦ **FFP** see Plasma, Fresh Frozen on page 851

♦ **FFP** see Plasma, Frozen, Donor Retested on page 851

♦ **FFP** see Plasma, Frozen, Solvent Detergent-Treated on page 851

♦ **Fibrin Glue** see Cryoprecipitate on page 838

♦ **Fibrinogen Therapy** see Cryoprecipitate on page 838

♦ **Filters, Blood Administration** see Filters for Blood on page 842

Filters for Blood

Related Information

Platelets, Apheresis, Donation on page 853
Red Blood Cells on page 857
Red Blood Cells, Leukocytes Reduced on page 858

Synonyms Clot Filters; Filters, Blood Administration; Filters, Leukocyte Reduction; Filters, Microaggregate; Leukocyte-Depletion Filters

Applies to Alloimmunization, Leukocyte; Febrile Transfusion Reaction; Transfusion Reaction, Febrile

Special Instructions Routine blood administration (or clot filters) and special blood filters (microaggregate and leukocyte reduction) are available, as a rule, at hospital transfusion services or from pharmacy and supplies services. Leukocyte reduction filters are designed to be component specific, thus, take care to select the appropriate filter for intended use. Prestorage leukocyte-reduced blood components may be available from the blood supplier. This negates the need for laboratory or bedside leukocyte reduction filtration.

Use All usual blood transfusions are given through an administration set which includes a filter. Clots may form in any unit of blood and are readily removed by the clot filters in all regular blood infusion sets.

Microaggregate filters remove debris composed of platelets with admixed granulocytes and fibrin in massive transfusions of older stored units of blood. Usage remains controversial as these filters cannot prevent HLA alloimmunization nor CMV transmission.

Leukocyte filters help reduce, but do not eliminate febrile nonhemolytic reactions. Two consecutive febrile reactions may be an indication for leukocyte-poor blood. Leukocyte reduction filters also reduce the likelihood of HLA alloimmunization and CMV transmission. The role of leukocyte reduction in altering the proposed immunomodulatory effects of allogeneic transfusion (tumor growth promotion, bacterial infection following surgery and transfusion-associated immunosuppression) is controversial.[1]

The importance of leukocyte reduction in platelet fractions is discussed in Platelet Transfusion on page 854 and in other monographs relevant to platelets. Leukocyte reduction by filtration and ultraviolet B irradiation of platelets were equally effective in prevention of refractoriness to platelets in a 1997 study.[2]

Limitations Do **not** use microaggregate or leukocyte reduction filters for granulocyte transfusions. Leukocyte reduction filtration after various periods of storage of RBCs or platelets may not be as effective as at the time of collection. Leukocyte reduction filters are not adequate to prevent graft-versus-host disease in susceptible blood recipients. Both microaggregate and leukocyte reduction filters have the potential to clog and become resistant to increased blood flow. Use of blood components leukocyte reduced prior to issue from the Blood Bank may alleviate this difficulty.[3]

Additional Information There are several different types of blood filters:

Clot filter (170 micron pore size): All blood and components must be given through this filter, intended to remove clots and fibrin shreds.[3]

Microaggregate filters (20-40 microns pore size). These filters remove the microaggregates of leukocytes and platelets that form in stored blood, particularly for blood that is recirculated in cardiac bypass devices.[3,4] The aim is to prevent microembolization and respiratory distress syndrome, although there is little support for routine use of microaggregate filters.[5] They have not been proven to influence development of the adult respiratory distress syndrome.[4]

Leukocyte-depletion filters (3-100 micron pore size).[6,7,8] These remove up to three logs (99.9%) of WBCs from platelets or RBCs. The purpose of leukocyte reduction is to prevent febrile nonhemolytic transfusion reactions, alloimmunization to HLA antigens, and transmission of viruses carried by leukocytes (eg, cytomegalovirus).[9,10] For such purposes, it appears that filtration must be so efficient that the platelet or RBC concentrates contain no more than 5×10^6 WBCs per transfusion. Since electronic particle counters are grossly inaccurate in those count ranges, quality control of leukocyte-reduced products requires special techniques. Cost and other practical matters are still evolving in the decision over universal leukocyte reduction and the manner (bedside filtration vs prestorage filtration) in which it will be achieved.[11] For optimal effect, all leukocyte reduction filters must be carefully used according to the manufacturer's instructions.

Footnotes

1. Blajchman MA, "Immunomodulatory Effects of Allogeneic Blood Transfusions: Clinical Manifestations and Mechanisms," Vox Sang, 1998, 75(Suppl 2):315-9.
2. Slichter S, "Leukocyte Reduction and Ultraviolet B Irradiation of Platelets to Prevent Alloimmunization and Refractoriness to Platelet Transfusions," The Trial to Reduce Alloimmunization to Platelets Study Group, N Engl J Med, 1997, 337(26):1861-9.
3. Triulzi DJ, Blood Transfusion Therapy: A Physician's Handbook, 6th ed, Bethesda, MD: American Association of Blood Banks Press, 1999, 82.
4. Snyder EL, "Transfusion Reactions," Hematology: Basic Principles and Practice, 3rd ed, Hoffman R, Benz EJ Jr, Shattil SJ, et al, eds, New York, NY: Churchill Livingstone, 2000, 2300-10.
5. Mollison PL and Engelfriet CP, "Some Unfavorable Effects of Transfusion," Blood Transfusion in Clinical Medicine, 10th ed, Oxford, UK: Blackwell Scientific Publications, 1997, 504-6.
6. Dzik S, "Prestorage Leukocyte Reduction of Cellular Blood Components," Transfus Sci, 1994, 15:131-9.
7. Freedman JJ, Blajchman MA, and McCombie N, "Canadian Red Cross Society Symposium on Leukoreduction: Report on Proceedings," Transfus Med Rev, 1994, 8:1-14.
8. Heddle NM, "The Efficacy of Leukoreduction to Improve Platelet Transfusion Response: A Critical Appraisal of Clinical Studies," Transfus Med Rev, 1994, 8:15-28.
9. Wenz B, "Clinical and Laboratory Precautions That Reduce the Adverse Reactions, Alloimmunization, Infectivity, and Possibly Immunomodulation Associated With Homologous Transfusions," Transfus Med Rev, 1990, 4(4 Suppl 1):3-7.
10. Przepiorka D, LeParc GF, Werch J, et al, "Prevention of Transfusion-Associated Cytomegalovirus Infection," Am J Clin Pathol, 1996, 106(2):163-9.
11. Sprogoe-Jakobsen U, Saetra AM, and Georgsen J, "Preparation of White Cell-Reduced Red Cells by Filtration: Comparison of a Bedside Filter and Two Blood Bank Filter Systems," Transfusion, 1995, 35(5):421-26.

References

Rossi EC, Simon TL, Moss GS, et al, eds, Principles of Transfusion Medicine, 2nd ed, Baltimore, MD: Lippincott Williams & Wilkins, 1996.

♦ **Filters, Leukocyte Reduction** see Filters for Blood on page 842

♦ **Filters, Microaggregate** see Filters for Blood on page 842

♦ **Forward Grouping** see Pretransfusion Testing on page 856

♦ **Fresh Blood** see Whole Blood on page 866

♦ **Fresh Frozen Plasma** see Plasma, Fresh Frozen on page 851

♦ **Fresh Frozen Plasma** see Plasma, Frozen, Donor Retested on page 851

♦ **Fresh Frozen Plasma** see Plasma, Frozen, Solvent Detergent-Treated on page 851

♦ **Frozen Blood** see Frozen Red Blood Cells on page 842

Frozen Red Blood Cells

Synonyms Frozen Blood; Red Blood Cells, Deglycerolized; Red Blood Cells, Frozen

Applies to Cryopreservation

Test Includes ABO, Rh, antibody screen, crossmatch, and antibody identification when screen is positive (ie, preparation as for other transfusions)

Abstract Glycerol serves as a cryoprotective agent when added to reasonably fresh or rejuvenated red blood cells, which can then be frozen at -80°C or lower. Freezing may be in mechanical freezers or in liquid nitrogen. After thawing and deglycerolization by washing, some 80% to 90% of the original red cells remain, as a more or less pure suspension in isotonic saline.[1] The hematocrit is usually about 60%. Platelets, leukocytes (except for a few lymphocytes), and plasma constituents are almost completely removed during processing. Frozen storage time can be up to 10 years, although some data support even longer periods.[2,3] Post-thaw storage time is 24 hours at 1°C to 6°C. Volume and hematocrit vary.

Patient Preparation As for transfusion of whole blood or red blood cells

Aftercare One unit should raise the hematocrit of an adult about 3 percentage points (or hemoglobin 1 g/dL). Monitor hemoglobin and hematocrit.

Specimen Blood

Container One red top tube or one lavender top (EDTA) tube

Collection (Of sample from intended recipient): At the patient's bedside, ask the patient to give his or her name. Compare with the patient's wristband. Label the sample tube with two unique forms of patient identification (eg, patient's full name, hospital number); also include date and initials of the collector. Further information may be required on a requisition form. Take extra care with identification of unresponsive patients.

Storage Instructions Deglycerolized red blood cells must be transfused within 24 hours after thawing or must be discarded.

Causes for Rejection If a crack is found in the frozen plastic of the container or if there is evidence of leakage, discard the unit.[1]

Turnaround Time Long processing time is a severe disadvantage in emergency settings.

Special Instructions After issue from the transfusion service, blood must be transfused within 4 hours.

Use Restores red cell volume. Frozen red cells are essentially free of plasma proteins; about 0.025% of the original plasma is present. Such properties have more to do with the washing, than with the freezing process itself. Frozen red cells are useful particularly for patients with very rare red cell types and antibodies to high frequency antigens or combinations of antigens.[1]

Long-term storage of autologous red cells.

Rare donor red cell depot.

Limitations About 10% to 15% of the original red cells are lost in processing; expensive - about two to three times the cost of a unit of conventional red blood cells; short dating after thawing - 24-hour shelf-life;[1] not always available even in larger cities; slow and complex freezing and deglycerolizing processes. Because of these problems, lack of stat availability for emergencies, and expense, frozen red cells have been somewhat of a disappointment.

Contraindications Sickling hemoglobinopathies in donors are contraindications to freezing, since red cell recovery in these conditions has been poor.[1] As for recipients, frozen red cells should generally not be used when anemia and/or hypoxia can be corrected with specific products (eg, iron, B_{12}, folic acid). Not suitable for correction of coagulation deficiencies.

Methodology A number of methods for freezing and thawing red cells are in use.

Additional Information Red blood cells, deglycerolized, must be ABO compatible. A crossmatch is necessary. Hepatitis and some other infectious diseases remain a hazard. See Risks of Transfusion on page 861. Red blood cells deglycerolized must be stored at 1°C to 6°C or no longer than 24 hours.

Footnotes
1. Mollison PL, Engelfriet CP, Contreras M, et al, *Blood Transfusion in Clinical Medicine*, 10th ed, Oxford, UK: Blackwell Scientific Publication, 1997, 300-4.
2. Umlas J, Jacobson M, and Kevy SV, "Suitable Survival and Half-Life of Red Cells After Frozen Storage in Excess of 10 Years," *Transfusion*, 1991, 31(7):648-9.
3. Valeri CR, Pivacek LE, Gray AD, et al, "The Safety and Therapeutic Effectiveness of Human Red Cells Stored at -80°C for as Long as 21 Years," *Transfusion*, 1989, 29(5):429-37.

References
Circular of Information for the Use of Human Blood and Blood Components, American Association of Blood Banks, America's Blood Centers, American Red Cross, 1998.
Vengelen-Tyler T, *Technical Manual*, 13th ed, Arlington, VA: American Association of Blood Banks Press, 1999, 85-6.

♦ **Galactocerebrosidase Deficiency** see Hematopoietic Progenitor Cells, Marrow on page 844

♦ **Granulocytapheresis** see Apheresis, Therapeutic on page 836

♦ **Granulocyte Agglutination Test** see Antineutrophil Antibody on page 835

♦ **Granulocyte Antibody** see Antineutrophil Antibody on page 835

♦ **Granulocyte-Colony-Stimulating Factor** see Hematopoietic Progenitor Cells, Peripheral Blood on page 845

♦ **Granulocyte-Colony-Stimulating Factor** see Neutrophils, Transfusion on page 847

♦ **Granulocyte Immunofluorescence Test** see Antineutrophil Antibody on page 835

♦ **Granulocytes, Apheresis, Donation** see Neutrophils, Apheresis, Donation on page 847

♦ **Granulocytes, Pheresis** see Neutrophils, Apheresis, Donation on page 847

♦ **Granulocytes, Transfusion** see Neutrophils, Transfusion on page 847

♦ **GTX** see Neutrophils, Transfusion on page 847

♦ **Hazards of Transfusion** see Risks of Transfusion on page 861

Hematopoietic Progenitor Cells, Cord Blood/Placental Blood

Related Information
CD34+ Hematopoietic Stem Cells by Flow Cytometry on page 413
Hematopoietic Progenitor Cells, Marrow on page 844
Hematopoietic Progenitor Cells, Peripheral Blood on page 845

Synonyms Placental Blood; Transplant, Cord Blood; Umbilical Cord Blood

Applies to Cryopreservation

Test Includes For unrelated allogeneic units, the following tests must be performed: ABO and Rh; HLA-A, -B, and -DR; HB$_s$Ag, anti-HTLV-I, anti-HTLV-II, anti-HIV-I, anti-HIV-II, HIV-I-Ag, anti-HCV, anti-HB$_c$, anti-CMV, and a serologic test for syphilis. A donor health history screen and a test for hemoglobin S will also be performed. Refer to appropriate Standards for additional specifications.[1,2]

Abstract Hematopoietic progenitor cells (HPC) can be obtained from the umbilical cord at the time of delivery, when umbilical cord blood is immediately placed in anticoagulant and cryopreserved to serve as a source of stem cells. Patients in need of allogeneic HPC transplant have a <85% chance of finding an HLA-matched donor, and umbilical cord blood stem cells may serve as the alternate source.

Patient Preparation Informed consent from the biologic mother must be obtained according to applicable laws.

Container Appropriate anticoagulated collection bag or syringe.

Collection Collect cord blood during the third stage of labor or after delivery of the placenta if the collection interferes with care of the mother or baby. After disinfecting the cord, a large-bore needle connected to a sterile blood collection bag containing CPDA is frequently used to collect the cord blood.[3] Approximately 65-70 mL of umbilical cord blood is typically collected in such a closed system. An attorney, writing an editorial in the *New England Journal of Medicine*, states that collection of placental blood has been considered more closely related to blood donation than to organ donation.[4]

Storage Instructions Since umbilical cord banks store large numbers of units, processing to reduce unit volume is usually employed prior to cryopreservation and storage in liquid nitrogen.[3]

Causes for Rejection Too small a volume collected, unsuitable donor medical condition. Legal issues of testing and privacy have been recently discussed.[4]

Special Instructions Coordination with appropriate HPC therapy service personnel is required.

Use While touting autologous cord blood HPC collection and storage, the chance of anyone requiring a cord blood transplant by age 20 is estimated to be 1 in 20,000.[4] Allogeneic cord blood HPC are used as a source of hematopoietic stem cells for both related and unrelated transplants.[5] HPC are for pediatric and adult patients, for certain neoplastic and non-neoplastic disease, including immunodeficiency states, Lesch-Nyhan syndrome, Hurler syndrome, and Diamond-Blackfan syndrome.[6] Engraftment of stem cells in recipients with neoplastic diseases can be achieved, given an adequate dose of nucleated cells. A decreased risk of graft-vs-host disease permits an increase in levels of histoincompatibility.

HPC are used for β-thalassemia, sickle cell anemia, and other lymphoid and hematopoietic genetic disorders.[7]

Limitations Repopulation of marrow depends on the number of stem cells in the collection. The relatively small number of HPC in cord blood may be inadequate to repopulate nonpediatric recipients. Success has been reported.[8]

Methodology For infusion of thawed, previously cryopreserved products: Hydrate patient and "alkalinize" urine 12 hours before HPC infusion. Immediately prior to infusion, premedicate patient with antihistamine (to prevent sudden and severe hypotension).[9] If the amount of DMSO infused exceeds 10 mL/kg, consider giving over 2 days.

Additional Information
- There may be reduced graft-vs-host disease in recipients of cord blood transplants.[5] Recipients of cord blood progenitor cells from HLA-identical siblings enjoy a lower incidence of graft-vs-host disease than recipients of bone marrow transplants from HLA-identical siblings.[10]
- Days to engraftment in unrelated transplants are routinely longer than other sources (eg, marrow or peripheral blood).
- Standards for HPC have been published by the American Association of Blood Banks, the Foundation for the Accreditation of Hematopoietic Cell Therapy, and the National Marrow Donor Program. The FDA may utilize voluntary standards in place of more comprehensive regulations.

(Continued)

Hematopoietic Progenitor Cells, Cord Blood/ Placental Blood (Continued)

- Complications include infectious diseases, hemorrhagic disorders, diffuse alveolar damage, hepatic veno-occlusive disease, and graft-vs-host disease.[6]
- Commercialism and market-based medicine, threatening to replace ethics as a cornerstone of medical practice, affect portions of the practice of placental blood collection.[4] Marketing practices for HPC from cord blood deserve close attention.[11]

A *Circular of Information for the Use of Hematopoietic Progenitor Cell Products* is available from blood banks or blood centers.[12]

Footnotes

1. *Standards for Hematopoietic Progenitor Cell Services*, 2nd ed, Bethesda, MD: American Association of Blood Banks Press, 2000, 45-51.
2. *Standards for Hematopoietic Progenitor Cell Collection, Processing and Transplantation*, 1st ed, Omaha, NE: Foundation for the Accreditation of Hematopoietic Cell Therapy, 1996, 22-3.
3. Rubinstein P, Dobrila L, Rosenfield RE, et al, "Processing and Cryopreservation of Placental/Umbilical Cord Blood for Unrelated Bone Marrow Reconstitution," *Proc Natl Acad Sci U S A*, 1995, 92(22):10119-22.
4. Annas GJ, "Waste and Longing - the Legal Status of Placental-Blood Banking," *N Engl J Med*, 1999, 340(19):1521-4.
5. Rubinstein P, Carrier C, Scaradovou A, et al, "Outcomes Among 562 Recipients of Placental-Blood Transplants From Unrelated Donors," *N Engl J Med*, 1998, 339(22):1565-77.
6. Nuckols JD, "Autopsy Findings in Umbilical Cord Blood Transplant Recipients," *Am J Clin Pathol*, 1999, 112(3):335-42.
7. Parkman R, "The Future of Placental-Blood Transplantation," *N Engl J Med*, 1998, 339(22):1628-9.
8. Laporte JP, Gorin NC, Rubinstein P, et al, "Cord-Blood Transplantation From an Unrelated Donor in an Adult With Chronic Myelogenous Leukemia," *N Engl J Med*, 1996, 335(6):167-70.
9. Rowley SD, "Storage of Hematopoietic Cells," *Marrow Transplantation: Practical and Technical Aspects of Stem Cell Reconstitution*, Sacher RA and AuBuchon JP, eds, Bethesda, MD: American Association of Blood Banks Press, 1992, 105-27.
10. Rocha V, Wagner JE, Sobocinski KA, et al, "Graft-Versus-Host Disease in Children Who Have Received a Cord Blood or Bone Marrow Transplant From and HLA-Identical Sibling," *N Engl J Med*, 2000, 342(25):1846-54.
11. Sugarman J, Kaalund V, Kodish E, et al, "Ethical Issues in Umbilical Cord Blood Banking," *JAMA*, 1997, 278(11):938-43.
12. *Circular of Information for the Use of Progenitor Cell Products*, American Association of Blood Banks, America's Blood Centers, American Red Cross, January 2000.

References

Ende N, Lu S, Mack R, et al, "The Feasibility of Using Blood Bank-Stored (4°C) Cord Blood, Unmatched for HLA for Marrow Transplantation," *Am J Clin Pathol*, 1999, 111(6):773-81.

Gluckman E, Rocha V, Boyer-Chammard A, et al, "Outcome of Cord-Blood Transplantation From Related and Unrelated Donors," *N Engl J Med*, 1997, 337(6):373-81.

Issaragrisil S, Visuthisakchai S, Suvatte V, et al, "Brief Report: Transplantation of Cord-Blood Stem Cells Into a Patient With Severe Thalassemia," *N Engl J Med*, 1995, 332(6):367-9.

Nash RA, "Hematopoietic Stem Cell Transplantation," *Wintrobe's Clinical Hematology*, Volume 1, Chapter 28, Lee GR, Foerster J, Lukens J, et al, eds, Baltimore, MD: Lippincott Williams & Wilkins, 1999, 875-93.

Rubin R, "A Hard Sell to Bank Your Baby's Blood," *US News World Rep*, 1996, 29:60-1.

Vengelen-Tyler V, "Hematopoietic Transplantation," *Technical Manual*, 13th ed, Chapter 25, Bethesda, MD: American Association of Blood Banks Press, 1999, 531-61.

Hematopoietic Progenitor Cells, Marrow

Related Information

CD34+ Hematopoietic Stem Cells by Flow Cytometry *on page 413*

Hematopoietic Progenitor Cells, Cord Blood/Placental Blood *on page 843*

Hematopoietic Progenitor Cells, Peripheral Blood *on page 845*

Synonyms Bone Marrow Transplant, Allogeneic; Bone Marrow Transplant, Autologous; Transplant, Bone Marrow

Applies to CD34 Analysis; Cryopreservation; Galactocerebrosidase Deficiency

Test Includes For autologous donors, the following tests must be performed: HB₀Ag, anti-HTLV-I, anti-HTLV-II, anti-HIV-I, anti-HIV-II, HIV-I-Ag, anti-HCV, and anti-HB_c. A donor health history screen, complete blood count, and pregnancy test (when applicable) will also be performed.

For allogeneic donors, the following tests must be performed: ABO, Rh, and antibody screen; HLA-A, -B, and -DR; HB₀Ag, anti-HTLV-I, anti-HTLV-II, anti-HIV-I, anti-HIV-II, HIV-I-Ag, anti-HCV, anti-HB_c, anti-CMV, and a serologic test for syphilis. A donor health history screen, complete blood, count and pregnancy test (when applicable) will also be performed. Refer to appropriate Standards for additional specifications.[1,2]

Abstract Bone marrow was the leading source of hematopoietic progenitor cells (HPC) for patients in need of transplantation before 1990. However, other stem cell sources (eg, peripheral blood) are replacing marrow as a sole source of HPC in both autologous and allogeneic transplantation. Human marrow contains mature as well as pluripotent cells which are capable of reconstituting the hematologic and lymphoid systems.

Patient Preparation Because of blood loss in marrow collection, it is customary to collect 2 units of autologous red cells 2-3 weeks prior to the scheduled collection.

Aftercare Red cell transfusions usually take place after the collection, if possible (avoids marrow dilution). Irradiate all blood fractions given during a collection for allogeneic transplantation.

Collection The volume of marrow collected is determined by the recipient's body weight and any postcollection product manipulation. Collection targets, in general, are as follows: 1.0×10^8 nucleated cells/kg for autologous transplant and 2.0×10^8 nucleated cells/kg for allogeneic transplant. The patient/donor is placed under general or spinal anesthesia and the procedure is performed under sterile conditions in the operating room. The posterior iliac crest provides the richest source. Collecting approximately 10-15 mL of marrow per kg of recipient body weight will achieve the target dose.[3] The aspirated marrow is anticoagulated, filtered to remove bony spicules and transported to the processing laboratory for quality assurance testing and any further manipulation or cryopreservation. Label the aspirated bone marrow with the same care needed in the preparation of other autologous blood components.

Storage Instructions Marrow may be processed prior to cryopreservation or infusion to remove plasma, red cells, or tumor. In an ABO-incompatible allogeneic transplant, processing to remove plasma or red cells prevents a hemolytic reaction. In an autologous transplant, processing to volume reduce means less dimethylsulfoxide (DMSO) required for cryopreservation. A number of manual or automated techniques are available for processing. Controlled-rate (-180°C storage) and noncontrolled rate (-80°C storage) cryopreservation techniques are available. An expiration date has not been defined, however, marrow stored for 11 years has been transplanted with resultant engraftment.[4]

Causes for Rejection Poor anesthesia risk, obesity, malignant involvement of bone marrow, fibrosis of marrow at usual sites of collection (usually caused by prior radiation therapy of the pelvis), and patient refusal. In these cases, consider using an alternative (peripheral blood) HPC collected by apheresis.

Special Instructions Coordination with appropriate HPC therapy service personnel is required.

Use Collection and storage of autologous bone marrow make it possible to treat malignant disease with heavy doses of chemotherapy and/or irradiation that would otherwise destroy the patient's marrow function. After such treatment, marrow is repopulated from the stored autologous supply. Allogeneic transplants are performed for indications such as marrow failure (eg, aplastic anemia), hemoglobinopathies, inborn errors of metabolism, and other disorders.

Central nervous system manifestations of globoid-cell leukodystrophy (deficiency of galactocerebrosidase) were reversed with allogeneic marrow and umbilical cord blood transplantation.[5]

Marrow transplantation from an HLA-identical donor or T-cell depleted haploidentical marrow from related donors provides life-sustaining therapy for severe combined immunodeficiency.[6]

Chemotherapy with stem cell transplantation is in use and/or in evaluation in neoplastic disease. Autologous stem cell transplantation is best with low tumor burden. A favorable impact is described with subsets of patients who have acute myelogenous leukemia, myelodysplasia, Hodgkin disease, and non-Hodgkin lymphoma.[7] Further trials are needed for some subgroups of carcinoma of ovary.[8]

Limitations Repopulation of marrow depends on the number of stem cells in the collection. Current enumeration is performed by CD34 analysis (1% to 3% of marrow cells). Numerous CD34 methods exist and site-to-site correlation may be unreliable.[9] Processing may result in loss of stem cells. Inadequacy of stem cells will mean failure of repopulation. Complications include graft-vs-host disease and death.[10] See Hematopoietic Progenitor Cells, Cord Blood/Placental Blood *on page 843*.

Methodology For thawed, previously cryopreserved marrow: Hydrate patients and "alkalinize" urine 12 hours before HPC infusion. Immediately prior to infusion, premedicate patient with antihistamine (to prevent sudden and severe hypotension).[11] If the amount of DMSO infused exceeds 10 mL/kg, consider administration of the component over 2 days.

Additional Information Elimination of T cells from the marrow graft is reported to prevent graft-vs-host disease in management of severe combined immunodeficiency. For patients treated with HLA haploincompatible marrow, graft-vs-host disease is a major determinant of outcome.[12] Standards for HPC have been published by the American Association of Blood Banks, the Foundation for the Accreditation of Hematopoietic Cell Therapy, and the National Marrow Donor Program. The FDA may utilize voluntary standards in place of more comprehensive regulations. A Circular of Information for the Use of Hematopoietic Progenitor Cell Products is available from blood banks or blood centers.[13]

Footnotes

1. "Standards for Hematopoietic Progenitor Cell Services," 2nd ed, Bethesda, MD: American Association of Blood Banks Press, 2000, 45-51.
2. "Standards for Hematopoietic Progenitor Cell Collection, Processing and Transplantation," 1st ed, Omaha, NE: Foundation for the Accreditation of Hematopoietic Cell Therapy, 1996, 22-3.
3. Patterson K, "Bone Marrow Harvesting," *Color Atlas and Text of Bone Marrow Transplantation*, Treleaven J and Wiernik P, eds, London: Mosby-Wolfe, 1995, 101-7.

4. Aird W, Labopin M, Gorin NC, et al, "Long-Term Cryopreservation of Human Stem Cells," *Bone Marrow Transplant*, 1992, 9(6):487-90.

5. Krivit W, Shapiro EG, Peters C, et al, "Hematopoietic Stem-Cell Transplantation in Globoid-Cell Leukodystrophy," *N Engl J Med*, 1998, 338(16):1119-26.

6. Buckley RH, Schiff SE, Schiff RI, et al, "Hematopoietic Stem-Cell Transplantation for the Treatment of Severe Combined Immunodeficiency," *N Engl J Med*, 1999, 340(7):508-16.

7. Sarosy GA and Reed E, "Autologous Stem-Cell Transplantation in Ovarian Cancer: Is More Better?" *Ann Intern Med*, 2000, 133(7):555-6.

8. Stiff PJ, Veum-Stone J, Lazarus HM, et al, "High-Dose Chemotherapy and Autologous Stem-Cell Transplantation for Ovarian Cancer: An Autologous Blood and Marrow Transplant Registry Report," *Ann Intern Med*, 2000, 133(7):504-15.

9. Brecher ME, Sims L, Schmitz J, et al, "North American Multicenter Study on Flow Cytometric Enumeration of CD34+ Hematopoietic Stem Cells," *J Hematother*, 1996, 5(3):227-36.

10. Platt OS and Guinan EC, "Bone Marrow Transplantation in Sickle Cell Anemia - The Dilemma of Choice," *N Engl J Med*, 1996, 335(6):426-8.

11. Rowley SD, "Storage of Hematopoietic Cells," *Marrow Transplantation: Practical and Technical Aspects of Stem Cell Reconstitution*, Sacher RA and AuBuchon JP, eds, Bethesda, MD: American Association of Blood Banks Press, 1992, 105-27.

12. Fischer A, "Thirty Years of Bone Marrow Transplantation for Severe Combined Immunodeficiency," *N Engl J Med*, 1999, 340(7):559-61.

13. *Circular of Information for the Use of Progenitor Cell Products*, American Association of Blood Banks, America's Blood Centers, American Red Cross, January, 2000.

References

Arico M, Valsecchi MG, Camitta B, et al, "Outcome of Treatment in Children With Philadelphia Chromosome-Positive Acute Lymphoblastic Leukemia," *N Engl J Med*, 2000, 342(14):998-1006.

Beatty PG, Kollman C, and Howe CW, "Unrelated-Donor Marrow Transplants: The Experience of the National Marrow Donor Program," *Clin Transpl*, 1995, 271-7.

Bensinger WI, Martin PJ, Storer B, et al, "Transplantation of Bone Marrow as Compared With Peripheral Blood Cells From HLA-Identical Relatives in Patients With Hematologic Cancers," *N Engl J Med*, 2001, 344(3):175-81.

Hansen JA, Gooley TA, Martin PJ, et al, "Bone Marrow Transplants From Unrelated Donors for Patients With Chronic Myeloid Leukemia," *N Engl J Med*, 1998, 338(14):962-8.

Walters MC, Patience M, Leisenring W, et al, "Bone Marrow Transplantation for Sickle Cell Disease," *N Engl J Med*, 1996, 335(6):369-76.

Hematopoietic Progenitor Cells, Peripheral Blood

Related Information

Alpha₁-Fetoprotein, Amniotic Fluid *on page 96*
Alpha₁-Fetoprotein, Serum *on page 97*
Breast Biopsy *on page 51*
CD34+ Hematopoietic Stem Cells by Flow Cytometry *on page 413*
Chorionic Gonadotropin, Human, Serum and Urine *on page 147*
Hematopoietic Progenitor Cells, Cord Blood/Placental Blood *on page 843*
Hematopoietic Progenitor Cells, Marrow *on page 844*

Synonyms Peripheral Blood Stem Cells, Autologous; Peripheral Stem Cells; Progenitor Cells; Stem Cell Collection

Applies to CD34; Cryopreservation; Granulocyte-Colony-Stimulating Factor

Test Includes For autologous units, the following tests must be performed: HB$_s$Ag, anti-HTLV-I, anti-HTLV-II, anti-HIV-I, anti-HIV-II, HIV-I-Ag, anti-HCV, and anti-HB$_c$. A donor health history screen, complete blood count, and pregnancy test (when applicable) will also be performed.

For allogeneic units, the following tests must be performed: ABO, Rh, and antibody screen; HLA-A, -B, and -DR; HB$_s$Ag, anti-HTLV-I, anti-HTLV-II, anti-HIV-I, anti-HIV-II, HIV-I-Ag, anti-HCV, anti-HB$_c$, anti-CMV, and a serologic test for syphilis. A donor health history screen, complete blood count, and pregnancy test (when applicable) will also be performed. Refer to appropriate Standards for additional specifications.[1,2]

Abstract Peripheral blood progenitor cells (PBPC) are collected after mobilizing hematopoietic stem cells from the marrow using hematopoietic growth factors (eg, G-CSF) and/or treatment with chemotherapy. PBPC are then collected using a stem-cell protocol with any suitable apheresis instrument. One to five apheresis procedures may be necessary to obtain the desired number of hematopoietic progenitor cells (HPC). If the desired number of HPC are obtained in 1-3 collections, transplants using PBPC are less expensive than a marrow transplant.[3]

Patient Preparation Excellent venous access is a daily requirement. Indwelling dual- or triple-lumen central venous catheters suitable for apheresis procedures are frequently necessary. Red cells may be required to prime the apheresis instrument for the pediatric donor.

Aftercare Complete blood counts should be performed to monitor hematocrit and platelet counts. Thrombocytopenia can be a complication.[4] A majority of G-CSF stimulated donors experience bone pain, headaches, and fatigue associated with cytokine therapy.[5]

Collection As described by the manufacturer of the apheresis instrument used. The optimal time to begin collection is controversial. Some institutions monitor using total white cell count, while others use CD34 count (*vide infra*). Collection target for engraftment ranges from a minimum total cell dose of 2-5 x 10⁶ CD34+ cells/kg.

Storage Instructions PBPC may be further processed prior to cryopreservation or infusion. A number of techniques for positive or negative selection are available to remove tumor cells or reduce the risk of graft-vs-host disease. Controlled rate (-180°C storage) and noncontrolled rate (-80°C

storage) cryopreservation techniques are available. An expiration date has not been defined, however, marrow stored for 11 years has been transplanted with resultant engraftment.[6]

Causes for Rejection Cancer or leukemia cells in peripheral blood

Special Instructions Coordination with appropriate HPC therapy service personnel is required.

Use Collection and storage of autologous PBPC make it possible to treat malignant disease with heavy doses of chemotherapy and/or irradiation that would otherwise destroy the patient's marrow function. After such treatment, marrow is repopulated from the stored autologous supply. Allogeneic peripheral blood cells used for hematopoietic rescue restored blood counts faster than allogeneic bone marrow, without an increase in risk of graft-vs-host disease, in subjects treated with high-dose chemotherapy with or without radiation in treatment of hematologic malignant disease.[7] Allogeneic transplants are also performed for indications such as marrow failure (eg, aplastic anemia), hemoglobinopathies or inborn errors of metabolism. The system is also useful for collecting stem cells for gene therapy.

Limitations Repopulation of marrow depends on the number of stem cells in the collection. Current enumeration is performed by CD34 analysis (0.01% to 0.1% of unstimulated peripheral blood cells). Numerous CD34 methods exist and site-to-site correlation may be unreliable.[8] (CD34 is a cell surface antigen which is expressed on hematopoietic progenitor cells and on vascular endothelium.[9]) Processing may result in loss of stem cells. Inadequacy of stem cells will mean failure of marrow repopulation.

Methodology For infusion of thawed, previously cryopreserved products: Hydrate patient and "alkalinize" urine 12 hours before HPC infusion. Immediately prior to infusion premedicate patient with antihistamine (to prevent sudden and severe hypotension).[10] If the amount of DMSO infused exceeds 10 mL/kg, administer HPC over 2 days.

Additional Information Compared to marrow or umbilical cord as the source of HPC, use of mobilized PBPC reduces the time to hematopoietic recovery.

Standards for HPC have been published by the American Association of Blood Banks, the Foundation for the Accreditation of Hematopoietic Cell Therapy, and the National Marrow Donor Program. The FDA may utilize voluntary standards in place of more comprehensive regulations.

A Circulator of Information for the Use of Hematopoietic Progenitor Cell Products is available from blood banks or blood centers.[11]

Footnotes

1. *Standards for Hematopoietic Progenitor Cell Services*, 2nd ed, Bethesda, MD: American Association of Blood Banks Press, 2000, 45-51.

2. *Standards for Hematopoietic Progenitor Cell Collection, Processing and Transplantation*, 1st ed, Omaha, NE: Foundation for the Accreditation of Hematopoietic Cell Therapy, 1996, 22-3.

3. Lane TA, "Mobilization of Hematopoietic Progenitor Cells," *Hematopoietic Progenitor Cell: Processing, Standards and Practice*, Brecher ME, Lasky LC, Sacher RA, et al, eds. Bethesda, MD: American Association of Blood Banks Press, 1995, 59-108.

4. Stroncek DF, Clay ME, Smith J, et al, "Changes in Blood Counts After the Administration of Granulocyte-Colony-Stimulating Factor and the Collection of Peripheral Blood Stem Cells From Healthy Donors," *Transfusion*, 1996, 36:596-600.

5. Stroncek DF, Clay ME, Petzoldt ML, et al, "Treatment of Normal Individuals With Granulocyte-Colony-Stimulating Factor: Donor Experience and the Effects on Peripheral Blood CD34+ Cell Counts and on the Collection of Peripheral Blood Stem Cells," *Transfusion*, 1996, 36(7):601-10.

6. Aird W, Labopin M, Gorin NC, et al, "Long-Term Cryopreservation of Human Stem Cells," *Bone Marrow Transplant*, 1992, 9(6):487-90.

7. Bensinger WI, Martin PJ, Storer B, et al, "Transplantation of Bone Marrow as Compared With Peripheral Blood Cells From HLA-Identical Relatives in Patients With Hematologic Cancers," *N Engl J Med*, 2001, 344(3):175-81.

8. Brecher ME, Sims L, Schmitz J, et al, "North American Multicenter Study on Flow Cytometric Enumeration of CD34+ Hematopoietic Stem Cells," *J Hematother*, 1996, 5(3):227-36.

9. Nash RA, "Hematopoietic Stem Cell Transplantation," *Wintrobe's Clinical Hematology*, Volume 1, Chapter 28, Lee GR, Foerster J, Lukens J, et al, eds, Baltimore, MD: Lippincott Williams & Wilkins, 1999, 875-93.

10. Rowley SD, "Storage of Hematopoietic Cells," *Marrow Transplantation: Practical and Technical Aspects of Stem Cell Reconstitution*, Sacher RA and AuBuchon JP, eds, Bethesda, MD: American Association of Blood Banks Press, 1992, 105-27.

11. *Circular of Information for the Use of Progenitor Cell Products*, American Association of Blood Banks, America's Blood Centers, American Red Cross, January, 2000.

References

Davis JM, Noga SJ, and Braine JG, "Apheresis and Hematopoietic Progenitor Cell Processing," *Apheresis: Principles and Practice*, McLeon BC, Price TH, and Drew MJ, eds, Bethesda, MD: American Association of Blood Banks Press, 1997, 453-63.

Lippman ME, "High-Dose Chemotherapy Plus Autologous Bone Marrow Transplantation for Metastatic Breast Cancer," *N Engl J Med*, 2000, 342(15):1119-20.

Neito Y and Shpall EJ, "Clinical Results of Autologous Stem Cell Transplantation for Solid Tumors in Adults," *Hematology: Basic Principles and Practice*, 3rd ed, Hoffman R, Benz EJ Jr, Shattil SJ, et al, eds, New York, NY: Churchill Livingstone, 2000, 1597-609.

Stadtmauer EA, O'Neil A, Goldstein L, et al, "Conventional-Dose Chemotherapy Compared With High-Dose Chemotherapy Plus Autologous Hematopoietic Stem-Cell Transplantation for Metastatic Brease Cancer," *N Engl J Med*, 2000, 342(15):1069-76.

Vengelen-Tyler V, "Hematopoietic Transplantation," *Technical Manual*, 13th ed, Chapter 25, Bethesda, MD: American Association of Blood Banks Press, 1999, 531-61.

Hemolytic Disease of the Newborn, Antibody Identification

Related Information

Antibody Detection/Identification, Red Cell *on page 834*
Antiglobulin Test, Indirect *on page 835*
Bilirubin, Amniotic Fluid, Delta A450 *on page 116*
Bilirubin, Neonatal, Serum *on page 117*
Cord Blood Screen *on page 838*
Newborn Crossmatch and Transfusion *on page 848*
Rh Genotype *on page 860*
Rh₀(D) Immune Globulin (Human) *on page 860*

Synonyms Newborn/Maternal Antibody Work-up

Applies to Exchange Transfusion

Test Includes Infant ABO group, Rh type; direct antiglobulin test; antibody elution, antibody identification. Mother ABO group, Rh type; antibody detection/identification.

Abstract Hemolytic disease of the newborn (HDN) takes place when fetal red cells cross the placenta and enter the maternal circulation, with immunization of the mother to a fetal red cell antigen absent from her own erythrocytes. Production of maternal IgG antibodies causes hemolysis of fetal red cells. Fetomaternal (transplacental) hemorrhage is detectable in about 5% of pregnant women. Other events that enhance the risk of transplacental hemorrhage include spontaneous and therapeutic abortion, ectopic gestation, amniocentesis, intrauterine surgery, abdominal trauma, and peripartum hemorrhage.[1]

Maternal antibody specificity influences therapeutic decisions, especially selection of blood for exchange transfusion and whether an Rh-negative mother is a candidate for Rh immunoprophylaxis. See Newborn Crossmatch and Transfusion *on page 848*.

Specimen Blood from infant and mother (collect maternal sample before administration of Rh immune globulin)

Container Lavender top (EDTA) tube and red top tube(s)

Causes for Rejection Gross hemolysis, sample collected in serum separator tube, improper labeling

Use Investigation of HDN, selection of blood for exchange transfusion

Limitations ABO HDN may not be detected by testing at birth. It may be indicated by subsequent clinical impression. Maternal antibody to a "private" paternal antigen may not be demonstrated with standard red cell antibody identification tests. Wharton's jelly may interfere with infant ABO tests. It may prove difficult to interpret results of Rh type of infant red cells heavily sensitized with IgG maternal antibodies. The presence of large numbers of maternal red cells in a cord blood sample can confuse interpretation of blood grouping results. Similarly, serological results can be complicated in newborns that received intrauterine blood transfusions. Administration of antenatal Rh immune globulin may complicate interpretation of cord blood DAT results.

Additional Information The fetal-maternal relationship presents special immunohematological problems for the Blood Bank Laboratory which are important for patient care. The results of initial cord blood screening tests will indicate need for additional studies to determine the likelihood of HDN or need for Rh immunoprophylaxis. Administration of postpartum Rh immune globulin will depend on maternal alloimmunization and the results of infant Rh type.

A positive DAT is an important indicator of HDN. A positive result will evolve into antibody identification studies of maternal serum or infant red cell eluate. Antibody specificity is an important guide to disease severity. Most severe HDN is caused by anti-D alone or in combination with other Rh antibodies, anti-C, or anti-E. The next grade of severity is associated with antibodies to other Rh antigens (notably anti-c) or with antibodies to antigens in other blood group systems (eg, anti-K).

IgG antibodies to antigens of the ABO system usually cause the lowest grade of HDN severity. ABO HDN can occur in any pregnancy, even the first. The DAT is often negative and the infant is rarely symptomatic at birth.

Blood group antibodies other than those in the ABO group and Rh type also cause HDN, which may be even more dangerous because they may be unsuspected.[2] They include antibodies directed against Duffy, Kidd, and MNSs systems.

Fetal genotyping can be performed.

Footnotes

1. Luban NLC, "Hemolytic Disease of the Newborn: Progenitor Cells and Late Effects," *N Engl J Med*, 1998, 338(12):830-1.
2. Bowman JM, Pollock JM, and Edmonds LD, "Epidemiology of Rh Disease of the Newborn in the United States," *JAMA*, 1991, 265(24):3270-4.

References

Garratty G, *Hemolytic Disease of the Newborn*, Arlington, VA: American Association of Blood Banks Press, 1984.
Issitt PD and Anstee DJ, *Applied Blood Group Serology*, 4th ed, Durham, NC: Montgomery Scientific Publications, 1998, 1045-95.
Judd WJ, Luban NLC, Ness PM, et al, "Prenatal and Perinatal Immunohematology: Recommendations for Serologic Management of the Fetus, Newborn, Infant, and Obstetric Patient," *Transfusion*, 1990, 30:175-83.
Lo YMD, Hjelm NM, Fidler C, et al, "Prenatal Diagnosis of Fetal RhD Status by Molecular Analysis of Maternal Plasma," *N Engl J Med*, 1998, 339(24):1734-8.
Saade GR, "Noninvasive Testing for Fetal Anemia," *N Engl J Med*, 2000, 342(1):52-3.
Vengelen-Tyler V, *Technical Manual*, 13th ed, Bethesda, MD: American Association of Blood Banks Press, 1999, 502-8.

♦ **Hemolytic Disease of the Newborn, Antibody Titer** *see* Antibody Titer *on page 834*

♦ **Hemolytic Disease of the Newborn, Crossmatch** *see* Newborn Crossmatch and Transfusion *on page 848*

♦ **Hemolytic Disease of the Newborn (HDN) Prognosis** *see* Rh Genotype *on page 860*

♦ **Hemophilia A Therapy** *see* Cryoprecipitate *on page 838*

♦ **IgA Antibodies** *see* Antibodies to IgA *on page 833*

♦ **Indirect Coombs Test** *see* Antiglobulin Test, Indirect *on page 835*

♦ **Intraoperative Cell Salvage** *see* Autologous Transfusion, Intraoperative Blood Salvage *on page 836*

♦ **Investigation of Hemolytic Disease of the Newborn** *see* Antibody Detection/Identification, Red Cell *on page 834*

Irradiated Blood Components

Related Information

Donation, Blood, Directed *on page 840*
Neutrophils, Transfusion *on page 847*
Newborn Crossmatch and Transfusion *on page 848*
Platelet Transfusion *on page 854*
Red Blood Cells *on page 857*
Whole Blood *on page 866*

Applies to Blood Components, Irradiated; Whole Blood, Irradiated

Test Includes Irradiation of blood components with a gamma radiation source, usually cesium-137 or cobalt-60

Abstract Transfusion associated graft-versus-host disease (TA-GVHD) may occur when donor T lymphocytes from transfused blood attack recipient tissues, beginning 2-30 days after transfusion. It is characterized by fever, maculopapular rash, diarrhea, hepatitis, and pancytopenia. Mortality is ~90%.

Patient Preparation Same as for other cellular component pretransfusion testing.

Aftercare Same as for transfused component.

Use Avoid TA-GVHD in blood recipients at risk for development of this condition. Indications for using irradiated blood components include immunocompromised transplant (stem cell or organ) recipients, allogeneic stem cell transplant candidates, intrauterine transfusions, neonatal exchange transfusion or extracorporeal membrane oxygenation, recipients with Hodgkin disease, recipients with congenital cell-mediated immunodeficiencies, recipients of directed donations from biologic relatives or HLA-matched donors, and recipients who are heterozygous at an HLA locus for which the donor is homozygous and shares an allele. Other possible indications include individuals receiving immunosuppressive therapy or who are immunosuppressed, patients undergoing high-dose chemotherapy, low birthweight infants/premature infants, and patients with AIDS who have opportunistic infections.[1] See table.

Indications for Gamma Irradiation of Cellular Blood Components

Well-Defined

Bone marrow or peripheral blood stem cell transplant

    Current or anticipated congenital cell-mediated immunodeficiencies (eg, severe combined immunodeficiency disease, Wiscott-Aldrich, DiGeorge)

Intrauterine or postintrauterine transfusions

Directed donations from blood relative or HLA-matched donors

Hodgkin disease

Adult/childhood acute lymphocytic leukemia

Immunocompromised organ transplant recipients

Relative (possible)

Malignancies and organ transplants treated with immunosuppressive chemotherapy or radiotherapy

Exchange transfusion or use of extracorporeal membrane oxygenation in neonates

Low-birth-weight neonates (<1200 g)

Neonates with possible immunodeficiency

Neonates receiving intrauterine transfusions

Human immunodeficiency virus-infected patients with opportunistic infections

Probably Not Indicated

Full-term neonates (exceptions noted above)

Human immunodeficiency virus-infected patients

Modified from "Practice Parameter for the Use of Red Blood Cell Transfusions. Developed by the Red Blood Cell Administration Practice Guideline Development Task Force of the College of American Pathologists," *Arch Pathol Lab Med*, 1998, 122(2):130-8.

Limitations Irradiation induces RBC membrane damage and causes higher potassium levels in the supernatant. Such increase in K+ is not clinically relevant except for exchange transfusions or when infants receive massive transfusions.[2] After irradiation, shelf-life is reduced to 28 days.

Methodology Irradiation of blood prevents proliferation of donor lymphocytes. The central portion of the canister should receive 2500 cGy, while no less than 1500 cGy should be delivered to the periphery of the canister.

Additional Information TA-GVHD occurs when viable lymphocytes are transfused into severely immunosuppressed patients. The patient is unable to destroy these incoming lymphocytes, which attack the host cells, recognizing them as foreign. TA-GVHD may occur in immunocompetent patients if they receive blood from a blood relative who is homozygous for an HLA haplotype for which the patient is heterozygous. Preventive irradiation is a wise resort in the case of directed donations from blood relatives, even if the HLA types are unknown. Available filtration methods of leukocyte removal are not adequate to prevent TA-GVHD. GVHD also occurs after allogeneic bone marrow transplantation, however, it is a distinct disease entity from TA-GVHD.[2] TA-GVHD results in pancytopenia, is resistant to therapy, and usually results in rapid death.

A molecular method has been described to demonstrate donor DNA in subjects with GVHD.[3]

Footnotes
1. Przepiorka D, LeParc GF, Stovall MA, et al, "Use of Irradiated Blood Components. Practice Parameter," *Am J Clin Pathol*, 1996, 106(1):6-11.
2. Mollison PL, Engelfriet CP, Contreras M, et al, "The Transfusion of Red Cells," *Blood Transfusion in Clinical Medicine*, 10th ed, Chapter 9, Oxford, UK: Blackwell Scientific Publications, 1997, 278-314.
3. Wang L, Juji T, Tokunaga K, et al, "Brief Report: Polymorphic Microsatellite Markers for the Diagnosis of Graft-Versus-Host Disease," *N Engl J Med*, 1994, 330(6):398-401.

References
Huston BM, Brecher ME, and Bandarenko N, "Lack of Efficacy for Conventional Gamma Irradiation of Platelet Concentrates to Abrogate Bacterial Growth," *Am J Clin Pathol*, 1998, 109(6):743-7.
Mollison PL, Engelfriet CP, Contreras M, et al, "Some Unfavorable Effects of Transfusion," *Blood Transfusion in Clinical Medicine*, 10th ed, Chapter 15, Oxford, UK: Blackwell Scientific Publications, 1997, 487-508.
Simon TL, Alverson DC, AuBuchon J, et al, "Practice Parameter for the Use of Red Blood Cell Transfusions. Developed by the Red Blood Cell Administration Practice Guideline Development Task Force of the College of American Pathologists," *Arch Pathol Lab Med*, 1998, 122(2):130-8.

Neutrophils, Apheresis, Donation

Related Information
Donation, Blood *on page 839*
Neutrophils, Transfusion *on page 847*

Synonyms Granulocytes, Apheresis, Donation; Granulocytes, Pheresis; Leukapheresis, Automated; Leukocytes, Apheresis

Test Includes As for regular blood donation. Many of the infectious disease tests, however, may not be completed prior to transfusion.

Abstract Granulocytes may be useful in septic patients with severe neutropenia (<0.5 x 10^9/L) who have not responded to appropriate antibiotic therapy and who have a reasonable chance of marrow recovery.

Patient Preparation The more granulocytes collected, the more effective the granulocyte transfusions (GTX). To increase granulocyte yields, donors may be stimulated with corticosteroids and granulocyte colony-stimulating factor (G-CSF). Neutrophilia is stimulated by giving the donor 300 μg G-CSF subcutaneously 12 hours before beginning leukapheresis, with three doses of oral prednisone, 20 mg, 18, 12, and 4 hours before leukapheresis

is begun. 7-10 L of donor blood is processed using a continuous-flow blood separator with citrated hydroxyethyl starch solution infused throughout the collection. Use of large volume leukapheresis with G-CSF makes it possible to collect large numbers of PMNs.[1] Donors should be questioned regarding history of hypertension, diabetes, or peptic ulcer disease before beginning corticosteroid stimulation. Use of growth factors for allogeneic granulocyte donation is not yet approved by the FDA. Thus, corticosteroids alone may be given to a donor to increase granulocyte yields.

Aftercare Donors receiving G-CSF experience bone pain, myalgia, headaches, and nausea/vomiting, which usually respond to acetaminophen. Headaches or peripheral edema from an increased circulatory volume may also occur secondary to the sedimenting agent used during the apheresis procedure.

Specimen Donor granulocytes including therapeutic doses of platelets

Collection A granulocyte unit should contain a minimum of 1 x 10^10 granulocytes per transfusion.[2,3] Thus, most collections are usually prepared from a single donor using an apheresis instrument. They may also be prepared as a "buffy coat" from a single unit of fresh whole blood for a neonatal transfusion.[4] During apheresis, a sedimenting agent is added which causes the red cells to aggregate and enhances the granulocyte harvest. A common sedimenting agent is hydroxyethyl starch (HES). Pentastarch, which has a shorter half-life, is now also available.

Selection of donors who are both red cell and leukocyte compatible is important.[1]

Storage Instructions Store granulocytes at 20°C to 24°C without agitation. Granulocyte concentrates should be transfused as soon as possible after collection. GTX should not be given when >24 hours old.

Causes for Rejection As for regular blood donation.

Special Instructions Donors selected for this procedure are often family members. ABO and Rh compatibility are desirable; HLA compatibility is desirable in the case of alloimmunized recipients but is seldom practical.

Use Severely neutropenic subjects with life-threatening infections should be considered for GTX provided in adequate doses.[1] Septic neonatal patients may also benefit from granulocyte transfusions. The importance of high patient doses of PMNs (≥1.7 x 10^10/day) is stressed.[1]

Limitations In the past, such concentrates contained inadequate numbers of PMNs. The interval between donations should be approved by the Blood Bank physician.

Contraindications Donors with intolerance to stimulating or sedimenting agents or donor reactions during apheresis procedure (see Platelets, Apheresis, Donation *on page 853* for a table listing donor reactions specific to leukapheresis).

Methodology Centrifugation leukapheresis; exact method depends upon apheresis instrument used. Filtration leukapheresis is no longer recommended.

Additional Information ABO and Rh compatibility are desirable; if more than 2 mL of red cells are present in the product, the component should be crossmatched. Many platelets are present in a granulocyte concentrate, which is beneficial because most neutropenic patients are also thrombocytopenic. Irradiate prior to infusing into immunocompetent recipients. Do **not** administer through a leukocyte-reduction filter.

Footnotes
1. Strauss RG, "Principles of Neutrophil (Granulocyte) Transfusions," *Hematology: Basic Principles and Practice*, 3rd ed, Chapter 137, Hoffman R, Benz EJ Jr, Shattil SJ, et al, eds, New York, NY: Churchill Livingstone, 2000, 2257-63.
2. Vamvakas EC and Pineda AA, "Meta-analysis of Clinical Studies of the Efficacy of Granulocyte Transfusions in the Treatment of Bacterial Sepsis," *J Clin Apheresis*, 1996, 11(1):1-9.
3. Menitove JE, *Standards for Blood Banks and Transfusion Services*, 20th ed, Bethesda, MD: American Association of Blood Banks Press, 2000, 35.
4. Rock G, Zurakowski S, Baxter A, et al, "Simple and Rapid Preparation of Granulocytes for the Treatment of Neonatal Septicemia," *Transfusion*, 1984, 24:510-2.

References
Blood Transfusion Therapy: A Physician's Handbook, 6th ed, Bethesda, MD: American Association of Blood Banks Press, 1999, 22-4.
Stroncek DF, Clay ME, Petzoldt ML, et al, "Treatment of Normal Individuals With Granulocyte-Colony-Stimulating Factor: Donor Experiences and the Effects on Peripheral Blood CD34+ Cell Counts and on the Collection of Peripheral Blood Stem Cells," *Transfusion*, 1996, 36(7):601-10.

Neutrophils, Transfusion

Related Information
Irradiated Blood Components *on page 846*
Neutrophils, Apheresis, Donation *on page 847*

Synonyms Granulocytes, Transfusion; GTX; Leukocyte Concentrate; Leukocytes, Transfusion; White Cells, Transfusion

Applies to Granulocyte-Colony-Stimulating Factor

Test Includes ABO and Rh type, antibody screen, and crossmatch; antibody identification if indicated

Abstract Granulocyte transfusions may be useful in septic patients with severe neutropenia (<0.5 x 10^9/L) as an adjunct to antimicrobial therapy, in treatment and/or possible prevention of infections. Severe neutropenia and disordered PMN function may lead to infections with bacteria, yeasts, and fungi. In neonates, WBC as high as 3.0 x 10^9/L may prompt candidacy for GTX, but GTX application in neonates is controversial.[1]
(Continued)

Neutrophils, Transfusion *(Continued)*

Patient Preparation Give daily for a minimum of 4 days to demonstrate clinical benefit.[2] Granulocytes obtained from granulocyte-colony-stimulating-factor (G-CSF) stimulated donors may allow for every-other-day transfusion.[3] However, use of growth factors for allogeneic granulocyte donation is not yet approved by the FDA.

Dosage and administration: Administer through a standard blood filter. Daily infusion of 4-8 x 10^{10} PMNs is advocated for patients with severe persistent neutropenia and infections which have not responded to reasonable courses of antibiotic therapy.[1] Slow the infusion rate or give an antihistamine, antipyretic, or steroid for the fever, chills, or allergic reactions that may occur with granulocyte infusions. Gamma irradiate the granulocyte component to prevent graft-vs-host disease if administering to an immunoincompetent recipient. Do not administer in conjunction with amphotericin, as severe pulmonary reactions may occur.[4]

Specimen Blood from recipient and donor

Container One red top tube or one lavender top (EDTA) tube

Collection (Of sample from intended recipient): As for other red-cell-containing blood components.

Storage Instructions Storage should be at 20°C to 24°C, without agitation, for a maximum of 24 hours.

Causes for Rejection (Of patient sample): Gross hemolysis, sample placed in a serum separator tube, specimen tube not properly labeled

Special Instructions Expiration date is 24 hours. Transfuse granulocytes as soon as possible after collection.

Use Granulocytes in adequate doses may be useful in therapy of serious infectious with bacteria, yeast, or fungi in patients with severe neutropenia (<0.5 x 10^9/L) as an adjunct to antimicrobial drugs, in subjects who have a reasonable chance of marrow recovery. Indications have included bacterial septicemia, pneumonia, serious localized infections, fever of unknown origin, and possibly invasive fungal and yeast infections. Especially, septic patients with persistent neutropenia caused by continuing marrow failure may be helped by GTX in adequate doses with antibiotic therapy.[1] Septic neonatal patients may also benefit from granulocyte transfusions.

Limitations There is a risk of viral transmission, particularly cytomegalovirus (CMV). Select appropriate CMV seronegative donors, if needed, since leukocyte reduction filters may not be used with these components to reduce the risk of CMV transmissions (see Filters for Blood *on page 842*). Granulocyte transfusions will not be of benefit to the patient whose bone marrow is unlikely to recover. They are expensive. GTX are recommended only for progressive infections uncontrolled with antimicrobials.

Risk of alloimmunization exists.

Contraindications Not indicated for infections that can be managed successfully with antibiotics.

Methodology Leukocyte crossmatching. See Neutrophils, Apheresis, Donation *on page 847*.

Additional Information Normal production of granulocytes is about 1 x 10^{11}/day in an adult. Only 5% to 10% of the PMN pool is in circulation.

ABO and Rh compatibility are desirable; if more than 2 mL of red cells are present in the product, the component should be crossmatched. Many platelets are present in a granulocyte concentrate, which is beneficial because most neutropenic patients are also thrombocytopenic.

Footnotes
1. Strauss RG, "Principles of Neutrophil (Granulocyte) Transfusions," *Hematology: Basic Principles and Practice*, 3rd ed, Hoffman R, Benz EJ Jr, Shattil SJ, et al, eds, New York, NY: Churchill Livingstone, 2000, 2257-63.
2. Dutcher JP, "Granulocyte Transfusion Therapy," *Am J Med Sci*, 1984, 287(2):11-7.
3. Adkins D, Spitzer G, Johnston M, et al, "Transfusions of Granulocyte-Colony-Stimulating-Factor Mobilized Granulocyte Components to Allogeneic Transplant Recipients: Analysis of Kinetics and Factors Determining Post-transfusion Neutrophil and Platelet Counts," *Transfusion*, 1997, 37(7):737-48.
4. Dutcher JP, Kendall J, Norris D, et al, "Granulocyte Transfusion Therapy and Amphotericin B: Adverse Reactions?" *Am J Hematol*, 1989, 31(2):102-8.

References
Blood Transfusion Therapy: A Physician's Handbook, 6th ed, Bethesda, MD: American Association of Blood Banks Press, 1999, 22-4.
Mollison PL, Engelfriet CP, and Contreras M, *Blood Transfusion in Clinical Medicine*, 10th ed, Oxford, UK: Blackwell Scientific Publications, 1997, 437-40.
Strauss RG, "Granulocyte Transfusion," *Apheresis: Principles and Practice*, McLeod BC, Price TH, and Drew MJ, eds, Bethesda, MD: American Association of Blood Banks Press, 1997, 195-209.

Newborn Crossmatch and Transfusion

Related Information
Bilirubin, Amniotic Fluid, Delta A450 *on page 116*
Bilirubin, Neonatal, Serum *on page 117*
Cord Blood Screen *on page 838*
Cytomegalovirus Serology *on page 600*
Hemolytic Disease of the Newborn, Antibody Identification *on page 846*
Irradiated Blood Components *on page 846*
Rh$_o$(D) Immune Globulin (Human) *on page 860*
Rosette Test for Fetomaternal Hemorrhage *on page 863*
Warming, Blood *on page 865*

Synonyms Exchange Transfusion; Neonatal Transfusion; Newborn Transfusion; Type and Crossmatch for Exchange Transfusion of Newborn

Applies to Cytomegalovirus Low Risk Blood; Hemolytic Disease of the Newborn, Crossmatch; Satellite Bags

Test Includes For exchange transfusion or routine transfusion, the unit should be compatible with the mother's ABO group and Rh type, and with any unexpected blood group antibodies present in mother's serum. Anti-A and anti-B may not correspond to the newborn's ABO blood group. For routine transfusions of nongroup O red cells, include an antiglobulin test when testing for the presence of anti-A and/or anti-B.[1] If the initial red cell antibody screen is negative, it is unnecessary to crossmatch donor red cells for the initial or subsequent transfusion and repeat testing may be omitted for an infant younger than 4 months of age.[2]

Abstract See Hemolytic Disease of the Newborn, Antibody Identification *on page 846*, Bilirubin, Neonatal, Serum *on page 117*, and Bilirubin, Amniotic Fluid, Delta A450 *on page 116*.

Patient Preparation For exchange transfusion, blood should be passed through a warming device to raise the temperature of the blood to about 37°C during administration. Neonates who have received intrauterine transfusions and those with known or suspected T-cell immune deficiencies should receive irradiated blood.[3] Irradiated blood is recommended for exchange transfusion in all neonates.[4] Neonates weighing less than 1200 grams should receive CMV-reduced-risk units; *vide infra*.[5] Consider selection of blood known to lack hemoglobin S for exchange transfusion.[2] For smaller, nonexchange transfusions, typically administer group O, Rh-specific blood, 10-15 mL/kg, over 2-3 hours.[6] The type of red cell storage medium is believed not to pose a risk to the neonate.[7]

Aftercare Fatal cardiac arrhythmias have been reported during exchange transfusion secondary to hyperkalemia.[8] Irradiation increases red cell potassium leakage. Irradiate blood as close to the time of transfusion as possible if large quantities of irradiated blood will be transfused. The quantity of potassium administered in routine (10-15 mL/kg) transfusions is comparatively insignificant. Hypocalcemia may be avoided by measurement of postexchange ionized calcium. It may be necessary to determine drug levels or repeat doses after exchange transfusion.

Specimen Blood from mother and infant

Container One red top tube or one lavender top (EDTA) tube from mother; appropriate pediatric tubes from newborn

Causes for Rejection (Of patient sample): Gross hemolysis, sample placed in a serum separator tube, specimen tube not properly labeled

Special Instructions Advance notice permits collection of appropriate donor blood into a bag with multiple attached satellite bags. This permits multiple small transfusions to be given to the infant from the same donor (ie, reduces donor exposure and reduces the risk of transfusion-transmitted infectious disease). Additional satellite bags may also be attached by means of a sterile-connecting device. Although many feel that washed red cells should be limited for low-volume transfusions in neonates to those, for example, with T-activation or in renal failure who would be harmed by the potassium load (see Red Blood Cells, Washed *on page 859*), others prefer washed red cells or fresh (<5 days old) red cells relevant to potassium load.[9] When needed, ABO-compatible plasma-containing fractions (eg, platelets, fresh-frozen plasma) are desirable for the neonate. If unavailable, platelets may be centrifuged and plasma removed.

Use Hemolytic disease of the newborn is due to transplacental passage of maternal antibodies - ABO, Rh (D, C, c), Kell, Duffy, Kidd, or other blood group system antibodies which are directed against antigens expressed on the neonate's red cells.

Immediate exchange laboratory criteria for term infants include significant anemia and rapidly increasing hyperbilirubinemia; see Bilirubin, Neonatal, Serum *on page 117*. The second indication for exchange is the presence of congestive heart failure secondary to severe anemia.[9] A classic indication for exchange transfusion in full-term infants is an indirect bilirubin level ≥20 mg/dL. At this level, brain damage may occur. In premature babies or those with other complications, brain damage may occur at lower levels of bilirubin.[1] An exchange transfusion may then be appropriate at levels <20 mg/dL. Severe bilirubinemia may also be seen in multiorgan failure. Consult pediatric literature for more detailed information.[10]

The blood volume of neonates is 85 mL/kg for full-term babies and 100-105 mL/kg for preterm infants. The anemia of prematurity responds to recombinant human erythropoietin.

Cytomegalovirus (CMV)-seronegative or leukocyte-reduced blood is indicated, and irradiated blood components are recommended.[11]

Limitations Relatively mild jaundice beginning 1-2 weeks after delivery with a weakly positive direct antiglobulin test in a baby of group A or B and a mother of group O usually indicates ABO hemolytic disease of the newborn. An eluate in these instances (group A or B infant born to a group O mother) is of no assistance in prediction of cases of hemolytic disease of the newborn. Exchange transfusion is seldom necessary in ABO hemolytic disease of the newborn.

Additional Information Red cell transfusions are not infrequently given to premature infants weighing less than 1300 g for anemia of prematurity and for loss from repeated blood sampling. The use of recombinant human erythropoietin in this group has been discussed.[12]

Use of blood components with low risk for CMV infection is advocated for intrauterine transfusion and transfusion in neonates with birth weight <1200 g, unless the mother is CMV antibody positive.

Blood components at low risk for CMV include those from CMV-negative donors. See Red Blood Cells, Leukocytes Reduced *on page 858*.[4]

Neonatal Red Blood Cell Transfusion Guidelines*

Transfuse with ≤20 mL/kg (not to exceed hematocrit of 0.45 or hemoglobin of 15 g/dL)
1. Hct ≤0.20 or Hb ≤7 g/dL and reticulocyte count <4% (or absolute <1000,000/mL)
2. Hct ≤0.25 or Hb ≤8 g/dL and any of the following conditions: a. Episodes of apnea/bradycardia ≥10 episodes/24 hours or ≥2 episodes requiring bag-mask ventilation   b. Sustained tachycardia (>180 beats/minute) or sustained tachypnea (>80 breaths/minute) (x 24 hours by averaging every 3-hour measurements)   c. Cessation of adequate weight gain x 4 days (≤10 g/24 hours despite ≥420 kJ/kg/24 hours)   d. Mild RDS + FiO_2 0.25-0.35 or nasal cannula 1/8-1/4 L/minute or IMV or NCPAP with Paw <6 cm H_2O
3. Hct ≤0.30 or Hb ≤10 g/dL with moderate RDS + FiO_2 >35% or nasal cannula O_2 or intermittent mandatory ventilation with Paw 6-8 cm + H_2O.
4. Hct ≤0.35 or Hb ≤12 g/dL with severe RDS requiring mechanical ventilation and Paw >8 cm H_2O and FiO_2 >50%, or severe congenital heart disease associated with cyanosis or heart failure.
5. Acute blood loss with shock: blood replacement to reestablish adequate blood volume and Hct of 0.40.
6. CMV-seronegative or leukocyte-reduced blood advocated in preterm infants and immunodeficient babies.
7. Irradiated blood components recommended, especially in preterm infants, those with possible immunodeficiency and possible transplant candidates, and those who are receiving intrauterine transfusions.

*RDS = respiratory distress syndrome; FiO_2 = inspired oxygen content; IMV = intermittent mandatory ventilation; NCPAP = nasal continuous positive airway pressure; Paw = mean airway pressure

Adapted from Simon TL, Alverson DC, AuBuchon J, et al, "Practice Parameter for the Use of Red Blood Cell Transfusions," *Arch Pathol Lab Med*, 1998, 122(2):130-8.

Footnotes

1. Chambers LA and Luban NC, "Neonatal and Intrauterine Transfusion," *Transfusion Therapy: Clinical Principles and Practice*, Mintz PD, ed, Bethesda, MD: American Association of Blood Banks Press, 1999, 299-311.

2. Menitove JE, *Standards for Blood Banks and Transfusion Services*, 20th ed, Bethesda, MD: American Association of Blood Banks Press, 2000, 48-50.

3. Parkman R, Mosier D, Umansky I, et al, "Graft-Versus-Host Disease After Intrauterine and Exchange Transfusions for Hemolytic Disease of the Newborn," *N Engl J Med*, 1974, 290:359-63.

4. Chambers LA, "Blood Transfusions in Infants," *Lab Med*, 1999, 30(4):254-61.

5. Smith DM and Shoos Lipton K, "Leukocyte Reduction for the Prevention of Transfusion-Transmitted Cytomegalovirus (TT-CMV)," Association Bulletin #97-2, Bethesda, MD: American Association of Blood Banks Press, 1997, 1-15.

6. Strauss RG, Burmeister LF, Johnson K, et al, "AS-1 Red Cells for Neonatal Transfusions: A Randomized Trial Assessing Donor Exposure and Safety," *Transfusion*, 1996, 36(10):873-8.

7. Luban NLC, Strauss RG, and Hume HA, "Commentary on the Safety of Red Blood Cells Preserved in Extended Storage Media for Neonatal Transfusions," *Transfusion*, 1991, 31:229-35.

8. Hall TL, Barnes A, Miller JR, et al, "Neonatal Mortality Following Transfusion of Red Cells With High Plasma Potassium Levels," *Transfusion*, 1993, 33:606-9.

9. Ness PM and Rothko K, "Principles of Red Blood Cell Transfusion," *Hematology: Basic Principles and Practice*, 3rd ed, Hoffman R, Benz EJ Jr, Shattil SJ, eds, New York, NY: Churchill Livingstone, 2000, 2241-8.

10. Anderson JM, "Hyperbilirubinemia," *Essentials of Pediatric Intensive Care*, 2nd ed, Levin DL and Morriss FC, eds, New York, NY: Churchill Livingstone, 1997, 829-44.

11. Simon TL, Alverson DC, AuBuchon J, et al, "Practice Parameter for the Use of Red Blood Cell Transfusions: Developed by the Red Blood Cell Administration Practice Guideline Development Task Force of the College of American Pathologists," *Arch Pathol Lab Med*, 1998, 122(2):130-8.

12. Obladen M and Maier RF, "Recombinant Erythropoietin for Prevention of Anemia in Preterm Infants," *J Perinat Med*, 1995, 23(1-2):199-26.

♦ **Newborn/Maternal Antibody Work-up** *see* Hemolytic Disease of the Newborn, Antibody Identification *on page 846*

♦ **Newborn Transfusion** *see* Newborn Crossmatch and Transfusion *on page 848*

♦ **Normal Serum Albumin (Human)** *see* Albumin and Plasma Protein Fraction for Infusion *on page 833*

♦ **Normovolemic Hemodilution** *see* Autologous Transfusion, Intraoperative Blood Salvage *on page 836*

♦ **Normovolemic Hemodilution** *see* Autologous Transfusion, Preoperative Deposit *on page 837*

♦ **Packed Red Cells, Transfusion** *see* Red Blood Cells *on page 857*

♦ **PAD** *see* Autologous Transfusion, Preoperative Deposit *on page 837*

♦ **Peripheral Blood Stem Cells, Autologous** *see* Hematopoietic Progenitor Cells, Peripheral Blood *on page 845*

♦ **Peripheral Stem Cells** *see* Hematopoietic Progenitor Cells, Peripheral Blood *on page 845*

♦ **Phlebotomy, Blood Donor** *see* Donation, Blood *on page 839*

Phlebotomy, Therapeutic

Related Information
Blood Gases and pH, Arterial *on page 119*
Blood Volume *on page 407*
Carboxyhemoglobin, Blood *on page 784*
Cobalamin, Serum *on page 150*
Donation, Blood *on page 839*
Erythropoietin, Serum *on page 169*
Ferritin, Serum *on page 173*
Hereditary Hemochromatosis DNA Test *on page 709*
Iron and Total Iron Binding Capacity/Transferrin, Serum *on page 203*
Leukocyte Alkaline Phosphatase *on page 455*
Liver Biopsy *on page 65*
Methemoglobin, Whole Blood *on page 800*
Porphyrins, Quantitative, Urine *on page 255*

Synonyms Therapeutic Phlebotomy

Abstract Blood may be electively removed via therapeutic phlebotomy in patients with erythrocytosis (eg, polycythemia vera or cyanotic heart disease) or to remove excess iron in patients with hemochromatosis. Phlebotomies are done for porphyria cutanea tarda. Phlebotomy may be necessary in acute pulmonary edema. Currently, such blood is not utilized for allogeneic transfusion, except for those units collected from individuals with hemochromatosis who have met the following criteria.[1]
- There is no charge to the individual for the therapeutic phlebotomy.
- The indication for the therapeutic phlebotomy is hemochromatosis.
- The Food and Drug Administration has approved the program.

Patient Preparation Before the elective removal of blood, the attending physician must document the request and specify the amount of blood to be withdrawn. Approval of the Blood Bank physician is also required.[1] Record prephlebotomy and postphlebotomy vital signs. The patient and physician should both understand that a therapeutic phlebotomy is an operative procedure and not a blood donation.

Aftercare Observe patient for at least 20 minutes for vasovagal and other adverse reactions. Local discomfort and, occasionally, hematoma occur at phlebotomy site. Avoid strenuous exercise for 24 hours. Tell patient whom to contact if adverse effects develop after discharge. Multiple phlebotomies may be necessary over a long time period.

Collection Phlebotomies for patients with hemochromatosis should remove 500 mL of blood weekly until the patient is iron deficient,[2] or until mild hypoferritinemia is found; then phlebotomy is done as required to maintain serum ferritin <50 μg/L.[3]

Only five to six phlebotomies are usually needed at 1- to 2-week intervals for porphyria cutanea tarda.[4]

Causes for Rejection Anemia, hematocrit at designated target, abnormal vital signs. Phlebotomy is contraindicated in stress polycythemia, in which plasma volume is contracted. Certain conditions may require the presence of the attending physician during phlebotomy (eg, hypertension, cardiac symptoms). The blood bank physician may decline to do the procedure on high-risk patients.

Special Instructions For polycythemia, evaluate the patient's hemoglobin, hematocrit, red cell count, platelet count, WBC count, leukocyte alkaline phosphatase, serum vitamin B_{12}, carboxyhemoglobin, and blood volume. In primary polycythemia, erythropoietin levels in blood and urine are decreased. Erythropoietin is increased in secondary polycythemia. Arterial blood gases may be helpful, with significantly decreased pO_2 and oxygen saturation pointing to secondary polycythemia.[2,5] Arterial blood oxygen saturation ≥92% is expected in polycythemia vera, and 75% have splenomegaly.

The diagnosis of **hemochromatosis** requires transferrin saturation >55% with serum ferritin >400 μg/L. The gold standard is liver biopsy with measured iron concentration.[6] The diagnosis of hereditary hemochromatosis can be confirmed by direct mutation analysis of the "HFE gene."[7] However, not all patients with hemochromatosis have mutations in the HFE gene.[3]

Each unit of 450-500 mL blood contains 200-250 mg iron.

The patient with hemochromatosis should be counseled to modify his/her diet as well.[3]

Use Removal of blood in polycythemia to maintain the hematocrit <45%; hypoxic lung disease or cyanotic heart disease; hemochromatosis, for which ferritin levels and/or transferrin saturation are used as monitors; therapy for porphyria cutanea tarda

Limitations Complications and deaths have been reported.[5] Very thin, elderly patients with active cardiopulmonary disease may not tolerate the 500 mL phlebotomy. Consider removing only 250 mL of blood in such patients. A crystalloid or colloid solution can be simultaneously infused as well.
(Continued)

Phlebotomy, Therapeutic (Continued)

Contraindications Lack of documented increase of red cell mass when polycythemia is considered. Hemoglobinopathies exist in which polycythemia occurs, the abnormal hemoglobin having increased oxygen affinity. Methemoglobinemias may relate to secondary polycythemias (see Methemoglobin, Whole Blood on page 800). Uncommonly, certain tumors induce erythrocytosis. Renal tumors are the most widely known cause of tumor erythrocytosis. These considerations must remain the responsibility of the clinical physician.

Additional Information Transfusional siderosis is a complication of long term transfusion therapy (eg, in management of thalassemia). The diagnosis is made with clinical history, liver biopsy, or magnetic-susceptibility evaluation; serum ferritin is less reliable in this setting. Phlebotomy is usually contraindicated.[3]

Footnotes

1. Menitove JE, *Standards for Blood Banks and Transfusion Services*, 20th ed, Bethesda, MD: American Association of Blood Banks Press, 2000, 28.
2. Brittenham GM, "Disorders of Iron Metabolism: Iron Deficiency and Overload," *Hematology: Basic Principles and Practice*, 3rd ed, Hoffman R, Benz EJ Jr, Shattil SJ, et al, eds, Philadelphia, PA: Churchill Livingstone, 2000, 397-428.
3. Andrews NC, "Disorders of Iron Metabolism," *N Engl J Med*, 1999, 341(26):1986-95.
4. Anderson KE, "The Porphyrias," *Cecil Textbook of Medicine*, 21st ed, Chapter 219, Goldman L and Bennett JC, eds, Philadelphia, PA: WB Saunders Co, 2000, 1123-30.
5. Kiraly JF, Feldman JE, and Whelby MS, "Hazards of Phlebotomy in Polycythemic Patients With Cardiovascular Disease," *JAMA*, 1976, 236:2080-1.
6. Edwards CQ and Kushner JP, "Screening for Hemochromatosis," *N Engl J Med*, 1993, 328(22):1616-20.
7. Feder JN, Gnirke A, Thomas W, et al, "A Novel MHC Class I-Like Gene Is Mutated in Patients With Hereditary Haemochromatosis," *Nat Genet*, 1996, 13(4):399-408.

References

Grima KM, "Therapeutic Apheresis in Hematological and Oncological Diseases," *J Clin Apheresis*, 2000, 15(1-2):28-52.

♦ **Photopheresis** see Apheresis, Therapeutic on page 836

♦ **Placental Blood** see Hematopoietic Progenitor Cells, Cord Blood/Placental Blood on page 843

Plasma Exchange

Related Information

Acetylcholine Receptor Antibody on page 502
Calcium, Ionized, Serum on page 130
Cholesterol, Total, Serum or Plasma on page 146
Cryoglobulin, Qualitative, Serum and Plasma on page 524
Low Density Lipoprotein Cholesterol on page 218
Plasma, Fresh Frozen on page 851
Plasmapheresis, Donor on page 852
Platelet Count on page 468

Synonyms Plasmapheresis; Plasmapheresis, Therapeutic

Test Includes ABO group is indicated if fresh frozen plasma must be selected and thawed for use as a replacement solution.

Abstract Selective removal of a pathologic component of a patient's plasma to assist in the treatment of a disease. Separation techniques are varied and include manual (whole blood bags) and automated instruments (eg, centrifugation and adsorption). With the numerous automated instruments available, manual techniques are seldom used.

Patient Preparation Excellent venous access is a daily requirement. Indwelling dual- or triple-lumen central venous catheters suitable for apheresis procedures are frequently necessary. Hypotension secondary to hypovolemia will become a concern if the extracorporeal volume exceeds 15% of the patient's blood volume. Patients taking angiotensin-converting-enzyme (ACE) inhibitors may be prone to marked hypotension prior to routine or adsorption treatment. Such therapy should be removed from their medication if possible.[1] Understanding which medications being given to the patient will be altered by the procedure is relevant so that dosage can be adjusted accordingly (withhold administration for 1 hour before and after procedure if possible). Obtain and document informed consent.

Aftercare Monitor patient for signs and symptoms of reduced plasma levels of ionized calcium (tingling, perioral paresthesias, cardiac arrhythmias) and hypotension secondary to hypovolemia. Hypocalcemia may be managed by decreasing the inlet flow rate or administering oral or intravenous calcium.[2]

Causes for Rejection Decision to perform this procedure is shared between Clinical and Blood Bank physicians. Guidelines for evidence of therapeutic efficacy have been developed by the American Association of Blood Banks and the American Society for Apheresis.[3]

Special Instructions Usually on a scheduled basis, but can be emergent. Consult with a Blood Bank physician. Typical plasma exchanges are 1-1.5 times plasma volume daily (40 mL/kg patient's body weight). Whenever possible, monitor efficacy of exchanges by monitoring levels of some marker that indicates progress or regression of the disease treated (eg, specific antibody, immunoglobulin, abnormal protein).

Use During therapeutic plasmapheresis, plasma containing the pathologic substance is removed and replaced with crystalloids, albumin, or fresh frozen plasma. Usually 1-1.5 plasma volumes are exchanged. Selective removal of pathologic substances in plasma via adsorption columns (eg, dextran sulfate removal of LDL cholesterol or staphylococcal protein A removal of IgG antibodies) eliminates the need for replacement fluid.[4,5] See the table for some established clinical indications for plasma exchange. Presently, they include hyperviscosity/Waldenström macroglobulinemia, thrombotic thrombocytopenic purpura, myasthenia gravis, and chronic inflammatory demyelinating polyneuropathy.[6]

Indications for Therapeutic Plasmapheresis

Generally Seems to Be Effective*
Hyperviscosity syndrome
Myasthenia gravis*
Goodpasture syndrome
Thrombotic thrombocytopenic purpura*
Cryoglobulinemia
Familial hypercholesterolemia (via selective adsorption)
Guillain-Barré syndrome*
Post-transfusion purpura
Efficacy Debatable or Controlled Studies Lacking
Systemic lupus erythematosus
Schizophrenia
Warm autoimmune hemolytic anemia
Amyotrophic lateral sclerosis
Rh hemolytic disease of the newborn
ABO-incompatible bone marrow transplantation
Renal transplant rejection
Thyroid storm

*Effective = producing significant clinical improvement that is better than transitory. Entities marked with * are among the most frequent indications for plasma exchange in the Canadian apheresis group study. Included among these are also Waldenström macroglobulinemia and chronic inflammatory demyelinating polyneuropathy.[4]

Adapted from Vengelen-Tyler V, *Technical Manual*, 13th ed, Bethesda, MD: American Association of Blood Banks Press, 1999, 136-7.

Contraindications The extent of each procedure is determined by the Blood Bank physician in consultation with the attending physician. Consultation is especially important if the patient is pediatric, elderly, clinically unstable, has poor vascular access, or has a condition for which apheresis is of unknown benefit.

Methodology Depends upon the type of apheresis instrument used. **Choice of replacement fluid:** Standard replacement fluid has been 5% albumin, although use with up to 50% normal saline has been reported successful.[7] Fresh frozen plasma should be used in thrombotic thrombocytopenic purpura, and may be considered in patients with a pre-existing bleeding diathesis. Use of hydroxyethyl starch instead of albumin has been reported.[8]

Additional Information The most common adverse effects are vasovagal reactions, hypovolemia, hypocalcemia, allergic reactions, and citrate toxicity. Allergic reactions (hives, dyspnea, wheezing) and symptoms of hypocalcemia (tingling, perioral paresthesias, cardiac arrhythmias) may occur more frequently when fresh frozen plasma is used as a replacement fluid. Allergic reactions may be treated with an antihistamine or, if symptoms progress, epinephrine. Symptoms of hypocalcemia may be treated by decreasing the inlet flow rate or replacing calcium during the procedure (taking care not to cause extracorporeal clotting). Symptoms of hypovolemia include hypotension, diaphoresis, and tachycardia and may be treated by administration of a saline bolus and placement of the patient in the Trendelenburg position.

Footnotes

1. Owen HG and Brecher ME, "Atypical Reactions Associated With the Use of Angiotensin-Converting Enzyme Inhibitors and Apheresis," *Transfusion*, 1994, 34:891-4.
2. Owen HG and Brecher ME, "Management of the Therapeutic Apheresis Patient," *Principles and Practice*, McLeod BC, Price TH, and Drew MJ, eds, Bethesda, MD: American Association of Blood Banks Press, 1997, 223-49.
3. Vengelen-Tyler V, *Technical Manual*, 13th ed, Bethesda, MD: American Association of Blood Banks Press, 1999, 136-7.
4. Knisel W, Pfohl M, Muller M, et al, "Comparative Long-Term Experience With Immunoadsorption and Dextran Sulfate Cellulose Adsorption for Extracorporeal Elimination of Low-Density Lipoproteins," *Clin Investig*, 1994, 72(9):660-8.
5. Felson D, Durst D, LaValley M, et al, "Results of a Randomized Double Blind Trial of the Prosorba Column for Treatment of Severe Rheumatoid Arthritis," *Arthritis Rheum*, 1998, 41:S364.
6. Clark WF, Rock GA, Buskard N, et al, "Therapeutic Plasma Exchange: An Update From the Canadian Apheresis Group," *Ann Intern Med*, 1999, 131(6):453-62.
7. Lewis EJ, Hunsicker LG, Lan SP, et al, "A Controlled Trial of Plasmapheresis in Severe Lupus Nephritis," *N Engl J Med*, 1992, 326:1371-9.
8. Owen HG and Brecher ME, "Partial Colloid Replacement for Therapeutic Plasma Exchange," *J Clin Apheresis*, 1997, 12(3):146-53.

References

"Clinical Applications of Therapeutical Apheresis," *J Clin Apheresis*, 2000, 15:1-159 (special issue).

McLeod BC, Price TH, and Drew MJ, *Apheresis Principles and Practice*, Bethesda, MD: American Association of Blood Banks Press, 1997.

Patel TC, Moore SB, Pineda AA, et al, "Role of Plasmapheresis in Thrombocytopenic Purpura Associated With Waldenström's Macroglobulinemia," *Mayo Clin Proc*, 1996, 71:597-600.

Womack EP Jr, "Treating Thrombotic Thrombocytopenic Purpura With Plasma Exchange," *Lab Med*, 1999, 30(4):276-9.

Plasma, Fresh Frozen

Related Information

Activated Partial Thromboplastin Time *on page 328*
Cryoprecipitate *on page 838*
Factor IX Concentrate *on page 841*
Factor VIII Concentrate *on page 841*
Factor XIII *on page 339*
Fibrinogen *on page 341*
Plasma, Frozen, Donor Retested *on page 851*
Plasma, Frozen, Solvent Detergent-Treated *on page 851*
Prothrombin Time *on page 354*
Warfarin *on page 770*

Synonyms FFP; Fresh Frozen Plasma

Applies to Cryopreservation; Factor IX Replacement; Factor VII Replacement; Factor V Replacement; Factor XI Replacement; Factor X Replacement; Thawed Plasma[1]

Test Includes ABO type[1]

Abstract Plasma from a unit of whole blood separated from the red blood cells and frozen at -18°C or lower within 8 hours of collection. The unit has a volume of 150-275 mL. FFP collected via apheresis has a volume of 500 mL. Both contain all labile and stable coagulation factors (each at 1 IU/mL), but are not concentrates. Does not contain platelets. A severe deficiency of coagulation factors cannot be corrected by giving FFP. Fluid overload would likely result.

Patient Preparation Use coagulation studies as a guide to transfusion of FFP.

Dosage and administration: FFP should be ABO compatible,[2] especially when it is to be given to infants. Depending on the ABO group, it may contain anti-A or anti-B. Rh need not be considered (but see Additional Information). Crossmatch is not necessary. Administer through a filter. The usual unit (prepared from one unit of whole blood) contains about 200 units of factor VIII,[1] and 250-400 mg of fibrinogen. It contains factor IX as well as other stable and labile coagulation factors. One unit of fresh frozen plasma will raise patient's plasma level of fibrinogen only about 10-13 mg/dL; cryoprecipitate is a better source of fibrinogen. Give FFP at about 10 mL/minute, to a total dose of about 10 mL/kg.[1]

Specimen Blood

Container One red top tube or one lavender top (EDTA) tube

Storage Instructions Frozen at -18°C or lower, FFP has a shelf-life of 1 year. Examine the frozen plastic bag for cracks, especially the seams. Thaw at 37°C with agitation in a waterbath, using a plastic overwrap.[3] Thawing requires 15-30 minutes depending on the number of units being thawed. Once thawed, store in Blood Bank refrigerator and transfuse within 24 hours.[3] Plasma ideally should be transfused within 2 hours after thawing when the patient requires labile coagulation factors. After 24 hours, a thawed unit of FFP becomes a unit of "thawed plasma".

Turnaround Time Usually available on request. Requires 15-30 minutes to thaw and issue.

Use Treatment of bleeding caused by multiple labile and stable coagulation factor deficiencies (eg, liver disease, DIC); with massive transfusion and abnormal coagulation assays, in severe warfarin overdosage before vitamin K can reverse the warfarin effect, with cardiac bypass surgery and as replacement medium in plasma exchange for thrombotic thrombocytopenic purpura (TTP).[1]

Limitations Transmission of infectious disease, including HIV, hepatitis A, B, and C, and parvovirus B19; circulatory overload; TRALI (transfusion-related acute lung injury); leukocytes 10^6 to 10^7 per bag with potential for reactions and allergic reactions are hazards of use of FFP. Patients with TTP may receive large volumes of plasma, which multiply their risks.

Considerable variation in coagulation factors per bag exists. **Fresh frozen plasma is grossly overused.**[4]

Contraindications Do not use FFP prophylactically to prevent dilutional coagulopathy in large transfusions. Do not use it as a plasma expander; albumin is better and safer. Do not use FFP if prothrombin time and activated partial thromboplastin time are less than 1.5 times normal and in the absence of abnormal bleeding. Coagulopathies in patients with hemophilia and von Willebrand disease are better treated with specific factor concentrates.

Additional Information Hazards: Risk of disease transmission (that of any single unit exposure), plasma volume overload, anaphylaxis in IgA deficient recipient is a remote hazard. One unit of FFP collected via apheresis contains the equivalent coagulation factor of ~2 units FFP while one exposing the patient to one donor. FFP contains anti-A or anti-B. Although FFP is basically cell-free, it is not without antigens. Recipients can have mild or severe allergic reactions and sometimes fever. Immunization can take place to soluble constituents as well as to Rh and other red cell antigens,[5] the latter presumably from cell fragments in the plasma. See also listings Cryoprecipitate *on page 838* and Plasma, Frozen, Solvent Detergent-Treated *on page 851*.

An alternative to increase the safety of plasma involves storage of the unit, while the donor is retested after a period longer than the window periods of known viruses. Negative results of such retesting would support lack of infectivity of the unit. This approach was approved by the FDA, September 1998, for units in which retesting takes place over a minimum of 112 days.[6]

Footnotes

1. *Circular of Information for the Use of Human Blood and Blood Components*, American Association of Blood Banks, American Blood Centers, American Red Cross, 1998, 15-22.
2. Menitove JE, *Standards for Blood Banks and Transfusion Services*, 20th ed, Bethesda, MD: American Association of Blood Banks Press, 2000, 47.
3. Vengelen-Tyler V, *Technical Manual*, 13th ed, Bethesda, MD: American Association of Blood Banks Press, 1999, 462-72.
4. Consensus Conference, "Fresh Frozen Plasma. Indications and Risks," *JAMA*, 1985, 253(4):551-3.
5. Ching EP, Poon MC, Neurath D, et al, "Red Blood Cell Alloimmunization Complicating Plasma Transfusion," *Am J Clin Pathol*, 1991, 96(2):201-2.
6. Goodnough LT, Brecher ME, Kanter MH, et al, "Transfusion Medicine. Second of Two Parts: Blood Conservation," *N Engl J Med*, 1999, 340(7):525-33.

References

Pehta JC, "Advances in Plasma Products Use," *Lab Med*, 2001, 32(1):26-31.
Triulzi DJ, *Blood Transfusion Therapy: A Physician's Handbook*, 6th ed, Bethesda, MD: American Association of Blood Banks Press, 1999.

Plasma, Frozen, Donor Retested

Related Information

Cryoprecipitate *on page 838*
Donation, Blood *on page 839*
Factor IX Concentrate *on page 841*
Factor VIII Concentrate *on page 841*
Plasma, Fresh Frozen *on page 851*

Synonyms FFP; Fresh Frozen Plasma

Applies to Cryopreservation; Factor IX Replacement; Factor VII Replacement; Factor V Replacement; Factor XI Replacement; Factor X Replacement

Test Includes ABO type

Abstract Donor retested (DR) plasma is collected and prepared in a similar manner to that as fresh frozen plasma (see Plasma, Fresh Frozen *on page 851*). However, DR plasma may reduce the risk of viral transmission for hepatitis C, hepatitis B, HIV, and HTLV because it is not released for transfusion until the donor returns for repeat testing. The plasma is then released if the donor tests negative for transfusion-transmitted infectious diseases.

Patient Preparation See Plasma, Fresh Frozen *on page 851*.

Container One red top tube or one lavender top (EDTA) tube

Storage Instructions See Plasma, Fresh Frozen *on page 851*.

Use See Plasma, Fresh Frozen *on page 851*.

Limitations As with fresh frozen plasma, circulatory overload, allergic reactions, and risk of infectious disease transmission continue to occur. **Fresh frozen plasma is grossly overused.**[1] Due to complex inventory management problems, DR plasma may not be available at every blood bank and at a constant supply.

Contraindications See Plasma, Fresh Frozen *on page 851*.

Methodology DR plasma may be prepared from a unit of whole blood by separating and freezing the plasma within 8 hours of phlebotomy or by apheresis (similar to fresh frozen plasma). The plasma is tested for routine infectious disease testing, but held for 90 or more days (usually at least 112 days) until the donor comes back a second time.[2] The first unit can be released once the donor tests negative the second time.

Additional Information DR plasma may be as safe as solvent detergent-treated plasma because the retesting helps verify that the donor is not in an infectious window period and DR plasma is not a pooled product.[3]

Hazards: See Plasma, Fresh Frozen *on page 851*.

Footnotes

1. Consensus Conference, "Fresh Frozen Plasma. Indications and Risks," *JAMA*, 1985, 253:551-3.
2. Triulzi DJ, *Blood Transfusion Therapy: A Physician's Handbook*, 6th ed, Bethesda, MD: American Association of Blood Banks Press, 1999, 24-6.
3. Vengelen-Tyler V, *Technical Manual*, 13th ed, Bethesda, MD: American Association of Blood Banks Press, 1999, 172.

References

"Fresh Frozen Plasma, Cryoprecipitate, and Platelets Administration Practice Guidelines Development Task Force of the College of American Pathologists. Practice Parameter for the Use of Fresh-Frozen Plasma, Cryoprecipitate and Platelets," *JAMA*, 1994, 271:777-81.
"Premium Plasma. Isn't Regular Blood Safe Enough?" *Consum Rep*, September 1999, 61-3.
Schreiber GB, Busch MP, Kleinman SH, et al, "The Risk of Transfusion-Transmitted Viral Infection," *N Engl J Med*, 1996, 334(26):1685-90.
Wallace EL, Churchill WH, Surgenor DM, et al, "Collection and Transfusion of Blood and Blood Components in the United States, 1994," *Transfusion*, 1998, 38(7):625-36.

Plasma, Frozen, Solvent Detergent-Treated

Related Information

Activated Partial Thromboplastin Time *on page 328*
Cryoprecipitate *on page 838*
(Continued)

Plasma, Frozen, Solvent Detergent-Treated
(Continued)

Factor IX Concentrate *on page 841*
Factor VIII Concentrate *on page 841*
Factor XIII *on page 339*
Fibrinogen *on page 341*
Plasma, Fresh Frozen *on page 851*
Plasma, Frozen, Donor Retested *on page 851*
Prothrombin Time *on page 354*
Warfarin *on page 770*

Synonyms FFP; Fresh Frozen Plasma; PLAS+®SD; S/D Plasma; Solvent Detergent-Treated Plasma

Applies to Cryopreservation; Factor IX Replacement; Factor VII Replacement; Factor V Replacement; Factor XI Replacement; Factor X Replacement

Test Includes ABO type

Abstract Solvent detergent-treated plasma (SD plasma), a pooled plasma product, is treated with the solvent tri-(n-butyl) phosphate and the detergent, Triton X-100, and refrozen in a uniform manner so as to preserve its content of labile coagulation factors. This solvent detergent treatment inactivates lipid-coated viruses such as HIV, HTLV, hepatitis B and hepatitis C, and reduces risks of transmission of such viruses to nearly zero.

Patient Preparation Use coagulation studies as a guide to transfusion of SD plasma.

Dosage and administration: For chronic users of blood products, patients should be prophylactically immunized against hepatitis A.[1] SD plasma should be ABO compatible with the recipient's red cells. One unit (standardized 200 mL volume) can increase the level of individual clotting factors by 2% to 3% in a normal 70 kg adult.[1] Thus, 4-6 units should increase factor levels 8% to 18%, which may be adequate for treatment of bleeding episodes or routine prophylaxis against spontaneous bleeding. A dose of 3 units in adults and 50-100 mL in children was found to be satisfactory at preventing relapse of chronic TTP.[1] Administer intravenously at room temperature.

Specimen Blood

Container One red top tube or one lavender top (EDTA) tube

Storage Instructions Frozen at -18°C or colder, SD plasma has a shelf life for 12 months at -18°C. Examine the frozen product for evidence of container thawing or breaking. Thaw between 30°C and 37°C using a plastic overwrap.[2] Fraction must not be refrigerated once thawed and should be transfused as soon as possible after thawing, but no more than 24 hours after thawing. Do not refreeze. Store thawed fraction at ambient temperature.

Turnaround Time Usually available on request. Requires 15-30 minutes to thaw and issue.

Use Treatment of bleeding caused by multiple acquired or inherited labile and stable coagulation factor deficiencies (eg, liver disease, DIC), with massive transfusion and abnormal coagulation assays, in severe warfarin overdosage before vitamin K can reverse the warfarin effect, and as replacement medium in plasma exchange for thrombotic thrombocytopenic purpura.[3,4] It is used in neonatal exchange transfusion and in open heart surgery.

Limitations Similar to Plasma, Fresh Frozen *on page 851*. Solvent detergent treatment will not inactivate nonlipid-enveloped viruses. Current licensed fraction is now tested for parvovirus B19 and hepatitis A via PCR technology.[5] Each unit is prepared from a pool containing plasma from no more than 2500 donors.

The cost of a 200 mL unit so treated is 2-5 times as high as the cost of a 250 mL unit of untreated plasma from a single donor. Costs and benefits of SD plasma versus untreated fresh frozen plasma were recently explained.[6]

Procoagulant activity is decreased about 15% and concentrations of large multimers of von Willebrand factor and certain other factors, including protein S, are diminished >50%.[7]

Additional Information Contains no leukocytes and lacks the largest von Willebrand multimers.[1]

Hazards: Adverse reactions are similar to those observed with infusion of Plasma, Fresh Frozen *on page 851* and include volume overload, allergic reaction, anaphylaxis in IgA deficient recipients, dyspepsia, citrate overload, hypothermia, and transfusion-related acute lung injury (TRALI).[1]

Footnotes
1. PLAS+®SD, Pooled Plasma, Solvent/Detergent Treated (package insert), The American National Red Cross, May 1998,
2. Vengelen-Tyler V, *Technical Manual*, 13th ed, Bethesda, MD: American Association of Blood Banks Press, 1999, 170-2.
3. *Circular of Information for the Use of Human Blood and Blood Components*, American Association of Blood Banks, America's Blood Centers, American Red Cross, 1998, 15-20.
4. Drohan WN and Clark DB, "Preparation of Plasma-Derived and Recombinant Human Plasma Proteins," *Hematology: Basic Principles and Practice*, 3rd ed, Chapter 139, Hoffman R, Benz EJ Jr, Shattil SJ, et al, eds, New York, NY: Churchill Livingstone, 2000, 2273-82.
5. "'Premium' Plasma - Isn't 'Regular' Blood Safe Enough?" *Consum Rep*, 1999, 64(9):61-3.
6. Blumberg N and Heal JM, et al, "Mortality Risks, Costs, and Decision Making in Transfusion Medicine," *Am J Clin Pathol*, 2000, 114(6):934-7.

7. Goodnough LT, Brecher ME, Kanter MH, et al, "Transfusion Medicine. Second of Two Parts: Blood Conservation," *N Engl J Med*, 1999, 340(7):525-33.

References
Jackson BR, AuBuchon JP, and Birkmeyer JD, "Update of Cost-Effectiveness Analysis for Solvent-Detergent-Treated Plasma," *JAMA*, 1999, 282(4):329.
Pehta JC, "Advances in Plasma Products Use," *Lab Med*, 2001, 32(1):26-31.
Pehta JC, "Clinical Studies With Solvent Detergent-Treated Products," *Transfus Med Rev*, 1996, 10(4):303-11.
Williamson LM, Llewelyn CA, Fisher NC, et al, "A Randomized Trial of Solvent/Detergent-Treated and Standard Fresh-Frozen Plasma in the Coagulopathy of Liver Disease and Liver Transplantation," *Transfusion*, 1999, 39(11-12):1227-34.

♦ **Plasmapheresis** *see* Apheresis, Therapeutic *on page 836*

♦ **Plasmapheresis** *see* Plasma Exchange *on page 850*

Plasmapheresis, Donor

Related Information
Donation, Blood *on page 839*
Plasma Exchange *on page 850*

Synonyms Donor Plasmapheresis

Test Includes As for regular whole blood donation, but may include total protein and serum protein electrophoresis, depending upon the donation interval.[1]

Abstract The expression, "**plasmapheresis**", means "taking away plasma" and indicates selective removal of the donor's plasma with return of all other components. Separation techniques are varied and include manual (whole blood bags) and automated instruments (centrifugation or membrane filtration). With the numerous automated instruments available, manual techniques are seldom used.

When sufficient plasma has been removed, it becomes advisable to infuse albumin or plasma as replacement; this is **plasma exchange**. Plasma exchange is used to remove a particular constituent.

Patient Preparation Obtain and document informed consent. Emergency medical care must be available.

For donors in the UK, prior blood donation is required with age older than 50 years, and normal CBC and total serum protein. Periodically CBC, total protein, and serum albumin are repeated and immunoglobulins, urine protein, and glucose are measured.

Aftercare Monitor total red cell losses during procedures. If red cells cannot be returned during a procedure, defer donor for 8 weeks.

Causes for Rejection (Of donor): As for regular whole blood donation, except for the donation interval.

Use Plasma is collected as fresh frozen plasma or for subsequent application into derivatives such as plasma protein fraction, albumin, immune globulins, and clotting factor concentrates. Plasma from particular donors hyperimmunized to particular antigens such as $Rh_o(D)$ is to provide certain specific immunoglobulins.

Limitations Must meet donor criteria specified by AABB and FDA.

Methodology May be separated manually from whole blood collections with return of RBCs to donors or may be prepared by use of automated apheresis instruments.

Additional Information A minimum of 48 hours should elapse between successive procedures. A donor should undergo no more than 2 procedures in 1 week.

Footnotes
1. *Code of Federal Regulations*. Title 21 CFR Part 640, Washington, DC: U.S. Government Printing Office, 1999.

References
Menitove JE, *Standards for Blood Banks and Transfusion Services*, 20th ed, Bethesda, MD: American Association of Blood Banks Press, 2000.
Mollison PL, Engelfriet CP, Contreras M, et al, "The Withdrawal of Blood," *Blood Transfusion in Clinical Medicine*, 10th ed, Chapter 1, Oxford, UK: Blackwell Scientific Publications, 1997, 1-36.
Vengelen-Tyler V, *Technical Manual*, 13th ed, Bethesda, MD: American Association of Blood Banks Press, 1999, 132-3.

♦ **Plasmapheresis, Therapeutic** *see* Plasma Exchange *on page 850*

♦ **Plasma Protein Fraction (Human) (PPF)** *see* Albumin and Plasma Protein Fraction for Infusion *on page 833*

♦ **PLAS+®SD** *see* Plasma, Frozen, Solvent Detergent-Treated *on page 851*

Platelet Antibody, Immunohematologic

Related Information
Platelet Antibodies *on page 349*
Platelet Count *on page 468*
Platelet Transfusion *on page 854*
Transfusion Reaction Work-up *on page 864*

Synonyms Antiplatelet Antibody; Platelet-Associated IgG; Platelet-Bound IgG; Platelet Serology

Abstract Like red cells, antigens on platelets may be the targets of antibody assault. The consequences of antiplatelet antibody action include refractoriness to platelet transfusion, neonatal alloimmune thrombocytopenia, autoimmune thrombocytopenic purpura, post-transfusion purpura, and drug-induced immune thrombocytopenia. Antibodies may be directed to antigens shared with red cells (eg, ABO), to antigens shared with white cells (eg, HLA), or to platelet glycoprotein antigens not found on other blood cells (eg, HPA).

Specimen Blood

Collection Methods for the collection of blood samples for platelet serology are very test specific - consult with the laboratory.

Storage Instructions Storage of blood for platelet serology is very test specific - consult with the laboratory.

Use Platelet serology is indicated in the investigation of thrombocytopenia and refractoriness to platelet transfusion. Platelet crossmatching may be indicated for refractory patients. Solid-phase antibody detection systems have proven to be the most practical for crossmatching. Many blood transfusion centers utilize both crossmatch and HLA-compatible platelets for transfusion to refractory patients. (See Platelet Transfusion *on page 854.*)

Limitations Platelet serology is an evolving discipline. A particular obstacle to the development of assays based on the detection of platelet-bound antibody is the inherent binding of inert IgG to the platelet through membrane Fc receptors. Methods that measure antibody binding to isolated platelet glycoproteins (radioimmunoprecipitation, immunoblotting, and antigen capture by monoclonal antibodies) represent attempts to overcome this. The significance of platelet-bound IgM and IgA has not been determined.

The collection of sufficient platelets for testing from thrombocytopenic patients may be problematic.

Methodology Current test systems are based on the detection of platelet-bound IgG. These include the enzyme-linked immunosorbent assay (ELISA) methods, platelet immunofluorescence test (PIFT), solid phase assays, radioimmunoprecipitation, immunoblotting, and monoclonal antibody immobilization of platelet antigen (MAIPA). Test systems that utilize fresh whole platelets can be employed to detect platelet-associated IgG. This is equivalent to the direct antiglobulin test on red cells. The tests used for platelet crossmatching are ELISA, PIFT, and solid-phase assays.

Platelet serology is in the development stage and new test modalities can be anticipated.

Additional Information Platelet serology is an evolving field. Consult with the laboratory for current recommendations. The availability of licensed test kits is providing laboratories with easier access to testing.

See Platelet Antibodies *on page 349.*

Platelets bear only class I, and not class II, HLA proteins. Simultaneously transfused WBCs in platelet and/or red cell fractions of fetal blood entering the maternal circulation in pregnancy cause primary immunization. Alloimmunization is almost eliminated by use of leukocyte-depleted fractions among recipients without prior WBC exposure.[1]

Footnotes
1. Kruskall MS, "The Perils of Platelet Transfusions," *N Engl J Med*, 1997, 337(26):1914-5.

References
Rachel JM, Sinor LT, Tawfik OW, et al, "A Solid-Phase Red Cell Adherence Test for Platelet Crossmatching," *Med Lab Sci*, 1985, 42(2):194-5.

The Trial to Reduce Alloimmunization to Platelets Study Group (TRAP Trial Study Group), "Leukocyte Reduction and Ultraviolet B Irradiation of Platelets to Prevent Alloimmunization and Refractoriness to Platelet Transfusions," *N Engl J Med*, 1997, 337(26):1861-9.

Vengelen-Tyler V, *Technical Manual*, 13th ed, Bethesda, MD: American Association of Blood Banks Press, 1999, 339-56.

♦ **Platelet-Associated IgG** *see* Platelet Antibody, Immunohematologic *on page 852*

♦ **Platelet-Bound IgG** *see* Platelet Antibody, Immunohematologic *on page 852*

♦ **Plateletpheresis** *see* Platelets, Apheresis, Donation *on page 853*

♦ **Platelet-Rich Plasma** *see* Platelet Transfusion *on page 854*

♦ **Platelets** *see* Platelet Transfusion *on page 854*

Platelets, Apheresis, Donation

Related Information
Donation, Blood *on page 839*
HLA Typing, Single Human Leukocyte Antigen *on page 529*
Neutrophils, Apheresis, Donation *on page 847*
Platelet Antibodies *on page 349*
Platelet Count *on page 468*
Platelet Transfusion *on page 854*
Transfusion Reaction Work-up *on page 864*

Synonyms Plateletpheresis; Platelets, Pheresis (FDA); Single-Donor Platelets

Applies to Platelets, Pheresis; Platelets, Single-Donor

Test Includes As for regular whole blood donation, but may donate more frequently. The donor's platelet count should be >150,000/μL if the donation interval is less than 4 weeks.[1]

Abstract Selective removal of the donor's platelets with return of all other components using automated apheresis instruments. Donors include

random volunteer donors, recipient's family members, and HLA-matched donors.

Patient Preparation Obtain and document informed consent. Emergency medical care must be available.

Aftercare Monitor total red cell losses during procedures. If red cells cannot be returned during a procedure, defer donor for 8 weeks.

Storage Instructions Store in the Blood Bank at 20°C to 24°C with continuous agitation for 5 days. Do not refrigerate.

Causes for Rejection (Of donor): As for regular blood donation. In addition, donors taking aspirin-containing medication within 36 hours of donation are usually deferred.

(Of units): Do not transfuse units containing excessive platelet aggregates. "Swirling" (observed while holding bag against a light source and gently squeezing) correlates well with adequate platelet *in vivo* viability.[2]

Special Instructions Single-donor platelets (platelets, pheresis) are available from most blood centers and larger hospital blood banks on a more or less regular basis. In some institutions they are reserved for patients who regularly receive platelet transfusions, or who may be refractory to regular platelet transfusions.

Use Single-donor platelets are suitable for any patient needing platelet transfusions. Single-donor platelets have the advantage of providing an entire platelet transfusion for an adult from one donor, hence with a single antigenic combination and a single donor exposure, decreasing the risk of alloimmunization or to infectious agents. Furthermore, the donor can be selected (eg, from a patient's relatives or by HLA type), providing easier selection of CMV-negative units when indicated.

Limitations A minimum of 48 hours should elapse between successive donation procedures and a maximum of 24 donations should take place in 1 year. Platelets, pheresis are more expensive than platelet concentrates, but were comparable in the TRAP study.[3] Adverse reactions to apheresis donation are given in the table.

Reactions Encountered in Apheresis Donors

Adverse Reactions	Prevention/Initial Treatment
General	
Vasovagal	Donor reassurance; Trendelenburg position; temporarily stop procedure
Hypovolemia	Avoid excessive extracorporeal volume; Trendelenburg position; saline administration
Hyperventilation	Donor reassurance; breathe into paper bag
Citrate	Decrease whole blood flow rate and/or citrate infusion; temporarily stop procedure
Hemolysis	Proper instrument set-up; monitor plasma color
Chills	Keep donor warm (use light blanket), use blood warmer
Air embolism	Proper instrument set-up; left-side in Trendelenburg position
Specific to Granulocyte Donation	
Headache, edema, hypervolemia	Avoid too frequent use of sedimenting agent
Hydroxyethylstarch accumulation	Consider use of Pentastarch as sedimenting agent
Steroid effect	Avoid excessive dosage
Growth factor effect	Usually relieved by acetaminophen

Adapted from Randels MJ, "Selection of Care of Apheresis Donors," *Apheresis: Principles and Practice*, McLeod RC, Price TH, and Drew MJ, eds, Bethesda, MD: American Association of Blood Banks Press, 1997, 113-22.

Methodology Exact procedure depends on apheresis instrument used. Use of a leukocyte reduction filter frequently is not necessary as the platelets produced by the instruments are leukocyte-reduced products. Platelet apheresis donation differs from leukocyte donation in that a sedimenting agent is not used and there is no need to stimulate the donor with steroids.

Additional Information One apheresis platelet unit may contain the equivalent in platelet dosage to four or five or more random donor platelet concentrates, containing at least 3.0×10^{11} platelets in ~300 mL of plasma. See Platelet Transfusion *on page 854* for transfusion information.

Footnotes
1. Menitove JE, *Standards for Blood Banks and Transfusion Services*, 20th ed. Bethesda, MD: American Association of Blood Banks Press, 2000, 23-4.
2. Bertolini F and Murphy S, "A Multicenter Inspection of the Swirling Phenomenon in Platelet Concentrates Prepared in Routine Practice," *Transfusion*, 1996, 36(2):128-32.
3. The Trial to Reduce Alloimmunization to Platelets Study Group (TRAP Trial Study Group), "Leukocyte Reduction and Ultraviolet B Irradiation of Platelets to Prevent Alloimmunization and Refractoriness to Platelet Transfusions," *N Engl J Med*, 1997, 337(26):1861-9.

References
Kruskall MS, "The Perils of Platelet Transfusions," *N Engl J Med*, 1997, 337(26):1914-5.

Silberman S, "Platelets: Preparations, Transfusion, Modifications, and Substitutes," *Arch Pathol Lab Med*, 1999, 123(10):889-94.

(Continued)

Platelets, Apheresis, Donation (Continued)

Vengelen-Tyler V, *Technical Manual*, 13th ed, Bethesda, MD: American Association of Blood Banks Press, 1999, 129-34.

♦ **Platelet Serology** see Platelet Antibody, Immunohematologic on page 852

♦ **Platelets, Pheresis** see Platelets, Apheresis, Donation on page 853

♦ **Platelets, Pheresis (FDA)** see Platelets, Apheresis, Donation on page 853

♦ **Platelets, Single-Donor** see Platelets, Apheresis, Donation on page 853

Platelet Transfusion

Related Information

Bleeding Time on page 334
HLA Typing, Single Human Leukocyte Antigen on page 529
Irradiated Blood Components on page 846
Platelet Aggregation on page 348
Platelet Antibodies on page 349
Platelet Antibody, Immunohematologic on page 852
Platelet Count on page 468
Platelet Hyperaggregation on page 350
Platelets, Apheresis, Donation on page 853
Platelet Sizing on page 471
Rh$_o$(D) Immune Globulin (Human) on page 860
Risks of Transfusion on page 861
Transfusion Reaction Work-up on page 864

Synonyms Platelet-Rich Plasma; Platelets; Pooled Platelets; Random Platelets

Applies to Antiglobulin-Augmented Lymphotoxicity Assay; Solid Phase Red Cell Adherence Assay

Test Includes ABO and Rh type

Abstract Two major types of platelet fractions have been available: **random donor platelets** or **platelets** and **platelets, pheresis** or **single-donor platelets**. Other types include **filtered, pooled platelet concentrates from random donors**, and **filtered platelets from apheresis from single random donors**.[1] Platelet concentrates (**platelets**) consist of platelets, suspended in about 50 mL of plasma, separated from whole blood collected from a single whole blood donation, known as **random donor platelets**. It contains at least 5.5×10^{10} platelets per unit. The platelets in a single bag of random donor platelets are insufficient to provide an adequate therapeutic dose in a thrombocytopenic adult. Storage life is 5 days. It contains stable coagulation factors, the presence of which may be significant, since a common dose is about 1 concentrate per 10 kg body weight. Thus, platelet concentrates from 4-10 donors are combined as **pooled concentrates**.

Platelets, pheresis contain at least 3×10^{11} platelets per unit. The dose is usually one unit per adult. The donor plasma should be ABO compatible with erythrocytes of the intended recipient, especially when the recipient is an infant.[2] When platelets of a specific antigenic type are needed, apheresis is especially useful. Use of leukocyte-depleted fractions should diminish the incidence of platelet transfusion reactions.[3]

Patient Preparation Follow standard transfusion patient identification procedures. It is not unusual for a platelet concentrate to have a pink tinge, indicating the presence of some RBCs. Despite this, a red cell crossmatch is not indicated. If the patient is likely to receive many platelet transfusions, it is wise to have the patient HLA-typed early, in case platelet refractoriness occurs. **Dosage and administration:** In a bleeding adult with a platelet count <20,000/mm³, 1 concentrate per 10 kg body weight or 1 unit of platelets, pheresis is a good dose. Use a 19-gauge needle or larger and administer through a routine administration filter designed for platelets. Give platelets rapidly, with an average of 10 minutes per platelet concentrate. Isotonic saline may be used to flush the container and filter. Do not warm platelets. Do not add any medications to platelet packs.

Causes of Refractoriness to Platelet Transfusions

Nonimmune	Immune
Infection, sepsis, fever	ABO
Hemorrhage, purpura, DIC	Prior transfusions
Splenomegaly	Pregnancy
Antibiotic therapy	HLA alloantibodies
Amphotericin B	Platelet-specific alloantibodies (uncommon)
Bone marrow transplant	Autoimmunity

Aftercare Close clinical/nursing observation for bleeding, petechiae is indicated. **To evaluate efficacy of platelet transfusions, get platelet counts prior to and within 1 hour after the transfusions are completed.** They are useful to evaluate the response to platelet transfusions and to calculate the corrected count increment (CCI). The latter expresses the platelet increment per 10^{11} platelets transfused per meter of body surface area (BSA). Where post = post-transfusion platelet count x 10³/mm³; pre = pretransfusion platelet count x 10³/mm³; and PTx = number of platelets transfused (x 10^{11}).

$$CCI \times 10^3 = (\text{post-pre}) \times BSA/PTx$$

A value above 7.5 is usually considered satisfactory. Thus, a patient with a BSA of 1.5 m² receives 6 platelet concentrates with a total of 4.2×10^{11} platelets. The pre- and postcounts are 10×10^3 and 40×10^3 respectively.

$$CCI = (40 - 10) \times 1.5/4.2 = 10.7 \times 10^3$$

That would be considered a good response. This formula is not needed if the raw increment is zero or close to it, or if the response is obviously satisfactory. But it is helpful when the platelet is small (eg, a child), or when the postcounts appear to show small or moderate increments. Poor response to platelet transfusions (refractoriness) is common,[4] usually from nonimmune causes (see table). When refractoriness seems to be due to alloimmunization, then it will be necessary to demonstrate the presence (and specificity, if possible) of those antibodies by antiglobulin-augmented lymphocytotoxicity assay (LCT) or solid phase red cell adherence assay (SPRCA). If the percentage of reactive antibody (PRA) is <70%, then the patient can receive either crossmatch compatible units or units which lack the antigen to which the patient has antibody. Patients with PRA >70% should be placed on a transfusion schedule because they need to receive "A" and "BU" crossmatch compatible units from donors who are selectively recruited from an HLA-typed donor pool.[5] Alloimmunization to platelets seems to be largely caused by contaminating leukocytes in the concentrates and may be prevented by the removal of leukocytes by special filtration (see Filters for Blood on page 842), or reduced experimentally by ultraviolet-B irradiation of platelets.

Fever within 6 hours of platelet transfusion may signal bacterial contamination. The organisms which contaminate platelets are often the same as those involved in catheter-related sepsis.[6]

Selection of Platelets for Immune-Refractory Patients

1. Recruit blood relatives of patient as donors, if available.

2. HLA type patient, if possible.

3. Test patient for cytotoxic antibodies.

4. Test patient for platelet-specific antibodies.

5. Select crossmatch compatible platelet units (check postplatelet counts).

6. Select donors by HLA type. The HLA does not have to be identical; a reasonable match by cross-reacting groups is usually as effective (check postplatelet counts).

7. Select patient donors lacking antigens corresponding to any antibodies detected in steps 3 and 4, if feasible (check postplatelet counts).

8. Check whether ABO compatibility affects outcome. Sometimes it does, especially type A platelets to an O patient and especially if no antibody is detected in steps 5 and 6.

9. If PRA is >70% or CCIs poor: Crossmatch antigen-negative units and selectively recruit 'A' and/or 'BU' donors.

10. Recognize that this is a thorny problem. Any or all of the above may work, not necessarily in the order given; or none of them may be effective.

Specimen Blood

Container One red top tube or one lavender top (EDTA) tube

Collection (Of sample from intended recipient): At the patient's bedside, ask the patient to give his or her name. Compare with the hospital wristband. Label the Blood Bank wristband (if there is one) with the patient's full name, hospital number, date, and initials of the collector. Label sample tube with the same information, including identification number from the wristband. Label requisition form with identification number. The collector signs the requisition, verifying the patient's identity with hospital wristband and Blood Bank wristband. Some hospitals require additional information. It is always best to stamp the requisition with the patient's identification plate to avoid transcription errors. Take extra care with identification of unresponsive patients.

Storage Instructions Platelets lose ability to aggregate at refrigerator temperature; such platelets become suboptimal for transfusion.[7] Store in the Blood Bank at 20°C to 24°C (room temperature) with continuous agitation for 5 days (agitation facilitates gas exchange). Pooled platelets must be transfused within 4 hours after pooling.

Special Instructions Do not refrigerate platelets.

Use Platelets may be used therapeutically to stop bleeding or prophylactically to prevent it. Treatment of bleeding, petechiae, and ecchymoses when platelet count is <20,000/mm³ or when platelets are functionally abnormal; prophylaxis against bleeding due to thrombocytopenia when platelet count is 5000-10,000/mm³, associated with chemotherapy or other marrow hypoplasias; in splenectomy for ITP when abnormal bleeding occurs; in acute blood loss or prior to invasive surgical procedures with platelet count <50,000/mm³. Platelets, pheresis can be used for any patient needing platelet transfusions. They have the advantage of providing an entire platelet transfusion for an adult from one donor, hence, a single donor exposure. Furthermore, the donor can be selected (eg, from a patient's relatives or by HLA type). Platelets, pheresis are available from most blood centers and larger hospital blood banks on a more or less regular basis. Some institutions reserve them for patients who regularly receive platelet transfusions or who may be refractory to regular platelet transfusions.

Limitations Hazards: As for transfusion of other blood components. Platelets may contain both red and white blood cells, and immunization to any of these antigens may occur. If feasible, Rh-negative women of childbearing age should receive Rh-negative platelets to avoid Rh immunization. Otherwise, consider giving them Rh immune globulin. The dosage can be calculated by knowing that platelets seldom contain more than 0.5 mL RBC each and platelets, pheresis rarely more than 5 mL each. Although ABO antigens are poorly developed on platelets, ABO-incompatible platelets sometimes have decreased post-transfusion survival.[8] ABO-incompatible platelet units have caused intravascular hemolysis by passive infusion of anti-A$_1$ or anti-B.[9]

Immunosuppressed patients, and rarely immunocompetent patients, receiving platelets from closely related donors can suffer graft-versus-host disease; this is prevented by irradiation of platelets (see Irradiated Blood Components *on page 846*). Bacterial contamination and growth during storage are a real risk, as platelets are stored at room temperature. Such contamination may derive from skin organisms of the donor or from occult bacteremia.

WBCs admixed with the platelets release interleukin-6, interleukin-8, tumor necrosis factor α, and other cytokines, causes of febrile reactions. White blood cells present in platelet units can cause febrile reactions, HLA alloimmunization, adverse immunomodulatory effects, and transmission of CMV and human T-lymphotropic virus 1.[10] Platelet-containing fractions are most often implicated in transmission of bacteria and caused 21 of 29 deaths reported to the FDA between 1986 and 1991.[11]

Contraindications Not usually useful in idiopathic or immune thrombocytopenia, thrombotic thrombocytopenic purpura or certain stages of disseminated intravascular coagulation. Not to be used if bleeding is not caused by thrombocytopenia or abnormal platelet function. Patients with hypersplenism or septicemia may also fail to respond.

Methodology Random donor platelets are obtained by centrifugation of whole blood within 8 hours of collection, at low centrifugal force, at room temperature, to provide platelet-rich plasma with or without contaminating white blood cells. Separation of such plasma from erythrocytes in a satellite bag and recentrifugation for platelet concentration follow. After most of the plasma is separated for use as fresh frozen plasma, the residual 50 mL of plasma is used to resuspend the platelets.[10] Platelets, pheresis are discussed in Platelets, Apheresis, Donation *on page 853*.

Leukocyte reduction by filtration and ultraviolet B irradiation are equally effective in prevention of alloantibody-mediated platelet refractoriness, respectively to remove or inactivate cells bearing alloantigens.[1] Ultraviolet B irradiation is not, however, available on a routine basis. See Platelet Antibodies *on page 349*.

Additional Information One unit of platelets usually increases the platelet count of an adult with a blood volume of 5000 mL by about 5000/mm^3. One unit of platelets, pheresis usually increases the platelet count of an adult by about 30,000-60,000/mm^3.

Neonatal and fetal[12] **alloimmune thrombocytopenia** are usually caused by Pl[A1] (HPA-1a) antigen inherited from the father by the baby, who then immunizes the mother so that she makes antibody to the baby's platelets (ie, anti-Pl[A1]).[12] The mother's platelet count is normal, but the baby's platelet count is low. It may not, however, be sufficiently low to cause symptoms, and so the diagnosis may be missed. The first born child may be affected.[13,14] The most serious complication is intracranial hemorrhage, which may occur during pregnancy,[15] but the risk is probably greatest during delivery. If the diagnosis is made after delivery and the baby is unharmed, remember that later babies are also at risk.

For confirmatory diagnosis, send mother's serum and father's platelets to a reference laboratory for antibody identification. See Platelet Antibodies *on page 349*.

Treatment: The most convenient and readily available source of compatible platelets is the mother. A large number of platelets, relative to the baby's size, can be obtained by maternal platelet apheresis. If maternal platelets are used, the antibody-containing plasma should be removed and the unit irradiated and leukocyte reduced.

Neonatal **autoimmune thrombocytopenia**, in which maternal thrombocytopenia also occurs, is treated by exchange transfusion or intravenous immune globulin.

Eight to 10 platelets may contain the equivalent amount of stable clotting factors found in two plasma units. This volume may need to be reduced for children.

Costs and benefits of apheresis versus random donor platelets were recently examined.[16]

Footnotes
1. Slichter S, "Leukocyte Reduction and Ultraviolet B Irradiation of Platelets to Prevent Alloimmunization and Refractoriness to Platelet Transfusions," The Trial to Reduce Alloimmunization to Platelets Study Group, *N Engl J Med*, 1997, 337(26):1861-9.
2. Vengelen-Tyler V, *Technical Manual*, 13th ed, Bethesda, MD: American Association of Blood Banks Press, 1999, 524.
3. Kruskall MS, "The Perils of Platelet Transfusions," *N Engl J Med*, 1997, 337(26):1914-5.
4. Benson K, Fields K, Hiemenz J, et al, "The Platelet-Refractory Bone Marrow Transplant Patient: Prophylaxis and Treatment of Bleeding," *Semin Oncol*, 1995, 5(Suppl 6):102-9.
5. Murphy S and Varma M, "Selecting Platelets for Transfusion of the Alloimmunized Patient: A Review," *Immunohematology*, 1998, 14:117-23.
6. Goodnough LT, Brecher ME, Kanter MH, et al, "Transfusion Medicine. First of Two Parts: Blood Transfusion," *N Engl J Med*, 1999, 340(6):438-48.

7. Xiao HY, Matsubayashi H, Bonderman DP, et al, "Generation of Annexin V-Positive Platelets and Shedding of Microparticles With Stimulus-Dependent Procoagulant Activity During Storage of Platelets at 4°C," *Transfusion*, 2000, 40(4):420-7.
8. Lee EJ and Schiffer CA, "ABO Compatibility Can Influence the Results of Platelet Transfusion. Results of a Randomized Trial," *Transfusion*, 1989, 29(5):384-9.
9. McManigal S and Sims KL, "Intravascular Hemolysis Secondary to ABO Incompatible Platelet Products: An Underrecognized Transfusion Reaction," *Am J Clin Pathol*, 1999, 111(2):202-6.
10. Silberman S, "Platelets: Preparations, Transfusion, Modifications, and Substitutes," *Arch Pathol Lab Med*, 1999, 123(10):889-94.
11. Popovsky MA, "Infection and America's Blood Supply: A 1999 Status Report," *Am J Clin Pathol*, 1998, 109(6):659-61.
12. Rothenberger SS and McCarthy LJ, "Neonatal Alloimmune Thrombocytopenia: From Prediction to Prevention," *Lab Med*, 1997, 28(9):592-6.
13. "Management of Alloimmune Neonatal Thrombocytopenia," *Lancet*, 1989, 1(8630):137-8.
14. Mueller-Eckhardt C, Grubert A, Weisheit M, et al, "348 Cases of Suspected Neonatal Alloimmune Thrombocytopenia," *Lancet*, 1989, 1(8634):363-7.
15. Bussel JB, Zabusky MR, Berkowitz RL, et al, "Fetal Alloimmune Thrombocytopenia," *N Engl J Med*, 1997, 337(1):22-6.
16. Blumberg N and Heal JM, "Mortality Risks, Costs, and Decision Making in Transfusion Medicine," *Am J Clin Pathol*, 2000, 114(6):934-7.

References
Circular of Information for the Use of Human Blood and Blood Components, American Association of Blood Banks, America's Blood Centers, American Red Cross, 1998.
Huston BM, Brecher ME, and Bandarenko N, "Lack of Efficacy for Conventional Gamma Irradiation of Platelet Concentrates to Abrogate Bacterial Growth," *Am J Clin Pathol*, 1998, 109(6):743-7.
Kickler TS and Herman JH, *Current Issues in Platelet Transfusion Therapy and Platelet Alloimmunity*, Bethesda, MD: American Association of Blood Banks Press, 1999.
Murphy S, "Platelet Transfusion Therapy," *Thrombosis and Hemorrhage*, 2nd ed, Loscalzo J and Schafer AI, eds, Baltimore, MD: Lippincott Williams & Wilkins, 1998, 1119-34.
Triulzi DJ, *Blood Transfusion Therapy: A Physician's Handbook*, 6th ed, Bethesda, MD: American Association of Blood Banks Press, 1999, 15-20.

♦ **Pooled Platelets** *see* Platelet Transfusion *on page 854*

♦ **Postoperative Cell Salvage** *see* Autologous Transfusion, Intraoperative Blood Salvage *on page 836*

♦ **Predeposit Autologous Donation** *see* Autologous Transfusion, Preoperative Deposit *on page 837*

Prenatal Screen, Immunohematology

Related Information
Antibody Titer *on page 834*
Antiglobulin Test, Indirect *on page 835*
Bilirubin, Amniotic Fluid, Delta A450 *on page 116*
Cord Blood Screen *on page 838*
Fetal Cell Detection by Flow Cytometry *on page 430*
Hemolytic Disease of the Newborn, Antibody Identification *on page 846*
Kleihauer-Betke *on page 453*
Polymerase Chain Reaction *on page 713*

Synonyms Prenatal Serology

Test Includes ABO group, Rh type, antibody screen, and antibody identification if antibody screen is positive

Abstract The purpose of prenatal serological screening is to identify mothers at risk for delivering an infant with hemolytic disease of the newborn (HDN). HDN occurs when the fetus possesses a paternal blood group antigen to which the mother is sensitized. The fetus may be affected by pre-existing maternal alloantibody as well as antibody provoked by the current pregnancy. Maternal alloantibodies, capable of causing HDN, can be detected. All positive antibody screens require identification of the antibody. Antibody specificity can be correlated with clinical significance. The prenatal serology report to the clinician should indicate the clinical significance of the antibody. Most severe HDN is caused by anti-Rh(D) alone or in combination with other Rh antibodies (eg, anti-C or anti-E). The next grade of severity is associated with antibodies to other Rh antigens (notably anti-c) or with antibodies to other blood group antigens (eg, anti-K). IgG antibodies to antigens of the ABO system cause the lowest grade of HDN severity.

Patient Preparation All pregnant women should be screened at the initial visit. Previous pregnancy or transfusion is an indication for follow-up antibody screens. Rh(D)-negative patients who are not immunized to Rh(D) should have antibody screening repeated at 28-30 weeks gestation before Rh immunoprophylaxis (Rh$_o$(D) immune globulin) is given. It is not necessary to repeat the antibody screen on Rh(D)-positive women unless antibodies associated with HDN other than anti-D are present. The presence of a clinically significant antibody in any patient is cause for evaluation of fetal risk (eg, coordination of antibody serial titration values with possible amniocentesis).

Specimen Blood

Container Red top tube

Causes for Rejection Gross hemolysis, improper labeling

Reference Interval Antibody screen negative (indirect antiglobulin test)

Use Identify women at risk for delivery of an infant with HDN: identify candidates for antenatal Rh immunoprophylaxis
(Continued)

Prenatal Screen, Immunohematology *(Continued)*

Limitations Antibody detection tests will not expose antibodies to "private" paternal antigens or predict HDN due to ABO fetal/maternal incompatibility. ABO HDN can occur in pregnancy, even the first. The direct antiglobulin test is often negative and the infant is rarely symptomatic at birth.

Methodology Methods to detect IgG alloantibodies, especially the indirect antiglobulin test

Additional Information Antibody screening tests are necessary to identify obstetric patients who may possess alloantibodies capable of causing HDN. Antibody screening should also be carried out on all Rh(D)-negative cases of ectopic pregnancy, incomplete abortion, or any situation that might immunize the mother to fetal Rh(D) antigen, in order to ascertain the need for Rh immunoprophylaxis.

Antepartum administration of $Rh_o(D)$ immune globulin causes positive antibody screens in most women, due to passively acquired anti-$Rh_o(D)$. This passively acquired antibody may remain detectable at the time of delivery. Its presence is not a contraindication for further $Rh_o(D)$ immune globulin administration.

Molecular biological techniques (eg, allele-specific polymerase chain reaction (PCR) or PCR-restriction fragment length polymorphisms) are beginning to be utilized in the clinical laboratory to predict the likelihood of HDN. Fetal DNA can be prepared from cells obtained by conventional invasive techniques (eg, amniocentesis or chorionic villus sampling) by noninvasive procedures from trophoblasts collected by transcervical sampling, or from fetal erythroblasts derived from the maternal circulation. These procedures will prove valuable in cases in which the maternal serum contains an antibody associated with HDN and the father's antigenic status is heterozygous, indeterminable, or unknown. Molecular biological techniques hold great promise to radically change approaches to prenatal laboratory testing.

References
Hartwell EA, "Use of Rh Immune Globulin. ASCP Practice Parameter," *Am J Clin Pathol*, 1998, 110(3):281-92.

Lo YMD, Hjelm NM, Fidler C, et al, "Prenatal Diagnosis of Fetal RhD Status by Molecular Analysis of Maternal Plasma," *N Engl J Med*, 1998, 339(24):1734-8.

Vengelen-Tyler V, *Technical Manual*, 13th ed, Bethesda, MD: American Association of Blood Banks Press, 1999, 495-501.

♦ **Prenatal Serology** *see* Prenatal Screen, Immunohematology *on page 855*

♦ **Prenatal Testing** *see* Rh Genotype *on page 860*

Pretransfusion Testing

Related Information
Antibody Detection/Identification, Red Cell *on page 834*
Antiglobulin Test, Direct *on page 834*
Antiglobulin Test, Indirect *on page 835*
Red Blood Cells *on page 857*
Rh Genotype *on page 860*
Risks of Transfusion *on page 861*
Uncrossmatched Blood, Emergency *on page 865*
Whole Blood *on page 866*

Applies to ABO Group and Rh Type; Blood Grouping and Rh Typing; Forward Grouping; Reverse Grouping; Rh(D) Typing; Type and Crossmatch; Type and Screen

Test Includes ABO group, Rh type, antibody screen (indirect antiglobulin test), crossmatch, and "type and screen"

Abstract Pretransfusion testing permits the appropriate selection of blood fractions which will have the intended therapeutic effect and cause no harm to the recipient. The *Standards* of the American Association of Blood Banks requires that the recipient be ABO and Rh grouped and screened for unexpected antibodies before transfusion.[1] Pretransfusion testing procedures may be modified in life-threatening situations (see Uncrossmatched Blood, Emergency *on page 865*).

Patient Preparation Procedures must be in place to positively identify the patient. Identification may include a wristband containing two unique identifiers, physically attached to the patient. Such identifiers should not be on the wall or clipped to the chart.

Specimen Blood

Container Red top tube, lavender top (EDTA) tube

Collection The vast majority of hemolytic transfusion reactions are the consequences of erroneous patient identification or sample labeling. The collection of a properly labeled blood sample from the intended recipient is the foundation of transfusion safety. Extra care must be taken with the identification procedure. At the patient's bedside, ask the patient to give his/her name and compare with the hospital wristband. Label the Blood Bank wristband (if there is one) with patient's full name, hospital number, date, and initials of the phlebotomist. Label sample tubes with the same information, including identification number from the wristband. Label requisition form with identification number. The sample collector must sign the requisition, verifying the patient's identity with hospital wristband and Blood Bank wristband. Some hospitals require additional information. It is always best to stamp the requisition with the patient's identification plate to avoid transcription errors. Ultimate safety in patient identification is achieved through bar coding.[2]

Causes for Rejection Hemolysis, improper labeling, sample collected in serum separator tube

Turnaround Time In life-threatening emergencies, group O RBCs can be issued immediately to patients whose blood group is unknown (see Uncrossmatched Blood, Emergency *on page 865*), but the more complete the pretransfusion testing, the safer the transfusion. In emergencies, the Blood Bank can issue blood at any stage of testing. The time requirements are shown in the table.

Timetable for Obtaining Emergency Blood From Blood Bank

Time Available (approx minutes)	Blood Bank Can Issue	Extent of Testing Done
<5	Type O RBCs, Rh-neg if possible	None
5-10	RBCs of patient's own ABO and Rh types	Patient's ABO and Rh typing, no crossmatch
45-60*	Serologically compatible RBCs	Full pretransfusion testing, including antibody screen

*Assuming no unexpected antibody detected.

Use Determine patient's blood group to enable blood selection before transfusion; detect and, if present, identify any unexpected blood group antibodies; detect any incompatibility with donor units before transfusion. ABO, Rh, and antibody screen are also used in prenatal testing to detect fetal-maternal incompatibility that might cause hemolytic disease of the newborn.

Limitations Abnormal plasma proteins, cold autoagglutinins, positive direct antiglobulin test, and in some cases, bacteremia may interfere. These tests do not assure normal red cell survival, will not detect all red cell antibodies or incompatibilities, do not prevent all transfusion reactions, and do not prevent reactions to blood components other than red cells. Clerical and technical competence is requisite. A great many pitfalls exist which may cause false-positive or false-negative reactions.

Contraindications See Risks of Transfusion *on page 861*.

Methodology Serologic pretransfusion testing attempts to reproduce *in vitro* biologic manifestations of incompatibility. The test systems involve reacting the patient's separated serum and red cells with known standardized antisera and phenotyped red cells. These procedures and reagents are common to ABO grouping and Rh typing, to testing of the serum for the presence of unexpected blood group antibodies, and to compatibility testing (crossmatching). All testing reagents are FDA licensed and procedures are subject to review and inspection by accrediting agencies, including any computerized programs for recording test results or for tracking of patients and donor blood components. Methods vary according to reagents, procedures, and equipment in use; testing may be in test tubes, microplates, or gel columns depending on testing techniques in use.[3]

ABO grouping consists of testing the patient's red cells with reagent anti-A, anti-B, and anti-AB (forward grouping). The patient's serum (other than infants) is also tested with reagent group A and B red cells (reverse grouping).

Rh typing is done by testing red cells with anti-D. Red cells positive for the Rh(D) antigen are referred to as Rh positive; those lacking Rh(D) are termed Rh negative. Because Rh(D) is by far the most antigenic of all the Rh antigens, this is the only distinction routinely necessary for transfusion. Do not be concerned about the numerous other Rh antigens unless the patient is immunized to one of them (which would usually become apparent from the results of antibody screening or crossmatching tests).

As a rule, the Blood Bank issues blood of the patient's own ABO and Rh types, but some leeway is permissible; see table. When difficulties occur in blood selection, consultation is necessary between the Blood Bank physician and the patient's physician.

Selection of Donor Red Cells (RBCs) for Transfusion to Recipients of Various ABO and Rh Types

Patient Blood Type	First Choice	Second Choice	Third Choice
O pos	O pos	O neg	
O neg	O neg	None	O pos
A pos	A pos	A neg, O pos, O neg	
A neg	A neg	O neg	O pos, A pos
B pos	B pos	B neg, O pos, O neg	
B neg	B neg	O neg	O pos, B pos
AB pos	AB pos	AB neg, A pos, B pos, A neg, B neg, O pos, O neg	
AB neg	AB neg	A neg, B neg, O neg	AB pos, A pos, B pos, O pos

Note: The technologist may always substitute Rh-negative donor RBC for Rh-positive patients, if supplies permit. **Physician approval is required for third choice donor blood selection in the event that first and second choice are unavailable.** In this table, "pos" and "neg" refer to Rh-positive and Rh-negative respectively.

Antibody screen: (See Antiglobulin Test, Indirect *on page 835*.) About 1.5% of patients possess unexpected blood group antibodies with the potential for causing hemolytic transfusion reactions. The antibody screening test is the procedure used to detect these antibodies. Antibody screening may be performed in advance of or simultaneous with crossmatching tests. A positive antibody screen indicates the need for further tests to determine the specificity of the antibody. Determination of antibody specificity permits the appropriate selection of donor blood, lacking the offending antigen, for compatibility tests.

Basically, the antibody screen can be thought of as a crossmatch against a small panel of red cells, selected to contain the clinically important antigens, instead of donor red cells. AABB *Standards* require that screening tests employ methods that detect clinically significant antibodies and include an indirect antiglobulin test preceded by incubation at 37°C. Antibody screening tests are not perfect and can miss antibodies to low-incidence antigens as well as weakly reacting antibodies. Transfusion of antigen-incompatible red cells to a patient with a weakly reactive, undetected, antibody can result in rapid immune recall of antibody leading to a hemolytic transfusion reaction.

Crossmatch: (See Antiglobulin Test, Indirect *on page 835* and Uncrossmatched Blood, Emergency *on page 865*.) The crossmatch is a direct test of compatibility between the patient's serum and donor red cells. Except for the source of the red cells, it is like the antibody screen. The crossmatch may utilize various techniques to detect IgG clinically significant antibodies, but its prime purpose is to detect ABO incompatibility. When antibody screening tests (both current and prior) have demonstrated no evidence of unexpected antibodies, the antiglobulin test may be omitted and the crossmatch restricted to a simple test for ABO incompatibility (eg, immediate spin test or computer-assisted crossmatch). The rarity of the exposure of a clinically significant antibody by the antiglobulin phase of the crossmatch, when the antibody screening test is negative, provides the rationale for the abbreviated crossmatch. The benefit of abbreviation of the crossmatch includes reduced turnaround time. It greatly lessens the amount of laboratory work per unit of blood, at little or no increase in risk.

Maximum Surgical Blood Order Schedule (MSBOS)

Procedure	Units*
General Surgery	
Breast biopsy	T/S
Colon resection	2
Exploratory laparotomy	2
Gastrectomy	2
Hernia repair	T/S
Laryngectomy	2
Mastectomy, radical	T/S
Splenectomy	2
Thyroidectomy	T/S
Cardiac-Thoracic	
Coronary artery bypass graft, adults	4
Coronary artery bypass graft, children	2
Lobectomy	2
Lung biopsy	T/S
Vascular	
Aortic bypass with graft	4
Endarterectomy	T/S
Femoral-popliteal bypass with graft	4
Orthopedics	
Arthroscopy	T/S
Laminectomy	T/S
Spinal fusion	3
Total hip replacement	3
Total knee replacement	2
Obstetrics	
Cesarean section	T/S
D& C	T/S
Hysterectomy, abdominal	T/S
Hysterectomy, radical	2
Urology	
Bladder, transurethral resection	T/S
Prostatectomy, perineal	2
Prostatectomy, transurethral	T/S
Renal transplant	2

*Numbers may vary with institutional practice.

T/S = Type and screen.

Adapted from Vengelen-Tyler V, *Technical Manual*, 13th edition, Bethesda MD: American Association of Blood Banks Press, 1999, 82.

Computer-assisted crossmatching: Under specified circumstances, accrediting agencies have sanctioned the use of the so-called "electronic or computer crossmatch".[2] This is not a serologic test at all, it is rather a computer check of donor and recipient ABO and Rh compatibility. The computer-assisted crossmatch may be employed when antibody screening and history review have detected no clinically significant antibodies. The computer program must be validated on site to ensure that only ABO compatible whole blood or red cells have been selected for transfusion. The program must verify correct entry of data prior to release of blood and contain logic to signal discrepancies. FDA approval of a variance to regulations on compatibility testing is required. The advantages of computer-assisted crossmatching include decreased laboratory workload and better utilization of blood.

Type and screen: When a patient is undergoing a procedure or treatment in which transfusion is very unlikely, it is wasteful to crossmatch blood and put it aside for that patient. Instead, it is more appropriate to order a "type and screen". The type and screen includes ABO and Rh typing and an antibody screen. If the antibody screen is negative and hemorrhage occurs, the Blood Bank may issue blood of the patient's type immediately, without awaiting the crossmatch. Of course, if the antibody screen detects an unexpected antibody, crossmatch becomes necessary, and the patient's physician is alerted to the situation beforehand. See Maximum Surgical Blood Order Schedule table for procedures in which Type and Screen is appropriate.

Additional Information Allow additional time for patients known to be immunized to red cell antigens. Unanticipated problems can occur with antibody reidentification and selection of blood of appropriate phenotype. Patients receiving a series of transfusions are at risk of forming red cell antibodies. For this reason, *Standards* require a new blood sample and repeat antibody screening every 3 days.

Footnotes
1. Menitove JE, *Standards for Blood Banks and Transfusion Services*, 20th ed, Bethesda, MD: American Association of Blood Banks Press, 2000, 42-52.
2. Beck ML and Tilzer LL, "Red Cell Compatibility Testing: A Perspective for the Future," *Transfusion Medicine Reviews*, 1996, 10(2):118-30.
3. Vengelen-Tyler V, *Technical Manual*, 13th ed, Bethesda, MD: American Association of Blood Banks Press, 1999, 375-88.

References
Linden JV, "Errors in Transfusion Medicine: Scope of the Problem," *Arch Pathol Lab Med*, 1999, 123(7):563-5.

♦ **Progenitor Cells** *see* Hematopoietic Progenitor Cells, Peripheral Blood *on page 845*

♦ **Prothrombin Complex Concentrates** *see* Factor IX Concentrate *on page 841*

♦ **Random Platelets** *see* Platelet Transfusion *on page 854*

Red Blood Cells

Related Information
Activated Partial Thromboplastin Time *on page 328*
Blood Gases and pH, Arterial *on page 119*
Coagulation Factor Assays *on page 335*
Cold Agglutinin Titer *on page 594*
Filters for Blood *on page 842*
Hematocrit *on page 441*
Hemoglobin *on page 442*
Hereditary Hemochromatosis DNA Test *on page 709*
Irradiated Blood Components *on page 846*
Oxygen Saturation, Blood *on page 240*
Pretransfusion Testing *on page 856*
Prothrombin Time *on page 354*
Red Blood Cells, Leukocytes Reduced *on page 858*
Red Blood Cells, Washed *on page 859*
Risks of Transfusion *on page 861*
Transfusion Reaction Work-up *on page 864*
Uncrossmatched Blood, Emergency *on page 865*
Warming, Blood *on page 865*
Whole Blood *on page 866*

Synonyms Packed Red Cells, Transfusion

Applies to Donor Blood Transfusion

Test Includes ABO and Rh type, antibody screen, crossmatch, antibody identification when screen is positive (ie, preparation as for other transfusions)

Abstract A unit of red blood cells has a volume of 230-350 mL. Red cells contain the same mass of red cells as does a unit of whole blood, ~200 mL with 15-30 mL of plasma. Red cells with CPDA-1 anticoagulant have a hematocrit of ~70% and expire 35 days after the date of collection, when stored continuously between 1°C to 6°C. With additional adenine supplementation after removal of plasma, AS-1 red blood cells have a hematocrit of 55% to 60% and a storage period of 42 days at 1°C to 6°C. If the hermetic seal is broken during preparation, the red blood cells must be infused within 24 hours.

Patient Preparation The patient should have an identification wristband. Emergency Departments (ERs) may use special or temporary identification. **Dosage and administration:** Give red cells through a standard 170 micron (Continued)

Red Blood Cells *(Continued)*

filter. Most transfusions should not exceed 4 hours duration; 2 hours or less per unit is preferable. Units collected with CPDA-1 anticoagulant can speed up the infusion by adding 50-100 mL of sterile isotonic sodium chloride solution, USP, just before administration.[1] **Do not add or transfuse with lactated Ringer's solution, 5% aqueous dextrose, 5% dextrose in 0.225% saline, or other calcium-containing, hypotonic, or glucose-containing fluids through the same tubing because clumping, hemolysis, or clotting may occur.**[1] **Drugs or medications may not be added to blood or blood components.**

Aftercare One unit should raise the hematocrit of a 70 kg adult about 3 percentage points (or hemoglobin 1 g/dL). Monitor hemoglobin and hematocrit.

Specimen Blood

Container One red top tube or one lavender top (EDTA) tube

Collection (Of sample from intended recipient): At the patient's bedside, ask the patient to give his or her name. Compare with the patient's wristband. Label the sample tube with two unique forms of patient identification (eg, patient's full name, hospital number), also include date and initials of the collector. Further information may be required on a requisition form. Take extra care with identification of unresponsive patients.

Storage Instructions Store in Blood Bank monitored refrigerator only until issue. When it is not possible to transfuse immediately after issue, return blood to Blood Bank within ~30 minutes. Otherwise, blood that has been out of monitored refrigeration must be discarded. Appropriate designated refrigeration includes specified storage conditions, temperature recorders, and alarm signals.[2] These conditions are regularly intensely inspected by regulatory agencies.

Beware of blood which appears darker than usual; it may be contaminated.[3]

If stored as packed red cells in CPDA-1 anticoagulant, red cells can be stored for up to 5 weeks. If stored as an additive system unit, unit can be stored for up to 6 weeks.[4]

Causes for Rejection (Of patient sample): Gross hemolysis, sample placed in a serum separator tube, specimen tube not properly labeled

Turnaround Time For routine situations, red blood cells can be ready for transfusion within 30-45 minutes from the time the Blood Bank gets the type and crossmatch sample, if blood of the appropriate type is on hand. Presence of unexpected antibodies may require hours to a day or two for identification.

Special Instructions Blood banks and hospital transfusion services hold crossmatched blood only for 24 hours, after which they make it available for other patients. There will be some exceptions. Notify the Blood Bank as soon as possible if the patient will not need transfusion so the blood can be available for some other patient.

Critical Values Perioperative patients almost always require transfusion at Hb <6 g/dL, but no magic number exists to trigger indication for transfusion for all patients. Thirty percent to 40% loss of blood volume is associated with increased signs of shock and >40% relates to severe shock.[4]

Possible Panic Range In otherwise stable patients, the risk of mortality without transfusion rises very significantly at hemoglobin levels of 3.5-4.0 g/dL.[4]

Use Replace red cell volume; rapid loss of >30% to 40% of blood volume or fall in Hb to <6 g/dL requires RBC transfusions in most subjects.[4] Hemoglobin >10 g/dL rarely indicates transfusion, whereas hemoglobin <6 g/dL almost always does.[5] Transfusion of patients with heart, liver, or renal disease in whom restriction of plasma volume or of sodium may be desirable, eg, to decrease the likelihood of volume overload (as compared with effect of whole blood); transfusion of patients with chronic anemias; replace blood lost in surgical operations. Type O RBCs may be given in emergencies to recipients of unknown ABO type (RBC units have less anti-A and anti-B than whole blood). Indications for transfusion include maintenance of perfusion, arterial oxygenation with augmentation of oxygen delivery to the tissues and maintenance of cardiac output and blood volume.

A major multicenter study recommends red cell transfusions for critically ill patients when Hb falls to <7 g/dL, and suggests that Hb should be maintained between 7-9 g/dL.[6] Others suggest a threshold for transfusion of Hb 7-8 g/dL in patients who are not critically ill and have no risk of ischemia, and 10 g for those at risk. Intraoperative or postoperative ischemia of myocardium is more likely to take place in patients whose hematocrits fall to <28%, especially in the presence of tachycardia.[3]

RBC transfusions are used in those patients with chronic anemias unresponsive to pharmacologic agents (eg, iron, cobalamin, folate, recombinant human erythropoietin). Neonates require a hematocrit >0.30-0.35 in the presence of respiratory distress.[4]

Special needs of patients with congenital and acquired hemolytic anemias are published.[4] See Red Blood Cells, Leukocytes Reduced *on page 858*.

A summary of transfusion guidelines is included in Whole Blood *on page 866*.

Limitations Red cells prepared in an "open" system expire in 24 hours. Most RBCs, however, are prepared in closed systems with full dating.

The potential problems of provision of blood essentially would nearly provide a glossary of the entire science of immunohematology. They include alloimmunization, autoimmunization, and requirements of competent professional credentialing and staffing at all levels, from phlebotomist through and inclusive of directorship.

Contraindications With the AIDS epidemic and increasing knowledge of the infectious disease risks of transfusion, as well as Transfusion Committee surveillance, documentation of the necessity for transfusion is required. Do not give blood transfusion when anemia and/or hypoxia can be corrected with specific and safer therapy such as iron, B$_{12}$, or folic acid. For correction of coagulation deficiencies, specific viral-inactivated concentrates are appropriate. Do not add medications to blood for transfusion; many are incompatible with stored blood.

Methodology Attention to electrolytes, blood gases and blood warmers is indicated with rapid and/or massive transfusion; see Warming, Blood *on page 865*.

Red cells should not be infused rapidly in elective situations; rather, they should be infused over a period not less than 2 hours or more than 4 hours/unit.

Additional Information Red blood cells must be ABO and Rh compatible. A crossmatch is necessary unless life-threatening urgency exists. See Risks of Transfusion *on page 861*. An advantage of RBCs as compared to whole blood is greater safety in treatment of patients likely to suffer complications of volume excess.

Problems of iron overload are partly addressed in Hereditary Hemochromatosis DNA Test *on page 709* and related monographs.

Anemia in pregnancy is defined as Hb <10 g/dL. The mean loss after vaginal delivery is 500 mL and after caesarean section, 1000 mL. CMV-seronegative or leukocyte-reduced blood is indicated when a CMV-negative or CMV status unknown pregnant patient requires transfusion.[4]

Footnotes

1. *Circular of Information for the Use of Human Blood and Blood Components*, American Association of Blood Banks, America's Blood Centers, American Red Cross, 1998, 20-2.
2. Menitove J, *Standards for Blood Banks and Transfusion Services*, 20th ed, Bethesda, MD: American Association of Blood Banks Press, 2000, 5-6.
3. Goodnough LT, Brecher ME, Kanter MH, et al, "Transfusion Medicine. First of Two Parts: Blood Transfusion," *N Engl J Med*, 1999, 340(6):438-48.
4. Simon TL, Alverson DC, AuBuchon J, et al, "Practice Parameter for the Use of Red Blood Cell Transfusions: Developed by the Red Blood Cell Administration Practice Guideline Development Task Force of the College of American Pathologists," *Arch Pathol Lab Med*, 1998, 122(2):130-8.
5. Stehling LC, Doherty DC, Faust RJ, et al, "Task Force on Blood Component Therapy: Practice Guidelines for Blood Component Therapy," A Report by the American Society of Anesthesiologists, *Anesthesiology*, 1996, 844:732-47.
6. Hebert PC, Wells G, Blajchman MA, et al, "A Multicenter, Randomized, Controlled Clinical Trial of Transfusion Requirements in Critical Care," *N Engl J Med*, 1999, 340(6):409-17.

References

Carson JL, Duff A, Berlin JA, et al, "Perioperative Blood Transfusion and Postoperative Mortality," *JAMA*, 1998, 279(3):199-205.
Carson JL, Poses RM, Spence RK, et al, "Severity of Anemia and Operative Mortality and Morbidity," *Lancet*, 1988, 1(8588):727-9.
Ely EW and Bernard GR, "Transfusions in Critically Ill Patients," *N Engl J Med*, 1999, 340(6):467-8.
Goodnough LT, Monk TG, and Andriole GL, "Erythropoietin Therapy," *N Engl J Med*, 1997, 336(13):933-8.
Thurer RL, "Evaluating Transfusion Triggers," *JAMA*, 1998, 279(3):238-9.
Vengelen-Tyler V, *Technical Manual*, 13th ed, Bethesda, MD: American Association of Blood Banks Press, 1999.
Weiskopf RB, Viele MK, Feiner J, et al, "Human Cardiovascular and Metabolic Response to Acute, Severe Isovolemic Anemia," *JAMA*, 1998, 279(3):217-21.

♦ **Red Blood Cells, Deglycerolized** *see* Frozen Red Blood Cells *on page 842*

♦ **Red Blood Cells, Frozen** *see* Frozen Red Blood Cells *on page 842*

Red Blood Cells, Leukocytes Reduced

Related Information
Filters for Blood *on page 842*
Frozen Red Blood Cells *on page 842*
Red Blood Cells *on page 857*
Red Blood Cells, Washed *on page 859*
Risks of Transfusion *on page 861*
Whole Blood *on page 866*

Synonyms Leukocyte-Reduced Red Blood Cells

Applies to Donor Blood Transfusion

Test Includes See Red Blood Cells *on page 857*.

Abstract The most common adverse effect of transfusion is the nonhemolytic febrile reaction.

AABB Standards specify that leukocyte-reduced red cells must contain <5 x 10^6 leukocytes per unit while retaining 85% of the original red cells.[1] This is usually accomplished by the use of a special, leukocyte-reduction filter (see Filters for Blood *on page 842*). Indications for use of leukocyte-reduced red cells include patients with repeated febrile transfusion reactions, to decrease the incidence of HLA alloimmunization,[2] prevention of alloimmunization to leukocyte antigens and hence, refractoriness to platelet transfusions, and prevention of cytomegalovirus transmission.[3,4]

Patient Preparation See Red Blood Cells *on page 857.*

Aftercare See Red Blood Cells.

Container One red top tube or one lavender top (EDTA) tube

Collection See Red Blood Cells.

Storage Instructions See Red Blood Cells.

Causes for Rejection (Of patient sample:) Gross hemolysis, sample placed in a serum separator tube, specimen tube not properly labeled

Special Instructions See Red Blood Cells.

Use See Red Blood Cells. Leukocyte-reduced red cells are specifically indicated for use in multitransfused patients and multiparous females with repeated febrile nonhemolytic transfusion reactions, to prevent alloimmunization to leukocyte antigens (HLA) (and, hence, refractoriness to platelet transfusions), and to prevent cytomegalovirus transmission.[5] Leukocyte-reduced red cells may provide benefits to patients with paroxysmal nocturnal hemoglobinuria. Leukocyte-reduced blood or CMV-seronegative blood is indicated, when pregnant patients known to be CMV negative or when CMV status is unknown, are to be transfused. See tables.

Table 1. Indications for Leukocyte-Reduced Red Blood Cells

Prevention of Alloimmunization

Congenital hemolytic anemias

Hypoproliferative anemias likely to need multiple transfusions

  Aplastic anemia

  Myelodysplasias

  Myeloproliferative syndrome

  Plasma cell dyscrasias

  Bone marrow/peripheral blood stem cell transplants

  Hematopoietic malignancies

Therapy in Pre-existing Conditions

Recurrent severe febrile hemolytic transfusion reaction

Known HLA alloimmunization

Possible Use

Alternative to cytomegalovirus-seronegative components; *vide infra*

Human immunodeficiency virus-infected patients

Adapted from Simon TL, Alverson DC, AuBuchon J, et al, "Practice Parameter for the Use of Red Blood Cell Transfusions," *Arch Pathol Lab Med*, 1998, 122(2):130-8.

Table 2. Indications for Prevention of Cytomegalovirus Transmission by Seronegative or Leukocyte-Reduced (<5 x 10⁶) Red Blood Cells

Well-Defined (patient seronegative for cytomegalovirus or status unknown)

Low-birth-weight neonates (<1200 g)

Human immunodeficiency virus-infected patients

Recipients of seronegative allogeneic, organ, marrow, or stem cell transplants or likely candidates for such transplants

Pregnant women

Intrauterine transfusion

Relative (patient seronegative for cytomegalovirus or status unknown)

Hodgkin disease and non-Hodgkin lymphoma

Recipients of immunosuppressive therapy

Candidates for autologous bone marrow/stem cell transplants

Hereditary or acquired cellular immunodeficiencies

Not Indicated

Seronegative full-term infants, birth weight >1200 g

Seropositive pregnant women

Adapted from Simon TL, Alverson DC, AuBuchon J, et al, "Practice Parameter for the Use of Red Blood Cell Transfusions," *Arch Pathol Lab Med*, 1998, 122(2):130-8.

Leukocyte-reduced RBCs reduce postoperative complications, morbidity, and mortality. Use of these fractions is highly cost effective in cardiac surgery.[6] Consultation with the Blood Bank physician is recommended.

Limitations Leukocyte reduction does **not** prevent graft-versus-host disease. It is an added expense.

Methodology Filtration is presently the most widely used method of leukoreduction, performed either in the Blood Bank or at the bedside. Personnel administering red cells through a bedside leukocyte reduction filter must be familiar with manufacturer's requirements for use in order to maximize leukocyte reduction and ensure against inordinate loss of red cells. Reproducibility and effectiveness is best sustained when filtration is performed in the laboratory.[7]

Additional Information The use of universal leukocyte reduction in preventing changes in host immune functions is controversial.[8] Animal models have supported the concept that early leukodepletion may prevent alloimmunization to HLA, a practice which may be especially relevant for candidates for bone marrow transplantation, and for other patients likely to need multiple transfusions (eg, those with certain hemoglobinopathies, lymphoplasmacytic and myeloproliferative diseases, and patients being treated for solid tumors with myelosuppressive adjuvant chemotherapy).

Early leukodepletion may diminish bacterial contamination, but further investigation is needed. The roles of transfused WBCs in other clinical settings require further studies.[5] Certain of the proposed roles for leukoreduced blood are controversial.[9]

Footnotes

1. Menitove JE, *Standards for Blood Banks and Transfusion Services*, 20th ed, Bethesda, MD: American Association of Blood Banks Press, 2000, 32.
2. Snyder EL, "Transfusion Reactions," *Hematology: Basic Principles and Practice*, 3rd ed, Hoffman R, Benz EJ Jr, Shattil SJ, et al, New York, NY: Churchill Livingstone, 2000, 2300-10.
3. Bowden RA, Cays MJ, Schoch F, et al, "Comparison of Filtered Blood (FB) to Seronegative Blood Products (SB) for Prevention of Cytomegalovirus (CMV) Infection After Marrow Transplant," *Blood*, 1995, 86:3598-603.
4. Lane TA, Anderson KC, Goodnough LT, et al, "Leukocyte Reduction in Blood Component Therapy," *Ann Intern Med*, 1992, 117(2):151-62.
5. LeParc GF, "Leukocyte Reduction in Cellular Blood Components," *Lab Med*, 1997, 28(5):328-31.
6. Blumberg N and Heal JM, "Mortality Risks, Costs, and Decision Making in Transfusion Medicine," *Am J Clin Pathol*, 2000, 114(6):934-7.
7. Lane TA, "Leukocyte Reduction of Cellular Blood Components. Effectiveness, Benefits, Quality Control and Costs," *Arch Pathol Lab Med*, 1994, 118(4):392-404.
8. Blajchman MA, "Allogeneic Blood Transfusion, Immunomodulation and Postoperative Bacterial Infection: Do We Have the Answers Yet?" *Transfusion*, 1997, 37(2):121-5.
9. Paxton A, "Universal Leukoreduction - Fix or Folly?" *CAP Today*, 2000, 14(10):1-46.

References

Ness PM and Rothko K, "Principles of Red Blood Cell Transfusion," *Hematology, Basic Principles and Practice*, 3rd ed, Hoffman R, Benz EJ Jr, Shattil SJ, et al, eds, New York, NY: Churchill Livingstone, 2000, 2241-8.

Triulzi DJ, *Blood Transfusion Therapy: A Physician's Handbook*, 6th ed, Bethesda, MD: American Association of Blood Banks Press, 1999, 10-3.

Red Blood Cells, Washed

Related Information

Antibodies to IgA *on page 833*

Ham Test *on page 439*

Red Blood Cells *on page 857*

Red Blood Cells, Leukocytes Reduced *on page 858*

Synonyms Washed Blood Cells

Applies to Transfusion Reaction, Allergic

Test Includes ABO and Rh type, antibody screen, crossmatch, and antibody identification when screen is positive, as for other transfusions.

Abstract Washed red cells are prepared using sterile saline to a final volume of 180 mL and a hematocrit of 70% to 80%.[1] The primary indications for use include 1) prevention of allergic or anaphylactic transfusion reactions; and 2) removal of antibodies in plasma which are harmful to the recipient.[1,2] Do not use when leukocyte reduction is indicated, as leukocyte reduction filters are more efficacious.

Patient Preparation Same as for other RBC transfusions.

Aftercare Same as for other RBC transfusions.

Specimen Blood

Container One red top tube or one lavender top (EDTA) tube

Collection (Of sample from intended recipient): Same as for other RBC transfusions.

Storage Instructions Once prepared, store in a monitored Blood Bank refrigerator only until issue. Same as for other RBC transfusions.

Causes for Rejection (Of patient sample): Gross hemolysis, sample placed in a serum separator tube, specimen tube not properly labeled

Turnaround Time Allow about 1 hour after selection of compatible red cells.

Special Instructions Must be used within 24 hours after preparation.

Use Useful for patients who have severe allergic reaction to conventional transfusion even with antihistamines. Prevention of transfusion reaction to plasma proteins, especially IgA, in patients with IgA immunoglobulin deficiency. In such subjects, with preformed anti-IgA, infusion of IgA-containing plasma can cause anaphylaxis. Washed red cells can be used for patients with paroxysmal nocturnal hemoglobinuria (PNH),[3] although for transfusion of patients with PNH,[4] leukocyte-reduced red cells may be preferable.

Limitations High outdating rate (24 hours). Cannot be ordered "on hold." Time consuming and expensive. There is up to 20% loss of red cells.

Methodology Various methods are available. The best is probably a system using a continuous-flow centrifuge and 2-3 L of isotonic saline per unit.

Additional Information This component is comparable to deglycerolized red blood cells, from which 99% of WBCs are removed. The washing process removes most of the plasma proteins, platelets, and leukocytes, including lymphocytes.[2] The effectiveness of washing depends on the method and on the volume of isotonic saline used. Red cells have been shown to have normal survival after washing. See also Filters for Blood *on page 842*. Use of washed RBCs has given way to leukocyte filters for removal of WBCs, but washed cells are appropriate for patients who have repeated allergic reactions or who have anti-IgA. Washing RBCs is not satisfactory for the prevention of graft-versus-host disease.

Footnotes

1. *Blood Transfusion Therapy: A Physician's Handbook*, 6th ed, Bethesda, MD: American Association of Blood Banks Press, 1999, 13-4.

(Continued)

Red Blood Cells, Washed *(Continued)*

2. *Circular of Information for the Use of Human Blood and Blood Components*, American Association of Blood Banks, America's Blood Centers, American Red Cross, 1998.

3. Bresher ME and Taswell HF, "Paroxysmal Nocturnal Hemoglobinuria and the Transfusion of Washed Red Cells. A Myth Revisited," *Transfusion*, 1989, 29(8):681-5.

4. Swisher SN and Petz LD, "Transfusion Therapy for Chronic Anemic States," *Clinical Practice of Transfusion Medicine*, 3rd ed, Petz LD, Swisher SN, Kleinman S, et al, eds, New York, NY: Churchill Livingstone, 1996, 451-67.

References
Ness PM and Rothko K, "Principles of Red Blood Cell Transfusion," *Hematology: Basic Principles and Practice*, 3rd ed, Chapter 135, Hoffman R, Benz EJ Jr, Shattil SJ, et al, eds, New York, NY: Churchill Livingstone, 2000, 2241-48.

♦ **Red Cell Exchange** *see* Apheresis, Therapeutic *on page 836*

♦ **Reverse Grouping** *see* Pretransfusion Testing *on page 856*

♦ **Rh(D) Typing** *see* Pretransfusion Testing *on page 856*

Rh Genotype

Related Information
Bilirubin, Amniotic Fluid, Delta A450 *on page 116*
Bilirubin, Neonatal, Serum *on page 117*
Cord Blood Screen *on page 838*
Hemolytic Disease of the Newborn, Antibody Identification *on page 846*
Newborn Crossmatch and Transfusion *on page 848*
Polymerase Chain Reaction *on page 713*
Pretransfusion Testing *on page 856*
Rh$_o$(D) Immune Globulin (Human) *on page 860*

Synonyms Rh Zygosity; Zygosity Rh

Applies to Hemolytic Disease of the Newborn (HDN) Prognosis; Prenatal Testing; Weak D

Test Includes Rh genotyping of male partners of pregnant, Rh-immunized women; testing of red cells with Rh antisera anti-D, C, E, c, e,

Abstract When a woman of childbearing age is found to have anti-D, it is important for prognostic purposes to know the husband's zygosity for the gene producing the Rh antigen D. A father homozygous for Rh(D) must produce Rh(D)-positive children, whereas a father heterozygous for Rh(D) has a 50% chance of producing Rh(D)-negative children.

Specimen Blood, amniotic fluid

Container Red top tube or lavender top (EDTA) tube

Causes for Rejection Gross hemolysis, improper labeling

Special Instructions Rh gene frequencies vary considerably with racial origins.[1] It is important that ethnic group of subject is recorded.

Reference Interval Rh gene frequencies vary considerably with different ethnic groups. Most published data are for European whites. It is important that the appropriate frequency table be utilized.

Incidence of the More Common Genotypes in D-Positive Persons

Phenotype	Genotype		Incidence (%)	
	DCE	Rh-hr	Whites	Blacks
DCce	DCe/ce	R^1r	31.1	8.8
	DCe/Dce	R^1R^0	3.4	15.0
	Ce/Dce	$r'R^0$	0.2	1.8
DCe	DCe/DCe	R^1R^1	17.6	2.9
	DCe/Ce	R^1r'	1.7	0.7
DcEe	DcE/ce	R^2r	10.4	5.7
	DcE/Dce	R^2R^0	1.1	9.7
DcE	DcE/DcE	R^2R^2	2.0	1.3
	DcE/cE	R^2r''	0.3	<0.1
DCcEe	DCe/DcE	R^1R^2	11.8	3.7
	DCe/cE	R^1r''	0.8	<0.1
	Ce/DcE	$r'R^2$	0.6	0.4
Dce	Dce/ce	R^0r	3.0	22.9
	Dce/Dce	R^0R^0	0.2	19.4

Adapted from Vengelen-Tyler V, *Technical Manual*, 13th edition, Bethesda, MD: American Association Blood Banks Press, 1999, 300.

Limitations Genotype frequencies are given for random populations. The partners of Rh-immunized women are a weighted population with a higher incidence of homozygosity.[2] On the other hand, if any or all of the subject's children or if either of his parents is Rh(D) negative, then the partner must be heterozygous.

Methodology The subject's red cells are tested with the range of Rh antisera indicated earlier. From the results, his Rh phenotype is determined. The most likely genotype can be determined by reference to a frequency table for the appropriate racial group. Fetal Rh(D) status can be determined from polymerase chain reaction (PCR) analysis of amniotic fluid, an invasive procedure.[3] Fetal Rh(D) status can be determined by analysis of maternal plasma, using a PCR assay.[4]

Additional Information Serologic results are often able to determine Rh phenotype only and genotype is assigned according to frequency tables.

Clearly, a significant number of "most probable genotypes" are incorrect. However, most clinically important blood groups have now been characterized at the gene level. This knowledge has permitted the development of noninvasive prenatal tests to identify the presence of fetal DNA in maternal plasma.[4] These procedures will prove valuable where the father's antigenic status is heterozygous, indeterminable, or unknown.[5] Furthermore, it is likely that in the near future, it will be feasible to screen Rh(D)-negative pregnancies by molecular biological methods, to select those requiring antenatal Rh immunoprophylaxis.[4,6]

The expression "D^u" is presently termed weak D. It indicates a weak expression of the D antigen in which red cells are not directly agglutinated by all anti-D sera. The frequency of weak D is about 0.2% in Caucasians.[7]

Footnotes
1. Mourant AE, Kopec A, and Domaniewska-Sobczak K, *The Distribution of the Human Blood Groups and Other Biochemical Polymorphisms*, 2nd ed, Oxford, UK: Oxford University Press, 1976.
2. Kanter MH, "Derivation of New Mathematic Formulas for Determining Whether a D-Positive Father Is Heterozygous or Homozygous for the D Antigen," *Am J Obstet Gynecol*, 1992, 166(1 Pt 1):61-3.
3. Bowman JM, "RhD Hemolytic Disease of the Newborn," *N Engl J Med*, 1998, 339(24):1775-6.
4. Lo YM, Hjelm NM, Fidler C, et al, "Prenatal Diagnosis of Fetal RhD Status by Molecular Analysis of Maternal Plasma," *N Engl J Med*, 1998, 339(24):1734-8.
5. Reid ME, Rios M, and Yazdanbakhsh K, "Applications of Molecular Biology Techniques to Transfusion Medicine," *Semin Hematol*, 2000, 37(2):166-76.
6. Saade GR, "Noninvasive Testing for Fetal Anemia," *N Engl J Med*, 2000, 342(1):52-3.
7. Hartwell EA, "Use of Rh Immune Globulin: ASCP Practice Parameter," *Am J Clin Pathol*, 1998, 110(3):281-92.

References
Domen RE, "Policies and Procedures Related to Weak D Phenotype Testing and Rh Immune Globulin Administration: Results From Supplementary Questions to the Comprehensive Transfusion Medicine Survey of the College of American Pathologists," *Arch Pathol Lab Med*, 2000, 124(8):1118-21.

♦ **RhIG** *see* Rh$_o$(D) Immune Globulin (Human) *on page 860*

♦ **Rh Immune Globulin** *see* Rh$_o$(D) Immune Globulin (Human) *on page 860*

Rh$_o$(D) Immune Globulin (Human)

Related Information
Antibody Detection/Identification, Red Cell *on page 834*
Antiglobulin Test, Direct *on page 834*
Cord Blood Screen *on page 838*
Fetal Cell Detection by Flow Cytometry *on page 430*
Hemolytic Disease of the Newborn, Antibody Identification *on page 846*
Kleihauer-Betke *on page 453*
Newborn Crossmatch and Transfusion *on page 848*
Rh Genotype *on page 860*
Rosette Test for Fetomaternal Hemorrhage *on page 863*

Synonyms RhIG; Rh Immune Globulin

Test Includes D/weak D type of mother and baby, test to detect excessive fetomaternal hemorrhage (rosette test followed by Kleihauer-Betke or flow cytometry), and, antibody screen on mother

Abstract Hemolytic disease of the newborn (HDN) is caused by an IgG maternal antibody which destroys the antigen-positive erythrocytes of the fetus and newborn. Anti-Rh$_o$(D) is the most important such alloantibody, produced by Rh$_o$(D) negative women exposed to Rh$_o$(D)-positive fetal/neonatal or transfused red cells. It is given to Rh$_o$(D) negative pregnant/postpartum women who have not developed anti-Rh$_o$(D); *vide infra*. Rh-immune globulin (RhIG) is an immune globulin, predominantly IgG anti-D prepared from pooled human plasma. Intramuscular (I.M.) or intravenous (I.V.) preparations are available for administration. I.M. RhIG is available in 300 µg and 50 µg doses. A 300 µg dose is sufficient to prevent immunization by 30 mL of D-positive whole blood or 15 mL of D-positive red cells. The 50 µg dose protects against fetal bleed during the first trimester only. Intravenous RhIG is available in 300 µg and 120 µg doses. The 300 µg dose can suppress the immunizing potential of ~17 mL of D-positive red cells. It is administered at 28-30 weeks gestation or after invasive procedures before 34 weeks gestation, unless the father is known to be Rh(D)-negative. The 120 µg dose can be administered to the mother within 72 hours of delivery or after invasive procedures associated with increased risk of Rh(D) isoimmunization after 34 weeks gestation.

Patient Preparation AABB Standards requires examination of a postpartum specimen from D-negative women to detect fetomaternal hemorrhage requiring >1 dose RhIG. The rosette test is an effective screening test (see Rosette Test for Fetomaternal Hemorrhage *on page 863*), which, if positive, must be followed by a quantitative test such as the Kleihauer-Betke test. The weak D test (formerly known as the D^u test) is not recommended to identify large fetomaternal hemorrhage.[1]

Specimen Blood from mother and infant

Container One red top tube or one lavender top (EDTA) tube

Collection Collected postpartum. Blood required from both mother and newborn. Label each specimen.

Storage Instructions RhIG must be stored at 2°C to 8°C.

Causes for Rejection (Of patient sample): Gross hemolysis, sample placed in a serum separator tube, specimen tube not properly labeled.

RhIG is not indicated when the newborn is Rh-negative, mother is Rh-positive or weak D-positive, or when anti-D is present in mother's serum when mother has not had prenatal Rh immune globulin.

Use Given to D-negative women postpartum, or after termination of pregnancy, ectopic pregnancy, abortion, threatened abortion, obstetric complications, tubal ligation, immune thrombocytopenic purpura, or any event associated with increased risk of fetomaternal hemorrhage to prevent development of anti-D. Anti-D antibody may cause erythroblastosis fetalis (hemolytic disease of the newborn) or years later lead to transfusion reaction if Rh-positive RBCs are transfused. RhIG is given to Rh-negative women after amniocentesis, percutaneous umbilical cord sampling, or chronic villus sampling. Give RhIG antepartum at 28-32 weeks, as well as within 3 days of delivery. When it is given antepartum, then after delivery there will still be anti-D in the maternal serum. Give a postpartum dose to the appropriate mother whether or not Rh immune globulin was given antepartum. Occasionally, RhIG is given to an Rh-negative person who received Rh-positive red blood cells or an Rh-positive component (eg, platelets, granulocytes). The I.V. RhIG is also approved for treatment of nonsplenectomized D-positive patients with immune thrombocytopenic purpura (ITP).

Limitations In instances of large fetomaternal hemorrhage, one dose is not sufficient. When a transplacental hemorrhage is >30 mL fetal blood (by Kleihauer-Betke) the dose of $Rh_o(D)$ immune globulin must be at least 10 µg/mL of fetal blood in the maternal circulation.[2] The weak D test is not recommended to identify large fetomaternal hemorrhage. The rosette test is more sensitive (see Rosette Test for Fetomaternal Hemorrhage *on page 863*). A smaller Rh immune globulin dose may be used after abortion or miscarriage up to 12 weeks gestation, but not beyond; after 12 weeks of gestation a conventional dose is indicated.

Failures occur. The most common cause of Rh immunization is failure to give RhIG when it is indicated. RhIG is sometimes forgotten in ectopic gestation and in abortion in Rh-negative women. However, 1% to 2% of term mothers develop anti-D in spite of postpartum RhIG properly administered. Postpartum failure may be secondary to fetomaternal hemorrhage in the third trimester (hence, antenatal RhIG)[3] and because of large fetomaternal hemorrhages at delivery.

The product contains small amounts of IgA.

Contraindications Do not give RhIG to an Rh-positive or weak D-positive[4] person (unless treating for ITP), or a person already immunized to the $Rh_o(D)$ blood factor whose serum contains anti-D. (However, if $Rh_o(D)$ immune globulin was given as an antenatal dose to mother, then anti-D detectable in her serum is not a contraindication to postnatal administration of RhIG.) (The usual antenatal dose of RhIG does not cause titers >4.) Women who deliver $Rh_o(D)$-negative infants are not candidates for RhIG. If there is certain documentation that the biologic father is Rh-negative, the RhIG is not needed. **Do not give RhIG to an infant.**

Methodology Read appropriate manufacturer's package inserts for dosage and administration instructions.

The product contains small amounts of IgA and other globulins.

Additional Information Give a full dose, 300 µg RhIG (I.M.) to an Rh-negative mother within 72 hours of delivery, miscarriage, or any event associated with increased risk of fetomaternal hemorrhage. If a fetomaternal hemorrhage >15 mL RBCs has taken place, then additional RhIG is indicated.

The **Kleihauer-Betke** test done on maternal blood after delivery estimates the volume of fetal-maternal hemorrhage. Calculate the dose of Rh_o immune globulin as follows.

- Percent of fetal red cells x 50 = mL fetal whole blood in maternal circulation.
- Although the usually recommended dose is 300 µg of RhIG per 30 mL of fetal blood, always give one more dose (300 µg) than that calculated because of the poor precision of the Kleihauer-Betke test. For example:
  1.8% fetal RBCs
  1.8 x 50 = 90 mL fetal whole blood
  90 mL/30 = 3 doses
  3 + 1 = 4
  four, 300 µg doses of RhIG administered

Give RhIG to Rh-negative mothers with negative screens when cord blood is not available (ectopic pregnancies, abortions, etc). If the patient refuses, she should sign an appropriate statement to that effect. Although **antenatal doses** may have been given at 28-32 weeks, give a postpartum dose anyway. Transmission of viral infections does not occur with this preparation.

Footnotes
1. Vengelen-Tyler V, *Technical Manual*, 13th ed, Bethesda, MD: American Association of Blood Banks Press, 1999, 501-8.
2. Bowman JM, "RhD Hemolytic Disease of the Newborn," *N Engl J Med*, 1998, 339(24):1775-6.
3. Bowman JM, "Antenatal Suppression of Rh Alloimmunization," *Clin Obstet Gynecol*, 1991, 34(2):296-303.
4. Judd WJ, Luban NLC, Ness PM, et al, "Prenatal and Perinatal Immunohematology: Recommendations for Serological Management of the Fetus, Newborn Infant and Obstetrical Patient," *Transfusion*, 1990, 30:175-83.

References
Domen RE, "Policies and Procedures Related to Weak D Phenotype Testing and Rh Immune Globulin Administration," Results From Supplementary Questions to the Comprehensive Transfusion Medicine Survey of the College of American Pathologists, *Arch Pathol Lab Med*, 2000, 124(8):118-21.
Hartwell EA, "Use of Rh Immune Globulin," ASCP Practice Parameter, *Am J Clin Pathol*, 1998, 110(3):281-92.
Mittendorf R and Williams MA, "$Rh_o(D)$ Immunoglobulin (RhoGAM™): How It Came Into Being," *Obstet Gynecol*, 1991, 77(2):301-3.
Rushin J, Rumsey DH, Ewing CA, et al, "Detection of Multiple Passively Acquired Alloantibodies Following Infusions of IV Rh Immune Globulin," *Transfusion*, 2000, 40(5):551-4.
Triulzi DJ, *Blood Transfusion Therapy: A Physician's Handbook*, 6th ed, Bethesda, MD: American Association of Blood Banks Press, 1999.
Snyder EL and Shoos Lipton K, "Prevention of Hemolytic Disease of the Newborn Due to Anti-D," *AABB Association Bulletin, 98-2. AABB News Briefs*, March 1998, 16-7.

♦ **Rh Zygosity** *see* Rh Genotype *on page 860*

Risks of Transfusion

Related Information
Alanine Aminotransferase, Serum *on page 87*
Antibodies to IgA *on page 833*
Babesiosis Serology *on page 561*
Chagas' Disease Serological Test *on page 588*
Coagulation Factor Assays *on page 335*
Cold Agglutinin Titer *on page 594*
Cytomegalovirus Serology *on page 600*
D-Dimers and Fibrin Degradation Products *on page 338*
Disseminated Intravascular Coagulation Screen *on page 338*
Hepatitis B Core Antibody *on page 622*
Hepatitis B Surface Antigen *on page 625*
Hepatitis C Virus RNA Detection and Quantitation *on page 626*
Hepatitis C Virus Serology *on page 627*
HIV-1/HIV-2 Antibody Screen and Western Blot *on page 636*
HIV p24 Antigen Detection *on page 637*
HTLV-I/II Antibody *on page 638*
Immunoglobulin A *on page 532*
Liver Disease: Laboratory Assessment, Overview *on page 216*
Parvovirus B19 DNA *on page 669*
Parvovirus B19 Serology *on page 669*
Platelet Antibodies *on page 349*
Platelet Antibody, Immunohematologic *on page 852*
Platelets, Apheresis, Donation *on page 853*
Platelet Transfusion *on page 854*
Pretransfusion Testing *on page 856*
Red Blood Cells *on page 857*
RPR *on page 677*
Transfusion Reaction Work-up *on page 864*
Uncrossmatched Blood, Emergency *on page 865*
VDRL, Serum *on page 688*
Whole Blood *on page 866*
Yersinia enterocolitica Antibody *on page 698*

Synonyms Adverse Effects; Adverse Reactions; Hazards of Transfusion; Transfusion Complications

Test Includes See Transfusion Reaction Work-up *on page 864* for a listing of tests performed for noninfectious complications of transfusion. Although blood is tested for the four major transfusion-transmitted viral diseases, hepatitis B, HIV, HTLV, and hepatitis C, transmission of these diseases can still occur through transfusion. Any cases of suspected transfusion-transmitted disease should be reported to the Blood Bank. Other agents known to be transmitted by transfusion include cytomegalovirus, malaria, babesiosis, and Chagas' disease.

Patient Preparation Obtain and document informed consent prior to transfusion.

Special Instructions Report all adverse effects of transfusion at once to the Blood Bank for follow-up and investigation (see Transfusion Reaction Work-up *on page 864*).

Use A physician's understanding of the estimated risks of transfusions plays a role in determining the need for transfusion and must be explained to the patient (in nonemergency situations) as part of the informed consent process. All transfusions carry risk, including autologous transfusions.

Additional Information

NONINFECTIOUS COMPLICATIONS:

Hemolytic transfusion reactions usually result from clerical and other identification errors and frequently result in ABO incompatibility.[1] This is why unlabeled or improperly labeled sample tubes are unacceptable to the Transfusion Service. Most blood errors in administration are caused by failure to correctly identify the recipient and blood unit, but phlebotomy errors and Blood Bank errors occur as well.[2] Chills, fever, dyspnea, chest or back pain, headache, abnormal bleeding, or shock can all characterize acute hemolytic reactions. Hemoglobinemia heralds **intravascular** hemolysis, followed by hemoglobinuria, then jaundice. This is usually mediated by anti-A or anti-B or both. **Extravascular** hemolysis takes place mostly in the spleen as a result of the action of IgG antibodies, such as those of the Rh system. With these, hemoglobinemia and hemoglobinuria seldom occur. (Continued)

Risks of Transfusion *(Continued)*

Some Risks of Allogeneic Transfusion

Reactions
Hemolytic, immediate, delayed
Febrile
Allergic, anaphylactic
Sepsis
Overload
Hypothermia, cold
Air embolism
Post-transfusion purpura
Disease Transmission
Hepatitis B, C, etc
Cytomegalovirus
Parvovirus B19
HTLV-I
HTLV-II
Syphilis
Malaria
Babesiosis
Yersinia
Chagas disease
AIDS
Other
Alloimmunization RBC, WBC, etc
Marrow suppression
Immunosuppression
Storage changes
Graft-vs-host disease
Dilutional coagulopathy
Nonimmune hemolysis
Siderosis (transfusional)

Renal shutdown, shock, or hemorrhage may be fatal. When this type of reaction occurs, stop the transfusion at once (see Transfusion Reaction Work-up *on page 864*). Treat shock. Give appropriate fluids and diuretics to maintain urinary output. Treat for incipient renal failure, if indicated. Rarely, passive transfer of alloantibodies can cause unanticipated hemolytic anemia.[3]

Delayed hemolytic reactions can occur in some patients with other serologically undetectable antibodies (frequently Kidd blood group system antibodies). Such reactions may come to the attention of the Blood Bank Staff when more blood is ordered a few days after an earlier transfusion of apparently compatible blood, usually with a poor clinical response to the prior transfusion. The Blood Bank finds a positive direct antiglobulin test and antibody that is now incompatible with the recently transfused RBCs. The antibody may be either in the patient's serum or in an eluate from the red cells. The diagnosis is easily missed. Delayed hemolytic reactions are not uncommon; they are usually mild and rarely severe.

Nonimmune hemolysis may occur secondary to inappropriate solutions running in the same tubing with blood components. With the exception of 0.9% sodium chloride, USP, drugs, or medications must not be added to blood unless they have been approved for this use by the FDA or unless records are available to show that such addition is safe and does not adversely affect the blood component.[4]

Other immune reactions include **febrile nonhemolytic** reactions.[5] Leukocyte-derived cytokines are a major cause of febrile reactions related to platelet transfusions. Leukocyte reduction by filtration is effective, but soluble mediators and cytokines are released in storage.[5,6,7] They are treated symptomatically with antipyretics and may be prevented by transfusion of leukocyte-reduced blood components. **Allergic transfusion reactions** usually appear in the form of hives (urticaria) without fever. Treatment and prevention is administration of antihistamine to the patient. Anaphylaxis is rare.

Bone marrow suppression of RBC production will occur after the transfusion of RBCs, another reason to avoid transfusions to patients whose anemia might respond to conventional medication.

Immunosuppression of varying degree follows allogeneic transfusion. Although it has been observed to improve renal allografts, survival concerns have been raised regarding the adverse effects of transfusion in other clinical settings, including increased rates of postoperative infections and tumor recurrence.[5] The usefulness of leukocyte-reduction in such clinical settings remains controversial.[8]

Transfusion-related acute lung injury ("TRALI") occurs within 4 hours following transfusion. It is caused by noncardiogenic pulmonary edema.[9] Clinically similar to adult respiratory distress syndrome, TRALI seems to be related to HLA or leukocyte antibodies in donor plasma, reacting with recipient's antigens, perhaps with release of complement.[10] Unlike ARDS, the condition usually improves quickly with pulmonary support.

Simple **volume overload** of the recipient's circulation may cause pulmonary edema without leukocyte antibodies.

Air embolism can result from any admission of air into intravenous tubing and can have serious consequences.

Anaphylactic reaction: See Immunoglobulin A *on page 532*. Nausea, chills, severe abdominal cramps, emesis, diarrhea, dyspnea, and flushing with hypotension may take place due to a generalized reaction associated with an IgA antibody. Washed cellular components or IgA-deficient plasma is available for these recipients.

Graft-versus-host disease (GVHD) can result from transfusion of blood components containing living donor lymphocytes that engraft and clonally expand in a susceptible host. GVHD usually occurs in immunocompromised individuals, but is occasionally seen in immunocompetent recipients. It has been seen when related directed donors are utilized, due to greater genetic homogeneity. While transfusion-associated GVHD is usually fatal, GVHD is preventable by irradiation of any blood component to be transfused to a patient at risk (see Irradiated Blood Components *on page 846*).

Immunosuppressed patients include recipients of hematopoietic stem-cell donations, recipients of other organ donations, others on immunosuppressive therapy, those with lymphomas and Hodgkin disease and leukemias undergoing chemotherapy, and those with AIDS. Such patients and other with immunodeficiency states are benefited by screening of blood fractions for CMV. See Red Blood Cells, Leukocytes Reduced *on page 858*. Immunosuppressed individuals are sensitive to bacterial contamination, an especially relevant problem when platelets are transfused. Graft-vs-host disease is a threat, prevented by irradiation.[11] See Irradiated Blood Components *on page 846*.

Complications of massive transfusion: Hemorrhagic diathesis may follow dilution and washout (dilutional coagulopathy) of coagulation factors and platelets.[12] DIC occurs in settings in which massive transfusions are given. Rapid laboratory evaluation of hemostasis can be vital. Treatment of abnormal bleeding in this situation is primarily with platelet concentrates, sometimes also with FFP, and less often with cryoprecipitate. If fluid balance is not carefully observed, fluid overload or adult respiratory distress syndrome may occur. 2,3-DPG depletion of stored RBCs is a theoretic problem, rarely of any clinical significance. Hypothermia, caused by rapid massive transfusion of cold blood, can be prevented with blood warmers (see Warming, Blood *on page 865*). Other possible problems faced with massive transfusions may include citrate toxicity and hyperkalemia.[13] With massive transfusions, particularly in trauma, there is often tumult and confusion, creating a setting which may promote likelihood of clerical error and increased possibility of incompatible blood transfusion. Avoiding errors in such settings is vital.

TRANSFUSION-ASSOCIATED INFECTIOUS DISEASES:

Viral hepatitis, the incidence of which is changing. Type A is very rare, B uncommon, and C decreasing significantly.[14] A causal relationship between hepatitis G virus and hepatitis has not been established.[15]

Cytomegalovirus (CMV) infection can be significant in premature newborns born to CMV-seronegative mothers and immunosuppressed CMV-seronegative adults, including transplant recipients.[16] Transfuse CMV-seronegative or leukocyte-reduced blood components.[16,17]

Bacterial contamination of blood components can cause septic shock and death and must be vigorously treated if observed. Gram-positive organisms are more frequently seen in components stored at room temperature; gram-negative organisms (eg, *Yersinia enterocolitica*[18]) can grow in refrigerated blood.

HIV/AIDS, as a transfusion hazard, is statistically rare,[19] but regarded by the public as a terrifying risk of transfusion. The onset of testing of the blood supply in 1985, beginning with a test for antibody to HIV and now including tests for HIV antigen and nucleic acid testing, has led to an extremely small estimated risk.

The following transfusion-associated infections should be considered rare in the U.S.: syphilis, malaria, babesiosis[20] (endemic in some areas of the East Coast), *Trypanosoma cruzi* (Chagas' disease),[21,22] and leishmaniasis. See table on following page.

The following information is provided for comparative purposes.[23,24]

	Deaths/Person/Year (Odds)
Smoking, 20 cigarettes per day	1 in 200
Motorcycling	1 in 50
Struck by automobile (U.S.)	1 in 20,000
Earthquake (California)	1 in 588,000
Tornado (Midwest)	1 in 455,000
Falling aircraft (U.S.)	1 in 10 million
DEATH from acute hemolytic reaction	1:633,000

Type of Outcome or Infectious Agent	Estimated Risk per Unit Transfused*
Acute hemolytic	1:12,000-1:33,000
Delayed hemolytic	1:100
Febrile, nonhemolytic	1:100-1:200
Allergic	1:33-1:100
Anaphylactic	1:18,000-1:170,000
Circulatory overload	1:100-1:10,000
Human immunodeficiency virus	1:1,000,000 (with nucleic acid testing)†
Hepatitis C virus	1:500,000-1:1,000,000 (with nucleic acid testing)†
Hepatitis A virus	1:1,000,000
Hepatitis B virus	1:63,000
Human T-cell lymphotropic virus	1:650,000
Bacteria, red cells	1:500,000
Bacteria, platelets	1:10,000-1:20,000
Trypanosoma cruzi	1:42,000
Malaria Babesia	<1:1,000,000

Modified from:

*Vengelen-Tyler V, Technical Manual, 13th ed, Bethesda, MD: American Association of Blood Banks Press, 1999, 578-81, 602.

†Wilkinson SL and Shoos Lipton K, NAT Implementation. Association Bulletin #99-3, Bethesda, MD: American Association of Blood Banks Press, February 1999.

Footnotes

1. Mollison PL, Engelfriet CP, and Contreras M, Blood Transfusion in Clinical Medicine, 10th ed, Chapter 11, Oxford, UK: Blackwell Scientific Publications, 1997, 358-89.
2. Linden JV, "Errors in Transfusion Medicine: Scope of the Problem," College of American Pathologists Conference XXXIII, August 20-22, 1998, Arch Pathol Lab Med, 1999, 123(7):563-5.
3. Garratty G, "Problems Associated With Passively Transfused Blood Group Alloantibodies," Am J Clin Pathol, 1998, 109(6):769-77.
4. Menitove JE, Standards for Blood Banks and Transfusion Services, 20th ed, Bethesda, MD: American Association of Blood Banks Press, 2000, 54.
5. Blumberg N and Heal JM, "Effects of Transfusion on Immune Function. Cancer Recurrence and Infection," Arch Pathol Lab Med, 1994, 118(4):371-9.
6. Heddle NM, Klama L, Singer J, et al, "The Role of Plasma From Platelet Concentrates in Transfusion Reactions," N Engl J Med, 1994, 331:625-8.
7. Sacher RA and Sandler SG, "Impact of Innovations on Transfusion Medicine," Arch Pathol Lab Med, 1999, 123(8):672-6.
8. Vamvakas EC and Blajchman MA, Immunomodulatory Effects of Blood Transfusion, Bethesda, MD: American Association of Blood Banks Press, 1999.
9. Goodnough LT, Brecher ME, Kanter MH, et al, "Transfusion Medicine. First of Two Parts: Blood Transfusion," N Engl J Med, 1999, 340(6):438-48.
10. Popovsky MA, Chaplin HC Jr, and Moore SB, "Transfusion-Related Acute Lung Injury: A Neglected, Serious Complication of Hemotherapy," Transfusion, 1992, 32(6):589-91.
11. Lichtiger B and Huh YO, "Transfusion Therapy for the Immunosuppressed Patient," Lab Med, 1997, 28(6):388-91.
12. Spence RK, Jeter EK, and Mintz PD, "Transfusion in Surgery and Trauma," Transfusion Therapy: Clinical Principles and Practice, Mintz PD, ed, Bethesda, MD: American Association of Blood Banks Press, 1999, 171-97.
13. Laine EP, Nelson JM, George FW IV, et al, "Hyperkalemia After Massive Blood Transfusion," Lab Med, 1997, 28(5):305-8.
14. Murphy EL, Bryzman S, and Williams AE, "Demographic Determinants of Hepatitis C Virus Seroprevalence Among Blood Donors," JAMA, 1996, 275(13):995-1000.
15. Alter HJ, Nakatsuji Y, Melpolder J, et al, "The Incidence of Transfusion-Associated Hepatitis G Virus Infection and Its Relation to Liver Disease," N Engl J Med, 1997, 336(11):747-54.
16. Przeporka D, LeParc GF, Werch J, et al, "Prevention of Transfusion-Associated Cytomegalovirus Infection," Am J Clin Pathol, 1996, 106(2):163-9.
17. Bowden RA, Slichter SJ, Sayers M, et al, "A Comparison of Filtered Leukocyte-Reduced and Cytomegalovirus (CMV) Seronegative Blood Products for the Prevention of Transfusion-Associated CMV Infection After Marrow Transplant," Blood, 1995, 86(9):3598-603.
18. Haverly RM, Harrison CR, and Dougherty TH, "Yersinia enterocolitica Bacteremia Associated With Red Blood Cell Transfusion," Arch Pathol Lab Med, 1996, 120(5):499-500.
19. Lackritz EM, Satten GA, Aberle-Grasse J, et al, "Estimated Risk of Transmission of the Human Immunodeficiency Virus by Screened Blood in the United States," N Engl J Med, 1995, 333(26):1721-25.
20. Dobroszycki J, Herwaldt BL, Boctor F, et al, "A Cluster of Transfusion-Associated Babesiosis Cases Traced to a Single Asymptomatic Donor," JAMA, 1999, 281(10):297-30.
21. Leiby DA, Lenes BA, Tibbals MA, et al, "Prospective Evaluation of a Patient With Trypanosoma cruzi Infection Transmitted by Transfusion," N Engl J Med, 1999, 341(16):1237-9.
22. Pan AA and Winkler MA, "The Threat of Chagas' Disease in Transfusion Medicine. The Presence of Antibodies to Trypanosoma cruzi in the U.S. Blood Supply," Lab Med, 1997, 28(4):269-74.
23. Dinman BD, "The Reality and Acceptance of Risk," JAMA, 1980, 244:1226-8.
24. Simon TL, Alverson DC, AuBuchon J, "Practice Parameter for the Use of Red Blood Cell Transfusions," Developed by the Red Blood Cell Administration Practice Guideline Development Task Force of the College of American Pathologists, Arch Pathol Lab Med, 1998, 122(2):130-8.

References

Blumberg N, "The Cost and Consequences of Management Fads and Politically Driven Regulatory Oversight. The Case of Blood Transfusion," Arch Pathol Lab Med, 1999, 123(7):580-4.

Brown P, Cervenáková L, McShane LM, et al, "Further Studies of Blood Infectivity in an Experimental Model of Transmissible Spongiform Encephalopathy, With and Explanation of Why Blood COmponents Do Not Transmit Creutzfeldt-Jakob Disease in Humans," Transfusion, 1999, 39(11-12):1169-78.

Chamberland M and Khabbaz RF, "Emerging Issues in Blood Safety," Infect Dis Clin North Am, 1998, 12(1):217-29.

Christensen PB, Groenbaek K, Krarup HB, et al, "Transfusion-Acquired Hepatitis C: The Danish Lookback Experience," Transfusion, 1999, 39(2):188-93.

Dry SM, Bechard KM, Milford EL, et al, "The Pathology of Transfusion-Related Acute Lung Injury," Am J Clin Pathol, 1999, 112(2):216-21.

Ely EW and Bernard GR, "Transfusions in Critically Ill Patients," N Engl J Med, 1999, 340(6):467-8.

Glynn SA, Kleinman SH, Schreiber GB, et al, "Trends in Incidence and Prevalence of Major Transfusion-Transmissible Viral Infections in US Blood Donors, 1991 to 1996," JAMA, 2000, 284(2):229-35.

Goodnough LT, Brecher ME, Kanter MH, et al, "Transfusion Medicine. Second of Two Parts: Blood Conservation," N Engl J Med, 1999, 340(7):525-33.

Hewlett IK and Epstein JS, "FDA Conference on the Feasibility of Genetic Technology to Close the HIV Window in Donor Screening," Transfusion, 1997, 37(3):346-51.

Myhre BA and McRuer D, "Human Error - A Significant Cause of Transfusion Mortality," Transfusion, 2000, 40(7):879-85.

Popovsky MA, "Infection and America's Blood Supply," Am J Clin Pathol, 1998, 109(6):659-61.

Sazama K, DeChristopher PJ, Dodd R, et al, "Practice Parameter for the Recognition, Management and Prevention of Adverse Consequences of Blood Transfusion," Arch Pathol Lab Med, 2000, 124(1):61-70.

Shulman IA, "Assessing Blood Administering Practices," Arch Pathol Lab Med, 1999, 123(7):595-8.

Rosette Test for Fetomaternal Hemorrhage

Related Information

Fetal Cell Detection by Flow Cytometry on page 430
Flow Cytometry, Overview on page 432
Kleihauer-Betke on page 453
Newborn Crossmatch and Transfusion on page 848
Rho(D) Immune Globulin (Human) on page 860

Synonyms Fetalscreen™

Applies to Acid Elution Test

Abstract A postdelivery qualitative test for fetomaternal hemorrhage, the rosette test detects small numbers of Rh(D)-positive fetal red cells in Rh(D)-negative mothers. A positive result must be followed by a quantitative procedure to identify mothers needing a greater than standard postpartum dose of Rh immune globulin.

Specimen Blood

Container One red top tube and one lavender top (EDTA) tube

Sampling Time Postdelivery - preferably within 1 hour of delivery

Causes for Rejection Specimen grossly hemolyzed, improper labeling

Reference Interval Specimens in which <2.5 mL of Rh_o(D)-positive fetal red cells are present yield negative results.

Use Determine if a fetomaternal hemorrhage of more than 15 mL has occurred

Limitations This is a screening test for detection of fetal Rh(D)-positive red cells in the circulation of Rh(D)-negative mothers. A positive result must be followed by a quantitative procedure such as an acid elution test, an enzyme-linked antiglobulin test, or flow cytometry to quantitate the number of fetal cells present. Weak D-positive (D^u) red cells do not react as strongly in the rosette test as normal D-positive genotypes.

The Kleihauer-Betke test is better when fetal red cells are the weak D phenotype; rosette test results are weak to negative in that circumstance. Strongly positive results are found with the rosette test when the maternal red cells are weak D phenotype, creating confusion with massive fetomaternal hemorrhage. Specific testing for fetal RBCs is recommended.[1]

Methodology A suspension of maternal red cells is incubated with human source polyclonal anti-D reagent. Any fetal Rh(D)-positive cells present will become sensitized with the anti-D. Coating of fetal red cells with anti-D is recognized by adding Rh(D)-positive indicator cells, which form rosettes around the fetal cells.

Additional Information The rosette test detects about 5 mL of Rh_o(D)-positive fetal red cells (about 10 mL of Rh_o(D)-positive whole blood). Positive results are only found in about 1% to 3% of women who are candidates for RhIG.[1]

The enzyme-linked antiglobulin test and flow cytometry are other methods to detect Rh_o(D)-positive erythrocytes.[1]

Footnotes

1. Hartwell EA, "Use of Rh Immune Globulin," Am J Clin Pathol, 1998, 110(3):281-92.

References

Issitt PD and Anstee DJ, Applied Blood Group Serology, 4th ed, Durham, NC: Montgomery Scientific Publications, 1998, 115-63, 1049.

Mollison PL, Engelfriet CP, and Contreras M, Blood Transfusion in Clinical Medicine, 10th ed, Oxford, UK: Blackwell Scientific Publications, 1997, 393-4.

Vengelen-Tyler V, Technical Manual, 13th ed, Bethesda, MD: American Association of Blood Banks Press, 1999, 507.

Transfusion Reaction Work-up

Related Information

Synonyms Adverse Effects; Adverse Reactions; Transfusion Complication Work-Up

Test Includes

Suspected acute hemolytic transfusion reaction work-up:[1] Clerical check (label on blood containers and all records examined for error in identification); postreaction patient specimen - perform direct antiglobulin test and examine for presence of hemolysis in serum/plasma. Compare to pretransfusion sample if present. Repeat serologic testing (ABO group and/or Rh type on patient and donor blood; crossmatch) as needed. Analyze urine for hemoglobinuria (intact red cells will pellet out of a centrifuged urine specimen - free hemoglobin will not; a dipstick does not differentiate between intact red cells and hemoglobin).

Delayed hemolytic transfusion reaction work-up: Direct antiglobulin test, eluate and antibody identification. Bilirubin may be elevated and hematocrit may be declining.

Transfusion-related acute lung injury (TRALI): Anti-HLA and/or antineutrophil antibody identification (from donor and recipient samples).

Anaphylactic/severe allergic: Evaluate for the presence of anti-IgA in an IgA deficient patient.

Platelet transfusion refractoriness, post-transfusion purpura, and problems of **alloimmunization** to platelets are addressed in the platelet monographs listed above under Related Information.

Use of leukocyte-depleted fractions almost eliminates alloimmunization among subjects without prior WBC exposure.[2]

Abstract Any adverse reaction event experienced by a patient in association with a transfusion is regarded as a suspected transfusion complication until proven otherwise and each transfusion service must have a system in place for detecting, reporting, and evaluating these complications.[1]

Aftercare

If a suspected acute transfusion reaction occurs:[3]
1. Stop transfusion immediately.
2. Verify that correct unit was given to the correct patient.
3. Maintain I.V. access. Ensure adequate urine output with an appropriate crystalloid or colloid solution.
4. Maintain blood pressure, pulse, adequate ventilation.
5. Notify Blood Bank and attending physician.
6. If sepsis is suspected, obtain a blood culture from the patient, and treat patient as needed.
7. Send the following to the Blood Bank for transfusion reaction work-up: blood bag and administration set and blood/urine samples.
8. Blood Bank performs work-up as follows:
   a. Clerical check of paperwork to ensure correct unit transfused to right patient.
   b. Perform direct antiglobulin test.
   c. Evaluate serum/plasma for presence of hemoglobinemia.
   d. Repeat other serologic testing as needed (ABO, Rh, antibody screen, crossmatch).
   e. Examine urine for hemoglobinuria.
   f. If sepsis is suspected, culture the unit and examine a Gram-stained smear from the unit.

If intravascular hemolytic transfusion reaction is confirmed:
9. Monitor renal status (BUN, creatinine).
10. Initiate a diuresis.
11. Monitor coagulation status (prothrombin time, activated partial thromboplastin time, platelet count).
12. Monitor for signs of hemolysis (lactate dehydrogenase, bilirubin, haptoglobin).

Specimen Blood, urine

Container Red top tube, lavender top (EDTA) tube, and plastic urine container

Causes for Rejection (Of patient sample): Specimen tube not properly labeled, sample placed in serum separator tube

Turnaround Time Examination of pretransfusion and current serum or plasma for hemolysis can be done very rapidly. A repeat ABO and Rh, direct antiglobulin test, and clerical check can be done in minutes.

Special Instructions If the only adverse event noted is mild urticaria, the transfusion may be temporarily interrupted and antihistamine administered (eg, diphenhydramine 25-50 mg). If symptoms promptly subside, the transfusion may be resumed. This **does not** apply to the anaphylactic-type reactions presenting with vasomotor instability or to a suspected acute hemolytic transfusion reaction. Mild allergic reactions, as well as circulatory overload, do not need to be evaluated as possible hemolytic transfusion reactions.[1]

Use Investigate cause of possible transfusion reactions. Some signs and symptoms are noted as follows:
- Acute hemolytic transfusion reaction: fever (1°C or 2°F) and/or chills, hemoglobinuria, renal failure, hypotension, DIC, back pain
- Febrile nonhemolytic transfusion reaction: fever (1°C or 2°F) and/or chills, headache, malaise
- Allergic: pruritus, urticaria, flushing
- Anaphylactic: urticaria, respiratory distress, hypotension, laryngeal edema
- TRALI: marked respiratory distress, fever (1°C or 2°F), hypoxia, hypotension, bilateral pulmonary edema
- Bacterial contamination: high fever, rigors, shock, hypotension

Limitations Two of the most common complications of transfusion are urticaria and fever. Fever (with or without chills) most frequently indicates a febrile nonhemolytic transfusion reaction (FNHTR). FNHTR is caused by either recipient antibody to donor leukocytes or to accumulated cytokines in the transfused unit. Treatment is either premedication with an antipyretic or use of leukocyte reduced blood products. FNHTR are rarely life-threatening. Unfortunately, signs and symptoms of this reaction mimic an acute hemolytic transfusion reaction, and a hemolytic transfusion reaction work-up will help differentiate the two.

Faulty blood warming blood apparatus, inappropriate storage of blood components before infusion or inappropriate medication added to blood are other causes of adverse effects of transfusion. These are not always detected by the transfusion reaction work-up. Most are prevented by properly functioning transfusion quality systems.

Additional Information Most fatal transfusion reactions involve clerical (labeling) error with resultant subsequent incompatibility in the ABO system, and intravascular hemolysis.

Fatal transfusion reactions must be reported to the Food and Drug Administration (FDA).

Delayed hemolytic transfusion reactions may not be considered in a differential diagnosis. They occur in patients with unexplained anemia and fever and may be detected by a positive direct antiglobulin test or by the detection of an unexplained blood group antibody which was absent when the type and screen was previously performed.

Transfusion-transmitted diseases: Although blood is tested for hepatitis B, HIV, HTLV, and hepatitis C, transmission of these diseases can still occur through transfusion. Any cases of suspected transfusion-transmitted disease should be reported to the Blood Bank to identify infectious donors. Other agents known to be transmitted include cytomegalovirus, malaria, babesiosis, Lyme disease, and Chagas' disease. See Risks of Transfusion *on page 861*.

Footnotes

1. Menitove JE, *Standards for Blood Banks and Transfusion Services*, 20th ed, Bethesda, MD: American Association of Blood Banks Press, 2000, 84-6.
2. Kruskall MS, "The Perils of Platelet Transfusions," *N Engl J Med*, 1997, 337(26):1914-5.
3. Triulzi DJ, *Blood Transfusion Therapy: A Physician's Handbook*, 6th ed, Bethesda, MD: American Association of Blood Banks Press, 1999, 108.

References

Lichtiger B and Huh YO, "Transfusion Therapy for the Immunosuppressed Patient," *Lab Med*, 1997, 28(6):388-91.

Mollison PL, Engelfriet CP, and Contreras M, *Blood Transfusion in Clinical Medicine*, 10th ed, Chapters 10 and 11, Oxford, UK: Blackwell Scientific Publications, 1997.

Uncrossmatched Blood, Emergency

Related Information

Blood Gases and pH, Arterial *on page 119*
Hematocrit *on page 441*
Hemoglobin *on page 442*
Oxygen Saturation, Blood *on page 240*
Pretransfusion Testing *on page 856*
Red Blood Cells *on page 857*
Risks of Transfusion *on page 861*
Transfusion Reaction Work-up *on page 864*
Warming, Blood *on page 865*
Whole Blood *on page 866*

Synonyms Emergency Blood; Emergency Transfusion; Universal Donor Blood; Urgent Transfusion

Applies to Emergency Issue of Uncrossmatched Blood; Exsanguinating Emergency; Massive Acute Blood Loss

Test Includes No testing is needed in the Transfusion Service if group O, Rh negative blood is issued. ABO group and Rh type can be completed in 5-10 minutes for issue of group specific blood. As soon as possible, complete antibody screen and crossmatch and other serologic tests (eg, antibody identification) if indicated.

Abstract The administration of a blood component, usually red cells, before the completion of routine pretransfusion testing, in an emergency situation when a delay in transfusion would harm the patient. Risks include those a physician must evaluate (eg, degree of atherosclerosis, nature of the disease, level of oxygenation, heart rate, blood pressure, and control or lack of control of bleeding).

Patient Preparation Proper patient identification is necessary. Emergency Department (ER) may use special or temporary identification. Care must be taken to follow transfusion protocols, especially when multiple trauma victims are being treated simultaneously, as errors in sample/patient identification may lead to fatal ABO hemolytic transfusion reactions.

Specimen Venous or arterial blood

Container One red top tube or one lavender top (EDTA) tube

Collection (Of sample from intended recipient): Identify patient by wristband(s) or other system specially set up for identification of unconscious or noncommunicating patients in emergencies. Label tube specimen with the same information, including identification number from the wristband; label requisition form with identification number. Requisition should be signed by collector, indicating that patient's identity has been verified. Positive identification of patient sample is important, even in an emergency. If it is impossible to get a blood sample, record this fact.

Causes for Rejection Nonemergent situations

Turnaround Time Although uncrossmatched O Rh-negative red blood cells can be issued immediately if available, ABO and Rh type can be done in only 5-10 minutes. Antibody screen and crossmatch require as much as 1 hour, longer if antibodies are detected. The process is much quicker if patient has already had a type and screen. See Pretransfusion Testing *on page 856* for a table of times needed for blood issuance in emergencies.

Special Instructions An emergency request for uncrossmatched blood should include name of physician requesting blood and signature of person authorized, name and location of patient, and nature of emergency. There should also be a statement that the situation was sufficiently urgent to require release of blood before completion of testing.

Critical Values 30% to 40% loss of blood volume is associated with increased signs of shock, and >40% relates to severe shock.[1]

Use Blood replacement in exsanguinating emergency, massive acute blood loss. See discussion of use in Red Blood Cells *on page 857*.

Limitations All parties involved need to understand that blood issued in life-threatening emergencies is clearly more dangerous than that in controlled circumstances.

Contraindications Do not use group O whole blood even in emergencies, for patients of other types, because the anti-A and anti-B can cause hemolysis of the recipient's RBCs. In life-threatening trauma or bleeding when the patient's type is unknown, group O RBCs should be used. Whenever possible, Rh-negative RBCs should be used in females of childbearing age.

Methodology When issuing uncrossmatched blood, apply a label indicating uncrossmatched status.

EMERGENCY RELEASE COMPATIBILITY TESTING INCOMPLETE

Additional Information There is no such thing as a "universal donor." Group O blood lacks A and B but has antigens of other blood group systems, any of which may be a problem for a given patient. Group O RBCs can be transfused when the blood type is unknown. A blood sample can be ABO and Rh typed in 5-10 minutes. Thus, the patient may then receive type-specific RBCs when their blood type is determined. If the patient's indirect antiglobulin test (screen for unexpected antibodies) is negative, transfusion of uncrossmatched but type-specific/compatible blood carries a very low risk of being incompatible.[2] Although volume can be made up temporarily with plasma expanders, possible adverse effects of albumin solutions have been noted in critically ill patients.[3] Artificial red cells,[4] which may be available in the near future, would be an ideal solution to use until compatible blood is available. See also Transfusions in Trauma and Other Emergencies in the Transfusion Service (Blood Bank) Introduction *on page 827*.

Footnotes

1. Simon TL, Alverson DC, AuBuchon J, et al, "Practice Parameter for the Use of Red Blood Cell Transfusions: Developed by the Red Blood Cell Administration Practice Guideline Development Task Force of the College of American Pathologists," *Arch Pathol Lab Med*, 1998, 122(2):130-8.
2. Oberman HA, Barnes BA, and Friedman BA, "The Risk of Abbreviating the Major Crossmatch in Urgent or Massive Transfusion," *Transfusion*, 1978, 18:137-41.
3. Cochrane Injuries Group Albumin Reviewers, "Human Albumin Administration in Critically Ill Patients: Systematic Review of Randomised Controlled Trials," *BMJ*, 1998, 317(7153):235-40.
4. Cohn SM, "Blood Substitutes in Surgery," *Surgery*, 2000, 127(6):599-602.

References

Goodnough LT, Brecher ME, Kanter MH, et al, "Transfusion Medicine. First of Two Parts: Blood Transfusion ," *N Engl J Med*, 1999, 340(6):438-48.

Hendrix NW, Chauhan SP, Mobley J, et al, "Risk Factors Associated With Blood Transfusion in Ectopic Pregnancy," *J Reprod Med*, 1999, 44(5):433-40.

Spence RK, Jeter EK, and Mintz PD, "Transfusion in Surgery and Trauma," *Transfusion Therapy: Clinical Principles and Practice*, Bethesda, MD: American Association of Blood Banks Press, 1999, 171-97.

Warming, Blood

Related Information

Cold Agglutinin Titer *on page 594*
Newborn Crossmatch and Transfusion *on page 848*
Red Blood Cells *on page 857*
Uncrossmatched Blood, Emergency *on page 865*
Whole Blood *on page 866*

Abstract Warming should take place, when necessary, using an FDA-approved device during passage through the transfusion set. A visible thermometer and a warning system are required.[1]

Use For very rapid, massive transfusion (>50 mL/kg/hour in adults or 15 mL/ kg/hour in children), patients with severe cold agglutinin disease and infants undergoing exchange transfusion.[2]

Limitations Uncontrolled warming of donor blood can severely damage RBCs. Although red cells must be heated to 44°C or higher to be damaged, it is probably best not to allow warming above 40°C. Warming must be done so as not to cause hemolysis.[1]

Contraindications When moderate volumes of blood are given at ordinary rates, warming is unnecessary. It is probably unnecessary also in most patients with cold agglutinin disease or paroxysmal cold hemoglobinuria who are not seriously ill.

Methodology A considerable variety of hardware is available for blood warming.[3] A simple system, not needing expensive equipment, is addition of an equal volume of 70°C isotonic saline to a unit of 4°C RBCs, which
(Continued)

Warming, Blood (Continued)

immediately results in a temperature about 37°C, without hemolysis or other damage.[4]

Additional Information Relatively large volumes of blood at refrigerator temperature, infused rapidly, can cause hypothermia and cardiac arrest. Blood subjected to excessive heat (ie, above 44°C) may be lethal. A quality assurance protocol is essential for all blood warmers and is required by accrediting agencies.[1] A standard operating procedure of any instrument should include instructions on performance of temperature and alarm checks, with instructions on what to do when the instrument is out of range.

Footnotes

1. Menitove JE, *Standards for Blood Banks and Transfusion Services*, 20th ed, Bethesda, MD: American Association of Blood Banks Press, 2000, 5-6.
2. *Blood Transfusion Therapy: A Physician's Handbook*, 6th ed, Bethesda, MD: American Association of Blood Banks Press, 1999, 80-8.
3. Iserson KV and Huestis DW, "Blood Warming: Current Applications and Techniques," *Transfusion*, 1991, 31(6):558-71.
4. Calhoun L, "Blood Product Preparation and Administration," *Clinical Practice of Transfusion Medicine*, 3rd ed, Petz LD, Swisher SN, Kleinman S, et al, eds, New York, NY: Churchill Livingstone, 1996, 305-33.

♦ **Washed Blood Cells** *see* Red Blood Cells, Washed *on page 859*

♦ **Weak D** *see* Rh Genotype *on page 860*

♦ **White Cells, Transfusion** *see* Neutrophils, Transfusion *on page 847*

Whole Blood

Related Information

Blood Gases and pH, Arterial *on page 119*
Donation, Blood *on page 839*
Irradiated Blood Components *on page 846*
Oxygen Saturation, Blood *on page 240*
Pretransfusion Testing *on page 856*
Red Blood Cells *on page 857*
Red Blood Cells, Leukocytes Reduced *on page 858*
Risks of Transfusion *on page 861*
Transfusion Reaction Work-up *on page 864*
Uncrossmatched Blood, Emergency *on page 865*
Warming, Blood *on page 865*

Applies to Fresh Blood; Massive Transfusions

Test Includes ABO and Rh type, antibody screen, crossmatch, and antibody identification when screen is positive, as for other transfusions

Abstract The primary indication for transfusion of whole blood is to provide both blood volume expansion and oxygen-carrying capacity. A unit of whole blood consists of about 450 mL (±10%) blood including plasma and about 63 mL of anticoagulant preservative such as citrate phosphate dextrose adenine solution (CPDA-1). A typical donor unit has a hematocrit of about 35% to 40%. The expiration date for CPDA-1 blood is 35 days after the date of collection if stored continuously at 1°C to 6°C. Storage and transportation temperatures and expiration dates of anticoagulants in use have been recently tabulated.[1]

Patient Preparation The patient should have an identification wristband. Emergency Departments (ERs) may use special or temporary identification. Measure blood loss if possible, as well as fluid intake and output. **Dosage and administration:** Give whole blood through a standard 170 micron filter. It can be warmed, if warming is clinically indicated, as with rapid infusion of large volumes of blood at refrigerator temperature. The blood should not be warmed above 38°C. The rate of infusion depends on clinical conditions but should not be slower than 4 hours per unit. **No medications or solutions should be added to blood. Never give Ringer's lactate, hypotonic, or dextrose-containing solutions through the same tubing as blood.** These solutions are incompatible with stored blood, causing clots, aggregates, and shortened cell survival.

Aftercare Same as for other RBC transfusions.

Specimen Blood

Container One red top tube or one lavender top (EDTA) tube

Collection (Of sample from intended recipient): At the patient's bedside, ask the patient to give his or her name. Compare with the patient's wristband. Label the sample tube with two unique forms or patient identification (eg, patient's full name, hospital number), also include date and initials of the collector. Further information may be required on a requisition form. Take extra care with identification of unresponsive patients.

Storage Instructions Store in Blood Bank monitored refrigerator only until issue. When it is not possible to transfuse immediately after issue, return blood to Blood Bank within approximately 30 minutes. Otherwise, blood that has been out of monitored refrigeration must be discarded. Appropriate designated refrigeration includes specified storage conditions, temperature recorders, and alarm signals.[1] These conditions are regularly intensely inspected by regulatory agencies.

Causes for Rejection (Of patient sample): Gross hemolysis, sample placed in a serum separator tube, specimen tube not properly labeled

Turnaround Time Because of required testing, the time from blood donation until the blood is available for transfusion varies from about 3-5 days. For routine situations, a unit can be ready for transfusion within 30-45 minutes from the time the Blood Bank gets the type and crossmatch

sample, if blood of the appropriate type is on hand. Presence of unexpected antibodies may require hours to a day or two for identification.

Special Instructions Blood Banks and hospital transfusion services hold crossmatched blood only for 24 hours, after which they usually must make it available from other patients. There will be some exceptions. Notify the Blood Bank as soon as possible if the patient will not need transfusion so the blood can be used for some other patient.

Use Replace red cell mass and plasma volume in patients in whom there is significant loss or depletion of both, improve oxygen transport (ie, treatment of acute blood loss). Therapy for acute bleeding, including massive transfusion in exsanguinating emergencies,[2,3] and some surgical cases. Exchange transfusion. See table and see Red Blood Cells *on page 857* for further discussion of medical indications for transfusion.

Summary of Transfusion Guidelines (Excluding Neonates)*

Acute Blood Loss

1. Evaluate for risk of ischemia and other concomitant disease
2. Estimate and/or anticipate degree of blood loss

   >30% to 40% rapid blood volume loss: transfuse RBCs, whole blood as available

   <30% to 40% rapid blood volume loss: RBCs usually not needed in previously healthy person
3. Measure hemoglobin

   >10 g/dL: RBCs rarely needed

   <6 g/dL: RBCs usually needed

   6-10 g/dL: RBC need depends on other factors
4. Measure vital signs and tissue oxygenation (most useful in 6-10 g/dL hemoglobin range when extent of blood loss is unknown)

   Tachycardia, hypotension not corrected by volume replacement alone: RBCs needed

   $P\bar{v} O_2$ <25 torr, extraction ratio >50%

   VO_2 <50% of baseline: RBCs often needed

Chronic Anemia

1. Treat with specific pharmacologic agents (eg, cobalamin, folic acid, recombinant human erythropoietin, iron) when diagnosis permits
2. Special strategies for sickle cell disease, thalassemia are needed
3. Transfuse to minimize symptoms and risk of anemia (usually at hemoglobin levels of 5-8 g/dL)

*RBCs = red blood cells; $P\bar{v} O_2$ = oxygen tension of pulmonary arterial blood at the completion of oxygen unloading; VO_2 = oxygen consumption.

Adapted from Simon TL, Alverson DC, AuBuchon J, et al, "Practice Parameter for the Use of Red Blood Cell Transfusions," *Arch Pathol Lab Med*, 1998, 122(2):130-8.

Limitations Usually in short supply because of demand for blood components. Although whole blood provides plasma proteins, other sources of oncotic/coagulation proteins are available. Some components, eg, platelets, factor V, factor VIII (AHF), are labile and not present in sufficient quantity in stored whole blood to provide adequate replacement therapy. Adenine, citrate, sodium, and antibodies are less in red blood cells, which are preferable to whole blood for patients with chronic renal or liver disease. The plasma in whole blood is unneeded in many situation.[4]

Contraindications Do not use whole blood for anemia that can be corrected with specific, safer products (eg, iron, B_{12}, folic acid). Whole blood is contraindicated in patients with congestive heart failure, uremia or hepatic failure, or with other chronic decrease of red cell mass. Such patients should receive red cells rather than whole blood if they require transfusion. For exchange transfusion, whole blood should preferably not be more than 5 days old. Replace blood volume deficits more safely and adequately with other volume expanders (saline, Ringer's lactate, albumin, plasma protein fraction). Treat coagulation factor deficiencies with appropriate factor-specific concentrates. The infusion of large volumes of blood may cause additional bleeding due to dilution of clotting factors or platelets. Donor and recipient must be ABO compatible.

Methodology Attention to electrolytes, blood gases and blood volumes is indicated with rapid and/or massive transfusion; see Warming, Blood *on page 865*.

Additional Information When whole blood is not available, red blood cells are substituted. **Fresh blood** is impossible to define and obtain except by reference to whatever labile component is needed. Requests for "fresh" blood necessitate consultation and are usually filled by provision of the appropriate components or fractions.

Footnotes

1. Menitove JE, *Standards for Blood Banks and Transfusion Services*, 20th ed, Bethesda, MD: American Association of Blood Banks Press, 2000, 61.
2. Velmahos GC, Chan L, Chan M, et al, "Is There a Limit to Massive Blood Transfusion After Severe Trauma?" *Arch Surg*, 1998, 133(9):947-52.
3. Laine EP, Nelson JM, George FW, et al, "Hyperkalemia After Massive Blood Transfusion," *Lab Med*, 1997, 28(5):305-8.
4. Simon TL, Alverson DC, AuBuchon J, et al, "Practice Parameter for the Use of Red Blood Cell Transfusions: Developed by the Red Blood Cell Administration Practice Guideline Development Task Force of the College of American Pathologists," *Arch Pathol Lab Med*, 1998, 122(2):130-8.

References

Circular of Information for the Use of Human Blood and Blood Components, American Association of Blood Banks, America's Blood Centers, American Red Cross, 1998.

Ely EW and Bernard GR, "Transfusions in Critically Ill Patients," *N Engl J Med*, 1999, 340(6):467-8.

Goodnough LT, Brecher ME, Kanter MH, et al, "Transfusion Medicine. First of Two Parts: Blood Transfusion," *N Engl J Med*, 1999, 340(6):438-48.

Hebert PC, Wells G, Blajchman MA, et al, "A Multicenter, Randomized, Controlled Clinical Trial of Transfusion Requirements in Critical Care," *N Engl J Med*, 1999, 340(6):409-17.

Petz LD, Swisher SN, Kleinman S, et al, *Clinical Practice of Transfusion Medicine*, 2rd ed, New York, NY: Churchill Livingstone, 1996, 312, 569-71.

Vengelen-Tyler V, *Technical Manual*, 13th ed, Bethesda, MD: American Association of Blood Banks Press, 1999.

URINALYSIS

David S. Jacobs, MD

Uri Alon, MD

Contributor: Wayne R. DeMott, MD

Analysis of urine dates to ancient times. Clinical microscopy has been practiced for several hundred years. Thus, many of the tests presented are among the most enduring in medicine. Other more recently developed tests, such as reagent strip screening procedures for urine glucose, protein, leukocyte esterase, and nitrite, yield significant clinical information rapidly and relatively inexpensively.

Urine testing is painless and, when competently performed, effective. It provides useful information for diagnosis and patient care.

A great many tests performed on urine are described in other chapters of this book, including monographs in Chemistry, Toxicology/Drugs of Abuse, Trace Elements, Infectious Disease, and Cytopathology. The sample for analysis for drugs of abuse is urine. Special needs exist for urine collection for this purpose. See the Toxicology/Drugs of Abuse Introduction *on page 773.*

Urine color has been of interest for centuries. Its color is determined by its concentration, the presence of drugs, exogenous and endogenous compounds, and its pH. **Colorless** urine may be normal or secondary to diuretic use, high fluid intake, diabetes insipidus, or diabetes mellitus. **Cloudy or hazy** urine may reflect the presence of phosphates, pyuria, bacteruria, chyluria, or radiographic dye. On oxidation, development of a **black** color is evidence for alkaptonuria.[1] Increased indican may cause the urine to blacken on standing. **Dark** urine is the second most common sign of acute intermittent porphyria; urine in porphyria has been described as port wine in color. Very rarely, dark urine may indicate the presence of malignant melanoma. **Green** urine may be produced by indigo carmine, methylene blue, phenol, and in some cases of iodochlorhydroxyquin (clioquinol)-induced subacute myelo-opticoneuropathy. Other causes of green urine are reported as *Pseudomonas* bacteremia, urinary bile pigments, amitriptyline hydrochloride or methocarbamol ingestion, and breath freshener abuse.[2] **Red** urine was described elegantly by Berman[3] and is described further in the listing, Blood, Urine. Chlorpromazine and haloperidol may cause pink, red, or red-brown discoloration. **Red to brown to tea** colored plasma and urine indicate hemoglobin or myoglobin; clear plasma with red urine may occur in congenital erythropoietic porphyria and cutanea tarda porphyria. **Red brown to brown black** urine may be caused by phenacetin, quinine, or methemoglobin, and **brown-black** urine can be caused by methemoglobin, homogentisic acid, or melanin. **Purple** urine, after standing, may be due to porphyrins.[4] The plastic urine bag may discolor **purple** in the presence of the indican produced by *Providencia* or *Klebsiella* species.[5] **Yellow** to **orange** urine may contain bile. Other causes of darker yellow to orange urine include increased concentration of urine or the presence of riboflavin, quinacrine (Atabrine®), rifampin (Rifadin®, Rimactane®), phenazopyridine (Pyridium®), or salicylazosulfapyridine (Azulfidine®). Color and appearance of urine were outlined well by Henry, Lauzon, and Shumann.[6] As in some examples above, **drugs** may cause unusual urine colors.[7,8]

Urine volume is not *per se* a laboratory test, although it is measured in 24-hour or other timed urine collections. It is relevant for nephrolithiasis.

Footnotes

1. Gaines JJ, "The Pathology of Alkaptonuric Ochronosis," *Hum Pathol*, 1989, 20:40-6.
2. Norfleet RG, "Green Urine," *JAMA*, 1982, 247:29.
3. Berman LB, "When the Urine Is Red," *JAMA*, 1977, 237:2753-4.
4. Nolan CR, McKinney TD, and Forland M, "Urinalysis and Renal Function Tests," *Internal Medicine*, 5th ed, Chapter 102, Stein JH, ed, St Louis, MO: Mosby, 1998, 742-56.
5. Dealler SF, Belfield PW, Belford M, et al, "Purple Urine Bags," *J Urol*, 1989, 142:769-70.
6. Henry JB, Lauzon RB, and Schumann GB, "Examination of Urine," *Clinical Diagnosis and Management by Laboratory Methods*, 19th ed, Chapter 18, Philadelphia, PA: WB Saunders Co, 1996, 411-56.
7. Lubran MM, "Effect of Drugs on Clinical Laboratory Tests," *Clinical Pathology in the Elderly*, Chapter 24, Rochman H, ed, 1988, 193-6.
8. Young DS, *Effect of Drugs on Clinical Laboratory Tests*, 5th ed, Volume 1: Listing by Test, Washington, DC: AACC Press, 2000. 24, Rochman H, ed, 1988, 193-6.

- **Acetest®** see Ketones, Urine on page 877

- **Acetoacetic Acid, Urine** see Ketones, Urine on page 877

- **Acetone, Semiquantitative, Urine** see Ketones, Urine on page 877

- **Albumin:Creatinine Ratio** see Microalbuminuria on page 879

- **Albumin Excretion** see Microalbuminuria on page 879

- **Albumin, Urine** see Protein, Semiquantitative, Urine on page 885

- **Bacteria Screen, Urine** see Leukocyte Esterase, Urine on page 878

- **Bacteria Screen, Urine** see Nitrite, Urine on page 882

- **Benedict Test** see Reducing Substances, Urine on page 885

- **Beta-Hydroxybutyric Acid, Urine** see Ketones, Urine on page 877

- **Bile, Urine** see Bilirubin, Urine on page 870

Bilirubin, Urine

Related Information

Bilirubin, Direct, Serum on page 117
Bilirubin, Total, Serum on page 118
Liver Disease: Laboratory Assessment, Overview on page 216
Urobilinogen, 2-Hour Urine on page 889

Synonyms Bile, Urine

Applies to Ictotest®; Urobilinogen, Urine

Abstract Urine bilirubin is a surrogate for increased serum conjugated bilirubin. Only conjugated bilirubin is passed into the urine; thus, a positive reaction is evidence of hepatocellular or biliary disease. Jaundice with negative urine bilirubin is evidence of unconjugated hyperbilirubinemia, commonly indicative of hemolytic anemia. Of heritable abnormalities of bilirubin metabolism, bilirubin is positive in Dubin-Johnson and Rotor types, but not in Gilbert or Crigler-Najjar disease.

Specimen Random urine. Sufficient bilirubin in urine causes a yellow-brown or green-brown color. When shaken, yellow foam may be seen if sufficient bilirubin is present. (A white foam is found when normal urine is shaken).

Storage Instructions Refrigeration. Specimen should not be permitted to stand; bilirubin glucuronide hydrolyzes, leading to false negatives. Light exposure breaks down bilirubin.

Special Instructions The specimen should be tested as soon as possible after voiding.

Reference Interval Negative (absent). (The chemical upper limit of normal, about 0.02 mg/dL is insufficient for detection by usual clinical testing).

Use Detect the presence of bilirubin in urine; screen for some instances of liver disease. In hepatocellular and obstructive disease of the biliary tract such as biliary calculi, carcinoma of pancreas or of bile ducts, urine bilirubin is frequently positive. See table.

Differential Diagnosis Using Urine Bilirubin and Urobilinogen Tests

Type of Jaundice	Urine Bilirubin	Urine Urobilinogen
Normal	0	0 - trace
Hepatocellular jaundice (eg, hepatitis, chemical, or drug injury)	↑	↑
Biliary obstruction (extrahepatic and intrahepatic); obstructive jaundice	↑	0
Hemolytic jaundice	0	↑

0 = absent; ↑ = increased

Limitations Reagent strips: Occasional false-positive are seen, predominantly in elderly patients. They commonly represent stool contamination of the urine sample. Ponstel® (mefenamic acid) administration, Thorazine®, Ormazine® (chlorpromazine), rifampin, and etodolac may result in false-positive reactions. Prolonged standing of the sample, especially at room temperature and in the light, may lead to false negatives. Increased urinary ascorbate causes false negatives. Sensitivity is decreased by increased urine nitrite. Pyridium® (phenazopyridine) and Serenium® (ethoxazene hydrochloride) and local anesthetic metabolites give bright reddish orange colors which may mask the reaction of small amounts of bilirubin. Indoxyl sulfate interferes both with negatives and positives. Specific urine bilirubin assays provide substantial numbers of false negatives when used as a screen for liver disease as determined by at least one abnormal serum liver function test abnormality. If just used to screen for the presence of raised serum bilirubin, the test is about 79% to 89% specific and has an 89% negative predictive value when used in an emergency room setting.[1] Indoxyl has been reported to interfere with dip-and-read testing for urine bilirubin sufficiently to mask a weak reaction.

Methodology Diazotization reaction in an acid medium yields a blue to purple color

Additional Information A more specific and sensitive **tablet** test, such as the Ictotest®, has been recommended when such dip-and-read results are inconclusive.[2] The manufacturer expresses need for proper storage of the reagent. The tablet method is more sensitive than dipsticks. It detects as little as 0.05-0.1 mg bilirubin/100 mL. The test is exquisitely sensitive for bilirubinuria. Rifampin and chlorpromazine metabolites may interfere, and metabolites of mefenamic acid and flufenamic acid may cause false positives. However, detection of bilirubinuria is not a sensitive indicator of hepatic disease. In uncomplicated hemolytic anemia serum bilirubin may be normal, or a minimal elevation of indirect bilirubin may be present; **indirect (unconjugated) bilirubin does not readily pass through the glomerulus. Therefore, bilirubin is not usually detectable in the urine in uncomplicated hemolytic anemia.** Because serum total bilirubin is not always increased with advanced liver disease, urine bilirubin may not be present in that circumstance. If jaundice is severe, renal excretion becomes significant; and if renal function deteriorates, serum direct bilirubin levels may increase.[3] Urine bilirubin, if positive, implies an elevated serum conjugated (direct) bilirubin, which should be confirmed by serum measurement.

The liver cell conjugates bilirubin with glucuronic acid to bilirubin glucuronide, which is water soluble and therefore can pass through the glomerulus.

Footnotes

1. Binder L, Smith D, Kupka T, et al, "Failure of Prediction of Liver Function Test Abnormalities With the Urine Urobilinogen and Urine Bilirubin Assays," Arch Pathol Lab Med, 1989, 113(1):73-6.

2. Skjold AC, Freitag JF, Stover LR, et al, "Indoxyl Sulfate Interferes With Dip-and-Read Urinary Bilirubin Estimate," Clin Chem, 1980, 26(9):1368-9.

3. Fleischner G and Arias IM, "Recent Advances in Bilirubin Formation, Transport, Metabolism and Excretion," Am J Med, 1970, 49:576-89.

References

Henry JB, Lauzon RB, and Schumann GB, "Basic Examination of Urine," Clinical Diagnosis and Management by Laboratory Methods, 19th ed, Chapter 18, Philadelphia, PA: WB Saunders Co, 1996, 411-56.

Kokk JP, "Approach to the Patient With Renal Disease," Cecil Textbook of Medicine, 21st ed, Chapter 100, Goldman L and Bennett JC, eds, Philadelphia, PA: WB Saunders Co, 2000, 526-32.

- **Blood, Occult, Urine** see Blood, Urine on page 870

Blood, Urine

Related Information

Anemia Flowchart on page 392
Antinuclear Antibody on page 507
Glomerular Basement Membrane Antibody on page 526
Hemoglobin, Qualitative, Urine on page 875
Hemosiderin Stain, Urine on page 876
Kidney Biopsy on page 64
Kidney Stone Analysis on page 877
Myoglobin, Qualitative, Urine on page 880
Ova and Parasites, Urine on page 667
Platelet Count on page 468
Protein, Quantitative, Urine on page 883
Prothrombin Time on page 354
Urinalysis on page 887
Urinalysis, Fractional on page 889
Urinary Tract Cytology on page 389

Synonyms Blood, Occult, Urine; Hemoglobin, Urine; Occult Blood, Urine

Applies to Dysmorphic Red Blood Cells; Urine Calcium:Creatinine Ratio; Urine Protein:Creatinine Ratio

Test Includes Dipstick method for occult blood is a part of urinalysis.

Abstract Positive dipstick usually indicates hematuria, hemoglobinuria, or myoglobinuria. When a dipstick is positive for blood, microscopy is indicated to search for RBCs. Evaluation of hematuria should always include microscopy as well as reagent strip testing.[1] A definition of pediatric hematuria is 2-5 RBCs/hpf in urine sediment, adult hematuria is 2-3 RBCs/hpf; each in sediment from 10-12 mL spun sample.

In adults, a definition of hematuria has included ≥5 RBCs/hpf. The presence of proteinuria is clinically relevant when hematuria is detected, as well as the presence of RBCs and casts.[2]

Both reagent strips and sediment microscopy are necessary.[3]

Specimen Random urine

Storage Instructions Refrigeration; examination of fresh urine is best.

Causes for Rejection Standing for more than 2 hours at room temperature may be a reason to consider a specimen unacceptable.

Reference Interval Negative by dipstick; up to 2-3 RBCs/hpf are generally accepted as normal by microscopy.

Use Detect myoglobin, hemoglobin, or red blood cells in urine (detect hematuria, microhematuria, hemoglobinuria, or erythrocyturia). See table.

Blood, Urine: Summary

Causes of Hematuria

Renal and ureteral diseases
glomerulonephritis
nephrotic syndrome
Goodpasture syndrome
hemolytic uremic syndrome
lupus nephritis
arteritis (vasculitis)
Wegener granulomatosis
stone/hypercalciuria/hyperuricosuria/hyperoxaluria
tumor (including renal cell carcinoma, carcinoma of renal pelvis and ureter)
polycystic kidney
infarct
infection (including pyelonephritis, necrotizing papillitis, tuberculosis)
trauma
renal vein thrombosis
Alport syndrome
thin-GBM disease
benign hematuria
loin-pain hematuria

Blood diseases
thrombocytopenia
thrombotic thrombocytopenic purpura
Henoch-Schönlein purpura
infective endocarditis
leukemia
hemophilias
sickle cell trait

Ureteral diseases
ureterolithiasis
carcinoma

Bladder entities
excessive exercise
cystitis
papilloma
carcinoma
tuberculosis

Prostatic diseases
prostatitis
BPH (benign nodular and glandular hyperplasia)
prostatic adenocarcinoma

Urethral diseases
urethritis
tumor

Trauma

Drugs
Coumadin®
heparin
salicylate
many others

Causes of Hemoglobinuria

Hemolysis associated with
G6PD deficiency
organisms (eg, malaria *Bartonella*)
drugs (eg, acetanilid)
chemicals
antibodies

Unstable hemoglobins

March hemoglobinuria
secondary to severe exercise

Transfusion reactions
incompatible blood

Burns

Crush injury (myoglobinuria)

Poisoning
snake or spide bite

Paroxysmal nocturnal hemoglobinuria

Paroxysmal cold hemoglobinuria

Myoglobin (may be detected as hemoglobin)

Limitations Reagent strips methods detect myoglobin as hemoglobin. Both intact erythrocytes and free hemoglobin give a positive reaction. Iodine solutions in urine, or applied to patient's skin, are reported to cause false positives.[4] Certain oxidizing agents such as hypochlorite (bleach) may produce false-positive results if present in the collection vessel. Microbial peroxidase, particularly that produced by gram-negative rods and staphylococci associated with urinary tract infection and leukocyte peroxidase, may cause a false-positive reaction. Pyridium® (phenazopyridine) and Serenium® (ethoxazene hydrochloride) metabolites may mask the dipstick reaction. Large amounts of nitrite may delay reactions. The sensitivity of the occult blood test is reduced in urines with high specific gravity and/or high ascorbic acid content.[5] Inhibition of the reagent in the dipstick by ascorbic acid is a common and important problem, especially if microscopy is omitted. High urine protein and formalin cause false negatives.[6] Prolonged air exposure of the strip (dipstick jar left uncapped) reduces the sensitivity of the dipstick for blood.[7] Transient hematuria can reflect menstruation, catheterization, or strenuous exercise. Urine sediment microscopy should be used to confirm a diagnosis of hematuria suggested by positive reagent strip. The dipstick sensitivity for detection of red cells was reported to be 75.3% and specificity 88.6% in a recent study; false-negative dipstick results can be substantial. Screening asymptomatic adults by use of microhematuria to detect urological cancers has not been recommended.

The clinical differential diagnosis of acute flank pain includes ureterolithiasis, torsion of an ovarian mass, appendicitis, diverticulitis, and common bile duct stone. The presence of hematuria in a patient with acute flank pain has been used to support the diagnosis of ureterolithiasis, especially in those with past medical history of stones. In a 1999 study, reagent strip urinalysis for hematuria provided sensitivity of 80%, specificity of 35%, positive predictive value of 54%, negative predictive value of 66%, and a diagnostic efficiency of only 57%. The presence of >5 RBCs/hpf in microscopic urinalysis provided only 67% sensitivity, 66% specificity, 65% positive predictive value, 68% negative predictive value, and 67% efficacy.[8]

Methodology Dipstick is based on the pseudoperoxidase activity of heme from hemoglobin or myoglobin. Microscopy is used for recognition of red blood cells and red cell casts.

Additional Information Clues to glomerular origin of hematuria include lack of pain, brown-colored urine, proteinuria, red cell casts and dysmorphic red cells, hypertension, and evidence of renal dysfunction.[9] The test will detect 0.03 mg/dL free hemoglobin or 10 intact red blood cells/μL. Further tests to work-up hematuria may include CBC, platelet count, urine culture, urine quantitative proteins, ESR, ANA, complements C3 and C4, prothrombin time, PTT, urea nitrogen, creatinine, and other examinations as appropriate, including evaluation of patient's blood pressure.[10] IgA nephropathy is the most common type of glomerular disease related to asymptomatic gross hematuria.[11,12] In children, asymptomatic microscopic hematuria is often associated with hypercalciuria. In adults, >3.5 g of protein in a 24-hour urine collection provides indication of glomerular disease;[13] >1 g of protein is suggestive. In children, random **urine protein:creatinine ratio** >2.0 is suggestive of glomerular disease.

The number of red cells (grade of microhematuria) does not necessarily correlate with the degree or significance of urologic pathologic findings (ie, a patient with >5 red cells in urine may have an important urologic lesion). Additional studies (such as urine culture, cytology, imaging studies of the urinary tract, cystoscopy) may be indicated. Patients on anticoagulants exhibiting gross or microscopic hematuria should be carefully evaluated for carcinoma and calculi.[14] Recognizable genitourinary tract disease is found in most anticoagulated individuals who have microscopic hematuria. Contemporary long-term anticoagulation protocols rarely cause hematuria;[15] microscopic hematuria in patients on anticoagulants is often caused by significant urologic abnormality and requires prompt investigation.[16] The use of nonsteroidal anti-inflammatory drugs including aspirin may be associated with hematuria.[17]

A positive dipstick test for blood without red cells in the urine sediment may indicate hemoglobinuria, myoglobinuria, or the presence of porphyrins. Algorithms for diagnosis of hematuria are published for children[18] and adults.[19] Phenytoin does not cause urine to appear red, but uric acid and urate crystals in acid urine may cause a pink to red-brown color.[20] See Urinalysis Introduction *on page 869* for further information on colored urine.

A statistically significant positive correlation exists between red cells in urine sediment, C-reactive protein, and disease activity in Wegener granulomatosis. 11-100 red cells/hpf with dysmorphism on first examination were described.[21]

The usual laboratory findings in renal tuberculosis are hematuria with sterile pyuria.[22]

In correlation between dipsticks and microscopy in abdominal trauma, some authors feel that microscopy is needed when the dipstick is positive to determine whether or not imaging studies are indicated. Others have recommended urine microscopy in all cases of blunt abdominal traumas.[23] Kennedy et al report false negatives and false positives but concluded that the safety of dipsticks for hematuria in subjects sustaining blunt or penetrating abdominal trauma is acceptable.[24] Messing and coworkers found that hematuria, even in the presence of significant disease such as urinary tract malignancy, often was intermittent. They have proposed home dipstick screening based upon their study of asymptomatic men older than 50 years of age;[25] others disagree.[26]
(Continued)

Blood, Urine (Continued)

Twenty percent of patients older than 40 years with asymptomatic hematuria have significant urologic lesions, of which half are malignant.[27] In children with asymptomatic microscopic hematuria, the only test with high yield is random **urine calcium:creatinine ratio**.[28]

Exercise-induced hematuria is a recognized clinical entity.[29]

An important response to a paper reporting inaccuracies of urine dipstick results[7] emphasizes the need for quality control and perceives the **need for laboratory testing to be performed by those well versed in good laboratory practice**.[30]

Footnotes

1. Misdraji J and Nguyen PL, "Urinalysis. When - and When Not - To Order," *Postgrad Med*, 1996, 100(1):173-6, 181-2, 185-8 passim.
2. Fitzwater DS and Wyatt RJ, "Hematuria," *Pediatr Rev*, 1994, 15(3):102-8.
3. Bartlett RC, Zern DA, Ratkiewicz I, et al, "Reagent Strip Screening for Sediment Abnormalities Identified by Automated Microscopy in Urine From Patients Suspected to Have Urinary Tract Disease," *Arch Pathol Lab Med*, 1994, 118(11):1096-101.
4. Said R, "Contamination of Urine With Povidone-Iodine. Cause of False-Positive Test for Occult Blood in Urine," *JAMA*, 1979, 242(8):748-9.
5. Jaffe RM, Lawrence L, Schmid A, et al, "Inhibition by Ascorbic Acid (Vitamin C) of Chemical Detection of Blood in Urine," *Am J Clin Pathol*, 1979, 72(3):468-70.
6. Brown SH, MacDougall ML, and Wiegmann TB, "Microscopic Hematuria," *Kans Med*, 1986, 87(4):99-101,113.
7. Cohen HT and Spiegel DM, "Air-Exposed Urine Dipsticks Give False-Positive Results for Glucose and False-Negative Results for Blood," *Am J Clin Pathol*, 1991, 96(3):398-400.
8. Bove P, Kaplan D, Dalrymple N, et al, "Reexamining the Value of Hematuria Testing in Patients With Acute Flank Pain," *J Urol*, 1999, 162(3 Pt 1):685-7.
9. Yadin O, "Hematuria in Children," *Pediatr Ann*, 1994, 23(9):474-8, 481-5.
10. McCarthy JJ, "Outpatient Evaluation of Hematuria: Locating the Source of Bleeding," *Postgrad Med*, 1997, 101(2):125-8, 131.
11. Scheinman JI, Trachtman H, Lin CY, et al, "IgA Nephropathy: To Treat or Not to Treat?" *Nephron*, 1997, 75(3):251-8.
12. Nolin L and Courteau M, "Management of IgA Nephropathy: Evidence-Based Recommendations," *Kidney Int Suppl*, 1999, 70:S56-62.
13. Abuelo JG, "The Diagnosis of Hematuria," *Arch Intern Med*, 1983, 143(5):967-70.
14. Schuster GA and Lewis GA, "Clinical Significance of Hematuria in Patients on Anticoagulant Therapy," *J Urol*, 1987, 137(5):923-5.
15. Culclasure TF, Bray VJ, and Hasbargen JA, "The Significance of Hematuria in the Anticoagulated Patient," *Arch Intern Med*, 1994, 154(6):649-52.
16. Thaller TR and Wang LP, "Evaluation of Asymptomatic Microscopic Hematuria in Adults," *Am Fam Phys*, 1999, 60(4):1143-52, 1154.
17. Kraus SE, Siroky MB, Babayan RK, et al, "Hematuria and the Use of Nonsteroidal Anti-inflammatory Drugs," *J Urol*, 1984, 132(2):288-90.
18. Lieu TA, Grasmeder HM 3d, and Kaplan BS, "An Approach to the Evaluation and Treatment of Microscopic Hematuria," *Pediatr Clin North Am*, 1991, 38(3):579-92.
19. Restrepo NC and Carey PO, "Evaluating Hematuria in Adults," *Am Fam Phys*, 1989, 40(2):149-56.
20. Derby BM and Ward JW, "The Myth of Red Urine Due to Phenytoin," *JAMA*, 1983, 249(13):1723-4.
21. Fujita T, Ohi H, Endo M, et al, "Level of Red Blood Cells in the Urinary Sediment Reflects the Degree of Renal Activity in Wegener's Granulomatosis," *Clin Nephrol*, 1998, 50(5):284-8.
22. Roberts JA, "Management of Pyelonephritis and Upper Urinary Tract Infections," *Urol Clin North Am*, 1999, 26(4):753-63.
23. Daum GS, Krolikowski FJ, Reuter KL, et al, "Dipstick Evaluation of Hematuria in Abdominal Trauma," *Am J Clin Pathol*, 1988, 89(4):538-42.
24. Kennedy TJ, McConnell JD, and Thal ER, "Urine Dipstick vs Microscopic Urinalysis in the Evaluation of Abdominal Trauma," *J Trauma*, 1988, 28(5):615-7.
25. Messing EM, Young TB, Hunt VB, et al, "Urinary Tract Cancers Found by Homescreening With Hematuria Dipsticks in Healthy Men Over 50 Years of Age," *Cancer*, 1989, 64(11):2361-7.
26. Woolhandler S, Pels RJ, Bor DH, et al, "Dipstick Urinalysis Screening of Asymptomatic Adults for Urinary Tract Disorders - I. Hematuria and Proteinuria," *JAMA*, 1989, 262(9):1214-9.
27. Chen HH, Shields RC, and Bardsley WT, "68-Year Old Man With Anemia and Renal Failure," *Mayo Clin Proc*, 1996, 71(2):197-200.
28. Feld LG, Meyers KE, Kaplan BS, et al, "Limited Evaluation of Microscopic Hematuria in Children," *Pediatrics*, 1998, 102:(4):E42.
29. Gambrell RC and Blount BW, "Exercise-Induced Hematuria," *Am Fam Phys*, 1996, 53(3):905-11.
30. Cadoff EM, "Inaccurate Results of Urine Dipstick Tests," *Am J Clin Pathol*, 1992, 98(2):269.

References

Abarbanel J, Benet AE, Lask D, et al, "Sports Hematuria," *J Urol*, 1990, 143(5):887-90.
Ahn JH, Morey AF, and McAninch JW, "Workup and Management of Traumatic Hematuria," *Emerg Med Clin North Am*, 1998, 16(1):145-64.
Alon US, Warady BA, and Hellerstein, "Assessment and Interpretation of Urinalysis and Routine Kidney Function Tests. Part I: Urinalysis," *Children's Hospital Quarterly*, 1990, 2:217-35.
Bonnardeaux A, Somerville P, and Kaye M, "A Study on the Reliability of Dipstick Urinalysis," *Clin Nephrol*, 1994, 41(3):167-72.
Campbell KL, "Blood, Urine, Saliva, and Dip-Sticks: Experiences in Africa, New Guinea, and Boston," *Ann N Y Acad Sci*, 1994, 709:312-30.
Feld LG, Waz WR, Perez LM, et al, "Hematuria. An Integrated Medical and Surgical Approach," *Pediatr Clin North Am*, 1997, 44(5):1191-210.

Grossfeld GD and Carroll PR, "Evaluation of Asymptomatic Microscopic Hematuria," *Urol Clin North Am*, 1998, 25(4):661-76.
Hiatt RA and Ordonez JD, "Dipstick Urinalysis Screening, Asymptomatic Microhematuria, and Subsequent Urological Cancers in a Population-Based Sample," *Cancer Epidemiol Biomarkers Prev*, 1994, 3(5):439-43.
Hricik DE, Chung-Park M, and Sedor JR, "Glomerulonephritis," *N Engl J Med*, 1998, 339(13):888-99.
Korman TM, Spelman DW, Perry GJ, et al, "Acute Glomerulonephritis Associated With Acute Q Fever: Case Report and Review of the Renal Complications of *Coxiella burnetii* Infection," *Clin Infect Dis*, 1998, 26(2):359-64.
Lam MH, "False Hematuria Due to Bacteriuria," *Arch Pathol Lab Med*, 1995, 119(8):717-21.
Rockall AG, Newman-Sanders AP, al-Kutoubi MA, et al, "Haematuria," *Postgrad Med J*, 1997, 73(857):129-36.
Smith RF, Mohr DN, Torres VE, et al, "Renal Insufficiency in Community Patients With Mild Asymptomatic Microhematuria," *Mayo Clin Proc*, 1989, 64(4):409-14.
Spitz A, Huffman JL, and Mendez R, "Autotransplantation as an Effective Therapy for the Loin Pain-Hematuria Syndrome: Case Reports and a Review of the Literature," *J Urol*, 1997, 157(5):1554-9.
Yoskikawa N, Iijima K, and Ito H, "IgA Nephropathy in Children," *Nephron*, 1999, 83(1):1-12.
Yoshikawa N, Matsuyama D, Iijima K, et al, "Benign Familial Hematuria," *Arch Pathol Lab Med*, 1988, 112(8):794-7.

♦ **Body Fluid, Specific Gravity** *see* Specific Gravity, Urine *on page 886*

♦ **Calculus Analysis** *see* Kidney Stone Analysis *on page 877*

♦ **Casts, Urine** *see* Urinalysis *on page 887*

♦ **Clinitest® for Sugar, Urine** *see* Reducing Substances, Urine *on page 885*

♦ **Concentrating Ability, Urine** *see* Concentration Test, Urine *on page 872*

Concentration Test, Urine

Related Information
Antidiuretic Hormone, Plasma *on page 107*
Calcium, Serum *on page 131*
Osmolality, Serum *on page 236*
Osmolality, Urine *on page 236*
Potassium, Serum or Plasma *on page 258*
Sodium, Serum or Plasma *on page 275*
Specific Gravity, Urine *on page 886*

Synonyms Concentrating Ability, Urine; Fishberg Concentration Test; Urine Concentration Test

Applies to Vasopressin Concentration Test

Test Includes Assessment of concentrating ability of the kidney by determination of specific gravity or osmolality following water deprivation and/or after administration of vasopressin

Abstract This testing protocol is done to evaluate polyuria. A random urine collected without water restriction (usually first morning urine) yielding a urine osmolality ≥850 mOsm/kg (SI: ≥850 mmol/kg) or a specific gravity ≥1.027 virtually excludes a defect in concentrating ability, and thus, may be done as a screening procedure before more elaborate deprivation studies are undertaken.[1] Patients with polyuria are sometimes difficult to evaluate, as some have polydipsia with resulting polyuria while others have polyuria with resultant mild or moderate hypernatremia and therefore polydipsia. To separate these groups, this test evaluates urine osmolality (and/or specific gravity) when water is withheld, sufficient to cause mild hypernatremia. Since the kidneys may abnormally excrete water in the face of hypernatremia or even hypovolemia, this test must be closely monitored to prevent patient injury (hyperosmolar state or dehydration).

Patient Preparation The evening meal must be high in protein and contain not more than 200 mL of liquid. Patient is to consume no fluids after the evening meal. On awakening in the morning, the patient voids and saves the specimen in container #1. All further urine passed until 1 hour later is included in specimen #2. All further urine then until 2 hours later is collected as specimen #3. If urine specific gravity plateaus but a specific gravity of 1.027 or urine osmolality of 850 mOsm/kg is not achieved, vasopressin can be administered.

Protein and radiographic dyes can increase specific gravity despite decreased concentrating ability. The patient must not be taking diuretics.

Aftercare Fluid restriction may decrease plasma volume and have an adverse effect on cardiac output in patients with compromised cardiac function. If diabetes insipidus is present, urine output may remain very high despite fluid deprivation. Body weight and blood pressure should be carefully followed throughout the procedure. If body weight is decreased by 5% or orthostatic hypotension occurs, the procedure should be terminated. Test should be supervised by the physician. Patients should also be watched to prevent them from unsupervised drinking (including drinking from toilet).

Specimen Urine

Container Three urine containers

Storage Instructions Refrigeration

Reference Interval Normal: specific gravity of at least one specimen should be >1.026 or >850 mOsm/kg (SI: >850 mmol/kg); severe renal disease: <400 mOsm/kg (SI: <400 mmol/kg). When fluids are withheld (overnight), the ratio of urine to serum osmolality >3.0 is considered normal.[2] Elevated urine osmolality in the face of hyponatremia may indicate the presence of the syndrome of inappropriate secretion of antidiuretic hormone (SIADH) or cerebral salt wasting.[3]

Use Evaluate renal concentrating ability, a test of tubular function; useful in the differential diagnosis of diabetes insipidus,[4] compulsive water drinking, and renal disease

Causes of Symptomatic (Polyuric) Deficiencies in Plasma Vasopressin

Decreased Secretion
Destruction of neurohypophysis (neurogenic diabetes insipidus)
Sporadic
Idiopathic
Trauma (surgical, accidental)
Malignancy
Primary (craniopharyngioma, dysgerminoma, meningioma, adenoma, glioma, astrocytoma)
Secondary (metastatic from lung or breast, lymphoma, leukemia, dysplastic pancytopenia)
Granuloma (sarcoid, histiocytosis, xanthoma disseminatum)
Infection (viral/bacterial meningitis, encephalitis)
Vascular (Sheehan syndrome, carotid aneurysm, hematoma, aortocoronary bypass, ischemic brain death)
Autoimmune disease
Dysplasia (septo-optic, microcephaly, porencephaly, etc)
Metabolic (anorexia nervosa)
Familial (autosomal dominant)
Excessive water intake (primary polydipsia)
Psychogenic (schizophrenia, ? neurosis)
Dipsogenic (abnormal thirst)
Idiopathic
Trauma
Granuloma (neurosarcoid, tuberculous meningitis)
Autoimmune (multiple sclerosis)
Chemical (lithium)
Increased Metabolism
Gestational

Adapted from Robertson GL and Berl T, "Pathophysiology of Water Metabolism," *The Kidney*, Brenner BM and Rector FC Jr, eds, Philadelphia, PA: WB Saunders Co, 1991, 695.

Causes of Defects in Antidiuretic Action of Vasopressin

Familial nephrogenic diabetes insipidus
X-linked recessive
Sporadic nephrogenic diabetes insipidus
Chemical (lithium, demeclocycline, methoxyflurane)
Metabolic (hypokalemia, hypercalcemia)
Mechanical (ureteral obstruction)
Vascular (sickle cell disease or trait)
Granulomatous (sarcoid)
Dysplastic (polycystic disease)
Infectious (pyelonephritis)
Infiltrative (amyloid)
Gestational
Malignant (fibrosarcoma)
Solute diuresis
Metabolic (glucosuria)
Iatrogenic (mannitol, diuretics, radiocontrast dyes, saline loading)
Mechanical (postureteral obstruction)

Adapted from Robertson GL and Berl T, "Pathophysiology of Water Metabolism," *The Kidney*, Brenner BM and Rector FC Jr, eds, Philadelphia, PA: WB Saunders Co, 1991, 699.

Limitations In polydipsic patients, the urine specific gravity may not rise to 1.026 until after many hours of deprivation. False-positive tests can be avoided by making sure serum sodium is 141-145 mmol/L before termination of the test. The test may have to be extended or adapted to the patient, and this is best done with a clear understanding of the physiology of vasopressin and of water metabolism. For details see Robertson and Berl footnote.[5]

Contraindications Glucosuria invalidates a concentration test by virtue of its diuretic effect; hypernatremia or orthostatic hypotension are contraindications.

Methodology Modified Fishberg procedure

Additional Information Glomerular disorders causing proteinuria result in decreased concentrating ability by producing an osmotic diuresis in the functioning nephrons. Even subtle renal interstitial disorders may impair concentrating ability. Hypokalemia and hypercalcemia decrease renal medullary tonicity and inhibit tubular reabsorption of water. Sickle cell disease decreases medullary blood flow and interferes with loop of Henle sodium transport. Achievement of normal maximal urinary concentration requires a normal or near normal glomerular filtration rate.[1] In central diabetes insipidus, administration of vasopressin will raise urine osmolality. In nephrogenic diabetes insipidus, the urine osmolality will not increase with vasopressin or water deprivation.

The urine:serum osmolality ratio is addressed in Osmolality, Serum *on page 236*.

Urine color may be used in athletic or industrial settings to determine whether humans are well hydrated, euhydrated, or hypohydrated. Urine osmolality and urine specific gravity can be utilized interchangeably to determine hydration status more accurately and precisely.[6]

Footnotes

1. Haycock GB, "Old and New Test of Renal Function," *J Clin Pathol*, 1981, 34(11):1276-81.
2. Pincus MR, Preuss HG, and Henry JB, "Evaluation of Renal Function, Water, Electrolytes, Acid-Base Balance, and Blood Gases," *Clinical Diagnosis and Management by Laboratory Methods*, 19th ed, Chapter 7, Philadelphia, PA: WB Saunders Co, 1996, 139-61.
3. Kappy MS and Ganong CA, "Cerebral Salt Wasting in Children: The Role of Atrial Natriuretic Hormone," *Adv Pediatr*, 1996, 43:271-308.
4. Price JD and Lauener RW, "Serum and Urine Osmolalities in the Differential Diagnosis of Polyuric States," *J Clin Endocrinol Metab*, 1966, 26(2):143-8.
5. Robertson GL and Berl T, "Pathophysiology of Water Metabolism," *Kidney*, Brenner BM and Rector FC Jr, eds, Philadelphia, PA: WB Saunders Co, 1991, 677-736.
6. Armstrong LE, Maresh CM, Castellani JW, et al, "Urinary Indices of Hydration Status," *Int J Sport Nutr*, 1994, 4(3):265-79.

References

Adam P, "Evaluation and Management of Diabetes Insipidus," *Am Fam Phys*, 1997, 55(6):2146-53.

Beuchat CA, "Structure and Concentrating Ability of the Mammalian Kidney: Correlations With Habitat," *Am J Physiol*, 1996, (1 Pt 2):R157-79.

Bichet DG, "Nephrogenic Diabetes Insipidus," *Am J Med*, 1998, 105(5):431-2.

Gupta AK, Kirchner KA, Nicholson R, et al, "Effects of α-Thalassemia and Sickle Polymerization Tendency on the Urine-Concentrating Defect of Individuals With Sickle Cell Trait," *J Clin Invest*, 1991, 88(6):1963-8.

♦ **Copper Reduction Tablet Test** *see* Reducing Substances, Urine *on page 885*

♦ **Crystals, Urine** *see* Urinalysis *on page 887*

♦ **Dysmorphic Red Blood Cells** *see* Blood, Urine *on page 870*

♦ **Dysmorphic Red Cells** *see* Urinalysis *on page 887*

♦ **Dysmorphic Red Cells** *see* Urinalysis, Fractional *on page 889*

Eosinophils, Urine

Related Information

Ova and Parasites, Urine *on page 667*
Protein, Quantitative, Urine *on page 883*
Urinalysis *on page 887*

Synonyms Eosinophiluria; Hansel's Stain of Urine; Urinary Eosinophils

Abstract A relatively nonspecific and poorly standardized marker for interstitial nephritis, eosinophilic cystitis, atheroembolic disease, and probably other entities.

Specimen Clean catch midstream urine specimen[1]

Storage Instructions Test should be done on a fresh specimen.

Causes for Rejection Urine more than 3 hours old from time of collection

Reference Interval <100 eosinophils/mL; using Hansel's stain, <1% eosinophils[2]

Use Eosinophils are sought in urine to help confirm suspected cases of allergic interstitial nephritis, eosinophilic cystitis, renal atheroemboli (cholesterol emboli syndrome), and schistosomiasis.

Limitations Eosinophiluria is not always present or prominent in interstitial nephritis and may be present in other disease entities. In one study, 6 of 15 patients with a confirmed diagnosis of acute interstitial nephritis (AIN) had eosinophiluria; however, 10 of 36 patients with other renal diagnosis also had eosinophiluria. Sensitivity was 40%, specificity 72%. Positive predictive value for AIN was only 38%.[2]

Methodology Centrifuged clean catch, midstream urine, stained with Hansel's stain.[3] It is methylene blue and eosin Y in methanol (Libe Labs, Florissant, MO). Wright stain is no longer recommended, as it is less sensitive, although still specific.

- Spin 10 mL of freshly voided urine at 2000 rpm, 5 minutes.
- Decant supernatant.
- Pipette sediment to a glass slide and air dry.
- Immerse slides in 95% methanol for 5 seconds.

(Continued)

Eosinophils, Urine (Continued)

- Apply Hansel's stain, 45 seconds.
- Add 20 drops of distilled water, allow to stand for 30 seconds.
- Remove excess stain with distilled water.
- Decolorize with four drops of methanol for 1-2 seconds.
- Rinse with distilled water.
- After drying, apply a coverslip with a drop of immersion oil.
- Following this protocol, 1% (or more) eosinophils is regarded as positive.[3]

Additional Information There is an uncertain relationship between eosinophiluria and peripheral blood eosinophilia. In only 33% of cases of drug-induced acute interstitial nephritis is the complete syndrome present. The complete syndrome includes fever, rash, eosinophiluria with acute renal failure.[3] Acute interstitial nephritis relates to penicillin derivatives, sulfa drugs, allopurinol, sulfinpyrazone, nitrofurantoin, and erythromycin. Methicillin is also frequently mentioned.[1] Eight of nine patients with biopsy proven atheroembolic renal failure demonstrated eosinophiluria by Hansel's stain. Six of eight of these patients had >5% of leukocytes as eosinophils.[4] Other diseases in which urinary eosinophilia is reported include contrast nephropathy, renal failure, glomerulonephritis, urinary tract infection,[5] and schistosomiasis.[6] Eosinophils are commonly bilobed.

Footnotes

1. Sutton JM, "Urinary Eosinophils," *Arch Intern Med*, 1986, 146(11):2243-4.
2. Ruffing KA, Hoppes P, Blend D, et al, "Eosinophils in Urine Revisited," *Clin Nephrol*, 1994, 41(3):163-6.
3. Nolan CR 3d, Anger MS, and Kelleher SP, "Eosinophiluria - A New Method of Detection and Definition of the Clinical Spectrum," *N Engl J Med*, 1986, 315(24):1516-8.
4. Wilson DM, Salazer TL, and Farkouh ME, "Eosinophiluria in Atheroembolic Renal Disease," *Am J Med*, 1991, 91(2):186-9.
5. Corwin HL, Korbet SM, and Schwartz MM, "Clinical Correlates of Eosinophiluria," *Arch Intern Med*, 1985, 145(6):1097-9.
6. Eltoum IA, Ghalib HW, Sualaiman S, et al, "Significance of Eosinophiluria in Urinary Schistosomiasis - A Study Using Hansel's Stain and Electron Microscopy," *Am J Clin Pathol*, 1989, 92(3):329-38.

References

Brunzel NA, *Fundamentals of Urine and Body Fluid Analysis*, Philadelphia, PA: WB Saunders Co, 1994, 214, 222.

Corwin HL, Bray RA, and Haber MH, "The Detection and Interpretation of Urinary Eosinophils," *Arch Pathol Lab Med*, 1989, 113(11):1256-8.

Nolan CR 3d and Kelleher SP, "Eosinophiluria," *Clin Lab Med*, 1988, 8(3):555-65.

♦ **Eosinophiluria** *see* Eosinophils, Urine *on page 873*

♦ **Esterase, Leukocyte, Urine** *see* Leukocyte Esterase, Urine *on page 878*

Fat, Urine

Related Information

Ethylene Glycol, Serum or Plasma *on page 790*
Glucose, Semiquantitative, Urine *on page 875*
Kidney Biopsy *on page 64*
Mercury, Blood *on page 797*
Mercury, Urine *on page 798*
Protein, Quantitative, Urine *on page 883*
Urinalysis *on page 887*

Synonyms Free Fat, Urine; Lipiduria

Test Includes Light and polarized microscopy of urine sediment and staining with Sudan III or IV

Abstract Lipiduria includes oval fat bodies, fatty casts, or free fat. These are found in nephrotic syndromes (proteinuria ≥3.5 g/24 hours).[1] Oval fat bodies are lipid-laden, pathologic, renal tubular epithelial cells which bear a strong association with marked proteinuria.

Patient Preparation Avoid contamination of the specimen with oils and lubricants from catheters and soaps. Avoid contamination with glove powder.

Specimen Random urine

Causes for Rejection Contamination of specimen with oils, soaps, and lubricants

Reference Interval Negative

Use Evaluate nephrotic syndrome, renal tubular necrosis, mercury poisoning, ethylene glycol ingestion (which may produce oval fat bodies), and fatty casts in the urine; evaluate bone marrow and fat embolism, which may produce gross fat globules in urine

Limitations Urinary fat globules, like air bubbles and yeasts, can be confused with erythrocytes if Sudan stain is not used. Structures resembling oval fat bodies may be from vaginal secretions, from the seminal vesicles, or as external contaminants.

Methodology Sudan III and IV or oil red O staining of urine sediment brings out triglycerides in lipiduria. Microscopically fat globules appear as spherical or ovoid dark glistening bodies. When they include substantial quantities of

cholesterol, under polarized light they appear doubly refractile and give a Maltese cross or cross pattée pattern. Maltese cross patterns may also be seen with some crystals, in particular starch granules found in some glove powders. Corn starch contamination may give rise to doubly refractile false urine lipid bodies[2] which are not as regular and round as are free urine lipid bodies. With polarized light the conical configuration of false lipid bodies tends to be off center, "French cross pattern."[3] True urine fat globules are usually seen in urines with increased protein. Lipiduria usually reflects glomerular abnormalities and/or multisystem disease states including diabetic glomerulopathy, amyloidosis, SLE, and cryoglobulinemia.[1]

Additional Information Urinary doubly refractile lipid bodies usually occur with heavy proteinuria. Refractile lipid bodies have been found in nonglomerular renal disease at relatively low levels of proteinuria and, rarely, even in patients without renal disease. The frequency of urine lipid bodies in patients with nonglomerular renal diseases include chronic interstitial nephritis (26%), polycystic kidney disease (38%), prerenal azotemia (20%), acute tubular necrosis (15%), and acute interstitial nephritis (33%). Presence of refractile urine lipid bodies in numbers >5 per 20 high power microscopic fields may be required to differentiate glomerular from nonglomerular renal disease.[4] See **Fatty casts** and **oval fat bodies ("lipiduria")** in Urinalysis *on page 887*.

Footnotes

1. Larson TS, "Evaluation of Proteinuria," *Mayo Clin Proc*, 1994, 69(12):1154-8.
2. Senécal PE and Rochette J, "Misidentification of Urine Lipid Bodies Owing to Use of Starch-Powdered Gloves," *Clin Chem*, 1988, 34(9):1926-7.
3. Hudson JB, Dennis AJ, and Gerhardt RE, "Urinary Lipid and the Maltese Cross," *N Engl J Med*, 1978, 299(11):586.
4. Braden GL, Sanchez PG, Fitzgibbons JP, et al, "Urinary Doubly Refractile Lipid Bodies in Nonglomerular Renal Diseases," *Am J Kidney Dis*, 1988, 11(4):332-7.

References

Streather CP, Varghese Z, Moorhead JF, et al, "Lipiduria in Renal Disease," *Am J Hypertens*, 1993, 6(11 Pt 2):353S-7S.

Yager HM and Harrington JT, "Urinalysis and Urinary Electrolytes," *The Principles and Practice of Nephrology*, Chapter 28, Jacobson HR, Striker GE, and Klahr S, eds, Philadelphia, PA: BC Decker Inc, 1991, 167-77.

♦ **Fishberg Concentration Test** *see* Concentration Test, Urine *on page 872*

♦ **Free Fat, Urine** *see* Fat, Urine *on page 874*

♦ **Glucose, Dipstick, Urine** *see* Glucose, Semiquantitative, Urine *on page 875*

♦ **Glucose, Qualitative, Urine** *replaced by* Glucose, Semiquantitative, Urine *on page 875*

Glucose, Quantitative, Urine

Related Information

Fructosamine, Serum *on page 177*
Glucose, Fasting, Plasma *on page 183*
Glucose, Postglucose Load, Plasma *on page 185*
Glucose, Random, Plasma *on page 186*
Glucose, Semiquantitative, Urine *on page 875*
Glucose Tolerance Test, Plasma *on page 186*
Glycated Hemoglobin (Hemoglobin A_{1c}), Blood *on page 188*
Ketone Bodies, Blood *on page 205*
Ketones, Urine *on page 877*
Microalbuminuria *on page 879*
Osmolality, Urine *on page 236*
Point-of-Care Testing *on page 43*
Reducing Substances, Urine *on page 885*
Urine Collection, 24-Hour *on page 47*

Synonyms Sugar, Quantitative, Urine; Urinary Sugar Test

Abstract Glucose can be assayed with excellent accuracy in urine. There are, however, very few indications for such testing.

Specimen 24-hour urine or other specific timed collections

Container Plain urine container, sodium fluoride preservative

Storage Instructions Refrigerate

Reference Interval ≤100 mg/24 hours (SI: ≤5.6 mmol/day); normal ranges are not available on random specimens.

Use This test may be useful in the evaluation of nondiabetic patients whose urine tests positive for reducing substances (see Reducing Substances, Urine *on page 885*). This test no longer has a place in the management of patients with diabetes mellitus.

Limitations With the advent of home glucose monitoring and the usefulness of glycosylated hemoglobin in following the degree of glucose control in a diabetic subject, the measurement of quantitative urine glucose is no longer used for control of diabetic patients.

Methodology Glucose oxidase

References

Knowles HC, "Evaluation of a Positive Urinary Sugar Test," *JAMA*, 1975, 234(9):961-3.

Glucose, Semiquantitative, Urine

Related Information

Synonyms Sugar, Qualitative, Urine; Urinary Sugar Test

Applies to Glucose, Dipstick, Urine; Glucose Tolerance Test Urines; Urines for Glucose Tolerance

Replaces Glucose, Qualitative, Urine

Test Includes Dipstick glucose is usually a part of urinalysis.

Abstract Clinistix®, among the first reagent strips, introduced in 1956, provided greater ease of use than did tablets and liquid reagents.[1] Screening for diabetes mellitus with reagent strips has been effective in detection of glycosuria. Glycosuria relates to the renal tubular threshold for glucose reabsorption, which is normally about 180 mg/dL, but which is variable.

Specimen Random urine, double-void technique preferred

Sampling Time Random or following a glucose load

Storage Instructions If the specimen cannot be processed promptly, it should be refrigerated.

Reference Interval None detected (by reagent strips). (Quantitative limits of normal are discussed by Li and Huang).[2]

Use This is a rapid test intended for detection of glucose (sugar) in the urine. The roles for reagent strip glucose testing in urine have evolved to two limited uses: 1) diagnostic evaluation of a comatose patient in an Emergency Department setting - and then it is only useful until the blood glucose measurement is available, possibly 5-10 minutes later; 2) diagnostic evaluation of a newborn who has a positive reducing substance test (see Reducing Substances, Urine *on page 885*).

Limitations Reagent strip methods are limited in usefulness as quantitative methods. Acquired color vision deficiency caused by diabetic retinopathy may cause erroneous reading of the strip by patients.[3] Each brand of commercial dipsticks lists interfering substances. Such package inserts should be reviewed. Home blood glucose testing has largely replaced qualitative and semiquantitative urine methods for long-term and outpatient monitoring of diabetic therapy. Glucose in urine is detected later in time than the hyperglycemia it indirectly represents by approximately one-half the time between voidings. In renal failure, the time delay may become excessive due to oliguria. Excessive urinary bladder residual volume further limits the test as a reflection of **current** hyperglycemia.

For diagnosis, fasting state urine glucose testing lacks sensitivity (17%) but provides 98% specificity. Such specificity will cause negative results in individuals with particular inherited metabolic diseases, such as galactosemia. Postload glucosuria provides only moderate sensitivity and specificity, 70% to 80%.

As a patient-based monitor of control in known diabetics, urine glucose determination does not provide reliable differentiation between current mild elevation, and normality or decrease of blood glucose. Urine glucose testing cannot detect hypoglycemia and lacks sufficient sensitivity for tight control. Urine glucose testing is considered inferior to self-monitoring of capillary glucose. Levels below the renal threshold of glucose are not subject to evaluation by urine glucose testing. The renal threshold for glucose is variable between different patients.

Large quantities of ketones and ascorbic acid (eg, after ingestion of vitamin C tablets) may depress the color reaction. Contamination of the collection container by hypochlorite, chlorine or peroxide may cause false positives. Pyridium® metabolites may mask the reaction.

The double enzyme (glucose-specific) method for urine sugar will not detect sugars in the urine other than glucose. For screening for other sugars, see Reducing Substances, Urine *on page 885*.

Urines negative for glucose with properly stored Multistix® (Miles Inc, Elkhart, IN) were trace positive following dipstick air exposure (jars left uncapped).[4]

Methodology Double sequential enzyme analysis, specific for glucose (glucose oxidase/peroxidase). Sensitivity is 50-100 mg glucose/dL (SI: 2.8-5.6 mmol/L) urine.

Seven types of urinary reagent strips for glycosuria were evaluated in a 1997 paper.[2]

Additional Information Glycosuria may occur in situations, such as pregnancy, in which the increased filtered load may exceed renal tubular reabsorption capacity. Rarely corticosteroid therapy may cause a combination of mild hyperglycemia and increased renal glomerular filtration, producing glycosuria. Renal glycosuria due to a low renal threshold for glucose occurs either as an isolated phenomenon or as part of tubular damage. Because these causes of glucosuria are rare and glucosuria usually indicates significant hyperglycemia, a positive screening test for urine glucose is significant and indicates a substantial likelihood of diabetes mellitus in the nonpregnant patient. In the pregnant patient, glucosuria has a 27% sensitivity and only a 7.1% predictive value for gestational diabetes. Its greatest value is to indicate which women should be screened with serum glucose after a 50 g oral glucose load **prior** to 24-28 weeks gestation, the usual recommended time of screening.[5] Urine glucose testing may be used as a monitor in diabetics in concert with plasma glucose and glycosylated hemoglobin. Bedside glucose monitoring has been advocated to replace urine testing for glucose, although these programs themselves may be wanting in performance characteristics.[6] Although the expense of blood testing, as well as its value, is questioned (in a 1997 BMJ paper),[7] Sherwin (in a 2000 text) describes urine glucose testing (as part of self-monitoring) as unreliable, writing that it should be used only in patients who cannot or will not apply self-monitoring of blood glucose or in whom the goal is only avoidance of symptomatic hyperglycemia.[8]

The renal threshold for glucose is 160-180 mg/dL (SI: 8.9-10.0 mmol/L). Thus, reasonable diabetic control can be maintained and the risk of hypoglycemia minimized if urine glucose screening tests are maintained at a trace to 1+ level. High urine specific gravity will decrease sensitivity.

It has been advocated that physicians examining ill-appearing dehydrated infants without any obvious cause for the dehydration should quickly screen the urine for glucose and ketones.[9]

Use of beta-blockers, bisoprolol, and atenolol, did not significantly show an increase in glycosuria in untreated noninsulin diabetics.[10]

Footnotes

1. Pugia MJ, "Technology Behind Diagnostic Reagent Strips," *Lab Med*, 2000, 31(2):92-6.
2. Li KL and Huang HS, "Comparing Urinary Reagent Strips for Detecting Glycosuria in Patients With Diabetes Mellitus," *Lab Med*, 1997, 28(6):397-401.
3. Bresnick GH, Groo A, Palta M, et al, "Urinary Glucose Testing Inaccuracies Among Diabetic Patients. Effect of Acquired Color Vision Deficiency Caused by Diabetic Retinopathy." *Arch Ophthalmol*, 1984, 102(10):1489-96.
4. Cohen HT and Spiegel DM, "Air-Exposed Urine Dipsticks Give False-Positive Results for Glucose and False-Negative Results for Blood," *Am J Clin Pathol*, 1991, 96(3):398-400.
5. Watson WJ, "Screening for Glycosuria During Pregnancy," *South Med J*, 1990, 83(2):156-8.
6. Jones BA, Bachner P, and Howanitz PJ, "Bedside Glucose Monitoring," *Arch Pathol Lab Med*, 1993, 117(11):1080-7.
7. Gallichan M, "Self Monitoring of Glucose by People With Diabetes: Evidence Based Practice," *BMJ*, 1997, 314(7085):964-7.
8. Sherwin RS, "Diabetes Mellitus," *Cecil Textbook of Medicine*, 21st ed, Chapter 242, Goldman L and Bennet JC, eds, Philadelphia, PA: WB Saunders Co, 2000, 1263-85.
9. Bland GL and Wood VD, "Diabetes in Infancy: Diagnosis and Current Management," *J Natl Med Assoc*, 1991, 83(4):361-5.
10. Vulpis V, Antonacci A, Prandi P, et al, "The Effects of Bisoprolol and Atenolol on Glucose Metabolism in Hypertensive Patients With Noninsulin Dependent-Diabetes Mellitus," *Minerva Med*, 1991, 82(4):189-93.

References

Gribble RK, Meier PR, and Berg RL, "The Value of Urine Screening for Glucose at Each Prenatal Visit," *Obstet Gynecol*, 1995, 86(3):405-10.

♦ **Glucose Tolerance Test Urines** *see* Glucose, Semiquantitative, Urine *on page 875*

♦ **Hansel's Stain of Urine** *see* Eosinophils, Urine *on page 873*

Hemoglobin, Qualitative, Urine

Related Information

Test Includes Dipstick screening of urine for hemoglobin

Abstract Test detects hemoglobin and myoglobin in urine. Urine sediment microscopy is needed as well.[1] Hemoglobinuria without hematuria (the presence of red cells in urine) implies intravascular hemolysis, while hematuria suggests a bleeding source (eg, tumor, stone) in the urinary tract. (Continued)

Hemoglobin, Qualitative, Urine *(Continued)*

Specimen Random urine

Reference Interval Negative

Use Hemoglobinuria, the presence of free hemoglobin in the urine, may result from hemolysis. It occurs if the serum haptoglobin binding capacity (100-200 mg/dL Hb (SI: 1.0-2.0 g/L)) is exceeded and if the renal threshold for tubular reabsorption of hemoglobin (90-140 mg/dL Hb (SI: 0.9-1.4 g/L)) is exceeded. The test may also be positive with hematuria or with myoglobinuria. Myoglobin may appear in the urine following severe physical exercise, trauma, and with rhabdomyolysis.

Limitations Menstrual or other uterine bleeding may appear as a contaminant in the urine. False positives may occur with oxidizing contaminants (eg, Betadine® (povidone-iodine)). False negatives occur with large amounts of ascorbic acid. Formalin in urine can cause false-negative results.[2] Urine dipsticks for blood that are exposed to air lose sensitivity over time. To prevent this, keep dipstick jar tightly capped.

Methodology The peroxidase-like activity of hemoglobin catalyzes the reaction of cumene hydroperoxide and 3,3',5,5'-tetramethylbenzidine. (Hemoglobin peroxidase catalyzes oxidation of a chromogen.)

Additional Information Hemoglobin is catabolized in the renal tubular cells, and the iron is stored as hemosiderin. See Hemosiderin Stain, Urine *on page 876.* The urine in hemoglobinuria may be clear red, clear redbrown, or dark brown. Myoglobinuria also produces a dark or red-orange urine. Both hemoglobin and myoglobin produce positive dipstick tests for blood and must be identified by additional tests,[3] including serum CK, aldolase, and myoglobin (see Myoglobin, Qualitative, Urine *on page 880*). In hematuria, red cells or ghosts (lysed red cells) are observed microscopically.

See Blood, Urine *on page 870.*

Footnotes

1. Bartlett RC, Zern DA, Ratkiewicz I, et al, "Reagent Strip Screening for Sediment Abnormalities Identified by Automated Microscopy in Urine From Patients Suspected to Have Urinary Tract Disease," *Arch Pathol Lab Med*, 1994, 118(11):1096-101.
2. Corwin HL and Silverstein MD, "Microscopic Hematuria," *Clin Lab Med*, 1988, 8(3):601-10.
3. Culclasure TF, Bray VJ, and Hasbargen JA, "The Significance of Hematuria in the Anticoagulated Patient," *Arch Intern Med*, 1994, 154(6):649-52.

♦ **Hemoglobin, Urine** *see* Blood, Urine *on page 870*

Hemosiderin Stain, Urine

Related Information

Anemia Flowchart *on page 392*
Antiglobulin Test, Direct *on page 834*
Autohemolysis Test *on page 405*
Blood, Urine *on page 870*
Cold Hemolysin Test *on page 418*
Glucose-6-Phosphate Dehydrogenase, Quantitative, Blood *on page 437*
Ham Test *on page 439*
Hemoglobin Electrophoresis *on page 444*
Hemoglobin, Qualitative, Urine *on page 875*
Hemoglobin, Unstable, Heat Labile Test *on page 447*
Iron and Total Iron Binding Capacity/Transferrin, Serum *on page 203*
Lactate Dehydrogenase, Serum *on page 207*
Red Blood Cell Enzyme Deficiency, Quantitative *on page 475*
Sickle Cell Tests *on page 486*
Sugar Water Test Screen *on page 488*

Synonyms Iron Stain, Urine; Prussian Blue Stain, Urine; Urine Hemosiderin

Abstract Hemosiderinuria is a marker for intravascular hemolysis including importantly chronic hemolytic anemia. With hemolysis, hemoglobin passes the glomerulus, is present in the glomerular filtrate, and is absorbed by renal tubular epithelial where it is converted to hemosiderin. Thus, hemosiderin may not be found in the urine at the onset of acute hemolysis or a hemolytic episode, even if hemoglobinemia and hemoglobinuria are present (unless there has been a previous hemolytic episode). On the other hand, a few days after a hemolytic attack, iron-containing granules may be present in the urine (hemosiderinuria), even in the absence of hemoglobinuria.

Specimen Random urine

Container Use iron-free container and centrifuge tubes if results of initial examination are difficult to interpret.

Storage Instructions Refrigeration

Reference Interval There should be absence of stainable iron in normal urine. Normal value for urinary iron excretion is <0.1 mg/day.[1]

Use A sign of recent intravascular hemolysis, hemosiderinuria is an important clue in the diagnosis of unexplained anemia. Urine sediment stained for hemosiderin is a screen for increased iron excretion, which can be quantitated and is increased in hemochromatosis, hemolytic anemia, and nephrotic syndrome.

Limitations Hemosiderin is first shed in the urine a few days after hemolysis begins. Hemosiderinuria declines slowly after hemolysis stops. Quantitatively, iron excretion remains slightly elevated for months after replacement of a cardiac valve which has caused hemolytic anemia, although hemosiderinuria is usually absent after a few weeks.

Methodology Microscopic examination of slide stained for hemosiderin (Prussian blue reaction). Environmental iron contaminants must be distinguished from true iron-positive granular deposits of intracellular origin. The inexperienced observer may generate a false-positive report. A true-positive test result shows blue-staining granules in an intracellular situation in intact tubular epithelial cells. Hemosiderin may appear as a brown coarsely granular pigment in tubular epithelial cells, epithelial cell casts, or free in the urine sediment.

Additional Information When haptoglobin is saturated, part of the hemoglobin in the plasma is filtered by the glomerulus and presented to the renal tubular cell. If tubular capacity is not exceeded, all hemoglobin in the urine may be absorbed by the proximal tubular cells, where hemoglobin iron is converted to hemosiderin. When these cells are shed, hemosiderin appears in urine sediment. Hemosiderinuria with or without hemoglobinuria may be seen in chronic hemolytic anemia, paroxysmal nocturnal hemoglobinuria, hemochromatosis, multiple transfusions, and other conditions which result in deposition of iron in the renal parenchyma. Hemosiderinuria may occur when the degree of hemolysis is at such a low level that hemoglobinuria is not detected.

With intravascular hemolysis, urinary iron values increase to between 3-11 mg/day.[1] Pernicious anemia and hereditary spherocytosis have normal values.

Footnotes

1. Lee GR, "Hemolytic Disorders: General Considerations," *Wintrobe's Clinical Hematology*, 10th ed, Volume 1, Chapter 40, Lee GR, Foerster J, and Lukens J, eds, Baltimore, MD: Lippincott Williams & Wilkins, 1999, 1119-20.

References

CRC Desk Reference for Hematology, Shinton NK, ed, Boca Raton, FL: CRC Press, 1998, 320-1.

Dacie Sir JV and Lewis SM, "Laboratory Methods Used in the Investigation of the Haemolytic Anaemias," *Practical Haematology*, 8th ed, Chapter 12, 1995, 204-5.

Tabbara IA, "Hemolytic Anemias. Diagnosis and Management," *Med Clin North Am*, 1992, 76(3):649-68.

♦ **Ictotest®** *see* Bilirubin, Urine *on page 870*

Indican, Semiquantitative, Urine

Synonyms Indoxyl Sulfate, Urine

Applies to Purple Urine Bags

Abstract This simple test has been used to screen for intestinal bacterial overgrowth, malabsorption due to intestinal or biliary obstruction, or Hartnup disease. It can confirm indican as the etiology for a dark or black urine.

Specimen Fresh random urine

Storage Instructions The test must be run on fresh urine specimens. Transport specimen to the laboratory immediately upon collection.

Reference Interval Indican is normally present in urine in small amounts (<100 mg/day). It is detected by a semiquantitative color reaction and is reported as "positive" or "negative" (normal).

Use Evaluate intestinal integrity, absorption, and protein catabolism

Limitations Diurnal variation is described in urinary indican excretion.[1] Presently, urine indican is rarely requested.

Methodology Detection of indican depends upon its decomposition and subsequent oxidation of the indoxyl to indigo blue and its absorption by chloroform.

Additional Information Indole is produced by intestinal bacterial action on unabsorbed tryptophan. Although most indole is eliminated in the feces, a small amount is absorbed and detoxified to be excreted as indican (indoxyl potassium sulfate) in the urine. Urinary indican may be increased in biliary obstruction, intestinal obstruction, malabsorption syndromes, and syndromes associated with achlorhydria (eg, gastric carcinoma, pernicious anemia). Hartnup disease patients also have high urine indican. Increased indican may cause the urine to blacken on standing.

Purple urine drainage bags have been reported in a few chronically catheterized, elderly, female patients with urinary tract infection caused by *Providencia* or *Klebsiella*. Urine indican excretion in such subjects was increased.[2]

There is experimental animal evidence that saccharin can induce increase in urinary indican[3] and provide a noninvasive indicator of trypsin inhibitor activity.[4]

Indoxyl sulfate can alter the dip-and-read strip reaction for urinary bilirubin in urines positive for bilirubin, sufficiently to mask a weak reaction. A more specific test such as the Ictotest® has been recommended when dip-and-read bilirubin testing is inconclusive.[5]

Footnotes

1. Kirkland JL, Vargas E, and Lye M, "Indican Excretion in the Elderly," *Postgrad Med J*, 1983, 59(697):717-9.
2. Dealler SF, Belfield PW, Bedford M, et al, "Purple Urine Bags," *J Urol*, 1989, 142(3):769-70.
3. Sims J and Renwick AG, "Diurnal Variation in the Excretion of Indican in Rats Fed Saccharin-Containing Diet," *Cancer*, 1984, 23(3):259-63.
4. Anderson RL, Maurer JK, Francis WR, et al, "Trypsin Inhibitor Ingestion-Induced Urinary Indican Excretion and Pancreatic Acinar Cell Hypertrophy," *Nutr Cancer*, 1986, 8(2):133-9.
5. Skjold AC, Freitag JF, Stover LR, et al, "Indoxyl Sulfate Interferes With Dip-and-Read Urinary Bilirubin Estimate," *Clin Chem*, 1980, 26(9):1368-9.

♦ **Indoxyl Sulfate, Urine** *see* Indican, Semiquantitative, Urine *on page 876*

♦ **Iron Stain, Urine** *see* Hemosiderin Stain, Urine *on page 876*

Ketones, Urine

Related Information
Amino Acids, Plasma *on page 100*
Ammonia, Plasma *on page 102*
Anion Gap, Serum, Plasma, or Urine *on page 106*
Bicarbonate, Blood *on page 115*
Ethylene Glycol, Serum or Plasma *on page 790*
Glucose, Postglucose Load, Plasma *on page 185*
Glucose, Quantitative, Urine *on page 874*
Glucose, Random, Plasma *on page 186*
Glucose, Semiquantitative, Urine *on page 875*
Ketone Bodies, Blood *on page 205*
Methylmalonic Acid, Serum, Plasma, Urine, or Amniotic Fluid *on page 224*
Osmolality, Calculated, Serum or Plasma *on page 234*
Osmolality, Serum *on page 236*
Reducing Substances, Urine *on page 885*
Urinalysis *on page 887*
Volatile Screen, Blood or Urine *on page 809*

Synonyms Acetest®; Nitroprusside Reaction for Ketones, Urine; Urine Ketones

Applies to Acetoacetic Acid, Urine; Acetone, Semiquantitative, Urine; Beta-Hydroxybutyric Acid, Urine

Abstract Classically associated with incomplete metabolic breakdown of fat, intermediary products called ketone bodies are detected in blood (ketosis) and urine (ketonuria). Ketonuria may warn of impending diabetic coma and signal the presence, in an infant, of an inborn metabolic error.

Specimen Random urine

Container Plastic urine container

Storage Instructions If sample cannot be tested immediately, it should be refrigerated. Standing for prolonged periods, specimens may yield false-negative reactions.

Special Instructions Transport specimen to the laboratory promptly following collection.

Reference Interval Negative; in very low carbohydrate diets or in instances of abnormal carbohydrate metabolism, ketones appear in the urine in excessively large amounts before serum ketones are elevated.

Use A semiquantitative test, it is used to evaluate ketonuria, detect acidosis, ketoacidosis of alcoholism and diabetes mellitus, fasting, starvation, high protein diets, and isopropanol ingestion. It remains useful as a monitor in known diabetics, in type I patients when ill and during marked hyperglycemia and in type II diabetics during acute illness. In pregnancy, the risk of ketosis is increased; all pregnant type I diabetics are advised to monitor urine for ketosis in first morning urine and when blood glucose is >150 mg/dL. A portion of initial assessment for inborn errors of metabolism in infancy and childhood.[1]

In infants and children, ketonuria can occur with febrile illnesses and toxic states with marked vomiting or diarrhea. Genetic disorders resulting in ketonuria include propionyl CoA carboxylase deficiency, glycogen storage disease, branched-chain ketonuria, and methylmalonic aciduria.

Limitations Specimens containing large amounts of ascorbic acid or levodopa metabolites, 2-mercaptoethane sulfonic acid, valproic acid, phenazopyridine (Pyridium®), PSP dye, phenylketones, or phthalein compounds such as are administered for liver and kidney function tests may cause false positives or apparent false positives. Beta-hydroxybutyric acid (the third of the three ketone bodies) is not detected by the nitroprusside method. N-acetylcysteine causes false-positive ketone results.[2,3]

Methodology Nitroprusside reaction, Ketostix® or Acetest®; acetoacetic acid and acetone react with nitroprusside to create a color change, especially the former.

Additional Information In adult healthy men, a fast of 18 hours or greater produces ketonemia at a level that would result in detectable ketonuria. Aging is associated with increased susceptibility to fasting-induced hyperketonemia.[4] Ketonuria may be noted in normal pregnancy.[5] Acetoacetic acid, beta-hydroxybutyric acid, and acetone are ketone bodies. In ketosis, usually 80% of total ketones are beta-hydroxybutyric acid. Acetoacetic acid comprises most of the remainder with acetone present in trace amounts. Urine ketones should generally be determined in patients with a positive urine test for urine glucose and followed during the management of diabetes mellitus and ketoacidosis. Ketones can depress the glucose oxidase reaction, providing falsely low results, on some glucose oxidase reagent strips.

Ketones detected by Multistix® correlated well with Acetest® results. Specificity 96%, sensitivity 87.5% (63.3% when trace ketonuria was regarded as positive ketonuria). Acetest® confirmation of Multistix® positive ketone results is only necessary for trace ketonuria.[6]

Footnotes
1. Lindor NM and Karnes PS, "Initial Assessment of Infants and Children With Suspected Inborn Errors of Metabolism," *Mayo Clin Proc*, 1995, 70:987-8.
2. Poon R, Hinberg I, and Peterson RG, "N-Acetylcysteine Causes False-Positive Ketone Results With Urinary Dipsticks," *Clin Chem*, 1990, 36(5):818-9.
3. Holcombe BJ, Hopkins AM, and Heizer WD, "False Positive Tests for Urinary Ketones," *N Engl J Med*, 1994, 330(8):578.
4. London ED, Margolin RA, Duara R, et al, "Effects of Fasting on Ketone Body Concentrations in Healthy Men of Different Ages," *J Gerontol*, 1986, 41(5):599-604.
5. Chez RA and Curcio FD, 3d, "Ketonuria in Normal Pregnancy," *Obstet Gynecol*, 1987, 69(2):272-4.
6. Abdelaziz HM and Billett HH, "Follow-up Testing for Ketonuria. Is it Necessary?" *Am J Clin Pathol*, 1994, 101(3):346-8.

References
Henry JB, Lauzon RB, and Schumann GB, "Basic Examination of Urine," *Clinical Diagnosis and Management by Laboratory Methods*, 19th ed, Chapter 18, Philadelphia, PA: WB Saunders Co, 1996, 411-56.

Schwab TM, Hendey GW, and Soliz TC, "Screening for Ketonemia in Patients With Diabetes," *Ann Emerg Med*, 1999, 34(3):342-6.

Kidney Stone Analysis

Related Information
Alkaline Phosphatase, Serum *on page 93*
Bacterial Culture, Urine *on page 578*
Blood, Urine *on page 870*
Calcium, Ionized, Serum *on page 130*
Calcium, Serum *on page 131*
Calcium, Urine *on page 133*
Carbon Dioxide, Total, Blood *on page 135*
Chloride, Serum, Plasma, or Blood *on page 144*
Chloride, Urine *on page 145*
Citrate, Serum, Plasma, or Urine *on page 149*
Creatinine Clearance *on page 160*
Creatinine, Serum or Plasma *on page 161*
Cryoprecipitate *on page 838*
Cystine, Urine *on page 164*
Electrolyte Panel, Serum *on page 168*
Magnesium, Serum *on page 221*
Magnesium, Urine *on page 222*
Oxalate, Urine *on page 238*
Parathyroid Hormone, Serum *on page 243*
Phosphorus, Serum *on page 251*
Phosphorus, Urine *on page 253*
pH, Urine *on page 882*
Potassium, Urine *on page 259*
Sodium, Urine *on page 278*
Urea Nitrogen, Serum or Plasma *on page 293*
Uric Acid, Serum *on page 293*
Uric Acid, Urine *on page 295*
Urinalysis *on page 887*
Vitamin D, Serum *on page 300*

Synonyms Calculus Analysis; Nephrolithiasis Analysis

Applies to Sulfate, Urine

Test Includes Analysis for calcium, carbonate, citrate, cystine, magnesium, oxalate, phosphates, and urates

Abstract Passage of a stone in the urinary tract is often accompanied by hematuria and usually by abrupt, severe, constant pain (acute renal colic). Infection may occur. Up to 80% of renal stones are calcium oxalate, of which about 30% include calcium phosphate (apatite); 3% to 5% are uric acid stones; ≤2% are cystine. Up to 20% are magnesium ammonium phosphate (struvite) (infection stones). Five percent to 20% of Americans will form kidney stones. Recurrence rate is ≤95% at 25 years. Diets rich in protein and salt bear association with nephrolithiasis. Risk factors for stone formation include positive family history, osteoporosis, pathologic fracture, urinary tract infections, gout, magnesium deficiency, and small bowel Crohn disease with prior resection, as well as age, sex, and climate. Diet and fluid intake are relevant. Low urine volume is a risk factor for nephrolithiasis. Rarely, genetic disorders (eg, cystinuria, xanthinuria, or oxaluria) can cause nephrolithiasis. Since the majority of individuals with nephrolithiasis suffer recurrence, prevention holds high priority, and therefore stone evaluation is needed for intelligent management.[1]

Specimen Kidney/ureteral stones

Collection Specimen should be washed free of tissue and blood, and submitted in a clean, dry container. If necessary, urine should be filtered to recover gravel or stone.

Storage Instructions Do **not** apply any tape to stones. Adhesives interfere with infrared spectroscopy.

Turnaround Time Usually several days
(Continued)

Kidney Stone Analysis (Continued)

Special Instructions Urinalysis can provide useful information including detection of crystalluria and presence of red blood cells. Urine culture is often indicated.

Use Evaluation of stone composition is indicated to decrease morbidity, prevent development of new stones, and support recognition of underlying abnormalities.

Limitations Chemical analysis is generally available in most laboratories while x-ray diffraction and infrared spectroscopy are reference laboratory procedures. The relative merits of stone analysis techniques are subject to debate. Chemical analysis is more readily available and has correlated with more sophisticated techniques,[2] but chemical analysis requires 5 mg of stone and is time consuming. X-ray diffraction can separately determine the composition of the nidus as well as the major portion of the stone. The composition of the nidus may be unlike that of the cortex.

Methodology Crystallographic analysis, chemical analysis, infrared spectroscopy, polarization microscopy, x-ray diffraction analysis

Additional Information Urine uric acid excretion reflects purine intake, usually from meats. Phosphate excretion reflects meat and dairy intake primarily. Sulfates reflect meat intake. Urine calcium is correlated with urine sulfate and urine sodium, giving clues to treatment. Decreased urine citrate excretion promotes calcium stone formation.

A **serum chemistry panel** which includes calcium and phosphorus (for hyperparathyroidism), alkaline phosphatase (for Paget disease of bone), uric acid, albumin, magnesium, BUN, and creatinine is usually needed. Serum sodium, potassium, chloride, and CO_2, and parathormone (PTH) levels, if indicated, may be useful additional investigations. CBC and vitamin D_3 levels may be helpful.

Urine culture is needed. Urine nitroprusside (for cystinuria), urine volume, and fasting morning urine pH (with electrolytes, for renal tubular acidosis) are generally indicated. **Twenty-four hour urine collections** for volume, creatinine clearance, uric acid, oxalate, calcium, sodium, chloride, potassium, citrate, ammonium, magnesium, and phosphate are commonly indicated but should be delayed about a month following stone passage or removal. Urine sulfate is a factor relevant to urine supersaturation, and may be useful to assess protein intake. A urine supersaturation profile has recently been announced by a major reference laboratory.[3]

See Citrate, Serum, Plasma, or Urine *on page 149.*

Cystinuria and xanthinuria are rare causes of renal calculi. See Cystine, Urine *on page 164.* Other uncommon causes of renal stones include sarcoidosis, Cushing syndrome, excessive calcium or vitamin D ingestion, steroids, immobilization, bone disease, Paget disease of bone, hyperthyroidism, and glycogen storage disease.[4] An increasing but still low rate of triamterene stones has been noted.[5] Most calcium stones relate to idiopathic hypercalciuria and hyperuricosuria, which may coexist. Hyperoxaluria is a factor requiring evaluation in patients with oxalate nephrolithiasis.[6]

Higher intake of calcium is associated with a reduced risk of oxalate nephrolithiasis. Such inverse relationship between dietary calcium and kidney stone is probably caused by increased binding of oxalate by ingested calcium.[7] Urinary oxalate excretion falls by 1.1–1.8 mg/day for each increase of 100 mg in calcium ingestion.[8] The risk of calcium nephrolithiasis is related to the free ion concentration product of oxalate and calcium. There are many urinary constituents which can complex calcium, but only calcium complexes and precipitates with oxalate.

Nephrolithiasis is a complication of magnesium deficiency. Decreased magnesium is found in patients with Crohn disease and in other states; see Magnesium, Serum *on page 221* and Magnesium, Urine *on page 222.* Magnesium supplements can diminish risk of calcium oxalate nephrolithiasis in subjects who have fat malabsorption.[9] Potassium and fluid intake are also associated with reduced risk, but intake of animal protein is directly related to risk of kidney stones,[7] probably because sulfated amino acids increase calciuria. Other dietary risk factors include ascorbic acid, oxalate-rich substances (eg, iced tea, chocolate, spinach), and sodium. High dietary potassium intake seems to decrease urine calcium excretion.[10] Males are two to three times more likely to develop stones than females. Whites are three to four times as likely as African-Americans to develop stones.[11]

Control of urine pH is an important facet of management of nephrolithiasis (eg, acid urine supports development of uric acid stones, while calcium carbonate stones develop in alkaline urine).

Careful microscopy of urine sediment may be helpful, especially when done on freshly voided, warm urine.

Footnotes

1. Wasserstein AG, "Nephrolithiasis: Acute Management and Prevention," *Dis Mon*, 1998, 44(5):196-213.
2. Moriss RH, Bedir MF, and Freeman JA, *Urinary Stone Analysis in Laboratory Medicine/Urinalysis and Medical Microscopy*, 2nd ed, Philadelphia, PA: Lea & Febiger, 1983, 341-4.
3. "For Your Information: Supersaturation Profile, Urine," *Mayo References Services Communique*, 2000.
4. Talente GM, Coleman RA, Alter C, et al, "Glycogen Storage Disease in Adults," *Ann Intern Med*, 1994, 120(3):218-26.
5. Carr MC, Prien EL Jr, and Babayan RK, "Triamterene Nephrolithiasis: Renewed Attention Is Warranted," *J Urol*, 1990, 144(6):1339-40.

6. Robertson WG and Peacock M, "The Cause of Idiopathic Calcium Stone Disease: Hypercalciuria or Hyperoxaluria?" *Nephron*, 1980, 26(3):105-10.
7. Curhan GC, Willett WC, Rimm EB, et al, "A Prospective Study of Dietary Calcium and Other Nutrients and the Risk of Symptomatic Kidney Stones," *N Engl J Med*, 1993, 328(12):833-8.
8. Lemann J Jr, "Composition of the Diet and Calcium Kidney Stones," *N Engl J Med*, 1993, 328(12):880-2.
9. Fleming CR, George L, Stoner GL, et al, "The Importance of Urinary Magnesium Values in Patients With Gut Failure," *Mayo Clin Proc*, 1996, 71(1):21-4.
10. Osorio AV and Alon US, "The Relationship Between Urinary Calcium, Sodium, and Potassium Excretion and the Role of Potassium in Treating Idiopathic Hypercalciuria," *Pediatrics*, 1997, 100(4):675-81.
11. Sarmina I, Spirnak JP, and Resnick MI, "Urinary Lithiasis in the Black Population: An Epidemiologic Study and Review of the Literature," *J Urol*, 1987, 138(1):14-7.

References

Baggio B, Plebani M, and Gambaro G, "Pathogenesis of Idiopathic Calcium Nephrolithiasis: Update 1997," *Crit Rev Clin Lab Sci*, 1998, 35(2):153-87.

Bushinsky DA, "Nephrolithiasis," *J Am Soc Nephrol*, 1998, 9(5):917-24.

Daudon M, Bader CA, and Jungers P, "Urinary Calculi: Review of Classification Methods and Correlations With Etiology," *Scanning Microsc*, 1993, 7(3):1081-106.

Heller HJ, "The Role of Calcium in the Prevention of Kidney Stones," *J Am Coll Nutr*, 1999, 18(5 Suppl):373S-378S.

Kingwatanakul P and Alon US, "Hypercalciuria and Urolithiasis in Childhood," *Pediatric Nephrology*, Trachtman H and Gauthier B, eds, Amsterdam: Harwood Academic Publishers, 1998, 231-52.

Klugman V and Favus MJ, "Diagnosis and Treatment of Calcium Kidney Stones," *Adv Endocrinol Metab*, 1995, 6:117-42.

Low RK and Stoller ML, "Uric Acid-Related Nephrolithiasis," *Urol Clin North Am*, 1997, 24(1):135-48.

Marangella M, Vitale C, Bagnis C, et al, "Idiopathic Calcium Nephrolithiasis," *Nephron*, 1999, 81(Suppl 1):38-44.

Messa P, Marangella M, Paganin L, et al, "Different Dietary Calcium Intake and Relative Supersaturation of Calcium Oxalate in the Urine of Patients Forming Renal Stones," *Clin Sci (Colch)*, 1997, 93(3):257-63.

Pak CY, "Southwestern Internal Medicine Conference: Medical Management of Nephrolithiasis - A New Simplified Approach for General Practice," *Am J Med Sci*, 1997, 313(4):215-9.

Ruml LA, Pearle MS, and Pak CY, "Medial Therapy, Calcium Oxalate Urolithiasis," *Urol Clin North Am*, 1997, 24(1):117-33.

Saklayen MG, "Medical Management of Nephrolithiasis," *Med Clin North Am*, 1997, 81(3):785-99.

Trivedi BK, "Nephrolithiasis: How It Happens and What to Do About It," *Postgrad Med*, 1996, 100(6):63-7, 71-2, 77-8.

Westbury EJ, "A Chemist's View of the History of Urinary Stone Analysis," *Br J Urol*, 1989, 64(5):445-50.

Leukocyte Esterase, Urine

Related Information

Bacterial Culture, Urine *on page 578*
Gram Stain *on page 617*
Nitrite, Urine *on page 882*
Urinalysis *on page 887*

Synonyms Bacteria Screen, Urine; Esterase, Leukocyte, Urine

Test Includes Screening of urine for leukocyte esterase activity by dipstick is usually a part of urinalysis

Abstract A rapid indirect test for detection of bacteriuria, it is a surrogate indicator for the presence of intact or lysed neutrophils. Evaluation of urinary tract infection includes nitrite (also on reagent strips) microscopy, Gram stain, urine culture with colony count, and other methods. **The best test for urinary tract infection is culture, which supports proper therapy.**

Specimen Random clean catch urine; preferably midstream, clean catch collection, catheterized specimen, bladder aspiration

Storage Instructions If the specimen cannot be processed within 2 hours, it should be refrigerated for other portions of urine evaluation.

Reference Interval Negative

Use Detect leukocytes in urine to screen for urinary tract infection. It will detect either intact or lysed white blood cells and therefore can be positive when WBCs are not found on microscopic examination. The lysis of leukocytes that occurs when urine is allowed to stand intensifies the color reaction from release of esterase. The test performs best for specimens in which colony counts are >10^5 CFU/mL and when combined with nitrite: together a specificity of 98.3%, sensitivity of 84%, positive predictive value of 84%, and negative predictive value of 98.3% was reported.[1] Sensitivity, however, was worse in a 1998 Belgian study.[2]

Limitations False positives may occur in specimens contaminated with vaginal secretions. False-positive results from trichomonads have been controversial. Cephalexin, cephalothin, nitrofurantoin, gentamicin, or large amounts of oxalic acid (eg, iced tea drinkers) may lead to decreases. High glucose or specific gravity may lead to decreased results. Sensitivity decreases with urinary tract infections characterized by 10^3-10^4 colony forming units/mL.[1] Albumin and ascorbic acid inhibit the method. Tetracycline may cause decreased reactivity or false negatives. Neutropenia can cause false-negative results. Leukocyte esterase is unacceptable as a screen unless combined at least with nitrite testing. Used with nitrite and leukocyte esterase, the urinalysis was not considered a sufficiently strong predictor of urinary tract infection to be utilized as the sole test.[3] Leukocyte esterase, even combined with nitrite, should not

replace microscopy and culture in symptomatic patients. Even combined with nitrite, when used in women having symptoms suggestive of acute cystitis, the selection of specimens for culture would miss approximately 1 in 5 patients who have positive cultures.[1] Urine culture is indicated for subjects with symptoms of urinary tract infection for whom laboratory testing is planned. Treatment of some patients with symptomatic urinary tract infection is straightforward, and laboratory testing may not be needed. Even with pyuria on microscopy, leukocyte esterase was found to be a poor predictor of positive urine cultures.[4]

The suitability of use of leukocyte esterase and nitrate reagent strips for screening for urinary tract infections has been questioned.[2]

Methodology Indoxyl is released by leukocyte esterase if present in the urine specimen. The substrate on the strip is indoxyl carbonic acid ester. Indoxyl is oxidized by atmospheric oxygen to indigo blue. The reaction time is 1 minute, but high sensitivity requires interpretation 5 minutes after immersion in the sample.[5] A package insert provides the following: "Granulocytic leukocytes contain esterases that catalyze the hydrolysis of the derivatized pyrrole amino acid ester to liberate 3-hydroxy-5-phenyl pyrrole. This pyrrole then reacts with a diazonium salt to produce a purple product," copyright Miles Inc.

Additional Information The principal advantage of the method is the ability to identify the presence of leukocyte esterase in dilute urine specimens and in specimens which have been subject to standing with lysis of white cells. When combined with the nitrite test, in some groups reagent strips provided sensitivity for both tests of up to 85% and specificity of 65%, for infections with 10^5 colony forming units/mL. Of 750 obstetric patients, five had negative screening tests and positive cultures, each a gram-positive organism.[6] Another study for detection of asymptomatic urinary tract infections in an obstetric population found Gram staining better than reagent strips or urinalysis.[4] Others support use of the Gram stain.[7,8] See Gram Stain *on page 617*. Urine culture remains the standard for the initial prenatal visit in some practices.[8] Dipstick screening has been compared to Gram stains of unspun urine[9] and to urine sediment microscopy[10,11,12,13] and culture.[12,14] A 1988 proposal indicates that for screening, a clear yellow specimen negative for blood, leukocyte esterase, nitrite, and with ≤30 mg/dL (SI: ≤0.3 g/L) of protein does not require microscopy, but even such samples should be examined by microscopy when from symptomatic subjects or persons with known renal disease.[13] Goldsmith and Campos found the leukocyte esterase comparable to urine sediment microscopy when negative but not positive with predictive accuracy for urines in the range of 10^4-10^5 bacteria/mL.[15]

The number of leukocytes/hpf used as a criterion of infection in urine sediment microscopy has been controversial in the literature.[16] Others would not do away with urine microscopy based on normal dipstick tests.[17,18,19] Sensitivity and specificity of leukocyte esterase and nitrite screening have been criticized.[2,4,20] Leukocyte esterase has been used for detection of sexually transmitted disease in males.[21,22,23] Its use for screening urethritis or urethral pathogens in asymptomatic patients is limited by lack of sufficient sensitivity.[24]

The **acute urethral syndrome** includes symptoms of urgency, frequency, and dysuria with low bacterial counts and with positive leukocyte esterase, indicating 8-10 WBC/hpf.[25]

E. coli is the most common cause of upper urinary tract infection. Complicated urinary tract infections include those associated with stones, diabetes mellitus, instrumentation, immunosuppression, and anatomic abnormalities.[26]

Footnotes

1. Semeniuk H and Church D, "Evaluation of the Leukocyte Esterase and Nitrite Urine Dipstick Screening Tests for Detection of Bacteriuria in Women With Suspected Uncomplicated Urinary Tract Infections," *J Clin Microbiol*, 1999, 37(9):3051-2.
2. Zaman Z, Borremans A, Verhaegen J, et al, "Disappointing Dipstick Screening for Urinary Tract Infection in Hospital Inpatients," *J Clin Pathol*, 1998, 51(6):471-2.
3. Van Nostrand JD, Junkins AD, and Bartholdi RK, "Poor Predictive Ability of Urinalysis and Microscopic Examination to Detect Urinary Tract Infection," *Am J Clin Pathol*, 2000, 113(5):709-13.
4. Bachman JW, Heise RH, Naessens JM, et al, "A Study of Various Tests to Detect Asymptomatic Urinary Tract Infections in an Obstetric Population," *JAMA*, 1993, 270(16):1971-4.
5. Shaw ST Jr, Poon SY, and Wong ET, "Routine Urinalysis, Is the Dipstick Enough?" *JAMA*, 1985, 253(11):1596-600.
6. Robertson AW and Duff P, "The Nitrite and Leukocyte Esterase Tests for the Evaluation of Asymptomatic Bacteriuria in Obstetric Patients," *Obstet Gynecol*, 1988, 71(6 Pt 1):878-81.
7. Keeler LL Jr, "Tests to Detect Asymptomatic Urinary Tract Infection," *JAMA*, 1994, 271(18):1399.
8. Bachman JW, "A Study of Various Tests to Detect Asymptomatic Urinary Tract Infections in an Obstetric Population," *JAMA*, 1994, 271(18):1399.
9. Sewell DL, Burt SP, Gabbert NJ, et al, "Evaluation of the Chemstrip 9™ as a Screening Test for Urinalysis and Urine Culture in Men," *Am J Clin Pathol*, 1985, 83(6):740-3.
10. Scheer WD, "The Detection of Leukocyte Esterase Activity in Urine With a New Reagent Strip," *Am J Clin Pathol*, 1987, 87(1):86-93.
11. Hamoudi AC, Bubis SC, and Thompson C, "Can the Cost Savings of Eliminating Urine Microscopy in Biochemically Negative Urines Be Extended to the Pediatric Population?" *Am J Clin Pathol*, 1986, 86(5):658-60.
12. Loo SY, Scottolini AG, Luanghpinith S, et al, "Performance of a Urine Screening Protocol," *Am J Clin Pathol*, 1986, 85(4):479-84.

13. High SR, Rowe JA, and Maksem JA, "Macroscopic Physiochemical Testing for Screening Urinalysis," *Lab Med*, 1988, 19:174-6.
14. Gutman SI and Solomon RR, "The Clinical Significance of Dipstick-Negative, Culture-Positive Urines in a Veterans Population," *Am J Clin Pathol*, 1987, 88(2):204-9.
15. Goldsmith BM and Campos JM, "Comparison of Urine Dipstick, Microscopy, and Culture for the Detection of Bacteriuria in Children," *Clin Pediatr (Phila)*, 1990, 29(4):214-8.
16. Wilson DM, "Tests to Detect Asymptomatic Urinary Tract Infection," *JAMA*, 1994, 271(18):1399.
17. Morrison MC and Lum G, "Dipstick Testing of Urine - Can It Replace Urine Microscopy?" *Am J Clin Pathol*, 1986, 85(5):590-4.
18. Nanji AA, Adam W, and Campbell DJ, "Routine Microscopic Examination of the Urine Sediment, Should We Continue?" *Arch Pathol Lab Med*, 1984, 108(5):399-400.
19. Propp DA, Weber D, and Ciesla ML, "Reliability of a Urine Dipstick in Emergency Department Patients," *Ann Emerg Med*, 1989, 18(5):560-3.
20. Wilkins EG, Ratcliffe JG, and Roberts C, "Leukocyte Esterase-Nitrite Screening Method for Pyuria and Bacteriuria," *J Clin Pathol*, 1985, 38(12):1342-5.
21. Sadof MD, Woods ER, and Emans SJ, "Dipstick Leukocyte Esterase Activity in First-Catch Urine Specimens: A Useful Screening Test for Detecting Sexually Transmitted Disease in the Adolescent Male," *JAMA*, 1987, 258(14):1932-4.
22. Shafer MA, Schacter J, Moscicki AB, et al, "Urinary Leukocyte Esterase Screening Test for Asymptomatic Chlamydial and Gonococcal Infections in Males," *JAMA*, 1989, 262(18):2562-6.
23. Tyndall MW, Nasio J, Maitha G, et al, "Leukocyte Esterase Urine Strips for the Screening of Men With Urethritis - Use in Developing Countries," *Genitourin Med*, 1994, 70(1):3-6.
24. Patrick DM, Rekart ML, and Knowles L, "Unsatisfactory Performance of the Leukocyte Esterase Test of First Voided Urine for Rapid Diagnosis of Urethritis," *Genitourin Med*, 1994, 70(3):187-90.
25. Sodeman TM, "A Practical Strategy for Diagnosis of Urinary Tract Infections," *Clin Lab Med*, 1995, 15(2):235-50.
26. Roberts JA, "Management of Pyelonephritis and Upper Urinary Tract Infections," *Urol Clin North Am*, 1999, 26(4):753-63.

References

Bartlett RC, Zern DA, Ratkiewicz I, et al, "Reagent Strip Screening for Sediment Abnormalities Identified by Automated Microscopy in Urine From Patients Suspected to Have Urinary Tract Disease," *Arch Pathol Lab Med*, 1994, 118(11):1096-101.

Carroll KC, Hale DC, Von Boerum DH, et al, "Laboratory Evaluation of Urinary Tract Infections in an Ambulatory Clinic," *Am J Clin Pathol*, 1994, 101(1):100-3.

Hurlbut TA, 3d and Littenberg B, "The Diagnostic Accuracy of Rapid Dipstick Tests to Predict Urinary Tract Infection," *Am J Clin Pathol*, 1991, 96(5):582-8.

Lachs MS, Nachamkin I, Edelstein PH, et al, "Spectrum Bias in the Evaluation of Diagnostic Tests: Lessons From the Rapid Dipstick Test for Urinary Tract Infection," *Ann Intern Med*, 1992, 117(2):135-40.

Nygaard IE and Johnson JM, "Urinary Tract Infections in Elderly Women," *Am Fam Phys*, 1996, 53(1):175-82.

Romero R, Emamian M, Wan M, et al, "The Value of the Leukocyte Esterase Test in Diagnosing Intra-Amniotic Infection," *Am J Perinatol*, 1988, 5(1):64-9.

Smalley DL, Kraus AP, and Baddour LM, "Clinical Use of the Leukocyte Esterase Test in Continuous Ambulatory Peritoneal Dialysis," *Lab Med*, 1988, 19:164-6.

Stamm WE and Hooton TM, "Management of Urinary Tract Infections in Adults," *N Engl J Med*, 1993, 329(18):1328-34.

White LV and Kunin CM, "Leukocyte Esterase Tests Detect Pyuria, Not Bacteriuria," *Ann Intern Med*, 1993, 118(3):230.

♦ **Lipiduria** *see Fat, Urine on page 874*

Microalbuminuria

Related Information

Glucose, Fasting, Plasma *on page 183*
Glucose, Postglucose Load, Plasma *on page 185*
Glycated Hemoglobin (Hemoglobin A_{1c}), Blood *on page 188*
Insulin, Serum *on page 201*
Protein Electrophoresis, Urine *on page 268*
Protein, Quantitative, Urine *on page 883*
Protein, Semiquantitative, Urine *on page 885*
Urinalysis *on page 887*
Urine Collection, 24-Hour *on page 47*

Synonyms Oligoalbuminuria

Applies to Albumin:Creatinine Ratio; Albumin Excretion

Test Includes Creatinine clearance may be advised from the same urine collection.

Abstract "Microalbumin" is not the name of a substance, but refers to the urinary excretion of a small, but diagnostically and prognostically important, quantity of protein. Specifically, the term, "microalbuminuria", refers to the urinary excretion of 30-300 mg/24 hours (or 200-200 μg/minute). This concentration is too low to be detected accurately by dipstick testing. It is very important for patients with diabetes mellitus to undergo microalbuminuria testing, because a positive result indicates early, but potentially reversible, diabetic nephropathy.[1,2]

Diabetic nephropathy includes glomerular disease, which is manifested as proteinuria. Small losses initially are detectable as microalbuminuria, developing after periods of hyperglycemia. Microalbuminuria is a test for early increase of proteinuria in diabetes mellitus and in preeclampsia, before proteinuria becomes evident by conventional urinalysis. Microalbuminuria may be considered a surrogate marker for renal disease,[3] an indicator of (Continued)

Microalbuminuria *(Continued)*

early, reversible glomerulopathy.[1] The leading cause of end-stage renal failure in the Western world is diabetic renal disease.[4] About 35% of subjects with type I (insulin-dependent diabetes mellitus) (IDDM) develop nephropathy, which is characterized by proteinuria with decreasing glomerular filtration rate.[5] Improvement in glycemic control exerts a beneficial effect on the rate of progression of microalbuminuria to macroalbuminuria.

Specimen A 24-hour urine specimen is best; timed overnight 10-hour collection, or spot AM urine after initial voiding may be used. Albumin:creatinine ratio in a random specimen is best done on a first-morning voiding.

Storage Instructions Refrigeration and freezing are usually acceptable; review instructions for the laboratory which will perform the test.[6]

Turnaround Time Often sent to a reference laboratory

Reference Interval <20 mg/L (SI: <0.02 g/L) or ≤30 mg/24 hours (SI: ≤0.03 g/day). For spot AM samples, <0.03 mg albumin/mg creatinine[7]

Critical Values "Microalbuminuria" is defined as albuminuria of 20-200 µg/minute, or 30-300 mg/24 hours.[1,8] Higher levels than these are regarded as diagnostic of diabetes nephropathy.[9] **Albumin:creatinine ratio** >30 mg/g predicts an overnight excretion rate >30 µg/minute.[1]

Use Microalbuminuria testing is used to detect albuminuria in diabetes mellitus, preeclampsia, hypertension, and systemic lupus erythematosus. Its major role is to attempt to predict subsequent development of proteinuria, diabetic nephropathy, serious extrarenal cardiovascular disease,[2] and early mortality in type I and/or II diabetes.[10] Time between appearance of microalbuminuria and full-blown proteinuria is typically in the range of 1-5 years.[2] This testing is proving useful in the management of patients with relatively early diabetes mellitus to try to avoid or delay the onset of diabetic renal disease. Intensive treatment, with tight control of diabetes, has delayed onset and reduced progression of microalbuminuria and albuminuria in subjects with IDDM.[8] The risk of microalbuminuria in such patients increases when hemoglobin A_1 exceeds 10.1% (which is equivalent to hemoglobin A_{1c} of 8.1%).[11]

Limitations The relationship between microalbuminuria and glycemia may not be linear.[12] The Clinitek® Microalbumin System reacts with Tamm-Horsfall mucoprotein. Diurnal variation in urine albumin excretion exists; it is 30% to 50% less at night.

Increased excretion may be secondary to exercise, pregnancy, febrile/inflammatory disorders, urinary tract infection, bleeding in the urinary tract, or benign postural proteinuria.[13]

Methodology Radial immunodiffusion (RID), enzyme-linked immunosorbent assay (ELISA), immunoturbidimetric methods,[12,14] radioimmunoassay (RIA).[10] Nephelometric and latex particle methods are described. A strip detection method is based on enzyme immunoassay. A test strip for low concentrations of albumin in urine has been developed ("Micral-Test") and tested.[9,15] It has excellent specificity (97.5%) but sensitivity of only 69.5% to 87.7%.[9] The Micral II test strip has become available, and is described as the most practical such system. The Clinitek® Microalbumin test strip bears an additional pad to estimate creatinine.[1] For spot AM sample, determine simultaneous urine creatinine.

Additional Information Of ~12 million Americans who have diabetes, 90% have noninsulin-dependent diabetes. Normal albuminuria is <20 mg/L, much lower than the sensitivity of current urinalysis with dipstick (150-300 mg/L). In insulin-dependent diabetes mellitus, detectable diabetic nephropathy begins with onset of microalbuminuria, 40-300 mg albumin in 24 hours. Such microalbuminuria may begin 5 years from onset of diabetes mellitus. In a 1995 study, the median duration from onset of microalbuminuria to development of diabetic nephropathy was 7 years.[16] In another study, 21% of patients developed end-stage kidney disease over 35 years of follow-up.[17] In addition to nephropathy, onset of increased hypertension and retinopathy is also preceded by microalbuminuria. The risk of cardiovascular disease is 30-40 times greater in those with nephropathy.[18] In IDDM, persistent increase of urine albumin excretion bears association with diabetic nephropathy and end-stage kidney disease in 80% of patients. In NIDDM, persistent increase of urine albumin excretion bears association with diabetic nephropathy in about 25%.[9]

Modifiable factors predict development of microalbuminuria and macroalbuminuria in subjects with NIDDM and IDDM with normal excretion of albumin. These include urine albumin excretion rate >15 mg/day, high levels of hyperglycemia, hypercholesterolemia, hypertension, and smoking.

See Glycated Hemoglobin (Hemoglobin A_{1c}), Blood *on page 188.*

Footnotes

1. Kutter D, "A Chemical Test Strip to Determine Low Concentration of Albumin and Creatinine in Urine," *Lab Med*, 1998, 29(12):769-72.
2. Hostetter TH, "Diabetes and the Kidney," *Cecil Textbook of Medicine*, 21st ed, Chapter 110, Goldman L and Bennett JC, eds, Philadelphia, PA: WB Saunders Co, 2000, 610-3.
3. Viberti G, "A Glycemic Threshold for Diabetic Complications?" *N Engl J Med*, 1995, 332(19):1293-4.
4. Viberti G, Mogensen CE, Groop LC, et al, "Effect of Captopril on Progression to Clinical Proteinuria in Patients With Insulin-Dependent Diabetes Mellitus and Microalbuminuria," *JAMA*, 1994, 271(4):275-9.
5. Remuzzi G and Ruggenenti P, "Slowing the Progression of Diabetic Nephropathy," *N Engl J Med*, 1993, 329(20):1496-7.
6. "For Your Information: Urine Testing Update - Preservatives for the Collection, Transportation, and Storage of Urine," *Mayo References Services Communique*, March 1999.

7. Ellis D, Coonrod BA, Dorman JS, et al, "Choice of Urine Sample Predictive of Microalbuminuria in Patients With Insulin-Dependent Diabetes Mellitus," *Am J Kidney Dis*, 1989, 13(4):321-8.
8. Jacobson HR and Striker GE, "Report on a Workshop to Develop Management Recommendations for the Prevention of Progression in Chronic Renal Disease," *Am J Kidney Dis*, 1995, 25(1):103-6.
9. Gossain VV, Gunaga KP, Carella MJ, et al, "Utility of Micral Test Strips in Screening for Microalbuminuria," *Arch Pathol Lab Med*, 1996, 120:1015-8.
10. Mogensen CE, "Microalbuminuria Predicts Clinical Proteinuria and Early Mortality in Maturity-Onset Diabetes," *N Engl J Med*, 1984, 310(6):356-60.
11. Krolewski AS, Laffel LM, Krolewski M, et al, "Glycosylated Hemoglobin and the Risk of Microalbuminuria in Patients With Insulin-Dependent Diabetes Mellitus," *N Engl J Med*, 1995, 332(19):1251-5.
12. Hindmarsh JT, "Microalbuminuria" *Clin Lab Med*, 1988, 8(3):611-6.
13. Emancipator K, "Laboratory Diagnosis and Monitoring of Diabetes Mellitus," *Am J Clin Pathol*, 1999, 112(5):665-74.
14. "Method Changes for Microalbuminuria Urine Tests," *Mayo Communique*, 1999, 24(11):3.
15. Jury DR, Mikkelsen DJ, Glen D, et al, "Assessment of Micral-Test Microalbuminuria Test Strip in the Laboratory and in Diabetic Outpatients," *Ann Clin Biochem*, 1992, 29(Pt 1):96-100.
16. Mathiesen ER, Ronn B, Storm B, et al, "The National Course of Microalbuminuria in Insulin-Dependent Diabetes: A 10-Year Prospective Study," *Diabet Med*, 1995, 12(6):482-7.
17. Krolewski M, Eggers PW, and Warram JH, "Magnitude of End-Stage Renal Disease in IDDM: A 35 Year Follow-up study," *Kidney Int*, 1996, 50(6):2041-6.
18. Nathan, DM, "Long-Term Complications of Diabetes Mellitus," *N Engl J Med*, 1993, 328(23):1676-85.

References

Campbell FM, "Microalbuminuria and Nephropathy in Insulin Dependent Diabetes Mellitus," *Arch Dis Child*, 1995, 73(1):4-7.

Chapman AB, Johnson AM, Gabow PA, et al, "Overt Proteinuria and Microalbuminuria in Autosomal Dominant Polycystic Kidney Disease," *J Am Soc Nephrol*, 1994, 5(6):1349-54.

Chavers BM, Bilous RW, Ellis EN, et al, "Glomerular Lesions and Urinary Albumin Excretion in Type 1 Diabetes Without Overt Proteinuria," *N Engl J Med*, 1989, 320(15):966-70.

Nelson RG, Bennett PH, Beck GJ, et al, "Development and Progression of Renal Disease in Pima Indians With Noninsulin-Dependent Diabetes Mellitus," *N Engl J Med*, 1996, 335(22):1636-42.

Parving HH, "Initiation and Progression of Diabetic Nephropathy," *N Engl J Med*, 1996, 335(22):1682-3.

Shihabi ZK, Konen JC, and O'Connor ML, "Albuminuria vs Urinary Total Protein for Detecting Chronic Renal Disorders," *Clin Chem*, 1991, 37(5):621-4.

Townsend JC, "Increased Albumin Excretion in Diabetes," *J Clin Pathol*, 1990, 43(1):3-8.

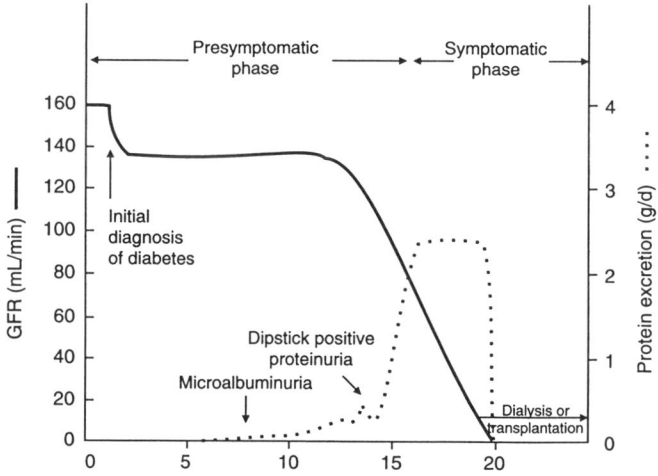

Adapted from Hostetter TH, "Diabetes and the Kidney," *Cecil Textbok of Medicine*, 21st ed, Chapter 110, Goldman L and Bennett JC, eds, Philadelphia, PA: WB Saunders Co, 2000, 610-3.

Myoglobin, Qualitative, Urine

Related Information

Blood, Urine *on page 870*
Carboxyhemoglobin, Blood *on page 784*
Cocaine (Cocaine Metabolite), Qualitative, Urine or Hair *on page 785*
Coccidioidomycosis Serology *on page 593*
Creatine Kinase, Serum *on page 158*
Hemoglobin, Qualitative, Urine *on page 875*
Lactate Dehydrogenase Isoenzymes, Serum *on page 206*
Malaria Smear and Tests *on page 458*
Muscle Biopsy *on page 69*
Myoglobin, Blood, Serum, or Plasma *on page 228*

Troponins, Serum *on page 291*

Synonyms Myoglobin Screen, Urine

Abstract Myoglobin facilitates movement of oxygen into striated muscle cells and facilitates its storage. It appears in plasma following damage to cardiac or striated muscle (eg, as in rhabdomyolysis). Release of large quantities of myoglobin into the circulation, especially in the presence of shock, can lead to acute renal failure[1] (eg, in massive crush injury).

The finding of dark red to dark brown to tea-colored urine positive on reagent strip for blood, without red cells on microscopy, suggests the presence of myoglobin or hemoglobin.

Specimen Random urine

Container Clean, chemical-free, plastic (preferable) urine container

Storage Instructions Stable for 12 days in urine when the pH is adjusted to between 8.0 and 9.5; stable for 1 month in serum.[2]

Reference Interval Negative (<5 ng/mL)

Use Assay for the presence of myoglobinuria is used to investigate myositis and other entities which damage muscle. Extensive injury to striated muscle is accompanied by high serum CK and may be accompanied by myoglobinuria.[3] See table.

Causes of Myoglobinuria: Summary

Metabolic – impaired substrate utilization for energy metabolism	Enzyme deficiencies (LD and others), substrate deficiency, hypokalemia, hypophosphatemia, hypomagnesemia
Excessive muscle use	Severe/unaccustomed exercise, seizures, march hemoglobinuria with myoglobinuria
Hyperpyrexia	Heat stroke, exertional hyperthermia, hyperthermia associated with drug use (eg, cocaine), heat injury
Postinfections	
viral	Influenza A, herpes simplex, Epstein-Barr, Coxsackie, AIDS
bacterial	Fever and sepsis, clostridial with gangrene; *Legionella*, *Streptococcus sp*, *Francisella tularemia*, *Salmonella sp*
Primary muscle disease	Muscular dystrophy, McArdle disease, polymyositis, dermatomyositis, familial paroxysmal myoglobinuria, steroids and other drugs
Poisoning	
drug	Carbon monoxide, alcohol, barbiturate, cocaine, amphetamine, phencyclidine, neuroleptic malignant syndrome
animal	Hoff disease (fish poisoning), sea snake bite (*Enhydrina schistosa*), trichinosis
Ischemia	Myocardial infarction, vascular occlusion (thromboembolism or external vascular compression); infarction of large muscle, anterior tibial syndrome
Traumatic	Crush injury, wounds, surgical muscle trauma, beatings, high voltage or lightning electrical injury, electrocution, limb compression with prolonged immobilization due to sleep, anesthesia, or coma

Limitations Presence of hypochlorite or microbial peroxidase or other oxidizing contaminants may cause false-positive reactions. Presence of ascorbic acid (high concentrations) may decrease sensitivity. **Serum testing is recommended.**

Methodology Qualitative or screening methods are based on the oxidation of a chromogen (eg, ortho-toluidine) with production of a colored compound. This reaction is catalyzed by hemoglobin or myoglobin. Test sensitivity is about 0.3 mg/dL (SI: 3 mg/L).[4] Specificity for myoglobin can be obtained by the ammonium sulfate test.[4] If initial testing is positive for blood (or myoglobin), preparation of an 80% saturated urine solution of ammonium sulfate will precipitate hemoglobin. On filtering or centrifugation myoglobin stays in solution. Color in the supernatant indicates presence of myoglobin pigment. Electrophoresis can provide definitive differentiation between hemoglobin and myoglobin. Immunoassays[1] (immunodiffusion (ID), isoelectric focusing (IEF), radioimmunoassay (RIA), immunoprecipitation, immunonephelometric, and hemagglutination inhibition (HAI)) can also be used in the determination of myoglobin. Four different immunoassays for serum and urine have been compared. Within run coefficients of variability from 5% to 13% with biases seen between assays was reported.[1]

Additional Information Myoglobin is released from cardiac/skeletal muscle, filtered by renal glomeruli and excreted in the urine. Resultant urine, depending upon the amount of excreted myoglobin varies in hue and intensity of red/brown/black color and is often referred to as cola colored. Myoglobin causes a false-positive reaction for urine hemoglobin on dipsticks. Plasma myoglobin, not bound to haptoglobin, has a renal threshold of 0.5-1.5 mg/dL.[5] Muscle injury (metabolic or traumatic, see table) releases myoglobin into the circulation, from which it is rapidly cleared into the urine. Plasma half-life of myoglobin is about 1-3 hours.[5]

Myoglobinuria has been associated with renal failure; rhabdomyolysis causes 5% to 7% of all instances of acute renal failure in the U.S.[5] Renal failure itself may cause high serum myoglobin level.[6] Myoglobinuric renal failure commonly complicates rhabdomyolysis of either traumatic and metabolic origin. The mechanism of renal injury is unknown but does not appear to be solely due to nephrotoxicity of myoglobin. The combined effects of toxic products released in rhabdomyolysis with hypotension, and electrolyte imbalance may play a role in pathogenesis of the renal failure. Recent studies have suggested that endothelin-1, a potent vasoconstrictor, is responsible, in part, for the massive tubular necrosis that can be observed in myoglobinuric nephropathy.[7]

Renal failure associated with the use of cocaine may develop as a result of cocaine-induced renal artery vasoconstriction, renal ischemia, and tubular damage.[8] Myoglobinuria may occur with myocardial infarction.[9] Myoglobin deposits in the kidney are demonstrable by immunofluorescent techniques.[10] There are a few reports of rhabdomyolysis-induced renal failure occurring in cases of child abuse.[11] Use of neuroleptic agents in individuals with or without predisposing factors (exhaustion, dehydration, others) may result in the neuroleptic malignant syndrome, a hyperpyrexic syndrome that may be fatal,[12] and associated with elevated creatine kinase concentrations and with myoglobinuria. The dark urine color associated with myoglobinuria develops on standing or in the bladder at acid pH.

The pathophysiology of cocaine- (and other drugs of abuse) induced rhabdomyolysis is not clearly established. In addition to presence of serum and urine myoglobin, there is striking increase in serum **CK** and elevations of **LD (LDH)**, **AST (SGOT)**, and **ALT (SGPT)**. Cocaine blocks presynaptic reuptake of neurotransmitters at postsynaptic receptor sites. In some cases, rhabdomyolysis subsequent to use of cocaine may relate to ischemia of arterial vasoconstriction, to muscle activity associated with dysphoric agitation, and/or to hyperthermia. The most common cause, however, of rhabdomyolysis related to use of abused drugs is limb compression during sleep or coma.[8] Serum CK is usually normal with hemolysis, in which serum LD is generally increased with high LD_1. With circulating myoglobin, serum CK is usually very high, serum LD may be moderately increased, but it is LD_5 that is usually elevated on LD isoenzyme electrophoresis. An isomorphic pattern of LD isoenzymes may also be seen. When no specific cause of rhabdomyolysis is apparent, or when precipitating physical exercise was not extreme, or when CPK does not return to baseline, muscle biopsy with measurement of specific muscle enzymes may be indicated. In 77 such muscle biopsies, enzyme deficiencies were noted in 36 patients.[13] A metabolic cause of myoglobinuria is carnitine palmitoyl-transferase II deficiency.[14] Psychiatric patients with autoaggressive behavior may represent a special risk group for the development of rhabdomyolysis and subsequent myoglobinuria.[15]

Alcoholics may suffer hypokalemic myopathy in which myoglobinuria may be found.

Rhabdomyolysis with myoglobinuria as well as hemoglobinuria may complicate *Plasmodium falciparum* malaria.[16]

Footnotes

1. Loun B, Astles R, Copeland KR, et al, "Adaptation of a Quantitative Immunoassay for Urine Myoglobin. Predictor in Detecting Renal Dysfunction," *Am J Clin Pathol*, 1996, 105(4):479-86.
2. Wu AH, Laios I, Green S, et al, "Immunoassays for Serum and Urine Myoglobin: Myoglobin Clearance Assessed as a Risk Factor for Acute Renal Failure," *Clin Chem*, 1994, 40(5):796-802.
3. Laios ID, Caruk R, and Wu AH, "Myoglobin Clearance as an Early Indicator for Rhabdomyolysis-Induced Acute Renal Failure," *Ann Clin Lab Sci*, 1995, 25(2):179-84.
4. Race GJ and White MG, "Urinary Pigments," *Basic Urinalysis*, Chapter 12, Hagerstown, MD: Harper & Row Publishers, 1979, 50-1.
5. Slater MS and Mullins RJ, "Rhabdomyolysis and Myoglobinuric Renal Failure in Trauma and Surgical Patients: A Review," *J Am Coll Surg*, 1998, 186(6):693-716.
6. Feinfeld DA, Briscoe AM, Nurse HM, et al, "Myoglobinuria in Chronic Renal Failure," *Am J Kidney Dis*, 1986, 8(2):111-4.
7. Karam H, Bruneval P, Clozel JP, et al, "Role of Endothelin in Acute Renal Failure Due to Rhabdomyolysis in Rats," *J Pharmacol Exp Ther*, 1995, 274(1):481-6.
8. Pogue VA and Nurse HM, "Cocaine-Associated Acute Myoglobinuric Renal Failure," *Am J Med*, 1989, 86(2):183-6.
9. Levine RS, Alterman M, Gubner RS, et al, "Myoglobinuria in Myocardial Infarction," *Am J Med Sci*, 1971, 262(3):179-83.
10. Kagen LJ, "Immunofluorescent Demonstration of Myoglobin in the Kidney. Case Report and Review of Forty-Three Cases of Myoglobinemia and Myoglobinuria Identified Immunologically," *Am J Med*, 1970, 48(5):649-53.
11. Mukherji SK and Siegel MJ, "Rhabdomyolysis and Renal Failure in Child Abuse," *AJR Am J Roentgenol*, 1987, 148(6):1203-4.
12. Guzé BH and Baxter LR Jr, "Current Concepts. Neuroleptic Malignant Syndrome," *N Engl J Med*, 1985, 313(3):163-6.
13. Tonin P, Lewis P, Servidei S, et al, "Metabolic Causes of Myoglobinuria," *Ann Neurol*, 1990, 27(2):181-5.
14. Venturini E and Pupeschi L, "Myoglobinuria Due to a Deficiency of Carnitine Palmitoyltransferase II. A Clinical Case Report," *Recenti Prog Med*, 1994, 85(5):282-3.
15. Zwettler U, Lippert J, Andrassy K, et al, "Acute Myoglobinuric Kidney Failure as a Consequence of Autoaggressive Behavior in Mental Retardation," *Deutsche Medizinische Wochenschrift*, 1994, 119(28-9):994-8.
16. Knochel JP and Moore GE, "Rhabdomyolysis in Malaria," *N Engl J Med*, 1993, 329(16):1206-7.

(Continued)

Myoglobin, Qualitative, Urine *(Continued)*

References

Henry JB, Lauzon RB, and Schumann GB, "Basic Examination of Urine," *Clinical Diagnosis and Management by Laboratory Methods*, 19th ed, Chapter 18, ed, Philadelphia, PA: WB Saunders Co, 1996, 411-56.

Thakur V, DeSalvo J, McGrath H Jr, et al, "Case Report: Polymyositis-Induced Myoglobinuric Acute Renal Failure," *Am J Med Sci*, 1996, 312(2):85-7.

Zager RA, "Rhabdomyolysis and Myohemoglobinuric Acute Renal Failure," *Kidney Int*, 1996, 49(2):314-26.

◆ **Myoglobin Screen, Urine** *see* Myoglobin, Qualitative, Urine *on page 880*

◆ **Nephrolithiasis Analysis** *see* Kidney Stone Analysis *on page 877*

Nitrite, Urine

Related Information

Bacterial Culture, Urine *on page 578*
Leukocyte Esterase, Urine *on page 878*
Urinalysis *on page 887*

Synonyms Bacteria Screen, Urine

Applies to Urinary Tract Infection Screen; UTI Screen

Test Includes This test is usually part of a routine urinalysis.

Abstract A rapid screening method for detection of bacteriuria, reacting with those bacteria which reduce urinary nitrate to nitrite. Urine dipstick testing is not consistently more sensitive than Gram stain and in some studies, does not compare favorably with Gram staining.[1] A lack of sensitivity for leukocyte esterase, nitrite, and presence of bacteria in urine microscopy as indicators of urinary tract infection provide support for the need culture.[2] **The best test for urinary tract infection is culture, which remains the definitive test to ascertain whether or not urinary tract infection is present.**

Specimen Urine, first morning specimen is preferred; random urine is acceptable; preferably midstream, clean catch collection; catheterized specimen; bladder aspiration

Storage Instructions Refrigeration is important if the specimen cannot be promptly processed.

Causes for Rejection A random urine is less likely to produce a positive reaction, in the presence of urinary tract infection, than an overnight specimen.

Reference Interval Negative

Use A reagent strip method is intended to detect the presence of potentially significant bacteriuria and aid in the diagnosis of cystitis, pyelonephritis, urinary tract infection in concert with leukocyte esterase. Dipstick screen for detection of bacteriuria performs best when there are $>10^5$ CFU/mL, when leukocyte esterase and urinary nitrite are used together; however, sensitivity when so used has been disappointing.[3,4]

Limitations The sensitivity of the nitrite test is decreased with high specific gravity and with high ascorbic acid content.[5] False negatives can occur when dipsticks are stored at ambient humidity.[6] False negatives are relatively common and relate to varying retention times of urine in the bladder, varying urinary nitrate concentrations (diet dependent) and the presence and quantity of nitrate reducing organisms present. Storage of sample at room temperature for excessive periods (more than 2 hours) may lead to reduction of nitrite to nitrogen. Some urinary tract infections are caused by organisms which do not contain reductase to convert nitrate to nitrite. (Negative results are found when infecting organisms do not convert nitrate to nitrite). These include infections caused by *Streptococcus faecalis* and other gram-positive cocci, *N. gonorrhoeae*, and *M. tuberculosis*.

In addition, the urine may not have been retained in the bladder for 4 hours or more to allow adequate reduction of nitrate to occur. In detection of asymptomatic urinary tract infections in obstetric patients, dipstick nitrite testing identified only 50% of the patients with such infections and was less sensitive than Gram staining. It was reported to be superior to urinalysis.[1]

Leukocyte esterase alone provides higher sensitivity than nitrite used alone.[3]

Methodology This reaction depends upon the conversion of nitrate to nitrite by the action of certain species of urinary bacteria. Nitrite from the urine reacts with *p*-arsanilic acid forming a diazonium compound. The diazonium compound couples with 1,2,3,4-tetrahydrobenzo(h)quinolin-3-ol. A color indicator produces a uniform pink color.[5]

Other Screening Methods for Detection of Urinary Tract Infection

	Sensitivity (%)	Specificity (%)
Microscopic analysis on spun urine	79	93
Methylene blue stain for pyuria	60	99
Gram stain for pyuria	45	93
Gram stain for bacteriuria	65	75

Adapted from Carroll KC, Hale DC, Von Boerum DH, et al, "Laboratory Evaluation of Urinary Tract Infections in an Ambulatory Clinic," *Am J Clin Pathol*, 1994, 101(1):100-3.

Additional Information A positive nitrite test is strongly suggestive of urinary tract infection (ie, $\geq 10^5$ organisms/mL). Therefore, when positive, a urine culture is recommended, but **urine culture is indicated in any case if the patient is symptomatic.** The use of nitrate and leukocyte esterase together is more extensively discussed in Leukocyte Esterase, Urine *on page 878*. See as well discussion in other tests noted in the related information field above.

For $>10^5$ colony counts/mL, the sensitivity of the nitrite test was recently reported as 27% and specificity 94%. The authors concluded that leukocyte esterase and nitrite dipstick tests are unsuitable for screening for urinary tract infections.[4]

Footnotes

1. Bachman JW, Heise RH, Naessens JM, et al, "A Study of Various Tests to Detect Asymptomatic Urinary Tract Infections in an Obstetric Population," *JAMA*, 1993, 270(16):1971-4.
2. Van Nostrand JD, Junkins AD, Bartholdi RK, "Poor Predictive Ability of Urinalysis and Microscopic Examination to Detect Urinary Tract Infection," *Am J Clin Pathol*, 2000, 113(5):709-13.
3. Semeniuk H and Church D, "Evaluation of the Leukocyte Esterase and Nitrite Dipstick Screening Tests for Detection of Bacteriuria in Women With Suspected Uncomplicated Urinary Tract Infections," *J Clin Microbiol*, 1999, 37(9):3051-2.
4. Zaman Z, Borremans A, Verhaegen J, et al, "Disappointing Dipstick Screening for Urinary Tract Infection in Hospital Inpatients," *J Clin Pathol*, 1998, 51(6):471-2.
5. Walters CS, "Why Can a Urine Specimen Have a Negative Nitrite Result on a Dipstick Reagent Test Yet Yield a Positive Urine Culture?" *Lab Med*, 1999, 30(1):22-3.
6. Gallagher EJ, Schwartz E, and Weinstein RS, "Performance Characteristics of Urine Dipsticks Stored in Open Containers," *Am J Emerg Med*, 1990, 8(2):121-3.

References

Alon US, Hellerstein S, and Warady BA, "Assessment and Interpretations of Urinalysis and Routine Kidney Function Tests. Part I: Urinalysis," *Children's Hospital Quarterly*, 1990, 2:317-23.

Bartlett RC, Zern DA, Ratkiewicz I, et al, "Reagent Strip Screening for Sediment Abnormalities Identified by Automated Microscopy in Urine From Patients Suspected to Have Urinary Tract Disease," *Arch Pathol Lab Med*, 1994, 118(11):1096-101.

Congdon DD and Fedorko DP, "Evaluation of Two Rapid Urine Screening Tests," *Lab Med*, 1992, 23(9):613-5.

Connoly A and Thorp JM Jr, "Urinary Tract Infections in Pregnancy," *Urol Clin North Am*, 1999, 26(4):779-87.

Hurlbut TA, 3d and Littenberg B, "The Diagnostic Accuracy of Rapid Dipstick Tests to Predict Urinary Tract Infection," *Am J Clin Pathol*, 1991, 96(5):582-8.

Lachs MS, Nachamkin I, Edelstein PH, et al, "Spectrum Bias in the Evaluation of Diagnostic Tests: Lessons From the Rapid Dipstick Test for Urinary Tract Infection," *Ann Intern Med*, 1992, 117(2):135-40.

Rippin KP, Stinson WC, Eisenstadt J, et al, "Clinical Evaluation of the Slide Centrifuge (Cytospin) Gram's Stained Smear for the Detection of Bacteriuria and Comparison With the Filtracheck-UTI and UTIscreen," *Am J Clin Pathol*, 1995, 103(3):316-9.

◆ **Nitroprusside Reaction for Ketones, Urine** *see* Ketones, Urine *on page 877*

◆ **Occult Blood, Semiquantitative, Urine** *see* Urinalysis *on page 887*

◆ **Occult Blood, Urine** *see* Blood, Urine *on page 870*

◆ **Oligoalbuminuria** *see* Microalbuminuria *on page 879*

pH, Urine

Related Information

Kidney Stone Analysis *on page 877*
Mexiletine, Serum *on page 757*
pH, Blood *on page 247*
Salicylate, Serum or Plasma *on page 806*
Urinalysis *on page 887*

Test Includes pH is part of a routine urinalysis.

Abstract Acids excreted by the renal glomeruli include sulfuric, phosphoric and hydrochloric with small quantities of pyruvic, citric, and lactic acids and when present, ketone bodies. Bicarbonate is reabsorbed. Sodium of the glomerular filtrate is exchanged for hydrogen ions. NH_4 is excreted.

Specimen Random urine

Storage Instructions If the specimen cannot be processed promptly, it should be refrigerated. (Bacterial proliferation shifts pH to >8.0, and carbon dioxide is lost on standing).

Reference Interval Normal kidneys can produce urine with pH from 4.6-8.0, but with ordinary diet, urine pH is about 6.0. Urine becomes more alkaline after meals because acid is secreted by gastric mucosa. Urine is most acidic fasting in the morning. Proteins cause lower pH, and citrus fruits induce higher pH.

Use pH is the negative of the log of the hydrogen ion (H^+) concentration. pH is related to the concentrations of undissociated acid and their corresponding anions. pH essentially is a measure of the potential difference which develops between the solution inside a pH electrode and the solution (in this case urine) being measured.

Urine pH is a crude measure of the acid-base balance of the body. It may be helpful in determination of renal tubular disease or pyelonephritis. Urine pH is useful for identification of crystals in urine and determination of predisposition to formation of a given type of stone. Control of urinary pH is important in management of nephrolithiasis. See table. When an accurate pH assessment of acid-base status and renal response is desired, the urine should be collected under circumstances more controlled than is usual. Attention is given to the time of day, the fasting status of the patient, and transfer of sample so as to prevent degassing of sample or growth of bacteria; rapid analysis by pH meter rather than dipstick is indicated. Simultaneous serum pH may also be ordered.

> **Conditions Associated With Acid Urine**
> Metabolic acidosis
> Diabetes mellitus
> Diarrhea
> Starvation
> Respiratory acidosis
> Emphysema
> Sleep
> Renal failure with lack of NH_3 buffer
> **Conditions Associated With Alkaline Urine**
> Respiratory alkalosis
> Metabolic alkalosis
> Urea-splitting bacteria (*Proteus* sp)
> Vegetable diet
> Gastric suction and vomiting
> Diuretic therapy
> Urine allowed to stand
> Postprandial alkaline tide (1 hour after meal)
> Alkali therapy (citrate, bicarbonate)
> Renal tubular acidosis

Limitations On standing urine becomes alkaline due to the action of urea splitting bacteria (*Proteus* sp). False decrease of pH occurs should urine spill from the protein region of the reagent strip.

Methodology Dipstick double indicator principle (methyl red and bromthymol blue) which gives a broad range of colors covering the urinary pH range 5-9 ±0.5 pH units. A pH meter is the back-up and most accurate method.

Additional Information Dietary factors affect urine pH. Alkaline urine is observed in persons who eat large quantities of citrus fruit and vegetables. Acid urine is observed with high meat intake. Pyridium® metabolites may mask the pH reaction. Urine pH >6.5 indicates presence of bicarbonate while pH <5.5 indicates absence of bicarbonate. Consistently acid urine, pH <5.5, is associated with xanthine, cystine, and uric acid stones. Calcium oxalate and apatite stones are not associated with any particular disturbance of urine pH. Alkaline urine (pH >7) is associated with calcium carbonate, calcium phosphate, and especially magnesium ammonium phosphate stones. In conjunction with serum pH and bicarbonate levels, urine pH may be applied to the study of renal tubular acidification.[1]

The capacity to exchange H^+ for cation is decreased with impaired renal tubular function. In renal tubular acidosis, the distal tubules cannot effectively exchange H^+ for cations. pH of the urine may reflect attempts at correction of metabolic acid-base disturbances. In chronic acidosis such as diabetic ketoacidosis, large amounts of H^+ are excreted. In metabolic alkalosis, high levels of bicarbonate are produced. Compensation of respiratory acidosis and respiratory alkalosis is also associated with increased excretion of H^+ and bicarbonate, respectively.

Urine pH is a part of a supersaturation profile intended to enhance management of patients with nephrolithiasis. Other relevant urinary analytes included by a reference laboratory for this profile include potassium, calcium, phosphorus, oxalate, uric acid, citrate, magnesium, sodium, chloride, and sulfate.[2] Urine volume is important, but is not usually regarded as an analyte.

Footnotes

1. Alon US, "Renal Tubular Acidosis: Clinical Assessment," *Pediatric Nephrology in Perspective*, Strauss J, ed, Coral Gables, FL: University of Miami Press, 1995, 33-44.

2. Mayo Reference Services Publication, "Supersaturation Profile, Urine, Test," *New Test Announcement*, #32029, Rochester, MN: Mayo Medical Laboratories, 2000.

References

Cogan MG and Rector FC Jr, "Acid-Base Disorders," *Kidney*, Chapter 18, Brenner BM and Rector FC Jr, eds, Philadelphia, PA: WB Saunders Co, 1991, 737-804.

Henry JB, Lauzon RB, and Schumann GB, "Basic Examination of Urine," *Clinical Diagnosis and Management by Laboratory Methods*, 19th ed, Chapter 18, Philadelphia, PA: WB Saunders Co, 1996, 411-56.

◆ **Protein:Creatinine Ratio** *see* Protein, Semiquantitative, Urine *on page 885*

Protein, Quantitative, Urine

Related Information

Applies to Tamm-Horsfall Protein

Test Includes Concomitant creatinine clearance is often indicated. Total urine creatinine should be **routinely** included to help assure that a complete 24-hour collection was tested.

Abstract Quantitation of urinary protein loss provides evaluation of renal diseases, including nephrotic syndromes. Favorable explanations for proteinuria include orthostatic proteinuria and benign persistent proteinuria. Persistent proteinuria may indicate serious disease requiring further evaluation.

Specimen 24-hour urine

Container Plain urine container; consult the laboratory performing the assay about whether or not there is a need for preservative.[1]

Collection Instruct patient to void at 8 AM and discard the specimen. Then collect all urine including the final specimen voided at the end of the 24-hour collection period (ie, 8 AM the next morning). Label the container with the patient's name and date and time collection started and finished.

Storage Instructions Refrigeration and freezing may be desirable; check with the laboratory performing the assay.

Reference Interval 30-150 mg/24 hours (SI: 0.03-0.15 g/day) (method dependent). Normal urine protein consists of albumin (up to 35 mg/24 hours), other plasma proteins (ie, immunoglobulins, lysozyme, transferrin, haptoglobin, beta₂-microglobulin, and light chains), and Tamm-Horsfall glycoprotein secreted by renal tubular cells (may contribute up to 50 mg/24 hours). Urinary protein normally tends to increase with age, exercise, and standing posture. Proteinuria has been defined as 24-hour urine protein excretion >150 mg/24 hours (SI: >0.15 g/day).[2] Infants and children: >100 mg/m²/day.[3]

Critical Values Nephrotic syndromes: children: >1.0 g/m²/day;[3] adults: ≥3.5 g/24 hours[4]

Use Evaluate proteinuria (eg, following urinalysis in which proteinuria is detected); evaluate renal diseases, including proteinuria complicating diabetes mellitus, the nephrotic syndromes (eg, lipoid nephrosis, membranous, proliferative glomerulopathies), metal poisoning (eg, gold, lead, and cadmium), renal vein thrombosis, systemic lupus erythematosus (SLE), constrictive pericarditis, and amyloidosis; work up other renal diseases including hypertension, glomerulonephritis, Goodpasture syndrome, Henoch-Schönlein purpura, thrombotic thrombocytopenic purpura, collagen diseases, cryoglobulinemia, preeclampsia, drug nephrotoxicity, hypersensitivity reactions, allergic reactions, and renal tubular lesions; management of myeloma and macroglobulinemia of Waldenström (Bence Jones proteinuria); evaluate hypoproteinemia; tubular proteinurias include Wilson disease and Fanconi syndrome. In the table shown, some renal lesions are not easily categorized (eg, the glomerular lesions of chrysotherapy) and of toxemia of pregnancy. All important entities are not shown in the table found on the following page, including for instance absence of one kidney and vasculitis.

Limitations Although evaluation for proteinuria may be the best single test to work up chronic renal disease, proteinuria may wax and wane. In preeclampsia, magnesium sulfate is used therapeutically, which may result in high urine magnesium levels, depending on methodology. Preeclampsia, characterized by hypertension, proteinuria, and edema in a woman more than 20 weeks pregnant, is a state in which urine protein excretion is commonly measured.[5]

Twenty-four hour urine collections are subject to collection errors. The laboratory method, depending on an aliquot and varying dilutions, is subject to calculation errors. When protein is determined by precipitation methods, x-ray contrast media, tolbutamide, penicillin or cephalosporin analogs and sulfonamides may cause false positives. Pyridium® interferes with the reaction by causing color interference. Functional and postural proteinuria occur.

Methodology A number of methods are in use including trichloroacetic acid, sulfosalicylic acid precipitation, biuret method with phosphotungstic acid, and Coomassie blue dye binding. The standard for most methodologies is albumin. Different methods are more or less sensitive to globulin than to albumin. Thus, for nonselective proteinurias, in which a variety of proteins are present, different methodologies yield different results.
(Continued)

Protein, Quantitative, Urine *(Continued)*

Some Causes of Proteinuria

Normal proteinuria	Albumin ≤35 mg/24 h	
	Tamm-Horsfall ≤50 mg/24 h	
Prerenal proteinuria	Congestive heart failure	
	Orthostatic proteinuria	
	Transient, associated with febrile illness, surgery, anemia, hyperthyroidism, stroke, exercise, seizures	
	Bence Jones proteinuria associated with myeloma, Waldenström macroglobulinemia, amyloidosis (light chain proteinuria)	
	Lysozyme associated with myelocytic leukemia	
Renal proteinuria	Renovascular hypertension	
	Malignant hypertension of any cause	
	Glomerular Proteinuria >3.5 g/24 h usually reflects a glomerular lesion (in children >1.0 g/m²/day)	Membranous nephropathy and proliferative glomerulonephritis
		Chronic pyelonephritis
		Polycystic disease
		Diabetic nephropathy
		Amyloidosis
		Lupus erythematosus (SLE)
		Goodpasture syndrome
		Renal vein thrombosis
		Minimal change nephropathy
		Focal segmental glomerulosclerosis
		HIV nephropathy
		Alport syndrome
		Preeclampsia
		High molecular weight proteinuria
	Tubular usually <1 g/24 h	Fanconi syndrome
		Wilson disease
		Renal tubular acidosis
		Heavy metal poisoning: lead mercury cadmium
		Galactosemia
		Low molecular weight (<60,000) proteinuria
		Beta₂-microglobulinemia (molecular weight 11,800)
	Interstitial	Bacterial pyelonephritis
		Uric acid, urate or calcium deposition
		Idiosyncratic drug reaction: methicillin phenindione sulfonamides phenytoin others
		Interstitial diseases generally reflected as tubular defects or mixed tubular interstitial
Postrenal proteinuria	Tumors of the bladder or renal pelvis	
	<1 g/24 h, IgM excretion significant marker, amount of proteinuria related to size and spread of tumor	
	Cystitis, severe	

Note that this brief outline is intended only to provide an overview, and is incomplete.

Additional Information

Lupus nephritis is not a single entity. A classification is available.[6]

Tests requiring a 24-hour urine collection with no preservative, such as creatinine, may also be performed on the same specimen. Although quantitative protein can be run on a random specimen or timed collections less than 24 hours, 24-hour collections are preferable for evaluation of the nephrotic states and inflammatory renal disorders. Creatinine, creatinine clearance, BUN, serum protein electrophoresis, ANA, anti-DNA antibodies, HIV, hepatitis C antibody, hepatitis B antigen, antineutrophil cytoplasmatic antibodies (ANCA), and complement levels (including C3 and C4) are among useful tests to work up patients with proteinuria. Serologic evaluation for hepatitis B and C is relevant. Urine electrophoresis, immunofixation and immunoelectrophoresis are useful in patients older than 35 years of age to investigate possible diagnosis of amyloidosis, myeloma, and Waldenström's macroglobulinemia.

Some patients exhibit orthostatic proteinuria (ie, recumbent urine protein 100-180 mg in a 12-hour overnight urine collection and up to 1 g in the subsequent 12 hours while ambulatory). The presence of urinary protein >200 mg in the overnight specimen or equally increased amounts of urine protein in both specimens indicates need for further work-up.[7]

In a study of blood pressure and the kidney, proteinuria was identified as an independent risk factor for progression of renal disease. Proteinuria was greater in subjects with glomerular disease entities, diabetes, and hereditary nephritis. Proteinuria is a predictor of decline of glomerular filtration rate.[8]

Nephrotic syndromes cause the most severe urinary protein losses. Nephrotic syndrome is defined now usually by presence of massive proteinuria (ie, proteinuria >50 mg/kg/day or ≥3.5 g/24 hours). After time, additional signs and symptoms occur including hypoproteinemia, hypoalbuminemia, elevation of alpha₂-globulin with decreased gamma globulin on electrophoresis, hyperlipidemia, and edema. Urinary albumin is a more sensitive marker of progression and regression of renal disease than urine total protein, especially when urine total protein is <300 mg/g creatinine.[9] In most laboratories, urine albumin is available from protein electrophoresis following concentration procedures. However, this method is not sensitive to low concentrations of albumin.[9]

For low concentrations, see Microalbuminuria *on page 879*. The relationship between long-term elevation of glycated hemoglobin, diabetic nephropathy, and protein loss is being addressed.[10,11] About 35% of subjects with insulin-dependent diabetes mellitus develop diabetic nephropathy, which is characterized by proteinuria with decreasing glomerular filtration rate. The risk of death is nine times greater than for diabetics who do not suffer this complication. End-stage renal failure may occur within 10 years from onset of proteinuria.[12] The leading cause of renal failure in the western world is diabetic kidney disease.[13] Urine electrophoresis may be helpful; see Protein Electrophoresis, Urine *on page 268*. See also **fatty casts** and **oval fat bodies ("lipiduria")** in Urinalysis *on page 887*.

Footnotes

1. "For Your Information: Urine Testing Update - Preservatives for the Collection, Transportation, and Storage of Urine," *Mayo References Services Communique*, March 1999.
2. Epstein M and Oster JR, "Proteinuria," *The Laboratory in Clinical Medicine: Interpretation and Application*, 2nd ed, Halsted JA and Halsted CH, eds, Philadelphia, PA: WB Saunders Co, 1981, 318-23.
3. Srivastava T, Simon SD, and Alon US, "High Incidence of Focal Segmental Glomerulosclerosis in Nephrotic Syndrome of Childhood," *Pediatr Nephrol*, 1999, 13(1):13-8.
4. Larson TS, "Evaluation of Proteinuria," *Mayo Clin Proc*, 1994, 69(12):1154-8.
5. Ludman J and Smith RN, "A 30-Year-Old Woman With Increasing Hypertension and Proteinuria," Case Records of the Massachusetts General Hospital, Case 30-1998, Scully RE, Mark EJ, McNeely WF, et al, eds, *N Engl J Med*, 1998, 339(13):906-13.
6. Madaio MP and McCluskey RT, "A 29-Year-Old Woman With Necrotizing Lymphadenitis, the Nephrotic Syndrome, and Acute Renal Failure," Case Records of the Massachusetts General Hospital, Case 33-1998, Scully RE, Mark EJ, McNeely WF, et al, eds, *N Engl J Med*, 1998, 339(18):1308-17.
7. Glassock RJ, "Postural (Orthostatic) Proteinuria: No Cause for Concern," *N Engl J Med*, 1981, 305(11):639-41.
8. Peterson JC, Adler S, Burkart JM, et al, "Blood Pressure Control, Proteinuria, and the Progression of Renal Disease. The Modification of Diet in Renal Disease Study," *Ann Intern Med*, 1995, 123(10):754-62.
9. Shihabi ZK, Konen JC, and O'Connor ML, "Albuminuria vs Urinary Tract Protein for Detecting Chronic Renal Disorders," *Clin Chem*, 1991, 37(5):621-4.
10. Kullberg CE and Arnqvist HJ, "Elevated Long-Term Glycated Haemoglobin Precedes Proliferative Retinopathy and Nephropathy in Type 1 (Insulin-Dependent) Diabetic Patients," *JAMA*, 1993, 36(10):961-5.
11. Viberti G, "A Glycemic Threshold for Diabetic Complications?" *N Engl J Med*, 1995, 332(19):1293-4.
12. Remuzzi G and Ruggenenti P, "Slowing the Progression of Diabetic Nephropathy," *N Engl J Med*, 1993, 329(20):1496-7.
13. Viberti G, Mogensen CE, Groop LC, et al, "Effect of Captopril on Progression to Clinical Proteinuria in Patients With Insulin-Dependent Diabetes Mellitus and Microalbuminuria," *JAMA*, 1994, 271(4):275-9.

References

Doumas BT and Peters T Jr, "Serum and Urine Albumin: A Progress Report on Their Measurement and Clinical Significance," *Clin Chim Acta*, 1997, 258(1):3-20.

Ettenger RB, "The Evaluation of the Child With Proteinuria," *Pediatr Ann*, 1994, 23(9):486-94.

Loghman-Adham M, "Evaluating Proteinuria in Children," *Am Fam Phys*, 1998, 58(5):1145-52, 1158-9 (published erratum *Am Fam Phys*, 1999, 59(3):540).

Magil AB, "Tubulointerstitial Lesions in Human Membranous Glomerulonephritis: Relationship to Proteinuria," *Am J Kidney Dis*, 1995, 25(3):375-9.

Maki DD, Ma JZ, Louis TA, et al, "Long-Term Effects of Antihypertensive Agents on Proteinuria and Renal Function," *Arch Intern Med*, 1995, 155(10):1073-80.

Morgensen CE, "Introduction: Nature of Microalbuminuria, Proteinuria, and Progressive Renal Disease," *J Diabetes Complications*, 1995, 9(1):2-6.

Orth SR and Ritz E, "The Nephrotic Syndrome," *N Engl J Med*, 1998, 338(17):1202-11.

Stephenson JM, Kenny S, Stevens LK, et al, "Proteinuria and Mortality in Diabetes: The WHO Multinational Study of Vascular Disease in Diabetes," *Diabet Med*, 1995, 12(2):149-55.

Trachtman H, Bergwerk A, and Gauthier B, "Isolated Proteinuria in Children. Natural History and Indications for Renal Biopsy," *Clin Pediatr (Phila)*, 1994, 33(8):468-72.

♦ **Protein, Screen, Urine** *see Protein, Semiquantitative, Urine on page 885*

Protein, Semiquantitative, Urine

Related Information
Chromium, Serum *on page 815*
Kidney Biopsy *on page 64*
Microalbuminuria *on page 879*
Osmolality, Urine *on page 236*
Protein Electrophoresis, Urine *on page 268*
Protein, Quantitative, Urine *on page 883*
Urinalysis *on page 887*

Synonyms Albumin, Urine; Protein, Screen, Urine; Protein, Urine, Sulfosalicylic Acid; Urine Screen for Albumin; Urine Screen for Protein

Applies to Protein:Creatinine Ratio

Test Includes Screening for urine protein by dipstick and, in some laboratories, sulfosalicylic acid method for confirmation is part of routine urinalysis.

Abstract The precipitation methods, including sulfosalicylic acid and trichloroacetic acid, are more sensitive to globulins including light chains, than are dipstick methods. Microscopic examination of urine sediment is essential to evaluate patients with proteinuria: the presence or absence of erythrocytes, red cell casts, leukocytes, white cell casts, eosinophiluria, oval fat bodies, fatty casts, and other abnormalities are important.[1] Other clinical facets (eg, patient history, age, findings on physical examination, and evaluation of renal function)[2] as well as microscopy of urinary sediment are relevant in interpretation.

Specimen Random urine

Collection Early morning specimen is recommended to provide maximally concentrated urine, when immunoglobulin light chain (Bence Jones protein) detection is important and when orthostatic proteinuria must be ruled out. For other renal disease, daytime urine is satisfactory or even preferred.[3,4] Transport specimen to the laboratory within 2 hours of collection. Container should state date and time of collection.

Storage Instructions If not run promptly, specimen should be refrigerated.

Reference Interval Dipstick results include grades negative and trace (10-20 mg/dL) (SI: 0.1-0.2 g/L). The sensitivity of the dipstick is in the range of 150-300 mg/L. It is sensitive mostly for albumin.

Critical Values Dipstick 1+ is about 30 mg/dL, 2+ 100 mg/dL, 3+ (300 mg/dL), or 4+ (1000 mg/dL)

Use Reagent strips for detection of urinary protein are used to screen for preeclampsia and other disorders, including nephrotic syndromes, complications of diabetes mellitus, glomerulonephritis, amyloidosis, and other entities. Some causes of proteinuria are found in the table in Protein, Quantitative, Urine *on page 883*. Proteinuria is probably the single most important indicator of renal disease and its severity.

Limitations The reagent strip method is sensitive to negatively charged proteins, but much less so to positively charged proteins; thus, dipsticks commonly will not detect immunoglobulin light chains (Bence Jones protein) or myeloma protein, to which sulfosalicylic acid procedures are usually sensitive. False negatives may be found with highly dilute urines. False negative rates for dipstick protein can be substantial. Both false negative and false positive reagent strip results are commonplace in testing pregnant patients.

False-positive results may be obtained with highly alkaline (pH ≥7) urines on dipsticks, with hematuria, and in highly concentrated urine. Positive protein dipstick results, especially in very alkaline urines, should be confirmed by sulfosalicylic acid testing. Contaminating quaternary ammonium groups or chlorhexidine present in disinfectants may also give false-positive dipstick results. The test area on dipsticks is more sensitive to albumin than to globulin, hemoglobin, Bence Jones protein, or mucoprotein. A negative result, therefore, does not rule out the presence of these other proteins. Pyridium® metabolites may mask the reaction. X-ray contrast media, tolbutamide, nafcillin, massive doses of penicillin, sulfisoxazole (Gantrisin®), para-aminosalicylic acid, and high levels of cephalosporins may cause false-positive reactions with the sulfosalicylic acid method. Dipstick methods may be unreliable in unusually colored urines or when a great deal of sediment is present. The detection limit of Albustix® (Ames Division, Miles Laboratories) is reported as 300 mg/L or 500 mg/day protein. Since normal albuminuria is <20 mg/L, the screening dipstick lacks sensitivity for early detection of protein loss in diabetic nephropathy.[5,6] See Microalbuminuria *on page 879*. Use of reagent strips is sometimes delegated to personnel whose level of training and whose supervision are limited.

Methodology Dipstick, and in some laboratories sulfosalicylic acid, are run on all urinalyses. The dipstick test is based on the color development of indicators, usually bromphenol blue in citric acid buffer. The sulfosalicylic acid test is based on the acid precipitation of protein. Immunofixation or immunoelectrophoresis is indicated when Bence Jones protein is suspected.

Additional Information The protein:creatinine ratio corrects protein concentration for urine creatinine, correcting for dilution effects in a random specimen. It provides a modicum of correlation with 24-hour collections for protein.[1] A ratio <0.20 is regarded as normal.

If the dipstick for protein is negative and the sulfosalicylic acid test is positive, immunoglobulin light chains may be present. If clinically indicated in this situation, a urine examination for electrophoresis and immunoelectrophoresis for light chains or immunofixation should be considered.

Normal newborns may have proteinuria during first 3 days of life.

Subclinical increased urinary albumin excretion is thought to be predictive of emergence subsequently of diabetic nephropathy[3] (see Microalbuminuria *on page 879*). In many situations beside diabetes, microalbumin determination is much more sensitive to progressing renal disease than is urinary total protein (eg, hypertension, systemic lupus erythematosus). Urine albumin is easier to standardize and should be more sensitive to specific glomerular disease.[7] Following exercise, proteinuria relates more to intensity of exercise than to its duration.[8] In low-risk women with no objective signs of hypertensive disorder, routine dipstick proteinuria screening at each prenatal visit did not provide any clinically important information regarding pregnancy outcome.[9] Asymptomatic mild/moderate proteinuria in a specimen obtained in an adolescent during daytime is most commonly due to orthostatic proteinuria.

Transient proteinuria may be secondary to fever, congestive heart failure, and following exercise or cold exposure. Repeat collection of first morning urine with sediment microscopy can direct further investigation.[1]

Proteinuria should be a portion of risk stratification for diabetics evaluated for cardiac revascularization procedures.[10]

Footnotes
1. Larson TS, "Evaluation of Proteinuria," *Mayo Clin Proc*, 1994, 69(12):1154-8.
2. Misdraji J and Nguyen PL, "Urinalysis. When - and When Not - To Order," *Postgrad Med*, 1996, 100(1):173-6, 181-2, 185-8 passim.
3. Risdon P and Shaw AB, "Which Urine Sample for Detection of Proteinuria?" *Br J Urol*, 1989, 63(2):209-10.
4. Harrison NA, Rainford DJ, White GA, et al, "Proteinuria - What Value Is the Dipstick?" *Br J Urol*, 1989, 63(2):202-8.
5. Hindmarsh JT, "Microalbuminuria," *Clin Lab Med*, 1988, 8(3):611-6.
6. Olivarius ND and Mogensen CE, "Danish General Practitioners' Estimation of Urinary Albumin Concentration in the Detection of Proteinuria and Microalbuminuria," *Br J Gen Pract*, 1995, 45(391):71-3.
7. Shihabi ZK, Konen JC, and O'Connor ML, "Albuminuria vs Urinary Total Protein for Detecting Chronic Renal Disorders," *Clin Chem*, 1991, 37(5):621-4.
8. Poortmans JR, "Postexercise Proteinuria in Humans - Facts and Mechanisms," *JAMA*, 1985, 253(2):236-40.
9. Gribble RK, Fee SC, and Berg RL, "The Value of Routine Urine Dipstick Screening for Protein at Each Prenatal Visit," *Am J Obstet Gynecol*, 1995, 173(1):214-7.
10. Marso SP, Ellis SG, Gurm HS, et al, "Proteinuria Is a Key Determinant of Death in Patients With Diabetes After Isolated Coronary Artery Bypass Grafting," *Am Heart J*, 2000, 139(6):939-44.

References
Hricik DE, Chung-Park M, and Sedor JR, "Glomerulonephritis," *N Engl J Med*, 1998, 339(13):888-99.
Schwab SJ, Christensen RL, Dougherty K, et al, "Quantitation of Proteinuria by the Use of Protein-to-Creatinine Ratios in Single Urine Samples," *Arch Intern Med*, 1987, 147(5):943-4.

♦ **Protein, Urine, Sulfosalicylic Acid** *see* Protein, Semiquantitative, Urine *on page 885*

♦ **Prussian Blue Stain, Urine** *see* Hemosiderin Stain, Urine *on page 876*

♦ **Purple Urine Bags** *see* Indican, Semiquantitative, Urine *on page 876*

Reducing Substances, Urine

Related Information
Ammonia, Plasma *on page 102*
Galactose-1-Phosphate Uridyl Transferase, Blood *on page 179*
Glucose, Fasting, Plasma *on page 183*
Glucose, Postglucose Load, Plasma *on page 185*
Glucose, Quantitative, Urine *on page 874*
Glucose, Random, Plasma *on page 186*
Glucose, Semiquantitative, Urine *on page 875*
Glucose Tolerance Test, Plasma *on page 186*
Ketone Bodies, Blood *on page 205*
Ketones, Urine *on page 877*
Newborn Screening Tests for Galactosemia *on page 232*

Synonyms Clinitest® for Sugar, Urine; Copper Reduction Tablet Test

Applies to Benedict Test

Test Includes Clinitest® testing of urine

Abstract Glucose is a substance which can reduce copper (cupric ion), and this fact was once the basis for urinary glucose detection. In contemporary practice, however, the copper reduction test has little role in the evaluation of diabetes mellitus. Many other carbohydrates, some amino acids, and a few other abnormal urinary substances also reduce copper and can be referred to as reducing substances, galactose among them.

Specimen Random urine

Container Plastic urine container

Storage Instructions If the specimen cannot be processed promptly by the laboratory, it should be refrigerated.

Reference Interval None detected

Use This test is no longer used to diagnose or monitor patients with diabetes mellitus. The differential diagnosis of a positive test for reducing substances in urine includes fructose, lactose, galactose, maltose, arabinose, xylose, ribose, uric acid, ascorbic acid, creatinine, cysteine, ketones, sulfanilamide, (Continued)

Reducing Substances, Urine *(Continued)*

oxalic acid, hippuric acid, homogentisic acid, glucuronic acid, formaldehyde, isoniazid, salicylates, cinchophen, and salicyluric acid, as well as glucose.[1]

It has been advocated that physicians examining ill-appearing dehydrated infants without any obvious cause for dehydration should quickly screen the urine for glucose and ketones.[2]

Methodology Copper sulfate reacts with reducing substances in urine, converting cupric sulfate to cuprous oxide. The lower limit of glucose detection by Clinitest® is 200 mg glucose/dL (SI: 11.1 mmol/L). Semiquantitation is accomplished by comparison of the color generated with a reference chart. Semiquantitation of urine glucose is also readily accomplished by urine dipstick. This reaction is also utilized in detection of reducing substances in stool.

Additional Information Positive urine samples from sick newborns and children that are negative for glucose can be further confirmed by carbohydrate chromatography. In this setting, even trace positive Clinitest® results should be recognized as abnormal.

Footnotes

1. Sacks DB, "Carbohydrates," *Tietz Textbook of Clinical Chemistry*, 3rd ed, Burtis CA and Ashwood ER, eds, Philadelphia, PA: WB Saunders Co, 1999, 750-808.
2. Bland GL and Wood VD, "Diabetes in Infancy: Diagnosis and Current Management," *J Natl Med Assoc*, 1991, 83(4):361-5.

References

Henry JB, Lanzon RB, and Schumann GB, "Basic Examination of Urine," *Clinical Diagnosis and Management by Laboratory Methods*, 19th ed, Chapter 18, Philadelphia, PA: WB Saunders Co, 1996, 411-56.

Lindor NM and Karnes PS, "Initial Assessment of Infants and Children With Suspected Inborn Errors of Metabolism," *Mayo Clin Proc*, 1995, 70:987-8.

McCue JD, Gal P, and Pearson RC, "Interference of New Penicillins and Cephalosporins With Urine Glucose Monitoring Tests," *Diabetes Care*, 1983, 6(5):504-5.

◆ **Refractive Index, Urine** *see* Specific Gravity, Urine *on page 886*

◆ **SG, Urine** *see* Specific Gravity, Urine *on page 886*

Specific Gravity, Urine

Related Information

Antidiuretic Hormone, Plasma *on page 107*
Concentration Test, Urine *on page 872*
Osmolality, Serum *on page 236*
Osmolality, Urine *on page 236*
Urinalysis *on page 887*

Synonyms Refractive Index, Urine; SG, Urine

Applies to Body Fluid, Specific Gravity

Test Includes Specific gravity is usually part of Urinalysis.

Abstract Specific gravity (SG) is a measure of the density of dissolved solids in a fluid. **Hyposthenuric urine** is urine with SG <1.007; **isosthenuric urine**, SG about 1.010, is that of fixed SG. (SG of the protein-free glomerular filtrate is about 1.010.) Loss of concentrating ability takes place in end-stage renal disease.

Specific Gravity, Urine

Increased >1.020
Water restriction
Dehydration
Fever
Sweating
Vomiting
Diarrhea
Diabetes mellitus (glycosuria)
Proteinuria
Congestive heart failure
X-ray dyes
Adrenal insufficiency
Inappropriate antidiuretic hormone secretion syndrome
Tumors-secreting antidiuretic hormone
Decreased <1.009
Excess water ingestion
Excess I.V. fluids
Diuresis
Hypothermia
Impaired renal concentrating ability
pyelonephritis
glomerulonephritis
diabetes insipidus (central, renal)
Fixed 1.010
Severe renal damage, urine concentration fixed at 1.010, the value of glomerular filtrate

Specimen Voided urine or body fluid. Refractometer requires only a few drops of urine. Other methods require considerably more.

Collection First morning specimen is recommended, unless part of complete urinalysis.

Storage Instructions Refrigeration

Reference Interval Range: 1.005-1.035; adult on normal fluid intake: 1.016-1.022. Following overnight fluid deprivation for 12 hours, urine SG should be ~1.022. Specific gravity decreases with increasing age.

Critical Values Although low values are not necessarily abnormal, they may reflect advanced kidney disease or diabetes insipidus.

Use SG provides evaluation of renal concentrating power and hydration status. Urine specific gravity test strips are effective in home use to help stone formers drink sufficient water to reduce risk of stone formation. The specific gravity of urine indicates the relative proportions of dissolved solid components to the total volume of the specimen. It reflects the relative degree of concentration or dilution of the specimen. Knowledge of the specific gravity is needed in interpretation of results of most tests in urinalysis. Specific gravity must be interpreted in light of presence or absence of glycosuria and/or proteinuria. Patients with diabetes insipidus have marked decrease in SG and osmolality of urine.[1] See table.

Limitations Radiographic dyes in urine increase the specific gravity by hydrometer or refractometer.[2] Glucose or protein also increase specific gravity out of proportion to osmolality, as measured by hydrometer or refractometer. **Strip method urine specific gravity** was reported as having a significant positive bias at urine pH ≤6 and negative bias at pH >7 compared to specific gravity by refractometer.[3] Urine osmolality is considered preferable in some settings. Benitez et al suggest that osmolality is the only accurate measure of urine concentration in newborn infants.[4]

Methodology Refractometer, urinometer, and colorimetric (reagent strip) methods.

When using the **refractometer**, cloudy urines or those with visible particles should be centrifuged, and the supernatant used for refractometer specific gravity determination. The refractometer is temperature corrected. Measuring the refractive index of a liquid, it is the method of choice for most patients in most circumstances.

Dipstick method responds to the ionic strength of urine (linear relation to osmolality due to electrolytes). The strip provides a polyionic polymer with binding sites saturated with hydrogen ions that with urine testing are replaced by sodium or potassium cations, consequent release of hydrogen ions (change of pH) affecting an indicator color change; apparent pKa change. Albumin, glucose, and osmotic effects are not measured, and as such a true specific gravity measurement may not be obtained.[5]

The **urinometer** is a hydrometer intended to measure urine SG. It is an obsolete method.

Additional Information Measurement of urine specific gravity is easier and more convenient than direct measurement of osmolality. The two methods correlate well. However, measured osmolality in newborns is generally lower than would be expected by refractometer specific gravity. In newborns, an elevated specific gravity should be confirmed by direct measurement of osmolality when the state of hydration and water balance are being assessed.[4]

Reagent strip methods for the determination of urine specific gravity employ a colorimetric method and are sensitive to ions but not undissociated solutes such as urea. The strip method requires a corrected reading for pH ≥6.5 and protein increases the reading.[5] Critical clinical decisions should be based on the more definitive methods. The strip methods are reported to be suitable for urine screening purposes, but not uniformly so. Strip methods are not described as showing a high degree of correlation with refractometer or urinometer methods.[6] Their additional cost as well as bias led Adams to conclude that strip specific gravity methods are neither cost-effective nor clinically useful[3] and Assadi and Fornell to conclude that the magnitude of observed discrepancies places important limitations on strip test SG measurement.[5]

In athletic and industrial settings or field studies urine color indicates hydration status. Urine osmolality as well as urine specific gravity is used to determine hydration status.[7]

Footnotes

1. Adam P, "Evaluation and Management of Diabetes Insipidus," *Am Fam Phys*, 1997, 55(6):2146-53.
2. Smith C, Arbogast C, and Phillips R, "Effect of X-ray Contrast Media on Results for Relative Density of Urine," *Clin Chem*, 1983, 29(4):730-1.
3. Adams LJ, "Evaluation of Ames Multistix®-SG for Urine Specific Gravity Versus Refractometer Specific Gravity," *Am J Clin Pathol*, 1983, 80(6):871-3.
4. Benitez OA, Benitez M, Stijnen T, et al, "Inaccuracy in Neonatal Measurement of Urine Concentration With a Refractometer," *J Pediatr*, 1986, 108(4):613-6.
5. Assadi FK and Fornell L, "Estimation of Urine Specific Gravity in Neonates With a Reagent Strip," *J Pediatr*, 1986, 108(6):995-6.
6. Ciulla AP, Newsome B, and Kaster J, "Reagent Strip Method for Specific Gravity: An Evaluation," *Lab Med*, 1985, 16:38-40.
7. Armstrong LE, Maresh CM, Castellani JW, et al, "Urinary Indices of Hydration Status," *Int J Sport Nutr*, 1994, 4(3):265-79.

References

Henry JB, Lauzon RB, and Schumann GB, "Basic Examination of Urine," *Clinical Diagnosis and Management by Laboratory Methods*, 19th ed, Chapter 18, Philadelphia, PA: WB Saunders Co, 1996, 411-56.

Maghnie M, Cosi G, Genovese E, et al, "Central Diabetes Insipidus in Children and Young Adults," *N Engl J Med*, 2000, 343():998-1007.

♦ **Sugar, Qualitative, Urine** *see* Glucose, Semiquantitative, Urine *on page 875*

♦ **Sugar, Quantitative, Urine** *see* Glucose, Quantitative, Urine *on page 874*

♦ **Sulfate, Urine** *see* Kidney Stone Analysis *on page 877*

♦ **Tamm-Horsfall Protein** *see* Protein, Quantitative, Urine *on page 883*

♦ **Three Glass Test, Urine** *see* Urinalysis, Fractional *on page 889*

♦ **Two Glass Test, Urine** *see* Urinalysis, Fractional *on page 889*

♦ **UA** *see* Urinalysis *on page 887*

Urinalysis

Related Information

Anion Gap, Serum, Plasma, or Urine *on page 106*
Anti-DNA *on page 504*
Ascorbic Acid, Serum or Plasma *on page 112*
Bacterial Culture, Urine *on page 578*
Blood, Urine *on page 870*
Chromium, Serum *on page 815*
Cystine, Urine *on page 164*
Eosinophils, Urine *on page 873*
Ethylene Glycol, Serum or Plasma *on page 790*
Fat, Urine *on page 874*
Glucose, Semiquantitative, Urine *on page 875*
Hemoglobin, Qualitative, Urine *on page 875*
Ibuprofen, Serum *on page 793*
Inherited Diseases of Metabolism and Cell Structure *on page 449*
Ketones, Urine *on page 877*
Kidney Biopsy *on page 64*
Kidney Stone Analysis *on page 877*
Leukocyte Esterase, Urine *on page 878*
Microalbuminuria *on page 879*
Mucopolysaccharides, Urine *on page 226*
Nitrite, Urine *on page 882*
Osmolality, Calculated, Serum or Plasma *on page 234*
Osmolality, Urine *on page 236*
Oxalate, Urine *on page 238*
pH, Urine *on page 882*
Primidone, Serum or Plasma *on page 762*
Protein, Quantitative, Urine *on page 883*
Protein, Semiquantitative, Urine *on page 885*
Specific Gravity, Urine *on page 886*
Urinalysis, Fractional *on page 889*
Urinary Tract Cytology *on page 389*

Synonyms UA

Applies to Casts, Urine; Crystals, Urine; Dysmorphic Red Cells; Occult Blood, Semiquantitative, Urine; Urine Crystals

Test Includes Opacity, color, appearance, specific gravity, pH, protein, glucose, occult blood, ketones, bilirubin, and in some laboratories, urobilinogen and microscopic examination of urine sediment. Some laboratories include screening for leukocyte esterase and nitrite and do not perform a microscopic examination unless one of the chemical screening (macroscopic) tests is abnormal or unless a specific request for microscopic examination is made.

Abstract The examination of urine is one of the oldest practices in medicine. A carefully performed urinalysis still provides a wealth of information about the patient, both in terms of differential diagnosis, and by exclusion of many conditions when the urinalysis is "normal." Its role in diagnosis and management of renal diseases is pivotal.

Patient Preparation Instructions should be given in method of collection. Both males and females need instruction in cleansing the urethral meatus. "Midstream collections" are performed by initiating urination into the toilet, then bringing the collection device into the urine stream to catch the midportion of the void. In infants and young children, urine specimens can be obtained by urine bag, bladder catheterization, or bladder aspiration.

Specimen Urine

Container Plastic urine container

Collection A voided specimen is usually suitable. If the specimen is likely to be contaminated by vaginal discharge or hemorrhage, a clean catch specimen is desirable. If the specimen is collected by catheter or bladder aspiration, it should be so labeled. The timing of urine collection will vary with the purpose of the test. To check for casts or renal concentration ability, a first voided morning specimen may be preferred. For screening purposes, this is also the best time, as a later and more dilute specimen may make small increases in protein, RBC, or WBC excretion harder to detect. The upright position increases protein excretion by hemodynamic factors. Midmorning urine is likely to give the highest albumin excretion, but early morning urine is best when attempting to detect Bence Jones protein.

Storage Instructions Transport specimen to the laboratory as soon as possible after collection. If the specimen cannot be processed immediately by the laboratory it should be refrigerated. Refrigeration preserves formed elements in the urine, but may precipitate crystals not originally present. **Examination is best done on freshly voided, warm urine.**

Preanalytic handling of urinalysis specimens has been evaluated and requires improvement.[1]

Causes for Rejection Specimen delayed in transport, fecal contamination, decomposition, or bacterial overgrowth

Reference Interval See table. **Crystals** are part of the morphologic evaluation and are interpreted by a physician or an experienced technologist. Warm, freshly voided urine sediment from normal subjects almost never contains crystals, despite maximal concentration. Xanthine, cystine, and uric acid crystal (and stone) formation is favored by a consistently acid urine (pH <5.5-6). Calcium oxalate and apatite stones are associated with no particular disturbance of urine pH. Calcium carbonate, calcium phosphate, and especially magnesium ammonium phosphate stones are associated with pH >7. Urine pH >7.5 may briefly follow meals (alkaline tide) but more commonly indicate systemic alkali intake ($NaHCO_3$, etc) or urine infected by bacteria which split urea to ammonia.

Urinalysis

Test	Reference Range
Specific gravity	1.003-1.029
pH	4.5-7.8
Protein	Negative/trace*
Glucose	Negative
Ketones	Negative
Bilirubin	Negative
Occult blood	Negative
Leukocyte esterase	Negative
Nitrite	Negative
Urobilinogen	0.1-1.0 EU/dL
WBCs	0-4/hpf
RBCs	male: 0-3/hpf female: 0-5/hpf
Casts	0-4/lpf hyaline
Bacteria	Negative

*In concentrated urine.
hpf = high power field
lpf = low power field
EU = Ehrlich units

Possible Panic Range The presence of massive amounts of oxalate crystals in fresh urine should be reported promptly to the physician, as this finding may represent ethylene glycol intoxication.

Use An extremely important laboratory examination is used to screen for abnormalities of urine to lead to diagnosis and management of renal diseases, urinary tract infection, urinary tract neoplasms, inflammatory or neoplastic entities adjacent to the urinary tract, and systemic disorders. Careful microscopy of urine sediment on freshly voided, warm urine is important whenever abnormalities are detected in urine protein, blood, leukocyte esterase or nitrite, or when checking for crystalluria. Microscopy of urinary sediment is especially important for those with urinary tract disease.[2]

Limitations Insufficient volume, less than 2 mL, may limit the extent of procedures performed. Metabolites of Pyridium® may interfere with the dipstick reactions by producing color interference. High vitamin C intake may cause an underestimate of glucosuria, or a false-negative nitrate test. Survival of WBCs is decreased by low osmolality, alkalinity, and lack of refrigeration. Formed elements in the urine including casts disintegrate rapidly, therefore the specimen should be analyzed as soon as possible after collection. Specific gravity is affected by glucosuria, proteinuria, mannitol infusion, or prior administration of iodinated contrast material for radiologic studies (IVP dye). Some brands of reagent strips give a "trace positive" protein indication if not stored in dry atmosphere (cap of test strip bottle not on tight). Ambient humidity exposure of the test strips over time also causes some reduction of sensitivity for occult blood and nitrate and increased sensitivity for glucose (false-positive). This can be detected by using tap water as a negative control. False-positive tests for protein can also be due to contamination of the urine by an ammonium-containing cleansing solution. Problems relevant to the sensitivity of protein detection have led to development of methods described in Microalbuminuria *on page 879*. All reagent strips are not time-independent; reading at incorrect times can lead to misleading results in some systems. Prolonged sample contact with a reagent pad can leach out chemical, altering reaction interpretation.[3]

Methodology The chemical portion of the urinalysis is done by reagent strip, with confirming chemical method for protein (sulfosalicylic acid precipitation). Such dipsticks were introduced for glucose (1956), protein (1957), ketone (1957), pH (1959), occult blood (1961), bilirubin (1969), urobilinogen (1969), nitrite (1972), specific gravity (1981), and for the presence of white blood cells. Most are colorimetric, read visually, but instruments are available. Avoid contamination of specimens with any additives.[3] See individual test entries for further information.
(Continued)

Urinalysis (Continued)

Additional Information

MICROSCOPY:

Crystalluria is frequently observed when urine temperature drops, in urine specimens stored at room temperature or refrigerated, *in vitro* crystal formation. Crystals are most diagnostically useful when observed in warm, fresh urine (*in vivo* crystal formation) in evaluation of hematuria, nephrolithiasis, or toxin ingestion. Intratubular fluid pH as well as decreased flow are relevant to solute concentration and crystallization. Polarizing microscopy and pH are useful in crystal identification.

Calcium oxalate crystals are classically fairly uniform small double pyramids, base to base, which under the microscope look like little crosses on a square, the octahedral shape of the dihydrate form. Ovoid and dumbbell shapes of oxalate crystals are more easily missed. Polarization helps: oxalate crystals are birefringent, but the red cells and yeasts with which the ovoid forms can be confused are not anisotropic. Acetic acid (3%) will lyse red cells but not oxalate crystals or yeasts. See Oxalate, Urine *on page 238* and Kidney Stone Analysis *on page 877*. In abundance, **calcium oxalate** and/or **hippurate crystals** may suggest ethylene glycol ingestion (especially if known to be accompanied by neurological abnormalities, appearance of drunkenness, hypertension, and a high anion gap acidosis.) Urine is usually supersaturated in calcium oxalate, often in calcium phosphate, and acid urine is often saturated in uric acid. Yet crystalluria is uncommon (in warm, fresh urine) because of the normal presence of crystal inhibitors, the lack of available nidus, and the time factor. When properly observed in fresh urine, crystals may provide a clue to the composition of renal stones even not yet passed, the nidus for such stones, or, as such, have been associated with hematuria.

Uric acid crystals are reddish brown, rectangular, rhomboidal, or flower-like structures of narrow rectangular petals. **Ammonium urates,** in alkaline urine, are irregular blobs and crescents, sometimes resembling fragmented red cell shapes.

Calcium phosphate crystallizes in urine as flowers of narrow rectangular needles.

Cystine crystals, uniquely in urine, form large irregular hexagonal plates, which may dissolve if alkalinized. They occur only in the urine of subjects with cystinuria. (See Cystine, Urine *on page 164*).

Calcium magnesium ammonium phosphate, or "triple phosphate," forms unique "coffin lid" angularly domed rectangles which may be present in massive quantities in alkaline urine. They usually are associated with urine infected by urea splitting bacteria which cause "infection," or "triple phosphate" stones.

Indinavir crystals are found in >30% of patients treated with this protease inhibitor. Manual microscopy detects such radial clusters, forming starburst shapes.[4,5]

Leukocyturia may indicate inflammatory disease in the genitourinary tract, including bacterial infection, glomerulonephritis, chemical injury, autoimmune diseases, or inflammatory disease adjacent to the urinary tract such as appendicitis[6] or diverticulitis. Pyuria predominating in the urinary sediment in renal failure is found even without superimposed usual bacterial infection with analgesic abuse nephropathy, renal tuberculosis, and polycystic kidney disease.

White cell casts indicate the renal origin of leukocytes, and are most frequently found in acute pyelonephritis. White cell casts are also found in glomerulonephritis such as lupus nephritis, and in acute and chronic interstitial nephritis. When nuclei degenerate, such leukocyte casts resemble renal tubular casts.

Red cell casts indicate renal origin of hematuria and suggest glomerulonephritis. Red cell casts may also be found in subacute bacterial endocarditis, renal infarct, vasculitis, Goodpasture syndrome, sickle cell disease, and in malignant hypertension. Degenerated red cell casts may be called **"hemoglobin casts"**. Orange to red casts may be found with myoglobinuria as well.

Dysmorphic red cells are observed in glomerulonephritis. "Dysmorphic" red cells refer to heterogeneous sizes, hypochromia, distorted irregular outlines and frequently small blobs extruding from the cell membrane. Phase contrast microscopy best demonstrates RBC and WBC morphology. Nonglomerular urinary red blood cells resemble peripheral circulating red blood cells.[7] The differentiation between glomerular and nonglomerular hematuria should, however, also be based on other clinical and laboratory findings.[8] See Urinalysis, Fractional *on page 889*.

Crenated RBCs provide no implication regarding RBC source.

Dark brown or smoky urine suggests a renal source of hematuria.

A **pink or red urine** suggests an extrarenal source.

Hyaline casts occur in physiologic states (eg, after exercise) and many types of renal diseases. They are best seen in phase contrast microscopy or with reduced illumination.

Renal tubular (epithelial) casts are most suggestive of tubular injury, as in acute tubular necrosis. They are also found in other disorders, including eclampsia, heavy metal poisoning, ethylene glycol intoxication, and acute allograft rejection.

Granular casts: Very finely granulated casts may be found after exercise and in a variety of glomerular and tubulointerstitial diseases.; coarse granular casts are abnormal and are present in a wide variety of renal diseases.

"Dirty brown" granular casts are typical of acute tubular necrosis.

Waxy casts are found especially in chronic renal diseases, and are associated with chronic renal failure; they occur in diabetic nephropathy, malignant hypertension, and glomerulonephritis, among other conditions. They are named for their waxy or glossy appearance. They often appear brittle and cracked.

Fatty casts and **oval fat bodies ("lipiduria")** are generally found in the nephrotic syndromes, usually glomerular diseases including minimal change disease, focal segmental glomerulosclerosis, membranous glomerulopathy, and membranoproliferative glomerulonephritis. Nephrotic range proteinuria is also found in multisystem diseases including amyloidosis, SLE, cryoglobulinemia, and diabetic nephropathy.[9] Fat droplets originate in renal tubular cells when they exceed their capacity to reabsorb protein of glomerular origin. See Fat, Urine *on page 874* and Protein, Quantitative, Urine *on page 883*.

Broad casts originate from dilated, chronically damaged tubules or the collecting ducts. They can be granular or waxy. **Broad waxy casts** are called "renal failure casts."

Spermatozoa may be seen in male urine related to recent or retrograde ejaculation. In female urine, the presence of spermatozoa may provide evidence of vaginal contamination following recent intercourse.

Automation of the urinalysis is routine in many laboratories.[10,11] Some authors wish to abandon microscopic evaluation of the urine, which is not easily automated, on urine samples testing "normal" by dipstick screening. A urine sample that is normal to inspection and dipstick will be normal to microscopic exam 95% of the time.[12] However, 5% remain. Two relevant published volumes may prove helpful.[13,14]

An instrument for automating the entire urinalysis, the Yellow IRIS®, includes a module that automates the microscopic sediment exam. This has been found to be more consistent than the manual method for routine urinalysis and has increased the number of abnormal urines detected.[10,11,15,16] Other instruments include the Cen-Slide, R/S 2000, Uri-Slide, KOVA, and Count-10.[17]

Tests for **inherited diseases of metabolism** involve blood as well as urine. These subjects are summarized in Inherited Diseases of Metabolism and Cell Structure *on page 449*.

Footnotes

1. Howanitz PJ, Saladino AJ, and Dale JC, "Timeliness of Urinalysis: A College of American Pathologists Q-Probes Study of 346 Small Hospitals," *Arch Pathol Lab Med*, 1997, 121(7):667-72.
2. Misdraji J and Nguyen PL, "Urinalysis. When - and When Not - To Order," *Postgrad Med*, 1996, 100(1):173-6, 181-2, 185-8 passim.
3. Pugia MJ, "Technology Behind Diagnostic Reagent Strips," *Lab Med*, 2000, 31(2):92-6.
4. Hortin GL, King C, Miller KD, et al, "Detection of Indinavir Crystals in Urine: Dependence on Method of Analysis," *Arch Pathol Lab Med*, 2000, 124(2):246-50.
5. Trainor LD, Steinberg JP, Austin GW, et al, "Indinavir Crystalluria: Identification of Patients at Increased Risk of Developing Nephrotoxicity," *Arch Pathol Lab Med*, 1998, 122(3):256-9.
6. Scott JH, Amin M, and Harty JI, "Abnormal Urinalysis in Appendicitis," *J Urol*, 1983, 129(5):1015.
7. Rizzoni G, Braggion F, and Zacchello G, "Evaluation of Glomerular and Nonglomerular Hematuria by Phase-Contrast Microscopy," *J Pediatr*, 1983, 103(3):370-4.
8. Ward JF, Kaplan GW, Mevorach R, et al, "Refined Microscopic Urinalysis for Red Blood Cell Morphology in the Evaluation of Asymptomatic Microscopic Hematuria in a Pediatric Population," *J Urol*, 1998, 160(4):1492-5.
9. Larson TS, "Evaluation of Proteinuria," *Mayo Clin Proc*, 1994, 69(12):1154-8.
10. Roe CE, Carlson DA, Daigneault RW, et al, "Evaluation of the Yellow IRIS®. An Automated Method for Urinalysis," *Am J Clin Pathol*, 1986, 86(5):661-5.
11. Wargotz ES, Hyde JE, Karcher DS, et al, "Urine Sediment Analysis by the Yellow IRIS® Automated Urinalysis Workstation," *Am J Clin Pathol*, 1987, 88(6):746-8.
12. Wenz B and Lampasso JA, "Eliminating Unnecessary Urine Microscopy - Results and Performance Characteristics of an Algorithm Based on Chemical Reagent Strip Testing," *Am J Clin Pathol*, 1989, 92(1):78-81.
13. Brunzel NA, *Fundamentals of Urine and Body Fluid Analysis*, Philadelphia, PA: WB Saunders Co, 1994.
14. Ringsrud KM and Linné JJ, *Urinalysis and Body Fluids: A ColorText and Atlas*, St Louis, MO: CV Mosby Co, 1995.
15. Carlson D and Statland BE, "Automated Urinalysis," *Clin Lab Med*, 1988, 8(3):449-61.
16. Bartlett RC, Zern DA, Ratkiewicz I, et al, "Reagent Strip Screening for Sediment Abnormalities Identified by Automated Microscopy in Urine From Patients Suspected to Have Urinary Tract Disease," *Arch Pathol Lab Med*, 1994, 118(11):1096-101.
17. Schumann GB and Friedman SK, "Comparing Slide Systems for Microscopic Urinalysis," *Lab Med*, 1996, 27(4):270-7.

References

Birch DF, Fairly KF, Becker GJ, et al, "A Color Atlas of Urine Microscopy," *Chapman & Hall Medical Atlas Series*, No. 13, 1994.

Brock DA and Hundley JM, "Identifying Calcium Oxalate Crystals in Urine," *Lab Med*, 1995, 26(11):733-5.

Cohen HT and Spiegel DM, "Air-Exposed Urine Dipsticks Give False-Positive Results for Glucose and False-Negative Results for Blood," *Am J Clin Pathol*, 1991, 96(3):398-400.

Geyer SJ, "Urinalysis and Urinary Sediment in Patients With Renal Disease," *Clin Lab Med*, 1993, 13(1):13-20.

Wilson DM, "Tests to Detect Asymptomatic Urinary Tract Infections," *JAMA*, 1994, 271(18):1399.

Urinalysis, Fractional

Related Information
Blood, Urine *on page 870*
Hemoglobin, Qualitative, Urine *on page 875*
Urinalysis *on page 887*

Synonyms Three Glass Test, Urine; Two Glass Test, Urine

Applies to Dysmorphic Red Cells

Test Includes Microscopic examination of each fraction

Abstract Sequential urinalysis is performed on the initial urine voided, the midstream urine, and the final passage of urine to attempt to gain information regarding the anatomic source of cellular elements in the urine.

Collection Patient voids and the specimen is collected in two or three containers without interrupting the flow of urine. If three containers are ordered, small amounts of urine are collected in the first and third while the second has the largest volume. Sometimes this method is modified by stopping the flow of urine after the second glass and the third glass is collected after prostatic massage. The exact collection procedure followed should be recorded on the requisition so that the results can be interpreted properly.

Reference Interval RBCs: 2-3 cells/hpf; WBCs: 0-5 cells/hpf

Use Fractional urinalysis may be useful to define the location of the source of red blood cells and white blood cells found in the urine of male patients. The primary intended use is in the differential diagnosis of urethritis vs cystitis and pyelonephritis. The test may also contribute to the differentiation of renal vs nonrenal hematuria.

Additional Information Initial hematuria, red blood cells in the first specimen, implies hematuria of urethral origin. Total hematuria, red cells in all three samples, implicates the upper urinary tract. Terminal hematuria, red cells in the last specimen, implies hematuria of prostatic or bladder neck origin. Phase contrast microscopy of urinary red blood cells may assist in differentiation of hematuria of glomerular vs nonglomerular origin.[1] Glomerular hematuria is characterized by "dysmorphic" urinary RBCs while red cells of nonglomerular origin are "eumorphic." Dysmorphic cells have irregular outlines, granular inhomogeneous cytoplasm (with phase microscopy), uneven cytoplasmic staining and hypochromia (with Wright stain), and often have small blob-like membrane extrusions (phase microscopy). Eumorphic cells have uniform size and are similar to normal circulating red cells. Nonglomerular hematuria may also be characterized by the presence of red cell "ghosts" (empty membranous sacks which have lost their hemoglobin).[2] Glomerular hematuria is likely when 10% of all urinary RBCs are dysmorphic.[1] One should be careful not to rely only on red blood cell morphology as an indicator of the source of hematuria.[3] If additional evidence of glomerulonephritis is present (edema, proteinuria, renal cellular casts), the glomerular nature of hematuria is essentially established. If all urine red cells are eumorphic, clinical evaluation for extraglomerular sources of hematuria is indicated. Glomerular hematuria does not exclude, in addition, bladder or prostate pathology or malignancy.

Footnotes
1. Stapleton FB, "Morphology of Urinary Red Blood Cells: A Simple Guide in Localizing the Site of Hematuria," *Pediatr Clin North Am*, 1987, 34(3):561-9.
2. Fairley KF and Birch DF, "Hematuria: A Simple Method for Identifying Glomerular Bleeding," *Kidney Int*, 1982, 21(1):105-8.
3. Ward JF, Kaplan GW, Mevorach R, et al, "Refined Microscopic Urinalysis for Red Blood Cell Morphology in the Evaluation of Asymptomatic Microscopic Hematuria in a Pediatric Population," *J Urol*, 1998, 160(4):1492-5.

References
Schramek P, Schuster FX, Georgopoulos M, et al, "Value of Urinary Erythrocyte Morphology in Assessment of Symptomless Microhaematuria," *Lancet*, 1989, 2(8675):1316-9.

♦ **Urinary Eosinophils** *see* Eosinophils, Urine *on page 873*

♦ **Urinary Sugar Test** *see* Glucose, Quantitative, Urine *on page 874*

♦ **Urinary Sugar Test** *see* Glucose, Semiquantitative, Urine *on page 875*

♦ **Urinary Tract Infection Screen** *see* Nitrite, Urine *on page 882*

♦ **Urine Calcium:Creatinine Ratio** *see* Blood, Urine *on page 870*

♦ **Urine Concentration Test** *see* Concentration Test, Urine *on page 872*

♦ **Urine Crystals** *see* Urinalysis *on page 887*

♦ **Urine Hemosiderin** *see* Hemosiderin Stain, Urine *on page 876*

♦ **Urine Ketones** *see* Ketones, Urine *on page 877*

♦ **Urine Protein:Creatinine Ratio** *see* Blood, Urine *on page 870*

♦ **Urine Screen for Albumin** *see* Protein, Semiquantitative, Urine *on page 885*

♦ **Urine Screen for Protein** *see* Protein, Semiquantitative, Urine *on page 885*

♦ **Urines for Glucose Tolerance** *see* Glucose, Semiquantitative, Urine *on page 875*

Urobilinogen, 2-Hour Urine

Related Information
Bilirubin, Direct, Serum *on page 117*
Bilirubin, Total, Serum *on page 118*
Bilirubin, Urine *on page 870*
Liver Disease: Laboratory Assessment, Overview *on page 216*
Phenothiazines, Serum or Urine *on page 760*
Porphobilinogen, Qualitative, Urine *on page 255*

Synonyms Urobilinogen, Quantitative, Urine

Replaces Urobilinogen, 24-Hour Urine

Abstract This urine screening test detects some but not all instances of hemolytic anemia and liver diseases, such as hepatitis and cirrhosis. Presently, it is not widely used.

Patient Preparation Alkalinization of the urine by sodium bicarbonate administration increases excretion of urobilinogen. A marked diurnal peak in excretion occurs; therefore an afternoon collection ideally should be scheduled. Patient should be hydrated.

Specimen 2-hour urine

Container Dark urine container or foil wrapped container

Collection Have patient void at 2 PM and discard urine. Give patient 500 mL of water to be ingested at once. Collect all urine from 2 PM - 4 PM. Transport promptly to the laboratory. Urobilinogen is sensitive to room temperature and light.

Storage Instructions Refrigerate specimen, protect from light.

Reference Interval Male: 0.3-2.1 mg/2 hours (SI: 0.5-3.6 µmol/2 hours); female: 0.1-1.1 mg/2 hours (SI: 0.2-1.9 µmol/2 hours). Results are often expressed in Ehrlich units, 1 mg urobilinogen = 1 EU, because what is measured is a mixture of compounds.

Use This inexpensive procedure provides a preliminary evaluation for biliary and liver disease, including obstructive jaundice. It is increased in hemolytic anemia, hepatitis, liver damage with or without jaundice (eg, cirrhosis, congestive heart failure). See table in Bilirubin, Urine *on page 870*.

Limitations Antibiotics suppressing intestinal flora may cause very low levels. Levels may be normal with incomplete obstructive jaundice. Patients with acute porphyria may have an increased value because porphobilinogen also gives a positive result with Ehrlich's aldehyde reagent, as does para-aminosalicylic acid. Sulfonamides and PABA also cause false positives. Fever and dehydration lead to urine concentration and increased values. The absence of or low urobilinogen cannot be determined by dipsticks, a serious drawback, since detection of decreased urine urobilinogen would enhance diagnosis of common duct obstruction. Like urine bilirubin detection, screen for increased urobilinogen in urine has fairly good specificity. However, the two tests lack great sensitivity when compared with a variety of serum tests related to liver disease.[1]

Methodology Urobilistix®, Watson's method, Ehrlich's aldehyde reagent. Para-dimethylaminobenzaldehyde reacts with urobilinogen in Multistix®; this reaction is not specific, reacting with substances which are detected by Ehrlich's reagent, including porphobilinogen, procaine, 5-HIAA, p-aminosalicylic acid metabolites, sulfonamides, indole, and methyldopa. Chemstrip® uses 4-methoxybenzene-diazonium-tetra fluoroborate. Specific for urobilinogen; nitrite or formalin can reduce the reaction.

Additional Information Urobilinogen is formed in the intestine by the action of bacteria on excreted conjugated (direct) bilirubin. A portion of the urobilinogen is absorbed from the gastrointestinal tract into the bloodstream. It returns to the liver where some is re-excreted in bile (enterohepatic circulation), and the rest (via the general circulation) is excreted into the urine. Urine urobilinogen can be increased as an early indicator of moderate hepatic parenchymal damage. Early toxic injury or hepatitis may also cause increased urine urobilinogen. However, if no bilirubin enters the bile no urobilinogen will be produced; thus, with high grade common bile duct obstruction, both urine and fecal urobilinogen will be decreased, but serum and urine bilirubin are greatly increased. Collection time is important because of diurnal variation in urobilinogen excretion. Alkaline pH of urine increases clearance of urobilinogen and increases reliability of results.

See Bilirubin, Urine *on page 870*.

Footnotes
1. Binder L, Smith D, Kupka T, et al, "Failure of Prediction of Liver Function Test Abnormalities With the Urine Urobilinogen and Urine Bilirubin Assays," *Arch Pathol Lab Med*, 1989, 113(1):73-6.

References
Henry JB, Lauzon RB, and Schumann GB, "Basic Examination of Urine," *Clinical Diagnosis and Management by Laboratory Methods*, 19th ed, Chapter 18, Philadelphia, PA: WB Saunders Co, 1996, 411-56.

♦ **Urobilinogen, 24-Hour Urine** *replaced by* Urobilinogen, 2-Hour Urine *on page 889*

♦ **Urobilinogen, Quantitative, Urine** *see* Urobilinogen, 2-Hour Urine *on page 889*

♦ **Urobilinogen, Urine** *see* Bilirubin, Urine *on page 870*

♦ **UTI Screen** *see* Nitrite, Urine *on page 882*

♦ **Vasopressin Concentration Test** *see* Concentration Test, Urine *on page 872*

ACRONYMS AND ABBREVIATIONS GLOSSARY

This glossary provides a useful listing of many acronyms and abbreviations commonly associated with laboratory medicine. We offer this glossary not as an exhaustive authoritative list, but more as a guide to assist in interpreting frequently used terminology.

a ... atto (10^{-18})
A ... apical; artery
A_1 ... blood group antigen
A_1AT ... alpha$_1$ antitrypsin
A_2 ... aortic second sound; blood group antigen
aa ... of each (ana)
AA ... arachidonic acid
aaa ... androgenic anabolic agent; aromatic amino acid
AAA ... abdominal aortic aneurysm; acquired aplastic anemia; acute anxiety attack
AAAAA ... aphasia, agnosia, apraxia, agraphia, and alexia
AAB ... action against burns; aminoazobenzene
AABB ... American Association of Blood Banks
AABCC ... alertness (consciousness), airway, breathing, circulation, and cervical spine
AAC ... antibiotic associated colitis
AACC ... American Association of Clinical Chemistry
AACSH ... adrenal androgen corticotropic stimulation hormone
AAE ... acute allergic encephalitis; annuloaortic ectasia
AaG ... alveolar arterial gradient
AAGS ... adult adrenogenital syndrome
AAIN ... acute allergic intestinal nephritis
AAL ... anterior axillary line
AAMS ... acute aseptic meningitis syndrome
AAN ... analgesic abuse nephropathy; analgesic associated nephropathy
AAO ... amino acid oxidase; awake to alert and oriented
$(A\text{-}a)O_2$ ... alveolar-arterial oxygen gradient
AAP ... American Academy of Pediatrics
AAPC ... antibiotic-associated pseudomembranous colitis
AAPCC ... American Association of Poison Control Centers
$A\text{-}aP_{co2}$ ... alveolar-arterial carbon dioxide difference
AAPF ... antiarteriosclerosis polysaccharide factor
AAPM ... antibiotic-associated pseudomembranous colitis
AAR ... active avoidance reaction; acute articular rheumatism; antigen-antiglobulin reaction; Australia antigen radioimmunoassay
AAS ... acute abdominal series; atomic absorption spectrometry
AASH ... adrenal androgen stimulating hormone
AASP ... acute atrophic spinal paralysis; ascending aorta synchronized pulsation
AAT ... alpha antitrypsin
AAU ... acute anterior uveitis
AAVV ... accumulated alveolar ventilatory volume
Ab ... antibody
AB ... abdominal; abort; antibiotic
A&B ... apnea and bradycardia
A/B ... acid-base ratio; apnea and bradycardia
ABA ... abscissic acid; allergic bronchopulmonary aspergillosis; antibacterial activity
ABB ... Albright-Butler-Bloomberg (syndrome)
ABC ... avidin-biotin complex
ABD ... after bronchodilator; aged, blind, and disabled; aggressive behavioral disturbance; average body dose
ABE ... acute bacterial endocarditis
ABG ... arterial blood gas
ABGT ... ancillary blood glucose testing
ABL ... abetalipoprotein
ABLB ... alternate binaural loudness balance
ABMT ... autologous bone marrow transplantation
ABO ... ABO blood group
ABPA ... allergic bronchopulmonary aspergillosis
ABR ... auditory brainstem response
ABS ... alkylbenzene sulfonate
ac ... before meals (ante cibum)
Ac ... actinium
AC ... air conduction; alternating current
ACA ... acute cerebellar ataxia; anticardiolipin antibody; Du Pont chemistry analyzer
ACC ... amylase creatinine clearance
ACD ... acid-citrate-dextrose; anemia of chronic disease
ACE ... angiotensin converting enzyme
AChR ... acetylcholine receptor antibody
ACIP ... Advisory Committee on Immunization Policies
ACL ... anterior cruciate ligament
ACLS ... advanced cardiac life support
ACOG ... American College of Obstetrics and Gynecology
ACOP ... Adriamycin (doxorubicin), cyclophosphamide, Oncovin (vincristine), and prednisone
ACOPP ... Adriamycin (doxorubicin), cyclophosphamide, Oncovin (vincristine), prednisone, and procarbazine
AcP ... acid phosphatase
ACPA ... anticytoplasmic antibodies
ACT ... activated clotting time
ACTH ... adrenocorticotropic hormone
ACTN ... adrenocorticotropin
ACV ... acyclovir; amifostine, cisplatin, and vinblastine
ACVB ... aortocoronary venous bypass
ACVD ... acute cardiovascular disease
ad ... right ear; up to (ad)
a.d. ... alternating days
AD ... admitting diagnosis; Alzheimer disease; atopic dermatitis; autosomal dominant
ADA ... adenosine deaminase
ADA# ... American Diabetes Association diet number
ADAS ... Alzheimer's Disease Assessment Scale
ADC ... Aid to Dependent Children
ADCA ... autosomal dominant cerebellar ataxia
ADCC ... antibody-dependent cell-mediated cytotoxicity
ADCONFU ... Adriamycin (doxorubicin), cyclophosphamide, Oncovin (vincristine), and 5-fluorouracil
ADD ... attention deficit disorder
ADDH ... attention deficit disorder with hyperactivity
ADH ... alcohol dehydrogenase; antidiuretic hormone
ADHD ... attention deficit hyperactive disorder
ADIC ... Adriamycin (doxorubicin) and dimethyltriazenylimidazole carboxamide (dacarbazine)
ADL ... active daily living
ad lib ... as desired (ad libitum)
ADM ... admission
ADME ... absorption, distribution, metabolism, and excretion
ADNase ... anti-DNAse
ADO ... adolescent medicine
ADP ... adenosine 5-diphosphate
ADPKD ... autosomal dominant polycystic kidney disease
ADR ... acceptable dental remedies; acute dystonic reaction; Adriamycin; adverse drug reaction
ADRs ... adverse drug reactions
ADT ... adenosine triphosphate; alternate-day treatment
AED ... anticonvulsant drugs
AEP ... acute edematous pancreatitis; auditory evoked potential; average evoked potential
AER ... acoustic evoked response; agranular endoplasmic reticulum; auditory evoked response; average evoked response
AES ... adult emergency service; antiembolic stockings
AF ... acid-fast; amniotic fluid; aortic flow; artrial fibrillation; atrial flutter
AFB ... acid-fast bacillus; aortofemoral bypass; aspirated foreign body
AFBG ... aortofemoral bypass graft
AFC ... adult foster care
AFCI ... acute focal cerebral ischemia
AFDC ... Aid to Families with Dependent Children
AFEB ... afebrile
aff ... afferent
AF/F ... atrial fibrillation and/or flutter
AFib ... atrial fibrillation
AFL ... atrial flutter
AFM ... atomic force microscopy
AFND ... acute febrile neutrophilic dermatosis
AFO ... ankle-foot orthrosis
aFP, AFP ... alpha-fetoprotein
AFRD ... acute febrile respiratory disease
AFRI ... acute febrile respiratory illness
AFS ... acid-fast smear
Ag ... antigen; silver
AG ... abdominal girth
A/G ... albumin/globulin ratio
AGA ... accelerated growth area; appropriate for gestational age; average for gestational age
AGF ... angle of greatest flexion
AGG ... aggregation
agit ... shake
agit ante us. ... shake before using
agit bene ... shake well
AGLT ... acidified glycerol lysis test
AGN ... acute glomerular nephritis
$AgNO_3$ ... silver nitrate
AGS ... adrenogenital syndrome
AGUS ... atypical glandular cells of indetermined significance
AH ... antihyaluronidase
A-H ... atrial-His
AHA ... acquired hemolytic anemia; acute hemolytic anemia; autoimmune hemolytic anemia
AHBC ... hepatitis B core antibody
AHC ... acute hemorrhagic conjunctivitis; acute hemorrhagic cystitis
AHE ... acute hemorrhagic encephalomyelitis
AHF ... acute heart failure; antihemophilic factor (factor VIII)
AHFS ... American Hospital Formulary Service
AHG ... antihemophilic globulin
AHLE ... acute hemorrhagic leukoencephalitis
AHP ... acute hemorrhagic pancreatitis
AHT ... antihyaluronidase titer
AI ... accidental injury; allergy index; aortic insufficiency; artificial insemination; atrial insufficiency
AICC ... anti-inhibitor coagulant complex
AID ... acquired immunodeficiency disease; acute infectious disease
AIDS ... acquired immunodeficiency syndrome
AIDS-KS ... acquired immunodeficiency syndrome with Kaposi's sarcoma
AIHA ... autoimmune hemolytic anemia
AIHD ... acquired immune hemolytic disease
AIMS ... abnormal involuntary movement scale; arthritis impact measurement scale
AIP ... acute intermittent porphyria; average intravascular pressure
AJ ... ankle jerk
AJR ... abnormal jugular reflex
AK ... adenylate kinase; above the knee
A/K ... above knee (amputation)
AKA ... above knee (amputation); all known allergies; also known as
AK amp ... above knee amputation
AKP ... alkaline phosphatase
Al ... aluminum
AL ... acute leukemia; arterial line
ALA ... aminolevulinic acid
ALAC ... antibiotic-loaded acrylic cement
ALAD ... abnormal left axis deviation
alb ... albumin
ALF ... acute liver failure
ALFT ... abnormal liver function test
A-line ... arterial catheter; arterial line
alk ... alkaline
AlkP ... alkaline phosphatase
alk phos, alk p'tase ... alkaline phosphates
all. ... allergic/allergy

ALL ... acute lymphoblastic leukemia; acute lymphocytic leukemia
ALMI ... anterior lateral myocardial infarction
ALO ... average lymphocyte output
$Al(OH)_3$ ... aluminum hydroxide
ALOMAD ... Adriamycin (doxorubicin), Leukeran (chlorambucil), Oncovin (vincristine), methotrexate, actinomycin D, and dacarbazine
ALOS ... average length of stay
AlP, ALP ... alkaline phosphatase
AlPI ... alkaline phosphatase isoenzymes
ALPS ... autoimmune lymphoproliferative syndrome
ALS ... acute lateral sclerosis; advanced life support; amyotrophic lateral sclerosis; antilymphocyte serum
ALT ... alanine aminotransferase
ALT/AST ... ratio of serum alanine aminotransferase to serum aspartate aminotransferase
Am ... americium
AM ... acute myelofibrosis; alveolar mucosa; morning
AMA ... against medical advice; American Medical Association; antimitrochondrial antibody
amb, AMB ... ambulate/ambulatory
AMBL ... acute myeloblastic leukemia
ambul ... ambulate/ambulatory
AMegL, AMEGL ... acute megakaryoblastic leukemia
AMI ... acute myocardial infarction
AML ... acute myeloblastic leukemia; acute myelogenous leukemia
AMOL ... acute monoblastic/monocytic leukemia
AMP ... adenosine monophosphate
AMPS ... acid mucopolysaccharide
AMPT ... alpha-methyl-p-tyrosine
AMS ... acute mountain sickness; altered mental status
AMT ... acute miliary tuberculosis
AN ... acanthosis nigricans; anorexia nervosa; aseptic necrosis; avascular necrosis
ANA ... antinuclear antibody
ANC ... absolute neutrophil count
ANCA ... antineutrophil cytoplasmic antibodies
ANDA ... Abbreviated New Drug Application
ANF ... antinuclear factor
ANH ... acute normovolemic hemodilution
ANLL ... acute nonlymphocytic leukemia
ANOVA ... analysis of variance
ANP ... atrial natriuretic peptide
anti-TB ... antituberculosis
ant. pit. ... anterior pituitary
ant. prand ... before parturition
AO ... abdominal aorta; aortic opening
A&O ... alert and oriented
AOD ... adult-onset diabetes
AODA ... alcohol and other drug abuse
AODM ... adult onset diabetes mellitus
aort sten ... aortic stenosis
AOS ... acridine orange staining
AOV ... aortic value
ap ... before dinner; prior to
AP ... acid phosphatase; adolescent psychiatry; antepartum; anteroposterior; appendectomy; appendicitis; assessment and plans
A&P ... anterior and posterior; assessment and plans
A/P ... ascites-plasma (ratio)
A-P ... anterior-posterior
APACHE ... acute physiology and chronic health evaluation (systems)
APAP ... acetaminophen
APB ... atrial premature beat
APCA ... antiparetial cell antibody
APCD ... adult polycystic kidney disease
APD ... acute polycystic disease; adult polycystic disease
APE ... doxorubicin (Adriamycin), cisplatin (Platinol), and etoposide
APGAR ... appearance, pulse, grimace, activity, and respiration (score of newbornphysical status)
aph ... aphasia
APhA ... American Pharmaceutical Association
APKD ... adult polycystic kidney disease
APP ... alum-precipitating pyridine
APR ... acute phase reactant
APSAC ... anisoylated plasminogen streptokinase activator complex
APTT ... activated partial thromboplastin time
APUD ... amine precursor uptake and decarboxylation
aq ... water (aqua)
aq ad ... add water
Ar ... argon
AR ... aortic regurgitation; apical-radial (pulse); autosomal recessive
A/R, A-R ... apical-radial (pulse)
ARA ... antireticulin antibody
araC-Hu ... arabinosylcytosine (cytarabine) and hydroxyurea
ARBD ... aluminum-related bone disease
ARC ... acquired immunodeficiency syndrome-related complex
ARD ... antimicrobial removal device; acute respiratory distress
ARDS ... adult respiratory distress syndrome
ARF ... acute renal failure
ARF/CRF ... acute renal failure/chronic renal failure
ARLD ... alcohol-related liver disease
ARM ... artificial rupture of membranes
ARN ... acute renal/retinal necrosis
AROM ... active range of motion; artificial rupture of membranes
Ars ... arylsulfatase
ART ... arterial line
ARV ... AIDS-associated retrovirus; AIDS-related virus; anterior right ventricular (wall)
as ... left ear
As ... arsenic
AS ... anal sphincter; ankylosing spondylitis; aortic stenosis; atrial septum; atrial stenosis
AsA ... arylsulfatase A
ASA ... acetylsalicylic acid
ASAP ... as soon as possible
ASAT ... aspartate aminotransferase
AsB ... arylsulfatase B
ASCP ... American Society of Clinical Pathologists
ASCVD ... arteriosclerotic cardiovascular disease
ASD ... Alzheimer senile dementia; atrial septal defect
ASDH ... acute subdural hematoma
ASHD ... arteriosclerotic/atherosclerotic heart disease; atrial septal heart disease
ASHP ... American Society of Health-System Pharmacists
ASK ... antistreptokinase
ASKA ... antiskeletal antibody
ASLO ... antistreptolysin O
ASLT ... antistreptolysin test
ASM ... American Society of Microbiology
ASMA ... antismooth muscle antibody
ASO ... antistreptolysin O; arterioselerosis obliterans
asp ... aspirate
ASP ... ankylosing spondylitis
AS-PCR ... allele-specific polymerase chain reaction
ASS ... acute serum sickness
AST ... alternate site testing; antistreptolysin titer; aspartate aminotransferase
ASVD ... arteriosclerotic vascular disease
At ... astatine
AT, A-T ... ataxia-telangiectasia
ATB ... atrial tachycardia with block; atypical tuberculosis
at. fib, At Fib ... atrial fibrillation
ATG ... antithymocyte globulin
AT-III ... antithrombin III
ATL ... adult T-cell leukemia
ATLL ... adult T-cell leukemia/lymphoma
ATLS ... advanced trauma life support
ATLV ... adult T-cell leukemia virus
ATN ... acute tubular necrosis
ATP ... adenosine triphosphate
ATPase ... adenosine triphosphatase
ATR ... Achilles tendon reflex
atr fib., ATR FIB ... atrial fibrillation
atrial flutter ... AFL
ATS ... American Thoracic Society
au ... each ear (auris utro)
Au ... gold
^{198}Au ... radioisotope of gold
AU ... both ears together
AUB ... abnormal uterine bleeding
AUC ... area under the curve
aud, AUD ... arthritis of unknown diagnosis
AUGIB ... acute upper gastrointestinal bleeding
AUL ... acute undifferentiated leukemia
aur fib., AUR FIB ... auricular fibrillation
AUS ... acute urethral syndrome
A-V ... arteriovenous; atrioventricular; audiovisual
AVA ... availability
AVB ... atrioventricular block
AVE ... aortic valve echocardiogram
AVH ... acute viral hepatitis
AVHB ... atrioventricular heart block
AVHD ... acquired valvular heart disease
AVM ... arteriovenous malformation
AVP ... aqueous vasopressin; arginine vasopressin
AVR ... accelerated ventricular rhythm; aortic valve replacement
AVSS ... afebrile, vital signs stable
A&W ... alive and well
Ax ... axillary
AZA-CR ... azacitidine
AZT ... zidovudine
B ... boron
Ba ... barium
BA ... Bachelor of Arts
B&A ... brisk and active
BAC ... blood alcohol concentration
BACON ... bleomycin, Adriamycin (doxorubicin), CCNU (lomustine), Oncovin (vincristine), and nitrogen mustard (mechlorethamine)
BACOP ... bleomycin, Adriamycin (doxorubicin), cyclophosphamide, Oncovin (vincristine), and prednisone
BACT ... bischloroethylnitrosourea, arabinosylcytosine, Cytoxan (cyclophosphamide), and 6-thioguanine; bleomycin, Adriamycin (doxorubicin), Cytoxan (cyclophosphamide), and tamoxifen citrate
BaE, BAE ... barium enema
BaEn ... barium enema
BAEP ... brainstem auditory evoked potential
BAER ... brainstem auditory evoked response
BAL ... bronchoalveolar lavage
B ALL ... B-cell acute lymphoblastic leukemia
BAN ... British approved name
BAND ... band neutrophil (stab)
BAO ... basal acid output
BAP ... bleomycin, Adriamycin (doxorubicin), and prednisone
BAVP ... balloon aortic valvuloplasty
BB ... Blood Bank
BBB ... blood-brain barrier; bundle-branch block
BBBB ... bilateral bundle-branch block
BBC ... basal cell carcinoma
BBF ... bronchial blood flow
BBPRL ... big big prolactin

BBT	basal body temperature
BB to MM	belly button to medial malleolus
B Bx	breast biopsy
BC	bone conduction
B&C	bed and chair
B-CAVE	bleomycin, CCNU (lomustine), Adriamycin (doxorubicin), and Velban (vinblastine)
BCC	basal cell carcinoma
BCCa	basal cell carcinoma
BCD	basal cell dysplasia; bleomycin, cyclophosphamide, and dactinomycin
BCE	basal cell epithelioma
BCG	bacillus Calmette-Guérin
BCH	basal cell hyperplasia/hypoplasia
BCLL	B-cell chronic lymphocytic leukemia
BCLS	basic cardiac life support (system)
BCM	bovine cervical mucus
BCNU	carmustine
BCP	birth control pills; blood cell profile
BCPs	birth control pills
bcr	breakpoint cluster region
BCSH	British Committee for Standards in Hematology
bd	twice a day (bis in die)
BD	bronchodilators
BDH-V	BCNU (carmustine), hydroxyurea, dacarbazine, and vincristine
BDM	black divorced male
B-DOPA	bleomycin, dacarbazine, Oncovin (vincristine), prednisone, and Adriamycin (doxorubicin)
Be	beryllium
BE	bacterial endocarditis; barium enema; below-elbow (amputation)
B/E	below-elbow (amputation)
BEA	below-elbow amputation
BEC	bacterial endocarditis
BEI	butanol-extractable iodine
benzodiazepine-GABA	gamma-aminobutyric acid
BEP	brainstem evoked potential
BERA	brainstem evoked response auditory
BF, B/F	black female
BFH	benign familial hematuria
BFS	blood fasting sugar
BFT	bentonite flocculation test
BFW	Bartlett-Farling-Wimbaly brush
BG	baby girl
B-G	Bender-Gestalt (test)
BGC	basal-ganglion calcification
BGL	blood glucose level
BGlu	blood glucose
BGP	bone GLA protein
BHAT	beta-blocker heart attack trial
BHB	beta-hydroxybutyrate
BHD	BCNU (carmustine), hydroxyurea, and dacarbazine
BHI	brain heart infusion
BHT	butylated hydroxytoluene
Bi	bismuth
bid, BID	twice a day (bis in die)
BIP	blood pressure
BJ	Bence Jones; biceps jerk; bone and joint
Bk	berkelium
BK	below knee
B/K	below-knee (amputation)
BKA	below-knee amputation
BKTT	below-knee to toe (cast)
BKWC	below-knee walking cast
BKWP	below-knee walking plaster
Bl	black
BLEO	bleomycin
BLEO-MOPP	bleomycin, mechlorethamine, Oncovin (vincristine), and prednisone
blk	black
BLL	below lower limit; bilateral lower lobe; brows, lids, and lashes
Bl Obs	bladder observation
bl pr, BL PR	blood pressure
BLS	basic life support
BM	black male; bone marrow; bowel movement; breast milk
B/M	black male
BMA	bone marrow arrest; bone marrow aspirate
BMD	bone mineral density
BMG	beta-2 microglobulin
BMI	body mass index
BMJ	bones, muscles, joints
BML	bone marrow lymphocytosis
BMMA	Bone Mass Measurement Act
BMR	basal metabolic rate
BMT	bone marrow transplantation
BNB	blood-nerve barrier
BNC	bladder neck contracture
BNO	bladder neck obstruction
BNR	bladder neck resection/retraction
B&O	belladonna and opium
BOLD	bleomycin, Oncovin (vincristine), lomustine, and dacarbazine
BOM	bilateral otitis media
BOMA	bilateral otitis media, acute
BOO	bladder outlet obstruction
BOOP	bronchiolitis obliterans organizing pneumonia
BOP	bleomycin, Oncovin (vincristine), and prednisone
BOPAM	bleomycin, Oncovin (vincristine), prednisone, Adriamycin (doxorubicin), and methotrexate
BP	back pressure; blood pressure
B/P	blood pressure
BPAC	Blood Product Advisory Committee
BPD	biparietal diameter
BPH	benign prostatic hyperplasia
bpm	beats per minute
BPO	bilateral partial oophorectomy
BPPP	bilateral pedal pulses present
BPR	blood per rectum
BPs	blood pressure, systolic
BPS	beats per secone; bilateral partial salpingectomy; breaths per second
BPT	benign paroxysmal torticollis
BPV	benign paroxysmal vertigo
Br	bromine; bromide
BR	bathroom; bedrest
BrdU	5-bromodeoxyuridine
BrM	breast milk
BRO	bromocriptine; bronchoscopy
broch	bronchoscopy
BRP	bathroom privileges
BRR	baroreceptor reflex response
BRU	bromide urine
BS	Bachelor of Science; blood sugar; bowel sounds; breath sounds
BSA	body surface area
BSEP	brainstem evoked potential
BSN	bowel sounds normal
BSNA	bowel sounds normal and active
BSO	bilateral salpingo-oophorectomy; bilateral serous otitis
BSOM	bilateral serous otitis media
BSP	bromsulfophthalein
BSR	basal skin resistance; blood sedimentation
BT	breast tumor
BTA	bladder tumor antigen
BTG	beta thromboglobulin
BTL	bilateral tubal ligation
BTPS	body temperature, ambient pressure, and saturated with water vapor (gas)
BTS	bradycardia-tachycardia syndrome
BU	bethesda units
BUN	blood urea nitrogen
BVAP	BCNU (carmustine), vincristine, Adriamycin (doxorubicin), and prednisone
BVL	bilateral vas ligation
BVP	blood volume pulse
bw, BW	birth weight; bite-wing (radiograph); body water; body weight
BWA	bed wetter admission
BWS	battered woman syndrome
BWt	birth weight
BWW	Biggers, Whitten, and Whittingham medium
bx, BX	biopsy
bz, BZ	benzodiazepine
BZD, BZDZ	benzodiazepine
c	with (cum)
C	carbon
C_2	second cervical vertebra
Ca	calcium
CA	cancer antigen; caproic acid; cardiac arrest; chronological age; Cocaine Anonymous
C&A	conscious and alert
CA 15-3	tumor marker antigen
CA 19-9	tumor marker antigen
CA 50	tumor marker antigen
CA 125	tumor marker antigen
CAA	computer-aided assessment; computer-assisted assessment
CAAT	computer-assisted axial tomography
CAB	coronary artery bypass
CABG	coronary artery bypass graft
CABGS	coronary artery bypass graft surgery
CABS	coronary artery bypass surgery
CAC	circulating anticoagulant
CaCl	calcium chloride
$CaCO_3$	calcium carbonate
CACX	cancer of cervix
Cad	cadaver
CAD	cadaver; computer-assisted diagnosis; coronary artery disease; cyclophosphamide, Adriamycin (doxorubicin), and dacarbazine; cytosine arabinoside and daunorubicin
CaEDTA	calcium disodium edetate
CAF	cyclophosphamide, Adriamycin (doxorubicin), and fluorouracil
CAFP	cyclophosphamide, Adriamycin (doxorubicin), fluorouracil, and prednisone
CAFVP	cyclophosphamide, Adriamycin (doxorubicin), fluorouracil, vincristine, and prednisone
CAG	cholangiogram; coronary angiogram/angiography
CAH	chronic active hepatitis; chronic aggressive hepatitis; combined atrial hypertrophy
CAHD	coronary arteriosclerotic heart disease; coronary atherosclerotic heart disease
CALD	chronic active liver disease
CALGB	cancer and leukemia group B
cALL	common null cell acute lymphocytic leukemia
CALLA	common acute lymphoblastic leukemia antigen
CAMB	cyclophosphamide, Adriamycin (doxorubicin), methotrexate, and bleomycin
CAMEO	cyclophosphamide, Adriamycin (doxorubicin), methotrexate, etoposide, and Oncovin (vincristine)
CAMF	cyclophosphamide, Adriamycin (doxorubicin), methotrexate, and fluorouracil
cAMP	cyclic AMP
CAMP	cyclophosphamide, Adriamycin (doxorubicin), methotrexate, and procarbazine
Can	cancer antigen
CAO	chronic airway obstruction
Ca_{o_2}	arterial oxygen concentration

CAOD . . . coronary artery occlusive disease
CAOM . . . chronic adhesive otitis media
CAP . . . cancer of prostate; community-acquired pneumonia; cyclophosphamide, Adriamycin (doxorubicin), and Platino (cisplatin); cyclophosphamide, Adriamycin (doxorubicin), and prednisone
CAPD . . . chronic ambulatory peritoneal dialysis
CAS . . . carotid artery stenosis; coronary artery spasm
CASA . . . computer-assisted semen analysis
CAST . . . cardiac arrhythmia suppression trial
CAT . . . computed axial tomography; cytosine arabinoside, Adriamycin (doxorubicin), and thioguanine
CATT . . . calcium tolerance test
CAV . . . cyclophosphamide, Adriamycin (doxorubicin), and vincristine
CAVB . . . complete atrioventricular block
CAVC . . . common arterioventricular canal
CAVD . . . complete atrioventricular dissociation; completion, arithmetic problems, vocabulary, following directions (battery)
CAVDH . . . continuous arteriovenous hemodialysis; continuous arteriovenous hemofiltration (with) dialysis
CAVE . . . CCNU (lomustine), Adriamycin (doxorubicin), and vinblastine
CAVH . . . continuous arteriovenous hemofiltration
CAVP . . . cyclophosphamide, Adriamycin (doxorubicin), vincristine, and prednisone
CAV-P-VP . . . cyclophosphamide, Adriamycin (doxorubicin), vincristine, Platino (cisplatin), and VP16-213 (etoposide)
CB . . . chair and bed; chest-back
C&B . . . chair and bed
C/B, C-B . . . chest-back
CBA . . . chronic bronchitis and asthma
CBAT . . . Coag battery; Coulter battery
CBAVD . . . congenital bilateral absence of the vas deferens
CBBB . . . complete bundle-branch block
CBC . . . complete blood count
CBCN . . . carbenicillin
CBD . . . common bile duct
CBDC . . . chronic bullous disease of childhood
CBDE . . . common bile duct ligation
CBE . . . clinical breast examination
CBF capillary blood flow; cerebral blood flow; coronary blood flow; cortical blood flow
CBFS . . . cerebral blood flow studies
CBFV . . . cerebral blood flow velocity
CBG . . . capillary blood gases; coronary bypass graft
CBH . . . chronic benign hepatitis
CBI . . . continuous bladder irrigation
CBIL . . . conjugated bilirubin
CBL . . . circulating blood lymphocytes
CBPPA . . . cyclophosphamide, bleomycin, procarbazine, prednisone, and Adriamycin (doxorubicin)
CBPS . . . coronary bypass surgery
CBS . . . chronic brain syndrome
CBT . . . circulating blood volume; cyclophosphamide, BCNU (carmustine), and VP16-213 (etoposide); computerized body tomography
CBVD . . . cerebrovascular disease
CBZ . . . carbamazepine
CC . . . chief complaint; closing capacity; colony count
C&C . . . cold and clammy
C/C . . . chief complaint
CCB . . . calcium channel blocker
CCCT . . . clomiphene citrate challenge test
CCH . . . chronic cholestatic hepatitis
CCI . . . chronic coronary insufficiency; corrected count increment
CCK . . . cholecystokinin
CCK-OP . . . cholecystokinin octapeptide
CCL . . . carcinoma cell line
CCl_4 . . . carbon tetrachloride
CCMS . . . clean-catch midstream (urine)
CCMSU . . . clean-catch midstream urine
CCMSUA . . . clean-catch midstream urinalysis
C_{cr} . . . creatinine clearance
CC&S . . . cornea, conjunctiva, and sclera
CCU . . . cardiac care unit; coronary care unit
CCUA . . . clean catch urinalysis
CCV . . . CCNU (lomustine), cyclophosphamide, and vincristine
CCVB . . . CCNU (lomustine), cyclophosphamide, vincristine, and bleomycin
CCVD . . . chronic cerebrovascular disease
CCVPP . . . CCNU (lomustine), cyclophosphamide, vinblastine, procarbazine, and prednisone
Cd . . . cadmium
C&D . . . curettage and desiccation
CDA . . . congenital dyserythropoietic anemia
CDC . . . carboplatin, doxorubicin, and cyclophosphamide; Centers for Disease Control
CDDP . . . cis-diaminedichloroplatinum
CDP . . . chlordiazepoxide; continuous distending pressure; cytidine diphosphate
CDT . . . carbohydrate-deficient transferrin
CDU . . . cumulative dose unit
CDX . . . chlordiazepoxide
CDZ . . . chlordiazepoxide
Ce . . . cerium
C&E . . . consultation and examination
CEA . . . carcinoembryonic antigen
CEBV . . . chronic Epstein-Barr virus
CERD . . . chronic end-stage renal disease
CES . . . conjugated estrogenic substances
CEV . . . cyclophosphamide, etoposide, and vincristine
Cf . . . californium
CF . . . cardiac failure; caucasian female; complement fixation; cystic fibrosis
C&F . . . curettage and fulguration
CFCL . . . continuous flow centrifugation leukapheresis
CFL . . . cisplatin, fluorouracil, and leucovorin calcium
CFM . . . cyclophosphamide, fluorouracil, and citoxantrone
CFTR . . . cystic fibrosis transmembrane conductance regulator
CFU . . . colony forming units
CFU-GM . . . colony forming units - granulocytic/monocytic
CG . . . chorionic gonadotropin
CGB . . . chronic gastrointestinal (tract) bleeding
CGD . . . chronic granulomatous disease
CGH . . . chorionic gonadotropic hormone
CGL . . . chronic granulocytic leukemia
CGRP . . . calcitonin gene-related peptide
CH . . . case history; congenital hypothyroidism
CHA . . . chronic hemolytic anemia
CHAM-OCA . . . cyclophosphamide, hydroxyurea, actinomycin D (dactinomycin), methotrexate, Oncovin (vincristine), citrovorum factor (leucovorin), and Adriamycin (doxorubicin)
CHAP . . . cyclophosphamide, hexamethylmelamine, Adriamycin (doxorubicin), and Platino (cisplatin)
CHBHA . . . congenital Heinz body hemolytic anemia
CHD . . Chediak-Higashi disease; congenital heart disease; congenital hip disease/dysplasia; congestive heart disease; coronary/cyanotic heart disease; cyclophosphamide, hexamethylmelamine, cisplatin
CHF . . . congenital hepatic fibrosis; congestive heart failure; cyclophosphamide, hexamethylmelamine, and 5-fluorouracil
CHI . . . closed head injury
CHO . . . cyclophosphamide, hydroxydaunorubicin, and Oncovin (vincristine)
CHOP . . . cyclophosphamide, hydroxydaunorubicin, Oncovin (vincristine), and prednisone
CHOR . . . cyclophosphamide, hydroxydaunorubicin, Oncovin (vincristine), and radiation
CHr . . . reticulocyte hemoglobin content
CHS . . . central hypoventilation syndrome
CHT . . . closed head trauma
CI . . . cardiac index; cardiac insufficiency; color index; confidence intervals; coronary insufficiency
CIBD . . . chronic inflammatory bowel disease
CIC . . . circulating immune complexes
cic-DDP . . . cis-diaminedichloroplatinum
CIE . . . counterimmunoelectrophoresis
CIF . . . clone-inhibiting factor
CIHD . . . chronic ischemic heart disease
CIN . . . cervical intraepithelial neoplasia; chronic interstitial nephritis
CIP . . . cellular immunocompetence profile
CIPD . . . chronic inflammatory polyradiculoneuropathy, demyelinating
circ & sen . . . circulation and sensation
CIRR . . . cirrhosis
CISCA . . . cisplatin, cyclophosphamide, and Adriamycin (doxorubicin)
CIVII . . . continuous intravenous insulin infusion
CIXU . . . constant infusion excretory urogram
CJD . . . Creutzfeldt-Jakob disease
CJS . . . Creutzfeldt-Jakob syndrome
CK . . . creatine kinase
CK-ISO . . . creatine kinase isoenzyme
Cl . . . chlorine
CL . . . cirrhosis of liver
Cla . . . clarithromycin
CLA . . . certified laboratory assistant
CLBB . . . complete left bundle-branch block
CLD . . . chronic liver disease
CLL . . . cholesterol-lowering lipid; chronic lymphocytic leukemia
CLO . . . cod liver oil
CLS . . . clinical laboratory scientist
CLSL . . . chronic lymphosarcoma (cell) leukemia
cm . . . centimeter
cm^2 . . . square centimeter
cm^3 . . . cubic centimeter
Cm . . . curium
CM . . . caucasian male; contrast media; culture media
C&M . . . cocaine and morphine
C/M . . . counts per minute
CMA . . . chronic metabolic acidosis; cow's milk allergy
C_{max} . . . maximum concentration of drug
CMB . . . carbolic methylene blue
CMBBT . . . cervical mucous basal body temperature
CMC . . . carboxymethylcellulose; cyclophosphamide, methotrexate, and CCNU (lomustine)
CMF . . . cyclophosphamide, methotrexate, and fluorouracil
CMFH . . . cyclophosphamide, methotrexate, fluorouracil, and hydroxyurea
CMFP . . . cyclophosphamide, methotrexate, fluorouracil, prednisone
CMF-TAM . . . cyclophosphamide, methotrexate, fluorouracil, and tamoxifen
CMFV . . . cyclophosphamide, methotrexate, fluorouracil, and vincristine
CMFVP . . . cyclophosphamide, methotrexate, fluorouracil, vincristine, and prednisone
CMG . . . congenital myasthenia gravis; cystometrogram
CMI . . . carbohydrate metabolism index; cell-mediated immunity
c/min . . . cycles per minute
C_{min} . . . minimum concentration of drug
CML . . . cell-mediated lymphocytotoxicity/lympholysis; cell-mediated lysis; chronic myelogenous leukemia
CMM . . . cell-mediated mutagenesis
CMML . . . chronic myelomonocytic leukemia
C-MOPP . . . cyclophosphamide, mechlorethamine, Oncovin (vincristine), procarbazine, and prednisone
cmp . . . counts per minute
CMP . . . cardiomyopathy; cervical mucus penetration
CMP-FX . . . complement fixation
CMPT . . . cervical mucous penetration test
CMSUA . . . clean, midstream urinalysis
CMV . . . cisplatin, methotrexate, and vinblastine; cytomegalovirus

CMVIG: cytomegalovirus immune globulin
CMV-IGIV: cytomegalovirus immune globulin intravenous
CMVS: culture midvoid specimen
CN: caudate nucleus; congenital nephrosis; cyanogen
CNDC: chronic nonspecific diarrhea of childhood
CNF: cyclophosphamide, Novantrone (mitoxantrone), and fluorouracil
CNHD: congenital nonspherocytic hemolytic disease
CNP: cranial nerve palsy
CNS: central nervous system; coagulase negative staph
CNSHA: congenital nonspherocytic hemolytic anemia
Co: cobalt
^{57}Co: radioisotope of cobalt
^{58}Co: radioisotope of cobalt
^{60}Co: radioisotope of cobalt
CO: carbon monoxide; cardiac output
CO_2: carbon dioxide
CO_3: carbonate
c/o: check out
C/O: check out; complaint of
CoA: coenzyme A
COAD: chronic obstructive airway/arterial disease
coag: coagulation
COAG: chronic open angle glaucoma
COAP: cyclophosphamide, Oncovin (vincristine), arabinosylcytosine, and prednisone
COB: chronic obstructive bronchitis; cisplatin, Oncovin (vincristine), and bleomycin; coordination of benefits
COBRA: Consolidated Omnibus Budget Reconciliation Act
COBS: chronic organic brain syndrome
COBT: chronic obstruction of biliary tract
COC: combined oral contraceptive
COD: cause of death
COEPS: cortical origination extrapyramidal system
COHb: carboxyhemoglobin
COLD: chronic obstructive lung disease
COM: chronic otitis media; cyclophosphamide, Oncovin (vincristine), and methotrexate; cyclophosphamide, Oncovin (vincristine), and methyl-CCNU (semustine)
COMA: cyclophosphamide, Oncovin (vincristine), methotrexate, and arabinosylcytosine
COMB: cyclophosphamide, Oncovin (vincristine), methyl-CCNU (semustine), and bleomycin
COMLA: cyclophosphamide, Oncovin (vincristine), methotrexate, leucovorin, and arabinosylcytosine
COMP: cyclophosphamide, Oncovin (vincristine), methotrexate, and prednisone
COMS: chronic organic mental syndrome
COMT: catechol-o-methyltransferase
CONPADRI I: cyclophosphamide, Oncovin (vincristine), L-phenylalanine mustard, and Adriamycin (doxorubicin)
CONPADRI II: CONPADRI I plus high dose methotrexate
CONPADRI III: CONPADRI I plus intensified doxorubicin
COP: capillary osmotic pressure; chronic obstructive pulmonary; cyclophosphamide, Oncovin (vincristine), and prednisone
COPA: cyclophosphamide, Oncovin (vincristine), prednisone, and Adriamycin (doxorubicin)
COP-BLAM: cyclophosphamide, Oncovin (vincristine), prednisone, bleomycin, Adriamycin (doxorubicin), and Matulane (procarbazine)
COPD: chronic obstructive pulmonary disease
COPE: chronic obstructive pulmonary emphysema
COPP: cyclophosphamide, Oncovin (vincristine), procarbazine, and prednisone
CORD: chronic obstructive respiratory disease
COT: continuous oxygen therapy
COTX: cast removed, take x-ray
CP: cardiac pacing; cardiac performance; cardiopulmonary; cerebral palsy; chest pain; cyclophosphamide and prednisone
C&P: compensation and pension; complete and pain-free (range of motion); cystoscopy and pyelogram
C/P: cardiopulmonary; cholesterol-phospholipid
CPA: carotid phonoangiography; cyclophosphamide
CPAP: continuous positive airway pressure
CPB: cardiopulmonary bypass
CPBV: cardiopulmonary blood volume
CPCS: clinical pharmacokinetics consulting service
CPD: childhood polycystic disease; chronic peritoneal dialysis; citrate phosphate dextrose; cyst disease protein
CPDA: citrate phosphate dextrose adenine
CPE: chronic pulmonary emphysema; cytopathogenic effects
CPEO: chronic progressive external ophthalmoplegia
CPH: chronic persistent hepatitis
CPI: coronary prognostic index
CPIP: chronic pulmonary insufficiency of prematurity
CPK: creatine phosphokinase
CPK-2: creatine phosphokinase MB fraction
CPK-BB: creatine phosphokinase BB fraction
CPKD: childhood polycystic kidney disease
CPK-MB: creatine phosphokinase of muscle band
cpm, CPM: counts per minute
CPmax: peak (maximum) serum concentration
CPmin: trough (minimum) serum concentration
CPMS: chronic progressive multiple sclerosis
CPP: cerebral perfusion pressure
CPPB: continuous positive pressure breathing
CPPD: calcium pyrophosphate dihydrate; chest percussion and postural drainage
CPR: cardiac and pulmonary rehabilitation; cardiopulmonary resuscitation; cortisol production rate
cps: counts per second; cycles per second
CPS: cardioplegic perfusion solution; cardiopulmonary support; characters per second; Compendium of Pharmaceuticals and Specialties
CPT: chest physiotherapy
CPUE: chest pain of unknown etiology
CQA: concurrent quality assurance
Cr: chromium
^{51}Cr: radioisotope of chromium
C&R: cardiac and respiratory; convalescence and rehabilitation; cystoscopy and retrograde
CRA: central retinal artery
CRAMS: circulation, respiration, abdomen, motor, and speech
CRAO: central retinal artery occlusion
CRC: colorectal carcinoma
CRD: childhood rheumatic disease; chronic renal disease; chronic respiratory disease
Cre: creatinine
creat: creatinine
CRF: chronic renal failure; chronic respiratory failure; corticotropin releasing factor
CRH: corticotropin-releasing hormone
crit, Crit: hematocrit
CRL: crown rump length
CRM: cross-reacting material
CROP: cyclophosphamide, rubidazone, Oncovin (vincristine), and prednisone
CRP: C-reactive protein
CRPD: chronic restrictive pulmonary disease
CRS: catheter related sepsis
CRST: calcinosis, Raynaud's phenomenon, sclerodactylia, telangiectasis
CRT: cadaver renal transplant; cardiac resuscitation team; cathode ray tube
CRTX: cast removed, take x-ray
CRU: cardiac rehabilitation unit; clinical research unit
CRV: central retinal vein
CRVF: congestive right ventricular failure
CRVO: central retinal vein occlusion
Cs: cesium
c/s: cycles per second
CS: cesarean section; coronary sclerosis
C&S: cough and sneeze; culture and sensitivity; culture and susceptibility
C/S: cesarean section; culture and sensitivity
C-S: cervical spine
CsA: cyclosporin A
CS&CC: culture, sensitivity, and colony count
CSD: cat scratch disease
C sect: cesarean section
CSF: cerebrospinal fluid; colony-stimulated factor
CSID: sucrase-isomaltase deficiency
CSII: continuous subcutaneous insulin infusion
CSIIP: continuous subcutaneous insulin infusion pump
CSNS: carotid sinus nerve stimulation
CSO: copied standing orders
CSOM: chronic serous/suppurative otitis media
CSP: carotid sinus pressure; chemistry screening profile
CSR: corrected sedimentation rate
CSS: carotid sinus stimulation; carotid sinus syndrome; coronary sinus stimulation
CST: cardiac stress test; cavernous sinus thrombosis; convulsive shock therapy
CSUF: continuous slow ultrafiltration
CT: cardiac tamponade; circulation time; clotting time; computerized tomography
C/T: compression to traction ratio; crossmatch to transfusion ratio
CTA: clear to auscultation; Committee on Thrombolytic Agents; computed tomoangiography
CTAB: cetyltrimethylammonium bromide
CTAP: computed tomography during arterial portography
CTAT: computed transaxial tomography
CTD: carpal tunnel decompression; chest tube drainage; congenital thymic dysplasia; connective tissue disease
CT&DB: cough, turn, and deep breath
CTDW: continues to do well
C/TG: cholesterol-triglyceride
CTGA: complete transposition of great arteries
CTM: *Chlamydia* transport media
C&TN BLE: color and temperature normal, both lower extremities
CTP: comprehensive treatment plan
C-TPN: cyclic total parenteral nutrition
CTPP: cerebral tissue perfusion pressure
CTPVO: chronic thrombotic pulmonary vascular obstruction
CTS: carpal tunnel syndrome
CTT: computerized transaxial tomography
CTUWSD: chest tube under water-seal drainage
CTV: cervical and thoracic vertebrae
CTX: cytoxan
Cu: copper
CU: cardiac unit; cause unknown
CUC: chronic ulcerative colitis
CUE: cumulative urinary excretion
CV: cardiovascular; cervical vertebra; coefficient of variation; conjugata vera
CVA: cardiovascular accident; cerebrovascular accident; cyclophosphamide, vincristine, and Adriamycin (doxorubicin)
CVA-BMP: cyclophosphamide, Oncovin (vincristine), Adriamycin (doxorubicin), BCNU (carmustine), methotrexate, and procarbazine
CVB: CCNU (lomustine), vinblastine, and bleomycin
CVC: central venous catheter
CVD: cardiovascular disease; cerebrovascular disease; cerebrovascular disorder; collagen vascular disease
CVE: cerebrovascular evaluation
CVEB: cisplatin, vinblastine, etoposide, and bleomycin
CVF: cardiovascular failure; central visual field; cervicovaginal fluid
CVHD: chronic valvular heart disease
CVI: cardiovascular insufficiency; cerebral vascular insufficiency; continuous venous infusion
CVM: cyclophosphamide, vincristine, and methotrexate

CVO ... central vein occlusion
CVOD ... cerebrovascular obstructive disease
CVP cardiac valve procedure; cardioventricular pacing; central venous pressure; cyclophosphamide, vincristine, and prednisone
CVPP ... cyclophosphamide, vincristine, prednisone, and procarbazine
CVR ... cardiovascular-renal (disease); cardiovascular resistance
CVRD ... cardiovascular-renal disease
CVS ... cardiovascular system; clean voided specimen
c/w, C/W ... compatible/consistent with
CW ... cardiac work
CWI ... cardiac work index
CWOP ... childbirth without pain
CWP ... childbirth without pain
CWS ... chest wall stimulation
Cx ... cervical; cervix
CXR ... chest x-ray
CXTX ... cervical traction
CyADIC ... cyclophosphamide, Adriamycin (doxorubicin), and DIC (dacarbazine)
CYT ... cyclophosphamide
Cy-VA-DIC ... cyclophosphamide, Oncovin (vincristine), Adriamycin (doxorubicin), DTIC (dacarbazine)
CZE ... capillary zone electrophoresis
d ... day
1/d ... daily, one per day
2/d ... twice a day
D_5W ... 5% dextrose in water solution
DA ... dopamine; ductus arteriosus
DAB ... days after birth
DAF ... delay accelerating factor
DALA ... delta aminolevulinic acid
D and C ... dilation and curettage
DAP ... Adriamycin (doxorubicin) and Platino (cisplatin)
DAT ... daunorubicin, arabinosylcytosine, and thioguanine; direct antiglobulin test
DAW ... dispense as written
db ... decibel
DB ... deep breath
D/B ... date of birth
DB&C ... deep breathing and coughing
DBE ... deep breathing exercise
DBF ... disturbed bowel function
DBI ... development at birth index
DBP ... diastolic blood pressure
DBS ... deep brain stimulation; diminished breath sounds
DC ... daily census; daunorubicin and cytarabine; dilation and curettage; direct current
D&C ... dilation and curettage
d/c ... discontinue
D/C ... diarrhea/constipation discharge; discontinue
DCAG ... double coronary artery graft
DC&B ... dilation, curettage, and biopsy
DCBE ... double contrast barium enema
DCBF ... dynamic cardiac blood flow
DCCMP ... daunomycin, cyclocytidine, 6-mercaptopurine, and prednisone
DCG ... dynamic electrocardiogram
DCH ... delayed and cutaneous hypersensitivity
DCIS ... ductal carcinoma *in situ*
DCMP ... daunomycin, cytarabine, 6-mercaptopurine, and prednisone
DCPM ... daunomycin, cytarabine, prednisone, and mercaptopurine
DCS ... decompression sickness
DCSA ... double-contrast shoulder arthrography
DCx ... double convex
DD ... differential diagnosis; discharge diagnosis
D&D ... diarrhea and dehydration
D/D ... differential diagnosis
dDAVP, DDAVP ... deamino-8-d-arginine vasopressin (desmopressin acetate)
DDD ... degenerative disc disease
DDI ... dideoxyinosine; dressing dry and intact
DDP ... diaminedichloroplatinum
DDS ... damaged disk syndrome; diaminodiphenylsulfone
DDT ... dichloro-diphenyltrichloroethane
DDVP ... dimethyldichlorovinyl phosphate (dichlorvos)
DDx, DDX ... differential diagnosis
D&E ... diet and elimination
DEA ... Drug Enforcement Agency
DEAE ... diethylaminoethyl
DEB ... diepoxybutane
DEC ... deceased
DED ... date of expected delivery
DER ... dermatome evoked response; disulfiram-ethanol reaction
DEXA ... dual energy x-ray absorptiometry
DF decapacitation factor (sperm); decayed and filled (permanent teeth); diastolic filling
DFA ... diet for age; direct fluorescent antibody
DFMO ... difluoromethylornithine
DFMR ... daily fetal movement
DFP ... diastolic filling period; diisopropylfluorophosphonate
dg ... decigram
DGE ... delayed gastric emptying
DGI ... disseminated gonococcal infection
DGM ... diffuse glomerulonephritis
DGS ... diabetic glomerulosclerosis
DH ... daily habits; dermatitis herpetiformis
DHA ... dehydroepiandrosterone
DHAD ... dihydroxybisaminoanthraquinone dihydrochloride
DHCA ... deep hypothermia and circulatory arrest
DHEA ... dehydroepiandrosterone
DHEA-S ... dehydroepiandrosterone sulfate
DHF ... dengue hemorrhagic fever
DHFR ... dihydrofolate reductase
DHFS ... dengue hemorrhagic fever shock (syndrome)
DHL ... diffuse histiocytic lymphoma
DHP ... dihydroxyacetone phosphate
DHR ... delayed hypersensitivity reaction
DHS ... delayed hypersensitivity; duration of hospital stay
DHST ... delayed hypersensitivity test
DHT ... dihydrotestosterone
DI ... date of injury; diabetes insipidus; dispensing information; dyspnea index
D&I ... debridement and irrigation; dry and intact
DIAGNO ... differential diagnosis
DIC ... disseminated intravascular coagulation
DIDMOAD ... diabetes insipidus, diabetes mellitus, optic atrophy, and deafness (syndrome)
dif ... differential (blood count)
diff ... difference; differential
Diff ... differential (blood count)
DIFF ... differential (blood count)
diff diag ... differential diagnosis
DIFP ... diffuse interstitial; fibrosing pneumonitis
dig, dig. ... digitalis
DIG ... digitalis; digitoxin; digoxin
dig. tox ... digitalis toxicity
DIH ... died in hospital
DILD ... diffuse interstitial lung
DILE ... drug-induced lupus erythematosus
DIMOAD ... diabetes insipidus, diabetes mellitus, optic atrophy, and deafness (syndrome)
DIP ... desquamative interstitial pneumonia/pneumonitis; dichlorophenolindophenol
DIPC ... diffuse interstitial pulmonary calcification
diph ... diphtheria
diph-tox ... diphtheria toxoid
DIRD ... drug-induced renal disease
DISIDA ... diisopropyl-iminodiacetic acid
DIVA ... digital intravenous angiography
DIVBC ... disseminated intravascular blood coagulation
DIVC ... disseminated intravascular coagulation
DJD ... degenerative joint disease
DK ... diabetic ketoacidosis
DKA ... diabetic ketoacidosis; did not keep appointment
DKB ... deep knee bends
DKP ... dibasic potassium phosphate
dL ... deciliter
D-L ... Donath-Landsteiner
DLB ... diffuse and lymphoblastic; direct laryngoscopy and bronchoscopy
DLC ... differential leukocyte count; double-lumen catheter
DLCO ... diffusing capacity of the lung for carbon monoxide
DLE ... discoid lupus erythematosus
DLF ... digoxin-like factors
DLS ... daily living skills
DLV ... defective leukemia virus
DLWD ... diffuse lymphocytic, well differentiated
dm ... decimeter
DM ... diabetes mellitus; diabetic mother; diastolic murmur
DMA ... dimethylarsine
DMAARD ... delayed-mechanism-of-action antirheumatic drug
DMARD ... disease-modifying antirheumatic drug
DMC ... dactinomycin, methotrexate, and cyclophosphamide
DMD ... Duchenne muscular dystrophy
DME ... degenerative myoclonus epilepsy
DMF ... decayed, missing, and filled (teeth)
DMKA ... diabetes mellitus ketoacidosis
DML ... diffuse mixed lymphoma
DMO ... dimethyloxazolidinedione
DMOOC ... diabetes mellitus out of control
DMS ... delayed microembolism syndrome; delayed muscle soreness; demarcation membrane system
DMSO ... dimethylsulfoxide
D,M,V,P ... disk, macula, vessels, periphery
D&N ... distance and near (vision)
D/N ... dextrose/nitrogen ratio
DNA ... deoxyribonucleic acid
DNase ... deoxyribonuclease
DNBT ... dinitroblue
DND ... died of natural death
DNI ... do not intubate
DNKA ... did not keep appointment
DNL ... diffuse nodular lymphoma; disseminated necrotizing leukoencephalopathy
DNP ... deoxyribonucleoprotein
DNPH ... dinitrophenylhydrazine
DNS ... do not substitute
DNT ... did not test
DO ... doctor's orders
D/O ... disorder
DOA ... date of admission; date of arrival; dead on arrival
DOA-DRA ... dead on arrival despite resuscitative attempts
DOAP ... daunorubicin, Oncovin (vincristine), araC (cytarabine), and prednisone
DOB ... date of birth
DOC ... date of conception; deoxycorticosterone; diabetes out of control; died of other causes; diet of choice; drug of choice
DOD ... date of death; date of discharge; died of disease
DOE ... date of examination; dyspnea on exertion
DOES ... disorders of excessive sleepiness
DOI ... date of injury; died of injuries
DOL ... day of life (followed by number)
DOOC ... diabetes out of control
dos ... dose (dosis)
DOS ... day of surgery
DOSS ... diocytl sodium sulfosuccinate
DOT ... date of transcription; date of transfer; died on (operating) table

DP	deep pulse; dental prosthodontics; diastolic pressure
DPE	dipivalyl epinephrine
DPFR	diastolic pressure-flow relationship
DPG	diphosphoglycerate
DPGN	diffuse proliferative glomerulonephritis
DPH	diphenhydramine; diphenylhydantoin
DPJ	dementia paralytica juvenilis
DPL	diagnostic peritoneal lavage
DPN	dermatosis papalosa nigra; diabetic polyneuropathy
DPPC	dipalmitoylphosphatidylcholine
DPT	diphtheria toxoid, pertussis vaccine, tetanus toxoid
DPTP	diphtheria, pertussis, tetanus, poliomyelitis (vaccines)
DPTPM	diphtheria, pertussis, tetanus, poliomyelitis, measles (vaccines)
DPU	delayed pressure urticaria
DPUD	duodenal peptic ulcer disease
DQ	developmental quotient
dr	diabetic retinopathy
Dr	doctor
DR	diabetic retinopathy; donor related; donor retested
DRE	digital rectal examination
DRG	diagnostic related group(s)
DRR	dorsal root reflex
D&S	dermatology and syphilology; dilation and suction
D/S	dextrose and sodium chloride; dextrose/saline
DSA	digital subtraction angiography
DSC	decussation superior cerebellar; differential scanning colorimeter
DSCG	disodium cromoglycate
DSD	discharge summary dictated; dry sterile dressing
DSDB	direct self-destructive behavior
ds-DNA	double-stranded DNA
DSE	digital subtraction echocardiogram
DSF	disulfiram
DSM	Diagnostic and Statistical Manual (of Mental Disorders)
DSP	decreased sensory perception
DST	dexamethasone suppression test
Dt	duration of tetany
DT	delirium tremons; duration tetany; dye test
D&T	diagnosis and treatment
D/T	date of treatment; deaths/total (ratio)
dtd	let such doses be given (dentur tales doses)
DTH	delayed-type hypersensitivity
DTM	dermatophyte test medium
DTO	deodorized opium tincture
DTP	diphtheria-tetanus pertussis; distal tingling on percussion
DTR	deep tendon reflex
DTs, DT's	delirium tremens
dU	deoxyuridine
DU	decubitus ulcer; diabetic urine; diagnosis undetermined; diffuse and undifferentiated; duodenal ulcer
DUI	driving under the influence
DUID	driving under the influence of drugs
DUL	diffuse undifferentiated lymphoma
DUR	Drug Usage Review
DV	deep vein
D&V	diarrhea and vomiting
DVA	desacetylvinblastine amide (vindesine)
DVLP	daunomycin, vincristine, L-asparaginase, and prednisone
DVPA	daunorubicin, vincristine, prednisone, and L-asparaginase
DVPL-ASP	daunorubicin, vincristine, prednisone, and L-asparaginase
DVR	double valve replacement
DVT	deep vein thrombosis
dw	dry weight
DWD	died with disease
DWDL	diffuse well-differentiated lymphocytic (lymphoma)
DWI	driving while intoxicated; driving while impaired
Dx	diagnosis
DXA	dual x-ray absorptiometry
DXR	deep x-ray
DXT	deep x-ray therapy
Dy	dysprosium
dysp	dyspnea
DZAPO	daunorubicin, azacytidine, araC (cytarabine), prednisone, and Oncovin (vincristine)
DZT	dizygotic twins
E	exa (10^{18})
EA	early antigen
E&A	evaluate and advise
EAC	external auditory canal
EACA	epsilon-aminocaproic acid
EAHF	eczema, asthma, and hay fever (complex)
EAR	electroencephalographic
EB, E-B	Epstein-Barr (virus)
EBA	epidermolysis bullosa acquisita/atrophicans
EBAB	equal breath sounds bilaterally
EBEA	Epstein-Barr early antigen
EBL	erythroblastic leukemia; estimated blood loss
EBMT	European blood and marrow transplantation
EBNA	Epstein-Barr nuclear antigen
EBS	epidermolysis bullosa simplex
EBV	Epstein-Barr virus
EBVCA	Epstein-Barr virus, capsid antigen
EBVEA	Epstein-Barr virus, early antigen
EBVNA	Epstein-Barr virus, nuclear antigen
EC	*Escherichia coli*; extracellular
ECA	external carotid artery
E-CABG	endarterectomy and coronary artery bypass grafting
ECBV	effective circulating blood volume
ECC	edema, clubbing, and cyanosis; embryonal cell carcinoma; endocervical curettage

ECG	electrocardiogram
Echo	echocardiogram; echoencephalogram
ECHO	echocardiogram; etoposide, cyclophosphamide, hydroxydaunomycin (Adriamycin), and Oncovin (vincristine); ultrasound
ECMO	extracorporeal membrane oxygenation
ECP	eosinophil catonic protein
ECPR	external cardiopulmonary resuscitation
ECS	ectopic corticotropin syndrome
ECT	electroconvulsive therapy; emission computed tomography
ECV	extracellular volume
ECVD	extracellular volume of distribution
ECVE	extracellular volume expansion
ECW	extracellular water
EDN	eosinophil derived neurotoxin
EDTA	ethylenediaminetetraacetic acid
EDWITH	end-diastolic wall thickness
EDX	electrodiagnosis
EE, E&E	eyes and ears
E-E	end to end (anastomosis); erythema-edema (reaction)
EEC	ectodactyly, ectodermal dysplasia, and facial clefts
EECG	electroencephalogram/electroencephalography
EEE	edema, erythema, and exudate
EEEP	end-expiratory esophageal pressure
EEG	electroencephalogram
EEGA	electroencephalographic audiometry
EENT	eyes, ears, nose, throat
EEP	end-expiratory pressure
EF	ejection fraction; extended-field
EFA	essential fatty acids
EFM	external fetal monitoring
EFV	extracellular fluid volume
EFVC	expiratory flow-volume curve
EF/WM	ejection fraction/wall motion
eg	example
EGA	estimated gestational age
EGC	early gastric cancer
EGD	esophagogastroduodenoscopy
EGFR	epidermal growth factor receptor
EH	enlarged heart; essential hypertension
EHBD	extrahepatic bile duct
EHBF	estimated hepatic blood flow; extrahepatic blood flow
EHDP	ethanehydroxydiphosphonic acid
EHEC	enterohemorrhagic *E. coli*
EHL	electrohydraulic lithotripsy
EHO	extrahepatic obstruction
EIA	enzyme immunoassay
EID	electroimmunodiffusion
EIEC	enteroinvasive *E. coli*
EJ	ejection (fraction); external jugular
EKG	electrocardiogram
ELAT	enzyme-linked antiglobulin test
ELISA	enzyme-linked immunosorbent assay
ELOS	estimated length of stay
ELT	euoglobulin lysis time
EM	electron microscopy
E&M	endocrine and metabolic
E/M	electron microscopy
EMA	endomysial antibody; epithelial membrane antigen
EMC	electron microscopy; encephalomyocarditis
EMC&R	emergency medical care and rescue
EMCV	encephalomyocarditis
EMG	electromyelogram; electromyogram
E-MICR	electron microscopy
EMIT	enzyme-multiplied immunoassay technique
EMM	erythema multiforme major
EMR	electromagnetic radiation; empty, measure, and record
EMRS	eosinophilic mucin rhinosinusitis
EMS	early morning specimen; early morning stiffness; electrical muscle stimulation; eosinophil myalgia syndrome
ENA	extractable nuclear antigen
ENG	electronystagmography
ENL	erythema nodosum leprosum
ENT	ear, nose, and throat
EO	ethylene oxide
EOD	early onset disease
EOG	electro-oculogram
EOJ	extrahepatic obstructive jaundice
eos	eosinophil
EP	ectopic pregnancy; electrophoresis; electrophysiologic
EPA	Environmental Protection Agency
EPBI	exercise penile-brachial index
EPEC	enteropathogenic *E. coli*
EPEG	etoposide
EPF	early pregnancy factor
EPI	exocrine pancreatic insufficiency
EPIS	episiotomy
EpoR	erythropoietin receptor
EPP	erythropoietic protoporphyria
EPS	electrophysiologic studies; extrapyramidal side effect; extrapyramidal symptom; extrapyramidal syndrome
EPSEs	extrapyramidal side effects
EPT	early pregnancy test; Eidetic Parents Test; endoscopic papillotomy
EPX	eosinophil peroxidase
Eq	equivalent
Er	erbium
ER	emergency room; estrogen receptors
E&R	equal and reactive; examination and report
ER+	estrogen receptor-positive
ERA	estrogen receptor assay; evoked response audiometry

ERC	(pupils) equal, reactive and contracting
ERCP	endoscopic retrograde cholangiopancreatography
ERE	external rotation in extension
ERF	external rotation in flexion
ERG	electroretinogram
ERPF	effective renal plasma flow
ERT	estrogen replacement therapy; external radiation therapy
ERV	expiratory reserve volume
Es	Einsteinium
ES	electrical stimulation
ESA	end-to-side anastomosis
ESAP	evoked sensory (nerve) action potention
ESB	electrical stimulation of brain
ESBL	extended-spectrum beta lactamases
ESLD	end-stage liver disease
ESP	extrasensory perception
ESR	erythrocyte sedimentation rate
ESRD	end-stage renal disease
ESRF	end-stage renal failure
ESRS	extra pyramidal symptom rating scale
EST	electroshock therapy
et	and (et)
ETA	endotracheal aspirates; estimated time of arrival
ETAAS	electrothermal atomic absorption spectroscopy
ETD	eustachian tube dysfunction
ETEC	enterotoxigenic *E. coli*
ETO	estimated time of ovulation; eustachian tube obstruction
EtOH	ethyl alcohol
ETOX	ethylene oxide
ETS-2	Educational Testing Service; electrical transcranial stimulation;
ETT	extrathyroidal thyroxine
EU	Ehrlich unit
EUL	expected upper limit
EUP	extrauterine pregnancy
EUS	endorectal ultrasound
EVI	endocardial, vascular, and interstitial
EVR	evoked visual response
EVS	endoscopic variceal sclerosis
EW	emergency ward
EWT	erupted wisdom teeth
ExEF	ejection fraction during exercise
Ez	eczema
f	femto (10^{-15})
F	fluorine
FA	false aneurysm; fatty acid; filterable agent; fluorescent antibody
F/A	fetus active
FAA	folic acid antagonist; formaldehyde, acetic acid, and alcohol (solution)
FAB	French-American-British
FAC	femoral arterial cannulation; fluorouracil, Adriamycin (doxorubicin), and cyclophosphamide
FACS	fluorescent-activated cell sorter
FAC-LEV	fluorouracil, Adriamycin (doxorubicin), cyclophosphamide, and levamisole
FACP	Fellow of the American College of Physicians; ftorafur, Adriamycin (doxorubicin), cyclophosphamide, and platinol (cisplatin)
FACS	fluorouracil, Adriamycin (doxorubicin), cyclophosphamide, and streptozocin
FAD	familial Alzheimer dementia; familial autonomic dysfunction; flavin adenine dinucleotide
FAM	fluorouracil, Adriamycin (doxorubicin), and mitomycin C
FAMA	fluorescent antibody to membrane antigen
FAME	fluorouracil, Adriamycin (doxorubicin), and methyl CCNU (semustine)
FAMMM	familiar atypical multiple mole melanoma (syndrome)
FAM-S	fluorouracil, Adriamycin (doxorubicin), mitomycin C, and streptozocin
FANA	fluorescent antinuclear antibody
FAP	familial polyposis
FAS	fetal alcohol syndrome
FB	finger breadths; foreign bodies
F/B	forward bending
FBA	fecal bile acid
FBC	full blood count; functional bactericidal concentration
FBCOD	foreign body of the cornea, oculus dexter (right eye)
FBCOS	foreign body of the cornea, oculus sinister (left eye)
FBD	fibrocystic breast disease
FBG	fasting blood glucose
FBH	familiar benign hypercalcemia
FBHH	familiar benign hypocalciuric hypercalcemia
FBL	fetal blood loss
FBM	fetal breathing movement
FBP	femoral blood pressure; fibrin breakdown product
FBS	fasting blood sugar
FBSS	failed back surgery syndrome
FBW	fasting blood work
Fc	portion of antibody molecule bound by membrane receptors
F&C	foam and condom
F/C	fever and chills
FCDB	fibrocystic disease of breast
FCE	fluorouracil, cisplatin, and etoposide
F-CL	fluorouracil and calcium leucovorin
FCM	flow cytometry
FCSNVD	fever, chills, sweating, nausea, vomiting, and diarrhea
FCT	fecal chymotrypsin test
FCVD	fracture complete and varus deformity
FD	food and drug
F&D	fixed and dilated
F/D	fracture/dislocation
FDA	Federal Drug Administration
FDBL	fecal daily blood loss
FD&C	Food, Drug, and Cosmetic (Act)
FDP	fibrin degradation product; fructose diphosphate
Fe	iron
FEC	fluorouracil, etoposide, and cisplatin; forced expiratory capacity
$FeCl_3$	ferric chloride
FEF	forced expiratory flow
FEFV	forced expiratory flow volume
FENa	fractional excretion of sodium (Na)
FEP	free erythrocyte protoporphyrin
FER	flexion, extension, and rotation
FES	functional electrical stimulation
FET	fecal elastase 1 test
FETI	fluorescent energy transfer immunoassay
Fe/TIBC	iron saturation of serum transferrin
FEUO	for external use only
FEV	forced expiratory volume
FEVB	frequency ectopic ventricular beat
FEV_t	forced expiratory volume
FEV_t/VC	ratio of one-second forced expiratory volume to vital capacity
FF	fat-free (diet); filtration fraction; force fluids
F&F	fixes and follows
FFA	free fatty acids
FFB	flexible fiberoptic bronchoscopy
FFD	fat-free diet
FFDCA	Food, Drug, and Cosmetic (Act)
FFP	fresh frozen plasma
FFROM	full, free range of motion
FFS	fat-free solid; fat-free supper
FFW	fat-free weight
fg	femtogram
FGF	father's grandfather
FGM	father's grandmother
FGS	focal glomerular sclerosis
FGT	female genital tract
FH	familial hypercholesterolemia; family history
FHA	familial hypoplastic anemia
FHD	family history of diabetes
FHH	familial hypocalciuric hypercalcemia; family history of hirsutism
FHIP	family health insurance plan
FHM	familial hemiplegic migraine
FHMI	family history of mental illness
FHP	family history positive
FHR	fetal heart rate; fetal heart rhythm
FHS	fetal heart sounds
FH_x	family history
FIC	functional inhibitory concentration
FID	father in delivery
FIF	forced inspiratory flow
FIH	fat-induced hyperglycemia
FIL	father-in-law
FIS	forced inspiratory spirogram
FISH	fluorescence *in situ* hybridization
FITC	fluorescein isothiocyanate
FIUO	for internal use only
FIV	forced inspiratory volume in one second
FIVC	forced inspiratory vital capacity
FJRM	full joint range of movement/motion
fL	femtoliter; fluid
FL	full liquids (diet)
FLA	left frontal anterior (position of fetus)
FLC	fatty liver cell
FLD	fatty liver disease
FLGA	full-term, large for gestational age
FLKS	fatty liver and kidney syndrome
FI_{O2}	force inspiratory oxygen; fraction of inspired oxygen
FLP	left frontal posterior (position of fetus)
FLS	fatty liver syndrome
FLU A	influenza A virus
Fm	fermium
FM	face mask
F&M	firm and midline (uterus)
FMC	fetal movement count
FMDV	foot-and-mouth disease virus
FME	foot-mouth extraction
FMEN	familial multiple endocrine neoplasia
FMH	family medical history
fmol	femtomole
FMTC	familial medullary thyroid carcinoma
FMULC	free monoclonal urinary light chains
FMV	fluorouracil, methyl-CCNU (semustine), and vincristine
FMX	full-mouth x-ray
FN	facial nerve; false-negative
F-N	finger-to-nose (coordination test)
FNA	fine needle aspiration
FNAB	fine needle aspiration biopsy
FNF	femoral neck fracture; finger-nose-finger (coordination test)
FNHTR	febrile nonhemolytic transfusion reaction
FOB	father of baby; fiberoptic bronchoscopy
FOC	father of child
FOD	free of disease
FOOB	fell out of bed
FOOSH	fell on outstretched hand
FOS	fiberoptic sigmoidoscopy
fp	forearm pronated
FP	false-positive; forearm pronated
F-P	femoral popliteal
FPB	femoral popliteal bypass
FPIA	fluorescence polarization immunoassay
FPN	ferric, perchloric, nitric
FPVB	demoral-popliteal vein bypass

Fr	francium
FR	failure rate
F&R	force and rhythm (of pulse)
FRA	fluorescent rabies antibody
FrBB, FRBB	fracture of both bones
FRC	frozen red cells; functional residual capacity
FRF	follicle-stimulating hormone-releasing factor
FRH	follicle-stimulating hormone-releasing hormone
FRM	full range of motion
FROM	full range of motion
FS	frozen section
F&S	full and soft (diet)
FSB	fetal scalp blood
FSBM	full-strength breast milk
FSG	focal sclerosing glomerulonephritis; focal segmental glomerulosclerosis
FSGA	full-term, small for gestational age
FSGHS	focal segmental glomerular hyalinosis and sclerosing
FSGN	focal sclerosing glomerulonephritis
FSGS	focal segmental glomerulosclerosis
FSH	follicle stimulating hormone
FSH/LR-RH	follicle-stimulating hormone and luteinizing hormone-releasing hormone
FSH-RF	follicle-stimulating hormone-releasing factor
FSH-RH	follicle-stimulating hormone-releasing hormone
FSI	foam stability index
FSL	fasting serum level
FSP	familial spastic paraplegia; fibrin split products
ft.	make (fiat, fiant)
FT	free thyroxine; full-term
FT$_3$I	free triiodothyronine index
FTA	fluorescent treponemal antibody
FTA-ABS	fluorescent treponemal antibody absorption
FTD	failure to descend
FTI	free thyroxine index
FTN	finger-to-nose (coordination test)
FTNB	full-term newborn
FTND	full-term normal delivery
FTP	failure to progress (in labor)
FTT	failure to thrive; fat tolerance test
FU	fluorouracil; follow-up
5-FU	5-fluorouracil
F&U	flanks and upper quadrants
F/U	follow-up
FUDR	floxuridine; fluorodeoxyuridine
FUDR-MP	floxuridine monophosphate
FUE	fever of unknown etiology
FUO	fever of unknown/undetermined origin
FUOV	follow-up office visit
FUR	fluorouracil riboside; fluorouridine
FURAM	ftorafur, Adriamycin (doxorubicin), and mitomycin
FVC	forced vital capacity
FVE	forced volume, expiratory
FVH	focal vascular headache
FVIC	forced inspiratory vital capacity
FVL	femoral vein ligation
Fx.	fracture
FX	factor X
FxBB	fracture of both bones
g.	gram
G+	gram-positive
G-	gram-negative
G6P	glucose 6 phosphate
G6PD	glucose 6-phosphate dehydrogenase
Ga	gallium
GABA	gamma-aminobutyric acid
GAD	generalized anxiety disorder
GAL	galactosemia
G and D	growth and development
GAS	gastric acid secretion
GAT	gelatin agglutination test
GAW	airway conductance
GAZT	glucuronide derivative of azidothymidine
GB	gallbladder
G&B	good and bad
GBD	gallbladder disease
GBM	glomerular basement membrane
GBS	gallbladder series; gastric bypass surgery
GC	geriatric chair; gonococcus; gonorrhea culture; gas chromatography
G+C	gram-positive cocci
GCA	gastric cancerous area; giant cell arteritis
GC/MS	gas chromatography/mass spectrometry
GCS	γ-glutamylcysteine synthetase
G-CSF	granulocyte colony-stimulating factors
GCSF	granulocyte cell-stimulating factor
GCU	gonococcal urethritis
GCV	ganciclovir
G&D	growth and development
Gd	gadolinium
g/dL	gram percent
gdw	gram dry weight
Ge	germanium
GE	gastroesophageal
GEN/ENDO	general anesthesia with endotracheal intubation
GER	gastroesophageal reflux
GEU	gestation, extrauterine
GF	gastric fistula; gastric fluid
GFAAS	graphite furnace atomic absorption spectrophotometry
GFM	good fetal movement
GFR	glomerular filtration rate
GFS	global focal sclerosis
GGCT	ground glass clotting time
GGT	gamma-glutamyltransferase
GH	growth hormone
GHB	glycohemoglobin
GHD	growth hormone deficiency
GHRH	growth hormone-releasing hormone
GHRIF	growth hormone release-inhibiting factor
GHRIH	growth hormone release-inhibiting hormone
GHRP-6	growth hormone-releasing peptide-6
GI	gastrointestinal; glucose intolerance; good impression
GIB	gastrointestinal bleeding
GIFT	gamete intrafallopian; granulocyte immunofluorescence test
GIH	gastric inhibitory hormone
GIP	gastric inhibitory polypeptide
GIS	gastrointestinal series
GIT	gastrointestinal tract
GITT	gastrointestinal transit time; glucose-insulin tolerance test
GK	galactokinase
GL	gastric lavage
GLC	gas-liquid chromatography
GM	gastric mucosa; geometric mean; grand mal; grandmother
GM+	gram-positive
GM-	gram-negative
GM-CFU	granulocyte-macrophage colony-forming unit
GMS	Grocott-Gomori methenamine-silver
Gn	gonadotropin
GN	gonococcus
G/N	glucose/nitrogen (ratio in urine)
GNR	gram-negative rod
GnRH	gonadotropin releasing hormone
GO	gonorrhea
GOT	glutamic-oxaloacetic transaminase
GP	glycoprotein
GPD	glucose-6-phosphate dehydrogenase
GPI	glycosylphosphatidyl inositol
GPK	guinea pig kidney
GPR	gram-positive rod
GPT	glutamic-pyruvic transaminase
GPUT	glactose phosphate uridyl transferase
GR	glutathione reductase
G+R	gram-positive rod
G-R	gram-negative rod
gr+	gram-positive
GR-FR	grandfather
GR-MO	grandmother
GrP	gram-positive
G/S	glucose and saline
GSA65	gross virus antigen
GSD	glycogen storage disease
GSH	glutathione; growth stimulating hormone
GSR	galvanic skin response; generalized Schwartzman reaction
GSSR	generalized Sandarelli-Shwartzman reaction
GSW	gunshot wound
GSWA	gunshot wound to abdomen
GT	gait training; gamma-glutamyltransferase
GTB	gastrointestinal tract bleeding
GTP	glutamyl transpeptidase
GTT	glucose tolerance test
gtt(s)	drop(s) (gutta)
GTX	granulocyte transfusion
GU	genitourinary; gastric ulcer; gonococcal urethritis
GVHD	graft-versus-host disease
GVHR	graft-versus-host reaction
GWA	gunshot wound of abdomen
GWT	gunshot wound of the throat
GXT	graded exercise test
gyn	gynecological
h.	hour (hora)
H	hydrogen
Ha	hahnium
HA	headache; hemagglutination; hemolytic anemia
H/A	headache
HAA	hepatitis-associated antigen
HAAA	human antianimal antibodies
HAART	highly activated antiretroviral therapy
HABA	hydroxybenzeneazobenzoic acid
HAI	hemagglutination inhibition
HAM	hexamethylmelamine, Adriamycin (doxorubicin), and melphalan; hypoparathyroidism, Addison disease, and mucocutaneous candidiasis (syndrome)
HANE	hereditary angioneurotic edema
HASCHD	hypertensive arteriosclerotic heart disease
HASCVD	hypertensive arteriosclerotic cardiovascular disease
HASHD	hypertensive arteriosclerotic heart disease
HAV	hepatitis A virus
HAVAB	hepatitis A virus antibody
Hb	hemoglobin
HBAb	hepatitis B antibody
HBAg	hepatitis B antigen
HB$_c$	hepatitis B core
HBD	hydroxybutric dehydrogenase
HBDH	hydroxybutyrate dehydrogenase
HB$_e$Ag	hepatitis B e antigen
HBF	hepatic blood flow
HBO	hyperbaric oxygen (therapy); hyperbaric oxygenation
HBOT	hyperbaric oxygenation
HBP	high blood pressure
HBs	Heinz body stain

HB$_s$Ag ... hepatitis B surface antigen
HBV ... hepatitis B vaccine; hepatitis B virus
HBW ... high birth weight
HC ... homocystinuria
H-CAP ... hexamethylmelamine, cyclophosphamide, Adriamycin (doxorubicin), and Platinol (cisplatin)
HCAP ... handicapped
HCFA ... Health Care Financing Administration
HCFSH ... human chorionic follicle-stimulating hormone
hCG ... human chorionic gonadotropin
HCl ... hydrochloric acid
HCL ... hairy-cell leukemia
HCO_3 ... bicarbonate
H'crit ... hematocrit
HCS ... human chorionic somatomammotropin
Hct, HCT ... hematocrit
HD ... Hodgkin's disease
HDAg ... hepatitis D antigen
HDL ... high density lipoprotein
HDLC ... high density lipoprotein cholesterol
HDLs ... high density lipoproteins
HDMP ... high-dose methylprednisolone
HDMTX ... high-dose methotrexate
HDMTX-CF ... high-dose methotrexate and citrovorum factor
HDMTX/LV ... high-dose methotrexate and leucovorin
HDN ... hemolytic disease of the newborn
HDP ... hydroxydimethylpyrimidine
He ... helium
HEENT ... head, ears, eyes, nose, and throat
HEG ... hemorrhagic erosive gastritis
HELLP ... hemolysis, elevated liver tests, low platelet count
hemat ... hematocrit
HEMPAS ... here. erythroblastic multinuclearity with positive acidified serum
hep ... hepatitis
HEp ... human epithelial cells
HEPT ... hamster egg penetration test
HES ... acute hypereosinophilic syndrome
Hf ... hafnium
HFHL ... high-frequency hearing loss
HFI ... hereditary fructose intolerance
HFR ... highly fluorescent reticulocyte
HFRS ... hemorrhagic fever with ernal symptoms
Hg ... mercury
^{197}Hg ... radioisotope of mercury
^{203}Hg ... radioisotope of mercury
HG ... herpes gestationis
HGA ... homogentisic acid
Hgb ... hemoglobin
HGE ... human granulocytic ehrlichiosis
hGG, HGG ... human gamma globulin
HGH ... human growth hormone
HGPRT ... hypoxanthine guanine phosphoribosyl transferase
Hgt ... height
HH ... hereditary hemochromatosis
H/H ... hemoglobin and hematocrit
HHC ... home health care
HHD ... hypertensive heart disease
HHH ... hyperornithinemia, hyperammonemia-homocitrullinuria
HHM ... humoral hypercalcemia of malignancy
HHS ... (Department of) Health and Human Services
HHT ... head holter traction
HHV-6 ... human herpesvirus 6
HHV-7 ... human herpesvirus 7
HHV-8 ... human herpesvirus 8
HI ... head injury; hydriodic acid
HIAA ... hydroxyindoleacetic acid
HIB ... *Haemophilus influenzae* B
HIDA ... acetanilidoiminodiacetic acid
HIDS ... hyperimmunoglobulin D syndrome
HIGM ... hyper-IgM syndrome
HIP ... humoral immunocompetence profile
HIT ... heparin-induced thrombocytopenia
HITB ... *Haemophilus influenzae* type B (meningitis)
HIV ... human immunodeficiency virus
HK ... hexokinase
H-K ... hand-to-knee (test); heel to knee (test)
HKAHO ... hip-knee-ankle-foot orthosis
HKAO ... hip-knee-ankle orthosis
HKO ... hip-knee orthosis (splint)
HKS ... hip-knee-shin (test)
HL ... half-life (of radioactive element); hearing level; Hickman line
H&L ... heart and lungs
H/L ... heparin lock
HLA ... histocompatibility leukocyte antigen; histocompatibility locus antigen; human leukocyte antigen
HLK ... heart, liver, and kidneys
H&L OK ... heart and lungs normal
HLT ... heart-lung transplantation
HLV ... herpes-like virus
HMB ... homatropine methylbromide
HME ... heat, massage, and exercise; human monocytic ehrlichiosis
HMETSC ... heavy metal screen
HMG-CoA ... hepatic hydroxymethylglutaryl coenzyme A
HMM ... hexamethylmelamine
HMO ... Health Maintenance Organization
HMS ... hexose monophosphate shunt
HMT ... hematocrit
HMW ... high molecular weight
HMWK ... high molecular weight kininogen
HMX ... heat, massage, and exercise
HN ... head nurse
H&N ... head and neck
HNPCC ... hereditary nonpolyposis colon cancer
HNS ... head and neck surgery
HNV ... has not voided
Ho ... holmium
HO ... house officer
H/O ... history of
HOA ... hip osteoarthritis
HOB ... head of bed
HOB UPSOB ... head of bed up for shortness of breath
HOH ... hard of hearing
HOP ... high oxygen pressure; hydroxydaunomycin (doxorubicin), Oncovin (vincristine), and prednisone
hor ... (L. *hora somni* hour of sleep) at bedtime
hor som ... (L. *hora somni* hour of sleep) at bedtime
HOS ... hypo-osmotic swelling test
HP ... hot packs
H&P ... history and physical
HPC ... hematopoietic progenitor cells
HPE ... history and physical examination
hpf ... high power field
HPFH ... hereditary persistence of fetal hemoglobin
HPI ... history of present illness
HPL ... human placental lactogen
HPLC ... high-performance liquid chromatography
HPN ... home parenteral nutrition
HPP ... human pancreatic polypeptide
HPPA ... hydroxyphenylpyruvic acid
HPPH ... hydroxyphenyl-phenylhydantoin
HPT ... hyperparathyroidism
hPTH ... human parathyroid hormone
HPTLC ... high performance thin layer chromatography
HPV ... *Haemophilus pertussis* vaccine; human papillomavirus
HR ... heart rate; hospital record
H&R ... hysterectomy and radiation
HRA ... health risk appraisal
HRANA ... histone reactive ANA
HRCT ... high resolution CT
HRL ... head rotation (to) left
HRLM ... high resolution light microscopy
HRP ... histidine-rich protein
HRR ... head rotation (to) right
HRs ... Hamilton Rating Scale
hs ... at bedtime (hora somni)
HS ... half strength; herpes simplex; hereditary spherocytosis
HSA ... human serum albumin
HSC ... hematopoietic stem cells
HSIL ... high-grade squamous intraepithelial lesions
h som ... (L. *hora somni* hour of sleep) at bedtime
HSV ... herpes simplex virus
HSVE ... herpes simplex virus encephalitis
ht ... height
HT ... hypertension; hypodermic tablet
3-HT ... 3-hydroxytyramine (dopamine)
5-HT ... 5-hydroxytyramine (serotonin)
H&T ... hospitalization and treatment
HTK ... heel to knee (test)
HTLV ... human T-lymphotropic virus
HTN ... hypertension
HTP ... hydroxytrytophan
HTVD ... hypertensive vascular disease
HUS ... hemolytic-uremic syndrome; hyaluronidase unit for semen
HV ... herpes virus
H&V ... hemigastrectomy and vagotomy
H-V ... His-ventricular
HVA ... homovanillic acid
HVLP ... high volume, low pressure
Hx ... history
HXM ... hexamethylmelamine
Hz ... hertz
I ... indeterminate; intermediate; iodine
^{125}I ... radioisotope of iodide
^{131}I ... radioisotope of iodide
Ia ... antigen
I&A ... irrigation and aspiration
IAA ... indole acetic acid
I-3-AA ... indole 3-acetic acid
IABC ... intra-aortic balloon catheter; intra-aortic balloon counterpulsation
IABCP ... intra-aortic balloon counterpulsation
IABP ... intra-aortic balloon pump
IACB ... intra-aortic counterpulsation balloon
IADH ... inappropriate antidiuretic hormone
IADHS ... inappropriate antidiuretic hormone syndrome
IAH ... idiopathic adrenal hyperplasis
I and O ... intake and output
IAO ... immediately after onset
IAP ... inhibitor of apoptosis
IARF ... ischemic acute renal failure
IAT ... indirect antiglobulin test
Ib ... a glycoprotein
IBBBB ... incomplete bilateral bundle-branch
IBC ... iron binding capacity
IBD ... infectious bowel disease; inflammatory bowel disease; irritable bowel disease; ischemic bowel disease
IBP ... intra-aortic balloon pumping
IBS ... irritable bowel syndrome
IBT ... Immunobead test

IBW ... ideal body weight
IC ... immune complexes; inspiratory capacity
ICA ... internal carotid artery
ICC ... intraclass coefficient; Indian childhood cirrhosis
ICD ... immune complex disease; isocitrate dehydrogenase
ICDH ... isocitrate dehydrogenase
ICF ... intracellular fluid
ICG ... indocyanine green
ICGN ... idiopathic crescentic glomerulonephritis
ICH ... intracranial hemorrhage; intracranial hypertension
ICL ... idiopathic C4D lymphocytopenia
ICN ... intensive care neonatal
ICPS ... inductively-coupled plasma spectrometry
ICS ... intercostal space
ICSH ... interstitial cell stimulating hormone
ICSI ... intracytoplasmic sperm injection
ICT ... indirect Coombs' test
ICU ... intensive care unit
ICVH ... ischemic cerebrovascular headache
I&D ... incision and drainage
ID ... identification; immunodiffusion; infectious disease; intradermal(ly)
IDA ... iron deficiency anemia; image display and analysis
IDAT ... indirect antiglobulin test
IDC ... idiopathic dilated cardiomyopathy
IDDF ... investigational drug data form
IDDM ... insulin dependent diabetes mellitus
IDDS ... implantable drug delivery system; investigational drug data sheet
IDL ... intermediate-density lipoprotein
IDM ... idiopathic disease of myocardium; intermediate-dose methotrexate
IDVC ... indwelling venous catheter
I&E ... internal and external
I/E ... inspiratory/expiratory
IEF ... isoelectric focusing
IEM ... inborn errors of metabolism
IEMA ... immunoenzymetric assay
IEP ... immunoelectrophoresis
IF ... immunofluorescence; inspiratory force; interstitial fluid; intrinsic factor
IFA ... indirect fluorescent antibody
IFCPC ... Internal Federation of Cervical Pathology and Colposcopy
IFIX ... immunofixation
IFLrA ... recombinant human leukocyte interferon A
IFOS ... ifosfamide
IFX ... ifosfamide
Ig ... immunoglobulin
IGH ... idiopathic growth hormone
IGIM ... immune globulin intramuscular
IGT ... impaired glucose tolerance
IHA ... indirect hemagglutination
IHSS ... idiopathic hypertrophic subaortic stenosis
IIb-IIIa ... glycoproteins found on platelet membranes
IIF ... indirect immunofluorescence
III-para ... tertipara (third pregnancy)
II-para ... secudipara (second pregnancy)
IK ... immobilized knee
I.M. ... intramuscular
IMAC ... ifosfamide, mesna uroprotection, Adriamycin (doxorubicin), and cisplatin
IMD ... inherited metabolic disorders
IMIG ... intramuscular immunoglobulin
IMP ... impression
IMV ... inferior mesenteric vein; intermittent mandatory ventilation
In ... indium
INB ... ischemic necrosis (of) bone
IND ... investigational new drug
INH ... isonicotinic acid hydrazide; isoniazid
Inh ... inhaler
INK ... injury not known
INR ... international normalized ratio
I&O ... in and out; intake and output
IOF ... intraocular fluid
IOFNA ... intraoperative fine needle aspiration
IOH ... idiopathic orthostatic hypotension
IOL ... intraocular lens
IOLI ... intraocular lens implantation
IOP ... intraocular pressure
IOT ... intraocular tension
IOUS ... intraoperative ultrasound
IOV ... initial office visit
IP ... intraperitoneal(ly)
I-PAO ... insulin induced peak acid output
I-para ... primipara (first pregnancy)
IPCD ... infantile polycystic disease
IPF ... idiopathic pulmonary fibrosis
IPG ... impedence phlebograph
IPPB ... intermittent positive pressure breathing
Ir ... iridium
I&R ... insertion and removal
IR ... infrared
IRB ... institutional review board
IRBBB ... incomplete right bundle-branch block
IRBC ... immature red blood cell
IRDS ... infant respiratory distress syndrome
IRF ... immature reticulocyte fraction
IRG ... immunoreactive glucose
IRGH ... immunoreactive growth hormone
IRI ... immunoreactive insulin
IRMA ... immunoradiometric assay
IRT ... immunoreactive trypsinogen
ISADH ... inappropriate secretion of antidiuretic hormone
ISD ... isosorbide dinitrate
ISDN ... isosorbide dinitrate
ISE ... ion-selective electrode
ISF ... interstitial fluid
ISFV ... interstitial fluid volume
ISI ... infarct size index
ISS ... Injury Severity Scale
IT ... inhalation therapy; intrathecal(ly)
ITCP ... immunogenic thrombocytopenic purpura
ITP ... idiopathic thrombocytopenic purpura; immunogenic thrombocytopenic purpura
ITT ... identical twins (raised) together; insulin tolerance test; iron tolerance test
IU ... International unit
IUD ... intrauterine death; intrauterine device
IUGR ... intrauterine growth retardation
IUI ... intrauterine insemination
IUP ... intrauterine pregnancy
IUPC ... intrauterine pressure catheter
IUPD ... intrauterine pregnancy, delivered
IUT ... intrauterine transfusion
I.V. ... intravenous
IVAC ... I.V. infusion control device
IVAD ... implanted vascular access device
IVB ... intraventricular block
IVBAT ... intravascular bronchoalveolar tumor
IVBC ... intravascular blood coagulation
IVC ... inferior vena cava; intravenous cholangiography
IVCP ... inferior vena cava pressure
IVCT ... inferior vena cave thrombosis
IVDU ... intravenous drug (use)
IVF ... *in vitro* fertilization
IVF-ET ... *in vitro* fertilization and embryonic transfer
IVH ... intravenous hyperalimentation; intraventricular hemorrhage
IVIG ... intravenous immune globulin; intravenous immunoglobulin
IVN ... intravenous nutrition
IVP ... intravenous push; intravenous pyelogram
IVPB ... intravenous piggyback
IVSA ... intravenous digital subtraction angiography
IVSD ... intraventricular septal defect
IVUS ... intravascular coronary ultrasound
IVV ... influenza virus vaccine
IWMI ... inferior wall myocardial infarct(ion)
JA ... juvenile atrophy
JD ... juvenile-onset diabetes
JDM ... juvenile-onset diabetes mellitus
JF ... joint fluid
JJ ... jaw jerk
JOD ... juvenile-onset diabetes
JODM ... juvenile-onset diabetes mellitus
JOMAC ... judgment, orientation, memory, abstraction, and calculation
JOMACI ... judgment, orientation, memory, abstraction, and calculation intact
JPB ... junctional premature beat
JRA ... juvenile rheumatoid arthritis
JVD ... jugular-venous distenion
JVP ... jugular-venous pressure; jugular vein/venous pulse
k ... kilo (10^3)
K ... potassium
KA ... alkaline phosphatase
KAFO ... knee-ankle-foot orthosis
KAO ... knee-ankle orthosis
KB, K-B ... Kleihauer-Betke
kcal ... kilocalorie
KCl ... potassium chloride
KCN ... potassium cyanide
KDA ... known drug allergies
kg ... kilogram
KGS ... ketogenic steroids
kL ... kiloliter
km ... kilometer
KO ... keep open
KOH ... potassium hydroxide
Kr ... krypton
KS ... ketosteroids; Kaposi's sarcoma
KSHV ... Kaposi sarcoma-associated herpesvirus
KS/OI ... Kaposi sarcoma and opportunistic infections
KU ... Karmen units
KUB ... kidney and urinary bladder
KUS ... kidney(s), ureter(s), and spleen
KVO ... keep vein open
KW ... Keith-Wagener
L ... left; liter; lumbar
L_2 ... second lumbar vertebra
La ... lanthanum
LA ... latex agglutination; left atrium; local anesthetic
L&A ... light and accommodation
LAD ... left anterior descending (artery)
LAH ... left atrial hypertrophy
LAHB ... left anterior hemiblock
LAI ... labioincisal
LAO ... left anterior oblique
Lap ... laparotomy
LAP laparoscopy; left atrial pressure; leucine aminopeptidase; leukocyte alkaline phosphatase
LASA ... lipid-associated sialic acid
LATS ... long-acting thyroid stimulating hormone
LATS-P ... long-acting thyroid-stimulation-protector
LB ... left bundle
L&B ... left and below
LBA ... left basal artery
LBB ... left breast biopsy; left bundle-branch

LBBB	left bundle-branch block
LBBsB	left bundle-branch system block
LBBX	left biopsy examination
LBCD	left border (of) cardiac dullness
LBM	lean body mass
LBO	large bowel obstruction
LBP	low back pain; low blood pressure
LBV	left brachial vein
LBW	lean body weight; low birth weight
LBWI	low birth weight infant
LC	lethal concentration
LCBF	local cerebral blood flow
LCI	lung clearance index
LCIS	lobular carcinoma *in situ*
LCM	lymphocytic choriomeningitis
LCO	low cardiac output
LCOS	low cardiac output syndrome
LCS	left coronary sinus; Leydig cell stimulation
LCT	lymphocytotoxicity assay
LD	labor and delivery; lactate dehydrogenase; lethal dose; light difference
LD₁	lactate dehydrogenase fraction 1
L&D	labor and delivery
LDH	lactate dehydrogenase
LDHI	LDH isoenzymes
LDL	low density lipoprotein
LDLC	low density lipoprotein cholesterol
LDLs	low density lipoproteins
LDT	lactate dehydrogenase total
LDV	lactate dehydrogenase virus
Le	Lewis antigen
LE	left ear; left eye; lens extraction; lower extremity; lupus erythematosus
LEA	lower extremity arterial
LEEP	loop electrosurgical excisional procedure
LEM	lateral eye movement
LER	lead excretion ratio
LES	lower esophageal sphincter
LETZ	loop excision of transformation
LEV	lower extremity venous
LFA	left femoral artery
LFC	left frontal craniotomy
LFD	lactose-free diet
LFT	liver function test
LGV	lymphogranuloma venereum
LH	luteinizing hormone
LHA	left hepatic artery
LHF	left heart failure
LHP	left hemiparesis; left hemiplegia
LHRF	luteinizing hormone releasing factor
LHRH	luteinizing hormone releasing hormone
LHV	left ventricular hypertrophy
Li	lithium
LIC	left iliac crest
LIO	left inferior oblique
LISS	low ionic strength saline
L-J	Löwenstein-Jensen
LKM	liver/kidney microsomes
LKS	liver, kidneys, spleen
LKSB	liver, kidneys, spleen, (and) bladder
LKS non.pal.	liver, kidneys, (and) spleen not palpable
LLA	lupus-like anticoagulant
LLDH	liver lactate dehydrogenase
LLETZ	large loop excision of transformation
LLL	left lower lobe
LLLE	lower lid, left eye
LLN	limit of normal
LLQ	left lower quadrant
LLRE	lower lid, right eye
LLSB	left lower scapular border; left lower sternal border
LLT	left lateral thigh
LM	light microscopy
LMD	left main disease
LMF	left middle finger
LMN	lower motor neuron
LMP	last menstrual period
LMT	lead mobilization test
LMW	low molecular weight
LMWH	low molecular weight heparin
LOA	leave of absence; left occipital anterior
LOC	laxative of choice
LOD	late onset disease
LOM	left otitis media; limitation of motion
LOP	leave on pass
LOS	length of stay; loss of sight; lower (o)esophageal sphincter
LOSP	lower (o)esophageal sphincter pressure
LP	light perception; lumbar puncture
LPA	lysophosphatidic acid
LPC	leukocyte-poor cells (leukocyte depleted)
lpf	low power field
LPHB	left posterior hemiblock
LPIH	left posterior-inferior hemiblock
LPO	left posterior oblique
LP&P	light perception and projection
LPRBC	leukocyte-poor red blood cells
LQTS	long QT syndrome
L&R	left and right
L/R	left-to-right (ratio)
LRC	Lipid Research Clinic
LRH	luteinizing releasing hormone
L&S	liver and spleen

L/S	lecithin/sphingomyelin ratio
LSD	lysergic acid diethylamide
LSG	labial salivary gland
LSIL	low-grade squamous intraepithelial lesions
LSN	left substantia nigra; left sympathetic nerve
LSO	lateral superior olive (of brain); left salpingo-oophorectomy
LSP	Laboratory Standardization Panel
LSVC	left superior vena cava
LTC	long-term care
LTCPs	L-tryptophan-containing products
LTE	leukotriene E
LTGA	left transposition (of) great artery
LTNP	long-term nonprogressors
LTT	lactose tolerance test; limited treadmill test; lymphocyte transformation test
Lu	lutetium
L&U	lower and upper (extremities)
LUL	left upper lobe
LUQ	left upper quadrant
LUS	laparoscopic ultrasound
LV	lung volume
LVET	left ventricular ejection time
LVH	left ventricular hypertrophy
LVOT	left ventricular outflow tract
LVW	lateral vaginal wall
Lw	lawrencium
L&W	living and well
Lytes	electrolytes
m	meter; milli (10^{-3})
m²	square meter
m³	cubic meter
M	mega (10^6); mix (misce)
M-2	vincristine, carmustine, cyclophosphamide, melphalan, and prednisone
mA	milliampere
MA	Master of Arts
M/A	mood and/or affect
MA-1	a type of respirator
MAA	microaggregatedalbumin
MABOP	Mustargen (nitrogen mustard), Adriamycin (doxorubicin), bleomycin, Oncovin (vincristine), and prednisone
MABP	mean arterial blood pressure
MACC	methotrexate, Adriamycin (doxorubicin), cyclophosphamide, and CCNU (lomustine)
MAH	malignancy-associated hypercalcemia
MAI	*Mycobacterium avium-intracellulare*
MAIGA	monoclonal antibody-specific immobilization of granulocyte antigens
MAIPA	monoclonal antibody immobilization of platelet antigens
MAO	maximal acid output; monoamine oxidase
MAP	mitomycin, Adriamycin (doxorubicin), and cisplatin
MAR	medication administration record; mixed antiglobulin reaction
MAT	multifocal atrial tachycardia
MB	a fraction of creatine kinase
MBA	Master of Business Administration
M-BACOD	methotrexate, bleomycin, Adriamycin (doxorubicin), cyclophosphamide, Oncovin (vincristine), and dexamethasone
MBC	methotrexate, bleomycin, and cisplatin; minimum bactericidal concentration; maximum breathing capacity
MB-CK	creatinine kinase isoenzyme containing M and B subunits
MBD	maximum bactericidal dilution; methotrexate, bleomycin, and diaminedichloroplatinum (cisplatin)
MBE	may be elevated
MBG	mean blood glucose
MBL	mannose-binding lectin
MBP	myelin basic protein
mc	millicurie
M&C	morphine and cocaine
MCA	major coronary artery; megestrol, cyclophosphamide, and Adriamycin (doxorubicin)
MC-Ab	monoclonal antibody
MCAD	medium chain ACYL CO-A dehydrogenase
MCBP	melphalan, cyclophosphamide, BCNU (bischloroethylnitrosourea), and prednisone
MCFA	medium-chain fatty acid
mcg	microgram
MCH	mean corpuscular hemoglobin
MCHC	mean corpuscular hemoglobin concentration
MCHCr	mean cell hemoglobin concentration
mCi	millicurie
MCI	mean cardiac index
MCL	midclavicular line; midcostal line
MCP	membrane cofactor protein
MCT	medium chain triglycerides
MCTD	mixed connective tissue disease
MCV	mean corpuscular volume
Md	mendelevium
MD	medical doctor
MDA	methylenedioxyamphetamine
MDIs	metered dose inhalers
MDM	mid-diastolic murmur; minor determinant mixture
MDMA	methylenedioxymethamphetamine
MDP	mentodextra posterior
MDR	minimum daily requirement
MDS	materials distribution system; myelodysplastic syndrome
MDUO	myocardial disease (of) unknown origin
MDV	multiple dose vial
MEA	mercaptoethylamine; multiple endocrine adenomatosis
MeCCNU	methylchloroethylcyclohexylnitrosourea (semustine)
MeCP	methyl-CCNU, cyclophosphamide, and prednisone
MECY	methyltrexate and cyclophosphamide

MED	minimal erythemal dose
MEET	multistage exercise electrocardiographics test
MEIA	microparticle enzyme immunoassay
MEN	multiple endocrine neoplasia
mEq	milliequivalent
methyl-CCNU	methylchloroethylcyclohexylmitrosourea (semustine)
METS	metastases
MF	mycosis fungoides
M&F	male and female; mother and father
M/F	male to female (ratio)
MFC	minimum fungicidal concentration
MFI	mean fluorescence intensity
MFISH	multicolor fluorescence *in situ* hybridization
MFR	mean flow rate
MFU	medical follow-up
MFVD	midforceps vaginal delivery
mg	milligram
mg%	milligrams per deciliter; milligrams per 100 milliliters; milligrams percent
Mg	magnesium
MG	myasthenia gravis
MgCl$_2$	magnesium chloride
MgCO$_3$	magnesium carbonate
MGDF	megakaryocyte growth and differentiation factor
MGP	methyl green pyronine
MgSO$_4$	magnesium sulfate
MGUS	monoclonal gammopathy of undetermined significance
MH	malignant hyperthermia; marital history; menstrual history; mental health
M/H	microcytic hypochromic (anemia)
MHA	microhemagglutination
MHA-TP	microhemagglutination *Treponema pallidum*
MHC	major histocompatibility complex
MHPG	methoxyhydroxyphenylglycol
MHz	megahertz
MI	myocardial infarction; maturation index
MIC	minimum inhibitory concentration
μ	micro (10^{-6})
μg	microgram
μL	microliter
μm	micrometer
μm^3	cubic micrometer
μmol	micromole
μmol/L	micromolar
μOsm	micro-osmolar
μU	microunit
MID	maximum bactericidal dilution
MIE	medical improvement expected
MIF	merthiolate-iodine-formalin; migration inhibitory factor
MIM	Mendelian Inheritance in Man
MIRL	membrane inhibitor of reactive lysis
MIT	migration inhibition test
MITO-C	mitomycin C
mIU	milli International unit
MJD	Machado-Joseph disease
mL	milliliter
MLAP	mean left atrial pressure
MLC	mixed leukocyte culture; mixed lymphocyte culture
MLD	metachromatic leukodystrophy; minimum lethal dose
mL/L	milliliters per liter
MLR	mixed lymphocyte reaction
MLT	medical laboratory technician
MLV	monitored live voice
mm	millimeter
mm^2	square millimeter
mm^3	cubic millimeter
mM	millimolar; millimole
MMA	methylmalonic acid
MMC	minimal medullary concentration
MMD	myotonic muscular dystrophy
MMEF	mean midexpiratory flow
MMF	maximal midexpiratory flow rate
mm Hg	millimeters of mercury
mmol	millimole
mmol/L	millimolar
MMPI	Minnesota multiple personality inventory
MMR	mass miniature radiography; mass miniature roentgenography; maternal mortality rate; measles, mumps, rubella
MMT	manual muscle test
Mn	manganese
M&N	morning and night
M/N	macrocytic/normochronic (anemia); microcytic/normochronic (anemia)
mNAP	membrane alkaline phosphatase
MNS	MNS blood group
Mo	molybdenum
MO	mesio-occlusal
MOA	mechanism of action
MOA-B	monoamine oxidase type-B inhibitor
MOAD	methotrexate, Oncovin (vincristine), L-asparaginase, and dexamethasone
MOB	mechlorethamine, Oncovin (vincristine), and bleomycin
MOB-PT	mitomycin C, Oncovin (vincristine), bleomycin, and cisplatin
MOCA	methotrexate, Oncovin (vincristine), Cytoxan (cyclophosphamide), and Adriamycin (doxorubicin)
MOD	maturity-onset diabetes
MODM	maturity-onset diabetes mellitus
MOF	mean osmotic fragility
MOFS	multiple-organ failure syndrome
mol	mole
mol/L	molar
mol/m^3	mole per cubic meter

mol/s	mole per second
MOMPs	major outer membrane proteins
MONO	mononucleosis
MOP-BAP	Mustargen (mechlorethamine), Oncovin (vincristine), prednisone, bleomycin, Adriamycin (doxorubicin), and procarbazine
MOPP	mustargen oncovin procarbazine and prednisone
MOPV	monovalent oral poliovirus
mOsm	milliosmole
mOsm/kg	milliosmoles per kilogram
MPC	mean platelet component concentration
MPD	myeloproliferative disease
MPDS	mandibular pain dysfunction syndrome
mph	miles per hour
MPH	Master of Public Health
MPHD	methoxyhydroxphenolglycerol
MPL	myeloproliferative leukemia
MPM	mean platelet mass
MPO	myeloperoxidase
MPPT	methylprednisolone pulse therapy
MPS	mucopolysaccharidosis
MPV	mean plasma volume; mean platelet volume
MR	moderately resistant
MRA	main renal artery
mrad	millirad
MRI	magnetic resonance imaging
MRM	modified radical mastectomy
MRP	multidrug-resistance program
MRS	methicillin-resistant *Staphylococcus aureus*
MRSA	methicillin-resistant *S. aureus*
MRVP	mean right ventricular pressure
m/s	meters per second
MS	mental status; mitral stenosis; multiple sclerosis
MSAFP	maternal serum alpha fetoprotein
MSAP	mean systemic arterial pressure
MSAT	modified slide agglutination test
MSD	metabolic screening disorders
msec	millisecond
m/sec	meters per second
MSH	melanocyte stimulating hormone
MSL	midsternal line
MSLT	multiple sleep latency test
MSOF	multiple systems organ failure
MST	metyrapone stimulation test
MSTA	mumps skin test antigen
MSTI	multiple soft tissue injuries
MSU	monosodium urate crystals
MSUD	maple syrup urine disease
mt	send of such (mitte talis)
MT	medical technologist; metallothionein
MTB	mycobacterium tuberculosis
MTC	mitomycin-C
mtDNA	mitochrondrial DNA
MTHF	5-methyl-tetrahydrofolate
MTR-O	mass, tenderness, rebound (abdominal examination)
MTR-O	no masses, tenderness, or rebound (abdominal examination)
MTRX	methotrexate
MTX	methotrexate
MTX's	methotrexate
mU	milliunit
MUGA	multiple gated scan
MUP	monitor unit potential
MV	minute volume
M-VAC	methotrexate, vinblastine, Adriamycin (doxorubicin), and cisplatin
MVB	mixed venous blood
MVC	maximal vital capacity; maximal voluntary contraction; myocardial vascular capacity
MVE	mitral valve echo
MVK	mevalonate kinase
MVOA	mitral valve orifice area
MVOS	mixed venous oxygen saturation
MVP	mean venous pressure; mitral valve prolapse
MVPP	mustine, vinblastine, procarbazine, and prednisone
MVR	mitral valve regurgitation; mitral valve replacement
MVS	mitral valve stenosis
MVV	maximum voluntary ventilation
MVVPP	Mustargen (nitrogen mustard), vincristine, vinblastine, procarbazine, and prednisone
MW	mean weight; molecular weight
MWP	mean wedge pressure
MyG	myasthenia gravis
MyMD	myotonic muscular dystrophy
MYO	myoglobin
MYOGLB	myoglobin
MZ	monozygotic
n	nano (10^{-9})
N	nitrogen; normal
Na	sodium
NA	not applicable; normal aggregation; nursing assistant
N&A	normal and active
Na$_2$CO$_3$	sodium carbonate
NACI	National Advisory Committee on Immunization
NaCl	sodium chloride
NAD	nicotinamide adenine dinucleotide; no acute distress; no apparent distress
NADH	reduced form of NAD
NADH-TR	nicotinamide adenine dinucleotide-tetrazolium reductase
NADP	nicotinamide adenine dinucleotide phosphate
NADPH	reduced form of NADP
NaF	sodium fluoride
NAF	nafcillin

NAIT — neonatal alloimmune thrombocytopenia
Na&K — sodium and potassium
NaOH — sodium hydroxide
NAPA — *N*-acetylprocainamide
NAS — no added salt
NASH — nonalcoholic steatohepatitis
NATP — neonatal autoimmune thrombocytopenic purpura
Nb — niobium
NBIL — neonatal bilirubin
NBT — nitro blue tetrazolium
NC — nerve conduction
NCA — National Certification Agency; nonspecific cross-reacting antigen
NCBI — National Center for Biotechnology Information
NCCLS — National Committee for Clinical Laboratory Standards
NCEP — National Cholesterol Education Program
NCI — National Cancer Institute
NCPR — no cardiopulmonary resuscitation
NCRC — nonchild-resistant container
NCS — nerve conduction study
NCV — nerve conduction velocity
NCVS — nerve condition velocity studies
Nd — neodymium
N&D — nodular and diffuse (lymphoma)
N/D — no defects
NDA — New Drug Application
NDC — National Drug Code Directory
NDD — no-dialysis days
Ne — neon
NEA — neoplasm embryonic antigen
NEC — necrotizing enterocolitis
NED — no evidence (of) disease
NEMD — nonspecific esophageal motility disorder; nonspecific esophageal motor dysfunction
NEOH — neonatal/high
NEOM — neonatal/medium
NERD — no evidence (of) recurrent disease
NETT — nasal endotracheal tube
NF — normal full-term delivery
ng — nanogram
NGT — nasogastric tube; normal glucose tolerance
NGU — nongonococcal urethritis
NH_4Cl — ammonium chloride
NH_4OH — ammonium hydroxide
NHANES — National Health and Nutrition Examination Survey
NHD — normal hair distribution
NHDL — non-high-density lipoprotein
Ni — nickel
NICU — neonatal intensive care unit
NIDDM — noninsulin-dependent diabetes mellitus
NIH — National Institutes of Health
NIOSH — National Institute for Occupational Safety and Health
NIRA — near-infrared reflectance
NIS — no inflammatory signs
NITD — non-insulin-treated disease
NK — natural killer
N/K — not known
NKA — no known allergies
NKDA — no known drug allergies
NKFA — no known food allergies
NKH — nonketotic hyperglycemia; nonketotic hyperosmolar; nonketotic hyperosmotic
NKHA — nonketotic hyperosmolar acidosis
NKHG — nonketotic hyperglycemia
NKHS — nonketotic hyperosmolar syndrome
NKMA — no known medication allergies
nL — nanoliter
NL — normal
NLB — needle liver biopsy
NLDL — normal low-density lipoprotein
NLE — neonatal lupus erythematosus
nm — nanometer
NMJ — neuromuscular junction disease
nmol — nanomole
nmol/L — millimicromolar
NMR — nuclear magnetic resonance
NMRI — nuclear magnetic resonance imaging
NMS — neuroleptic malignant syndrome
NND — neonatal death
NNE — neonatal necrotizing enterocolitis
NNO — no new orders
NNS — neonatal screen (hematocrit, total bilirubin, and total protein)
NNT — neonatally tolerant
No — nobelium
NO — nasal oxygen
noc — in the night (nocturnal)
NOF — National Osteoporosis Foundation
NOII — nonocclusive intestinal ischemia
NOK — next of kin
NOM — nonsuppurative otitis media
NONF — nonfasting
non rep — do not repeat; no refills
NOOB — not out of bed
NOR-EPI — norepinephrine
NOS — no organisms seen
NOT — nocturnal oxygen therapy
NOTT — nocturnal oxygen therapy trial
Np — neptunium
NP — nasal prongs; nasopharynx
NPA — nasal pharyngeal airway
NPAT — nonparoxysmal atrial tachycardia
NPC — nasopharyngeal cancer; nasopharyngeal carcinoma
NPF — no predisposing factor
NPO — nothing by mouth
NPO/HS — nothing by mouth at bedtime
NPT — nocturnal penile tumescence
NPTM — nocturnal penile tumescence monitoring
NPV — negative pressure ventilation
nr — do not repeat (non repetatur)
N/R — not remarkable
NRBCs — normal red blood cells; nucleated red blood cells
NRC — National Research Council; Nuclear Regulatory Commission
NREM — nonrapid eye movement
NRM — normal range (of) motion
nRNP — nuclear ribonucleoprotein
NROM — normal range of motion
NS — normal saline; not seen; not significant
N/S — normal saline
NSA — normal serum albumin; no salt albumin
NSAID — nonsteroidal anti-inflammatory drug
NSDA — nonsteroid-dependent asthmatic
NSE — neuron specific enolase
NSM — nonsmoker
NSR — normal sinus rhythm
NST — nonstress test
NSU — nonspecific urethritis
NSV — nonspecific vaginitis
NSVD — normal spontaneous vaginal delivery
NSVT — nonsustained ventricular tachycardia
NT — nasotracheal
N&T, N+T — nose and throat
NTA — natural thymocytotoxic autoantibody
NTG — nitroglycerine
NTI — nonthyroidal illness; nonthyroidal index
NTMI — nontransmural myocardial infarction
NTN — nephrotoxic nephritis
NTND — not tender, not distended
NTR — negative therapeutic reaction
NTS — nasotracheal suction
NTT — nasotracheal tube
NTX — naltrexone
NU — name unknown
N&V — nausea and vomiting
NVA — near visual acuity; normal visual acuity
NVAF — nonvalvular atrial fibrillation
NVD — nausea, vomiting, diarrhea; neck vein distention
NYD — not yet diagnosed; not yet discovered
nyst — nystagmus
O — oxygen
O&A — observation and assessment
OAG — open-angle glaucoma
OAH — ovarian androgenic hyperfunction
OAR — orientation/alertness remediation
OB — obstetrics; occult blood
O&B — opium and belladonna
OBS — organic brain syndrome
OC — on call; oral contraceptive
O&C, O+C — onset and course (of disease)
OCAD — occlusive carotid disease
OCD — obsessive-compulsive disorder
OCG — oral cholecystogram
OCs — oral contraceptives
OCT — ornithine carbamyl transferase
od — right eye (oculus dexter)
OD — overdose
ODAP — Oncovin (vincristine), dianhydrogalactitol, Adriamycin (doxorubicin), and Platinol (cisplatin)
ODC — oxygen dissociation curve
ODE — O-desmethylencainide
ODm — ophthalmodynamometry
O&E — observation and examination
O/E — (ratio of) observed to expected; on examination
OEC — outer ear canal
OGT — oral glucose tolerance
OGTT — oral glucose tolerance test
OH — hydroxide; hydroxyl
OHCS — hydroxycorticosteroid
17-OHCS — 17-hydroxycorticosteroids
OHG — oral hypoglycemic
OHL — oral hairy leukoplakia
OHP — oxygen under high pressure
OHS — occipital horn syndrome
O-I — outer-to-inner
OIF — oil immersion field
oint — ointment
OKT — a group of monoclonal antibodies for typing lymphocytes
OL — left eye
OLD — obstructive lung disease
OM — otitis media
OMAC — otitis media, acute, catarrhal
OMAD — Oncovin (vincristine), methotrexate, Adriamycin (doxorubicin), and dactinomycin
OMAS — otitis media, acute, suppurating
OMC — open mitral commissurotomy
OMCA — otitis media, catarrhal, acute
OMCC, OMCCH — otitis media, catarrhal, chronic
OME — otitis media (with) effusion
OMN — oculomotor nerve
OMPA — otitis media, purulent, acute

OMPC, OMPCh ... otitis media, purulent, chronic
OMSA ... otitis media, suppurative, acute
OMSC, OMSCh ... otitis media, secretory, chronic; otitis media, suppurative, chronic
OMVC ... open mitral valve commissurotomy
ONTG ... oral nitroglycerin
ONTR ... orders not to resuscitate
OO ... oophorectomy
O&O ... off and on
O-O ... outer-to-outer
OOB ... out of bed; out-of-body (experience)
OOBBRP ... out of bed (with) bathroom privileges
OOC ... onset of contractions
OOL ... onset of labor
O&P ... ova and parasites (stool exam)
OPE ... outpatient evaluation
OPG ... ocular plethysmography
OPLL ... ossification (of) posterior longitudinal ligament
OPP ... Oncovin (vincristine), procarbazine, and prednisone; osmotic
OPV ... oral (attenuated) poliovirus vaccine; oral polio vaccine; outpatient visit
O.R. ... operating room
ORAC ... oxygen radical absorbance capacity
ORS ... oral rehydration solution
OR x1 ... oriented to time
OR x2 ... oriented to time and place
OR x3 ... oriented to time, place, and person
os ... left eye (oculus sinister)
Os ... osmium
OSA ... obstructive sleep apnea
OSAS ... obstructive sleep apnea syndrome
Osm/kg ... osmole per kilogram (osmolality)
Osm/L, Osm/l ... osmole per liter (osmolality)
OSM S ... osmolarity serum
OSM U ... osmolarity urine
OT ... objective test; old tuberculin
O/T ... oral temperature
OTA ... open to air
OTC ... ornithine transcarbamylase
OTC Rx ... over-the-counter prescription
OTD ... oral temperature device
OTH ... other
OTT, OT(T) ... orotracheal tube
ou ... each eye (oculus uterque)
OULQ ... outer upper left quadrant
OURQ ... outer upper right quadrant
OUZ ... upper outer zone (quadrant)
ov ... ovarian
o/w ... otherwise
O/W ... oil in water (emulsion)
OWNK ... out of wedlock (and) not keeping (child)
OWR ... ovarian wedge resection
P ... L. *post* after; mean pressure
p ... pico (10^{-12})
P ... peta (10^{15}); phosphorus; pulse
^{32}P ... radioisotope of phosphorus
/P ... partial lower denture
P/ ... partial upper denture
p_2, P-2 ... pulmonic secod (heart) sound
$P_2=A_2$ ... pulmonic second heart sound equal to aortic second heart sounds
$P_2<A_2$ ... pulmonic heart sound less than aortic second heart sound
$P_2>A_2$ ... pulmonic second heart sound greater than aortic second heart sound
p24 ... antigen in HIV infection
p50 ... half saturation (oxygen)
Pa ... arterial pressure; protactinium; pulmonary arterial (pressure); pulmonary artery (line)
PA ... alveolar pressure; panic attack; partial pressure; passive aggressive; pernicious anemia; phenylalinine; photo-allergy; physical assistance; pituitary-adrenal; platelet associated
P&A ... percussion and auscultation
P/A ... percussion (and) auscultation
P-A ... posteroanterior
PABA ... para-aminobenzoic acid
PAC ... phenacetin (acetophenetidin), aspirin, and caffeine; Platinol (cisplatin), Adriamycin (doxorubicin), and cyclophosphamide); premature atrial contraction
PAC-V ... Platinol (cisplatin), Adriamycin (doxorubicin), and cyclophosphamide
PAd ... pulmonary artery diastolic
PAD ... preoperative autologous donation
PADP ... pulmonary artery diastolic pressure
PA&F ... percussion, auscultation, and fremitus
PAF ... paroxysmal atrial fibrillation
PAF-A ... platelet-activating factor of anaphylaxis
PAFI ... platelet-aggression factor inhibitor
PAFIB ... paroxysmal atrial fibrillation PAF
PAH ... phenylalanine hydroxylase; pulmonary artery hypertension; pulmonary artery hypotension
PAHA ... *para*-aminohippuric acid
PAHVC ... pulmonary alveolar hypoxic vasoconstriction
PAI ... plasminogen activator inhibitor
PA-LS-ID ... pernicious anemia-like syndrome (and) immunoglobulin deficiency
PAM ... periodic acid-methanamine silver
PAMP ... pulmonary artery mean pressure
PAN ... periarteritis nodosa
P_{ao} ... airway opening pressure
Pao ... ascending aortic pressure
PaO_2 ... partial pressure of arterial oxygen
PAo ... pulmonary artery occlusion (pressure)
PAO ... peak acid output; peripheral airway obstruction
PAO_2 ... partial pressure of oxygen in alveoli
PAO_2-PaO_2 ... alveolar-arterial difference in partial pressure of oxygen
PAOD ... peripheral arterial occlusive disease; peripheral arteriosclerotic occlusive disease
PAOP ... pulmonary artery occlusion pressure
Pap ... Papanicolaou's stain
PAP ... peroxidase antiperoxidase; pri. atypical pneum.; prostate acid phosphatase
PA/PS ... pulmonary atresia/pulmonary stenosis
PAR ... pulmonary arteriolar resistance
Para ... paraplegic; parous (having borne one or more children)
para ... number of pregnancies producing viable offspring; paraplegia/paraplegic
para I ... unipara (having borne one child)
para II ... bipara (having borne two children)
para III ... tripara (having borne three children)
para IV ... quadripara (having borne four children)
para O ... nullipara (no child borne)
parasym ... parasympathetic (division of antonomic nervous system)
PARR ... postanesthesia recovery room
PAS para-aminosalicylic acid; periodic acid Schiff stain; preadmission screening; pulmonary arterial stenosis; pulmonary artery systolic
Pas Ex ... passive exercise
PAT ... paroxysmal atrial tachycardia; paroxysmal auricular tachycardia; preadmission testing
PATCO ... prednisone, araC, thioguanine, cyclophosphamide, and Oncovin (vincristine)
pat. T ... patellar tenderness
p aur ... behind the ear
PAV ... partial atrioventricular
Paw ... mean airway pressure
PAW ... peak airway pressure; pulmonary artery wedge
PAWP ... pulmonary arterial wedge pressure
Pb ... lead
P&B ... pain and burning; phenobarbital and belladonna
P_{BA} ... brachial arterial pressure
PBA ... percutaneous bladder aspiration
Pb-B ... lead level in blood
PBC ... peripheral blood cell; pregnancy and birth complications; primary biliary cirrhosis
PBF ... peripheral blood flow; placental blood flow; pulmonary blood flow
PB-Fe ... protein-bound iron
PBG ... porphobilinogen
Pbl ... lead intoxication
PBI ... phenformin; protein-bound iodine
PBL ... peripheral blood leukocytes; peripheral blood lymphocytes
PBLI ... premature birth, live infant
PBLT ... peripheral blood lymphocyte transformation
PBM ... peripheral basement membrane; peripheral blood mononuclear
PBMC ... peripheral blood mononuclear cell
PBMV ... pulmonary blood mixing volume
PBP ... peak blood pressure
PBPC ... peripheral blood progenitor cells
PBPs ... penicillin-binding proteins
PBS ... peripheral blood smear
PBSC ... peripheral blood stem cells
PBZ ... phenoxybenzamine; Pyribenzamine (tripelennamine)
pc ... after meals (post cibum)
PC ... porto-caval; present complaint
pc1 ... platelet count pretransfusion
pc2 ... platelet count post-transfusion
PCA ... parietal cell antibody; percutaneous coronary angioplasty
PCB ... polychlorinated biphenyls
PCD ... paroxysmal cerebral dysrhythmia; platelet component distribution width; polycystic disease; posterior corneal deposits
PCDW ... platelet component distribution width
PCE ... pseudocholinesterase
PCG ... pneumocardiogram
PCH ... paroxysmal cold hemoglobinuria
PCHE ... pseudocholinesterase
PCI ... prothrombin consumption index
PCK ... polycystic kidney
PCKD ... polycystic kidney disease
PCM ... primary cutaneous melanoma
PCMX ... parachlorometaxylenol
PCN ... penicillin; platelet-neutrophil complex
PCNS ... penicillins
pCO_2 ... carbon dioxide partial pressure (tension)
Pco, P_{co} ... carbon monoxide pressure or tension
PCoA ... posterior communicating artery
PCOD ... polycystic ovarian disease
PCOS ... polycystic ovary syndrome
PCP ... phencyclidine
PCR ... polymerase chain reaction
PCR-SBT ... polymerase chain reaction sequence-based typing
PCR-SSCP ... polymerase chain reaction single-strand conformation polymorphism
PCR-SSOP ... polymerase chain reaction sequence-specific oligonucleotide blot hybridization
PCR-SSP ... polymerase chain reaction sequence-specific primers
P c/s ... primary cesarean section
PCT ... platelet-crit; postcoital test; prothrombin consumption test
PCTA ... percutaneous coronary transluminal angioplasty
PCU ... patient care unit
p cut ... percutaneous
PCV ... packed cell volume
PCW ... pulmonary capillary wedge (pressure)
PCWP ... pulmonary capillary wedge pressure
PCZ ... procarbazine; prochlorperazine
p/d ... packs per day (cigarettes)
Pd ... palladium
PD ... patent ductus; percutaneous drain; peritoneal dialysis; postural drainage

P(D+) — probability of having disease
P(D-) — probability of not having disease
P/D — packs per day (cigarettes)
PD$_{50}$ — median paralyzing dose
PDA — patent ductus arteriosus; posterior descending (coronary) artery; pulmonary disease anemia
PDB — *para*-dichlorobenzene
PD&C — postural drainage and clapping
PDCB — *para*-dichlorobenzene
PDCD — primary degenerative cerebral disease
PDD — platinum diamminodichloride (cisplatin); pyridoxine-deficient diet
PDE — paroxysmal dyspnea (on) exertion
PDF — peritoneal dialysis fluid
PDFC — premature dead female child
PDH — past dental history
PDI — periodontal disease index
PDL — poorly differentiated lymphocyte
PDLC — poorly differentiated lung cancer
PDLD — poorly differentiated lymphocytic-diffuse
PDLL — poorly differentiated lymphocytic lymphoma
PDLN — poorly differentiated (lymphocytic) lymphoma-nodular
PDM — polymyositis (and) dermatomyositis
PDMC — premature dead male child
PD&P — postural drainage and percussion
PDR — peripheral diabetic retinopathy; *Physician's Desk Reference*
PDS — pain-dysfunction
PDT — photodynamic therapy
PDW — platelet distribution width
PE — partial epilepsy; physical examination; physical exercise; pleural effusion; pulmonary edema; pulmonary embolism
PEARLA — pupils equal and react to light and accommodation
PEB — Platinol (cisplatin), etoposide, and bleomycin
PEEP — peak end-expiratory pressure; positive end-expiratory pressure
PEF — peak expiratory flow; pulmonary edema fluid
PEFR — peak expiratory flow rate
PEFT — peak expiratory flow time
PEFV — partial expiratory flow volume
PEG — polyethylene glycol
pen., Pen — penicillin
PEN — parenteral (and) enteral nutrition
PEP — phosphoenolpyruvate
PEPI — pre-ejection period index
PEPP — positive expiratory pressure plateau
PER — peak ejection rate
perf — perforation
PERF — peak expiratory flow rate
PERK — prospective evaluation (of) radial keratomy
PERL — pupils equal (and) react (to) light (and) accommodation
PERLA — pupils equal, reactive to light and accommodation
PERR — pattern evoked retinal response
PERRLA — pupils equal, round, react (to) light (and) accommodation
PET — peak flow; pericardial fluid; peritoneal fluid; pleural fluid; positron emission tomography; pre-eclamptic toxemia
PeV — peripheral vein
PEWV — pulmonary extravascular water volume
PF — platelet factor; preservative free
PFA — phosphonoformatic acid; profunda femoris artery
PFG — peak-flow gauge
PFGE — pulse-field gel electrophoresis
PFK — phosphofructoaldolase
PFM — peak flow meter
PFO — patent foramen ovale
PFR — peak flow rate; pericardial friction rub
PFS — penile flow study; prefilled syringe
PFT — prednisone, fluorouracil, and tamoxifen; pulmonary function test
PFU — plaque forming units
pg — picogram
PG — parotid gland; phosphatidyl glycine
P$_G$ — plasma glucose
PGD — phosphogluconate dehydrogenase
PGE — primary generalized epilepsy; prostaglandin E
pgf — paternal grandfather
PGH — pituitary growth hormone; prostaglandin H
PGI — phosphoglucose isomerase; potassium, glucose, and insulin; prostaglandin I
PGK — phosphoglycerokinase
pgm — paternal grandmother
PGM — paternal grandmother
PGN — proliferative glomerulonephritis
PgR — progesterone receptor
PGs — prostaglandin; pyoderma gangrenosum
PGTR — plasma glucose tolerance rate
PGTT — prednisolone glucose tolerance test
PGU — peripheral glucose uptake; postgonococcal
pH — measurement of acidity or alkalinity
PH — past history; persistent hepatitis; personal history
pHa — arterial blood pH
PHA — phytohemagglutinin activation
PHCC — primary hepatocellular carcinoma
PhD — Doctor of Philosophy
pheo, Pheo — pheochromocytoma
PHHI — persistent hyperinsulinemic hypoglycemia of infancy
PHI — phosphohexoseisomerase
PHIS — posthead injury syndrome
PHK — postmortem human kidney
PHP — persistent hyperphenylalaninemia
pHPT — primary hyperparathyroidism
PHR — peak heart rate
PHT — peroxide hemolysis test; portal hypertension; primary hyperthyroidism; pulmonary hypertension
PHTN — portal hypertension
PHx — past history
pi — platelet count increment
PI — phosphatidylinositol; protamine insulin; pulmonary infarction
PICC — peripherally inserted central catheter
PICD — primary irritant contact dermatitis
PID — pelvic inflammatory disease
PIE — postinfectious encephalomyelitis; prosthetic infectious endocarditis
PIF — peak inspiratory flow
PIFT — platelet immunofluorescence test
PIH — pregnancy-induced hypertension
PIHH — postinfluenza-like hyposmia and hypogeusia
PIIP — portable insulin infusion pump
PIM — penicillamine-induced myasthenia
PIMS — programmable implantable medication system
PIO — progesterone in oil
PIO$_2$ — inspired oxygen tension; partial pressure of inspiratory oxygen
PIV — parainfluenza virus
PIWT — partially impacted wisdom teeth
PJS — Peutz-Jeghers syndrome
PJT — paroxysmal junctional tachycardia
PJVT — paroxysmal junctional-ventricular tachycardia
P$_K$ — plasma potassium
PK — pyruvate kinase
PKD — polycystic kidney disease
PKN — parkinsonism
PKU — phenylketonuria
PLCC — primary liver cell cancer
PLL — peripheral light loss
PLR — pupillary light reflex
PLS — primary lateral sclerosis
Plt — platelet
PLT — psittacosis-lymphogranuloma venereum trachoma
PLV — live poliomyelitis vaccine
Pm — promethium
PM — afternoon; pacemaker
PM-1 — polymorph; postmortem
PMC — premature mitral closure; pseudomembranous colitis
PMD — primary myocardial disease; progressive muscular dystrophy
PMDW — platelet mass distribution width
PMEC — pseudomembranous enterocolitis
PMH — past medical history
PMI — past medical illness
PMIS — postmyocardial infarction syndrome
PM-I — platelet membrane antigen
pML — posterior mitral valve leaflet
PMN — polymorphonuclear neutrophil
PMO — postmenopausal osteoporosis
pmol — picomole
PMP — pain management program; previous menstrual period
PM&R — physical medicine and rehabilitation
PMR — perinatal morbidity rate; perinatal mortality rate
PMS — premenstrual syndrome
PMTS — premenstrual tension syndrome
PN — parenteral nutrition
P$_{N2}$ — partial pressure of nitrogen
P$_{Na}$ — plasma sodium
PNC — penicillin
PNH — paroxysmal nocturnal hemoglobinuria
PNP — nonprotein nitrogen
PNPB — positive-negative pressure breathing
pNPP — paranitrophenylphosphate
PNPR — positive-negative pressure respiration
Pnx — pneumothorax
po — by mouth (per os)
pO$_2$ — oxygen partial pressure (tension)
Po — polonium
P&O — parasites and ova
P-O — postoperative
POA — pancreatic oncofetal antigen
POC — point-of-care
POCT — point-of-care testing
PODx — preoperative diagnosis
POEMS — polyneuropathy, organomegaly, endocrinopathy, M protein, skin changes
POHI — physically (or) otherwise health-impaired
POHS — presumed ocular histoplasmosis syndrome
POL — premature onset (of) labor
POM — pain on motion
POMP — prednisone, Oncovin (vincristine), methotrexate, and Purinethol (mercaptopurine)
POMR — problem oriented medical record
POP — pain on palpation
POR — physician of record; problem oriented record
POS — polycystic ovary syndrome
POVT — puerperal ovarian vein thrombophlebitis
PP — paradoxical pulse; pedal pulse; peripheral pulse; postprandial
PPA — phenylpropanolamine
PPAS — peripheral pulmonary artery stenosis
PPB — platelet-poor blood; positive pressure breathing
PPBE — postpartum breast engorgement
PPBS — postprandial blood sugar
PPCM — postpartum cardiomyopathy
P&PD — percussion and postural drainage
PPD — packs per day (cigarettes); purified protein derivative
PPF — plasma protein fraction
PPG — photoplethysmography

PPH	persistent pulmonary hypertension; postpartum hemorrhage
PPK	palmoplantar keratosis
PPL	penicilloye-polylysine
PPLO	pleuropneumonia-like organisms
ppm	parts per million
PPP	palmoplantar pustulosis; pedal pulse present; peripheral pulse palpable
PPROM	prolonged premature rupture of membranes
ppt	precipitate
Pr	praseodymium; presbyopia
PR	per rectum
P&R	pelvic and rectal (examination); pulse and respiration
P/R	productivity to respiration (ratio)
P-R	time between P wave and beginning of QRS complex in electrocardiography
PRA	percentage of reactive antibody; plasma renin activity; progesterone receptor assay
pRB	retinoblastoma gene product
PRBC	packed red blood cells
PRBCs	packed red blood cells
PRED	prednisone
PRERLA	pupils round, equal, react to light (and) accommodation
PRF	progressive renal failure
PRFM	premature rupture (of) fetal membranes; prolonged rupture (of) fetal membranes
PRG	phleborheography
PRH	past relevant history
PRL	prolactin
PRLA	pupils react to light and accommodation
prn	as needed (pro re nata)
PROM	passive range of motion; premature rupture of membranes; prolonged rupture of membranes
PRP	polyribophosphate
PRRE	pupils round, regular, (and) equal
PRSM	peripheral smear
PS	periodic syndrome; phosphatidylserine; population sample; Porter-Silber; pulmonary stenosis; pyloric stenosis
P&S	pain and suffering
PSA	prostate specific antigen
PSBO	partial small bowel obstruction
PSG	polysomnography
PSIS	posterior/superior iliac spine
PSP	phenolsulfonphthalein
PSRBOW	premature spontaneous rupture (of) bag of waters
PSRO	Professional Standards Review Organization
PSS	progressive systemic sclerosis
PS-VER	pattern shift - visual evoked response
PSVT	paroxysmal supraventricular tachycardia
PSW	past sleepwalker
Pt	platinum
PT	pericardial tamponade; physical therapy; prothrombin time
P&T	Pharmacy & Therapeutics
PTA	platelet thromboplastin antecedent; prothrombin activity
PTAH	phosphotungstic acid hematoxylin
PTBA	percutaneous transluminal balloon angioplasty
PTBD	percutaneous transhepatic biliary drainage
PTBD-EF	percutaneous transhepatic biliary drainage-enteric feeding
PTBS	post-traumatic brain syndrome
PTC	phenylthiocarbamide; plasma thromboplastin component
PTCA	percutaneous transluminal coronary angioplasty
PTCR	percutaneous transluminal coronary recanalization
PTD	percutaneous transluminal dilatation
PTED	pulmonary thromboembolic disease
PTH	parathyroid hormone
PTHBD	percutaneous transhepatic biliary drain(age)
PTMDF	pupils, tension, media, disc, fundus
PTP	prothrombin-proconvertin
PTPN	peripheral (vein) total parenteral nutrition
PTR	patella tendon reflex; peripheral total resistance
PTRA	percutaneous transluminal renal angioplasty
PTS	pneumatic tube system
PTT	partial thromboplastin time
PTV	posterior tibial vein
PTWTKG	patient's weight (in) kilograms
Pu	plutonium
PU	peptic ulcer
PUBS	percutaneous umbilical blood sampling
PuD	pulmonary disease
PUD	peptic ulcer disease; pulmonary disease
PUE	pyrexia (of) unknown etiology
pulv	a powder (pulvis)
PUNL	percutaneous ultrasonic nephrolithotripsy
PUO	pyrexia (of) undetermined/unknown origin
PUP	percutaneous ultrasonic pyelolithotomy
PUPPP	pruritic urticarial papules and plaques of pregnancy
PUVA	pulsed ultraviolet actinotherapy
PV	peripheral vein; plasma volume
PVA	polyvinyl alcohol
PVB	Platinol (cisplatin), vinblastine, and bleomycin; premature ventricular beat
PVC	premature ventricular contraction
PVD	peripheral vascular disease
PVE	prosthetic valve endocarditis
PVF	portal venous flow; primary ventricular fibrillation
PVH	pulmonary vascular hypertension
PVI	peripheral vascular insufficiency
PVO	peripheral vascular occlusion; pulmonary venous obstruction; pulmonary venous occlusion
PVOD	peripheral vascular occlusive disease
PVP	penicillin V potassium
PVR	pulse volume recording
PVT	paroxysmal ventricular tachycardia
PWM	pokeweed mitogen
Px	physical
PYP	pyrophosphate
q.	every (quaque)
QALE	quality-adjusted life expectancy
QALY	quality-adjusted life years
QBCA	quantitative buffy coat analysis
qd	every day (quaque die)
qh	every hour (quaque hora)
qhr	every hour (quaque hora)
qid	four times a day (quarter in die)
QMI	Q-wave myocardial infarction
QNS	quantity not sufficient
qod	every other day
Qp	pulmonary blood
qs	sufficient quantity (quantum sufficiat)
qs ad	sufficient quantity to make (quantum sufficiat ad)
QTC	quantitative tip culture
QUIGS	quantitative immune globulins
QUS	quantitative ultrasound
qv	as much as you will (quam volveris)
R	respiration; right
Ra	radium
RA	refractory anemia; rheumatoid arthritis; right atrium
RABG	room air blood gas
RAC	right atrial catheter
RAD	radiation absorbed dose
RADCA	right anterior descending coronary artery
RADS	reactive airway disease syndrome
RAEB	refractory anemia with excess blasts
RAEB-T	refractory anemia with excess blasts in transformation
RAF	rheumatoid arthritis factor
RAI	radioactive iodine
RAO	right anterior oblique
RAP	rheumatoid arthritis precipitins
RAR	renal-aortic ratio
RAW	airway resistance
Rb	rubidium
RBB	right breast biopsy; right bundle-branch
RBBB	right bundle-branch block
RBBX	right breast biopsy examination
RBC	red blood cell
RBP	resting blood pressure; retinol binding protein
RBS	random blood sugar
RC	red cell; retrograde cystogram
RC100	red cell; red cell casts
RCM	radiographic contrast media; right costal margin
RCMI	red cell morphology index
RCS, R/CS	repeat cesarean section
rd	rutherford
RDOD	retinal detachment, oculus dexter (right eye)
RDOS	retinal detachment, oculus sinister (left eye)
RDS	respiratory distress syndrome
RDVT	recurrent deep vein thrombosis
RDW	red cell distribution width
Re	rhenium
R&E	rest and exercise; round and equal
REM	rapid eye movement
REMS	rapid eye movement sleep
repet	to be repeated (repetatur)
Rf	rutherfordium
RF	renal failure; rheumatoid factor
RFLP	restriction fragment length polymorphism
RFOL	results to follow
rGM-CSF	granulocyte-macrophage colony stimulating factor
Rh	antigen; blood group; rhesus; rhodium
RHA	right hepatic artery
RHBV	right-heart blood volume
RhIG	$Rh_o(D)$ immune globulin
RHL	recurrent herpes labialis; right hepatic lobe
$Rh_o(D)$	red cell antigen
rHuEPO	recombinant human erythropoietin
RI	reticulocyte index
RIA	radioimmunoassay
RID	radial immunodiffusion
RIPA	radioimmunoprecipitation
RISA	radioiodinated serum albumin
RK	radial keratotomy
RL, R-L, R/L	right to left (shunt)
RLL	right liver lobe; right lower lobe
RLQ	right lower quadrant
RMCA	right main coronary artery; right middle cerebral artery
RMI	reticulocyte maturity index
RMSF	Rocky Mountain spotted fever
Rn	radon
RN	registered nurse
RNA	ribonucleic acid
RNP	ribonucleoprotein
RO	routine order
R/O	rule out
ROAD	reversible obstructive airway disease
RODAC	replicate organism detection and counting
ROM	range of motion; range of movement; right otitis media; rupture of membrane
ROS	review of symptoms; review of systems
ROT	right occipital transverse
RPBI	resting penile-brachial index
RPF	renal plasma flow

RPGN	rapidly progressive glomerulonephritis
RPI	reticulocyte production index
RPLT	reticulated platelets
rpm	revolutions per minute
RPO	right posterior oblique
RPR	rapid plasma reagin
RQ	respiratory quotient
RR	recovery room; respiratory rate
R&R	rate and rhythm; recent and remote; rest and recuperation
R/R	rales/ronchi
RRA	right renal artery
RRI	ribonucleotide reductase inhibitor
RROM	resistive range of motion
RSV	respiratory syncytial virus
RSVC	right superior vena cava
RT	reverse transcriptase
R/T	rectal temperature
rT$_3$	reverse T$_3$
rT$_3$U	reverse T$_3$ uptake
RTA	renal tubular acidosis
RTH	resistance to thyroid hormone
RTL	reactive to light (pupils)
RTM	routine medical care
RTN	renal tubular necrosis
RT-PCR	reverse transcriptase polymerase chain reaction
Ru	ruthenium
RUG	right upper quadrant
RUL	right upper lobe
RUOQ	right upper outer quadrant
RUQ	right upper quadrant
RV	reserve volume
RVA	right vertebral artery
RVH	renovascular hypertension; right ventricular hypertrophy
RVHD	rheumatic valvular heart disease
RVVT	Russell viper venom test
Rx	a recipe; drug; medication; prescribe/prescription; prescription drug
s	without (sine)
S	sulfur
S$_1$	first heart sound
S$_2$	second heart sound
SA	sinoatrial; surface area
S-A	sinoatrial
SAAG	serum ascites albumin gradient
SACE	serum angiotensin converting enzyme
SADD	Standardized Assessment of Depressive Disorders
SADR	suspected adverse drug reaction
SAH	subarachnoid hemorrhage
SAL	suction assisted lipectomy
SAMHSA	Substance Abuse and Mental Health Services Administration
SAO	small airway obstruction
SASA	sulfapyridine and 5-aminosalicylic acid
SAZ	sulfasalazine
Sb	antimony
SBB	small bowel biopsy; specialist in Blood Bank technology
SBE	subacute bacterial endocarditis
SBL	serum bactericidal level
SBP	systemic blood pressure; systolic blood pressure
SBS	shaken baby syndrome; short bowel syndrome
SBT	sequence-based testing
Sc	scandium
SC	sickle cell; subclavian; subcutaneous
S-C	sickle cell
SCA	sickle-cell anemia
SCAT	sheep cell agglutination test
SCC	squamous cell carcinoma
SCCB	small cell carcinoma (of) bronchus
SCCHN	squamous cell carcinoma (of) head (and) neck
SCCL	small cell carcinoma (of) lung
SCD	sickle cell disease
SCE	sister chromatid exchange
SCh	succinylcholine chloride
SCID	severe combined immunodeficiency
SCIV	subclavian intravenous; subcutaneous intravenous
Scl	scleroderma; scleroderma antibody
SCL	scleroderma
SCPK, S-CPK	serum creatine phosphokinase
SCr	serum creatinine
SCV	squamous cell carcinoma (of) vulva; subclavian vein
SCV-CPR	simultaneous compression ventilation-cardiopulmonary resuscitation
SD	senile dementia; spontaneous delivery; standard deviation
S&D	stomach and duodenum
S/D	sharp/dull; systolic/diastolic (ratio)
S-D	sickle cell-(hemoglobin) D (disease); strength duration
SDA	same day admission
SDAS	same day admission for surgery
SDAT	senile dementia, Alzheimer type
SDB	sleep-disordered breathing
SD&C	suction, dilation, and curettage
SDFP	single donor frozen plasma
SDH	succinate dehydrogenase
SDHD	sudden death heart disease
SDIHD	sudden death ischemic heart disease
SDS	same day surgery
SD-SK	streptodornase-streptokinase
Se	selenium
S&E	safety and efficiency
SED	sedimentation (rate); skin erythema dose
SEM	scanning electron microscopy; standard error of the mean
SEP	serum electrophoresis; somatosensory evoked potential
SER	somatosensory evoked response
SF-EMG	single fiber electromyography
SFLE	Stress From Life Experience
SG	specific gravity
SGA	small for gestational age
SGOT	serum glutamic oxaloacetic transaminase
SGPT	serum glutamic pyruvic transaminase
SGS	second generation sulfonylurea
SGTT	standard glucose tolerance test
SH	serum hepatitis
S&H	speech and hearing
S/H	sample and hold
SHAA	serum hepatitis-associated antigen
SHBG	sex hormone binding globulin
Si	silicon
SI	Système International (SI) units
S&I	suction and irrigation
SIADH	syndrome of inappropriate antidiuretic hormone
SID	sudden infant death; systemic inflammatory disease
SIDS	sudden infant death syndrome
Sig	mark, write (signa)
SIL	squamous intraepithelial lesions
SIRF	severely impaired renal function
SIS	saliine infusion sonography
SISI	short increment sensitivity index
SIT	sperm immobilization test
SK	streptokinase
SKAB	skeletal antibody
SKSD, SK-SD	streptokinase-streptodornase
SKY	spectral karyotyping
SL	sublingual(ly)
S/L	slip lamp (examination)
S:L	sucrase to lactase (ratio)
SLCG	sulfolithoecholylglycine
SLE	systemic lupus erthyematosus
SLN	sentinel lymph node
Sm	samarium; Smith antigen
SMA	sequential/serial multiple analysis; smooth muscle antibody
SMX	sulfamethoxazole
SMZ	sulfamethoxazole
Sn	tin
SND	sinus node dysfunction
SNF	skilled nursing facility
SO, S&O, S-O	salpingo-oophorectomy
SOAP	subjective, objective, assessment, and plans
SOAPIE	subjective (data), objective (data), assessment, plan, implementation, (and) evaluation (problem-oriented record)
SOB	short of breath
SOBOE	shortness of breath on exertion
SOD	superoxide dismutase
sos	if there is need (si opus sit)
SPA	sperm penetration assay
SPC	standard plate count
SPCA	serum prothrombin conversion accelerator
SPE	septic pulmonary edema
SPECT	single-photon emission tomography
SPEP	serum protein electrophoresis
SPF	S-phase fraction
SPI	selective protein index
SPL	sound pressure level
SPMI	status postmyocardial infarction
SPO	status postoperative
SPOD	spouse's perception of disease
SPRCA	solid phase red cell adherence assay
SPS	sodium polyanetholsulfonate; sulfite polymyxin sulfadiazine
SPT	secretin and pancreozymes test
SQ	subcutaneous(ly)
SQA	sperm quality analyzer
SqCCA	squamous cell carcinoma
sq cell ca	squamous cell carcinoma
Sr	strontium
SR	sedimentation rate; sustained release; systems review
S&R	seclusion and restraint(s)
SRAW	specific airway resistance
SRC	sedimented red cell
SRF	severe renal failure
SRF-A	slow-reacting factor of anaphylaxis
SRI	severe renal insufficiency
SRIF	somatotropin releasing inhibiting factor
SR/NE	sinus rhythm, no ectopy
SRNG	sustained release nitroglycerin
SROM	spontaneous rupture of membranes
SRSA, SRS-A	slow-reacting substance (of) anaphylaxis
SRT	sedimentation rate test; speech reception threshold
SRU	side rails up
ss	one-half (semis)
SS	*Salmonella-Shigella*; saturated solution; subaortic stenosis
S&S	shower and shampoo; signs and symptoms
S/S	signs and symptoms
SS-A	Sjögren's syndrome A antibody
SS-B	Sjögren's syndrome B antibody
SSD	sickle cell disease; silver sulfadiazine
SS-DNA	single-stranded DNA
SSEP	somatosensory evoked potential
SSKI	saturated solution of potassium iodide
SSN	severely subnormal
SSOP	sequence-specific oligonucleotide blot hybridization
SSP	sequence-specific primers
SSPE	subacute sclerosing panencephalitis

S-T	sickle-cell thalassemia
St AE	standard above-elbow (cast)
stat	at once (statim); immediately
STD	sexually transmitted disease; skin test dose
STDH	skin test (for) delayed-type hypersensitivity
sTfR	soluble transferrin receptor
STH	somatotropic hormone
STI	systolic time intervals
STIC	serum trypsin inhibitory capacity
STLOM	swelling, tenderness, limitation of motion
STP	standard temperature and pressure
STS	serologic test for syphillis
S&U	supine and upright
supp	suppository (suppositorium)
SVAS	subvalvular aortic stenosis
SVBG	saphenous vein bypass graft
SVC	slow vital capacity
SVCO	superior vena cava obstruction
SVC-PA	superior vena cava-pulmonary artery (shunt)
SVCS	superior vena cava syndrome
SVD	single vessel disease
SVPB	supraventricular premature beat
SVPC	supraventricular premature contraction
SVR	systemic vascular resistance
SVT	sinoventricular tachyarrhythmia; subclavian vein thrombosis; supraventricular tachyarrhythmia; supraventricular tachycardia
SW	short wave
SWI	sterile water injection
Sx	signs; symptom(s)
syr	syrup (syrupus)
SYS BP	systolic blood pressure
T	temperature; tera (10^{12})
T+1, T+2, T+3	first, second, and third stages of increased intraocular tension
T_1	monoiodotyrosine; tricuspid first heart sound
T1-T12	first to twelfth thoracic vertebrae or nerves
T_2	diiodothyronine
T_3	triiodothyronine
T_3RU	triiodothyronine redin uptake
T_3UP	triiodothyronine uptake
T_3UR	triiodothyronine uptake ratio
T_4	levothyroxine; thyroxine
Ta	tantalum
TA	thyroglobulin autoprecipitins
T&A	tonsillectomy and adenoidectomy
TAA	thoracic aortic aneurysm
tab	tablet (tabella)
TAb	therapeutic abortion
TAD	tricyclic antidepressant drug
TA-GVHD	transfusion-associated graft-vs-host disease
TAH	total abdominal hysterectomy; transabdominal hysterectomy
tal	such
tal dos	such doses
TAM	tamoxifen
TAT	thematic apperception test; toxin-antitoxin; tray agglutination test; turnaround time
Tb	terbium
TB	tuberculosis
TBA	to be administered; to be admitted
TBB	transbronchial biopsy
TBC	total body calcium
TBD	total body density
TBE	tick-borne density
TBF	total body fat
TBFB	tracheobronchial foreign body
TBG	thyroxine binding globulin
TBGI	thyroid binding globulin index
TBH	total-body hematocrit
TBI	thyroid binding index; thyroxine binding index; total-body irradiation
TBL	total body load
TBM	tuberculous meningitis
TBN	total body nitrogen
TBNA	transbronchial needle aspiration
TBPA	thyroxine binding prealbumin
TBR	total bed rest
TBSA	total body surface area
TBTT	tuberculin tine test
TBW	total body water
TBWA	total body water
TBV	total blood volume
TBX	total-body irradiation
Tc	technetium
^{99m}Tc	radioisotope of technetium Tc 99m
TC	throat culture; total cholesterol
T&C	type and crossmatch
TCA	trichloracetic acid; tricyclic antidepressant
TCABG	triple coronary artery (bypass) graft
TCAD	tricyclic antidepressant
TCAG	triple coronary artery (bypass) graft
TCBS	thiosulfate citrate bile salts sucrose
TCC	transitional cell carcinoma
TCCB	transitional cell carcinoma (of) bladder
TCE	trichloroethanol
TCM	tissue culture medium
TCT	thrombin clotting time
TDK	tardive dyskinesia
TDM	therapeutic drug monitoring
TdT	terminal deoxynucleotidyl transferase
Te	tellurium; tetanus
TE	tetanus
T&E	testing and evaluation
TEA	total elbow arthroplasty
TEAC	tetraethylammonium chloride
TeBG	testosterone-estradiol-binding globulin
TEE	transesophageal echocardiography
TEG	thromboelastogram
TEN	toxic epidermal necrolysis; toxic epidermal necrosis
TENS	transcutaneous electrical nerve stimulation; transelectrical nerve stimulator
ter	terminal
TER	total elbow replacement
term.	full-term (infant); terminal
tet	tetanus
Tet	tetralogy of Fallot
TET	tetanus; treadmill exercise test
TF	tetralogy (of) Fallot
TFEV	timed forced expiratory volume
TFPI	tissue factor pathway inhibitor
TfR	transferrin receptor
TG	triglyceride
TGF	transforming growth factor
TGT	thromboplastin generation test
TGV	thoracic gas volume
th	thoracic
Th	thorium
THA	transient hemispheric attack
THb	total hemoglobin
THC	tetrahydrocannabinol
THR	targeted heart rate; total hip replacement
Ti	titanium
TI	total iron
TIA	transient ischemic attack
TIBC	total iron binding capacity
tid	three times a day (ter in die)
TIF	tumor-inducing factor; tumor-inhibiting factor
TIT	triiodothyronine
TIUV	total intrauterine volume
TJA	total joint arthroplasty
TJR	total joint replacement
TK	through (the) knee; transketolase
TKA	total knee arthroplasty
TKO	to keep open
TKR	total knee replacement
TKVO	to keep vein open
Tl	thallium
TL	tubal ligation
TLA	translumbar aortogram
TLC	tender loving care; thin-layer chromatography; total lung capacity
TLW	total lung water
Tm	thulium
TM	temporomandibular (joint)
t_{max}	time of maximal concentration
TMB	transient monocular blindness
TMD	transmembrane domain
TMET	treadmill exercise test
TMJ	temporomandibular joint
TMJ-PDS	temporomandibular joint-pain dysfunction syndrome
TMJS	temporomandibular joint syndrome
TMO	total motile oval count
TMP	trimethoprim
TMP-SMX	trimethoprim-sulfomethoxazole
TMP-SMZ	trimethoprim-sulfomethoxazole
TMX	tamoxifen
TNF	tumor necrosis factor
TNS	transcutaneous nerve stimulation
TNTC	too numerous to count
T&O	tubes and ovaries
TOAP	thioguanine, Oncovin (vincristine), araC (cytarabine), and prednisone
TOB	tobramycin
TOF	tetralogy of Fallot
TOGV	transposition of great vessels
TOL	trial of labor
TOS	thoracic outlet syndrome
TP	total protein
TPA	tissue plasminogen activator; *Treponema pallidum* agglutination
TPC	telescoping plugged catheter
TPCV	total packed cell volume
TPI	*Treponema* immobilization test; triose phosphate isomerase
TPN	total parenteral nutrition
TPO	thyroperoxidase
TPP	thiamine pyrophosphate
TPR	temperature, pulse, respiration
TPVR	total peripheral vascular resistance
TR	turbidity-reducing
TRALI	transfusion-related acute lung injury
TRAP	tartrate resistance leukocyte acid phosphatase
TRCV	total red cell volume
TRH	thyroid releasing hormone
TRIC	trachoma inclusion conjunctivitis
trig	triglycerides
TRIS	tris(hydroxymethyl)aminomethane
trit	triturate (tritura)
Trml, TRML	terminal
TRP	tubular reabsorption of phosphorus
TS	Tay-Sachs; total solids
TSAT	tube-slide agglutination test
TSB	trypticase soy broth
TSE	testicular self-examination

TSH	thyroid stimulating hormone
TSH-RF	thyroid-stimulating hormone-releasing factor
TSH-RH	thyroid-stimulating hormone-releasing hormone
TSI	thyroid stimulating immunoglobulin; total serum iron
tsp	teaspoon
TSS	toxic shock syndrome
TSST	toxic shock syndrome toxin
TST	thermal sensitivity test
TT	tablet triturate; thrombin time
T&T	time and temperature
TT₄	total thyroxine
TTP	thrombotic thrombocytopenic purpura
TTS	tarsal tunnel syndrome
TTUTD	tetanus toxoid up-to-date
TU	thiouracil; Todd unit; toxic unit; tuberculin unit
TUD	total urethral discharge
TUN	total urinary nitrogen
TUNEL	terminal dUTP nick end labeling
TUPR	transurethral prostatic resection
TUR	transurethral resection
TURB	transurethral resection (of) bladder (tumor)
TURBN	transurethral resection (of) bladder neck
TURBT	transurethral resection (of) bladder tumor
TURP	transurethral prostatectomy; transurethral resection of prostate
TURV	transurethral resection (of) valves
TV	tidal volume; total volume
TVC	triple voiding cystogram
TVU	total volume (of) urine
TVUS	transvaginal ultrasound
TWG	total weight gain
Tx	therapy; treatment
T&X	type and crossmatch
TXM	type and crossmatch
Txn	transplant
TZ	transformation zone
U	uranium
UA, U/A	uric acid; urinalysis
UAO	upper airway obstructions
UB12BC	unsaturated B₁₂ binding capacity
UBBC	unsaturated vitamin B₁₂ binding capacity
UBBST	universal blood and body substance technique
UBC	unsaturated binding capacity
UBW	usual body weight
UC	ulcerative colitis
U&C	urethral and cervical (cultures)
U/C	urine culture
UCB	umbilical cord blood
UCCI	urinary cortisol/creatinine increment
UCD	urine collection device
UCG	urinary chorionic gonadotropin
UCI	urethral catheter in; urinary catheter in
UCO	urethral catheter out; urinary catheter out
UCRE	urine creatinine
ud	as directed (ut dictum)
UDP	uridine diphosphate
UDPG	uridinediphosphoglucose
UE	under elbow; upper extremity
U/E	upper extremity
UEA	upper extremity arterial
UES	upper esophageal sphincter
UFC	urinary free cortisol
UGA	under general anesthesia
UGI	upper GI
UIBC	unbound iron binding capacity
U-I-S	uroporphyrinogen-I-synthetase
UK	urokinase
Umax	maximal urinary osmolality
UMN	upper motor neuron
UNa	urinary sodium
ung	ointment (unguentum)
UO	under observation
UOP	urinary output
UOQ	upper outer quadrant
UOsm	urinary osmolality
UP	universal precautions
U/P	urine-plasma (ratio)
URI	upper respiratory illness; upper respiratory infection
URQ	upper right quadrant (of abdomen)
URT	upper respiratory tract
US	ultrasound
U.S.	United States
USAN	United States Adopted Names
USB	upper sternal border
USP	United States Pharmacopeia
UTBG	unbound thyroxin-binding globulin
ut dict	as directed (ut dictum)
UTI	urinary tract infection
UTO	unable to obtain
UUN	urine urea nitrogen
UV	ultraviolet; umbilical vein
UVA	midrange spectrum; ultraviolet
UVI	ultraviolet irradiation
V	vanadium
VA	visual activity
VAB	vincristine, actinomycin D, and bleomycin
VABP	ventroarterial bypass pumping
VAD	vascular access device; venous admixture
VADA	vincristine, Adramycin (doxorubicin), dexamethasone, and actinomycin D
VADH	vincristine, Adramycin (doxorubicin), and cyclophosphamide

vas., VAS	vasectomy
VB₁	first voided bladder specimen
VB₂	second midstream bladder specimen
VB₃	third midstream bladder specimen
VBAP	vincristine, BCNU (carmustine), Adriamycin (doxorubicin), and prednisone
VBC	vincristine, bleomycin, and cisplatin
VBG	venous blood gases
VBL	vinblastine
VBM	vinblastine, bleomycin, and methotrexate
VBMCP	vincristine, BCNU (carmustine), melphalan, cyclophosphamide, and prednisone
VBP	vinblastine, bleomycin, and Platinol (cisplatin)
VC	vena cava; vital capacity
VCA	vancomycin, colistin, and anisomycin; viral capsid antigen
VCA-EB	viral capsid antigen, Epstein-Barr
VCAP	vincristine, cyclophosphamide, Adriamycin (doxorubicin), and prednisone
VCG	vectorcardiogram
VCMP	vincristine, cyclophosphamide, melphalan, and prednisone
VCN	vancomycin, colistomethane, and nystatin
VCP	vincristine, cyclophosphamide, and prednisone
VCR	vincristine
VCT	venous clotting time
VCU	voiding cystourethrogram
VCUG	voiding cystourethrogram
VD	vascular disease; venereal disease
V&D	vomiting and diarrhea
VDAC	vaginal delivery after cesarean
VDG, VD-G	venereal disease, gonorrhea
VDP	vinblastine, decarbazine, and cisplatin; vincristine, daunorubicin, and prednisone
VDRL	test for syphilis; Venereal Disease Research Laboratory
VDS	vindesine
VE	vaginal examination; visual efficiency
VEMP	vincristine, Endaxan (cyclophosphamide), mercaptopurine, and prednisone
VEP	visual evoked potential
VER	visual evoked response
VF	ventricular fibrillation; vision field
VFAM	vincristine, 5-fluorouracil, Adriamycin (doxorubicin), and mitomycin C
vFW	von Willebrand factor
V&G	vagotomy and gastroenterotomy
VGH	very good health
VHD	valvular heart disease
VHDL	very high density lipoprotein
VIP	vasoactive intestinal polypeptide
VLBW	very low birth weight
VLD	very low density
VLDL	very low density lipoprotein
VLDLC	very low density lipoprotein cholesterol
VLDLP	very low density lipoprotein
VLDL-TG	very low density lipoprotein triglyceride
VLM	visceral larva migrans
VMA	vanillylmandelic acid
VMO	vastus medialis oblique (muscle)
vo	verbal order
VP	venous pressure
VPA	valproic acid
VPCs	ventricular premature complexes
VPRBC	volume (of) packed red blood cells
VS	vital signs
VSD	ventricular septal defect
VSS	vital signs stable
VSV	vesicular stimatitis virus
VT	ventricular tachyarrhythmia; ventricular tachycardia
V tach, V-TACH	ventricular tachycardia
VTE	venous thromboembolism
VTM	virus transport media
VU	voltage unit
VV	varicose vein
V&V	vulva and vagina
vW, VW	von Willebrand (disease)
vWD	von Willebrand disease
vWf, vWF	von Willebrand factor
vWS, vWs	von Willebrand syndrome
VZ, V-Z	varicella-zoster (virus)
VZIG	varicella-zoster immune globulin
VZV	varicella-zoster virus
W	tungsten
wa	while awake
WB	weight-bearing; whole blood
WBAT	weight-bearing as tolerated
WBC	white blood cell; white blood cell (count)
WBC/hpf	white blood cells per high power field
WBTT	weight-bearing to tolerance
WD	warm dry; well developed; well differentiated; wet dressing
W/D	warm (and) dry
WDF	white divorced female
WDHA	watery diarrhea-hypokalemia-achlorhydria
WDHH	watery diarrhea-hypokalemia-hypochlorhydria
WDLL	well-differentiated lymphatic lymphoma
WDM	white divorce male
WEE	Western equine encephalitis/encephalomyelitis
WF	white female
W-F	Weil-Felix
WFI	water for injection
WFL	within functional limits
WG	Wegener granulomatosis
WIC	women, infants, (and) children
WLS	wet lung syndrome

ACRONYMS AND ABBREVIATIONS GLOSSARY

WM	white male
WN	well nourished
WNL	within normal limits
WP	whirlpool
WPW	Wolff-Parkinson-White syndrome
W&S	wound and skin
WSF	white single female
WSM	white single male
WSR	Westergren sedimentation rate
w/u, W/U	work-up
WWAC	walk with aid (of) cane
WWidF	white widowed female
WWidM	white widowed male
X&D	examination and diagnosis
Xe	xenon
XKO	not knocked out
XN	night blindness
XO	gonadal dysgenesis of Turner type
XOM	extraocular movement
X-Prep	bowel evacuation prior to radiography
y	year
Y	yttrium
YAG	yttrium-argon-garnet - a type of laser
Yb	ytterbium
y/o, Y/O	years old
YOB	year of birth
YORA	younger-onset rheumatoid arthritis
Z-E	Zollinger-Ellison
ZES	Zollinger-Ellison syndrome
Z/G	zoster (serum) immunoglobulin
ZIg, ZIG	zoster (serum) immunoglobulin
ZIP	zoster immune plasma
Zn	zinc
ZPP	zinc protophorhyrin
Zr	zirconium
ZSR	zeta sedimentation rate

KEY WORD INDEX

The Key Word Index is not intended in any way to suggest patterns of physicians' orders, nor is it complete. Rather, it is the intent of the authors and editors to make information easier to find and utilize in order to support better patient care.

The Key Word Index provides a reference to test names based on a diagnostic property, disease entity, organ system, or syndrome for which the test may be useful. It provides lists of specific tests. Some may support possible clinical diagnoses or help to rule out other diagnostic possibilities.

Each laboratory test which may be relevant to the indexed diagnosis is listed and weighted. Two symbols (••) indicate that the test strongly supports a diagnosis or entity, that is, it significantly contributes to documentation of the diagnosis if the expected result is found. A single symbol (•) indicates a test frequently used in the diagnosis or management of the particular disease. The other listed tests may be useful on a selective basis with consideration of clinical factors and specific aspects of the case. A negative laboratory test result can be, and frequently is, highly relevant in the practice of medicine.

Clinical diagnosis is determined following history, physical examination, and usual laboratory investigation with selected additional tests. Complete blood count (CBC) with differential, urinalysis, and a basic chemistry profile are not only good medicine, they are in fact cost effective. Thus, these basic tests are excluded from much of the Key Word Index.

Diagnoses with *International Classification of Disease—Ninth Revision—Clinical Modification* (ICD-9-CM) codes are indicated within the [ ] symbol.

ABSCESS (LUNG) [513.0] *see also* ALCOHOLISM; BRONCHIECTASIS; DRUG ABUSE/DEPENDENCE; EMPYEMA; FUNGI; INFECTIVE ENDOCARDITIS; PNEUMONIA; SEIZURES; SEPTICEMIA; TUBERCULOSIS

An abscess within lung parenchyma, the expression usually is not intended to include cavitary lesions caused by mycobacterial, fungal, or parasitic diseases. Causes include tricuspid valve infective endocarditis in intravenous drug users, in whom septic pulmonary embolism may cause multiple lung abscesses. Lung abscess secondary to aspiration is usually solitary. Culture is best obtained by bronchoalveolar lavage or by protected specimen brush.

ACANTHOCYTOSIS *see* ABETALIPOPROTEINEMIA

ACETAMINOPHEN TOXICITY [965.4] *see also* ALCOHOLISM; DRUG ABUSE/DEPENDENCE; POISONING

In the alcohol-acetaminophen syndrome, coagulopathy and extremely abnormal transaminases are found. ALT >3500 units/L may be seen.

ACHLORHYDRIA *see* ATROPHIC GASTRITIS

ACIDOSIS/ALKALOSIS (ACID-BASE BALANCE) [276.2; 276.3; 775.7] *see also* ALCOHOL INTOXICATION; ALDOSTERONISM; CUSHING SYNDROME; DEHYDRATION/HYPOVOLEMIA; DIABETES MELLITUS; DIARRHEA; ETHYLENE GLYCOL POISONING; FANCONI SYNDROME; HEMOPTYSIS; METHANOL POISONING; PARALDEHYDE POISONING; RENAL FAILURE; RESPIRATORY FAILURE; SALICYLISM; VOMITING; WILSON DISEASE

ACIDOSIS (LACTIC) [276.2] *see also* ACIDOSIS/ALKALOSIS (ACID-BASE BALANCE)

ACIDOSIS (METABOLIC) *see* ACIDOSIS/ALKALOSIS (ACID-BASE BALANCE)

ACIDURIA (ARGININOSUCCINIC) *see* ARGININOSUCCINIC ACIDURIA

ACQUIRED IMMUNODEFICIENCY SYNDROME (AIDS) [042] *see also* CANDIDIASIS; COCCIDIOIDOMYCOSIS; CRYPTOCOCCOSIS; CRYPTOSPORIDIOSIS; CYTOMEGALOVIRUS; DIARRHEA; FEVER UNDETERMINED ORIGIN (FUO); FUNGEMIA; FUNGI; HEMOPHILIA; HEPATITIS; HERPESVIRUS INFECTION; HISTOPLASMOSIS; HUMAN T-CELL LYMPHOTROPIC VIRUS-I/II (HTLV-I/II); IDIOPATHIC THROMBOCYTOPENIC PURPURA (ITP); IMMUNE COMPLEX DISEASE; KAPOSI SARCOMA; LYMPHADENOPATHY; LYMPHOCYTES/LYMPHOPROLIFERATIVE DISORDERS; LYMPHOMA; MALABSORPTION/MALDIGESTIVE DISEASES; MENINGITIS (ASEPTIC); MYCOBACTERIAL INFECTION (ATYPICAL); NOCARDIOSIS; *PNEUMOCYSTIS CARINII*; SEPTICEMIA; SYPHILIS; TOXOPLASMOSIS; TUBERCULOSIS; VARICELLA-ZOSTER

ANEMIA (HYPOCHROMIC) *see* ANEMIA (MICROCYTIC)

ANEMIA (HYPOPLASTIC) [284.9]

ANEMIA (IRON DEFICIENCY) [280.9] *see also* BLEEDING (GASTROINTESTINAL); CARCINOMA (COLORECTAL); CARCINOMA (DUODENUM); CARCINOMA (GASTROINTESTINAL TRACT); CARCINOMA (STOMACH); CYSTIC FIBROSIS; HOOKWORM INFESTATION; MENORRHAGIA; PEPTIC ULCER
See the Anemia Flowchart in the introduction to the Hematology chapter.

ANEMIA (MACROCYTIC/MEGALOBLASTIC) [281.9] *see also* ALCOHOLISM; ATROPHIC GASTRITIS
See the Anemia Flowchart in the introduction to the Hematology chapter.

ANEMIA (MICROANGIOPATHIC HEMOLYTIC) [283.19] *see also* RENAL VEIN THROMBOSIS
See the Anemia Flowchart in the introduction to the Hematology chapter.

ANEMIA (MICROCYTIC) [280.9]
See the Anemia Flowchart in the introduction to the Hematology chapter.

ANEMIA (SICKLE CELL AND VARIANT SICKLING HEMOGLOBINS) [282.60] *see also* ASPLENIA; HEMOGLOBINOPATHY
See the Anemia Flowchart in the introduction to the Hematology chapter.

922

CARDIAC ARRHYTHMIAS *see* ARRHYTHMIAS (DYSRHYTHMIAS)

CARDIAC TAMPONADE *see* PERICARDIAL EFFUSION/PERICARDITIS

CARDIOMYOPATHY [425.4] *see also* ACQUIRED IMMUNODEFICIENCY SYNDROME (AIDS); ALCOHOLISM; AMYLOIDOSIS; CONGESTIVE HEART FAILURE; DERMATOMYOSITIS; DIPHTHERIA; DUCHENNE MUSCULAR DYSTROPHY; GAUCHER DISEASE; GLYCOGEN STORAGE DISEASE; HEART; HEMOCHROMATOSIS; HEMOLYTIC-UREMIC SYNDROME; HYPERTENSION; HYPERTHYROIDISM; HYPOTHYROIDISM; INBORN ERRORS OF METABOLISM; LYME DISEASE; MYOCARDITIS; NIEMANN-PICK DISEASE; PHEOCHROMOCYTOMA; REYE SYNDROME; RICKETTSIAL INFECTION/ROCKY MOUNTAIN SPOTTED FEVER; SARCOIDOSIS; SCLERODERMA; SYSTEMIC LUPUS ERYTHEMATOSUS (SLE); TAY-SACHS DISEASE; THYROID; UREMIA; VASCULITIS

CATARACT [366.9]

CAT BITE *see* BITES

CATECHOLAMINE *see* PHEOCHROMOCYTOMA

CAT SCRATCH DISEASE [078.3] *see also* MYCOBACTERIAL INFECTION (ATYPICAL); TUBERCULOSIS; TULAREMIA

CD *see also* LYMPHOCYTES/LYMPHOPROLIFERATIVE DISORDERS

Refer to the Hematology introduction for the table, Cluster of Differentiation (CD) Antigens. Consult the listing, Immunophenotypic Analysis of Tissues by Flow Cytometry, in the Anatomic Pathology chapter for the table, Frequently Used Lymphocyte Differentiation Antigens for Flow Cytometry.

CD *see* LYMPHOCYTES/LYMPHOPROLIFERATIVE DISORDERS

CELIAC DISEASE [579.0] *see also* CYSTIC FIBROSIS; DIARRHEA; LACTOSE INTOLERANCE; MALABSORPTION/MALDIGESTIVE DISEASES; MALNUTRITION; PROTEIN-LOSING ENTEROPATHY

After antiendomysial antibodies and endoscopic biopsies, other relevant laboratory studies include the presence of hypochromic anemia, iron <60 µg/dL, ferritin <50 ng/dL, and cholesterol <156 mg/dL.

CELL BLOCK

CELLULAR IMMUNE RESPONSE *see also* ACQUIRED IMMUNODEFICIENCY SYNDROME (AIDS); IMMUNE STATUS

CELLULITIS [682.9]

CELLULITIS (*S. AUREUS*, METHICILLIN-RESISTANT)

CENTRAL NERVOUS SYSTEM *see also* ALZHEIMER DISEASE; CEREBRAL INFARCTION/CEREBRAL THROMBOSIS/CEREBROVASCULAR ACCIDENT (CVA); COMA; DEMENTIA; ENCEPHALITIS; INBORN ERRORS OF METABOLISM; LEAD POISONING; MENINGITIS; MENINGITIS (ASEPTIC); MULTIPLE SCLEROSIS

CEREBRAL INFARCTION/CEREBRAL THROMBOSIS/ CEREBROVASCULAR ACCIDENT (CVA) [434.0; 434.91; 436]
see also BLEEDING; COMA; EMBOLISM; ENCEPHALITIS; THROMBOSIS; THROMBOSIS (VENOUS)

CERVICITIS [616.0] *see also* CARCINOMA (CERVIX); CARCINOMA (ENDOCERVIX); GONORRHEA; HERPES (GENITAL); SEXUALLY TRANSMITTED DISEASES; UROGENITAL INFECTIONS

CHAGAS DISEASE [086.2]

CHÉDIAK-HIGASHI SYNDROME [288.2] *see also* GENETIC COUNSELING

CHEST PAIN [786.50] *see also* ANGINA; CORONARY ARTERIAL DISEASE; DYSPNEA; ESOPHAGITIS; HEART; HEMOPTYSIS; MYOCARDIAL INFARCT; PANCREATITIS; PLEURAL EFFUSION/EXUDATE/ PLEURISY/PLEURITIS; PULMONARY EMBOLISM

CHIARI-FROMMEL SYNDROME *see* HYPERPROLACTINEMIA/CHIARI-FROMMEL SYNDROME

CHICKENPOX *see* VARICELLA-ZOSTER

CHLAMYDIA INFECTION [079.98] *see also* CONJUNCTIVITIS; PNEUMONIA; PNEUMONITIS

CHLAMYDIA TRACHOMATIS

CHOLANGITIS (PRIMARY SCLEROSING) [576.1] *see also* BILIARY FUNCTION TESTS; BILIARY OBSTRUCTION; CARCINOMA (CHOLANGIOCARCINOMA); CIRRHOSIS (PRIMARY BILIARY); HEPATITIS (AUTOIMMUNE)

Typically, look for marked increase in serum alkaline phosphatase with slight increases of aminotransferase concentrations.

CHOLECYSTITIS/CHOLEDOCHOLITHIASIS/CHOLELITHIASIS [574.2; 574.5; 575.1] *see also* ANEMIA (SICKLE CELL AND VARIANT SICKLING HEMOGLOBINS); ANEMIA (SPHEROCYTOSIS); APPENDICITIS; BILIARY OBSTRUCTION; CYSTIC FIBROSIS; JAUNDICE; PANCREATITIS; PEPTIC ULCER

COMPLEMENT *see also* ANGIONEUROTIC EDEMA; GLOMERULONEPHRITIS; SYSTEMIC LUPUS ERYTHEMATOSUS (SLE)

CONDYLOMA ACUMINATUM [078.11]

CONGENITAL ADRENAL HYPERPLASIA [255.2] *see also* ADENOMA (ADRENAL); CARCINOMA (ADRENAL); HIRSUTISM; INTERSEXUALITY; POLYCYSTIC OVARY SYNDROME; VIRILIZATION

See text in listing, Testosterone, Total and Free, Serum or Plasma.

CONGENITAL RUBELLA SYNDROME [771.0]

CONGESTIVE HEART FAILURE [428.0] *see also* ALCOHOLISM; AMYLOIDOSIS; ARSENIC POISONING; ASCITES; CARDIAC ACTIVE DRUGS; DIABETES MELLITUS; EDEMA; EFFUSIONS/TRANSUDATES/ EXUDATES; HEART; HEMOCHROMATOSIS; HYPERTENSION; LEAD POISONING; LIVER; LYME DISEASE; MYOCARDIAL INFARCT; MYOCARDITIS; PLEURAL EFFUSION/EXUDATE/PLEURISY/ PLEURITIS; RENAL FAILURE; RHEUMATIC FEVER; SARCOIDOSIS; SCLERODERMA; UREMIA

Chest x-ray, EKG, echocardiography, or radionucleotide ventriculography are among studies recommended. Myocarditis should be ruled out in selected patients.

CONJUNCTIVITIS [372.30] *see also* CHLAMYDIA INFECTION; CORNEAL ULCER; GONORRHEA; LYME DISEASE; SJÖGREN SYNDROME

HEINZ BODY ANEMIA *see* ANEMIA (HEINZ BODY)

HELICOBACTER PYLORI [041.86]

HELLP SYNDROME [642.5] *see also* DISSEMINATED INTRAVASCULAR COAGULATION (DIC); FATTY LIVER OF PREGNANCY, ACUTE; HEMOLYTIC-UREMIC SYNDROME; IDIOPATHIC THROMBOCYTOPENIC PURPURA (ITP); LIVER; PREECLAMPSIA; THROMBOTIC THROMBOCYTOPENIC PURPURA (TTP)

Characterized by right upper quadrant pain, nausea and vomiting, microangiopathic hemolytic anemia, elevated concentrations of liver-related enzymes, and low platelets (thrombocytopenia), the HELLP syndrome is a cause of maternal and fetal morbidity and mortality. It is found with severe pre-eclampsia or eclampsia. Other types of liver disease unique to pregnancy are hyperemesis gravidarum, cholestasis, and acute fatty liver.

HEMATEMESIS *see* BLEEDING; CARCINOMA (STOMACH); CIRRHOSIS; ESOPHAGEAL VARICES

HEMATEMESIS [578.0]

HEMATEMESIS *see* PEPTIC ULCER

HEMATURIA [599.7] *see also* BLEEDING; CARCINOMA (BLADDER); CYSTITIS/PYELONEPHRITIS; GLOMERULONEPHRITIS; GOODPASTURE SYNDROME; HEMOGLOBINOPATHY; HEMOGLOBINURIA; HEMOGLOBINURIA (PAROXYSMAL NOCTURNAL) (PNH); KIDNEY; MALARIA; PURPURA (HENOCH-SCHÖNLEIN); RENAL INFARCT; SYSTEMIC LUPUS ERYTHEMATOSUS (SLE); THROMBOCYTOPENIA; WEGENER GRANULOMATOSIS; WILMS TUMOR

HEMOCHROMATOSIS [275.0] *see also* CARCINOMA (LIVER); CIRRHOSIS; HEMOSIDEROSIS; JAUNDICE; SIDEROSIS (TRANSFUSIONAL)

Ferritin concentrations >1000 µg/L, transferrin saturation >60% (men) or 50% (women) provide evidence of hemochromatosis.

HEMOGLOBIN F *see* HEREDITARY PERSISTENCE OF HEMOGLOBIN F

HEMOGLOBINOPATHY [282.7] *see also* ANEMIA; ANEMIA (HEMOLYTIC); ANEMIA (SICKLE CELL AND VARIANT SICKLING HEMOGLOBINS); ANEMIA (SPHEROCYTOSIS); HEMOGLOBINURIA; HEMOLYSIS; THALASSEMIA

HEMOGLOBINURIA [791.2] *see also* ANEMIA (HEMOLYTIC); BLEEDING; GLOMERULONEPHRITIS; HEMATURIA; HEMOLYSIS; HEMOSIDERINURIA

HEMOGLOBINURIA (PAROXYSMAL COLD) [283.2] *see also* ANEMIA (HEMOLYTIC)

HYPEREMESIS GRAVIDARUM [643.0]

Occurring in the first trimester of pregnancy, symptoms are nausea and vomiting.

HYPERGAMMAGLOBULINEMIA [289.8] *see also* CIRRHOSIS; HEPATITIS (AUTOIMMUNE); LEISHMANIASIS; LEPROSY; MACROGLOBULINEMIA OF WALDENSTRÖM; MALARIA; MYELOMA; SARCOIDOSIS; SYSTEMIC LUPUS ERYTHEMATOSUS (SLE)

HYPERGLYCEMIA [790.6] *see also* COMA; DIABETES MELLITUS; PANCREATITIS; PHEOCHROMOCYTOMA

HYPERGLYCINEMIAS [270.7]

HYPER-IGE SYNDROME

HYPER-IGM SYNDROME

HYPERKALEMIA [276.7] *see also* ADDISON DISEASE; AMYLOIDOSIS; DEHYDRATION/HYPOVOLEMIA; HYPERGLYCEMIA; HYPEROSMOLALITY; RENAL FAILURE; RHABDOMYOLYSIS; UREMIA

HYPERLIPIDEMIA [272.4] *see also* ATHEROSCLEROSIS; CIRRHOSIS (PRIMARY BILIARY); CORONARY ARTERIAL DISEASE; DIABETES MELLITUS; HYPERTRIGLYCERIDEMIA; NEPHROSIS/NEPHROTIC SYNDROME

HYPERMAGNESEMIA [275.2; 775.5] *see also* UREMIA

HYPERMENORRHEA *see* MENORRHAGIA

HYPERNATREMIA [276.0] *see also* ALDOSTERONISM; CUSHING SYNDROME; DEHYDRATION/HYPOVOLEMIA; DIABETES INSIPIDUS; DIABETES INSIPIDUS (NEPHROGENIC); DIARRHEA; HYPEROSMOLALITY; VOMITING

HYPEROSMOLALITY [276.0] *see also* ACIDOSIS/ALKALOSIS (ACID-BASE BALANCE); HYPERGAMMAGLOBULINEMIA; HYPERKALEMIA; HYPERLIPIDEMIA; HYPERNATREMIA

The nonketotic hyperosmolar syndrome includes hyperglycemia, plasma osmolality >320 mOsm/L without ketonemia. See individual monographs.

HYPERPARATHYROIDISM [252.0] *see also* CARCINOMA (LUNG); ENDOCRINE TUMORS; HYPERCALCEMIA; MEDULLARY CARCINOMA OF THYROID; MULTIPLE ENDOCRINE NEOPLASIA (MEN 1, MEN 2); PANCREATITIS; PHEOCHROMOCYTOMA; RENAL FAILURE; TUMOR MARKERS

KIDNEY see also AMYLOIDOSIS; CYSTITIS/PYELONEPHRITIS; GLOMERULONEPHRITIS; GOODPASTURE SYNDROME; HYPERTENSION; KIDNEY STONE; LEAD POISONING; LEPTOSPIROSIS (WEIL SYNDROME); MYELOMA; NEPHROSIS/NEPHROTIC SYNDROME; NEPHROTOXICITY; POLYCYSTIC DISEASE (KIDNEY); PRERENAL AZOTEMIA; RENAL FAILURE; RENAL INFARCT; RENAL VEIN THROMBOSIS; TRANSPLANTATION; UREMIA; VASCULITIS
Refer to the Urinalysis chapter.

KIDNEY STONE [592.0] see also COLITIS (ULCERATIVE); CROHN DISEASE; CUSHING SYNDROME; CYSTINOSIS/CYSTINURIA; GOUT; HYPERPARATHYROIDISM; HYPERTHYROIDISM; IMMOBILIZATION (PROLONGED); INBORN ERRORS OF METABOLISM; OXALURIA; RENAL FAILURE; SARCOIDOSIS; UREMIA; HYPERVITAMINOSIS D; WILSON DISEASE
Although not an analyte, urine volume is relevant.

KIKUCHI DISEASE
(Histiocytic necrotizing lymphadenitis)

KIMMELSTIEL-WILSON DISEASE see DIABETIC NEPHROPATHY
***KLEBSIELLA* [041.3]**

KLINEFELTER SYNDROME [758.7] see also GENETIC COUNSELING; HYPOGONADISM

LABOR AND DELIVERY see FETAL MATURITY; RESPIRATORY DISTRESS SYNDROME

LACTIC ACIDOSIS see ACIDOSIS (LACTIC)

LACTOSE INTOLERANCE [271.3] see also ABDOMINAL PAIN; CELIAC DISEASE; IGA DEFICIENCY

LANGERHANS CELL (EOSINOPHILIC) GRANULOMATOSIS see also DIABETES INSIPIDUS

LARYNGOTRACHEITIS [464.20] see also ANGIONEUROTIC EDEMA; CROUP; DIPHTHERIA; PARAINFLUENZA VIRUS INFECTION

LEAD POISONING [984.9] see also ANEMIA (HEMOLYTIC); NEUROPATHY; PORPHYRIA

LEGIONNAIRES' DISEASE [482.83] see also HYPONATREMIA; *MYCOPLASMA* INFECTION; PNEUMONIA; PSITTACOSIS; Q FEVER; SYNDROME OF INAPPROPRIATE SECRETION OF ANTIDIURETIC HORMONE (SIADH)

LEIOMYOMA

LEISHMANIASIS [085.9] see also PARASITIC INFESTATIONS

LEPROSY [030.9] see also AMYLOIDOSIS; MYCOBACTERIAL INFECTION (ATYPICAL); TUBERCULOSIS

MULTIPLE SCLEROSIS [340] *see also* ALZHEIMER DISEASE; AMYOTROPHIC LATERAL SCLEROSIS (ALS); ATAXIA; DEMENTIA; NERVOUS SYSTEM (DEGENERATIVE DISORDERS); NEUROSYPHILIS

MUMPS [072.9]

MUSCLE DISEASE [359.9] *see also* DERMATOMYOSITIS; MIXED CONNECTIVE TISSUE DISEASE (MCTD); MUSCULAR DYSTROPHY; MYASTHENIA GRAVIS; MYOSITIS

MUSCULAR DYSTROPHY [359.1] *see also* AMYOTROPHIC LATERAL SCLEROSIS (ALS); DUCHENNE MUSCULAR DYSTROPHY; MUSCLE DISEASE; MYOSITIS

MYASTHENIA GRAVIS [358.0] *see also* BOTULISM; GUILLAIN-BARRÉ SYNDROME; MUSCULAR DYSTROPHY; THYMOMA; TICK PARALYSIS

MYCOBACTERIAL INFECTION *see* TUBERCULOSIS

MYCOBACTERIAL INFECTION (ATYPICAL) [031.9] *see also* ACQUIRED IMMUNODEFICIENCY SYNDROME (AIDS); CAT SCRATCH DISEASE; LEPROSY; TUBERCULOSIS; TULAREMIA

MYCOBACTERIUM AVIUM-INTRACELLULARE (MAI) *see* MYCOBACTERIAL INFECTION (ATYPICAL)

MYCOPLASMA INFECTION [041.81] *see also* BRONCHITIS; HYPOGAMMAGLOBULINEMIA; LEGIONNAIRES' DISEASE; PHARYNGITIS; PNEUMONIA

MYELODYSPLASTIC SYNDROME [238.7]

Patients have a disorder of hematopoietic stem cells (CD34 positive) characterized by variation from normal development and morphology of bone marrow cells with dyserythropoiesis, dysgranulopoiesis, and dysmegakaryopoiesis in various combinations and which may predispose to the development of leukemia.

MYELOFIBROSIS [238.7A] *see also* LEUKEMIA

MYELOID METAPLASIA *see* MYELOFIBROSIS

MYELOMA [203.0] *see also* AMYLOIDOSIS; HYPERPROTEINEMIA; MACROGLOBULINEMIA OF WALDENSTRÖM; MONOCLONAL GAMMOPATHY; MYELOMA

RENAL INFARCT [593.81]

RENAL VEIN THROMBOSIS [453.3] see also ANEMIA (MICROANGIOPATHIC HEMOLYTIC); DISSEMINATED INTRAVASCULAR COAGULATION (DIC); EMBOLISM; HEMOLYTIC-UREMIC SYNDROME; NEPHROSIS/NEPHROTIC SYNDROME; RENAL FAILURE; THROMBOSIS

Sudden flank pain with macroscopic hematuria is seen in acute renal vein thrombosis.

RESPIRATORY DISTRESS SYNDROME [769] see also FETAL MATURITY; NEONATAL TESTING; PNEUMONIA

RESPIRATORY DISTRESS SYNDROME (ADULT) [518.5] see also FAT EMBOLISM; GOODPASTURE SYNDROME; PANCREATITIS; PNEUMONIA; POISONING; SEPTICEMIA; SHOCK; SYSTEMIC LUPUS ERYTHEMATOSUS (SLE)

RESPIRATORY FAILURE [518.81] see also PNEUMONIA; RESPIRATORY DISTRESS SYNDROME (ADULT)

RESPIRATORY FAILURE (NEONATE) [770.8] see also NEONATAL TESTING; PNEUMONIA

RESPIRATORY SYNCYTIAL VIRUS INFECTION [519.8] see also BRONCHIOLITIS; BRONCHITIS; PNEUMONIA (VIRAL)

RETINITIS [363.20] see also ANEMIA (SICKLE CELL AND VARIANT SICKLING HEMOGLOBINS); SYSTEMIC LUPUS ERYTHEMATOSUS (SLE)

RETINOBLASTOMA [190.5]

REYE SYNDROME [331.81] see also COMA; HEPATITIS; HYPOGLYCEMIA; JAUNDICE; LIVER; SALICYLISM; SYNDROME OF INAPPROPRIATE SECRETION OF ANTIDIURETIC HORMONE (SIADH)

ALPHABETICAL INDEX

The most expedient method for locating a given test is the Alphabetical Index. Test names and synonyms are listed and the page number on which the test description many be found is indicated.

NOTES

NOTES

NOTES

NOTES

NOTES

NOTES

Other titles offered by

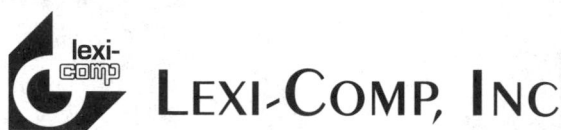
LEXI-COMP, INC

DRUG INFORMATION HANDBOOK (International edition available)
by Charles Lacy, RPh, PharmD, FCSHP; Lora L. Armstrong, RPh, PharmD, BCPS; Morton P. Goldman, PharmD, BCPS; and Leonard L. Lance, RPh, BSPharm

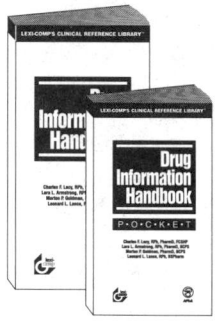

Specifically compiled and designed for the healthcare professional requiring quick access to concisely-stated comprehensive data concerning clinical use of medications.

The Drug Information Handbook is an ideal portable drug information resource, providing the reader with up to 29 key points of data concerning clinical use and dosing of the medication. Material provided in the Appendix section is recognized by many users to be, by itself, well worth the purchase of the handbook.

All medications found in the *Drug Information Handbook,* are included in the abridged *Pocket* edition (select fields were extracted to maintain portability).

DRUG INFORMATION HANDBOOK FOR THE ALLIED HEALTH PROFESSIONAL by Leonard L. Lance, RPh, BSPharm; Charles Lacy, RPh, PharmD, FCSHP; Lora L. Armstrong, RPh, PharmD, BCPS; and Morton P. Goldman, PharmD, BCPS

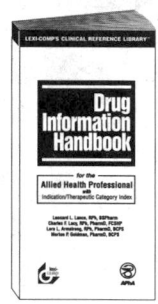

Working with clinical pharmacists, hospital pharmacy and therapeutics committees, and hospital drug information centers, the authors have assisted hundreds of hospitals in developing institution-specific formulary reference documentation.

The most current basic drug and medication data from those clinical settings have been reviewed, coalesced, and cross-referenced to create this unique handbook. The handbook offers quick access to abbreviated monographs for generic drugs.

This is a great tool for physician assistants, medical records personnel, medical transcriptionists and secretaries, pharmacy technicians, and other allied health professionals.

PEDIATRIC DOSAGE HANDBOOK (International edition available)
by Carol K. Taketomo, PharmD; Jane Hurlburt Hodding, PharmD; and Donna M. Kraus, PharmD

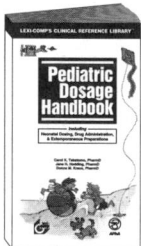

Special considerations must frequently be taken into account when dosing medications for the pediatric patient. This highly regarded quick reference handbook is a compilation of recommended pediatric doses based on current literature, as well as the practical experience of the authors and their many colleagues who work every day in the pediatric clinical setting.

Includes neonatal dosing, drug administration, and (in select monographs) extemporaneous preparations for medications used in pediatric medicine.

GERIATRIC DOSAGE HANDBOOK
by Todd P. Semla, PharmD, BCPS, FCCP; Judith L. Beizer, PharmD, FASCP; and Martin D. Higbee, PharmD, CGP

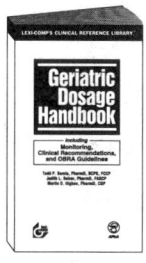

Many physiologic changes occur with aging, some of which affect the pharmacokinetics or pharmacodynamics of medications. Strong consideration should also be given to the effect of decreased renal or hepatic functions in the elderly, as well as the probability of the geriatric patient being on multiple drug regimens.

Healthcare professionals working with nursing homes and assisted living facilities will find the drug information contained in this handbook to be an invaluable source of helpful information.

An International Brand Name Index with names from 22 different countries is also included.

DRUG-INDUCED NUTRIENT DEPLETION HANDBOOK
by Ross Pelton, RPh, PhD, CCN; James B. LaValle, RPh, DHM, NMD, CCN; Ernest B. Hawkins, RPh, MS; Daniel L. Krinsky, RPh, MS

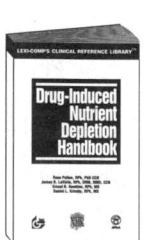

A complete and up-to-date listing of all drugs known to deplete the body of nutritional compounds.

This book is alphabetically organized and provides extensive cross-referencing to related information in the various sections of the book. Drug monographs identify the nutrients depleted and provide cross-references to the nutrient monographs for more detailed information on Effects of Depletion Symptoms, of Deficiencies, RDA, Dosage Range, and Dietary Sources. This book also contains a Studies & Abstracts section, a valuable Appendix, and Alphabetical & Pharmacological Indexes.

NATURAL THERAPEUTICS POCKET GUIDE
by James B. LaValle, RPh, DHM, NMD, CCN; Daniel L. Krinsky, RPh, MS; Ernest B. Hawkins, RPh, MS; Ross Pelton, RPh, PhD, CCN; Nancy Ashbrook Willis, BA, JD

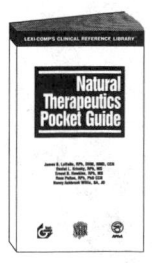

Provides condition-specific information on common uses of natural therapies. Each condition discussed includes the following: review of condition, decision tree, list of commonly recommended herbals, nutritional supplements, homeopathic remedies, lifestyle modifications, and special considerations.

Provides herbal/nutritional/nutraceutical monographs with over 10 fields including references, reported uses, dosage, pharmacology, toxicity, warnings & interactions, and cautions & contraindications.

The Appendix includes: drug-nutrient depletion, herb-drug interactions, drug-nutrient interaction, herbal medicine use in pediatrics, unsafe herbs, and reference of top herbals.

To order call toll free anywhere in the U.S.: 1-800-837-LEXI (5394)
Outside of the U.S. call: 330-650-6506 or online at www.lexi.com

Other titles offered by

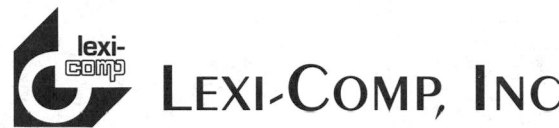
LEXI-COMP, INC

DRUG INFORMATION HANDBOOK for PHYSICIAN ASSISTANTS

by Michael J. Rudzinski, RPA-C, RPh and J. Fred Bennes, RPA, RPh

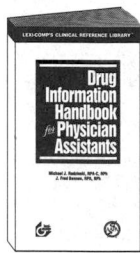

This comprehensive and easy-to-use handbook covers over 4100 drugs and also includes monographs on commonly used herbal products. There are up to 26 key fields of information per monograph, such as Pediatric and Adult Dosing With Adjustments for Renal/Hepatic Impairment, Labeled and Unlabeled Uses, Drug & Alcohol interactions, and Education & Monitoring Issues. Brand (U.S. and Canadian) and generic names are listed alphabetically for rapid access. It is fully cross-referenced by page number and includes alphabetical and pharmacologic indexes.

DRUG INFORMATION HANDBOOK for ADVANCED PRACTICE NURSING

by Beatrice B. Turkoski, RN, PhD; Brenda R. Lance, RN, MSN; and Mark F. Bonfiglio, PharmD Foreword by: Margaret A. Fitzgerald, MS, RN, CS-FNP

1999 "Book of the Year" — American Journal of Nursing
Advanced Practice Nursing Category

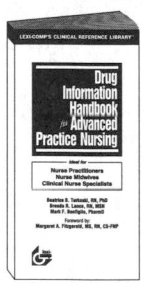

Designed specifically to meet the needs of nurse practitioners, clinical nurse specialists, nurse midwives, and graduate nursing students. The handbook is a unique resource for detailed, accurate information, which is vital to support the advanced practice nurse's role in patient drug therapy management. Over 4750 U.S., Canadian, and Mexican medications are covered in the 1000 monographs. Drug data is presented in an easy-to-use, alphabetically organized format covering up to 46 key points of information (including dosing for pediatrics, adults, and geriatrics). Cross-referenced to Appendix of over 230 pages of valuable comparison tables and additional information. Also included are two indexes, Pharmacologic Category and Controlled Substance, which facilitate comparison between agents.

DRUG INFORMATION HANDBOOK for NURSING

by Beatrice B. Turkoski, RN, PhD; Brenda R. Lance, RN, MSN; and Mark F. Bonfiglio, PharmD

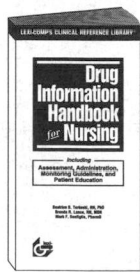

Registered Professional Nurses and upper-division nursing students involved with drug therapy will find this handbook provides quick access to drug data in a concise easy-to-use format.

Over 4000 U.S., Canadian, and Mexican medications are covered with up to 43 key points of information in each monograph. The handbook contains basic pharmacology concepts and nursing issues such as patient factors that influence drug therapy (ie, pregnancy, age, weight, etc) and general nursing issues (ie, assessment, administration, monitoring, and patient education). The Appendix contains over 230 pages of valuable information.

DRUG INFORMATION HANDBOOK for CARDIOLOGY

by Bradley G. Phillips, PharmD and Virend K. Somers, MD, Dphil

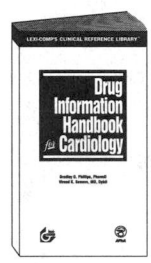

An ideal resource for physicians, pharmacists, nurses, residents, and students. This handbook was designed to provide the most current information on cardiovascular agents and other ancillary medications.
- Each monograph includes information on Special Cardiovascular Considerations and I.V. to Oral Equivalency
- Alphabetically organized by brand and generic name
- Appendix contains information on Hypertension, Anticoagulation, Cytochrome P-450, Hyperlipidemia, Antiarrhythmia, and Comparative Drug Charts
- Special Topics/Issues include Emerging Risk Factors for Cardiovascular Disease, Treatment of Cardiovascular Disease in the Diabetic, Cardiovascular Stress Testing, and Experimental Cardiovascular Therapeutic Strategies in the New Millenium, and much more . . .

DRUG INFORMATION HANDBOOK for ONCOLOGY

by Dominic A. Solimando, Jr, MA; Linda R. Bressler, PharmD, BCOP; Polly E. Kintzel, PharmD, BCPS, BCOP; and Mark C. Geraci, PharmD, BCOP

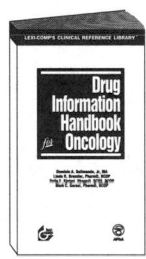

Presented in a concise and uniform format, this book contains the most comprehensive collection of oncology-related drug information available. Organized like a dictionary for ease of use, drugs can be found by looking up the brand or generic name!

This book contains individual monographs for both Antineoplastic Agents and Ancillary Medications.

The fields of information per monograph include: Use, U.S. Investigational, Bone Marrow/Blood Cell Transplantation, Vesicant, Emetic Potential. A Special Topics Section, Appendix, and Therapeutic Category & Key Word Index are valuable features to this book, as well.

ANESTHESIOLOGY & CRITICAL CARE DRUG HANDBOOK

by Andrew J. Donnelly, PharmD; Francesca E. Cunningham, PharmD; and Verna L. Baughman, MD

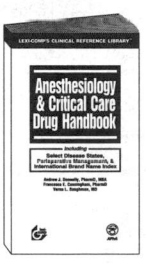

Contains the most commonly used drugs in the perioperative and critical care setting. This handbook also contains the following Special Issues and Topics: Allergic Reaction, Anesthesia for Cardiac Patients in Noncardiac Surgery, Anesthesia for Obstetric Patients in Nonobstetric Surgery, Anesthesia for Patients With Liver Disease, Chronic Pain Management, Chronic Renal Failure, Conscious Sedation, Perioperative Management of Patients on Antiseizure Medication, and Substance Abuse and Anesthesia.

The Appendix includes Abbreviations & Measurements, Anesthesiology Information, Assessment of Liver & Renal Function, Comparative Drug Charts, Infectious Disease-Prophylaxis & Treatment, Laboratory Values, Therapy Recommendations, Toxicology information, and much more.

International Brand Name Index with names from over 22 different countries is also included.

To order call toll free anywhere in the U.S.: 1-800-837-LEXI (5394)
Outside of the U.S. call: 330-650-6506 or online at www.lexi.com

Other titles offered by

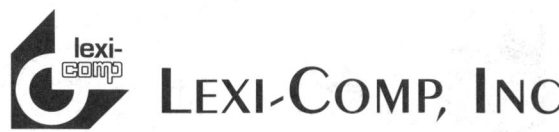

LEXI-COMP, INC

DIAGNOSTIC PROCEDURE HANDBOOK by Frank Michota, MD

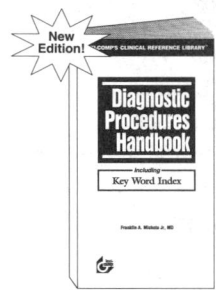

A comprehensive, yet concise, quick reference source for physicians, nurses, students, medical records personnel, or anyone needing quick access to diagnostic procedure information. This handbook is an excellent source of information in the following areas: allergy, rheumatology, and infectious disease; cardiology; computed tomography; diagnostic radiology; gastroenterology; invasive radiology; magnetic resonance imaging; nephrology, urology, and hematology; neurology; nuclear medicine; pulmonary function; pulmonary medicine and critical care; ultrasound; and women's health.

POISONING & TOXICOLOGY HANDBOOK
by Jerrold B. Leikin, MD and Frank P. Paloucek, PharmD

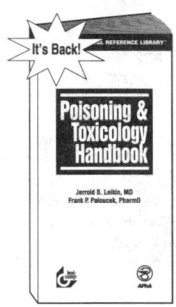

It's back by popular demand! The small size of our Poisoning & Toxicology Handbook is once again available. Better than ever, this comprehensive, portable reference contains 80 antidotes and drugs used in toxicology with 694 medicinal agents, 287 nonmedicinal agents, 291 biological agents, 57 herbal agents, and more than 200 laboratory tests. Monographs are extensively referenced and contain valuable information on overdose symptomatology and treatment considerations, as well as, admission criteria and impairment potential of select agents. Designed for quick reference with monographs arranged alphabetically, plus a cross-referencing index. The authors have expanded current information on drugs of abuse and use of antidotes, while providing concise tables, graphics, and other pertinent toxicology text.

CLINICIAN'S GUIDE TO LABORATORY MEDICINE—A Practical Approach by Samir P. Desai, MD and Sana Isa-Pratt, MD

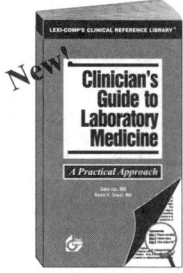

When faced with the patient presenting with abnormal laboratory tests, the clinician can now turn to the *Clinician's Guide to Laboratory Medicine: A Practical Approach*. This source is unique in its ability to lead the clinician from laboratory test abnormality to clinical diagnosis. Written for the busy clinician, this concise handbook will provide rapid answers to the questions that busy clinicians face in the care of their patients. No longer does the clinician have to struggle in an effort to find this information - *it's all here.*

CLINICIAN'S GUIDE TO DIAGNOSIS—A Practical Approach
by Samir Desai, MD

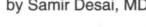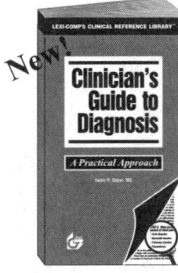

Symptoms are what prompt patients to seek medical care. In the evaluation of a patient's symptom, it is not unusual for healthcare professionals to ask "What do I do next?" This is precisely the question for which the *Clinician's Guide to Diagnosis: A Practical Approach* provides the answer. It will lead you from symptom to diagnosis through a series of steps designed to mimic the logical thought processes of seasoned clinicians. For the young clinician, this is an ideal book to help bridge the gap between the classroom and actual patient care. For the experienced clinician, this concise handbook offers rapid answers to the questions that are commonly encountered on a day-to-day basis. Let this guide become your companion, providing you with the tools necessary to tackle even the most challenging symptoms.

INFECTIOUS DISEASES HANDBOOK
by Carlos M. Isada, MD; Bernard L. Kasten Jr., MD; Morton P. Goldman, PharmD; Larry D. Gray, PhD; and Judith A. Aberg, MD

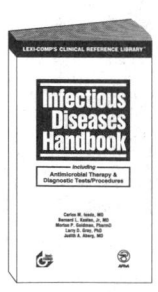

This four-in-one quick reference is concerned with the identification and treatment of infectious diseases. Each of the four sections of the book (disease syndromes, organisms, laboratory tests, and antimicrobials) contain related information and cross-referencing to one or more of the other three sections.

The disease syndrome section provides the clinical presentation, differential diagnosis, diagnostic tests, and drug therapy recommended for treatment of more common infectious diseases. The organism section presents the microbiology, epidemiology, diagnosis, and treatment of each organism. The laboratory diagnosis section describes performance of specific tests and procedures. The antimicrobial therapy section presents important facts and considerations regarding each drug recommended for specific diseases of organisms. Also includes an International Brand Name Index with names from 22 different countries.

LABORATORY TEST HANDBOOK & CONCISE version
by David S. Jacobs MD, FACP; Wayne R. DeMott, MD, FACP; Harold J. Grady, PhD; Rebecca T. Horvat, PhD; Douglas W. Huestis, MD; and Bernard L. Kasten Jr., MD, FACP

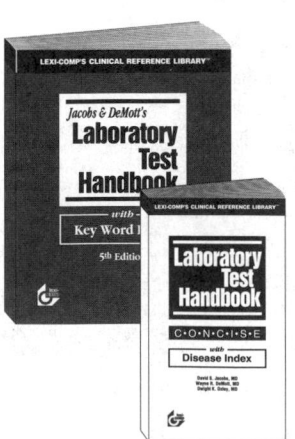

Contains over 900 clinical laboratory tests and is an excellent source of laboratory information for physicians of all specialties, nurses, laboratory professionals, students, medical personnel, or anyone who needs quick access to most routine and many of the more specialized testing procedures available in today's clinical laboratory.

Including updated AMA CPT coding, each monograph contains test name, synonyms, patient care, specimen requirements, reference ranges, and interpretive information with footnotes and references.

The *Laboratory Test Handbook Concise* is a portable, abridged (800 tests) version and is an ideal, quick reference for anyone requiring information concerning patient preparation, specimen collection and handling, and test result interpretation.

To order call toll free anywhere in the U.S.: 1-800-837-LEXI (5394)
Outside of the U.S. call: 330-650-6506 or online at www.lexi.com

Other titles offered by

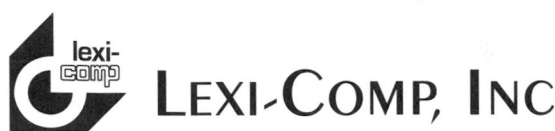

DRUG INFORMATION FOR MENTAL HEALTH
by Matthew A. Fuller, PharmD and Martha Sajatovic, MD

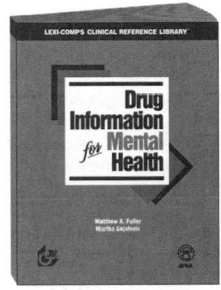

Formerly titled Drug Information Handbook for Psychiatry, this desk reference is a complete guide to psychotropic and nonpsychotropic drugs. The new 8 ½ x 11 size, presents information on all medications in a double column format. It is specifically designed as a tool for mental health professionals when assessing a client's medication profile with emphasis on a drug's Effect on Mental Status, as well as considerations for psychotropic medications.

A special topics/issues section includes psychiatric assessment, major psychiatric disorders, major classes of psychotropic medications, psychiatric emergencies, special populations, patient education information, and DSM-IV classification. Also contains a valuable appendix section, Pharmacologic Index, Alphabetical Index, and International Brand Name Index.

PSYCHOTROPIC DRUG INFORMATION HANDBOOK
by Matthew A. Fuller, PharmD and Martha Sajatovic, MD

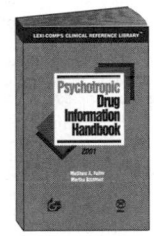

This portable, yet comprehensive guide to psychotropic drugs provides healthcare professionals with detailed information on use, drug interactions, pregnancy risk factors, warnings/precautions, adverse reactions, mechanism of action, and contraindications. Alphabetically organized by brand and generic name this concise handbook provides quick access to the information you need and includes patient education sheets on the psychotropic medications. It is the perfect pocket companion to the Drug Information for Mental Health.

RATING SCALES IN MENTAL HEALTH
by Martha Sajatovic, MD and Luis F. Ramirez, MD

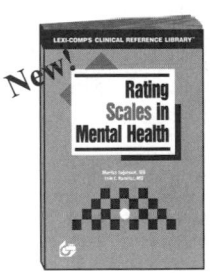

A basic guide to the rating scales in mental health, this is an ideal reference for psychiatrists, nurses, residents, psychologists, social workers, healthcare administrators, behavioral healthcare organizations, and outcome committees. It is designed to assist clinicians in determining the appropriate rating scale when assessing their client. A general concepts section provides text discussion on the use and history of rating scales, statistical evaluation, rating scale domains, and two clinical vignettes. Information on over 80 rating scales used in mental health organized in 6 categories. Appendix contains tables and charts in a quick reference format allowing clinicians to rapidly identify categories and characteristics of rating scales.

Coming Soon! *RATING SCALES TRAINING VIDEOS*
by Martha Sajatovic, MD and Luis F. Ramirez, MD

A PATIENT GUIDE TO MENTAL HEALTH ISSUES

New!

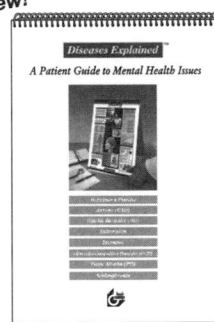

Patient Education Desk Chart
▶ Alzheimer's Disease
▶ Anxiety (GAD)
▶ Bipolar Disorder (BD)
▶ Depression
▶ Insomnia
▶ Obsessive-Compulsive Disorder (OCD)
▶ Panic Attacks (PD)
▶ Schizophrenia

DRUG INFORMATION HANDBOOK FOR THE CRIMINAL JUSTICE PROFESSIONAL
by Marcelline Burns, PhD; Thomas E. Page, MA; and Jerrold B. Leikin, MD

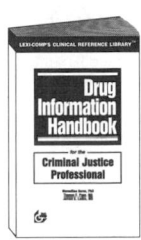

Compiled and designed for police officers, law enforcement officials, and legal professionals who are in need of a reference which relates to information on drugs, chemical substances, and other agents that have abuse and/or impairment potential. Contains over 450 medications, agents, and substances. Contains up to 33 fields of information including Scientific Name, Commonly Found In, Abuse Potential, Impairment Potential, Use, When to Admit to Hospital, Mechanism of Toxic Action, Signs & Symptoms of Acute Overdose, Drug Interactions, Reference Range, and Warnings/Precautions. There is a glossary of medical terms for the layman along with a slang street drug listing and an Appendix includes Chemical, Bacteriologic, and Radiologic Agents - Effects and Treatment; Controlled Substances - Uses and Effects; Medical Examiner Data; Federal Trafficking Penalties, and much more.

POISONING & TOXICOLOGY COMPENDIUM
by Jerrold B. Leikin, MD and Frank P. Paloucek, PharmD

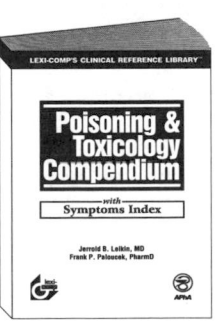

A six-in-one reference wherein each major entry contains information relative to one or more of the other sections. This compendium offers comprehensive, concisely-stated monographs covering 645 medicinal agents, 256 nonmedicinal agents, 273 biological agents, 49 herbal agents, 254 laboratory tests, 79 antidotes, and 222 pages of exceptionally useful appendix material.

A truly unique reference that presents signs and symptoms of acute overdose along with considerations for overdose treatment. Ideal reference for emergency situations.

To order call toll free anywhere in the U.S.: 1-800-837-LEXI (5394)
Outside of the U.S. call: 330-650-6506 or online at www.lexi.com

Other titles offered by

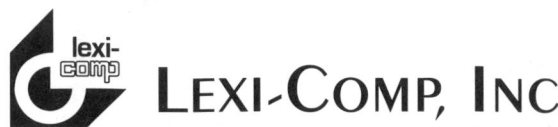

DRUG INFORMATION HANDBOOK FOR DENTISTRY
(International edition available) by Richard L. Wynn, BSPharm, PhD; Timothy F. Meiller, DDS, PhD; and Harold L. Crossley, DDS, PhD

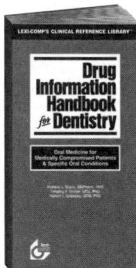

For all dental professionals requiring quick access to concisely-stated drug information pertaining to medications commonly prescribed by dentists and physicians.
Designed and written by dentists for all dental professionals as a portable, chair-side resource. Includes drugs commonly prescribed by dentists or being taken by dental patients and written in an easy-to-understand format. There are 24 key points of information for each drug including **Local Anesthetic/Vasoconstrictor, Precautions, Effects on Dental Treatment, and Drug Interactions.** Includes information on dental treatment for medically compromised patients and dental management of specific oral conditions.

An International edition contains an index with brand names from 22 countries.

ORAL SOFT TISSUE DISEASES
by J. Robert Newland, DDS, MS; Timothy F. Meiller, DDS, PhD; Richard L. Wynn, BSPharm, PhD; and Harold L.Crossley, DDS, PhD

New!

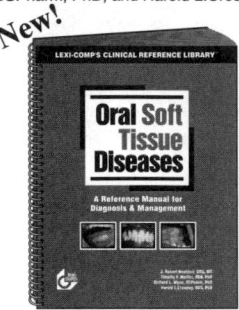

Designed for all dental professionals a pictoral reference to assist in the diagnosis and management of oral soft tissue diseases, (over 160 photos).

Easy-to-use, sections include:

Diagnosis process: obtaining a history, examining the patient, establishing a differential diagnosis, selecting appropriate diagnostic tests, interpreting the results, etc.; White lesions; Red lesions; Blistering-sloughing lesions; Ulcerated lesions; Pigmented lesions; Papillary lesions; Soft tissue swelling (each lesion is illustrated with a color representative photograph); Specific medications to treat oral soft tissue diseases; Sample prescriptions; and Special topics.

CLINICIAN'S ENDODONTIC HANDBOOK
by Thom C. Dumsha, MS, DDS and James L. Gutmann, DDS, FACD, FICD

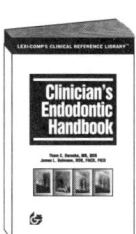

Designed for all general practice dentists.

- A quick reference addressing current endodontics
- Easy-to-use format and alphabetical index
- Latest techniques, procedures, and materials
- Root canal therapy: Why's and Why Nots
- A guide to diagnosis and treatment of endodontic emergencies
- Facts and rationale behind treating endodontically-involved teeth
- Straight-forward dental trauma management information
- Pulpal Histology, Access Openings, Bleaching, Resorption, Radiology, Restoration, and Periodontal / Endodontic Complications
- Frequently Asked Questions (FAQ) section and "Clinical Note" sections throughout.

DENTAL OFFICE MEDICAL EMERGENCIES
by Timothy F. Meiller, DDS, PhD; Richard L. Wynn, BSPharm, PhD; Ann Marie McMullin, MD; Cynthia Biron, RDH, EMT, MA; and Harold L. Crossley, DDS, PhD

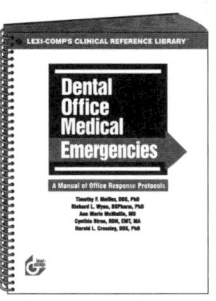

Designed specifically for general dentists during times of emergency. A tabbed paging system allows for quick access to specific crisis events. Created with urgency in mind, it is spiral bound and drilled with a hole for hanging purposes.

- Basic Action Plan for Stabilization
- Allergic / Drug Reactions
- Loss of Consciousness / Respiratory Distress / Chest Pain
- Altered Sensation / Changes in Affect
- Management of Acute Bleeding
- Office Preparedness / Procedures and Protocols
- Automated External Defibrillator (AED)
- Oxygen Delivery

New! Patient Education Dental Desk Charts

A PATIENT GUIDE TO ROOT THERAPY
Contributor Thom C. Dumsha, M.S., D.D.S., M.S.

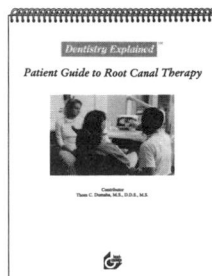

- An ideal tool used to educate and explain to your patients about root canals

- 8 1/2" x 11" colorful tabbed flip chart explaining each of the steps involved in a root canal

- Actual clinical photographs, radiographs, and diagrams

"Take home" patient education pamphlets also included.

A PATIENT GUIDE TO DENTAL IMPLANTS
Contributor Marvin L. Baer, D.D.S., M.Sc.

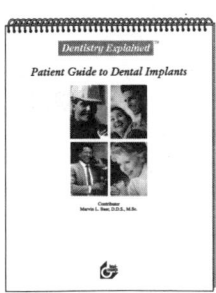

- An ideal tool used to educate and explain to your patients about dental implants

- 8 1/2" x 11" colorful tabbed flip chart explaining each of the steps involved in:

  1.) Single tooth restoration
  2.) Replacement of several teeth
  3.) Implants supported overdenture (4 implants/2 implants)
  4.) Screw-retained denture

"Take home" patient education pamphlets also included.

**To order call toll free anywhere in the U.S.: 1-800-837-LEXI (5394)
Outside of the U.S. call: 330-650-6506 or online at www.lexi.com**

Introducing . . . Diseases Explained™

by

LEXI-COMP, INC

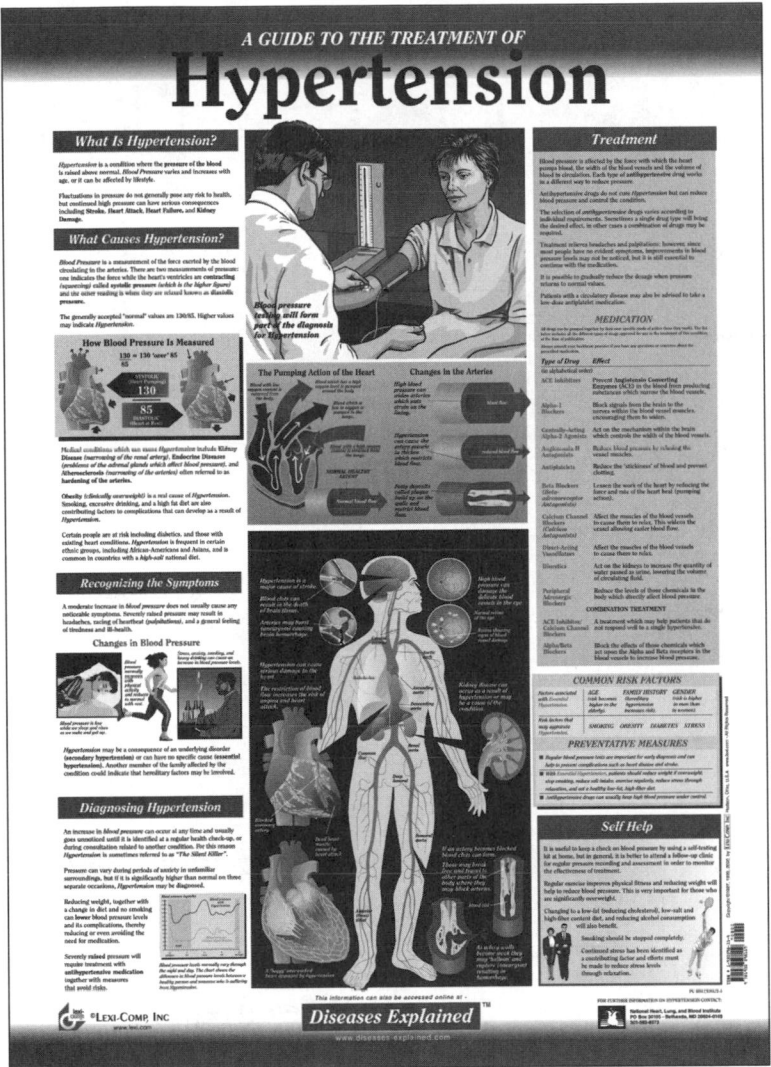

Lexi-Comp is proud to introduce Diseases Explained™, our new series of patient education material. Written in a language a patient can easily understand, each product will help the healthcare professional explain to patients about their specific medical condition. Available now in a wall chart format and soon to be released as booklets, leaflets, and desk flip charts, this series will help you educate the patient about the cause, symptoms, diagnosis, treatment, and self-help concerning their condition.

Available now:

- Alzheimer's Disease
- Anemia
- Angina
- Asthma
- Anxiety
- Cholesterol
- COPD
- Depression
- Diabetes
- Enlarged Prostate
- Epilepsy
- Essential Tremor
- Glaucoma
- Heart Attack
- Hypertension
- Incontinence
- Insomnia
- Irritable Bowel Syndrome
- Menopause
- Migraine
- Multiple Sclerosis
- Obsessive-Compulsive Disorder
- Osteoporosis
- Otitis
- Panic Disorder
- Parkinson's Disease
- Schizophrenia
- Spasticity
- Stroke
- Thyroid Disease

To order call toll free anywhere in the U.S.: 1-800-837-LEXI (5394)
Outside of the U.S. call: 330-650-6506 or online at www.lexi.com

LEXI-COMP'S CLINICAL REFERENCE LIBRARY™

Accurate, Up-To-Date, Clinically Relevant Information

Available on:

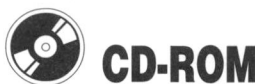 **CD-ROM**   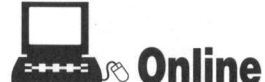 **Online**   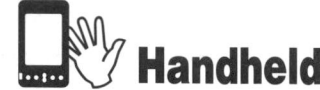 **Handheld**

Lexi-Comp's Clinical Reference Library™ (CRL™) offers a series of clinical databases as portable handbooks, integrated on CD-ROM for use with Microsoft Windows or available through CRLOnline, our new Internet application. CRL provides you with quick access to current lab, diagnostic and treatment information where you need it most, at the Point-of-Care.

CRL™ on CD-ROM and CRLOnline™ provide:
- A user-friendly interface
- Licensing for Individual, Academic or Institutional use
- CD-ROM updates or real-time online updates
- Drug Interactions with detailed information
- Over 3,000 Drug Images
- Patient Education Leaflets
- Currently, the following Clinical Decision Support Modules are available only for CRL™ on CD-ROM (coming soon for CRLOnline™):
  - ➤ Stedman's Electronic Medical Dictionary
  - ➤ Calculations:
    Ideal Body Mass, Estimated Creatinine Clearance, Body Surface Area and Temperature Conversion
  - ➤ Symptoms Analysis for Toxicity

Visit our website to sign up for a **FREE** 30-day trial of CRLOnline™

www.lexi.com

....

Also access your favorite Lexi-Comp databases from the ***"palm of your hand"!***

Running on Palm or Windows CE operating system version 2.0 or higher

Ask about other newly available and soon to be available databases

Now available for your handheld device:

✓ **LexiDrugs**™
(Drug Information Handbook)

✓ **CardioDrugs**™
(Drug Information Handbook for Cardiology)

✓ **NursingDrugs**™
(Drug Information Handbook for Nursing)

✓ **PediatricDrugs**™
(Pediatric Dosage Handbook)

✓ **OncologyDrugs**™
(Drug Information Handbook for Oncology)

✓ **Apothecarium:** Add this interaction program to any available palm database

✓ **GeriatricDrugs**™
(Geriatric Dosage Handbook)

✓ **AnesthesiaDrugs**™
(Anesthesiology & Critical Care Drug Handbook)

✓ **5 Minute Clinical Consult**

✓ **PsychDrugs**™
(Drug Information for Mental Health)

✓ **DentalDrugs**™
(Drug Information Handbook for Dentistry)

**To order call toll free anywhere in the U.S.: 1-800-837-LEXI (5394)
Outside of the U.S. call: 330-650-6506 or online at www.lexi.com**